AF690975

DIRECTORY OF BIOMEDICAL AND HEALTH CARE GRANTS 2010

21st Edition

Schoolhouse Partners LLC
Nashville, Indiana

Why 'Partners'? Partners work together as a team, with each person contributing different skills and expressing his or her individual interests and opinions to the unity and efficiency of the group in order to achieve common goals. Our aim is to make worthwhile resources available to you so that you and your institution or organization can and will achieve those goals.

Schoolhouse Partners, Post Office Box 2059, Nashville, IN 47448
www.schoolhousepartners.net
Published 1985, 21st edition 2010

Printed and bound in the United States of America

ISBN 978-0-9841725-4-2
0-9841725-4-8

Table of Contents

Introduction iv
How to Use This Directory.......... v
Government and Organization Acronyms viii
Grant Programs.......... 1
Subject Index.......... 535
Program Type Index.......... 681
Geographic Index.......... 757

Introduction

For over three decades the GRANTS Database and its print complements, including the annual Directory of Re- Biomedical and Health Care Grants, have provided the research community with current, accurate information regarding funding for research-related programs and projects, scholarships, fellowships, conferences, and internships. To meet the increased information needs of professionals, the GRANTS Database, researched and edited by members of the Schoolhouse Partners editorial staff, has grown significantly. This 21st edition of the annual Directory of Biomedical and Health Care Grants offers factual and concise descriptions of more than 3,500 funding programs. With this new edition both experienced and novice grantseekers will be better able to target only the most applicable programs for their biomedical and healthcare needs.

Directory of Biomedical and Health Care Grants 2010

The *Directory of Biomedical and Healthcare Grants 2010* features listings of programs that offer non-repayable funding for projects ranging from laboratory investigations to those designed to study the needs of society in healthcare delivery. Listings in the main section of the *Directory* contain annotations describing each program's focuses and goals, program requirements explaining eligibility, funding amounts, deadlines, *Catalog of Federal Domestic Assistance* program number (for U.S. government programs only), sponsor name and address, contact information, and the sponsor's Internet Web address. Grantseekers with access to the Internet can use the addresses to locate further information about the organizations and their application procedures. Internet addresses are also provided, when available, within listings. Some of the grant programs listed in the main section have geographic restrictions for applicants.

The following people have devoted a great deal of patience, hard work and thought to keep this project and the database an informative service for the user. It is especially important to mention the GrantSelect team – Louis S. Schafer, Ed.S., Anita Schafer and Joy Blakeley – for their diligent research, editorial work, development and assignment of index terms, and production – as well as all Schoolhouse Partners staff who contribute to the GRANTS effort.

Indexes. The Subject Index of this *Directory* lists all program titles—with accession numbers—under their applicable subject terms. Other indexes follow, including the Sponsoring Organizations Index, which lists program sponsors alphabetically along with their programs; the Grants by Program Type Index, which lists 38 program categories, such as Basic Research, Fellowships, Travel Grants, etc., with the grants that fall within their scope; and the Geographic Index, which lists programs that have state, regional, or international focus. See How to Use This Directory on pages v-vii for sample index entries.

Using the *Directory* for Grantseeking

By using the *Directory of Biomedical and Health Care Grants*, grantseekers can match the needs of their particular programs with those sponsors offering funding in the researchers' area of interest. The information listed here is meant to eliminate the costs incurred by both grantseekers and grantmakers when inappropriate proposals are submitted for a sponsor's funding program. However, because the GRANTS Database is updated daily basis, with program listings continually added, deleted, and revised, grantseekers using this *Directory* may also search the GRANTS database online through *GrantSelect* (www.grantselect.com).

All new and revised information has been taken from (1) the sponsor's updated of previously published program statements included in earlier editions of GRANTS publications, (2) questionnaires sent to sponsors whose programs were not listed in previous editions, or (3) other materials published by the sponsor and furnished to Schoolhouse Partners. Updated information for U.S. government programs includes new and revised program information published in the *Federal Register*; the latest edition of the *Catalog of Federal Domestic Assistance*; the *NIH Guide*, published weekly by the National Institutes of Health; and the *NSF E-Bulletin*, a monthly publication of the National Science Foundation. Included in this edition are identifying document numbers from the NIH and NSF publications. Located at the ends of the program descriptions in certain entries, the numbers indicated the ongoing NIH program number (PA) or the request for applications number (RFA). For programs of the National Science Foundation, the *NSF Bulletin* number appears. This information will help users identify the programs when seeking additional information from program staff.

While Schoolhouse Partners has made every effort to verify that all information is both accurate and current within the confines of format and scope, the publisher does not assume and hereby disclaims any liability to any party for loss or damages caused by errors or omissions in this *Directory*, whether such errors or missions result from accident, negligence, or any other cause. Anyone having questions regarding the content, format, or any other aspect of the *Directory of Biomedical and Health Care Grants 2010*, GrantSelect, or the GRANTS Database should contact the Editors, GRANTS, Schoolhouse Partners or editor@schoolhousepartners.net.

How to Use This Directory

The *Directory of Biomedical and Health Care Grants 2010* is designed to allow the user quick and easy access to information regarding funding programs in a researcher's specific area of interest. This *Directory* is composed of a main section, Grant Programs, which lists grant programs in alphabetical order, and three indexes: the Subject Index, the Grants by Program Type Index, and the Geographic Index.

GRANT PROGRAMS

Each listing in this section consists of the following elements: an annotation describing each program's focus and goals, requirements explaining eligibility, funding amounts, application and renewal dates, the *Catalog of Federal Domestic Assistance* program number (for U.S. government programs only), sponsor information, contact information, and Internet address.

GRANT TITLE — **Paul G. Allen Family Foundation Grants** **4298** — ACCESSION NUMBER

The single foundation, created through the consolidation of Allen's six previous foundations (The Allen Foundation for the Arts, The Paul G. Allen Charitable Foundation, The Paul G. Allen Foundation for Medical Research, The Paul G. Allen Forest Protection Foundation, The Allen Foundation for Music, and The Paul G. Allen Virtual Education Foundation), will continue to focus on the Allen family's philanthropic interests in the areas of arts and culture, youth engagement, community development and social change, and scientific and technological innovation. The Arts and Culture Program fosters creativity and promotes critical thinking by helping strong arts organizations become sustainable and supporting projects that feature innovative and diverse artistic forms. — GRANT DESCRIPTION
The Youth Engagement Program improves the way young people learn by supporting organizations that use innovative teaching strategies and provide opportunities for children to address issues relevant to their lives. The Community Development and Social Change Program promotes individual and community development by supporting initiatives and organizations that provide access to resources and opportunities. The Scientific and Technological Innovation Program advances promising scientific and technology research that has the potential to enhance understanding and stewardship of the world in which we live. Organizations may only receive one grant per year. Organizations must not have any delinquent final reports due to any of the Paul G. Allen Foundations for previous grants. Grantseekers are encouraged to apply through the online application process, where basic organizational and project information will be requested. Guidelines are available online.

REQUIREMENTS — *Requirements* 501(c)3 tax-exempt organizations, status from the Internal Revenue government entities, and IRS-recognized tribes are eligible. Eligible organizations must be located in, or serving populations of, the Pacific Northwest, which includes Alaska, Idaho, Montana, Oregon, and Washington.

RESTRICTIONS — *Restrictions* In general, the foundation will not consider requests for general fund drives, annual appeals, or federated campaigns; special events or sponsorships; direct grants, scholarships, or loans for the benefit of specific individuals; projects of organizations whose policies or practices discriminate on the basis of race, ethnic origin, sex, creed, or sexual orientation; contributions to sectarian or religious organizations whose principle activity is for the benefit of their own members or adherents; loans or debt retirement; projects that will benefit the students of a single school; general operating support for ongoing activities; or projects not aligned with the foundation's specified program areas. 509(a) private foundations are ineligible.

APPLICATION/ DUE DATE — *Date(s) Application Is Due* Mar 31; Sep 30.

Contact Grants Administrator, (206) 342-2030; fax: (206) 342-3030; email: info@pgafamilyfoundation.org — CONTACT

INTERNET ADDRESS — *Internet* http://www.pgafamilyfoundation.org

Sponsor Paul G. Allen Family Foundation — SPONSOR INFORMATION
505 Fifth Ave S, Ste 900
Seattle, WA 98104

SUBJECT INDEX

The most effective way to access specific funding programs is through the Subject Index. This index lists the subject terms with applicable grants program titles – and their accession numbers – alphabetically under each term. Terms were assigned to target the specific area of research designated in the description of each program. Cross-references are used to link subjects and assist the user in finding specific grant information.

Following are general guidelines that can make your search of this index more successful. First, check under the specific topic of interest rather than a more general term. For instance, if you are interested in chemical engineering, look under "Chemical Engineering" rather than "Engineering." Items indexed under "Engineering" indicate funding in broad areas of engineering.

Use general headings when you want grants covering broader areas or if you can't find a specific topic. For example, many grants list funding for humanities research, health programs, or science and technology. To find these grants use such headings as "Humanities," "Medical Programs," "Science," or "Technology." For additional grant information on more specific humanities research opportunities, such as in American History or Cultural Anthropology, also check under the topics "United States History" and "Anthropology, Cultural."

Many of the grant programs provide funding for research-related scholarships, faculty fellowships, dissertations, undergraduate education, conferences, or internships. If grant funds are designated for specific disciplines, you will find the items under the specific subject. Scholarships and fellowships are also listed under the terms "Native American Education," "African Americans (Student Support)," "Hispanic Education," "Minority Education," and "Women's Education."

Grants concerning study of a particular country are listed under the name of the country. Grants concerning the history, literature, art and language of a country are listed under the name of the country also, e.g., "Chinese Art" and "Chinese Language/Literature."

SUBJECT TERM ——— **Education**

A.L. Mailman Family Foundation Grants, 5
AAAS Science & Technology Policy Fellowships - Health, Education & Human Services, 22
AARP Andrus Foundation Grants, 104
Abbott Laboratories Fund Grants, 125
ACIE Host University Edmund S. Muskie/Freedom Support Act Graduate Fellowships, 156
ACT Awards, 189
Akonadi Foundation Anti-Racism Grants, 351 ——— **PROGRAM TITLE**
Akron Community Foundation Grants, 352
Albert and Margaret Alkek Foundation Grants, 370
Albuquerque Community Foundation Grants, 379
Alcoa Foundation Grants, 380
Alcon Foundation Grants Program, 382

GEOGRAPHIC INDEX

This index lists programs that have state, regional, or international geographic focus. The Geographic Index is arranged by state, followed by Canadian programs, then by international programs by country, and lists grant program titles and their corresponding accession numbers.

COUNTRY ——— **United States**

Alabama ——— **STATE**

3M Fndn Grants, 2
Alabama Humanities Fndn Grants Program, 368
Arkema Inc. Fndn Science Teachers Program, 705
CDC Injury Control Research Centers Grants, 1198
PROGRAM TITLE ——— DOE Experimental Program to Stimulate Competitive Research (EPSCoR), 1653
Hill Crest Fndn Grants, 2293
Linn-Henley Charitable Trust Grants, 2777
NOAA Community-Based Restoration Program (CRP) Grants, 3843
Southern Company's Longleaf Pine Reforestation Fund, 4726

PROGRAM TYPE INDEX

This index is broken into 38 categories according to the type of program funded:

- Adult Basic Education
- Adult/Family Literacy Training
- Awards/Prizes
- Basic Research
- Building Construction and/or Renovation
- Capital Campaigns
- Centers: Research/Demonstration/Service
- Citizenship Instruction
- Community Development
- Consulting/Visiting Personnel
- Cultural Outreach
- Curriculum Development/Teacher Training
- Demonstration Grants
- Development (Institutional/Departmental)
- Dissertation/Thesis Research Support
- Educational Programs
- Environmental Programs
- Exhibitions, Collections, Performances, Video/ Film Production
- Faculty/Professional Development
- Fellowships
- General Operating Support
- Graduate Assistantships
- International Exchange Programs
- International Grants
- Job Training/Adult Vocational Programs
- Matching/Challenge Funds
- Materials/Equipment Acquisition (Computers, Books, Tapes, etc.)
- Preservation/Restoration
- Publishing/Editing/Translating
- Religious Programs
- Scholarships
- Seed Grants
- Service Delivery Programs
- Symposia, Conferences, Workshops, Seminars
- Technical Assistance
- Training Programs/Internships
- Travel Grants
- Vocational Education

Government and Organization Acronyms

AAAAI	American Academy of Allergy Asthma and Immunology
AAAS	American Association for the Advancement of Science
AACAP	American Academy of Child and Adolescent Psychiatry
AACN	American Association of Critical Care Nurses
AACR	American Association of Cancer Research
AAFCS	American Association of Family and Consumer Sciences
AAFP	American Academy of Family Physicians Foundation
AAFPRS	American Academy of Facial Plastic and Reconstructive Surgery
AAR	American Academy in Rome
AAS	American Antiquarian Society
AASL	American Association of School Libraries
AAUW	American Association of University Women
ACC	Asian Cultural Council
ACLS	American Council of Learned Societies
ACM	Association for Computing Machinery
ACS	American Cancer Society
ADA	American Diabetes Association
ADHF	American Digestive Health Foundation
AF	Arthritis Foundation
AFAR	American Federation for Aging Research
AFOSR	Air Force Office of Scientific Research
AFUD	American Foundation for Urologic Disease
AFUW	Australian Federation of University Women
AGS	American Geriatrics Society
AHA	American Heart Association
AHAF	American Health Assistance Foundation
AFHMR	Alberta Heritage Foundation for Medical Research
AHRQ	Agency for Healthcare Research and Quality
AICR	American Institute for Cancer Research
AIIS	American Institute for Indian Studies
AJA	American Jewish Archives
ALA	American Library Association
ALISE	Association for Library and Information Science Education
AMNH	American Museum of Natural History
AMS	American Musicological Society
ANL	Argonne National Library
ANS	American Numismatic Society
AOA	American Osteopathic Association
APA	American Psychological Association
APSA	American Political Science Association
ARIT	American Research Institute in Turkey
ARO	Army Research Office
ASA	American Statistical Association
ASCSA	American School of Classical Studies at Athens
ASECS	American Society for Eighteenth-Century Studies
ASF	American-Scandinavian Foundation
ASHRAE	American Society of Heating, Refrigerating, and Air Conditioning Engineers
ASME	American Society of Mechanical Engineers
ASNS	American Society for Nutritional Sciences
ASPRS	American Society of Photogrammetry and Remote Sensing
AWU	Associated Western Universities
AWWA	American Water Works Association
BA	British Academy
BWF	Burroughs Wellcome Fund
CBIE	Canadian Bureau for International Education
CCFF	Canadian Cystic Fibrosis Foundation
CDC	Centers for Disease Control and Prevention
CES	Council for European Studies
CF	The Commonwealth Fund
CFF	Cystic Fibrosis Foundation
CFPC	College of Family Physicians of Canada
CFUW	Canadian Federation of University Women
CHEA	Canadian Home Economics Association
CIES	Council for International Exchange of Scholars
CIUS	Canadian Institute of Ukrainian Studies
CLA	Canadian Lung Association
CLF	Canadian Liver Foundation
CRI	Cancer Research Institute
DAAD	Deutscher Akademische Austauschdienst (German Academic Exchange Service)
DHHS	Department of Health and Human Services
DOA	Department of Agriculture
DOC	Department of Commerce
DOD	Department of Defense
DOE	Department of Energy
DOI	Department of the Interior
DOJ	Department of Justice
DOL	Department of Labor
DOS	Department of State
DOT	Department of Transportation
EFA	Epilepsy Foundation of America
EPA	Environmental Protection Agency
ESF	European Science Foundation
ETS	Educational Testing Service
FCAR	Formation de Chercheurs et L'Aide a la Recherche
FDA	Food and Drug Administration
FIC	Fogarty International Center
GAAC	German American Academic Council

HHMI Howard Hughes Medical Institute
HRSA Health Resources and Services Administration
HUD Department of Housing and Urban Development
IRA International Reading Association
IREX International Research and Exchanges Board
IUCP Indiana University Center on Philanthropy
JDF Juvenile Diabetes Foundation International
JMO John M. Olin Foundation
JSPS Japan Society for the Promotion of Science
KFC Kidney Foundation of Canada
LSA Leukemia Society of America
MHRC Manitoba Health Research Council
MLA Medical Library Association
MMA Metropolitan Museum of Art
MSSC Multiple Sclerosis Society of Canada
NAACP National Association for the Advancement of Colored People
NARSAD National Alliance for Research on Schizophrenia and Depression
NASM National Air and Space Museum
NATO North Atlantic Treaty Organization
NCCAM National Center for Complementary and Alternative Medicine
NCI National Cancer Institute
NCIC National Cancer Institute of Canada
NCRR National Center for Research Resources
NEH National Endowment for the Humanities
NEI National Eye Institute
NFID National Foundation for Infectious Diseases
NFWF National Fish and Wildlife Foundation
NHGRI National Human Genome Research Institute
NHLBI National Heart, Lung and Blood Institute
NIA National Institute on Aging
NIAAA National Institute on Alcohol Abuse and Alcoholism
NIAF National Italian American Foundation
NIAID National Institute of Allergy and Infectious Diseases
NIAMS National Institute of Arthritis and Musculoskeletal Skin Diseases
NICHD National Institute of Child Health and Human Development
NIDA National Institute on Drug Abuse
NIDCD National Institute on Deafness and Other Communication Disorders
NIDCR National Institute of Dental and Craniofacial Research
NIDDK National Institute of Diabetes, and Digestive and Kidney Diseases
NIDRR National Institute on Disability and Rehabilitation Research
NIEHS National Institute of Environmental Health Sciences
NIGMS National Institute of General Medical Sciences
NIH National Institutes of Health
NIJ National Institute of Justice
NIMH National Institute of Mental Health
NINDS National Institute of Neurological Disorders and Stroke
NINR National Institute of Nursing Research
NIOSH National Institute for Occupational Safety and Health
NIST National Institute of Standards and Technology
NKF National Kidney Foundation
NL Newberry Library
NLM National Library of Medicine
NMF National Medical Fellowships, Inc.
NMSS National Multiple Sclerosis Society
NOAA National Oceanic and Atmospheric Administration
NRC National Research Council
NSERC Natural Sciences and Engineering Research Council of Canada
NSF National Science Foundation
OAH Organization of American Historians
ONF Oncology Nursing Foundation
ONR Office of Naval Research
OREF Orthopaedic Research and Education Foundation
ORISE Oak Ridge Institute for Science and Education
OSI Open Society Institute
PDF Parkinson's Disease Foundation
PhRMA Pharmaceutical Research and Manufacturers of American Foundation
PHSC The Photographic Historical Society of Canada
RCPSC Royal College of Physicians and Surgeons of Canada
RSC Royal Society of Canada
RWJF Robert Wood Johnson Foundation
SLA Special Libraries Association
SSHRC Social Sciences and Humanities Research Council of Canada
SSRC Social Science Research Council
STTI Sigma Theta Tau International
USHMM United States Holocaust Memorial Museum Research Institute
USIA United States Information Agency
USIP United States Institute of Peace
WAWH Western Association of Woman Historians

and education materials, sponsors meetings and scientific workshops, funds research, and provides referrals to chapters and support groups. Seed grants and research grants are available.
Amount of Grant: $35,000-$255,000
Contact: Pamela Smith, President; (818) 906-2861; fax: (818) 906-2870; email: becca4435@aol.com or atmrf@aol.com
Sponsor: Ataxia Telangiectasia Medical Research Foundation
16224 Elisa Place
Encino, CA 91436-3320

A. Gary Anderson Family Foundation Grants 17
The foundation supports nonprofits in its areas of interest, including arts and culture, higher education, children and youth, and social services. Requests from California receive priority. There are no application deadlines with which to adhere, but application forms are required. Applicants should begin by initially forwarding a letter outlining the proposed project.
Requirements: Funding is primarily for higher education, and arts and culture in California.
Restrictions: Grants are not made to individuals.
Geographic Focus: California
Amount of Grant: $1,000-$25,000 average
Contact: Erin J. Lastinger, President; (714) 685-3990; fax: (714) 685-3994
Sponsor: A. Gary Anderson Family Foundation
300 S. Harbor Boulevard, Suite 1010
Anaheim, CA 92805-3721

A.O. Smith Community Grants 18
The foundation supports nonprofit organizations in communities where A.O. Smith Corporation has facilities. The foundation supports elementary and secondary school projects that focus on the quality of educational programs and curriculum development; civic, cultural, and social welfare of communities; and medical research and improved local health services. Types of support include continuing support, annual campaigns, building/renovation, scholarship funds, and employee matching gifts. Proposals should describe the project's benefits and constituency, budget information including other sources of funding, and how results will be reported. There is no deadline for applications, although proposals to be considered for the following year's foundation budget must be received by October 30.
Requirements: Nonprofit organizations in company areas may apply.
Restrictions: Grants do not support political organizations or organizations whose chief purpose is to influence legislation.
Amount of Grant: $500-$20,000 typically; $2,000 average
Date(s) Application is Due: Oct 30
Contact: Edward J. O'Connor; (414) 359-4000; fax: (414) 359-4064
Internet: http://www.aosmith.com/About/Detail.aspx?id=132
Sponsor: A.O. Smith Foundation
P. O. Box 245008
Milwaukee, WI 53224-9510

A/H Foundation Grants 19
The A/H Foundation was established in California in 1996, and was named after the initials of its two founders, Albert Friedman and Harvey Friedman. Its primary mission is to support: cancer research, community and economic development; law enforcement and police agencies; community health organizations; public and private universities; human services; and Jewish agencies and synagogues. There are no specific deadlines with which to adhere, and initial approach should be by letter.
Requirements: Giving is primarily in the State of California to 501(c)3 organizations (although there is some giving outside of California).
Geographic Focus: California
Amount of Grant: $25,000 maximum
Contact: Keith Rosen; (818) 920-9888; fax: (818) 920-9388; email: info@wantacpa.com
Sponsor: A/H Foundation
15545 Devonshire Street, Suite 210
Mission Hills, CA 91345

AAAAI / Schering Allergy/Immunology Fellowship of Excellence Training Awards 20
The Award will support the two years of training (MDs and DOs) for a fellow at an ACGME-accredited allergy/immunology training program who is a member of an underrepresented minority community, a graduate of a U.S. medical school certified in Internal Medicine or Pediatrics, and a U.S. citizen. The application must be received no later than April 1, and should be completed by the fellow who will start training July 1.
Requirements: Receipt of the Award does not preclude the applicant from obtaining grant support from other sources
Restrictions: Funds may not be used for institutional indirect costs
Amount of Grant: $50,000 per year for two years
Date(s) Application is Due: Apr 1
Contact: Jerome Schultz; (414) 272-6071; fax: (414) 276-6070; email: jschultz@aaaai.org or info@aaaai.org
Internet: http://www.aaaai.org/members/grants%5Fawards/immunology_fellowship/
Sponsor: American Academy of Allergy, Asthma, and Immunology
555 East Wells Street, Suite 1100
Milwaukee, WI 53202-3823

AAAAI Allergy, Asthma and Immunology Education and Research Trust (ART) Allied Health Travel Grants 21
The AAAAI abstract submission and travel grant application provides a new process for growth and learning. The Program includes: presentation of original research; attendance at AAAAI Annual Meeting postgraduate program and symposia; participation in a special program that includes basic research presentations by AAAAI members who are NIH funded researchers in allergy/immunology; information about career opportunities in allergy, asthma and immunology research; and funds for travel (including a stipend for ground transportation), hotel accommodation, and meeting registration.
Requirements: Eligible candidates include first-, second-, and third-year RNs in training.
Restrictions: Individuals with a faculty appointment will not be considered.
Samples: Consuelo M. Carcel, RN, Children's Hospital of Orange County—for The Impact of Home Visits on Retention in a Low-Income School Based Mobile Asthma Clinic, $750 (2007); Patricia S. Hutcheson, Saint Louis University Medical School—for Is Allergic Fungal Sinusitis A Distinct Form Of Chronic Rhinosinusitis?, $750, (2007); Carrie L. Vibbert, RN, University of Maryland School of Medicine—for Does Use of Asthma Controllers Really Indicate Asthma Control?, $750 (2007).
Amount of Grant: $750 maximum
Contact: Mikelle Johnson, Program Manager; (414) 272-6071; fax: (414) 276-3349; email: mjohnson@aaaai.org
Internet: http://www.aaaai.org/members/allied_health/abstractstravelgrants.stm
Sponsor: American Academy of Allergy, Asthma, and Immunology (AAAAI)
555 East Wells Street, Suite 1100
Milwaukee, WI 53202-3823

AAAAI Allergy, Asthma and Immunology Education and Research Trust (ART) Clinical Research Grants 22
Formerly the Education and Research Trust (ERT), training program directors, deans, department chairpersons, and sponsors are invited to nominate promising investigators involved in research dealing with asthma for this grant. The award is a grant in aid provided to the program sponsoring the applicant and is intended to provide salary support. Application should include a biographical sketch, including a curriculum vita, an outline of past accomplishments, a summary of a current research project, and plans for future research.
Requirements: Applicants must be MDs or PhDs who are fellows in training or residents associated with an approved allergy and immunology program and are AAAAI members (or individuals who have submitted applications for membership by September 1).
Restrictions: Individuals with a faculty appointment and past AAAAI research award recipients will not be considered.
Samples: Seema Sharma Aceves, MD, PhD, Children's Hospital San Diego—for Evaluating Disease Severity and Tissue Remodeling in Pediatric Patients with Eosinophilic Esophagitis, $10,000 (2006); Kevin P. O'Brien, MD, Parker, Colorado—for Prevention of Atopy by Combination of Lactobacillus Supplements (pro-TH1) and Omega-3 Supplements (anti-TH2) During Pregnancy and Breastfeeding: A Randomized, Placebo-controlled Trial, $10,000 (2005).
Contact: Angela Gade, Development Senior Project Manager; (414) 272-6071; fax: (414) 276-6070; email: agade@aaaai.org or info@aaaai.org
Internet: http://www.aaaai.org/members/grants_awards
Sponsor: American Academy of Allergy, Asthma, and Immunology
555 East Wells Street, Suite 1100
Milwaukee, WI 53202-3823

AAAAI Allergy, Asthma and Immunology Education and Research Trust (ART) Faculty Development Award 23
The award offers an individual three years of financial support to concentrate his/her research efforts in either basic or clinical allergy and immunology. The objectives of this award are to recognize and support young researchers and promote the specialty of allergy/immunology. The recipient is expected to participate in a seminar at the AAAAI annual meeting, where awardees present their research.
Requirements: The award is open to researchers of junior faculty status—either instructor, assistant professor, or the equivalent grade. This award is directed toward MDs, but in unusual circumstances PhDs will be considered. Applicants must be U.S. or Canadian citizens or permanent residents who are AAAAI members (or have applied for membership by September 1).
Restrictions: Past recipients are ineligible.
Samples: Christine Seroogy, MD, University of Wisconsin School of Medicine and Public Health—for The role of toll-like receptors (TLRs) in CD25+ T regulatory cell development and function, $300,000 over three years (2007); Jordan S. Orange, MD, PhD, Children's Hospital of Philadelphia—for Directed Secretion Through the Immunological Synapse, $300,000 over three years (2005); Sanjeev Jain, MD, PhD, University of Washington—for Development of Structure Based Inhibitors of Nitric Oxide Synthase for the Treatment of Asthma, $300,000 over three years (2003).
Amount of Grant: $100,000 per year for three years
Date(s) Application is Due: Nov 15
Contact: Angela Gade, Development Senior Project Manager; (414) 272-6071; fax: (414) 276-6070; email: agade@aaaai.org or info@aaaai.org
Internet: http://www.aaaai.org/art/
Sponsor: American Academy of Allergy, Asthma, and Immunology
555 East Wells Street, Suite 1100
Milwaukee, WI 53202-3823

AAAAI Phoenix Program Award 24

Funded by the ERT, the AAAAI Allergy Educational Forum and the AAAAI, the grant is a critical element in the development of new allergy/immunology training programs. This grant award can be utilized to effectively increase the size of programs, increase research staff, increase the number of fellows being trained and to develop future faculty members. It is hoped that such additions will increase research quantity and quality, teaching and training mission, and the delivery of health care. Awards average $50,000 to $100,000 per year for three successive years.
Requirements: U.S. college and university medical centers are eligible to apply.
Samples: Penn State University College of Medicine, $150,000 over three years (2006); University of Mississippi Medical Center, $250,000 over three years (2005); University of North Carolina-Chapel Hill, $250,000 over three years (2004).
Amount of Grant: $250,00 over three years maximum
Contact: Angela Gade, Development Senior Project Manager; (414) 272-6071; fax: (414) 276-6070; email: agade@aaaai.org or info@aaaai.org
Internet: http://www.aaaai.org/art/
Sponsor: American Academy of Allergy, Asthma, and Immunology
555 East Wells Street, Suite 1100
Milwaukee, WI 53202-3823

AAAAI Research Award Grants 25

The organization promotes and stimulates research and study in allergy, asthma and immunology. The goal of this program is to support the research by a fellow-in-training, resident, and post-doctoral scholar at an allergy and immunology or a clinical and laboratory immunology training program.
Requirements: Fellow-in-training, resident, or post-doctoral scholar affiliated with an allergy and immunology or clinical and laboratory immunology training program that is in good standing with Residency Review Committee and is fully-accredited by the Accreditation Council of Graduate Medical Education may apply. Applicants must be an AAAAI member or must submit a membership application with the award application.
Restrictions: Applicants with faculty status will not be considered. Past AAAAI research award recipients are not eligible.
Amount of Grant: $25,000 for one year
Contact: Angela Gade, Development Senior Project Manager; (414) 272-6071; fax: (414) 276-6070; email: agade@aaaai.org or info@aaaai.org
Internet: http://www.aaaai.org/members/grants_awards
Sponsor: American Academy of Allergy, Asthma, and Immunology
555 East Wells Street, Suite 1100
Milwaukee, WI 53202-3823

AAAAI STAR Program Grants 26

The goal of the Program is to provide U.S. and Canadian Ph.D. candidates and Ph.D. postdocs with an opportunity to consider research opportunities in the field of allergy and immunology. The AAAAI Annual Meeting provides a forum for those interested in translating basic science advances into clinical practice to network with basic scientists, translational clinical researchers, and clinical experts in allergy/ immunology U.S. and Canadian Ph.D. candidates and Ph.D. postdocs are invited to submit abstracts for presentation at the AAAAI Annual Meeting. Up to 40 selected participants will be invited to participate in the STAR Program, which will include: presentation of original research at the STAR Program; attendance at AAAAI Annual Meeting postgraduate program and symposia; participation in a special STAR Program that includes basic research presentations by AAAAI members who are NIH funded researchers in allergy/ immunology; information about career opportunities in allergy, asthma and immunology research; and funds for travel (including a stipend for ground transportation), hotel accommodation, and meeting registration.
Requirements: Eligible candidates include first-, second-, and third-year MD fellows in training in either an allergy and immunology or a clinical and laboratory immunology training program approved by the Accreditation Council of Graduate Medical Education or a clinical immunology and allergy training program approved by the Royal College of Physicians and Surgeons of Canada.
Restrictions: Individuals with a faculty appointment will not be considered.
Contact: Mikelle Johnson, Program Manager; (414) 272-6071; fax: (414) 276-3349; email: mjohnson@aaaai.org
Internet: http://www.aaaai.org/members/allied_health/abstractstravelgrants.stm
Sponsor: American Academy of Allergy, Asthma, and Immunology
555 East Wells Street, Suite 1100
Milwaukee, WI 53202-3823

AAAAI Summer Clinical Research Fellowship Medical Student Grants 27

The Program goal is to award grants to medical students wishing to conduct clinical research in allergy/immunology during their summer recess in order to encourage their consideration of careers as a clinician in allergy/immunology. Grants will be awarded to outstanding medical students who wish to pursue clinical research. Clinical topics for research examples include optimizing health care of asthma, collecting a series of cases with an interesting diagnosis and preparing a literature review of the topic, a case report with a literature review, reviewing practice parameters related to management of a problem in allergy/immunology and applying to care in a clinic or office, as well as other topics of interest in the practice of allergy/immunology.
Requirements: Applicant must be a full-time medical student residing in the U.S. or Canada and will have completed at least 8 months of medical school by May 15.
Restrictions: Past Summer Fellowship Grant recipients are not eligible.
Amount of Grant: $2,000
Date(s) Application is Due: Mar 3
Contact: Program Administrator; (414) 272-6071; fax: (414) 276-6070; email: info@aaaai.org
Internet: http://www.aaaai.org/members/grants%5Fawards/
Sponsor: American Academy of Allergy, Asthma, and Immunology (AAAAI)
555 East Wells Street, Suite 1100
Milwaukee, WI 53202-3823

AAAAI Summer Research Fellowship Medical Student Grants 28

Fellowships are awarded on an annual basis to assist medical students interested in pursuing research in allergy and immunology during their summer recess. The fellowships will be awarded to outstanding individuals who wish to pursue research in the following areas: physiology of allergic diseases, pharmacology of allergy and inflammation, basic cellular and molecular immunology, AIDS, and other topics pertinent to the understanding of allergic and immune mechanisms of disease.
Requirements: Applicant must be a full time medical student residing in the U.S. or Canada and must have successfully completed at least eight months of medical school by May 15.
Restrictions: Past recipients are ineligible.
Samples: Jason Konner, Aaron Diamond AIDS Research Ctr (New York, NY)—summer fellowship recipient, $1500.; Goron Lai, Johns Hopkins Asthma and Allergy Ctr (Baltimore, MD)—summer fellowship recipient, $1500.
Amount of Grant: $2,000
Date(s) Application is Due: Mar 3
Contact: Program Administrator; (414) 272-6071; fax: (414) 276-6070; email: info@aaaai.org
Internet: http://www.aaaai.org/members/grants%5Fawards/
Sponsor: American Academy of Allergy, Asthma, and Immunology (AAAAI)
555 East Wells Street, Suite 1100
Milwaukee, WI 53202-3823

AAAS Science & Technology Policy Fellowships - National Defense and Global Security 29

Fellows spend one year contributing external perspective and expertise on technology in defense policy, national and international security and systems analysis, and assisting with project and program oversight. Fellows will be placed in one of the following: Federal Bureau of Investigation (FBI), Nuclear Regulatory Commission, U.S. Department of Defense or U.S. Department of Homeland Security. Fellows will work on a variety of issues related to defense policy, national security, weapons of mass destruction, technology applications, defense systems analysis and support, and program oversight and management. Assignments may involve significant interagency, congressional or international activity. The program includes an orientation on international affairs and executive branch and congressional operations, and a year-long seminar series on issues involving science, technology and public policy. Fellows should not expect to work specifically on technical issues related to their dissertations or previous post-doctoral appointments, but rather to apply their technical, organizational, and communication skills to technical and policy issues in the placement agency. Additionally, Fellows help increase the awareness of the placement agency and its departments as a challenging and rewarding career environment for scientists and engineers.
Requirements: All applicants must have a doctoral-level degree (PhD, MD, DVM, DSc, PharmD, and other terminal degrees), in any physical, biological, health/medical or social science, any field of engineering, or any relevant interdisciplinary field (individuals with a master's degree in engineering and at least three years of post-degree professional experience also may apply). Note: All requirements for the degree must be completed by the application deadline. A prospective fellow must demonstrate exceptional competence in their specialty appropriate to their career stage, and have the strong endorsement of three references. Show an understanding of the opportunities for science and engineering to support a broad range of non-scientific issues, and display a commitment to apply their scientific or technical expertise to serve society; Exhibit awareness and sensitivity to the political, economic and social issues that influence policy; Be articulate communicators, both verbally and in writing, to decision-makers and non-scientific audiences, and have the ability to work effectively with individuals and groups outside the scientific community; Demonstrate integrity and good judgment, and the flexibility and willingness to address policy issues outside their scientific realm.
Restrictions: Federal employees are ineligible. All applicants must be U.S. citizens (dual citizenship from the United States and another country is acceptable). Some program areas and host agencies seek additional qualifications. Holding a Title 42 position is considered federal employment and therefore renders an applicant ineligible for a AAAS Science & Technology Policy Fellowship. Individuals working in postdoctoral positions at government labs or agencies, for private contractors, and in state government posts are not federal employees and therefore are eligible for the AAAS Fellowships.
Amount of Grant: Stipend: (depending on degree level and post-degree experience) $67,000-$87,000. Plus professional development, travel and relocation reimbursement and health insurance
Date(s) Application is Due: Dec 15
Contact: Rick Kempinski, Senior Program Manager; (202) 326-6700; fax: (202) 289-4950; email: rkempinski@aaas.org or fellowships@aaas.org
Internet: http://fellowships.aaas.org/02_Areas/02_index.shtml
Sponsor: American Association for the Advancement of Science
1200 New York Avenue, NW
Washington, DC 20005

AACAP Beatrix A. Hamburg Award for the Best New Research Poster by a Child and Adolescent Psychiatry Resident 30

This award recognizes the author of the best new research poster presented at the AACAP Annual Meeting. The award provides a $1,000 honorarium. The recipient will receive a plaque at the Young Leader Awards Ceremony during the AACAP Annual Meeting. There is no application process for this award. The AACAP Program Committee will review all new research poster submissions by child and adolescent psychiatry residents to determine the recipient of this award. The recipient will be notified through an acceptance letter. Non-recipients will not be notified.

Requirements: The author must be a child and adolescent psychiatry resident at an accredited institution and AACAP member. Applicants must: be a child and adolescent psychiatry resident; attend an accredited institution; be an AACAP member; and attend and present a new research poster at the AACAP Annual Meeting.

Amount of Grant: $1,000 honorarium

Date(s) Application is Due: Jun 14

Contact: Stacie Hall, Director; (202) 966-7300, ext. 113; fax: (202) 966-2891; email: shall@aacap.org

Internet: http://www.aacap.org/cs/root/research_and_training_awards/aacap_beatrix_a_hamburg_award_for_the_best_new_research_poster_by_a_child_and_adolescent_psychiatry_resident_at_the_aacap_annual_meeting

Sponsor: American Academy of Child and Adolescent Psychiatry
3615 Wisconsin Avenue, NW
Washington, DC 20016-3007

AACAP Child and Adolescent Psychiatry (CAP) Teaching Scholarships 31

The program is offered through the Harvard Macy Institute for Physician Educators Program, and is designed to fashion master teachers who will inspire medical students and residents to become child and adolescent psychiatrists. To facilitate this objective, the field of child and adolescent psychiatry needs educators trained in state-of-the-art teaching principles, methodologies, and technologies of adult education and learning. The AACAP Teaching Scholars Program addresses this challenge by creating a group of highly trained medical educators. This program is an opportunity for CAP faculty who are committed to teaching careers to train at the prestigious Harvard Medical School, gain research and teaching experience, and to give back to future generations of CAP faculty.

Requirements: Applicants must: have a mid-level academic appointment (Senior Assistant Professor, Associate Professor or early Professor); have a commitment to an active career in medical student/resident teaching; have been accepted by the joint AACAP-Harvard Macy Institute admissions group; attend at two meetings in Boston, MA (12 days in January and 6 days in May); have active participation in a collaborative CAP project spanning January through May; be potential participants as program faculty during a subsequent second year; participate in AACAP Annual Meetings and Mid-Year Institutes to bring modern teaching and educational methods to the AACAP membership; participate in an AACAP College of Teaching Scholars; and possess strong support from the applicant's School of Medicine, Department of Psychiatry and Division of Child and Adolescent Psychiatry (letter of institutional commitment and some release time required).

Amount of Grant: $8,500 maximum over two years

Date(s) Application is Due: Jul 15

Contact: Gabe Robbins; (202) 966-7300, ext. 117; fax: (202) 966-2891; email: grobbins@aacap.org

Internet: http://www.aacap.org/cs/root/research_and_training_awards/child_and_adolescent_psychiatry_teaching_scholars_program

Sponsor: American Academy of Child and Adolescent Psychiatry
3615 Wisconsin Avenue, NW
Washington, DC 20016-3007

AACAP Congressional Fellowships 32

The Program is designed to educate policy makers and Congressional staff about child and adolescent psychiatry and to foster awareness of children's mental health issues. This experience will allow the Fellow to develop a keen understanding of how public policy affects patient care, education, and health insurance issues. The AACAP Congressional Fellow will be placed with a Congressional office or Committee where they will gain invaluable experience as they assist in the development of legislative and public policy initiatives. The award includes an $85,000 stipend, up to $3,000 in relocation or moving expenses, and health insurance for the length of the fellowship program.

Requirements: Successful applicants must: be an AACAP member; be a PGY-4 psychiatry resident or beyond; have completed training in or be scheduled to complete training in one of the child and adolescent psychiatry programs (CAP training program, Combined General Psychiatry/CAP Program, or Triple Board Program); have a demonstrated interest in public policy issues; exhibit an interest in applying medical and scientific knowledge to the resolution of public policy issues; and be a U.S. citizen or permanent resident.

Amount of Grant: $85,000 stipend; up to $3,000 in relocation or moving expenses

Date(s) Application is Due: Feb 1

Contact: Gabe Robbins; (202) 966-7300, ext. 117; fax: (202) 966-2891; email: grobbins@aacap.org

Internet: http://www.aacap.org/cs/root/legislative_action/2008_congressional_fellowship_program

Sponsor: American Academy of Child and Adolescent Psychiatry
3615 Wisconsin Avenue, NW
Washington, DC 20016-3007

AACAP Educational Outreach Program for Child and Adolescent Psychiatry Residents 33

The Educational Outreach Program (EOP) funding provides the opportunity for up to 50 child and adolescent psychiatry residents to receive a formal overview to the field of child and adolescent psychiatry, establish child and adolescent psychiatrists as mentors and experience the AACAP Annual Meeting. Participants will be exposed to the breadth and depth of the field of child and adolescent psychiatry, including research opportunities, access to mentors, and various networking opportunities. Participation in this program provides up to $750 for travel expenses.

Requirements: Applicants must: be child and adolescent psychiatry residents at the time of the AACAP Annual Meeting; be currently enrolled in a residency program in the United States; be residents in their first or second year of child fellowship training are eligible (Triple Boarders in their fourth or fifth year of training in their triple board programs are eligible); either be members of the AACAP or have a membership application pending at the time of application; and attend all AACAP Annual Meeting events specified by AACAP.

Amount of Grant: $750 maximum

Date(s) Application is Due: Jul 12

Contact: Gabe Robbins; (202) 966-7300, ext. 117; fax: (202) 966-2891; email: grobbins@aacap.org

Internet: http://www.aacap.org/cs/residents/eop-capfellows

Sponsor: American Academy of Child and Adolescent Psychiatry
3615 Wisconsin Avenue, NW
Washington, DC 20016-3007

AACAP Educational Outreach Program for General Psychiatry Residents 34

The Educational Outreach Program (EOP) for General Psychiatry residents provides the opportunity for up to 20 general psychiatry residents to receive a formal overview to the field of child and adolescent psychiatry, establish child and adolescent psychiatrists as mentors and experience the AACAP Annual Meeting. Participants will be exposed to the breadth and depth of the field of child and adolescent psychiatry, including research opportunities, access to mentors, and various networking opportunities. Participation in this program provides up to $1,500 for travel expenses to the AACAP Annual Meeting.

Requirements: Applicants must: be general psychiatry residents at the time of the AACAP Annual Meeting; be currently enrolled in a residency program in the United States; be residents in their first, second or third year of general psychiatry training (Triple Boarders in their first, second or third year of training in their triple board programs are eligible); either be members of the AACAP or have a membership application pending at the time of application; and attend all AACAP Annual Meeting events specified by AACAP.

Amount of Grant: $1,500 maximum

Date(s) Application is Due: Jul 12

Contact: Gabe Robbins; (202) 966-7300, ext. 117; fax: (202) 966-2891; email: grobbins@aacap.org

Internet: http://www.aacap.org/cs/residents/eop-generalresidents

Sponsor: American Academy of Child and Adolescent Psychiatry
3615 Wisconsin Avenue, NW
Washington, DC 20016-3007

AACAP Elaine Schlosser Lewis Award for Research on Attention-Deficit Disorder 35

This annual award acknowledges outstanding leadership and continuous contributions in the field of research by giving $5,000 for the best paper published in the Journal on attention-deficit disorder written by a child and adolescent psychiatrist. The award winner will be recognized at a Distinguished Awards Luncheon and make an Honors Presentation about his or her work during the AACAP Annual Meeting.

Requirements: Nomination letters must be accompanied by a CV for the individual nominated.

Samples: Margaret Weiss, M.D., Children's Hospital Vancouver, BC—Sleep Hygiene and Melatonin Treatment for Children and Adolescents With ADHD and Initial Insomnia (2006).

Amount of Grant: $5,000

Date(s) Application is Due: May 7

Contact: Alyssa Sommer, Research Coordinator; (202) 966-7300, ext. 157; fax: (202) 364-5925; email: asommer@aacap.org

Internet: http://www.aacap.org/cs/root/research_and_training_awards/aacap_journal_awards

Sponsor: American Academy of Child and Adolescent Psychiatry
3615 Wisconsin Avenue, NW
Washington, DC 20016-3007

AACAP George Tarjan Award for Contributions in Developmental Disabilities 36

This award recognizes a child and adolescent psychiatrist and Academy member who has made significant contributions in a lifetime career or single seminal work to the understanding or care of those with mental retardation and developmental disabilities. These contributions must have national and/or international stature and clearly demonstrate lasting effects. The contributions may be in areas of teaching, research, program development, direct clinical service, advocacy or administrative commitment. A cash prize of up to $1,000 will be awarded. The award winner will be recognized at a Distinguished Awards Luncheon and make an Honors Presentation about his or her work during the AACAP Annual Meeting.

Requirements: Nomination letters must be accompanied by a CV for the individual nominated.

Amount of Grant: $1,000
Date(s) Application is Due: Apr 30
Contact: Edwin Cook, Jr., M.D. or Byron King, M.D., Co-Chairs; (202) 966-7300; fax: (202) 966-2891; email: training@aacap.org
Internet: http://www.aacap.org/cs/distinguishedmembers
Sponsor: American Academy of Child and Adolescent Psychiatry
3615 Wisconsin Avenue, NW
Washington, DC 20016

AACAP Irving Philips Award for Prevention 37

This award recognizes a child and adolescent psychiatrist and Academy member who has made significant contributions in a lifetime career or single seminal work to the prevention of mental illness in children and adolescents. These contributions must have national and/or international stature and clearly demonstrate lasting effects. The contributions may be in the areas of teaching, research, program development, direct clinical service, advocacy or administrative commitment. The award pays $2,500 to the winner and a $2,000 donation to a prevention program or center of the awardee's choice. The award winner will be recognized at a Distinguished Awards Luncheon and make an Honors Presentation about his or her work during the AACAP Annual Meeting.
Requirements: Nomination letters must be accompanied by a CV for the individual nominated.
Samples: Charles Zeanah, M.D., Tulane University New Orleans, LA—Preventing Adverse Outcomes for Abandoned Children: The Bucharest Early Intervention Project (2006).
Amount of Grant: $2,500 to winner, plus $2,000 donation
Date(s) Application is Due: Apr 30
Contact: Harry H. Wright, M.D. Chair, Prevention Committee; (202) 966-7300; fax: (202) 966-2891; email: training@aacap.org
Internet: http://www.aacap.org/cs/distinguishedmembers
Sponsor: American Academy of Child and Adolescent Psychiatry
3615 Wisconsin Avenue, NW
Washington, DC 20016

AACAP Jeanne Spurlock Lecture and Award on Diversity and Culture 38

The lecture and award reflects the spirit of the nomination for outstanding contributions to diversity and culture and in some way encourages individuals from diverse cultural backgrounds to become child and adolescent psychiatrists. Nominees should be individuals who have made contributions in the areas of social awareness including: civil rights; spirituality and/or religion; social welfare; public information; scientific research; education and mentoring; and the arts (literature, theatre, music, painting, sculpture or photography). The award includes an honorarium of $2,500, with the award winner being recognized at a Distinguished Awards Luncheon where he or she will make an honors award presentation about his or her work during the AACAP Annual Meeting.
Amount of Grant: $2,500
Date(s) Application is Due: May 1
Contact: Jennifer Mecidus, Clinical Practice Manager; (202) 966-7300, ext. 137; fax: (202) 966-9518; email: jmedicus@aacap.org
Internet: http://www.aacap.org/cs/awards
Sponsor: American Academy of Child and Adolescent Psychiatry
3615 Wisconsin Avenue, NW
Washington, DC 20016-3007

AACAP Jeanne Spurlock Minority Medical Student Clinical Fellowship in Child and Adolescent Psychiatry 39

Up to fourteen (14) fellowships are available each year for minority medical students to explore a career in child and adolescent psychiatry, gain valuable work experience, and meet leaders in the child and adolescent psychiatry field. The fellowship opportunity provides up to $3,500 for 12 weeks of clinical training under a child and adolescent psychiatrist mentor. Research assignments may include responsibility for part of the observation or evaluation, developing specific aspects of the research mechanisms, conducting interviews or tests, use of rating scales, and psychological or cognitive testing of subjects. Contact AACAP for applications.
Requirements: African American, Asian American, Native American, Alaskan Native, Mexican American, Hispanic, and Pacific Islander students in accredited U.S. medical schools are eligible.
Amount of Grant: $3,500 each, plus expenses to attend the annual meeting
Date(s) Application is Due: Mar 1
Contact: Gabe Robbins; (202) 966-7300, ext. 117; fax: (202) 966-2891; email: grobbins@aacap.org
Internet: http://www.aacap.org/cs/students/opportunities/SpurlockClinical
Sponsor: American Academy of Child and Adolescent Psychiatry
3615 Wisconsin Avenue, NW
Washington, DC 20016

AACAP Jeanne Spurlock Research Fellowship in Substance Abuse and Addiction for Minority Medical Students 40

The Fellowship offers a unique opportunity for minority medical students to explore a research career in substance abuse in relation to child and adolescent psychiatry, gain valuable work experience, and meet leaders in the child and adolescent psychiatry field. The fellowship opportunity provides up to $3,500 for 12 weeks of summer research under a child and adolescent psychiatrist researcher/mentor. The research training plan must provide for significant contact between the student and the mentor and for exposure to state-of-the-art drug abuse and addiction research. The plan should include program planning discussions, instruction in research planning and implementation, regular meetings with the mentor, laboratory director, and the research group, and assigned readings. Research assignments may include responsibility for part of the observation or evaluation, developing specific aspects of the research mechanisms, conducting interviews or tests, use of rating scales, and psychological or cognitive testing of subjects.
Requirements: All fellowship participants must attend the AACAP Annual Meeting. Applications are considered from African-American, Native American, Alaskan Native, Mexican American, Hispanic, Asian, and Pacific Islander students in accredited U.S. medical schools.
Amount of Grant: $3,500 maximum
Date(s) Application is Due: Mar 1
Contact: Gabe Robbins; (202) 966-7300, ext. 117; fax: (202) 966-2891; email: grobbins@aacap.org or apartner@aacap.org
Internet: http://www.aacap.org/cs/students/opportunities/SpurlockResearch
Sponsor: American Academy of Child and Adolescent Psychiatry
3615 Wisconsin Avenue, NW
Washington, DC 20016

AACAP Junior Investigator Awards 41

The AACAP Junior Investigator Award offers two awards of up to $30,000 a year for two years for child and adolescent psychiatry junior faculty (assistant professor level or equivalent). The program is intended to facilitate innovative research. The research may be basic or clinical in nature but must be relevant to our understanding, treatment and prevention of child and adolescent mental health disorders. The award also includes the cost of attending the AACAP Annual Meeting for five days.
Requirements: Recipients are required to submit a poster or oral presentation on his or her research for the AACAP's Annual Meeting. Applicants must: be board eligible or certified in child and adolescent psychiatry; have a doctoral level degree and be in a faculty or independent research position; and have an on-site mentor who has had experience in the type of research that is being proposed that will normally include work with children and adolescents. Candidates must either be AACAP members or have a membership application pending (not paid by the award).
Restrictions: Applicants who have served as Principal Investigator on an NIH R01 grant are not eligible.
Amount of Grant: $30,000 maximum per year for two years
Date(s) Application is Due: Mar 1
Contact: Alyssa Sommer, Research Coordinator; (202) 966-7300, ext. 157; fax: (202) 364-5925; email: asommer@aacap.org
Internet: http://www.aacap.org/cs/root/research_and_training_awards/aacap_junior_investigator_awards
Sponsor: American Academy of Child and Adolescent Psychiatry
3615 Wisconsin Avenue, NW
Washington, DC 20016-3007

AACAP Klingenstein Third Generation Foundation Award for Research in Depression or Suicide 42

This annual award acknowledges outstanding leadership and continuous contributions in the field of research by giving $5,000 for the best paper on suicide and/or depression published in the Journal during the past year. The award winner will be recognized at a Distinguished Awards Luncheon and make an Honors Presentation about his or her work during the AACAP Annual Meeting.
Requirements: Nomination letters must be accompanied by a CV for the individual nominated.
Samples: David DeMaso, M.D., Children's Hospital Boston, MA—Depression Experience Journal: A Computer-Based Intervention for Families Facing Childhood Depression (2006).
Amount of Grant: $5,000
Date(s) Application is Due: May 7
Contact: Gabe Robbins; (202) 966-7300, ext. 117; fax: (202) 966-2891; email: grobbins@aacap.org
Internet: http://www.aacap.org/cs/root/research_and_training_awards/aacap_journal_awards
Sponsor: American Academy of Child and Adolescent Psychiatry
3615 Wisconsin Avenue, NW
Washington, DC 20016-3007

AACAP Norbert and Charlotte Rieger Award for Scientific Achievement 43

This award is given annually for the most significant article published in the Journal of the American Academy of Child and Adolescent Psychiatry (JAACAP) in the past year (July-May). The article must be written by a psychiatrist specializing in child and/or adolescent psychiatry and cannot be a review.
Requirements: The only submissions accepted are papers from child and adolescent psychiatrists that have been published in the Journal during the past year.
Amount of Grant: $4,500 maximum
Date(s) Application is Due: May 7
Contact: Gabe Robbins; (202) 966-7300, ext. 117; fax: (202) 966-2891; email: grobbins@aacap.org
Internet: http://www.aacap.org/cs/root/research_and_training_awards/aacap_journal_awards
Sponsor: American Academy of Child and Adolescent Psychiatry
3615 Wisconsin Avenue, NW
Washington, DC 20016-3007

AACAP Norbert and Charlotte Rieger Psychodynamic Psychotherapy Award 44

The Award recognizes the best published or unpublished paper, written by an AACAP member that addresses the use of psychodynamic psychotherapy in clinical practice and fosters development, teaching, and practice of psychodynamic psychotherapy within child and adolescent psychiatry. Papers that express a novel hypothesis, raise questions about existing theory, or integrate new neuroscience and developmental psychotherapy research with psychodynamic principles may be nominated. Unpublished, new papers and papers published within the last three years may be submitted by their authors. Published papers may be nominated by any member of the AACAP. Authors may be senior or junior faculty members or residents. Delivery of the winning paper will be made at the AACAP Annual Meeting Honors Presentation.
Amount of Grant: $4,500
Date(s) Application is Due: May 7
Contact: Gabe Robbins; (202) 966-7300, ext. 117; fax: (202) 966-2891; email: grobbins@aacap.org
Internet: http://www.aacap.org/cs/2007_press_releases/rachel_seidel_md_wins_aacap_2007_norbert_and_charlotte_rieger_psychodynamic_psychotherapy_award
Sponsor: American Academy of Child and Adolescent Psychiatry
3615 Wisconsin Avenue, NW
Washington, DC 20016-3007

AACAP Pilot Research Award for Attention-Deficit Disorder, Supported by the Elaine Schlosser Lewis Fund 45

The Award for Attention-Deficit Disorder is available for a junior faculty or child psychiatry resident, and is supported by the Elaine Schlosser Lewis Fund. The award recipient will be encouraged to work with a child and adolescent psychiatric investigator with expertise in his or her particular area of interest. Work must be completed within one year of receipt of the award.
Requirements: Candidates must be board eligible, certified in child and adolescent psychiatry, or enrolled in a child psychiatry residency or fellowship program. Candidates must also have a faculty appointment in an accredited medical school or be in a fully accredited child and adolescent psychiatry clinical research or training program.
Restrictions: At the time of application, candidates may not have more than two years experience following graduation from residency/fellowship training. Candidates must not have any previous significant, individual research funding in the field of child and adolescent mental health. These include the following: NIMH/NIH Funding (Small Grants, T Award or R-01) or similar foundation or industry research funding.
Amount of Grant: $15,000
Date(s) Application is Due: May 7
Contact: Alyssa Sommer, Research Coordinator; (202) 966-7300, ext. 157; fax: (202) 364-5925; email: asommer@aacap.org
Internet: http://www.aacap.org/cs/root/research_and_training_awards/pilot_research_award_for_attention_disorder_for_a_junior_faculty_or_child_psychiatry_resident_supported_by_the_elaine_schlosser_lewis_fund
Sponsor: American Academy of Child and Adolescent Psychiatry
3615 Wisconsin Avenue, NW
Washington, DC 20016-3007

AACAP Pilot Research Award for Learning Disabilities, Supported by the Elaine Schlosser Lewis Fund 46

The Award for Learning Disabilities and Psychiatric Disorders is available for a junior faculty or child psychiatry resident, and is supported by the Elaine Schlosser Lewis Fund. The award encourages work with a child and adolescent psychiatric investigator with expertise in his or her particular area of interest. Work must be completed within one year of receipt of the award. Please note that travel to both the Annual Meeting and the Research Update Luncheon is not included in the award and is the responsibility of the recipient.
Requirements: Candidates must be board eligible, certified in child and adolescent psychiatry, or enrolled in a child psychiatry residency or fellowship program. Candidates must also have a faculty appointment in an accredited medical school or be in a fully accredited child and adolescent psychiatry clinical research or training program.
Restrictions: Candidates must not have any previous significant, individual research funding in the field of child and adolescent mental health. These include the following: NIMH/NIH Funding (Small Grants, T Award or R-01) or similar foundation or industry research funding. The recipient must be an AACAP member at the time of application and agree to present his or her research.
Amount of Grant: $15,000
Date(s) Application is Due: May 7
Contact: Alyssa Sommer, Research Coordinator; (202) 966-7300, ext. 157; fax: (202) 364-5925; email: asommer@aacap.org
Internet: http://www.aacap.org/cs/root/research_and_training_awards/pilot_research_award_for_learning_disabilities_for_a_junior_faculty_or_child_psychiatry_resident_supported_by_the_elaine_schlosser_lewis_fund
Sponsor: American Academy of Child and Adolescent Psychiatry
3615 Wisconsin Avenue, NW
Washington, DC 20016-3007

AACAP Pilot Research Awards, Supported by Eli Lilly and Company 47

Eight awards are available each year to junior faculty and child psychiatry fellows for pilot research with child and adolescent psychiatric researchers. Award recipients will be matched with child and adolescent psychiatric investigators working in their particular area of interest to act as consultants or mentors during the course of the award. Work must be completed within one year of receipt of the award.
Requirements: Candidates must be board eligible, certified in child and adolescent psychiatry, or enrolled in a child psychiatry residency or fellowship program. Candidates must have a faculty appointment in an accredited medical school or be in a fully accredited child and adolescent psychiatry clinical research or training program.
Restrictions: At the time of application, candidates may not have more than two years experience following graduation from residency/fellowship training. Candidates must not have any previous significant, individual research funding in the field of child and adolescent mental health. These include the following: NIMH/NIH Funding (Small Grants, T Award or R-01) or similar foundation or industry research funding.
Amount of Grant: $15,000
Date(s) Application is Due: May 7
Contact: Alyssa Sommer, Research Coordinator; (202) 966-7300, ext. 157; fax: (202) 364-5925; email: asommer@aacap.org
Internet: http://www.aacap.org/cs/root/research_and_training_awards/aacap_pilot_research_award_for_junior_faculty_and_child_psychiatry_fellows_supported_by_lilly_usa_llc
Sponsor: American Academy of Child and Adolescent Psychiatry
3615 Wisconsin Avenue, NW
Washington, DC 20016-3007

AACAP Quest for the Test Bipolar Disorder Pilot Research Award 48

The AACAP Quest for the Test Bipolar Disorder Pilot Research Award, supported by The Ryan Licht Sang Bipolar Foundation, offers $15,000 for child and adolescent psychiatry residents and junior faculty who have an interest in beginning a career in child and adolescent mental health research. Proposed research projects should address questions concerning the pathology or diagnosis of children and adolescents with bipolar disorder. The award also includes the cost of attending the AACAP Annual Meeting for five days.
Requirements: The recipient is required to submit a poster presentation on his or her research for the AACAP's Annual Meeting. Candidates must be board eligible, certified in child and adolescent psychiatry, or enrolled in a child psychiatry residency or fellowship program. Candidates must also have a faculty appointment in an accredited medical school or be in a fully accredited child and adolescent psychiatry clinical research or training program.
Restrictions: At the time of application, candidates may not have more than two years experience following graduation from residency/fellowship training. Candidates must not have any previous significant, individual research funding in the field of child and adolescent mental health. These include the following: NIH Funding (K or R level grants) or similar foundation or industry research funding.
Amount of Grant: $15,000
Date(s) Application is Due: May 7
Contact: Alyssa Sommer, Research Coordinator; (202) 966-7300, ext. 157; fax: (202) 364-5925; email: asommer@aacap.org
Internet: http://www.aacap.org/cs/root/research_and_training_awards/aacap_quest_for_the_test_bipolar_disorder_pilot_research_award
Sponsor: American Academy of Child and Adolescent Psychiatry
3615 Wisconsin Avenue, NW
Washington, DC 20016-3007

AACAP Rieger Service Program Award for Excellence 49

This award recognizes innovative programs that address prevention, diagnosis, or treatment of mental illnesses in children and adolescents, and serve as model programs to the community. This award of $4,500 is shared among the awardee and his or her service program. The award winner will be recognized at a Distinguished Awards Luncheon and make an Honors Presentation about his or her work during the Annual Meeting.
Requirements: Nomination letters must be accompanied by a CV and any support materials for the individual or organization nominated.
Samples: Bradley Stein, M.D., Ph.D., Rand Corporation, Pittsburgh, PA—The Development, Implementation, and Dissemination of an Effective School-based Program for Children Exposed to Violence (2006).
Amount of Grant: $4,500
Date(s) Application is Due: Apr 30
Contact: Kaye McGinty, M.D., and Mark Chenven, M.D., Co-Chairs; (202) 966-7300; fax: (202) 966-2891; email: aboccanelli@aacap.org
Internet: http://www.aacap.org/cs/distinguishedmembers
Sponsor: American Academy of Child and Adolescent Psychiatry
3615 Wisconsin Avenue, NW
Washington, DC 20016

AACAP Robert Cancro Academic Leadership Award 50

This award recognizes a currently serving General Psychiatry Training Director, Medical School Dean, CEO of a Training Institution, Chair of a Department of Pediatrics or Chair of a Department of Psychiatry for his or her contributions to the promotion of child and adolescent psychiatry. Named in honor of Robert Cancro, M.D., Chairman at New York University, this award offers $500 to the awardee. Nominations for the award may be made by Child and Adolescent Training Directors or Division Directors. The recipient of this award will receive a plaque and be recognized at the AACAP Annual Meeting. The award recipient will be honored at the Distinguished Awards Luncheon, Training Directors Dinner, and will provide an Honors Presentation on his or her work during the Annual Meeting.
Requirements: Nominations must include a CV for the individual nominated
Amount of Grant: $500
Date(s) Application is Due: Apr 30

Contact: Jeffrey Hunt, M.D. and Dorothy Stubbe, M.D., Co-Chairs; (202) 966-7300; fax: (202) 966-2891; email:
Internet: http://www.aacap.org/cs/distinguishedmembers
Sponsor: American Academy of Child and Adolescent Psychiatry
3615 Wisconsin Avenue, NW
Washington, DC 20016

AACAP Sidney Berman Award for the School-Based Study and Intervention for Learning Disorders and Mental Ilness 51
This award recognizes an individual or program that has shown outstanding achievement in the school-based study or delivery of intervention for learning disorders and mental illness. A cash prize of $4,500 will be awarded. The award winner will be recognized at a Distinguished Awards Luncheon and make an Honors Presentation about his or her work during the AACAP Annual Meeting.
Requirements: Nomination letters must be accompanied by a CV for the individual nominated or program information.
Amount of Grant: $4,500
Date(s) Application is Due: Apr 30
Contact: Steven Adelsheim, M.D. and Richard Mattison, M.D., Co-Chairs; (202) 966-7300; fax: (202) 966-2891; email: aboccanelli@aacap.org
Internet: http://www.aacap.org/cs/distinguishedmembers
Sponsor: American Academy of Child and Adolescent Psychiatry
3615 Wisconsin Avenue, NW
Washington, DC 20016

AACAP Simon Wile Leadership in Consultation Award 52
This annual award acknowledges outstanding leadership and continuous contributions in the field of liaison child and adolescent psychiatry. Nomination letters must be accompanied by a CV for the individual nominated. The award winner will be recognized at a Distinguished Awards Luncheon and make an Honors Presentation about his or her work during the AACAP Annual Meeting.
Requirements: Practicing child and adolescent psychiatrists are eligible for nomination.
Amount of Grant: $500 honorarium and duty of presentation at annual meeting
Date(s) Application is Due: Apr 30
Contact: Richard Martini, M.D., David DeMaso, M.D., and Read Sulik, M.D., Co-Chairs; (202) 966-7300; fax: (202) 966-2891; email: aboccanelli@aacap.org
Internet: http://www.aacap.org/cs/distinguishedmembers
Sponsor: American Academy of Child and Adolescent Psychiatry
3615 Wisconsin Avenue, NW
Washington, DC 20016

AACAP Summer Medical Student Fellowships 53
The American Academy of Child and Adolescent Psychiatry (AACAP) is offering summer fellowships for work with a child and adolescent psychiatrist mentor in a clinical or research setting. Sponsored by the AACAP Campaign for America's Kids, the Fellowships offer a chance for up to 6 medical students to explore a career in child and adolescent psychiatry, gain valuable work experience, and meet leaders in the child and adolescent psychiatry field. The fellowship opportunity provides up to $3,500 for 12 weeks of clinical or research training under a child and adolescent psychiatrist mentor.
Requirements: Applicants must be students enrolled in accredited U.S. medical schools.
Amount of Grant: $3,500
Contact: Gabe Robbins; (202) 966-7300, ext. 117; fax: (202) 966-2891; email: grobbins@aacap.org or apartner@aacap.org
Internet: http://www.aacap.org/cs/students/summerfellowship
Sponsor: American Academy of Child and Adolescent Psychiatry
3615 Wisconsin Avenue, NW
Washington, DC 20016

AACAP Systems of Care Special Program Scholarships 54
The scholarship includes up to $750 for travel expenses to the AACAP's Annual Meeting. Residents may apply to both the Special Program Scholarship and the Educational Outreach Program (EOP); however, individuals cannot receive both awards at the same time. This includes airfare, hotel, and meals, maximum $75 per day.
Amount of Grant: $750
Date(s) Application is Due: Jul 13
Contact: Adriano Boccanelli, Clinical Practice Assistant; (202) 966-7300, ext. 133; fax: (202) 966-2891; email: aboccanelli@aacap.org
Internet: http://www.aacap.org/cs/root/medical_students_and_residents/residents/2009_systems_of_care_special_program_scholarship
Sponsor: American Academy of Child and Adolescent Psychiatry
3615 Wisconsin Avenue, NW
Washington, DC 20016

AACAP-NIDA K12 Career Development Awards 55
The grant provides up to five years of salary support and mentored addiction research training for qualified child and adolescent psychiatrists (CAPs) who intend to establish careers as independent investigators in mental health and addiction research. Letters of Intent are required and due on or before January 5. Full applications are due March 30, with new grants awarded on June 1. Applicants are strongly encouraged to contact program staff regarding the program and candidate qualifications before submitting Letters of Intent.
Requirements: Eligible applicants must be a child and adolescent psychiatrist with a commitment and goal of becoming an independent investigator in addiction-related research focused on children and adolescents. Applicants must also be U.S. citizens, non-citizen nationals, and/or individuals with permanent residence status. Women and minority candidates are especially encouraged to apply.
Amount of Grant: $140,000 maximum
Date(s) Application is Due: Jan 5
Contact: Stacia Fleisher; (202) 966-7300; fax: (202) 966-2891; email: sfleisher@aacap.org or research@aacap.org
Internet: http://www.aacap.org/cs/root/research_and_training_awards/aacap_nida12
Sponsor: American Academy of Child and Adolescent Psychiatry
3615 Wisconsin Avenue, NW
Washington, DC 20016

AACN Clinical Inquiry Fund Grants 56
The fund provides small awards to qualified individuals carrying out clinical research projects that directly benefit patients and/or families. Interdisciplinary projects are encouraged. Funds may be awarded for new projects, projects in progress, and projects required for an academic degree as long as all other project criteria are met. The funds may be used to cover direct project expenses—i.e., printed materials, small equipment, and supplies including computer software.
Requirements: Principal Investigators must be nurses holding current AACN membership and must remain AACN members throughout the life of the grant funding.
Restrictions: Funds may not be used to pay salaries or institutional overhead or augment funding from formal grants.
Amount of Grant: $500
Date(s) Application is Due: Oct 1
Contact: Pamela Shellner, Clinical Practice Specialist; (949) 362-2050, ext. 321 or (800) 394-5995, ext. 321; fax: (949) 362-2020; email: research@aacn.org or info@aacn.org
Internet: http://www.aacn.org/WD/Practice/Docs/Grant_Table09-10.pdf
Sponsor: American Association of Critical-Care Nurses
101 Columbia
Aliso Viejo, CA 92656-4109

AACN Clinical Practice Grants 57
This $6,000 grant supports research focused on one or more AACN Research priorities. Research conducted in fulfillment of an academic degree is acceptable. Funds may be awarded for new projects, projects in progress and projects required for an academic degree as long as all other project criteria are met. Eligible projects may include research utilization studies, CQI projects or outcomes evaluation projects. Interdisciplinary and collaborative projects are encouraged and may involve interdisciplinary teams, multiple nursing units, home health, subacute and transitional care, other institutions or community agencies. Funds may be used to cover direct project expenses, such as printed materials, small equipment or supplies including computer software. Six awards are available each year. One award is funded up to $6,000 each year.
Requirements: Principal Investigators must be nurses holding current AACN membership and must remain AACN members throughout the life of the grant funding.
Restrictions: Funds may not be used to pay salaries or institutional overhead or augment funding from formal grants. Principal investigators who have received funding from AACN are ineligible to receive additional funding from AACN during the lifetime of the original award.
Amount of Grant: $6,000 maximum
Date(s) Application is Due: Oct 1
Contact: Pamela Shellner, Clinical Practice Specialist; (949) 362-2050, ext. 321 or (800) 394-5995, ext. 321; fax: (949) 362-2020; email: research@aacn.org or info@aacn.org
Internet: http://www.aacn.org/WD/Practice/Content/grant-CP.pcms?pid=1@menu=practice
Sponsor: American Association of Critical-Care Nurses
101 Columbia
Aliso Viejo, CA 92656-4109

AACN Critical Care Grants 58
AACN's research agenda promotes the creation of cultures of inquiry, broad sharing and evidence-based practice. This $15,000 grant supports research focused on one or more of AACN Research priorities. Research priority areas include: effective and appropriate use of technology to achieve optimal patient assessment, management, and/or outcomes; creating a healing, humane environment; processes and systems that foster the optimal contribution of critical care nurses; effective approaches to symptom management; and prevention and management of complication.
Requirements: Principal Investigators must be nurses holding current AACN membership and must remain AACN members throughout the life of the grant funding.
Restrictions: The proposed research may not be used to meet the requirements of an academic degree. Funds may not be used to pay salaries or institutional overhead or augment funding from formal grants. Principal investigators who have received funding from AACN are ineligible to receive additional funding from AACN during the lifetime of the original award.
Amount of Grant: $15,000
Date(s) Application is Due: Oct 1
Contact: Pamela Shellner, Clinical Practice Specialist; (949) 362-2050, ext. 321 or (800) 394-5995, ext. 321; fax: (949) 362-2020; email: research@aacn.org or info@aacn.org
Internet: http://www.aacn.org/WD/Practice/Content/grant-CC.pcms?pid=1@menu=practice
Sponsor: American Association of Critical-Care Nurses
101 Columbia
Aliso Viejo, CA 92656-4109

AACN End of Life/Palliative Care Small Projects Grants 59
The end of life/palliative care grant provides an award to a qualified individual(s) carrying out a project focusing on end of life and/or palliative care outcomes in acute and/or critical care settings. Eligible projects may focus on any age group (neonatal to elderly) in the acute or critical care arena. They may include patient education programs, staff development programs, competency-based educational programs, CQI/outcomes evaluation projects, or small clinical research studies. Funds may be awarded for new projects, projects in progress and projects required for an academic degree as long as all other project criteria are met. Collaborative projects are encouraged and may involve interdisciplinary teams, multiple nursing units, home health, subacute and transitional care, other institutions or community agencies. Funds may be used to cover direct project expenses, such as printed materials, small equipment, supplies including computer software. Two awards are available each year. Each proposal can be funded for up to $500.
Requirements: Principal Investigators must be nurses holding current AACN membership and must remain AACN members throughout the life of the grant funding.
Restrictions: Funds may not be used to pay for salaries, speaker honorarium or costs, institutional overhead nor augment funding from formal large grants.
Amount of Grant: $500 maximum
Date(s) Application is Due: Oct 1
Contact: Pamela Shellner, Clinical Practice Specialist; (949) 362-2050, ext. 321 or (800) 394-5995, ext. 321; fax: (949) 362-2020; email: research@aacn.org or info@aacn.org
Internet: http://www.aacn.org/WD/Practice/Content/grant-EOL.pcms?pid=1@menu=Practice
Sponsor: American Association of Critical-Care Nurses
101 Columbia
Aliso Viejo, CA 92656-4109

AACN Evidence-Based Clinical Practice Grants 60
The Evidence-Based Clinical Practice Grant provides awards to grants that stimulate the use of patient-focused data and/or previously generated research findings to develop, implement and evaluate changes critical and acute care nursing practice. Funds may be awarded for new projects, projects in progress and projects required for an academic degree as long as all other project criteria are met. Eligible projects may include research utilization studies, CQI projects or outcomes evaluation projects. Interdisciplinary and collaborative projects are encouraged and may involve interdisciplinary teams, multiple nursing units, home health, subacute and transitional care, other institutions or community agencies. Funds may be used to cover direct project expenses, such as printed materials, small equipment or supplies including computer software. Six awards are available each year. Each proposal can be funded for up to $1,000.
Requirements: Principal Investigators must be nurses holding current AACN membership and must remain AACN members throughout the life of the grant funding.
Restrictions: Funds may not be used to pay salaries or institutional overhead or augment funding from formal grants. Principal investigators who have received funding from AACN are ineligible to receive additional funding from AACN during the lifetime of the original award.
Amount of Grant: $1,000 maximum
Date(s) Application is Due: Oct 1
Contact: Pamela Shellner, Clinical Practice Specialist; (949) 362-2050, ext. 321 or (800) 394-5995, ext. 321; fax: (949) 362-2020; email: research@aacn.org or info@aacn.org
Internet: http://www.aacn.org/WD/Practice/Content/grant-EBP.pcms?pid=1@menu=Practice
Sponsor: American Association of Critical-Care Nurses
101 Columbia
Aliso Viejo, CA 92656-4109

AACN Mentorship Grant 61
This award, cosponsored by Mallinckrodt Inc. and AACN, facilitates critical care nursing practice research between a novice and an experienced researcher. The novice researcher is a beginning researcher with limited or no research experience in the area of the proposed investigation. The novice researcher is also a registered nurse with current AACN membership. The grant may be used to fund research for an academic degree. The mentor must show strong evidence of research expertise in the proposed area of research to be pursued by the novice investigator.
Requirements: Principal Investigators must be nurses holding current AACN membership and must remain AACN members throughout the life of the grant funding.
Restrictions: The mentor may not be designated mentor in two consecutive years and may not be conducting research as part of an academic degree.
Amount of Grant: $10,000 maximum
Date(s) Application is Due: Oct 1
Contact: Pamela Shellner, Clinical Practice Specialist; (949) 362-2050, ext. 321 or (800) 394-5995, ext. 321; fax: (949) 362-2020; email: research@aacn.org or info@aacn.org
Internet: http://www.aacn.org/WD/Practice/Content/grant-Mentor.pcms?pid=1@menu=practice
Sponsor: American Association of Critical-Care Nurses
101 Columbia
Aliso Viejo, CA 92656-4109

AACN Physio-Control Small Projects Grants 62
The program provides awards to qualified individuals carrying out projects focusing on aspects of acute myocardial infarction, resuscitation, or sudden cardiac death. Such projects may include the use of defibrillation, synchronized cardioversion, noninvasive pacing, or interpretive 12-lead electrocardiogram. Eligible projects may include patient education programs, staff development programs, competency-based educational programs, continuous quality improvement projects, outcomes evaluation projects, or small clinical research studies. Funds may be awarded for new projects, projects in progress, and projects required for an academic degree as long as all other project criteria are met. Collaborative projects are encouraged and may involve interdisciplinary teams, multiple nursing units, home health, subacute and transitional care, other institutions, or community agencies. Funds may be used to cover direct project expenses, such as printed materials, small equipment, or supplies including computer software.
Requirements: Principal Investigators must be nurses holding current AACN membership and must remain AACN members throughout the life of the grant funding.
Restrictions: Funds may not be used to pay for salaries, speaker honorarium or costs, institutional overhead nor augment funding from formal large grants.
Amount of Grant: $1,500 maximum
Date(s) Application is Due: Oct 1
Contact: Pamela Shellner, Clinical Practice Specialist; (949) 362-2050, ext. 321 or (800) 394-5995, ext. 321; fax: (949) 362-2020; email: research@aacn.org or info@aacn.org
Internet: http://www.aacn.org/WD/Practice/Docs/Grant_Table09-10.pdf
Sponsor: American Association of Critical-Care Nurses
101 Columbia
Aliso Viejo, CA 92656-1491

AACN-Edwards Lifesciences Nurse-Driven Clinical Practice Outcomes Grants 63
Co-sponsored by Edwards Lifesciences and the American Association of Critical-Care Nurses, each grant supports a nurse experienced in research who is conducting a clearly articulated research study that relates to use of protocol-based care driven by nurses. A commitment is required to produce results that will be available and disseminated in a short timeframe. Proposals submitted by an interdisciplinary team or an experienced researcher mentoring a novice will also be considered. Funds may be used for original research or replication of existing research. Especially desirable are proposals that focus on any of the following at any point in the continuum of acute or critical care: implementation of nurse-driven protocols using technology, including minimally invasive devices, with evaluation of patient outcomes and nurses' role in implementing the protocols; or development and clinical evaluation of nurse-driven protocols. Two awards are available each year. Each proposal can be funded up to of $5,000.
Requirements: Principal Investigators must be nurses holding current AACN membership and must remain AACN members throughout the life of the grant funding.
Restrictions: Funds may not be used to pay salaries or institutional overhead or augment funding from formal grants. Principal investigators who have received funding from AACN are ineligible to receive additional funding from AACN during the lifetime of the original award.
Amount of Grant: $5,000 maximum
Date(s) Application is Due: Oct 1
Contact: Pamela Shellner, Clinical Practice Specialist; (949) 362-2050, ext. 321 or (800) 394-5995, ext. 321; fax: (949) 362-2020; email: research@aacn.org or info@aacn.org
Internet: http://www.aacn.org/WD/Practice/Content/grant-Edwards.pcms?pid=1@menu=practice
Sponsor: American Association of Critical-Care Nurses
101 Columbia
Aliso Viejo, CA 92656-4109

AACN-Philips Medical Systems Clinical Outcomes Grants 64
Co-sponsored by Philips Medical Systems and the American Association of Critical-Care Nurses, each grant supports experienced nurses in conducting clearly articulated research studies. The research must be relevant to clinical nursing practice in acute or critical care. Proposals submitted by an interdisciplinary team or an experienced researcher mentoring a novice will also be considered. Funds may be used for original research or replication of existing research. Qualified proposals should seek to achieve improved outcomes and/or system efficiencies in care of acute or critically ill individuals of any age. Especially desirable are proposals for hospital-based inquiry that focuses on any of the following: intervention strategies addressing technology integration into patient care; use of computerized medical record systems in assessing patient outcomes and managing care; improving specific patient care outcomes (e.g., clinical, safety, financial); use of simulation in clinical education of nurses; and one or more of the 2006 National Patient Safety Goals issued by the Joint Commission on Accreditation of Healthcare Organizations.
Requirements: Principal Investigators must be nurses holding current AACN membership and must remain AACN members throughout the life of the grant funding.
Restrictions: Funds may not be used to pay salaries or institutional overhead or augment funding from formal grants. Principal investigators who have received funding from AACN are ineligible to receive additional funding from AACN during the lifetime of the original award.
Amount of Grant: $10,000 maximum
Date(s) Application is Due: Oct 1
Contact: Pamela Shellner, Clinical Practice Specialist; (949) 362-2050, ext. 321 or (800) 394-5995, ext. 321; fax: (949) 362-2020; email: research@aacn.org or info@aacn.org
Internet: http://www.aacn.org/WD/Practice/Content/grant-Philips.pcms?pid=1@menu=practice
Sponsor: American Association of Critical-Care Nurses / Philips Medical Systems
101 Columbia
Aliso Viejo, CA 92656-4109

AACN-Sigma Theta Tau Critical Care Grant 65
The grant, cosponsored by AACN and Sigma Theta Tau International, supports critical care nursing research and is awarded annually for a study relevant to critical care nursing practice. The proposed study may be used to meet requirements of an academic degree.
Requirements: Principal investigators must be a member of AACN and/or of Sigma Theta Tau International. The PI must have a minimum Masters Degree.
Restrictions: Funds may not be used to pay salaries or institutional overhead or augment funding from formal grants. Principal investigators who have received funding from AACN are ineligible to receive additional funding from AACN during the lifetime of the original award.
Amount of Grant: $10,000 maximum
Date(s) Application is Due: Oct 1
Contact: Pamela Shellner, Clinical Practice Specialist; (949) 362-2050, ext. 321 or (800) 394-5995, ext. 321; fax: (949) 362-2020; email: research@aacn.org or info@aacn.org
Internet: http://www.aacn.org/WD/Practice/Content/grant-STT.pcms?pid=1@menu=practice
Sponsor: American Association of Critical-Care Nurses
101 Columbia
Aliso Viejo, CA 92656-4109

AACR Award for Lifetime Achievement in Cancer Research 66
The AACR Award for Lifetime Achievement in Cancer Research was established and first given in 2004 to honor an individual who has made significant fundamental contributions to cancer research, either through a single scientific discovery or a body of work. These contributions, whether they have been in research, leadership, or mentorship, must have had a lasting impact on the cancer field and must have demonstrated a lifetime commitment to progress against cancer. Nominations may be made by any scientist, whether an AACR member or nonmember, who is now or has been affiliated with any institution involved in cancer research, cancer medicine, or cancer-related biomedical science. Nominations for the Award must be submitted electronically to the AACR no later than 4:00 p.m. United States Eastern Time on November 16.
Requirements: Nominations may be made on behalf of individuals who are living at the time of the nomination. Candidates need not be members of the AACR. Candidates need not be currently engaged in cancer research.
Restrictions: Institutions or organizations are not eligible for the Award. Paper nominations will not be accepted.
Date(s) Application is Due: Nov 16
Contact: Monique P. Eversley, Staff Associate; (267) 646-0576 or (215) 440-9300, ext. 1400; fax: (215) 440-9372; email: monique.eversley@aacr.org or awards@aacr.org
Internet: http://www.aacr.org/home/scientists/scientific-achievement-awards/lifetime-achievement-award.aspx
Sponsor: American Association for Cancer Research
615 Chestnut Street, 17th Floor
Philadelphia, PA 19106-4404

AACR Award for Outstanding Achievement in Cancer Research 67
This award is given in recognition of a young investigator on the basis of meritorious achievement in cancer research. The winner receives an honorarium of $5,000, presents a 50-minute lecture, and is given full support for the winner and a guest to attend the AACR Annual Meeting.
Requirements: Candidacy is open to all cancer researchers who are affiliated with any institution involved in cancer research, cancer medicine, or cancer-related biomedical science anywhere in the world. Such institutions include those in academia, industry, or government. In accordance with the wishes of the donor, the recipient must be no more than 40 years of age by the time the award is received.
Restrictions: Institutions or organizations are not eligible for the Award.
Amount of Grant: $5,000 honorarium
Date(s) Application is Due: Oct 15
Contact: Monique P. Eversley, Program Associate; (267) 646-0576; email: monique.eversley@aacr.org
Internet: http://www.aacr.org/home/scientists/scientific-achievement-awards/outstanding-achievement-award.aspx
Sponsor: American Association for Cancer Research
615 Chestnut Street, 17th Floor
Philadelphia, PA 19106-4404

AACR Award for Outstanding Achievement in Chemistry in Cancer Research 68
The Award will be given for outstanding, novel, and significant chemistry research, which has led to important contributions to the fields of basic cancer research; translational cancer research; cancer diagnosis; the prevention of cancer; or the treatment of patients with cancer. Such research may include, but is not limited to, drug discovery and design; structural biology; proteomics, metabolomics and biological mass spectrometry; chemical aspects of carcinogenesis; imaging agents and radiotherapeutics; and chemical biology. The winner of the award will give a 50-minute lecture during the AACR Annual Meeting, will receive a commemorative plaque and a $10,000 honorarium, and receive support for the winner and a guest to attend the Annual Meeting. Nominations for the Award must be submitted electronically no later than 4:00 p.m. United States Eastern Time on October 15.
Requirements: Candidacy is open to all researchers who are affiliated with any institution involved in cancer research, cancer medicine, or cancer-related biomedical science anywhere in the world. Institutions include those in academia, industry, or government.
Restrictions: Institutions or organizations are not eligible for the Award. Paper nominations will not be accepted.
Amount of Grant: $10,000 honorarium
Date(s) Application is Due: Oct 15
Contact: Lauren Medvetz, Program Coordinator; (267) 646-0689; fax: (215) 440-9372; email: lauren.medvets@aacr.org
Internet: http://www.aacr.org/home/scientists/scientific-achievement-awards/chemistry-in-cancer-research-award.aspx
Sponsor: American Association for Cancer Research
615 Chestnut Street, 17th Floor
Philadelphia, PA 19106-4404

AACR Brigid G. Leventhal Scholar in Cancer Research Awards 69
The purpose of this award program is to enhance the education and training of early career scientists by providing financial support for their participation in AACR Annual Meetings and Special Conferences. The AACR-WICR Brigid G. Leventhal Scholar Award Committee makes selection for these competitive awards after careful consideration of the candidate's application and accompanying materials.
Requirements: Candidates must be: Women in Cancer Research members; full time scientists in training who are graduate students, medical students, residents, clinical fellows or equivalent, or postdoctoral fellows; and first authors on abstracts submitted for consideration for presentation at the AACR Annual Meeting or Special Conference which the applicant wants to attend.
Date(s) Application is Due: Sep 10
Contact: Mona E. Shater, Staff Assistant; (215) 440-9300 or (267) 646-0654; fax: (215) 440-9372; email: mona.shater@aacr.org or wicr@aacr.org
Internet: http://www.aacr.org/home/membership-/association-groups/women-in-cancer-research.aspx
Sponsor: American Association for Cancer Research
615 Chestnut Street, 17th Floor
Philadelphia, PA 19106-4404

AACR Career Development Awards for Pediatric Cancer Research 70
Two Career Development Awards will be presented, the AACR-Aflac Incorporated Career Development Award for Pediatric Cancer Research and the AACR Centennial Career Development Award for Childhood Cancer Research. These Awards are open to junior faculty who are in their first full-year, faculty appointment. The Awards provide two-year grants of $100,000 ($50,000 per year) for direct research expenses and/or salary support. Research projects must have direct applicability to pediatric cancer.
Requirements: Candidates must have acquired a doctoral degree and have completed postdoctoral studies or clinical fellowships on or after July 2 (two years prior to the start of the grant term). Candidates must be in their first full-time, faculty appointment and hold the title of Instructor, Research Assistant Professor, Assistant Professor, or an equivalent full-time faculty appointment at the start of the grant term (July 1).
Restrictions: Non AACR members must submit a satisfactory application for Active Membership with the grant application by December 10th. Employees or subcontractors of a government or a for-profit private industry are not eligible.
Amount of Grant: two-year grant $100,000 ($50,000 per year)
Date(s) Application is Due: Dec 18
Contact: Julia Laurence, Program Assistant; (267) 646-0655; fax: (215) 440-9372; email: julia.laurence@aacr.org or awards@aacr.org
Internet: http://www.aacr.org/home/scientists/research-funding—fellowships/career-development-awards.aspx
Sponsor: American Association for Cancer Research
615 Chestnut Street, 17th Floor
Philadelphia, PA 19106-4404

AACR Centennial Postdoctoral Fellowships in Cancer Research 71
AACR Centennial Postdoctoral Research Fellowships in Cancer Research will provide $60,000 per year for up to three years to provide salary support and research funding for clinical and postdoctoral fellows in the first, second, or third year of their fellowship status. In addition to financial flexibility these fellowships also provide career flexibility. Fellowship funds may be transferred to move with the grantee if the grantee's fellowship is completed during the grant term - a valuable commodity for a newly-independent investigator. Under this award mechanism, the postdoctoral trainee is considered the Lead Investigator and should write the proposal independently with appropriate direction from the mentor. Proposals may be submitted in any area of cancer research whether laboratory-based, translational, clinical, epidemiological, behavioral, or other. Applications must be completed online using the proposalCENTRAL website, with one paper copy submitted to the AACR office. Application instructions and program guidelines are available online.
Requirements: Applicants must: be in the 1st, 2nd, or 3rd year of their postdoctoral training at the start of the fellowship term; be members of the AACR or must submit an application for membership prior to the fellowship application deadline; have acquired a doctoral degree in a biological sciences-related field; and hold the title of Postdoctoral Fellow or Clinical Research Fellow at an academic facility, teaching hospital, or research institution.
Restrictions: Employees, trainees, or subcontractors of a national government or private industry are not eligible.
Amount of Grant: $60,000 per year for up to 3 years
Date(s) Application is Due: Feb 1
Contact: Hanna Hopfinger, Program Assistant; (267) 646-0665; fax: (215) 440-9372; email: hanna.hopfinger@aacr.org
Internet: http://www.aacr.org/home/scientists/research-funding—fellowships/research-funding.aspx

Sponsor: American Association for Cancer Research
615 Chestnut Street, 17th Floor
Philadelphia, PA 19106-4404

AACR Centennial Pre-doctoral Fellowships in Cancer Research 72

The AACR Centennial Pre-doctoral Research Fellowships will provide full-time graduate students a rare opportunity to invest in their future cancer research careers. The grant terms are flexible, allowing applicants to tailor their grant funds to fit their individual research funding and salary needs. Grantees may also transfer their funds to a postdoctoral fellowship position, should they advance in their careers during the grant term. Under this award mechanism, the pre-doctoral trainee is considered the Lead Investigator and should write the proposal independently with appropriate direction from the mentor. Proposals may be submitted in any area of cancer research whether laboratory-based, translational, clinical, epidemiological, behavioral, or other. A grant of $30,000 per year over a maximum period of three years will be awarded for salary support and research funding.
Requirements: Applicants must: be full-time graduate students who are pursuing a doctoral degree and engaged in a program of cancer research; be members of the AACR or must submit an application for membership prior to the fellowship application deadline; have completed at least one year of research training at the graduate level or have equivalent research experience; and be engaged in basic, clinical, translational or epidemiological cancer research. At the time of award acceptance the awardee must have advanced to degree candidacy.
Restrictions: Summer student positions and undergraduate summer studentships do not qualify. Employees, trainees, or subcontractors of a national government or private industry are not eligible.
Amount of Grant: $30,000 per year over a maximum period of three years
Date(s) Application is Due: Feb 1
Contact: Hanna Hopfinger, Program Assistant; (267) 646-0665; fax: (215) 440-9372; email: hanna.hopfinger@aacr.org
Internet: http://www.aacr.org/home/scientists/research-funding—fellowships/research-funding.aspx
Sponsor: American Association for Cancer Research
615 Chestnut Street, 17th Floor
Philadelphia, PA 19106-4404

AACR Clinical and Translational Research Fellowships 73

The AACR Clinical and Translational Research Fellowships consist of three different Fellowships: AACR-Astellas U.S.A Foundation Fellowship in Clinical/Translational Cancer Research, which is a one-year grant of $30,000; AACR-AstraZeneca Fellowship for Translational Lung Cancer Research, which is a two-year grant of $90,000; and, AACR-Bristol-Myers Squibb Oncology Fellowship in Clinical Cancer Research, which is a one-year grant of $40,000. These fellowships support the salary and benefits of the Fellow. A partial amount of funds may be designated for direct research support. The AACR requires applicants to submit both an online and a paper application. The online application deadline is December 10th, the application must be submitted using the proposalCENTRAL website at https://proposalcentral.altum.com. The paper application with original signatures and all supporting documents must be postmarked and sent no later then December 15.
Requirements: Applications are open to Postdoctoral Fellows and Clinical Research Fellows at an academic facility, teaching hospital, or research institution who will be in the 1st, 2nd, or 3rd year of their postdoctoral training at the start of the fellowship.
Restrictions: Academic faculty holding the rank of assistant professor or higher, graduate or medical students, government employees, and employees of private industry are not eligible.
Amount of Grant: $30,000-$90,000 range
Date(s) Application is Due: Dec 10; Dec 15
Contact: Hanna Hopfinger; (267) 646-0665 or (215) 440-9300; fax: (215) 440-9372; email: hanna.hopfinger@aacr.org or awards@aacr.org
Internet: http://www.aacr.org/home/scientists/research-funding—fellowships/postdoctoral-fellowships.aspx
Sponsor: American Association for Cancer Research
615 Chestnut Street, 17th Floor
Philadelphia, PA 19106-4404

AACR Fellows Grants 74

The Fellowship program supports innovative research by a meritorious young investigator by presenting the Fellow with research funds to pursue an independent line of investigation within the context of his/her current Fellowship placement. By allowing a Fellow to acquire the equipment and supplies needed to pursue a new direction in his/her research program, the Fellows Grant assists the Fellow in developing preliminary data to support a future project or investigating a new technique that otherwise would not be possible in the absence of this funding. The Selection Committee favors proposals that provided evidence of an applicant's research initiative and creativity, and the support of a scientific mentor. The Committee also weighed the potential of the candidate to make meaningful contributions to the field, and promise of success as a cancer researcher in future years.
Requirements: Candidates must be, at the start of the grant term, in their third, fourth, or fifth year of their fellowship status.
Amount of Grant: $30,000-$40,000 per year
Date(s) Application is Due: Dec 18
Contact: Julia Laurence, Staff Assistant; (267) 646-0655; fax: (215) 440-9372; email: julia.laurence@aacr.org or awards@aacr.org
Internet: http://www.aacr.org/home/scientists/research-funding—fellowships/fellows-grants.aspx
Sponsor: American Association for Cancer Research
615 Chestnut Street, 17th Floor
Philadelphia, PA 19106-4404

AACR G.H.A. Clowes Memorial Award 75

The AACR and Eli Lilly and Company established this Award in 1961 to honor Dr. G.H.A. Clowes, who was a founding member of the AACR and a research director of Eli Lilly. The Clowes Award recognizes an individual with outstanding recent accomplishments in basic cancer research. Nominations for the Award must be submitted electronically to the AACR no later than 4:00 p.m. United States Eastern Time on October 15. Paper nominations will not be accepted.
Requirements: Candidacy is open to all cancer researchers who are affiliated with any institution involved in cancer research, cancer medicine, or cancer-related biomedical science anywhere in the world. Such institutions include those in academia, industry, or government.
Restrictions: Institutions or organizations are not eligible for the Award. Paper nominations will not be accepted.
Amount of Grant: $10,000 honorarium
Date(s) Application is Due: Oct 15
Contact: Monique P. Eversley, Staff Associate; (267) 646-0576 or (215) 440-9300, ext. 1400; fax: (215) 440-9372; email: monique.eversley@aacr.org or awards@aacr.org
Internet: http://www.aacr.org/home/scientists/scientific-achievement-awards/clowes-award.aspx
Sponsor: American Association for Cancer Research
615 Chestnut Street, 17th Floor
Philadelphia, PA 19106-4404

AACR Gertrude Elion Cancer Research Award 76

This prestigious award provides a one-year research grant to an assistant professor at an academic or nonprofit research institute worldwide for salary and benefits, laboratory supplies, and limited domestic travel to support research in cancer etiology, diagnosis, treatment, or prevention (basic, translational, or clinical cancer research). The AACR requires applicants to submit both an online and a paper application. The online application must be submitted by 12:00 noon (United States Eastern Daylight Time) on February 27, using the proposalCENTRAL website at https://proposalcentral.altum.com. The paper application with original signatures and all supporting documents must be postmarked and sent no later then March 3.
Requirements: Candidates must be nominated by an AACR member and submit a detailed application. Candidates must have completed postdoctoral studies or clinical fellowships no later than July 1 of the award year and ordinarily not more than five years earlier. Candidates must be tenure-tracked scientists at the level of assistant professor at an academic institution anywhere in the world.
Restrictions: Tenured faculty in academia, employees of a national government, and employees of private industry are not eligible.
Amount of Grant: $50,000
Date(s) Application is Due: Feb 27; Mar 3
Contact: Julia Laurence, Staff Assistant; (215) 440-9300, ext. 102 or (267) 646-0655; fax: (215) 440-9372; email: laurence@aacr.org
Internet: http://www.aacr.org/home/scientists/research-funding—fellowships/elion-award.aspx
Sponsor: American Association for Cancer Research
615 Chestnut Street, 17th Floor
Philadelphia, PA 19106-4404

AACR Henry Shepard Bladder Cancer Research Grants 77

These two-year Grants will provide up to $250,000 in total support for innovative cancer research projects designed to accelerate the discovery, development, and application of new agents to treat bladder cancer and/or for pre-clinical research with direct therapeutic intent. Laboratory-based projects must present plans with clinical collaborators indicating how the work will be translated into the clinic. Similarly, clinical studies must show how the work was derived from basic preclinical work and how results will be channeled back to laboratory-based collaborators. Four grants will be awarded. The submission deadline is July 25, at 12:00 noon, U.S. Eastern Time.
Requirements: Independent investigators who are affiliated with any institution involved in cancer research, cancer medicine, or cancer-related biomedical science anywhere in the world may apply. There are no geographic, national, or residency status restrictions. Applicants must have acquired a doctoral degree in a related field.
Restrictions: Pre- and Postdoctoral fellows are not eligible. Employees or subcontractors of a national government or the for-profit private industry are not eligible to serve as the Principal Investigator for the purpose of these Grants. However, collaborations with such individuals are encouraged. Neither the members of the Scientific Review Committee nor the members of their individual laboratories are eligible for these Grants.
Amount of Grant: $250,000 maximum over two years
Date(s) Application is Due: Jul 25
Contact: Hanna Hopfinger, Program Assistant; (267) 646-0665; fax: (215) 440-9372; email: hanna.hopfinger@aacr.org
Internet: http://www.aacr.org/home/scientists/research-funding—training-grants/research-funding/research-funding—fellowships/bladder-cancer-research-grants.aspx
Sponsor: American Association for Cancer Research
615 Chestnut Street, 17th Floor
Philadelphia, PA 19106-4404

AACR Joseph H. Burchenal Memorial Award 78

This Award was established in 1996 to recognize outstanding achievements in clinical cancer research. It is named for the late Dr. Joseph H. Burchenal, Honorary Member and Past President of the AACR, and a major figure in clinical cancer research and chemotherapy. The winner of the Award for Outstanding Achievement in Clinical Cancer Research will give a 50-minute lecture during the AACR Annual Meeting, and receive an honorarium and support for attendance at the meeting.

Requirements: Candidacy is open to all cancer researchers who are affiliated with any institution involved in cancer research, cancer medicine, or cancer-related biomedical science anywhere in the world, including those in academia, industry, or government.

Restrictions: Institutions or organizations are not eligible for the Award. Candidates may not nominate themselves.

Samples: Joseph R. Bertino, M.D., Interim Director & Chief Scientific Officer, The Cancer Institute of New Jersey (2008).

Date(s) Application is Due: Oct 15

Contact: Monique P. Eversley, Program Associate; (267) 646-0576; email: monique.eversley@aacr.org

Internet: http://www.aacr.org/home/scientists/scientific-achievement-awards/burchenal-award.aspx

Sponsor: American Association for Cancer Research
615 Chestnut Street, 17th Floor
Philadelphia, PA 19106-4404

AACR Judah Folkman Career Development Award for Anti-Angiogenesis Research 79

The AACR Judah Folkman Career Development Award for Angiogenesis Research is open to junior faculty who completed postdoctoral studies or clinical fellowships no more then three years prior to the start of the grant term (Dec 1); who are in their first full-time, faculty appointment and hold the title of Instructor, Research Assistant Professor, Assistant Professor, or an equivalent full-time faculty appointment; and who are at an academic, medical, or research Institution. The Career Development Award provides a two-year grant of $100,000 ($50,000 per year) for direct research expenses and/or salary support. One Award will be presented.

Requirements: Applicants must have acquired a medical degree or hold a combined M.D./Ph.D and may not currently be a candidate for a further doctoral or professional degree. The Award is open to AACR members. Non-members must submit a satisfactory application for Active Membership and additional Curriculum Vitae with the grant application.

Restrictions: Employees, trainees, or subcontractors of a national government or private industry are not eligible. Exceptions may apply if an applicant holds a full-time position at a Veterans' Hospital or national laboratory in the U.S. Current recipients of any AACR grant are also not eligible.

Amount of Grant: two-year grant $100,000 ($50,000 per year)

Date(s) Application is Due: Aug 10

Contact: Julia Laurence, Program Assistant; (267) 646-0655; fax: (215) 440-9372; email: julia.laurence@aacr.org or awards@aacr.org

Internet: http://www.aacr.org/home/scientists/research-funding—fellowships/career-development-awards.aspx

Sponsor: American Association for Cancer Research
615 Chestnut Street, 17th Floor
Philadelphia, PA 19106-4404

AACR Kirk A. Landon and Dorothy P. Landon Foundation Prizes 80

These two major international awards recognize outstanding scientists who have made seminal basic and translational cancer research discoveries at the cutting edge of scientific novelty and significance, which have accelerated progress against cancer and have implications for future discoveries and contributions to cancer research. The Kirk A. Landon-AACR Prize for Basic Cancer Research recognizes significant, fundamental contributions to laboratory research. The Dorothy P. Landon-AACR Prize for Translational Cancer Research recognizes extraordinary achievement in translational cancer research—the interface between basic research and its application to the clinic in the areas of diagnosis, treatment, or the prevention of cancer. Both prizes bring heightened public attention to landmark achievements in the continuing effort to prevent and cure cancer through the presentation of dynamic lectures during the AACR annual meeting; and promote and reward continued, productive cancer research.

Requirements: The prizes are open to all cancer researchers who are affiliated with any institution involved in cancer research, cancer medicine, or cancer-related biomedical science anywhere in the world. Such institutions include those in academia, industry, or government. Candidates must be active researchers and have recent publications.

Restrictions: Institutions or organizations are ineligible.

Samples: Arnold J. Levine, Ph.D., Professor, The Cancer Institute of New Jersey—Kirk A. Landon-AACR Prize for Basic Cancer Research (2008); John Mendelsohn, M.D., President, UT M.D. Anderson Cancer Center, Houston, Texas—Dorothy P. Landon-AACR Prize for Translational Cancer Research (2008).

Amount of Grant: $100,000 each

Date(s) Application is Due: Aug 25

Contact: Monique P. Eversley, Staff Associate; (267) 646-0576 or (215) 440-9300, ext. 1400; fax: (215) 440-9372; email: monique.eversley@aacr.org or awards@aacr.org

Internet: http://www.aacr.org/home/scientists/scientific-achievement-awards/landon-prizes.aspx

Sponsor: American Association for Cancer Research
615 Chestnut Street, 17th Floor
Philadelphia, PA 19106-4404

AACR Margaret Foti Award for Leadership and Extraordinary Achievements in Cancer Research 81

This Award will recognize a true champion of cancer research, who embodies the sustained commitment of Margaret Foti to the prevention and cure of cancer. The Award will be given to an individual whose leadership and extraordinary achievements in cancer research have made a major impact in the field. Such achievements may include contributions to the acceleration of progress in cancer research; raising national or international awareness of cancer research; or in other ways demonstrating a sustained commitment to cancer research. Nominations for the Award must be submitted electronically no later than 4:00 p.m. U.S. Eastern Time on November 16. The recipient will receive an honorarium, a commemorative plaque, and support for the winner to attend the AACR Annual Meeting.

Requirements: Candidacy is open to all individuals who are affiliated with any organization whose mission supports cancer research or any institution involved in cancer research, cancer medicine, or cancer-related biomedical science anywhere in the world. Such institutions include those in academia, industry, or government.

Restrictions: Institutions or organizations are not eligible for the Award. Paper nominations will not be accepted.

Date(s) Application is Due: Nov 16

Contact: Monique P. Eversley, Program Associate; (267) 646-0576 or (215) 440-9300, ext. 1400; fax: (215) 440-9372; email: monique.eversley@aacr.org or awards@aacr.org

Internet: http://www.aacr.org/home/scientists/scientific-achievement-awards/margaret-foti-award.aspx

Sponsor: American Association for Cancer Research
615 Chestnut Street, 17th Floor
Philadelphia, PA 19106-4404

AACR Minority Scholar in Cancer Research Awards 82

The AACR administers this award program that is supported by a grant from the Comprehensive Minority Biomedical Branch of the National Cancer Institute to provide funds for participation of meritorious minority scientists in the AACR Special Conferences Series (U.S. domestic conferences only). These awards are intended to enhance the education and training of minority researchers and to increase the visibility and recognition of minorities involved in cancer research.

Requirements: Candidates must be full-time graduate students, medical students, residents, clinical or postdoctoral fellows, or junior faculty members who are either engaged in cancer research or who have the training and potential to make contributions to this field. Candidates must also be citizens or permanent residents of the United States or Canada.

Restrictions: This program applies only to racial/ethnic minority groups identified by the National Cancer Institute as being traditionally underrepresented in cancer and biomedical research. These groups include African Americans/Blacks, Alaskan Natives, Hispanic Americans, Native Americans, and Native Pacific Islanders. Only citizens of the United States or Canada or scientists who are permanent residents of these countries may receive one of these awards.

Samples: Irene Alvarez, B.S., University of Arizona, Tucson, Arizona (2008); Cristina M. Contreras, B.S., UT Southwestern Medical Center, Dallas, Texas (2008).

Date(s) Application is Due: Jul 20

Contact: Mona E. Shater, Staff Assistant; (215) 440-9300 or (267) 646-0654; fax: (215) 440-9372 or (215) 440-9412; email: mona.shater@aacr.org or micr@aacr.org

Internet: http://www.aacr.org/home/scientists/meetings—workshops/special-conferences/metabolism-and-cancer/financial-support-for-attendance.aspx

Sponsor: American Association for Cancer Research
615 Chestnut Street, 17th Floor
Philadelphia, PA 19106-4404

AACR Minority-Serving Institution Faculty Scholar in Cancer Research Awards 83

The AACR is pleased to announce the availability of Scholar Awards in Cancer Research for full-time faculty members of Minority-Serving Institutions [Historically Black Colleges and Universities (HBCUs), Hispanic Serving Institutions (HSIs), and Tribal Colleges and Universities and other post-secondary institutions as defined by the U.S. Department of Education]. The purposes of this Award program is to increase the scientific knowledge base of faculty members at Minority-Serving Institutions, and to encourage them and their students to pursue careers in cancer research. AACR Minority-Serving Institution Faculty Scholar in Cancer Research Awards are presented by the American Association for Cancer Research to scientists at the level of Assistant Professor or above at a Minority-Serving Institution, who are engaged in meritorious basic, clinical, or translational cancer research.

Requirements: Candidates must have completed doctoral studies or clinical fellowships and hold full-time faculty status at an institution designated as a Minority-Serving Institution. Candidates must have acquired doctoral degrees in fields relevant to cancer research. Candidates must be citizens or permanent residents of the U.S. or Canada.

Samples: Joseph Agyin, Ph.D., UT Health Science Center, San Antonio, Texas (2008); Wellington Ayensu, M.D., Jackson State University, Jackson, Mississippi (2008); Rebecca Hartley, Ph.D., University of New Mexico, Albuquerque, New Mexico (2008).

Date(s) Application is Due: Jul 20

Contact: Mona E. Shater, Staff Assistant; (215) 440-9300 or (267) 646-0654; fax: (215) 440-9372 or (215) 440-9412; email: mona.shater@aacr.org or micr@aacr.org

Internet: http://www.aacr.org/home/scientists/meetings—workshops/special-conferences/metabolism-and-cancer/financial-support-for-attendance.aspx

Sponsor: American Association for Cancer Research
615 Chestnut Street, 17th Floor
Philadelphia, PA 19106-4404

AACR Outstanding Investigator Award for Breast Cancer Research 84

The AACR Outstanding Investigator Award for Breast Cancer Research, funded by Susan G. Komen for the Cure, will recognize an investigator of no more than 50 years of age whose novel and significant work has had or may have a far-reaching impact on the etiology, detection, diagnosis, treatment, or prevention of breast cancer. Such work may involve any discipline across the continuum of biomedical research, including basic, translational, clinical, and epidemiological studies. The recipient of the Award will receive a $10,000 honorarium and present a 25-minute lecture at the Annual San Antonio Breast Cancer Symposium. Nominations may be made by any scientist, whether an AACR member or nonmember, who is now or has been affiliated with any institution involved in cancer research, cancer medicine, or cancer-related biomedical science. Candidates may not nominate themselves. Nominations must be submitted online at https://proposalcentral.altum.com, no later than 4:00 p.m. United States Eastern Time on May 15th.

Requirements: All cancer researchers who are affiliated with any institution involved in cancer research, cancer medicine, or cancer-related biomedical science anywhere in the world may be nominated. Such institutions include those in academia, industry, or government. Candidates must be no more than 50 years of age at the time the Award is received.

Restrictions: Institutions or organizations are not eligible for the Award. Paper nominations will not be accepted.

Amount of Grant: $10,000 honorarium

Date(s) Application is Due: May 15

Contact: Monique P. Eversley, Program Associate; (267) 646-0576 or (215) 440-9300, ext. 1400; fax: (215) 440-9372; email: monique.eversley@aacr.org or awards@aacr.org

Internet: http://www.aacr.org/home/scientists/scientific-achievement-awards/outstanding-investigator-award.aspx

Sponsor: American Association for Cancer Research
615 Chestnut Street, 17th Floor
Philadelphia, PA 19106-4404

AACR Princess Takamatsu Memorial Lectureship 85

This Lectureship will recognize an individual scientist whose novel and significant work has had or may have a far-reaching impact on the detection, diagnosis, treatment, or prevention of cancer, and who embodies the dedication of the Princess to multinational collaborations. The Lecturer will receive an unrestricted cash award of $10,000, support to attend the AACR Annual Meeting, and a commemorative item serving as tangible witness to the singular honor of his/her selection. Nominations must be submitted electronically no later than 4:00 p.m. U.S. Eastern Time on November 16.

Requirements: Candidacy is open to all cancer researchers who are affiliated with any institution involved in cancer research, cancer medicine, or cancer-related biomedical science anywhere in the world. Such institutions include those in academia, industry, or government.

Restrictions: Institutions or organizations are not eligible for the Lectureship. Paper nominations will not be accepted.

Amount of Grant: $10,000

Date(s) Application is Due: Nov 16

Contact: Monique P. Eversley, Staff Associate; (267) 646-0576 or (215) 440-9300, ext. 1400; fax: (215) 440-9372; email: monique.eversley@aacr.org or awards@aacr.org

Internet: http://www.aacr.org/home/scientists/scientific-achievement-awards/takamatsu-lectureship.aspx

Sponsor: American Association for Cancer Research
615 Chestnut Street, 17th Floor
Philadelphia, PA 19106-4404

AACR Richard and Hinda Rosenthal Memorial Awards 86

AACR and the Rosenthal Family Foundation established this Award in 1977 to recognize research that has made, or promises to soon make, a notable contribution to improved clinical care in the field of cancer. In its desire to honor and provide incentive to investigators relatively early in their careers, the Foundation has stipulated that recipients not be more than 50 years of age at the time the Award is received. The winner of the AACR Richard and Hinda Rosenthal Memorial Award will receive an honorarium of $10,000, give a 50-minute lecture during the AACR Annual Meeting and be given support for the winner and a guest to attend the Annual Meeting.

Requirements: Candidacy is open to cancer researchers, engaged in the practice of medicine, who are affiliated with any institution involved in cancer research, cancer medicine, or cancer-related biomedical science. Such institutions include those in academia, industry, or government.

Restrictions: Candidates may not nominate themselves. Nominations must be submitted online at https://proposalcentral.altum.com, no later than 4:00 p.m. United States Eastern Time on October 15th. Paper nominations will not be accepted. Institutions or organizations are not eligible for the Award.

Amount of Grant: $10,000 honorarium

Date(s) Application is Due: Oct 15

Contact: Monique P. Eversley, Staff Associate; (267) 646-0576 or (215) 440-9300, ext. 1400; fax: (215) 440-9372; email: monique.eversley@aacr.org or awards@aacr.org

Internet: http://www.aacr.org/home/scientists/scientific-achievement-awards/clowes-award.aspx

Sponsor: American Association for Cancer Research
615 Chestnut Street, 17th Floor
Philadelphia, PA 19106-4404

AACR Scholar-in-Training Awards 87

Scholar-in-Training Awards provide financial support for early-career scientists to attend the AACR Annual Meeting. Since its inception in 1986, the program has provided over 3,200 grants and has received support from more than 30 cancer research foundations, corporations, individuals, and other organizations dedicated to the fight against cancer. A stipend (from $400-$2,000 depending on the geographic location of the recipient or the type of award) will be presented to recipients on-site. Recipients may pick up their a check and welcome package at the Associate Member Resource and Career Center.

Requirements: Eligible candidates are graduate students, medical students and residents, clinical fellows or equivalent, and postdoctoral fellows. Eligible candidates must be the presenter of a proffered paper. Eligible candidates may be traveling within the U.S. or from abroad. Some awards are specifically designated for those traveling from Asia, Europe, and countries with emerging economies.

Restrictions: Employees or subcontractors of private industry are not eligible.

Amount of Grant: $400-$2,000

Date(s) Application is Due: Jul 20

Contact: Mona E. Shater, Staff Assistant; (215) 440-9300 or (267) 646-0654; fax: (215) 440-9372; email: mona.shater@aacr.org

Internet: http://www.aacr.org/home/scientists/meetings—workshops/special-conferences/metabolism-and-cancer/financial-support-for-attendance.aspx

Sponsor: American Association for Cancer Research
615 Chestnut Street, 17th Floor
Philadelphia, PA 19106-4404

AACR Scholar-in-Training Awards - Special Conferences 88

The AACR offers Scholar-in-Training Awards to enhance the education and training of early career scientists by providing financial support for their attendance at AACR Special Conferences. These awards are provided to offset a portion of the registration, travel, and subsistence expenses incurred in attending these conferences. A stipend (typically $400–$1,400) will be presented to award recipients at the conference.

Requirements: All graduate and medical students, postdoctoral fellows, and physicians-in-training who submit abstracts may be considered for a Scholar-in-Training Award.

Restrictions: Employees or subcontractors of private industry are not eligible.

Amount of Grant: $400-$1,400

Contact: Mona E. Shater, Staff Assistant; (215) 440-9300 or (267) 646-0654; fax: (215) 440-9372 or (215) 440-9412; email: mona.shater@aacr.org or programs@aacr.org

Internet: http://www.aacr.org/home/scientists/meetings—workshops/travel-grants/scholar-in-training-awards—-special-conferences.aspx

Sponsor: American Association for Cancer Research
615 Chestnut Street, 17th Floor
Philadelphia, PA 19106-4404

AACR Team Science Award 89

The Award has been established by the AACR and Eli Lilly and Company to acknowledge and catalyze the growing importance of interdisciplinary teams to the understanding of cancer and/or the translation of research discoveries into clinical cancer applications. In addition, through the presentation of this Award, the AACR and Eli Lilly seek to effect change within the traditional cancer research culture by recognizing those institutions that value and foster interdisciplinary team science. These institutions will have demonstrated their support of a team science environment by creating mechanisms to enhance the required infrastructure, such as through pilot funding, technology transfer offices, shared resources, etc., and by presenting awards, honors, appointments, and promotions to those who participate in interdisciplinary teams. Nominations for the 2009 Award will be accepted until November 16.

Requirements: For the purpose of this Award, a team is defined as a group of individuals representing interdisciplinary expertise, each of whom have made substantive and quantifiable contributions to the research being recognized. Team members may be working within the same institution or at several institutions. Candidacy is open to all cancer researchers who are affiliated with any institution involved in cancer research, cancer medicine, or cancer-related biomedical science anywhere in the world. Such institutions include those in academia, industry, or government.

Amount of Grant: $50,000

Date(s) Application is Due: Nov 16

Contact: Monique P. Eversley, Program Associate; (267) 646-0576 or (215) 440-9300, ext. 1400; fax: (215) 440-9372; email: monique.eversley@aacr.org or awards@aacr.org

Internet: http://www.aacr.org/home/scientists/scientific-achievement-awards/team-science-award.aspx

Sponsor: American Association of Cancer Research
615 Chestnut Street, 17th Floor
Philadelphia, PA 19106-4404

AACR Thomas J. Bardos Science Education Awards 90

AACR-Thomas J. Bardos Science Education Awards for Undergraduate Students are available to full-time third-year undergraduate students majoring in science. The purpose of these awards is to inspire young science students to enter the field of cancer research. The award consists of a waiver of registration fees for two annual AACR meetings and $1500/year for research and travel expenses. The award is for a two-year period.

Requirements: Candidates must be full-time, third year undergraduate students majoring in science. Applications from students who are not yet committed to cancer research are welcome.

Amount of Grant: $1,500 plus a wave of registration fee

Date(s) Application is Due: Dec 7

Contact: Mona E. Shater, Staff Assistant; (215) 440-9300 or (267) 646-0654; fax: (215) 440-9412; email: mona.shater@aacr.org or scienceeducation@aacr.org
Internet: http://www.aacr.org/home/scientists/meetings—workshops/travel-grants/aacr-thomas-j-bardos-science-education-awards-for-undergraduate-students-.aspx
Sponsor: American Association for Cancer Research
615 Chestnut Street, 17th Floor
Philadelphia, PA 19106-4404

AACR-American Cancer Society Award for Research Excellence in Cancer Epidemiology and Prevention 91

The AACR and the American Cancer Society established this Award in 1992 to honor outstanding research accomplishments in the fields of cancer epidemiology, biomarkers, and prevention. Nominations may be made via letter from any scientist, whether an AACR member or nonmember, who is now or has been affiliated with any institution involved in cancer research, cancer medicine, or cancer-related biomedical science. The winner will receive an honorarium of $5,000 and give a 50-minute lecture during the AACR Annual Meeting.
Requirements: Candidacy is open to all cancer researchers who are affiliated with any institution involved in cancer research, cancer medicine, or cancer-related biomedical science anywhere in the world. Such institutions include those in academia, industry, or government.
Restrictions: Institutions or organizations are not eligible for the Award. Candidates may not nominate themselves.
Amount of Grant: $5,000 honorarium
Date(s) Application is Due: Oct 15
Contact: Monique P. Eversley, Program Associate; (267) 646-0576; email: monique.eversley@aacr.org
Internet: http://www.aacr.org/home/scientists/scientific-achievement-awards/acs-award.aspx
Sponsor: American Association for Cancer Research
615 Chestnut Street, 17th Floor
Philadelphia, PA 19106-4404

AACR-Colorectal Cancer Coalition Fellows Grant 92

The Fellowship program supports innovative research by a meritorious young investigator by presenting the Fellow with research funds to pursue an independent line of investigation within the context of his/her current placement. This is a one-year grant of $30,000. Research projects are restricted to translational or clinical cancer research that has an ultimate goal of developing or improving therapeutic interventions for patients with metastatic colorectal cancer. One grant will be awarded this cycle.
Requirements: Candidates must be, at the start of the grant term, in their third, fourth, or fifth year of their fellowship status.
Amount of Grant: $30,000
Date(s) Application is Due: Dec 18
Contact: Hanna Hopfinger, Grants Program Assistant; (267) 646-0665; fax: (215) 440-9372; email: hanna.hopfinger@aacr.org
Internet: http://www.aacr.org/home/scientists/research-funding—fellowships/fellows-grants.aspx
Sponsor: American Association for Cancer Research
615 Chestnut Street, 17th Floor
Philadelphia, PA 19106-4404

AACR-FNAB Fellows Grant for Translational Pancreatic Cancer Research 93

The AACR-FNAB Fellows Grant for Translational Pancreatic Cancer Research provides a one-year grant of $35,000. Research projects are restricted to translational pancreatic cancer research that includes the use of human tissue and has implications for therapeutic application and individualized medicine. Proposed research must have implications for individualized cancer treatment and must make use of human biopsies or samples, such as needle biopsies or circulating cancer cells. In vivo primary tumor explants meet these criteria, but xenografts from established cell lines do not. One grant will be awarded this cycle.
Requirements: Candidates must hold the title of Postdoctoral Fellow or Clinical Research Fellow at an academic facility, teaching hospital, or research institution. Candidates must hold this title at the start of the fellowship term on July 1, and continue to hold it during the entire fellowship term.
Samples: Sarat Chandarlapaty, M.D., Ph.D., Memorial Sloan-Kettering Cancer Center, New York, NY (2007); Sibele I. Meireles, Ph.D., Fox Chase Cancer Center, Philadelphia, PA (2006); Daniel C. Cho, M.D., Beth Israel Deaconess Medical Center, Boston, MA (2006).
Amount of Grant: $35,000
Date(s) Application is Due: Dec 18; Dec 23
Contact: Hanna Hopfinger, Program Assistant; (267) 646-0665 or (215) 440-9300; fax: (215) 440-9372; email: hanna.hopfinger@aacr.org or awards@aacr.org
Internet: http://www.aacr.org/home/scientists/research-funding—fellowships/fellows-grants.aspx
Sponsor: American Association for Cancer Research
615 Chestnut Street, 17th Floor
Philadelphia, PA 19106-4404

AACR-FNAB Fellows Grant for Translational Pancreatic Cancer Research 94

The Fellows Grants support innovative research by a meritorious young investigator by presenting the Fellow with research funds to pursue an independent line of investigation within the context of his/her current placement. This is a one-year grant of $35,000. Research projects are restricted to translational pancreatic cancer research that includes the use of human tissue and has implications for therapeutic application and individualized medicine.
Requirements: Candidates must be, at the start of the grant term, in their third, fourth, or fifth year of their fellowship status.
Amount of Grant: $35,000
Date(s) Application is Due: Dec 18
Contact: Julia Laurence, Staff Assistant; (215) 440-9300, ext. 102 or (267) 646-0655; fax: (215) 440-9372; email: laurence@aacr.org
Internet: http://www.aacr.org/home/scientists/research-funding—fellowships/fellows-grants.aspx
Sponsor: American Association for Cancer Research
615 Chestnut Street, 17th Floor
Philadelphia, PA 19106-4404

AACR-FNAB Foundation Career Development Award for Translational Cancer Research 95

Career development awards are two-year awards that support research by scientists who are engaged in meritorious cancer research at academic institutions. These awards provide important transitional support for direct research expenses as researchers move from the ranks of early career scientists to faculty status. The Awards are open to junior faculty who completed postdoctoral studies or clinical fellowships between specified dates and who are at an academic or medical institution. Research projects in this area should have direct applicability to translational cancer and be focused on any individualized therapeutic area. Projects should have implications for individualized cancer treatment and make use of human biopsies or samples, such as needle biopsies or circulating cancer cells. One grant will be presented annually. The submission deadline is December 3, with the decision date March 31.
Requirements: Candidates must have acquired a doctoral degree in a related field and may not currently be a candidate for a further doctoral or professional degree. If a candidate has obtained an equivalent degree at a foreign institution, information on the nature of the degree must be provided at the time of application.
Restrictions: Awards are restricted to investigators or institutions within the U.S. Employees of a national government and employees of private industry are ineligible.
Samples: Tara A. Young, M.D., Ph.D., University of California, Los Angeles, Los Angeles, CA, $50,000 - Project: High Resolution Cytogenetic Study of Archival Metastatic Choroidal Melanoma (2008-2010).
Amount of Grant: $50,000 per year for two years
Date(s) Application is Due: Dec 3
Contact: Julia Laurence, Staff Assistant; (267) 646-0655; fax: (215) 440-9372; email: julia.laurence@aacr.org or awards@aacr.org
Internet: http://www.aacr.org/home/scientists/research-funding—fellowships/research-funding/research-funding—fellowships/career-development-award-recipients.aspx
Sponsor: American Association for Cancer Research
615 Chestnut Street, 17th Floor
Philadelphia, PA 19106-4404

AACR-Genentech BioOncology Career Development Award for Cancer Research on the HER Family Pathway 96

Career development awards are two-year awards that support research by scientists who are engaged in meritorious cancer research at academic institutions. These awards provide important transitional support for direct research expenses as researchers move from the ranks of early career scientists to faculty status. The Awards are open to junior faculty who completed postdoctoral studies or clinical fellowships between specified dates and who are at an academic or medical institution. Research projects in this area should have direct applicability to basic, translational, or clinical cancer research focused on the HER Family Pathway. One grant will be presented annually. The submission deadline is December 3, with the decision date March 31.
Requirements: Candidates must be affiliated with an institution in the U.S. and must hold an M.D. or combined M.D./Ph.D. If a candidate has obtained an equivalent degree at a foreign institution, information on the nature of the degree must be provided at the time of application.
Restrictions: Employees of a national government and employees of private industry are ineligible.
Amount of Grant: $50,000 per year for two years
Date(s) Application is Due: Dec 3
Contact: Julia Laurence, Staff Assistant; (267) 646-0655; fax: (215) 440-9372; email: julia.laurence@aacr.org or awards@aacr.org
Internet: http://www.aacr.org/
Sponsor: American Association for Cancer Research
615 Chestnut Street, 17th Floor
Philadelphia, PA 19106-4404

AACR-Genentech BioOncology Fellowship for Cancer Research in Angiogenesis 97

AACR Research Fellowships are open to Postdoctoral Fellows and Clinical Research Fellows at an academic facility, teaching hospital, or research institution who will be in the 1st, 2nd, or 3rd year of their postdoctoral training at the start of the fellowship term on July 1. This is a two-year term with a grant of $35,000 per year. One Fellowship will be awarded.
Requirements: The recipients of the Fellowships must attend the AACR Annual Meeting to accept the award.
Restrictions: Research projects are restricted to cancer research with direct applicability to angiogenesis.

Amount of Grant: $35,000 per year for two years
Date(s) Application is Due: Dec 3
Contact: Hanna Hopfinger, Program Assistant; (267) 646-0665; fax: (215) 440-9372; email: hanna.hopfinger@aacr.org
Internet: http://www.aacr.org/
Sponsor: American Association for Cancer Research
615 Chestnut Street, 17th Floor
Philadelphia, PA 19106-4404

AACR-GlaxoSmithKline Clinical Cancer Research Scholar Awards **98**
These awards provide support of $4,000 which may be used by the recipient to support attendance at the Annual Meeting and any other AACR meeting within a two-year period. Up to $2,000 per meeting may be used, and reimbursement checks are provided after the meeting upon submission of proper documentation of travel, housing, registration, and/or subsistence expenses. Award recipients are still required to pay the Annual Meeting registration fee and make their own travel and housing arrangements. Selection is made by the Program Committee based upon the novelty, quality, and significance of the abstract submitted. Award recipients will receive notification separate from abstract acceptance and scheduling information.
Requirements: Graduate students, medical students and residents, clinical fellows or equivalent, and postdoctoral fellows (AACR members and nonmembers) who are presenters of a meritorious abstract in clinical cancer research are eligible.
Restrictions: Employees or subcontractors of private industry are not eligible.
Samples: Manisha Bhutani, M.D., UT M.D. Anderson Cancer Center (2008); David W. Cescon, M.D., Princess Margaret Hospital, University of Toronto (2008); Zeshaan A. Rasheed, M.D., Ph.D., Sidney Kimmel Comprehensive Cancer Center, Johns Hopkins University School of Medicine (2008).
Amount of Grant: $2,000-$4,000
Date(s) Application is Due: Nov 28
Contact: Mona E. Shater, Staff Assistant; (215) 440-9300 or (267) 646-0654; fax: (215) 440-9372; email: mona.shater@aacr.org
Internet: http://www.aacr.org/home/scientists/meetings—workshops/travel-grants/aacr-glaxosmithkline-clinical-cancer-research-scholar-awards.aspx
Sponsor: American Association for Cancer Research
615 Chestnut Street, 17th Floor
Philadelphia, PA 19106-4404

AACR-Minorities in Cancer Research Jane Cooke Wright Lectureship Awards **99**
The AACR-Minorities in Cancer Research Jane Cooke Wright Lectureship was first presented in 2006. The Lectureship is intended to give recognition to an outstanding scientist who has made meritorious contributions to the field of cancer research and who has, through leadership or by example, furthered the advancement of minority investigators in cancer research. The recipient will present the AACR-Minorities in Cancer Research Jane Cooke Wright Lectureship during the AACR Annual Meeting, receive an honorarium and commemorative plaque, and receive support for the winner and a guest to attend the Annual Meeting.
Requirements: Candidacy is open to all cancer researchers who are affiliated with any institution involved in cancer research, cancer medicine, or cancer-related biomedical science anywhere in the world. Such institutions include those in academia, industry, or government. Nominations may be made by any scientist, whether an AACR member or nonmember, who is now or has been affiliated with any institution involved in cancer research, cancer medicine, or cancer-related biomedical science. Candidates may not nominate themselves. Nominations must be submitted online at https://proposalcentral.altum.com, no later than 4:00 p.m. United States Eastern Time on October 15th. Paper nominations will not be accepted.
Restrictions: Institutions or organizations are not eligible for the Lectureship.
Date(s) Application is Due: Oct 15
Contact: Monique P. Eversley, Staff Associate; (267) 646-0576 or (215) 440-9300, ext. 1400; fax: (215) 440-9372; email: monique.eversley@aacr.org or awards@aacr.org
Internet: http://www.aacr.org/home/scientists/scientific-achievement-awards/micr-wright-lectureship.aspx
Sponsor: American Association for Cancer Research
615 Chestnut Street, 17th Floor
Philadelphia, PA 19106-4404

AACR-National Brain Tumor Foundation Fellows Grant **100**
The AACR-National Brain Tumor Society Fellowship, in memory of Bonnie Brooks, is open to Postdoctoral Fellows and Clinical Research Fellows at an academic facility, teaching hospital, or research institution. This fellowship provides a one-year grant of $40,000 to support the salary and benefits of Fellows engaged in Glioblastoma multiforme (GBM) research. A partial amount of funds may be designated for research support. It is anticipated that two fellowships will be awarded. The AACR requires applicants to submit both an online and a paper application. The online application must be submitted by 12:00 noon (United States Eastern Time) on August 10, the application must be submitted using the proposalCENTRAL website at https://proposalcentral.altum.com. The paper application with original signatures and all supporting documents must be postmarked and sent no later then August 12.
Requirements: Candidates must be, at the start of the grant term, in their third, fourth, or fifth year of their fellowship status.
Restrictions: Investigators holding the rank of Instructor, Adjunct Professor, Assistant Professor, Research Assistant Professor, the equivalent or higher are not eligible.
Amount of Grant: $40,000
Date(s) Application is Due: Aug 10; Aug 12
Contact: Hanna Hopfinger, Grants Program Assistant; (267) 646-0665; fax: (215) 440-9372; email: hanna.hopfinger@aacr.org
Internet: http://www.aacr.org/home/scientists/research-funding—fellowships/postdoctoral-fellowships.aspx
Sponsor: American Association for Cancer Research
615 Chestnut Street, 17th Floor
Philadelphia, PA 19106-4404

AACR-NCI International Investigator Opportunity Grants **101**
Recognizing that there is no substitute for the collegial interaction and scholarly discussion that is a cornerstone of scientific advancement, these grants provide significant financial support for meeting registration, housing, travel, and incidentals to attend the annual American Association for Cancer Research Meeting. Grants are available for ten cancer researchers from countries where such opportunities are limited.
Requirements: Applicants must be nationals or permanent residents of, and must reside and conduct cancer research within, low and middle-income countries as defined by the World Bank. Applicants should also hold an doctorate or equivalent degree and be actively engaged in a program of cancer research with a record of cancer-focused publications in peer-reviewed scientific journals.
Restrictions: Funds may not be used for entertainment expenses (such as for tours or in-room movies), meals for other individuals, souvenirs, and other non-meeting expenses.
Samples: Hakan Akbulut, M.D., Professor, Medical Oncology, Ankara University, Ankara, Turkey (2008); Soo H. Teo, D.Phil., Chief Executive, Cancer Research Initiatives Foundation, Subang Jaya, Malaysia (2008); Jozsef Tovari, Ph.D., Lab Head, Department of Tumor Progression, National Institute of Oncology, Budapest, Hungary (2008).
Date(s) Application is Due: Sep 28;
Contact: Susan Waskey, Program Assistant; (215) 440-9300 or (866) 423-3965; fax: (215) 440-9313; email: susan.waskey@aacr.org
Internet: http://www.aacr.org/home/scientists/meetings-workshops/travel-grants.aspx
Sponsor: American Association for Cancer Research and the National Cancer Institute
615 Chestnut Street, 17th Floor
Philadelphia, PA 19106-4404

AACR-Pancreatic Cancer Action Network Career Development Award for Pancreatic Cancer Research **102**
The Pancreatic Cancer Action Network-AACR Career Development Award represents a joint effort to encourage and support early career scientist who are in the first four years of a faculty appointment to conduct pancreatic cancer research and establish successful career paths in this field. The research proposed for funding may be basic, translational, clinical or epidemiological in nature and must have direct applicability and relevance to pancreatic cancer. The Award provides a two year grant of $200,000 ($100,000 per year) for direct research expenses, which may include salary and benefits of the grant recipient, postdoctoral or clinical research fellows, and/or research assistants, research/laboratory supplies and equipment. It is anticipated that three Career Development Awards will be funded.
Requirements: Candidates must have acquired a doctoral degree in a related field and may not currently be a candidate for a further doctoral or professional degree. If a candidate has obtained an equivalent degree at a foreign institution, information on the nature of the degree must be provided at the time of application.
Restrictions: Awards are restricted to investigators or institutions within the U.S. Employees of a national government and employees of private industry are ineligible.
Amount of Grant: $200,000 per year for two years
Date(s) Application is Due: Oct 28
Contact: Julia Laurence, Program Assistant; (267) 646-0655; fax: (215) 440-9372; email: julia.laurence@aacr.org or awards@aacr.org
Internet: http://www.aacr.org/home/scientists/research-funding—fellowships/career-development-awards.aspx
Sponsor: American Association for Cancer Research
615 Chestnut Street, 17th Floor
Philadelphia, PA 19106-4404

AACR-Pancreatic Cancer Action Network Innovative Grants **103**
The AACR-PanCAN Pilot Grants represent a joint effort of the AACR and the Pancreatic Cancer Action Network to support innovative research focusing on the early detection or treatment of pancreatic cancer. Research projects may have direct application to pancreatic cancer or may demonstrate relevance to pancreatic cancer in order to encourage investigators with experience in other areas of research to apply their ideas to this challenging field. Proposals will be accepted for innovative research projects that have a direct application or demonstrate relevance to the early detection or treatment of pancreatic cancer; projects may be in any discipline of basic, translational, clinical, or epidemiological cancer research. Proposals that will develop preliminary data necessary to prepare and submit a competitive research grant application to a major federal funding agency will also be accepted. Special emphasis will be placed on research that is not duplicative of other efforts and has the potential for national application. Researchers who are affiliated with any institution involved in cancer research, cancer medicine, or cancer-related biomedical science within the United States may apply. There are no residency status restrictions. Each grantee will be awarded a total of $200,000, paid over the two-year term.
Requirements: Applicants must have acquired a doctoral degree in a related field. If an applicant has obtained an equivalent degree at a foreign institution, information on the nature of the degree must be provided at the time of application.

Restrictions: Employees or subcontractors of a national government or the for-profit private industry are not eligible to apply. Members of the Scientific Review Committee are not eligible for these grants. Current or past recipients of a PanCAN Pilot Grant are not eligible.
Amount of Grant: $200,000 over two years
Date(s) Application is Due: Oct 5; Nov 30
Contact: Julia Laurence, Program Assistant; (215) 440-9300, ext. 102 or (267) 646-0655; fax: (215) 440-9372; email: julia.laurence@aacr.org
Internet: http://www.aacr.org/home/scientists/research-funding—fellowships/pancreatic-cancer-action-network-aacr-innovative-grants.aspx
Sponsor: American Association for Cancer Research
615 Chestnut Street, 17th Floor
Philadelphia, PA 19106-4404

AACR-Prevent Cancer Foundation Award for Excellence in Cancer Prevention Research **104**
he Award for Excellence in Cancer Prevention Research will be given to a scientist residing in any country in the world for his or her seminal contributions to the field of cancer prevention. Such investigations must have been conducted in basic, translational, clinical, epidemiological, or behavioral science in cancer prevention research. Further, these studies must have had not only a major impact on the field, but must also have stimulated new directions in this important area. The recipient of the Award will receive a $5,000 honorarium and will present a lecture at the Annual AACR International Conference. Nominations for the Award must be submitted electronically no later than 4:00 p.m. United States Eastern Time on Monday, July 31.
Requirements: All cancer researchers who are affiliated with any institution involved in cancer research, cancer medicine, or cancer-related biomedical science anywhere in the world. Such institutions include those in academia, industry, or government may be nominated for the Award. Candidates must currently maintain an active research program, have a record of recent publications, and be able to present the Award lecture at the Conference.
Restrictions: Institutions or organizations are not eligible for the Award. Paper nominations will not be accepted.
Amount of Grant: $5,000 honorarium
Date(s) Application is Due: Jul 31
Contact: Monique P. Eversley, Staff Associate; (267) 646-0576 or (215) 440-9300, ext. 1400; fax: (215) 440-9372; email: monique.eversley@aacr.org or awards@aacr.org
Internet: http://www.aacr.org/home/scientists/scientific-achievement-awards/prevent-cancer-award.aspx
Sponsor: American Association for Cancer Research / Prevent Cancer Foundation
615 Chestnut Street, 17th Floor
Philadelphia, PA 19106-4404

AACR-WICR Scholar Awards **105**
AACR-WICR Scholar Awards are awarded to ten members of Women in Cancer Research who are scientists-in-training and presenters of meritorious scientific papers at AACR Annual Meetings.
Requirements: Eligible candidates for these awards must fit the following criteria, candidates must be: members of Women in Cancer Research (WICR); full time scientists-in-training who are graduate students, medical students, residents, clinical fellows or equivalent, or postdoctoral fellows; travelling from within the United States or abroad; first authors on abstracts submitted for consideration for presentation at the AACR Annual Meeting.
Date(s) Application is Due: Dec 1
Contact: Lauren Medvetz, Program Coordinator; (267) 646-0689; fax: (215) 440-9372; email: lauren.medvets@aacr.org
Internet: http://www.aacr.org/home/scientists/meetings—workshops/travel-grants/wicr-scholar-awards.aspx
Sponsor: American Association for Cancer Research and Women in Cancer Research (WICR)
615 Chestnut Street, 17th Floor
Philadelphia, PA 19106-4404

AACR-Women in Cancer Research Charlotte Friend Memorial Lectureships **106**
The AACR-Women in Cancer Research Charlotte Friend Memorial Lectureship was established in 1998 in honor of renowned virologist and discoverer of the Friend virus, Dr. Charlotte Friend, for her pioneering research on viruses, cell differentiation, and cancer. The lecture is intended to give recognition to an outstanding female or male scientist who has made meritorious contributions to the field of cancer research and who has, through leadership or by example, furthered the advancement of women in science. The winner of the Lectureship will present a 50-minute lecture during the AACR Annual Meeting, receive an honorarium and commemorative plaque, and receive support for the winner and a guest to attend the Annual Meeting.
Requirements: Candidacy is open to all cancer researchers who are affiliated with any institution involved in cancer research, cancer medicine, or cancer-related biomedical science anywhere in the world. Such institutions include those in academia, industry, or government.
Restrictions: Nominations may be made by any scientist, whether an AACR member or nonmember, who is now or has been affiliated with any institution involved in cancer research, cancer medicine, or cancer-related biomedical science. Candidates may not nominate themselves. Nominations must be submitted online at https://proposalcentral.altum.com, no later than 4:00 p.m. United States Eastern Time on October 15th. Paper nominations will not be accepted. Institutions or organizations are not eligible.
Date(s) Application is Due: Oct 15
Contact: Lauren Medvetz, Program Coordinator; (267) 646-0689; fax: (215) 440-9372; email: lauren.medvets@aacr.org
Internet: http://www.aacr.org/home/scientists/scientific-achievement-awards/wicr-friend-lectureship.aspx
Sponsor: American Association for Cancer Research
615 Chestnut Street, 17th Floor
Philadelphia, PA 19106-4404

AACR Basic Cancer Research Fellowships **107**
The AACR Basic Cancer Research Fellowships consist of two Fellowships, each one-year grants. The AACR Anna D, Barker Fellowship in Basic Cancer Research, funds $40,000, and the AACR-Astellas U.S.A Foundation Fellowships in Basic Cancer Research provides funding in the amount of $30,000. These grants are for salary and benefits to the Fellows. A partial amount of funds may be designated for direct research support. The recipients must attend the AACR Annual Meeting to accept the grants. The AACR requires applicants to submit both an online and a paper application. The online application must be completed by 12:00 noon (United States Eastern Time) on December 10, using the proposalCENTRAL website at http://propasalcentral.altum.com. The paper application with original signatures and all supporting documents must be postmarked and sent no later then December 15.
Requirements: Applications are open to Postdoctoral Fellows and Clinical Research Fellows at an academic facility, teaching hospital, or research institution who will be in the 1st, 2nd, or 3rd year of their postdoctoral training at the start of the fellowship.
Restrictions: Academic faculty holding the rank of assistant professor or higher, graduate or medical students, government employees, and employees of private industry are not eligible.
Amount of Grant: $30,000 - $40,000 range
Date(s) Application is Due: Dec 10; Dec 15
Contact: Hanna Hopfinger, Grants Program Assistant; (267) 646-0665; fax: (215) 440-9372; email: hanna.hopfinger@aacr.org
Internet: http://www.aacr.org/home/scientists/research-funding—fellowships/postdoctoral-fellowships.aspx
Sponsor: American Association for Cancer Research
615 Chestnut Street, 17th Floor
Philadelphia, PA 19106-4404

AAFA Investigator Research Grants **108**
AAFA is dedicated to finding the causes, new treatments and cures for asthma and allergic diseases. AAFA offers a program that sponsors seed grants for investigators wishing to explore new areas of scientific merit related to asthma and allergic diseases. Support has enabled 80% of the researchers who have received the AAFA research grant to win additional research funding from other sources totaling more than $18 million. The Asthma and Allergy of Foundation of America is the only patient organization in the United States that funds research grants for both asthma and allergies. At this time, the application process for grants is through an NIH referral system.
Contact: Mary Brasler, Director of Programs and Services; (202) 466-7643, ext. 238; email: mbrasler@aafa.org
Internet: http://www.aafa.org/display.cfm?id=6⊠=64
Sponsor: Asthma and Allergy Foundation of America
1233 20th Street, NW, Suite 402
Washington, DC 20036

AAFCS International Graduate Fellowships **109**
The Association encourages graduate study in family and consumer sciences and its subspecialties, such as textiles and clothing, nutrition, institutional management/food service systems administration, consumer studies, Cooperative Extension, and family and consumer sciences communication, education, and administration. International graduate fellowships are awarded to individuals who have exhibited the potential to make contributions to the family and consumer sciences profession.
Requirements: Applicants must be citizens or permanent residents of the United States. Applicant must show clearly defined plans for full-time graduate or undergraduate study during the time for which the fellowship is awarded. Each request for appropriate application form must be accompanied by an application fee of $40.
Contact: Fellowships and Awards Committee; (703) 706-4600; fax: (703) 706-4663; email: staff@aafcs.org
Internet: http://www.aafcs.org/programs/scholarships.htm
Sponsor: American Association of Family and Consumer Sciences
400 N. Columbus Street, Suite 202
Alexandria, VA 22314

AAFCS National Graduate Fellowships **110**
AAFCS annually awards national graduate fellowships to support graduate study in areas such as family and consumer sciences, nutrition, textiles, and home economics. The fellowships are awarded to individuals who have exhibited the potential for making contributions to these professions. It is recommended that applicants first complete at least one year of professional family and consumer science experience.
Requirements: Applicants must be citizens or permanent residents of the United States. Applicant must show clearly defined plans for full-time graduate or undergraduate study during the time for which the fellowship is awarded. Each request for appropriate application form must be accompanied by an application fee of $40.
Amount of Grant: $5,000 maximum
Date(s) Application is Due: Jan 7

Contact: Fellowships and Awards Committee; (703) 706-4600; fax: (703) 706-4663; email: staff@aafcs.org
Internet: http://www.aafcs.org/programs/fellowshipseven.html
Sponsor: American Association of Family and Consumer Sciences
400 N. Columbus Street, Suite 202
Alexandria, VA 22314

AAFCS National Undergraduate Scholarships 111
The Association encourages undergraduate study in family and consumer sciences and its subspecialties, such as textiles and clothing, nutrition, institutional management/food service systems administration, consumer studies, Cooperative Extension, and family and consumer sciences communication, education, and administration. Scholarships are awarded to individuals who have exhibited the potential to make contributions to the family and consumer sciences profession.
Requirements: Applicants must be citizens or permanent residents of the United States. Applicant must show clearly defined plans for full-time graduate or undergraduate study during the time for which the fellowship is awarded. Each request for appropriate application form must be accompanied by an application fee of $40.
Amount of Grant: $5,000
Date(s) Application is Due: Jan 7
Contact: Scholarships and Awards Committee; (703) 706-4600; fax: (703) 706-4663; email: staff@aafcs.org
Internet: http://www.aafcs.org/programs/scholarships.htm
Sponsor: American Association of Family and Consumer Sciences
400 N. Columbus Street, Suite 202
Alexandria, VA 22314

AAFP Foundation Health Literacy State Grants 112
The AAFP Foundation recognizes that nearly half of all American adults (90 million people) have difficulty reading, understanding and acting upon all types of health information. They are often ashamed and devise methods to mask their difficulty or may be reluctant to ask questions for fear of being perceived as ignorant. To help address literacy concerns, the AAFP Foundation has developed the Health Literacy State Grant Awards Program. The purpose of the program is to support collaborative projects that address health literacy concerns at the state and local level. Five awards in the amount $10,000 each will be offered.
Amount of Grant: $10,000
Date(s) Application is Due: Mar 26
Contact: Susie Morantz, Senior Program Manager; (913) 906-6000, ext. 4470 or (800) 274-2237; fax: (913) 906-6095; email: smorantz@aafp.org
Internet: http://www.aafpfoundation.org/x821.xml
Sponsor: American Academy of Family Physicians Foundation
11400 Tomahawk Creek Parkway, Suite 440
Leawood, KS 66211-2672

AAFP Foundation Joint Grants 113
The foundation supports clinical research projects within family practice that ultimately will result in improved patient care. This program includes a research grant stimulation program that is designed to stimulate research in family practice by supporting small and first-time research projects. Longer research proposals must be prepared in accordance with standard guidelines for grant proposals.
Requirements: Eligible to apply are individual family physicians, residents in family practice, and medical students planning to pursue the specialty of family practice; educational and health care institutions or organizations that will use the grant exclusively for programs or projects directly involved with family practice or family medicine; departments of family practice; family practice residency programs; and family practice organizations or associations. Research stimulation proposals may be reviewed at any time during the year depending on availability of funds.
Restrictions: Proposals seeking support for the cost of instituting programs or support for such activities as videotape production, designing curriculum, or implementing a project, etc., will be denied.
Amount of Grant: $30,000 maximum
Contact: Susie Morantz, Senior Program Manager; (913) 906-6000, ext. 4470 or (800) 274-2237; fax: (913) 906-6095; email: smorantz@aafp.org
Internet: http://www.aafpfoundation.org/x270.xml
Sponsor: American Academy of Family Physicians Foundation
11400 Tomahawk Creek Parkway, Suite 440
Leawood, KS 66211-2672

AAFP Foundation Pfizer Teacher Development Awards 114
The purpose of the awards is to honor community-based physicians who give up time from their practice to teach family medicine students and/or residents part time. Eligible candidates may serve as preceptors or as volunteer teachers at other sites, including family medicine teaching centers. Guidelines are available online.
Requirements: Applicant must have graduated from an ACGME-approved family practice residency program within the last seven years; have entered family medicine; be a member of the American Academy of Family Physicians; have entered or plan to enter part-time family medicine teaching (not less than four hours per month and no more than 32 hours per month—averaged over a year); and teach voluntarily or receive no more than $18,000 compensation for the educational time devoted to residents and/or students.
Amount of Grant: $2,000
Contact: Sondra Goodman, Grants Program Manager; (913) 906-6000, ext. 4457 or (800) 274-2237; fax: (913) 906-6095; email: sgoodman@aafp.org
Internet: http://www.aafpfoundation.org/x269.xml
Sponsor: American Academy of Family Physicians Foundation
11400 Tomahawk Creek Parkway, Suite 440
Leawood, KS 66211-2672

AAFP Foundation Wyeth Immunization Awards 115
This program offers family medicine residency programs the opportunity to receive recognition for identifying and developing creative solutions to overcoming barriers to childhood immunizations, thus increasing immunization rates, and to share the best practices that have benefited the communities in which they live. Applications are accepted annually for one of the following award track categories: Best Practices Award—overall achievement with systems already in place to overcome immunization barriers and achieve high rates within a certain time frame; Most Improved Award—overcame barriers and other challenges to greatly enhance immunization rates; and Implement New System Grant—residency programs seeking to implement a new system to help increase immunization rates in under-served children. Grant winners will receive: one of 10 monetary awards (four at $5,000 and six at $10,000) determined by rank of application as scored by review panel; an education scholarship for $1,000 to send a resident to the annual AAFP National Conference of Family Medicine Residents and Medical Students; an additional travel scholarship to send a resident to the AAFP Scientific Assembly (top six); and a plaque of recognition.
Requirements: Family medicine residency programs that have increased immunization rates within a defined time frame and can demonstrate the best practices implemented to achieve the higher compliance are eligible.
Amount of Grant: $1,000-$10,000
Date(s) Application is Due: Apr 21
Contact: Sondra Goodman, Grants Program Manager; (913) 906-6000, ext. 4457 or (800) 274-2237; fax: (913) 906-6095; email: sgoodman@aafp.org
Internet: http://www.aafpfoundation.org/x655.xml
Sponsor: American Academy of Family Physicians Foundation
11400 Tomahawk Creek Parkway, Suite 440
Leawood, KS 66211-2672

AAFP Research Stimulation Grants 116
This Program provides relatively small grants to stimulate research in family practice in the areas of preliminary efforts leading to a larger research project, pilot projects, and data collection for a larger research project. The applicant must include a discussion of how the proposed project is anticipated to lead to a larger project. Grant applications will be accepted twice a year: by March 1 and September 1.
Requirements: Eligible to apply are individual family physicians, family practice/medicine organizations or associations, residents in family practice, departments of family medicine, and educational and health care institutions directly involved in family practice/medicine.
Amount of Grant: $7,500
Date(s) Application is Due: Mar 1; Sep 1
Contact: Susie Morantz, Senior Program Manager; (913) 906-6000, ext. 4470 or (800) 274-2237; fax: (913) 906-6095; email: smorantz@aafp.org
Internet: http://www.aafpfoundation.org/x446.xml
Sponsor: American Academy of Family Physicians Foundation
11400 Tomahawk Creek Parkway, Suite 440
Leawood, KS 66211-2672

AAFPRS Ben Shuster Memorial Award 117
This award is given annually for the best paper based on clinical work or research in the field of facial plastic surgery by a resident or fellow in training. The paper must have been delivered at a national meeting (or its equivalent) within the preceding two years prior to the February 1 date of submission. Studies prepared during the first year after completion of residency training will be considered provided that the research was conducted during the author's residency training program or fellowship. A certificate and an award of $1,000 are presented.
Requirements: The competition is open to U.S. or Canadian residents or fellows in otolaryngology who are members of AAFPRS. Each entrant must be the sole or senior author and an AAFPRS member.
Amount of Grant: $1,000
Date(s) Application is Due: Feb 1
Contact: Coordinator; (703) 299-9291; fax: (703) 299-8898; email: info@aafprs.org
Internet: http://www.aafprs.org/physician/awards_grants/awards.html
Sponsor: American Academy of Facial, Plastic, and Reconstructive Surgery
310 S Henry Street
Alexandria, VA 22314

AAFPRS Bernstein Grant 118
The purpose of the grant is to encourage original research projects that will advance facial plastic and reconstructive surgery. The grant may be used as seed money for research projects. Applicants should submit an application, a detailed proposal, the investigator's curriculum vita, and letters from the appropriate institutional review committees certifying institutional conformity to the U.S. government guidelines for human and animal experiments. The recipient should complete his or her work within three (3) years with interim reports due each year. All research grant monies awarded are intended to fund direct costs related to the research as described in the grant proposal.
Requirements: Applicants should be U.S. or Canadian AAFPRS fellow members. The primary criteria are that the research be original and have direct application to facial plastic and reconstructive surgery.

Amount of Grant: $25,000
Date(s) Application is Due: Jan 15
Contact: Research Grant Coordinator; (703) 299-9291; fax: (703) 299-8898; email: info@aafprs.org
Internet: http://www.aafprs.org/physician/awards_grants/bernstein_grant.html
Sponsor: American Academy of Facial, Plastic, and Reconstructive Surgery
310 South Henry Street
Alexandria, VA 22314

AAFPRS Fellowships 119
The Educational and Research Foundation for the American Academy of Facial Plastic and Reconstructive Surgery fellowship program provides postgraduate training in facial plastic surgery. The objectives of the fellowship program are to: provide an outstanding academic opportunity for the acquisition of specialized knowledge and skills in facial plastic surgery; develop trained specialists who will contribute to the ongoing development of facial plastic and reconstructive surgery; foster development of facial plastic and reconstructive surgery educators, especially in residency programs; and encourage the development of new skills and knowledge in facial plastic and reconstructive surgery through basic research and clinical trials. Eligible physicians may apply for 40 positions available each year.
Requirements: Applicants to the Fellowship Program must be physicians who are in or have completed an otolaryngology or plastic surgery residency program accredited by the Accreditation Council for Graduate Medical Education (ACGME) or Royal College of Physicians and Surgeons of Canada (RCPSC) or board-certified in otolaryngology-head and neck surgery or plastic surgery. Applicants must be members of the AAFPRS before submitting an application.
Restrictions: Applicants should not be full-time faculty members holding the rank of assistant professor or higher at the institution where the fellowship will take place.
Date(s) Application is Due: Feb 1
Contact: Fellowship Coordinator; (703) 299-9291; fax: (703) 299-8898; email: info@aafprs.org or fsanders@aafprs.org
Internet: http://www.aafprs.org/physician/benefits/ben_fellow.html
Sponsor: American Academy of Facial, Plastic, and Reconstructive Surgery
310 South Henry Street
Alexandria, VA 22314

AAFPRS Investigator Development Grant 120
The purpose of the Investigator Development Grant is to support the work of a young faculty member in facial plastic surgery conducting significant clinical or laboratory research and involved in the training of resident surgeons in research. One $15,000 grant may be awarded each year upon receipt of the signed agreement. Recipients should complete their work within three (3) years with interim reports due each year. An extension is possible upon written request to the Research Committee. The original proposal and all other requirements should be submitted to C.O.R.E. no later than January 15 or the next business day thereafter.
Requirements: An applicant must be an AAFPRS member at any level involved in the training of resident surgeons.
Amount of Grant: $15,000 maximum
Date(s) Application is Due: Jan 15
Contact: Research Grant Coordinator; (703) 299-9291; fax: (703) 299-8898; email: info@aafprs.org
Internet: http://www.aafprs.org/physician/awards_grants/investigator_grant.html
Sponsor: American Academy of Facial, Plastic, and Reconstructive Surgery
310 South Henry Street
Alexandria, VA 22314

AAFPRS Ira J. Tresley Research Award 121
This annual award is given to a U.S. or Canadian academy member for the best paper based on any research study in the field of facial plastic surgery. The competition is open to any U.S. or Canadian physician who is an AAFPRS member and who has been board certified for at least three years. The paper must have been presented at a national meeting or its equivalent within the preceding two years prior to the February 1 date of submission. A certificate and an award of $1,000 are presented.
Amount of Grant: $1,000
Date(s) Application is Due: Feb 1
Contact: Coordinator; (703) 299-9291; fax: (703) 299-8898; email: info@aafprs.org
Internet: http://www.aafprs.org/physician/awards_grants/awards.html
Sponsor: American Academy of Facial, Plastic, and Reconstructive Surgery
310 South Henry Street
Alexandria, VA 22314

AAFPRS John Orlando Roe Award 122
This award, named for John Orlando Roe, the surgeon who accomplished the first rhinoplasty in 1887, includes a certificate and an award of $1,000 to be presented each year to an AAFPRS Fellow in an AAFPRS Foundation Fellowship Program who submits the best clinical research paper written during the current fellowship year.
Amount of Grant: $1,000
Date(s) Application is Due: Feb 1
Contact: Coordinator; (703) 299-9291; fax: (703) 299-8898; email: info@aafprs.org
Internet: http://www.aafprs.org/physician/awards_grants/awards.html
Sponsor: American Academy of Facial, Plastic, and Reconstructive Surgery
310 S. Henry Street
Alexandria, VA 22314

AAFPRS Leslie Bernstein Resident Research Grants 123
Two resident research grants, tenable in the United States or Canada, may be awarded each year to stimulate resident research in facial plastic surgery on projects that are well conceived and scientifically valid. Residents are encouraged to enter early in their training so that their applications may be revised and resubmitted if not accepted the first time. This award may be integrated with other funding to complete a project. Interested residents should write for entry guidelines.
Requirements: U.S. and Canadian residents at any level who are AAFPRS members are eligible to apply, even if the research work will be done during their fellowship year. Grant recipients must complete their work in one (1) to two (2) years with interim reports due each year.
Amount of Grant: $5,000
Date(s) Application is Due: Dec 15; Jan 15
Contact: Coordinator; (703) 299-9291; fax: (703) 299-8898; email: info@aafprs.org
Internet: http://www.aafprs.org/physician/awards_grants/grants.html
Sponsor: American Academy of Facial, Plastic, and Reconstructive Surgery
310 South Henry Street
Alexandria, VA 22314

AAFPRS Residency Travel Awards 124
Two Residency Travel Awards may be given each year for two outstanding papers in facial plastic and reconstructive surgery primarily authored by a resident or medical student in training. The paper must be submitted by February 1 for consideration, which will be presented at the Annual Fall Meeting. Entries should conform to the guidelines of the Archives of Facial Plastic Surgery, the official journal of the AAFPRS. Papers submitted will be judged anonymously. Only the cover page should contain the applicant's name or institutional identification.
Date(s) Application is Due: Feb 1
Contact: Coordinator; (703) 299-9291; fax: (703) 299-8898; email: info@aafprs.org
Internet: http://www.aafprs.org/physician/awards_grants/awards.html
Sponsor: American Academy of Facial, Plastic, and Reconstructive Surgery
310 South Henry Street
Alexandria, VA 22314

AAFPRS Sir Harold Delf Gillies Award 125
This award is named for Sir Harold Delf Gillies, a British otolaryngologist who in September 1917 described the tubed pedicle flap. Dr. Gillies frequently visited the U.S. and lectured widely to surgeons of various specialties and was given the title Father of Plastic Surgery. A certificate and an award of $1,000 will be presented each year to an AAFPRS Fellow in an AAFPRS Foundation Fellowship Program who submits the best basic science research paper written during the current fellowship year.
Amount of Grant: $1,000
Date(s) Application is Due: Feb 1
Contact: Coordinator; (703) 299-9291; fax: (703) 299-8898; email: info@aafprs.org
Internet: http://www.aafprs.org/physician/awards_grants/awards.html
Sponsor: American Academy of Facial, Plastic, and Reconstructive Surgery
310 South Henry Street
Alexandria, VA 22314

AAHN Grant for Historical Research 126
The American Association for the History of Nursing is offering a research grant of $3,000 for new researchers. (Indirect costs of 8% are also available). It is expected that the research and new materials produced by the award winner will help ensure the growth of scholarly work focused on the history of nursing. The deadline for submission of applications is April 1. The AAHN Panel will make its decision about the award by May 15 and the recipient will be notified by June 1 of each year. Funding will start July 1 of the grant year and last for one year. A no-cost extension may be granted on request.
Requirements: Applicants must be members of AAHN and hold the doctorate. They may be faculty members or independent researchers.
Amount of Grant: $3,000
Date(s) Application is Due: Apr 1
Contact: David Stumph, Executive Director; (303) 422-2685; fax: (303) 422-8894; email: aahn@aahn.org
Internet: http://www.aahn.org/grants.html
Sponsor: American Association of the History of Nursing
10200 W. 44th Avenue, Suite 304
Wheat Ridge, CO 80033

AAHN Pre-Doctoral Research Grant 127
This grant is designed to encourage and support graduate training and historical research at the Masters and Doctoral levels. The grant will be in the amount of $2,000. Proposals will focus on a significant question in the history of nursing. Selection criteria include the scholarly merit of the proposal, consideration of the student's preparation for this study, the advisor's qualifications for guiding the study and the project's potential for contributing to scholarship in the field of nursing history.
Requirements: The student must be: enrolled in an accredited masters program or doctoral program; and a member of AAHN. The research advisor must be doctorally prepared with scholarly activity in the field of nursing history and prior experience in guidance of research training.
Amount of Grant: $2,000
Date(s) Application is Due: Apr 1
Contact: David Stumph, Executive Director; (303) 422-2685; fax: (303) 422-8894; email: aahn@aahn.org

Internet: http://www.aahn.org/grants.html
Sponsor: American Association of the History of Nursing
10200 W. 44th Avenue, Suite 304
Wheat Ridge, CO 80033

AAHPERD Ruth Abernathy Presidential Scholarships 128

The Ruth Abernathy Presidential Scholarship, developed by the past presidents of AAHPERD to honor deserving students, is awarded to three undergraduate students and two graduate students in January of each year. All scholarships are presented at the AAHPERD National Convention & Exposition held in the spring. Undergraduate awards are $1,250 each and graduate awards are $1,750 each. Recipients also receive a complimentary three-year AAHPERD membership.
Requirements: Applicants must be enrolled in a full-time program at the time that the scholarship recipients are selected and must be majoring in a field related to one or more of the disciplines represented by AAHPERD and its associations (i.e., health, physical education, recreation, dance, sport – see the list of interest areas at the website). Applicants will be asked to describe the field of study/degree area and its relationship to the HPERDS-related fields. Application forms containing detailed application criteria and procedures for submission are available at the website.
Restrictions: Individuals in the following medical programs are not eligible: Nursing, Pharmacology, Physical Therapy, Occupational Therapy, Athletic Training, and Acupuncture and Oriental Medicine. Students pursuing teaching licensure, national board certification, or completing prerequisite coursework in preparation for admission to a master's degree program are are also not eligible to apply.
Amount of Grant: $1,750 - $1,250
Date(s) Application is Due: Oct 15
Contact: Deb Callis, Director; (703) 476-3400; email: dcallis@aahperd.org
Internet: http://www.aahperd.org/whatwedo/scholarships/Abernathy_Scholarship.cfm
Sponsor: American Alliance for Health, Physical Education, Recreation and Dance
1900 Association Drive
Reston , VA 20191

AAHPERD-AAHE Barbara A. Cooley Scholarships 129

The award will be $1,000 per scholarship. Recipients may spend the award in any manner they desire. The awarded scholarship will be recognized at the annual Awards Luncheon at the AAHE/AAHPERD annual meeting. Recipients will also receive a one-year complimentary student membership in AAHE. Additional guidelines and application are available at the AAHPERD website. Application materials must be received by November 15.
Requirements: The award is open to a master's level student who is currently enrolled in a health education program at an accredited college/university in the United States or a U.S. territory. To be eligible, the applicant must have a minimum current overall grade point average of 3.0 on a 4.0 scale.
Restrictions: Prior AAHE scholarship recipients are not eligible.
Amount of Grant: $1,000
Date(s) Application is Due: Nov 15
Contact: Linda Moore, Program Administrator; (703)476-3437; fax: (703) 476-6638; email: aahe@aahperd.org
Internet: http://www.aahperd.org/aahe/events/Barbara-Cooley.cfm
Sponsor: American Alliance for Health, Physical Education, Recreation and Dance (AAHPERD)
1900 Association Drive
Reston , VA 20191-1599

AAHPERD-AAHE Delbert Oberteuffer Scholarships 130

The award will be $1,500, which may be used at the discretion of the recipient. The scholarship recipient will be recognized at the annual Awards Luncheon at the AAHE/AAHPERD convention. Additional guidelines and application are available at the AAHPERD website. Application materials must be received by November 15.
Requirements: The award is open to a doctoral level student who is currently enrolled in a health education program in the United States or a U.S. territory. To be eligible to apply, you must be an AAHE member and a graduate student at an accredited college/university in a doctoral level course of study leading to preparing you to develop, implement and/or evaluate health education programs for children and youth. The applicant must also have a minimum cumulative grade point average of 3.5 in graduate courses.
Amount of Grant: $1,500
Date(s) Application is Due: Nov 15
Contact: Linda Moore, Program Administrator; (703)476-3437; fax: (703) 476-6638; email: aahe@aahperd.org
Internet: http://www.aahperd.org/aahe/events/awards/Delbert-Oberteuffer.cfm
Sponsor: American Alliance for Health, Physical Education, Recreation and Dance
1900 Association Drive
Reston , VA 20191-1599

AAHPERD-AAHE Undergraduate Scholarships 131

AAHE Undergraduate Scholarships are available to an outstanding student officially recognized as an undergraduate health education major at any four-year university/college. These are one year scholarships.
Requirements: Open to undergraduate students who are enrolled full time in a health education program at a 4-year college or university. Applicants must a GPA of 3.25 or higher and be active in health education professional activities and organizations at their school and/or in their community. They must submit a list of extracurricular service activities; an official transcript; 3 letters of recommendation; and an essay that includes what they hope to accomplish as a health educator (during training and in the future) and attributes and aspirations brought to the field of health education. Financial need is not considered in the selection process.
Contact: Linda Moore, Program Administrator; (703)476-3437; fax: (703) 476-6638; email: aahe@aahperd.org
Internet: http://www.aahperd.org/whatwedo/scholarships/Abernathy_Scholarship.cfm
Sponsor: American Alliance for Health, Physical Education, Recreation and Dance
1900 Association Drive
Reston , VA 20191-1599

AAHPM Hospice and Palliative Medicine Fellowships 132

The program offers training programs to prepare physicians for careers in academic or community-based palliative medicine. Fellowships provide clinical experience and supervision for palliative medicine in hospitals, homes, hospices, chronic care institutions, and outpatient settings, and include consultational and longitudinal care exposure, as well as training in bereavement care. Some programs also provide opportunities for mentored research or teaching. Most programs begin in July, and clinical training generally lasts one year, allowing for board eligibility upon successful completion. For a complete list of U.S. palliative medicine fellowship training programs, members should visit the web site.
Requirements: Trainees must have already completed residency training in a primary specialty, such as internal or family medicine, or have similar clinical training and experience.
Contact: Director; (847) 375-4712; fax: (847) 375-6475; email: info@aahpm.org
Internet: http://www.aahpm.org/fellowship/index.html
Sponsor: American Academy of Hospice and Palliative Medicine
4700 W. Lake Avenue
Glenview, IL 60025-1485

AAMC Abraham Flexner Award 133

The Abraham Flexner Award for Distinguished Service to Medical Education is granted annually to an individual for extraordinary contributions to the medical education community. The award was first presented by the Association in 1958 and is the AAMC's most prestigious honor. The Flexner Award recognizes the highest standards in medical education and honors individuals whose impact on medical education is national in scope. Nominations may be made by any faculty or staff member of a medical school or teaching hospital or by any member of an academic society. The Award Review Committee may also solicit nominations.
Requirements: Any individual who has made a significant contribution to academic medicine is eligible for nomination.
Amount of Grant: $10,000
Date(s) Application is Due: May 1
Contact: Sandra D. Gordon; (202) 828-0472; fax: (202) 828-1125; email: sgordon@aamc.org
Internet: http://www.aamc.org/about/awards/flexner.htm
Sponsor: Association of American Medical Colleges
2450 N Street NW
Washington, DC 20037-1127

AAMC Alpha Omega Alpha Robert J. Glaser Distinguished Teacher Awards 134

The award recognize the significant contributions to medical education made by gifted teachers. Up to four awards will be granted each year. Each awardee will receive a $10,000 grant. The awardee's nominating institution will receive $2,500 for teaching activities, and, if the nominating institution has an AOA chapter, the chapter will receive a stipend of $1,000 toward its activities. The awards will be presented during the AAMC Annual Meeting in Washington, D.C.
Requirements: The nomination must be made by the Dean of the nominating institution.
Amount of Grant: $10,000 recipient and $2,500 nominating institution
Date(s) Application is Due: May 1
Contact: Henry M. Sondheimer, M.D.; (202) 828-0680; fax: (202) 828-1125; email: hsondheimer@aamc.org
Internet: http://www.aamc.org/about/awards/aoa.htm
Sponsor: Association of American Medical Colleges
2450 N Street NW
Washington, DC 20037-1127

AAMC Award for Distinguished Research 135

The Award for Distinguished Research in the Biomedical Sciences honors outstanding biomedical research related to health and disease. The research recognized should have contributed to the substance of medicine. Nominations may be made by anyone on the faculty or staff of a medical school or teaching hospital or by a member of an academic society.
Requirements: The nominee must be an individual who serves on the faculty of an AAMC member medical school or teaching hospital.
Amount of Grant: $5,000
Date(s) Application is Due: May 1
Contact: Sandra D. Gordon; (202) 828-0472; fax: (202) 828-1125; email: sgordon@aamc.org
Internet: http://www.aamc.org/about/awards/research.htm
Sponsor: Association of American Medical Colleges
2450 N Street NW
Washington DC 20037-1127

AAMC Caring for Community Grants 136

The association, with the support of the Pfizer Medical Humanities Initiative, conducts an institutional grant program to encourage the development of student-initiated services and programs to the community. Eligible programs may range from those that promote awareness about sexually transmitted diseases, to vaccination and literacy programs, to any program that fulfills an unmet need within the community. Grant awards will also be offered to eligible service programs that are currently underway. Up to 10 grant awards are made each year. Program requirements and applications are available online.
Requirements: Medical schools are eligible to receive support for community service-oriented projects in which they explore new ways to serve their local communities.
Amount of Grant: $2,000-$15,000
Date(s) Application is Due: Mar 12
Contact: Ally Anderson; (202) 828-0682; fax: (202) 828-1125; email: aanderson@aamc.org
Internet: http://www.aamc.org/about/awards/cfc/start.htm
Sponsor: Association of American Medical Colleges
2450 N Street NW
Washington, DC 20037-1127

AAMC David E. Rogers Award 137

The Award honors Dr. David Rogers, a former president of the Foundation and an exemplar of academic medicine's commitment to meeting the health care needs of our country. The award is granted annually to a member of a medical school faculty who has made major contributions to improving the health and health care of the American people. Presentation of the award and a will be made at the association's annual meeting. Nomination guidelines are available online.
Requirements: Nominations may be made by any faculty or staff member of a medical school or teaching hospital or by any member of an academic society. The award is limited to an individual who has spent the majority of his or her career in academic medicine in the United States.
Amount of Grant: $10,000
Date(s) Application is Due: May 1
Contact: Sandra D. Gordon; (202) 828-0472; fax: (202) 828-1125; email: sgordon@aamc.org
Internet: http://www.aamc.org/about/awards/rogers.htm
Sponsor: Association of American Medical Colleges
2450 N Street NW
Washington, DC 20037-1127

AAMC Herbert W. Nickens Award 138

The annual award is given to an individual who has made outstanding contributions to promoting justice in medical education and health care for people in the United States. The recipient receives a monetary award and presents the Nickens Memorial Lecture at the association's annual meeting. Nomination guidelines are available online.
Requirements: Nominees may come from a wide range of fields including medicine, public health, education, law, nursing, and the social sciences.
Amount of Grant: $10,000
Date(s) Application is Due: May 1
Contact: Juan Amador; (202) 862-6149; fax: (202) 828-1125; email: jamador@aamc.org
Internet: http://www.aamc.org/about/awards/nickensaward.htm
Sponsor: Association of American Medical Colleges
2450 N Street NW
Washington, DC 20037-1127

AAMC Herbert W. Nickens Faculty Fellowship 139

The award recognizes an outstanding junior faculty member who has demonstrated leadership in the United States in addressing inequities in medical education and health care; demonstrated efforts in addressing educational, societal, and health care needs of minorities; and is committed to a career in academic medicine. Funding for the fellowship begins on the year after the fellowship is awarded, and it can be used over a two year period. The recipient is required to submit final narrative and financial reports. Nomination guidelines are available onnline.
Requirements: A medical school may nominate one faculty member for this award. A candidate must: be a U.S. citizen or permanent resident; hold the rank of full-time assistant professor in a LCME-accredited U.S. medical school department; have held a faculty position for no more than three years; have received only one appointment as assistant professor; and hold a M.D., Ph.D., or have earned another doctoral degree.
Amount of Grant: $15,000
Date(s) Application is Due: May 1
Contact: Juan Amador; (202) 862-6149; fax: (202) 828-1125; email: jamador@aamc.org or nickensawards@aamc.org
Internet: http://www.aamc.org/about/awards/nickensfellowships.htm
Sponsor: Association of American Medical Colleges
2450 N Street NW
Washington, DC 20037-1127

AAMC Herbert W. Nickens Medical Student Scholarships 140

The association makes scholarship awards that are given to outstanding third-year medical students who have demonstrated leadership in efforts to eliminate inequities in medical education and health care, and who have demonstrated leadership efforts in addressing educational, societal, and health care needs of minorities in the United States. Each recipient receives a scholarship and an award certificate. Institutions that have a pass/fail grading system and do not assign honor grades should fully discuss the applicant's academic accomplishments in the nomination letter. Nomination guidelines are available online.
Requirements: A medical school may nominate one student. A candidate must be: a U.S. citizen or permanent resident; and entering the third year of study in a LCME-accredited U.S. medical school in the fall semester. Students enrolled in combined degree programs (such as M.D./Ph.D.) are eligible when they are entering their third year of medical school.
Samples: Nehkonti Adams, Eastern Virginia Medical School (2006); Dora Cristina Castaneda, Stanford University School of Medicine (2006).
Amount of Grant: $5,000
Date(s) Application is Due: May 1
Contact: Juan Amador; (202) 862-6149 or (202) 828-0400; fax: (202) 828-1125; email: jamador@aamc.org or nickensawards@aamc.org
Internet: http://www.aamc.org/about/awards/nickensscholarships.htm
Sponsor: Association of American Medical Colleges
2450 N Street NW
Washington, DC 20037-1127

AAMC Humanism in Medicine Award 141

The award recognizes a medical school faculty physician who exemplifies the qualities of a caring and compassionate mentor in the teaching and advising of medical students. The goal of the award is to emphasize and reinforce among medical school faculty and students the importance of humanistic qualities in physicians, and to enhance interactions between medical school faculty and students. Nominations and award information were sent to medical school's organization of student representatives and student affairs deans. The award will be presented at the association's annual meeting.
Requirements: Each medical school in the United States may nominate one physician faculty member.
Samples: Yasmin S. Meah, M.D., Assistant Professor of Medical Education and Medicine, The Mount Sinai Visting Doctors Program, Mount Sinai School of Medicine (2007); Robert J. Paeglow, M.D., Albany Medical College (2006); Melissa A. Warfield, M.D., Eastern Virginia Medical School (EVMS) (2005); Sharad Jain, M.D., University of California, San Francisco School of Medicine (2004).
Amount of Grant: $5,000 to recipient; $1,000 to recipient's institution
Date(s) Application is Due: Apr 16
Contact: Denine Hales; (202) 828-0681; fax: (202) 828-1125; email: dhales@aamc.org
Internet: http://www.aamc.org/about/awards/humanism.htm
Sponsor: Association of American Medical Colleges
2450 N Street NW
Washington, DC 20037-1127

AANS Neurosurgery Research and Education Foundation Young Clinician Investigator Award 142

This one-year, renewable award is available to North American neurosurgeons who are full-time faculty in teaching institutions and are in the early years of their careers. The purpose of the program is to fund pilot studies that could provide preliminary data to be used for strengthening applications for more permanent funding from other sources. Applications related to any field of neurosurgery are encouraged. The NREF encourages both patient-oriented clinical research and basic science research projects. The one-year award totals $40,000.
Restrictions: Applicant may not accept another award for the same project during the same period. No more than one award per year will be awarded to the same institution.
Amount of Grant: $40,000
Date(s) Application is Due: Oct 31
Contact: Michele S. Gregory, Director of Development; (847) 378-0540 or (847) 378-0500; fax: (847) 378-0600; email: msg@aans.org or info@aans.org
Internet: http://www.aans.org/research/fellowship/nref_y.asp
Sponsor: Research Foundation of the American Association of Neurological Surgeons
5550 Meadowbrook Drive
Rolling Meadows, IL 60008-3852

AANS Neurosurgery Research and Education Foundation/Spine Section Young Clinician Investigator Award 143

Established by the Neurosurgery Research and Education Foundation (NREF) of the American Association of Neurological Surgeons (AANS), the Joint Section on Disorders of the Spine and Peripheral Nerves Award grants support to young faculty who are pursuing careers in the area of spinal cord, vertebral column or peripheral nerve disorders. The purpose of the award is to fund pilot studies that provide preliminary data used to strengthen applications for more permanent funding from other sources. The one-year award totals $40,000.
Requirements: Applicants must be physicians or neurosurgeons who are full-time faculty in North American teaching institutions and in the early years of their careers.
Restrictions: Applicant may not accept another award for the same project during the same time period. No more than one award per year will be awarded to the same institution.
Date(s) Application is Due: Oct 31
Contact: Michele S. Gregory, Director of Development; (847) 378-0540 or (847) 378-0500; fax: (847) 378-0600; email: msg@aans.org or info@aans.org
Internet: http://www.aans.org/research/fellowship/nref_y.asp
Sponsor: Research Foundation of the American Association of Neurological Surgeons
5550 Meadowbrook Drive
Rolling Meadows, IL 60008-3852

AAO-HNS Medical Student Research Prize 144

The Medical Student Research Prize is given annually for a manuscript submitted to the Editor of Otolaryngology-Head and Neck Surgery for review and consideration for publication in the journal. An award winning manuscript will be automatically accepted as an oral or poster presentation at the Translational and Basic Research Presentations Program (previously called the Research Forum). First prize is $1,000, and the award is available in both clinical and basic science categories.
Requirements: All manuscripts submitted for this competition must have a medical student as senior author and must describe work that has not been placed under active consideration for publication other than in Otolaryngology-Head and Neck Surgery.
Amount of Grant: $1,000
Date(s) Application is Due: Mar 9
Contact: Stephanie L. Jones, Assistant Director; (703) 519-1586 or (703) 836-4444; email: sljones@entnet.org
Internet: http://www.entnet.org/educationandresearch/grantsandfellowships.cfm
Sponsor: American Academy of Otolaryngology-Head and Neck Surgery
1650 Diagonal Road
Alexandria, VA 22314-2857

AAO-HNS Resident Research Prizes 145

Resident Research Prizes are given annually for manuscripts submitted to the Editor of Otolaryngology-Head and Neck Surgery for review and consideration for publication in the journal. All award winning manuscripts will be automatically accepted as oral or poster presentations at the Translational and Basic Research Presentations Program. First prize is $2,000, second prize is $1,500, and third prize is $1,000. All awards are available in both clinical and basic science categories.
Requirements: All manuscripts submitted for this competition must have a resident as senior author and must describe work that has not been placed under active consideration for publication other than in Otolaryngology-Head and Neck Surgery.
Amount of Grant: $1,000-$2,000
Date(s) Application is Due: Mar 9
Contact: Stephanie L. Jones, Assistant Director; (703) 519-1586 or (703) 836-4444; email: sljones@entnet.org
Internet: http://www.entnet.org/educationandresearch/grantsandfellowships.cfm
Sponsor: American Academy of Otolaryngology-Head and Neck Surgery
1650 Diagonal Road
Alexandria, VA 22314-2857

AAO-HNSF CORE Research Grants 146

CORE Research Grants are available in three different categories: Research Project Grants—an independent or assisted project using existing skills and resources, and is hypothesis-based, with specific aims and timetable; Research Training Grants—a research project that is designed to help you refine existing research skill set or acquire new skills, and requires mentor and evidence of training process; and Career Development Grants—a formal, mentored period of research combined with coursework, designed to help researcher become independent researcher. Applicants should complete a Letter of Intent by December 15th, using the online application system, and should then submit the completed application before 12 o'clock midnight EST on January 15.
Date(s) Application is Due: Dec 15; Jan 15
Contact: Stephanie L. Jones, Assistant Director; (703) 519-1586 or (703) 836-4444; email: sljones@entnet.org
Internet: http://www.entnet.org/EducationAndResearch/coreGrants.cfm
Sponsor: American Academy of Otolaryngology-Head and Neck Surgery
1650 Diagonal Road
Alexandria, VA 22314-2857

AAO-HNSF Health Services Research Grants 147

The purpose of the Health Services Research Grant is to foster research that will improve the effectiveness and appropriateness of medical practice. Projects supported under this program will develop and disseminate scientific information on the effects of otolaryngology services and procedures on patients' survival, health status, functional capacity, and quality of life. The award is intended to promote increased participation by otolaryngologists in the rapidly expanding area of health services research. Proposed projects may be related to any area of otolaryngology-head and neck surgery, but must have direct or potential clinical significance for patients seen by otolaryngologist-head and neck surgeons. Grants range up to $10,000 maximum, are for one year, and are not renewable. Projects must be completed within two years of the award date; no-cost extensions are available upon written request. Letters of intent must be received by December 15, and completed applications must be submitted by January 15.
Requirements: Any otolaryngologist in the United States or Canada is eligible to apply for the Health Services Research Grant. Applicants may be independent practitioners, residents or fellows in an approved training program, or practitioners affiliated with academic or similar institutions. All applicants must be members in good standing of AAO-HNSF; Associate and Corresponding Members are not eligible to apply as Principal Investigator, but may participate actively in the proposed project.
Amount of Grant: $10,000 maximum total (direct and indirect) costs
Date(s) Application is Due: Dec 15; Jan 15
Contact: Stephanie L. Jones, Assistant Director; (703) 519-1586 or (703) 836-4444; email: sljones@entnet.org
Internet: http://www.entnet.org/EducationAndResearch/coreGrants.cfm
Sponsor: American Academy of Otolaryngology-Head and Neck Surgery Foundation
One Prince Street
Alexandria, VA 22314-3357

AAO-HNSF Maureen Hannley Research Training Awards 148

The purpose of the Maureen Hannley Research Training Award program is to foster the acquisition of contemporary basic or clinical research skills among new full-time academic otolaryngologist-head and neck surgeons. The award is intended as a preliminary step in clinical investigator career development and is expected to facilitate the recipient's preparation of a more comprehensive individualized research training plan suitable for submission to one of the National Institutes of Health Clinical Investigator Career Development Award (CIA) programs (K series). Grants range up to $15,000 maximum. The award is one year, and is non-renewable. Projects must be completed within two years of the award date; no-cost extensions are available upon written request. Letters of intent must be received by December 15, and completed applications must be submitted by January 15.
Requirements: Applicants in the United States or Canada and members in good standing of the AAO-HNSF are welcome. Applicants must have demonstrated potential for excellence in research and teaching and a serious commitment to an academic research career in otolaryngology-head and neck surgery. Priority will be given to senior residents, fellows or faculty who have completed residencies or fellowships within two years of the application receipt date. All candidates must be sponsored by the Chairperson of his/her Division or Department and by an official representative of the institution which would administer the Award and in whose name the application is formally submitted.
Amount of Grant: $15,000 maximum total (direct and indirect) costs
Date(s) Application is Due: Dec 15; Jan 15
Contact: Stephanie L. Jones, Assistant Director; (703) 519-1586 or (703) 836-4444; email: sljones@entnet.org
Internet: http://www.entnet.org/EducationAndResearch/coreGrants.cfm
Sponsor: American Academy of Otolaryngology-Head and Neck Surgery Foundation
One Prince Street
Alexandria, VA 22314-3357

AAO-HNSF Percy Memorial Research Award 149

The Percy Memorial Research Award is an annual grant-in-aid of a worthy research project proposed in any area within the scope of otolaryngology-head and neck surgery. The Award was established in memory of A. Edward Percy, Jr., M.D. and his parents. Projects must have direct or potential clinical significance for patients seen by otolaryngologists-head and neck surgeons. They must be designed so as to yield useful information within the period of award, but priority will be given to projects which are also innovative and promise to develop into new long range research programs which will attract funding from other sources. Grants range up to $10,000 maximum, are for one year, and are not renewable. Letters of intent must be received by December 15, and completed applications must be submitted by January 15.
Requirements: Applicants in the United States or Canada and members in good standing of AAO-HNSF are welcome to apply. Applicants should be experienced independent otolaryngologist investigators affiliated with academic or similar institutions eligible to apply for and administer Federal research awards. Fellows with substantial research experience are eligible to apply, as are individuals who have already competed successfully for independent research grant support from a private or Federal funding agency.
Restrictions: Funds may not be requested to pay any portions of the salaries of the principal investigator or of any support personnel with strictly secretarial or clerical responsibilities. Funds may also not be used for the purchase of any item of equipment costing more than $500.
Amount of Grant: $25,000 maximum total (direct and indirect) costs
Date(s) Application is Due: Dec 15; Jan 15
Contact: Stephanie L. Jones, Assistant Director; (703) 519-1586 or (703) 836-4444; email: sljones@entnet.org
Internet: http://www.entnet.org/EducationAndResearch/coreGrants.cfm
Sponsor: American Academy of Otolaryngology-Head and Neck Surgery Foundation
One Prince Street
Alexandria, VA 22314-3357

AAO-HNSF Rande H. Lazar Health Services Research Grant 150

The purpose of the Rande H. Lazar Health Services Research Grant is to support the gathering of socioeconomic data for otolaryngology. The award is intended to promote increased participation by otolaryngologists in the rapidly expanding area of health services research. Proposed projects may be related to any area of otolaryngology-head and neck surgery, but must have direct or potential clinical significance for patients seen by otolaryngologist-head and neck surgeons. Grants range up to $10,000 maximum, are for one year, and are not renewable. Letters of intent must be received by December 15, and completed applications must be submitted by January 15.
Requirements: Any otolaryngologist in the United States or Canada is eligible to apply for the Rande H. Lazar Health Services Research Grant. Applicants may be independent practitioners, residents or fellows in an approved training program, or practitioners affiliated with academic or similar institutions. All applicants must be members in good standing of AAO-HNSF; Associate and Corresponding Members are not eligible to apply as Principal Investigator, but may participate actively in the proposed project.
Amount of Grant: $10,000 maximum total (direct and indirect) costs
Date(s) Application is Due: Dec 15; Jan 15
Contact: Stephanie L. Jones, Assistant Director; (703) 519-1586 or (703) 836-4444; email: sljones@entnet.org
Internet: http://www.entnet.org/EducationAndResearch/coreGrants.cfm
Sponsor: American Academy of Otolaryngology-Head and Neck Surgery Foundation
One Prince Street
Alexandria, VA 22314-3357

AAO-HNSF Resident Research Awards 151

The purpose of this grant is to stimulate original resident research in otolaryngology projects that are well-conceived and scientifically valid, with the potential to advance otolaryngology. Proposed projects may be related to any area of otolaryngology-head and neck surgery, and should be designed in collaboration with a preceptor investigator and approved by the candidate's department chairperson and institution. Grants range up to $10,000 maximum. Projects must be completed within one year of the award date; no-cost extensions are available upon written request. Letters of intent must be received by December 15, and completed applications must be submitted by January 15. Up to eight awards are available annually.
Requirements: The award is open to any AAO-HNS member in good standing who is a resident in an accredited otolaryngology - head and neck surgery training program in the U.S. and Canada.
Amount of Grant: $10,000 maximum
Date(s) Application is Due: Dec 15; Jan 15
Contact: Stephanie L. Jones, Assistant Director; (703) 519-1586 or (703) 836-4444; email: sljones@entnet.org
Internet: http://www.entnet.org/EducationAndResearch/coreGrants.cfm
Sponsor: American Academy of Otolaryngology-Head and Neck Surgery Foundation
One Prince Street
Alexandria, VA 22314-3357

AAOA Foundation/AAO-HNSF Combined Research Grants 152

The purpose of this award is to support a collaborative AAOA Foundation research project by fostering basic or clinical research related to otolaryngic allergy, rhinology, or related immunology by otolaryngologists-head and neck surgeons. Grants range up to $10,000 maximum. Projects must be completed within two years of the award date; no-cost extensions are available upon written request. Letters of intent must be received by December 15, and completed applications must be submitted by January 15.
Requirements: Applicants must have demonstrated potential for excellence in research. There are no restrictions on career stage, education, or country of residence. AAOA members are preferred but not required. All candidates must be sponsored by the Chairperson of his/her Division or Department and by an official representative of the institution that would administer the Award and in whose name the application is formally submitted.
Amount of Grant: $10,000 maximum
Date(s) Application is Due: Dec 15; Jan 15
Contact: Stephanie L. Jones, Assistant Director; (703) 519-1586 or (703) 836-4444; email: sljones@entnet.org
Internet: http://www.entnet.org/EducationAndResearch/coreGrants.cfm
Sponsor: American Academy of Otolaryngic Allergy (AAOA) Foundation
One Prince Street
Alexandria, VA 22314-3357

AAOHN Foundation Experienced Researcher Grants 153

The foundation funds research focused on improving the health and safety of the nation's workforce. Research grants are awarded to support research in the field of occupational and environmental health by an experienced occupational and environmental health registered nurse. Proposals may be submitted that are in the early stages of development (prior to data collection). Two $10,000 grants are awarded annually.
Requirements: Experienced occupational and environmental health registered nurse researchers are eligible to apply.
Restrictions: Completed research projects will not be accepted for consideration.
Amount of Grant: $10,000
Date(s) Application is Due: Dec 1
Contact: Ann Cox, Executive Director; (770) 455-7757; fax: (770) 455-7271; email: ann@aaohn.org
Internet: http://www.aaohn.org/foundation/grants/index.cfm
Sponsor: American Association of Occupational Health Nurses Foundation
2920 Brandywine Road, Suite 100
Atlanta, GA 30341

AAOHN Foundation New Investigator Researcher Grants 154

The foundation funds research, scholarship, and leadership development grants focused on improving the health and safety of the nation's workforce. Grants are awarded to encourage research in the field of occupational and environmental health by a new or novice registered nurse principal investigator. Proposals may be submitted that are in the early stages of development (prior to data collection).
Restrictions: Completed research projects are ineligible.
Amount of Grant: $3,000
Date(s) Application is Due: Dec 1
Contact: Ann Cox, Executive Director; (770) 455-7757; fax: (770) 455-7271; email: ann@aaohn.org
Internet: http://www.aaohn.org/foundation/grants/index.cfm
Sponsor: American Association of Occupational Health Nurses Foundation
2920 Brandywine Road, Suite 100
Atlanta, GA 30341

AAOHN Foundation Professional Development Scholarships 155

Annually, the AAOHN Foundation awards grants to support professional development (academic and continuing education) and leadership development in occupational and environmental health. Leadership development scholarship applications, due August 1, support volunteer leadership development in occupational and environmental health nursing. Scholarship applications for academic study, due December 1, are offered to provide opportunities to further professional education for occupational and environmental health professionals. To support occupational and environmental health professionals in attending and successfully completing continuing education activities that will further their professional development and continued competence, the AAOHN Foundation offers continuing education scholarships, with applications due December 1.
Restrictions: These grants are not intended to supplement tuition in an academic program.
Amount of Grant: $3,000
Date(s) Application is Due: Dec 1
Contact: Ann Cox, Executive Director; (770) 455-7757; fax: (770) 455-7271; email: ann@aaohn.org
Internet: http://www.aaohn.org/foundation/scholarships/index.cfm
Sponsor: American Association of Occupational Health Nurses Foundation
2920 Brandywine Road, Suite 100
Atlanta, GA 30341

AAP Anne E. Dyson Child Advocacy Awards 156

The AAP Resident Section Anne E. Dyson Child Advocacy Award, supported by the Dyson Foundation, celebrates the efforts of pediatricians-in-training as they work in their communities to improve the health of children. This award seeks to showcase projects that are designed and implemented by residents, which aim to improve the lives of children. The Award includes: $300 in funds to advance the winning projects' goals; travel and lodging expenses for up to 2 residents per project to the AAP National Conference and Exhibition (NCE); and presentation of the Advocacy Award plaque during the Resident Section assembly meeting.
Requirements: Any resident-sponsored and/or resident led project that seeks to advocate on behalf of children is eligible for this award.
Amount of Grant: $300, plus travel and lodging expense
Date(s) Application is Due: Jul 15
Contact: Kimberley VandenBrook, Grants Administrator; (800) 433-9016, ext. 7134; email: kvandenbrook@core.com
Internet: http://www.aap.org/sections/ypn/r/funding_awards/anne_dyson.html
Sponsor: American Academy of Pediatrics
P.O. Box 927, 141 Northwest Point Boulevard
Elk Grove Village, IL 60007-1098

AAP Community Access To Child Health Advocacy Training Grants 157

The Program supports five pediatric faculty-resident pairs (10 people) to attend the AAP Legislative Conference in Washington, DC each year. Each faculty-resident pair is required to implement an educational activity on child advocacy in coordination with their local AAP chapter following the conference. Local chapters will receive up to $1,000 toward completing the educational activity in conjunction with the faculty-resident pairs. The next call for applications will be available each fall.
Amount of Grant: $1,000 maximum
Date(s) Application is Due: Nov 9
Contact: Kathy Kocvara, Program Coordinator; (847) 434-7085 or (800) 433-9016, ext. 7632; email: kkocvara@aap.org or catch@aap.org
Internet: http://www.aap.org/commpeds/cpti/Opportunities.htm
Sponsor: American Academy of Pediatrics
P.O. Box 927, 141 Northwest Point Boulevard
Elk Grove Village, IL 60007-1098

AAP Community Access To Child Health Implementation Grants 158

This program supports pediatricians in the initial and/or pilot stage of developing and implementing a community-based child health initiative. Grants of up to $12,000 are awarded each year on a competitive basis to pediatricians who want to address the local needs of children in the community. Priority will be given to projects serving communities with the greatest demonstrated health care access needs and health disparities. Strong collaborative community partnerships and future sustainability of the project are encouraged.
Requirements: A pediatrician must lead the project and be significantly involved in proposal development and project activities.
Restrictions: Only applicants from the United States and its territories are eligible to apply.
Amount of Grant: $12,000 maximum
Date(s) Application is Due: Jan 29
Contact: Kathy Kocvara, Program Coordinator; (847) 434-7085 or (800) 433-9016, ext. 7632; email: kkocvara@aap.org or catch@aap.org
Internet: http://www.aap.org/catch/implementgrants.htm
Sponsor: American Academy of Pediatrics
P.O. Box 927, 141 Northwest Point Boulevard
Elk Grove Village, IL 60007-1098

AAP Community Access to Child Health Planning Grants 159

The program awards competitive grants to pediatricians who want to plan community-based initiatives to increase access to children's health care. Proposed initiatives must be broad-based community partnerships. Priority will be given to proposals promoting medical homes for under-served children and those with special health care needs; collaborating with SCHIP or Medicaid, and representing new initiatives within the community. Grant funds must be used for planning, not implementation. Planning activities may include needs assessments and community asset mapping, feasibility

studies, community meetings, focus groups, and development of grant proposals. If an applicant is not an AAP member, a letter of support from the AAP chapter president in his/her area must be obtained. Applicants must contact their chapter CATCH facilitators for approval of applications prior to submission. Technical assistance for applicants is available from CATCH staff and facilitators. Annual deadline dates may vary; contact program staff for exact dates.
Requirements: U.S. pediatricians and those in U.S. territories are eligible. Every program must be led by, facilitated by, or have the significant involvement of a pediatrician. During the planning phase, the involvement of other community members should be secured in order to ensure local support for the program. Applicants are encouraged to demonstrate collaboration with state child health insurance programs and/or state Medicaid programs.
Restrictions: Only applicants from the United States and its territories are eligible.
Amount of Grant: $2,500-$12,000
Date(s) Application is Due: Jul 30
Contact: Kathy Kocvara, Program Coordinator, CATCH; (847) 434-7632; fax: (847) 228-6432; email: kkocvara@aap.org
Internet: http://www.aap.org/catch/planninggrants.htm
Sponsor: American Academy of Pediatrics
P.O. Box 927, 141 Northwest Point Boulevard
Elk Grove Village, IL 60007-1098

AAP Community Access To Child Health Residency Training Grants **160**
The Community Pediatrics Training Initiative (CPTI) partners with the Community Access to Child Health (CATCH) Program to provide this grant opportunity targeting pediatric residency training programs. The mission of the program is to provide support to residency programs to build sustainable opportunities for residents to gain experience working on community-based child health initiatives that increase access to medical homes or specific health services not otherwise available. Grants of up to $15,000 will be awarded on a competitive basis to pediatric residency programs which submit proposals to plan and implement community-based child health initiatives as part of the training curriculum over the course of 16 months. The next Call for Proposals will be available in September.
Requirements: A pediatric faculty member must oversee the project and provide mentorship for residents participating in project activities.
Amount of Grant: $15,000 maximum
Date(s) Application is Due: Nov 18
Contact: Kathy Kocvara, Program Coordinator; (847) 434-7085 or (800) 433-9016, ext. 7632; email: kkocvara@aap.org or catch@aap.org
Internet: http://www.aap.org/commpeds/cpti/Opportunities.htm
Sponsor: American Academy of Pediatrics
P.O. Box 927, 141 Northwest Point Boulevard
Elk Grove Village, IL 60007-1098

AAP Community Access To Child Health Resident Grants **161**
The Community Access to Child Health (CATCH) Resident Funds program supports pediatric residents in the planning of community-based child health initiatives. Grants of up to $3,000 are awarded twice each year on a competitive basis for pediatric residents to address the needs of children in their communities. CATCH Resident Funds grant projects must include planning activities and also may include some implementation activities. Resident grants are available twice a year—May to July, during the CATCH Planning Funds grant cycle, and November to January, during the CATCH Implementation Funds grant cycle.
Requirements: A pediatric resident must lead the project and be significantly involved in proposal development and project activities.
Restrictions: Only pediatric residents from the United States and its territories are eligible to apply for CATCH Resident Funds grants.
Amount of Grant: $3,000 maximum
Date(s) Application is Due: Jan 31; Jul 31
Contact: Kathy Kocvara, Program Coordinator; (847) 434-7085 or (800) 433-9016, ext. 7632; email: kkocvara@aap.org or catch@aap.org
Internet: http://www.aap.org/catch/residentgrants.htm
Sponsor: American Academy of Pediatrics
P.O. Box 927, 141 Northwest Point Boulevard
Elk Grove Village, IL 60007-1098

AAP International Travel Grants **162**
The AAP has set aside a minimum of twelve (12) five-hundred dollar ($500.00) grants to be awarded to categorical pediatric or combined-training pediatric residents who wish to complete a clinical pediatric elective in the developing world during residency. The selection committee is composed of members from the AAP Section on International Child Health and the Section on Residents. After the selection committee reviews the applications the recipients will be notified mid-May and mid-November.
Requirements: Must be a categorical pediatric or combined-training pediatric resident at a U.S. or Canadian university.
Samples: Gunjan Kamdar, New York Presbyterian (2006); Bill Finn, University of Rochester (2006); Raina Paul, Boston Combined Residency Program (2006).
Amount of Grant: $500
Date(s) Application is Due: Mar 15; Sep 15
Contact: Kimberley VandenBrook, Grants Administrator; (800) 433-9016, ext. 7134; email: kvandenbrook@core.com
Internet: http://www.aap.org/sections/ypn/r/funding_awards/international_travel.html
Sponsor: American Academy of Pediatrics
P.O. Box 927, 141 Northwest Point Boulevard
Elk Grove Village, IL 60007-1098

AAP Legislative Conference Scholarships **163**
The American Academy of Pediatrics Legislative Conference Scholarships is specifically designed to help allay financial difficulties for members interested in attending the annual Legislative Conference, typically help each March. The Academy grants annually a number of scholarships varying from $1,000 to $2,000 on average. Each applicant will be reviewed carefully and awards will be granted to the most deserving.
Internet: http://www.aap.org/sections/ypn/r/funding_awards/
Sponsor: American Academy of Pediatrics
601 13th Street, NW, Suite 400
Washington, DC 20005

AAP Leonard P. Rome Community Access to Child Health Visiting Professorships **164**
The purpose of the Leonard P. Rome Community Access to Child Health (CATCH) Visiting Professorships Program is to promote advocacy for children and advance the field of community pediatrics. Beginning with the 2008 grant cycle, CATCH will be collaborating with the Community Pediatrics Training Initiative (CPTI) to implement this program. Four accredited pediatric residency programs will receive up to $4,500 each to fund a 2-or 3-day educational program focusing on the field of community pediatrics. District CATCH Facilitators (DCFs) and Chapter CATCH Facilitators (CCFs) are available to provide technical assistance.
Amount of Grant: $4,500 maximum
Contact: Alanna Bailey Whybrew; (847) 434-7085 or (800) 433-9016, ext. 7397; email: awhybrew@aap.org or catch@aap.org
Internet: http://www.aap.org/catch/vp.htm
Sponsor: American Academy of Pediatrics
P.O. Box 927, 141 Northwest Point Boulevard
Elk Grove Village, IL 60007-1098

AAP Nutrition Award **165**
One award is given annually for outstanding achievements in research relating to nutrition of infants and children. The award is made to an individual or for one project. There is no age restriction for the award; however, it is hoped that younger persons will be considered. The award is made possible by a grant from the Infant Formula Council. In addition to the honorarium, the award includes round-trip airfare and two days' lodging for the recipient and a guest to attend the annual meeting and receive the award.
Requirements: The competition is open to residents of the United States or Canada whose research has been completed and publicly reported. Separate letters should be written for each individual nominated; a letter should contain a description of the nominee's achievements, stating clearly the basis for the recommendation, including references to the literature that describes her/his work. Nominee's bibliography is to be submitted with the nominating letter together with copies of available reprints. Letters supporting the nomination are to be screened by the nominator and forwarded with the nomination.
Restrictions: An individual may not submit more than five letters supporting the nomination. Current members of the AAP Committee on Nutrition are not eligible for this award.
Samples: Virginia A Stallings (2008); Dennis M Bier (2007); William Dietz (2006); William W. Hay, Jr. (2005).
Amount of Grant: $3,000 plus round-trip tourist class airfare and lodging for two days
Date(s) Application is Due: Mar 1
Contact: Debra Burrows, Manager; (847) 434-4000; fax: (847) 434-8000; email: research@aap.org
Internet: http://www.aap.org/visit/nutrannouncemts.htm
Sponsor: American Academy of Pediatrics
P.O. Box 927, 141 Northwest Point Boulevard
Elk Grove Village, IL 60009-0927

AAP Program Delegate Awards **166**
The travel grants are available to residents who serve as program delegates to the AAP. This grant serves to support the program delegate's travel to the AAP Resident Section meeting at the annual National Conference and Exhibition (NCE). The travel grant is available to both categorical and combined-training pediatric residents. However, there is only one grant available per institution. The AAP Program Delegate will automatically receive the $300 travel grant.
Amount of Grant: $300
Date(s) Application is Due: Sep 14
Contact: Kimberley VandenBrook, Grants Administrator; (800) 433-9016, ext. 7134; email: kvandenbrook@core.com
Internet: http://www.aap.org/sections/ypn/r/funding_awards/nce.html
Sponsor: American Academy of Pediatrics
P.O. Box 927, 141 Northwest Point Boulevard
Elk Grove Village, IL 60007-1098

AAP Resident Initiative Fund Grants **167**
The Program is offering twenty-five (25) grants of up to $1,000 each. The funding will enable residents to educate fellow residents and/or parents on a specific aspect of one of the Academy's national child health priorities (Special Health Care Needs – Foster Care, Oral Health, Disaster Preparedness, Mental Health, Obesity, and Immunizations). The Academy hopes that this program will: increase the number of new, creative and innovative opportunities for residents to apply their leadership and advocacy skills

within the AAP structure; increase residents' knowledge of the Academy's child health priorities; and increase resident collaboration with national AAP and its chapters.
Amount of Grant: $1,000
Date(s) Application is Due: Mar 31
Contact: Kimberley VandenBrook, Grants Administrator; (800) 433-9016, ext. 7134; email: kvandenbrook@core.com
Internet: http://www.aap.org/sections/ypn/r/funding_awards/res_initiative.html
Sponsor: American Academy of Pediatrics
P.O. Box 927, 141 Northwest Point Boulevard
Elk Grove Village, IL 60007-1098

AAP Resident Research Grants 168
The Program is designed to give pediatric residents with limited research experience an opportunity to initiate and complete research projects related to their professional interests. Projects may be related to the full spectrum of child health research, such as behavioral sciences, biomedical sciences, epidemiology, health services, perinatal/neonatal health, prevention, public health, quality improvement, quality measurement, or basic laboratory-based science. Research projects can be conducted for a maximum of 2 years and should be completed during the residency program.
Requirements: Applicants must be legal residents of the United States or Canada. Although awards are primarily intended for support of first- and second-year pediatric residents, individuals who have secured a position for a third or fourth year of residency beginning in July may also apply.
Amount of Grant: $2,000 maximum
Date(s) Application is Due: Feb 27;
Contact: Jeannine Hess, Grants Administrator; (800) 433-9016, ext. 7876; fax: (847) 434-8000; email: jhess@aap.org
Internet: http://www.aap.org/sections/ypn/r/funding_awards/research_grants.html
Sponsor: American Academy of Pediatrics
P.O. Box 927, 141 Northwest Point Boulevard
Elk Grove Village, IL 60007-1098

AAPD Henry B. Betts Award 169
Each year the award honors an individual whose work and scope of influence has significantly improved the quality of life for people with disabilities in the past, and will be a force for change in the future. It is named for Henry B. Betts, MD, in recognition of his pioneering leadership in the field of physical medicine and rehabilitation and decades of dedicated service to the Rehabilitation Institute of Chicago. The awardee receives an unrestricted cash award and a commemorative crystal piece, which is presented publicly at AAPD's Leadership Gala in Washington, DC.
Requirements: Successful nominees will have demonstrated a strong vision and understanding of how to improve the quality of life for Americans with disabilities; possess a record of efforts and accomplishments that have affected a wide disability population; and have served as a powerful force for change, enhancing the opportunities for people with disabilities to participate fully in all aspects of society.
Amount of Grant: $50,000 cash award
Date(s) Application is Due: Oct 9
Contact: Tracey Murray, Leadership Coordinator; (800) 840-8844 or (770) 232-9001; email: murr9001@bellsouth.net
Internet: http://www.aapd-dc.org
Sponsor: American Association of People with Disabilities
1629 K Street, NW, Suite 503
Washington, DC 20006

AAPD Paul G. Hearne Leadership Award 170
The awards are presented to people with disabilities who are emerging as leaders in their respective fields to help them continue their progress as leaders. They will also have an opportunity to meet and network with national disability leaders at the AAPD Leadership Gala in Washington, DC. Winners of the Award must demonstrate all of the following: leadership achievements that show a positive impact on the community of people with disabilities or within their area of disability interest; connections they have made between individuals with disabilities and others in their communities; a positive vision for the disability community and a continuing commitment to their leadership activities; and potential to contribute at a national level. AAPD encourages emerging leaders with disabilities of any age to apply. Previous awardees represent a diverse group of people with disabilities aged 11 to 56.
Requirements: U.S. residents with any type of disability are eligible to apply.
Samples: Claudia Gordon, a consultant to the National Council on Disability (Washington, DC)—award winner, the first black deaf female lawyer in the United States and a long-time advocate for the rights of deaf people, $10,000.; Peter Cody Hunt—award winner, a graduate student in rehabilitation science and technology in Pittsburgh, who has developed outreach programs for Asian-Americans with disabilities, $10,000.; Sarah Louise Triano—award winner, director of the Yield the Power to the Youth program at Access Living (Chicago), who works to mobilize and educate disabled people and increase their ability to influence public and social policy, $10,000.
Amount of Grant: $10,000
Date(s) Application is Due: Oct 1
Contact: David Hale, Program Manager; (202) 521-4306; email: dHale@aapd.com or awards@aapd.com
Internet: http://www.aapd.com/DMD/PaulHearneAward.html
Sponsor: American Association of People with Disabilities
1629 K Street, NW , Suite 503
Washington, DC 20006

Aaron & Cecile Goldman Family Foundation Grants 171
The Aaron and Cecile Goldman Family Foundation, established in 1962 in the District of Columbia, offers its primary support to Jewish and local agencies, including education and human services, and to local children's programs and camps. Fields of interest include: arts and humanities; children and youth services; education; human services; Jewish agencies and synagogues; Jewish federated giving programs; recreational programs; and camps. Types of support include building and renovation, capital campaigns, emergency funding, endowments, equipment purchase, fellowships, matching/challenge grants, support for professions, program development, and scholarships. Applicants should forward a letter of proposal to the Foundation office, whose board members meet in the spring and fall of each year.
Requirements: One copy of the proposal letter is required. 501(c)3 organizations supporting the residents of Washington, DC, and its surrounding area are eligible to apply.
Restrictions: No grants are offered to individuals.
Geographic Focus: District of Columbia
Samples: The Institute for Jewish Leadership and Values, Rockville, Maryland, $18,000 (2008); Ethiopian Community Services and Development Council, Washington, DC, $15,000 (2008); Save a Childs Heart Foundation, Potomac, Maryland, $10,000 (2008).
Amount of Grant: $20,000 maximum
Contact: Jennifer Margolius Fisher; (202) 332-6600; fax: (202) 332-1800; email: jennifer@themargoliusfirm.com
Sponsor: Aaron & Cecile Goldman Family Foundation
3000 Connecticut Avenue NW, Suite 100
Washington, DC 20008-2509

Aaron & Freda Glickman Foundation Grants 172
The Aaron and Freda Glickman Foundation, established in New York, offers grant support primarily in the State of New York. Funding typically comes in the form of general operating support for health organizations and associations, as well as Jewish agencies and synagogues. There are no specific deadlines or application forms with which to adhere, and applicants should contact the Foundation in writing, outlining the need and a description of the program.
Requirements: 501(c)3 organizations and Jewish agencies serving the residents of New York are eligible to apply.
Geographic Focus: New York
Amount of Grant: $2,500 maximum
Contact: Edwin J. Glickman, Secretary; (561) 470-1434
Sponsor: Aaron & Freda Glickman Foundation
3080 N. 36th Avenue, V-61
Hollywood, FL 33021

Aaron Foundation (California) Grants 173
The Aaron Foundation, established in California in 1987 by the Aaron Mortgage Corporation, supports programs for children and youth, health care facilities, and human services agencies. Giving is primarily centered in the Bakersfield, California, region. Applicants should submit: a copy of current year's organizational budget and/or project budget; a copy of IRS Determination Letter; a detailed description of project and amount of funding requested; a statement of the problem that the project will address; and a brief history of organization and description of its mission.
Requirements: The project must benefit the residents of Bakersfield, California.
Geographic Focus: California
Date(s) Application is Due: Nov 30
Contact: Hal E. Aaron; (661) 322-6353; fax: (661) 322-6120
Sponsor: Aaron Foundation
651 H Street, Suite 100
Bakersfield, CA 93304-1305

Aaron Foundation (Massachusetts) Grants 174
The foundation awards grants to eligible nonprofit organizations in its areas of interest, including: arts and culture; health care; higher education; Jewish services and temples; health care; social services; and youth. There are no application deadlines or forms. Applicants should submit: results expected from proposed grant; a copy of IRS Determination Letter; copy of most recent annual report/audited financial statement or 990; a listing of board of directors, trustees, officers and other key people and their affiliations; and a copy of current year's organizational budget and/or project budget.
Requirements: Connecticut, Massachusetts, and Rhode Island nonprofit organizations are eligible.
Restrictions: Individuals are ineligible to apply.
Geographic Focus: Connecticut; Massachusetts; Rhode Island
Samples: Boston Latin School Foundation (MA)—to support the capital campaign, $10,000.; United Way of Massachusetts Bay (Boston, MA)—for the annual campaign, $20,000.
Amount of Grant: $1,000-$190,000 range
Contact: Avram J. Goldberg, Trustee; (617) 695-1300 or (617) 695-1946
Sponsor: Aaron Foundation
225 Franklin Street, Suite 1450
Boston, MA 02110

AARP Foundation Gerontology Graduate Scholarships and Fellowships 175
The association awards graduate scholarships and fellowships for research on aging. Gerontology and aging studies faculty are invited to nominate qualified students. This

program is funded by the AARP Andrus Foundation. Faculty nomination and student application forms are available online. Annual deadline dates may vary; contact program staff for exact dates.
Requirements: Gerontology and aging studies faculty are invited to nominate qualified students for these awards.
Amount of Grant: $15,000; $7000 graduate scholarships
Contact: Derek Stepp, Director, (202) 289-9806 ext 122; fax: (202) 289-9824; email: dstepp@aghe.org
Internet: http://www.aghe.org/site/aghewebsite/section.php?id=8183
Sponsor: Association for Gerontology in Higher Education
1030 15th St NW, Suite 240
Washington, DC 20005

Abbott Fund Access to Health Care Grants **176**
Abbott's Access to Health Care programs seek innovative solutions to improve and expand access to health care services for disadvantaged populations. Specific areas of focus include cardiovascular health, diabetes, nutrition, maternal and child health and neonatal care. Many Abbott Fund programs are engaged in closing gaps in ethnic and minority communities, promoting health and nutrition education for families, training health workers, and improving delivery of health services.
Requirements: Grants are made to tax-exempt organizations supporting access to health care.
Restrictions: Contributions will not be made to individuals; for-profit entities; purely social organizations; political parties or candidates; sectarian religious organizations; advertising; symposia, conferences, and meetings; ticket purchases; memberships; business-related purposes; volunteer efforts of non-Abbott employees; or marketing sponsorships.
Geographic Focus: Arizona; California; Illinois; Kansas; Massachusetts; Michigan; New Jersey; New York; North Carolina; Ohio; Puerto Rico; Texas; Utah; Virginia
Amount of Grant: $20,000-$100,00
Contact: Cindy Schwab, Vice President; (847) 937-7075; fax: (847) 935-5051; email: cindy.schwab@abbott.com
Internet: http://www.abbottfund.org/sections/what.html
Sponsor: Abbott Fund
Department 379, Building 6D, 100 Abbott Park Road
Abbott Park, IL 60064-3500

Abbott Fund Community Vitality Grants **177**
The Abbott Fund Community Vitality Grant program is active in communities around the world where Abbott has a significant presence. It pursues local partnerships and creative programs that address unmet needs of a community. Emphasis is placed on improving access to health care and promoting science education. The program also supports major civic, arts and other cultural institution programming, primarily in the Chicago metropolitan area where Abbott is headquartered.
Requirements: Grants are made to tax-exempt organizations supporting company operating areas in Arizona, California, Illinois, Kansas, Massachusetts, Michigan, New Jersey, New York, North Carolina, Ohio, Puerto Rico, Texas, and Virginia, and Utah. It also supports the communities of: Abingdon, England; Brockville, Canada; Campoverde, Italy; Clonmel, Ireland; Cootehill, Ireland; Delkenheim, Germany; Kanata, Canada; Katsuyama, Japan; Ludwigshafen, Germany; Queenborough, England; Rio de Janeiro, Brazil; Sligo, Ireland; and Zwolle, the Netherlands.
Restrictions: Contributions will not be made to individuals; for-profit entities; purely social organizations; political parties or candidates; sectarian religious organizations; advertising; symposia, conferences, and meetings; ticket purchases; memberships; business-related purposes; volunteer efforts of non-Abbott employees; or marketing sponsorships.
Geographic Focus: Arizona; California; Illinois; Kansas; Massachusetts; Michigan; New Jersey; New York; North Carolina; Ohio; Puerto Rico; Texas; Utah; Virginia
Amount of Grant: $10,000-$100,00
Contact: Cindy Schwab, Vice President; (847) 937-7075; fax: (847) 935-5051; email: cindy.schwab@abbott.com
Internet: http://www.abbottfund.org/sections/what.html
Sponsor: Abbott Fund
Department 379, Building 6D, 100 Abbott Park Road
Abbott Park, IL 60064-3500

Abbott Fund Global AIDS Care Grants **178**
Abbott Global AIDS Care programs focus on four key areas: strengthening health care systems, helping children affected by HIV/AIDS, preventing mother-to-child transmission of HIV, and expanding access to testing and treatment. Together with our implementing partner organizations, Abbott and Abbott Fund are pioneering innovative model programs, and sharing progress and lessons learned to encourage the adaptation of successful programs.
Requirements: Grants are made to tax-exempt organizations supporting global HIV/AIDS programs.
Restrictions: Contributions will not be made to individuals; for-profit entities; purely social organizations; political parties or candidates; sectarian religious organizations; advertising; symposia, conferences, and meetings; ticket purchases; memberships; business-related purposes; volunteer efforts of non-Abbott employees; or marketing sponsorships.
Geographic Focus: Arizona; California; Illinois; Kansas; Massachusetts; Michigan; New Jersey; New York; North Carolina; Ohio; Puerto Rico; Texas; Utah; Virginia
Amount of Grant: $10,000-$100,000
Contact: Cindy Schwab, Vice President; (847) 937-7075; fax: (847) 935-5051; email: cindy.schwab@abbott.com
Internet: http://www.abbottfund.org/sections/what.html
Sponsor: Abbott Fund
Department 379, Building 6D, 100 Abbott Park Road
Abbott Park, IL 60064-3500

Abbott Fund Science and Medical Innovation Grants **179**
The Abbott Fund Science and Medical Innovation program supports new approaches to learning that are designed to foster a better understanding of science and medical innovation and the value they bring to improving human health. Partnerships support K-12 education through postgraduate level research including funding and volunteer assistance for student and educator workshops and programs; career development; and educational grants for college and university science facilities, scholarships and fellowships.
Requirements: Grants are made to tax-exempt organizations supporting company operating areas in Arizona, California, Illinois, Kansas, Massachusetts, Michigan, New Jersey, New York, North Carolina, Ohio, Puerto Rico, Texas, and Virginia, and Utah. It also supports the communities of: Abingdon, England; Brockville, Canada; Campoverde, Italy; Clonmel, Ireland; Cootehill, Ireland; Delkenheim, Germany; Kanata, Canada; Katsuyama, Japan; Ludwigshafen, Germany; Queenborough, England; Rio de Janeiro, Brazil; Sligo, Ireland; and Zwolle, the Netherlands.
Restrictions: Contributions will not be made to individuals; for-profit entities; purely social organizations; political parties or candidates; sectarian religious organizations; advertising; symposia, conferences, and meetings; ticket purchases; memberships; business-related purposes; volunteer efforts of non-Abbott employees; or marketing sponsorships.
Geographic Focus: Arizona; California; Illinois; Kansas; Massachusetts; Michigan; New Jersey; New York; North Carolina; Ohio; Puerto Rico; Texas; Utah; Virginia
Amount of Grant: $20,000-$100,00
Contact: Cindy Schwab, Vice President; (847) 937-7075; fax: (847) 935-5051; email: cindy.schwab@abbott.com
Internet: http://www.abbottfund.org/sections/what.html
Sponsor: Abbott Fund
Department 379, Building 6D, 100 Abbott Park Road
Abbott Park, IL 60064-3500

Abbott-ASM Lifetime Achievement Award **180**
The award, sponsored by Abbott Laboratories, is given to honor a distinguished scientist for a lifetime of outstanding contributions in fundamental biomedical research in any of the microbiological sciences. The award consists of a cash prize, framed certificate, medallion, and national or international travel expenses incidental to receiving the award at the ASM general meeting. Guidelines are available online. All nomination materials must be submitted electronically.
Requirements: Mature scientists, both active and retired, from all areas of microbiology are eligible.
Restrictions: Self-nominations are not be accepted.
Samples: Norman R. Pace, $20,000—award recipient (2007); R. John Collier, $20,000—award recipient (2006); Jonathan Beckwith, $20,000—award recipient (2005).
Amount of Grant: $20,000, a commemorative piece, and travel to the ASM General Meeting
Date(s) Application is Due: Oct 1
Contact: Awards Committee, (202) 942-9226; fax: (202) 942-9353; email: awards@asmusa.org
Internet: http://www.asm.org/Academy/index.asp?bid=2587
Sponsor: American Society for Microbiology
1752 N Street, NW
Washington, DC 20036-2804

Abel Foundation Grants **181**
The foundation awards grants to eligible Nebraska nonprofit organizations in its areas of interest, including environmental programs and natural resource conservation, health care, higher education, Protestant religion and churches, and social services. Types of support include building construction/renovation, capital campaigns, general operating support, and program grants. Contact the office for application forms. Applications qualifying for review will be considered within 1 to 3 months of receipt.
Requirements: Nebraska nonprofit organizations are eligible. Preference is given to requests from Licoln, Nebraska, and the state's southeastern area.
Restrictions: The Foundation does not accept applications from organizations: that have had requests approved or declined in the past 12 months; or that are currently received payments for a multi-year grant.
Geographic Focus: Nebraska
Amount of Grant: $50-$40,000 range
Date(s) Application is Due: Apr 15; Jul 31; Oct 31
Contact: J. Ross McCown, Vice President, (402) 434-1212; fax: (402) 434-1799; email: rossm@nebcoinc.com
Internet: http://www.abelfoundation.org/grant.htm
Sponsor: Abel Foundation
1815 Y Street, P.O. Box 80268
Lincoln, NE 68501-0268

Abell Foundation Health and Human Services Grants 182

Through grants awarded in this area, the Foundation seeks to address societal issues associated with family disintegration, family planning, child support, teenage parenting, domestic violence, children's health and well-being, child abuse and neglect, hunger, food self-sufficiency and homelessness. The Foundation also supports advocacy programs for better health care and social services for children and youth as well as for a comprehensive system of universal health care. Of particular concern is the support of efforts to combat childhood lead paint poisoning and mental health disorders. Furthermore, the Foundation continues to provide opportunities for low-income families to live in quality housing in good neighborhoods in the region. While the Foundation's primary focus is on the development of permanent housing, it also will consider emergency and transitional housing.
Requirements: 501(c)3 organizations serving Maryland communities, especially in the Baltimore area, may apply. The foundation prefers grantees that show strong fiscal management, their project's benefit to the community, ability to achieve goals, unique work, and other sources of financial support.
Restrictions: Grants are not given to individuals, or for sponsorships, deficit financing, operating budgets, annual sustaining funds, travel, or loans. The foundation currently does not fund housing projects, hospitals, or medical research.
Geographic Focus: Maryland
Samples: Advocates for Children and Youth, Baltimore, MD, $120,000 - toward support of a community outreach program designed to improve quality-of-life outcomes for Baltimore City children (2008); Harlem Park Buckeyes, Baltimore, MD, $5,000 - toward the purchase of uniforms and equipment for 150 youth participating in the Harlem Park football program (2008); Health Care for the Homeless, Inc., Baltimore, MD, $75,000 - costs for expansion of the Baltimore Housing First pilot project for homeless persons with physical and mental disabilities (2008).
Amount of Grant: $5,000-$50,000 range
Date(s) Application is Due: Jan 1; Mar 1; May 1; Aug 1; Sep 1; Nov 1
Contact: Melanie Styles, Program Officer; (410) 547-1300; fax: (410) 539-6579; email: styles@abell.org
Internet: http://www.abell.org/programareas/health.html
Sponsor: Abell Foundation
111 S. Calvert Street, Suite 2300
Baltimore, MD 21202-6174

Abell-Hanger Foundation Grants 183

The foundation makes grants to nonprofit Texas organizations, other than private foundations, that are involved in such undertakings for the public/society benefit including arts, cultural, and humanities; education; health; human services; and religion. Types of support include general operating support, continuing support, annual campaigns, capital campaigns, building construction/renovation, equipment acquisition, endowment funds, program development, seed funds, scholarship funds, research grants, and matching funds. Block scholarship grants are made only to institutions of higher education located in Texas. Recipient colleges and universities are free to administer the grants. Education grants are limited generally to institutions of higher education, including religious institutions (Baptist, Christian, Lutheran, Methodist, and Presbyterian). Applicants must seek funding for the same proposal from various sources because sole sponsorship of programs is rarely undertaken. Grant requests are considered and awarded throughout each year. The trustees prefer to consider only one request per applicant each fiscal year. Unsuccessful proposals may not be resubmitted for at least 12 months. Applicant organizations that have never received funding from the foundation should request a preproposal questionnaire; the trustees will review the request to determine whether it warrants a complete proposal.
Requirements: Applicant organizations must be located in Texas and be 501(c)3 tax-exempt. National organizations with significant operations in, or providing material benefits to the citizens of, Texas will be considered based on the degree of operations/benefits within the state.
Restrictions: The foundation does not offer funding to individuals.
Geographic Focus: Texas
Samples: Church on Wheels, Inc. (Midland, TX), $36,000 for operating expenses; Rock the Desert Ministries, Inc. (Midland, TX), $15,000 for operating expenses for the 2006 Christian music rock concert to reach teenagers; St. Andrew's Presbyterian Mission (Midland, TX), $37,500 for the utility bill assistance program.
Amount of Grant: $6.2 million total; $20,000-$50,000 typically
Contact: David Smith, Executive Director; (432) 684-6655; fax: (432) 684-4474; email: ahf@abell-hanger.org
Internet: http://www.abell-hanger.org
Sponsor: Abell-Hanger Foundation
P.O. Box 430
Midland, TX 79702-0430

Abington Foundation Grants 184

The foundation awards grants to Ohio nonprofit organizations serving Cuyahoga County in its areas of interest, including pre-primary and higher education, geriatric healthcare and nursing, the promotion or sustenance of individual and family economic independence, and cultural activities. Current priority for the Foundations resources is given to funding requests for specific programs or projects that represent critical periods in a childs development from birth to age 5 and to early adolescence, ages 10-15. Requests for endowment or general operating support are discouraged. Foundation staff is available for consultation during the proposal preparation process.
Requirements: Ohio nonprofit organizations serving Cuyahoga County are eligible.
Geographic Focus: Ohio
Samples: Hard Hatted Women (OH)—to recruit welfare clients into its training program and increase programming, $10,000. Boys and Girls Clubs of Cleveland (OH)—to build a new facility, $75,000. Regina High School (OH)—to renovate the science lab, $15,000.
Date(s) Application is Due: May 1; Sep 1; Dec 1
Contact: Janet Narten, Consultant, c/o Foundation Management Services, (216) 621-2901; fax: (216) 621-8198
Internet: http://www.fmscleveland.com/abington
Sponsor: Abington Foundation
1422 Euclid Avenue, Suite 627
Cleveland, OH 44115-1952

Able To Serve Grants 185

Able to Serve Inc. is a public charity, providing services and opportunities for persons with mental and physical disabilities. Able primarily serves Wake and Johnston counties in North Carolina with some services extended to surrounding counties when resources are available. There are currently four programs that cover the services Able fund within the local community; Local Ministry Network, Community Partnerships, Van Transportation Services, and Computer Learning/Donations.
Requirements: Able to Serve provides each service and program at no charge to the individual or family receiving services within the Wake and Johnston counties of North Carolina.
Geographic Focus: North Carolina
Contact: Carlton S. McDaniel, Jr., President; (919) 779-5545; email: carlton@abletoserve.com
Internet: www.abletoserve.com
Sponsor: Able To Serve, Inc.
P.O. Box 334
Garner, NC 27529-0334

Able Trust Vocational Rehabilitation Grants for Individuals 186

The trust supports individuals and non-profit vocational rehabilitation programs throughout Florida with fund-raising, grant making and public awareness of disability issues. Created by the Florida Legislature in 1990, the Florida Endowment Foundation for Vocational Rehabilitation, parent organization of The Able Trust, is 501(c)3 non-profit public/private partnership with a goal of assisting Floridians with disabilities in achieving employment. The trust provides grant funds to Florida not-for-profit agencies and Floridians with disabilities for a wide array of projects leading to the employment of individuals with disabilities. To be considered for funding a proposal must address the employment individuals with disabilities and priority is given to those projects with direct employment placement outcomes during the grant time period. Grants to individuals are typically around $2,500. Historically grants have been made between $500-$4,000 for job accommodations.
Requirements: Individuals currently residing in the state of Florida that need emergency on-the-job accommodations to accept an employment offer, retain or receive a promotion at their current employment and are not currently open clients with a state agency provider may apply to be considered for assistance. There are no deadlines; guidelines, helpful tips and forms can be found at the sponsor's website.
Restrictions: Grants funds may not be used to purchase: Vehicles, property, building improvements, capital campaigns, endowments, fellowships, scholarships, travel grants, tuition where state and federal aid is available, lobbying, medical items, incurred debt, and proposed expenses prior to grant approval.
Geographic Focus: Florida
Amount of Grant: $500 - $4,000
Contact: Guenevere Crum, Vice President of Grant Programs; (850) 224-4493; fax: (850) 224-4496; email: guenevere@abletrust.org
Internet: http://www.abletrust.org/grant
Sponsor: Able Trust
3320 Thomasville Road, Suite 200
Tallahassee, FL 32308

Abney Foundation Grants 187

The foundation makes grants for innovative and creative projects, and to programs that are responsive to changing community needs in the areas of health, social service, education, and cultural affairs in South Carolina. The foundation's primary focus is on higher education. All requests must be in writing and in accordance with foundation guidelines, which are available upon request, and from the Web site. Applicants may submit a Letter of Intent (LOI) briefly describing the project before submitting a proposal in order to find out if their ideas are potentially supported by the foundation.
Requirements: Agencies applying for funds should be serving the citizens of South Carolina.
Restrictions: The foundation does not generally fund requests for operating expenses.
Geographic Focus: South Carolina
Samples: Anderson College (Anderson, SC)—for scholarships, $100,000.; Anderson College (Anderson, SC)—to establish a scholarship fund, $100,000.
Amount of Grant: $5,000-$100,000
Date(s) Application is Due: Nov 15
Contact: Carl T. Edwards, Executive Director; (864) 964-9201; fax: (864) 964-9209; email: info@abneyfoundation.org
Internet: http://www.abneyfoundation.org/guideline.htm
Sponsor: Abney Foundation
100 Vine Street
Anderson, SC 29621-3265

Abramson Family Foundation Grants 188

The foundation awards grants nationwide to Jewish organizations, educational institutions, and health associations in its areas of interest, including arts, education, higher education; hospitals (general); Israel; Jewish agencies, temples, and charitable giving; and social services delivery. The foundation also sponsors a scholarship program. Contact the office for application forms.

Samples: U of Pennsylvania (PA)—for the Abramson Family Cancer Research Institute, $9.1 million (2005).

Contact: Judith Abramson Felgoise, c/o Foundation Grant Committee

Sponsor: Abramson Family Foundation
376 Regatta Drive
Jupiter, FL 33477

ACAAI Foundation Research Grants 189

The Foundation develops, promotes and funds clinical research and educational programs related to allergy, asthma & immunology. The Foundation is dedicated to: strengthening, supporting and funding allergy/immunology training programs; heightening awareness of the critical role of the allergist in cost-effective treatment of asthma and other allergic and immunologic diseases; and supporting asthma camp programs to teach children and their parents how to live with asthma. Programs include clinical fellowship stipends, fellow-in-training research grants, young faculty support awards, scholar's return awards, and support for asthma camps.

Amount of Grant: $250,000 maximum

Contact: Program Administrator, (847) 427-1200; fax: (847) 427-1294; email: mail@acaai.org

Internet: http://www.acaai.org/Member/ACAAI_Foundation/ACAAI_Foundation.htm

Sponsor: American College of Allergy, Asthma & Immunology Foundation
85 West Algonquin Road, Suite 550
Arlington Heights, IL 60005

AcademyHealth Alice S. Hersh New Investigator Awards 190

The Alice S. Hersh New Investigator Award recognizes the contribution of new scholars to the field of health services research. Eligible nominees are those whose first research appointments were no earlier than January 1, 2002. Post-doctoral positions will be considered research appointments unless these years provided training necessary for entry into the field. In addition, the eligibility period may be extended for a nominee who has taken a formal leave of absence from their employer. The awards will be presented at the Annual Research Meeting in June. All awardees receive complimentary registration and lodging to attend the meeting and a $2,500 prize from the Alice S. Hersh Memorial Fund.

Requirements: Nominators must be members of AcademyHealth although nominees need not be. Nominees from academic and non-academic institutions are encouraged. Nominations must include one letter of nomination (no more than two pages) that reviews the nominee's contribution to the field and specifies the date of the nominee's first research appointment, and must include curriculum vitae.

Amount of Grant: $2,500

Date(s) Application is Due: Mar 2

Contact: Jennifer Muldoon, Director; (202) 292-6770; fax: (202) 292-6870; email: jennifer.muldoon@academyhealth.org

Internet: http://www.academyhealth.org/content.cfm?ItemNumber=954@navItemNumber=2342

Sponsor: AcademyHealth
1150 17th Street NW, Suite 600
Washington, DC 20036

AcademyHealth Alice S. Hersh Student Scholarships 191

AcademyHealth is pleased to announce a new scholarship program, The Alice S. Hersh Student Scholarship, which provides two free registrations to the National Health Policy Conference (NHPC) and four free registrations to the Annual Research Meeting (ARM). The scholarship is designed to encourage professional and educational development in health services research and policy among student members. This scholarship commemorates the dedication of Alice S. Hersh, the founding executive director of the Association for Health Services Research (AHSR), to supporting the next generation of health services researchers. Application deadline dates are: November 15, for the National Health Policy Conference Scholarships; and March 15, for the Annual Research Meeting Scholarships.

Requirements: Applicants must be current student members of AcademyHealth and must be enrolled in a masters or doctoral program at the time of application. To apply, students must submit the following: a completed scholarship application form (available on the AcademyHealth website); essay outlining how attendance at the ARM or NHPC will assist in your educational and professional pursuits in health services research or policy; current resume; letter from faculty advisor or project coordinator (optional).

Date(s) Application is Due: Nov 15; Mar 15

Contact: Jennifer Muldoon, Director; (202) 292-6770; fax: (202) 292-6870; email: jennifer.muldoon@academyhealth.org

Internet: http://www.academyhealth.org/Training/content.cfm?ItemNumber=2064&navItemNumber=2341

Sponsor: AcademyHealth
1150 17th Street NW, Suite 600
Washington, DC 20036

AcademyHealth Awards 192

AcademyHealth's awards programs recognize individuals who have made significant contributions to the fields of health services research and health policy. Nominations are requested for four awards: Distinguished Investigator Award; Article-of-the-Year; Alice S. Hersh New Investigator Award; and the Dissertation Award. These awards will be presented at the Annual Research Meeting in June. To obtain a description of each award and guidelines, see AcademyHealth website at: http://www.academyhealth.org/content.cfm?ItemNumber=954@navItemNumber=2342.

Requirements: Nominators must be members of AcademyHealth although nominees need not be. Self-nominations are acceptable. All nominations must include the name and contact information for the nominator and nominee, as well as any additional information specified under the description of each award. Complete nominations must be received at AcademyHealth by March 2. Nominations may be submitted by email or postal mail. All awardees receive complimentary registration and lodging to attend the Annual Research Meeting. The Alice S. Hersh New Investigator Awardee receives a $2,500 prize from the Alice S. Hersh Memorial Fund.

Date(s) Application is Due: Mar 2

Contact: Jennifer Muldoon, Director; (202) 292-6770; fax: (202) 292-6870; email: jennifer.muldoon@academyhealth.org

Internet: http://www.academyhealth.org/content.cfm?ItemNumber=954@navItemNumber=2342

Sponsor: AcademyHealth
1150 17th Street NW, Suite 600
Washington, DC 20036

AcademyHealth HSR Impact Awards 193

The program requests nominations of health services research that has made a positive impact on health policy and/or practice. The winning impacts will be disseminated widely as part of AcademyHealth's ongoing efforts to promote the field of health services research and communicate its value for health care decision-making. Nominated research may be published or unpublished, a single study or a body of work, the work of an individual or a team. The time frame for when the research was conducted is open, but the impact should have occurred recently. Nominators and nominees are not required to be AcademyHealth members. Self-nominations are accepted. Award winners are announced at the National Health Policy Conference, February 6 and 7, and the winners receive complimentary registration, travel, and lodging to the conference.

Requirements: Each nomination must include a summary describing the research used, the method of translation, and the impact on policy and/or practice (no more than 500 words); a letter of recommendation from the user of this research discussing the impact the research has had; contact information for the lead researcher; and contact information for the nominator (may be the lead researcher).

Amount of Grant: $2000

Date(s) Application is Due: Jul 29

Contact: Jennifer Muldoon, Director; (202) 292-6770; fax: (202) 292-6870; email: jennifer.muldoon@academyhealth.org

Internet: http://www.academyhealth.org/awards/hsrimpacts.htm

Sponsor: AcademyHealth
1150 17th Street NW, Suite 600
Washington, DC 20036

AcademyHealth Nemours Child Health Services Research Awards 194

The Nemours Child Health Services Research Award recognizes the scientific work of emerging scholars in the field of child health services research, particularly research on quality improvement of pediatric health services. Recipients must be within seven years of entry into the field of child health services research as of December 31, 2007. Year of entry will be judged by the nominee's first publication in child health services research. The winner will receive $1,000 in recognition of his/her contribution to child health services research, and the award will be presented at the Child Health Services Research Meeting, held in in Washington, D.C., in conjunction with AcademyHealth's Annual Research Meeting in June.

Requirements: Nominations should include: Letter of nomination that identifies when the candidate first entered the field (i.e., title and year of first publication in child health services research); Curriculum vitae that includes a detailed list of accomplishments that merit this recognition. Self-nominations will be accepted.

Amount of Grant: $1,000

Date(s) Application is Due: Apr 15

Contact: Jennifer Muldoon, Director; (202) 292-6770; fax: (202) 292-6870; email: jennifer.muldoon@academyhealth.org

Internet: http://www.academyhealth.org/content.cfm?ItemNumber=982&navItemNumber=2342

Sponsor: AcademyHealth
1150 17th Street NW, Suite 600
Washington, DC 20036

AcademyHealth PHSR Interest Group Student Scholarships 195

Public Health Systems Research (PHSR) is a field of inquiry examining the organization, financing, performance, and impact of health systems, defined as the constellation of governmental and non-governmental actors that influence population health, including health care providers, insurers, purchasers, public health agencies, community-based organizations, and entities that operate outside the traditional sphere of health care. The Student Scholarships recognize graduate students who demonstrate potential to contribute to the field of PHSR through promising research. Scholarship recipients will receive $1,000 to be put toward registration and travel to attend AcademyHealth's

Annual Research Meeting (ARM) and the PHSR IG Annual Meeting. Additionally, students will have an opportunity to present their research during the PHSR IG Meeting's poster session.
Requirements: Masters or doctoral students engaged in research that shows potential to advance the understanding of public health systems are encouraged to apply. The deadline for applications is April 15. Applications may be submitted by email or postal mail. To apply, students must submit the following: completed Student Scholarship Form (available at the AcademyHealth website); an abstract for a poster to be presented at the PHSR Interest Group Meeting (this research maybe in-progress); a letter of recommendation from a faculty member or research project director.
Amount of Grant: $1,000
Date(s) Application is Due: Apr 15
Contact: Jennifer Muldoon, Director; (202) 292-6770; fax: (202) 292-6870; email: jennifer.muldoon@academyhealth.org
Internet: http://www.academyhealth.org/Communities/content.cfm?ItemNumber=2535&navItemNumber=2035
Sponsor: AcademyHealth
1150 17th Street NW, Suite 600
Washington, DC 20036

AcademyHealth PHSR Research Article of the Year Awards **196**
Public Health Systems Research (PHSR) is a field of inquiry examining the organization, financing, performance, and impact of health systems – defined as the constellation of governmental and non-governmental actors that influence population health, including health care providers, insurers, purchasers, public health agencies, community-based organizations and entities that operate outside the traditional sphere of health care. The Article of the Year Award recognizes the best scientific work that the field of PHSR has produced and published in the previous year. The awardee will receive complimentary registration for both the PHSR Interest Group Annual Meeting and AcademyHealth's Annual Research Meeting, travel assistance, and a $1,000 cash award. Nominated articles must have been published in a peer-reviewed journal between January 1 and December 31 of the previous year, using either qualitative or quantitative techniques, articles must present, analyze, and comment on new data or synthesize and analyze data that have already been collected. The selection will be based on the article's contribution to the understanding of public health systems; provision of new insights to the field of PHSR; and potential to advance the field and/or challenge current thinking. Nominators must be members of AcademyHealth, although nominees need not be. Self-nominations are acceptable.
Requirements: Nominations must: be received at AcademyHealth by April 15; include the name and contact information for both the nominator and nominee and a copy of the article(s). Nominations may be submitted by email or postal mail. email to: PHSR@academyhealth.org. Mail to: AcademyHealth, Attention: PHSR Article of the Year Committee, 1150 17th Street, NW, Suite 600, Washington, DC 20036.
Amount of Grant: $1,000
Date(s) Application is Due: Apr 15
Contact: Jennifer Muldoon, Director; (202) 292-6770; fax: (202) 292-6870; email: jennifer.muldoon@academyhealth.org
Internet: http://www.academyhealth.org/Communities/content.cfm?ItemNumber=2536
Sponsor: AcademyHealth
1150 17th Street NW, Suite 600
Washington, DC 20036

ACCP Anticoagulation Training Program Grants **197**
The Anticoagulation Traineeship is a minimum of a four-week intensive training program for pharmacy students, residents, and fellows that includes a structured didactic component; extensive clinical experience and participation in ongoing clinical research. The training period can be extended 1 or 2 weeks if needed to meet academic requirements of the trainee's academic institution. Under the current system, the trainee spends five half-days per week actively involved in clinics providing patient care under the direct supervision of one of the ACNA clinicians. Trainees whose usual residence is outside the metropolitan San Antonio area will receive a grant-in-aid of $1000 to partially offset travel and living expenses incurred in conjunction with the traineeship.
Requirements: The program is targeted to doctoral-level pharmacy students enrolled in their final year of professional study, residents, and fellows. The necessary arrangements will be made with the student's home institution so the traineeship qualifies for academic and clerkship credit. Students actively enrolled in a Pharm.D. degree program need not be members of ACCP to be eligible. Residents and fellows must be current members of ACCP to be eligible.
Amount of Grant: $1,000 for non-residents of San Antonio
Date(s) Application is Due: Nov 1
Contact: Cathy Englund, Executive Secretary; (913) 492-3311; fax: (913) 492-0088; email: cenglund@accp.com
Internet: http://www.accp.com/frontiers/research.php#resfel
Sponsor: American College of Clinical Pharmacy
13000 W. 87th Street Parkway
Lenexa, KS 66215-4530

ACCP Heart Failure Training Program Grants **198**
Funded through an educational grant from Scios this heart failure training program is conducted at six different sites within the U.S; the University of Illinois Medical Center, the University of Michigan Health System, the University of North Carolina Heart Failure Program, the Ohio State University, the University of Southern California Medical Center, and the University of Utah Medical Center UTAH Affiliated Heart Failure Program. Depending on the specific site, the Traineeship is a two to four week, intensive training program that includes extensive clinical experience in either the ambulatory care and/or inpatient setting(s), a structured didactic component, and exposure to ongoing clinical research. The primary goals of the heart failure traineeship are to provide pharmacy practitioners, fellows, and residents with specific knowledge and skills central to the management of patients with heart failure. For practitioners, the traineeship will provide sufficient knowledge and experience such that they should have the basis to establish a heart failure clinic or disease management program within their own practices.
Requirements: Residents, fellows, or practicing clinical pharmacists must be current members of ACCP at the time of application to be eligible.
Amount of Grant: $1,000
Date(s) Application is Due: May 1; Sep 1
Contact: Kathy Lemons, Administrative Assistant, Professional Development; (913) 492-3311; fax: (913) 492-0088; email: klemons@accp.com
Internet: http://www.accp.com/
Sponsor: American College of Clinical Pharmacy
13000 W. 87th Street Parkway
Lenexa, KS 66215-4530

ACE Charitable Foundation Grants **199**
ACE supports the communities around the world in which its employees live and work through its established ACE Foundations and through company-sponsored volunteer initiatives. They focus their philanthropic support in the areas of education, poverty and health, and the environment. Particular consideration is given to opportunities where ACE employees' time and expertise can be utilized in addition to financial support. ACE encourages the development of local and regional initiatives, which reflect their employees' commitment to the needs of the communities in which they live and work. ACE employees direct a significant portion of the company's charitable giving.
Requirements: The mission of the ACE Charitable Foundation is to assist less fortunate individuals and communities in achieving and sustaining productive and healthy lives in geographic areas where ACE employees live and work. The ACE Charitable Foundation strives to accomplish this by focusing the majority of its funds on clearly defined projects that have measurable objectives and outcomes and solve problems in the areas of education, the environment and poverty and health. Submit a brief letter of introduction to the Executive Director for consideration.
Geographic Focus: Arizona; Arkansas; California; Colorado; Connecticut; Delaware; District of Columbia; Florida; Georgia; Hawaii; Illinois; Indiana; Kansas; Louisiana; Maryland; Massachusetts; Michigan; Minnesota; Nevada; New Jersey; New York; North Carolina; Ohio; Oregon; Pennsylvania; Puerto Rico; South Carolina; Texas; Virginia; Washington
Samples: The following is a partial list of organizations with which the ACE Charitable Foundation is associated: American Red Cross.; City of Hope Cancer Center.; Fairmount Park Conservancy.; Kids' Chance.; Need in Deed.; Philadelphia Cares.; Philadelphia Museum of Art.; Philadelphia Academies, Inc..; United Way
Contact: Eden Kratchman, Executive Director; email: acefoundation@acegroup.com
Internet: http://www.acelimited.com/AceLimitedRoot/About+ACE/ACE+Philanthropy+Worldwide/The+ACE+INA+Foundation+One+Column.htm
Sponsor: ACE Charitable Foundation
436 Walnut Street, WA 08G
Philadelphia, PA 19106

ACF Ethnic Community Self-Help Grants **200**
The Office of Refugee Resettlement (ORR) invites the submission of applications for funding, on a competitive basis, to connect newcomer refugees and their communities with community resources. The objective of this program is to strengthen organized ethnic communities comprised and representative of refugee populations to ensure ongoing support and services to refugees after initial resettlement. Ethnic Community Self-Help applications are for project periods of up to three years (36 months). Awards, on a competitive basis, will be for twelve (12)-month budget periods although project periods may be up to thirty-six (36) months. Applications for continuation grants funded under these awards, beyond the twelve (12)-month budget period but within the thirty-six (36) month project period, will be entertained in subsequent years on a non-competitive basis subject to availability of funds, satisfactory progress of the grantee and determination that continued funding would be in the best interest of the government.
Requirements: Public or private nonprofit agencies are eligible applicants. Faith-based and community organizations that meet the statutory eligibility requirements are also eligible to apply. ORR is interested in applications from national, regional (multi-state) or local refugee community organizations that address community building, facilitate cultural adjustment and integration of refugees, and deliver mutually supportive functions such as information exchange, civic participation, resource enhancement, orientation and support to newly arriving refugees (and other refugees that maybe in need of such assistance regardless of their resettlement date) and public education to the larger community on the background, needs and potential of refugees. Applicants to this program will be of two general types: (1) National or Multi-site ethnic organizations that propose to develop or strengthen local ethnic groups and/or a national network of ethnic entities for purposes of linking refugees to community resources and promoting and strengthening community participation; or (2) Emerging local ethnic communities that seek to function as bridges between newly arrived refugees and mainstream local resources and organizations.
Restrictions: Foreign entities are not eligible under this announcement.
Amount of Grant: $50,000 - $200,000

Date(s) Application is Due: Feb 24
Contact: Thomas Giossi; Program Manager, Division of Community Resettlement; (202) 401-5720; email: Thomas.Giossi@acf.hhs.gov
Internet: http://www.acf.hhs.gov/grants/open/HHS-2008-ACF-ORR-RE-0117.html
Sponsor: Administration for Children and Families (ACF) - Office of Refugee Resettlement
370 L'Enfant Promenade, S.W., 5th Floor
Washington, DC 20447

ACF Preferred Communities Grants 201

The purpose and objectives of the Preferred Communities program are to support resettlement of newly arriving refugees with the best opportunities for their self-sufficiency and integration into new communities, and to support refugees with special needs that require more intensive case management. Applicants may apply to support resettlement in new communities targeted to geographic sites or special populations agreed to in consultation with the Department of State/Bureau for Population, Refugees and Migration (BPRM) and ORR. There are two types of Preferred Communities programs for the purposes of this grant. The first type of Preferred Communities program should expect to receive a minimum of 100 new refugees annually. ORR will consider exceptions to this standard where the applicant provides substantial justification for the request and documents the community's history of arrivals, the period of time needed to reach a level of 100 new refugees and the record of outcomes for achieving self-sufficiency soon after arrival. The second type of Preferred Communities program will expect to receive a proposed number of cases that will need intensive case management. If the Preferred Community plans to focus resources on special needs cases, a history of its qualifications and experience with serving special needs cases should be provided.
Requirements: Eligible applicants are ten national voluntary agencies that currently resettle refugees under a Reception and Placement Cooperative Agreement with the Department of State or with the Department of Homeland Security. The Preferred Communities program is restricted to these agencies because placements of new arrivals occur under the terms of the cooperative agreements, and no other agencies place new arrivals or participate in determining their resettlement sites. The ten eligible applicants are the following: Church World Service, Inc.; Domestic and Foreign Missionary Society; Ethiopian Community Development Council, Inc.; Hebrew Immigrant Aid Society, Inc.; International Rescue Committee; Lutheran Immigration and Refugee Service; State of Iowa; U.S. Conference of Catholic Bishops; U.S. Committee for Refugees and Immigrants; and World Relief Corporation. Faith-based and community organizations that meet the statutory eligibility requirements are eligible to apply under this announcement. Preferred Communities are those localities that support populations where refugees have excellent opportunities to achieve early employment and sustained economic independence without public assistance. Preferred Communities should have a history of low welfare utilization by refugees. In addition, refugees should have the potential for earned income at a favorable level relative to the cost of living and to public assistance benefits. Characteristics of these communities include: (1) A moderate cost of living; (2) excellent employment opportunities in a strong, entry-level labor market; (3) affordable housing and transportation accessible for employment; (4) low secondary out-migration rates for refugees; (5) communities that meet the religious needs of arriving populations; (6) local community support and positive reception for the refugees; (7) receptive school environments; and (8) other related community features that contribute to a favorable quality of life for arriving refugees, such as excellent medical facilities.
Restrictions: Foreign entities are not eligible under this announcement.
Amount of Grant: $100,000 - $300,000
Date(s) Application is Due: Feb 24
Contact: Susan S. Benjamin; (202) 401-4851; email: Susan.Benjamin@acf.hhs.gov
Internet: http://www.acf.hhs.gov/grants/open/HHS-2008-ACF-ORR-RP-0112.html
Sponsor: Administration for Children and Families (ACF) - Office of Refugee Resettlement
370 L'Enfant Promenade, S.W., 5th Floor
Washington, DC 20447

ACF Standing Announcement for Unaccompanied Alien Children Grants 202

One of the functions of the Office of Refugee Resettlement (ORR) Division of Unaccompanied Children's Services (DUCS) is to provide temporary shelter care and other related services to children in ORR custody. This program seeks to fund providers for basic shelter and/or group homes, staff secure, secure and more specialized types of care. There are two priority areas for funding and applicants can apply to both priority areas under separate applications.
Requirements: Eligibility is open to all types of domestic applicants other than individuals. Non-profit organizations (including faith-based and community organizations) and for-profit organizations are eligible to apply. Organizations must be appropriately licensed (at the time of submission of the application) as facilities for the provision of shelter care and other related services to dependent children. For-profit organizations must clearly demonstrate that they are only charging the program actual costs incurred. Program Services: The provision of services will include a structured, safe and productive environment that meets or exceeds respective State guidelines, the Flores Settlement Agreement, and ORR service requirements. Applicants shall provide or arrange for the services listed below for each child in their care. Service delivery shall be accomplished in a manner that is sensitive to the age, culture, religion, dietary needs, native language, and the individual needs of each child. These critical services and assessments must be administered even during the shortest length of stay. Staffing *Requirements:* Applicants shall hire and retain direct care staff that has experience in child welfare, youth work, child care or a related field. A majority of staff that are responsible for direct care delivery shall be bilingual in English and the major language of the children under their care. While Spanish is the primary language of the majority of UAC, access to other languages should be available, if necessary. Applicants are encouraged to identify direct care staff with a minimum level of education equivalent to a high school diploma or higher. Applicants shall screen all employees for criminal background including past history of child sexual abuse. Additionally, applicants shall demonstrate a commitment to comply with state mandatory reporting requirements for child sexual abuse. This requirement includes but is not limited to children who have been victims of commercial sexual exploitation. Program Location: Applicants must plan for the delivery of the minimum services as described in Program Services (above). The shelter/s should be located in areas easily accessible to immigration courts, pro bono legal services, national airports, and community mental health and medical services. Geographic priority consideration and discretion will be given based on overall program capacity and services delivery considerations. Applicants must designate their application in one of the following priority areas: Priority 1 Mega Grants (National Network Applicant)— Priority will be given to applicants who have large national network capability to assist ORR with building capacity and who will be able to accommodate volume fluctuations in the UAC population. Applicants will also be required to provide oversight and monitoring of the facilities within their networks. Clarity of plan for maintaining minimum capacity, as well as their ability to expand capacity in response to program fluctuations and serve specialized types of care (such as staff secure and/or therapeutic care) in addition to primary shelter care. All identified capacity must be appropriately licensed to ensure immediate accessibility as the program necessitates. Priority 2 Micro Grants (Individual Applicants)— ORR may also seek applications from individual care providers or partnerships between two entities to provide specialized services.
Restrictions: Foreign entities are not eligible under this announcement. The U.S. Government is opposed to prostitution and related activities, which are inherently harmful and dehumanizing, and contribute to the phenomenon of trafficking in persons. U.S. non-governmental organizations, and their sub-grantees, cannot use U.S. Government funds to lobby for, promote, or advocate the legalization or regulation of prostitution as a legitimate form of work. It is the responsibility of the primary grantee to ensure these criteria are met by its sub-grantees. Accordingly, the grant application must ensure that no monies, if awarded, will be used for these unallowable purposes.
Amount of Grant: $2,000,000 - $40,000,000
Date(s) Application is Due: Mar 24
Contact: Belinda Rochelle, Division of Unaccompanied Children Services; (202) 401-5269; email: belinda.rochelle@acf.hhs.gov
Internet: http://www.acf.hhs.gov/grants/open/HHS-2008-ACF-ORR-ZU-0119.html
Sponsor: Administration for Children and Families (ACF) - Office of Refugee Resettlement
370 L'Enfant Promenade, S.W., 5th Floor
Washington, DC 20447

ACF Supplemental Services for Recently Arrived Refugees Grants 203

The purpose and objectives ORR seeks to achieve through Supplemental Services for Recently Arrived Refugees are to provide additional resources to communities where the refugee services are insufficient. Under these circumstances, resources are needed to provide additional service capacity to accommodate an increase of refugees. Through Supplemental Services for Recently Arrived Refugees, ORR intends to offer to communities the resources to respond to the needs of newly arrived refugees with adequate and culturally and linguistically appropriate social services. This grant program is intended to provide services to arriving refugees or sudden and unexpected large secondary migration of refugees where communities are not sufficiently prepared in terms of linguistic or culturally appropriate services. In providing services to refugees who have arrived in country less than three years, applicants should view these resources as a temporary solution to insufficient services currently available to meet emerging needs of recently arrived refugees in a specific community. ORR formula social service funds are awarded to States to provide services proportionate to the number of refugee arrivals during the previous three years. ORR invites applications that propose seventeen (17) month projects for a minimum of 100 refugees annually. Examples of situations for which applicants may request funds for grants under Supplemental Services for Recently Arrived Refugees are as follows: (1) Refugee services do not presently exist or the service capacity is not sufficient to accommodate significant increases in arrivals; and (2) the existing service system does not have culturally and linguistically compatible staff.
Requirements: Public or private nonprofit agencies are eligible applicants. Faith-based and community organizations that meet the statutory eligibility requirements are eligible to apply. Allowable activities in the Supplemental Services for Recently Arrived Refugees program are social services for refugees that are appropriate and accessible in language and culture. Examples of allowable social or emergency services to recently arrived refugees include: information and referral services, outreach services, social adjustment services, emergency services, health-related services, home management services, day care for children, transportation, translation and interpretation, case management, citizenship and naturalization preparation services, employment services, employability assessment, on-the job training, English language instruction, vocational training, skills recertification and any additional services approved by the Director of ORR as supporting the objectives of this program.
Restrictions: Foreign entities are not eligible under this announcement.
Amount of Grant: $75,000 - $500,000
Date(s) Application is Due: Feb 24
Contact: Susan S. Benjamin; (202) 401-4851; email: Susan.Benjamin@acf.hhs.gov
Internet: http://www.acf.hhs.gov/grants/open/HHS-2008-ACF-ORR-RU-0113.html
Sponsor: Administration for Children and Families - Office of Refugee Resettlement
370 L'Enfant Promenade, S.W., 5th Floor
Washington, DC 20447

ACGT Investigators Grants 204

The Investigators Award in Clinical Translation of Gene Therapy for Cancer distributes funds over 3-5 years, inclusive of a maximum of 10% indirect costs. Funds may be used at the recipient's discretion for salary, technical assistance, supplies, animals or capital equipment, but may not support staff not directly related to the project, e.g. secretaries or administrative assistants. Purchase of equipment is not allowed in the final year of the grant. ACGT is accepting grant applications to produce and release-testing of the clinical trial agents under cGMP, conduct the necessary pre-clinical pharmacological and toxicological studies in appropriate animal models, and/or conducting the clinical translational trials in patients in support of an Investigative New Drug application to the FDA.

Requirements: The candidate must hold an MD, PhD, or equivalent degree and be a tenure-track or tenured faculty. The investigator must be conducting original research as an independent faculty member. ACGT has no citizenship restrictions, and research supported by the award must be conducted at medical schools and research centers only in the United States. While the unambiguous demonstration of preclinical efficacy in cancer treatment by gene therapy is a pre-requisite, entering into the clinical trial during the funding period is also a requirement.

Amount of Grant: $1 million maximum over three to five years

Contact: Grace Pedersen, Foundation Administrator; (203) 358-8000, ext. 495; email: aneslage@acgtfoundation.org

Internet: http://www.acgtfoundation.org/grants.html

Sponsor: Alliance for Cancer Gene Therapy
96 Cummings Point Road
Stamford, CT 06902

ACGT Young Investigator Grants 205

The alliance funds research aimed at furthering the development of gene therapy approaches to the treatment of cancer. The overall objectives of this grant are to advance gene therapy into the causes, treatment, and prevention of all types of cancer by promoting development of novel and innovative studies by young investigators. The emphasis of this initiative is to promote basic, and preclinical research approaches utilizing cells and genes as medicine. The six main areas of research ACGT will support are: tumor-specific replicating viruses and bacteria, anti-angiogenesis, immune-mediated gene therapy and cancer vaccines, oncogenes/suppressor oncogenes/apoptosis, tumor targeting and vector development, and other cancer gene therapy research. The three-year grant may be used at the recipient's discretion for salary, technical assistance, supplies, animals or capital equipment, but may not support staff not directly related to the project, e.g. secretaries or administrative assistants. Purchase of equipment is not allowed in the third year of the grant. Continued support is contingent upon submission and approval of a noncompetitive renewal application each year. Guideline and applications are available online.

Requirements: Candidates must hold an MD, MPH, PhD, or equivalent degree and be a tenure-track assistant professor within five years of their initial appointment to this rank, at the time of award activation. The investigator must be conducting original research as an independent faculty member. ACGT has no citizenship restrictions, and research supported by the award must be conducted at medical schools and research centers only in the United States.

Amount of Grant: $500,000 maximum over three years

Date(s) Application is Due: Sep 21

Contact: Grace Pedersen, Foundation Administrator; (203) 358-8000, ext. 495; email: aneslage@acgtfoundation.org

Internet: http://www.acgtfoundation.org/grants.html

Sponsor: Alliance for Cancer Gene Therapy
96 Cummings Point Road
Stamford, CT 06902

Achelis and Bodman Foundations Grants 206

Both Foundations concentrate their grant programs in New York City, although The Bodman Foundation also makes grants in northern New Jersey. Funding is concentrated in six program areas: Arts and Culture, Education, Employment, Health, Public Policy, and Youth and Families.

Requirements: Nonprofit organizations based in New York City and northern New Jersey that are tax-exempt under Section 501(c)3 of the Internal Revenue Code and fall within the program areas of the foundations are welcome to submit an inquiry or proposal letter by regular mail. Do not send initial inquiries by email or fax; also do not send CDs, DVDs, computer discs, video tapes, or proposals through the Internet or by facsimile. An initial inquiry to the foundations should include only the following items: (1) A proposal letter that briefly summarizes the history of the project, need, research, objectives, time period, key staff, project budget, and evaluation plan. (2) Latest annual report. (3) Latest complete audited financial statements. (4) IRS 501(c)3 tax-exemption letter. There are no deadlines and applications may be submitted at any time during the year. Each request is reviewed by staff and will usually receive a written response within thirty days. Those requests deemed consistent with the interests and resources of the Foundations will be evaluated further and more information will be requested. Staff may request a site visit, conference call, or meeting. All grants are reviewed and approved by the Trustees at one of their three board meetings in May, September, or December.

Restrictions: The foundations generally do not make grants for the following purposes or program areas: Nonprofit organizations outside of New York and New Jersey; Annual appeals, dinner functions, and fundraising events; Endowments and capital campaigns; Loans and deficit financing; Direct grants to individuals; Individual day-care and after-school programs; Housing; Organizations or projects based outside the U.S.; Films or video projects; Small art, dance, music, and theater groups; Individual K-12 schools (except charter schools); National health and mental health organizations; Government agencies or nonprofit organizations significantly funded or reimbursed by government agencies. Limited resources prevent the foundations from funding the same organization on an ongoing annual basis.

Geographic Focus: New Jersey; New York

Samples: Foundation for Cultural Review - (Achelis, 2007) $35,000 toward the redesign of the website of the New Criterion magazine.; High 5 Tickets to the Arts - (Bodman, 2006) $15,000 for the Take 5 Program for disadvantaged youth.; Coalition for Educational Freedom - (Bodman, 2007) $50,000 toward the creation of a state-wide school choice organization in Connecticut.; Center for Alternative Sentencing and Employment Services - (Achelis, 2007) $35,000 toward the Career Exploration Program for young ex-offenders in New York City.; Jericho Project - (Achelis, 2007) $50,000 toward the Vocational and Educational Program for those with substance abuse or mental health problems.; Brain Trauma Foundation - (Achelis, 2007) $50,000 for the Veterans Information Initiative.; Children of Bellevue - (Bodman, 2007) $25,000 for the Frances L. Loeb Child Protection and Development Center at Bellevue Hospital Center

Contact: John B. Krieger, Executive Director; (212) 644-0322; fax: (212) 759-6510; email: main@achelis-bodman-fnds.org

Internet: http://foundationcenter.org/grantmaker/achelis-bodman/guidelines.html

Sponsor: Achelis and Bodman Foundations
767 Third Avenue, 4th Floor
New York, NY 10017

ACOG History of American Obstetrics and Gynecology Fellowship 207

ACOG and Ortho-McNeil Pharmaceutical Corporation jointly sponsor the fellowship in the History of American Obstetrics and Gynecology each year. The recipient of the fellowship spends one month in the Washington, DC, area working full-time to complete their specific historical research project. Although the fellowship will be based in the ACOG History Library, the fellow is encouraged to use other national, historical, and medical collections in the Washington, DC, area. The results of this research must be disseminated through either publication or presentation at a professional meeting. Application and guidelines are available online.

Requirements: ACOG junior fellows and fellows are encouraged to apply.

Amount of Grant: $5000

Date(s) Application is Due: Oct 1

Contact: Debra Scarborough, (202) 863-2578; fax: (202) 484-1595; email: history@acog.org

Internet: http://www.acog.org/from_home/departments/dept_notice.cfm?recno=21&bulletin=254

Sponsor: American College of Obstetricians and Gynecologists
409 12th St SW
Washington DC 20024-2588

ACS Master's Training Grants in Clinical Oncology Social Work 208

These grants are awarded annually to qualifying institutions that train clinical oncology social workers to provide cancer patients and their families with psychosocial services. Grants are available to second-year students in a master's program and post-master's social workers within five years of graduation. The master's training must introduce social workers to the special needs of cancer patients and their families. Contact the society for application forms.

Requirements: Applications will be considered from institutions that identify clinical oncology social work training activities, cancer programs with defined psychosocial support services, and relationships with schools accredited by the Council on Social Work Education.

Amount of Grant: $12,000 maximum

Date(s) Application is Due: Oct 15

Contact: Extramural Grants Department, (404) 329-7558; fax: (404) 321-4669; email: grants@cancer.org;; Virginia Krawiec, Program Director; (404) 329-5734; email: Ginger.Krawiec@cancer.org

Internet: http://www.cancer.org/docroot/RES/content/RES_5_2x_Masters_Training_Grants_in_Clinical_Oncology_Social_Work.asp?sitearea=RES

Sponsor: American Cancer Society
1599 Clifton Rd NE
Atlanta, GA 30329-4251

ACS Cancer Control Career Development Awards for Primary Care Physicians 209

ACS annually awards three three-year career development awards to physicians specializing in primary care (e.g., family practice, internal medicine, pediatrics, and obstetrics and gynecology). These awards are intended to encourage and assist in the development of promising candidates who will pursue academic careers in primary care specialties. It is anticipated that physicians trained under these awards will improve cancer control through involvement in primary care practice, education, and research activities related to cancer control. Awards are made for three years with progressive stipends.

Requirements: Candidates must be U.S. citizens or permanent residents; must hold an MD, DO, or equivalent degree; and must have completed residency requirements of the appropriate primary care specialty board. Candidate must hold academic rank from instructor to assistant professor and must not be more than 10 years out of training.

Restrictions: Applicants may not have academic rank above that of assistant professor and must not be tenured or be the section head (or equivalent) in his/her discipline. Additionally, the applicant may not be training as a fellow at the time of the award.

Amount of Grant: $100,000 maximum per year

Date(s) Application is Due: Oct 15

Contact: Extramural Grants Department, (404) 329-7558 or (800) 875-2562; fax: (404) 321-4669; email: grants@cancer.org
Internet: http://www.cancer.org/docroot/RES/content/RES_5_2x_Cancer_Control_Career_Development_Awards_for_Primary_Care_Physicians.asp?sitearea=RES
Sponsor: American Cancer Society
1599 Clifton Rd NE
Atlanta, GA 30329-4251

ACS Clinical Research Professor Grants **210**
The American Cancer Society offers a limited number of grants to established investigators in mid-career who have made seminal contributions that have changed the direction of clinical, psychosocial, behavioral, health policy or epidemiologic cancer research. Furthermore, it is expected that these investigators will continue to provide leadership in their research area. Up to two awards are made annually for a five-year term that can be renewed once. The award of up to $80,000 per year (direct costs only) may be used for salary or research project support. Interested individuals should submit their curriculum vitae with a complete bibliography and a letter of intent that briefly describes their seminal contributions to research. This information must be submitted via the Research Professor letter of intent on proposalCENTRAL at: https://proposalcentral.altum.com. The Letter of Intent for the Clinical Research Professor Award must be submitted no later than August 1. Upon receipt, the ACS will provide appropriate guidance either by telephone or email. Clinical Research Professor candidates whose Letter of Intent has been approved must submit their application for the award before the October 15 deadline.
Amount of Grant: $80,000 maximum per year
Date(s) Application is Due: Aug 1; Oct 15
Contact: John J. Stevens, Vice President Extramural Grant; (404) 329-7550; email: john.stevens@cancer.org
Internet: http://www.cancer.org/docroot/RES/content/RES_5_2x_Clinical_Research_Professorships.asp?sitearea=RES
Sponsor: American Cancer Society
1599 Clifton Rd NE
Atlanta, GA 30329-4251

ACS Doctoral Degree Scholarships in Cancer Nursing **211**
Awarded to graduate students pursuing doctoral study in the field of cancer nursing research, and preparing for careers as nurse scientists. Initial awards are made for up to two years with the possibility of a two-year renewal. There is a stipend of $15,000 per year.
Requirements: The applicant must: be currently enrolled in or applying to a doctoral degree program in nursing or a related field of research; meet requirements for doctoral study and must have been accepted by the institution to which s/he has applied at the time of funding; have a current license to practice as a registered nurse; project a program of study that integrates cancer nursing and provides evidence of faculty support for the program of study. Scholarship recipients must take a minimum of 18 credit hours or 6 courses per year (unless coursework has been completed and the student accepted to candidacy).
Restrictions: Students in programs that award the doctorate of nursing practice (DNP) are not eligible for this program.
Amount of Grant: $15,000 stipend
Date(s) Application is Due: Oct 15
Contact: Virginia Krawiec, MPA Director; (404) 329-7612; fax: (404) 321-4669; email: ginger.krawiec@cancer.org
Internet: http://www.cancer.org/docroot/RES/content/RES_5_2x_Doctoral_Degree_Scholarships_in_Cancer_Nursing.asp?sitearea=RES
Sponsor: American Cancer Society
1599 Clifton Rd NE
Atlanta, GA 30329-4251

ACS Doctoral Scholarships in Cancer Nursing **212**
Doctoral degree scholarships in cancer nursing are awarded to graduate students pursuing doctoral study in the following cancer nursing fields: research, education, administration, or clinical practice. Awards are made for up to four years.
Requirements: Applicants must be currently enrolled in or applying to a doctoral degree program and have current licensure to practice as a registered nurse. American citizens or permanent residents are eligible.
Amount of Grant: $15,000 per year
Date(s) Application is Due: Oct 15
Contact: Extramural Grants Department, (404) 329-7558; fax: (404) 321-4669; email: grants@cancer.org
Internet: http://www.cancer.org/docroot/RES/content/RES_5_2x_Doctoral_Degree_Scholarships_in_Cancer_Nursing.asp?sitearea=RES
Sponsor: American Cancer Society
1599 Clifton Rd NE
Atlanta, GA 30329-4251

ACS Doctoral Training Grants in Oncology Social Work **213**
This grant is awarded to qualifying doctoral students at schools of social work that train individuals to conduct research related to the psychosocial needs of persons with cancer and their families. Initial 2-year grant providing a stipend of $20,000 per year with possibility of a 2-year competitive renewal.
Requirements: The following eligibility requirements must be met: the applicant must have master's degree in social work; at least one year of social work experience in a health care setting (oncology/cancer control experience preferred, but not required); a demonstrated commitment to a career in oncology social work as evidenced by recent experience, education, and/or research; the applicant must be currently enrolled in or applying to a doctoral degree program in social work; if an applicant is not yet enrolled in a Ph.D. program, the applicant must meet requirements for doctoral study and must have been accepted by the institution to which s/he has applied at the time of funding; the applicant must project a full-time program of study that integrates oncology social work and provides evidence of faculty support for the program of study; to qualify for funding for the dissertation phase of the doctoral program, the applicant must conduct a dissertation relevant to Oncology Social Work. Successful applicants must also agree to attend the American Cancer Society activities at the annual Society for Social Work Research meeting. (Recipients at the dissertation phase will be expected to present their research at this meeting.)
Amount of Grant: $20,000 per year
Date(s) Application is Due: Oct 15
Contact: Virginia Krawiec, MPA Director; (404) 329-7612; fax: (404) 321-4669; email: ginger.krawiec@cancer.org
Internet: http://www.cancer.org/docroot/RES/content/RES_5_2x_Post-Masters_Training_Grants_in_Clinical_Oncology_Social_Work.asp?sitearea=RES
Sponsor: American Cancer Society
1599 Clifton Rd NE
Atlanta, GA 30329-4251

ACS Graduate Scholarships in Cancer Nursing Practice **214**
This award supports graduate students pursuing a master's degree in cancer nursing or doctorate of nursing practice (DNP). Awards may be for two years, with stipend of $10,000 per year. The goal of this program is to strengthen nursing practice by providing assistance for advanced preparation in the following fields of cancer nursing: clinical practice, education, and administration.
Requirements: The applicant must: be currently enrolled in or applying to a master's or DNP degree graduate program with demonstrated integration of cancer content; meet requirements for graduate study and at the time of funding have been accepted by the institution to which s/he has applied. The institution must verify the applicant's acceptance into the master's or DNP program; be pursuing an advanced degree and not solely a post master's certificate. All applicants must have a current license to practice as a registered nurse. Students in "bridge" programs must have passed the N-CLEX examination by the time the award begins.
Amount of Grant: $10,000 stipend
Date(s) Application is Due: Feb1
Contact: Virginia Krawiec, MPA Director; (404) 329-7612; fax: (404) 321-4669; email: ginger.krawiec@cancer.org
Internet: http://www.cancer.org/docroot/RES/content/RES_5_2x_Masters_Degree_Scholarships_in_Cancer_Nursing.asp?sitearea=RES
Sponsor: American Cancer Society
1599 Clifton Rd NE
Atlanta, GA 30329-4251

ACS Institutional Research Grants **215**
The IRG program provides seed money for the initiation of promising new projects by independent junior investigators so they may obtain preliminary results that will enable them to compete successfully for national research grants.
Requirements: Only full-time, tenure-track JHU faculty members at the ranks of Instructor or Assistant Professor or equivalent who are within the first six years of their first independent research or faculty appointment may apply. Relevance to the cancer problem is important and must be well documented. Within this research scope, a wide breadth of research approaches will be considered; these include basic laboratory studies and clinical research.
Restrictions: Senior investigators, postdoctoral fellows and junior investigators who have competitive national research grants or who have received prior support form the IRG are not eligible.
Amount of Grant: $90,000 per year
Date(s) Application is Due: Apr 1
Contact: Grace Bigelow, Research Projects Administration; (410) 516-5256; fax: (410) 516-7775; email: graceb@jhu.edu
Internet: http://www.cancer.org/docroot/RES/content/RES_5_2x_Institutional_Research_Grants.asp?sitearea=RES
Sponsor: American Cancer Society
3100 Wyman Park Drive, Suite W400
Baltimore, MD 21211

ACS MEN2 Thyroid Cancer Professorship Grants **216**
The Professorship award is intended for an outstanding senior investigator who is well known for their contributions to the understanding and/or management of MEN2. Appropriate areas of investigation include, but are not limited to: understanding consequences of RET mutations, molecular events underlying the development of MEN2-related tumors, improved animal models of MEN2, new screening and monitoring tools, new imaging approaches, and new pharmacologic and other strategies to blunt the effects of mutations in RET and other genes associated with medullary thyroid cancer. This person will serve as the leader for a consortium consisting of up to seven (7) investigators with Research Scholar and/or Mentored Research Scholar grants and up to five (5) Postdoctoral Fellows. Responsibilities primarily involve serving as the chairman of an annual research meeting of MEN2 investigators. The amount of the award is $80,000 per year for five years and can be budgeted at the recipient's discretion.

Only one award will be made and a letter of intent must be submitted. The awardee must be willing to be an occasional spokesperson for the American Cancer Society and for the Consortium. Interested individuals must electronically submit their curriculum vitae with a complete bibliography and a letter of intent that briefly describes their seminal contributions to thyroid cancer research. This information must be submitted via Access Electronic Grant application process at proposalCENTRAL no later than December 31, by applying for the American Cancer Society – MEN2 Thyroid Cancer Professorship. Qualified candidates will be invited no later than January 15 to submit full applications by April 1.
Requirements: Candidates must be American citizens or permanent residents with at least 10 years of experience beyond receipt of their terminal degree and in general are expected to hold the rank of full professor. Department chairs or individuals with equivalent administrative positions are eligible.
Amount of Grant: $80,000 per year
Date(s) Application is Due: Dec 31
Contact: Charles Saxe, Program Director; (404) 929-6919; email: charles.saxe@cancer.org
Internet: http://www.cancer.org/docroot/RES/content/RES_5_2x_RFA_for_The_American_Cancer_Society_MEN2_Thyroid_Cancer_Consortium_Professorship.asp?sitearea=RES
Sponsor: American Cancer Society
1599 Clifton Rd NE
Atlanta, GA 30329-4251

ACS Mentored Research Scholar Grant in Applied and Clinical Research **217**
This funding opportunity supports mentored research by full-time faculty, typically within the first four years of their appointment, with the goal of becoming independent investigators in clinical, cancer control and prevention, epidemiologic, psychosocial, behavioral, health services and health policy research. Awards are made up to five years and for up to $135,000 per year (direct costs) plus 8% allowable indirect costs. A maximum of $10,000 per year for the mentor(s) (regardless of the number of mentors) is included in the $135,000. These grants are not renewable.
Amount of Grant: $135,000
Date(s) Application is Due: Apr 1; Oct 15
Contact: Ronit Elk, Program Director; (404) 417-5957; fax: (404) 321-4669; email: ronit.elk@cancer.org;; Extramural Grants Department, (404) 329-7558; fax: (404) 417-5974; email: grants@cancer.org
Internet: http://www.cancer.org/docroot/RES/content/RES_5_2x_Mentored_Research_Scholar_Grant_in_Applied_and_Clinical_Research.asp?sitearea=RES
Sponsor: American Cancer Society
1599 Clifton Rd NE
Atlanta, GA 30329

ACS Physician Training Awards in Preventive Medicine **218**
The Physician Training Award in Preventive Medicine (PTAPM) is intended to encourage and assist the development of promising individuals who will pursue careers in preventive medicine. This program is designed to create a cadre of preventive medicine specialists who are expert in cancer prevention and control, and with the potential to become leaders in research, education, and intervention in this area. Through the Physician Training Award in Preventive Medicine, the Society seeks to support physicians in accredited residency programs that will lead to eligibility for certification in preventive medicine; such programs must provide cancer prevention and control research and practice opportunities. Awards are for four years in the total amount of $300,000, based on an average of $50,000 per resident training year. These grants are renewable.
Requirements: Requirements for the institution are available on the ACS website. Eligibility requirements for the residents are: nominated residents must be citizens or non-citizen nationals of the United States or its possessions and territories, or must have been lawfully admitted to the United States for permanent residence at the time of application; must have an MD, DO, or equivalent degree; must have completed the clinical year of a residency program in preventive medicine, or have at least one year of postgraduate clinical training; must be accepted by or applying to the sponsoring residency program. It is preferred that the candidates not have completed more than half of the required academic work at the beginning of the award period. Residents that have completed the MPH degree will be considered on a case-by-case basis, and must propose course work in cancer prevention and control.
Amount of Grant: $300,000 maximum
Date(s) Application is Due: Apr 1
Contact: Extramural Grants Department, (404) 329-7558; fax: (404) 417-5974; email: grants@cancer.org;; Virginia Krawiec, MPA, Program Director; (404) 329-7612; email: ginger.krawiec@cancer.org
Internet: http://www.cancer.org/docroot/RES/content/RES_5_2x_Physician_Training_Awards_in_Preventive_Medicine.asp?sitearea=RES
Sponsor: American Cancer Society
1599 Clifton Rd NE
Atlanta, GA 30329-4251

ACS Pilot and Exploratory Projects in Palliative Care of Cancer Patients and Their Families Grants **219**
This request for application (RFA) provides funding for investigators performing pilot and exploratory research studies whose purpose is to test interventions, develop research methodologies, and explore novel areas of research in palliative care of cancer patients and their families. A condition of funding is a clearly defined plan as to how the investigator will use the results of the project to develop larger, extramurally funded research projects. This RFA is limited to applications that focus on palliative care research projects for seriously ill cancer patients and their families in three specific areas: exploring the relationship of pain and other distressing symptoms on quality and quantity of life, independence, function, and disability and developing interventions directed at their treatment in patients with advanced and chronic illnesses; studying methods of improving communication between adults living with serious illness, their families and their health care providers; evaluating models and systems of care for patients living with advanced illness and their families. As a condition of accepting the award, each recipient of this grant, will agree to: attend the required meetings of the NPCRC in Fall during the award period; present results of the funded research at this required NPCRC meeting; prepare annual progress reports for each year of funding and a final report at the conclusion of the award period; list the American Cancer Society as funding this study on all publications and presentations.
Requirements: Applications may be submitted by not-for-profit institutions located within the United States, its territories and the Commonwealth of Puerto Rico. Applicants must: be United States citizens, non-citizen nationals or permanent residents of the United States; hold a doctorate degree (MD, PhD, or equivalent) and have a full-time faculty position or equivalent at a college, university, medical school, or other fiscally responsible not-for-profit organization within the United States. Independent investigators at all stages of their career are eligible to apply. Applicants must submit their full application electronically and in paper format per guidelines on cancer.org no later than 5pm (Eastern) on October 15th.
Restrictions: Awards may not exceed $60,000 per year (direct costs) plus 20% indirect costs. Salary support for the Principal Investigator may not exceed 20% of the direct costs. Awards may not exceed a period of one to two years duration.
Amount of Grant: $60,000 maximum per year
Date(s) Application is Due: Oct 15
Contact: Ronit Elk, Program Director; (404) 417-5957; fax: (404) 321-4669; email: ronit.elk@cancer.org
Internet: http://www.cancer.org/docroot/RES/content/RES_5_2x_RFA__Pilot_and_Exploratory_Projects_in_Palliative_Care_of_Cancer_Patients_and_Their_Families.asp?sitearea=RES
Sponsor: American Cancer Society
1599 Clifton Rd NE
Atlanta, GA 30329-4251

ACS Postdoctoral Fellowships **220**
Fellowships are designed to enable a new investigator to qualify for an independent career in cancer research. Postdoctoral fellowships may be made for one, two, or three years. Stipend payments are made directly to the individual, or the institution if requested, at the beginning of each month. Travel funds are paid to the individual. Institutional allowances are paid annually at the start of the grant and on the anniversary date thereafter. Awards are made for one to three years with progressive stipends.
Requirements: Applicants must be citizens or permanent residents of the United States (the latter must provide notarized evidence of their legal resident alien status) and shall have been awarded a doctoral degree prior to the activation date of the grant. Application must be endorsed by applicant's mentor and the head of the department in which the training will be received. A plan of training must be formulated and agreed upon by the mentor and the applicant and described in detail in the application.
Restrictions: Awards will not be made to applicants who have completed five or more years of postdoctoral training prior to the start date of the fellowship.
Amount of Grant: $44,000, $46,000, and $48,000 for the first, second, and third years, respectively, and $4,000 maximum per year institutional allowance
Date(s) Application is Due: Apr 1; Oct 15
Contact: Extramural Grants Department, (404) 329-7558; fax: (404) 321-4669; email: grants@cancer.org
Internet: http://www.cancer.org/docroot/RES/content/RES_5_2x_Postdoctoral_Fellowships.asp?sitearea=RES
Sponsor: American Cancer Society
1599 Clifton Rd NE
Atlanta, GA 30329-4251

ACS Research Professor Grants **221**
The American Cancer Society offers a limited number of grants to investigators in mid-career who have made seminal contributions that have changed the direction of cancer research. Furthermore, it is expected that these investigators will continue to provide leadership in their research area. Up to two awards are made annually for a five-year term that can be renewed once. The award of up to $80,000 per year (direct costs only) may be used for salary or research project support. Interested individuals should submit their curriculum vitae with a complete bibliography and a letter of intent that briefly describes their seminal contributions to research. This information must be submitted no later then February 1, via the Research Professor letter of intent on proposalCENTRAL at: https://proposalcentral.altum.com. Upon receipt, ACS will provide appropriate guidance either by telephone or email.
Amount of Grant: $80,000 maximum per year
Date(s) Application is Due: Feb 1; Apr 1
Contact: John J. Stevens, Vice President Extramural Grant; (404) 329-7550; email: john.stevens@cancer.org
Internet: http://www.cancer.org/docroot/RES/content/RES_5_2x_Research_Professorships.asp?sitearea=RES
Sponsor: American Cancer Society
1599 Clifton Rd NE
Atlanta, GA 30329-4251

ACS Research Scholar Grants for Health Services and Health Policy Research 222
The grants support research projects centered on health services and health policy initiated by investigators at any stage in their careers. The initial award includes 20 percent for indirect costs for up to four years, and may be renewed once for up to four years.
Amount of Grant: $200,000 maximum per year
Date(s) Application is Due: Apr 1; Oct 15
Contact: Extramural Grants Department, (404) 329-7558; fax: (404) 321-4669; email: grants@cancer.org
Internet: http://www.cancer.org/docroot/RES/content/RES_5_2x_Research_Scholar_Grants_For_Health_Services_and_Health_Policy_and_Outcomes_Research.asp?sitearea=RES
Sponsor: American Cancer Society
1599 Clifton Rd NE
Atlanta, GA 30329-4251

ACS Research Scholar Grants in Basic, Preclinical, Clinical and Epidemiology Research 223
This grant supports investigator-initiated research projects in basic, preclinical, clinical and epidemiologic research. Awards are for up to four years and for up to $200,000 per year (direct costs), plus 20% allowable indirect costs.
Amount of Grant: $200,000
Date(s) Application is Due: Apr 1; Oct 15
Contact: Extramural Grants Department, (404) 329-7558; fax: (404) 417-5974; email: grants@cancer.org;; William Chambers, Program Director; (404) 329-7552; email: william.chambers@cancer.org
Internet: http://www.cancer.org/docroot/RES/content/RES_5_2x_Research_Scholar_Grants_for_Beginning_Investigators.asp?sitearea=RES
Sponsor: American Cancer Society
1599 Clifton Rd NE
Atlanta, GA 30329-4251

ACS Research Scholar Grants in Psychosocial and Behavioral and Cancer Control Research 224
The grants support research projects focusing on the psychosocial and behavioral aspects of cancer by independent investigators at any stage in their careers. Applications are encouraged in which an individual at an early career stage is coprincipal investigator with an established researcher. The initial award supports four years of research and may be renewed once for four additional years.
Requirements: Individuals must not have held an independent position for more than six years at the time the application is submitted.
Amount of Grant: $200,000 maximum per year
Date(s) Application is Due: Apr 1; Oct 15
Contact: Extramural Grants Department, (404) 329-7558; fax: (404) 417-5974; email: grants@cancer.org;; Ronit Elk, Program Director; (404) 417-5957; fax: (404) 321-4669; email: Ronit.Elk@cancer.org
Internet: http://www.cancer.org/docroot/RES/content/RES_5_2x_Research_Scholar_Grants_in_Psychological_and_Behavioral_Research_for_Beginning_and_Senior_Investigators.asp?sitearea=RES
Sponsor: American Cancer Society
1599 Clifton Rd NE
Atlanta, GA 30329-4251

Actors Fund Social Services and Financial Assistance 225
The Actors Fund Social Services offer comprehensive programs designed to meet the critical needs of entertainment professionals throughout their lives. Social workers provide crisis intervention, individual and family needs assessments, and develop long-term plans include ongoing support, education, information and referrals. In addition, financial assistance can be provided for essential living expenses such as rent, utilities or medical costs.
Requirements: Eligibility for financial assistance varies by program. You are encouraged to call and speak with an Intake Social Worker who can best determine how the program may be of assistance. Overall eligibility for financial assistance is based on: a minimum of five years of industry employment with earnings of at least $6,500 for three out of the last five years and financial need. To apply for financial assistance, an application with supporting documentation and an interview is required. There are no specific deadlines.
Contact: Eastern Region, (212) 221-7300 ext. 119, intakeny@actorsfund.org; Central Region, (312) 372-0989, dtowne@actorsfund.org; Western Region, (323) 933-9244 ext. 55, intakela@actorsfund.org
Internet: http://new.actorsfund.org/services/Social_Services_and_Financial_Assistance/index_html
Sponsor: Actors Fund
729 7th Avenue, 10th floor
New York, NY 10019

Acushnet Foundation Grants 226
The foundation awards one-year, renewable grants to eligible Massachusetts nonprofit organizations in its areas of interest, including community, hospitals and health care, family, and youth and at-risk youths. Types of support include capital grants (building funds and materials), seed money grants, annual campaigns, and emergency funds. Applicants should submit a letter of inquiry.
Requirements: Massachusetts 501(c)3 tax-exempt organizations serving the New Bedford area are eligible.
Restrictions: Grants are not made to individuals.
Geographic Focus: Massachusetts
Amount of Grant: $1000-$95,000 range
Contact: William Blasdale, c/o Seamark Financial Services Inc, (508) 758-6159
Sponsor: Acushnet Foundation
P.O. Box 1498
Mattapoisett, MA 02739

ACVIM Foundation Clinical Investigation Grants 227
The Foundation improves the health and well-being of animals by funding humane studies and communicating information about this work to the veterinary community and the general public. It supports leading veterinary scientists as they take on a range of critical animal health issues within the specialties of small and large animal internal medicine, cardiology, neurology, and oncology. This work, in turn, holds promise for better preventive care, better nutrition, and more sensitive screening and improved treatment for such devastating diseases as cancer, epilepsy, cardiomyopathy, and kidney failure. The Foundation's main goal is to support clinical investigations that lead to new diagnostic, treatment, and prevention techniques. Resident applicants may request up to $12,500 per year, while diplomate applicants may request up to $15,000. One $20,000 grant will be awarded to a collaborative/multi-center proposal, with preference toward private practice/academia partnerships. Funding for multi-year projects up to 3 years will be considered, subject to annual non-competitive renewal based on availability of funds and demonstration of adequate progress on the project. The foundation will consider funding for multi-year projects up to three years.
Samples: Dr. Jill Beech, University of Pennsylvania School of Veterinary Medicine—Evaluation of Endogenous Alpha MSH Concentrations at Different Seasons and in Response to TRH in Normal Horses and Those with Pituitary Hyperplasia (2006); Dr. Stephanie Kottler, University of Missouri-Columbia College of Veterinary Medicine—Prevalence of Staphylococcus aureus and MRSA carriage in three populations (2006).
Amount of Grant: $20,000 maximum
Date(s) Application is Due: Sep 15
Contact: Angela E. Frimberger, Executive Director; (303) 231-9933 or (800) 245-9081; email: info@acvimfoundation.org
Internet: http://www.acvimfoundation.org/grants/info.html
Sponsor: American College of Veterinary Internal Medicine (ACVIM)
997 Wadsworth Boulevard, Suite A
Lakewood, CO 80214

ADA Foundation Dental Education Grants 228
In an effort to stimulate innovation in dental education, the foundation is looking for submissions for innovative projects or programs that promote a stronger, more dynamic dental education system. Submissions may describe projects, both in progress and in the planning stages, or projects that would be implemented if resources were available. Project ideas should address one or more of the following criteria: new teacher training models; new faculty practice models; incentives or recognition programs for teachers in dental schools; reformed school business and curriculum structure; innovative faculty recruitment or retention programs; reformed school business infrastructures that enhance delivery of care; pooling resources among dental schools or other institutions; and addressing financial problems of renewed capital for schools and high student indebtedness. To be considered, the submission must address how the innovative project/program will enhance the delivery of dental education; demonstrate why the project/program meets a critical need in dental education; address how the project/program will enhance or complement existing programs; and describe any challenges that currently inhibit the applicant organization from implementing the innovative project/program and identify the resources needed to overcome those challenges. Grantees will receive an unrestricted grant, which may or may not be used on the projects described. Application and guidelines are available online.
Requirements: Dental schools, nonprofit organizations, and other organizations in the United States and its territories are eligible.
Amount of Grant: $25,000
Date(s) Application is Due: Nov 1
Contact: Lisa Barron, Director of Programs, (800) 621-8099 ext 4639; email: barronl@ada.org
Internet: http://www.adafoundation.org/prof/resources/pubs/adanews/adanewsarticle.asp?articleid=1532
Sponsor: American Dental Association Foundation
211 E Chicago Avenue
Chicago, IL 60611-2678

ADA Foundation Dental Literature Grants 229
The foundation will award grants to applicants who submit competitive proposals to complete a systematic literature review on a high-priority research topic supporting evidence-based dentistry. The program focuses on available dental literature addressing four specific clinical questions. Applicants are asked to choose one of the following questions for a systematic literature review. At what frequency is dental prophylaxis effective in preventing periodontitis in individuals with and without known risk factors? Does correcting malocclusion in children and adults reduce the risk of periodontal disease? What are the clinical, biological, psychosocial, and/or economic outcomes of treating a pulpally involved (periodontally sound) single tooth through: endodontic care, extraction and implant placement, fixed partial denture, and/or extraction without implant placement? What are the longitudinal beneficial and harmful effects of endodontic services compared to extraction and implant placement? Proposals must be submitted in hard copy. Guidelines are available online.

Requirements: Applicants must be affiliated with a dental school or advanced education program accredited by the Commission on Dental Accreditation, a dental specialty organization or a national dental related organization; should be knowledgeable and experienced in systematic review; have a demonstrated track record in research; and have published studies in clinical dental research.
Amount of Grant: $50,000 maximum
Date(s) Application is Due: Jan 30
Contact: Lisa Barron, at (312) 440-4639; email: barronl@ada.org
Internet: http://www.adafoundation.org/prof/resources/pubs/adanews/adanewsarticle.asp?articleid=1640
Sponsor: American Dental Association Foundation
211 E Chicago Avenue
Chicago, IL 60611-2616

Adam Richter Charitable Trust Grants 230
The Trust, which is administered by the Bank of America in Dallas, Texas, was established in California in 1994. Offering grants on a national basis, its primary fields of interest include: the arts; animal welfare; Christian agencies and churches; the environment; health organizations; higher education; hospitals; and human services. There are no formal applications or deadlines, and interested applicants should begin by
Samples: Habitat for Humanity International, San Francisco, CA, $13,082 (2007); Greenpeace, Washington, DC, $2,000 (2007); Sonoma Land Trust, Santa Rosa, CA, $12,000 (2007).
Contact: c/o Michael Schlebach, Specialty Asset Manager; (214) 922-9290
Sponsor: Adam Richter Charitable Trust
411 N. Akard Street
Dallas, TX 75201-3307

Adams County Foundation Grants - Pennsylvania 231
The Community Foundation, established in 1985, offers funding that is limited to Adams County, Pennsylvania. The foundation gives to organizations that assist, promote and improve the moral, mental, social and physical well-being of area residents. Fields of interest include: arts; Christian agencies and churches; community and economic development; education; and health organizations. Letters of Intent (LOIs) are due by June 31st. An application form is required and, if invited, is due by the end of July.
Requirements: Applicants must serve residents living in Adams County, Pennsylvania.
Geographic Focus: Pennsylvania
Amount of Grant: $2,000 maximum
Date(s) Application is Due: Jun 31; Jul 31
Contact: John W. Phillips, Executive Director; (717) 337-0060 or (717) 337-3353; fax: (717) 337-1080; email: info@adamscountycf.org
Internet: http://www.adamscountycf.org/learn.html
Sponsor: Adams County Foundation
P.O. Box 4565, 101 W. Middle Street
Gettysburg, PA 17325-2109

Adaptec Foundation Grants 232
The corporate contributions program is primarily directed, although not exclusively, to organizations and programs serving the communities where its employees work and live, with special emphasis in the Silicon Valley area. Funding priorities include education and research—programs that lower the drop-out rate of youth in accredited schools and colleges, address career development and preparation, job training and placement, educational scholarship assistance, and investment in higher education (primarily in engineering-related university programs); health and human services—research cures for devastating diseases, emergency shelter and subsistence for the homeless, treatment and assistance for abused spouses and children, drug and alcohol rehabilitation, and supporting organizations that strengthen youths and families; helping people enjoy life more fully through music, dance, art museums, opera, theater, and performing arts groups; and $25-$500 employee matching gifts. The Corporate Contributions Committee meets quarterly to consider requests.
Restrictions: In general, Adaptec does not make contributions to any organization that does not have 501(c)3 or comparable status; individuals, except through the Adaptec Scholarship program; churches, synagogues, and other religious groups. (Requests are considered from religious-sponsored and other groups whose activities do not support any specific religious doctrine or ethnic/cultural group.); political or fraternal organizations; underwrite or assist with the development of films, television, or video/radio productions, whether for commercial, independent, or nonprofit ventures, unless such activity is in support of the computer I/O software/hardware industry and is directly related to the business of the company; tickets for raffles, contests, or other fundraising activities (except requests from major fundraising organizations that meet the defined objectives of the contribution program, such as United Way, the Silicon Valley Charity Ball and the San Jose Symphony); organizations whose primary objective is to assist, benefit, and address animal welfare or environmental issues, such as the preservation of endangered species and plants or conservation efforts to preserve the quality of wildlife, water, soil, or air; reduce debts, fund general operating expenses or capital improvement projects, or retroactively fund activities or programs that are already completed; and school sports leagues and events, and other non-educational related activities such as band, debate teams, and goodwill trips.
Amount of Grant: $250-$2,500
Contact: Corporate Contributions; (408) 945-8600; fax: (408) 262-2533
Internet: http://cms.adaptec.com/ko-KR/company/about/_corporate/adaptec_corpcontributions.htm?nc=/ko-KR/company/about/_corporate/adaptec_corpcontributions.htm
Sponsor: Adaptec Foundation
691 South Milpitas Boulevard, MS-15
Milpitas, CA 95035-5473

Addison H. Gibson Foundation Medical Grants 233
The Foundation's principal philanthropic interest is to provide medical care; specifically, to enable working people to continue their employment without the burden of untreated illness, or the financial hardship resulting from loss of income associated with untreated illness. The funds provide such medical treatment to needy, self-supporting, long-term western Pennsylvania residents who otherwise cannot afford the medical aid which they require. Physicians, social service and hospital administrators may apply on behalf of their patients.
Requirements: Applicants for medical grants must be referred by their attending physicians, or via social service or hospital administrators. Medical grants are applied for in advance of prescribed treatment. Previously incurred medical expenses are not eligible for consideration. Patients with a correctable condition only will be considered.
Restrictions: Recipients who benefit from these grants must be long-term residents of western Pennsylvania. Grant monies are paid directly to the providers, never to the patients.
Geographic Focus: Pennsylvania
Contact: Rebecca Wallace, Director; (412) 261-1611; fax: (412) 261-5733
Internet: http://www.gibson-fnd.org/Docs/Medical_Grants.htm
Sponsor: Addison H. Gibson Foundation
One PPG Place, Suite 2230
Pittsburgh, PA 15222-5401

Adelaide Breed Bayrd Foundation Grants 234
The foundation supports programs and projects of nonprofit organizations serving the Malden, MA, area. Areas of interest include adult/continuing education, aging, centers/services, arts, children/youth services, community development, education, family services, health care, health organizations, hospitals (general), human services, libraries/library science, residential/custodial care, hospices. The foundation supports projects and programs and requests for capital and seed money. Grants have been awarded in the past to support public libraries, hospitals, and the Girl Scouts. There are no application forms; applicants should submit a letter describing the request and organization.
Requirements: 501(c)3 organizations serving the Malden, MA, area are eligible.
Restrictions: The foundation does not award grants to individuals or the performing arts in general, matching or challenge grants, demonstration projects, conferences, publications, research or endowments.
Geographic Focus: Massachusetts
Amount of Grant: $200-$63,000 range
Contact: Dr. Russell Watts, President, (781) 662-7342 or (781) 662-7971
Sponsor: Adelaide Breed Bayrd Foundation
28 Pilgrim Road
Melrose, MA 02176

Administaff Community Affairs Grants 235
Five areas qualify for Administaff corporate contribution consideration: the elderly, education, social service, environment, and health. Administaff will consider four types of requests: volunteers and grants; grants; event sponsorships; and in-kind donations—equipment such as computers, copiers and furniture. All contribution requests must be made in writing. Guidelines and sample cover letter are available online.
Requirements: Charitable organizations must have 501(c)3 status, according to IRS standards; operate in one of Administaff's district markets; and submit a written request. Qualifying organizations also must submit a financial statement to the Better Business Bureau before consideration.
Restrictions: Ineligible entities include: religious organizations (i.e., churches, temples, and other houses of worship, or those whose main purpose is to promote a particular faith or creed); political organizations; individuals; athletic groups; or school clubs.
Amount of Grant: $5,000 average
Contact: Betty Collins, Community Involvement, (281) 358-8986; fax: (281) 312-3559; email: community_involvement@administaff.com
Internet: http://www.administaff.com/about_asf/grants.asp
Sponsor: Administaff Corporation
19001 Crescent Springs Drive
Kingwood, TX 77339-3802

Administration on Aging Senior Medicare Patrol Project Grants 236
The goal of SMP Projects is to empower beneficiaries/consumers to prevent health care fraud through outreach and education. Program coverage must target vulnerable, hard-to-reach population beneficiaries, their families and other consumers. The purpose of this competition is to provide the opportunity to fund one (1) Project in each of 26 eligible states including the District of Columbia for a project period of up to three (3) years.
Requirements: Domestic public or private and non-profit entities including state, local and Indian tribal governments (American Indian/Alaskan Native/Native American), faith-based organizations, community-based organizations, hospitals, and institutions of higher education are eligible to apply. Through this competition, AoA plans to fund one project in each of the following 26 states and the District of Columbia: Alaska, Arizona, Arkansas, Colorado, Delaware, the District of Columbia, Florida, Georgia, Idaho, Kansas, Kentucky, Maine, Massachusetts, Michigan, Montana, New Jersey, New Mexico, Ohio, Oklahoma, Oregon, Puerto Rico, Tennessee, Texas, Virginia, Washington, and West Virginia.
Amount of Grant: $345,000 per year for up to three years

Date(s) Application is Due: Apr 11
Contact: Barbara Lewis, Project Officer; (202) 357-3532; email: Barbara.Lewis@aoa.hhs.gov
Internet: http://www.aoa.dhhs.gov/doingbus/fundopp/fundopp.asp
Sponsor: Administration on Aging (AoA)
330 Independence Avenue SW
Washington, DC 20201

Adobe Community Investment Grants **237**
Adobe supports strategic programs and partnerships that help make its communities better, stronger, and more vibrant places to live, work and do business. Adobe's focus areas for giving and grants programs are designed to: increase Adobe's impact in the community through support of more organizations; and strengthen Adobe's role as a corporate partner by creating deeper, stronger, and richer partnerships. The Adobe Community Investment Grant program provides multi-year (with annual review), comprehensive support, including cash, software, volunteers, and facilities use through an Adobe-initiated, RFP application process. Grant amounts are at least $20,000 and can be for up to three years. Organizations selected become Adobe Community Investment Partners and are required to sit out one year after the grant ends before reapplying.
Requirements: Adobe is currently accepting grant proposals in the following communities: San Jose/Silicon Valley, California (southern San Mateo County, Santa Clara County, southern Alameda County); San Francisco, California; Seattle/King County, Washington; and Ottawa, Ontario, Canada.
Geographic Focus: California; WashingtonCanada
Contact: Lesley Dierks, Community Relations; (408) 536-6000 or (408) 536-3993; fax: (408) 537-6000 or (408) 537-6313; email: ldierks@adobe.com or community_relations@adobe.com
Internet: http://www.adobe.com/aboutadobe/philanthropy/commgivingprgrm.html#Community%20giving%20programs
Sponsor: Adobe Systems, Inc.
345 Park Avenue
San Jose, CA 95110-2704

Adolph Coors Foundation Grants **238**
The foundation's grant program supports programs in the area of health that are preventive in nature, promote wellness and/or can demonstrate a reduction in health-care costs. The support in education is directed to institutions and programs that foster excellence in the knowledge of free enterprise, science, technology and ethics. The Foundation is generally supportive of community and human services agencies that assist the disadvantaged in their efforts to be self-sufficient and productive and that nurture the development of integrity and leadership. Civic and cultural programs attracting the Foundation's attention are typically those that enhance our culture and heritage, demonstrate our creativity as a people and are likely to be of economic benefit to and broadly used by the communities they serve. Past grants have supported boys and girls clubs and inner-city health programs. Types of support include building funds, general operating budgets, seed money, and special projects. Application guidelines are available from the foundation; there is no formal application form. Applications are not accepted by fax or email.
Requirements: Only tax-exempt, nonprofit organizations in or benefiting Colorado that do not also receive tax money are eligible to apply.
Restrictions: Individuals are ineligible. The foundation does not support preschools or day-care centers.
Geographic Focus: Colorado
Samples: Colorado College (Colorado Springs, CO)—to renovate Palmer Hall, an academic building that was constructed in 1904, $400,000 (2004).
Contact: Jeanne Bistranin, (303) 388-1636; email: generalinfo@acoorsfdn.org
Internet: http://www.coorsfoundation.org/guidelines.html
Sponsor: Adolph Coors Foundation
4100 E Mississippi Avenue, Suite 1850
Denver, CO 80246

Advanced Micro Devices Community Affairs Grants **239**
AMD awards grants to nonprofit organizations and schools that serve the communities in which it operates: Sunnyvale, CA, and Austin, TX, and in Europe and Asia. AMD grants funds to agencies that serve the community's health and human service, education and civic needs. AMD K-12 initiatives target programs that increase student interest and/or proficiency in literacy, math, science, and computer technology. AMD also funds programs aimed at developing and supporting effective classroom instruction. AMD also funds basic needs programs to local health and human services organizations. In addition, AMD matches employee gifts to organizations whose activities fall within one of the approved funding areas. AMD also supports engineering education at universities throughout the United States. Generally, funds are granted for specific projects, not for general operating expenses. Requests must be submitted in writing, using appropriate forms, and must include a description of the applicant organization with a statement of its purposes and objectives, a statement regarding the need the grant will address and the geographic area and population served, the names and qualifications of the person(s) who will administer the grant, and amount requested with an explanation of how the funds will be used. Awards are made on a quarterly basis.
Requirements: IRS 501(c)3 tax-exempt organizations and schools based in Sunnyvale, CA, and Austin, TX, are eligible.
Restrictions: AMD will not fund political activities, national programs, advocacy programs, religious or fraternal organizations, individuals, fund-raising events, conferences, seminars, door prizes, registration fees, advertising, or sports leagues.
Geographic Focus: California; TexasAsia; Europe; Germany
Date(s) Application is Due: May 1
Contact: Community Affairs, (408) 749-5373;
Internet: http://www.amd.com/us-en/Corporate/AboutAMD/0,,51_52_7697_7702,00.html
Sponsor: Advanced Micro Devices
P.O. Box 3453
Sunnyvale, CA 94088-3453

Advancing Colorado's Mental Health Care Project Grants **240**
This project, a joint venture of the foundation, the Colorado Trust, the Denver Foundation, and HealthOne Alliance, focuses on improving the integration and coordination of mental health services for adults with serious mental illness and children with severe emotional disturbances. The project will support the integration of mental health services in five to eight Colorado communities so that people with significant mental health needs can be treated across agencies, regardless of funding sources, organizational structures, or policy and practice differences. Applicant communities propose the target population(s), local approaches for accomplishing improved system integration, and specific strategies and structures for integrating services. Complete program information is available online.
Requirements: Applicants must have the following qualifications and characteristics: a fiscal agent that has 501(c)3 tax-exempt status or is a governmental entity; and an existing collaborative identified to oversee project policy and funding that includes members from agencies and provider organizations serving persons with mental health needs, as well as recipients of mental health services and their families.
Restrictions: Applicants may not propose the use of grant or match funds for new construction or renovation; grants to individuals; retirement of debt; institutional indirect cost recovery; lobbying or political purposes; religious purposes; activities other than charitable activities; replacement of existing or lost funds; or payment for individual services that could be covered by existing funding sources or that falls outside the intent of the grant (i.e., hospital or medication expenses).
Geographic Focus: Colorado
Amount of Grant: $375,000-$650,000 for five years
Date(s) Application is Due: May 31
Contact: Rachel Mondragon, (303) 837-1200 or (888) 847-9140; email: rachel@coloradotrust.org
Internet: http://www.coloradotrust.org/index.cfm?fuseAction=Grantmaking.FundingOpportunities
Sponsor: Caring for Colorado Foundation
4855 Riverbend Road, Suite 100
Boulder, CO 80301

Advocate HealthCare Post Graduate Administrative Fellowship **241**
The program is open to recent graduates from programs in Healthcare Administration or Business Administration, and is designed to provide its fellows with an educational working environment that enables them to use their analytical, project management and communication skills in team-based setting. Under the supervision of senior leaders, fellows complete projects in operational and/or strategic areas. Project assignments are adapted to the individual's needs and interests. The postgraduate fellowship is a one-year program designed to enables the graduate to develop leadership skills and management skills. Fellows are given the opportunity for exposure across Advocate's eight hospitals, three physician practice organizations, home health care agency and corporate offices.
Requirements: In order to be considered, the following must be submitted no later than November 1, the year previous to entry in to the program: (1) Personal statement of interest from explaining qualifications and career objectives; (2) Statement of community involvement; (3) A current resume; (4) Letters of recommendation from applicant's program director and at least one other professional recommendation; and, (5) Copy of unofficial undergraduate transcripts and most recent graduate school transcripts.
Date(s) Application is Due: Nov 1
Contact: Melissa O'Neill, Director; (630) 572-9393
Internet: http://www.advocatehealth.com/body.cfm?id=888
Sponsor: Advocate HealthCare
2025 Windsor Drive
Oak Brook, IL 60523

AEC Trust Grants **242**
The trust awards grants to eligible nonprofits in Colorado, Florida, Georgia, Massachusetts, and Wisconsin in its areas of interest, including AIDS, arts and culture, community development, elementary education, the environment, health care, higher education, social services, and women. Types of support include building construction/renovation, capital campaigns, challenge/matching grants, equipment acquisition, general operating support, land acquisition, project support, and publications. Request guidelines in writing.
Requirements: 501(c)3 nonprofit organizations in the communities of Boulder, Colorado, Gainesville, Florida, Atlanta, Georgia, Amherst, Massachusetts, and Green Bay, Wisconsin, are eligible.
Restrictions: Grants do not support individuals, international organizations, political organizations, religious organizations, school districts, special events/benefit dinners, state and local government agencies, United Way agencies, national public charities, endowments, sponsorships, or annual fund campaigns.
Geographic Focus: Colorado; Florida; Georgia; Massachusetts; Wisconsin
Amount of Grant: $10,000-$50,000 range
Date(s) Application is Due: Apr 1; Sep 1

Contact: Julia Beisel, c/o Foundation Source; (800) 839-1754 or (401) 881-3409; email: requests@foundationsource.com
Internet: https://online.foundationsource.com/public/home/aec
Sponsor: AEC Trust
191 Peachtree Street, Suite 2300
Atlanta, GA 30309-7676

AEGON Transamerica Foundation Grants **243**
The foundation supports organizations involved with arts and culture, education, cancer, ALS research, hunger, human services, and the disabled. Giving on a national basis in areas of company operations, with some emphasis on Little Rock, Arkansas, California, Atlanta, Georgia, Cedar Rapids, Iowa, Louisville, Kentucky, Baltimore, Maryland, Charlotte, North Carolina, New York, Pennsylvania, and Fort Worth, Texas.
Requirements: Grant recipient must be a 501(c)3 organization.
Restrictions: Grants are not awarded to individuals. Unsolicited proposals not accepted.
Geographic Focus: Arkansas; California; Georgia; Iowa; Kentucky; Maryland; New York; North Carolina; Pennsylvania; Texas
Samples: Johns Hopkins University, Baltimore, MD, $2,500,000 (2008); United Way of Central Carolinas, Charlotte, NC, $46,676 (2008); Theater Cedar Rapids, Cedar Rapids, IA, $150,000 (2008).
Amount of Grant: $50 - $ 2,500,000 range
Contact: Grants Administrator, (319) 398-8935
Sponsor: AEGON Transamerica Foundation
4333 Edgewood Road, NE
Cedar Rapids, IA 52499-3210

Aetna Foundation Health Grants in Connecticut **244**
The Aetna Foundation is the independent charitable and philanthropic arm of Aetna Inc. Founded in 1972, the Foundation helps build healthy communities by promoting volunteerism, forming partnerships and funding initiatives that improve the quality of life where our employees and customers live and work. With its Health Grants in Connecticut, the foundation supports programs designed to enhance the quality of health care, and address disabilities and chronic diseases. Support is limited to Hartford and Middletown, Connecticut. Grants of up to $35,000 are awarded.
Requirements: 501(c)3 tax-exempt organizations serving the residents of Hartford and Middletown, Connecticut, are eligible.
Restrictions: The Foundation does not support grants or scholarships to individuals; religious organizations in support of their sacramental or theological functions; advertising; political causes and events; multi-year requests; or fund raising activities, including tables, tickets, dinners, walks, sporting events, etc.
Geographic Focus: Connecticut
Amount of Grant: $35,000 maximum
Date(s) Application is Due: Apr 10
Contact: Marilda L. Gandara, President; (860) 273-6382 or (860) 273-0123; fax: (860) 273-4764; email: aetnafoundation@aetna.com
Internet: http://www.aetna.com/foundation/grants_ct/
Sponsor: Aetna Foundation
151 Farmington Avenue
Hartford, CT 06156

Aetna Foundation Quality of Care Grants **245**
Aetna is committed to enhancing the quality of health care for all Americans through its business practices and charitable giving. Aetna will support philanthropic initiatives focused on: disparities in health—programs to improve the quality of health care delivered to racial and ethnic populations; and end-of-life care—programs to enhance care and services for both caregivers and patients at the end of life. Priority consideration will be given to programs that address both areas of interest (i.e., end-of-life care for racially and ethnically diverse populations). The listed application deadline is for proposal abstracts; full proposals are by invitation.
Requirements: Grants will be made only to nonprofit organizations with evidence of IRS 501(c)3 designation or de facto tax-exempt status.
Restrictions: The program does not support grants and scholarships to individuals, fundraising activities, advertising, and political or religious activities.
Amount of Grant: $25,000-$100,000 typically
Contact: Marilda L. Gandara, President; (860) 273-6382 or (860) 273-0123; fax: (860) 273-4764; email: aetnafoundation@aetna.com
Internet: http://www.aetna.com/foundation/grants_qc/index.html
Sponsor: Aetna Foundation
151 Farmington Avenue
Hartford, CT 06156

Aetna Foundation Quality of Care Grants for Depression **246**
With its Quality of Care Grants for Depression, the foundation supports programs designed to provide screening and outreach efforts to enhance early identification, diagnosis, and treatment of depression, with a particular emphasis on children and women; integrate mental health services with general medical and preventive health services; provide public education and awareness programs to enhance understanding and treatment of depression and reduce the stigma associated with mental illness; and provide training and education that enhances the ability of health care professionals to communicate and deliver culturally sensitive mental health care and services. Special emphasis is directed toward programs designed to focus on depression for racially and ethnically diverse populations. Grants range from $50,000 to $300,000. Depression Grant abstracts are due on October 15, with full proposals (by invitation from abstracts) due on February 15 of the following year.
Requirements: 501(c)3 tax-exempt organizations are eligible.
Restrictions: The Foundation does not support grants or scholarships to individuals; religious organizations in support of their sacramental or theological functions; advertising; political causes and events; multi-year requests; or fund raising activities, including tables, tickets, dinners, walks, sporting events, etc.
Amount of Grant: $50,000-$300,000 range
Date(s) Application is Due: Oct 15; Feb 15
Contact: Marilda L. Gandara, President; (860) 273-6382 or (860) 273-0123; fax: (860) 273-4764; email: aetnafoundation@aetna.com
Internet: http://www.aetna.com/foundation/grants_qc/overview.html
Sponsor: Aetna Foundation
151 Farmington Avenue
Hartford, CT 06156

Aetna Foundation Quality of Care Grants for End of Life Care **247**
With its Quality of Care Grants for End of Life Care, the foundation supports programs designed to provide training and education, including cultural competency, for professionals across the health care continuum to enhance communication and care at the end of life; provide support services and resources for caregivers to help them deal more effectively with complex and emotionally charged end of life care issues; and reduce barriers and increase use of palliative and home care services for patients at the end of life. Special emphasis is directed toward programs designed to focus on end of life care for racially and ethnically diverse populations. Grants range from $50,000 to $300,000. End of Life Care Grant abstracts are due on September 15, with full proposals (by invitation from abstracts) due on February 15 of the following year.
Requirements: 501(c)3 tax-exempt organizations are eligible.
Restrictions: The Foundation does not support grants or scholarships to individuals; religious organizations in support of their sacramental or theological functions; advertising; political causes and events; multi-year requests; or fund raising activities, including tables, tickets, dinners, walks, sporting events, etc.
Amount of Grant: $50,000 to $300,000
Date(s) Application is Due: Sep 15; Feb 15
Contact: Marilda L. Gandara, President; (860) 273-6382 or (860) 273-0123; fax: (860) 273-4764; email: aetnafoundation@aetna.com
Internet: http://www.aetna.com/foundation/grants_qc/overview.html
Sponsor: Aetna Foundation
151 Farmington Avenue
Hartford, CT 06156

Aetna Foundation Regional Community Health General Support Grants **248**
The Aetna Foundation is the independent charitable and philanthropic arm of Aetna Inc. Founded in 1972, the Foundation helps build healthy communities by promoting volunteerism, forming partnerships and funding initiatives that improve the quality of life where our employees and customers live and work. The foundation awards Regional Community Health General Support Grants to nonprofit organizations that have discussed possibilities with a local Aetna Representative, received an invitation to apply, and are involved with arts and culture, education, health, human services, and economic development.
Requirements: 501(c)3 tax-exempt organizations in regionally designated communities are eligible (list available online).
Restrictions: Restrictions include: grants to individuals; scholarships; tables or tickets for sporting events; fund-raising activities, e.g., dinners, walks, golf tournaments or similar events; religious organizations in support of their sacramental or theological functions; advertising; multiyear requests; or political causes and events.
Amount of Grant: $25,000-$50,000 average
Date(s) Application is Due: Mar 15; Apr 15; May 15
Contact: Marilda L. Gandara, President; (860) 273-6382 or (860) 273-0123; fax: (860) 273-4764; email: aetnafoundation@aetna.com
Internet: http://www.aetna.com/foundation/grants_reg/overview.html#2
Sponsor: Aetna Foundation
151 Farmington Avenue
Hartford, CT 06156

Aetna Foundation Regional Community Health Grants **249**
The foundation's grants focus on reducing disparities in health care among racial and ethnic populations. Areas of interest include cultural competency—training and education for health care professionals, including culturally appropriate end-of-life care training; disease prevention, awareness, and delivery of culturally sensitive care and services related to children's oral health—community-based screening, treatment, and/or family education initiatives regarding the importance of dental care; diabetes—initiatives targeting individuals and families with prevention and healthy behavior modification messages to help combat the growing incidence of type 2 diabetes in children and adults; and depression—screening, education, and outreach efforts to enhance early identification, diagnosis, and treatment of depression in youth and adults. Applicants may submit only one application per regional program. Guidelines are available online.
Requirements: 501(c)3 tax-exempt organizations in regionally designated communities are eligible (list available online).
Restrictions: Restrictions include: grants to individuals; scholarships; tables or tickets for sporting events; fund-raising activities, e.g., dinners, walks, golf tournaments or similar events; religious organizations in support of their sacramental or theological functions; advertising; multiyear requests; or political causes and events.

Amount of Grant: $25,000-$50,000
Date(s) Application is Due: Mar 31
Contact: Marilda L. Gandara, President; (860) 273-6382 or (860) 273-0123; fax: (860) 273-4764; email: aetnafoundation@aetna.com
Internet: http://www.aetna.com/foundation/grants_reg/
Sponsor: Aetna Foundation
151 Farmington Avenue
Hartford, CT 06156

Aetna Foundation Regional Community Health Outreach Grants 250
Awards will be granted to nonprofit organizations to support grassroots efforts that increase awareness of critical health initiatives through health walks, health fairs and health education outreach. Grants of up to $25,000 will be considered. Applicants should provide all levels of event sponsorships on the application. Funding decisions and notifications will be made throughout the year while all notifications will be made by November 1.
Requirements: 501(c)3 tax-exempt organizations in regionally designated communities are eligible (list available online).
Restrictions: Restrictions include: grants to individuals; scholarships; tables or tickets for sporting events; fund-raising activities, e.g., dinners, walks, golf tournaments or similar events; religious organizations in support of their sacramental or theological functions; advertising; multiyear requests; or political causes and events.
Amount of Grant: $25,000 maximum
Contact: Marilda L. Gandara, President; (860) 273-6382 or (860) 273-0123; fax: (860) 273-4764; email: aetnafoundation@aetna.com
Internet: http://www.aetna.com/foundation/grants_reg/overview.html#2
Sponsor: Aetna Foundation
151 Farmington Avenue
Hartford, CT 06156

Aetna Foundation Sponsorships Grants in Connecticut 251
The Aetna Foundation is the independent charitable and philanthropic arm of Aetna Inc. Founded in 1972, the Foundation helps build healthy communities by promoting volunteerism, forming partnerships and funding initiatives that improve the quality of life where our employees and customers live and work. With its Sponsorships Grants in Connecticut, the foundation awards grants to nonprofit organizations to sponsor fundraising and other events, including walks, dinners, health fairs, or similar events, with an emphasis on health-related issues. Support is limited to Hartford and Middletown, Connecticut. Grants of up to $10,000 are awarded on a quarterly basis.
Requirements: 501(c)3 tax-exempt organizations serving the residents of Hartford and Middletown, Connecticut, are eligible.
Restrictions: The Foundation does not support grants or scholarships to individuals; religious organizations in support of their sacramental or theological functions; advertising; political causes and events; multi-year requests; or fund raising activities, including tables, tickets, dinners, walks, sporting events, etc.
Geographic Focus: Connecticut
Amount of Grant: $10,000 maximum
Date(s) Application is Due: Feb 27; Jul 24; Oct 30
Contact: Marilda L. Gandara, President; (860) 273-6382 or (860) 273-0123; fax: (860) 273-4764; email: aetnafoundation@aetna.com
Internet: http://www.aetna.com/foundation/grants_ct/
Sponsor: Aetna Foundation
151 Farmington Avenue
Hartford, CT 06156

Aetna Foundation Voice Of Conscience Award 252
The program was created in memory of Arthur Ashe Jr., tennis great, citizen of the world, member of Aetna's board of directors for more than 10 years, and chairman of the Aetna Foundation at the time of his death. The award is made to a citizen/leader who emulates the selfless commitment to education, civil rights, health and human services that Arthur had. The award winner will receive a grant to the nonprofit(s) organizations of his/her choice. Characteristics of the award recipient include: advancing human rights, opportunity, and dignity; commitment to serve other, regardless of personal benefit; devotion to achieving humanitarian ideals; accomplishments in civil rights, education, health care, and social equity; willingness to take risks for challenging causes; and breaking boundaries across race, culture, class, faith, and ethnicity. Guidelines and nomination form are available online.
Samples: Marie Alfano, case management nurse consultant, Cranbury, New Jersey (2008).
Amount of Grant: $50,000
Date(s) Application is Due: Jun 15
Contact: Marilda L. Gandara, President; (860) 273-6382 or (860) 273-0123; fax: (860) 273-4764; email: aetnafoundation@aetna.com
Internet: http://www.aetna.com/foundation/award/index.html
Sponsor: Aetna Foundation
151 Farmington Avenue
Hartford, CT 06156

AF Doctoral Dissertation Award for Arthritis Health Professionals 253
The award provides one or two years of salary and/or research support to projects related to arthritis management and/or comprehensive patient care in rheumatology practice, research, or education. A dissertation project is preferred. Suitable studies include, but are not limited to, functional, behavioral, nutritional, occupational, or epidemiological aspects of patient care and management. Drug studies and laboratory in vitro studies are not appropriate. Application and guidelines are available online. Annual deadline dates may vary; contact program staff for exact dates.
Requirements: The awards are designed for predoctoral students entering the research phase of their programs. The doctoral chairperson must approve the project. A candidate must have membership or eligibility for membership in his/her professional organization. Applicants must be U.S. citizens or have permanent residence.
Restrictions: The award does not support laboratory research.
Amount of Grant: $30,000 per year
Date(s) Application is Due: Sep 1
Contact: Research Department, (404) 965-7537
Internet: http://www.arthritis.org/research/ProposalCentral.asp
Sponsor: Arthritis Foundation
1330 W Peachtree Street, Suite 100
Atlanta, GA 30309

AFAR CART Fund Grants 254
The goal of the CART Fund is to encourage exploratory and developmental AD research projects within the United States by providing support for the early and conceptual plans of those projects that may not yet be supported by extensive preliminary data but have the potential to substantially advance biomedical research. This proposal should be distinct from those projects designed to increase knowledge in a well established area unless it is intended to extend previous discoveries toward new directions or applications. Applications may encompass a project period of up to two years with a combined budget for direct cost up to $250,000. No indirect costs are allowed. Domestic public and private institutions are eligible, such as universities, colleges, hospitals and laboratories. This is for NEW projects only. Up to two $250,000 awards will be available this year. Dr. John Trojanowski will chair a scientific review group that will triage the Letters-of-Intent and select a maximum of fifteen deemed to have the highest merit. Those selected will be invited to submit a subsequent standard grant application from which the final recommendation will be made by the review group. The final selection will be made by the CART Fund selection committee. Notifications of the finalists (maximum of 15) will be mailed by January 7th. Investigators whose proposals are accepted for further consideration will be sent a full application form which must be completed and returned by February 16th.
Requirements: The CART Fund is inviting interested applicants from within the United States to submit a Letter-of-Intent that includes sufficient detail to communicate the importance of your study as well as information on its feasibility. Submit email questions and Letters-of-Intent to Dr. James B. Puryear, Chairman, CART Grants Program: jimpuryear@comcast.net.
Restrictions: Applications will be deemed ineligible from for-profit organizations as well as those already supported by regular or program grants.
Amount of Grant: $250,000
Date(s) Application is Due: Feb 16
Contact: Grants Manager; (212) 703-9977 or (888) 582-2327; fax: (212) 997-0330; email: grants@afar.org or info@afar.org
Internet: http://www.afar.org/CART.html
Sponsor: American Federation for Aging Research
55 West 39th Street, 16th Floor
New York, NY 10018

AFAR Medical Student Training in Aging Research Program 255
The Medical Student Training in Aging Research Program (MSTAR) provides medical students, early in their training, with an enriching experience in aging related research and geriatrics, under the mentorship of top experts in the field. This program introduces students to research and academic experiences that they might not otherwise have during medical school. Students participate in an eight to twelve week structured research, clinical, and didactic program in geriatrics, appropriate to their level of training and interests. Students may train at a National Training Center supported by the National Institute on Aging or, for a limited number of medical schools, at their own institution. Refer to the AFAR website for a complete listing of the participating institutions.
Requirements: Any allopathic or osteopathic medical student in good standing, who will have successfully completed one year of medical school at a U.S. institution by June, may apply. Applicants must be citizens or non-citizen nationals of the United States, or must have been lawfully admitted for permanent residence (i.e., in possession of a currently valid Alien Registration Receipt Card I-551, or some other legal verification of such status.)
Restrictions: Individuals on temporary or student visas and individuals holding PhD, MD, DVM, or equivalent doctoral degrees in the health sciences are not eligible.
Date(s) Application is Due: Feb 6
Contact: Grants Manager; (212) 703-9977 or (888) 582-2327; fax: (212) 997-0330; email: grants@afar.org or info@afar.org
Internet: http://www.afar.org/medstu.html
Sponsor: American Federation for Aging Research
55 West 39th Street, 16th Floor
New York, NY 10018

AFAR Paul Beeson Career Development Awards in Aging Research for the Island of Ireland 256
The Paul Beeson Career Development Awards In Aging Research Program offers faculty development awards to outstanding junior physician faculty committed to academic careers in aging-related research, teaching, and practice. The goals of the program are: to encourage and assist the development of future leaders in the field of aging by supporting

faculty members early in their careers to gain additional research training as needed and to establish independent programs in aging research; to deepen the commitment of research institutions to academic research in aging and to translating research outcomes to geriatric medicine by involving mentor and recipient in establishing and advancing the recipient's career in aging research; to expand medical research on aging broadly defined as including the biology of aging, maintenance of health and independence in old age, diseases and disabilities of old age and issues in their clinical management, and systems of care for the elderly. To maximize the educational/training opportunities of this fellowship program, Beeson Ireland Scholars are encouraged to spend three to six months abroad with a research team in the U.S. in the second or the third year of the award. The goals of this rotation are varied and can be for purposes of training in techniques, data collection, data analysis, etc. to enhance the Scholars' transition to independence. This is unique to the Beeson Ireland Program. To date, the program has provided awards to 149 very promising junior faculty at institutions in the United States as well as 3 junior faculty on the Island of Ireland. The program was established in 1994 by The Atlantic Philanthropies, The John A. Hartford Foundation, The Commonwealth Fund and The Starr Foundation, and administered by the American Federation for Aging Research (AFAR.) In 2004, The Atlantic Philanthropies, The John A. Hartford Foundation, The Starr Foundation and AFAR entered a partnership with The National Institute on Aging (NIA.) Until 2006, the program soley funded Scholars at U.S.-based institutions but beginning in 2007, with support from The Atlantic Philanthropies, Scholars are also funded in Ireland (The Republic of Ireland and Northern Ireland.) The scholar will receive a grant for three years. The salary will be at specialty registrar/clinical lecturer level to protect a minimum of 75% of the scholar's time for research, with the remainder available annually for research support, including an institutional overhead on the research support component.
Requirements: Nominations for the Paul Beeson Career Development Awards In Aging Research Program are to be made by the deans of medical schools (or equivalent) in Ireland (the Republic of Ireland and Northern Ireland.) Institutions may submit as many applications as they wish. To be eligible for nomination, a candidate must: be a U.S. physician or an Irish citizen physician of the Republic of Ireland, a United Kingdom citizen of Northern Ireland, an EU citizen living and working in the Island of Ireland or a non-EU citizen resident in the island of Ireland with a valid work permit; commit at least 75% of his/her full-time professional effort to the goals of this award; be a medical graduate who has recently completed or is about to complete a doctoral degree (PhD/MD) and be undertaking or have recently completed higher clinical training; have at least one research publication in a high-impact journal. If the candidate is not the first author, he/she must provide a short description of his/her contribution to the research and the writing of the paper; this should be substantial. For each scholar, a senior faculty member at the scholar's institution must be selected to serve as a mentor to help guide the scholar's research and career planning and provide access to organizations, programs, and colleagues helpful to the scholar's efforts. More than one mentor may be selected. Letters of endorsement including specific information on institutional support for the scholar should be provided by the dean, the relevant department chairperson (or equivalent - may be one person), and the mentor. In addition, three letters of reference should be provided by other faculty members and/or senior professionals with whom the scholar has worked and who are well acquainted with his/her capabilities, potential, accomplishments, and commitment. All candidates must submit applications endorsed by the Dean of School of Medicine (or equivalent).
Date(s) Application is Due: Jan 22
Contact: Grants Manager; (212) 703-9977 or (888) 582-2327; fax: (212) 997-0330; email: beeson@afar.org
Internet: http://afar.org/BeesonIreland.html
Sponsor: American Federation for Aging Research
55 West 39th Street, 16th Floor
New York, NY 10018

AFAR Research Grants **257**
The major goal of this program is to assist in the development of the careers of junior investigators committed to pursuing careers in the field of aging research. Of particular interest are research projects concerned with understanding the basic mechanisms of aging; projects investigating age-related diseases, especially if approached from the point of view of how basic aging processes may lead to these outcomes; and projects concerning mechanisms underlying common geriatric functional disorders, as long as these include connections to fundamental problems in the biology of aging. Examples of promising areas of research include: aging and immune function; genetic control of longevity; neurobiology and neuropathology of aging; invertebrate or vertebrate animal models; cardiovascular aging; aging and cellular stress resistance; metabolic and endocrine changes; age-related changes in cell proliferation; caloric restriction and aging; DNA repair and control of gene expression; biology of the menopause; and aging and apoptosis. Application and instruction sheet are available online.
Requirements: The applicant must be an independent investigator with assigned independent space and must be within the first four years of a junior faculty appointment (instructor, assistant professor or equivalent) by July 1st.
Restrictions: The program does not provide support for postdoctoral fellows in the laboratory of a senior investigator; investigators who have already received major independent funding for research on aging, such as an R01 grant or a grant of equal to or greater than $100,000 from another private funding source; senior faculty, i.e., at the rank of associate professor level or higher; and projects that deal strictly with clinical problems, such as the diagnosis and treatment of disease, health outcomes, or the social context of aging. Former AFAR grant recipients are not eligible to reapply. Applicants for the Glenn/AFAR Breakthroughs in Gerontology (BIG) program cannot also submit an application for this research grant.
Amount of Grant: $75,000
Date(s) Application is Due: Dec 16
Contact: Grants Manager; (212) 703-9977 or (888) 582-2327; fax: (212) 997-0330; email: grants@afar.org or info@afar.org
Internet: http://afar.org/afar99.html
Sponsor: American Federation for Aging Research
55 West 39th Street, 16th Floor
New York, NY 10018

Affymetrix Corporate Contributions Grants **258**
Affymetrix makes charitable donations to nonprofit organizations through its corporate philanthropy program. The company focuses its giving in three main areas: education—programs that support science and math education, focusing on K-12 students and their teachers; ethics—organizations that help foster an ongoing public dialog about genetic-related ethics; and cancer research and advocacy—nonprofit organizations working in the areas of disease research and advocacy, with a specific emphasis on cancer. Requests are reviewed four times per year. The average grant size is approximately $2500.
Requirements: 501(c)3 nonprofit organizations are eligible.
Restrictions: The corporation does not provide funding for advertising journals or booklets; fundraising events such as telethons, walkathons, and races; specific performances or concerts; sporting events; endowment campaigns; film, video, television, or radio projects; grants to individuals; political causes or candidates; or organizations that practice discrimination or limit membership on the basis of race, creed, gender, age, sexual orientation, or national origin.
Contact: Contributions Manager, email: outreach@affymetrix.com
Internet: http://www.affymetrix.com/corporate/outreach/corporate.affx
Sponsor: Affymetrix
3420 Central Expwy
Santa Clara, CA 95051

AFG Industries Grants **259**
The corporation awards general operating grants to nonprofits in its headquarters area in the categories of arts and humanities, civic and public affairs, education at all levels, health care, and social services. There are no application deadlines. Submit a brief letter of inquiry.
Requirements: Tennessee nonprofits are eligible.
Geographic Focus: Tennessee
Amount of Grant: $100,000-$250,000
Contact: Human Resources, (800) 251-0441or (423) 229-7200; fax: (423) 229-7459
Internet: http://www.afgglass.com
Sponsor: AFG Industries Inc
P.O. Box 929
Kingsport, TN 37662

African American Fund of New Jersey Grants **260**
The fund concentrates on providing significant funding to New Jersey's African American communities to promote and enhance human services delivery and community empowerment. Program areas that will receive primary funding consideration are in the areas of pre-school through high school education initiatives, technology-oriented initiatives, health-related programs, community issues, and building wealth. Programs that emphasize positive family values, traditions, social customs, and family practices that have contributed to the survival of the African American family are encouraged. Types of support include general operating grants, program development grants, and technical assistance. Proposals must demonstrate the intention to commit the necessary financial and human resources to a program that is well coordinated with related human services within the respective communities. All applicants will be notified of approval or disapproval of their proposals. Annual deadline dates may vary; contact program staff for exact dates.
Requirements: New Jersey 501(c)3 nonprofit, tax-exempt agencies, community-based organizations, and schools are eligible.
Geographic Focus: New Jersey
Amount of Grant: $1000-$5000 range
Contact: Sondra Clark, President, (973) 676-5283; fax: (973) 672-5030; email: sclark@aafnj.org
Internet: http://www.aafnj.org/HBW_Grants.htm
Sponsor: African American Fund of New Jersey
132 S Harrison Street
East Orange, NJ 07018

Agnes B. Hunt Trust Grants **261**
The trust awards grants to eligible Georgia nonprofit organizations in the general areas of health, welfare, and education for the poor and needy in its local community. Apply online; complete guidelines are provided.
Requirements: 501(c)3 nonprofit organizations in Griffin and Spalding County, GA, are eligible.
Geographic Focus: Georgia
Amount of Grant: $500-$5000 average
Date(s) Application is Due: Nov 1
Contact: c/o Joseph Walker
Internet: http://www.agnesbhunttrust.org
Sponsor: Agnes B. Hunt Trust
P.O. Box 1610
Griffin, GA 30224-1610

Agnes Gund Foundation Grants 262

The foundation awards general operating grants in its areas of interest, including health organizations, higher education, and performing arts (dance, music). There are no application deadlines or forms. Submit a letter of inquiry.

Requirements: Although there are no restrictions there is a focus on New York City.

Restrictions: Applicants must be a tax-exempt organization.

Geographic Focus: New York

Samples: Museum of Modern Art (New York, NY)—for general operating support, $1 million.; Cleveland Museum of Art (OH)—for general operating support, $200,000.; Virginia Museum of Fine Arts (Richmond, VA)—for general operating support, $100,000.; Creative Capital Foundation (New York, NY)—for general operating support, $75,000.

Amount of Grant: $5000-$100,000 average

Contact: Agnes Gund, (330) 385-3400

Sponsor: Agnes Gund Foundation
517 Broadway, 3rd Floor
East Liverpool, OH 43920

Agnes M. Lindsay Trust Grants 263

The trust makes grants to nonprofit organizations in the New England states to improve the quality of life. Areas of interest include higher education, students from rural areas, health and welfare agencies, health projects, special needs groups (e.g., blind, deaf, learning disabled, and elderly), children's hospitals and homes, youth and family organizations, and summer camps. Types of support include capital campaigns and items, renovation, equipment acquisition, and seed grants. Proposals should contain a brochure of purposes and programs, recent financial figures and statement of income and expenses for the last two years, copy of current budget, list of capital items with costs, copy of 501(c)3 determination letter, and federal tax identification number. The trustees meet and review proposals on a monthly basis.

Requirements: 501(c)3 Maine, Massachusetts, New Hampshire, and Vermont tax-exempt organizations are eligible.

Restrictions: The trustees rarely, if ever, approve grants for general operating funds. They do not fund grant requests from public entities, municipalities, sectarian organizations, do not fund grant requests from individuals, and do not fund endowments.

Geographic Focus: Maine; Massachusetts; New Hampshire; Vermont

Samples: College of the Atlantic (Bar Harbor, ME)—to provide scholarships for students from rural New England, with an emphasis on Maine, Massachusetts, New Hampshire, and Vermont, $50,000 over five years.; Marlboro College (Marlboro, VT)—for scholarships for students from rural New England, $50,000 over five years.

Amount of Grant: $1000-$15,000 range

Contact: Susan Bouchard, Administrative Director, (603) 669-1366; fax: (603) 665-8114; email: admin@lindsaytrust.org

Internet: http://www.lindsaytrust.org/index.html

Sponsor: Agnes M. Lindsay Trust
660 Chestnut Street
Manchester, NH 03104

AGS Dennis W. Jahnigen Career Development Scholars Awards 264

The awards are designed to address the urgent need to create a structure for developing leaders in geriatrics in academic surgery and such related specialties as anesthesiology, emergency medicine, general surgery, gynecology, ophthalmology, orthopedic surgery, otolaryngology, physical medicine and rehabilitation, thoracic surgery, and urology. Awards are for two years. Nomination may be made online.

Requirements: Nominations may be made by department chairs in any of the specialty areas listed. Departments may submit one application; institutions may submit more than one application. To be eligible, a candidate must be a physician who is a U.S. citizen or permanent resident, and be certified or board eligible to practice in one of the targeted specialty areas; have a primary academic appointment in a U.S. institution in one of the targeted specialty departments; and have completed his/her training (residency and/or fellowship) on or after June 30, 1995. (Exceptions to this limit will be considered for compelling reasons and must be reviewed and approved prior to application submission.)

Amount of Grant: $75,000 per year salary and fringe benefits plus $25,000 per year research costs

Date(s) Application is Due: Dec 6

Contact: Amy Tam-Liao, (212) 308-1414; fax: (212) 832-8646; email: atamliao@americangeriatrics.org

Internet: http://www.americangeriatrics.org/hartford/jahnigen.shtml

Sponsor: American Geriatrics Society
350 Fifth Avenue, Suite 801
New York, NY 10118

Agway Foundation Grants 265

The primary goal of the foundation is to support organizations dedicated to serving the interests of farmers and rural communities in the Northeast, including health care, children and youth services, rural youth organizations, and agriculture. The foundation also supports organizations that contribute to the quality of life in the Agway headquarters area and it actively promotes employee volunteer involvement in community service.

Requirements: 501(c)3 nonprofit organizations are eligible for grant support.

Restrictions: The foundation funds are not used for individuals; political, religious, or labor organizations; scholarships; matching gift programs or capital campaigns of educational institutions; memberships in professional societies or trade associations; or the general operating funds of health care facilities.

Geographic Focus: Northeast

Amount of Grant: $1000 to $10,000

Contact: Stephen Hoefer, Chairman, (315) 449-6474; email: info@agway.com or chairman@agway.com

Internet: http://www.colebrook-nh.com/Public_Documents/ColebrookNH_BBoard/I008D1C75

Sponsor: Agway Foundation
P.O. Box 4933
Syracuse, NY 13221

AHAF Alzheimer's Disease Research Grants 266

AHAF funds outstanding scientists and physicians in neurobiology, physiology, pathology, molecular and developmental biology, chemistry, pharmacology, epidemiology, and surgery who are conducting research to better understand and/or treat Alzheimer's disease. Junior or senior investigators will be considered. Grants are awarded for up to two years and are renewable. Grant applications are reviewed by a scientific review committee on a competitive peer-review system.

Requirements: Grants are awarded to universities, medical centers, and independent research institutions. AHAF funds grants for research at nonprofit organizations only. The principal investigator must hold the academic rank of assistant professor (or equivalent) or higher.

Restrictions: Funding is not provided for overhead, construction, or building expenses.

Amount of Grant: $300,000 maximum per year

Date(s) Application is Due: Oct 19

Contact: Kara Hurst, Grants Coordinator; (800) 437-2423 or (301) 948-3244; fax: (301) 258-9454; email: khurst@ahaf.org

Internet: http://www.ahaf.org/alzdis/research/grants.htm

Sponsor: American Health Assistance Foundation
22512 Gateway Center Drive
Clarksburg, MD 20871

AHAF Macular Degeneration Research Grants 267

The foundation awards research grants to advance study of macular degeneration. Applications are evaluated based on the scientific merit of the proposal, the feasibility of the proposed research, the potential of the research to lead to better understanding and treatment of eye diseases, and the demonstrated ability of the investigator to complete the research. Application materials are available on the Web site.

Amount of Grant: $50,000 maximum per year

Date(s) Application is Due: July 10; Oct 29

Contact: Kara Hurst, Grants Coordinator; (800) 437-2423 or (301) 948-3244; fax: (301) 258-9454; email: khurst@ahaf.org

Internet: http://www.ahaf.org/macular/research/grants.htm

Sponsor: American Health Assistance Foundation
22512 Gateway Center Drive
Clarksburg, MD 20871

AHAF National Glaucoma Research Grants 268

AHAF funds outstanding scientists and physicians with expertise in cell and molecular biology, physiology, biochemistry, endocrinology, and pharmacology. Grants are awarded on the basis of scientific merit of the proposal, the relevance of the research, and the potential impact of the proposed study on better understanding and/or treatment of glaucoma. Applications are reviewed by a scientific review committee on a competitive peer-review system. AHAF is interested in receiving focused research grant applications from investigators at all stages of their careers. AHAF is particularly interested in new investigators with little or no previous grant support and established investigators with new ideas or directions for their research.

Requirements: AHAF grants are awarded to universities, medical centers, and independent research institutions. AHAF provides grants for research at nonprofit organizations only.

Restrictions: Grants are not made to individuals. Funding is not provided for overhead costs, construction, or building expenses.

Samples: Teri Belecky-Adams, Ph.D., Trustees of Indiana University, Indianapolis, IN, $100,000.; David Calkins, Ph.D., Vanderbilt University Medical Center, Nashville, TN, $100,000.; Mortimer Civan, M.D., University of Pennsylvania, Philadelphia, PA, $100,000.

Amount of Grant: $100,000 maximum

Date(s) Application is Due: Oct 27

Contact: Kara Hurst, Grants Coordinator; (800) 437-2423 or (301) 948-3244; fax: (301) 258-9454; email: khurst@ahaf.org

Internet: http://www.ahaf.org/glaucoma/research/glresrch.htm

Sponsor: American Health Assistance Foundation
22512 Gateway Center Drive
Clarksburg, MD 20871

AHFMR Clinical Fellowships 269

The program is designed for highly qualified individuals who hold an M.D. or D.D.S. degree, and who anticipate undertaking a career in health related or clinical research in Alberta. The awards consist of a stipend and a research allowance. A Clinical Fellowship award is normally tenable for a maximum of 3 years. However, if the trainee is registered in a graduate program, the term may be extended.

Requirements: Normally, an award will be held within the Province of Alberta; however, candidates who are Canadian citizens or permanent residents with records of outstanding performance in postgraduate training may seek research training elsewhere, if sponsored

by an Alberta faculty with an expressed interest in future recruitment of the candidate. Candidates must hold an MD or DDS degree and have received a significant portion of their postgraduate training in Alberta.
Amount of Grant: $20,000-$50,000
Date(s) Application is Due: Mar 1; Oct 1
Contact: Pamela Valentine, Director of Grants and Awards; (780) 423-5727; fax: (780) 429-3509; email: pamela.valentine@ahfmr.ab.ca
Internet: http://www.ahfmr.ab.ca/grants/Clin-fellow.php
Sponsor: Alberta Heritage Foundation for Medical Research
10104-103 Avenue, Suite 1500
Edmonton, Alberta T5J 4A7 Canada

AHFMR Clinical Investigator Awards 270
The Award allows highly qualified clinicians in the early stages of their careers in health research to commit the majority of their time (greater than 75%) to research. This award includes a $110,000 annual contribution toward salary and benefits, a $10,000 annual research prize, a $35,000 annual research allowance, and additional funds for renovations, operations, relocation, and equipment. In all cases, the relevance of the applicant's proposed research to human health should be apparent. All applicants must name a mentor or group of mentors who will foster their early career development.
Requirements: Canadian citizens or permanent residents of Canada who hold an MD or DDS degree, have completed all requirements for clinical specialty recognition, and qualify to hold a full-time position in a clinical department of the sponsoring institution are eligible to apply.
Amount of Grant: $155,000
Date(s) Application is Due: Sep 15
Contact: Pamela Valentine, Director of Grants and Awards; (780) 423-5727; fax: (780) 429-3509; email: pamela.valentine@ahfmr.ab.ca
Internet: http://www.ahfmr.ab.ca/grants/ClinInvest.php
Sponsor: Alberta Heritage Foundation for Medical Research
10104-103 Avenue, Suite 1500
Edmonton, Alberta T5J 4A7 Canada

AHFMR Community Support Grants 271
Community support program grants will provide two types of awards: Community Health Research Visiting Lecturer Awards and Community Health Research Travel Grants. The former (Community Health Research Visiting Lecturer Awards) are intended to assist Alberta's non-profit organizations in attracting outstanding health researchers to the province. The latter (Community Health Research Travel Grants) facilitate contact among health researchers in Alberta, as well as with national and international colleagues. Candidates from a wide variety of disciplines may apply as long as the purpose of the travel is to promote community health research.
Requirements: The Community Health Research Visiting Lecturer Awards program is open to community organizations that are directly involved in health research. The Universities of Alberta, Calgary and Lethbridge are not eligible to apply to this program but must submit requests to the AHFMR Visiting Lecturer Program. The Community Health Research Travel Grants program is open to independent investigators actively engaged in health research in a non-profit organization in Alberta are eligible to apply.
Restrictions: University faculty are not eligible to apply for these awards.
Date(s) Application is Due: Jan 9; Apr 14; Jul 10; Oct 9
Contact: Pamela Valentine, Director of Grants and Awards; (780) 423-5727; fax: (780) 429-3509; email: pamela.valentine@ahfmr.ab.ca
Internet: http://www.ahfmr.ab.ca/grants/commsupp.php
Sponsor: Alberta Heritage Foundation for Medical Research
10104-103 Avenue, Suite 1500
Edmonton, Alberta T5J 4A7 Canada

AHFMR Dr. Lionel E. McLeod Health Research Scholarship 272
The award enables academically superior graduate students to undertake full-time training in medical or health research. The Scholarship is tenable through the Faculty of Medicine in any area related to health including: medicine; health services research; social and behavioral sciences (sociology, anthropology, psychology, economics, or political science); quantitative and population sciences (epidemiology and biostatistics, operations research, decision sciences, or computer sciences); and the humanities (philosophy, history, or theology).
Requirements: Candidates must be students at the University of Alberta, the University of Calgary, or the University of British Columbia and sponsored by the Faculty of Medicine.
Amount of Grant: $21,500
Contact: Pamela Valentine, Director of Grants and Awards; (780) 423-5727; fax: (780) 429-3509; email: pamela.valentine@ahfmr.ab.ca
Internet: http://www.ahfmr.ab.ca/grants/mcleod.php
Sponsor: Alberta Heritage Foundation for Medical Research
10104-103 Avenue, Suite 1500
Edmonton, Alberta T5J 4A7 Canada

AHFMR Establishment and Independent Establishment Grants 273
The two types of grants available include: Establishment Grants—AHFMR provides funds to assist reseachers (newly recruited to Alberta) in the start-up of their laboratories and/or research projects; and Independent Establishment Grants—open to new Alberta Investigators who are not candidates for Heritage personnel awards (it is understood that these investigators will commit much of their time to medical or health research). Those sponsoring investigators for these awards must notify the Foundation of their intent to do so at least four months in advance of the application deadline, and request a determination of the eligibility of the candidate. The Foundation will not accept applications for which advanced notice has not been received. There are two categories of grant funding: Operating Funds and Major Equipment Funds.
Requirements: Eligibility to apply for these grants is restricted to applicants recruited to leadership positions (such as Department Head or Director of a centre, institute or division), where the recruitment is expected to stimulate the development of research in a field or discipline of interest to the Foundation.
Date(s) Application is Due: Sep 15
Contact: Pamela Valentine, Director of Grants and Awards; (780) 423-5727; fax: (780) 429-3509; email: pamela.valentine@ahfmr.ab.ca
Internet: http://www.ahfmr.ab.ca/grants/EstabIndep.php
Sponsor: Alberta Heritage Foundation for Medical Research
10104-103 Avenue, Suite 1500
Edmonton, Alberta T5J 4A7 Canada

AHFMR Fast-Track Studentships and Fellowships 274
AHFMR will accept, at any time, applications from Alberta-based institutions for full-time Studentship or Fellowship awards for outstanding candidates currently training outside of Alberta. The fast-track program is intended to assist these institutions in recruiting highly qualified trainees to the province. Up to a maximum of 10 awards per calendar year will be awarded through the fast-track review process in each category. Applications to the program will be reviewed on a first come-first serve basis.
Requirements: Applications must include a letter from the Dean/designate of the faculty indicating that the proposal for a fast-track award has been reviewed and stating why a fast-track application should be considered for the candidate in question. Please refer to the sections on Full-Time Fellowships or Full-Time Studentships for further details regarding eligibility for training awards.
Amount of Grant: $20,000-$23,000 for studentships; $35,000-$50,000 for fellowships
Contact: Pamela Valentine, Director of Grants and Awards; (780) 423-5727; fax: (780) 429-3509; email: pamela.valentine@ahfmr.ab.ca
Internet: http://www.ahfmr.ab.ca/grants/fasttrack.php
Sponsor: Alberta Heritage Foundation for Medical Research
10104-103 Avenue, Suite 1500
Edmonton, Alberta T5J 4A7 Canada

AHFMR Forefront Internship Program Grants 275
The Internship Program addresses the need for highly trained staff and management of the Alberta-based health, medical products and biotechnology industries. This Program is intended to support technology commercialization training and experience for individuals with an appropriate background in science and/or business. Although the work plan should identify the specific area of focus, the intern should receive a broad exposure to all of the following areas: product development; intellectual property strategy; regulatory requirements; market research and strategy; and business planning and development. Interns are awarded a $5,000 training allowance, which may be used for expenses related to educational workshops/seminars/courses necessary for relevant commercialization training, plus a $45,000 to $50,000 stipend.
Requirements: The applicant must hold, or be in the final year of a degree in business, management, or science. The applicants should have some relevant experience in the business or private sector. Applicants must be sponsored by an Alberta organization actively engaged in the commercialization of medical or health related technology. The organization must have the experience and resources to provide an appropriate training environment, and designate one person within the organization who will be the primary supervisor for the intern. The organization must agree to provide direct and continuous supervision.
Amount of Grant: $45,000-$50,000 per year
Date(s) Application is Due: Feb 15
Contact: Carla Weyland, ForeFront Officer; (780) 423-5727; fax: (780) 429-3509; email: carla.weyland@ahfmr.ab.ca
Internet: http://www.ahfmr.ab.ca/forefront/internship.php
Sponsor: Alberta Heritage Foundation for Medical Research
10104-103 Avenue, Suite 1500
Edmonton, Alberta T5J 4A7 Canada

AHFMR Full-Time Fellowships 276
The program is designed to enable highly qualified doctoral graduates to prepare for careers in medical or health research as independent investigators. A fellowship award will provide to the host institution funding for one year's stipend, its associated benefits, and a research allowance. Fellows may engage in teaching activities related to their research discipline a maximum of 20 percent of their time.
Requirements: Candidates must have a Ph.D., M.D., D.D.S., D.V.M. or D.Pharm. degree. Normally, support will not be provided beyond 6 years after receipt of the Ph.D. degree, or beyond 8 years after receipt of the M.D., D.D.S., D.V.M. or D.Pharm. degrees.
Amount of Grant: $35,000-$50,000
Date(s) Application is Due: Mar 1; Oct 1
Contact: Pamela Valentine, Director of Grants and Awards; (780) 423-5727; fax: (780) 429-3509; email: pamela.valentine@ahfmr.ab.ca
Internet: http://www.ahfmr.ab.ca/grants/FT-fellow.php
Sponsor: Alberta Heritage Foundation for Medical Research
10104-103 Avenue, Suite 1500
Edmonton, Alberta T5J 4A7 Canada

AHFMR Full-Time M.D./Ph.D. Studentships 277

Full-Time M.D./Ph.D. Studentships are intended to provide an opportunity for exceptional candidates, who wish to pursue careers as Clinical Investigators, to study for the M.D. and the Ph.D. degrees simultaneously. AHFMR support is complementary to the formal M.D./Ph.D. programs at the University of Alberta and the University of Calgary. M.D./Ph.D. studentship awards are tenable only at an Alberta-based university.

Requirements: Applicants are limited to those students that formally enter the MD/PhD program not later than the start of their second year of PhD studies at either the University of Alberta or the University of Calgary. AHFMR's offer of support is contingent on the granting of complementary stipend support from the Faculty of not less than 15% of the value of the AHFMR award, for the duration of the award. Furthermore, it is expected that the universities will undertake to provide administrative support to the offices of the coordinators of the M.D./Ph.D. programs.

Amount of Grant: $20,000

Date(s) Application is Due: Mar 1; Oct 1

Contact: Pamela Valentine, Director of Grants and Awards; (780) 423-5727; fax: (780) 429-3509; email: pamela.valentine@ahfmr.ab.ca

Internet: http://www.ahfmr.ab.ca/grants/FT-student.php#MPS

Sponsor: Alberta Heritage Foundation for Medical Research
10104-103 Avenue, Suite 1500
Edmonton, Alberta T5J 4A7 Canada

AHFMR Full-Time Studentships 278

AHFMR Full-time Studentships enable academically superior students to undertake full-time research training in the basic biomedical sciences or in clinical research. The award consists of a stipend and a research allowance. Approved uses of the research allowance include: the purchase of scientific materials, supplies and expendables; the purchase of minor equipment; computer software programs; costs for the use of libraries, or computers; costs associated with the publication of research results; travel expenses to attend scientific meetings; and purchase of books, periodicals and journals.

Requirements: Candidates must have been accepted into, or be currently engaged in, a full-time, thesis-based, graduate program at an Alberta-based university in a health-related discipline leading to a Master's or doctoral degree.

Restrictions: This award is not available to students registered in a course-based program. Normally, support will not be provided beyond 6 years of enrollment in graduate school. Candidates who have interrupted their training for parenting or other reasons and who have consequently exceeded this time limit, may apply for studentship support. In such cases, however, the candidate is advised to clearly explain the nature of his/her particular circumstances at the time of application.

Amount of Grant: $20,000 plus research allowance

Date(s) Application is Due: Mar 1; Oct 1

Contact: Pamela Valentine, Director of Grants and Awards; (780) 423-5727; fax: (780) 429-3509; email: pamela.valentine@ahfmr.ab.ca

Internet: http://www.ahfmr.ab.ca/grants/FT-student.php

Sponsor: Alberta Heritage Foundation for Medical Research
10104-103 Avenue, Suite 1500
Edmonton, Alberta T5J 4A7 Canada

AHFMR Health Research Career Renewal Awards 279

Research Career Renewal Awards allow qualified Alberta-based faculty members to obtain rigorous training in any of the following disciplines: epidemiology; biostatistics; psychosocial sciences; and clinical experimental method and design. Training must be undertaken in a center that is renowned for the quality of research and training in the particular area of study. The Career Renewal award will provide a contribution to stipend and/or a research allowance (which can be applied toward offsetting tuition costs, for example).

Requirements: An Alberta-based institution must propose and sponsor the candidate (who must be a full-time faculty member) in addition to committing to provide an adequate research environment upon the trainee's return.

Date(s) Application is Due: Mar 1; Oct 1

Contact: Pamela Valentine, Director of Grants and Awards; (780) 423-5727; fax: (780) 429-3509; email: pamela.valentine@ahfmr.ab.ca

Internet: http://www.ahfmr.ab.ca/grants/CareerAward.php

Sponsor: Alberta Heritage Foundation for Medical Research
10104-103 Avenue, Suite 1500
Edmonton, Alberta T5J 4A7 Canada

AHFMR Health Research Full-Time Studentships 280

The Full-Time Health Research Studentship program enables academically superior students to undertake full-time training in health research. The award supports training in: research on the organization and delivery of health care; technology assessment; community health; health promotion; disease prevention; and related disciplines. The Health Research Studentship consists of a stipend and a research allowance.

Requirements: Candidates must have been accepted into, or be currently studying in, a full-time, thesis-based, graduate program at an Alberta-based university in a health-related discipline leading to a Master's or doctoral degree. This award is not available to students registered in a course-based program. Normally, support will not be provided beyond 6 years of enrollment in graduate school. Candidates who have interrupted their training for parenting or other reasons and who have consequently exceeded this time limit, may apply for studentship support. In such cases, however, the candidate is advised to clearly explain the nature of his/her particular circumstances.

Amount of Grant: $20,000 plus research allowance

Date(s) Application is Due: Mar 1; Oct 1

Contact: Pamela Valentine, Director of Grants and Awards; (780) 423-5727; fax: (780) 429-3509; email: pamela.valentine@ahfmr.ab.ca

Internet: http://www.ahfmr.ab.ca/grants/FT-student.php#HRS

Sponsor: Alberta Heritage Foundation for Medical Research
10104-103 Avenue, Suite 1500
Edmonton, Alberta T5J 4A7 Canada

AHFMR Health Research Fund Grants 281

The Health Research Fund (HRF), an operating grant program that has been in existence for over ten years, is a collaborative program with the funding originating from Alberta Health and Wellness and with AHFMR doing the program administration. The Fund supports relevant, high quality health research studies in the areas of: health services; population health; health technology assessment. There are no specific deadlines.

Requirements: The HRF competition is aimed at investigative teams which include both researchers and decision-makers or users of health research information working together on issues relating to the appropriate research areas. Proposals that do not include a relevant decision-maker and /or user of health research information as part of the investigative team are not eligible for funding. Applications may be sponsored by either non-profit decision-making organizations (health agencies, associations, service provider organizations, regional or provincial health authorities, Ministry of Health and Wellness) or non-profit research organizations (universities, hospitals, research institutions or centers). The sponsoring organization must be Alberta-based and have been in existence for at least one year.

Restrictions: Funding will not be provided for the following activities/items: projects consisting strictly of basic biomedical or clinical research (such as clinical trials); projects that are limited to program development or evaluation; projects that involve issues not related to human health; projects that duplicate services already provided; staff training, unless such training is required for the proposed project; purchase of furniture, or renting/leasing space and office equipment, (unless such items are not provided for by existing organizations).

Amount of Grant: $50,000 - $75,000 for two years

Contact: Pamela Valentine, Director of Grants and Awards; (780) 423-5727; fax: (780) 429-3509; email: pamela.valentine@ahfmr.ab.ca

Internet: http://www.ahfmr.ab.ca/grants/HRF/hrfguide.php

Sponsor: Alberta Heritage Foundation for Medical Research
10104-103 Avenue, Suite 1500
Edmonton, Alberta T5J 4A7 Canada

AHFMR Heritage Summer Studentships 282

AHFMR Summer Studentships offer motivated students with exceptional academic records an opportunity to participate in medical or health research in Alberta during the summer months. The award is meant to encourage students to consider pursuing formal training and a career in health research. The award is tenable for a minimum of 2 months, and a maximum of 4 months during the period of May to August. The award consists of a $1300 per month stipend only.

Requirements: Those candidates who meet one of the following criteria are eligible to apply: registered in an Alberta-based undergraduate degree program in a medical or health-related field; registered in an undergraduate degree program outside of Alberta, and desiring to engage in research during the summer at an Alberta institution; registered in an M.D. program, and who may also hold an undergraduate or graduate degree; exceptional high school students with records of participation in the health care system, and a clear interest in pursuing a health research career; or currently in the last term of their undergraduate degrees and who have applied either to Medical School or to a graduate program that would start in the coming Fall.

Amount of Grant: $2,600-$5,200 stipend

Date(s) Application is Due: Feb 1

Contact: Christina Van Gelderen; (780) 423-5727; fax: (780) 429-3509; email: christina.van.gelderen@ahfmr.ab.ca

Internet: http://www.ahfmr.ab.ca/grants/Sum-student.php

Sponsor: Alberta Heritage Foundation for Medical Research
10104-103 Avenue, Suite 1500
Edmonton, Alberta T5J 4A7 Canada

AHFMR Infrastructure Funding Grants 283

AHFMR has developed a program to support infrastructure costs associated with the Canada Research Chairs (CRC) program. Infrastructure support for the Chairs comes from the Canada Foundation for Innovation (CFI), which covers 40% of total eligible costs. The remaining costs come from other funding partners. AHFMR has developed a program that will provide a contribution to the 60% of the cost of the CFI-eligible projects that normally comes from the universities and their funding partners.

Requirements: The Program provides support for successful CRC holders who are: faculty members at an Alberta institution, who are ineligible to apply for AHFMR Establishment awards and are principal investigators on active Canadian Institute for Health Research (CIHR) Operating Grants: or are currently recipients of unconditional AHFMR Personnel Awards and are principal investigators on non-AHFMR peer-reviewed operating grants.

Restrictions: Investigators being recruited to the province, and who are eligible to apply for, or have received AHFMR Establishment grants are not eligible for consideration under this program.

Amount of Grant: $62,500 average

Contact: Pamela Valentine, Director of Grants and Awards; (780) 423-5727; fax: (780) 429-3509; email: pamela.valentine@ahfmr.ab.ca

Internet: http://www.ahfmr.ab.ca/grants/crcinfo.php#1
Sponsor: Alberta Heritage Foundation for Medical Research
10104-103 Avenue, Suite 1500
Edmonton, Alberta T5J 4A7 Canada

AHFMR Interdisciplinary Team Grants 284
The Alberta Heritage Foundation for Medical Research (AHFMR) Interdisciplinary Team Grants Program provides opportunities for high-quality, internationally recognized teams of investigators to complete research initiatives with defined health outcomes. Funds available in this competition are to support collaborative, interdisciplinary and multi-institutional teams that address important research questions, health problems or issues in defined areas of research that are aligned with strategic research priorities of the Foundation and Alberta. The Program will provide up to $1 million per year per team for up to five years. Funding can be used for a broad range of research-related costs including research infrastructure, research operating costs, core administrative/management costs, scientific support for the team (including the costs for recruitment of new investigators to the team), collaborative/linkage activity and knowledge exchange/translation activity.
Requirements: Each eligible AHFMR Interdisciplinary Team Grant application will include: A Team Leader—the Team Leader must be an established researcher with proven leadership skills and experience who will act as research program director and who will assume administrative responsibility for the grant. It is expected that the Team Leader will devote a significant and appropriate portion of her/his time to these tasks. The Team Leader will have their primary academic appointment at an Alberta-based university; at least two additional independent investigators with established research track records. Teams with a nucleus of experienced investigators are encouraged to include promising new investigators as part of their group; team members who collectively have an extensive record of success, are creative and original in their approach to research and its translation, and who have experience working in research teams. The specific contribution of each team member and end-user partner, where applicable, must be described; representation from more than one research discipline and from more than one "research pillar" (i.e. biomedical; clinical science; health systems and services; and the social, cultural and other factors that affect the health of populations.); and representation from more than one Alberta-based university. Multi-institutional collaboration is strongly encouraged in this Program.
Amount of Grant: $1,000,000 maximum
Date(s) Application is Due: Nov 14
Contact: Pamela Valentine, Director of Grants and Awards; (780) 423-5727; fax: (780) 429-3509; email: pamela.valentine@ahfmr.ab.ca
Internet: http://www.ahfmr.ab.ca/grants/team_guidelines.php
Sponsor: Alberta Heritage Foundation for Medical Research
10104-103 Avenue, Suite 1500
Edmonton, Alberta T5J 4A7 Canada

AHFMR Major Equipment Grants 285
AHFMR holds an annual competition to assist Alberta's medical or health researchers in obtaining major scientific equipment (defined as equipment costing more than $10,000 per unit or setup). It is AHFMR's expectation that large requests (e.g. greater than $100,000) will include contribution from other sources. Major equipment funds may be applied toward the purchase of the equipment, as well as toward the following expenses: installation; freight; transportation; duty; sales tax; and GST.
Requirements: An Alberta-based institution must sponsor applications on behalf of full-time, competitively-funded, productive faculty members.
Amount of Grant: $10,000-$100,000 per unit
Date(s) Application is Due: Mar 1
Contact: Pamela Valentine, Director of Grants and Awards; (780) 423-5727; fax: (780) 429-3509; email: pamela.valentine@ahfmr.ab.ca
Internet: http://www.ahfmr.ab.ca/grants/equipment.php
Sponsor: Alberta Heritage Foundation for Medical Research
10104-103 Avenue, Suite 1500
Edmonton, Alberta T5J 4A7 Canada

AHFMR Medical or Health Scholars Investigator Grants 286
Heritage Medical or Health Scholars are investigators who have recently completed their postdoctoral research training, and are currently seeking their first faculty-level appointments, or who are at the Heritage Population Heath Investigator or Heritage Clinical Investigator levels. Candidates must demonstrate an ability to initiate and conduct independent and collaborative research, as well as an interest and ability, or potential ability, to train future investigators. The Scholarship award includes a contribution toward salary and benefits, and may also include a research allowance and funds for renovations, and relocation.
Requirements: Candidates for the Heritage Scholar award must possess a M.D., D.D.S., D.V.M., Ph.D. or equivalent qualification. Furthermore, they must be eligible to hold a full-time appointment with the sponsoring institution.
Amount of Grant: $20,000
Date(s) Application is Due: Sep 15
Contact: Pamela Valentine, Director of Grants and Awards; (780) 423-5727; fax: (780) 429-3509; email: pamela.valentine@ahfmr.ab.ca
Internet: http://www.ahfmr.ab.ca/grants/scholars.php
Sponsor: Alberta Heritage Foundation for Medical Research
10104-103 Avenue, Suite 1500
Edmonton, Alberta T5J 4A7 Canada

AHFMR Medical or Health Scientist Awards 287
The Heritage Medical or Health Scientist Award is the most senior personnel award offered by AHFMR. Heritage Scientists must be established, internationally recognized scientific leaders in their fields of study. Their stature should be apparent by: the quality of their publication records; the originality and vision of their research proposals; the quality and number of their trainees; their ability to attract and retain research grants; and the leadership qualities they exhibit locally, nationally, and internationally. The Scientist award includes a contribution toward salary and benefits, and may also include a research allowance and funds for renovations, and relocation.
Requirements: Candidates for the Heritage Scientist award must possess a M.D., D.D.S., D.V.M., Ph.D. or equivalent qualification. Furthermore, they must be eligible to hold a full-time appointment with the sponsoring institution. AHFMR expects a time commitment of not less than 75% to health research activities. The department chair and the dean will designate the time expected for teaching, clinical duties, examining, and other activities.
Amount of Grant: $10,000-$40,000
Date(s) Application is Due: Sep 15
Contact: Pamela Valentine, Director of Grants and Awards; (780) 423-5727; fax: (780) 429-3509; email: pamela.valentine@ahfmr.ab.ca
Internet: http://www.ahfmr.ab.ca/grants/scientists.php
Sponsor: Alberta Heritage Foundation for Medical Research
10104-103 Avenue, Suite 1500
Edmonton, Alberta T5J 4A7 Canada

AHFMR Part-Time Fellowships 288
AHFMR Part-Time Fellowships enable highly qualified doctoral graduates to prepare for careers in medical or health research as independent investigators doing part-time research training during the regular academic year while enrolled in a full-time professional degree program in Alberta. Part-time awards will consist of a stipend only and will be pro-rated to the amount of time the candidate is prepared to commit to research. The full-time fellowship rate will be used as the basis for this calculation.
Requirements: Candidates must hold a PhD and must be engaged in a professional degree program (usually the MD program).
Restrictions: Part-time fellowship awards are tenable only at an Alberta-based university.
Amount of Grant: $5,000-$30,000
Date(s) Application is Due: Mar 1; Oct 1
Contact: Pamela Valentine, Director of Grants and Awards; (780) 423-5727; fax: (780) 429-3509; email: pamela.valentine@ahfmr.ab.ca
Internet: http://www.ahfmr.ab.ca/grants/PT-fellow.php
Sponsor: Alberta Heritage Foundation for Medical Research
10104-103 Avenue, Suite 1500
Edmonton, Alberta T5J 4A7 Canada

AHFMR Part-Time Studentships 289
AHFMR Part-Time Studentships enable students enrolled in a full-time professional degree program (usually the M.D. program) in Alberta to engage in part-time research training during the regular academic year. The award consists of a stipend only. Part-time students may elect to engage in full-time research during the summer; these students should contact AHFMR to request that full-time summer trainee status be implemented.
Requirements: Candidates must normally have been accepted into, or be currently engaged in, a full-time graduate program at an Alberta-based university in a health-related discipline leading to a Master's or doctoral degree. It is expected that the amount of time the candidate will commit to research will not be less than the equivalent of 1 day per week, taken either as 1 full day or 2 half days.
Restrictions: The award is tenable at an Alberta-based university only.
Date(s) Application is Due: Mar 1; Oct 1
Contact: Pamela Valentine, Director of Grants and Awards; (780) 423-5727; fax: (780) 429-3509; email: pamela.valentine@ahfmr.ab.ca
Internet: http://www.ahfmr.ab.ca/grants/PT-student.php
Sponsor: Alberta Heritage Foundation for Medical Research
10104-103 Avenue, Suite 1500
Edmonton, Alberta T5J 4A7 Canada

AHFMR Personnel Funding Grants 290
AHFMR has developed a program to support personnel costs associated with the Canada Research Chairs (CRC) program. In general, support will be given to Heritage personnel who receive CRC awards consistent with AHFMR guidelines concerning competitive personnel funding contributions from other agencies. Though it does not duplicate personnel funding, the Foundation has approved stipend incentives to partner with other personnel awards received. Currently the stipend incentive program provides funding to about 50 AHFMR researchers who have been successful in both AHFMR Personnel Award competitions and the personnel award competitions of other agencies.
Requirements: Researchers recruited to Alberta with a CRC award are eligible to apply for AHFMR Personnel Awards. If they are successful, the latter may be used as a contribution to matching the CFI allocation for CRC awards.
Contact: Pamela Valentine, Director of Grants and Awards; (780) 423-5727; fax: (780) 429-3509; email: pamela.valentine@ahfmr.ab.ca
Internet: http://www.ahfmr.ab.ca/grants/crcinfo.php#1
Sponsor: Alberta Heritage Foundation for Medical Research
10104-103 Avenue, Suite 1500
Edmonton, Alberta T5J 4A7 Canada

AHFMR Polaris Awards 291

The Alberta Heritage Foundation for Medical Research (AHFMR) Polaris Award was established as a means to help Alberta universities recruit outstanding mid-career health researchers of exceptional international calibre to the province. Individuals supported via this program will be known as AHFMR Polaris Investigators. The goal of this Award is to accelerate research activity in key areas that are priorities for Albertans. AHFMR will provide up to $1 million per year per award for up to ten years. This funding is to be at least matched by the institution nominating the AHFMR Polaris Investigator. The institutional support can include funding provided from other partners including government, the private sector and non-profit agencies. It generally cannot include funding originating from standard grants and awards programs of research organizations such as CFI, CIHR, and NSERC. The first AHFMR Polaris Award will be made in 2008. It is anticipated that initially up to three awards will be available.
Requirements: AHFMR Polaris Investigators must meet a number of eligibility criteria, including being: mid-career investigators with outstanding records of accomplishments in health research. Investigators active in any one (or more) of the four pillars of health research (basic, clinical, health services research, population health) are eligible for consideration; leaders who have histories of accomplishment in science and research demonstrated via executive positions in scientific societies, editorship of a prestigious journal, and invitations to speak at international conferences (they would be recognized as candidates for, or would have recently received, a major international recognition award); nominated by the University of Alberta, the University of Calgary, or the University of Lethbridge. Nominations may also be considered for individuals to be based within an Alberta Regional or Provincial Health Authority, but it is anticipated that they will have academic appointments at one of the universities as well; currently based outside Alberta and prepared to relocate to Alberta full-time for the duration of the AHFMR Polaris Award; and prepared to commit a majority of their time to research.
Amount of Grant: $1,000,000
Contact: Pamela Valentine, Director of Grants and Awards; (780) 423-5727; fax: (780) 429-3509; email: pamela.valentine@ahfmr.ab.ca
Internet: http://www.ahfmr.ab.ca/grants/polaris.php
Sponsor: Alberta Heritage Foundation for Medical Research
10104-103 Avenue, Suite 1500
Edmonton, Alberta T5J 4A7 Canada

AHFMR Population Health Investigator (PHI) Awards 292

The Award allows independent investigators in the early stages of their careers in health research to commit the majority of their time (greater than 75%) to research. This award includes a $110,000 annual contribution toward salary and benefits, a $10,000 annual research prize, a $15,000 annual research allowance, and additional funds for renovations, operations, relocation, and equipment. Potential areas of research are: quantitative and population sciences (epidemiology and biostatistics, operations research, decision sciences, and computer sciences); health services research; social and behavioural sciences (sociology, anthropology, psychology, economics, and political science); and the humanities (law, philosophy, history, and theology). In all cases, the relevance of the applicant's proposed research to human health should be apparent.
Requirements: Canadian citizens or permanent residents who hold an MD or DDS, have completed all requirements for clinical specialty recognition, and qualify to hold a full-time position in a clinical department of the sponsoring institution are eligible.
Amount of Grant: $135,000
Date(s) Application is Due: Sep 15
Contact: Pamela Valentine, Director of Grants and Awards; (780) 423-5727; fax: (780) 429-3509; email: pamela.valentine@ahfmr.ab.ca
Internet: http://www.ahfmr.ab.ca/grants/PopHealthInvest.php
Sponsor: Alberta Heritage Foundation for Medical Research
10104-103 Avenue, Suite 1500
Edmonton, Alberta T5J 4A7 Canada

AHFMR Proposals for Special Initiatives 293

AHFMR welcomes proposals for innovative initiatives that accelerate the achievement of its overall objectives. Institutions recruiting internationally-recognized researchers to lead new initiatives should consult AHFMR, if current programs are inappropriate. AHFMR will also consider proposals for pilot projects in patient or population-based research. These projects must have the potential to develop information, and the investigators must have the expertise to attract grants from other agencies. The review process and financial support for special initiatives may be shared by AHFMR and other agencies.
Restrictions: Applications that are normally eligible for regular operating grants from other agencies will NOT be considered under this program.
Contact: Pamela Valentine, Director of Grants and Awards; (780) 423-5727; fax: (780) 429-3509; email: pamela.valentine@ahfmr.ab.ca
Internet: http://www.ahfmr.ab.ca/grants/initiatives.php
Sponsor: Alberta Heritage Foundation for Medical Research
10104-103 Avenue, Suite 1500
Edmonton, Alberta T5J 4A7 Canada

AHFMR Research Prize 294

The AHFMR Research Prize is intended to maintain and improve AHFMR Personnel Awards as a potent vehicle for the recruitment and retention of highly qualified, internationally competitive investigators at Alberta institutions. The Prize will be made to every eligible investigator supported by AHFMR through the AHFMR Personnel Support Programs (Population Health Investigator, Clinical Investigator, Scholar, Senior Scholar, Scientist).
Requirements: To be eligible, the investigator must be currently supported by an unconditional AHFMR investigator award. Investigators receiving AHFMR Terminal support or those on Leaves of Absence are not eligible to receive the Research Prize. The Research Prize is not determined by institutional rank and salary scale. It is provided in recognition of the individual investigator's research accomplishments, and of his/her success in obtaining an AHFMR Independent Investigator award. The Research Prize is a personal prize to the recipient.
Restrictions: Successful applicants for an Independent Establishment Grant are not eligible to receive the AHFMR Research Prize.
Amount of Grant: $10,000-$20,000
Contact: Pamela Valentine, Director of Grants and Awards; (780) 423-5727; fax: (780) 429-3509; email: pamela.valentine@ahfmr.ab.ca
Internet: http://www.ahfmr.ab.ca/grants/resprize.php
Sponsor: Alberta Heritage Foundation for Medical Research
10104-103 Avenue, Suite 1500
Edmonton, Alberta T5J 4A7 Canada

AHFMR Scholar Awards 295

The Scholars grant allows independent researchers in the early stages of their careers in health research to commit the majority of their time (greater than 75%) to research. Scholars are defined as investigators who have recently completed their postdoctoral research training, and are currently seeking their first faculty-level appointments, or who are completing their term as AHFMR Population Heath Investigator or Clinical Investigator awards. This award includes a $110,000 annual contribution toward salary and benefits, a $10,000 to $20,000 annual research prize, a $35,000 annual research allowance, and additional funds for renovations, operations, relocation, and equipment. Potential areas of research are: quantitative and population sciences (epidemiology and biostatistics, operations research, decision sciences, and computer sciences); health services research; social and behavioral sciences (sociology, anthropology, psychology, economics, and political science); and the humanities (law, philosophy, history, and theology). In all cases, the relevance of the applicant's proposed research to human health should be apparent. All new awards are for seven years.
Requirements: Candidates must possess a M.D., D.D.S., D.V.M., Ph.D. or equivalent qualification. Furthermore, they must be eligible to hold full-time faculty appointments with the sponsoring institutions.
Amount of Grant: $155,000 minimum per year for seven years
Date(s) Application is Due: Sep 15
Contact: Pamela Valentine, Director of Grants and Awards; (780) 423-5727; fax: (780) 429-3509; email: pamela.valentine@ahfmr.ab.ca
Internet: http://www.ahfmr.ab.ca/grants/scholars.php
Sponsor: Alberta Heritage Foundation for Medical Research
10104-103 Avenue, Suite 1500
Edmonton, Alberta T5J 4A7 Canada

AHFMR Scientist Awards 296

The Scientist award is the most senior investigator award offered by AHFMR. Scientists must be established, internationally recognized scientific leaders in their fields of study. Their stature should be demonstrated through: the quality of their publications; the originality and vision of their research proposals; the quality and number of their trainees; their ability to attract and retain research grants; and the leadership qualities they exhibit locally, nationally, and internationally. This award includes a $160,000 annual contribution toward salary and benefits, a $20,000 annual research prize, a $50,000 annual research allowance, and additional funds for renovations, operations, relocation, and equipment. In all cases, the relevance of the applicant's proposed research to human health should be apparent. All new awards are for seven years.
Requirements: Candidates for the award must possess a M.D., D.D.S., D.V.M., Ph.D. or equivalent qualification. Furthermore, they must be eligible to hold full-time faculty appointments with the sponsoring institutions. At time of implementation, candidates will typically have ten to fifteen years experience as independent investigators and are expected to have attained full professor level faculty appointments.
Amount of Grant: $230,000 minimum
Date(s) Application is Due: Sep 15
Contact: Pamela Valentine, Director of Grants and Awards; (780) 423-5727; fax: (780) 429-3509; email: pamela.valentine@ahfmr.ab.ca
Internet: http://www.ahfmr.ab.ca/grants/scientists.php
Sponsor: Alberta Heritage Foundation for Medical Research
10104-103 Avenue, Suite 1500
Edmonton, Alberta T5J 4A7 Canada

AHFMR Senior Investigator Awards 297

Like the Scientist Award, this is the most senior investigator award offered by AHFMR. Applicants must be established, internationally recognized scientific leaders in their fields of study. Their stature should be demonstrated through: the quality of their publications; the originality and vision of their research proposals; the quality and number of their trainees; their ability to attract and retain research grants; and the leadership qualities they exhibit locally, nationally, and internationally. This award includes a $160,000 annual contribution toward salary and benefits, a $40,000 annual research prize, a $20,000 annual research allowance, and additional funds for renovations, operations, relocation, and equipment. In all cases, the relevance of the applicant's proposed research to human health should be apparent. All new awards are for seven years.
Requirements: Candidates for the award must possess a M.D., D.D.S., D.V.M., Ph.D. or equivalent qualification. Furthermore, they must be eligible to hold full-time faculty appointments with the sponsoring institutions. At time of implementation, candidates

will typically have ten to fifteen years experience as independent investigators and are expected to have attained full professor level faculty appointments.
Amount of Grant: $220,000 minimum
Contact: Pamela Valentine, Director of Grants and Awards; (780) 423-5727; fax: (780) 429-3509; email: pamela.valentine@ahfmr.ab.ca
Internet: http://www.ahfmr.ab.ca/grants/independent-investigator-revised.php
Sponsor: Alberta Heritage Foundation for Medical Research
10104-103 Avenue, Suite 1500
Edmonton, Alberta T5J 4A7 Canada

AHFMR Senior Medical or Health Scholars Investigator Grants **298**
The Heritage Senior Medical or Health Scholars must have an excellent track record of independent research over several years. They are more senior than Heritage Scholars and have usually been previously supported via an external salary support award (e.g. as an AHFMR Scholar, CIHR New Investigator, or equivalent). At the time of application, candidates for a Senior Scholar Award will typically have four to six years as an independent investigator and will be appointed at either the Assistant Professor or Associate Professor level. The Senior Scholarship award includes a contribution toward salary and benefits, and may also include a research allowance and funds for renovations, and relocation.
Requirements: Candidates for the Heritage Senior Scholar award must possess a M.D., D.D.S., D.V.M., Ph.D. or equivalent qualification. Furthermore, they must be eligible to hold a full-time appointment with the sponsoring institution. AHFMR expects a time commitment of not less than 75% to health research activities. The department chair and the dean will designate the time expected for teaching, clinical duties, examining, and other activities.
Amount of Grant: $30,000 maximum
Date(s) Application is Due: Sep 15
Contact: Pamela Valentine, Director of Grants and Awards; (780) 423-5727; fax: (780) 429-3509; email: pamela.valentine@ahfmr.ab.ca
Internet: http://www.ahfmr.ab.ca/grants/seniorscholars.php
Sponsor: Alberta Heritage Foundation for Medical Research
10104-103 Avenue, Suite 1500
Edmonton, Alberta T5J 4A7 Canada

AHFMR Senior Scholar Awards **299**
The Senior Scholars award allows independent researchers in the later stages of their careers in health research to commit the majority of their time (greater than 75%) to research. Applicants are more senior than Scholars and have usually been previously supported via salary support awards (e.g. as an AHFMR Scholar, CIHR New Investigator, or equivalent). At time of implementation, candidates for a Senior Scholar award will typically have five to ten years experience as independent investigators and are expected to have attained an associate professor level faculty appointment. This award includes a $135,000 annual contribution toward salary and benefits, a $20,000 annual research prize, a $50,000 annual research allowance, and additional funds for renovations, operations, relocation, and equipment. In all cases, the relevance of the applicant's proposed research to human health should be apparent. All new awards are for seven years.
Requirements: Candidates must possess a M.D., D.D.S., D.V.M., Ph.D. or equivalent qualification. Furthermore, they must be eligible to hold a full-time faculty appointment with the sponsoring institution.
Amount of Grant: $205,000 minimum
Contact: Pamela Valentine, Director of Grants and Awards; (780) 423-5727; fax: (780) 429-3509; email: pamela.valentine@ahfmr.ab.ca
Internet: http://www.ahfmr.ab.ca/grants/seniorscholars.php
Sponsor: Alberta Heritage Foundation for Medical Research
10104-103 Avenue, Suite 1500
Edmonton, Alberta T5J 4A7 Canada

AHIMA Dissertation Assistance Grants **300**
The Dissertation Assistance Award program supports research undertaken as part of an academic program to qualify for a doctorate in areas relevant to health information management (HIM). Each recipient shall be limited to one funded grant per year. Ordinarily, the scope of the proposal shall be such that it can be completed within 18 months from the date of funding. There are no minimum or maximum grant request expectations, but the range of grants historically has been between $5,000 and $10,000. Submissions that address one or more of the AHIMA research priorities will receive priority consideration for funding.
Requirements: To qualify for an award under this program the student (principal investigator) must be enrolled in an accredited doctoral degree program in an area related to HIM (computer science, business management, education, public health, and so forth) and must be an active, associate, or student member of AHIMA. All requirements for the doctoral degree, other than the dissertation, must be completed by the award date.
Samples: Ellen Jacobs, MEd, RHIA—titled In Search of a Message to Promote the Personal Health Record (2007); Melinda Wilkins, MEd, RHIA—titled Adoption of Electronic Health Records: Perceptions of Health Information Managers (2007); Rebecca Reynolds, MHA, RHIA—titled The Intentions of First Year Medical Students to use Electronic Health Records (2007).
Amount of Grant: $5,000-$10,000
Date(s) Application is Due: Oct 31
Contact: Carol Nielsen; (312) 233-1175; email: carol.nielsen@ahimafoundation.org
Internet: http://www.ahimafoundation.org/Scholarships/dissertation.aspx
Sponsor: Foundation of Research and Education (FORE) of the American Health Information Management Association (AHIMA)
233 N. Michigan Avenue, 21st Floor
Chicago, IL 60601

AHIMA Faculty Development Stipends **301**
FORE Faculty Development Stipends are intended to encourage excellence in effective teaching and leadership in areas related to e-HIM. Program goals are to: expedite curriculum innovation and development in e-HIM content areas; research and develop new methods of teaching, evaluation, and assessment in the HIM learning process; support faculty in maintaining the highest standards of knowledge and practice in e-HIM; integrate new technologies effectively into the HIM learning process; and strengthen the capacity of HIM academic programs to address emerging issues in design and implementation of the electronic health record at all levels of health care delivery, in support of an electronic health information infrastructure.
Requirements: Application should be for activity planned during the four (4) month period following the expected notification date.
Date(s) Application is Due: Mar 14; Jul 11; Oct 3
Contact: Susan H. Fenton, PhD, RHIA, Director of Research; (312) 233-1532 or (312) 233-1100; fax: (210) 479-1043; email: susan.fenton@ahima.org or fore@ahima.org
Internet: http://www.ahimafoundation.org/Scholarships/Faculty.aspx
Sponsor: Foundation of Research and Education (FORE) of the American Health Information Management Association (AHIMA)
233 N. Michigan Avenue, 21st Floor
Chicago, IL 60601

AHIMA Grant-In-Aid Research Grants **302**
The FORE Grant-in-Aid program is directed toward supporting the development of HIM professionals as leaders in defining and validating the unique body of knowledge encompassed by HIM. The results of these studies not only provide information for the HIM professional to apply in meeting current and future challenges, but also support policy initiatives and the redefinition of the roles of HIM practitioners. Ordinarily, the scope of the proposal shall be such that it can be completed within 18 months from the date of funding. There are no minimum or maximum grant request expectations, but the range of grants historically has been between $15,000 and $40,000. Submissions that address one or more of the AHIMA research priorities will receive priority consideration for funding.
Requirements: The primary or secondary investigator must be an active, associate, or student member of AHIMA. Each recipient is limited to one funded grant per year.
Amount of Grant: $15,000-$40,000 average range
Date(s) Application is Due: Sep 19
Contact: Susan H. Fenton, PhD, RHIA, Director of Research; (312) 233-1532 or (312) 233-1100; fax: (210) 479-1043; email: susan.fenton@ahima.org or fore@ahima.org
Internet: http://www.ahima.org/fore/research/grantinaid.asp
Sponsor: Foundation of Research and Education (FORE) of the American Health Information Management Association (AHIMA)
233 N. Michigan Avenue, 21st Floor
Chicago, IL 60601

Ahmanson Foundation Grants **303**
The Foundation reviews grant requests from 501(c)3 organizations that are based in and serving Los Angeles County in the areas of education (elementary and secondary education, higher education, nursing school education, and adult literacy and basic skills), the arts and humanities (including libraries and cultural programs), disadvantaged, domestic violence, health and medicine, human services including youth, and religion (Christian, Episcopal, interdenominational, Jewish, Lutheran, Methodist, Presbyterian, Roman Catholic, and Salvation Army). Types of grant support include capital campaigns, challenge, building/renovations, equipment, endowment funds, matching funds, program development, scholarship funds, and seed money. There are no application forms; the board meets four times annually to consider requests. Full proposals will be invited. Letters of inquiry are to be sent through the postal service following the guidelines listed.
Requirements: 501(c)3 nonprofit organizations that serve or are based in Los Angeles County, California, may apply.
Restrictions: Grants are not awarded to individuals or for continuing support, annual campaigns, professorships or internships, fellowships, or film production.
Geographic Focus: California
Samples: Optimist Youth Homes and Family Services (Los Angeles, CA)—to help construct its new facility that will expand and enhance academic and therapeutic programs for at-risk youngsters, $100,000 (2005); California Lutheran U (Thousand Oaks, CA)—to equip the Exercise Physiology/ Biomechanics Laboratory in the new Gilbert Sports and Fitness Center, $500,000 (2005).
Amount of Grant: $10,000-$50,000 average
Contact: Leonard Walcott Jr., Vice President & Managing Director; (310) 278-0770; email: info@theahmansonfoundation.org
Internet: http://www.theahmansonfoundation.org/fund.html
Sponsor: Ahmanson Foundation
9215 Wilshire Boulevard
Beverly Hills, CA 90210

Ahn Family Foundation Grants **304**
The Ahn Family Foundation, established by Sangwoo and Laura Ahn in 1997, has as its primary purposes to support aging, religion, human and social services, art,

culture, education, and the environment. Giving is primarily limited to Connecticut, Massachusetts, and New York, although the Foundation has also supported projects in Maryland and Washington. There are no particular guidelines or deadlines with which to adhere, and applicants should begin by contacting the Foundation in writing. This letter of inquiry should outline the purpose for the request, the mission of the applicant organization, and the amount requested.
Geographic Focus: Connecticut; Massachusetts; New York
Samples: Holy Apostles Soup Kitchen, New York, New York, $20,000 (2006); Saint Lukes LifeWorks, Stamford, Connecticut, $20,000 (2006); All Saints Church, Chevy Chase, Maryland, $5,000 (2006).
Amount of Grant: $1,000-$20,000 range
Contact: Alison D. Ahn, Treasurer; (203) 869-4875
Sponsor: Ahn Family Foundation
901 Hillsboro Mile
Hillsboro Beach, FL 33062-2801

AHNS Alando J. Ballantyne Resident Research Pilot Grant 305
The purpose of this award is to support basic, translational, or clinical research projects in head and neck oncology. Clinical or translational research studies are strongly encouraged and should be specifically related to the prevention, diagnosis, treatment, outcomes, or pathophysiology of head and neck neoplastic disease. Research supported by this award should be specifically directed toward the pathogenesis, pathophysiology, diagnosis, prevention, or treatment of head and neck neoplastic disease, and may be either basic or clinical/translational in approach. While not specifically required, proposals which aim to introduce new knowledge and methodology from other disciplines to research in head and neck disease, or which demonstrate collaborative effort with members of other related disciplines are encouraged. Grants range up to $10,000 maximum, are for one year, and are not renewable. Letters of intent must be received by December 15, and completed applications must be submitted by January 15.
Requirements: This grant is open to resident in U.S. or Canadian training programs. Previous AHNS or AAO-HNS Foundation research grant recipients are eligible to compete for this grant. However, candidates who have successfully obtained funding from a private or federal funding agency for the same research are ineligible. Candidates who have applied for support of the same research from other funding sources, and who are notified of an award from both another agency and from AHNS must choose only one of the awards.
Amount of Grant: $10,000 maximum
Date(s) Application is Due: Dec 15; Jan 15
Contact: Stephanie L. Jones, Assistant Director; (703) 519-1586 or (703) 836-4444; email: sljones@entnet.org
Internet: http://www.headandneckcancer.org/research/grants.php
Sponsor: American Head and Neck Society (AHNS)
11300 W. Olympic Boulevard, Suite 600
Los Angeles, CA 90064

AHNS Pilot Grant 306
The purpose of this award is to support basic, translational, or clinical research projects in head and neck oncology. Clinical or translational research studies are strongly encouraged and should be specifically related to the prevention, diagnosis, treatment, outcomes, or pathophysiology of head and neck neoplastic disease. Research supported by this award should be specifically directed toward the pathogenesis, pathophysiology, diagnosis, prevention, or treatment of head and neck neoplastic disease, and may be either basic or clinical/translational in approach. While not specifically required, proposals which aim to introduce new knowledge and methodology from other disciplines to research in head and neck disease, or which demonstrate collaborative effort with members of other related disciplines are encouraged. Grants range up to $10,000 maximum, are for one year, and are not renewable. Letters of intent must be received by December 15, and completed applications must be submitted by January 15.
Requirements: Candidates for this award should reside in the U.S. or Canada, be medical students, residents, Ph.D.s or faculty members at the rank of associate professor or below.
Amount of Grant: $10,000 maximum
Date(s) Application is Due: Dec 15; Jan 15
Contact: Stephanie L. Jones, Assistant Director; (703) 519-1586 or (703) 836-4444; email: sljones@entnet.org
Internet: http://www.headandneckcancer.org/research/grants.php
Sponsor: American Head and Neck Society (AHNS)
11300 W. Olympic Boulevard, Suite 600
Los Angeles, CA 90064

AHNS/AAO-HNSF Surgeon Scientist Combined Award 307
The Grant is open to surgeons beginning a clinician-scientist career track to support research in the pathogenesis, pathophysiology, diagnosis, prevention, or treatment of head and neck neoplastic disease. This grant is only available during odd numbered years. Awards are two year, nonrenewable, with a possible $70,000 maximum total costs ($35,000 per year). One award available per year. Letters of intent must be received by December 15, and completed applications must be submitted by January 15.
Requirements: Applicants must be members or candidate members of the American Academy of Otolaryngology-Head and Neck Surgery and/or the American Head and Neck Society.
Amount of Grant: $70,000 maximum total costs ($35,000 per year)
Date(s) Application is Due: Dec 15; Jan 15
Contact: Stephanie L. Jones, Assistant Director; (703) 519-1586 or (703) 836-4444; email: sljones@entnet.org
Internet: http://www.headandneckcancer.org/research/grants.php
Sponsor: American Head and Neck Society (AHNS)
11300 W. Olympic Boulevard, Suite 600
Los Angeles, CA 90064

AHNS/AAO-HNSF Young Investigator Combined Award 308
The purpose of this award is to support a collaborative AHNS/AAO-HNSF research project by fostering the development of contemporary basic or clinical research skills focused on neoplastic disease of the head and neck among new full-time academic surgeons. The award is intended as a preliminary step in clinical investigator career development and is expected to facilitate the recipient's preparation of a more comprehensive individualized research plan suitable for submission to the National Institutes of Health or comparable funding agency. This is a two year, non-renewable award, offering $40,000 maximum ($20,000 per year). One award is available annually. Letters of intent must be received by December 15, and completed applications must be submitted by January 15.
Requirements: Applicants must be physicians with demonstrated potential for excellence in research and teaching and serious commitment to an academic research career in head and neck surgery. Applicants must be members or candidate members of the American Academy of Otolaryngology-Head and Neck Surgery and/or the American Head and Neck Society. Priority will be given to fellows or junior faculty who have completed residencies or fellowships within four years of the application receipt date. All candidates must be sponsored by the Chair of his/her Division or Department and by an official representative of the institution which would administer the Award and in whose name the application is formally submitted.
Amount of Grant: $40,000 maximum ($20,000 per year)
Date(s) Application is Due: Dec 15; Jan 15
Contact: Stephanie L. Jones, Assistant Director; (703) 519-1586 or (703) 836-4444; email: sljones@entnet.org
Internet: http://www.headandneckcancer.org/research/grants.php
Sponsor: American Head and Neck Society (AHNS)
11300 W. Olympic Boulevard, Suite 600
Los Angeles, CA 90064

AHRF Eugene L. Derlacki, M.D. Research Grants 309
The Eugene L. Derlacki, M.D. Grant is awarded for excellence in the field of hearing research. This grant provides $25,000 per year for two years, for a total award of $50,000. It is dedicated to hearing research and is intended for more significant research projects requiring funding that extends beyond the normal AHRF grant of $25,000. Researchers are invited to apply for this grant using the Research Grant Application Guidelines. According to the rules of the grant, the recipient will receive the first year funding of $25,000. After the first year, a progress report must be submitted to the Research Committee. If the report is approved, the second year funding of $25,000 will then be awarded.
Amount of Grant: $25,000 per year for two years
Date(s) Application is Due: Aug 3
Contact: Kristen Madhuizen, Development and Communication Associate; (312) 726-9670; fax: (312) 726-9695; email: kristen.madhuizen@american-hearing.org or ahrf@american-hearing.org
Internet: http://www.american-hearing.org/research/derlacki_grant.html
Sponsor: American Hearing Research Foundation (AHRF)
8 South Michigan Avenue, Suite 814
Chicago, IL 60603-4539

AHRF Georgia Birtman Grant 310
The American Hearing Research Foundation (AHRF), together with the Northwestern Memorial Foundation (NMF) give the Georgia Birtman Grant, named in honor of long-time supporter of the AHRF. The one-year $75,000 grant ($25,000 each from the Birtman Fund, the AHRF and Northwestern Memorial Foundation) supports the advancement of research and education in otology and neurotology. The grant is awarded to an exceptional researcher in audiology, otology or neurotology who will work in a lab at Northwestern University. The research topic involves some aspect of the diagnosis, treatment, and rehabilitation of hearing and balance disorders related to the inner ear. The research has the potential to generate clinical care innovations, facilitate translational clinical studies, and develop creative educational programs.
Samples: Timothy C. Hain, M.D., Northwestern University, Feinberg School of Medicine, Chicago, Illinois—for Vestibular Evoked Myogenic Potentials (2007); Claus-Peter Richter, M.D., Ph.D., Northwestern University, Feinberg School of Medicine, Chicago, Illinois—for Electrical Stimulation of Spiral Ganglion Cells (2006).
Amount of Grant: $75,000 maximum
Date(s) Application is Due: Aug 3
Contact: Kristen Madhuizen, Development and Communication Associate; (312) 726-9670; fax: (312) 726-9695; email: kristen.madhuizen@american-hearing.org or ahrf@american-hearing.org
Internet: http://www.american-hearing.org/research/birtman_grant.html
Sponsor: American Hearing Research Foundation (AHRF)
8 South Michigan Avenue, Suite 814
Chicago, IL 60603-4539

AHRF Regular Research Grants 311

The American Hearing Research Foundation funds five to ten $20,000 research grants each year. Research Grants should relate to the hearing or balance functions of the ear. Both basic and clinical studies may be proposed. Priority is given to providing start-up funds for new projects. Applications are reviewed by a Research Committee and awards begin in January. Applications are due no later that noon on August 3 of the previous year.

Amount of Grant: $20,000 maximum
Date(s) Application is Due: Aug 3
Contact: Kristen Madhuizen, Development and Communication Associate; (312) 726-9670; fax: (312) 726-9695; email: kristen.madhuizen@american-hearing.org or ahrf@american-hearing.org
Internet: http://www.american-hearing.org/research/grant_guidelines.html
Sponsor: American Hearing Research Foundation (AHRF)
8 South Michigan Avenue, Suite 814
Chicago, IL 60603-4539

AHRF Wiley H. Harrison Memorial Research Award 312

The purpose of this award is to support clinical research projects in otology or neurotology designed to increase understanding of hearing disorders. Research supported by this award should be specifically directed toward the clinical identification, diagnosis, prevention, or treatment of diseases, disorders, or conditions of the ear. While not specifically required, proposals which aim to introduce new knowledge and methodology from other disciplines to research in otology or neurotology, or which demonstrate collaborative effort with members of other related disciplines are encouraged. This is a one year, non-renewable grant of $25,000 maximum, with only one award available annually. Completed applications must be submitted by August 3.

Requirements: Candidates for this award should be physicians (M.D.) at the resident, fellow, or junior faculty stage, or PhD scientists. Previous AHRF or AAO-HNS Foundation research grant recipients are eligible to compete for this grant.
Amount of Grant: $25,000 maximum
Date(s) Application is Due: Aug 3
Contact: Kristen Madhuizen, Development and Communication Associate; (312) 726-9670; fax: (312) 726-9695; email: kristen.madhuizen@american-hearing.org
Internet: http://www.american-hearing.org/research/harrisongrant.html
Sponsor: American Hearing Research Foundation (AHRF)
8 South Michigan Avenue, Suite 814
Chicago, IL 60603-4539

AHRQ Independent Scientist Award 313

The award is a special salary-only grant designed to provide protected time for newly independent scientists who currently have non-research obligations such as heavy teaching loads, clinical work, committee assignments, service, and administrative duties that prevent them from having a period of intensive research focus. The award is targeted to persons with doctoral degrees who have completed their research training, have independent peer-reviewed research support, and who need a period of protected research time in order to foster their research career development. New applications are due February 12, June 12, and October 12, while renewal applications are due March 12, July 12, and November 12. Up to $90,000 per year of base salary plus fringe benefits is available. No other research development support funds are provided.

Requirements: The following organizations and institutions are eligible to apply: public/state controlled institutions of higher education; private institutions of higher education; nonprofits with 501(c)3 IRS status; nonprofits without 501(c)3 IRS status; small businesses; for-profit organizations; State governments; U.S. territories or possessions; Indian/Native American tribal governments (Federally recognized and other than Federally recognized); Indian/Native American tribally designated organizations; Hispanic-serving institutions; historically Black colleges and universities (HBCUs); tribally controlled colleges and universities (TCCUs); Alaska Native and Native Hawaiian serving institutions; regional organizations; and faith-based or community based organizations. The candidate must have a doctoral degree and peer-reviewed, independent research support at the time the award is made. The candidate must spend a minimum of 75 percent effort conducting research during the period of the award.
Restrictions: The award is not intended for investigators who already have full time to perform research, or have substantial publication records or considerable research support indicating that they are well established in their fields. Foreign institutions are not eligible to apply.
Amount of Grant: Up to $90,000 annually, plus associated fringe benefits.
Date(s) Application is Due: Feb 12; Mar 12; Jun 12; Jul 12; Oct 12; Nov 12
Contact: Kay Anderson, Ph.D.; (301) 427-1555; fax: (301) 427-1562; email: Kay.Anderson@ahrq.hhs.gov
Internet: http://grants.nih.gov/grants/guide/pa-files/PAR-07-444.html
Sponsor: Agency for Healthcare Research and Quality
540 Gaither Road
Rockville, MD 20850

AHRQ Individual Awards for Postdoctoral Fellows Ruth L. Kirschstein National Research Service Awards (NRSA) 314

The purpose of the postdoctoral fellowship award is to provide support to promising postdoctoral applicants who have the potential to become productive and successful independent research investigators. The proposed postdoctoral training must offer an opportunity to enhance the applicant's understanding of health services research and must be responsive to AHRQ's mission, which is to improve the quality, safety, efficiency, and effectiveness of health care for all Americans. The research sponsored and conducted by AHRQ develops and presents scientific evidence regarding all aspects of health care. It addresses issues of organization, delivery, financing, utilization, patient and provider behavior, outcomes, effectiveness and cost. It evaluates both clinical services and the system in which these services are provided. These scientific results improve the evidence base to enable better decisions about health care, including such areas as disease prevention, appropriate use of medical technologies, improving diagnosis and treatment utilizing comparative effectiveness research, and reducing racial and ethnic disparities. In addition, AHRQ is interested in the application of health information technology (health IT), as well as reducing medical errors and improving patient safety.

Requirements: The following organizations and institutions are eligible to apply: public or non-profit private institutions, such as a university, college, or a faith-based or community-based organization; units of local or State government; eligible agencies of the Federal government; Indian/Native American tribal governments (Federally recognized); Indian/Native American tribal governments (other than Federally recognized); and Indian/Native American tribally designated organizations.
Restrictions: Awards for fellowship training may only be made to domestic institutions.
Date(s) Application is Due: Apr 8; Aug 8; Dec 8
Contact: Shelley M. Benjamin; (301) 427-1528; fax: (301) 427-1562; email: Shelley.Benjamin@ahrq.hhs.gov
Internet: http://grants.nih.gov/grants/guide/pa-files/PA-09-229.html
Sponsor: Agency for Healthcare Research and Quality (AHRQ)
540 Gaither Road
Rockville, MD 20850

AIDS Vaccine Advocacy Coalition (AVAC) Fund Grants 315

The Fund functions as a small-scale emergency fund to assist needy clinical sites that require immediate help with purchases such as additional medical or lab supplies not covered by grants or contracts for vaccine research. All AIDS vaccine clinical trial sites in resource-limited countries or needy communities, regardless of sponsor, can apply for grants up to $2,000. A committee consisting of HIV vaccine investigators from around the world reviews proposals and makes recommendations to a special Fund Committee of the AVAC Board.

Samples: Kenya AIDS Vaccine Initiative, Department of Medical Microbiology, Nairobi University, $2,000—for HIV Rapid Test Kits and Emergency Medicines.; Brooke Bond Tea Plantation Hospital, $2,000—for general health screenings.
Amount of Grant: $2,000
Contact: Marie Semmelbeck; (212) 367-1188 or (212) 367-1279; fax: (646) 365-3452; email: fund@avac.org
Internet: http://www.avac.org/ht/d/sp/i/962/pid/962
Sponsor: AIDS Vaccine Advocacy Coalition
101 West 23rd Street, #2227
New York, NY 10011

AIG American General Corporation Grants 316

Corporate contributions support organizations that make the greatest impact in its operating communities in the areas of education, health and human services, arts and culture, and community development. The program also recognizes employee volunteer efforts with its Community Spirit Awards program. Award recipients each designate a grant to the organizations they served. Contact the office for application procedures.

Requirements: 501(c)3 nonprofits, particularly those located in the corporation's operating communities, may apply.
Restrictions: Contributions will generally not be made to organizations without 501(c)3 status; United Way agencies (except through an annual employee-giving campaign and corporate gift); veterans groups, along with labor, religious, political, fraternal or external athletic groups, except in specific cases in which such groups provide needed benefits or services to the community at large; national organizations; private foundations; individuals; hospitals, unless it is a teaching institution; and international organizations.
Samples: Anti-Defamation League—to support its No Place for Hate campaign, $115,000.; America's Promise—for youth programs, $1.5 million.
Amount of Grant: $25,000 average; $2500 Community Spirit Awards
Date(s) Application is Due: Mar 31; Jun 30; Sep 30; Dec 31
Contact: Christina Minkley; Christina_Minkley@aigag.com
Internet: http://www.aigag.com/life/life.nsf/contents/aboutus_community_givingguidelines
Sponsor: AIG American General Corporation
2929 Allen Pkwy, A35-00
Houston, TX 77019

AIHP Sonnedecker Visiting Scholar Grants 317

The Sonnedecker Visiting Scholar Program offers assistance for short-term historical research related to the history of pharmacy, including the history of drugs, at the University of Wisconsin-Madison. The program provides assistance for travel, maintaining temporary residence in Madison, and meeting research expenses associated with utilizing the collection. A brochure is available on request that describes the pharmaco-historical collections, which have been developed in Madison during more than a century by the University of Wisconsin-Madison, the State Historical Society of Wisconsin, and the American Institute of the History of Pharmacy. At least $1,000 becomes available annually to defray part of the expenses of a recipient, for whatever period of residence is appropriate. Grants are made throughout the year on the basis of the merit of previous historical work and on the appropriateness of historical resources on the University of Wisconsin campus to the research proposed.

Requirements: Eligible applicants are: Historians, Pharmacists, and other scholars working in the Pharmacy field.
Amount of Grant: $1,000
Contact: Gregory Higby, Director; (608) 262-5378; email: grants@aihp.org
Internet: http://cms.pharmacy.wisc.edu/aihp/programs/sonnedecker
Sponsor: American Institute of the History of Pharmacy
777 Highland Avenue
Madison, WI 53705-2222

AIHP Thesis Support Grants **318**
The Program offers a grant-in-aid totaling $2,000 or more annually to a graduate student to reinforce historical investigations of some aspect of pharmacy, whether ancient or modern, to pay research expenses not normally met by the university granting the degree. Any thesis project devoted to the history of pharmacy, history of drugs, or other humanistic study utilizing a pharmaco-historical approach, is eligible if based in an institution of higher learning of the U.S.A. The maximum grant in this program of the Institute will be $2,500.
Requirements: Any graduate student in good standing at an institution of the United States may apply, regardless of the department through which the Doctor of Philosophy degree will be granted. The graduate student need not be an American citizen; nor does the research topic need to be in the field of American history.
Restrictions: Examples of ineligible expenses would be: living expenses of the applicant at the home university; routine typing to produce research notes or the thesis manuscript; routine illustrations for the manuscript; and publication of research results. Indirect expenses, such as overhead and other institution-related costs, may not be included in a grant application.
Amount of Grant: $2,500 maximum
Date(s) Application is Due: Feb 1
Contact: Gregory Higby, Director; (608) 262-5378; email: grants@aihp.org
Internet: http://cms.pharmacy.wisc.edu/aihp/programs/thesisgrant
Sponsor: American Institute of the History of Pharmacy
777 Highland Avenue
Madison, WI 53705-2222

Air Products and Chemicals Grants **319**
The foundation supports nonprofit organizations in company-operating areas in the fields of precollege and higher education; fitness, health, and welfare; community and economic development, arts and culture; and the environment and safety. Types of support include capital grants, employee matching gifts, general operating support, multiyear-continuing grants, project grants, seed grants, fellowships, employee-related scholarships, and donated equipment. There are no application forms; requests must be in writing. Guidelines are available online.
Requirements: 501(c)3 nonprofit organizations in company-operating areas are eligible.
Restrictions: Grants are not made to/for individuals, sectarian or denominational organizations, political candidates or activities, veterans organizations, organizations receiving United Way support, labor groups, elementary or secondary schools, capital campaigns of national organizations, hospital operating expenses, national health organizations, or goodwill advertising.
Contact: Kassie Hilgert, Manager of Community Relations & Philanthropy, email: hilgerk@airproducts.com
Internet: http://www.airproducts.com/Responsibility/SocialResponsibility
Sponsor: Air Products and Chemicals Corporation
7201 Hamilton Boulevard
Allentown, PA 18195-1501

AJCC Cancer Staging Grants **320**
AJCC seeks proposals to develop and evaluate improved staging algorithms for specific cancer sites and types. Successful proposals will present new approaches and utilize data sets available to the applicant to test and validate current or revised staging algorithms. Applicants may use elements currently used for AJCC/UICC TNM staging, additional or modified anatomic and non-anatomic factors to define prognosis, and incorporate validated factors that identify response to treatment. Proposals that address and validate the use of non-anatomic factors to improve the utility of staging and define the response to therapy are encouraged. The AJCC will provide funding to a number of groups for a variety of disease sites to promote innovative strategies for enhancing the clinical utility of staging while maintaining compatibility with current staging data collection systems. The listed application deadline is for letters of intent. Guidelines are available online.
Requirements: Eligible institutions include for-profit and nonprofit organizations; public or private institutions, such as universities, colleges, laboratories, and hospitals; units of state and local government; eligible agencies of the federal government; and domestic or foreign institutions/organizations.
Amount of Grant: $150,000 maximum
Date(s) Application is Due: Dec 15
Contact: Valerie Vesich, (312) 202-5420; fax: (312) 202-5009; email: AJCC@facs.org
Internet: http://www.cancerstaging.org/initiatives/rfp.html#
Sponsor: American Joint Committee on Cancer
633 N Saint Clair Street
Chicago, IL 60611

Alabama Power Foundation Grants **321**
The foundation's mission is to improve the lives and circumstances of Alabama residents and to strengthen the communities in which they live. It supports programs that will improve education (by supporting innovative programs and assisting teachers in their crucial responsibilities), strengthen communities, promote arts and culture or restore and enhance the environment. The project must meet several of the guidelines to be considered. The majority of grants are made to support targeted efforts with specific objectives. The foundation also provides general operating assistance to organizations, capital grants for endowment and building, and scholarship funds. Applications should be sent to the local Alabama Power Company office for review and recommendation to the foundation. The amount of the request determines the review frequency.
Requirements: Applications are accepted from Alabama nonprofit organizations whose programs fall within foundation guidelines.
Restrictions: Grants are not made to individuals, for sectarian religious purposes, or for political activities.
Geographic Focus: Alabama
Amount of Grant: $1,000-$100,000 average
Date(s) Application is Due: Feb 1; May 1; Aug 1; Nov 1
Contact: William Johnson, President, (205) 257-2508; fax: (205) 257-1860
Internet: http://www.alabamapower.com/foundation/grantsandinitiatives.asp
Sponsor: Alabama Power Foundation
P.O. Box 2641, 600 N. 18th Street
Birmingham, AL 35291-0011

Aladdin Industries Foundation Grants **322**
The foundation awards grants, primarily in Tennessee, in its areas of interest, including arts and culture, youth services, health and human services, education, business, drug abuse, and the elderly. Types of support include general operating support, seed grants, and employee-related scholarships. Proposals are reviewed quarterly.
Requirements: Most grants are awarded in Tennessee. Proposals are reviewed quarterly.
Geographic Focus: Tennessee
Contact: L.B. Jenkins, Secretary & Treasurer, (615) 748-3360
Sponsor: Aladdin Industries Foundation Inc
703 Murfreesboro Road
Nashville, TN 37210-4521

Alaska Airlines Corporate Giving Grants **323**
Alaska Airlines and Horizon Air Corporate Giving support health and human services, arts and cultural programs, as well as education, environmental, and civic organizations. The program focuses on communities served now or in the near future and where a significant number of its employees live or work. When considering requests, the corporation favors organizations and efforts that are most likely to enhance a community's cultural and economic vitality and improve the quality of life for its citizens. Objectives of the Corporate Giving Program are to: provide support to charitable and cultural organizations within our communities; and maintain a reasonable balance of contributions supporting a wide range of organizations.
Requirements: Giving is on a national and international basis in areas of company operations, with emphasis on Alaska and Washington; some further giving occurs in Canada and Mexico.
Restrictions: Alaska Airlines or Horizon Air do not provide support for: loans and grants to individuals or private business; groups that discriminate; endowments; religious organizations (if for sacramental purposes); pageants; capital projects; multi-year commitment or automatic renewal grants; general operating expenses; publicly or privately funded educational institutions; or organizations whose prime purpose is to influence legislation.
Geographic Focus: Alaska; WashingtonCanada; Mexico
Contact: Susan Bramstedt, Director of Public Affairs (Alaska); (907) 266-7230; fax: (907) 266-7229; email: susan.bramstedt@alaskaair.com;; Donna R. Hartman, Manager; (206) 392-5383; email: donnahartman@alaskaair.com
Internet: http://www.alaskaair.com/as/www2/company/csr/social-responsibility.asp
Sponsor: Alaska Airlines, Inc.
4750 Old International Airport Road
Anchorage, AK 99502

Alaska Airlines Foundation Grants **324**
A small number of cash grants ranging on average from $5,000 to $15,000 are given to 501©(3) non-profit organizations classified as public charities in Alaska and Washington. These grants should focus on educational efforts that address a unique need or value to a community. The Foundation supports health and human services, arts and cultural programs, as well as education, environmental, and civic organizations.
Requirements: 501(c)3 organizations based in Alaska and Washington are eligible to apply.
Restrictions: Alaska Airlines or Horizon Air do not provide support for: loans and grants to individuals or private business; groups that discriminate; endowments; religious organizations (if for sacramental purposes); pageants; capital projects; multi-year commitment or automatic renewal grants; general operating expenses; publicly or privately funded educational institutions; or organizations whose prime purpose is to influence legislation.
Geographic Focus: Alaska; Washington
Amount of Grant: $5,000-$15,000 range
Contact: Susan Bramstedt, Director of Public Affairs (Alaska); (907) 266-7230; fax: (907) 266-7229; email: susan.bramstedt@alaskaair.com;; Donna R. Hartman, Manager; (206) 392-5383; email: donnahartman@alaskaair.com
Internet: http://www.alaskaair.com/as/www2/company/csr/as-foundation.asp
Sponsor: Alaska Airlines Foundation
4750 Old International Airport Road
Anchorage, AK 99502

Albany Medical Center Prize in Medicine and Biomedical Research 325

The prize recognizes a physician or biomedical scientist (or group of physicians or scientists) who has made extraordinary and sustained leadership contributions to improving healthcare and patient care; or who has successfully pursued innovative biomedical research with demonstrated translational benefits applied to improved patient care. Each year's prize winner will have demonstrated significant outcomes that offer medical value of national or international importance. Prize winner activities will include but not be limited to disease and injury management, clinical research, and basic science investigations of diseases and injuries, leading to new discoveries and improved clinical outcomes. Nomination guidelines are available online.

Requirements: Any physician or scientist or group whose work has led to significant advances in the fields of health care and scientific research with demonstrated translational benefits applied to improved patient care may be nominated. Those honored will be practitioners and/or scientists whose accomplishments and outcomes have been demonstrated in the past quarter century, with preference to demonstrated accomplishments in the past decade.

Amount of Grant: $500,000

Date(s) Application is Due: Jan 8

Contact: Teri A. Cerveny, Secretary; (518) 262-8043; fax: (518) 262-4769; email: AMCprize@mail.amc.edu

Internet: http://www.amc.edu/Academic/AlbanyPrize/prize_criteria.html

Sponsor: Albany Medical Center
Center Building, 628 Madison Avenue - 1st Floor
Albany, NY 12208

Albert and Margaret Alkek Foundation Grants 326

The foundation awards grants to Texas nonprofit organizations to support charitable, religious, scientific (primarily medical), literary, cultural and educational organizations and programs. Preference will be given to research and education-related projects that will pay lasting dividends in terms of new discoveries and improved quality of life. One application per 12-month period will be considered. There are no application deadlines or forms. Applicants should submit a one- to two-page letter of inquiry that includes a brief description of the organization and the project for which funds are being considered, and the amount of funding need in total as well as the amount being requested. Inquiries should be sent via U.S. postal mail; fax or email applications are not accepted.

Requirements: Texas nonprofit organizations are eligible.

Restrictions: The foundation does not make grants to individuals or loans of any type. The foundation does not make direct scholarships to students. All scholarship programs are administered through educational institutions. The foundation prefers not to fund: organizations that in turn make grants to others; grants intended to influence legislation or to support candidates for political office; fund-raising events such as luncheons, dinners, galas, advertising in programs, or other similar activities; charities operated by service clubs; memorials for individuals; student organizations; or purchase of uniforms, equipment, or trips for school-related organizations or sports teams.

Geographic Focus: Texas

Contact: Grants Administrator, (713) 951-0019; fax: (713) 951-0043; email: info@alkek.org

Internet: http://www.alkek.org/grantguidelines.htm

Sponsor: Albert and Margaret Alkek Foundation
1221 McKinney, Suite 4525
Houston, TX 77010-2023

Albert and Mary Lasker Foundation Awards 327

The major purpose of the awards is to honor the individual(s) who have made significant contributions in basic or clinical research in diseases that are the main cause of death and disability. Three categories of awards are made. The Basic Medical Research Award honors the scientist or scientists who have made fundamental investigations that open new areas of biomedical science. The Clinical Medical Research Award honors the scientist(s) whose contributions, directly or indirectly, have led to the improvement of the clinical management or treatment of patients and to the alleviation or elimination or one of the major medical causes of disability or death. The Special Achievement Award in Medical Science honors a scientist whose contributions to research are of unique magnitude and immeasurable influence on the course of science, health, or medicine, and whose professional career has engendered extreme respect within the biomedical community. Nomination forms are available online. Nominations must be received by the listed application deadline.

Amount of Grant: $50,000 medical research award; $50,000 clinical medical research award; $25,000 special achievement award

Date(s) Application is Due: Feb 1

Contact: David Keegan, (212) 286-0222; fax: (212) 286-0924; email: dkeegan@laskerfoundation.org

Internet: http://www.laskerfoundation.org/awards/awards.html

Sponsor: Albert and Mary Lasker Foundation
110 E 42nd Street, Suite 1300
New York, NY 10017

Albert Pick Jr. Fund Grants 328

The fund contributes to organizations in the following categories: culture, education, health and human services, civic and community organizations. The fund will consider assistance to new and creative programs within these areas and to operating support. Support will be given to requests from organizations that conduct their programs in Chicago, IL, only. The fund functions on a calendar year; applications are considered four times a year based on dates of board meetings. The fund prefers that prospective grantees call or write for guidelines prior to sending their proposals.

Requirements: Only Illinois organizations may apply.

Restrictions: Funds will not be provided for reduction or liquidation of debts, religious purposes, endowments, long-term commitments, building programs, individuals, political purposes, or advertising/program books.

Geographic Focus: Illinois

Samples: Children First Fund/CPS Foundation (Gale Academy Links to Literacy Program) $6900 (2006); Art Resources in Teaching (Chicago, IL)—for general operating support, $7500 (2003); Chicago Academy of Sciences/Peggy Notebaert Nature Museum (Chicago, IL)—for general operating support, $10,000 (2003); Chicago Opera Theater (Chicago, IL)—for general operating support, $10,000 (2003).

Amount of Grant: $3000 minimum

Date(s) Application is Due: Jan 21; Apr 1; Jul 1; Oct 1

Contact: Cleopatra Alexander, Executive Director, (312) 236-1192; email: cleopatra@albertpickjrfund.org

Internet: http://www.albertpickjrfund.org

Sponsor: Albert Pick Jr. Fund
30 N Michigan Avenue, Suite 1002
Chicago, IL 60602

Alberto Culver Corporate Contributions Grants 329

The company prefers to make small donations to a large number of organizations rather than substantial contributions to a few institutions. Major areas of support are civic and community programs, health and welfare, education, culture and art, and youth activities. Special consideration is given to proposals that benefit a large number of people; directly or indirectly assist women's groups or other purchasers or potential customers of Alberto-Culver products; are involved in programs that rehabilitate, train, teach skills or employ the underprivileged, handicapped or minorities; have received support from Alberto-Culver in the past; and received matching grants for donations. Grants are awarded for one year and may be renewed.

Requirements: Only 501(c)3 organizations are eligible. Requests should be in writing on organization letterhead and should state amount requested, and whether the donation will be used for operating funds, capital expansion, supplies or special projects. The objectives and programs of the organization should be clearly defined. Additional requirements are available from the company.

Restrictions: Grants are not awarded to support United Way affiliates, religious groups, preschools, K-12 schools, tax-supported colleges, projects that duplicate other efforts, and multiyear commitments.

Contact: Corporate Communications, (708) 450-3000; fax: (708) 450-3435

Internet: http://www.alberto.com

Sponsor: Alberto Culver
2525 Armitage Avenue
Melrose Park, IL 60160

Albertson's Charitable Giving Grants 330

Albertson's Inc invests in its operating communities and makes corporate contributions to support nonprofits. Areas of charitable giving include health and hunger relief—food banks, churches, and other community-based relief groups; health and nutrition—medical services, flu shots, health screening for diseases such as diabetes and heart disease; and education and development of youth—academic excellence or nurturing efforts. Submit requests in writing and include information about the organization's goals, accomplishments, evaluation plans, leadership, and finances. Requests are accepted throughout the year.

Requirements: Tax-exempt organizations in Arizona, Arkansas, California, Colorado, Delaware, Florida, Georgia, Idaho, Illinois, Indiana, Iowa, Kansas, Louisiana, Maine, Maryland, Massachusetts, Michigan, Minnesota, Mississippi, Missouri, Montana, Nebraska, Nevada, New Hampshire, New Jersey, New Mexico, North Dakota, Oklahoma, Oregon, Pennsylvania, South Dakota, Tennessee, Texas, Utah, Vermont, Washington, Wisconsin, and Wyoming are eligible. Applicants must pass an online eligibility test. Preference will be given to requests that offer volunteerism opportunities.

Restrictions: Contributions cannot be made to churches or religious organizations for purposes of religious advocacy.

Geographic Focus: Arizona; Arkansas; California; Colorado; Delaware; Florida; Georgia; Idaho; Illinois; Indiana; Iowa; Kansas; Louisiana; Maine; Maryland; Massachusetts; Michigan; Minnesota; Mississippi; Missouri; Montana; Nebraska; Nevada; New Hampshire; New Jersey; New Mexico; North Dakota; Oklahoma; Oregon; Pennsylvania; South Dakota; Tennessee; Texas; Utah; Vermont; Washington; Wisconsin; Wyoming

Contact: Community Relations; (877) 932-7948 or (208) 395-6200; fax: (208) 395-4382; email: albertsonscustomercare@albertsons.com

Internet: http://www.albertsons.com/abs_inthecommunity

Sponsor: Albertson's Inc
250 E Parkcenter Boulevard
Boise, ID 83706

Albuquerque Community Foundation Grants 331

The foundation seeks to improve the quality of life in the greater Albuquerque, New Mexico, area by providing support for projects and organizations that serve the community in arts and culture, education, environmental and historic preservation, children and youth, and health and human services. Through its grant program, the foundation supports projects that are innovative, meet the needs of underserved segments of the community, encourage matching funds or additional gifts, promote cooperation among agencies, empower the disadvantaged and disabled, and enhance the effectiveness

of local charitable organizations. Types of support include continuing support, general operating support, program development, publication, seed grants, scholarships funds and scholarships to individuals, and technical assistance.
Requirements: IRS 501(c)3 organizations based in Albuquerque, NM, are eligible. Proposals are reviewed on the basis of the following priorities: impact, innovation, leverage, management, and nonduplication.
Restrictions: Grants are generally not made to or for individuals, political or religious purposes, debt retirement, payment of interest or taxes, annual campaigns, endowments, emergency funding, to influence legislation or elections, scholarships, awards, or to private foundations and other grantmaking organizations.
Geographic Focus: New Mexico
Amount of Grant: $10,000 maximum
Date(s) Application is Due: Apr 16; Aug 15
Contact: R. Randall Royster, Executive Director; (505) 883-6240; fax: (505) 883-3629; email: rroyster@albuquerquefoundation.org
Internet: http://www.albuquerquefoundation.org/grants/grant-home.htm
Sponsor: Albuquerque Community Foundation
P.O. Box 36960
Albuquerque, NM 87176-6960

Alcatel-Lucent Technologies Corporate Contributions Grants 332
Alcatel-Lucent is committed to enhancing and serving the communities where its employees and customers live and work. The corporation demonstrates that commitment through employee volunteerism in community service projects around the world and Foundation grant making. It is building on that heritage as it develops plans for future Alcatel-Lucent corporate sponsorship and philanthropic endeavors. The company's dedication supports programs to improve education and youth development. And Alcatel-Lucent continues to support photography worldwide as well as citizenship initiatives, especially those that use information and communication technologies which enable social inclusion.
Requirements: Government recognized public charities with appropriate tax-exempt identification, such as 501(c)3 status or the international equivalent, are eligible.
Restrictions: The program does not support fund raisers or events; individuals, including awards, sponsorships such as walk-a-thons, or any form of personal financial assistance; endowments; conferences, seminars, trips, tours, etc.; multiyear pledges; capital campaigns, including construction/renovation; ads in fundraising publications or journals; religious programs; veterans, labor, or political organizations; fraternal, athletic, and social clubs or programs; operating expenses of organizations supported by United Way; national health organizations other than United Way; or local chapters of organizations receiving Lucent support at the national level.
Contact: Michele Donato, Manager; (908) 582-7906; fax: (908) 508-2576; email: foundation@alcatel-lucent.com
Internet: http://www.alcatel-lucent.com/wps/portal/!ut/p/kcxml/04_Sj9SPykssy0xPLMnMz0vM0Y_QjzKLd4y3NA0FSYGYRq6m-pEoYgbxjgiRIH1vfV-P_NxU_QD9gtzQiHJHR0UAvqLryQ!!/delta/base64xml/L3dJdyEvd0ZNQUFzQUMvNElVRS82X0FfNDZP
Sponsor: Alcatel-Lucent Technologies Corporation
600 Mountain Avenue, Room 6F430C
Murray Hill, NJ 07974-2008

Alcatel-Lucent Technologies Foundation Grants 333
The Alcatel-Lucent Foundation is the philanthropic arm of Alcatel-Lucent and it leads the company's charitable activities. With a focus on volunteerism, the Foundation's mission is to support the commitment of Alcatel-Lucent to social responsibility by serving and enhancing the communities where its employees and customers live and work. To accomplish its mission, the Foundation manages grants and employee volunteerism on a global level. It receives its income from the corporation - Alcatel-Lucent - whose name it bears. However, legally the Foundation is an independent, charitable, non-profit and private entity and is governed by its own board of trustees that is separate from the corporate board of directors. Global Foundation grants are dedicated to the main focus areas of the Foundation and are managed by the Foundation.
Requirements: Giving is on an international basis.
Amount of Grant: $500-$5,000 typically
Contact: Michele Donato, Manager; (908) 582-7906; fax: (908) 508-2576; email: foundation@alcatel-lucent.com
Internet: http://www.alcatel-lucent.com/wps/portal/foundation
Sponsor: Alcatel-Lucent Technologies Foundation
600 Mountain Avenue, Room 6F4
Murray Hill, NJ 07974-2008

Alcoa Foundation Grants 334
General priorities of the foundation include safe and healthy children and families—ensuring that children and their families have the tools, the knowledge and the services to remain healthy and safe at home, in the community and in the workplace; conservation and sustainability—educating young leaders on conservation issues, protecting forests, promoting sound public policy research, and understanding the linkages between business and the environment; skills today for tomorrow—providing individuals with critical skills and services to be economically connected, workplace-ready, and productive in a changing economy; business and community partnerships—strengthening the nonprofit sector and developing meaningful partnerships among nonprofits, the private sector, and local government; and global education in science, engineering, technology and business—broadening student participation in areas central to Alcoa to prepare a diverse cross-section of our communities for a global workplace. Types of support include capital grants, building funds, challenge grants, matching gifts, general support, research grants, scholarships, and seed money. Initial contact should be a letter of inquiry.
Requirements: The foundation awards grants to nonprofit public charities in communities where Alcoa has a presence. Local Alcoans work within their communities to evaluate organizations and make recommendations for funding to Alcoa Foundation. Nonprofit organizations that serve localized communities should find the Alcoa facility nearest to them and write a one-page letter describing their mission, nature of request, connection to the areas of excellence and offering contact information. If interested, the Alcoa location contact will notify the requesting organization and invite them to submit more information. Areas of operation include western Pennsylvania; Davenport, Iowa; Evansville, Indiana; Massena, New York; New Jersey; Cleveland, Ohio; Knoxville, Tennessee; and Rockdale, Texas.
Restrictions: The foundation does not make gifts to local projects other than those near Alcoa plant or office locations; endowment funds, deficit reduction, or operating reserves; hospital capital campaign programs unless the hospital presents a comprehensive area analysis that justifies, on a regional rather than an individual institutional basis, the need for the capital improvement; individuals, except for the scholarship program for children of Alcoa employees; tickets and other promotional activities; trips, tours, or student exchange programs; or documentaries and videos.
Amount of Grant: $1,000-$50,000 average
Contact: Meg McDonald, President and Treasurer; (412) 553-2348; fax: (412) 553-4498; email: alcoa.foundation@alcoa.com
Internet: http://www.alcoa.com/global/en/community/foundation.asp
Sponsor: Alcoa Foundation
201 Isabella Street
Pittsburgh, PA 15212-5858

Alcohol Misuse and Alcoholism Research Grants 335
The foundation's research interests include factors influencing transitions in drinking patterns and behavior, effects of moderate use of alcohol on health and well-being, mechanisms underlying the behavioral and biomedical effects of alcohol, biobehavioral/interdisciplinary research on the etiology of alcohol misuse. Applications may be obtained from the Web site or by contacting the office. Grantees are usually notified within two weeks following the advisory council meetings, held in April and November.
Requirements: Applications may be submitted by public or private nonprofit organizations such as universities, colleges, hospitals, research institutes and organizations, and governmental research agencies and laboratories in the United States and Canada.
Restrictions: Non-research activities such as education projects, public awareness efforts and treatment or referral services are not eligible for support. The Foundation also does not support the training of pre- and post-doctoral fellows, undergraduates, graduate students, medical students, interns or residents. It does not fund thesis or dissertation research. The Foundation does not encourage applications on treatment of the complications of advanced alcoholism. However, research involving treatment intended to elucidate the pathogenesis of alcohol-related problems will be considered.
Samples: Boston U (MA)—to study alcohol abuse among college students, $38,500.; Bowman School of Medicine (Winston-Salem, NC)—for research on mechanisms in the transition and development of chronic alcohol consumption-induced cardiomyopathy, $39,000.; Cleveland Clinic Foundation (OH)—for research in sub-cellular homeostasis in the heart: effects of chronic ethanol consumption, $40,000.
Amount of Grant: $100,000 maximum over two years
Date(s) Application is Due: Feb 1; Sep 1
Contact: Research Grants Administrator, (410) 821-7066; fax: (410) 821-7065; email: info@abmrf.org
Internet: http://www.abmrf.org/grants.htm
Sponsor: Alcoholic Beverage Medical Research Foundation (ABMRF)
1122 Kenilworth Drive, Suite 407
Baltimore, MD 21204

Alcon Foundation Grants Program 336
The foundation supports organizations in the fields of health care, leadership programs, research, education and community responsibility. Programs that advance the education and skill levels of eye care professionals are given special consideration. General operating grants to organizations and institutions improving education and research in the areas of specialization of Alcon Laboratories—ophthalmology and vision care. Grants are also awarded to community activities that benefit company employees. Applications may be submitted at any time.
Requirements: Grants are not made for building programs.
Restrictions: Non 501(c)3organizations, individuals and scholarship programs, religious, veterans or fraternal organizations, political causes, capital campaigns, matching gifts, trips, tournaments and tours, and endowments are not supported.
Samples: National Sjogrens Syndrome Assoc (Phoenix, AZ)—for general operating support, $2500.
Amount of Grant: $100-$50,000 average
Contact: Mary Dulle, Chair, (817) 293-0450; email: Mary.Dulle@Alconlabs.com
Internet: http://www.alconlabs.com/corporate-responsibility/alcon-foundation.asp
Sponsor: Alcon Foundation
6201 S Freeway
Fort Worth, TX 76134

Alex Brown and Sons Charitable Foundation Grants 337
The foundation awards one-year renewable grants to U.S. nonprofit organizations in its areas of interest, including arts and culture, community affairs, education, medicine, and science. Types of support include annual campaigns, capital grants, endowment funds,

general operating grants, program development grants, and scholarship funds. Applicants should submit a letter of intent that briefly outlines the purpose of the grant.
Requirements: 501(c)3 tax-exempt organizations in Maryland are eligible.
Restrictions: No support for private schools or churches. Grants are not made to individuals.
Geographic Focus: Maryland
Samples: Baltimore Symphony Orchestra (MD)—for discretionary use, $1 million.; Johns Hopkins Hospital (Baltimore, MD)—for discretionary use, $1 million.; Baltimore Zoo (MD)—for discretionary use, $1 million.
Amount of Grant: $1000-$100,000 range
Contact: Margaret Preston, Secretary, c/o Deutsche Bank Alex Brown Inc
Sponsor: Alex Brown and Sons Charitable Foundation
P.O. Box 2257
Baltimore, MD 21203

Alexander & Baldwin Foundation Hawaiian and Pacific Island Grants **338**
The foundation awards grants to eligible Hawaii nonprofit organizations in its areas of interest, including health and human services, education, the community, culture and arts, the maritime arena and the environment. Grant preferences are given to organizations and projects that address significant community needs, have the active support of A&B employees, are preventive in nature, and have demonstrated support of the community. Start-up, general operating and special project needs, as well as major and minor capital requests are considered. Deadlines listed are for organizations in Hawaii and the Pacific Islands. Although the majority of grants range between $1,000 and $5,000, the Foundation considers request upward of $20,000.
Requirements: The foundation gives funding to community-based projects and organizations that qualify with 501(c)3 status.
Restrictions: Grants are not awarded to support United Way agencies for operating support, individuals, events, travel expenses, or scholarships.
Geographic Focus: Hawaii
Amount of Grant: $1,000-$5,000 average
Date(s) Application is Due: Dec 1; Feb 1; Apr 1; Jun 1; Aug 1; Oct 1
Contact: Linda Howe; (808) 525-6642; fax: (808) 525-6677; email: lhowe@abinc.com;; Nami Nielipinski; (808) 525-6641; fax: (808) 525-6677; email: nnielipinski@abinc.com
Internet: http://www.alexanderbaldwinfoundation.org/appguide.htm
Sponsor: Alexander & Baldwin Foundation
P.O. Box 3440
Honolulu, HI 96801-3440

Alexander & Baldwin Foundation Mainland Grants **339**
The foundation awards grants to eligible U.S. nonprofit organizations in its areas of interest, including health and human services, education, the community, culture and arts, the maritime arena and the environment. Grant preferences are given to organizations and projects that address significant community needs, have the active support of A&B employees, are preventive in nature, and have demonstrated support of the community. Start-up, general operating and special project needs, as well as major and minor capital requests are considered. Although the majority of grants range between $1,000 and $5,000, the Foundation considers request upward of $20,000.
Requirements: The foundation gives funding to community-based projects and organizations that qualify with 501(c)3 status.
Restrictions: Grants are not awarded to support United Way agencies for operating support, individuals, events, travel expenses, or scholarships.
Amount of Grant: $1,000-$5,000 average
Date(s) Application is Due: Jan 1; Feb 1; Mar 1; Apr 1; May 1; Jun 1; Jul 1; Aug 1; Sep 1; Oct 1; Nov 1; Dec 1
Contact: Paul Merwin; (707) 421-8121; fax: (707) 421-1835; email: plmifm@aol.com
Internet: http://www.alexanderbaldwinfoundation.org/appguide.htm
Sponsor: Alexander & Baldwin Foundation
555 12th Street
Oakland, CA 94607

Alexander and Margaret Stewart Trust Grants **340**
The trust awards grants in the greater Washington, DC, area for cancer treatment, especially equipment used in diagnosis and treatment; and caring for children who are physically ill, mentally ill, or disabled. Grants also support research, education, and prevention of common childhood diseases, including negative societal behavioral patterns that impact children. Proposals for projects aiding the economically deprived receive preference. The trust awards start-up funding. Applications may be submitted at any time; requests received by the listed deadline are reviewed by the end of the year.
Requirements: Nonprofits in the greater District of Columbia area are eligible.
Restrictions: Support of endowments, buildings, or capital campaigns are denied.
Geographic Focus: District of Columbia
Samples: Childrens National Medical Center, Washington, DC, $420,000—for Center for Cancer and Blood Disorders (2007); DC Campaign to Prevent Teen Pregnancy, Washington, DC, $75,000—for general support (2007).
Amount of Grant: $50,000-$150,000 average
Date(s) Application is Due: Sep 15
Contact: William J. Bierbower; (202) 785-9892; fax: (202) 785-0918; email: wbierbower@stewart-trust.org
Internet: http://www.stewart-trust.org/guidelines.htm
Sponsor: Alexander and Margaret Stewart Trust
888 17th Street NW, Brawner Building, Suite 610
Washington, DC 20006-3321

Alexander Eastman Foundation Grants **341**
The purposes of the Alexander Eastman Foundation are served through grant support to organizations awarded in response to proposals and special initiative commitments planned collaboratively by the Foundation with local service providers. Grants are awarded to support the capital, special projects and operations needs of qualifying organizations. In considering proposals, priority is given to funding activity which serves the Foundation's priority interests. The Alexander Eastman Foundation supports: Education - provide information and community education to improve the health and well-being of residents of the greater Derry area; address goals for healthy individuals and families through a long-term commitment to prevention, health promotion and education of consumers and providers; foster individual responsibility, independence, self-care and healthy life-style choices; Family Systems - strengthen families as the critical unit for community health and well-being; recognize the changing nature of families and provide resources and assistance to reduce stress on families and improve family function; Access - expand access to quality health care and prevention services for people with financial need. Applications are available at the Foundations website.
Requirements: Nonprofit organizations serving Derry, Londonderry, Windham, Chester, Hampstead, and Sandown, NH, are eligible.
Restrictions: Grants are made neither to individuals nor to qualifying organizations to support the cost of services to particular individuals, except through the Alexander Eastman Scholarship Program.
Geographic Focus: New Hampshire
Samples: Community Caregivers of Greater Derry, Derry, NH, $10,000 - to support the volunteer-driven program of quality client care in the greater Derry community (2009); The Upper Room, A Family Resource Center, Derry, NH, $28,000 - to support prevention and intervention for families at risk of having a child placed in foster care (2009); Child and Family Services of New Hampshire, Manchester, NH, $19,760 - to support services to twelve non-Medicaid-eligible teens in the Healthy Family Home Visiting program, to support tuition assistance for low-income, at risk greater Derry area youth to attend a session of residential summer camp at Camp Spaulding (2009).
Date(s) Application is Due: Apr 1; Oct 1
Contact: Amy Lockwood, Director of Grants; (888) 228-1821 ext. 80; email: alockwood@alexandereastman.org
Internet: http://www.alexandereastman.org/02grants.html
Sponsor: Alexander Eastman Foundation
26 South Main Street, PMB 250
Concord NH 03301

Alexander Foundation Cancer, Catastrophic Illness and Injury Grants **342**
The program is intended to provide support to lesbian, gay, bisexual and transgendered people who are at risk of losing their ability to provide basic life needs due to treatment or complications related to cancer, a catastrophic illness, or a serious illness. Some examples of basic life needs are medical care, housing, food, clothing, phones, utilities, and so on. Unlike the one grant payment provided through the Emergency Grant Program, this program provides a fixed monthly grant for up to 12 months. The amount of the grant is determined by the recipients' needs but not to exceed $2,400.
Requirements: Applicants must have diagnosis and treatment of any form of cancer, catastrophic illness, or serious injury except those occurring simultaneously with HIV/AIDS. Recipients must be gay, lesbian, bisexual or transgendered, diagnosed with AIDS or HIV positive, demonstrate a perceived financial need and have been recommended by a recognized referral agency. Additionally, recipients must reside in Colorado.
Restrictions: Recipients must demonstrate financial need and cannot have received financial assistance from the Foundation during the previous 6 months. The Alexander Foundation will only accept applications from an approved referring agency or source.
Geographic Focus: Colorado
Amount of Grant: $2,400 maximum
Contact: Jack Heruska, President; (303) 331-7733; fax: (303) 331-1953; email: egrants@thealexanderfoundation.org
Internet: http://www.thealexanderfoundation.org/cancer.html
Sponsor: Alexander Foundation
P.O. Box 1995
Denver, CO 80201-1995

Alexander Foundation Insurance Continuation Grants **343**
The program provides funds on a monthly basis to pay medical insurance premiums for those individuals who have been diagnosed with AIDS or HIV positive. After a recipient has been accepted into the program, they remain in the program as long as they can demonstrate a continued need. New applicants may be added to a waiting list until such time as funds become available.
Requirements: Recipients must be gay, lesbian, bisexual or transgendered, diagnosed with AIDS or HIV positive, demonstrate a perceived financial need and have been recommended by a recognized referral agency. Additionally, recipients must reside in Colorado.
Geographic Focus: Colorado
Contact: Jack Heruska, President; (303) 331-7733; fax: (303) 331-1953; email: egrants@thealexanderfoundation.org
Internet: http://www.thealexanderfoundation.org/insurance.html
Sponsor: Alexander Foundation
P.O. Box 1995
Denver, CO 80201-1995

Alexander von Humboldt Foundation Georg Forster Fellowships for Experienced Researchers 344

Fellowships are available to scholars from developing countries in humanities and social sciences; political science and economics; projects in the public health sector and in the fields of agriculture, forestry, and geosciences; and interdisciplinary projects relating to environmental and resource protection. Fellowships are designed to promote the transfer of knowledge and methods and to contribute to further development in fellows' home countries. Applications may be submitted for long-term research stays of between six and 18 months. The fellowship is flexible and can be divided up into as many as three stays within three years. The Foundation grants up to 60 Fellowships for postdoctoral researchers and experienced researchers annually.

Requirements: Scholars from developing countries (excluding Turkey, India, and the Peoples' Republic of China) may apply. Applicants must have completed their doctorates less than twelve years ago. Scholars in the humanities or social sciences and physicians must have a good knowledge of German if it is necessary to carry out the project successfully; otherwise a good knowledge of English; scientists and engineers must have a good knowledge of German or English.

Restrictions: Short-term study tours, participation in conferences, or educational visits cannot be funded. Applications for extension of research stays already commenced in Germany cannot be considered.

Amount of Grant: 2,450 EUR

Contact: Program Contact; (+49) 0228-833-0; fax: (+49) 0228-833-199; email: info@avh.de

Internet: http://www.humboldt-foundation.de/web/georg-forster-research-fellowship-experienced.html

Sponsor: Alexander von Humboldt Foundation
Jean-Paul-St 12
Bonn D-53173 Germany

Alexander von Humboldt Foundation Georg Forster Fellowships for Postdoctoral Researchers 345

Fellowships for postdoctoral researchers are the instrument with which the Foundation enables highly-qualified scientists and scholars who are just embarking on their academic careers and who completed their doctorates less than four years agol to spend extended periods of research (6-24 months) in Germany. Scientists and scholars from all disciplines from developing and threshold countries (excluding People's Republic of China, India and Turkey) may apply. The research proposal must deal with issues of major relevance to the future development of the candidate's country of origin and, in this context, particularly suited to transferring knowledge and methods to developing and threshold countries. Research projects are carried out in cooperation with academic hosts at research institutions in Germany. Candidates choose their own research projects and their host in Germany and prepare their own research plan.

Amount of Grant: 2,250 EUR

Contact: Contact; (+49) 0228-833-0; fax: (+49) 0228-833-199; email: info@avh.de

Internet: http://www.humboldt-foundation.de/web/georg-forster-research-fellowship-postdoc.html

Sponsor: Alexander von Humboldt Foundation
Jean-Paul-Street 12
Bonn D-53173 Germany

Alexander von Humboldt Foundation Institutional Academic Cooperation Grants346

Under the follow-up program of the Foundation, institutional partnerships for long-term research collaboration can be created by combining various sponsorship opportunities. Special emphasis is placed on the exchange of younger scientists. The aim is to give these scientists access to the world-wide network of scholars sponsored by the Foundation and to alert them to the Humboldt Research Fellowship Program. The program includes: reciprocal research visits by applicants and their co-workers at the partner institutes (including travel and living expenses); jointly hosted academic conferences and workshops (including travel and living expenses for participants from the partner institutes, as well as expenses for organizing and realizing the events); and funds for the purchase of scientific equipment and additional material (for the foreign institutes).

Requirements: Young scientists and scholars who are involved in the co-operation should preferably have completed a PhD or should at least be doctoral candidates and must be under 35 years of age.

Restrictions: Funds up to a maximum of 50,000 Euro. Funds for material costs (scientific equipment and additional material) are limited to a maximum of 50% of the total funds requested. The purchase price of scientific equipment may not exceed a total amount of 20,000 Euro.

Amount of Grant: 55,000 EUR maximum

Contact: Program Coordinator; (+49) 0228-833-0; fax: (+49) 0228-833-199; email: info@avh.de

Internet: http://www.humboldt-foundation.de/web/31390.html

Sponsor: Alexander von Humboldt Foundation
Jean-Paul-Street 12
Bonn D-53173 Germany

Alexander von Humboldt Foundation Research Fellowships for Experienced Researchers 347

These Fellowships for experienced researchers are the instrument with which the Foundation enables highly-qualified scientists and scholars from abroad, who completed their doctorates less than twelve years ago to spend extended periods of research (6-18 months; may be divided up into a maximum of three blocks) in Germany. Candidates are expected to have their own, clearly defined research profile. This means they should usually be working at least at the level of Assistant Professor or Junior Research Group Leader or be able to document independent research work over a number of years. Scientists and scholars from all disciplines and countries may apply. The fellowship is worth 2,450 EUR per month. This includes a mobility lump sum and a contribution towards health and liability insurance.

Requirements: Application requirements include: a doctorate or comparable academic degree (Ph.D., C.Sc. or equivalent), completed less than twelve years prior to the date of application; the candidate's own research profile documented by a comprehensive list of academic publications reviewed according to international standards and printed in journals and/or by publishing houses; and a good knowledge of German if it is necessary to carry out the project successfully (otherwise a good knowledge of English; scientists and engineers must have a good knowledge of German or English).

Restrictions: Short-term visits for study and training purposes or for attending conferences are not eligible for sponsorship.

Amount of Grant: 2,450 EUR per month

Contact: Coordinator; (+49) 0228-833-0; fax: (+49) 0228-833-199; email: info@avh.de

Internet: http://www.humboldt-foundation.de/web/humboldt-research-fellowship-experienced.html

Sponsor: Alexander von Humboldt Foundation
Jean-Paul-Street 12
Bonn D-53173 Germany

Alexander von Humboldt Foundation Research Fellowships for Postdoctoral Researchers 348

These Fellowships for postdoctoral researchers are the instrument with which the Foundation enables highly-qualified scientists and scholars from abroad who are just embarking on their academic careers and who completed their doctorates less than four years ago to spend extended periods of research (6-24 months) in Germany. Scientists and scholars from all disciplines and countries may apply. Research projects are carried out in cooperation with academic hosts at research institutions in Germany. Candidates choose their own research projects and their host in Germany and prepare their own research plan. Details of the research project and the time schedule must be agreed upon with the prospective host in advance. Candidates are selected solely on the basis of their academic record. There are no quotas for individual disciplines or countries. The fellowship is worth 2,250 EUR per month. This includes a mobility lump sum and a contribution towards health and liability insurance.

Requirements: Application requirements include: a doctorate or comparable academic degree (Ph.D., C.Sc. or equivalent), completed less than twelve years prior to the date of application; the candidate's own research profile documented by a comprehensive list of academic publications reviewed according to international standards and printed in journals and/or by publishing houses; and a good knowledge of German if it is necessary to carry out the project successfully (otherwise a good knowledge of English; scientists and engineers must have a good knowledge of German or English).

Restrictions: Short-term visits for study and training purposes or for attending conferences are not eligible for sponsorship.

Amount of Grant: 2,250 EUR per month

Contact: Coordinator; (+49) 0228-833-0; fax: (+49) 0228-833-199; email: info@avh.de

Internet: http://www.humboldt-foundation.de/web/humboldt-research-fellowship-postdoc.html

Sponsor: Alexander von Humboldt Foundation
Jean-Paul-Street 12
Bonn D-53173 Germany

Alexis Gregory Foundation Grants 349

The Foundation, established in 1986, gives primarily for education purposes. Interests include: AIDS and AIDS research; arts; France; health organizations; human services; Italy; Jewish agencies and temples; libraries and library science; museums; performing arts; and the United Kingdom. Types of support include program development and scholarships to individuals. The primary region of giving is New York, though grants are sometimes approved for out-of-state organizations. Though there is no specific deadline date, the board generally reviews applications in January. An application form is not required. Applicants should initially send a letter or full proposal.

Geographic Focus: New York

Amount of Grant: $15,000 maximum

Contact: Alexis Gregory, President; (212) 737-5297; fax: (212) 737-5340

Sponsor: Alexis Gregory Foundation
1334 York Avenue, 3rd Floor
New York, NY 10021

Alfred Bader Award in BioInorganic or BioOrganic Chemistry 350

This award is given annually to recognize outstanding contributions to bioorganic or bioinorganic chemistry. The award will be granted for outstanding research accomplishments without regard to age or nationality. The award is intended to recognize significant accomplishments that are at the interface between biology and organic or inorganic chemistry. Special consideration will be given to applications of the fundamental principles and experimental methodology of chemistry to areas of biological significance. The award consists of $5,000 and a certificate.

Requirements: Any individual, except a member of the awards committee, may submit one nomination or seconding letter for the award in any given year. The nominating documents consist of a letter of not more than 1000 words containing an evaluation of the nominee's accomplishments and a specific identification of the work to be recognized, a biographical sketch including date of birth, and a list of publications and patents authored by the nominee.

Restrictions: Self-nominations are not accepted.
Samples: Kevin M. Smith—award recipient, $5,000 (2009); Lawrence Que, Jr.—award recipient, $5,000 (2008); Eckard Munck—award recipient, $5,000 (2007).
Amount of Grant: $5,000 and reimbursement of travel expenses to award meeting
Date(s) Application is Due: Nov 1
Contact: Felicia Dixon, Awards Administrator; (800) 227-5558 or (202) 872-4408; fax: (202) 776-8008; email: f_dixon@acs.org or awards@acs.org
Internet: http://portal.acs.org/portal/acs/corg/content?_nfpb=true&_pageLabel=PP_ARTICLEMAIN&node_id=1319&content_id=CTP_004490&use_sec=true&sec_url_var=region1
Sponsor: American Chemical Society
1155 Sixteenth Street, NW
Washington, DC 20036

Alfred Burger Award in Medicinal Chemistry **351**
This award, supported by GlaxoSmithKline in 1978, is awarded biennially in even-numbered years to recognize outstanding contributions to research in medicinal chemistry. The award is granted without regard to age or nationality, and the recipient presents an award address at the spring meeting of the ACS Division of Medicinal Chemistry. Applications are accepted in odd-numbered years. The award consists of $3,000 and a certificate.
Requirements: Any individual, except a member of the award committee, may submit one nomination or seconding letter for the award in any given year. The nominating documents consist of a letter of not more than 1000 words containing an evaluation of the nominee's accomplishments and a specific identification of the work to be recognized, a biographical sketch including date of birth, and a list of publications and patents authored by the nominee.
Restrictions: Self-nominations are not accepted.
Samples: Magid Abou-Gharbia—award recipient, $3,000 (2008); Joel R. Huff—award recipient, $3,000 (2006); William Greenlee—award recipient, $3,000 (2004).
Amount of Grant: $3,000 and travel to award meeting
Date(s) Application is Due: Nov 1
Contact: Felicia Dixon, Awards Administrator; (800) 227-5558 or (202) 872-4408; fax: (202) 776-8008; email: f_dixon@acs.org or awards@acs.org
Internet: http://portal.acs.org/portal/acs/corg/content?_nfpb=true&_pageLabel=PP_ARTICLEMAIN&node_id=1319&content_id=CTP_004491&use_sec=true&sec_url_var=region1
Sponsor: American Chemical Society
1155 Sixteenth Street, NW
Washington, DC 20036

Alfred P. Sloan Foundation History of Science and Technology Grants **352**
The goal of this program is to preserve the raw material of history by supporting archival projects now centered on Charles Darwin, Thomas A. Edison, and Kurt G'del, and via new projects based on the World Wide Web. Two specific areas are of interest: the archival program; and recent history of science and engineering on the web. Grant requests can be made at any time for support of activities related to Foundation program areas and interests. The Foundation is generally limited to supporting tax-exempt organizations. The Foundation has no deadlines or standard forms. The Foundation accepts proposals sent by email. A brief letter of inquiry, rather than a fully developed proposal, is an advisable first step for an applicant, conserving his or her time and allowing for a preliminary response regarding the possibility of support.
Requirements: Concise, well-organized proposals are preferred. In no case should the body of the proposal exceed 20 double-spaced pages.
Restrictions: The Foundation's activities do not normally extend to religion, the creative or performing arts, elementary or secondary education, medical research or health care, the humanities or to activities outside the United States. Grants are not made for endowments or for buildings or equipment.
Contact: Doron Weber, Program Director; (212) 649-1649; fax: (212) 757-5117; email: weber@sloan.org;; Jesse H. Ausubel, Program Director; (212) 649-1649; fax: (212) 757-5117; email: ausubel@sloan.org
Internet: http://sloan.org/programs/scitech_historysci.shtml
Sponsor: Alfred P. Sloan Foundation
630 Fifth Avenue, Suite 2550
New York, NY 10111

Alfred P. Sloan Foundation Research Fellowships **353**
Fellowships stimulate fundamental research by young scholars of outstanding promise at a time in their careers when their creative abilities are especially high and when government or other support is difficult to obtain. Fellows are free to pursue whatever lines of inquiry that are of the most compelling interest to them. Funds are awarded directly to the fellow's institution and may be used by the fellow for such purposes as equipment, technical assistance, professional travel, trainee support, or activities directly related to the fellow's research. The foundation welcomes nominations of all candidates who meet the traditional high standards of this program and strongly encourages the participation of women and members of underrepresented minority groups. Awards are made in the fields of physics, chemistry, neuroscience, economics, pure mathematics, applied mathematics, computer science, and computational and evolutionary molecular biology. Fellowships are awarded for a two-year period, with possible extension for another two years. Each year 118 fellows are selected from the nominations received. Nominations are due September 15 for awards to begin the following September. Nomination forms are available upon request.
Requirements: Candidates must hold a PhD or equivalent in chemistry, physics, mathematics, computer science, economics, neuroscience or computational and evolutionary molecular biology, or in a related interdisciplinary field, and must also be a faculty member at a U.S. or Canadian university. Candidates must be no more than six years from the completion of the most recent PhD or equivalent as of the year of their nomination.
Restrictions: Direct applications are not accepted. Candidates must be nominated by department heads or other senior scholars.
Amount of Grant: $45,000 for two years
Date(s) Application is Due: Sep 15
Contact: Michael Teitelbaum, Program Director; (212) 649-1649; fax: (212) 757-5117; email: teitelbaum@sloan.org
Internet: http://sloan.org/programs/scitech_fellowships.shtml
Sponsor: Alfred P. Sloan Foundation
630 Fifth Avenue, Suite 2550
New York, NY 10111

Alfred W. Bressler Prize in Vision Science **354**
The Prize recognizes a professional in the field of vision science whose leadership, research and service have resulted in important advancements in the treatment of eye disease or rehabilitation of persons with vision loss. A panel of distinguished vision science professionals will select the winner who receives a prize of $40,000.
Requirements: The application process is open to established professionals in the field of vision science whose contributions have advanced vision care, the treatment of eye disease, or the rehabilitation of persons with visual disabilities or blindness and whose further work is expected to contribute significantly. Candidates from the United States and countries around the world are eligible for the award.
Samples: Roy W. Beck, MD, PHD, University of South Florida, Tampa, FL— for his work in the field of Epidimiology (2009); Jonathan C. Horton, MD, PhD, University of California, San Francisco— for his work in the field of Neuro - Ophthalmology (2008).
Amount of Grant: $40,000
Date(s) Application is Due: Dec 31
Contact: Program Administrator, (212) 769-7801; email: bressler@jgb.org
Internet: http://www.jgb.org/programs_bressler.asp
Sponsor: Jewish Guild for the Blind
15 West 65th Street
New York, NY 10023

Alice C. A. Sibley Fund Grants **355**
The purpose of the Alice C.A. Sibley Fund is to provide medical eye care to vulnerable populations of all ages in Worcester including: hospital and surgical fees; medical equipment; and eye glasses and corrective treatment. Approximately $24,000 in grants will be awarded annually to one or more organizations that directly support people's eye health.
Requirements: Applicants must be tax-exempt, nonprofit organizations as recognized by IRS code 501(c)3, and must be located in or providing services to residents of Worcester, Massachusetts.
Geographic Focus: Massachusetts
Amount of Grant: $24,000 maximum
Date(s) Application is Due: Apr 15
Contact: Lois Smith, Senior Program Officer; (508) 755-0980, ext. 107; email: lsmith@greaterworcester.org
Internet: http://www.greaterworcester.org/grants/Sibley.htm
Sponsor: Greater Worcester Community Foundation
370 Main Street, Suite 650
Worcester, MA 01608-1738

Alice Fisher Society Fellowships **356**
The Barbara Bates Center for the Study of the History of Nursing offers a fellowship of $2,500 to support two weeks in residence at the Center and ongoing collaboration with Center historians. Selection of Alice Fisher Society scholars will be based on evidence of interest in and aptitude for historical research related to nursing. It is expected that the research and new materials produced by Alice Fisher Society scholars will help ensure the growth of scholarly work focused on the history of nursing. Fisher scholars will participate in Center activities and will present their research at a Center seminar.
Requirements: The scholarships are open to individuals with master's and doctoral level preparation. The application should be sent via email to either Patricia D'Antonio, PhD, RN, FAAN (dantonio@nursing.upenn.edu) or Barbra Mann Wall, PhD, RN (wallbm@nursing.upenn.edu).
Amount of Grant: $2,500
Date(s) Application is Due: Dec 31
Contact: Dr. Karen Buhler-Wilkerson, Director; (215) 898-4725; fax: (215) 573-2168; email: karenwil@nursing.upenn.edu
Internet: http://www.nursing.upenn.edu/history/Pages/Alice_Fisher_Fellowship.aspx
Sponsor: University of Pennsylvania
School of Nursing, 418 Curie Boulevard
Philadelphia, PA 19104-6020

Alice Tweed Tuohy Foundation Grants Program **357**
The foundation promotes organizations that promote young people; that provide outstanding opportunities for performance, growth, and creativity; that nurture personal integrity and ambition; and that reward high achievement. The foundation

assists organizations offering services to children whose choices might otherwise be unfairly restricted by need; supported are activities both academic and extracurricular that challenge young people while encouraging the growth of responsibility and personal integrity. Organizations dedicated to improving the quality of life by meeting the vital needs of the community are also supported. Types of support include building construction/ renovation, scholarship funds, and matching funds. Financing priority is accorded those organizations with the least in-house capacity to raise capital, assisting these groups to surmount critical monetary obstacles and continue productive service to the community. Proposals may be submitted annually between July 1 and September 15. However, the foundation has announced that a three-year partial moratorium period on awarding grants will commence July 1, 2009.
Requirements: Applications are considered only from Santa Barbara, CA public, tax-exempt organizations. Priority consideration is given to applications from organizations serving young people, education, health and medicine, community affairs, and the arts.
Restrictions: Excluded from consideration are applications for the benefit of specific individuals, organizations outside the Santa Barbara area, organizations in overpopulated nonprofit areas, national campaigns, fund-raising normally carried out by the organization, operating expenses, or budgetary support.
Geographic Focus: California
Samples: Scholarship Foundation of Santa Barbara (Santa Barbara, CA)—for general support, $97,125 (2004); Mental Health Association of Santa Barbara (Santa Barbara, CA)—for capital campaign, $25,000 (2004).
Amount of Grant: $750-$98,000 range
Date(s) Application is Due: Sep 15
Contact: Program Contact; (805) 962-6430; fax: (805) 962-7135; email: atuohyfdn@aol.com
Sponsor: Alice Tweed Tuohy Foundation
P.O. Box 1328, 205 E. Carrillo Street, Room 219
Santa Barbara, CA 93102-1328

Allegan County Community Foundation Grants 358
The foundation awards one-year grants to eligible Michigan charitable organizations to improve the quality of life in Allegan County. Areas of interest include education, health, and social services. Types of support include youth grants, general grants, matching/challenge grants, building construction/renovation, program development, and emergency funds. A copy of the IRS tax-exemption letter must be submitted with application. Any youth group, club, school or class can apply for the T.A.G. awards but must have an adult leader who oversees the project and any funds awarded.
Requirements: 501(c)3 tax-exempt organizations serving Allegan County, Michigan, residents are eligible. All applicants are required to schedule an appointment with foundation staff prior to submitting an application.
Restrictions: Individuals are ineligible. All T.A.G. mini-grants must be handwritten by youth 18 or younger.
Geographic Focus: Michigan
Samples: Martin Area Resource Center, $1,000 - general operating funds (2009); Safe Harbor Children's Advocacy Center, $5,000 – forensic interviewer (2009); Allegan Ministerium Central Food, $7,000 - food for pantry (2009).
Date(s) Application is Due: Dec 4
Contact: Theresa Bray, Executive Director; (269) 673-8344; fax: (269) 673-8745
Internet: http://www.alleganfoundation.org/grants.htm
Sponsor: Allegan County Community Foundation
524 Marshall Street
Allegan, MI 49010

Allegheny Technologies Charitable Trust 359
The corporation awards one-year renewable grants to nonprofit organizations to enhance the quality of life for people in company operating locations. Areas of interest include arts and culture, civic and public affairs, education, health, and social services. Types of support include capital grants, general operating grants, program development grants, and employee matching gifts. Applicants should submit a letter of inquiry that describes the organization, purpose of grants, and funds sought. No particular form or information is required. Potential applicants are requested to provide proof of exempt public charity status. There are no deadlines.
Requirements: 501(c)3 tax-exempt organizations in company-operating areas are eligible.
Restrictions: Contributions are made only to public charities. Individuals and private foundations are excluded.
Geographic Focus: Pennsylvania
Samples: Pittsburgh Symphony Society (Pittsburgh, PA)—grant recipient, $55,000.
Amount of Grant: $1000-$35,000 average
Contact: Jon D. Walton, Jr. Trustee, (412) 394-2800; fax: (412) 394-3034
Internet: http://www.alleghenytechnologies.com
Sponsor: Allegheny Technologies
1000 Six PPG Pl
Pittsburgh, PA 15222

Allegis Group Foundation Grants 360
The foundation awards grants to support organizations providing services or programs in the areas of education, health, and underprivileged children. Giving is national in scope, with an emphasis on Baltimore. There are no application deadlines or forms. Send a letter of inquiry as the initial approach.
Samples: Leukemia and Lymphoma Society (San Jose, CA)—$1000.; Odyssey School (Baltimore, MD)—$4000.; Heart to Heart International (Olathe, KS)—$15,000.
Contact: Hillary Murray, (410) 579-3509
Internet: http://www.allegisgroup.com
Sponsor: Allegis Group Foundation
7301 Parkway Drive
Hanover, MD 21076

Allen P. and Josephine B. Green Foundation Grants 361
The mission of the foundation is to improve the quality of life in Missouri. Grants support programs to bring health care services to people; counseling and educational services for children and adults with physical, mental, or behavioral problems; innovative developmental and educational programs for children; cultural and preservation projects to safeguard our heritage and to promote broader awareness and understanding of such programs and activities on the part of Missourians; and environmental and conservation projects based in Missouri. Grants will be made for one year only. Priority will be given to new projects and to those that have not been funded for at least one year. The board meets in May and November. Guidelines are available online.
Requirements: Grants are awarded to 501(c)3 nonprofit organizations in Missouri.
Restrictions: Grants are not awarded to individuals; to projects and programs located outside of the United States; to charities that are not publicly supported; for social causes or for social activism; for lobbying, propagandizing, or for political campaigns; or to requests deemed as inappropriate for a variety of other reasons. Grant requests that probably will not be approved include projects and programs located outside of Missouri; commitment of funds for more than one year; funding to the same organization for two years in a row; grants for operating funds and annual budgets; unspecified general funds; other than to specific projects or programs; projects with a perceived small chance of success; programs that would seem unlikely to continue without further funding from the Green Foundation; large capital fund drives; large building fund drives; large endowments; to an organization whose primary mission is to raise and distribute funds; or to federated giving programs.
Geographic Focus: Missouri
Samples: Childhaven (Saint Louis, MO)—for a computer system, $5000.; Cardinal Ritter Institute Adult Day Care Ctr (Saint Louis, MO)—toward purchase of bus to transport elderly, $20,000.; Ctr for Environmental Studies, Mineral Area College (Park Hills, MO)—to support the environmental action plan, $10,000.
Date(s) Application is Due: Mar 15; Jun 15; Sep 15; Dec 15
Contact: Walter Staley, Jr., Secretary-Treasurer, (573) 581-5568; fax: (573) 581-1714; email: wstaley@greenfdn.org
Internet: http://www.greenfdn.org
Sponsor: Allen P. and Josephine B. Green Foundation
P.O. Box 523
Mexico, MO 65265

Alliance Healthcare Foundation Grants 362
The Foundation provides a public voice for the critical health care needs of its communities. Areas of interest include: Access to Health, Mental Health, Community Health, and HIV Health Care programs. Grants to local organizations support a wide range of programs and services. Priority is given to program and financing strategies that can produce discernible outcomes. All grant applicants should start by submitting a Letter of Intent (LOI), written and addressed according to the Foundation's guidelines. The LOI is the only form of application the Foundation accepts. Letters are reviewed on a monthly basis. Each is carefully evaluated by program staff in relation to other funding requests. Applicants will be notified about the results of the review within four to six weeks.
Restrictions: The Foundation does not fund projects and programs outside San Diego and Imperial Counties. In addition, the Foundation does not fund: research; lobbying; underwriting of medical expenses; general operating expenses we deem to be excessive; construction or renovation; the purchase of costly equipment; development activities, such as fundraising events, capital campaigns or annual fund drives; projects or proposals from individuals; or organizations that do not have 501(c)3 status.
Geographic Focus: California
Samples: Imperial County Office of Education (El Centro, CA)—to establish a family-resource center on the grounds of Seeley Elementary School, $450,000; Point Loma Nazarene U (San Diego, CA)—for its free clinic that provides health services to uninsured residents of San Diego's City Heights neighborhood, $122,880; Shakti Rising (San Diego, CA)—for strategic planning at this organization that uses holistic health practices and counseling to assist women struggling with abuse, addiction, and unhealthy relationships and behavior patterns, $159,415 over two yars;.
Contact: Karen Romero; (858) 614-4888; fax: (858) 874 3656; email: kromero@alliancehf.org;; Hamse Warfa, Program Officer; (858) 614-4892 or (858) 874-3788; fax: (858) 874-3656; email: hwarfa@alliancehf.org
Internet: http://www.alliancehf.org/grants_prog/what_we_fund/access_healthcare.html
Sponsor: Alliance Healthcare Foundation
9325 Sky Park Court, Suite 350
San Diego, CA 92123

Allstate Corporate Giving Grants 363
Allstate is a company of energized people with great ideas. The Corporate Giving program is committed to supporting the communities where company employees live and work by contributing to programs where its experience, partnership and leadership will have the greatest impact. The company offers financial support to a variety of programs and organizations throughout the country that help create strong and vital communities.
Requirements: The Allstate Corporation makes grants to nonprofit, tax-exempt groups under Section 501(c)3 of the Internal Revenue Code.

Contact: Executive Director; (847) 402-5000 or (847) 402-5502; fax: (847) 326-7517; email: allfound@allstate.com
Internet: http://www.allstate.com/social-responsibility/corporate/corporate-giving.aspx
Sponsor: Allstate Corporation
2775 Sanders Road, Suite F4
Northbrook, IL 60062

Allstate Corporate Hometown Commitment Grants 364

Allstate takes a special interest in the greater Chicagoland community, the company's hometown for more than 75 years. The corporation is particularly invested in this community because it recognizes that a thriving hometown is critical to Allstate's success. The company recruits local talent, relies on local infrastructure, and depends on the city's vibrancy to ensure that its associates have a rich quality of life. By supporting organizations that build strong Chicagoland communities, the company contributes to the city's position as a center of global culture, education and business.
Requirements: The Allstate Corporation makes grants to Chicago area nonprofit, tax-exempt groups under Section 501(c)3 of the Internal Revenue Code.
Geographic Focus: Illinois; Indiana
Samples: Chicago Children's Museum, Chicago, Illinois, $15,000,000 (2008).
Contact: Executive Director; (847) 402-5000 or (847) 402-5502; fax: (847) 326-7517; email: allfound@allstate.com
Internet: http://www.allstate.com/social-responsibility/corporate/corporate-giving.aspx
Sponsor: Allstate Corporation
2775 Sanders Road, Suite F4
Northbrook, IL 60062

Allyn Foundation Grants 365

The mission of the Allyn Foundation is to improve the quality of life in Central New York. To accomplish this, the foundation focuses its grant making in the following areas: health facilities and services: promote the delivery of quality health care in our communities; higher education in the Onondaga and Cayuga counties: expand access and success in education beyond high school, particularly for students of low income or other underrepresented backgrounds; basic human services: work to ensure that all people have basic daily needs of food, clothing, and shelter and enable the means to provide for themselves; family planning medical and educational services: promote education in family planning and improved access to service; quality of life for youth: improve quality of life for children and families through organizations that are focused on at risk youth and families.
Requirements: Nonprofit organizations in Onondaga and Cayuga Counties, NY, may submit grant applications.
Restrictions: Grants are not awarded for religious purposes, endowment funds, loans, or to individuals.
Geographic Focus: New York
Samples: Auburn Memorial Hospital, $350,000 (2008); Frank Hiscock Legal Aid Society, $18,000 (2008); Child Care Council of the Finger Lakes, $4,000 (2008).
Contact: Margaret O'Connell, Executive Director; (315) 685-5059; email: info@allynfoundation.org
Internet: http://www.allynfoundation.org/apply.html
Sponsor: Allyn Foundation
14 West Genesee Street, P.O. Box 22
Skaneateles, NY 13152

Alpha Omega Foundation Grants 366

The Foundation was established to advance the dental profession through research, grants, and scholarships. Fields of interest include: dental care, dental education, and medical research. Grants are given to individuals, program development, and higher education institutions. The application, which can be found at the web site, must be typed and submitted via email by September 1 each year. Notification will be completed by the following December.
Amount of Grant: $1,000-$36,000 range
Date(s) Application is Due: Sep 1
Contact: Ben Williamowsky; (877) 368-6326 or (301) 294-2773; fax: (301) 738-6403; email: bawilly@verizon.net or foundation@ao.org
Internet: http://www.ao.org/index.php?option=com_content&task=view&id=80&Itemid=147
Sponsor: Alpha Omega Foundation
50 W. Edmonston Drive, Suite 404
Rockville, MD 20852-1274

Alpha Research Foundation Grants 367

The primary purpose of the Foundation is to encourage and support biomedical research for the welfare of the general public. There are no specific deadlines or application formats with which to adhere. Applicants should contact the foundation prior to submission, in order to discuss their proposed project. If approved, applicants should then submit an outline of the proposed research along with a proposed budget.
Geographic Focus: Maryland
Amount of Grant: $2,000 maximum
Contact: Barry Rueben Fierst; (301) 762-8872; fax: (301) 762-8874; email: bfierst@aol.com
Sponsor: Alpha Research Foundation
7118 Glenbrook Road
Bethesda, MD 20814-1238

Alpine Winter Foundation Grants 368

Established in California in 1963, the Alpine Winter Foundation's primary purpose is to support alpine safety, health programs, and education within the Tahoe-Donner, California, region. Applications should be in the form of a written request, and should include the specific purpose and history of the requesting organization. There are no specific deadlines with which to adhere.
Requirements: Giving is limited to organizations described in Section 170(b)(1)(a) and Section 501(c)3(a) that promote alpine safety, heath, and education within the Tahoe-Donner area of California,
Geographic Focus: California
Samples: Donner Trail School, Soda Springs, California, $1,500—for winter survival training programs (2008); Sugar Bowl Ski Team Foundation, Norden, California, $37,500—for need-based scholarships and a building fund *2008).
Amount of Grant: $40,000 maximum
Contact: Mary S. Tilden, President; (415) 221-7762
Sponsor: Alpine Winter Foundation
P.O. Box 591659, 3863 Jackson Street
San Francisco, CA 94118-1610

ALSAM Foundation Grants 369

The foundation awards grants in its areas of interest, including agriculture, Christian agencies and churches, higher education, health care and medical research, human services, minorities, and the economically disadvantaged. Types of support include building construction/renovation, general operating costs, and scholarships. The board meets in January and October. Contact the office for application forms.
Requirements: Higher education institutions, nonprofit organizations, religious organizations, and research institutions are eligible.
Restrictions: No grants to individuals.
Samples: University of Utah, Moran Eye Center (Salt Lake City, UT)—for building fund, $2.5 million (2003); Saint George Catholic Church (Saint George, UT)—for building fund, $200,000 (2003); Harvard University (Cambridge, MA)—for research of Neurofibromatosis and Allied Disorders, $600,000.; Verbum Dei High School (Los Angeles, CA)—for conversion, $2,374,378.
Amount of Grant: $5000-$50,000 average
Contact: Ron Cutshall, Chair, (801) 266-4950
Sponsor: ALSAM Foundation
6190 Moffat Farm Lane
Salt Lake City, UT 84121

Alternatives Research and Development Foundation Alternatives in Education Grants 370

The mission of the Alternatives Research and Development Foundation is to fund and promote the development, validation and adoption of non-animal methods in biomedical research, product testing and education. ARDF has announced a special grant initiative seeking proposals to replace traditional use of animals for education and training purposes. Up to $10,000 in funding is available to support individual projects. the deadline for Letters of Intent is January 8, while invited full proposals are due March 12.
Requirements: Grants from the Foundation are made only to individuals affiliated with a non-profit, tax-exempt, institution, organization, or foreign equivalent.
Amount of Grant: $10,000 maximum
Date(s) Application is Due: Jan 8; Mar 12
Contact: Sue A. Leary, President and Executive Director; (215) 887-8076; fax: (215) 887-0771; email: grants@ardf-online.org or info@ardf-online.org
Internet: http://www.ardf-online.org/
Sponsor: Alternatives Research and Development Foundation
801 Old York Road, Suite 316
Jenkintown, PA 19046

Alternatives Research and Development Foundation Grants 371

The foundation awards grants to research centers, educational institutions, and other nonprofit organizations exploring non-animal testing. Grants will be awarded for research projects that use human, rather than nonhuman, vertebrae tissue; do not use intact, vertebrae animals; and can be completed within one year. Multiyear projects are considered on a case-by-case basis. The foundation often provides partial grants to initiate projects, with continuation funding available at a later date. The foundation will not consider proposals if program staff uses animals acquired from a shelter, or if individuals are employed who use such animals in their personal research programs. Winners are announced on July 15. Telephone inquiries are discouraged.
Requirements: Individuals attending or employed by U.S. universities and research institutions may apply. Applications from non-U.S. institutions or investigators may be considered.
Restrictions: The foundation does not make grants for in vitro projects that use nonhuman animal serum, indirect costs, purchase of personal computers, salary supplements, fringe benefits, travel expenses, or publication costs for the principal investigators. Phone calls to the foundation are discouraged. Guidelines and application are available online.
Samples: Dr. Anthony Hickey, School of Pharmacy, U of North Carolina at Chapel Hill (NC)—for research, Physiologically Relevant Lung Model of Regional Aerosol Deposition and Drug Transport Utilizing Human Respiratory Tract Cells.; Dr. Katherine Ralls, Department of Conservation Biology, Smithsonian Institution (Washington, DC)—for research, Dogs, Scats, and DNA: A Noninvasive Approach for Carnivore Field Studies.; Dr. Carol Reinisch, Marine Biological Laboratory (Woods Hole, MA)—for research, Regulation of p53 Gene Family Expression in Clam Leukemia Cells.;

Dr. Bingfang Yan, Department of Biomedical Sciences, U of Rhode Island (Kingston, RI)—for research, Prediction of Human CYP3A Induction by a Receptor-Activator Based Method.
Amount of Grant: $40,000 maximum
Date(s) Application is Due: Apr 30
Contact: Sue A. Leary, President and Executive Director; (215) 887-8076; fax: (215) 887-0771; email: grants@ardf-online.org or info@ardf-online.org
Internet: http://www.ardf-online.org
Sponsor: Alternatives Research and Development Foundation
801 Old York Road, Suite 316
Jenkintown, PA 19046

Altman Foundation Health Care Grants 372
The Altman Foundation's mission is to support programs, and institutions that enrich the quality of life in New York City, with a particular focus on initiatives that help individuals, families, and communities benefit from the services and opportunities that will enable them to achieve their full potential.
Requirements: IRS 501(c)3 organizations in New York are eligible.
Restrictions: Grants are not awarded to individuals. As a general rule, the foundation does not consider requests for bricks and mortar funds or the purchase of capital equipment.
Geographic Focus: New York
Samples: Literacy Assistance Venter, Inc., N.Y., $200,000 - to provide support for the Health Literacy Resource Center (2007); The Boys' Club of New York, N.Y., $50,000 - to renew support for the After School Academy (2007); The New York Community Trust, N.Y., to help support the New York City Workforce Development Funders Group $50,000 (2007).
Amount of Grant: $10,000-$100,000 average
Contact: Karen L. Rosa, Vice President and Executive Director; (212) 682-0970; email: krosa@altman.org
Internet: http://www.altmanfoundation.org/guide.html
Sponsor: Altman Foundation
521 Fifth Avenue, 35th Floor
New York, NY 10175

Alton Ochsner Award 373
The Award is presented to one or more clinical or basic science investigators, without regard to age, race, gender, or nationality, for outstanding and exemplary original scientific investigations that relate tobacco consumption and health. This scientific work may be clinical, fundamental, epidemiological or preventive in scope. The prime criterion for award selection is its scientific impact on this major health threat. The $15,000 award is presented at the Annual Convocation of the American College of Chest Physicians.
Requirements: All nominations, whatever the category of scientific inquiry, must be supported by letters and copies of peer-reviewed scientific publications.
Amount of Grant: $15,000
Date(s) Application is Due: Mar 31
Contact: Edward D. Frohlich, Alton Ochsner Distinguished Scientist, (504) 842-3000; fax: (504) 842-3258
Internet: http://www.ochsner.org/homepage.cfm
Sponsor: Ochsner Clinic Foundation
1514 Jefferson Highway
New Orleans, LA 70121

ALVRE Casselberry Award 374
The Casselberry Award has been established to encourage the advancement of the art and science of Laryngology and Rhinology. The award is given for outstanding manuscripts or accomplishments in Laryngology and Rhinology and consists of a $1,000 award and a certificate from the Association. Competition for this award will be limited to those persons whose abstracts are selected in consideration for inclusion in the Annual Scientific Program.
Amount of Grant: $1,000
Date(s) Application is Due: Nov 30
Contact: Maxine Cunningham, Administrator; (615) 322-6326; fax: (615) 322-9102; email: Maxine@alahns.org or ala-hns@comcast.net
Sponsor: American Laryngological Association / American Laryngological Voice and Research Education Foundation
1215 21st Avenue South, 7302 MCE South
Nashville, TN 37232-8783

ALVRE Grant 375
The purpose of this award is to support basic, translational, or clinical research projects in laryngology, voice, outcomes, and related subjects. Research supported by this award should be specifically directed toward the pathogenesis, pathophysiology, diagnosis, prevention, or treatment of diseases, disorders, or conditions of the larynx and may be either basic or clinical/translational in approach. While not specifically required, proposals which aim to introduce new knowledge and methodology from other disciplines to research in laryngology or neurolaryngology, or which demonstrate collaborative effort with members of other related disciplines are encouraged. Projects must be designed so as to yield useful information within the period of award, but priority will be given to projects that are also innovative with promise to develop into new long-range or expanded research programs capable of attracting funding from other sources. A single, one-year, non-renewable award of $25,000 maximum is available annually. The foundation will consider requests to cover travel expenses up to $1,000 for the principal investigator to present his/her results at the ALA annual meeting.
Requirements: Candidates for this award should be otolaryngologists in the U.S. or Canada who have completed their training at an ACGME accredited program in otolaryngology—head and neck surgery. The prinicipal investigator should be a physician faculty member of a recognized department, division, or section of otolaryngology-head and neck surgery.
Amount of Grant: $25,000 maximum
Contact: Maxine Cunningham, Administrator; (615) 322-6326; fax: (615) 322-9102; email: Maxine@alahns.org or ala-hns@comcast.net
Internet: http://www.entnet.org/EducationAndResearch/coreGrants.cfm
Sponsor: American Laryngological Association / American Laryngological Voice and Research Education Foundation
1215 21st Avenue South, 7302 MCE South
Nashville, TN 37232-8783

ALVRE Seymour R. Cohen Award 376
The Seymour R. Cohen Award was established with a bequest by the Cohen family during Dr. Cohen's presidency in 1989. In order to qualify for the Award, the candidate must perform basic science research in the area of pediatric laryngology and/or pediatric neurolaryngology and be a citizen of the United States or Canada. The material must be approved and accepted for presentation at the Annual Meeting. Should multiple candidates collaborate in the research, all authors must comply with the citizenship requirements. Dr. Cohen wishes this Award only to be used for the funding of research in pediatric laryngology and/or pediatric neurolaryngology. The Award is to be presented bi-annually.
Requirements: The scope of the Award is limited to citizens of the United States of America and Canada.
Contact: Maxine Cunningham, Administrator; (615) 322-6326; fax: (615) 322-9102; email: Maxine@alahns.org or ala-hns@comcast.net
Internet: http://www.alahns.org/i4a/pages/index.cfm?pageid=3332
Sponsor: American Laryngological Association / American Laryngological Voice and Research Education Foundation
1215 21st Avenue South, 7302 MCE South
Nashville, TN 37232-8783

Alzheimer's Association Everyday Technologies for Alzheimer Research Grants 377
Everyday Technologies for Alzheimer Care (ETAC) is a cooperative research funding initiative sponsored by the Alzheimer's Association and Intel Corporation. ETAC seeks proposals on personalized diagnostics, preventive tools and interventions for adults coping with the spectrum of cognitive aging and neurodegenerative disease, particularly Alzheimer's disease. ETAC is designed to support exploratory multidisciplinary research that would not typically be funded by national health and science granting foundations. Minor iterations in testing plans or populations will not be considered for funding. Collaboration between social science/medical/public health and computer science/engineering researchers is valued. Mobile computing, high bandwidth sensing, robotics, imaging, face recognition, natural language processing, statistical modeling and a host of other technology advances allow unprecedented opportunities to study disease progression and therapeutic strategies in the context of everyday life. ETAC supports research that integrates such emerging technology capabilities with leading directions in behavioral science and biomedical research. Grants that merely create Internet-based versions of existing services or paper tools will not be considered. Submissions must be original ideas, not continuations of previously funded ETAC projects. Please see links provided below for examples of studies that have been funded by ETAC. Letters of Intent (LOIs) must be received by December 1, with completed applications due by January 8.
Requirements: Researchers with full-time staff appointments are encouraged to apply.
Restrictions: The Alzheimer's Association will not accept new research grant applications from currently funded Alzheimer's disease investigators who are delinquent in submitting interim/final scientific or interim/final financial reports on active grants. ETAC applications from post-doctoral candidates will not be accepted.
Samples: Alex Mihailidis, Ph.D., University of Toronto, Toronto, Ontario, Canada—Toward a Pervasive Prompting System: Improving and Expanding the COACH, $196,324 over three years (2008); Arlene Astell, Ph.D., University of St. Andrews, St. Andrews, United Kingdom—Prompting to Support Independence in Dementia, $179,634 over two years (2008).
Amount of Grant: $200,000 maximum
Date(s) Application is Due: Dec 1; Jan 8
Contact: Nico Stanculescu; (312) 335-5747 or (312) 335-5729; fax: (312) 335-4034; email: Nico.Stanculescu@alz.org or grantsapp@alz.org
Internet: http://www.alz.org/professionals_and_researchers_everyday_technologies_for_alzheimer_care.asp
Sponsor: Alzheimer's Association
225 N. Michigan Avenue, Floor 17, Suite 1700
Chicago, IL 60601-7633

Alzheimer's Association Investigator-Initiated Research Grants 378
The program is structured to provide one to three years of sustained project support for independent, ongoing research. Proposals are solicited for basic, clinical, and social/behavioral research relevant to degenerative brain diseases such as Alzheimer's disease. Allowable costs for this award include the purchase and care of laboratory animals; small pieces of laboratory equipment and laboratory supplies; and salary for the principal investigator, scientific (including postdoctoral fellows) and technical staff (including laboratory technicians and modest secretarial support). It is required that most of the

funds awarded under this program be used for direct research support. Letters of Intent (LOIs) must be received by December 1, with completed applications by January 8.
Requirements: Public, private, domestic and foreign research laboratories, medical centers and hospitals, and universities are eligible to apply. Investigators from all stages of their research career development are encouraged to apply.
Restrictions: This program does not support travel to scientific and professional meetings, computer hardware or software, or construction or renovation costs.
Samples: Mathieu Lesort, Ph.D., University of Alabama at Birmingham, Birmingham, Alabama—Pathological Interactions in Diabetes and Alzheimer's Disease, $200,000 over three years (2008); David H. Cribbs, Ph.D., University of California, Irvine, Irvine, California—Reducing the Risk of Cerebral Vascular Adverse Events in Alzheimer's Disease, $240,000 over three years (2008).
Amount of Grant: $240,000 total for up to three years; $100,000 maximum per year
Date(s) Application is Due: Dec 1; Jan 8
Contact: Nico Stanculescu; (312) 335-5747 or (312) 335-5729; fax: (312) 335-4034; email: Nico.Stanculescu@alz.org or grantsapp@alz.org
Internet: http://www.alz.org/professionals_and_researchers_investigatorinitiated.asp
Sponsor: Alzheimer's Association
225 N. Michigan Avenue, Floor 17, Suite 1700
Chicago, IL 60601-7633

Alzheimer's Association Mentored New Investigator Research Grants to Promote Diversity 379
The Mentored New Investigator Research Grant to Promote Diversity (MNIGD) is a three-year award intended to be a research-based and mentoring investment in the process of closing the health disparities gap between diverse and non-diverse investigator populations. The Alzheimer's Association feels strongly that the mentoring and involvement of diverse researchers in independently funded Alzheimer's research is a pressing need. The MNIRGD is intended to enhance the capacity of diverse and non-diverse scientists to conduct basic, clinical and social/behavioral research. Each MNIRGD award is limited to $170,000. A total of $150,000 will be awarded for costs related to the proposed research for up to three years (direct and indirect costs). Letters of Intent must be received by December 1, with completed applications due by January 8.
Requirements: Eligibility for this grant competition is restricted to investigators who have less than 10 years of research experience after receipt of their terminal degree.
Amount of Grant: $170,000 maximum
Date(s) Application is Due: Dec 1; Jan 8
Contact: Nico Stanculescu; (312) 335-5747 or (312) 335-5729; fax: (312) 335-4034; email: Nico.Stanculescu@alz.org or grantsapp@alz.org
Internet: http://www.alz.org/professionals_and_researchers_mentored_new_investigator_promote_diversity_grant.asp
Sponsor: Alzheimer's Association
225 N. Michigan Avenue, Floor 17, Suite 1700
Chicago, IL 60601-7633

Alzheimer's Association Molecular Imaging Grants 380
The Alzheimer's Association is launching an initiative to stimulate further research and development of new approaches to image molecular changes associated with early neurodegenerative processes in living humans, animal models and cells. The Association's Request for Applications (RFAs) is aimed at supporting new high-risk exploratory approaches to stimulate new directions of research in molecular imaging. The RFA is designed to enable preliminary pilot research or proof-of-principle studies that can provide data for further research support by other funding agencies. The Association anticipates funding up to 3 Molecular Imaging awards. Each award is limited to $400,000 (direct and indirect costs) for two to three years. Letters of Intent (LOIs) must be received by December 1, with completed applications due by January 8.
Requirements: Researchers with full-time staff or faculty appointments are encouraged to apply. Molecular Imaging applications from post-doctoral candidates will not be accepted.
Amount of Grant: $400,000 (direct and indirect costs) for two to three years
Date(s) Application is Due: Dec 1; Jan 8
Contact: Nico Stanculescu; (312) 335-5747 or (312) 335-5729; fax: (312) 335-4034; email: Nico.Stanculescu@alz.org or grantsapp@alz.org
Internet: http://www.alz.org/professionals_and_researchers_molecular_imaging_grant.asp
Sponsor: Alzheimer's Association
225 N. Michigan Avenue, Floor 17, Suite 1700
Chicago, IL 60601-7633

Alzheimer's Association New Investigator Research Grants 381
The purpose of this program is to provide new investigators with funding that will allow them to develop preliminary or pilot data, to test procedures, and develop hypotheses which will then underpin the preparation of research grant applications to NIH, NSF, and other funding agencies and groups, including the Alzheimer's Association. All applications submitted to the program must focus on a question or questions in interventions for Alzheimer's disease to be considered responsive to the program announcement. Thirty awards will be made under this program. Letters of Intent (LOIs) must be received by December 1, with completed applications due by January 8.
Requirements: Public, private, domestic and foreign research laboratories, medical centers and hospitals, and universities are eligible to apply. Eligibility is restricted to investigators who have less than 10 years of research experience, including postdoctoral fellowships or residencies, after receipt of the doctoral degree. Applications from graduate and doctoral students for research projects will be accepted.
Samples: Valentina Echeverria Moran, Ph.D., Bay Pines Foundation, Bay Pines, Florida— Molecular Mechanisms Underlying the Neuroprotective Actions of Cotinine, $100,000 over two years (2008); Grace Stutzmann, Ph.D., Rosalind Franklin University of Medicine and Science, North Chicago, Illinois—Neuronal Ca2+ Dysregulation as a Pathogenic Factor in Alzheimer's Disease, $100,000 over two years (2008).
Amount of Grant: $100,000 maximum for two years; $60,000 maximum per year
Date(s) Application is Due: Dec 1; Jan 8
Contact: Nico Stanculescu; (312) 335-5747 or (312) 335-5729; fax: (312) 335-4034; email: Nico.Stanculescu@alz.org or grantsapp@alz.org
Internet: http://www.alz.org/professionals_and_researchers_new_investigator_research_grants.asp
Sponsor: Alzheimer's Association
225 N. Michigan Avenue, Floor 17, Suite 1700
Chicago, IL 60601-7633

Alzheimer's Association New Investigator Research Grants to Promote Diversity 382
The New Investigator Research Grant to Promote Diversity (NIRGD) in Alzheimer's research is a two-year award to investigators who are currently underrepresented at academic institutions in Alzheimer's or related dementias research. The objective of this award is to increase the number of highly trained investigators from diverse backgrounds whose basic, clinical and social/behavioral research interests are grounded in the advanced methods and experimental approaches needed to solve problems related to Alzheimer's and related dementias in general and in health disparities populations. Each NIRGD award is limited to $100,000 (direct and indirect costs) for up to two years. Requests in any given year may not exceed $60,000 (direct and indirect costs). Letters of Intent (LOIs) must be received by December 1, with completed applications due by January 8.
Requirements: Eligibility to apply is restricted to investigators who have less than 10 years of research experience after receipt of their terminal degree.
Amount of Grant: $60,000 maximum per year; $100,000 for two years
Date(s) Application is Due: Dec 1; Jan 8
Contact: Nico Stanculescu; (312) 335-5747 or (312) 335-5729; fax: (312) 335-4034; email: Nico.Stanculescu@alz.org or grantsapp@alz.org
Internet: http://www.alz.org/professionals_and_researchers_new_investigator_promote_diversity_grant.asp
Sponsor: Alzheimer's Association
225 N. Michigan Avenue, Floor 17, Suite 1700
Chicago, IL 60601-7633

Alzheimer's Association Senator Mark Hatfield Award 383
The Hatfield Award is aimed at those investigators whose goal is to establish research careers focused on clinical issues in Alzheimer's disease. The Alzheimer's Association recognizes the need to increase the number of scientists from underrepresented groups in the research enterprise. Researchers from these groups are encouraged to apply. The Association anticipates funding one award under this program. The total award is limited to $225,000 (direct and indirect costs) for up to three years. Requests in any given year may not exceed $112,500 (direct and indirect costs). Indirect costs are capped at 10 percent (rent for laboratory/office space is expected to be covered by indirect costs paid to the institution). Letters of Intent (LOIs) must be received by December 1, with completed applications due by January 8.
Requirements: It is required that most of the funds awarded under this program be used for direct research support.
Samples: Ken A. Paller, Ph.D., Northwestern University, Evanston, Illinois—Memory Processing During Sleep in Alzheimer's Disease, $240,000 over three years (2008).
Amount of Grant: $225,000 maximum
Date(s) Application is Due: Dec 1; Jan 8
Contact: Nico Stanculescu; (312) 335-5747 or (312) 335-5729; fax: (312) 335-4034; email: Nico.Stanculescu@alz.org or grantsapp@alz.org
Internet: http://www.alz.org/professionals_and_researchers_mark_hatfield_award.asp
Sponsor: Alzheimer's Association
225 N. Michigan Avenue, Floor 17, Suite 1700
Chicago, IL 60601-7633

Alzheimer's Association Zenith Fellows Awards 384
Five awards will be granted to talented scientists who have already contributed substantially to the advancement of Alzheimer's research and who are likely to continue to make significant contributions for many years. Proposals are solicited for basic, biomedical research only, and research should address fundamental problems related to early detection, etiology, pathogenesis, treatment, and prevention of Alzheimer's disease. Awardees receive a two-year grant, with a provision for possible competitive renewal upon review of research progress. Applications will be evaluated by an expert panel of senior scientists, already well recognized for their own accomplishments in Alzheimer's research. Letters of Intent (LOIs) must be received by December 1, with completed applications due by January 8.
Requirements: Only established independent investigators are eligible as evidenced by (examples are for illustrative purposes only) academic appointment; major, peer-reviewed, external multi-year grant support on which the applicant is the principal investigator (PI); independent laboratory operation; and quality and independence of publication record.
Restrictions: Previous recipients of Zenith Awards, Alzheimer's Disease Center Directors (P50 and P30), Medical and Scientific Advisory Council, and members of the National Board of the Alzheimer's Association are not eligible to apply.

Samples: Mary Jo LaDu, Ph.D., University of Illinois, Chicago, Illinois—The Effect of ApoE Isoform on Intraneuronal ApoE/Abeta42 Interactions, $450,000 over three years (2008); Michael S. Wolfe, Ph.D., Brigham and Women's Hospital, Boston, Massachusetts—Regulation of RNA Splicing in Alzheimer's and Related Dementias, $450,000 over three years (2008).
Amount of Grant: $250,000 maximum for two years; $150,000 maximum for one year
Date(s) Application is Due: Dec 1; Jan 8
Contact: Nico Stanculescu; (312) 335-5747 or (312) 335-5729; fax: (312) 335-4034; email: Nico.Stanculescu@alz.org or grantsapp@alz.org
Internet: http://www.alz.org/professionals_and_researchers_zenith.asp
Sponsor: Alzheimer's Association
225 N. Michigan Avenue, Floor 17, Suite 1700
Chicago, IL 60601-7633

Alzheimer's Association Conference Grants 385

The Alzheimer's Association has a long history of supporting scientific conferences that advance research on Alzheimer's disease. One of the principal goals of the Association from its inception has been to increase public awareness and to facilitate the exchange of information through the scientific and clinical communities. The support of conferences, workshops and meetings has been a key vehicle in achieving this goal. The objectives for conference support are to: facilitate and speed the exchange of information relevant to Alzheimer's disease research; convene experts to address emerging issues in Alzheimer's disease research; offer opportunities for new investigators and graduate students to participate in scientific meetings; facilitate the creation of networks among investigators in related areas; and increase visibility of the research interests and programs of the Alzheimer's Association.
Requirements: Requests for conference support may be submitted at any time. It is recommended that requests be submitted at least three months before the conference.
Amount of Grant: $10,000 maximum
Contact: Rachel Souris; (312) 335-5807; fax: (312) 335-4034; email: rachel.souris@alz.org
Internet: http://www.alz.org/professionals_and_researchers_conference_grants.asp
Sponsor: Alzheimer's Association
225 N. Michigan Avenue, Floor 17, Suite 1700
Chicago, IL 60601-7633

AMA Foundation Arthur N. Wilson, MD, Scholarship 386

The Arthur N. Wilson, MD Scholarship provides a $5,000 tuition assistance scholarship to a currently enrolled medical student who graduated from a high school in Southeast Alaska. This scholarship highlights the importance of supporting future physicians in rural communities. The majority of Southeast Alaska is part of the Tongass National Forest, the United States' largest national forest. Major cities are Juneau, Sitka, and Ketchikan. Due to the rural nature of Southeast Alaska, many communities have no road connections, so aircraft and boats are a major means of transport.
Geographic Focus: Alaska
Amount of Grant: $5,000
Date(s) Application is Due: Jun 15
Contact: Steven W. Churchill, Executive Director; (312) 464-4200; fax: (312) 464-4142; email: Steven.Churchill@ama-assn.org
Internet: http://www.ama-assn.org/ama/pub/about-ama/ama-foundation/our-programs/medical-education/arthur-n-wilson.shtml
Sponsor: American Medical Association Foundation
515 N. State Street
Chicago, IL 60654

AMA Foundation Dr. Nathan Davis International Awards in Medicine 387

Named for the founder of the AMA, the Dr. Nathan Davis International Award in Medicine recognizes physicians whose influence reach the international patient population and change the future of their medical care. By treating, educating and counseling patients beyond the U.S. border, the physician's work is having a positive impact on health care in the global arena. A $2,500 grant will be given to the institution or organization with which the recipient works. The recipient will also receive travel expenses and accommodations to the Excellence in Medicine Awards Banquet, and the AMA National Advocacy Conference in Washington D.C.
Requirements: To qualify, nominees must: have improved dramatically medical practice, medical education or medical research outside of the United States; embody the values of the medical profession through leadership, service, excellence, integrity and ethical behavior; during a lifetime of service or in a current initiative, has benefited the health and well-being of a specific patient population.
Amount of Grant: 2,500
Date(s) Application is Due: Nov 16
Contact: Steven W. Churchill, Director; (312) 464-2593 or (312) 464-4200; fax: (312) 464-4142; email: Steven.Churchill@ama-assn.org or amafoundation@ama-assn.org
Internet: http://www.ama-assn.org/ama/pub/about-ama/ama-foundation/our-programs/public-health/excellence-medicine-awards.shtml
Sponsor: American Medical Association Foundation
515 N. State Street
Chicago, IL 60654

AMA Foundation Fund for Better Health Grants 388

The philosophy of the AMA Foundation Fund for Better Health begins with the idea that local communities and organizations have great knowledge and insight into their community's health care issues. Based on this thought, the AMA Foundation, with support from the AMA Alliance, created the Fund for Better Health. Through this program, the AMA Foundation provides seed grants for grassroots, public health projects in communities throughout America. Over the years, the fund has provided over 200 grants totaling nearly $300,000 to projects that address healthy lifestyles, domestic violence prevention, substance abuse prevention, health literacy, patient safety and care for the uninsured. A maximum of $5,000 will be distributed to each grant recipient. The number of grant recipients will be determined by the AMA Foundation after all applications have been received. Typically, the number of grants awarded does not exceed twenty.
Requirements: Organizations are eligible to apply for grants which further the charitable and educational purposes of the AMA Foundation. Grants made in 2009 support programs addressing the issue of healthy lifestyles in the areas of nutrition and physical fitness, alcohol, substance abuse and smoking prevention (and cessation), and violence prevention. The three types of organizations eligible to apply are organizations with annual operating budgets of $1 million or less; new organizations begun in the last 5 years; or established organizations starting a new service or expanding a current service to an underserved population.
Restrictions: None of the funds awarded are to pay for staff salary or overhead expenses.
Amount of Grant: $5,000 maximum
Date(s) Application is Due: Jul 15
Contact: Dina Lindenberg, Program Officer; (312) 464-4193; email: dina.lindenberg@ama-assn.org
Internet: http://www.ama-assn.org/ama/pub/about-ama/ama-foundation/our-programs/public-health/fund-better-health.shtml
Sponsor: American Medical Association Foundation
515 N. State Street
Chicago, IL 60654

AMA Foundation Health Literacy Grants 389

The foundation awards grants to programs that promote clearer communication between patients and their physicians and other health care providers. They are given to four groups: medical students; residents and fellows; physicians, hospital staffs and medical societies; and AMA Alliance groups and community organizations.
Amount of Grant: $500-$4,000
Contact: Steven W. Churchill, Executive Director; (312) 464-2593 or (312) 464-4200; fax: (312) 464-4142; email: Steven.Churchill@ama-assn.org or healthliteracy@ama-assn.org
Internet: http://www.ama-assn.org/ama/pub/about-ama/ama-foundation/our-programs/public-health/health-literacy-program.shtml
Sponsor: American Medical Association Foundation
515 N. State Street
Chicago, IL 60654

AMA Foundation Healthy Communities/Healthy America Grants 390

Through the Healthy Communities/Healthy America program, the AMA Foundation awards $10,000-$25,000 grants to physician-led free clinics. Grants will be awarded to free clinics that: are requesting funds for specific projects, not for activities such as routine operations, maintenance or facility repairs; have regular and considerable operating hours; have significant physician involvement; and provide medical services. Preference will be given to applicants who demonstrate how grant dollars will be leveraged to provide the greatest amount of care.
Restrictions: Clinics that provide both medical and dental services, but are requesting funds for a project that is dental care-specific will not be considered.
Amount of Grant: $10,000-$25,000 range
Contact: Steven W. Churchill, Executive Director; (312) 464-2593 or (312) 464-4200; fax: (312) 464-4142; email: Steven.Churchill@ama-assn.org or healthliteracy@ama-assn.org
Internet: http://www.ama-assn.org/ama/pub/about-ama/ama-foundation/our-programs/public-health/healthy-communities-healthy.shtml
Sponsor: American Medical Association Foundation
515 N. State Street
Chicago, IL 60654

AMA Foundation Jack B. McConnell, MD Awards for Excellence in Volunteerism 391

The Jack B. McConnell, MD, Award for Excellence in Volunteerism recognizes the work of senior physicians who provides treatment to U.S. patients who lack access to health care. After a full career of practice, these physicians remain dedicated to the future of medicine through the spirit of volunteerism. A $2,500 grant will be given to the institution or organization with which the recipient works. The recipient will also receive travel expenses and accommodations to the Excellence in Medicine Awards Banquet, and the AMA National Advocacy Conference in Washington D.C.
Requirements: To qualify, nominees must: have volunteered a significant portion of their medical services while over the age of 55; demonstrate their commitment to health care access by assisting underserved U.S. patients.
Amount of Grant: $2,500
Date(s) Application is Due: Nov 16
Contact: Steven W. Churchill, Director; (312) 464-2593 or (312) 464-4200; fax: (312) 464-4142; email: Steven.Churchill@ama-assn.org or amafoundation@ama-assn.org
Internet: http://www.ama-assn.org/ama/pub/about-ama/ama-foundation/our-programs/public-health/excellence-medicine-awards.shtml
Sponsor: American Medical Association Foundation
515 N. State Street
CHicago, IL 60654

AMA Foundation Joan F. Giambalvo Memorial Scholarships 392

The American Medical Association (AMA) Women Physicians Congress (WPC) has established the Joan F. Giambalvo Memorial Scholarship Fund and partners with the AMA Foundation with the goal of advancing the progress of women in the medical profession and strengthening the AMA's ability to identify and address the needs and interests of women physicians and medical students.

Requirements: Applicants shall be: Female or male; Working alone or collaboratively on the specific research project; Physicians, medical students, other health professionals, or individuals working or doing graduate work in an applicable profession such as public health, sociology, psychology, etc. Proposals will be evaluated and awardee(s) selected based on a variety of factors, including, but not limited to: the innovation, quality and/or feasibility of the idea; project/research methodology; potential to produce action, change or more comprehensive studies; and career goals of the applicant. AMA membership is not required in order to be eligible for this award.

Restrictions: Members of the AMA-WPC Governing Council, AMA Foundation Board of Directors, AMA Board of Trustees and Joan F. Giambalvo Memorial Scholarship Fund selection committee, and AMA and AMA Foundation staff are not eligible for this award.

Samples: 2008 Recipients: Sue Yom, MD, PhD, Assistant Professor of Radiation Oncology at the University of California San Francisco.; Maurice Clifton, MD, MSEd, Associate Dean for Admissions and Student Affairs with the Mercer University School of Medicine.

Amount of Grant: $10,000 maximum

Date(s) Application is Due: Feb 15

Contact: Alice Reed; (312) 464-5523; email: alice.reed@ama-assn.org

Internet: http://www.ama-assn.org/ama/pub/category/15566.html

Sponsor: American Medical Association Foundation
515 N. State Street
Chicago, IL 60654

AMA Foundation Jordan Fieldman, MD, Awards 393

The Jordan Fieldman, MD Award was established in the name of Dr. Jordan Fieldman and is sponsored by the AMA Resident and Fellow Section in association with the AMA Foundation. Dr. Jordan Fieldman was an outstanding physician and deeply concerned with helping his patients and making the world of medicine a better place. Unfortunately, Jordan lost his battle with cancer in June 2004. In establishing this award, the AMA-RFS desires to continue to create physicians like Dr. Fieldman and give them the skills and means to do so. The award money will cover resident travel to both the Annual and Interim meeting during the year of the award and necessary expenses while attending these meetings. This award will give a young doctor an opportunity that he or she may otherwise never be able to experience.

Requirements: The Awardee must be: a first-time delegate or attendee to the AMA-RFS meetings; from a state or district that does not have funding available to support resident or fellow travel to attend the AMA-RFS Meetings; interested and active in patient advocacy efforts; involved in organized medicine. Additional guidelines, as well as, an online application are available at, http://www.ama-assn.org/ama/pub/about-ama/ama-foundation/our-programs/public-health/jordan-fieldman-md.shtml.

Contact: Sharyn Grose, Program Administrator; (312) 464-4978 or (800) 621-8335; fax: (312) 464-5845; email: sharyn.grose@ama-assn.org or rfs@ama-assn.org

Internet: http://www.ama-assn.org/ama/pub/about-ama/ama-foundation/our-programs/public-health/jordan-fieldman-md.shtml

Sponsor: American Medical Association Foundation
515 N. State Street
CHicago, IL 60654

AMA Foundation Leadership Awards 394

An exceptional medical professional goes beyond the medical practice to positively influence health care. Through organized medicine and community activities, individuals from each stage of the physician lifecycle can, and do, make a difference in the quality of health care and the medical environment. The Leadership Awards are presented to 15 medical students, 10 residents/fellows and 5 early career physicians to recognize their strong, nonclinical leadership skills in advocacy, community service and/or education. Award recipients will be invited to attend leadership development training in Washington, D.C. This training will strengthen leadership skills and result in a greater effort to advance health care in America. Directly following the training, recipients will attend the Excellence in Medicine Awards Banquet and stay for the AMA National Advocacy Conference. Airfare and accommodations are provided, in addition to a nominal reimbursement to help defray additional travel-related costs.

Requirements: All Leadership Awards are self-nominated, with applicants responsible for submitting all appropriate materials and documentation. To qualify, applicants must demonstrate outstanding leadership in the areas of advocacy, community service and/or education and be either: a medical student enrolled in an accredited medical school; a resident physician enrolled in an accredited residency program; a fellow physician enrolled in a fellowship program; an early-career physician under the age of 40 or in his or her first eight years of practice following residency/fellowship.

Date(s) Application is Due: Nov 16

Contact: Steven W. Churchill, Director; (312) 464-2593 or (312) 464-4200; fax: (312) 464-4142; email: Steven.Churchill@ama-assn.org or amafoundation@ama-assn.org

Internet: http://www.ama-assn.org/ama/pub/about-ama/ama-foundation/our-programs/public-health/excellence-medicine-awards.shtml

Sponsor: American Medical Association Foundation
515 N. State Street
CHicago, IL 60654

AMA Foundation Minority Scholars Awards 395

The AMA Foundation, in collaboration with the AMA Minority Affairs Consortium (MAC), with support from Pfizer Inc, offers the Minority Scholars Award. Approximately twelve Minority Scholars Awards are awarded annually, each in the amount of a $10,000 scholarship.

Requirements: You must be a current first or second-year student and a permanent resident or citizen of the U.S. Eligible students of minority background include African American/Black, American Indian, Native Hawaiian, Alaska Native and Hispanic/Latino. Each medical school is invited to submit up to two nominees. Contact your medical school if you are interested in being nominated for the Minority Scholars Award.

Samples: 2007 Recipients: Chuck Branch, University of Minnesota Medical School, Duluth.; Michael Nevarez, Harvard Medical School.

Amount of Grant: $10,000

Date(s) Application is Due: Apr 15

Contact: Steven W. Churchill, Executive Director; (312) 464-4200; fax: (312) 464-4142; email: Steven.Churchill@ama-assn.org

Internet: http://www.ama-assn.org/ama/pub/category/20116.html

Sponsor: American Medical Association Foundation
515 N. State Street
Chicago, IL 60654

AMA Foundation Physicians of Tomorrow Scholarships 396

These $10,000 scholarships reward current third-year medical students, who are entering their fourth-year of study. There will be 12 Physicians of Tomorrow scholarships funded by the AMA Foundation. Multiple scholarships, funded by the AMA Foundation, the Audio-Digest Foundation and the Johnson F. Hammond, MD Fund will be awarded in 2009.

Requirements: The selection of the recipients will be based on academic achievement and financial need. The recipient of the one Physicians of Tomorrow Scholarship funded by the Audio-Digest Foundation should have an interest in 'the communication of science.' Activities such as mentoring and/or teaching are examples of 'communication of science.' The recipient of the one Physicians of Tomorrow Scholarship funded by the Johnson F. Hammond, MD Fund should have an interest in and commitment to a career in medical journalism. Contact your medical school if you are interested in being nominated for the Physicians of Tomorrow Scholarships. Each medical school may submit one nomination for each of these scholarship opportunities. Thus, each school may submit up to three nominations in total.

Samples: 2008: Puya Alikhani, Texas A&M Health Science Center College of Medicine.; Diana Badillo, Stanford University School of Medicine.; Andrew Barina, Saint Louis University School of Medicine.; Karl Bezak, Vanderbilt University School of Medicine.; Rozalina Grubina, Johns Hopkins University School of Medicine.; Nadia Hernandez, University of Texas Health Science Center at Houston.; Stephanie Hu, Harvard Medical School.; Arman Kilic, University of Pittsburgh School of Medicine.; Youssra Marjoua, Yale University School of Medicine.; Monica Patton, University of Vermont College of Medicine.; Janae Phelps, Howard University College of Medicine.; Dominic Sanford, University of Missouri Columbia.; Javay Ross, Charles Drew University/UCLA Medical Education Program.; Matthew Bivens, George Washington University School of Medicine and Health Sciences.; Helena Hart, University of California, San Francisco School of Medicine.

Amount of Grant: $10,000

Date(s) Application is Due: May 29

Contact: Steven W. Churchill, Executive Director; (312) 464-4200; fax: (312) 464-4142; email: Steven.Churchill@ama-assn.org

Internet: http://www.ama-assn.org/ama/pub/category/20119.html

Sponsor: American Medical Association Foundation
515 N. State Street
Chicago, IL 60654

AMA Foundation Pride in the Profession Grants 397

The Pride in the Profession Awards honor physicians whose lives encompass the true spirit of being a medical professional: caring for people. By practicing medicine in areas of challenge or crisis, or by devoting their time to volunteerism or public service, these physicians serve as the voice of patients in the United States who otherwise might not be heard. A $2,500 grant will be given to the institution or organization with which the recipient works. The recipient will also receive travel expenses and accommodations to the Excellence in Medicine Awards banquet, and the AMA National Advocacy Conference in Washington D.C.

Requirements: To qualify, nominees must: promote the art and science of medicine and the betterment of the public health; embody the values of the medical profession through leadership, service, excellence, integrity and ethical behavior; enrich patients, colleagues and the community through dedicated medical practice or service; offer better access to quality health care for an underserved patient population in the U.S.

Amount of Grant: $2,500

Date(s) Application is Due: Nov 16

Contact: Steven W. Churchill, Director; (312) 464-2593 or (312) 464-4200; fax: (312) 464-4142; email: Steven.Churchill@ama-assn.org or amafoundation@ama-assn.org

Internet: http://www.ama-assn.org/ama/pub/about-ama/ama-foundation/our-programs/public-health/excellence-medicine-awards.shtml

Sponsor: American Medical Association Foundation
515 N. State Street
Chicago, IL 60654

AMA Foundation Seed Grants for Research 398

The AMA Foundation established the Seed Grant Research Program to encourage medical students, physician residents and fellows to enter the research field. The program provides $2,500-$5,000 grants to help them conduct small basic science, applied, or clinical research projects. These funds will round out new project budgets, rather than sustain current initiatives. One-year grants will be awarded in the following research categories: Cardiovascular/pulmonary diseases; HIV/AIDS; Leukemia; Neoplastic diseases; Secondhand smoke. Grants in Cardiovascular/Pulmonary Diseases, HIV/AIDS, Leukemia, and Neoplastic Diseases will be $2,500. Grants in the Secondhand smoke category will be $5,000.
Requirements: Applicants must be a medical student, physician resident or fellow of an accredited U.S. medical school or institution; they must also be either a U.S. citizen or a permanent resident of the U.S.. Projects must be applicant-conceived, rather than ongoing research of their mentor or Principal Investigator.
Restrictions: Seed grant funds cannot be used for salary or stipend, indirect/administrative costs, to hire a consultant or contractor, and solely for travel expenses. Seed grants will not be awarded to any applicant who has previously received an AMA Foundation seed grant in the research category in which they are applying.
Amount of Grant: $2,500 - $5,000
Date(s) Application is Due: Dec 15
Contact: Seed Grants Program; (312) 464-4200; fax: (312) 464-5973; email: seedgrants@ama-assn.org
Internet: http://www.ama-assn.org/ama/pub/category/7785.html
Sponsor: American Medical Association Foundation
515 N. State Street
Chicago, IL 60654

AMA Foundation Worldscopes Program 399

WorldScopes collects stethoscopes from U.S. physicians and distributes them, with the help of humanitarian organizations, to communities around the world where medical supplies are scarce. A stethoscope donation will help a colleague in diagnosing and treating diseases that deprive so many of health, life, and human dignity.
Contact: Ethical Force Program Office; (312) 464-4075; fax: (312) 464-4799; email: WorldScopes@ama-assn.org
Internet: http://www.ama-assn.org/ama/pub/category/12768.html
Sponsor: American Medical Association Foundation
515 N. State Street
Chicago, IL 60654

AMA Virtual Mentor Theme Issue Editor Grants 400

Virtual Mentor [www.virtualmentor.org] is the American Medical Association's online ethics journal. Its mission is to promote the ethical and professional development of tomorrow's physicians, and its primary audiences are medical students, residents, other physicians, and medical educators. VM serves as an educational resource for a rapidly growing number of readers. VM invites medical students and residents to apply to serve as theme issue editors. Each theme issue editor undertakes, with help from VM staff editors, responsibility for: (1) selecting a theme for one issue and defining the ethical and professionalism concerns inherent in that theme, (2) generating case narratives that provide opportunities for examining those concerns in clinical and educational contexts, (3) identifying, securing, and corresponding with contributors to the issue, (4) editing copy and reviewing page proofs before the issue goes live on the first working day of the month. These tasks will be accomplished at each editor's "home" location. Theme issue editors, selected in late November, will be flown to Chicago to meet with Virtual Mentor staff some time in February. Each theme issue editor receives a $1,000-stipend.
Requirements: Experience in editing or journalism is desirable. The abilities to critique an argument or article, work well with authors, and meet deadlines are essential. To apply, send a short letter stating your current medical student or resident program status and your reason for wishing to be a theme issue editor for VM. Attach to the letter, the following: a curriculum vitae; a writing sample of not more than 1,000 words; your response to this exercise in 500 words or fewer. Additional guidelines available at: http://virtualmentor.ama-assn.org/site/issue-edscall.html. Send your letter of application and attachments by email to: Faith.Lagay@ama-assn.org. The deadline for applications is midnight CST on November 13.
Amount of Grant: $1,000 stipend
Date(s) Application is Due: Nov 13
Contact: Faith Lagay, Managing Editor of the Virtual Mentor Staff; (312) 464-5438 or (312) 464-5260; fax: (312) 464-4799; email: Faith.Lagay@ama-assn.org or virtualmentor@ama-assn.org
Internet: http://www.ama-assn.org/ama/pub/about-ama/our-people/member-groups-sections/medical-student-section/opportunities/internships-fellowships.shtml
Sponsor: American Medical Association
515 N. State Street
Chicago, IL 60654

AMA-MSS Chapter Involvement Grants 401

The AMA-MSS Chapter Involvement Grant (CIG) Program provides each MSS chapter with up to $1,000 per academic year for chapter activities including recruitment and retention, chapter development, education, and community service events. A maximum of $250 or $500 is available for each event, depending on the type of event. Applications are due at least 30 days prior to the event.
Amount of Grant: $250-$500 range per event
Contact: Rebecca Gierhahn, Director; (800) 262-3211 ext. 4753; email: rebecca.gierhahn@ama-assn.org or mss@ama-assn.org
Internet: http://www.ama-assn.org/ama/pub/about-ama/our-people/member-groups-sections/medical-student-section/opportunities/grants-awards-scholarships.shtml
Sponsor: American Medical Association - Department of Medical Student Services
515 N. State Street
Chicago, IL 60654

AMA-MSS Chapter of the Year (COTY) Award 402

The AMA-MSS Chapter of the Year (COTY) Award recognizes the true strength of the AMA-MSS organization, the local chapters. Applicant chapters are judged in a number of areas, including membership, community service, advocacy, innovation, and collaboration. The winning chapter is awarded a $500 grant to be used toward chapter activities and is recognized at the MSS Annual Meeting. All MSS chapters are encouraged to apply.
Samples: University of Texas Medical School at Houston (2008); University of Arkansas for Medical Sciences College of Medicine (2007).
Amount of Grant: $500
Date(s) Application is Due: Apr 30
Contact: Rebecca Gierhahn, Director; (800) 262-3211 ext. 4753; email: rebecca.gierhahn@ama-assn.org or mss@ama-assn.org
Internet: http://www.ama-assn.org/ama/pub/about-ama/our-people/member-groups-sections/medical-student-section/opportunities/grants-awards-scholarships.shtml
Sponsor: American Medical Association - Department of Medical Student Services
515 N. State Street
Chicago, IL 60654

AMA-MSS Government Relations Advocacy Fellowship 403

The AMA-MSS Government Relations Advocacy Fellowship (GRAF) for medical students is currently in its fifth year. One Fellow is selected each spring to work in Washington, D.C., as a full-time paid member of the AMA's Federal advocacy team for one year. The Fellow is responsible for working with the AMA's federal advocacy team to advance the Association's legislative agenda and policies on behalf of physicians, patients and medical students. A key goal for the fellowship is to educate medical student, resident and young physician AMA members about issues in public health and health policy in order to encourage activism and leadership in local communities. Applicants are not expected to be proficient advocates and managers at the start of the fellowship. It is meant to be a learning experience where proficiencies will be developed or enhanced. Prior health policy, legislative, or political experience is helpful. For additional information, please contact the Department of Medical Student Services at mss@ama-assn.org.
Requirements: Any AMA-MSS member in good standing at a medical school in the United States is eligible to apply.
Date(s) Application is Due: Jan 31
Contact: Rebecca Gierhahn, Director; (800) 262-3211 ext. 4753; email: rebecca.gierhahn@ama-assn.org or mss@ama-assn.org
Internet: http://www.ama-assn.org/ama/pub/about-ama/our-people/member-groups-sections/medical-student-section/opportunities/internships-fellowships.shtml
Sponsor: American Medical Association - Department of Medical Student Services
515 N. State Street
Chicago, IL 60654

AMA-MSS Government Relations Internship Programs 404

The Department of Medical Student Services, in conjunction with the Washington, D.C., office of the American Medical Association, offer assistance to students seeking to increase their involvement and education in national health policy and in the national legislative activities of organized medicine. The Government Relations Internship Program (GRIP) provides stipends to assist selected students who are completing summer health policy internships in the Washington, D.C., area. Medical students report that their credibility as AMA-sponsored interns allows them to pursue issues in depth, and in many cases, become experts on a specific topic. Similarly, internship sponsors welcome the enthusiasm and unique perspective that medical students bring to discussions about issues that require medicine's point of view. All students selected to participate in GRIP will receive a stipend. Additionally, GRIP participants completing internships with non-governmental organizations will benefit from attendance at weekly seminars conducted at the AMA Washington Office. These seminars are designed to increase the continuity of the internship experience, promote camaraderie among medical students working in health policy, and facilitate continuing education on important political issues. Upon completion of the program, all GRIP participants will be required to complete and submit a report on their internship experiences. The GRIP application deadline is February 15. However, late applications (through April 15) will be considered on a rolling basis if space remains.
Requirements: To be eligible for the GRIP program, students must be AMA members who have secured policy internships in the Washington, DC, area during the summer. Eligible internship sites include: National specialty societies seated in the AMA House of Delegates; Public health advocacy groups; Non-clinical international health policy programs (limited spots); Congressional offices*; Federal agencies*.
Restrictions: Please note that internships with narrowly focused lobbying organizations or with specialty organizations that are not seated in the AMA House of Delegates are strongly discouraged. *Due to new Congressional lobbying disclosure rules, interns in Congressional offices or federal agencies will not be able to participate in the weekly educational seminars at the AMA's Washington, D.C., office.
Date(s) Application is Due: Feb 15
Contact: Rebecca Gierhahn, Director; (800) 262-3211 ext. 4753; email: rebecca.gierhahn@ama-assn.org or mss@ama-assn.org

Internet: http://www.ama-assn.org/ama/pub/about-ama/our-people/member-groups-sections/medical-student-section/opportunities/internships-fellowships.shtml
Sponsor: American Medical Association - Department of Medical Student Services
515 N. State Street
Chicago, IL 60654

AMA-MSS Research Poster Award 405

The MSS/RFS Joint Research Poster Symposium is held annually at the MSS Interim Meeting (November). Research is presented in eight categories (biochemistry/cell biology, cancer biology, cardiology/vascular biology, clinical/epidemiological/health care, immunology/microbiology, neurobiology/neuroscience, radiology/imaging, surgery). The overall winner receives a free trip to the MSS Annual Meeting in Chicago.
Date(s) Application is Due: Sep 1
Contact: Rebecca Gierhahn, Director; (800) 262-3211 ext. 4753; email: rebecca.gierhahn@ama-assn.org or mss@ama-assn.org
Internet: http://www.ama-assn.org/ama/pub/about-ama/our-people/member-groups-sections/medical-student-section/opportunities/grants-awards-scholarships.shtml
Sponsor: American Medical Association
515 N. State Street
Chicago, IL 60654

AMA-RFS and AMA Foundation Medical Student & Resident/Fellow Elective-Medicine & the Media 406

Discovery Communications, the leading global real-world media company, is offering an exclusive four to six week elective for American Medical Association (AMA) medical student and resident/fellow members. As part of Discovery's ongoing dedication to education, Discovery Channel produces continuing medical education (CME) programs that air on the Discovery Channel weekly. During the elective, one AMA medical student and one AMA resident/fellow will each work closely with all members of the Discovery team to develop a medical education program that will air on the network and be viewed by over 2 million people. This exciting opportunity gives the student and resident/fellow hands-on experience in the translation of rigorous scientific data into an entertaining and informational program. The student and resident/fellow will work primarily at Discovery Communications headquarters in Silver Spring, MD, but will also travel to relevant on-site and studio shoots for the program. A stipend will be provided to cover living expenses based on length of rotation ($3,000 for four-week rotation). Dates and length of rotation are flexible. Applications for the Winter elective are due September 30. Applicants not selected for the Winter elective must resubmit for the Summer elective if they wish to be considered for it. Summer applications are due March 15.
Requirements: All medical student and resident/fellow members of the American Medical Association (AMA) are eligible to apply for an exclusive elective in health communications with Discovery Channel in Silver Spring, MD. One AMA medical student and one AMA resident/fellow will be selected.
Amount of Grant: $3,000+ based on length of elective
Date(s) Application is Due: Sep 30; Mar 15
Contact: Jon Fanning, Director; (800) 262-3211 ext. 4978; fax: (312) 464-5845; email: Jon.Fanning@ama-assn.org or rfs@ama-assn.org
Internet: http://www.ama-assn.org/ama/pub/about-ama/our-people/member-groups-sections/resident-fellow-section/awards-grants.shtml
Sponsor: AMA Foundation and AMA Resident and Fellow Services
515 N. State Street, 14th Floor
Chicago, IL 60654

AMA-RFS Legislative Awareness Internships 407

The Department of Resident and Fellow Services, in conjunction with the Washington, DC office of the American Medical Association, is sponsoring a two-week legislative internship program in the spring. Two residents and/or fellows will be selected. The program will afford residents and fellows the unique opportunity to participate in the political process of organized medicine at the national level. Each resident or fellow will receive a $1,000 stipend to help defray program-related expenses (e.g., airfare, hotel, cabs); all other expenses are the responsibility of the resident or fellow. The selected resident or fellow is also responsible for securing his or her own housing accommodations.
Requirements: Applicants must be members of the AMA.
Restrictions: The selected resident or fellow must obtain permission to participate in the program from their program director prior to the selection process.
Amount of Grant: $1,000 stipend
Contact: Jon Fanning, Director; (800) 262-3211 ext. 4978 or (312) 464-4978; fax: (312) 464-5845; email: Jon.Fanning@ama-assn.org or rfs@ama-assn.org
Internet: http://www.ama-assn.org/ama/pub/about-ama/our-people/member-groups-sections/resident-fellow-section/awards-grants.shtml
Sponsor: American Medical Association Resident and Fellow Services
515 N. State Street, 14th Floor
Chicago, IL 60654

AMA-WPC Joan F. Giambalvo Memorial Scholarships 408

The American Medical Association (AMA) Foundation in association with the AMA Women Physicians Congress (WPC) has established the Joan F. Giambalvo Memorial Scholarship Fund with the goal of advancing the progress of women in the medical profession and strengthening the ability of the AMA to identify and address the needs of women physicians and medical students. Proposals for the Joan F. Giambalvo Memorial Scholarship Fund will be accepted between Nov. 1 and Feb. 15. The AMA-WPC Joan F. Giambalvo Memorial Scholarship seeks innovative research proposals focusing on professional work/practice issues that affect women physicians, including, but not limited to: part-time working strategies; leadership training protocols; gender-based physician practice patterns; physician satisfaction or burnout; retention incentives; practice re-entry issues. Proposals for projects with concurrent/complementary funding and/or plans to use this grant as seed money for larger studies to follow will be received favorably, as will proposals for independent new projects. This award is for a maximum of $10,000. A budget submitted with each applicant's proposal should reflect the anticipated use of funds for the amount requested. Proposals will be evaluated and awardee(s) selected based on a variety of factors, including, but not limited to: the innovation, quality and/or feasibility of the idea; project/research methodology; potential to produce action, change or more comprehensive studies; and career goals of the applicant.
Requirements: Applicants/awardees shall be: female or male; working alone or collaboratively on the specific research project; physicians, medical students, other health professionals, or individuals working or doing graduate work in an applicable profession such as public health, sociology, psychology, etc.
Restrictions: Members of the AMA-WPC Governing Council, AMA Foundation Board of Directors, AMA Board of Trustees and Joan F. Giambalvo Memorial Scholarship Fund selection committee, and AMA and AMA Foundation staff are not eligible.
Amount of Grant: $10,000 maximum
Date(s) Application is Due: Feb 15
Contact: Alice Reed, Scholarships; (312) 464-5523; email: alice.reed@ama-assn.org
Internet: http://www.ama-assn.org/ama/pub/about-ama/our-people/member-groups-sections/women-physicians-congress/about-wpc/joan-f-giambalvo-memorial-scholarship.shtml
Sponsor: American Medical Association
515 N. State Street
Chicago, IL 60654

Amador Community Foundation Grants 409

The foundation supports organizations that enhance the quality of life for the people of Amador County by: encouraging private giving for the public good by providing a flexible, cost-effective and tax-exempt vehicle for donors with varied charitable interests and abilities to give; building and maintaining a permanent endowment fund in order to provide a continuing source of income for grants; making grants that are innovative, strategic and relevant in the support of nonprofit sectors; and serving as a catalyst to address changing and challenging community issues. There are no set project or program areas for funding.
Restrictions: The Foundation does not award grants for political or religious purposes, to retire long-term indebtedness, to influence legislation or elections, to private foundations and other grant-making organizations.
Geographic Focus: California
Contact: (209) 223-2148; fax: (209) 223-4569; email: acf@amadorcommunityfoundation.org
Internet: http://www.amadorcommunityfoundation.org/grant.html
Sponsor: Amador Community Foundation
P.O. Box 1154, 21-B Main Street
Jackson, CA 95642

Amarillo Area/Harrington Foundations Grants 410

The community foundation seeks to improve the quality of life in the 26 northernmost counties of the Texas Panhandle. Grants are awarded to nonprofits in support of arts and culture, education, health care, and social services. Types of support include research, building construction/renovation, equipment acquisition, program development, seed grants, scholarship funds, and matching funds.
Requirements: Nonprofit 501(c)3 organizations located in the northernmost 26 counties of the Texas Panhandle, including Dallam, Sherman, Hansford, Ochiltree, Lipscomb, Hartley, Moore, Hutchinson, Roberts, Hemphill, Oldham, Potter, Carson, Gray, Wheeler, Deaf Smith, Randall, Armstrong, Donley, Collingsworth, Parmer, Castro, Swisher, Briscoe, Hall, and Childress, are eligible.
Restrictions: The foundation does not make grants to or for religious activities; political lobbying or legislative activities; endowments; debt retirement; deficit financing, reduction of operating deficit, etc.; private or parochial schools; national, state, or local fund-raising activities; general operating expenses for United Way agencies; or umbrella funding organizations that would distribute requested funds at their own discretion.
Geographic Focus: Texas
Date(s) Application is Due: Jan 5; Jul 6
Contact: Kathy Grant, (806) 376-4521; email: kathie@aaf-hf.org
Internet: http://aaf-hf.org/grants/guidelines.htm
Sponsor: Amarillo Area/Harrington Foundations
801 S Fillmore Street, Suite 700
Amarillo, TX 79101

AMD Corporate Contributions Grants 411

AMD has established two global focus areas: strengthening community and strengthening education. Priority is given to basic needs (food, shelter, and basic health care), education (math and science, teacher development, and college and career awareness), and university education. The k-12 initiatives target programs that increase student interest and/or proficiency in literacy, match, science, and computer technology. AMD also funds programs aimed at developing and supporting effective classroom instruction.
Requirements: Most contributions are made to accredited schools and 501(c)3 nonprofit agencies operating in Austin, Texas (Travis Couunty) or Sunnyvale, California (Santa Clara County) with which AMD has a strong established relationship.

Restrictions: AMD does not consider unsolicited applications for programs outside of the communities in which they operate or outside their focus areas. Also excluded are individuals, medical research, religious, political, service or fraternal organizations, arts or cultural programs, advocacy groups, athletic teams, recreational programs, or individual scouting troops. Organization must be non-discriminatory.
Amount of Grant: $2.5 million total
Date(s) Application is Due: May 1
Contact: Community Affairs, 1 (800) 538-8450, ext 45373; (408) 749-5373
Internet: http://www.amd.com/us-en/Corporate/AboutAMD/0,,51_52_7697_7702,00.html
Sponsor: AMD Corporation
P.O. Box 3453, M/S 42, 1 AMD Pl
Sunnyvale, CA 94088

American Academy of Dermatology Camp Discovery Scholarships 412
Every year, the academy sponsors a week of fishing, boating, swimming, water skiing, arts and crafts for young people with a serious skin condition. Under the expert care of dermatologists and nurses, the camp offers the opportunity of spending a week among other young people who have similar skin conditions. Many of the counselors have serious skin conditions as well, and can provide support and advice to campers. The camp fee is covered by full scholarships, including transportation.
Requirements: Campers may attend at any one of four locations selected each year. Campers must meet the age criteria at time of camp (generally between the ages of 8 and 16). Campers must also get a recommendation from a dermatologist who is an academy member. Registration can be completed online at the website.
Contact: Jill Mueller; (847) 240-1737; fax: (847) 330-8907; email: jmueller@aad.org
Internet: http://www.campdiscovery.org/
Sponsor: American Academy of Dermatology
930 E. Woodfield Road
Schaumburg, IL 60173

American Academy of Dermatology Shade Structure Grants 413
The program awards grants to support the purchase of shade structures designed to provide shade and ultraviolet radiation protection for outdoor areas. Locations can include any area where children and adults gather and are exposed to the harmful rays of the sun, such as playgrounds, pools, bleachers, and eating or recreation areas.
Requirements: The program is open to non-profit organizations or educational institutions that serve children and teenagers, ages 18 and younger. Applicants will be reviewed based on the following: demonstrated commitment to sun safety within the organization and community; sponsorship of application by an academy member dermatologist; and ability to meet the build timeline outlined in grant criteria. Application and guidelines are available online.
Restrictions: Faxed nor emailed applications will not be accepted.
Samples: Amelia Earhart Elementary, Goddard, Kan. (2009); Anthony Wayne Rehabilitation Center for Handicapped and Blind Inc., Fort Wayne, Ind. (2009); Bear Exploration Center, Montgomery, Ala. (2009).
Amount of Grant: $8000 maximum
Date(s) Application is Due: Apr 12
Contact: Jennifer Allyn, Program Director; (847) 240-1730; email: jallyn@aad.org
Internet: http://www.aad.org/public/sun/grants.html
Sponsor: American Academy of Dermatology
930 E .Woodfield Road
Schaumburg, IL 60173

American Academy of Nursing Building Academic Geriatric Nursing Capacity (BAGNC) Scholarships 414
The Foundation's overall goal is to increase the nation's capacity to provide effective and affordable care to its rapidly increasing older population. Specifically, the Foundation seeks to enhance the training of physicians, nurses, social workers and other health professionals who care for older adults, and promote innovations in the integration and delivery of services. The goal of the Scholarship program is to increase academic geriatric nursing capacity in the United States. BAGNC focuses on the development of academic leadership in gerontological nursing through strong mentorship in the components of academic geriatric nursing (research, teaching and community service); leadership development, a national network of scholars and academic geriatric nurses; and exposure to a wide range of experts in gerontology and geriatrics. Scholars in collaboration with their identified mentor will design and implement a tailored professional development plan designed to support development of new competencies and enhanced effectiveness as an academic leader.
Requirements: Registered nurses who are U.S. citizens or U.S. permanent residents and who hold a degree(s) in nursing are eligible. Predoctoral applicants must: be registered nurses; hold degree(s) in nursing; be United States citizens or permanent U.S. residents; plan an academic and research career; and demonstrate potential for long-term contributions to geriatric nursing.
Amount of Grant: $50,000 maximum per annum for two years
Date(s) Application is Due: Jan 15
Contact: Patricia Archbold, Program Director; (202) 777-1172; fax: (202) 777-0107; email: parchbold@aannet.org
Internet: http://www.aannet.org/i4a/pages/Index.cfm?pageID=3295
Sponsor: American Academy of Nursing / John A. Hartford Foundation
888 17th Street, NW Suite 800
Washington, DC 20006

American Academy of Nursing Claire M. Fagin Fellowships 415
The Fellowship supports two years of full time advanced research and leadership training for doctorally prepared faculty committed to careers in academic geriatric nursing by providing $120,000 for the 2-year fellowship ($60,000 per annum). Program focuses on the development of academic leadership in gerontological nursing through such activities as: research; focused study; networking among scholars, mentors and colleagues in other fields; demonstration of growth in ability to transform self and organizations by moving outside of traditional modes of success; completion and write-up of a significant research project; and by success in achieving funding from other sources. Selected fellows, in collaboration with their mentor, will design and implement an individual professional development plan that will support them in developing new competencies and enhanced effectiveness as an academic leader and researcher. Award programs must begin between July 1st and September 1st of the award year. The program is committed to advancing well-qualified applicants from under-represented minority groups to improve the nation's ability to provide culturally competent care to its increasingly diverse aging population.
Requirements: Applicants must: be doctorally-prepared registered nurses; hold degree(s) in nursing; be United States citizens or permanent U.S. residents; be doctorally-prepared registered nurses,; have the potential to develop into independent investigators; and demonstrate potential for long-term contributions to geriatric nursing. Applications will be accepted from doctoral students who will complete their doctoral program prior to the award. Faculty members in accredited Schools of Nursing who hold the rank of assistant professor or associate professor may apply for fellowships.
Amount of Grant: $120,000 for the 2-year fellowship ($60,000 per annum)
Date(s) Application is Due: Jan 13
Contact: Patricia Archbold, Program Director; (202) 777-1172; fax: (202) 777-0107; email: parchbold@aannet.org
Internet: http://www.geriatricnursing.org/applications/cmf-fellowship.asp
Sponsor: American Academy of Nursing / John A. Hartford Foundation
888 17th Street, NW Suite 800
Washington, DC 20006

American Academy of Nursing Mayday Fund Grants 416
The Foundation's overall goal is to increase the nation's capacity to provide effective and affordable care to its rapidly increasing older population. Specifically, the Foundation seeks to enhance the training of physicians, nurses, social workers and other health professionals who care for older adults, and promote innovations in the integration and delivery of services. This program is aimed at candidates whose research includes the study of pain in the elderly. Award programs must begin between July 1st and September 1st.
Requirements: Predoctoral applicants must: be registered nurses; hold degree(s) in nursing; be United States citizens or permanent U.S. residents; plan an academic and research career; and demonstrate potential for long-term contributions to geriatric nursing.
Amount of Grant: $5,000 maximum
Date(s) Application is Due: Jan 9
Contact: Patricia Archbold, Program Director; (202) 777-1172; fax: (202) 777-0107; email: parchbold@aannet.org
Internet: http://www.geriatricnursing.org/applications/applications.asp
Sponsor: American Academy of Nursing / John A. Hartford Foundation
888 17th Street, NW Suite 800
Washington, DC 20006

American Academy of Nursing MBA Scholarships 417
The Program seeks nurse applicants pursuing a Masters of Business Administration (including Executive MBA) at a highly ranked school of business, and committed to a career focus on the management/leadership of institutions serving older persons. The Scholarship offers grant-funded scholarship support of $50,000 over the period of one or two years to successful candidates who will commence or continue full-time in an MBA program. The Scholarship program includes additional leadership development experiences.
Requirements: Scholarship applicants must: be registered nurses; hold degree(s) in nursing; and be United States citizens or permanent U.S. residents. Applicants must be accepted to, or be currently enrolled in, a highly ranked business school. Applicants must provide specific examples of ability to understand organizational and management challenges as well as strategic approaches to such challenges and provide evidence of previous commitment to gerontology.
Amount of Grant: $50,000 per year for up to two years
Date(s) Application is Due: Jan 15
Contact: Patricia Archbold, Program Director; (202) 777-1172; fax: (202) 777-0107; email: parchbold@aannet.org
Internet: http://www.geriatricnursing.org/applications/mba-scholarship.asp
Sponsor: American Academy of Nursing / John A. Hartford Foundation
888 17th Street, NW Suite 800
Washington, DC 20006

American Academy of Nursing Media Awards 418
The Award is presented to the individual(s) or organization(s) whose use of media has highlighted the unique contribution of nursing and: increased public awareness of the value nursing plays in promoting health and providing health care to the public and/or the need to address the growing nursing shortage; reported the impact of specific public policies on the health status of individuals, communities or the general population; been responsible for motivating specific actions to improve healthcare for diverse groups of people; disseminated nursing research findings nationally (and possibly internationally)

using both interdisciplinary and public media; and depicted specific examples of health-enhancing interactions, culturally sensitive health care, health care addressing health disparity issues of under-served and vulnerable populations, health promoting activities or healing actions. Examples of items that may be submitted for the Academy's Media Awards Program include, but are not limited to: newspaper articles, radio programs, motion pictures, public service announcements, books, feature films, television shows, magazine articles, novels, documentaries, popular literature, creative endeavors, and multimedia. Entries are encouraged to highlight nursing practice and/or nursing issues.
Requirements: A non-refundable entry fee of $50.00 is required.
Date(s) Application is Due: Jul 27
Contact: Patricia Archbold, Program Director; (202) 777-1172; fax: (202) 777-0107; email: parchbold@aannet.org;; Liz Perry, Media Contact; (202) 777-1174
Internet: http://www.aannet.org
Sponsor: American Academy of Nursing
888 17th Street, NW, Suite 800
Washington, DC 2006

American Chemical Society Claude S. Hudson Awards **419**
This award, supported by the National Starch and Chemical Company, is given biennially in odd-numbered years to recognize outstanding contributions to carbohydrate chemistry, whether in education, research, or application. The award is granted without regard to age or nationality. Applications are accepted in even-numbered years. The award consists of $5,000 and a certificate. Up to $1,000 for travel expenses to the meeting at which the award will be presented will be reimbursed.
Requirements: Any individual, except a member of the award committee, may submit one nomination or seconding letter for the award in any given year. Nominating documents consist of a letter of not more than 1000 words containing an evaluation of the nominee's accomplishments and a specific identification of the work to be recognized, a biographical sketch including date of birth, and a list of publications and patents authored by the nominee.
Restrictions: Self-nominations are not accepted.
Samples: Peter H. Seeberger—award recipient, (2009); Pierre Sinay—award recipient, (2007); David Bundle—award recipient, (2005).
Amount of Grant: $5,000 and up to $1,000 for travel expenses to award meeting
Date(s) Application is Due: Nov 1
Contact: Felicia Dixon, Awards Administrator; (202) 872-4408; fax: (202) 776-8008; email: f_dixon@acs.org or awards@acs.org
Internet: http://portal.acs.org/portal/acs/corg/content?_nfpb=true&_pageLabel=PP_ARTICLEMAIN&node_id=1319&content_id=CTP_004501&use_sec=true&sec_url_var=region1
Sponsor: American Chemical Society
1155 Sixteenth Street, NW
Washington, DC 20036

American Chemical Society GCI Pharmaceutical Roundtable Research Grants **420**
The Roundtable is a partnership with the ACS GCI (Green Chemistry Institute) and pharmaceutical corporations united by a shared commitment to integrate the principles of green chemistry and engineering into the business of drug discovery and production. The program was created to support research in the key green chemistry research areas. (Ten chemical transformations and two process related operations were identified and subsequently published - download the list from the sponsor's website). The primary purpose of this grant is to publish research to make information publicly available.
Requirements: Proposals will only be accepted from public and private institutions of higher education. The grant is not limited to institutions in the United States. Proposals must be submitted through the appropriate institutional office for external funding. Proposed research must focus on the key targeted areas identified by the Roundtable. Proposals must clearly describe how the proposed research will provide improvements over existing technology that are consistent with the goals of Green Chemistry including improved atom economy, use of less hazardous reagents, more energy efficient processes, elimination of by-products, reduced waste generation, improved environmental, health, and safety and life cycle impacts, catalytic versus stoichiometric methods, and development of inherently safer transformations. Illustrations of the relevance of the proposed technology to synthetic and process related problems within the pharmaceutical industry are encouraged. Complete guidelines can be downloaded at the sponsor's website.
Restrictions: Applicants may have only one research grant with the ACS GCI Pharmaceutical Roundtable at a time. Current research grant holders may not apply for a new grant until their active grant or no-cost time extension officially expires.
Amount of Grant: up to $130,000
Date(s) Application is Due: Sep 9
Contact: Michael Bernstein; (202) 872-4400 or (202) 872-6102; fax: (202) 776-8009; email: m_bernstein@acs.org or gcipr@acs.org
Internet: http://portal.acs.org/portal/acs/corg/content?_nfpb=true&_pageLabel=PP_TRANSITIONMAIN&node_id=1456&use_sec=false&sec_url_var=region1
Sponsor: American Chemical Society
1155 Sixteenth Street, NW
Washington, DC 20036

American College of Rheumatology Fellows-in-Training Travel Scholarships **421**
The American College of Rheumatology Fellows-in-Training (FIT) Travel Scholarship is designed to provide funding to assist Fellows- In-Training at U.S. and Canadian programs in rheumatology attend the Annual Meeting. Preference will be given to those applicants who are currently a first or second year adult or first, second or third year pediatric fellows in a training program approved by the Accreditation Council of Graduate Medical Education or the Royal College of Physicians and Surgeons of Canada. Applicants in a third year of an adult or fourth year of a pediatric fellowship will be given consideration after the registration deadline, space permitting on a first come first serve basis.
Requirements: Applicant must be first or second year adult or first, second or third year pediatric fellows in a training program approved by the Accreditation Council of Graduate Medical Education or the Royal College of Physicians and Surgeons of Canada. Applicants must be in an accredited fellowship position at the time of the Annual Meeting.
Restrictions: Individuals with a faculty appointment will not be considered.
Date(s) Application is Due: Jul 24
Contact: Fellowship Coordinator; (404) 633-3777; fax: (404) 633-1870; email: fittravel@rheumatology.org
Internet: http://www.rheumatology.org/fellows/fitscholarship.asp
Sponsor: American College of Rheumatology (ACR)
1800 Century Place, Suite 250
Atlanta, GA 30345-4300

American College of Surgeons and The Triological Society Clinical Scientist Development Awards **422**
The Triological Society (TRIO) and the American College of Surgeons (ACS) announce a competitive research career development program that will provide supplemental funding to otolaryngologist-head and neck surgeons who receive NIH Mentored Clinical Scientist Development Awards (K08) or Mentored Patient-Oriented Research Development Awards (K23). The TRIO and ACS are offering these awards as a means to facilitate the research career development of otolaryngologists-head and neck surgeons, with the expectation that awardees will have sufficient pilot data to submit a competitive R01 proposal prior to the conclusion of the K awards. Awards will use the K08 or K23 mechanisms. Planning, direction, and execution of the program will be the responsibility of the candidate and her/his mentor on behalf of the applicant institution. The project period will be for a period of up to five years with a minimum of three years. Awards are not renewable. TRIO and ACS will provide salary and fringe benefits for the NIH K08/K23 recipient. A combined total of $80,000 per year in direct costs will be awarded to the institution of the awardee.
Requirements: Applicants must be MD otolaryngologist-head and neck surgeons and members of the American College of Surgeons. Applicants must meet all requirements as set forth in the K08 and K23 application criteria and must be recipients of a new K08 or K23 award or have an existing K08/K23 award with a minimum of three years remaining in the funding period as of June.
Restrictions: Pre-existing applications and awards are not eligible for consideration.
Amount of Grant: $80,000
Date(s) Application is Due: Apr 15
Contact: Kate Early, Administrative Assistant; (312) 202-5281; email: kearly@facs.org
Internet: http://www.facs.org/memberservices/acstriol.html
Sponsor: American College of Surgeons / Triological Society
633 N. Saint Clair Street
Chicago, IL 60611-3211

American College of Surgeons Australia and New Zealand Chapter Travelling Fellowships **423**
The International Relations Committee of the American College of Surgeons announces the availability of a traveling fellowship, the Australia and New Zealand Chapter of the American College of Surgeons Travelling Fellowship. The purpose of this fellowship is to encourage international exchange of information concerning surgical science, practice, and education and to establish professional and academic collaborations and friendships. The Chapter and the College will provide the sum of $8,000 to the successful applicant, who will also be exempted from registration fees for the Annual Scientific Congress. He/she must meet all travel and living expenses.
Requirements: The scholarship is available to a Fellow of the American College of Surgeons in any of the surgical specialties who meets the following requirements: has a major interest and accomplishment in clinical and basic science related to surgery; holds a current full-time academic appointment in Canada or the United States; is under 45 years of age on the date the application is filed; and is enthusiastic and personable and possesses good communication skills. The Fellow is required to spend a minimum of two weeks in Germany. The Fellow is required to spend a minimum of two or three weeks in Australia and New Zealand.
Amount of Grant: $8,000
Date(s) Application is Due: Nov 16
Contact: Kate Early, Administrative Assistant; (312) 202-5281; email: kearly@facs.org
Internet: http://www.facs.org/memberservices/traveling.html
Sponsor: American College of Surgeons
633 N. Saint Clair Street
Chicago, IL 60611-3211

American College of Surgeons Co-Sponsored K08/K23 NIH Supplement Awards **424**
The American College of Surgeons announces a program that will provide supplemental funding to up to five individuals who receive a Mentored Clinical Scientist Development Award (K08/K23). It is directed at surgeon-scientists working in the early stages of their research careers. The award requires co-sponsorship with an approved surgical society of a three, four or five year period of supervised research experience that may integrate didactic studies with laboratory or clinically based research. This award program will offer a means to facilitate the career development of individuals pursuing careers in

surgical research by enhancing salary support over and above that offered by the K08/ K23 mechanism. The application deadline is June 12, with funding to begin July 1.
Requirements: Awardees must be members in good standing of both the College and a co-sponsoring surgical society. Participating surgical societies include American Association of Plastic Surgeons (AAPS), American Head and Neck Society (AHNS), American Society of Transplant Surgeons (ASTS), American Vascular Association (AVA), Society of Gynecologic Oncologists (SGO), Society of University Surgeons (SU. S.), and Thoracic Surgery Foundation for Research and Education (TSFRE).
Date(s) Application is Due: Jun 12
Contact: Kate Early, Administrative Assistant; (312) 202-5281; email: kearly@facs.org
Internet: http://www.facs.org/memberservices/acs-nih.html
Sponsor: American College of Surgeons
633 North Saint Clair Street
Chicago, IL 60611-3211

American College of Surgeons Faculty Career Development Award for Neurological Surgeons 425
The American College of Surgeons (ACS) and the Neurosurgery Research and Education Foundation of the American Association of Neurological Surgeons (NREF-AANS) are offering a two-year faculty career development award to neurological surgeons. The award is to support the establishment of a new and independent research program in an area of neurological surgery. The award is $40,000 per year for each of two years, to support the research, and is not renewable thereafter.
Requirements: The award is open to surgeons who are members or candidate members in good standing of both the American College of Surgeons (ACS) and the American Association of Neurological Surgeons (AANS); and have completed specialty training within the preceding five years and have received a full-time faculty appointment at a medical school accredited by the Liaison Committee on Medical Education in the United States or by the Committee for Accreditation of Canadian Medical Schools in Canada.
Restrictions: Applicants may not be current recipients of major research grants.
Amount of Grant: $40,000 per year for two years
Date(s) Application is Due: Dec 1
Contact: Michele S. Gregory, Director of Development; (847) 378-0540 or (847) 378-0500; fax: (847) 378-0600; email: msg@aans.org or info@aans.org
Internet: http://www.facs.org/memberservices/acsnrefaans07.pdf
Sponsor: American College of Surgeons
633 N. Saint Clair Street
Chicago, IL 60611-3211

American College of Surgeons Faculty Research Fellowships 426
The American College of Surgeons is offering two-year faculty research fellowships to surgeons entering academic careers in surgery or a surgical specialty. The fellowship is to assist a surgeon in the establishment of a new and independent research program. Applicants should have demonstrated their potential to work as independent investigators. The fellowship award is $40,000 per year for each of two years, to support the research.
Requirements: The fellowship is restricted to surgeons who have recently (usually within three years) completed formal surgical education and entered the field of full-time academic surgery and received a faculty appointment in a department of surgery, or one of the surgical specialties, at an approved medical school in the United States or Canada. Preference will be given to applicants who directly enter academic surgery following residency or fellowships. Approval of the application is required from the administration (dean or fiscal officer) and the head of the department under whom the recipient will be studying during the fellowship.
Amount of Grant: $40,000 per year
Date(s) Application is Due: Nov 2
Contact: Kate Early, Administrative Assistant; (312) 202-5281; email: kearly@facs.org
Internet: http://www.facs.org/memberservices/acsfaculty.html
Sponsor: American College of Surgeons
633 North Saint Clair Street
Chicago, IL 60611-3211

American College of Surgeons Health Policy Scholarships 427
The American College of Surgeons, in partnership with a number of other organizations, is offering annual scholarships to subsidize attendance and participation in the Executive Leadership Program in Health Policy and Management at Brandeis University. The awards are in the amount of $8,000, to be used toward the cost of tuition, travel, housing, and subsistence during the period of the course. The closing date for receipt of all applications is February 2. All applicants will be notified of the outcome of the selection process by March 31.
Requirements: The award is open to surgeons who are members in good standing of both the American College of Surgeons (ACS) and the specific partnering organization for each award. These include: the American Association of Neurological Surgeons (AANS); the American Academy of Ophthalmology (AAO); the American Academy of Otolaryngology, Head and Neck Surgery Foundation (AAO-HNS); the American Association for the Surgery of Trauma (AAST); the American Pediatric Surgical Association (APSA); the American Surgical Association (ASA); the American Society of Breast Surgeons (ASBrS); the American Society of Colon and Rectal Surgeons (ASCRS); the American Society of Plastic Surgeons (ASPS); the American Urogynecologic Society (AUGS); the Society of Thoracic Surgeons (STS); and the Society for Vascular Surgery (SVS). Applicants must be at least 30 years old, but under 55, on the date that the completed application is filed.
Restrictions: Indirect costs are not paid to the recipient or to the recipient's institution.
Amount of Grant: $8,000
Date(s) Application is Due: Feb 2
Contact: Michele S. Gregory, Director of Development; (847) 378-0540 or (847) 378-0500; fax: (847) 378-0600; email: msg@aans.org or info@aans.org
Internet: http://www.facs.org/memberservices/acsaans.html
Sponsor: American College of Surgeons
633 North Saint Clair Street
Chicago, IL 60611-3211

American College of Surgeons Health Policy Scholarships for General Surgeons 428
The American College of Surgeons is offering an annual scholarship to subsidize attendance and participation in the Executive Leadership Program in Health Policy and Management at Brandeis University. The award is in the amount of $8,000, to be used toward the cost of tuition, travel, housing, and subsistence during the period of the course. The closing date for receipt of applications is February 2. All applicants will be notified of the outcome of the selection process by March 31
Requirements: The award is open to general surgeons who are members in good standing of the American College of Surgeons (ACS). Applicants must be at least 30 years old, but under 55, on the date that the completed application is filed. The scholarship must be used in the year for which it is designated.
Restrictions: Indirect costs are not paid to the recipient or to the recipient's institution.
Amount of Grant: $8,000
Date(s) Application is Due: Feb 2
Contact: Administrator, Scholarships Division; (800) 621-4111 or (312) 202-5000; fax: (312) 202-5001
Internet: http://www.facs.org/memberservices/acshealthpolicy.html
Sponsor: American College of Surgeons
633 North Saint Clair Street
Chicago, IL 60611-3211

American College of Surgeons International Guest Scholarships 429
The American College of Surgeons offers International Guest Scholarships to competent young surgeons from countries other than the United States or Canada who have demonstrated strong interests in teaching and research. The scholarships, in the amount of $8,000 each, provide the Scholars with an opportunity to visit clinical, teaching, and research activities in North America and to attend and participate fully in the educational opportunities and activities of the American College of Surgeons Clinical Congress.
Requirements: Applicants must: be graduates of schools of medicine; be at least 35 years old, but under 45, on the date that the completed application is filed; submit their applications from their intended permanent location; and have demonstrated a commitment to teaching and/or research in accordance with the standards of the applicant's country.
Amount of Grant: $8,000
Date(s) Application is Due: Jul 1
Contact: Kate Early, Administrative Assistant; (312) 202-5281; fax: (312) 202-5021; email: kearly@facs.org
Internet: http://www.facs.org/memberservices/igs.html
Sponsor: American College of Surgeons
633 North Saint Clair Street
Chicago, IL 60611-3211

American College of Surgeons Nizar N. Oweida, MD, FACS, Scholarships 430
The Board of Governors of the American College of Surgeons announces the availability of a scholarship for young rural surgeons, the Nizar N. Oweida, MD, FACS, Scholarship of the American College of Surgeons. The Scholarship provides an award of $5,000 to subsidize the participation of a young rural-based Fellow or Associate Fellow in attendance at the annual Clinical Congress of the American College of Surgeons. This amount is to be used to help defray travel expenses for the Clinical Congress, postgraduate course fees, hotel costs, and per diem expenses during the Clinical Congress.
Requirements: The Oweida Scholarship is available to a member of the American College of Surgeons in any of the surgical specialties who meets the following requirements: serves a rural community in the U.S. or Canada; is a Fellow or Associate Fellow in good standing; and is under 45 years of age on the date the application is filed.
Amount of Grant: $5,000
Date(s) Application is Due: Dec 15
Contact: Kate Early, Administrative Assistant; (312) 202-5281; email: kearly@facs.org
Internet: http://www.facs.org/memberservices/oweida.html
Sponsor: American College of Surgeons
633 North Saint Clair Street
Chicago, IL 60611-3211

American College of Surgeons Resident and Associate Society (RAS-ACS) Leadership Scholarships 431
The Resident and Associate Society of the American College of Surgeons (RAS-ACS) is accepting applications for its leadership scholarship for Resident Members and Associate Fellows of the College. The RAS Scholarship will be awarded competitively to young surgeons who exemplify an important goal the RAS has set for itself—developing future leaders in the field of surgery. The award is for the purpose of allowing the young surgeon awardee to attend one of several courses that will be offered for this scholarship. The courses are intended to engage young surgeons and expose them to opportunities to

improve their abilities in areas such as leadership, communications skills, and research, skills that are necessary to succeed as leaders in surgery.
Date(s) Application is Due: Jan 30
Contact: Peg Haar, Member Services; (312) 202-5312; email: phaar@facs.org
Internet: http://www.facs.org/ras-acs/resources/scholarship.html
Sponsor: American College of Surgeons
633 North Saint Clair Street
Chicago, IL 60611-3211

American College of Surgeons Resident Research Scholarships 432
ACS scholarships will be awarded each year to encourage residents to pursue careers in academic surgery. Priority will be given to residents beginning full-time investigative activities, with no clinical responsibilities, for the two-year period of the scholarship. Study outside the United States or Canada is permissible. The scholarship is for the personal use of the recipient and is not to diminish or replace the usual or expected compensation; award is made directly to the scholar and not to the institution. Renewal for the second year is contingent upon acceptable progress and study protocol for the second year.
Requirements: The applicant must have completed two postdoctoral years in an accredited surgical training program in the United States or Canada at the time the scholarship is awarded and shall not complete formal residency training before the end of the scholarship. Approval of the application is required from the administration and the head of the department under whom the recipient will be studying.
Restrictions: Only in exceptional circumstances will more than one ACS scholarship be granted in a single year to applicants from the same institution.
Amount of Grant: $30,000 per year
Date(s) Application is Due: Sep 1
Contact: Administrator, Scholarships Division; (800) 621-4111 or (312) 202-5000; fax: (312) 202-5001
Internet: http://www.facs.org/memberservices/acsresident.html
Sponsor: American College of Surgeons
633 N. Saint Clair Street
Chicago, IL 60611-3211

American College of Surgeons Wound Care Management Award 433
The American College of Surgeons is offering a two-year faculty research award through KCI U.S.A, to a general surgeon engaged in a research project addressing wound care management. The purpose of this fellowship will be to acquire knowledge leading to new clinical applications or projects that will provide the medical community with a better understanding of the use of advanced wound healing therapies. The fellowship award is $85,000 per year, with the possibility of an extension for a second year if satisfactory progress is made. Specifically, translational projects such as new methods to mechanically stimulate wound healing, design of clinically applicable skin substitutes, methods to enhance specific, difficult-to-heal wounds related to general or extremity trauma, various soft-tissue injuries, quality limb salvage, or methods to reduce surgical intervention to heal a variety of wounds, are being sought. This award may be used by the recipient for support of his/her research or academic enrichment in any fashion that the recipient deems maximally supportive of his/her investigations. This may include faculty salary replacement, support for clinical research personnel, supplies directly related to the research activity, consumable equipment, and research related travel costs up to $2,000 per year.
Requirements: The fellowship is open to Fellows or Associate Fellows of the College who have: (1) completed the chief residency year or accredited fellowship training within the preceding 10 years; and (2) received a fulltime faculty appointment in a department of surgery or a surgical specialty at a medical school accredited by the Liaison Committee on Medical Education in the United States or by the Committee for Accreditation of Canadian Medical Schools in Canada. Preference will be given to applicants who directly enter academic surgery following residency or fellowship.
Amount of Grant: $85,000 per year
Date(s) Application is Due: May 1
Contact: Administrator; (800) 621-4111 or (312) 202-5000; fax: (312) 202-5001
Internet: http://www.facs.org/memberservices/woundcareposter2008.pdf
Sponsor: American College of Surgeons
633 North Saint Clair Street
Chicago, IL 60611-3211

American Electric Power Grants 434
The corporate contributions program awards grants to nonprofit organizations in company-operating areas. Contributions are made principally in the areas of education, the environment, and human services (i.e., hunger, housing, health, safety). Priority is based on the perceived overall benefit to communities in the company's service area. In the area of education, preference is given to grades pre-K through 12 in the fields of science, technology and math. Multiyear commitments to capital campaigns generally do not exceed five years. AEP and its employees provide strong support to many annual United Way campaigns within its service territory; therefore, additional support to United Way agencies is extremely limited. There is no formal application form or deadline. Each request should include evidence of tax-exempt status; amount of funds requested; description of intended use of requested funds, who will benefit, and how they will benefit; overall budget of related program; and description of how the organization will measure results and report outcome of the use of funds being requested. Written requests for local or statewide projects may be submitted to the appropriate AEP state office. Electronic requests in MS Word format may be submitted to the corresponding email address. Guidelines are available online.
Requirements: 501(c)3 nonprofit organizations in Arkansas, Indiana, Kentucky, Louisiana, Michigan, Ohio, Oklahoma, Tennessee, Texas, Virginia and West Virginia are eligible. Grant-seekers should first approach their local AEP operating company.
Restrictions: Grants are not awarded to religious, fraternal, service, and veteran organizations, except for nonsectarian social service activities available to the broader community; organizations with a purpose that is solely athletic in nature; or to individuals.
Geographic Focus: Arkansas; Indiana; Kentucky; Louisiana; Michigan; Ohio; Oklahoma; Tennessee; Texas; Virginia; West Virginia
Contact: Contributions Administrator, (614) 716-1000; email: mkwalsh@aep.com or corpcomm@aep.com
Internet: http://www.aep.com/about/community/corpGive/Default.htm
Sponsor: American Electric Power
AEP Community Relations, 1 Riverside Plaza, 19th Floor
Columbus, OH 43215

American Express Foundation Community Service Grants 435
Whether it is feeding the hungry, mentoring students, building homes for the homeless or cleaning up the environment, tens of thousands of American Express employees serve their communities through volunteerism and personal financial contributions, and the Foundation views this activity as an extension of the service ethic that lies at the heart of its business. It encourages good citizenship by supporting organizations that cultivate meaningful opportunities for civic engagement by employees and members of the community. The Foundation also serves its communities by supporting immediate and long-term relief and recovery efforts to help victims of natural disasters. Funding also goes to support preparedness programs that allow relief agencies to be better equipped in responding to emergencies as they occur.
Requirements: Eligible organizations must: certify tax-exempt status under Section 501(c)3 and 509(a)(1), (2) or (3) of the U.S. Internal Revenue Code. Organizations outside the U.S. must be able to document not-for-profit status.
Restrictions: The program does not fund: individual needs, including scholarships, sponsorships and other forms of financial aid; fund-raising activities, such as galas, benefits, dinners and sporting events; goodwill advertising, souvenir journals or dinner programs; travel for individuals or groups; sectarian activities of religious organizations; political causes, candidates, organizations or campaigns; or books, magazines or articles in professional journals.
Samples: Arizona Foundation for Women, Phoenix, AZ (2007); The Points of Light & Hands On Network, Washington, DC (2007).
Contact: Manager, Philanthropic Program; (212) 640-5661; fax: (212) 693-1033
Internet: http://home3.americanexpress.com/corp/gb/comm_serv.asp
Sponsor: American Express Foundation
3 World Financial Center, mail code 01-48-04
New York, NY 10285-4804

American Foundation for Suicide Prevention Grants 436
The research grants are awarded to investigators conducting clinical, biological, or psychosocial research on the problem of suicide, for one- or two-year periods, and for up to three years for research fellowships. Grant applicants compete in five categories: Pilot Grants provide seed money for new projects and are awarded to individual investigators without regard to academic rank or pervious research experience with suicide; Young Investigator Grants are awarded for two years of support to investigators at the level of assistant professor or lower; Standard Research Grants are awarded to individual investigators for a two-year period; Distinguished Researcher Awards are awarded to investigators at the level of associate professor or higher with a proven history of research in the area of suicide (to fund new directions and initiatives in suicidology); Postdoctoral Research Fellowships are awarded for full-time training projects by investigators who have received a PhD degree within the preceding three years and have not had more than three years of fellowship support. Application deadlines are December 15 for Young Investigator Grants, Standard Research Grants, Distinguished Researcher Awards, and Postdoctoral Fellowships; and April 15, August 15, and December 15 for Pilot Grants. Guidelines and application forms are available online.
Amount of Grant: $20,000 maximum Pilot Grants; $70,000 maximum Young Investigator Grants; $60,000 maximum Standard Research Grants; $100,000 maximum Distinguished Researcher Awards
Date(s) Application is Due: Apr 15; Aug 15; Dec 15
Contact: Grants Administrator, (888) 333-2377 or (212) 363-3500; fax: (212) 363-6237; email: bkoestner@afsp.org
Internet: http://www.afsp.org/research/grants.htm
Sponsor: American Foundation for Suicide Prevention
120 Wall Street, 22nd Floor
New York, NY 10005

American Jewish World Service Grants 437
AJWS' grantmaking supports community-based organizations in the developing world that are undertaking holistic community development programs. These groups design and implement projects that creatively and effectively address economic development, education, healthcare, and sustainable agriculture. All of the initiatives also have strong components of strengthening civil society and/or promoting women's empowerment. Grantmaking links human rights and sustainable development.
Requirements: Grassroots organizations are eligible.
Restrictions: Grants are not awarded to individuals.
Samples: Cross-Cultural Solutions (New Rochelle, NY)—to provide food to rescue workers and to coordinate volunteer efforts at the site of the World Trade Center,

$5000.; Independent Press Assoc (New York, NY)—to place advertisements in New York ethnic publications on the availability of disaster resources in the wake of the September 11 attacks, $25,500.; Mount Sinai Hospital, Disaster Psychiatry Outreach (New York, NY)—to work with the New York City Department of Mental Health in its outreach efforts to counsel rescue workers and victims of the World Trade Center collapse, $10,000.
Amount of Grant: $3000-$30,000
Contact: Grants Administrator, (800) 889-7146 or (212) 792-2100; fax: 212.792.2930; email: grants@ajws.org
Internet: http://www.ajws.org/index.cfm?section_id=3
Sponsor: American Jewish World Service
45 W 36th Street, 10th Floor
New York, NY 10018-7904

American Legacy Foundation National Calls for Proposals Grants 438
The American Legacy Foundation provides grants to support innovations in tobacco control. National calls for proposals, such as the Priority Populations Initiative, are issued annually to address a variety of tobacco prevention and control issues. Comprehensive assistance and training are provided to the foundation's grantees as well as to state and local tobacco programs. Application forms, guidelines, and procedures are available online. There are no application deadlines.
Requirements: Funding is available only to state or local political subdivisions and legally constituted tax-exempt 501(c)3 organizations based in the 46 states, the District of Columbia, and five territories (American Samoa, Guam, Northern Mariana Islands, Puerto Rico, and the Virgin Islands) identified in the MSA with tobacco product manufacturers. An Indian reservation, Indian tribe, or tribal organization located within the 46 settling states or a non-governmental entity that serves such a reservation may also apply for funding.
Restrictions: The foundation will not award grants to applicants that are in current receipt of grant monies or in-kind contributions from any tobacco manufacturer, distributor, or other tobacco-related entity.
Contact: Katherine Wilson, Assistant Vice President of Grants; (202) 454-5555; fax: (202) 454-5599; email: grantsinfo@americanlegacy.org
Internet: http://www.americanlegacy.org/64.aspx
Sponsor: American Legacy Foundation
1724 Massachusetts Avenue, NW
Washington, DC 20036

American Legacy Foundation Small Innovative Grants 439
The program supports projects that advance creative, promising solutions based on sound principles of tobacco control to remedy the harm caused by tobacco use in America. The program was created to seed new projects or enable an organization to pilot a new idea or approach. The proposed project must demonstrate an element of creativity, ingenuity or innovation and must distinguish itself from the large number of solid programs proposed to the foundation in each grant round.
Requirements: Funding is available only to state or local political subdivisions and legally constituted tax-exempt 501(c)3 organizations based in the 46 states, the District of Columbia, and five territories (American Samoa, Guam, Northern Mariana Islands, Puerto Rico, and the Virgin Islands) identified in the MSA with tobacco product manufacturers. An Indian reservation, Indian tribe, or tribal organization located within the 46 settling states or a nongovernmental entity that serves such a reservation may also apply for funding. Successful applications submitted under the Small Innovative Grants Program must: address one or both of Legacy's goals; demonstrate innovative or new tobacco prevention or cessation efforts; demonstrate a strong likelihood for a sustainable effort after the grant period; demonstrate that the project may be replicated; address the Healthy People 2010 risk reduction objectives related to tobacco use, and; incorporate the CDC's Best Practices for Comprehensive Tobacco Control Programs as appropriate. The foundation will give special consideration to applications addressing these current areas of interest.
Restrictions: The foundation will not award a grant to any applicant that is in current receipt of any grant monies or in-kind contribution from any tobacco manufacturer, distributor, or other tobacco-related entity. In addition, the foundation expects that a grantee will not accept any grant monies or in-kind contribution from any tobacco manufacturer, distributor, or other tobacco-related entity over the duration of the grant. Additionally, will not consider applications for: Projects focusing on youth prevention, cessation, activism, or education (up to 18 years old); Nicotine replacement therapy (NRT) and pharmaceuticals (as the sole or primary focus of the grant); Conference support (as the sole or primary focus of the grant); Media or marketing campaigns (as the sole or primary focus of the grant); Research projects EXCEPT community-based participatory research, which is allowed; Projects focusing on substances other than tobacco; Replication of an existing program; Expansion of an existing program; and Replacement funds; Grants to individuals, for religious activities, to build endowments, to support operating deficits, to retire debt, for capital purchases for building improvements, for construction, for lobbying, or for real estate purchase or development.
Amount of Grant: $20,000-$100,000 annually
Date(s) Application is Due: Feb 27; Aug 8
Contact: Katherine Wilson, Assistant Vice President of Grants; (202) 454-5555; fax: (202) 454-5599; email: grantsinfo@americanlegacy.org
Internet: http://www.americanlegacy.org/2530.aspx
Sponsor: American Legacy Foundation
1724 Massachusetts Avenue, NW
Washington, DC 20036

American Medical Association Awards 440
The American Medical Association recognizes excellence through the following AMA Awards: Distinguished Service Award; Citation for Distinguished Service; AMA Medal of Valor; Scientific Achievement Award; Benjamin Rush Award for Citizenship and Community Service; President's Citation for Service to the Public; Joseph B. Goldberger Award in Clinical Nutrition; Dr. William Beaumont Award in Medicine; AMA Foundation Award for Health Education; Isaac Hays, MD and John Bell, MD Award for Leadership in Medical Ethics and Professionalism; Medical Executive Lifetime Achievement Award; and Medical Executive Meritorious Achievement Award. Candidates may be nominated for more than one award. Nominations should be emailed by February 23 each year.
Date(s) Application is Due: Feb 23
Contact: Roger Brown; (312) 464-4344; fax: (312) 464-4505; email: roger.brown@ama-assn.org
Internet: http://www.ama-assn.org/ama/pub/about-ama/awards/about-ama-awards-program.shtml
Sponsor: American Medical Association (AMA)
515 N. State Street
Chicago, IL 60610

American Philosophical Society Daland Fellowships in Clinical Investigation 441
A limited number of fellowships are awarded annually for research in clinical medicine including the fields of internal medicine, neurology, psychiatry, pediatrics, and surgery. Patient-oriented research is emphasized. Essentially 100 percent of the fellow's time will be devoted to research. Teaching or clinical service of a limited amount is permitted. Additional salary may be granted by the institution at which the fellow is located, from another fellowship, or from a similar award during the tenure of the fellowship. The term of the fellowship is one year, with possible renewal for another year. Applications are available on the Web site, or may be obtained by written request, stating when the MD or MD/PhD degree was awarded; include a self-addressed mailing label.
Requirements: These fellowships are designed for qualified persons who have held an MD, or MD/PhD degree for less than eight years. The fellowship is generally intended to be the first post-clinical fellowship; but each case will be decided on its merits. Preference is generally given to candidates who have not more than two years of post-doctoral training and research. Applicants must expect to perform their research at an institution in the United States, under the supervision of a scientific adviser. Candidates are to be nominated by their department chairman, in a letter providing assurance that the nominee will work with the guidance of a scientific adviser of established reputation who has guaranteed adequate space, supplies, etc. for the Fellow. The adviser need not be a member of the department nominating the Fellow, nor need the activities of the Fellow be limited to the nominating department. As a general rule, no more than one fellowship will be awarded to a given institution in the same year of competition.
Restrictions: The society does not provide funds for institutional overhead.
Amount of Grant: $40,000 per year for up to two years
Date(s) Application is Due: Sep 1
Contact: Linda Musumeci, Research Administrator; (215) 440-3429; email: LMusumeci@amphilsoc.org
Internet: http://www.amphilsoc.org/grants/daland.htm
Sponsor: American Philosophical Society
104 South Fifth Street
Philadelphia, PA 19106-3387

American Psychiatric Association Award for Research in Psychiatry 442
The Award is given in recognition of a single distinguished contribution, a body of work, or a lifetime contribution that has had a major impact on the field and/or altered the practice of psychiatry. The Award is intended to cover the full spectrum of psychiatric research. The Award consists of a $5,000 prize and an honorary plaque to be presented at APA's Annual Meeting. The Award also includes an honorary lecture by the awardee.
Requirements: Candidates for the Award must be citizens of the United States or Canada and be nominated by a sponsor. Sponsors must be members of the American Psychiatric Association.
Restrictions: Members of the Award Committee are excluded from submitting nominations.
Amount of Grant: $5,000
Date(s) Application is Due: Aug 28
Contact: Harold Goldstein; (703) 907-8623; email: goharold@psych.org
Internet: http://www.psych.org/research/apire/training_fund/psychaward.cfm
Sponsor: American Psychiatric Association
1000 Wilson Boulevard, Suite 1825
Arlington, VA 22209-3901

American Psychiatric Association Minority Fellowships Program 443
The APA offers psychiatric residents one-year fellowships in the APA organization to increase the knowledge of cultural factors influencing psychiatric diagnosis and treatment, provide opportunities for these residents to participate in the deliberations and decision-making processes, and provide role models for the fellows. Each fellow is appointed to a component of the APA's organizational structure and attends the association's annual meeting as an observer and active participant. Fellows are selected on the basis of their commitment to serving underrepresented populations, demonstrated leadership abilities, and interest in the interrelationship between mental health/illness and transcultural factors.
Requirements: Psychiatric residents who are starting their second year of psychiatric training, or third year if they are in a four-year residency program, are eligible to apply.

Contact: Marilyn King, Fellowship Coordinator; (703) 907-8653; fax: (703) 907-7849; email: mking@psych.org
Internet: http://www.psych.org/Resources/OMNA/MFP.aspx
Sponsor: American Psychiatric Association
1000 Wilson Boulevard, Suite 1825
Arlington, VA 22209-3901

American Psychiatric Association Minority Medical Student Fellowship in HIV Psychiatry 444

The APA invites ethnic minority medical students who have an interest in psychiatric issues to apply. The program is intended to identify minority medical students who have primary interests in services related to HIV/AIDS and substance abuse and its relationship to the mental health or psychological well being of ethnic minorities.
Requirements: These programs are open to ethnic minority medical students who are U.S. citizens or permanent residents currently enrolled in a U.S. medical school.
Date(s) Application is Due: Mar 31
Contact: Diane Pennessi, Project Manager; (703)907-8668; email: dpennessi@psych.org.
Internet: http://www.psych.org/Resources/OMNA/MFP/HIV-Information-10.aspx
Sponsor: American Psychiatric Association
1000 Wilson Boulevard, Suite 1825
Arlington, VA 22209-3901

American Psychiatric Association Minority Medical Student Summer Externship in Addiction Psychiatry 445

The APA invites ethnic minority medical students who have an interest in psychiatric issues to apply. This clinical shadowing program identifies minority medical students who may have a specific interest in services related to substance abuse treatment/prevention and provide a setting where the student can work closely with a mentor who specializes in addiction psychiatry for one month.
Requirements: These programs are open to ethnic minority medical students who are U.S. citizens or permanent residents currently enrolled in a U.S. medical school.
Amount of Grant: $1,500
Date(s) Application is Due: Feb 28
Contact: Marilyn King, Assistant Program Director; (703) 907-8653; fax: (703) 907-7852; email: mking@psych.org
Internet: http://www.psych.org/Resources/OMNA/MFP/minoritymedicalstudent summerexternshipinaddictionpsychiatry.aspx
Sponsor: American Psychiatric Association
1000 Wilson Boulevard, Suite 1825
Arlington, VA 22209-3901

American Psychiatric Association Minority Medical Student Summer Mentoring Program 446

The APA invites ethnic minority medical students who have an interest in psychiatric issues to apply. This program is intended to identify ethnic minority medical students who have an interest in psychiatric issues and expose students to a setting where they can work closely with a psychiatrist mentor for one month.
Requirements: These programs are open to ethnic minority medical students who are U.S. citizens or permanent residents currently enrolled in a U.S. medical school.
Amount of Grant: $1,500
Date(s) Application is Due: Feb 28
Contact: Marilyn King, Assistant Program Director; (703) 907-8653; fax: (703) 907-7852; email: mking@psych.org
Internet: http://www.psych.org/Resources/OMNA/MFP/minoritymedicalstudentsu mmermentoringprogram.aspx
Sponsor: American Psychiatric Association
1000 Wilson Boulevard, Suite 1825
Arlington, VA 22209-3901

American Psychiatric Association Program for Minority Research Training in Psychiatry (PMRTP) 447

The program is designed to increase the number of underrepresented minority men and women in the field of psychiatric research. Research training offers the opportunity to engage in scientific investigation across the full array of disciplines, from basic neuroscience, genetics, and pharmacology to the cognitive behavioral, and social sciences, clinical psychiatry, and mental health services research. Research exposure can help students and trainees develop sound skills for clinical assessment and treatment planning. The program provides funding for short and long-term training opportunities at three levels: Medical School, Residency and Post-residency. National competitions also enable qualified mini-fellows to attend research-oriented meetings of psychiatric organizations. For medical students and residents, the duration can be two months to one year. For post-residency fellows, the duration is generally two years. A third year of fellowship support may be available if appropriate to a trainee's career development. Support from PMRTP falls into three categories: stipends, travel, and tuition and fees. Stipends are based on the trainee's years of relevant experience and the length of the research training experience.
Requirements: Preference in selection is given to underrepresented minorities such as American Indians, Asian-Americans, Blacks/African-Americans, Hispanics, Pacific Islanders, or other ethnic or racial group members found to be underrepresented in biomedical or behavioral research.
Amount of Grant: $20,772-$51,036
Date(s) Application is Due: Dec 1; Apr 1
Contact: Ernesto Guerra, (703) 907-7300; fax: (703) 907-1085; email: eguerra&@psych.org or apa@psych.org
Internet: http://www.psych.org/MainMenu/Research/ResearchTrainingandFunding/ResearchFellowships/ProgramforMinorityResearchTraininginPsychiatry.aspx
Sponsor: American Psychiatric Association
1000 Wilson Boulevard, Suite 1825
Arlington, VA 22209-3901

American Psychiatric Association Research Colloquium for Junior Investigators 448

The purpose of the colloquium is to provide guidance, mentorship and encouragement to young investigators in the early phases of their training. Junior investigators will have an opportunity to obtain feedback about their past, present, and future research interests from mentors who are tops in their field in a small group setting as well as general information about research career development and grantsmanship. Candidates whose research interests are similar to those listed below are also encouraged to apply. An all-day workshop for junior psychiatric investigators will focus on these three areas: childhood disorders including autism, ADHD, conduct, eating, and mood disorders; genomics, epigenetics, and proteomics; and treatment of major psychiatric disorders: from substance abuse to schizophrenia.
Requirements: Psychiatrists who are senior residents, fellows, or junior faculty, and who have an interest and potential in developing research careers in the areas of research listed above. Participants should hold a medical degree or be a member of the APA; or be eligible to become members of the APA.
Restrictions: Those with individual federal research awards are not eligible.
Amount of Grant: $1,000 stipend
Date(s) Application is Due: Nov 16
Contact: Ernesto Guerra; (703) 907-7300; fax: (703) 907-1085; email: eguerra@psych.org or apa@psych.org
Internet: http://psych.org/MainMenu/Research/ResearchTrainingandFunding/ResearchColloquiumforJuniorInvestigators.aspx
Sponsor: American Psychiatric Association
1000 Wilson Boulevard, Suite 1825
Arlington, VA 22209-3901

American Psychiatric Association Travel Scholarships for Minority Medical Students 449

The APA invites ethnic minority medical students who have an interest in psychiatric issues to apply. The program supports travel and related costs for approximately 10 minority medical students interested in psychiatric to attend either the APA annual meeting in May or the Institute on Psychiatric Services (IPS) meeting in October. This program is a way for medical students to witness organized psychiatry at work and to learn more about the field. Not only will students attend sessions for experts and trainees alike, but they will be assigned to a mentor who will help them maximize their annual meeting or IPS experience and discuss career plans and resident training programs.
Requirements: These programs are open to U.S. ethnic minority medical students who are U.S. citizens or permanent residents currently enrolled in a U.S. medical school. Ethnic minorities are: American-Indian, Alaska Native, Native Hawaiian, Asian-American, African-American, and Hispanic/Latino.
Date(s) Application is Due: Jan 29
Contact: Marilyn King, Assistant Program Director; (703) 907-8653; fax: (703) 907-7852; email: mking@psych.org
Internet: http://www.psych.org/Resources/OMNA/MFP/MedicalStudent TravelScholarships.aspx
Sponsor: American Psychiatric Association
1000 Wilson Boulevard, Suite 1825
Arlington, VA 22209-3901

American Psychiatric Association/AstraZeneca Young Minds in Psychiatry International Awards 450

The program recognizes and supports promising international young psychiatrists within five years of completing a psychiatric residency. Four unrestricted career development awards of $45,000 (U.S.D) will be available. Awards will be made to two promising physicians from the U.S. with one in Bipolar Disorder research and one on research in Schizophrenia. An additional two awards will be made to promising physicians from countries outside the U.S., with one in Bipolar Disorder research and one on research in Schizophrenia. Three other awards of $30,000 (U.S.D) in either Bipolar Disorder or Schizophrenia research will specifically focus on applicants from developing countries whose economies are classified by the World Bank as low income or lower middle income.
Requirements: The U.S. applicants must be citizens or permanent residents of the United States. Applications are evaluated based on evidence of academic promise; how the proposal will advance the applicant's career; and innovative or original concepts, approaches, or methods for developing the applicant's career.
Amount of Grant: $45,000
Date(s) Application is Due: Nov 30
Contact: Ernesto Guerra, (703) 907-7300; fax: (703) 907-1085; email: eguerra@psych.org or apa@psych.org
Internet: http://psych.org/MainMenu/Research/ResearchTrainingandFunding/ResearchFellowships/APAAstraZenecaYoungMindsinPsychiatryInternationalAward.aspx
Sponsor: American Psychiatric Association
1000 Wilson Boulevard, Suite 1825
Arlington, VA 22209-3901

American Psychiatric Association/Bristol-Myers Squibb Fellowships in Public Psychiatry 451

This important collaborative venture between the American Psychiatric Association and the Bristol-Myers Squibb Company provides for the selection of ten residents in psychiatry, based on recommendations from their Departments and evidence of a track record of commitment to and accomplishment in public psychiatry. The purposes of the APA/Bristol-Myers Squibb Fellowship are twofold: (1) to heighten psychiatric residents' awareness of the many activities of psychiatry in the public sector and of the career opportunities in this work, and (2) to provide experiences which will contribute to the professional development of those residents who will play leadership roles within the public sector in future years.
Requirements: Nomination Procedure and Eligibility Criteria: One outstanding resident who has a substantial interest in any area of public sector psychiatry and a significant potential for a leadership role in such work may be nominated by a psychiatric residency training program that is accredited by the Accreditation Council for Graduate Medical Education or the Royal College of Physicians and Surgeons of Canada; submission of a nomination represents an explicit commitment by the residency program to permit the candidate, if selected, time off to attend APA meetings in their entirety during the fellowship term, as well as the candidate's willingness to do so; Psychiatric residents who will be in the PG-3 year of training during the fellowship term are eligible to participate in the program; residents who will be in their PG-4 year will also be considered if they are in a 5-year psychiatric training program; nominee must be an APA member or in the process of becoming a member.
Restrictions: Residents who have received (or are scheduled to receive) other APA fellowships or comparable outside fellowships (e.g., Ginsberg, Laughlin) are not eligible. Those residents who currently serve on APA's Committee of Residents and Fellows are not eligible for the fellowship.
Date(s) Application is Due: Mar 31
Contact: Nancy Delanoche, APA Office of Graduate and Undergraduate Education; (703) 907-8635; email: ndelanoche@psych.org
Internet: http://www.psych.org/Departments/EDU/ResidentMIT/fellowshipinpublicpsychiatry.aspx
Sponsor: American Psychiatric Association
1000 Wilson Boulevard, Suite 1825
Arlington, VA 22209-3901

American Psychiatric Association/Janssen Resident Psychiatric Research Scholars 452

The program is intended to identify promising PGY-1, PGY-2, and PGY-3 psychiatric residents with the potential to become leaders in clinical and health services research in all areas of psychiatric research. Emphasis will be placed on special mentoring and career enrichment programs both at the APA Annual Meeting and throughout the year. An individual research mentor will be assigned to oversee the resident's fellowship. The mentors will be chosen among nationally known leaders in clinical and health services research. The mentor will advise and encourage the Scholar during the two-year fellowship. The scholar will receive $2,500 during the second year of the fellowship, to assist in their research career development (e.g., for use in developing a pilot research project, obtaining statistical consultation, or visiting potential research training programs). The program also provides funding for travel to the American Psychiatric Association (APA) Annual Meeting during both years of the fellowship.
Amount of Grant: $2,500
Date(s) Application is Due: Jan 15
Contact: Ernesto Guerra, (703) 907-7300; fax: (703) 907-1085; email: eguerra@psych.org or apa@psych.org
Internet: http://psych.org/MainMenu/Research/ResearchTrainingandFunding/ResearchFellowships/APIREJanssenResidentPsychiatricResearchScholars.aspx
Sponsor: American Psychiatric Association
1000 Wilson Boulevard, Suite 1825
Arlington, VA 22209-3901

American Psychiatric Association/Merck Early Academic Career Research Award 453

The Award is intended to help support the research of a junior faculty member with an interest in sleep disorders or schizophrenia. Two separate awards will be made to candidates who have completed a psychiatry residency, at least one year of a psychiatry research fellowship, and are seeking to make a commitment to a research career with the end goal of successfully transitioning to that of an independent investigator. The Award is intended to assist in this key transition period by providing one year of funding of $45,000. Salary support provided by this award will allow junior faculty in departments of psychiatry at U.S. academic institutions to devote more time to research.
Requirements: Candidates must be citizens or permanent residents of the U.S. and should also be APA members. Eligible candidates will be trained psychiatrists with an MD, MD/Ph.D. or DO degree who have completed residency training in general psychiatry or child psychiatry in the U.S. Candidates also should have completed at least one year of a psychiatry research fellowship but are not 3 or more years post fellowship completion, and do not currently hold an academic rank higher than Assistant Professor.
Restrictions: Individuals who have obtained K-awards or are considered an independent Principal Investigator on R-01 or R-21 research grants from NIH are not eligible.
Amount of Grant: $45,000
Date(s) Application is Due: Oct 14
Contact: Ernesto Guerra, (703) 907-7300; email: eguerra@psych.org or apa@psych.org
Internet: http://www.psych.org/research/apire/res_careerdev/apamerck.cfm
Sponsor: American Psychiatric Association
1000 Wilson Boulevard, Suite 1825
Arlington, VA 22209-3901

American Schlafhorst Foundation Grants 454

The foundation awards grants to eligible North Carolina nonprofit organizations in its areas of interest, including arts, children and youth, elderly, education, health care, science, and social services delivery. Types of support include building construction/renovation, equipment acquisition, general operating grants, research grants, scholarships, and seed money grants.
Requirements: 501(c)3 tax-exempt organizations serving the greater Charlotte, NC, area are eligible.
Restrictions: Individuals are not eligible.
Geographic Focus: North Carolina
Amount of Grant: $1000-$40,000
Contact: Grants Administrator, (704) 554-0800; email: info@schlafhorst.com
Sponsor: American Schlafhorst Foundation
8801 South Boulevard
Charlotte, NC 28224

American Society on Aging Graduate Student Research Award 455

The award is presented annually to a graduate student for research relevant to aging and applicable to practice. The winner will be expected to attend the joint conference of the ASA and the National Council on the Aging to present the winning paper. The award comprises a certificate, complimentary registration and one-night's lodging for the conference, presentation of research findings at a highlighted session at the conference, and complimentary one-year membership in ASA. Submission guidelines and application are available online.
Requirements: Only graduate-level research will be considered. Findings must be from completed research; submission of the conceptual framework alone is not sufficient. Applicants must either be currently enrolled in a graduate degree program or must have completed their studies no more than one year before the time of submission. Applicants must be sponsored by a faculty member. Applicants and faculty sponsors need not be ASA members.
Restrictions: Papers that have been published are not eligible for submission.
Date(s) Application is Due: Oct 1
Contact: Nancy Decia, Coordinator, Education & Training; (415) 974-9610; fax: (415) 974-0300; email: awards@asaging.org
Internet: http://www.asaging.org/asav2/awards/description_grad.cfm?submenu1=grad
Sponsor: American Society on Aging
833 Market Street, Suite 511
San Francisco, CA 94103-1824

American Society on Aging Mental Health and Aging Awards 456

The awards are made to organizations that have demonstrated high-quality, innovative programs that enhance the health-related quality of life in older adults. The program recognizes outstanding intervention programs developed in recent years to improve the health and health care of the aging. Model programs can include, but are not limited to, wellness/health promotion programs, community-based care, dementia care, mental health, caregiver supports, medication management, chronic illness care, end-of-life care, and programs that expand access to underserved groups of older adults. Winning programs will be honored at the Conference of The National Council on the Aging (NCOA) and the American Society on Aging (ASA). Up to six programs will receive cash awards, one-night's lodging for one person at the conference, and a one-year complimentary membership to ASA and the Healthcare and Aging Network.
Requirements: Applicants must be ASA members. The program must have at least one year's worth of program results and cannot have been in existence longer than five years (or must represent a substantially new program model in the past five years) by the date of submission.
Restrictions: Organizations that have won this award within the past two years are not eligible to apply.
Amount of Grant: $2,500 cash award
Date(s) Application is Due: Oct 31
Contact: Nancy Decia, Coordinator, Education & Training; (415) 974-9610; fax: (415) 974-0300; email: awards@asaging.org;; Tobi Abramson; (516) 596-0073; email: tabramson@excite.com
Internet: http://www.asaging.org/asav2/awards/description_mhan.cfm?submenu1=mhan
Sponsor: American Society on Aging
833 Market Street, Suite 511
San Francisco, CA 94103-1824

American Society on Aging NOMA Award for Excellence in Multicultural Aging 457

Awards will be given to organizations that have demonstrated high-quality, innovative programs that enhance the lives of a multicultural aging population. Using the framework that supports the broader vision of diversity at the American Society on Aging, the NOMA Award for Excellence in Multicultural Aging seeks to identify and recognize best practices in developing and implementing programs and/or services that meet the needs of a multicultural aging population. Up to three programs will receive cash awards of $1,500, one complimentary conference registration, one night's lodging for one person at the conference and a one-year complimentary membership to ASA and the Network on Multicultural Aging (NOMA).
Requirements: Eligible applicants must: be an organization or have an affiliation with an organization that focuses on providing information and services to an aging population; have a program and/or service targeted to a multicultural aging population that has been tested, has a proven and successful track record, and has been in existence for a minimum of one year; and have a membership with ASA.
Amount of Grant: $1,500

Date(s) Application is Due: Dec 15
Contact: Mahi Sadeghi, Coordinator, Diversity & Education; (415) 974-9602; fax: (415) 974-0300; email: awards@asaging.org
Internet: http://www.asaging.org/asav2/awards/description_noma.cfm?submenu1=noma
Sponsor: American Society on Aging / Network on Multicultural Aging
833 Market Street, Suite 511
San Francisco, CA 94103-1824

American Sociological Association Minority Fellowships **458**
Through its Minority Fellowship Program (MFP), the American Sociological Association (ASA) supports the development and training of sociologists of color in mental health and drug abuse research. Funded by a training grant sponsored by the National Institute of Mental Health (NIMH) and co-funded by the National Institute of Drug Abuse (NIDA), MFP seeks to attract talented doctoral students to ensure a diverse and highly trained workforce is available to assume leadership roles in research related to the nation's mental health and drug abuse research agendas.
Requirements: American citizens and permanent visa residents including, but not limited to, persons who are African American, Latino/Hispanic (e.g., Chicano, Cuban, Puerto Rican), Native American, and Asian American (e.g., Chinese, Japanese, Korean), and Pacific Islanders (e.g., Hawaiian, Guamanian, Samoan, Filipino) are eligible. The program is open to students beginning or continuing study in graduate sociology departments. New students must qualify for acceptance at accredited institutions of higher learning and express a commitment to sociological research on mental health. Upon completion of their support, recipients are expected to engage in behavioral research or teaching, or a combination thereof, for a period equal to the period of support beyond 12 months.
Amount of Grant: $20,000-$25,000 stipend
Date(s) Application is Due: Jan 31
Contact: Margaret Weigers Vitullo, Director; (202) 383-9005, ext. 323; fax: (202) 638-0882; email: spivack@asanet.org or apap@asanet.org
Internet: http://www.asanet.org/cs/root/leftnav/funding/minority_fellowship_program
Sponsor: American Sociological Association
1430 K Street NW, Suite 600
Washington, DC 20005

American-Italian Cancer Foundation Fellowships **459**
The mission of the program is to further the advancement of cancer research by sponsoring the research and training of promising young scientists in Italy and in the United States. A major activity is the award of fellowships to Italian and American scientists so that they might spend a period of research and advanced training in preclinical or clinical research centers in the United States or Italy. The fellowships are intended to augment the training of motivated scientists who have the potential to conduct path-breaking original research upon the return to their respective countries. The one-year fellowships are renewable for an additional year.
Requirements: Individuals in the United States and Italy who have been awarded the degrees of PhD, MD, DSc, or DVM may apply in conjunction with a host institution. Candidates must have received their degree no more than three years prior to the date of application.
Amount of Grant: $25,000 Italian fellowships; $30,000 U.S. fellowships
Date(s) Application is Due: Mar 1
Contact: Franca Gaudio, (212) 628-9090; fax: (212) 517-6089; email: fgaudio@aicfonline.org
Internet: http://www.aicfonline.org
Sponsor: American-Italian Cancer Foundation
112 E 71st Street, Suite 2B
New York, NY 10021

American-Scandinavian Foundation Visiting Lectureship Grants **460**
The ASF invites U.S. colleges and universities to apply for funding to host a visiting lecturer from Norway or Sweden. The $20,000 awards are for appointments of one semester. Lectureships should be in the areas of: public policy, conflict resolution, health care, environmental studies or multiculturalism. Letters of Intent are due by November 6, with full applications postmarked by February 5.
Requirements: The competition is open to all American colleges and universities. The award is appropriate not just for Scandinavian studies departments, but for any department or inter-disciplinary program with an interest in incorporating a Scandinavian focus into its course offerings. The lecturer must be a Norwegian or Swedish citizen, and a scholar or expert in a field appropriate to the host department or program.
Amount of Grant: $20,000
Date(s) Application is Due: Nov 6; Feb 5
Contact: Ellen McKey, Director of Fellowships and Grants; (212) 879-9779; fax: (212) 249-3444; email: grants@amscan.org
Sponsor: American-Scandinavian Foundation
58 Park Avenue
New York, NY 10016

Amerisure Insurance Community Service Grants **461**
The company awards grants nationwide to nonprofit organizations in the areas of education and health. There are no application forms. Send proposals to the headquarters office or the nearest facility. Proposals should contain a detailed description of the project and the amount requested. Junior achievement is supported especially in K-12 classrooms in the Farmington Hills, MI school system.
Requirements: Nonprofit organizations are eligible.
Date(s) Application is Due: Dec 31
Contact: Human Resources, (248) 615-9000
Internet: http://www.amerisure.com/au_1d_community.cfm
Sponsor: Amerisure Insurance Company
26777 Halsted Road
Farmington Hills, MI 48331-3586

amfAR Fellowships **462**
An amfAR fellowship is a grant that encourages the postdoctoral (M.D., Ph.D., or equivalent) investigator with limited experience in the field to advance a career in HIV/AIDS research. Fellowships are awarded for two years and may not be renewed for additional funding. amfAR fellows and mentors must be affiliated with the same nonprofit institution. The applicant's interest in a career in HIV/AIDS will be demonstrated by previous relevant work at the postdoctoral fellow or instructor level and will be carefully evaluated. Each fellowship is funded at a total of up to $125,000: a maximum of $110,000 is allowed for personnel (salary and fringe benefits) and other research-related direct costs. It is expected that a fellow will devote the decided majority of his or her time to the approved fellowship project. Personnel costs supported by the fellowship must represent a minimum of 85% effort and be consistent with institution policy for other institution personnel of similar rank and title, regardless of source(s) of support. An additional $3,636 is provided to support attendance at amfAR-approved professional development activities, for a direct cost maximum of $113,636. The period of performance for fellowships awarded under this RFP will be for two years starting January 1.
Requirements: The fellowship applicant must be mentored by an experienced investigator who: is qualified to oversee the proposed research; has successfully supervised postdoctoral fellows; and is at the associate professor level or higher.
Restrictions: Institutional indirect costs may not exceed 10% of direct costs.
Amount of Grant: $125,000 total
Date(s) Application is Due: Jul 7
Contact: Grant Administrator; (212) 806-1696 or (212) 806-1600; fax: (212) 806-1601; email: grants@amfar.org
Internet: http://www.amfar.org/lab/grants/default.aspx?id=7455&terms=Fellowships
Sponsor: American Foundation for AIDS Research
120 Wall Street, 13th Floor
New York, NY 10005-3908

amfAR Global Initiatives Grants **463**
Since awarding its first international grant in 1986, amfAR has supported HIV/AIDS research, prevention, education, and training programs in dozens of countries across the developing world. Today, amfAR's international grant making supports two important initiatives. Formed in 2001, TREAT Asia is a network of clinics, hospitals, and research centers working with civil society to ensure the safe and effective delivery of HIV/AIDS treatments across Asia and the Pacific. And through a newly established MSM Initiative, amfAR awards grants to grassroots groups in support of innovative HIV/AIDS services for men who have sex with men in resource-limited countries.
Amount of Grant: $15,000 maximum
Date(s) Application is Due: 7/21/09
Contact: Grant Administrator; (212) 806-1696 or (212) 806-1600; fax: (212) 806-1601; email: grants@amfar.org
Internet: http://www.amfar.org/world/grants/default.aspx?id=192
Sponsor: American Foundation for AIDS Research
120 Wall Street, 13th Floor
New York, NY 10005-3908

amfAR Mathilde Krim Fellowships in Basic Biomedical Research **464**
amfAR, The Foundation for AIDS Research, is pleased to announce the availability of support for Mathilde Krim Fellowships in Basic Biomedical Research. Each fellowship is funded at a total of up to $125,000 (phase I): a maximum of $110,000 is allowed for personnel (salary and fringe benefits) and other research-related direct costs. It is expected that a Krim fellow will devote the decided majority of his or her time to the approved fellowship project. Personnel costs supported by the fellowship must represent a minimum of 85% effort and be consistent with institution policy for other institution personnel of similar rank and title, regardless of source(s) of support. An additional $3,636 is provided to support attendance at amfAR-approved professional development activities, for a direct cost maximum of $113,636. Contingent upon subsequent application and peer review, phase II funding for an additional consecutive year may be approved to support basic biomedical HIV/AIDS research costs (up to $50,000 total) during the first year of a tenure-track position at any U.S. or international nonprofit research institution. The period of performance for Mathilde Krim Fellowships awarded under this RFP will be from January 1 to December 31 of the following year.
Restrictions: Institutional indirect costs may not exceed 10% of direct costs.
Amount of Grant: $125,000 total
Date(s) Application is Due: Jul 7
Contact: Grant Administrator; (212) 806-1696 or (212) 806-1600; fax: (212) 806-1601; email: grants@amfar.org
Internet: http://www.amfar.org/lab/grants/default.aspx?id=7455&terms=Fellowships
Sponsor: American Foundation for AIDS Research
120 Wall Street, 13th Floor
New York, NY 10005-3908

amfAR Public Policy Grants **465**
AmfAR's public policy grants support the advancement of evidence-based AIDS-related public policies. Many of these awards facilitate the study and implementation of

HIV prevention methods, such as harm reduction programs, that are based on sound science and help save lives. Public policy grants also help fund policy-related educational programs, including conferences.
Samples: Ronald Bayer, Ph.D., The Evolving Ethics and Politics for HIV Testing, Columbia University, Joseph L. Mailman School of Public Health, New York, NY, $66,000 (2008); Paula Santiago, 7th National Harm Reduction Conference, Harm Reduction Coalition, New York, NY, $10,000 (2008).
Contact: Grant Administrator; (212) 806-1696 or (212) 806-1600; fax: (212) 806-1601; email: grants@amfar.org
Internet: http://www.amfar.org/hill/article.aspx?id=3920
Sponsor: American Foundation for AIDS Research
120 Wall Street, 13th Floor
New York, NY 10005-3908

amfAR Research Grants 466
Grants are awarded to support basic and clinical research projects in biomedical, humanistic, and social sciences research relevant to AIDS. In general, funds are applied to direct costs of salaries and fringe benefits for professional and technical personnel, laboratory supplies and equipment, travel, and the publication of findings. Research grants are awarded for one year without assurance of continued funding. $100,000 in direct costs plus up to 20% for indirect costs is available. Investigators are required to submit a pre-application letter of intent (LOI). Any postdoctoral investigator who is affiliated with a nonprofit institution may submit an LOI.
Requirements: Principal investigators for research grants must be faculty-level researchers affiliated with a nonprofit institution. Research grants are given to nonprofit institutions worldwide to support investigator-led projects approved by the Foundation.
Samples: Columbia U (New York, NY)—to support the work of Susana Valente, for studies on microbicide development and AIDS-related research, $90,000.
Amount of Grant: $100,000
Contact: Grant Administrator; (212) 806-1696 or (212) 806-1600; fax: (212) 806-1601; email: grants@amfar.org
Internet: http://www.amfar.org/rfp/
Sponsor: American Foundation for AIDS Research
120 Wall Street, 13th Floor
New York, NY 10005-3908

Amgen Foundation Grants 467
Amgen seeks to: advance science education, improve quality of care and access for patients, and support resources that create sound communities where Amgen staff members live and work. Requests must be received at least 90 days in advance of the desired contribution date. Guidelines are available online.
Requirements: 501(c)3 tax-exempt organizations located in Amgen communities are eligible. Eligible grantees may include public elementary and secondary schools, as well as public colleges and universities, public libraries and public hospitals.
Restrictions: In general, Amgen does not consider requests for the following: support to individuals, fundraising or sports-related events, corporate sponsorship requests, religious organizations unless the program is secular in nature and benefits a broad range of the community, political organization or lobbying activity, labor unions, fraternal, service or veterans' organizations, private foundations, or organizations that are discriminatory.
Samples: California State U (Camarillo, CA)—for scientific equipment, $950,000 (2005); Institute for Systems Biology (Seattle, WA)—for the endowment and operations, $3 million (2005); International Federation of the Red Cross and Red Crescent Societies (Geneva)—for relief efforts in South Asia and Africa, $1 million (2005).
Contact: Program Contact, (805) 447-4056 or (805) 447-1000; fax: (805) 447-1010
Internet: http://wwwext.amgen.com/citizenship/apply_for_grant.html
Sponsor: Amgen Foundation
1 Amgen Center Drive, MS 38-3-B
Thousand Oaks, CA 91320

AMI Semiconductors Corporate Grants 468
The company makes grants to nonprofit organizations in support of the performing arts, economic development, business education, health cost containment, and social services for senior citizens. Types of support include conferences and seminars, general operating support, matching grants, multiyear grants, professorships, research, and scholarships. There are no application deadlines. Submit a letter of inquiry that includes a description of the organization and program, amount of funds requested, purpose of the request, recently audited financial statement, and proof of tax-exempt status. Contact office for grant availability.
Restrictions: The company does not support political or lobbying groups.
Amount of Grant: $1000-$2500
Contact: TAMERA DRAKE, (208) 234-6890; fax: (208) 234-6795 email: tamera_Drake@amis.com
Internet: http://www.amis.com/about
Sponsor: AMI Semiconductors
2300 Buckskin Road
Pocatello, ID 83201

AMSSM Foundation Research Grants 469
The purpose of the AMSSM Foundation Research Grant Awards is to foster original scientific investigations by members of AMSSM. in this program, the Foundation welcomes research grant proposals that investigate issues within the broad discipline of sports medicine, including clinical practice, injury prevention and rehabilitation, basic science, epidemiology, and education. Grant awards are designed to provide partial support of research projects. Grantee institutions are expected to provide all necessary basic facilities and services that normally would be expected to exist in any institution qualified to undertake such research. Overhead or indirect costs will be supported to a maximum of 10% of direct costs. It is anticipated that the requested support will fall into one of three ranges. 1) $500 to $2,500 total costs annually for mailings, supplies, equipment, and technical support of small or pilot projects; 2) $2,500 to $10,000 total costs annually for a project larger in scope than the previous category and may provide partial support of research assistants or study coordinators; and 3) $10,000 to $25,000 total costs annually for a significant project that includes well documented pilot or previous studies and may provide partial salary support for key investigators. The maximum grant award is $25,000.
Requirements: The primary investigator of the grant must be an AMSSM member at the time of grant submission. Resident and fellow AMSSM members may apply as the principal investigator but must have at least one full AMSSM member listed as a co-investigator at the time of application.
Amount of Grant: $25,000 maximum
Date(s) Application is Due: Oct 1
Contact: Grants Administrator; (913) 327-1415; fax: (913) 327-1491; email: office@amssm.org
Internet: http://www.newamssm.org/Research%20Grant%20Information.html
Sponsor: American Medical Society for Sports Medicine
11639 Earnshaw
Overland Park, KS 66210

Andersen Corporate Foundation 470
The Foundation contributes to: organizations that enhance self-sufficiency for people living in poverty, senior citizens, and people with disabilities; organizations that promote safe and healthy environments, as well as organizations that seek to improve health through prevention and education programs, primarily for young people, senior citizens, and people in vulnerable situations; organizations that offer intellectual and social opportunities with a focus primarily on young people, senior citizens, and people with disabilities; and support that builds, promotes, and preserves communities. Complete guidelines are available online.
Requirements: All grant recipients must meet these giving guidelines: the organization's programs and services are consistent with Andersen Corporate Foundation's mission and values; the organization's purpose and programs fit within Andersen Corporate Foundation's defined program focus areas; the organization can demonstrate sound fiscal management and effective delivery of services; nonprofit corporation is registered under section 501(c)3 of the IRS Code in the United States or for Canadian Charities with the Canadian Revenue Agency.
Restrictions: The Foundation avoids making grants in organizations that are in competition with each other to provide the same service to the community. The Foundation does not support endowments or make grants to individuals. Funding is not granted to national research organizations.
Geographic Focus: Iowa; Minnesota; Virginia; WisconsinCanada
Date(s) Application is Due: Apr 15; Jul 15; Oct 15; Dec 15
Contact: Program Director, (888) 439-9508 or (651) 439-1557; fax: (651) 439-9480; email: andersencorpfdn@srinc.biz
Internet: http://www.scenicriver.org/bp/index.html
Sponsor: Andersen Corporate Foundation
342 5th Avenue N.
Bayport, MN 55003

Andersen Foundation Grants 471
The corporate foundation awards one-year renewable grants to educational institutions, mainly colleges and universities; social services; health; and religious causes (Baptist, Christian, Lutheran, nondenominational, Presbyterian, and Salvation Army). Specific areas of interest include arts/culture—arts centers, historic preservation, libraries, performing arts, and public radio/TV; education—colleges and universities, education funds, K-12, minority, religious, and special; health—general, clinics/centers, cancer, vision, heart, kidney, and mental health; religious services—churches, religious organizations and religious welfare; and social services—animal welfare, child welfare, family services, domestic violence, aging, and substance abuse. Types of support include capital grants, general operating grants, program development grants, and seed money grants. Emphasis is placed on Minnesota, with some national giving.
Requirements: 501(c)3 tax-exempt organizations are eligible. Giving is on a national basis although preference is given to requests from Minnesota.
Restrictions: The foundation does not make grants to institutions that receive federal funding.
Samples: Dallas Baptist U (TX)—to construct a chapel building, $250,000 (2003).
Amount of Grant: $5000-$500,000 average range
Contact: Mary Gillstrom, Director, (651) 264-5150
Sponsor: Andersen Foundation
100 Fourth Ave N
Bayport, MN 55003-1096

Angel Kiss Foundation Grants 472
Angel Kiss Foundation (AKF) is a nonprofit organization dedicated to helping families with children who are being treated for cancer. The Foundation provides financial assistance to families to help with the astronomical expenses associated with the disease. The Foundation works with families on an individual basis and reviews the needs of each family. It provides financial assistance for a variety of expenses including: medical

expenses, insurance deductibles, uncovered procedures, household living expenses, mortgage payments, rent, food, utilities, travel expenses related to treatment and other family expenses causing hardship during the child's cancer treatment. Families can work with their social worker and medical doctor for a referral to Angel Kiss Foundation, call Angel Kiss Foundation for guidance in the application procedure, or access the Web site for an online application.
Contact: Donna Breen, President; (775) 323-7721 or (888) 589-5477; fax: (775) 323-2161; email: donna@dlbreen.com
Internet: http://angelkissfoundation.org/About/FAQ.html
Sponsor: Angel Kiss Foundation
150 Ridge Street, Suite 3
Reno, NV 89501

Angels Baseball Foundation Grants 473
Since its inception in 2004, the Angels Baseball Foundation has awarded many grants to worthy organizations throughout the community, ranging from music programs to at-risk youth shelters. Currently, it focuses on initiatives aimed to create and improve education, health care, arts and sciences, and community related youth programs, in addition to providing children the opportunity to experience the game of baseball. Giving is limited to the greater Los Angeles, California, area. Fields of interest include: the arts, athletics/sports activities, children and youth, cancer detection, cancer research, community and economic development, education (at all levels), health care, and community service programs. Applicants should begin by contacting the Foundation directly.
Requirements: Applicants must serve the residents of the greater Los Angeles area.
Geographic Focus: California
Contact: Anne Bafus, Community Relations; (714) 940-2174 or c; fax: (714) 940-2244
Internet: http://losangeles.angels.mlb.com/ana/community/baseball_foundation.jsp
Sponsor: Angels Baseball Foundation
2000 E. Gene Autry Way
Anaheim, CA 92806-6100

Anheuser-Busch Foundation Grants 474
Support is provided almost exclusively to causes that are located in communities in which the company has manufacturing facilities. Contributions are made for education, health, social services, minorities and youth, cultural enrichment, and environmental protection programs. Types of support include capital grants, employee matching gifts, equipment and material acquisition, general support, and donated products. Full proposals are accepted throughout the year. At the Web site, click on Guidelines for Charitable Giving.
Requirements: 501(c)3 tax-exempt organizations in St. Louis, MO; Baldwinsville, N.Y.; Cartersvile, Ga.; Columbus, Oh; Fairfield, Ca.; Fort Collins, Co.; Houston, Tx.; Jacksonville, Fl.; Los Angeles, Ca.; Merrimack, N.H.; Newark, N.J.; Williamsburg, Va., Orlando, Fl.; Tampa, Fl.; San Antonio, Tx.; San Diego, Tx.
Restrictions: Grants are not made to individuals; political, social, fraternal, religious, or athletic organizations; or hospitals for operating funds.
Geographic Focus: California; Colorado; Florida; Georgia; Missouri; New Hampshire; New Jersey; New York; Ohio; Texas; Virginia
Amount of Grant: $16.6 million total; $25,000-$100,000 typically
Contact: Assistant Manager, Charitable Contributions; (314) 577-2453; fax: (314) 557-3251
Internet: http://www.anheuser-busch.com/CharitableGivingIndex.html
Sponsor: Anheuser-Busch Foundation
One Busch Place
Saint Louis, MO 63118-1852

Ann and Robert H. Lurie Family Foundation Grants 475
Founded in 1986, the foundation initially had set up six categories: medical services and research; child-related medical organizations; basic services including food and shelter; education; the arts; and so-called wild things. When Ann Lurie's husband, Robert, died in 1990, she was left with a fortune worth hundreds of millions and six kids — ages 5 to 15. She has given away well over $100-million since Robert H. Lurie died at age 48, generally spurning requests from nonprofit groups with undistinguished records and concentrating her gifts on some of the world's biggest problems, including hunger, cancer, and inadequate health care. Today, the foundation supports educating and providing resources to children so they are better prepared for the future.
Requirements: There are no specific deadlines or application forms to fill out. An organization requesting funding should have finances in good order, demonstrating that it is making good use of its resources. Note: Ann Lurie has a preference for identifying her own projects, rather than responding to solicitations.
Geographic Focus: Illinois; Michigan
Samples: University of Michigan College of Engineering (Ann Arbor, Michigan) - $2,500,000.; University of Michigan Entrepreneurial Institute (Ann Arbor, Michigan) - $1,000,000.; Africa Infectious Disease Village Clinic (Chicago, Illinois) - $403,429
Contact: Ann Lurie, President; (312) 466-3750; fax: (312) 466-3700
Sponsor: Ann and Robert H. Lurie Family Foundation
2 N. Riverside Plaza, Suite 1500
Chicago, IL 60606-2600

Ann Arbor Area Community Foundation Grants 476
The foundation is interested in funding projects that will improve the quality of life for citizens of the Ann Arbor, Michigan, area. Eligible projects generally fall within the categories of education, culture, social service, community development, environmental awareness, health and wellness, and youth and senior citizens. Types of support include: emergency funds, program development, conferences and seminars, publication, seed grants, scholarship funds, research, and matching funds. Higher priority is given to programs that are preventive rather than remedial, increase individual access to community resources, examine and address the underlying causes of local problems, promote independence and personal achievement, attract volunteer resources and support, strengthen the private nonprofit sector, encourage collaboration with other organizations, and build the capacity of the applying organization. Organizations interested in applying are strongly encouraged to discuss their project with the program director prior to submitting an application.
Requirements: 501(c)3 nonprofit organizations in the Ann Arbor area, which is the area that falls within the boundaries of the Ann Arbor public schools district, are eligible.
Restrictions: The foundation usually does not make grants for construction projects, annual giving campaigns or capital campaigns, normal operating expenses (except for start-up purposes), religious or sectarian purposes, computer hardware equipment, individuals, advocacy or political purposes, multiyear funding, or regranting.
Geographic Focus: Michigan
Samples: Jazzistry, $9,139 for Finding Your Place in the Jazz Story; Community Respite Center, Inc., $14,079 for development of a Lifespan Respite Center for Washtenaw County; Jewish Family Services, $9,000 for a database implementation project; Washtenaw United Way, $25,000 for a 2-1-1 Call Center; Vineyard Church of Ann Arbor, $8,000 or a mentoring ministry for single parent families; University of Michigan-Turner Geriatric Clinic, $3,500 for the Senior Unmet Needs Fund (all 2006).
Date(s) Application is Due: Feb 11; Oct 7
Contact: Phil D'Anieri, Program Director; (734) 663-0401; fax: (734) 663-3514; email: pdanieri@aaacf.org
Internet: http://www.aaacf.org/grants.asp
Sponsor: Ann Arbor Area Community Foundation
301 North Main Street, Suite 300
Ann Arbor, MI 48104

Ann Jackson Family Foundation Grants 477
The foundation awards grants to eligible nonprofit organizations in its areas of interest, including secondary education, healthcare, child welfare, animal welfare, and the disabled. Types of support include building construction/renovation, capital campaigns, and general operating grants. Most grants are awarded to nonprofits in Santa Barbara, California. There are no application forms or deadlines. Contact the foundation for document attachments required.
Geographic Focus: California
Samples: Albany Institute of History & Art (NY)—$25,000; American Heart Association (CA)—$5,000; Blind Babies Foundation (CA)—$3,000; Carondelet High School (CA)—$1,000; Cottage Hospital Foundation (CA)—$200,000; Family Service Agency (CA)—$10,00; Humane Society of Santa Barbara (CA)—$1,000; Seedlings-Braille Books for Children (MI)—$3,000.
Amount of Grant: $5000-$50,000 average
Contact: Palmer Jackson, President, (805) 969-2258
Sponsor: Ann Jackson Family Foundation
P.O. Box 5580
Santa Barbara, CA 93150-5580

Ann Peppers Foundation Grants 478
The foundation awards grants to eligible California nonprofit organizations in its areas of interest, including arts and cultural programs, disabled, elderly, health care, private education, and social services. Types of support include capital grants, general operating grants on a temporary basis, matching grants, scholarships, and research grants. Grants are initiated by the foundation manager. There are no application deadlines; the board meets quarterly to consider requests.
Requirements: Southern California 501(c)3 nonprofits, colleges, and universities are eligible. Preference is given to requests from Los Angeles County.
Geographic Focus: California
Samples: Boys Republic (Chino Hills, CA)—for kitchen renovation at residential facility , $5,000.; Pepperdine University (Malibu, CA)—for scholarships, $25,000.; Huntington Medical Research Institute (Pasadena, CA)—to purchase imaging technology for preclinical breast cancer, $5,000.; Marymount College (Rancho Palos Verdes, CA)—for scholarships, $10,000.
Amount of Grant: $2000-$50,000 range
Contact: Jack Alexander, Secretary, (626) 449-0793
Sponsor: Ann Peppers Foundation
625 S Fair Oaks Avenue
South Pasadena, CA 91030

Annenberg Foundation Grants 479
The foundation provides support for projects within its grantmaking interests of education and youth development, arts and culture, civic, community and the environment, and health and human services. It encourages the development of more effective ways to share ideas and knowledge. Letters of inquiry may be submitted at all times during the year and there are no deadlines. Please review the grants database for additional types of grants given.
Requirements: 501(c)3 tax-exempt organizations are eligible.
Restrictions: Full proposals are not accepted unless requested by a Foundation representative. The foundation is not presently considering inquiries for: individuals, individual K-12 schools, for-profit organizations, political activities or attempts to influence specific legislation, individual scholarships, projects focused exclusively on research, or programs outside of its grant-making interests.

Samples: Centro Latino De Educacion Popular, Los Angeles, CA, $50,000 - for the Spanish Literacy Campaign to mobilize, train, equip, and support Spanish speakers to teach their non-literate friends and family members to read and write using an online literacy program (2009); American Patrons of the Tate Gallery Foundation, Inc., New York, NY, $50,000 - to support special exhibitions and education programs at the Tate Modern (2009); National Public Radio, Inc., Washington, DC, $500,000 - for the programs of NPR West to broaden the creation and distribution of high-quality public radio programming (2009).
Contact: Leonard Aube, Executive Director; (310) 209-4560; fax: (310) 209-1631; email: info@annenbergfoundation.org
Internet: http://www.annenbergfoundation.org/grants
Sponsor: Annenberg Foundation
2000 Avenue of the Stars, Suite 1000
Los Angeles, CA 90067

Annie Sinclair Knudsen Memorial Fund/Kaua'i Community Grants Program 480
The priorities of the Fund are projects and services that benefit the Kaua'i community including: culture and arts; education; environment; and health and human services. Priority will be given to programs that are well-defined and likely to be successful, address a community need, demonstrate an ability to deliver, and have an adequate budget. Application information is available online.
Requirements: Any 501(c)3 organization, neighborhood group or project is eligible.
Geographic Focus: Hawaii
Amount of Grant: $2,000-$15,000
Date(s) Application is Due: July 16
Contact: Deborah Rice, (808) 245-4585; email: drice@hcf-hawaii.org
Internet: http://www.hawaiicommunityfoundation.org/index.php?id=71&categoryID=22
Sponsor: Hawaii Community Foundation
Attn: Annie Sinclair Knudsen Memorial Fund, 1164 Bishop Street, Suite 800
Honolulu, HI 96813

Annunziata Sanguinetti Foundation Grants 481
The foundation supports charitable organizations in San Francisco, CA, that are devoted wholly or partially to the care, treatment, rehabilitation, and education of children with physical or mental defects or illnesses. Applicants are requested to submit with the application a copy of federal and state tax-exempt status and exemption letters, current financial statement, budget for the grant request, and a description of the program for which funding is sought. Application accepted between July 1 and October 31.
Restrictions: Restricted to organizations which benefit the children residing in San Francisco County.
Geographic Focus: California
Amount of Grant: $3000-$10,000 average
Date(s) Application is Due: Oct 31
Contact: Eugene Ranghiasci, Vice President, (415) 396-3215; fax: (415) 834-0604
Sponsor: Annunziata Sanguinetti Foundation
420 Montgomery Street, 5th Floor
San Francisco, CA 94106

ANS Neurotology Fellows Award 482
The Neurotology Fellows Award was established by the American Neurotology Society in 1996 to reward scientific excellence. The award has been generously endowed through royalties received for the textbook Neurotology, Mosby Publishers, D. Brackmann and R. Jackler, editors. One or more awards of $500 each is intended to subsidize travel expenses incurred while giving a scientific presentation at the Annual Spring Meeting of the American Neurotology Society. The material presented need not have been performed during the Fellowship year; it may derive from earlier work performed during the residency or extracurricular research experience. Applicants should submit electronically a cover letter, a supporting letter from the Fellowship director to verify qualifications, and electronic submission of the abstract by October 15.
Requirements: Applicants must be full-time participants in a post-residency Neurotology Fellowship in the United States or Canada. In addition, the Fellow must be both podium presenter and first author of the paper submitted for publication.
Amount of Grant: $500
Date(s) Application is Due: Oct 15
Contact: Shirley Gossard, Administrator; (352) 751-0932 or (217) 414-4868; fax: (352) 751-0696; email: segossard@aol.com
Internet: http://www.americanneurotologysociety.com/funding.html
Sponsor: American Neurotology Society
3096 Riverdale Road
The Villages, FL 32162

ANS Nicholas Torok Vestibular Award 483
The Nicholas Torok Vestibular Award, established under the aegis of the American Neurotology Society instituting a yearly lecture, is to be presented at the Annual Scientific Spring Meeting of the Society. The subject should be an innovative observation, experience or technique in the field of vestibular basic science or clinical science. The candidate shall be selected preferably from the membership of the Society or upon specific merit of any M.D. or Ph.D. A yearly award of $1,500 will be given for the selected manuscript.
Requirements: The manuscript must be presented electronically in the publication format recommended by Otology & Neurotology, the official journal of the American Neurotology Society.
Amount of Grant: $1,500
Date(s) Application is Due: Oct 15
Contact: Shirley Gossard, Administrator; (352) 751-0932 or (217) 414-4868; fax: (352) 751-0696; email: segossard@aol.com
Internet: http://www.americanneurotologysociety.com/funding.html
Sponsor: American Neurotology Society
3096 Riverdale Road
The Villages, FL 32162

ANS Trainee Award 484
The American Neurotology Society offers an award for the best clinical or basic science paper in Neurotology submitted by a Resident or Fellow in training in the field of Otolaryngology-Head and Neck Surgery. A clinical study or basic research study is acceptable. The Society has established a cash award of $1,000 for the winning paper. The author will be expected to attend the Annual ANS Spring Meeting and present the paper personally.
Requirements: Residents from any approved residency program or Fellows in Neurotology in the United States or Canada are eligible to compete. The Resident or Fellow must be the primary author. He or she must provide the main inspiration for the paper and do the literature search, data collection, original and final drafts of the article, the discussion, and the conclusions.
Restrictions: The paper must be an original contribution, not previously published.
Amount of Grant: $1,000
Date(s) Application is Due: Oct 15
Contact: Shirley Gossard, Administrator; (352) 751-0932 or (217) 414-4868; fax: (352) 751-0696; email: segossard@aol.com
Internet: http://www.americanneurotologysociety.com/funding.html
Sponsor: American Neurotology Society
3096 Riverdale Road
The Villages, FL 32162

ANS/AAO-HNSF Herbert Silverstein Otology and Neurotology Research Award 485
The purpose of this award, which is jointly sponsored by the AAO-HNS Foundation and the American Neurotology Society, is to support a clinical or translational research project focused on diseases, disorders, or conditions of the peripheral or central auditory and/or vestibular system among new full-time academic surgeons. The award is intended as a preliminary step in clinical investigator career development and is expected to facilitate the recipient's preparation of a more comprehensive individualized research plan suitable for submission to the National Institutes of Health or comparable funding agency.
Requirements: Applicants must be physicians in the United States or Canada with demonstrated potential for excellence in research and teaching and serious commitment to an academic research career in otology or neurotology. Priority will be given to fellows or junior faculty, who have completed residencies or fellowships within four years of the application receipt date, although otolaryngology-head and neck surgery residents are eligible. All candidates must be sponsored by the Chair of his/her Division or Department and by an official representative of the institution which would administer the Award and in whose name the application is formally submitted.
Amount of Grant: $25,000 maximum ($12,500 per year)
Contact: Stephanie L. Jones, Assistant Director; (703) 519-1586 or (703) 836-4444; email: sljones@entnet.org
Internet: http://www.americanneurotologysociety.com/funding.html
Sponsor: American Neurotology Society / American Academy of Otolaryngology-Head and Neck Surgery Foundation
One Prince Street
Alexandria, VA 22314-3357

Anschutz Family Foundation Grants 486
The foundation makes grants in Colorado's rural and urban communities, to assist the elderly, the young, and the economically disadvantaged. Support is given to programs and projects that strengthen families and enable individuals to become productive and responsible citizens of society. Religious organizations, including Christian, Lutheran, Presbyterian, Roman Catholic, and the Salvation Army, also are eligible for funding. Types of support include special projects, general operating budgets, continuing support, seed money, emergency funds, technical assistance, and publications.
Requirements: Nonprofit organizations in Colorado may apply.
Restrictions: Grants are not awarded to individuals, programs outside of Colorado, graduate and post-graduate research, religious organizations for religious purposes, special events, promotions or conferences, candidates for political office, endowments, debt reduction, multi-year grants, and capital campaigns.
Geographic Focus: Colorado
Samples: The Center for Hearing, Speech, and Language (Denver, CO)—to support Kidscreen, a vision, hearing, speech and language developmental screening service for low-income families, $5,000.; The Learning Source for Adults and Families (Denver, CO)—general operating support for neighborhood literacy programs for adults and families, $7,500.
Amount of Grant: $2,500-$10,000
Date(s) Application is Due: Jan 15; Aug 1
Contact: Sue Anschutz-Rodgers, President & Executive Director, (303) 293-2338; fax: (303) 299-1235; email: info@anschutzfamilyfoundation.org
Internet: http://www.anschutzfamilyfoundation.org/info.htm
Sponsor: Anschutz Family Foundation
555 17th Street, Suite 2400
Denver, CO 80202

Ansell, Zaro, Grimm & Aaron Foundation Grants **487**

The Ansell, Zaro, Grimm and Aaron Foundation was established in New Jersey in 2007 by a leading law firm of the same name. Funding is offered primarily in the State of New Jersey to Jewish agencies and synagogues, health research, and social service agencies in support of the economically disadvantaged. There are no specific deadlines or application forms, and applicants should initially approach the Foundation with a letter of request detailing the purpose of the grant and verification of tax exempt status. The maximum amount given is $5,000.

Requirements: 501(c)3 organizations supporting residents of New Jersey are eligible.
Geographic Focus: New Jersey
Samples: Monmouth University, West Long Branch, New Jersey, $2,750 (2008); Shore Builders Association of Central New Jersey, Lakewood, New Jersey, $200 (2008); Juvenile Diabetes Research Foundation, Shrewsbury, New Jersey, $4,000 (2008).
Amount of Grant: $5,000 maximum
Contact: Jerold Zaro; (732) 922-1000; fax: (732) 922-6161; email: jlz@ansellzaro.com
Internet: http://www.ansellzaro.com/index_contact.html
Sponsor: Ansell, Zaro, Grimm & Aaron Foundation
1500 Lawrence Avenue
Ocean, NJ 07712-4023

Anthem Blue Cross and Blue Shield Grants **488**

As a multistate entity, the program supports charitable, civic, and nonprofit groups in company operating areas. Categories of giving include healthy minds (educational), healthy bodies (health oriented), and healthy communities (community projects and human services initiatives). Joint sponsorships with hospitals and providers for programs that benefit the community are encouraged. Requests must be submitted in writing. Contact the office for guidelines.

Requirements: 501(c)3 organizations in corporate communities are eligible.
Restrictions: Grants do not support individuals; political organizations/candidates; religious groups; fraternal, military, or labor organizations; or providers/hospitals.
Geographic Focus: Colorado; Connecticut; Indiana; Kentucky; Maine; Missouri; Nevada; New Hampshire; Ohio; Virginia; Wisconsin
Contact: Vicki Perkins, (317) 488-6216
Internet: http://www.anthem.com/wps/portal/ahpculdesac?content_path=shared/noapplication/f4/s0/t0/pw_018991.htm&na=aboutanthem&rootLevel=3&label=Charity%20Guidelines
Sponsor: Anthem Blue Cross and Blue Shield
120 Monument Circle
Indianapolis, IN 46204

Anthem Blue Cross and Blue Shield School Nurse Grants **489**

The mission of the project is to promote cardiovascular health among school-age children. Anthem's goals are to assist school nurses in initiating programs that may encourage a healthy lifestyle, reduce cardiovascular risk factors, promote physical activity, and encourage healthy eating behaviors; and facilitate the development of innovative school health programs that are based on research. No awards will be made to individuals, but will be awarded to the school. To apply, the school nurse representing the school must submit a completed application form with the appropriate attachments by the listed application deadline. Guidelines, including program contacts in Kentucky and Indiana, and application are available online.

Requirements: Eligible applicants include school nurses who are licensed in the state in which they practice and who represent a public or private school (elementary, junior high, middle, or high school) in Ohio, Kentucky, or Indiana.
Restrictions: Funds cannot be used for the salary or wages of any staff or employee.
Geographic Focus: Indiana; Kentucky; Ohio
Amount of Grant: $500-$1000
Date(s) Application is Due: Feb 1
Contact: Gabrielle Karpowicz, (614) 529-5068; email: gkarpowicz@aol.com
Internet: http://oasn.org/Awards_Grants/awards.htm
Sponsor: Ohio Association of School Nurses
6167 Heritage Point Ct
Hilliard, OH 43026

Anthony R. Abraham Foundation Grants **490**

For more than 30 years, the Anthony R. Abraham Foundation mission has been to help non-profit organizations worldwide. The foundations strives to: provide programs and services to help people around the world become self-productive and give back to their communities; ensure that no child is denied medical treatment due to a lack of insurance; provide education that breaks barriers; guarantee that research into the cure of catastrophic diseases continues; help raise the quality of life. It's been a privilege for Foundation to be able to help ease poverty, raise hospitals, build orphanages and further medical research and the Foundation looks forward to doing even more. Some of the organizations helped include: Domestic organizations -St. Jude Children's Research Hospital; Camillus House; Miami Rescue Mission; Habitat for Humanity of Greater Miami; America's Second Harvest; Miami Children's Hospital; Jackson Memorial Hospital; Florida Heart Research Institute; Big Brothers/Big Sisters; Alonzo Mourning Charities; Honey Shine Mentoring Program; Cancer Link; The Miami Lighthouse for the Blind; Overtown Youth Center. International organizations: Brothers of the Good Shepherd; School for the Blind, Lebanon; Rene Moawad Foundation; Haitian Foundation; Children's International Network; Doctors without Borders; Little Sisters of Nazareth; Maronite Order of the Holy Family.

Requirements: Non-profit 501(c)3 organization requesting funding should fill out a funds-request form and submit it at the Foundation's website. The Foundation will contact you, if your organization qualifies under the Foundation's guidelines and the law.
Restrictions: Grants are not made to individuals.
Amount of Grant: $100-$50,000 range average
Contact: Anthony R. Abraham, Chairman; (305) 665-2222
Internet: http://www.abrahamfoundation.com/about
Sponsor: Anthony R. Abraham Foundation
1320 S. Dixie Highway, Suite. 241
Coral Gables, FL 33146-2937

AON Foundation Grants **491**

AON funds community-based initiatives that focus on youths' development through health, education, the arts and cultural activities to schools, school districts and other nonprofit organizations in communities where the company operates, especially the Chicago area. Supported initiatives include community-based projects that focus on youths' development mentally, physically, and academically, and demonstrate positive intervention by including an outcome-evaluation component. The foundation supports higher and other education, social services, community funds, and hospitals and health associations. The board meets three times each year to consider requests. There is no specific application. A letter is acceptable.

Requirements: Nonprofit organizations in AON Corporation domestic and international operating communities, especially organizations in the Chicago area, may apply.
Restrictions: Awards are restricted or limited to charitable, educational (excluding the operation of a secondary educational institution or vocational school) and scientific organizations that qualify as 501(c)3 or 509(a)(1),(2), or (3).
Samples: Achievement Centers for Children—$5,000.; After-school Matters, Inc.—$25,000.;
Amount of Grant: $1,000-$10,000 average
Date(s) Application is Due: Apr 1; Jul 1; Oct 1
Contact: Carolyn Labutka, Executive Director, (312) 381-3549; fax: (312) 701-4533
Internet: http://edreform.com/info/grant.htm
Sponsor: AON Foundation
200 East Randolph Street
Chicago, IL 60601

APA Congressional Fellowships **492**

The fellowships afford an opportunity for the recipient psychologists to participate in the policy-making process of the U.S. Congress. Trained scientists and practitioners work with the staff members of Congress or congressional committees and are involved in the process of relating social and behavioral science to public policy. The fellowships are sponsored by APA in cooperation with American Association for the Advancement of Science (AAAS). The fellowship is for a period of one year beginning in September. The Fellowship stipend ranges from $60,000 to $75,000, depending upon years of post-doctoral experience. In addition, APA provides $375 per month for health insurance and funding may also be available for professional development and relocation expenses during the Fellowship year.

Requirements: Applicants must have a doctorate in psychology and be members of APA. Persons who are receiving sabbatical funds are also eligible to apply.
Amount of Grant: 60,000 - $75,000 stipend
Date(s) Application is Due: Jan 7
Contact: Micah Haskell-Hoehl, Program Administrator; (202) 336-5935; email: mhaskell-hoehl@apa.org
Internet: http://www.apa.org/ppo/fellows/
Sponsor: American Psychological Association
750 First Street NE
Washington, DC 20002-4242

APA Culture of Service in the Psychological Sciences Award **493**

The Award recognizes departments that demonstrate a commitment to service in the psychological sciences. Departments selected for this award will show a pattern of support for service from faculty at all levels, including a demonstration that service to the discipline is rewarded in faculty tenure and promotion. Successful Departments will also demonstrate that service to the profession is an integral part of training and mentoring. Service to the discipline includes such activities as departmental release time for serving on boards and committees of psychological associations; editing journals; serving on a review panel; or chairing an IRB. Other culture of service activities that a department would encourage include mentoring students and colleagues; advocating for psychological science's best interests with state and federal lawmakers; and promoting the value of psychological science in the public eye. The focus of this award is a department's faculty service to the discipline and not their scholarly achievements. Both Undergraduate and Graduate Departments of Psychology are eligible. Self-nominations are encouraged.

Amount of Grant: $5,000
Contact: Suzanne Wandersman, Director for Governance Affairs; (202) 336-6000; fax: (202) 336-5953; email: swandersman@apa.org
Internet: http://www.apa.org/science/dept_award.html
Sponsor: American Psychological Association
750 First Street, NE
Washington, DC 20002-4242

APA Dissertation Research Awards **494**

Dissertation awards are granted to graduate students in psychology programs to help offset the costs associated with dissertation research. The research may be done in any area of psychology. Applicants who have already defended their dissertations are eligible to apply for these funds, as long as they have not yet received doctoral degrees as of the application deadline. APA provides dissertation research awards to approximately 50

students annually. Dissertations must be approved by the students' committees before application. The application deadline falls in mid-September of each year. Awards are announced in late December.
Requirements: APA student affiliates enrolled in a psychology graduate program are eligible to apply.
Restrictions: Departments may not nominate more than three students per year for dissertation awards.
Amount of Grant: $1000, $3000, $5000
Date(s) Application is Due: Sep 15
Contact: APA Science Directorate, (800) 374-2721 or (202) 336-5500; fax: (202) 336-5953; email: science@apa.org
Internet: http://www.apa.org/science/dissinfo.html
Sponsor: American Psychological Association
750 First St NE
Washington, DC 20002-4242

APA Distinguished Scientific Award for Early Career Contribution to Psychology 495
The Distinguished Scientific Award for Early Career Contribution to Psychology recognizes excellent young psychologists. Nominations of persons who received doctoral degrees during and since 1998 are being sought in these five areas: animal learning and behavior, comparative; cognition/human learning; developmental psychology; health; and psychopathology. These categories should be interpreted broadly and are not meant to be exclusive; all of psychology is of sufficient merit to be considered for awards. The Award consists of a citation and a cash prize, which are presented at the APA Annual Convention.
Samples: Robert D. Gray, PhD (applied research), Department of Applied Psychology, Arizona State University (2007); Patrik O. Vuilleumier, MD (behavioral /cognitive neuroscience), Department of Neurology, University of California, Davis (2007); R. Chris Fraley, PhD (individual differences), Department of Psychology at University of Illinois at Urbana-Champaign (2007); Jorn Diedrichsen, PhD (perception/motor performance), School of Psychology, Adeilad Brigantia University, Wales (2007); Matthew D. Lieberman, PhD (social), University of California, Los Angeles (2007).
Contact: Suzanne Wandersman, Director for Governance Affairs; (202) 336-6000; fax: (202) 336-5953; email: swandersman@apa.org
Internet: http://www.apa.org/science/sciaward.html
Sponsor: American Psychological Association
750 First Street, NE
Washington, DC 20002-4242

APA Distinguished Scientific Award for the Applications of Psychology 496
The Distinguished Scientific Award for the Applications of Psychology honors psychologists who have made distinguished theoretical or empirical advances in psychology leading to the understanding or amelioration of important practical problems. The Award consists of a citation and a cash prize, which are presented at the APA Annual Convention.
Samples: Karl G. Joreskog, PhD, Emeritus Professor, University of Upssala, Sweden (2007),; Peter M. Bentler, PhD, UCLA Psychology Department, Los. Angeles, CA (2007).
Contact: Suzanne Wandersman, Director for Governance Affairs; (202) 336-6000; fax: (202) 336-5953; email: swandersman@apa.org
Internet: http://www.apa.org/science/sciaward.html
Sponsor: American Psychological Association
750 First Street, NE
Washington, DC 20002-4242

APA Distinguished Scientific Contribution Award 497
The Distinguished Scientific Contribution Award honors psychologists who have made distinguished theoretical or empirical contributions to basic research in psychology. The Award consists of a citation and a cash prize, which are presented at the APA Annual Convention.
Samples: Marilynn B. Brewer, PhD, Department of Psychology, Ohio State University, Columbus, OH (2007); Jean M. Mandler, PhD, Research Professor, Department of Cognitive Science, University of California, San Diego (2007); Paul Rozin, PhD, Professor of Psychology, University of Pennsylvania (2007).
Contact: Suzanne Wandersman, Director for Governance Affairs; (202) 336-6000; fax: (202) 336-5953; email: swandersman@apa.org
Internet: http://www.apa.org/science/sciaward.html
Sponsor: American Psychological Association
750 First Street, NE
Washington, DC 20002-4242

APA Distinguished Service to Psychological Science Award 498
This Award recognizes individuals who have made outstanding contributions to psychological science through their commitment to a culture of service. Award recipients will receive an honorarium of $1,000. Nominees will have demonstrated their service to the discipline by aiding in association governance; serving on boards, committees and various psychological associations; editing journals; reviewing grant proposals; mentoring students and colleagues; advocating for psychological science's best interests with state and federal lawmakers; and promoting the value of psychological science in the public eye. Nominees may be involved in one service area, many of the areas, or all of the service areas noted above. An individual's service to the discipline and not a person's scholarly achievements are the focus of this award.
Amount of Grant: $1,000
Contact: Suzanne Wandersman, Director for Governance Affairs; (202) 336-6000; fax: (202) 336-5953; email: swandersman@apa.org
Internet: http://www.apa.org/science/serv_award.html
Sponsor: American Psychological Association
750 First Street, NE
Washington, DC 20002-4242

APA Meritorious Research Service Commendation 499
The Commendation recognizes individuals who have made outstanding contributions to psychological science through their service as employees of the federal government or other organizations. Contributions are defined according to service to the field that directly or indirectly advances opportunities and resources for psychological science. This may include staff at federal or non-federal research funding, regulatory or other agencies. Nominees may be active or retired but ordinarily will have a minimum of 10 years of such service. The individual's personal scholarly achievements (i.e., research, teaching, and writing) are not considered in the selection process independent of their service contributions.
Samples: Robert B. Huebner, National Institute on Alcohol Abuse and Alcoholism (2008); Jack D. Maser, University of California, San Diego (2008); Robert S. Ruskin, Consortium Research Fellows Program, Universities of the Washington (2008).
Contact: Suzanne Wandersman, Director for Governance Affairs; (202) 336-6000; fax: (202) 336-5953; email: swandersman@apa.org
Internet: http://www.apa.org/science/meritorious.html
Sponsor: American Psychological Association
750 First Street, NE
Washington, DC 20002-4242

APA Scientific Conferences Grants 500
The program seeks proposals for research conferences in psychology. The purpose of this program is to promote the exchange of important new contributions and approaches in scientific psychology. Conference formats include festschrifts—conferences organized as tributes to distinguished scholars; stand-alone conferences—usually two days long, involves psychologists as the primary organizers; and add-a-day conference—meetings that occur at the beginning or end of a scientific conference other than APA (e.g., Society for Ingestive Behavior or Psychonomics Society). The conference must also be supported by the host institution with direct funds, in-kind support, or a combination of the two.
Requirements: One of the primary organizers must be a member of APA. Only academic institutions accredited by a regional body may apply. Independent research institutions must provide evidence of affiliation with such an accredited institution. Joint proposals from cooperating institutions are encouraged. Conferences may be held only in the United States, its possessions, or Canada.
Restrictions: APA governance groups, APA divisions, and related entities are not eligible for funding under this program.
Amount of Grant: $500-$20,000
Date(s) Application is Due: Jun 1; Dec 1
Contact: Deborah McCall, Science Directorate, (202) 336-6000; fax: (202) 336-5953; email: dmccall@apa.org
Internet: http://www.apa.org/science/psa/sep07ann.html
Sponsor: American Psychological Association
750 First Street, NE
Washington, DC 20002-4242

APA Travel Awards 501
The purpose of the travel award program is to help psychology graduate students travel to the annual APA convention to present their research. The APA awards up to 100 travel awards annually. Multiple authors are accepted, but the student applicant must be the designated presenter of the research. The application deadline falls in mid-April of each year. Awards will be announced in mid-June. Applications are available on the Web site.
Requirements: Applicants must be student affiliates of the APA; students who are not affiliates may apply for affiliation at the time of application.
Restrictions: Departments may not endorse more than three students per year for travel awards.
Amount of Grant: $300
Date(s) Application is Due: Apr 12
Contact: Science Directorate, (800) 374-2721 or (202) 336-5500; fax: (202) 336-5963; email: science@apa.org
Internet: http://www.apa.org/science/funding.html
Sponsor: American Psychological Association
750 First Street, NE
Washington, DC 20002-4242

APA Young Investigator Grant Program 502
The program provides financial support to teaching, research, and health care delivery projects in general pediatrics. The number of awards is dependent on available funds and the size of grant requests of selected projects. Proposals should address the goal of the association: to encourage, promote, and facilitate improved patient care, teaching, and research in general pediatrics.
Requirements: The principal investigator must be a member of the APA or have submitted an application for membership. Preference will be given to new investigators, including those in training.
Restrictions: Multiple year funding requests will not be considered.
Amount of Grant: $10,000 maximum

Date(s) Application is Due: Oct 25
Contact: Grants Administrator, (703) 556-9222; fax: (703) 556-8729; email: info@academicpeds.org
Sponsor: Ambulatory Pediatric Association
6728 Old McLean Village Drive
McLean, VA 22101

APF Alexander Gralnick, MD, Award for Research in Schizophrenia **503**
The award will annually acknowledge research achievements in the treatment of schizophrenia, emphasizing early diagnosis and treatment and psychosocial aspects of the disease process. Additional preference will be given to researchers working in a psychiatric facility. The applicant should submit a statement summarizing the nature of the research relevant to the award, emphasizing its internal consistency and scientific implications; a list of publications (or articles accepted for publication) relevant to the award; a current curriculum vita; and a current bibliography. Four copies and the original application should be submitted. The $4,000 award will be presented at the annual meeting.
Samples: Robert E. Drake, M.D., $4,000 (2008); William R. McFarlane, M.D., $4,000 (2007); Gerard E. Hogarty, M.S.W., $4,000 (2006).
Amount of Grant: $4,000
Date(s) Application is Due: Nov 2
Contact: Thomas H. McGlashan, M.D., Chair; (703) 907-8512; fax: (703) 907-7851; email: srubloff@psych.org
Internet: http://www.psychfoundation.org/GrantAndAwards/AwardsandFellowships/AlexanderGralnickMDAward.aspx
Sponsor: American Psychiatric Foundation
1000 Wilson Boulevard, Suite 1825
Arlington, VA 22209

APF Awards for Advancing Minority Mental Health **504**
The program was established by the foundation, with support of Otsuka America Pharmaceutical, to recognize psychiatrists, other health professionals, mental health programs, and other organizations that have undertaken innovative and supportive efforts to raise awareness of mental illness in minority communities, the need for early recognition, the availability of treatment and how to access it, and the cultural barriers to treatment; increase access to quality mental health services for minorities; and improve the quality of care for minorities, particularly those in the public health system or with severe mental illness. The awards, although given to mental health professionals, will focus on patient issues such as raising awareness of mental illness, the need for treatment, and how to access treatment. Programs or efforts that reduce language and cultural barriers, enhance direct community understanding of mental illness, expand efforts to reach out to their community, and support community reintegration are just a few examples of the types of activities that could be recognized by these awards. Winning programs will be featured in publications such as Psychiatric News, and on American Psychiatric Association and American Psychiatric Foundation Web sites. In addition, award winners and their programs will be recognized at the APA Annual Meetings each May. Guidelines are available online.
Requirements: Psychiatrists, other health professionals, mental health programs, and other organizations are eligible. Psychiatrists and other health professionals must be licensed and/or accredited in the state in which you practice. Mental health programs and other organizations must have been in operation for at least two years before the application deadline.
Samples: Asian Community Mental Health Services, Oakland, CA (2006); Los Angeles Child Guidance Clinic, Los Angeles, CA (2006); La Clinica del Pueblo, Washington, D.C. (2006).
Amount of Grant: $5,000
Date(s) Application is Due: Nov 1
Contact: Barbara Matos, Director; (703) 907-8517; fax: (703) 907-7851; email: bmatos@psych.org
Internet: http://www.psychfoundation.org/GrantAndAwards/AwardsandFellowships/AAMMH.aspx
Sponsor: American Psychiatric Foundation
1000 Wilson Boulevard, Suite 1825
Arlington, VA 22209

APF Call for Proposals **505**
The program is intended to fund public education programs, as well as information and outreach initiatives that promote the early recognition and treatment of mental illness. Up to $750,000 in grant funds are available over the course of three years. Average grants are in the $50,000 range. Grant making under this program has been temporarily suspended while a new Call for Proposals is being developed. Contact the office for further updates.
Requirements: Organizations that have been in existence for at least two years and currently maintain a 501(c)3 charitable status and American Psychiatric Association District Branches and subsidiaries. Organizations need not be mental health programs.
Amount of Grant: $50,000 average
Contact: Barbara Matos, Director; (703) 907-8517; fax: (703) 907-7851; email: bmatos@psych.org
Internet: http://www.psychfoundation.org/GrantAndAwards/Grants/CallforProposals.aspx
Sponsor: American Psychiatric Foundation
1000 Wilson Boulevard, Suite 1825
Arlington, VA 22209-3901

APF Disaster Recovery Fund for Psychiatrists **506**
The Grant is intended to assist psychiatrists and psychiatric residents who have been adversely affected by disasters such as hurricanes Katrina, Rita and Wilma. Psychiatrists and psychiatric residents who have been affected by disasters are eligible to apply for grant funding up to $2500. Grants will be made to allow psychiatric residents to continue their medical training and to help psychiatrists rebuild their practices in order to serve the mental health needs of the people in their communities.
Amount of Grant: $2,500 maximum
Contact: Barbara Matos; (703) 907-8517; fax: (703) 907-7851; email: bmatos@psych.org
Internet: http://www.psychfoundation.org/GrantAndAwards/Grants/DisasterRecoveryFund.aspx
Sponsor: American Psychiatric Foundation
1000 Wilson Boulevard, Suite 1825
Arlington, VA 22209

APF Helping Hands Grants **507**
The program was established to encourage medical students to participate in community mental health service activities, particularly those focused on underserved populations. The program seeks to raise awareness of mental illness and the importance of early recognition and builds an interest among medical students in psychiatry and working in underserved communities. The foundation makes grants to medical schools for mental health service projects that are created and managed by medical students. Projects can be new initiatives conducted in partnership with community agencies or in conjunction with ongoing medical school outreach activities. Examples of fundable activities include screening in community health centers or homeless shelters; outreach and community education about mental health; and health literacy programs.
Requirements: Medical schools are eligible to apply. All projects must be conducted under the supervision of medical faculty. Medical students who participate in the program must be in their second, third, or fourth year of medical school at the time they are engaged in community service. Funds must be expended within one year. Unused funds must be returned to the foundation.
Restrictions: Grants will not fund services beyond basic mental health screenings and referrals.
Amount of Grant: $5,000
Date(s) Application is Due: May 26
Contact: Barbara Matos; (703) 907-8517; fax: (703) 907-7851; email: bmatos@psych.org
Internet: http://www.psychfoundation.org/GrantAndAwards/Grants/HelpingHands.aspx
Sponsor: American Psychiatric Foundation
1000 Wilson Boulevard, Suite 1825
Arlington, VA 22209-3901

APF James H. Scully Jr., M.D., Educational Fund Grants **508**
The fund supports education and research within the APA, its subsidiary organizations, or affiliated organizations, including district branches, state associations, or other psychiatric organizations that are in partnership with the APA. The fund can be used to support activities that improve the quality of care for patients with mental illness, advance the prevention of mental illness, raise awareness of mental illness and its treatments, and increase access to mental health services. Requests for funding should be sent in writing to the foundation and include the following: identification and significance of need; description of program/activity to address that need; expected outcomes and evaluation process; budget and time line; and background of key project personnel. Funding decisions are made by the foundations board of directors.
Restrictions: The fund will not support public policy or lobbying activities.
Contact: Barbara Matos; (703) 907-8517; fax: (703) 907-7851; email: bmatos@psych.org
Internet: http://www.psychfoundation.org/GrantAndAwards/Grants/JamesHScullyEducationalFund.aspx
Sponsor: American Psychiatric Foundation
1000 Wilson Boulevard, Suite 1825
Arlington, VA 22209-3901

APF Jeanne Spurlock Congressional Fellowships **509**
The fellowship provides general psychiatry and child psychiatry residents an opportunity to work in a congressional office or committee on federal health policy, particularly policy related to child and minority issues. The recipient will serve a ten-month fellowship in Washington, DC. The fellow will be introduced to the structure and development of federal and congressional health policy procedures, with a focus on mental health issues affecting minorities and under-served populations, including children. Fellows traditionally help develop legislative proposals, track and analyze legislative initiatives, arrange hearings, and brief Members of Congress and their staff, and interact with their constituents. During the fellowship, recipients have opportunities to interact with health policymakers and advocacy/professional groups, including the APA.
Requirements: PGY-II and III general psychiatry residents, child psychiatry residents, or child psychiatrists who will be out of training for less than one year at the time of the fellowship may apply. Applicants must be U.S. citizens or permanent residents. The recipient will be required to submit a written summary of the Fellowship experience at the end of the fellowship and may make recommendations or suggestions for improving the fellowship.
Amount of Grant: $35,000 stipend; $2,500 maximum moving expenses
Date(s) Application is Due: Mar 14
Contact: Marilyn King; (703) 907-8653; email: mking@psych.org
Internet: http://www.psychfoundation.org/GrantAndAwards/AwardsandFellowships/SpurlockFellowship.aspx

Sponsor: American Psychiatric Foundation
1000 Wilson Boulevard, Suite 1825
Arlington,VA 22209-3901

APF Typical or Troubled School Mental Health Education Grants 510
The Grant Program provides funding to implement the Typical or Troubled School Mental Health educational model in communities nationwide. Community organizations, high schools and school districts are eligible to receive funding. The educational program is designed for school personnel (teachers, coaches guidance counselors, etc.) to raise their awareness of mental disorders in teens. The program focuses on promoting the importance of early recognition and treatment, recognizing the early warning signs of mental health problems, and encouraging action and appropriate referral to a mental health professional.
Amount of Grant: $5,000 maximum
Date(s) Application is Due: Mar 30
Contact: Barbara Matos; (703) 907-8517; fax: (703) 907-7851; email: bmatos@psych.org
Internet: http://www.psychfoundation.org/GrantAndAwards/Grants/TypicalorTroubled.aspx
Sponsor: American Psychiatric Foundation
1000 Wilson Boulevard, Suite 1825
Arlington, VA 22209-3901

APF/COGDOP Graduate Research Scholarships in Psychology 511
The American Psychological Foundation (APF) and the Council of Graduate Departments of Psychology (COGDOP) jointly offer graduate research scholarships, including the Clarence J. Rosecrans Scholarship ($2000), the Ruth G. and Joseph D. Matarazzo Scholarship ($3000), as well as a number of $1,000 scholarships. The scholarships will be given directly to the individual graduate students enrolled in an interim master's program or doctoral program. If a student is currently enrolled in a terminal master's program, the student must intend to enroll in a PhD program. Several fellowships have been reserved for students who, at the time of application, are within the first two years of graduate study in psychology. The purpose of the scholarship program is to assist graduate students of psychology with research costs. The scholarships are administered by APA. Application and guidelines are available online.
Requirements: Each graduate department of psychology that is a member of COGDOP may submit nominations. The number of candidates that each member department is allowed to nominate depends upon the total number of students enrolled in the graduate program. Departments that have 100 or fewer students enrolled in their graduate programs may nominate one candidate; departments that have 101-200 graduate students enrolled may nominate up to two candidates; and departments that have more than 200 graduate students enrolled may nominate up to three candidates.
Samples: Arathi Sethumadhavan, Texas Tech University —$3,000 (2008); Kristen M. Culbert, Michigan State University—$2,000 (2008); Jennifer M. Brielmaier, George Mason University—$1,000 (2008).
Amount of Grant: $1,000-$3,000
Date(s) Application is Due: Jun 15
Contact: Science Directorate, (202) 336-6000; fax: (202) 336-5953; email: science@apa.org
Internet: http://www.apa.org/science/apf-cogdop.html
Sponsor: American Psychological Association / Council of Graduate Departments of Psychology
750 First Street, NE
Washington, DC 20002-4242

APhA Foundation Incentive Grants 512
The incentive grants provide seed funding to help pharmacists in all practice settings explore new methods and services that enhance their role as pharmaceutical care providers, and to encourage them to share their experiences with other pharmacists. This year, the incentive grants program will continue to expand to include project proposals specifically for pharmacists interested in establishing or supporting an already existing practice model in the area of pain management. Projects should concentrate on new, innovative patient care service that is of significance to pharmacy care settings and that can be evaluated for its relevance. Application and guidelines are available online.
Requirements: Applicants must be members of APhA, currently licensed, and actively engaged in ambulatory pharmacy practice. Recipients are encouraged to attend the APhA annual meeting and submit present findings, if applicable.
Restrictions: Indirect costs will not be funded. Salaries for recipients are not funded; however, consultant fees, fees for reseach/technician services, and expenses for adminsitrative services may be allowable if essential if essential to development/implementation of the project.
Amount of Grant: $1000
Date(s) Application is Due: Oct 3
Contact: Grants Administrator, email: info@aphafoundation.org
Internet: http://www.aphafoundation.org/IncentiveGrants/incentive.htm
Sponsor: American Pharmacists Association
2215 Constitution Ave NW
Washington, DC 20037-2985

APPEAL Social Justice and Tobacco Control Grants 513
This national initiative will provide resources for organizations to promote policy change in tobacco control among Asian American and Pacific Islander communities through community organizing and advocacy policy. Previous experience with tobacco-related work is not necessary. Application and guidelines are available online.
Requirements: Qualified applicants must be experienced in grassroots community organizing and have 501(c)3 nonprofit status.
Amount of Grant: $20,000-$50,000 per year for two years
Date(s) Application is Due: Apr 25
Contact: Lisa Fu, (510) 272-9536 ext 104; fax: (510) 272-0817; email: lfu@aapcho.org
Internet: http://www.appealforcommunities.org/pages/Call_for_Proposals44.php?project_id=44
Sponsor: Asian Pacific Partners for Empowerment and Leadership
300 Frank H Ogawa Plz, Suite 620
Oakland, CA 94612

APSA Congressional Fellowships Health and Aging Policy Fellows Program 514
Supported by the Atlantic Philanthropies and administered by Columbia University, this national program seeks to provide professions in health and aging with the experience and skills necessary to make a positive contribution to the development and implementation of health policies that affect older Americans. The program will offer two different tracks for individual placement: a residential track that includes a nine-to-12-month placement in Washington, D.C. or at a state agency (as a legislative assistant in Congress, a professional staff member in an executive agency or in a policy organization; and a non-residential track that includes a health policy project and brief placement(s) throughout the year at relevant sites. Core program components focused on career development and professional enrichment are provided for fellows in both tracks.
Requirements: The program is open to physicians, nurses and social workers at all career stages (early, mid, and late) with demonstrated commitment to health and aging issues and a desire to be involved in health policy at the federal, state or local level. Other professionals with clinical backgrounds (e.g. pharmacists, dentists, clinical psychologists) working in the field of health and aging are also eligible to apply.
Contact: Harold Alan Pincus M.D., Director; (212) 543-6213; email: pincush@pi.cpmc.columbia.edu;; Jeffrey R. Biggs, Program Director; (202) 483-2512; fax: (202) 483-2657; email: jbiggs@apsanet.org or cfp@apsanet.org
Internet: http://www.apsanet.org/content_50835.cfm
Sponsor: American Political Science Association
1527 New Hampshire Avenue, NW
Washington, DC 20036-1206

APSA Robert Wood Johnson Foundation Health Policy Fellowships 515
The purpose of this fellowship is to give outstanding mid-career health professionals in academic and community-based settings an opportunity to learn more about the legislative process through direct participation. Fellows actively contribute to the formulation of national health policies and accelerate their careers as leaders in health policy. Initiated in 1973, the program is funded by The Robert Wood Johnson Foundation (RWJF)and conducted by the Institute of Medicine (IOM) of the National Academy of Sciences. The application process typically opens in September and the application deadline typically occurs in mid-November of each year.
Date(s) Application is Due: Nov 14
Contact: Jeffrey R. Biggs, Program Director; (202) 334-1506 or (202) 483-2512; fax: (202) 483-2657; email: jbiggs@apsanet.org or info@healthpolicyfellows.org
Internet: http://www.apsanet.org/content_3544.cfm
Sponsor: American Political Science Association
1527 New Hampshire Avenue, NW
Washington, DC 20036-1206

APSAA Fellowships 516
The mission of the Fellowship Program is to encourage interest and involvement in psychoanalysis among the future leaders, researchers and educators of mental health and academia. Early-career psychiatrists, psychologists, social workers and academics are eligible for to apply for the Fellowship. The Fellowship offers the opportunity to attend the biannual meetings of APSAA, to meet analysts and Fellows from across the country, to have a Mentor, and to present their clinical work or research at the meetings. The application for the Fellowship Program is available online September 15.
Requirements: Psychiatrists, psychologists, social workers, and academics who meet the specific eligibility requirements (available online) are eligible. Applicants may be nominated by their department chairs or program directors if applicable. When not applicable, self-nominations are encouraged. Applicants must be training or working in the United States during the fellowship year. All applicants should have demonstrated leadership ability in their discipline, or have special aptitude in research, teaching, and/or clinical endeavors; and have special interest in psychodynamics, psychoanalysis, or applied psychoanalysis.
Contact: James Guimaraes, Fellowship Coordinator; (212) 752-0450; fax: (212) 593-0571; email: jguimaraes@apsa.org or info@apsa.org
Internet: http://www.apsa.org/FELLOWSHIPPROGRAM/GENERALINFORMATION/tabid/298/Default.aspx
Sponsor: American Psychoanalytic Association
309 East 49th Street
New York, NY 10007-1601

APSAA Foundation Grants 517
The mission of the APF Committee is to raise funds and sponsor programs promoting a better understanding of psychoanalysis and encouraging effective and innovative dissemination of psychoanalytic ideas and services to the public. The APF Committee's objective is to educate the public, the community of mental health workers, and allied disciplines about the relevance of psychoanalysis as a powerful therapeutic and research instrument whose applications span a wide range of understanding of individual behavior

and cultural phenomena. One or several of the following elements should be a part of the proposal in order to be considered: community outreach; national focus—not a program that is generally put on as a regular activity by a society or institute; fund raising element—seeks co-funding, matching or other sources of support for project (grant money may be used as seed money for helping Grantee to get other sources of funding); transportable—broad applicability to other psychoanalytic institutes, societies and foundations; and creative and original.
Samples: Washington Center for Psychoanalysis—to enable the design and implementation of a system of psychodynamic support for Jubilee JumpStart, a new child care and education facility for low-income families, $5,000 (2007); Allen Creek Preschool, Ann Arbor, Michigan—to support the Early Childhood Training Initiative, a new outreach program designed to nurture the growth of early childhood educators and day care workers through professional training, workshops, and consultations, $4,000 (2007).
Amount of Grant: $1,000-$5,000 range
Contact: Dean K. Stein, Executive Director; (212) 752-0450; fax: (212) 593-0571; email: deankstein@apsa.org or info@apsa.org
Internet: http://www.apsa.org/AmericanPsychoanalyticbrFoundationCommittee/tabid/70/Default.aspx
Sponsor: American Psychoanalytic Association
309 East 49th Street
New York, NY 10007-1601

APSAA Mini-Career Grants **518**
The Fund conceives of psychoanalytic research along the broadest lines, including: scholarly and empirical investigative contributions that can advance knowledge of psychoanalytic theory, practice, and links between psychoanalysis and neighboring disciplines such as developmental psychology or neuroscience. Awards of up to $15,000 annually for up to two years are intended to support the beginning career of a psychoanalytic investigator. These mini-career awards are intended, for example, to buy time for a junior faculty member or clinician just starting a practice so that they may consult with other investigators, join an investigative team, or attend year long seminars on research methodology or specific methods relevant to their research. Applicants for these awards must provide a year-long career development plan with letters from appropriate faculty and mentors describing the candidate's career development plan and how the award will facilitate the candidate's goals.
Requirements: Applicants should meet the following criteria: proposal relevant to psychoanalysis; applicant is either a new applicant to the Fund or resubmitting a previously reviewed application; applicant has a masters degree or higher; and human subject protection and consent procedures must be specified for research studies involving ongoing data collection.
Restrictions: Applicants who have received $80,000 total from the Fund are ordinarily not eligible to apply again.
Amount of Grant: $15,000 maximum annually
Date(s) Application is Due: Apr 1; Nov 1
Contact: Dean K. Stein, Executive Director; (212) 752-0450; fax: (212) 593-0571; email: deankstein@apsa.org or info@apsa.org
Internet: http://www.apsa.org/RESEARCH/FUNDFORPSYCHOANALYTICRESEARCH/GRANTS/tabid/137/Default.aspx
Sponsor: American Psychoanalytic Association
309 East 49th Street
New York, NY 10007-1601

APSAA Research Grants **519**
The Fund conceives of psychoanalytic research along the broadest lines, including: scholarly and empirical investigative contributions that can advance knowledge of psychoanalytic theory, practice, and links between psychoanalysis and neighboring disciplines such as developmental psychology or neuroscience. Grants of one or two years duration at a maximum of $20,000 yearly are intended for a specific project building upon psychoanalytic principles or directly investigating the process and/or outcome of psychoanalytically informed treatments. The Board recognizes that this amount of money is not sufficient usually to cover the costs of a large research study, particularly one that may involve a large number of subjects or a longitudinal design. Hence, the Board encourages applicants to consider feasibility of their request, that is, what they can achieve for this amount of money, and also to think about this type of award as supporting the beginning stages of a research project, the gathering of pilot data, or the refinement of design and methods.
Requirements: Applicants should meet the following criteria: proposal relevant to psychoanalysis; applicant is either a new applicant to the Fund or resubmitting a previously reviewed application; applicant has a masters degree or higher; and human subject protection and consent procedures must be specified for research studies involving ongoing data collection.
Restrictions: Applicants who have received $80,000 total from the Fund are ordinarily not eligible to apply again.
Amount of Grant: $20,000 maximum
Date(s) Application is Due: Apr 1; Nov 1
Contact: Dean K. Stein, Executive Director; (212) 752-0450; fax: (212) 593-0571; email: deankstein@apsa.org or info@apsa.org
Internet: http://www.apsa.org/RESEARCH/FUNDFORPSYCHOANALYTICRESEARCH/GRANTS/tabid/137/Default.aspx
Sponsor: American Psychoanalytic Association
309 East 49th Street
New York, NY 10007-1601

APSAA Small Beginning Scholar Pre-Investigation Grants **520**
The Fund conceives of psychoanalytic research along the broadest lines, including: scholarly and empirical investigative contributions that can advance knowledge of psychoanalytic theory, practice, and links between psychoanalysis and neighboring disciplines such as developmental psychology or neuroscience. These small grants of less than $5,000 for one year are intended to permit a beginning scholar to gather pilot data in preparation for the submission of a full grant to the Fund or to another agency. The Fund accepts revisions of a previously submitted application up to four years after the previous submission date. Up to two revised submissions may be submitted within four years of the original submission date.
Requirements: Applicants should meet the following criteria: proposal relevant to psychoanalysis; applicant is either a new applicant to the Fund or resubmitting a previously reviewed application; applicant has a masters degree or higher; and human subject protection and consent procedures must be specified for research studies involving ongoing data collection.
Restrictions: Applicants who have received $80,000 total from the Fund are ordinarily not eligible to apply again.
Amount of Grant: $5,000 maximum for one year
Date(s) Application is Due: Apr 1; Nov 1
Contact: Dean K. Stein, Executive Director; (212) 752-0450; fax: (212) 593-0571; email: deankstein@apsa.org or info@apsa.org
Internet: http://www.apsa.org/RESEARCH/FUNDFORPSYCHOANALYTICRESEARCH/GRANTS/tabid/137/Default.aspx
Sponsor: American Psychoanalytic Association
309 East 49th Street
New York, NY 10007-1601

APSAA Small Beginning Scholar Visiting and Consulting Grants **521**
The Fund conceives of psychoanalytic research along the broadest lines, including: scholarly and empirical investigative contributions that can advance knowledge of psychoanalytic theory, practice, and links between psychoanalysis and neighboring disciplines such as developmental psychology or neuroscience. Small grants of $3,000 are intended to permit a beginning scholar to spend time visiting and consulting with a more experienced, senior investigator who has agreed to help the junior investigator begin their investigative work. Typically these awards are made to permit the beginning scholar the funds to travel and/or to reimburse the senior investigator for travel and consultation. These grants may also be used to support travel to a research training seminar in the U.S. or abroad. The Fund accepts revisions of a previously submitted application up to four years after the previous submission date. Up to two revised submissions may be submitted within four years of the original submission date.
Requirements: Applicants should meet the following criteria: proposal relevant to psychoanalysis; applicant is either a new applicant to the Fund or resubmitting a previously reviewed application; applicant has a masters degree or higher; and human subject protection and consent procedures must be specified for research studies involving ongoing data collection.
Restrictions: Applicants who have received $80,000 total from the Fund are ordinarily not eligible to apply again.
Amount of Grant: $3,000 maximum
Date(s) Application is Due: Apr 1; Nov 1
Contact: Dean K. Stein, Executive Director; (212) 752-0450; fax: (212) 593-0571; email: deankstein@apsa.org or info@apsa.org
Internet: http://www.apsa.org/RESEARCH/FUNDFORPSYCHOANALYTICRESEARCH/GRANTS/tabid/137/Default.aspx
Sponsor: American Psychoanalytic Association
309 East 49th Street
New York, NY 10007-1601

AptarGroup Foundation Grants **522**
The foundation awards grants to Illinois nonprofit organizations in its areas of interest, including in order of priority, health and social services, cultural activities and programs, and higher education.
Requirements: Illinois nonprofit organizations are eligible.
Restrictions: Grants do not support nursing homes, animal welfare groups, national or international relief organizations, primary, secondary, or theological schools, or religious, civic, fraternal, veterans', social, or political organizations. Individuals, testimonial dinners, fundraising events, courtesy advertising, or trips or tours will not be supported.
Geographic Focus: Illinois
Date(s) Application is Due: Mar 15; Oct 15
Contact: Lawrence Lowrimore, Secretary, (815) 477-0424; fax: (815) 477-0481; email: info@aptargroup.com
Sponsor: AptarGroup Charitable Foundation
475 W Terra Cotta Avenue, Suite E
Crystal Lake, IL 60014-9695

Aratani Foundation Grants **523**
The foundation awards grants to nonprofits in its areas of interest, including education, health care, museums, recreation, and religion. Preference is given to Japanese-American cultural organizations. Types of support include annual campaigns, building construction/renovation, capital campaigns, conferences and seminars, continuing support, curriculum development, endowments, exchange programs, fellowships, general operating support, program development, scholarship funds, and seed grants. Application forms are not required, but application outlines are available.

Requirements: Giving primarily in California.
Restrictions: Grants are not made to individuals.
Geographic Focus: California
Amount of Grant: $100-$150,000 average range
Contact: George Aratani, President
Sponsor: Aratani Foundation
23505 Crenshaw Boulevard, No 230
Hollywood, CA 90505

Arcadia Foundation Grants 524

The foundation awards grants to Pennsylvania nonprofit organizations to improve the quality of life. Areas of interest include hospitals and hospital building funds, health agencies and services, nursing, hospices, early childhood, adult and higher education, libraries, child development and welfare agencies, youth organizations, and social service and general welfare agencies, including care of the handicapped, aged, and hungry. Also supported are family services, environment and conservation, wildlife and animal welfare, religious organizations, historical preservation, and music organizations. Types of support include general operating support, continuing support, annual campaigns, capital campaigns, building construction/renovation, equipment acquisition, endowment funds, program development, scholarship funds, and research. Applications are accepted between September 1 and November 1.
Requirements: Eastern Pennsylvania organizations whose addresses have zip codes of 18000-19000 are eligible. Application form not required. The initial approach should be a letter or proposal—not exceeding two pages.
Restrictions: Grants are not awarded to support individuals, deficit financing, land acquisition, fellowships, demonstration projects, publications, or conferences.
Geographic Focus: Pennsylvania
Date(s) Application is Due: Nov 1
Contact: Marilyn Lee Steinbright, President, fax: (610) 275-8460
Sponsor: Arcadia Foundation
105 E Logan Street
Norristown, PA 19401

Archer Daniels Midland Foundation Grants Program 525

The foundation prefers to fund programs that will directly impact the communities where operating units are located. Nearly a third of the funding is directed toward educational institutions, including elementary, secondary, and higher education. The advocacy category covers world affairs and foreign relations groups that deal with international trade; also supported are projects stressing free enterprise and assistance for women. Support of social services goes to minority group development, cultural activities, and hospital and youth agencies. Health service funding supports hospital and disease association programs. Conservation funding supports programs for protecting the environment and beautification as well as conservation. Religion grants support Christian, Jewish, and Roman Catholic organizations, such as churches, colleges and universities, international ministries/missions, Jewish welfare, and the Salvation Army. Applications are accepted at any time; initial contact by letter of inquiry is encouraged.
Requirements: Tax-exempt organizations are eligible. Current United Way recipients and national organizations are also eligible.
Restrictions: Grants are restricted to public, religious, charitable, philanthropic, benevolent, scientific, literary, artistic, and educational groups, or for the prevention of cruelty to children and animals.
Samples: The German Coast Farmers' Market (LA) to add new location to its farmers market—award recipient 2006; The Audrain County 4-H Foundation (MO) to build a replacement for its 45-year-old building and fulfill its commitments to the children and families in the area—award recipient 2006; The Girl Scouts of U.S.A-Kickapoo Council (IL) to construct a lab for girls from local schools and outreach agencies to learn about career opportunities in agriculture.
Amount of Grant: $10,000 per award
Contact: Brian Peterson, Program Contact, (217) 424-5413
Internet: http://www.admworld.com/naen/
Sponsor: Archer Daniels Midland Foundation
P.O. Box 1470
Decatur, IL 62526

ARCO Foundation Education Grants 526

The foundation will concentrate its aid to education in support of the following: precollege programs to improve the quality of teaching and learning in urban public education; programs aimed at decreasing attrition rates among low-income and minority students; programs to motivate low-income and minority students to succeed in college, especially in mathematics-based careers of engineering, science, and business; support for laboratory renovation and scientific equipment in academic disciplines of interest at major research universities; programs to retain the most talented young faculty in academic careers in selected disciplines; selected liberal arts programs at colleges and universities of interest; state associations of private colleges in the states where the company has interests; academic programs relevant to energy interests at regional universities and colleges; and national education associations and organizations that seek to improve education in public high schools and at higher academic levels. Grants are awarded for operating budgets, seed money, equipment, land acquisition, matching funds, employee matching gifts, employee related scholarships, special projects, and technical assistance. Applications are accepted at any time; annual report should be obtained prior to submitting a formal proposal.
Requirements: The foundation is a regional organization funding nonprofit organizations in states where ARCO has facilities and personnel, including Alaska, Arizona, California, Colorado, Nevada, Texas, and Washington. Requests from those states and those nearby should be addressed to the local community affairs managers.
Restrictions: The foundation discourages applications from the following: programs not focused on promoting self-sufficiency and economic development of minority populations; historic preservation or urban development projects not tied to neighborhood economic revitalization; proposals from religious organizations; or funding requests from federal, state, county, and municipal agencies, including school districts. The foundation does not generally consider support of hospital building or endowment campaigns, medical equipment, medical research programs, single-issue health organizations, or health services not directed at low-income people.
Geographic Focus: Alaska; Arizona; California; Colorado; Nevada; Texas; Washington
Samples: U of Montana (Butte, MT)—to help retain and graduate minority students pursuing engineering degrees, $16,500.; U of California (Davis, CA)—to help retain and graduate minority students pursuing engineering degrees, $47,000.
Amount of Grant: $1500-$360,000
Contact: Grants Administrator, (213) 486-3342; fax: (213) 486-0113
Internet: http://www.ntlf.com/html/grants/5977.htm
Sponsor: ARCO Foundation
151 S Flower Street
Los Angeles, CA 90071

Argyros Foundation Grants Program 527

The foundation annually awards grants for cultural activities, higher education, religious projects, social services, recreation, and health services. Types of support include general operating support and program development. Proposals must give a detailed outline of the project for which funds are requested.
Requirements: Giving is primarily made to organizations in Orange County, CA.
Geographic Focus: California
Samples: Estell Doheny Eye Institute (Los Angeles, CA)—for operating support, $110,000.; South Coast Repertory Theater (Costa Mesa, CA)—for program support, $20,000.; Boy Scouts of America, Orange County (Santa Ana, CA)—for operating support, $7000.
Amount of Grant: $5000-$50,000 average
Date(s) Application is Due: Jun 1
Contact: Daniel Russo, Argyros Charitable Trusts, (714) 481-5000
Sponsor: Argyros Foundation
949 S Coast Drive, No 600
Costa Mesa, CA 92626

Arie and Ida Crown Memorial Grants 528

The program supports programs that offer opportunities to the disadvantaged, strengthens the bond of families, and improves the quality of people's lives. As a general rule, the Foundation funds organizations that serve the greater Chicago area as well as organizations that serve the broader Jewish community. Most grants are awarded to organizations within the city of Chicago. Organizations are supported in the areas of arts and culture (concentrating on educational and enrichment programs for youth), civic affairs, education, health (stressing access to services, hospice and health promotion), and human service (focusing on programs which offer assistance for children and families).
Requirements: Nonprofit organizations in Chicago and Cook County, IL, may apply for grant support.
Restrictions: Grants are not made to support individuals, conference expenses, film projects, government programs (50 percent government funded), or research projects.
Geographic Focus: Illinois
Amount of Grant: $1000-$200,000 average
Date(s) Application is Due: Jan 31; Jul 31
Contact: Susan Crown, President, (312) 236-6300; fax: (312) 984-1499; email: AICM@crown-Chicago.com
Internet: http://www.crownmemorial.org/
Sponsor: Arie and Ida Crown Memorial
222 N LaSalle Street, Suite 2000
Chicago, IL 60601

Arizona Cardinals Grants 529

The National Football League franchise supports programs designed to improve the quality of life and enhance opportunities for children, women, and minorities in the state of Arizona. Specific areas of interest include arts and culture, civic affairs, education, health, science, and social services. The foundation is interested in expanding its giving and looks for new charities to fund. First-time applicant organizations generally will receive grants of $5000 or less.
Requirements: Applicants must be exempt under 501(c)3 of the Internal Revenue Service code.
Geographic Focus: Arizona
Samples: AZCenters for Comprehensive Education and Life Skills; Chrysalis Shelter for Victims of Domestic Violence; Child crisis Center-East Valley; Jewish Family and Children's Services; Juvenile Diabetes Research Foundation; United Food Bank.
Amount of Grant: $2000-$5000
Date(s) Application is Due: Aug 1
Contact: Pat Tankersley, (602) 379-0101; fax: (480) 785-7327
Internet: http://www.azcardinals.com/community/charities.php
Sponsor: Arizona Cardinals
P.O. Box 888
Phoenix, AZ 85001-0888

Arizona Diamondbacks Charities Grants 530

The major-league baseball franchise awards grants in Arizona to support as wide as possible a variety of charitable causes. Priority will to be given to organizations that fall under the foundation's focus areas of health care for the indigent, homelessness and youth education. Types of support include general support, project grants, donated equipment, employee matching gifts, corporate sponsorships, and speakers. Organizations wishing to apply for a grant can fax a request to the community affairs department.
Requirements: Applicants must be 501(c)3 Arizona-based organizations committed to spending grant proceeds in Arizona.
Geographic Focus: Arizona
Samples: Arizona's Children (Phoenix, AZ)—for a program to provide behavioral health services to children and their families.; Golden Gate Community Ctr (Phoenix, AZ)—to help replace evaporative coolers in the center's gymnasium.; Make Way for Books (Tucson, AZ)—to promote early literacy in low-income area preschools.
Contact: Contact, Communities Affairs, (602) 462-6500; fax: (602) 462-6575
Internet: http://arizona.diamondbacks.mlb.com/ari/community/foundation.jsp
Sponsor: Arizona Diamondbacks
P.O. Box 2095
Phoenix, AZ 85001

Arizona Public Service Corporate Giving Program Grants 531

Grants are awarded to support Arizona nonprofit organizations in the areas of health and human services, community development, arts and culture, education, and environment. The foundation awards support for project grants, capital building funds, research, employee matching gifts, in-kind services, conferences and seminars, and operating support. Applications are accepted on an ongoing basis.
Requirements: Arizona 501(c)3 nonprofits are eligible.
Restrictions: APS Corporate Giving does not fund individual request, charter or private schools, religious, political fraternal, legislative or lobbying efforts to organizations, travel-related or hotel expenses, private or family foundation, private non-profit organizations, salaries and/or debt reduction.
Geographic Focus: Arizona
Samples: Hospice of the Valley (Phoenix, AZ)—for operating support, $10,000.; Arizona Bridge to Independent Living (Phoenix, AZ)—for program support, $3000.; Arizona Wolf Trap—to sponsor a series of field trips for children to visit performing arts centers.
Contact: Cindy Slick, Manager; (602) 250-4707; fax: (602) 250-2113; email: Cindy.Slick@aps.com
Internet: http://www.aps.com/main/community/dev/default.html
Sponsor: Arizona Public Service Corporation
P.O. Box 53999, MS 8010
Phoenix, AZ 85072-3999

Arkansas Community Foundation Arkansas Black Hall of Fame Grants 532

Grants support programs and projects that address problems, challenges, and opportunities in black communities in Arkansas. Categories of interest include education; health and wellness; youth development; and small business and/or economic development. Priority goes to proposals that show multiple sponsoring agencies/organizations; include evidence of local financial support; demonstrate collaborative ventures among community organizations; and have promise for sustainability beyond the period of the grant.
Requirements: Tax-exempt entities such as schools, churches, or government entities are eligible. Preference is given to applications submitted by 501(c)3 nonprofit organizations.
Restrictions: Funds cannot be allocated for adult salary support in carrying out the duties of the project; used to support general operating budgets outside of the specific proposal or project; or for scholarships for formal education at any level.
Geographic Focus: Arkansas
Amount of Grant: $5,000 maximum; $1,000-$2,500 typically
Date(s) Application is Due: Apr 10
Contact: Cecilia Patterson, Program Director; (501) 372-1116; fax: (501) 372-1166; email: cpatterson@arcf.org or arcf@arcf.org
Internet: http://www.arcf.org/page27973.cfm
Sponsor: Arkansas Community Foundation (ARCF)
1400 West Markham, Suite 206
Little Rock, AR 72201

Arkansas Community Foundation Grants 533

The Arkansas Community Foundation (ARCF) serves philanthropic donors and supports non-profits in Arkansas. ARCF makes grants from charitable funds established by individuals, families, corporations, and non-profit organizations. From among over 1100 funds, its donors make grants in the following areas of interest: animal welfare, arts and humanities, community development, education, environment, health, human services, and religion. While the Foundation's discretionary grant cycles are few, grants are usually modest and, generally, fund capital or building campaigns are not funded.
Requirements: 501(c)3 Arkansas nonprofit organizations are eligible.
Geographic Focus: Arkansas
Amount of Grant: $500-$2,500
Contact: Cecilia Patterson, Program Director; (501) 372-1116; fax: (501) 372-1166; email: cpatterson@arcf.org or arcf@arcf.org
Internet: http://www.arcf.org/page12714.cfm
Sponsor: Arkansas Community Foundation (ARCF)
1400 West Markham, Suite 206
Little Rock, AR 72201

Arkell Hall Foundation Grants 534

The primary mission of the foundation is the operation and maintenance of a home for elderly women. Funds that may become available above the needs of the home may be distributed annually to tax-exempt organizations providing services in the target community—Western Montgomery County, NY—with preference given to those active in service to senior citizens, education (higher education, medical education, adult basic education and literacy), religion (Christian, Christian Reformed Church, Lutheran, Methodist, Roman Catholic, the Salvation Army, and United Methodist), and health care. Types of support include capital, challenge, endowment, general support, matching, and seed money grants. Grants are made on a single-year basis and are awarded annually in October or November. It is recommended that requests be submitted between July 1 and September 15. Initial review of requests is performed upon receipt. Results are forwarded to the applicant within one month.
Requirements: IRS 501(c)3 organizations directly impacting the Western Montgomery County, NY, community are eligible.
Restrictions: Requests that do not include written proof of 501(c)3 status will not be considered. Projects or organizations with large service areas, such as national or regional, will not qualify for funding, nor will projects in which the target community is not the primary area of focus.
Geographic Focus: New York
Samples: Cornell University, College of Human Ecology (Ithaca, NY)—for general support, $20,000.; College of Saint Rose (Albany, NY)—to support scholarships for single mothers, $3000.
Amount of Grant: $1000-$50,000 average
Date(s) Application is Due: Oct 1
Contact: Joseph Santangelo, Vice President & Treasurer, (518) 673-5417; fax: (518) 673-5493
Sponsor: Arkell Hall Foundation, Inc.
68 Front Street, P.O. Box 240
Canajoharie, NY 13317-0240

Arkema Foundation Science Teachers Program 535

This program is an intensive week-long session for elementary and secondary school teachers. Armed with innovative science experiment kits and the guidance of chemical engineers and scientists, teachers learn new and fascinating ways to illustrate scientific concepts. Scientific topics explored include life, earth and physical science and technology. School principals are asked to nominate two teachers in grades three through six, who are then chosen by the corporate committee to participate in the program. Application forms and contact information are available on the Web site.
Requirements: Teachers in the following geographic areas may participate: Alabama (Mobile county); Kentucky (Graves, Livingston, Lyon, Marshall, McCracken, Carroll, Gallatin, Trimble, Jefferson counties); Michigan (Wayne county); Minnesota (Didge, Mower, Steele counties); New Jersey (Burlington, Camden, Gloucester, and Salem counties); New York (Genesee, Livingston counties); Pennsylvania (Berks, Bucks, Chester, Delaware, Montgomery, and Philadelphia counties); Tennessee (Shelby county); Texas (Jasper, Newton, Jefferson, Orange, Harris, and Brazos counties).
Geographic Focus: Alabama; Kentucky; Michigan; Minnesota; New Jersey; New York; Pennsylvania; Tennessee; Texas
Amount of Grant: $500
Contact: Jane Crawford, (215) 419-7614; email: jane.crawford@arkemagroup.com
Internet: http://www.products.arkemagroup.com/index.cfm?pag=190
Sponsor: Arkema Inc. Foundation
2000 Market Street
Philadelphia, PA 19103-3222

Arlington Community Foundation Grants 536

The foundation awards grants in Arlington to educators and nonprofit organizations for innovative projects that supplement and enrich the learning environment for preschool to adult students. The focus is curriculum enrichment, the arts (musical, dramatic, visual), pursuit of higher education, vocational education, after school and summer programs, life-long learning, environmental issues, parent involvement, and community involvement. The community enhancement grants support arts and humanities, children & families, community improvement, health, housing/homeless & hunger, legal, social services, and senior enrichment. The purpose of the Prompt Response Fund is to enable nonprofit groups in Arlington respond quickly to unanticipated opportunities or unexpected, urgent community needs. Deadlines may vary. Guidelines and applications are available online.
Requirements: Organizations and individuals with projects designed to meet educational needs of Arlington residents are encouraged to apply.
Restrictions: The foundation does not make grants for endowments, capital campaigns, religious purposes, individual debts, or political lobbying.
Geographic Focus: Virginia
Contact: Wanda L. Pierce, Executive Director, (703) 243-4785; fax: (703) 243-4796; email: info@arlcf.org
Internet: http://www.arlcf.org/grants.html
Sponsor: Arlington Community Foundation
2525 Wilson Boulevard
Arlington, VA 22201

Armstrong McDonald Foundation Grants 537

The foundation awards grants to eligible nonprofit organizations in its areas of interest, including animal welfare, children and youth, education, special needs, health, and relief and social.

Requirements: 510(c)3 nonprofit organizations, colleges and universities, schools, and school districts are eligible. Application must be downloaded from website.
Restrictions: Grants do not support advocacy organizations, individuals, international organizations, political organizations, or state and local government agencies. The foundation does not fund capital campaigns, salaries/stipends, and multi-year projects. Organization must have received a grant from the foundation within the last five years unless it is located within the states of Arizona or Nebraska. No organization east of the Mississippi is eligible for a grant.
Samples: San Diego Zoo (San Diego, CA) $40,000.; Tucson Children's Museum (Tucson, AZ) $20,000; Omaha Street School (Omaha, NE) $17,500; UofA Found for Steele Children (Tucson, AZ) $72,900; Saddlebrook Community Outreach (Tucson, AZ) $10,000; Canine Co-Pilots (Flagstaff, AZ) $10,000; NW School for Hearing Impaired (Seattle, WA) $7,500.
Amount of Grant: $1000-$80,000 range
Date(s) Application is Due: Sep 30
Contact: Laurie Bouchard, Vice President, (520) 878-9627; email: info@ArmstrongMcDonaldFoundation.org
Internet: http://www.armstrongmcdonaldfoundation.org/
Sponsor: Armstrong McDonald Foundation
P.O. Box 70110
Tucson, AZ 85737.0110

ARS Foundation Grants **538**
The mission of the foundation is to make a positive difference in the lives of others. They support human and social services, the arts, children and the elderly, and health care but will consider other organizations. Giving is focused in New York City and Fairfield County, CT, areas. Applicants should submit a cover letter containing a brief history and description of the organization, the program(s), the needs/goals to be addressed, and a description of the project; an itemized budget, current organizational annual budget, and recent audited financial statement; annual report; other funding sources; and 501(c)3 determination letter. There are no application deadlines or forms.
Requirements: Qualified 501(c)3 charitable organizations in the New York City and Fairfield County, CT, areas are eligible.
Restrictions: The foundation does not give grants to individuals, private foundations, or organizations not qualified as charitable organizations.
Geographic Focus: Connecticut; New York
Contact: Grants Administrator, (212) 986-1533; fax: (212) 972-2303; email: info@arsfoundation.com
Internet: http://www.arsfoundation.com
Sponsor: Adolph and Ruth Schnurmacher Foundation
551 Fifth Avenue, Suite 1210
New York, NY 10176

ARS New Investigator Award **539**
The purpose of this award is to support basic, translational, or clinical research projects in rhinology. Proposed projects may be related to any area of rhinology. Proposed project shall be designed in collaboration with a preceptor investigator and approved by the candidate's department chairperson and institution. One award of up to $25,000 over a two-year period will be given annually. Letters of Interest should be received no later than December 15, with full proposals due on January 15.
Requirements: Any member of the American Rhinologic Society who has not received previous, significant outside funding is eligible. The applicant must have, as a mentor, an established researcher who will provide a letter of support stating the extent of involvement in the project and provide a summary of his/her research experience.
Amount of Grant: $25,000 maximum total (direct and indirect) costs
Date(s) Application is Due: Dec 15; Jan 15
Contact: Stephanie L. Jones, Assistant Director; (703) 519-1586 or (703) 836-4444; email: sljones@entnet.org
Internet: http://www.entnet.org/EducationAndResearch/coreGrants.cfm
Sponsor: American Rhinology Society (ARS)
One Prince Street
Alexandria, VA 22314-3357

ARS Resident Research Grants **540**
The purpose of this award is to support basic, translational, or clinical research projects in rhinology. Proposed projects may be related to any area of rhinology. Proposed project shall be designed in collaboration with a preceptor investigator and approved by the candidate's department chairperson and institution. Two awards of up to $8,000 over a one-year period will be given annually. Letters of Interest should be received no later than December 15, with full proposals due on January 15.
Requirements: Any resident in training in an approved program in the U.S. or Canada is eligible to apply for the American Rhinologic Society Research Grant. Resident applicants must have as a co-investigator a supervising faculty who is a member in good standing in the American Rhinologic Society (ARS).
Amount of Grant: $8,000 maximum
Date(s) Application is Due: Dec 15; Jan 15
Contact: Stephanie L. Jones, Assistant Director; (703) 519-1586 or (703) 836-4444; email: sljones@entnet.org
Internet: http://www.entnet.org/EducationAndResearch/upload/2009-ARS-Resideint-Research-Grant.pdf
Sponsor: American Rhinology Society (ARS)
One Prince Street
Alexandria, VA 22314-3357

Arthritis Foundation of Australia Grants **541**
The foundation awards grants in the fields of medicine and health, with emphasis on arthritis research and education. Types of awards include grants-in-aid, fellowships, and scholarships. Grants are awarded in Australia, the United Kingdom, and the United States. Annual deadline dates may vary; contact program staff for exact dates.
Requirements: Awards are available to clinical, scientific, and allied health professionals who are Australian citizens or permanent residents. Scholarships, fellowships, and grants may only be held in universities, hospitals, or recognized research institutes.
Amount of Grant: $A10,000-$A15,000 grants-in-aid
Date(s) Application is Due: Jun 30
Contact: Grant Coordinator, 61 (0)2 9552 6085; fax: 61 (0)2 9552 6078; email: info@arthritisaustralia.com.au
Internet: http://arthritisaustralia.com.au/Research%20Grants
Sponsor: Arthritis Foundation of Australia
P.O. Box 121
Sydney 2001 Australia

Arthur and Rochelle Belfer Foundation Grants **542**
The foundation awards grants to nonprofit organizations of the Jewish faith, with a focus on New York. Grants are targeted toward programs supporting the elderly and women; education/higher education; institutions such as seminaries, synagogues, and temples; hospitals; Jewish welfare; and medical centers. Types of support include general support grants and fellowships. There are no application deadlines. Applicants should send a brief letter of inquiry describing the program.
Restrictions: Grants are not made to individuals.
Geographic Focus: New York
Samples: Joan S. Brugge, PhD, chair, Department of Cell Biology, arvard Medical School—for breast cancer studies (2006); Dana-Farber Cancer Institute (Boston, MA)—for general support, $1 million.; Anti-Defamation League of B'nai B'rith (New York, NY)—for operating support, $22,000.
Amount of Grant: $1000-$100,000 average
Contact: Robert Belfer, President; 212-508-6020
Sponsor: Arthur and Rochelle Belfer Foundation, Inc
767 Fifth Avenue, 46th Floor
New York, NY 10153-0002

ArvinMeritor Foundation Health Grants **543**
The foundation provides grants primarily in company-operating locations in the areas of education and training, civic and health, youth organizations, and arts and culture. In the area of Health, the foundation supports programs designed to promote health research, treatment, education, and awareness; and reduce the cost of illness. Types of support include general operating budgets, building funds, continuing support, equipment, and projects. The committee foundation meets every six to eight weeks to review grant requests. Contact program staff for current guidelines.
Requirements: Nonprofit 501(c)3 organizations should submit a one- to two-page letter outlining the purpose and needs of the program, its budget, duration, goals, leadership, and amount requested.
Restrictions: Ineligibility applies to individuals; organizations that limit participation or services based on race, gender, religion, color, creed, age, or national origin; projects without ties to a community that is home to an ArvinMeritor facility; organizations that pose any conflict with the goals and mission of ArvinMeritor, its employees, communities, or products; operating expenses for United Way local agencies, except through the foundation's support of annual United Way campaigns; sponsorships of fund raising activities by individuals (i.e., walk-a-thons); requests for loans or debt retirement; religious or sectarian programs for religious purposes; labor, political, or veterans organizations; fraternal, athletic, or social clubs; or seminars, conferences, trips, and tours.
Contact: Jerry Rush, Senior Director, Government and Community Affairs; (248) 435-7907; fax: (248) 245-1031; email: jerry.rush@arvinmeritor.com
Internet: http://www.arvinmeritor.com/community/community.asp
Sponsor: ArvinMeritor Foundation
2135 W. Maple Road
Troy, MI 48084

ArvinMeritor Grants **544**
ArvinMeritor???s philanthropic programs focus on education and the communities where its employees live and work. Grants support engineering and technical schools worldwide to increase the number of engineers and scientists in the field of automotive engineering, and to stimulate technological development and innovation in this field. The corporation also partners with local, private, and public agencies in order to improve the quality of life in the areas of education, cultural programs, civic responsibility, and health and human services. There are no application deadlines.
Requirements: Nonprofit organizations in ArvinMeritor communities are eligible.
Restrictions: Grants do not support organizations without nonprofit status; individuals; organizations that limit participation or services based on race, gender, religion, color, creed, age, or national origin; projects without ties to a community that is home to an ArvinMeritor facility; organizations that pose any conflict with the goals and mission of ArvinMeritor, its employees, communities, or products; operating expenses for United Way local agencies, except through support of annual United Way campaigns; sponsorships of fund-raising activities by individuals; requests for loans or debt retirement; religious or sectarian programs for religious purposes; labor, political, or veterans organizations; fraternal, athletic, or social clubs; or seminars, conferences, trips, and tours.

Amount of Grant: $1000-$100,000
Contact: Jerry Rush, Community Relations, (248) 435-7907; fax: (248) 245-1031; email: jerry.rush@arvinmeritor.com
Internet: http://www.arvinmeritor.com/community/guidelines.asp
Sponsor: ArvinMeritor Inc
2135 W Maple Road
Troy, MI 48084-7186

ASA Metlife Foundation MindAlert Awards 545
The awards were established to recognize innovations in mental fitness programming for older adults. Awards recognize programs, products, or tools that promote cognitive fitness in later life. One award will be made to a program in each of three categories: lifelong learning and third age learning programs where mental fitness is implicit; educational programs focused on enhancing mental fitness for the general population of older adults; and programs specifically designed to enhance mental fitness for cognitively-impaired older adults. Applications are judged for their innovation, their basis in research, demonstration of their effectiveness, potential for replicability and the extent to which the programs are accessible to diverse populations of elders. Guidelines and application are available online.
Requirements: Programs and products or tools that promote cognitive function in later life are eligible.
Amount of Grant: $1,500 cash award
Date(s) Application is Due: Oct 1
Contact: Nancy Decia, Coordinator, Education & Training; (415) 974-9610; fax: (415) 974-0300; email: awards@asaging.org
Internet: http://www.asaging.org/asav2/mindalertaward/index.cfm
Sponsor: American Society on Aging
833 Market Street, Suite 511
San Francisco, CA 94103-1824

ASCO Improving Cancer Care Grants 546
The ASCO Cancer Foundation Improving Cancer Care Grant, funded by Susan G. Komen for the Cure, will provide extramural research funding to address important issues regarding access to healthcare, quality of care, and delivery of care, with general applicability to breast cancer. The goal of this program is to encourage multi-disciplinary research that will have a major impact on cancer care, with general applicability in the breast cancer arena. This grant opportunity is part of the Susan G. Komen for the Cure/ASCO Cancer Foundation Research Initiative. Susan G. Komen for the Cure and The ASCO Cancer Foundation expect to award up to three research grants, each totaling 1.35 million dollars. This money will be distributed as $450,000 total costs per year over three years. Applicants must submit their letter of intent in the online application system by 5:00 PM EDT on September 1st. Only online applications will be accepted. After review by the Research Initiative Grant Review Subcommittee, applicants will be notified about the status of their letter of intent. Only applicants who have submitted an approved letter of intent will be eligible to submit the full proposal. Applicants can expect to be notified on October 1st.
Requirements: Eligible research teams: will focus on implementing and/or evaluating new solutions to existing problems in quality of, access to, and delivery of care, with general applicability to breast cancer; will be led by a single Principal Investigator, who must be an active ASCO member (or have submitted a membership application) with an MD, DO, PhD or equivalent degree. All categories of active ASCO members are eligible; will have a multidisciplinary team of investigators that may include clinicians, nurses, pharmacists, statisticians, epidemiologists, information technologists, and other research experts; will be allowed to obtain expertise not represented in the core team through consultants and/or sub-contracts.
Amount of Grant: 1.35 million dollars total
Date(s) Application is Due: Sep 1; Dec 1
Contact: Nancy R. Daly, Executive Director; (571) 483-1432; email: dalyn@asco.org
Internet: http://www.ascocancerfoundation.org/TACF/Grants/Grant+Opportunities/Improving+Cancer+Care+Grant
Sponsor: American Society of Clinical Oncology
2318 Mill Road, Suite 800
Alexandria, VA 22314

ASCO State Affiliate Grants 547
The State Affiliate Grant Program enables state/regional affiliates to engage in activities that will benefit their members, ASCO members, other state societies and the oncology community at large. The purpose of the State Affiliate Grant Program is to provide financial support to help state/regional affiliates to implement specific activities, such as conducting an educational meeting, developing an informational brochure or newsletter, creating a state clinical trials network, or taking part in a quality cancer care initiative collaborating with a patient advocacy group on an awareness campaign. For more information about the State Affiliate Grant Program, email stateaffiliates@asco.org. Applications are available online, with a submission deadline of November 17.
Requirements: All 48 Affiliates are eligible to apply for a grant.
Samples: Denali (Alaska) Oncology Group, $10,000 (2009); Georgia Society of Clinical Oncology, $10,000 (2009); Maryland/DC Society of Clinical Oncology, $10,000 (2009); New York State Society of Medical Oncologists & Hematologists, $10,000 (2009); Northern New England Society of Clinical Oncology, $10,000 (2009).
Amount of Grant: $10,000
Contact: Nancy R. Daly, Executive Director; (571) 483-1432; email: dalyn@asco.org
Internet: http://www.ascocancerfoundation.org/TACF/Professional+Education+and+Support/Cancer+Policy
Sponsor: American Society of Clinical Oncology
2318 Mill Road, Suite 800
Alexandria, VA 22314

ASCO Advanced Clinical Research Award in Colorectal Cancer 548
The Advanced Clinical Research Award (ACRA) in Colorectal Cancer is designed to fund investigators who are committed to clinical cancer research and who wish to conduct original research not currently funded. The grant totals $450,000 and is paid in 3 annual increments of $150,000 made on or about July 1 of each year of the grant term. The grant funds will be directed to the sponsoring institution and should be used towards salary support, supplies, equipment, travel, etc. necessary for the pursuit of the recipient's research project.
Requirements: Appplicants must meet the following criteria: be a physician (MD, DO, or international equivalent) who is in the fourth to ninth year of a full-time, primary faculty appointment in a clinical department at an academic medical institution at the time of grant submission; have completed productive post doctoral/post fellowship research and demonstrated the ability to undertake independent investigator-initiated clinical research; be an active member of ASCO or have submitted a membership application with the grant application; be able to commit to 75% of full-time effort in research (applies to total research, not just the proposed project) during the award period.
Amount of Grant: $450,000
Date(s) Application is Due: Nov 3
Contact: Nancy R. Daly, Executive Director; (571) 483-1432; email: dalyn@asco.org
Internet: http://www.ascocancerfoundation.org/TACF/Grants/Grant+Opportunities/Advanced+Clinical+Research+Award+in+Colorectal+Cancer
Sponsor: American Society of Clinical Oncology
2318 Mill Road, Suite 800
Alexandria, VA 22314

ASCO Advanced Clinical Research Awards in Breast Cancer 549
The ASCO Foundation and Genentech BioOncology invite physicians with full-time faculty appointments to apply for a clinical oncology research award in Breast Cancer. The program funds clinical investigators who are committed to clinical cancer research. Their research must have a direct patient-oriented focus including clinical trials and/or translational research involving human subjects. The Advanced Clinical Research Award is designed to provide funding beyond the Clinical Research Career Development Award (CDA). By continuing to support proven clinical researchers who are post-CDA but at a critical stage in their early career, the foundation hopes to expand the cadre of expert clinical oncology researchers who are developing promising research initiatives.
Requirements: The applicant must meet the following criteria at the time of grant award: be a physician (MD or DO) who is 5-10 years post final sub-specialty training; have a full-time faculty appointment in a clinical department at an academic medical center; have completed productive postdoctoral/post-fellowship research and demonstrated the ability to undertake independent investigator-initiated clinical research; be an active member of the American Society of Clinical Oncology (ASCO); and expect to spend 75% of time during the award period dedicated to research.
Amount of Grant: $450,000
Date(s) Application is Due: Oct 20
Contact: Nancy R. Daly, Executive Director; (571) 483-1432; email: dalyn@asco.org
Internet: http://www.ascocancerfoundation.org/TACF/Grants/Grant+Opportunities/Advanced+Clinical+Research+Award+in+Breast+Cancer
Sponsor: American Society of Clinical Oncology
2318 Mill Road, Suite 800
Alexandria, VA 22314

ASCO Advanced Clinical Research Awards in Sarcoma 550
The Advanced Clinical Research Award (ACRA) in Sarcoma is designed to fund investigators who are committed to clinical cancer research and who wish to conduct original research not currently funded. The award is intended to support proposals with a patient-oriented focus, including a clinical research study and/or translational research involving human subjects. The grant totals $450,000 and is paid in three annual increments of $150,000 made on or about January 1 of each year of the grant term. Preference will be given to proposals involving therapeutic vaccine or immunotherapeutic approaches for sarcoma.
Requirements: Applicants must meet the following criteria: be a physician (MD, DO, or international equivalent) who is in the fourth to ninth year of a full-time, primary faculty appointment in a clinical department at an academic medical institution at the time of grant submission; have completed productive post doctoral/post fellowship research and demonstrated the ability to undertake independent investigator-initiated clinical research; be an active member of ASCO or have submitted a membership application with the grant application; be able to commit to 75% of full-time effort in research (applies to total research, not just the proposed project) during the award period.
Restrictions: Proposals with a predominant focus on in vitro or animal studies (even if clinically relevant) are not allowed.
Amount of Grant: $450,000
Date(s) Application is Due: Aug 6
Contact: Nancy R. Daly, Executive Director; (571) 483-1432; email: dalyn@asco.org
Internet: http://www.ascocancerfoundation.org/TACF/Grants/Grant+Opportunities/Advanced+Clinical+Research+Award+in+Sarcoma
Sponsor: American Society of Clinical Oncology
2318 Mill Road, Suite 800
Alexandria, VA 22314

ASCO Career Development Award 551

The program provides funds to clinical investigators who have received their initial faculty appointment to establish an independent clinical cancer research program. Since many awards are supported with restricted grants from outside organizations, the ASCO is particularly interested in identifying young researchers working in the following sub-specialties and emerging disciplines: breast cancer; cancer survivorship; geriatric oncology; health disparities; kidney cancer; multiple myeloma; ovarian cancer; pancreatic cancer; sarcoma; survivorship; and young adult cancer. However, The ASCO Foundation welcomes application submissions in all oncology sub-specialties.
Requirements: Clinical investigators who have received their initial faculty appointment to establish an independent clinical cancer research program are eligible.
Amount of Grant: $200,000 (paid over three years)
Date(s) Application is Due: Sep 9
Contact: Nancy R. Daly, Executive Director; (571) 483-1432; email: dalyn@asco.org
Internet: http://www.ascocancerfoundation.org/TACF/Grants/Grant+Opportunities/Career+Development+Award/Career+Development+Award
Sponsor: American Society of Clinical Oncology
2318 Mill Road, Suite 800
Alexandria, VA 22314

ASCO Community Oncology Research Grants 552

The Community Oncology Research Grant is open to all eligible, community-based practices. The award is intended to support community-based practices, in their efforts to enhance their clinical trials program. Areas of improvement are based on the American Society of Clinical Oncology Statement on Minimum Standards and Exemplary Attributes of Clinical Trial Sites (Journal of Clinical Oncology, May 20 2008). The grant period begins July 1 and concludes June 30, in addition to a six-month follow-up period for evaluation. Progress reports are required at six and twelve months. A final report is due at eighteen months. Eligible practices are encouraged to apply for the award by completing an online application. Grant proposals will be entertained up to $30,000, including no more than $26,000 for grant support, $1,500 for travel to the ASCO Annual Meeting, and $2,500 for overhead costs. The grant funds will be directed to the community practice, not to an individual. A total of three awards will be presented at the ASCO's Annual Meeting in Chicago, IL.
Requirements: CORG eligibility is based on the following criteria, practices must: have at least one member of ASCO involved in the research program; have at least one member of an ASCO State/Regional Affiliate Program involved in the research program; meet basic standards for a quality clinical trials site (based on Good Clinical Practice standards, the accepted international ethical and scientific quality standard for designing, conducting, recording, and reporting trials); be community-based, with high-quality audit reports and investigators in good standing.
Samples: Billings Clinic Cancer Center, Billings, MT (2009); Marion L Shepard Cancer Center, Washington, NC (2009); Nebraska Cancer Specialists, Omaha, NE (2009).
Amount of Grant: $30,000
Contact: Nancy R. Daly, Executive Director; (571) 483-1432; email: dalyn@asco.org
Internet: http://www.ascocancerfoundation.org/TACF/Grants/Grant+Opportunities/Community+Oncology+Research+Grant
Sponsor: American Society of Clinical Oncology
2318 Mill Road, Suite 800
Alexandria, VA 22314

ASCO Comparative Effectiveness Research Professorship n Breast Cancer 553

The Comparative Effectiveness Research Professorship (CERP) in Breast Cancer is intended to provide support to qualified individuals to investigate comparative effectiveness in breast cancer and to train future generations of researchers in this field. The CERP will provide funding to outstanding researchers who have made and are continuing to make significant contributions that have changed the direction of breast cancer research and who will provide mentorship to junior researchers. The award totals $500,000 and is paid in five annual increments of $100,000 made on or about July 1 of each year of the grant term. The award is not designed to cover the total cost of a research project or the investigator's entire compensation, but can be used at the discretion of the awardee to support their overall research activities.
Requirements: Applications focusing on all aspects of breast cancer including prevention, diagnosis, treatment, delivery of care, and health economics will be accepted. Applicants must: have an MD, DO, PhD or equivalent degree; have the rank of full professor (or equivalent). If current rank is not that of a full professor but meets all other eligibility criteria, a written explanation must be provided for equivalency of current rank; have a full-time faculty appointment at an academic medical center; have made significant contributions that have changed the direction of breast cancer research; be serving as a research mentor to one or more researcher(s) in training, and must be planning to continue to provide leadership in this area throughout the award period; lead a research team in conducting research on comparative effectiveness in breast cancer; be an active member of ASCO or have submitted a membership application with the grant application; commit to spending 75% of time during the award period dedicated to research (applies to total research, not just the proposed project) including leading a team of researchers (in the lab and/or the clinic) and mentoring physician-scientists. Individuals with an endowed professorship from their own institution are eligible to apply for this award. Individuals with administrative responsibilities (such as a Division or Department Chair) must clearly document their time commitment for performing research activities and mentoring activities. The sponsoring institution must be a not-for-profit institution.
Amount of Grant: $500,000
Date(s) Application is Due: Nov 3
Contact: Nancy R. Daly, Executive Director; (571) 483-1432; email: dalyn@asco.org
Internet: http://www.ascocancerfoundation.org/TACF/Grants/Grant+Opportunities/Comparative+Effectiveness+Research+Professorship
Sponsor: American Society of Clinical Oncology
2318 Mill Road, Suite 800
Alexandria, VA 22314

ASCO International Development and Education Awards (IDEA) 554

The award provides support for oncologists in developing countries to attend the ASCO annual meeting and spend additional time at a comprehensive cancer center. The grants are designed to provide continuing medical education, assist in career development, and help establish strong relationships with leading ASCO members who serve as scientific mentors to each recipient. The strongest consideration will be given to candidates who: have submitted an abstract for the most recent Annual Meeting; and have less than 10 years of experience in the field of oncology. Guidelines are available online.
Requirements: Applicants must: complete an application, which includes a 250-word essay, letter of recommendation, and submission of the applicant's CV; be able to travel to the United States and have no visa restrictions or anticipate having any difficulty obtaining a U.S. visa; be citizens of a country identified by ASCO as one of greatest need or with limited resources; and either be or meet the requirements of being either an ASCO Active Member, Active-Junior Member, or an Associate Member.
Restrictions: Applicants cannot: have received one year or more of formal training (for instance, attended medical school, participated in internships, fellowships, or residency programs) in the United States, Western Europe, Australia, New Zealand, Canada, or the United Kingdom; be a previous recipient of the IDEA (formally known as ITG) program; or have previously attended more that one (1) ASCO Annual Meeting.
Date(s) Application is Due: Jan 13
Contact: Amanda Woodell, International Affairs Department; (571) 483-1501; email: idea@asco.org
Internet: http://www.ascocancerfoundation.org/TACF/Awards/Award+Opportunities/International+Development+and+Education+Award+%28IDEA%29
Sponsor: American Society of Clinical Oncology
2318 Mill Road, Suite 800
Alexandria, VA 22314

ASCO Loan Repayment Grants 555

The ASCO Diversity in Oncology Initiative, funded by Susan G. Komen for the Cure, is designed to facilitate the recruitment and retention of individuals from populations underrepresented in medicine to cancer careers, with particular attention to the development of clinical practitioners and investigators. The ASCO Loan Repayment Program, funded by Susan G. Komen for the Cure (LRP), provides repayment of qualifying educational debt to oncologists, or to oncology fellows upon completion of training, who commit to practicing oncology in a medically underserved region of the United States. The LRP will repay up to $35,000 per year for two years (up to $70,000 total) of qualifying education loans. The application period opened September 16, and will close December 16. Applications are available online. Awardees will be announced in early April.
Requirements: To qualify to receive LRP loan assistance, applicants must have completed an approved oncology fellowship training program in the United States by July 1. Candidates must be U.S. citizens, U.S. nationals, or permanent residents. Candidates must have an M.D., D.O., or equivalent medical doctoral degree from an accredited institution. An applicant must be an Associate or Active ASCO member or submit an ASCO membership application with the LRP application.
Amount of Grant: $35,000 per year for two years
Date(s) Application is Due: Sep 16
Contact: Nancy R. Daly, Executive Director; (571) 483-1432; email: dalyn@asco.org;; Kimberly Head, Policy & Clinical Affairs Department; (571) 483-1654; email: DOI@asco.org
Internet: http://www.ascocancerfoundation.org/TACF/Awards/Award+Opportunities/ASCO+Diversity+in+Oncology+Initiative+funded+by+Susan+G.+Komen+for+the+Cure/The+ASCO+Loan+Repayment+Program%2C+funded+by+Susan+G.+Komen+for+the+Cure®
Sponsor: American Society of Clinical Oncology
2318 Mill Road, Suite 800
Alexandria, VA 22314

ASCO Long-Term International Fellowships 556

The ASCO Cancer Foundation Long Term International Fellowship (LIFe) provides young oncologists in developing nations the support and resources needed to advance their training by deepening their relationship with a U.S. or Canadian colleague and his or her institution. Through a one or two year fellowship the recipient will earn valuable training and experience with which they can affect change in cancer care in their home country. Recipients must return to their home institutions after completing their fellowship and are expected to disseminate the knowledge they have gained. The ASCO Cancer Foundation (TACF) will administer fundraising and grant distribution for the fellowships. Funds will be sent from TACF to the host institution in January of the award year. The host institution will then be responsible for financial management of the fellowship. Any funds not spent on the fellowship will be returned to TACF. Recipients must attend the ASCO Annual Meeting that falls during the first year of their award term where they will be honored at The ASCO Cancer Foundation Grants Brunch. Recipients will also be expected to submit their research to ASCO via an abstract or publication submission following their fellowship. Applications are due to ASCO by October 15 for the fellowship to begin anytime in the next calendar year. Applications

should be completed and returned jointly by the prospective host and fellow. A decision will be distributed by December 15.
Requirements: Hosts must: be an ASCO member in good standing; be employed at a U.S. or Canadian institution with sufficient infrastructure to provide for a 1 year fellowship; independently identify fellowship applicants; agree to cover any costs in excess of ASCO's contribution; complete the host section of the LIFe Application; complete fellowship evaluations as requested by ASCO. Applicants must: be an ASCO member in good standing; reside in a country identified by the World Bank as income level low, lower middle, and upper middle; have the support of their home institution including a letter of support from their supervisor; be a medical doctor who has finished a fellowship in clinical oncology or the equivalent; have less than 10 years experience in the field of oncology; complete the applicant section of the LIFe application including submission of a CV of up to 3 pages in length; commit to return to country of origin at the completion of their fellowship.
Date(s) Application is Due: Oct 15
Contact: Nancy R. Daly, Executive Director; (571) 483-1432; email: dalyn@asco.org
Internet: http://www.ascocancerfoundation.org/TACF/Awards/Award+Opportunities/Long-term+International+Fellowship+%28LIFe%29
Sponsor: American Society of Clinical Oncology
2318 Mill Road, Suite 800
Alexandria, VA 22314

ASCO Medical Student Rotation Grants **557**
The ASCO Diversity in Oncology Initiative, funded by Susan G. Komen for the Cure, is designed to facilitate the recruitment and retention of individuals from populations underrepresented in medicine to cancer careers, with particular attention to the development of clinical practitioners and investigators. The ASCO Medical Student Rotation, funded by Susan G. Komen for the Cure, provides 8 - 10 week clinical or clinical research oncology rotations for U.S. medical students from populations underrepresented in medicine who are interested in pursuing oncology as a career. Recipients receive a $5,000 stipend for the rotation plus $1,500 for future travel to the ASCO Annual Meeting. An additional $2,000 will be provided to support the student's mentor. The application period opened October 7 and will close January 7. Awardees will be announced in early April.
Requirements: To qualify, applicants must be enrolled in an MD or DO, U.S. medical school program and be of an underrepresented population as defined by the program eligibility criteria. Applicants self-identify and recipients are drawn from this pool. Candidates must be U.S. citizens, U.S. nationals, or permanent residents. Candidates also must demonstrate an interest in pursuing oncology as a career and have a record of good academic standing.
Amount of Grant: $8,500 total
Date(s) Application is Due: Jan 7
Contact: Nancy R. Daly, Executive Director; (571) 483-1432; email: dalyn@asco.org
Internet: http://www.ascocancerfoundation.org/TACF/Awards/Award+Opportunities/ASCO+Diversity+in+Oncology+Initiative+funded+by+Susan+G.+Komen+for+the+Cure/The+ASCO+Medical+Student+Rotation%2C+funded+by+Susan+G.+Komen+for+the+Cure®
Sponsor: American Society of Clinical Oncology
2318 Mill Road, Suite 800
Alexandria, VA 22314

ASCO Merit Awards **558**
The Merit Awards are designed to further promote clinical research by young scientists and to provide fellows with an opportunity to present their research and interact with other clinical cancer investigators at ASCO scientific meetings. A select number of Merit Awards are given annually to recognize outstanding abstracts submitted for consideration for presentation at an ASCO scientific meeting. The awards are given to oncology fellows who are first authors on selected abstracts.
Requirements: The first author of an abstract must meet the following requirements to be considered for an Award: be a physician (MD or DO) in an oncology fellowship training program or a doctoral degree candidate (such as PharmD or PhD) enrolled in an approved oncology specialty training program at the time of abstract submission; work in an oncology laboratory or clinical research setting; agree to present the abstract at the ASCO scientific meeting; check the Merit Award consideration box on the online abstract submitter; provide a letter of support from the Training Program Director indicating eligibility for the award; and submit a two-page curriculum vitae.
Contact: Nancy R. Daly, Executive Director; (571) 483-1432; email: dalyn@asco.org
Internet: http://www.ascocancerfoundation.org/TACF/Awards/Award+Opportunities/Merit+Award
Sponsor: American Society of Clinical Oncology
2318 Mill Road, Suite 800
Alexandria, VA 22314

ASCO Resident Travel Awards **559**
The ASCO Diversity in Oncology Initiative, funded by Susan G. Komen for the Cure, is designed to facilitate the recruitment and retention of individuals from populations underrepresented in medicine to cancer careers, with particular attention to the development of clinical practitioners and investigators. The ASCO Resident Travel Award, funded by Susan G. Komen for the Cure, provides financial support for residents from underrepresented populations to attend ASCO's Annual Meeting. The intention of this award is to attract residents from under-represented populations to a possible career in one of the oncology specialties. This travel award will allow the recipients to travel to the ASCO Annual Scientific Meeting, where they will have an opportunity to meet oncologists and to understand the career possibilities in this area. The Resident Travel Award includes a $1,500 travel advance, complimentary Annual Meeting registration, and access to the Annual Meeting housing block and ASCO's travel agent. The application period opened October 7 and close January 7. Awardees will be announced in early April. Applications are available online.
Requirements: To qualify, applicants must be enrolled in an ACGME-accredited residency program required for future training in a cancer related subspecialty (i.e., Internal Medicine considering Med/Onc, Surgery considering Surg/Onc) and be of an underrepresented population as defined by the program eligibility criteria. Candidates must be U.S. citizens, U.S. nationals or permanent residents. Candidates must demonstrate an interest in pursuing oncology as a career as well as a record of good academic standing.
Amount of Grant: $1,500
Date(s) Application is Due: Jan 7
Contact: Nancy R. Daly, Executive Director; (571) 483-1432; email: dalyn@asco.org
Internet: http://www.ascocancerfoundation.org/TACF/Awards/Award+Opportunities/ASCO+Diversity+in+Oncology+Initiative+funded+by+Susan+G.+Komen+for+the+Cure/The+ASCO+Resident+Travel+Award%2C+funded+by+Susan+G.+Komen+for+the+Cure®
Sponsor: American Society of Clinical Oncology
2318 Mill Road, Suite 800
Alexandria, VA 22314

ASCO State Affiliate Grants **560**
The Program is designed to enable State/Regional Affiliates to engage in activities that will have an overall benefit to their members, ASCO members, other state societies, and the oncology community at-large. The purpose of the Program is to provide financial support to State/Regional Affiliates, which will assist them in implementing specific activities. The grant Program allows ASCO to utilize its strength and expertise in raising funds, taking advantage of resources not available on the state level, and demonstrates ASCO's commitment to strengthening state societies. Possible projects include, but are not limited to, conducting an educational meeting, developing an informational brochure or newsletter, creating a state clinical trials network, taking part in a quality cancer care initiative, or collaborating with a patient advocacy group on an awareness campaign.
Requirements: Grant applicants must be either the current President of Administrator/Executive Director of a state society that is formally affiliated with ASCO. Applications must illustrate a commitment by society leadership in carrying out the requested activities.
Restrictions: Funds should not be used for general operating costs of the state society. Grants will also not be provided for State/Regional Affiliates to carry out lobbying activities.
Amount of Grant: $10,000 maximum
Date(s) Application is Due: Nov 17
Contact: Nancy R. Daly, Executive Director; (571) 483-1432; email: dalyn@asco.org
Internet: http://www.ascocancerfoundation.org/TACF/Grants/Grant+Opportunities/State+Affiliate+Grant+Program
Sponsor: American Society of Clinical Oncology
2318 Mill Road, Suite 800
Alexandria, VA 22314

ASCO Translational Research Professorships **561**
The Translational Research Professorship is designed to provide flexible funding to outstanding translational researchers who have made and are continuing to make significant contributions that have changed the direction of cancer research and who provide mentorship to future translational researchers. The award is intended to support qualified individuals who are dedicated to bringing advances in basic sciences into the clinical arena and to mentoring other translational researchers. The award totals $500,000 and is paid in 5 annual increments of $100,000 throughout the award period. Only online applications will be accepted. In order to complete an application, a Letter of Intent must first be submitted by November 20th. Completed applications must be submitted by January 22nd.
Requirements: The applicant must meet the following criteria at the time of grant award (July 1): be a physician (MD, DO or international equivalent) with a full-time faculty appointment in a clinical department at an academic medical center; currently hold the rank of full professor (or equivalent) at an academic medical center. If applicant does not hold the rank of full professor, but meets all other eligibility criteria, he/she must provide written explanation of why his/her current rank at their institution should be considered equivalent; made significant contributions that have changed the direction of cancer research; be serving as a research mentor to one or more translational researcher(s) in training, and must be planning to continue to provide leadership in this area throughout the award period Lead a research team in the conduct of translational research; be a member of the American Society of Clinical Oncology (ASCO); expect to spend 75% of time during the award period dedicated to translational research activities, leading a team of translational researchers (both in the lab and in the clinic) and mentoring physician-scientists. Individuals with an endowed professorship from their own institution are eligible to apply for this award. Individuals with administrative responsibilities (such as a Division or Department Chair) must clearly document their time commitment for performing research activities and mentoring activities. The application must originate jointly from the sponsoring institution and the applicant. The sponsoring institution must be a not-for-profit institution.
Samples: Merrill Egorin, MD, The Hillman Cancer Institute, Pittsburgh, PA—Preclinical and Clinical Studies of PARP Inhibitors as Cancer Therapy (2009).
Amount of Grant: $500,000 over five years
Date(s) Application is Due: Nov 20; Jan 22

Contact: Nancy R. Daly, Executive Director; (571) 483-1432; email: dalyn@asco.org
Internet: http://www.ascocancerfoundation.org/TACF/Grants/Grant+Opportunities/Translational+Research+Professorship
Sponsor: American Society of Clinical Oncology
2318 Mill Road, Suite 800
Alexandria, VA 22314

ASCO Young Investigator Award **562**
This grant provides funding to promising investigators to encourage and promote quality research in clinical oncology. The purpose of this award is to fund physicians during the transition from a fellowship program to a faculty appointment. Priority consideration will be given to proposals that include patient-oriented and, ultimately, clinical research. Since many awards are supported with restricted grants from outside organizations, the ASCO is particularly interested in identifying young researchers working in the following sub-specialties and emerging disciplines: breast cancer; cancer survivorship; geriatric oncology; health disparities; kidney cancer; multiple myeloma; ovarian cancer; pancreatic cancer; sarcoma; survivorship; and young adult cancer. However, The ASCO Foundation welcomes application submissions in all oncology subspecialties.
Requirements: The recipient must be a physician (MD or DO) who, at the time of grant award is in the final year of his/her final sub-specialty training program or in the first year post his/her final sub-specialty training. The sponsoring facility must be an academic medical institution. The primary mentor must be in the candidate's proposed research field, must assume responsibility, and provide guidance for the research. The applicant must either be a member of ASCO or submit a membership application with the grant application. The applicant should spend at least 60 to 75% of his or her time in research during the award period.
Amount of Grant: $50,000
Date(s) Application is Due: Sep 9
Contact: Nancy R. Daly, Executive Director; (571) 483-1432; email: dalyn@asco.org
Internet: http://www.ascocancerfoundation.org/TACF/Grants/Grant+Opportunities/Young+Investigator+Award
Sponsor: American Society of Clinical Oncology
2318 Mill Road, Suite 800
Alexandria, VA 22314

ASCO/UICC International Cancer Technology Transfer Fellowships **563**
The scholarships are intended primarily for researchers in the early stages of their career as well as for experienced clinical oncologists. The ICRETT objective is to facilitate rapid international transfer of cancer research and clinical technology, and it allows fellows to exchange knowledge and enhance skills in basic, clinical, behavioral and epidemiological areas of cancer research, and cancer control and prevention. Through the program fellows also acquire appropriate clinical management, diagnostic and therapeutic expertise for effective application and use in home organizations upon return. The UICC has also developed the ICRETT for teaching faculty which funds experts to teach at host institutions throughout the world for a duration of 1 week to 1 month.
Requirements: The candidate must possess the appropriate professional qualifications and experience according to the specifications of each fellowship described on the website and must currently be engaged in cancer research, clinical oncology practice, or cancer society work. To permit effective communication at the host institute, the candidate must have adequate fluency in a common language. The candidate must also be on the staff payroll of a university, research laboratory or institute, hospital, oncology unit, or voluntary cancer society (or be accredited volunteers of such societies) to where they will return at the end of a fellowship.
Restrictions: Candidates attached to commercial entities, going to a profit organization or have associations with the tobacco industry not eligible.
Amount of Grant: $3,400
Contact: Nancy R. Daly, Executive Director; (571) 483-1432; email: dalyn@asco.org
Internet: http://www.ascocancerfoundation.org/TACF/Awards/Award+Opportunities/ASCO+%26+UICC+ICRETT+Fellowship
Sponsor: American Society of Clinical Oncology
2318 Mill Road, Suite 800
Alexandria, VA 22314

ASGE / ConMed Award for Outstanding Manuscript by a Fellow/Resident **564**
The American Society for Gastrointestinal Endoscopy and ConMed Endoscopic Technologies sponsor the annual ASGE/ConMed Outstanding Manuscript Award. The prize consists of $10,000 cash award to the Fellow or Resident in training in a gastroenterology or a surgical gastrointestinal endoscopic program whose manuscript is accepted in for publication in Gastrointestinal Endoscopy. The award is presented during Digestive Disease Week, the largest and most prestigious meeting in the world for the GI professional.
Amount of Grant: $10,000
Contact: Chair, ASGE Research Committee, (630) 573-0600; fax: (630) 573-0691; email: grants@asge.org;; GIE Office, (630) 570-5640; email: gie@asge.org
Internet: http://www.asge.org/index.aspx?id=4892&terms=ConMed+Award
Sponsor: American Society for Gastrointestinal Endoscopy and ConMed Endoscopic Technologies
1520 Kensington Road, Suite 202
Oak Brook, IL 60523

ASGE Don Wilson Award **565**
The Award provides Advanced Fellows or Junior Faculty with the opportunity to train outside of their home country with a premier GI endoscopist or group in order to advance their training. The award assists in underwriting reasonable and customary travel and living expenses for a period of one to three months. The award includes a $7,500 cash stipend prior to the recipient's travel. In addition, a 20% disbursement will be made to the host institution. A total of three awards will be available annually for North American and International ASGE members. Note: One training must take place in the United States.
Requirements: Applicants must be the equivalent of Junior Faculty or Advanced Fellows and be proficient in the English Language. Applicants must also: be a current ASGE Member; be a Junior Faculty or Advanced Fellow (3rd or 4th year or international equivalent); have permission from their own institution to undertake the travel; and have permission from an ASGE member at the host institution to accept the application for training.
Restrictions: Individuals applying for 1-2 year advanced fellowships do not qualify for this award.
Amount of Grant: $7,500
Date(s) Application is Due: Sep 1
Contact: Chair, ASGE International Committee, (630) 573-0600; fax: (630) 573-0691; email: membership@asge.org
Internet: http://www.asge.org/nspages/research/applications/donWilson.cfm
Sponsor: American Society for Gastrointestinal Endoscopy
1520 Kensington Road, Suite 202
Oak Brook, IL 60523

ASGE Endoscopic Research Awards **566**
These research awards are offered to physicians for projects in basic and clinical endoscopic technology research, outcomes and effectiveness of endoscopy research. The primary objective is to foster research in gastrointestinal endoscopy both within and outside of academic centers. Two categories of grants may be used for up to two years of study: grants of $1-15,000 (category A) and grants of $15,001 - 50,000 (category B). Requests for funding seed projects that will lead to further research as well as larger requests for definitive clinical trials will be considered. Funding requests may also include: personnel expenses for research assistant and/or faculty salary support (percentage of time for study should be specified and appropriately justified); study supplies; and equipment essential for study.
Requirements: Candidate must be: an ASGE member; an MD (or have equivalent degree); and current in a gastroenterology-related and endoscopic practice in academic institutions or private practice in North America.
Restrictions: Funding will not be provided for: salary support for trainees; computer purchases (unless a unique application is proposed); standard equipment and supplies needed for appropriate patient care; travel to meetings; or indirect costs.
Amount of Grant: $50,000 maximum per year for ywo years
Date(s) Application is Due: Sep 12
Contact: Chair, ASGE Research Committee, (630) 573-0600; fax: (630) 573-0691; email: grants@asge.org
Internet: http://www.asge.org/index.aspx?id=4892&terms=ConMed+Award
Sponsor: American Society for Gastrointestinal Endoscopy
1520 Kensington Road, Suite 202
Oak Brook, IL 60523

ASGE Endoscopic Research Career Development Awards **567**
These awards provide the salary and/or research support necessary for the investigator to enhance his/her career development. The award must be used to acquire new skills for furthering a career in endoscopic research. Examples of such skills include advanced training in endoscopic procedures, training in outcomes research relevant to endoscopy, training in use of large databases such as CORI, and new endoscopic research techniques, including animal models.
Requirements: Applicants must be ASGE members and hold full-time faculty positions at North American (U.S., Canada, or Mexico) universities or professional institutions at the time of application. The award is intended for faculty who have demonstrated promise and have some record of accomplishment in research. Candidates must devote at least 30 percent of their effort to research related to gastrointestinal endoscopy during the period of the award.
Restrictions: The award is not available for fellows. Faculty with principle investigator current federal funding or other concurrent career development support still active at the time of this award are not eligible. Recipients of the ASGE Career Development Awards may not be granted an ASGE Research & Outcomes & Effectiveness Award during their two-year award period.
Amount of Grant: $75,000 per year for two years
Date(s) Application is Due: Dec 12
Contact: Chair, ASGE Research Committee, (630) 573-0600; fax: (630) 573-0691; email: grants@asge.org
Internet: http://www.asge.org/index.aspx?id=4892&terms=ConMed+Award
Sponsor: American Society for Gastrointestinal Endoscopy
1520 Kensington Road, Suite 202
Oak Brook, IL 60523

ASGE Given Capsule Endoscopy Research Award **568**
These research awards are offered to physicians for projects specific to capsule endoscopy both within and outside of academic centers. The award must be used for projects directly relating to capsule endoscopy. Requests for funding seed projects that will lead to further research as well as requests for definitive clinical trials will be considered. Funding requests may include: personnel (research assistant and/or faculty salary support—

percentage of time for study should be specified and appropriately justified); study supplies; and equipment essential for study.
Requirements: Candidate must be an ASGE member, be an MD (or have equivalent degree), and be current in a gastroenterology-related and endoscopic practice in academic institutions or private practice in North America.
Restrictions: Funding will not be provided for: salary support for trainees; computer purchases (unless a unique application is proposed); standard equipment and supplies needed for appropriate patient care (for example, sclerotherapy needles); travel to meetings; publication costs; or indirect costs.
Amount of Grant: $25,000 maximum
Date(s) Application is Due: Dec 7
Contact: Chair, ASGE Research Committee, (630) 573-0600; fax: (630) 573-0691; email: grants@asge.org
Internet: http://www.asge.org/nspages/research/applications/ceapp.cfm
Sponsor: American Society for Gastrointestinal Endoscopy
1520 Kensington Road, Suite 202
Oak Brook, IL 60523

ASHA Advancing Academic-Research Careers (AARC) Award 569
This award is given to new faculty in higher education to support their academic and research endeavors in the field of communication sciences and disorders (CSD). Up to five awards of $5,000 each will be granted to support activities such as: Improving teaching skills; Mentoring graduate students; Participating in research activities; Preparing a grant application; Preparing a manuscript or publication; Presenting at a professional meeting (e.g., the ASHA Convention).
Requirements: Candidates must possess: A research doctoral degree (PhD, ScD, CScD, or equivalent, e.g., EdD), which must be conferred by August 1; A full-time faculty appointment; Primary responsibilities of teaching and conducting research; Less than six years of teaching/research experience or are below the level of associate professor; A tenure or non-tenure track appointment. A list of required documents and a downloadable application form are available at the website.
Restrictions: Postdoctoral fellows are not eligible. Only students attending a university in the U.S. are eligible to apply for the award.
Amount of Grant: $5,000
Date(s) Application is Due: May 15
Contact: Margaret Rogers, PhD, Chief Staff Officer for Science & Research; (800) 498-2071 or (301) 296-5706; email: mrogers@asha.org
Internet: http://www.asha.org/students/awards.htm#aarc
Sponsor: American Speech-Language-Hearing Association (ASHA)
2200 Research Boulevard, #245
Rockville, MD 20850-3289

ASHA Minority Student Leadership Program Awards 570
The MSLP is a leadership development program established for undergraduate seniors and graduate students who are enrolled in communication sciences and disorders programs. Aditionally, ASHA's Focused Initiative on the PhD Shortage in Higher Education will provide funding for 10 eligible candidates enrolled in a research doctoral program. The award package includes complimentary registration to the ASHA Convention held annually; up to five nights lodging; meal stipend; and, program materials. Forty students are chosen to participate – 5 undergraduate seniors, 20 master's students, 5 entry level clinical doctoral students and 10 PhD students.
Requirements: Undergraduate seniors and graduate students who are or will be enrolled in the fall communication sciences and disorders programs and are not members of ASHA are eligible. Preference will be given to students who are members of racial/ethnic minority groups historically under-represented within ASHA, including American Indian or Alaska Native, Asian, Black or African American, Native Hawaiian or other Pacific Islander, and/or Hispanic/Latino. For Graduate Study – The student must be enrolled in, or accepted for, graduate study in a communication sciences and disorders program in the United States. Master's degree candidates and entry level clinical doctoral candidates must be in a program accredited by the Council of Academic Accreditation (CAA). PhD Track – You must be enrolled in a research doctoral degree program. ASHA members may apply. The required application packet is available for download at the website (http://www.asha.org/students/awards.htm#MSLP).
Restrictions: Program participants are responsible for transportation expenses to and from the convention city and personal incidentals.
Date(s) Application is Due: May 18
Contact: Melanie Johnson; (301) 296-8681; email: mjohnson@asha.org
Internet: http://www.asha.org/students/awards.htm#MSLP
Sponsor: American Speech-Language-Hearing Association (ASHA)
2200 Research Boulevard
Rockville, MD 20850-3289

ASHA Multicultural Activities Projects Grants 571
The program is open to clinical and/or school-based speech, language, and hearing programs; university programs, state associations, allied and related professional organizations, and ASHA's Special Interest Divisions. ASHA has allocated funding for projects on multicultural activities with a maximum of $18,000 awarded for a single grant. It is expected that the average individual award given will be between $7,000 and $10,000. Applications must be postmarked by April 4. Proposals receiving funding will be announced in July.
Requirements: Proposals must have a multicultural focus. Multicultural is defined to include issues dealing with race, ethnicity, language, gender or gender identification, age, sexual orientation, and disability. There is particular interest in, but not limited to, proposals that respond to one or more of ASHA's Strategic Initiatives from ASHA's Strategic Pathway to Excellence. Projects must: be compatible with ASHA's mission and vision; have a clear high-quality plan for meeting its objectives; be completed, including evaluation, within 12 months of initiation of the project; be adaptable by other clinical and/or school-based programs, university programs, state associations, and associated and related professional organizations for their own use; and describe what will happen to the project once ASHA funding has ended. Criteria for evaluating proposals and the required downloadable forms are available at the website.
Restrictions: An ASHA member must serve as project director. Grants will not be awarded for fund raising, governmental lobbying, or awards ceremonies.
Samples: 2007-2008: Development of Standard and Multifrequency Tympanometry Norms for Native American Children (Birth – 5 years) and Young Adults - Samuel R. Atcherson & Paul Brueggeman, University of South Dakota; Digital Treatment Materials for Intervention in Spanish and English - Steven Long, Marquette University; The Validation of a Language Use Questionnaire across Bilingual Clinical Populations - Swathi Kiran, The University of Texas at Austin
Amount of Grant: $18,000 maximum
Contact: Karen Beverly-Ducker; (800) 638-8255; fax: (301) 296-8580; email: OMAGrants@asha.org
Internet: http://www.asha.org/about/leadership-projects/multicultural/funding/rfp.htm
Sponsor: American Speech-Language-Hearing Association (ASHA)
2200 Research Boulevard
Rockville, MD 20850-3289

ASHA Research Mentoring-Pair Travel Award 572
This award is designed to foster the professional development of students, clinicians, and emerging scientists who have expressed an interest in research in communication sciences and disorders. Up to 10 travel awards of $1,000 each will be granted to eligible mentor mentee pairs (mentee= $750; mentor= $250) to help defray the cost of attending the annual research symposium. Special consideration will be given to individuals whose research or research interests are (a) relevant to the symposium topic, (b) interdisciplinary in nature, (c) translational in nature, or (d) related to issues of cultural or linguistic diversity.
Requirements: Mentees must be (a) a current student at the bachelor's, master's, AuD, or PhD level, (b) a postdoctoral fellow, (c) a junior level faculty member (less than 6 years teaching/research experience in a tenure-track position or below the level of associate professor), or (d) a clinician. Mentors must be a seasoned investigator in an academic or health care environment. Download the Mentee and Mentory Application Forms at the website.
Amount of Grant: $1,000
Date(s) Application is Due: Jun 22
Contact: Margaret Rogers, PhD, Chief Staff Officer for Science & Research; (800) 498-2071 or (301) 296-5706; fax: (301) 296-8580; email: mrogers@asha.org
Internet: http://www.asha.org/students/awards.htm#2008%20Research%20Mentoring-Pair%20Travel%20Award
Sponsor: American Speech-Language-Hearing Association (ASHA)
2200 Research Boulevard, #245
Rockville, MD 20850-3289

ASHA Student Research Travel Award 573
The awards are intended to highlight the research activities of budding scientists and encourage careers in science and research. Approximately 40 student research travel awards of $500 each are available for undergraduate, Master's, and doctoral students who are first authors on a paper (all session types are acceptable: technical, poster, one hour seminar, two hour seminar, or short course). Identification of prospective awardees will be based on the recommendation of Convention co-chairs and topic coordinators. Awardees will receive a $500 travel award; have their exceptional paper highlighted in the convention program; and, be recognized at the Researcher-Academic Town Meeting and other designated events.
Requirements: Each award recipient will be required to: register for the Convention at his or her own expense; present his or her paper at the assigned time (as noted in the Convention program booklet); secure a mentor to shadow throughout the convention; and, attend selected research-related sessions during the convention. In order to apply, students must: submit an abstract summarizing their research through the normal Call for Papers process; check the appropriate box (when prompted) indicating that their paper is 'student-authored'; and, check the appropriate box (when prompted) indicating that they desire to have this abstract considered for the Student Research Travel Award.
Restrictions: Papers must be submitted online by the deadline date and must be designated as a student-authored paper.
Amount of Grant: $500
Date(s) Application is Due: Mar 31
Contact: Margaret Rogers, PhD, Chief Staff Officer for Science & Research; (800) 498-2071 or (301) 296-5706; email: mrogers@asha.org
Internet: http://www.asha.org/students/awards.htm#research
Sponsor: American Speech-Language-Hearing Association (ASHA)
2200 Research Boulevard
Rockville, MD 20850-3289

ASHA Students Preparing for Academic & Research Careers (SPARC) Award 574
The goal of SPARC is to foster students' interest in the pursuit of PhD education and careers in academia in order to fill faculty/researcher vacancies in communication sciences and disorders (CSD). Students will identify a primary faculty mentor and propose a one-year CSD Career Mentoring Plan. As many as ten students will be awarded up to $1,500

each to be used for teaching and research enhancement activities, such as travel to a research, pedagogy conference, or meeting; travel for a visit to an off-campus site that provides learning opportunities in a research lab and/or a college classroom setting; or course registration to support the mentoring plans outlined in the application.
Requirements: Eligible applicants include junior or senior undergraduates, 1st year master's students, and 1st and 2nd year entry-level clinical doctoral (e.g., AuD) students enrolled part-time or full-time in a CSD program in the United States. At the time of the award, eligible recipients' education status for the upcoming academic year must be undergraduate senior, 1st or 2nd year master's, or 1st, 2nd or 3rd year entry-level clinical doctoral (i.e., AuD) in a full-time or part-time CSD program in the United States. Master's degree and entry-level clinical doctoral students must be in a program accredited by the Council for Academic Accreditation in Audiology and Speech-Language Pathology (CAA). Full requirements (essay question, documentation, etc.) are listed at the website, along with the downloadable application form.
Amount of Grant: $5,000
Date(s) Application is Due: May 15
Contact: Arlene A. Pietranton, Executive Director; email: apietranton@asha.org or academicaffairs@asha.org
Internet: http://www.asha.org/students/awards.htm#sparc
Sponsor: American Speech-Language-Hearing Association (ASHA)
2200 Research Boulevard
Rockville, MD 20850-3289

ASHFoundation Clinical Research Grants **575**
These $50,000–$75,000 grants support scientists with a research doctorate within the discipline of communication sciences and disorders to support investigations that will advance knowledge of the efficacy of treatment and assessment practices. Project funding is available for mentored treatment research, independent treatment research, or collaborative treatment research as specified in grant guidelines.
Samples: Swathi Kiran, Assistant Professor, University of Texas at Austin—Semantic Feature Analysis in the Treatment of Lexical Retrieval Deficits in Spanish-English and French-English Bilingual Aphasia, $50,000 (2008); Tiffany Johnson, Assistant Professor, University of Kansas Center for Research, Inc.—New Directions in Clinical Applications of Otoacoustic Emissions. $50,000 (2008); Andrea Pittman, Assistant Professor, Arizona State University—Evaluating Advanced Signal Processing in Children with Hearing Loss, $75,000 (2008); Nancy Pearl Solomon, Research Speech Pathologist, Walter Reed Army Medical Center—Treating Dysphagia in Blast-Injured Patients. $50,000 (2008).
Amount of Grant: $50,000 - $75,000 range
Contact: Emily Diaz, Project Assistant; (301) 296-8703; email: ediaz@asha.org
Internet: http://www.ashfoundation.org/Foundation/grants/research_grants.htm
Sponsor: American Speech-Language-Hearing Foundation
2200 Research Boulevard
Rockville, MD 20850-3289

ASHFoundation Graduate Student International Scholarship **576**
One award is available for a full-time international graduate student who has demonstrated outstanding academic achievement. Applicants must be studying communications sciences and disorders at a U.S. institution accredited by ASHA's Council of Academic Accreditation. All scholarship recipients will be announced and recognized at the ASHA convention.
Requirements: Applicants must be full-time students.
Samples: Beverly A. Collisson, PhD Candidate, University of Connecticut, $5,000 (2008); Beula M. Magimairaj, PhD Candidate, Ohio University, $5,000 (2008); Maria V. Ivanova, PhD candidate, Ohio University, $4,000 (2007); Victoria Lee, AuD candidate, Northwestern University, $4,000 (2006).
Amount of Grant: $4,000 maximum
Contact: Emily Diaz, Project Assistant; (301) 296-8703; email: ediaz@asha.org
Internet: http://www.ashfoundation.org/Foundation/grants/GraduateScholarships.htm
Sponsor: American Speech-Language-Hearing Foundation
2200 Research Boulevard
Rockville, MD 20850-3289

ASHFoundation Graduate Student Scholarships **577**
The foundation invites full-time graduate students to submit applications in competition for one of seven scholarships. Full-time master's or doctoral students in communication sciences and disorders programs demonstrating outstanding academic achievement are eligible to compete for these $4,000 awards. Supported in part by Psi Iota Xi National Philanthropic Organization and the Marni Reisberg Memorial Fund. All scholarship recipients will be announced and recognized at the annual convention held in November.
Requirements: Applicants must be accepted for graduate study in a communication sciences and disorders program (master's degree candidates must be in an ASHA Educational Standards Board accredited program; this is not mandatory for doctoral degree candidates); be enrolled for full-time study (12 or more credit hours or the full-time standard); submit official university transcripts of academic coursework, credits, and grades; and be recommended by a committee of two or more past or present college faculty and colleagues (at least one supervisor) at the student's current place of employment. Annual deadline dates may vary; contact program staff for exact dates.
Restrictions: Applicants must not have received a prior scholarship from the foundation.
Samples: Tracy Conner, MA candidate, University of Massachusetts--Amherst Minority Scholarship, Minority Fund (2008); Beverly A. Collisson, PhD Candidate, University of Connecticut—International Scholarship, Kala Singh Memorial Fund (2008); Stephanie Cochran, MA Candidate, Duquesne University—Disability Scholarship, Leslie Londer Fund (2008).
Amount of Grant: $4,000
Contact: Emily Diaz, Project Assistant; (301) 296-8703; email: ediaz@asha.org
Internet: http://www.ashfoundation.org/Foundation/grants/GraduateScholarships.htm
Sponsor: American Speech-Language-Hearing Foundation
2200 Research Boulevard
Rockville, MD 20850-3289

ASHFoundation Graduate Student Scholarships for Minority Students **578**
Racial/ethnic minority students who are U.S. citizens, who are accepted for graduate study in speech-language pathology or audiology, and who demonstrate outstanding academic achievement are eligible to compete for this scholarship. Applicants should submit a formal paper, such as a term paper, in competition for this award. The paper must be either an integrative literature review or an opinion paper on a current professional issue. All scholarship recipients will be announced and recognized at the ASHA convention.
Requirements: Candidates must be U.S. citizens and members of a racial/ethnic minority, including Native American and Alaska Native, Asian and Pacific Islander, African American, and Hispanic. Applicants must be accepted for master's or doctoral study in a speech-language pathology or audiology program for the upcoming academic year. The student must be enrolled for full-time (12 or more credit hours) study.
Restrictions: Applicants may not have received a prior scholarship from the foundation.
Samples: Tracy Conner, MA candidate, University of Massachusetts–Amherst, $5,000 (2008); Rhona Galera, CScD candidate, University of Pittsburgh, $5,000 (2008); Derek E. Daniels, PhD candidate, Bowling Green State University, $4,000 (2006).
Amount of Grant: $2,000-$4,000
Contact: Emily Diaz, Project Assistant; (301) 296-8703; email: ediaz@asha.org
Internet: http://www.ashfoundation.org/Foundation/grants/GraduateScholarships.htm
Sponsor: American Speech-Language-Hearing Foundation
2200 Research Boulevard
Rockville, MD 20850-3289

ASHFoundation Graduate Student with a Disability Scholarship **579**
Full-time graduate students with a disability who are enrolled in a communication sciences and disorders program and demonstrate outstanding academic achievement are eligible to compete for a $4,000 scholarship. Applicants must demonstrate superior academic achievement and submit transcripts, essay and references with official application. The Award is intended for the blind, hearing impaired, physically handicapped, or learning impaired. Master's, but not doctoral, students must be enrolled in an ASHA Council on Academic Accreditation approved program.
Requirements: Candidates must be U.S. citizens and either blind, hearing impaired, physically handicapped, or learning impaired. Applicants must be accepted for master's study in a speech-language pathology or audiology program for the upcoming academic year. The student must be enrolled for full-time (12 or more credit hours) study.
Samples: Stephanie Cochran, MA Candidate, Duquesne University (2008); Stephanie P. Hirsh, MA candidate, Northwestern University (2006); Alexandra Eng, MS candidate, University of the Pacific (2003).
Amount of Grant: $4,000
Contact: Emily Diaz, Project Assistant; (301) 296-8703; email: ediaz@asha.org
Internet: http://www.ashfoundation.org/Foundation/grants/GraduateScholarships.htm
Sponsor: American Speech-Language-Hearing Foundation
2200 Research Boulevard
Rockville, MD 20850-3289

ASHFoundation New Century Scholars Program Doctoral Scholarships **580**
The Program is a special funding initiative resulting from the ASHFoundation's Dreams and Possibilities Campaign. The Award is for students accepted or currently enrolled in a research doctoral program in communications sciences and disorders. Full-time study will be given priority; part-time status will be considered. Students should be committed to a teacher-investigator career in communication sciences and disorders in the United States.
Requirements: The Award is available to U.S. citizens only. Applicants must be accepted or currently enrolled in a research doctoral program.
Samples: Sophie Ambrose, PhD Candidate, University of Kansas (2008); Megha Bahl, PhD Candidate, University of Arizona (2008); Angela Yarnell Bonino, PhD candidate, University of North Carolina at Chapel Hill (2008); Deanna Britton, PhD Candidate, University of Washington (2008); Jamie L. Desjardins, PhD Candidate, Syracuse University (2008).
Amount of Grant: $10,000 minimum
Contact: Emily Diaz, Project Assistant; (301) 296-8703; email: ediaz@asha.org
Internet: http://www.ashfoundation.org/Foundation/grants/GraduateScholarships.htm
Sponsor: American Speech-Language-Hearing Foundation
2200 Research Boulevard
Rockville, MD 20850-3289

ASHFoundation New Century Scholars Research Grant **581**
The Program is a special funding initiative resulting from the ASHFoundation's Dreams and Possibilities Campaign. The Grant is a one-time award intended to advance the knowledge base in communication sciences and disorders. Applicants must have a PhD

or equivalent research doctorate within the discipline. Priority will be given to studies that are innovative, groundbreaking, or that meet research needs not yet addressed.
Restrictions: Students enrolled in a degree program or working on dissertation research are not eligible.
Samples: Jungmee Lee, Assistant Professor, University of Arizona—Proposal: Correlation Between Cochlear Tuning and Otoacoustic Emissions: Exploring Scientific and Clinical Implications, $10,000 (2008); Chang Liu, Assistant Professor, University of Texas at Austin—Auditory Processing: Comparing Phonologically Disordered and Typically Developing Children, $10,000 (2008); John McCarthy, Assistant Professor, Ohio University—Improving Auditory Scanning Interfaces in AAC Devices, $10,000 (2008); Valeriy Shafiro, Assistant Professor, Rush University Medical Center—Effects of Environmental Sound Training on the Perception of Environmental Sounds and Speech in Cochlear Implant Patients, $10,000 (2008).
Amount of Grant: $10,000
Contact: Emily Diaz, Project Assistant; (301) 296-8703; email: ediaz@asha.org
Internet: http://www.ashfoundation.org/Foundation/grants/research_grants.htm
Sponsor: American Speech-Language-Hearing Foundation
2200 Research Boulevard
Rockville, MD 20850-3289

ASHFoundation Research Grant for New Investigators 582

The grants are designed to help further research activities of new investigators and should have particular clinical relevance to speech-language pathology and audiology. The awards are designed to encourage research activities of new scientists who earned their latest degree within the last five years. Proposals, while not limited in topic, are encouraged in the area of treatment research, particularly efficacy and outcome studies. Include abstract, research plan, bibliography, management plan, and budget with application.
Requirements: The individual must have received the master's or doctoral level degree in the last five years; must not have received prior funding for research, with the exception of internal university funding; and the proposal must be for research to be initiated.
Restrictions: Open to individuals with a Master's degree or doctoral degree who are not currently enrolled in a degree program.
Samples: Nina C. Capone, Associate Professor, Seton Hall University—The Effects of Gesture Cues on Object Word Learning by Children with Language Impairments (2008); Gayle L. DeDe Assistant Professor, University of Arizona—On-Line Sentence Comprehension in Aphasia: Is Reading Different than Listening? (2008).
Amount of Grant: $5,000
Contact: Emily Diaz, Project Assistant; (301) 296-8703; email: ediaz@asha.org
Internet: http://www.ashfoundation.org/Foundation/grants/research_grants.htm
Sponsor: American Speech-Language-Hearing Foundation
2200 Research Boulevard
Rockville, MD 20850-3289

ASHFoundation Research Grant in Speech Science 583

ASLH, in conjunction with the Acoustical Society of America, invites new researchers to submit proposals in competition for one grant every other year. The grant is designed to further research activities of new investigators and promulgate the work of the late Dennis Klatt, a noted researcher and scientist in the area of speech communication. Priority will be given to areas reflecting Dr. Klatt's broad interests, such as proposals studying speech perception, synthesis, and acoustics, with an emphasis on an interdisciplinary research approach. The grant can be used to initiate new research or supplement an existing research project. Funds may be requested for a variety of purposes, i.e., equipment, subjects, research assistants, or research-related travel. The grant recipient will be announced at the ASHA convention.
Requirements: Individuals having received a doctoral degree within the last five years and who wish to further research activities in the areas of speech communication are eligible to compete for the grant.
Amount of Grant: $5,000
Contact: Emily Diaz, Project Assistant; (301) 296-8703; email: ediaz@asha.org
Internet: http://www.ashfoundation.org/Foundation/grants/research_grants.htm
Sponsor: American Speech-Language-Hearing Foundation
2200 Research Boulevard
Rockville, MD 20850-3289

ASHFoundation Student Research Grants in Audiology 584

Each year the foundation awards one grant for support of research to be initiated in the area of clinical and/or rehabilitative audiology. One $2,000 award to a master's or doctoral student for research to be initiated in the area of audiology. Applicants must submit up to a ten-page research plan, one-page abstract, two-page management plan and budget, and letter of support. All study must be done in the United States.
Requirements: The competition open to master's or doctoral degree students enrolled in, or accepted for, graduate study in a communication sciences and disorders program in the United States. Master's degree candidates must be in a program accredited by the Council on Academic Accreditation in Audiology and Speech-Language Pathology (CAA); this is not mandatory for doctoral degree candidates. Applicants must be enrolled for full-time study for the full academic year.
Amount of Grant: $2,000
Contact: Emily Diaz, Project Assistant; (301) 296-8703; email: ediaz@asha.org
Internet: http://www.ashfoundation.org/Foundation/grants/research_grants.htm
Sponsor: American Speech-Language-Hearing Foundation
2200 Research Boulevard
Rockville, MD 20850-3289

ASHFoundation Student Research Grants in Early Childhood Language Development 585

One $2,000 grant per year is awarded to a graduate or postgraduate student to support research in early childhood language development. The applicant must submit up to a ten-page research plan, one-page abstract, two-page management plan and budget, and letter of support. All study must be done in the United States. The recipient and the recipient's mentor will be announced and recognized at the ASHA Convention.
Requirements: The competition is open to graduate or postgraduate students in the area of communication sciences and disorders. Applicants must submit a proposal according to foundation guidelines, to be received by the indicated deadline date for applications.
Samples: Kathryn Wright Brady, University of Missouri, Mentor: Judith C. Goodman—Clues to Meaning: Exploring Potential Effects of Paired, Congruent Cues on Toddlers' Word Learning (2008); Dawn Vogler-Elias, University of Buffalo, Mentor: Geralyn Timler—A Shared Storybook Reading Intervention for Preschoolers with Autism (2008); Jonathan L. Preston, Syracuse University, Mentor: Mary Louise Edwards—Preliminary Investigation of a Weighted Measure of Speech Sound Accuracy (2007).
Amount of Grant: $2,000
Contact: Emily Diaz, Project Assistant; (301) 296-8703; email: ediaz@asha.org
Internet: http://www.ashfoundation.org/Foundation/grants/research_grants.htm
Sponsor: American Speech-Language-Hearing Foundation
2200 Research Boulevard
Rockville, MD 20850-3289

Ashland Corporate Contributions Grants 586

The foundation awards grants to eligible Kentucky, Ohio, and West Virginia nonprofit organizations in its areas of interest, including education, arts, communities/civic, disaster relief, environment, and health and human services. Types of support include seed money grants, project grants, endowments, matching gifts, and employee volunteers. The foundation does not provide an application. Most giving is centered on programs that best address the needs of Ashland???s employees, stockholders, customers, and other constituencies, and the communities in which they live. Funding requests are not solicited but will be considered. The primary focus is on education, with an emphasis on mentoring, literacy and/or diversity.
Requirements: 501(c)3 tax-exempt organizations in Boyd and Greenup Counties, KY; Lawrence County, OH; and Cabell and Wayne Counties, WV; are eligible. Charitable groups within church or religious organizations are eligible.
Restrictions: The foundation does not support individuals, capital campaigns for building or equipment, endowments, travel, film or video production, tickets, religious or political activities, or goodwill advertising.
Geographic Focus: Kentucky; Ohio; West Virginia
Contact: Program Contact, (859) 815-3333; email: community@ashland.com
Internet: http://www.ashland.com/commitments/contributions.asp
Sponsor: Ashland Inc
P.O. Box 391, 50 E Rivercenter Boulevard
Covington, KY 41012-0391

ASM Abbott Laboratories Award in Clinical and Diagnostic Immunology 587

The ASM Abbott Laboratories Award in Clinical and Diagnostic Immunology honors a distinguished scientist in clinical or diagnostic immunology for outstanding contributions to those fields.
Requirements: The nominee must demonstrate significant contributions to the understanding of the functioning of the host immune system in human disease, clinical approaches to diseases involving the immune system or development or clinical application of immunodiagnostic procedures.
Restrictions: Self-nominations will not be accepted.
Amount of Grant: A cash prize of $2,000, a commemorative piece, and travel to the ASM General Meeting
Date(s) Application is Due: Oct 1
Contact: Awards Committee, (202) 942-9226; fax: (202) 942-9353; email: awards@asmusa.org
Internet: http://www.asm.org/Academy/index.asp?bid=2301
Sponsor: American Society for Microbiology
1752 N Street, NW
Washington, DC 20036-2804

ASM BD Award for Research in Clinical Microbiology 588

The ASM BD Award for Research in Clinical Microbiology honors a a distinguished scientist for research accomplishments that form the foundation for important applications in clinical microbiology.
Requirements: The nominee must be a distinguished clinical microbiologist. All nomination components must be emailed to awards@asmusa.org. Nominations must consist of the following: curriculum vitae; letter of nomination; letters of support.
Restrictions: Self-nominations will not be accepted.
Amount of Grant: A cash prize of $2,000, a commemorative piece, and travel to the ASM General Meeting
Date(s) Application is Due: Oct 1
Contact: Awards, (202) 942-9226; fax: (202) 942-9353; email: awards@asmusa.org
Internet: http://www.asm.org/Academy/index.asp?bid=2304
Sponsor: American Society for Microbiology
1752 N Street, NW
Washington, DC 20036-2804

ASM bioMerieux Sonnenwirth Award for Leadership in Clinical Microbiology 589
Given in memory of Alexander Sonnenwirth, Ph.D., this award recognizes a distinguished microbiologist for the promotion of innovation in clinical laboratory science, dedication to ASM, and the advancement of clinical microbiology as a profession.
Requirements: Nominations will be considered without updating for three years. email (see contact info.) all nomination components. Nominations must consist of the following: curriculum vitae, including a list of nominee's publications; letter of nomination, describe the nominee's innovation in clinical laboratory science, dedication to ASM, role as a leader in the field of diagnostic microbiology, and the advancement of clinical microbiology as a profession; letters of support, two letters of support must come from persons, other than the nominator, who are familiar with the nominee's qualifications and accomplishments. No more than one of the three letters may be from the nominee's institution or the same institution.
Restrictions: Self-nominations will not be accepted.
Amount of Grant: A cash prize of $2,000, a commemorative piece, and travel to the ASM General Meeting, where the laureate delivers the Sonnenwirth Award Lecture.
Date(s) Application is Due: Oct 1
Contact: Awards, (202) 942-9226; fax: (202) 942-9353; email: awards@asmusa.org
Internet: http://www.asm.org/Academy/index.asp?bid=36368
Sponsor: American Society for Microbiology
1752 N Street, NW
Washington, DC 20036-2804

ASM Congressional Science Fellowships 590
The program will select a postdoctoral to mid-career microbiologist to spend one year on the staff of an individual congressman, congressional committee, or with some other appropriate organizational unit of Congress. The purpose of the program is to make practical contributions to more effective use of scientific knowledge in government, to educate the scientific communities regarding public policy, and to broaden the perspective of both the scientific and governmental communities regarding the value of such science-government interaction. The ASM Fellow will function as special legislative assistant within the congressional staff. The American Association for the Advancement of Science will arrange a carefully structured orientation program, guide the placement process, and coordinate weekly seminars throughout the year for the ASM Fellow, as well as other Congressional Fellows. The period of appointment is from September 1 and extends for one year. The award will include a $60,000 stipend plus health care benefits. The stipend is supported by the Martin Frobisher Fund.
Requirements: Prospective Fellows must be citizens of the United States, be members of ASM for at least one year and must have completed their Ph.D. by the time the fellowship begins in September. Candidates are expected to show competence in some aspect of microbiology, have a broad background in science and technology, and have interest and some experience in applying scientific knowledge toward the solution of social problems. Candidates are expected to be articulate, literate, adaptable, interested in work on a range of public policy problems, and able to work with a variety of people from diverse professional backgrounds. A Complete Application for the Fellowship must include: a letter from the candidate indicating a desire to apply and listing three references; three letters of references; a statement from the candidate about his or her qualifications and career goals.
Restrictions: Candidates selected for interviews must provide travel to and from Washington at their own expense. The candidate is responsible for soliciting the required references, providing the six guidelines for the reference response and seeing that the references are forwarded before the deadline.
Amount of Grant: $60,000
Date(s) Application is Due: Feb 20
Contact: Heather Garvey, Program Assistant, (202) 942-9209; fax: (202) 942-9335; email: hgarvey@usmusa.org
Internet: http://www.asm.org/Policy/index.asp?bid=12335
Sponsor: American Society for Microbiology
1752 N Street, NW
Washington, DC 20036-2804

ASM Corporate Activities Program Student Travel Grants 591
The Corporate Activities Program Student Travel Grant is a $500 grant given a maximum of 160 students who are ASM members and who are the presenting author of a poster at the General Meeting. Students are selected based on a review of their abstract submission for the meeting. The awards are highly competitive and only about 25-30% of those seeking grants will receive them. If a grant recipient cannot present the accepted poster, the grant money must be returned to ASM.
Requirements: To qualify for consideration the student must: be an ASM Member and the presenting author; be accepted to present a poster at the General Meeting; be an undergraduate/pre-doctoral student, or; be a Ph.D. or M.D. whose degree has been or will be awarded after May of the current year and before May of the meeting year; have indicated a desire to be considered for the grant on the abstract submission, and submit a letter of nomination from a faculty member or department head on official letterhead. The letter must state that the student is expected to be active in the training or degree program at the time of the meeting. If the student will complete their terminal degree between the date of submission and the meeting, the letter must indicate the expected date of completion. The abstract tracking number must be included in the body of the letter. The letter should be submitted to ASM not later than December of each year. Exact date will be published in the Call for Abstracts for the General Meeting.
Amount of Grant: $500
Contact: Awards, (202) 942-9226; fax: (202) 942-9353; email: awards@asmusa.org
Internet: http://www.asm.org/Awards/index.asp?bid=14968
Sponsor: American Society for Microbiology
1752 N Street, NW
Washington, DC 20036-2804

ASM D.C. White Research and Mentoring Award 592
The ASM D.C. White Research and Mentoring Award recognizing distinguished accomplishments in interdisciplinary research and mentoring in microbiology, this award honors D.C. White, who was known for his interdisciplinary scientific approach and for being a dedicated and inspiring mentor.
Requirements: Consideration will be given to the breadth of the nominee's contributions, as well as their originality and overall impact. There are no age restrictions, but the nominee must have a distinguished record of accomplishments in microbiological research. Nominees in all areas of microbiology will be considered. Nominations must consist of the following: curriculum vitae, including a list of publications; list of those mentored; letter of nomination, describe the nominee's accomplishments of unusual merit in interdisciplinary research in the field of microbiology; letters of support, two letters of support must come from persons, other than the nominator, who are familiar with the nominee's qualifications and accomplishments. One letter should be from someone who can comment specifically on the nominee's mentoring. No more than one of the three letters may be from the nominee's institution or the same institution.
Restrictions: Self nominations will not be accepted.
Amount of Grant: A cash prize of $5,000, a commemorative medal, and travel to the ASM General Meeting, where the laureate delivers the D.C. White Research and Mentoring Award Lecture.
Date(s) Application is Due: Oct 1
Contact: Awards, (202) 942-9226; fax: (202) 942-9353; email: awards@asmusa.org
Internet: http://www.asm.org/Academy/index.asp?bid=50931
Sponsor: American Society for Microbiology
1752 N Street, NW
Washington, DC 20036-2804

ASM Early-Career Faculty Travel Award 593
SM offers travel awards to attend the ASM Conference for Undergraduate Educators (ASMCUE) to increase the participation of early-career undergraduate faculty, post-doctoral scientists or senior level graduate students interested in teaching careers.
Requirements: Eligibility: accepted to present a poster at both ASM General Meeting in any division and ASMCUE; be an active ASM member; teach an undergraduate microbiology course or participates in outreach activities related to microbiology; have an interest in pursuing a teaching career at an undergraduate institution; not be a recipient of substantial federal funding or any other ASM faculty enhancement or travel award.
Amount of Grant: $500
Date(s) Application is Due: Mar 20
Contact: Awards, (202) 942-9226; fax: (202) 942-9353; email: awards@asmusa.org
Internet: http://www.asm.org/Education/index.asp
Sponsor: American Society for Microbiology
1752 N Street, NW
Washington, DC 20036-2804

ASM Eli Lilly and Company Research Award 594
ASM's oldest and most prestigious prize, it rewards fundamental research of unusual merit in microbiology or immunology by an individual on the threshold of his or her career.
Requirements: The nominee's work is not judged by comparison with the research of more experienced scientists, and special consideration is given to originality and independence of thought. The nominee must not have reached his or her 45th birthday by April 30 of the year the award is given. The nominee must be working in the United States or Canada and be actively engaged in the line of research for which the award is to be made.
Restrictions: Nominations must consist of the following: curriculum vitae, including a list of publications; verification of date of birth. Photocopy or scanned file of driver's license, passport or birth certificate; letter of nomination, describe the nominee's fundamental research of unusual merit in microbiology or immunology; letters of support, two letters of support must come from persons, other than the nominator, who are familiar with the nominee's qualifications and accomplishments. No more than one of the three letters may be from the nominee's institution or the same institution.
Amount of Grant: A cash prize of $5,000, a commemorative piece, and travel to the ASM General Meeting where the laureate delivers the Eli Lilly Award Lecture.
Date(s) Application is Due: Oct 1
Contact: Awards, (202) 942-9226; fax: (202) 942-9353; email: awards@asmusa.org
Internet: http://www.asm.org/academy/index.asp?bid=2281
Sponsor: American Society for Microbiology
1752 N Street, NW
Washington, DC 20036-2804

ASM Faculty Ehancement Program -Travel Awards 595
ASM offers travel awards to attend the ASMCUE to faculty who teach microbiology at 2- or 4-year institutions with a large percentage of historically excluded and underrepresented students.
Requirements: Eligibility: accepted to present a poster at both ASM General Meeting in any division and ASMCUE; be an active ASM member; teach an undergraduate microbiology course or participates in outreach activities related to microbiology; have an interest in pursuing a teaching career at an undergraduate institution; not be a recipient of substantial federal funding or any other ASM faculty enhancement or travel award.
Amount of Grant: $500
Date(s) Application is Due: Mar 20

Contact: Awards, (202) 942-9226; fax: (202) 942-9353; email: awards@asmusa.org
Internet: http://www.asm.org/Education/index.asp
Sponsor: American Society for Microbiology
1752 N Street, NW
Washington, DC 20036-2804

ASM Founders Distinguished Service Award **596**

The Founders Distinguished Service Award honors a member of the ASM for outstanding contributions and commitment to the ASM as a volunteer at the national level.
Requirements: Selection is based on commitment to furthering the goals of the ASM, ability to inspire commitment from others, and significance of contributions to the membership of ASM and its various audiences. The nominee must be an ASM member in good standing who has served in a volunteer capacity for ASM at the national level (e.g., as a member of committees or editorial boards or as a workshop leader) for a minimum of five years, and has not held office as ASM President, Secretary, Treasurer, or Chair of a CPC Board or the American Academy of Microbiology. Nominations must consist of the following: curriculum vitae; letter of nomination, describe the nominee's ASM service and contributions on which the nomination is based; letters of support, two letters of support must come from persons, other than the nominator, who are familiar with the nominee's service and contributions to the ASM. No more than one of the three letters may be from the nominee's institution or the same institution.
Amount of Grant: A commemorative piece and travel to the ASM General Meeting.
Date(s) Application is Due: Oct 1
Contact: Awards, (202) 942-9226; fax: (202) 942-9353; email: awards@asmusa.org
Internet: http://www.asm.org/Academy/index.asp?bid=2324
Sponsor: American Society for Microbiology
1752 N Street, NW
Washington, DC 20036-2804

ASM Gen-Probe Joseph Public Health Award **597**

The ASM Gen-Probe Joseph Public Health Award honors a distinguished microbiologist who has exhibited exemplary leadership and service in the field of public health. This award has been established in memory of J. Mehsen Joseph, Ph.D., who dedicated his life toward the advancement of both microbiology and public health.
Requirements: The nominee must be a microbiologist identified with public health. The recipient will be recognized for significant achievements in integrating the science of microbiology into the practice of public health and for promoting the importance of linking these two disciplines. Nominations must consist of the following: curriculum vitae, including a list of nominee's publications; letter of nomination, describe the nominee's leadership and service in the field of public health; letters of support, two letters of support must come from persons, other than the nominator, who are familiar with the nominee's qualifications and accomplishments, citing in particular the nominee's leadership and service in the field of public health. No more than one of the three letters may be from the nominee's institution or from the same institution.
Amount of Grant: A cash prize of $2,000, a commemorative piece, and travel to the ASM General Meeting where the laureate is the ASM Division Y Lecturer.
Date(s) Application is Due: Oct 1
Contact: Awards, (202) 942-9226; fax: (202) 942-9353; email: awards@asmusa.org
Internet: http://www.asm.org/Academy/index.asp?bid=36040
Sponsor: American Society for Microbiology
1752 N Street, NW
Washington, DC 20036-2804

ASM General Meeting Minority Travel Grants **598**

The American Society for Microbiology (ASM) will offer travel grants to increase the participation of underrepresented minority (URM) groups in the ASM General Meeting. The ASM will select post-doctoral scholars from URM groups in the microbiological sciences or faculty from Minority Serving Institutions. Each grantee will be offered up to $1500 to defray expenses associated with travel to the ASM General Meeting.
Requirements: Eligibility: ASM Member; U.S. citizen or permanent resident; faculty member from a Minority Serving Institution (MSI), Historically Black Colleges and Universities (HBCU), Hispanic Serving institutions (HSI), Tribal Colleges and Universities (TCU) and other institutions with substantial enrollments of minority students are considered to be Minority Serving Institutions (MSI); post-doctoral Scholars from an URM Group
Amount of Grant: up to $1,500
Date(s) Application is Due: Jan 30
Contact: Awards, (202) 942-9226; fax: (202) 942-9353; email: awards@asmusa.org
Internet: http://www.asm.org/Awards/index.asp?bid=38173
Sponsor: American Society for Microbiology
1752 N Street, NW
Washington, DC 20036-2804

ASM GlaxoSmithKline International Member of the Year Award **599**

The ASM GlaxoSmithKline International Member of the Year Award honors a distinguished microbiologist who exhibited exemplary leadership in the international microbiological community. It recognizes an international ASM member for education, communication, research, and advancement of the profession to the international microbiology community while demonstrating a commitment to the ASM.
Requirements: The nominee can be any international member of ASM who has made major contributions toward the advancement of the microbiological sciences within the international community through education, research, communication, and leadership. The nominee must not have served on the International Board, the International Education Committee or the International Membership Committee within the past two years. Nominations must consist of the following: curriculum vitae, including a list of publications; letter of nomination, describe the nominee's contributions towards the advancement of the microbiological sciences within the international community through education, research, communication, and leadership. Emphasis should be on the nominee's creativity and originality, as well as the nominee's role in ASM-sponsored activities; letters of support, two letters of support must come from persons, other than the nominator, who are familiar with the nominee's contributions and accomplishments. No more than one of the three letters may be from the nominee's institution or the same institution.
Restrictions: Self-nominations will not be accepted.
Amount of Grant: A commemorative piece and travel to the ASM General Meeting where the laureate delivers the ASM International Member of the Year Award lecture.
Date(s) Application is Due: Oct 1
Contact: Awards, (202) 942-9226; fax: (202) 942-9353; email: awards@asmusa.org
Internet: http://www.asm.org/Academy/index.asp?bid=36033
Sponsor: American Society for Microbiology
1752 N Street, NW
Washington, DC 20036-2804

ASM Intel Awards **600**

ASM sponsors a special prize in microbiology at the Intel International Science and Engineering Fair. The fair recognizes excellence in science and technology by high school students. Ten cash prizes are given and all laureates receive a one-year student membership in ASM and access to members-only web resources. The first place laureate receives a cash prize of $2,000, the second place laureate receives a cash prize of $1,250, the thrid place laureate receives a cash prize of $750, and the fourth place laureate receives a cash prize of $500. Six honorable mentions of $250 are also awarded.
Amount of Grant: $250 - $2,000 range
Contact: Awards, (202) 942-9226; fax: (202) 942-9353; email: awards@asmusa.org
Internet: http://www.asm.org/Academy/index.asp?bid=36845
Sponsor: American Society for Microbiology
1752 N Street NW
Washington, DC 20036-2804

ASM International Fellowship for Latin America and the Caribbean **601**

Funded by ASM this award offers fellowships to promising young investigators in South and Central America and the Caribbean who are within five years of obtaining, or are in the process of obtaining, their Masters, PhD, or other equivalent academic degree, and who are working in any of the microbiology disciplines, to visit a host scientist in the U.S.. The International Fellowship Program provides funding to meet the costs of a visit to one institution for between 6 weeks to 6 months. The International Fellowship Program provides funding to meet the costs of a visit to one institution for between 6 weeks to 6 months.
Requirements: The application must be made jointly between a host institution and the visiting fellow. The Investigator must be:a member of ASM or any other national microbiological society; actively involved in research in the microbiological sciences; have obtained, or be in the process of obtaining, their masters, PhD, or other equivalent academic degree within the last five years; a national of a resource-limited Africa, Asian or Latin American country submitting the application from an institution in their home region. Investigators from developed nations, as defined by BOTH the UN high HDI group and the World Bank high income economy group, are ineligible. Investigators submitting an application from the U.S. where they are spending a training period are ineligible; sufficiently proficient in the use of the English language. The Host Scientist must be: an ASM member; actively involved in research in the microbiological sciences in the U.S.; actively involved in teaching in the microbiological sciences in the U.S.; interested in sustaining international collaborations Preference will be given to: applicants who can prove three years of membership in ASM or any other national microbiological society, and; applicants who have not previously had the opportunity to travel to a facility in another country. The application should demonstrate to the Review Committee: academic excellence of the applicant - Honors & Awards, CV, and Letters of Recommendation; depth of the applicant's research experience - Statement of prior Research Experience; quality and originality of work proposed during the Fellowship - Potential Collaboration and Proposed Research Plan; relevance of the work proposed to the applicant's locale - Potential Collaboration and Proposed Research Plan; excellence of the host, and the research and training environment
Amount of Grant: $4,000
Date(s) Application is Due: Apr 15; Oct 15
Contact: International Fellowship Program, (202) 942-9368; fax: (202) 942-9328; email: international@asmusa.org
Internet: http://www.asm.org/International/index.asp?bid=2778
Sponsor: American Society for Microbiology
1752 N Street NW
Washington, DC 20036-2804

ASM International Fellowships for Asia and Africa **602**

Funded by ASM this award offers a maximum of one fellowship to a promising young investigator in Asia, as well as to one young investigator in Africa who is within five years of obtaining, or in the process of obtaining, his/her Masters, PhD, or other equivalent academic degree, and who is working in any of the microbiology disciplines, to visit a host scientist in the U.S.. Both International Fellowships will award a maximum grant of $5,500. The award is not intended to provide travel to obtain a degree at the host institution.

Requirements: The application must be made jointly between a host institution and the visiting fellow. The Investigator must be: a member of ASM or any other national microbiological society; actively involved in research in the microbiological sciences; have obtained, or be in the process of obtaining, their masters, PhD, or other equivalent academic degree within the last five years; a national of a resource-limited Africa, Asian or Latin American country submitting the application from an institution in their home region. Investigators from developed nations, as defined by BOTH the UN high HDI group and the World Bank high income economy group, are ineligible. Investigators submitting an application from the U.S. where they are spending a training period are ineligible; sufficiently proficient in the use of the English language. The Host Scientist must be: an ASM member; actively involved in research in the microbiological sciences in the U.S.; actively involved in teaching in the microbiological sciences in the U.S.; interested in sustaining international collaborations Preference will be given to: applicants who can prove three years of membership in ASM or any other national microbiological society, and; applicants who have not previously had the opportunity to travel to a facility in another country.
Amount of Grant: $5,500
Date(s) Application is Due: Apr 15; Oct 15
Contact: International Fellowship Program, (202) 942-9368; fax: (202) 942-9328; email: international@asmusa.org
Internet: http://www.asm.org/International/index.asp?bid=2778
Sponsor: American Society for Microbiology
1752 N Street NW
Washington, DC 20036-2804

ASM International Professorship for Latin America **603**
The program provides funding support to an ASM member from the U.S. who is scientifically recognized in his/her area to teach a hands-on, highly interactive short course on a single topic in the microbiological sciences at a Latin American institution of higher learning. Up to five Teaching Professorships offered per program year.
Requirements: The application must be made jointly between a hosting institution and the visiting professor. Eligibility for Host Institution: institution with graduate students enrolled in a masters, doctoral or equivalent program, post-doctoral fellows or residents, and teaching faculty; institution where at least 12 students will be enrolled full-time in the short course; commitment to maximizing use of the course, as demonstrated by the applicability of the course's contents to existing programs at the institution or to the field of research of the Research Professor. demonstrated commitment to international collaborations and partnerships; demonstrated commitment to advancing the microbiological sciences through interactions with professional organizations; institutions in developed nations, as defined by the UN high HDI group, are ineligible. Eligibility for Visiting Teaching Professor: scientifically recognized their area of microbiological expertise; actively engaged in teaching at the post-secondary level; commitment to international collaborations and partnerships; must be an ASM member during the term of the Professorship. Preference will be given to: applicants who will be able to make maximal use of the course, as demonstrated either by the applicability of the course's contents to existing programs at the host institution or to the field of research of the visiting Professor; applications that demonstrate a commitment to building an ongoing institutional relationship. It is strongly recommended that the course include a hands-on component, such as a wet lab or other practical activity.
Amount of Grant: $4,000
Date(s) Application is Due: Apr 15; Oct 15
Contact: International Professorship Program, (202) 942-9368; fax: (202) 942-9328; email: international@asmusa.org
Internet: http://www.asm.org/International/index.asp?bid=57785
Sponsor: American Society for Microbiology
1752 N Street NW
Washington, DC 20036-2804

ASM International Professorships for Asia and Africa **604**
Each program provides funding support to an ASM member from the U.S. who is scientifically recognized in his/her area to teach a hands-on, highly interactive short course on a single topic in the microbiological sciences at an institution of higher learning in Asia and in Africa. The Teaching Professorship for both programs is limited to one per program year.
Requirements: The application must be made jointly between a hosting institution and the visiting professor. Eligibility for Host Institution: institution with graduate students enrolled in a masters, doctoral or equivalent program, post-doctoral fellows or residents, and teaching faculty; institution where at least 12 students will be enrolled full-time in the short course; commitment to maximizing use of the course, as demonstrated by the applicability of the course's contents to existing programs at the institution or to the field of research of the Research Professor. demonstrated commitment to international collaborations and partnerships; demonstrated commitment to advancing the microbiological sciences through interactions with professional organizations; institutions in developed nations, as defined by the UN high HDI group, are ineligible. Eligibility for Visiting Teaching Professor: scientifically recognized their area of microbiological expertise; actively engaged in teaching at the post-secondary level; commitment to international collaborations and partnerships; must be an ASM member during the term of the Professorship. Preference will be given to: applicants who will be able to make maximal use of the course, as demonstrated either by the applicability of the course's contents to existing programs at the host institution or to the field of research of the visiting Professor; applications that demonstrate a commitment to building an ongoing institutional relationship. It is strongly recommended that the course include a hands-on component, such as a wet lab or other practical activity.
Amount of Grant: $5,500
Date(s) Application is Due: Apr 15; Oct 15
Contact: International Professorship Program, (202) 942-9368; fax: (202) 942-9328; email: international@asmusa.org
Internet: http://www.asm.org/International/index.asp?bid=57785
Sponsor: American Society for Microbiology
1752 N Street NW
Washington, DC 20036-2804

ASM Maurice Hilleman/Merck Award **605**
The award is presented in memory of Maurice R. Hilleman, whose work in the development of vaccines has saved the lives of many throughout the world.
Requirements: The nominee must have made outstanding achievements in pathogenesis, vaccine discovery, vaccine development, and/or control of vaccine-preventable diseases. Nominations must consist of the following: curriculum vitae, including a full list of publications; letter of nomination, describe the nominee's remarkable contributions to pathogenesis, vaccine discovery, vaccine development, and/or the control of vaccine-preventable diseases, including a list of the ten publications most relevant to the award; letters of support, two letters of support must come from persons, other than the nominator, who are familiar with the nominee's achievements. No more than one of the three letters may be from the nominee's institution or the same institution.
Restrictions: Self-nominations will not be accepted.
Amount of Grant: A cash prize of $20,000, a commemorative medal, and travel to the ASM General Meeting where the laureate delivers the Maurice Hilleman/Merck Award Lecture.
Date(s) Application is Due: Oct 1
Contact: Awards, (202) 942-9226; fax: (202) 942-9353; email: awards@asmusa.org
Internet: http://www.asm.org/Academy/index.asp?bid=57948
Sponsor: American Society for Microbiology
1752 N Street, NW
Washington, DC 20036-2804

ASM Merck Irving S. Sigal Memorial Awards **606**
The ASM Merck Irving S. Sigal Memorial Awards recognize and award excellence in basic research in medical microbiology and infectious diseases. The awards are presented in memory of Irving S. Sigal, who was instrumental in the early discovery of therapies to treat HIV/AIDS.
Requirements: The nominee must be no more than five years beyond completion of postdoctoral research training in microbiology or infectious diseases at the time of the nomination deadline. Nominations must consist of the following: curriculum vitae, including a list of publications; letter of nomination, describe the nominee's excellence in basic research in medical microbiology and infectious diseases; letters of support, two letters of support must come from persons, other than the nomination, who are familiar with the nominee's qualifications and accomplishments. No more than one of the three letters may be from the nominee's institution or the same institution.
Amount of Grant: A cash prize of $2,500 and a commemorative piece.
Date(s) Application is Due: Oct 1
Contact: Awards, (202) 942-9226; fax: (202) 942-9353; email: awards@asmusa.org
Internet: http://www.asm.org/academy/index.asp?bid=15056
Sponsor: American Society for Microbiology
1752 N Street, NW
Washington, DC 20036-2804

ASM Microbiology Undergraduate Research Fellowship **607**
The goal of the Microbiology Undergraduate Research Fellowship (MURF) program is to increase the number of underrepresented undergraduate students who wish to, and have demonstrated the ability to pursue graduate careers (Ph.D. or M.D./Ph.D.) in microbiology. Students will have the opportunity to conduct full time summer research with an ASM member at a host institution, and present research results at the Annual Biomedical Research Conference for Minority Students and the ASM General Meeting. Students will: agree to participate in an undergraduate summer research program at a U.S. based institution; conduct a research project for a minimum of 10 weeks; work with a faculty mentor who is an ASM member; submit a research abstract to the Annual Biomedical Research Conference for Minority Students (ABRCMS); submit a research abstract to ASM for presentation at the ASM General Meeting. Students decide the institution, research area, and level of activity for the summer. Based on interests, independence, and ability, students will be placed at a host U.S. Institution of the student's choice to conduct basic science research. From a list provided on the application, students interested in conducting research at a host institution will select three institutions where they would like to conduct their summer research. Every effort will be made to place fellows at their first choice.
Requirements: Eligible student candidates for the fellowship must be from groups that have been determined by the applicant's institution to be underrepresented in the microbiological sciences. The ASM encourages institutions to identify individuals that have been historically underrepresented, and remain underrepresented today in the microbiological sciences nationally. These groups include African-Americans, Hispanics, Native Americans, Alaskan Natives, and Pacific Islanders. In addition, applicants must also: be U.S. citizen or permanent U.S. resident; be enrolled as full-time matriculating undergraduate students during the academic year at an accredited U.S. institution; be either freshmen with college level research experience, sophomores, juniors, or seniors who will not graduate before the completion date of the summer program; be members of an underrepresented group in microbiology; have taken introductory courses in biology, chemistry, and preferably microbiology prior to submission of the application; have

strong interests in obtaining a Ph.D., or M.D./Ph.D. in the microbiological sciences, and have lab research experience.
Restrictions: Travel funds are contingent upon acceptance of an abstract for the General Meeting.
Amount of Grant: $5,850
Date(s) Application is Due: Feb 1
Contact: Fellowship Committee, (202) 942-9283; fax: (202) 942-9329; email: fellowships-careerinformation@asmusa.org
Internet: http://www.asm.org/Education/index.asp?bid=4322
Sponsor: American Society for Microbiology
1752 N Street, NW
Washington, DC 20036-2804

ASM Millis-Colwell Postgraduate Travel Grant **608**
This new grant, negotiated between the American Society for Microbiology (ASM U.S.A) and the Australian Society for Microbiology (ASM Australia), allows for the exchange of one student member from each society to present an abstract at the annual General Meeting of the other society and to spend a week at nearby research laboratory. The grant aims to create a long lasting bond between ASM U.S.A and ASM Australia and is designed to benefit PhD students in both countries by giving them the opportunity to travel overseas to present their work and experience the best of microbiology in the partner country. ASM U.S.A will submit the successful applicant's abstract for an oral or poster presentation to ASM Australia for their Annual Scientific Meeting & Exhibition. The applicant will also have negotiated an agreement to visit the research laboratory of an Australian scientist in the period either immediately before or immediately after the ASM Australia annual meeting. The award will be conditional upon ASM Australia's acceptance of the submitted abstract.
Requirements: The successful applicant will be: a U.S. citizen or permanent resident of the U.S.; a student member of the American Society for Microbiology; and enrolled in a PhD program at an American University. The award will cover roundtrip economy airfare between the U.S. and Australia, and any necessary internal flights; per diem living allowance for up to 14 days; and, registration fee for the Australian Society for Microbiology's Annual Scientific Meeting & Exhibition.
Amount of Grant: up to $5,000
Date(s) Application is Due: Jan 1
Contact: Education Programs/Resources; (202) 942-9282; fax: (202) 942-9329
Internet: http://www.asm.org/International/index.asp?bid=53729
Sponsor: American Society for Microbiology
1752 N St NW
Washington, DC 20036

ASM Procter & Gamble Award in Applied and Environmental Microbiology **609**
The ASM Procter & Gamble Award in Applied and Environmental Microbiology recognizes distinguished achievement in research and development in applied (non-clinical) and environmental microbiology.
Requirements: The nominee must demonstrate outstanding accomplishment in research or development in an appropriate field and be actively engaged in research or development at the time that the award is presented. Nominations must consist of the following: curriculum vitae, including a list of publications; letter of nomination, describe the nominee's outstanding accomplishments in research or development in the appropriate field, including a list of the ten most relevant publications to the award; letters of support, two letters of support must come from persons, other than the nominator, who are familiar with the nominee's outstanding accomplishments. No more than one of the three letters may be from the nominee's institution or the same institution.
Restrictions: Self-nominations will not be accepted.
Amount of Grant: A cash prize of $2,000, a commemorative piece,
Date(s) Application is Due: Oct 1
Contact: Awards Committee, (202) 942-9226; fax: (202) 942-9353; email: awards@asmusa.org
Internet: http://www.asm.org/academy/index.asp?bid=2288
Sponsor: American Society for Microbiology
1752 N Street, NW
Washington, DC 20036-2804

ASM Promega Biotechnology Research Award **610**
The ASM Promega Biotechnology Research Award honors outstanding contributions to the application of biotechnology through fundamental microbiological research and development.
Requirements: A nomination can be a single exceptionally significant achievement or the aggregate of a number of exemplary achievements. Nominations must consist of the following: curriculum vitae, including a list of publications; letter of nomination, describe the nominee's outstanding accomplishments in microbiological research and development, including a list of the ten most relevant publications to the award; letters of support, two letters of support must come from persons, other than the nominator, who are familiar with the nominee's accomplishments. No more than one of the three letters may be from the nominee's institution or the same institution.
Restrictions: Neither self-nominations nor co-nominations will be accepted.
Amount of Grant: A cash prize of $5,000, a commemorative piece, and travel to the ASM General Meeting where the laureate delivers the Promega Biotechnology Research Award Lecture.
Date(s) Application is Due: Oct 1
Contact: Awards, (202) 942-9226; fax: (202) 942-9353; email: awards@asmusa.org
Internet: http://www.asm.org/academy/index.asp?bid=2291
Sponsor: American Society for Microbiology
1752 N Street, NW
Washington, DC 20036-2804

ASM Public Communications Award **611**
The ASM Public Communications Award, sponsored by ASM, recognizes outstanding achievement in increasing public awareness, knowledge and understanding of microbiology. Microbiology is concerned with issues such as the environment, prevention and treatment of infectious diseases, laboratory and diagnostic medicine, and food and water safety, among others.
Requirements: Eligibility is limited to primary authors of information concerning the microbiological sciences appearing in mass media, including print (newspapers and periodicals only) and broadcast media readily available to the general public. Individual items and series are both eligible. Applicants may nominate themselves. International entries are accepted but must be translated into English prior to submission.
Restrictions: Books, websites, and institutionally sponsored publications are not eligible.
Amount of Grant: The award consists of a $2,500 cash prize, a commemorative plaque, and travel expenses to attend the ASM General Meeting for presentation of the award.
Date(s) Application is Due: Jan 31
Contact: Garth Hogan, Office of Communications, (202) 942-9226; fax: (202) 942-9353; email: ghogan@asmusa.org
Internet: http://www.asm.org/Media/index.asp?bid=2676
Sponsor: American Society for Microbiology
1752 N Street, NW
Washington, DC 20036-2804

ASM Raymond W. Sarber Awards **612**
The ASM Raymond W. Sarber Awards recognize students at the undergraduate and predoctoral levels for research excellence and potential. The awards honor Raymond W. Sarber for his contributions to the growth and advancement of ASM.
Requirements: Nominees must be a student at the undergraduate or predoctoral level, attending an accredited institution in the United States, in an academic program involving microbiology. Two awards are presented at the ASM General Meeting, one to an undergraduate and one to a graduate student. They will be judged separately.
Restrictions: Nominations must consist of the following: curriculum vitae; statement, no longer than two pages, from the student outlining academic achievements, research accomplishments, and future career goals; letter of nomination, describe the nominee's research excellence and potential; letters of support, two letters of support: one from a supervisor or mentor, and the other letter may be from an academic advisor or colleague.
Amount of Grant: A framed certificate and cash prize of $1,500.
Date(s) Application is Due: Oct 1
Contact: Awards, (202) 942-9226; fax: (202) 942-9353; email: awards@asmusa.org
Internet: http://www.asm.org/academy/index.asp?bid=2294
Sponsor: American Society for Microbiology
1752 N Street, NW
Washington, DC 20036-2804

ASM Richard and Mary Finkelstein Travel Grant **613**
The Richard and Mary Finkelstein Travel Grant is a $500 grant given to 6 students who are ASM members and who are the presenting author of a poster at the General Meeting. Selection criteria for this award are the same as the Corporate Activities Program Student Travel Grant but the research presented must be in the area of microbial pathogenesis. Potential nominees must first be selected to receive a Corporate Activities Program Student Travel Grant and then the abstracts are reviewed again to establish the quality of the research in the additional area of microbial pathogenesis.
Requirements: To qualify for consideration the student must: be presenting research in the area of microbial pathogenesisbe; be an ASM Member and the presenting author; be accepted to present a poster at the General Meeting; be an undergraduate/pre-doctoral student, or; be a Ph.D. or M.D. whose degree has been or will be awarded after May of the current year and before May of the meeting year; have indicated a desire to be considered for the grant on the abstract submission, and submit a letter of nomination from a faculty member or department head on official letterhead. The letter must state that the student is expected to be active in the training or degree program at the time of the meeting. If the student will complete their terminal degree between the date of submission and the meeting, the letter must indicate the expected date of completion. The abstract tracking number must be included in the body of the letter. The letter should be submitted to ASM not later than December of each year. Exact date will be published in the Call for Abstracts for the General Meeting.
Amount of Grant: $500
Contact: Awards, (202) 942-9226; fax: (202) 942-9353; email: awards@asmusa.org
Internet: http://www.asm.org/Awards/index.asp?bid=14968h
Sponsor: American Society for Microbiology
1752 N Street, NW
Washington, DC 20036-2804

ASM Robert D. Watkins Graduate Research Fellowship **614**
The goal of the fellowship is to increase the number of underrepresented groups completing doctoral degrees in the microbiological sciences. The ASM Robert D. Watkins Graduate Research Fellowship is aimed at highly competitive graduate students who are enrolled in a Ph.D. program and who have completed their graduate course work in the microbiological sciences. The fellowship encourages students to continue

and complete their research project in the microbiological sciences. Students will be required to submit an abstract each year to ASM for presentation at the annual ASM General Meeting and attend the ASM Kadner Institute one time during the three-year tenure of the fellowship.
Requirements: Eligible candidates must be from groups that have been determined by the applicant's institution to be underrepresented in the microbiological sciences. The ASM encourages institutions to identify individuals that have been historically underrepresented, and remain underrepresented today in the microbiological sciences nationally. These groups include African-Americans, Hispanics, Native Americans, Alaskan Natives, and Pacific Islanders. In addition, applicants must: be formally admitted to a doctoral program in the microbiological sciences in an accredited U.S. institution; have successfully completed the first year of the graduate program (first year graduate students cannot apply); have successfully completed all graduate coursework requirements for the doctoral degree by the date of activation of the fellowship; be a student member of ASM; be mentored by an ASM member; be a U.S. citizen or a permanent resident; not have funding or have funding that will expire by the start date of the fellowship(fellowship cannot run concurrently with other national fellowships from NIH, NSF, HHMI, etc.); three letters of recommendations must be submitted with your application. One letter must be from your research advisor/mentor; Official transcripts from all colleges and universities attended.
Amount of Grant: a total stipend of $63,000 ($21,000 a year) for a three year period
Date(s) Application is Due: May 1
Contact: Education Board, (202) 942-9283; fax: (202) 942-9329; email: fellowships-careerinformation@asmusa.org
Internet: http://www.asm.org/Education/index.asp?bid=6278
Sponsor: American Society for Microbiology
1752 N Street, NW
Washington, DC 20036

ASM Roche Diagnostics Alice C. Evans Award 615
The ASM Roche Diagnostics Alice C. Evans Award recognizes contributions toward the full participation and advancement of women in microbiology. This award was established by the ASM's Committee on the Status of Women in Microbiology, and is given in memory of Alice C. Evans, the first woman to be ASM President in 1928.
Requirements: The nominee can be any member of ASM who has made major contributions toward fostering the inclusion, development, and advancement of women in careers in microbiology. The nominee must demonstrate commitment to women in science through mentorship and advocacy and by setting an example through scientific and professional achievement. Nominations must consist of the following: curriculum vitae, including a list of nominee's publications; letter of Nomination, describe the nominee's major contributions toward fostering the inclusion, development, and advancement of women in careers in microbiology; letters of support, two letters of support must come from persons, other than the nominator, who are familiar with the nominee's qualifications and accomplishments. No more than one of the three letters may be from the nominee's institution or from the same institution.
Restrictions: Self-nominations will not be accepted.
Amount of Grant: A plaque and travel to the ASM General Meeting.
Date(s) Application is Due: Oct 1
Contact: Awards, (202) 942-9226; fax: (202) 942-9353; email: awards@asmusa.org
Internet: http://www.asm.org/Academy/index.asp?bid=2332
Sponsor: American Society for Microbiology
1752 N Street, NW
Washington, DC 20036-2804

ASM sanofi-aventis ICAAC Award 616
ASM's premier award in antimicrobial chemotherapy research; it stimulates research and honors outstanding accomplishment in antimicrobial chemotherapy.
Requirements: The nominee must be actively engaged in research involving development of new agents, investigation of antimicrobial action or resistance to antimicrobial agents, and/or the pharmacology, toxicology or clinical use of those agents. The nominee must not have served on the ICAAC Program Committee within the past two years. Nominations must consist of the following: curriculum vitae, including a list of publications; letter of nomination, describe the nominee's outstanding accomplishment in antimicrobial chemotherapy, including a list of the ten most relevant publications to the award; letters of support, two letters of support should come from two people, other than the nominator, who are familiar with the nominee's accomplishments. No more than one of the three letters may be from the nominee's institution or the same institution.
Restrictions: Self-nominations will not be accepted.
Amount of Grant: A cash prize of $20,000, a commemorative medal, and travel to ICAAC where the laureate delivers the sanofi-aventis ICAAC Award Lecture.
Date(s) Application is Due: Apr 1
Contact: Awards, (202) 942-9226; fax: (202) 942-9353; email: awards@asmusa.org
Internet: http://www.asm.org/academy/index.asp?bid=2268
Sponsor: American Society for Microbiology
1752 N Street, NW
Washington, DC 20036-2804

ASM Scherago-Rubin Award 617
The ASM Scherago-Rubin Award recognizes an outstanding, bench-level clinical microbiologist. The award was established by the late Sally Jo Rubin, an active member of ASM's Clinical Microbiology Division, in honor of her grandfather, Morris Scherago.
Requirements: The nominee must be a non-doctoral-level clinical microbiologist involved primarily in routine diagnostic work, rather than in research, who has distinguished himself or herself with excellent performance in the clinical laboratory. Nominations must consist of the following: curriculum vitae, including a list of the nominee's publications; letter of nomination, a letter from the supervisor describing how the nominee's routine diagnostic work, rather than research, has distinguished himself or herself in the clinical laboratory; letters of support, two letters of support preferably from individuals from different institutions who are familiar with the nominee's laboratory accomplishments.
Restrictions: Self-nominations will not be accepted.
Amount of Grant: A cash prize of $1,500 and a framed certificate.
Date(s) Application is Due: Oct 1
Contact: Awards, (202) 942-9226; fax: (202) 942-9353; email: awards@asmusa.org
Internet: http://www.asm.org/academy/index.asp?bid=2335
Sponsor: American Society for Microbiology
1752 N Street, NW
Washington, DC 20036-2804

ASM Siemens Healthcare Diagnostics Young Investigator Award 618
The ASM Siemens Healthcare Diagnostics Young Investigator Award honors outstanding laboratory research in clinical microbiology or antimicrobial agents and is intended to further the career development of a young clinical scientist and promote awareness of clinical microbiology as a career.
Requirements: The nominee should be conducting outstanding research in clinical microbiology, automation in clinical laboratories, development of novel antimicrobial agents, mechanisms of action of antimicrobial agents or mechanisms of resistance to antimicrobial agents. The nominee must be no more than five years beyond completion of postdoctoral research training in microbiology, infectious diseases or related disciplines at the time of the nomination deadline. Nominations must consist of the following: curriculum vitae, including a list of publications, abstracts, and manuscripts in preparation; letter of nomination, describe the nominee's outstanding clinical research and potential; letters of support, two letters of support must come from persons, other than the nominator, who are familiar with the nominee's qualifications and accomplishments. No more than one of the three letters may be from the nominee's institution or from the same institution.
Restrictions: Self-nominations will not be accepted.
Amount of Grant: A cash prize of $2,000, commemorative piece, and travel to the ASM General Meeting.
Date(s) Application is Due: Oct 1
Contact: Awards, (202) 942-9226; fax: (202) 942-9353; email: awards@asmusa.org
Internet: http://www.asm.org/Academy/index.asp?bid=2307
Sponsor: American Society for Microbiology
1752 N Street, NW
Washington, DC 20036-2804

ASM Student and Post Doctoral Fellow Travel Grants 619
The ICAAC Program Committee will award travel grants worth at least $500, to support students' attendance at the 43rd ICAAC. Travel grants are selected on the basis of the scientific quality of the submitted abstracts. Preference is given to students who have not received a travel grant in the past two years, and the Committee strives to award only one travel grant per laboratory. They are sponsored by the ASM Corporate Partners.
Requirements: Criteria: ASM membership at time of application; undergraduate or pre-doctoral student; Ph.D. or M.D. within two years of graduation at the time of the meeting; or an M.D. in a residency or fellowship program within six years of receipt of the M.D. degree at the time of the meeting; cover letter from the applicant, including their contact information, accompanied by letter of nomination from a faculty member on department letterhead, stating that the applicant is expected to be active in the training or degree program at the time of the meeting. If the applicant will have attained their terminal degree at the time of the meeting, the date of graduation must be included in this letter; submission of an abstract for the ICAAC, which is accepted for presentation; letter of nomination, copy of the abstract, and submission control number.
Amount of Grant: $500 range
Date(s) Application is Due: May 30
Contact: Awards, (202) 942-9226; fax: (202) 942-9353; email: awards@asmusa.org
Internet: http://www.asm.org/Meetings/index.asp?bid=15264
Sponsor: American Society for Microbiology
1752 N Street, NW
Washington, DC 20036-2804

ASM Student Travel Grants 620
ASM has provided funds for the awarding travel grants of $500 each to predoctoral students.
Requirements: To qualify, applicants must be: a member of ASM (student membership in ASM is only $15); a presenter on an accepted abstract; and must be at the predoctoral level at the time of abstract submission. Applicants submitting an abstract via the ASM web site should check the box on the screen when filling out the electronic submission form where indicated. In addition, selected recipients must return a confirmation form sent with notice of award selection, including proof of predoctoral status, either in the form of a copy of the validated student identification card, or a letter on departmental letterhead from their departmental chair which verifies their student status.
Amount of Grant: $500
Contact: Awards, (202) 942-9226; fax: (202) 942-9353; email: awards@asmusa.org
Internet: http://www.asm.org/Meetings/index.asp?bid=15264
Sponsor: American Society for Microbiology
1752 N Street, NW
Washington, DC 20036-2804

ASM TREK Diagnostic ABMM/ABMLI Professional Recognition Award 621

The ASM TREK Diagnostic ABMM/ABMLI Professional Recognition Award recognizes a Diplomate of the American Board of Medical Microbiology (ABMM) or the American Board of Medical Laboratory Immunology (ABMLI) for outstanding contributions to the professional recognition of certified microbiologists and/or immunologists and the work they do. Primary consideration will be given to ABMM or ABMLI Diplomates who have made significant contributions to the advancement and public recognition of the profession over and above scientific achievements or board-related activities.

Requirements: Nominations must consist of the following: curriculum vitae, including a list of nominee's publications; letter of nomination, describe the nominee's outstanding contributions to the professional recognition of clinical microbiologists and/or immunologists; letters of support, two letters of support must come from persons, other than the nominator, who are familiar with the nominee's qualifications and accomplishments. No more than one of the three letters may be from the nominee's institution or from the same institution.

Restrictions: Self-nominations will not be accepted.

Amount of Grant: A commemorative piece and travel to the ASM General Meeting where the laureate delivers the keynote lecture at the ABMM/ABMLI session.

Date(s) Application is Due: Oct 1

Contact: Awards, (202) 942-9226; fax: (202) 942-9353; email: awards@asmusa.org

Internet: http://www.asm.org/Academy/index.asp?bid=2321

Sponsor: American Society for Microbiology
1752 N Street, NW
Washington, DC 20036-2804

ASM Undergraduate Research Fellowship 622

The ASM Undergraduate Research Fellowship (URF) is aimed at highly competitive students who wish to pursue graduate careers (Ph.D. or MD/Ph.D) in microbiology. Students will have the opportunity to conduct full time research at their home institutions with an ASM member and present research results at the ASM General Meeting the following year. Students will: conduct a research project for a minimum of 10 weeks beginning in the summer; work with faculty mentors who are ASM members and who are employed at the students home institutions, and submit a research abstract for presentation at the ASM General Meeting. The Fellowship provides: up to $4000 for student stipend; two-year ASM student membership, and up to $1000 in travel support for students to present the results of the research project at the ASM General Meeting. Travel funds are contingent upon acceptance of an abstract for the General Meeting.

Requirements: Eligible student candidates for the fellowship must: be enrolled as full-time matriculating undergraduate students during the academic year at an accredited U.S. Institution; be involved in a research project; have an ASM member at their home institutions willing to serve as a mentor, and not receive financial support for research during the fellowship. Applicants who do not meet all eligibility requirements will not be considered.

Restrictions: The program requires a joint application from both the student and a faculty mentor. It is student's responsibility to submit a completed application.

Amount of Grant: $4,000 - $5,000 range

Date(s) Application is Due: Feb 1

Contact: Fellowship Committee, (202) 942-9283; fax: (202) 942-9329; email: fellowships-careerinformation@asmusa.org

Internet: http://www.asm.org/Education/index.asp?bid=4319

Sponsor: American Society for Microbiology
1752 N Street, NW
Washington, DC 20036-2804

ASM U.S.FCC/J. Roger Porter Award 623

This award recognizes outstanding efforts by a scientist who has demonstrated the importance of microbial biodiversity through sustained curatorial or stewardship activities for a major resource used by the scientific community. It honors the memory of Dr. Porter and his remarkable contributions to science.

Requirements: The nominee will have greatly aided other scientists by demonstrating the fundamentals of culture collections and related resources and the rich biodiversity that such collections preserve. These resources may include collections of cells or microorganisms, databases or tools, or major reference works or services as an essential aspect of either one or more major publications or an extensive work effort.

Restrictions: Nominations must consist of the following: curriculum vitae, including a list of publications; letter of nomination, describe the nominee's outstanding efforts demonstrating the importance of microbial biodiversity through sustained curatorial or stewardship activities for a major resource used by the scientific community; letters of support, two letters of support must come from persons, other than the nominator, who are familiar with the nominee's outstanding efforts. No more than one of the three letters may be from the nominee's institution or the same institution.

Samples: Self-nominations will not be accepted.

Amount of Grant: A cash prize of $2,000, commemorative piece, and travel to the ASM General Meeting where the laureate delivers the U.S.FCC/J. Roger Porter Award Lecture.

Date(s) Application is Due: Oct 1

Contact: Awards Committee, (202) 942-9226; fax: (202) 942-9353; email: awards@asmusa.org

Internet: http://www.asm.org/academy/index.asp?bid=2297

Sponsor: American Society for Microbiology
1752 N Street, NW
Washington, DC 20036-2804

ASM William A Hinton Research Training Award 624

The ASM William A Hinton Research Training Award honors outstanding contributions toward fostering the research training of underrepresented minorities in microbiology. It is given in memory of William A. Hinton, a physician-research scientist and one of the first African-Americans to join the ASM.

Requirements: The nominee must contribute to the research training of undergraduate students, graduate students, postdoctoral fellows or health professional students and efforts leading to the increased participation of underrepresented minorities in microbiology. Nominations must consist of the following: curriculum vitae, including a list of nominee's publications; letter of nomination, describe the nominee's training of undergraduate students, graduate students, postdoctoral fellows, or health professional students. Detail specific examples of excellence in training and mentoring of underrepresented minorities. Describe the duration, extent, and impact of the nominee's training of underrepresented minority students, graduate students, postdoctoral fellows, or health professional students; letters of support, two letters of support must come from persons, other than the nominator, who are familiar with the nominee's outstanding contributions to the training of underrepresented minorities. No more than one of the three letters may be from the nominee's institution or from the same institution.

Amount of Grant: A cash prize of $2,000, a commemorative piece, and travel to the ASM General Meeting.

Date(s) Application is Due: Oct 1

Contact: Awards Committee, (202) 942-9226; fax: (202) 942-9353; email: awards@asmusa.org

Internet: http://www.asm.org/Academy/index.asp?bid=2317

Sponsor: American Society for Microbiology
1752 N Street, NW
Washington, DC 20036-2804

ASM-PAHO Infectious Diseases Epidemiology and Surveillance Fellowships 625

Funded by the Pan American Health Organization and ASM, this award offers fellowships to young scientists from Bolivia, Colombia, Costa Rica, Dominican Republic, Ecuador, El Salvador, Guatemala, Honduras, Nicaragua, Panama, Paraguay, or Peru, who have obtained their Masters, PhD, or other equivalent academic degree, and who have at least five years of laboratory experience in the area of antimicrobial resistance, to visit a host scientist in the U.S.. The ASM-PAHO Infectious Diseases Epidemiology and Surveillance Fellowship will award a maximum grant of $4,000. The award is not intended to provide travel to obtain a degree at the host institution.

Requirements: The application must be made jointly between a host institution and the visiting fellow. The Investigator must be: a member of ASM or any other national microbiological society; actively involved in research in the microbiological sciences; have obtained, or be in the process of obtaining, their masters, PhD, or other equivalent academic degree within the last five years; a national of a resource-limited Africa, Asian or Latin American country submitting the application from an institution in their home region. Investigators from developed nations, as defined by BOTH the UN high HDI group and the World Bank high income economy group, are ineligible. Investigators submitting an application from the U.S. where they are spending a training period are ineligible; sufficiently proficient in the use of the English language. The Host Scientist must be: an ASM member; actively involved in research in the microbiological sciences in the U.S.; actively involved in teaching in the microbiological sciences in the U.S.; interested in sustaining international collaborations Preference will be given to: applicants who can prove three years of membership in ASM or any other national microbiological society, and; applicants who have not previously had the opportunity to travel to a facility in another country. The application should demonstrate to the Review Committee: academic excellence of the applicant - Honors & Awards, CV, and Letters of Recommendation; depth of the applicant's research experience - Statement of prior Research Experience; quality and originality of work proposed during the Fellowship - Potential Collaboration and Proposed Research Plan; relevance of the work proposed to the applicant's locale - Potential Collaboration and Proposed Research Plan; excellence of the host, and the research and training environment

Amount of Grant: $4,000

Date(s) Application is Due: Apr 15; Oct 15

Contact: International Fellowship Program, (202) 942-9368; fax: (202) 942-9328; email: international@asmusa.org

Internet: http://www.asm.org/International/index.asp?bid=2778

Sponsor: American Society for Microbiology
1752 N Street NW
Washington, DC 20036-2804

ASM-UNESCO Leadership Grant for International Educators 626

This new program, sponsored jointly by ASM and UNESCO, has been developed to enable a select group of educators from resource-limited countries to attend the ASM Conference for Undergraduate Educators (ASMCUE) and a pre-conference workshop to provide leaders in education with the resources to build innovative teaching modules that engage students and lead to enduring understandings in microbiology. Successful applicants will receive financial support to cover airfare (economy class), room, board and registration to the pre-conference workshop and ASMCUE. Participants will be reimbursed for airfare via wire transfer upon submission of a confirmed invoice. Room, board and registration will be arranged by ASM.

Requirements: Preference will be given to ASM members. Applicants must be a citizen of, and residing in, a resource-limited country in Latin America, Asia, Africa, and Central and Eastern Europe. Resource-limited countries are classified as upper-middle income and below by the World Bank Development Group. (To find out if your country fits this criteria, visit http://tinyurl.com/7he3u.) Participants must have a minimum of eight

years teaching in microbiology/biology at a university level and must also have regular and sustained access to the Internet.
Restrictions: Members of the ASM International Board, International Education Committee, International Membership Committee, International Laboratory Capacity Building Committee, and the ASM International Ambassador Network are not eligible for this program.
Date(s) Application is Due: Dec 1
Contact: Michelle Godinez, Coordinator, Education Programs and Events; (202) 942-9317; fax: (202) 942-9328; email: mgodinez@asmusa.org
Internet: http://www.asm.org/International/index.asp?bid=61306
Sponsor: American Society for Microbiology
1752 N St NW
Washington, DC 20036

ASM/CCID Fellowships 627
The program is sponsored by the American Society for Microbiology (ASM) and the Coordinating Center for Infectious Diseases (CCID), formerly known as the National Center for Infectious Diseases (NCID). The goal of ASM/CCID Fellowship is to support the development of new approaches, methodologies and knowledge in infectious disease prevention and control in areas within the public health mission of the CDC. The fellowship allows one to perform research in residence at the CCID which is headquartered at the Centers for Disease Control and Prevention (CDC) in Atlanta, GA. Eligible fields of study include: bacterial and Mycotic Diseases; viral and Rickettsial Infections; nosocomial Infections; HIV/AIDS; vector-borne Infectious Diseases; parasitic Diseases. The Fellowship provides an annual stipend (up to $42,188), health benefits (up to $3000 annually) for a maximum of 2 years, relocation benefits (up to $500), and (up to $2000 annually) for professional development for a maximum of 2 years.
Requirements: The program is intended for individuals who either earned their doctorate degree or completed a primary residency within three years of their proposed start date. Applicants may not have a faculty position or be enrolled in a graduate degree program during the fellowship. Considerations will be given to individuals with more experience if there are compelling reasons. Qualified applicants will receive consideration without regard to race, creed, color, age, sex, or national origin.
Amount of Grant: $41,000 - $42,000 range
Date(s) Application is Due: Jan 15
Contact: Fellowship Committee, (202) 942-9283; fax: (202) 942-9329; email: fellowships-careerinformation@asmusa.org
Internet: http://www.asm.org/Education/index.asp?bid=15497
Sponsor: American Society for Microbiology
1752 N Street NW
Washington, DC 20036-2804

ASMCUE/GM Travel Assistance Grants 628
ASM offers travel awards to attend the 2009 ASMCUE to ASM Members who have been accepted to present a poster at ASM General Meeting and ASMCUE.
Requirements: Eligibility: accepted to present a poster at both ASM General Meeting in any division and ASMCUE; be an active ASM member; teach an undergraduate microbiology course or participates in outreach activities related to microbiology; have an interest in pursuing a teaching career at an undergraduate institution; not be a recipient of substantial federal funding or any other ASM faculty enhancement or travel award.
Amount of Grant: $500
Date(s) Application is Due: Mar 20
Contact: Awards Committee, (202) 942-9226; fax: (202) 942-9353; email: awards@asmusa.org
Internet: http://www.asm.org/Education/index.asp
Sponsor: American Society for Microbiology
1752 N Street, NW
Washington, DC 20036-2804

ASPEN C. Richard Fleming Grant 629
The Foundation provides annual grant support to nutrition researchers at all stages of their careers. This grant, funded by the donations of ASPEN members, is intended to assist a nutrition investigator by providing preliminary funding for promising new research in the field of nutrition and metabolic support and related areas of clinical nutrition. Applicants still in training positions may apply. Corporate employees are eligible to receive grants if the research project is not part of their normal duties and they have at least a part-time academic appointment or are associated with a professional institute that conducts nutrition research. In making choices among otherwise high-quality applicants, the reviewers will take into account the geographic distribution of grant winners; their ethnic background and gender, should the applicant choose to supply such information; their professional discipline; and other criteria as appropriate to ensure an equitable system. Funds may be used only for technician salary, equipment, supplies, animals, clinical research costs or other expenses directly related to the conduct of the proposed research.
Requirements: Applicants must submit a letter from their supervisor or department head at the institution confirming his/her commitment to the project. If the project involves human subjects, a letter pledging support in recruiting patients from the primary care provider and the institutional review board overseeing human studies is required. For junior faculty and applicants who do not hold faculty positions, three letters of reference are required.
Restrictions: This grant is not intended to support pursuit of an additional degree. Grant funds may not be used for: comparison of commercial products; indirect costs or overhead; costs of patient care; constructing or renovating facilities; furniture or office equipment; secretarial services; honoraria or membership dues; textbooks or periodicals; repair or service contract costs on institutional equipment; entertainment; travel; or salary support for the Principal Investigator.
Amount of Grant: $3,500
Date(s) Application is Due: Sep 8
Contact: Paula Bowen, Research Program Administrator; (301) 587-6315, ext. 132 or (301) 920-9132; fax: (301) 587-2365; email: paulab@aspen.nutr.org
Internet: http://www.nutritioncare.org/wcontent.aspx?id=784
Sponsor: American Society for Parenteral and Enteral Nutrition (ASPEN) Rhoads Research Foundation
8630 Fenton Street, Suite 412
Silver Spring, MD 20910

ASPEN Douglas Wilmore Grant 630
The Foundation provides annual grant support to nutrition researchers at all stages of their careers. The grant is intended to assist a nutrition investigator by providing preliminary funding for promising new research in the field of nutrition and metabolic support and related areas of clinical nutrition. Priority consideration is given to applications that involve a multidisciplinary team or that investigate the efficacy of parenteral or enteral nutrition. Applicants still in training positions may apply for the Fleming Grant. Corporate employees are eligible to receive grants if the research project is not part of their normal duties and they have at least a part-time academic appointment or are associated with a professional institute that conducts nutrition research. In making choices among otherwise high-quality applicants, the reviewers will take into account the geographic distribution of grant winners; their ethnic background and gender, should the applicant choose to supply such information; their professional discipline; and other criteria as appropriate to ensure an equitable system. Funds may be used only for technician salary, equipment, supplies, animals, clinical research costs or other expenses directly related to the conduct of the proposed research. The grant can be renewed for a second year of funding, assuming satisfactory progress.
Requirements: Applicants must submit a letter from their supervisor or department head at the institution confirming his/her commitment to the project. If the project involves human subjects, a letter pledging support in recruiting patients from the primary care provider and the institutional review board overseeing human studies is required. For junior faculty and applicants who do not hold faculty positions, three letters of reference are required.
Restrictions: Individuals who have received other research grants in excess of $25,000 are ineligible to apply, as are those who completed training more than 5 years prior to the start of the grant period. This grant is not intended to support pursuit of an additional degree. Grant funds may not be used for: comparison of commercial products; indirect costs or overhead; costs of patient care; constructing or renovating facilities; furniture or office equipment; secretarial services; honoraria or membership dues; textbooks or periodicals; repair or service contract costs on institutional equipment; entertainment; travel; or salary support for the Principal Investigator.
Amount of Grant: $25,000 maximum
Date(s) Application is Due: Sep 8
Contact: Paula Bowen, Research Program Administrator; (301) 587-6315, ext. 132 or (301) 920-9132; fax: (301) 587-2365; email: paulab@aspen.nutr.org
Internet: http://www.nutritioncare.org/wcontent.aspx?id=784
Sponsor: American Society for Parenteral and Enteral Nutrition (ASPEN) Rhoads Research Foundation
8630 Fenton Street, Suite 412
Silver Spring, MD 20910

ASPEN Dudrick Research Scholar Award 631
A.S.P.E.N. members are invited to nominate individuals to be considered by the Dudrick Award Committee for the Stanley Dudrick Research Scholar Award. A.S.P.E.N. presents this annual award to recognize and support a mid-career investigator who has shown significant achievements in nutrition support, is an A.S.P.E.N. member, and demonstrates exceptional research productivity and the potential to continue to make contributions in the field of nutrition therapy. The award includes $5,000, plus recognition during the Rhoads Lecture and Awards Symposium.
Requirements: The applicant should: be an A.S.P.E.N. member; have an advanced degree (MD, PharmD, MS, PhD, or equivalent); currently be in a training program or have completed formal training in nutritional research/therapy within the past 10-15 years, e.g. mid-career; have demonstrated exceptional research productivity during and/or following formal training.
Amount of Grant: $5,000
Date(s) Application is Due: Oct 15
Contact: Paula Bowen, Research Program Administrator; (301) 587-6315, ext. 132 or (301) 920-9132; fax: (301) 587-2365; email: paulab@aspen.nutr.org
Internet: http://www.nutritioncare.org/wcontent.aspx?id=878
Sponsor: American Society for Parenteral and Enteral Nutrition
8630 Fenton Street, Suite 412
Silver Spring, MD 20910

ASPEN Harry M. Vars Award 632
The Award is made annually for the best research presentation by an investigator at Nutrition Week. The recipient of the award is selected by the Vars Award Selection Subcommittee based upon a review of manuscripts submitted by qualified candidates. The author of the best paper presents his or her paper at the Premier Paper Session and is given a $1,000 cash prize, a travel grant and a plaque during the Research Awards

Ceremony at Nutrition Week. The winning manuscript is published in the Journal of Parenteral and Enteral Nutrition (JPEN). The Award is open to all disciplines.
Amount of Grant: $1,000
Contact: Michelle Spangenburg, Program Director for Education; (301) 587-6315, ext. 127; fax:(301) 587-2365; email: michelles@aspen.nutr.org
Internet: http://www.nutritioncare.org/wcontent.aspx?id=878
Sponsor: American Society for Parenteral and Enteral Nutrition
8630 Fenton Street, Suite 412
Silver Spring, MD 20910

ASPEN Maurice Shils Grant **633**

The Foundation provides annual grant support to nutrition researchers at all stages of their careers. This grant, funded by a donation from Baxter Health Care and Nestle Clinical Nutrition, is intended to assist a nutrition investigator by providing preliminary funding for promising new research in the field of nutrition and metabolic support and related areas of clinical nutrition. Persons applying for the grant must be in a post-training position and commit at least 20% of their time to research. Corporate employees are eligible to receive grants if the research project is not part of their normal duties and they have at least a part-time academic appointment or are associated with a professional institute that conducts nutrition research. In making choices among otherwise high-quality applicants, the reviewers will take into account the geographic distribution of grant winners; their ethnic background and gender, should the applicant choose to supply such information; their professional discipline; and other criteria as appropriate to ensure an equitable system. Funds may be used only for technician salary, equipment, supplies, animals, clinical research costs or other expenses directly related to the conduct of the proposed research. Grants can be renewed for a second year of funding, assuming satisfactory progress.
Requirements: Applicants must submit a letter from their supervisor or department head at the institution confirming his/her commitment to the project. If the project involves human subjects, a letter pledging support in recruiting patients from the primary care provider and the institutional review board overseeing human studies is required. For junior faculty and applicants who do not hold faculty positions, three letters of reference are required.
Restrictions: Individuals who have received other research grants in excess of $25,000 are ineligible to apply, as are those who completed training more than 5 years prior to the start of the grant period. This grant is not intended to support pursuit of an additional degree. Grant funds may not be used for: comparison of commercial products; indirect costs or overhead; costs of patient care; constructing or renovating facilities; furniture or office equipment; secretarial services; honoraria or membership dues; textbooks or periodicals; repair or service contract costs on institutional equipment; entertainment; travel; or salary support for the Principal Investigator.
Amount of Grant: $18,000
Date(s) Application is Due: Sep 8
Contact: Paula Bowen, Research Program Administrator; (301) 587-6315, ext. 132 or (301) 920-9132; fax: (301) 587-2365; email: paulab@aspen.nutr.org
Internet: http://www.nutritioncare.org/wcontent.aspx?id=784
Sponsor: American Society for Parenteral and Enteral Nutrition (ASPEN) Rhoads Research Foundation
8630 Fenton Street, Suite 412
Silver Spring, MD 20910

ASPEN Norman Yoshimura Grant **634**

The Foundation provides annual grant support to nutrition researchers at all stages of their careers. This grant, supported by B. Braun Medical, Inc. funding, is intended to assist a nutrition investigator by providing preliminary funding for promising new research in the field of nutrition and metabolic support and related areas of clinical nutrition. Applicants still in training positions may apply. Corporate employees are eligible to receive grants if the research project is not part of their normal duties and they have at least a part-time academic appointment or are associated with a professional institute that conducts nutrition research. In making choices among otherwise high-quality applicants, the reviewers will take into account the geographic distribution of grant winners; their ethnic background and gender, should the applicant choose to supply such information; their professional discipline; and other criteria as appropriate to ensure an equitable system. Funds may be used only for technician salary, equipment, supplies, animals, clinical research costs or other expenses directly related to the conduct of the proposed research.
Requirements: Applicants must submit a letter from their supervisor or department head at the institution confirming his/her commitment to the project. If the project involves human subjects, a letter pledging support in recruiting patients from the primary care provider and the institutional review board overseeing human studies is required. For junior faculty and applicants who do not hold faculty positions, three letters of reference are required.
Restrictions: This grant is not intended to support pursuit of an additional degree. Grant funds may not be used for: comparison of commercial products; indirect costs or overhead; costs of patient care; constructing or renovating facilities; furniture or office equipment; secretarial services; honoraria or membership dues; textbooks or periodicals; repair or service contract costs on institutional equipment; entertainment; travel; or salary support for the Principal Investigator.
Amount of Grant: $15,000
Date(s) Application is Due: Sep 8
Contact: Paula Bowen, Research Program Administrator; (301) 587-6315, ext. 132 or (301) 920-9132; fax: (301) 587-2365; email: paulab@aspen.nutr.org
Internet: http://www.nutritioncare.org/wcontent.aspx?id=784
Sponsor: American Society for Parenteral and Enteral Nutrition (ASPEN) Rhoads Research Foundation
8630 Fenton Street, Suite 412
Silver Spring, MD 20910

ASPEN Nutrition Research Grants **635**

The Foundation provides annual grant support to nutrition researchers at all stages of their careers. This grant, funded by a donation from the Abbott Foundation, is intended to assist a nutrition investigator by providing preliminary funding for promising new research in the field of nutrition and metabolic support and related areas of clinical nutrition. Persons applying for the grant must be in a post-training position and commit at least 20% of their time to research. Corporate employees are eligible to receive grants if the research project is not part of their normal duties and they have at least a part-time academic appointment or are associated with a professional institute that conducts nutrition research. In making choices among otherwise high-quality applicants, the reviewers will take into account the geographic distribution of grant winners; their ethnic background and gender, should the applicant choose to supply such information; their professional discipline; and other criteria as appropriate to ensure an equitable system. Funds may be used only for technician salary, equipment, supplies, animals, clinical research costs or other expenses directly related to the conduct of the proposed research. Grants can be renewed for a second year of funding, assuming satisfactory progress.
Requirements: Applicants must submit a letter from their supervisor or department head at the institution confirming his/her commitment to the project. If the project involves human subjects, a letter pledging support in recruiting patients from the primary care provider and the institutional review board overseeing human studies is required. For junior faculty and applicants who do not hold faculty positions, three letters of reference are required.
Restrictions: Individuals who have received other research grants in excess of $25,000 are ineligible to apply, as are those who completed training more than 5 years prior to the start of the grant period. This grant is not intended to support pursuit of an additional degree. Grant funds may not be used for: comparison of commercial products; indirect costs or overhead; costs of patient care; constructing or renovating facilities; furniture or office equipment; secretarial services; honoraria or membership dues; textbooks or periodicals; repair or service contract costs on institutional equipment; entertainment; travel; or salary support for the Principal Investigator.
Amount of Grant: $25,000 maximum
Date(s) Application is Due: Sep 8
Contact: Paula Bowen, Research Program Administrator; (301) 587-6315, ext. 132 or (301) 920-9132; fax: (301) 587-2365; email: paulab@aspen.nutr.org
Internet: http://www.nutritioncare.org/wcontent.aspx?id=784
Sponsor: American Society for Parenteral and Enteral Nutrition (ASPEN) Rhoads Research Foundation
8630 Fenton Street, Suite 412
Silver Spring, MD 20910

ASPEN Scientific Abstracts Awards for Papers or Posters **636**

ASPEN will consider all Scientific Abstract submissions for awards. Applicants will be notified if their abstract is a candidate. The first authors of the three highest ranked abstracts from this category (paper or poster) will receive travel grants to attend the Research Workshop, and to present their work at Clinical Nutrition Week. In addition, cash awards in the amounts of $750, $500 and $250 will be offered to the presenters of the three best papers. Awards are presented during the Rhoads Lecture and Research Awards Ceremony at Clinical Nutrition Week.
Amount of Grant: $250-$750 plus travel expenses
Contact: Paula Bowen, Research Program Administrator; (301) 587-6315, ext. 132 or (301) 920-9132; fax: (301) 587-2365; email: paulab@aspen.nutr.org
Internet: http://www.nutritioncare.org/Index.aspx?id=724
Sponsor: American Society for Parenteral and Enteral Nutrition
8630 Fenton Street, Suite 412
Silver Spring, MD 20910

ASPEN Scientific Abstracts Promising Investigator Awards **637**

ASPEN will consider all Scientific Abstract submissions for awards. Applicants will be notified if their abstract is a candidate. These awards are presented to the top three Scientific Abstract authors, who are also in the early stages of their careers. Winners receive $750 in travel funds to offset their travel expenses to and from Clinical Nutrition Week. Vars Award winners are eligible for these awards if they are in the early stages of their careers.
Amount of Grant: $750 in travel funds
Contact: Paula Bowen, Research Program Administrator; (301) 587-6315, ext. 132 or (301) 920-9132; fax: (301) 587-2365; email: paulab@aspen.nutr.org
Internet: http://www.nutritioncare.org/wcontent.aspx?id=878
Sponsor: American Society for Parenteral and Enteral Nutrition
8630 Fenton Street, Suite 412
Silver Spring, MD 20910

ASPET Benedict R. Lucchesi Award in Cardiac Pharmacology **638**

The Benedict R. Lucchesi Award in Cardiac Pharmacology was established to honor Dr. Lucchesi's lifelong scientific contributions to our better understanding and appreciation of pharmacological treatment and prevention of cardiovascular disease and for his mentoring of countless prominent functional (in vivo) cardiovascular pharmacologists. The Benedict R. Lucchesi Award is a biennial award, consisting an honorarium of $1,000, a custom-designed crystal bowl depicting the named Lectureship, and up to

$2,000 travel expenses including registration to the annual spring ASPET meeting. A recipient will be selected and invited to deliver a state-of-the-art lecture on recent advances in the field of cardiac and electropharmacology at the spring ASPET meeting (Division's programming session). The presentation of his/her research should be of broad interest and contribute to the growth of the Cardiovascular Pharmacology Division.
Requirements: There are no restrictions on institutional affiliation, nationality, or age of the candidate, but the recipient must be a member of the ASPET. Nominations must be made by a member of the ASPET, and no member may nominate more than one candidate per year.
Amount of Grant: $1,000 honorarium; $2,000 maximum for travel
Date(s) Application is Due: Sep 15
Contact: Christine Carrico, Ph.D., Executive Officer; (301) 634-7060; fax: (301) 634-7061; email: ccarrico@aspet.org or info@aspet.org
Internet: http://www.aspet.org/public/divisions/cardiovascular/lucchesi_award.htm
Sponsor: American Society for Pharmacology and Experimental Therapeutics
9650 Rockville Pike
Bethesda, MD 20814-3995

ASPET Bernard B. Brodie Award in Drug Metabolism **639**
This biennial award (even-numbered years), established by CIBA-GEIGY Corporation to honor the fundamental contributions of Bernard B. Brodie, is presented to recognize outstanding original research contributions in drug metabolism and disposition, particularly those having a major impact on future research in the field. Only one nominator is necessary although more are acceptable. The award consists of a $2,000 honorarium, a commemorative medal, hotel and economy airfare to the award ceremony at the annual meeting. Nominations must be received by deadline prior to the award year.
Requirements: Nominees must be members of ASPET; nominators need not be members of ASPET.
Restrictions: Supporting research accomplishments must not have been used to win any other major award.
Amount of Grant: $2,000
Date(s) Application is Due: Sep 15
Contact: Christine Carrico, Ph.D., Executive Officer; (301) 634-7060; fax: (301) 634-7061; email: ccarrico@aspet.org or info@aspet.org
Internet: http://www.aspet.org/public/awards/brodie_award.html
Sponsor: American Society for Pharmacology and Experimental Therapeutics
9650 Rockville Pike
Bethesda, MD 20814-3995

ASPET Division for Drug Metabolism Early Career Achievement Award **640**
The ASPET Division for Drug Metabolism Early Career Achievement Award has been established to recognize excellent original research by early career investigators in the area of drug metabolism and disposition. The award is presented biennially in odd-numbered years. The award consists of $1,000, a plaque, and complimentary registration plus travel expenses (to a maximum of $1,000) for the winner to attend the award ceremony at the annual meeting. The awardee will deliver a lecture at the annual meeting describing their relevant research accomplishments. The awardee will be invited to publish a review article on the subject matter of the award lecture in Drug Metabolism and Disposition.
Requirements: Nominees for this award must have a doctoral degree (e.g. Ph.D., M.D., Pharm. D., D.V.M.) and must be within 15 years of having received their final degree, as of December 31 of the year of the award. There are no restrictions on institutional affiliation and a candidate need not be a member of ASPET.
Amount of Grant: $1,000 honorarium; $1,000 maximum for travel
Date(s) Application is Due: Sep 15
Contact: Christine Carrico, Ph.D., Executive Officer; (301) 634-7060; fax: (301) 634-7061; email: ccarrico@aspet.org or info@aspet.org
Internet: http://www.aspet.org/public/divisions/drugmetab/early_achievement_award.htm
Sponsor: American Society for Pharmacology and Experimental Therapeutics
9650 Rockville Pike
Bethesda, MD 20814-3995

ASPET Epilepsy Research Award for Outstanding Contributions to the Pharmacology of Antiepileptic Drugs **641**
The International League Against Epilepsy (ILAE) has sponsored this biennial award of $2,000 and a Certification of Citation to be awarded by the American Society for Pharmacology and Experimental Therapeutics, for the purpose of recognizing and stimulating outstanding research leading to better clinical control of epileptic seizures. This research may include the basic screening and testing of new therapeutic agents, studies on mechanisms of action, metabolic disposition, pharmacokinetics, and clinical pharmacology studies. The recipient will be selected by the Epilepsy Award Committee appointed by the President of ASPET, with representation of ILAE.
Requirements: Nominations for the Award may be submitted by members of any recognized scientific association, domestic or foreign.
Amount of Grant: $2,000
Date(s) Application is Due: Sep 15
Contact: Christine Carrico, Ph.D., Executive Officer; (301) 634-7060; fax: (301) 634-7061; email: ccarrico@aspet.org or info@aspet.org
Internet: http://www.aspet.org/public/awards/epilepsy_award.html
Sponsor: American Society for Pharmacology and Experimental Therapeutics
9650 Rockville Pike
Bethesda, MD 20814-3995

ASPET Goodman and Gilman Award in Drug Receptor Pharmacology **642**
This award is given biennially (even-numbered years) to recognize and stimulate outstanding research in the pharmacology of biological receptors. It is the hope that such research might provide a better understanding of the mechanism of biological processes and potentially provide the basis for the discovery of drugs useful in the treatment of diseases. The award includes a monetary prize and travel support for winner and spouse to attend the award ceremony. Nominations must be received September 15 of the year prior to the year in which the award will be made.
Requirements: Nominations must be made by ASPET members; however, there are no restrictions as to age, sex, nationality, or institutional affiliation. Nominee need not be a member of ASPET.
Amount of Grant: $2,500 honorarium
Date(s) Application is Due: Sep 15
Contact: Christine Carrico, Ph.D., Executive Officer; (301) 634-7060; fax: (301) 634-7061; email: ccarrico@aspet.org or info@aspet.org
Internet: http://www.aspet.org/awards/goodman_and_gilman/
Sponsor: American Society for Pharmacology and Experimental Therapeutics
9650 Rockville Pike
Bethesda, MD 20814-3995

ASPET John J. Abel Award in Pharmacology **643**
This award, sponsored by Eli Lilly and Company and administered by ASPET, is given annually to stimulate original and outstanding fundamental research in pharmacology and experimental therapeutics by young investigators. Candidates may not have passed their 39th birthday as of April 30 of the year of the award, or previously received an award from the sponsor for the same technical accomplishment.
Requirements: Candidates need not be members of the society; however, nominations must be made by ASPET members.
Amount of Grant: $2,500
Date(s) Application is Due: Sep 15
Contact: Christine Carrico, Ph.D., Executive Officer; (301) 634-7060; fax: (301) 634-7061; email: ccarrico@aspet.org or info@aspet.org
Internet: http://www.aspet.org/public/awards/abel_award.html
Sponsor: American Society for Pharmacology and Experimental Therapeutics
9650 Rockville Pike
Bethesda, MD 20814-3995

ASPET Julius Axelrod Award in Pharmacology **644**
The Julius Axelrod Award is presented annually for significant contributions to understanding the biochemical mechanisms underlying the pharmacological actions of drugs and for contributions to mentoring other pharmacologists. The award consists of an honorarium of $5,000, a medal, hotel and economy airfare for the winner and spouse to the annual meeting. The formal presentation of this award and medal will be made at the annual meeting of ASPET. The recipient will be invited by the President of the Society to deliver the Julius Axelrod Lecture and organize the Julius Axelrod Symposium at the annual meeting a year hence. The recipient will also be invited by the Catecholamine Club to give a less formal presentation at its annual dinner meeting that year of the award.
Amount of Grant: $5,000 honorarium
Date(s) Application is Due: Sep 15
Contact: Christine Carrico, Ph.D., Executive Officer; (301) 634-7060; fax: (301) 634-7061; email: ccarrico@aspet.org or info@aspet.org
Internet: http://www.aspet.org/public/awards/axelrod_award.html
Sponsor: American Society for Pharmacology and Experimental Therapeutics
9650 Rockville Pike
Bethesda, MD 20814-3995

ASPET P. B. Dews Lifetime Achievement Award for Research in Behavioral Pharmacology **645**
ASPET's Division of Behavioral Pharmacology sponsors the P. B. Dews Award for Research in Behavioral Pharmacology to recognize outstanding lifetime achievements in research, teaching and professional service in the field of Behavioral Pharmacology and to honor Peter Dews for his seminal contributions to the development of behavioral pharmacology as a discipline. The Award consists of $750, a plaque, and partial travel expenses to the award ceremony at the ASPET annual meeting. The recipient will be invited by the Chair of the Division of Behavioral Pharmacology to deliver a special lecture on this occasion. The lecture will be published subsequently in an appropriate ASPET-sponsored publication.
Requirements: Nominations may be made by members of ASPET or of any relevant scientific society.
Restrictions: There are no restrictions on nominees for this award.
Amount of Grant: $750
Date(s) Application is Due: Sep 15
Contact: Christine Carrico, Ph.D., Executive Officer; (301) 634-7060; fax: (301) 634-7061; email: ccarrico@aspet.org or info@aspet.org
Internet: http://www.aspet.org/public/awards/dews_award.html
Sponsor: American Society for Pharmacology and Experimental Therapeutics
9650 Rockville Pike
Bethesda, MD 20814-3995

ASPET Paul M. Vanhoutte Award **646**
The Paul M. Vanhoutte Award in Vascular Pharmacology was established to honor Dr. Vanhoutte's lifelong scientific contributions to our better understanding and appreciation

of the importance of endothelial cells and vascular smooth muscle function in health and disease and for his mentoring of countless prominent endothelial and vascular biologists and pharmacologists. This is a biennial award, consisting an honorarium of $1,000, a custom-designed crystal bowl depicting the named Lectureship, and up to $2,000 travel expenses including registration to the annual spring ASPET meeting.
Requirements: There are no restrictions on institutional affiliation, nationality, or age of the candidate, but the recipient must be a member of the ASPET.
Amount of Grant: $1,000 honorarium; $2,000 maximum for travel
Date(s) Application is Due: Sep 15
Contact: Christine Carrico, Ph.D., Executive Officer; (301) 634-7060; fax: (301) 634-7061; email: ccarrico@aspet.org or info@aspet.org
Internet: http://www.aspet.org/public/divisions/cardiovascular/vanhoutte_award.htm
Sponsor: American Society for Pharmacology and Experimental Therapeutics
9650 Rockville Pike
Bethesda, MD 20814-3995

ASPET Torald Sollmann Award in Pharmacology **647**
This award, established by Wyeth-Herst Labs, is given in odd-numbered years to commemorate the pioneer work in the United States of Dr. Torald Sollmann in the fields of pharmacological investigation and education. The award is made to a nominee for significant contributions over many years to the advancement and extension of knowledge in the field of pharmacology. The award consists of an honorarium of $3,500, a medal, hotel and economy airfare for the winner and spouse to the annual meeting. The formal presentation of this biennial award and medal will be made at the annual meeting of ASPET. The recipient will be invited by the President of the Society to deliver a lecture to the membership that may be published in an appropriate ASPET journal.
Requirements: Nominations must be made by ASPET members; however, the nominee need not be a member. There are no restrictions as to age or institutional affiliation.
Amount of Grant: $3,500
Date(s) Application is Due: Sep 15
Contact: Christine Carrico, Ph.D., Executive Officer; (301) 634-7060; fax: (301) 634-7061; email: ccarrico@aspet.org or info@aspet.org
Internet: http://www.aspet.org/public/awards/sollmann_award.html
Sponsor: American Society for Pharmacology and Experimental Therapeutics
9650 Rockville Pike
Bethesda, MD 20814-3995

ASPET Travel Awards **648**
Graduate Student Travel Awards, Minority Graduate Student Travel Awards, and Summer Undergraduate Student Travel Awards are a fixed sum of $600 plus registration. Young Scientist Travel Awards and Minority Young Scientist Travel Awards are a fixed sum of $600 plus registration. All travel awards are inclusive of registration and are given to partially defray the costs of travel and housing. The check for the award and an award certificate will be presented at the annual ASPET Opening Awards Ceremony. Applications will be available in late September.
Requirements: Applications must be submitted electronically online or as email attachments.
Amount of Grant: $600
Date(s) Application is Due: Dec 1
Contact: Christine Carrico, Ph.D., Executive Officer; (301) 634-7060; fax: (301) 634-7061; email: ccarrico@aspet.org or travelawards@aspet.org
Internet: http://www.aspet.org/public/awards/awards_fellowships.html#Travel_Awards
Sponsor: American Society for Pharmacology and Experimental Therapeutics
9650 Rockville Pike
Bethesda, MD 20814-3995

ASPET-Astellas Awards in Translational Pharmacology **649**
The ASPET-Astellas Awards in Translational Pharmacology are intended to extend fundamental research closer to applications directed towards improving human health. The awards will be given to: recognize those individuals whose research has the potential to lead to the introduction of novel pharmacologic approaches or technologies that may offer significant advances in clinical medicine in the future; and to facilitate that translational process. Three (3) awards of $30,000 each will be made to individuals. The money may be used for supplemental research funding, travel, training, or in any way that furthers the goals of the organization. Nominations should be made electronically.
Requirements: Any ASPET member in good standing may nominate an individual for this award.
Restrictions: Self-nominations will not be accepted.
Amount of Grant: $30,000
Date(s) Application is Due: Sep 15
Contact: Christine Carrico, Ph.D., Executive Officer; (301) 634-7060; fax: (301) 634-7061; email: ccarrico@aspet.org or info@aspet.org
Internet: http://www.aspet.org/public/awards/Astellas_awards.html
Sponsor: American Society for Pharmacology and Experimental Therapeutics
9650 Rockville Pike
Bethesda, MD 20814-3995

ASPO Daiichi Innovative Technology Grant **650**
The Daiichi Innovative Technology Grant will fund exploratory or hypothesis-generating projects that are not well-suited to a formal grant application (eg, based on statistical analysis and sample size specification) such as: development of new surgical or diagnostic instruments; survey or quality of life measures; new use of internet technology or computer software such as CDs or DVDs; educational brochures, materials, software for patients or physicians; and other applications of innovative technology for education or research in pediatric otolaryngology. Full patent and copyright control must be retained by the applicant and the applicant's institution. If patented innovations funded by this award generate more than $5,000, the applicant may be required to return funds to the Society. One award of up to $5,000, to be used over a one-year period, will be given annually. Letters of Intent should be received no later than December 15, with full proposals due on January 15.
Requirements: Researchers (MD, PhD, DMD, DO) in disciplines who will conduct research directly relevant to innovative technology in pediatric otolaryngology are eligible to apply. Applications submitted by otolaryngologists or demonstrating collaborations with otolaryngologists are preferred. Participation of an ASPO member is not required, but is preferred.
Amount of Grant: $5,000
Date(s) Application is Due: Dec 15; Jan 15
Contact: Stephanie L. Jones, Assistant Director; (703) 519-1586 or (703) 836-4444; email: sljones@entnet.org
Internet: http://www.aspo.us/information.php?info_id=12
Sponsor: American Society for Pediatric Otolaryngology (ASPO)
One Prince Street
Alexandria, VA 22314-3357

ASPO Fellowships **651**
ASPO exists to foster excellence in the care of children with otorhinolaryngologic disorders through education and research and thereby enhance the profession of Pediatric Otolaryngology. Its fellowship program intends to: facilitate the creation and dissemination of knowledge about the care of infants and children with ORL disorders; serve as an advocate for infants and children with ORL disorders, ASPO members and others with shared goals; and preserve and promote dedication to excellent and humane care for infants and children with ORL disorders. See the web site for details and all available fellowships.
Contact: Stephanie L. Jones, Assistant Director; (703) 519-1586 or (703) 836-4444; email: sljones@entnet.org
Internet: http://www.aspo.us/fellowships.php
Sponsor: American Society for Pediatric Otolaryngology (ASPO)
One Prince Street
Alexandria, VA 22314-3357

ASPO Research Grants **652**
The American Society of Pediatric Otolaryngology (ASPO) awards funds annually to support innovative research in pediatric otolaryngology. ASPO will consider applications from both individuals and institutions. Preference is given to proposed projects that are to be completed within one year, although exceptional proposals that have duration in excess of one year will be considered. Two awards of up to $15,000, to be used over a one-year period, will be given annually. Letters of Intent should be received no later than December 15, with full proposals due on January 15.
Requirements: Researchers (MD, PhD, DMD) in disciplines who will conduct research directly relevant to pediatric otolaryngology are eligible to apply.
Restrictions: No portion of any grant may be used for travel expenses or for principal investigator salaries.
Amount of Grant: $15,000
Date(s) Application is Due: Dec 15; Jan 15
Contact: Stephanie L. Jones, Assistant Director; (703) 535-3747 or (703) 836-4444; email: sljones@entnet.org
Internet: http://www.aspo.us/information.php?info_id=12
Sponsor: American Society for Pediatric Otolaryngology (ASPO)
One Prince Street
Alexandria, VA 22314-3357

Assisi Foundation Grants **653**
The foundation supports organizations in its areas of interest, including health and human services—promote the health and well-being of the Mid-South community and help the healthcare system respond more effectively to community needs; education and literacy—projects/programs that build organizational capacity of provider agencies, provide professional development to service providers, promote collaboration among provider agencies, and leverage resources (local, state, and federal); social justice/ethics—projects/programs that strengthen ethical values among Mid-South citizens and promote social justice leading to a better understanding of and a more effective response to economic or social threats to the community; and cultural enrichment and the arts—projects/programs that foster an appreciation of the arts in the Greater Memphis community. Religious organizations seeking funding for religious programs also are eligible. Types of support include general grants, mini grants, and capital project grants. Deadlines are set to coordinate with quarterly meetings of the Board of Directors of the Foundation. Information and application are available online.
Requirements: Memphis-area and Shelby, Fayette, and Tipton Counties, TN, Crittenden County, AK, and Desota County, Mississippi nonprofit organizations are eligible.
Restrictions: Grants are not made for individuals, national fundraising drives, projects that address the needs of only one congregation, tickets for benefits, political organizations or candidates for public office, lobbying activities, recurring budget deficits, or tournament fees and/or travel for athletic competitions.
Geographic Focus: Tennessee
Samples: National Ornamental Metal Museum (Memphis, TN)—for a new library, $75,000 (2004); Memphis Urban League (TN)—to provide basic-skills, workplace-behavior, and computer training, $25,000 (2004); Christian Brothers U (Memphis,

TN)—for its LaSallian Assoc of New Catholic Educators Program, $90,000 over three years (2004); Saint Jude Children's Research Hospital (Memphis, TN)—for research in cell and gene therapy, $750,000 (2004).
Amount of Grant: $20,000 maximum
Contact: Jan Young, Director, (901) 684-1564; email: joung@assisifoundation.org
Internet: http://www.assisifoundation.org/generalgrants.html
Sponsor: Assisi Foundation
515 Erin Drive
Memphis, TN 38117

Assurant Foundation Grants **654**
The Foundation awards approximately 15 grants per year to improve the quality of life in the New York metropolitan community. The Foundation is committed to fulfilling the basic needs of the community, be they educational, health, nutrition, or housing.
Requirements: 501(c)3 nonprofits in the New York City metropolitan area are eligible.
Restrictions: As a general policy the foundation does not make grants to individuals; political parties, candidates or lobbying activities; religious organizations; or fundraising events.
Geographic Focus: New York
Amount of Grant: $5000 maximum
Contact: Kristy Hall, (212) 859-7000; email: Kristy.Hall@assurant.com
Internet: http://www.assurant.com/inc/assurant/community/new-york.html
Sponsor: Assurant Foundation
1 Chase Manhattan Pl, 41st Floor
New York, NY 10005

Assurant Health Foundation Grants **655**
The foundation awards grants in Wisconsin in its areas of interest, including health care access and promotion, disease prevention, the arts and education, as well as the foundation's national public policy initiatives. Types of support include capital campaigns, consulting services, continuing support, employee matching gifts, employee-related scholarships, in-kind gifts, matching/challenge support, and program development.
Requirements: Wisconsin nonprofit organizations are eligible. Preference is given to requests serving southeastern Wisconsin.
Restrictions: Unsolicited requests for funds not accepted. Requests for funds only accepted after the foundation sends out requests for proposals.
Geographic Focus: Wisconsin
Samples: Gerald Ignace Clinic (WI)—$10,000 (2005); Task Force on Family Violence (WI)—$10,000 (2005); Latino Arts Organization (WI)—$5000 (2005).
Contact: Grants Administrator, (414) 299-1348; email: megan.hindman@assurant.com
Internet: http://www.newsroom.eassuranthealth.com/corp/news/newsroom/articles/press_06092005.htm
Sponsor: Assurant Health Foundation
501 W Michigan Street
Milwaukee, WI 53203

Astellas Foundation Research Grants **656**
The Foundation was established with the objectives of contributing to the improvement of national health and welfare, and to the progress of therapeutic medicines. In fulfilling the objectives, the Foundation aims to conduct pioneering research in new fields of diseases and metabolisms of medicines, by elucidating the mechanism of diseases and their treatment, in particular the relationship between therapeutic medicines and in-situ metabolisms. Major activities include: subsidizing research on metabolic disorders related to the diagnosis of diseases and therapeutic medicine; publication and editing of periodicals for research achievements; supporting and production of educational movies; and other projects to achieve the objectives of the Foundation.
Contact: Grants Manager; +81-3-3244-3397; fax: +81-3-5201-8512
Sponsor: Astellas Foundation
2-3-11 Nihonbashihoncho, Chuo-ku
Tokyo 103-8411 Japan

AT&T Excelerator **657**
AT&T Excelerator helps nonprofit organizations better serve their communities by improving technology resources — including hardware, software and networking tools. These grants also fund resources, such as Internet access and computer training, to assist organizations with various programs, many aimed to increase educational learning and job skills development.
Requirements: The AT&T Foundation prefers to work with 501(c)3 public charity or government instrumentalities that have clearly stated objectives, long-range planning, active participation of the governing board and strategies that incorporate diversified sources of support. The Foundation also considers grants to organizations that qualify as government instrumentalities, including public libraries, police and fire departments and publicly funded social services agencies. The project you are seeking funding for should fall within at least one of the following four foundation funding priorities: Education, Community Development, Health & Human Services, Arts & Cultural Assets.
Restrictions: While unsolicited grant applications are accepted, few receive funding.
Geographic Focus: Alabama; Arkansas; California; Connecticut; Florida; Georgia; Illinois; Indiana; Kansas; Kentucky; Louisiana; Michigan; Mississippi; Missouri; Nevada; North Carolina; Ohio; Oklahoma; South Carolina; Tennessee; Texas; Wisconsin
Samples: Leader Dogs for the Blind (Rochester, Mich.) — Leader Dogs for the Blind received a $25,000 grant to launch a program geared toward blind and visually impaired individuals. The program will show individuals how to use specific hardware and software programs, along with technology devices, including Braille embossers and vocal bar readers.; Women's Intercultural Network Inc. (San Francisco) — Women's Intercultural Network received $25,000 for its Connecting California Women's Voices program. The program will use technology to reach out to low-income women in surrounding counties, and support its public policy advocacy.; Friends of the Dallas Public Library Inc. (Dallas) — Friends of the Dallas Public Library received a $25,000 grant to support a Teen Center with technology tools and training in South Dallas.
Amount of Grant: $1,000 to $25,000; One-time grants are the norm, and multi-year awards are given under special circumstances.
Date(s) Application is Due: May 4
Contact: Chris Chavez, AT&T PR Director; cchavez@attmail.com, 800-591-9663
Internet: http://www.att.com/excelerator
Sponsor: AT&T Foundation
AT&T Public Relations, 1875 Lawrence Street, Suite 825
Denver, CO 80202

AT&T Foundation Civic and Community Service Program Grants **658**
The foundation supports programs that enhance education by integrating new technologies and increasing learning opportunities, improve economic development through technology and local initiatives, provide vital assistance to key community-based organizations, support cultural institutions that make a community unique, and advance the goals and meet the needs of diverse populations.
Requirements: The foundation makes 501(c)3 grants to tax-exempt, nonprofit organizations in certain states. Requirements are available online.
Samples: Leader Dogs for the Blind (Rochester, Mich.) received a $25,000 grant for blind and visually impaired individuals. Communities in Schools of San Antonio - received a grant to enhance the technology infrastructure to reach more young people at risk of dropping out of school.
Contact: Marilyn Reznick; (212) 387-6555; fax: (212) 387-5097; email: reznick@att.com
Internet: http://www.att.com/gen/corporate-citizenship?pid=7736&DCMP=att_foundation
Sponsor: AT&T Foundation
32 Avenue of the Americas, 24th Floor
New York, NY 10013

Atherton Family Foundation Grants **659**
The foundation supports the establishment, maintenance, or promotion of such religious, charitable, educational, benevolent, scientific, or other like purposes in Hawaii. Types of support include general operating grants, equipment acquisition, capital fund projects, seed grants, and theology scholarships to children of ministers in the state. The grant period generally is one year, though some multiyear grants will be awarded. Applications are due one month prior to board meetings. Contact the office for application procedures.
Requirements: Hawaii nonprofit organizations are eligible.
Restrictions: Requests for annual operating support or mature programs, an organization that has already received a grant in the same calendar year (with some exceptions), individuals or for the benefit of specific individuals, loans, grants to endowment funds, private foundations, purpose of lobbying, conferences, festivals and one-time events, re-granting, or individual Department of Education schools not typically funded.
Geographic Focus: Hawaii
Amount of Grant: $2,000-$75,000 average
Date(s) Application is Due: Feb 1; Apr 1; Aug 1; Oct 1; Dec 1
Contact: Grant Coordinator; (808) 566-5524 or (888) 731-3863 ext. 524; fax: (808) 521-6286; email: foundations@hcf-hawaii.org
Internet: http://www.Athertonfamilyfoundation.org
Sponsor: Atherton Family Foundation
1164 Bishop Street, Suite 800
Honolulu, HI 96813

Athwin Foundation Grants **660**
Areas of interest include arts and humanities, education, human services, the natural environment, and organizational capacity building. General operating grants, capital grants, and special project grants will be awarded. Applications are accepted throughout the year.
Requirements: Tax-exempt organizations in the Twin Cities area of Minnesota and Western Montana are eligible.
Restrictions: Grants do not support individuals, scholarships, fellowships, or loans.
Geographic Focus: Minnesota; Montana
Samples: Claremont McKenna College (CA)—for program support, $30,000.; Minnesota Children's Museum (Saint Paul, MN)—to support the capital campaign, $5000.
Amount of Grant: $1000-$100,000 range
Date(s) Application is Due: Mar 1: Oct 1
Contact: Bruce Bean, Trustee, (952) 915-6165
Sponsor: Athwin Foundation
5200 Wilson Road, Suite 307
Minneapolis, MN 55424

Atkinson Foundation International Grants **661**
International grants are awarded to contribute to the efforts of U.S. nonprofits working to assist people toward economic, social, and physical self-sufficiency and well-being. The foundation also awards grants in San Mateo County, CA. Primary areas of interest include the disadvantaged and the homeless, child welfare, family planning, and the disabled. Grants support social services, including youth and the elderly, education,

AIDS programs, and the United Methodist Church. Organizations should contact the foundation by phone prior to applying. Listed application deadlines are for international programs; there are no deadlines for domestic grants.
Requirements: International grants are awarded to organizations working in the Caribbean, Central America, and Mexico; domestic grants are awarded in San Mateo County, CA. Organizations should contact the foundation by phone prior to applying.
Restrictions: The fund does not make grants to organizations without proof of tax-exempt status; grants to organizations chartered outside the United States; grants, scholarships, or loans to individuals; grants designed to influence legislation; grants for doctoral study or research; grants for travel to conferences or events; grants for media presentations; donations to annual campaigns or special fund-raising events; sponsorship of sports groups; or grants to national or statewide umbrella organizations.
Geographic Focus: CaliforniaCaribbean; Central America; Mexico
Samples: Community Career Education Ctr (San Mateo, CA)—to upgrade computer training equipment, $4000.
Amount of Grant: $5000-$10,000 range
Date(s) Application is Due: Feb 1; May 1; Aug 1; Nov 1
Contact: Elizabeth Curtis, Administrator, (650) 357-1101; email: atkinfdn@aol.com
Internet: atkinsonfdn.org
Sponsor: Atkinson Foundation
1720 Amphlett Boulevard, Suite 100
San Mateo, CA 94402

Atlanta Foundation Grants **662**
Grants are awarded to assist Georgia charitable and educational institutions to improve the quality of life in Fulton and DeKalb Counties. Primary areas of interest include education, cultural programs, housing, and other charitable giving. Additional areas of support include adult basic education and literacy training; higher education; health care organizations; recreation; and youth, family, and human services. The board meets in August to consider requests.
Requirements: Nonprofit organizations in Georgia's DeKalb and Fulton Counties may apply for grant support.
Restrictions: Grants are not awarded to individuals or for scholarships, fellowships, or loans.
Geographic Focus: Georgia
Amount of Grant: $2500-$50,000 range
Date(s) Application is Due: Mar 1; Sep 1
Contact: Trustee, Wachovia Bank of Georgia, email: grantinquiriesga@wachovia.com
Internet: http://www.wachovia.com/corp_inst/charitable_services/0,,4269_3296,00.html
Sponsor: Atlanta Foundation
3414 Peachtree Road, 5th Fl, MC GA8023
Atlanta, GA 30326

Atran Foundation Grants **663**
The foundation supports Jewish nonprofits with a focus on New York and Israel in the areas of higher education, Jewish education, religious education, community services, Jewish welfare, temples, international ministries and missions, temples, medical centers, and women's affairs. Types of support include conferences and seminars, endowment funds, general support, matching funds, multiyear/continuing support, project support, research, scholarships, and seed money grants. The foundation requires that proposals be in writing. Proposals should include the nature of the project, its objectives and significance, time estimate, and budget.
Requirements: 501(c)3 tax-exempt Jewish organizations are eligible.
Restrictions: Grants are not made to individuals.
Samples: Yivo Institute for Jewish Research (New York, NY)—for project support, $90,000.; Brandeis University (Waltham, MA)—for operating support, $28,000.; Folksbiene Yiddish Theater (New York, NY)—for operating support, $15,000.
Amount of Grant: $250-$100,000 average
Date(s) Application is Due: Sep 30
Contact: Diane Fischer, President, (212) 505-9677
Sponsor: Atran Foundation
23-25 E 21st Street, 3rd Floor
New York, NY 10010

Auburn Foundation Grants **664**
The purpose of the Foundation is to stimulate giving and cooperative leadership among the citizens of Auburn; help improve the lives of all community residents, especially those who are most vulnerable; and enrich the cultural environment and community life. Of special interest are projects that bring together all ages and sections of the town, or that contribute to healthy, active living. Application is available online.
Requirements: Any nonprofit organization that serves residents of Auburn can apply.
Restrictions: Grants will not be awarded to for-profit businesses or expenses already incurred by the applicant.
Geographic Focus: Massachusetts
Samples: Bancroft School (Worcester, MA)—for general support, $45,000.; New England Science Ctr, Rutland House (Worcester, MA)—for repairs, $20,000.; Tower Hill Botanic Garden (Boylston, MA)—for general support, $30,000.
Amount of Grant: $5,000
Date(s) Application is Due: Apr 15
Contact: Lois Smith, Senior Program Officer; (508) 755-0980, ext. 107; email: lsmith@greaterworcester.org
Internet: http://www.greaterworcester.org/grants/Auburn.htm
Sponsor: Auburn Foundation
370 Main Street, Suite 650
Worcester, MA 01608-1738

Audrey and Sydney Irmas Charitable Foundation Grants **665**
The foundation awards grants to eligible nonprofit organizations in its areas of interest, including arts and culture, higher education, homeless and urban issues, hospitals, and Jewish welfare. Grants support long-term, nonrenewable pledges and general operating grants. Most grants are made to Los Angeles County, CA, nonprofits.
Requirements: 501(c)3 nonprofit organizations are eligible.
Geographic Focus: California
Samples: Childrens Hospital of Los Angeles (Los Angeles, CA)—$2810.65.; Jewish Family Services (Los Angeles, CA)—$500.; Downtown Womens Center (Los Angeles, CA)—$200.; Carnegie Museum of Art (Pittsburg, PA)—$25,000.
Amount of Grant: $1000-$75,000 average
Contact: Robert Irmas, (818) 382-3313; fax: (818) 382-3315; email: robirm@aol.com
Sponsor: Audrey and Sydney Irmas Charitable Foundation
16830 Ventura Boulevard, Suite 364
Encino, CA 91436-2797

AUPHA Baxter International Foundation Prize for Health Services Research **666**
The prize acknowledges national or international contributions of health services research, defined as a product of the application of analytic methods to the organization, financing, and/or delivery of health services. An individual's specific contribution or a career-long achievement may be recognized. The prize recognizes a person who has made significant and demonstrable contributions to the health of the public in three primary focus areas: health services management, health policy development, and health care delivery.
Requirements: Nominations must include a letter of nomination, two letters of recommendation, and a current curriculum vita. Nominations should focus on the nominee's contribution in the areas of health services management, health policy development, and health care delivery. Nominations should be sent to and further information can be obtained from the Secretary, HSR Prize Committee, AUPHA, 2000 N. 14th Street, Suite 780, Arlington, VA 22201.
Amount of Grant: $10,000 personal award and $15,000 to a nonprofit institution designated by the recipient, to support his or her work
Date(s) Application is Due: Dec 15
Contact: Lydia Reed, (703) 894-0940; email: lydia.reed@aupha.org
Internet: http://www.e-guana.net/organizations.php3?action=printContentItem&orgid=75&typeID=506&itemID=3744
Sponsor: Association of University Programs in Health Administration
2000 14th St N, Suite 780
Arlington, VA 22201

Aurora Foundation Grants **667**
The foundation provides grants to eligible nonprofit organizations in the following categories: education, social services, health care, and the arts and humanities. In general, grants are made for capital purposes only, not for operating expenses. Evidence of tax-exempt status must be submitted with all applications. Preference will be given to requests that demonstrate the most urgent and immediate need for funding. Grants are ordinarily made for one year only.
Requirements: 501(c)3 and 170(b)1a nonprofit agencies located in the foundation's service area, which includes the City of Aurora, southern Kane County, and Kendall County in Illinois, are eligible.
Restrictions: The foundation rarely provides the entire support of a project. Grants are not generally available for those agencies and institutions that are funded primarily through tax support. Telephone the office prior to submitting a formal proposal.
Geographic Focus: Illinois
Date(s) Application is Due: Aug 1
Contact: Grants Administrator, (630) 896-7800; email: grant@aurorafdn.org
Internet: http://www.aurorafdn.org/grantmaking.html
Sponsor: Aurora Foundation
111 W Downer Pl, Suite 312
Aurora, IL 60506

Austin College Leadership Award **658**
The award honors an outstanding individual who through his/her life's work has demonstrated the principles of servant leadership by: taking a courageous stand on a public policy issue that advances a humanitarian or educational purpose; serving the youth of a state, nation, or international community to improve the quality of health, educational, or community services; or creating opportunities for young people that help them enhance their educational experience and move to a new level of service to society. The recipient also will visit Austin College to speak to community leaders and interact with students and faculty. Nomination form and guidelines are available online.
Requirements: Nominees will be leaders from all levels whose leadership position will have placed him/her in a unique and special position among leaders throughout the world.
Amount of Grant: $100,000
Date(s) Application is Due: Jun 1
Contact: Award Administrator, (903) 813-2000
Internet: http://www.austincollege.edu/category.asp?3523
Sponsor: Austin College
900 N Grand Avenue
Sherman, TX 75090-4400

Austin-Bailey Health and Wellness Foundation Grants 669

The foundation awards grants to Ohio nonprofit organizations to support programs that promote the physical and mental well-being of the citizens of Holmes, Stark, Tuscarawas and Wayne Counties in the state of Ohio. The Foundation emphasizes healthcare affordability concerns of the uninsured adn underinsured, the poor, children, single parents and the aging. It also advocates programs that speak to the mental health needs of the individuals and families. Opportunities to work with other foundations and organizations to promote the principles of health and wellness are welcome.
Requirements: Applicant organizations must provide a current copy of IRS determination indicating 501(c)3 and 509(a) tax-exempt status; serve part or all of the four county area of Holmes, Stark, Tuscarawas, and Wayne; provide a description of the organization and its activities; state the need to be addressed; and provide a brief description of the project or program and how it will address the health and wellness needs of the community.
Restrictions: The foundation generally does not support annual appeals or membership drives; fund-raising events, program advertising, lobbying activities, endowment funds or organizations not classified as tax exempt by the IRS.
Geographic Focus: Ohio
Amount of Grant: $1000-$15,000
Date(s) Application is Due: Jun 30; Dec 30
Contact: Grants Administrator, (330) 580-2380; fax: (330) 580-2381; email: abfdn@sbcglobal.net
Internet: http://fdncenter.org/grantmaker/austinbailey/guide.html
Sponsor: Austin-Bailey Health and Wellness Foundation
2719 Fulton Rd NW, Suite D
Canton, OH 44718

Australian Academy of Science Grants 670

The objectives of the Academy are to promote science through a range of activities. It has defined four major program areas as their focus. The Academy focus is on recognition of outstanding contributions to science, education and public awareness, science policy, and international relations. Guidelines are available online.
Contact: Executive Secretary, 61-2-6201-9400; fax: 61-2-6201-9494; email: eb@science.org.au
Internet: http://www.science.org.au
Sponsor: Australian Academy of Science
GP.O. Box 783
Canberra, ACT 2601 Australia

Autodesk Community Relations Grants 671

Autodesk plays an active role in the communities where employees live and work. Grants are awarded to local nonprofit organizations in the program's areas of interest, including community development, arts, the disabled, education, environment, health and human services, science and technology, and civic affairs. Grants are awarded on a national basis. Preference is given to organizations where Autodesk does business. There are no application deadlines. Written proposal requirements are available online.
Requirements: 501(c)3 tax-exempt organizations are eligible.
Restrictions: Grants do not support sporting events or athletic teams, churches or religious organizations, political parties or organizations, general advertising, video, film or television productions, individuals, subscription fees or admission tickets, fraternal, veteran or sectarian groups or direct funds to Autodesk employees participating in fund-raising events.
Amount of Grant: $1000-$3000 average
Contact: Community Relations, fax: (415) 507-6138
Internet: http://usa.autodesk.com/adsk/servlet/index?siteID=123112&id=1064603
Sponsor: Autodesk Inc
111 McInnis Pkwy
San Rafael, CA 94903

Autzen Foundation Grants 672

The foundation awards grants to Oregon nonprofit organizations in its areas of interest of arts, children/youth, services, environment, health care, higher education, human services, and performing arts. Types of support include building construction/renovation, continuing support, matching/challenge grants, program development, and seed grants.
Requirements: Nonprofit organizations in the Pacific Northwest are eligible with an emphasis on those in Oregon.
Restrictions: Grants do not support individuals, scholarships, fellowships, or loans.
Geographic Focus: Oregon; Pacific Northwest
Samples: Northwest Habitat Institute (Corvalis, OR)—$1000.; American Business Women's Assoc (Beaverton, OR)—$2000.; Gearhart Volunteer Fire Department (OR)—$2000.; American Lung Assoc (Portland, OR)—$5000.
Amount of Grant: $200-$27,000 range
Date(s) Application is Due: Apr 15; Aug 15; Nov 15
Contact: Robin Stewart, Administrator, (503) 226-6051
Sponsor: Autzen Foundation
P.O. Box 3709
Portland, OR 97208

AVDF Health Care Grants 673

This program supports efforts to encourage caring attitudes in the delivery of patient care. Projects should have potential for widespread practical application and should be of interest to other groups. New ideas are encouraged, especially if they facilitate communication between patients (and their families) and doctors, nurses and other caregivers; ameliorate patient anxieties; strengthen trust and cooperation; and foster caring attitudes. Proposals, must have potential for wide application and not merely local improvement of requesting institutions or their communities.
Requirements: Proposals should be submitted by the head of the institution under whose auspices the project would be accomplished.
Samples: Southern Illinois U School of Medicine (IL)—for a program designed to foster caring attitudes toward aging patients, $195,523 (2005); U of Chicago, Pritzker School of Medicine (IL)—to expand the community-based teaching of cross-cultural patient-doctor communication, $199,986 (2005); U of Massachusetts Medical School (Worcester, MA)—for efforts to identify the unique attributes of a caring attitude in health-care settings, $198,314 (2005).
Amount of Grant: $100,000-$200,000
Contact: Dr. Jonathan Howe, Executive Director, (904) 359-0670; email: arthurvining@msn.com
Internet: http://jvm.com/davis/PROGRAMS.HTM#health
Sponsor: Arthur Vining Davis Foundations
225 Water Street, Suite 1510
Jacksonville, FL 32202-5185

Avon Foundation Breast Care Fund Grants 674

The fund awards grants for the development of breast cancer education and outreach activities, particularly breast health education and early detection services for underserved women. AFBCF supports programs that: recruit women for both first time screening and annual screening; develop partnerships between community-based outreach providers and local medical providers; work with health care providers to ensure proper clinical follow-up of abnormal screening results; and educate older women (65+ years old) about Medicare coverage of annual screening mammograms and assist them in obtaining the service from providers who accept Medicare.
Requirements: Private, non-government, nonprofit organizations in the United States and Puerto Rico are eligible. Grants are awarded to community-based programs and/or health care agencies that provide medically under-served women aged 40 and older with direct access to breast cancer education, annual clinical screening services, and prompt follow-up care. All programs must utilize the three-part approach to breast cancer early detection including regular screening mammography, clinical breast examination, and monthly breast self-examination.
Samples: Family Services Center of Coffee County, Enterprise, AL (2007); The Witness Project, University of Arkansas for Medical Sciences, Little Rock, AR (2007); Latino Community Development Agency, Oklahoma City, OK (2007).
Amount of Grant: $30,000-$50,000
Date(s) Application is Due: Aug 28
Contact: Coordinating Center; (212) 244-5368; fax: (212) 695-3081; email: admin@avonbreast care.org
Internet: http://www.avonbreastcare.org/fundinginfo.htm
Sponsor: Avon Foundation
505 Eighth Avenue, Suite 1601
New York, NY 10018-6505

Avon Products Foundation Grants 675

The foundation's two-fold focus is to support education, community and social services, and arts organizations and programs that provide economic opportunities for women and girls; and to support breast cancer and other women's health organizations and programs. The foundation awards grants in cities and regions with a large concentration of representatives and business operations, with the majority of funds going to U.S.-based institutions. National, international, and New York metropolitan area programs are administered through the foundation's headquarters in New York.
Requirements: Applying organizations must be tax-exempt; national and municipal organizations are eligible. Request the guidelines brochure prior to submitting a formal proposal.
Restrictions: Grants do not support individuals; memberships; lobbying organizations; political activities and organizations; religious, veteran, or fraternal organizations; fundraising events; and journal advertisements.
Samples: World Trade Ctr Memorial Foundation (new York, NY)—to build the World Trade Center Memorial and a museum to remember the September 11, 2001, and February 26, 1993, terrorist attacks, $325,000 (2005); Red Cross and Red Crescent Societies (Geneva, Switzerland) and U.S. Fund for UNICEF (New York, NY)—to assist tsunami-relief efforts, $500,000 jointly (2005); Family Violence Prevention Fund (San Francisco, CA)—to develop an educational program available online and in print on relationship violence, $100,000 (2004); Georgetown U, Lombardi Cancer Ctr (Washington, DC)—to provide breast-health education and care at the Capital Breast Care Ctr, $500,000 (2004).
Amount of Grant: $2.3 million total
Contact: Grants Administrator, (866) 505-2866; email: info@avonfoundation.org
Internet: http://www.avoncompany.com/women/avonfoundation
Sponsor: Avon Products Foundation
1345 Avenue of the Americas
New York, NY 10105

Award for Creative Advances in Environmental Science and Technology 676

The purpose of the Award is to encourage creativity in research and technology or methods of analysis to provide a scientific basis for informed environmental control decision-making processes, or to provide practical technologies that will reduce health risk factors. The award consists of $5,000 and a certificate. Reasonable travel expenses to the meeting at which the award will be presented will be reimbursed.

Requirements: Any individual, except a member of the award committee, may submit one nomination or seconding letter for the award in any given year. The nominating documents consist of a letter of not more than 1000 words containing an evaluation of the nominee's accomplishments and a specific identification of the work to be recognized, a biographical sketch including date of birth, and a list of publications and patents authored by the nominee.
Restrictions: The award will be granted without regard to age or nationality. Self-nominations are not accepted.
Samples: Margaret A. Tolbert—award recipient, $5,000 (2009); Susan D. Richardson—award recipient, $5,000 (2008); Richard C. Flagan—award recipient, $5,000 (2007).
Amount of Grant: $5,000 and allowance of up to $1000 for travel expenses to award meeting
Date(s) Application is Due: Nov 1
Contact: Felicia Dixon, Awards Administrator; (800) 227-5558 or (202) 872-4408; fax: (202) 776-8008; email: f_dixon@acs.org or awards@acs.org
Internet: http://portal.acs.org/portal/acs/corg/content?_nfpb=true&_pageLabel=PP_ARTICLEMAIN&node_id=1319&content_id=CTP_004504&use_sec=true&sec_url_var=region1
Sponsor: American Chemical Society
1155 Sixteenth Street, NW
Washington, DC 20036

Award in Separations Science and Technology **677**

This award is given annually to recognize outstanding accomplishments in fundamental or applied research directed to separations science and technology. The award shall be granted to an individual without regard to age or nationality. The scope of the award is to be as broad as possible, covering all fields where separations science and technology is practiced, including but not limited to biology, chemistry, engineering, geology, and medicine.
Requirements: Any individual, except a member of the award committee, may submit one nomination or seconding letter for the award in any given year. The nominating documents consist of a letter of not more than 1000 words containing an evaluation of the nominee's accomplishments and a specific identification of the work to be recognized, a biographical sketch including date of birth, and a list of publications and patents authored by the nominee.
Restrictions: Self-nominations are not accepted.
Samples: Abraham M. Lenhoff—award recipient, $5,000 (2009); Allan S. Myerson—award winner, $5,000 (2008); William H. Pirkle—award winner, $5,000 (2004).
Amount of Grant: $5,000 and reimbursement of travel expenses to award meeting
Date(s) Application is Due: Nov 1
Contact: Felicia Dixon, Awards Administrator; (800) 227-5558 or (202) 872-4408; fax: (202) 776-8008; email: f_dixon@acs.org or awards@acs.org
Internet: http://portal.acs.org/portal/acs/corg/content?_nfpb=true&_pageLabel=PP_ARTICLEMAIN&node_id=1319&content_id=CTP_004552&use_sec=true&sec_url_var=region1
Sponsor: American Chemical Society
1155 Sixteenth Street, NW
Washington, DC 20036

Axe-Houghton Foundation Grants **678**

The foundation operates in the New York City metropolitan area exclusively for charitable, educational, and scientific purposes to foster and encourage an appreciation of the English language, with major emphasis on the spoken language. Priority is given to projects for the improvement of speech and its uses in the areas of public affairs, education, theater, poetry, debate, and the oral interpretation of literature. A portion of available funds is devoted to speech remediation and to scientific research pertaining to speech. Types of support include program grants and seed money grants.
Requirements: Initial inquiries should be by full proposal and should contain a brief statement of objective, duration of time required to complete this objective, qualifications of personnel responsible for conducting the project, and the general amounts of funds needed. The proposal should also indicate the degree of internal support committed.
Restrictions: Grants are made only to tax-exempt institutions and not to individuals, private foundations or organizations outside of the United States. Grants are not made for scholarships, fellowships, capital, or general support programs.
Geographic Focus: New York
Amount of Grant: $1000-$7500
Date(s) Application is Due: Sep 1
Contact: Claire Brook, President, (212) 909-8304
Internet: http://www.foundationcenter.org/grantmaker/axehoughton/index.html
Sponsor: Axe-Houghton Foundation
919 3rd Avenue, 2nd Floor
New York, NY 10022

Bacon Family Foundation Grants **679**

The foundation awards grants to Colorado nonprofit organizations in its areas of interest, including arts and culture, community development, disabilities, economic development, education, food distribution, environment, health care, historic preservation, homelessness, housing, literacy, recreation/parks, religion, social services, and youth. Types of support include capital campaigns, challenge/matching grants, equipment acquisition, general operating support, project grants, and seed grants. A letter should outline the project or program in brief but sufficient detail for the Foundation to initially evaluate the proposal. There are no application deadlines. The Bacon Family Foundation meets quarterly to consider applications.
Requirements: Colorado nonprofit organizations are eligible. Preference will be given to requests from western Colorado.
Restrictions: No grants are made to individuals.
Geographic Focus: Colorado
Contact: Linda Simpson; (970) 243-3767; email: lsimpson@wc-cf.org
Internet: http://www.wc-cf.org/bacon.htm
Sponsor: Bacon Family Foundation
P.O. Box 4570
Grand Junction, CO 81502-4570

Bailey Foundation Grants **680**

The foundation supports South Carolina nonprofits, primarily in Laurens County, its areas of interest, include: health clinics and organizations involved with theater, education, human services, business promotion, Christianity and awards college scholarships to students graduating from public high schools in Laurens County, South Carolina. Support is offered in the form of : capital campaigns; employee matching gifts; endowments; matching/challenge support; scholarship funds, including individual scholarships; annual campaigns; building/renovation grants. Initial contact may be by telephone or letter. Deadline for scholarship applications is April 15, contact Foundation to request an application form.
Requirements: Nonprofit organizations in Laurens County, South Carolina are eligible.
Restrictions: No grants to individuals (except scholarships), or for general operating support.
Geographic Focus: South Carolina
Samples: YMCA of Greater Clinton South Carolina, Clinton, SC, $50,000 (2007); South Carolina Independent Colleges and Universities, Columbia, SC, $20,000 (2007); Thornwell Home and School for Children, Clinton, SC, $25,500 (2007).
Amount of Grant: $2,500-$50,000 range
Date(s) Application is Due: Apr 15; Oct 1
Contact: Robert S. Link, Jr., Administration, Carolina First Bank, (864) 938-2632; fax: (864) 938-2669
Sponsor: Bailey Foundation
P.O. Box 494
Clinton, SC 29325-0494

Balance Bar Sports Individual/Team Grants **681**

The program awards grants to enable amateur athletes and teams to pursue a sport or recreational activity that enhances physical health. Past grants have supported equipment costs, training, and other activities related to archery, cycling, hiking, the martial arts, rock climbing, running, yoga, and other pursuits. Complete guidelines and application, which must be submitted online, are available on the Web site.
Requirements: U.S. citizens who are at least 18 years old and are amateur athletes/enthusiasts/hobbyists who have not competed in athletic activities as their main source of income are eligible. Amateur teams also may apply, provided that all members meet the above qualifications.
Amount of Grant: $500-$10,000
Date(s) Application is Due: Mar 15; Aug 30
Contact: Hunter PR, (212) 679-6600; fax: (212) 481-6076; email: atucker@hunterpr.com
Internet: http://www.balance.com/grants/default.aspx
Sponsor: Balance Bar
41 Madison Avenue, 5th Floor
New York, NY 10010

Balfe Family Foundation Grants **682**

The Balfe Family Foundation, established in Florida in 1999, has as its primary fields of interest: education, health care and research, human services, and social services. Types of support are typically in the form of general operations, service delivery support, and seed funding. There are particular application forms or deadlines with which to adhere. Applicants should contact the Foundation in writing, outlining the program and funding need.
Samples: Crystal Cathedral, Garden Grove, California, $1,200—religious contribution (2006); Greater Lafayette Community Foundation, Lafayette, Indiana, $48,594—for a general contribution (2006).
Amount of Grant: $50-$50,000 range
Contact: Opal M. Balfe, President; (954) 462-6300; fax: (954) 462-4607
Sponsor: Balfe Family Foundation
2731 N.E. 14 St. Causeway No. 829
Pomano Beach, FL 33062-3562

Ball Brothers Foundation General Grants **683**

Ball Brothers Foundation offers funding opportunities for initiatives that have one of the six broad subject areas: education; arts; culture and humanities; human services; public/society benefit; health; and environment. For those interested in school or community wellness, application must be submitted through application found under Ball Wellness Grants in the application materials.
Requirements: Ball Brothers Foundation is restricted by its charter to grants to nonprofit institutions and organizations within Indiana.
Restrictions: Applications are limited to organization and institutions within in the State of Indiana. The Foundation will not support: direct assistance to individuals or scholarships; applications coming from outside of Indiana; booster organizations; on-going salary requests of staff personnel to support an organization; services that the community-at-large should normally underwrite (i.e. roads, bus transportation,

etc.0; capital building projects; research projects (except for philanthropic studies); or unsolicited proposals (all requests must begin with a preliminary proposal).
Geographic Focus: Indiana
Amount of Grant: $5,000 - $100,000 range
Date(s) Application is Due: Feb 15; Jul 15
Contact: Donna Munchel; (765) 741-5500; fax: (765) 741-5518; email: donna.munchel@ballfdn.org
Internet: http://www.ballfdn.org/index/staff/generalinfo.asp
Sponsor: Ball Brothers Foundation
222 South Mulberry Street
Muncie, IN 47305

Ball Brothers Foundation Grants 684
The foundation seeks to build and sustain a high quality of life in Indiana by awarding grants to nonprofit organizations in broad subject areas, including elementary, secondary, higher, and adult basic education and literacy skills; cultural activities; community betterment; and health and human services. Usually Muncie and Delaware Counties receive a higher priority for funding than requests from within East Central Indiana or across the state. Types of support include general operations, annual campaigns, capital campaigns, building construction/renovation, program development, conferences and seminars, professorships, publication, curriculum development, research, fellowships, matching funds, seed grants, and technical assistance. Preference will be given to catalytic grants that will stimulate others to participate in problem solving or in matching fund programs and to innovative approaches for addressing either traditional or emerging community needs. Applications are reviewed by the board of directors in January, May, and September of each calendar year. Proposals are encouraged to be submitted from February to May. Grant seekers may send a preliminary proposal, complete proposal, or ask for a personal visit to discuss a potential grant request.
Requirements: Indiana nonprofit institutions and organizations are eligible.
Restrictions: The Foundation will not support: direct assistance to individuals or scholarships; applications coming from outside of Indiana; booster organizations; on-going salary requests of staff personnel to support an organization; services that the community-at-large should normally underwrite (i.e. roads, bus transportation, etc.); capital building projects; research projects (except for philanthropic studies); or unsolicited proposals (all requests must begin with a preliminary proposal).
Geographic Focus: Indiana
Samples: Muncie Center for the Arts (Muncie, IN)—for general operating support, $15,000.; Ball State U (Muncie, IN)—for the university's museum, $2 million and artwork valued at $8 million.; Minnetrista Cultural Foundation (IN)—for general support, $2.6 million.
Contact: Donna Munchel; (765) 741-5500; fax: (765) 741-5518; email: donna.munchel@ballfdn.org
Internet: http://www.ballfdn.org
Sponsor: Ball Brothers Foundation
222 South Mulberry Street
Muncie, IN 47305

Baltimore Washington Center Adult Psychoanalysis Fellowships 685
The Adult Psychoanalysis Fellowship Program is a one-year program designed for individuals who have a significant interest in psychoanalysis as a body of knowledge and as a framework with which to understand and carry out therapeutic efforts. Intended for advanced graduate students and residents as well as recent graduates in Psychiatry, Psychology and Social Work, the program at its core consists of monthly seminars presented by psychoanalysts on clinically-related topics. Fellows are also welcome to attend Forums on Psychoanalysis and other conferences offered by the Institute and Society.
Date(s) Application is Due: Jul 15
Contact: Elizabeth Manne, Executive Director; (301) 470-3635 or (410) 792-8060; fax: (410) 792-4912; email: admin@bwanalysis.org
Internet: http://www.bwanalysis.org/Fellowship%20Program-Adult.html
Sponsor: Baltimore Washington Center for Psychoanalysis
14900 Sweitzer Lane, Suite 102
Laurel, MD 20707

Baltimore Washington Center Child Psychotherapy Fellowships 686
The Child Psychotherapy Fellowship program is a one-year program specifically designed for child mental health professionals who are interested in deepening their understanding of working with children from a psychoanalytic or psychodynamic perspective. The program is tuition-free. Detailed discussions of actual clinical work with children and reviews of relevant psychoanalytic literature will be used as a framework to enhance understanding and ability to carry out therapeutic work. Fellowship meetings will be held monthly, September through May, on the second Wednesday of every month, at the homes of Baltimore and Washington faculty members.
Requirements: Professionals, including psychiatrists, psychologists, social workers, and counselors currently working with children in psychotherapy should apply. Recent graduates of training programs should also apply.
Date(s) Application is Due: Jul 15
Contact: Elizabeth Manne, Executive Director; (301) 470-3635 or (410) 792-8060; fax: (410) 792-4912; email: admin@bwanalysis.org
Internet: http://www.bwanalysis.org/Fellowship%20Program-Child.html
Sponsor: Baltimore Washington Center for Psychoanalysis
14900 Sweitzer Lane, Suite 102
Laurel, MD 20707

Banfi Vintners Foundation Grants 687
The foundation awards general operating grants to nonprofits in its areas of interest, including higher education, civic and public affairs, arts and humanities, wildlife protection, health (hospitals and disease research/prevention), religion, science, social services, and international. Grants are made nationwide, with preference given to requests from Massachusetts and the New York, NY, area.
Geographic Focus: Massachusetts; New York
Samples: Colgate U (Hamilton, NY)—for operating support, $75,000.; Friends for Long Island's Heritage (Syosset, NY—for operating support, $25,000.; Huntington Hospital Assoc (Huntington, NY)—for operating support, $25,000.; Cornell U (Ithaca, NY)—for operating support, $465,000.
Amount of Grant: $100-$465,000 range
Contact: Philip Calderone, Executive Director, (516) 626-9200
Sponsor: Banfi Vintners Foundation
1111 Cedar Swamp Road
Glen Head, NY 11545

Bank of America Charitable Foundation Anchor Institutions Grants 688
Bank of America's local leaders, working within their communities, look for opportunities to support community stakeholders; opportunities that will further economic and community development, that will do more than put bricks and mortar on your block. When it does find those opportunities, the Foundation invites anchor institutions to apply for a grant. Such institutions might include: arts and cultural institutions such as museums, zoos, and performance halls; colleges, universities, and community colleges that attract and educate the workforce; and hospitals that provide excellent health care.
Samples: Apollo Theater, New York, New York (2007); Children's Hospital, Boston, Massachusetts (2007); Cook Children's Hospital, Fort Worth, Texas (2007); New Jersey Performing Arts Center, Newark, New Jersey (2007).
Contact: Anne Finucane; (800) 218-9946 or (617) 434-9405; email: anne.m.finucane@bankofamerica.com;; Andrew Plepler, President; (800) 218-9946 or (800) 432-1000; email: andrew.plepler@bankofamerica.com
Internet: http://www.bankofamerica.com/foundation/index.cfm?template=fd_anchorinstitutions
Sponsor: Bank of America Charitable Foundation
100 North Tryon Street
Charlotte, NC 28202

Bank of America Charitable Foundation National Programs and Partners Grants 689
Part of the Foundation's philanthropic objective is to sustain community efforts and provide funding flexibility so nonprofits can distribute funds as they know will best serve their clients and build their organizations. Its national partners are an integral part of the neighborhoods they serve. These are organizations that complement what the Foundation is able to do in a local community and collectively impact hundreds of neighborhoods across the country. It's possible an organization needs funding for capacity building or operating support at the national level; it may be just as possible the funding needs to be directed to the local level to strengthen that office's reach. And when disaster strikes, the Foundation is prepared to respond nationally when need overwhelms local capabilities to respond.
Requirements: To be considered for a local grant, an organization must be: tax-exempt under section 501(c)3 of the Internal Revenue Code; must be based and serve communities in particular markets; and must be aligned with funding priorities for those markets. A map of markets is available online.
Restrictions: The following organizations are not eligible for funding: organizations that deny service to a potential client or beneficiary on the basis of race, religion, color, sex, sexual orientation, age, national origin, ancestry, citizenship, veteran, or disability status; individuals, including those seeking scholarships or fellowship assistance; political, labor, fraternal organizations, or civic clubs; religious organizations (for example, churches and synagogues). Some secular community service programs such as soup kitchens, shelters for the homeless, and job banks are eligible, even when sponsored by religious groups; individual pre-K-12 schools (public or private); sports, athletic events, or athletic programs; travel-related events, including student trips or tours; development or production of books, films, videos, or television programs; or memorial campaigns.
Contact: Program Administrator; (800) 218-9946
Internet: http://www.bankofamerica.com/foundation/index.cfm?template=fd_nationalprograms
Sponsor: Bank of America Charitable Foundation
100 North Tryon Street
Charlotte, NC 28255

Bank of America Client Foundation Grants 690
The Foundation gives primarily to the arts, education, human services, natural science, youth and family organizations, and historic preservation. Fields of interest include: adult education; aging; AIDS; arts; children and youth services; community and economic development; crime and violence prevention; economically disadvantaged; education; the environment; family services; health care; historic preservation and historical societies; human services; marine science; media; mental health/crisis services; museums; performing arts; recreation; and urban/community development.
Requirements: Giving is limited to organizations operating in or providing services to residents of Sarasota County, Florida.
Restrictions: Generally the Foundation will not provide grants for: endowments, deficit financing, debt reduction, or ordinary operating expenses; conferences, seminars, workshops, travel, surveys, advertising, fund-raising costs or research; annual giving

campaigns; individuals; projects that have already been completed; public or private schools; or child care facilities.
Geographic Focus: Florida
Samples: Jewish Family and Children's Service of Sarasota-Manatee, Inc., $50,000 - to purchase conference room equipment and Brain Fitness Center technology and furnishings (2008); Pines of Sarasota Foundation, Inc., $45,000 - to renovate sections of The Garden - The Pines Alzheimer's/Dementia Facility (2008); Forty Carrots of Sarasota, Inc., $50,000 - Capital Campaign to purchase building and property and create a reserve to cover long-term maintenance (2008).
Amount of Grant: $35,000 average
Date(s) Application is Due: Apr 15; Sep 15
Contact: Renee Armbruster, CTFA Senior Vice President; (941) 952-2804; fax: (941) 952-2768; email: renee.armbruster@ustrust.com
Sponsor: Bank of America Client Foundation
c/o Renee Armbruster, Bank of America Private Wealth Management, 1605 Main Street, Suite 800
Sarasota, FL 34236

Baptist Community Ministries Grants **691**
BCM funds grants primarily in four major areas of interest: health; education; public safety; and governmental oversight. Applications not falling in these four major areas of interest are not typically considered. BCM funds transom grants and strategic grants. Transom grants are unsolicited grant proposals submitted by qualified, nonprofit organizations during our two semi-annual open transom cycles, and encourage the development of new ideas and nurture inventive solutions to community problems. Strategic grants generally target the long-range goals in each area of interest and are longer in duration. Strategic grants are usually generated through Request for Proposals or by invitation.
Requirements: Grants are made to eligible organizations in one or more of the five Louisiana parishes of Orleans, Jefferson, St. Bernard, St. Tammany and Plaquemines. Beneficiaries of grants should reside in one or more of the five parishes. It is preferred that the organization receiving a grant also be located in the same five-parish region and be overseen by unpaid volunteers living in the area.
Restrictions: Grants are not made to private foundations described in Section 509(a) of the Internal Revenue Code, private or publicly held corporations, limited liability corporations, partnerships, or sub-chapter S corporations. Funding requests not supported are: capital projects; general operating expenses; projects of national or statewide scope; single-disease charities; direct support to individuals or fraternal bodies.
Geographic Focus: Louisiana
Amount of Grant: $50,000 minimum
Date(s) Application is Due: Mar 15; Sep 15
Contact: Joanne M. Schmidt, Grants Manager; (504) 593-2345 or (504) 593-2323; fax: (504) 593-2301; email: jschmidt@bcm.org or info@bcm.org
Internet: http://www.bcm.org/grantmaking/
Sponsor: Baptist Community Ministries
400 Poydras Street, Suite 2950
New Orleans, LA 70130-3245

Baptist-Trinity Lutheran Legacy Foundation Grants **692**
The Foundation provides support in the greater Kansas City area for crisis related medical assistance, neighborhood school health grants, and health education programs and services in the service area of Baptist Medical Center and Trinity Lutheran Hospital. Funding priorities include: emergency medical assistance; health education; and health education in neighborhood schools. Highest consideration will be given for funding programs or services that demonstrate diversity, have measurable outcomes and can document continued existence after grant funding. Health Education Grant requests will be reviewed in January, March, May, July, September and November.
Requirements: All applicants must be non-profit, tax exempt organizations.
Restrictions: No grants will be made to individuals, political parties, candidates or political activities. Grants will not be given for special events, annual campaigns, endowments, or construction projects.
Geographic Focus: Missouri
Contact: Becky Schaid, Executive Director; (816) 276-7515 or (816) 276-7555; fax: (816) 926-2261; email: becky@btllf.org
Internet: http://www.btllf.org/funding.html
Sponsor: Baptist-Trinity Lutheran Legacy Foundation
6601 Rockhill Road
Kansas City, MO 64131

Barberton Community Foundation Grants **693**
The foundation awards grants to improve the quality of life for the citizens of Barberton. In addition to the regular grants program quarterly deadlines, the Foundation's Small Grant Program accepts applications monthly for grants up to $1,000. Areas of interest include charitable endeavors, education, public health, and public recreation.
Requirements: The eligibility requirements for small grants and large grants differ. See the Application Guidelines for specific requirements.
Restrictions: Grants are not given to: individuals; endowments housed at institutions other than the Barberton Community Foundation; religious organizations for religious purposes; projects that do not exclusively benefit the citizens of Barberton; fund debt reductions, deficits, or previous obligations; fund annual fund raising drives; fund ongoing operating expenses; fund political projects, sabbatical leaves or scholarly research; or fund venture capital for competitive profit-making activities.
Geographic Focus: Ohio
Samples: Barberton All-Town Little League (OH)—to refurbish two ball fields and construct two fields at the U.L. Light Middle School, $14,075.; City of Barberton (OH)—for summer concert programs at Lake Anna Park, $55,000.; Metro Regional Transit Authority (Akron, OH)—for a transit center in Barberton, $102,000.; Barberton Area United Way (OH)—to help needy residents make utility and rent payments, $60,000.
Amount of Grant: $1,000 maximum for Small Grant Program
Date(s) Application is Due: Jan 2; Apr 1; Jul 1; Oct 1
Contact: Chuck Sandstrom, Executive Director; (330) 745-5995; fax: (330) 745-3990; email: csandstrom@bcfcharity.org
Internet: http://www.bcfcharity.org/bcf/grant/grants.shtml
Sponsor: Barberton Community Foundation
460 W. Paige Avenue
Barberton, OH 44203

Barker Foundation Grants **694**
The foundation offers funding to New Hampshire non-profit organizations in the areas of: children/youth services; education; health organizations, association; hospitals (general); and human services. Giving primarily for health associations, social services and youth. Grants are awarded in the following types: Annual campaigns building/renovation; capital campaigns; continuing support; equipment; general/operating support and; program development.
Requirements: New Hampshire nonprofit organizations are eligible for funding. The Foundation accepts written requests only. No formal application form is required. Send a 1 page concept paper and request for guidelines to the Foundation with a SASE for response.
Restrictions: Grants are not made to individuals.
Geographic Focus: New Hampshire
Samples: Boys and Girls Club of Greater Nashua, Nashua, NH, $10,000 (2007); Senior Activity Center, Nashua, NH, $2,000 (2007); Nashua Soup Kitchen and Shelter, Nashua, NH, $13,000 (2007).
Amount of Grant: $2,000-$13,000 range
Contact: Allan Barker, Treasurer
Sponsor: Barker Foundation
P.O. Box 328
Nashua, NH 03061-0328

Barker Welfare Foundation Grants **695**
The mission of the foundation is to make grants to qualified charitable organizations whose initiatives improve the quality of life, with an emphasis on strengthening youth and families and to reflect the philosophy of Catherine B. Hickox, the Founder. Consideration will be given to applications from institutions and agencies operating in the fields of health, welfare, education and literacy, cultural activities, and civic affairs, primarily serving the metropolitan area of New York, NY, and Michigan City, IN. The foundation board meets twice per year to consider requests.
Requirements: In advance of submitting a request, a brief letter or telephone call is suggested to determine if the organization seeking to apply for a grant falls within the current general policy of the Foundation. Before the Foundation sends out its application form, a brief 2-3 page letter describing the organization, the purpose and amount requested should be sent. A copy of the first page of the most recent 990 filed with the IRS and a current budget for the whole organization and a budget for program/project (if requesting program/project support) including income and expense should be sent with the letter of inquiry. Grants are made to tax-exempt organizations which have received a ruling by the Internal Revenue Service that they are organizations described in Section 501(c)3 and classified in Section 509(a)(1),(2), or (3) of the Internal Revenue Code (publicly supported organizations and their affiliates).
Restrictions: Appeals for the following will be declined: organizations not located in nor directly serving the defined areas; national health; welfare; or education agencies; institutions or funds; scholarships; fellowships; loans; student aid; appeals from individuals; medical and scientific research; private elementary and secondary schools; colleges; universities; professional schools; trade organizations; films; program advertising; conferences; seminars; benefits and fund raising costs; start-up organizations; emergency funds; and deficit financing; lobbying-related or legislative activities; endowment funds; and intermediary organizations.
Geographic Focus: Indiana; New York
Amount of Grant: $7500-$15,000 range
Date(s) Application is Due: Feb 1; Aug 1
Contact: Sarane Ross, President; (516) 759-5592; email: BarkerSMD@aol.com
Internet: http://www.barkerwelfare.org
Sponsor: Barker Welfare Foundation
P.O. Box 2
Glen Head, NY 11545

Barnes Group Foundation Grants **696**
The foundation awards grants in the following areas of interest: Education; Health and Welfare; Hospitals; Culture and Art and Civic and Youth Organizations. Highest priority is given to the support of organizations and projects in communities where the company has its executive office, group headquarters offices, plants and other facilities. There are no deadlines for submitting requests. Initial contact should be by letter.
Requirements: In order to be considered for support by the Foundation, a grant seeker must furnish a copy of its ruling from the Internal Revenue Service determining that it is an organization described in Section 501(c)3 and Section 509(a)(1), (2), (3), or (4) of the Internal Revenue Code.

Restrictions: No grants are made to organizations located outside the United States. The Foundation will consider only one grant request per organization during any one year period. The Foundation will not contribute directly or indirectly to any political activities or legislative lobbying efforts.
Geographic Focus: Connecticut; Maine; Massachusetts; New Hampshire; Rhode Island; Vermont
Amount of Grant: $500 to $3,500
Contact: Secretary, (860) 973-2112; fax: (860) 589-7466
Internet: http://www.barnesgroupinc.com/about/foundation.html
Sponsor: Barnes Group Foundation
123 Main Street, P.O. Box 489
Bristol, CT 06011-0489

Barr Fund Grants **697**
The fund awards grants to Illinois nonprofits in its areas of interest, including services for children and youth, orchestras, higher education, mental health/crisis services, Jewish temples and organizations, and social services. Grants are awarded for general operating support. There are no application forms or deadlines. Submit a letter of request.
Requirements: Illinois nonprofits are eligible.
Restrictions: Individuals are not eligible.
Geographic Focus: Illinois
Samples: Rush University Medical Center, Chicago, IL, $10,000 (2008); New Israel Fund, Washington, DC, $1,000 (2008); Highland Park Community Foundation, Highland Park, IL, $1,000 (2008); The Barr Harris Center of the Institute For Psychoanalysis, Chicago, IL, $50,000 (2008).
Amount of Grant: $100-$75,000
Contact: Donald Lubin, President, c/o Philip C. Ravid, Ravid & Bernstein, LLP; (312) 782-4710 (312) 876-8000
Sponsor: Barr Fund
230 West Monroe Street, Suite 330
Chicago, IL 60606-4701

Barra Foundation Community Fund Grants **698**
Community Fund grants provide unrestricted contributions to qualified organizations primarily in the Greater Philadelphia area. These grants are generally in amounts between $1,000 and $10,000 per year. The Foundation's categories of funding for these grants are: human services; arts and culture; health; and education. These grants are made at certain times of the year, depending on the category of grant. The categories and time frames for each are as follows: human services—March 1 with grants made in the Spring of each year; arts and culture—June 1 with grants made in the Summer of each year; and health and education—September 1 with grants made in the fall of each year.
Requirements: Applications are welcome from 501(c)3 organizations serving the greater Philadelphia region.
Geographic Focus: Pennsylvania
Amount of Grant: $2,000 - $15,000 range
Date(s) Application is Due: Mar 1; Jun 1; Sep 1
Contact: William Harral, III, President; (215) 233-5115; fax: (215) 836-1033; email: william.harral@verizon.net
Internet: http://www.barrafoundation.org/grants/index.html
Sponsor: Barra Foundation
8200 Flourtown Avenue, Suite 12
Wyndmoor, PA 19038-7976

Barra Foundation Project Grants **699**
Project grants are one-time grants generally for amounts above $10,000. The Foundation considers grants for innovative projects that aid research in advancing the frontiers of human services, arts and culture, health and education. Grants are not made for ongoing or expanding programs where substantial initial support was previously provided from other sources. Three principal criteria are strictly adhered to in judging the merits of a proposed project. They are: innovation; evaluation; and dissemination. Proposals may be submitted at any time of the year. Initial requests for project grants should be in the form of a preliminary concept paper, generally not to exceed two pages, summarizing: the principal focus and objectives of the proposed project; uniqueness of the concept; the overall methodology; estimated timetable; preliminary budget data; and other sources of support for the project.
Restrictions: The foundation does not provide grants for: ongoing operating budgets; staff salaries; budget deficits; endowments; capital campaigns and projects; international programs; environmental and religious organizations; scholarships and fellowships; or audio/video projects, publications, catalogs, and exhibitions.
Geographic Focus: Pennsylvania
Samples: U of Pennsylvania (Philadelphia, PA)—to build a facility to house the Center for Early American Studies at the School of Arts and Sciences, and to endow the building's operating costs, $2.5 million.; Woodmere Art Museum (Philadelphia, PA)—to endow the position of curator of education, $1 million.
Amount of Grant: $10,000-$500,000 range
Contact: William Harral, III, President; (215) 233-5115; fax: (215) 836-1033; email: william.harral@verizon.net
Internet: http://www.barrafoundation.org/grants/index.html
Sponsor: Barra Foundation
8200 Flourtown Avenue, Suite 12
Wyndmoor, PA 19038-7976

Barth Syndrome Foundation Research Grants **700**
Barth syndrome is a serious X-linked recessive condition associated with cardiomyopathy, neutropenia, skeletal muscle weakness, exercise intolerance, growth delay, and diverse biochemical abnormalities (including defects in mitochondrial metabolism and phospholipid biosynthesis). Because many clinical and biochemical abnormalities of Barth syndrome remain poorly understood, the program is seeking proposals for research that will advance knowledge on any aspect of the syndrome. The foundation prefers to award seed grants to experienced investigators for testing of initial hypotheses and collection of preliminary data leading to successful long-term funding by NIH and other major granting institutions. The foundation also encourages investigators new to the field of Barth Syndrome research. Send an electronic version of the full application and all the attachments by the listed application deadline. The Foundation anticipates awarding several one- or two-year grants of up to $40,000 each. Funds will be available as soon as the successful grant applicants have been notified.
Requirements: Principal investigators who are affiliated with nonprofit institutions are eligible.
Amount of Grant: $10,000-$40,000
Date(s) Application is Due: Oct 31
Contact: Matthew J. Toth, Ph.D., Science Director; (617) 469-6769; fax: (617) 849-5695; email: mtoth@barthsyndrome.org
Internet: http://www.barthsyndrome.org/english/View.asp?x=1635
Sponsor: Barth Syndrome Foundation
675 VFW Parkway, #372
Chestnut Hill, MA 02467

Batchelor Foundation Grants **701**
The foundation supports food banks and organizations involved with arts and culture, education, the environment, animals and wildlife, health, human services, and economically disadvantaged people. Special emphasis is directed toward programs designed to engage in medical research and provide care for childhood diseases; and promote study, preservation, and public awareness of the natural environment. Funding is available in the form of: capital campaigns; continuing support; endowments; general/operating support; and program development grants. There are no application forms. Initial approach should be a letter that details the grant proposal.
Requirements: Florida area nonprofits are eligible.
Restrictions: Individuals are not eligible.
Geographic Focus: Florida
Samples: Community Partnership for Homeless, Miami, FL, $1,056,600—for general operating support and endowment (2008); Fairchild Tropical Botanic Garden, Coral Gables, FL, $540,000— For general operating support (2008); University of Miami, Miami, FL, $525,000— for general operating support (2008).
Amount of Grant: $1,000-$1,000,000 range
Contact: Anne Batchelor-Robjohns, Co-C.E.O.; (305) 416-9066 or (305) 534-5004; email: jbatchelor@bellsouth.net
Sponsor: Batchelor Foundation Inc
111 NE 1st Street, Suite 820
Miami, FL 33132

Baton Rouge Area Foundation Grants **702**
The foundation seeks to enhance the quality of life for all citizens of Baton Rouge, Louisiana. The foundation concentrates on projects and programs in the areas of community development, education, environment, health and medical, and religion. Applicants should call the office to determine if their project or program is consistent with the foundation's goals before sending an application.
Requirements: Only nonprofits that are registered as 501(c)3 corporations working in the service region of East and West Baton Rouge Parish, East and West Feliciana, Ascension, Livingston, Iberville and Pointe Coupee can apply for grants.
Geographic Focus: Louisiana
Samples: Louisiana Art and Science Museum, Baton Rouge, LA., $125,835 (2008); Rhode Island School of Design, Providence, RI, $10,000 (2008); Friends of Hilltop Arboretum, Inc., Baton Rouge, LA., $5,450 (2008).
Contact: Angela Fitzgerald, Executive Assistant; (225) 387-6126 or (877) 387-6126; fax: (225) 387-6153 or (225) 408-8125; email: afitzgerald@braf.org
Internet: https://www.braf.org/braf/GRANTS/tabid/103/Default.aspx
Sponsor: Baton Rouge Area Foundation
402 North Fourth Street
Baton Rouge, LA 70802

Battle Creek Community Foundation Grants **703**
The Battle Creek Community Foundation focuses on the greater Battle community, and is most interested in projects that focus on education, health, human services, arts and culture, public affairs or community development. In general, priority is given to those grant ideas that: increases the capacity of the community to participate in identifying needs and developing and implementing solutions; encourages cooperation; demonstrates a clean and convincing need; develops self-reliance; avoids unnecessary duplication of services; targets gaps in services; Mirrors the diversity of our community; promotes equity among its various segments; and has clean, defined goals and/or measurable outcomes. Grant applications and guidelines are available on the Web site.
Requirements: Grants will be considered only from 501(c)3 nonprofit agencies in Michigan offering services to the residents of Battle Creek.
Restrictions: Individuals are not eligible to receive grants.
Geographic Focus: Michigan

Samples: Drug Free Workplace (Battle Creek, MI)—program support.; Battle Creek Health System (Battle Creek, MI)—program support.
Amount of Grant: $5,000-$10,000 average
Contact: Kelly Boles Chapman, Vice President of Programs; (269) 962-2181; fax: (269) 962-2182; email: bccf@bccfoundation.org
Internet: http://www.bccfoundation.org/grants/
Sponsor: Battle Creek Community Foundation
One Riverwalk Centre, 34 West Jackson Street
Battle Creek, MI 49017-3505

Batts Foundation Grants 704

The foundation supports organizations involved with arts and culture, K-12 and higher education, disease, and human services. Grants will be awarded primarily in western MI area. There are no application forms or deadlines. Submit a one page letter summarizing your project.
Requirements: Michigan nonprofit organizations are eligible.
Restrictions: Individuals are ineligible.
Geographic Focus: Michigan
Amount of Grant: $250-$25,000 range
Contact: Robert Batts, Director; (616) 956-3053
Sponsor: Batts Foundation
3777 Sparks Drive, SE, Suite 100
Grand Rapids, MI 49546

Baxter International Foundation Grants 705

The foundation supports the development of more accessible and affordable healthcare. The foundation funds initiatives that improve the access, quality and cost-effectiveness of healthcare. Focusing on these priorities, the foundation focusing on communities where Baxter has a corporate presence. In Illinois, grants are restricted to Lake, McHenry and Cook counties. The foundation also funds in Asia, Australia, Canada, Europe, Latin America and Mexico.
Requirements: U.S. nonprofits in Lake, McHenry and Cook counties of Illinois are eligible to apply. Internationally, the following countries are eligible to apply: Asia, Australia, Canada, Europe, Latin America and Mexico.
Restrictions: In general, The Baxter International Foundation does not make grants to: capital and endowment campaigns (includes requests for infrastructure of any kind, equipment, vehicles, etc.); disease or condition-specific organizations or programs; educational grants/continuing professional education scholarships; educational institutions, except in instances where a grant would help achieve other goals, such as increasing community-based direct health services or the skills and availability of community health-care providers, in areas where there are Baxter facilities; general operating support or maintenence of effort; hospitals; individuals, including scholarships for individuals; lobbying and political organizations; magazines, professional journals, documentary, film, video, radio or website productions; medical missions; organizations seeking travel support for individuals or groups, medical missions or conferences; organizations soliciting contributions for advertising space, tickets to dinners, benefits, social and fund-raising events, sponsorships and promotional materials; organizations with a limited constituency, such as fraternal, veterans or religious organizations; research.
Geographic Focus: Illinois;Asia; Australia; Canada; Europe; Mexico
Samples: Abraham Low Self-Help Systems, Chicago, IL, $70,000—for staff to initiate veterans' mental health support groups at the North Chicago VA facility (2008); Fundacao Julita, Sao Paulo, Brazil, $51,700—to expand and stabilize mental health services to highly disadvantaged children, youth and families in Jardim Sao Luis neighborhood of Sao Paulo, Brazil (2008); Charities Aid Foundation for the Chronic Care Foundation, New Delhi, India, $240,000—to expand programs to prevent non-communicable chronic diseases in India (2008); The Irish Hospice Foundation, Dublin, Ireland, $109,390—for a pilot program to train healthcare specialists in palliative care to expand access to non-cancer patients in Dublin, Ireland (2008).
Date(s) Application is Due: Jan 21; Apr 13; Jul 13; Sep 29
Contact: Foundation Contact, (847) 948-4605; email: fdninfo@baxter.com
Internet: http://www.baxter.com/about_baxter/foundation/index.html
Sponsor: Baxter International Foundation
Baxter International Foundation, One Baxter Parkway - DF2-2E
Deerfield, IL 60015-4625

Bayer Clinical Scholarship Award 706

This award is intended to facilitate the development of specific clinical expertise in the field of hemophilia for applicants who have completed medical training and have an interest in pursuing a career as a hemophilia treater/researcher. The award will support a mentored physician in training for two years. Clinical duties will encompass diagnosis, evaluation, and the planning of management strategies for patients with hereditary bleeding disorders. In addition to the clinical experience, the applicant may pursue a research project in the field of hemostasis. Clinical scholarships will provide funding for two years. Up to five new awards will be made each year. Guidelines and application are available online.
Requirements: The applicant should have earned his/her medical degree within the previous eight years. The commitment of the mentor to the grantee and the research project (if applicable) is a vital element of the application, as is the quality of the clinical environment at which the applicant will undertake the scholarship.
Amount of Grant: $70,000 annually for two years
Contact: Program Administrator, email: programadministrator@bayer-hemophilia-awards.com
Internet: http://www.bayer-hemophilia-awards.com/awards.cfm#clinical
Sponsor: Bayer HealthCare Corporation
100 Bayer Road
Pittsburgh, PA 15205-9741

Bayer Hemophilia Caregivers Education Award 707

This award recognizes the essential role of caregivers and allied health professionals in the care of patients with hemophilia. It is designed to support their role by promoting continuing education. Awards will be provided for education activities in the field of hemophilia. This may include, but is not limited to, the development of educational seminars/symposia, mentored experiences, or training workshops. The Award is not designed for the development of materials for patients and parents. Applications will be judged by: Educational merit of the proposed initiative; Innovation of study rationale and techniques; Impact on the development of the professional and his/her ability to deliver care; Educational environment. The duration of the award is one year. Up to six Awards of up to $25,000 will be made annually. Part of the award may fund salary support. The candidate must spend at least 25% of his/her time on the project in order to request salary support.
Requirements: Requests for these grants must come from caregivers and allied health professionals involved in the care of patients with hemophilia. These may include nurses and nurse practitioners, physical therapists, pharmacists, psychiatrists, psychologists, genetic counselors, social workers, clinical dieticians, dentists and dental hygienists, among others. The Award is not designed for medically qualified hematologists who treat patients with bleeding disorders.
Restrictions: Unauthorized expenses are: Salaries, travel and/or housing related to sabbaticals; Purchase or rental of office equipment; Fees for tuition; Membership dues, congress/meeting registrations, subscriptions.
Amount of Grant: $25,000
Contact: Program Administrator, email: programadministrator@bayer-hemophilia-awards.com
Internet: http://www.bayer-hemophilia-awards.com/awards.cfm#caregivers
Sponsor: Bayer HealthCare Corporation
100 Bayer Road
Pittsburgh, PA 15205-9741

BCBS of Massachusetts Catalyst Fund Grants 708

The program provides small grants to support capacity building in community-based organizations. Grants will assist with one-time expenses needed to strengthen an organization's ability to fulfill its mission. Examples of activities that could be supported include community outreach for health insurance enrollment, health prevention activities, or health care education convening; hiring a grant writer; community meetings to engage stakeholders and constituents; leadership development opportunities; strategic planning activities; and board development and staff training.
Requirements: Grants will only be made to Massachusetts-based organizations that serve the health care needs of uninsured and low-income residents of the state.
Restrictions: Grants will not be made to individuals, for-profit entities, hospitals, or public agencies. Grants are not intended to cover recurring general operating funds, such as salaries, overhead, or membership dues.
Amount of Grant: $500-$2500
Contact: Grants Administrator, (617) 246-3744; email: bcbsmafoundation.org
Internet: http://www.bcbsmafoundation.org/foundationroot/en_U.S./documents/catalystFundguidelines.pdf
Sponsor: Blue Cross Blue Shield of Massachusetts Foundation
401 Park Drive
Boston, MA 02115-3326

BCBS of Massachusetts Foundation Grants 709

With a mission to expand access to health care, the foundation awards grants intended to make a significant impact on the health of Massachusetts's low income and uninsured residents. Grant programs include Innovation Fund for the Uninsured; Connecting Consumers with Care; Strengthening the Voice for Access; Pathways to Culturally Competent Health Care; Catalyst Fund; Building Bridges in Children's Mental Health; and Policy Research and Analysis. Grant awards in particular focus areas are made during specific grant cycles. Deadlines and additional information are available online.
Requirements: Massachusetts 501(c)3 nonprofit organizations or government agencies with a mission that includes improving access and removing barriers to healthcare for low-income or uninsured Massachusetts's residents are eligible.
Restrictions: The foundation will not fund individuals; for-profit organizations; capital campaigns, endowments, or building drives; fundraising drives and events; retiring debt or operating deficits; direct political or lobbying activity; projects outside of Massachusetts; or religious organizations for religious purposes (proposals for secular programs of faith-based organizations that meet funding criteria will be considered). Grants are rarely made for curriculum development, conferences, film or video production, or scholarships.
Geographic Focus: Massachusetts
Samples: Beth Israel Deaconess Medical Ctr (Boston, MA)—to help managers select, retain, and promote highly qualified, diverse staff members, $40,000 (2004); Boston U, Goldman School of Dental Medicine (Boston, MA)—to develop policy recommendations designed to increase access to fluoridated water, with a focus on uninsured and low-income people and minorities, $46,716 (2004); John Snow Research and Training Institute (Boston, MA)—to study the extent to which a subsidized health-insurance program for people in the Massachusetts fishing industry can be duplicated in other industries, $50,000 (2004); Massachusetts Department of Mental Health (Boston,

MA)—to integrate primary care and mental-health services for underserved Hispanics in the Worcester, MA, area, $50,000 (2004).
Date(s) Application is Due: Jan 20; Sep 7
Contact: Grant Requests, (617) 246-3744; fax: (617) 246-3992; email: grantinfo@bcbsmafoundation.org
Internet: http://www.bcbsmafoundation.org/foundationroot/en_U.S./grants/focusArea.jsp#aInnovation%20Fund%20for%20the%20Uninsured
Sponsor: Blue Cross Blue Shield of Massachusetts Foundation
401 Park Drive
Boston, MA 02215

BCBS of Massachusetts Health Coverage Fellowships 710
The fellowship, the first of its kind in the country, is designed to help New England media do a better job covering critical health care issues. Ten reporters and editors from newspapers, radio stations, and television outlets are chosen each year to participate in a nine-day intensive program to deepen their understanding of the complex and changing world of medicine and health care. Throughout the remainder of the year, fellows participate in half-day retreats and can consult on stories and projects with former Boston Globe medical reporter Larry Tye. Application is available online.
Requirements: New England health-care journalists are eligible. Reporters must have an editor's approval.
Geographic Focus: New England
Date(s) Application is Due: Dec 1
Contact: Larry Tye, email: info@bcbsmafoundation.org
Internet: http://www.bcbsmafoundation.org/foundationroot/en_U.S./policyAndPrograms/policyPresent.jsp?repositoryId=/foundationroot/en_U.S./repositories/commonMainContent/policyAndPrograms/healthCoverageFellowship.xml
Sponsor: Blue Cross Blue Shield of Massachusetts Foundation
401 Park Drive
Boston, MA 02115-3326

BCBS of Minnesota Growing Up Healthy Grants 711
Growing Up Healthy: Kids and Communities is a statewide initiative to improve the health of Minnesota's children through a focus on social and environmental determinants of health. The goal is to build strong and connected communities where children can thrive and grow up healthy by working at the intersection of health and two or more of the following health determinants: early childhood development; stable, affordable housing; and the physical environment.
Requirements: Eligible applicants include community- and faith-based organizations; state, county and municipal agencies; tribal governments and agencies; professional associations or collaboratives; and policy and research organizations. Applicants must be located in Minnesota or serve Minnesotans. Eligible applicants include units of government as well as organizations designated as nonprofit under section 501(c)3 of the IRS code.
Geographic Focus: Minnesota
Date(s) Application is Due: Apr 13
Contact: Lisa Simer, program officer, (651) 662-0188; email Lisa_K_Simer@bluecrossmn.com.
Internet: http://www.bluecrossmn.com/bc/wcs/groups/bcbsmn/@mbc_foundation/documents/public/mbc2_index.hcsp
Sponsor: Blue Cross Blue Shield of Minnesota Foundation
3535 Blue Cross Road, Rte M459
Eagan, MN 55122

BCBS of Minnesota Healthy Together Grants 712
Healthy Together: Creating Community with New Americans is a grantmaking initiative designed to reduce health disparities for immigrants and improve the health and vitality of the entire community. The foundation awards grants to projects that foster exchanges and interactions between newcomers and the receiving community, strengthen the capacity of immigrant-led organizations and their attention to health, and address social adjustment and mental health.
Requirements: Eligible applicants include community- and faith-based organizations; state, county and municipal agencies; tribal governments and agencies; professional associations or collaboratives; and policy and research organizations. Applicants must be located in Minnesota or serve Minnesotans. Eligible applicants include units of government as well as organizations designated as nonprofit under section 501(c)3 of the IRS code.
Geographic Focus: Minnesota
Amount of Grant: $1200-$250,000
Date(s) Application is Due: Feb 1
Contact: Jocelyn Ancheta, program officer, (651) 662-2894; email, Jocelyn_L_Ancheta@bluecrossmn.com.
Internet: http://www.bluecrossmn.com/public/foundation/index.html
Sponsor: Blue Cross Blue Shield of Minnesota Foundation
3535 Blue Cross Road, Rte M459
Eagan, MN 55122

BCBSM Building Healthy Communities Engaging Elementary Schools and Community Partners Grants 713
BCBSM (Blue Cross Blue Shield of Michigan) is offering this grant program to strengthen school and community efforts to reduce the risk and prevalence of childhood obesity through prevention and partnership. With this request for proposals Blue Cross invited Michigan elementary schools to collaborate with students, parents and community partners to address childhood obesity's root causes by promoting awareness of and education about physical activity and nutrition. See BCBSM website for all required forms.
Requirements: Electronic notice of intent is to be submitted no later then April 3. The application must be postmarked by April 24 to be eligible and be submitted with three copies of the proposal.
Geographic Focus: Michigan
Amount of Grant: $40,000 - $60,000 range
Date(s) Application is Due: Apr 3; Apr 24
Contact: BHC Director; (800) 658-6715; email: buildhealth@bcbsm.com
Internet: http://www.bcbsm.com/buildhealth/index.shtml
Sponsor: Blue Cross Blue Shield of Michigan
600 East Lafayette Boulevard, MC B718
Detroit, MI 48226-2998

BCBSM Claude Pepper Award 714
The Claude Pepper Award is presented annually to two outstanding senior citizen advocates who demonstrate a strong concern for the special needs of the elderly. The BCBSM (Blue Cross Blue Shield of Michigan) named the award after the late U.S. Congressman who campaigned for senior citizens' rights. Blue Cross Blue Shield of Michigan's Senior Advisory Council selects two individuals, a retiree volunteer over age 55 and another person of any age who's employed in the senior advocacy field. Each award recipient receives a $1,000 donation for the nonprofit organization of his or her choice. Candidates for this award will have clearly demonstrated their dedication to Michigan's seniors through work that positively impacts older adults, particularly those who don't receive adequate health services due to mental, physical, financial or geographical limitations. To nominate someone for a Claude Pepper Award, submit the nomination online using the form provided at the BCBSM website.
Requirements: Nomination Criteria: awards are given to individuals, not groups or teams of people. However, you may nominate a person for their individual work on behalf of a group to which he or she belongs; volunteers are defined as people who freely choose to provide a service that contributes to the well-being of an individual or a community; nominees can be paid workers; however, the committee is looking for efforts that go above and beyond job responsibilities; the candidate must have performed the services in the State of Michigan; monetary contributions can only be made to 501(c)3 nonprofits.
Restrictions: Employees of Blue Cross Blue Shield of Michigan, its subsidiaries and members of all selection committees are not eligible for this award, nor are their family members or elected political office holders.
Geographic Focus: Michigan
Amount of Grant: $1,000
Contact: Community Affairs Hotline; (800) 733-2583
Internet: http://www.bcbsm.com/home/commitment/claude_pepper_award.shtml
Sponsor: Blue Cross Blue Shield of Michigan
600 E Lafayette Boulevard, MC 0250
Detroit, MI 48226

BCBSM Community Health Matching Grants 715
The Community Health Matching Program Grants focuses on access to care for the uninsured and under insured. The program's purpose is to encourage nonprofit community based organizations to form partnerships with health care organizations, research organizations, or governmental agencies to develop and rigorously evaluate new ways of increasing access to care for the under and uninsured, in Michigan. Up to $50,000 per year for 2 years is available, contingent on a 25% match. See the BCBSM Foundation website to obtain the application form.
Requirements: Nonprofit 501 (c)(3) organizations based in Michigan are eligible. Nonprofits do not need a firm commitment of matching support prior to the submission of the proposal (letters from potential funding partners are encouraged, indicating their support for the project and interest in possible funding partnership(s)).
Restrictions: Grants under this program do not pay for the cost of equipment (e.g., personal computers), hardware or software.
Geographic Focus: Michigan
Amount of Grant: $50,000
Contact: Ira Strumwasser, Director; (313) 225-8706; fax: (313) 225-7730; email: foundation@bcbsm.com
Internet: http://www.bcbsm.com/foundation/grant.shtml
Sponsor: Blue Cross Blue Shield Michigan Foundation
600 East Lafayette Boulevard, X520
Detroit, MI 48226-2998

BCBSM Corporate Contributions Grants 716
The BCBSM (Blue Cross Blue Shield of Michigan) corporate giving program supports nonprofit 501(3)(c) organizations throughout Michigan. BCBSM invests in local communities by supporting organizations that share a commitment to Michigan. BCBSM charitable contributions support programs that: address health issues specific to Michigan's youth and seniors; extend a nonprofit organization's reach through effective use of volunteers; emphasize collaboration across regions within Michigan. Contribution requests are accepted year round and are reviewed monthly by BCBSM's director of community affairs.
Requirements: To be considered for a charitable contribution from the BCBSM, an organization must be: nonprofit 501(3)(c) status; Michigan based and focused. Requests for contributions must be submitted in writing, and include: Corporate Contributions

Cover Sheet (available on BCBSM website); IRS 501(c)3 tax exemption documentation; organization's annual report. Submit requests for contribution one of three ways: mail; fax and; email.
Restrictions: Contributions are not made to: individuals; political organizations, campaigns or candidates; extracurricular school activities; endowments; alumni associations; scholarship programs; research projects; multi-year pledges; operational expenses; group travel expenses; capital campaigns.
Geographic Focus: Michigan
Contact: Cathy Mozham; (313) 225-0539; fax: (313) 225-9693; email: cmozham@bcbsm.com
Internet: http://www.bcbsm.com/home/commitment/corporate_contributions.shtml
Sponsor: Blue Cross Blue Shield of Michigan
600 East Lafayette Boulevard, MC 1808
Detroit, MI 48226

BCBSM Foundation Excellence in Research Awards for Students **717**
The annual Excellence in Research Award for Students acknowledges doctoral candidates or medical students enrolled in Michigan universities who have published research papers that represent significant contributions to health policy or clinical care. Entries will be judged based on the subject matter's potential to make a contribution to health policy and medical care as well as the quality and originality of the research. There will be three awards: 1st place - $1,000; 2nd place - $750; 3rd place - $500.
Requirements: Doctoral candidates or medical students enrolled in Michigan universities are eligible. The nomination must be made by a faculty member at the student's university. If the paper has multiple authors, the student must be the first author.
Restrictions: Basic research papers are not eligible.
Geographic Focus: Michigan
Amount of Grant: $500 - $1,000 range
Date(s) Application is Due: Jan 1
Contact: Ira Strumwasser, Director; (313) 225-8706; fax: (313) 225-7730; email: foundation@bcbsm.com
Internet: http://www.bcbsm.com/foundation/grant.shtml
Sponsor: Blue Cross Blue Shield of Michigan Foundation
600 East Lafayette Boulevard, X520
Detroit, MI 48226

BCBSM Foundation Physician Investigator Research Awards **718**
The Physician Investigator Research Award program provides $10,000 in seed money to physicians who a propose a pilot, feasibility or small research study related to quality, cost or appropriate access to health and medical care for Michigan residents. See BCBSM Foundation website to obtain application form.
Requirements: Applicants must be a physician interested in research, who is licensed and domiciled in the state of Michigan. Applicants may include physicians working in research environments such as medical schools or university-affiliated hospitals, health care systems, or nonprofit agencies.
Restrictions: The program does not support basic science, biomedical research including drug studies, or studies using animals.
Geographic Focus: Michigan
Amount of Grant: $10,000
Contact: Nora Maloy, Senior Program Officer; (313) 225-8706; fax: (313) 225-7730; email: foundation@bcbsm.com
Internet: http://www.bcbsm.com/foundation/grant.shtml
Sponsor: Blue Cross Blue Shield of Michigan Foundation
600 East Lafayette Boulevard, X520
Detroit, MI 48226

BCBSM Foundation Primary and Clinical Prevention Grants **719**
The Blue Cross Blue Shield of Michigan Foundation requests letters of interest from Michigan physicians and members of the research community interested in preventing the three leading causes of death in Michigan: heart disease, cancer and stroke. The purpose of this grant initiative is to increase the use of evidence-based prevention efforts to improve the health of Michigan residents. The BCBSM Foundation has allocated $500,000 to fund several projects for up to two years. Funds will be available for salary support, program costs, supplies, office operations and other costs related to the proposed project. Computer equipment expenses, including PC hardware and software, will not be supported. In addition to the overall quality of the project, the feasibility and appropriateness of the budget is a factor in the funding decisions. The required application cover page and the terms and conditions may be downloaded for the BCBSM web site.
Requirements: Applicants must be doctoral level researchers (including physicians) based at Michigan universities, academic medical settings, community hospitals, health systems and community based nonprofit organizations. The principal investigator must have appropriate research and clinical credentials.
Geographic Focus: Michigan
Date(s) Application is Due: Sep 1
Contact: Nora Maloy, Senior Program Officer; (313) 225-8706; fax: (313) 225-7730; email: nmaloy@bcbsm.com
Internet: http://www.bcbsm.com/foundation/grant.shtml
Sponsor: Blue Cross Blue Shield Michigan Foundation
600 East Lafayette Boulevard, X520
Detroit, MI 48226

BCBSM Foundation Proposal Development Awards **720**
The BCBSM Foundation's Proposal Development Award is intended to help Michigan based nonprofit community organizations develop grant proposals for new health care initiatives. This award of up to $3,500 is available to help nonprofits obtain grant writing resources so they may secure the funding they need to bring creative community based health care programs to life. Expenditure of award funds is restricted to proposal development costs, such as technical assistance, freelance proposal writers and related proposal development costs.
Requirements: Applicants must be Michigan based nonprofit community organizations that deliver health services.
Restrictions: Award funds are not intended to support any type of project activity or to supplement operational expenses.
Geographic Focus: Michigan
Amount of Grant: $3,500
Contact: Nora Maloy, Senior Program Officer; (313) 225-8706; fax: (313) 225-7730; email: foundation@bcbsm.com
Internet: http://www.bcbsm.com/foundation/grant.shtml
Sponsor: Blue Cross Blue Shield Michigan Foundation
600 East Lafayette Boulevard, X520
Detroit, MI 48226

BCBSM Foundation Student Award Program **721**
The program offers a one year stipend to fund a wide range of health care projects, including applied research, pilot programs, or demonstration and evaluation projects.
Requirements: All doctoral and medical students enrolled in Michigan universities are eligible. For consideration, the proposed project must focus geographically on the state of Michigan and address the BCBSM Foundation's objectives.
Restrictions: Completed or substantially completed dissertations or research projects are not eligible. Students who previously received this award are not eligible. Blue Cross and Blue Shield of Michigan affiliates and subsidiaries are not eligible. Investigation of pharmaceutical efficacy, basic research or research involving non-human subjects is not eligible. Grant monies are not intended to support field placements, practica or internships.
Geographic Focus: Michigan
Amount of Grant: $3000
Date(s) Application is Due: Apr 30
Contact: Ira Strumwasser, Director; (313) 225-8706; fax: (313) 225-7730; email: foundation@bcbsm.com
Internet: http://www.bcbsm.com/foundation/
Sponsor: Blue Cross Blue Shield of Michigan Foundation
600 Lafayette East-X520
Detroit, MI 48226

BCBSM Frank J. McDevitt, DO, Excellence in Research Awards **722**
The Frank J. McDevitt Excellence in Research Awards for Health Services, Policy and Clinical Care recognize Michigan-based researchers and physicians who have published research in research journals that contributes to improving health and medical care in Michigan. The BCBSM Foundation will award $10,000 for unrestricted research to physician and doctoral level researchers for research on: health policy; health services; clinical care.
Requirements: Applicants must be from Michigan based researchers with terminal research degrees (e.g. PhD, DrPH) and from Michigan based physicians (MD or DO). In the case of multiple authorship, the nominee must be the first author. All authors will be nominated and will constitute one team nomination. The nomination research must have been published, or accepted for publication in a refereed health or medical care journal, within the previous two years. The financial award will be made to the recipient's 501 (c)(3) non-profit or educational organization.
Restrictions: Only one article per nominee will be accepted for consideration each year.
Geographic Focus: Michigan
Amount of Grant: $10,000
Date(s) Application is Due: Jan 1
Contact: Nora Maloy, Senior Program Officer; (313) 225-8706; fax: (313) 225-7730; email: nmaloy@bcbsm.com
Internet: http://www.bcbsm.com/foundation/grant.shtml
Sponsor: Blue Cross Blue Shield of Michigan Foundation
600 Lafayette E, X520
Detroit, MI 48226

BCBSM Investigator-Initiated Research Program Grants **723**
This program encourages Michigan-based applied research projects designed to improve health care in the state of Michigan. Projects that focus on the quality and cost of health care and appropriate access are considered priority and include: organization and delivery of health care services; evaluation of new methods or approaches to containing health care costs; evaluation of new methods or approaches to providing access to high quality health care; assessment and assurance of quality care; identification and validation of clinical protocols and evidence based practice guidelines. Applications are excepted at any time and are reviewed at the next possible Board of Directors meeting.
Requirements: Applications will be accepted from medical and doctoral-level researchers based in hospitals, university settings, non-profit health care organizations, health systems, medical or nursing schools, schools of public health, or other relevant academic disciplines. A complete application must include the original (unbound) and four copies of the supporting documents.

Restrictions: This program does of support basic science or biomedical research, including drug studies or studies using animals.
Geographic Focus: Michigan
Amount of Grant: $50,000-$75,000 per year
Contact: Grants Administrator, (313) 225-8706; fax: (313) 225-7730; email: foundation@bcbsm.com
Internet: http://www.bcbsm.com/foundation/gp_iip.shtml
Sponsor: Blue Cross Blue Shield of Michigan Foundation
600 Lafayette East, X520
Detroit, MI 48226

BCBSNC Foundation Fit Together Grants 724
The program provides funding and technical assistance to rural North Carolina communities that seek to improve community health by implementing innovative and integrated strategies to increase physical activity. Up to five grantees will be chosen to develop and maintain interdisciplinary community partnerships that seek to implement programs, policies, physical projects, and promotional strategies that increase access and reduce barriers to opportunities for active living.
Requirements: North Carolina nonprofit or government organizations are eligible.
Geographic Focus: North Carolina
Amount of Grant: $40,000 per year for three years
Date(s) Application is Due: Dec 16
Contact: Polly Leousis, (919) 765-4102
Internet: http://www.bcbsnc.com/foundation/fitogether_grants.html
Sponsor: Blue Cross Blue Shield of North Carolina Foundation
5901 Chapel Hill Road
Durham, NC 27707-0718

BCBSNC Foundation Grants 725
The foundation's primary objective is to fund clearly defined, innovative grants that further the foundation mission of improving the health and well-being of North Carolinians. The foundation funds programs typically possessing the following characteristics: programs and/or services designed to produce measurable, long-term impact; programs that are sustainable and designed to be ongoing, rather than one-time or sporadic events; programs and/or services that are replicable. The three primary focus areas include health of vulnerable populations, healthy active communities and community impact through nonprofit excellence.
Requirements: Applicants must meet the following criteria to be eligible for funding: organization is located within North Carolina; organization is a 501(c)3 organization or an educational or governmental entity with tax-exempt status, that is not a private foundation or Type III supporting organization; organization must be able to provide its most recent IRS Form 990. Depending on the type of grant and the size of the organization, an audit may be required as part of the submitted proposal.
Restrictions: The foundation will not provide funding for annual campaigns, political campaigns, religious purposes, individuals, endowments, purchase of advertisements, or for the sole purpose of receiving goods or entitlements from a charitable organization.
Geographic Focus: North Carolina
Contact: Grant Review Committee, (919) 765-7347; email: foundation@bcbsnc.com
Internet: http://www.bcbsnc.com/foundation/grants.html?previouslyOver=true&currentlyOver=true
Sponsor: Blue Cross Blue Shield of North Carolina Foundation
P.O. Box 2291
Durham, NC 27702

BCRF Research Grants 726
The goal of the grant process is a serious peer review of all proposals. Proposals are invited by the Medical Advisory Board, rather than accepted as unsolicited requests. The MAB generally reviews proposals in the late summer. There is no set format, but the BCRF requests a brief narrative (no more than 4-5 pages), lay language summary, annual budget (no more than $225,000 initially, with a maximum of 20% in indirect costs) and budget narrative. Considerable latitude is given to the investigators in terms of the work proposed. Both the Board of Directors and the Medical Advisory Board concur that some of the most important advances in understanding the disease will most likely occur by enabling brilliant minds to pursue some of their most creative theories.
Restrictions: While most of the grants are unrestricted, the Foundation has donors requesting restricted grants for specific purposes. When this occurs, the Medical Advisory Board will meet to determine whether the area of interest merits further exploration. If so, they will identify various research projects meeting the donor's criteria.
Amount of Grant: $225,000 maximum
Contact: Administrator, (646) 497-2600; fax: (646) 497-0890; email: bcrf@bcrfcure.org
Internet: http://www.bcrfcure.org/action_grantguidelines.html
Sponsor: Breast Cancer Research Foundation
60 East 56th Street, 8th Floor
New York, NY 10022

BCRF-AACR Grants for Translational Breast Cancer Research 727
The grants will provide direct support for innovative cancer research projects designed to accelerate the discovery, development, and application of new agents to treat breast cancer and/or for pre-clinical research with direct therapeutic intent. Special emphasis will be placed on research that holds promise for leading to individualized therapeutic options for treatment in the near future.
Requirements: Researchers who are affiliated with any institution involved in cancer research, cancer medicine, or cancer-related biomedical science anywhere in the world may apply. There are no geographic, national, or residency status restrictions. Applicants must have acquired a doctoral degree in a related field. If an applicant has obtained an equivalent degree at a foreign institution, information on the nature of the degree must be provided at the time of application.
Restrictions: Employees or subcontractors of a national government or the for-profit private industry are not eligible to serve as the Principal Investigator for the purpose of these grants. However, collaborations with such individuals are encouraged. Neither the members of the Scientific Review Committee nor the members of their individual laboratories are eligible for these grants.
Amount of Grant: $200,000
Date(s) Application is Due: May 20; Jul 20
Contact: Hanna Hopfinger, Program Assistant; (267) 646-0665 or (215) 440-9300; fax: (215) 440-9372; email: hanna.hopfinger@aacr.org or awards@aacr.org
Internet: http://www.aacr.org/home/scientists/research-funding—fellowships/bcrf-aacr-grants.aspx
Sponsor: Breast Cancer Research Foundation and the American Association for Cancer Research
615 Chestnut Street, 17th Floor
Philadelphia, PA 19106-4404

Bearemy's Kennel Pals Grants 728
The program provides direct support for animals in domestic pet programs including animal welfare organizations, pet rescue and rehabilitation organizations, and therapeutic and humane education pet programs. Grants will be a one-time contribution and generally range from $1,000 to $10,000, but the average grant tends to be $4,000. Programs that will be funded include: (1) Individual Project grants – generally for one-time purchases or to fulfill a short-term need. Examples include equipment purchases or spay/neuter events, etc; (2) Organization Program grants – start-up or operational costs for ongoing programs. Examples include spay/neuter programs, humane education initiatives, and service dog training programs.
Requirements: While the geographic focus of the program is broad (United States and Canada), priority is given to organizations located near Build-A-Bear Workshop stores. United States applicants must be a tax-exempt organization under Section 501(c)3 of the IRS Code, and not a private foundation, within the meaning of Code Sections 509(a)(1) or 509(a)(2), or a state college or university within the meaning of Code Section 511(a)(2)(B) (a Public Charity). In addition, grant recipients must certify that they are not a supporting organization within the meaning of Code Section 509(a)(3). Canadian applicants must be a registered Canadian charity.
Restrictions: Grant types not funded: (1) Capital Campaigns; (2) Construction or new facility expenses; (3) Fundraising or Event Sponsorships; (4) Political Activities; (5) Religious organizations for religious purposes.
Samples: Animal Advocates of South Carolina (Barnwell, SC); Bunny Castle Rabbit Rescue (Bishop, CA); EquiFriends (Snohomish, WA); Hearing and Service Dogs of Minnesota (Minneapolis, MN); Pet Adoption Fund (Canoga Park, CA).
Amount of Grant: $1,000 - $10,000
Date(s) Application is Due: Mar 31; Jun 30; Sep 31; Dec 31
Contact: Maxine Clark, President; (314) 423-8000; email: giving@buildabear.com
Internet: http://www.buildabear.com/aboutus/community/bearhugs.aspx
Sponsor: Build-A-Bear Workshop Bear Hugs Foundation
1954 Innerbelt Business Center Drive
Saint Louis, MO 63114

Beatrice Laing Trust Grants 729
The trust was founded for the relief of poverty and for the advancement of the evangelical faith internationally. Grants are awarded for general charitable purposes at the discretion of the Trustees, with an emphasis on social services and relief, and medical aid and research. Grant recipients typically are charities working in deprived sections of the community in the United Kingdom, to missionary societies and, less frequently, to individuals working in the field of missions in United Kingdom and abroad.
Samples: ActionAid, 10,000 pounds to improve access to education for pastoralist families in Somaliland; OxFam, 10,000 pounds to the "You Are Here" program; Sense International, 15,000 pounds for work with deaf-blind people in Romania.
Contact: Trust Administrator, 020 8238 8890; fax: 020 8238 8897
Sponsor: Beatrice Laing Trust
33 Bunns Lane
London NW7 2DX United Kingdom

Beazley Foundation Grants 730
The foundation makes grants to Virginia nonprofit organizations engaged in educational, charitable, and religious activities. The focus of support is within the South Hampton Roads cities and counties. Past awards include: music appreciation; educational outreach and mentoring programs; health and wellness; equipment and operating expenses; environmental education programs; renovations and repairs; literacy and community development. Grant applications can be found online.
Requirements: 501(c)3 nonprofit organizations in Virginia are eligible.
Restrictions: Individuals are ineligible.
Geographic Focus: Virginia
Samples: The Tidewater Winds, Norfolk, VA, $7,500—operating expenses (2008); The Union Mission Ministries, Norfolk, VA, $125,000—capital campaign (2008); Virginia College Fund, Richmond, VA, $50,000—Beazley Scholarship Endowments (2008).
Date(s) Application is Due: Jan 4; Mar 1; Jun 1; Oct 1
Contact: Donna Russell, Associate Director; (757) 393-1605; fax: (757) 393-4708; email: info@beazleyfoundation.org

Sponsor: Beazley Foundation
3720 Brighton Street
Portsmouth, VA 23707-3902

Bechtel Group Foundation Building Positive Community Relationships Grants 731
Bechtel Group Foundation was created in 1954 to respond to the needs of the communities around the world in which Bechtel has offices or major projects. These grants support educational, civic and cultural, and social service programs in the communities that host major Bechtel offices and projects. These grants are typically under U.S. $5,000.
Geographic Focus: Arizona; California; Maryland; Tennessee; Texas; Virginia; Washington; Australia; Brazil; Canada; China; Japan; Peru; Philippines; Poland; Russia; United Kingdom
Amount of Grant: $1,000-$5,000 range
Contact: Susan Grisso, Manager; (415) 768-5444; email: becfoun@bechtel.com
Internet: http://www.bechtel.com/foundation.html
Sponsor: Bechtel Group Foundation
50 Beale Street
San Francisco, CA 94105

Beckley Area Foundation Grants 732
The Foundation makes annual discretionary grants to charitable organizations in the areas of education, health and human services, the arts, public recreation and civic beautification. Using several general unrestricted endowments which generate income, BAF makes these grants to address the community's current most pressing needs and promising opportunities.
Requirements: To be eligible for a grant from the Beckley Area Foundation, applicants must be a non-profit organizatiion tax-exempt under section 501(c)3 of the Internal Revenue Code, or they must be a public institution. Programs funded through this annual grant must be located in Raleigh County.
Restrictions: As a Community Foundation, BAF cannot accept requests on behalf of individuals or groups that do not have official recognition as a non-profit charity or public entity. Grants are for one year only. Generally grants are not made for: annual campaigns; endowments; sectarian religious programs; political purposes or lobbying; ongoing operating expenses; expenses outside the grant period.
Geographic Focus: West Virginia
Amount of Grant: $10,000
Date(s) Application is Due: Dec 15
Contact: Grants Administrator, (304) 253-3806; fax: (304) 253-7304; email: funds@beckleyareafoundation.com
Internet: http://beckleyareafoundation.com/id7.html
Sponsor: Beckley Area Foundation
129 Main Street, Suite 203
Beckley, WV 25801

Beckman Coulter Community Relations Grants 733
The corporation funds nonprofit organizations, charities and educational institutions that support and promote progress and interest in the areas of science, research-related health care and science education in our plant and customer communities.
Requirements: Organizations seeking funding should submit a letter of request providing the following information: full legal name of the organization; brief description of the organization, including a mission statement and services provided; amount requested; description of how the funds will be used. Additional attachments should include: history of previous support by Beckman Coulter; description of any involvement by Beckman Coulter employees; statement as to why you consider Beckman Coulter an appropriate donor; list of governing board members.
Restrictions: Grants do not fund golf events, galas, or religious or political activities.
Contact: Cathy Doherty, Community Relations, (714) 961-4478
Internet: http://www.beckman.com/hr/ourcompany/oc_communityRelations.asp#
Sponsor: Beckman Coulter Corporation
Community Relations, Beckman Coulter, Inc., 200 S. Kraemer Boulevard
Brea, CA 92821

Beckman Scholars Program Grants 734
The Program is an invited program for accredited universities and four-year colleges in the United States. It provides scholarships that contribute significantly in advancing the education, research training and personal development of select students in chemistry, biochemistry, and the biological and medical sciences. The sustained, in-depth undergraduate research experiences and comprehensive faculty mentoring are unique in terms of program scope, content and level of scholarship awards. The amount given is $19,300 for two summers and one academic year.
Samples: Christa Jordan Laser, Arizona State University—Photosynthetic Reaction Center Mutagenesis (2007-08); Diana Ahn Tran, Harvey Mudd College—Characterization of Conserved Regulatory Elements in the Telomerase Promoter in Primates (2007-08); Donald Bungum, University of Chicago—Synthesis of 61Ni Compounds for Mossbauer Spectroscopy (2007-08).
Amount of Grant: $19,300
Contact: Program Administrator, (949) 721-2222; fax: (949) 721-2225; email: beckmanscholars@beckman-foundation.com or k.williams@beckman-foundation.com
Internet: http://www.beckman-foundation.com/bsp.html
Sponsor: Arnold and Mabel Beckman Foundation
100 Academy Drive
Irvine, CA 92617

Beckman Young Investigators Program Grants 735
The foundation makes grants to nonprofit research institutions to promote research in chemistry and the life sciences, broadly interpreted, and particularly to foster the invention of methods, instruments, and materials that will open up new avenues of research in science. The program is intended to provide research support to the most promising young faculty members in the early stages of academic careers in the chemical and life sciences. The program is open to persons with tenure-track appointments in academic and nonprofit institutions that conduct fundamental research in the chemical and life sciences. The program is intended primarily for U.S. institutions. Only proposals of exceptional merit from foreign institutions will receive consideration. Projects are normally funded for a period of two years. When extraordinary circumstances warrant, support may be provided over a one-year or three-year period. Application materials are available on the Web site.
Requirements: To be eligible, an applicant should not have completed more than three full years in his or her tenure-track or other comparable independent research appointment on the anniversary date of initial appointment in the year in which application is to be made. Individuals may not apply more than three times.
Restrictions: Funding will not be considered for general institutional expenses or general fund-raising campaign expenses such as dinners and mass mailings. The foundation does not provide funds for overhead or indirect costs.
Amount of Grant: $264,000 average
Date(s) Application is Due: Sep 28
Contact: Administrator, (949) 721-2222; fax: (949) 721-2225; email: younginvestigators@beckman-foundation.com or k.williams@beckman-foundation.com
Internet: http://www.beckman-foundation.com/byi_guides.html
Sponsor: Arnold and Mabel Beckman Foundation
100 Academy Drive
Irvine, CA 92617

Becton Dickinson and Company Grants 736
The company supports national and international activities in keeping with its commitment to advance the quality of medical practice and patient care in four areas: the global healthcare fund; the local initiatives fund; the matching gifts program; and the BD product donation program. Call for guidelines.
Contact: Community Relations, (201) 847-6800
Internet: http://www.bd.com/responsibility/contributions
Sponsor: Becton Dickinson and Company
1 Becton Drive
Franklin Lakes, NJ 07417

Beirne Carter Foundation Grants 737
The Foundation places an emphasis on health, education, local history, nature, ecology and youth. Except in rare instances, grants are limited to institutions and organizations located in the Commonwealth of Virginia. Requests that are not of a recurring nature are given preference. Any organization that has been awarded a grant is encouraged to wait at least three years before submitting a new grant request. Any organization seeking grant consideration must complete a Preliminary Proposal form which is online. Its content should be limited to the two page format provided online.
Requirements: The Foundation is organized exclusively for charitable purposes. Grants are made only to institutions and organizations which qualify under IRS regulations as tax exempt and which are not private operating foundations as defined by the IRS.
Restrictions: Grants will not normally be made: to endowment funds (including scholarship funds); to organizations supported primarily by government funds (such as public secondary schools and colleges and local municipalities); to churches and related organizations; for ongoing operating expenses (such as salaries, rent, office supplies, etc.); for existing deficits; or for debt reduction. Grants are not made to individuals.
Geographic Focus: Virginia
Date(s) Application is Due: Feb 1; Aug 3
Contact: Peter C. Toms, Executive Director, (804) 521-0272; fax: (804) 521-0274; email: bcarterfn@aol.com
Internet: http://www.bcarterfdn.org
Sponsor: Beirne Carter Foundation
1802 Bayberry Court, Suite 401
Richmond, VA 23226-3773

Beldon Fund Grants 738
The fund focuses project and general support grants in two programs: human health and the environment, and key states. Human health and the environment—the fund seeks proposals that engage new constituencies in exposing the connection between toxic chemicals and human health and in promoting public policies that prevent or eliminate environmental risks to people's health. The program focuses grant making in three areas: new advocates, human exposure to toxic chemicals, and environmental justice. Key states—the fund believes that states hold the key to bringing about rapid, real change on environmental issues and policy in the United States. By strengthening public support for environmental protection in several of these key states, the fund hopes to transform the nation's approach to environmental protection. The fund is currently accepting proposals from Florida, Michigan, Minnesota, Wisconsin, and North Carolina for this program. Proposals do not need to be tied to any particular issue or set of issues, but targeted issues must be those that will build active public support for the environment. From time to time, the fund will add and remove states from this program. Types of support include special projects, seed money, general operating budgets, and technical assistance. One-year and multiyear grants are awarded. Due date applies to the letter of intent; full proposals are by invitation.By supporting effective, nonprofit advocacy organizations, the

Beldon Fund seeks to build a national consensus to achieve and sustain a healthy planet. The Fund plans to invest its entire principal and earnings by 2009 to attain this goal.
Requirements: 501(c)3 tax-exempt organizations are eligible.
Restrictions: Grants do not support international efforts, academic or university efforts, school-based environmental education, land acquisition, wildlife or habitat preservation, film or video production, deficit reduction, endowments, capital campaigns, acquisitions of museums, service delivery, scholarshp, publications, or arts/culture.
Geographic Focus: Florida; Michigan; Minnesota; North Carolina; Wisconsin
Samples: Ctr for Public Interest Research (Boston, MA)—for its Campaign Staff Training Institute Program to ameliorate the shortage of skilled activists, $75,000 (2004); Institute for Conservation Leadership (Takoma Park, MD)—for its outreach and hands-on support efforts, along with Environmental Support Ctr, $10,000 (2004); State Environmental Leadership Program (Madison, WI)—for general support, $175,000 (2004); Washington Environmental Alliance for Voter Education (Seattle, WA)—for general support, $50,000 (2004).
Amount of Grant: $5000-$100,000
Date(s) Application is Due: Feb 28; Jun 13
Contact: Holeri Faruolo, Grants Manager, (800) 591-9595 or (212) 616-5600; fax: (212) 616-5656; email: info@beldon.org
Internet: http://www.beldon.org
Sponsor: Beldon Fund
99 Madison Avenue, 8th Floor
New York, NY 10016

Belk Foundation Grants 739

The Foundation makes grants to a wide variety of community-based nonprofit organizations and institutions whose missions and actions support the advancement of Christian causes and the up-building of mankind. The Foundation supports local and regional organizations by: assisting secondary schools, colleges and universities and their programs; assisting religious institutions and organizations and their programs; supporting area arts and other cultural organizations and their programs; supporting community-based human services organizations and their programs; and aiding hospitals and health care organizations and their programs.
Requirements: 501(c)3 nonprofits in communities in the 14 states where Belk stores are located. Preference is given to organizations in North Carolina.
Restrictions: Grants are not awarded to: individuals, including students; public, government or quasi-governmental programs, agencies or organizations (excluding certain public secondary schools, colleges and universities); or international programs and/or organizations. Additionally, the Foundation does not provide door prizes, gift certificates, merchandise or other giveaways.
Geographic Focus: Alabama; Arkansas; Florida; Georgia; Kentucky; Louisiana; Maryland; Mississippi; North Carolina; South Carolina; Tennessee; Texas; Virginia; West Virginia
Date(s) Application is Due: Apr 15; Oct 15
Contact: Susan C. Blount, Foundation Administrator; (704) 426-8396; email: susan_blount@belk.com
Internet: http://www.belk.com/AST/Misc/Belk_Stores/About_Us/Belk_Community/Belk_Foundation.jsp
Sponsor: Belk Foundation
2801 W. Tyvola Road
Charlotte, NC 28217-4500

Bella Vista Foundation Grants 740

The foundation has two main focus areas: early childhood—healthy emotional development in children during the first years of their lives, and parents involvement to help their children deal with the internal issues of attachment and independence; and environment restoration—restoration of land, streams, wetlands, habitat, etc., and acquisition of land for the purpose of preservation, particularly requests that include restoration efforts. Deadlines are January 30 and June 15 for environmental restoration grants, and January 15 and June 15 for early childhood grants. Guidelines are available online.
Requirements: Early childhood grants support public charities located in California's San Francisco, Marin, San Mateo, and Santa Clara counties. Environmental restoration grants support projects in California or Oregon.
Restrictions: Grants will not be made to or for the arts, sectarian religious purposes, individuals, or benefit events, and will only be made for medical research, health care, publications, or video production under special circumstances and only in the early childhood development focus area. The foundation does not make multiyear grants.
Geographic Focus: California; Oregon
Amount of Grant: $2.79 million total
Date(s) Application is Due: Jan 15; Jan 30; Jun 15
Contact: Mary Gregory, Executive Director, (415) 561-6540; fax: (415) 561-6477; email: mgregory@pfs-llc.net
Internet: http://www.pfs-llc.net/bellavista/index.html
Sponsor: Bella Vista Foundation
P.O. Box 29906, Presidio Building 1016, Suite 300
San Francisco, CA 94129-0906

Ben B. Cheney Foundation Grants 741

The foundation organizes its grant making into eight categories: charity—programs providing for basic needs such as food, shelter, and clothing; civic— programs improving the quality of life in a community as a whole such as museums and recreation facilities; culture—programs encompassing the arts; education—programs supporting capital projects and scholarships, primarily for 14 pre-selected colleges and universities in the Pacific Northwest; elderly—programs serving the social, health, recreational, and other needs of older people; health—programs related to providing health care; social services—programs serving people with physical or mental disabilities or other special needs; and youth—programs helping young people to gain the skills needed to become responsible and productive adults. All inquiries must be submitted as a two to three page proposal letter. There are no deadlines. The foundation accepts proposal letters throughout the year.
Requirements: The foundation sets a priority on projects serving the people of Tacoma/Pierce County and southwestern Washington, southern Oregon—particularly the area around Medford—and portions of Del Norte, Humboldt, Lassen, Shasta, Siskiyou, and Trinity counties in California.
Restrictions: The foundation generally does not make grants to support general operating budgets or annual campaigns; projects that are primarily or normally financed by tax funds; religious organizations for sectarian purposes; basic research; endowment funds; individuals; produce books, films, or videos; conferences, seminars, or attendance at same; or individual students or student groups raising money for school-related trips.
Geographic Focus: California; Oregon; Washington
Samples: Whitman College (Walla Walla, WA)—to construct a new science building and to renovate the current facility, $40,000 (2002); Gonzaga U (Spokane, WA)—to equip two multimedia classrooms in the Herak Ctr for Engineering, $35,000.
Contact: Brad Cheney, Executive Director, (253) 572-2442; email: info@benbcheneyfoundation.org
Internet: http://www.benbcheneyfoundation.org
Sponsor: Ben B. Cheney Foundation
3110 Ruston Way, Suite A
Tacoma, WA 98402-5307

Bender Foundation Grants 742

The foundation supports projects for higher education, health agencies, Jewish welfare funds and organizations, Christian youth organizations, and social welfare. Emphasis is support for programs to assist the elderly and aging, children and parenting, and environmental programs. Grants are awarded for challenge/matching grants, endowments, general operations, and scholarships.
Requirements: Grants are made to organizations and institutions in Maryland and Washington, DC. An applicant should initially send a brief letter of intent. Full proposals are by invitation.
Restrictions: Grants are not made to individuals.
Geographic Focus: District of Columbia; Maryland
Samples: Jewish Community Center of Greater Washington (Rockville, MD)—for fitness center, $87,500.; Discovery Creek Childrens Museum (Washington, DC)—general support, $50,000.; Anti-Defamation League of Bnai Brith(Washington, DC)—for Concert Against Hate, $25,000.
Amount of Grant: $100-$100,000 range
Date(s) Application is Due: Nov 30
Contact: Julie Bender Silver, President, (202) 828-9000; fax: (202) 785-9347
Sponsor: Bender Foundation
1120 Connecticut Ave NW, Suite 1200
Washington, DC 20036

Benton Community Foundation Grants 743

Benton Community Foundation holds one grant making cycle each year. Public announcement is made in the local press and on the website under news and events. The Foundation address's the broad needs of residents of Benton County which fall generally into five categories: civic affairs; cultural affairs; education; health and safety; and social services. The deadline for grant applications is August 1st and awards are announced by mid-September. Priority is given to programs that: reach as many people as possible; improve the ability of the organization to serve the community over the long term; serve Benton County residents; and are run by nonprofit organizations. Benton Community Foundation also administers several scholarship programs including the Lilly Endowment Community Scholarship Program which is funded by Lilly Endowment Inc. The application procedures and selection criteria vary for each of the scholarships, see Foundations website for further guidelines.
Restrictions: The Foundation generally does not fund: political organizations or candidates; endowments; ongoing operating expenses; individuals (except scholarships from scholarship funds); programs already completed; special events such as parades, festivals, and sporting events; multi-year programs; or debt reduction or elimination.
Geographic Focus: Indiana
Date(s) Application is Due: Aug 1
Contact: Ashley Bice, Executive Director; (765) 884-8022; fax: (765) 884-8023; email: ashley@bentoncf.org or info@bentoncf.org
Internet: http://www.bentoncf.org/grants.html
Sponsor: Benton Community Foundation
P.O. Box 351
Fowler, IN 47944

Benton County Foundation Grants 744

The Foundation's investment philosophy is built on the precepts of diversification, long-term strategic focus, and prudent risk management. The mission is to establish endowments, manage the funds received, and distribute a portion of the earnings each year to benefit youth and community. The Foundation focuses on funding programs that enhance youth education and/or provide positive character building and life skills experience.

Requirements: Organizations must be located in Benton County, Oregon.
Geographic Focus: Oregon
Date(s) Application is Due: Mar 13
Contact: Dick Thompson, Executive Director; (541) 753-1603 or (541) 231-7604; email: BCF@peak.org
Internet: http://www.bentoncountyfoundation.org/grants/
Sponsor: Benton County Foundation
P.O. Box 911
Corvallis, OR 97330

Berks County Community Foundation Grants **745**
The foundation supports a broad range of community projects in this Pennsylvania county, including the arts and culture, economic development, education, the environment, and health and human services. Types of support include general operating grants, capital campaigns, demonstration grants, seed grants, and program grants. Although applicants do not have to be located in Berks County, they must provide programs and services within the county.
Requirements: Tax exempt or public benefit organizations, individuals, associations and private or public agencies are eligible to apply. The grant must be used for charitable purposes only. Organizations are eligible to apply to more than one grant program in the same year.
Geographic Focus: Pennsylvania
Contact: Richard Mappin, Vice President for Grantmaking; (610) 685-2223; fax: (610) 685-2240; email: info@bccf.org
Internet: http://www.bccf.org/pages/grants.html
Sponsor: Berks County Community Foundation
P.O. Box 212, 501 Washington Street, Suite 801
Reading, PA 19603-0212

Bernard and Audre Rapoport Foundation Grants **746**
The mission of the foundation is to support programs that have the broadest possible impact in meeting important human needs and aspirations, with an emphasis on the needs of the least advantaged members of society. Preference is given to five primary areas: education, including early learning through the elementary years, adult education and training initiatives, and programs that enhance the capabilities of teachers and other professionals in public schools; arts and culture, especially activities that encourage the participation and enrich the lives of children and disadvantaged members of the community; healthcare— especially services to women, children, and those who do not have access to conventional medical resources; community-based outreach initiatives such as immunization programs; community building and social services—i.e., programs that build grassroots neighborhood networks, provide job training and job opportunities for the unemployed and underemployed, or provide a comprehensive safety net of social services for the least advantaged citizens; democracy and civic participation—efforts to make government more responsive, encourage citizens to take an active interest and role in political life, encourage intergovernmental cooperation, broaden public awareness of public policy issues and alternatives, build skills necessary for political leadership, and provide opportunities for community service; and Rapoport Service Scholarships at the University of Texas at Austin. There are no deadlines for proposals.
Requirements: Applicant must provide proof of tax exempt status.
Geographic Focus: Texas
Contact: Carole Jones, (254) 741-0510; fax: (254) 741-0092; email: carole@rapoportfdn.org
Internet: http://www.rapoportfdn.org/priorities.asp
Sponsor: Bernard and Audre Rapoport Foundation
5400 Bosque Boulevard, Suite 245
Waco, TX 76710

Bernard F. and Alva B. Gimbel Foundation Grants **747**
The foundation's areas of interest are currently education, workforce and economic development, civil legal services, criminal justice, reproductive rights, and the environment. In most program areas, the Foundation seeks to fund both direct services programs and advocacy efforts. The Foundation's support for direct services programs is limited to those operating in New York City.
Requirements: Grants are made only to tax-exempt 501(c)3 organizations.
Restrictions: The Foundation does not make grants to: individuals; direct service programs outside of New York City; individual schools; short-term educational programs and workshops; mentoring programs; after-school and summer programs; youth development programs. Unsolicited proposals for the Environment program are not accepted.
Geographic Focus: New York
Contact: Leslie Gimbel, Executive Director, (212) 895-8050; fax: (212) 895-8052
Internet: http://www.gimbelfoundation.org/index.html
Sponsor: Bernard F. and Alva B. Gimbel Foundation
271 Madison Avenue, Suite 605
New York, NY 10016

Bernard Van Leer Foundation Grants **748**
The foundation operates in 34 countries in Europe, the Far East, Australia, Central and South America, the United States, and Africa to further the holistic development of young children. Grantmaking focuses on thematic initiatives, which may include partners from countries where the foundation does not otherwise have a grantmaking program. Current themes are: children affected by HIV/AIDS; respect for diversity; and growing up in indigenous societies. The foundation funds projects that promote a holistic approach to early childhood development; the enhancement of parental capacity to support their children's development; a development strategy that is rooted in the local context and is culturally, socially, and economically appropriate; and the building of capacity, local ownership, and working in partnership. Unsolicited proposals are rarely funded. To be considered, submit information about the organization; the project's objectives, strategies, beneficiaries, scope, location, and duration; and the overall budget and the amount required.
Requirements: Grants are made to governmental and nongovernmental organizations located in the list of eligible countries, which include: Brazil, Colombia, the East Caribbean region, Germany, Greece, India, Indonesia, Israel, Kenya, Mexico, Morocco, the Netherlands, Peru, Poland, South Africa, Tanzania, Thailand, Turkey, Uganda, United States of America and Zimbabwe.
Restrictions: The foundation does not offer support to individual children; projects that concentrate solely on one aspect of children's development or learning; projects that specifically focus on children with special needs such as mental and/or physical handicap; proposals for the construction and maintenance of buildings, or the purchase of equipment and materials; isolated requests for scholarships, conferences, media or theatre events; or general support, or requests to cover recurrent costs or deficits
Contact: Peter Laugharn, Executive Director; 31-70-351-20-40; fax: 31-70-350-23-73; email: proposal.administration@bvleerf.nl
Internet: http://www.bernardvanleer.org/about/Applications_for_funding
Sponsor: Bernard Van Leer Foundation
Eisenhowerlaan 156, P.O. Box 82334
The Hague 2508 EH Netherlands

Berrien Community Foundation Grants **749**
The community foundation awards grants to nonprofits in Berrien County, Michigan, that address community needs. The Foundation is very interested in providing start-up funding for programs that address our focus areas of nurturing children, building community spirit/arts and culture and youth leadership and development. Higher priority is given to requests that demonstrate community-based collaborative solutions likely to stay in place after Foundation funding concludes. Low priority is given to requests for bricks and mortar, operational funds on a repetitive basis, annual fund drives, equipment, and ongoing programs where alternative funding is not planned to carry a program/project forward following a Foundation grant. Low priority is also given to advertising and capital campaigns and grants to cover deficits or other previously incurred obligations. Applicants must first call the Foundation's program director to discuss the proposed program/project.
Requirements: Grant applications will only be accepted from nonprofit 501(c)3 and grass roots organizations serving Berrien County residents.
Restrictions: Grants are not made for sectarian religious purposes, national fundraising efforts, political organizations or campaigns. Grants are not made to individuals, and form letters/emails are neither reviewed nor acknowledged.
Geographic Focus: Michigan
Amount of Grant: $10,000 maximum
Date(s) Application is Due: Sep 1
Contact: Anne McCausland, Program Director: (269) 983-3304, ext. 2; fax: (269) 983-4939; email: AnneMcCausland@BerrienCommunity.org
Internet: http://www.berriencommunity.org
Sponsor: Berrien Community Foundation
2900 South State Street, Suite 2 East
Saint Joseph, MI 49085

Bert W. Martin Foundation Grants **750**
The foundation awards grants to eligible nonprofit organizations in its areas of interest, including higher education, healthcare, sports, and general charitable giving. There are no application forms or deadlines. Proposal letters are accepted by postal mail only. No email proposals accepted.
Requirements: Nonprofit organizations in Florida and Arizona.
Geographic Focus: Arizona; Florida
Samples: Columbia U (New York, NY)—to enable undergraduate students to attend the Earth Semester program, a series of studies in earth systems and policy designed to foster an understanding of critical global issues, at its Biosphere 2 Center, $800,000.
Contact: Grants Administrator, c/o Northern Trust Co
Sponsor: Bert W. Martin Foundation
50 S. LaSalle Street, B-3
Chicago, IL 60675-0002

Bertha Russ Lytel Foundation Grants **751**
The foundation awards grants to eligible California nonprofit organizations in its areas of interest, including civic affairs; cultural programs, libraries and museums; elementary education; higher education, including agricultural and nursing scholarships; health organizations, including hospitals and hospice; and social services for the elderly and disabled. The primary focus of the Foundation is programs for seniors. Types of support include building construction/renovation, continuing support, equipment acquisition, general operating grants, matching grants, scholarship funds, and seed grants. Contact the Foundation Manager for guidelines and application information.
Requirements: California nonprofit organizations in Humboldt County are eligible.
Geographic Focus: California
Contact: Don Hindley, Manager, (707) 786-9236
Sponsor: Bertha Russ Lytel Foundation
P.O. Box 893
Ferndale, CA 95536

Besser Foundation Grants 752

The foundation limits its giving to nonprofits in the Alpena, MI area. Areas of interest include education, social services, civic affairs, arts and culture, religion, and international. Types of support include scholarship funds, matching funds, operating budgets, and continuing support. The board meets quarterly to consider requests.
Requirements: Only nonprofits in Michigan may apply.
Restrictions: Unless specifically requested by a Trustee, the Foundation will not consider grant requests from organizations outside of Alpena; nor for endowment funds, to defray meeting or conference expenses, or to pay for travel of individuals or groups. We will not relieve organizations or the public of their responsibilities, nor make grants to individuals for any purpose.
Geographic Focus: Michigan
Samples: Jesse Besser Museum, Alpena, MI, $220,00 (2006); Alpena Community College, Alpena, MI, $100,000 (2006); Child and Family Services of Northeast Michigan, Alpena, MI, $40,000 (2006).
Contact: J. Richard Wilson, President; (989) 354-4722; fax: (517) 354-8099; email: besserfoundation@verizon.net
Sponsor: Besser Foundation
123 North Second Avenue, Suite 3
Alpena, MI 49707-2801

BHHS Legacy Foundation Grants 753

BHHS Legacy Foundation funds efforts that enhance and improve the quality of life and health of children, families and senior citizens that are primarily low-income and under-served in the greater Phoenix and Tri-State regions. The Foundation places a high priority on collaborative projects and programs with other foundations, government agencies and nonprofit entities seeking to strengthen communities and support systemic change in health care access, health improvement and delivery. It also places a strong emphasis on funding nonprofit community organizations to increase their capacity to serve. These may include projects and programs offered by established nonprofit entities as well as those provided by start-up nonprofit organizations. Types of grants include: program/project; education; capacity building; capital equipment; operating; transition; and : Community Assistance Relief for Emergencies (CARE) funding. The foundation recommends discussing project or program concept and proposal with a foundation representative prior to submitting a written request for funding.
Restrictions: Giving is primarily restricted to the greater Phoenix and Bullhead/Laughlin regions, Arizona.
Geographic Focus: Arizona
Samples: Assistance League of Phoenix, Arizona, $15,000—for Operation School Bell Program to strengthen communities (2009); Alhambra Foundation for the Future, $150,000—for the Alhambra Foundation, for the Future Scholarships, a healthcare workforce development funding priority (2009).
Amount of Grant: $25,000 - $75,000 range
Date(s) Application is Due: Apr 3; Aug 7; Dec 4
Contact: Karen E. Orth, Grants Manager; (602) 778-1200; fax: (602) 778-1255; email: korth@bhhslegacy.org or info@bhhslegacy.org
Internet: http://bhhslegacy.org/access_healthcare.aspx
Sponsor: BHHS Legacy Foundation
2999 N. 44th Street, Suite 530
Phoenix, AZ 85018

BibleLands Grants 754

The organization was founded to support Christian missions in the lands of the Bible. The program awards grants to hospitals and schools in the Middle East. BibleLands supports schools and colleges that offer good quality Christian-based education for children whose families could not otherwise afford it.
Requirements: Projects must be Christian led.
Restrictions: Grants are not made to individuals or to projects outside the Middle East.
Contact: N. Edward-Few, 01494 897 950; fax: 01494 897 951; email: info@biblelands.org.uk
Internet: http://www.biblelands.org.uk/index2.htm
Sponsor: BibleLands
P.O. Box 50
High Wycombe, Buckinghamshire HP15 7QU United Kingdom

Bildner Family Foundation Grants 755

The foundation awards grants to nonprofit organizations in its areas of interest, including arts and performing arts, health care and health organizations, Jewish and social service delivery. Types of support include continuing support, general operating support, and program support. The majority of grants are awarded in New Jersey and New York. There are no application forms or deadlines.
Restrictions: The foundation does not support private foundations or individuals.
Geographic Focus: New Jersey; New York
Amount of Grant: $2000-$300,000 range
Contact: Allen Bildner, President
Sponsor: Bildner Family Foundation
293 Eisenhower Pkwy, Suite 150
Livingston, NJ 07039

Bill and Melinda Gates Foundation Grants 756

The foundation awards grants in its areas of interest, including increasing access to innovations in technology, education, libraries, and global health. Education grants are intended to provide teachers with opportunities to learn together the best ways to use technology to enhance student learning. Global health grants are awarded to improve the health of women and children, particularly in developing countries, by expanding services to enable women to safely carry and deliver babies and to prevent cervical cancer. Grants to libraries bridge the digital divide between those who have access to computers and the Internet and those who lack such access.
Requirements: 501(c)3 tax-exempt organizations are eligible. Priority is given to requests in the Pacific Northwest, including Idaho, Oregon, and Washington.
Samples: CARE (Atlanta, GA)—for relief efforts following tsunamis in South Asia and Africa, $750,000 (2005); Experience Music Project (Seattle, WA)—for general operating support, $250,000 (2005); CARE (Atlanta, GA)—to assist victims of flooding in eastern Nepal, $300,000 (2005); Korean Women's Assoc (Tacoma, WA)—for its capital campaign for a domestic-violence shelter, $200,000 (2005).
Contact: Program Contact, (206) 709-3140; email: info@gatesfoundation.org
Internet: http://www.gatesfoundation.org/ForGrantSeekers
Sponsor: Bill and Melinda Gates Foundation
P.O. Box 23350
Seattle, WA 98122

Binney and Smith Community Grants 757

Awards include cash and product donations to nonprofit organizations that address the needs of children and young adults through projects in the arts, education, health and welfare, and civic areas. Special consideration is given to nonprofit organizations with which employees serve in a volunteer capacity. Funding is concentrated on specific programs or capital campaign projects rather than general operational support, galas and other fundraising events and event sponsorship. Direct funding and product donations are limited to non-profit organizations in Lehigh and Northampton Counties along with the cities of Kutztown, PA and Phillipsburg, N.J.
Requirements: Eastern Pennylvania nonprofit organizations are eligible.
Restrictions: Grants do not support: nonprofit organizations outside the Lehigh Valley; individuals; religious organizations; fraternal organizations; political organizations; national or international organizations; individual child care centers; nursing and convalescent homes; prisoners; conventions; hospitals; endowment funds; labor groups; social clubs; veterans organizations; athletic organizations. In addition, organizations eligible for support generally will not be funded when the purpose is to cover any of the following: past operating deficits; travel; conferences; non-product goodwill advertising; undefined operational support; tickets for or tables to special events; advertising in programs.
Geographic Focus: Pennsylvania
Contact: Community Affairs Manager, (800) 272-9652
Internet: http://www.binney-smith.com/page.cfm?id=17&hasFlash=false
Sponsor: Binney and Smith Corporation
P.O. Box 431, 1100 Church Lane
Easton, PA 18044-0431

Biogen Corporate Giving Grants 758

The corporate giving program gives back to Biogen communities through grants awarded to nonprofit, community-based organizations, most of which are dedicated to education, community service, healthcare, and culture and the arts. There are no application forms or deadlines; guidelines are available online. See submission information for proposal mailing instructions.
Requirements: To be eligible for funding, an organization must be: a non-profit agency with tax-exempt status under section 501(c)3 of the Internal Revenue Service code; serving residents of Cambridge or the Greater Boston area, San Diego or San Diego County, and Raleigh-Durham, NC.
Restrictions: Eligible organizations must not: advocate, support or practice discrimination based on race, religion, age, national origin, language, gender, sexual preference or physical limitation; include the promotion of any particular religious faith as an explicit and primary goal; have the nomination or election of candidates to political office as an explicit goal, be government agencies, political organizations or individuals. Grants should not cover fundraising or capital campaign activities.
Geographic Focus: California; Massachusetts; North Carolina
Amount of Grant: $500 to $2,500
Contact: Kathryn Bloom, Communications, (617) 679-2000; fax: (617) 679-2617
Internet: http://www.biogen.com/site/014.html
Sponsor: Biogen Inc
14 Cambridge Center
Cambridge, MA 02142

Birds Eye Foods Foundation Grants 759

The Foundation provides grants to not-for-profit organizations operating in communities where Birds Eye Foods has facilities. Giving areas for the Foundation are limited to organizations whose primary mission revolves around healthy eating, feeding the hungry and/or dealing with issues of hunger.
Requirements: Applicants must submit a letter on the organization's letterhead. Include the following information: background of the organization and the work they do; the dollar amount that the organization is attempting to raise; a description of the project for which the funds will be used; a copy of the IRS 501(c)3 determination letter.
Restrictions: Grants are not available for: land acquisitions; start-up funds; internships; pilot projects; publications; conferences/seminars; matching grants/gifts; loans; individuals; multiple year funding.
Geographic Focus: Michigan; Minnesota; New York; Pennsylvania; Washington; Wisconsin
Contact: Susan Riker, (585) 264-3155

Internet: http://www.birdseyefoods.com/corp/about/foundation.asp
Sponsor: Birds Eye Foods Foundation
P.O. Box 20670
Rochester, NY 14602-0670

Birmingham Foundation Grants **760**

The Birmingham Foundation is a private, independent foundation, dedicated to health-related and human services grant-making in the south neighborhoods of Pittsburgh, Pennsylvania, which are part of the 15203, 15210 and 15211 zip code areas. The Board of Directors meets three times a year, in March, June and November.
Requirements: 501(c)3 nonprofits in South Pittsburgh communities including Allentown, Arlington, Arlington Heights, Beltzhoover, Bon Air, Carrick, Duquesne Heights, Knoxville, Mount Oliver, Mount Washington, Saint Clair Village, and South Side are eligible.
Restrictions: Grants are not normally made for operating budgets, deficits, fund-raising campaigns, general research, overhead costs, scholarships, political campaigns, or loans. Grants are not made to individuals, to other private foundations, for sectarian religious activities, or for the efforts to influence legislation unless grant-related.
Geographic Focus: Pennsylvania
Samples: Strong Women Strong Girls, $15,000 - mentoring program (2009); SIDS of PA, $10,000 - SIDS outreach program (2009); Saltworks Theater, $10,000 - bully/drug prevention program (2009).
Amount of Grant: $2,500-$50,000 typically
Contact: Chris Mason, Administrative Assistant; (412) 481-2777; fax: (412) 481-2727; email: info@birmfoundpgh.org
Internet: http://www.birminghamfoundation.org
Sponsor: Birmingham Foundation
2005 Sarah Street, 2nd Floor
Pittsburgh, PA 15203

BJ's Charitable Foundation Grants **761**

Established with the goal of creating a positive, long-lasting impact on the communities BJ's serves, the mission of BJ's Charitable Foundation is to enhance and enrich community programs that primarily benefit children and families. The majority of the foundation's giving is focused on organizations that: (a) Promote the safety, security and well-being of children and families; (b) Support education and health programs; (c) Provide community service opportunities; or, (d) Aid in hunger and disaster relief.
Requirements: Organizations that are tax-exempt under 501(c)3 of the Internal Revenue Code and recognized as a 'public charity' by the IRS may apply. The program must align with the foundation's mission of supporting children and families in the specific areas of safety, security and well-being, education, health, community service, hunger/homelessness and disaster relief. And, the program must positively impact communities where BJ's Clubs are located. All organizations are limited to one (1) application per 12-month period. Additional applications will not be considered.
Restrictions: The foundation does not provide funding for: (1) Organizations that discriminate on the basis of race, color, gender, sexual orientation, age, religion, national or ethnic origin or physical disability. (2) Political organizations, fraternal groups or social clubs that engage in any kind of political activity. (3) Religious organizations, unless they serve the general public in a significant non-denominational way. (4) Programs that have been in place for less than one (1) year. (5) Individuals. (6) Organizations located outside BJ's markets. (7) Capital campaigns. (8) Private foundations. (9) Sponsorships for music, film and art festivals. (10) Business expositions/conferences. (11) Journal or program advertisements.
Geographic Focus: Connecticut; Delaware; Florida; Georgia; Maine; Maryland; Massachusetts; New Hampshire; New Jersey; New York; North Carolina; Ohio; Pennsylvania; Rhode Island; South Carolina; Virginia
Date(s) Application is Due: Dec 30; Mar 6; Jul 10; Dec 6
Contact: Community Relations; (508) 651-7400; fax: (508) 651-6623
Internet: http://www.bjs.com/about/community/charity.shtml
Sponsor: BJ's Charitable Foundation
1 Mercer Road, P.O. Box 9614
Natick, MA 01760

Black River Falls Area Foundation Grants **762**

Grant applications are evaluated with consideration to the policies, funding objectives and the mission statement of the Foundation. General categories of support include: education, health services, cultural activities, social services and civic projects. Grants to be considered are those that meet charitable needs of: a new or innovative nature to fulfill unmet needs; one-time projects; capital improvements; equipment needs; start-up expenses; special programs; and emergency funding. Applications will be accepted April 1 through May 15.
Requirements: Any non-profit organization in Jackson County, Wisconsin, may apply for a grant. A copy of the organization's tax-exempt status is required.
Restrictions: Requests to support endowments, operating expenses, debt repayment, religious purposes, individuals, and lobbying expenses are usually discouraged.
Geographic Focus: Wisconsin
Date(s) Application is Due: May 15
Contact: Beth Overlien, Administrative Assistant; (715) 284-3113;; Gilbert Homstad, Chairman; (715) 284-5341
Internet: http://www.brfareafoundation.org/application
Sponsor: Black River Falls Area Foundation
P.O. Box 99
Black River Falls, WI 54615

Blackford County Community Foundation Grants **763**

The Blackford County Community Foundation and its supporting organizations award numerous grants annually. Primary areas of interest include: community and economic development; education; community services planning and coordination; and human services. The Blackford County Community Foundation also offers several scholarships including the Lilly Scholarship, contact Foundation for guidelines.
Requirements: Nonprofit 501 (C)(3) organizations, coalitions, community associations, and other civic groups may apply if it provides services in Blackford County, Indiana.
Restrictions: The Blackford County Community Foundation generally does not fund: profit-making enterprises; political activities; operating budgets of organizations, except for limited experimental or demonstration periods; sectarian or religious purposes or to sectarian or religious organizations operated primarily for the benefit of their own members; endowment purposes; Capital grants to building campaigns will only be made when there is evidence that such support is vital to the success of a program meeting priority needs of the community. Payments of such grants are made only after a significant percentage of the total campaign requirements have been raised.
Geographic Focus: Indiana
Date(s) Application is Due: Jan 20; Mar 20; Jul 20; Sep 20
Contact: Ben Oswalt, Executive Director; (765) 348-3411; fax: (765) 348-4945; email: boswalt@blackfordcounty.org
Internet: http://www.blackfordcofoundation.org/pages.asp?PageIndex=377
Sponsor: Blackford County Community Foundation
P.O. Box 327, 121 North High Street
Hartford City, IN 47348

Blanche and Irving Laurie Foundation Grants **764**

The foundation makes charitable gifts to institutions and nonprofits in broad areas of interest, including arts, especially theater and music; children, with emphasis on health care and education; elderly, including social services and long-term residential needs; education at all levels; medical care needs of a community; and needs and concerns of the Jewish community. Capital grants, grants for programs/projects, and scholarships are awarded. Applicants should submit seven copies of a written proposal containing a statement of project objectives, detailed budget, plans for publicizing the project, plans for maintaining the project, relevant background information concerning the organization, and a copy of the organization's IRS tax-exemption letter.
Requirements: Nonprofit organizations in New Jersey are eligible.
Restrictions: The foundation denies requests for general endowments, operating expenses, or budget deficits.
Geographic Focus: New Jersey
Samples: Roundabout Theater Company (New York, NY)—for general support, $207,500.; Rutgers U, Ctr for the Study of Jewish Life (New Brunswick, NJ)—to endow a chair in Jewish history, $1 million.; Saint Barnabas Medical Ctr (Livingston, NJ)—to establish the Women's Pavilion for Breast and Gynecological Diseases, $250,000 over five years.
Amount of Grant: $250-$350,000 range
Contact: Gene Korf, Esquire, (973) 993-1583
Sponsor: Blanche and Irving Laurie Foundation
P.O. Box 53
Roseland, NJ 07068-5788

Blanche and Julian Robertson Family Foundation Grants **765**

The Blanche and Julian Robertson Family Foundation is totally committed to the goal of improving the quality of life in Salisbury and Rowan County. The general direction of the Foundation's interest is: programs which address social problems and nurture positive social relationships; efforts aimed at enriching lives through exposure to the cultural arts; neighborhood revitalization programs, especially when such programs encourage development of transitional housing and enable first-time homeowners to purchase homes; programs that improve opportunities for youth at risk and families in crisis; efforts to improve broad-based educational, recreational, and athletic opportunities; efforts which address health and the environment. The Foundation is also interested in programs and projects that demonstrate the attributes of leverage (where a grant will attract matching gifts or other funding), as well as innovation, thoroughness, passion, and commitment. Contact the office for application and guidelines.
Requirements: North Carolina nonprofit organizations serving Salisbury and Rowan County.
Restrictions: Foundation does not make grants outside Salisbury and Rowan County.
Geographic Focus: North Carolina
Samples: Rowan Regional Medical Ctr Foundation (Salisbury, NC)—for its capital campaign for a new emergency department, patient-care facility, and community-education center, $1 million (2005).
Date(s) Application is Due: Mar 30
Contact: David Setzer, Executive Director, (704) 637-0511; fax: (704) 637-0177; email: bjrfoundation@aol.com
Sponsor: Blanche and Julian Robertson Family Foundation
P.O. Box 4242, 141 East Council Street
Salisbury, NC 28145-4242

Blowitz-Ridgeway Foundation Early Childhood Development Research Award **766**

The foundation supports nonprofit organizations and programs in the areas of medicine, psychology, residential care, and education, and for research in medicine, psychology, social science, and education. Types of support include capital grants, endowments, program development grants, research grants, and scholarships. The Foundation prefers prospective grantees whose programs or services benefit persons who have not yet reached

their majority and/or are for the care of individuals or elderly persons who lack sufficient resources to provide for themselves. Although grants may be made to organizations outside the state of Illinois, preference will generally be given to applicants from Illinois. Application information is available on the Web site.
Requirements: Applicants must be classified as 501(c)3 by the IRS.
Restrictions: Grants will not be made for religious or political purposes, nor generally for the production or writing of audio-visual materials.
Contact: Laura Romero, Program Associate; (847) 330-1020; fax: (847) 330-1028; email: laura@blowitzridgeway.org
Internet: http://www.blowitzridgeway.org/information/information.html
Sponsor: Blowitz-Ridgeway Foundation
1701 East Woodfield Road, Suite 201
Schaumburg, IL 60173

Blowitz-Ridgeway Foundation Grants 767

The foundation supports nonprofit agencies that provide medical, psychiatric, and psychological care to economically disadvantaged children and adolescents. Program and capital grants are awarded, primarily in Illinois, in support of medical, psychiatric, psychological, and/or residential care; and research programs in medicine, psychology, social science, and education. The foundation supports operating budgets, and applicants may request commitments that extend beyond one year, but requests for annual funding will not be considered. Applications are accepted throughout the year and are reviewed in the order in which they are received. Guidelines and applications are available online.
Requirements: 501(c)3 nonprofit organizations that offer services to people who lack resources to provide for themselves may apply.
Restrictions: Grants will not be awarded to government agencies or to organizations that subsist mainly on third-party funding and have demonstrated no ability or expended little effort to attract private funding. Grants will not be made for religious or political purposes or for the production or writing of audio-visual materials.
Geographic Focus: Illinois
Samples: Elizabeth Ann Seton Program, $5,000 in general operating support of programs for pregnant and parenting mothers; The Enterprising Kitchen, $15,000 for programs improving self-sufficiency and employability of low-income women; Faith in Action of McHenry County, $7,000 to recruit volunteers; Gospel Rescue Mission, $10,000 for children's social and recreational activities; Guardian Angel Community Services, $5,000 for the Groundwork Domestic Violence Program (2006).
Amount of Grant: $5000-30,000
Contact: Serena Moy, Administrator, (847) 330-1020; fax: (847) 330-1028; email: serena@blowitzridgeway.org
Internet: http://www.blowitzridgeway.org/information/information1.html
Sponsor: Blowitz-Ridgeway Foundation
1701 E Woodfield Road, Suite 201
Schaumburg, IL 60173

Blue Grass Community Foundation Grants 768

The foundation awards grants to nonprofits in central Kentucky in its areas of interest, including arts and culture, housing, employment support and education. Types of support include building construction/renovation, equipment acquisition, seed grants, matching grants, and scholarships to individuals. Grants will range from approximately $5,000 to $20,000. To apply, submit a letter of inquiry of no more than three pages by 4:00 pm, August 17. Applicants will then be invited to submit full proposals, which are due by October 14.
Requirements: Central Kentucky nonprofit organizations are eligible.
Geographic Focus: Kentucky
Samples: The Nest, a Center for Women, Children and Families, $7500 - to replenish the emergency food bank (2008); Central Music Academy, $5000 - for operating funds and programs benefitting disadvantaged youth (2008); Ruby Bailey Family Services Inc., $7000 - to expand free meal programs between school terms (2008).
Amount of Grant: $5,000 - $20,000
Date(s) Application is Due: Aug 17; Oct 14
Contact: Barbara A. Fischer, Grants Officer; (859) 225-3343; fax: (859) 243-0770; email: bfischer@bgcf.org
Internet: http://www.bgcf.org/page27526.cfm
Sponsor: Blue Grass Community Foundation
250 West Main Street, Suite 1220
Lexington, KY 40507-1714

Blue Mountain Community Foundation Grants 769

The Foundation administers charitable funds to benefit people of the Blue Mountain Area. Most of the money for discretionary grants is designated by donors for use by agencies serving Walla Walla County. The Foundation's grant making policies are generally directed toward the fields of social and community services, the arts and humanities, education and health. In reviewing grant applications, careful consideration will be given to: potential impact of the program/project on the community and the number of people who will benefit; local volunteer involvement and support; commitment of the organization's Board of Directors; degree to which the applicant works with or complements the services of other community organizations; organization's fiscal responsibility and management skills; possibility of using the grant as seed money for matching funds from other sources; ability of the organization to obtain additional funding and to provide ongoing funding after the term of the grant.
Requirements: Nonprofit organizations serving the Walla Walla Valley, from Dayton to Milton-Freewater are encouraged to submit proposals.
Restrictions: Grants usually will not be made for the following: programs outside the Blue Mountain Area, operating expenses, annual fund drives, field trips, travel to or in support of conferences. No grants will be made for sectarian religious purposes nor to influence legislation or elections.
Geographic Focus: Oregon; Washington
Samples: Blue Mountain Action Council, WA, $7,000 - Volunteer Adult Literacy Program (2008); Walla Walla Community College Foundation, WA, $1,500 - Parent Education Program Scholarships (2008); Carnegie Art Center, WA, $3,000 - general support (2008).
Amount of Grant: $125-$4,000 range
Date(s) Application is Due: Jul 1
Contact: Lawson F. Knight, Executive Director; (509) 529-4371; fax: (509) 529-5284; email: BMCF@bluemountainfoundation.org
Internet: http://www.bluemountainfoundation.org/grant-making-programs.php
Sponsor: Blue Mountain Community Foundation
P.O. Box 603, 8 South Second, Suite 168
Walla Walla, WA 99362-0015

Blue River Community Foundation Grants 770

The Blue River Community Foundation is a community-based philanthropic organization that identifies, promotes, supports, and manages programs that will enhance the quality of life in Shelby County, Indiana, for this generation and future generations. To this end, the Foundation has established five areas of interest for the competitive grant making program: community and civic—support for community programs designed to improve life in Shelby County; arts and culture—support for programs and facilities that offer wide-spread opportunities for participation and appreciation; education—support for programs at all levels of education; health—support for the promotion of health and well-being for Shelby County residents; and social services—support of human service organization programs. Organizations interested in submitting a grant request should first submit the grant interest form found on the website. If the grant request meets the Foundation's funding guidelines, the organization will be invited to submit our formal Grant Application Form. Grant applications may be submitted at any time, but will only be reviewed during the next upcoming grant cycle.
Requirements: Any 501(c)3 organization serving residents of Shelby County, Indiana, may apply.
Geographic Focus: Indiana
Date(s) Application is Due: Feb 1; Jun 1; Oct 1
Contact: Lynne Ensminger, Program Administrator; (317) 392-7955; fax: (317) 392-4545; email: lensminger@blueriverfoundation.com or brf@blueriverfoundation.com
Internet: http://blueriverfoundation.com/main.asp?SectionID=6&TM=34321.26
Sponsor: Blue River Community Foundation
54 W. Broadway Street, Suite 1, P.O. Box 808
Shelbyville, IN 46176

Blue Shield of California Grants 771

Consideration for funding will be given exclusively to organizations that pursue activities directly related to the foundation's program goals, including domestic violence prevention through service provision, education, and outreach; research and education regarding medical best practices and health technologies; and direct or indirect provision of medical insurance or health care to those populations that are uninsured or underinsured, and related policy development.
Requirements: The Foundation funds organizations that are non-profit and tax-exempt under 501(c)3 of the Internal Revenue Service Code (IRC) and defined as a public charity under 509(a)1, 2, or 3 (types I, II, or a functionally integrated type III); accredited schools; units of government/public agencies; tribal governments. The foundation will only support projects that meet the following criteria: the mission of the grantee organization is consistent with the goals and mission of the foundation; the grant is used primarily to serve Californians; the grant seeking organization has a reputation for credibility and integrity; the grant seeking organization is pursuing activities directly related to one of the Foundation's three Program Areas: Health Care and Coverage, Health and Technology and Blue Shield Against Violence.
Restrictions: The foundation does not fund award dinners, athletic events, competitions, special events, or tournaments; conferences or seminars; capital construction; television/film/media production; religious organizations for religious purposes; political causes, candidates, organizations or campaigns; capital projects over $50,000; multi-year projects (generally); grants to individuals (with the exception of the regulated Blue Shield of California Employee Scholarship Program); grants to 509(a) 3, type III supporting organizations that are not "functionally integrated".
Geographic Focus: California
Contact: Grants Administrator, (415) 229-5785; fax: (415) 229-6268
Internet: http://blueshieldcafoundation.org/grant-center/index.cfm
Sponsor: Blue Shield of California
50 Beale Street
San Francisco, CA 94105-1808

Blum-Kovler Foundation Grants 772

The foundation awards general operating grants to eligible Illinois nonprofit organizations in its areas of interest, including child welfare, civic affairs, cultural programs, health care, higher education, hospitals, medical research, and social services. Grants are awarded primarily in the Chicago metropolitan area. There are no application forms or deadlines. Submit a letter of request.
Requirements: Illinois nonprofit organizations are eligible.
Geographic Focus: Illinois

Amount of Grant: $2500-$50,000 average
Contact: Hymen Bregar, Secretary, (312) 664-5050
Sponsor: Blum-Kovler Foundation
875 N. Michigan Avenue, Suite 3400
Chicago, IL 60611

Blumenthal Foundation Grants 773

The foundation focuses the majority of its grants on programs and projects that have an impact on Charlotte, and the state of North Carolina. The foundation also believes that it is important to provide basic operational funding for non-profits, not just support for special programs or projects. The philanthropic efforts of the Foundation are focused in nine areas of grantmaking: arts, science and culture; civic and community; education; environment; foundation affiliates; health; Jewish institutions and philanthropies; religious and interfaith; social sciences.
Requirements: Nonprofit, tax-exempt charitable organizations and institutions that are exempt under Section 501(c)3 of the Internal Revenue code, or governmental agencies are eligible.
Restrictions: Grants are not made to individuals for any purpose.
Geographic Focus: North Carolina
Contact: Philip Blumenthal, (704) 688-2305; fax: (704) 688-2401; email: foundation@gunk.com
Internet: http://www.blumenthalfoundation.org/BFGrantListings.htm
Sponsor: Blumenthal Foundation
P.O. Box 34689
Charlotte, NC 28234-4689

Bob and Delores Hope Charitable Foundation Grants 774

The foundation is primarily focusing its efforts on the economically disadvantaged populations of California and Texas. Projects of strong interest will be programs designed to help those living at or below the poverty guidelines. Other fields of interest include: the arts; Catholic agencies and churches; education; higher education; human services; medical research; and treatments for substance abuse. There are no specific application forms or deadlines, and applicants should send a letter of inquiry.
Requirements: Proposals are only accepted upon request. Applicants should submit the following: listing of additional sources and amount of support; timetable for implementation and evaluation of project; results expected from proposed grant; brief history of organization and description of its mission; and a detailed description of project and amount of funding requested.
Restrictions: No grants are given to/for: individuals; capital construction; fund raising; deficit financing; conferences; seminars; media events or workshops (unless they are an integral part of a broader program); or loans.
Geographic Focus: California; Texas
Amount of Grant: $50,000 average; $100,000 maximum
Contact: Linda Hope, Vice-President; (818) 841-2020
Sponsor: Bob and Delores Hope Charitable Foundation
10346 Moorpark Street
North Hollywood, CA 91602-2407

Bodenwein Public Benevolent Foundation Grants 775

The foundation awards grants to Connecticut nonprofit organizations to support social service and health agencies, including AIDS support, mental health services, health associations, and cancer and AIDS research; arts and culture, including performing arts and fine arts; youth and child welfare agencies; community development; education, including early childhood education, adult basic education, and continuing education; libraries and literacy and reading programs; the environment; animal rights and welfare; legal services; children, youth, women, and family services; religion; and minority services. Types of support include capital campaigns, building/renovations, equipment, program/project development, conferences and seminars, publication, seed money, scholarship funds, research, consulting services, and matching funds. The board meets in January and July of each year to consider requests. Applicants may submit one grant application per calendar year.
Requirements: Nonprofit organizations in Lyme, Old Lyme, East Lyme, Waterford, New London, Montville, Groton, Ledyard, Stonington, and North Stonington, CT, are eligible to apply.
Geographic Focus: Connecticut
Date(s) Application is Due: May 15; Nov 15
Contact: Grants Administrator, c/o Bank of America (800) 841-4000
Sponsor: Bodenwein Public Benevolent Foundation
777 Main Street, CTEH40222B
Hartford, CT 06115

Bodman Foundation Grants Program 776

The Foundation concentrates its programs in New York City, but also makes some grants in northern New Jersey. Funding is concentrated in six program areas: Arts and Culture, Education, Employment, Health, Public Policy, and Youth and Families. In both Health and Arts and Culture, the Foundation tends to focus its grants on leading institutions, generally where there is a longstanding relationship. In other areas, special consideration is given to competition, self-help, volunteerism, leadership and character development, parental involvement, consumer choice, economic empowerment, independent living, prevention and earlier intervention, independent research, faith-based programs, free markets, social entrepreneurship, advancing the state of the art, measuring participant outcomes and programs results, and strengthening traditional marriages and families.
Requirements: Nonprofit organizations based in New York City and northern New Jersey that are tax-exempt under Section 501(c)3 of the Internal Revenue Code and fall within the program areas of the Foundations are welcome to submit an inquiry or proposal letter. Initial contact should only include: an inquiry or proposal letter briefly summarizing the history of the project, need, research, objectives, time period, key staff, project budget, and evaluation plan emphasizing measurable outcomes and specific program results; latest annual report; current and complete audited financial statements; copy of IRS 501(c)3 tax-exemption letter.
Restrictions: The Foundations generally do not offer the following types of support, nor participate in the following program areas: nonprofit organizations outside of New York and New Jersey; annual appeals, dinner functions, and fundraising events; endowments and capital campaigns; loans and deficit financing; direct grants to individuals (such as scholarships and financial aid); individual day-care and after-school programs; housing; international; films and travel; projects for the elderly; small art, dance, music, and theater groups; independent or public K-12 schools (except charter schools); national health and mental health organizations; government agencies and nonprofit programs and services significantly funded or substantially reimbursed by government.
Geographic Focus: New Jersey; New York
Samples: Catholic Relief Services (Baltimore, MD)—for relief efforts for refugees and other victims of the fighting in Afghanistan, $20,000.; STRIVE/East Harlem Employment Services (New York, NY)—for its Community Partnership, a citywide job training and placement effort by 15 nonprofit groups to assist workers displaced by the terrorist attacks and the economic recession, $75,000 (2001); Manhattan Institute for Policy Research (New York, NY)—for research, articles, panels, and other events on rebuilding New York, as part of a round of grants responding to the September 11 attacks and their aftermath, $100,000.; New York Historical Society (NY)—for an exhibition and public program series in collaboration with the Skyscraper Museum on the conception, design, engineering, building, and destruction of the World Trade Center, $20,000.
Amount of Grant: $10,000-$100,000 average
Contact: Joseph S. Dolan, Executive Director, (212) 644-0322; fax: (212) 759-6510; email: main@achelis-bodman-fnds.org
Internet: http://fdncenter.org/grantmaker/achelis-bodman
Sponsor: Bodman Foundation
767 Third Avenue, 4th Floor
New York, NY 10017-2023

Boeing Company Contributions Program Grants 777

The Boeing U.S. contributions program welcomes applications in five focus areas: education; health and human services; arts and culture; civic and the environment. Education is a priority for Boeing. The largest single block of charitable contributions goes toward supporting programs and projects related to education. Boeing also believes that the health of a community is measured by the well being of all its citizens. Boeing locks for innovative initiatives that promote the economic well-being of the community and neighborhood revitalization. Boeing invests in programs that promote participation in arts and cultural activities and experiences, programs that increase public understanding of and engagement in the processes and issues that affect communities and programs that protect and conserve the natural environment. Boeing accepts applications for cash grants, in-kind donations, and services.
Requirements: To apply for support you must be a U.S. based IRS 501(c)3 qualified charitable or educational organization or an accredited K-12 educational institution. U.S. grant guidelines and applications are available online.
Restrictions: Grants do not support: an individual person or families; adoption services; political candidates or organizations; religious activities, in whole or in part, for the purpose of further religious doctrine; memorials and endowments; travel expenses; nonprofit and school sponsored walk-a-thons, athletic events and athletic group sponsorships other than Special Olympics; door prizes or raffles; U.S. hospitals and medical research; school-affiliated orchestras, bands, choirs, trips, athletic teams, drama groups, yearbooks and class parties; general operating expenses for programs within the United States; organizations that do not follow our application procedures; follow-on applications from past grantees that have not met our reporting requirements or satisfactorily completed the terms of past grants; fundraising events, annual funds, galas and other special-event fundraising activities; advertising, t-shirts, giveaways and promotional items; documentary films, books, etc.; debt reduction; dissertations and student research projects; loans, scholarships, fellowships and grants to individuals; for-profit businesses; gifts, honoraria, gratuities; capital improvements to rental properties.
Samples: Mercy Corps (Portland, OR)—to expand its disaster-relief efforts to provide food, water, and other supplies to people in Pakistan affected by the recent earthquake, $1 million (2005); Muntu Dance Theatre of Chicago (IL)—to provide this African-dance company with a permanent performance space, $3 million (2005); Millennium Park (Chicago, IL)—to construct two outdoor art-exhibition spaces, $5 million (2005); Mercy Corps (Portland, OR)—to assist tsunami-relief efforts, $300,000 (2005).
Contact: Corporate Contributions Manager, (312) 544-2000
Internet: http://www.boeing.com/companyoffices/aboutus/community/charitable.htm
Sponsor: Boeing Company Contributions Program
100 North Riverside
Chicago, IL 60606

Boettcher Foundation Grants 778

Grant support is given to promote the general well-being of humanity. Grants are awarded for arts and culture, community and social service, education and healthcare. Organizations seeking support from the Foundation should send a preliminary letter, describing the organization that wishes to submit a proposal and the project for which

funding is being requested. The letter should be signed by the head of the applicant agency and should include a statement related to the priority of the project within the organization's overall plans. Letters of inquiry should be mailed or emailed.
Requirements: Capital grants are made in the form of challenges, conditional on an applicant agency's ability to raise the balance of the funds needed for a project. Although no absolute guidelines have been established, 50 to 75 percent of the goal should already be in hand before the grant request will be considered.
Restrictions: The Foundation does not accept proposals, or provide grants, for the following giving interests: operations; gymnasiums/athletic fields; housing; purchase of tables or tickets for dinner/events; individuals; large urban hospitals; out-of-state projects; media presentations; small business start-ups; open space/parks; conferences, seminars, workshops; organizations that primarily serve animals; debt reduction; pilot programs; endowments; religious groups or organizations for their religious purposes; scholarships; travel.
Geographic Focus: Colorado
Contact: Grants Administrator, (800) 323-9640 or (303) 534-1937; email: grants@boettcherfoundation.org
Internet: http://www.boettcherfoundation.org/grants/index.html
Sponsor: Boettcher Foundation
600 Seventeenth Street, Suite 2210 South
Denver, CO 80202-5422

Bonfils-Stanton Foundation Grants 779
Colorado nonprofit organizations are eligible to apply, and funds must be used within the state for the benefit of Colorado citizens. The focus of the foundation is to advance excellence in the areas of arts and culture, community service, and science and medicine. Types of support include operating grants, capital campaigns, and capacity-building grants. Proposals will be reviewed at quarterly meetings. Guidelines and forms are available online.
Requirements: Colorado 501(c)3 organizations are eligible.
Restrictions: Areas generally not eligible for funding include loans, grants, or scholarships to individuals; events, media productions, seminars, conferences, or travel expenses related to meetings; activities or initiatives that have a religious purpose or objective; endowment funding, fellowships, endowed chairs; funding to retire operating debt; requests from organizations outside the State of Colorado or that are not for the benefit of Colorado citizens.
Geographic Focus: Colorado
Samples: ArtReach (CO)—for a Web-based ticket reservation system (2003); Capitol Hill Community Services (CO)—to fund meal sites for the homeless (2003); Kids in Need of Dentistry (CO)—to develop a comprehensive technology plan (2003).
Date(s) Application is Due: Jan 31; Apr 30; Jul 31; Oct 31
Contact: Susan France, Vice President of Programs, (303) 825-3774; fax: (303) 825-0802; susan@bonfils-stanton.org
Internet: http://www.bonfils-stantonfoundation.org
Sponsor: Bonfils-Stanton Foundation
1601 Arapahoe Street, Suite 500
Denver, CO 80202

Booth-Bricker Fund Grants 780
The Foundation makes contributions for the purposes of promoting, developing and fostering religious, charitable, scientific, literary and educational programs. Requests are welcomed for capital needs, special projects and other one-time requirements. Applications should be made by letter. There are no forms or deadlines. Requests should include complete information about the applicant organization, including its history, purpose, finances, current operations, governing board and tax status. A detailed explanation of the proposed use of the funds must be provided.
Requirements: Requests are accepted for the funding of projects within the state of Louisiana. Priority is given to the New Orleans area.
Restrictions: The Foundation generally does not provide sustaining (operations and maintenance) funding. No grants are made to individuals.
Geographic Focus: Louisiana
Samples: YMCA (New Orleans, LA)—program support, $51,700.; Tulane U (New Orleans, LA)—for the Medical Ctr Cerise Chair, $30,000.; Saint Dominic School (New Orleans, LA)—program support, $15,000.
Amount of Grant: $5000-$50,000
Contact: Gray S. Parker, Chairperson, (504) 581-2430
Sponsor: Booth-Bricker Fund
826 Union Street, Suite 300
New Orleans, LA 70112

Borkee-Hagley Foundation Grants 781
The foundation awards grants in a wide range of interests, including social services to children and families, religious organizations, and environmental programs. Delaware nonprofits receive preference. The board meets in December to consider requests.
Requirements: Delaware nonprofits are eligible to apply.
Restrictions: No support for specific churches or synagogues. Grants are not made to individuals.
Geographic Focus: Delaware
Samples: Artistic Productions Inc (Hockessin, DE)—$1000.; Delaware Hospice (Wilmington, DE)—$13,000.; Better Life Outreach Ministries (Newport, DE)—$5000.; Children and Families First (Wilmington, DE)—$13,000.
Amount of Grant: $1000-$25,000
Date(s) Application is Due: Nov 1
Contact: Henry H. Silliman Jr., President, (302) 652-8616
Sponsor: Borkee-Hagley Foundation
P.O. Box 4590
Wilmington, DE 19807-4590

Bosque Foundation Grants 782
The foundation gives primarily for higher education, human services, Baptist & Protestant agencies/churches and, medical research in Texas. Types of support include capital campaigns, building/renovation and research grants. There are no application forms or deadlines. Applicants should submit a one-page letter of intent that describes the program and request.
Requirements: Texas nonprofit and for-profit organizations are eligible.
Restrictions: Individuals are not eligible.
Geographic Focus: Texas
Samples: Midland Community Theater, Midland, TX, $1,000 (2007); Peoples Missionary Baptist Church, Detroit, MI, $20,000 (2007); Dallas Baptist University, Dallas, TX, $10,000 (2007).
Amount of Grant: $5000-$20,000 average
Contact: Louis A. Beecherl, Jr., Trustee; (214) 956-6732; fax: (214) 956-6733
Sponsor: Bosque Foundation
5950 Cedar Springs Boulevard, Suite 210
Dallas, TX 75235-6803

Boston Foundation Grants 783
The Boston Foundation has a particular concern for low income and disenfranchised communities and residents and supports organizations and programs whose work helps advance the Foundation's high priorities in a variety of subject areas: Arts and Culture; Civic Engagement; Community Safety, Economic Development; Education/Out-of-School Time, Health and Human Services; Housing and Community Economic Development; the Nonprofit Sector, Urban Environment and Workforce Development. The Foundation generally makes the following types of grants: Project or program support for community-based efforts that improve the quality of life in the community, test new models, and promote collaborative and innovative ventures; advocacy and public policy research that is linked to specific action; support for planning to enable organizations and residents to assess community needs, respond to new challenges and opportunities, and provide for the inclusion of new populations; organizational support to develop and build the capacity of nonprofit organizations - support that helps organizations keep pace with the changing requirements and demands of their communities and broader environments; small grants awarded on a rolling basis for one-time organizational development needs through the Vision Fund. In addition, on a very limited basis, the Foundation will consider development grants and strategic alliances.
Requirements: Grants are made only to tax-exempt organizations in Massachusetts.
Restrictions: The committee does not consider more than one proposal from the same organization within a 12-month period. Discretionary grants are generally not made to the following applicants: city or state government agencies or departments; individuals; medical research; endowments; equipment; replacement of lost/expired government funding or gap funding to cover the full cost of providing services; scholarships and fellowships; video and film production; construction and renovation projects and capital campaigns; programs with religious content; travel; summer camps and lobbying. Activities that are generally lower priorities for the Foundation are conferences, lectures, one-time events, programs benefiting only a small number of participants or routine service delivery and/or operating expenses.
Geographic Focus: Massachusetts
Samples: Raw Art Works in Lynn, MA, $75,000 - for arts-based youth development programs to young people in Lynn (2009); Boston Private Industry Council, Boston, MA, $200,000 - to administer the Accuplacer assessment to all program participants to determine the need for remedial writing support, and provide college transition coaching to 75 participating students headed to Bunker Hill and Roxbury Community College (2009);
Date(s) Application is Due: Jan 5; Jul 1
Contact: Corey Davis; (617) 338-1700; fax: (617) 338-1604; email: info@tbf.org
Internet: http://www.tbf.org
Sponsor: Boston Foundation
75 Arlington Street, 10th Floor
Boston, MA 02116

Boston Globe Foundation Grants 784
The foundation concentrates on three focus areas: strengthen the reading, writing, and critical thinking of young people, while fostering their inherent love of learning; strengthen the roads that link people to culture; and strengthen the civic fabric of the city. The foundation also sponsors the Neighbor to Neighbor Initiative, which funds exceptional Dorchester focused nonprofits.
Requirements: Massachusetts nonprofits in the greater Boston area are eligible.
Restrictions: The Foundation will only review one proposal per year from any organization.
Geographic Focus: Massachusetts
Amount of Grant: $5,000
Contact: Leah P. Bailey, (617) 929-2895; email: foundation@globe.com
Internet: http://bostonglobe.com/foundation
Sponsor: Boston Globe Foundation
P.O. Box 55819
Boston, MA 02205-55819

Boston Jewish Community Women's Fund Grants 785

The fund, a project of Combined Jewish Philanthropies, invites letters of intent for projects that benefit women and girls. Grants are made in the areas of health, abuse, hunger, education, and empowerment. In Massachusetts, projects funded are sponsored by organizations both within the Jewish community and from the community at large. In Israel, proposals from programs that serve the Haifa community or have a documented history of funding from other North American organizations are invited to apply. Letters of intent should not be more than two pages long and must contain: your organization's mission; a statement of need for the project, how the project will address it, and how it meets BJCWF objectives; a budget narrative including the amount of funding requested, projected major expenditures, and use of BJCWF funds.

Requirements: Grants are made to 501(c)3 organizations in Massachusetts or comparable organizations in Israel.

Geographic Focus: MassachusettsIsrael

Amount of Grant: $25,000 maximum

Date(s) Application is Due: Oct 15

Contact: Susan Ebert, (617) 457-8500; email: susane@cjp.org

Internet: http://www.cjp.org/section_display.html?ID=572

Sponsor: Boston Jewish Community Women's Fund
126 High Street
Boston, MA 02110

Boston Psychoanalytic Society and Institute Fellowship in Child Psychoanalytic Psychotherapy 786

The Child Fellowship Program offers participants an intensive, one year course of study in psychoanalytic approaches to child and adolescent psychotherapy. The curriculum includes both a theoretical course and a clinical course to be taught weekly. The theory courses will introduce the fundamentals of child analytic theories and will review historical as well as modern theoretical approaches. The clinical courses are organized around different developmental stages of childhood. Those who complete the program and wish to continue on in the Child and Adolescent Advanced Training Program will receive credit for their participation and can apply for advanced standing. A printable application form is available for download.

Requirements: The program is open to mental health clinicians who have completed or are in an advanced phase of their clinical training (residency, graduate internship) and who are interested in further didactic and clinical education in psychoanalytic work with children. Other professionals who work with children and their families such as pediatricians, teachers, and ancillary therapists are also encouraged to apply.

Date(s) Application is Due: May 15

Contact: Elizabeth Jordan, Program in Psychoanalytic Studies; (617) 266-0953; fax: (617) 266-3466; email: office@bostonpsychoanalytic.org

Internet: http://www.bostonpsychoanalytic.org/child_fellowship

Sponsor: Boston Psychoanalytic Society and Institute
15 Commonwealth Avenue
Boston, MA 02116

Boston Psychoanalytic Society and Institute Fellowship in Psychoanalytic Psychotherapy 787

The Fellowship is a one-year program designed to enhance participants' grasp of the principles and practice of psychoanalytic psychotherapy. It is also well suited for clinicians considering more extensive training in psychoanalytic psychotherapy or training in psychoanalysis, but who are either uncertain or not yet ready for a multi-year training commitment. The Fellowship offers two seminars weekly, one theoretical and one clinical, led by outstanding teachers from the Boston Psychoanalytic Society and Institute. The theoretical seminar focuses on Fundamental Concepts of Psychoanalytic Psychotherapy for the first term, on Comparative Theories of Psychotherapeutic Technique for the second term and on Selected Topics in Psychoanalytic Psychotherapy for the third term. The clinical seminar consists of discussion of case material presented by instructors and class members, with senior faculty as discussants. The seminars meet on Thursday evenings for 30 weeks starting in September. Each Fellow is matched with a faculty advisor who is available to discuss individual training goals and options. There is also an opportunity for individual supervision at reduced fees with a wide choice of experienced supervisors from the Boston Psychoanalytic Society and Institute. Tuition will be $1,677 for the academic year. The application fee is $25.

Requirements: The Fellowship is designed especially for mental health clinicians who have completed or are in an advanced phase of their requisite clinical training (psychiatric residency, psychology internship, MSW, masters in psychiatric nursing, etc.) and who desire further didactic and clinical education in psychoanalytic psychotherapy.

Amount of Grant: $1,677

Date(s) Application is Due: May 15

Contact: Elizabeth Jordan, Program in Psychoanalytic Studies; (617) 266-0953; fax: (617) 266-3466; email: office@bostonpsychoanalytic.org

Internet: http://www.bostonpsychoanalytic.org/fellowship

Sponsor: Boston Psychoanalytic Society and Institute
15 Commonwealth Avenue
Boston, MA 02116

Boyd Gaming Corporation Contributions Program 788

From giving generously to a variety of worthy charitable organizations to continually enhancing the effectiveness of our diversity programs, Boyd Gaming Corp. has a long-standing commitment to responsible gaming, and concern for the plantet, Boyd strives to make a positive differences in the communities in which it operates. The type of support offered is in: employee volunteer services; general/operating support; in-kind gifts

Requirements: All charitable requests must originate from a 501(c)3 non-profit organization and be from a state in which the company operates.

Restrictions: Boyd Gaming is not unable to act favorably on any request: for an individual, team or school-sponsored endeavor; for programs that discriminate for any reason, including race, color, creed, religion, age, sex or national origin

Geographic Focus: Hawaii; Illinois; Indiana; Louisiana; Mississippi; Nevada; New Jersey

Contact: Corporate Office, (702) 792-7200

Internet: http://www.boydgaming.com/about-boyd/corporate-responsibility

Sponsor: Boyd Gaming Corporation
3883 Howard Hughes Parkway, Ninth Floor
Las Vegas, NV 89169

Bradley Turner Foundation Grants 789

The foundation has a special interest in endeavors related to family and children services, education, religion (Baptist, Christian, interdenominational, Methodist, Presbyterian, Salvation Army, and United Methodist), health, and culture and the arts. Major focus is placed on the vitality and quality of life in Columbus, Georgia, though compelling programs beyond the city's boundaries will also be considered. The foundation is particularly interested in projects that have a broad base of community support. There are no application forms. Applicants are asked to submit a letter of three to five pages describing the project. Grants are reviewed quarterly, in February, May, August, and November, when the board meets.

Requirements: IRS 501(c)3 tax-exempt organizations in Georgia are eligible. Heavily focuses on the southern region of the United States, but the Foundation is not solely limited to this area. It has also donated in Massachusetts, Illinois, and Colorado.

Restrictions: Grants are not made to individuals or to for-profit businesses or corporations.

Geographic Focus: Georgia

Amount of Grant: $2500-$250,000 average

Contact: Tom B. Black, Administrator; (706) 571-6040; fax: (706) 571-3408

Internet: http://www.wcbradley.com/divisions.asp

Sponsor: Bradley-Turner Foundation
P.O. Box 140
Columbus, GA 31902-0140

Breast Cancer Fund Grants 790

Traditionally, the fund has awarded three types of grants: innovative research grants support projects investigating cutting-edge scientific approaches to the detection, treatment, and prevention of breast cancer; community model grants (non-research grants) to encourage and support the start-up of truly creative, innovative, and replicable U.S. programs that are developing new methods for addressing the support, education, health care access, and advocacy needs of women affected by breast cancer; and discretionary grants that generally fund smaller education, support, and advocacy initiatives. The fund gives preference to projects that address the needs of an ethnically, economically, and geographically diverse representation of women, including persons who are underserved or have low incomes. Initial application for research and community model grants is by letter of intent. If interested, the fund will invite a full proposal. Applicants for discretionary grants may submit an abbreviated application form available from the fund. Contact program staff for project availability.

Requirements: The fund will consider applications from individuals or organizations, whether public or private, for-profit or nonprofit.

Restrictions: No support is available for the direct cost of medical services, and no funds may be used for any lobbying efforts or political expenditures.

Contact: Jeanne Rizzo, Executive Director: (415) 346-8223; fax: (415) 543-2975; email: ed@breastcancerfund.org or info@breastcancerfund.org

Internet: http://www.breastcancerfund.org

Sponsor: Breast Cancer Fund
1388 Sutter Street, Suite 400
San Francisco, CA 94109-5400

Brian G. Dyson Foundation Grants 791

The Foundation, established in Atlanta in 1994 by former Coca-Cola Bottling executive, Brian G. Dyson, offers funding to community foundations, higher education, and federated programs in the Atlanta region and throughout Georgia. Grants typically range up to $20,000, and funding supports general operating costs. There are no specific guidelines, application formats, or deadlines with which to adhere, and initial contact should be made in writing.

Requirements: Applicants must be colleges, public or private schools, or other non-profit organizations located within the State of Georgia.

Geographic Focus: Georgia

Amount of Grant: $20,000 maximum

Contact: Brian G. Dyson, Director; (404) 364-2940

Sponsor: Brian G. Dyson Foundation
3060 Peachtree Road, NW, Suite 1465
Atlanta, GA 30305-2241

Bridgestone/Firestone Trust Fund Grants 792

The trust supports programs and projects of nonprofit organizations in the areas of education, child welfare, and environment and conservation in communities where the company has operations. While primary consideration is given to organizations and causes related to the three major focus points, the Fund recognizes the importance and value in supporting all types of civic, community and cultural activities. Assistance is regularly given for: community and neighborhood improvements; civil rights and equal

opportunity; voter registration and education; job training; performing arts programs; public radio and television; cultural programs; non-academic libraries; and museums. Types of support include: annual campaigns; building/renovation; capital campaigns; continuing support; donated equipment; emergency funds; employee matching gifts; employee-related scholarships; endowments; exchange programs; fellowships; general/operating support; matching/challenge support; program development; research; scholarship funds; and sponsorships. Applications must be submitted in writing and should include a description of the organization (two-page maximum) and its record of accomplishment, objectives of the program, whom the program benefits, and proposed method to evaluate the program's success; amount sought from the trust in relation to the total need; exactly how trust fund money would be used; copy of IRS 501(c)3 confirmation letter; list of board of directors and their professional affiliations; previous year's financial report; current year's operating budget; Form 990; list of other contributors and the amount of their donations; and copy of recent audit if available. Proposals are reviewed upon receipt.
Requirements: IRS 501(c)3 nonprofit tax-exempt organizations in Alabama, Arkansas, Colorado, Connecticut, Florida, Kentucky, Illinois, Indiana, Iowa, Louisiana, Michigan, Minnesota, Mississippi, North Carolina, Ohio, Pennsylvania, South Carolina, Tennessee, Texas, Utah, and Wisconsin are eligible. Schools, governmental agencies or other nonprofit, civic organizations are included. Grant proposals should be sent directly to the management of the local Bridgestone Firestone facility.
Restrictions: It is essential that all organizations receiving grants be equal opportunity employers who will operate their programs in support of equal opportunity objectives. Contributions will not be made to groups that discriminate on the basis of race, color, religion, gender, mental or physical disabilities, sexual orientation, national origin, age, citizenship, veteran/reserve/national guard status, or other protected status; partisan political organizations; or groups limited to members of a single religious organization.
Geographic Focus: Alabama; Arkansas; Colorado; Connecticut; Florida; Illinois; Indiana; Iowa; Kentucky; Louisiana; Michigan; Minnesota; Mississippi; Nevada; North Carolina; Ohio; Pennsylvania; South Carolina; Tennessee; Texas; Utah; Wisconsin
Amount of Grant: $50-$50,000 average
Contact: Bernice Csaszar, Administrator; (615) 937-1415 or (615) 937-1000; fax: (615) 937-1414; email: CsaszarBernice@bfusa.com or bfstrustfund@bfusa.com
Internet: http://www.bridgestone-firestone.com/trustfund.asp
Sponsor: Bridgestone/Firestone Trust Fund
535 Marriott Drive, P.O. Box 140990
Nashville, TN 37214-0990

Bright Family Foundation Grants 793
The foundation awards grants to eligible California nonprofit organizations in its areas of interest, including children and youth, education (medical, business, and other), health, medical research, and religion. Types of support include general operating support, building construction/renovation, scholarship funds, and special projects. Grants are awarded for one year, with possible renewal.
Requirements: Stanislaus County, CA, 501(c)3 tax-exempt organizations within 30 miles of Modesto, CA, are eligible.
Geographic Focus: California
Samples: California Youth Soccer (CA)—$200.; Slavic Gospel Assoc (CA)—$7500.; Big Valley Grace Church (CA)—$10,000.; Ctr for Human Services (CA)—$2500.
Amount of Grant: $377,500 total
Date(s) Application is Due: Dec 1
Contact: Calvin Bright, President, (209) 526-8242
Sponsor: Bright Family Foundation
1620 N Carpenter Road, Building B
Modesto, CA 95351

Brinson Foundation Grants 794
The foundation supports education, public health, and scientific research programs that engage, inform, and inspire committed citizens to confront the challenges that face humanity. Grantmaking priorities are education—awareness and outreach, democracy and citizenship, economically disadvantaged, and libraries and literacy; public health—awareness and outreach, and economically disadvantaged; and scientific research—astrophysics, cosmology, geophysics, medical research (i.e., Alzheimer's disease, cancer, Lou Gehrig's Disease (ALS), and stroke). Types of support include general operating grants and project grants. The foundation does not accept unsolicited grant applications. Grantseekers are asked to review the foundation's mission, vision, beliefs, priorities (accessed from the Who We Are link), and guidelines. If a grantseeker believes the request would match one or more of the foundation's grantmaking priorities, they can make an inquiry by completing the online Grantseeker Information Form. The completed form should be emailed to the office. Further application is by invitation.
Requirements: The foundation will consider inviting grant applications from organizations: whose request matches one or more of the Foundation's grantmaking priorities; located in the United States of America that are exempt from tax under Section 501(c)3 of the Internal Revenue Code and are defined as charitable organizations as described in Section 509(a)(1), (2) or (3) or 170(b)(1)(A); located outside the United States of America provided they produce a written legal opinion stating that they are a charitable equivalency to a qualifying U.S. organization and/or a written affidavit containing sufficient information for the Foundation to make a reasonable judgment that the organization is charitable.
Restrictions: The Foundation will not consider grant inquiries from organizations that: discriminate on the basis of race, gender, religion, ethnicity or sexual orientation. The Foundation will not consider grant inquiries that request funding for: activities that attempt to influence public elections; voter registration; political activity; lobbying efforts; promotion of a specific religious faith; medical research involving human cloning. The Foundation discourages grant inquiries requesting funds for: capital improvements; endowments; fundraising events.
Samples: University of Chicago, Department of Astronomy and Astrophysics, Chicago, IL, $100,000—Brinson Lectureship Program (2008); Children's Research Foundation, Clarendon Hills, IL. $15,000—Pediatric Disease Research (2008); Eisenhower Medical Center, Palm Desert, CA, $50,000—nursing retention and development programs (2008).
Contact: Cheryl A. Heads, Grants Manager; (312) 799-4500; fax: (312) 799-4310; email: mail@brinsonfoundation.org
Internet: http://www.brinsonfoundation.org/grant_seekers/grantseekers.shtml
Sponsor: Brinson Foundation
737 North Michigan Avenue, Suite 1850
Chicago, IL 60611

Bristol-Myers Squibb / Meade Johnson Award for Distinguished Achievement in Nutrition Research 795
The Award was first presented in 1978. The Award includes a $50,000 cash prize and a silver commemorative medallion. The winners are selected by an independent peer-review selection committee whose members are grant administrators of current Bristol-Myers Squibb/Mead Johnson Unrestricted Nutrition Research Grants. The annual application deadline is in late April.
Amount of Grant: $50,000
Date(s) Application is Due: Apr 24
Contact: John Damonti, President; (212) 546-4000; fax: (212) 546-9574
Internet: http://www.bms.com/aboutbms/grants/data/nutrit.html
Sponsor: Bristol-Myers Squibb Foundation
345 Park Avenue, Suite 4364
New York, NY 10154-0037

Bristol-Myers Squibb Foundation Global HIV/AIDS Initiative Grants 796
The intent of the Program is to develop new models in awareness, in medical care, in community development and in prevention and treatment in poor and resource-limited areas of the world, where the need for all such efforts is greatest. Health care infrastructures must be developed and enhanced, stigmatization must be overcome, health care worker capacity must be built and preserved and local people must be empowered to generate and sustain local solutions to this global problem.
Requirements: The Bristol-Myers Squibb Foundation considers requests for support only from tax-exempt organizations that satisfy the requirements of section 501(c)3 of the U.S. Internal Revenue Code.
Restrictions: The Foundation does not award funds to: individuals; political, fraternal, social or veterans' organizations; religious or sectarian organizations unless engaged in a significant project benefiting the entire community; organizations receiving support through United Way or other federated campaigns; endowments; courtesy advertising; or conferences/special events/videos.
Contact: John Damonti, President; (212) 546-4000; fax: (212) 546-9574
Internet: http://www.bms.com/sr/philanthropy/data/globhiv.html
Sponsor: Bristol-Myers Squibb Foundation
345 Park Avenue, Suite 4364
New York, NY 10154-0037

Bristol-Myers Squibb Foundation Health Disparities Grants 797
One mission of the Foundation is to reduce health disparities by strengthening community-based health care worker capacity, integrating medical care and community-based supportive services, and mobilizing communities to fight disease. To this end, this Program attempts to address health disparities in four strategic disease areas representing major public health burdens and in four highly affected geographies: hepatitis in Asia, HIV/AIDS in Africa, serious mental illness in the U.S., and cancer in Europe. Additional areas of concern include: metabolic diseases, infectious diseases; rheumatoid arthritis; cardiovascular diseases; substance abuse; women's health issues; and overal health care giving.
Requirements: Nonprofit organizations in communities where Bristol-Myers Squibb maintains a facility should submit their requests for company contributions directly to that location. Contact persons are listed at the company website.
Restrictions: The foundation does not support individuals; conferences, special events, or videos; political, fraternal, social, or veterans organizations; religious or sectarian activities, unless they benefit the entire community; organizations funded through federated campaigns; endowments; or courtesy advertising.
Geographic Focus: Connecticut; Indiana; Massachusetts; New Jersey; New York
Contact: John Damonti, President, (212) 546-4000; fax: (212) 546-9574
Internet: http://www.bms.com/foundation/reducing_health_disparities/Pages/default.aspx
Sponsor: Bristol-Myers Squibb Foundation
345 Park Avenue, Suite 4364
New York, NY 10154-0037

Bristol-Myers Squibb Foundation Health Education Grants 798
The Program supports the development and replication of novel approaches aimed at individuals in the community to learn more about their health and wellbeing so that they can become more informed decision makers about health care and they can actively participate in disease prevention and management. In many of the grants, the Foundation seeks to be a catalyzing force for changes in government or social policies, supporting

programs that can demonstrate the value of new approaches to health care through educational efforts. Nearly all the education programs focus on taking on major diseases, like hepatitis B or cancer – and creating model programs for either preventing them or helping treat aspects of them in community settings.
Requirements: The Bristol-Myers Squibb Foundation considers requests for support only from tax-exempt organizations that satisfy the requirements of section 501(c)3 of the U.S. Internal Revenue Code.
Restrictions: The Foundation does not award funds to: individuals; political, fraternal, social or veterans' organizations; religious or sectarian organizations unless engaged in a significant project benefiting the entire community; organizations receiving support through United Way or other federated campaigns; endowments; courtesy advertising; or conferences/special events/videos.
Samples: Children's Health Fund, $300,000 over two years—to establish a comprehensive health resource center at the Harlem Children's Zone's Promise Academy (2006); World Walk Foundation, $300,000 over four years—to establish a model program to improve prevention and treatment of diabetic wounds by educating health care professionals, other health workers, family care givers and the patients themselves at rural health clinics in Central America and the Caribbean (2006).
Contact: John Damonti, President; (212) 546-4000; fax: (212) 546-9574
Internet: http://www.bms.com/sr/philanthropy/data/healthed.html
Sponsor: Bristol-Myers Squibb Foundation
345 Park Avenue, Suite 4364
New York, NY 10154-0037

Bristol-Myers Squibb Foundation Product Donations Grants 799
The Foundation partners with designated non-governmental organizations, donating medical products to support long term health care programs in developing countries as well as addressing immediate needs to provide emergency health care disaster relief. Through this Program, it addresses health disparities and community infrastructure building alongside other Foundation and company charitable contributions programs. There are three main areas where the company's donations of products are used: the Medical Mission Box program; health care infrastructure support; and disaster relief.
Samples: Pillatre, Haiti, in support of a mission trip to serve the rural poor of Northern Haiti.; Karigiri, India, to conduct primary care outreach in conjunction with Karigiri Hospital (Schieffeline Leprosy Research and Training Center).
Contact: John Damonti, President; (212) 546-4000; fax: (212) 546-9574
Internet: http://www.bms.com/foundation/reducing_health_disparities/donations/Pages/default.aspx
Sponsor: Bristol-Myers Squibb Foundation
345 Park Avenue, Suite 4364
New York, NY 10154-0037

Bristol-Myers Squibb Foundation Women's Health Grants 800
Bristol-Myers Squibb Women's Health Program supports projects that enhance women's health with strategies that improve education, prevention, diagnosis, treatment and access to care for women worldwide. Support has been given to projects that test innovative outreach programs, cultivate multi-sectoral partnerships and add new information to the existing body of knowledge to help define and achieve improved health for women around the world. The goal of the program is to generate initiatives that will help enhance women's health through novel interdisciplinary strategies that improve education, prevention, diagnosis, treatment and access to care for women worldwide. Since its inception, significant resources have been invested in programs that educate women about diseases and conditions that particularly threaten them as women.
Requirements: The Foundation considers requests for support from tax-exempt organizations that satisfy the requirements of section 501(c)3 of the Internal Revenue Code.
Restrictions: The Foundation does not award funds to: individuals; political, fraternal, social or veterans' organizations; religious or sectarian organizations unless engaged in a significant project benefiting the entire community; organizations receiving support through United Way or other federated campaigns; endowments; courtesy advertising; or conferences/special events/videos.
Contact: John Damonti, President; (212) 546-4000; fax: (212) 546-9574
Internet: http://www.bms.com/Documents/foundation/women2002.pdf
Sponsor: Bristol-Myers Squibb Foundation
345 Park Avenue, Suite 4364
New York, NY 10154-0037

Bristol-Myers Squibb Patient Assistance Program 801
The Foundation was established to provide temporary assistance to qualifying patients with a financial hardship who generally have no private prescription drug insurance and are not enrolled in a prescription drug coverage plan through Medicaid or any other federal, state or local health program. The program provides free medications to indigent patients who qualify in all 50 states, Puerto Rico and the U.S. Virgin Islands. All patients and their health care providers must complete a program application to be considered for assistance. A printable version of the application is available online. Applications can also be obtained by calling the toll free telephone number.
Requirements: Applicants are required to provide information regarding household income, prescription insurance coverage, and citizenship, along with both patient and health care provider signatures.
Contact: Program Coordinator; (800) 736-0003
Internet: http://www.bmspaf.org/program0.html
Sponsor: Bristol-Myers Squibb Patient Assistance Foundation
345 Park Avenue, Suite 4364
New York, NY 10154-0037

Bristol-Myers Squibb Virology and Oncology M.D. Research Fellowships 802
The Program provides support for fellows to gain experience in epidemiological and clinical research as it relates to the care of individuals infected with HIV/AIDS and/or HBV. Goals of the Program include: support of studies that will further strengthen the science and knowledge of HIV/AIDS and HBV; development of a foundation for future prospective and retrospective studies; to provide a forum to share research findings; and support of the development of future clinical researchers. Up to 18 fellows will be selected annually, with grant awards up to $20,000 to support research-related expenses for a one-year research period. Applications must be submitted online.
Requirements: Candidates must: be an active Fellow in good standing in an ACGME-accredited Fellows training program; be a senior Fellow not in the first years of the fellowship; desire to enhance knowledge and skill development in the area of HIV/AIDS, HBV, or Oncology research; and identify a faculty member as the project mentor.
Restrictions: Total grant amount is inclusive of indirect costs and associated IRB fees and is not permitted for use towards travel to conferences or for durable equipment.
Amount of Grant: $20,000 maximum
Date(s) Application is Due: Feb 26
Contact: John Damonti, President, Bristol Myers Squibb Foundation, (212) 546-4000; fax: (212) 546-9574
Internet: http://www.bms.com/clinical_trials/investigator_sponsored_trials/fellows_research_program/Pages/default.aspx
Sponsor: Bristol-Myers Squibb Company
345 Park Avenue
New York, NY 10154

Broad Foundation IBD Research Grants 803
The program seeks to stimulate innovative research that will lead to both the prevention and successful therapy of inflammatory bowel disease (IBD), including Chrohn's disease and ulcerative colitis. The foundation's goal is to fund basic or clinical research projects that are in the early stages of exploration; propose new directions or ideas; are creative, novel, cutting edge, and imaginative; and are not ready for funding by other more traditional granting agencies. All proposals must be based on sound scientific evidence and careful evaluation of current knowledge in IBD research. Requests must be preceded by a brief (one to three pages)letter of interest, which may be submitted at any time. Funding will be granted for one year; continued funding is based on progress reports and the perceived value of the findings.
Requirements: Nonprofit institutions worldwide, such as universities, hospitals, and research institutes, are eligible.
Restrictions: It is anticipated that the foundation will not fund projects after sufficient progress and maturity have made them fundable by other agencies.
Samples: Charles N. Bernstein, M.D., University of Manitoba, Winnipeg, Manitoba, Canada—Project Title: A population-based characterization of potential microbial etiologies of inflammatory bowel disease using geographically defined high and low rate prevalence/incidence areas in Manitoba (2009); Cucchiara, Salvatore, M.D., Ph.D., Sapienza University of Rome, Rome, Italy—Project Title: Molecular characterization of mucosa-associated intestinal microbiota and intestinal innate immune response: searching for additional mechanisms in pediatric Crohn's disease (2009); Huang, Emina, M.D., University of Florida, Gainesville, Florida—Project Title: Colitis derived tumorigenic stem cells and the inflammatory bowel (2009).
Amount of Grant: $100,000 average
Contact: Heather Kubinec, Senior Research Administrator; (310) 954-5091; fax: (310) 954-5092; email: info@broadmedical.org
Internet: http://www.broadmedical.org/funding.htm
Sponsor: Broad Foundation
10900 Wilshire Boulevard, 12th Floor
Los Angeles, CA 90024-6532

Brook J. Lenfest Foundation Grants 804
The foundation primarily supports programs and organizations operating in urban areas of southeastern and south central Pennsylvania, southern New Jersey, and northern Delaware. Nonprofit organizations in Philadelphia receive preference. The foundation is dedicated to making people aware of positive life choices and providing support and opportunities for those motivated to pursue them. The Foundation will focus mainly on education, job training, mentoring programs, wellness based healthcare and the arts. The Foundation considers grant requests twice annually. To apply, send a short (two to four page) letter of inquiry that includes: amount requested; description of the program; date by which funding should be received; short and long term outcomes information for existing programs; expected outcomes and how the results of the program will be evaluated for new programs; description of how the program will support the mission and interests of the Foundation; total program budget involved in the request; other support for the program received, requested or expected from foundations, corporation, government or other revenue sources.
Requirements: Nonprofit organizations operating in urban areas of southeastern and south central Pennsylvania, southern New Jersey, and northern Delaware with a particular interest in Philadelphia are eligible.
Geographic Focus: Delaware; New Jersey; Pennsylvania
Contact: Grants Administrator, (610) 828-4510; fax: (610) 828-0390; email: lenfestfoundation@lenfestfoundation.org
Internet: http://www.brookjlenfestfoundation.org
Sponsor: Brook J. Lenfest Foundation
Five Tower Bridge, Suite 450, 300 Barr Harbor Drive
West Conshohocken, PA 19428

Brookdale Foundation Leadership in Aging Fellowships 805

The Leadership in Aging Fellowship provides two years of support to junior academics to focus on a project that will help establish them in an area of aging research. The fellowship is open to a broad range of disciplines including, but not limited to, medical, biological and basic sciences, nursing, social sciences, the arts and humanities. The award is a two-year grant paid to the candidate's sponsoring institution in support of the candidate's research project. The grant amount of up to $125,000 each year is intended to cover 75% of the fellow's time, base salary and fringe benefits. The award could also be used to include the support of a graduate assistant if necessary as long as the total amount does not exceed $125,000.

Requirements: The fellowship is open to all professionals in the field of aging. Candidates must have: (1) leadership potential; (2) an ongoing commitment to a career in aging; (3) a mentor (or mentors); (4) and, a willingness to commit at least 75% of his or her time for career development during each of the two years of the fellowship.

Samples: (2008) Kate de Medeiros, Ph.D. - Johns Hopkins University School of Medicine.; Jennifer Hagerty Lingler, PhD, MA, FNP - University of Pittsburgh Schools of Nursing and Medicine.; Teresita M Hogan MD, FACEP - Department of Emergency Medicine at the University of Illinois Chicago.; Brie A. Williams, MD, MS - Division of Geriatrics at the University of California, San Francisco.

Amount of Grant: up to $125,000 each year

Contact: Cara Kenien, Fellowship Contact; (212) 308-7355; fax: (212) 750-0132; email: cjk@brookdalefoundation.org

Internet: http://www.brookdalefoundation.org/Leadership/Fellows/fellows.html

Sponsor: Brookdale Foundation
950 Third Avenue, 19th Floor
New York, NY 10022

Brookdale Foundation National Group Respite and Early Memory Loss Grants 806

The Group Respite Program and the specialized Early Memory Loss Program are both community-based, social model, day service programs that provide dementia-specific group activities for participants and respite from caregiving tasks for family caregivers. Programs are open a minimum of one day a week for at least four hours per session, offering people with AD and other memory disorders regularly scheduled opportunities for socialization and group activities in a supportive environment. At least one paid professional staff member and a core of trained volunteers, students and program assistants, provide staffing for sites. In addition, programs offer access to other services for participants and their families, such as individual counseling for caregivers, information and referral to other health and social services, and support group meetings for family members. Additional program guidelines are available at the Foundations website.

Requirements: Applicants must be non-profit organizations with tax-exempt status under Section 501(c)(30 of the Internal Revenue Code or public agencies as defined under Section 509(a).

Samples: Alzheimer's Association, South Central, Madison, WI (2008); First United Methodist Church of Magnolia, Magnolia, AR (2008); Friends of Salem Senior Center, Salem, OR (2008).

Date(s) Application is Due: Jul1

Contact: Carmen Mendieta, Director; (212) 308-7355; fax: (212) 750-0132; email: cm@ brookdalefoundation.org

Internet: http://www.brookdalefoundation.org/Respite/respiteprogram2008.html

Sponsor: Brookdale Foundation
950 Third Avenue, 19th Floor
New York, NY 10022-3668

Brown County Community Foundation Grants 807

The Brown County Community Foundation exists for the purpose of enhancing the lives of the citizens and organizations of the community. It is a non-profit enterprise that seeks to provide the mechanism through which those who desire to help others in the community may carry out their philanthropy. By supporting charitable organizations in broad areas of community need – education, social services, health care, arts and humanities, and environment – it helps build a stronger, healthier Brown County. In general, grants shall be made for capital purposes only, not for operating expenses. Grant applications are generally available in April. Applications are due late May, with decisions announced in late June, or July.

Requirements: Evidence of 501(c)3 and/or 170(b)(1)(A) tax status must be submitted with all applications. Proposals must serve the residents of Brown County, Indiana.

Geographic Focus: Indiana

Contact: Judy Bowling; (812) 988-4882; fax: (812) 988-0299; email: judy@ browncountycommunityfoundation.org

Internet: http://www.browncountycommunityfoundation.org/grants.html

Sponsor: Brown County Community Foundation
P.O. Box 191, 96 S. Jefferson Street
Nashville, IN 47448

Bruce and Adele Greenfield Foundation Grants 808

The Foundation offers funding primarily in the forms of ongoing support and capital campaigns. Focus areas include: the arts; community development; health care; higher education; environmental issues; human/social service programs that support families and seniors; and science. Of particular interest are the performing arts, including dance, music, and theater. Though the geographic focus is Florida and Pennsylvania, support is also occasionally given outside of these two states. Initial approach should be by Letter of Interest (LOI), with no specific application forms or deadlines.

Requirements: Grantees must be 501(C)(3) organizations with a sound track record.

Restrictions: Generally the Foundation will not provide grants for individuals.

Geographic Focus: Florida; Pennsylvania

Amount of Grant: $100-$3,000

Contact: Adele G. Greenfield; (508) 428-1762; fax: (508) 428-0607

Sponsor: Bruce and Adele Greenfield Foundation
575 Mistic Drive
Marstons Mills, MA 02648-1405

Bullitt Foundation Grants 809

The foundation functions to protect and restore the environment of the Pacific Northwest, including Washington, Oregon, Idaho, western Montana, coastal rainforests in Alaska, and British Columbia, Canada. Program priorities include aquatic ecosystems; terrestrial ecosystems; conservation and stewardship in agriculture; energy and climate change; growth management and transportation; toxic and radioactive substances; training, organizational development, and unique opportunities (including education and public outreach). Areas of interest include air pollution, climate change, endangered species, energy conservation, environmental education and justice, human health, transportation, and tribal communities. The foundation supports challenge/matching, general operating, project/program, seed money, demonstration, and development grants, as well as requests for conferences/seminars and technical assistance support. Grants will be awarded for one year with possible renewal.

Requirements: Nonprofit organizations in the Pacific Northwest, including Washington, Oregon, Idaho, western Montana, coastal rainforests in Alaska, and British Columbia, Canada are eligible.

Geographic Focus: Alaska; Idaho; Montana; Oregon; Pacific Northwest; WashingtonCanada

Samples: North Seattle Community College Foundation (WA)—to support a model project for watershed educational activities, $10,000.; Washington's National Park Fund (WA)—to support a program for youth from local school districts, $5000.

Date(s) Application is Due: May 1; Nov 1

Contact: Officer , (206) 343-0807; fax: (206) 343-0822; email: info@bullitt.org

Internet: http://www.bullitt.org

Sponsor: Bullitt Foundation
1212 Minor Avenue
Seattle, WA 98101-2825

Burden Trust Grants 810

The trust supports international nonprofit organizations in the fields of medical research and hospitals; schools and training institutions; and care of and homes for the elderly, children, and other individuals in need. Preference will be given to organizations affiliated with the Anglican Church.

Date(s) Application is Due: Mar 31

Contact: Patrick O'Conor, 0117 9628611; email: p.oconor@netgates.co.uk

Sponsor: Burden Trust
51 Downs Park W
Bristol BS6 7QL United Kingdom

Burlington Industries Foundation Grants 811

This is a company-sponsored foundation, giving primarily in areas of company operations in North Carolina, South Carolina, and Virginia. The foundation supports organizations involved with arts and culture, education, health, youth development, community development, and civic affairs.

Requirements: 501(c)3 organizations in Burlington communities (North Carolina, South Carolina, and Virginia), are eligible for grant support. Requests for funding must be accompanied by: proof of 501(c)3 tax-exempt status; description of the organization and its objective; justification for the project; evidence that the organization is well established; information about the organization's reputation, efficiency, management ability, financial status and sources of income.

Restrictions: No support for: sectarian or denominational religious organizations, national organizations, private secondary schools, historic preservation organizations, individuals (except for employees in distress), conferences, seminars, workshops, endowments, outdoor dramas, films, documentaries, medical research, loans.

Geographic Focus: North Carolina; South Carolina; Virginia

Samples: Greensboro Day School, Greensboro, NC, $12,450 (2007); United Way of Alamance County, Burlington, NC, $3,000 (2007); Independent College Fund of North Carolina, Raleigh, NC, $15,000 (2007).

Amount of Grant: $1,000-$50,000

Contact: Delores Sides, Executive Director; (336) 379-2903; email: delores.sides@itg-global.com

Sponsor: Burlington Industries Foundation
P.O. Box 26540
Greensboro, NC 27415-6540

Burlington Northern Santa Fe Foundation Grants 812

The foundation is focused on the communities where the company operates and areas where its railways pass. The foundation supports education, including scholarships for Native Americans and scholarships for children of employees in conjunction with the National Merit Scholarships program; the arts, including museums, performing arts, and libraries; and civic and public affairs. Support goes to the Nature Conservancy and for local fire departments and law enforcement. Types of support include general operating support, continuing support, annual campaigns, capital campaigns, and program development. Health and human services funding concentrates on the United Way. Awards are made for a single year and for continuing support. The company also matches employee funds given to public and private colleges and universities, cultural

organizations, and hospitals in the United States. Requests for applications should describe the purpose for the grant. Requests are reviewed every six weeks.
Requirements: Any 501(c)3 organization located in Schaumburg, IL, and communities where the corporation operates, including 28 states and two Canadian provinces, are eligible to apply.
Samples: Texas Christian University, Fort Worth, TX, $600,000 - for Career Services Center and Neeley Schools Next Generation Leadership Program (2007); Hastings Rural Fire District, Glenvil, NE, $20,000 - for replacement of rescue truck and grass firefighting rig (2007); Foss Waterway Seaport, Tacoma, WA, $50,000 - for restoration and development of waterfront cultural center and maritime museum (2007).
Contact: Deanna Dugas, Manager Corporate Contributions; (817) 867-6407; fax: (817) 352-7924; email: Deanna.dugas@bnsf.com
Sponsor: Burlington Northern Santa Fe Foundation
2650 Lou Menk Drive, 2nd Floor, P.O. Box 961057
Fort Worth, TX 76131-2830

Burton G. Bettingen Grants 813
The fields of activity of the corporation are education at all levels, mental health, crime and abuse victims and public protection programs, religion (Christian, Roman Catholic, and Salvation Army), environment, and welfare. Top funding priority is children and youth. The current focus is on child prostitutes, runaways, and abandoned children. Nonprofits servicing the economically disadvantaged also may apply. The corporation provides broad types of support, including operating, capital, research, challenge/matching grants, and endowments. A letter of inquiry stating the applicant's background, goals and objectives, and the specific need for funding is welcome. Unsolicited submissions are considered but receive low priority.
Requirements: IRS 501(c)3 organizations are eligible. Giving primarily, but not limited to, Southern California.
Restrictions: The corporation does not award grants to individuals; for general fund-raising events, dinners, or mass mailings; or to grantmaking organizations.
Geographic Focus: California
Amount of Grant: $5000-$200,000 average
Contact: Patricia Brown, Executive Director, (323) 938-8478; fax: (323) 938-8479; email: burtonbet@aol.com
Sponsor: Burton G. Bettingen Corporation
134 S Mansfield Avenue
Los Angeles, CA 90036-3019

Bush Foundation Health & Human Services Grants 814
The foundation responds to a broad range of human services proposals. Proposals are reviewed on a case-by-case basis; applicant organizations take the lead in identifying promising solutions to the challenges faced by people who use their programs. In recent years, most grant dollars given to human services organizations have been for programs serving children, youth, and families. The foundation also considers program proposals that will improve the quality, accessibility, and efficiency of health care services in the region.
Requirements: The foundation is most interested in proposals that: (1) Promote opportunities for individuals and communities to become fully contributing members of society by supporting organizational projects that remove barriers to effective education, economic security and good health; (2) Improve the abilities of immigrant and refugee organizations, groups and individuals to obtain basic needs and rights, promote refugee and immigrant civic engagement and enhance their contribution to economic and cultural life; (3) The foundation will also consider proposals for comprehensive capital campaigns for building purchases, major building renovations and new construction to improve physical facilities. To be eligible for consideration, your organization must be a 501(c)3 nonprofit, tax-exempt organization, located in Minnesota, North Dakota or South Dakota, and able to demonstrate that you can take the lead in identifying promising solutions to challenges faced by people who use your programs. The two-step application process begins with a letter of inquiry. Guidelines for writing the letter of inquiry are on the information sheet which is available by contacting the sponsor or by download at the website.
Restrictions: The foundation does not make grants to: Individuals; Government agencies (except in special cases dictated by foundation priorities); Projects not benefiting the three-state region of Minnesota, North Dakota and South Dakota; Or, projects outside the United States. Download the Grant Restrictions file from the website for more details.
Geographic Focus: Minnesota; North Dakota; South Dakota
Amount of Grant: varies
Date(s) Application is Due: Mar 1; Jul 1; Nov 1
Contact: Program Officer; (651) 227-0891; email: grants@bushfoundation.org
Internet: http://www.bushfoundation.org/grants/human_services.asp
Sponsor: Bush Foundation
332 Minnesota Street, Suite East 900
St. Paul, MN 55101

Bush Foundation Medical Fellowships 815
The program was established to enhance community health care in Minnesota, North Dakota, South Dakota through the professional and personal development of selected physician leaders. Each year, the program awards approximately 13 fellowships that enable physicians to take a leave of absence from their practices to pursue professional and personal goals that address the health care needs of their communities. Their programs are self designed and self managed; they may last from three to 12 months. During this time, the fellowship provides a monthly stipend, as well as other financial aid.
Requirements: Applicants to the program must be: Physicians currently practicing in Minnesota, North Dakota or South Dakota; At least 35 years old and at least 10 years out of medical or osteopathic college; Able to state clearly their needs and opportunities for application of new skills and knowledge, both for the communities they serve and their own career development; and, able to explain how their programs will benefit an underserved population or need. All applications and references should be submitted via postal or express service. emailed applications and references must be followed by hard copy.
Restrictions: Previous Bush Medical Fellows may not reapply. If a physician (or his or her spouse/partner) is an elected official or public policymaker, the applicant may receive a grant for a degree-granting program only.
Geographic Focus: Minnesota; North Dakota; South Dakota
Date(s) Application is Due: Dec 1
Contact: Michael R. Wilcox, M.D., Program Director; (952) 442-2420 or (952) 758-4144; fax: (952) 442-5841; email: bushmed@bushfoundation.org
Internet: http://www.bushfellows.org/medical
Sponsor: Bush Foundation
Medical Fellows Program, 299 Lakeview Terrace Boulevard
Waconia, MN 55387

Bushrod H. Campbell and Adah F. Hall Charity Fund Grants 816
Grants are awarded to organizations in the Boston area devoted to basic needs for the elderly, projects relating to medicine and medical research, health care, hospitals, the blind and deaf, and certain discretionary projects. Grants are also awarded countrywide for projects addressing population control. Types of support include capital grants, general operating grants, program grants, and research grants.
Requirements: Tax-exempt organizations located within Boston and neighboring communities and U.S. tax-exempt organizations devoted to population control are eligible.
Restrictions: Grants are not awarded to individuals.
Geographic Focus: Massachusetts
Amount of Grant: $3000-$7500 average
Date(s) Application is Due: Jan 15; Apr 15; Aug 15; Oct 15
Contact: Brenda Taylor, c/o Palmer & Dodge, (617) 239-0556; fax: (617) 227-4420
Sponsor: Bushrod H. Campbell and Adah F. Hall Charity Fund
111 Huntington Ave at Prudential Ctr
Boston, MA 02199-7613

Business Bank of Nevada Community Grants 817
Business Bank of Nevada contributes financial assistance to nonprofit institutions and organizations that enhance the quality of life and promote public interest where the company conducts its business. The four main areas of giving include education, health and human services, community development, and arts and culture.
Requirements: Nevada 501(c)3 tax-exempt organizations in communities where the Bank has a presence. Community Grants are part of Business Bank of Nevada's grants program and must comply with the Bank's overall charitable funding guidelines. Requests must include the following information: a copy of the IRS letter of nonprofit tax-exempt 501C(3) status; a statement of purpose of the organization; the purpose and amount of the grant; the geographic area served; the project budget; a list of current board members with affiliations; a list of sources and amounts of other funding obtained, pledged, or requested; a copy of the latest audited or board approved financial statement.
Geographic Focus: Nevada
Amount of Grant: $250-$2,500
Contact: Paul Stowell, Public Relations, (702) 952-4415; email: pstowell@bbnv.com
Internet: http://www.bbnv.com/charitable_giving.php
Sponsor: Business Bank of Nevada
6085 West Twain Avenue
Las Vegas, NV 89103

BWF Ad Hoc Grants 818
To complement the competitive award programs, BWF also makes modest grants on an ad hoc basis to nonprofit organizations conducting activities intended to improve the general environment for science. These noncompetitive grants are for activities closely related to the Foundation's focus areas. The Foundation places special priority on working with non-profit organizations, including government agencies, to leverage financial support for targeted areas of research, and on encouraging other foundations to support biomedical research. Proposals should be brief and include a description of the focus of the activity, the expected outcomes, qualifications of the organization or individuals involved; provide certification of the sponsor's Internal Revenue Service tax-exempt status; and give the total budget for the activity, including any financial support obtained or promised. Proposals are given careful preliminary review, and those deemed appropriate are presented for consideration by BWF's board of directors.
Contact: Nancy S. Sung,
Senior Program Officer; (919) 991-5100; fax: (919) 991-5160; email: info@bwfund.org
Internet: http://204.85.36.154/page.php?mode=privateview&pageID=79&navID=110
Sponsor: Burroughs Wellcome Fund
P.O. Box 13901, 21 T. W. Alexander Drive
Research Triangle Park, NC 27709-3901

BWF Career Awards at the Scientific Interface 819
This initiative supports the early career development of postdoctoral scientists in the physical and computational sciences, whose work addresses biological questions and who are dedicated to pursuing careers in academic research. Research methods may

include any combination of experiment, computation, mathematical modeling, statistical analysis, or computer simulation. Areas of interest include: chemistry, computer sciences, engineering, mathematics, and physics. Awards provide a stipend over five years to support up to two years of advanced postdoctoral training and the first three years of a faculty appointment. During both the postdoctoral and the faculty periods, grants must be made to degree-granting institutions in the United States or Canada on behalf of the award recipient. Award recipients must complete at least one year of postdoctoral training during the period of the award, usually at the institution that nominates the candidate.
Requirements: U.S. and Canadian academic institutions, including medical schools, graduate schools, affiliated hospitals, and research institutes are eligible. Candidates must hold a PhD degree in the fields of mathematics, physics, chemistry (physical, theoretical, or computational), computer science, statistics, or engineering. Exceptions will be made only if the applicant can demonstrate significant expertise in one of these areas, evidenced by publications or advanced course work. Candidates must have completed at least six months but not more than 48 months of postdoctoral training at the time of application.
Restrictions: Candidates must not hold or have accepted a faculty appointment as a tenure-track assistant professor at the time of application.
Amount of Grant: $500,000 total over five years
Contact: Dr. Nancy S. Sung, Senior Program Officer; (919) 991-5100; fax: (919) 991-5160; email: info@bwfund.org
Internet: http://204.85.36.154/page.php?mode=privateview&pageID=129&navID=160
Sponsor: Burroughs Wellcome Fund
P.O. Box 13901, 21 T. W. Alexander Drive
Research Triangle Park, NC 27709-3901

BWF Career Awards for Medical Scientists (CAMS) 820

The program proved five-year, $700,000 awards for physician-scientists bridge advanced postdoctoral/fellowship training and the early years of faculty service. Proposals must be in the area of basic biomedical, disease-oriented, translational, or molecular, genetic, or pharmacological epidemiology research. Proposals in the area of epidemiology should contact BWF to determine their eligibility. Proposals in health services research or involving large-scale clinical trials are ineligible. Awards are made to degree granting institutions in the U.S. or Canada on behalf of the awardee. The postdoctoral/fellowship portion of the award may last up to two years, and allows the awardee the use of up to $95,000 per year ($65,000 per year salary support).
Requirements: Candidates must hold an M.D., D.D.S., D.V.M., Pharm.D., or equivalent clinical degree.
Amount of Grant: $700,000 over five years
Contact: Rolly L. Simpson Jr., Program Officer; (919) 991-5100; fax: (919) 991-5160; email: info@bwfund.org
Internet: http://204.85.36.154/page.php?mode=privateview&pageID=189&navID=191
Sponsor: Burroughs Wellcome Fund
P.O. Box 13901, 21 T. W. Alexander Drive
Research Triangle Park, NC 27709-3901

BWF Clinical Scientist Awards in Translational Research 821

The Clinical Scientist Awards in Translational Research program supports established independent physician-scientists who are dedicated to translational research—the two-way transfer between work at the laboratory bench and patient care. The program is intended to help protect award recipients' time to pursue the vital link between basic and clinical research. Importantly, the program aims to identify and reward proven mentors and to increase their capacity to train the next generation of investigators skilled in translational research. In this way, BWF hopes to increase the ranks of experienced physician-scientists critically positioned to bridge the gap between bench and bedside. Selection criteria include the candidate's qualifications, quality of the proposed activities, the ability to conduct innovative research, originality of the proposed research, and the potential to advance research in the scientific fields of study.
Requirements: U.S. or Canadian nonprofit hospitals and educational, scientific, research, or health institutions may submit applications. Candidates must have an MD or MD/PhD degree; hold an appointment or a joint appointment in a sub-specialty of clinical medicine; present evidence of an established research career; and be investigators at the assistant-professor level, associate-professor level, or an equivalent tenure-track position. Institutions may nominate up to four candidates, as long as at least one of the candidates is female, and at least one of the candidates is a member of an underrepresented minority group (Hispanic-American, African-American, Native American).
Samples: Gilbert Chu, Stanford U Medical Ctr (Palo Alto, CA)—to support researchers working to bridge the gap between basic research and patient treatment and care, $750,000 over five years.
Amount of Grant: $750,000 average over five years ($150,000 per year)
Contact: Nancy S. Sung, Ph.D., Senior Program Officer; (919) 991-5100; fax: (919) 991-5160; email: info@bwfund.org
Internet: http://204.85.36.154/page.php?mode=privateview&pageID=177&navID=180
Sponsor: Burroughs Wellcome Fund
P.O. Box 13901, 21 T. W. Alexander Drive
Research Triangle Park, NC 27703-8472

BWF Institutional Program Unifying Population and Laboratory Based Sciences 822

The program offers five-year institutional training awards of $500,000 per year to bridge the gap between the population and computational sciences and the laboratory-based biological sciences. The award will support the training of researchers between existing concentrations of research strength in population approaches to human health and in basic biological sciences. The goal is to establish training programs by partnering researchers working in schools of medicine and schools of public health.
Requirements: Degree-granting institutions in the U.S. or Canada may submit applications.
Restrictions: For-profit companies may not participate in the application, but could be valuable partners in such training programs.
Amount of Grant: $500,000 per year for five years
Contact: Victoria McGovern, Ph.D., Senior Program Officer; (919) 991-5100; fax: (919) 991-5160; email: info@bwfund.org
Internet: http://204.85.36.154/page.php?mode=privateview&pageID=159&navID=164
Sponsor: Burroughs Wellcome Fund
P.O. Box 13901, 21 T. W. Alexander Drive
Research Triangle Park, NC 27709-3901

BWF Investigators in the Pathogenesis of Infectious Disease 823

These five-year awards provide $500,000 for opportunities for accomplished investigators at the assistant professor level to study pathogenesis, with a focus on the intersection of human and microbial biology. The program is intended to shed light on the overarching issues of how human hosts handle infectious challenge. The awards are intended to give recipients the freedom and flexibility to pursue new avenues of inquiry and higher-risk research projects that hold potential for advancing significantly the biochemical, pharmacological, immunological, and molecular biological understanding of how infectious agents and the human body interact.
Requirements: Candidates must: generally have an M.D., D.V.M., or Ph.D. degree; have an established record of independent research and hold a tenure-track position as an assistant professor or equivalent at a degree-granting institution; and be nominated by accredited, degree-granting institutions in the United States or Canada.
Restrictions: Applications from non-tenure track investigators at tenure-offering, degree-granting institutions will not be accepted.
Amount of Grant: $500,000 over five years
Contact: Victoria McGovern, Ph.D., Senior Program Officer; (919) 991-5100; fax: (919) 991-5160; email: info@bwfund.org
Internet: http://204.85.36.154/page.php?mode=privateview&pageID=105&navID=135
Sponsor: Burroughs Wellcome Fund
P.O. Box 13901, 21 T. W. Alexander Drive
Research Triangle Park, NC 27709-3901

Byron W. and Alice L. Lockwood Foundation Grants 824

The foundation awards grants to Washington nonprofit organizations in its areas of interest, including arts, biomedical research, higher education, hospitals and health care organizations, housing and homelessness, museums, religion and religious welfare programs, and social services. Types of support include capital improvements, continuing support, general operating grants, professorships, projects grants, and research grants. There are no application forms; submit a letter of request.
Requirements: Washington nonprofit organizations are eligible. Grants are awarded primarily in Washington's Seattle and Puget Sound areas.
Samples: Seattle's Union Gospel Mission (Seattle) for capital improvements at the men's shelter, $50,000; Youth Suicide Prevention Plan for Washington State, (2006).
Amount of Grant: $900-$56,000 range
Date(s) Application is Due: Oct 31
Contact: Lee Kraft, Executive Director, (206) 230-8489
Sponsor: Byron W. and Alice L. Lockwood Foundation
P.O. Box 4
Mercer, WA 98040

C.R. Bard Foundation Grants 825

The foundation's areas of interest are health care; arts, cultural, and community life; and education and research in company-operating areas. In the area of health care, the foundation supports organizations and programs specializing in vascular medicine, urology, and oncology. In the arts/cultural/community category, the foundation considers requests from local civic, recreational, youth, and art and cultural organizations. In the area of education and research, the foundation considers requests from institutions of higher education that offer medical and managerial curricula, as well as organizations whose programs and services benefit the health care industry. Types of support include program development, scholarship funds, and employee matching gifts. Requests for funding must be in writing. Contact the office for application requirements.
Requirements: 501(c)3 organizations in primarily New Jersey, Massachusetts, and California may apply for grant support.
Geographic Focus: California; Massachusetts; New Jersey
Amount of Grant: $1.4 million total
Contact: Program Contact, (908) 277-8182, (800) 367-2273; fax: (908) 277-8240
Internet: http://www.crbard.com/about/com_relations/foundations/index.cfm
Sponsor: C.R. Bard Foundation
730 Central Avenue
Murray Hill, NJ 07974

C.W. Titus Foundation Grants 826

The foundation awards grants to eligible nonprofit organizations in Missouri and Oklahoma for programs in its areas of interest, including arts and culture, healthcare and health organizations, and social services. Types of support include building construction/renovation, general operating support, and materials/equipment acquisition. There are no application forms or deadlines.
Requirements: Missouri and Oklahoma nonprofit organizations are eligible.

Geographic Focus: Missouri; Oklahoma
Samples: Southwest Missouri State U Foundation (Springfield, MO)—to construct and equip a new master-control facility for the university's Ozarks Public Television station, $1 million.
Amount of Grant: $1000-$10,000 average
Contact: Grants Administrator
Sponsor: C.W. Titus Foundation
950 Philtower Building, Suite 950
Tulsa, OK 74103-4123

Cable Positive's Tony Cox Community Fund Grants **827**
Cable Positive's Tony Cox Community Fund is a national grant program that exists to encourage community-based AIDS Service Organizations (ASOs) and cable outlets to partner in joint community outreach efforts, or to produce and distribute new, locally focused HIV/AIDS-related programs and Public Service Announcements (PSAs). Grants are available up to $7,000 for 501(c)3 organizations, with special consideration given to AIDS Service Organizations (ASOs) and cable systems and producers partnering with ASOs. Eligible local community outreach projects include, but are not limited to: World AIDS Day and National HIV Testing Day events, AIDS Rides/Walks, other joint efforts between AIDS organizations and local cable operators, etc. Funding is also available for production costs of HIV/AIDS-related programs and PSAs.
Requirements: In order to be considered, you must partner with a cable system. To find your local cable partner go to www.cableyellowpages.com. If you do not have an existing relationship with your local cable system, contact their Public Affairs or Community Relations department. Successful applicants usually demonstrate the following tactics: PSA or program production; Community partnering-third party participation; Local government involvement; Media outreach (press kits & promotion); and, Marketing campaign. The following funding levels are available: $3,000-Alpha Cable System (up to 150,000 television households); $5,000-Beta Cable System (150,001 - 300,000 television households); $7,000- Gamma Cable System (more than 300,000 television households).
Amount of Grant: up to $7,000
Date(s) Application is Due: Sep 12
Contact: Jennifer Medina; (212) 459-1504; email: Jennifer@cablepositive.org
Internet: http://www.cablepositive.org/programs-tonycox.html
Sponsor: Tony Cox Community Fund
1775 Broadway, Suite 443
New York, NY 10019

Caddock Foundation Grants **828**
The foundation supports nonprofit national and international Evangelical Christian religious organizations including churches and religious institutions, community groups, hospitals, international missions and ministries, religious centers and facilities, and youth organizations. Types of support include conferences/seminars, fellowships, and general operating support. Application must be made in writing and include a description of the organization and its objectives and the purpose of the grant. There are no deadlines.
Restrictions: Grants are made to Evangelical Christian organizations. Grants are not made to individuals.
Samples: Set Free Prison Ministries (Riverside CA)—for operating support, $152,000.; Grace Evangelical Society (Roanoke, TX)—for operating support, $40,000.
Amount of Grant: $1800-$390,000 range
Contact: Richard E. Caddock, Jr., Treasurer, (951) 683-5361
Sponsor: Caddock Foundation
1717 Chicago Avenue
Riverside, CA 92507

Cailloux Foundation Grants **829**
The foundation awards grants to nonprofit organizations in its areas of interest, including civic and cultural, education and youth, family and community service, and health and rehabilitation. Requests for specific projects or programs, technical assistance, and capital projects are considered; general operations are less common and usually small; challenge grants are awarded occasionally; and endowment grants are rare. The general policy of the foundation is not to make grants to an organization more than once within any 12-month period. Applicants must submit a letter of inquiry; instructions are available online.
Requirements: 501(c)3 tax-exempt organizations are eligible. Only grant proposals originating in Kerr and the surrounding communities (Gillespie, Bandera, Edwards, Real, and Kimble Counties) will be considered.
Restrictions: In general, grants are not made for fund raising events, professional conferences, membership drives, competition expenses, or programs/projects normally funded by governmental entities. The foundation does not fund church or seminary construction, or church related entities or activities other than ecumenically oriented projects/programs that otherwise meet foundation guidelines. Grants or loans to individuals are never made.
Contact: Grants Administrator; (830) 895-5222; email: info@caillouxfoundation.org
Internet: http://www.caillouxfoundation.org/grant_guidelines.htm
Sponsor: Cailloux Foundation
P.O. Box 291276
Kerrville, TX 78029-1276

Caleb C. and Julia W. Dula Educational and Charitable Foundation Grants **830**
Grants are given in the areas of the arts and humanities (particularly museums and libraries), child welfare, the aged, community funds and appeals, health care, religion, and historical preservation. Most groups receiving foundation grants have an established reputation in their particular field. There are no set requirements.
Requirements: Grants are given to support projects of tax-exempt organizations.
Restrictions: Support is not available to individuals.
Amount of Grant: $5,000-$50,000 average
Date(s) Application is Due: Apr 1; Oct 1
Contact: James Mauze; (314) 726-2800; fax: (314) 863-3821; email: jfmauze@msn.com
Sponsor: Caleb C. and Julia W. Dula Educational and Charitable Foundation
112 S. Hanley Road
Saint Louis, MO 63105

California Community Foundation Health Care Grants **831**
The foundation strives to ensure that low-income adults and children have access to regular, sustainable, affordable and quality health care. Priorities include: efforts that serve federally designated Medically Underserved Areas or Health Professional Shortage Areas, and that deliver comprehensive health services (e.g., medical, dental, mental health, etc.) to low-income and underserved populations; efforts that enroll people in health care coverage and connect them with a source of regular care; efforts that integrate strong prevention and early intervention strategies into their health services; and requests that clearly demonstrate knowledge of the health conditions that affect the specific population to be served.
Requirements: Tax-exempt organizations (not private foundations) located within or serving primarily residents of Los Angeles County are eligible.
Restrictions: Grants will not be considered for annual campaigns or special fund-raising events; building campaigns, with the exception of community development grants; endowments; existing obligations; equipment, unless it is an integral part of an eligible project; incurring a debt liability; individuals, with the exception of arts and culture grants; routine operating expenses; sectarian purposes; or programs that will in turn make grants.
Geographic Focus: California
Samples: Northeast Valley Health Corporation, San Fernando and Santa Clarita Valleys, CA, $150,000 (2009); Planned Parenthood of Pasadena, Northern San Gabriel Valley, CA $125,000 (2009); American Heart Association Inc, Los Angeles County, CA, $80,633 (2009).
Amount of Grant: $100,000-$1,000,000
Date(s) Application is Due: Jun 1; Oct 1; Feb 1
Contact: Tamu Jones, Program Officer; (213) 413-4130, ext. 250; fax: (213) 383-2046; email: tjones@ccf-la.org
Internet: http://www.calfund.org/receive/health_care.php
Sponsor: California Community Foundation
445 South Figueroa Street, Suite 3400
Los Angeles, CA 90071

California Community Foundation Human Development Grants **832**
The human development program aims to expand support services for special populations that enable them to acquire the resources and skills that will lead to self-sufficiency. Special populations include aging adults, developmentally and/or physically disabled children and adults, at-risk youth and foster youth. Priorities include: support services for aging adults, developmentally and/or physically disabled children and adults, at-risk youth and foster youth; and efforts that promote civic dialogue and advocate for critical issues affecting aging adults, developmentally and/or physically disabled children and adults, at-risk youth and foster youth.
Requirements: IRS 501(c)3 tax-exempt organizations (not private foundations) located within or serving primarily residents of Los Angeles County are eligible.
Restrictions: Grants will not be considered for annual campaigns or special fund-raising events; building campaigns, with the exception of community development grants; endowments; existing obligations; equipment, unless it is an integral part of an eligible project; incurring a debt liability; individuals, with the exception of arts and culture grants; routine operating expenses; sectarian purposes; or programs that will in turn make grants.
Geographic Focus: California
Samples: Alliance for Leadership and Education, Los Angeles County, CA, $102,000 - two-year core operating support for a statewide advocacy organization that provides public education and supports public policies that advance adult day services throughout California (2009); Exceptional Children's Foundation, Los Angeles County, CA, $90,000 - one-year core operating support for a comprehensive education, rehabilitation, social service, and advocacy agency that assists children and adults with developmental disabilities throughout most of Los Angeles County (2009).
Amount of Grant: $50,000-$300,000 range
Date(s) Application is Due: Jun 1; Oct 1; Feb 1
Contact: Robert Lewis, Program Officer; (213) 413-4130, ext. 273; fax: (213) 383-2046; email: rlewis@ccf-la.org
Internet: http://www.calfund.org/receive/human_development.php
Sponsor: California Community Foundation
445 South Figueroa Street, Suite 3400
Los Angeles, CA 90071

California Endowment CommunitiesFirst Grants **833**
The endowment supports California nonprofits in the provision of programs and services promoting the health of all California residents. Favorable consideration is given to programs serving women, children, the elderly, and minorities. Areas of support include community innovation, which encourages communities to explore new ways to upgrade access to care; health and well-being, which promotes prevention strategies for all populations; and multicultural health, which addresses sociocultural barriers to improve health. Preference will be given to letters of intent that show that the project

is community-driven, takes an innovative approach, benefits underserved populations, demonstrates cultural competency, builds partnerships, and addresses persistent problems.
Requirements: California 501(c)3 nonprofits may apply.
Restrictions: Requests are denied for biomedical or nonapplied research, overhead costs, annual fund drives, endowments, operating deficits, general support, or scholarships.
Geographic Focus: California
Samples: Asian Pacific Environmental Network (Oakland, CA)—to encourage Asian immigrant workers to advocate workplace health and safety in the high-tech industry in Alameda County, CA, $102,438 (2005); San Francisco Senior Action Network (San Francisco, CA)—to develop and implement advocacy and education activities to counter the high costs of prescription drugs for older people, $264,996 (2005); Liberty Hill Foundation (Santa Monica, CA) and Seventh Generation Fund for Indian Development (Arcata, CA)—to support advocacy designed to improve the health and well-being of American Indians and lesbian, gay, bisexual, and transgender people, $150,000 each (2005); Afghan Coalition (Fremont, CA)—for culturally appropriate, collaborative advocacy and outreach efforts to help people from Afghanistan who are living in Alameda County, CA, gain access to health and mental-health services, $318,924 (2005).
Amount of Grant: $50-$60 million total
Contact: Grants Administrator, (818) 703-3311 or (800) 449-4149 ext 3311 (California only); fax: (818) 703-4193; email: CommunitiesFirst@calendow.org
Internet: http://www.calendow.org/opportunities/communitiesfirst.stm
Sponsor: California Endowment
1000 N Alameda Street
Los Angeles, CA 90012

California Wellness Foundation Work and Health Program Grants **834**

The foundation focuses its activities on specific priority areas where it has a significant, long-term commitment. Within each priority area, the foundation allocates the majority of its funds toward initiatives. Initiatives are targeted grantmaking programs with distinct objectives and are generally announced through requests for proposals. The foundation awards general grants and project grants. Under general grants, requests for core operating support for organizations that provide direct services to Californians for disease prevention or health promotion are of primary interest. Priority areas under general grants are diversity in the health professions, environmental health, healthy aging, mental health, teenage pregnancy prevention,, violence prevention, women's health, and work and health. Special projects grants are awarded to areas that fall outside the priority areas. Of particular interest are proposals to help California communities respond to cutbacks in federally funded programs. Activities commonly supported under special projects include strengthening traditional safety-net providers, educating consumers about changes in health care systems, advocating for underserved communities in health policy debates, and informing public decision making through policy analysis.
Requirements: Eligible applicants are California 501(c)3 nonprofit organizations, or organizations with a preapproved fiscal sponsor. An organization should first write a succinct letter of interest (one to two pages) that describes the organization, its leadership, the region and population(s) served, and the activities for which funding is needed, including the amount requested.
Geographic Focus: California
Amount of Grant: $5000-$200,000 over one to three years
Contact: Grants Administrator, (818) 702-1900; fax: (818) 593-6614
Internet: http://www.tcwf.org/grants_program/index.htm
Sponsor: California Wellness Foundation
6320 Canoga Avenue, Suite 1700
Woodland Hills, CA 91367-7111

Callaway Foundation Grants **835**

The foundation awards grants to eligible Georgia nonprofit organizations in its areas of interest, including arts and entertainment, elementary, higher, and secondary education; libraries; health and hospitals; community funds; care for the aged; community development; historic preservation; and church support. Types of support include annual campaigns, building construction/renovation, capital campaigns, continuing support, equipment acquisition, general operating support, land acquisition, and matching/challenge support. There are no application deadlines or forms. The board meets in January, April, July, and October.
Requirements: Georgia nonprofit organizations are eligible. Preference is given to requests from La Grange, GA, and Troup County. Preference is given to enduring construction projects and capital equipment.
Geographic Focus: Georgia
Samples: La Grange College (GA)—to endow its Callaway campus, which includes an auditorium, tennis courts, athletic field, and a multipurpose athletic and educational building, $5.75 million.
Amount of Grant: $1000-$200,000 average
Contact: Program Contact, (706) 884-7348; fax: (706) 884-0201; email: hsburdette@callaway-foundation.org
Internet: http://www.callawayfoundation.org/grant_policies.php
Sponsor: Callaway Foundation
P.O. Box 790
La Grange, GA 30241

Callaway Golf Company Foundation Grants **836**

The foundation strives to support initiatives in communities where Callaway Golf Company employees live and work. The focus is to improve the lives of young people and provide access to essential health services. The geographic area of focus is primarily North San Diego County, CA. The foundation supports youth—improving the lives of young people in need primarily through the building of life-skills; health—providing access to essential health services; military—PGA Tour Birdies for the Brave Program. Types of support include matching funds, special projects, and general operating budgets. The foundation does not require the completion of a formal application document but requests a description of the organization and its history, the project at issue including goals and time lines, the qualifications of the leadership personnel involved in the project, and a detailed project budget. Grants are awarded semiannually. The Callaway Golf Company Foundation is not accepting unsolicited requests for grants.
Requirements: IRS 501(c)3 nonprofit organizations in California are eligible.
Restrictions: The foundation will not fund applicants that illegally discriminate on the basis of gender, race, color, religion, national origin, ancestry, age, marital status, medical condition, or physical disability, either in the services they provide or in the hiring of staff; or promote political or particular religious doctrines.
Geographic Focus: California
Amount of Grant: $500-$10,000 average
Date(s) Application is Due: Feb 1; May 1; Aug 1
Contact: Paul Thompson, Executive Director, (760) 930-8686; fax: (760) 930-5021; email: cgcfoundation@callawaygolf.com
Internet: http://www.callawaygolf.com/en/corporate.aspx?pid=foundation
Sponsor: Callaway Golf Company Foundation
2180 Rutherford Road
Carlsbad, CA 92008-7328

Cambridge Community Foundation Grants **837**

Cambridge Community Foundation is dedicated to improving the quality of life for the residents of Cambridge, Massachusetts. The CCF serves Cambridge through our support of nonprofit community organizations, by making direct financial grants, providing technical assistance, and forming partnerships among organizations to coordinate services, address gaps, and highlight emerging issues. CCF primarily supports work in: early childhood services; youth service; senior services; community services; emergency outreach; arts; and the environment.
Requirements: To be eligible to apply, the agency must be tax-exempt 501(c)3 under the IRS code), and the program must serve the people of Cambridge, Massachusetts.
Restrictions: Support is not provided to municipal, state, or federal agencies. Grants for individuals, scholarships, research studies, conferences, films, capital fund drives, or loans are not eligible.
Geographic Focus: Massachusetts
Samples: Family First, Cambridge, MA — funding for the Family First parenting education and support programs for low-income and homeless families living in Cambridge (2008); Big Sister Association of Greater Boston, Boston, MA — funding to support Cambridge girls who participate in Big Sister's traditional one-to-one community-based mentoring program (2008); YNA Care Network, Inc./Hospice of Cambridge, Cambridge, MA — funding to support the patient care needs and running of the Chilton House, Cambridge's hospice, as well as bereavement support groups and counseling services to patient family members (2008).
Amount of Grant: $500-$60,000 range
Date(s) Application is Due: Apr 1; Oct 1
Contact: Robert S. Hurlbut, Jr., Executive Director; (617) 576-9966; fax: (617) 876-8187; email: RHurlbut@CambridgeCF.org or info@cambridgecf.org
Internet: http://www.cambridgecf.org
Sponsor: Cambridge Community Foundation
99 Bishop Richard Allen Drive
Cambridge, MA 02139

Camp-Younts Foundation Grants **838**

The foundation supports social services, higher and secondary education, youth organizations, Protestant religion, and hospitals and other health organizations in Florida, Georgia, North Carolina, and Virginia. Applicants should submit a letter describing the program, a copy of the 501(c)3 tax-determination letter, listing of board members, and an audited budget for the previous year.
Requirements: Nonprofit organizations in Florida, Georgia, North Carolina, and Virginia may request grant support.
Geographic Focus: Florida; Georgia; North Carolina; Virginia
Samples: Virginia Baptist General Board (Richmond, VA)—for operating support, $40,000.; Saint Edwards School (Bon Air, VA)—for operating support, $25,000.
Amount of Grant: $1000-$55,000 average
Date(s) Application is Due: Sep 1
Contact: Bobby Worrell, Executive Director, (757) 562-3439
Sponsor: Camp-Younts Foundation
P.O. Box 4655
Atlanta, GA 30302

Campbell Foundation HIV/AIDS Research Grants **839**

The foundation awards grants for research projects on ways to prevent and treat HIV, AIDS, and related conditions or illnesses. Proposals focusing on alternative, nontraditional avenues of study receive preference. Most grants support clinical research, although other types of work are considered. After initial screening, requests are reviewed by a peer review board of noted HIV/AIDS physicians and then sent to the board for final decisions. There are no application deadlines, but as all grants are handled chronologically, the foundation suggests submitting grant requests as early as possible.
Requirements: U.S. nonprofit organizations are eligible.
Amount of Grant: $20,000-$80,000 average

Contact: Contact, (954) 493-8822; fax: (954) 493-8801; email: campfound@aol.com
Internet: http://members.aol.com/campfound
Sponsor: Campbell Foundation
5975 N Federal Hwy, Suite 126
Fort Lauderdale, FL 33308

Campbell Hoffman Foundation Grants **840**

The mission of the Campbell Hoffman Foundation is to promote and fund efforts to increase access to comprehensive health care for underserved and uninsured populations in the Northern Virginia region. Northern Virginia is defined as the counties of Arlington, Fairfax, Loudoun and Prince William and the cities of Alexandria, Falls Church, Fairfax, Manassas and Manassas Park. A letter of Inquiry should be submitted, as the initial approach, when approaching the Foundation for funding. Upon review, if the letter of inquiry meets with Foundations criteria, the applicant will be asked to submit a proposal; guidelines will be provided to them when the proposal is requested.
Requirements: Eligible organizations include nonprofit 501(c)3 organizations, government agencies and faith-based organizations. Eligible organizations must be both located in and serve the target populations of Northern Virginia.
Restrictions: The Foundation will not provide funding for capital campaigns, endowment campaigns, special events and/or conferences (including travel to and participation in same) , emergency funding, loans, capital projects (including but not limited to building, construction or renovation), land purchases, lawsuits, films, video or publications. The Foundation may choose to provide general operating support.
Geographic Focus: Virginia
Samples: Northern Virginia Family Service, $12,200—expand Dentral Resource Recruitment Program (2008); Arlington Free Clinic, $30,000—continue integration of mental health into primary care setting (2008); Loudoun Community Health Center, $45,000—initiate mental heatlh program; integrate w/ primary care; create community mental health provider coalition (2008).
Contact: Lyn S. Hainge, Executive Director; (703) 749-1794; fax: (703) 442-0846; email: lhainge@campbellhoffman.org
Internet: http://www.campbellhoffman.org/applicants/default.aspx
Sponsor: Campbell Hoffman Foundation
1420 Spring Hill Road, Suite 600
McLean, VA 22102

CampusRN/AACN Nursing Scholarship Fund **841**

The scholarship program supports students who are seeking a baccalaureate, master's, or doctoral degree in nursing. Special consideration will be given to students enrolled in a master's or doctoral program with the goal of pursuing a nursing faculty career; completing an RN to baccalaureate program (BSN); or enrolled in an accelerated baccalaureate or master's degree nursing program. Applicants must submit an online application and create a complete profile on CampusRN. All applicants must already be enrolled (not just accepted) at an AACN member institution. Applications are accepted only by email.
Requirements: Nursing students enrolled in a baccalaureate, master's or doctoral degree program in nursing are eligible.
Amount of Grant: $2500
Date(s) Application is Due: Jan 1; Mar 1; May 1; Jul 1; Sep 1; Nov 1
Contact: Scholarship Administrator, (202) 463-6930; fax: (202) 785-8320; email: info@campuscareercenter.com
Internet: http://aacn.campusrn.com/scholarships/scholarship_rn.asp
Sponsor: American Association of Colleges of Nursing
One Dupont Circle NW, Suite 530
Washington, DC 20036

CAN Autism Treatment-Related Study Awards **842**

The organization recognizes the urgent need to develop effective therapies to treat both core and domain specific features of autism. Research proposals focused on all aspects of treatment, from basic research models, to clinical trials, to biomarker identification, are acceptable for submission. Due to the current lack of effective treatment and absence of known biomarkers, applications are reviewed as they are received. Funding amount and duration is determined per individual proposal. Indirect costs are limited to 10 percent of the total amount. Letters of intent are required prior to invitation of full proposals.
Amount of Grant: $60,000 per year for one, two, or three years
Date(s) Application is Due: Sep 1
Contact: Therese Finazzo, Grants Officer, (888) 828-8476 or (323) 549-0500 ext 18; fax: (323) 549-0500; email: therese@cureautismnow.org
Internet: http://www.cureautismnow.org/research/funding/3523.jsp
Sponsor: Cure Autism Now
5455 Wilshire Boulevard, Suite 715
Los Angeles, CA 90036

CAN Pilot Research Projects **843**

Pilot research programs will provide funding for investigators at any stage in their career to work on innovative pilot projects. The purpose of these awards is to encourage innovative approaches towards elucidating the causes, prevention, and appropriate therapy of autism. They are intended to provide support for innovative research that may not have reached a stage where funding can be obtained from federal sources. Annual deadline dates may vary; contact program staff for exact dates.
Requirements: Investigators whose focus has been outside the field of autism as well as innovative investigators from within the field are encouraged to apply.
Restrictions: Members of CAN's Board of Directors are not eligible as investigators in CAN supported research. Members of CAN's Scientific Advisory Committee are eligible, provided they comply with foundation policies regarding the avoidance of conflict of interest.
Amount of Grant: $120,000 maximum two-year award
Date(s) Application is Due: Mar 3; Jun 9
Contact: Therese Finazzo, Grants Officer, (888) 828-8476 or (323) 549-0500 ext 18; fax: (323) 549-0500; fax: (323) 549-0547; email: therese@cureautismnow.org
Internet: http://www.cureautismnow.org/research/funding/3522.jsp
Sponsor: Cure Autism Now
5455 Wilshire Boulevard, Suite 715
Los Angeles, CA 90036-4234

CAN Young Investigator Awards **844**

The purpose of these awards is to encourage innovative approaches towards elucidating the causes, prevention, and appropriate therapy of autism. These awards are designed to support outstanding projects that involve innovative approaches and the application of cutting-edge technologies. All proposals must have direct and immediate relevance to autism and related disorders.
Requirements: Awards provide for the work of outstanding candidates to be carried out under the supervision of a mentor who is an established investigator. The investigator need not be directly involved in autism research but must provide an environment in which the CAN fellow can pursue a project with relevance to autism or related disorders.
Restrictions: Applicants should be no more than four years out of a MD or PhD program on the date the fellowship would begin.
Amount of Grant: $40,000 and $1000 travel allowance per year for two years
Date(s) Application is Due: Mar 3; Jun 9
Contact: Therese Finazzo, Grants Officer, (323) 549-0500 ext 18 or (888) 828-8476; fax: (323) 549-0500; email: therese@cureautismnow.org
Internet: http://www.cureautismnow.org/research/funding/3522.jsp
Sponsor: Cure Autism Now
5455 Wilshire Boulevard, Suite 715
Los Angeles, CA 90036-4234

Canada Graduate Scholarships and NSERC Postgraduate Scholarships **845**

Canada Graduate Scholarships and NSERC Postgraduate Scholarships provide financial support to high-calibre scholars who are engaged in master's or doctoral programs in the natural sciences or engineering. The Canada Graduate Scholarships will be offered to the top-ranked applicants at each level (master's and doctoral) and the next tier of meritorious applicants will be offered an NSERC Postgraduate Scholarship. This support allows these scholars to fully concentrate on their studies and to seek out the best research mentors in their chosen fields. NSERC encourages interested and qualified Aboriginal students to apply.
Requirements: To be considered eligible for support, applicants must: (1) be a Canadian citizen or a permanent resident of Canada; (2) hold, or expect to hold (at the time you take up the award), a degree in science or engineering from a university whose standing is acceptable to NSERC (if you have a degree in a field other than science or engineering, NSERC may accept your application at its discretion); (3) intend to pursue in the following year full-time graduate studies and research at the master's or doctoral level in an eligible program in one of the areas of the natural sciences and engineering supported by NSERC; and (4) have obtained a first-class average (a grade of 'A-') in each of the last two completed years of study (full-time equivalent). Any exceptions to this requirement must be accompanied by supporting comments that justify the submission.
Restrictions: Scholarships are not available to students entering graduate studies in a qualifying year. Students who, after receiving an NSERC scholarship, change their field of study and research to a field that is not supported by NSERC, cease to be eligible and their awards will be cancelled.
Amount of Grant: $17,300 - $35,000 CAN per year
Date(s) Application is Due: Oct 15
Contact: Program Officer; (613) 995-5521; fax: (613) 996-2589; email: schol@nserc.ca
Internet: http://www.nserc-crsng.gc.ca/Students-Etudiants/PG-CS/BellandPostgrad-BelletSuperieures_eng.asp
Sponsor: Natural Sciences and Engineering Research Council of Canada
350 Albert Street, 14th Floor
Ottawa, ON K1A 1H5 Canada

Canada-U.S. Fulbright New Century Scholars Program Grants **846**

The Fulbright New Century Scholars Program allows scholars who have attained a level of national or international recognition for demonstrated professional accomplishments pertaining to higher education and its role in national and global economic development. The deadline for this specific award is October 30 for an award to be taken up from May of the following year and conclude the next April. The New Century Scholar award carries a value of U.S.$30,000.
Requirements: Eligibility requirements include: Canadian or American citizenship at time of application (permanent resident status or landed immigrant status are not sufficient); a Ph.D. or equivalent professional/terminal degree by December 31 of the application year or equivalent professional experience; and English language proficiency.
Restrictions: Applicants are not eligible for a Canada-U.S. Fulbright Award if he or she: currently holds permanent residency status in the intended host country; is currently residing in or enrolled at a university in the intended host country; has resided abroad for five or more consecutive years in the six year period immediately preceding the date of application; has received a Fulbright Award within the last five years; has had recent substantial experience in the intended host country (recent substantial experience is

defined as study, teaching, research or employment for a period of more than an academic year (nine months) during the past five years); or is a Canadian applicant and you are a dual citizen of Canada and the United States.
Amount of Grant: $30,000 per year
Date(s) Application is Due: Oct 30
Contact: Jennifer Regan, Senior Program Officer & NNASC Coordinator; (613) 688-5517 or (613) 688-5540; fax: (613) 237-2029; email: jregan@fulbright.ca
Internet: http://www.fulbright.ca/en/award.asp
Sponsor: Foundation for Educational Exchange between Canada and the United States of America
350 Albert Street, Suite 2015
Ottawa, ON K1R 1A4 Canada

Canada-U.S. Fulbright Senior Specialists Program Grants 847
The Fulbright Senior Specialists Program is designed to provide U.S. and Canadian faculty and professionals with opportunities to collaborate on curriculum and faculty development, institutional planning and a variety of other activities. During the course of their grant, Fulbright Senior Specialists may engage in any of the following activities at their Canadian host institution: conduct needs assessments, surveys, institutional or programmatic research; take part in specialized academic programs and conferences; consult with administrators and instructors of post-secondary institutions on faculty development; present lectures at graduate and undergraduate levels; participate in or lead seminars or workshops at overseas academic institutions; develop and/or assess academic curricula or educational materials; and conduct teacher-training programs at the tertiary level. These are short-term grants of two to six weeks offered on a continuous basis.
Requirements: Eligibility requirements include: Canadian or American citizenship at time of application (permanent resident status or landed immigrant status are not sufficient); a Ph.D. or equivalent professional/terminal degree by December 31 of the application year or equivalent professional experience; and English language proficiency.
Restrictions: Applicants are not eligible for a Canada-U.S. Fulbright Award if he or she: currently holds permanent residency status in the intended host country; is currently residing in or enrolled at a university in the intended host country; has resided abroad for five or more consecutive years in the six year period immediately preceding the date of application; has received a Fulbright Award within the last five years; has had recent substantial experience in the intended host country (recent substantial experience is defined as study, teaching, research or employment for a period of more than an academic year (nine months) during the past five years); or is a Canadian applicant and you are a dual citizen of Canada and the United States.
Contact: Jennifer Regan, Senior Program Officer & NNASC Coordinator; (613) 688-5517 or (613) 688-5540; fax: (613) 237-2029; email: jregan@fulbright.ca
Internet: http://www.fulbright.ca/en/seniorspecialists.asp
Sponsor: Institute of International Education
350 Albert Street, Suite 2015
Ottawa, ON K1R 1A4 Canada

Canadian Dental Research Foundation Award 848
This research award is offered biennially to encourage research related to dentistry conducted by graduate or postgraduate students in Canada. The monetary prize will be presented to the student who will have submitted the best report on a research project at the CDA annual meeting and the paper will be presented at the ACFD/CADR biennial meeting.
Requirements: Research papers entered are limited to graduate or postgraduate students who have conducted their work in association with the dental faculty of a Canadian university.
Contact: Richard Munro, Executive Director, (613) 236-4763; fax: (613) 236-3935; email: Information@dcf-fdc.ca
Internet: http://www.dcf-fdc.ca
Sponsor: Dentistry Canada Fund
427 Gilmour Street
Ottawa, ON K2P OR5 Canada

Canadian Foundation for Dietetic Research Awards 849
Within the broad category of practice-based dietetic research, the foundation prefers to support research that is of direct relevance to the nutritional well-being of populations within Canada. Priority research directions are outcomes of intervention, new roles for dietitians in meeting the health needs of all Canadians, identification of vulnerable groups and their nutritional needs, and determinants of food choice. An active member of Dietitians of Canada must be a member, if not the leader, of the research team. Applications for projects extending beyond one year will not be considered. The researchers must be associated with an institution or agency with charitable status (such as a teaching hospital or university) that will administer the funds awarded. Grants are intended to finance the direct operating costs of dietetic practice-based research projects.
Requirements: Applications will only be considered where a practicing dietitian who is an active member of Dietitians of Canada and who is delivering direct or indirect client/patient/public care of service is the principal investigator or a co-investigator.
Amount of Grant: $C10,000 maximum for large projects; $C5000 maximum for small projects
Date(s) Application is Due: Sep 30
Contact: Manager, (416) 642-9307; fax: (416) 596-0603; email: cfdr@dietitians.ca
Internet: http://www.dietitians.ca/cfdr/grants.htm
Sponsor: Canadian Foundation for Dietetic Research
480 University Avenue, Suite 604
Toronto, ON M5G 1V2 Canada

Canadian Friends of Hebrew University Research and Study Grants 850
Grants are awarded for one year of undergraduate or graduate study to Canadian citizens or residents of Canada who are able to fulfill the entrance requirements of the Hebrew University in Jerusalem in their chosen fields of study, which may include law, dentistry, social sciences and economics, humanities, arts, science, agriculture, pharmacy, and library science.
Amount of Grant: $C1000-$C4000
Date(s) Application is Due: May 1
Contact: Dina Wachtel, National Director, (416) 485-8000; fax: (416) 485-8565; email: dwachtel@cfhu.org
Internet: http://www.cfhu.org
Sponsor: Canadian Friends of Hebrew University
3080 Yonge Street, Suite 5024
Toronto, ON M4N 3P4 Canada

Canadian Liver Foundation Grants 851
The foundation awards organization grants, fellowships, and studentships to support research into nephrology, hepatic function or disease, and other related disciplines.
Requirements: Canadian citizens and organizations are eligible.
Date(s) Application is Due: Mar 31
Contact: Billie Potkonjak, (800) 563-5483; fax: (416) 491-4952; email: bpotkonjak@liver.ca
Internet: http://www.liver.ca/Research/Grant_Program
Sponsor: Canadian Liver Foundation
2235 Sheppard Ave E, Suite 1500
Toronto, ON M2J 5B5 Canada

Canadian Nurses Foundation Study Awards 852
Grants provide funding for nurses undertaking university studies in nursing and health care and for research related to nursing practice and health care. Awards are given for university study at the baccalaureate, master's, and doctoral levels. Priority will be given to nurses studying in programs with a nursing focus. Once recipients have completed their degrees, they must return to nursing and assist in the development of improved nursing and health care in Canada.
Requirements: Applicants must be members of the Canadian Nurses Foundation and must have gained acceptance into a university program of study; applicants must identify the practice area in which they plan to study and have definite career goals.
Amount of Grant: $C3000-$C6000
Contact: Linda Piazza, Executive Director, (613) 237-2159 ext 250; fax: (613) 237-3520; email: lpiazza@cna-aiic.ca orcnf@cnursesfdn.ca
Internet: http://www.canadiannursesfoundation.com/welcome.htm
Sponsor: Canadian Nurses Foundation
50 Driveway
Ottawa, ON K2P 1E2 Canada

Canadian Optometric Education Trust Fund Grants 853
Since 1980, the COETF has received applications and awarded funding to projects covering a vast and varied scope of research. The fund supports quality vision and eye care services for Canadians of all ages. Projects have been funded for improving optometrical education, professional development, and research. The Awards Committee meets annually (generally in March) to consider applications. The deadline for applications is typically in early February. Interested applicants should secure forms from the fund.
Restrictions: The fund customarily does not provide support for travel to and from sites where the results of a project are intended to be presented, i.e., a symposium or continuing education seminar.
Amount of Grant: $C3000-$C5000 average
Contact: Glenn Campbell, Executive Director; (888) 263-4676 or (613) 235-7924; fax: (613) 235-2025; email: gcampbell@opto.ca or info@opto.ca
Internet: http://www.opto.ca/en/public/03_optometry/03_06_coetf.asp#apply
Sponsor: Canadian Optometric Education Trust Fund
234 Argyle Avenue
Ottawa, ON K2P 1B9 Canada

Canadian Patient Safety Institute (CPSI) Patient Safety Studentships 854
The Canadian Patient Safety Institute (CPSI) is inviting applications from organizations/supervisors interested in enabling students to participate in patient safety work. Funding is to support the work of students in any healthcare profession, as well as other disciplines (including but not limited to social sciences, human kinetics, psychology and human factors engineering) interested in patient safety. The goal is to create new collaborative learning opportunities aligned with the mandate of CPSI. Students are required to be the major resource in carrying out the work for each patient safety project. Any person from organizations such as universities, health regions, and hospitals, non-governmental or not-for-profit private organizations who will provide supervision for a student project may apply for this award. The student selected can be a student of any health care profession as well as other disciplines (including but not limited to social sciences, human kinetics, psychology and human factors) with an interest in patient safety, who are registered in an undergraduate or graduate program (part-time or full-time), and who will be a student during the period of the award. The value of the award from CPSI is $6,000.
Requirements: Applying organizations/supervisors that are interested in accessing these resources must provide matching funding to augment studentship funding that will enable students to participate in patient safety work. Matched funding must be in actual dollars and cannot be in-kind contributions.

Restrictions: CPSI funding is to be used for student stipends only. CPSI will not make funds available for administrative or overhead purposes.
Amount of Grant: $6,000
Date(s) Application is Due: Dec 12
Contact: Laurel Taylor, Director of Operations; (866) 421-6933 or (780) 409-8090; fax: (780) 409-8098; email: ltaylor@cpsi-icsp.ca
Internet: http://www.patientsafetyinstitute.ca/education/Patientsafetystudentship2009.html
Sponsor: Canadian Patient Safety Institute (CPSI)
10235 - 101 Street
Edmonton, AB T5J 3G1 Canada

Canadian Patient Safety Institute (CPSI) Research Grants 855
The Canadian Patient Safety Institute (CPSI) announces its annual Research Competition to continue its strategic mandate of increasing the scope and scale of research and evaluation activities in patient safety. The primary goal for CPSI Research Competition is to develop knowledge about patient safety that can be helpful in a variety of settings and circumstances in organizations across Canada. It is the applicant team's responsibility to identify and secure matching funding from other contributing organization(s). Applicant teams may obtain matching funding from universities, foundations, voluntary health charities, provider associations, provincial government departments, regional health authorities, hospitals, research centers or the private sector.
Requirements: A 1:1 funding ratio is the acceptable minimum required for any project over $20,000.
Amount of Grant: $120,000
Date(s) Application is Due: Dec 2
Contact: Laurel Taylor, Director of Operations; (866) 421-6933 or (780) 409-8090; fax: (780) 409-8098; email: ltaylor@cpsi-icsp.ca
Internet: http://www.patientsafetyinstitute.ca/news/2008researchcompetition.html
Sponsor: Canadian Patient Safety Institute (CPSI)
10235 - 101 Street
Edmonton, AB T5J 3G1 Canada

Cancer Research Postdoctoral Fellowships for Basic and Physician Scientists 856
This program grants initial postdoctoral fellowships to support promising young investigators pursuing careers in cancer research. The fund encourages all theoretical and experimental research that is relevant to the study of cancer and the search for cancer causes, mechanisms, therapies, and prevention. Candidates must apply for the fellowships under the guidance of a sponsor—a senior member of the scientific research community. The sponsor should be actively engaged in the planning, execution, and supervision of the proposed research and should encourage the fellow to report the results of the research in scientific journals and meetings. Awards are made to institutions for the support of the fellow under direct supervision of the sponsor.
Requirements: Candidates must have completed one or more of the following degrees or equivalent: MD, PhD, DDS, or DVM. For level one funding, basic and physician scientist applicants must have received their degrees no more than one year prior to the SAC meeting at which their applications are to be considered and DVM applicants no more than three years. For level two funding, physician scientists (MD, DDS, DVM, or the equivalent) must have completed their residencies and clinical training no more than three years prior to the SAC meeting at which their applications are to be considered.
Restrictions: Only one application will be accepted from a given sponsor or fellow per review session; there is no limit, however, on the number of applications from an institution. No more than two Runyon-Winchell Fellows will be funded to work with the same sponsor at any time.
Amount of Grant: $41,000 first year, $43,000 second year, $44,000 third year for level 1; $55,000 first year, $56,000 second year, $57,000 third year for level 2
Date(s) Application is Due: Mar 15; Aug 15
Contact: Lorraine Egan, Executive Director, (212) 455-0541; fax: (212) 697-4950; email: lorraine.egan@drcrf.org or fellowship@cancerresearchfund.org
Internet: http://www.drcrf.org/apFellowship.html
Sponsor: Cancer Research Fund of the Damon Runyon-Walter Winchell Foundation
675 Third Avenue, 25th Floor
New York, NY 10017

Cancer Research Society Fellowships and Grants 857
Grants and fellowships are supported for projects researching the cause and cure of cancer. Recipients are selected annually by the society's medical advisory board on the basis of the scientific value of the research projects submitted.
Requirements: Research projects supported must be carried out in Canada.
Date(s) Application is Due: Feb 15
Contact: Program Director, (514) 861-9227; fax: (514) 861-9220; email: grants@cancerresearchsociety.ca
Internet: http://src-crs.ca/main.php?lang=2&id=305
Sponsor: Cancer Research Society
402-625 Av Du President-Kennedy
Montreal, QC H3A 3S5 Canada

Cancer Research United Kingdom Fellowships 858
The fund operates in the United Kingdom and worldwide to investigate all matters connected with or bearing on the causes, prevention, treatment, and cure of cancer. Principal disciplines include cellular and molecular biology, clinical cancer research, and epidemiology. Types of support include research fellowships, visiting fellowships, clinical research fellowships, and graduate studentships.
Contact: Grants Administrator, 020 7242 0200; fax: 020 7269 3100; email: research_enquiries@cancer.org.uk
Internet: http://science.cancerresearchuk.org/fandm/grantapplications/?version=1
Sponsor: Cancer Research United Kingdom
P.O. Box 123, Lincoln's Inn Fields
London WC2A 3PX United Kingdom

Cancer Research United Kingdom Grants 859
The organization supports cancer research throughout the United Kingdom. Grants are awarded to universities, medical schools, and hospitals in support of research projects. Additional types of support include life fellowships, career development awards, clinical and nonclinical scientists fellowships, and capital grants for new research buildings and major items of equipment.
Contact: Grants Administrator, 020 7242 0200; fax: 020 7269 3100; email: research_enquiries@cancer.org.uk
Internet: http://science.cancerresearchuk.org/gapp/?version=3
Sponsor: Cancer Research United Kingdom
P.O. Box 123, Lincoln's Inn Fields
London WC2A 3PX United Kingdom

Cancer Society of New Zealand Grants 860
The society supports cancer research through grants to individuals and organizations in New Zealand. Types of support include research grants and traveling fellowships to enable New Zealand graduates to travel abroad for study.
Date(s) Application is Due: Nov 1
Contact: Grants Administrator, (04) 494 7270; fax: (04) 494 7271; email: admin@cancernz.org.nz
Internet: http://www.cancernz.org.nz
Sponsor: Cancer Society of New Zealand
P.O. Box 10847
Wellington New Zealand

Cancer Treatment Research Foundation Clinical Investigation Grants 861
The grants support new and pilot feasibility clinical projects in cancer therapy. Grants are intended to stimulate innovative research relevant to cancer therapy, such as new agents, innovative anticancer therapies, biological response modifiers, immunotherapy, and gene therapy; and quality of life, cancer education, and nutritional oncology. Funds may be used for salaries, supplies, and nonreimbursable research-related patient care costs, including extraordinary laboratory and imaging studies. There are no application deadlines. Preliminary grant request forms are available on the foundation's Web site. The foundation will invite a formal application.
Requirements: New and established investigators are encouraged to apply: young investigators working in established research programs relevant to clinical research who are without support from NIH or other cancer research agencies; and established, clinical researchers who wish to embark on innovative studies directly relevant to the foundation's mission with novel, new, or pilot projects distinctly removed from their currently funded research projects.
Amount of Grant: $25,000-$300,000 range
Date(s) Application is Due: Aug 15
Contact: Kristine Nelson, Administrator, (847) 342-7450; email: grants@ctrf.org
Internet: http://www.ctrf.org/grantapp.cfm
Sponsor: Cancer Treatment Research Foundation
1336 Basswood Road
Schaumburg, Illinois 60173

Capital Region Community Foundation Grants 862
The foundation awards grants to eligible Michigan nonprofit organizations in its areas of interest, including education, environment, health care, human services, humanities, and public benefit. Types of support include capital grants, program development grants, and seed money grants. Grants are awarded for one year and are nonrenewable. Guidelines and application are available on-line. Application must be made on-line. Program deadlines vary: Youth Fund grant deadline is January 31; Eaton County Community Foundation grant deadline is March 1; and Capital Region Community Foundation grant deadline is April 1.
Requirements: Michigan 501(c)3 tax-exempt organizations in Clinton, Eaton, and Ingham Counties are eligible. Churches in the tri-county area are eligible for programs including food banks, after-school programs, programs assisting the needy, and charitable work benefiting the community, there grant applications are due June 1st.
Restrictions: Grants do not support sectarian or religious programs; individuals; international organizations; endowment funds; administrative costs of fund raising campaigns; annual meetings; routine operating expenses; or existing obligations, debts, or liabilities.
Geographic Focus: Michigan
Amount of Grant: $25,000 large grant; $2,000-$5,000 typically
Date(s) Application is Due: Jan 31; Mar 1; Apr 1
Contact: Brad Patterson, Vice President of Program; (517) 272-2870; fax: (517) 272-2871; email: bpatterson@crcfoundation.org
Internet: http://crcfoundation.org/grantmaking/grants
Sponsor: Capital Region Community Foundation
6035 Executive Drive, Suite 104
Lansing, MI 48901

Cardiac Arrhythmias Research and Education Foundation Research Grants **863**
The foundation's two primary goals are to raise funds for clinical research of cardiac arrhythmias and to educate the public and the medical community about sudden death. Awards will be granted to promising young investigators working on the genetics, mechanisms, therapy, and prevention of sudden death due to cardiac arrhythmias. Two research grants are awarded each year.
Samples: Johns Hopkins U—to support the research of David Charles Johns on the mechanisms and treatment of cardiac arrhythmias and the prevention of sudden death caused by heart rhythm disorders, $100,000 over two years.
Amount of Grant: $50,000
Contact: Grants Administrator, (800) 404-9500 or (425) 788-1987; fax: (425) 788-1927; email: care@longqt.org
Internet: http://www.longqt.org/fundingmedical.html
Sponsor: Cardiac Arrhythmias Research and Education Foundation
P.O. Box 369, 26425 NE Allen Street, Suite 103
Duvall, WA 98019

Cardinal Health Foundation Grants **864**
The foundation's mission is to support employees' interests and to advance and fund programs that improve access to and delivery of health care services in CardinalHealth communities. Additional areas of interest include arts and culture, education, and youth development. Application forms are not required; submit a project summary of no more than three pages. Proposals are by invitation.
Requirements: 501(c)3 tax-exempt organizations in CardinalHealth communities are eligible.
Restrictions: Capital campaigns, endowments, religious organizations or sectarian programs for religious purposes, veteran, labor, and political organizations or campaigns, fraternal, athletic or social clubs, requests for loans or debt retirements, individual endeavors or needs, organizations that discriminate on the basis of age, disability, religion, ethnic origin, gender, or sexual orientation, or organizations with divisive or litigious public agendas will not be supported.
Amount of Grant: $250-$450,000
Contact: Debra Hadley, (614) 757-7450; email: cardinalfoundation@cardinal.com
Internet: http://www.cardinal.com/us/en/aboutus/what/community/request/index.asp#nonprofit
Sponsor: Cardinal Health Foundation
7000 Cardinal Pl
Dublin, OH 43017

Cargill Citizenship Fund-Corporate Giving Grants **865**
Cargill's purpose is to be the global leader in nourishing people. Cargill measures their performance through engaged employees, satisfied customers, profitable growth and enriched communities. Corporate giving is one important way Cargill works to enrich the 1,000 communities where they conduct business. With 149,000 employees in 63 countries, Cargill people are working everyday to nourish the lives of those around us. The Cargill Citizenship Fund provides strategic grants to organizations serving communities where Cargill has a presence. The Fund provides direct grants for regional, national and global partnerships and provides matching grants for selected local projects supported by our businesses. Cargill seeks to build sustainable communities by focusing our human and financial resources in three areas: Nutrition and Health-support for programs and projects that address long-term solutions to hunger, increase access to health education and/or basic health care in developing and emerging countries, and improve youth nutrition and wellness; Education-support for innovative programs that improve academic achievement, develop logic and thinking skills, promote leadership development, and/or increase access to education for socio-economically disadvantaged children. Cargill also supports mutually beneficial partnerships with selected higher education institutions; Environment-support for projects that protect and improve accessibility to water resources; promote biodiversity conservation in agricultural areas; and educate children about conservation and/or proper sanitation. Application and additional guidelines are available at: http://www.cargill.com/wcm/groups/public/@ccom/documents/document/doc-giving-funding-app.pdf
Requirements: Applicants must have 501(c)3 status or the equivalent; and they must be located in communities where Cargill has a business presence. Only under special circumstances will Cargill consider general operating or capital support. Organizations requesting capital or operating support should contact the Cargill Citizenship Fund staff before applying.
Restrictions: Cargil will not fund: organizations without 501(c)3 status or the equivalent; organizations that do not serve communities where Cargill has a business presence; individuals or groups seeking support for research, planning, personal needs or travel; public service or political campaigns; lobbying, political or fraternal activities; benefit dinners or tickets to the same; fundraising campaigns, walk-a-thons, or promotions to eliminate or control; specific diseases; athletic scholarships; advertising or event sponsorships; religious groups for religious purposes; publications, audio-visual productions or special broadcasts; endowments; medical equipment.
Amount of Grant: $500-$100,000 average
Contact: Michelle Grogg, Director, Corp Contributions; (952) 742-2931; email: michelle_grogg@cargill.com;; Stacey Smida, Grants Administrator; (952) 742-4311; email: stacey_smida@cargill.com
Internet: http://www.cargill.com/wcm/groups/public/@ccom/documents/document/doc-giving-funding-app.pdf
Sponsor: Cargill Corporation
Cargill Citizenship Fund, P.O. Box 5650
Minneapolis, MN 55440-5650

Caring Foundation Grants **866**
Blue Cross and Blue Shield of Alabama, Incorporated sponsors The Caring Foundation. The Foundation was established in 1990 in Alabama and focuses it's support primarily in the region. The foundation supports organizations involved with education, federated giving programs, health, hospitals, safety education, children and youth services. The Foundation offers support of a general/operating nature as well, as program development.
Requirements: There is no formal application form, submit a proposal containing the following: name, address and phone number of organization; brief history of organization and description of its mission; detailed description of project and amount of funding requested.
Restrictions: Grants aren't available to individuals, or for capital campaigns.
Geographic Focus: Alabama
Samples: Alabama Child Caring Foundation, Birmingham, AL, $900,000 (2007); Ronald McDonald House Charities of Alabama, Birmingham, AL, $15,500 (2007); Auburn University Foundation, Auburn, AL, $105,000 (2007); Salvation Army of Birmingham, Birmingham, AL, $100,400 (2007);
Amount of Grant: $10,000 - $900,000 range
Contact: James M. Brown, Sr. V.P., Blue Cross and Blue Shield of Alabama, Inc.; (205) 220-2500
Sponsor: The Caring Foundation
450 Riverchase Parkway, East
Birmingham, AL 35244-2858

Carl and Eloise Pohlad Family Foundation Grants **867**
The mission of the foundation is to improve the lives of economically disadvantaged children and youth and participate in projects that positively impact the quality of life in the Minneapolis/St.Paul area. The foundation awards grants to Minnesota nonprofits in its areas of interest, including arts and culture, economic development, education, environment, health care, housing, and social services. Types of support include general operating support, continuing support, capital campaigns, building construction/renovation, endowments, emergency funds, scholarship funds, and research.
Requirements: Minnesota nonprofits are eligible.
Restrictions: Individuals are not eligible. Capital request are considered only for physical plant improvements or significant technology investments. Capital requests for housing construction, endowment, program start-up or expansion or to establish operating reserves are not considered.
Geographic Focus: Minnesota
Samples: Abbott Northwestern Hospital (Minneapolis, MN)—to construct a cardiology hospital, $3 million.
Amount of Grant: $3.2 million total
Contact: Rose Peterson, Program Manager, (612) 661-3903; fax: (612) 661-3715; email: rpeterson@pohladfamilygiving.org
Internet: http://www.pohladfamilyfoundation.org/pff/pff_default.aspx
Sponsor: Carl and Eloise Pohlad Family Foundation
60 S Sixth Street, Suite 3900
Minneapolis, MN 55402

Carl and Lily Pforzheimer Foundation Grants **868**
The foundation awards grants to U.S. nonprofit organizations in its areas of interest, including higher and secondary education, cultural activities and programs, public affairs, and healthcare. Types of support include capital campaigns, fellowships, internship funds, matching grants, professorships, program development, publication, scholarship funds, and seed grants. There are no application forms or deadlines. The board meets in April, June, October, and December to consider requests.
Restrictions: Grants are not awarded to individuals or for building construction/renovation.
Samples: Bank Street College of Education (New York, NY)—for scholarships and unrestrictd support, $2 million.
Amount of Grant: $10,000-$150,000 average
Contact: Grants Administrator, (212) 223-6500
Sponsor: Carl and Lily Pforzheimer Foundation
950 Third Avenue, 30th Floor
New York, NY 10022

Carl B. and Florence E. King Foundation Grants **869**
The lives of Carl B. and Florence E. King were marked by warmth, compassion, and generosity. As they prospered, they believed in giving back. With gracious benevolence, they dedicated themselves to the betterment of individuals, communities, and society through informed giving. Today, the Carl B. and Florence E. King Foundation honors their memory, continues their tradition, and builds upon their vision. The Foundation is principally interested in the following areas: aging population; arts, culture, and history; children and youth; education; indigent; and to build non-profit capacity. The Foundation awards grants twice each year. Applicants must first submit a letter of inquiry, and then a full grant proposal only upon invitation.
Requirements: The King Foundation distributes grants only to entities that serve residents of Arkansas and Texas. Within Texas, the Foundation is principally interested in the Dallas-Fort Worth area and West Texas. Within Arkansas, the foundation focuses on the southern and eastern portions of the state. Applicants must also have a letter of determination from the Internal Revenue Service acknowledging tax-exempt status as described in Section 501(c)3 of the Internal Revenue Code.
Restrictions: The Foundation does not award grants: to individuals; to organizations or programs that do not serve residents of our geographic focus areas in Texas or Arkansas;

to organizations that are not tax exempt; for general operating support, annual fund drives, or funds to offset operating losses (including retiring debt incurred to cover operating losses); to create endowments; toward balls, events, or galas benefiting charitable organizations; to efforts to treat or cure a single disease or condition; to church or seminary construction, or religious programs (other than social service-based initiatives); toward the cost of hosting or attending professional conferences or symposia, or participating in amateur sports competitions or similar activities.
Geographic Focus: Arkansas; Texas
Samples: The Dallas Foundation, Dallas, TX, $50,000 - support for the funding pool for the Zero-to-Five Funders' Collaborative project in the Bachman Lake area of Dallas (2009); Amon Carter Museum, Fort Worth, TX, $25,000 - program support for professional development programs for North Texas educators (2009); Learning Center Jonesboro, AR, $25,000 - capital support to purchase and install a playground for young children with physical and developmental disabilities (2009).
Amount of Grant: $100,000 maximum funding
Date(s) Application is Due: Dec 15; Jun 15
Contact: Michelle D. Monse, President; (214) 750-1884; fax: (214) 750-1651; email: michellemonse@kingfoundation.com
Internet: http://www.kingfoundation.com/Grants/King-Foundation-Grants.aspx
Sponsor: The Carl B. & Florence E. King Foundation
The Oaks at Turtle Creek, 2929 Carlisle, Suite 222
Dallas, TX 75204

Carl C. Icahn Foundation Grants **870**
The foundation awards grants to New York and New Jersey nonprofits in the areas of education, arts and culture, health care, child welfare, and Jewish temples and organizations. Types of support include general operating support, annual campaigns, building construction/renovation, and matching funds. There are no application deadlines or forms.
Requirements: New York and New Jersey nonprofits are eligible to apply.
Restrictions: No grants are provided to individuals.
Geographic Focus: New Jersey; New York
Amount of Grant: $1000-$500,000 range
Contact: Gail Golden, Secretary-Treasurer, c/o Icahn Associates, (212) 702-4300
Sponsor: Carl C. Icahn Foundation
767 5th Avenue, 47th Floor
New York, NY 10153-0023

Carl Gellert and Celia Berta Gellert Foundation Grants **871**
The foundation funds religious, charitable, scientific, literary or educational purposes restricted in the nine counties of the greater San Francisco Bay Area (Alameda, Contra Costa, Marin, Napa, San Francisco, San Mateo, Santa Clara, Solano and Sonoma). No grants are made to individuals. Types of support include general operations, annual and capital campaigns, building construction/ renovation, equipment acquisition, debt reduction, program/project development, medical research, publication, and scholarships.
Requirements: California 501(c)3 tax-exempt nonprofit organizations that are not private foundations are eligible.
Restrictions: Grants are not awarded to individuals.
Geographic Focus: California
Samples: U of San Francisco, School of Business and Management (CA)—to renovate and add a new wing to the McLaren Center, home of the School of Business and Management, $500,000.
Amount of Grant: $1000-$10,000 typically
Date(s) Application is Due: Aug 15 at noon
Contact: Jack Fitzpatrick, Executive Director, (415) 255-2829
Internet: http://home.earthlink.net/~cgcbg
Sponsor: Carl Gellert and Celia Berta Gellert Foundation
1169 Market Street, Suite 808
San Francisco, CA 94103

Carl J. Herzog Foundation Grants **872**
The foundation awards grants, primarily in Connecticut, for research and general operating support in its areas of interest, including medical research, dermatology research, hospitals, and education. There are no application deadlines or forms.
Requirements: 501(c)3 tax-exempt organizations are eligible.
Geographic Focus: Connecticut
Samples: Meharry Medical College (Nashville, TN)—for scholarships for minority students, $250,000 (2005).
Amount of Grant: $1000-$200,000; $5000-$50,000 average
Contact: David Babson, (203) 629-2424
Sponsor: Carl J. Herzog Foundation
321 Railroad Avenue
Greenwich, CT 06836-0788

Carl W. and Carrie Mae Joslyn Trust Grants **873**
Grants support activities providing services to resident children, elderly, and the disabled in El Paso County, CO. Areas of interest include education, medical care, rehabilitation, children and youth services, and aging centers and services. Types of support include general operating support, annual campaigns, building construction/renovation, equipment acquisition, endowment funds, and program development. Application must be in writing and must specifically describe the use of the funds. Grants are not sustaining and new applications must be submitted semiannually for renewal.
Requirements: Nonprofit organizations in El Paso County, CO, are eligible.
Restrictions: Grants are not made to individuals or for research, scholarships, fellowships, loans, or matching gifts.
Geographic Focus: Colorado
Samples: Colorado School for the Deaf and Blind (Colorado Springs, CO)—for equipment and dormitory furnishings, $18,330.; Junior Achievement of Colorado Springs (CO)—for materials, $1000.; Pikes Peak Hospice (Colorado Springs, CO)—for respiratory equipment, $2800.; Goodwill Industries of Colorado Springs (CO)—for the endowment fund, $1800.
Amount of Grant: $500-$15,000 average
Date(s) Application is Due: Apr 30; Oct 31
Contact: Grants Administrator, c/o Bank One, (719) 227-6435
Sponsor: Carl W. and Carrie Mae Joslyn Charitable Trust
P.O. Box 1699, Trust Dept
Colorado Springs, CO 80942

Carlisle Foundation Grants **874**
The foundation prefers to support proposals that are new, innovative, and/or demonstrate promise as models that might be replicated in other sites. In many instances, grants act as venture capital or seed money through which the applicant organization can demonstrate a new concept or expand its own capacity to deliver services. Although the foundation reviews a wide range of proposals, several areas receive high priority, including substance abuse; domestic and community violence; homelessness/housing; economic development; and services for children, youth, and families. The foundation prefers to make grants for restricted project support rather than general operating support. Applicant organizations should submit a one-page concept paper accompanied by a copy of the 501(c)3 determination letter.
Requirements: Connecticut, Vermont, Rhode Island, Massachusetts, New Hampshire and Maine C501(c)3 organizations are eligible. Applicant organizations should submit a one-page concept paper accompanied by a copy of the 501(c)3 determination letter.
Restrictions: Requests for capital support are rarely considered; requests for support of endowments are never considered. The foundation does not usually support programs with a primary focus on day care, disabilities, education, health services, legal services, mental retardation, or older adults. The foundation also does not provide direct support for individuals.
Geographic Focus: Connecticut; Maine; Massachusetts; New Hampshire; Rhode Island; Vermont
Contact: Richard Goldblatt, Executive Director; (401) 284-0368; fax:(401) 284-0390; email: rag@carlislefoundation.org
Internet: http://www.carlislefoundation.org/annualgrants.htm
Sponsor: Carlisle Foundation
P.O. Box 5549
Wakefield, RI 02880-5549

Carlos and Marguerite Mason Trust Grants **875**
The trust awards grants in Georgia with a focus on organ transplants. The trust's interests are patient services—needs relating to the transplantation process for the patient and the immediate family members, as well as donor family members and living donors; donation and transplantation—related education (donor education, professional education, and technical education for transplantation providers; programs to improve consent rates; and programs to promote living organ donations); and research—medical research relating to the area of transplantation. Types of support include capital improvements, start-up grants for new projects, and challenge/matching grants. Grants will be awarded for up to three years. Applicants are encouraged to contact the trustee for an appointment prior to submitting a grant request.
Requirements: Georgia nonprofit organizations are eligible.
Restrictions: Requests for general operating or administrative funds are discouraged. The trust generally does not fund endowment, nor does it fund general goodwill advertising; make grants that would replace existing sources of funding; or pay indirect overhead expenses for projects at colleges, universities, governmental units, or other established organizations.
Geographic Focus: Georgia
Amount of Grant: $1.5 million maximum
Date(s) Application is Due: Jun 1
Contact: Randy Karesh, c/o Wachovia Bank of Georgia, (404) 332-6677; email: grantinquiriesga@wachovia.com
Internet: http://www.wachovia.com/corp_inst/charitable_services/0,,4269_3300,00.html
Sponsor: Carlos and Marguerite Mason Trust
3414 Peachtree Road, 5th Fl, MC GA8023
Atlanta, GA 30326

Carls Foundation Grants **876**
The foundation has broadly defined charitable purposes, but the principal purpose and mission of the foundation is as follows: children's welfare (primarily in Michigan), including health care facilities and programs, with special emphasis on the prevention and treatment of hearing impairment; recreational, educational, and welfare programs especially for children who are disadvantaged for economic and/or health reasons; and preservation of natural areas, open space, and historic buildings and areas having special natural beauty or significance in maintaining America's heritage and historic ideals, through assistance to land trusts and land conservancies and directly related environmental educational programs. Types of grants include capital grants, limited budget support, start up/seed money, and multi-year grants. The foundation has no

formal application for grant requests. The Trustees meet minimally three times per year. Requests are accepted at all times, but organizations are encouraged to submit requests well in advance of scheduled board meetings, in January, May, and September. A letter of inquiry is not required and phone calls are welcome. Guidelines are available online.
Requirements: 501(c)3 tax-exempt organizations are eligible.
Restrictions: Grants are not awarded to individuals or for endowments, publications, conferences, seminars, film, fellowships, educational loans, travel, research, playground structures or athletic facilities, or underwriting special events.
Geographic Focus: Michigan
Amount of Grant: $5,000-$50,000 range
Date(s) Application is Due: Nov 1; Mar 1; Jul 1
Contact: Kathy Stenman, Program Officer; (313) 965-0990; fax: (313) 965-0547
Internet: http://www.carlsfdn.org
Sponsor: Carls Foundation
333 W Fort Street, Suite 1940
Detroit, MI 48226

Carlsbad Charitable Foundation Grants **877**
The mission of the Carlsbad Charitable Foundation is to advance philanthropy in its service region in order to: build community excellence; stimulate innovation; and enhance capacity of nonprofits. Its primary purpose is to: meet emerging needs by encouraging and increasing responsible and effective philanthropy by and for the benefit of all who live, work and play in Carlsbad; build a Carlsbad community endowment; provide funding annually to Carlsbad organizations and causes; and give Carlsbad community members a vehicle for legacy planning and gifts that will benefit Carlsbad now and forever. The field of grant giving focus changes annually, so applicants should contact the office directly for specific details. Most recently, the Foundation was interested in funding Senior Health and Human Services programs managed by non-profit or government agencies.
Requirements: Any 501(c)3 organization serving the residents of Carlsbad, California, are eligible to apply. Projects must specifically target seniors over the age of 55 who live in the City of Carlsbad.
Restrictions: The Carlsbad Charitable Foundation does not make grants for: annual campaigns and fund raising events for non-specific purposes; capital campaigns for buildings or facilities; stipends for attendance at conferences; endowments or chairs; for-profit organizations or enterprises; individuals unaffiliated with a qualified fiscal sponsor; projects that promote religious or political doctrine; research projects (medical or otherwise); scholarships; or existing obligations or debt.
Geographic Focus: California
Date(s) Application is Due: Jan 12
Contact: Kerry Helmer; (619) 814-1384; email: kerry@sdfoundation.org;; Trudy Amstrong, Regional Manager; (619) 814-1384; email: trudy@sdfoundation.org
Internet: http://www.endowcarlsbad.org/grants.html
Sponsor: Carlsbad Charitable Foundation / San Diego Foundation
2508 Historic Decatur Road, Suite 200
San Diego, CA 92106

Carnahan-Jackson Foundation Grants **878**
The foundation's areas of interest include higher and other education, libraries, hospitals, youth, the disabled, drug abuse programs, ecology, housing, community development, dance and other performing arts groups, and churches. Types of support include general operating support, continuing support, capital campaigns, building construction/renovation, equipment acquisition, programs/projects, seed grants, curriculum development, scholarship funds, and matching funds.
Requirements: IRS 501(c)3 organizations serving western New York, particularly Chautauqua County, are eligible.
Geographic Focus: New York
Amount of Grant: $2500-$125,000 range
Contact: Stephen E. Sellstrom; (716) 483-1015
Sponsor: Carnahan-Jackson Foundation
13 East 4th Street, P.O. Box 3326
Jamestown, NY 14701-3326

Carnegie Corporation of New York Grants **879**
The foundation provides research, study, and support for projects to improve government at all levels, to increase public understanding of social policy issues, to equalize opportunities for minorities and women, and to increase participation in political and civic life. Also supported are projects that promote electoral reform; education reform from early childhood through higher education; early childhood development; and urban school reform. The foundation will also fund research on the increasing availability and success of after-school and extended service programs for children and teenagers, particularly those in urban areas, that promote high academic achievement. Dissemination of best practices in teacher education will also be emphasized. There is no formal procedure for submitting a proposal. To apply under any of the corporation's grantmaking programs, applicants should submit a full proposal that describes the project's aims, duration, methods, amount of financial support required, and key personnel. The board meets four times a year, in October, February, April, and June.
Restrictions: Grants are not made for construction or maintenance of facilities or endowments. The Corporation does not generally make grants to individuals except through the Carnegie Scholars Program, that supports the work of select scholars and experts conducting research in the foundation's fields of interest.
Samples: American Academy of Arts and Sciences, Cambridge, Massachusetts, $500,000—an initiative on minimizing the risks of nuclear energy expansion (2009); George Washington University, Washington, DC, $349,900— research and writing on the effects of domestic foreign policy debates on U.S. global engagement (2009).
Amount of Grant: $80 million total approximately annually
Contact: Sarina Cipriano, Grants Manager; (212) 371-3200; fax: (212) 754-4073
Internet: http://www.carnegie.org/sub/program/grant.html
Sponsor: Carnegie Corporation of New York
437 Madison Avenue
New York, NY 10022

Carolyn Foundation Grants **880**
Priorities for funding include community and environmental grantmaking. In the community focus area needs are addressed only in the communities of interest to the foundation: Minneapolis, MN, and New Haven, CT. There are two community focus areas for funding: economically disadvantaged children and youth; and community and cultural vitality. The foundation works to empower economically disadvantaged children and youth by supporting their families and others to inspire, nurture, educate and guide them to achieve long-term stability and well-being. The environmental program area is divided between responsive for which unsolicited requests are considered, and foundation initiated requests for which unsolicited requests will not be considered.
Requirements: IRS 501(c)3 nonprofit organizations in Minnesota and Connecticut may apply for the community grants. All 501(c)3 organizations are eligible for the environmental grants. The foundation encourages use of Carolyn Foundation Application Form adapted from the Minnesota Common Grant Application Form. Applicants choosing not to use the common grant form must address the same information as required by the common grant. All proposals must use the Carolyn Foundation Coversheet, found on the web page.
Restrictions: Grants are not awarded to individuals, political organizations or candidates, veterans??? organizations, fraternal societies or orders, annual fund drives, umbrella organizations, or to deficits already incurred. The foundation does not generally make grants to religious organizations for religious purposes or to organizations in support of operations carried on in foreign countries.
Geographic Focus: Connecticut; Minnesota
Samples: Environmental Law & Policy Center of the Midwest (Chicago, IL)—$50,000 for the Farm Bill-Clean Energy Development Initiative.; Great River Greening (St. Paul, MN)—$20,000 for the partnership to recover healthy water, shores, and bluffs of the St. Croix River.; Admission Possible (St. Paul, MN)—$25,000 for general operating support to help disadvantaged youth successfully transition to post secondary education.; Neighborhood Involvement Program (Minneapolis, MN)—$12,000 for the Teachable Moment child abuse prevention program.
Amount of Grant: $5000-$50,000
Date(s) Application is Due: Jan 15; Jul 15
Contact: Becky Erdahl, Executive Director, (612) 596-3266; fax: (612) 338-2084; email: BErdahl@carolynfoundation.org
Internet: http://www.carolynfoundation.org/guidelines.html
Sponsor: Carolyn Foundation
706 2nd Ave S, Suite 760
Minneapolis, MN 55402

Carpenter Foundation Grants **881**
The foundation's primary areas of interest include the arts, education, public interest, and human services. The foundation is deeply concerned with the well-being of children and families and their relationship to their neighborhoods and communities. Also of concern is the health of the web of agencies and organizations which serve them. Grants are awarded for general operating support, program development, capital campaigns, equipment acquisition, scholarship funds, seed money, matching funds, and technical support. Deadlines are generally about six weeks before the quarterly board meetings, held in January, March, June, and September.
Requirements: Tax exempt agencies in the Jackson and Josephine Counties of Oregon may submit proposals.
Restrictions: Grants are not made to individuals. The foundation rarely makes grants for historical applications, hospital construction or equipment, group or individual trips, or activities for religious purposes.
Geographic Focus: Oregon
Samples: Community Health Center (Medford, OR)—fir a program to provide discounted medications to low-income/uninsured patients, $15,000.; Science Works Hands-On Museum, (Ashland, OR)—in support of a life science hands-on exhibition for local schools and students, $6,000.; Southern Oregon State College (Ashland, OR)—for faculty development opportunities which improve teaching, $25,000.; Oregon Water Trust, (Portland, OR)—for a community outreach and education project to locally distribute the General Elections Voter's Guide, $12,000.
Amount of Grant: $250-$25,000 range
Contact: Polly Williams, Program Officer, (541) 772-5732; fax: (541) 773-3970; email: carpfdn@internetcds.com
Internet: http://www.carpenter-foundation.org
Sponsor: Carpenter Foundation
711 E Main Street, Suite 10
Medford, OR 97504

Carrie E. and Lena V. Glenn Foundation Grants **882**
Established in 1971, the Glenn Foundation provides annual grants in the following areas of interest: arts; children/youth, services; Christian agencies & churches; Elementary/secondary education; Environment; and Human services.

Requirements: Federally tax-exempt institutions and not-for-profit agencies that serve Gaston County, NC. agencies or out-of-county agencies whose projects have an impact on Gaston County citizens are eligible to apply.
Restrictions: Funding is not available for: planning grants; grants to individuals; scholarships; capital campaigns; umbrella campaigns; and multi-year grants.
Geographic Focus: North Carolina
Samples: Community Foundation of Gaston County, Gastonia, NC., $25,000 - for purchase and installment of This Little Light of Mine, a painting by John Biggers, recreated as mosaic time mural (2007); Gastonia Potters House, Lowell, NC., $10,000 - for operating expenses for residential drug rehabiliation program for women.; Alliance for Children and Youth, Gastonia, NC., $8,885 - for Strengthening Families program for parents and their children (2007);
Amount of Grant: $3,000-$25,000 range
Date(s) Application is Due: Mar 1
Contact: Barbara H. Voorhees, Executive Director; (704) 867-0296; fax: (704) 867-4496; email: glennfnd@bellsouth.net
Sponsor: Carrie E. and Lena V. Glenn Foundation, inc.
1552 Union Road, Suite D
Gastonia, NC 28054

Carrie Estelle Doheny Foundation Grants 883
The foundation primarily funds local, not-for profit organizations endeavoring to advance education, medicine and religion, to improve the health and welfare of the sick, aged, incapacitated, and to aid the needy. Educational funding includes support of inner city Catholic schools, and scholarship funds for Catholic high schools and universities. Adult education programs and religious education are also supported. Medical funding is focused in two areas: research and care of the disadvantaged. Religious funding is directed to support the gospel values as expressed in the Roman Catholic faith. Health and welfare funding is directed to organizations who assist individuals to lead independent satisfying lives. Specific areas of interest include adoption and foster care service groups, programs for the disabled, health education programs, and senior programs. Aiding the needy funding includes inner city youth clubs, summer camps, and food banks. No formalized application or proposal format is required. The board reviews appropriate proposals monthly. Submitted proposals should be concise and contain a brief description of what is planned and a clear statement of objectives sought. Support is given mainly to those in the Southern California area.
Requirements: U.S. nonprofit tax-exempt organizations in California are eligible. An application form is required for submission and may be downloaded from the web site.
Restrictions: Grant requests are not considered from individuals or from tax-supported entities. Areas also excluded from consideration include support for individuals, endowment funds, publishing books, television or radio programs, travel funds, advertisement, scholarships, or political purposes in any form.
Geographic Focus: California
Amount of Grant: $5000-$150,000 average
Contact: Shirley Bernard, Senior Grants Administrator, (213) 488-1122; fax: (213) 488-1544; email: doheny@dohenyfoundation.org or shirley@dohenyfoundation.org
Internet: http://www.dohenyfoundation.org/grant/grant.htm
Sponsor: Carrie Estelle Doheny Foundation
707 Wilshire Boulevard, Suite 4960
Los Angeles, CA 90017

Carrier Corporation Contributions Grants 884
Carrier donates approximately $2 million around the world to registered nonprofit organizations. In the United States, Carrier funds only qualified 501(c)3 organizations that meet its eligibility criteria and operate in locations where the company has a significant employee base. Carrier believes in helping people in the communities where they live, work and do business. To better serve those communities and to better align its corporate contributions with mission and values, it focuses giving on the following these areas: environment and sustainability; civic & community; education; arts & culture; health & human services. All U.S. non-profits are required to complete an online grant application. Applications are accepted from March 1 through June 1 of each year, and are reviewed for funding to be paid the following year. Applicants will receive notification in the first quarter of the calendar year in which funding will occur.
Requirements: Carrier funds only qualified 501(c)3 organizations that meet eligibility criteria and operate in locations where it has a significant employee base.
Restrictions: Carrier will not fund: individuals; religious organizations; alumni groups, sororities or fraternities; booster clubs; political groups; any organization determined by Carrier to have a conflict of interest; any organization whose practices are inconsistent with the company's Code of Ethics
Geographic Focus: Alabama; Arizona; Connecticut; Georgia; Illinois; Indiana; Michigan; Nevada; New York; North Carolina; South Carolina; Tennessee; Texas
Date(s) Application is Due: Jun 1
Contact: Rajan Goel, VP; (860) 674-3420; fax: (860) 622-0488
Internet: http://www.corp.carrier.com/vgn-ext-templating/v/index.jsp?vgnextoid=6afa80757d7e7010VgnVCM100000cb890b80RCRD
Sponsor: Carrier Corporation
One Carrier Place
Farmington, CT 06034-4015

Carroll County Community Foundation Grants 885
This foundation is the catalyst for stimulating and funding initiatives that improve the quality of life for citizens of Carroll County. The Community Foundation is a not-for-profit charitable corporation. In order to most effectively fulfill its philanthropic responsibilities in Carroll County within the limits of its resources, the Foundation's grants program will emphasize change-oriented and focused types of grants. Areas of interest include: social services; education; cultural affairs; civic affairs; health & medical. It is the general policy of the Carroll Community Foundation to operate without discrimination as to age, race, religion, sex or national origin in the overall administration of the Foundation and in the consideration of grant requests from agencies and organizations.
Requirements: See website for grant guidelines, policies & evaluation criteria.
Restrictions: Must be a citizen of Carroll County.
Geographic Focus: Indiana
Date(s) Application is Due: As a general rule, a grant decision will be made within ninety days from date of submission.
Contact: Ron Harper, President, (765) 454-7298 or (800) 964-0508; email: ron@cfhoward.org
Internet: http://cfcarroll.org/newsite/grantprogram.shtml
Sponsor: Carroll County Community Foundation
215 W. Sycamore
Kokomo, IN 46901

Carylon Foundation Grants 886
The foundation awards general support grants to nonprofits of the Christian, interdenominational, Jewish, and Presbyterian faiths. Higher education institutions, health care organizations, international missions/ministries, medical centers, religious organizations, and temples receive support. Application may be made by submitting a brief letter describing the organization and program. There are no application deadlines.
Amount of Grant: $50-$50,000 range
Contact: Marcie Mervis, Trustee, (312) 666-7700
Sponsor: Carylon Foundation
2500 W Arthington
Chicago, IL 60612-4108

Cass County Community Foundation Grants 887
The Cass County Community Foundation honors the spirit of giving and assists donors in building enduring sources of charitable assets to promote education, enhance humanity and advance community development throughout Cass County. The Foundation operates on an annual grant cycle, with applications due each June 30. All applications are reviewed by a committee comprised of CCCF Board members and other volunteers from the community.
Requirements: Those eligible to apply for a grant are non-profit organizations with documentation of 501(c)3 status, whose projects directly impact the lives of Cass County, Indiana residents.
Restrictions: Public schools, while non-profit, are not 501(c)3 and therefore are not eligible.
Geographic Focus: Indiana
Date(s) Application is Due: Jun 30
Contact: Deanna Crispen, Executive Director; (574) 722-2200; fax: (574) 753-7501; email: cccf@cassfoundation.com
Internet: http://www.casscountycf.org/applyGrant.htm
Sponsor: Cass County Community Foundation
P.O. Box 441 417 North Street, Suite 102
Logansport, IN 46947

Castle Rock Foundation Grants 888
The foundation's grants are awarded to promote a better understanding of the free-enterprise system; preserve principles on which democracy was founded, ensure a limited role for government, and protect individual rights; encourage personal leadership; and uphold traditional American values. Types of support include general operating grants and special project grants.
Requirements: U.S. 501(c)3 organizations are eligible.
Restrictions: Grants requests from human service agencies, museums, organizations primarily supported by tax-derived funding, endowments, scientific or medical research, publications or media projects, churches, debt retirement, special events, or individuals will be denied.
Samples: College Fund/United Negro Fund, Fairfax, VA, $40,000 for scholarships; Congressional Medal of Honor Society, Mt. Pleasant, SC, $20,000 for general operating expense; Foundation for Research on economics and the Environment, $50,000 for general operating expense; Fund for American Studies, Washington, DC, $25,000 for general operating expense (2006).
Amount of Grant: $25,000-$75,000 average
Date(s) Application is Due: Mar 15
Contact: Sally W. Rippey, Executive Director, (303) 388-1683; fax: (303) 388-1684; email: generalinfo@castlerockfdn.org
Internet: http://www.castlerockfoundation.org
Sponsor: Castle Rock Foundation
4100 E Mississippi Avenue, Suite 1850
Denver, CO 80246

Catherine Holmes Wilkins Foundation Grants 889
The foundation awards grants in Washington's Puget Sound region to nonprofit organizations in its areas of interest. Funding priorities include medical research and education—medical and academic centers conducting research and training in areas such as cancer, heart disease, and mental illness; physically handicapped and mentally ill—community nonprofit agencies providing direct social services to people

with physical disabilities or mental illness; services for the needy—community-based programs providing immediate support to the needy, with particular emphasis on services for abused women and children. Preference will be given to project support, rather than ongoing operating expenses. Proposals are accepted throughout the year. Grants are awarded quarterly.
Requirements: 501(c)3 organizations that operate within or significantly affect the residents of the greater Seattle region are eligible.
Restrictions: Grants are not made for multi-year projects, debt retirement, operational deficits, or to individuals or for scholarships.
Amount of Grant: $3000-$10,000
Contact: c/o Bank of America, Charitable Investment Services
Internet: http://fdncenter.org/grantmaker/wilkins
Sponsor: Catherine Holmes Wilkins Foundation
P.O. Box 24565
Seattle, WA 98124

Catherine Kennedy Home Foundation Grants 890
The Catherine Kennedy Home Foundation established in 2001, supports nonprofit organizations involved with Aging, centers/services; Christian agencies & churches; developmentally disabled, centers & services; family services; domestic violence; food distribution, meals on wheels; residential/custodial care, hospices; YM/YWCAs & YM/YWHAs. Giving primarily in Wilmington, North Carolina.
Requirements: Initial approach should be made through a letter to the Foundation requesting an application form.
Restrictions: Funding not available outside of North Carolina.
Geographic Focus: North Carolina
Amount of Grant: $1,000-$30,000 range
Date(s) Application is Due: Feb 28
Contact: Garry A. Garris, Director; (910) 452-0611;
Sponsor: The Catherine Kennedy Home, Inc.
P.O. Box 4782
Wilmington, NC 28406-1782

Catholic Campaign for Human Development Community Organizing Grants 891
CCHD is committed to supporting groups of low-income individuals as they work to break the cycle of poverty and improve their communities. By helping the poor to participate in the decisions and actions that affect their lives, CCHD empowers them to move beyond poverty. The organization's efforts should directly benefit a relatively large number of people rather than a few individuals. The organization should generate cooperation among and within diverse groups in the interest of a more integrated and mutually understanding society. An applicant organization seeking 'seed' or 'matching monies' will also be considered. (If requesting these monies, applicants should present positive documentation that other public and/or private sources will commit their funds to support the organization's efforts.)
Requirements: Only organizations that are not now receiving an organizing grant are required to submit an Eligibility Quiz. Eligibility Quizzes are accepted on a rolling basis between September 1st and November 1st. The sponsor recommends submitting your Eligibility Quiz well in advance of the November 1st deadline, to help with processing and to give eligible applicants more time with the next step in application. To be eligible for CCHD funds, an organization must satisfy ALL the following criteria and guidelines: (1) The activity for which funding is requested must conform to the moral and social teachings of the Catholic Church. (2) The applicant organization must demonstrate both the intention and capacity to effectively work toward the elimination of the root causes of poverty and to enact institutional change. (3) The organization's efforts must benefit people living in poverty. At least 50 percent of those benefiting from the organization's efforts must be people experiencing poverty. (4) People living in poverty must have the dominant voice in the organization. At least 50 percent of those who plan, implement and make policy, hire and fire staff (e.g., the Board of Directors, etc.) should be persons who are involuntarily poor (clergy, VISTA volunteers, students, etc. are considered by CCHD to be voluntarily poor). (5) The organization should demonstrate ongoing leadership development because it is considered essential to the strength, depth and sustainability of the organization. (6) The organization should demonstrate a clear vision for development of financial capacity that might include membership dues, grassroots fundraising, foundation and/or corporate support. (7) The organization must be fully nonpartisan when engaging in political activities. Organizations engaged in partisan political activity are not eligible. See the website for further explanations.
Restrictions: The following general classifications do not meet CCHD criteria and/or guidelines for community organizing grants: (1) Organizations with primary focus on direct service ; (2) Advocacy efforts where only staff, a few individuals or middle to upper-income people are speaking for a particular low income constituency without the direct involvement and leadership of low income individuals; (3) Organizations controlled by governmental (federal, state, local), educational, or ecclesiastical bodies; (4) Research projects, surveys, planning and feasibility studies, etc.; (5) Individually owned, for-profit businesses. (6) Organizations that would use CCHD money for re-granting purposes or to fund other organizations.
Amount of Grant: $25,000 - $50,000
Date(s) Application is Due: Sep 1; Nov 1
Contact: See http://www.usccb.org/cchd/fieldreps.shtml to find the Grant Specialist in your area.
Internet: http://www.usccb.org/cchd/grants/criteria.shtml
Sponsor: United States Conference of Catholic Bishops (U.S.CCB)
3211 Fourth Street, NE
Washington DC 20017-1194

CCFF Clinic Incentive Grants 892
The grants are intended to enhance the standard of clinical care available to Canadians with cystic fibrosis by providing funds to initiate a comprehensive program for cystic fibrosis patient care, research, and teaching; or to strengthen an existing program. Clinic incentive grants are awarded for a term of one year, and are renewable on an annual basis. The grants provide an honorarium for the clinic director, as compensation for his or her administrative responsibilities. Requests may be made for salary support for other nonphysician clinic personnel. A component of the grants is allocated to travel.
Requirements: Canadian hospitals and/or medical schools are eligible to apply.
Date(s) Application is Due: Oct 3
Contact: Grants Administrator, (416) 485-9149; fax: (416) 485-0960; email: info@cysticfibrosis.ca
Internet: http://www.ccff.ca/page.asp?id=87
Sponsor: Canadian Cystic Fibrosis Foundation
2221 Yonge Street, Suite 601
Toronto, ON M4S 2B4 Canada

CCFF Fellowships 893
A limited number of competitive fellowships are offered by the foundation each year for basic or clinical research training in areas of the biomedical or behavioral sciences pertinent to cystic fibrosis. Fellowships are tenable at approved universities, hospitals, and research institutes in Canada. Initial fellowships are awarded for a two-year period. Fellows may apply for a one-year renewal. No one may receive more than three years of support under a CCFF fellowship. Canadian fellowship applicants of exceptional quality requesting funding to study abroad will be considered. Applicants are expected to demonstrate that comparable training is not available in Canada. Equitable consideration is given to applicants from outside of Canada who intend to return to their own country on completion of the fellowship.
Requirements: Individuals who hold MD or PhD degrees are eligible to apply.
Restrictions: Applicants who have already completed six or more years of postgraduate study or training are not eligible.
Date(s) Application is Due: Oct 1
Contact: Grants Administrator, (416) 485-9149; fax: (416) 485-0960; email: info@cysticfibrosis.ca
Internet: http://www.ccff.ca/page.asp?id=87
Sponsor: Canadian Cystic Fibrosis Foundation
2221 Yonge Street, Suite 601
Toronto, ON M4S 2B4 Canada

CCFF Research Grants 894
Research grants are intended to facilitate the scientific investigation of all aspects of cystic fibrosis. Applications may be submitted by groups of individuals who plan to collaborate. Grants are awarded for up to three years. Investigators are eligible to hold more than one research grant. Research grants may be allocated to personnel (research assistant(s), technicians, and specified other personnel); materials and supplies; equipment not in excess of $10,000; and travel.
Requirements: A principal investigator should hold a recognized, full-time faculty appointment in a relevant discipline at a Canadian university or hospital.
Restrictions: Research grants do not provide support for graduate students, postdoctoral fellows, or summer students; construction costs; institutional overheads for laboratory facilities; or purchase of equipment in excess of $10,000.
Date(s) Application is Due: Oct 1
Contact: Grants Administrator, (416) 485-9149; fax: (416) 485-0960; email: info@cysticfibrosis.ca
Internet: http://www.ccff.ca/page.asp?id=87
Sponsor: Canadian Cystic Fibrosis Foundation
2221 Yonge Street, Suite 601
Toronto, ON M4S 2B4 Canada

CCFF Scholarships 895
Scholarships provide salary support to gifted investigators in CF research, offering them the opportunity to develop outstanding cystic fibrosis research programs. Scholarships are held in conjunction with a CCFF research grant. Applications are available online.
Requirements: Applications are accepted from candidates who have received their first faculty appointment within the preceding five calendar years.
Date(s) Application is Due: Oct 1
Contact: Grants Administrator, (416) 485-9149; fax: (416) 485-0960; email: info@cysticfibrosis.ca
Internet: http://www.ccff.ca/page.asp?id=87
Sponsor: Canadian Cystic Fibrosis Foundation
2221 Yonge Street, Suite 601
Toronto, ON M4S 2B4 Canada

CCFF Small Conference Grants 896
Small conference grants are offered to support medical/scientific conferences which focus on subjects of direct relevance to cystic fibrosis. Such grants will be up to a maximum of $C2500 and are intended to supplement other funding sources. The small conference grants will also support inter-clinic exchanges which are used to facilitate the exchange of special expertise between larger, university-based CF clinics and smaller, more remote clinics. Requests of this type will involve fewer individuals, and will not normally exceed $C1000. Applications may be submitted at any time, but the foundation should be consulted in advance with respect to the availability of funds. Grants are on a first-come, first-served basis.

Requirements: CF clinic directors and CCFF-funded investigators are eligible to apply.
Amount of Grant: $C2500 for medical/scientific conferences; $C1000 for inter-clinic exchanges
Contact: Grants Administrator, (416) 485-9149; fax: (416) 485-0960; email: info@cysticfibrosis.ca
Internet: http://www.ccff.ca/page.asp?id=87
Sponsor: Canadian Cystic Fibrosis Foundation
2221 Yonge Street, Suite 601
Toronto, ON M4S 2B4 Canada

CCFF Studentships 897
A limited number of competitive studentships are offered by the foundation each year to highly qualified graduate students who are registered for a higher degree and who are undertaking full-time research training in areas of the biomedical or behavioral sciences relevant to cystic fibrosis. Students are expected to spend at least 75 percent of their time on the research training described in their application.
Requirements: Awards are tenable only at Canadian universities.
Date(s) Application is Due: Apr 1; Oct 1
Contact: Grants Administrator, (416) 485-9149; fax: (416) 485-0960; email: info@cysticfibrosis.ca
Internet: http://www.ccff.ca/page.asp?id=87
Sponsor: Canadian Cystic Fibrosis Foundation
2221 Yonge Street, Suite 601
Toronto, ON M4S 2B4 Canada

CCFF Summer Studentship 898
Summer studentships are intended to provide support to students engaged in summer research projects in areas of the biomedical or behavioral sciences relevant to cystic fibrosis, under the direction of CF clinic directors or principal investigators. The research project should be attainable within the three-month term of the award.
Requirements: Full-time students pursuing an undergraduate degree in an appropriate discipline are eligible to receive this award. Under certain circumstances, other special academic situations, may be considered for a summer studentship.
Restrictions: Applications must be made by the proposed supervisor on behalf of a student. Applications directly from students cannot be accepted.
Date(s) Application is Due: Feb 1
Contact: Grants Administrator, (416) 485-9149; fax: (416) 485-0960; email: info@cysticfibrosis.ca
Internet: http://www.ccff.ca/page.asp?id=87
Sponsor: Canadian Cystic Fibrosis Foundation
2221 Yonge Street, Suite 601
Toronto, ON M4S 2B4 Canada

CCFF Transplant Center Incentive Grants 899
The grants are intended to enhance the quality of care available to cystic fibrosis transplant candidates by providing eligible centers with supplementary funding for support of personnel directly involved in the provision of patient services; travel to the annual North American Cystic Fibrosis conference; and administrative costs associated with providing data to the Canadian Cystic Fibrosis Lung Transplant Registry. Grants are renewable on an annual basis.
Requirements: Canadian lung transplant centers that currently have one or more individuals with cystic fibrosis listed for transplant may apply.
Date(s) Application is Due: Oct 1
Contact: Grants, (416) 485-9149; fax: (416) 485-0960; email: info@cysticfibrosis.ca
Internet: http://www.ccff.ca/page.asp?id=87
Sponsor: Canadian Cystic Fibrosis Foundation
2221 Yonge Street, Suite 601
Toronto, ON M4S 2B4 Canada

CCFF Visiting Scientist Awards 900
Awards are made to senior investigators from abroad who are invited to engage in CF research at a Canadian institution; or junior and senior Canadian investigators who wish to work in another laboratory in Canada or abroad. It is intended that this experience as a CCFF visiting scientist will, in some way, benefit the Canadian CF research effort. Applications may be submitted at any time, but the foundation should be consulted in advance with respect to the availability of funds.
Requirements: Senior investigators from abroad or junior and senior Canadian investigators who wish to work in another laboratory in Canada or abroad are eligible to apply.
Contact: Grants Administrator, (416) 485-9149; fax: (416) 485-0960; email: info@cysticfibrosis.ca
Internet: http://www.ccff.ca/page.asp?id=87
Sponsor: Canadian Cystic Fibrosis Foundation
2221 Yonge Street, Suite 601
Toronto, ON M4S 2B4 Canada

CDC Evidence-Based Laboratory Medicine: Quality/Performance Measure Evaluation 901
The purpose of the program is to evaluate clinical laboratory practice by identifying evidence-based laboratory medicine quality/performance measures associated with the pre- and post-analytic stages of the total testing process, and to identify and address gaps and opportunities for improvement consistent with national health care priorities to improve public health. The primary objectives are to: provide an evidence base which systematically identifies and defines important gaps in laboratory medicine quality related to individuals or populations and/or patient safety health outcomes with demonstrated impacts (i.e., clinical and/or economic); identify, develop, and define laboratory medicine performance/quality measures that can be broadly implemented to evaluate performance associated with patient outcomes; and identify interventions to improve performance.
Requirements: Eligible applicants include: public nonprofit organizations; private nonprofit organizations; small, minority, women-owned businesses; universities; colleges; research institutions; hospitals; community-based organizations; faith-based organizations; federally recognized Indian tribal governments; Indian tribes; Indian tribal organizations; state and local governments or their Bona Fide Agents (this includes the District of Columbia, the Commonwealth of Puerto Rico, the Virgin Islands, the Commonwealth of the Northern Marianna Islands, American Samoa, Guam, the Federated States of Micronesia, the Republic of the Marshall Islands, and the Republic of Palau); and political subdivisions of States (in consultation with States).
Restrictions: Recipients may: not use funds for research; not use funds for clinical care; only expend funds for reasonable program purposes, including personnel, travel, supplies, and services, such as contractual. Awardees may not generally use HHS/CDC/ATSDR funding for the purchase of furniture or equipment (any such proposed spending must be identified in the budget). The direct and primary recipient in a cooperative agreement program must perform a substantial role in carrying out project objectives and not merely serve as a conduit for an award to another party or provider who is ineligible. Reimbursement of pre-award costs is not allowed.
Amount of Grant: $100,000-$500,000
Date(s) Application is Due: Jul 17
Contact: Yolanda Sledge, Grants Specialist, (770) 488-2787; email: yiso@cdc.gov
Internet: http://www.cdc.gov/od/pgo/funding/FOAs.htm
Sponsor: Centers for Disease Control and Prevention
2920 Brandywine Road, Mail stop: E-14
Atlanta, GA 30341-3717

CDC Antimicrobial Resistance in Hospital-Acquired Infections Among Intensive Care Unit Patients 902
CDC offers funds to conduct studies on antimicrobial resistance in hospital-acquired infections among intensive care unit patients. Grants will be awarded to conduct both economic and outcome evaluations on the extent of the problem, as well as on factors that lead to different outcomes.
Requirements: Applications may be submitted by public and private nonprofit organizations and by governments and their agencies.
Amount of Grant: $60,000-$100,000
Contact: Nealean Austin, Centers for Disease Control and Prevention, (770) 488-2700
Internet: http://edocket.access.gpo.gov/2004/04-9808.htm
Sponsor: Centers for Disease Control and Prevention
2920 Brandywine Road, Room 3000
Atlanta, GA 30341

CDC Cancer Prevention and Control Programs 903
The purpose of the program is to improve and to promote health among at-risk cancer populations and to reduce cancer morbidity and mortality.
Requirements: Assistance will be provided only to the organizations listed. The Healthcare Association of New York to develop an integrated model for the delivery of comprehensive breast cancer services; the Health Choice Network, Miami/Dade County, Florida to administer the Jesse Trice Cancer Prevention Project; the East Tennessee State University, Cancer Prevention Research Center, James H. Quillen College of Medicine to address cancer care in the rural Appalachian region; the University of Rhode Island, Cancer Prevention Research Center to provide interactive interventions to at-risk populations; the Sisters of Charity Health Care System, to ensure that patients have access to early detection of gastrointestinal cancers; and Marin County, California to evaluate high incidence of breast cancer in the San Francisco Bay Area.
Geographic Focus: California; Florida; New York; Rhode Island; Tennessee
Amount of Grant: $4.1million total
Contact: Grants Administrator, (770) 488-4751; email: cancerinfo@cdc.gov
Internet: http://www.cdc.gov/cancer
Sponsor: Centers for Disease Control and Prevention
4770 Buford Hwy NE, MS K-64
Atlanta, GA 30341-3717

CDC Cooperative Agreement for Continuing Enhanced National Surveillance for Prion Diseases in the United States 904
The purpose of the funding is to continue an active surveillance program similar to that conducted by the National Prion Disease Pathology Surveillance Center since 1997 to monitor the occurrence of potentially emerging human TSEs in the United States. This program addresses the Healthy People 2010 focus area(s) of Immunizations and Infectious Diseases. Eligible applicants should have experience in conducting prion disease surveillance and must be capable of fulfilling the ongoing needs for enhancing such surveillance at the national level.
Requirements: Eligible applicants include: public nonprofit organizations; private nonprofit organizations; small, minority, women-owned businesses; universities; colleges; research institutions; hospitals; community-based organizations; faith-based organizations; federally recognized Indian tribal governments; Indian tribes; Indian tribal organizations; state and local governments or their Bona Fide Agents (this includes the District of Columbia, the Commonwealth of Puerto Rico, the Virgin Islands, the Commonwealth of the Northern Marianna Islands, American Samoa, Guam, the Federated States of Micronesia, the Republic of the Marshall Islands, and the Republic of Palau); and political subdivisions of States (in consultation with States).

Restrictions: Recipients may: not use funds for research; not use funds for clinical care; only expend funds for reasonable program purposes, including personnel, travel, supplies, and services, such as contractual. Awardees may not generally use HHS/CDC/ATSDR funding for the purchase of furniture or equipment (any such proposed spending must be identified in the budget). The direct and primary recipient in a cooperative agreement program must perform a substantial role in carrying out project objectives and not merely serve as a conduit for an award to another party or provider who is ineligible.
Amount of Grant: $2,550,000.00 first year; $12,750,000.00 over five years
Date(s) Application is Due: Jun 30
Contact: Mattie Jackson, Grants Specialist, (770) 488-2696; email: MIJ3@cdc.gov
Internet: http://www.cdc.gov/od/pgo/funding/FOAs.htm
Sponsor: Centers for Disease Control and Prevention
2920 Brandywine Road, Mail stop: E-14
Atlanta, GA 30341-3717

CDC Coop Agreement for Partnership to Enhance Public Health Informatics **905**
The purpose of the program is to strengthen the breadth and depth of the public health workforce by providing training in public health informatics and encouraging new explorations of innovations at the intersection of public health and health informatics. CDC wants to partner with a national organization that is established as a leader in clinical and health informatics and with established tutorials and other training in informatics. This program addresses the Healthy People 2010 focus area of Public Health Infrastructure and the CDC's Healthy Protection Goal of People Prepared for Emerging Health Threats to develop and measure how well public health systems perform in critical times.
Requirements: Assistance will be provided only to national non-profit organizations (a national non-profit, tax-exempt Section 501(c)3 agency. Eligible national organizations must have a web-based training and in person tutorials in clinical and public health informatics. These resources should have been established, fully operational, and deemed successful before application is submitted. Additionally, applicants are required to have an active national and international professional membership in informatics. Limiting assistance to national non-profit organizations is necessary to produce the maximum possible enhancement, given available resources.
Restrictions: The following restrictions apply: recipients may not use funds for research; recipients may not use funds for clinical care; recipients may only expend funds for reasonable program purposes, including personnel, travel, supplies, and services, such as contractual; awardees may not generally use HHS/CDC/ATSDR funding for the purchase of furniture or equipment; the direct and primary recipient in a cooperative agreement program must perform a substantial role in carrying out project objectives and not merely serve as a conduit for an award to another party or provider who is ineligible; reimbursement of pre-award costs is not allowed; and these funds may not be used to set up or support lobbying by interest/advocacy groups.
Amount of Grant: $500,000 current fiscal year; $2,500,000 over a five-year period
Date(s) Application is Due: Jul 2
Contact: Kaleema McLean, Grants Specialist, (770) 488-2742, email: kmclean@cdc.gov
Internet: http://www.cdc.gov/od/pgo/funding/FOAs.htm
Sponsor: Centers for Disease Control and Prevention
2920 Brandywine Road, Mail stop: E-14
Atlanta, GA 30341

CDC Cooperative Agreement for the Development, Operation, and Evaluation of an Entertainment Education Program **906**
The purpose of this program is raise awareness and behavioral change concerning public health issues through the use of the television media as means of accessing the television viewing public by providing: accurate public health information and public health issues, as well as accurate depictions of healthy living at all stages of life, to entertainment industry leadership for possible inclusion in television story lines; assistance with public health outreach, including providing additional information concerning public health topics depicted on television story lines, and assistance with public service announcements and informational short videos to be aired in conjunction with drama presentations; and evaluation of public health television story lines and the effect on the viewing public.
Requirements: Eligible applicants include: public nonprofit organizations; private nonprofit organizations; universities; colleges; research institutions; federally recognized Indian tribal governments; Indian tribes; Indian tribal organizations; state and local governments or their Bona Fide Agents (this includes the District of Columbia, the Commonwealth of Puerto Rico, the Virgin Islands, the Commonwealth of the Northern Marianna Islands, American Samoa, Guam, the Federated States of Micronesia, the Republic of the Marshall Islands, and the Republic of Palau); and political subdivisions of States (in consultation with States).
Date(s) Application is Due: Jun 7
Contact: Sharon Robertson, Grants Management Officer, (770) 488-2748; email: SRobertson1@cdc.gov
Internet: http://www.cdc.gov/od/pgo/funding/FOAs.htm
Sponsor: Centers for Disease Control and Prevention
2920 Brandywine Road, Mail stop: E-14
Atlanta, GA 30341

CDC Core Capacity Program Grants **907**
This program seeks to develop basic cardiovascular health promotions and strategies at the state level. It should include statewide partnerships and program coordination among health agencies aimed at primary and secondary heart disease prevention.
Requirements: State health agencies, the District of Columbia, Puerto Rico, and U.S. territories are eligible to apply.
Restrictions: Funds may not be used to supplant state or local funds, to provide inpatient care or personal health services, nor to support construction or renovation of facilities.
Amount of Grant: $250,000-$500,000 range; $300,000 average
Contact: Nealean Austin, Team Lead, (770) 488-2754
Internet: http://www.cdc.gov
Sponsor: Centers for Disease Control and Prevention
2920 Brandywine Road
Altanta, GA 30341

CDC Emerging Infectious Diseases Fellowships **908**
The goal of this program is to attract and prepare laboratory scientists for careers in public health. The two-track program (Training and Research Fellowships) will recruit and train qualified candidates (bachelor's and master's levels) to support public health initiatives and provide opportunities for doctoral level scientists to conduct high-priority infectious disease research in public health laboratories.
Requirements: Applicants must have completed a bachelor's- or master's-level degree in microbiology, virology or a related discipline and/or completed and accredited medical technologist program by program initiation to be eligible for the training fellowship and applicants must have received a PhD, MD, or DVM, or have completed all requirements for such a degree prior to program initiation to be eligible for the research fellowship. All applicants must be U.S. citizens.
Date(s) Application is Due: Feb 17
Contact: Program Contact, (202) 822-5227; fax: (202) 887-5098; email: fellowships@aphl.org
Internet: http://www.cdc.gov/ncidod/eidlfp.htm
Sponsor: Centers for Disease Control and Prevention
2025 M St NW, Suite 550
Washington, DC 20036

CDC Epidemiology and Laboratory Capacity Infectious Diseases Grants **909**
The program grants funds to states and eligible local public health agencies in strengthening basic epidemiologic and laboratory capacity to address infectious disease threats with a focus on notifiable diseases, food-, water-, and vector-borne diseases, vaccine-preventable diseases, and drug-resistant infections. Awards are intended to support activities that enhance the ability of a community to identify and monitor outbreaks of infectious diseases and other infectious disease emergencies, characterize disease determinants, use public health data to develop policy, and assess the effectiveness of these activities. Matching funds are not required. Funding preference will be given to competing continuation applications over new applications. Annual deadline dates may vary; contact program staff for exact dates.
Requirements: Eligible are state health departments, the District of Columbia, Puerto Rico and U.S. territories, and city and county public health agencies.
Restrictions: States that already have ELC projects are ineligible to apply.
Amount of Grant: $300,000 maximum
Contact: Nealean Austin, Grants Management Branch, Centers for Disease Control and Prevention, (770) 488-2700
Internet: http://www.cdc.gov/epo/index.htm
Sponsor: Centers for Disease Control and Prevention
2920 Brandywine Road
Atlanta, GA 30341

CDC Evaluation of the Use of Rapid Testing For Influenza in Outpatient Medical Settings **910**
The purpose of this project is to evaluate how rapid tests for influenza are being implemented and used in clinical practice in outpatient medical settings such as community clinics, solo and group practice physician offices, and hospital emergency rooms across the United States. This evaluation will include a determination of the scope of rapid influenza test use, the types of tests in use and how they are selected, the personnel performing testing, the extent to which good laboratory practices and testing guidelines are being followed, how results are reported and interpreted, how results are used for patient care and antiviral and antibiotic prescribing practices, and the presence of linkages between these outpatient settings and the public health system. Additionally, this project may identify potential opportunities to provide guidance to assist sites in making decisions on the appropriate use of these tests and ways to enhance the connectivity with the public health system. Connectivity with public health is especially important in light of the possibility of an influenza pandemic. This project will identify and evaluate practices used in outpatient settings related to processes such as specimen collection, testing, reporting and referral for influenza.
Requirements: Eligible applicants include: public nonprofit organizations; private nonprofit organizations; small, minority, women-owned businesses; universities; colleges; research institutions; hospitals; community-based organizations; faith-based organizations; federally recognized Indian tribal governments; Indian tribes; Indian tribal organizations; state and local governments or their Bona Fide Agents (this includes the District of Columbia, the Commonwealth of Puerto Rico, the Virgin Islands, the Commonwealth of the Northern Marianna Islands, American Samoa, Guam, the Federated States of Micronesia, the Republic of the Marshall Islands, and the Republic of Palau); and political subdivisions of States (in consultation with States).
Restrictions: Recipients may: not use funds for research; not use funds for clinical care; only expend funds for reasonable program purposes, including personnel, travel, supplies, and services, such as contractual. Awardees may not generally use HHS/CDC/ATSDR funding for the purchase of furniture or equipment (any such proposed spending must be identified in the budget). The direct and primary recipient in a cooperative agreement program must perform a substantial role in carrying out project objectives and not

merely serve as a conduit for an award to another party or provider who is ineligible. Reimbursement of pre-award costs is not allowed. Reimbursement of construction costs is not allowed.
Amount of Grant: $200,000
Date(s) Application is Due: Aug 6
Contact: Yolanda Sledge, Grants Specialist, (770) 488-2787; email: yiso@cdc.gov
Internet: http://www.cdc.gov/od/pgo/funding/FOAs.htm
Sponsor: Centers for Disease Control and Prevention
2920 Brandywine Road, Mail stop: E-14
Atlanta, GA 30341-3717

CDC Hepatitis Education for Inmates and Correctional Staff Program Grants 911
CDC announces the availability of funds for a cooperative agreement with one or more national voluntary organizations involved with correctional facilities to develop and distribute materials to educate inmates and correctional staff about the risks of transmission and acquisition of viral hepatitis, as well as prevention, counseling, testing, and treatment of viral hepatitis, with an emphasis on hepatitis A, B, and C prevention and counseling.
Requirements: Applications may be provided only to organizations currently providing health education materials to correctional populations and health related training materials to staff of correctional institutions at a national or regional level.
Amount of Grant: $242,614 average
Contact: Nealean Austin, Grants Management Branch, Procurement and Grants Office, Centers for Disease Control and Prevention (CDC), Department of Health and Human Services, (770) 488-2700
Internet: http://www.cdc.gov
Sponsor: Centers for Disease Control and Prevention
2920 Brandywine Road, Room 3000
Atlanta, GA 30341

CDC Increasing Breast and Cervical Cancer Screening Services for Urban American Indian/Alaska Native Women 912
The purpose of this program is to: increase the number of urban American Indian/Alaska Native (AI/AN) women receiving BCCED screening; decrease time to access diagnosis and treatment; increase participation of Urban Indian Health Organizations (UIHOs) in state BCCEDP & Comprehensive Cancer Control (CCC) coalitions; and to provide a model for other state health department programs to work with UIHOs in a collaborative, culturally appropriate manner.
Requirements: Eligible applicants that can apply for this funding are non-profit organizations with experience and expertise in addressing the health care needs of urban Indian populations and providing culturally competent services to them. These include, but are not limited to organizations such as: Indian health boards; inter-tribal councils; American Indian/Alaska native health tribal organizations; inter-tribal councils; inter-tribal consortia; urban organizations; and other non-profit organizations, if incorporated for the primary purpose of improving AI/AN health and represent such interests for the tribes, or urban Indian communities throughout the United States.
Restrictions: Recipients may: not use funds for research; not use funds for clinical care; only expend funds for reasonable program purposes, including personnel, travel, supplies, and services, such as contractual. Awardees may not generally use HHS/CDC/ATSDR funding for the purchase of furniture or equipment (any such proposed spending must be identified in the budget). The direct and primary recipient in a cooperative agreement program must perform a substantial role in carrying out project objectives and not merely serve as a conduit for an award to another party or provider who is ineligible. Reimbursement of pre-award costs is not allowed.
Amount of Grant: $350,000 first year; $1,050,000 over three years
Date(s) Application is Due: Jul 23
Contact: Stephanie Lankford, Grants Specialist, (770) 488-2936, email: fzi8@cdc.gov
Internet: http://www.cdc.gov/od/pgo/funding/FOAs.htm
Sponsor: Centers for Disease Control and Prevention
2920 Brandywine Road, Mail stop: E-14
Atlanta, GA 30341-3717

CDC Injury Control Research Centers Grants 913
Grants are intended to support injury control research and demonstrations on priority issues; to integrate aspects of engineering, public health, behavioral sciences, medicine, and other disciplines to prevent and control injuries more effectively; to rigorously apply and evaluate current and new interventions, methods, and strategies that focus on the prevention and control of injuries; to stimulate and support injury control research centers in academic institutions that will develop a comprehensive and integrated approach to injury control research and training; and to bring the knowledge and expertise of injury control research centers to bear on the development of effective public health programs for injury control. Refer to announcement number 01007. Annual deadline dates may vary; contact the office for exact dates.
Requirements: Any nonprofit or for-profit organization in eligible regions may apply. Eligible regions include 34 states as well as the District of Columbia, the Virgin Islands, and Puerto Rico.
Restrictions: Grantees may not award subgrants but may enter into contracts as necessary to achieve the aims of the program.
Geographic Focus: Alabama; Alaska; Arizona; Arkansas; California; Delaware; District of Columbia; Florida; Georgia; Hawaii; Idaho; Illinois; Indiana; Kentucky; Louisiana; Maryland; Michigan; Minnesota; Mississippi; Nevada; New Jersey; New Mexico; New York; North Carolina; Ohio; Oklahoma; Oregon; Pennsylvania; South Carolina; Tennessee; Texas; Virginia; Washington; West Virginia; Wisconsin
Amount of Grant: $905,500 average
Contact: Program Manager, National Center for Injury Prevention and Control, (770) 488-1506; email: OHCINFO@cdc.gov
Internet: http://www.cdc.gov/ncipc/profiles/icrcs/default.htm
Sponsor: Centers for Disease Control and Prevention
4770 Buford Hwy NE, MS K65
Atlanta, GA 30341-3724

CDC Injury Prevention and Control Research and State and Community Based Programs 914
Research grants support injury control research on priority issues; projects that integrate aspects of engineering, public health, behavioral sciences, medicine, and other disciplines in order to prevent and control injuries more effectively; projects that rigorously apply and evaluate current and new interventions, methods, and strategies that focus on the prevention and control of injuries; projects that stimulate and support Injury Control Research Centers (ICRC) in academic institutions which will develop a comprehensive and integrated approach to injury control research and training; and projects that bring the knowledge and expertise of ICRC's to bear on the development of effective public health programs for injury control. State and Community Program grants are to develop and evaluate new methods or to evaluate existing methods and techniques used in injury surveillance by public health agencies; and to develop, expand, or improve injury control programs to reduce morbidity, mortality, severity, disability, and cost from injuries.
Requirements: Applications may be submitted by all public and private nonprofit and for-profit organizations and by governments and their agencies.
Contact: Program Officer, Injury Prevention and Control Research Projects, (770) 488-1506; fax: (770) 488-1667; email: OHCINFO@cdc.gov
Internet: http://www.cdc.gov/ncipc/profiles/icrcs/default.htm
Sponsor: Centers for Disease Control and Prevention
4770 Buford Hwy NE, MS K65
Atlanta, GA 30341-3724

CDC Intervention Epidemiologic Research Studies of HIV/AIDS 915
CDC announces the availability of funds for a cooperative agreement program to support intervention epidemiologic research studies of AIDS and HIV infection. These awards will help support researchers in two areas: the development and evaluation of innovative interventions for preventing and reducing the transmission of HIV infection in young and recently initiated injection drug users (IDUs); and the development and evaluation of an intervention study to improve access to antiretroviral therapy in HIV-infected disadvantaged populations.
Requirements: Applications may be submitted by public and private nonprofit organizations and by governments and their agencies.
Amount of Grant: $5000-$270,000 range; $200,265 average
Contact: Allyn Nakashima, Epidemiology Branch, Center for Disease Control and Prevention, (404) 639-0900
Internet: http://www.cdc.gov/epo
Sponsor: Centers for Disease Control and Prevention
1600 Clifton Rd NE, MS-E-45
Atlanta, GA 30333

CDC Minority Health Statistics Dissertation Research Grants 916
The purpose of the program is to make awards for the conduct of special surveys or studies on the health of racial and ethnic populations or subpopulations; analysis of data on ethnic and racial populations and subpopulations; and research on improving methods for developing statistics on ethnic and racial populations and subpopulations. The deadline date listed is for letters of intent. Annual dates may vary; contact the program office for exact dates.
Requirements: Eligible applicants may be public or private nonprofit institutions that will administer the grant on behalf of the proposed principal investigator. The proposed principal investigator must be a registered doctoral candidate in resident or nonresident status. All requirements for the doctoral degree other than the dissertation must be completed by the time of the award. Students seeking a doctorate in any relevant research discipline are eligible. An applicant institution may be either the degree-granting institution or another nonprofit institution with which the proposed principal investigator is professionally affiliated.
Amount of Grant: $15,000-$30,000; $20,000 average
Contact: Program Contact, Minority Health Statistics Grants, National Center for Health Statistics (3311 Toledo Road, Hyattsville, MD 20782); (301) 458-4000; email: MGP@cdc.gov
Internet: http://www.cdc.gov/nchswww/about/grants/grants.htm
Sponsor: Centers for Disease Control and Prevention
1600 Clifton Road
Atlanta, GA 30333

CDC National Breast and Cervical Cancer Early Detection Program 917
The purpose of this program is to apply a state, territorial, or tribal public health approach to increase access to and use of screening services. Funded programs will establish a comprehensive breast and cervical cancer early detection screening program that includes breast and cervical cancer screening, tracking, follow-up and case management; public education and outreach; professional education; quality assurance and improvement; surveillance and evaluation; coalitions and partnerships; and management.
Requirements: Assistance will be provided only to the official health departments of states or their bona fide agents, including the District of Columbia, the Commonwealth of

Puerto Rico, the Virgin Islands, the Commonwealth of the Northern Mariana Islands, the Republic of Palau, and federally recognized Indian Tribal governments.
Restrictions: Alaska, Arizona, Arkansas, American Samoa, California, Colorado, Connecticut, Florida, Georgia, Illinois, Iowa, Kansas, Louisiana, Maine, Maryland, Massachusetts, Michigan, Minnesota, Missouri, Nebraska, New Jersey, New Mexico, New York, North Carolina, Ohio, Oklahoma, Oregon, Pennsylvania, Rhodes Island, South Carolina, Texas, Utah, Vermont, Washington, West Virginia, Wisconsin, Puerto Rico, and Guam are not eligible for funding. See announcement for complete listing.
Amount of Grant: $145,000-$8.4 million; $2.1 million average
Contact: Carlos Smiley, Grants Management Branch, Procurement and Grants Office, (770) 488-2754
Internet: http://www.cdc.gov/cancer/nbccedp/index.htm
Sponsor: Centers for Disease Control and Prevention
2920 Brandywine Road
Atlanta, GA 30341-4146

CDC National Poison Prevention and Control Program Grants 918
The purpose of the program is to support an integrated system of poison prevention and control services including: coordination of all poison control centers (PCCs) through development, implementation, and evaluation of standardized public education; and development of a plan to improve national toxicosurveillance and development of a single, nationwide toll-free telephone number and related public service media campaign.
Requirements: Applications may be submitted by public and private nonprofit organizations, governments and their agencies, other public and private nonprofit organizations, state and local governments or their bona fide agents, and federally recognized American Indian tribal governments, American Indian tribes, or American Indian tribal organizations.
Contact: Cheryl Maddux, Grants Management Officer, Centers for Disease Control and Prevention, (770) 488-2645
Internet: http://www.cdc.gov
Sponsor: Centers for Disease Control and Prevention
4770 Buford Hwy NE
Atlanta, GA 30341

CDC National Programs That Build the Capacity of Schools To Prevent Foodborne Illness Through Coordinated School Health Programs 919
The purpose of this program is to develop a national program to build the capacity of state and local education and health agencies, and others to prevent foodborne illness and other important health problems as part of a coordinated school health program.
Requirements: Assistance will be provided to national organizations that are private health, education, or social service agencies (professional, or voluntary); qualify as a nonprofit 501(c)3 entity; have the capacity and experience to assist their local affiliates; and have affiliate offices or local, state, or regional membership constituencies in a minimum of ten states and territories.
Restrictions: National organizations that are funded currently by CDC/Division of Adolescent and School Health (DASH) under program announcements 99023, 97065, 00026, 00081, 00109, 00719, 98885, 99072, 00079 or 00618 are not eligible for this program announcement.
Amount of Grant: $299,000 average
Contact: Nealean Austin, Grants Management Officer, (770) 488-2754
Internet: http://www.cdc.gov/healthyyouth
Sponsor: Centers for Disease Control and Prevention
2920 Brandywine Road, MS E-18
Atlanta, GA 30341-4146

CDC National Training Information and Exchange Program 920
The purpose of this program is to make data and information on trauma care in the United States more accessible to a broad spectrum of individuals and organizations, including trauma care professionals and professional associations, trauma centers and other acute care hospitals, trauma care systems, emergency medical services (EMS) systems, injury researchers and research organizations, public health agencies, health care payers, and the general public.
Requirements: Applications may be submitted by public and private nonprofit organizations and by governments and their agencies.
Contact: Cheryl Maddux, Grants Management Officer, (770) 488-2645
Internet: http://www.cdc.gov
Sponsor: Centers for Disease Control and Prevention
2920 Brandywine Road, Suite 3000
Atlanta, GA 30341

CDC Oral Diseases Prevention and Oral Health Promotion Grants 921
The purpose of the program is to develop initiatives related to oral disease prevention and related chronic disease and health promotion capacity; and, to coordinate the dissemination of comprehensive oral disease information and health promotion programmatic expertise among state and local agencies, public and private sector organizations, and health care professionals in the United States. The purpose of this program includes conducting projects that promote the development of leadership and infrastructure to establish sustainable oral health programs at the state and local levels; advance tobacco control programs, especially smokeless tobacco; advance school oral health education and targeted oral disease and oral injury prevention efforts (e.g., athletic mouth guards); and develop and carry out oral health education and disease prevention programs for high-risk adults.
Requirements: Assistance will be provided only to dental health organizations that are 501(c)3 private, nonprofit organizations. Eligible applicants must have established working relationships with public advocacy coalitions and national, state, and local organizations.
Amount of Grant: $70,000 approximately
Contact: Scott Presson, Program Director, Division of Oral Health, (770) 488-6056; email: skp4@cdc.gov
Internet: http://www.cdc.gov/oralhealth
Sponsor: Centers for Disease Control and Prevention
4770 Buford Hwy NE
Atlanta, GA 30341

CDC Prevention Education and Access to Care Services for Persons Infected and Affected by HIV 922
The goal of this program is to provide prevention education and access to care services for persons infected and affected by HIV. The purpose of this program is to support the establishment of a national program to provide education and prevention programs for persons infected with HIV to reduce risk for transmitting HIV and facilitate access to care services; and to provide technical assistance to other CDC grantees to enhance their capacity to serve persons living with HIV and involve them in HIV prevention programs and planning efforts.
Requirements: National 501(c)3 nonprofit organizations that have established policies and a documented record for at least three years of providing HIV prevention technical assistance and education nationally, serving as a national prevention and education resource, and facilitating access to care services for all people infected by HIV/AIDS are eligible to apply.
Amount of Grant: $50,000-$1 million
Contact: Cheryl Maddux, Grants Officer, (770) 498-1911; email: info@cdc.gov
Internet: http://www.cdc.gov/hiv/dhap.htm
Sponsor: Center for Disease Control and Prevention
2920 Brandywine Road
Atlanta, GA 30341

CDC Preventive Health Services-Sexually Transmitted Diseases Control Grants 923
The objective of the grants is to reduce morbidity and mortality by preventing cases and complications of sexually transmitted diseases. Grant funds may be used for sexually transmitted disease (STD) surveillance activities, including reporting, screening, and follow-up of diagnostic tests for, and diagnosed cases of, STD; STD case finding and case follow-up activities, including notification of sex partners to infectious cases of STD and follow-up systems; interstate epidemiologic referral and follow-up activities; program-specific professional (including appropriate allied health personnel) STD education, training, and clinical skills improvement activities as authorized under section 318(b) of the PHS Act; program-specific STD education and information activities as authorized under section 318(b) of the PHS Act; special studies or demonstrations to evaluate or test STD prevention activities; and control strategies and activities as may be prescribed by the program.
Requirements: Any state, state health authority, or political subdivision of a state may apply.
Amount of Grant: $19,000-$5.1 million; $850,000 average
Contact: Sevgi Aral, Director, Division of STD Prevention, (404) 639-8259; fax: (4404) 639-8608; Gladys Gissentanna, Grants Management Officer, CDC, (770) 498-1912
Internet: http://www.cdc.gov
Sponsor: Centers for Disease Control and Prevention
2920 Brandywine Road
Atlanta, GA 30341

CDC Program to Prevent Smoking Among Urban Youth 924
The program supports youth smoking and prevention services with a focus on urban communities, particularly in the District of Columbia and states where the 2004 KOOL MIXX DJ Competitions were held (California, Florida, Georgia, Illinois, Louisiana, Maryland, Michigan, Missouri, New York, Ohio, Pennsylvania, and Texas). Twelve- to 24-month grants are awarded to support ongoing programs that can be enhanced or expanded. Interested applicants should submit a letter of intent by the listed deadline; full proposals are by invitation.
Requirements: 501(c)3 tax-exempt organizations and faith-based organizations qualifying as churches under the code are eligible.
Restrictions: New programs are ineligible.
Amount of Grant: $75,000-$200,000
Date(s) Application is Due: May 6
Contact: Dacia LaDonis, Program Officer, (404) 653-0790; fax: (404) 653-0330; email: DLaDonis@cdc.gov
Internet: http://www.cdcfoundation.org/pages.html?page=488
Sponsor: CDC Foundation
50 Hurt Plz, Suite 765
Atlanta, GA 30303

CDC Promoting Prevention in Managed Care Cooperative Agreements 925
CDC announces the availability of funds for a cooperative agreement program for promoting prevention in managed care. This announcement relates to all of the priority areas of Healthy People 2010. Its purpose is to promote the attainment of the objectives outlined in Healthy People 2010 through strengthening the infrastructure supporting the science and practice of prevention in managed care. Annual deadline dates may vary; contact program staff for exact dates.

Requirements: Applications may be submitted by private sector, nonprofit, managed care membership organizations who provide an array of services and products (e.g., technical support, publications, training and continuing education, communication and information sharing, etc.) to member plans in at least 20 states; and whose member plans and affiliated entities can demonstrate past and current experience conducting public domain, prevention research (i.e., research in the areas of health promotion, disease prevention, and chronic disease management) in the managed care environment.
Samples: (1) Cooperative agreements to states for the Behavioral Risk Factor Surveillance system, (2) Public Health Conference support grants, (3) cooperative agreements to states for core capacity building for Tobacco Prevention and Control Programs, (4) cooperative agreements to states for the National Program of Cancer Registries, (5) cooperative agreements for Community Coalition Partnerships for the prevention of teen pregnancy, (6) cooperative agreements to states for the Pregnancy Risk Assessment Monitoring System, (7) cooperative agreement for epilepsy program activities, and (8) cooperative agreement for Oral Disease Prevention.
Amount of Grant: $242,614 average
Contact: Nealean Austin, Grants Management Branch, (770) 488-2700
Internet: http://www.cdc.gov/nchs/hphome.htm
Sponsor: Centers for Disease Control and Prevention
2920 Brandywine Road, Room 3000
Atlanta, GA 30341

CDC Public Health Conference Support Grant Program 926

The purpose of the grants is to provide partial support for specific non-federal conferences in the areas of health promotion and disease prevention information/education programs. Funds may be used for direct cost expenditures, such as salaries, speaker fees, rental of necessary equipment, registration fees, and transportation costs (not to exceed economy-class fare) for non-federal individuals. The program continues through March 8, 2009.
Requirements: Public and private organizations, including colleges and universities, and units of state and local government are eligible to apply. Applicants must provide a portion of the conference cost.
Restrictions: Funds may not be used for indirect costs, equipment purchases, honoraria, entertainment, or personal expenses.
Contact: Sharon Robertson, Grants Management Officer, (770) 488-2748; email: SRobertson1@cdc.gov
Internet: http://www.cdc.gov/od/pgo/funding/FOAs.htm
Sponsor: Centers for Disease Control and Prevention
2920 Brandywine Road, Room 3000
Atlanta, GA 30341

CDC Research, Treatment, and Education Programs on Lyme Disease in the United States Cooperative Agreements 927

The objective of the program is to develop and implement practical and effective measures for the primary and secondary prevention of Lyme disease. Funds will be available to develop disease surveillance, conduct ecological and epidemiological studies, develop prevention and control activities, develop better diagnostic tests, and develop and disseminate educational materials and programs. Cooperative agreements are usually awarded for a three-year project period. Initial awards are made for a one-year budget period with continuation awards for up to an additional two years. Contact the office listed for application deadline dates. PA-04-008
Requirements: Public and nonprofit organizations able to provide services to geographical areas where Lyme disease is endemic or found to be newly emerging are eligible to apply. Funding preference will be given to proposals that incorporate evaluation of effectiveness, cost, and acceptability of strategies, or combinations of strategies, for population-based control of tick-borne diseases.
Samples: Examples of some funded projects include: development of materials for education intervention; conducting studies in integrated pest management; conducting studies on the pathogenesis of Lyme neuroborreliosis using the monkey model; implementation of active surveillance systems; and studies to improve serologic diagnostic techniques.
Amount of Grant: $100,000-$700,000; $350,000 average
Contact: Dr. Brian Mahy, National Center for Infectious Diseases, (404) 639-0043; fax: (404) 639-2469; email: bxm1@cdc.gov
Internet: http://www.cdc.gov/od/pgo/funding/Expired/04008.htm
Sponsor: Centers for Disease Control and Prevention
P.O. Box 2087
Fort Collins, CO 80522

CDC School Health Programs to Prevent the Spread of HIV Coop Agreements 928

The objective of the program is to support the development and implementation of effective health education for HIV and other important health problems for school-age populations (elementary- through college-age youth); parents; and relevant school, health, and education personnel. Cooperative agreement funds may be used to support personnel, their training and travel, and to purchase supplies and services for planning, organizing, and conducting activities directly related to the objectives of this program. These activities may include obtaining baseline data and establishing a system to monitor the availability and adequacy of HIV education in schools; increasing the number of schools providing HIV education; monitoring the levels of HIV-related knowledge, beliefs, and behaviors among students; collaborating with state and local health agencies in carrying out HIV education programs in the schools; establishing policies, guidelines, advisory committees, and/or standards to increase the number of schools providing HIV education; integrating HIV education within a more comprehensive program of school health education; disseminating information about accessibility, availability, and quality of educational strategies, materials, and curricula to local education agencies and schools; and providing technical assistance to local school districts and schools in implementing HIV education. The maximum project period is five years. Contact the office for deadline dates.
Requirements: Eligible state education agencies in U.S. states and territories, nonprofit organizations, and universities may apply.
Restrictions: Funds may not be spent for research activities, surveys, or questionnaires except as may be needed to collect basic evaluation requirements. In addition, funds may not be used for purchasing computer equipment, office equipment or furnishings, renting or leasing office space, or financing construction or renovation unless specifically approved.
Amount of Grant: $87,000-$650,000 range; $299,000 average
Contact: Mary Sue Lancaster, Program Development and Services, (770) 488-6130, fax: (770) 488-6163; email: msl0@cdc.gov
Internet: http://www.cdc.gov
Sponsor: Centers for Disease Control and Prevention
255 E Paces Ferry Rd NE
Atlanta, GA 30305

CDC Sexually Transmitted Diseases Research, Demonstration, Public Information, and Education Grants 929

The grants are meant to develop, improve, apply, and evaluate methods for the prevention and control of syphilis, gonorrhea, and other sexually transmitted diseases through demonstration and applied research. Also, the grants are meant to develop, improve, apply, and evaluate methods and strategies for public information and education about these diseases; to support professional (including appropriate allied health personnel) education, training, and clinical skills improvement activities; and to support particularly deserving public information and education programs that cannot be supported through other grant programs. Grant funds may be used for the costs associated with planning, organizing, and conducting applied research, demonstrations and education programs, and to reimburse individuals asked to be participants in the applied research. Contact the program office for deadline dates.
Requirements: Any state, political subdivision of a state, or any other public or private nonprofit institution may apply.
Amount of Grant: $125,000-$450,000; $313,809 average
Contact: Sevgi Aral, Director, Division of STD Prevention, (404) 639-8259; Gladys Gissentanna, Grants Management Officer, (770) 498-1912
Internet: http://www.cdc.gov
Sponsor: Centers for Disease Control and Prevention
255 E Paces Ferry Rd NE
Atlanta, GA 30305

CDC Suicide Prevention Research Center 930

The purpose of this grant is to establish a Suicide Prevention Research Center. The recipient of the grant will conduct, evaluate, and publish suicide prevention research; design, implement, and evaluate suicide prevention programs; collaborate with outside agencies; develop a curricula and graduate training programs in disciplines relevant to suicide prevention; and disseminate findings.
Requirements: Eligible applicants must demonstrate expertise in some form of suicide prevention research. Applicant must provide a director/Principal Investigator.
Amount of Grant: $500,000 approximately
Contact: Dr. Thomas Shires, Director, Trauma Institute, (702) 671-2297; fax: (702) 385-9399; email: DVPINFO@cdc.gov
Internet: http://www.cdc.gov/ncipc/dvp/suinevada.htm
Sponsor: Centers for Disease Control and Prevention
455 E Paces Ferry Rd NE
Atlanta, GA 30305

CDC Tech Translation and Transfer of Effective HIV Behavioral Interventions 931

HIV/AIDS researchers have developed and tested prevention interventions that aim to reduce sex-related and drug-related risk behaviors. A number of these interventions have credible evidence of effectiveness, defined as reporting positive and significant results on an HIV-relevant behavioral or health outcome. The purposes of this cooperative agreement project are to: translate effective HIV prevention interventions whose original research was conducted with methodological rigor, preferably at multiple sites with multiple populations at risk; develop packages of materials in collaboration with health departments, community-based organizations, and/or other prevention providers and consumers, that prevention providers can use to replicate the interventions in nonresearch field situations; and study the process of technology transfer using the prevention packages in at least one field setting supported by training, quality assurance, and technical assistance.
Requirements: Applications may be submitted by public and private nonprofit organizations and governments and their agencies.
Amount of Grant: $50,000-$1 million; $293,253 average
Contact: Allyn Nakashima, National Center for HIV, STD, and TB Prevention, (404) 639-0900; Cheryl Maddux, Grants Management Officer, (770) 498-1911
Internet: http://www.cdc.gov/od/pgo/funding/grantmain.htm
Sponsor: Centers for Disease Control and Prevention
1600 Clifton Rd NE
Atlanta, GA 30333

CDC Using Genetic Info to Prevent Disease & Improve Health Research Grants 932

The purpose of this program is to strengthen science for public health action, collaborate with health care partners for prevention, and promote healthy living at every stage of

life. The program will provide funding for conducting population-based research to assess how risk for disease and disability in well-defined populations is influenced by the interaction of human genetic variation with modifiable risk factors, and ensure that genetic tests and services are incorporated in population-based interventions that promote health and prevent disease and disability. Annual deadline dates may vary; contact the program office for exact dates.
Requirements: Applications may be submitted by public and private nonprofit organizations and by governments and their agencies, other public and private nonprofit organizations, state and local governments or their bona fide agents, and federally recognized American Indian tribal governments, American Indian tribes, or American Indian tribal organizations.
Contact: Nealean Austin, Grants Management Branch, Centers for Disease Control and Prevention, (770) 488-2700
Internet: http://www.cdc.gov
Sponsor: Centers for Disease Control and Prevention
4770 Buford Hwy NE
Atlanta, GA 30341

Cemala Foundation Grants 933
The foundation awards grants to charitable organizations in North Carolina, with emphasis on Guilford County, to improve the quality of life. Areas of interest include the performing arts, arts and culture, education associations (higher education and adult basic skills/literacy), health associations and hospices, crime and law enforcement, housing development, and services for children and families. Grants will be awarded in support of new initiatives, special projects, expansion of current programs, and capital improvements. The foundation will consider operating support grant requests for projects that fall under the 'Special Interest Areas.' Occasionally the Foundation will fund emergency operating support of an organization if the applicant organization has taken responsible action on its own to assume its economic viability but has experiences adversity due to economic turndown or other extraordinary circumstances. The board meets in April and October to consider requests. Application can be submitted online.
Requirements: Giving is limited to Guilford County, NC, and to projects with statewide benefit. The organization must be a 501(c)3 or a public governmental unit.
Restrictions: Annual campaigns, endowments, sectarian religious activities, or requests under $1000 will not be considered. Grants are not made to individuals.
Geographic Focus: North Carolina
Amount of Grant: $5000-$200,000 average
Date(s) Application is Due: Mar 1; Sep 1
Contact: Susan S. Schwartz, Executive Director, (336) 274-3541; fax: (336) 272-8153; email: cemala@cemala.org
Internet: http://www.cemala.org/grant/guidelines.php
Sponsor: Cemala Foundation
330 S Greene Street, Suite 101
Greensboro, NC 27401

Center for Alternatives to Animal Testing Grants 934
The center seeks to develop innovative non-whole animal methods to evaluate fully commercial and/or therapeutic products to ensure the health and safety of the public. The program funds research that will lead to the refinement, replacement, or reduction of animals in toxicity testing and by disseminating scientifically correct information about these methods and their applications. The center encourages the development of in vitro approaches to toxicity evaluation including, but not limited to, methods using human cells/cell lines and studies in the areas of skin hypersensitivity/toxicity, phototoxicity, target organ toxicity, and structure-activity relationships. Grants support one year of research with possible renewal for another year. Preproposals must meet the application deadline; full proposals are invited.
Requirements: Applicants must have an established mechanism for handling private funding.
Restrictions: Projects focusing on mutagenicity or carcinogenicity are not funded.
Amount of Grant: $25,000 maximum per year
Contact: Alan Goldberg, Center Director, (410) 223-1692; fax: (410) 223-1603; email: caat@jhsph.edu or goldberg@jhsph.edu
Internet: http://caat.jhsph.edu/programs/grants/grants.htm
Sponsor: Johns Hopkins University
111 Market Pl, Suite 840
Baltimore, MD 21202-6709

Center for Science in the Public Interest Internships 935
The center is a national consumer organization that focuses on health and nutrition issues. CSPI offers internships for a small number of qualified students in undergraduate, graduate, law, and medical schools each summer and during the school year. Generally, an internship is for 10 weeks. The specific dates of internship are flexible and depend on the center's needs and the applicant's schedule. Application materials should include a cover letter indicating issues of interest, future plans, available dates; resume; writing sample; two letters of recommendation; and official transcript of courses and grades. Application materials should be submitted as early as possible.
Amount of Grant: $6 per hour undergraduates; $7 per hour graduates
Contact: Human Resources Manager, (202) 332-9110; fax: (202) 265-4954; email: cspi@cspinet.org
Internet: http://www.cspinet.org/about/jobs_internship_2005_2006.html
Sponsor: Center for Science in the Public Interest
1875 Connecticut Ave NW, Suite 300
Washington, DC 20009-5728

Central Carolina Community Foundation Community Impact Grants 936
The Foundation's Community Impact grants fund programmatic initiatives of nonprofit organizations. In order to support positive community change and help ensure a program's success, the Grants have a maximum request amount of $10,000. The grant making process is a bi-annual process. Proposals are accepted, April 1 - September 30, for the Fall cycle, October 1 - March 31 for the Spring cycle.
Requirements: Nonprofit organizations serving South Carolina are eligible.
Restrictions: Grants do not support routine operating expenses, fund raising projects, debt reduction, endowment development, medical research, conference travel, or conference underwriting or sponsorship. LOIs or proposals may not be submitted by email or fax.
Geographic Focus: South Carolina
Samples: Cooperative Ministry, Columbia, SC, $10,000—for the Helping Hands of Hope program, which provides assistance to individuals and families for rent, utilities, food/household, hygiene, transportation and furniture (2007); Project Life: Positeen, Orangeburg, SC, $10,000—to expand its services into two new sites, Rivelon and Bethune-Bowman Elementary Schools in Orangeburg County (2007).
Amount of Grant: $10,000 maximum
Date(s) Application is Due: Mar 31; Sep 30
Contact: Veronica L. Pinkett-Barber, Program Officer; (803) 254-5601, ext. 331; fax: (803) 799-6663; email: veronica@yourfoundation.org
Internet: http://www.yourfoundation.org/nonprofits/foundationgrants/impactgrants.aspx
Sponsor: Central Carolina Community Foundation
2711 Middleburg Drive, Suite 213
Lancaster, SC 29204

Central Okanagan Foundation Grants 937
The foundation seeks to enhance the quality of life in Canada and awards grants to nonprofit organizations in its areas of interest, including arts and culture, children, youth, families, education, health, community services, environmental conservation, and heritage preservation. Types of support include emergency funds, equipment acquisition, program development, scholarship funds, and seed money. Contact the foundation by phone to discuss the proposed project. Guidelines and application form will be sent if the project falls within the foundation's guidelines.
Requirements: Nonprofit British Columbia organizations in the Central Okanagan region as defined by the boundaries of BC School District 23 are eligible.
Restrictions: Grants are not awarded to individuals or religious organizations for religious purposes. Grants do not support capital campaigns, debt retirement, endowments, building construction/renovation, or operating expenses.
Date(s) Application is Due: May 1; Oct 1
Contact: Cheryl Miller, Grants Manager; (250) 861-6160; fax: (250) 861-6156; email: cheryl@centralokanaganfoundation.org
Internet: http://www.centralokanaganfoundation.org/pages/grants/cof-grants.php
Sponsor: Central Okanagan Foundation
217-1889 Springfield Road
Kelowna, BC V1Y 5V5 Canada

Cessna Foundation Grants Program 938
Grants are made to organizations primarily in the areas where the company operates. Support is given for projects that take a creative approach to such fundamental issues as education, health and human services, youth enrichment, and arts and culture. The foundation values projects which take a creative approach to such fundamental issues as education, neighborhood improvement, youth development, community problem-solving, assistance to people who are disadvantaged, environmental conservation and cultural enrichment. Grants cover projects, building, equipment, capital campaigns, program development, employee matching gifts, and employee-related scholarships. All proposals must be in writing and should include the following information: needs statement and project objectives; purpose of organization; constituency; board members, community, and volunteer involvement; how results of the project will be measured; plans for continued funding of the project, if applicable; one-page project budget and an organizational chart; and primary source of funds. Proposals are accepted at any time.
Requirements: Giving limited to areas of company operations, with emphasis on Wichita.
Restrictions: Grants are not awarded to individuals; national or regional organizations, unless their programs address specific local community needs; programs or initiatives where the primary purpose is the promotion of religious doctrine or tenets; elementary or secondary schools (except to provide special initiatives or programs not provided by regular school budgets); political action or legislative advocacy groups; operational funds; medical or other research organizations; organizations located in or benefiting nations other than the United States and its territories; or fraternal groups, athletic teams, bands, veterans organizations, volunteer firefighters, or similar groups.
Amount of Grant: $300-$10,000
Contact: Rhonda Fullerton, Secretary-Treasurer; (316) 517-7810; fax: (316) 517-7812
Internet: http://www.cessna.com/about/corporate-citizenship.html
Sponsor: Cessna Foundation
P.O. Box 7706
Wichita, KS 67277

Cetana Educational Foundation Scholarships 939
Cetana selects a limited number of scholars, simply because the foundation has limited resources. Scholars from all religious and ethnic groups in Myanmar are eligible for scholarships. Support for scholars covers the cost of education, room and board, travel to and from the university, and associated expenses for the duration of their study abroad. Cetana also provides mentors who are available to offer the scholars advice and practical support in bridging cultures. The Outreach Committee in Myanmar assists the graduate

in finding rewarding employment upon return. Once they have finished their studies, scholars return to Myanmar for a period of at least three years so that they may share their new knowledge and experience. Most scholarships are for graduate studies in neighboring SE Asian countries. Only a few scholarships are available in the U.S. where colleges provide full tuition grants.
Requirements: Applicants must be living in Myanmar. Those living outside the country will not be considered. Scholars must be studying in majors that have application to work opportunities in country. Students must pledge to return home for a minimum of 3 years after completion of studies. If the recipient breaks the pledge, he or she must pay back full scholarship so that another student may take his or her place.
Contact: Tin May Thein, Executive Director; (240) 242-3997; email: tinmaythein@cetana.org
Internet: http://www.cetana.org/Cetana/Scholarship_Program.html
Sponsor: Cetana Educational Foundation
12817 Twinbrook Pkw., #207
Rockville, MD 20851

CF Clinical Research Trainee Awards **940**
This is a training program for physicians enrolled in a U.S. or Canadian subspecialty training program. Ten awards will be granted for clinical research in thrombosis, asthma, critical care, lung cancer, and women's health. Applicants may apply for only one type of clinical research award, and each program director may support only one applicant for an award in each area. Requests should be written to include goals and objectives that may be accomplished within one year of the starting date (July 1) of the research project. Research funding may be used as the research mentor and program director deem appropriate (e.g., salary support and supplies directly related to the research project).
Requirements: Applicants must be citizens of the United States or Canada or have a J-1 or H-1 visa and be working in a certified U.S. or Canadian institution and enrolled in a subspecialty training program at the time of application; hold an MD degree or its equivalent; be enrolled in a U.S. or Canadian subspecialty training program in allergy/immunology, cardiac electrophysiology, critical care anesthesiology, critical care intensive care, critical care medicine, infectious disease, cardiology, pediatric critical care, pediatric pulmonary disease, pulmonary disease, surgical critical care, or thoracic surgery; be affiliate members of the American College of Chest Physicians (contact Angela Popa-Padilla at 847/ 498-1400 for an application); show promise of significant contribution to his/her specialty; and apply for only one type of award and be the sole applicant from the subspecialty program to apply for that type of award.
Restrictions: Awards are to support clinical research, not basic or bench level research.
Amount of Grant: $10,000
Date(s) Application is Due: Jun 30
Contact: Sue Ciezadlo, Grants Administrator, (847) 498-8363; fax: (847) 498-5460; email: sciezadlo@chestnet.org
Internet: http://www.chestfoundation.org/researchAwards/index.php
Sponsor: Chest Foundation
3300 Dundee Road
Northbrook, IL 60062-2348

CF Roger C. Bone Award for Advances in End-of-Life Care **941**
The award was created to annually recognize members of the American College of Chest Physicians who have demonstrated leadership in end-of-life care. Recipients of this award have shown substantial improvement in the care of patients as documented in the related sections of the application form. Application forms and guidelines are available online.
Requirements: Applicants must be members of the American College of Chest Physicians and have the endorsement of another ACCP member.
Amount of Grant: $10,000
Date(s) Application is Due: Apr 29
Contact: Sue Ciezadlo, Senior Project Coordinator, (847) 498-8363; fax: (847) 498-5460; email: sciezadlo@chestnet.org
Internet: http://www.chestfoundation.org/criticalCare/index.php
Sponsor: Chest Foundation
3300 Dundee Road
Northbrook, IL 60062-2348

CFF Clinical Research Grants **942**
These awards offer support of clinical research projects directly related to cystic fibrosis. Projects may address diagnostic or therapeutic methods related to cystic fibrosis or the pathophysiology of cystic fibrosis. However, studies performed in animal models or cell/tissues removed from patients will not be supported under this award. Applicants must demonstrate access to a sufficient number of cystic fibrosis patients and appropriate controls. A letter of intent to apply must be submitted by June 1 with applications required by December 1.
Amount of Grant: $80,000 maximum per year for single center; $150,000 maximum for multicenter
Date(s) Application is Due: Jun 1; Dec 1
Contact: Office of Grants Management, (800) 344-4823 or (301) 951-4422; fax: (301) 951-6378; email: grants@cff.org
Internet: http://www.cff.org/research/cystic_fibrosis_foundation_grants/research_grants
Sponsor: Cystic Fibrosis Foundation
6931 Arlington Road, 2nd Floor
Bethesda, MD 20814

CFF First- and Second-Year Clinical Fellowships **943**
The foundation offers competitive clinical fellowships for up to three years for physicians interested in cystic fibrosis and other chronic pulmonary and gastrointestinal diseases of children and adolescents/adults. The intent of this award is to encourage specialized training early in a physician's career and to prepare well-qualified candidates for careers in academic medicine. Training must take place in one of the foundation's accredited centers and must provide thorough grounding in diagnostic and therapeutic procedures, comprehensive care, and cystic fibrosis-related research. All first- and second-year programs must commit a significant portion (at least 30 percent over two years) to research training. Fellows funded by other sources for their first year of training may apply to the foundation for subsequent training support. Third-year fellowships are available for additional basic and/or clinical research training. Research fellowships are also available from the foundation to support physicians beyond the fellowship experience; salary will be commensurate with experience.
Requirements: Applicants must be U.S. citizens or have permanent U.S. resident visas, and must have completed pediatric training and be eligible for board certification in pediatrics by the time the fellowship begins. Candidates with prior training in internal medicine may also apply but must have completed at least two years of an approved adult pulmonary or GI fellowship; be jointly sponsored by the departments of medicine and pediatrics; and be willing to commit at least 75 percent of their time to cystic fibrosis and related problems of young adults.
Amount of Grant: $42,000 stipends first year, $43,750 second year
Date(s) Application is Due: Oct 1
Contact: Office of Grants Management, (800) 344-4823 or (301) 951-4422; fax: (301) 951-6378; email: grants@cff.org
Internet: http://www.cff.org/research/cystic_fibrosis_foundation_grants/training_grants
Sponsor: Cystic Fibrosis Foundation
6931 Arlington Road, 2nd Floor
Bethesda, MD 20814

CFF Leroy Matthews Physician-Scientist Awards **944**
This award will provide up to six years of support for outstanding newly trained pediatricians and internists (MDs and MD/PhDs) to complete subspecialty training, develop into independent investigators, and initiate research programs. Institutional and individual grants are available.
Requirements: U.S. citizenship or permanent resident status is required.
Amount of Grant: $42,000 stipend plus $10,000 for research and development in years one to five; up to $70,000 stipend plus $15,000 for research and development for year six
Date(s) Application is Due: Sep 1
Contact: Office of Grants Management, (800) 344-4823 or (301) 951-4422; fax: (301) 951-6378; email: grants@cff.org
Internet: http://www.cff.org/research/cystic_fibrosis_foundation_grants/research_grants
Sponsor: Cystic Fibrosis Foundation
6931 Arlington Road, 2nd Floor
Bethesda, MD 20814

CFF Pilot and Feasibility Awards **945**
These grants are for developing and testing new hypotheses and/or new methods, and to support promising new investigators as they establish themselves in research areas relevant to cystic fibrosis. Proposed work must be hypothesis driven and must reflect innovative approaches to critical questions in cystic fibrosis research. Two years of support may be requested.
Restrictions: The award is not meant to support continuation of programs begun under other granting mechanisms. Electronic submission is required.
Amount of Grant: $40,000 per year maximum
Date(s) Application is Due: Sep 1
Contact: Office of Grants Management, (800) 344-4823 or (301) 951-4422; fax: (301) 951-6378; email: grants@cff.org
Internet: http://www.cff.org/research/cystic_fibrosis_foundation_grants/research_grants
Sponsor: Cystic Fibrosis Foundation
6931 Arlington Road, 2nd Floor
Bethesda, MD 20814

CFF Postdoctoral Research Fellowships **946**
Competitive postdoctoral fellowships in basic or clinical research are made on an annual basis, renewable for a second year. The fellowships are awarded in areas of basic cellular and metabolic research or in other problem areas pertinent to cystic fibrosis and related chronic and recurrent pulmonary and gastrointestinal diseases of childhood. Preference is shown to recent graduates or those just beginning their investigative careers. A third year is offered on a limited basis to highly qualified candidates. Interested individuals are encouraged to contact the foundation for application procedures and/or to discuss the potential relevance of their work to the objectives of the foundation.
Requirements: These awards are offered to MDs, PhDs, and MD/PhDs interested in conducting basic or clinical research related to cystic fibrosis.
Restrictions: Electronic submission only.
Amount of Grant: $33,000 first year, $34,100 second year, $36,300 optional third year
Date(s) Application is Due: Sep 1
Contact: Office of Grants Management, (800) 344-4823 or (301) 951-4422; fax: (301) 951-6378; email: kcurley@cff.org
Internet: http://www.cff.org/research/cystic_fibrosis_foundation_grants/training_grants
Sponsor: Cystic Fibrosis Foundation
6931 Arlington Road, 2nd Floor
Bethesda, MD 20814

CFF Research Grants 947

Grants are offered in support of high-quality research projects ranging from basic cellular and metabolic mechanisms to therapy of cystic fibrosis and related chronic and recurrent pulmonary and gastrointestinal diseases of childhood. These grants are broadly oriented to the support of projects for developing and initially testing new hypotheses and/or new methods, or those being applied to problems of cystic fibrosis for the first time. The intent of this award is to enable the investigator to collect sufficient data to compete successfully for long-term support from NIH. Interested individuals are encouraged to contact the foundation for guidelines and/or to discuss the potential relevance of their work to the objectives of this program.
Requirements: Applications may be submitted by established investigators or new investigators starting their independent research careers but may not represent support for continuation of a line of research already established by the applicant.
Amount of Grant: $90,000 maximum per year for a two-year period
Date(s) Application is Due: Sep 1
Contact: Office of Grants Management, (800) 344-4823 or (301) 951-4422; fax: (301) 951-6378; email: grants@cff.org
Internet: http://www.cff.org/research/cystic_fibrosis_foundation_grants/research_grants
Sponsor: Cystic Fibrosis Foundation
6931 Arlington Road, 2nd Floor
Bethesda, MD 20814

CFF Student Traineeships 948

The traineeships are offered to qualified students to introduce them to cystic fibrosis research. Each recipient must work with a faculty sponsor on a research project related to cystic fibrosis. Interested individuals are encouraged to contact the foundation for application procedures and/or to discuss the potential relevance of their work to the objectives of the program. Applications are accepted throughout the year. A maximum of $300 of the award may be used for laboratory expenses with the remainder used as a stipend for the trainee.
Requirements: Applicants must be students in or about to enter a doctoral program (MD, PhD, or MD/PhD); senior-level undergraduates planning to pursue graduate training may also apply.
Amount of Grant: $1500
Contact: Office of Grants Management, (800) 344-4823 or (301) 951-4422; fax: (301) 951-6378; email: grants@cff.org
Internet: http://www.cff.org/research/cystic_fibrosis_foundation_grants/training_grants
Sponsor: Cystic Fibrosis Foundation
6931 Arlington Road, 2nd Floor
Bethesda, MD 20814

CFF Therapeutics Development Program 949

The purpose of this program is to provide funds to businesses that will develop commercial products to benefit individuals with cystic fibrosis. Structured as a matching grants program, funds will be awarded only if they are matched by the recipient. First, the grantee will examine the scientific potential of new products under component 1. Component 2 studies will involve support for the continuation of component 1 developments and the initiation of patient clinical studies. Component 1 and component 2 awards each will receive a maximum of two years of support. Funds will be provided for research prior to, but not including, phase 3 clinical trials. Applications are accepted on an ongoing basis.
Amount of Grant: $100,000 maximum per year for component I; up to $750,000 per year for component II
Contact: Office of Grants Management, (800) 344-4823 or (301) 951-4422; fax: (301) 951-6378; email: grants@cff.org
Internet: http://www.cff.org/research/cystic_fibrosis_foundation_therapeutics
Sponsor: Cystic Fibrosis Foundation
6931 Arlington Road, 2nd Floor
Bethesda, MD 20814

CFF Third-Year Clinical Fellowships 950

The foundation offers competitive clinical fellowships for up to three years for physicians interested in cystic fibrosis and other chronic pulmonary and gastrointestinal diseases of children and adolescents/adults to encourage specialized training early in a physician's career and to prepare well-qualified candidates for careers in academic medicine. The third-year fellowship award offers support for additional intense basic and/or clinical research training related to cystic fibrosis.
Requirements: Applicants and sponsors must submit proposals of the research studies to be undertaken and other specialized training that will be offered during this year. Preference will be given to applicants whose training was supported by the foundation.
Restrictions: Recipients who do not enter a career of academic medicine will be subject to payback provisions.
Amount of Grant: $62,600 maximum; $52,600 stipend for fellow and up to $10,000 for research costs
Date(s) Application is Due: Oct 1
Contact: Office of Grants Management, (800) 344-4823 or (301) 951-4422; fax: (301) 951-6378; email: grants@cff.org
Internet: http://www.cff.org/research/cystic_fibrosis_foundation_grants/training_grants
Sponsor: Cystic Fibrosis Foundation
6931 Arlington Road, 2nd Floor
Bethesda, MD 20814

CFF-NIH Funding Grants 951

The objective of this award is to support excellent cystic fibrosis-related research projects that have been submitted to and approved by NIH but cannot be supported by available NIH funds. Applications must fall within the upper 40th percentile with a priority score of 200 or better. Investigators will be required to resubmit applications to NIH. Interested individuals are encouraged to contact the foundation for application procedures and/or to discuss the potential relevance of their work to the objectives of this program. Applications may be submitted on an ongoing basis.
Amount of Grant: $75,000-$125,000 per year for up to two years
Contact: Office of Grants Management, (800) 344-4823 or (301) 951-4422; fax: (301) 951-6378; email: grants@cff.org
Internet: http://www.cff.org/research
Sponsor: Cystic Fibrosis Foundation
6931 Arlington Road, 2nd Floor
Bethesda, MD 20814

CFFVR Opportunity Grants 952

The mission of the community foundation includes making prudent, sensitive, and creative grants to help solve community problems and to address opportunities for improvement. Funding categories include arts/culture, community development, education, environment, health, and human services. Listed application deadlines are for letters of intent. Guidelines and forms are available online.
Requirements: Wisconsin 501(c)3 tax-exempt organizations serving residents of Outagamie, Calumet, Waupaca, and northern Winnebago counties are eligible.
Restrictions: The foundation typically does not fund operating expenses of well-established organizations, except those directly related to a project; annual fund drives; existing or new endowment funds; capital projects such as the acquisition of land or buildings; medical or scientific research; travel for individuals or groups such as bands, sports teams, or classes; reimbursement for previously incurred expenses; or expenses typically considered as overhead, unless crucial to the survival and success of the program or project proposed for funding.
Geographic Focus: Wisconsin
Amount of Grant: $15,000 maximum
Date(s) Application is Due: Mar 10; Jun 10; Aug 30; Dec 10
Contact: Grants Administrator, (920) 830-1290; fax: (920) 830-1293; email: cffvr@cffoxvalley.org
Internet: http://www.cffoxvalley.org/grantseekers.html
Sponsor: Community Foundation for the Fox Valley Region
P.O. Box 563, 4455 W Lawrence Street
Appleton, WI 54912-0563

CFPC Family Medicine Resident Leadership Awards 953

The CFPC Research and Education Foundation honors outstanding educational and research initiatives in the area of family medicine through conferral of Family Medicine Resident Awards. Canadian Research Awards for Family Medicine Residents provide national recognition for original research carried out by postgraduate trainees. The Murray Stalker Memorial Lecture Award is given to promote and recognize scholarly activities of family medicine residents. The Nadine St. Pierre Award recognizes the outstanding achievement of a francophone family practice resident. Award recipients receive return air fare, complimentary registration for the Section of Teachers Annual Workshop, and a stipend for expenses. Deadline dates vary between programs; contact program staff for exact dates.
Amount of Grant: $C250-$C1000
Date(s) Application is Due: Jun 1
Contact: Kiki Ziten, Coordinator, (905) 629-0900 ext 432; fax: (905) 629-0893; email: kziten@cfpc.ca
Internet: http://www.cfpc.ca/English/cfpc/programs/awards%20program/default.asp?s=1
Sponsor: College of Family Physicians of Canada
2630 Skymark Avenue
Mississauga, ON L4W 5A4 Canada

CFPC Family Physician of the Year Award 954

The annual award recognizes an individual for outstanding contribution to family medicine. Criteria for the award include excellence in family practice over time, community medical service, contribution to the community, and involvement with CFPC. The award is presented at the time of the CFPC Convocation in conjunction with the National Annual Scientific Assembly in Halifax, Nova Scotia. The recipient will present a short addresss at the time of convocation and will be involved as a spokesperson for Canadian family medicine throughout the year following receipt of the award. The recipient will receive return air fare, complimentary registration, and a stipend for expenses. The deadline for submission varies according to each Provincial Chapter. Please contact the Provincial Chapter of your nominee to confirm the deadline date.
Requirements: Each provincial chapter may select a nominee for the award. Names must be submitted to the National Honours and Awards Committee.
Amount of Grant: $C2000
Contact: Kiki Ziten, Coordinator, Honours and Awards Program, (905) 629-0900 ext 432; fax: (905) 629-0893; email: kziten@cfpc.ca
Internet: http://www.cfpc.ca/English/cfpc/programs/awards%20program/members%20can%20apply%20for/default.asp?s=1#Perkinawards
Sponsor: College of Family Physicians of Canada
2630 Skymark Avenue
Mississauga, ON L4W 5A4 Canada

CFPC Fellowships 955

The program awards fellowships to CFPC members to recognize achievement in the discipline of family medicine. The conferral of fellowships will take into consideration the nominee's exemplary performance as a family physician and exceptional contributions to community activities that enhance health in its broadest sense; outstanding leadership in the academic discipline of family medicine and major administrative responsibilities within a university department of family medicine; and significant elected or appointed executive positions at the national or chapter level of the CFPC or involvement in major committee or other college activities.

Requirements: Nominees must hold certification in family medicine, have a minimum of 10 years continuous membership, and be members in good standing at the time of nomination.

Date(s) Application is Due: Feb 15

Contact: Kiki Ziten, Coordinator, (905) 629-0900 ext 432; fax: (905) 629-0893; email: kziten@cfpc.ca

Internet: http://www.cfpc.ca/English/cfpc/research/section%20of%20researchers/home/default.asp?s=1

Sponsor: College of Family Physicians of Canada
2630 Skymark Avenue
Mississauga, ON L4W 5A4 Canada

CFPC Research and Education Foundation Grants 956

The program is supported by the CFPC Research and Education Foundation and industry partners and comprises research grants, scholarships, and training programs for educational and research initiatives in the area of family medicine. The Royal Canadian Legion One-Month Traineeship grants are awarded to improve the quality of medical education and the provision of care to elderly patients. The Hollister King grant provides an opportunity for a practicing family physician to attain or enhance special skills in the delivery of rural medical care. The Douglas M. Robb research grant is given to a community-based member who plans to conduct research on a topic relevant to the practice of family medicine. Research/development grants provide seed money to members to initiate or complete research/development projects in family medicine. Practice Enrichment grants enable members in active practice to participate in a course of study under the direction of a Canadian university for a minimum of three months in fields related to family medicine. Traveling Scholarship grants enable members to pursue clinical studies for a minimum of three weeks under the direction of a clinical department at a Canadian university. Graduate Study grants enable members to pursue a course of study at a Canadian university for a period of at least six months on a part-time basis.

Amount of Grant: $C1000-$C5000

Contact: Kiki Ziten, (905) 629-0900 ext 432; fax: (905) 629-0893; email: kziten@cfpc.ca

Internet: http://www.cfpc.ca/English/cfpc/programs/awards%20program/awardshome%20pdf/default.asp?s=1

Sponsor: College of Family Physicians of Canada
2630 Skymark Avenue
Mississauga, ON L4W 5A4 Canada

CFPC Special Recognition Awards 957

The CFPC Research and Education Foundation with support of industry partners honors outstanding educational and research initiatives in the area of family medicine through conferral of Special Recognition Awards. The W. Victor Johnston Oration award is presented each year at convocation by a renowned leader in family medicine; the orator is selected by the CFPC executive committee. The Donald I. Rice Merit Award allows a nationally or internationally renowned leader in family medicine the opportunity to travel and engage in educational activities. The Ian McWhinney Family Medicine Education Award is presented to an outstanding family medicine teacher. The Irwin Bean Award is presented annually to the practice-eligible candidate who achieves the highest standing in the Certification Examination in Family Medicine. The Janssen-Ortho Literary Awards are given annually to authors of articles published in Canadian Family Physician that are judged to be the best sumbission in English and in French. The Canadian Family Physician Research Award promotes research and publication by family physicians. Annual deadline dates may vary; contact program staff for exact dates.

Amount of Grant: $C500-$C5000

Contact: Kiki Ziten, (905) 629-0900 ext 432; fax: (905) 629-0893; email: kziten@cfpc.ca

Internet: http://www.cfpc.ca/English/cfpc/programs/awards%20program/awardshome%20pdf/default.asp?s=1

Sponsor: College of Family Physicians of Canada
2630 Skymark Avenue
Mississauga, ON L4W 5A4 Canada

Challenged Athletes Foundation Grants 958

The foundation awards grants to individuals with physical disabilities who need funding for sport-specific training, competition, or athletic equipment needs. All sports are eligible. Applications are accepted year round with a December 1st postmarked deadline.

Requirements: People of all ages with permanent disabilities are eligible. Disabilities must be recognized by the International Paralympic Committee

Date(s) Application is Due: Dec 1

Contact: Virginia Tinley, Executive Director, (858) 793-9293; fax: (858) 793-9291; email: execdir@challengedathletes.org

Internet: http://www.challengedathletes.org

Sponsor: Challenged Athletes Foundation
2148 Jimmy Durante Boulevard, Suite B
Del Mar, CA 92014

Champ-A Champion Fur Kids Grants 959

Grants for children's health and wellness are awarded twice each year. The program provides direct support for children in the areas of health and wellness such as childhood disease research foundations, child safety organizations and organizations that serve children with special needs. The goal is to provide grants to help many programs that are working hard to make the world a healthier and happier place for kids. Programs funded include: (a) Individual Project grants (generally for one-time purchases or to fulfill a short-term need, such as the purchase of materials or equipment); or, (b) Organization Program grants (start-up or operational costs for ongoing programs. Examples include funds for research, health and wellness educational programs, or financial assistance for children and families in-need.)

Requirements: United States applicants must be a tax-exempt organization under Section 501(c)3 of the IRS Code, and 'not a private foundation,' within the meaning of Code Sections 509(a)(1) or 509(a)(2), or a state college or university within the meaning of Code Section 511(a)(2)(B) (a 'Public Charity'). In addition, grant recipients must certify that they are not a supporting organization within the meaning of Code Section 509(a)(3). Canadian applicants must be a registered Canadian charity.

Restrictions: Programs that will not be funded include: Annual Appeals or Capital Campaigns; Construction or New Facility expenses; Fundraising or Event Sponsorships; Political Activities; or Religious organizations for religious purposes.

Samples: Angels with Special Needs (Columbia, SC); Building A Generation (Redlands, CA); Hearts and Noses Hospital Clown Troupe (Needham, MA); Catholic Charities of the Diocese of Santa Rosa (Santa Rosa, CA); Hole in the Wall Gang Fund (New Haven, CT); St. Patrick Center (St. Louis, MO); The Children's Hospital Foundation (Omaha, NE); Youth in Need (St. Charles, MO)

Amount of Grant: $1,000 - $10,000

Date(s) Application is Due: Feb 28; Aug 30; Nov 30

Contact: Maxine Clark, President; (314) 423-8000; email: giving@buildabear.com

Internet: http://www.buildabear.com/aboutus/community/bearhugs.aspx

Sponsor: Build-A-Bear Workshop Bear Hugs Foundation
1954 Innerbelt Business Center Drive
Saint Louis, MO 63114

Champlin Foundations Grants 960

The Champlin Foundations are comprised of three foundations, the first established in 1932 by George S. Champlin, Florence C. Hamilton and Hope C. Neaves, who also created The Second Champlin Foundation in 1947. Both of these trusts are administered by the same Distribution Committee. The Third Champlin Foundation was established by George S. Champlin in 1975 and is administered by a separate Distribution Committee. All three foundations share the same management and PNC Bank/Delaware is the trustee of each. The Champlin Foundations are private foundations as defined in Section 509(a) of the Internal Revenue Code and are exempt from Federal income tax under Section 501(c)3. The Foundations areas of interest include: Youth/Fitness; Hospitals/Healthcare; Open Space/Conservation/Environment; Education; Libraries; Social Services; Historic Preservation; Cultural/Artistic; Animal Humane Societies. The Foundations make direct grants to tax exempt organizations, substantially all in Rhode Island, mostly for capital needs. Capital needs may consist of equipment, construction, renovations, the purchase of real property and reduction of mortgage indebtedness. One important goal is to fund tax exempt organizations within Rhode Island that will have the greatest impact on the broadest possible segment of the population. Another important goal is to provide "hands on" equipment and facilities for those being served by these tax-exempt organizations. Grant applications are accepted March 1st through April 30th. No applications will be accepted via facsimile or email. Applications must be postmarked no later than April 30th, or in the case of April 30th falling on a weekend, then the first business day thereafter.

Requirements: 501(c)3 tax exempt organizations of Rhode Island are eligible to apply.

Geographic Focus: Rhode Island

Samples: RiverzEdge Arts Project, Woonsocket, RI, $3,045—technology equipment (2008); Broad Rock Middle School, Wakefield, RI, $91,145— equip a Cardio Fitness Center (2008); Home & Hospice Care of RI, Pawtucket, RI, $500,000— towards constructing a new headquarters building with a 24 bed inpatient hospice unit in Providence (2008); Preservation Society of Newport County, Newport, RI, $100,000— towards the completion of the restoration of the roof at Chateau-sur-Mer (2008); Blackstone Parks Conservancy, Providence, RI, $10,000— towards the repair of the historic trolley shelter on Blackstone Boulevard (2008).

Amount of Grant: $25,000-$65,000 average

Date(s) Application is Due: Apr 30

Contact: Keith Lang, Executive Director; (401) 736-0370; fax: (401) 736-7248; email: champlinfdns@worldnet.att.net

Internet: http://www.fdncenter.org/grantmaker/champlin

Sponsor: Champlin Foundations
300 Centerville Road, Suite 300S
Warwick, RI 02886-0226

CharityWorks Grants 961

Each year, CharityWorks seeks a partner whose programs improve the quality of life for children and families in the Washington metropolitan area. CharityWorks contributes manpower and money to qualified nonprofit organizations in the Washington Metropolitan area that make a significant impact on the area???s most urgent societal and educational needs. Specific focus areas are education, health, and poverty reduction. The beneficiary will receive 80 percent of the proceeds of CharityWork's fundraising efforts. The remaining 20 percent of the proceeds will be divided among the other two finalists.

Geographic Focus: District of Columbia
Date(s) Application is Due: Apr 18
Contact: Grants Administrator, (703) 286-0758; fax: (703) 286-0791; email: charityworks@aol.com
Internet: http://www.charityworksdc.org
Sponsor: CharityWorks
P.O. Box 3294
McLean, VA 22103

Charles A. Frueauff Foundation Grants 962
The foundation considers proposals 501(c)3 organizations that support private four-year colleges and universities, social service agencies, and health-related agencies and institutions. Types of support include building construction/renovation, capital campaigns, equipment acquisition, general operating support, matching/challenge grants, annual campaigns, and emergency funds. Consideration will be given to programs that support persons leaving welfare, preparing students for employment in non-profit agencies, tutoring at-risk youth, and revitalizing neighborhoods. Applicants are requested to send via postal service a one-page letter of inquiry and include the following information: very brief agency mission and purpose; agency location; brief purpose of request and amount requested; and email address if you wish to receive notification via email.
Requirements: Applicants must be private nonprofit corporations with 501(c)3 status.
Restrictions: The foundation funds nationwide except: Arizona, Alaska, California, Hawaii, Idaho, Iowa, Michigan, Minnesota, Montana, Nevada, New Mexico, North Dakota, Ohio, Oregon, Utah, Washington, Wisconsin, and Wyoming. K-12 schools are ineligible. Grants are not awarded to individuals, provide emergency funds, fund research, or for loans. Multi-year grants, international projects, state supported colleges or universities, primary and secondary schools, churches, or fund raising drives and special events are not supported.
Geographic Focus: Alabama; Arkansas; Colorado; Connecticut; Delaware; District of Columbia; Florida; Georgia; Illinois; Indiana; Kansas; Kentucky; Louisiana; Maine; Maryland; Massachusetts; Mississippi; Missouri; Nebraska; New Hampshire; New Jersey; New Mexico; New York; North Carolina; Oklahoma; Pennsylvania; Rhode Island; South Carolina; South Dakota; Tennessee; Texas; Vermont; Virginia; West Virginia
Samples: Melmark Home (Berwyn, PA)—for classroom and office renovation, $50,000.; Stetson U (Deland, FL)—to provide scholarships to students majoring in the natural sciences, $100,000.
Date(s) Application is Due: Mar 15; Sep 15
Contact: Sue Frueauff; (501) 324-2233; fax: (501) 324-2236
Internet: http://www.frueaufffoundation.com/application/default.asp
Sponsor: Charles A. Frueauff Foundation
200 South Commerce, Suite 100
Little Rock, AR 72201

Charles Delmar Foundation Grants 963
Established in 1957, the Foundation supports organizations involved with inter-American studies, higher, secondary, elementary, and other education, underprivileged youth, the disadvantaged, the aged, the homeless and housing issues, general welfare organizations, and fine and performing arts. Giving primarily in the Washington, DC area in the U.S., and in Europe and South America. There are no specific deadlines with which to adhere. Contact the Foundation for further application information and guidelines.
Restrictions: No grants to individuals, or for building or endowment funds, or matching gifts; no loans.
Geographic Focus: District of Columbia; Maryland; Virginia; West VirginiaEurope; South America
Samples: James River Association, Mechanicsville, VA, $4,000 - for general support (2006); Pan American Development Foundation, Washington, DC, $5,000 - for environmental operations (2006); College of Wooster, Wooster, OH, $9,000 - for general support (2006);
Amount of Grant: $500 - $10,000 range
Contact: Mareen D. Hughes, President; (703) 534-9109
Sponsor: The Charles Delmar Foundation
5205 Leesburg Pike, Suite 209
Falls Church, VA 22041-3858

Charles Edison Fund Grants 964
The Charles Edison Fund (the "Fund") is an endowed philanthropic institution dedicated to the support of worthwhile endeavors generally within the areas of medical research, science education and historic preservation. Funding is available on a national level but, the majority of institutions and, organizations assisted are based principally in the New York-New Jersey Metropolitan area. This concentration of interest facilitates the efforts of the Trustees to evaluate the work of recipient groups, frequently accomplished by personal visitations.
Requirements: Public and private schools, universities and colleges, and nonprofits are eligible.
Contact: Fund Administrator, (973) 648-0500; fax: (973) 648-0400; email: info@charlesedisonfund.org
Internet: http://www.charlesedisonfund.org/thefund.html
Sponsor: Charles Edison Fund
One Riverfront Plaza, 4th Floor
Newark, NJ 07102

Charles G. Koch Charitable Foundation Grants 965
The foundation provides funding for academic and public policy research directed at solving social problems through voluntary action and free enterprise. In the area of research, the foundation primarily funds organizations working with doctorate-level investigators in disciplines such as economics, history, philosophy, political science, and organizational behavior. Types of support include general operating, scholarship funds, conferences and seminars, research, special projects, and seed money. There are no application deadlines. Submit preproposal letters (three-page limit).
Samples: George Mason U (Fairfax, VA)—to recruit faculty members, and for programs in experimental economics, $3 million.
Amount of Grant: $25,000-$300,000 average
Contact: Kelly Young, Vice President, (202) 393-2354; fax: (202) 393-2355; email: email@cgkfoundation.org
Internet: http://www.cgkfoundation.org
Sponsor: Charles G. Koch Charitable Foundation
655 15th St NW, Suite 445
Washington, DC 20005-2001

Charles H. Dater Foundation Grants 966
The foundation makes grants to private, nonprofit organizations and public agencies in Greater Cincinnati for programs that benefit children in the region in the areas of arts/culture, education, healthcare, social services, and other community needs. Grants are usually made for one year, and subsequent grants for an extended or ongoing program are based on an evaluation of annual results. Multiple grants to an organization in the foundation's same fiscal year (September through August) are possible, but rare. The foundation looks favorably on applications that leverage a grant to seek additional funding and resources. The foundation directors meet monthly to review grant applications.
Requirements: Nonprofit organizations in the greater Cincinnati area are eligible. This area is defined as the eight-county metropolitan area made up of the counties of Hamilton, Butler, Warren and Clermont in Ohio; Boone, Kenton and Campbell in Northern Kentucky; and Dearborn in Indiana.
Restrictions: The foundation does not make grants to individuals, for scholarships for individuals, for debt reduction, and, with rare exception, for capital fund projects.
Geographic Focus: Indiana; Kentucky; Ohio
Samples: SON Ministries (Cincinnati, OH)—to provide school supplies and clothing to underprivileged children, $30,000.; Children's Home of Cincinnati (OH)—for a summer day camp designed to enhance the creativity and social skills of disadvantaged children, $10,000.; Children's Hospital Medical Ctr (Cincinnati, OH)—for salary support of a chaplain in the psychiatry department's Adolescent Medicine Psychiatric Service units, $28,000.
Amount of Grant: $10,000-$20,000 average
Contact: Beth Broomall, Grants Coordinator; (513) 241-2658: fax: (513) 274-2731; email: bb@DaterFoundation.org
Internet: http://www.daterfoundation.org/grants.php
Sponsor: Charles H. Dater Foundation
602 Main Street, Suite 302
Cincinnati, OH 45202

Charles H. Farnsworth Trust Grants 967
Grants are awarded to nonprofits whose programs and activities provide services to seniors in their residences for health care, homemaker services, nutrition, services to elderly persons in collective/supportive housing, and research and communication to better inform individuals and institutions of ways to improve the quality and quantity of housing and support services for the elderly. Types of support include equipment, general operating budgets, renovation projects, seed money, research, and building funds. Applicants should submit a letter of intent (three-page limit).
Requirements: Only nonprofits in Massachusetts are eligible to apply.
Amount of Grant: $80,000 maximum
Contact: Grants Administrator, (617) 451-0049 ext 702; fax: (617) 423-4619; email: research@tmfnet.org
Sponsor: Charles H. Farnsworth Trust
95 Berkeley Street, Suite 201
Boston, MA 02116

Charles H. Hood Foundation Child Health Research Grants 968
The grants assist in the promotion of child health in New England. Interest areas include pediatrics, pediatric surgery, pediatric medical and surgical subspecialties, and perinatal obstetrics. Emphasis is on medical research contributing to a reduction of the health problems and health needs of large numbers of children. The foundation seeks innovative, start-up projects that are not yet candidates for government or large foundation support. Guidelines are published twice each year.
Requirements: Applicants must have completed postdoctoral training and must not be receiving salary support from training funds, including fellowships, at the time of the grant award. Giving is limited to Connecticut, Massachusetts, Maine, New Hampshire, Rhode Island, and Vermont.
Restrictions: Grants are not given for building funds, endowments, regular budgets, or public fund-raising campaigns. Grants are not awarded to individuals.
Geographic Focus: Connecticut; Maine; Massachusetts; New England; New Hampshire; Rhode Island; Vermont
Samples: Dr. David Ludwig, Beth Israel Hospital (Boston, MA)—for research on the neuroendocrine regulation of obesity, $50,000.; Dr. Samuel Varghese, Saint Francis Hospital and Medical Ctr (Hartford, CT)—for research on regulation of collagenase gene, $49,994.

Amount of Grant: $75,000 average
Contact: Raymond Considine, Executive Director, (617) 695-9439; fax: (617) 423-4619; email: chhoodfdn@tmfnet.org
Sponsor: Charles H. Hood Foundation
95 Berkeley Street, Suite 201
Boston, MA 02116

Charles H. Revson Foundation Grants **969**
The foundation awards grants nationwide in its areas of interest, including urban affairs and public policy, education and higher education, biomedical research policy, and Jewish education and philanthropy. Types of support include capital campaigns, continuing support, fellowships, internship funds, program development, and research. Preference is given to requests serving New York, NY. There are no application forms or deadlines. The board meets in April, June, October, and December.
Restrictions: Grants do not support local or national health appeals or direct service programs, individuals, building construction/renovation, book projects, charity events, travel expenses, or budgetary support.
Samples: The Legal Aid Society, New York, NY, $100,000—to support the Economic Security Initiative, which provides essential legal assistance to meet the current economic challenges (2009); Jewish Theological Seminary of America, New York, NY, $500,000—to support the creation of the Center for Pastoral Education (2009); Albert Einstein Collefe of Medicine of Yeshiva University, New York, NY, $170,619—to support a fellow in the Charles H. Revson Senior Fellowships in the Life Sciences Program (2009); Fiscal Policy Institute, Somerville, MA, $200,000—to support research, public education, and advocacy work on budget, economic, and related policy issues that affect low- and moderate-income New Yorkers (2009).
Contact: Maria Marcantonio, Grants Administrator; (212) 935-3340; fax: (212) 688-0633; email: info@revsonfoundation.org
Internet: http://www.revsonfoundation.org/guidelines.html
Sponsor: Charles H. Revson Foundation
55 E 59th Street, 23rd Floor
New York, NY 10022

Charles Lafitte Foundation Grants **970**
The foundation is committed to helping groups and individuals foster lasting improvement on the human condition by providing support to education, children's advocacy, medical research, and the arts. Children's advocacy grants support organizations working to improve the quality of life for children, particularly in relation to child abuse, literacy, foster housing, hunger, and after-school programs. Education grants support innovative programs that work to resolve social service issues, address the needs of students with learning disabilities, provide technology and computer-based education, offer leadership skills education, and support at-risk students. Colleges and universities also receive support for research and conferences. The foundation's medical issues and research grants support healthcare studies, with emphasis on cancer research and treatment, children's health, health education, and promoting healthy living and disease prevention. Art grants support emerging artists and educational art programs.
Requirements: 501(c)3 tax-exempt organizations are eligible.
Contact: Jennifer Vertetis, President, email: jennifer@charleslafitte.org
Internet: http://www.charleslafitte.org
Sponsor: Charles Lafitte Foundation
29520 2nd Ave SW
Federal Way, WA 98023

Charles M. and Mary D. Grant Foundation Grants **971**
The foundation awards grants primarily in the U.S. southeast in its areas of interest, including community and economic development, health and human services, education, and literacy. The foundation prefers to support projects, but may consider requests for operating support from organizations with budgets of less than $1 million. Grants are made in September. A minimum of three years must elapse between grant awards.
Requirements: Southeast U.S. 501(c)3 tax-exempt organizations are eligible.
Restrictions: Individuals are ineligible, and loans are not awarded.
Samples: Free Clinic of Danville (VA)—for building renovations, $15,000 (2005); United Negro College Fund (New York, NY)—for the Faculty Advancement Program of the technology enhancement capital campaign, $30,000 (2005); Mountain Assoc for Community Economic Development (Berea, KY)—for general support, $35,000 (2005); Atlanta Legal Aid Society (GA)—for the Health Law Partnership, $25,000 (2005).
Amount of Grant: $10,000-$50,000 average
Date(s) Application is Due: Apr 30
Contact: Jacqueline Elias, JPMorgan Private Bank Philanthropic Services NY1-N040
Internet: http://fdncenter.org/grantmaker/grant
Sponsor: Charles M. and Mary D. Grant Foundation
345 Park Avenue, 4th Floor
New York, NY 10154

Charles M. Bair Family Trust Grants **972**
The trust awards general support grants to Montana nonprofits in its areas of interest, including museums, performing arts, arts and culture, higher education, youth, and social services. Application forms are required.
Requirements: Montana nonprofit organizations are eligible, with emphasis on Yellowstone, Meagher and Wheatland counties.
Restrictions: Funding is not provided for: churches, conventions, or associations of churches; individuals; conferences; symposiums; or for fundraising events.
Geographic Focus: Montana
Amount of Grant: $2000-$300,000
Date(s) Application is Due: Jan 15; Aug 1
Contact: Grants Administrator, c/o U.S. Bank, Tax Department
Sponsor: Charles M. Bair Family Trust
P.O. Box 20678
Billings, MT 59115

Charlotte County (FL) Community Foundation Grants **973**
The foundation awards grants from its unrestricted funds to support innovative solutions for the citizens of Charlotte County through the implementation of projects and programs that address specific identified needs of the community and demonstrate a wide-spread positive impact on its residents. The foundation places priority on funding requests from nonprofit organizations whose project can: Provide an unduplicated value and/or service; Leverage dollars and/or people power; Match foundation funds with funds from other sources; Establish cooperative efforts of two or more organizations where such synergy is likely to demonstrate superior results and/or lower costs; Enhance, expand and/or improve the organization's capabilities; Show visible end results within a specific timeline for completion; Demonstrate that the Foundation grant will play an important role; Provide a meaningful outcomes evaluations process with a project completion report; Reach a large number of Charlotte County residents; and, be completed within one year with a request of less than $7,500.
Requirements: Foundation grants are made to tax exempt organizations that have been in existence for at least two years and whose focus is in one of the following areas of interest: Animal Welfare; Arts and Culture; Community Development; Education; Environment; Health, Human, and Social Services; Historic Preservation; Nonprofit Organization Capacity Building. Additionally, organizations must also show that they have: a Board of Directors composed of individuals of diverse backgrounds, at least half of whom reside in Charlotte County; Strong management and leadership qualities; Demonstrated fiscal responsibility; Submitted its prior year IRS Form 990; Benefited Charlotte County residents. To apply, submit a Letter of Intent (LOI) summarizing your request. (See instructions at the foundation's website.) If the foundation feels that the proposed project has merit, you will be asked to complete a grant proposal package to be submitted as your formal request for funding.
Restrictions: The foundation is generally not interested in requests for: General operating support; Building or capital campaigns; Deficit financing and debt reduction; Endowment funds; Fraternal organizations, societies or orders; Loans or assistance to individuals; Religious organizations for sectarian purposes; Lobbying legislators or influencing elections; Political organizations or campaigns; Fund raising events; Basic scientific research; Start up organization funding; Travel expenses for individuals or groups; or, Re-granting.
Geographic Focus: Florida
Amount of Grant: up to $7,500
Date(s) Application is Due: Apr 5; May 5; Jul 6; Sep 16
Contact: Gregory C. Bobonich, J.D.
Chief Executive Officer; (941) 637-0077; email: gbobonich@charlottecommunityfoundation.org
Internet: http://www.charlottecommunityfoundation.org/index.php?subcat=20&articleid=68&page_num=1#
Sponsor: Charlotte County Community Foundation
1675 West Marion Avenue
Punta Gorda, FL 33950

Charlotte Geyer Foundation Cancer Research Grants **974**
The foundation supports research into the cause, prevention, and treatment of cancer. The purpose of the awards is to provide one year's funding to exceptional proposals to give investigators the opportunity of advancing and improving projects to the point where they are able to successfully compete for an NCI RO1 or other award. Proposals are reviewed three times per year.
Requirements: The foundation will review recent proposals—either the original proposal, a revised proposal, or a portion of the original proposal deemed to have special merit—that were submitted to NCI; received a peer-review ranking in the 10 percentiles above the NCI payline; and did not receive funding.
Amount of Grant: $100,000 maximum
Date(s) Application is Due: Feb 1; Jun 1; Oct 1
Contact: Nancy Falletta, Executive Director, (716) 632-6448; fax: (716) 632-6098
Internet: http://www.charlottegeyer.org
Sponsor: Charlotte Geyer Foundation
P.O. Box 1276
Williamsville, NY 14231-1276

Chase Paymentech Corporate Giving Grants **975**
The corporation awards grants to nonprofit organizations that provide needed services in the areas of education, health and human services. Preference for funding is given to organizations whose work impacts the citizens of those areas in which Paymentech offices are located, including Westerville, OH; Dallas, TX; Salem, NH; Silver Springs, MD; Tampa, FL; Tempe, AZ; and Toronto, Canada. The Corporate Giving Committee meets each quarter. Organizations are notified about funding status after each meeting.
Requirements: 501(c)3 non-profit organizations that provide needed services in the areas of education and health and human services are eligible. Applicants submit a written request on the organization's letterhead detailing the organization's mission, the amount requested and a detailed explanation of the purpose for which the funds would be used. Organizations should also submit proof of non-profit status.

Restrictions: Paymentech does not make grants to individuals; religious, fraternal, political, or veterans organizations; or colleges and universities. Nor is funding provided for the following purposes: or deficit spending or debt liquidation; annual capital campaigns of hospitals, colleges, universities, grade schools, or high schools.
Geographic Focus: Arizona; Florida; Maryland; New Hampshire; Ohio; TexasCanada
Amount of Grant: $5000 maximum
Date(s) Application is Due: Mar 30; Jun 29; Sep 28; Dec 31
Contact: Corporate Giving Director at each local facility
Internet: http://www.chasepaymentech.com/portal/community/chase_paymentech/public/public_website/about_us/company_information_pages/corporate_giving_program
Sponsor: Chase Paymentech
14221 Dallas Parkway, Building Two
Dallas, TX 75254

Chateaubriand Exact Sciences, Engineering, and Medicine Research Scholarships 976
Individuals currently pursuing the PhD or who have completed it in the last three years may qualify for a scholarship from the French government to conduct research at a French university, school of engineering, or state-funded laboratory. Candidates must contact the host institution to secure a position before applying. Scholarships are available for periods of six to 18 months and carry a stipend, health insurance, and round-trip travel expenses. Application forms are available on the Web site.
Requirements: Applicants must be U.S. citizens and registered in a U.S. university, and must be PhD candidates or recent PhD holders. Applicants must obtain written agreement from the French hosting institution before applying; an online registration form is available on the Web site.
Amount of Grant: Ff8700 minimum per month
Date(s) Application is Due: Jan 15
Contact: Chateaubriand Fellowship Program, Mission pour la Science et la Technologie, Ambassade de France, (202) 944-6246; fax: (202) 944-6244; email: Chateaubriand@amb-wash.fr
Internet: http://www.frenchculture.org/education/support/chateaubriand/
Sponsor: French Embassy Cultural Services
4101 Reservoir Rd NW
Washington, DC 20007-2176

Chatlos Foundation Grants 977
The Chatlos Foundation supports nonprofit organizations in the U.S.A and around the globe. Support is provided to organizations currently exempt by the Internal Revenue Service of the United States. The Foundation's areas of interest are: Bible Colleges/Seminaries, Religious Causes, Medical Concerns, Liberal Arts Colleges and Social Concerns.
Requirements: Applicants must be U.S. tax-exempt, nonprofit organizations that provide services in the following areas: bible colleges, religious causes, medical concerns, liberal arts colleges, and social concerns. Proposals must include cover letter, specific request, tax-exemption letter, and budget. If proposal is to be considered at board level, additional information will be requested.
Restrictions: The foundation will not accept requests from individual church congregations, individuals, organizations in existence for less than two years as indicated by IRS tax-exempt letter of determination, for education below the college level, for medical research projects, or for support of the arts.
Amount of Grant: $10,000-$25,000 range
Contact: C. J. Leff, Administrator: (407) 862-5077; email: cj@chatlos.org
Internet: http://www.chatlos.org/AppInfo.htm
Sponsor: Chatlos Foundation
P.O. Box 915048
Longwood, FL 32791-5048

Chazen Foundation Grants 978
The foundation awards grants nationwide to eligible nonprofit organizations in its areas of interest, including arts; business education; higher education; hospitals; human services; Israel; Jewish agencies, temples, and federated giving programs; museums; and music performance. Types of support include building construction/renovation, capital campaigns, general operating support, grants and scholarships to individuals, professorships, and scholarship funds. Education grants are awarded to students of the Rockland County, NY, area. There are no application deadlines.
Contact: Grants Administrator, (212) 750-6600
Internet: http://www.chazenscholar.com/project.php3
Sponsor: Chazen Foundation
767 5th Avenue, 26th Floor
New York, NY 10153-2696

CHCF Grants 979
The foundation's mission is to expand access to affordable, quality health care for underserved individuals and communities in California and to promote fundamental improvements in the health status of Californians. The foundation has five funding areas: improving care delivery, business of healthcare, healthcare quality, California health policy, and California's uninsured. The one-year, renewable grants will focus on areas where the foundation's resources can initiate meaningful policy recommendations, innovative research, and the development of model programs. Philanthropic activities include foundation-initiated projects, requests for proposals, and unsolicited proposals. emailed letters of inquiry should include, in two to three pages, a brief description of the proposed project, along with an estimated time line and budget. A full proposal may be requested.
Requirements: California 501(c)3 nonprofit organizations are eligible.
Restrictions: The foundation does not generally support the cost of direct clinical care, ongoing general operating expenses, capital campaigns, annual appeals or other fund-raising events, construction, purchase or renovation of facilities, or purchase of equipment.
Geographic Focus: California
Date(s) Application is Due: Oct 14
Contact: Grants Administrator, (510) 238-1040; fax: (510) 238-1388; email: grants@chcf.org
Internet: http://www.chcf.org/grantinfo
Sponsor: California HealthCare Foundation
476 Ninth Street
Oakland, CA 94607

CHCF Health Care Affordability Grants 980
The program awards grants to support initiatives that reduce rising health care costs in the short term. Instead of merely shifting costs from one part of the health care sector to another, the goal of these projects will be to achieve net cost savings for the overall health system. Projects funded under this RFP may include efforts to reduce health care costs by streamlining information exchange, improving efficiency, and decreasing costs; collaborating to reduce duplication and achieve economies of scale; aligning incentives among players in the health care system; and increasing transparency and promoting informed decision making. Initial funding will support grantees as they develop ideas, partnerships, and plans for implementing appropriate strategies. Based on the success of Phase I, CHCF anticipates a future funding phase that would support implementation of selected California-based interventions. Complete details, including submission instructions, are available online.
Requirements: Nonprofit and for-profit organizations are eligible. Proposals from outside of California need to clearly demonstrate applicability of the strategy to the California health care system; a partnership that would allow the cost-saving strategy to be introduced in California; and a specific plan for coordinating the project.
Amount of Grant: $25,000-$75,000
Date(s) Application is Due: Dec 1
Contact: Grants Administrator, (510) 238-1040; fax: (510) 238-1388
Internet: http://www.chcf.org/grantinfo/rfps/view.cfm?itemid=115045
Sponsor: California Healthcare Foundation
476 Ninth Street
Oakland, CA 94607

CHCF Local Coverage Expansion Initiative 981
This initiative supports California counties and local coalitions seeking to expand coverage to uninsured children and adults that are ineligible for public insurance programs. This solicitation will fund two types of technical assistance grants: planning grants will assist coverage expansion efforts with activities such as coalition strengthening, better defining the target population's needs, and/or developing an implementation plan; and implementation grants will provide funding for specific unmet needs associated with launching a local coverage program. Grants will be awarded for period up to one year. Application and guidelines are available online.
Requirements: Any type of organization may apply, but the program will focus on public programs seeking to expand coverage, primarily through the use of public funds. It is anticipated that successful proposals will either come from public or quasi-public agencies, or include a plan for close collaboration with public sector entities.
Amount of Grant: $25,000-$50,000 planning grants; $100,000-$200,000 implementation grants
Date(s) Application is Due: Oct 14
Contact: Grants Administrator, (510) 238-1040; fax: (510) 238-1388; email: localcoverage@chcf.org
Internet: http://www.chcf.org/grantinfo/rfps/index.cfm?itemID=21263
Sponsor: California Healthcare Foundation
476 Ninth Street
Oakland, CA 94607

Chesapeake Corporation Foundation Grants 982
The foundation supports U.S. and international nonprofits in its areas of interest, including civic affairs, community development, cultural programs, higher education, and health. Types of support include endowments, capital grants, matching gifts, and scholarships. Grants are awarded for one year with the possibility of renewal.
Requirements: Nonprofits internationally are eligible.
Restrictions: Grants do not support athletic purposes or individuals, except for employee-related scholarships.
Amount of Grant: $1000-$10,000 typically
Contact: J.P. Causey Jr., (804) 697-1000; fax: (804) 697-1199
Internet: http://www.cskcorp.com
Sponsor: Chesapeake Corporation Foundation
P.O. Box 2350
Richmond, VA 23218-2350

Chest Foundation Eli Lilly and Company Distinguished Scholar in Critical Care Medicine Award 983
The Eli Lilly and Company Distinguished Scholar in Critical Care Medicine will have a 3-year opportunity to examine issues that relate to critically ill patients. The award is

intended to permit the investigation of issues that are not easily supported by traditional funding, such as clinical trials or basic science. Rather, the award would support activities such as the development of public policy, patient education models, or economic analysis of treatment or care delivery in this patient group. A stipend of $50,000 annually over the 3-year term of the program will be provided. A fourth year stipend of $10,000 will also be awarded to the individual who will serve in a mentorship role to the fourth Distinguished Scholar position during his/her inaugural year of service.
Requirements: An applicant must be: an FCCP and hold the degree of MD, DO, MBChB, MBBCh, MBBS, DNSc, PharmD, PhD, or EdD; board-certified in critical care medicine; and a recognized clinician and/or scientist with a specialty in sepsis and/or critical care as evidenced by publications, presentations, and/or peers.
Amount of Grant: $50,000 per year for first three years, $10,000 for fourth year
Date(s) Application is Due: Apr 30
Contact: Sue Ciezadlo, Senior Project Coordinator; (847) 498-8363; fax: (847) 498-5460; email: sciezadlo@chestnet.org
Internet: http://www.chestfoundation.org/foundation/clinical/dsCriticalCare.php
Sponsor: Chest Foundation
3300 Dundee Road
Northbrook, IL 60062-2348

Chest Foundation Geriatric Development Research Awards 984

The two-year award is intended to provide the impetus required for long-term career development focused on integrating geriatrics into the sub-specialties of internal medicine. The program awards the grant to an academic internist to develop and implement a basic, clinical, or health services research project focused on a geriatric aspect of chest medicine. The funding can support the salary of the award recipient and/or the purchase of supplies, the salaries of technical personnel, and other resources necessary for the completion of the research project. The award also includes a one-time travel grant to attend the meetings of the American Geriatrics Society and the American College of Chest Physicians in the second year of the award.
Requirements: To be eligible for the award, applicants must: have U.S. citizenship or permanent resident status; hold a degree of MD or its equivalent; have completed a sub-specialty internal medicine fellowship leading to certification in his/her sub-specialty by the American Board of Internal Medicine and be within the first three years of his/her faculty appointment; possess a faculty appointment by July 1 (this faculty appointment should be documented in the required letters of recommendation from the applicant's department chair and division director); be a member of the American College of Chest Physicians; commit 75 percent of his/her professional effort to research activities; develop and implement a basic, clinical, or health services research project focused on a geriatric aspect of chest medicine; and generate and implement a career development plan focused on the geriatrics aspects of chest medicine. This plan must include organizing and interacting with a mentorship team made up of a minimum of four members—the applicant's research mentor as the leader of the research team, a sub-specialist in the applicant's field of chest medicine, a geriatrician, and one other member at the applicant's discretion.
Restrictions: The funding cannot be used to acquire administrative or clerical support. Funding is to cover total costs; no indirect cost funds will be provided.
Amount of Grant: $50,000 per year for two years plus $3,000 travel grant
Date(s) Application is Due: Apr 30
Contact: Sue Ciezadlo, Senior Project Coordinator; (847) 498-8363; fax: (847) 498-5460; email: sciezadlo@chestnet.org
Internet: http://www.chestfoundation.org/foundation/clinical/geriatricAward.php
Sponsor: Chest Foundation
3300 Dundee Road
Northbrook, IL 60062-2348

Chest Foundation Grant in Venous Thromboembolism 985

The Chest Foundation is issuing this Request for Proposal (RFP) that will fund two projects with up to a total grant amount of $180,000 each for a 1-year period. The goal of the grant process is to confer awards to projects that include evidence-based replicable programs and tools to address the current gaps in the management and prophylaxis in venous thromboembolism (VTE). The deadline is February 20.
Requirements: To be considered a candidate for The Chest Foundation Grant in Venous Thromboembolism, an individual must: be a current ACCP member and hold the degree of MD, DO, MBChB, MBBCh, MBBS, DNSc, PharmD, PhD, or EdD; and be a recognized scientist focused on an area of VTE or clinical decision making as evidenced by academic productivity and/or publications and presentations.
Amount of Grant: $180,000 maximum
Date(s) Application is Due: Feb 20
Contact: Sue Ciezadlo, Senior Project Coordinator; (847) 498-8363; fax: (847) 498-5460; email: sciezadlo@chestnet.org
Internet: http://www.chestfoundation.org/foundation/clinical/VT_Grant.php
Sponsor: Chest Foundation
3300 Dundee Road
Northbrook, IL 60062-2348

Chest Foundation/LUNGevity Foundation Clinical Research Grants 986

The goal of this joint clinical research program is, ultimately, to save the lives of those people afflicted with lung cancer by funding innovative research designed to treat and cure lung cancer. A clinical research award of $75,000 will be granted to a single award recipient for clinical research in lung cancer over a period of 2 years. The amount of $37,500 will be granted after July 1. Upon receipt of the Progress Report received before July 15, the remaining $37,500 will be granted.
Requirements: To be considered a candidate for The Chest Foundation/LUNGevity Foundation Clinical Research Award in Lung Cancer, an individual must: be an ACCP member who has completed at least 2 years of pulmonary or oncology fellowship and be within 5 years of fellowship or no more than 5 years in practice; hold a degree of MD, DO, MB,BCh, PharmD, PhD or its equivalent; can be a citizen of the United States, or have a J-1 or H-1 visa, and be working in a certified United States institution or organization, or be a Canadian or international member who is working in a certified institution or organization in his/her country; and be a clinician in lung cancer research.
Amount of Grant: $75,000
Date(s) Application is Due: Apr 30
Contact: Sue Ciezadlo, Senior Project Coordinator; (847) 498-8363; fax: (847) 498-5460; email: sciezadlo@chestnet.org;; Beth Ida Stern, Executive Director; email: bstern@lungevity.org
Internet: http://www.chestfoundation.org/foundation/clinical/LUNGevityAward.php
Sponsor: Chest Foundation / LUNGevity Foundation
3300 Dundee Road
Northbrook, IL 60062-2348

Chestnut Hill Charitable Foundation, Inc Grants 987

The foundation awards grants to nonprofit organizations in the greater Boston, MA, area in support of medical research, children and youth, and arts and education. Specifically, the foundation's interests include visual arts, museums, humanities, arts and culture, early childhood education and development, education at all levels, hospitals and medical research (cancer, heart and lungs, AIDS, and diabetes), social services, and general charitable giving. Types of support include general operating support, annual campaigns, capital campaigns, building construction/renovations, programs and projects, seed grants, curriculum development, research, and matching funds. There are no application forms; submit a letter of request.
Requirements: Nonprofit organizations in the greater Boston area may submit requests.
Restrictions: Grants are not awarded to support individuals or political or religious organizations.
Geographic Focus: Massachusetts
Samples: Leslie Berg, U of Massachusetts Medical Ctr (Worcester, MA)—for the Chestnut Hill Award for Excellence in Medical Research, administered by the Medical Foundation, in Boston, $15,000 (2003).
Amount of Grant: $1000-$15,000 average
Contact: Kay Kilpatrick, Director Corporate Giving, (617) 630-2415
Sponsor: Chestnut Hill Charitable Foundation, Inc
27 Boylston Street
Chestnut Hill, MA 02167-1700

Chicago Board of Trade Foundation Grants 988

The foundation provides grant support to organizations in the metropolitan Chicago, IL, area in its areas of interest: arts and culture, including libraries and museums; education, including higher education, adult basic education and literacy training, and science and technology; health care, including mental health services, cancer research, and rehabilitation; child and youth development; minorities; the economically disadvantaged; wildlife; and media and communication. Grants are awarded for general operating support, continuing support, annual campaigns, capital campaigns, and endowments. An application form is not required; the initial approach should be by letter, or via the CBOT Foundation form on the Web site. The board meets during the first quarter annually to consider requests.
Requirements: Nonprofit organizations in a 75-mile radius of the metropolitan Chicago, IL, area may apply for grant support.
Restrictions: Support is not given to hospitals or foundations. Loans and program-related investments will also be denied.
Geographic Focus: Illinois
Date(s) Application is Due: Oct 1
Contact: Grants Administrator, (312) 435-3456; fax: (312) 341-3306
Internet: http://www.cbot.com/cbot/pub/page/0,3181,948,00.html
Sponsor: Chicago Board of Trade Foundation
141 W Jackson Boulevard, Suite 600-A
Chicago, IL 60604

Chicago Community Trust Grants 989

The community trust supports charitable programs that provide mental, moral, intellectual and physical improvement, assistance, and relief for people in Cook County, IL. Grants are made in the areas of education—teaching and learning in public schools, with emphasis on improved literacy rates, professional development for teachers and administrators, and alternative educational models; arts and humanities—arts education, dance, and leadership transitions at arts groups; basic human needs—food, shelter, and related needs; community development—job training, criminal and juvenile justice, and strengthening nonprofits; and health—violence prevention, health and the environment, and healthful lifestyles. From time to time, guidelines are developed for specific programs or areas of grantmaking. In considering grants for either general operating support of a continuing program or for a specific time-limited program or project, the initial grant usually will be for one or two years. Consecutive funding, including the initial grant, rarely will extend beyond five years. The listed application deadlines are for letters of intent; full proposals are by invitation.
Requirements: Trust funds support 501(c)3 charitable organizations that serve residents of Cook, DuPage, Kane, Lake, McHenry, or Will Counties, IL. In general, grant requests from organizations that do not directly serve this geographic area will not be considered.

Restrictions: The trust generally will not make grants for scholarships, individuals, religious purposes, endowments, or operating support of government agencies.
Geographic Focus: Illinois
Samples: Hyde Park Art Center—for integrated audience development for its family programming, $40,000 (2007); La Casa Norte—for its Solid Ground Supportive Housing Program, $25,000 (2007); The Chicago Community Foundaation—for the planning and development of a public arts high school in Chicago, $50,000 (2007).
Date(s) Application is Due: Mar 17; Jul 15; Nov 11
Contact: Sandy Phelps, Grant Manager, (312) 616-8000; fax: (312) 616-7955; email: info@cct.org
Internet: http://www.cct.org/page28925.cfm
Sponsor: Chicago Community Trust
111 E Wacker Drive, Suite 1400
Chicago, IL 60601

Chicago Institute for Psychoanalysis Fellowships 990
This is a program for advanced trainees in psychiatry, social work, and psychology who have significant interest in psychoanalysis as a body of knowledge and as a framework with which to understand and carry out therapeutic work. It is jointly sponsored by the Chicago Psychoanalytic Society and the Institute for Psychoanalysis. A mentor is assigned to each Fellow, who is available throughout the year-long program to discuss cases, papers, research, etc. In addition, Fellows are guests at Society meetings and conferences held locally. Opportunities are provided for the Fellows to discuss presented papers with their mentors. A monthly conference is held to acquaint Fellows with basic psychoanalytic clinical concepts through readings and discussion. Each Fellow receives a copy of the Annual of Psychoanalysis and other publications.
Date(s) Application is Due: Aug 15
Contact: Christine Susman, Director; (312) 922-7474 ext. 324; email: csusman@chicagoanalysis.org or admin@chicagoanalysis.org
Internet: http://www.chicagoanalysis.org/fellow.php
Sponsor: Chicago Institute for Psychoanalysis
122 South Michigan Avenue
Chicago, IL 60603

Chicago Tribune's Corporate Contributions Grants 991
The foundation's mission is to promote public knowledge and strengthen the Chicago metropolitan community by encouraging journalistic excellence, diversity and liberty; supporting diverse cultural institutions; and promoting civic efforts. Program areas for the foundation are civic, culture, and journalism. Grants in the civic program area support business, nonprofit or educational initiatives. These grants are considered by invitation only and are accepted throughout the year. The range is $2,500 to $20,000. Grants in the culture area support cultural organizations within the Chicago metropolitan area that provide educational programs in the arts for children from low-income communities or that foster diverse art. The range for these grants is $5,000 to $7,500. Proposals are due February 1. Grants in the journalism are support organizations on a national level that offer programs for professional journalists that lead to journalistic excellence, promote diversity in the newspaper industry and protect freedom of the press. Support is considered for journalism programs in the metropolitan Chicago area that promote diversity. Support is not provided to high school or college newspapers. The grant range is $5,000 to $20,000. Proposals are due June 1. Types of support include general operating grants, matching gifts, and program development grants. A brief summary proposal should be sent; if interested, the foundation will request a full proposal.
Requirements: Grants are made to Chicago-area tax-exempt organizations.
Restrictions: Grants are not made to individuals nor for fund-raising events.
Geographic Focus: Illinois
Samples: Innovations for Learning (Evanston, IL)—for its reading programs for first graders supported by online tutors, $10,000.; Chicago History Museum (Chicago, IL)—for curriculum development for Great Chicago Stories for schools, $5,000.; Young Chicago Authors (Chicago, IL)—for in-school and after-school creative writing programs, $5,000.; Association for Women Journalists-Chicago (Chicago, IL)—a survey about careers of women employed in the news media in the Chicago area.; McCormick Tribune YMCA—Kids Need Heroes campaign, $1,000.
Amount of Grant: $5000-$25,000 average
Date(s) Application is Due: Feb 1; Jun 1
Contact: Community Relations, (312) 222-4300; fax: (312) 222-3751; email: ctcommunityrelations@tribune.com
Internet: http://about.chicagotribune.com/community/foundation.htm
Sponsor: Chicago Tribune Foundation
435 N Michigan Avenue, 2nd Floor
Chicago, IL 60611-4041

Chicago White Metal Charitable Foundation Grants 992
The charitable foundation awards grants to Chicago-area nonprofits in its areas of interest, including community development, government/public administration, human services, performing arts, opera, recreation, scholarships/financial aid, and youth development. Grants are awarded for one year and are renewable for a second year.
Requirements: Chicago, IL, 501(c)3 organizations are eligible.
Restrictions: Religious organizations and individuals are ineligible.
Geographic Focus: Illinois
Contact: Grants Administrator, (630) 595-4424; fax: (630) 595-4474
Sponsor: Chicago White Metal Charitable Foundation
Rte 83 and Fairway Drive
Bensenville, IL 60106-9806

Child Nutrition Foundation School Community Kitchens Grants 993
The program awards seed grants for local school community kitchen projects. School community kitchens are school-community partnerships that help people move into foodservice jobs while providing meals for those in need.
Requirements: Applicants must represent a school foodservice or nutrition department at the district or school building level and be a current American School Food Service Association (ASFSA) member.
Amount of Grant: $10,000
Date(s) Application is Due: Oct 15
Contact: Grants Aministrator, (703) 739-3900; fax: (703) 739-3915; email: cnf@schoolnutrition.org
Internet: http://www.schoolnutrition.org/CNF.aspx?id=1133
Sponsor: Child Nutrition Foundation
700 S Washington Street, Suite 300
Alexandria, VA 22314

Children Affected by AIDS Foundation Camp Network Grants 994
The mission of the CAAF Camp Network is to increase the number of children that attend camp every year by providing grants; to foster communication among agencies providing camp experiences for children and their families; and to support the development of new camps. Members of the network gain access to the competitive funding process from the CAAF's yearly financial allocation to the Camp Network.
Requirements: For consideration for membership, Camp Service Providers need to provide proof of the following: (a) Proof of 501(c)3 Not-for-Profit Status; (b) 990 IRS form if applicable; (c) Experience with children infected with or affected by HIV/AIDS and providing camp services. Camps seeking funding from CAAF need to provide proof of the following: (1) Proof of minimum Insurance Coverage's as recommended by the Camp Network; (2) Indemnity for CAAF (Camp Network) from camp agencies, including any employment related claims (Contractual provision, prior to receiving a CAAF grant award.); (3) Compliance with applicable laws such as: employment, health and safety laws and the Americans with Disabilities Act. This will be a contractual provision of the grant agreement, before receiving a CAAF grant award.; (4) Release of Liability from Parent or Guardians and Children, using unique identifiers; and, (5) Evidence that the Camp has policies and procedures in place for: (a) Children's safety and emergencies; (b) Pre-screening of paid and non-paid staff; (c) Other information as needed.
Amount of Grant: $1,000 - $15,000 range
Date(s) Application is Due: May 16
Contact: Rolla Bedford; (310) 258-0850, ext. 14; email: rolla.bedford@caaf4kids.org
Internet: http://www.caaf4kids.org/
Sponsor: Children Affected by AIDS Foundation
6033 W. Century Boulevard, Suite 603
Los Angeles, CA 90045

Children Affected by AIDS Foundation Domestic Grants 995
The foundation awards grants to nonprofit organizations that provide for the medical, emotional, social, and basic needs of children who are infected with HIV or affected by AIDS. Organizations can request funds for their programs that directly impact the lives of children affected by AIDS by submitting a proposal during the foundation's once-a-year application period. Special needs requests are considered throughout the year, depending on funding availability. Funding categories include Basic Needs (clothing, formula, food, diapers, burial services, transportation to/from appointments, emergency child care, and respite services); Social & Recreational (social activities such as arts and crafts, sports, holiday parties, field expeditions, and other forms of recreation); Psychosocial Support (intended to benefit direct services related only to the provision of psychosocial services to children which may include individual and family therapy/counseling, support groups, and life skills classes); Guidelines and application are available online.
Requirements: 501(c)3 nonprofit organizations that provide direct care, support, and assistance to children, ages birth to 13 years, who are HIV-positive or otherwise affected by HIV/AIDS are eligible. This includes children who are HIV-infected, those who are or may become orphaned as a result of losing parents to HIV disease, and those who have siblings, parents, or caregivers who are infected with HIV.
Restrictions: Individuals, research activities, fraternal groups, political or religious activities, and organizations not in good standing with CAAF are not eligible. Additionally, CAAF will not grant funds to pass-through organizations.
Amount of Grant: $1000-$25,000
Date(s) Application is Due: May 16
Contact: Rolla Bedford; (310) 258-0850 ext 14; fax: (310) 258-0851; email: rolla.bedford@caaf4kids.org
Internet: http://www.caaf4kids.org
Sponsor: Children Affected by AIDS Foundation
6033 W. Century Boulevard, Suite 280
Los Angeles, CA 90045

Children Affected by AIDS Foundation Family Assistance Emergency Grants 996
The foundation is making available its Emergency Fund to help HIV/AIDS Service Organizations in the U.S. to meet the needs of HIV-impacted children and their families. Funds can be accessed by qualified HIV/AIDS non-profits with IRS 501(c)3 status. The Foundation will only provide grants to organizations that do not discriminate on the basis of race, color, religion, gender, gender identity, gender expression, age, sexual orientation, marital status, national origin, disability, or other characteristics protected by law. The goal of the Emergency Fund is to meet the pressing, unanticipated needs in

the day-to-day life of children, up to 13 years of age, and their families. Requests may be submitted at any time, and will be reviewed shortly after being received.
Requirements: Funds requested must directly improve the well-being of children in the household. Funds can be accessed by qualified HIV/AIDS non-profits with IRS 501(c)3 status. Eligible requests include: Food; Utility assistance; School uniforms, clothing; Transportation to medical/social service appointments; Medications and medical co-pays; Transitional housing assistance; Burial expenses. Other needs not listed may be considered-please contact the Foundation Program staff prior to sending a request. To download the Emergency Fund's guidelines, go to the sponsor's site, click on 'Initiatives' on the home page, then 'Family Assistance.'
Restrictions: The emergency fund cannot be accessed by or for the following purposes: political or fraternal organizations, or for research or religious purposes.
Amount of Grant: $50 - $2,000
Contact: Rolla Bedford; (310) 258-0850, ext. 14; email: rolla.bedford@caaf4kids.org
Internet: http://www.caaf4kids.org/
Sponsor: Children Affected by AIDS Foundation
6033 W. Century Boulevard, Suite 280
Los Angeles, CA 90045

Children's Advocacy Center Grants **997**

The program supports the establishment and expansion of children's advocacy centers, with the goal of helping to prevent child abuse. One-year grants are awarded in the following categories: program support, research, member training, prevention, associate member program development, nonmember training, and recognized chapters. Applicants must designate a steering committee that comprises child-welfare workers, law-enforcement officials, medical doctors, and mental-health professionals. Application and guidelines are available online.
Requirements: 501(c)3 tax-exempt organizations are eligible.
Amount of Grant: $4.989 million total; $5000-$50,000
Date(s) Application is Due: Sep 13
Contact: Grants Administrator, (800) 239-9950 ext 116
Internet: http://www.nca-online.org
Sponsor: National Children's Alliance
516 C St NE
Washington, DC 20002

Children's Brain Tumor Foundation Research Grants **998**

Science grants are awarded for basic laboratory research on pediatric brain and central nervous system tumors. Priority will be given to research that relates to: priorities I and II of the Research and Scientific Priorities for Pediatric Brain Tumors, as listed in the Report of the Brain Tumor Progress Review Group, which can be found at: http://prg.nci.nih.gov/brain/pediatrics.Submission of a two-page, preapplication form, equivalent to a letter of intent, is required. An original, signed form must be submitted along with five copies. The listed deadline is for preapplication forms; full proposals are by invitation.
Requirements: Funding is currently restricted to principal investigators at institutions within the United States.
Restrictions: The foundation does not award grants to individuals or to private foundations, and does not fund debt reduction, capital improvements, or travel expenses. Overhead expenses are not to exceed 10 percent of the total project cost.
Amount of Grant: $75,000 per year
Contact: Judy Hurley, Executive Director, (212) 448-9494; fax: (212) 448-1022; email: JHurley@cbtf.org
Internet: http://www.cbtf.org/grant_info.html
Sponsor: Children's Brain Tumor Foundation
274 Madison Avenue, Suite 1301
New York, NY 10016-0701

Children's Leukemia Research Association Research Grants **999**

The association supports research efforts into the causes and cure of leukemia and gives patient aid to families in need while meeting the expenses incurred in leukemia treatment. A medical advisory committee consisting of prominent internationally known and respected hematologists reviews grant proposals submitted for consideration of projects that are not otherwise funded. Grants are available for start-up funding for laboratory or clinical investigations in leukemia. Although the association prefers to fund new investigators, applications from established investigators for new initiatives are also solicited. Renewal for a second year is considered if other funding for promising projects has not been obtained.
Restrictions: Previously funded projects are not usually considered for additional funding.
Amount of Grant: $20,000 maximum per year
Date(s) Application is Due: Jun 30
Contact: Executive Director, (516) 222-1944; fax (516) 222-0457; email: info@childrensleukemia.org
Internet: http://www.childrensleukemia.org/ResearchPast%20Pres.htm
Sponsor: Children's Leukemia Research Association Inc
585 Stewart Avenue, Suite LL-18
Garden City, NY 11530

Children's Medical Research Institute Grants **1000**

The program, which is designed to promote pediatric research as a career, supports summer scholarships for first- and second-year Oklahoma University College of Medicine students. Each year students are awarded grants to support their pediatric research interests as they assist OU Medical Center Department of Pediatrics physicians. The program also awards small research grants/short-term projects to individual scientists at the OU Medical Center, who often use the funds as seed money to finance pilot research projects.
Contact: Sana Rettig, (405) 271-8001 option 1, ext 42389; fax: (405) 271-1175; email: sana-rettig@ouhsc.edu
Internet: http://www.cmri.net/scholarships.html
Sponsor: Children's Medical Research Institute
800 Research Pwy, Suite 150
Oklahoma City, OK 73104

Children's Trust Fund of Oregon Grants **1001**

The trust's mission is to support the establishment of community-based direct service programs to provide primary prevention program to reduce the incidence of child abuse and neglect and to promote healthy families. Preference is given to programs that help children by increasing caretaker skills and the knowledge of child development. The trust prefers projects that focus on underserved minorities or geographic areas, and efforts that can be replicated as proven models. There are no deadline dates; proposals are reviewed twice each year.
Requirements: Oregon public and private nonprofit organizations are eligible.
Amount of Grant: $20,000 maximum
Date(s) Application is Due: Apr 1
Contact: Cindy Thompson, Executive Director, (503) 222-7102; fax: (503) 222-6975; email: cindy@ctfo.org
Internet: http://www.ctfo.org
Sponsor: Children's Trust Fund of Oregon
1410 SW Morrison Street, Suite 501
Portland, OR 97205

Children's Cardiomyopathy Foundation Research Grants **1002**

The foundation awards funds to support research related to all forms of cardiomyopathy affecting children under the age of 18 years. The goal of CCF's research program is to advance medical knowledge on the disease and develop more accurate diagnostic methods, life-improving therapies and ultimately a cure. The grant program is designed to provide seed funding to investigators for the testing of initial hypotheses and collecting of preliminary data to help secure long-term funding by the National Institutes of Health and other major granting institutions.
Requirements: Proposals will be accepted on an annual basis for innovative basic, clinical or translational research relevant to the cause or treatment of cardiomyopathy in children. Principal investigators must hold a MD, PhD or equivalent degree and reside in the United States or Canada. The investigator must have a faculty appointment at an accredited U.S. or Canadian institution and have the proven ability to pursue independent research as evidenced by original research in peer-reviewed journals. Guidelines and application forms can be downloaded at the website.
Samples: 2007: Tain-Yen Hsia, MD, Medical University of South Carolina - ($50,000) Extracellular Mechanisms in Pediatric Cardiomyopathy; Anne I. Dipchand, MD, Hospital for Sick Children, Toronto, Canada - ($42,642) Outcome of pediatric patients with cardiomyopathy: a multi-centre review of pediatric patients listed for transplant in the Pediatric Heart Transplant Study. 2006: Tracie Miller, MD, University of Miami, Miami, FL - ($45,000) Exercise Intervention in a Pediatric Population with Cardiomyopathy
Amount of Grant: $25,000 - $50,000
Date(s) Application is Due: Oct 5
Contact: Lisa Yue, Executive Director; (866) 808-2873; fax: (201) 227-7016; email: lyue@childrenscardiomyopathy.org info@childrenscardiomyopathy.org
Internet: http://www.childrenscardiomyopathy.org/site/grants.php
Sponsor: Children's Cardiomyopathy Foundation (CCF)
P.O. Box 547
Tenafly, NJ 07670

Chiles Foundation Grants **1003**

The foundation has a deep concern for and confidence in the future of Oregon and the Pacific Northwest. Although the foundation has made a steady commitment to the improvement of the quality of life for those who live and work in this area, it is not restricted in its grant making to the Pacific Northwest. The foundation has traditionally made grants to certain select institutions of higher education for business schools, scholarships, and athletics; supports basic research in certain select medical institutions; supports religion through divinity schools and religious education; and believes that the arts and cultural activities of a community are important and supports certain select, established institutions. Types of support include building construction/renovation, equipment acquisition, and scholarship funds. Annual deadline dates may vary; contact Foundation by a letter of Inquiry. The Foundation does not accept unsolicited proposals.
Requirements: The preferred initial method of contact is a phone call to the grants administration office to determine whether a prospective proposal is within guidelines; if so, an applicant will be invited to submit a one-page written preliminary proposal. An application form will be sent after approval of the preliminary proposal by the executive committee.
Restrictions: No support for projects involving litigation. Grants are not made to individuals, for deficit financing, mortgage retirement, or projects and conferences already completed.
Geographic Focus: California; OregonGermany

Samples: Boston Symphony Orchestra, Boston, MA, $100,000— general operating support (2008); Stanford University, Stanford, CA, $159,000—scholarship assistance (2008); Ludwig-Maximilians University, Munich, Germany, $180,000—support continuing clinical and experimental research (2008).
Amount of Grant: $1000-$270,000 range
Contact: Earle M. Chiles, President; (503) 222-2143; fax: (503) 228-7079; email: cf@uswest.net
Sponsor: Chiles Foundation
111 South West Fifth Avenue, Suite 4050
Portland, OR 97204-3643

Chiron Foundation Community Grants **1004**
The foundation's focus areas are health and medicine, education, and community. Four imperatives guide health-care giving: accelerating progress toward the prevention and cure or successful management of cancer through research, education, early detection, and public-policy debate; combating infectious disease through prevention-related programs, educational efforts, and therapeutics targeting at-risk populations, with emphasis on the special needs of children and families; ensuring the availability and safety of the blood supply and promoting the highest standards of care for blood donors and recipients; and supporting initiatives in the international medical community to provide vaccines and immunization services to protect at-risk populations, especially children, against the devastation of crippling and lethal diseases. Four imperatives guide education giving: providing training and professional development opportunities to enable classroom teachers to teach science and math more effectively; increasing opportunities for economically disadvantaged students to continue on to postsecondary education; supporting community-based training programs to prepare underrepresented minorities and underprivileged groups for careers in the biosciences; and encouraging and assisting promising scholars to pursue advanced research in the biosciences and medicine. Four imperatives guide community giving: providing early diagnosis, intervention, and support for children with disabilities or other special physical or emotional needs; providing essential social services such as meals and housing to those in greatest need; empowering individuals to achieve self-sufficiency through employment training and job-skill development; and enriching the character and celebrating the distinctives of local communities. Requests are accepted anytime, and proposals are reviewed quarterly.
Requirements: 501(c)3 tax-exempt organizations in Chiron communities (San Francisco East Bay Area, including Alameda, Contra Costa, and Solano Counties; Seattle; and Philadelphia) are eligible.
Restrictions: In general, Chiron does not support organizations that do not have 501(c)3 tax status; religious, fraternal, service, or veterans' organizations; civic or cultural organizations that do not serve the areas in which Chiron is located; alumni drives and teacher organizations; memorials; municipal and for-profit hospitals; labor unions; city, municipal, or federal government departments; organizations or causes that do not support the company's commitment to non-discrimination and diversity; projects of national scope or from national organizations not related to health care; matching gifts; individuals, including scholarships (other than those awarded as part of the company-sponsored college scholarship program); travel support; fund-raising activities related to individual sponsorship; and fund-raising dinners other than those for health care or medical research organizations aligned with company research and product interests.
Geographic Focus: California; Pennsylvania; Washington
Amount of Grant: $5000-$30,000 average, education and community; $15,000-$75,000 health and medicine
Contact: Community Relations, fax: (510) 601-6952; email: Chiron_foundation@chiron.com
Internet: http://www.chiron.com/foundation/index.html
Sponsor: Chiron Foundation
4560 Horton Street
Emeryville, CA 94608

Christine O. Gregoire Youth/Young Adult Award for Outstanding Use of Tobacco Industry Documents **1005**
The award recognizes a person 24 years of age or younger who has made a contribution to the health of the public in the recent past through use of tobacco documents. The award also honors innovation in the use and application of tobacco industry documents to improve the public's health and, where applicable, to further the goals of tobacco prevention and control in order to help build a world where young people reject tobacco and anyone can quit. Those nominated should be individuals who have made a notable impact through innovative use of tobacco industry documents as applied to research, policy, or advocacy.
Requirements: At least one of the following two criteria must be met by the nominated individual: Nominees must have made a remarkable research, policy, or advocacy contribution with the use of tobacco industry documents, and/or; Nominees must have employed innovative, creative approaches to the employment of tobacco industry documents that result in an improvement in the health or public awareness of a community or nation. Nominations may be made by individuals such as colleagues, peers, coworkers, instructors/professors, governments, or CBOs that are qualified to make such a nomination because of their familiarity with the nominee's work and contribution.
Restrictions: Nominees must not have any affiliation with the tobacco industry. Members of the awards committee may not nominate potential recipients, although they may provide written support as part of a nomination package. Employees and directors of the American Legacy Foundation and their relatives are not eligible.
Amount of Grant: $7,500
Date(s) Application is Due: Feb 6
Contact: Virginia Lockmuller, Grant Coordinator; (202) 454-5555; fax: (202) 454-5599; email: awards@americanlegacy.org
Internet: http://www.legacyforhealth.org/awards/
Sponsor: American Legacy Foundation
Legacy Awards, 724 Massachusetts Avenue, NW
Washington, DC 20036

Christopher Reeve Paralysis Foundation Individual Research Grants **1006**
The mission of the foundation is to support cutting-edge research to develop effective treatments and cures for paralysis caused by spinal cord injury and other central nervous system disorders. International individual grants support research that seeks to promote neuronal growth and survival, encourage the formation of synapses, enhance the production of myelin, and restore conduction capabilities in the acutely and chronically injured spinal cord; evaluate drugs or other interventions that protect against secondary neuronal injury or provide insight into the mechanisms causing such damage; elucidate the biological mechanisms underlying approaches to improve concomitant function; and understand anatomical characteristics of injury in both animals and human spinal cord, documenting neuronal systems that are most vulnerable to injury and resultant losses in function. The program is designed to encourage promising new investigators to undertake research on spinal cord regeneration and recovery; encourage researchers who are well-established in other areas to transfer their efforts to spinal cord research; and enable researchers with novel ideas to test their ideas and develop pilot data for seeking larger awards from NIH and other funding sources.
Requirements: Senior scientists, young investigators, and postdoctoral fellows are eligible to serve as principal investigators.
Samples: 13 reseachers nationwide—for research on paralysis resulting from spinal-cord injuries, $1.976 million divided (2003).
Amount of Grant: $75,000 maximum per year, senior scientists and young investigators; $60,000 maximum per year postdoctoral fellowships
Date(s) Application is Due: Jun 15; Dec 15
Contact: Dr. Douglas Landsman, (800) 225-0292; email: dlandsman@crpf.org
Internet: http://www.christopherreeve.org/research/researchmain.cfm
Sponsor: Christopher Reeve Paralysis Foundation
500 Morris Avenue
Springfield, NJ 07081

Christopher Reeve Paralysis Foundation Quality of Life and Health Promotions Grants **1007**
The foundation awards grants to organizations nationwide that help improve opportunities, access, and day-to-day quality of life for individuals living with disabilities—primarily paralysis—and their families. This program recognizes the unique and numerous needs of these individuals and the importance of providing services and programs that enable them to participate in all areas of life. Quality of Life grants are given to programs or projects that improve the daily lives of people living with disabilities, particularly spinal cord injuries. Funding is awarded twice yearly to programs that provide assistance through access, advocacy, education, recreation, and technology, among others. Health Promotion Grants seek to remove societal and environmental barriers that limit the abilities of individuals with paralysis to participate in life activities. Participation in these activities improves physical and emotional health and prevents secondary conditions for persons living with paralysis. Priority funding goes to programs that focus on paralysis generally and are not specific to one condition or disease that results in paralysis. Complete guidelines are available online.
Requirements: 501(c)3 tax-exempt organizations are eligible.
Restrictions: No grants will to individuals, for benefit tickets, or for courtesy advertising.
Samples: To be distributed among 126 nonprofit groups nationwide—for awards through the Quality of Life program, which seeks to improve the well-being of people who are paralyzed, $779,321 (2004).
Amount of Grant: $5000-$25,000 quality of life grants; $25,000 program awards (health promotion); $5000-$10,000 direct impact awards (health promotion)
Date(s) Application is Due: Mar 1; Sep 1
Contact: Donna Valente, Quality of Life Grants Coordinator, (800) 539-7309 or (973) 467-8270 ext 211; email: qol@crpf.org
Internet: http://www.christopherreeve.org/qlgrants/qlgrantsmain.cfm
Sponsor: Christopher Reeve Paralysis Foundation
500 Morris Avenue
Springfield, NJ 07081

Christy-Houston Foundation Grants **1008**
The foundation awards grants to nonprofits in Rutherford County, TN, for health, education, arts and culture, and community development. Areas of interest include hospitals, nursing care, health care and health associations, nutrition, hospice care, and community development. Types of support include building construction/renovation, equipment acquisition, scholarship funds, and matching funds. Application forms are not required, and there are no application deadlines. The board meets in March, June, September, and December to consider requests.
Requirements: 501(c)3 nonprofits in Rutherford County, TN, are eligible.
Restrictions: Grants are not awarded to: religious organizations for religious purposes, veterans organizations, historical societies, individuals, operating expenses or endowments.
Geographic Focus: Tennessee
Samples: City of Murfreesboro, Murfreesboro,TN, $1,000,000—Chambers of Commerce Building (2007); City of Murfreesboro, Murfreesboro,TN, $88,000-fitness program (2007); Easter Seals, $5,050—camp scholarships (2007).

Amount of Grant: $50,000-$200,000 average
Contact: Robert B. Mifflin, Executive Director; (615) 898-1140; fax: (615) 895-9524
Sponsor: Christy-Houston Foundation
1296 Dow Street
Murfreesboro, TN 37130-2413

Chula Vista Charitable Foundation Grants **1009**
Community leaders throughout Chula Vista are partnering with the San Diego Foundation to create and sustain a local foundation to serve solely the community of Chula Vista. Endow Chula Vista is a community-specific effort to focus on endowment building for Chula Vista, now and for generations to come. It is part of The San Diego Foundation's region-wide initiative, Endow San Diego, to inform and inspire San Diegans regarding the benefits of endowment.
Requirements: Any 501(c)3 organization serving the residents of Chula Vista, California, are eligible to apply.
Restrictions: The Chula Vista Charitable Foundation does not make grants for: annual campaigns and fund raising events for non-specific purposes; capital campaigns for buildings or facilities; stipends for attendance at conferences; endowments or chairs; for-profit organizations or enterprises; individuals unaffiliated with a qualified fiscal sponsor; projects that promote religious or political doctrine; research projects (medical or otherwise); scholarships; or existing obligations or debt.
Geographic Focus: California
Contact: Kerry Helmer; (619) 814-1384; email: kerry@sdfoundation.org;; Jennifer Quijano; (619) 814-1384; email: jquijano@chulavistaca.gov
Internet: http://www.endowchulavista.org/
Sponsor: Chula Vista Charitable Foundation / San Diego Foundation
2508 Historic Decatur Road, Suite 200
San Diego, CA 92106

CICF Legacy Fund Community Foundation Grants **1010**
The fund awards grants to Hamilton County nonprofits to enhance the quality of life through support of arts and culture, civic affairs, education, health, and social services. Types of support include program development grants and scholarships. Application forms are available on the Web site.
Requirements: In reviewing grant applications, the Foundation gives careful consideration to: The potential impact of the grant and the number of Hamilton County individuals who will benefit; Programs and projects which promote inclusiveness and diversity; Programs and projects which are responsive to basic human needs; Programs and project which connect individuals and families to our community; The extent of commitment and capacity of the organization's directors, trustees, and volunteers to carry out the program or project; The degree to which the applicant works with or complements the services of other organizations in an attempt to eliminate duplication of services; The organization's fiscal responsibility and management qualifications; The possibility of using the grant to match funds from other sources; The ability of the organization to obtain the necessary additional funding to implement the project and to provide or obtain ongoing funding after the grant has been expended.
Restrictions: Limited to not-for-profit organizations and for the benefit of the people of Hamilton County, Indiana.
Geographic Focus: Indiana
Amount of Grant: $1,500-$20,000
Date(s) Application is Due: Mar 1; May 1; Sep 1; Nov 1
Contact: Liz Tate; (317) 843-2479, ext. 302; fax (317) 848-5463; email: lizt@cicf.org
Internet: http://www.cicf.org/newsarticle.cfm?articleid=9842&ptsidebaroptid=0&returnto=page26437.cfm&returntoname=How%20To%20Apply&siteid=1824&pageid=26545&sidepageid=26437&banner1img=banner%5F1%2EJPG&banner2img=banner%5F2%2EJPG&bannerbg=bannerbg%2Egif
Sponsor: Central Indiana Community Foundation
515 E. Main Street, Suite 100
Carmel, IN 46032

CIGNA Foundation Grants **1011**
CIGNA Foundation has identified four areas for grant consideration—health and human services, education, community and civic affairs, and culture and the arts. Health and education are of primary concern and receive priority. Under education, priority is placed on public secondary education, higher education for minorities, and adult basic education/literacy. The foundation also considers requests from U.S. cultural, educational, and public policy organizations that have international components. Requests are accepted and reviewed throughout the year. Consideration will be given to requests for general operating support, program development, annual campaigns, conferences and seminars, fellowships, scholarship funds and employee-related scholarships, and matching gifts and funds.
Requirements: Organizations with 501(c)3 tax-exempt status are eligible.
Restrictions: The foundation will not consider applications for grants to individuals, organizations operating to influence legislation or litigation, political organizations, or religious activities. In general, the foundation will not consider applications from organizations receiving substantial support through the United Way or other CIGNA-supported federated funding agencies; hospitals' capital improvements; or research, prevention, and treatment of specific diseases.
Samples: Susan G. Komen Breast Cancer Foundation (Dallas, TX)—for the work of this organization, which supports research and awareness programs to help combat breast cancer, $25,000 (2005).
Amount of Grant: $5000-$50,000 average
Contact: Program Contact, email: communityrelations@cigna.com
Internet: http://www.cigna.com/general/about/community/grant_information.html
Sponsor: CIGNA Foundation
1601 Chestnut Street, TL06B
Philadelphia, PA 19192-1540

CIIT Postdoctoral Fellowships **1012**
Ten to 15 fellowships are offered annually to support persons holding recently earned PhD, MD, or DVM degrees during further training in genetic toxicology, immunotoxicology, biochemical toxicology, pathology, reproductive toxicology, epidemiology, teratology, and carcinogenesis. Fellowships are tenable at the institute for two to three years. The institute holds 501(c)6 status. Applications are available on the Web site.
Requirements: Applicants who recently were awarded PhD degrees in a discipline related to toxicology are eligible to apply; those holding recently awarded DVM or MD degrees are expected to have substantial research experience.
Restrictions: Traineeships and fellowships are awarded only for research conducted at the CIIT. Awardees may not use their stipends to supplement funds from other awards.
Amount of Grant: $27,000 first year; $28,500 second year
Contact: Rusty Bramlage, Human Resources Manager, (919) 558-1331; fax: (919) 558-1300; email: bramlage@ciit.org
Internet: http://www.ciit.org/careers/openings_postdoc.asp
Sponsor: Chemical Industry Institute of Toxicology
P.O. Box 12137
Research Triangle Park, NC 27709

Cinergy Foundation Grants **1013**
The Cinergy corporate contributions program was developed to reinvest in southwest Ohio, northern Kentucky, and Indiana communities. The mission of the foundation is to be a national leader in community development by creating proactive, innovative partnerships that improve the quality of life in Indiana, Ohio, and Kentucky, especially within the electric utility's 69-county service area. Grant categories include arts and culture; lifelong learning—K-12 (BASICS) and higher education; and healthy communities—environment and youth. Applicants are requested to submit grant applications to the district office closest to them; contact program staff for office locations. The board meets in April, July, October, and December to consider requests.
Requirements: The foundation supports projects and programs of 501(c)3 tax-exempt organizations located in 10 southwestern Ohio counties, six northern Kentucky counties, and sixty nine Indiana counties.
Restrictions: Grants do not support advertising; capital and endowment campaigns; competitions (scholastic or athletic); construction/renovation projects; equipment purchases of any type (playground, computers, etc.); golf events; K-12 schools outside the BASICS program; membership dues; organizations without 501(c)3 status; programs that pose a potential conflict of interest; projects/organizations benefiting an individual or a few persons; requests outside the Cinergy service territory; scholarship programs; sponsorships for athletic teams; travel expenses for individuals or groups; uniforms; or veterans, labor, religious, political, or fraternal groups.
Geographic Focus: Indiana; Kentucky; Ohio
Amount of Grant: $50,000 maximum
Contact: Karol King, Foundation Manager, (800) 262-3000 ext 1251 or (513) 287-1251; email: kking@cinergy.com
Internet: http://www.cinergy.com/Community/Cinergy_Foundation/default.asp
Sponsor: Cinergy Foundation Inc
139 E Fourth Street
Cincinnati, OH 45202

CIT Corporate Giving Grants **1014**
The corporate giving program focuses its giving to programs that substantially strengthen the communities where CIT has a significant presence; provide services that benefit employees, their families, and communities; and support employee volunteerism. Funding priorities include organizations, institutions, or programs that work to foster excellence in education, particularly among at-risk and underprivileged youth; support local health and social welfare issues; help stabilize and improve neighborhoods by providing viable economic and educational growth opportunities to the community; and support the arts, and their accessibility, as a means of enhancing personal and social development. Proposals are reviewed on an ongoing basis and must be formally submitted by mail.
Requirements: 501(c)3 tax-exempt organizations and Canadian charities registered with the Canada Customs and Revenue Agency (CCRA) are eligible.
Restrictions: The following will not be considered for funding: political organizations, campaigns, or candidates; conferences, memberships, or sports competitions; organizations that discriminate in any way with national equal opportunity policies; organizations whose chief purpose is to influence legislation; veteran and fraternal organizations; religious organizations, unless engaged in a significant, nonsectarian project that benefits a broad base of the community; or individuals.
Contact: Stacy Papas, Manager, Community Affairs, email: stacy.papas@cit.com
Internet: http://www.cit.com/main/about-cit/corporate-giving/
Sponsor: CIT Group Inc
11 W. 42 Street
New York, NY 10036

Citizens Bank Mid-Atlantic Charitable Foundation Grants **1015**
Charitable grants are made only to qualified 501(c)3 Rhode Island-based organizations serving Rhode Island residents. Citizens look for opportunities where moderate funding can affect significant results in the community. Priority consideration is given to programs

that encourage the development of innovative responses to basic human needs; promote fair housing and focus on community issues of neighborhood development and economic self-sufficiency; support the availability of quality, cost-effective, community-based health care, particularly for low-income families and children who are at risk; promote new ways to provide a quality education to populations that are underserved, including job training; promote availability and accessibility in the area of culture and the arts; and promote citizen participation in the development of new and workable solutions for improving and maintaining a healthy environment. Charitable grants are usually for capital funding (to build or renovate a facility) or implementation of a specific program.
Requirements: 501(c)3 Rhode Island-based nonprofits are eligible.
Restrictions: Grants do not support individuals, single disease/issue research organizations, religious organizations for religious purposes, labor or fraternal or veterans groups, political organizations or projects, operating deficits, underwriting of conferences and seminars, governmental public agencies, endowments, annual operating support, trips and tours, payment on bank loans, advertising, or fund-raising events.
Geographic Focus: Rhode Island
Amount of Grant: $1000-$100,000 average
Contact: Jeanne Cola, Charitable Grants, (401) 456-7038; fax: (401) 456-7366
Sponsor: Citizens Bank Mid-Atlantic Charitable Foundation
870 Westminster Street
Providence, RI 02903

CJ Foundation for SIDS Express Grants 1016
The foundation addresses the special needs of the SIDS community. This program provides a simple manner for organizations to apply for funding. Areas considered for funding are: Programmatic: funding for specific programs/projects including support/bereavement services, education and public awareness, sponsorship of relevant meetings and conferences; Administrative/Management: includes general operating support directly associated with the effective delivery of services and/or efficient management of the organization; and Staffing Needs: salary support for staff positions (full-time or part-time) and/or project consultants.
Amount of Grant: $500 minimum; $5000 maximum
Contact: Program Director, (866) 314-7437; email: wendy@cjsids.com
Internet: http://www.cjsids.com/grant_programs.htm
Sponsor: CJ Foundation for SIDS
30 Prospect Avenue
Hackensack, NJ 07601

CJ Foundation for SIDS Support Services Grants 1017
The foundation addresses the special needs of the SIDS community. Support services grants comprise program support—funding for support services, education and public awareness, and sponsorship of relevant meetings and conferences; administrative/management support— general operating support directly associated with efficient management of the grantee's organization (may include the purchase of equipment); temporary staffing needs—grants for full- or part-time staff positions; and special projects—i.e., initial underwriting associated with new programs and innovative pilot or demonstration projects.
Samples: Tomorrow's Child/Michigan SIDS (Lansing, MI)—to upgrade its systems in order to better support families who have lost a child because of sudden infant death syndrome or other causes, $15,000 (2003).
Amount of Grant: $5000 maximum
Date(s) Application is Due: Mar 15
Contact: Program Director, (866) 314-7437; email: wendy@cjsids.com
Internet: http://www.cjsids.com/grant_programs.htm
Sponsor: CJ Foundation for SIDS
30 Prospect Avenue
Hackensack, NJ 07601

CLA Nurses Respiratory Society Fellowships 1018
The objective of the fellowships is to permit nurses to pursue graduate study so that they may be better able to contribute to the Canadian field of respiratory illness and health care. Applicants may register in any master's or doctoral program where knowledge, skill, and expertise may develop toward this objective. The program should show evidence of a plan to foster theory, research, and either a clinical or functional area of specialization. Application forms may be obtained from the association.
Requirements: Applicant must be a Canadian citizen or permanent Canadian resident, be a registered nurse, be enrolled full-time in a graduate program at the master's or doctoral level, and be a member of CNRS.
Amount of Grant: $C3750-$C7500
Date(s) Application is Due: Feb 1
Contact: Grants Administrator, (416) 864-9911; fax: (416) 864-9916; email: orcs@on.lung.ca
Internet: http://www.on.lung.ca/orcs/fellowships.html
Sponsor: Canadian Lung Association
1900 City Park Drive, Suite 508
Gloucester, ON K1J 1A3 Canada

CLA Nurses Respiratory Society Nursing Research Grants 1019
Research grants are offered to those studying respiratory nursing, chronic or acute lung disease, which will result in improved quality of patient care. Research may include clinical investigation of any nursing-related phenomenon; be pertinent to illness assessment, management, or responses; or be aimed at health promotion and prevention issues. Studies may use either quantitative or qualitative methodologies.
Requirements: Applicant must be a Canadian citizen or permanent Canadian resident; a registered nurse; hold an appointment in, or have an affiliation with, a health care agency, educational institution, or other organization in Canada that can administer the funds in an approved manner; and be a member of CNRS.
Amount of Grant: $C3000-$C30,000
Date(s) Application is Due: Nov 1
Contact: Grant Administrator, (613) 747-6776; fax: (613) 747-7430; email: dhogg@cha.ab.ca
Internet: http://www.lung.ca/resp/Fellowships/Fellow_Grants.htm
Sponsor: Canadian Lung Association
1900 City Park Drive, Suite 508
Gloucester, ON K1J 1A3 Canada

CLA Physiotherapy Cardio-Respiratory Society Fellowships 1020
The purpose of the research program is to pursue increased scientific knowledge in the area of cardio-respiratory physiotherapy practice. Fellowships are offered to physiotherapists pursuing postgraduate training, with respiratory research as the major component. The award period is one year.
Requirements: Applicants must be Canadian citizens or permanent Canadian residents, be registered physiotherapists, be enrolled or accepted for full-time study in a graduate program at the master's or doctoral level, and be a member of the Canadian Physiotherapy Cardio-Respiratory Society.
Amount of Grant: $C6000-$C12,000
Date(s) Application is Due: Nov 1
Contact: Administrator, Societies & Special Projects, (613) 569-6411; email: nprt@lung.ca
Internet: http://www.lung.ca/crhp/index.html
Sponsor: Canadian Lung Association
1900 City Park Drive, Suite 508
Gloucester, ON K1J 1A3 Canada

Clarcor Foundation Grants 1021
Clarcor, through its foundation, seeks to improve the quality of life in the communities in which the company operates. Grants support nonprofits in the categories of health, human services, education, culture and art, and civic activities. Types of support include general operating support, annual campaigns, capital campaigns, and employee matching gifts. There are no application deadlines. The board meets in February, May, August, and November.
Requirements: Tax-exempt organizations in company-operating areas in Rockford, IL; Louisville, KY; Kearney and Gothenburg, NE; Cincinnati, OH; Oklahoma, and Lancaster, PA; are eligible.
Restrictions: Grants are not made to support individuals, endowment funds, research, scholarships, fellowships, or loans.
Geographic Focus: Illinois; Kentucky; Nebraska; North Carolina; Ohio; Oklahoma; Pennsylvania
Samples: Boys & Girls Assoc of Rockford (IL)—to support the Crime Prevention program, $3000.; New American Theater (Rockford, IL)—for educational outreach, $6000.; Lancaster Theological Seminary (Lancaster, PA)—to fund creation of a computerized card catalog system, $2500.; Boy Scouts of America (Kearney, NE)—to support the annual campaign, $1000.
Amount of Grant: $500-$50,250 range
Contact: Pete Nangel, (815) 962-8867; fax: (815) 962-0417
Sponsor: Clarcor Foundation
840 Crescent Centre Drive, Suite 600
Franklin, TN 37067

Clarence E. Heller Charitable Foundation Grants 1022
The charitable foundation supports nonprofit organizations, with priority given to proposals from California, in its areas of interest, including environment and health—to prevent serious risk to human health from toxic substances and other environmental hazards by supporting programs in research, education, and policy development; management of resources—to protect and preserve the earth's limited resources by assisting programs that demonstrate how natural resources can be managed on a sustainable and an ecologically sound basis, and supporting initiatives for sustainable agriculture, and for promoting the long-term viability of communities and regions; music—to encourage the playing, enjoyment, and accessibility of symphonic and chamber music by providing scholarship and program assistance at selected community music organizations and schools, and by helping community-based ensembles of demonstrated quality implement artistic initiatives, diversify and increase audiences, and improve fund-raising capacity; and education—to focus on support for programs that improve the teaching skills of educators and artists in environmental and arts education. Types of support include continuing support, general operating expenses, publications, research, seed money, and special projects. The foundation's board meets typically in March, June, and October. Letters of inquiry are accepted at any time.
Requirements: 501(c)3 tax-exempt organizations are eligible.
Restrictions: Grants are not made to individuals.
Geographic Focus: California
Samples: Crossroads School, Santa Monica, CA, $50,000— to support the Elizabeth Mandell Music Institute (2008); Brentwood Agricultural Land Trust, Brentwood, CA, $50,000—for a program to save productive agricultural lands on the urban edge and market farm products from family-scale farms (2008); Graduate School of Education,

UC Berkeley, Berkeley, CA, $10,000—for the Principal Leadership Institute Scholarship Endowment Fund (2008).
Amount of Grant: $5,000-$600,000 range
Contact: Bruce Hirsch, Executive Director; (415) 989-9839; fax: (415) 989-1909; email: info@cehcf.org
Internet: http://cehcf.org/app_info.html
Sponsor: Clarence E. Heller Charitable Foundation
44 Montgomery Street, Suite 1970
San Francisco, CA 94104

Clarian Health Critical / Progressive Care Internships **1023**
The Clarian Health Critical / Progressive Care Internship Program is a 12 week individualized program. The Internship is offered year round, complete with salary. The program provides experience in the following specialized services: adult critical care; cardiac; comprehensive critical care; cardiovascular critical care; medical intensive care; neuro/trauma critical care; neuro-surgery intensive care; progressive care; surgical intensive care
Requirements: Contact Julie Ruschhaupt, Critical Care Recruiter, to begin application process
Geographic Focus: Indiana
Contact: Julie Ruschhaupt, Critical Care Recruiter, (317) 278-7082 or (877) 354-2996; email: jruschhaupt@clarian.org
Internet: http://www.clarian.org/clarianjobs/nursing/internships_externships.htm#top
Sponsor: Clarian Health Partners, Inc.
950 North Meridian Street, Gateway Plaza
Indianapolis, IN 46204

Clarian Health Multi-Specialty Internships **1024**
The Clarian Health Multi-Specialty Internship is a 7 to 8 week individualized program, that is offered year round.
Requirements: Contact Joy Fay for additional information to apply.
Geographic Focus: Indiana
Contact: Joy Fay, RN, (317) 962-3788; email: jfay@clarian.org
Internet: http://www.clarian.org/clarianjobs/nursing/internships_externships.htm#multi
Sponsor: Clarian Health Partners, Inc.
950 North Meridian Street, Gateway Plaza
Indianapolis, IN 46204

Clarian Health OR Internships **1025**
The Clarian Health OR Internship Program is offered twice a year, for a duration of 6 months. The program provides experience in the following specialized services: general; cardio thoracic; cardiovascular; endoscopies; ENT; GYN; laser; neurosurgery; ophthalmology; orthopedics; pediatrics; plastic / Reconstructive; transplants; trauma; urology
Geographic Focus: Indiana
Contact: Shalunda Tyler, Clarian Health Nurse Recruiter, (317) 962-9083; email: styler1@clarian.org
Internet: http://www.clarian.org/clarianjobs/nursing/internships_externships.htm#multi
Sponsor: Clarian Health Partners, Inc.
950 North Meridian Street, Gateway Plaza
Indianapolis, IN 46204

Clarian Health Scholarships for LPNs **1026**
The Clarian Health Scholarships for LPNs Program provides an award of $750 per semester. The scholarship does require a post graduate commitment of 6 months full-time employment for each semester of funding.
Requirements: Applicant must: be employed as an LPN at Clarian; be in good standing to receive the scholarship. A participant whose job performance does not meet the standards of Clarian's performance review program during any time of the employment period/year that the scholarship is in effect will jeopardize his/her opportunity for future funding; be actively involved in Clinical Unit Operations (i.e., attend staff meetings, keep mandatory education requirements up to date, etc.); must maintain a competitive GPA. To complete the application process, you must: complete the online application; schedule appointment to complete paperwork; submit proof of enrollment in an approved nursing school; submit 2 professional recommendations; one from current manager, one from RN co-worker; submit a one-page narrative on why you should be awarded the scholarship
Geographic Focus: Indiana
Amount of Grant: $750 per semester
Date(s) Application is Due: Jul 1 - Jul 31, Nov 1 - Nov 30
Contact: Clarian Nurse Recruitment Line, (877) 354-2996
Internet: http://www.clarian.org/clarianjobs/nursing/lpnscholarship.htm
Sponsor: Clarian Health Partners, Inc.
950 North Meridian Street, Gateway Plaza
Indianapolis, IN 46204

Clarian Health Student Nurse Extern Scholarships **1027**
The Clarian Health Student Nurse Extern Scholarship Program offers scholarships for each semester worked as a student nurse extern (SNE) at one of the three downtown Clarian hospitals: Methodist Hospital, Indiana University Hospital and Riley Hospital for Children. The SNE Scholarship Program offers several options to meet scheduling and financial needs. See website for details.
Requirements: Any nursing student in good standing and actively enrolled in a program that results in a RN degree may apply. A nursing student must meet the requirements of the SNE job description by completing at least one semester of nursing clinicals and remain actively enrolled and a student in good standing in the school of nursing they are attending. To apply for a Student Nurse Extern position at Clarian health, please send resume to dspilker@clarian.org. In a cover letter or the objective section of your resume, indicate your interest in the Student Nurse Extern position.
Geographic Focus: Indiana
Amount of Grant: $250 - $1,000 range per semester
Contact: Clarian Recruitment Line, (877) 354-2996; email: dspilker@clarian.org
Internet: http://www.clarian.org/portal/patients/education?clarianContentID=/education/nursing_education/SNE.xml
Sponsor: Clarian Health Partners, Inc.
950 North Meridian Street, Gateway Plaza
Indianapolis, IN 46204

Clark County Community Foundation Grants **1028**
Clark County Community Foundation will award grants to 501(c)3 charitable organizations, schools, and exempt governmental units or their subdivisions serving Clark County, Kentucky. Areas of interest include arts and culture, housing, employment support and education. Grants will range from approximately $5,000 to $10,000. To apply, submit a letter of inquiry of no more than three pages by 4:00 pm, March 15. Applicants will then be invited to submit full proposals, which are due by May 15.
Requirements: Clark County, Kentucky, nonprofit organizations are eligible.
Geographic Focus: Kentucky
Amount of Grant: $5,000-$10,000
Date(s) Application is Due: Mar 15; May 15
Contact: Barbara A. Fischer, Grants Officer; (859) 225-3343; fax: (859) 243-0770; email: bfischer@bgcf.org
Internet: http://www.bgcf.org/page27526.cfm
Sponsor: Clark County Community Foundation
250 West Main Street, Suite 1220
Lexington, KY 40507

Clark Foundation Grants **1029**
The foundation awards grants in New York, NY, and upstate New York for charitable and educational purposes and in support of health care, youth, cultural, environmental, and community organizations. Types of support include general operating support, continuing support, annual campaigns, capital campaigns, building construction/renovation, equipment acquisition, program development, seed money, and scholarships to Cooperstown County residents.
Requirements: Nonprofits in upstate New York and New York, NY, are eligible.
Geographic Focus: New York
Samples: Harlem RBI (New York, NY)—for general operating support, $100,000 (2004); Partnership with Children (New York, NY)—for general support, $150,000 (2003).
Amount of Grant: $20,000-$200,000 average range
Date(s) Application is Due: Jan 1; Apr 1; Jul 15; Oct 1
Contact: Charles Hamilton, Executive Director, (212) 977-6900
Sponsor: Clark Foundation
1 Rockefeller Plz, 31st Floor
New York, NY 10020

Clark-Winchcole Foundation Grants **1030**
The foundation awards grants to nonprofit organizations in the District of Columbia, with an emphasis on higher education, hospitals and health care, cultural programs, youth, the disabled, and religion. Types of support include general operating support, scholarships, and building construction/renovation. Applicants should submit a letter of inquiry that includes a description of the project, amount requested, audited financial report, budget, and proof of tax-exempt status. Further information will be requested by the foundation if interested.
Requirements: Only nonprofits in the District of Columbia are eligible to apply.
Geographic Focus: District of Columbia
Samples: Wolf Trap Foundation for the Performing Arts, Vienna, VA — $200,000 to assist in the capital campaign for the Center for Education; Washington Jesuit Academy, Washington, DC — $75,000 towards general operating support; District of Columbia College Access Program (DC)—$100,000 for general operating support.
Amount of Grant: $5000-$50,000 average
Contact: Vincent Burke, President, (301) 654-3607
Sponsor: Clark-Winchcole Foundation
3 Bethesda Metro Ctr, Suite 550
Bethesda, MD 20814

Claude Bennett Family Foundation Grants **1031**
Established in Alabama in 1993, the Claude Bennett Family Foundation has as its primary interest areas: health care, health organizations, higher education, human services, and Protestant churches and agencies. The range of funding is up to $15,000, and the Foundation has supported agencies across the U.S. There are no specific applications or deadlines with which to adhere, and applicants should contact the Foundation in writing, stating the purpose of their request and offering a detailed budget.
Samples: Food Bank of Larimer County, Fort Collins, Colorado, $1,500 (2007); Poudre School District, Fort Collins, Colorado, $3,000 (2007); South Highland Presbyterian Church, Birmingham, Alabama, $11,025 (2007); Penguin Project, East Peoria, Illinois, $1,000 (2007).

Amount of Grant: $15,000 average
Contact: Harold I. Apolinsky, Treasurer; (205) 930-5122; fax: (205) 212-3888; email: hapolinsky@sirote.com
Sponsor: Claude Bennett Family Foundation
P.O. Box 130804, 2311 Highland Avenue, S
Birmingham, AL 35213-0804

Claude Pepper Foundation Grants 1032
The foundation makes grants primarily to support the work of the Claude Pepper Center and the Pepper Institute on Aging and Public Policy, both located at Florida State University, Tallahassee, FL. The foundation makes limited grants to other organizations to continue the work and vision of Claude and Mildred Pepper. The foundation also supports a visiting scholars program and an oratory competition for Florida students. Grants are usually made for a period of one year and except in rare instances no grant will be made for longer than a three-year period of time. Guidelines are available online.
Requirements: 501(c)3 tax-exempt organizations are eligible.
Samples: Florida Council on Aging - To support Special Plenary Sessions at the Annual Aging Network Conferences; National Academy of Social Insurance - To sponsor the Academy's annual conference opening dinner in Washington, D.C., which addressed issues surrounding Social Security reform; Tallahassee Senior Center - To co-sponsor the Claude Pepper Senior Walk/Run, which consists of a competition for walkers over the age of 60, and one for runners, with prizes and refreshments.
Contact: John T. Herndon, Executive Director; 850) 644-9309; fax: (850) 644-9301; email: herndon@claudepepperfoundation.org
Internet: http://www.claudepepperfoundation.org/programs_grants.cfm
Sponsor: Claude Pepper Foundation
636 West Call Street
Tallahassee, FL 32306-1122

Claude Worthington Benedum Foundation Grants 1033
Grants are made in the areas of education, health and human services, community and economic development, environment, and the arts. Grants have been awarded to support education reform, teacher education, higher education, workforce development, rural health, professional developing in healthcare, human services, affordable housing, and economic development. Grants are awarded to organizations in West Virginia and southwestern Pennsylvania. Funds are provided for general operations for projects, sometimes including building and equipment, in West Virginia, and for projects in Pittsburgh that address regional problems and needs, that establish demonstration projects with strong potential for replication in West Virginia, or make outstanding contributions to the area. Additional types of support include matching funds, consulting services, technical assistance, capital campaigns, conferences and seminars, research, and seed grants. Organizations wishing to apply should request a copy of the annual report, which includes application guidelines. Applications may be submitted at any time; the board meets for review in March, June, September, and December.
Requirements: Southwestern Pennsylvania and West Virginia nonprofit organizations may apply.
Restrictions: Support is not given for national health and welfare campaigns, medical research, religious activities, fellowships, scholarships, annual campaigns, or travel.
Geographic Focus: Pennsylvania; West Virginia
Contact: Margaret M. Martin, Grants Administrator; (800) 223-5948 or (412) 246-3636; fax: (412) 288-0366; email: mmartin@benedum.org
Internet: http://www.benedum.org/pages.cfm?id=10
Sponsor: Claude Worthington Benedum Foundation
1400 Benedum-Trees Building, 223 Fourth Avenue
Pittsburgh, PA 15222

Clay Foundation Grants 1034
The primary mission of the foundation is to promote and enhance the quality of life of the citizens of West Virginia. Initially, grants will be confined to organizations or projects within the greater Kanawha Valley that significantly affect its residents. The foundation considers a broad range of organizations, though special interest is given to programs in the field of aging; health care, research, and education; vocational education; and services to disadvantaged youth and their families. Applicants are asked to submit a preliminary letter. If foundation priorities and resources permit consideration of the request, a detailed formal proposal may be requested. There are no deadline dates for the submission of preliminary letters. The board meets four times annually, generally in January, April, July, and October, at which times applications are considered and grants made.
Requirements: IRS 501(c)3 tax-exempt organizations in West Virginia are eligible.
Restrictions: Grants are not made for ongoing normal operations, debt retirement or operational deficits, contributions to endowment or scholarship funds, annual appeals or other fund-raising events, national fund-raising campaigns, religious organizations for religious purposes, or grants to conduit organizations.
Geographic Focus: West Virginia
Samples: U of Charleston (WV)—to construct the Buckner and Lyell Clay Ctr, $1.15 million.; Charleston Catholic High School (Charleston, WV)—for the science wing, $60,000.; Fund for the Arts (Charleston, WV)—challenge grant, $60,000. West Virginia State Museum—for renovation, $350,000.
Amount of Grant: $5000-$75,000 average
Contact: Charles Avampato, President, (304) 344-8656; fax: (304) 344-3805
Sponsor: Clay Foundation
1426 Kanawha Blvd E
Charleston, WV 25301

Cleo Foundation Grants 1035
The foundation supports public charities in San Francisco, San Benito, Mendocino, and southern Monterey counties, with primary interest in supporting organizations that benefit at-risk and/or low-income children, youth, and adults. The foundation is most interested in programs that can make good use of relatively small grants. Types of support include building construction/renovation, capital campaigns, continuing support, operating support, and program development. Applications are due 12 weeks before board meetings in March and September. Request guidelines in writing.
Requirements: 501(c)3 organizations in San Francisco, San Benito, Mendocino, and southern Monterey counties in California may apply.
Geographic Focus: California
Amount of Grant: $1000-$20,000
Contact: Mary Gregory, Executive Director, (415) 561-6540; fax: (415) 561-6477; email: mgregory@pfs-llc.net
Internet: http://www.pfs-llc.net/cleo.html
Sponsor: Cleo Foundation
P.O. Box 29906, Presidio Building 1016, Suite 300
San Francisco, CA 94129-0906

Cleveland Browns Foundation Grants 1036
The foundation supports the northeast Ohio community by funding programs that improve the lives of disadvantaged children. The foundation's four focus areas are education, arts and culture, health, and career development as they relate to children. There are no application deadlines.
Requirements: Northern Ohio nonprofit organizations are eligible. Applications sold be submitted by mail
Restrictions: Organizations and causes that will not be considered for funding include fund-raising, sponsorship events, or donation requests; religious organizations for sectarian religious purposes; general or annual operation expenses; capital or building funds; or staff salaries or stipends.
Geographic Focus: Ohio
Contact: Grant Program, (440) 891-5063; fax, (440) 891-7529.
Internet: http://www.clevelandbrowns.com/community/foundation
Sponsor: Cleveland Browns Foundation
Community Relations Department, 76 Lou Groza Boulevard
Berea, OH 44017

CLF Fellowships 1037
The fellowships provide support for specialized clinical or experimental training in hepatic function or disease to individuals who have already completed the basic graduate program. The value of the fellowship is based on the qualifications and seniority of the applicant and will include, if applicable, a travel grant equivalent to return economy airfare for the grantee and spouse between the university of origin and the place of training. Guidelines and application forms are available from the office and in medical schools through the office of the Dean of the Faculty of Medicine.
Requirements: Candidates must hold an MD or PhD degree or equivalent. Canadian citizens and landed immigrants who are resident in Canada at the time of application or Canadian citizens who are normally resident in Canada are eligible. Applications must be sponsored by a Canadian Faculty of Medicine or Health Sciences and accompanied by a letter of support from the Dean (or designee).
Amount of Grant: $C30,000 maximum per year
Date(s) Application is Due: Mar 31
Contact: Research Awards Administrator, (800) 563-5483 or (416) 491-3353; fax: (416) 491-4952; email: clf@liver.ca
Internet: http://www.liver.ca/Research/Grant_Program
Sponsor: Canadian Liver Foundation
2235 Sheppard Ave E, Suite 1500
Toronto, ON M2J 5B5 Canada

CLF Graduate Studentships 1038
Studentships enable academically superior students to undertake full-time studies in Canadian universities in disciplines relevant to liver function, structure, and disease. Awards are for one academic year and may be renewed three times for a total of four years of support. Registrants in an MS program are restricted to a maximum of three years of support. Guidelines are available from the office or at medical schools through the office of the Dean of the Faculty of Medicine.
Requirements: The candidate must be accepted into a full-time university graduate science program in a medically related discipline related to a master's or doctoral degree; hold a record of superior academic performance; and be sponsored by a faculty supervisor with a record of productive medical research and sufficient, competitively acquired research funding to ensure the satisfactory conduct of the student's research during the term of the award.
Amount of Grant: $C16,500 per year
Date(s) Application is Due: Mar 31
Contact: Billie Potkonjak, (800) 563-5483; fax: (416) 491-4952; email: bpotkonjak@liver.ca
Internet: http://www.liver.ca/Research/Grant_Program
Sponsor: Canadian Liver Foundation
2235 Sheppard Ave E, Suite 1500
Toronto, ON M2J 5B5 Canada

CLF Operating Grants 1039

The grants provide funding to help fully qualified and trained hepatologists and basic scientists begin liver research projects in their own laboratories at Canadian universities. Candidates must be prepared to spend 80 percent of their time in research and to commit the remaining time to active participation in teaching and/or patient care.

Requirements: Candidates must hold an MD or PhD or equivalent and have a proven interest in liver structure, function, or disease. The applicant must have completed a minimum of two and preferably three years of formal research training (post medical specialty training in the case of MDs) and have obtained additional research experience as a clinical investigator or postdoctoral fellow under the supervision of a well-established, competitively funded, senior basic or clinical scientific faculty colleague who holds a faculty level position.

Amount of Grant: $C60,000 maximum per year for two years

Date(s) Application is Due: Mar 31

Contact: Research Awards Administrator, (416) 964-1953; fax: (416) 964-0024; email: bpotkonjak@liver.ca

Internet: http://www.liver.ca/Research/Grant_Program

Sponsor: Canadian Liver Foundation
2235 Sheppard Ave E, Suite 1500
Toronto, ON M2J 5B5 Canada

CLIF Bar Family Foundation Grants 1040

The foundation's mission is to support nonprofits — grassroots organizations in particular — working to promote environmental restoration and conservation, sustainable food and agriculture, people's health, and a wide range of social concerns. It focuses on organizations whose missions support environmental restoration and conservation, sustainable food and agriculture, people's health and youth.

Requirements: The foundation funds nonprofit organizations working on projects that are well informed, have clearly defined objectives, demonstrate strong community ties, and promote values such as compassion, inclusiveness, patience, and positive development both in the program and in its implementation. Emphasis is on grassroots organizations that have the ability to engage local groups, positively impact their communities, and focus most of their resources on useful and positive actions.

Restrictions: Applications that require funding in less then 12 weeks will not be accepted. The foundation will not fund: Deficit financing; Loans or grants to individuals; Capital construction; Research projects, conferences, seminars, media events or workshops, unless they are an integral part of a broader program; State agencies; Religious groups; Individual Sponsorships; Fundraising events for your organization such as fun runs, bike rides, etc. If you are a local/regional branch of a national organization they will not fund grants to local chapters if they fund the national organization. Otherwise, they only take into consideration local offices in Northern California.

Samples: (2007) The Alameda County Community Food Bank.; American Farmland Trust Breast Cancer Fund.; New Leaders Initiative/Earth Island Institute.; Center for Food Safety.; Center for Rural Affairs.; Circle of Life.; City Slicker Farms.; Community Alliance with Family Farmers.; Community Resources for Science.; Diabetic Youth Foundation.; Disability Rights Education & Defense Fund.; Ecological Farming Association.; Ecology Center.; Focus the Nation: Global Warming Solutions for America.; Food Alliance Green Belt Movement.; Greentreks Grid Alternatives.; Habitat for Humanity.; Healthy Child Healthy World.; Heifer International.; The Land Institute.; Leave No Trace.; Leukemia & Lymphoma Society.; Luna Kids Dance.; Lungevity Foundation.; KIPP Bay Area.; Marin Agricultural Land Trust.

Contact: Kit Crawford, President; (510) 859-2283; fax: (510) 588-5490; email: familyfoundation@clifbar.com

Internet: http://clifbarfamilyfoundation.org/subtemplate.php?s=1

Sponsor: CLIF Bar Family Foundation
1610 5th Street
Berkeley, CA 94710

Clowes Jointly Sponsored Mentored Clinical Scientist Development Award 1041

The American College of Surgeons and American Association for the Surgery of Trauma announce a program that will provide supplemental salary funding of up to $75,000 per year to an individual who has received a Mentored Clinical Scientist Development Award (K08/K23) from the National Institute for General Medical Science (NIGMS). This award is directed at surgeon-scientists working in the early stages of their research careers. The award supports a three-, four-, or five-year period of supervised research experience that may integrate didactic studies with laboratory or clinical research. The award program offers a means to facilitate the career development of individuals pursuing careers in trauma surgery research by enhancing salary support over and above that offered by the K08/K23 mechanism.

Requirements: Awardees must be members in good standing of the College and eligible for membership in AAST.

Restrictions: Pre-existing applications and awards are not eligible for consideration.

Amount of Grant: $75,000 per year maximum

Date(s) Application is Due: Oct 12

Contact: Kate Early, Administrative Assistant; (312) 202-5281; email: kearly@facs.org

Internet: http://www.facs.org/memberservices/acs-aast-nigms.html

Sponsor: American College of Surgeons
633 N. Saint Clair Street
Chicago, IL 60611-3211

CMA Foundation Grants 1042

The foundation seeks to improve the quality of life for central Ohio residents through the promotion of wellness, prevention of disease, and delivery of services and research. The foundation will review funding requests for matching or challenge grants, multiyear commitments, and capital expenditures on a project-by-project basis. The foundation is the leading local source of funding for health care projects benefiting the local community. Application may be made online.

Requirements: Nonprofit organizations in central Ohio, including Franklin, Delaware, Fairfield, Licking, Madison, Pickaway, and Union Counties, are eligible.

Geographic Focus: Ohio

Samples: Children's Hunger Alliance (Columbus, OH)—to promote school-breakfast programs, $30,000 (2003); Educational Council Foundation (Columbus, OH)—to train middle- and high-school educators to provide information about positive health behaviors, $50,000 maximum (2003); Franklin County Health Dept (Columbus, OH)—to expand its anti-tobacco activities, $30,000 maximum (2003); Mount Carmel Health Systems Foundation (Columbus, OH)—to provide education, information, and self-care skills training to people who have experienced heart failure, $90,000 (2003).

Contact: Contact, (614) 240-7410; email: yourthoughts@goodhealthcolumbus.org

Internet: http://www.cmaf-ohio.org/cmaf/grants.html

Sponsor: Columbus Medical Association Foundation
431 E Broad Street
Columbus, OH 43215

CMAP Physician Advocacy Fellowship 1043

This program supports doctors to develop or enhance their advocacy skills by implementing a project in partnership with an advocacy organization. The fellowship seeks to make advocacy a core professional value for physicians by developing a cadre of advocates with expertise in achieving system or policy-level social change at the local, state, and national level. Projects must be focused within the United States and should identify system or policy level changes as the outcomes of the fellowship work. Application guidelines are available online. Deadline listed is for short proposals; full proposals are by invitation.

Requirements: U.S. physicians at all stages of their careers are eligible; however, the most competitive applicants are practicing physicians. Prospective applicants must secure the commitment of an advocacy organization that is prepared to house, mentor, and support them throughout the fellowship period. A list of advocacy organizations that are interested in participating in the fellowship is available online. Applicants also may apply with organizations other than those listed online.

Samples: Robert Goodman—for efforts to minimize the influence of commercial interests, particularly those of the pharmaceutical industry, in medical education and training, $111,804.

Amount of Grant: $40,000-$80,000 salary support; $2000 travel funds to MAP-sponsored meetings; $5000 maximum overhead support to organizations

Date(s) Application is Due: Oct 7

Contact: Claudia Calhoon, Program Manager, (212) 342-4769; email: cmc100@columbia.edu

Internet: http://www.cmap.columbia.edu/research_fellowship.shtml

Sponsor: Columbia University
630 W 168th Street, P&S Box 11
New York, NY 10032

CMS Historically Black Colleges and Universities Health Services Grants 1044

The purpose of the grant program is to support researchers in implementing health services research activities to meet the needs of diverse CMS beneficiary populations. The goals of the grant program are to: 1) encourage HBCU health services researchers to pursue research issues which impact the Medicare, Medicaid, and SCHIP (State Children's Health Insurance Program) programs, 2) assist CMS in implementing its mission focusing on health care quality and improvement for its beneficiaries, 3) assist HBCU researchers by supporting extramural research in health care capacity development activities for the African American communities, 4) increase the pool of HBCU researchers capable of implementing the research, demonstration, and evaluation activities of CMS, and 5) assist in fostering interuniversity communication and collaboration regarding African American health disparity issues. Funding is available for grants to implement research related to health care delivery and health financing issues affecting African American communities, including issues of access to health care, utilization of health care services, health outcomes, quality of services, cost of care, health and racial disparities, socio-economic differences, cultural barriers, managed care systems, and activities related to health screening, prevention, outreach, and education.

Requirements: To be eligible for grants under this program, an organization must be an HBCU (Historically Black College or University) and meet one of the following three requirements: 1) offer a Ph.D. or Master's Degree Program in one or more of the following disciplines - Allied Health, Gerontology, Health Care Administration, Health Education, Health Management, Nursing, Nutrition, Pharmacology, Public Health, Public Policy, Social Work; or 2) have a School of Medicine; or 3) a member of the National HBCU Network for Health Services and Health Disparities. All proposals should describe research to be conducted with relevance to the CMS Medicare, Medicaid, and SCHIP programs and which area of Healthy People 2010 is served by this project. Applications must be submitted electronically (via grants.gov). CMS will accept a hard copy if the applicant is unable to access grants.gov or is having serious problems in sending the application electronically.

Restrictions: Grant funds may not be used for any of the following: to provide direct services to individuals except as explicitly permitted under the grant solicitation; to match any other Federal funds; to provide services, equipment, or supports that are already the legal responsibility of another party under Federal law.

Amount of Grant: $200,000 - $250,000

Date(s) Application is Due: Jul 2
Contact: Joi Grymes, (410) 786-7251; email: Joi.Grymes@cms.hhs.gov
Internet: http://www.cms.hhs.gov/ResearchDemoGrantsOpt/02_Historically_Black_Colleges_and_Universities.asp#TopOfPage
Sponsor: Centers for Medicare & Medicaid Services
Office of Acquisition and Grants Management, 7500 Security Boulevard, C2-21-15
Baltimore, MD 21244-1850

CMS Research and Demonstration Grants **1045**
The general purpose of the Centers for Medicare & Medicaid Services' (CMS) research and demonstration program is to conduct and support projects to develop, test, and implement new health care financing and payment policies and to evaluate the impact of the agency's programs on its beneficiaries, providers, States, and other customers and partners. The scope of the agency's activities embraces all areas of health care: costs, access, quality, service delivery models, and financing and payment approaches.
Requirements: The following themes represent the agency's current priorities in research. Note that all projects must fall into the agency's statutory authorities to operate and improve Medicare, Medicaid, and other CMS programs and activities: (1) Monitoring and Evaluating CMS Programs; (2) Strengthening Medicaid, State Children's Health Insurance Program (SCHIP), and State Programs; (3) Expanding Beneficiaries' Choices and Availability of Managed Care Options; (4) Developing FFS Payment and Service Delivery Systems; (5) Improving Quality of Care and Performance Under CMS Programs; (6) Improving the Health of Our Beneficiary Population; (7) Prescription Drugs; (8) Building Research Capacity. Application packet is available online.
Restrictions: Applicants are expected to contribute towards the project costs. Generally 5 percent of the total project costs is considered acceptable. CMS rarely approves grants or cooperative agreements for research or demonstration projects in which the Federal Government covers 100 percent of the project's costs. The budget may not include costs for construction or remodeling or for project activities that take place before the applicant has received official notification of our approval of the project.
Amount of Grant: $25,000 - $1,000,000; avg. $235,000
Date(s) Application is Due: none
Contact: Grant Officer, Office of Acquisition and Grants Management; (410) 786-5130; email: Jnorris1@cms.hhs.gov
Internet: http://www.cms.hhs.gov/ResearchDemoGrantsOpt/04_Other_CMS-Grant_Opportunities.asp
Sponsor: Centers for Medicare & Medicaid Services
Office of Acquisition and Grants Management, 7500 Security Boulevard, C2-21-15
Baltimore, MD 21244-1850

CNA Foundation Grants **1046**
The foundation serves as the principal funding entity for CNA social investments. It makes charitable contributions to community priorities primarily where CNA has a presence. Areas of interest include education, health and human services, culture and the arts, and civic and community. Types of support include donated equipment, employee matching gifts, general operating support, in-kind gifts, multiyear support, and continuing support. The foundation encourages activities that meet the needs of special populations such as the disadvantaged, the young, the elderly, the gifted, people with disabilities, minorities, and women. Requests for funding are accepted year-round. Generally, only one request for funding per organization will be considered during the calendar year. Potential applicants should obtain a copy of the foundation guidelines.
Requirements: IRS 501(c)3 tax-exempt organizations are eligible.
Restrictions: Grants are not made to/for individuals; political causes, candidates, or organizations; veterans, labor, alumni, military, athletic clubs, or social clubs; sectarian organizations or denominational religious organizations; capital improvement or building projects; endowed chairs or professorships; United Way-affiliated agencies; or national groups whose local chapters have already received support.
Geographic Focus: Illinois
Amount of Grant: $5000-$50,000 average
Contact: Gina Lockhart, Manager, (312) 822-2828; email: gina.lockhart@cna.com
Internet: http://www.cna.com/cnaeportal/eportal/site/cna/menuitem.7204aaf0316757e8715f09f6556631a0/?vgnextoid=b1e 940fa11056010VgnVCM1000005566130aRCRD#CNA%20FOUNDATION
Sponsor: CNA Foundation
333 S Wabash Avenue
Chicago, IL 60604

CNCS Engaging Persons with Disabilities in National and Community Service Grants **1047**
The program funds innovative national or regional (operating in at least three or more states) partnership models in which persons with disabilities are engaged in service that results in measurable impact on the community served. The opportunity will engage more Americans with disabilities in national and community service. The following categories are of particular interest: using service as a strategy to assist in the transition of young persons with disabilities from school to adult life; and providing adults with disabilities, preferably disabled veterans, the opportunity to engage in service. Grants are awarded covering a period not to exceed three years, with continued funding beyond year one contingent on satisfactory performance. Proposals may be submitted through the eGrants system (April 12 deadline) or by postal mail (April 14 deadline). Guidelines and additional information are available online.
Requirements: Public or private nonprofit organizations, including faith-based and other community-based organizations, are eligible. Applicant organizations must be national or regional (operating in at least three or more states) in scope.
Amount of Grant: $1 million-$5.1 million
Date(s) Application is Due: Apr 12; Apr 14
Contact: Grants Administrator, (202) 606-5000; TTY: (202) 565-2799; email: disabilityoutreach@cns.gov
Internet: http://www.nationalservice.org/funding_initiatives
Sponsor: Corporation for National and Community Service
1201 New York Ave NW
Washington, DC 20525

CNCS Foster Grandparent Projects Grants **1048**
Dual purposes of the program are to provide part-time volunteer service opportunities for income-eligible persons age 60 and over and to give supportive person-to-person service in health, education, human services, and related settings to help address the physical, mental, and emotional needs of infants, children, or youth having special or exceptional needs. The grants may be used for low-income foster grandparent stipends, transportation, physical examinations, and meals; staff salaries and fringe benefits; staff travel; equipment; and space costs; etc. An amount equal to 90 percent of the federal share must be used for foster grandparent direct benefits. Assignment of foster grandparents to children and youth may occur in residential and nonresidential facilities including preschool establishments and to children living in their own homes. In addition, eligible agencies or organizations may, under a Memorandum of Agreement with the Corporation for National Service, receive technical assistance and materials to aid in establishing and operating a noncorporation-funded foster grandparent program project using local funds.
Requirements: Grants are made only to state and local government agencies and private nonprofit organizations.
Restrictions: Volunteers are not to supplant hiring or displace employed workers or impair existing contracts for service. No agency supervising volunteers shall request or receive compensation for services of the volunteers. Volunteers are not to be involved in and funds are not to be used for religious activities, labor or antilabor organization, lobbying, or partisan or nonpartisan political activities.
Amount of Grant: $12,000-$1.9 million; $318,333 average
Contact: Ruth Archie, Foster Grandparent Program, National Senior Service Corps, (202) 606-5000 ext 289 or (800) 424-8867; email: rarchie@cns.gov
Internet: http://www.nationalservice.gov/about/search/search_results.asp?strSearchWords=foster%20grandparent
Sponsor: Corporation for National and Community Service
1201 New York Ave NW
Washington, DC 20525

CNCS Next Generation Grants **1049**
The program supports innovative and demonstrative national and community service proposals throughout the country. The intent of this funding is to help organizations implement innovative strategies or programs through service. Applicant's proposals must fall under at least one of three service areas: programs that engage individuals in an intensive commitment to service in communities (defined as serving at least 40 hours per week); volunteer programs for seniors (minimum age 55); and programs that connect service with education. Concept papers may address community needs in one of the following issues areas: education, environment, health and human services, homeland security, public safety, or another compelling community need.
Requirements: Eligible applicants are nonprofit charitable organizations, such as public charities, community organizations (faith-based and secular), private foundations, and individual schools. Applicants other than individual schools generally will have an annual operating budget of $500,000 or less.
Restrictions: Applicants cannot have received a previous grant from the Corporation.
Amount of Grant: $4 million total; $400,000 maximum
Contact: Marci Hunn, (202) 606-5000 ext 309; TDD: (202) 565-2799; email: nextgeneration@cns.gov
Internet: http://www.nationalservice.gov/about/programs/initiatives.asp
Sponsor: Corporation for National and Community Service
1201 New York Ave NW, Box NGG
Washington, DC 20525

Coastal Bend Community Foundation Grants **1050**
The community foundation awards grants to nonprofit organizations in the Aransas, Bee, Jim Wells, Kleberg, Nueces, Refugio and San Patricio counties of Texas. Grants are usually made to provide seed money for innovative and start-up programs that will generate additional future funding or revenues. Capital projects will also receive favorable consideration. The board of directors approves grant recipients in early November after considering recommendations presented by the Grants Committee. Areas of interest include alcohol and drug abuse, libraries and literacy, arts and culture, higher and other education, adult basic education, child welfare, hospitals, community development, animal welfare, human services, and general charitable giving. Grants are awarded for general operating support, program and project development, equipment, seed money, scholarship funds, and fellowships. Application forms are not required.
Requirements: Nonprofit organizations in Texas in Aransas, Bee, Jim Wells, Kleberg, Nueces, Refugio, and San Patricio counties, may submit grant proposals.
Geographic Focus: Texas
Samples: Texas A&M U (Corpus Christi, TX)—for program support, $10,000.;HIV/AIDS Housing Ctr (Corpus Christi, TX)—for operating support, $12,500.
Amount of Grant: $3.4 million total; $250-$50,000
Date(s) Application is Due: Sep 1

Contact: Jim Moloney, Executive Vice President, (361) 882-9745; fax: (361) 882-2865; email: jmoloney@cbcfoundation.org
Internet: http://www.cbcfoundation.org/grant.html
Sponsor: Coastal Bend Community Foundation
600 Building, Suite 1716
Corpus Christi, TX 78473

Coastal Community Foundation of South Carolina Grants **1051**
The foundation awards grants to South Carolina nonprofit organizations in its areas of interest, including arts and culture, education, environment, health, religion, justice and equity, and social services. Types of support include general operating support, emergency funds, program development, publication, seed money, scholarship funds, and technical assistance. Deadlines vary per program; check website for exact dates.
Requirements: 501(c)3 South Carolina nonprofits located in the following coastal counties are eligible to apply: Beaufort, Berkeley, Charleston, Colleton, Dorchester, Georgetown, Hampton and Jasper.
Restrictions: Grants do not support individuals (except for designated scholarship funds), endowments, deficit financing, dinners, and rarely building funds.
Geographic Focus: South Carolina
Samples: To each, a $15,000 annual grant for 3 years: Boys & Girls Clubs for Rural Units; Child Abuse Prevention Association; Citizens Opposed to Domestic Abuse; Colleton County Arts Council; Friends of Caroline Hospice; Hope Haven of the Lowcountry (formerly Hope Cottage); Literacy Volunteers of the Lowcountry; Lowcountry Food Bank; Second Helpings; (2006).
Amount of Grant: $500-$10,000
Date(s) Application is Due: Jun 1
Contact: George C. Stevens, President-CEO, (843) 723-3635; fax: (843) 577-3671; email: gstevens@tcfgives.org or info@ccfgives.org
Internet: http://www.ccfgives.org
Sponsor: Coastal Community Foundation of South Carolina
90 Mary Street
Charleston, SC 29403

Coca-Cola Foundation Grants **1052**
The foundation has established education as its philanthropic focus and set aside most of its funds to support educational initiatives that address pressing needs. To help prepare youth for life, the foundation gives in three areas: higher education—pipeline programs that connect various levels of education and help students stay in school, scholarships, and minority advancement; classroom teaching and learning—innovative K-12 projects, teacher development, and small projects that deal with classroom activities; and global education—projects that encourage international studies, global understanding, and student exchange. Grants are awarded to both public and private institutions at all levels of education: universities, colleges, and secondary and elementary schools. International educational institutions and health care organizations also receive consideration. Types of support include annual campaigns, donated equipment, employee matching gifts, operating budgets, special projects, capital campaigns, continuing support, fellowships, internships, endowment funds, matching funds, and scholarship funds. Proposals may be submitted at any time.
Requirements: IRS 501(c)3 nonprofits are eligible.
Restrictions: The foundation does not make grants to individuals, religious endeavors, political or fraternal organizations, or organizations without 501(c)3 status.
Samples: Archdiocese of New Orleans, $200,000 for Hurricane Katrina recovery; Churchill Center and School for learning Disabilities, St. Louis, $25,000 for outreach to student with learning disabilities; Fundacion Escolares, Buenos Aires, $30,000 for rural school development; Global Environment & Technology Foundation, $1.5 million for the Community Watershed Partnership; Hispanic Scholarship Fund, San Francisco, $250,000 for first generation college students; St. Pius Catholic High School, Atlanta, $50,000 for scholarships for students of color; University of the South, Sewanee, TN, $250,000 for student scholarships (all 2006).
Amount of Grant: $25,000-$200,000 average
Date(s) Application is Due: Mar 1; Jun 1; Sep 1; Dec 1
Contact: Executive Director, (404) 676-2568; fax: (404) 676-8804
Internet: http://www2.coca-cola.com/citizenship/foundation_guidelines.html
Sponsor: Coca-Cola Foundation
P.O. Box 1734
Atlanta, GA 30301

Cockrell Foundation Grants **1053**
The Cockrell Trust was established in 1957 with funds donated by Ernest and Virginia Cockrell. The Foundation's special emphasis is The University of Texas at Austin. Other fields of interest are: youth services, arts, health care, cultural programs, civic, religious and social services. The Foundation awards grants to support: annual campaigns, building funds, capital campaigns, endowment funds, general purposes, matching funds, and special projects. There are no deadlines for making a request to The Cockrell Foundation. The Foundation meetings are in the late spring and late Fall. An application form is not required. See website for recommended guidelines in making a proposal: http://www.cockrell.com/foundation/grant_guidelines.asp .
Requirements: Texas 501(c)3 nonprofit organizations in Houston are eligible.
Restrictions: The Foundation generally makes grants for only one-year periods. An organization should apply only once during any calendar year. If a grant request is denied, the applicant must wait until the following year before submitting a new request. The Foundation does not participate in feasibility studies and generally does not make grants for the following: individuals; mass appeal solicitations; medical or scientific research projects; organizations outside of Houston, Texas and the United States. Grant requests sent via email or fax will not be accepted.
Geographic Focus: Texas
Samples: The University of Texas, M.D. Anderson Cancer Center, $20,000—support for the Cord Blood Bank Program (2008); Greater Houston Community Foundation, $100,000—support for the Mayor's Gulf Coast Ike Relief Fund (2008); Houston Museum of Natural Science, $2,500—to support the HMNS student enrichment and teacher training programs for Houston schools (2008).
Contact: M. Nancy Williams, Executive Vice President; (713) 209-7500; email: foundation@cockrell.com
Internet: http://www.cockrell.com/foundation/grant_guidelines.asp
Sponsor: Cockrell Foundation
1000 Main Street, Suite 3250
Houston, TX 77002

Coeta and Donald Barker Foundation Grants **1054**
The foundation awards grants to California and Oregon nonprofit organizations in its areas of interest, including arts, children and youth, community development, disabled, environmental conservation, family services, federated giving, health care and health organizations, heart and circulatory research, higher education, hospitals, mental health, and secondary school education. Types of support include building construction/renovation, equipment acquisition, general operating support, program development, and scholarship funds.
Requirements: California and Oregon nonprofit organizations are eligible.
Restrictions: Grants do not support sectarian religious purposes, federal and tax-dependent organizations, individuals, or endowment funds.
Geographic Focus: California; Oregon
Samples: Santa Barbara Zoological Gardens (Santa Barbara, CA), $5000.
Amount of Grant: $100-$20,450 range
Date(s) Application is Due: Mar 1; Aug 1
Contact: Nancy Harris, Executive Administrator, (760) 324-2656; fax: (760) 321-8662
Sponsor: Coeta and Donald Barker Foundation
P.O. Box 936
Rancho Mirage, CA 92270

Coleman Foundation Cancer Care Grants **1055**
Since the 1980's, the Foundation has been an active advocate for raising the standards of cancer care in the Midwest region. Cancer care including support services, treatment and research are primary initiatives of the Foundation. The Foundation has funded specific health care programs, community-based and psychosocial support services, cancer research, development of new treatments, and improvement of direct patient services. Additionally, the Foundation has supported both cancer-specific and general health patient programs.
Requirements: Nonprofits across the Midwest are eligible. Preference is given to requests from Illinois and Chicago.
Restrictions: The program does not fund for-profit businesses, individuals, individual scholarships, ad books, tickets, equipment purchases (including computer hardware or software), or advertising.
Geographic Focus: Illinois; Midwest
Samples: Sinai Health System, Illinois, $328,000—towards capital support for Oncology Infusion Center and OB Triage & Ante partum Testing, to improve oncologic and obstetric facilities, enhance direct patient service areas, and streamline delivery of health care (2008); Wellness House , Illinois, $3,000—to support the 2008 Psychosocial Conference for medical and psychosocial oncology professionals to understand the implication of the Cancer Care for the Whole Patient report published by the Institute of Medicine and discuss ways to improve comprehensive care of cancer patients (2008).
Contact: Michael Hennessy, President; (312) 902-7120; fax: (312) 902-7124; email: info@colemanfoundation.org
Internet: http://www.colemanfoundation.org/cancer.html
Sponsor: Coleman Foundation, Inc.
651 West Washington Boulevard, Suite 306
Chicago, IL 60661

Colin Higgins Foundation Grants **1056**
The foundation supports organizations that help people respond to a variety of life challenges, with a focus on responding to the AIDS pandemic by supporting innovative programs in the areas of education, service, and advocacy for people infected, affected, and at risk for HIV; and empowering lesbian, gay, bisexual, and transgender peoples by supporting community-based organizations that combat homophobia and foster leadership. The foundation is particularly interested in organizations that have a significant impact working in underserved, rural areas with traditionally underserved constituencies. The process of applying consists of two stages: submission of a letter of inquiry, and, if requested, a full proposal.
Requirements: The foundation only considers organizations with overall budgets under $2 million, or project budgets under $500,000.
Restrictions: Grants do not support projects that had previously fallen within its funding priorities, including any organizations or programs based in urban areas (population over 1 million); film and video projects; or organizations with overall budgets of over $2 million, or project budgets over $500,000. The one exception to the exclusion of programs in urban areas is those organizations and projects working with underserved communities (i.e., communities of color, low-income communities, transgender people, etc.). The foundation does not accept letters of inquiry from universities, schools, individuals, or corporations. It does not support political or legislative activities, endowments,

or deficit budgets. Additionally, the foundation does not support capital campaigns, although it will consider requests for capital improvements, and does not award grants to organizations outside the United States.
Samples: The AIDS Mastery Fund (New York, NY)—for general support, $15,000.; Archdiocese of San Francisco (CA)—for the Today's Students, Tomorrow's Leaders Program, $2500.; Intersect: The HIV/Violence Against Women Project (New York, NY)—for general support, $5000.; Unity Fellowship Church (Los Angeles, CA)—for the It Starts With Us Outreach Program, $5000.
Amount of Grant: $5000-$15,000
Date(s) Application is Due: Jul 1
Contact: Grants Administrator, (415) 561-6346; fax: (415) 561-6401; email: info@colinhiggins.org
Internet: http://www.colinhiggins.org/grantmaking
Sponsor: Colin Higgins Foundation
P.O. Box 29903
San Francisco, CA 94129-0903

Collins C. Diboll Private Foundation Grants **1057**
The foundation awards grants to Louisiana nonprofit organizations in the areas of higher education, human services, and youth. Field of interest include: Catholic churches and agencies; education; higher education; human services; museums (art); and protestant agencies and churches. Types of support include building construction/renovation, capital campaigns, endowment funds, and general operating support. Applicants should submit a detailed description of the project and the amount of funding requested, along with a copy of an IRS determination letter.
Requirements: Louisiana nonprofit organizations are eligible.
Restrictions: Individuals are not eligible to apply.
Geographic Focus: Louisiana
Samples: Alton Ochsner Medical Foundation (New Orleans, LA)—for Golden Jubilee/Initiative Campaign, $100,000.; New Orleans Museum of Art (New Orleans, LA)—$100,000.; Junior Achievement of New Orleans (New Orleans, LA)—$35,000.; Preservation Resource Ctr of New Orleans (New Orleans, LA)—for renovations, $11,000.
Amount of Grant: $500-$200,000 average
Contact: Donald W. Diboll, Chair; (504) 582-8103
Sponsor: Collins C. Diboll Private Foundation
201 Saint Charles Avenue, 50th Floor
New Orleans, LA 70170-5100

Collins Foundation Grants **1058**
Grants are awarded to organizations in Oregon with emphasis on higher education, youth and health agencies, social welfare, natural resource and wildlife conservation, religion, and arts and cultural programs. A special area of support includes building and medical equipment, and programs for those who are physically or mentally disabled. Challenge/matching grants, general operating support, scholarships, and internships also are awarded. The annual report, which includes application guidelines, is available upon request. Applications may be submitted at any time.
Requirements: Grants are made to 501(c)3 nonprofit agencies domiciled in Oregon. The proposed project must directly benefit the citizens of Oregon.
Restrictions: Grants are not made to individuals or to organizations sponsoring requests intended to be used by or for the benefit of an individual. Grants normally are not made to elementary, secondary, or public higher education institutions; or to individual religious congregations. Grants normally are not made for development office personnel, annual fundraising activities, endowments, operational deficits, financial emergencies, or debt retirement.
Geographic Focus: Oregon
Contact: Cynthia G. Adams, Director of Programs, (503) 227-7171; fax: (503) 295-3794; email: information@collinsfoundation.org
Internet: http://www.collinsfoundation.org
Sponsor: Collins Foundation
1618 SW First Avenue, Suite 505
Portland, OR 97201

Colonel Stanley R. McNeil Foundation Grants **1059**
The foundation awards grants to eligible Illinois nonprofit organizations in its areas of interest, including child welfare, education, health care, and youth. Types of support include building construction/renovation, equipment acquisition, general operating support, matching grants, research, and special projects. There are no application deadlines or forms.
Requirements: Illinois nonprofit organizations serving the Chicago metropolitan area are eligible.
Restrictions: Grants are not made to individuals.
Geographic Focus: Illinois
Samples: ChildServ (Chicago, IL)—to support ChildServ's Lake County Family Service Center, $45,000 (2005).
Amount of Grant: $7000-$250,000 range
Contact: Charles Slamar, Jr., Vice President, Bank of America, (312) 828-8028
Sponsor: Colonel Stanley R. McNeil Foundation
231 S LaSalle Street
Chicago, IL 60697-0246

Colorado Interstate Gas Grants **1060**
Nonprofits in communities served by the company are eligible to apply for grants in the categories of education, including early child development, K-12, and higher education; civic; health and welfare; minorities; cultural programs; environmental programs, particularly those focusing on air quality; and youth groups that concentrate on improving areas where CIG employees live and work. The company also supports special event sponsorships, corporate memberships, joint projects with other organizations, and employee participation in volunteer activities.
Requirements: Colorado, Wyoming, Texas, Utah, and Kansas 501(c)3 tax-exempt organizations where the company has pipelines are eligible.
Geographic Focus: Colorado
Amount of Grant: $200-$20,000
Date(s) Application is Due: Aug 1
Contact: Richard Wheatley, Media Relations, (713) 420-6828
Internet: http://www.cigco.com
Sponsor: Colorado Interstate Gas Company
P.O. Box 1087
Colorado Springs, CO 80944

Colorado Springs Community Trust Fund Grants **1061**
Grants are awarded to El Paso and Teller Counties in Colorado. The community trust supports Colorado nonprofits with an emphasis on community funds, youth agencies, health, and child welfare. Fields of interest include the arts and cultural programs (visual arts, performing arts, museums), education (elementary education, higher education, adult basic education, literacy, and reading), health care and health organizations, substance abuse and mental health services, crime and law enforcement, human services, and community development. Continuing support for programs/projects will be awarded, as well as support for annual campaigns, building/renovations, equipment, emergency funds, and seed money. There are no application forms; initial approach should be by letter. The board meets four times each year to consider requests.
Requirements: Colorado nonprofits, with an emphasis on El Paso and Teller Counties, are eligible for grant support.
Restrictions: Grants are not awarded to individuals or for operating budgets, deficit financing, endowment funds, matching gifts, scholarships, fellowships, research, demonstration projects, publications, conferences, or loans.
Geographic Focus: Colorado
Samples: Adult Literacy Network (Colorado Springs, CO)—program support, $2000.; YMCA, Parks Peak (Colorado Springs, CO)—program support, $10,807.; Ctr for the Prevention of Domestic Violence (Colorado Springs, CO)—program support, $5000.
Amount of Grant: $500-$5000 average
Date(s) Application is Due: Mar 1; Aug 1; Nov 1
Contact: Michael Hannigan, Executive Director, (719) 389-1251; fax: (719) 389-1252; email: mhannigan@PPCF.org
Sponsor: Colorado Springs Community Trust Fund
P.O. Box 1443
Colorado Springs, CO 80901

Colorado Trust Grants **1062**
The Trust's strategic grantmaking supports the development of a coordinated system of policies, programs and services that, expand health coverage, improve and expand health care. The Trust issues Requests for Proposals (RFP) and welcomes responses from nonprofit organizations and governmental entities across Colorado. When a competitive funding opportunity is available, a detailed RFP with related instructions and specific application deadlines is posted to the Funds website. On occasion, The Trust also asks organizations that are focused on strategies specific to achieving access to health to submit individual, non-competitive proposals.
Requirements: The following types of organizations are eligible to apply for grants: nonprofit organizations that are exempt under Section 501(c)3 of the Internal Revenue Code and are classified as "not a private foundation" under Section 509(a); independent sponsored projects of a nonprofit 501(c)3 organization acting as a fiscal agent; government and public agencies.
Restrictions: The Trust asks for proposals through a Request for Proposal process, rather than accepting unsolicited proposals. Announcements of Requests for Proposals are posted at the website. Grant seekers also may register with the Trust to receive notification of new funding opportunities. The Colorado Trust does not make grants for the following: political campaigns or voter registration drives; capital funding for the purchase, construction or renovation of any facilities or other physical infrastructure; operating deficits or retirement of debt; indirect allocations (excluding fiscal agent fees); religious purposes.
Geographic Focus: Colorado
Contact: Ed Lucero, Senior Program Officer; (888) 847-9140 or (303) 837-1200; fax: (303) 839-9034; email: ed@coloradotrust.org
Internet: http://www.coloradotrust.org
Sponsor: Colorado Trust
1600 Sherman Street
Denver, CO 80203-1200

Colorado Trust Partnerships for Health Initiative **1063**
The trust supports this statewide initiative to improve the coordination of health services at the community level. The program will support new or existing community health partnerships, consisting of local health departments, county nursing services, community-based organizations, and other interested organizations, businesses, and community members. Each partnership will identify a Healthy People 2010 focus area

important to its community and will develop and implement a coordinated plan to address that health issues. Grants will be awarded to help partnerships build, strengthen, and sustain the public health infrastructure of Colorado communities by proactively addressing public health issues. The complete RFP is available online.
Requirements: Partnerships must have a 501(c)3 fiscal agent or be a governmental entity; strong community support including representatives from the public, private, and nonprofit sectors; ability to develop strategic partnerships; knowledge of the the public health system and health promotion/disease prevention issues; ability to design a service approach to meet targeted Health People 2010 needs; cultural competency and a demonstrated commitment to diversity; sound fiscal management; and willingness to work in partnership with the Colorado Trust in the planning and implementation phases of the initiative.
Geographic Focus: Colorado
Amount of Grant: $10,000-$15,000 planning grants; $30,000-$75,000 per year implementation grants
Date(s) Application is Due: Nov 17
Contact: Susan Downs-Karkos, (888) 847-9140 or (303) 837-1200; fax: (303) 839-9034; email: susan@coloradotrust.org
Internet: http://www.coloradotrust.org
Sponsor: Colorado Trust
1600 Sherman Street
Denver, CO 80203

Columbus Foundation Allen Eiry Fund Grants **1064**
The Fund provides support to organizations that serve older adults in Seneca County. Projects supported by the fund include transportation, recreation, homemaker services, hot meals, court ordered guardianships, information and referral programs, library programs for nursing homes, support for capital projects, and other projects that enhance the lives of needy elderly.
Requirements: The Fund welcomes requests from organizations having recognition under Section 501(c)3 of the Internal Revenue Code that serve older adults in Seneca County.
Restrictions: The Fund makes no grants to individuals. Requests for religious purposes, budget deficits, endowments, conferences, scholarly research, or projects that are normally the responsibility of a public agency are generally not funded.
Geographic Focus: Ohio
Date(s) Application is Due: Nov 5
Contact: Dottie Henderson, Executive Assistant; (614) 251-4000; fax: (614) 251-4009; email: dhenderson@columbusfoundation.org
Internet: http://www.columbusfoundation.org/gogrants/targeted_needs/specialized_grants.aspx
Sponsor: Columbus Foundation
1234 East Broad Street
Columbus, OH 43205

Columbus Foundation Ann Ellis Fund Grants **1065**
The Fund is used for eye research, with primary emphasis on sponsoring scientific research on the diagnosis, prevention, and treatment of glaucoma. Once this is accomplished, the fund will assist in the research of other hidden eye problems.
Restrictions: Individuals are ineligible. Requests for religious purposes, budget deficits, endowments, conferences, or projects that are normally the responsibility of a public agency are generally not funded.
Date(s) Application is Due: Oct 1
Contact: Dottie Henderson, Executive Assistant; (614) 251-4000; fax: (614) 251-4009; email: dhenderson@columbusfoundation.org
Internet: http://www.columbusfoundation.org/gogrants/targeted_needs/specialized_grants.aspx
Sponsor: Columbus Foundation
1234 East Broad Street
Columbus, OH 43205

Columbus Foundation Competitive Grants **1066**
The foundation's competitive grants are made in the following fields: advancing philanthropy, arts and humanities, conservation, education, health, social services, and urban affairs. The Governing Committee approves distributions from unrestricted and field of interest funds through competitive grants. Competitive grants are the most common way nonprofit organizations request funding from the Foundation. Submit a Letter of Intent or a Full Proposal by accessing our online grant application system.
Requirements: Central Ohio, tax-exempt public charities under Section 501(c)3 of the Internal Revenue Service Code may submit grant requests.
Restrictions: Individuals are ineligible. Requests for religious purposes, budget deficits, endowments, conferences, scholarly research, or projects that are normally the responsibility of a public agency are generally not funded. Funding is not available for projects when funds are available elsewhere.
Geographic Focus: Ohio
Contact: Emily Savors, Director of Community Research and Grants Management; (614) 251-4000; fax: (614) 251-4009; email: esavors@columbusfoundation.org
Internet: http://www.columbusfoundation.org/gogrants/index.aspx
Sponsor: Columbus Foundation
1234 East Broad Street
Columbus, OH 43205

Columbus Foundation Estrich Fund Grants **1067**
The Fund is designed to provide home health care and/or inpatient services to the terminally ill. Funds may be used to provide medical services (excluding doctor visits, in-hospital costs, or care facilities), medical supplies and equipment, transportation and physical and occupational therapy. Funds may also be used to make available emotional, social, and spiritual support through the use of professionals and/or trained volunteers.
Requirements: Central Ohio, tax-exempt public charities under Section 501(c)3 of the Internal Revenue Service Code may submit grant requests.
Restrictions: Requests for religious purposes, budget deficits, endowments, conferences, scholarly research, or projects that are normally the responsibility of a public agency are generally not funded.
Geographic Focus: Ohio
Samples: Fisrtlink, Columbus, OH, $18,725—to support the Dental Options Program, which provides free or low cost dental care to residents of central Ohio; Central Ohio Diabetes Association, Columbus, OH—to support outreach and education programs for the Hispanic community; Impact Safety Programs, Columbus, OH, $20,000—to provide a violence prevention program for residents of Amethyst; Columbus AIDS Task Force (CATF), Columbus, OH, $22,000—to support outreach offices at Neighborhood House and Just For Today.
Date(s) Application is Due: Apr 20
Contact: Sandi Smith, (614) 251-4000; fax: (614) 251-4009; email: ssmith@columbusfoundation.org
Internet: http://www.columbusfoundation.org/GD/Templates/Pages/TCF/TCFSecondary.aspx?page=66
Sponsor: Columbus Foundation
1234 East Broad Street
Columbus, OH 43205

Columbus Foundation J. Floyd Dixon Memorial Fund Grants **1068**
The purpose of the Fund is to provide educational programs for children, health programs for the elderly, and social services programs in Jackson County. An individual grant seldom exceeds $10,000. Applications must be received by May 28, and decisions will be announced three to four months after the application deadline.
Requirements: The fund welcomes requests from organizations having recognition under Section 501(c)3 of the Internal Revenue Code that serves residents of Jackson County.
Restrictions: The Fund makes no grants to individuals, and generally does not fund governmental agencies. Requests for religious purposes, budget deficits, endowments, conferences, scholarly research, or projects that are normally the responsibility of a public agency are generally not funded.
Geographic Focus: Ohio
Amount of Grant: $10,000 maximum
Date(s) Application is Due: May 28
Contact: Dottie Henderson, Executive Assistant for Community Research and Grants Management; (614) 251-4000; fax: (614) 251-4009; email: dhenderson@columbusfoundation.org
Internet: http://www.columbusfoundation.org/gogrants/targeted_needs/specialized_grants.aspx
Sponsor: Columbus Foundation
1234 East Broad Street
Columbus, OH 43205

Columbus Foundation Mary Eleanor Morris Fund Grants **1069**
The Fund supports quality-of-life projects, with a focus on the arts, civic affairs, conservation, education, health, and social services that benefits the residents of Logan County. Deadlines are the first Friday in January and the first Friday in July.
Requirements: The fund welcomes requests from organizations having recognition under Section 501(c)3 of the Internal Revenue Code that services the residents of Logan County, as well as public and private schools.
Restrictions: The Fund makes no grants to individuals. Requests for religious purposes, budget deficits, endowments, conferences, scholarly research, or projects that are normally the responsibility of a public agency are generally not funded.
Geographic Focus: Ohio
Date(s) Application is Due: Jan 1; Jul 2
Contact: Emily Savors, Director of Community Research and Grants Management; (614) 251-4000; fax: (614) 251-4009; email: esavors@columbusfoundation.org
Internet: http://www.columbusfoundation.org/gogrants/targeted_needs/small_grants.aspx
Sponsor: Columbus Foundation
1234 East Broad Street
Columbus, OH 43205

Columbus Foundation Robert E. and Genevieve B. Schaefer Fund Grants **1070**
The purpose of the Fund is to benefit the residents of Chillicothe and/or Ross County. The funding supports programs that enhance the community in three broad areas: cultural development, health and human welfare, and economic development.
Requirements: The Fund welcomes applications from organizations recognized under Section 501(c)3 of the Internal Revenue Code that serves the residents of Chillicothe and/or Ross County. All organizations with budgets over $75,000 must provide an audit, and those with budgets less than $75,000 must provide their most recent form 990 and compiled financial statements.
Restrictions: The Fund makes no grants to individuals, churches, governmental agencies, or school districts.
Geographic Focus: Ohio
Date(s) Application is Due: Oct 29

Contact: Dottie Henderson, Executive Assistant for Community Research and Grants Management; (614) 251-4000; fax: (614) 251-4009; email: dhenderson@columbusfoundation.org
Internet: http://www.columbusfoundation.org/gogrants/targeted_needs/specialized_grants.aspx
Sponsor: Columbus Foundation
1234 East Broad Street
Columbus, OH 43205

Columbus Foundation Traditional Grants **1071**
The Traditional Grants Program creates quality opportunities and meets community need by focusing on three areas: Basic Needs funds programs and projects that provide food, shelter, and clothing. Priority will be given to programs and projects that meet current needs and simultaneously integrate services designed to support long-term stability; Disadvantaged Children funds programs and projects that meet the diverse needs of at-risk children. Priority will be given to programs and projects that are in the home, build relationships with the family, and create a support network around and for the families of disadvantaged children; Developmental Disabilities funds programs and projects that address the needs of children and adults with physical or cognitive disabilities that impair functions or behavior and that occurred before a person reaches the age of 22. (Blindness/visual impairments and deafness/hearing impairments are not considered within this category.) If you are implementing your project in a Columbus City School building, or collaborating with the district on a project, and asked to submit a full application, you must request a letter of endorsement from the Office of Development.
Requirements: Central Ohio, tax-exempt public charities under Section 501(c)3 of the Internal Revenue Service Code may submit grant requests .If you are implementing your project in a Columbus City School building, or collaborating with the district on a project, and asked to submit a full application, you must request a letter of endorsement from the Office of Development. Letter of Intent deadlines are twice a year on the first Friday in February and September. See Foundations website for further guidelines.
Restrictions: Operating support will only be considered when the applicant demonstrates continuous innovation that enhances services.
Geographic Focus: Ohio
Date(s) Application is Due: Feb 5; Sep 3
Contact: Emily Savors, Director of Community Research and Grants Management; (614) 251-4000; fax: (614) 251-4009; email: esavors@columbusfoundation.org
Internet: http://www.columbusfoundation.org/gogrants/targeted_needs/traditional_grants.aspx
Sponsor: Columbus Foundation
1234 East Broad Street
Columbus, OH 43205

Comer Foundation Grants **1072**
The foundation awards grants to U.S. nonprofits in its areas of interest, including needle-exchange programs grounded in harm-reduction practice and programs providing direct services addressing health related to drug use; education—AIDS education, job training, and career guidance for low-income groups; health, with an emphasis on AIDS; social services—temporary shelters for homeless people and organizations offering diverse child, youth, and family services; and arts, culture, and humanities—to make programs of established organizations accessible to the public at large. Types of support include operating budgets, special projects, and staff development. There are no deadlines.
Restrictions: Individuals are ineligible for grant support.
Geographic Focus: Illinois
Amount of Grant: $5000-$30,000 average
Date(s) Application is Due: Mar 1; Jul 1; Nov 1
Contact: Stephanie Comer, (415) 256-9917; fax: (415) 256-9918; email: scomer@comer-foundation.org
Internet: http://www.comer-foundation.com/home.html
Sponsor: Comer Foundation
P.O. Box 78154
San Francisco, CA 94107

Comerica Charitable Foundation Grants **1073**
The Comerica Charitable Foundation funding priorities support community needs in it's primary markets within Texas, Michigan, California, Arizona, and Florida. Applications are accepted for program support and capital expense of those non-profit organizations that support the foundation's priorities. Economic self-sufficiency for low and moderate income individuals and families will be supported in the areas of financial literacy, job readiness, job creation and retention, small business training and development, and transitional and supportive housing. Neighborhood revitalization areas to be supported are affordable housing and neighborhood business development. Financial literacy programs (K-12 and adult) and scholarships for students with income needs for studies in business, finance and growth industries will be supported. Also a priority is access to health care to include preventive care for the uninsured and under-insured. Also a priority are programs that support diversity and inclusion. Funding deadlines vary according to region. See the Foundation's website for regional offices.
Requirements: 501(c)3 nonprofits are eligible.
Restrictions: Grants are not awarded for United Way organizations, religious and fraternal groups, political parties, charitable golf events, athletic programs, multiyear pledges, or endowment funds.
Geographic Focus: Arizona; California; Florida; Michigan; Texas
Date(s) Application is Due: Mar 15; Jun 15; Sep 15; Nov 15
Contact: Program Contact, Corporate Contributions, (313) 222-7356;
Internet: http://www.comerica.com/vgn-ext-templating/v/index.jsp?vgnextoid=374970d75d994010VgnVCM1000004502a8c0RCRD
Sponsor: Comerica Charitable Foundation
MC 3390, P.O. Box 75000
Detroit, MI 48275-3390

Commission on Religion in Appalachia Grants **1074**
The commission supports Christian and interdenominational nonprofits in U.S. Appalachian regions. Churches and ministries and nonprofits in the areas of parochial education, religious welfare, civil rights, health care, and social services (domestic violence, housing, women's affairs, and food distribution) are awarded grants. The commission strongly encourages applicants to obtain guidelines prior to submitting proposals.
Requirements: Nonprofits in the Appalachian regions of Mississippi, Alabama, Georgia, South Carolina, North Carolina, Tennessee, Kentucky, Virginia, West Virginia, Ohio, Pennsylvania, Maryland, and New York are eligible.
Geographic Focus: Mississippi
Amount of Grant: $5000-$15,000
Date(s) Application is Due: Jan 31
Contact: Grant Administrator, (304) 720-2672; fax: (304) 720-2673; email: corainappa@aol.com
Internet: http://www.geocities.com/appalcora/About.html
Sponsor: Commission on Religion in Appalachia
P.O. Box 11908
Charleston, WV 25339-1908

Commonweal Foundation Community Assistance Grants **1075**
The foundation supports educational programs and projects assisting disadvantaged, at-risk youth. The foundation focuses on secondary and, to a lesser extent, elementary education. The foundation also considers grants for educational research and, to a limited extent, health care. Guidelines are available online.
Requirements: 501(c)3 tax-exempt organizations located in the District of Columbia, Maryland, or Northern Virginia are eligible. Applicant organizations should have an annual budget not exceeding $1 million.
Geographic Focus: District of Columbia; Maryland; Virginia
Amount of Grant: $25,000 maximum
Date(s) Application is Due: Mar 1; Aug 1
Contact: Gloria Dairsow, (240) 450-0000; fax: (240) 450-4115; email: gdairsow@cweal.org
Internet: http://www.cweal.org/cag.htm
Sponsor: Commonweal Foundation
10770 Columbia Pike, Suite 150
Silver Spring, MD 20901

Commonweal Foundation Grants **1076**
The foundation awards grants to eligible nonprofit organizations serving disadvantaged youth in the area comprising the corridor between Baltimore, MD, and Washington, DC. It also offers some assistance to elementary education, educational research, and some health care causes. Programs include Partners in Learning (address low literacy skills of economically disadvantaged children), community assistance grants (i.e., after-school tutoring, parenting classes, and shelters for the homeless or abused women), and learning disabilities support program (special education services to economically disadvantaged children). Contact the office for application procedures.
Requirements: 501(c)3 tax-exempt organizations serving disadvantaged youth in the corridor between Baltimore, MD, and Washington, DC, are eligible.
Geographic Focus: District of Columbia; Maryland; Virginia
Amount of Grant: $10,000-$25,000
Date(s) Application is Due: Feb 1; May 1; Aug 1; Nov 1
Contact: Renee Cottman-Reyes, (240) 450-0000; fax: (240) 450-4115; email: gdairsow@cweal.org
Internet: http://www.commonweal-foundation.org/index.html
Sponsor: Commonweal Foundation
10770 Columbia Pke, Suite 150
Silver Spring, MD 20901

Commonwealth Fund Affordable Health Insurance Grants **1077**
The Program on Affordable Health Insurance envisions an efficient and equitable health insurance system that makes available to all Americans comprehensive, continuous, and affordable coverage. In support of that vision, the program seeks to: analyze changes in employer-based, private and public insurance coverage for people under age 65, and determine how those changes may affect the affordability and comprehensiveness of coverage, the number of uninsured, the number of under-insured, and churning in and out of coverage; document the consequences of being uninsured, under-insured, and unstably insured, with regard to access to care, health status, personal financial security, and economic productivity; and develop and evaluate federal and state policies to expand and stabilize health insurance, make it more affordable and aligned with incentives to access appropriate and high quality care, and enhance the efficiency with which it is administered.
Requirements: The Commonwealth Fund requests letters of inquiry to initiate the grant application process, and does not wish to review full proposals at this stage. Applicants are encouraged to submit letters of inquiry using our online form.

Restrictions: The Fund makes grants only to tax-exempt organizations and public agencies and does not support: general planning and ongoing activities or existing deficits; endowment or capital costs, including construction, renovation, or equipment; basic biomedical research; conferences, symposia, major media projects, or documentaries, unless they are an outgrowth of one of the Fund's programs; individuals; scholarships; churches or other religious organizations unless the project for which they seek funding is entirely secular in nature; and work for which achievements cannot be measured.
Contact: Sara R. Collins, Ph.D., Assistant Vice-President; (212) 606-3838 or (212) 606-3800; fax: (212) 606-3500; email: src@cmwf.org
Internet: http://www.commonwealthfund.org/Content/Program-Areas/Affordable-Health-Insurance.aspx
Sponsor: Commonwealth Fund
One East 75th Street
New York, NY 10021-2692

Commonwealth Fund Australian-American Health Policy Fellowships 1078
The Australian Government Department of Health and Aging hopes to enrich health policy thinking as Australian-American Health Policy Fellows study how Australia approaches health policy issues, share lessons learned from the United States, and develop an international perspective and network of contacts to facilitate policy exchange and collaboration that extends beyond the fellowship experience. Australian-American Health Policy Fellowships are open to accomplished, mid-career health policy researchers and practitioners, including, academics, physicians, decision makers in managed care and other private sector health care organizations, federal and state health officials, and journalists. The Fellowship provides up to $55,000 (AUD) for terms of six to ten months, with a minimum stay of six months in Australia required. Focused on issues of common concern to Australian and U.S. policymakers, the fellowships are structured around areas of mutual policy interest, for example: health care quality and safety, the private/public mix of insurance and providers, the fiscal sustainability of health systems, the health care workforce, management and efficiency of health care delivery, and investment in preventive care strategies.
Requirements: All applicants must also meet the following criteria: be a citizen of the United States; be a mid-career health services researcher or practitioner (e.g., a physician, decision maker in a managed care organization or other private health care organization, government official or policy analyst, or journalist); have a demonstrated expertise in health policy issues and track record of informing health policy through research, policy analysis, health services, or clinical leadership; have completed a master's degree or doctorate (or the equivalent thereof) in health services research, health administration, health policy, or a related discipline, such as economics or political science; and if academically based, be at a mid-career level (e.g., research fellow to associate professor).
Restrictions: Fellowships are not awarded to support basic research or study for an academic degree.
Amount of Grant: $55,000 maximum (AUD)
Date(s) Application is Due: Aug 15
Contact: Robin Osborn, Director; (212) 606-3809 or (212) 606-3800; fax: (212) 606-3875; email: ro@cmwf.org
Internet: http://www.commonwealthfund.org/Fellowships/Australian-American-Health-Policy-Fellowships.aspx
Sponsor: Commonwealth Fund
One East 75th Street
New York, NY 10021-2692

Commonwealth Fund Harkness Fellowships in Health Care Policy and Practice 1079
The Harkness Fellowships in Health Care Policy and Practice provide an opportunity for professionals from the Australia, Germany, the Netherlands, New Zealand, Norway, Switzerland, and the United Kingdom to spend four to 12 months in the United States conducting a research study that is relevant to health care policy and practice in both the United States and the fellow's home country, and that is focused on the issues of greatest concern to the fund. Fellowship awards provide up to $107,000, which covers round trip airfare to the United States, a living allowance, funds for project-related travel, research, and conferences, travel to attend the Commonwealth Fund program of fellowship seminars, health insurance, and U.S. and state taxes. A family supplement - including airfare, living allowance, and health insurance - is also provided to Fellows accompanied by a partner and/or children up to age 18.
Requirements: Applicants must be citizens of Australia, Germany, the Netherlands, New Zealand, Norway, Switzerland, and the United Kingdom in their late 20s to early 40s with broad educational backgrounds, not just those in research or academic careers. In order to apply, applicants must be nominated by their institution and submit a formal application, which is available from The Commonwealth Fund in New York City or its representatives in their home country.
Amount of Grant: $107,000 maximum
Date(s) Application is Due: Sep 15
Contact: Robin Osborn, Director; (212) 606-3809 or (212) 606-3800; fax: (212) 606-3875; email: ro@cmwf.org
Internet: http://www.commonwealthfund.org/Fellowships/Minority-Health-Policy-Fellowship.aspx
Sponsor: Commonwealth Fund
One East 75th Street
New York, NY 10021-2692

Commonwealth Fund Health Care Quality Improvement and Efficiency Grants 1080
The goal of the Fund's Program on Health Care Quality Improvement and Efficiency is to improve the quality and efficiency of health care in the United States. To that end, the program supports projects that: promote the development and widespread adoption of health care quality and efficiency measures; assess and enhance the capacity of health care organizations to provide better care more efficiently; and promote the development and adoption of payment and incentive models that encourage providers to improve quality and efficiency.
Requirements: The Commonwealth Fund requests letters of inquiry to initiate the grant application process, and does not wish to review full proposals at this stage. Applicants are encouraged to submit letters of inquiry using our online form.
Restrictions: The Fund makes grants only to tax-exempt organizations and public agencies and does not support: general planning and ongoing activities or existing deficits; endowment or capital costs, including construction, renovation, or equipment; basic biomedical research; conferences, symposia, major media projects, or documentaries, unless they are an outgrowth of one of the Fund's programs; individuals; scholarships; churches or other religious organizations unless the project for which they seek funding is entirely secular in nature; and work for which achievements cannot be measured.
Contact: Anne-Marie J. Audet, M.D.; (212) 606-3800; fax: (212) 606-3500; email: ama@cmwf.org
Internet: http://www.commonwealthfund.org/Content/Program-Areas/Health-Care-Quality-Improvement-and-Efficiency.aspx
Sponsor: Commonwealth Fund
One East 75th Street
New York, NY 10021-2692

Commonwealth Fund Patient-Centered Coordinated Care Program Grants 1081
As defined by the Institute of Medicine, patient-centered care is health care that establishes a partnership among practitioners, patients, and their families (when appropriate), to ensure that decisions respect patients' needs and preferences, and that patients have the education and support they need to make decisions and participate in their own care. In primary care, such care is best provided in a medical home - a primary care practice or health center that ensures patients have enhanced access to their clinicians (for example, through the availability of evening or weekend appointments), coordinates care, and engages in continuous quality improvement. The goal of The Commonwealth Fund's Patient-Centered Coordinated Care Program, established in 2005, is to improve the quality of primary care by making it more patient- and family-centered. The initiative supports projects that: promote the collection of information on patient-centered care and the delivery of care to facilitate public reporting and quality improvement; stimulate adoption of effective practices, models, and tools to make primary care practices patient- and family-centered; and improve policy to encourage patient- and family-centered care in medical homes.
Requirements: The Commonwealth Fund requests letters of inquiry to initiate the grant application process, and does not wish to review full proposals at this stage. Applicants are encouraged to submit letters of inquiry using our online form.
Restrictions: The Fund makes grants only to tax-exempt organizations and public agencies and does not support: general planning and ongoing activities or existing deficits; endowment or capital costs, including construction, renovation, or equipment; basic biomedical research; conferences, symposia, major media projects, or documentaries, unless they are an outgrowth of one of the Fund's programs; individuals; scholarships; churches or other religious organizations unless the project for which they seek funding is entirely secular in nature; and work for which achievements cannot be measured.
Contact: Melinda Abrams; (212) 606-3800; fax: (212) 606-3500; email: mka@cmwf.org
Internet: http://www.commonwealthfund.org/Content/Program-Areas/Patient-Centered-Coordinated-Care.aspx
Sponsor: Commonwealth Fund
One East 75th Street
New York, NY 10021-2692

Commonwealth Fund Payment System Reform Grants 1082
To achieve a high performing health system, the U.S. must curb spending growth and improve the way health care is provided. Payment system reform is critical to accomplishing these objectives. As a nation, we need to align incentives so that health care providers are rewarded for high-value care rather than a high volume of services. Rewarding value over volume will also encourage the development of a more integrated health care delivery system. The Commonwealth Fund, through its Program on Payment System Reform, supports analysis and the development of policy options to accomplish these goals. Areas of interest include: reforming the existing payment structure to improve the alignment of incentives and to provide a base for more comprehensive payment reform; modeling and analyzing the potential impact of alternative options for payment reform in Medicare and throughout the health system; using payment reform to encourage the development of new models of health care delivery that provide better and more coordinated care; and using comparative effectiveness research to support better decision-making by providers, payers, and patients.
Requirements: The Commonwealth Fund requests letters of inquiry to initiate the grant application process, and does not wish to review full proposals at this stage. Applicants are encouraged to submit letters of inquiry using our online form.
Restrictions: The Fund makes grants only to tax-exempt organizations and public agencies and does not support: general planning and ongoing activities or existing deficits; endowment or capital costs, including construction, renovation, or equipment; basic biomedical research; conferences, symposia, major media projects, or documentaries, unless they are an outgrowth of one of the Fund's programs; individuals; scholarships;

churches or other religious organizations unless the project for which they seek funding is entirely secular in nature; and work for which achievements cannot be measured.
Contact: Heather Drake, Program Associate; (212) 606-3800; fax: (212) 606-3500; email: hd@cmwf.org;; Stuart Guterman; (202) 292-6735 or (212) 606-3800; fax: (212) 606-3500; email: sxg@cmwf.org
Internet: http://www.commonwealthfund.org/Content/Program-Areas/Payment-System-Reform.aspx
Sponsor: Commonwealth Fund
One East 75th Street
New York, NY 10021-2692

Commonwealth Fund Quality of Care for Frail Elders Grants **1083**
The Commonwealth Fund Program on Quality of Care for Frail Elders aims to transform the nation's nursing homes and other long-term care facilities into resident-centered organizations that are good places to live and work, capable of providing the highest-quality care. The projects it supports aim to: identify, evaluate, and spread models of resident-centered care, or care delivered in accordance with the needs and desires of the people who live in nursing homes; equip nursing home operators to lead transformational change; and promote policy options that support resident-centered care.
Requirements: The Commonwealth Fund requests letters of inquiry to initiate the grant application process, and does not wish to review full proposals at this stage. Applicants are encouraged to submit letters of inquiry using our online form.
Restrictions: The Fund makes grants only to tax-exempt organizations and public agencies and does not support: general planning and ongoing activities or existing deficits; endowment or capital costs, including construction, renovation, or equipment; basic biomedical research; conferences, symposia, major media projects, or documentaries, unless they are an outgrowth of one of the Fund's programs; individuals; scholarships; churches or other religious organizations unless the project for which they seek funding is entirely secular in nature; and work for which achievements cannot be measured.
Contact: Mary Jane Koren; (212) 606-3800; fax: (212) 606-3500; email: mjk@cmwf.org
Internet: http://www.commonwealthfund.org/Content/Program-Areas/Quality-of-Care-for-Frail-Elders.aspx
Sponsor: Commonwealth Fund
One East 75th Street
New York, NY 10021-2692

Commonwealth Fund Small Grants **1084**
The fund awards small grants for projects in its major program areas, which include: affordable health insurance; international health care policy and practice; improving the quality of health care services; and improving insurance coverage and access to care. Types of support include employee-matching gifts, program development, program evaluation, and research. Preference is given to projects that seek to solve problems, especially those affecting vulnerable groups; that analyze the effects of policies and trends on well-defined health issues; and that develop and test practical solutions. Prospective grantees should submit a letter of inquiry via regular or electronic mail. Program staff will contact applicants if more detailed information is required. Proposals recommended by fund staff are reviewed and voted upon by the board of directors, which meets in July, April, and November. Letters of inquiry should be brief, no more than two pages.
Requirements: The fund makes grants only to tax-exempt organizations and public agencies.
Restrictions: The fund does not support general planning and ongoing activities or existing deficits; endowment or capital costs, including construction, renovation, or equipment; basic biomedical research; conferences, symposia, major media projects or documentaries, unless they are an outgrowth of one of the fund's programs; individuals; scholarships; churches or other religious organizations, unless the project is entirely secular in nature; or work for which achievements cannot be measured.
Contact: Andrea Landes, Director of Grants Management; (212) 606-3800; fax: (212) 606-3508; email: acl@cmwf.org
Internet: http://www.commonwealthfund.org/Grants-And-Programs/Applicant-and-Grantee-Resources/Applying-for-a-Grant.aspx
Sponsor: Commonwealth Fund
One East 75th Street
New York, NY 10021-2608

Commonwealth Fund State High Performance Health Systems Grants **1085**
The Commonwealth Fund's State High Performance Health Systems program is designed to help states develop the infrastructure needed to improve health care quality and outcomes - and to draw out and share lessons of national import from the experience of states that are moving toward comprehensive health care reforms. To enable states to help local health care providers better meet the needs of their patient populations, the program will support approaches that offer providers shared access to the clinical support and practice-management services essential to achieving high performance. Such resources will often be developed though state-initiated, public–private partnerships. To inform and support state health care leaders, additional projects will facilitate information-sharing among states working toward health care reform.
Requirements: The Commonwealth Fund requests letters of inquiry to initiate the grant application process, and does not wish to review full proposals at this stage. Applicants are encouraged to submit letters of inquiry using our online form.
Restrictions: The Fund makes grants only to tax-exempt organizations and public agencies and does not support: general planning and ongoing activities or existing deficits; endowment or capital costs, including construction, renovation, or equipment; basic biomedical research; conferences, symposia, major media projects, or documentaries, unless they are an outgrowth of one of the Fund's programs; individuals; scholarships; churches or other religious organizations unless the project for which they seek funding is entirely secular in nature; and work for which achievements cannot be measured.
Contact: Edward L. Schor, Vice President; (212) 606-3800; fax: (212) 606-3500; email: els@cmwf.org
Internet: http://www.commonwealthfund.org/Content/Program-Areas/State-High-Performance-Health-System.aspx
Sponsor: Commonwealth Fund
One East 75th Street
New York, NY 10021-2692

Commonwealth Fund/Harvard University Fellowship in Minority Health Policy **1086**
The Commonwealth Fund/Harvard University Fellowship in Minority Health Policy is a one-year, full-time, academic degree-granting program designed to create physician-leaders, particularly minority physician-leaders, who will pursue careers in health policy, public health practice, and academia. It is designed to incorporate the critical skills taught in schools of public health, government, business, and medicine with leadership forums and seminar series conducted by Harvard senior faculty and nationally recognized leaders in minority health and public policy; supervised practicums and shadowing opportunities; and site visits, conferences, and travel. Each fellowship provides: $50,000 stipend; full tuition; health insurance; books; travel; and related program expenses, including financial assistance for a practicum project.
Requirements: Applicants are required to complete applications to both the Commonwealth Fund/Harvard University Fellowship in Minority Health Policy and the Harvard School of Public Health. Applicants must have finished residency and be U.S. citizens.
Amount of Grant: $50,000 stipend
Date(s) Application is Due: Jan 4
Contact: Joan Y. Reede; (617) 432-2922; email: mfdp_cfhuf@hms.harvard.edu
Internet: http://www.commonwealthfund.org/Fellowships/Minority-Health-Policy-Fellowship.aspx
Sponsor: Commonwealth Fund
164 Longwood Avenue, 2nd Floor
Boston, MA 02115-5818

Community Campus Partnerships for Health Fellowships **1087**
Community-based professionals, academic administrators, and faculty with significant knowledge and expertise in building and sustaining service-learning, community-based participatory research, and community-campus partnerships are encouraged to apply for a fellowship with CCPH. The expected outcome of the program is to advance and support these concepts in the context of health professions education and practice. Fellows will receive a stipend for a one-year fellowship period, with the potential for a second year of funding. Funding provides support for time spent participating in fellow-related activities. Fellows also receive a certificate of recognition upon completing the fellowship. Application procedures and additional information are available online.
Requirements: CCPH members and nonmembers are eligible.
Amount of Grant: $5000
Contact: Sarena Seifer, Executive Director, (206) 616-4305; fax: (206) 685-6747; email: sarena@u.washington.edu or ccphuw@u.washington.edu
Internet: http://depts.washington.edu/ccph
Sponsor: Community Campus Partnerships for Health
UW Box 354809
Seattle, WA 98195-4809

Community Foundation AIDS Endowment Awards **1088**
The foundation administers an annual special grants program called the AIDS Endowment Awards. Grants of $1,000 will be awarded to one or two organizations that demonstrate a commitment to working towards the prevention, education and treatment of AIDS so that they may continue their efforts. Services provided could include education programs for the prevention of HIV/AIDS, medical and social services for those living with HIV/AIDS, housing services for those living with HIV/AIDS and medical research for the treatment and prevention of HIV/AIDS.
Requirements: Selected organizations in the metropolitan Richmond area interested in the field of AIDS education, research or community service and care are encouraged to apply. Organizations interested in applying should submit a brief proposal to foundation which should be no more than two single-spaced pages and include: [1] a description of the organization's mission; and [2] a description of the agency's work in the field of AIDS. Include a list of Board of Governors, a copy of the most recent IRS Form 990, an audited financial statement if available, and an IRS Tax Exempt Letter designating your organization a 501(c)3 non-profit.
Geographic Focus: Virginia
Amount of Grant: $1,000
Date(s) Application is Due: Feb 15
Contact: Susan Hallett, Program Officer, (804) 330-7400; fax: (804) 330-5992; email: shallett@tcfrichmond.org
Internet: http://www.tcfrichmond.org/Page2954.cfm
Sponsor: Community Foundation Serving Richmond and Central Virginia
7501 Boulders View Drive, Suite 110
Richmond, VA 23225

Community Foundation Alliance City of Evansville Endowment Fund Grants **1089**
The City of Evansville Endowment Fund originated in 1994, when former Mayor Frank McDonald II proposed that $5 million of revenue from the gaming boat be invested in a way that would serve the City of Evansville, Indiana, forever. The City of Evansville Endowment Fund's earnings allow for grant making year after year. During its most

recent grant cycle, the Fund allowed for grants totaling more than $180,000 to 21 nonprofit organizations serving the City of Evansville. The Foundation's grant cycle runs from May through October each year. Funding requests are accepted only during the grant cycle. The CEEF grants committee will consider funding requests of any amount. Requests of at least $1,000 are preferred.
Requirements: CEEF serves to provide funds to organizations that qualify as tax-exempt organizations under sections 501(c)3 and 509(a) of the Internal Revenue Code. The organization must serve within the city limits of Evansville, Indiana. At least sixty percent (60%) of grant funding will be distributed for activities that will support or benefit the 4th and 6th wards of the City of Evansville.
Restrictions: Not more than thirty percent (30%) of any grant request may be for personnel costs, travel costs, office supplies and other program operating costs.
Geographic Focus: Indiana
Samples: Ark Crisis Child Care Center—to purchase and install fencing to enclose the playground, $3,200 (2008); Evansville Junior Football League—to assist with the construction of a handicap accessible restroom and storage building on the football field grounds in Howell Park, $5,000 (2008); Little Lambs of Evansville—for the purchase and installation of shelving units and for a rolling cart, clothes racks, and storage containers, $1,700 (2008).
Date(s) Application is Due: Oct 31
Contact: Melinda Waldroup, Program Director; (812) 429-1191 or (877) 429-1191; fax: (812) 429-0840; email: mwaldroup@alliance9.org
Internet: http://www.alliance9.org/city-of-evansville-endowment-fund
Sponsor: Community Foundation Alliance
123 N.W. Fourth Street, Suite 322
Evansville, IN 47708-1712

Community Foundation for Greater Buffalo Grants **1090**
Grants are made to organizations in and for the benefit of Erie County, NY, residents. The foundation supports charitable, educational, and civic purposes and awards grants for educational institutions, scholarships, family and child health and welfare, and community development. Highest priority is given to projects that support creative and innovative responses to existing or emerging community problems.
Requirements: IRS 509(a) organizations in or benefiting residents of Allegany, Cattaraugus, Chautauqua, Erie, Genesee, Niagara, Orleans, and Wyoming Counties, NY, are eligible.
Restrictions: Grant requests are not considered for endowment funds, religious purposes, projects outside the western New York region, or schools not registered with the state education department.
Geographic Focus: New York
Samples: Greater Buffalo Opera Comp (Buffalo, NY)—to refurbish and renovate a set for a production of Carmen, $10,000.; Bison Fund-Buffalo Inner-City Scholarship Opportunity Network (Buffalo, NY)—for elementary school students, to provide low-income, inner-city parents with the option of choosing a private or parochial school for their children, $10,000.
Amount of Grant: $1000-$25,000 typically
Date(s) Application is Due: Feb 1; Aug 1
Contact: Jean McKeown, Program Officer, (716) 852-2857, ext. 204; fax: (716) 852-2861; email: jeanm@cfgb.org
Internet: http://www.cfgb.org/page17000.cfm
Sponsor: Community Foundation for Greater Buffalo
712 Main Street
Buffalo, NY 14202

Community Foundation for Greater New Haven Grants **1091**
The foundation is interested in all fields of community activity—education, health, basic human needs, programs for children and youth, and community vitalization. It seeks to strengthen existing Connecticut organizations and to assist in the development of new programs and services in direct response to a need in the community. Types of support include general operating budgets, continuing support, seed money, emergency funds, building funds, equipment, matching funds, consulting services, technical assistance, special projects, loans, scholarship funds, and endowment funds. Capital projects or requests for building funds are a low priority. Interested organizations should discuss the proposed project with foundation staff prior to application. Annual deadline dates may vary; contact program staff for exact dates.
Requirements: IRS 501(c)3 nonprofit organizations in the greater New Haven area, which includes the area from Wallingford to Long Island Sound, shoreline communities from Milford to Madison, and towns in the lower Naugatuck Valley, are eligible.
Restrictions: Grants are not made to support religious activities, lobbying, or travel. Only in rare instances does the foundation support research projects, publications, scholarship programs, or single event/activities.
Geographic Focus: Connecticut
Samples: Saint Rose Parish (CT)—support for maintenance and improvements to a garden used by residents of the area as a tool to teach science to children attending Saint Rose School.; Long Wharf Theater (New Haven, CT)—to refurbish and expand this 32-year-old theater, $500,000.
Date(s) Application is Due: Mar 9; Jun 15
Contact: Grants Administrator, (203) 777-2386; fax: (203) 787-6584; email: contactus@cfgnh.org
Internet: http://www.cfgnh.org/page9075.cfm
Sponsor: Community Foundation for Greater New Haven
70 Audubon Street
New Haven, CT 06510-9755

Community Foundation for Monterey County Grants **1092**
The community foundation supports nonprofits in Monterey, CA, in the areas of social services, education, environment, arts, health, historic preservation, and general charitable giving. Collaboratives are highly encouraged. The foundation awards grants through its General Endowment. Technical Assistance grants and Neighborhood Grants also are awarded. Types of support include seed money, emergency funds, general operating support, building funds, equipment acquisition, land acquisition, matching funds, projects, consulting services, and technical assistance. Information on how to apply for each type of grant can be accessed online.
Requirements: 501(c)3 tax-exempt organizations in Monterey may submit applications.
Restrictions: The foundation does not support individuals, religious activities, scholarships, fellowships, travel, research, salaries and other operating expenses of schools and public agencies, annual campaigns, or special events; create or add to endowment funds; or pay off debt.
Geographic Focus: California
Amount of Grant: $20,000 maximum, $40,000 maximum for collaboratives; $5000-$9000 typically
Date(s) Application is Due: Jan 3; May 2; Aug 1
Contact: Jackie Wendland, Grants Administrator, (831) 375-9712 ext 11; fax: (831) 375-4731; email: jackie@cfmco.org
Internet: http://www.cfmco.org/grantsOverview.php
Sponsor: Community Foundation for Monterey County
2354 Garden Road
Monterey, CA 93940

Community Foundation for Muskegon County Grants **1093**
The community foundation was established to serve the needs of the people of Muskegon County and nearby western Michigan. The foundation's strategic plan for grant making focuses on the prevention of problems rather than the cure; encourages programs that are collaborative, comprehensive, and have the potential to be continuous; encourages leveraging and matching grant opportunities from multiple funders; and supports seed money opportunities for innovative projects. Major grant interest areas include the arts, community development and urban revitalization, education, environment, health/human services, and needs of young children (ages 0-3). Types of support include seed money grants, special projects, matching funds, equipment, scholarship funds, loans, research, publications, conferences and seminars, endowment funds, consulting services, continuing support, emergency funds, internships, professorships, and renovation projects. Although the foundation generally makes one-year grant commitments, it will consider making longer term commitments for new efforts that show strong promise for positive impact. Applications are accepted on specific dates each year; it is recommended that the applicant contact the foundation to discuss their interests and to obtain the next grant application deadline.
Requirements: IRS 501(c)3 organizations and institutions in Muskegon County and nearby western Michigan are eligible.
Restrictions: Support will not be provided for routine operating expenses; capital equipment, computer hardware and software, and motor vehicles; conferences, publications, videos, films, television, or radio programs; endowment campaigns; special fund-raising events; religious programs that serve specific denominations; existing obligations or debts; individual schools or districts; or individuals.
Geographic Focus: Michigan
Samples: Camp Bluebird, $5,000 to support the participation of Muskegon residents at a retreat for cancer patients; Michigan State University—Muskegon County extension Office, $5,000 to support a local match for the Land Use Education Program; West Shore Symphony Orchestra, $3,000 to support year three of the Carnegie LinkUP; First Congregational Church, $3,200 to support the Saturday Morning Breakfast program; Muskegon County Museum, $5,000 for an exhibit of the history of medicine in Muskegon.
Amount of Grant: $250-$50,000 average
Contact: Gina Van Bruggen or Arn Boezaart, Program Officers, (231) 722-4538; fax: (231) 722-4616; email: gvanbruggen@cffmc.org or aboezaart@cffmc.org
Internet: http://www.cffmc.org/grantapply.php
Sponsor: Community Foundation for Muskegon County
425 W Western Avenue, Suite 200
Muskegon, MI 49440

Community Foundation for Southeastern Michigan Grants **1094**
The community foundation's grantmaking activity focuses on a seven-county region and supports a wide variety of activities benefiting arts and culture, education, health, human services, civic affairs, neighborhood and regional economic development, workforce development, and environment and land use. Usually grants provide start-up or short-term funding for innovative projects that meet new needs or demonstrate new solutions for old ones. Additional types of support include scholarship funds, technical assistance, and general operating support. Priority will be given to applications that develop or test new solutions to community challenges, increase the effectiveness or efficiency of nonprofit activities, enhance the quality of an organization's efforts and its stature, facilitate cooperation and collaboration among organizations, increase the diversity and competitiveness of the region's economy, and encourage civic development and volunteerism. Grant proposals may be submitted at any time. The application must be in writing and include a cover letter outlining purpose, background, amount requested, and time limits of the proposed activity.
Requirements: 501(c)3 nonprofits in the following seven Michigan counties are eligible to apply: Livingston, Macomb, Montclair, Monroe, Oakland, Washtenaw, Wayne.

Restrictions: Normally, grants will not be made for buildings or equipment, general operating support (except in the first few years of an organization's existence), endowments, sectarian religious programs, fund-raising campaigns, grants to individuals, conferences and annual meetings, or projects outside the seven-county region.
Geographic Focus: Michigan
Amount of Grant: $10,000-$75,000; $30,000 average
Date(s) Application is Due: Mar 1; Jun 1; Sep 1; Dec 1
Contact: Grant Administrator, (313) 961-6675; fax: (313) 961-2886; email: cfsem@cfsem.org
Internet: http://www.cfsem.org/grants/index.html
Sponsor: Community Foundation for Southeastern Michigan
333 W Fort Street, Suite 2010
Detroit, MI 48226-3134

Community Foundation for Southern Arizona Grants **1095**
The foundation awards grants in southern Arizona for a broad array of charitable purposes in the areas of arts and humanities, education, the environment, health, social services. Types of support include challenge/matching grants, conferences and seminars, scholarships, equipment acquisition, fellowships, general support, multiyear support, project development, publications, research, seed funding, and technical assistance. Priority is given to proposals that promote collaboration and build on the strengths of individuals and communities. Deadlines are determined on a yearly basis.
Requirements: Nonprofit and grassroots organizations in southern Arizona communities are eligible. Southern Arizona communities include all of Cochise, Santa Cruz, and Pima Counties; and the areas of Yuma, Mariposa, Pinal, Graham, and Greenlee Counties that lie south of the Gila River.
Restrictions: Funds are generally not available for ongoing operating or capital campaigns, debt retirement, endowments, individuals, individual schools, sectarian activities, or underwriting of fund-raising events.
Geographic Focus: Arizona
Samples: Arizona's Children Association (AZ)—for KARE legal services, $7200 (2005); Tucson Clean and Beautiful (Tucson, AZ)—for Adopt-A-Park Program, $2000 (2005); Tucson Children's Museum, Inc (Tucson, AZ)—to cover admission costs for low-income children, $2250 (2004); Tucson Cinema Foundation Inc (Tucson, AZ)—funding for a ten-month program for high school students, $5600 (2004).
Amount of Grant: $1000-$10,000 average range
Contact: Barbara Brown, Executive Vice President, (520) 770-0800 ext 107; fax: (520) 770-1500; email: bbrown@CFSoAZ.org
Internet: http://www.cfsoaz.org/page17480.cfm
Sponsor: Community Foundation for Southern Arizona
2250 E Broadway Boulevard
Tucson, AZ 85719

Community Foundation of Bartholomew County Heritage Fund Grants **1096**
The goal of the Heritage Fund's grant program is to achieve the maximum impact with the available resources. The Fund will consider grant applications that: are change-orientated and problem-solving in nature; strive to anticipate the changing needs of the community and to be flexible in responding to them; address the needs of a significant number of community residents and provide the greatest benefit per dollar granted; encourage support from the community by using matching, challenge and other grant techniques; have a broad funding base, with additional support being sought from the government, foundations, associations and other funders; enable grant recipients to achieve certain objectives such as capacity building, and/or increasing efficiency, effectiveness and fund-raising capabilities; request technical assistance or specialized help with projects that respond to community needs; or positively impact the Heritage Fund's Areas of Initiative.
Requirements: Grants are made to not-for-profit organizations whose programs benefit the residents of Bartholomew County, Indiana.
Restrictions: The Heritage Fund provides seed money or support for the pilot phase of a program. The Heritage Fund does not generally provide operating support.
Geographic Focus: Indiana
Amount of Grant: $3,000 maximum
Date(s) Application is Due: Mar 1; Jun 1; Sep 1; Dec 1
Contact: Lynda J. Morgan, Program Officer; (812) 376-7772; fax: (812) 376-0051; email: lmorgan@heritagefundbc.org
Internet: http://www.heritagefundbc.com/grants/process_guidelines_deadlines.php
Sponsor: Community Foundation of Bartholomew County
538 Franklin Street, P.O. Box 1547
Columbus, IN 47202-1547

Community Foundation of Bartholomew County James A. Henderson Award for Fund-Raising **1097**
This award recognizes the invaluable role volunteer fund-raisers play in advancing the quality of life within Bartholomew County, Indiana. Not-for-profit organizations in the county are invited to nominate volunteers who have performed outstanding fund-raising for their organizations. A committee will review the nominations and select the person to be honored. The committee will consider such criteria as innovation, sustainability, creativity, effectiveness, effort, ability to engage others, outreach to new donors, etc. Generally the amount raised will not be a major factor in the scoring. Efforts will be made to recognize unsung heroes in fund-raising. The successful nominee will be recognized at the Heritage Fund's Annual Report to the Community. He/she will receive a small gift and the nominating organization will receive a $2,500 grant in honor of the winner.
Geographic Focus: Indiana
Amount of Grant: $2,500 honorarium
Contact: Lynda J. Morgan, Program Officer; (812) 376-7772; fax: (812) 376-0051; email: lmorgan@heritagefundbc.org
Internet: http://www.heritagefundbc.com/grants/award_james_henderson.php
Sponsor: Community Foundation of Bartholomew County
538 Franklin Street, P.O. Box 1547
Columbus, IN 47202-1547

Community Foundation of Bloomington and Monroe County Grants **1098**
Grants will be made for a wide variety of programs and purposes in support of the arts and cultural activities, social and health concerns, educational activities, beautification projects, and for other community development needs that will benefit the citizens of Bloomington and Monroe County, Indiana. Start-up funds for special projects reflecting incremental growth possibilities will be given particular attention. Additional types of support include building construction and renovation, equipment acquisition, program development, seed grants, and scholarship funds. Projects that provide leverage for generating other funds and community resources or are seed money for new programs will also receive special attention. It is expected that the majority of grants will be made for one time only; however, multi-year grants may be considered in unusual circumstances. Applications are reviewed in March, June, September, and December.
Requirements: Grants are made only to nonprofit organizations and programs in Bloomington or Monroe County, Indiana.
Restrictions: Grants will not be made for general operating support purposes; endowment campaigns or for previously incurred debts; or for political purposes.
Geographic Focus: Indiana
Samples: Camerata (IN)—to underwrite musical performances for children, $2000.; Shelter Inc (IN)—to replace locks on temporary shelter homes, $1500.; Bloomington Fire Department (IN)—to underwrite a fire safety program for children, $200.; Bloomington Parks and Recreation (IN)—for historic park development, $9000.
Contact: Renee M. Chambers, Program Director; (812) 333-9016; fax: (812) 333-1153; email: renee@cfbmc.org
Internet: http://www.communityfoundation.ws
Sponsor: Community Foundation of Bloomington and Monroe County
101 W. Kirkwood Avenue, Suite 321
Bloomington, IN 47404

Community Foundation of Boone County Grants **1099**
Generally, the Community Foundation of Boone County provides grants in the following areas: youth, human services, arts, culture, health, civic affairs, environment, recreation, education and the elderly. Applications for grants of $10,000 or less should be submitted on the Short Form (found at the website); applications for more than $10,000 should follow instructions in the Content and Format section of the website. There are no particular deadlines with which to adhere.
Requirements: Awards will be made to nonprofit organizations exempt from federal taxation under section 501 (C)(3) of the Internal Revenue Code. Grants may be allowed to individuals and to non-501(C)(3) organizations if there is documented charitable activity benefiting or serving the residents of Boone County, or if the Community Foundation is acting as fiscal agent for the project or program.
Restrictions: Non-allowable expenses include support of pre-award costs (i.e., project costs generated during the preparation of a proposal for the same project); existing general fund operating expenses; regular salaries of pre-award permanent staff (unless overload compensation is justified during the life of the funded project); international travel; first-class air fare; luxury accommodations; hospitality for purposes other than those directly related to meeting program objectives as defined in the proposal; alcohol; and indirect or regular existing administrative costs (e.g., telephone, utilities, general maintenance, etc.) of the applicant organization.
Geographic Focus: Indiana
Contact: Barbara J. Schroeder, Program Director; (317) 873-0210 or (765) 482-0024; fax: (317) 873-0219; email: barb@CommunityFoundationBC.org
Internet: http://www.communityfoundationbc.org/grants.html
Sponsor: Community Foundation of Boone County
P.O. Box 92, 60 East Cedar Street
Zionsville, IN 46077

Community Foundation of Broward Grants **1100**
Through its competitive grantmaking process, the foundation supports programs that strengthen families within low socioeconomic communities in Florida's Broward County. Grantmaking priorities include the arts, foster care, out-of-school time, and technology. Proposals also are accepted in specific areas of interest, including animal welfare—protect and educate; cancer and arthritis research—finding a cure; patient care—relief and assistance to individuals with cancer or other terminal diseases; literacy—opening worlds through language, an AIDS/HIV—through issued RFP. Proposals are accepted anytime throughout the year. Application and guidelines are available online.
Requirements: 501(c)3 organizations, public charities as defined by the IRS code, and governmental agencies located in Broward County or directly benefiting the residents of Broward County are eligible.
Restrictions: Grants are not awarded in the following areas: annual fundraising, capital campaign/improvements, deficit financing, endowment efforts, grants to individuals, religious purposes, or routine operating needs.
Geographic Focus: Florida
Amount of Grant: $10,000 average
Contact: Sheri Brown, Vice President of Strategic Community Initiatives, (954) 761-9503 ext 103; fax: (954) 761-7102; email: jbull@cfbroward.org

Internet: http://www.cfbroward.org/new/grant.html
Sponsor: Community Foundation of Broward
1401 E Broward Boulevard, Suite 100
Fort Lauderdale, FL 33301

Community Foundation of Central Illinois Grants **1101**
The foundation funds programs in the fields of education, arts, human services, community service, or community development, and that advance one or more of the following objectives: address and help resolve important existing or emerging community issues; support new and creative projects and organizations offering the greatest opportunity for positive and significant change; promote cooperation and collaboration among organizations; identify, enhance, and develop leadership in the community through creative and innovative activities that empower individuals; and improve the quality or scope of charitable works in our community. Application guidelines are available online.
Requirements: Nonprofits within a 50-mile radius of Peoria, IL, are eligible.
Restrictions: The foundation will not fund annual campaigns, individuals, or endowments, or make grants for sectarian religious purposes.
Geographic Focus: Illinois
Amount of Grant: $2500-$3000 average range
Date(s) Application is Due: Jan 15; Apr 15; Sep 15
Contact: Kerri Foutch, Program Officer, (309) 674-8730; fax: (309) 674-8754; email: kerri@communityfoundationci.org
Internet: http://www.communityfoundationci.org/grant_guidelines.asp
Sponsor: Community Foundation of Central Illinois
331 Fulton Street, Suite 310
Peoria, IL 61602

Community Foundation of Champaign County Grants **1102**
The community foundation awards grants from its unrestricted funds to Champaign County, IL, nonprofit organizations to use for charitable purposes. Representative categories include arts and humanities, environmental concerns, education, health, human services, research, urban affairs, church, and youth programs. Types of support include continuing support, annual campaigns, building/renovation, equipment, publication, consulting services, and scholarships.
Requirements: Champaign County, IL, nonprofit organizations are eligible.
Geographic Focus: Illinois
Amount of Grant: $1000-$2000 typically
Date(s) Application is Due: Aug 31
Contact: Joan Dixon, (217) 359-0125; fax: (217) 352-6494; email: cfcc@soltec.net
Sponsor: Community Foundation of Champaign County
404 W Church Street
Champaign, IL 61820

Community Foundation of Crawford County Grants and Scholarships **1103**
The CFCC's community grant program reflects the needs of the community. The CFCC maintains an effective relationship as grantor, and community organizations (as grantees), which is based on mutual respect and partnership. Since 1998 the CFCC has awarded over $5.5million in programming/grants and scholarships. Fields of interest are: animal Protection; arts; community development; education; environment; health & safety; human services; historical preservation; emergency recovery; infants & children; literacy; parks & recreation; public radio; public service; religion; technology; youth; women & girls. Grant, as well as scholarship requests are made by first contacting the President & CEO of the foundation.
Requirements: Grantees are required to provide ongoing status reports. CFCC Board members are assigned grant projects to mentor. Additionally, grantees are required to report on the actual outcomes of the funding versus the original anticipated outcomes.
Restrictions: Funding opportunities are generally restricted to the Crawford County.
Geographic Focus: Indiana
Contact: Bonita Embry Coots, President & CEO, (812) 633-2077; fax: (812) 633-2429; email: BECoots@cf-cc.org
Internet: http://www.cf-cc.org/page31105.cfm
Sponsor: Community Foundation of Crawford County
9430 East State Road 64 or P.O. Box 205
Milltown, IN 47145

Community Foundation of Grant County Grants **1104**
The Community Foundation of Grant County Indiana intends to address the needs of the county, in the following fields of interest: community development; education; health; human services
Requirements: Nonprofit 501 (C)(3) organizations, coalitions, community associations, and other civic groups may apply if it provides serves in Grant County, Indiana.
Restrictions: To be eligible for a grant, the project must be located in, or directly serve the people and natural resources in Grant County Indiana.
Geographic Focus: Indiana
Date(s) Application is Due: Deadlines for applications are prior to noon on the last Friday in April, July, October, and January.
Contact: Sherrie Stahl, Office and Program Director; (765) 662-0065; email: sstahl@comfdn.org
Internet: http://www.comfdn.org/grants.htm
Sponsor: Community Foundation of Grant County
505 West Third Street
Marion, IN 46952

Community Foundation of Grant County Scholarships **1105**
The mission of the Community Foundation of Grant County has always been to enhance an improved quality of life in Grant County. The Foundation provides scholarships in the following areas: agriculture, medical field, religion/philosophy, math sciences, environment, sports
Requirements: The foundation has one standard form for all scholarships, which is available at the foundations office, website, the Grant County Library or from your guidance counselors.
Restrictions: Must be a resident of Grant County to apply.
Geographic Focus: Indiana
Contact: Sherrie Stahl, Program Director; (765) 662-0065; email: sstahl@comfdn.org
Internet: http://www.comfdn.org/scholarships.htm
Sponsor: Community Foundation of Grant County
505 West Third Street
Marion, IN 46952

Community Foundation of Greater Birmingham Grants **1106**
The community foundation serving the greater Birmingham, AL, area awards grants in arts and culture, education, environment, health, and welfare. Types of support include capital campaigns, operating support, building/renovation, equipment, program development, publication, seed money, curriculum development, and matching funds. Grant requests are considered twice a year at distribution committee meetings. The foundation requires that grant requests be submitted in writing. There is no application form. Applicants are asked to submit a cover letter and a complete statement of the purpose of the grant, including the need for the project and population and number of people to be served, project budget, other funding sources, length of time for which foundation aid is needed, a method to evaluate the project's success, description of applicant organization including annual budget, copy of IRS determination letter, and names of the board of directors or trustees.
Requirements: 501(c)3 organizations that provide services in greater Birmingham metrop area (Jefferson, Shelby, St. Clair, Blount and Walker counties) are eligible.
Restrictions: Grants are not made to or for individuals, operating expenses of organizations, religious organizations for religious purposes, national fund-raising drives, conference or seminar expenses, tickets for benefits, political organizations or candidates for public office, organizations with IRS 501(h) status, budget deficits, replacement of government funding cuts, or scholarships or endowment funds.
Geographic Focus: Alabama
Samples: Exchange Club Family Skills Center, $2,200—program support (2009); Catholic Family Services, $4,600— to expand outpatient psychiatric care for uninsured women and children in metro Birmingham (2009); Birmingham Civil Rights Institute, $20,000— toward operating costs as the institute continues to serve the general public, tourists and students, particularly in kindergarten through second grade (2009).
Date(s) Application is Due: Mar 15; Sep 15
Contact: James McCrary, Senior Program Officer; (205) 327-3812 or (205) 327-3800; fax: (205) 328-6576; email: jmccrary@foundationbirmingham.org or guidelines@foundationbirmingham.org
Internet: http://www.foundationbirmingham.org/page30508.cfm
Sponsor: Community Foundation of Greater Birmingham
2100 First Avenue, North, Suite 700
Birmingham, AL 35203-4223

Community Foundation of Greater Flint Grants **1107**
The community foundation is interested in funding charitable organizations that are able to demonstrate they have planned their projects with respect to the community's needs in the areas of arts and humanities, community services, education, environment and conservation, ethics, health, human and social services, and philanthropy. The foundation's current objectives for the allocation of discretionary funds give top priority to programs that: advance the health and well-being of children; and/or improve the capacity of public education. Types of support include general operating support, program development, seed money, scholarship funds, and technical assistance. Applications are available on the Web site.
Requirements: IRS 501(c)3 organizations with programs of direct relevance to the residents of Genesee County, Michigan are eligible. Types of support include general operating support.
Restrictions: Grants will not be made to individuals. In general, requests for sectarian religious purposes, budget deficits, routine operating expenses of existing organizations, litigation, endowments, and other capital fund drives or projects are not funded.
Geographic Focus: Michigan
Samples: Greater Flint Health Coalition, $40,000—towards the Flint Healthcare Employment Opportunities (FHEO) program, which helps unemployed or low-income individuals in Genesee County to obtain employment opportunities or to advance in the healthcare industry (2009); Genesee Chamber Foundation,$30,000— towards the Summer Youth Initiative, a summer employment and leadership development program for Genesee County youth ages 14-18 (2009); United Way of Genesee County, $66,000-in support of the BEST Project (Building Excellence, Sustainability and Trust) BEST provides technical assistance and resources designed to build the capacity of area nonprofit organizations (2009).
Contact: Lynn Larkin, Senior Program Officer; (810) 767-8270; fax: (810) 767-0496; email: llarkin@cfgf.org
Internet: http://www.cfgf.org/page32610.cfm
Sponsor: Community Foundation of Greater Flint
500 South Saginaw Street
Flint, MI 48502-1206

Community Foundation of Greater Fort Wayne: Community Endowment & Clarke Endowment Fund Grants 1108

The Foundation encourages projects or programs that are developed in consultation with other agencies and planning groups that increase coordination and cooperation among agencies and reduce unnecessary duplication of services. Preference is given to projects or programs that: address priority community concerns; encourage more effective use of community resources; test or demonstrate new approaches and techniques in the solution of community problems; are intended to strengthen the management capabilities of agencies; promote volunteer participation and citizen involvement in community affairs. Contact program staff for current guidelines and deadlines. The deadlines listed are for concept letters, with final invited proposals due by dates provided by the Foundation.
Requirements: Nonprofit organizations in the greater Fort Wayne, Indiana, area are eligible to apply.
Restrictions: Grants do not support: annual fund drives; operating deficits or after-the-fact support; endowment funds, except for endowment-building matching grants for funds held at the Community Foundation; direct or grassroots lobbying; religious purposes; hospitals, medical research, or academic research; public, private, or parochial educational institutions except in special situations when support is essential to projects/programs that meet critical community needs; governmental agencies, including public school systems, except in special situations when support is essential to projects/programs that meet critical community needs; limited, special interest organizations except when such support significantly benefits the disadvantaged; and funding for sponsorships, special events, commercial advertising, films or videos, television programs, conferences, group uniforms, or group trips.
Geographic Focus: Indiana
Samples: Salvation Army of Fort Wayne (Fort Wayne, Indiana)—for remodeling of building, $50,000.; United Way of Allen County (Fort Wayne, Indiana)—for diversity and special urban initiatives, $100,000.; Local Education Fund (Fort Wayne, IN)—for training materials, $38,314.
Date(s) Application is Due: Jan 12; Apr 13; Oct 14
Contact: Christine Meek, Senior Program Officer; (260) 426-4083; fax: (260) 424-0114; email: cmeek@cfgfw.org
Internet: http://www.cfgfw.org/
Sponsor: Community Foundation of Greater Fort Wayne
555 East Wayne Street
Fort Wayne, IN 46802

Community Foundation of Greater Greensboro Grants 1109

The foundation supports community projects that strengthen the community, embrace the diversity of the community, demonstrate community support and in-kind investment, outline well-established proposed plans, and focus on collaborative efforts. Grants are awarded in the areas of community building, cultural and civic programs, arts, community development, health, environment, and social services. Types of support include general support, program development, seed grants, and emergency community funding. Annual deadline dates may vary; contact program staff for exact dates.
Requirements: Nonprofit organizations in Greensboro, NC, are eligible.
Restrictions: The Foundation does not award grants from the Community Grants Program for individuals, debt retirement, political organizations or campaigns, for-profit entities, capital campaigns, programming that promotes religious instruction or doctrine, or endowments.
Geographic Focus: North Carolina
Amount of Grant: $10,000 average
Date(s) Application is Due: Feb 15; Jun 15; Oct 15
Contact: Melissa Johnson, Program Officer, (336) 379-9100 ext 124; fax: (336) 378-0725; email: mjohnson@cfgg.org
Internet: http://www.cfgg.org/guidelines-new.htm
Sponsor: Community Foundation of Greater Greensboro
P.O. Box 20444
Greensboro, NC 27420

Community Foundation Of Greater Lafayette Grants 1110

An important part of The Community Foundation of Greater Lafayette's mission is realized though the use of grants to meet the ever-changing needs of the community. The foundation achieves this by carrying out the wishes of our donors through restricted dollars and by using discretionary funds to award grants to address community needs. Some of the areas funded include arts and humanities, health, education, housing and homelessness, child care, substance abuse, mental health, community beautification, and conservation — helping you help your community. Grant seekers are encouraged to submit proposals that include diverse financial support and that do not rely on the community foundation for 100% of the funding. There are three separate funding tiers and deadlines for discretionary grant proposals: tier 1, proposals requesting $15,000 or more, with a deadline of noon on April 1; tier 2, proposals requesting $7,500 - $14,999 with a deadline of noon on September 1; tier 3, proposals requesting less than $7,500, with a deadline of noon on December 1.
Requirements: Charitable organizations that serve Tippecanoe and the surrounding counties are eligible to apply for grants. Most of our grants are awarded to organizations that are located in and serve Tippecanoe County.
Restrictions: The foundation generally doesn't fund political organizations or candidates, government agencies or public institutions, programs that taxpayers would normally support, or individuals (except scholarships from scholarship funds).
Geographic Focus: Indiana
Date(s) Application is Due: Apr 1; Sep 1; Dec 1
Contact: Cheryl Ubelhor, Program Director; (765) 742-9078; fax: (765) 742-2428; email: cheryl@cfglaf.org
Internet: http://www.glcfonline.org/grantseekers/index.htm
Sponsor: Community Foundation of Greater Lafayette
1114 East State Street
Lafayette, IN 47905-1219

Community Foundation of Greater New Britain Grants 1111

Grants from the Community Foundation of Greater New Britain support organizations and programs benefiting the residents of Berlin, New Britain, Plainville and Southington, Connecticut. The foundation supports organizations involved with arts, culture and heritage; community and economic development; early childhood development; education; health and human services.
Requirements: Grants are available to non-profit organizations that have tax-exempt status under Section 501(c)3 of the IRS Code or that are a qualified entity eligible to receive grants from community foundations under the IRS Code. The foundation will also consider funding a grassroots group if it consists of at least five people, has a governing body and a fiscal agent with the appropriate tax status. All grant applications must begin with a one or two page Letter of Intent summarizing the program or project for which funding is being sought. Submitted Letters of Intent will be reviewed by staff. Applicants selected by staff to submit complete, formal applications will be contacted directly to begin the proposal.
Restrictions: The Foundation does not make grants for: sectarian or religious activities; previously incurred expenses; annual or endowment campaigns; sponsorships or fundraisers; political activities; direct support of individuals; camperships or scholarships for academic and/or enrichment programs. In addition, the Foundation generally does not make grants for performances or one-time events, conferences or advertising.
Geographic Focus: Connecticut
Samples: New Britain Museum of American Art, New Britain, Connecticut, $60,000 - fund for support of the Museum's Education and Outreach program (2008); Municipal Economic Development Agency, New Britain, Connecticut, $15,000 - to develop an economic development website for the City of New Britain featuring economic development tools and information that will promote business in New Britain (2008); New Britain Public Library/Jefferson Family Resource Center, New Britain, Connecticut, $12,000 - for the "Raise a Reader" program, aimed at improving literacy skills among hard-to-reach New Britain families with children under age five. (2008);
Amount of Grant: $5,000 - $25,000 range
Date(s) Application is Due: Feb 15; Jun 15; Oct 15;
Contact: Joeline Wruck, Program Director; (860) 229-6018, ext. 307; email: jwruck@cfgnb.org
Internet: http://www.cfgnb.org/GrantsScholarships/tabid/68/Default.aspx
Sponsor: Community Foundation of Greater New Britain
74A Vine Street
New Britain, CT 06052

Community Foundation of Greater Tampa Grants 1112

The Community Foundation of Tampa Bay is a nonprofit, tax-exempt organization which administers funds established by individuals, corporations, private foundations, and nonprofit organizations to support the charitable needs of the Tampa Bay area. Program interests of the Foundation include: arts and culture, community development, education, environment, animals, health and, human services.
Requirements: Florida 501(c)3 organizations based in and serving communities in Hillsborough, Pasco, Pinellas and/or Hernando counties are eligible.
Restrictions: The Foundation is generally not interested in requests for: funding of ongoing operating costs; grants for capital campaigns or expenditures; tickets for any fundraising event, conference, or advertising space in programs or other publications; legislative lobbying or political campaigns; medical research; religious or sectarian purposes; loans or assistance to individuals; a multiple year funding commitment.
Geographic Focus: Florida
Samples: Bay Springs—for the equipment, uniforms, shoes, and transportation of adolescent boys in foster care to participate in city and community sports leagues (2009); Salesian Youth Center/Boys and Girls Club—for the Literacy and Technology Initiative at the Salesian Youth Center to offer reading comprehension and computer skills training to children 5-18 (2009).
Amount of Grant: $7,500 maximum
Date(s) Application is Due: Mar 1; Sep 1
Contact: Ann Berg, Vice President of Grants; (813) 282-1975; fax; (813) 282-3119; email: aberg@cftampabay.org
Internet: http://www.cftampabay.org/nonprofit_resources/grant_app_guidelines.html
Sponsor: Community Foundation of Greater Tampa
550 North Reo Street, Suite 301
Tampa, FL 33609

Community Foundation of Greenville Community Enrichment Grants 1113

The Community Foundation of Greenville supports qualified nonprofit organizations in the areas of the arts and humanities, education, early childhood education, religion, and environmental programs. The Foundation is committed to the responsible allocation of the Foundation's unrestricted funds. As an organization, the Foundation seeks ways to make meaningful, sustained differences in the quality of life for the citizens of Greenville County. The goal is to seek out community-based projects where a modest grant can make a significant impact. The Foundation encourages proposals that: propose practical solutions to community problems; promote cooperation among agencies without duplicating services; use modest funds to make a significant impact; address prevention

as well as remediation; make use of matching funds; strengthen an agency's effectiveness and stability; generate community support, both professional and volunteer; state project objectives in measurable terms. The application deadline is 4:00 pm on Friday, March 5.
Requirements: All 501(c)3 non-profit groups can apply for Community Foundation grants to fund innovative projects that have a direct relevance to the Greenville County, South Carolina area. An agency can receive one community enrichment grant per year.
Restrictions: The Foundation will: not make grants to individuals; not fund capacity building; will give low grant making priority to capital fund projects.
Geographic Focus: South Carolina
Date(s) Application is Due: Mar 5
Contact: Debbie Cooper, Director of Donor Services; (864) 331-8414 or (864) 233-5925; fax: (864) 242-9292; email: dcooper@cfgg.com or Cfgg@cfgg.com
Internet: http://www.cfgreenville.org/page18740.cfm
Sponsor: Community Foundation of Greenville Inc
27 Cleveland Street, Suite 101
Greenville, SC 29601

Community Foundation of Greenville Hollingsworth Program/Project Grants 1114
The Hollingsworth Funds, Inc. has a competitive grant process that is administered by the Community Foundation. Consistent with the purposes established by its benefactor, John D. Hollingsworth, Jr., an astute textile executive and real estate investor. The Hollingsworth Funds will serve a broad range of charitable, educational, religious, literary and cultural purposes. The Hollingsworth Funds has adopted initial guidelines in order to assist its evaluation of charitable organizations for funding. The Hollingsworth Funds will make grants: to health and human service agencies dedicated to improving quality of life for residents of Greenville County and particularly for those which deliver services to the poor, homeless, and illiterate; to interdenominational faith-based programs that benefit a broad cross-section of the community; to a wide variety of arts and education related initiatives including high quality preschool and after school programs; for grants for capital projects that provide a public benefit on a nondiscriminatory basis; to increase the organizational capacity of a non-profit organization; to public/private partnerships. The Hollingsworth Funds will give priority to new and innovative projects that are outside of the scope of an organization's ongoing operating budget. To submit a request for funding, a charitable organization must deliver or mail two (2) complete application packets to the Community Foundation of Greenville by 4:00 pm on September 3. All applicants will be notified of their status by December 31.
Requirements: A 501(c)3 charitable organization can submit one grant application per year for an amount not to exceed $50,000 to fund innovative projects for the benefit of charitable uses within Greenville County, South Carolina, or for the benefit of residents of Greenville County.
Restrictions: The Hollingsworth Funds will not make grants: to sponsor special fundraising events, celebration functions, dinners or annual meetings; for areas that are traditionally the primary responsibility of local, state or federal governments; for core operating expenses of public, private or parochial schools; that primarily benefit the religious activities of a church, synagogue, mosque or other house of worship; to pay off existing debts; scholarship awards or grants to individuals.
Geographic Focus: South Carolina
Amount of Grant: $50,000 maximum
Date(s) Application is Due: Sep 3
Contact: Debbie Cooper, Director of Donor Services; (864) 331-8414 or (864) 233-5925; fax: (864) 242-9292; email: dcooper@cfgg.com or Cfgg@cfgg.com
Internet: http://www.cfgreenville.org/page18741.cfm
Sponsor: Community Foundation of Greenville
27 Cleveland Street, Suite 101
Greenville, SC 29601

Community Foundation of Greenville-Greenville Women Giving Grants 1115
Greenville Women Giving (GWG) is a special initiative of Community Foundation of Greenville. GWG is a philanthropic organization, founded on the idea that women, informed about philanthropy and the needs in their community, collectively can make a real difference. GWG is committed to strengthening the community through the collective resources of it's members by awarding high-impact grants in five areas: arts and culture, education, health, human services, and environment. GWG will award grants ranging from a minimum of $40,000 to $100,000 to community organizations in Greenville County, South Carolina. Consideration will be given to applications requesting that funding be spent over a two year period. Additional guidelines and application are available on the GWG website: http://greenvillewomengiving.org/faq.aspx. The completed application should be mailed or delivered to Greenville Women Giving, c/o Community Foundation of Greenville on or before January 15, at 4 p.m.
Requirements: Applicants must qualify as tax-exempt under Section 501(c)3 of the Internal Revenue Code or be classified as a unit of government, located and providing services in Greenville County, South Carolina. Organizations must not discriminate on the basis of age, race, national origin, ethnicity, gender, physical ability, sexual orientation, political affiliation or religious belief.
Restrictions: Support is not available for the following: endowment campaigns; travel expenses and conferences; individuals; projects or programs that promote religious or political views; organizations for re-granting purpose.
Geographic Focus: South Carolina
Samples: Camp Opportunity, $25,000—to fund a week of summer camp for children in DSS protective custody (2009); Greenville Literacy Association, $29,000—for their young adult job-readiness program (2009); Graduate Greenville, $50,000—for meeting its aim to increase the high school graduation percentage of Greenville County students (2009).
Amount of Grant: $40,000-$100,000 range
Date(s) Application is Due: Jan 15
Contact: Debbie Cooper, Director of Donor Services; (864) 233-5925; fax: (864) 242-9292; email: dcooper@cfgg.com
Internet: http://greenvillewomengiving.org/guidelines.aspx
Sponsor: Greenville Women Giving, c/o The Community Foundation of Greenville
27 Cleveland Street, Suite 101
Greenville, SC 29601

Community Foundation of Howard County Grants 1116
The mission of the Community Foundation of Howard County, Inc. is to serve the interest of donors of enduring charitable gifts. Through vision, effective organization and good stewardship, the Foundation is a catalyst for stimulating and funding initiatives that improve the quality of life for citizens of Howard County, Clinton County and Carroll County of Indiana. In Howard County, the Foundation addresses needs that generally fall into the following categories: health & medical; social services; education; cultural affairs; and civic affairs.
Requirements: Grants will be made only to organizations: whose programs benefit the residents of Howard County and preference will be given to those projects that have high visibility in the community; which provide for a responsible fiscal agent and adequate accounting procedures, and preference will be given to those projects that generate revenue and/or that have plans that sustain the project. Final grant evaluation reports will be required to be submitted by the grantees. Grant applications from a previous grantee will not be considered if final reports have not been received for previous grants. Grants may be made to previous grantees. In a competitive situation with grants of equal value, preference may be given to organizations that have not received a recent grant. In a competitive situation quality of the application will be used in the selection between grants that are otherwise equal. All applicants must receive pre-qualification prior to submitting an application. Pre-qualification will consist of attendance at one community grants meeting annually and a letter of inquiry. The Community Foundation of Howard County utilizes a formal grant application which can be obtained at the Foundation's office. When submitting an application include, one original application, plus the twenty (20) copies.
Restrictions: The Community Foundation of Howard County typically does not award grants for: normal operating expenses and/or salaries; solely to individuals but grants can be made for the benefit of certain individuals for such purposes as scholarships and special programs through educational institutions and other sponsoring recipient organizations; enabling individuals or groups of individuals to attend seminars or take trips except where there are special circumstances which will benefit the larger community; sectarian religious purposes but can be made to religious organizations for general community programs; endowment purposes of recipient organizations; projects which have been proposed by individuals or organizations responsible to advisory bodies or persons unless letters of recommendation or approval from those advisory bodies or persons accompany the grant proposals; new projects and/or equipment which were purchased prior to the grant application being approved.
Geographic Focus: Indiana
Date(s) Application is Due: Mar 5; May 7; Sep 3; Nov 5
Contact: LaCinda Chapman, Secretary; (765) 454-7298 or (800) 964-0508
Internet: http://www.cfhoward.org/newsite/grantsapplications.shtml
Sponsor: Community Foundation of Howard County, Inc.
215 W. Sycamore
Kokomo, IN 46901

Community Foundation of Madison & Jefferson County Grants/Scholarships 1117
The Community Foundation of Madison and Jefferson County was established in 1991 by a group of local volunteers. Since its birth, more than 100 permanent funds have been established in the Foundation. The main interest are: animals, community conservation and beautification, community service, education, the elderly, fine arts, religion, health and youth. The Community Foundation has over 30 scholarships available to graduating seniors of Jefferson County high schools. To see what scholarships are available at your school, visit the Foundations website. The deadline for most scholarships is in March. Because of the current economic climate, the Board of Directors of the Community Foundation of Madison and Jefferson County has started a special "Help Your Neighbor" campaign instead of conducting its traditional competitive Spring and Fall Grants programs. The Foundation's Help Your Neighbor initiative will make grants to 501 (c)(3) charities that assist Jefferson County residents struggling to meet day-to-day expenses. Up to $30,000 is available. Awards of up to $2,000 each will be made. Contact the Foundation for more information about Help Your Neighbor grants.
Requirements: Grants given to 501(c)3 charities that assist Jefferson County residents.
Geographic Focus: Indiana
Contact: Louise Markel, Executive Director, (812) 265-3327; fax: (812) 273-0181: email: jeffcom@cfmjc.org
Internet: http://www.cfmjc.org/index.html
Sponsor: Community Foundation of Madison and Jefferson County, Inc.
214 E. Main Street or P.O. Box 306
Madison, IN 47250

Community Foundation of Morgan County Grants/Scholarships 1118
The foundation supports student education, builds community, improves health care services, develops programs for youth, preserves the environment, supports the arts, and strengthens the nonprofit sector. Several scholarship programs assist Morgan County students in achieving their educational goals. Scholarship amounts and deadlines vary. Information is available online.

Requirements: Morgan County nonprofit organizations are eligible for grants. Morgan County high school graduates are available to apply for scholarships.
Geographic Focus: Indiana
Contact: Edward Thiebe, Executive Director; (877) 822-6958, (317) 831-1232; fax: (317) 831-2854; email: ethiebe@cfmconline.org
Internet: http://cfmconline.org/GrantsScholarships/Grants/tabid/63/Default.aspx
Sponsor: Community Foundation of Morgan County
250 N Monroe Street
Mooresville, IN 46158

Community Foundation of Mount Vernon and Knox County Grants 1119
The Community Foundation of Mount Vernon/Knox County, awards grants and scholarships from a variety of funds. The Foundations mission is to improve the quality of life in Mount Vernon and, Knox County through charitable giving. To assess and respond to emerging and changing community needs in the fields of: education, youth services, recreation, arts and culture, social services, and civic and community development. All grant applications are considered by the Foundation board at regularly scheduled meetings in the months of February, April, June, August, October and December. Applicants should be aware grants are awarded on a competitive basis, and that deadlines for submission of requests must be strictly observed. See the Foundations website for additional guidelines, deadline dates and two different grant applications (small and major.)
Requirements: Most grants are made to tax-exempt, private agencies classified as 501 (c)(3) organizations, and to public charities as defined by the U.S. Internal Revenue Service. Public schools, governmental entities and Knox County colleges and universities are also eligible to apply for Foundation grants.
Restrictions: Certain projects and organizations are not eligible for funding, including but not limited to: grants to individuals; endowment campaigns; ongoing operating expenses; religious organizations (for religious purposes); purchase of computers or other equipment (that is not part of a broader project); existing obligations, debts or liabilities; police and fire protection; staff positions for government agencies travel (when it is the proposal's primary focus) organizations that do not operate programs in Knox County, or for the benefit of Knox County residents; political campaigns.
Geographic Focus: Ohio
Samples: Knox County Historical Society, $30,000— for a building addition project (2005); Hospice of Knox County, $75,000— for its new administrative and training facility (2005); City of Mount Vernon, $3,000— for its historic district street sign placement project (2005).
Contact: Sam Barone, Executive Director; (740) 392-3270; fax: (740) 399-5296; email: thefoundation@firstknox.com or sbarone@mvkcfoundation.org
Internet: http://www.mvkcfoundation.org/Grant/index.html
Sponsor: Community Foundation of Mount Vernon and Knox County
One South Main Street, P.O. Box 1270
Mount Vernon, OH 43050

Community Foundation of Muncie and Delaware County Grants 1120
The foundation contributes to improving the quality of life in the city of Muncie, IN, and in Delaware County for this and future generations. Areas of interest include cultural programs, charitable institutions, economic development, educational programs, and community betterment. The foundation will focus on capital needs of community institutions and organizations, the emerging needs of the city of Muncie and Delaware County, the establishment of community priorities, the monitoring of community services to avoid duplication and ineffective programs, and acting as a catalyst for action and community participation. Types of support include general operating support, building construction/renovation, equipment acquisition, program development, conferences and seminars, seed grants, scholarship funds and scholarships to individuals, technical assistance, in-kind gifts, and matching funds. The foundation seeks to fund new and innovative projects and programs for which there is a demonstrable need or community benefit. Grant applications may be submitted at any time. The grant policy committee and the board of directors will review applications on a quarterly basis, in January, April, July, and October. Deadlines are the second Friday of January, April, July, and October.
Requirements: 501(c)3 tax-exempt organizations in Muncie and Delaware County, IN, are eligible.
Restrictions: The foundation does not make grants to individuals or for religious purposes, budget deficits, endowments, or projects normally the responsibility of a public agency.
Geographic Focus: Indiana
Amount of Grant: $3.5 million total
Date(s) Application is Due: Second Friday of Jan, Apr, Jul, Oct
Contact: Suzanne Kadinger, Program Officer, (765) 747-7181; fax: (765) 289-7770; email: commfound@cfmdin.org
Internet: http://www.cfmdin.org
Sponsor: Community Foundation of Muncie and Delaware County
201 E Jackson Street
Muncie, IN 47305

Community Foundation of Randolph County Grants 1121
The Community Foundation of Randolph County, Inc. seeks to bring people and resources together to enrich the lives of Randolph County, Indiana residents. The Foundation makes grants to increase the capacity of Randolph County's not-for-profit organizations to respond effectively to the needs of the community. In general, the Foundation prefers funding for: start-up costs for new programs; one-time projects or needs; capital needs beyond an applicant's capabilities and means. Historically the Foundation has funded projects in the areas of community betterment, art and culture, health and human services, youth, economic development and education.
Requirements: The Foundation makes grants to tax-exempt 501 (c)(3) organizations operating or proposing to operate programs for the benefit of Randolph County residents. Proposals shall include: completed application cover; one original and 10 copies of completed application; one list of your organization's/agency's officers or governing body; one copy of your federal tax exemption 501 (c)(3) letter; one copy of your last financial statement showing income and expenses (annual report); one copy of the total project budget; one copy of all pertinent supporting information. Applications can be obtained by contacting the Foundation office or downloading the form from the Foundation's website. Completed typewritten applications forms should be sent or delivered to the Foundation's office, applications cannot be submitted online.
Geographic Focus: Indiana
Date(s) Application is Due: Sep 30; Mar31
Contact: Ruth Mills, Executive Director; (765) 584-9077; fax: (765) 584-7710; email: rmills@cfrandolphcounty.org
Internet: http://cfrandolphcounty.org/cfrc/jsp/AboutUs/TypesofFunds/main.jsp
Sponsor: Community Foundation of Randolph County, Inc.
213 South Main Street
Winchester, IN 47394

Community Foundation of Santa Cruz County Grants 1122
The foundation promotes philanthropy to make greater Santa Cruz County a better place to live, now and in the future. Grants are designed to develop and strengthen services delivered by the nonprofit sector. Fields of interest include arts and humanities; community development; education; environment; health; historic preservation; human services; youth-led projects (11 to 14 years olds); lesbian, gay, bisexual, transgender community; and Vecinos project, to support residents' capacity to improve their neighborhoods. Management assistance grants are available for projects that strengthen the ability of an organization to fulfill its mission through improved governance and management practices. The listed application deadlines are for program grants; management assistance grants have no deadline. Complete guidelines are available online.
Requirements: To be eligible, an organization must be a nonprofit 501(c)3 organization or public agency, not classified as a private foundation; have a board-approved policy regarding staff employment, electing a governing board, and providing services without discrimination on the basis of race, religion, gender, sexual orientation, age, disability, or national origin; provide direct benefits to residents of Santa Cruz County, the Summit, or the Pajaro Valley and include representation of Santa Cruz County residents on its board of directors; and be current on all reports due to the community foundation for any previous grants.
Geographic Focus: California
Samples: Actors Theatre (CA)—to support the continuation of marketing and audience development efforts, $10,000 (2005); The Beat Within (CA)—to support a music education and recording program for county youth, ages 7 through 18, $5000 (2005).
Amount of Grant: $1000-$5000 management assistance grants; $5000-$15,000 project grants
Date(s) Application is Due: Feb 18; Apr 29
Contact: Christina Cuevas, (831) 477-0800 ext 213; fax: (831) 477-0991; email: christina@cfsscc.org
Internet: http://www.cfscc.org/page17117.cfm
Sponsor: Community Foundation of Santa Cruz County
2425 Porter Street, Suite 17
Soquel, CA 95073

Community Foundation of South Alabama Grants 1123
The community foundation provides grant support to South Alabama nonprofit organizations in four major program areas: community and civic affairs, education, arts and recreation, and social services (health and human services). Priority consideration is given to projects that clearly provide innovative responses to community needs, are collaborative in nature when appropriate, and potentially affect broad segments of the community. Types of support include general operating support, capital campaigns, endowment funds, program development, and scholarship funds. The board of directors meets annually to consider grant requests.
Requirements: Nonprofit organizations that have a 501(c)3, government entities and religious organizations that are located in Mobile, Baldwin, Clarke, Conecuh, Washington, Choctaw, Escambia and Monroe counties are eligible.
Restrictions: Grants generally are not provided for or to individuals, recurring requests for the same purpose for which foundation grant funds have already been awarded, research that is noncommunity-related or that does not have short-range results, films, conferences and workshops, lobbying activities, and tickets to fund-raising events.
Geographic Focus: Alabama
Amount of Grant: $2,500-$28,000 range
Contact: Thomas H. Davis, Jr., President; (334) 438-5591; fax: (334) 438-5592; email: info@communityendowment.com
Internet: http://communityendowment.com/grants/grants.htm
Sponsor: Community Foundation of South Alabama
P.O. Box 990
Mobile, AL 36601-0990

Community Foundation of South Puget Sound Grants 1124
The foundation awards grants to a variety of charitable, cultural, education, health, and welfare organizations. Grants from the unrestricted funds are considered for general operational or program support. Typical grants range from $1,000 to $7,500. Emergency

grants may be considered on a case-by-case basis. Application and guidelines for grants and scholarships are available online.
Requirements: The foundation awards grants to Washington tax-exempt organizations primarily for use in Thurston, Mason, and Lewis Counties, except on instructions of the donor at the time of the gift or bequest.
Restrictions: Grants do not support religious organizations for religious purposes; individuals; annual campaigns of organizations (direct mail or special events); political or lobbying activities; organizations that discriminate based on race, creed, or ethnic group; capital campaigns for bricks and mortar or endowment funds; or for multiple year commitments.
Geographic Focus: Washington
Samples: Rochester Organization of Families, $7,000—to help maintain ROOF's "Kid's Place" academic enrichment program for 50 low -income, at-risk children in the first through fifth grades (2008); Harmony Hill, $4,500—to purchase a computer server to maintain its extensive database of clients and donors; which in turn supports their mission to improve the quality of life for those affected by cancer (2008); Thurston Mason Project Access, $4,000—to make donated medical services available to uninsured, low-income Thurston County residents with acute, urgent conditions (2008).
Amount of Grant: $1,000-$7,500 typically
Date(s) Application is Due: Apr 3; Oct 2
Contact: Norma Schuiteman, Executive Director; (360) 705-3340; fax: (360) 705-2656; email: legacy@thecommunityfoundation.com
Internet: http://www.thecommunityfoundation.com/grants.php
Sponsor: Community Foundation of South Puget
111 Market Street NE, Suite 375
Olympia, WA 98501

Community Foundation of Southeastern Connecticut Grants 1125

Within its geographic area, comprising the 11 towns of southeastern Connecticut, the community foundation awards grants to assist charitable, educational, and civic institutions; promote health and general welfare; support environmental programs; provide human care services for the needy; secure the care of children and families; encourage artistic and cultural endeavors; and initiate planning of appropriate projects within these areas. High-priority programs include those that strengthen families; improve access to area resources, especially for underserved populations; encourage residents to participate in the cultural life of the community; demonstrate collaborative efforts and inclusive practices; reinforce best practices or show innovative approaches; and add to the general well being of the community. Types of support include building/ renovation, equipment, emergency funds, program development, conferences and seminars, publication, seed grants, scholarship funds, technical support, and scholarships to individuals. Applications requesting support of normal operating expenses will not be considered. Proposals may be submitted between April 1 and November 15 each year.
Requirements: IRS tax-exempt organizations serving the towns of East Lyme, Groton, Ledyard, Lyme, Montville, New London, North Stonington, Old Lyme, Salem, Stonington, and Waterford, CT, including inner-city, suburban, and rural areas, are eligible.
Restrictions: The foundation does not consider requests for direct financial assistance to individuals; religious or sectarian programs; political or lobbying purposes; fundraising events; or debt retirement.
Geographic Focus: Connecticut
Samples: Thames River Family Program (Norwich, CT)—to support the Parents as Advocates program, $3937.; East Lyme Youth Services Assoc (East Lyme, CT)—to support the DARE Challenge eight-hour ropes course, $2700.; Science Ctr of Eastern Connecticut (New London, CT)—to help establish a museum store, $5000.; Lyme Academy of Fine Arts (Old Lyme, CT)—to support library acquisition, $5000.
Amount of Grant: $2000-$10,000 average
Date(s) Application is Due: Nov 15
Contact: Jennifer O'Brien, Program Officer, (860) 442-3572; fax: (860) 442-0584; email: jennob@cfsect.org
Internet: http://www.cfsect.org/grant.html
Sponsor: Community Foundation of Southeastern Connecticut
P.O. Box 769
New London, CT 06320

Community Foundation of St. Joseph County Special Project Challenge Grants 1126

The purpose of the program is to assist public and other 501(c)3 agencies in their efforts to serve community needs. For every $1 raised by the chosen agency, the Community Foundation will match $1. The foundation encourages projects in the following areas (listed alphabetically): Community Development & Urban Affairs; Health & Human Services; Parks, Recreation, & Environment; Youth & Education
Requirements: Public agencies and 501(c)3 agencies in St. Joseph County, IN are eligible to apply. The project should benefit a significant constituency within the community. The agency must exhibit the ability to raise the required matching funds. Only cash gifts will be matched. Forms and application guidelines are available from the website.
Restrictions: Grants are not made to fund: a) Operational phases of established programs; b) Endowment campaigns; c) Religious organizations for religious purposes; d) Individuals directly; e) Development or public relations activities (e.g. literature, videos, etc.); f) Retirement of debts; g) Camperships; h) Annual appeals or membership contributions; i) Travel for bands, sports teams, classes, etc.; j) Computers (unless presented as a necessary component of larger program or objective); k) Post-event or after-the-fact situations.
Geographic Focus: Indiana
Date(s) Application is Due: Mar 1; Oct 1
Contact: Angela Butiste, Senior Program Officer; (574) 232-0041; fax: (574) 233-1906; email: angela@cfsjc.org
Internet: http://www.cfsjc.org/grants/sproj/special_project_grants.html
Sponsor: Community Foundation of St. Joseph County
205 W. Jefferson Boulevard, P.O. Box 837
South Bend, IN 46624

Community Foundation of Switzerland County Grants 1127

The Community Foundation of Switzerland County is a nonprofit organization created by and for the people of the Switzerland County area with one goal, making our community a better place to live, now and for future generations. Organizations applying for a grant may request up to $1,000. In addition, the Community Foundation will give priority to grant applications that focus on the basic needs of the community. While the term "basic needs" can be interpreted differently, in general, the Community Foundation uses the term to describe food, housing, shelter, health care, clothing, personal care, transportation services and other essential needs that people in our community may not have due to the weakened economy. While grant applications addressing basic needs of the community will be given priority, the Community Foundation still welcomes applications for other programs and projects that benefit Switzerland County. To make grant dollars available on a timely basis, there are no deadlines. Grant letters will be reviewed and decided upon monthly. Any request in by the 1st of each month will be notified of a decision by the end of that month.
Requirements: Any organization with a 501(c)3 or any organization that provides a program with charitable intent and has a fiscal agent is eligible to apply. To apply for a grant, an organization must write a one page letter explaining: who will be doing the requested program/project; what will be done (program, purchase, training, etc); when it will be done; where it will be done; and how much it will cost (short budget). If the cost is more than being requested from the Community Foundation, indicate where the rest of the money will come from. There will be no match required for these grants, so a program or project can be totally funded by a request or it may be part of a larger project.
Geographic Focus: Indiana
Amount of Grant: $1,000
Contact: Pam Acton, Grant Program DIrector, (812) 427-9160; fax: (812) 427-4033; email: pacton@cfsci.org
Internet: http://www.cfsci.org/
Sponsor: Community Foundation of Switzerland County, Inc.
03 Ferry Street or P.O. Box 46 Vevay, IN
Vevay, IN 47043

Community Foundation of Tampa Bay Grants 1128

The Community Foundation of Tampa Bay awards creative grants from its community fund with the goal of fostering positive changes in the lives of their citizens. The areas of interest include: arts and culture, community development, education, environment and animals, and health and human services. See the Foundations website for the Grant Application Form and guidelines: http://www.cftampabay.org/nonprofit_resources/grant_app_guidelines.html
Requirements: Non-profit organizations based in and serving communities in Hillsborough, Pasco, Pinellas and Hernando counties, with a 501(c)3 status in good standing from the IRS are eligible to apply.
Restrictions: The Foundation is generally not interested in requests for: funding of ongoing operating costs; grants for capital campaigns or expenditures; tickets for any fundraising event or advertising space in programs or other publications; legislative lobbying or political campaigns; medical research; religious or sectarian purposes; loans or assistance to individuals; a multiple year funding commitment, although in exceptional cases, such funding will be considered not to exceed three years.
Geographic Focus: Florida
Amount of Grant: $7,500 maximum award
Date(s) Application is Due: Mar 1; Sep 1;
Contact: Ann Berg, Vice President of Grants; (813) 282-1975; fax: (813) 282-3119; email: aberg@cftampabay.org
Internet: http://www.cftampabay.org/nonprofit_resources/grant_app_guidelines.html
Sponsor: Community Foundation of Tampa Bay, Inc.
550 North Reo Street, Suite 301
Tampa, FL 33609

Community Foundation of the Eastern Shore Community Needs Grants 1129

The Community Foundation of the Eastern Shore awards grants from its discretionary fund, known as the Lower Shore Fund for Community Needs. Monetary grants are awarded to a wide range of tax exempt organizations in Somerset, Wicomico and Worcester Counties of Maryland, whose programs benefit: health; human services; arts and culture; community affairs; environmental conservation; and historic preservation. Through this grant program, the Foundation identifies high priority needs and seeks opportunities where a relatively modest amount of grant money can make a significant difference in the community. Often the grants provide start-up or short-term funding for innovative, potentially replicable projects that meet newly identified needs or demonstrate new solutions for previously identified needs.
Requirements: To be eligible for a grant from this program, an organization must meet two fundamental criteria: it must be a governmental unit, a religious organization engaged in a non-sectarian activity, or a non-profit, tax exempt "public charity," as defined in Section 501(c)3 of the Internal Revenue Code; and it must provide services to benefit the residents of the lower three counties of Maryland's Eastern Shore: Worcester, Wicomico, and Somerset. Programs are not required to serve all three counties, but regional projects are encouraged.

Restrictions: The Community Needs Grant Program does not fund: endowment funds; ongoing/operating expenses; fundraising campaigns; sectarian religious programs; playground equipment; building campaigns; operational deficits; debt retirement; capital requests; political/lobbying programs; office equipment/staff training; and school-based programs. Grants through this program are made to organizations, not individuals.
Geographic Focus: Maryland
Amount of Grant: $500 - $7,500 range
Date(s) Application is Due: Aug 1; Feb 1
Contact: Erica N. Joseph, Program Officer; (410) 742-9911; fax: (410) 742-6638; email: joseph@cfes.org
Internet: http://www.cfes.org/grants_community_needs.php
Sponsor: Community Foundation of the Eastern Shore
1324 Belmont Avenue, Suite 401
Salisbury, MD 21804

Community Foundation of the Ozarks Grants 1130
Grants from unrestricted funds of the community foundation are made to qualified nonprofit organizations that serve the Greene County area of Missouri. Areas of interest include arts, community betterment, education, and social justice. Preference will be given to projects that are exclusive of the ongoing operation of the organization; provide seed money for new programs; open the possibility of receiving matching funds; and offer the community foundation the opportunity to meet needs in full in diverse problem areas. Agencies are encouraged to ask for funding amounts that reflect their true needs. Submittal of a one-page concept letter is the first step in applying. Concept letters must be received by the August deadline for grants awarded in November, by the December deadline for grants awarded in March, and by the March deadline for grants awarded in June. Concept letters may be submitted to dmyers@cfozarks.org.
Requirements: IRS 501(c)3 organizations that serve the Greene County area in Missouri are eligible.
Restrictions: Capital campaigns and grants to individuals are not allowed.
Geographic Focus: Missouri
Samples: Skate Park (Springfield, MO)—to complete construction of skate park for youth, $25,000.; Congretional Health Ministries (Springfield, MO)—start up money, $5000.; Springfield Symphony (Springfield, MO)—to purchase tickets for the elderly to the symphony, $3000.
Date(s) Application is Due: Mar 1; Aug 1; Dec 1
Contact: Gary Funk, President, (417) 864-6199; fax: (417) 864-8344; email: gfunk@cfozarks.org
Internet: http://www.cfozarks.org/grantseekers.html
Sponsor: Community Foundation of the Ozarks
901 Saint Louis Street, Suite 701
Springfield, MO 65806

Community Foundation of Wabash County Grants 1131
The Foundation endeavors to enrich the quality of life in Wabash County, Indiana, by responding to emerging and changing needs and by sustaining existing organizations and institutions through grants in support of the following categories: arts and culture; community and civic development; education; environment; health and human services; and recreation. Types of support include: building or renovation; continuing support; curriculum development; endowments; equipment; general operating support; matching/challenge support; program development; program evaluation; scholarship funds; scholarships to individuals; seed money; and technical assistance. Applicants should forward the entire proposal with attachments.
Requirements: Proposals are accepted from organizations serving Wabash County that are defined as tax exempt under Section 501(c)3 of the Internal Revenue Service code or have comparable status and charitable causes. Faith-based organizations may apply for program funding, provided there is not a requirement to participate in religious instruction and/or take part in religious activities.
Restrictions: The following are not eligible for funding: national organizations (except for local chapters serving Wabash County); annual fund campaigns; or programs or products produced for resale.
Geographic Focus: Indiana
Amount of Grant: $3,000 or less average
Date(s) Application is Due: Mar 15; Jul 15; Nov 15
Contact: Tracy Trump, Executive Director; (260) 982-4824; fax: (260) 982-8644; email: tracy@cfwabash.org
Internet: http://grants.cfwabash.org/
Sponsor: Community Foundation of Wabash County
218 E. Main Street, P.O. Box 98
North Manchester, IN 46962-0098

Community Foundation of Western North Carolina Grants 1132
The foundation serves an 18-county area, including Cherokee, Graham, Clay, Swain, Macon, Jackson, Haywood, Transylvania, Madison, Buncombe, Henderson, Yancey, McDowell, Rutherford, Polk, Burke, Mitchell, and Avery Counties. The community foundation awards grants for projects in the areas of arts and culture, children and youth, community development, education, environment, health, human services, and social justice. The foundation awards seed money grants to new or existing programs and technical assistance grants to strengthen nonprofit organizations. A workshop for grant applicants is held one month prior to the deadline at which time the guidelines are reviewed and questions are addressed; contact the foundation for date and times.
Requirements: 501(c)3 organizations serving areas within the 18-county region are eligible. Applicants must obtain foundation approval in order to apply for signature grants.
Restrictions: Grants are not made for the following: operating support (except for start-up); activities taking place before grant decisions are made; capital requests (except for modest budget items, such as equipment); endowments; sectarian purposes; private schools and clubs; political purposes; veteran affairs; deficit funding or debt retirement; and individuals except through scholarships. Multiple-year grants are not made. The foundation is only occasionally able to fund the second phase of a project. Organizations may not submit more than one application at a time; it is suggested that no more than one request be submitted during a 12-month period.
Geographic Focus: North Carolina
Samples: Asheville Area Chamber of Commerce Community Betterment Foundation—for an expanded, outdoor Mountain Dance and Folk Festival, $5000.; Citizens for Media Literacy—to produce a video to show nonprofits and local governments how to utilize public access television, $8000.
Amount of Grant: $10,000 maximum seed grants ($5000 average); $20,000 maximum signature grants
Date(s) Application is Due: Feb 1; Sep 1
Contact: Tara Scholtz, Program Officer, (828) 254-4960; fax: (828) 251-2258; email: scholtz@cfwnc.org
Internet: http://www.cfwnc.org/grants.html
Sponsor: Community Foundation of Western North Carolina
P.O. Box 1888
Asheville, NC 28802

Community Foundation Silicon Valley Grants 1133
The foundation supports California nonprofits in its areas of interest, including arts and cultural participation, education and lifelong learning, self-reliant individuals and family, and neighborhood and civic projects. The foundation also supports the Youth in Philanthropy program and early literacy grants. Preference is given to proposals that focus on the prevention of problems rather than the cure, equip people to become self-sufficient, encourage programs that take a comprehensive approach to addressing interrelated problems, promote cooperation and collaboration among agencies, encourage leveraging and matching grant opportunities, and provide seed funding for innovative projects. Additional types of support include program development, technical assistance, consulting services, and general operating grants. Grants generally are made for one year of support; long-term commitments are contingent upon annual review of progress and available funds. Guidelines and application are available online.
Requirements: Nonprofit organizations benefiting Santa Clara County and southern San Mateo County, CA, are eligible.
Restrictions: In general, the foundation does not consider fundraising events, capital equipment and endowment campaigns, on-going operating expenses, existing debts/obligations, for-profit schools, or individuals.
Geographic Focus: California
Amount of Grant: $25,000 maximum
Contact: Jeff Sunshine, Director of Programs, (408) 278-2200; fax: (408) 278-0280; email: jsunshine@cfsv.org or info@cfsv.org
Internet: http://www.cfsv.org/grants_focusareas.html
Sponsor: Community Foundation Silicon Valley
60 S Market Street, Suite 1000
San Jose, CA 95113

Community Health Scholars Program Fellowships 1134
The Community Health Scholars Program (CHSP) is a postdoctoral fellowship program designed to meet the growing needs of schools of public health and other health professions for faculty with community competency. The 12-month fellowship enables scholars to develop and enhance skills in working with communities and engaging in participatory community-based research at institutions where these skills are present. Applications are welcome from junior faculty as well as those recently completing doctoral-level training so long as the above eligibility requirements are met. Women and other underrepresented groups are encouraged to apply.
Requirements: Applicants must be U.S. citizens located at one of three training sites (Johns Hopkins, University of Michigan, or University of North Carolina) and have completed all formal requirements for professional and postprofessional training (e.g., internships or residencies) at the doctoral level (e.g., PhD, MD, JD, or DrPH) by the date of entry into the program.
Restrictions: Scholars may not hold other training fellowships or be enrolled full time in another degree program during their tenure in this program.
Amount of Grant: $50,000 fellowship award plus $10,000 research fund
Contact: Saundra Bailey, Program Administrator, (734) 647-3065; fax: (734) 936-0927; email: chsp@umich.edu
Internet: http://www.sph.umich.edu/chsp
Sponsor: University of Michigan
109 Observatory Street, M4142
Ann Arbor, MI 48109-2029

Community Impact Fund 1135
The foundation awards grants aimed at meeting the needs and enhancing the lives of individuals in California's Riverside and San Bernardino Counties. Funding categories include health and human services—promoting access to healthcare for all residents and helping individuals and families obtain basic services to promote an improved quality of life; youth and families—enhancing opportunities that promote academic achievement and positive youth development and developing family support services that foster learning and growth; arts and culture—encouraging creative expression and providing opportunities for enjoyment of cultural activities and art forms; civic

and public benefit—building a sense of community and promoting civic participation. Preference is given to projects that are perceived as a high need in the community being served; fill a gap in service; benefit a large number of residents; enhance collaboration and/or make the delivery of services more effective and efficient; have clear objectives and can document successful outcomes; expand successful programs to serve additional residents or new geographic areas within the two counties; serve remote areas or areas that have received little funding from the foundation. Contact the office for application deadlines and forms.
Requirements: The foundation will only accept applications from 501(c)3 organizations that can document on-going operations and nonprofit status for at least three years. Organizations may only apply once very 12 months.
Restrictions: Grants are generally not made for on-going operating expenses; retroactive funding for cost already incurred; paying off deficits or existing obligations; endowment, capital fund, or annual fund appeals; capital projects, i.e. construction of new buildings; direct support of individuals; sectarian programs or fraternal organizations; event sponsorships; research or development activities; school or college-based extracurricular activities; partisan activities; or re-granting purposes.
Amount of Grant: $10,000 maximum
Contact: Celia Cudiamat, Vice President of Grant Programs, (951) 684-4194; email: ccudiamat@thecommunityfoundation.net
Internet: http://www.thecommunityfoundation.net/grants/grant_commImpact_04.html
Sponsor: Community Foundation Serving Riverside and San Bernardino Counties
3880 Lemon Street, Suite 300
Riverside, CA 92501

Community Technology Foundation of California Building Communities Through Technology Grants 1136
The foundation awards grants to eligible California nonprofit organizations in support of programs that bring communications technologies to traditionally underserved populations, including low-income, inner-city, minority, disabled, limited-English speaking, and low-income senior communities. Areas of support include community building, community economic development, education, and health. Current grantmaking focuses on the development and maintenance of—as well as the removal of barriers to—digital media, communications, and outreach for underserved Californians. Successful grantees will be those who effectively utilize ICT in a manner that enables their target communities to become more active and engaged participants in civic action. Types of support include fellowships, matching/challenge grants, and leveraged gifts. Applications for proposals are accepted on a rolling basis, with funding decisions made at quarterly meetings (usually held in January, April, July, and October).
Requirements: California nonprofit organizations are eligible.
Restrictions: CTFC will specifically not fund projects in the following areas: general operating expenses (unless an applicant organization's sole mission and purpose is to conduct work that falls within the grantmaking guidelines); grants to individuals; grants to non-501(c)3 organizations (unless such organizations have a commitment in writing from a 501(c)3 sponsoring fiscal agent); requests for only distribution or dissemination of completed media projects; media projects used solely for distribution at agency special events, memorials, annual fundraisers, anniversary celebrations, etc.; requests that are solely for equipment or software purchases without a corresponding content-based component; ICT projects that are only for organizational internal infrastructure upgrades or administrative/operational support; or any project that does not have a media, information, or communications technology component.
Geographic Focus: California
Amount of Grant: $10,000-$50,000
Contact: Grants Administrator, (415) 371-8808; fax: (415) 371-8818; TTY: (415) 371-8823; email: info@zerodivide.org
Internet: http://www.zerodivide.org
Sponsor: Community Technology Foundation of California
101 Spear Street, Suite 218
San Francisco, CA 94105

Community Toolbox for Children's Environmental Health Grants 1137
Grants are awarded to community-based groups working on children's environmental health and on lead poisoning prevention. Priority will be given to requests from organizations serving children at the highest risk of lead poisoning, including children in urban, low income, and minority communities living in areas with older housing stock. The majority of grants will be awarded for capacity building only. The request for proposal and grant application are available on the Web site, as well as from the office. Applications for round one are due by September 13; invited applications for round two are due by January 21.
Requirements: Nonprofit, community-based organizations are eligible to apply.
Restrictions: Grants do not support organizations with annual budgets greater than $250,000 for the past year and the current year; federal, state, or local government agencies; international organizations; academic institutions; for-profit businesses; or programs that seek to influence legislation.
Samples: Echo Park Community Coalition (Los Angeles, CA)—to develop leadership skills, to conduct workshops on preventing lead poisoning, and to create a strategic plan, $40,000 over two years (2003); Friends of McKinley (Los Angeles, CA)—to organize parents and teachers to advocate lead abatement in schools, $10,000 (2003); Josiah Hill III Clinic (P.O.rtland, OR)—for community education and outreach, strategic planning, and the development of a fundraising strategy, $12,000 (2003); Justus WeCare (Louisville, KY)—to build awareness about lead poisoning and risk reduction through home visits, screenings, and resident surveys, $30,000 over two years (2003).
Date(s) Application is Due: Jan 21; Sep 13
Contact: Program Contact, (800) 220-7630 or (415) 614-9533; fax: (415) 614-9537; email: info@communitytoolbox.org
Internet: http://www.communitytoolbox.org/grantmk.htm
Sponsor: Community Toolbox for Children's Environmental Health
999 Sutter Street, 4th Floor
San Francisco, CA 94109

Compass Bank Foundation Grants 1138
The Foundation, established in 1981, supports organizations involved with arts and culture, higher and law education, health, heart disease, multiple sclerosis, medical research, youth development, human services, and philanthropy. Giving is primarily centered in the states of Alabama, Arizona, Colorado, Florida, New Mexico, and Texas. There are no specific deadlines with which to adhere. Contact the Foundation for further application information and guidelines.
Restrictions: No support is provided for religious organizations, and there are no grants to individuals (except for employee-related scholarships).
Geographic Focus: Alabama; Arizona; Colorado; Florida; New Mexico; Texas
Contact: Jerry W. Powell, Treasurer; (205) 297-3960
Sponsor: Compass Bank Foundation
P.O. Box 10566, M.C. AL/BI/CH/ACT
Birmingham, AL 35296-0002

Comprehensive Health Education Foundation Grants 1139
The foundation awards grants to support programs that address health inequities. The initial grantmaking effort will focus on Clark, Pierce, and Spokane Counties in Washington State. One-year grants of up to $20,000 each will be awarded to culturally appropriate, community-led collaborations to test their best idea on how to make it easier for people who suffer from health inequities to move more and eat healthier. Health inequities are defined as differences in the incidence, prevalence, mortality, and burden of diseases that exist for specific populations in the United States. Low-income individuals and people of color within the United States generally have higher rates of poor health and injury than those who are in higher-income groups and are Caucasian.
Requirements: 501(c)3 tax-exempt organizations located in Clark, Pierce, and Spokane Counties in Washington State and units of government that are nondiscriminatory in policy and practice regarding disabilities, age, sex, sexual orientation, race, ethnic origin, or creed are eligible.
Restrictions: Support will not be provided for building or land acquisitions; equipment or furniture purchases; endowment funds; emergency funds; grants to individuals; fellowships/scholarships; research; debt retirement; fundraising activities; general fund drives; indirect overhead; or CHEF programs or products.
Geographic Focus: Washington
Amount of Grant: $500-$20,000 typically
Contact: Kari L. Lewis, Grant Coordinator; (800) 323-2433, ext. 1899; fax: (206) 824-3072; email: KariL@chef.org
Internet: http://www.chef.org/about/grants.php
Sponsor: Comprehensive Health Education Foundation
159 S Jackson Street, Suite 510
Seattle, WA 98104

ConAgra Foods Foundation Grants 1140
The foundation supports projects of U.S.-based nonprofits with an international focus and international organizations through its foreign subsidiaries in the areas of education, health and human services, arts and culture, and civic and community betterment in communities where the company operates. The foundation is committed to fighting childhood hunger in America. Support is given to organizations or projects that address specific community needs and suggest solutions designed to meet those needs; organizations or projects seeking self-support or broad-based community support as their ultimate goal; and well-managed organizations staffed and supervised by people who are adept at stating goals, selecting measurements, and setting and meeting deadlines. Types of support include general operating support, project support, continuing support, annual campaigns, building construction/renovation, matching/challenge grants, and employee matching gifts. In some cases, ConAgra operating companies match ConAgra Foundation contributions in their communities. Requests for funding should be written; no phone or fax requests will be accepted.
Requirements: Eligible organizations must have been in existence for at least one year, have 501(c)3 tax-exempt status, and be located in California, Colorado, Illinois, Minnesota, Nebraska, or Wisconsin.
Restrictions: The foundation does not support individuals; fundraising and testimonial events/dinners; organizations with a limited constituency, such as clubs, fraternal, athletic, or social organizations; religious organizations for religious endeavors; travel or tours; advertising; K-12 education institutions; radio or TX programming; emergency operating support; or for-profit organizations.
Geographic Focus: California; Colorado; Illinois; Minnesota; Nebraska; Wisconsin
Amount of Grant: $7.5 million total; $500-$25,000 typically
Date(s) Application is Due: Jan 31; Apr 30; Jul 31; Oct 31
Contact: Kori Reed, (402) 595-6303
Internet: http://company.conagrafoods.com/phoenix.zhtml?c=202310&p=irol-foundation1
Sponsor: ConAgra Foods Foundation
The ConAgra Foods Foundation, CC-304, One ConAgra Drive
Omaha, NE 68102-5001

Connecticut Community Foundation Grants **1141**

The Connecticut Community Foundation serves the people of Greater Waterbury and Northwest Connecticut by supporting public and nonprofit organizations providing programs and services including those for the arts, human services, health care, environment, youth development and education. The Foundation gives priority to efforts that prevent problems, encourage community solutions or improve the organizational capability and financial stability of nonprofit agencies.
Requirements: Nonprofit organizations in Beacon Falls, Bethlehem, Bridgewater, Cheshire, Goshen, Litchfield, Middlebury, Morris, Naugatuck, New Milford, Oxford, Prospect, Roxbury, Southbury, Thomaston, Warren, Watertown, Washington, Wolcott, and Woodbury, CT, may submit applications.
Restrictions: Grants are not awarded for religious purposes, political activities, deficit financing, continuing support, fund-raising events, annual campaigns, newly established arts organizations, commissioning of new works of art, general operating support, or endowments.
Geographic Focus: Connecticut
Amount of Grant: $8000-$10,000 average
Date(s) Application is Due: Jan 9; Mar 27; Aug 28
Contact: Carol O'Donnell, Associate CEO/Director of Grants; (203) 753-1315; fax: (203) 756-3054; email: info@conncf.org
Internet: http://www.conncf.org/grants/grants.htm
Sponsor: Connecticut Community Foundation
43 Field Street
Waterbury, CT 06702

Connecticut Health Foundation Health Initiative Grants **1142**

The foundation awards grants to organizations and institutions that directly respond to its current priority areas and result in improving the health status of Connecticut's underserved and unserved populations. Program priorities include children???s mental health—projects related to children???s mental health, including research, community grants, creating resources for clinical effective practices, and parent advocacy groups; oral health—improving oral health care access, quality, and utilization; and racial and ethnic health disparities—improving the diversity of the health care workforce, and increasing cultural competency in the existing workforce. The foundation awards two major types of grants: strategic and responsive. Application and guidelines are available online.
Requirements: Connecticut state and local units of government, community health centers, health advocacy organizations, community-based organizations, community and cultural groups, schools, and faith-based organizations are eligible. Applicants must have IRS 501(c)3 tax-exempt status or be public entities. Unincorporated organizations may apply through 501(c)3 fiscal agents.
Restrictions: Foundation grants do not support awards to individuals; construction of buildings; capital projects, endowments, or chairs associated with universities, and medical schools; conferences (unless part of a greater project or program); projects that do not benefit Connecticut residents; lobbying or influencing the outcomes of a proposed piece of legislation or election; and indirect cost for discretionary grants.
Geographic Focus: Connecticut
Samples: 1000 Friends of Connecticut, $10,000 to improve public health through the "Smart Growth Education and Communications Campaign"; Asian Family Services, Inc., Hartford $25,000 to integrate health-related policy issues into the community dialogue during the political season in 2006; Asian Family Services, Inc., Hartford, $10,000 to merge their services with Community Renewal Team, an anti-poverty multi-service agency that serves families and people throughout the Connecticut River Valley; Association of Yale Alumni in Public Health, New Haven, $30,000 to conduct an assessment of the policy, practices and procedures for recruiting and retaining historically under-represented faculty members at the Yale University School of Public Health.
Amount of Grant: $50,000-$200,000 typically
Date(s) Application is Due: Mar 15; Jun 15; Sep 15; Dec 15
Contact: Onell Jesus Calderas, Grants Administrator, (860) 224-2200; fax: (860) 224-2230; email: onell@cthealth.org
Internet: http://www.cthealth.org/matriarch
Sponsor: Connecticut Health Foundation
74B Vine Street
New Britain, CT 06052

Connelly Foundation Grants **1143**

To achieve its mission to foster learning and improve the quality of life, Connelly Foundation provides grants toward costs associated with programs, direct services, general operations and capital projects to non-profit organizations and institutions working in the following fields: education; health and human services; arts and culture and civic enterprise. The Foundation supports non-profits with strong leadership, sound ideas, future viability, and attainable and well defined goals. It directs its philanthropy toward 501(c)3 organizations and institutions based in and serving Philadelphia and the counties of Bucks, Chester, Delaware, Montgomery and the City of Camden. The Foundation values the proposal process. Given its preference to review a comprehensive package as a primer for discussion, letters of inquiry or requests for pre-proposal discussions are not deemed necessary. Written proposals from nonprofit organizations are accepted and reviewed by the Connelly Foundation throughout the year, there are no deadlines.
Requirements: 501(c)3 organizations and institutions based in and serving in Philadelphia and its surrounding counties of Bucks, Chester, Delaware, and Montgomery in Pennsylvania and in the City of Camden, New Jersey are eligible to apply. There are determined parameters to the Foundation's financial support. It provides non-profit organizations only one grant within a twelve month period. As a general practice, it does not fund advocacy, annual appeals, charter schools, conferences, environmental projects, feasability or planning studies, general solicitations, historic preservation projects, national organizations, organizations focused on a single disease, public schools or research.
Restrictions: The foundation does not award grants to individuals, or political or national organizations; Nor does it respond to annual appeals or general letters of solicitation.
Geographic Focus: Pennsylvania
Contact: Emily C. Riley, Executive Vice President; (610) 834-3222; fax: (610) 834-0866; email: info@connellyfdn.org
Sponsor: Connelly Foundation
One Tower Bridge, Suite 1450
West Conshohocken, PA 19428

ConocoPhillips Foundation Grants **1144**

The foundation makes charitable grants (primarily in the communities where it has operations) in support of education, medical programs, human services, civic, cultural, youth, and other services. Contributions will be considered for organizations such as: federated organizations; educational institutions, both public and private, primarily at the college level; youth organizations; hospital and medical facilities and programs such as hospital buildings and equipment, improvement campaigns and other medical facilities; cultural organizations; civic services; and human service organizations. Applicants may download the application form from the Web site. There are no application deadlines.
Requirements: 501(c)3 tax-exempt organizations and, where appropriate 170(c) organizations, and international nonprofit organizations are eligible. Proof of the exemption must be submitted with grant applications.
Restrictions: Grants do not support religious organizations for religious purposes; war veterans and fraternal service organizations; endowment funds; national health organizations and programs; grants or loans to individuals; fund-raising events; corporate memberships or contributions to chambers of commerce, taxpayer associations and other bodies whose activities are expected to directly benefit the company; or political organizations, campaigns and candidates.
Geographic Focus: Alaska; California; Illinois; Louisiana; Montana; New Jersey; Oklahoma; Pennsylvania; Texas; Washington
Samples: Christian Community Service (Houston, TX)—$25,000.; Jewish Day School of Metropolitan Seattle (Seattle, WA)—$25,000.; YMCA of Greater Seattle (Seattle, WA)—$15,000.
Amount of Grant: $4.6 million total
Date(s) Application is Due: Applications accepted Jun 1 through Aug 1
Contact: Community Relations, ConocoPhillips (see list at internet site)
Internet: http://www.conocophillips.com/about/Contribution+Guidelines/index.htm
Sponsor: ConocoPhillips Foundation Grants
600 N. Dairy Ashford
Houston, TX 77079

Constantin Foundation Grants **1145**

The foundation awards grants to nonprofit organizations in Texas, with an emphasis on higher and other education, including secondary school education, vocational education, and adult continuing education. Grants also support human, family, and social service agencies; hospitals and health organizations, including substance abuse; community development; and arts and culture. Grants are awarded for continuing support, capital campaigns, building construction/renovation, equipment acquisition, challenge/matching funds, and to develop programs. Request guidelines prior to applying.
Requirements: Nonprofit organizations in Dallas County, TX, may submit applications.
Restrictions: No support for tax-supported institutions, theater groups, churches, debt retirement, political organizations or second party requesters. No grants to individuals, or for endowments, research, debt retirement, operations, research, special events, fundraisers, or second party requests; no loans.
Geographic Focus: Texas
Amount of Grant: $1,000-$100,000 range
Date(s) Application is Due: Sep 15
Contact: Cathy Doyle, Executive Director; (214) 522-9300 or (214) 522-9305; fax: (214) 521-7023; email: constantinfdn@sbcglobal.net
Sponsor: Constantin Foundation
4809 Cole Avenue, LB 127
Dallas, TX 75205-3578

Constellation Energy Group and Baltimore Gas & Electric Corp Contributions **1146**

The program is based on the recognition that the company's vitality as an organization depends on the well-being of the communities in which it operates. Grants are allocated in a few key program areas, including energy assistance/poverty solutions; education; economic development; and environment. It is important that organizations demonstrate a broad base of community support as well as support from other local corporations and/or foundations. All requests must be made in writing and include a cover letter, narrative, and attachments. Requests for $10,000 or more should be submitted by the listed application deadlines.
Requirements: The company makes charitable donations to 501(c)3 tax-exempt, nonprofit organizations.
Restrictions: The company does not contribute to individuals, churches, religious causes, organizations that actively oppose the company's position on issues, nor does it provide funds for start-up funding. hospitals capital campaigns will not be supported.
Samples: Maryland Food Bank (Baltimore, MD)—campaign for new warehouse $30,000 (2005); JK Group (Princeton, NJ)—for Tsunami relief, EXE matching gifts, matching

gifts for higher education $408,069 (2005); American Red Cross Calvert County (MD)—support for victims in Calvert and Charles Counties of April 29, 2002 toronado, $10,000; Baltimore???s Festival of the Arts (MD)—sponsorship of ARTSCAPE???s 21st annual celebration, $7500.
Date(s) Application is Due: May 1; Sep 1
Contact: Malinda Small, Corporate Contributions Committee, (410) 234-7481; fax: (410) 234-7471; email: corporate.contributions@constellation.com
Internet: http://www.bge.com/portal/site/constellation/menuitem.94939662e40191875fb60610025166a0/#corpgiving
Sponsor: Constellation Energy Group and Baltimore Gas & Electric Company Foundation
750 East Pratt Street, 16th Floor
Baltimore, MD 21202

Consumers Energy Foundation **1147**
Since its creation in 1990, the Consumers Energy Foundation has touched countless lives and communities through it's grant programs, corporate giving and employee volunteers. The Foundation accepts grant applications from nonprofit organizations for innovative projects and activities creating measurable impact in five areas: Social Welfare, Michigan Growth and Environmental Enhancement, Education, Community and Civic, and Culture/Arts. The Foundation's areas of support include, operating budgets and capital funds.
Requirements: The Consumers Energy Foundation provides financial support primarily to Michigan organizations classified by the Internal Revenue Service as tax-exempt under section 501(c)3 of the Internal Revenue Code.
Restrictions: The following are ineligible for funding: individuals; individual scholarships; individual sponsorship related to fund-raising; organizations that do not qualify as charitable organizations as defined by the Internal Revenue Service; organizations that practice discrimination on the basis of sex, age, height, weight, marital status, race, religion, sexual orientation, creed, color, national origin, ancestry, disability, handicap, or veteran status; organizations whose operating activities are already supported by the United Way (except when the request is approved by the appropriate community United Way organization); political organizations and political campaigns; religious organizations when the contribution will be used for denominational or sectarian purposes; labor or veterans organizations; fraternal orders; social clubs; sports tournaments; talent or beauty contests; loans for small business; debt reduction campaigns.
Geographic Focus: Michigan
Samples: Saginaw Basin Land Conservancy, $6,000—for educational outreach efforts supporting wetlands preservation and land conservation within the Saginaw Bay Watershed (2009); American Red Cross Mid-Michigan Chapter, $10,000—for a disaster response vehicle (2009); Kalamazoo Department of Public Safety, $15,000—for development of a Kalamazoo Regional Police and Fire Training Center (2009).
Amount of Grant: $500-$10,000 average
Contact: Carolyn Bloodworth, Secretary/Treasurer; (517) 788-0432; fax: (517) 788-2281; email: foundation@consumersenergy.com
Internet: http://www.consumersenergy.com/welcome.htm
Sponsor: Consumers Energy
1 Energy Place, Room EP8-210
Jackson, MI 49201-2276

Cooke Foundation Grants **1148**
Grants are awarded primarily for culture and the arts, social services, education, programs for youth and the elderly, humanities, health, and the environment. Organizations receiving grants must be located in Hawaii or serve the people of Hawaii. Preference will be given to requests from Ohau. Types of support include general operating support, capital campaigns, building and renovations, program development, seed money, and matching funds.
Requirements: Grant making is limited to the state of Hawaii.
Restrictions: Grants are not made to individuals, churches, or religious organizations, or for endowment funds, scholarships, or fellowships.
Geographic Focus: Hawaii
Samples: Maui Community Arts and Cultural Ctr (HI)—to support the capital campaign to complete construction, $10,000.; Honolulu Dance Theatre (HI)—for a ballet performance, $2500.; Kauai Historical Society (HI)—to support the lecture series, $2500.; Honolulu Academy of Arts (HI)—annual grant, $100,000.
Amount of Grant: $5,000-$25,000 average
Date(s) Application is Due: Mar 2; Sep 1
Contact: Carrie Shoda-Sutherland, Senior Program Officer; (808) 566-5524 or (888) 731-3863, ext. 524; fax: (808) 521-6286; email: csutherland@hcf-hawaii.org;; Christel Wuerfel, Philanthropic Services Assistant; (808) 566-5524 or (888) 731-3863; email: cwuerfel@hc
Internet: http://www.cookefdn.org/
Sponsor: Cooke Foundation, Limited
1164 Bishop Street, Suite 800
Honolulu, HI 96813

Cooley's Anemia Research Fellowships **1149**
The grants-in-aid program supports research that will add to current knowledge about Cooley's anemia and related disorders. The ultimate goal is to find the cause and cure or effective treatment of these diseases. This involves a great deal of basic research in hematology, pathology, physiology, biochemistry, physical chemistry, and related sciences. Fellowships are also available and are awarded for one year, with possible renewal for a second year upon reapplication. The deadline for both fellowships and grants in aid of research is mid-March each year; awards are announced by June 1.
Requirements: Grants are made to institutions and researchers of any country. Individual applicant must have a doctoral degree and no more than five years postdoctoral training.
Amount of Grant: $40,000 maximum stipend per year
Date(s) Application is Due: Mar 1
Contact: Chairperson, Medical Advisory Board, (718) 321-2873 or (800) 522-7222; fax: (718) 321-3340; email: info@cooleysanemia.org
Internet: http://www.cooleysanemia.org/sections.php?sec=58
Sponsor: Cooley's Anemia Foundation
129-09 26th Avenue, Suite 203
Flushing, NY 11354

Cooper Industries Foundation Grants **1150**
Cooper and the Cooper Industries Foundation annually donate more then $3 Million to nonprofit organizations serving the communities where their employees live and work. The Cooper Industries Foundation accepts and reviews grant requests throughout the year. There is no deadline; however, budgets are compiled annually each fall for the following year. Applicants must submit a brief letter explaining the purpose of the request with: concise description of organization and its mission; purpose and amount of request; budget information and other funding sources; evidence of 501(c)3 tax-exempt status; current listing of board members.
Requirements: Only 501(c)3 tax-exempt-status organizations are eligible. Programs must: benefit a community where Cooper is a significant employer; be endorsed by local Cooper management when applicable; not duplicate the efforts of the four Cooper-created programs; fulfill an important community need. Program objectives must coincide with that of the company.
Restrictions: The following types of organizations are generally ineligible for funding: United Way-funded organizations; national and state organizations; religious organizations; veterans organizations; political candidates, labor and lobbying organizations; hospitals; primary and secondary schools; scholarship organizations (except National Merit).
Geographic Focus: Alabama; Georgia; Illinois; Missouri; New York; North Carolina; South Carolina; Texas; WisconsinUnited Kingdom
Contact: Victoria B. Guennewig, VP Public Affairs, (713) 209-8800; fax: (713) 209-8982; email: info@cooperindustries.com
Internet: http://www.cooperindustries.com/common/aboutCooper/corporateGiving.cfm?CFID=160327&CFTOKEN=61243618
Sponsor: Cooper Industries Foundation
P.O. Box 4446
Houston, TX 77210

Coors Brewing Corporate Contributions Grants **1151**
The company has a firm commitment to giving back to its home-market communities—including Denver, CO; Memphis, TN; and Elkton, VA—and supports grassroots, nonprofit organizations that address community, civic and industry issues. The primary focus is on programs that enhance the quality of life. Vehicles of support include cash grants, Coors products for events, Coors logo items for fund-raisers, volunteer hours by Coors employees or retirees, or used equipment or in-kind services. Preference will be given to groups that focus on issues of national scope. Corporate Contributions usually reviews requests the first Wednesday of every month. A minimum of two months lead time is required before the event or funding need.
Requirements: IRS 501(c)3 nonprofit organizations located in Denver, CO; Memphis, TN; and Elkton, VA; are eligible.
Restrictions: Requests will not be considered for individuals in personal programs; individual scholarships; teams, groups, or races; travel expenses; third-party fund-raisers or sales promotions; political activities; or requests by telephone.
Geographic Focus: Colorado; Tennessee; Virginia
Contact: Buck Boze, Corporate Contributions Manager; (800) 642-6116 or (303) 277-5953; fax: (303) 277-6132
Internet: http://www.coors.com
Sponsor: Coors Brewing Company
P.O. Box 4030, Dept NH420
Golden, CO 80401

Cornerstone Foundation of Northeastern Wisconsin Grants **1152**
The community foundation supports nonprofit organizations primarily in Brown County, Wisconsin. The foundations area of interest are: education, cultural programs, social service and, youth agencies. With an additional interest in supporting healthcare facilities. The foundation offers the following types of support: annual campaigns; building/renovation; capital campaigns; continuing support; debt reduction; emergency funds; endowments; equipment; general/operating support; matching/challenge support; program; development. Contact the foundation by telephone for guidelines before submitting a proposal, no application form is required.
Requirements: Nonprofit organizations in Green Bay and northeastern Wisconsin may submit applications for grant support. The primary focus is Brown County.
Restrictions: No grants are available to individuals, religious, or political organizations.
Geographic Focus: Wisconsin
Samples: Green Bay Symphony Orchestra, Green Bay, WI, $10,000—for youth orchestra program (2007); Boys and Girls Club of Green Bay, Green Bay, WI, $400,000—for capital campaign (2007); Salvation Army of Green Bay, Green Bay, WI, $24,900—for transitional housing program (2007).
Amount of Grant: $10,000-$400,000 range
Date(s) Application is Due: Jan 15; Sep 15

Contact: Sheri Prosser, Executive Director; (920) 490-8290; fax: (920) 490-8620; email: cornerstone@cfnew.org
Sponsor: Cornerstone Foundation of Northeastern Wisconsin
111 North Washington Street, Suite 450
Green Bay, WI 54301-4208

Covenant Foundation Grants (Iowa) **1153**
Covenant Foundation, Inc. was created in 1988 through the merger of the Schoitz and St. Francis Hospital Foundations. The Foundation seeks to bring together the gifts and resources of the community to help meet the health care needs of those who are served in all areas of the hospital. Since its creation, the Foundation has served patients and families through the purchase of technical and specialized equipment, the construction and improvement of physical facilities, and community education program that promote health and illness prevention.
Requirements: 501(c)3 organizations of northeast Iowa are eligible to apply.
Geographic Focus: Iowa
Contact: Heather Bremer-Miller, Executive Director; (319) 272-7678; email: Heather.BremerMiller@wfhc.org
Internet: http://www.covhealth.com/covenant_foundation.asp
Sponsor: Covenant Foundation, Inc.
3421 West Ninth Street
Waterloo, IA 50702

Covenant Matters Foundation Grants **1154**
The Covenant Matters Foundation, established in 2003, is the non-profit arm of Strategic Health Policy International, a group that organizes chaos and solves complex problems in health care. The Foundation supports research, strategic planning, marketing, sales, public affairs and other business operations, and it helps to fund, facilitate, negotiate, analyze, strategize, and mentor health care policy-makers. Currently, there are no specific application forms or deadlines, and potential applicants should contact the foundation in writing.
Contact: Glenna M. Crooks, President; (215) 646-8182 or (215) 646-0542; fax: (215) 646-7368; email: GMC@strategichealthpolicy.com
Internet: http://www.strategichealthpolicy.com/OPENSOURCE/Grantseeking/tabid/123/Default.aspx
Sponsor: Covenant Matters Foundation
1075 Fort Washington Avenue
Fort Washington, PA 19034-1617

Cowles Charitable Trust Grants **1155**
The foundation awards grants, primarily in New York, Florida, and on the East Coast, for the arts and culture, including museums and the performing arts; environment; education, including early childhood education, secondary and higher education, medical school education, adult basic education and literacy, and adult continuing education; hospitals and AIDS programs, including research; social services, including family planning, human services, and federated giving; and community funds, including leadership development, civil rights, and race relations. Types of support include general operating support, capital campaigns, annual campaigns, equipment acquisition, endowment funds, continuing support, seed money, building construction/renovation, matching funds, professorships, and program development. Application forms are required; initial approach should be by letter. The board meets in January, April, July, and October.
Requirements: Nonprofit organizations may apply for grant support. Grants are awarded primarily along the Eastern Seaboard.
Geographic Focus: Florida; New York
Samples: Church of the Holy Comforter, Burlington, NC, $53,200 (2006); Miami Art Museum of Dade County, Miami, FL, $30,000 (2006); Allen-Stevenson School, New York, NY, $27,500 (2006).
Amount of Grant: $1000-$40,000 range
Date(s) Application is Due: Mar 1; Jun 1; Sep 1; Dec 1
Contact: Mary Croft, Treasurer; (732) 936-9826
Sponsor: Cowles Charitable Trust
P.O. Box 219
Rumson, NJ 07760

CPhA Centennial Award **1156**
The objective of these awards is to give firsthand information to qualified pharmacy students to improve and develop their knowledge of their chosen profession. The awards provide travel, accommodation, and registration for the CPhA annual conference. One student per university is selected on the basis of achievement up to midterm period of the particular year, the achievement especially related to student activity involvement, and leadership coupled with academic qualifications. Nine awards are made each year.
Requirements: Honors students in their second-last year of study from each faculty or school of pharmacy in Canada who have actively promoted the profession and faculty of pharmacy, and who have a good academic standing.
Amount of Grant: $C300 plus travel expenses
Date(s) Application is Due: Jan 31
Contact: Nancy Shurtleff, Manager of Board Affairs, (613) 523-7877; fax: (613) 523-0445; email: Nshurtleff@cdnpharm.ca
Internet: http://www.pharmacists.ca/content/about_cpha/who_we_are/awards/centennial.cfm
Sponsor: Canadian Pharmaceutical Association
1785 Alta Vista Drive
Ottawa, ON K1G 3Y6 Canada

Crail-Johnson Foundation Grants **1157**
The Crail-Johnson Foundation (CJF) has defined itself as a children's charity, and the vast majority of grant-making is directed toward programs benefiting children, youth and families in the greater Los Angeles area. Proposals, which are not relevant to the foundation's mission and funding priorities, will not be considered. CJF provides grants for program initiatives and enhancements, general operating support and capital projects as well as selected endowments. CJF provides technical assistance to selected community-based initiatives benefiting children and families. The majority of Crail-Johnson Foundation funding supports organizations located in the greater Los Angeles area and projects that directly benefit Los Angeles area residents. National organizations providing services in Los Angeles are also considered. Occasionally, grants are made to programs and projects that are regional or national in scope, where potential benefits to children and families in Los Angeles can be clearly demonstrated. Initial contact with the Crail-Johnson Foundation should be in the form of a letter of inquiry, letters are accepted October through December each year for the following year's grant cycle and are generally considered in the order in which they are received. Organizations selected to submit proposals will be asked to complete a Grant Application Form provided by the Foundation.
Requirements: The foundation provides financial support primarily through grants to public non-profit organizations that are exempt under Section 501(c)3of the Internal Revenue code and are not a private foundation under Section 509(a).
Restrictions: Support is not granted for programs and projects benefiting religious purposes, university level education, research, events recognizing individuals or organizations, political causes or programs attempting to influence legislation. No grants are made directly to individuals.
Geographic Focus: California
Samples: Heart of Los Angeles Youth, Los Angeles, CA, $25,000—Smart Start Elementary Education Program (2009); Mentor LA, Los Angeles, CA, $25,000—staffing and special program enrichment (2009); Strive Foundation, Houston, TX, $20,000—expansion of academic and arts Program (2009).
Amount of Grant: $5000-$50,000 average
Contact: Pat Christopher, Program Officer; (310) 519-7413; fax: (310) 519-7221; email: pat-christopher@crail-johnson.org
Internet: http://www.crail-johnson.org/grants-application.htm
Sponsor: Crail-Johnson Foundation
222 West Sixth Street, Suite 1010
San Pedro, CA 90731

Cranston Foundation Grants **1158**
The foundation directs most of its grants to the geographic areas where Cranston Print Works Company has operations and a large number of employees, including Rhode Island, Massachusetts, Louisiana, and New York. Targeted priority areas are education, health and welfare, culture and the arts, and civic and community programs. Types of support include general operating support, employee matching gifts, and employee-related scholarships. All requests should be made in writing and should contain details and funding requirements pertaining to the project. The February deadline is for scholarships; the August deadline is for grants.
Requirements: IRS 501(c)3 organizations serving Rhode Island, Massachusetts, Louisiana, and New York are eligible.
Geographic Focus: Massachusetts; New York; Rhode Island
Amount of Grant: $200-$5000
Date(s) Application is Due: Feb 15; Aug 31
Contact: Trustees, (401) 943-4800
Sponsor: Cranston Foundation
1381 Cranston Street
Cranston, RI 02920

Crestlea Foundation Grants **1159**
The foundation supports Delaware nonprofits in its areas of interest, including secondary education, higher education, natural resource conservation, health care, housing development, community development, social services, and public affairs. Types of support include annual campaigns, general operating support, capital campaigns, building construction/renovation, and equipment acquisition. There are no application forms.
Requirements: Delaware nonprofits are eligible.
Geographic Focus: Delaware
Samples: Philadelphia Museum of Art (Philadelphia, PA)—for operating support, $82,500.; Archmere Academy (Claymont, DE)—for capital campaign, $20,000.
Amount of Grant: $5000-$50,000 average
Date(s) Application is Due: Nov 1
Contact: Stephen Martinenza, Secretary-Treasurer, (302) 654-2477
Sponsor: Crestlea Foundation
100 W 10th Street, Suite 1109
Wilmington, DE 19801

CRH Foundation Grants **1160**
The foundation awards general operating grants to U.S. nonprofit organizations in its areas of interest, including health and human services. Religious organizations also are eligible. Preference is given to requests from New Jersey and New York. Applications are accepted each year between May 1 and October 31. Inquiries must be in writing.
Requirements: U.S. 501(c)3 nonprofit organizations may apply.
Amount of Grant: $74,000 total
Date(s) Application is Due: Oct 31

Contact: Grants Administrator, (201) 568-9300; fax: (201) 568-6374
Sponsor: CRH Foundation
175 N Woodland Street
Englewood, NJ 07631

CRI Clinical Investigator Award in Cancer Immunology **1161**
Investigator awards are available to six qualified scientists at the assistant professor level who are working in the field of clinical cancer immunology. The four-year award may be used at the recipient's discretion for salary, technical assistance, supplies, or capital equipment. CRI has no citizenship restrictions, and research supported by the award may be conducted anywhere in the United States or abroad, excluding for-profit institutions. Applications may be downloaded from the Web site.
Requirements: Candidate must hold a doctoral degree and be a tenure-track assistant professor or equivalent rank at the time of the award.
Amount of Grant: $50,000 a year for four years for each investigator
Date(s) Application is Due: Mar 1
Contact: Lynne Harmer, Grants Administrator, (212) 688-7515; fax: (212) 832-9376; email: grants@cancerresearch.org
Internet: http://www.cancerresearch.org/clinical.html
Sponsor: Cancer Research Institute
681 Fifth Avenue
New York, NY 10022-4209

CRI Postdoctoral Fellowships **1162**
Each year the institute awards postdoctoral fellowships to qualified individuals in the formative stages of their career who wish to receive training in cancer immunology with special emphasis on tumor immunology. Work may be carried out in the United States or abroad. The fellowships are awarded for a period of two years, with the possibility of renewal for one additional year. CRI requires all fellowship applicants to complete an electronic application as well as a paper application.
Requirements: Applicant of any nationality must have a doctoral degree and must conduct research under a sponsor who holds a formal appointment at the sponsoring institution.
Amount of Grant: $40,000 first year, $42,000 second year, $44,000 third year; plus $1500 institutional allowance per year
Date(s) Application is Due: Apr 1; Oct 1
Contact: Brian Brewer, Grants Administrator, (212) 688-7515 ext 242 or (800) 992-2623; fax: (212) 832-9376; email: grants@cancerresearch.org
Internet: http://www.cancerresearch.org/postdoc.html
Sponsor: Cancer Research Institute
681 Fifth Avenue
New York, NY 10022-4209

CRI Prostate Cancer Initiative Grants **1163**
The program supports Phase I and Phase I/II clinical trials that test novel therapies for advanced prostate cancer, with particular emphasis on hormonal therapy and immunotherapy. CRI does not provide funds for indirect costs. The completed application consists of 15 sets of the following items collated in the order specified: application form; biographical sketches for all key personnel; abstract of proposed project explaining the importance of the proposed research and ramifications; five-page description of research program, including summary of past work and future plans; and IRB-approved protocol. Applications must be typed or printed (using both sides of the paper, if possible). In addition, a self-addressed, stamped postcard is required if applicant would like to receive notification of receipt of application. Annual deadline dates may vary; contact the program office for exact dates.
Amount of Grant: $150,000 over two years
Date(s) Application is Due: Apr 15
Contact: Grants Administrator, (212) 688-7515 or (800) 992-2623; fax: (212) 832-9376; email: info@cancerresearch.org
Internet: http://www.cancerresearch.org/pciinit.html
Sponsor: Cancer Research Institute
681 Fifth Avenue
New York, NY 10022-4209

Crohn's Disease and Colitis Research Fellowships **1164**
Three-year fellowships are awarded to encourage the development of individuals with research potential to help them prepare for careers of independent research in the areas of Crohn's disease and ulcerative colitis. Yearly renewal is dependent on the receipt of satisfactory progress reports. Application forms must be obtained from the foundation. Letters of intent are due May 1 and November 1. Submission deadlines for full applications are January 14 and July 1 of each year. Annual deadline dates may vary; contact program staff for exact dates.
Requirements: The applicant must hold an MD, PhD, or equivalent degree and be currently employed by an institution engaged in health care and/or health-related research within the United States. Candidates who have obtained MD degrees must have at least two years of postdoctoral experience, one year of which must be documented research experience relevant to inflammatory bowel disease. Candidates holding PhD degrees must have one year of postdoctoral experience and at least one year of documented research experience relevant to IBD.
Amount of Grant: $58,250 maximum salary per year
Date(s) Application is Due: Jan 14; May 1; Jul 1; Nov 1
Contact: Carol Cox, Director of Research and Scientific Programs, (212) 685-3440 or (800) 932-2423; fax: (212) 779-4098; email: ccox@ccfa.org
Internet: http://www.ccfa.org/research/?LMI=4
Sponsor: Crohn's & Colitis Foundation of America Inc
386 Park Ave S, 17th Floor
New York, NY 10016-8804

Crohn's Disease and Ulcerative Colitis Senior Research Grants **1165**
Grants are awarded to individuals for up to two years for research in the basic biomedical and clinical sciences that will increase the understanding of the cause, mechanisms of symptoms, and treatment of inflammatory bowel disease including Crohn's disease and ulcerative colitis. Support for additional one-year periods will be by competitive renewal. Application forms must be secured from the foundation. Submission deadlines for letters of intent are November 1 and May 1.
Requirements: Applicants must be established researchers in the field of inflammatory bowel disease.
Amount of Grant: $115,000 maximum
Date(s) Application is Due: Jan 14; May 1; Jul 1; Nov 1
Contact: Carol Cox, Research and Scientific Programs, (212) 685-3440 or (800) 932-2423; fax: (212) 779-4098; email: ccox@ccfa.org
Internet: http://www.ccfa.org/research/?LMI=4
Sponsor: Crohn's & Colitis Foundation of America Inc
386 Park Ave S, 17th Floor
New York, NY 10016-8804

Cruise Industry Charitable Foundation Grants **1166**
The foundation awards grants to improve the quality of life in U.S. cities and towns where the cruise industry maintains vessel operations, employs a significant number of individuals, and purchases products and services. Areas of interest include civic and community development, educational assistance and training programs, public health programs, and environmental initiatives. There are no application deadlines, see Foundation's website for application guidelines.
Requirements: U.S. 501(c)3 organizations are eligible to apply.
Restrictions: Requests will not be considered from individuals, fraternal groups, religious organizations, political groups, or organizations that conduct lobbying activity.
Samples: American Heart Association—Public Health Program (2009); Armed Forces Foundation—Civic and Community Development Program (2009); Page Ahead—Educational Assistance and Training Program (2009).
Contact: Cynthia Colenda; (703) 522-3160; fax: (703) 522-3161; email: cicf@iccl.org
Internet: http://www.cruisefoundation.org/requirements-and-guidelines.php
Sponsor: Cruise Industry Charitable Foundation
2111 Wilson Boulevard, 8th Floor
Arlington, VA 22201

CSL Behring Local Empowerment for Advocacy Development Grants **1167**
CSL Behring Local Empowerment for Advocacy Development (LEAD) Grants are community-based grants of approximately $10,000. These grants are intended to help local patient organizations achieve their advocacy objectives. CSL Behring will award LEAD Grants to organizations that submit proposals demonstrating that financial assistance would help them address important local and state advocacy issues and initiatives. Local patient organizations have already demonstrated significant leadership in tackling complex legislative and regulatory public policy issues. Advocacy can, however, be costly. CSL Behring LEAD Grants will help defray these costs. Moreover, CSL Behring will work with the grant recipients to advance their objectives in order to obtain success.
Requirements: In order to qualify, a local organization must be: a recognized patient advocacy organization representing individuals who use plasma/recombinant therapies to treat bleeding disorders, immune disorders, Alpha-1 deficiency or other conditions; a non-profit organization with 501(c)3 tax status; and an organization currently addressing a specific advocacy issue or intending to address such an issue.
Amount of Grant: $10,000 maximum
Date(s) Application is Due: Apr 30; Oct 31
Contact: Patrick Collins, Sr. Manager, Public Affairs; (610) 878-4311; email: Patrick.Collins@cslbehring.com;; Christine Kuhinka; (610) 878-4387; email: Christine.Kuhinka@cslbehring.com
Internet: http://www.cslbehring.com/s1/cs/enco/1199979063088/content/1199979062780/content.htm
Sponsor: CSL Behring
P.O. Box 61501, 1020 First Avenue
King of Prussia, PA 19406-0901

CSRA Community Foundation Grants **1168**
The foundation awards grants to organizations that provide programs and services to the Greater Augusta area, including Richmond, Columbia, McDuffie, Burke, Aiken and Edgefield counties. Areas of interest include arts and cultural; children, youth, and family services; civic affairs; community development; economic development, education; environmental; health; and human services. Types of support include annual campaigns, capital campaigns, seed grants, scholarship funds, and matching funds. The board meets quarterly to consider requests.
Requirements: Georgia 501(c)3 organizations, providing programs and services to the Greater Augusta area, including one or more of the following counties : Richmond, Columbia, McDuffie, Burke, Aiken and Edgefield are eligible to apply.
Restrictions: The Community Foundation discourages applicants from submitting applications in support of the following: computer/word processing hardware not directly related to project or services; grants for individuals; building campaigns;

deficit financing and debt retirement; endowments; fraternal organizations, societies or orders; professional/association conferences or seminars (support for or attendance at); political organization or campaigns; lobbying legislators or influencing elections; special fundraising events/celebration functions; surveys, feasibility studies, marketing endeavors and personal research; travel for individuals or groups such as bands, sports teams, and classes; core operating expenses for public and private elementary and secondary schools and public and private colleges and universities; projects that are typically the funding responsibility of federal, state or local governments; fifteen passenger vans.
Geographic Focus: Georgia
Samples: Full Circle Refuge, Inc., $15,000—for the support of the Gang Prevention Youth Mentoring Program (2009); Georgia Committee on Employment of People with Disabilities, $9,600—to purchase equipment for 45 students with disabilities who are enrolled in the High School High Tech programs (2009); Gertrude Herbert Institute of Art, $4,100—to present a collaborative project, Hidden Thoughts: Visual Communication, a yearlong program for children under the age of 18 who are victims of domestic violence and child abuse (2009).
Amount of Grant: $15,000 maximum
Date(s) Application is Due: Jul 31
Contact: Cindy Arrant, Manager of Finance & Administration; (706) 724-1314; fax: (706) 724-1315; email: info@csracf.com
Internet: http://www.cfcsra.org/common/content.asp?PAGE=336
Sponsor: CSRA Community Foundation Inc
P.O. Box 31358
Augusta, GA 30903

CSX Corporate Contributions Grants 1169
The program is focusing its support on personal safety education and community safety. In an effort to keep kids safe, CSX will support nonprofit organizations and school programs which help educate children and their parents on issues of personal safety, help keep children safe on the internet, teach railroad saety to children, teens and adults, and provide safe havens that keep children and adults safe from abuse. First responders are the key to a timely and effective manner of keeping a community safe. Safety, disaster, high alert and Hazmat training, equipment requirements of first responders, and projects and activities that keep communities safe, such as a fence around a neighborhood playground are supported. Programs that protect air, land and water resources in the communities in which CSX operates, preserve natural resources, and teach environmental stewardship to children and adults. A limited number of grants to local social service agencies and arts and culture organizations will be supported. Organizations in the targeted cities must submit an on-line application for sponsorship.
Requirements: 501(c)3 charities and government institutions, such as schools and libraries in their areas of operations are eligible.
Restrictions: Grants do not support individuals; galas, concerts, sports tournaments, auctions, lunches, banquets or dinners; film and video projects; churches or faith-based organizations whose projects benefit wholly their members or adherents; or organizations geographically falling outside of CSX's targeted giving areas. Operating costs or capital improvements are seldom supported.
Geographic Focus: Alabama; Connecticut; Delaware; Florida; Georgia; Illinois; Indiana; Kentucky; Louisiana; Maryland; Massachusetts; Michigan; Mississippi; New Jersey; New York; North Carolina; Ohio; Pennsylvania; South Carolina; Tennessee; Virginia; West Virginia
Contact: Ellen M. Fitzsimmons, Corporate Secretary; (904) 359-3200; email: corporatecontributionsd@csx.com
Internet: http://www.csx.com/?fuseaction=general.csxog_giving
Sponsor: CSX Corporation
Office of the Corporate Secretary, 500 Water Street, C160
Jacksonville, FL 32202

CTCRI Idea Grants 1170
Idea Grants are designed to encourage unique or original research that has the potential to advance knowledge in tobacco control. Grants will allow investigators with innovative ideas and observations to conduct pilot studies, to perform secondary analysis of data sets or to gather new evidence necessary to determine the viability of research directions or hypotheses. Innovative projects are a priority for the Idea Grant program. Preference will be given to proposals that address research priorities identified by the Canadian Tobacco Control Research Summit. Research employing new or unconventional methodologies is encouraged. Proposed methods must be appropriate to the research question(s). Each successful proposal may receive a one-time grant of up to $50,000.
Requirements: Research proposals must meet the following eligibility criteria: The Principal Applicant (PA) is a Canadian citizen or legal resident (Co-applicants may be citizens or residents of other countries); The research proposal demonstrates basic relevance to tobacco abuse / nicotine addiction / tobacco control and addresses research priorities identified by the Canadian Tobacco Control Research Summit; Applicant(s) has disclosed other sources of funding; Commercial interests have been disclosed or applicant(s) has indicated no commercial interests; Applicant(s) has affirmed lack of support from the tobacco industry; Applicant(s) can demonstrate that he/she works in an environment that adequately supports research through ethical review, administration of funds, provision of space and equipment, etc.; Research plans include gender analysis, or it has been demonstrated that this is not appropriate; Proposal avoids duplication of previous research, unless it can be demonstrated that replication is of value; Research proposal involves pilot testing of research methods, tools, or hypotheses by a research team in order to strengthen proposals prepared for submission to traditional funding sources; Proposal articulates preliminary plans for development of a full research proposal -OR- Research proposal constitutes a novel idea which falls outside the normal scope of traditional research, either in topic or methodology; Proposal demonstrates that adequate funding is not available from other sources for this purpose.
Restrictions: Members of the staff or Board of Directors of the CTCRI, or a staff member of any CTCRI funding partner organization are not eligible to apply.
Amount of Grant: up to $50,000
Date(s) Application is Due: Apr 1; Oct 1
Contact: Carol Bishop, Assistant Director, Research Operations; (416) 934-5640; email: cbishop@cancer.ca
Internet: http://www.ctcri.ca/en/index.php?option=com_content&task=view&id=25&Itemid=44
Sponsor: Canadian Tobacco Control Research Initiative
10 Alcorn Avenue, Suite 200
Toronto, ON M4V 3B1 Canada

Cudd Foundation Grants 1171
The foundation awards grants to eligible nonprofit organizations in its areas of interest, including arts, culture, performing arts, children and youth, education, environment, health care, historic preservation, and social services. Types of support include annual campaigns, building construction/renovation, capital campaigns, continuing support, curriculum development, emergency grants, endowments, program development, research, and scholarship funds. The listed application deadline is for letters of intent; full proposals are by invitation.
Requirements: Louisiana and New Mexico nonprofit organizations are eligible.
Geographic Focus: Louisiana; New Mexico
Amount of Grant: $250-$222,088 range
Contact: Amanda Stuermer, (505) 986-8416; fax: (505) 986-8427; email: cuddfdn@aol.com
Sponsor: Cudd Foundation
P.O. Box 2322
Santa Fe, NM 87504

Cullen Foundation Grants 1172
The foundation awards grants to eligible Texas nonprofit organizations in its areas of interest, including arts and culture, education, health, and public service programs. There are no application deadlines or forms. Proposals should detail the purpose and scope of the grant; the amount requested; other sources of anticipated funding; a list of trustees, directors, and staff; financial statements and tax returns of the last two years; and anticipated project budgets. Preference is given to requests from Houston.
Requirements: Texas 501(c)3 or 170(c) nonprofit organizations are eligible.
Restrictions: The board prefers not to consider galas, testimonials, and various other types of fundraising events; organizations that in turn make grants to others; activities whose sole purpose is the promotion or support of a specific religion, denomination, or church; purchase of uniforms, equipment, or trips for school-related organizations or amateur sports teams; applications from an organization more frequently than once every 12 months, whether the previous application was approved or denied; applications from an organization that has received a multi-year grant from the foundation, until all payments of that grant have been made; or oral presentations from potential applicants.
Geographic Focus: Texas
Samples: Reasoning Mind (Houston, TX)—Bringing the internet-based 5th grade math curriculum to Houston students, $50,000 (2005); Child Advocates, Inc. (TX)—Operating support, $20,000 (2005); The Heritage Society (Houston, TX)—for the relocation and restoration of the 1868 Pilot House, $25,000 (2005); Camp for All Foundation (Houston, TX)—Improvements to the camp's drainage system and main thoroughfare, $72,950 (2005);
Amount of Grant: $3.01 million total
Contact: Sue Alexander, Grant Administrator, (713) 651-8837; email: salexander@cullenfdn.org
Internet: http://www.cullenfdn.org
Sponsor: Cullen Foundation
601 Jefferson, 40th Floor
Houston, TX 77002

Cultural Society of Filipino Americans Grants 1173
The CSFA is a non-profit organization dedicated to the promotion and preservation of Filipino culture. Grants are made to local, regional, foreign or international organizations engaged in non-profit activities designed to improve the economic, social, emotional, physical, educational and mental well-being of members of stated organizations in fulfillment of the prescribed responsibility of CSFA.
Requirements: Grants will be made only to organizations that have evidence of 501(c)3 tax-exempt status or to organizations with the endorsement and support of a fiscal agent. In general, the Charitable Committee will look for projects or programs that: (1) fill a real need; (2) have clear, attainable, measurable objectives; (3) are likely to produce results which can be replicated or marketed; (4) are likely to reduce costs, increase revenues or otherwise pay for themselves over time; (5) propose activities which will continue after the grant period without additional funding; and, (6) contain a simple, workable, evaluation plan. The committee will give special consideration to project/programs which propose collaboration with other community organization.
Restrictions: Funds will not be given to individuals; organizations whose primary function is to influence legislation or the local, state or federal levels of government; political parties or candidates; churches or sectarian organizations; however, funds may be given to provide humanitarian aid/services on completely non-sectarian reasons.
Amount of Grant: $500-$1,000
Contact: Jose Rivera, President; email: webmaster@csfamn.org

Internet: http://www.csfamn.org
Sponsor: Cultural Society of Filipino Americans
P.O. Box 2773
St. Paul, MN 55102

CUNA Mutual Group Foundation **1174**
The corporation makes grants to programs and organizations that are of benefit to its subsidiaries; communities in which associates reside; and programs that are of benefit to Waverly, Bremer/Butler Counties, and Iowa (in that order). Priority areas include education, urban/civic services, human services, and the arts. Some multiyear grants will be awarded. The committee gives preference to programs in which associates and their families are involved and those involving more than just monetary funding.
Requirements: Iowa 501(c)3 organizations are eligible.
Restrictions: The committee will not consider grants for individuals; political parties, candidates, and partisan political campaigns; professional associations; operating expenses for organizations receiving United Way funding; or religious groups for religious purposes.
Geographic Focus: Iowa
Amount of Grant: $2500 minimum
Contact: Executive Director, (608) 231-7908
Internet: http://www.cunamutual.com/cmg/freeFormDetail/0,1248,888,00.html
Sponsor: CUNA Mutual Group
P.O. Box 391
Madison, WI 53701

CVS All Kids Can Grants **1175**
CVS Caremark and the CVS Caremark Charitable Trust will support nonprofit organizations that provide innovative programs and services that are focused on helping children with disabilities learn, play and succeed in life. The goals of CVS Caremark All Kids Can are to provide medical rehabilitation and related services to children with disabilities, to build barrier-free playgrounds so children of all abilities can play side-by-side; and to raise awareness in school and in local communities about the importance of inclusion.
Amount of Grant: $1,000
Date(s) Application is Due: Nov 30
Contact: Jennifer Veilleux, Director of Community Relations; (401) 770-4517 or (401) 770-4209; email: jhveilleux@cvs.com or CommunityMailbox@cvs.com
Internet: http://info.cvscaremark.com/community/our-impact/all-kids-can
Sponsor: CVS Charitable Trust, Inc
One CVS Drive
Woonsocket, RI 02895

CVS Caremark Charitable Trust Grants **1176**
The trust has a goal of positively impacting the culturally diverse populations in the communities where CVS stores are located. Health programs that serve children (under the age of 18) with disabilities and address awareness, accessibility, early intervention, health and rehabilitative services are funded. Public schools (grades pre-K through 12) that are expanding programs promoting inclusion of children with disabilities in all aspects of school functions, including: student academic activities, extracurricular programs, and physical activity/play will be considered. Disabilities are impairments that limit one or more routine activities of daily living. Physical, developmental, and sensory disabilities are supported. The primary focus is on children with disabilities and health care for the uninsured. Application must be submitted online.
Requirements: 501(c)3 public charities as determined by the IRS are eligible. Organizations must benefit the customers and communities in the areas where the corporation operates, and demonstrate the specific ways that the organization benefits the community. Religious organizations are eligible for nonsectarian, nondenominational programs.
Restrictions: The trust does not provide funding for sectarian and religious organizations that do not serve the general public on a nondenominational basis; organizations that discriminate on the basis of race, color, gender, sexual orientation, age, religion, national or ethnic origin or physical disability; political or fraternal groups, social clubs, or any other organization that engages in any kind of political activity; sponsorship of sports teams; journal or program advertisements; organizations geographically located outside of CVS markets; sponsorships for music, film, and art festivals; or business expositions/conferences.
Date(s) Application is Due: Jun 15
Contact: Jennifer Veilleux, Director of Community Relations; (401) 770-4517 or (401) 770-4209; email: jhveilleux@cvs.com or CommunityMailbox@cvs.com
Internet: http://info.cvscaremark.com/community/our-impact/charitable-trust
Sponsor: CVS Pharmacy Corporation
One CVS Drive
Woonsocket, RI 02895

CVS Community Grants **1177**
CVS Caremark Pharmacy Community Grants target effective and innovative programs. Grants support programs that promote independence among children with disabilities including physical and occupational therapies, speech and hearing therapies, technology that will assist and recreational therapies. They also support public schools that promote inclusive programs in student activities and extracurricular programs and enrich the lives of children with disabilities. The Community Grants Program works to ensure that students are not left behind in school. Proposed programs must be fully inclusive where children with disabilities are full participants in early childhood, adolescent, or teenage programs along side their typically developing peers. CVS is also devoted to the principle of free play. The unstructured, spontaneous, voluntary activity that is so engaging for children—has long been recognized as the most beneficial form. Proposed programs may include either physical activities or play opportunities and should address the specific needs of the population served.
The CVS/pharmacy Community Grants Program assures that more uninsured people receive needed care that the care received is of higher quality, and that the uninsured are served by providers who participate in accountable community health care programs. There is no age limit on proposed programs that create greater access to health care services.
Restrictions: An EIN number must be provided before beginning the eligibility quiz for all non-profit organizations applying for a Community Grant for children under age 18 with disabilities. All public schools applying for a Community Grant for this type of program are not required to provide an EIN number. An EIN number must be provided before beginning the eligibility quiz for all non-profit organizations applying for a Community Grant for health care for uninsured people.
Amount of Grant: $5,000
Date(s) Application is Due: Oct 31
Contact: Jennifer Veilleux, Director of Community Relations; (401) 770-4517 or (401) 770-4209; email: jhveilleux@cvs.com or CommunityMailbox@cvs.com
Internet: http://info.cvscaremark.com/community/our-impact/community-grants
Sponsor: CVS Caremark Pharmacy Corporation
One CVS Drive
Woonsocket, RI 02895

Cyrus Eaton Foundation Grants **1178**
The foundation awards grants to eligible Ohio nonprofit organizations in its priority areas of arts, conservation and restoration, education, health and social welfare, public affairs, and science. The Foundation supports both well-known regional art institutions and up-and-coming organizations, which broaden the audience for the arts. Organizations that utilize hands-on learning, foster academic skills, and design programs which stimulate the learner's understanding of diversity, invention, and risk-taking are also supported. Programs that nourish creativity and enhance artistic skills are encouraged. Programs that encourage students to hypothesize, test theories, seek multiple ways to solve problems, and design inventions are also encouraged. Programs that cultivate curiosity, encourage scientific inquiry, and exhibit scientific discoveries are also supported. Hands-on experimentation and the development of quality resources are also encouraged. Public Affairs involve the civic-mindedness of citizens as they work together to solve social, political and economic issues. Free speech is essential to the exchange of diverse ideas. The Foundation promotes the distribution of information to help citizens make informed decisions. Community responsibility and debate of ideas are encouraged. Conservation not only preserves our architectural and environmental history, but it also works toward ensuring a healthy environment. The Foundation considers programs that educate people about the past and the future development of our region. Programs whose aim is to control urban sprawl, preserve historical landmarks, and protect our natural habitats are supported. The health and social welfare of the community require commitment to the care of the mental, physical and social well being of the diverse populations of the community. Shelter, medical treatment, counseling, and one-on-one attention are only a few of the ingredients that help people live a healthier life and become more self-reliant. The Foundation supports institutions that provide free medical and social services to the citizens without discrimination. Innovative and caring solutions to community problems are encouraged.
Requirements: Cleveland and northeast Ohio nonprofit organizations are eligible.
Restrictions: The foundation does not consider more than one proposal from the same organization within a twelve-month period, unless that organization is applying for an Impact Grant. Tickets or tables for events, municipalities or individuals will not be funded.
Geographic Focus: Ohio
Samples: Beck Ctr for the Arts (Lakewood, OH)—$3000.; Cleveland Playhouse (OH)—$2000.; Hoospice of the Western Reserve (OH)—$15,000.
Date(s) Application is Due: May 1; Oct 1
Contact: Raymond Szabo, President, (216) 320-2285; fax: (216) 320-2287; email: r.szabo@deepcove.org or cyrus.eaton.foundation@deepcove.org
Internet: http://www.deepcove.org/index.html
Sponsor: Cyrus Eaton Foundation
2475 Lee Boulevard, Suite 2B
Cleveland Heights, OH 441118

Cystic Fibrosis Research Grants **1179**
The trust was founded to find a complete solution for cystic fibrosis and to improve upon current methods of treatment. Research grants are awarded in the United Kingdom and internationally in the fields of science and medicine.
Requirements: Only researchers from recognized academic institutions are eligible to apply.
Contact: Research Administrator, Research Administrator, 020 8290 7906; email: researchgrants@cftrust.org.uk
Internet: http://www.cftrust.org.uk/scope/page/view.go?layout=cftrust&pageid=54
Sponsor: Cystic Fibrosis Trust
11 London Road
Bromley BR1 1BY United Kingdom

D. W. McMillan Foundation Grants **1180**
The D. W. McMillan Foundation, established in 1956, supports organizations involved with youth services, health care, health organizations, homelessness, hospitals, human

services, mental health/crisis services, residential/custodial care, hospices, people with disabilities, and the economically disadvantaged population. Giving is primarily centered in the states of Alabama, and Florida. There are no specific deadlines with which to adhere. Contact the Foundation for further application information and guidelines.
Geographic Focus: Alabama; Florida
Samples: Manna Food Bank, Pensacola, FL, $20,000 (2007); Baptist Health Care Foundation, Pensacola, FL, $76,000 (2007); Boy Scouts of America, Pensacola, FL, $20,000 (2007);
Contact: Ed Leigh McMillan II, Treasurer; (251) 867-4881
Sponsor: D. W. McMillan Foundation
329 Belleville Avenue
Brewton, AL 36426-2039

D.F. Halton Foundation Grants **1181**
The foundation awards grants to nonprofit organizations in Charlotte, NC, and San Miguel County, CO, primarily in the areas of youth, education, social services, and the performing arts. Additional areas of interest include historical preservation, education, vocational education, business school education, substance abuse, cancer research, heart/circulatory diseases and research, human and family services, and community development. Grants are awarded for general operating support, annual campaigns, capital campaigns, and scholarship funds. There are no application deadlines or forms.
Requirements: Nonprofit organizations in North Carolina counties, including Mecklenburg, Union, Cleveland, Cabarrus, Stanly, Lincoln, and Gaston, may submit proposals. Nonprofit organizations in San Miguel county, CO. may also submit proposals.
Restrictions: No grants will be awarded to individuals.
Geographic Focus: Colorado; North Carolina
Contact: Dale Halton, President
Sponsor: D.F. Halton Foundation
P.O. Box 834
Ophir, CO 81426

D.V. and Ida J. McEachern Charitable Trust Grants **1182**
The Trust was established to give a better start in life to all children, both educationally and physically. Most grants are made to social service agencies addressing basic human needs for children and youth. The Trust is also interested in providing creative and positive opportunities to enhance the lives of the region's children through a variety of artistic and cultural programs. The Advisory Committee prefers proposals from groups that clearly describe how their program makes a positive difference in the lives of children, provides a unique service, or addresses problems that are not being met by other agencies in the area. Grants will be made solely for capital projects and items of immediate and direct service to children. There is no letter of inquiry process. If your project fits the guidelines, submit a proposal letter with a narrative no longer than four pages.
Requirements: Grant organizations should: request capital support only (McEachern grants will generally not exceed 5% of a capital campaign budget); provide services to a broad cross-section of the population up to age 18; be established for at least five years (exceptions may be made for groups with strong community leadership and reputation, offering unique enrichment programs for children); serve Puget Sound region (particularly King, Pierce, and Snohomish Counties); have a secure and diverse funding base, with a majority of budget income derived from non-governmental sources.
Restrictions: Grants will generally not be made to endowment campaigns, individuals, private schools, public schools, day-care programs, political candidates, or religious institutions.
Geographic Focus: Washington
Samples: Burke Museum (Seattle, WA)—for renovation and development of a Natural History Demonstration Lab for students, $25,000 (2004); Highline Community Hospital Foundation (Tukwila, WA)—for children's area of a new cancer care center, $15,000 (2004); Salish Sea Expeditions (Bainbridge, WA)—equipment upgrades for the inquiry-based marine education science program, $2500 (2004); YMCA Tacoma Pierce County (Tacoma, WA)—for sports equipment replacement for youth programs, $5000 (2004).
Amount of Grant: $15,000-$25,000
Date(s) Application is Due: Mar 8; Sep 8; Dec 8
Contact: Therese Ogle, Grants, (206) 781-3472; email: OgleFounds@aol.com
Internet: http://fdncenter.org/grantmaker/mceachern/guide.html
Sponsor: D.V. and Ida J. McEachern Charitable Trust
P.O. Box 3123
Seattle, WA 98114

DAAD Research Stays for University Academics and Scientists **1183**
These grants and scholarships aim to provide foreign academics and scientists working in higher education or at research institutes with an opportunity to carry out a research project at a state (public) or state-recognized higher education institution or non-university research institute in Germany. Depending on the applicant's work schedule, the research stay will last between one and three months. Depending on the applicant's academic status, the monthly award will amount to 1,840 Euros for assistant lecturers, assistant professors and young lecturers, and 1,990 Euros for professors. In some rare exceptions, 2,240 Euros may be available. In addition to these payments, the DAAD generally will pay an appropriate flat-rate travel allowance, unless these costs are covered by the home country or by another funding source. Applications for research grants are decided twice a year. Applications must have been submitted by 1 August or 15 January. At the earliest, grants can begin 4 months after the date of application.
Requirements: Applications for DAAD research stays are open to excellently-qualified academics and scientists who should generally hold a doctorate/PhD. All applicants must be working in higher education or at a research institute in their home country. Besides their previous academic achievements (for example, recent publications), the most important selection criterion is a convincing and well-planned research project to be completed during the stay in Germany. The application must provide proof of a workplace being provided at the host institute.
Restrictions: DAAD support for a research stay can only be awarded once in any three-year period. No travel expenses can be paid from the grant.
Amount of Grant: Euro 1,840 - Euro 2,240 per month
Contact: Scholarship Administrator, (212) 758-3223; fax: (212) 755-5780; email: kim@daad.org or daadny@daad.org
Internet: http://www.daad.de/deutschland/foerderung/stipendiendatenbank/00462.en.html?detailid=39&fachrichtung=15&land=44&status=4&seite=1&daad=1
Sponsor: German Academic Exchange Service (DAAD)
871 United Nations Plaza
New York, NY 10017

Dade Community Foundation Community AIDS Partnership Grants **1184**
The Community AIDS Partnership, is a special funding initiative established in 1990 through the National AIDS Fund and local funders to increase the availability of private funds to address gaps in the local HIV/AIDS service system, particularly in the area of prevention. The Community AIDS Partnership represents one of the major sources of private philanthropic funds for HIV prevention in Miami-Dade County. As the result of a public/private partnership with Miami-Dade County, the Foundation also awards $350,000 in county funds, which represents a significant increase in the local public sector's commitment to funding HIV prevention. Through the Community AIDS Partnership, the Foundation supports quality programs that respond to the local population risk profile and that incorporate strategies with the greatest potential to effectively address the priority populations, communities and service needs related to HIV prevention in Miami-Dade County. Grant Size: $30,000 Single Organization, $60,000 for Collaborations.
Requirements: Eligible applicants include nonprofit tax-exempt organizations, as defined by the Internal Revenue Code, which are serving the residents of Miami-Dade County. Preference will be given to organizations based in Miami-Dade County or if located outside the county, are working in partnership with a group based in Miami-Dade.
Geographic Focus: Florida
Samples: Camillus House, $30,000 - to support a comprehensive HIV/AIDS program that targets homeless members of racial/ethnic minority communities who are either HIV positive or are at very high risk for HIV infection due to injection drug use and/or heterosexual contact (2007); MUJER, $30,000 - to continue the Nosotras Viviremos project which seeks to increase awareness about HIV/AIDS in migrant farmworker communities in South Miami-Dade County (2007);
Amount of Grant: $30,000 - $60,000
Contact: Gianne Ewing-Chow, Senior Program Officer; (305) 371-2711; fax: (305) 371-5342; email: gianne.ewingchow@dadecommunityfoundation.org
Internet: http://www.dadecommunityfoundation.org/Site/wc/wc145.jsp
Sponsor: Dade Community Foundation
200 South Biscayne Boulevard, Suite 505
Miami, FL 33131-5330

Dade Community Foundation Grants **1185**
The funding for this program is made available through the Foundation's unrestricted and field of interest funds. This program is designed to honor both the donors interests and address significant community issues such as: education; health; human services; arts and culture; environment; economic development; at-risk youth; abused and neglected children; living with HIV/AIDS; homelessness; social justice; care of animals; heart disease and more.
Requirements: Eligible applicants include nonprofit tax-exempt organizations, as defined by the Internal Revenue Code, which are serving the residents of Miami-Dade County. Preference will be given to or- ganizations based in Miami-Dade County or if located outside the county, are working in partnership with an group based in Miami-Dade.
Restrictions: The Foundation does not provide grants to individuals, for memberships, fundraising events or memorials. Grants to government agencies are made on a very restricted basis.
Geographic Focus: Florida
Amount of Grant: $7,500
Date(s) Application is Due: Nov 15
Contact: Charisse Grant, Vice President for Programs; (305) 371-2711; fax: (305) 371-5342; email: charisse.grant@dadecommunityfoundation.org
Internet: http://www.dadecommunityfoundation.org/Site/programs/overview.jsp
Sponsor: Dade Community Foundation
200 South Biscayne Boulevard, Suite 505
Miami, FL 33131-5330

DaimlerChrysler Corporation Fund Grants **1186**
The fund contributes to organizations grouped under the general categories of education, health and human services, civic and community, religion, and culture and the arts. Within these categories, grants are made available for public welfare or for charitable, scientific, educational, environmental, safety, building, and affirmative action purposes. Higher education grants largely support science and engineering education and business management. A major interest of the corporation is the establishment of national certification standards for elementary and secondary teachers. Another area of concern

is the encouragement of early reading skills, and a pilot project has been funded for research in this area. The fund earmarks funds for its future workforce initiatives, which support business and engineering departments, community-based job-skill training, and entry-level work preparation. Types of support include matching gifts, program grants, scholarships, annual campaigns, building construction/renovation, general support, and employee matching gifts. In considering requests, the fund evaluates each applicant organization on its own merits; considered are the programs in which it is engaged, constituencies served, operation procedures, services offered, quality of management, its accountability, finances, and fund-raising practices. A

Requirements: Eligible for support are nonprofit, tax-exempt educational, health, civic, and cultural organizations primarily in locations where the greatest number of employees of Chrysler and its U.S.-based subsidiaries live and work (Alabama, Delaware, Illinois, Indiana, Michigan, Missouri, New York, Ohio, and Wisconsin). Some support is targeted for national organizations as well.

Restrictions: Grants are not awarded to support endowments, conferences, trips, direct health care delivery, multiyear pledges, capital campaigns, fund-raising activities related to sponsorships, advertising, or debt retirement.

Contact: Brian Glowiak, (248) 512-2502; fax: (248) 512-2503; email: mek@dcx.com

Internet: http://www.fund.daimlerchrysler.com

Sponsor: DaimlerChrysler Corporation Fund
1000 Chrysler Drive
Auburn Hills, MI 48326-2766

Dairy Queen Corporate Contributions Grants **1187**

The Foundation's philosophy toward awarding contribution grants is to assist those organizations which have an impact on the company's home state of Minnesota and its communities and have programs geared toward children. Foundation focus is on: culture and the performing arts, education, health care and hospitals, and social welfare and community services. Application information is available online.

Requirements: U.S. nonprofits are eligible. Priority is given to Minnesota organizations.

Restrictions: Funds are not available for: strictly sectarian or denominational religious organizations; direct or indirect use for political purposes; lobbying activities; benefits and fund-raisers; commemorative, courtesy, institutional or any other form of advertising; organizations that tend to be for the benefit of the individual members, rather than the general public, such as fraternities, sororities, social clubs, labor organizations, parties and banquets; conferences, seminars or meetings; individuals or scholarships to individuals.

Geographic Focus: Minnesota

Date(s) Application is Due: Sep 1

Contact: Janelle Ianfolla, Corporate Contributions Manager; (952) 830-0207; fax: (952) 830-0480; email: janelle.ianfolla@idq.com

Internet: http://www.dairyqueen.com/us-en/community/

Sponsor: Dairy Queen Corporation
7505 Metro Boulevard
Minneapolis, MN 55439-0286

Daisy Marquis Jones Foundation Grants **1188**

The mission of the Foundation is to improve the well being of residents in Yates and Monroe counties, New York in particular, the City of Rochester. A central concern is disadvantaged children and families and the neighborhoods in which they live. The Foundation believes it can best serve those in need by granting time-limited support with programs or projects that provide access to health care, attend to the needs of young children, assist senior citizens, or help families develop economic security. The Foundation also looks for programs that: give people the tools they need to help themselves; encourage collaboration among agencies and between individuals and agencies; have measurable outcomes; and make long-term commitments to specific neighborhoods. A letter of inquiry is the first step to application and is available on line. The board reviews letters of inquiry once a month except July and August.

Requirements: Grants are awarded to qualified 501(c)3 nonprofit organizations that are located in Monroe and Yates Counties, NY.

Restrictions: Grants are not awarded to fund the arts, endowments, local chapters of national health-related organizations, private schools, religious projects, research, scholarships, projects by individuals, or organizations, projects not in Yates or Monroe Counties, or non 501(c)3 organizations.

Geographic Focus: New York

Samples: Advertising Council of Rochester, $10,000— to help support the Ad Council Academy, "Enhancing Professional Know How," an educational program for non-profits; Community Partners for Youth, Inc., $45,000—to help support the Big Brothers Big Sisters program.; George Eastman House, $10,000—to support the Senior Citizens Matinee Series at the Dryden Theatre.

Contact: Roger Gardner, President, (585) 461-4950; fax (585) 461-9752; email: mail@dmjf.org

Internet: http://www.dmjf.org/funding.asp

Sponsor: Daisy Marquis Jones Foundation
1600 South Avenue, Suite 250
Rochester, NY 14620

Dale and Edna Walsh Foundation Grants **1189**

The foundation joins hands with effective charitable organizations to meet human need and promote the common good worldwide. Grants support ministries, religious activities, health, relief efforts, education, community services, and arts organizations. Guidelines are available online.

Requirements: Tax-exempt, nonprofit charities are eligible.

Restrictions: The foundation does not contribute toward normal church operation; culturally liberal activist causes or organizations that primarily seek to influence legislation or government spending; or political parties or associated political organizations.

Contact: Grants Administrator, (847) 230-0056; fax: (847) 901-9193; email: Info@dewfoundation.org

Internet: http://dewfoundation.org

Sponsor: Dale and Edna Walsh Foundation
6461 Valley Wood Drive
Reno, NV 89523

Dallas Mavericks Foundation Grants **1190**

The foundation of this National Basketball Association franchise makes grants in the Dallas, Texas, area for projects that provide education, good health, and leadership skills for kids. The foundation supports the programs and organizations in the Dallas-Fort Worth Metroplex that address the community's most pressing problems involving youth, specifically education, good health, and community service activity. Application guidelines are available online.

Requirements: To apply for an award, complete a grant application form which can be obtained on line. Include the supporting data: copy of IRS 501(c)3 final determination letter; fact sheet; current board roster; project timeline; project line-item detail budget; general operating budget. There is one grant cycle annually.

Restrictions: Grants will not be made to individuals, churches, public/private schools, or national organizations that do not have locally, financially independent chapters. Grants also will not be made for medical research, travel, salaries, operational phases of established programs, political campaigns or fundraising events, including the purchase of tables, tickets or advertisements. The Foundation would prefer not to commit funds for continued support of long-term programs lasting more than one year, endowment campaigns, administrative costs, advertising/fund raising drives, salaries for staff/individuals, intermediary funding agencies and/or research. The Foundation does not fund multi-year-grants.

Geographic Focus: Texas

Date(s) Application is Due: Jun 30

Contact: Dawn Holgate, (214) 658-7170

Internet: http://www.nba.com/mavericks/news/00405573.html

Sponsor: Dallas Mavericks Foundation
2909 Taylor Street
Dallas, TX 75226

Dallas Women's Foundation Grants **1191**

The Foundation promotes women's philanthropy and raises money to support community programs that help women and girls realize their full potential. Priority will be given to funding programs that include elements of the following: effect long-term, positive changes to help women succeed in reaching their full potential; expanded choices and opportunities for women and girls; evaluation tools that include measurement for effectiveness with clean definition of program success; and programs specifically designed to take into consideration the gender-specific needs and differences of women and girls. The Foundation also encourages projects developed in consultation and collaboration with other agencies, and which promote coordination, cooperation and sharing among organizations. Effective use of volunteers, as well as Board diversity and involvement, are equally encouraged.

Requirements: To be eligible to receive a grant from the Foundation, applicants must meet all of the following criteria: be in receipt of a current 501(c)3 tax-exempt designation from the Internal Revenue Service (dated within the last 10 years); at least 50% of the population served must be residents of Dallas, Denton, or Collin County, with priority given to organizations serving residents of Dallas County; 75% of the clients benefiting from the grant funding must be women and/or girls.

Geographic Focus: Texas

Contact: Pat Alexander, (214) 965-9977; fax: (214) 526-3633; email: palexander@dallaswomensfoundation.org

Internet: http://www.dallaswomensfoundation.org/grants/highlights.html

Sponsor: Dallas Women's Foundation
4300 MacArthur Avenue, Suite 255
Dallas, TX 75209

Dammann Fund Grants **1192**

The fund is committed to using its resources for the support of qualified charitable organizations operating programs in New York City, Southwestern Connecticut and Charlottesville, VA with a focus in any one or more of two areas: mental health - programs that foster living or independent living for the mentally ill; teen parenthood - programs that enable development of parenting skills in young parents. Grant recipients are eligible to receive funding for a single program for up to three consecutive years.

Requirements: Nonprofits in the greater New York City, Southwestern Connecticut and Charlottesville, Virginia, are eligible.

Restrictions: Grants are not made to individuals and they are not made for capital or annual campaigns, endowments, loans, conferences or travel.

Geographic Focus: Connecticut; New York; Virginia

Samples: Institute for Community Living (New York, NY)—to support residential and rehabilitation services for people with mental and physical disabilities, $12,000.; Boston Medical Ctr Corp (Boston, MA)—for the Domestic Violence Guardian and Litem Program, $30,000.; Louise Wise Services (New York, NY)—for the Teen Dad Program, $30,000.; Northside Ctr for Child Development (New York, NY)—for therapeutic and educational programs for the Harlem community, $25,000.

Date(s) Application is Due: Jun 30

Contact: Administrator, (212) 956-4118; fax: (212) 262-9321; email: df@engelanddavis.com
Internet: http://www.thedammannfund.com/
Sponsor: Dammann Fund
521 Fifth Avenue, 31st Floor
New York, NY 10175

Damon Runyon Cancer Foundation Fellowships **1193**
The foundation encourages all theoretical and experimental research relevant to the study of cancer and the search for cancer causes, mechanisms, therapies, and prevention. Candidates must apply for the fellowships under the guidance of a sponsor—a senior member of the scientific research community. The sponsor should be actively engaged in the planning, execution, and supervision of the proposed research and should encourage the fellow to report the results of the research in scientific journals and meetings. Awards are made to institutions for the support of the fellow under direct supervision of the sponsor.
Requirements: Applicants must have completed one or more of the following degrees or its equivalent: MD, PhD, DDS, and DVM.
Amount of Grant: $41,000 and $55,000 year one (level I and level II); $43,000 and $56,000 year two; $44,000 and $57,000 year three; $2000 in expenses each year
Date(s) Application is Due: Mar 15; Aug 15
Contact: Fellowship Administrator, (212) 455-0520; email: awards@drcrf.org
Internet: http://www.drcrf.org/apFellowship.html
Sponsor: Damon Runyon Cancer Research Foundation
675 Third Avenue, 25th Floor
New York, NY 10017

Dana Brown Charitable Trust Grants **1194**
The trust awards grants to eligible Missouri nonprofit organizations in its areas of interest, including children and youth, health care, the arts, and human services.
Requirements: Missouri nonprofit organizations are eligible. Preference is given to requests from the greater Saint Louis metropolitan area.
Geographic Focus: Missouri
Samples: KETC/Channel 9 (Saint Louis, MO)—to develop and implement a three-part educational program for children, $1.2 million.; Saint Vincent Home for Children (Saint Louis, MO)—for the Day Treatment program, which provides education and counseling to help children overcome emotional and behavioral problems and return to community schools; and for a temporary-placement program for children in crisis situations, $100,000.
Amount of Grant: $5000-$100,000 average
Date(s) Application is Due: Feb 15; May 15; Aug 15; Nov 15
Contact: Carol Eaves, c/o U.S. Bank, N.A., P.O. Box 387, St. Louis, MO 63166
Sponsor: Dana Brown Charitable Trust
12935 N Outer Forty Drive
Saint Louis, MO 63141-8695

Dana Clinical Hypotheses in Brain and Immuno-Imaging Research Grants **1195**
The program focuses on improving human brain and immune system functioning in health and disease. The program consists of two tracks. Track A is for conventional systems imaging of brain tissues (imaging white or gray matter in the brain). Track B is for the evolving field of cellular and molecular imaging of brain cells, or immune cells, or their interactions (imaging at the level of cells rather than tissues). Applicants undertaking cellular and molecular imaging also can employ systems imaging in their proposals to view the actions of cells within their system. Institutions may submit only one application per track. Both tracks are designed to support pilot-testing of promising but high-risk innovative ideas that have direct clinical application and that, when successful, could be supported on a larger scale by other funders. Although one goal of the program is to make support available to researchers early in their careers, any researcher with a promising new hypothesis is eligible. Guidelines are available online.
Requirements: Each U.S. medical school dean, and the presidents of the few selected biomedical research institutions that have been invited by letter, may nominate a total of two applicants, one for Track A, conventional brain systems imaging research, and one application for Track B, using cellular and molecular imaging techniques alone or in combination with brain tissue (systems) imaging techniques. Each application must be countersigned by the medical school dean or invited biomedical institution's president.
Amount of Grant: $100,000 maximum per year
Date(s) Application is Due: May 27
Contact: Rebecca Husman, email: danainfo@dana.org
Internet: http://www.dana.org/grants/health/proposals/brainimaging.cfm
Sponsor: Charles A. Dana Foundation
745 Fifth Avenue, Suite 900
New York, NY 10151

Dana Corporation Foundation Grants **1196**
The foundation gives to communities throughout the country. Social services and education are top priorities. Most education grants are awarded to colleges and universities through a matching gifts program. Other grants go to civic affairs, environmental, youth, and health organizations with the smallest percentage awarded in the areas of culture and arts. Types of support include annual campaigns, building construction/renovation, continuing support, equipment acquisition, land acquisition, operating budgets, seed grants, and capital campaigns.
Requirements: 501(c)3 organizations in communities where Dana Corporation facilities are located are eligible.
Restrictions: The foundation does not make grants to individuals or to organizations that practice discrimination, religious groups for denominational purposes, political activities, or United Way-supported organizations for operating expenses. The foundation does not purchase tickets to charitable or fund-raising events or support goodwill advertising.
Amount of Grant: $1000-$20,000 average
Contact: Ed McNeal, (419) 535-4500
Internet: http://www.dana.com
Sponsor: Dana Corporation Foundation
P.O. Box 1000
Toledo, OH 43697

Dana Foundation Science and Health Grants **1197**
The Foundation supports research in neuroscience, immunology, and the effects of arts training on cognition. Areas of focus are: Brain and Immuno-imaging; Human Immunology; Neuroimmunology; Clinical Neuroscience Research; and Arts and Cognition. All other Science and Health Grants are made solely by invitation.
Requirements: The Foundation requires institutions, in many cases, to share the cost of a project or raise matching funds.
Restrictions: The foundation makes no grants directly to individuals; does not support annual operating budgets of organizations, deficit reduction, capital campaigns, or individual sabbaticals; and does not schedule meetings with applicants, other than by specific invitation initiated by the foundation.
Contact: Grants Administrator, (212) 223-4040; fax: (212) 317-8721; email: danainfo@dana.org
Internet: http://www.dana.org/grants
Sponsor: Charles A. Dana Foundation
745 Fifth Avenue, Suite 900
New York, NY 10151-0002

Danellie Foundation Grants **1198**
The foundation's primary areas of interest include services for the financially disadvantaged, including housing and social services. The types of support offered are: building/renovation; capital campaigns; continuing support; general/operating support; program development; scholarship funds and; sponsorships. Contact foundation for application guidelines. New York/New Jersey Area Common Application Form and New York/New Jersey Common Report Form accepted. Application form required.
Requirements: Nonprofit organizations in Southern New Jersey, (including Mercer and portions of Monmouth counties), the Greater Philadelphia, Pennsylvania area and, the Balimore, Maryland region are eligible to apply. The foundation also has an international interest in Guatemala and Haiti.
Restrictions: No support for political organizations or professional sports, libraries or museums. No grants to individuals, or for endowments or radio and television.
Geographic Focus: Maryland; New Jersey
Samples: University of Medicine and Dentistry, Stratford, NJ, $71,000 - for Latino health clinic (2007); Doctors of the World U.S.A, New York, NY, $65,000 - for medical needs in Third World countries (2007); Aid for Friends, Philadelphia, PA, $20,000 - for needy, disabled, and the elderly homebound (2007).
Amount of Grant: $4,000-$180,000 range
Contact: Nancy Dinsmore, (856) 810-8320; email: danelliefoundation@verizon.net
Sponsor: Danellie Foundation
P.O. Box 376
Marlton, NJ 08053

Daniel Mendelsohn New Investigator Award **1199**
The Daniel P. Mendelsohn award is intended to encourage new investigators whose work is compatible with this mission. New investigators in the field of research or education whose work relates to health and well being are eligible for the award. Candidates, who may or may not be members of the FRI organization, must have demonstrated scholarly research potential compatible with the mission of FRI. They must show future promise, evidenced by energy and enthusiasm in research that addresses prevention, treatment or education activities. Candidates for the biennial award are reviewed by the Awards Review Committee of FRI that presents their recommendation to the Board of Directors at their October Annual Meeting. Deadline for recommending candidates is May 1 of even numbered years. The Award is a check for $5000 payable to the recipient for her or his personal or professional use. The award will be presented in the fall of the awarding year.
Samples: Michael S.Gordon, D.P.A., University of Baltimore, Baltimore, MD, $5,000—drug abuse treatment for criminal justice populations (2008).
Amount of Grant: $5,000
Date(s) Application is Due: May 1
Contact: Janet Klein Brown, Chair; (410) 823-5116; fax: (410) 823-5131; email: fri@friendsresearch.org
Internet: http://www.friendsresearch.org/mendelsohn_award.htm
Sponsor: Friends Research Institute
505 Baltimore Avenue, P.O. Box 10676
Baltimore, MD 21285

Daniels Fund Grants **1200**
The fund focuses its efforts on providing a better life and greater opportunities to thousands of individuals in Colorado, New Mexico, Utah, and Wyoming. The fund also supports national programs. The grants program addresses the following areas of need: aging, alcoholism and substance abuse, amateur sports, disabilities, education, homeless and disadvantaged, and youth development. Generally, national grants are reserved for

projects with national impact, rather than projects in a single state. Grant applications are accepted at any time throughout the year, however, decisions are made quarterly.
Requirements: 501(c)3 nonprofit organizations in Colorado, New Mexico, Utah, and Wyoming—as well as nationwide—are eligible.
Restrictions: The fund generally will not support medical or scientific research; arts and cultural programs; candidates for public office; endowments; special events or fundraising events; or debt elimination.
Geographic Focus: Colorado; New Mexico; Utah; Wyoming
Contact: Grants Program Officer, (303) 393-7220; fax: (303) 393-7339; email: grantsinfo@danielsfund.org
Internet: http://www.danielsfund.org/Grants/index.asp
Sponsor: Daniels Fund
101 Monroe Street
Denver, CO 80206

Daphne Seybolt Culpeper Memorial Foundation Grants 1201
The Foundation, established in 1983, supports organizations involved with education, health care and human services. Giving is limited to Fairfield County, Connecticut and Palm Beach County, Florida. There are no specific deadlines with which to adhere. Contact the Foundation for further application information and guidelines.
Requirements: Nonprofits in Connecticut and Florida are eligible.
Restrictions: No grants to individuals, or for endowments, forums, conferences, seminars, gratuities, honorariums, travel, meals or lodging.
Geographic Focus: Connecticut; Florida
Samples: Bethesda Hospital Foundation, Boynton Beach, FL, $100,000 - funding for new therapy system (2008); Advent Lutheran Church, Boca Raton, FL, $50,000 - funding for a new school bus (2008).
Amount of Grant: $1,000-$100,000 range
Contact: Nicholas Nardi, Secretary; (203) 762-3984
Sponsor: Daphne Seybolt Culpeper Memorial Foundation
P.O. Box 206, 129 Musket Ridge Road
Norwalk, CT 06852-0206

David Geffen Foundation Grants 1202
The foundation supports nonprofits in Los Angeles, California, and New York, New York, with some giving in Israel as well. The Foundation offers support in its five principal funding areas: AIDS/HIV, civil liberties, the arts, issues of concern to the Jewish community, and health care. Support is provided for general operations and special projects. There are no application deadlines. Applicants are asked to submit a letter of request.
Requirements: 501(c)3 tax-exempt organizations in Los Angeles, CA, and New York, NY, may submit a proposal letter (without folder or binder) including description of the project, objectives, constituents served, evaluation criteria; background on the organization including key staff, volunteers, and board; copy of IRS letter confirming tax-exempt status; financial information including line-item budget for the project; and copy of non-discrimination policy from the organization's hiring guidelines.
Restrictions: The Foundation does not fund individuals, or organizations based outside of the United States. The foundation generally does not support documentaries or other types of audio-publication of books or magazines.
Geographic Focus: California; New YorkIsrael
Samples: Natural Resources Defense Council, New York, NY, $50,000 (2006); Childrens Diabetes Foundation at Denver, Denver, CO, $25,000 (2006); Morehouse College, Atlanta, GA, $50,000 (2006).
Contact: J. Dallas Dishman, Program Director; (310) 581-5955; fax: (310) 581-5949; email: ddishman@geffenco.com
Sponsor: David Geffen Foundation
12011 San Vicente Boulevard, Suite 606
Los Angeles, CA 90049-4926

Daviess County Community Foundation Health Grants 1203
The Foundation considers proposals for grants on a yearly cycle, which begins each June. At the start of each cycle, a notice is mailed to nonprofit organizations that have applied for grants in the past, have received grants in the past, or have otherwise requested notification of the start of each cycle. Grants in the area of Health include activities that: improve and promote health outcomes; provide general and rehabilitative health services; offer mental health services; provide crisis intervention programs; strengthen associations or services associated with specific diseases, disorders, and medical disciplines; and support medical research. Applications are due by August 4, and all organizations that have submitted grant proposals will be notified of the outcome of the grants committee's deliberation in writing no later than November 1.
Requirements: The Foundation welcomes proposals from nonprofit organizations that are deemed tax-exempt under sections 501(c)3 and 509(a) of the Internal Revenue Code and from governmental agencies serving the County of Daviess, Indiana. Proposals from nonprofit organizations not classified as a 501(c)3 public charity may be considered provided the project is charitable and supports a community need.
Geographic Focus: Indiana
Samples: Mental Health America of Daviess County—for the Bridges out of Poverty program, $1,780 (2008); Pregnancy Care Cente—for the Essentials for Newborns parenting project, $6,000 (2008).
Amount of Grant: $5,000-$10,000 average
Date(s) Application is Due: Aug 4
Contact: Jeanne Fields, Director; (812) 254-9354; fax: (812) 254-9355; email: jeanne@daviesscommunityfoundation.org
Internet: http://www.daviesscommunityfoundation.org/program-areas
Sponsor: Daviess County Community Foundation
320 E. Main Street, P.O. Box 302
Washington, IN 47501

Davis Family Foundation Grants 1204
The foundation provides grants primarily to Maine-based educational, medical, and cultural/arts charitable organizations in support of a wide variety of worthwhile projects. Eligible educational organizations include: colleges, universities, and other educational institutions. Eligible medical organizations include: hospitals, clinics and medical research organizations (grant requests will also be considered from other similar health organizations for programs designed to increase the effectiveness or decrease the cost of medical care). Eligible cultural and arts organizations include: those agencies whose customary and primary activity is to promote music, theater, drama, history, literature, the arts or other similar cultural activities. Further guidelines are available online.
Requirements: Eligible educational organizations include colleges, universities, and other educational institutions (grants are not made to public elementary and secondary schools, nor to schools whose financial support is derived primarily from a church or other religious organization. Trustees will consider grant requests from other educational organizations whose purpose is to promote systemic change in education or to provide innovative programs whose objectives are to improve education). Medical organizations eligible for support include hospitals, clinics, and medical research organizations. Grant requests will also be considered from other similar health organizations for programs designed to increase the effectiveness or decrease the cost of medical care. Eligible cultural/arts organizations include organizations whose customary and primary activity is to promote music, theater, drama, history, literature, the arts, or other similar cultural activities.
Restrictions: The Foundation does not make grants to individuals, religious programs, fellowships, or in the form of loans. The Foundation does not normally provide support for annual giving campaigns or general operating needs. Grants to endowment campaigns have a low priority.
Geographic Focus: Maine
Samples: Arthur L. Mann Memorial Library, West Paris, ME, $15,000 - expansion and renovation project (2008); Maine Archaeological Society, Inc., Augusta, ME, $8,300 - Maine Archaeology Classroom Initiative (2008); South Bristol Historical Society, South Bristol, ME, $20,000 - schoolhouse restoration (2008).
Date(s) Application is Due: Feb 10; May 10; Aug 10; Nov 10
Contact: Anne Vaillancourt, Executive Director; (207) 781-5504; email: info@davisfoundations.org
Internet: http://www.davisfoundations.org/site/family.asp
Sponsor: Davis Family Foundation
4 Fundy Road
Falmouth, ME 04105

Dayton Power and Light Foundation Grants 1205
The foundation contributes general operating grants to nonprofit organizations in the greater Dayton, OH, area in support of education and charitable activities and programs. Education grants are made to support adult basic education/literacy-skills development and engineering school education. Direct donations are made to civic, cultural, and health and welfare organizations that do not participate in community funds, such as United Way or community chests, but serve a real need. There is no official application form. Requests should be made in writing and must include a description of the history, structure, purpose, and program of the organization and a summary of the support needed and how it will be used. Contributions are planned a year in advance and based on a calendar-year budget. The distribution committee normally meets quarterly.
Requirements: 501(c)3 organizations in the greater Dayton, OH, area are eligible.
Restrictions: The foundation prefers not to support capital campaigns; college fund-raising associations; conduit organizations; endowment or development funds; fraternal, labor, or veterans organizations; hospital operating budgets; individual members of federated campaigns; individuals; national organizations outside the DP&L service territory; religious organizations; sports leagues; or telephone or mass-mail solicitations. Grants are rarely made to tax-supported institutions.
Geographic Focus: Ohio
Samples: Dayton Art Institute (OH)—to support the capital campaign, $25,000.; United Way of the Greater Dayton Area (OH)—to support the annual campaign, $200,000.
Amount of Grant: $1000-$20,000 average
Contact: Ginny Strausburg, Executive Director, (937) 259-7925; fax: (937) 259-7923
Internet: http://www.waytogo.com/cc/cc.phtml
Sponsor: Dayton Power and Light Company Foundation
1065 Woodman Drive
Dayton, OH 45432

Daywood Foundation Grants 1206
The Foundation distributes available funds primarily to community service organizations focusing on the arts, and health and human services. Grants are available in the following types: annual campaigns; building/renovation; capital campaigns; continuing support; debt reduction; emergency funds; equipment; general/operating support; matching/challenge support; seed money.
Requirements: Nonprofit 501(c)3 organizations situated in, and benefiting Charleston, Lewisburg, Barbour, Greenbrier and Kanawha counties of West Virginia are eligible. There is no standardized grant application form.
Restrictions: Grants do not support endowment funds, research, individuals, or individual scholarships or fellowships.

Geographic Focus: West Virginia
Samples: Clay Center for the Arts and Sciences of West Virginia, Charleston, WV, $150,000—for endowment (2007); University of Charleston, Charleston, WV, $125,000— for pharmacy school (2007); West Virginia Symphony Orchestra, Charleston, WV, $100,000- for endowment (2007).
Date(s) Application is Due: Sep 15
Contact: William W. Booker, Treasurer; (304) 343-4841
Sponsor: Daywood Foundation
707 Virginia Street, East, Suite 1600
Charleston, WV 25301

Deaconess Community Foundation Grants **1207**
The foundation awards grants to eligible Ohio nonprofit organizations in its areas of interest, including health, education, welfare, community, and social service activities. Proposals that are of greatest interest to the Foundation are those that have the strongest fit to the mission statement and that have some or all of the following characteristics: projects that have specific measurable outcomes and a tangible ability to evaluate results and measure success; projects that are supported by other funding sources; and projects that have identified potential for ongoing support beyond the life of the grant. Application information is available online.
Requirements: Only qualified non-profit organizations located in Cuyahoga County which are classified by the Internal Revenue Code as tax-exempt 501(c)3 organizations are eligible for funding consideration.
Restrictions: Grant requests for the following will not be considered: individuals, governmental agencies or any other organization that is not a tax exempt 501(c)3 organization; internal operations and capital campaigns of churches; research projects; or endowments. Grant funds may not be used to carry on propaganda or otherwise attempt to influence legislation, participate in, or intervene in, any political campaign on behalf of or in opposition to any candidate for public office, or to conduct, directly or indirectly, any voter registration drive (within the meaning of Section 4945(d)(2) of the Internal Revenue Code).
Geographic Focus: Ohio
Samples: Junior Achievement, $10,000—Workforce Readiness & Entrepreneurship programs (2008); Magnolia Clubhouse, $35,000—part-time senior development consultant, $2,000 —general operating support (2008); The Intergenerational School, $28,000—establishment of a development department (2008).
Date(s) Application is Due: Jan 15; May 15; Sep 15
Contact: Deborah Vesy, Executive Director; (216) 741-4077; fax: (216) 741-6042; email: dvesy@deacomfdn.org
Internet: http://www.deacomfdn.org/guidelines.html
Sponsor: Deaconess Community Foundation
7575 Northcliff Avenue, Suite 203
Brooklyn, OH 44144

Deafness Research Foundation Research Grants **1208**
The grants are intended for research directed to any aspect of the ear, e.g., investigation of function, physiology, biochemistry, genetics, anatomy, or pathology. Grants cover a range of subjects from basic neuroscience research to studies on corrective hearing/speech testing and training. Grants may be renewed for one to two years.
Requirements: Current policy favors awarding grants in support of projects directed by new investigators, so-called seed money support for studies in generally unexplored areas of research. It does not exclude grant support for new research by established researchers. Application should state whether the same project is receiving support from another source and whether an application has been submitted to another source of funding. The principal investigator and grantee institution must notify the DRF when and if this same project receives support from another granting agency.
Amount of Grant: $20,000
Date(s) Application is Due: Dec 1
Contact: Administrator, (800) 829-5934 or (703) 610-9025; email: grants@drf.org
Internet: http://www.drf.org/grants/grants.htm
Sponsor: Deafness Research Foundation
8201 Greensboro Drive, Suite 300
McLean, VA 22102

Dean Foods Community Involvement Grants **1209**
The company's community support efforts are focused in three main areas: health/nutrition (including hunger); education/arts; and environmental stewardship/conservation. It supports worthy organizations both at the corporate level and locally through its network of processing facilities nationwide. Preference is given to supporting and participating in a meaningful way with a limited number of organizations that support these three focus areas, rather than spreading limited resources more broadly. Specifically, funding goes to programs that provide direct service to individuals and communities in need. The corporation places special emphasis on supporting organizations that assist children, particularly at-risk children or children with disabilities, or that are dedicated to serving their needs. As a point of contact, the corporate headquarters requests that no phone calls be made regarding its giving programs.
Requirements: 501(3)3 tax-exempt organizations are eligible. Applications must provide background information on the organization as well as how it relates to the mission of Dean Foods. The corporation supports initiatives only in the communities in which they operate and where employees live and work.
Geographic Focus: Alabama; California; Colorado; Connecticut; Florida; Georgia; Hawaii; Idaho; Illinois; Indiana; Kentucky; Louisiana; Maine; Maryland; Massachusetts; Michigan; Minnesota; Montana; Nebraska; Nevada; New Jersey; New Mexico; New York; North Carolina; North Dakota; Ohio; Oklahoma; Pennsylvania; South Carolina; South Dakota; Tennessee; Texas; Utah; Virginia; Wisconsin
Contact: Gregg Engles, Chief Executive Officer; (214) 303-3400; fax: (214) 303-3499
Internet: http://www.deanfoods.com/our-company/about-us/corporate-responsibility.aspx
Sponsor: Dean Foods
2515 McKinney Avenue, Suite 1200
Dallas, TX 75201

Dearborn Community Foundation City of Lawrenceburg Community Grants **1210**
The City of Lawrenceburg has generously allocated grant funds specifically for not-for-profit organizations that provide a benefit, direct or indirect, to the Lawrenceburg community and Dearborn County. The Dearborn Community Foundation is pleased to administer this program. The program consists of two phases, Phase I: grants requesting $5,000 or less will be accepted. Applications will be considered as long as funds are available. Phase II: grants requesting $5,001 - $100,000 will be excepted to the grant application deadlines. Applications will be considered as long as funds are available.
Requirements: The maximum grant award is $100,000 per organization per calendar year; grant funds are not granted to sustain ongoing programs/projects; and grant applications will be considered as long as funds are available.
Restrictions: Funds specifically for not-for-profit organizations that provide a benefit, direct or indirect, to the Lawrenceburg community and Dearborn County.
Geographic Focus: Indiana
Amount of Grant: $5,000 - $100,000 range
Date(s) Application is Due: Feb 3, May 5, Aug 4, Oct 6
Contact: Jerri Worthington, DCF Program Director, (812) 539-4115; fax: (812) 539-4119; email: dcfgrants@comcast.net
Internet: http://www.dearborncf.org/grants/G_Lawrence.aspx
Sponsor: Dearborn Community Foundation, Inc.
322 Walnut Street
Lawrenceburg, IN 47025

Dearborn Community Foundation County Progress Grants **1211**
The Dearborn Community Foundation, Inc. (DCF) has been working to build the community's philanthropic resources since it was founded in December of 1997. The DCF County Progress Grant Program supports the interests of the community from non-profit organizations for charitable purposes in the fields of community service, social service, education, health, environment, and the arts. The maximum grant award allotted is $10,000 per organization per calendar year. To be considered, grant applications must be received in the DCF office no later than noon on the deadline date. All questions relating to available scholarship/educational grant opportunities should be directed to the DCF Program Director.
Requirements: Grants are awarded only to organizations whose programs benefit the residents of Dearborn County Indiana and which provide for a responsible fiscal agent and adequate accounting procedures.
Restrictions: Submitted grant applications shall contain one original application and ten copies. This must be done for each grant program from which the organization is seeking grant funds. (Absolutely no binders or folders). Applicants should also retain a copy for their records.
Geographic Focus: Indiana
Samples: Dillsboro Elementary School, Outdoor Learning Center, IN, $5,073 .;2007.; Hamline Chapel United Methodist Church, Restoration of Boy Scout cabin, IN $2,500 .;2007.;
Amount of Grant: $10,000
Date(s) Application is Due: Feb 3, May 5, Aug 4, Oct 6
Contact: Jerri Worthington, DCF Program Director, (812) 539-4115; fax: (812) 539-4119; email: dcfgrants@comcast.net
Internet: http://www.dearborncf.org/grants/G_Progress.aspx
Sponsor: Dearborn Community Foundation, Inc.
322 Walnut Street
Lawrenceburg, IN 47025

DeBakey Medical Foundation Fellowships and Scholarships **1212**
The foundation fosters and encourages medical education and graduate training and promotes medical research in any field of medicine, but it is especially interested in investigations that have direct clinical application, particularly those concerned with cardiovascular disease. Financial aid may be extended to persons in the form of scholarships or fellowships and to institutions in the form of grants or funds for hospital care. Applications are accepted at any time.
Contact: Director, (713) 798-8600; fax: (713) 793-1192; email: pa@bcm.tmc.edu
Sponsor: DeBakey Medical Foundation
1 Baylor Plz, Baylor College of Medicine
Houston, TX 77030

Del E. Webb Foundation Grants **1213**
The Foundation applies its resources only for the benefit of the residents of Arizona, California and Nevada for improved and expanded medical services, medical research and education. Within these broad areas of interest, the Foundation draws upon the talent and experience of leaders from many walks of life to select organizations of demonstrated competence which have sound programs that will be able to reach and sustain high levels of performance. In choosing particular projects for support, the Foundation's Board acts on the basis of how the public welfare most effectively may be served. Application information is available online.

Requirements: Grants are confined to the support of nonpartisan, non-profit organizations that are operated in the public interest and have tax-exempt status as charitable organizations granted by the Internal Revenue Service and the states in which the respective organizations are incorporated and/or engage in activities.
Restrictions: Grants are not made to the following: governmental agencies or subdivisions; sectarian or religious organizations whose principle activity is exclusively for the benefit of their own members; organizations soliciting funds in support of projects or programs operated by organizations other than the applicant; expenditures before the recipient incurs and makes such expenditures, and, in the absence of compelling circumstances, the Foundation does not make grants to recipients to liquidate or reduce previously incurred obligations or operating deficits. No grants or loans are awarded or made to individuals for any purpose. Grants are not made for scholarships, student aid or medical assistance. Grants may be made to organizations that provide scholarships, student aid or medical assistance when the organization selects recipients in conformity with accepted standards. The Foundation does not participate in the administration of program(s) that the Foundation funds through the award of the application. The Foundation does not fund or underwrite: galas or gala-like events, testimonial or fund-raising luncheons or dinners, advertising in programs or similar fund-raising activities; organizations that in turn make grants to others; purchase of uniforms, equipment, or trips for school related organizations or amateur sports teams; honoraria for guest speakers or panelists; charities operated by service clubs; or educational seminars.
Geographic Focus: Arizona; California; Nevada
Amount of Grant: $5000-$100,000 average
Date(s) Application is Due: Nov 30; Feb 28; May 31; Aug 31
Contact: Program Contact, (928) 684-7223; fax: (928) 684-5665
Internet: http://www.dewf.com/DEFAULT.shtml
Sponsor: Del E. Webb Foundation
300 E. Willis, Suite C
Prescott, AZ 86301-3110

Deland Fellowships in Health Care and Society **1214**
This one-year fellowship provides a training opportunity for graduates interested in pursuing careers in health care management. Appointees will explore the most challenging issues of health care delivery today, including problems of access to quality health care for the poor, uninsured, and underinsured; the changing roles of physicians, nurses, social workers, administrators, and allied health professionals; ethical, legal, and human considerations arising from new biomedical technologies; the impact of for-profit ventures on the work of teaching and community hospitals; and development of integrated delivery systems in the health care marketplace. Stipends are commensurate with the seniority, prior educational experience, and living requirements of the appointees. Fellowship tenure begins in July. For current deadline information, please email Kevin Gahagan at kgahagan@partners.org.
Requirements: It is anticipated that candidates will come from a variety of careers and educational backgrounds including business, law, economics, public policy, and medicine. Candidates are required to have an advanced degree.
Contact: Kevin Gahagan, (617) 732-5500; TTY/TTD: (617) 732-6458; email: kgahagan@partners.org
Internet: http://www.brighamandwomens.org/general/Deland_Fellowship.asp
Sponsor: Brigham and Women's Hospital
75 Francis Street
Boston, MA 02115

Delaware Community Foundation Grants **1215**
The Foundation supports organizations and programs throughout the State of Delaware that address a wide range of community needs, including, but not limited to, health and human services, the arts, humanities and culture, the environment, housing and community development. The foundation awards capital grant and program grants. Capital grants are for construction, major renovation or repair of buildings and/or the purchase of land; and also may include requests for equipment purchases. Capital grants typically range from $5,000 to $20,000, with a maximum award of $25,000. Equipment grants generally range from $2,000 to $7,000, with a maximum award of $10,000. Grant proposals must be submitted on the appropriate DCF application form (capital projects or equipment). One application per organization will be accepted. Application forms may be obtained from the DCF office or at the DCF Web site.
Requirements: IRS 501(c)3 non-profit organizations in Delaware are eligible to apply.
Restrictions: Ineligible for support: endowment; debt reduction; religious organizations for sectarian purposes (However, projects that serve the entire community, regardless of religious affiliation, are eligible for support); annual fundraising campaigns or general operating expenses; projects completed before June 30; sports clubs or leagues; educational institutions; purchase of vehicles; individuals.
Geographic Focus: Delaware
Amount of Grant: $2,000-$25,000 range
Date(s) Application is Due: Jan 29
Contact: Beth Bouchelle, Director; (302) 504-5239; email: bbouchelle@delcf.org
Internet: http://www.delcf.org/Apply_4_1.htm
Sponsor: Delaware Community Foundation
P.O. Box 1636
Wilmington, DE 19899

Delaware Community Foundation-Youth Philanthropy Board for Kent County **1216**
The Youth Philanthropy Board (YPB) for Kent County of the Delaware Community Foundation is composed of 19 students from public, independent and diocesan high schools in Kent County. The Board is studying youth issues in their neighborhoods and schools, learning about community service and grant making, and will award a total of $10,000 to schools and qualified 501(c)3 organizations to carry out youth programs for residents of Kent County. This year, the Youth Philanthropy Board for Kent County will consider programs that provide support for minors who are affected by abusive situations. Additional consideration will be given to programs that encompass reinforcement of academic achievement and/or extracurricular activities.
Requirements: 501(c)3 organizations in Kent County, Delaware are eligible to apply.
Restrictions: Programs completed prior to May 1, are ineligible for funding.
Geographic Focus: Delaware
Date(s) Application is Due: Jan 7
Contact: Ann Frazier, Administrative Assistant; (302) 856-4393; fax: (302) 856-4367; email: frazier@delcf.org
Internet: http://www.delcf.org/Apply_4_1.htm
Sponsor: Youth Philanthropy Board for Kent County c/o Delaware Community Foundation
Southern Delaware Office, 36 The Circle
Georgetown, DE 19947

Dell Foundation Healthy Communities, Literate Communities, and Connected Communities Grants **1217**
Healthy Communities Grants: Through two-year partnerships with organizations, Dell helps empower its communities to address basic needs for children, such as food, shelter, safety, and healthcare. (March 15 deadline). Literate Communities Grants: Through two-year partnerships with organizations, Dell helps empower its communities to address basic needs of quality education, particularly in math, science, and literacy (May 15 deadline). Connected Communities Grants: Through two-year partnerships with organizations, Dell helps empower its communities to address technology access needs through computer labs for areas of the community with limited access to technology (July 15 deadline).
Requirements: Middle Tennessee and Central Texas 501(c)3 tax-exempt organizations are eligible.
Geographic Focus: Tennessee; Texas
Amount of Grant: $50,000
Date(s) Application is Due: Mar 15; May 15; Jul 15
Contact: Grants Administrator, (512) 338-4400; email: the_dell_foundation@dell.com
Internet: http://www1.us.dell.com/content/topics/global.aspx/corp/foundation/en/index?c=us&l=en&s=corp
Sponsor: Dell Foundation
1 Dell Wy
Round Rock, TX 78682

Dell Foundation Open Grants **1218**
The foundation, the giving arm of Dell Computer, seeks to fund collaborative and innovative solutions to community and children's issues addressing youth (ages newborn to high-school seniors) in Texas, Tennessee, Idaho, and Oregon. Through these efforts, Dell strives to effect change in its local community, while providing lessons and best practices for communities everywhere. Funded areas include arts, education, social services, and health. The foundation supports specific, preventative, and measurable programs with cash, in-kind, and volunteer contributions. Grants are awarded quarterly. An online application form is available on the Web site.
Requirements: Eligibility is open to 501(c)3 nonprofit organizations in Texas—Travis, Williamson County, and McLennan County; Tennessee—Wilson, Davidson County; Idaho—Twin Falls County; and Oregon—Roseburg, Douglas County.
Restrictions: Grants do not support individuals; academic or research projects; civic, religious, or political institutions; school fundraisers; marketing opportunities; or sports events and organizations.
Geographic Focus: Idaho; Oregon; Tennessee; Texas
Samples: Various rescue and relief organizations—to assist organizations providing disaster-relief services related to the September 11 terrorist attacks, $1 million in cash and products.
Amount of Grant: $5000 maximum
Date(s) Application is Due: Jan 15; Apr 15; Jul 15; Oct 15
Contact: Grants Administrator, (512) 338-4400; email: the_dell_foundation@dell.com
Internet: http://www1.us.dell.com/content/topics/global.aspx/corp/foundation/en/open_grants?c=us&l=en&s=corp
Sponsor: Dell Foundation
1 Dell Wy
Round Rock, TX 78682

Della Martin Foundation Grants **1219**
The foundation awards grants to organizations located in southern California for research seeking to find the causes of and cures for mental illness. Types of support include challenge/matching grants, endowments, fellowships, professorships, and research grants. There is no application deadline, but the foundation usually makes grants for mental health research at the year's end.
Requirements: Grants are made only to California 501(c)3 organizations.
Geographic Focus: California
Amount of Grant: $263,000
Contact: Laurence Gould Jr., Director, (213) 617-4143; fax: (213) 620-1398
Sponsor: Della Martin Foundation
333 S Hope Street, 48th Floor
Los Angeles, CA 90071

Delta Air Lines Foundation Grants 1220

The foundation awards grants to nonprofits in the areas of: Community Enrichment - focusing on involvement and participation in volunteer, civic, and social activities; Health and Wellness - with support to organizations that dedicate their efforts to the health and well-being of communities with a focus on broad-reaching research for cures and education around diseases that affect all walks of life; Youth Development - offering support to organizations focusing on keeping young people interested in math and science and helping them develop leadership skills and positive self esteem; and Arts and Culture to include fine art, theatre, music, or other creative endeavors which enhance a community's quality of life.

Requirements: For proposals which meet the foundation's area of focus, priority will be given to: programs meeting compelling needs in communities where Delta has a presence; proposals that exhibit clear, reasonable goals, and measurable outcomes; distinctive projects where the foundation's involvement will leave a legacy; projects that include collaboration or cooperation with other nonprofit organizations; projects that offer opportunities for Delta employee involvement. The foundation Board of Trustees reviews and approves funding in March, June, September, and November. The deadline for receiving completed proposals is the first day of each of these months.

Restrictions: The foundation will generally not consider: individual applicant's request for support of personal needs; religious activities; political organizations or campaigns; specialized single-issue health organizations; annual or automatic renewal grants; general operating expenses; endowment campaigns; capital campaigns; multi-year commitments; fraternal organizations, professional associations, or membership groups; fundraising events such as benefits; charitable dinners, or sporting events.

Contact: Administrator; (404) 715-5487; fax: (404) 715-3267

Internet: http://www.delta.com/about_delta/community_involvement/delta_foundation/

Sponsor: Delta Air Lines

P.O. Box 20706, Dept 979

Atlanta, GA 30320-6001

DeMatteis Family Foundation Grants 1221

The foundation makes grants in the New York metropolitan area to eligible institutions whose mission involves education, health and human services, medical research, social services, and the arts. Types of support include facilities construction, expansion, renovation; acquisition of capital equipment; scientific/medical research; projects and programs that enable the applicant to expand its mission through new or expanded programs to reach a greater segment of the community served; project-oriented capital campaigns. In general, most grants are made to cover projects that can be accomplished within one year. For construction and longer duration projects, grants may be structured to conform to identified milestones. For major projects, the payment of the grant may be over a number of years.

Requirements: Metropolitan New York 501(c)3 tax-exempt agencies, institutions, and organizations are eligible.

Restrictions: In general, the foundation does not support grants for operating deficits; general operating support; endowments; loans, or financing of any kind; annual appeals, dinner functions, and other special fund raising events; or unrestricted funds.

Geographic Focus: New York

Contact: Grants Administrator, (516) 705-4974

Internet: http://fdncenter.org/grantmaker/dematteis/about.html

Sponsor: DeMatteis Family Foundation

P.O. Box 25

Glen Head, NY 11545

Dennis and Phyllis Washington Foundation Grants 1222

The foundation supports a broad spectrum of worthy causes benefiting people of all ages primarily serving the State of Montana and surrounding states where the Washington Companies are located. Priorities for funding are direct service, youth oriented programs and the advancement of educational opportunities through scholarships to units of higher education in Montana. The Foundation also focuses on the needs of economical and socially disadvantaged people, troubled or at-risk youth and individuals with special needs.

Requirements: Eligible applicants must be a charitable, nonprofit entity with tax exempt status under Section 501(c)3. Organizations applying for support must be categorized in one of the four giving areas of education, health and human services, community service and arts and culture. The Foundation places particular emphasis on those organizations and programs that provide a direct service to economically and socially disadvantaged youth and their families, at-risk or troubled youth, and individuals with special needs. Preference is given to applicants who are able to demonstrate that a majority, if not all, of Foundation funds will be used for direct services. The Foundation prefers giving to organizations with no or low administrative costs. Organizations may apply for funding only in the year in which funds will be used. The Foundation prefers that organizations show evidence of substantial financial support from their community, constituency groups or other funding sources prior to applying.

Restrictions: Applications will not be considered for the following organizations or purposes: organizations that, in policy or practice, unfairly discriminate against race, ethnic origin, sex, creed, or religion; to fund loans, debt retirement or operational deficits; to fund on-going, general operations; to individuals, unless under an approved educational scholarship program; to sectarian or religious organizations for religious purposes where the principal activity is for the benefit of their own members or adherents; to veterans or fraternal organizations, unless their programs are available to members of the community as a whole; for travel expenses or trips; to general endowment funds, private or public foundations and most capital campaigns; for operation expenses of tax-supported groups; for sponsorships including auctions, dinners, tickets, advertising, or annual fundraising events; for political action or legislative advocacy groups or influencing legislation or elections; for operational costs or curriculum development at educational institutions; the purchase of motor vehicles or other forms of transportation; to organizations acting on behalf of, but without the authority of, qualified tax exempt organizations.

Geographic Focus: Montana

Contact: Mike Halligan, Executive Director, (406) 523-1325

Internet: http://www.dpwfoundation.org/home.htm

Sponsor: Dennis and Phyllis Washington Foundation

P.O. Box 16630

Missoula, MT 59808-6630

Dental Laboratory Technology Scholarships 1223

The current shortage of trained dental laboratory technicians hampers our nation's ability to meet the increased public demand for dental services and products. To fulfill this need, up to 25 scholarships are awarded each year to individuals who wish to follow careers in dental laboratory technology.

Requirements: Resident citizens of the United States enrolled full time in a dental laboratory technology program accredited by the American Dental Association are eligible to apply.

Amount of Grant: $1000

Date(s) Application is Due: Aug 15

Contact: Administrator, (312) 440-2547; fax: 312-440-3526; email: adaf@ada.org

Internet: http://www.ada.org/ada/prod/adaf/index.asp

Sponsor: American Dental Association

211 E Chicago Avenue

Chicago, IL 60611

Dental Teaching and Research Fellowships 1224

Fellowships are awarded to individuals who plan to become dental teachers and/or researchers in dental schools in Canada and who must guarantee to pursue careers in teaching and research at a university for a minimum of two years following fellowship tenure. A formal application form must be filed with official transcripts and letters of support. The award is given for one year with possible renewal for a second year based on satisfactory progress.

Requirements: Candidates must be Canadian citizens or permanent residents who have completed an undergraduate course in dentistry, a dental hygiene program, or a program in science and who are also eligible for admission to a graduate or other advanced education program.

Amount of Grant: $C1800-$C8000

Date(s) Application is Due: Feb 1

Contact: Richard Munro, Executive Director, (613) 236-4763; fax: (613) 236-3935; email: Information@dcf-fdc.ca

Internet: http://www.dcf-fdc.ca/grants.html

Sponsor: Dentistry Canada Fund

427 Gilmour Street

Ottawa, ON K2P OR5 Canada

Denton A. Cooley Foundation Grants 1225

The foundation awards grants in Texas in support of health care, health education, hospitals, and medical research. Types of support include endowments, general operating grants, program grants, and research grants. There are no application forms or deadlines.

Restrictions: Grants do not support conferences, loans, individuals, scholarships, fellowships, or publication.

Geographic Focus: Texas

Samples: U of Texas Medical Branch at Galveston (TX)—to establish a professorship in the division of cardiothoracic surgery, $250,000 (2003).

Amount of Grant: $100-$250,000

Contact: Grants Administrator, (713) 799-2700

Sponsor: Denton A. Cooley Foundation

6624 Fannin, Suite 1640

Houston, TX 77030

Denver Broncos Charities Fund Grants 1226

The fund supports qualified non-profit organizations that work to impact the quality of life for youth, health and the hungry and homeless. The emphasis of the fund is on programs designed to assist young people in the areas of education and youth football with a particular emphasis on programs aimed at disadvantaged and at-risk youth. The fund will also consider programs devoted to health and hunger issues. Grants may be stand-alone grants or magnet grants that attract other corporate dollars.

Requirements: Nonprofit organizations in the state of Colorado are eligible.

Geographic Focus: Colorado

Samples: Denver Public Schools Foundation, $50,000—Prep League Football Program (2008); Inner City Health Center, $50,000—Denver Rescue Mission (2008); Meeker School District, $50,000—Community Fields Project (2008); Darrent Williams Memorial Teen Center, $50,000—Darrent Williams Memorial Grant (2008).

Date(s) Application is Due: Jun 1

Contact: Charities Fund Manager, (720) 258-3000

Internet: http://www.denverbroncos.com/page.php?id=1157

Sponsor: Denver Broncos Charities Fund

1701 Bryant Street, Suite 1400

Denver, CO 80204

Denver Foundation Community Grants 1227

The Denver Foundation carries out its mission of improving life in Metro Denver by investing in the vision, passion and expertise of hundreds of nonprofit organizations. The Community grants program awards hundreds of grants annually to nonprofit organizations in the seven-county Metro Denver area, which includes: Adams, Arapahoe, Boulder, Broomfield, Denver, Douglas, and Jefferson counties. Grants are awarded in the four major focus areas of arts and culture, health, human services and civics and education.

Requirements: To qualify for a grant an organization must be a 501(c)3 tax-exempt nonprofit organization, serve residents in seven specific Denver counties, and provide a service that falls under one of the four funding areas.

Restrictions: The Foundation will not consider requests to fund the following: requests from organizations that have received funding from the program for the three previous consecutive calendar years; organizations with fund balance deficits in their most recently completed fiscal year; organizations that discriminate on the basis of race, color, religion, gender, age, national origin; disability, marital status, sexual orientation, or military status; debt retirement; endowments or other reserve funds; membership or affiliation campaigns, dinners, or special events; conferences and symposia and related travel; grants that further political doctrine; grants that further religious doctrine; grants to individuals; scholarships or sponsorships; individual medical procedures; medical, scientific, or academic research; grants to parochial or religious schools; grants to governmental agencies, except public schools; requests from individual public schools that have not coordinated the request with their central school district administration; requests from foundations/organizations that raise money for individual public schools; creation or installation of art objects; development, production, or distribution of books, newspapers, or video productions; grants for re-granting programs; requests for capital campaigns that have not met 75% of their goal; activities, projects, or programs that will have been completed before funding becomes available; and multi-year funding requests.

Geographic Focus: Colorado

Date(s) Application is Due: Feb 2; Jun 1; Oct 1

Contact: Jeff Hirota, Vice President of Programs; (303) 300-1790, ext. 129; fax: (303) 300-6547; email: jhirota@denverfoundation.org

Internet: http://www.denverfoundation.org/page17823.cfm

Sponsor: Denver Foundation
55 Madison, 8th Floor
Denver, CO 80206

Dept of Ed College Assistance Migrant Program (CAMP) 1228

The College Assistance Migrant Program (CAMP) assists students who are migratory or seasonal farmworkers (or children of such workers) enrolled in their first year of undergraduate studies at an IHE. The funding supports completion of the first year of studies. Competitive five-year grants for CAMP projects are made to IHEs or to nonprofit private agencies that cooperate with such institutions. The grants funded under CAMP grantee serve approximately 2,400 participants each year.

Requirements: Institutions of higher education or private nonprofit agencies in cooperation with institutions of higher education may apply.

Restrictions: Institutions of higher education or a nonprofit private agency in cooperation with an IHE may apply.

Contact: David De Soto, (202) 260-8103; fax: (202) 205-0089; email: david.de.soto@ed.gov

Internet: http://web99.ed.gov/GTEP/Program2.nsf/b39cd123fd4a045b8525644400514f2b/07783e5ad0636ec5852563bc00540495?OpenDocument

Sponsor: Department of Education
400 Maryland Avenue S.W., Room 3E225, FB-6
Washington, DC 20202-6135

Dept of Ed Rehabilitation Training Grants 1229

The purpose of this program is to ensure that skilled personnel are available to serve the rehabilitation needs of individuals with disabilities assisted through vocational rehabilitation (VR), supported employment and independent living programs. The program supports training and related activities designed to increase the number of qualified personnel trained in providing rehabilitation services. Grants and contracts are awarded to states and public and nonprofit agencies and organizations, including institutions of higher education, to pay all or part of the cost of conducting training programs.

Requirements: Institutions of Higher Education (IHEs), Nonprofit Organizations, Other Organizations and/or Agencies may apply. Applicants may include state and public or nonprofit agencies and organizations and Indian tribes.

Contact: Ruth Brannon, Program Contact; (202) 245-7278; fax: (202) 245-7591; email: ruth.brannon@ed.gov

Internet: http://www.ed.gov/programs/rsatrain/index.html

Sponsor: Department of Education
400 Maryland Avenue, S.W., Room 5052, PCP
Washington, DC 20202-2800

Dept of Ed Safe and Drug-Free Schools and Communities State Grants 1230

This program provides support to SEAs for a variety of drug and violence prevention activities focused primarily on school-age youths. Activities may include: developing instructional materials; providing counseling services and professional development programs for school personnel; implementing community service projects and conflict resolution, peer mediation, mentoring and character education programs; establishing safe zones of passage for students to and from school; acquiring and installing metal detectors; and hiring security personnel.

Requirements: State Education Agencies may apply. Local Education Agencies or intermediate education agencies or consortia must apply to the State Education Agency.

Contact: Paul Kesner, Office of Safe and Drug-Free Schools, (202) 205-8134; fax: (202) 260-7767; email: paul.kesner@ed.gov

Internet: http://www.ed.gov/programs/dvpformula/index.html

Sponsor: Department of Education
400 Maryland Avenue, S.W., Room 3E230, FB-6
Washington, DC 20202-6450

Dept of Ed Special Education—Personnel Development to Improve Services and Results for Children with Disabilities 1231

The objectives of this program are to help address state-identified needs for highly qualified personnel in special education, related services, early intervention, and regular education, to work with children with disabilities; and ensure that those personnel have the skills and knowledge, derived from practices that have been determined, through research and experience, to be successful, that are needed to serve those children. Awards are made to train personnel in the areas of: leadership; early intervention and early childhood; low-incidence; high-incidence; related services, speech/language, and adapted physical education; and programs in minority institutions.

Requirements: Institutions of Higher Education, Local Education Agencies, Nonprofit Organizations, Other Organizations and/or Agencies and State Education Agencies are eligible to apply. In addition to these categories, public charter schools that are LEAs under state law, other public agencies, private nonprofit organizations, for-profit organizations, outlying areas (American Samoa, Guam, the Northern Mariana Islands, and the U.S. Virgin Islands), freely associated states, and Indian tribes or tribal organizations are eligible to apply.

Contact: Patricia Wright, (202) 245-7620; fax: (202) 245-7619; email: patricia.wright@ed.gov

Internet: http://www.ed.gov/programs/osepprep/index.html

Sponsor: Department of Education
400 Maryland Avenue, S.W., Room 4113, PCP
Washington, DC 20202-2600

Dept of Ed Special Education—Studies and Evaluations 1232

This program is designed to assess progress in implementing IDEA, including the effectiveness of state and local efforts to provide: free appropriate public education to children with disabilities; and early intervention services to infants and toddlers with disabilities. This program supports studies, evaluation, and assessments.

Requirements: Institutions of higher education, local education agencies, nonprofit organizations, other organizations and/or agencies, and state education agencies are eligible. Public agencies, outlying areas (American Samoa, Guam, the Northern Mariana Islands, and the U.S. Virgin Islands), freely associated states, Indian tribes, tribal organizations, and for-profit organizations, if appropriate, may apply.

Contact: Jeffrey Payne, Office of Special Education Programs, (202) 245-7473; fax: (202) 245-7617; email: jeffrey.payne@ed.gov

Internet: http://www.ed.gov/programs/osepsae/index.html

Sponsor: Department of Education
400 Maryland Avenue, S.W., Room 4064, PCP
Washington, DC 20202-2500

Dept of Ed Special Education—Technical Assistance and Dissemination to Improve Services and Results for Children with Disabilities 1233

The purpose of this program is to promote academic achievement and improve results for children with disabilities by providing technical assistance, model demonstration projects, dissemination of useful information, and implementation activities that are supported by scientifically based research. The program supports technical assistance and dissemination activities. Annual deadline dates may vary; contact the office for exact dates.

Requirements: Institutions of Higher Education, Local Education Agencies, Nonprofit Organizations, Other Organizations and/or Agencies, and State Education Agencies are eligible to apply. Public charter schools that are LEAs under state law, for profit organizations, outlying areas (American Samoa, Guam, the Northern Mariana Islands, and the U.S. Virgin Islands), freely associated states, and Indian tribes or tribal organizations may also apply.

Amount of Grant: $200,000-$2 million range

Contact: Claudette Carey, Office of Special Education and Rehabilitative Services, (202) 245-7291; fax: (202) 245-7617; email: claudette.carey@ed.gov

Internet: http://web99.ed.gov/GTEP/Program2.nsf/a5b8d6c38fdd4ca08525644400514f2c/02df9c7d71171b1785256571007ce61c?OpenDocument

Sponsor: Department of Education
400 Maryland Ave SW, Room 4098, PCP
Washington, DC 20202

Dept of Ed Special Education-National Activities-Technology and Media Services for Individuals with Disabilities 1234

The purpose of this program is designed to: improve results for children with disabilities by promoting the development, demonstration, and use of technology; support educational media services activities designed to be of education value in the classroom setting to children with disabilities; and provide support for captioning and video description that is appropriate for use in the classroom setting.

Requirements: State Education Agencies; Local Education Agencies; public charter schools that are LEAs under state law; Institutions of Higher Education; other public agencies; private nonprofit organizations; outlying areas (American Samoa, Guam, the Northern Mariana Islands, The U.S. Virgin Islands); freely associated states; Indian tribes or tribal organizations; and for-profit organizations may apply.
Contact: Jeffrey Payne, Office of Special Education Programs, (202) 245-7473; fax: (202) 245-7617; email: jeffrey.payne@ed.gov
Internet: http://www.ed.gov/programs/oseptms/index.html
Sponsor: Department of Education
400 Maryland Avenue, S.W., Room 4064, PCP
Washington, DC 20202-2500

Dermatology Clinical Career Development Awards **1235**
The purpose of this award is to enhance the academic careers of clinician-scientists in the early stages of their career development. The program is aimed at junior investigators with significant creativity in clinically relevant research. Research must be conducted in the United States. Such studies could include research on diagnostic and/or prognostic indicators, as well as outcome and/or epidemiologic studies. Creativity in developing new treatment modalities, including novel pharmacologic approaches and clinical trials, is encouraged. Studies need not involve direct laboratory investigation. The primary criteria for selection of a successful awardee are the quality of the research proposal, the environment of the candidate, and ability of the proposal to clarify the place of dermatologic practice in a changing health care environment. Award recipients are expected to spend at least 75 percent of their time in clinical research. Awardees are encouraged to seek simultaneous grant support from other agencies.
Requirements: Applications are accepted from faculty members in a department or division of dermatology who have completed clinical training in a U.S. dermatology residency program. Applicants must demonstrate a strong commitment to skin research and have already had appropriate initial training (a two- to three-year research fellowship or postdoctoral training) in relevant research.
Restrictions: The foundation does not fund awards to be performed as part of the U.S. government research program (with the exception of the Veterans Administration) or awards to private foundations without an academic affiliation to dermatology.
Amount of Grant: $55,000
Date(s) Application is Due: Oct 17
Contact: Sandra Rahn Benz, Executive Director, (847) 328-2256; fax: (847) 328-0509; email: dfgen@dermatologyfoundation.org
Internet: http://www.dermfnd.org
Sponsor: Dermatology Foundation
1560 Sherman Avenue, Suite 870
Evanston, IL 60201

Dermatology Foundation Grants **1236**
Limited funds are available for investigators at the early stages of their career development to initiate research projects in dermatology and cutaneous biology. Applications are reviewed by the Medical and Scientific Committee and awarded on a competitive basis for projects not funded from other sources. The research has to be performed under the sponsorship of a division or department of dermatology. The maximum period of funding is for one year. Only one grant application will be considered from a single academic center.
Restrictions: Awards cannot be used for payment of indirect costs.
Amount of Grant: $10,000 average
Date(s) Application is Due: Oct 17
Contact: Sandra Rahn Benz, Executive Director, (847) 328-2256; fax: (847) 328-0509; email: dfgen@dermatologyfoundation.org
Internet: http://dermatologyfoundation.org
Sponsor: Dermatology Foundation
1560 Sherman Avenue, Suite 870
Evanston, IL 60201

Dermatology Postdoctoral Research Fellowships **1237**
Financial support is available to postdoctoral fellows with commitments to careers in academic dermatology who desire research training. Applications will be accepted in two categories. Dermatologist Investigator Research Fellowships are designed to support dermatologists who desire research training and have commitments to careers in academic dermatology. Research Fellowships support training in research skills relevant to dermatology and cutaneous biology. Highest priority will be given to new applicants. A limited number of second-year awards may be given. Although it is recognized that fellowships will encompass specific research projects, they are intended primarily for the support of research training. Fellowship recipients must spend at least 75 percent of their total effort in cutaneous research.
Requirements: Applications for Dermatologist Investigator Research Fellowships are accepted from individuals holding the MD, MD-PhD, or DO degree who have completed their clinical training in U.S. dermatology residency programs. Research Fellowship applications are accepted from individuals holding the MD or PhD or equivalent.
Restrictions: In general, investigators at more than four years past their terminal degrees or two years beyond their residencies at the time of the initial application are not eligible. (Consideration will be given to individuals with substantial training in other areas and who are entering into skin research.) Individuals with academic appointments at the level of assistant professor or above are not ordinarily eligible.
Amount of Grant: $25,000 maximum for one year
Date(s) Application is Due: Oct 17
Contact: Sandra Rahn Benz, Executive Director, (847) 328-2256; fax: (847) 328-0509; email: dfgen@dermatologyfoundation.org
Internet: http://dermatologyfoundation.org/rap
Sponsor: Dermatology Foundation
1560 Sherman Avenue, Suite 870
Evanston, IL 60201

Dermatology Research Career Development Awards **1238**
Awards are available to assist in the transition from fellowship to established investigator in cancer and other diseases of the skin, hair, and nails. The intent of the program is to advance the research careers of young individuals in dermatology and cutaneous biology, with the emphasis on research benefiting the dermatology community at large. Award recipients are expected to spend at least 75 percent of their time in cutaneous research. Awardees are encouraged to seek simultaneous grant support from other agencies to provide for the nonsalary components of the research being performed under the auspices of this award.
Requirements: Applicants must be faculty members in a department or division of dermatology who demonstrate a strong commitment to skin research and have already had appropriate initial training (a two- to three-year research fellowship or postdoctoral training) in biomedical research.
Restrictions: The foundation does not fund awards to be performed as part of the U.S. government research program (with the exception of the Veterans Administration) or awards to private foundations without an academic affiliation to dermatology.
Amount of Grant: $55,000
Date(s) Application is Due: Oct 17
Contact: Sandra Rahn Benz, Executive Director, (847) 328-2256; fax: (847) 328-0509; email: dfgen@dermatologyfoundation.org
Internet: http://dermatologyfoundation.org/rap
Sponsor: Dermatology Foundation
1560 Sherman Avenue, Suite 870
Evanston, IL 60201

DeRoy Testamentary Foundation Grants **1239**
Established in 1979, the Foundation gives primarily in the state of Michigan. Giving primarily for youth development and services, education, human services, health care, and the arts. The Foundation offers support in the form of: scholarship funds; annual campaigns; building/renovation; continuing support; general/operating support; program development grants. There are no application deadlines. The board meets monthly.
Requirements: Michigan nonprofit organizations are eligible.
Restrictions: Grants are not made to individuals.
Geographic Focus: Michigan
Samples: National Bone Marrow Transplant Link, Southfield, MI, $10,000 (2007); Oakland Family Services, Pontiac, MI, $65,000 (2007); Interlochen Center for the Arts, Interlochen, MI, $300,000 (2007).
Amount of Grant: $10,000-$300,000 range
Contact: Julie Rodecker Holly, Vice President; (248) 827-0920; fax: (248) 827-0922; email: deroyfdtn@aol.com
Sponsor: DeRoy Testamentary Foundation
26999 Central Park Boulevard, Suite 160N
Southfield, MI 48076

Detlef Schrempf Foundation Grants **1240**
The focus of the foundation is on children, youth and families in the Pacific Northwest. This foundation seeks supporting organizations that can help underwrite the costs of events, enabling the maximum amount of proceeds to go directly to the benefiting charity.
Requirements: Typically, a qualifying charity partner will have a $5-million, or smaller, operating budget.
Geographic Focus: Pacific Northwest
Contact: Nicole Morrison, Executive Director, (206) 464-0826; fax: (206) 464-8020; email: info@detlef.com
Internet: http://www.detlef.com
Sponsor: Detlef Schrempf Foundation
1904 Third Avenue, Suite 339
Seattle, WA 98101

Detroit Lions Charities Grants **1241**
The organization supports charitable and community causes in Michigan. Funding interests include child abuse and domestic violence prevention, youth recreation, and spinal cord injury research. Grants have been awarded to support the Never, Never Shake a Baby billboard campaign; Pigskin Geography, a learning initiative for youth; Big Brothers/Big Sisters; Grand Rapids Metropolitan YMCA—for swimming lessons for inner-city youth; and Saint Joseph Mercy Hospital—for a domestic violence education program. Requests are accepted between October 1 and December 31.
Geographic Focus: Michigan
Samples: Dominion Family Services (MI)— to battle child abuse and domestic violence in Michigan, $210,000.
Date(s) Application is Due: Dec 31
Contact: Detroit Lions Community Affairs Information Hotline, (313) 216-4056
Internet: http://detroitlions.com/community/index.cfm?cont_id=49715
Sponsor: Detroit Lions Charities
222 Republic Drive
Allen Park, MI 48101

DHHS Abandoned Infants Assistance Grants 1242

Funds are provided to prevent the abandonment of infants and young children including the provision of services; to identify and address their needs, especially those who have been infected with the human immunodeficiency virus or who have been prenatally exposed to the virus or a dangerous drug; to assist such children to reside with their natural families or in foster care, as appropriate; to conduct residential programs for abandoned infants and young children who are unable to reside with their families; to provide respite care for families and caregivers; to recruit, train, and obtain foster families; and to recruit and train health and social services personnel to work with families. Contact the office for deadline dates.

Requirements: Eligible applicants are state or local governments, federally recognized Native American tribal governments, U.S. territories and possessions, and nonprofit organizations.

Amount of Grant: $475,000 maximum

Date(s) Application is Due: Aug 12

Contact: Patricia Campiglia, Children's Bureau, (202) 205-8060; email: pcampiglia@acf.hhs.gov

Internet: http://a257.g.akamaitech.net/7/257/2422/01jan20051800/edocket.access.gpo.gov/2005/05-11592.htm

Sponsor: Department of Health and Human Services
330 C St SW, Room 2428
Washington, DC 20447

DHHS Adolescent Family Life Demonstration Projects 1243

This program has multiple components of prevention, care and research. The prevention component focuses on development and testing of abstinence based programs designed to delay the onset of sexual activity reducing the incidence of adolescent pregnancy, STD transmission and HIV/AIDS. The care component is focused on providing comprehensive health, education and social services to pregnant adolescents, adolescent parents, their infants, male partners and their families. The primary focus of research is to improve understanding of the issues surrounding sexuality, pregnancy and parenting by examining the factors that influence adolescent sexual, contraceptive and fertility behaviors, the nature and effectiveness of care services for pregnant and parenting adolescents and why adoption is a little-used alternative among pregnant adolescents. Deadlines are announced in the Federal Register and on the Office of Population Affairs Web site (http://opa.osophs.dhhs.gov).

Requirements: Public and private non-profit organizations may apply.

Contact: Andrea Brandon, Chief Grants Management Officer, (301) 594-6554

Internet: http://aspe.hhs.gov/SelfGovernance/inventory/OPA/111.htm

Sponsor: Department of Health and Human Services
4350 East West Highway, Suite 200
Bethesda, MD 20814

DHHS AIDS and HIV Epidemiologic Research Studies Grants 1244

The purpose of this program is to encourage studies using the new rapid HIV tests in different settings (Operational Research), specifically focused on African American, Latino, and other racial and ethnic minorities that are underserved and/or disproportionally affected by the HIV epidemic, and conducted by researchers who have experience working with these populations; to learn more about the effects of rapid HIV testing on motivators and barriers to HIV testing at the individual, provider, and system levels; and to foster collaborations between organizations serving minority communities and their respective state and local health departments in the design and implementation of innovative practical strategies using rapid HIV tests to increase knowledge of HIV serostatus and facilitate entry into prevention and care systems. The research should contribute to the health services knowledge base from which empirically based information can be derived by policy makers, both immediately and over the coming decades. Assistance is available for a 12-month budget period within project periods ranging from one to five years. Contact the office for deadline dates.

Requirements: Applications may be submitted by public and private nonprofit organizations; community-based, national, and regional organizations; state and local governments or their bona fide agents or instrumentalities; federally recognized Indian tribal governments; and Indian tribes or organizations.

Amount of Grant: $5000-$270,000; $200,265 average

Contact: JAllyn Nakashima, Epidemiology Branch, Division of HIV/AIDS Prevention/Surveillance and Epidemiology, (404) 639-0900; Cheryl Maddux, Grants Management, (770) 498-1911

Internet: http://www.dhhs.gov

Sponsor: Department of Health and Human Services
1600 Clifton Rd NE, MS-E-45
Atlanta, GA 30333

DHHS AIDS Project Grants 1245

The grants are intended to fund programs that develop and implement surveillance, epidemiological research, health education, school health, and risk reduction activities of AIDS in states and major cities. The program also gives support for cooperative agreements for AIDS activities. The funding period will be from one to five years, renewable. Applicants should contact the CDC for deadline information.

Requirements: Public and private organizations, both nonprofit and for profit, state and local governments, U.S. territories and possessions, small and minority businesses, and businesses owned by women are encouraged to apply.

Amount of Grant: $45,000-$2 million; $390,174 average

Contact: Allyn Nakashima , Division of HIV/AIDS Prevention, (404) 639-0900; Cheryl Maddux, Grants Management Branch, (770) 498-1911

Internet: http://www.dhhs.gov

Sponsor: Department of Health and Human Services
2920 Brandywine Road
Atlanta, GA 30341

DHHS Chiropractic Demonstration Project Grants 1246

The objective of the program is to make grants and enter into contracts with schools, colleges, and universities of chiropractic for the purposes of carrying out demonstration projects in which chiropractors and physicians collaborate to identify and provide effective treatment for spinal and lower back conditions. Grant funds may be used for personnel, equipment, supplies, domestic travel, consultants and guest lecturers, rental of space, renovations, and other costs directly related to the project as described in the approved application. Application materials are available on the World Wide Web at address: http://www.hrsa.gov/bhpr/grants.html.

Requirements: Public or private nonprofit schools, colleges, and universities of chiropractic medicine are eligible to apply.

Restrictions: Grant funds may not be used for construction of facilities, acquisition of land, foreign travel, or support of students, including fellowships, stipends, tuition, fees, or travel allowances.

Amount of Grant: $381,048 -$389,214; $386,456 average

Contact: Jennifer Hannah, (301) 443-0908

Internet: http://bhpr.hrsa.gov/interdisciplinary/chiro.html

Sponsor: Department of Health and Human Services
5600 Fishers Ln, Parklawn Building
Rockville, MD 20857

DHHS Comprehensive Community Mental Health Services Grants for Children with Serious Emotional Disturbances 1247

This program provides community-based systems of care for children and adolescents with serious emotional disturbances and their families. The program will ensure that services are provided collaboratively across child-serving systems; that each child or adolescent served through the program receives an individualized service plan developed with the participation of the family; that each individualized plan designates a case manager to assist the child and family; and that funding is provided for mental health services required to meet the needs of youngsters in these systems.

Requirements: States; political subdivisions of a state, such as county or local governments; and federally recognized Native American tribal governments are eligible to apply.

Amount of Grant: $200,064-$3.5 million; $1.85 million average

Contact: Gary Blau, Chief, Child Adolescent and Family Branch, (301) 443-1333

Internet: http://mentalhealth.samhsa.gov/publications/allpubs/CA-0013/default.asp

Sponsor: Department of Health and Human Services
5600 Fishers Ln, Parklawn Building
Rockville, MD 20857

DHHS Developmental Disabilities University Affiliated Programs Grants 1248

Grants assist with the cost of administration and operation of facilities for providing interdisciplinary training for personnel concerned with developmental disabilities, demonstrations of the provision of exemplary services related to the developmentally disabled, demonstration of technical assistance for generic and specialized agencies, dissemination of findings related to the provision of services to researchers and government agencies, and generation of information on the need for further service-related research. Grants may cover salaries for administrators, coordinators, and others needed to operate a training facility, such as clerical and financial personnel, and maintenance and housekeeping personnel; overhead expenses and expenses required to start up new programs; and faculty for training programs that will meet critical personnel shortages and are not eligible for support from other sources. Deadline dates are available from the office.

Requirements: Public and private nonprofit organizations are eligible to apply.

Amount of Grant: $480,000

Date(s) Application is Due: Sep 1

Contact: Jennifer Johnson, (202) 690-5982

Internet: http://www.dhhs.gov

Sponsor: Department of Health and Human Services
370 L'Enfant Promenade, SW
Washington, DC 20447

DHHS Emergency Medical Services for Children (EMSC) Program 1249

The purpose of this program is to support demonstration projects for the expansion and improvement of emergency medical services for children who need treatment for trauma or critical care. It is expected that maximum distribution of projects among the states will be made and that priority will be given to projects targeted toward populations with special needs, including Native Americans, minorities, and the disabled. Annual deadline dates may vary; contact program staff for exact dates.

Requirements: States and accredited schools of medicine are eligible to apply.

Amount of Grant: $200,000 average

Contact: Dan Kavanaugh, (301) 443-1321; email: dkavanaugh@hrsa.gov

Internet: http://mchb.hrsa.gov/programs/emsc

Sponsor: Department of Health and Human Services
5600 Fishers Lane
Rockville, MD 20857

DHHS Geriatric Training for Physicians and Dentists Grants 1250

These grants are intended to assist in the operation of postdoctoral training preparing current and future faculty for leadership roles in geriatric medicine and dentistry and to provide support, including traineeships and fellowships, for geriatric medicine training projects to train physicians and dentists who plan to teach geriatric medicine or geriatric dentistry. Geriatric training is to be provided through one or both of the following projects: one grant is offered for a one-year retraining program in geriatrics for physicians who are faculty members in departments of internal medicine, family medicine, gynecology, geriatrics, and psychiatry at schools of medicine and osteopathy; and dentists who are faculty members at schools of dentistry or at hospital departments of dentistry. A grant is offered for a two-year internal medicine or family medicine fellowship program with emphasis in geriatric research for physicians who have completed graduate medical education programs in internal medicine, family medicine, psychiatry, neurology, gynecology, geriatrics, or rehabilitation medicine; and dentists who have completed postdoctoral dental education programs. Each project for which a grant is made must be staffed by full-time teaching physicians who have experience or training in geriatric medicine, be staffed by full-time or part-time teaching dentists who have experience or training in geriatric dentistry, and be based in a graduate medical education program in a department of internal medicine or family medicine or a department of geriatrics that has been in existence over a year. Each project must provide participants with exposure to a diversified population of elderly individuals and provide training in geriatrics and exposure to the physical and mental disabilities of elderly individuals through a variety of service rotations, such as geriatric consultation services, acute care services, dental services, geriatric psychiatry units, day and home care programs, rehabilitation services, extended care facilities, geriatric ambulatory care and comprehensive evaluation units, and community care programs for elderly mentally retarded individuals. Applications and deadline date information can be obtained on the Web site or by contacting the office.
Requirements: Grants will be made to accredited public or private nonprofit schools of medicine, schools of osteopathic medicine, teaching hospitals, and graduate medical education programs.
Amount of Grant: $178,721-$632,825; $374,575 average
Contact: Kathleen Bond, Department of Health and Human Services, (301) 443-8681
Internet: http://www.dhhs.gov
Sponsor: Department of Health and Human Services
5600 Fishers Ln, Parklawn Building
Rockville, MD 20857

DHHS Grants for Dental Public Health 1251

The purpose of this program is to promote the postgraduate education of dentists in public health. Grants are intended to assist in meeting the costs of planning and developing new dental public health residency training programs and providing financial assistance to trainees enrolled in the programs. Grants may not be used for construction or for providing direct patient services. Annual deadline dates may vary; contact program staff for exact dates.
Requirements: Any accredited public or private school of public health or dentistry may apply. Applicants must demonstrate that it has or will have available full-time faculty members with training and experience in the field of preventive dental public health and support from other faculty members trained in public health and other relevant specialties and disciplines.
Amount of Grant: $46,962-$153,323; $73,758 average
Contact: Raymond Lala, (301) 443-1707; email: rlala@hrsa.gov
Internet: http://www.dhhs.gov
Sponsor: Department of Health and Human Services
5600 Fishers Lane
Rockville, MD 20857

DHHS Health Care Systems Cost and Access Research & Development Grants 1252

Grants are made to support health services research to create new knowledge and better understanding of the process by which health services are made available and how they may be provided more efficiently and effectively. The AHCPR has a broad legislative mandate to support general health services research on problems related to health care cost, quality, and access to health services. Major categories of research issues include consumer decision making, managed care and the health care marketplace, primary care, rural health services, and AIDS.
Requirements: Government agencies (federal, state, and local), federally recognized tribal governments, U.S. territories, sponsored organizations, nongovernment organizations, minority groups, specialized groups, public or private institutions of higher education, and other public or nonprofit private agencies, institutions, or organizations are eligible. Research project grants may also be awarded to individuals.
Restrictions: Profit-making organizations are not eligible for grants.
Amount of Grant: $5000-$2.8 million; $310,000 average
Date(s) Application is Due: Feb 1; Jun 1; Oct 1
Contact: Mable Lam, Grants Management Officer, (301) 427-1447
Internet: http://www.dhhs.gov
Sponsor: Department of Health and Human Services
2101 E Jefferson Street, Executive Office Ctr
Rockville, MD 20852

DHHS Health Careers Opportunity Grants 1253

The grants award funds to identify, recruit, and select individuals from disadvantaged backgrounds for education/training in a health or allied health professions school; facilitate their entry into such a school; provide counseling or other services designed to assist selected individuals so that they may successfully complete their education/training; provide preliminary education for a period prior to entry into the regular course of health or allied health professions education, designed to assist students in completing successfully regular course of education or to refer the appropriate individuals to institutions providing preliminary education; and publicize existing sources of financial aid. Annual deadline dates may vary; contact program staff for exact dates.
Requirements: Eligible to apply are health professions schools and public or nonprofit private health or educational entities including schools of medicine, osteopathy, public health, dentistry, veterinary medicine, optometry, pharmacy, allied health, chiropractic and podiatry, public and nonprofit private schools that offer graduate programs in clinical psychology, and other public or private nonprofit health or educational entities.
Restrictions: Grant funds may not be used for tuition and fees, training of program staff or retraining of health professionals, sectarian instruction, religious purposes, construction, land acquisition, or foreign travel.
Amount of Grant: $116,237-$1 million; $399,000 average
Contact: Lawrence Poole, Director, Division of Grants Management, (301) 443-2385
Internet: http://www.dhhs.gov
Sponsor: Department of Health and Human Services
5600 Fishers Ln, Parklawn Building
Rockville, MD 20857

DHHS Health Centers Grants for Residents of Public Housing 1254

Grants are awarded to improve minority access to primary care services and reduce infant mortality by enabling grantees, directly or through contracts, to provide to public housing residents, especially pregnant residents and their infants, primary health services, including health screening, education, and counseling. Applications should be designed to improve the availability, accessibility, and provision of primary health care services, including comprehensive perinatal care, to residents of public housing.
Requirements: Eligible applicants are public and nonprofit private entities that have the capacity to administer a grant and are located in a high infant mortality area as determined by the Healthy Start Initiative criteria. Preference is given to community health centers, health care for the homeless programs, and resident management corporations.
Amount of Grant: $140,000-$400,000 range; $270,000 average
Contact: Director, Division of Programs for Special Populations, Bureau of Primary Health Care, (301) 594-4420; Office of Grants Management, Bureau of Primary Health Care, (301) 594-4235
Internet: http://www.federalgrantswire.com/health_centers_grants_for_residents_of_public_housing.html
Sponsor: Department of Health and Human Services
4350 East-West Hwy
Bethesda, MD 20814

DHHS Health Conference Support for Toxic Substances and Disease Registry 1255

Funds are available through this program for partial support for nonfederal conferences on disease prevention, health promotion, and projects related to hazardous substances. The purpose of this program is to work closely with state, local, and other federal agencies to reduce or eliminate illness, disability, and death resulting from exposure of the public and workers to toxic substances at spill and waste disposal sites.
Amount of Grant: $130,000-$300,000; $200,000 average
Contact: Caroline McDonald, Agency for Toxic Substances and Disease Registry, (404) 498-0270; fax: (404) 498-0059; email: COS4@cdc.gov; Mildred Garner, Grants Management Branch, (770) 488-2745, fax: (770) 488-2777
Internet: http://www.dhhs.gov
Sponsor: Department of Health and Human Services
1600 Clifton Rd NE
Atlanta, GA 30333

DHHS Health Education and Training Centers Project Grants 1256

The objective of this program is to provide assistance for planning, developing, establishing, maintaining, and operating health education and training centers (HETC). Grants are to assist in meeting costs of the program that cannot be met from other sources. Not less than 75 percent of the total funds provided to a school or schools of allopathic medicine or osteopathic medicine will be expended in the development and operation of the HETC in the service area of such program. To the maximum extent feasible, the schools of medicine are to obtain from nongovernmental sources the amount of the total operating funds for such programs that are not provided by DHHS. Grants or contracts will not provide funds solely for the planning or development of a HETC program for a period in excess of two years, not more than 10 percent of the annual budget of each program may be utilized for the renovation and equipping of clinical teaching sites, and grants or contracts shall not provide funds to be used outside the United States except as the DHHS may prescribe for travel and communications purposes related to the conduct of a border HETC. The first project period will be up to three years to allow for the development of the HETC.
Requirements: Accredited schools of allopathic or osteopathic medicine, or the parent institution on behalf of such schools or a consortium of such schools, may apply.
Amount of Grant: $92,228-$525,094 border HETC, $376,004 average; $152,199-$241,211 nonborder HETC, $214,865 average
Contact: Louis Coccodrilli, Division of Medicine, (301) 443-6950
Internet: http://www.dhhs.gov
Sponsor: Department of Health and Human Services
5600 Fishers Ln, Parklawn Building
Rockville, MD 20857

DHHS Health Professions Preparatory Scholarship Program for Indians 1257

The program makes scholarship grants for a maximum of two years to individuals of Native American or Alaskan Native descent for the purpose of completing compensatory preprofessional education to enable the recipient to qualify for enrollment or re-enrollment in a health professions school. Grants for stipends and books are made directly to the individual applicant; tuition payments are made to the college or university. New applications are usually available in February with an annual submission deadline in April. Annual deadline dates may vary; contact program staff for exact dates.

Requirements: Scholarship awards are made to individuals of Native American or Alaskan Native descent who have successfully completed high school education or high school equivalency and who have been accepted for enrollment in a compensatory, preprofessional general education course or curriculum.

Amount of Grant: $17,500-$26,019; $17,366 average

Date(s) Application is Due: Apr 1

Contact: Harold Jess Brier, Chief, Scholarship Branch, (301) 443-6197; Lois Hodge, Grants Management Officer, (301) 443-0243

Internet: http://www.ihs.gov

Sponsor: Department of Health and Human Services
12300 Twinbrook Pkwy, Twinbrook Metro Plz
Rockville, MD 20852

DHHS Health Professions Scholarship Program 1258

The program makes scholarship grants to Native Americans and other students for the purposes of completing health professional education—nursing; medicine including allopathic, osteopathic, and veterinary medicine; dentistry; x-ray technology; optometry; pharmacy; public health nutrition (graduate); medical social work (graduate); speech pathology/audiology (graduate); podiatry; health care administration; and other allied health professions—to obtain health professionals to serve Native Americans. Not all disciplines participate each year. Upon completion, grantees are required to fulfill an obligated service payback. Maximum length of funding is four years. Grants for stipends and books are made directly to the individual applicant; tuition payments are made to the college or university. New applications are available in February with a submission deadline in April.

Requirements: Priority consideration for scholarship awards is granted to persons of Native American or Alaskan Native descent. Applicants for new awards must be accepted by an accredited U.S. educational institution for a full-time course of study leading to a degree in medicine, osteopathy, dentistry, or other participating health profession that is deemed necessary by the Indian Health Service; be eligible for or hold an appointment as a commissioned officer in the regular or reserve corps of the Public Health Service; or be eligible for civilian service in the Indian Health Service.

Amount of Grant: $24,128-$38,222; $24,694 average

Date(s) Application is Due: Apr 1

Contact: Harold Jess Brier, Chief, Scholarship Branch, (301) 443-6197; Lois Hodge, Grants Management Officer, (301) 443-0243

Internet: http://www.dhhs.gov

Sponsor: Department of Health and Human Services
12300 Twinbrook Pkwy, Twinbrook Metro Plz
Rockville, MD 20852

DHHS Health Professions Training in Geriatrics Grants 1259

Grants provide funds to develop regional resource centers focused on strengthening multidisciplinary training of health professionals in geriatric health care. Annual deadline dates may vary; contact program staff for exact dates.

Requirements: Any accredited health professions school or school of allied health or any program for the training of physician assistants may apply.

Restrictions: Grant funds may not be used for trainee costs, construction of buildings, initial equipment, additions, extensions, or the acquisition of land. Grants may not be spent for sectarian instruction or for any religious purpose.

Amount of Grant: $47,072-$432,000; $316,950 average

Contact: Jennifer Hannah, (301) 443-0908

Internet: http://www.dhhs.gov

Sponsor: Department of Health and Human Services
5600 Fishers Ln, Parklawn Building
Rockville, MD 20857

DHHS Health Promotion and Disease Prevention Research and Demonstration Centers Grants 1260

Grants are awarded to qualified schools to establish, maintain, and operate academic-based centers for high-quality research and demonstration with respect to health promotion and disease prevention; to establish linkages between ongoing basic research in a wide array of fields and applied research in disease prevention and health promotion; to bring the knowledge and expertise of academic health centers to bear on practical public health problems; to field test and rigorously evaluate more cost-effective methods and strategies for preventing unnecessary illness and promoting good health; and to shorten the time lag between the development of new and proven effective disease prevention and health promotion techniques and their widespread application. The length of assistance will be from one to five years, renewable based on competitive applications and availability of funds. Deadlines will be announced in the Federal Register.

Requirements: Eligible applicants are schools of medicine, schools of osteopathy, and schools of public health.

Restrictions: Grantees may not award subgrants but may enter into consortia agreements or contracts as necessary to achieve the aims of the program.

Amount of Grant: $740,000-$770,000; $755,000 average

Contact: Dr. Eduardo Simoes, Program Director, National Center for Chronic Disease Prevention and Health Promotion, (770) 488-5919; Carlos Smiley, Grants Management Officer, (770) 488-2754

Internet: http://www.cdc.gov/prc

Sponsor: Department of Health and Human Services
4770 Buford Hwy, K-45
Atlanta, GA 30333

DHHS Healthy Tomorrows Partnership for Children 1261

This program encourages community-based partnerships to coordinate health resources for pregnant women, infants, and children. Grantees are encouraged to seek additional support from the private sector and foundations. Applicants must provide a dollar for dollar cash match after the end of the first year of the grant.

Requirements: Eligible applicants include public and private entities, community-based organizations, Indian tribes, and tribal organizations. Priority is given to projects in all U.S. territories and in Alabama, Delaware, Florida, Georgia, Hawaii, Idaho, Indiana, Iowa, Kansas, Louisiana, Maine, Maryland, Massachusetts, Mississippi, Missouri, Montana, Nevada, New Hampshire, New Jersey, North Carolina, North Dakota, South Carolina, Texas, West Virginia, Wisconsin, and Wyoming.

Geographic Focus: Alabama; Delaware; Florida; Georgia; Hawaii; Idaho; Indiana; Iowa; Kansas; Louisiana; Maine; Maryland; Massachusetts; Mississippi; Missouri; Montana; Nevada; New Hampshire; New Jersey; North Carolina; North Dakota; South Carolina; Texas; West Virginia; Wisconsin; Wyoming

Amount of Grant: $50,000 maximum

Contact: Lawrence Poole, Director, Division of Grants Management, (301) 443-2385

Internet: http://mchb.hrsa.gov/programs/training/healthytomorrows.htm

Sponsor: Department of Health and Human Services
200 Independence Avenue, SW
Washington, DC 20201

DHHS HIV Demonstration Program for Children, Adolescents, and Women 1262

Grants are awarded to support, improve, and expand the system of comprehensive care services for children, youth, women, and families who are infected with or affected by HIV and AIDS and to link comprehensive care systems with clinical research. Projects should promote collaboration between research institutions and primary care medical and social service programs. Funding priority will be given to projects that demonstrate established models of care that are comprehensive and coordinated, sensitive to differing cultural needs, and family and community based. Grants may be made for up to three-year project periods, renewable competitively after the first year.

Requirements: All public and private nonprofit organizations that provide or arrange for primary health care are eligible for grants. This includes state or local health departments, hospitals, community health centers, drug abuse treatment agencies, school-based clinics, tribal health programs, colleges, and hemophilia treatment centers.

Amount of Grant: $230,384-$2.5 million; $766,222 average

Contact: Dr. Jose Rafael Morales, Division of Community Based Programs/Title IV, HIV/AIDS Bureau, (301) 443-9051

Internet: http://www.dhhs.gov

Sponsor: Department of Health and Human Services
5600 Fishers Ln, Parklawn Building
Rockville, MD 20857

DHHS Maternal and Child Health Projects Grants 1263

The goal of the program is to improve the quality and use of genetic services in maternal and child health care, integrate services for children with special health care needs, support state fetal and infant mortality review centers, and enhance the use of data in problem solving for maternal and child health. The four grant programs currently accepting applications are genetic services, integrated services for children with special health care needs, state fetal/infant mortality review support centers, and data utilization and enhancement for state/community infrastructure building and managed care. Genetic services projects should improve the quality, availability, accessibility, and use of genetic services as an integral part of comprehensive maternal and child health care. Integrated services for children with special health care needs should demonstrate innovative and replicable models of community-based services. State fetal/infant mortality review support centers should provide training and technical assistance to state maternal and child health agencies on their particular needs. Data utilization and enhancement for state/community infrastructure building and managed care projects should enhance the use of qualitative and quantitative analytic methods in solving health problems for women and children. Contact the office for deadlines.

Requirements: Eligible applicants are public and private nonprofit agencies, including hospitals, Native American tribes, and social service agencies. The bureau will give extra attention to applications from historically black colleges and universities and Hispanic-serving institutions.

Amount of Grant: $14,000-$1.5 million; $179,248 average

Contact: Program Contact, (301) 443-2170; fax: (301) 443-1797

Internet: http://mchb.hrsa.gov/programs/default.htm

Sponsor: Department of Health and Human Services
5600 Fishers Ln, Parklawn Building
Rockville, MD 20857

DHHS Maternal and Child Health Research and Training Programs Grants 1264

Grants fund special projects that develop new data and improve the professional development of health practitioners who serve women and children. Research grants will fund projects that address minority and disadvantaged populations, health-promoting

behaviors, quality outcome measures, and systems integration and reform. Long-term training grants will be awarded to train health professionals at the graduate and postgraduate levels. Training should focus on family-centered, community-based care. Continuing education grants support continuing education for workers in the maternal and child health field. Priority will be given to projects focusing on emergency medical services for children, violence prevention in schools, and core public health. Application kits may be obtained by calling toll-free (877) 477-2123.
Requirements: Training grants may be made to public or nonprofit private institutions of higher learning. Research grants may be made to public or nonprofit institutions of higher learning and public or nonprofit private agencies and organizations engaged in research, maternal and child health, or programs for children with special health care needs.
Amount of Grant: $14,000-$1.5 million; $179,248 average
Contact: Program Contact, (301) 443-2170; Lawrence Poole, Director, Division of Grants Management Operations, (301) 443-2385
Internet: http://www.dhhs.gov
Sponsor: Department of Health and Human Services
5600 Fishers Ln, Parklawn Building
Rockville, MD 20857

DHHS National Health Service Corps Loan Repayment Awards 1265
To help ensure an adequate supply of trained health professionals for the National Health Service Corps, this program provides for the repayment of educational loans for participants who agree by written contract to serve an applicable period of time in a health-related workforce shortage area or in an Indian health program or facility. Awards provide payments toward participants' qualified government and commercial health professions education loans during each year of practice at a selected NHSC loan repayment service site with a two-year service minimum. Health professions given priority for selection are those determined by the workforce needs of the NHSC and the Indian Health Service. Beneficiaries include primary care physicians; dentists; certified nurse midwives; certified nurse practitioners; physicians assistants; clinical psychologists; clinical social workers; psychiatric nurse specialists; marriage and family therapists; licensed professional counselors; and dental hygienists. Deadline dates are published in the Federal Register.
Requirements: U.S. citizens who are enrolled as full-time students in the final year of study in an accredited health profession education institution or possess a health professions degree and are either enrolled in postgraduate health professions training or are in professional practice are eligible to apply. They must hold an unrestricted health professions license in a state and be eligible for or hold an appointment as a commissioned officer in the regular or reserve corps of the Public Health Service or be eligible for selection for a federal civil service appointment.
Amount of Grant: $25,000 maximum per year plus a tax assistance payment of 39 percent
Date(s) Application is Due: Mar 26
Contact: Chief, Loan Repayment Programs Branch, Division of Health Services Scholarships, (301) 594-4400; Public Information Phone, (800) 435-6464
Internet: http://www.hrsa.gov
Sponsor: Department of Health and Human Services
4350 East-West Hwy
Rockville, MD 20857

DHHS National Health Service Corps Scholarships Program 1266
To obtain adequate numbers of trained physicians, dentists, and other health-related specialists for the National Health Service Corps, scholarships are given in exchange for service in health personnel shortage areas within the United States. Disciplines have included allopathic and osteopathic medicine, dentistry, nursing (baccalaureate and graduate), public health nutrition (graduate), medical social work (graduate), speech pathology/audiology (graduate), veterinary medicine, optometry, podiatry, and pharmacy. Not all disciplines participate each year. Deadlines for receipt of applications for each academic year are the last Friday in March. A student may not receive more than a total of four years of support. Each award covers one academic year of support (including monthly living stipend, tuition, and fees), as specified by signed contracts, with annual continuation awards if funds are available.
Requirements: Applicants for new awards must be accepted by accredited U.S. educational institutions for full-time courses of study leading to degrees in medicine, osteopathy, or dentistry; be former recipients of the federal scholarship program for first-year students of exceptional financial need; be eligible for or hold appointments as commissioned officers in the regular or reserve corps of PHS or be eligible for civilian service in the NHSC; and submit applications and signed contracts to accept payment of scholarships and to serve for the applicable period of obligated service in health workforce shortage areas.
Restrictions: Each year of scholarship support incurs a year of federal service obligation with the minimum obligation being two years. Failure to fulfill the service obligation incurs financial damages, payable in one year, calculated at three times the scholarship benefits plus interest.
Amount of Grant: $1128 plus tuition, fees and other reasonable costs
Contact: Division of National Health Service, (301) 594-4400 or (800) 221-9393
Internet: http://www.dhhs.gov
Sponsor: Department of Health and Human Services
4350 East-West Hwy
Bethesda, MD 20814

DHHS Native American Health Service Loan Repayment Awards 1267
To help ensure an adequate supply of trained health professionals for IHS facilities, the program provides for the repayment of educational loans for participants who agree by written contract to serve an applicable period of time at a facility IHS has designated as a retention/recruitment priority site or in a designated specialty at a site with an appropriate position. Recipients must agree to serve an applicable period of time in such a site with a minimum period of participation of two years. Contact the program office for deadline dates.
Requirements: Eligible applicants must be individuals who are enrolled as full-time students in the final year of a course of study or program leading to a degree in allopathic or osteopathic medicine, dentistry, or other health profession in a state; are enrolled in an approved graduate training program in allopathic or osteopathic medicine, dentistry, or other health profession; or have a degree in allopathic or osteopathic medicine, dentistry, or other health profession and have completed an approved graduate training program and have a current and valid license to practice such health profession in a state. In addition, applicants must be eligible for appointment as commissioned officers in the regular or reserve corps of Public Health Service (PHS) or be eligible for selection for civilian service in IHS, submit an application to participate in the loan repayment program, and sign and submit it to DHHS at the time of agreeing to accept repayment of educational loans, and serve for the applicable period of service in a retention/recruitment site as determined by DHHS.
Amount of Grant: $3000-$48,000 for a 2-year obligation
Contact: Jackie Sanitago, Chief, Loan Repayment Program, IHS, (301) 443-3396
Internet: http://www.dhhs.gov
Sponsor: Department of Health and Human Services
12300 Twinbrook Pkwy
Rockville, MD 20852

DHHS Neurodevelopmental Test Methods Research Grants 1268
The purpose of the program is to determine and validate a battery of neurodevelopmental tests for use in assessing the effects of prenatal or postnatal exposure to developmental toxicants. The battery of tests should be applicable to a wide range of potential neurodevelopmental toxicants found at waste sites and in the environment including metals and solvents; be applicable to a wide range of exposure levels found in the environment; and cover a broad range of developmental domains including cognitive function, sensory function, motor function, and complex multi-tasking performance. These research methods will address an agency goal to develop methods and tools for evaluating human health consequences from exposure to toxic substances in the environment.
Requirements: Applications may be submitted by official public health agencies of the states, or their bona fide agents. This includes the District of Columbia, American Samoa, the Commonwealth of Puerto Rico, the Virgin Islands, the Federated States of Micronesia, Guam, the Northern Mariana Islands, the Republic of the Marshall Island, the Republic of Palau, federally recognized Indian tribal governments, public and private nonprofit and for-profit universities, colleges, and research institutions.
Amount of Grant: $130,000-$300,000; $200,000 average
Date(s) Application is Due: Jul 15
Contact: Mildred Garner, Grants Management Officer, (770) 488-2745; fax: (770) 488-2777; email: info@cdc.gov
Internet: http://www.cdc.gov
Sponsor: Department of Health and Human Services
2920 Brandywine Road
Atlanta, GA 30341-4146

DHHS Oral Health Promotion Research Across the Lifespan 1269
The National Institute of Dental and Craniofacial Research has invited proposals for improving the oral health of people of all ages. The research team must include someone with extensive experience in health promotion, behavioral and/or social science research. The health promotion intervention proposed for funding must be based on a previously conducted assessment of the epidemiology, social, behavioral and/or environmental factors related to the disease or condition under study. Research could focus on maternal and child health, adolescent and young adult health, or health of adults with complex diseases. For example, an applicant might propose to study approaches to involving families, social networks, communities, or neighborhoods in behaviors that promote and improve oral health; improving patient-provider communication related to oral preventive measures; or effective ways to train oral health professional students to communicate with diverse patient populations.
Requirements: Any person with the skills, knowledge, and resources necessary to carry out the proposed research as the project director/principal investigator (PD/PI) is invited to work with his/her organization to develop an application for support. Applications must be submitted electronically through Grants.gov (http://www.grants.gov) using the SF424 research and related forms and the SF424 application guide.
Date(s) Application is Due: Mar 5; Jul 5; Nov 5
Contact: Maria Teresa Canto, (301) 594-5497; fax: (301) 480-8322; email: maria.canto@nih.gov
Internet: http://grants.nih.gov/grants/guide/pa-files/PA-07-225.html
Sponsor: National Institute of Dental and Craniofacial Research (NIDCR)
Building 45, Room 4AS43D, 45 Center Drive MSC 6401
Bethesda, MD 20892

DHHS Podiatric Primary Care Residency Training Grants 1270
This program intends to promote the postgraduate education of podiatrists in primary care podiatric practice. Grants are to assist in meeting the costs of the program that cannot be met from other sources. Grants may include support for the program only, residents only, or support for both the program and residents but are not intended to absorb costs of existing or new positions that can be supported from other available funds.

Project period is a maximum of 36 months; a noncompeting continuation application is required at the end of each budget period. Contact the office for deadline dates.
Requirements: Public or nonprofit private accredited schools of podiatric medicine and teaching hospitals may apply.
Amount of Grant: $205,291-$286,362; $245,826 average
Contact: Chris McLaughlin, (301) 443-1568; email: cmclaughlin@hrsa.gov
Internet: http://www.dhhs.gov
Sponsor: Department of Health and Human Services
5600 Fishers Ln, Parklawn Building
Rockville, MD 20857

DHHS Preventive Medicine 1271
The grants promote the postgraduate education of physicians in preventive medicine. Grants are intended to assist in meeting the costs of planning and developing new preventive medicine programs; maintaining or improving existing residency training programs in preventive medicine; and providing financial assistance to trainees enrolled in such programs. Contact the office for deadlines and application materials.
Requirements: Any accredited public or private school of medicine, osteopathy, or public health may apply. To be eligible for a grant, the applicant must demonstrate that it has or will have available, full-time faculty members with training and experience in the fields of preventive medicine.
Restrictions: Grants may not be used for construction or patient services.
Amount of Grant: $101,897-$430,188; $206,768 average
Contact: Dr. Douglas Lloyd, Public Health and Dental Education, (301) 443-0157
Internet: http://www.dhhs.gov
Sponsor: Department of Health and Human Services
5600 Fishers Ln, Parklawn Building
Rockville, MD 20857

DHHS Primary Medical Care National Research Service Awards (NRSA) 1272
This program is intended to promote postdoctoral research training programs in primary medical care. NRSAs are made directly to individuals for research training in primary medical care; in addition, grants may be made to institutions to enable them to award NRSAs to individuals selected by them. Each individual who receives an NRSA is obligated, upon termination of the award, to comply with certain service and payback provisions. Recipients agree to engage in primary medical care research and/or teaching for a period equal to the period of the NRSA support in excess of 12 months. Contact the office for deadline dates.
Requirements: Domestic public or private nonprofit organizations may apply for training grants. States or local governments and U.S. territories are eligible. Individual applicants for fellowships must have received doctoral degrees. All persons supported as fellows or trainees must be citizens or noncitizen nationals of the United States or have been lawfully admitted for permanent residence. Eligibility is limited to individuals affiliated with entities having received grants or contracts under Sections 780, 784, or 786 of the Public Health Service Act.
Amount of Grant: $258,100-$538,167; $389,688 average
Contact: Christopher McLaughlin and Anne Patterson, (301) 443-6785
Internet: http://www.dhhs.gov
Sponsor: Department of Health and Human Services
5600 Fishers Ln, Parklawn Building
Rockville, MD 20857

DHHS Priority Health Conditions Studies Initiative 1273
The primary purpose of this program is to solicit scientific proposals designed to study the occurrence of and risk factors for priority adverse health conditions. The priority health conditions are birth defects and reproductive disorders, cancers, immune function disorders, kidney dysfunction, liver dysfunction, lung and respiratory diseases, and neurotoxic disorders. Each fiscal year, one of the seven priority health conditions will be emphasized; however, applications may address any of the seven. This will improve recipients' ability to address potential public health problems related to exposure to hazardous substances. Contact the office for deadline dates.
Requirements: Eligible applicants are state health departments and the District of Columbia; the Commonwealth of Puerto Rico; the Virgin Islands; Guam; the Federated States of Micronesia; the Republic of the Marshall Islands; the Republic of Palau; the Northern Mariana Islands; American Samoa; the political subdivisions thereof, which may include state universities, state colleges, and state research institutions; and federally recognized Native American tribal governments.
Amount of Grant: $50,000-$500,000; $100,000 average
Contact: Caroline McDonald, Division of Health Studies, (404) 498-0270; fax: (404) 498-0059; email: COS4@cdc.gov
Internet: http://www.dhhs.gov
Sponsor: Department of Health and Human Services
1600 Clifton Rd NE
Atlanta, GA 30333

DHHS Professional Nurse Traineeships Program 1274
Grants are awarded to eligible institutions to provide financial support through traineeships for registered nurses enrolled in advanced education nursing programs to prepare nurse practitioners, clinical nurse specialists, nurse midwives, nurse anesthetists, nurse administrators, nurse educators, public health nurses and nurses in other specialties determined by the Secretary to require advanced education.
Requirements: Schools of nursing and public health, public or nonprofit private hospitals, and other public or nonprofit entities are eligible for funds. Trainees are selected by participating institutions. A candidate must be a U.S. citizen or have been lawfully admitted to the United States for permanent residence; a graduate of a state-approved school of nursing; licensed as a professional nurse in a state or territory; and able to enroll full-time in a course of study.
Amount of Grant: $1000-$235,000; $45,000 average
Contact: Karen Breeden, Division of Nursing, (301) 443-6333
Internet: http://www.dhhs.gov
Sponsor: Department of Health and Human Services
5600 Fishers Ln, Parklawn Building
Rockville, MD 20857

DHHS Grants for Renovation or Construction of Nonacute Health Care Facilities 1275
Grants are intended to be used to renovate, expand, repair, equip, or modernize nonacute care intermediate and long-term care facilities for patients with AIDS. Contact the program office for deadline dates.
Requirements: Applicants must be public or nonprofit entities.
Amount of Grant: $1.16 million average
Contact: Paul Murhy, Division of Facilities Compliance and Recovery, (301) 443-5656; Neal Meyerson, Grants Management Specialist, (301) 443-5906
Internet: http://www.dhhs.gov
Sponsor: Department of Health and Human Services
5600 Fishers Ln, Parklawn Building
Rockville, MD 20857

DHHS Promoting Safe and Stable Families Grants 1276
The National Center on Child Abuse and Neglect is interested in research on the impact of community-based family support and family preservation programs on child abuse and neglect. Research should focus on expanding the current knowledge base, build on previous research, and provide insights into new approaches to preventing child maltreatment and preserving families through support and preservation services. The center is particularly interested in projects that address specific populations and outcomes. The populations are families who receive family support services but have had no previous contact with child protective services; families who have been referred to child protective services whose cases were unsubstantiated but were found to need services and were referred to family support programs; families who have been in the system whose child abuse or neglect cases were substantiated, who received family preservation or support services, and whose cases are now closed; and families who have open cases whose children have not been removed and who are receiving family preservation services. Outcomes of interest are case finding, which involves families who were not referred to child protective services, and the impact of family support and/or preservation services on prevention, recidivism, and removal of children. Applicants should plan and design the proposed research in collaboration with state and local CPS and Title IV-B agencies as well as community-based entities providing family support services, such as family resource centers. Contact the office for deadline dates.
Requirements: Agencies of state and local governments, public and private nonprofit agencies, and institutions engaged in child and family welfare activities and research are eligible for these grants.
Amount of Grant: $194,000-$48 million range
Contact: Joseph Bock, Deputy Associate Commissioner, (202) 205-8618
Internet: http://www.acf.hhs.gov/programs/cb/programs/fpfs.htm
Sponsor: Department of Health and Human Services
330 C Street, SW
Washington, DC 20447

DHHS Public Health Students Traineeships and Other Graduate Public Health Programs 1277
The programs support traineeships for students in graduate educational programs in schools of public health or other public or nonprofit educational entities that offer graduate programs for training in biostatistics or epidemiology; health administration, health planning, or health policy analysis and planning; environmental or occupational health; dietetics or nutrition; maternal and child health; or approved residency training in preventive medicine or dentistry. Deadlines and application kits are forwarded to all eligible applicants.
Requirements: Accredited schools of public health and other public or nonprofit educational entities providing graduate or specialized training in public health may apply. Trainees must be U.S. citizens or noncitizen nationals possessing visas permitting permanent residence in the United States and must be pursuing a graduate degree in an eligible school of public health or be enrolled in an eligible program.
Amount of Grant: $8109-$148,850; $50,150 average
Contact: Cecelia Maryland, Public Health Branch, Division of State, Community and Public Health, (301) 443-1973
Internet: http://www.dhhs.gov
Sponsor: Department of Health and Human Services
5600 Fishers Ln, Parklawn Building
Rockville, MD 20857

DHHS Residency Training in Family Practice, General Internal Medicine, or General Pediatrics Grants 1278
Grants are awarded to assist graduate training programs in family medicine, general internal medicine and/or general pediatrics to expand and improve the quality of residency training programs that prepare graduates to enter primary care practice.

Residency training programs should emphasize national innovations aimed at primary care residency education across disciplines.
Requirements: An accredited public or private nonprofit school of medicine, a school of osteopathic medicine, and a public or private nonprofit hospital or other entity located in a state is eligible to apply. Each allopathic program must be fully or provisionally approved by the Accreditation Council for Graduate Medical Education. Each osteopathic program must be approved by the American Osteopathic Association.
Restrictions: Grants may not be used for construction, patient services, or student assistance.
Amount of Grant: $27,000-$657,344; $178,803 average
Contact: Dr. P. Preston Reynolds, Division of Medicine and Dentistry of the Bureau of Health Professions, (301) 443-1467
Internet: http://www.dhhs.gov
Sponsor: Department of Health and Human Services
5600 Fishers Ln, Parklawn Building
Rockville, MD 20857

DHHS Rural Telemedicine Grants **1279**
The objective of this program is to demonstrate and collect information on the feasibility, costs, appropriateness, and acceptability of telemedicine for improving access to health services for rural residents and reducing the isolation of rural practitioners, and to demonstrate how telemedicine can be used as an effective tool for the development of integrated systems of health care for rural areas. Annual deadline dates may vary; contact program staff for exact dates.
Requirements: Eligible applicants are nonprofit public (nonfederal) or private health care providers or a consortium of providers, nonprofit or for profit, that are members of an existing or proposed telemedicine network.
Restrictions: Not more than 40 percent of grant funds may be expended for equipment. Not more than 20 percent of grant funds may be expended for direct costs. Grant funds may not be used for purchasing and installing telecommunications equipment.
Amount of Grant: $250,000 maximum
Contact: Monica Cowan, Administrative Assistant, Office for the Advancement of Telehealth, (301) 443-1730
Internet: http://www.telehealth.hrsa.gov
Sponsor: Department of Health and Human Services
4350 East-West Hwy
Rockville, MD 20814

DHHS Technical and Non-Financial Assistance to Health Centers **1280**
The grants assist community health centers in the areas of collaborative activities on state or regional issues; promotion of support and involvement of state agencies in primary care; provision of, or arrangement for, training and technical assistance; and development of shared services and joint purchasing arrangements—for purposes including, but not limited to, primary care provider retention and recruitment, clinical development, assessment of community health needs, expertise in dealing with maternal and child health and other special populations, and management and maximization of nonfederal sources. Recipients will be expected to provide certain technical and nonfinancial assistance to community health centers. Support is recommended for a specified project period, not in excess of five years. Deadlines are specified in application instructions.
Requirements: Grants will be made to private nonprofit entities, including state and regional primary care associations.
Amount of Grant: $580,000 average
Contact: Cicely Nelson, (301) 594-4300; email: cnelson@hrsa.gov
Internet: http://www.hrsa.gov/grants/preview/primary.htm
Sponsor: Department of Health and Human Services
4350 East-West Hwy
Bethesda, MD 20814

DHHS Thimerosal Pharmacokinetics: Assessment of the Distribution, Metabolism, and Excretion **1281**
The purpose of this program is to define and characterize the appropriate pharmacokinetics of both methyl mercury and thimerosal distribution, metabolism, and elimination that are needed to accurately characterize the comparative neurotoxicity of these substances and develop recommendations for future extrapolation of these results to possible human exposure scenarios.
Requirements: Applications may be submitted by official public health agencies of the states, or their bonafide agents. This includes the District of Columbia, American Samoa, Guam, the Commonwealth of Puerto Rico, the Commonwealth of the Northern Mariana Islands, the Federated States of Micronesia, the Virgin Islands, the Federated States of Marshall Island, the Republic of Palau, federally-recognized Indian tribal governments, public and private nonprofit universities and colleges.
Amount of Grant: $130,000-$300,000; $200,000 average
Date(s) Application is Due: Aug 15
Contact: Mildred Garner, Grants Management, (770) 488-2745; fax: (770) 488-2777
Internet: http://www.dhhs.gov
Sponsor: Department of Health and Human Services
200 Independence Ave SW
Washington, DC 20201

DHHS Universal Newborn Hearing Screening and Intervention **1282**
This program supports the implementation of universal physiologic newborn hearing screening prior to hospital discharge with linkages to medical home, ongoing family-to-family support, diagnostic evaluation by three months of age, and enrollment in a program of early intervention by six months of age for those infants identified with hearing loss. Applicants are expected to notify the Maternal and Child Health Bureau's Division of Services for Children with Special Health Care Needs by November 10; the deadline for receipt of applications is December 8.
Requirements: This program is open to state agencies with the capacity to implement a statewide universal newborn hearing screening and intervention program for all newborn infants in the state.
Amount of Grant: $43,650-$515,382; $161,017. average
Contact: Irene Forsman, Integrated Services Branch, Division of Services for Children with Special Health Needs, (301) 443-2370; email: iforsman@hrsa.gov; Lawrence Poole, Director, Division of Grants Management Operations, (301) 443-0354
Internet: http://www.dhhs.gov
Sponsor: Department of Health and Human Services
5600 Fishers Ln, Parklawn Building
Rockville, MD 20857

DHL Charitable Shipment Support **1283**
The corporation provides free shipment of materials supporting charitable programs. Applicants must submit a complete web questionnaire.
Requirements: Application by internet only.
Restrictions: Religious organizations are ineligible for religious sectarian activities, and political organizations are not eligible for political purposes.
Contact: Technical Support, (800) 527-7298
Internet: http://www.dhl-usa.com
Sponsor: DHL International, Ltd.
DHL Express, 1220 South Pine Island Road, Suite 600
Plantation, FL 33324

Dickson Foundation Grants **1284**
The foundation awards grants primarily to local nonprofit organizations in its areas of interest, including education (secondary schools, higher education),and health care. Types of support include building construction/renovation and general operating support. There are no application deadlines or forms. Submit a letter of interest for consideration.
Requirements: Giving is primarily in the Southeast.
Restrictions: Grants are not awarded to individuals, or for building or endowment funds.
Geographic Focus: North Carolina
Contact: Susan Patterson, (704) 372-5404; fax: (704) 372-6409
Sponsor: Dickson Foundation
301 S. Tryon Street, Suite 1800
Charlotte, NC 28202

Dietetic Outcomes Research Study Grants **1285**
The program seeks proposals for a prospective, controlled trial study on the effectiveness of nutrition services. The objective is to investigate the cost and clinical effectiveness of nutrition services provided by registered dietitians compared to other health practitioners or health care teams with and without dietitians in an ambulatory setting. The study must focus on one of four disease states: diabetes, hyperlipidemia, congestive heart failure, or obesity with metabolic complications. Key personnel requirements include an experienced research dietitian and ADA members as a principal or co-principal investigator. Specifications are contained in the RFP posted on the Web site.
Amount of Grant: $225,000 maximum
Contact: Elisabeth Puga, (800) 877-1600 ext 4803; email: epuga@eatright.org
Internet: http://www.eatright.org/Public/7713_7808.cfm
Sponsor: American Dietetic Association Foundation
120 S Riverside Plz, Suite 2000
Chicago, IL 60606

Disable American Veterans Charitable Grants **1286**
The trust is dedicated to building better lives for U.S. disabled veterans and their families. Grants support physical and psychological rehabilitation programs, aid efforts to meet the special needs of veterans with specific disabilities such as amputation and blindness, and support programs and shelters for homeless veterans. Priority is given to long-term service projects providing direct assistance to disabled veterans and their families. The trust also awards grants to service programs that assist veterans suffering from substance abuse and post traumatic stress disorder, health promotion programs for aging disabled veterans, and nursing and health programs designed to ensure quality healthcare for veterans.
Requirements: Nonprofit organizations are eligible.
Restrictions: Grants generally do not support individuals; goodwill advertising, souvenir journals, or dinner programs; political causes, candidates, organizations, or campaigns; or endowments or capital campaigns.
Date(s) Application is Due: Jan 31; May 1; Aug 1; Nov 1
Contact: Grants Administrator, (877) 426-2838, ext. 2057; fax: (859) 442-2088; email: cst@davmail.org
Internet: http://www.dav.org/cst/index.html
Sponsor: Disabled American Veterans Charitable Service Trust
3725 Alexandria Pike
Cold Spring, KY 41076

Do Something BR!CK Awards 1287

The awards honor dynamic young people for service in the areas of community building, health, and the environment. BR!CK winners are leaders who identify and realize solutions to problems facing local communities across America. Nine winners will receive a minimum of $10,000 in community grants and scholarships (if applicable). Of those nine winners, 1 will be selected by a national, online vote as a Golden BR!CK Award winner. That Golden BR!CK Award winner receives a total of $100,000 in community grants. Winners are announced and recognized at an annual gala in New York City. Application and guidelines are available online.

Requirements: Applicants must be 25 years old or younger. Only winners who are age 18 and under are eligible for a scholarship of $5,000 and a $5,000 community grant (total= $10,000 BR!CK Award). Winners age 19-25 receive their entire award in the form of a community grant.

Samples: Ashley Rhodes-Courter (21) - GOLDEN BR!CK - North American Council on Adoptable Children.; William Hwang (22) - United InnoWorks Academy.; Kelly Voigt (14) - Prevent the Bite.; Kimmie Weeks (25) - GOLDEN BR!CK - Youth Action International.; Cheryl Perera (21) - OneChild Network & Support Systems Inc.; Ruth DeGolia (24) - Mercado Global.; Jennifer Staple (25) - GOLDEN BR!CK - Unite For Sight.; Jennifer Zwilling (16) - Tourette Syndrome Association Youth Ambassador Program.; David Fajgenbaum (21) - National Students of AMF (Ailing Mothers & Fathers); Divine Bradley (24) - GOLDEN BR!CK - Team Revolution.; Jacob Komar (14) - Computers for Communities.; Hannah Taylor (11) - The Ladybug Foundation, Inc.

Amount of Grant: $10,000 - $100,000

Date(s) Application is Due: Dec 15

Contact: Jordyn Wells; (212) 254-2390 ext. 238; email: jwells@dosomething.org

Internet: http://www.dosomething.org/programs/awards

Sponsor: Do Something
32 Union Square E, Suite 4L
New York, NY 10003-3209

DOA Distance Learning and Telemedicine Grant Program 1288

The purpose of the program is to encourage and improve the use of telemedicine, telecommunications, computer networks, and related advanced technologies to provide educational and medical benefits through distance learning and telemedicine projects to people living in rural areas and to improve rural opportunities. Funds may be used for telecommunications, computer networks, and related advanced technologies that provide educational and/or medical benefits to students, teachers, medical professionals, and rural residents. Annual deadline dates may vary; contact program staff for exact dates. Application materials are available on the Web site.

Requirements: To be eligible for a grant your organization must: currently deliver or propose to deliver distance learning or telemedicine services for the term of the grant; be legally organized as an incorporated organization or partnership, an Indian tribe or tribal organization, a state or local unit of government, a consortium, or other legal entity including a private corporation organized on a for profit or not-for profit basis; operate a rural community facility or deliver distance learning or telemedicine services to entities that operate a rural community facility or to residents of rural areas at rates calculated to ensure that the benefit of the financial assistance passes through to such entities or to residents of rural areas.

Restrictions: Grants are ineligible for: salaries, wages, or employee benefits to medical or educational personnel; salaries or administrative expenses of the applicant or the project; acquiring, installing or constructing telecommunications transmission facilities; medical equipment not having telemedicine as its essential function; purchasing equipment that will be owned by a local exchange carrier or another telecommunications service provider unless that service provider is the applicant; duplicating facilities already in place which provide distance learning or telemedicine services; reimbursing your organization or others for costs incurred prior to the date application was received; DLT application preparation costs; projects that only provide links between people located at the same physical facility; site development, or the destruction or alteration of buildings; purchasing land or building or for building construction; projects located in areas covered by the Coastal Barrier Resources Act; or recurring or operating project expenses or costs such as monthly fees for telecommunications and electric service.

Amount of Grant: $50,000-$500,000

Contact: Director, (202)-720-0413; email: dltinfo@usda.gov or dltinfo@wdc.usda.gov

Internet: http://www.usda.gov/rus/telecom/dlt/dlt.htm

Sponsor: Department of Agriculture
STOP 1550, Room 2845, 1400 Independence Avenue, S.W.
Washington, DC 20250-1550

DOA National Integrated Food Safety Initiative 1289

The purpose of this program is to support competitive projects that address selected priority issues in food safety that are best solved using an integrated approach. Special emphasis is given to research describing multi-functional activities (i.e., research that contains research, education, and extension components). The research component of the National Integrated Food Safety Initiative focuses on applied food safety research. The education component focuses on education and training in a formal classroom setting, which may include elementary, secondary, undergraduate, or graduate education. The extension component addresses education and training outside of the classroom. Where there is no extension program, outreach activities that deliver science-based and informational education to people in a variety of non-formal settings are appropriate. The RFP is usually announced in the Federal Register in February or March of each year, and proposals are due eight weeks following the release of the RFP. Funding opportunity number: U.S.DA-GRANTS-090304-001

Requirements: Faculty at all four year accredited colleges and universities are eligible to apply.

Amount of Grant: $500,000 maximum

Contact: Chris Wozniak , Food Science and Food Safety, (202) 401-6020; fax: (202) 401-6156; email: cwozniak@csrees.usda.gov

Internet: http://www.csrees.usda.gov/fo/fundview.cfm?fonum=1087

Sponsor: Department of Agriculture
1400 Independence Ave SW
Washington, DC 20250

DOD Breast Cancer Center of Excellence Award 1290

The award mechanism supports multidisciplinary, multi-institutional teams of gifted scientists, clinicians, and consumer advocates in making groundbreaking advances toward the eradication of breast cancer. The Breast Cancer Research Program (BCRP) encourages highly accomplished scientists renowned for their contributions to the proposed areas of research and promising young investigators who can provide fresh insight to work together to accelerate the solution of a central, overarching research problem in a way that could not be accomplished by a single investigator or group. In addition, the BCRP strongly endorses the integration of scientists from nontraditional disciplines such as computer science, mathematics, economics, physics, and other quantitative disciplines. The BCRP also encourages centers of excellence to incorporate study components addressing ethical issues in breast cancer research. Breast cancer consumer/survivor groups must be active participants in all aspects of these awards. The listed application deadline is for preproposals; full proposals are by invitation. Preproposals must be submitted through the CDMRP eReceipt system. Guidelines are available online.

Requirements: All individuals, regardless of ethnicity, nationality, or citizenship status, may apply as long as they are employed by, or affiliated with, an eligible institution. Eligible institutions include for-profit, nonprofit, public, and private organizations. Agencies of local, state, and federal governments are eligible to the extent that proposals do not overlap with their fully funded intramural programs. Federal agencies will be expected to explain how their proposals do not overlap with their intramural programs.

Amount of Grant: $20 million maximum

Date(s) Application is Due: Apr 5

Contact: Commander, U.S. Army Medical Research and Materiel Command, (301) 619-7079; fax: (301) 619-7792; email: cdmrp.pa@det.amedd.army.mil

Internet: http://cdmrp.army.mil/funding/bcrp.htm

Sponsor: Department of Defense
1077 Patchel St (Building 1077), MCMR-ZB-C (BC05-COE)
Fort Detrick, MD 21702-5024

DOD Clinical Translational Research Grants 1291

The award is designed to sponsor innovative research that will result in substantial improvements over current approaches to breast cancer chemoprevention and therapy by accelerating the progression of recent, highly promising findings in preclinical breast cancer research from the laboratory to the clinic. These awards are intended to support both new and established scientists across a broad spectrum of disciplines. Partnerships between academic institutions and biotechnology companies are encouraged. Proposals are being sought only in the areas of chemoprevention and therapeutics. Successful applicants must initiate a prospective clinical trial and accrue participants for a minimum of one year during the award period. They must also include preliminary data to support the feasibility of their hypotheses and approaches. Funding for these awards may be requested for up to five years. The listed application deadline is for preproposals; full proposals are by invitation. Preproposals must be submitted through the CDMRP eReceipt system. Guidelines are available online.

Requirements: All individuals, regardless of ethnicity, nationality, or citizenship status, may apply as long as they are employed by, or affiliated with, an eligible institution. Eligible institutions include for-profit, nonprofit, public, and private organizations. Agencies of local, state, and federal governments are eligible to the extent that proposals do not overlap with their fully funded intramural programs. Federal agencies will be expected to explain how their proposals do not overlap with their intramural programs.

Restrictions: This award is not intended to support early drug discovery or development, correlative studies, or new combinations of standard breast cancer therapies.

Amount of Grant: $20 million total

Date(s) Application is Due: Apr 5

Contact: Commander, U.S. Army Medical Research and Materiel Command, (301) 619-7079; fax: (301) 619-7792; email: cdmrp.pa@det.amedd.army.mil

Internet: http://cdmrp.army.mil/funding/bcrp.htm

Sponsor: Department of Defense
1077 Patchel St (Building 1077), MCMR-ZB-C (BC05-CTR)
Fort Detrick, MD 21702-5024

DOD Era of Hope Scholar Award 1292

The Breast Cancer Research Program sponsors this grant to identify individuals with high potential for innovation in breast cancer research early in their careers. Candidates should be exceptionally talented, early-career scientists who have demonstrated that they are the best and brightest in their field(s) through extraordinary creativity, vision, and productivity. They should also exhibit strong potential for leadership in the breast cancer research community that supports a vision for the eradication of breast cancer. These individuals should challenge current dogma and demonstrate an ability to look beyond tradition and convention. Award recipients will be expected to successfully challenge the status quo through creative, high-risk research that may lead ultimately to the eradication of breast cancer. Proposals must focus on the candidate's emerging record of creative and

original accomplishments and potential for leadership in the field. Experience in breast cancer is not a requirement; however, the proposal must focus on breast cancer, and the applicant must commit a minimum of 50 percent effort during the award period to breast cancer research. All nominations must be converted into an electronic PDF file for electronic submission. Nominations guidelines are available online.
Requirements: Applicants must be nominated to be considered for this award. Applicants must be independent, nonmentored investigators within six years of their last training position. All individuals, regardless of ethnicity, nationality, or citizenship status, may apply as long as they are employed by, or affiliated with, an eligible institution. Eligible institutions include for-profit, nonprofit, public, and private organizations. Agencies of local, state, and federal governments are eligible to the extent that proposals do not overlap with their fully funded intramural programs.
Restrictions: Self-nominations will not be accepted. Postdoctoral fellows, clinical fellows (including residents and interns), and other mentored researchers are not eligible.
Amount of Grant: $2.5 million for up to five years
Date(s) Application is Due: Apr 5
Contact: Commander, U.S. Army Medical Research and Materiel Command, (301) 619-7079; fax: (301) 619-7792; email: cdmrp.pa@det.amedd.army.mil
Internet: http://cdmrp.army.mil/bcrp/era/default.htm
Sponsor: Department of Defense
1077 Patchel St (Building 1077), MCMR-ZB-C (BC05-EHSA)
Fort Detrick, MD 21702-5024

DOD HBCU/MI Partnership Training Award 1293
This program's goal challenges the scientific community to design innovative research that will foster new directions for, address neglected issues in, and bring new investigators to the field of breast cancer research. The program focuses its funding on innovative projects, particularly those involving multidisciplinary and/or multi-institutional collaborations and alliances that have the potential to make a significant impact on breast cancer. Proposals that address the needs of minority, low-income, rural, and other underrepresented and/or medically underserved populations are strongly encouraged. The listed application deadline is for preproposals. Preproposals must be submitted through the CDMRP eReceipt system. Guidelines are available online.
Requirements: Applicants must be HBCU/MI doctoral-level faculty members. All individuals, regardless of ethnicity, nationality, or citizenship status, may apply as long as they are employed by, or affiliated with, an eligible HBCU/MI institution. Eligible institutions are those approved as HBCU/MIs by the Department of Education.
Contact: Commander, U.S. Army Medical Research and Materiel Command, (301) 619-7079; fax: (301) 619-7792; email: cdmrp.pa@det.amedd.army.mil
Internet: http://cdmrp.army.mil/bcrp/default.htm
Sponsor: Department of Defense
1077 Patchel Street (Building 1077), MCMR-ZB-C (BC05-HPT)
Fort Detrick, MD 21702-5024

DOD Idea Award for Breast Cancer Research 1294
The award supports innovative, high-risk/high-reward breast cancer research. Proposals should describe new paradigms and challenge existing dogma in the study of breast cancer. The award also supports efforts to examine existing problems from a new perspective; however, these proposals will face a greater burden to demonstrate innovation. Special consideration will be given to proposals that focus on biological signal integration, and/or systems implications. Proposals must be submitted electronically.
Requirements: All individuals, regardless of ethnicity, nationality, or citizenship status, may apply as long as they are employed by, or affiliated with, an eligible institution. Eligible institutions include for-profit, nonprofit, public, and private organizations. Agencies of local, state, and federal governments are eligible to the extent that proposals do not overlap with their fully funded intramural programs.
Amount of Grant: $300,000 maximum for up to three years; $625,000 maximum for population-based studies
Date(s) Application is Due: May 24
Contact: Commander, U.S. Army Medical Research and Materiel Command, (301) 619-7079; fax: (301) 619-7792; email: cdmrp.pa@det.amedd.army.mil
Internet: http://cdmrp.army.mil/bcrp/default.htm
Sponsor: Department of Defense
1077 Patchel St (Building 1077), MCMR-ZB-C (BC05-IDEA)
Fort Detrick, MD 21702-5024

DOD Multidisciplinary Postdoctoral Award for Breast Cancer Research 1295
The award is designed to identify and fund exceptionally talented recent doctoral graduates committed to broadening the scope of their research by adding significant, mentored training in more than one major discipline. Mentors should be identified for each discipline represented in the proposed project. Major disciplines for this award include, but are not limited to, laboratory, clinical, social/behavioral science, and public health research. The Breast Cancer Research Program is especially interested in proposals that integrate training in disciplines currently underrepresented in breast cancer, such as engineering, physics, and mathematics; however, innovative proposals that incorporate any combination of the major disciplines listed above will be considered. Proposals must be submitted electronically at https://cdmrp.org. Guidelines are available online.
Requirements: Eligible applicants should have been in the laboratory or research setting in which the proposed research is to be performed for no longer than two years at the time of submission and should have a total of less than five years of postdoctoral research experience (excluding clinical residency or fellowship training). All individuals, regardless of ethnicity, nationality, or citizenship status, may apply as long as they are employed by, or affiliated with, an eligible institution as defined below. Eligible institutions include for-profit, nonprofit, public, and private organizations. Agencies of local, state, and federal governments are eligible to the extent that proposals do not overlap with their fully funded intramural programs.
Amount of Grant: $375,000 maximum
Date(s) Application is Due: May 24
Contact: Commander, U.S. Army Medical Research and Materiel Command, (301) 619-7079; fax: (301) 619-7792; email: cdmrp.pa@det.amedd.army.mil
Internet: http://cdmrp.army.mil/funding/bcrp.htm
Sponsor: Department of Defense
1077 Patchel St (Building 1077), MCMR-ZB-C (BC05-MPA)
Fort Detrick, MD 21702-5024

DOD Predoctoral Traineeship in Breast Cancer Research 1296
The award prepares promising graduate students with a strong commitment to breast cancer research for successful and competitive careers. This award promotes creative approaches to training breast cancer investigators. Successful trainees will be selected for their talent, potential, and commitment to breast cancer research; the mentor's qualifications and experience in breast cancer research; the strong breast cancer research training program at the trainee's institution; the innovative research environment; and the institution's commitment to training future leaders in breast cancer research. The proposed training must focus on breast cancer research. Historically Black Colleges and Universities/Minority Institutions are highly encouraged to apply. Proposals must be submitted electronically at https://cdmrp.org. Guidelines are available online.
Requirements: Applicants must be graduate students under the guidance of a designated mentor. Individuals enrolled in a PhD or MD/PhD program are encouraged to apply. All individuals, regardless of ethnicity, nationality, or citizenship status, may apply as long as they are employed by, or affiliated with, an eligible institution. Eligible institutions include for-profit, nonprofit, public, and private organizations. Examples include universities, colleges, hospitals, laboratories, and companies. Agencies of local, state, and federal governments are eligible to the extent that proposals do not overlap with their fully funded intramural programs.
Amount of Grant: $30,000 per year for a maximum of three years
Date(s) Application is Due: May 24
Contact: Commander, U.S. Army Medical Research and Materiel Command, (301) 619-7079; fax: (301) 619-7792; email: cdmrp.pa@det.amedd.army.mil
Internet: http://cdmrp.army.mil/funding/archive/05bcrppredoc_pa.pdf
Sponsor: Department of Defense
1077 Patchel St (Building 1077), MCMR-ZB-C (BC05-PREDOC)
Fort Detrick, MD 21702-5024

DOE Environmental Remediation Grants 1297
The objectives of the program relate to environmental processes affected by energy production and use. The program develops information on the physical, chemical, and biological processes that cycle and transport energy-related material, particularly contaminates that arose during nuclear weapons production, through the earth's surface and subsurface. Emphasis is put on the development of a strong basis for understanding and implementing the appropriate and efficient use of bioremediation, particularly at the department's sites. Applications are accepted at any time.
Amount of Grant: $10,000-$2 million range; $200,000 average
Contact: Martin Rubinstein, Grants and Contracts Division, Office of Science, (301) 903- 5212
Internet: http://www.science.doe.gov/production/grants/grants.html
Sponsor: Department of Energy
19901 Germantown Road
Germantown, MD 20874

DOE Health Effects and Life Sciences Research Grants 1298
The objectives of this program of basic and biological research are to create and apply new technologies and resources in mapping, sequencing, and information management for characterizing the molecular nature of the human genome; to develop and support DOE national user facilities for use in fundamental structural biology; to use model organisms to understand human genome organization, human gene function and control, and the functional relationships between human genes and proteins; to characterize and exploit the genomes and diversity of microbes with potential relevance for energy, bioremediation, or global climate; to understand and characterize the risks to human health from exposures to low levels of radiation and chemicals; to develop novel technologies for high throughput determination of protein structure; and to anticipate and address ethical, legal, and social implications arising from genome research.
Requirements: Unsolicited research proposals should be preceded by an information preproposal of no more than two or three pages that briefly describes the research project and the proposed level of funding.
Amount of Grant: $10,000-$2 million range; $200,000 average
Contact: Martin Rubinstein, Grants and Contracts Division, (301) 903- 5212
Internet: http://www.science.doe.gov/production/grants/grants.html
Sponsor: Department of Energy
19901 Germantown Road
Germantown, MD 20874

DOE Human Genome Program—Ethical, Legal, and Social Implications 1299
DOE announces its interest in receiving applications in support of the Ethical, Legal, and Social Implications (ELSI) subprogram of the Human Genome Program (HGP). Applications should focus on issues of genetics and the workplace, storage of genetic information and tissue samples, education, or complex or multigenic traits. The HGP is

a coordinated, multidisciplinary, directed research effort aimed at obtaining a detailed understanding of the human genome at the molecular level.
Amount of Grant: $10,000-$2 million range; $200,000 average
Contact: Martin Rubinstein, Grants and Contracts Division, (301) 903-5212
Internet: http://www.sc.doe.gov/production/grants/grants.html
Sponsor: Department of Energy
19901 Germantown Road
Germantown, MD 20874

DOE Low Dose Radiation Research Program 1300
Research is specifically sought for pilot projects that involve innovative collaborations between experimentalists and modelers to model the mechanisms of key radiation-induced biological responses and to describe or identify strategies for developing biologically-based risk models that incorporate information on mechanisms of radiation-induced biological responses. Potential applicants should submit a one-page preapplication referencing Program Notice 01-17 by February 1; formal applications are due May 1. Annual deadline dates may change; contact program staff for exact dates.
Amount of Grant: $10,000-$2 million range; $200,000 average
Date(s) Application is Due: Feb 1; May 1
Contact: Martin Rubinstein, Grants and Contracts Division, (301) 903-5212
Internet: http://www.science.doe.gov/grants
Sponsor: Department of Energy
19901 Germantown Road
Germantown, MD 20874

DOE Medical Applications and Measurement Science Grants 1301
The objectives of this program are to develop technologies for the beneficial applications of radiation and in-vivo radiotracer detection in the study, diagnosis, and treatment of human diseases and disorders; to develop new instrumentation for biological and medical research; and to develop new concepts and techniques for detecting and measuring the hazardous agents of biochemical, physical, and environmental consequences related to energy production. Applications are accepted at any time.
Amount of Grant: $10,000-$2 million range; $200,000 average
Contact: Martin R. Rubinstein, Grants and Contracts Division, (301) 903- 5212
Internet: http://www.er.doe.gov/production/grants/guide.html
Sponsor: Department of Energy
19901 Germantown Road
Germantown, MD 20874

DOI Biological Resource Division Brucellosis Program 1302
Applications are invited for a research project on the improvements in ballistic delivery systems for brucellosis vaccination of free-ranging elk and bison of the Greater Yellowstone area. The purpose of this project is to develop methods of ballistic delivery that improve the distance, reliability, ease, and/or rapidity of brucella vaccine parenteral delivery.
Requirements: Applications may be submitted by educational institutions, private firms, private foundations, individuals, and agencies of state and local governments.
Amount of Grant: $1000-$582,000; $50,000 average
Contact: Branch of Acquisition and Federal Assistance; (703) 648-7478 or (703) 648-7361
Internet: http://www.usgs.gov/contracts
Sponsor: Department of the Interior
P.O. Box 25046, MS 204B
Denver, CO 80225

DOJ Gang-Free Schools and Communities Intervention Grants 1303
The objectives of the program include support to prevent and reduce the participation of juveniles in the activities of gangs that commit crimes. Such programs and activities may include individual, peer, family, and group counseling, including provision of life skills training and preparation for living independently, which shall include cooperation with social services, welfare, and health care programs; education and social services designed to address the social and developmental needs of juveniles; crisis intervention and counseling to juveniles, who are particularly at risk of gang involvement, and their families; the organization of the neighborhood and community groups to work closely with parents, schools, law enforcement, and other public and private agencies in the community; and training and assistance to adults who have significant relationships with juveniles who are or may become members of gangs, to assist such adults in providing constructive alternatives to participating in the activities of gangs. Deadlines are published in program announcements.
Requirements: Public or private nonprofit organizations or individuals may apply.
Contact: Heidi Hsia, Office of Juvenile Justice and Delinquency Prevention, (202) 307-5924; email: Hsiah@ojp.usdoj.gov
Internet: http://www.ojp.usdoj.gov/FinGuide/part4chap2.htm#ojjdp
Sponsor: Department of Justice
633 Indiana Avenue, N.W.
Washington, DC 20531

DOJ Mental Health and Juvenile Justice 1304
The purpose of this initiative is to substantially improve knowledge about the nature and prevalence of mental health and co- occurring substance abuse disorders among youth in the juvenile justice system and to develop and test a service delivery model based on theoretical and empirical information regarding best practices for meeting the needs of this population. The model will incorporate both current theory and best practices in the areas of screening, assessment, service provision, and quality assurance. The model should include youth at all stages of the juvenile justice system, including, but not limited to, arrest, intake, adjudication, detention, secure corrections, probation, and community-based treatment.
Requirements: Public or private agencies or organizations with a demonstrated capacity to carry out the requirements of this initiative may apply. Private, for-profit organizations must agree to waive any profit or fee. The organization must have demonstrated experience in conducting extensive literature reviews, conducting in-depth sample surveys of juvenile or criminal justice offenders and facilities, carrying out research and program development, and writing reports.
Amount of Grant: $1 million
Contact: Demonstration Division, Office of Juvenile Justice and Delinquency Prevention, (202) 307-5940
Internet: http://ojjdp.ncjrs.org/funding/funding.html
Sponsor: Department of Justice
2277 Research Boulevard, MS 2K
Rockville, MD 20850

DOL Occupational Safety and Health—Susan Harwood Training Grants 1305
Grants provide funds for programs to train workers and employers to recognize, avoid, and prevent safety and health hazards in their workplaces. The program emphasizes three areas: educating workers and employers in small businesses; training workers and employers about new OSHA standards; and training workers and employers about high risk activities or hazards identified by OSHA through its Strategic Management Plan, or as part of an OSHA special emphasis program.
Requirements: Nonprofit organizations, including community-based and faith-based organizations, that are not an agency of a State or local government are eligible to apply. State or local government supported institutions of higher education are eligible to apply in accordance with 29 CFR part 95. Eligible organizations can apply independently for funding or in partnership with other eligible organizations, but in such a case, a lead organization must be identified. Sub-contracts must be awarded in accordance with 29 CFR 95.40-48, including OMB circulars requiring free and open competition for procurement transactions.
Restrictions: Grants may not be used for: any activity that is inconsistent with the goals and objectives of the Occupational Safety and Health Act of 1970; training individuals not covered by the Occupational Safety and Health Act; training workers or employers from workplaces not covered by the Occupational Safety and Health Act; training on topics that do not cover the recognition, avoidance, and prevention of unsafe or unhealthy working conditions; assisting workers in arbitration cases or other actions against employers, or assisting employers and workers in the prosecution of claims against Federal, State or local governments; duplicating services offered by OSHA, a State under an OSHA approved State Plan, or consultation programs provided by State designated agencies under section 21(d) of the Occupational Safety and Health Act; generating membership in the grantee's organization; administrative costs exceeding 25% of the total grant budget.
Contact: Cynthia Bencheck, (847) 297-4810; email: bencheck.cindy@dol.gov
Internet: http://www.osha.gov/dcsp/ote/sharwood.html
Sponsor: Department of Labor
U.S. Department of Labor, 2020 S. Arlington Heights Road
Arlington Heights, IL 60005-4102

Dolan Foundation Grants 1306
The foundation awards community service grants with a focus on Long Island, NY. Areas of support include human services, disability services, mental health, schools, rehabilitation, hospitals, and health facilities. Grants provide program support. There are no application deadlines.
Requirements: Schools and other nonprofits in New York are eligible. Applicants outside New York should call or write prior to submitting proposals.
Geographic Focus: New York
Amount of Grant: $25,000-$375,000 average range
Date(s) Application is Due: Mar 1; Jun 1; Sep 1; Nov 1
Contact: Robert Vizza , President, (516) 629-2103; fax: (516) 629-2183
Sponsor: Dolan Foundations
1 Media Crossways
Woodbury, NY 11797

Dole Food Company Charitable Contributions 1307
Dole's charitable program is dedicated to bringing about positive change in the area of nutrition education for children. The goal of the program is to help the next generation of adults prevent many diseases by teaching the value of good nutrition to children through improved and interactive teaching curriculum for schools nationwide.
Requirements: Dole's program makes grants based on the following guidelines: the program is restricted to funding 501(c)3 charitable organizations only; documentation from the I.R.S. confirming 501(c)3 status must be provided; and the organization should provide nutrition education programs that benefit schools on a nationwide basis as opposed to assisting an individual school.
Restrictions: Grants are restricted for the following: individuals; religious, fraternal, sports or political groups; legislative or lobbying efforts or groups who have a primary focus of changing laws; and sporting events and sponsorships.
Contact: Corporate Contributions, (818) 879-6600; fax: (818) 879-6615
Internet: http://dolecsr.com/Principles/CharitableGiving/tabid/410/Default.aspx
Sponsor: Dole Food Company Inc
P.O. Box 5132
Westlake Village, CA 91361

Dominion Educational Partnership Grant 1308

The Foundation is accepting applications to encourage the development of new programs to strengthen math and science education in kindergarten through grade 12. Successful proposals should represent innovative and promising ideas, teach math and/or science skills, reach a significant number of students and demonstrate broad-based community support.
Requirements: Accredited public and private elementary and secondary schools, public school divisions, institutions of higher education, state agencies and 501(c)3 non-profit organizations are invited to apply.
Restrictions: Awards are throughout a 10-state area to include: Connecticut, Maryland, Massachusetts, North Carolina, Ohio, Pennsylvania, Rhode Island, Texas, Virginia and West Virginia. Information pertaining to the specific counties served in each state is on the website.
Geographic Focus: Connecticut; Maryland; Massachusetts; North Carolina; Ohio; Pennsylvania; Rhode Island; Texas; Virginia; West Virginia
Amount of Grant: $10,000
Contact: Educational Partnerships Coordinator; (800) 730-7217; fax: (412) 690-7608; email: Educational_Grants@dom.com
Internet: http://www.dom.com/about/education/grants/index.jsp
Sponsor: Dominion Foundation
625 Liberty Avenue, 21st Floor
Pittsburgh, PA 15222-3199

Donaghue Practical Benefit Initiatives Grants 1309

The foundation initiates research projects showing particular promise for producing practical benefit to human health and works in an interactive process with prospective investigators to develop projects for funding. Organizations with project ideas aimed at productive ways to deliver practical benefit to the public through health research should submit a short summary letter. There is no specific timeline for application or designated grant award amount.
Contact: Director of Operations, (860) 521-9011; fax: (860) 521-9018; email: office@donaghue.org
Internet: http://www.donaghue.org
Sponsor: Patrick and Catherine Weldon Donaghue Medical Research Foundation
18 N Main Street
West Hartford, CT 06107-1919

Donald and Sylvia Robinson Family Foundation Grants 1310

The foundation awards grants to U.S. nonprofit organizations in its areas of interest, including animal and wildlife protection, arms control, arts (general, performing arts, and visual arts), environmental conservation and protection, eye diseases and eye research, family planning and human reproductive health, food distribution, international affairs, Israel, Jewish social services, and social service delivery programs. Types of support include annual campaigns, building construction/renovation, capital campaigns, and general operating support. There are no application deadlines or forms.
Requirements: National nonprofit organizations are eligible to apply.
Restrictions: Individuals are ineligible.
Geographic Focus: Pennsylvania
Amount of Grant: $500-$5,000 range
Contact: Donald Robinson, Treasurer; (412) 661-1200; fax: (412) 661-4645
Sponsor: Donald and Sylvia Robinson Family Foundation
6507 Wilkins Avenue
Pittsburgh, PA 15217

Dora Roberts Foundation Grants 1311

The foundation awards general operating grants to eligible Texas organizations in its areas of interest, Arts, Social Services, Health and Education. Most grants are awarded in Big Spring, TX. There are no application forms. Trustees meet annually in the Fall to review all requests received prior to the deadline.
Requirements: The Foundation can distribute grants only to qualified charitable organizations in the State of Texas. Persons who represent an organization which they believe might qualify for our support are welcome to submit an application in letter form containing: a brief narrative history of the organization's purpose and work; a specific description of the program or project for which support is asked; a statement of the amount of funds requested; proof of tax exempt status; a list of Trustees or Directors and principal staff; and budgetary information pertaining to the requested grant.
Restrictions: The Foundation does not give or lend money to individuals.
Geographic Focus: Rhode Island
Date(s) Application is Due: Sep 30
Contact: Konnie Darrow, c/o JP Morgan Chase Bank, N.A., (817) 884-4772
Sponsor: Dora Roberts Foundation
P.O. Box 2050
Fort Worth, TX 76113

Doreen Kronick Scholarship 1312

This scholarship is awarded annually to a graduate student in a program that will lead to the recipient's being able to assist persons with learning disabilities. Application forms are available from the association or the faculty of graduate studies at Canadian universities.
Requirements: Any student, 18 or older, enrolled in any graduate program of any university in Canada is eligible.
Restrictions: Scholarship recipients will not be eligible to reapply for three years.
Amount of Grant: $C500
Date(s) Application is Due: May 15
Contact: Kronick Scholarships, (613) 238-5721; fax: (613) 235-5391; email: information@ldac-taac.ca
Internet: http://www.ldac-taac.ca/Scholarships/scholarships-e.asp
Sponsor: Learning Disabilities Association of Canada
323 Chapel Street, Suite 200
Ottawa, ON K1N 7Z2 Canada

Doris and Victor Day Foundation Grants 1313

The foundation supports local community organizations providing food, shelter, clothing, medical care, and education in Illinois/Iowa Quad Cities region. Preference will be given to preventive programs and projects that foster pride in the local community. Types of support include general operating support, building/renovation, equipment, emergency funds, seed grants, and scholarship funds.
Requirements: Illinois/Iowa Quad Cities region nonprofit organizations may apply.
Restrictions: The Foundation is committed to programs that are non-sectarian, and therefore, will not contribute toward programs and capital projects for religious purposes, except for modest contributions to the churches in which the Days held membership. However, clearly non-sectarian, community serving programs of religious organizations will be considered for funding.
Geographic Focus: Illinois; Iowa
Date(s) Application is Due: May 1
Contact: Program Contact, (309) 788-2300; email: info@dayfoundation.org
Internet: http://www.dayfoundation.org/guide.htm
Sponsor: Doris and Victor Day Foundation Grants
1800 3rd Avenue, Suite 302
Rock Island, IL 61201-8019

Doris Duke Charitable Foundation Clinical Interfaces Award Program 1314

The program seeks to catalyze activity at the interface of clinical and other research disciplines by: supporting the formation of new collaborations and strengthening existing collaborations of outstanding scientists across disciplines; demonstrating successful models for clinical research at the interface of multiple disciplines; and supporting interdisciplinary and inter-institutional endeavors that go beyond the program project mindset. Full grants, awarded over five years, are made to established teams with key investigators from at least three disciplines. Planning grants are awarded to new teams for the development of full proposals over 18 months. The listed application deadline is for pre-proposals; full proposals are by invitation. Though new grants are not being offered continually, potential applicants can sign up to be notified of future competitions.
Requirements: Teams of at least three key investigators whose primary expertise lie in different disciplines are eligible to apply. Key investigators must have advanced degrees (MD, PhD, MD/PhD, or the equivalent), and one of the key investigators must be a clinical researcher. The team leader must work in a U.S. nonprofit institution, such as an academic medical center. The team may include investigators at other institutions in the United States and overseas.
Restrictions: Planning grants will not be awarded in the current competition.
Amount of Grant: $2.25 million maximum over 5 years
Date(s) Application is Due: Nov 2
Contact: Elaine K. Gallin, Program Director; (212) 974-7104; fax: (212) 974-7590; email: egallin@ddcf.org
Internet: http://www.ddcf.org/page.asp?pageId=299
Sponsor: Doris Duke Charitable Foundation
650 Fifth Avenue, 19th Floor
New York, NY 10019

Doris Duke Charitable Foundation Clinical Research Fellowships for Medical Students 1315

The fellowship program is designed to encourage medical students to pursue careers in clinical research by giving exceptional students the opportunity to take a year to experience clinical research first hand. The CRF program is available at the following medical schools: Columbia University College of Physicians and Surgeons; Harvard Medical School; Mount Sinai School of Medicine; University of California at San Francisco School of Medicine; University of Iowa Roy J. and Lucille A. Carver College of Medicine; University of North Carolina at Chapel Hill School of Medicine; University of Pennsylvania School of Medicine; University of Texas Southwestern Medical Center at Dallas; Washington University Medical School; and Yale University School of Medicine. An additional 11-12 fellowships will be available to medical students interested in conducting clinical research in Africa. Each participating medical school provides medical students with a one-year fellowship experience in clinical research that includes both didactic and research components; matches students to outstanding clinical research mentors; and offers fellowships to at least five students per year.
Requirements: Medical students matriculated at any U.S. medical school who have completed two or more years of medical school prior to the start of the fellowship and who have completed some clinical experience are eligible to apply to any of the participating schools.
Amount of Grant: $27,000 plus health insurance
Date(s) Application is Due: Jan 18
Contact: Elaine K. Gallin, Program Director; (212) 974-7104; fax: (212) 974-7590; email: egallin@ddcf.org
Internet: http://www.ddcf.org/page.asp?pageId=292
Sponsor: Doris Duke Charitable Foundation
650 Fifth Avenue, 19th Floor
New York, NY 10019

Doris Duke Charitable Foundation Clinical Scientist Development Award 1316

Grants are awarded to junior physician-scientists to facilitate their transition to independent clinical research careers. The program is designed to help prepare and support new investigators with an MD or MD/PhD as they begin their careers as independent clinical researchers. The program is aimed at conducting clinical research in any disease area. The listed application deadline is for preproposals, which must be submitted electronically.

Requirements: Applicants must: be a physician-scientist conducting clinical research in any disease area; have received an M.D. or a foreign equivalent from an accredited institution; be working in a U.S. degree-granting institution, but do not have to be a U.S. citizen; have a full-time faculty level position not higher than the Assistant Professor level; and have been appointed to their first full-time faculty level position between January 31, 2002 and January 31 of the grant year. (All full-time post-fellowship Instructor level positions will be considered full-time faculty level appointments).

Restrictions: Funds cannot be used on experiments that utilize animals or primary tissues derived from animals. An award will not be made if, prior to the commencement of the award, the applicant becomes the principal investigator on a federal government, peer-reviewed, research or career development award or any non-government award averaging more than $126,000 per year in direct costs and of a duration of three or more years.

Amount of Grant: $125,000 (direct costs) per year and $10,000 (indirect costs) per year for three years

Date(s) Application is Due: Jan 23

Contact: Elaine K. Gallin, Program Director; (212) 974-7104; fax: (212) 974-7590; email: egallin@ddcf.org

Internet: http://www.ddcf.org/page.asp?pageId=291

Sponsor: Doris Duke Charitable Foundation
650 Fifth Avenue, 19th Floor
New York, NY 10019

Doris Duke Charitable Foundation Clinical Scientist Development Award Bridge Grants 1317

The purpose of the bridge grant is to help Doris Duke Clinical Scientist Development Award (CSDA) recipients successfully transition to independent National Institutes of Health (NIH) R01 funding. The Medical Research Program created these grants to bridge the time between when a CSDA investigator learns of a very strong but unfunded score on an NIH application to when s/he is able to successfully obtain an R01 grant. The bridge grants provide protected time and support for CSDA recipients to continue their research projects, collect supportive data, keep patients enrolled if applicable, and strengthen their proposals to resubmit to the NIH. The foundation hopes that the bridge grants will help keep promising physician-scientists committed to clinical research careers by providing stable support during their critical transition to independent R01 funding. The foundation will award up to four bridge grants of $135,000 each to be spent only on direct costs over 12 to 18 months. Eligible CSDA recipients are invited to submit applications throughout the year up to the deadline of September 1.

Requirements: This competition is open only to former CSDA grantees or current CSDA grantees in the last year of their award (or in a no-cost extension period).

Amount of Grant: $135,000 maximum

Date(s) Application is Due: Sep 1

Contact: Elaine Gallin, Program Director for Medical Research; (212) 974-7104; fax: (212) 974-7590; email: egallin@ddcf.org

Internet: http://www.ddcf.org/page.asp?pageId=291

Sponsor: Doris Duke Charitable Foundation
650 Fifth Avenue, 19th Floor
New York, NY 10019

Doris Duke Charitable Foundation Distinguished Clinical Scientist Award 1318

The purpose of the program is to recognize outstanding physician-scientists who are engaged in applying the latest basic science advances to the prevention, diagnosis, treatment, and cure of disease, and to enable the physician-scientist to support and mentor the next generation of physician-scientists conducting translational clinical research. Awards will be granted to physician-scientists conducting translational clinical research in any disease area; this award cycle is not limited to specific disease areas.

Requirements: Grantees must hold an M.D. degree from an accredited institution in the United States (holders of M.D./Ph.D. degrees are also eligible, as are holders of M.D.-equivalent degrees from non-U.S. institutions); hold a full-time university faculty appointment at the level of Associate Professor or above as of the date of nomination; have been appointed to their first full-time, faculty-level position for no more than 15 years; and have an established translational clinical research program.

Restrictions: Experiments that utilize animals or primary tissues derived from animals are not eligible for support through this award program. An award will not be made if, prior to the commencement of the foundation's award, the applicant becomes the principal investigator of a federal government, peer-reviewed, research or career development award or of any nongovernment award averaging $100,000 or more per year and of three years or more duration.

Amount of Grant: $1.5 million maximum

Date(s) Application is Due: Feb 14

Contact: Elaine Gallin, Program Director for Medical Research; (212) 974-7104; fax: (212) 974-7590; email: egallin@ddcf.org

Internet: http://www.ddcf.org/page.asp?pageId=297

Sponsor: Doris Duke Charitable Foundation
650 Fifth Avenue, 19th Floor
New York, NY 10019

Doris Duke Charitable Foundation Operations Research on AIDS Care and Treatment in Africa (ORACTA) Grants 1319

The Program seeks to improve the care and treatment of AIDS patients in resource-limited settings, inform antiretroviral therapy (ART) policy and practice, and improve outcomes of the roll-out and scale-up of ART in Africa. ORACTA grants provide two-year grants of up to $100,000 per year to teams of investigators conducting health operations research on AIDS care and treatment in Africa. Though new grants are offered only periodically, applicants should sign up for the Medical Research Program's mailing list.

Restrictions: Indirect costs are not supported by this award.

Amount of Grant: $100,000 per year for two years

Contact: Elaine Gallin, Program Director for Medical Research; (212) 974-7104; fax: (212) 974-7590; email: egallin@ddcf.org

Internet: http://www.ddcf.org/page.asp?pageId=486

Sponsor: Doris Duke Charitable Foundation
650 Fifth Avenue, 19th Floor
New York, NY 10019

Dorothea Haus Ross Foundation Grants 1320

The foundation awards grants to eligible nonprofit organizations that work to relieve suffering among children who are sick, handicapped, injured, disfigured, orphaned, or otherwise vulnerable. Types of support include direct services, medical research, equipment and supplies, and small renovation projects. There are no application deadlines. Grants have supported projects for children in Native American schools and schools that serve populations of children who are disadvantaged or underserved.

Requirements: U.S. Charities may apply if: they have 501(c)3 status; they are listed in the current edition of the Cumulative List of Charities published by the U.S. Department of the Treasury; they are a Catholic organization listed in the current edition of the Catholic Director; or they are listed in the Free Methodist Yearbook, or other Protestant Denomination Directory that has a group ruling for tax exemption from the IRS. Although grants are made internationally, Foundation by-laws prohibit sending money directly to foreign charities.

Restrictions: The Foundation does not fund day-to-day operations, individuals, conferences, day care, or public education. Although the Foundation makes international grants, there are restrictions in some countries for the following reasons: war, widespread violence, or breakdown of law and order; or countries where grants are restricted by the U.S. Government due to a boycott or other reason.

Contact: Wayne Cook, Executive Director, (716) 473-6006; fax: (716) 473-6007; email: rossfoundation@frontiernet.net

Internet: http://www.dhrossfoundation.org/index.html

Sponsor: Dorothea Haus Ross Foundation
1036 Monroe Avenue
Rochester, NY 14620

Dorothy Hooper Beattie Foundation Grants 1321

The Foundation primarily supports higher education, health care, and religious programs in and around the Greenville, South Carolina, region. Its program interests include: camps; cancer treatment; Catholicism; children and youth programs; higher education; health services; literacy; and the environment. Grants range from $620 to $6,500, and there are no specific deadlines or application forms. Initial approach should be by letter, with telephone contacts discouraged. Mail applications to: Bank of America, 7 North Laurens Street, Greenville, SC 29601.

Geographic Focus: South Carolina

Samples: The Bernardine Fund St. Francis, Greenville, SC, $620 (2006); Upstate Forever, Greenville, SC, $1,345 (2006); Greenville Free Medical Clinic, Greenville, SC, $4,000 (2006); United Ministries, Greenville, SC, $6,500 (2006).

Amount of Grant: $620-$6,500 range

Contact: Mary W. Green, Bank of America; (864) 271-5789

Sponsor: Dorothy Hooper Beattie Foundation
101 South Tryon Street
Charlotte, NC 28255

Dorothy Rider Pool Health Care Grants 1322

The Foundation's intent is to serve as a means to improve the quality of life in the Lehigh Valley community, to build on community strengths and add to its vitality, and to increase the capacity of the community to serve the needs of all its citizens. Within this objective the Foundation's funding program is focused on education, health and welfare, culture and art and community development. Interested applicants should submit a letter of intent of five pages or less.

Requirements: Allentown, PA, nonprofit organizations are eligible.

Restrictions: The Foundation is restricted from providing funds to individuals, legislative or lobbying efforts, political or fraternal organizations or organizations outside the United States and its territories. The Foundation as a policy does not provide operating or capital funds to Sectarian institutions, organizations or programs in which funds will be used primarily for the propagation of religion, hospitals or United Way member agencies. Further, the Foundation does not underwrite charitable or testimonial dinners, fund-raising events or related advertising or the subsidization of books, mailings or articles in professional journals.

Geographic Focus: Pennsylvania

Samples: Lehigh Valley Hospital and Health (Allentown, PA)—for its department of obstetrics and gynecology, $225,000 over three years.; Lehigh Valley Hospital and Health Network (Allentown, PA)—for the department of emergency medicine's sexual assault response team, $150,000 over three years.; Lehigh Valley Hospital and Health

Network (Allentown, PA)—for the Physician Leaders in the Lehigh Valley program, $120,000 over three years.
Amount of Grant: $100,000
Date(s) Application is Due: Apr 1; Aug 15
Contact: Ronald Dendas, Program Manager, (610) 770-9346; fax: (610) 770-9361; email: drpool@ptd.net
Internet: http://www.pooltrust.com
Sponsor: Dorothy Rider Pool Health Care Trust
1050 S. Cedar Crest Boulevard, Suite 202
Allentown, PA 18103

Dorrance Family Foundation Grants **1323**
The Dorrance Family Foundation was founded by Bennett Dorrance, co-owner of the Campbell Soup Company. The Foundation gives primarily in the state of Arizona, offering support in the areas of : education; national resources; arts and museums.
Requirements: No formal application form is required, non-profits operating in Arizona are eligible to apply for these grants. Applicants should submit a proposal consisting of a detailed description of project and amount of funding requested.
Restrictions: No funding available to individuals.
Geographic Focus: Arizona
Contact: Carolyn O'Malley, Program Officer, (480) 367-7000
Sponsor: Dorrance Family Foundation
7600 East Doubletree Ranch Road, Suite 300
Scottsdale, AZ 85258

DPA Promoting Policy Change Advocacy Grants **1324**
The program seeks to broaden public and political support for drug policy reform and will fund strategic and innovative approaches to increase such support. Proposals should be designed to: educate the public and policymakers about the negative consequences of current local, state or national drug policies; promote better awareness and understanding of alternatives to current drug policies; and broaden awareness and understanding of the extent to which punitive prohibitionist policies are responsible for most drug-related problems around the country.
Requirements: 501(c)3 tax-exempt organizations and organizations with 501(c)3 fiscal sponsors are eligible. All grantmaking will be directed to organizations working within the United States, and possibly Canada, with particular emphasis on state-based activity.
Amount of Grant: $50,000
Date(s) Application is Due: Jun 15
Contact: Asha Bandele, (212) 613-8020; fax: (212) 613-8021; email: abandele@drugpolicy.org
Internet: http://www.drugpolicy.org/about/jobsfunding/grants/index.cfm
Sponsor: Drug Policy Alliance
70 West 36th Street, 16th Floor
New York, NY 10018

Dr. Bob and Jean Smith Foundation Grants **1325**
The foundation awards grants to Texas nonprofit organizations in its areas of interest, including arts and culture, higher education, medical education, medical research, and health care. Types of support include annual campaigns, building construction/renovation, capital campaigns, general operating support, matching/challenge grants, and scholarship funds. There are no application deadlines; the board meets quarterly.
Requirements: Texas nonprofit organizations are eligible. Preference is given to Dallas-based organizations.
Restrictions: Individuals are ineligible.
Geographic Focus: Texas
Contact: Sally Smith, Grants Administrator, (214) 521-3461
Sponsor: Dr. Bob and Jean Smith Foundation
3811 Turtle Creek Ctr, No 2150 LB 53
Dallas, TX 75219

Dr. Courtney W. Shropshire Scholarship Grant **1326**
All qualified applicants will be considered without regard to race, creed, sex, or national origin. The grant is to be used only for tuition and approved purposes that are invoiced from the school. Necessary forms are available annually after September 1 from the Civitan International Foundation; please include a self-addressed business envelope with postage to cover two-ounce U.S. mailing.
Requirements: Candidates must be a Civitan member (or a Civitan's immediate family member) and must have been a Civitan for at least two years and/or must be or have been a junior Civitan for no less than two years. Candidates must be enrolled in a degree or certificate program at an accredited community college, vocational school, four-year college, or graduate school.
Amount of Grant: $1000 maximum
Date(s) Application is Due: Jan 31
Contact: Shropshire Scholarship Grant, (205) 591-8910; fax: (205) 592-6307; email: civitan@civitan.org
Internet: http://www.civitaninternational.com/templates/cuscivitan/details.asp?id=23844&PID=155457
Sponsor: Civitan International Foundation
P.O. Box 130744
Birmingham, AL 35213-0744

Dr. John T. Macdonald Foundation Grants **1327**
The foundation awards grants to eligible Florida nonprofit organizations in Miami-Dade County for medical and health-related programs with priority given to those serving children, youth, and economically disadvantaged individuals. The foundation supports medical rehabilitation, disease prevention, and health education. Types of support include capital grants, matching/challenge grants, program development grants, seed money grants, and training grants. Deadline listed is for letters of intent; full proposals are by request. Annual deadline dates may vary; contact program staff for exact dates.
Requirements: Florida nonprofit organizations serving the health care needs of people in Miami-Dade County are eligible. Priority will be given to projects in the Coral Gables community.
Restrictions: Grants do not support national projects, multiyear funding requests, for-profit organizations, political candidates or campaigns, religious projects, individuals, or other grantmaking foundations.
Geographic Focus: Florida
Samples: Voices for Children Foundation (Hollywood, FL)—to hire a case coordinator for the Guardian Ad Litem Program, which provides advocacy for abused, neglected, and abandoned children, $30,000.; U of Miami (Coral Gables, FL)—to create a new genetics-research center, and for a public school health program that will serve as a national model for school-based health centers, $12.5 million over five years.
Date(s) Application is Due: Apr 15
Contact: Kim Greene, Executive Director, (305) 667-6017; fax: (305) 667-9135; email: info@jtmacdonaldfdn.org
Internet: http://www.jtmacdonaldfdn.org
Sponsor: Dr. John T. Macdonald Foundation
1550 Madruga Avenue, Suite 215
Coral Gables, FL 33146

Dr. Leon Bromberg Charitable Trust Fund Grants **1328**
The trust awards grants to U.S. nonprofit organizations in its areas of interest, including arts, education, hospitals and health organizations, and social services. Types of support include building construction/renovation, capital campaigns, conferences and seminars, equipment acquisition, professorships, scholarship funds, and social services. Preference will be given to requests from Texas nonprofits in Bryan, Galveston, Crockett, and Houston. Applications must be received by the 10th of each month for consideration; the board meets monthly.
Requirements: U.S. nonprofit organizations are eligible.
Restrictions: Grants are not awarded to individuals or for operating grants, endowment funds, or debt reduction.
Samples: U of Texas Medical Branch (Galveston, TX)—to endow a mentor program in the sciences that pairs graduate students, postdoctoral students, and faculty members with high-school students, $250,000.
Contact: Program Contact, (409) 762-5890
Sponsor: Dr. Leon Bromberg Charitable Trust Fund
2200 Market Street, Suite 710
Galveston, TX 77550-1532

Dr. Scholl Foundation Grants Program **1329**
Applications are considered in the following areas: private education, including elementary, secondary, college and university level; programs for children, developmentally disabled, senior citizens, civic and cultural institutions, social service agencies, hospitals and health care, environmental organizations and religious institutions. The general areas of interest are not intended to limit the interest of the foundation from considering other worthwhile projects. An application form is required and may be obtained from the foundation office. All grant applications must be requested in writing. Telephone, email or fax requests will not be accepted.
Requirements: Grants are awarded on an annual basis to valid IRS 501(c)3 organizations. Non-U.S. applicants without a 501(c)3 must complete a notarized affidavit.
Restrictions: Funding is not available for: organizations that do not have a valid IRS 501(c)3 determination letter; political organizations, political action committees, or individual campaigns whose primary purpose is to influence legislation; foundations that are themselves grantmaking bodies; grants to individuals, endowments or capital campaigns; grants for loans, operating deficit reduction, the liquidation of a debt, or general support; event sponsorships including the purchase of tables, tickets or advertisements; or more than one request from the same organization in the same year.
Date(s) Application is Due: Mar 1
Contact: Pamela Scholl, President, (847) 559-7430
Internet: http://www.drschollfoundation.com/procedures.htm
Sponsor: Dr. Scholl Foundation
1033 Skokie Boulevard, Suite 230
Northbrook, IL 60062

Dr. Stanley Pearle Scholarships **1330**
OneSight Research Foundation (formerly known as the Pearle Vision Foundation) will award ten (10) scholarships in the amount of $2,000 each through the Dr. Stanley Pearle Scholarship Fund. Invitation to apply is extended to second, third, and fourth year full-time students pursuing graduate studies leading to a Doctor of Optometry degree. Scholarships will be awarded on a competitive basis, based on scholastic performance and potential and evidence of commitment to a career in the optometric profession and to community service. Applicants will be required to describe accomplishments they believe would qualify them for recognition in general, and specifically, accomplishments in the areas of leadership, community service, and extracurricular activities.

Requirements: Students accepted to, or enrolled in, a fully accredited college or university that is an Approved Educational Institution pursuing full-time graduate studies in an optometry program accredited by the Accreditation Council on Optometric Education of the American Optometric Association ("ACOE") are eligible to apply. Scholarships are not renewable, but an individual may re-apply for a Scholarship. OneSight values diversity. Members of racial and ethnic minorities are especially encouraged to apply. All scholarships will be awarded on an objective, non-discriminatory basis.
Restrictions: Limited to students in graduating class 2010, 2011 or 2012.
Amount of Grant: $2,000
Date(s) Application is Due: Apr 15
Contact: Trina Parasiliti, Administrator; (972) 277-6191; fax: (972) 277-6414; email: tparasil@onesight.org
Internet: http://www.onesight.org/northamerica/na/
Sponsor: OneSight Research Foundation
2465 Joe Field Road
Dallas, TX 75229

Dr. Sydney Segal Research Grants **1331**
Research grants are awarded to enable students to pursue full-time higher degree studies at a Canadian institution researching the possible causes, effects, and/or prevention of sudden infant death syndrome. The research grants are awarded for one year in any discipline—medical, psychological, biological, sociological, nursing, or other. Contact the foundation for applications.
Requirements: Applications are invited from suitably qualified graduate students who are undertaking full-time training in research in the health sciences leading to an MSC, PhD, or equivalent degree.
Amount of Grant: $C35,000 maximum
Date(s) Application is Due: Jun 1
Contact: Executive Director, (800) 363-7437 or (416) 488-3260; fax: (416) 488-3864; email: sidsinfo@sidscanada.org
Internet: http://www.sidscanada.org/segal_research_grants.htm
Sponsor: Canadian Foundation for the Study of Infant Deaths
586 Eglinton Ave E, Suite 308
Toronto, ON M4P 1P2 Canada

Dreitzer Foundation Grants **1332**
The foundation awards general operating grants to nonprofit organizations in its areas of interest, including health, homeless, social services, and youth programs. Grants are awarded nationally, with preference given to New York nonprofits. Applications are available by mail or fax. Phone calls are strongly discouraged.
Requirements: 501(c)3 tax-exempt organizations in New York are eligible.
Geographic Focus: New York
Samples: Partnership for the Homeless (New York, NY)—grant recipient, $50,000.; Ethical Culture Society of Queens (Bayside, NY)—grant recipient, $25,000.
Amount of Grant: $5000-$65,000 range
Date(s) Application is Due: Jul 1
Contact: Alan Seget, (212) 557-7700; fax: (212) 286-8513
Sponsor: Dreitzer Foundation
60 E 42nd Street, 38th Floor
New York, NY 10165

Drs. Bruce and Lee Foundation Grants **1333**
The Foundation's goal is to advance the general welfare and the quality of all life in the Florence, S.C. area by providing economic support to qualified programs and non-profit organizations. The Foundation will support a broad range of charitable purposes including, but not limited to: medical; health; human services; education; arts; religion; civic affairs; and the conservation, preservation and promotion of cultural, historical and environmental resources. There are no application deadlines.
Requirements: Florence, SC, nonprofit organizations are eligible.
Restrictions: The Foundation does not purchase tickets for fundraising events. Grants to individuals will not be considered.
Geographic Focus: South Carolina
Samples: Francis Marion U (Florence, SC)—to construct a facility for the new bachelor's-degree nursing program, $5 million (2004).
Contact: L. Bradley Callicott, Executive Director, (843) 664-2870; email: blfound@bellsouth.net
Sponsor: Drs. Bruce and Lee Foundation
181 East Evans Street, BTC Box 022
Florence, SC 29506

DSO Controlling Pathogen Evolution Workshop Grants **1334**
The goal of the workshop is to explore: the potential of computational methods to precisely predict pathogen evolution; and vaccination and/or therapeutic strategies to control direction of pathogen evolution. The workshop will investigate tools for predicting protective epitopes, pathogen evolution and protein structure, and then review strategies to force pathogens into an evolutionary trap that prevents escape through mutation. From there, vaccines and therapies can be developed against the particular pathogen strain. Workshop participants are strongly encouraged to prepare posters describing previous or potential research in the area in order to facilitate discussions and/or formation of well-rounded teams.
Requirements: Attendees should have specific expertise in infectious disease, epitope prediction (computational and/or immunomic), vaccinology, mathematical modeling, protein structure, pathogen evolution, drug design, and/or animal modeling.
Date(s) Application is Due: Mar 16
Contact: Dr. Michael V. Callahan, Program Manager; (571) 218-4596; fax: (571) 218-4553; email: michael.callahan@darpa.mil
Internet: http://www.darpa.mil/baa/SN07-21.html
Sponsor: Defense Sciences Office within the Defense Advanced Research Projects Agency (DARPA)
3701 North Fairfax Drive
Arlington, VA 22203-1714

DSO Radiation Biodosimetry (RaBiD) Grants **1335**
The DSO is seeking proposals for new technologies for rapid, high-throughput, portable and low-cost biodosimeters to determine radiation dose to individuals after acute radiation exposure. This technology would provide rapid identification of individuals who have been exposed to high-dose radiation in order to accurately assess radiation exposure levels. The Program is a single phase, 15-month program with a goal of revolutionizing radiation exposure detection. The first 12 months consist of scientific research and development during which the proposer will develop a non- or minimally-invasive radiological biodosimeter and demonstrate accurate radiological detection from biological samples into quartiles of doses for humans with a detection time less than 10 minutes. This will include radiological dose/detection curves, as well as multipoint data regarding decay of biological signal as a function of time after radiation exposure. A successful proposal will demonstrate a clear path to these deliverables, including a timeline for technology development, experimentation, and delivery of results.
Requirements: All proposers must provide evidence of a competent team capable of developing a new radiation biodosimetry technology meeting all program objectives and milestones. The Program requires that each proposal include a team with demonstrated (or established) capability. At a minimum, proposers are expected to possess expertise or demonstrate collaboration with professionals in the following areas: radiation biologist/radiation oncologist—with expertise in radiation exposure to animal models; and engineering—with developmental expertise needed to translate biological sampling to radiation readout.
Restrictions: Only unclassified proposals will be accepted in response.
Date(s) Application is Due: Jul 9
Contact: Dr. Mildred Donlon, Program Manager; (703) 696-2289; fax: (703) 741-3896; email: mildred.donlon@darpa.mil
Internet: http://www.darpa.mil/dso/solicitations/baa07-29.htm
Sponsor: Defense Sciences Office within the Defense Advanced Research Projects Agency (DARPA)
3701 North Fairfax Drive
Arlington, VA 22203-1714

Dubois County Community Foundation Grants **1336**
The central purpose of the community foundation is to serve the needs of Dubois County, Indiana and the philanthropic aims of donors who wish to better their community. The Foundations fields of interests are: arts, education, environment, beautification programs, health care, human services, recreation, youth development.
Requirements: Application: obtain grant application form from the Dubois County Community Foundation offices. Completed "Grant Application Form," "Grant Agreement,"and "Grant Application Certification." Attachments: Program Narrative - expansion upon the summary including program procedures, indication of whom the program will serve and an estimated number of individuals so served, personnel involved, anticipated results, and internal evaluation procedures; IRS 501(c)3 Determination Letter; Governing Body Information - names of the organization's officers, directors, and key project personnel; Detailed Project Budget - identification of all projected expenses AND anticipated income associated with the program in justification of the amount being requested; Most recent Audit Report and/or Financial Report; Visual materials may be submitted as appendices. Submit one original and 11 copies of your complete application (a total of 12)
Restrictions: Giving concentrated in Dubois County, Indiana. No support for the operational expenses of government units or agencies. No grants for operating expenses of nonprofits, funding after the fact, annual fund raising, sponsorship of events, or debt retirement, no loans.
Geographic Focus: Indiana
Date(s) Application is Due: Sep 15
Contact: Marilyn Rumbach Weisheit, Executive Director, (812) 482-5295; fax (812) 482-7461; email: dccf@fullnet.com
Internet: http://www.duboiscountycommunityfoundation.org/grant process.htm
Sponsor: Dubois County Community Foundation
323 East Sixth Street or P.O. Box 269
Jasper, Indiana 47547-0269

Duchossois Family Foundation Grants **1337**
The foundation focuses its efforts in the Chicago metropolitan area and gives primary consideration to nonprofit organizations that contribute to the community in the area of health. The foundation supports organizations involved with mental health/crisis services, cancer, HIV/AIDS, cancer research, AIDS research and, human services. A one-page summary-request letter should include a description of the organization and its specific needs and purposes, the amount requested, and a list of members of the board of directors and their business/professional affiliations.
Requirements: 501(c)3 tax-exempt public charities serving the Chicago metropolitan area are eligible.
Geographic Focus: Illinois

Samples: American Cancer Society, Chicago, IL, $50,000 (2008); Metropolitan Family Services, Chicago, IL, $125,000 (2008); Barrington Area Council on Aging, Barrington, IL, $2,500 (2008).
Contact: Iris Krieg, Executive Director; (312) 641-5765; email: iriskriegl@aol.com
Sponsor: Duchossois Family Foundation
203 North Wabash, Suite 1800
Chicago, IL 60601

Duke Endowment Health Care Grants **1338**
The purpose of the program is to: improve the quality and safety of health care in the areas of patient quality and safety programs/intervention, workforce development, and health information technology; improve access to health care in the areas of care for the medically indigent/uninsured, mental health care, and where racial disparities are evident; and expand prevention and early intervention in the areas of child health and early intervention programs, wellness and healthy lifestyle programs, and disease management.
Requirements: The endowment awards grants in North Carolina and South Carolina to: not-for-profit hospitals; academic health centers; health education centers; and select health organizations in counties without an eligible hospital.
Geographic Focus: North Carolina; South Carolina
Date(s) Application is Due: Dec 15; Jun 15
Contact: Mary L. Piepenbring, Director; (704) 376-0291; fax: (704) 376-9336; email: mpiepenbring@tde.org
Internet: http://www.dukeendowment.org/program-areas/health-care
Sponsor: Duke Endowment
100 N. Tryon Street, Suite 3500
Charlotte, NC 28202-4012

Duke Energy Foundation Grants **1339**
The Duke Energy Foundation gives primarily in areas of company operations in Indiana, Kentucky, North Carolina, Ohio and South Carolina. At the core of The Duke Energy Foundation is its commitment to the community, with a focus in three areas: Environment and Energy Efficiency; Economic Development; and Community Vitality.
Requirements: Organizations with a 501(c)3 verification from the IRS or are a part of a governmental entity are eligible. All organizations applying for a grant must have: completed the Online Grant Application; a clear reason for making the contribution that relates to the areas of focus; regular reports on the measurable results of the project.
Restrictions: Foundation funds are not provided for: organizations that discriminate by race, creed, gender, age or national origin; political activities and organizations; grants to individual agencies of the United Way or the Charlotte Arts and Science Council; capital campaigns and endowments, except in extremely rare and specialized situations that relate directly to our areas of expertise in business; individuals; athletics, including individual sports teams and all-star teams; underwriting of films, video and television productions; reducing the cost of utility service; sectarian or religious activities; conferences, trips or tours; fraternal, veteran or labor groups serving only their members; advertising; membership fees or association fees, either personal or corporate; dinners or tables at fund-raisers are rarely considered; family foundations.
Geographic Focus: Indiana; Kentucky; North Carolina; Ohio; South Carolina
Samples: Arts and Science Council of Charlotte-Mecklenburg, Charlotte, NC., $1,250,000 - for capital support (2007); United Way of Cleveland County, Shelby, NC., $12,610 - for operating support (2007); Greater Cincinnati Arts and Education Center, Cincinnati, OH., $550,000 - for capital support (2007);
Amount of Grant: $1,000-$1,250,000 range
Contact: Deanita McCall, Vice President; (704) 382-7200; fax: (704) 382-7600;
Internet: http://www.duke-energy.com/community/foundation.asp
Sponsor: Duke Energy
P.O. Box 35469
Charlotte, NC 28254

Duke University Adult Cardiothoracic Anesthesia and Critical Care Medicine Fellowships **1340**
Nine one year fellowship positions are available each year in the ACGME Accredited Fellowship. Second year research and clinical fellowship opportunities are available; programs are individualized to meet the goals of successful applicants. Generally clinical experience is the focus of the first fellowship year, along with involvement in clinical research. Fellows opting for a two year fellowship continue with one clinical day per week in their second year, in addition to a structured plan involving laboratory and/or clinical research and teaching. Second year clinical specialization in pediatric cardiac anesthesiology or intensive care is also available. The Adult cardiothoracic Anesthesia Fellowship is highly recommended as formal training for specialization in cardiac and/or thoracic anesthesiology. The Fellowship is designed to develop clinical, consultant, and in-depth research expertise. Applications are usually considered starting 18 months prior to the start date
Requirements: Complete application (see Duke University website), in addition to the references required, include a letter from your Chairperson/Program Director and two letters from other faculty members who have worked with you closely.
Contact: Mark S. Smith, Director; (919) 681-5046 or (919) 416-3853; fax: (919)681-8993
Internet: http://medschool.duke.edu/modules/som_rt/index.php?id=1
Sponsor: Duke University Medical Center, Department of Anesthesiology
P.O. Box 3094
Durham, NC 27710

Duke University Ambulatory and Regional Anesthesia Fellowships **1341**
The Fellowship in Ambulatory/Regional Anesthesia is designed to provide advanced training in anesthesia in the ambulatory surgery setting. This program will be an extension to the previous training with an emphases on the continued educational component to include research, clinical and teaching responsibilities.
Requirements: The selection process for fellows includes the completion of a Fellowship Application (see website) which is to be substantiated by three letters of recommendation from experts in the field. In addition to the letters of reference the application is to include a current CV and a letter of affirmation stating interest in the program.
Date(s) Application is Due: Aug 15
Contact: Stephen M. Klein, Director; (919) 668-2056; email: klein006@mc.duke.edu;; LuAnne Latta, Staff Assistant to Dr. Stephen M. Klein; (919) 681-9941; email: latta005@mc.duke.edu
Internet: http://anesthesiology.duke.edu/modules/anes_flwshp/index.php?id=1
Sponsor: Duke University Medical Center, Department of Anesthesiology
P.O. Box 3094 #4
Durham, NC 27710

Duke University Clinical Cardiac Electrophysiology Fellowships **1342**
The Clinical Cardiac Electrophysiology fellowship training program is a comprehensive two-year program including training in catheter ablation of supraventricular tachycardias, ventricular tachycardias, and complex arrhythmias such as atrial fibrillation, ischemic VT, and arrhythmias associated with congenital heart disease. Comprehensive training is also provided in lead extraction and device therapy including permanent pacing, implantable defibrillators, and bi-ventricular devices. Fellows are provided with significant opportunity for research activity through protected block time and are expected to participate in and complete a research project with a faculty mentor. Applicants must have completed at least three years in an ACGME approved Cardiology fellowship program.
Requirements: Applications for training to begin July 1, will be accepted beginning January 1; the application deadline will be September 1. To apply, please include with the completed CCE (EP) Application form (available on the Duke University website), a current curriculum vitae, personal statement (not to exceed 250 words), and the $40 (check or money/order no cash please) processing fee.
Date(s) Application is Due: Sep 1
Contact: Dr. Patrick Hranitzky, Program Director; (919) 684-2304; fax: (919) 684-4322; email: Patrick.hranitzky@duke.edu
Internet: http://fellowships.medicine.duke.edu/modules/fellows_cardio/index.php?id=8
Sponsor: Duke University School of Medicine
P.O. Box 3878
Durham, NC 27710

Duke University Hyperbaric Center Fellowships **1343**
The clinical Hyperbaric fellow works in the Hyperbaric Center and F.G. Hall Environmental Laboratory, both of which are an integral part of Duke University Medical Center. Fellowships are available for 12 months although they may be extended for additional time. During the period of training the Hyperbaric fellow will be trained in the clinical use of hyperbaric oxygen. This includes the emergency treatment of clostridial myonecrosis, necrotizing fasciitis, arterial gas embolism, decompression sickness, carbon monoxide poisoning and certain other less common conditions such as acute vasculitis with ischemia. The fellow will receive training in the appropriate critical care interventions necessary for the treatment of these patients. This will include hemodynamic monitoring, ventilatory support, fluid resuscitation and the interpretation of arterial blood gases during hyperbaric therapy. The fellow will also receive training in the use of hyperbaric oxygen therapy for non-emergency conditions. The fellow will be responsible for all inpatient and outpatient consults, under the direction of the clinical Hyperbaric faculty. During the training period the fellow will also be required to complete a research project. This will be completed under the guidance of one of the faculty members in the Hyperbaric Center. Part of the didactic program includes regular hyperbaric conferences. The fellow will participate in these and normally be required to present at least one topic during his year of training. The fellow will also have the opportunity to attend the annual two-week course in Hyperbaric and Diving Medicine given by the National Oceanic and Atmospheric Administration in Seattle, Washington. In addition to these activities the applicant may participate in numerous other teaching activities within Duke Medical Center, for example those sponsored by the Departments of Anesthesiology, Medicine, Surgery and Emergency Medicine. Clinical participation under the aegis of those departments can be arranged in some cases, depending upon the training of the individual concerned.
Requirements: Applicants must be eligible for license as a trainee in the state of North Carolina. The Duke Hyperbaric Center Fellowship Application can be downloaded at: http://hyperbaric.mc.duke.edu/education.htm
Contact: John J. Freiberger M.D., Program Director; (919) 668-0005; email: freib002@mc.duke.edu;; Ms. Tonya Manning, Assistant; (919) 681-1685 or (919) 684-6726
Internet: http://hyperbaric.mc.duke.edu/education.htm
Sponsor: Duke University Medical Center for Hyperbaric Medicine and Environmental Physiology
P.O. Box 3823
Durham, NC 27710

Duke University Interventional Cardiology Fellowships **1344**
The Interventional Cardiology Fellowship Training Program at Duke University Medical Center focuses on training leaders in Interventional Cardiology committed to a career in academic cardiology. The length of the fellowship is 12 months. During the fellowship,

all fellows will develop both clinical and technical skills in interventional cardiology. All fellows will gain experience in diagnosing, selecting therapies, performing diagnostic and interventional procedures, and judging the effectiveness of treatments for inpatients and outpatients with chronic ischemic heart disease, acute ischemic syndromes, and valvular heart disease. All fellows are expected to participate in research efforts. During the fellowship, each fellow will work with a mentor on a research project which will help foster their long-term goals.
Requirements: Individuals applying for only a 1 year Interventional Cardiology Fellowship position will be required to provide his/her own funding resources for salary support during their training. This funding must be institutional funding (no personal or private funds). A processing fee of $40 (check or money/order made payable to Duke University- no cash please), letter documenting funding support, current curriculum vitae, and personal statement will be required to accompany the completed Interventional Cardiology Application (see Duke University website for application).
Date(s) Application is Due: Feb 1
Contact: Sherolyn Patterson, Fellowship Program Coordinator; (919) 684-2304; fax: (919) 684-4322; email: sherolyn.patterson@duke.edu
Internet: http://fellowships.medicine.duke.edu/modules/fellows_cardio/index.php?id=8
Sponsor: Duke University School of Medicine
P.O. Box 3878
Durham, NC 27710

Duke University Obstetric Anesthesia Fellowships **1345**
The Department of Anesthesiology at Duke University Medical Center offers 1 - 2 positions of a one year Fellowship in Obstetric Anesthesia. Emphasis is on clinical research, advanced clinical training and teaching. Duke University is a tertiary center with approximately 3,000 deliveries per year. The division is currently made up of 8 faculty staff with diverse international pedigree.
Contact: Yemi Olufolabi, Fellowship Director; (919) 681-6535 or (919) 668-6266; fax: (919) 668-6265; email: olufo001@mc.duke.edu
Internet: http://anesthesiology.duke.edu/modules/anes_flwshp/index.php?id=1
Sponsor: Duke University Medical Center, Department of Anesthesiology, Division of Women's Anesthesia
P.O. Box 3094
Durham, NC 27710

Duke University Pain Management Fellowships **1346**
The Fellowship Program is based in the Duke Health Center at Morreene Road (MRC). Fellows will: cover the Pain Clinic and Durham VAMC, and Acute Pain Service at Duke North; evaluate new patients; perform comprehensive or neurologic studies; formulate diagnosis and plan; become familiar with procedures; learn intervention of the lumbar spine and its application e.g. facet rhizotomy, discography, and intradiscal annuloplasty; implantation therapies; dictation of clinic and procedure notes. Fellows will be asked to participate in research, journal clubs, round table discussions, grand rounds and lectures. There are opportunities for the fellow to become involved in research projects already in progress or to develop an original project. The clinical objectives are to build knowledge, skills and professionalism.
Requirements: Applicants must meet eligibility specified by the ACGME. Acceptance into the program is based on demonstrated academic qualification, interpersonal skills, and evidence of ability to function in a multidisciplinary setting. Fellowship applications may be downloaded from http://anesthesia.duhs.duke.edu/. Submit application, CV and three letters of reference.
Date(s) Application is Due: Jun 30
Contact: Dianne L. Scott, M.D., Fellowship Director; (919) 684-6736;
Internet: http://anesthesiology.duke.edu/modules/anes_flwshp/index.php?id=1
Sponsor: Duke University, Duke Pain Clinic
932 Morreene Road, RM 232
Durham, NC 27705

Duke University Pediatric Anesthesiology Fellowship **1347**
The pediatric anesthesia fellowship program provides an opportunity for one anesthesia to develop skills in pediatric anesthesia. The goals of the program are to foster the development of the following for the fellow: a broad clinical experience in pediatric anesthesia to allow proficiency in providing care for neonates, infants, children, and adolescents undergoing a wide variety of surgical, diagnostic, and therapeutic procedures; technical skills in pediatric airway management; technical expertise in pediatric invasive monitoring; a comprehensive understanding of the developmental, pharmacological, anatomic, physiologic, and psychological changes that occur with age and disease; an understanding of pediatric pain and its management; an understanding of critical perioperative care and advanced life support; and competence as a perioperative pediatric anesthesiologist and consultant. The goals of the program will be met by providing fellows with: graded clinical experiences; didactic lectures, seminars, and conferences; and clinical electives and research opportunities.
Requirements: The fellowship application can be downloaded from : http://anesthesia.duhs.duke.edu/education/fellows/fellowapp.pdf. Fellowship selection is based on the process used for application to the core residency program. All applicants are considered without regard to race, color, religion, gender, or national origin and must have completed an ACGME accredited program in Anesthesiology or it's equivalent. Documentation of completion will be required. In addition to the completed application, all candidates are required to submit: completed fellowship application; three letters of recommendation; curriculum vitae; one page personal statement; medical school transcript; letter of completion from the Anesthesiology residency chairman or program director or copy of Anesthesiology training certificate.
Contact: B. Craig Weldon M.D., Director; (919) 668-0976 or (919) 668-4208; fax: 919-668-4228; email: weldo@mc.duke.edu
Internet: http://anesthesiology.duke.edu/modules/anes_flwshp/index.php?id=1
Sponsor: Duke University Medical Center
Department of Anesthesiology, DUMC 3094
Durham, NC 27710

Duke University Postdoctoral Research Fellowships in Aging **1348**
The goal of the postdoctoral research training program is to produce highly skilled research scientists who have the potential for leadership in gerontological research. In the Duke Research Training Program (RTP), much of the training for each fellow is provided by that person's faculty mentor(s) in a research apprenticeship program. A fellow carries out his/her own research as a junior colleague in the mentor's research program or laboratory. In addition to working in their mentor's programs, all fellows attend a weekly interdisciplinary didactic seminar. The stipend amount is determined by years of relevant postdoctoral experience. The program also provides health insurance for the fellow (using the University's insurance plan), and partial travel support when presenting research at a professional meeting.
Requirements: Applicants must be citizens of the United States, or have been lawfully admitted to the United States for permanent residence. Applicants must have a completed doctoral degree when joining the program. All course work must be completed, and if applying as a Ph.D., final orals must be passed, and the dissertation signed before an applicant can begin the program.
Date(s) Application is Due: May 1
Contact: James A. Blumenthal, Ph.D.; (919) 660-7517; fax: (919) 684-8569; email: blume003@mc.duke.edu
Internet: http://www.geri.duke.edu/post_doc/
Sponsor: Duke University School of Medicine
Box 3003
Durham, NC 27710

Duncan L. Gordon Fellowships **1349**
Fellowships are available for research in pediatric medicine including nutrition, infectious diseases, mental retardation, environmental health, and clinical pharmacology, tenable in any agreed institution within Canada for one or two years. Candidates should be nominated by the head of the department in which they are employed or in which they will be employed upon completion of the fellowship. Nominating institutions must affirm their intention to employ the fellow upon completion of studies and to continue or establish a program in the field concerned. Award includes a full-time stipend, paid on a quarterly basis, plus a modest transportation allowance to take up the fellowship if required.
Requirements: Fellowships are available to Canadian citizens or landed immigrants at a post-doctoral level and who are of outstanding academic achievement in a pediatric related health care field and who can provide evidence of aptitude for pediatric patient care, teaching, and research.
Amount of Grant: $C47,500 maximum
Date(s) Application is Due: Oct 1
Contact: Pam Gilliland, Coordinator, National Grants Program, (416) 813-6166 ext 2354; fax: (416) 813-7311; email: national.grants@sickkids.ca
Internet: http://www.sickkidsfoundation.com
Sponsor: Sick Kids Foundation
555 University Avenue
Toronto, ON M5G 1X8 Canada

Duneland Health Council Incorporated Grants **1350**
The Duneland Health Council, Inc. is a private foundation focused on improving the health and general welfare of the greater Michigan City, Indiana community.
Restrictions: Funding limited primarily in the metropolitan Michigan City, IN area. No support for religious organizations. No grants to individuals, or for fund-raising, endowments or advertising.
Geographic Focus: Indiana
Contact: Norm Steider, Director, (219) 874-4193; fax: (219) 873-2416; email: normsteider@yahoo.com
Sponsor: Duneland Health Council Incorporated
P.O. Box 9327
Michigan City, IN 46361-9327

Dunspaugh-Dalton Foundation Grants **1351**
The foundation awards grants to eligible nonprofit organizations in the areas of higher, secondary, and elementary education; social services; youth; health associations and hospitals; cultural programs; and civic affairs. Types of support include capital campaigns, continuing support, endowment funds, matching funds, operating support, professorships, and special projects. The board meets monthly to consider requests.
Requirements: U.S. nonprofit organizations are eligible. The foundation primarily supports programs in California, Florida, and North Carolina.
Restrictions: Individuals are not eligible.
Geographic Focus: California; Florida; North Carolina
Amount of Grant: $5000-$50,000
Contact: William Lane Jr, (305) 668-4192; fax: (305) 668-4247
Sponsor: Dunspaugh-Dalton Foundation
1533 Sunset Drive, Suite 150
Coral Gables, FL 33143-5700

DuPage Community Foundation Grants 1352

The DuPage Community Foundation is a community-based philanthropic organization that identifies, promotes, and supports programs that raise the quality of life in DuPage County for this generation and future generations. To this end, the Foundation seeks to address the broad needs of DuPage County through grants in support of the following program categories: Arts and Culture, Education, Environmental, Health, and Human Services.

Requirements: Grant applications will be accepted from non-profit charitable organizations that: are classified as exempt from federal income taxes under section 501(c)3 of the Internal Revenue Code; and are located in DuPage County. Previous grantees must have complied with all reporting requirements and be in good standing before submitting another grant request.

Restrictions: The Foundation does not generally award grants to: organizations located outside of DuPage County (exceptions, if any, will be made by the director of grants); individuals; governmental agencies, including supporting foundations; programs for religious purposes; endowments; disease-specific organizations; private foundations and private operating foundations; or public, parochial, private or charter schools (pre-K through 12th grade).

Geographic Focus: Illinois

Samples: To be divided among 44 organizations in DuPage County (IL)—to support nonprofit groups working in the fields of the arts and culture, civic affairs, education, health, and human services, and for two special projects, $288,000 (2005); Willowbrook Wildlife Foundation (Glen Ellyn, IL)—to help establish a permanent endowment at the foundation, $10,000 challenge grant (2005).

Date(s) Application is Due: Feb 2; Aug 3

Contact: Bonnie Heydorn, (630) 665-5556; fax: (630) 665-9571; email bheydorn@dcfdn.org

Internet: http://www.dcfdn.org

Sponsor: DuPage Community Foundation
2100 Manchester Road, Building A, Suite 303
Wheaton, IL 60187-4584

Dysautonomia Research Grants 1353

Grants are awarded to promote research into control and/or cure for familial dysautonomia with particular emphasis on genetic screening; prenatal and/or carrier tests are necessary. Funds awarded are variable and depend on research proposed.

Requirements: Postdoctoral candidates must be connected with a recognized medical and/or teaching institution. There are no geographic limitations.

Amount of Grant: $100,000

Date(s) Application is Due: Nov 30

Contact: Grants Administrator, (212) 949-6644; fax: (212) 682-7625; email: info@familialdysautonomia.org

Internet: http://www.familialdysautonomia.org/researchgrantprogram.htm

Sponsor: Dysautonomia Foundation
633 Third Avenue, 12th Floor
New York, NY 10017

Dyson Foundation Mid-Hudson Valley General Operating Support Grants 1354

General operating support grants are sometimes referred to as core support or unrestricted grants. Many organizations use general operating support grants to cover day-to-day activities or ongoing expenses such as administrative salaries, utilities, office supplies, technology maintenance, etc. Other organizations use this type of funding to cover project costs, capital, technology purchases, and professional development. The use of these funds is totally at the discretion of the organization's board and/or executive staff, although the Foundation expects all organizational expenditures to be part of a board-approved annual budget. The first step in applying for a general operating support grant is to submit a letter of inquiry.

Restrictions: The Foundation places no restrictions on the use of these funds, unlike project or management technical assistance grants that are restricted by the Foundation to a particular project or activity. Colleges and universities, hospitals, faith-based institutions, and organizations with annual budgets in excess of $15 million dollars are not eligible to apply for general operating support grants.

Geographic Focus: New York

Amount of Grant: $1,000-$1,000,000; $80,000 average and $20,000 median

Contact: Diana M. Gurieva, Executive Vice President; (845) 677-0644; fax: (845) 677-0650; email: dgurieva@dyson.org or info@dyson.org

Internet: http://www.dysonfoundation.org/programareas/programareas_show.htm?doc_id=328141

Sponsor: Dyson Foundation
25 Halcyon Road
Millbrook, NY 12545-9611

Dystonia Medical Research Grants and Fellowships 1355

The research grants provide assistance in supporting investigations in specified areas of biomedical research pertinent to dystonia and related disorders. Research grants are being sought to develop important tools for DYT1 dystonia research; these include cell culture models, proteomics, genetic animal models of DYT1 dystonia, including transgenic and knock-in/ knock-out mice, Drosophila, C. elegans, and Zebrafish models. Grants are also being sought to develop new assays suitable for high throughput drug screening. Funding is available up to $40,000 for one-year pilot studies. A limited number of two-year grants are also available for larger studies with funding up to $75,000 per year. Fellowships assist post-doctoral students in establishing careers in dystonia research.

Requirements: Eligible for research grants are all nonprofit organizations or institutions. Eligible for research fellowships are investigators with MD or PhD degrees. For all investigations involving humans, approval by the institution's human subject protection committee is necessary. The regulations pertaining to recombinant DNA research and animal welfare as established by PHS have been adopted by DMRF.

Restrictions: Grant support will not be given for medical care of dystonia patients or for constructions and alterations.

Amount of Grant: $50,000 per year for two years for fellowships; $75,000 per year for two years for research grants and contracts

Date(s) Application is Due: Dec 30

Contact: Dr. Robert McAlister, Executive Director, (312) 755-0198; fax: (312) 803-0138; email: dystonia@dystonia-foundation.org

Internet: http://www.dystonia-foundation.org/research/other.asp?id=1

Sponsor: Dystonia Medical Research Foundation
One E Wacker Drive, Suite 2430
Chicago, IL 60601-2001

E. Rhodes and Leona B. Carpenter Foundation Grants 1356

The Foundation considers grant requests from: public charities which had direct relationships with Leona or Rhodes Carpenter during their lifetime; requests in support of graduate theological education from U.S. and Canadian organizations which are public charities; public charities in communities where Carpenter Co. has had long-time manufacturing facilities; museums which have a permanent collection for the purchase, restoration and conservation of Asian art; charities involved in providing hospice care; and projects (e.g., programs, conferences, resources, etc.) offering support to lesbian, gay, bisexual and transgender persons of faith, or endeavoring to insure faith communities' understanding, affirmation, and inclusion of such persons.

Requirements: IRS 501(c)3 organizations are eligible.

Restrictions: Generally, the Foundation will not consider grant requests to support private secondary education, individuals or large public charities and will not transfer funds from its endowment to the endowment of another organization.

Date(s) Application is Due: Jan 31; Jul 31

Contact: Grants Administrator, (215) 979-3221

Sponsor: E. Rhodes and Leona B. Carpenter Foundation
1735 Marker Street, Suite 3420
Philadelphia, PA 19103

E.A. Baker Foundation for the Prevention of Blindness Grants 1357

The foundation awards grants to Canadian hospitals and universities conducting research in ophthalmology and eye diseases and awards fellowships for advanced training for Canadian ophthalmologists. The advanced training may be undertaken outside of Canada, but the ophthalmologist must return to Canada to teach or practice, particularly in remote areas.

Amount of Grant: $C40,000 average

Date(s) Application is Due: Dec 1

Contact: Barbara Marjeram, Canadian National Institute for the Blind, (416) 486-2500 ext 7586; email: barbara.marjeram@cnib.ca

Internet: http://www.cnib.ca/eng/eabaker/eabf

Sponsor: E.A. Baker Foundation for the Prevention of Blindness
1929 Bayview Avenue
Toronto, ON M4G 3E8 Canada

E.B. Hershberg Award for Important Discoveries in Medicinally Active Substances 1358

This award, supported by Schering-Plough Corporation, is given biennially in odd-numbered years to recognize and encourage outstanding discoveries in the chemistry of medicinally active substances. The discovery for which the award is given should have been made during the past two decades. Nominations are accepted in even-numbered years, and the award consists of $3,000 and a certificate.

Requirements: Any individual, except a member of the award committee, may submit one nomination or seconding letter for the award in any given year. The nominating documents consist of a letter of not more than 1000 words containing an evaluation of the nominee's accomplishments and a specific identification of the work to be recognized, a biographical sketch including date of birth, and a list of publications and patents authored by the nominee.

Restrictions: Self-nominations are not accepted.

Amount of Grant: $3,000 and reimbursement of up to $1,000 for travel expenses to award meeting

Date(s) Application is Due: Nov 1

Contact: Felicia Dixon, Awards Administrator; (800) 227-5558 or (202) 872-4408; fax: (202) 776-8008; email: f_dixon@acs.org or awards@acs.org

Internet: http://portal.acs.org/portal/acs/corg/content?_nfpb=true&_pageLabel=PP_ARTICLEMAIN&node_id=1319&content_id=CTP_004515&use_sec=true&sec_url_var=region1

Sponsor: American Chemical Society
1155 Sixteenth Street, NW
Washington, DC 20036

E.D.Thomas Fellowship 1359

The foundation supports research into the diagnosis, prevention, and cure of leukemia and related hematological malignancies. The fellowship is awarded for one year, renewable yearly for two additional years upon satisfactory performance. The award supports costs

not to exceed 8% and salary not to exceed $35,000 including fringe benefits, with the remainder for supplies and/or equipment. Applications must be requested by October 15.
Requirements: Candidates must hold an MD or PhD degree and have completed at least three years postdoctoral training but must be less than 10 years post their first doctoral degree when the award begins. There are no restrictions based on nationality, but only one application will be considered from each sponsoring institution. Candidates must be committed to the research goals of the foundation, must be able to devote at least 80% of their time to the project and must have a sponsoring institution with the academic environment to provide adequate support for the proposed project.
Amount of Grant: $50,000
Date(s) Application is Due: Nov 2
Contact: Grants Administrator, 34 93 414 55 66; fax: 34 93 201 0588; email: fundacio@fcarreras.es
Internet: https://www.fcarreras.org/eng/seccio.php?opcion=5
Sponsor: Jose Carreras International Leukemia Foundation
Muntaner, 383 2n
Barcelona 08021 Spain

E.J. Grassmann Trust Grants **1360**
The trust awards grants in Georgia and Union County, NJ, in support of higher and secondary education, hospitals and health organizations, historical associations, environmental conservation, and social welfare. Types of support include capital campaigns, building construction/renovation, equipment acquisition, and endowment funds. Groups with low administrative costs, that have outside funding, and that encourage self-help are preferred. Grants are awarded in May and November. Written proposals should not be longer than four pages.
Restrictions: Grants are not awarded to individuals or for operating expenses, current scholarship funds, conferences, or workshops.
Geographic Focus: Georgia
Amount of Grant: $5000-$20,000 average
Date(s) Application is Due: Apr 20; Oct 15
Contact: William Engel, Executive Director, (908) 753-2440
Sponsor: E.J. Grassmann Trust
P.O. Box 4470
Warren, NJ 07059

E.L. Wiegand Foundation Grants **1361**
The foundation provides grants to develop and strengthen programs and projects at Arizona, California, the District of Columbia, Idaho, Nevada, New York, Oregon, Utah, and Washington educational institutions in the academic areas of science, business, fine arts, and law; and medicine and health organizations in the areas of heart, eye, and cancer surgery, treatment, and research. The foundation also considers requests for projects that enrich children, communities, public policy, and art. Grants for education, including funds for computers and scientific equipment, are awarded. The board of trustees meets in February, June, and October to choose recipients, but applications may be submitted at any time. Application guidelines are available upon request.
Requirements: Nonprofit organizations in Arizona, California, District of Columbia, Idaho, Nevada, New York, Oregon, Utah, and Washington State are eligible.
Geographic Focus: Arizona; California; District of Columbia; Idaho; Nevada; New York; Oregon; Utah; Washington
Amount of Grant: $10,000-$200,000 average
Contact: Kristen Avansino, Executive Director, (775) 333-0310; fax: (775) 333-0314
Sponsor: E.L. Wiegand Foundation
165 W Liberty Street, Suite 200
Reno, NV 89501

Eastman Chemical Company Foundation Grants **1362**
The Foundation supports organizations and programs that help to promote its efforts of enhancing the quality of life in Eastman communities. Contributions are concentrated on the following areas: education, health and human services, civic and community, and culture and the arts. Grants may be considered outside of these areas.
Requirements: Contributions are generally restricted to organizations which have been granted 501(c)3 tax exempt status and are usually directed toward the communities in which the company has operating units.
Restrictions: Contributions will not be made to the following: individuals, athletic teams or sports related events, choirs, bands, drill teams, labor, veteran, fraternal, social or political organizations; individual agencies supported by the area United Way organization, except capital fund drives which are normally supported by the community, not the United Way; organizations that discriminate on the basis of race, color, sex or national origin; national organizations whose programs do not directly serve the region's needs; places of worship and institutions devoted solely to religious instruction; travel related, including student trips or tours.
Geographic Focus: Pennsylvania; South Carolina; Tennessee; Texas
Contact: CeeGee McCord, Contributions Manager; (423) 229-2000; fax: (423) 229-6974; email: CeeGeeMcCord@kingsporthousing.org
Internet: http://www.eastman.com/Company/Sustainability/communities/Philanthropy/Pages/Philanthropy.aspx
Sponsor: Eastman Chemical Company
P.O. Box 431
Kingsport, TN 37662

eBay Foundation Community Grants **1363**
The mission of the Foundation is to make investments that improve the economic and social well-being of local communities. The Foundation works to fulfill its mission by collaborating with non-profit organizations and funding innovative programs primarily in microenterprise development. The Foundation also provides support to community organizations in areas where employees are located.
Requirements: 501(c)3 nonprofit organizations in communities where eBay has a major employment base, which includes San Jose, CA, and Salt Lake City, UT, are eligible.
Geographic Focus: California; Utah
Samples: Friends of Farm Drive (San Jose, CA)—for operating support of this organization, which is dedicated to improving the quality of life for residents of a neighborhood rampant with drug dealing and gang activity.; U Research Expedition Program (U of California)—for scholarships to send California elementary and high school teachers on UREP trips, where they learn by working with university scientists and local residents in countries around the world, to increase awareness of current events and to foster understanding of different cultures among both students and teachers.
Amount of Grant: $1000-$15,000 average
Contact: Grants Administrator, email: ebayfdn@cfsv.org
Internet: http://pages.ebay.com/community/aboutebay/foundation/grantapp.html
Sponsor: eBay Foundation
60 South Market Street, Suite 1000
San Jose, CA 95113

Eberly Foundation Grants **1364**
The foundation awards grants to eligible nonprofit organizations in the areas of: undergraduate educational opportunities; arts programming and institutions; health and human services projects; primary and secondary supplemental educational programming; and economic development activities and organizations that benefit the residents of Fayette County. The initial approach should be submittal of a letter of request.
Requirements: Nonprofit organizations in Pennsylvania are eligible.
Geographic Focus: Pennsylvania
Samples: Pennsylvania State U (University Park, PA)—to construct a community center on the Fayette campus that will house performance spaces, a cafeteria and dining hall, a fitness center, an auditorium, and other features needed for large gatherings, $6.9 million.; Indiana U of Pennsylvania, College of Business (PA)—to support technology initiatives, $599,000 challenge grant.; Western Pennsylvania Conservancy (Pittsburgh, PA)—for restoration and protection of Fallingwater, $1 million.
Contact: Carolyn Blaney, President, (724) 438-3789; fax: (724) 438-3856
Sponsor: Eberly Foundation
2 West Main Street, Suite 101
Uniontown, PA 15401-3448

Echoing Green Fellowships **1365**
The program awards full-time fellowships to emerging entrepreneurs to create innovative domestic or international public service projects that seek to catalyze positive social change. The proposed project may be in any public service area, including but not limited to, the environment, arts, education, health, youth service and development, civil and human rights, and community and economic development. The fellowship provides a two-year stipend, health care benefits, online connectivity, access to Echoing Green's network of social entrepreneurs, training, and technical assistance.
Requirements: Applicants must be at least 18 years old and commit to leading the project for at least two years. Partnerships of up to two individuals also are eligible.
Restrictions: Faith-based and research projects and lobbying activities are not eligible.
Amount of Grant: $30,000 per year for two years, individual fellowships; $45,000 per year (per project, not per individual) for two years, partnership fellowships
Date(s) Application is Due: Dec 2
Contact: Maritza Martinez, Senior Associate;(212) 400-3958; fax: (212) 689-9010; email: Maritza@echoinggreen.org or apply@echoinggreen.org
Internet: http://www.echoinggreen.org/index.cfm?fuseaction=Page.viewPage&pageId=41
Sponsor: Echoing Green Foundation
494 Eighth Avenue, Second Floor
New York, NY 10001

Eckerd Corporation Foundation Grants **1366**
The Foundation's philanthropic mission is to monetarily support nonprofit organizations that directly benefit health care, education, women and children through programs and events. Funding proposals are submitted to the board for review on a quarterly basis.
Requirements: Nonprofit organizations in company operating areas are eligible.
Contact: Tami Alderman, Public Relations, (727) 395-7091; fax: (727) 395-7934; email: service@eckerd.com
Internet: http://www.eckerd.com/content.asp?content=company/news/presscontact
Sponsor: Eckerd Corporation
8333 Bryan Dairy Road
Largo, FL 33777

Eddie C. and Sylvia Brown Family Foundation Grants **1367**
The Brown Family Foundation will focus its grant making in three general areas: the arts, education, and health (HIV/AIDS and cancer). The foundation's grant making will support programs that: provide opportunities for youth involvement in meaningful art experiences—this can include support for arts organizations or youth serving organizations that have developed programs which expose young people to the arts (programs that infuse the arts as a tool for leadership development, academic enrichment,

and are built on strong youth development principles are encouraged to apply); provide access to educational opportunities for disadvantaged children and youth—this can include local organizations that work to improve PreK-12 public education and to offer enhancement and enrichment opportunities to Baltimore City students (educational opportunities are defined in the broadest sense to include, but are not limited to afterschool programs, mentoring, alternative education, computer technology, scholarship support, as well as traditional in-school K-12 programs); address the impact of HIV/AIDS on the African American community—programs that provide direct services and intervention including testing and counseling, case management strategies, and access to treatment will be considered; and address the prevention and treatment of cancer—this can include local organizations that provide cancer screening, prevention education, and treatment modalities.
Requirements: Organizations (or their fiscal agents) serving the Baltimore area that qualify as public charities under section 501(c)3 of the Internal Revenue Code and do not discriminate on the basis of race, creed, national origin, color, physical handicap, gender or sexual orientation can apply.
Restrictions: The Foundation does not make grants for: start-up programs; capital campaigns; individuals; multiple years; institutions of higher education; and organizations outside the Baltimore region.
Geographic Focus: Maryland
Amount of Grant: $2,500 typical
Date(s) Application is Due: Sep 26
Contact: Maya Smith, Program Administrative Assistant; (410) 332-4172, ext. 142; fax: (410) 837-4701; email: msmith@bcf.org
Internet: http://www.bcf.org/ourgrants/ourgrantsdetail.aspx?grid=2
Sponsor: Eddie C. and Sylvia Brown Family Foundation
2 East Read Street, 9th Floor
Baltimore, MD 21202

Eden Hall Foundation Grants **1368**
Eden Hall Foundation is a private foundation established pursuant to the will of Sebastian Mueller, a Pittsburgh philanthropist and vice president and director of the H. J. Heinz Company. During his lifetime, Mr. Mueller gave substantial support to improve conditions of the poor and disadvantaged, the promotion of sound education, and the support of health facilities and projects. Today, the trustees of Eden Hall Foundation continue his stewardship in the areas of social welfare, health, education and the arts. Eden Hall Foundation seeks to improve the quality of life in Pittsburgh and western Pennsylvania through support of organizations whose missions address the needs and concerns of the area. Proposals and projects of primary interest to the Foundation are: educational programs dedicated to the advancement and dissemination of useful knowledge. Support of schools is generally confined to four-year privately funded and controlled colleges, universities and other educational institutions; social welfare, women's issues, and the improvement of conditions of the poor and disadvantaged; and the advancement of better health through support of organizations dedicated to health issues. Eden Hall Foundation will entertain grant proposals for capital projects, scholarship funds, research projects, programming and, in limited cases, endowments directed toward these objectives. A specific application form is not required. Therefore, grant requests should be submitted by letter proposal to the Foundation. Acknowledgements will be made promptly, advising applicants whether or not their requests meet Eden Hall Foundation's criteria.
Requirements: Requests for grants should include: a brief statement of the background and purpose of the requesting organization; a copy of that organization's most recent financial statements, as prepared by its certified public accountants; the specific purpose for which the requested grant is to be used, including a detailed budget, timetable for implementation and proposed method of evaluation; IRA certification of tax-exempt and charitable status under sections 501(c)3 and 509(c) of the Internal Revenue Code; information concerning the status of grants solicited from other foundations in the past twelve-month period (indicating the name of each foundation and amount requested); and a listing of the organization's officers and directors, their primary occupations and the responsibilities to the organization.
Restrictions: Grants cannot be made to individuals or private foundations. Not eligible for funding are sectarian or denominational religious organizations, except those providing direct educational or health care services to the public, tax-supported organizations, political parties and fraternal organizations. Requests to cover operating expenses, endowments or accumulated deficits are discouraged.
Geographic Focus: Pennsylvania
Contact: Sylvia Fields, Executive Director; (412) 642-6697; fax: (412) 642-6698
Internet: http://www.edenhallfdn.org
Sponsor: Eden Hall Foundation
600 Grant Street, Suite 3232
Pittsburgh, PA 15219

Edina Realty Foundation Grants **1369**
The Foundation extends financial support to organizations primarily in Minnesota, which provide housing and related services such as counseling and medical care to homeless children, families and individuals. Application forms may be submitted at anytime, see Foundations website for Grant Application forms: http://www.edinarealty.com/Content/Content.aspx?ContentID=148855
Requirements: Nonprofits 501(C)(03) operating in Minnesota are eligible.
Geographic Focus: Minnesota
Samples: Home of the Good Shepherd, MN, $15,000 - operates two transitional housing programs in St. Paul for homeless and at-risk women (2008); Spare Key of Minnesota, MN, $13,000 - provides mortgage assistance to Minnesota homeowners with critically ill or seriously injured children by making a mortgage payment directly to the lender on behalf of the family (2008);
Amount of Grant: $500-$2,000 range
Contact: Susan Cowsert, Director; (952) 928-5900; email: susancowsert@edinarealty.com
Internet: http://www.edinarealty.com/Content/Content.aspx?ContentID=187015
Sponsor: Edina Realty Foundation
6800 France Avenue South, Suite 670
Edina, MN 55435-2017

Edna G. Kynett Memorial Foundation Grants **1370**
The purpose of the Foundation is to improve cardiovascular health. Grants support programs and services that educate primary care practitioners and community members and promote cardiovascular health. Grants are made to medical schools, hospitals and other nonprofit health organizations. Programs that have received support in recent years include innovative curricula, lectures and seminars, a tobacco prevention program, a summer Community Health Internship program and clinical research projects. Innovative projects are preferred.
Requirements: Applicants must be nonprofit organizations in the Delaware Valley, including Philadelphia, Bucks, Delaware, Chester, Montgomery, Berks, Lehigh and Camden counties and New Castle County, Delaware. Applicants must be either public entities or tax-exempt under Section 501(c)3 of the Internal Revenue Code and not private foundations as defined under Section 509(a).
Geographic Focus: Pennsylvania
Samples: Penn Presbyterian Medical Center, Philadelphia, PA, $5,000 - Cardiology update (2009); Drexel University College of Medicine, Philadelphia, PA, $40,000 - Cardiovascular CME programs (2008); FOCU.S. on Health and Leadership for Women (Trustees of the University of Pennsylvania) Philadelphia, PA, $39,000 - Junior Faculty Investigators and Medical Student Fellowship in cardiovascular health (2008).
Amount of Grant: $50,000 maximum
Contact: Judith L. Bardes, Manager; (610) 828-8145; fax: (610) 834-8175; email: judy1@aol.com
Sponsor: Edna G. Kynett Memorial Foundation
P.O. Box 540
Plymouth Meeting, PA 19462-0540

EDS Foundation Grants **1371**
The Foundation wishes to ensure information technology champions cultural and civic change which will enrich the education of current and future generations, while enhancing the communities they serve. The Foundation is interested in supporting comprehensive technology solutions that increase performance and productivity in educational institutions and community organizations globally. Grant seekers must complete the EDS Foundation Application for Funding and have a current EDS employee volunteer partnership.
Requirements: Eligible applicants must be verified as a non-profit charitable organization (or equivalent) according to each country's rules and regulations. For the U.S., the organization must have a 501(c)3 IRS tax-exempt code.
Restrictions: Funding will not be provided for: individuals; operating deficits; foundations that are grant-making institutions; sponsorships; trips or tours; local athletic teams or events; fraternal, social or labor organizations; political or partisan organizations; journal or program advertising; private foundations; or organizations that do not comply with all applicable laws prohibiting discrimination and EDS Equal Opportunity policy.
Geographic Focus: California; Colorado; Georgia; Illinois; Michigan; Texas; Virginia
Contact: Diane Spradlin, Executive Director; (972) 605-8429; email: diane.spradlin-eds@eds.com
Internet: http://www.eds.com
Sponsor: EDS Foundation
5400 Legacy Drive, H3-6F-47
Plano, TX 75024

Educational Foundation of America Grants **1372**
The foundation makes grants only for specific projects in its areas of interest, including, but not limited to, the environment, reproductive freedom, theatre, education, medicine, drug policy reform, democracy, peace & national security issues and human services. Important characteristics considered by EFA are an organization's record of achievement, intended broad impact, sound financial practices, increasing independence, and correspondence with EFA objectives.
Requirements: U.S. nonprofits are eligible for grant support. Applicants are required to send the EFA Inquiry Form via email as the first step.
Restrictions: Grants are not made for endowment or endowed faculty chairs, building/capital programs, religious purposes, grants to individuals, annual fund-raising campaigns, indirect costs, overhead or general support. The Foundation prefers not to fund projects located outside the U.S..
Contact: Diane Allison, Executive Director, (203) 226-6498; email: dallison@efaw.org
Internet: http://www.efaw.org/Inquiry%20Guidelines.htm
Sponsor: Educational Foundation of America
35 Church Lane
Westport, CT 06880

Edward Bangs Kelley and Elza Kelley Foundation Grants **1373**
The Foundation's interest is primarily in Barnstable County, Massachusetts. The Foundation has been the leader in improving the health and welfare of the community. Grants are made to a great variety of health, social and human service agencies, as well

as to cultural and environmental organizations. Town libraries, theatre and art groups, and musical organizations have been supported. Grants are sometimes utilized as seed money by young organizations.

Requirements: Grant applicants must be tax-exempt organizations which are not private foundations and must be located in Barnstable County. The proposed project/program must have a direct benefit to the inhabitants of Barnstable County. If the tax-exempt organization is located outside of Barnstable, but the proposed project/program will have a direct and substantial benefit to the inhabitants of Barnstable, the grant application may be eligible for funding.

Restrictions: Applicants must be residents of Barnstable County, Massachusetts, or must demonstrate very significant ties to Barnstable County.

Geographic Focus: Massachusetts

Contact: Henry Murphy Jr., Administrative Manager, (508) 775-3117; email: contact@kelleyfoundation.org

Internet: http://www.kelleyfoundation.org

Sponsor: Edward Bangs Kelley and Elza Kelley Foundation
243 South Street, P.O. Drawer M
Hyannis, MA 02601

Edward S. Moore Foundation Grants 1374

The foundation awards grants to nonprofits in Connecticut and New York in its areas of interest, including youth, hospitals, education, cultural programs, museums, and Christian religion. Types of support include operating budgets, continuing support, annual campaigns, seed money, emergency funds, building funds, equipment, land acquisition, endowment funds, matching funds, internships, scholarship funds, special projects, and research. There are no application deadlines. The board meets in January, April, July, and October to consider proposals.

Requirements: Nonprofits in Connecticut and New York may submit proposals.

Restrictions: Grants are not awarded to individuals or for deficit financing, publications, or conferences.

Geographic Focus: Connecticut; New York

Samples: Children's Aid Society (New York, NY)—$50,000.; Metropolitan Opera (New York, NY)—$35,000.; Stamford Hospital Foundation (Stamford, CT)—$430,000.

Amount of Grant: $10,000-$50,000 average

Contact: John W. Cross III, President, (203) 629-4591

Sponsor: Edward S. Moore Foundation
30 Lismore Lane
Greenwich, CT 06831

Edwards Memorial Trust Grants 1375

The trust awards grants to eligible Minnesota nonprofit organizations in support of health care for people without health insurance or who are underinsured, preventive health care for children, and programs for the disabled. Areas of support include health care and hospitals, mental health crisis services, social services, children and youth, and the disabled. Types of support include building construction/renovation, equipment acquisition, general operating grants, and program development. A copy of the tax determination letter and most recent audited financial statements must accompany applications.

Requirements: Minnesota 501(c)3 tax-exempt organizations in the greater Saint Paul area are eligible.

Geographic Focus: Minnesota

Amount of Grant: $2000-$50,000 range

Date(s) Application is Due: May 1; Nov 1

Contact: Cheryl Nelson, c/o U.S. Bank, (651) 466-8441; fax: (651) 244-4267

Sponsor: Edwards Memorial Trust
P.O. Box 64713
Saint Paul, MN 55164-0713

Edwin S. Webster Foundation Grants 1376

The policy of the foundation is to support charitable organizations that are well known to the trustees, with emphasis on special projects and capital programs, or operating income for hospitals, medical research, education, youth agencies, cultural activities, and programs addressing the needs of minorities. Types of support include operating budgets, continuing support, annual campaigns, building funds, equipment, land acquisition, endowment funds, matching funds, scholarship funds, professorships, internships, fellowships, special projects, and research.

Requirements: The Foundation confines its grants primarily to the New England area. Grantees must provide evidence of their tax-exempt status. The AGM common proposal format, available on the Internet at http://agmconnect.org is suitable for submission of proposals but not required. There are no set deadlines, but for consideration at the spring meeting, proposals should arrive by May 1 and by November 1 for consideration at the fall meeting. Proposals received after the trustees meet will be held for consideration at the next meeting.

Restrictions: Grants are not made to organizations outside the United States or to individuals.

Geographic Focus: Massachusetts

Samples: Massachusetts Institute of Technology, Office of Minority Education, Cambridge, MA, $40,000 - Mentor Advocate Partnership (2008); Eastern Virginia Medical School, Norfolk, VA, $25,000 - general operations and interdisciplinary research (2008); Museum of Science, Boston, MA, $50,000 - capital support for the Hayden Planetarium (2008).

Amount of Grant: $15,000-$50,000 average

Date(s) Application is Due: May 1; Nov 1

Contact: Michelle Jenney, Administrator; (617) 391-3087; fax: (617) 426-7080; email: mjenney@gmafoundations.com

Sponsor: Edwin S. Webster Foundation
c/o GMA Foundations,
77 Summer Street, 8th Floor
Boston, MA 02110-1006

Edwin W. and Catherine M. Davis Foundation Grants 1377

The foundation awards grants to U.S. nonprofit organizations in its areas of interest, including arts, elderly, environment, higher education, housing, mental health, religion, social services,and youth. Types of support include annual campaigns, endowment funds, fellowships, operating grants, research grants, and scholarship funds. There are no application deadlines. The board meets in May or June; submit a proposal that is three pages or less in length.

Requirements: U.S. nonprofit organizations are eligible.

Geographic Focus: Washington

Amount of Grant: $1,000-$10,000 average

Contact: Gayle Roth, Grants Administrator; (651) 228-0935; fax: (651) 228-0776

Sponsor: Edwin W. and Catherine M. Davis Foundation
30 East 7th Street, Suite 2000
Saint Paul, MN 55101-1394

Edyth Bush Charitable Foundation Grants 1378

The Foundation is operated exclusively for charitable, religious, literary, and other exempt purposes. Grants are available for challenge and development purposes, construction and renovation, equipment and expansion of functions, pilot projects and seed start-up of new programs, and study or planning grants. The Foundation has broad interests in human service, education, health care and a limited interest in the arts. Requests for grants or other funds should be submitted in writing. Contact the Program Officer before beginning any proposals or applications.

Requirements: The Foundation welcomes grant requests from otherwise eligible tax-exempt organizations under IRS Sections 501(c)3 and Section 509(a) headquartered within the Orlando MSA of Orange, Seminole, and Osceola Counties, Florida. Other grant requests should have special interest or support from one or more of our Directors.

Restrictions: The Foundation will ordinarily deny grant requests: from chiefly tax-supported institutions, or their support foundations; for individual scholarships or for individual research grants even if through an exempt or otherwise qualified educational organization; for alcoholism or drug abuse programs or facilities; for routine operating expenses; to pay off deficits or pre-existing debt; for foreign organizations or for foreign expenditure; for travel projects or fellowships; for chiefly church, sacramental, denominational or inter-denominational purposes, except outreach projects for elderly, indigents, needy, youth, or homeless regardless of belief, race, color, creed, or sex; for endowment funds or other purely revenue generating funds; advocacy organizations or advocacy component funding; for cultural or arts organizations unless their collections, exhibits, projects or performances are of demonstrated nationally recognized quality; from organizations having receipts of revenues from memberships and/or contributions of less than $25,000 in the previous year, or from any organization whose IRS Sec. 509(a) publicly supported status will need renewal in the next six (6) months.

Geographic Focus: Florida

Samples: Jewish Community Ctr of Greater Orlando (Maitland, FL)—to renovate its playground for toddlers and to help raise additional funds for a project to renovate the elementary school playground, $75,867 partial challenge grant (2005); Community Communications, Inc., WMFE-TV/FM (Orlando, FL)—for hurricane emergency relief effort, $12,000 (2005); Holocaust Memorial Resource and Education Center (Maitland, FL)—to support work in addressing intolerance, $2500 (2005); Winter Garden Heritage Foundation (Winter Garden , FL)—for leadership training, $350 (2005).

Amount of Grant: $5,000-$50,000

Contact: Deborah Hessler, Program Officer, (888) 647-4322 or (407) 647-4322; fax: (407) 647-7716; email: dhessler@edythbush.org

Internet: http://www.edythbush.org

Sponsor: Edyth Bush Charitable Foundation
P.O. Box 1967
Winter Park, FL 32790-1967

EF Behavioral Sciences Student Fellowships 1379

This fellowship stimulates individuals to pursue careers in epilepsy in either research or practice settings. Appropriate fields include sociology, social work, psychology, anthropology, nursing, economics, vocational rehabilitation, counseling, political science, and others relevant to epilepsy research or practice. Annual deadline dates may vary; contact program staff for exact dates.

Requirements: Applicant must be actively enrolled in a degree program at the time the fellowship is to be undertaken. The fellowship must be undertaken during a free period in the student's year, e.g., during the summer. Both graduate and undergraduate students are eligible provided all other eligibility criteria are met. The project must be carried out at an approved facility.

Samples: Cathleen Buchanan, U of Wisconsin, Madison (WI)—for an examination of attention deficit hyperactivity disorder in children with epilepsy.; David Sbarra, U of Virginia (VA)—for an assessment of patterns of self-reliance, social and emotional adaptation, and parent-child interactions and how they affect children with epilepsy.

Amount of Grant: $3000 stipend

Date(s) Application is Due: Mar 1

Contact: Fellowship Programs, Research and Professional Education, (301) 459-3700; fax: (301) 577-2684; email: grants@efa.org
Internet: http://www.epilepsyfoundation.org/research/grants.cfm
Sponsor: Epilepsy Foundation
4351 Garden City Drive, Suite 406
Landover, MD 20785-7223

EF Health Sciences Student Fellowships **1380**

Three-month fellowships are awarded to medical and health science students for work on epilepsy study projects. The project may be carried out at the U.S. institution of the student's choice where there are ongoing programs of research, training, or service in epilepsy. Application forms and guidelines are available upon request. Annual deadline dates may vary; contact program staff for exact dates.
Requirements: Predoctoral training students in the Health Sciences may be accepted at any point in their schooling-following acceptance but before beginning the first year, or in the period immediately following their final year. A supervisor or preceptor must accept responsibility for the supervision of the student program and for the submission of a full report to the institute upon completion of the program.
Samples: Rosalind Carter Brown, U of Virginia Medical School (VA)—for an examination of the mechanisms of action of diazepam (Valium) in the treatment of status epilepticus, prolonged seizures.; Daniel Campbell, Pennsylvania State U College of Medicine (PA)—for an analysis of the role played by one type of calcium-related molecule in a genetic model of epilepsy.
Amount of Grant: $3000 stipend
Date(s) Application is Due: Mar 1
Contact: Fellowship Programs, Research and Professional Education, (301) 459-3700; fax: (301) 577-2684; email: grants@efa.org
Internet: http://www.epilepsyfoundation.org/research/grants.cfm
Sponsor: Epilepsy Foundation
4351 Garden City Drive, Suite 406
Landover, MD 20785

EF Making a Difference Award **1381**

The award recognizes women with epilepsy who have contributed in a significant way at the local, regional, or national level to support and advance quality of life for women with epilepsy; or inspire people with epilepsy and those with other chronic disabilities; or enhance public understanding of epilepsy and its impact on women. The winner will receive a monetary award and expense-paid trip to the foundation's national conference, in October. Information and nomination form are available online.
Amount of Grant: $1500
Contact: Making a Difference Award, fax: (301) 577-4941
Internet: http://www.epilepsyfoundation.org/programs/wei/index.cfm
Sponsor: Epilepsy Foundation
4351 Garden City Drive
Landover, MD 20785-7223

EF Postdoctoral Research Training Fellowships **1382**

The foundation awards grants and fellowships for cutting-edge research into the causes of epilepsy. Program goals include understanding basic mechanisms, developing new therapeutic approaches, understanding the behavioral and psychosocial aspects of having epilepsy, and encouraging the professional development of scientists and healthcare professionals. The purpose of the fellowship is to support predoctoral students with dissertation research related to epilepsy. Applications from all fields of research pertinent to epilepsy will be considered.
Requirements: Physicians or PhD neuroscientists who desire postdoctoral research experience are eligible for these fellowships, which must be carried out at an approvable facility where there is an ongoing epilepsy research program. Applicants must be licensed to practice medicine in the United States or Canada.
Restrictions: Individuals holding faculty appointments at the level of assistant professor or higher are ineligible.
Samples: Dr. Jon Backstrom, Vanderbilt U School of Medicine (TN)—for an investigation of the anatomical interaction between GABA and seratonin, and its effect on seizures.; Dr. Sarah Caddick, Duke U Medical Ctr (NC)—for an investigation of the function of zinc in certain systems of the brain that exhibit high concentrations of ion zinc and are highly prone to seizures.
Amount of Grant: $40,000 maximum
Date(s) Application is Due: Sep 1
Contact: Research and Professional Education, (301) 459-3700; fax: (301) 577-2684
Internet: http://www.epilepsyfoundation.org/research/grants.html
Sponsor: Epilepsy Foundation
4351 Garden City Drive, Suite 406
Landover, MD 20785

EF Predoctoral Research Training Fellowship **1383**

The predoctoral research training fellowship supports predoctoral students with dissertation research related to epilepsy, thus strengthening their interest in establishing epilepsy research as a career direction. Annual deadline dates may vary; contact program staff for exact dates.
Requirements: Graduate students pursuing a PhD degree in neuroscience, physiology, pharmacology, psychology, biochemistry, genetics, nursing, or pharmacy may apply.
Amount of Grant: $20,000 ($19,000 stipend plus $1000 travel allowance)
Date(s) Application is Due: Sep 1
Contact: Research and Professional Education, (301) 459-3700; fax: (301) 577-2684; email: grants@efa.org
Internet: http://www.epilepsyfoundation.org/research/grants.cfm
Sponsor: Epilepsy Foundation
4351 Garden City Drive, Suite 406
Landover, MD 20785

EF Research and Training Fellowships for Clinicians **1384**

These fellowships offer qualified individuals the opportunity to develop expertise in epilepsy research through a one-year training experience and involvement in an epilepsy research project. The purpose of the fellowships is to develop academic clinicians to teach patient care of persons with epilepsy and advance knowledge about epilepsy through clinical investigation. Applications from individuals interested in acquiring experience in the conduct of human clinical studies and who plan to study epilepsy as a human disorder are encouraged. Emphasis is placed on individuals who will be trained in clinical research in epilepsy rather than use epilepsy as a tool in their research in other fields. Applications from women, members of minority groups, and people with disabilities are especially encouraged.
Requirements: Individuals with the MD or DO degree who will have completed residency training in neurology, neurosurgery, pediatrics, internal medicine, or psychiatry by the time the fellowship commences and desire additional postdoctoral clinical research experience are eligible. Applicants planning to work in the United States receive preference.
Restrictions: These are training fellowships and will not be granted to individuals who have received faculty appointments at the level of assistant professor or higher. Individuals may not receive concurrent support for more than one EFA or AES grant or fellowship.
Amount of Grant: $50,000
Date(s) Application is Due: Oct 14
Contact: Research and Professional Education, (301) 459-3700; fax: (301) 577-2684
Internet: http://www.epilepsyfoundation.org/research/grants.cfm
Sponsor: Epilepsy Foundation
4351 Garden City Drive, Suite 406
Landover, MD 20785

Effie and Wofford Cain Foundation Grants **1385**

The foundation gives primarily for higher and secondary education, medical research, and public service organizations. Grants also are awarded to religious organizations (Baptist, Christian, Episcopal, Presbyterian, Salvation Army, and United Methodist), and for aid for the handicapped. Additional fields of interest include elementary and secondary education, early childhood development and education, medical school education, nursing school education, hospitals and general health care and health organizations, religious federated giving programs, government and public administration, African Americans, Latinos, the disabled, the aging, and economically disadvantaged and homeless. Types of support include general operating support, continuing support, annual campaigns, capital campaigns, building/renovations, equipment acquisition, endowment funds, program development, seed money, curriculum development, fellowships, internships, scholarship funds, research, and matching funds. Organizations may reapply for funding every other fiscal year.
Requirements: The foundation only makes grants to 501(c)3 tax-exempt organizations in Texas.
Restrictions: Individuals are ineligible.
Geographic Focus: Texas
Samples: U of Texas at Austin (TX)—to acquire works of art for its collection, $500,000 (2004); Texas College (Tyler, TX)—for its concert choir, $100,000 over four years (2004).
Amount of Grant: $1000-$100,000 average
Contact: Lynn Fowler, Executive Director, (512) 346-7490; fax: (512) 346-7491
Sponsor: Effie and Wofford Cain Foundation
4131 Spicewood Springs Road, Suite A-1
Austin, TX 78759

EIF Community Grants **1386**

Grants are made in the greater Los Angeles area for education and prevention programs, creative and performing arts, environmental programs, literacy and education, family care and welfare, substance abuse prevention, and youth welfare. Applicants must apply annually and an organization may submit only one application per year. Grants fund only specific programs or special projects of an organization. Applicants must call the foundation to have an application sent to their organization.
Requirements: Grants are made to nonprofit 501(c)3 organizations in the greater Los Angeles area. Organizations must be responsive to the changing needs of the constituents served and the local community.
Restrictions: The foundation does not give funds for political organizations, capital campaigns, public or private schools, fund-raising events, or religious or sectarian purposes.
Geographic Focus: California
Amount of Grant: $3000-$15,000
Contact: Grants Administrator, (818) 760-7722; fax: (818) 760-7898; email: info@eifoundation.org
Internet: http://www.eifoundation.org/grants/wp_grants/how_to_apply.asp
Sponsor: Entertainment Industry Foundation
11132 Ventura Boulevard, Suite 401
Studio City, CA 91604-3156

Eisner Foundation Grants 1387

The Eisner Foundation exists to provide access and opportunity for disadvantaged children and the aging of Los Angeles County. The Eisner Foundation has been funding innovative and effective non-profit organizations that improve and enrich the lives of underserved children in Southern California since 1996. In 2008, the Foundation recognized that many of the same attributes that the children unfortunately possess—physical and emotional vulnerability, extreme poverty, lack of advocacy on their behalf, minimal access to the arts, and general powerlessness—also applied to many members of our rapidly aging population in the community. The Foundation elected to broaden the funding focus to include those at both ends of the spectrum of life, the young and the old. The Foundation's now dedicated to bringing about lasting changes in the lives of disadvantaged and vulnerable people starting and ending their lives in Los Angeles County.

Requirements: California nonprofit organizations serving Los Angeles and Orange Counties are eligible to apply. Applicants can apply at any time, but should know that these proposals will be reviewed and approved at the June or December board meetings. Applying to the Foundation is a two step process. The first step is to submit a Letter of Inquiry (see Eisner Foundation website for guidelines). If Letter of Inquiry meets the Foundation's criteria, a full application will be sent to the applicant for completion and submission, completing the second step.

Restrictions: Proposals for endowments are rarely excepted.

Geographic Focus: California

Samples: LA Scores, Los Angeles, CA, $100,000—to provide project support for an after-school program that combines creative writing, soccer, and community service (2008); California Institute of the Arts, Los Angeles, CA, $1,250,000—to support the Community Arts Partnership program which provides new media arts education programs to local youth (2008); Friendship Circle, Los Angeles, CA, $25,000—to provide support for an organization that addresses the challenges of families with special-needs children in the South Bay (2008); Eisner Pediatric & Family Medical Center, Los Angeles, CA, $1,000,000—to support the endowment campaign for a pediatric and family medical center serving low-income, uninsured and under-insured families (2008); Aquarium of the Pacific, Los Angeles, CA, $100,000—to provide support for a project that increases science learning access to Title I school communities in the South Bay (2008); St. Barnabas Senior Center, Los Angeles, CA, $75,000—to support a program that provides education on sustained nutrition, adult day care, and other health promotion services for 3,000 seniors in the greater downtown Los Angeles area (2008).

Amount of Grant: $5,000-$100,000

Contact: Trent Stamp, Executive Director; (310) 228-6808; email: trent.stamp@eisnerfoundation.org

Internet: http://www.eisnerfoundation.org/what_we_do/

Sponsor: Eisner Foundation
233 South Beverly Drive
Beverly Hills, CA 90212

El Paso Community Foundation Grants 1388

The Foundation is a facilitator linking the generosity of the region's donors to local non-profit organizations to meet the charitable needs of the El Paso area. In this capacity, the Foundation helps to provide funding for programs and initiatives of these organizations for the broader good of the El Paso Community. Major areas of interest are arts and humanities, education, public benefit, health and disabilities, environment and animals and human services. Priority is given to: more effective ways of doing things; projects where a moderate amount of grant money can have an impact; and projects that show collaboration with other organizations.

Requirements: Grant requests will be considered only from agencies located within or offering services to the citizens of our community, which includes far west Texas, southern New Mexico and northern Chihuahua, Mexico. Applicants must be exempt from income taxes under Section 501(c)3 of the Internal Revenue Service Code.

Restrictions: Grants will generally not be made for academic research; capital campaigns; fundraising events or projects; projects of a religious nature; medical or academic research; travel for individuals or groups; annual appeals and membership contributions; ongoing requests for general operating support; initiatives that are political or partisan in purpose; and requests from organizations outside the El Paso geographic area.

Geographic Focus: Texas

Amount of Grant: $3,000-$10,000 average

Date(s) Application is Due: Feb 1; Aug 1

Contact: Bonita Johnson, Program Officer, (915) 533-4020; fax: (915) 532-0716; email: info@epcf.org

Internet: http://www.epcf.org/grants_scholarships.sstg

Sponsor: El Paso Community Foundation
P.O. Box 272
El Paso, TX 79943

El Paso Corporate Foundation Grants 1389

El Paso Corporate Foundation funds initiatives that strengthen the communities where employees live, work, and volunteer. The primary focus areas of the foundation are education, health and human services and the community. The Foundation's secondary focus areas are the environment and arts and culture. Organizations must be invited by the Foundation to submit a letter of inquiry for funding consideration.

Requirements: Giving is limited to nonprofits in Alabama, Colorado and Texas.

Restrictions: The following are ineligible requests for funding: organizations without 501(c)3 status; organizations that already have an active El Paso Corporate Foundation grant; capital campaigns; multi-year commitments; religious organizations for religious purposes; individuals; hospitals and medical research; athletics or youth sports organizations; national or state-wide initiatives; war veterans and fraternal service organizations; endowment funds; pass-through grants; fundraising events, such as dinners, luncheons, and golf tournaments; political organizations, campaigns, and candidates; and technology grants, i.e. computers, software, or related hardware.

Geographic Focus: Alabama; Colorado; Texas

Date(s) Application is Due: Jan 31; May 31; Sep 30

Contact: Community Relations, (713) 420-2878; fax: (713) 420-5312; email: foundation@elpaso.com

Internet: http://www.elpaso.com/community/default.shtm

Sponsor: El Paso Corporate Foundation
P.O. Box 2511
Houston, TX 77252-2511

El Pomar Foundation Awards and Grants 1390

The Foundation is one of the largest and oldest private foundations in the Rocky Mountain West and contributes annually through direct grants and Community Stewardship Programs to support Colorado nonprofit organizations. The Foundation's primary focus is in health, human services, education, arts and humanities, and civic and community initiatives.

Requirements: The foundation makes grants to 501(c)3 nonprofit Colorado organizations and for activities that take place within the state.

Restrictions: The Foundation does not accept grant applications for: other foundations or nonprofits that distribute money to recipients of its own selection; endowments; individuals; organizations that practice discrimination of any kind; organizations that do not have fiscal responsibility for the proposed project; organizations that do not have an active 501(c)3 nonprofit IRS determination letter; camps, camp programs, or other seasonal activities; religious organizations for support of religious programs; cover deficits or debt elimination; cover travel, conferences, conventions, group meetings, or seminars; influence legislation or support candidates for political office; produce videos or other media projects; fund research projects or studies; primary or secondary schools.

Geographic Focus: Colorado

Samples: Four Miles Historical Park (Denver, CO)—to construct a visitors center on the history of Denver, $50,000 (2003); Saint Paul Catholic Church (Colorado Springs, CO)—to construct a community center, $333,333 (2003); Pikes Peak Hospice and Palliative Care (Colorado Springs, CO)—for a new system for managing patient information, $75,000 (2003); Colorado Assoc of Nonprofit Organizations (Denver, CO)—for general operating support for statewide nonprofit programs, $20,000 (2003).

Amount of Grant: $500-$500,000 typically

Contact: Executive Office, (719) 633-7733 or (800) 554-7711; fax: (719) 577-5702 email: grants@elpomar.org

Internet: http://www.elpomar.org/grant2.html

Sponsor: El Pomar Foundation
10 Lake Circle
Colorado Springs, CO 80906

Eli Lilly & Company Welcome Back Awards 1391

The awards annually recognize excellence and courage in the mental health community and are designed to help fight the stigma associated with mental illness and show others that depression is treatable. The awards acknowledges individuals whose accomplishments in the areas of psychiatry, primary care, community service, and destigmatization have helped give new hope to those suffering from clinical depression. The program also presents a Lifetime Achievement Award to honor those people who have overcome depression to lead fulfilling and productive lives. A donation is made to the nonprofit organization of each awardee's choice.

Requirements: Nominations may be made by anyone wishing to recognize an individual for outstanding contributions to the depression community. Anyone may be nominated, including mental health consumers, advocates, physicians, research scientists, and employees of corporate, civic or academic institutions.

Amount of Grant: $15,000 lifetime achievement award; $10,000 destigmatization award; $10,000 community service award; $10,000 primary care award; $10,000 psychiatry award

Date(s) Application is Due: Nov 14

Contact: Welcome Back Awards, (800) 463-6440; fax: (212) 884-0628

Internet: http://www.lilly.com/about/awards/wba/index.html

Sponsor: Eli Lilly & Company
P.O. Box 845
New York, NY 10268-0845

Elisabeth Severance Prentiss Foundation Grants Program 1392

The foundation awards the majority of its support in the field of health and medicine. Scientific and medical research, hospitals, health projects, medical education, and care and support of the elderly are funded. Types of support include building programs, equipment needs, research, operating budgets, continuing support, seed grants, endowment funds, and projects/programs. Decision makers favor specific projects over general operating support. The maximum term of a commitment is five years, with preference for proposals for three years or less. Special consideration will be given to requests from applicants in the Cuyahoga County area. The board meets in June and December.

Requirements: Grants are awarded to promote and improve medical services in the greater Cleveland, OH, area.

Restrictions: Grants are not awarded to individuals for scholarships, fellowships, or grants in aid; or to organizations for fund-raising campaigns, surveys, assessments, studies, or planning activities.

Geographic Focus: Ohio
Samples: University Hospitals of Cleveland (OH)—to create an inpatient psychiatric unit for children and adolescents at Rainbow Babies and Children's Hospital, $5 million (2005).
Amount of Grant: $10,000-$100,000 average
Date(s) Application is Due: May 15; Nov 15
Contact: Michael Galland, c/o National City Bank, (216) 222-2736
Sponsor: Elisabeth Severance Prentiss Foundation
P.O. Box 94651
Cleveland, OH 44104

Elizabeth Glaser Pediatric AIDS Foundation International Leadership Awards 1393
The Award program is designed to invest in trained individuals in resource-poor countries who have the potential to develop programs which will have a direct impact on the pediatric HIV epidemic in their country, but that lack the resources to do so. This program will complement existing training programs by providing support after training is completed. The Award specifically seeks to identify individuals who are likely to have an enduring impact on control of the epidemic. Applicants may apply for support to create and or scale-up effective pediatric HIV/AIDS research and/or implementation programs including those addressing epidemiology, prevention of mother-to-child transmission, treatment of infected mothers and infants, continuum of care and scale up of prevention services to include care and treatment, development of national policies or strategies to combat pediatric HIV, assessment of the economic impact of disease and its prevention, or to help train additional in-country and regional scientists and program leaders. Award recipients will be asked to mentor a minimum of three additional people who would benefit from the experience and could help them achieve their goals. These are individuals who would be hired and trained to work on the project proposed by the applicant. The Award provides up to $100,000 in total costs per year for three years for a total of $300,000. Funding in years 2 and 3 is dependent on progress in year one and is not guaranteed. Letters of Intent are due by August 24th, with full applications solicited by August 31st and full applications due on September 28th. Awards are made to institutions on behalf of individuals.
Requirements: Applicants must be from either Africa or India, and performing work in either Africa or India in order to apply. Special interested will be given to applications from the African nations of South Africa and Tanzania, but the foundation will consider applicants from other African countries as well. Applicants must demonstrate commitment to continuing to work in a developing country on HIV/AIDS when the award is complete, which is a requirement of the award. Applicants are expected to be in the process of establishing successful careers and programs. Most applicants will have completed training within the past 5 years. Senior investigators such as Full Professors will usually not be eligible for the award. Applicants must hold a position at a public or private non-profit institution that will allow him or her adequate time and provide appropriate facilities to perform the work proposed.
Restrictions: U.S. citizens or European citizens living in these countries are not eligible to apply. Previous International Leadership Award recipients will not be eligible for this round of funding. Grants can not be made directly to individuals.
Amount of Grant: $100,000 in total costs per year for three years
Date(s) Application is Due: Mar 20
Contact: Chris Hudnall, Senior Program Coordinator; (310) 491-3154 or (310) 314-1459, ext. 154; fax: (310) 314-1469; email: Chris@pedaids.org or research@pedaids.org
Internet: http://www.pedaids.org/GrantsandAwards/Awards/International-Leadership-Award.aspx
Sponsor: Elizabeth Glaser Pediatric AIDS Foundation
11150 Santa Monica Boulevard, Suite 1050
Los Angeles, CA 90025

Elizabeth Glaser Pediatric AIDS Foundation Operations Research Grants 1394
The Foundation, in its commitment to improve programs to prevent mother-to-child transmission of HIV (PMTCT), announces the availability of a second and final round of funding for operations research (OR) projects under the new Operations Research for Enhancing PMTCT Program. The RFP will further develop an OR program that is designed to utilize Foundation-supported sites and data to generate studies capable of ultimately improving PMTCT program activities. For the purposes of this EGPAF Request for Proposals (RFP), Operations Research is defined broadly and includes the use of analytical techniques to achieve better health outcomes, assessment of the relative contribution of components of service delivery to achieve desired outcomes, and the measurement of cost-effective systems to achieve desired goals. One year awards will be funded up to a maximum of $150,000 inclusive of 5% (maximum) indirect costs. Two year awards will provide up to $125,000 per year to a total of $250,000 in research support per 2 year award including 5% indirect costs. Letters of Intent (LOIs) are due April 14th, with full applications due at the Foundation office by June 6.
Requirements: Proposals will be accepted from investigators who are working with health care teams that are providing PMTCT services to EGPAF-supported sites around the world. Foundation staff, Foundation partners including host-country government and non-governmental organizations and/or combinations of the above are eligible.
Amount of Grant: $150,000-$250,000
Contact: Chris Hudnall, Senior Program Coordinator; (310) 491-3154 or (310) 314-1459, ext. 154; fax: (310) 314-1469; email: Chris@pedaids.org or research@pedaids.org
Internet: http://www.pedaids.org/GrantsandAwards/Awards/Operations-Research-Award.aspx
Sponsor: Elizabeth Glaser Pediatric AIDS Foundation
11150 Santa Monica Boulevard, Suite 1050
Los Angeles, CA 90025

Elizabeth Glaser Pediatric AIDS Foundation Pediatric HIV Vaccine Grants 1395
The Foundation's Pediatric HIV Vaccine Research Program seeks to address basic and pre-clinical research relevant to pediatric HIV vaccine design and development, including, but not limited to, the following topics: the study of breast-milk transmission of HIV; pediatric immune responses to HIV; identification of potential vaccines for pediatric populations; and identification of obstacles to the conduct of clinical trials in infants.
Samples: Marylyn Addo, M.D., Ph.D., Massachusetts General Hospital, Charlestown, Massachusetts (2008); Grace Aldrovandi, M.D. Children's Hospital, Los Angeles, U.S.C Los Angeles, California (2008).
Contact: Chris Hudnall, Senior Program Coordinator; (310) 491-3154 or (310) 314-1459, ext. 154; fax: (310) 314-1469; email: Chris@pedaids.org or research@pedaids.org
Internet: http://www.pedaids.org/GrantsandAwards/Awards/Pediatric-HIV-Vaccine-Program.aspx
Sponsor: Elizabeth Glaser Pediatric AIDS Foundation
11150 Santa Monica Boulevard, Suite 1050
Los Angeles, CA 90025

Elizabeth Glaser Pediatric AIDS Foundation 2-Year International Scholar Award 1396
The Foundation is offering a postdoctoral fellowship for clinicians/scientists from developing countries. The program is aimed at health care professionals who have specific training or experience with HIV/AIDS and hold an M.D. or Ph.D. Applicants must demonstrate commitment to continuing to work in a developing country on HIV/AIDS when the award is complete, as the emphasis of this program is on building long-term scientific capacity in developing countries. The subjects for these projects could include, but are not limited to, the following: epidemiology; issues related to implementation of either prevention or therapy programs; transmission of the HIV virus from mother to infant, including breast-milk transmission and prevention; pediatric HIV vaccine development; antiretroviral drug treatment including pharmacology, complications, and resistance; and microbicide research.
Requirements: Applicants must be from a developing country, and performing work in a developing country. The Foundation encourages those who are determined to improve care in the international setting, as well as those interested in basic science, to apply.
Restrictions: United States or European citizens living in developing countries are not eligible to apply.
Amount of Grant: $57,225
Contact: Chris Hudnall, Senior Program Coordinator; (310) 491-3154 or (310) 314-1459, ext. 154; fax: (310) 314-1469; email: Chris@pedaids.org or research@pedaids.org
Internet: http://www.pedaids.org/GrantsandAwards/Awards/Two-Year-International-Award.aspx
Sponsor: Elizabeth Glaser Pediatric AIDS Foundation
11150 Santa Monica Boulevard, Suite 1050
Los Angeles, CA 90025

Elizabeth Glaser Pediatric AIDS Foundation Two-Year Scholar Awards 1397
The Awards are postdoctoral fellowships that provide two years of salary support, plus supplies and/or travel costs toward medical research on pediatric HIV/AIDS. Annual salaries—based on years of postdoctoral experience—range from $30,000 to $46,000. These awards provide a powerful incentive for a new generation of scientists to take an early professional interest in studying pediatric HIV/AIDS. Scientists are supported by a mentor experienced in HIV/AIDS research. Through this mentoring relationship, a growing number of talented investigators are focusing their efforts on helping to bring an end to HIV/AIDS in children.
Requirements: Scholars must select an experienced sponsor with appropriate qualifications to oversee the proposed research. The sponsor should be a faculty member with an advanced degree (M.D. or Ph.D.) who will oversee the research, provide guidance to the applicant, and can provide evidence of the institution's commitment to the career development of the applicant.
Samples: Melissa Farrow, Ph.D., College of the Holy Cross—Investigation of the Expression of Anti-HIV AP.O.BEC3 Family Members (2005); Vandana Kalia, Ph.D., Emory University School of Medicine—Development of CD8 T Cell Immunological Memory (2005); Surojit Sarkar, Ph.D., Emory University School of Medicine—Immune Reconstitution and Reversal of T Cell Exhaustion During Chronic Infection (2005).
Amount of Grant: $60,000 maximum
Contact: Chris Hudnall, Senior Program Coordinator; (310) 491-3154 or (310) 314-1459, ext. 154; fax: (310) 314-1469; email: Chris@pedaids.org or research@pedaids.org
Internet: http://www.pedaids.org/GrantsandAwards/Awards/Two-YearScholar.aspx
Sponsor: Elizabeth Glaser Pediatric AIDS Foundation
11150 Santa Monica Boulevard, Suite 1050
Los Angeles, CA 90025

Elizabeth Glaser Scientist Award 1398
The Award is the Foundation's highest scientific honor, and is an investment in the most promising HIV/AIDS researchers at a critical stage in their careers. These scientists, who represent the best and brightest investigators from the international medical science community, are selected on the basis of their knowledge, innovation, and dedication. By providing up to $682,500 in research funding over a five-year period, this award enables recipients to focus their long-term efforts on issues specific to pediatric HIV/AIDS. The Award fosters an unprecedented spirit of collaboration among these scientists. Each year, the Elizabeth Glaser Scientists meet with our internationally renowned advisory board to stimulate ideas, report on current programs, and plan future research. Since the program's inception, the Foundation has built an invaluable network of scientists whose work in vaccine development, immune response, breast milk transmission, and other

critical areas impacts the entire field of HIV/AIDS research. Interested applicants must contact the foundation to request a letter of intent cover sheet. Letters of intent are due by the listed deadline date; full applications are by invitation.
Requirements: Candidates must have an MD, PhD, DDS, or DVM degree and be at the assistant professor level or above.
Restrictions: The foundation will not fund large therapeutic trials or the pharmocologic development of drugs.
Samples: David Evans, Ph.D., Department of Microbiology and Molecular Genetics, New England National Primate Research Center—Oral Transmission of Single-Cycle SIV in Neonates (2006); Margaret Feeney, M.D., M.Sc., Massachusetts General Hospital—The Immune Response to Acute Perinatal HIV Infection (2006); Alexandra Trkola, Ph.D., Division of Infectious Diseases and Hospital Epidemiology, University Hospital Zurich—The Humoral Immune Response to HIV (2006).
Amount of Grant: $682,500 maximum for a period of five years
Contact: Chris Hudnall, Senior Program Coordinator; (310) 491-3154 or (310) 314-1459, ext. 154; fax: (310) 314-1469; email: Chris@pedaids.org or research@pedaids.org
Internet: http://www.pedaids.org/GrantsandAwards/Awards/ElizabethGlaserScientist.aspx
Sponsor: Elizabeth Glaser Pediatric AIDS Foundation
11150 Santa Monica Boulevard, Suite 1050
Los Angeles, CA 90025

Elizabeth McGraw Foundation Grants 1399

The foundation awards grants nationally, with a focus on the U.S. Northeast, in its areas of interest, including cancer research, elementary and secondary education, art museums, performing arts (opera and theater), and culture. There are no application deadlines or specific guidelines. Send letter containing a detailed description of project and amount of funding requested to: John McGraw, Pres., 157 Eel River Road, Osterville, MA 02655
Geographic Focus: Florida; Massachusetts; New York
Contact: Paul J. Bisset, V.P., Deutsche Bank Trust Co. of NY; (212) 454-8607
Sponsor: Elizabeth McGraw Foundation
c/o Deutsche Bank Trust Co. of NY, P.O. Box 1297
New York, NY 10008-1297

Elizabeth Morse Genius Charitable Trust Grants 1400

The trust awards grants to eligible Illinois nonprofit organizations in its areas of interest, including the arts, health and human services, and children and youth services. Types of support include continuing support, general operating grants, matching/challenge grants, program development, seed grants, and technical assistance. There are no application forms or deadlines.
Requirements: Nonprofit organizations in the Chicago metropolitan area are eligible.
Restrictions: Grants are not awarded to individuals, religious or political organizations, or for capital campaigns, endowments, scholarships, or loans.
Geographic Focus: Illinois
Samples: Art Encounter (Evanston, IL)—to conduct art-appreciation programs and workshops at Chicago's North Kenwood-Oakland Charter School, and to track students' progress, $30,000 over three years (2005).
Amount of Grant: $10,000-$300,000 range
Contact: Charles Salmar, Jr., c/o Bank of America, N.A., (312) 828-5554
Sponsor: Elizabeth Morse Genius Charitable Trust
231 S LaSalle Street
Chicago, IL 60697

Elkhart County Community Foundation Grants 1401

The foundation is looking for innovative programs or projects that address problems to be solved or opportunities to be seized in Indiana's Elkhart County. Community collaboration where organizations work together toward a shared goal with shared responsibility, shared resources, and shared accountability is encouraged. Support generally will not be given for continuing operating costs of established programs, projects, and agencies. Grants also are awarded for continuing support, technical assistance, and matching funds. Grants are awarded in the areas of arts and culture, community development, education, and health and human services. Most grants are single-year awards; however, multiyear grants also will be considered, subject to performance review. The staff is available for advice in the preparation of a proposal. Letters of interest are due to the Foundation by January 1st, April 1st, June 1st and August 1st.
Requirements: Elkhart County 501(c)3 organizations, or those seeking such status, and some governmental agencies, such as the public library or public school system, are eligible.
Restrictions: The foundation does not offer support for religious or sectarian purposes. No grants are awarded to individuals (other than scholarships), or for operating budgets or budget deficits, annual funds, conferences, scholarly research, endowments, personal travel, or films.
Geographic Focus: Indiana
Amount of Grant: $250-$5000
Date(s) Application is Due: Jan 1, Apr 1, Jun 1 and Aug 1
Contact: Jim Siegmann, Program Officer, (574) 295-8761; fax: (574) 389-7497; email: jim@elkhartccf.org
Internet: http://www.elkhartccf.org/static/grant_seekers/index.shtml
Sponsor: Elkhart County Community Foundation
P.O. Box 2932, 101 S. Main Street
Elkhart, IN 46615

Elliot Foundation Inc Grants 1402

The Elliot Foundation Inc. formerly known as Elliot Foundation for Medical Research and Education, Inc. is a independent foundation, operating primarily in the state of Indiana. The foundation offers funding in the form of general/operating support. The fields of interest include: Christian agencies & churches; crime/violence prevention; environment; natural resources; child abuses; education.
Requirements: Contact Foundation for more information.
Geographic Focus: Indiana
Contact: Richard E. Bond, Secretary, (575) 293-1165
Sponsor: Elliot Foundation, Inc.
2210 East Jackson Boulevard
Elkhart, IN 46516-1165

Ellison Medical Foundation/AFAR Julie Martin Mid-Career Award in Aging Research 1403

The Ellison Medical Foundation and AFAR developed this program for outstanding mid-career scientists who propose novel directions of high importance to biological gerontology. Proposals in areas where NIH awards or other traditional sources are unlikely because the research is high risk, are particularly encouraged if they have the potential for leading to major new advances in our understanding of basic mechanisms of aging. Projects investigating age-related diseases are also supported, but only if approached from the point of view of how basic aging processes may lead to these outcomes. Projects concerning mechanisms underlying common geriatric functional disorders are also encouraged, as long as these include connections to fundamental problems in the biology of aging. Two four-year awards of $500,000 will be given, at the level of $125,000 per year. In addition, up to 10% ($50,000) may be requested for administrative/indirect costs. Recipients of this award are expected to attend the AFAR Grantee Conference. The purpose of the meeting is to promote scientific and personal exchanges among recent AFAR grantees and experts in aging research.
Requirements: The applicant must be an Associate Professor who achieved tenured status after December 1st. Non-tenured Associate Professors at institutions with tenure (even if tenure is only offered at the Full Professor level) are not eligible. Applicants at institutions that do not offer tenure must demonstrate that their appointment is equivalent to that of an Associate Professor who received tenure status after December 1st. The proposed research must be conducted at any type of not-for-profit setting in the United States. The deadline of receipt of applications and all supporting materials is December 16th at 5:00 p.m. EST.
Restrictions: Projects that deal strictly with clinical problems such as the diagnosis and treatment of disease, health outcomes, or the social context of aging are not eligible. Applicants who are employees in the NIH Intramural program are not eligible.
Amount of Grant: $125,000 per year
Date(s) Application is Due: Dec 16
Contact: Grants Manager; (212) 703-9977 or (888) 582-2327; fax: (212) 997-0330; email: grants@afar.org or info@afar.org
Internet: http://afar.org/Ellison%20Mid-Career.html
Sponsor: American Federation for Aging Research
55 West 39th Street, 16th Floor
New York, NY 10018

Ellison Medical Foundation/AFAR Postdoctoral Fellows in Aging Research 1404

The Ellison Medical Foundation, in partnership with the American Federation for Aging Research (AFAR), created the Ellison/AFAR Postdoctoral Fellows in Aging Research Program to encourage and further the careers of postdoctoral fellows with outstanding promise in the basic biological and biomedical sciences relevant to understanding aging processes and age related diseases and disabilities. The award is intended to provide significant support to permit these postdoctoral fellows to become established in the field of aging. Projects concerned with understanding the basic mechanisms of aging will be considered. Projects investigating age related diseases are also supported, if approached from the point of view of how basic aging processes may lead to these outcomes. Projects concerning mechanisms underlying common geriatric functional disorders are also considered. It is anticipated that up to 15 one year grants will be awarded, ranging from $44,850 for a first year fellow, up to $58,850 for a fellow with more than 7 years of training. Of the award, up to $7,850 may be requested for expenses such as research supplies, equipment, health insurance and travel to scientific meetings. Refer to the Ellison/AFAR instruction sheet and application on the AFAR website for complete application procedures. Recipients of this award are expected to attend the AFAR Grantee Conference. The purpose of the meeting is to promote scientific and personal exchanges among recent AFAR grantees and experts in aging research.
Requirements: The applicant must be a postdoctoral fellow (MD and/or PhD degree) at the start date of the award (July 1). Any former Ellison/AFAR postdoctoral award recipient may apply for this award. All candidates must submit applications endorsed by their institutions. The proposed research must be conducted at any type of not-for-profit setting in the United States.
Restrictions: Employees in the NIH Intramural program are not eligible. Fellows may not hold any concurrent foundation or not-for-profit funding.
Amount of Grant: $44,000 - $58,000 range
Date(s) Application is Due: Dec 16
Contact: Grants Manager; (212) 703-9977 or (888) 582-2327; fax: (212) 997-0330; email: grants@afar.org or info@afar.org
Internet: http://www.afar.org/ellisonpostdoc.html
Sponsor: American Federation for Aging Research
55 West 39th Street, 16th Floor
New York, NY 10018

Ellison Medical Foundation/AFAR Senior Postdoctoral Fellows Research 1405

The program seeks to encourage and further the careers of senior postdoctoral fellows with outstanding promise in the basic biological and biomedical sciences relevant to understanding aging processes and age-related diseases and disabilities. The award is intended to provide significant support to permit these postdoctoral fellows to become established in the field of aging. Projects concerned with understanding the basic mechanisms of aging will be considered. Projects investigating age-related diseases are also supported, if approached from the point of view of how basic aging processes may lead to these outcomes. Projects concerning mechanisms underlying common geriatric functional disorders are also considered. It is anticipated that three two-year grants will be awarded each year.

Requirements: Postdoctoral fellows, both MDs and PhDs, are eligible. Fellows with at least three and not more than five years of prior postdoctoral training are eligible.

Amount of Grant: $100,000

Date(s) Application is Due: Dec 15

Contact: Grants Manager, (212) 703-9977; fax: (212) 997-0330; email: grants@afar.org

Internet: http://www.afar.org/ellison.html

Sponsor: American Federation for Aging Research
70 W 40th Street, 11th Floor
New York, NY 10018

Elmer L. and Eleanor J. Andersen Foundation Grants 1406

The foundation exists to enhance the quality of the civic, cultural, educational, environmental, and social aspects of life in Minnesota, primarily in the metropolitan area of Saint Paul and Minneapolis. Types of support include general operating support, continuing support, annual campaigns, capital campaigns, building construction/renovation, endowment funds, program development, deficit reduction, publication, seed money, curriculum development, research, technical assistance, and matching funds. The board meets four times annually.

Requirements: Minnesota nonprofit organizations are eligible.

Geographic Focus: Minnesota

Amount of Grant: $500-$75,000 range

Date(s) Application is Due: Feb 1; May 1; Aug 1; Nov 1

Contact: Mari Oyanagi Eggum, Foundation Administrator, (651) 642-0127; fax: (651) 645-4684; email: eandefdn@mtn.org

Sponsor: Elmer L. and Eleanor J. Andersen Foundation
2424 Territorial Road
Saint Paul, MN 55114

Elsa U. Pardee Foundation Grants 1407

The foundation has three main grantmaking focuses: ongoing research grants to established institutions for cancer research, the funding of worthwhile new cancer research projects, and grants to committees providing financial assistance to cancer victims in specified areas. The foundation particularly welcomes innovative, small-scale, short-term projects that may be difficult to fund elsewhere until some interesting results are obtained. Application forms are available on written request and must accompany all project proposals. Applications are accepted at any time.

Requirements: Application must include completed form, description of project, itemized budget, approval from the institution where the project will be done, amount requested, duration of project, and any other supportive material deemed helpful.

Restrictions: Grants are limited to research toward the cure and control of cancer and in general do not provide for building funds, equipment (except that used in a specific project), fellowships, or fund-raising campaigns.

Samples: U of Maryland (MD)—for the study of synthetic, conformational, and enzymatic factors of asn-linked glycoproteins, $34,760.; John Muir Foundation (CA)—for chemotherapy program for cancer patients in Contra Costa County, CA, $150,000.

Amount of Grant: $50,000-$200,000 average

Contact: James Kendall, Secretary, (989) 832-3691; email: info@pardeefoundation.org

Internet: http://www.pardeefoundation.org

Sponsor: Elsa U. Pardee Foundation
P.O. Box 2767
Midland, MI 48641-2767

Elsie Lee Garthwaite Memorial Foundation Grants 1408

Established in 1943, the Foundation supports organizations primarily in Philadelphia, Chester, Montgomery and Delaware counties of Pennsylvania. Giving to organizations that: provide for the physical and emotional well-being of children and young people; seek to enable young people, particularly the needy, to reach their fullest potential through education, empowerment, and exposure to the arts; are smaller organizations, with budgets under $1 million per year.

Requirements: Non-profits are eligible in the Philadelphia, Chester, Montgomery and Delaware counties, PA. Contact the Foundation at least 30 days prior to deadlines with a Letter of Intent. An application form can be obtained from the Foundation after reviewing the Letter of Intent, unsolicited applications will not be excepted. Contact the Foundation for further guidelines.

Restrictions: No grants to individuals, public, private, or parochial schools, colleges and universities.

Geographic Focus: Pennsylvania

Samples: United States Fund for UNICEF, New York, NY, $15,000 - for Pakistan earthquake victim relief (2005); Citizen Schools, Boston, MA, $10,000 - for program support (2005); Center for Grieving Children, Teens and Families, Philadelphia, PA, $3,000 - for general operating support (2005);

Amount of Grant: $3,000-$16,000 range

Date(s) Application is Due: Mar 31; Aug 31

Contact: Thomas Kaneda, Secretary; (610) 527-8101; fax: (610) 527-7808

Sponsor: Elsie Lee Garthwaite Memorial Foundation
1234 Lancaster Avenue, P.O. Box 709
Rosemont, PA 19010-0709

EMBO Installation Grants 1409

The aim of this scheme is to strengthen science in participating EMBC member states. At present applications are accepted from Croatia, the Czech Republic, Estonia, Hungary, Portugal, Poland and Turkey. Additional member states have expressed an interest to join in the near future. Grants will help scientists to relocate, set up their labs and rapidly establish a reputation in the European scientific community. The program is entirely funded by the participating EMBC member states and successful applicants receive an annual support of Euro $50,000 for three to five years. Each participating country sets an upper limit to the number of grants available per year. Application forms should be completed by the individual scientists and the receiving institute.

Requirements: Eligible scientists should: have an excellent publication record; have spent at least two consecutive years prior to the application deadline, outside the country in which they are applying to establish their lab; and be negotiating a full-time position at an institute/university in participating member states by the date of application. No age limit applies.

Amount of Grant: $50,000 Euro per year for 3-5 years

Date(s) Application is Due: Apr 15

Contact: Hermann Bujard, Executive Director; +49 (if outside Germany) (0) 6221-8891, ext. 101; fax: +49 (if outside Germany) (0) 6221 8891-200; email: embo@embo.org

Internet: http://www.embo.org/sdig/index.html

Sponsor: European Molecular Biology Organization
Meyerhofstrasse 1
Heidelberg D-69117 Germany

EMBO Long-Term Fellowships 1410

Long-Term Fellowships are awarded for prolonged visits (12 to 24 months) and are intended for advanced training through research. As the aim of the EMBO is to promote international research, it follows that mobility is a crucial element in deciding the eligibility of an application. All applications must involve a laboratory of origin or a receiving institute or applicant's nationality from one of the member states. Stipend rates depend on the country being visited, marital status, etc.

Requirements: Applicants must hold a doctorate degree or equivalent before the start of the fellowship but not necessarily when applying. For clarity, it is deemed that this requirement is fulfilled only when the thesis has been stamped as submitted for final examination by the university. As a minimum, applicants must have at least one first author publication in press or published in an international peer reviewed journal at the time of application.

Restrictions: Applications are only considered from candidates with a maximum of 3 years postdoctoral experience.

Date(s) Application is Due: Feb 15; Aug 15

Contact: Liselott Maidment; +49 (if outside Germany) (0) 6221-8891, ext. 116; fax: +49 (if outside Germany) (0) 6221 8891-200; email: fellowships@embo.org

Internet: http://www.embo.org/fellowships/long_term.html

Sponsor: European Molecular Biology Organization
Meyerhofstrasse 1
Heidelberg D-69117 Germany

EMBO Short-Term Fellowships 1411

Short-term fellowships are established to advance molecular biology research by helping scientists to visit another laboratory with a view to applying a technique not available in the home laboratory. Such fellowships are not awarded for exchanges between two laboratories within the same country, and are intended for joint research work rather than consultations. The fellowships cover travel plus subsistence of the fellow only and not of any dependents. These fellowships are intended for visits of one week to three months duration (for non-European applicants the short-term fellowships are intended for a fixed duration of 90 days). Stipends vary widely from country to country,

Requirements: Applicants must be either: post-doctoral scientists with less than 10 years of professional experience since finishing their Ph.D. degree (or the equivalent); or pre-doctoral scientists who have not yet completed a Ph.D. degree (or the equivalent).

Restrictions: All applications must involve either a laboratory of origin or a receiving institute from one of the EMBC member states.

Contact: Agnes Visser-de Matteis; +49 (if outside Germany) (0) 6221-8891, ext. 115; fax: +49 (if outside Germany) (0) 6221 8891-200; email: fellowships@embo.org

Internet: http://www.embo.org/fellowships/short_term.html

Sponsor: European Molecular Biology Organization
Meyerhofstrasse 1
Heidelberg D-69117 Germany

Emerson Charitable Trust Grants 1412

Established in 1944 in Missouri as the Emerson Electric Manufacturing Company Charitable Trust, the Foundation supports: arts and culture—fine arts and cultural institutions to enrich the diversity, creativity, and liveliness of the community; education—programs designed to promote educational systems at all levels; health and human services—programs designed to help individuals and families in times of need,

including sickness, old age, family crisis, and natural disasters; civic affairs—programs designed to protect citizenry; further economic health of the community; and build and maintain assets such as parks and zoos; and youth—programs designed to give young people the opportunity to recognize their potential, confidence, and skills to achieve their dreams. The foundation awards college scholarships to children and step-children of employees of Emerson Electric. No specific application form is required, and initial approach should be the complete proposal,
Samples: Alvin J. Siteman Ctr, Washington U School of Medicine and Barnes-Jewish Hospital (Saint Louis, MO)—for a new cancer-research facility and for cancer research, $6 million challenge grant.
Amount of Grant: $5,000-$300,000 average
Contact: Jo Ann Harmon, Senior Vice President; (314) 553-3722; fax: (314) 553-1605
Internet: http://www.emerson.com/en-us/about_emerson/company_overview/pages/our_approach_to_corporate_philanthropy.aspx
Sponsor: Emerson Charitable Trust
P.O. Box 4100, 8000 W. Florissant Avenue
Saint Louis, MO 63136

Emerson Electric Company Contributions Grants 1413
Emerson believes it is important to help support organizations and institutions that play significant roles in enhancing the quality of life in the communities where its facilities are located and where its employees and their families live and work. As a complement to its foundation, Emerson makes charitable contributions to nonprofit organizations directly. Support is given on a national basis in areas of company operations, with emphasis on St. Louis, Missouri. Its primary fields of interest include the arts, education, health care, and public affairs. An application form should be obtained from the nearest company facility.
Contact: Robert M. Cox, Senior Vice President; (314) 553-2000; (314) 553-1605
Internet: http://www.emerson.com/en-us/about_emerson/company_overview/pages/our_approach_to_corporate_philanthropy.aspx
Sponsor: Emerson Electric Company
P.O. Box 4100, 8000 W. Florissant Avenue
Saint Louis, MO 63136

Emily Davie and Joseph S. Kornfeld Foundation Grants 1414
The Foundation's selection criteria for all programs are: evidence of strong and visionary leadership; development of new initiatives that are replicable and sustainable; creation of new ways to address existing critical issues; interest in building connections and creative partnerships; desire to improve and enrich lives of individuals (rather than capital improvements); and original, unusual, dynamic and focused proposals. Proposal letters should include a background on the organization, a detailed description of the proposed project and financial information.
Requirements: Eligible applicants must provide a copy of a 501(c)3 determination letter.
Date(s) Application is Due: Mar 1; Jul 15; Nov 15
Contact: Bobye List, Executive Director, (718) 624-7969; fax: (718) 834-1204; email: office@kornfeldfdn.org
Internet: http://fdncenter.org/grantmaker/kornfeld
Sponsor: Emily Davie and Joseph S. Kornfeld Foundation
41 Schermerhorn Street, Suite 208
Brooklyn, NY 11021

Emma B. Howe Memorial Foundation Grants 1415
The Emma B. Howe Memorial Foundation makes grants through the Minneapolis Foundation. The focus of all grants is to improve: the health and well-being of children, youth and families; opportunities for educational achievement; access to quality affordable housing; and economic vitality throughout the region. Information on the application process is available online.
Requirements: Eligible organizations include 501(c)3 nonprofits, public institutions; and emerging groups organized for nonprofit purposes.
Restrictions: Funds are not available for: individuals; organizations/activities outside of Minnesota; conference registration fees; memberships; direct religious activities; political organizations or candidates; direct fundraising efforts; telephone solicitations; courtesy advertising; financial deficits.
Geographic Focus: Minnesota
Contact: Community Philanthropy, (612) 672-3836; email: grants@mplsfoundation.org
Internet: http://www.mplsfoundation.org/partners/emma.htm
Sponsor: Emma B. Howe Memorial Foundation
80 South Eighth Street
Minneapolis, MN 55402

Ensworth Charitable Foundation Grants 1416
The Foundation, established in 1948, supports organizations involved with health and welfare programs, youth activities, enjoyment of the natural environment, relief of human suffering, education, religion, and the arts, particularly music. Giving is limited to Hartford, CT, and contiguous surrounding areas.
Requirements: Non-profits operating in the Harford, CT and contiguous surrounding areas are eligible to apply. Send a Letter of Intent to begin the application process.
Restrictions: No grants to individuals, or for operating budgets, annual campaigns, deficit financing, building or endowment funds, equipment and materials, land acquisition, scholarships, fellowships, research, or publications; no loans.
Geographic Focus: Connecticut
Samples: Southside Institutions Neighborhood Alliance, Hartford, CT, $25,000 - for Civic Youth Leadership Program (2006); Habitat for Humanity, Hartford Area, Hartford, CT, $15,000 - for construction of home in Hartford(2006); Almada Lodge-Times Farm Camp Corporation, Andover, CT, $10,400 - for overnight summer camping program (2006);
Amount of Grant: $1,000-$25,000
Date(s) Application is Due: Jan 15; Jul 15
Contact: Amy R. Lynch, V.P., Bank of America; fax: (860) 952-7395;
Sponsor: The Ensworth Charitable Foundation
777 Main Street, CT2-102-22-02
Hartford, CT 06115-2303

Entergy Community Partnership Grants 1417
The Foundation will bestow a monetary award for projects that effectively impact arts and culture, community improvement/enrichment, education and literacy, or healthy families. Organizations must be located within Entergy's service territory in Arkansas, Louisiana, Mississippi, or Texas. Applications should be submitted online before midnight on March 31. The application will be available January 26 through March 31.
Requirements: 501(c)3 organizations, schools, hospitals, governmental units, and religious institutions are eligible. Each organization may submit only one application per year.
Restrictions: The Foundation will not fund: groups without 501(c)3 or similar non-profit status; administrative expenses (e.g., salaries, office equipment), or recurring expenses that exceed 15% of the requested amount; capital project funding (i.e., building campaigns); political candidates or groups; purchase of uniforms or trips for school-related organizations; amateur sports teams; activities whose sole purpose is promotion or support of a specific religion, denomination, or religious institution; grants to individuals or loans of any type; any organization owned or operated by an employee of Entergy.
Geographic Focus: Arkansas; Louisiana; Mississippi; Texas
Amount of Grant: $1,000 maximum
Date(s) Application is Due: Mar 31
Contact: Christine Jordan; (504) 576-7705 or (504) 576-6980; fax: (504) 576-2190; email: cminor@entergy.com;; Jennifer Quezergue; (504) 576-2674 or (504) 576-6980; email: jquezer@entergy.com
Internet: http://www.entergy.com/our_community/cpGrant_Guidelines.aspx
Sponsor: Entergy Corporation
P.O. Box 61000
New Orleans, LA 70160

Entergy Corporation Open Grants for Healthy Families 1418
Entergy's Open Grants Program focuses on improving communities as a whole. The Corporation believes that children need a good start to grow into healthy, well-adjusted adults. With that in mind, it gives to programs that have a direct impact on children educationally and emotionally. The Corporation is also interested in family programs, like those that better prepare parents to balance the demands of work and home. In considering requests for grants, priority is placed on programs in specific counties/parishes, including areas of: Arkansas, Louisiana, Massachusetts, Michigan, Mississippi, New Hampshire, New York, Texas, and Vermont. Applicants should contact the contributions coordinator in their region, which are listed on the web site. Open grant applications are accepted on an ongoing basis.
Requirements: Grants from Entergy will only be made to the following types of organizations: non-profit organizations that are tax exempt under section 501(c)3 of the Internal Revenue Code; or schools, hospitals, governmental units and religious institutions that hold nonprofit status similar to that of 501(c)3 organizations.
Restrictions: Entergy will not fund: groups without 501(c)3 or similar non-profit status; administrative expenses (e.g., salaries, office equipment) or recurring expenses that exceed 15% of the requested amount; capital project funding (i.e., building campaigns); political candidates or groups; purchase of uniforms or trips for school-related organizations; amateur sports teams; activities whose sole purpose is promotion or support of a specific religion, denomination, or religious institution; grants to individuals or loans of any type; or any organization owned or operated by an employee of Entergy.
Geographic Focus: Arkansas; Louisiana; Massachusetts; Michigan; Mississippi; New Hampshire; New York; Texas; Vermont
Contact: Christine Jordan; (504) 576-7705 or (504) 576-6980; fax: (504) 576-2190; email: cminor@entergy.com;; Jennifer Quezergue; (504) 576-2674; email: jquezer@entergy.com
Internet: http://www.entergy.com/our_community/Grant_Guidelines.aspx
Sponsor: Entergy Corporation
P.O. Box 61000; Mail Unit: L-ENT-8A
New Orleans, LA 70161

EPA Baseline Assessment of Risks of Exposure to Lead Poisoning of Native American Children 1419
This program supports efforts to identify the risks of lead poisoning among children by conducting a baseline assessment of potential lead exposures. Tribes may then use this data to determine whether there is a need to implement an a lead-reduction program.
Requirements: Federally recognized Indian tribes, tribal consortia, and tribal organizations are eligible to apply.
Restrictions: Funds may not be used to purchase property, provide lead hazard reduction activities, conduct renovation or construction activities, or cover case management.
Amount of Grant: $75,000 maximum
Contact: Darlene Watford, (202) 566-0516; fax: (202) 566-0469; email: Watford.Darlene@epa.gov
Internet: http://www.epa.gov/lead
Sponsor: Environmental Protection Agency
1200 Pennsylvania Avenue, NW
Washington, DC 20460

EPA Children's Health Protection Grants 1420

The objectives of this program are to catalyze community-based and regional projects and other actions that enhance public outreach and communication; assist families in evaluating risks to children and in making informed consumer choices; build partnerships that increase a community's long-term capacity to advance the protection of children's environmental health and safety; leverage private and public investments to enhance environmental quality by enabling community efforts to continue past EPA's ability to provide assistance to communities; and promote protection of children from environmental threats through lessons learned. There are no deadline dates.

Requirements: Eligible applicants include community groups, public nonprofit institutions/organizations, tribal governments, specialized groups, profit organizations, private nonprofit institutions/organizations, and municipal and local governments. Potential applicants are strongly encouraged to discuss proposed projects with or submit preapplications to program staff prior to the completion of a full proposal.

Amount of Grant: $5000-$250,000 average

Contact: Bettina Fletcher, Office of Children's Health Protection, (202) 564-2188; fax: (202) 564-2733; email: fletcher.bettina@epa.gov

Internet: http://yosemite.epa.gov/ochp/ochpweb.nsf/content/grants.htm

Sponsor: Environmental Protection Agency

1200 Pennsylvania Ave NW, Mail Code 1107A, Room 2512 Ariel Rios N

Washington, DC 20004

EPA Lead Awareness Outreach for Native American Tribes 1421

This program provides financial assistance to tribes to launch outreach efforts that would educate Native American families about the dangers of exposure to lead-based paint hazards among children, distribute educational information and encourage families to have their children screened and homes tested for lead hazards. Activities may include providing medical training, developing culturally specific lead outreach materials, distributing pamphlets and establishing an in-home education program.

Requirements: Federally recognized Indian tribes, tribal consortia, and tribal organizations are eligible to apply.

Restrictions: Funds may not be used to purchase property, provide lead hazard reduction, conduct renovation or construction activities, or cover case management costs.

Amount of Grant: $50,000 maximum per outreach project

Contact: Darlene Watford, Office of Pollution Prevention and Toxics, (202) 566-0516; fax: (202) 566-0469; email: Watford.Darlene@epa.gov

Internet: http://www.epa.gov/lead

Sponsor: Environmental Protection Agency

1200 Pennsylvania Avenue, NW

Washington, DC 20460

Epilepsy Postdoctoral and Clinical Research Fellowships 1422

A few fellowships will be awarded to scientists (PhD or MD) wishing to carry out full-time research projects in the field of epilepsy. The period of support may begin at any time between May and October. The grant will be for one year but will be renewable once and exceptionally twice, upon request.

Requirements: Fellowships are available to Canadian citizens or for projects conducted in Canada.

Amount of Grant: $C30,000

Date(s) Application is Due: Jan 15

Contact: Caroline Savoy, (450) 358-9779; fax: (450) 346-1045; email: epilepsy@savoy-foundation.ca

Internet: http://www.savoy-foundation.ca/eng/mission/defaut.htm

Sponsor: Savoy Foundation

230 Foch Street

St Jean Sur Richelieu, PQ J3B 2B2 Canada

Epilepsy Research Foundation New Therapy Grants 1423

The foundation supports innovative research leading to new insights into a cure for epilepsy. The primary focus of this program is to bring new approaches and therapies to patients through translational research. Other areas of consideration include but are not limited to: meaningful grants to senior-level scientific and clinical investigators on the brink of new discoveries, working at the nation's leading academic and research institutions, and in private industry; seed funding for preliminary work necessary to explore novel approaches; building innovative platform technologies; research to bring new approaches and therapy to children; innovative cutting edge projects that could lead to breakthrough discoveries; support for applying work in other areas with potential for promise in epilepsy; research programs that might not otherwise be funded through traditional sources; projects that encourage collaboration among scientists and industry; and proposals dealing with commercializing academic research projects. Grant funds may be used to support the direct costs of research such as salary support for personnel directly engaged in the project, consumable supplies and services, and travel essential to the conduct of the research. Multi-year awards will be considered.

Requirements: Investigators must hold a relevant advanced degree (MD and/or PhD) and have completed all research training. The program is open to investigators at corporations as well as the academic/university arena. All applications will be judged on a competitive basis, without regard to the academic rank or title of the investigator. Applicants whose research will involve patient care or direct involvement with patients must be licensed to practice their profession at their institution and must obtain Institutional Review Board (IRB) approval of their research. IRB approval must be included with the original application.

Restrictions: Grant funds may not be used for indirect costs or institutional overhead, or purchase of equipment that exceeds 10% of the budget without prior approval.

Amount of Grant: $100,000-$200,000

Date(s) Application is Due: Apr 1; Oct 1

Contact: Research Department, (800) 332-1000 or (301) 459-3700; email: grants@efa.org or EpilepsyCure@aol.com

Internet: http://www.epilepsytdp.org/sec/support_translational

Sponsor: Epilepsy Research Foundation

4351 Garden City Drive

Landover, MD 20785-7223

Eppendorf & Science Prize for Neurobiology 1424

The Eppendorf & Science Prize for Neurobiology acknowledges the increasingly active and important role of neurobiology in advancing our understanding of the functioning of the brain and the nervous system — a quest that seems destined for dramatic expansion in the coming decades. This international prize, established in 2002, encourages the work of promising young neurobiologists by providing support in the early stages of their careers. It is awarded annually for the most outstanding neurobiological research by a young scientist, as described in a 1,000-word essay based on research performed during the past three years. The winner is awarded money and publication of his or her essay in 'Science'. The essay and those of up to three finalists are also published on 'Science Online'. The award is announced and presented at a ceremony at the annual meeting of the Society for Neuroscience. Eppendorf provides financial support to help enable the grand prize winner to attend the meeting.

Requirements: Entrants must be a neurobiologist with an advanced degree and not older than 35 years. The research described in the entrant's essay must be based on the methods of molecular and cell biology. The entrant must have performed or directed the work described in the essay. The research must have been performed during the previous three years.

Restrictions: Employees of Eppendorf AG, its subsidiaries, Science and AAAS, and their relatives are not eligible for the prize.

Samples: Mauro Costa, $25,000- for essay "Mattioli Switching Memories ON and OFF" (2008); Rachel Wilson, $25,000- for essay "Neural Circuits Underlying Chemical Perception" (2007); Doris Tsao, $25,000- for essay "A Dedicated System for Processing Faces" (2006).

Amount of Grant: $25,000 and publication of his or her essay in 'Science'.

Date(s) Application is Due: Jun 15

Contact: Maryrose Madrid, email: mmadrid@aaas.org or eppendorfscienceprize@aaas.org

Internet: http://www.sciencemag.org/feature/data/prizes/eppendorf/eppenprize.dtl

Sponsor: American Association for the Advancement of Science

1200 New York Avenue, NW, Room 1049B

Washington, DC 20005

Eppley Foundation Postdoctoral Grants 1425

The foundation supports research in advanced scientific subjects, both in the biological and physical sciences, and is interested in supporting research where federal support is not available or to provide seed money toward larger undertakings. Work must be original and independent. Approximately 12 grants are awarded each year.

Requirements: Individuals who have several years of postdoctoral research experience in the biological and physical sciences are eligible. Grant proposals from foreign countries are considered only when a U.S. institution will administer the grant on their behalf.

Restrictions: Grants are not made to individuals and rarely for support of newly awarded PhDs or MDs. Social sciences, computer sciences, and education programs will not be supported. Under most circumstances, the foundation will not support heart, HIV, cancer, or DNA research.

Amount of Grant: $15,000 average

Contact: Huyler Held, Secretary-Treasurer, (212) 448-1100 or (212) 371-1660; fax: (212) 448-6260; email: bblauner@Mclaughlinstern.com

Sponsor: Eppley Foundation for Research

260 Madison Avenue

New York, NY 10016

Eric Berne Fund for the Future Grants 1426

Grants support research or projects that demonstrate an interest in the evaluation of the effectiveness of various applications of transactional analysis (TA) theory. Preference is given to projects that are expected to generate particular benefits within a region or community, that extend TA to new areas of the world, support development of measurable professional standards of competency, and/or build bridges between TA and other disciplines. The deadline for making nominations for the EBMA is December 1 of the year preceding the award.

Requirements: Grants are open to individuals or nonprofit organizations. If profit-making organizations wish to submit proposals, special royalty or profit-sharing agreements may be required.

Contact: Eric Berne Fund Distribution Committee, (925) 600-8110; fax: (925) 600-8112

Internet: http://www.itaa-net.org/itaa/grants.htm

Sponsor: International Transactional Analysis Association

2186 Rheem Dr #B-1

Pleasanton, CA 94588

Erie Community Foundation Grants 1427

The Erie Community Foundation is a collection of charitable endowments operating under the administrative umbrella of a single public charity. Grants will be awarded in four program areas: quality of life; human services; health; and education. The Foundation's goal is to help local charities more effectively and efficiently accomplish their

missions. Application information is available online. Applicants are strongly encouraged to contact the Foundation's program officer prior to submitting an application.
Requirements: Erie, PA, 501(c)3 tax-exempt organizations are eligible.
Restrictions: The Foundation does not fund: program ads; fund raising events/ sponsorships; more than 50 percent of the cost of a vehicle; deficit reduction; sectarian religious activities; government funding cuts; start-up organizations; school playgrounds; fire departments or nursing homes.
Geographic Focus: Pennsylvania
Amount of Grant: $2,000-$15,000
Date(s) Application is Due: Feb 2; Aug 3; Oct 16
Contact: David Gonzalez, Program Officer; (814) 454-0843; fax: (814) 456-4965; email: mbatchelor@eriecommunityfoundation.or
Internet: http://www.eriecommunityfoundation.org/for-grant-seekers/
Sponsor: Erie Community Foundation
459 West 6th Street
Erie, PA 16507

Essex County Community Foundation Discretionary Fund Grant **1428**
The grant awards funds across the broad areas of nonprofit activity, including arts and culture, education, environment, health, social and community services and youth services. The fund will assist nonprofits with projects which strengthen the capacity of the organization to perform its work. Application information is available online.
Requirements: Eligible organizations must be Massachusetts 501(c)3 agencies that serve Essex County citizens with operating budgets of less than $500,000.
Restrictions: Funds are not available for: individuals; costs associated with programs or services provided to citizens outside of Essex County; sectarian or religious purposes; political purposes; debt or deficit reduction; capital campaigns for buildings, land acquisition or endowment; or to support academic research.
Geographic Focus: Massachusetts
Amount of Grant: $1,000-$5,000
Date(s) Application is Due: Jan 12
Contact: Julie Bishop, Coordinator of Grants and Nonprofit Services, (978) 777-8876; email: j.bishop@eccf.org
Internet: http://www.eccf.org/newsarticle.cfm?articleid=118119&PTSidebarOptID=19642&returnTo=page30910.cfm&returntoname=Overview&SiteID=1890&pageid=30910&sidepageid=30910&thetitle=Discretionary%20Fund&banner1img=banner_1.JPG&banner2img=banner_2.JPG&bannerbg=bannerb
Sponsor: Essex County Community Foundation
15 Cherry Street
Danvers, MA 01923

Estee Lauder Grants **1429**
The company has long supported numerous institutions and programs that reflect the interests and concerns of their consumers and employees around the world. Over the years, corporate and brand philanthropy programs and community initiatives have focused on advancing the activities and growth of numerous organizations dedicated to health and human services, education, the environment and the arts. Contributions take many forms, both global and local. Submit a letter of request on company letterhead that describes the request, organization, and intended use of funds.
Amount of Grant: $8.5 million total
Contact: Corporate Contributions, (212) 572-4200; fax: (212) 527-7955
Internet: http://www.elcompanies.com/citizenship/corporate_responsibility/corporate_philanthropy.asp
Sponsor: Estee Lauder
767 Fifth Avenue, Box 100
New York, NY 10153

Ethel S. Abbott Charitable Foundation Grants **1430**
The Foundation, established in 1972, offers support for art and culture, education, health, federated giving, and human service programs. The Board of Trustees will generally consider grant requests for capital projects and endowment projects more favorably than grant requests for operating funds. However, the Board will occasionally make an operating grant for the start up of a new 501(c)3 or a program which will become self-sustaining after the start up period. The application and its guidelines can be downloaded from the web site.
Requirements: The primary grant areas are: Lincoln, Nebraska and the surrounding 50 mile radius; Omaha, Nebraska and the surrounding 50 mile radius up to the Missouri River; and Western, Nebraska, which is defined as all parts of the state in the Mountain Time Zone.
Geographic Focus: Nebraska
Samples: University of Nebraska Foundation, Lincoln, Nebraska $1,000,000—endowment fund for program development for the Sheldon Art Gallery (2007); Quality Living, Omaha, Nebraska, $500,000—for endowment fund for handicap accessible housing in Omaha, Nebraska (2007).
Amount of Grant: $250,000 maximum
Contact: Del Lienemann, Sr., President; (402) 435-4369; fax: (402) 435-4371; email: info@abbottfoundation.org
Internet: http://www.abbottfoundation.org/request_a_grant/index.html
Sponsor: Ethel S. Abbott Charitable Foundation
P.O. Box 81407
Lincoln, NE 68501-1407

Ethical Research Grants and Fellowships **1431**
Graduate fellowships are available for investigations into the discovery, development, validation, and implementation of alternatives to the use of live animals in research, testing, and teaching. Areas of interest include tissue cultures, bacteria cultures, protozoan studies, gas chromatography, mass spectrometry, radioimmunoassay, mathematical and computer models, quantum pharmacology, mechanical models, and clinical and epidemiological surveys. Awards include stipend plus supplies. Students from all over the world are eligible to apply.
Requirements: Nonprofit educational and research institutions are eligible for grants. Students who are enrolled in master's and PhD programs in the sciences, humanities, psychology, and journalism are eligible for graudate fellowships.
Amount of Grant: $15,000 maximum
Date(s) Application is Due: Mar 15
Contact: Peter O'Donovan, Executive Director, (312) 427-6025; fax: (312) 427-6524; email: ifer@navs.org
Internet: http://www.ifer.org
Sponsor: International Foundation for Ethical Research
53 W Jackson Boulevard, Suite 1552
Chicago, IL 60604

Eugene and Agnes E. Meyer Foundation Grants **1432**
The Foundation awards grants to nonprofit organizations that serve the people and communities in the Washington, D.C. region. Grants are awarded in ten program areas: arts; heritage, and culture; children, youth and families; civic engagement; education; employment and skills training; health and mental health; homelessness and hunger; housing and community development; immigrant communities; and law and justice. Candidates are required to first submit a letter of inquiry. Instructions for completion of LOI are available online.
Requirements: Eligible applicants must be a nonprofit organization with tax-exempt status and be located within and primarily serve the Washington, D.C. region which is defined as: the District of Columbia; the Maryland counties of Montgomery, Prince George's, Calvert, Charles, and St. Mary's; and the Virginia counties of Arlington, Fairfax, Loudoun, Prince William, and Stafford and cities of Alexandria, Falls Church, Manassas, and Manassas Park in Virginia.
Restrictions: The Foundation generally will not consider requests to fund: individuals, either through scholarships or other forms of financial assistance; scientific or medical research; sectarian purposes (programs that promote religious doctrine); special events or conferences; endowments.
Geographic Focus: District of Columbia; Maryland; Virginia
Samples: Theatre Downtown, Washington Stage Guild (Washington, DC)—for general operating support, $20,000.; Empower Program (Washington, DC)—to support local youth-services programs, $20,000.; Community Family Life Services (Washington, DC)—to revamp and document its financial accounting and reporting systems, $10,000.; Independent Sector (Washington, DC)—for its conference program, $10,000.
Date(s) Application is Due: Feb 9; Jun 8; Oct 1
Contact: Julie Rogers, President, (202) 483-8294; fax: (202) 328-6850; email: jrogers@meyerfdn.org
Internet: http://www.meyerfoundation.org
Sponsor: Eugene and Agnes E. Meyer Foundation
1400 16th Street, N.W., Suite 360
Washington, DC 20036

Eugene B. Casey Foundation Grants **1433**
The foundation awards grants to nonprofit organizations in the District of Columbia and Maryland. Nonprofit organizations of the Christian and Roman Catholic faiths also are eligible. Organizations receiving grants include colleges and universities, community service organizations, government agencies, medical centers, parochial schools, and religious groups. Types of support include capital grants and general support grants. There are no application forms or deadlines. Applicants should submit written proposals that include an annual report, the purpose for which the funds are requested, and the amount requested compared with the total sought.
Requirements: Nonprofits in Maryland or the District of Columbia are eligible to apply.
Geographic Focus: District of Columbia; Maryland
Samples: Redlands Christian Migrant Association, Immokalee, FL, $10,000—for general operating support (2008); Cystic Fibrosis Foundation, Bethesda, MD, $20,000—for general operating support (2008); United States Department of State, Washington, DC, $50,000—for general operating support (2008).
Amount of Grant: $10,000-$100,000 average
Contact: Betty Brown Casey, Treasurer; (301) 948-4595
Sponsor: Eugene B. Casey Foundation
800 South Frederick Avenue, Suite 100
Gaithersburg, MD 20877-1701

Eugene M. Lang Foundation Grants **1434**
The foundation awards grants in New York and Pennsylvania in its areas of interest, including education (early childhood education and higher education), medical and health programs, arts, health organizations, medical research, minorities, and performing arts. Types of support include annual campaigns, conferences and seminars, continuing support, fellowships, general operating support, internship funds, professorships, program development, scholarship funds, and seed money. The foundation favors social services such as those helping homeless or single mothers. Locally based groups wanting support must involve a Lang family member. There are no application deadlines; initial approach should be by letter.

Requirements: Organizations in New York and Pennsylvania are eligible to apply.
Restrictions: Grants are not made to individuals, or for building funds, equipment and materials, capital or endowment funds, deficit financing, publications, or matching gifts.
Geographic Focus: New York; Pennsylvania
Samples: New York-Presbyterian Hospital (New York, NY)—for a six-year health-sciences education program for selected inner-city youths, designed to boost their academic success and facilitate their entry into health careers, $1.25 million (2003).
Amount of Grant: $500-$50,000 average
Contact: Program Contact, (212) 949-4100
Sponsor: Eugene M. Lang Foundation
535 5th Avenue, Suite 906
New York, NY 10017

Eugene McDermott Foundation Grants **1435**
The foundation awards grants to Texas nonprofit organizations in its areas of interest, including children and youth, community development, education (early childhood through higher education), health care/organizations, international human rights, medical research, minorities, and social service delivery programs. Types of support include annual campaigns, building construction/renovation, capital campaigns, equipment/land acquisition, general operating grants, matching/challenge grants, professorships, programs/project support, research grants, scholarship funds, and seed grants. There are no application deadlines or forms. The board meets quarterly to consider requests.
Requirements: Texas nonprofit organizations are eligible.
Geographic Focus: Texas
Samples: Nasher Sculpture Center (Dallas, TX)—for endowment, $500,000 (2004); U of Texas Southwestern Medical Center (Dallas, TX)—to refurbish Medical School, $400,000 (2004); U of Texas Southwestern Medical Ctr (Dallas, TX)—to establish a chair in cardiothoracic anesthesiology, $1 million (2003).
Amount of Grant: $1000-$25,000 average
Contact: Grants Administrator, (214) 521-2924
Sponsor: Eugene McDermott Foundation
3808 Euclid Avenue
Dallas, TX 75205

Eva L. and Joseph M. Bruening Foundation Grants **1436**
The Foundation gives priority to grant requests that address one of the four program areas: services for vulnerable older adults; services for physically and mentally impaired individuals; secondary/higher education; and social services for the economically disadvantaged. There is no application or proposal form. Information regarding the application process is available online. Applicants are encouraged to contact the office for further clarification of the Foundation's grantmaking policies.
Requirements: Grants are awarded only to tax-exempt, nonprofit organizations located within Cuyahoga County, OH, usually for program, capital, and start-up operating support.
Restrictions: Grants are not awarded for endowment, general operating support, research, symposia or seminars. No grants are awarded to individuals, nor does the Foundation respond to mass mailings or annual campaign solicitations.
Geographic Focus: Ohio
Samples: Jewish Family Service Assoc (OH)—to create a centralized, relational database system, $50,000 (2004); Youth Opportunities Unlimited (OH)—to help match Workforce Investment Act funds for the Jobs for Ohio's Graduates program in East Cleveland, $25,000 (2004); Towards Employment, Inc (OH)—to integrate Cleveland Works' legal assistance and ex-offender employment programs into Towards Employment's program structure, $50,000 (2004); Lutheran Chaplaincy Service (OH)—to support the full-time development director position, $25,000 (2004).
Date(s) Application is Due: Mar 1; Jul 1; Oct 1
Contact: Janet Narten, Executive Director, (216) 621-2632; fax: (216) 621-8198
Internet: http://www.fmscleveland.com/bruening
Sponsor: Eva L. and Joseph M. Bruening Foundation
1422 Euclid Avenue, Suite 627
Cleveland, OH 44115-1952

Evan and Susan Bayh Foundation Grants **1437**
Established in 2002 by Senator Evan Bayh and his wife Susan, the foundation gives to various education and human services programs mostly in Indiana.
Requirements: There are no deadlines and no specific forms to use. It is suggested that you contact the foundation prior to submitting an application.
Geographic Focus: Indiana
Samples: Indiana University, Matching the Promise Campaign - $50,000.; (2007) American Cancer Society, Atlanta, GA - $2,500.; Deaconess Hospital, Evansville, IN - $5,000.; Fisher House Foundation, Rockville, MD - $5,000.; Munster Medical Research Foundation, Munster, IN - $5,000.; Nature Conservancy, Arlington, VA - $2,500.; St. Albans School of Public Service, Washington, DC - $5,000.; Salvation Army, Indianapolis, IN - $2,500.; United Way of Central Indiana, Indianapolis, IN - $2,500.
Amount of Grant: $2,500 - $5,000
Contact: G. Frederick Glass; (317) 237-0300; email: fred.glass@bakerd.com
Sponsor: Evan and Susan Bayh Foundation
c/o G. Frederick Glass, 300 N. Meridian Street, Suite 2700
Indianapolis, IN 46204-1750

Evanston Community Foundation Grants **1438**
Grants awarded by the Foundation: encourage and support new initiatives and innovative approaches to addressing community needs; build the capacity of local nonprofit organizations to fulfill their missions more effectively; encourage collaborative ventures that will strengthen the community; provide initial support of projects that will have impact beyond the scope and timeline of the proposed project; build community partnerships and resources; and strengthen the area's nonprofit community. Grants typically provide initial seed money to launch new projects, capstone dollars for a larger project that will grow over a longer period, and support a one-time activity or initial phase of a new program. The Foundation's area of interests include: arts and culture; basic human needs; community development; education; environment; health; women and girls and youth and families. The Foundation's RFP and application instructions are available online.
Requirements: IRS 501(c)3 organizations serving the Evanston, IL, community are eligible.
Geographic Focus: Illinois
Samples: Evanston Youth Bank (Evanston, IL)—for Northwestern University Undergraduate Leadership Program, $1000 (2003).
Date(s) Application is Due: Feb 26
Contact: Sara Schastok, Executive Director, (847) 492-0990; fax: (847) 492-0904; email: schastok@evcommfdn.org or info@evcommfdn.org
Internet: http://www.evcommfdn.org/grant_making.htm
Sponsor: Evanston Community Foundation
1007 Church Street, Suite 108
Evanston, IL 60201

Evjue Foundation Grants **1439**
The Foundation contributes each year to worthy educational, cultural and charitable organizations that contribute to the quality of life in Madison and Dane County. The Foundation's interests include: theater, hunger, troubled youth, and universities. The Foundation looks favorably upon projects responding to overall community needs and priorities that do not duplicate existing services. Application and guidelines are available online.
Requirements: Grants are only made to nonprofit organizations.
Restrictions: Grants are not made to individuals. All grants for scholarships are given to educational institutions, which have full responsibility for selecting the individual recipients. Grants are not usually made to establish or add to endowment funds. Grants are not ordinarily made to fund specific medical or scientific research inquiries, nor to support operating expenses and general administrative expenses of organizations.
Geographic Focus: Wisconsin
Samples: U of Wisconsin at Madison (WI)—to endow a professorship at its school of journalism, $1 million (2005).
Date(s) Application is Due: Mar 12
Contact: Arlene Hornung, Executive Director, (608) 252-6401; email: ahornung@madison.com
Internet: http://www.madison.com/tct/evjue/policy/index.php
Sponsor: Evjue Foundation
1901 Fish Hatchery Road
Madison, WI 53713

Ewing Halsell Foundation Grants **1440**
The foundation awards grants to eligible Texas nonprofit organizations in its areas of interest, including education, environment, health care and health organizations, medical research, social services, and youth services. Types of support include annual campaigns, building construction/renovation, equipment acquisition, land acquisition, publication, research, seed grants, and technical assistance. There are no application deadlines or forms.
Requirements: Texas nonprofit organizations are eligible. Preference is given to requests from southwestern Texas, particularly San Antonio.
Restrictions: The foundation's grants do not support individuals or requests for deficit financing, emergency funds, general endowments, matching gifts, scholarships, fellowships, demonstration projects, general purposes, conferences, or loans.
Geographic Focus: Texas
Samples: San Antonio Botanical Society (TX)—to endow the Lucile Halsell Conservatory, $1 million matching grant (2005).
Contact: Grants Administrator, (210) 223-2640
Sponsor: Ewing Halsell Foundation
711 Navarro Street, Suite 537
San Antonio, TX 78205

Express Scripts Foundation Grants **1441**
The Foundation provides financial and volunteer support for numerous causes. Requests are considered from organizations that advance medical and health-related causes, particularly those intended to support youth and strengthen families. Educational activities that enrich education and help create tomorrow's leaders are of particular interest. Programs designed to provide support that enables at-risk children to complete their educations are considered. The Foundation will consider requests from organizations that fall outside the established criteria if they enhance the communities in which the Foundation operates and make strong appeals for community support. Interested applicants should complete an expression of interest form provided online.
Requirements: All projects or programs requesting funding must be tax-exempt as described in both sections 501(c)3 and 509(a)1, 509(a)3 of the Internal Revenue Code. Organizations and programs must have broad community support and a record of fiscal

and administrative stability. Preference is given to innovative projects that develop or expand services, or improve the quality of an organization's program. Typically, support will be awarded only for a term of one year; organizations must reapply for any subsequent year in which they are seeking funding.
Restrictions: The Foundation does not fund: organizations that discriminate on the basis of race, color, sex, or national origin; political causes, candidates, organizations or campaigns; fundraising activities such as benefits, charitable dinners, galas, social clubs; athletic teams or events; individual needs, including scholarships, sponsorships and other forms of financial aid; and endowment funds or capital-fund drives.
Samples: Parents as Teachers National Ctr (Saint Louis, MO)—to provide child-rearing education and information about early-childhood development to families in Missouri, $50,000 (2004).
Contact: Grants Administrator
Internet: http://www.express-scripts.com/ourcompany/aboutus/foundation
Sponsor: Express Scripts Foundation
13900 Riverport Drive, Suite 20S
Maryland Heights, MO 63043

ExxonMobil Grants 1442
The corporation favors grants that relate to the conduct of U.S. business in general and the conduct of the petroleum and chemical industries in particular. The company is also concerned about social and economic conditions in corporate areas. Philanthropic giving is concentrated in the areas of the environment, public policy and public research; health; united appeals and civic and community-service organizations; minority- and women-oriented service organizations; arts, museums, and historical associations; and education. There are no application forms; submit a letter of inquiry that includes a brief history of the organization, the operating budget, a list of the board of directors and contributors, and a copy of the tax-exemption letter.
Requirements: Grants are made to tax-exempt organizations within principal company-operating areas.
Restrictions: Grants are not made to individuals for scholarships, fellowships, research, or travel. Organizations that are primarily religious in nature are ineligible.
Samples: U of Oklahoma (Norman, OK)—for a new facility that will enable engineering students to apply what they have learned in the classroom to real-world scenarios, $5 million (2005); Path Malaria Vaccine Initiative (Bethesda, MD)—for its efforts to increase financial and political support for the development of a malaria vaccine, $500,000 (2005); To be divided among 13 organizations—for 24 community projects intended to prevent, control, and treat malaria in nine African countries; to promote the research in development of new medicines; and to advocate international support for such efforts, $5 million (2005); American National Red Cross (Washington, DC)—for relief efforts in South Asia and Africa, $5 million (2005).
Amount of Grant: $126 million total
Contact: Public Affairs, Contributions, Exxon Mobil Corporation, (972) 444-1103; fax: (972) 444-1405; email: contributions@exxonmobil.com
Internet: http://www.exxon.mobil.com
Sponsor: ExxonMobil
5959 Las Colinas Boulevard
Irving, TX 75039-2298

F.M. Kirby Foundation Grants 1443
Foundation grants are made to a wide range of nonprofit organizations in education, health and medicine, the arts and humanities, civic and public affairs, as well as religious, welfare and youth organizations. Grantees are largely in geographic areas of particular interest to the Kirby family. The Foundation has no required application format and applications will be accepted throughout the year. No solicitations by fax or email.
Requirements: North Carolina, New Jersey, and Pennsylvania tax-exempt organizations are eligible.
Restrictions: Grants are not made to individuals, public foundations or to underwrite fund-raising activities such as benefits, dinners, theater or sporting events.
Geographic Focus: New Jersey; North Carolina; Pennsylvania
Samples: Wake Forest U (Winston-Salem, NC)—to construct a wing at the Wayne Calloway School of Business and Accountancy, $5 million.; Children's Hospital of Boston, Division of Neuroscience (Boston, MA)—for research on cerebral palsy, epilepsy, Alzheimer's disease, and other diseases and degenerative disorders, $2 million.
Date(s) Application is Due: Oct 31
Contact: S. Dillard Kirby, Executive Director, (973) 538-4800
Internet: http://www.fdncenter.org/grantmaker/kirby
Sponsor: F.M. Kirby Foundation
17 DeHart Street, P.O. Box 151
Morristown, NJ 07963-0151

FACES Assistance Grants 1444
The grants provide financial aid toward travel to and from comprehensive medical centers for families of patients with severe facial deformities resulting from birth defects, accidents, or disease. Applicants should submit a medical history, recent photograph, and financial statement with their request for assistance. Applications are accepted at any time.
Contact: Lynne Mayfield, Executive Director, (800) 332-2373; fax: (423) 267-3124; email: faces@faces-cranio.org
Internet: http://www.faces-cranio.org
Sponsor: National Association for the Craniofacially Handicapped (FACES)
P.O. Box 11082
Chattanooga, TN 37401

FACHE Albert W. Dent Scholarships 1445
These scholarships have been established to provide financial aid and to increase the enrollment of minority students in health care management graduate programs and to encourage students, through structured, formalized study, to obtain positions in middle and upper levels of health care management. Applications are accepted between January 1 and March 31, and scholarship awards are announced in July. Interested persons should request application forms from the director of their graduate program in health care administration or from the foundation.
Requirements: To be eligible, an applicant must be a U.S. or Canadian student associate in good standing in the ACHE, a minority student who has been enrolled for full-time study for the upcoming fall term, which is his/her final year in a health care management graduate program. Financial need also must be demonstrated.
Restrictions: Previous recipients are ineligible.
Amount of Grant: $3500
Date(s) Application is Due: Mar 31
Contact: Membership, (312) 424-2800; fax: (312) 424-0023; email: membership1@ache.org
Internet: http://www.ache.org/Faculty_Students/dent_scholarship.cfm
Sponsor: Foundation of the American College of Healthcare Executives
1 N Franklin Street, Suite 1700
Chicago, IL 60606-3491

Fairfield County Community Foundation Grants 1446
As a community foundation, FCCF makes discretionary grants to nonprofits in the broad program areas of economic opportunity (including affordable housing, neighborhood development, and workforce development); children, youth and families; health and human services; the environment; arts and culture; and nonprofit organizational effectiveness. The Foundation is particularly interested in proposals focused on: economic opportunity; education and youth development; advancing school readiness in Fairfield County; organizational effectiveness; and regionalism. Applicants must first submit a letter of inquiry. Application information is available online.
Requirements: Nonprofit organizations in Fairfield County, CT, are eligible.
Restrictions: Funds are not used to provide support for religious or political purposes, deficit financing, annual appeals, fundraising events, open space purchases, for-profit, parochial, charter or private schools, or nonprofit endowments. Grants are not given to individuals.
Geographic Focus: Connecticut
Samples: Cardinal Shehan Center, Bridgeport, CT, $20,000—to support the Made for Talent Program that offers youth arts education throughout the year (2008); ACORN Housing Corporation, Bridgeport, CT, $30,000—to support ACORN's foreclosure counseling program in Bridgeport that prevents mortgage foreclosures as well as assists homeowners impacted by the subprime loan crisis (2008); Danbury Youth Services, Danbury, CT, $20,000—to support the Target After School Program that offers after-school education to children who live in Danbury public housing (2008).
Contact: Karen Brown, Vice President of Programs; (203) 750-3200; fax: (203) 750-3232; email: kbrown@fccfoundation.org
Internet: http://www.fccfoundation.org/cm/grantseekers/what_we_fund.html
Sponsor: Fairfield County Community Foundation
383 Main Avenue
Norwalk, CT 06851-1543

Fairlawn Foundation Grants 1447
The Foundation is dedicated to supporting excellence and innovation in health care delivery, education and research in the Worcester area. The Foundation was established to: provide financial support to organizations, both public and private, that have specific, well-defined proposals to improve and/or expand the practice and delivery of medical and allied health care services in the Worcester area; and to support the education of Worcester area residents in health care related areas.
Requirements: Funding preference is given to institutions involved in higher education, medical or scientific research, hospitals and health care providers, and other organizations capable of making a long-term impact on health care through innovation or research. Applicants must be tax-exempt, nonprofit organizations as recognized by IRS code 501(c)3.
Restrictions: Except in unusual circumstances, the Foundation generally will not approve grants: to any program or individual in excess of $120,000; to programs that require more than five years to complete; for projects supported by other funds in which the Fairlawn Foundation contribution would comprise less than half of total funding; or for pre-existing projects as a minor participant.
Geographic Focus: Massachusetts
Amount of Grant: $120,000 maximum
Date(s) Application is Due: Mar 15; Sep 15
Contact: Lois Smith, Senior Program Officer; (508) 755-0980, ext. 107; email: lsmith@greaterworcester.org
Internet: http://www.greaterworcester.org/grants/Fairlawn.htm
Sponsor: Greater Worcester Community Foundation
370 Main Street, Suite 650
Worcester, MA 01608-1738

Fairview Lutheran Foundation Grants 1448
The foundation's mission is to advance the health and well-being of the Cleveland community by supporting Fairview and Lutheran Hospitals in their commitment to provide superior health-care services. The foundation also awards grants to Cleveland-area agencies and organizations that contribute to those efforts to meet the health-

care needs of Cleveland's West Side. Grants are awarded usually for one year only. Application and guidelines are available online.
Requirements: Ohio 501(c)3tax-exempt organizations located in the greater western Cleveland area are eligible.
Restrictions: No funding is available for capital needs, endowments, or individuals.
Geographic Focus: Ohio
Date(s) Application is Due: Feb 16; May 18; Aug 24; Nov 16
Contact: Grants Administrator, (216) 476-7060; fax: (216) 476-9730; email: linda@flfonline.org
Internet: http://www.flfonline.org/highlights.htm
Sponsor: Fairview Lutheran Foundation
20545 Center Ridge Road, Suite 448
Rocky River, OH 44116

Fallon OrNda Community Health Fund Grants **1449**
The purpose of the health fund is to advance projects that increase access to health care or health promotion services that improve the health status of vulnerable populations. Of particular interest are projects that result in: the support or creation of primary care outreach services to vulnerable populations; the development of continuing managed care services rather than episodic or uncoordinated care; and the removal of barriers that prevent people from receiving services such as lack of transportation, cultural competency of providers, language differences, or others. Grants may be for operational expenditures such as personnel costs, or for construction, renovation, equipment purchase or other physical improvements. Past grants have ranged from $6,500 to $30,000.
Requirements: Funding will not be provided for long-term underwriting of operational costs for any one program.
Geographic Focus: Massachusetts
Amount of Grant: $6,500-$30,000
Date(s) Application is Due: Feb 15
Contact: Lois Smith, Senior Program Officer; (508) 755-0980, ext. 107; email: lsmith@greaterworcester.org
Internet: http://www.greaterworcester.org/grants/Fallon.htm
Sponsor: Greater Worcester Community Foundation
370 Main Street, Suite 650
Worcester, MA 01608-1738

Families U.S.A Wellstone Fellowship for Social Justice **1450**
The annual, one-year fellowship is designed to foster the advancement of social justice through participation in health care advocacy work that focuses on the unique challenges facing many communities of color. The fellowship, from August through July, will be based in the Families U.S.A office in Washington, DC, and will afford the fellow the opportunity to learn about Medicare, Medicaid, efforts to achieve universal coverage, and other important health policy issues. At the same time, the fellow will learn about conducting health care campaigns through communication and collaboration with a network of state grassroots advocates and organizations. The goals of the program are to address disparities in access to health care; inspire fellows to continue to work for social justice throughout their lives; and increase the number and racial and ethnic diversity of up-and-coming social justice advocates and leaders. Guidelines are available online.
Requirements: Candidates must demonstrate an interest in both health care and grassroots organizing and a commitment to contributing to social justice work following their year of hands-on experience as a fellow. Preference will be given to applicants who have experience with, or demonstrate a keen interest in, working with communities of color. While there is no bias in favor of any specific academic discipline, a college degree is preferred.
Amount of Grant: $35,000 stipend plus health benefits
Date(s) Application is Due: Jan 7
Contact: Melissa Rosenblatt, (202) 628-3030; fax: (202) 347-2417; email: wellstonefellowship@familiesusa.org
Internet: http://www.familiesusa.org/site/PageServer?pagename=Wellstone_Fellowship_About
Sponsor: Families U.S.A
1334 G St NW
Washington, DC 20005

Fan Fox and Leslie R. Samuels Foundation Grants Program **1451**
The foundation's areas of funding are the performing arts and healthcare. Healthcare funding supports patient-based and social service activities that directly help the elderly of New York City. The foundation supports performing arts organizations in the City of New York, principally, but not exclusively, in the borough of Manhattan. The foundation's primary mission is to support major performing arts institutions of national or international eminence. In addition to providing direct support, the foundation also assists presenting entities that have the requisite expertise, knowledge, and artistic judgment to present groups or individuals, new works, varied repertoire, and arts-in-education projects that will be contributions to the aesthetic and intellectual life of New York. Application guidelines are available on the Web site or upon request.
Requirements: The foundation funds organizations in the New York City area only. Only 501(c)3 tax-exempt organizations are invited to apply.
Restrictions: The foundation does not give grants to individuals or for scholarships, and does not support research, film, or video, nor does it fund education or social services. The foundation no longer actively solicits applications for support of arts-in-education programs at the primary and secondary level.
Geographic Focus: New York
Amount of Grant: $25,000-$250,000 average
Date(s) Application is Due: Mar 1; Jun 1: Sep 1; Dec 1
Contact: Joseph Mitchell, President , (212) 239-3030; fax: (212) 239-3039; email: info@samuels.org
Internet: http://www.samuels.org
Sponsor: Fan Fox and Leslie R. Samuels Foundation
350 Fifth Avenue, Suite 4301
New York, NY 10118

Fannie E. Rippel Foundation Grants **1452**
The foundation aids, assists, funds, equips, and provides maintenance for corporations, institutions, associations, organizations, or societies maintained for the relief and care of aged women; provides funds for the building, equipping, and maintenance of hospitals; and provides funds for corporations, institutions, and other organizations existing for treatment of and/or research on heart disease or cancer. The foundation gives emphasis to the equipment and programmatic needs of major teaching medical centers and local rural hospitals, particularly where opportunities exist for leveraging the expertise or capabilities of the medical centers/rural hospitals. Programs should reach underserved rural and urban groups, advocate preventive care, present strategies to change behaviors of the people served, and promote humanistic medicine and mind-body-spirit connections in the healing process. Preference also is given to proposed projects where the benefits can be leveraged through challenge grants.
Requirements: Organizations, associations, institutions, and hospitals in the Northeast are eligible.
Restrictions: Grants are not awarded to individuals.
Geographic Focus: Northeast
Amount of Grant: $50,000-$300,000 average
Contact: (973) 540 -0101; fax: (973) 540-0404; email: pmacbain@rippelfoundation.org
Internet: http://fdncenter.org/grantmaker/rippel
Sponsor: Fannie E. Rippel Foundation
14 Maple Avenue, Suite 200
Morristown, NJ 07960

FAR Fund **1453**
The Fund focuses its resources in three domains: improving and expanding services and systems for people on the autistic spectrum; preventing violence against youth; and preventing homelessness. The Fund encourages the creation of projects that operate across domains. The Fund also encourages projects that increase the participation and influence of consumers in shaping the service system that affect their lives. Particular interest is in projects that incorporate psychodynamic thinking in their program philosophy and service delivery. Proposal information is available on the website.
Requirements: The application proposal should be brief and describe the following: the organization where the project will be located; the problem; the project, including the project title; the expected impact; a plan for project evaluation, including outcome indicators; plans for the project beyond the grant period; project staff; project expense budget and income budget, and an organization expense and income budget; the percentage of the project budget that would be supported by the Fund; a monitorable work plan; and the name of the tax-exempt organization that would receive the grant.
Geographic Focus: New York
Amount of Grant: $25,000
Date(s) Application is Due: Feb 1; Jun 1; Oct 1
Contact: Kaajal Shah, Program Officer
Internet: http://www.farfund.org/
Sponsor: Fund for Social Change
135 East 15th Street
New York, NY 10003

Fargo-Moorhead Area Foundation Grants **1454**
The Foundation awards grants each year according to current and emerging community needs. The Board also prioritizes grants that: effect a broad segment of our community; leverage support from other sources; promote collaboration, without duplicating services; strengthen organization, self-sufficiency and long term stability; focus on problem solving; and show realistic planning and management. The Foundation's focus is on arts and culture, education, environment and animals, health, human services and public/society benefit. Applicants are required to use the FMAF grant application forms available online.
Requirements: The foundation welcomes grant requests from 501(c)3 organizations in Cass and Clay Counties in North Dakota and Minnesota or those serving residents of these counties.
Restrictions: Grants are not normally funded for: annual appeals or membership drives; capital debt reduction; capital campaigns; individuals or for-profit organizations; organizations with outstanding final reports from previous FMAF grants; organizations with outstanding due diligence reports from FMAF; political projects; religious groups for religious purposes; travel for groups and retroactive funding for any project expenses incurred before the decision date.
Geographic Focus: Minnesota; North Dakota
Date(s) Application is Due: Feb 16
Contact: Wendy DeLane Milligan, Gifts & Grants Specialist, (701) 234-0756; fax: (701) 234-9724; email: wendy@areafoundation.org
Internet: http://www.areafoundation.org
Sponsor: Fargo-Moorhead Area Foundation
502 First Avenue North, Suite 202
Fargo, ND 58102

Farmers Insurance Group of Companies Grants **1455**

The corporate community relations program awards grants in the areas of education, public safety, arts and culture, civic improvement, and health and human services. Education giving focuses on literacy programs, mentoring programs, adopt-a-school programs, employee matching grants, and aid-to-education undergraduate scholarships. Public safety awards support tougher laws against drunk driving, drug/alcohol-free graduation night parties, neighborhood crime prevention, highway safety, and earthquake relief. Arts and culture funding supports children's programs and public television. Civic improvement focuses on recognizing exemplary youth, voter registration drives, adopt-a-highway programs, and community paint-a-thons. Health and human services giving supports March of Dimes, United Way, aid for families with cancer, aid to migrant farmworkers, and feeding the hungry. There are no application deadlines. Requests for contributions should be in the form of a letter outlining the purpose of the organization or program. The letter also should include the amount requested, its intended use, and a description of how Farmers' support will be recognized. Additional information should include a budget, annual report, proof of tax-exempt status, and a roster of the board of directors.

Requirements: 501(c)3 tax-exempt organizations are eligible.

Restrictions: Farmers does not make charitable contributions to individuals, political candidates, or religious groups or for sports events, advertising or raffle tickets, construction projects, or international programs.

Samples: John Wayne Institute for Cancer Treatment and Research (Santa Monica, CA)—for its cancer research and treatment programs, $50,000.; Los Angeles Urban League (Los Angeles, CA)—to upgrade the Information Training Ctr, which teaches computer skills to low-income, minority residents, $10,000.

Amount of Grant: $4.3 million total

Contact: Angela Easton, Director of Community Affairs and Sponsorship, (213) 932-3518

Internet: http://www.farmers.com/FarmComm/content/CC010153.jsp

Sponsor: Farmers Insurance Group of Companies
4680 Wilshire Boulevard
Los Angeles, CA 90010

Faye McBeath Foundation Grants **1456**

Grants are made within the state of Wisconsin and principally to support projects or programs having primary focus on the welfare of the residents of the greater Milwaukee community including Milwaukee, Waukesha, Ozaukee and Washington counties. Generally, the Foundation supports programs for children, aging and elders, health, health education, and civic and governmental affairs. Capital grants are limited to projects with community-wide impact that reflect the program interests of the Foundation. There are no published deadlines for proposals. The common application form is available online.

Requirements: 501(c)3 nonprofit organizations in the metropolitan Milwaukee area are eligible. The Foundation requires its grant applicants to use the Milwaukee-area common application form when submitting a full proposal.

Restrictions: The Foundation does not consider or acknowledge general solicitation letters. Basic health sciences research is not funded. The Foundation does not award grants for annual fund drives, scholarships, support of individuals, or provide funds on an emergency basis.

Geographic Focus: Wisconsin

Samples: Penfield Children's Ctr (Milwaukee, WI)—to redesign and upgrade a playground for children with special needs, $15,000 (2005); Leaders Forum (Milwaukee, WI)—for its African American Fund-Development Institute, which trains executives and civic leaders for civic and nonprofit leadership positions, $15,000 over two years (2005); Friends of Boerner Botanical Garden (Milwaukee, WI)—for the Horticultural Therapy Program, which serves elderly people, $15,000 (2005); Latino Health Organization (Milwaukee, WI)—for its Health Awareness Program, a series of health-education presentations for children and families, $20,000 (2005).

Amount of Grant: $12.5 million total; $10,000-$50,000 average

Contact: Sarah Dean, Executive Director, (414) 272-2626; fax: (414) 272-6235; email: info@fayemcbeath.org

Internet: http://www.fayemcbeath.org

Sponsor: Faye McBeath Foundation
1020 N Broadway
Milwaukee, WI 53202

Fayette County Foundation Grants **1457**

Founded in 1986, the Fayette County Foundation is the community's resource for charitable giving. The Foundation serves the entire Fayette County by assisting donors and meeting community needs. To be eligible to receive funding from the Fayette County Foundation a letter of intent must be submitted by March 1, July 1 or October 1 and followed by a completed grant application by the appropriate grant deadline. All grant seekers must have prior governing board approval for the project seeking funding. The approval of signed minutes and a signed letter from governing board must be available to the Fayette County Foundation. Faith-based organizations may apply as long as the project does not mandate participation in a religious activity as a condition for receiving services.

Requirements: Projects must have public access for all people. Completed grant application (original plus eight copies) must be received by the Foundation by the last Friday in March, the last Friday in July or the last Friday in October at Noon to be considered for funding.

Restrictions: Legal requirements forbid staff, trustees, directors, committee members and their families from profiting financially from any philanthropic grant. All persons actively connected with the Foundation will consistently strive to avoid self-interest in the processing and disposition of grant request. Only one successful application per 12 months will be considered. Repeat funding for the same project may be considered five years after the initial project on a case by case basis.

Geographic Focus: Indiana

Samples: Crossroads Shelter, to replace roof and siding — $10,000.00 (2008); Fayette County Cancer Society, medicine, dietary needs, wigs — $6,000.00 (2008)

Date(s) Application is Due: Mar 1, Jul 1, Oct 1

Contact: Loree Crowe, Program Officer, (765) 827-9966; fax: (765) 827-5836; email: info@fayettefoundation.com

Internet: http://www.fayettefoundation.com/default.asp?PageIndex=128

Sponsor: Fayette County Foundation
P.O. Box 844 or 521 N. Central Avenue, Suite A
Connersville, IN 47331

FCD Child Development Grants **1458**

The foundation awards grants to support programs for children, particularly the disadvantaged, and promote their well-being through basic and policy-relevant research about the factors that promote optimal development of children and adolescents, policy analysis, advocacy, services, and public education to enhance the discussion and adoption of social policies that support families in their important child-raising responsibilities; and leadership development activities linked to the programmatic focus of the foundation. Grants focus on the integration of research, policy, and advocacy in two areas: the availability of and access to early childhood education programs and health care for children. Most grants support research, but a small number of direct service grants are made for New York City-based projects that advance the foundation's research and policy analysis efforts. There are no application deadlines; submit a brief letter of inquiry. Full proposals are by invitation.

Requirements: Nonprofit organizations are eligible.

Restrictions: The foundation does not consider requests for scholarships or support for individuals, capital campaigns, building purchase or renovation, or equipment purchase. The foundation does not make grants outside the United States.

Samples: Barnard College (New York, NY)—to create an internship program that will encourage and prepare undergraduate students to pursue public-service careers that benefit children and their families, $30,000 (2005); Harvard Education Letter (Cambridge, MA)—to produce and distribute nine articles, including a special edition, on the most effective ways to educate children age three to eight, $120,750 (2005); U of Wisconsin at Madison (WI)—to prepare a working paper that describes and assesses issues related to the structure, financing, and implementation of Chicago Parent-Child Centers, $30,000 (2005); National Education Assoc (Washington, DC)—to survey existing contract language, develop a policy brief on the survey results, and recommend strategies for bargaining units of the NEA to use contract language to support improved educational opportunities for children in pre-kindergarten through third grade, $104,479 (2005).

Contact: Grants Administrator, (212) 213-8337; fax: (212) 213-5897; email: info@fcd-us.org

Internet: http://www.ffcd.org/ourwork/g-how.html

Sponsor: Foundation for Child Development
145 E 32nd Street, 14th Floor
New York, NY 10016

FCER Chiropractic Research Grants **1459**

The grants support basic and clinical research and research program development related to chiropractic. Types of support include awards/prizes, challenge/matching grants, conferences and seminars, demonstration grants, fellowships, research grants, residencies, and research contracts. Fellowships are for a maximum of five years.

Amount of Grant: $10,000-$130,000 per year

Date(s) Application is Due: Mar 1; Oct 1

Contact: Dr. Anthony Rosner, Director of Research, (617) 734-3397; fax: (617) 734-0989; email: rosnerfcer@aol.com

Internet: http://www.fcer.org/html/Research/Grants/guidelines.htm#Instructions%20for%20Application

Sponsor: Foundation for Chiropractic Education and Research
1330 Beacon Street, Suite 315
Brookline, MA 02446-3202

FCER Research Grants and Fellowships **1460**

The fellowships support research training primarily for graduate chiropractors enrolled in academic programs in basic sciences and clinical health-related areas. Grants are for basic research and related expenses.

Requirements: Priority for funding will be based on merit and the relevance/importance of the proposed research of chiropractic theory and practice, as well as the ability of the investigator and sponsoring institutions to bring the project to successful completion.

Samples: Robert Maust, Research Dimensions—for research on referral rates to chiropractors, $80,502.; Deborah Callahan, Foundation for Chiropractic Education and Research—for research on the treatment of back pain, $9961.

Amount of Grant: $10,000-$120,000 range

Contact: Dr. Anthony Rosner, Director of Research & Education, (617) 734-3397; fax: (617) 734-0989; email: rosnerfcer@aol.com

Internet: http://www.fcer.org/research.htm

Sponsor: Foundation for Chiropractic Education and Research
1330 Beacon Street, Suite 315
Brookline, MA 02446-3202

FCNY Union Square Awards 1461

The awards seek to encourage grassroots activism as a means of strengthening communities throughout New York City, and they recognize notable contributions to the educational, economic, and cultural life of New York City. The awards honor individuals who have initiated and developed projects/organizations in the areas of homelessness and hunger; HIV/AIDS prevention, education and treatment; conflict resolution; economic self-sufficiency; and youth and family development. Awards are made once a year through the generosity and commitment of the Union Square Fund.
Requirements: Anyone may submit a nomination. To do so, provide a description of the candidate and their project with the names of two references. Only individuals who have demonstrated extraordinary initiative and commitment and who have not yet received substantial funding will be considered.
Geographic Focus: New York
Amount of Grant: $50,000 maximum
Contact: Iris Morales, Director, (212) 925-6675; fax: (212) 925-5675
Internet: http://www.fcny.org/unionsquare
Sponsor: Fund for the City of New York
121 Sixth Avenue, 6th Floor
New York, NY 10013

FDA Orphan Products Clinical Studies Grants 1462

The objective of the grants is to support clinical trials on the safety and effectiveness of products to treat a rare disease or condition. These include conditions for which no current therapy exists or the therapy that does exist is in need of improvement. The FDA provides grants to conduct clinical studies intended to provide data that will either result in or substantially contribute to approval of these medical products. All studies of new drugs and biological products must be conducted under the FDA's investigational new drug procedure. Studies of medical devices must be conducted under the investigational device exemption procedures.
Requirements: Public or private for-profit or nonprofit organizations may apply. Profit organizations must commit to excluding fees or profit in their request for support.
Amount of Grant: $100,000 maximum for new awards; $200,000 maximum for continuation awards
Contact: Rosemary Springer, Chief Grants Management Officer, (301) 827-7182; fax: (301) 827-7101; email: rspringe@oc.fda.gov
Internet: http://www.fda.gov
Sponsor: Food and Drug Administration
5630 Fishers Ln, HFA-520, Room 2129
Rockville, MD 20857

FDA Scientific Conferences Grants 1463

The FDA accepts applications for grants for scientific conferences held in the United States and Canada on topics relating directly to the agency's mission and funding priorities. This initiative is intended to support and encourage state food regulatory agencies to establish (or provide support of existing) regularly scheduled Food Safety Task Force meetings. These meetings should foster communication and cooperation within the state among state and local food safety regulatory agencies and is part of the President's Food Safety Initiative (FSI).
Requirements: Awards can be made to any public or private nonprofit university, college, hospital, laboratory, or other institution, including state and local units of government. Commercial and nonprofit organizations are also eligible.
Amount of Grant: $5000-$3 million; $225,970 average
Contact: Rosemary Springer, Chief, Grants and Agreements Management Branch, Division of Contracts and Assistance Management, (301) 827-7182; fax: (301) 827-7101; email: rspringe@oc.fda.gov
Internet: http://www.fda.gov
Sponsor: Food and Drug Administration
5600 Fishers Ln, HFA-520, Room 2129
Rockville, MD 20857

FDHN Bridging Grants 1464

Awards of $50,000 each are available to assist investigators were not awarded their first R01 or the first renewal of their R01 to continue their gastroenterology related research. Two awards will be made following each of the three annual NIH review cycles and availability of Summary Statements. The primary objective of the award is to provide interim support to AGA Members who have submitted grants to NIH that were approved on the basis of scientific merit, but received priority scores out of the funding range.
Requirements: Applicants must: be AGA members who are applying for their first R01 or their second R01 either as a competitive renewal or a new R01 (this includes investigators going from a K award to their first R01); hold an MD, PhD, or equivalent degree (e.g., MB, ChB, MBBS, DO); hold full-time faculty positions at North American universities or professional institutes at the time of application; and have submitted a proposal to NIH that has undergone the peer review process and was either approved and not funded or received high commendation but not funded.
Restrictions: Applicants cannot receive more than $75,000 of any additional extramural research support. Up to 25% of total amount the award may be used for salary support of the Principal Investigator. Indirect costs, including travel are not allowed.
Amount of Grant: $50,000
Date(s) Application is Due: Feb 14; Jun 14; Oct 14
Contact: Research Awards Manager, (301) 222-4012; fax: (301) 652-3890; email: awards@fdhn.org
Internet: http://www.fdhn.org/wmspage.cfm?parm1=119
Sponsor: Foundation for Digestive Health and Nutrition
4930 Del Ray Avenue
Bethesda, MD 20814

FDHN Centocor International Research Fellowship in Gastrointestinal Inflammation & Immunology 1465

This award provides $50,000 to enable promising young investigators from outside the United States to spend a year at a U.S. institution engaged full-time in research related to the fundamental processes in gastrointestinal inflammation and immunology. The primary objectives of the award are: to provide the opportunity for young investigators from outside the U.S. to participate in basic research on inflammatory disease processes at prominent institutions in the U.S. (the award provides salary support for fulltime research); to initiate future international collaborative research efforts in inflammatory digestive diseases; and to address an important question in such a way as to provide a meaningful answer.
Requirements: Candidates must hold an MD or equivalent degree (eg, MB. ChB, MBBS). Applicants should currently be on the faculty of an academic institution outside the U.S. Applicants must be AGA members or be eligible for and submit an application for membership.
Restrictions: At the time of application, candidates are not allowed to hold any other similar research grant. These awards may not be renewed. No more than one application will be accepted from any institution in a given year.
Samples: Bo-In Lee, MD, PhD, Cleveland Clinic Foundation Cleveland, OH (2007); Seamus J. Murphy, BSc, PhD, MB, BCh, Mount Sinai School of Medicine New York, NY (2006).
Amount of Grant: $50,000
Date(s) Application is Due: Jan 14
Contact: Research Awards Manager, (301) 222-4012; fax: (301) 652-3890; email: awards@fdhn.org
Internet: http://www.fdhn.org/wmspage.cfm?parm1=105
Sponsor: Foundation for Digestive Health and Nutrition
4930 Del Ray Avenue
Bethesda, MD 20814

FDHN Designated Outcomes Award in Geriatric Gastroenterology 1466

Two awards in the amount of $35,000 for one year are available to support investigator-initiated outcomes research in geriatric gastroenterology. In general, outcomes studies examine clinical outcomes, patient satisfaction, quality of life, economic evaluation, quality of care, functional status, appropriateness of care, conformance of recommended/desirable standards of performance, or change in practice patterns. The objective of this award is to promote research by young investigators in the area of outcomes, broadly defined above, as it relates to geriatric gastroenterology. Please review the AGA Future Trends Committee Report: Effects of Aging of the Population on Gastroenterology Practice, Education and Research to learn more about research topics encouraged for study. Funds may be used for salary support of personnel and technicians only, supplies and/or equipment/services. Women and minorities are strongly encouraged to apply.
Requirements: Investigators must possess an MD, PhD or equivalent and must hold faculty positions at accredited North American academic institutions by the time of the start date of the award. MD applicants: No more than five years should elapse following the completion of your clinical training (GI fellowship or equivalent) and the start date of this award. Applicants must be AGA Members.
Restrictions: The award is intended for junior faculty; therefore, established investigators are not eligible. Candidates may not hold awards on a similar topic from other agencies. Indirect costs are not allowed.
Amount of Grant: $35,000
Date(s) Application is Due: Sep 5
Contact: Research Awards Manager, (301) 222-4012; fax: (301) 652-3890; email: awards@fdhn.org
Internet: http://www.fdhn.org/wmspage.cfm?parm1=234
Sponsor: Foundation for Digestive Health and Nutrition
4930 Del Ray Avenue
Bethesda, MD 20814

FDHN Designated Research Award in Geriatric Gastroenterology 1467

This award provides $75,000 per year for three years (total $225,000) for young investigators working toward independent careers in academic research related to geriatric gastroenterology. The overall objective is to enable young investigators to develop independent and productive research careers, with a focus on research related to geriatric gastroenterology, by ensuring that a major proportion of their time is protected for research. Non-recipient applicants for this award will be considered for the Research Scholar Awards. Applicants should review the AGA Future Trends Committee Report: Effects of Aging of the Population on Gastroenterology Practice, Education and Research to learn more about research topics encouraged for study. The award is not intended for fellows, but for young faculty who have demonstrated unusual promise and have some record of accomplishment in research.
Requirements: Candidates must hold an MD, PhD, or equivalent degree (e.g., MB, ChB, MBBS, DO). Applicants must hold full-time faculty positions at North American universities or professional institutes at the time award begins. Applicants must be Members of the AGA. # MD applicants: no more than five years shall have elapsed following the completion of your clinical training (GI fellowship or its equivalent) and the start date of this award. PhD applicants: no more than five years shall have elapsed from the completion of your postdoctoral training and the start date of this award.

Candidates must devote at least 70 percent of their efforts to research related to geriatric gastroenterology.
Restrictions: Candidates should be in the beginning years of their careers; therefore, established investigators are not appropriate candidates.
Amount of Grant: $75,000 per year for three years
Date(s) Application is Due: Sep 15
Contact: Research Awards Manager, (301) 222-4012; fax: (301) 652-3890; email: awards@fdhn.org
Internet: http://www.fdhn.org/wmspage.cfm?parm1=224
Sponsor: Foundation for Digestive Health and Nutrition
4930 Del Ray Avenue
Bethesda, MD 20814

FDHN Designated Research Award in Research Related to Pancreatitis **1468**
The overall objective of this Award is to enable young investigators to develop independent and productive research careers, with a focus on pancreatic disease, by ensuring that a major proportion of their time is protected for research. The Award provides $75,000 per year for three years (total $225,000) for young investigators working toward independent careers in academic research related to understanding, improving treatments or curing Pancreatitis.
Requirements: Candidates must hold an MD, PhD, or equivalent degree (e.g., MB, ChB, MBBS, DO). Applicants must hold full-time faculty positions at North American universities or professional institutes at the time award begins. Applicants must also be members of the AGA. The award is not intended for fellows, but for young faculty who have demonstrated unusual promise and have some record of accomplishment in research. Candidates should be in the beginning years of their careers; therefore, established investigators are not appropriate candidates. MD applicants: No more than five years shall have elapsed following the completion of your clinical training (GI fellowship or its equivalent) and the start date of this award. PhD applicants: No more than five years shall have elapsed from the completion of your postdoctoral training and the start date of this award.
Amount of Grant: $75,000 per year for three years
Date(s) Application is Due: Apr 17
Contact: Research Awards Manager, (301) 222-4012; fax: (301) 652-3890; email: awards@fdhn.org
Internet: http://www.fdhn.org/wmspage.cfm?parm1=100
Sponsor: Foundation for Digestive Health and Nutrition
4930 Del Ray Avenue
Bethesda, MD 20814

FDHN Fellow Abstract Prizes **1469**
Two awards of $1000 each will be given to fellows who have submitted abstracts chosen to be presented during Digestive Disease Week®. Awards will be presented at a ceremony during DDW. The primary objective of this award is to stimulate interest in GI research careers through competition and recognition
Requirements: Qualified candidates are MD or PhD postdoctoral fellows who are trainee members the AGA. Women and minority investigators are strongly encouraged to apply. Applicants must: be sponsored by an AGA member; and be the first author of an abstract accepted for presentation at DDW and provide evidence of abstract acceptance. Individuals with faculty appointments are not eligible. Applicants may only submit one abstract for consideration.
Restrictions: Fellows who have been awarded must present the abstract. No substitute presenters are allowed. Abstracts must have been selected for presentation at DDW. A letter of recommendation from the sponsor is required.
Amount of Grant: $1,000
Date(s) Application is Due: Mar 21
Contact: Research Awards Manager, (301) 222-4012; fax: (301) 652-3890; email: awards@fdhn.org
Internet: http://www.fdhn.org/wmspage.cfm?parm1=124
Sponsor: Foundation for Digestive Health and Nutrition
4930 Del Ray Avenue
Bethesda, MD 20814

FDHN Fellowship to Faculty Transition Awards **1470**
This award provides $40,000 per year for two years for current trainees in gastroenterology related fields so they may gain additional research training in gastrointestinal, liver function or related diseases. The objective is to prepare physicians for independent research careers in digestive diseases. The award provides salary support for additional full-time research training in basic science to acquire modern laboratory skills. The additional two years of research training provided by this award should broaden and expand the scope of investigative tools available to the recipient, generally in basic disciplines such as cell or molecular biology or immunology.
Requirements: Applicants must be MDs or MD/PhDs currently in a gastroenterology-related fellowship at an accredited North American institution, committed to academic careers. They will have completed two years of research training at the start of this award. Applicants must be AGA Trainee Members and be sponsored by an AGA Member.
Restrictions: Individuals who hold a PhD are ineligible. Although the institution may supplement the award, the applicant may not concurrently hold a similar training award or grant from another organization, such as the NIH, ALF, CCFA, or the Glaxo Institute of Digestive Health.
Samples: John Chang, MD, Fellow in Gastroenterology University of Pennsylvania, Philadelphia, PA (2007); Lee Peng, MD, PhD, Massachusetts University, Boston, MA (2007); Carl B. Rountree, Jr., MD, Children's Hospital, Los Angeles, CA (2006).
Amount of Grant: $40,000 per year for two years
Date(s) Application is Due: Sep 5
Contact: Research Awards Manager, (301) 222-4012; fax: (301) 652-3890; email: awards@fdhn.org
Internet: http://www.fdhn.org/wmspage.cfm?parm1=102
Sponsor: Foundation for Digestive Health and Nutrition
4930 Del Ray Avenue
Bethesda, MD 20814

FDHN Funderburg Research Scholar Award in Gastric Biology Related to Cancer **1471**
This grant of $25,000 per year for two years (total $50,000) is awarded to an established investigator working on novel approaches in gastric cancer, including the fields of gastric mucosal regeneration and regulation of cell growth (not as they relate to peptic ulcer disease inflammation (including Helicobacter pylori) as precancerous lesions; genetics of gastric oncogenes in gastric epithelial malignancies; epidemiology of gastric cancer; etiology of malignancies; or clinical research in the diagnosis or treatment of gastric carcinoma. The primary objective of the award is to support an active, established investigator in the field of gastric biology who enhances the fundamental understanding of gastric cancer pathobiology in order to ultimately develop a cure for the disease.
Requirements: Applicants must hold faculty positions at accredited North American institutions and must have established themselves as independent investigators in the field of gastric biology. Women and minority investigators are strongly encouraged to apply. Applicants must be Members of the AGA.
Samples: Xiaolu Yang, PhD, Associate Professor, Department of Cancer Biology, Associate Investigator, Abramson Family Cancer Research Institute, University of Pennsylvania School of Medicine, PA (2007); Steven Itzkowitz, MD, FACP, FACG The Dr. Burrill B. Crohn Professor of Medicine, Director, Gastroenterology Fellowship Program, Associate Director, Division of Gastroenterology, Mount Sinai School of Medicine, New York City, NY (2006); JeanMarie Houghton, PhD, University of Massachusetts Medical School, Worchester, MA (2005).
Amount of Grant: $25,000 per year for two years
Date(s) Application is Due: Sep 5
Contact: Research Awards Manager, (301) 222-4012; fax: (301) 652-3890; email: awards@fdhn.org
Internet: http://www.fdhn.org/wmspage.cfm?parm1=90
Sponsor: Foundation for Digestive Health and Nutrition
4930 Del Ray Avenue
Bethesda, MD 20814

FDHN Graduate Student Awards **1472**
Two awards of $20,000 a year for two years are offered to fund graduate students undertaking research in the biology and epidemiology of diseases of the gastrointestinal tract, liver or pancreas. The award includes $18,000 for stipend and $2,000 to be used towards fringe benefits such as medical insurance and travel to a national meeting. The primary objective of the award is to provide a salary stipend for graduate students performing doctoral research related to the gastrointestinal tract, liver or pancreas.
Requirements: Applicants should have completed at least one year and no more than three years of training towards the doctoral degree and have selected and confirmed the laboratory or department in which they will conduct doctoral research. Research is to be conducted at an accredited academic institution within North America and the research advisor must be a Member of the AGA. Applicants should be U.S. citizens, permanent residents or overseas students who have a current visa to pursue education within North America.
Restrictions: Indirect costs, excluding travel, are not allowed. Tuition costs are expected to be covered by the institution or host department and laboratory.
Amount of Grant: $20,000 per year for two years
Date(s) Application is Due: Mar 14
Contact: Research Awards Manager, (301) 222-4012; fax: (301) 652-3890; email: awards@fdhn.org
Internet: http://www.fdhn.org/wmspage.cfm?parm1=154
Sponsor: Foundation for Digestive Health and Nutrition
4930 Del Ray Avenue
Bethesda, MD 20814

FDHN Jon I. Isenberg International Research Scholar Award **1473**
This award provides a total of $50,000 for one year of study, $25,000 from the AGA and $25,000 in matching funds from the applicant's national GI society. The award provides for non-U.S. citizen young investigators to spend one year performing GI-related research at an American institution under the tutelage of an AGA member. Four awards will be given annually. The primary objective of this award is to promote international scholarship, increase AGA's involvement within the international GI community and foster international collaboration in training GI investigators.
Requirements: An eligible candidate must be nominated by his or her national GI Society. The national GI society must match the $25,000 contribution from the AGA. Before submitting an application, a candidate must identify a sponsoring American institution and a research preceptor who agrees in writing to supervise his or her training and research. Qualified candidates must possess a doctoral degree, either an MD, or equivalent degree, and/or a PhD degree. In keeping with the intent to support the career development of young investigators, the candidate must be within five (5) years of completing GI training or, if a PhD, within five (5) years of the receipt of the degree, at the time of initiation of the award. A documented parental leave of absence will not be counted towards the five (5) years of eligibility.

Amount of Grant: $50,000
Date(s) Application is Due: Mar 1
Contact: Research Awards Manager, (301) 222-4012; fax: (301) 652-3890; email: awards@fdhn.org
Internet: http://www.fdhn.org/wmspage.cfm?parm1=101
Sponsor: Foundation for Digestive Health and Nutrition
4930 Del Ray Avenue
Bethesda, MD 20814

FDHN June & Donald O. Castell MD, Esophageal Clinical Research Award 1474

One award of $35,000 is made annually to provide research and/or salary support for junior faculty involved in clinical research in esophageal diseases. This award is funded by the June and Donald O. Castell, MD, Gastroenterology Research and Education Trust. The primary objective of the award is to support investigators who have demonstrated high potential to develop independent, productive research careers.
Requirements: Candidates must hold a MD or PhD or equivalent. Applicants must hold a full-time faculty position at a North American universities or professional institute. Applicants must be members of the AGA. The recipient must be at or below the level of assistant professor, and his/her initial appointment to the faculty position must have been within seven (7) years of the time of application. This award is not intended for fellows, but for junior faculty who have demonstrated unusual promise; have some record of accomplishment in research; and have established independent research programs at the time of the award. Candidates must devote at least 50 percent of their efforts to research related to esophageal function or diseases.
Restrictions: If an award recipient receives notification of another award with overlapping scientific objectives, prior to the start date of an AGA or FDHN award, the applicant must choose between the two awards.
Samples: John Pandolfino, MD, Northwestern University, Chicago, IL (2007); Marcelo Vela, MD, Medical University of South Carolina, Charleston, SC (2006); Braden Kuo, MD, Massachusetts General Hospital Boston, MA (2005).
Amount of Grant: $35,000
Date(s) Application is Due: Jan 14
Contact: Research Awards Manager, (301) 222-4012; fax: (301) 652-3890; email: awards@fdhn.org
Internet: http://www.fdhn.org/wmspage.cfm?parm1=104
Sponsor: Foundation for Digestive Health and Nutrition
4930 Del Ray Avenue
Bethesda, MD 20814

FDHN Moti L. & Kamla Rustgi International Travel Awards 1475

This program awards grants to young basic, translational and clinical investigators to support their travel and related expenses to attend Digestive Disease Week®. Two awards of $500 each will be given to selected individuals residing outside North America. The primary objective of the award is to enable young investigators outside of North American (U.S. or Canada) institutions to attend Digestive Disease Week and encourage international trainees to become more involved in digestive tract, pancreatic and liver disease research.
Requirements: Candidates must: be MD or PhD or MD PhD postdoctoral fellows who are international trainee members of the AGA; be sponsored by an International member of AGA; be 35 years of age or younger at the time of the meeting; be fluent in English; and have a sufficient number of scientific papers (impact factor) published and/or poster presentations.
Amount of Grant: $500
Date(s) Application is Due: Mar 21
Contact: Research Awards Manager, (301) 222-4012; fax: (301) 652-3890; email: awards@fdhn.org
Internet: http://www.fdhn.org/wmspage.cfm?parm1=126
Sponsor: Foundation for Digestive Health and Nutrition
4930 Del Ray Avenue
Bethesda, MD 20814

FDHN Non-Career Research Awards 1476

This award provides approximately $10,000 (per symposia) for travel support for young investigators and selected established investigators to participate in symposia on gastrointestinalrelated topics. The primary objective of the award is to foster interactions and enhance the exchange of information between clinical and basic science investigators, and established and junior investigators working in gastrointestinal research. Eligibility women and minority organizers are strongly encouraged to apply. Travel support may be provided for: junior investigators who are within 5 years of completing their clinical training in GI or from completion of their PhD doctoral thesis and are at or below the rank of assistant professor; and up to two established investigators who are invited speakers. Biosketches of these individuals and a letter addressing their contribution to the scientific content and atmosphere of the meeting should be submitted with the application.
Requirements: Within 60 days of the conclusion of the meeting, a one-page summary of the highlights of the meeting and an accounting of the use of funds must be submitted. The names of participants and speakers in the symposium, addresses, dates of birth and academic ranks of the attending scientists and their itemized expenses, must be sent to the Foundation. Any unexpended funds must be returned.
Restrictions: Indirect costs are not allowed.
Amount of Grant: $10,000 average
Date(s) Application is Due: Feb 1; May 1; Oct 1
Contact: Research Awards Manager, (301) 222-4012; fax: (301) 652-3890; email: awards@fdhn.org
Internet: http://www.fdhn.org/wmspage.cfm?parm1=123
Sponsor: Foundation for Digestive Health and Nutrition
4930 Del Ray Avenue
Bethesda, MD 20814

FDHN Non-Career Research Grants 1477

A research initiative grant of $25,000 for one year is offered to investigators to support pilot research projects in gastroenterology- or hepatology-related areas. The primary objective of the award is to provide non-salary funds for new investigators to help them establish their research careers or to support pilot projects that represent new research directions for established investigators. The intent is to stimulate research in gastroenterology- or hepatology-related areas by permitting investigators to obtain new data that can ultimately provide the basis for subsequent grant applications of more substantial funding and duration.
Requirements: Investigators must possess an MD or PhD degree or equivalent and must hold faculty positions at accredited North American institutions. Candidates may not hold awards on a similar topic from other agencies. Applicants must be AGA Members. Applicants for this award may not simultaneously apply for the AGA/Miles and Shirley Fiterman Foundation Basic Research Award or the AGA June and Donald O. Castell, MD, Esophageal Clinical Research Award.
Restrictions: If an award recipient receives notification of another award with overlapping scientfic objectives, prior to the start date of an AGA or FDHN award, the applicant must choose between the two awards.
Amount of Grant: $25,000
Date(s) Application is Due: Jan 14
Contact: Research Awards Manager, (301) 222-4012; fax: (301) 652-3890; email: awards@fdhn.org
Internet: http://www.fdhn.org/wmspage.cfm?parm1=121
Sponsor: Foundation for Digestive Health and Nutrition
4930 Del Ray Avenue
Bethesda, MD 20814

FDHN Research Scholar Awards 1478

These awards provide salary support for young investigators working in any area of gastrointestinal, liver function, or related diseases. The primary intent of the program is to support physician-investigators who have a high potential to develop independent, productive research careers in gastroenterology and hepatology. Candidates must devote at least 70 percent of their effort to research related to the gastrointestinal tract or liver. There must be a strong commitment from the candidate's division and department to support the candidate by protecting time for research and providing adequate laboratory space and facilities.
Requirements: Applicants must hold full-time faculty positions at North American universities or professional institutes. Nonphysician candidates with a PhD will also be considered. Candidates should be early in their research careers and commonly will have recently completed their fellowship training.
Restrictions: Indirect costs are not allowed. Candidates who have been at the assistant professor level or equivalent for more than five years are not eligible. Nor can applicants hold, or have held, an RO1, R29, K11, K08, or VA research award or any award with similar objectives from nonfederal sources (such as ALF, CCFA, or Glaxo Institute of Digestive Health). However, awards or grants obtained after receipt of this award need not be surrendered.
Samples: Michael Beyak, BSc, MD, Queen's University at Kingston—Ion channels underlying the actions of the satiety hormone CCK on gastrointestinal vagal afferents (2007); Sean Koppe, MD, Northwestern University Feinberg School of Medicine—The Role of Fatty Acids in the Pathogenesis of Non-Alcoholic Steatohepatitis (NASH) (2007).
Amount of Grant: $75,000 per year for three years
Date(s) Application is Due: Sep 5
Contact: Research Awards Manager, (301) 222-4012; fax: (301) 652-3890; email: awards@fdhn.org
Internet: http://www.fdhn.org/wmspage.cfm?parm1=103
Sponsor: Foundation for Digestive Health and Nutrition
4930 Del Ray Avenue
Bethesda, MD 20814

FDHN Student Abstract Prizes 1479

Ten travel awards of $500 each will be given to high school, college, graduate and medical students who have submitted abstracts chosen to be presented during Digestive Disease Week. The three best student abstracts submitted will receive a $1,000 prize. Awards will be presented at a ceremony during DDW. The primary objective of the award is to stimulate interest in gastroenterology research careers through competition and recognition.
Requirements: Any high school, undergraduate medical, premedical, pre-doctoral student or medical resident (up to and including postgraduate year three) who has performed original research related to gastroenterology or hepatology. Applicants must be sponsored by an AGA member.
Restrictions: Post doctoral fellows, technicians, visiting scientists and MD research fellows are not eligible for this award. Applicants may only submit one abstract for consideration and must be the designated presenter or first author of the abstract.
Amount of Grant: $500-$1,000
Date(s) Application is Due: Mar 21

Contact: Research Awards Manager, (301) 222-4012; fax: (301) 652-3890; email: awards@fdhn.org
Internet: http://www.fdhn.org/wmspage.cfm?parm1=152
Sponsor: Foundation for Digestive Health and Nutrition
4930 Del Ray Avenue
Bethesda, MD 20814

FDHN Student Research Fellowships **1480**

This program offers financial support for students to spend a minimum of 10 weeks performing research in digestive diseases or nutrition and is intended to stimulate interest in research careers in these areas. The work may take place at any time during the year. Up to 20 fellowships will be available for full-time research with a preceptor, who must be a faculty member who directs a research project in a gastroenterology-related area at an accredited North American institution. A complete financial statement and scientific progress report are required upon completion of the program. The AGA has recognized the need to attract and encourage minority individuals to enter and pursue gastroenterology research careers. In response to this concern, seven of the student research fellowship awards will be reserved for underrepresented minority students. For the purpose of this award, minorities have been defined as African American, Hispanic, Native American/Alaskan Native, and Pacific Islander.
Requirements: Candidates may be high school, undergraduate, medical, or graduate students (not yet engaged in thesis research) in accredited North American institutions. Women and minority students are strongly encouraged to apply. The preceptor must be a faculty member who directs a research project in a gastroenterology-related area at an accredited North American institution.
Restrictions: Candidates may not hold similar salary support from other agencies: e.g., American Liver Foundation, Crohn's and Colitis Foundation.
Samples: Joanna M. Peloquin, Mayo Medical School (2006); Alexandra Berger, University of California, Los Angeles, CA (2006); Jeremy Thoms Hetzel, University of Chicago, Chicago, IL (2006).
Amount of Grant: $2,000-$3,000
Date(s) Application is Due: Mar 5
Contact: Research Awards Manager, (301) 222-4012; fax: (301) 652-3890; email: awards@fdhn.org
Internet: http://www.fdhn.org/wmspage.cfm?parm1=115
Sponsor: Foundation for Digestive Health and Nutrition
4930 Del Ray Avenue
Bethesda, MD 20814

FDHN TAP Endowed Designated Research Award in Acid-Related Diseases **1481**

This award provides $75,000 per year for three years (total $225,000) for young investigators working toward independent careers in acid-related diseases. The overall objective is to enable young investigators to develop independent and productive careers in acid-related research by ensuring that a major proportion of their time is protected for research.
Requirements: Candidates must hold an MD, PhD, or equivalent degree (e.g., MB, ChB, MBBS, DO). Applicants must hold full-time faculty positions at North American universities or professional institutes at the time award begins. Applicants must be Members of the AGA. The award is not intended for fellows, but for young faculty who have demonstrated unusual promise and have some record of accomplishment in research. Candidates should be in the beginning years of their careers; therefore, established investigators are not appropriate candidates. Candidates must devote at least 70 percent of their efforts to research related to geriatric gastroenterolgy.
Restrictions: MD applicants: no more than five years shall have elapsed following the completion of your clinical training (GI fellowship or its equivalent) and the start date of this award. PhD applicants: no more than five years shall have elapsed from the completion of your postdoctoral training and the start date of this award.
Amount of Grant: $75,000 per year for three years
Date(s) Application is Due: Sep 5
Contact: Research Awards Manager, (301) 222-4012; fax: (301) 652-3890; email: awards@fdhn.org
Internet: http://www.fdhn.org/wmspage.cfm?parm1=132
Sponsor: Foundation for Digestive Health and Nutrition
4930 Del Ray Avenue
Bethesda, MD 20814

FDHN Translational Research Awards **1482**

One award of $100,000 per year for two years will be made annually to support translational research in gastroenterology and/or hepatology. Translational research will be defined as the process of applying ideas, insights and discovery generated through basic science research to the diagnosis, treatment or prevention of human disease. The primary objective of the award is to enhance interaction between researchers with basic science and clinical backgrounds with the goal of accelerating the pace of discovery that is directly applicable to patient care. The creation of teams including both a Ph.D. and an M.D. researcher is particularly encouraged.
Requirements: This award must be applied for jointly by a team of researchers (typically consisting of two members), including at least one researcher with significant training and experience in a basic science discipline (including areas outside the traditional biomedical sciences, such as physical sciences and engineering) and at least one researcher who is qualified to provide direct clinical care to patients. Junior investigators in either or both categories are particularly encouraged to apply. Applicants must be members of the AGA. Research must be conducted at an accredited North American institution.
Restrictions: Candidates may not hold support for the same project from another agency. If a proposed award recipient receives notification of another award with overlapping scientific objectives prior to the start date of an AGA or FDHN award, the applicant must choose only one of the awards to accept.
Amount of Grant: $100,000 per year for two years
Date(s) Application is Due: Mar 14
Contact: Research Awards Manager, (301) 222-4012; fax: (301) 652-3890; email: awards@fdhn.org
Internet: http://www.fdhn.org/wmspage.cfm?parm1=148
Sponsor: Foundation for Digestive Health and Nutrition
4930 Del Ray Avenue
Bethesda, MD 20814

Federal Express Corporate Contributions Program **1483**

The mission of the FedEx Social Responsibility department is to actively support the communities served and to strengthen global reputation through strategic investment of people, resources, and network. The foundation directs its philanthropic efforts to health and welfare programs, education, cultural/arts and civic assistance. Charitable shipping is limited to emergency, disaster or life-threatening situations coordinated through a nonprofit organization, disaster relief agency, or agency of the federal, state, or local government. FedEx is especially interested in supporting nonprofit organizations that request 5 percent or less of a total project budget; contingency grants; or seed monies with the thought that other sources will contribute matching amounts. Organizations must show evidence of competent management, low administrative/fundraising expense ratios, and a nondiscriminatory program benefiting broad segments of the community. FedEx Community Relations responds to all requests in writing. Requests are accepted year-round and generally are reviewed within three weeks of receipt.
Requirements: Charities must be registered 501(c)3 organizations in good financial and public standing.
Samples: St. Jude Children's Research Hospital (Memphis, TN)—to improve medical care for children worldwide with illnesses such as pediatric cancers and AIDS, $2 million.
Contact: Grants Administrator, Community Relations, (901) 369-3600
Internet: http://www.fedex.com/us/about/responsibility/community/guidelines.html?link=4
Sponsor: Federal Express Corporation
3610 Hacks Cross Road, Building A
Memphis, TN 38125

Feldman Foundation Grants Program **1484**

Giving is concentrated in the areas of community development, social welfare, and Jewish causes. Types of support include annual campaigns, building construction/renovation, general operating support, program development, research, and scholarship funds. Initial contact should be by proposal letter. Foundation trustees meet in the spring and fall to review proposals under serious consideration. Applications are accepted at any time.
Requirements: Organizations based in New York and Texas are eligible to apply.
Restrictions: Grants will not be awarded to individuals.
Geographic Focus: New York; Texas
Amount of Grant: $10,000-$50,000 average
Contact: Robert Feldman, Trustee, (214) 689-4337
Sponsor: Feldman Foundation
P.O. Box 1046
Dallas, TX 75221

Fellowships in Infectious Diseases **1485**

The program encourages and assists young qualified physicians to become specialists and investigators in the field of infectious diseases. The fellowship will be awarded to individuals who do not or will not have training or research grant support during the period of this grant and who are seeking support for one to three years of postdoctoral fellowship experience. Preference will be given to those applying for the third year of such support. The applicant must be sponsored by a university affiliated medical center. A letter from the chair of the infectious diseases department expressing a willingness to assume responsibility for training the applicant must accompany the application. In addition, each application must be accompanied by a letter from the host laboratory and signed by the laboratory director or appropriate department chair attesting willingness to accept the applicant and provide guidance, research space, and necessary research equipment. One thousand dollars of the award amount may be used for travel and supplies.
Requirements: Applicants must be U.S. physicians who have satisfactorily completed three or more years of postgraduate medical training (internal medicine, surgery, pediatrics, epidemiology, etc.).
Restrictions: The fellowship will not be awarded if the applicant has received or will receive a major fellowship, research grant, or traineeship in excess of the amount of this award from the federal government or another foundation.
Amount of Grant: $25,000 stipend
Date(s) Application is Due: Feb 15
Contact: Senior Executive Director, (301) 656-0003; fax: (301) 907-0878; email: info@nfid.org
Internet: http://www.nfid.org/fellow
Sponsor: National Foundation for Infectious Diseases
4733 Bethesda Avenue, Suite 750
Bethesda, MD 20814-5278

Ferree Foundation Grants 1486

The foundation is a private family foundation dedicated to promoting and supporting excellence in the arts, culture and history, education, youth engagement, health, human services, and local economic and community development. Paul W. Ware is the Chairman of Ferree Foundation and continues the Ware family tradition of using philanthropy to enhance the lives of families and institutions primarily throughout Lancaster County and, occasionally, Southeastern Pennsylvania and beyond. Grant requests should be in writing and mailed to the executive director. Guidelines are available online.

Requirements: 501(c)3 nonprofit organizations are eligible. Preference is given to organizations serving Pennsylvania's Chester and Lancaster Counties.

Restrictions: The foundation does not make grants to individuals.

Geographic Focus: Pennsylvania

Date(s) Application is Due: Sep 15

Contact: Philip Calhoun, Executive Director, (717) 735-8288; email: pcalhoun@Ferree-Foundation.org

Internet: http://www.ferree-foundation.org

Sponsor: Ferree Foundation
229 N. Duke Street
Lancaster, PA 17602

FIC International Cooperative Biodiversity Groups Grants 1487

Funding for this program has been provided by six components of the National Institutes of Health (NIH), the Biological Sciences Directorate of the National Science Foundation (NSF) and the Foreign Agriculture Service of the U.S.DA. The cooperating NIH components are the Fogarty International Center (FIC), National Cancer Institute (NCI), National Institute of Allergy and Infectious Diseases (NIAID), National Institute of Mental Health (NIMH), National Institute on Drug Abuse (NIDA) and the National Heart, Lung, and Blood Institute (NHLBI). The purpose of these groups will be to address the interdependent issues of biodiversity conservation, sustained economic growth, and human health in terms of drug discovery for cancer, infectious diseases including AIDS, cardiovascular diseases, mental disorders, and diseases of primary concern to developing countries. A group, under a single group leader (principal investigator), is expected to be a consortium of associate programs working together to form a multidisciplinary and/or multi-institutional team from academic, nonprofit, and/or commercial organizations. At least one of the group's associate programs must be located in a developing country. It is strongly advised that applicants contact program staff early in the planning process to discuss prospective applications and to obtain supplemental clarifying information and instructions. RFA-TW-04-004

Requirements: Public and private nonprofit institutions, governments and their agencies, and foreign institutions are eligible. Applicant institutions must be in the United States or in a participating developing country. For-profit institutions may participate as members of the group.

Amount of Grant: $500,000-$600,000 per year

Contact: Dr. Joshua Rosenthal, Director, (301)496-1653; fax: (301) 402-2056; email: Joshua_Rosenthal@nih.gov

Internet: http://www.fic.nih.gov/programs/grants.html#research

Sponsor: Fogarty International Center
31 Center Dr MSC 2220, Building 31, B2C39
Bethesda, MD 20892-2220

FIC International Malaria Research Training Program Award 1488

FIC invites applications to train or expand the capabilities of scientists and health professionals from malaria endemic developing countries to engage in malaria research. Proposals are requested that would create innovative, collaborative malaria research training programs and that would contribute to the long-term goal of harnessing scientific knowledge and skills to enhance efforts to prevent malaria-related morbidity and mortality and to control malaria transmission in endemic developing countries. To develop sustainable research capacity in endemic developing countries, FIC will support malaria research training efforts as part of ongoing, productive malaria research projects in collaboration with internationally recognized research institutions in Africa and other highly endemic regions of the world.Annual deadlines may vary; contact program staff for exact dates. RFA: TW-00-006

Requirements: Applications may be submitted by U.S. nonprofit public and private institutions, such as universities, colleges, hospitals, laboratories, and eligible agencies of the federal government capable of meeting the objectives of the RFA.

Restrictions: Principal Investigators currently supported by other FIC malaria focused research training awards (D43) are not eligible to apply.

Amount of Grant: $45,000 maximum stipend per year

Contact: Administrator, (301) 496-2075; fax: (301) 594-1211; email: ficinfo@nih.gov

Internet: http://www.fic.nih.gov/programs/malaria.html

Sponsor: Fogarty International Center
31 Center Drive, Building 31
Bethesda, MD 20892

FIC International Research and Training in Population and Health Grants 1489

FIC, NICHD, and NIA have developed this program to support international research and training in population-related sciences and to enable NIH grant recipients to extend the geographic base of research and training efforts to developing nations, in support of international population priorities. Types of training for foreign scientists or health professionals may include predoctoral training in research related to population; postdoctoral training in laboratory procedures and research projects and techniques conducted at the host U.S. institutions or in the trainee's home country; and participation in advanced research training conducted by U.S. faculty in the host country and also short-term in-country training for foreign scientists and health professionals in the host country. A letter of intent is requested by December 13; full application is due January 13. Annual deadline dates may vary; contact program staff for exact dates.

Requirements: Applicants must be U.S. principal investigators on at least one NIH-sponsored research grant, cooperative agreement, or contract. The grantee institution must be a U.S. nonprofit private or public institution.

Amount of Grant: $139,000-$185,000

Date(s) Application is Due: Jan 13; Dec 13

Contact: Dr. Jeanne McDermott , Division of International Training and Research, (301) 496-1492; fax: (301) 402-0779; email: mcdermoj@mail.nih.gov

Internet: http://grants.nih.gov/grants/guide/rfa-files/RFA-TW-05-002.html

Sponsor: Fogarty International Center
31 Center Dr MSC 2220, Building 31, Room B2C39
Bethesda, MD 20892-2220

FIC International Research Fellowship Program 1490

The program provides opportunities for non-U.S. postdoctoral biomedical or behavioral scientists in the formative stages of their research careers to gain further research experience by working in the laboratories of distinguished U.S. scientists on problems of mutual interest. Nominations are made by the national nominating committee in each participating country. These committees submit applications to the Fogarty International Center. More than 50 countries or regions in the Americas, Africa, Asia, the Far East, Australia, Europe, and New Zealand participate in the program. Fellowships are awarded for a minimum of 12 months and provide stipend, travel, and institutional allowance. Fellowships provide round-trip travel for the fellow only. In addition, the host institution receives a modest allowance to cover such costs as the fellow's health insurance, supplies, equipment, and travel to scientific meetings or laboratories in the United States or Canada.

Requirements: Candidate must hold a doctoral degree or equivalent in a health science field at the time of submission of application to a nominating committee, have demonstrated the ability to engage in independent basic or clinical research, have a sponsor in the United States at a nonprofit institution who has accepted the applicant for research on his/her proposed project, and have assurance from a nonprofit institution in the home country that there is a position for him/her upon return. Applicant must be proficient in spoken and written English.

Contact: Program Officer, (301) 496-1653; fax: (301) 402-0779/2056; email: nugentr@mail.nih.gov

Internet: http://www.fic.nih.gov/programs/grants.html#fellowships

Sponsor: Fogarty International Center
31 Center Drive, Building 31
Bethesda, MD 20892

FIC International Research Scientist Development Award 1491

The award supports basic research for behavioral and clinical scientists who are committed to a career in international health research and would benefit from an additional period of mentored research as part of a strong, established collaboration between a U.S. sponsor and leading scientists at a developing country center of scientific excellence. The specific research training may be new to the candidate or in an area that would demonstrably enhance the candidate's pursuit of a career focusing on international research pertinent to health in developing countries. Applications are encouraged to address one of the global health research priorities defined by the World Health Organization (http://www.who.ch), which include both infectious and chronic/degenerative conditions and mental health disorders. It is expected that following this experience, the candidate will be able to pursue an independent and productive international research career involving ongoing collaboration with developing country scientists to more effectively pursue research relevant to stemming a major global health problem. Annual deadlines may vary; contact program staff for exact dates. PAR-04-058

Requirements: An applicant must be a U.S. citizen or non-citizen national; hold doctoral or medical degree or the equivalent in a health science field; have earned the relevant degree within seven years of the application receipt date (not including clinical training); have demonstrated a commitment and competence in international health research as well as the potential to engage in independent and productive basic biomedical, behavioral, or epidemiological/clinical research in the period following the award; and have a sponsor in an internationally recognized developing country research institution addressing one or more of that country's major health problems. Eligible countries are in regions that include Africa, Asia (except Japan, Singapore, South Korea, and Taiwan), Central and Eastern Europe, Latin America and the Caribbean, the Middle East (except Israel) and the Pacific Ocean Islands (except Australia and New Zealand). Contact the program office or visit the Web site for full eligibility requirements.

Amount of Grant: $70,000 maximum direct costs per year

Date(s) Application is Due: Feb 16

Contact: Dr. Rachel Nugent, Division of International Training and Research, (301) 496-8733; fax: (301) 402-0779; email: nugentra@mail.nih.gov

Internet: http://www.fic.nih.gov/programs/irsda.html

Sponsor: Fogarty International Center
31 Center Drive, Building 31
Bethesda, MD 20892

FIC International Training & Research in Emerging Infectious Diseases Grants 1492

The Fogarty Center and NIAID have developed this program to train laboratory scientists and public health workers in developing countries and the United States in emerging and re-emerging infectious diseases research, control, and prevention strategies and their implementation and evaluation; facilitate international collaboration on emerging

infectious diseases research, including the conduct of research in developing countries; enhance domestic infectious diseases research programs and improve the protection of the U.S. population from infectious diseases by early detection and response to epidemics internationally and nationally; and develop international leaders in science and public health. Training will include predoctoral and postdoctoral programs, participation in advanced and/or short-term in-country training conducted by U.S. faculty in the host country; and participation in training of health workers in the diagnosis, patient management, control, and prevention of disease. RFA: TW-96-001
Requirements: Applicant must be a U.S. principal investigator of at least one NIH-sponsored research grant related to infectious diseases.
Contact: Dr. Joel Breman, International Training and Research, (301) 496-0815; email: Joel_Breman@.nih.gov
Internet: http://www.fic.nih.gov/programs/erid.html
Sponsor: Fogarty International Center
31 Center Drive, Building 31
Bethesda, MD 20892

FIC International Training and Research in Environmental and Occupational Health 1493
This program, sponsored by the Fogarty International Center, NIEHS, NIOSH, and CDC, was developed to train foreign health scientists, clinicians, epidemiologists, toxicologists, engineers, industrial hygienists, chemists, and allied health workers from developing countries and emerging democracies in both general environmental health and occupational health. Types of training may include training in epidemiology concepts and methods, environmental monitoring, industrial hygiene, field studies, and other research related to environmental and occupational health that will lead to the MS or PhD degree for individuals with previous field research experience; short-term comprehensive courses in epidemiology, toxicology, chemistry, industrial hygiene, and environmental and safety engineering, with an emphasis on control of occupational injuries and illnesses, for health and safety professionals to be given in the United States; training in laboratory procedures and research techniques related to environmental and occupational health for individuals with the MS or PhD degree to be given in the United States; and postdoctoral research training for foreign scientists who want to expand their abilities in the epidemiology, diagnosis, prevention, and treatment of environmental and occupational disease and injury. Postdoctoral training can take place both in the United States and in foreign countries. RFA: TW-01-002.
Requirements: The grantee institution must be a U.S., nonprofit private or public institution. Although most applications will be from academic institutions, a nonacademic, nonprofit institution may apply.
Contact: Dr. Christopher Schonwalder, Senior Environmental Health Advisor to the Director, (919) 541-4794; fax: (919) 541-2583; email: cs64c@nih.gov
Internet: http://www.fic.nih.gov/programs/environ.html
Sponsor: Fogarty International Center
31 Center Drive, Building 31
Bethesda, MD 20892

FIC Israeli Ministry of Health Postdoctoral Research Fellowships 1494
The program provides postdoctoral fellowships to U.S. health scientists to conduct biomedical research in Israel. The purpose is to enhance the exchange of research experience and information in the biomedical and behavioral sciences with emphasis on heart diseases, aging, cancer, human reproduction, and child development. Short- and long-term fellowships are available for appointments at Hebrew University, Hadassah Medical School; Sackler Faculty of Medicine, Tel Aviv University; Weizmann Institute of Science; Technion-Israel Institute of Technology; and Ben Gurion University of the Negev. Information and applications are available from NIH Fogarty International Center; funding is from the Israeli Ministry of Health.
Requirements: Applicants must be citizens or permanent residents of the United States; have doctorates in one of the clinical, biomedical, or behavioral sciences; and have professional experience in the proposed area.
Restrictions: Support is not provided for brief observational visits, attendance at scientific meetings, or independent study.
Contact: Bruce Butrum, Grants Management Officer, (301) 496-1653
Internet: http://www.fic.nih.gov
Sponsor: Fogarty International Center
31 Center Drive, Building 31
Bethesda, MD 20892

FIC Swedish Medical Research Council Fellowships 1495
The Swedish Medical Research Council (SMRC) provides a limited number of research fellowships to U.S. health scientists to conduct research in Sweden and to enhance the exchange of research experience and information in the biomedical and behavioral sciences. Activities supported include collaboration in basic or clinical research and the familiarization with or utilization of special techniques and equipment not otherwise available to the applicant. The program is administered by the Fogarty International Center and funded by the SMRC; applications may be obtained from the center.
Requirements: Candidate must be a citizen or permanent resident of the United States; have a doctorate in clinical, behavioral, or biomedical science; have 10 years or less of postdoctoral experience; and have professional experience in the health sciences for at least two of the last four years. A letter of invitation from the host sponsor is required.
Restrictions: Support is not provided for brief observational visits, attendance at scientific meetings, or independent study.
Amount of Grant: $30,000-$45,000 per year; $41,000 average
Contact: Bruce Butrum, Grants Management Officer, (301) 496-1653
Internet: http://www.fic.nih.gov/programs/grants.html#fellowships
Sponsor: Fogarty International Center
31 Center Drive, Building 31
Bethesda, MD 20892

FIC/NIH AIDS International Training and Research Program 1496
The primary goal of this program is to build research capacity. This program is intended to complement ongoing HIV/AIDS and TB research efforts of the NIH and to the extent possible, of other government, nongovernment, and international organizations. Programs are encouraged to develop human resources in those developing and other participating countries that currently are or are likely to be sites of HIV/AIDS-related research on HIV and/or TB vaccines, anti-HIV and TB drugs, and other HIV and TB interventions. A letter of intent is requested by November 21; full application is due December 21.
Requirements: Countries in Central and Eastern Europe and the New Independent States are eligible to participate, as are countries in Africa, the Americas, Asia, and the Pacific Region. The grantee institution must be a U.S. nonprofit private or public institution capable of meeting the objectives in this RFA.
Restrictions: Institutions that currently hold an award are not eligible to submit a second application.
Date(s) Application is Due: Nov 21; Dec 21
Contact: Dr. Jeanne McDermott, Program Officer, (301) 496-1653; fax: (301) 402-0779; email: mcdermoj@mail.nih.gov
Internet: http://www.fic.nih.gov/programs/aitrp/aitrp.html
Sponsor: Fogarty International Center
31 Center Drive, Building 31
Bethesda, MD 20892

FIC/ORMH Minority International Research Training Grants 1497
FIC and ORMH jointly support scientific training programs that offer international research training opportunities to qualified minority undergraduates and graduate/medical students underrepresented in biomedical and behavioral research careers. Applications are invited from innovative programs that provide international research and training to encourage underrepresented minority students to pursue biomedical research careers, broaden minority research efforts and scientific training to encompass international health problems, stimulate novel approaches to studying health problems that disproportionately affect underserved groups in the United States or in developing countries, and assist minority scientists to participate in international collaborative relationships and work effectively in the rapidly evolving global scientific environment. A letter of intent is requested by December 10; full application is due January 14. Annual deadline dates may vary; contact program staff for exact dates. RFA: TW-00-001
Requirements: Applicant institution and its associated consortia institutions must be colleges or universities that offer baccalaureate degrees in fields relevant to biomedical science. Only one application per institution will be accepted. Priority is given to consortia which include historically black colleges and universities, hispanic serving institutions, or tribal colleges and universities. Participant students and faculty must be U.S. citizens or permanent residents.
Amount of Grant: $1.8 million total
Date(s) Application is Due: Jan 14; Dec 10
Contact: Dr. Barbara Sina, Division of International Training and Research, (301) 496-1653; fax: (301) 402-0779; email: barbara_sina@nih.gov
Internet: http://www.fic.nih.gov/programs/mirt.html
Sponsor: Fogarty International Center
31 Center Drive, Building 31
Bethesda, MD 20892

Fidelity Foundation Grants 1498
The foundation awards grants to nonprofits in community-operating areas working in the fields of community development, cultural affairs, education, and health. Fields of interest include arts and cultural programs, education, health care and health organizations, medical research, and community development. Types of support include capital campaigns, building/renovations, endowment funds, program development, technical assistance, and employee matching gifts.
Requirements: Nonprofit organizations in community-operating areas, particularly in Covington, KY, Boston and Marlborough, MA; Merrimack, NH; New York, NY; Cincinnati, OH; Smithfield, RI; Dallas/Fort Worth, TX; Salt Lake City, UT; and Toronto, Canada, are eligible.
Restrictions: Grants are not awarded to support sectarian organizations, disease-specific associations, or public school systems. Support does not go to individuals or for scholarships, civic or start-up organizations, corporate memberships, operating support, or participation in benefit events, film, or video projects. Multiyear requests will be denied.
Geographic Focus: Kentucky; Massachusetts; New Hampshire; New York; Ohio; Rhode Island; Texas; UtahCanada
Samples: Ctr for Information and Crisis Services (Lantana, FL)—for organizational development and to improve their volunteer programs, $50,000.; YMCA of Metropolitan Dallas (Dallas, TX)—for capital support of the new Irving Family YMCA at North Lake, $40,000.
Contact: Margaret Morton, Senior Vice President, Program, (617) 563-6806
Internet: http://www.fidelityfoundation.org
Sponsor: Fidelity Foundation
82 Devonshire Street, S2
Boston, MA 02109

Field Foundation of Illinois Grants 1499

The Foundation awards grants only to institutions and agencies operating in the fields of urban and community affairs, culture, education, community welfare, health, and environment, primarily serving the people of Chicago with extremely limited grant making in the metropolitan area. Preference will be given to funding innovative approaches for addressing program areas.

Requirements: Applicants must reside in Illinois. Grant applications are not provided; however, a formal proposal is required. The Foundation does not accept grant requests via email or fax.

Restrictions: No grants will be made to support: endowments; individuals; medical research or national health agency appeals; propaganda organizations or committees whose efforts are aimed at influencing legislation; printed materials, video or computer equipment; fund-raising events or advertising; appeals for religious purposes; other granting agencies or foundations for ultimate distribution to agencies or programs of its own choosing; custodian afterschool programs or tutoring; most disease specific programs, research or activities; or operating support of established neighborhood health centers or clinics, day care centers for children, or small cultural groups. Requests for computer equipment will not be considered.

Geographic Focus: Illinois

Samples: Catholic Charities of the Archdiocese of Chicago (IL)—to support expansion of the Emergency Assistance Services program, $15,000 (2005); Jobs for Youth/Chicago (IL)—to support the Workforce Advancement Initiative, $10,000 (2005); Palliative Care Center and Hospice of the North Shore (IL)—to support the capital campaign for a new community facility, $25,000 (2005); Puerto Rican Alliance (IL)—to support the Community Arts Program, $10,000 (2005).

Amount of Grant: $50,000

Date(s) Application is Due: Jan 15; May 15; Sep 15

Contact: Joann Ross, (312) 831-0910; fax: (312) 831-0961; email: jross@fieldfoundation.org

Internet: http://www.fieldfoundation.org

Sponsor: Field Foundation of Illinois, Inc
200 S. Wacker Drive, Suite 3860
Chicago, IL 60606

Field Psychology Research Grants 1500

Grants support promising graduate students exploring the history, contributions, and further development of perceptual (field) psychology in relationship to the research and writings of Arthur W. Combs, PhD. Applications of Dr. Combs's theoretical position to the improvement of educational, community, conflict-resolution, therapeutic efforts, etc. are also encouraged.

Amount of Grant: $500-$1500

Date(s) Application is Due: Jan 31; Oct 5

Contact: Anne Richards, Trustee, (770) 834-8143; email: arichard@westga.edu

Internet: http://www.fieldpsychtrust.org/application.asp

Sponsor: Field Psychology Trust
301 Dixie Street
Carrollton, GA 30117

Fifth Third Foundation Grants 1501

The foundation awards grants to eligible nonprofit organizations in its areas of interest, including community development, education, health and human services, and arts and culture. Proposals are favored that are likely to make a substantial difference in the quality of community life; strengthen families and communities; expand meaningful civic engagement and build social capital; use volunteers; help nonprofit organizations build capacity and become more effective; include financial and other strategic commitments from other funding organizations; and leverage change in the capacity of community-wide systems rather than individual organizations. Interested applicants should initially contact the Foundation via a brief letter detailing the organization, its mission, the project it seeks funding for, and an approximate grant amount to be requested. Guidelines are available online.

Requirements: 501(c)3 nonprofit, tax-exempt organizations operating in Fifth Third's geographic regions—Ohio, Kentucky, Indiana, Michigan, Illinois, Tennessee, West Virginia, and Florida— are eligible.

Restrictions: Capital campaigns for individual churches; publicly supported entities, such as public schools or government agencies; elementary schools; and individuals are ineligible.

Geographic Focus: Florida; Illinois; Indiana; Kentucky; Michigan; Ohio; Tennessee; West Virginia

Samples: Athenaeum of Ohio (Cincinnati, OH)—to renovate the Eugene H. Maly Library, which houses more than 500 rare books, religious texts, and manuscripts, $500,000 (2005).

Contact: Grants Administrator, (513) 534-7001

Internet: http://www.53.com/wcm/connect/FifthThirdSite/About+53/In+the+Community/Foundation+Office/

Sponsor: Fifth Third Foundation
38 Fountain Square Plaza, MD 1090CA
Cincinnati, OH 45263

Fight for Sight Research Grants 1502

Grants support basic or clinical research of high scientific merit into diseases of the eye. The award may cover salaries, equipment, necessary travel, and/or research expenses. Awards are tenable at the Institute of Ophthalmology or other institutes or universities in the United Kingdom for up to three years.

Requirements: Awards are open to all medical and scientific researchers.

Samples: To be distribute among 19 universities—for research into the causes of blindness and vision disorders, through the grants-in-aid program, $223,000 (2004).

Contact: Janice Benson, Grants Manager, (212) 679-6060; fax: (212) 679-4466; email: janice@fightforsight.com

Internet: http://www.fightforsight.com

Sponsor: Fight for Sight
381 Park Ave S, Suite 809
New York, NY 10016

Fight for Sight Research Grants and Fellowships 1503

The primary purpose of the program is to encourage and finance research in ophthalmology, vision, and related sciences. The goal is to restore and preserve sight through research in detection, prevention, treatment, and curing of visual disorders, as well as diseases leading to impaired sight and partial or total blindness. Funding priority is given to pilot projects for research relating to clinically important eye diseases. Fight for Sight will continue to support younger investigators, promoting the development of scientific skills that will lead to more substantial funding from other sources. Preference will be given to clinical and disease-oriented grants and training fellowships in the areas of age-related macular degeneration, diabetic retinopathy, retinitis pigmentosa, glaucoma, amblyopia, strabismus, AIDS-related eye disorders, cataract, and uveal and corneal inflammation. Award mechanisms include grants in aid, postdoctoral fellowships, and student fellowships.

Requirements: Applicant must have a doctoral degree in medicine, optometry, or basic science and have less than one year of postdoctoral training. Fellowships are available to U.S. and Canadian residents and are not offered for study abroad. Undergraduate, graduate, and medical students may apply for student fellowships.

Restrictions: An applicant may not currently be financed by other research funds.

Amount of Grant: $25,000-$50,000

Date(s) Application is Due: Mar 1

Contact: Program Coordinator, Fight for Sight Research Division, (847) 843-2020; fax: (847) 843-8458; email: info@preventblindness.org

Internet: http://www.preventblindness.org/research

Sponsor: Prevent Blindness America
500 E Remington Road
Schaumburg, IL 60173

Fireman's Fund Foundation Grants 1504

Program interests are primarily in support of education, human needs, arts and culture, and civic community activities, especially programs for youth, the elderly, and minority groups. Support is provided primarily to organizations in Marin County in the San Francisco Bay area. Limited funding is provided to Sonoma County. There is no deadline for applications. Proposals are reviewed four times a year. Once an application is submitted, a decision is usually made within 90 days. Guidelines and application are available online.

Requirements: To apply, a nonprofit, tax-exempt organization should send a letter to the director setting forth the request for funding and the amount desired, enclosing a financial statement, IRS letter, and a list of board members. Support is provided primarily to organizations in Marin County in the San Francisco Bay area.

Restrictions: The foundation does not make grants for capital campaigns; endowment funds; general operating expenses; individuals; religious organizations; fraternal, veteran, or sectarian groups; medical research and health organizations; trips or tours; advertising; video, television, or film productions; fundraising events; sporting events; political organizations; subscription fees or admission tickets; or public sector services (with the exception of some school district programs).

Geographic Focus: California

Samples: North Bay Children's Ctr (CA)—for program support, $15,000.; Youth in Arts (CA)—for program support, $5000.

Amount of Grant: $5000-$15,000

Date(s) Application is Due: Apr 1; Oct 1

Contact: Phyllis Secosky, Executive Director, Fireman's Fund Foundation, (415) 899-2757 or (415) 899-2000; email: phyllis_secosky@ffic.com

Internet: http://www.firemansfund.com/servlet/dcms?c=about&rkey=131

Sponsor: Fireman's Fund Foundation
777 San Marin Drive
Novato, CA 94998-1406

FirstEnergy Foundation Community Grants 1505

The Foundation believes it takes commitment to help make communities strong, resilient, and responsive to the needs of citizens. It also takes vision, cooperation, and financial support. The Foundation considers grants in the following areas that: ensure the safety and overall health of the community; support employee involvement and investment; promote economic development; and advance professional development and education. Interested applicants should submit a one or two page proposal letter. Guidelines are available online.

Requirements: 501(c)3 organizations within the FirstEnergy Corp. operating companies' service areas - Ohio Edison, The Illuminating Company, Toledo Edison, Penn Power, Met-Ed, Penelac, and Jersey Central Power and Light are eligible to apply.

Restrictions: Funding is not considered for: direct grants to individuals, political or legislative activities; organizations that receive sizable public tax funding; fraternal, religious, labor, athletic, social or veterans organizations - unless the contribution is earmarked for an eligible program or campaign open to all beneficiaries, including those not affiliated with the host organization; national or international organizations;

organizations supported by federated campaigns, such as United Way; research; equipment purchases; loans or second party giving, such as endowments, debt retirement, or foundations; or public or private schools.
Geographic Focus: New Jersey; Ohio; Pennsylvania
Samples: United Way Services (Cleveland, OH)—for operating support, $493,000.; Musical Arts Assoc (Cleveland, OH)—for operating support, $43,394.; Cleveland Initiative for Education (Cleveland, OH)—for operating support, $40,000.
Contact: Mary Beth Carroll, President, (330) 761-4246
Internet: http://www.firstenergycorp.com/community
Sponsor: FirstEnergy Foundation
76 South Main Street
Akron, OH 44308

Fisa Foundation Grants **1506**
The foundation's mission is to build a culture of respect and improve the quality of life for three populations in southwestern Pennsylvania: women, girls, and people with disabilities. Emphasis is given to addressing gaps and unmet needs in the community. The foundation will consider support for new and ongoing programs and projects, operating needs, capacity building, equipment, and capital expenditures. Applicants are encouraged to submit a letter of inquiry outlining the needs to be addressed, a brief description of the proposed project or program, and the amount of the request. Letters of inquiry are reviewed on a monthly basis; full proposals are by invitation.
Requirements: 501(c)3 and 509(a) nonprofit organizations in the 10-county southwestern Pennsylvania area, including Allegheny, Armstrong, Beaver, Butler, Fayette, Greene, Indiana, Lawrence, Washington and Westmoreland Counties, are eligible.
Restrictions: The foundation does not make grants in support of individuals; political campaigns or lobbying; religious organizations for religious purposes; travel, study and scholarships; services for people with disabilities that result from the aging process; renovations to improve physical accessibility of buildings; programs with the primary mission of serving individuals with mental illness; clinical research; or parenting programs, unless they specifically relate to parents with disabilities.
Geographic Focus: Pennsylvania
Amount of Grant: $5000 to $75,000 typically
Contact: Mary Delaney, (412) 456-5550; fax: (412) 456-5551; email: info@fisafoundation.org
Internet: http://www.fisafoundation.org/grtmk.ivnu
Sponsor: Fisa Foundation
1001 Liberty Avenue, Suite 650
Pittsburgh, PA 15222

Fischelis Grants for Research in the History of American Pharmacy **1507**
The institute supports a wide range of scholarly activities as long as they promise to contribute significantly to historical understanding and are clearly related to the modern practice of pharmacy in the United States. Projects must be connected directly to American pharmacy practice. Preference will be given to 20th-century topics, although studies of earlier periods will be considered. Historical discussions of current practice issues are also eligible. An application received after the deadline date will be evaluated individually if any funds remain unawarded; otherwise it will be considered in the next year's program.
Requirements: Each application is referred for evaluation to a committee of the institute. Principal criteria used in evaluating an application are a candidate's qualifications and record relevant to the intended purpose, relevance to the history of modern American pharmacy, and the adequacy of resources to fulfill the stated purpose.
Amount of Grant: $5,000 maximum
Date(s) Application is Due: Mar 1
Contact: Gregory Higby, Director; (608) 262-5378; email: grants@aihp.org
Internet: http://www.pharmacy.wisc.edu/aihp
Sponsor: American Institute of the History of Pharmacy
777 Highland Avenue
Madison, WI 53705-2222

Fisher Foundation Grants **1508**
The foundation awards grants to Connecticut nonprofits that benefit education, health and human services, housing, community needs, and arts and culture. The majority of grants are single year awards. Before submitting an application, a letter of inquiry or conversation with staff to discuss the specific purpose for which the funds are being requested is strongly recommended. Application information and guidelines are available online. Do not submit applications by fax or email.
Requirements: Nonprofits located in, and/or serving the residents of the Greater Hartford area, including: Andover, Avon, Bloomfield, Bolton, Canton, East Hartford, East Granby, East Windsor, Ellington, Enfield, Farmington, Glastonbury, Granby, Hartford, Hebron, Manchester, Marlborough, Newington, Rocky Hill, Simsbury, Somers, South Windsor, Suffield, Tolland, Vernon, West Hartford, Wethersfield, Windsor, and Windsor Locks are eligible.
Restrictions: Foundation policy does not allow funding for: organizations which are not tax-exempt under IRS Code section 501(c)3; organizations which have the IRS private foundation designation; individuals; performances, conferences, retreats, one-time events, trips; annual campaigns.
Geographic Focus: Connecticut
Date(s) Application is Due: Jan 15; Apr 15; Sep 15
Contact: Beverly Boyle, Executive Director; (860) 570-0221; fax: (860) 570-0225; email: bboyle@fisherfdn.org
Internet: http://www.fisherfdn.org/application/instructions.htm
Sponsor: Fisher Foundation
36 Brookside Boulevard
West Hartford, CT 06107

Fisher House Foundation Newman's Own Awards **1509**
Grants are made to implement innovative programs to improve the quality of life for military families and their communities. This program is administered by Fisher House, a charitable organization that provides a home-like place to stay for United States military families while a family member is receiving treatment at a major military or Veterans Administration medical facility. One award will be given to an organization supporting the Army, Navy, Air Force, Marines, or Coast Guard The organization with the most innovative project submitted will receive up to $15,000. The other four organizations will receive lesser amounts, as determined by the judges. Annual deadline dates may vary; contact program staff for exact dates.
Requirements: Eligible applicants must support an Active Duty, National Guard, or Reserve unit or installation, and be tax-exempt, a private organization, or a volunteer organization. Private, nonprofit organizations as defined in Department of Defense (DoD) Instruction 1000.15 and approved for operation on a DoD installation by the installation commander are eligible.
Amount of Grant: $1,000-$15,000
Date(s) Application is Due: Apr 30
Contact: James D. Weiskopf, Executive Vice President; (888) 294-8560 or (301) 294-8560; fax: (301) 294-8562; email: info@fisherhouse.org
Internet: http://www.fisherhouse.org/programs/newmans.shtml
Sponsor: Fisher House Foundation
1401 Rockville Pike, Suite 600
Rockville, MD 20852

Fishman Family Foundation Grants **1510**
The Foundation considers grants for: research, education, and cultural development of and for the community; scholarships related to Jewish services, education, social, and community activities; medical and scientific research; providing resources to meet critical needs in Israel; and educational grants and scholarships. Proposals are reviewed in April and October. Application information is available online.
Requirements: 501(c)3 nonprofits are eligible.
Date(s) Application is Due: Mar 31; Sep 30
Contact: Betty Fishman, President, email: info@fishman.org
Internet: http://www.fishman.org/apply.html
Sponsor: Fishman Family Foundation
730 E. Cypress Avenue
Monrovia, CA 91016

Flinn Foundation Grants Programs **1511**
The foundation's grantmaking programs, limited to Arizona, include enhancing community-based solutions to local health care needs, especially those for children and youth; strengthening medical education and biomedical research programs in Arizona; strengthening Arizona's universities through an undergraduate scholarship program for outstanding Arizona high school students; and enhancing the visibility and long-term artistic mission of Arizona's principal visual and performing arts organizations. Types of support include program development, seed money, scholarships, and research grants.
Requirements: Arizona-based institutions or organizations whose programs are operated for the benefit of Arizona institutions and individuals are eligible to apply. Applications are accepted at any time. There is no application form, but a preliminary letter of inquiry or phone call is requested to determine the appropriateness of a full submission.
Restrictions: The foundation rarely provides grants to individuals, building projects (capital campaigns), purchase of equipment, endowment projects, annual fund-raising campaigns, ongoing operating expenses, or deficit needs. Requests to support conferences and workshops, publications, or the production of films and video are considered only when these activities are an integral component of a larger foundation initiative.
Geographic Focus: Arizona
Samples: Northern Arizona U (Flagstaff, AZ)—to expand teacher-preparation programs in the biological sciences, $517,100 over three years.; Homeward Bound (Phoenix, AZ)—to coordinate access to health care services for disadvantaged children, $10,000.; Ballet Arizona (Phoenix, AZ)—for 15 months of support, $200,000.
Amount of Grant: $2500-$150,000 average
Contact: JoAnn Fazio, Grants Coordinator, (602) 744-6800; fax: (602) 744-6815; email: info@flinn.org
Internet: http://www.flinn.org/about/grants.cms
Sponsor: Flinn Foundation
1802 N Central Avenue
Phoenix, AZ 85004-1506

Florida BRAIVE Fund of Dade Community Foundation **1512**
The Florida BrAIve Fund at Dade Community Foundation will award grants to non-profits to assist eligible military personnel and family members residing in Miami-Dade, Monroe, Broward, Palm Beach and Martin counties. BRAIVE Fund grants will address needs of military personnel and their families in the target population related to pre-deployment, during deployment, and their return from duty. To obtain more information and the application forms, go to http://www.dadecommunityfoundation.org/Site/wc/wc143.jsp.
Requirements: General criteria for evaluating applications to The Florida BrAIve Fund of Dade Community Foundation: applicant is a 501(c)3 organization; applicant organization has a proven record of effective service to its clientele; applicant organization demonstrates

the management and financial capacity to efficiently achieve the grant purpose; grants will be made to nonprofit organizations, not individuals; programs or services can only benefit current and former military personnel serving in Iraq or Afghanistan and their families; program services must be provided in the area of Florida to be covered by Dade Community Foundation as indicated in The Florida BrAIve Fund map; successful organizations will demonstrate that the agency is currently serving military personnel and their families in Florida or has the experience to address an unmet need.
Geographic Focus: Florida
Date(s) Application is Due: Jun 8
Contact: Claudianna Williams, Foundation's administrative assistant; (305) 371-2711; fax: (305) 371-5342; email: claudianna.williams@dadecommunityfoundation.org
Internet: http://www.dadecommunityfoundation.org/Site/wc/wc143.jsp
Sponsor: Dade Community Foundation
200 South Biscayne Boulevard, Suite 505
Miami, FL 33131-5330

Florida BRAIVE Fund of Gulf Coast Community Foundation of Venice **1513**
Through the Florida BrAIve Fund the Foundation seeks to support efforts of existing nonprofit organizations who have established relationships with the military community and who currently serve Operation Iraqi Freedom and Operation Enduring Freedom personnel and their families in Central and Southwest Florida. Funding priorities will include the following for military personnel before, during, and after their deployment to Afghanistan or Iraq. Submit an application any time between November 11, 2008, and July 31, 2010. The Foundation will accept and review applications on a rolling basis. Application form and additional guidelines are available at the Foundations website.
Requirements: The Foundation will provide grants to nonprofit organizations with a 501(c)3 designation from the Internal Revenue Service in the counties of Brevard, Charlotte, Citrus, Collier, DeSoto, Glades, Hardee, Hendry, Hernando, Highlands, Hillsborough, Indian River, Lake, Lee, Manatee, Okeechobee, Orange, Osceola, Pasco, Pinellas, Polk, Sarasota, Seminole, Sumter, and St. Lucie.
Geographic Focus: Florida
Samples: Special Operations Warrior Foundation, $500,000 - immediate financial assistance for special operations personnel, who have been severely wounded, to have his/her family travel and be bedside (2009); Charlotte Behavioral Health Care, $200,000 - addressing mental health, substance abuse, and related psychosocial needs of veterans and their families (2009);
Contact: Kirstin Fulkerson, Program Officer; (941) 486-4600; fax: (941) 486-4699; email: floridabraive@gulfcoastcf.org or info@gulfcoastcf.org
Internet: http://www.gulfcoastcf.org/page10003300.cfm
Sponsor: Gulf Coast Community Foundation of Venice
601 Tamiami Trail South
Venice, FL 34285

Florida BRAIVE Fund of The Community Foundation in Jacksonville **1514**
The Florida BrAIve Fund of The Community Foundation in Jacksonville was created to provide assistance to North Florida military personnel and families affected by deployment to Afghanistan or Iraq. Grants will be made to non-profit agencies in North Florida to support services that assist military personnel and their families before, during, and after deployment. Specific priority target populations include: military personnel returning from deployment to Afghanistan or Iraq and their families; military personnel with physical or mental health needs as a result of deployment to Afghanistan or Iraq; families of military personnel currently deployed or preparing for imminent (within 120 days) deployment to Afghanistan or Iraq; families of those killed in action during deployment to Afghanistan or Iraq; and individual augmentees or others deployed without a typical support structure. Grant applications for The Florida BrAIve Fund of The Community Foundation in Jacksonville will be considered on a rolling basis as they are received. You may submit an application at any time. Once the Foundation have received your application and all supplemental materials, you may expect to receive a decision from The Community Foundation in Jacksonville within 60 days. See the Foundations website for a application form and additional guidelines.
Requirements: Nonprofit 501(c)3organization providing services to meet the unmet needs of North Florida military personnel and families affected by deployments to Iraq and Afghanistan as part of Operation Enduring Freedom or Operation Iraqi Freedom, may be eligible to apply for a grant.
Geographic Focus: Florida
Contact: Cheryl Riddick, Vice President of Grantmaking Services; (904) 356-4483; email: info@jaxcf.org
Internet: http://www.jaxcf.org/NetCommunity/Page.aspx?pid=430
Sponsor: The Community Foundation in Jacksonville
121 West Forsyth Street, Suite 900
Jacksonville, FL 32202

Florida High School/High Tech Project Grants **1515**
The purpose of the program is to assist an existing high school/high tech project to provide a transition program to motivate and prepare high school students with disabilities for college, jobs, and careers. The goal of the program is to help reduce the dropout rate of youth with disabilities, increase their enrollment in college, and improve participation in education/vocational/employment related activities. The program provides step-down funding while the program is gaining independent funding for the future of their program.
Requirements: Any established, Florida nonprofit corporation, agency, organization or association that has been granted exemption from federal income tax under Section 501(c)3 of the IRS Tax Code is eligible to submit a proposal for review.
Geographic Focus: Florida
Contact: Grants Administrator, (850) 224-4493; fax: (850) 224-4496; email: info@abletrust
Internet: http://www.abletrust.org
Sponsor: Able Trust
106 E. College Avenue, Suite 820
Tallahassee, FL 32301

Floyd A. and Kathleen C. Cailloux Foundation Grants **1516**
The foundation awards grants in the areas of civic and cultural, education and youth, family and community service, and health and rehabilitation. Grants support specific projects or programs, technical assistance, and capital projects. Grants for general operations are less common and usually small. Endowment grants are rare. The foundation only reviews grant proposals from applicants whose letters of inquiry have been approved. Applications are taken online.
Requirements: Grants support 501(c)3 nonprofit organizations. Preference is given to requests from Texas Hill Country.
Restrictions: The Foundation does not fund church or seminary construction, or church related entities or activities other than ecumenically oriented projects/programs that otherwise meet Foundation guidelines. The general policy of the Foundation is not to make grants to an organization more than once within any 12-month period. Grants or loans to individuals are never made.
Contact: Grants Administrator; (830) 895-5222; email: info@caillouxfoundation.org
Internet: http://www.caillouxfoundation.org/grant_guidelines.htm
Sponsor: Floyd A. and Kathleen C. Cailloux Foundation
P.O. Box 291276
Kerrville, TX 78029-1276

Fluor Foundation Grants **1517**
The Fluor Corporation achieves its contribution objectives through the Fluor Foundation and corporate giving. The Foundation's areas of interest are: education; human services; cultural outreach; and public/civic affairs. The Foundation considers requests for operating, program, capital or endowment support. Priority is given to funding organizations with employee volunteer participation. Application information is available online.
Requirements: Fluor's giving programs focus on community organizations in those locations around the world where the company has a presence. See website for local contact information: http://www.fluor.com/sustainability/community/fluor_giving/Pages/applying_for_fluor_foundation_grants.aspx
Restrictions: Funding is not available for: film production/publishing activities; individuals; sports organizations/programs; veterans, fraternal, labor or religious organizations; or lobbying/political organizations or campaigns.
Geographic Focus: Alaska; California; Louisiana; New Jersey; New York; North Carolina; Pennsylvania; South Carolina; Tennessee; Texas; Virginia; WashingtonAsia; Australia; Belgium; Canada; Caribbean; China; Europe; Japan; Mexico; New Zealand; Peru; Philippines; Poland; Russia; United Kingdom; Venezuela
Contact: Suzanne Esber, Executive Director of Community Relations; (949) 349-7847; fax: (949) 349-7694; email: suzanne.esber@fluor.com
Internet: http://www.fluor.com/sustainability/community/fluor_giving/Pages/applying_for_fluor_foundation_grants.aspx
Sponsor: Fluor Foundation
3 Polaris Way
Aliso Viejo, CA 92698

FMC Foundation Grants **1518**
The foundation supports education, community improvement, urban affairs, health and human services, and public issues/economic education. Higher education is supported through scholarships and employee matching gifts. Education support tends to be in business, engineering, chemistry, and some minority education programs. Eligible applicants need to contact the FMC in their geograhic area. Each individual FMC location determines how their contributions will be given.
Requirements: Grants are awarded to 501(c)3 organizations in FMC-plant communities. U.S.-based organizations with an international focus are also eligible.
Restrictions: Grants are not made to individuals.
Geographic Focus: Arizona; California; Delaware; Florida; Illinois; Louisiana; Maine; Maryland; Missouri; New Jersey; New York; North Carolina; Pennsylvania; Tennessee; Texas; West Virginia; WyomingCanada
Contact: Program Contact, (215) 299-6000; fax: (215) 299-6140
Internet: http://www.fmc.com
Sponsor: FMC Foundation
1735 Market Street
Philadelphia, PA 19103

Foellinger Foundation Grants **1519**
The foundation awards grants primarily in Fort Wayne and Allen County, IN, to improve the quality of life in the areas of early child development, youth development, strengthening family services, strengthening organizations, and community concerns. Special emphasis is given to projects/programs that help children and their families, particularly those with the greatest economic need and least opportunity. By doing so, the Foundation hopes to help children and their families move from dependence to independence. In addition to programs and projects, the foundation also awards grants for general operating, capital, seed money, renovation projects, conferences and seminars, consulting services, equipment, challenge/matching, and planning purposes.

Requirements: Indiana organizations are eligible to apply.
Restrictions: The foundation does not fund scholarships, travel assistance, conference fees, religious groups, public or private elementary or secondary schools, sponsorships, special events, advertising, or endowments.
Geographic Focus: Indiana
Samples: Public Broadcasting of Northeast Indiana (IN)—for general operating support.; Arthur J. Blaising Social Services (IN)—for its after-school program and its 10-week summer day camp, $75,585.; Turnstone (IN)—for a transportation program that serves elderly and disabled people, $187,500 over 18 months.; Taylor U—for the Allen County Postsecondary Education Consortium, $219,690 over two years.
Amount of Grant: $10,000-$100,000 average
Date(s) Application is Due: Feb 1; May 1; Nov 1
Contact: Cheryl Taylor, President, (219) 422-2900; fax: (219) 422-9436; email: info@foellinger.org
Internet: http://www.foellinger.org
Sponsor: Foellinger Foundation
520 E. Berry Street
Fort Wayne, IN 46802

Fondren Foundation Grants **1520**
The foundation awards grants to Texas-based programs in the areas of education, youth services, health care, and human services. The board meets quarterly to consider requests.
Requirements: Texas nonprofit organizations, with an emphasis on Houston and the Southwest are eligible to apply.
Restrictions: The Foundation does not allow funding to individuals, or for operating or annual fund drives.
Geographic Focus: Texas
Amount of Grant: $10,000-$100,000
Contact: Melanie Scioneaux, Assistant Secretary
Internet: http://www.tcc.state.tx.us/cancerfunding/regional/05.html
Sponsor: Fondren Foundation
7 TCT 37, P.O. Box 2558
Houston, TX 77252-8037

Food, Pharmaceutical, and Bioengineering Division Award in Chemical Engineering **1521**
This award is given to recognize outstanding chemical engineering contributions and achievements by an individual in those industries involved in food, pharmaceutical, and bioengineering activities. The recipient need not be a member of AIChE, and there is no age limit. The individual's contributions may have been made in industrial, governmental, or academic areas, or with other organizations.
Requirements: All members, as well as other interested persons, are urged to nominate deserving candidates.
Amount of Grant: $4000
Date(s) Application is Due: Mar 25
Contact: AIChE Awards Programs, (212) 591-7107; fax: (212) 591-8890; email: awards@aiche.org
Internet: http://www.aiche.org/awards/awarddtl.asp?AwardID=36
Sponsor: American Institute of Chemical Engineers
3 Park Avenue
New York, NY 10016-5910

Ford Motor Company Fund Grants **1522**
The fund supports not-for-profit organizations in three major areas: innovation and education; community development and American legacy, and auto-related safety education. The fund seeks to build partnerships with organizations that have a well-defined sense of purpose, a demonstrated commitment to maximizing available resources, and a reputation for meeting objectives and delivering quality programs and services. Priority is placed on the support and development of organizations that promote diversity and inclusion. Requests for support are accepted and reviewed throughout the year. The fund now implements an online application system. Details are available online.
Restrictions: Ford does not fund: advocacy-directed programs; animal-rights organizations; beauty or talent contests; day-to-day business operations; debt reduction; donation of vehicles; efforts to influence legislation, or the outcome of any elections or any specific election of candidates to public office or to carry on any voter registration drive; endowments; fraternal organizations; general operating support to hospitals and health care institutions; individual sponsorship related to fundraising activities; individuals; labor groups; loans for small businesses; loans to program-related investments; organizations that do not have 501(c)3 status; organizations that unlawfully discriminate in their provision of goods and services based on race, color, religion, gender, gender identity or expression, ethnicity, sexual orientation, national origin, physical challenge, age, or status as a protected veteran; political contributions; private K-12 schools; profit-making enterprises; religious programs or sectarian programs for religious purposes; species-specific organizations; sports teams.
Samples: American Red Cross, Southeastern Michigan Chapter (Detroit, MI)—for disaster-relief efforts in Florida related to Hurricane Charley, $50,000 (2004).
Contact: Ford Fund Coordinator, (888) 313-0102; email: Fordfund@ford.com
Internet: http://www.ford.com/en/goodWorks/fundingAndGrants/fordMotorCompanyFund/default.htm
Sponsor: Ford Motor Company Fund
P.O. Box 1899
Dearborn, MI 48121-1899

Forrest C. Lattner Foundation Grants **1523**
The Foundation's primary objectives are in six areas of interest: arts and humanities; education; environment; health and social services; historic preservation; and medical research. The Foundation also wishes to encourage the development of innovative model programs. Application guidelines are available online.
Restrictions: The foundation is unable to fulfill grant requests to individuals, or to support programs that are the primary responsibility of the public sector.
Geographic Focus: Florida; Georgia; Kansas; Rhode Island; Texas
Samples: Woodmere Art Museum (Philadelphia, PA)—for programs and exhibitions at the Helen Millard Children's Gallery, $20,000.
Date(s) Application is Due: Mar 1; Sep 1
Contact: Susan Lattner Lloyd, President, (561) 278-3781; fax: (561) 278-3167; email: lattner@bellsouth.net
Internet: http://www.lattnerfoundation.org
Sponsor: Forrest C. Lattner Foundation Inc
777 E. Atlantic Avenue, Suite 317
Delray Beach, FL 33483

Foster Foundation Grants **1524**
The Foundation funds effective, nonprofit organizations that can provide tangible benefits and ongoing support to improve the quality of life for individuals, families and communities within the Pacific Northwest. The Foundation's primary field of interests are: basic human welfare issues, education, medical research, treatment and care and cultural activities. The Foundation places special emphasis on meeting the needs of the underserved and disadvantaged segments of the population, especially children, women and seniors.
Requirements: Eligible applicants must: be a nonprofit located in or serving the populations of the Pacific Northwest; address as their mission or project intent one of the Foundation's priority issues for funding; not have any delinquent final reports due to the Foundation from previous grant cycles.
Restrictions: The Foundation will not consider requests for: direct grants, scholarships or loans for the benefit of specific individuals; projects of organizations whose policies or practices discriminate on the basis of race, ethnic origin, sex, creed or sexual orientation; contributions or program support for sectarian or religious organizations whose activities benefit only their members; or loans.
Geographic Focus: Alaska; Idaho; Montana; Oregon; Pacific Northwest; Washington
Samples: U of Washington (Seattle, WA)—to design and build a new facility for the business school, $10 million (2005).
Contact: Jill Goodsell, Grants Administrator, (206) 726-1815; fax: (206) 903-0628; email: info@thefosterfoundation.org
Internet: http://thefosterfoundation.org/Grants_Guide.asp
Sponsor: Foster Foundation
601 Union Street, Suite 3707
Seattle, WA 98101

Foster G. McGaw Prize **1525**
This prize, established by the Baxter Foundation and administered by the Hospital Research and Educational Trust, the research and development affiliate of the American Hospital Association, is awarded to a community hospital that has undertaken an identifiable program or project that improves the status or enhances the quality of life of community members, particularly the poor. The winner will receive a monetary prize; trophy; recognition at a special awards ceremony at the AHA annual meeting; and coverage in AHA News, Hospitals and Health Networks, and other health care publications. Up to three finalists will each receive a monetary prize and mention in AHA News, Hospitals and Health Networks, and other health care publications. Application and guidelines are available online.
Requirements: Nominations can be made by either the hospitals themselves or by other community organizations.
Amount of Grant: $100,000 to the winner; $10,000 to finalists
Date(s) Application is Due: Apr 8
Contact: AHA Member Relations, (312) 422-3932
Internet: http://www.aha.org/aha/awards-events/foster/application/application.html#o
Sponsor: Hospital Research and Educational Trust
1 N Franklin, 32nd Floor
Chicago, IL 60606

Foundation Fighting Blindness Marjorie Carr Adams Women's Career Development Awards **1526**
The Program's primary purpose is to support female clinical research scientists of superior dedication and talent to pursue vigorous research programs to find the cures for retinal degenerative diseases research (RDD) i.e. inherited orphan retinal degenerative diseases and dry age-related macular degeneration. The goal of this program is to facilitate advances in the laboratory and clinical research, to elucidate the mechanisms for the etiology and pathogenesis of RDDs and to develop innovative strategies to prevent, treat and cure these diseases. This award provides support for mentored study and research for clinically trained biomedical research professionals who have the potential to assume leadership roles as clinician-scientists in RDD research.
Requirements: Female clinical scientists possessing an, M.D., D.O., or recognized equivalent foreign degrees and who are in their first, second or third year of a junior faculty appointment are eligible to apply for the Adams WCDA. Applicants do not have to be U.S. citizens.
Amount of Grant: $65,000 annually; $325,000 over five years
Date(s) Application is Due: Nov 14

Contact: Cindy Settar; (410) 568-0150 or (800) 683-5555; email: csettar@Fightblindness.org or grants@Fightblindness.org
Internet: http://www.blindness.org/index.php?option=com_content&view=section&id=9&Itemid=107#career-development
Sponsor: Foundation Fighting Blindness
11435 Cronhill Drive
Owings Mills, MD 21117-2220

Foundation for a Healthy Kentucky Grants **1527**
The foundation seeks to address the unmet health care needs of the people of Kentucky through strategic grants designed to improve health status and access to care with influencing public policy as a key component for permanent change. Funding is concentrated in the following areas: health education and prevention programs focused on fitness and nutrition for children and families, youth smoking prevention, and youth substance abuse prevention; and initiatives to enhance access to health services and care for all ages, with emphasis on access to health care for low-income and the uninsured populations, access to health care for rural populations, and access to integrated mental health services. Guidelines are available online.
Requirements: Kentucky nonprofit organizations are eligible.
Restrictions: Grants do not support direct patient care, except as part of demonstration or replication projects; capital campaigns or requests for bricks and mortar (although project related equipment may be included in requests); overhead expenses except in limited amounts for specific projects; organizations that discriminate on the basis of race, gender, age, religion, national origin, sexual orientation, disability, military, or marital status in hiring; multiyear commitments; expenses related to registered legislative agents for the purpose of lobbying; endowment funds; individuals; private, for-profit entities; religious organizations for religious purposes; political causes; or retroactive expenses, deficit reduction, or forgiveness.
Contact: Susan Zepeda, Executive Director, (502) 326-2583; fax: (502) 326-5748; email: szepeda@healthyky.org
Internet: http://www.healthyky.org
Sponsor: Foundation for a Healthy Kentucky
9300 Shelbyville Road, Suite 1305
Louisville, KY 40222

Foundation for Medical Research Grants **1528**
The foundation promotes all forms of scientific medical research, in particular clinical research and that connected with the basic biological sciences directly or indirectly related to medicine. Grants are awarded to individuals and institutions in France and on an international basis. Types of support include subsidies for travel and study abroad and equipment acquisition. Major annual awards include the Rosen Prize for Cancer Research and the Delahautemaison Prize, which is awarded every two years, alternately for research in nephrology and cancer; the annual Grand Prix; and five prizes for molecular biology, endocrinology, immunology, clinical investigation, and neurobiology.
Amount of Grant: $10 million total annually
Contact: Program Contact, 33-1-44-39-75-75; fax: 33-1-44-39-75-99; email: frm@frm.org
Internet: http://www.frm.org
Sponsor: Foundation for Medical Research
54 rue de Varenne
Paris 75007 France

Foundation for Physical Therapy Mary McMillan Doctoral Scholarships **1529**
The purpose of this program is to assist physical therapists with outstanding potential for doctoral studies in the first year of graduate studies towards a doctorate.
Requirements: Applicants must be entering post professional full-time or part-time doctoral study during the current academic year. Applicants must possess a license to practice physical therapy in a U.S. jurisdiction or have met all the requirements for licensure in a U.S. jurisdiction, including having received a passing score on the licensure exam.
Samples: Mark Diehl, PT, MPT, Virginia Commonwealth, $5000 (2004); Shauna D Dudley-Javoroski, PT, MPT, U of Iowa (IA)—scholarship recipient, $5000 (2004); Jill Stewart, PT, MPT, MS, NCS, University of Southern California CA)—scholarship recipient, $5000 (2004).
Amount of Grant: $5000
Date(s) Application is Due: Aug 15
Contact: Lucy Dickson, (800) 999-2782 ext 8505; email: foundation@apta.org
Internet: http://www.apta.org/AM/Template.cfm?Section=Awards_and_Scholarships&TEMPLATE=/CM/ContentDisplay.cfm&CONTENTID=23362
Sponsor: Foundation for Physical Therapy
1055 N Fairfax Street, Suite 350
Alexandria, VA 22314

Foundation for Physical Therapy Research Grants **1530**
The foundation provides sole support or matching funds to individuals and groups of researchers to pursue scientifically based and clinically related physical therapy research, focused on studies initiated by emerging investigators. Emerging investigators are individuals who have had some previous research experience, may or may not have completed graduate or postgraduate work, or are beginning a new field of research or making strategic changes in research direction within an existing line of research. Proposed studies should add to or refine the body of theoretical, scientific, and clinical knowledge on which physical therapy practice is based, using any of a variety of recognized investigative methods such as experimental, descriptive, or correlational. Annual deadline dates may vary; contact program staff for exact dates.
Requirements: Proposals may be submitted by individuals or groups of investigators independently or through a sponsoring institution or organization with which they are affiliated. Groups must designate one member as the principal investigator responsible for directing the project. This person must be eligible for licensure as a physical therapist. Other members of the group may be physical therapists, physical therapist assistants, or persons from other fields that are relevant to the proposed study.
Amount of Grant: $40,000 maximum per year for up to two years
Date(s) Application is Due: Aug 15
Contact: Lucy Dickson, (800) 999-2782 ext 8505; email: foundation@apta.org
Internet: http://www.apta.org/AM/Template.cfm?Section=Awards_and_Scholarships&TEMPLATE=/CM/ContentDisplay.cfm&CONTENTID=23363
Sponsor: Foundation for Physical Therapy
1111 N Fairfax Street
Alexandria, VA 22314-1488

Foundation for Psychocultural Research Postdoctoral Fellowships **1531**
The foundation funds research aimed at advancing interdisciplinary research projects and scholarship at the intersection of psychology, culture, neuroscience, and psychiatry, with emphasis on psychocultural factors as central, not peripheral. The current topical focus is Interdisciplinary Approach to Post Traumatic Stress and Resilience. The research will integrate cultural and neuroscientific approaches to the study of PTSD, in its design and/or clinical application. Candidates must conduct their proposed research under a sponsor who holds an academic appointment at an accredited U.S. university or institution. The fellowship may be extended up to the maximum of three years, based on the evaluation of the previous year's performance. An institutional allowance is allotted monthly to the host institution, to be used at the sponsor's discretion to help pay for the fellow's research supplies, travel to scientific meetings, or health insurance. If a deadline falls on a weekend, applications will be accepted on Monday. Guidelines are available online.
Requirements: Applicants must have a doctoral or MD degree and should have interest in pursuing a career involving interdisciplinary research in neuroscience, culture, and psychiatry.
Amount of Grant: $40,000 stipend; $1500 per-year for supplies, travel or health insurance
Date(s) Application is Due: Feb 15
Contact: Director, email: foundationpsycul@aol.com
Internet: http://www.thefpr.org/programs_funding/applications/post_doctoral_app.html
Sponsor: Foundation for Psychocultural Research
P.O. Box 826
Pacific Palisades, CA 90272

Foundation for Science and Disability Grant Program for Physically Disabled Students in the Sciences **1532**
A grant may be awarded annually to a disabled student who is interested in obtaining a graduate degree in science, mathematics, medicine, engineering, or computer science. Selection is based on financial need, sincerity of purpose, and scholarship and/or research ability. Funds may be used for an assistive device or instrument, or as financial support to work with a professor on an individual research project, or for some other special need. The number of grants awarded each year varies depending on funds available. Application must include a 250-word essay on professional goals and objectives, as well as the specific purpose for which the grant monies will be used, and two letters of recommendation from faculty members, one of whom must be the student's academic research advisor.
Requirements: College seniors who have some physical or sensory disability and who have been accepted to graduate or professional school, as well as students already in graduate or professional schools, are eligible to apply.
Restrictions: Undergraduate students are not eligible.
Amount of Grant: $1000
Date(s) Application is Due: Dec 1
Contact: Dr. Richard Mankin, Co-Chair, Science Student Grant Committee, (352) 374-5774; fax: (352) 374-5804; email: rmankin@nervm.nerdc.ufl.edu
Internet: http://www.as.wvu.edu/~scidis/organize/fsdinfo.html
Sponsor: Foundation for Science and Disability
503 NW 89th Street
Gainesville, FL 32607

Foundation for Seacoast Health Grants **1533**
The mission of the foundation is to invest its resources to improve the health and well being of Seacoast residents. The foundation considers a very limited number of new grant initiatives which address one or more of the following prioritized health needs; access to affordable mental health services; access to preventative and restorative dental services; access to affordable child care and after school care; access to affordable primary medical care; and coordination and dissemination of health information related to identified priority needs. The deadline for the submission of the letter of intent is March 1 for Infants, Children and Adolescence and June 1 for Promoting Health and Preventing Disease. Annual deadline dates may vary; contact program staff for exact dates.
Requirements: Nonprofit organizations in cities and towns in the New Hampshire/Maine Seacoast area, including Greenland, New Castle, Newington, North Hampton, Portsmouth, and Rye, NH; and Eliot, Kittery, and York, ME, may submit applications.
Restrictions: Grants do not support ongoing general operating expenses, deficit elimination, political activities, travel, conferences, or lodging.

Geographic Focus: Maine; New Hampshire
Date(s) Application is Due: Mar 1; Jun 1
Contact: Susan Bunting, (603) 422-8200; email: ffsh@communitycampus.org
Internet: http://www.ffsh.org/grants.cfm
Sponsor: Foundation for Seacoast Health
100 Campus Drive, Suite 1
Portsmouth, NH 03801

Foundation for Spirituality and Medicine Grants 1534

The foundation awards grants to nonprofit organizations in its areas of interest, including health, health education, and religious leaders. Preference is given to requests for matching funds. Awards are made primarily in Maryland. As part of the application process, the foundation may request an oral presentation to the board.
Requirements: Nonprofit organizations whose mission is the training of professionals in the health care field, the delivery of health care, or the provision of spiritual services are eligible.
Amount of Grant: $50,000-$100,000 total
Date(s) Application is Due: Jan 15; Jul 15
Contact: Grants Administrator, (410) 938-3309
Sponsor: Foundation for Spirituality and Medicine
19 Glenbrook Drive
Phoenix, MD 21131

Foundation for the Carolinas Grants 1535

The foundation supports nonprofit organizations in North and South Carolina, especially in the greater Charlotte, NC, area. The foundation awards grants in the following program areas: education, religion, human services, the environment, historic preservation, public and civic affairs, health, the arts, youths, and senior citizens. Building Youth grants help school-age children make the transition from youth to adulthood.
Requirements: The foundation awards grants to nonprofit organizations serving the following areas in North Carolina: Cebarrus, Cleveland, Iredell, Lincoln, Mecklenburg, Richmond, Stanley, and Union Counties and the cities of Lexiington and Salisbury; and Cherokee, Lancaster, and York Counties in South Carolina.
Restrictions: Grants are not awarded for capital campaigns, operating budgets, endowments, publications, equipment, videos, or conferences, nor to individuals.
Geographic Focus: North Carolina; South Carolina
Contact: Dr. Don Jonas, Senior Vice President of Community Philanthropy, (704) 973-4500 or (800) 973-7244; fax: (704) 973-4599; email: djonas@fftc.org
Internet: http://www.fftc.org/grants
Sponsor: Foundation for the Carolinas
P.O. Box 34769
Charlotte, NC 28234-4769

Foundation for the Mid-South Grants 1536

The Foundation for the Mid South invests in people and strategies that build philanthropy and promote racial, social and economic equality in Arkansas, Louisiana, and Mississippi. The Foundation is focused on four priorities: community development; education; health and wellness; and wealth building. Types of funding include: general support; project support; and planning.
Requirements: To be eligible for grants, the applying organization or institution, as well as the purpose of the proposed project, must meet both of the following criteria: possess tax-exempt status under section 501(c)3 of the Internal Revenue Code; possess a certificate from the Mississippi Secretary of State that designates it as a public charity or exempt for the state of Mississippi. For those applying to the Foundation for the Mid South—regardless of the state where your organization is established or operates: All organizations MU.S.T register and receive a certificate that designates it as a public charity or exempt for the state of Mississippi when submitting a full proposal. The application—Form URS—to apply to the Mississippi Secretary of State is available on their website: http://www.sos.state.ms.us/forms/forms.asp?Unit=Charities. An eligible organization may submit an initial inquiry using the Grant Inquiry Form, which is available on The Foundation for the Mid South website. If the review of the initial inquiry is favorable, applicants will be contacted by the appropriate program officer to discuss the request in greater detail. Inquiries are reviewed throughout the year. Within six weeks of the Foundation's receipt of your unsolicited Grant Inquiry Form, you will receive one of the following: a request to submit a full proposal; a request for more information; a letter informing you that your project will not be supported at this time.
Restrictions: The Foundation do not award grant funds to individuals or make grants for personal needs or business assistance. Additionally, funds are not awarded for lobbying activities; ongoing general operating expenses or existing deficits; endowments,; capital costs including construction, renovation, or equipment; or international programs.
Geographic Focus: Arkansas; Louisiana; Mississippi
Contact: Denise Ellis, Grants & Technology Officer; (601) 355-8167; fax: (601) 355-6499; email: bdellis@fndmidsouth.org
Internet: http://www.fndmidsouth.org/grants_funding.htm
Sponsor: Foundation for the Mid South
134 East Amite Street
Jackson, MS 39201

Foundation Northwest Grants 1537

Grants are awarded to organizations in the Inland Northwest—eastern Washington and northern Idaho—for charitable and educational purposes in the fields of music and drama; education; civic categories which include culture, education, civic and community development; and human services. The foundation has five distinct grant programs and types of support include matching funds, special projects, seed money, and occasional operating support and capital funding. Deadlines vary according to area and contributing sponsorship; contact program support for exact dates.
Requirements: Grant applications are accepted for projects that will enrich the quality of life in the communities of eastern Washington and northern Idaho. Eligible Washington counties include Adams, Asotin, Columbia, Ferry, Garfield, Lincoln, Pend Oreille, Spokane, Steven, and Whitman. Eligible Idaho counties include Benewah, Bonner, Boundary, Clearwater, Idaho, Kootenai, Latah, Lewis, Nez Perce, and Shoshone.
Restrictions: Grants do not support endowments, debt retirement, lobbying, sectarian religious purposes, individuals, travel, sports teams and classes, projects that taxpayers or commercial interests normally support, fundraising campaigns, publications or films (unless an integral part of a foundation-supported program), or nondonor-supported research.
Geographic Focus: Idaho; Washington
Amount of Grant: $2500-$7500 average
Contact: Program Contact, (509) 624-2606; fax: (509) 624-2608; email: admin@foundationnw.org
Internet: http://www.foundationnw.org
Sponsor: Foundation Northwest
221 Wall St N, Suite 624
Spokane, WA 99201-0826

Foundation of CVPH April LaValley Fund Grants 1538

In December of 1997, Mrs. Caroline LaValley announced the creation of the April LaValley Endowment Fund. She said that it was April's wish that money which was donated to her family to assist them with expenses related to April's care should be used for other families battling cystic fibrosis. Income generated by the fund is used to help pay for transportation and lodging expenses incurred by immediate family members who travel to be with a family member receiving care for cystic fibrosis. Expenses associates with travel and lodging of family members are allowed.
Requirements: Residents of Clinton, Essex and Franklin counties in New York are eligible for consideration. The person for whom medical expenses are incurred must have a diagnosis of cystic fibrosis.
Restrictions: Funds are not intended to be used for direct medical expenditures.
Geographic Focus: New York
Contact: Roger G. Ahrens, Executive Director; (518) 562-7168 or (518) 561-2000; fax: (518) 561-0881; email: rahrens@cvph.org
Internet: http://www.cvph.org/Foundation/NamedFunds/AprilLaValleyFund/
Sponsor: Foundation of Champlain Valley Medical Center
75 Beekman Street
Plattsburgh, NY 12901

Foundation of CVPH Chelsea's Rainbow Fund Grants 1539

In December of 1999, the Kinblom family announced the creation of the Chelsea's Rainbow Fund. Their seven year old daughter, Chelsea, fought a long courageous battle against brain cancer. Friends throughout the North Country contributed to a fund to assist with expenses not covered by health insurance. The Kinblom family wishes to help other families that face similar battles against childhood cancer. Income generated by this fund will be used to help pay for transportation, food and housing expenses incurred by immediate family members who travel with a child receiving care for cancer. Expenses associates with travel and lodging of family members are allowed.
Requirements: Residents of Clinton, Essex, and Franklin counties in New York are eligible for consideration. Families that have children 18 years old and younger who are battling cancer are eligible for assistance.
Restrictions: Funds are not intended to be used for direct medical expenditures.
Geographic Focus: New York
Contact: Roger G. Ahrens, Executive Director; (518) 562-7168 or (518) 561-2000; fax: (518) 561-0881; email: rahrens@cvph.org
Internet: http://www.cvph.org/Foundation/NamedFunds/ChelseasRainbow/
Sponsor: Foundation of Champlain Valley Medical Center
75 Beekman Street
Plattsburgh, NY 12901

Foundation of CVPH Melissa Lahtinen-Penfield Organ Donor Fund Grants 1540

The Fund was created in memory of Melissa Lahtinen-Penfield, whose wish was to assist families with expenses related to organ donation and educate the community of its vital importance. In July 2000, William Santa and members of the Hometown WIRY team, established the annual Melissa Lahtinen-Penfield (MLP) Organ Donor Golf Tournament in her memory. Proceeds of the tournament, together with donations made directly to the fund, are used to promote organ donation awareness and defray those costs associated with organ transplants which are not covered by health insurance. Expenses considered for reimbursement include medical expenses not covered by insurance, travel and lodging expenses, and meals not including alcohol. Financial need will be the primary determinant upon which the application will be weighed. The size of grants is limited to the income generated by the fund.
Requirements: Residents of Clinton County, New York, are eligible to receive consideration for grants of up to $2,500/annually for expenses associated with organ transplants not covered by health insurance.
Restrictions: Funds are not intended to be used for direct medical expenditures.
Geographic Focus: New York
Amount of Grant: $2,500 maximum
Contact: Roger G. Ahrens, Executive Director; (518) 562-7168 or (518) 561-2000; fax: (518) 561-0881; email: rahrens@cvph.org

Internet: http://www.cvph.org/Foundation/NamedFunds/OrganDonor/
Sponsor: Foundation of Champlain Valley Medical Center
75 Beekman Street
Plattsburgh, NY 12901

Foundation of CVPH Rabin Fund Grants 1541

In December of 2000, Pearlie and Mark Rabin established a fund to assist patients with fundamentals of care at CVPH Medical Center. With a gift which endowed the fund, they outlined their wish to offer patients who experience financial hardship, services such as essential articles of clothing and other inexpensive incidentals, which might make their stay in the hospital more pleasant. Throughout the year, CVPH staff takes care of patients who are not able to afford these types of items. In the past, staff members pooled their personal resources and purchased the item or the patient managed without it. The Rabin's Fund provides about $3,500 annually, which assists friends and neighbors from throughout the North Country.
Requirements: Residents of Clinton, Essex, and Franklin counties in New York are eligible for consideration.
Restrictions: Funds are not intended to be used for direct medical expenditures.
Geographic Focus: New York
Contact: Roger G. Ahrens, Executive Director; (518) 562-7168 or (518) 561-2000; fax: (518) 561-0881; email: rahrens@cvph.org
Internet: http://www.cvph.org/Foundation/NamedFunds/RabinFund/
Sponsor: Foundation of Champlain Valley Medical Center
75 Beekman Street
Plattsburgh, NY 12901

Foundation of CVPH Roger Senecal Endowment Fund Grants 1542

The Roger Senecal Endowment Fund exists because of the North Country's love for children, particularly when a child is in need. Income generated by the fund is used to help pay for transportation and housing expenses incurred by an ill or injured child's family in order to be near the child when vital care is being given. Applications will be evaluated and approved by a committee appointed by the Foundation of CVPH Medical Center. Financial need is the primary determinant upon which application will be weighed. The size of the grants is limited to the income generated by the endowment fund on a quarterly basis.
Requirements: Residents of Clinton, Essex, and Franklin counties in New York are eligible for consideration. The person for whom medical expenses are incurred must be 19 years of age or younger.
Restrictions: Funds are not intended to be used for direct medical expenditures.
Geographic Focus: New York
Contact: Roger G. Ahrens, Executive Director; (518) 562-7168 or (518) 561-2000; fax: (518) 561-0881; email: rahrens@cvph.org
Internet: http://www.cvph.org/Foundation/NamedFunds/RogerSenecal/
Sponsor: Foundation of Champlain Valley Medical Center
75 Beekman Street
Plattsburgh, NY 12901

Foundation of CVPH Travel Fund Grants 1543

In 2001, the Board of Directors of the Foundation decided to provide funding for adults who need to travel outside the community to receive health care. The fund provides reimbursement for travel, food and lodging expenses. In many ways, it mimics the Roger Senecal Endowment Fund established in the mid 1980s to assist the families of children who need to leave the North Country to receive health care.
Requirements: Residents of Clinton, Essex, and Franklin counties in New York are eligible for consideration. The person for whom medical expenses are incurred must be 19 years of age or older.
Restrictions: Only one adult may apply for travel funds in addition to the patient. The fund will not provide funds for children to travel. No health care expenses, medications or medical equipment will be funded. Maximum income for the family is limited to $45,000.
Geographic Focus: New York
Amount of Grant: $1,000 maximum per year
Contact: Roger G. Ahrens, Executive Director; (518) 562-7168 or (518) 561-2000; fax: (518) 561-0881; email: rahrens@cvph.org
Internet: http://www.cvph.org/Foundation/NamedFunds/TravelFund/
Sponsor: Foundation of Champlain Valley Medical Center
75 Beekman Street
Plattsburgh, NY 12901

Fourjay Foundation Grants 1544

The Foundation supports only those organizations whose chief purpose is to improve health and/or promote education, within Philadelphia, Montgomery, and Bucks counties in southeastern Pennsylvania. The Fourjay Foundation requires no specific application form. It will consider proposals that address a well-defined need, offer a concrete plan of action, and request a specific amount, from organizations whose staff has the ingenuity, commitment, and motivation to carry out the proposal's objectives. Requests may be for operating support, project specific funds, or capital funds.
Requirements: Organizations serving Philadelphia, Montgomery, and Bucks Counties in southeastern Pennsylvania are eligible.
Restrictions: Funding is not available for: charities operating outside Montgomery, Bucks, or Philadelphia counties; individuals; elementary or secondary educational institutions; museums, musical groups, theaters, or cultural organizations; religious organizations in support of their sacramental or theological functions; political groups or related think tanks; athletic organizations or alumni associations; libraries; public radio or television; United Way or the YMCA; civic organizations; organizations that have applied or been funded within the last 12 month period.
Geographic Focus: Pennsylvania
Amount of Grant: $1,000-$10,000 range
Date(s) Application is Due: Mar 1; Jun 1; Sep 1; Dec 1
Contact: Ann T. Bucci, Grant Coordinator; (215) 830-1437; fax: (215) 830-0157; email: abucci@fourjay.org
Internet: http://www.fourjay.org/grantGuidelines.asp
Sponsor: Fourjay Foundation
2300 Computer Avenue, Building G, Suite 1
Willow Grove, PA 19090-1753

Fragile X Syndrome Postdoctoral Research Fellowships Program 1545

The purpose of this program is to promote research aimed at finding a specific treatment for fragile X syndrome, the primary inherited cause of mental retardation. The foundation is particularly interested in preclinical studies of potential pharmacological and genetic treatments for fragile X and studies aimed at understanding the function of the FMR1 gene. The goal is to bring practical treatment into current medical practice as quickly as possible; therefore, preference will be given to research projects that have a clear practical application and the results of which will be shared with other qualified researchers in a timely fashion. Fellowships are awarded for one year and may be renewed for a second.
Requirements: Tax-exempt 501(c)3 institutions are eligible for funding. Individuals are nominated by applicant institutions for the fellowships and should have training and experience at least equal to the PhD or MD level.
Amount of Grant: $40,000 maximum
Date(s) Application is Due: May 1; Dec 1
Contact: Katie Clapp, (978) 462-1866; fax: (978) 463-9985; email: kclappFRAXA@comcast.net
Internet: http://www.fraxa.org/research_howtoapply.aspx
Sponsor: FRAXA Research Foundation
45 Pleasant Street, 2nd Floor
Newburyport, MA 01950

Frances and John L. Loeb Family Fund Grants 1546

The fund is committed to improving the quality of American life. To that end, its grant-making program seeks to address significant issues of society. The fund has chosen as its initial priorities the fields of education, health and family planning, including the public policy questions relating to them. In making grants, the fund favors proposals that offer new knowledge of and innovative approaches to problems rather than palliative measures. It also prefers applications that call for challenge grants and provide evaluation of results. There is no formal application form. Interested applicants should submit a preliminary request in letter form.
Requirements: Funding is directed primarily to organizations and institutions operating in the New York City metropolitan area that are tax exempt under the provisions of Section 501(c)3 of the Internal Revenue Code. Exceptions to this geographical limitation will be made for proposals that have the promise of national implication or extensive replication.
Restrictions: The fund will not consider proposals for annual or capital campaigns, building or renovation projects or loan or emergency funds. Neither will it make grants to individuals or for sectarian or religious purposes or political activities such as lobbying or propaganda. It will not fund any organization that discriminates on the basis of race, sex, religion, national origin or sexual preference.
Contact: John L. Loeb, Jr., President and Treasurer; (212) 588-9052; fax: (212) 838-6470; email: loebff@aol.com
Internet: http://www.geocities.com/CapitolHill/5601/family_fund_brochure.html
Sponsor: Frances and John L. Loeb Family Fund
375 Park Avenue, Suite 801
New York, NY 10152

Frances L. and Edwin L. Cummings Memorial Fund Grants 1547

The foundation supports nonprofits in New York City and northern New Jersey in the areas of education, especially programs that serve public school children from disadvantaged backgrounds; social welfare concerns; and campaigns to build endowments through establishment of challenge grants. Other areas of interest include elementary education, secondary education, vocational education, adult basic education and literacy, and higher education; hospitals, medical care, AIDS, and cancer; children, youth, and human services; and community development. Support is provided for endowment funds, seed money, consulting services, matching funds, technical assistance, professorships, and program development. The board meets in June and December. Application forms are not required.
Requirements: Grants are awarded to nonprofit organizations in the metropolitan New York, NY, area, with emphasis on New York City, southern Westchester County, and northern New Jersey.
Restrictions: Grants are not awarded to individuals or for capital building campaigns, general operating support, moving expenses, conferences, surveys, annual fund-raising campaigns, or research conducted by individuals or private institutions.
Geographic Focus: New Jersey; New York
Samples: Little Sisters of the Assumption Family Health Service (New York, NY)—to establish an endowment fund, $100,000.; Neighborhood Initiatives (Bronx, NY)—for staff support to expand a teen center program, $30,000.; Korean Community Service of Metropolitan New York (Woodside, NY)—to support a health educator and outreach worker for an HIV/AIDS prevention and education program, $40,000.

Amount of Grant: $10,000
Contact: Elizabeth Costas, Director, (212) 286-1778; fax: (212) 682-9458
Sponsor: Frances L. and Edwin L. Cummings Memorial Fund
501 Fifth Avenue, Suite 708
New York, NY 10017-6103

Frances W. Emerson Foundation Grants 1548

The Foundation, in the care of Goldman Tax Service of Bellingham, Massachusetts, offers grants throughout Massachusetts and Vinalhaven, Maine. Its primary fields of interest include community development, economic development, education, and health care. There is no application form required or deadlines to adhere to, and applicants should send a letter or the full proposal to Eaton Vance management in Boston.
Geographic Focus: Maine; Massachusetts
Contact: Thomas Huggins, Vice President; Eaton Vance Management; (617) 482-8260;; Donald M. Harding, Treasurer; c/o Goldman Tax Service; (508) 966-4020
Sponsor: Frances W. Emerson Foundation
255 State Street
Boston, MA 02109

Francis L. Abreu Charitable Trust Grants 1549

The trust supports Atlanta-area nonprofit organizations in its areas of interest, including arts and cultural programs, secondary education, higher education, health associations, human services, and children and youth services. Types of support include capital campaigns, seed money, program development, and matching funds. Requests are reviewed at April and October trustee meetings.
Requirements: Georgia nonprofits serving the greater Atlanta area are eligible.
Restrictions: The foundation does not approve requests for operating or grants to individuals.
Geographic Focus: Georgia
Date(s) Application is Due: Mar 31; Sep 30
Contact: Peter Abreu, (770) 649-7381
Internet: http://www.abreufoundation.org
Sponsor: Francis L. Abreu Charitable Trust
P.O. Box 502407
Atlanta, GA 31150

Francis T. & Louise T. Nichols Foundation Grants 1550

The Foundation gives primarily in the areas of education, health care, and human services. Its major fields of interest include: children and youth services; distaster relief; fire prevention and control; elementary and secondary education programs; health care; hospital support; and human/community service programs. There are no deadlines.
Requirements: Applicants should approach the Foundation initially by letter.
Restrictions: Giving primarily in Hancock County, Maine. There are no grants made to individuals.
Geographic Focus: Maine
Amount of Grant: $80,000 maximum
Contact: Calvin E. True, Treasurer, (207) 947-0111
Sponsor: Francis T. & Louise T. Nichols Foundation
P.O. Box 1210
Bangor, ME 04402-1210

Frank E. and Seba B. Payne Foundation Grants 1551

The foundation awards grants in the Chicago, IL, area and in Pennsylvania in its areas of interest, including AIDS prevention, children and youth, cultural activities, education, and hospitals. Types of support include building construction/renovation, equipment acquisition, and general operating support.
Requirements: Nonprofit organizations in the greater Chicago, IL, metropolitan area and in Pennsylvania are eligible.
Restrictions: Grants are not made to individuals.
Geographic Focus: Illinois; Pennsylvania
Contact: M. Catherine Ryan, c/o Bank of America, (312) 828-1785
Sponsor: Frank E. Payne and Seba B. Payne Foundation
231 South LaSalle Street
Chicago, IL 60697

Frank G. and Freida K. Brotz Family Foundation Grants 1552

The Foundation supports Wisconsin nonprofits of the Christian, Lutheran, and Roman Catholic faiths, including Salvation Army. Types of support include capital support and general support. Organizations receiving support include colleges and universities, community service groups, hospitals, ministries, parochial schools and religious education organizations, religious welfare organizations, and youth organizations. There are no application deadlines. Applicants should submit a brief letter of inquiry that contains a description of the organization, its purpose, purpose of grant, and proof of tax-exempt status.
Requirements: Grants are awarded to publicly supported, Sec. 170(c) IRC qualified organizations, primarily in the State of Wisconsin.
Restrictions: No grants are awarded to individuals or organizations that require expenditure responsibility under Treasury Regulations.
Geographic Focus: Wisconsin
Contact: Stuart W. Brotz, Grants Committee; (920) 458-2121; fax: (920) 458-1923
Sponsor: Frank G. and Freida K. Brotz Family Foundation
3518 Lakeshore Road, P.O. Box 551
Sheboygan, WI 53082-0551

Frank Stanley Beveridge Foundation Grants 1553

The foundation welcomes proposals in the areas of: animal care; arts, culture and humanities; civil rights, social action, advocacy; education; employment/jobs; environmental quality, protection and beautification; food, nutrition and agriculture; health; housing; human services; medical research; mental health; philanthropy; safety; recreation; religion; science; social services; and youth development. The board meets in October and April to consider requests. Multiyear grants are rare. Contact the foundation via the Web site only. No phone or written inquiries will be accepted.
Requirements: Applicants must be 501(c)3 nonprofit organizations or foundations in Massachusetts's Hampden and Hampshire Counties.
Restrictions: The Foundation prefers not to support: awards or prizes; commissioning of new artistic work; conferences/seminars; curriculum development; debt reduction; employee matching gifts; employee-related scholarships; endowment funds; exhibitions; faculty/staff development; fellowship funds; fellowships to individuals; film/video/radio production; foundation administered programs; general operating support; grants to individuals; income development; internship funds; management development; performance/production costs; professorships; program-related investment/loans; publications; scholarships to individuals; student aid; technical assistance.
Geographic Focus: Massachusetts
Amount of Grant: $50,000
Date(s) Application is Due: Feb 1; Aug 1
Contact: Philip Caswell, President; (800) 229-9667; fax: (561) 748-0644; email: administrator@beveridge.org or caswell@beveridge.org
Internet: http://www.beveridge.org/
Sponsor: Frank Stanley Beveridge Foundation
1340 U.S. Highway 1, Suite 102
Jupiter, FL 33469

Franklin County Community Foundation Grants 1554

The foundation was established in 1998 in Indiana. The Franklin County Foundation seeks to build permanent partnerships in giving that effectively connect donors and community projects to promote an enriched future for all citizens of Franklin County, Indiana. The Foundation also administers separate scholarship funds established by individuals, families, corporations, and organizations to assist local students in pursuit of advanced education. Together, these scholarships make up our Community Scholarship Program. Eligibility, criteria, and supplemental requirements are different for each scholarship. To apply for one these scholarships contact the Foundation's office.
Geographic Focus: Indiana
Contact: Shelly Lunsford, Director; (765) 647-6810; fax: (765) 647-0238; email: fcfoundation@yahoo.com
Internet: http://www.franklincountyindiana.info/2005%20Grants.htm
Sponsor: Franklin County Community Foundation, Inc.
527 Main Street
Brookville, IN 47012-1284

Fraser-Parker Foundation Grants 1555

The foundation awards general operating grants in its areas of interest, including Christian religion organizations, education and higher education, and hospitals. There are no application forms.
Geographic Focus: Georgia
Amount of Grant: $5000-$50,000 average
Date(s) Application is Due: Apr 15; Oct 15
Contact: John Stephenson, Executive Director, (404) 658-9066
Sponsor: Fraser-Parker Foundation
50 Hurt Plz, Suite 850
Atlanta, GA 30303

Fred Baldwin Memorial Foundation Grants 1556

The Foundation supports programs and projects that benefit the people of Maui County. Projects in the arts, education, environment, health, and human services are of greatest interest. Funding is available for capital improvement projects. There are two annual deadlines, which fall on the first business day in February and August. Application information is available online.
Requirements: Eligible applicants must have 501(c)3 status, or must apply through a fiscal sponsor with 501(c)3 status.
Restrictions: The Foundation does not fund loans or debt service, endowments, funds for re-granting, scholarships, grants to individuals or units of government, or activities that have already occurred.
Geographic Focus: Hawaii
Amount of Grant: $10,000
Date(s) Application is Due: Feb 1; Aug 1
Contact: Carrie Shoda-Sutherland, Senior Program Officer; (808) 566-5524 or (888) 731-3863, ext. 524; email: csutherland@hcf-hawaii.org;; Christel Wuerfel, Philanthropic Services Assistant; (808) 566-5524 or (888) 731-3863; email: cwuerfel@hcf-hawaii.org
Internet: http://www.fredbaldwinfoundation.org/
Sponsor: Fred Baldwin Memorial Foundation
1164 Bishop Street, Suite 800
Honolulu, HI 96813

Fred L. Emerson Foundation Grants 1557

The foundation gives grants to nonprofits in Auburn, Cayuga County, and upstate New York to improve the quality of life in the areas of education (primarily private, higher education), hospital and health programs, community agencies, churches, cultural

institutions, youth and community service programs and social welfare agencies. An application form is not required. Proposals may be submitted in letter form detailing the project for which support is being sought.
Requirements: New York nonprofit organizations in Auburn, Cayuga County, and the upstate area are eligible.
Restrictions: Grants do not support individuals, operating budgets, or loans.
Geographic Focus: New York
Amount of Grant: $200-$250,000
Contact: Daniel J. Fessenden, Executive Director; (315) 253-9621; email: dan@emersonfoundation.com
Sponsor: Fred L. Emerson Foundation
5654 South Street Road, P.O. Box 276
Auburn, NY 13021-9602

Freddie Mac Foundation Grants **1558**
The Foundation focus is on children whose families have limited resources and who are vulnerable to poor outcomes. The Foundation emphasizes the integration of services that focus on family strengthening and youth development in order to maximize the benefit to children and their families. Grants will be made for direct service projects, general operating support, capacity building, public awareness, planning and capital projects. The following funding priorities will be considered: the early years; elementary school years; junior high and high school years; children and families in crisis; and public awareness education. Proposals must be submitted online.
Requirements: Eligible organizations must be tax exempt under IRS code 501(c)3 and defined as a public charity. The Foundation's grantmaking program services the following metropolitan Washington, DC areas: District of Columbia; Virginia - the counties of Arlington, Fairfax, Loudoun and Prince William and the cities of Alexandria, Falls Church, Manassas Park, and Leesburg; Maryland - the counties of Charles, Frederick, Howard, Montgomery, and Prince George's.
Restrictions: The Foundation will not fund organizations that discriminate in the provision of services or in employment practices based on race, color, religion, ethnicity, sex, age, national origin, disability, sexual orientation, marital status, and any other characteristics protected by applicable law. Unless approved by the board, the Foundation does not fund: individuals; training in/promotion of religious doctrine; incurring a debt liability; endowment campaigns.
Geographic Focus: District of Columbia; Maryland; Virginia
Samples: Distributed among nonprofit organizations to aid support-relief efforts following Hurricane Katrina, $10 million (2005); CrossChildren's Law Ctr (Washington, DC)—to support the caregivers of children in the Washington, DC, foster-care system who are seeking adoption and guardianship, $90,000 (2005); Ctr for Multicultural Human Services (Falls Church, VA)—to acquire five transitional-housing units that will provide 16 homeless families in northern Virginia, many of whom are recent immigrants, with safe housing and intensive support services, $550,000 (2005); American National Red Cross (Washington, DC)—to assist tsunami-relief efforts, $150,000 (2005).
Amount of Grant: $5,000-$50,000
Date(s) Application is Due: Sep 9
Contact: Ralph F. Boyd, Jr., President and CEO; (703) 918-8888; email: freddie_mac_foundation@freddiemac.com
Internet: http://www.freddiemacfoundation.org
Sponsor: Freddie Mac Foundation
8250 Jones Branch Drive, MS A40
McLean, VA 22102-3110

Frederic Stanley Kipping Award in Silicon Chemistry **1559**
This award, supported by Dow Corning Corporation, is given biennially in even-numbered years to recognize distinguished achievement in research in silicon chemistry and to stimulate the creativity of others toward further advancement of this field of chemistry. A nominee must have accomplished distinguished achievement in research in silicon chemistry during the preceding 10 years. The measure of this achievement should focus primarily on the nominee's significant publications in the field of silicon chemistry but may include consideration of contributions to the related field of organometallic chemistry. There are no limits on age or nationality. Applications are accepted in odd-numbered years. The award consists of $5,000 and a certificate.
Requirements: Any individual, except a member of the award committee, may submit one nomination or seconding letter for the award in any given year. Nominating documents consist of a letter of not more than 1000 words containing an evaluation of the nominee's accomplishments and a specific identification of the work to be recognized, a biographical sketch including date of birth, and a list of publications and patents authored by the nominee.
Restrictions: Self-nominations are not accepted.
Samples: T. Don Tilley—award winner, $5,000 (2008); Akira Sekiguchi—award winner, $5,000 (2006); James E. Mark—award winner, $5,000 (2004).
Amount of Grant: $5,000 and allowance for travel expenses to award meeting
Date(s) Application is Due: Nov 1
Contact: Felicia Dixon, Awards Administrator; (800) 227-5558 or (202) 872-4408; fax: (202) 776-8008; email: f_dixon@acs.org or awards@acs.org
Internet: http://portal.acs.org/portal/acs/corg/content?_nfpb=true&_pageLabel=PP_ARTICLEMAIN&node_id=1319&content_id=CTP_004523&use_sec=true&sec_url_var=region1
Sponsor: American Chemical Society
1155 Sixteenth Street, NW
Washington, DC 20036

Frederick Gardner Cottrell Foundation Grants **1560**
Giving primarily in Woods Hole, Massachusetts, Hunt Valley, Maryland, Brunswick, Maine, and Houston, Texas. The foundation awards grants to educational and scientific organizations to advance research and chair teaching positions. The foundation's areas of interest include eye research, higher education, marine science, and science. There are no application deadline. Submit a written request for application.
Geographic Focus: Maine; Maryland; Massachusetts; Texas
Amount of Grant: $100,000-$300,000 average
Contact: Gary Munsinger, President; (520) 748-4400; fax: (520) 748-0025; email: munsinger@rctech.com
Sponsor: Frederick Gardner Cottrell Foundation
5210 East Williams Circle, Suite 240
Tucson, AZ 85711-4410

Fremont Area Community Foundation Grants **1561**
The community foundation welcomes grant requests for projects that benefit the residents of Newaygo County, MI, by providing opportunities in the areas of education, community health, human services, arts and culture, the environment, and community development. The Foundation's grantmakiing principals are: to build on prior investments; to respond to community and identify priorities; to focus resources and increase impact; and to remain consistent with our mission, values, and capacities. Grant application forms are available online.
Requirements: Michigan 501(c)3 organizations in Newaygo County are eligible.
Restrictions: The foundation typically does not fund requests for projects that have previously been denied, grants to individuals, programs that advocate specific religions, or services which are government or school obligations.
Geographic Focus: Michigan
Samples: Arts Center for Newaygo County, Fremont, MI, For community contributions for construction of Dogwood Center for the Performing Arts, $943,773.; Grand Rapids Symphony Society (Grand Rapids, MI)—for performances at schools in Newaygo County, $10,000.; Newaygo County Sheriffs Department (White Cloud, MI)—for staff support of a team to respond to domestic-violence calls, $15,437.
Amount of Grant: $9 million total
Date(s) Application is Due: Feb 15; May 15; Sep 15
Contact: Jeff Jahr, Senior Program Officer, (231) 924-5350; fax: (231) 924-5391; email: jjahr@tfacf.org
Internet: http://www.tfaf.org/grants.html
Sponsor: Fremont Area Community Foundation
P.O. Box B
Fremont, MI 49412

Frey Foundation Grants **1562**
The foundation is committed to excellence and accountability in its role as a catalyst for productive social change and makes grants to nonprofit organizations based in and serving residents of Kent, Emmet, and Charlevoix Counties in Michigan. Primary areas of interest include enhancing the lives of children and families, protecting natural resources, encouraging civic progress, nurturing community art, capital projects, and philanthropy. Community-based projects receive priority consideration. Types of support include program development, seed money, technical assistance, program evaluation, and employee matching gifts. Send a one- to two-page letter of inquiry. Requests for less than $30,000 are reviewed monthly; requests over $30,000 must be approved by the board. Guidelines are available online.
Requirements: Nonprofit organizations based in and serving residents of Kent, Emmet, and Charlevoix Counties in Michigan are eligible.
Restrictions: Individuals are not eligible to apply.
Geographic Focus: Michigan
Samples: Nature Conservancy, Michigan Chapter (Lansing, MI)—for the Northern Great Lakes Project, which will protect 271,000 acres across eight counties in Michigan's Upper Peninsula and link more than 2.5 million acres of protected federal, state, and natural areas, $1 million (2005).
Date(s) Application is Due: Feb 15; May 15; Aug 15; Nov 15
Contact: Teresa Crawford, Grants Manager, (616) 451-4565; fax: (616) 451-8481; email: freyfdn@freyfdn.org
Internet: http://www.freyfdn.org
Sponsor: Frey Foundation
40 Pearl St NW, Suite 1100
Grand Rapids, MI 49503

Frist Foundation Grants **1563**
The foundation supports a variety of organizations in the fields of health, human services, civic affairs, education, and the arts. Grants support building the capacity of nonprofit organizations by strengthening their management structure and systems. Types of support include capital, management, operating, project, and technology grants. Deadline listed is for technology grants.
Requirements: 501(c)3 nonprofits in Davidson County, TN, area may apply.
Restrictions: The foundation does not support: individuals or their projects, private foundations, political activities, or advertising or sponsorships. The foundation does not ordinarily support: projects, programs, or organizations that serve a limited audience or a relatively small number of people; organizations during their first three years of operation; disease-specific organizations seeking support for national projects and programs; biomedical or clinical research; hospitals; organizations whose principal impact is outside of Middle Tennessee; endowments; social events or similar fund-raising activities; or religious organizations for religious purposes.

Geographic Focus: Tennessee
Samples: Domestic Violence Intervention Ctr (TN)—to translate domestic violence educational materials into Spanish, $3000.; Mockingbird Theatre (TN)—for general support, $5000.; Metropolitan Nashville Public Schools (TN)—to establish a pilot reading program at Haywood Elementary School, $65,000.; Faith Family Medical Clinic of Nashville (TN)—to help establish a medical clinic for low-income working people, $105,000.
Amount of Grant: $6.5 million total; $500-$10,000 average
Date(s) Application is Due: Apr 1
Contact: Peter Bird, (615) 292-3868; fax: (615) 292-5843; email: askfrist@fristfoundation.org
Internet: http://www.fristfoundation.org/grants/general.asp
Sponsor: Frist Foundation
3100 W End Avenue, Suite 1200
Nashville, TN 37203

Fritz B. Burns Foundation Grants **1564**
The foundation supports nonprofit organizations primarily in southern California by awarding grants for education, with an emphasis on buildings, equipment, endowments (except for ordinary operating expenses), student scholarship and loan funds, and faculty fellowships; to/for hospitals, hospital equipment, and medical research; and religious organizations (Christian, Jewish, Latter-day Saints, nondenominational, Presbyterian, Protestant, Roman Catholic, and Salvation Army). Proposals should be concise, containing a brief description of what is planned, with a clear statement of the objective sought; IRS letter certifying tax exemption; financial statements; and a list of officers and directors. No formalized application or proposal format is required. Proposals are considered on a quarterly basis.
Requirements: Nonprofit, tax-exempt organizations in southern California may apply.
Restrictions: Requests are not considered from individuals or tax-supported entities.
Geographic Focus: California
Samples: Brigham Young University, Provo, UT, $1,025,000 (2008); Valley Presbyterian Hospital, Van Nuys, CA, $250,000 (2008); Little Sisters of the Poor, Los Angeles, CA, $150,000 (2008).
Amount of Grant: $10,000-$250,000 range
Date(s) Application is Due: Sep 30
Contact: Joseph Rawlinson, President, (818) 840-8802
Sponsor: Fritz B. Burns Foundation
4001 West Alameda Avenue, Suite 203
Burbank, CA 91505-4338

Fuji Film Grants **1565**
Grants are awarded to proposals that have relevance to Fujifilm's strategic interests which are: environment; education; arts and culture and health and human services. Organizations are limited to one grant per calendar year. Applications are reviewed monthly and applicants should anticipate an award or decline within six to eight weeks after submitting a request.
Requirements: 501(c)3 tax-exempt organizations are eligible. Organizations must serve or be located within the communities where Fujifilm is a member. Preference is given to those proposals that have relevance to the company's strategic interests.
Restrictions: The program does not fund: individuals or personal use; political organizations, causes, candidates or campaigns; legislative advocacy groups; religious groups; military agencies; fraternal, veterans or social organizations.
Samples: Sea World and Busch Gardens Conservation Fund (Clayton, MO)—for the Environmental Excellence Awards program, $125,000 (2003); Westchester Community College (Valhalla, NY) and Rhode Island School of Design (Providence, RI)—for scholarships, $25,000 and $50,000, respectively (2003).
Amount of Grant: $1000-$5000
Contact: Corporate Contributions, (800) 755-3854; email: contributions@fujifilm.com
Internet: http://www.fujifilm.com/JSP/fuji/epartners/givingGuidelines.jsp?nav=2
Sponsor: Fuji Photo Film U.S.A
200 Summit Lake Drive, Floor 2
Valhalla, NY 10595

Fulbright Alumni Initiatives Awards Program Grants **1566**
The objective of the AIA program is to help translate the individual Fulbright experience into long-term institutional impact. To this end, the program provides small institutional grants to Fulbright alumni to develop innovative projects that will foster institutionally supported linkages and sustainable, mutually beneficial relationships between the Fulbright scholar's home and host institutions. Just about any activity resulting in the creation or fostering of a sustainable institutional relationship that will have an impact on both the Fulbright alum's home institution and the Fulbright host institution abroad and which both institutions are prepared to support in both the long and short terms will be considered. The program has been temporarily suspended, and applicants should check back for updates.
Requirements: Applicants must be U.S. citizens. The program is open to eligible alumni whose grants occurred at any time from the 1998/1999 academic year through the present academic year.
Restrictions: This program is limited to application by a Fulbright alum (whether U.S. or Visiting Scholar) in partnership with his/her host institution colleague. However, other faculty members from both applicants' institutions may be part of the proposal and participate in the project.
Contact: Stacey Bustillos; (202) 686-6252; email: sbustillos@cies.iie.org;; Hajra Zahid, Senior Program Associate; (202) 686-6250; email: hzahid@cies.iie.org
Internet: http://www.cies.org/aia/
Sponsor: Council for International Exchange of Scholars
3007 Tilden Street, NW, Suite 5L
Washington, DC 20008-3009

Fulbright Distinguished Chairs Program Grants **1567**
The Fulbright Distinguished Chairs Program comprises approximately forty distinguished lecturing, distinguished research and distinguished lecturing/research awards ranging from three to 12 months. Awards in the Fulbright Distinguished Chairs Program are viewed as among the most prestigious appointments in the Fulbright Scholar Program. Candidates should be senior scholars and have a significant publication and teaching record. Applicants should submit hard copies of the Distinguished Chairs Application Form (one page), a letter of interest (about three pages), a curriculum vitae (maximum eight pages) and, if required, a sample syllabus (maximum four pages). Chairs are available in Australia, Austria, Brazil, Canada, Denmark, Finland, France, Germany, Hungary, Ireland, Israel, Italy, Netherlands, Poland, Portugal, Russia, and Sweden. Because an objective of the Fulbright Program is to provide an educational exchange experience for those not previously afforded such an opportunity, preference will usually be given to candidates who have not had substantial recent experience in the country to which they are applying.
Requirements: Applicants must meet all of the following eligibility requirements: U.S. citizenship at the time of application (permanent resident status is not sufficient); possess a Ph.D. or equivalent professional terminal degree at the time of application (for professionals and artists outside academe, recognized professional standing and substantial professional accomplishments); have college or university teaching experience at the level and in the field of the proposed lecturing activity as specified in the award description (for Distinguished Chairs awards, candidates should be senior scholars with a significant publication and teaching record); have foreign language proficiency only if specified in the award description or required for the completion of the proposed project; be of sound physical and mental health; and disclose prior conviction or current indictment for commission of a felony.
Restrictions: Previous Fulbright scholar grantees are eligible to apply only if five years will have elapsed between the ending date of one scholar award and the beginning date of the new scholar award. This rule does not apply if the previous grant was for less than two months. Employees, spouses or dependent children of the United States Department of State or public and private organizations under contract to the United States Department of State are ineligible to apply for a Fulbright grant until one year after the employee's termination.
Date(s) Application is Due: Aug 3
Contact: Maria Bettua; (202) 686-6245; email: mbettua@cies.iie.org;; Abby Greenwell; (202) 686-6232; email: agreenwell@cies.iie.org
Internet: http://www.cies.org/Chairs/
Sponsor: Council for International Exchange of Scholars
3007 Tilden Street, NW, Suite 5L
Washington, DC 20008-3009

Fulbright German Studies Seminar Grants **1568**
The program allows participation in a group seminar on current German society and culture. The program will begin in Berlin and include visits to other cities in Germany. The focus will be on the formation of policies in current issues at the core of modern society such as climate change, food technology, gene technology, stem cell research and the broad scope of education. The seminar will explore how Germany and its European neighbors view the role of science in their societies, examining the factors that result in differing approaches to these issues and the challenges of harmonizing different standards under a uniform EU-policy umbrella. With an eye to the global marketplace and worldwide competition in science, the seminar will further examine the multiple interests which structure relations between national governments, economic corporations, political and supranational bodies as well as research and development institutions. Scholars from U.S. universities, colleges, and community colleges who hold full-time teaching appointments and meet other academic requirements (Ph.D., Ph.D. candidacy or other equivalent degree or qualifications) are eligible. The seminar lasts two weeks, typically during the month of June.
Requirements: Applicants must be U.S. citizens with permanent residence in the United States at the time of application.
Date(s) Application is Due: Nov 1
Contact: Maria Bettua, Assistant Director; (202) 686-6245; email: mbettua@cies.iie.org;; Abby Greenwell; (202) 686-6232; email: agreenwell@cies.iie.org
Internet: http://www.iie.org/cies/us_scholars/us_awards/GSS/index.html
Sponsor: Council for International Exchange of Scholars
3007 Tilden Street, NW, Suite 5L
Washington, DC 20008-3009

Fulbright International Education Administrators Seminar Program Grants **1569**
The IEA seminars are designed to introduce participants to the society, culture and higher education systems of these countries through campus visits, meetings with foreign colleagues and government officials, attendance at cultural events and briefings on education. Participants in the International Education Administrators Program gain a firsthand look into the host country's academic infrastructure and culture. They gain new perspective on the need to internationalize U.S. campuses and insight into how it can be done. The deadline for the German program is February 1, while the deadline for both Japan and Korea is November 1.
Requirements: To be eligible, applicants must: be U.S. citizens; be international education professionals and senior university administrators (e.g., deans, provosts, vice presidents)

with significant responsibility for international programs and activities; have an affiliation with an accredited college or university or nonprofit international exchange organization administering postsecondary student or faculty exchange; and have a minimum of three years of work experience in international education. Applicants for the Japan program must be affiliated with a four-year college or university, while Germany and Korea will consider applicants from both two- and four-year institutions.
Restrictions: Employees, spouses or dependent children of the United States Department of State or public and private organizations under contract to the United States Department of State are ineligible to apply for a Fulbright grant until one year after the employee's termination. TEFL administrators are ineligible for these seminar programs, but they are encouraged to view a listing of other Fulbright opportunities.
Date(s) Application is Due: Feb 1; Nov 1
Contact: Maria Bettua, Program Officer for Germany; (202) 686-6245; email: mbettua@cies.iie.org;; David B.J. Adams, Senior Program Officer for Japan and Korea, (202) 686-4021; email: dadams@cies.iie.org
Internet: http://www.cies.org/IEA/
Sponsor: Council for International Exchange of Scholars
3007 Tilden Street, NW, Suite 5L
Washington, DC 20008-3009

Fulbright New Century Scholars (NCS) Program Grants 1570
The NCS Program brings 30 top academics and professionals from around the world together each year to collaborate on an issue of global importance. Of the thirty, approximately one-third will be U.S. citizens while the remaining two thirds will be visiting scholars from countries with an operational Fulbright Scholar Program. NCS will provide a platform for scholars from the U.S. and around the world to engage in debate and dialogue based on multidisciplinary research and to develop new global models for understanding the social context within which nations and communities shape their responses to the many challenges of the 21st century. This particular aspect of the New Century Scholars program is a unique feature that distinguishes it from the core Fulbright Scholar Program.
Requirements: Applicants must be conducting current research relevant to the program's theme and objectives, be open to exploring and incorporating comparative, interdisciplinary approaches in their investigations, and interested in developing collaborative activities with other NCS Scholars. U.S. applicants must have U.S. citizenship and be residing permanently in the United States. For academic applicants, a Ph.D. or equivalent terminal degree in a relevant field is required. For applicants in the professional fields, the appropriate terminal degree in a relevant field is required. Non-U.S. applicants must be citizens or permanent residents of and residing in the country from which they are applying at the time of application. All applicants must have fluency in English.
Restrictions: Non-U.S. applicants holding permanent residency green cards, whether or not they reside in the U.S., are not eligible.
Contact: Jonathan Looper, Program Associate; (202) 686-6235; fax: (202) 362-3442; email: jlooper@cies.iie.org
Internet: http://www.cies.org/NCS/
Sponsor: Council for International Exchange of Scholars
3007 Tilden Street, NW, Suite 5L
Washington, DC 20008-3009

Fulbright Specialists Program Grants 1571
The Program is designed to provide short-term academic opportunities (two to six weeks) for U.S. faculty and professionals. Shorter grant lengths give specialists greater flexibility to pursue a grant that works best with their current academic or professional commitments. Applications for the Program are accepted on a rolling basis, and peer review of applications is conducted eight times per year. Program goals include: to increase the participation of leading U.S. scholars and professionals in Fulbright academic exchanges; to encourage new activities that go beyond the traditional Fulbright activities of lecturing and research; and to promote increased connections between U.S. and non-U.S. post-secondary academic institutions.
Requirements: Applicants must: be U.S. citizen at the time of application (permanent resident status is not sufficient; if a naturalized citizen, applicant must provide actual date of naturalization); possess a Ph.D. or equivalent professional/terminal degree at the time of application; have a minimum of five years of post-doctoral teaching or professional experience in the field in which you are applying (for professionals and artists outside academe, recognized professional standing and substantial professional accomplishments plus a minimum of five years of professional experience in the field in which you are applying); disclose prior conviction or current indictment for commission of a felony; and be residing in the United States at the time they are approved for a grant and intend to return to their U.S. institution after the grant's completion.
Restrictions: Employees, spouses or dependent children of the United States Department of State or public and private organizations under contract to the United States Department of State exchange programs are ineligible to apply for a Fulbright grant until one year after the employee's termination.
Date(s) Application is Due: Jan 28; Feb 24; Mar 25; Apr 21; May 20; Jul 15; Sep 9; Nov 4; Dec 30
Contact: Ryan Hathaway, Senior Program Coordinator; (202) 686-4026; email: rhathaway@cies.iie.org
Internet: http://www.cies.org/specialists/#top
Sponsor: Council for International Exchange of Scholars
3007 Tilden Street, NW, Suite 5L
Washington, DC 20008-3009

Fulbright Traditional Scholar Program in Europe and Eurasia 1572
The traditional Fulbright Scholar Program sends 800 U.S. faculty and professionals abroad each year. Grantees lecture and conduct research in a wide variety of academic and professional fields. Distribution of awards to countries in the region will vary annually according to the caliber of the applicants. Grants are available to: Albania, Andorra, Armenia, Austria, Azerbaijan, Belarus, Belgium, Bosnia and Herzegovina, Bulgaria, Croatia, Cyprus, Czech Republic, Denmark, Estonia, European Union, Finland, France, Georgia, Germany, Greece, Hungary, Iceland, Ireland, Italy, Latvia, Lithuania, Luxembourg, Macedonia, Moldova, Netherlands, Norway, Poland, Portugal, Romania, Russia, Slovakia (Slovak Republic), Slovenia, Spain, Sweden, Switzerland, Turkey, Ukraine, and United Kingdom. Only countries Considered to be in the Eastern Europe or Eurasia regions may be part of a multi-country application (2 to 3 countries). Multi-country proposals are not permitted for Western Europe. Language requirements vary by country, and prior knowledge of the local language may not be required, particularly where language is not commonly taught in the U.S.
Requirements: Applicants must: be U.S. citizens at the time of application (permanent residents are not eligible); be in good health (grantees will be required to submit a satisfactory Medical Certificate of Health from a physician); have sufficient proficiency in the written and spoken language of the host country (where required) to communicate with the people and to carry out the proposed study; and hold a B.A. degree or the equivalent before the start of the grant (applicants who have not earned a B.A. degree or the equivalent, but who have extensive professional study and/or experience in fields in which they wish to pursue a project, may be considered). In the creative and performing arts area, four years of professional study and/or experience meets the basic eligibility requirement. All candidates for the Europe and Eurasia region are required to obtain their own affiliations, generally established with an educational and/or research institution in the host country or countries. Candidates are responsible for securing their own research clearance as required by the host country.
Restrictions: The following persons are ineligible: anyone who has already held a U.S. Department of State-funded Fulbright student grant of any type; anyone who has previously received a Department of Education-funded Doctoral Dissertation Research Abroad (Fulbright Hays grant); employees of the U.S. Department of State, and their immediate families, for a period ending one year following termination of such employment; employees of private and public agencies (excluding educational institutions) under contract to the U.S. Department of State to perform administrative or screening services on behalf of the U.S. Department of State's exchange program, for a period ending one year following the termination of their services for the U.S. Department of State provided such employees have been directly engaged in performing services related to the exchange programs; applicants holding a doctoral degree at the time of application; applicants seeking enrollment in a medical degree program abroad; or applicants currently residing in the countries of Australia, Belgium/Luxembourg, Canada, Chile, Finland, Hungary, Mexico, Netherlands, New Zealand, Sweden, or Switzerland.
Date(s) Application is Due: Aug 1
Contact: Rachel Holskin, Program Manager; (212) 984-5326; email: rholskin@iie.org
Internet: http://us.fulbrightonline.org/program_regions_countries.php?id=3
Sponsor: Institute of International Education
809 United Nations Plaza
New York, NY 10017-5330

Fulbright Traditional Scholar Program in Sub-Saharan Africa 1573
The traditional Fulbright Scholar Program sends 800 U.S. faculty and professionals abroad each year. Grantees lecture and conduct research in a wide variety of academic and professional fields. Selection for countries in sub-Saharan Africa, with the exception of South Africa, will be made based on the quality of the applications, rather than per-country quotas. Distribution of awards to countries in the region will vary annually according to the caliber of the applicants. Grants are available to: Benin, Botswana, Burkina Faso, Cameroon, Chad, Eritrea, Ethiopia, Ghana, Guinea, Ivory Coast, Kenya, Madagascar, Malawi, Mali, Mauritius, Mozambique, Namibia, Niger, Nigeria, Senegal, South Africa, Swaziland, Tanzania, Togo, Uganda, Zambia, and Zimbabwe. All countries within the sub-Saharan Africa Region, with the exception of South Africa, may be part of a multi-country application (2 to 3 countries). For unlisted countries, applications may be considered on a case-by-case basis for dissertation research only.
Requirements: Applicants must: be U.S. citizens at the time of application (permanent residents are not eligible); be in good health (grantees will be required to submit a satisfactory Medical Certificate of Health from a physician); have sufficient proficiency in the written and spoken language of the host country to communicate with the people and to carry out the proposed study; and hold a B.A. degree or the equivalent before the start of the grant (applicants who have not earned a B.A. degree or the equivalent, but who have extensive professional study and/or experience in fields in which they wish to pursue a project, may be considered). In the creative and performing arts area, four years of professional study and/or experience meets the basic eligibility requirement. All candidates for Africa are required to obtain their own affiliations, generally established with an educational and/or research institution in the host country or countries.
Restrictions: Grants are not available to: Burundi, Central African Republic, Guinea-Bissau, Liberia, Somalia, or Sudan. The following persons are ineligible: anyone who has already held a U.S. Department of State-funded Fulbright student grant of any type; anyone who has previously received a Department of Education-funded Doctoral Dissertation Research Abroad (Fulbright Hays grant); employees of the U.S. Department of State, and their immediate families, for a period ending one year following termination of such employment; employees of private and public agencies (excluding educational institutions) under contract to the U.S. Department of State to perform administrative or screening services on behalf of the U.S. Department of State's exchange program,

for a period ending one year following the termination of their services for the U.S. Department of State provided such employees have been directly engaged in performing services related to the exchange programs; applicants holding a doctoral degree at the time of application; applicants seeking enrollment in a medical degree program abroad; or applicants currently residing in the countries of Australia, Belgium/Luxembourg, Canada, Chile, Finland, Hungary, Mexico, Netherlands, New Zealand, Sweden, or Switzerland.
Date(s) Application is Due: Aug 1
Contact: Jermaine Jones, Program Manager; (212) 984-5341; email: jjones@iie.org
Internet: http://us.fulbrightonline.org/program_regions_countries.php?id=1
Sponsor: Institute of International Education
809 United Nations Plaza
New York, NY 10017-3580

Fulbright Traditional Scholar Program in the East Asia/Pacific Region 1574
The traditional Fulbright Scholar Program sends 800 U.S. faculty and professionals abroad each year. Grantees lecture and conduct research in a wide variety of academic and professional fields. Distribution of awards to countries in the region will vary annually according to the caliber of the applicants. Grants are available to: Australia, Cambodia, China, Hong Kong, Indonesia, Japan, Korea, Laos, Macau, Malaysia, Mongolia, New Zealand, Philippines, Singapore, Taiwan, Thailand, and Vietnam. All countries within the East Asia/Pacific region, with the exception of China, may be part of a multi-country application (2 to 3 countries). For unlisted countries, applications may be considered on a case-by-case basis, but for dissertation research only. Language requirements vary by country, and prior knowledge of the local language may not be required, particularly where language is not commonly taught in the U.S.
Requirements: Applicants must: be U.S. citizens at the time of application (permanent residents are not eligible); be in good health (grantees will be required to submit a satisfactory Medical Certificate of Health from a physician); have sufficient proficiency in the written and spoken language of the host country to communicate with the people and to carry out the proposed study; and hold a B.A. degree or the equivalent before the start of the grant (applicants who have not earned a B.A. degree or the equivalent, but who have extensive professional study and/or experience in fields in which they wish to pursue a project, may be considered). In the creative and performing arts area, four years of professional study and/or experience meets the basic eligibility requirement. All candidates for the East Asia/Pacific region are required to obtain their own affiliations, generally established with an educational and/or research institution in the host country or countries. Candidates are responsible for securing their own research clearance as required by the host country.
Restrictions: Grants are not available to: Brunei, the Cook Islands, East Timor, Fiji, Myanmar, the Pacific Island Nations, Papua New Guinea, or Western Samoa. The following persons are ineligible: anyone who has already held a U.S. Department of State-funded Fulbright student grant of any type; anyone who has previously received a Department of Education-funded Doctoral Dissertation Research Abroad (Fulbright Hays grant); employees of the U.S. Department of State, and their immediate families, for a period ending one year following termination of such employment; employees of private and public agencies (excluding educational institutions) under contract to the U.S. Department of State to perform administrative or screening services on behalf of the U.S. Department of State's exchange program, for a period ending one year following the termination of their services for the U.S. Department of State provided such employees have been directly engaged in performing services related to the exchange programs; applicants holding a doctoral degree at the time of application; applicants seeking enrollment in a medical degree program abroad; or applicants currently residing in the countries of Australia, Belgium/Luxembourg, Canada, Chile, Finland, Hungary, Mexico, Netherlands, New Zealand, Sweden, or Switzerland.
Date(s) Application is Due: Aug 1
Contact: Jonathan Akeley, Program Manager; (212) 984-5487; email: jakeley@iie.org
Internet: http://us.fulbrightonline.org/program_regions_countries.php?id=2
Sponsor: Institute of International Education
809 United Nations Plaza
New York, NY 10017-3580

Fulbright Traditional Scholar Program in the Near East and North Africa Region 1575
The traditional Fulbright Scholar Program sends 800 U.S. faculty and professionals abroad each year. Grantees lecture and conduct research in a wide variety of academic and professional fields. Selection for countries in the Near East and North Africa region will be made based on the quality of the applications, rather than per-country quotas. Distribution of awards to countries in the region will vary annually according to the caliber of the applicants. Grants are available to: Bahrain, Egypt, India, Jordan, Kuwait, Morocco, Oman, Qatar, Syria, Tunisia, United Arab Emirates, and Yemen. Multi-country applications (2 to 3 countries) are available, except in Egypt, India, Jordan, and Morocco. For unlisted countries, applications will be considered on a case-by-case basis.
Requirements: Applicants must: be U.S. citizens at the time of application (permanent residents are not eligible); be in good health (grantees will be required to submit a satisfactory Medical Certificate of Health from a physician); have sufficient proficiency in the written and spoken language of the host country to communicate with the people and to carry out the proposed study; and hold a B.A. degree or the equivalent before the start of the grant (applicants who have not earned a B.A. degree or the equivalent, but who have extensive professional study and/or experience in fields in which they wish to pursue a project, may be considered). In the creative and performing arts area, four years of professional study and/or experience meets the basic eligibility requirement. Candidates are responsible for securing research clearance, as required. In countries with Fulbright Commissions, assistance may be provided.
Restrictions: Grants are not available to: Algeria, Iran, Iraq, Lebanon, Saudi Arabia, the West Bank, or Gaza. The following persons are ineligible: anyone who has already held a U.S. Department of State-funded Fulbright student grant of any type; anyone who has previously received a Department of Education-funded Doctoral Dissertation Research Abroad (Fulbright Hays grant); employees of the U.S. Department of State, and their immediate families, for a period ending one year following termination of such employment; employees of private and public agencies (excluding educational institutions) under contract to the U.S. Department of State to perform administrative or screening services on behalf of the U.S. Department of State's exchange program, for a period ending one year following the termination of their services for the U.S. Department of State provided such employees have been directly engaged in performing services related to the exchange programs; applicants holding a doctoral degree at the time of application; applicants seeking enrollment in a medical degree program abroad; or applicants currently residing in the countries of Australia, Belgium/Luxembourg, Canada, Chile, Finland, Hungary, Mexico, Netherlands, New Zealand, Sweden, or Switzerland.
Date(s) Application is Due: Aug 1
Contact: Jermaine Jones, Program Manager; (212) 984-5341; email: jjones@iie.org
Internet: http://us.fulbrightonline.org/program_regions_countries.php?id=4
Sponsor: Institute of International Education
809 United Nations Plaza
New York, NY 10017-3580

Fulbright Traditional Scholar Program in the South and Central Asia Region 1576
The traditional Fulbright Scholar Program sends 800 U.S. faculty and professionals abroad each year. Grantees lecture and conduct research in a wide variety of academic and professional fields. Selection for countries in the South and Central Asia region will be made based on the quality of the applications, rather than per-country quotas. Distribution of awards to countries in the region will vary annually according to the caliber of the applicants. Grants are available to: Bangladesh, India, Kazakhstan, Kyrgyz Republic, Nepal, Sri Lanka, Tajikistan, and Uzbekistan. Multi-country applications (2 to 3 countries) are not available. Language requirements vary by country. Applicants to India who are recommended for final review will need to submit research visa applications in January or February.
Requirements: Applicants must: be U.S. citizens at the time of application (permanent residents are not eligible); be in good health (grantees will be required to submit a satisfactory Medical Certificate of Health from a physician); have sufficient proficiency in the written and spoken language of the host country to communicate with the people and to carry out the proposed study; and hold a B.A. degree or the equivalent before the start of the grant (applicants who have not earned a B.A. degree or the equivalent, but who have extensive professional study and/or experience in fields in which they wish to pursue a project, may be considered). In the creative and performing arts area, four years of professional study and/or experience meets the basic eligibility requirement. Candidates are responsible for securing research clearance, as required. In countries with Fulbright Commissions, assistance may be provided.
Restrictions: Grants are not available to: Afghanistan, Bhutan, Pakistan, Republic of Maldives, or Turkmenistan. The following persons are ineligible: anyone who has already held a U.S. Department of State-funded Fulbright student grant of any type; anyone who has previously received a Department of Education-funded Doctoral Dissertation Research Abroad (Fulbright Hays grant); employees of the U.S. Department of State, and their immediate families, for a period ending one year following termination of such employment; employees of private and public agencies (excluding educational institutions) under contract to the U.S. Department of State to perform administrative or screening services on behalf of the U.S. Department of State's exchange program, for a period ending one year following the termination of their services for the U.S. Department of State provided such employees have been directly engaged in performing services related to the exchange programs; applicants holding a doctoral degree at the time of application; applicants seeking enrollment in a medical degree program abroad; or applicants currently residing in the countries of Australia, Belgium/Luxembourg, Canada, Chile, Finland, Hungary, Mexico, Netherlands, New Zealand, Sweden, or Switzerland.
Date(s) Application is Due: Aug 1
Contact: Jonathan Akeley, South Asia Program Manager; (212) 984-5487; email: jakeley@iie.org;; Jon Adler, Central Asia Program Manager; (212) 984-5326; email: jadler@iie.org
Internet: http://us.fulbrightonline.org/program_regions_countries.html?id=6
Sponsor: Institute of International Education
809 United Nations Plaza
New York, NY 10017-3580

Fulbright Traditional Scholar Program in the Western Hemisphere 1577
The traditional Fulbright Scholar Program sends 800 U.S. faculty and professionals abroad each year. Grantees lecture and conduct research in a wide variety of academic and professional fields. Selection for countries in Central America and the Caribbean will be made based on the quality of the applications, rather than per-country quotas. Distribution of awards to countries in the region will vary annually according to the caliber of the applicants. Grants are available to: Argentina, Barbados and the Eastern Caribbean, Bolivia, Brazil, Canada, Chile, Colombia, Costa Rica, Dominican Republic, Ecuador, El Salvador, Guatemala, Honduras, Jamaica, Mexico, Nicaragua, Panama, Paraguay, Peru, Trinidad and Tobago, Uruguay, and Venezuela. English Teaching Assistantships are available in Argentina, Brazil, Chile, Uruguay and Venezuela. Language proficiency

may be preferred or required. Applicants for English Teaching Assistantships can apply to only one country. Multi-country applications (2 to 3 countries) are available in all other disciplines throughout the Western Hemisphere. For unlisted countries, applications may be considered on a case-by-case basis, but for dissertation research only.
Requirements: Applicants must: be U.S. citizens at the time of application (permanent residents are not eligible); be in good health (grantees will be required to submit a satisfactory Medical Certificate of Health from a physician); have sufficient proficiency in the written and spoken language of the host country to communicate with the people and to carry out the proposed study; and hold a B.A. degree or the equivalent before the start of the grant (applicants who have not earned a B.A. degree or the equivalent, but who have extensive professional study and/or experience in fields in which they wish to pursue a project, may be considered). In the creative and performing arts area, four years of professional study and/or experience meets the basic eligibility requirement. Candidates are responsible for securing research clearance, as required. In countries with Fulbright Commissions, assistance may be provided.
Restrictions: Grants are not available to: Bahamas, Belize, Cuba, French Guiana, Guyana, Haiti, Martinique, or Suriname. The following persons are ineligible: anyone who has already held a U.S. Department of State-funded Fulbright student grant of any type; anyone who has previously received a Department of Education-funded Doctoral Dissertation Research Abroad (Fulbright Hays grant); employees of the U.S. Department of State, and their immediate families, for a period ending one year following termination of such employment; employees of private and public agencies (excluding educational institutions) under contract to the U.S. Department of State to perform administrative or screening services on behalf of the U.S. Department of State's exchange program, for a period ending one year following the termination of their services for the U.S. Department of State provided such employees have been directly engaged in performing services related to the exchange programs; applicants holding a doctoral degree at the time of application; applicants seeking enrollment in a medical degree program abroad; or applicants currently residing in the countries of Australia, Belgium/Luxembourg, Canada, Chile, Finland, Hungary, Mexico, Netherlands, New Zealand, Sweden, or Switzerland.
Date(s) Application is Due: Aug 1
Contact: Jody Dudderar, Program Manager in South America, Mexico and Canada; (212) 984-5565; fax: (212) 984-5325; email: jdudderar@iie.org;; Cara Wolinsky, Program Manager in Central America and the Caribbean; (212) 984-5366; email: cwolinsky@iie.org
Internet: http://us.fulbrightonline.org/program_regions_countries.php?id=5
Sponsor: Institute of International Education
809 United Nations Plaza
New York, NY 10017-3580

Fuller E. Callaway Foundation Grants **1578**
The foundation awards grants to nonprofit organizations and individuals in LaGrange and Troup County, GA. Grants are awarded in the areas of religion, higher and other education, social services, youth, and health. Types of support include general operating budgets, annual campaigns, building funds, equipment, matching funds, and student aid. Letters of application from organizations are accepted and have deadlines at the end of December, March, June, and September. Application forms are required for the scholarship program. Scholarship deadlines are February 15 and June 30 for law school scholarships. The board meets in January, April, July, and October to consider scholarship requests.
Requirements: Nonprofit organizations and individuals in LaGrange and Troup County, GA, are eligible for support.
Geographic Focus: Georgia
Samples: First Baptist Church of Fannin Street (LaGrange, GA)—for permanent improvements, $267,296.
Amount of Grant: $500-$25,000 average for organizations; $500-$10,000 average for individuals
Contact: H. Speer Burdette, General Manager, (706) 884-7348; fax: (706) 884-0201; email: hsburdette@callaway-foundation.org
Sponsor: Fuller E. Callaway Foundation
P.O. Box 790
LaGrange, GA 30241

Fulton County Community Foundation Grants **1579**
Fulton County Community Foundation is a part of the Northern Indiana Community Foundation (NICF). The NICF allows the Foundation to maximize its investment benefits and be more cost efficient. This way Fulton County donations can do more in Fulton County and the communities thereof. The Fulton County Community Foundation makes grant determinations in November of each year. Applications are due October 3rd each year. Applications received after the due date will not be considered for that particular grant cycle. Grant making areas of interest are: education; health; human services; arts and culture; environment; and civic and recreation. Contact the Program Coordinator at Northern Indiana Community Foundation, to discuss your project before applying for a grant. The Foundation favors activities that: reach a broad segment of the community, especially those citizens whose needs are not being met by existing services that are normally expected to be provided by private rather than government sources; request seed money to realize innovative opportunities to meet needs in the community; stimulate and encourage additional funding; promote cooperation and avoid duplication of effort; help make charitable organizations more effective and efficient and better able to be self-sustaining; and one time projects or needs.
Requirements: Grant seekers must use the application form provided by the Foundation. Funding is limited to Fulton County and the communities thereof.
Restrictions: The foundation will not consider grants for: religious organizations for the sole purpose of furthering that religion; political activities or those designated to influence legislation; national organizations (unless the monies are to be used solely to benefit citizens of Fulton County); grant that directly benefit the donor or the donor's family; fund-raising projects; contributions to endowments
Geographic Focus: Indiana
Date(s) Application is Due: Oct 3
Contact: Corinne Becknell Lucas, Program/Scholarship Coordinator; (574) 223-2227 or (877) 432-6423; fax: (574) 224-3709; email: corinne@nicf.org
Internet: http://www.nicf.org/fulton/index.html
Sponsor: Fulton County Community Foundation
P.O. Box 807 or 715 Main Street
Rochester, IN 46975

Fyssen Foundation Postdoctoral Study Grants **1580**
The foundation awards postdoctoral research grants for research on cognitive mechanisms, including thought and reasoning, that underlie animal and human behavior; their biological and cultural bases; and phylogenetic and ontogenetic development. Research should be in ethology and psychology, neurobiology, anthropology/ethnology, and human paleontology. Grants support French scientists for research abroad and foreign researchers conducting research in France. Annual deadline dates may vary; contact program staff for exact dates.
Date(s) Application is Due: Mar 31
Contact: Postdoctoral Study Grants, 331 42975316; fax: 331 42601795; email: secretariat@fondation-fyssen.org
Internet: http://www.fondation-fyssen.org
Sponsor: Fyssen Foundation
194 rue de Rivoli
Paris 75001 France

G.N. Wilcox Trust Grants **1581**
The trust provides partial support to programs and projects of tax-exempt, public charities in Hawaii to improve the quality of life in the state, particularly the island of Kauai. Grants of one year's duration are awarded in categories of interest to the trust, including education, literacy programs and adult basic education, health, Protestant religion, delinquency and crime prevention, social services, youth services, and culture and the performing arts. Types of support include general operating grants, capital grants, equipment acquisition, seed grants, scholarship funds, and challenge/matching grants.
Requirements: Giving is limited to Hawaii, with emphasis on the island of Kauai.
Restrictions: Grants are not awarded to support government agencies (or organizations substantially supported by government funds), individuals, or for endowment funds, research, deficit financing, or student aid in scholarships or loans.
Geographic Focus: Hawaii
Samples: Save our Seas (HI)—to support scholarships for youth to participate in the Second Annual Clean Oceans Conference, $2954.; Church of the Crossroads (HI)—to support the capital campaigns for renovations, $10,000.; Hawaii Public Radio (HI)—to support the membership challenge grant, $3000.
Contact: Paula Boyce, c/o Bank of Hawaii, (808) 538-4944; fax: (808) 538-4647; email: pboyce@boh.com or emoniz@boh.com
Sponsor: G.N. Wilcox Trust
P.O. Box 3170
Honolulu, HI 96802-3170

Gamble Foundation Grants **1582**
The Foundation is primarily interested in supporting organizations that serve disadvantaged children and youth in San Francisco, Marin and Napa counties. Within the field of youth development, the Foundation focuses on educational and personal enrichment programs designed to open doors of opportunity for at-risk youth in order to help them succeed in school and become productive, self-sufficient members of society. The Foundation is particularly interested in agricultural/environmental education, vocational training, and programs that prevent substance abuse and teen violence. The Foundation also supports environmental organizations that focus on land preservation and sustainability, animal welfare and management, and pollution control. Application information is available online.
Requirements: Northern California 501(c)3 nonprofit organizations, with an emphasis on San Francisco, Marin, and Napa Counties, are eligible.
Restrictions: Grants do not support religious organizations, individuals, medical research, endowment funds, capital improvements, or annual appeals.
Geographic Focus: California
Amount of Grant: $5,000-$20,000
Contact: Eric Sloan, (415) 561-6540, ext. 205; fax: (415) 561-6477; email: esloan@pfs-llc.net
Internet: http://www.pfs-llc.net/gamble/gamble.html
Sponsor: Gamble Foundation
1660 Bush Street, Suite 300
San Francisco, CA 94109

Gates Global HIV/AIDS Vaccine Grants **1583**
The program seeks research proposals to apply new technologies, concepts, and approaches to the design of safe and effective preventive vaccines against HIV/AIDS, in the context of the Scientific Strategic Plan of the Global HIV/AIDS Vaccine Enterprise. The foundation will fund a number of consortia or centers targeting three different priority areas identified in the Scientific Strategic Plan of the Global HIV/AIDS

Vaccine Enterprise: Design of Immunogens that Induce Broadly Reactive Neutralizing Antibodies (RFP: GH-HTR-05-01); Design of Immunogens that Induce Persistent High Levels of Cell-mediated Immunity (RFP: GH-HTR-05-02); and Standardization and Development of Laboratory Assays to Comparatively Measure the Immunogenicity of HIV Vaccine Candidates in Pre-clinical and Clinical Trials (RFP: GH-HTR-05-03). The complete RFPs are available online. The listed application deadline is for letters of intent; full proposals are by invitation.
Requirements: Governmental entities and 501(c)3 tax-exempt organizations are eligible. Foreign governmental agencies and equivalent organization also are eligible.
Restrictions: Grants are not awarded to support individuals or projects that serve an exclusively religious purpose.
Date(s) Application is Due: Apr 1
Contact: Grants Administrator, (206) 709-3140; email: info@gatesfoundation.org
Internet: http://www.gatesfoundation.org/GlobalHealth/Grantseekers/GrantmakingAreas/default.htm
Sponsor: Bill and Melinda Gates Foundation
P.O. Box 23350
Seattle, WA 98102

GE & Science Prize for Young Life Scientists **1584**
The GE & Science Prize for Young Life Scientists has been established to provide support to scientists at the beginning of their careers, because Science/AAAS and GE Healthcare believe that such support is critical for continued scientific progress. The prize will recognize outstanding graduate students in molecular biology from all regions of the world. This international prize will be awarded for the outstanding thesis in the general area of molecular biology as described in a 1000-word essay. The winning essay will be published in Science; essays of the regional award winners will appear in the online version of Science. For judging purposes, the essays will be grouped according to the geographic location of the degree-granting institution: North America, Europe, Japan, and all other countries. Initial screening of the submissions will be done by regional judges. Essays will be judged on the quality of the research and the entrant's ability to articulate the contribution of the research to the field of molecular biology. The top five essays from each geographic region will be forwarded to a panel of judges. All regional winners will compete for the grand prize of U.S.$25,000. The regional winners who do not receive the grand prize will be awarded U.S.$5,000. Winners will be announced in Science and the prize will be awarded in a location to be announced. The grand prize essay will be published in 'Science', and essays of the regional winners will be published on the online version of 'Science'.
Requirements: Entrants must have been awarded their Ph.D. between January, 1 and, December 31, of the previous year. Candidates for M.D./Ph.D. degrees are eligible to compete for the prize in either the year the Ph.D. is awarded or the year the final degree is awarded. The research described in the entrant's thesis must be in the field of molecular biology as described above. The prize will recognize only work that was performed while the entrant was a graduate student. The prize will be awarded without regard to sex, race, or nationality.
Restrictions: Employees of GE, Science and AAAS, and their relatives are not eligible for the prize.
Samples: Ethan Garner, a North American regional winner, $25,000—for his essay "Understanding a Minimal DNA-Segregating Machine" (2008); Xu Tan, regional winner, $5,000—for his essay "Plant Hormone Auxin Functions as Novel Molecular Glue" (2008); Sabrina Buttner, regional winner, $5,000—for her essay "Endonuclease G Regulates Cellular Fate" (2008)
Amount of Grant: $25,000
Date(s) Application is Due: Aug 1
Contact: Sylvia Kihara, Prize Coordinator, (202) 326-6507; fax: (202) 289-7562; email: skihara@aaas.org or gescienceprize@aaas.org
Internet: http://www.sciencemag.org/feature/data/prizes/ge/index.dtl
Sponsor: American Association for the Advancement of Science
1200 New York Avenue, NW, Room 1049B
Washington, DC 20005

Gebbie Foundation Grants **1585**
The Foundation's mission is to support appropriate charitable and humanitarian programs to improve the quality of life, primarily in Chautauqua County, by focusing on: children, youth and education; arts; human services; and community development. The Board meets quarterly and proposals are accepted throughout the year. Before preparing a complete proposal, applicants are urged to submit a letter of inquiry addressed to the Executive Director.
Requirements: Proposals should be consistent with the Foundation's strategic focus. The Foundation prefers not to be the primary or sole funding source. Organizations requesting funding must be approved as (or sponsored by) a 501(c)3 organization.
Restrictions: Grants are not made to individuals or sectarian or religious organizations.
Geographic Focus: New York
Samples: Fund for the Arts in Chautauqua County—to support an annual campaign, $90,000.; Berry College (Mount Berry, GA)—toward renovations of Blackstone Hall, $25,000.; WCA Hospital—to purchase exercise equipment, $3055.; Chautauqua Watershed Conservancy—for seed money to expand operations, $28,580.
Contact: Executive Director , (716) 487-1062; fax: (716) 484-6401; email: info@gebbie.org or info@gebbie.org
Internet: http://www.gebbie.org
Sponsor: Gebbie Foundation
111 West Second Street, Suite 1100
Jamestown, NY 14701

GEICO Public Service Awards **1586**
This program observes the many accomplishments of federal employees. These employees are making tremendous differences in the quality and efficiency of services and are responsible for the success of many scientific, medical, and technical programs. The foundation recognizes four active and one retired federal employee who have made outstanding achievements in one of the four fields of endeavor: Substance Abuse Prevention and Treatment, Fire Prevention and Safety, Physical Rehabilitation, and Traffic Safety and Accident Prevention. Nomination information is available online.
Requirements: All career civil service employees are eligible, including employees of the Library of Congress, the General Accounting Office, the Office of the Architect of the Capital, the Government Printing Office, the Administrative Office of the U.S. Courts, the Smithsonian Institution, the Botanic Garden, and the Office of Homeland Security.
Amount of Grant: $2,500
Contact: Program Contact, (877) 206-0215; email: federal@geico.com
Internet: http://www.geico.com/insproducts/fedpsa.html
Sponsor: GEICO Philanthropic Foundation
One GEICO Plaza
Washington, DC 20076

GenCorp Foundation Grants **1587**
The Foundation is dedicated to supporting the communities where our employees live, work and volunteer. While the Foundation's primary focus is education, it also supports human services, civic and arts organizations. Emphasis is on science education. Funding preference is given to projects that involve issues important to employees and requests that are recommended by Foundation coordinators at company facilities. Interested applicants should submit a letter of inquiry.
Requirements: Non-profit organizations are eligible to apply. Priority is given to organizations that are in the GenCorp communities: Huntsville, AL; Camden, AR; Sacramento, CA; Socorro, NM; Jonesborough, TN; Clearfield, UT; Gainesville and Orange, VA; or Redmond, WA.
Geographic Focus: Alabama; Arkansas; California; New Mexico; Tennessee; Utah; Virginia; Washington
Samples: Keep Akron Beautiful (Akron, OH)—for continued support, $1000.; Challenger Ctr for Space Science Education (Sacramento, CA)—for funding of space science education at the Sacramento Science Ctr, $20,000.
Contact: Program Contact, (916) 355-3600; email: gencorp.foundation@gencorp.com
Internet: http://www.gencorp.com/pages/gcfound.html
Sponsor: GenCorp Foundation
P.O. Box 15619
Sacramento, CA 95852-0619

Genentech Corporate Charitable Contributions Grants **1588**
The Foundation's primary focus areas are health science education, patient education/advocacy, and community. The Foundation supports nonprofits through its contributions in two primary ways: project-specific or general support funding to organizations whose mission aligns with the Foundation's focus areas; and sponsorships of selected events that fall into the Foundation's focus areas. Interested applicant's are encouraged to submit applications online.
Requirements: Nonprofit organizations recognized by the IRS as tax exempt, public charities, located in the United States are eligible to apply. Eligible grantees may include public elementary and secondary schools, as well as public colleges and universities and public hospitals.
Restrictions: The Foundation does not provide funding to organizations that discriminate on the basis of age, political affiliation, race, national origin, ethnicity, gender, disability, sexual orientation or religious beliefs. Funding is not provided for: advertising journals or booklets; alumni drives; capital campaigns/building funds; continuing medical education; infrastructural requests (e.g. salaries, equipment); memorial funds; memberships; organizations based outside of the United States; political or sectarian organizations; professional sports events or athletes; religious organizations; scholarships; yearbooks.
Geographic Focus: California
Samples: To be distributed among 19 organizations (CA)—for science programs for students in the San Francisco Bay area, $1 million (2003).
Contact: Community & Patient Programs, (650) 467-9494; email: give@gene.com
Internet: http://www.gene.com/gene/about/community/overview.jsp
Sponsor: Genentech Inc
1 DNA Way
South San Francisco, CA 94080-4990

General Mills Champions for Healthy Kids Grants **1589**
The program aims to improve youth nutrition and fitness in the United States through grants to community-based groups. The initiative consists of grants to community-based groups as well as three additional components: sponsorship of the President's Active Lifestyle Awards, developing nutrition and fitness mentoring models, and sharing best practices. Grants are intended to encourage the improvement of eating and physical activity patterns of young people, ages two to 20. Priority is given to programs that demonstrate significant potential impact on youth groups with special needs or for having an impact on large populations of youth. Guidelines are available online.
Requirements: U.S. 501(c)3 and 509(a) tax-exempt organizations are eligible. Proposed projects should reflect the practices and concepts recommended by the Dietary Guidelines for American 2000 and the American Dietetic Association, and should include at least one nutritional behavioral objective and at least one physical activity behavioral objective.

Samples: Adams Park Community Ctr (Saint Louis, MO)—for Healthy Futures, a diabetes- prevention curriculum that inspires eight- to 11-year olds, from a low-income African-American community to maintain eating habits and physical activity conducive to a healthy lifestyle, $10,000 (2005); Fitness Forward Foundation (Durham, NC)—a program in which students earn points by meeting four daily behaviors: limiting TV and computer time to one hour, being physically active for one hour, not drinking sugar-sweetened beverages and getting eight to 11 hours of sleep, $10,000 (2005).
Amount of Grant: $10,000 maximum
Date(s) Application is Due: Jan 15
Contact: Beth Labrador, Program Contact; (800) 877-1600, ext. 4821; fax: (763) 764-4114; email: blabrador@eatright.org
Internet: http://www.generalmills.com/corporate/commitment/champions.aspx
Sponsor: General Mills Foundation
Number One General Mills Boulevard, P.O. Box 1113
Minneapolis, MN 55440

General Mills Foundation Grants 1590
The Foundation was created to focus its philanthropic resources on community needs. Strategic objectives are to: demonstrably improve the quality of life in communities with GM facilities and employees; initiate innovative solutions and approaches to improve youth nutrition and fitness; and to support GM employees and retirees giving to United Way, education, and arts and culture organizations through gift matching. Funding priorities include: social services; youth nutrition and fitness; education; and arts and culture. Priority is given to organizations meeting the following criteria: their mission is closely related to the Foundation's priorities; programs or activities are based in communities with GM operations and employees; programs or activities involve GM employees and retirees; and services create sustainable community improvement. Applications are accepted at any time.
Requirements: U.S. and Canadian charitable 501(c)3 and 509(a) nonprofits in communities where General Mills operates (California, Georgia, Illinois, Indiana, Iowa, Maryland, Massachusetts, Missouri, Minnesota, Missouri, Montana, New Jersey, New York, Ohio, Oklahoma, Pennsylvania, Tennessee and Wisconsin) are eligible.
Restrictions: The Foundation does not support: organizations without 501(c)3 and 509(a) status; organizations that do not comply with the Foundation's non-discrimination policy; individuals; social, labor, veterans, alumni or fraternal organizations serving a limited constituency; travel by groups; recreational, sporting events or athletic associations; religious organizations for religious purposes; basic research; organizations seeking underwriting for advertising; political causes, candidates or legislative lobbying efforts; conferences, seminars and workshops; campaigns to eliminate or control specific diseases; publications, films or television programs; underwriting for program sponsorship.
Geographic Focus: Arizona; Arkansas; California; Georgia; Illinois; Indiana; Iowa; Maryland; Massachusetts; Michigan; Minnesota; Missouri; Montana; New Jersey; New Mexico; New York; Ohio; Oklahoma; Pennsylvania; Tennessee; Wisconsin
Contact: Christina L. Shea, President; (763) 764-2211; fax: (763) 764-4114
Internet: http://www.generalmills.com/corporate/commitment/foundation.aspx
Sponsor: General Mills Foundation
Number One General Mills Boulevard, P.O. Box 1113
Minneapolis, MN 55440

General Motors Foundation Grants Support Program 1591
With a strong commitment to diversity in all areas, the targeted areas of focus for the Foundation are: education; health and human services; civic and community; public policy; arts and culture; and environment and energy. Primary consideration is given to requests that meet the following criteria: exhibit a clear purpose and defined need in one of the foundation's areas of focus; recognize innovative approaches in addressing the defined need; demonstrate an efficient organization and detail the organization's ability to follow through on the proposal; and, explain clearly the benefits to the foundation and the plant city communities. Paper applications are no longer accepted. Completion of an online eligibility quiz is the first step in the application process.
Requirements: Nonprofit, tax-exempt organizations and institutions are eligible to apply. Applications must be made online.
Restrictions: The Foundation not not support organizations that discriminate on the basis of race, religion, creed, gender, age, veteran status, physical challenge or national origin. Contributions are generally not provided for: individuals; religious organizations; political parties or candidates; U.S. hospitals and health care institutions (general operating support); capital campaigns; endowment funds; conferences, workshops or seminars not directly related to GM's business interests.
Contact: Grant Coordinator, (313) 556-5000
Internet: http://www.gm.com/company/gmability/community/guidelines/index.html
Sponsor: General Motors Foundation
P.O. Box 300, 300 Renaissance Center
Detroit, MI 48265-3000

General Service Foundation Reproductive Health and Rights Grants 1592
The foundation is concerned with the related issues of rapid population growth and unintended pregnancies, particularly the availability of high-quality reproductive health care and access to that care. The foundation funds research for policy analysis, litigation, public education, and advocacy. Grants are made for programs in the United States and Latin America that address the needs of low-income women, women of color, adolescents, and the issue of access. Apply online.
Requirements: Grants are made to organizations that are tax-exempt under U.S. laws. The foundation prefers projects and/or programs that give promise of significant contribution and that are new, innovative, demonstrational, and/or research in nature.
Restrictions: Generally, grants are not made for service delivery, contraceptive development, or university-based research. In addition, contributions are not made to operating budgets or to annual campaigns of established organizations. The foundation ordinarily does not contribute to capital (physical plant, equipment, endowment), to individuals, nor for relief.
Amount of Grant: $3.1 million total; $2500-$35,000 average
Date(s) Application is Due: Feb 1
Contact: Holly Bartling, Program Contact, (202) 232-1005 or (970) 920-6834; fax: (970) 920-4578; email: holly@generalservice.org or rhr@generalservice.org
Internet: http://www.generalservice.org/Reproductive%20Health.htm
Sponsor: General Service Foundation
557 N Mill Street, Suite 201
Aspen, CO 81611

Genesis Foundation Grants 1593
The Foundation funds projects and program in the areas of health and formal education, benefiting children 0 to 18 years old, as well as training programs in these two areas. Capital, operating, program and general grants are funded. Approximately eighty percent of grant-making is devoted to Colombian entities, with the remainder devoted to projects in the U.S., specifically in Southern Florida, Washington, DC and the New York Metropolitan area.
Requirements: Preliminary criteria to apply for a grant include: must be located in Colombia, Southern Florida, Washington, DC or the New York Metropolitan Area; must be incorporated as a non-profit, charitable institution in the appropriate jurisdiction; must have been in operation for a minimum of two (2) full years; must include at least three (3) people in decision-making process at all times; must benefit a minimum of 50 people per year; in Colombia, must have raised at a minimum the equivalent of U.S. $10,000 in the previous two years; in the U.S. must have raised a minimum of $20,000 in the previous two years; must have an independent financial auditor; must be able to provide audited financial statements for the previous three years; must be able to provide a budget for the organization and the project for which the grant is sought; must not be a political organization; and must not have a religious purpose.
Restrictions: Individuals and political or religious causes are ineligible.
Geographic Focus: District of Columbia; Florida; New YorkColombia
Samples: Asociacion Social Popular (Bello, Colombia)—to purchase an educational facility, $35,000 (2005); Fundacion Estructurar (Bucaramanga, Colombia)—to provide education to working children, with an emphasis on training in design and graphic arts, $15,000 (2005); Fundacion Neumologica Colombiana (Bogota, Colombia)—to create an asthma center for children, $240,000 (2005); Nutrir (Bogota, Colombia)—to construct an additional facility that will provide nutritional and social services to underserved children, $40,000 (2005).
Amount of Grant: $10,000-$100,000 typically
Date(s) Application is Due: Mar 15; Sep 15
Contact: Grants Administrator, (212) 763-3703; fax: (917) 591-7858; email: genesis@genesid-foundation.org
Internet: http://www.genesis-foundation.org
Sponsor: Genesis Foundation
140 East 45th Street, 2 Grant Central Tower 18th Floor, Suite A
New York, NY 10017

Genuardi Family Foundation Grants 1594
The Foundation supports direct providers of services in the areas of education, health, human services, and culture. The Foundation gives preference to projects which receive broad-based community support and provides for reasonable costs associated with conducting the proposed project or program. Grant proposals may include the allocation of a reasonable percentage of grant monies towards general support of the recipient organization. On a limited basis, the Foundation will also consider grants in support of capital campaigns for facilities or equipment, and organizational capacity building.
Requirements: The Foundation only considers grant requests from organizations designated as tax exempt under Section 501(c)3 of the Internal Revenue Code. Preference will be given to non-profit organizations based in the Greater Philadelphia Area.
Restrictions: The Foundation's funding will not process grant requests from: individuals; fraternal and/or civic organizations; political candidates or to influence legislation; other foundations; general fund raising and endowment drives; debt reduction; environmental issues or initiatives; annual appeals or letters of solicitation; or public, private or parochial schools that serve the general public.
Geographic Focus: Pennsylvania
Amount of Grant: $5,000-$50,000
Date(s) Application is Due: Aug 1
Contact: Meredith A. Huffman, Executive Director; (610) 834-2030; email: info@genuardifamilyfoundation.org
Internet: http://www.genuardifamilyfoundation.org/genuardi_priorities.html
Sponsor: Genuardi Family Foundation
Blue Bell Executive Campus, 470 Norristown Road, Suite 300
Auburn, NY 13021

George and Ruth Bradford Foundation Grants 1595
The foundation awards grants to local nonprofit organizations in a broad range of interest areas, including children and youth, families, education and higher education, environmental and wildlife conservation, housing, and social services. Types of support include general operating support and scholarship funds. Letters of inquiry may be submitted throughout the year.

Requirements: California nonprofit organizations in the San Francisco peninsula are eligible.
Geographic Focus: California
Samples: Environmental Traveling Companions (San Francisco, CA)—operating support, $10,000.; Terwilliger Nature Education Ctr (San Rafael, CA)—operating support, $10,000.
Contact: Robert Bradford, Director, (650) 344-0422
Sponsor: George and Ruth Bradford Foundation
P.O. Box 720
Ukiah, CA 95482

George B. Storer Foundation Grants **1596**
The foundation awards grants, primarily in Florida, in its areas of interest, including higher education, social services—particularly for the blind, youth organizations, conservation, hospitals, and cultural programs. Types of support include building construction/renovation, capital campaigns, general operating support, matching/challenge grants, and research grants. There are no application forms. Applications should be submitted between October 15 and the listed deadline.
Samples: U of Miami (FL)—for marine-science and business-education programs, $205,000 (2005).
Date(s) Application is Due: Nov 15
Contact: Grants Administrator, c/o Thomas McDonald, CPA
Sponsor: George B. Storer Foundation
P.O. Box 1040
Tavernier, FL 33070

George F. Baker Trust Grants **1597**
Grants are awarded nationwide, with preference given to nonprofits in the eastern United States, primarily for K-12, higher, and secondary education; hospitals; social services; civic affairs; environmental conservation; religion; and international affairs. Types of support include general operating support and matching funds. There are no application forms or deadlines. The board meets in June and November to consider requests.
Restrictions: Grants are not made to individuals.
Samples: West Granville Christian Academy (West Granville, MA)—for operating support, $25,000.; Saint Paul's Community Development Corp (Patterson, NJ)—for operations and program support, $20,000.
Amount of Grant: $10,000-$100,000 average
Contact: Rocio Suarez, Executive Director, (212) 755-1890; fax: (212) 319-6316; email: rocio@bakernye.com
Sponsor: George F. Baker Trust
477 Madison Avenue, Suite 1650
New York, NY 10022

George Family Foundation Grants **1598**
The mission of the Foundation is to foster wholeness in mind, body, spirit, and community in order to enhance the development of human potential. The Foundation's areas of interest are: integrative medicine, leadership development, educational opportunities, social justice and spirituality. Non- solicited proposals will not be accepted. Invited applicants are encouraged to submit a letter of inquiry or to discuss their request with staff before submitting an application.
Requirements: 501(c)3 tax-exempt organizations are eligible. Primary giving is restricted to the Twin Cities metropolitan area.
Restrictions: Grants do not support endowment or capital campaigns, programs in which the family has no active interest or involvement; individuals; memberships, special events, or other fundraisers; or programs that address debt retirement or recovery of operating losses.
Geographic Focus: Minnesota
Samples: WATCH (Minneapolis, MN) for efforts to improve the criminal-justice system's handling of cases involving domestic violence and sexual assault, $15,000.; Twin Cities RISE (Minneapolis, MN)—for scholarships for participants in its skills-training and job-acquisition programs, $50,000.; Plymouth Congregation Church (Minneapolis, MN)—to add an outreach worker to the church's staff roster, $17,000.; Sigma Chi Foundation (Evanston, IL)—for the Horizons Leadership project, $25,000.
Amount of Grant: $1000-$200,000 range
Date(s) Application is Due: May 30; Oct 30
Contact: Grants Administrator, (612) 377-8400; fax: (612) 377-8407
Internet: http://www.georgefamilyfoundation.org/
Sponsor: George Family Foundation
1818 Oliver Avenue South
Minneapolis, MN 55405

George Frederick Jewett Foundation Grants Program **1599**
The foundation is concerned primarily with people and values. The grants program focuses on the future and on stimulating and supporting activities and projects of established, voluntary, nonprofit organizations that are of importance to human welfare. Grants are made in the fields of arts and humanities, conservation and preservation, education, health care and medical services, population, religion, and social welfare. The foundation may support research on and studies of important problems of public concern solely for the purpose of aiding in the gathering and presenting of facts that may assist the public to better understand such problems and to arrive at realistic and effective solutions to them. From time to time, support may be given to the scholarship, fellowship, and research programs of established institutions when sufficient evidence is available to establish clearly that the applicant organization is awarding such grants in accordance with the regulations established by the IRS. Grants are awarded to support activities in progress, research into potential projects, building and equipment, general operations, program development, seed funding, research, technical assistance, and matching funds. Inquiries for clarification of the foundation's policy and program emphasis are encouraged.
Requirements: Preference is given to public charities or nonprivate foundations. The foundation confines its grants largely to requests from eastern Washington and the San Francisco Bay area.
Restrictions: Grants do not support advertising; advocacy, athletic, international, religious, political, or veterans organizations; or individuals.
Geographic Focus: California; Washington
Samples: American U of Beirut (New York, NY)—general support, $15,000.; Committee to Restore the Opera House (San Francisco, CA)—for a three-year commitment for restoration of the San Francisco War Memorial Opera House, $120,000.
Amount of Grant: $5000-$50,000
Contact: Ann Gralnek, (415) 421-1351; fax: (415) 421-0721; email: ADGjewettf@aol.com or tfbjewettf@aol.com
Sponsor: George Frederick Jewett Foundation
235 Montgomery Street, Suite 612
San Francisco, CA 94104

George H. Hitchings New Investigator Award in Health Research **1600**
Provides awards to provide flexible support for young researchers in their second year of graduate school. Students planning to follow a career path in academic teaching and research that is closely tied to the health of North Carolinians and the strength of North Carolina Science are particularly encouraged to apply.
Requirements: Applications/nominations must be submitted by the institution on behalf of the student(s). Nomination applications are accepted from Duke, NCCU, NCSU, and UNC-Chapel Hill.
Restrictions: Only one nomination/application per graduate program/department within the university will be accepted.
Geographic Focus: North Carolina
Amount of Grant: $10,000
Date(s) Application is Due: Mar 5
Contact: Libby Long, Scholarships and Special Projects Coordinator: (919) 474-8370 ext. 134; fax: (919) 941-9208; email: libby@trialglecf.org
Internet: http://www.trianglecf.org/DatasetRecord.cfm?recordID=10001417&returnURL=%2Fpage10000237%2Ecfm&returntoname=View%20all%20Scholarships&sidepageid=10000237&thetitle=George%20H.%20Hitchings%20New%20Investigator%20Award%20in%20Health%20Research&Ds_PagepropId=1
Sponsor: Triangle Community Foundation
324 Blackwell Street, Suite 1220
Durham, NC 27701

George Kress Foundation Grants **1601**
The foundation awards grants to eligible Wisconsin nonprofit organizations in its areas of interest, including arts and culture, children and families, Christian churches and organizations, health care/health organizations/hospitals, historical preservation, human and social services, and sports and recreation. Types of support include building construction and renovation, capital campaigns, emergency services, professorships, program development, research grants, and scholarship funds. There are no application deadlines or forms.
Requirements: Wisconsin nonprofit organizations are eligible. Preference is given to requests benefiting Green Bay and Madison
Geographic Focus: Wisconsin
Samples: Saint Mary's Medical Ctr (Green Bay, WI)—to construct an addition that will house an expanded emergency-services department and improved facilities for surgery, $1 million (2005).
Contact: John Kress, Secretary, (920) 433-3109
Sponsor: George Kress Foundation
P.O. Box 408
Neenah, WI 54957-0408

George S. and Dolores Dore Eccles Foundation Grants **1602**
The foundation awards grants to eligible Utah organizations in its areas of interest, including arts, children and youth, economics, higher education, hospitals, medical research, performing arts, visual arts, and social services. Types of support include building construction/renovation, capital campaigns, equipment acquisition, general operating grants, matching/challenge grants, professorships, program development, research grants, and scholarship funds. A request for application is available online.
Requirements: Giving primarily in Utah.
Restrictions: Funding requests will not be considered from the following types of organizations: those that have not received a tax exemption letter establishing 501(c)3 status from the Internal Revenue Service, unless they are a unit of government, in which case such a letter is not required; other private foundations; those of a political nature that attempt to influence legislation and/or candidacy of persons for elected public office; conduit organizations, unified funds, or those that use funds to make grants to support other organizations; those that do not have fiscal responsibility for the proposed project. Funds will also not be considered for: contingencies, deficits, or debt reduction; general endowment funds; direct aid to individuals; conferences, seminars, or medical research; requests which do not fall within the Foundation's specified areas of interest.
Geographic Focus: Utah
Samples: Westminster College of Salt Lake City (UT)—for undergraduate scholarships, $1.2 million over three years.

Contact: Director, (801) 246-5340; fax: (801) 350-3510; email: gseg@gseccles.org
Internet: http://www.gsecclesfoundation.org
Sponsor: George S. and Dolores Dore Eccles Foundation
79 South Main Street, 12th Floor
Salt Lake City, UT 84111

Georgia Power Foundation Grants **1603**

Giving is focused on issues that directly affect customers, employees, business and shareholders. These include: improving the quality of education by partnering with organizations to assist students with personal development, mentoring and career exploration; protecting the environment by promoting programs to improve air and water quality, preserve natural resources and protect endangered species; preventing cancer; and promoting diversity. The Foundation gives strong preference to Georgia-based organizations and programs that seek to improve the quality of life for the state's residents. Applicants may apply online or with a written proposal.
Requirements: The foundation makes grants to tax-exempt organizations that seek to improve the quality of life for Georgia's residents.
Restrictions: The Foundation does not provide grants to individuals, private elementary or secondary schools, and religious organizations, nor political campaigns or causes. The Foundation does not provide multi-year funding commitments.
Geographic Focus: Georgia
Amount of Grant: $10,000
Date(s) Application is Due: Feb 15; May 15; Aug 15; Nov 15
Contact: Grants Administrator, (404) 506-6784; email: gpfoundation@southernco.com
Internet: http://www.georgiapower.com/community/apply.asp
Sponsor: Georgia Power Foundation
241 Ralph McGill Boulevard, N.E., Bin 10131
Atlanta, GA 30308-3374

Georgiana Goddard Eaton Memorial Fund Grants **1604**

Established in 1917, the Trust supports organizations involved with improving the lives of low-income individuals of Boston, Massachusetts. The fields of interest are: education; employment; family services; homelessness; housing/shelter; human services; legal services; urban/community development. Contact the Foundation for further application information and guidelines.
Requirements: Non-profits in the Boston, MA area are eligible. Applications should be addressed to: c/o Grants Mgmt. Assocs., 77 Summer Street, 8th Floor, Boston, MA 02110-1006
Restrictions: No grants to individuals (except former employees of Community Workshops, Inc.), or for endowment funds, or matching gifts; no loans.
Geographic Focus: Massachusetts
Date(s) Application is Due: Mar 1; Sep 1
Contact: Philip Hall, Administrator; (617) 426-7080; fax: (617) 426-7087; email: phall@grantsmanagement.com
Sponsor: Georgiana Goddard Eaton Memorial Fund
c/o Welch & Forbes LLC, 45 School Street
Boston, MA 02108-3206

Geraldine R. Dodge Foundation Morris County Grants **1605**

To help foster a more livable Morristown area, the Foundation will support organizations that help their neighbors and build community by doing one or more of the following: serve those whose needs and potential are great, especially children and youth; foster meaningful connections among people of diverse ethnicities, cultures, ages, and socio-economic groups; build collaborations among government, the business sector and nonprofit organizations that generate entrepreneurial solutions to current challenges; and help create a sustainable Morristown for the future through efforts such as inclusive community visionary processes, the development and promotion of local assets, and/or the promotion of green design. The Foundation also invites proposals for mini-grants in the range of $3,000 to $5,000 that feature new or recent connections and collaborations. These can be stand-alone proposals from two or more groups, or part of a broader proposal from a single organization.
Requirements: The foundation awards grant to 501(c)3 nonprofits in Morristown New Jersey.
Restrictions: Grants are not made to individuals or for the support of religion, higher education, health, international programs, conduit organizations, capital projects, deficit financing, or endowment funds.
Geographic Focus: New Jersey
Amount of Grant: $150,000 maximum
Date(s) Application is Due: May 1
Contact: David Grant, President; (973) 540-8442; fax: (973) 540-1211; email: info@grdodge.org
Internet: http://www.grdodge.org/morriscounty/index.htm
Sponsor: Geraldine R. Dodge Foundation
14 Maple Avenue, P.O. Box 1239
Morristown, NJ 07962-1239

Gerber Foundation Grants **1606**

The foundation awards grants to support national programs that have a significant impact on issues facing infants and young children. Areas of interest include pediatric health—promoting health and preventing disease, including projects geared toward research or interventions that will reduce the incidence of serious chronic illnesses (e.g., diabetes, heart disease, obesity, or cancer) or improve cognitive, social, and emotional aspects of development; pediatric nutrition—assuring adequate nutrition for infants and young children through projects of research or interventions; and the effects of environmental hazards. The listed deadlines are for letters of inquiry. Guidelines and application are available online.
Requirements: 501(c)3 nonprofit organizations are eligible. Priority is given to projects that improve infant and young children nutrition, care, and development from the first year before birth to three years of age.
Restrictions: The foundation does not make grants or loans to individuals. Outside the West Michigan area, the foundation does not support capital campaigns, operating support, national child welfare programs, international based programs, or food/baby products giveaway programs.
Samples: Children's Hospital of Michigan (Detroit, MI)—to evaluate a pain-assessment technique for use in infants, $59,798 (2005); Cincinnati Children's Hospital (OH)—to evaluate a potential treatment for necrotizing enterocolitis, $247,331 (2005); U of Minnesota-Twin Cities (Minneapolis, MN)—for a study evaluating oxygen therapy in neonates and oxidative stress, $223,288 (2005); Van Andel Research Institute (Grand Rapids, MI)—for a study involving protein profiling in congenital abnormalities of infants, $743,665 (2005).
Amount of Grant: $1 million maximum; $20,000-$500,000 typically
Date(s) Application is Due: Jun 1; Dec 1
Contact: Contact; (231) 924-3175; fax: (231) 924-7906; email: cobits@ncresa.org
Internet: http://www.gerberfoundation.org
Sponsor: Gerber Foundation
4747 W 48th Street, Suite 153
Fremont, MI 49412-8119

Gertrude and William C. Wardlaw Fund Grants **1607**

The fund awards general operating grants to Georgia nonprofit organizations in its areas of interest, including cultural activities, community development, education and higher education, and health and hospitals.
Requirements: Georgia nonprofit organizations are eligible.
Geographic Focus: Georgia
Amount of Grant: $675,546 total
Date(s) Application is Due: Feb 15
Contact: Mark Drake, Secretary
Sponsor: Gertrude and William C. Wardlaw Fund
P.O. Box 4655, MC 217
Atlanta, GA 30302

Gertrude B. Elion Mentored Medical Student Research Awards **1608**

An annual award granted to support women medical students interested in pursuing health-related research projects.
Requirements: Students must have the support of a faculty mentor and must conduct their research at one of the four medical schools in North Carolina. Applications are accepted from Duke University Medical Center, East Carolina University School of Medicine, UNC-Chapel Hill School of Medicine or Wake Forest University Baptist Medical Center only.
Restrictions: Candidates must be women, enrolled as full-time students, and will have completed at least one year of medical school prior to the start of the award. They must conduct their research at the applying institution. Candidates must be citizens or permanent residents of the United States or Canada at the time of application. Documentation of permanent residency status must be provided with the application. Persons who have applied for permanent residency but have not received their government documentation by the time of application are not eligible.
Geographic Focus: North Carolina
Amount of Grant: $10,000
Date(s) Application is Due: Mar 5
Contact: Libby Long, Scholarships and Special Projects Coordinator; (919) 474-8370 ext. 134; fax: (919) 941-9208; email: libby@trianglecf.org
Internet: http://www.trianglecf.org/page10000237.cfm
Sponsor: Triangle Community Foundation
324 Blackwell Street, Suite 1220
Durham, NC 27701

Gertrude E. Skelly Charitable Foundation Grants **1609**

The primary mission of the Foundation is to provide educational opportunities, primarily at colleges and universities, and needed medical care for those who cannot afford them. The advisory committee will meet in October to review applications. There is no formal application. Interested applicants will contact the Foundation to receive application instructions and guidelines.
Requirements: 501(c)3 tax-exempt organizations, including colleges and universities, are eligible.
Restrictions: Funding is not available for endowments or capital projects. Multi-year commitments are generally not favored. Grants will not be made to private foundations, non-charitable organizations or directly to individuals.
Amount of Grant: $50,000 maximum
Date(s) Application is Due: Jul 31
Contact: Bettee M. Collister, Esq., Executive Director, (561) 276-1008; fax: (561) 272-2793; email: skelly@erikjoh.com
Sponsor: Gertrude E. Skelly Charitable Foundation
4600 North Ocean Boulevard, Suite 206
Boynton Beach, FL 33435-7365

Gheens Foundation Grants 1610

The Foundation makes grants in Metro Louisville, Kentucky and LaFourche and Terrebonne Parishes in Louisiana. The Foundation supports a wide variety of endeavors at all levels, including education, economic development, medical, arts, social/health services, handicapped, and mental health programs. Foundation focus is on education and Christian works. There are no deadlines for applications. Guidelines and application information are available online.
Requirements: The Foundation contributes only to 501(c)3 organizations that are not private foundations.
Restrictions: The Foundation does not give to individuals.
Geographic Focus: Kentucky; Louisiana
Samples: Western Kentucky U (Bowling Green, KY)—to provide scholarships to minority teacher-education students who are committed to teaching in Jefferson County, KY, public schools, $80,000 over four years.; Louisville Seminary (Louisville, KY)—to construct the seminary's new academic building, $625,000 (2000); U of Louisville (KY)—to create a center where scientists will work to develop new gene-based technologies for studying a wide variety of age-related diseases, $2.5 million over five years.
Contact: Carl Thomas, Executive Director, (502) 584-4650; fax: (502) 584-4652; email: carl@gheensfoundation.org
Internet: http://gheensfoundation.org/grant_application
Sponsor: Gheens Foundation
705 One Riverfont Plaza, 401 West Main Street
Louisville, KY 40202

Giant Eagle Foundation Grants 1611

The foundation awards grants in Pennsylvania in its areas of interest, including community development; health and human services; Jewish agencies, charitable organizations, and temples; performing arts; and philanthropy. Types of support include project grants and employee-related scholarship. There are no application deadlines. The board meets four times each year to review requests.
Requirements: Pennsylvania nonprofit organizations are eligible. Preference will be given to requests from Pittsburgh.
Geographic Focus: Ohio; Pennsylvania
Samples: U of Pittsburgh (PA)—for educational and community-outreach programs of the Cancer Institute, the College of Arts and Sciences, the Graduate School of Business, the School of Pharmacy, and the School of Social Work, $1.4 million (2003).
Amount of Grant: $1000-$2000 range
Contact: David Shapira, c/o Giant Eagle, Inc., (412) 963-6200
Sponsor: Giant Eagle Foundation
101 Kappa Drive
Pittsburgh, PA 15238

Gibson Foundation Grants 1612

The Foundation is committed to making the world a better place for children by creating, developing and supporting programs and other non-profit organizations in their efforts to advance education, music and the arts, the environment and health & welfare causes. The Foundation actively seeks out programs that will be a direct mission-fit and further its goals.
Requirements: Applicants must be 501(c)3 organizations.
Restrictions: The Foundation does not support religious or political affiliations, and does not award individual scholarships.
Contact: Nina Miller, Executive Director; (615) 871-4500, ext. 2114; fax: (615) 884-9597; email: nina.miller@gibson.com
Internet: http://www.gibson.com/en-us/Lifestyle/GibsonFoundation/
Sponsor: Gibson Foundation
309 Plus Park Boulevard
Nashville, TN 37217

Gill Foundation - Gay and Lesbian Fund Grants 1613

In partnership with grantees, the Fund works to create a vibrant, healthy Colorado, where all families can thrive, while being a vehicle for cultural change toward equality for all. Programs of interest are: arts and culture; civic leadership; healthy families; and public broadcasting. Grantmaking is carried out in three ways: events sponsorship; invitation only; and opportunity grants. Requests may not exceed 15% of an organization's total budget, or for event sponsorships, may not exceed 50% of the event budget. Application information is available online.
Requirements: Eligible recipients must: be a 501(c)3 public charity organization; have a board-approved employment nondiscrimination policy in the organization's by-laws, employee manual or other official source stating explicitly that employees will not be discriminated against based on sexual orientation; provide services or programming within the state of Colorado.
Restrictions: Funding is not available for: organizations that are not a 501(c)3 public charity; lesbian, gay, bisexual, and transgender, or HIV/AIDS organizations; housing developments; emergency requests; endowments; individuals; major capital campaigns or projects; golf tournaments; film production or promotion.
Geographic Focus: Colorado
Samples: National Assoc of People With AIDS (Washington, DC)—for programs related to HIV/AIDS, $15,000 (2003); Human Rights Campaign Foundation (Washington, DC)—for programs supporting lesbian, gay, bisexual, and transgender people, $100,000 (2003); Gay and Lesbian Fund of Colorado (CO)—for leadership-development activities, $26,500 distributed among seven organizations (2003); AIDS Resource Ctr of Wisconsin (Milwaukee, WI)—for HIV/AIDS prevention and human services programs, $60,000 (2003).
Contact: Grants Manager, Gay & Lesbian Fund for Colorado, (800) 964-5643 or (719) 473-4455 fax: (719) 473-2254; email: info@gayandlesbianfund.org
Internet: http://www.gillfoundation.org/glfc_grants/glfc_grants_show.htm?doc_id=408610&cat_id=1394
Sponsor: Gill Foundation
315 East Costilla Street
Colorado Springs, CO 80903

Gilroy and Lillian P. Roberts Charitable Foundation Grants 1614

The foundation awards grants to eligible nonprofit organizations in its areas of interest, including arts and fine arts, health care and health organizations, higher education, Jewish temples and organizations, and social services. Types of support include annual campaigns, capital campaigns, continuing support, fellowships, general operating grants, professorships, program development, and scholarships. Most grants are awarded in Montgomery and Delaware Counties, PA. There are no application deadlines or forms.
Restrictions: Individuals are not eligible.
Geographic Focus: Pennsylvania
Samples: Temple University (Philadelphia, PA)—for Merves Professorship in Accounting, $155,000 (2003).
Amount of Grant: $408,750 total
Contact: Stanley Merves, Treasurer, (610) 668-1998
Sponsor: Gilroy and Lillian P. Roberts Charitable Foundation
101 W Elm Street, Suite 500
Conshohocken, PA 19428

Gina Finzi Memorial Student Summer Fellowship 1615

Fellowships are awarded to encourage clinical, basic or psychosocial research related to the causes, treatments, prevention, or cure of lupus. Awards are made in May to the top 10 applicants for support during the summer months. Application materials are available in December of each year. There are no renewals; applicant must submit a new proposal.
Requirements: Junior investigators, defined as assistant professor and below rank if in academic medicine, are eligible to apply.
Amount of Grant: $2000
Date(s) Application is Due: Mar 15
Contact: Grants Coordinator, (202) 349-1155; fax: (202) 349-1156; email: Finzifellowship@lupus.org
Internet: http://www.lupus.org/research/studentannounc.html
Sponsor: Lupus Foundation of America
2000 L St NW, Suite 710
Washington, DC 20036-4916

Ginn Foundation Grants 1616

The foundation's mission is to address educational and community-based health care needs through supporting effective programs and services that bring about long-term solutions for individuals and the community, principally in Cuyahoga County, OH. The Foundation will consider not only grants to academic institutions, but also to organizations that meet non-academic educational needs, such as, programs that address issues of disease avoidance, child and family counseling, after-school training, arts, housing, and employment. Preference in all of these areas will be given to organizations and programs that serve low-income recipients. Faxed applications will not be considered. Application information is available online.
Requirements: Nonprofit organizations in Cuyahoga County, OH, may apply. Consideration will also be given to trustee-sponsored grants to similar types of organizations in the Chicago, Washington, DC, and Minneapolis-St. Paul metropolitan areas.
Restrictions: The foundation will not fund requests for support of advocacy activities. Nor will it make grants to endowment, capital, or annual fund campaigns. The foundation will not fund special events or attendance at conferences or symposia.
Geographic Focus: District of Columbia; Illinois; Minnesota; Ohio
Samples: Bellflower Center for the Prevention of Abuse, Cleveland, OH, $10,000—general operating support for support services directly addressing healthy child development through the prevention & treatment of child abuse (2008); Cleveland Playhouse, Cleveland, OH, $15,000—collaboration with Cleveland School of the Arts (2008); Cleveland Hearing & Speech, Cleveland, OH, $15,000—Speech-Language Pathology Program (2008).
Amount of Grant: $5,000-$30,000 average
Date(s) Application is Due: Mar 15; Sep 15
Contact: Walter Pope Ginn, Trustee; email: info@ginnfoundation.org
Internet: http://www.ginnfoundation.org/index.html
Sponsor: Ginn Foundation
13938 A Cedar Road, P.O. Box 239
Cleveland Heights, OH 44118

Giving in Action Society Children & Youth with Special Needs Grants 1617

Giving in Action Society is a charitable organization established by Vancouver Foundation in 2006. The Society provides grants directly to individuals and families in B.C. The Children and Youth with Special Needs Fund provides grants to families who have children or youth (newborn to 19 years) with special needs living at home. The Fund offers one-time capital grants to help enhance or improve the individual's health, development or ability to participate in daily activities at home, in school and in the community. Eligible expenses may include such things as home renovations and vehicle modifications. This Fund defines children and youth with special needs as those who have significant impairments in one or more of the following areas: health,

cognition, communication, sensory motor, social/emotional/behavioural or self help. The Children and Youth with Special Needs Fund helps address family needs that are not currently met through government-funded programs. If a family receives support from other government-funded programs, they can apply to the Fund for grants but only if the funds will complement — versus duplicate — the government support. The Fund was established with financial assistance from the B.C. Ministry of Children and Family Development.
Requirements: Only residents of B.C. are eligible to apply. The Children and Youth with Special Needs Fund provides grants to families who have children or youth (newborn to 19 years) with special needs living at home. There is a two-stage application process. The first stage, submit a Letter of Inquiry, consisting of an informal proposal to determine basic suitability and eligibility. The second stage is a full application. If your Letter of Inquiry fits within the funding guidelines you will be sent a grant application form with specific instructions for completion. You have 6 months to submit your application.
Contact: Faye Wightman President and CEO, Vancouver Foundation; (866) 523-3157 or (604) 683-3157; fax: (604) 683-3134
Internet: http://www.givinginaction.ca/ourprograms/specialneeds.htm
Sponsor: Giving in Action Society, Vancouver Foundation
Suite 1200-555 West Hastings Street, Box 12132 Harbour Centre
Vancouver BC V6B 4N6 Canada

Giving in Action Society Family Independence Grants **1618**
Giving in Action Society is a charitable organization established by Vancouver Foundation in 2006. The Society provides grants directly to individuals and families in B.C. The Family Independence Fund helps families throughout the province who have children or adults with developmental disabilities living at home. Grants from the Family Independence Fund help with the ongoing care of the relative by providing support for projects such as home renovations — including lifts, elevators, ramps, flooring, door widening or vehicle modifications — that enable the individual with the developmental disability to live in the family home and access their community. Preference is given to families that indicate their request for support is part of a long- term plan for their relative. Note that families who receive support from other government-funded programs are still eligible for Family Independence Fund grants. However these additional funds must complement — versus duplicate — the government support.
Requirements: Only residents of B.C. are eligible to apply. The Family Independence Fund supports a child/relative who has a developmental disability, defined as: concurrent with impaired adaptive functioning; low IQ; manifests before the age of 18. There is a two-stage application process. The first stage, submit a Letter of Inquiry, consisting of an informal proposal to determine basic suitability and eligibility. The second stage is a full application. If your Letter of Inquiry fits within the funding guidelines you will be sent a grant application form with specific instructions for completion. You have 6 months to submit your application.
Contact: Faye Wightman President and CEO, Vancouver Foundation; (866) 523-3157 or (604) 683-3157; fax: (604) 683-3134
Internet: http://www.givinginaction.ca/ourprograms/familyindependencefund.htm
Sponsor: Giving in Action Society, Vancouver Foundation
Suite 1200-555 West Hastings Street, Box 12132 Harbour Centre
Vancouver BC V6B 4N6 Canada

Giving Sum Annual Grant **1619**
Giving Sum is an organization of next generation givers working together to identify challenges in the community and to address them through education, engagement, inspiration and grants. Giving Sum is a charitable giving vehicle pooling resources raised through memberships, sponsorships, and fundraisers to establish annual grants for recipients selected by the organization and its members. Each year Giving Sum will grant 100 percent of its membership contributions to a nonprofit organization in Indianapolis working towards change. Members will be proactive in searching out these organizations in the greater Indianapolis area and having them apply.
Requirements: To be eligible, organizations must be recognized by the Internal Revenue Service as a public charity under sections 501(c)3 and 509(a)(1), (2), or (3) of the Internal Revenue Code, and provide a copy of their determination letter from the Internal Revenue Service. Organizations or the proposed project must serve audiences within the greater Indianapolis area, including the counties of: Boone, Hamilton, Hancock, Hendricks, Johnson, Marion, Morgan and Shelby. Eligible nonprofit organizations may submit only one application to request a grant of $50,000 (Money), volunteer hours (Time) and advocacy efforts (Voice) from Giving Sum to support general operations or special projects in one of Giving Sum's five Focus Areas (Arts, Culture & Humanities, Civic & Community Development, Education, Environment, and Health & Human Services). Each organization must select one of the above focus areas in which to apply. Applicants should select the focus area which best describes the primary operations or mission of their organization. If your organization and/or request is multi-disciplinary, select the category which best describes the activities that will be carried out using the Giving Sum grant. Preliminary review of the applications occurs within each of the five focus areas. Preference will be given to applications that meaningfully and creatively engage Giving Sum members in innovative, high-impact initiatives.
Restrictions: Grant funds may not be used to lobby or otherwise attempt to influence legislation, to influence the outcome of any public election, or to carry on any voter registration drive.
Geographic Focus: Indiana
Samples: 2009 - Starfish Initiative: $50,000 grant for a leadership camp for up to 300 academically promising, economically disadvantaged high school students, attending more than 30 different high schools in greater Indianapolis. 2008 - Coburn Place: $50,000 toward a playground for the children of Coburn Place.
Amount of Grant: $50,000
Contact: Ryan Brady, Senior Donor Services Advisor; Central Indiana Community Foundation; (317) 634-2423; email: grants@givingsum.org
Internet: http://givingsum.org/grants.asp
Sponsor: Giving Sum
c/o CICF, 615 N. Alabama Street, Suite 119
Indianapolis, IN 46204-1498

Gladys Brooks Foundation Grants **1620**
At the beginning of each year, the Foundation Board determines a limited scope of activities for which it will consider grant applications. Current giving will be in the fields of libraries, education, hospitals, and clinics. Applications will be considered where: outside funding (including governmental) is not available; the project will be largely funded by the grant unless the grant request covers a discrete component of a larger project; and the funds will be used for capital projects including equipment or endowments. The Foundation's application form must be used and is available online. Electronic submissions are not acceptable.
Requirements: The foundation makes grants to nonprofit, private, publicly supported, tax-exempt organizations located in Connecticut, Delaware, Florida, Illinois, Indiana, Louisiana, Maine, Maryland, Massachusetts, New Hampshire, New Jersey, New York, Ohio, Pennsylvania, Rhode Island, Tennessee, and Vermont.
Restrictions: Applications for direct salary support will not be accepted. No portion of grants shall be appropriated as an administrative or processing fee, for overseeing the project or for its general overhead.
Geographic Focus: Connecticut; Delaware; Florida; Illinois; Indiana; Louisiana; Maine; Maryland; Massachusetts; New Hampshire; New Jersey; New York; Ohio; Pennsylvania; Rhode Island; Tennessee; Vermont
Samples: Hobart and William Smith College (Geneva, NY)—for endowed arts scholarships, $100,000.
Amount of Grant: $50,000-$100,000
Date(s) Application is Due: Jun 1
Contact: Jessica Rutledge, (516) 746-6103
Internet: http://www.gladysbrooksfoundation.org
Sponsor: Gladys Brooks Foundation
1055 Franklin Avenue, Suite 208
Garden City, NY 11530

Glaucoma Foundation Grants **1621**
The foundation funds research initiatives to determine the causes of glaucoma, to improve methods of treatment, and to develop cures for the various kinds of glaucoma. Two areas of particular focus are: optic nerve rescue and restoration—research into new approaches designed to protect the optic nerve against glaucomatous damage, to restore vision lost to glaucoma and eventually reverse blindness by restoring or regenerating the function of the optic nerve cells, and to explore the feasibility of achieving transplantation of optic nerve cells; and molecular genetics—research into the genetic causes of the various forms of glaucoma, particularly the identification of the responsible genes, with the long-term goal of finding ways to reverse these genetic defects. Grants are awarded for a one-year period and are renewable. Guidelines and application are available online.
Requirements: Applicants must have a full time faculty position or the equivalent.
Restrictions: The foundation does not provide funds for investigator salaries, travel, overhead, or other indirect costs.
Amount of Grant: $40,000 - $50,000 range
Date(s) Application is Due: Mar 1; Sep 1
Contact: Kira A. Zmuda, Director of Research Programs: (212) 651-2509; email: kzmuda@glaucomafoundation.org
Internet: http://www.glaucomafoundation.org/Grant_Application.htm
Sponsor: Glaucoma Foundation Grants
80 Maiden Lane, Suite 700
New York, NY 10038

Glaucoma Research Pilot Project Grants **1622**
These grants provide funds to encourage innovative and pilot research, as well as to aid ongoing studies that seek to protect and restore the optic nerve, accurately monitor glaucoma's progression, find the genes responsible for the glaucoma, understand the intraocular pressure system and develop better treatments, and determine the risk factors for glaucoma damage.
Requirements: Applicants must have a graduate degree.
Restrictions: Funding is not granted for equipment purchases, overhead commercial applications, or indirect costs.
Amount of Grant: $40,000
Date(s) Application is Due: Aug 1
Contact: Jennifer Rulon; (800) 826-6693 or (415) 986-3162; fax: (415) 986-3763; email: research@glaucoma.org
Internet: http://www.glaucoma.org/research/index.php
Sponsor: Glaucoma Research Foundation
251 Post Street, Suite 600
San Francisco, CA 94108

GlaxoSmithKline Corporate Grants **1623**
In the United States, GlaxoSmithKline Corporate makes charitable contributions through its U.S. Contributions Committee. Requests for U.S.-based community partnerships with nonprofit organizations should address issues in one of four general areas: education—science education, K-12 literacy, teacher professional development;

health and human services—child health or prevention and access to health care for women related to breast or gynecologic cancers, targeting the needs of underserved and diverse populations; arts and culture—local organizations in the Greater Philadelphia and the Research Triangle Park areas, based on local needs, focusing on public school educational outreach; and civic and community—local organizations in the Greater Philadelphia and the Research Triangle Park areas, based on local needs.
Requirements: Organizations based in the United States that have a 501(c)3 IRS designation and that meet GSK's corporate criteria for funding may complete an application. Funding for the arts and civic programs is concentrated exclusively in the Greater Philadelphia and Research Triangle Park areas where employees live and work.
Restrictions: As a matter of policy, grants are not provided for general operating expenses or capital building costs, and they are not made to individuals. Grants are not given to political, religious, fraternal, profit-making, discriminatory, hobby-oriented, or tax-subsidized organizations.
Geographic Focus: Pennsylvania
Amount of Grant: $15.3 million total
Contact: Mary Anne Rhyne, Corporate Press; (919) 483-2319; fax: (919) 483-8765; email: community.partnership@gsk.com
Internet: http://us.gsk.com/html/community/community-grants-corporate.html
Sponsor: GlaxoSmithKline Corporation
P.O. Box 7929, 1 Franklin Plaza, FP2130
Philadelphia, PA 19101-7929

GlaxoSmithKline Foundation IMPACT Awards **1624**
The awards reward excellence in the delivery of nonprofit community health care. Awards are made to small and mid-size community-based health care organizations in the greater Philadelphia area and, the Research Triangle Park, North Carolina area. Selection criteria include: commitment to serving people in need; facilitating access to health care delivery, education, creative partnerships, and policy development; and demonstration of a solid record of achievement, management, and leadership. The application process for the GlaxoSmithKline 1st Annual IMPACT Awards in the Research Triangle Park, North Carolina region closed on May 15. July 15 is the deadline date for the greater Philadelphia region.
Requirements: Nominees in the following Philadelphia counties are eligible: Berks, Bucks, Chester, Delaware, Lancaster, Montgomery, or Philadelphia or in the City of Camden, NJ. Nominees in the following Research Triangle Park, North Carolina counties are: Chatham, Durham, Orange and Wake Counties. Organizations must have an operating or program budget of under $2 million and have been in existence at least five years. Nonprofit healthcare organizations must be nominated by individuals knowledgeable of the complexities and challenges of healthcare delivery in their communities.
Geographic Focus: Pennsylvania
Amount of Grant: $40,000
Date(s) Application is Due: May 15; Jul 15
Contact: Mary Anne Rhyne, Corporate Press; (919) 483-2319; fax: (919) 483-8765; email: community.partnership@gsk.com
Internet: http://www.gsk-us.com/html/community/community-healthcare-awards.html
Sponsor: GlaxoSmithKline Foundation
P.O. Box 7929, 1 Franklin Plaza, FP2130
Philadelphia, PA 19101-7929

Glazer Family Foundation Grants **1625**
The foundation awards grants to eligible Florida nonprofit organizations for programs focused on youth and families in the areas of general health, safety, education, and recreation. Types of support include grants, contributions, tickets, and special programs. Proposals are accepted May 1 through July 1 and September 1 through November 1. Annual deadline dates may vary; contact program staff for exact dates.
Requirements: Florida nonprofit organizations serving the greater Tampa Bay and West Central areas are eligible.
Restrictions: Grants do not support general fundraising drives, celebrations, administrative/training costs, capital expenditures, sponsorships, individual medical needs, scholarships, research, political activities, conferences, and university capital campaigns.
Geographic Focus: Florida
Amount of Grant: $5000 maximum
Date(s) Application is Due: Jul 1; Nov 1
Contact: Grants Administrator, (813) 870-2700 ext 275; fax: (813) 554-1324
Internet: http://www.glazerfamilyfoundation.com/GuidelinesforGrants.aspx
Sponsor: Glazer Family Foundation
One Buccaneer Pl
Tampa, FL 33607

Glendale Community Foundation Grants **1626**
The Foundation awards grants in the following areas of interest: arts and culture; civic; disabled/handicapped; education programs; health; homeless services; human services; senior services; student aid; and youth services. Application information is available online.
Requirements: Nonprofit, tax-exempt organizations that serve the Glendale areas (La Crescenta, La Canada Flintridge, Montrose, and Verdugo City) are eligible.
Restrictions: Other than student loans or scholarships, the foundation generally does not make grants to individuals, funding for religious or political purposes, or for budget deficits or projects that usually are the responsibility of a public agency.
Geographic Focus: California
Samples: Camp Fire Council of the Foothills (Glendale, CA)—to purchase a computer and printer, $1250.; VNACare (Glendale, CA)—to purchase handheld computers for nurses, $3500.; YMCA (Glendale, CA)—to purchase computers and peripherals in the first phase of a two-year technology upgrade, $10,000.
Date(s) Application is Due: Feb 1; Apr 2; Jun 1; Aug 1; Oct 1; Dec 3
Contact: Executive Director, (818) 241-8040; fax: (818) 241-8045; email: info@glendalecommunityfoundation.org
Internet: http://www.glendalecommunityfoundation.org/grants.htm
Sponsor: Glendale Community Foundation
P.O. Box 313
Glendale, CA 91209-0313

Glenn/AFAR Breakthroughs in Gerontology Awards **1627**
The goal of the program is to provide timely support to a small number of pilot research programs that may be of high risk but offer significant promise of yielding transforming discoveries in the fundamental biology of aging. The hope is that one or more of the funded research projects will lead to major new insights into the molecular factors that coordinate aging in multiple cells and tissues, and the ways in which the aging process is differentially timed in long-lived species. Projects that focus on genetic controls of aging and longevity, on delay of aging by pharmacological agents or dietary means, or that elucidate the mechanisms by which alterations in hormones, anti-oxidant defenses, or repair processes promote longevity are all well within the intended scope of this competition. Projects that focus instead on specific diseases or on assessment of health care strategies will receive much lower priority, unless the research plan makes clear and direct connections to fundamental issues in the biology of aging. Studies of invertebrates, mice, human clinical materials, or cell lines are all potentially eligible for funding. Although preliminary data are always helpful for evaluating the feasibility of the experiments proposed, the emphasis in review will be on creativity and the likelihood that the findings will open new vistas and approaches to aging research that might merit intensive follow-up studies. Applications from individuals not previously engaged in aging research are particularly encouraged, as long as the research proposals show high promise for leading to important new discoveries in biological gerontology. The proposed research must be conducted at any type of nonprofit setting in the United States. Guidelines are available online.
Requirements: Applicants must at the time they submit their proposal be full-time faculty members at the rank of assistant professor or higher. A strong record of independent publication beyond the postdoctoral level is a requirement.
Restrictions: Applicants who are employees in NIH Intramural are not eligible.
Amount of Grant: $200,000
Date(s) Application is Due: Dec 16
Contact: Grants Manager; (212) 703-9977 or (888) 582-2327; fax: (212) 997-0330; email: grants@afar.org or info@afar.org
Internet: http://afar.org/grants.html
Sponsor: American Federation for Aging Research
55 West 39th Street, 16th Floor
New York, NY 10018

Glenn/AFAR Research Grants for Postdoctoral Fellows **1628**
AFAR funds research projects concerned with understanding the basic mechanisms of aging. Projects investigating age-related diseases are also supported, especially if approached from the point of view of how basic aging processes may lead to these outcomes. Projects concerning mechanisms underlying common geriatric functional disorders are also encouraged. Examples of promising areas of research include aging and immune function; genetic control of longevity; neurobiology and neuropathology of aging; invertebrate or vertebrate animal models; cardiovascular aging; aging and cellular stress resistance; metabolic and endocrine changes; age-related changes in cell proliferation; caloric restriction and aging; DNA repair and control of gene expression; biology of the menopause; aging and apoptosis; and biodemographic analysis of aging. Funding begins July 1. Guidelines and application are available online.
Requirements: Postdoctoral fellows (MDs and PhDs) who will have had at least two and not more than five years of prior postdoctoral training at the time of the award are eligible.
Restrictions: Funds may not be requested for overhead or indirect costs. Fellows may not hold any concurrent foundation or not-for-profit funding.
Amount of Grant: $60,000
Date(s) Application is Due: Dec 15
Contact: Grants Manager, (212) 703-9977; fax: (212) 997-0330; email: amfedaging@aol.com
Internet: http://www.afar.org/grants.html
Sponsor: American Federation for Aging Research
70 W 40th Street
New York, NY 10018

Global Fund for Children Grants **1629**
The Fund's mission is to advance the dignity of children and youth around the world through small grants to innovative community-based organizations working with some of the world's most vulnerable children and youth. The Fund selects its grantee partners based on their potential to grow in effectiveness and to become valuable resources or models for others. Selection criteria include exceptional leadership, sound management, strong community participation, innovative and effective programs, and direct engagement with the most vulnerable children. Fund focus is on four specific issues: learning, enterprise, safety, and healthy minds and bodies. Application information is available online.

Requirements: Nonprofit organization worldwide are eligible.
Amount of Grant: $5,000-$20,000
Contact: Grants Administrator, (202) 331-9003; fax: (202) 331-9004; email: info@globalfundforchildren.org
Internet: http://www.globalfundforchildren.org/applyforagrant/index.html
Sponsor: Global Fund for Children
1101 Fourteenth Street, N.W., Suite 420
Washington, DC 20005

Goddess Scholars Grants 1630
The purpose of these grants is to develop young researchers at the entry faculty level (Instructor or Assistant Professor) who will focus a research career on studying the unique aspects of stroke in women. Such research may be basic or clinical in orientation, including areas such as mechanisms of ischemic brain injury, neuroprotective treatments, primary or secondary stroke prevention, epidemiological studies, educational programs for patients or health care providers, rehabilitation, and outcome research. The grant provides funding for two years, with potential non-competitive renewal for a third year should satisfactory progress be demonstrated. These grants are intended to provide bridging funds for individuals who are finishing or have completed residency or postdoctoral training and require additional support before their subsequent establishment as independent investigators.
Requirements: Goddess Scholar grants are targeted at individuals who: hold an M.D., Ph.D., or equivalent degree; are at the fellow, instructor, or assistant professor rank; and are within 5 years of completion of residency or post-doctoral fellowship at the time of grant activation. Individuals who are currently enrolled in a fellowship program may apply if there is assurance of a faculty position at the time of the grant's activation.
Amount of Grant: $65,000 direct salary plus research costs (e.g. research or laboratory assistant, materials, small equipment)
Contact: Erin Tower, Program/Operations Assistant; (212) 713-6789; fax: (212) 288-2160; email: erin@thegoddessfund.org
Internet: http://www.thegoddessfund.org/grants.html
Sponsor: Hazel K. Goddess Fund for Stroke Research in Women
785 Park Avenue
New York, NY 10021-3552

Godfrey Foundation Grants 1631
The Foundation, established in Wisconsin in 1945 and supported by a donation from the Fleming Companies, Inc., offers grants primarily in the Milwaukee and Waukesha, Wisconsin, region. Its major field of interest include: education; health care; human services; community development and services; and youth development programs. The major type of support comes in the form of general operations funding. An application form is required, and interested organizations should contact the Foundation for a copy. There are no particular deadlines with which to adhere, and grant amounts have ranged from $500 to $30,000.
Requirements: Applicants must be 501(c)3 organizations serving the residents of Wisconsin.
Geographic Focus: Wisconsin
Amount of Grant: $500-$30,000
Contact: Terry L. Daniels, Director; (262) 275-0458
Sponsor: Godfrey Foundation
680 Kenosha Street, P.O. Box 810
Walworth, WI 53184-0810

GoGirlGo! Ambassador Team Awards 1632
The program awards grants to teams that demonstrate leadership in their communities by inspiring girls to get involved in sports and physical activity. Its aim is to get one million inactive girls to participate in physical activity and keep another one million currently active girls from dropping out of physical activity. A total of $50,000 in grants will be awarded in recognition of the outstanding efforts of 20 teams throughout the country.
Requirements: School, amateur, community, and/or nonprofit affiliated teams whose members are all of the following are eligible: female; enrolled in 9th through 12th grade; at least 13 years old; and residents of the United States, its territories, or protectorates. Grants will be made payable to the school, nonprofit institution or 501(c)3 organization. Proof of nonprofit status and/or 501(c)3 status is required (if applicable). Complete guidelines and entry forms can be downloaded at the sponsor's website.
Restrictions: Projects must be original, current work and not previously submitted.
Amount of Grant: $2,500
Date(s) Application is Due: Jul 17
Contact: Marjorie Snyder, Chief Programs Officer; (516) 542-4700; fax: (516) 542-4716; email: info@womenssportsfoundation.org
Internet: http://www.womenssportsfoundation.org/Content/Grants-And-Scholarships/Grants/GoGirlGo-Ambassador-Team-Awards.aspx
Sponsor: Women's Sports Foundation
1899 Hempstead Turnpike, Suite 400
East Meadow, NY 11554

Golden State Warriors Foundation Grants 1633
The foundation committed to positively impacting the communities of Oakland and the greater San Francisco Bay Area by providing financial assistance and opportunities to other non-profit civic and community organizations that benefit and enrich the lives of children, youth and those in need. By providing financial support and unique resources, the Foundation endeavors to meet the social, educational and cultural needs of the community. Although the Warriors Foundation will not be accepting grant applications until the beginning of the 2007-08 fiscal year, it remains committed to providing assistance and in-kind support to Bay Area nonprofit organizations through the donation of tickets, autographed memorabilia, promotional items, sponsorships, and player and talent appearances. Application information and forms are available on the Web site.
Requirements: 501(c)3 nonprofit organizations that provide programs and services in the greater San Francisco Bay area are eligible.
Restrictions: Grants do not support individuals; schools; political, labor, religious, or fraternal activities; endowments; fundraising events; government agencies; or organizations with discriminatory or unlawful practices.
Geographic Focus: California
Amount of Grant: $375,000 total
Contact: Angela Cohan, President, (510) 986-5307; email: community_web@gs-warriors.com
Internet: http://www.nba.com/warriors/community/Warriors_Foundation-011024.html
Sponsor: Golden State Warriors Foundation
1011 Broadway
Oakland, CA 94607-4019

Goldhirsh Foundation Brain Tumor Research Grants 1634
The Goldhirsh Foundation is interested in providing strategic investment in both pediatric and adult brain tumor research to accelerate progress toward more effective treatment for malignant diffuse glioma tumors. Applications are encouraged from investigators working in the continuum between basic research and clinical application, integrating and translating knowledge in various disciplines into meaningful progress for patients. The Initial Proposal Application must be submitted by Thursday, January 7, 12:00 Noon, U.S. and Canada Eastern Time (GMT-5), to the online application system. Applicants who are invited to submit Full Proposals will be notified by email in early March. Up to three investigators will receive grants of $400,000 U.S.D (inclusive of 10% indirect costs) over two years at $200,000 U.S.D per year. The Foundation also makes awards of $100,000 U.S.D (inclusive of 10% indirect costs) for one-year pilot studies. Please note that The Goldhirsh Foundation is not offering the three-year $600,000 U.S.D award for the 2010 Grant Cycle.
Requirements: The Goldhirsh Foundation is accepting Initial Proposal Applications from applicants who meet the following eligibility requirements: have an M.D. and/or Ph.D. degree(s) or equivalent degree; hold a faculty appointment at a nonprofit academic, medical or research institution in the United States, Canada or Israel. The applicant may collaborate with investigators from other institutions and these institutions may include for-profit companies; preference will be given to originality of ideas, regardless of applicant seniority; eligibility is not limited to those investigators currently working in brain tumor research. Investigators from other fields are encouraged to apply with proposals directly relevant to malignant diffuse glioma tumors; projects must be relevant to tumors within the category of malignant diffuse gliomas, i.e., glioblastomas, diffuse astrocytomas (WHO grade III), oligoastrocytomas (WHO grade III), and oligodendrogliomas (WHO grade III).
Restrictions: Projects focusing on WHO grade I-II gliomas, non-glial neuroepithelial tumors, meningeal tumors, nerve sheath tumors, CNS lymphomas, germ-cell tumors and tumors of the sella region are beyond the scope of the grant program. Projects that characterize genes and gene products of normal cellular development are not eligible, nor are epidemiological studies.
Samples: Lara Collier, Ph.D., University of Wisconsin-Madison, $600,000— Genetic Approaches to Identify and Characterize Potential Drug Targets for High-grade Gliomas (2009); Al Charest, Ph.D., Tufts Medical Center, $100,000—Targeting Cancer Stem Cells in a Pre-Clinical Mouse Model of Glioblastoma Multiforme Using Therapeutic Nanoparticles (2009).
Amount of Grant: $600,000 maximum
Date(s) Application is Due: Jan 7
Contact: Sally E. McNagny, Director; (617) 279-2254; fax: (617) 423-4619; email: smcnagny@goldhirshfoundation.org
Internet: http://www.goldhirshfoundation.org/application_information.htm
Sponsor: Goldhirsh Foundation
95 Berkeley Street, Suite 201
Boston, MA 02116

Goldman Philanthropic Partnerships Program 1635
Since its founding, the Program has solicited, validated and helped donors co-fund innovative research with the potential to quickly find cures for life-altering diseases, and supported these donors using for-profit business tools to insure that the research and philanthropic goals are met through proper project and resource management. The Program provides funding research for cures for a range of catastrophic diseases by exploring groundbreaking research in all disciplines of medicine, including those areas of research outside of conventional medicine such as alternative medicine. The Program usually co-funds a venture with at least one organizational, institutional, or corporate partner. The Partnerships maintains a strong interest in diseases of children and young adults, although it will fund research into any patient population where it believes there is a high likelihood of return on disease prevention, treatment or cure.
Contact: Dr. Bruce E. Bloom, President; (312) 601-8856 or (312) 780-3440; fax: (312) 780-3459; email: bruce@goldmanpartnerships.org
Internet: http://www.goldmanpartnerships.org/aboutus.html
Sponsor: Goldman Philanthropic Partnerships
70 West Madison Street, Suite 1500
Chicago, IL 60602

Good Samaritan Foundation Inc Grants 1636

The foundation supports health care projects aimed at the low-income population in Kentucky. It generally supports primary and preventive care and professional training for medical personnel who will work in an underserved area, and limits its grants to charitable and educational activities related to health care, health education, and research in Kentucky. Preference is given to activities serving Lexington, and central and eastern Kentucky. Grants should be used to make significant contributions to a community or area by improving access, delivery, affordability, and the quality of health care in Kentucky. Guidelines are available on the Web site.

Requirements: An applicant must be 501(c)3 tax-exempt organization or an appropriate public charity in Kentucky.

Restrictions: The foundation does not support staff funding within an organization; individuals; endowment funds; indirect costs; major organizations (e.g. heart funds, cancer societies, etc.); hospitals, colleges, or universities; activities that serve a small number of people or have a high per person cost; activities that compete with or duplicate a publicly supported program such as Medicare, Medicaid, Health Department, or other; building/capital improvement projects; custodial care, adult or child day care, retirement facilities, or nursing homes; benefit fund-raisers, testimonials, recognition dinners, or events; program advertising, tickets, or raffles.

Geographic Focus: Kentucky

Date(s) Application is Due: Jan 10

Contact: Joyce Triantafilou, Administrative Assistant , (859) 255-1691; fax: (859) 254-7337; email: joyce@gsfky.org

Internet: http://www.gsfky.org/grants.htm

Sponsor: Good Samaritan Foundation Inc
270 S Limestone Street
Lexington, KY 40508-2566

Good Samaritan Inc Grants 1637

Good Samaritan, Inc. is an independent foundation, which was incorporated in 1938, in Delaware. This foundation gives primarily in the northeastern region of the United States: Pennsylvania, New Jersey, Delaware and Maryland. The foundation field of interest include: higher education; cancer research; secondary school/education; human services; hospitals (general); and the economically disadvantaged. Support is offered in the form of: endowments; professorships; program development; seed money: and general/operating support grants.

Requirements: 501(c)3 nonprofit organizations are eligible.

Restrictions: No grants to individuals, or for building funds, capital assets or conferences.

Amount of Grant: $10,000-$200,000 range

Date(s) Application is Due: Apr 1; Oct 1

Contact: Edmund Carpenter II, President, (302) 654-7558; fax: (302) 654-2376

Sponsor: Good Samaritan Inc
600 Center Mill Road
Wilmington, DE 19807-1502

Goodrich Corporation Foundation Grants 1638

The Foundation makes charitable grants in four categories: education; arts and culture; civic and community; and health and human services. Preference shall be given to requests for projects or programs in areas having a significant number of employees, employees serving on boards of charitable organizations or other noticeable corporate presence. The Foundation staff accepts and reviews grant requests quarterly. To request funding, applicants will need to complete the application form which is available online. Telephone and email requests or inquiries are not accepted.

Requirements: 501(c)3 tax-exempt organizations are eligible.

Restrictions: The foundation generally will not support: multiyear grants in excess of five years; individuals, private foundations, endowments, churches or religious programs, fraternal/social/ labor/veterans organizations; groups with unusually high fundraising or administrative expenses; political parties, candidates, or lobbying activities; travel funds for tours, exhibitions, or trips by individuals or special interest groups; organizations that discriminate because of race, color, religion, national origin, or areas covered by applicable federal, state, or local laws; local athletic/sports programs or equipment, courtesy advertising benefits, raffle tickets and other fundraising events; organizations that receive sizable portions of their support through municipal, county, state, or federal dollars; individual United Way agencies that already benefit from Goodrich contributions to the United Way; or international organizations.

Date(s) Application is Due: Feb 1; Aug 1

Contact: Foundation Contact, fax: (704) 423-7011

Internet: http://www.goodrich.com/CDA/GeneralContent/0,1136,59,00.html

Sponsor: Goodrich Foundation
Four Coliseum Centre, 2730 West Tyvola Road
Charlotte, NC 28217-4578

Goodyear Tire Grants 1639

Requests for charitable gifts are required to meet guidelines of strategic giving based on safety by focusing on safety programs plus at least one additional category (civic and community; culture and the arts, education, or health and human services) of giving and/or provide volunteer opportunities for company associates which are appropriately aligned with the company's strategy.

Requirements: 501(c)3 tax-exempt organizations in Goodyear communities are eligible. Organizations in the greater Akron, OH area should send requests to: Faith Stewart, Director, Goodyear Tire and Rubber Company, 1144 East Market Street, D/798, Akron, OH, 44316. Organizations in U.S. communities where Goodyear has plants and major facilities should contact the local plant manager's office for mailing instructions.

Restrictions: Grants cannot be made to: organizations outside of communities in which plants or principal offices are located; individuals or to organizations on behalf of an individual; national, political, labor, fraternal, social, veterans organizations; individual schools within public or private school systems; athletic programs/extracurricular activities, travel or exchange programs; endowments or for debt reduction; religious organizations or endeavors; major hospitals or medical center; second parties except specialized organizations.

Contact: Faith Stewart, Director, Global Community Enterprise, Diversity & Philanthropy

Internet: http://www.goodyear.com/corporate/about/about_community.html

Sponsor: Goodyear Tire and Rubber Company
1144 East Market Street D/798
Akron, OH 44316

Google Grants Beta 1640

The Google Grants program supports organizations sharing their philosophy of community service to help the world in areas such as science and technology, education, global public health, the environment, youth advocacy, and the arts. Google Grants has awarded AdWords advertising to non-profit groups whose missions range from animal welfare to literacy, from supporting homeless children to promoting HIV education. Recipients use their award of free AdWords advertising on Google.com to raise awareness and increase traffic. Application available online only.

Requirements: In the United States – Organizations must have current 501(c)3 status, as assigned by the Internal Revenue Service to be considered for a Google Grant. Outside the U.S – currently accepting applications from eligible charitable organizations based in Australia, Brazil, Canada, Denmark, France, Germany, India, Ireland, Italy, Japan, the Netherlands, Spain, Sweden, Switzerland and the United Kingdom.

Restrictions: Organizations already participating in the Google AdSense program are not eligible for Google Grants consideration. In addition, organizations that are either religious or political in nature are not eligible, including those groups focused primarily on lobbying for political or policy change.

Samples: Three award recipients have achieved these results: - Room to Read, which educates children in Vietnam, Nepal, India and Cambodia, attracted a sponsor who clicked on its AdWords ad. He has donated funds to support the education of 25 girls for the next 10 years. - The U.S. Fund for UNICEF's e-commerce site, Shop UNICEF, has experienced a 43 percent increase in sales over the previous year. - CoachArt, supporting children with life-threatening illnesses through art and athletics programs, has seen a 60 to 70 percent increase in volunteers.

Amount of Grant: Each organization awarded a Google Grant receives at least three months of in-kind advertising.

Contact: Google Grants Team, email: googlegrants@google.com

Internet: http://www.google.com/grants/

Sponsor: Google
1600 Amphitheatre Parkway
Mountain View, CA 94043

GPP Charles E. Culpeper Foundation Biomedical Pilot Initiative Grants 1641

The initiative is designed to encourage the investigation of novel ideas in cures for disease, particularly in the areas of molecular genetics, bio-engineering, and molecular pharmacology. Research into complimentary and alternative medicine will also be considered. Grants will be made on a one-time basis with the possibility for renewal for a second year upon reapplication. No more than 8 percent of the grant may be allocated to cover indirect costs. The purpose of these grants is to explore new and even untested hypotheses, thus substantial preliminary information is not required. Proposals are accepted throughout the year and each successful

Requirements: Nonprofit health care organizations, accredited medical schools, and universities in the United States are eligible.

Samples: Dr. Natalia Broude, Boston U (MA)—to support a study that will develop an innovative test for SARS, which would hook a molecule that glows in the dark to a protein that would attach a specific spot on the SARS gene, $25,000 (2005); Ji-Xin Cheng, PhD, Purdue University (West Lafayette, IN)—to support a project that will develop a new highly sensitive microscope for the imaging of molecules using vibrational imaging, $25,000 (2005); Dr. Gregory Crawford, Brown U (Providence, RI)—to create a device that will take a photo of the lining of the lower eyelid using a small camera, resulting in accuracy similar to the current lab test when the physician draws blood from the patient, $25,000 (2005). .

Amount of Grant: $25,000 maximum

Date(s) Application is Due: Nov 16

Contact: Grants Administrator, (847) 948-5512; fax: (847) 948-5516

Internet: http://www.goldmanpartnerships.org/Culpeper/CulpeperBiomedicalPilotInitiativegrants.htm

Sponsor: Goldman Philanthropic Partnerships
155 N Pfingsten Road, Suite 109
Deerfield, IL 60015

Graco Foundation Grants 1642

The Foundation's goal is to help organizations grow their ability to serve community needs through grants specifically aimed at expanding or enhancing services to clients, with particular focus on capital projects and technology needs. The Foundation addresses the needs of the community in the following areas: self-sufficiency - emphasizing educational programs, human service programs that promote self-sufficiency, and sports/

youth development programs; and civic projects - focusing on healthy communities. Projects that improve the community will be given special consideration. Application information is available online.
Requirements: IRS 501(c)3 organizations in company-operating areas may apply.
Restrictions: Grants are not awarded for: organizations or causes that do not directly impact Graco communities; political campaigns; individuals; religious organizations for religious purposes; fund-raising; travel; special events, dinners, courtesy advertising; fraternal organizations; national or local campaigns for disease research; first time general operating grants; or product donations.
Geographic Focus: Minnesota; Ohio; South Dakota
Samples: Minneapolis Neighborhood Employment Network—for operating support, $3000.; United Negro College Fund—for scholarships, $5000.; City Inc—for renovations of its north Minneapolis facility, $125,000.
Date(s) Application is Due: Feb 1; May 1; Aug 1; Nov 1
Contact: Kristin R. Ridley, Grants Administration Manager, (612) 623-6684; email: kridley@graco.com
Internet: http://www.graco.com/Internet/T_Corp.nsf/SearchView/Foundation2006
Sponsor: Graco Foundation
P.O. Box 1441
Minneapolis, MN 55440-1441

Grammy Foundation Grants **1643**
The foundation awards grants in two program areas. Research Projects grants are made to organizations and individuals to support efforts that advance the research and/or broad- reaching implementations of original research projects related to the impact of music study on early childhood development, the human development, and the medical and occupational well-being of music professionals. Archiving and Preservation Projects grants are made to organizations and individuals to support efforts that advance the archiving and preservation of the music and recorded sound heritage of the Americas. The foundation funds preservation of original, preexisting media and source material; preservation projects that follow the recommended methodology; projects of historical, artistic, cultural, and or/national significance; and archiving projects including the rescue, organization of, and access to preexisting media and materials. Application and guidelines are available online.
Restrictions: The foundation does not fund Recording Academy chapters, trustees, governors, officers, or staff; organizations that discriminate on the basis of race, sex, religion, national origin, disability, or age; projects promoting advocacy issues; a single organization or individual for more than three consecutive years; organizations or individuals not based in the Americas; purchase of collections; recording projects, demo tapes, or performance events; proposals for commercial purposes (i.e., CD reissue or textbook/ A/V package); purchase of repairs of equipment; purchase or repairs of musical instruments; maintenance or upgrading of computer systems; competitions or any expense associated with competitions; work toward academic degrees; music education or in-residence programs; documentaries; endowments and fundraising; buildings and facilities; marketing, publicity, design costs; or projects where copyright status is unknown.
Samples: The Institute for Music & Brain Science, Boston, MA, $20,000 - this project will test whether music decreases behavioral, neurophysiological and endocrinological pain and stress caused by medically-necessary procedures. In addition, the hypothesis that humans innately prefer consonant over dissonant music will be tested (2009); Elliott Leib, San Diego, CA, $5,000 - a plan will be developed to digitally preserve material from the Trade Roots Reggae Collection (2009); Bob Moog Memorial Foundation for Electronic Music, Asheville, N.C., $15,000 - musical and historical content relative to the unique legacy of synthesizer pioneer Dr. Robert Moog will be cleaned, restored, re-housed and transferred to digital format for accessibility and long-term storage (2009).
Amount of Grant: $10,000-$40,000
Date(s) Application is Due: Oct 1
Contact: Kristin Murphy, (310) 392-3777 ext. 8662; fax: (310) 392-2188; email: grants@grammy.com
Internet: http://www.grammy.com/GRAMMY_Foundation/Grants/
Sponsor: Grammy Foundation
3030 Olympic Boulevard
Santa Monica, CA 90405

Grand Haven Area Community Foundation Grants **1644**
The community Foundation awards grants to meet the changing and emerging needs of residents of the tri-cities area in such fields as arts, education, health, the environment, youth, social services and other human needs. The Foundation encourages programs which: are collaborative, comprehensive and have potential for continuity; encourage leveraging and matching grant opportunities involving multiple funding sources; support seed money requests to assist innovative projects; encourages programs and projects focused on problem prevention rather than cure. Applicants are encouraged to call and talk with a staff member before beginning a proposal. Application information is available online.
Requirements: IRS 501(c)3 organizations working to enhance the quality of life for residents in the Tri-Cities area of Grand Haven, Spring Lake and Ferrysburg in West Michigan.
Restrictions: The Foundation does not generally fund: general operating expenses; private individuals; profit making organizations; elimination of existing financial obligations/debts/liabilities; religious programs that serve, or appear to serve, specific religious denominations; fund raising events.
Geographic Focus: Michigan
Samples: City of Grand Haven, $20,000 - restoration of the Boardwalk for the 25th Anniversary of the Connector Park Boardwalk (2008); Grand Haven Area Public Schools, $5,000 - to support pre-school scholarships (2008); Tri-Cities Area Habitat for Humanity, $39,719 - seed money for the Grand Haven ReStore (2008).
Date(s) Application is Due: Jan 7; Mar 13; Jun 26; Oct 10
Contact: Carol Bedient, Grants and Programs Director; (616) 842-6378; fax: (616) 842-9518; email: cbedient@ghacf.org or bpost@ghacf.org
Internet: http://www.ghacf.org/grants.htm
Sponsor: Grand Haven Area Community Foundation
One South Harbor Drive
Grand Haven, MI 49417

Grand Rapids Area Community Foundation Grants **1645**
The Foundation enables donors to make a difference in the community through grants, scholarships and programs. The deadline for applications is September 15th, and grants are distributed during the month of October. Specific funds include: Alzheimer's Family Support Fund; Fund for the Arts; Fund for the Community; Betty Kauppi Music Fund; Streufert Peace and Safety Fund; Warren Youngdahl Memorial Fund; and the Fund for Women. Amount of funding ranges from $500 to $3,000
Restrictions: No funding is available for individuals.
Geographic Focus: Minnesota
Amount of Grant: $3,000 maximum
Date(s) Application is Due: Sep 15
Contact: Wendy Roy, Executive Director; (218) 999-9100; fax: (218) 999-7430; email: wroy@gracf.org
Internet: http://www.gracf.org/index.php/grants-and-programs
Sponsor: Grand Rapids Area Community Foundation
350 NW First Avenue, Suite E
Grand Rapids, MN 55744

Grand Rapids Area Community Foundation Nashwauk Area Endowment Fund Grants **1646**
The Fund is interested in supporting innovative and effective ideas that support the greater Nashwauk, Minnesota area. This area includes the areas of: Nashwauk, Nashwauk Township, Buck Lake and Pengilly. The main cycle offers grants of up to $15,000, with a deadline for application November 15th. The Mini-Grant cycle offers grants of up to $5,000, with the deadline for applications being September 15th. Nonprofit organizations that serve or benefit these areas are encouraged to submit a Letter of Inquiry.
Restrictions: Grants can only be made to charitable organizations, and cannot be made to individuals.
Geographic Focus: Minnesota
Amount of Grant: $5,000-$15,000
Date(s) Application is Due: Sep 15
Contact: Wendy Roy, Executive Director; (218) 999-9100; fax: (218) 999-7430; email: wroy@gracf.org
Internet: http://www.gracf.org/index.php/grants-and-programs
Sponsor: Nashwauk Area Endowment Fund
350 NW First Ave , Suite E
Grand Rapids, MN 55744

Grand Rapids Community Foundation Grants **1647**
The Foundation impacts a wide range of nonprofit organizations in the communities they serve. Funding is in six broad categories: academic achievement; high quality of life; healthy people; economic prosperity; vibrant neighborhoods; and environmental integrity.
Requirements: IRS 501(c)3 organizations supporting residents of Kent County are eligible to apply, applications are available at the Foundation's website.
Restrictions: The Foundation does not fund one-time, special or annual events, annual operating funds, political or religious causes, or endowments.
Geographic Focus: Michigan
Contact: Marcia Rapp, Vice President, Programs; (616) 454-1751, ext. 104; fax: (616) 454-6455; email: mrapp@grfoundation.org or grfound@grfoundation.org
Internet: http://www.grfoundation.org/grants.php
Sponsor: Grand Rapids Community Foundation
185 Oakes Street SW
Grand Rapids, MI 49503

Grass Foundation Marine Biological Laboratory Fellowships **1648**
The foundation awards fellowships to encourage independent research for scientific discovery by investigators early in their careers and to increase research opportunities for persons trained for careers in neurobiological investigation. Neurobiological approaches supported include neurophysiology, membrane biophysics, integrative neurobiology and neuroethology, neuroanatomy, neuropharmacology, systems neuroscience, cellular and developmental neurobiology, and computational approaches to neural systems. Fellowships provide funds to support an investigator, his/her spouse or domestic partner, and dependent children for one summer at the Marine Biological Laboratory in Woods Hole, MA. Laboratory research space, equipment, housing and board, and travel expenses to and from the MBL are covered. Guidelines and application are available online.
Requirements: Applicants may be researchers in the late stages of predoctoral training or postdoctoral researchers. Priority is given to applicants who have demonstrated a commitment to a research career, who have no more than five years of postdoctoral research and who have no prior research experience at the Marine Biological Laboratory. All U.S. citizens, permanent residents, and foreign applicants with or able to obtain J-1

Visas for the duration of the fellowship are eligible to participate in this program. The foundation must have a copy of the J-1 Visa prior to participation in the program.
Restrictions: Applicants should not attempt to combine a fellowship at the Marine Biological Laboratory with writing a dissertation (PhD thesis).
Date(s) Application is Due: Dec 15
Contact: Fellowship Administrator, (781) 843-0219; fax: (781) 843-0474; email: grassfdn@aol.com
Internet: http://www.grassfoundation.org/fellowships/grass_fellowship/index.html
Sponsor: Grass Foundation
400 Franklin Street, Suite 302
Braintree, MA 02184

Great-West Life Grants **1649**

The program's objectives are to support organizations that meet the most vital needs in the greater Denver metro community, including access to affordable health care, shelter, nutrition and education, and to support our employees' involvement in their communities. Funding priorities are on preventive and ongoing health services, homeless shelters, food services, and keeping children in school. Support is limited to organizations providing direct services, free or charge or on a sliding scale basis, that demonstrate effectiveness in addressing the communities vital issues. There is no formal application process. Interested applicants should submit a brief concept paper.
Requirements: To be eligible for support an organization: must be a U.S. based, charity and tax-exempt under 501(c)3 of the Internal Revenue Code; must not discriminate on the basis of race, religion, gender, age, national origin, disability, or sexual orientation; must show demonstrated success in meeting the program's objectives and fall within the program's focus areas; must serve residents in areas with a Great-West presence.
Restrictions: Funding is not provided for: capital campaigns; debt financing; endowments; advertising; grant-making foundations; individuals; political organizations; exclusively religious organizations; veterans organizations; fraternal organizations.
Contact: Corporate Community Support, Human Resources, (800) 537-2033; email: greatwestcomments@gwl.com
Internet: http://www.greatwest.com/about/community_supp.htm
Sponsor: Great-West Life and Annuity Insurance Company
8515 East Orchard Road
Greenwood Village, CO 80111

Greater Bridgeport Area Foundation Community Impact Grants **1650**

The Foundation's grantmaking is guided by five key principles. The Foundation seeks to: support programs which respond effectively to current needs and emphasize community strengths; encourage collaboration and build or strengthen bridges among stakeholders; build nonprofit capacity; increase access to opportunities and resources, and improve and enrich the lives of individuals and the communities in which they work and live; and increase community knowledge regarding effective programs and strategies. The Foundation awards grants in the following areas: arts; community and economic development; education; environment; and health and human services. Instructions for submitting a LOI are available online.
Requirements: Organizations with IRS 501(c)3 status serving the Greater Bridgeport Area Foundation's nine town region - Bridgeport, Easton, Fairfield, Milford, Monroe, Shelton, Stratford, Trumbull and Westport - are eligible to submit letters of inquiry.
Restrictions: Funding is not available for: religious purposes; political campaigns; annual appeals; building fund/capital, endowments, memorial campaigns; loans or deficit financing; federal, state, or municipal agencies or departments supported by taxation; or individuals.
Geographic Focus: Connecticut
Date(s) Application is Due: Jan 15
Contact: Anne Watkins , Director of Programs, (203) 334-7511; fax: (203) 333-4652; email: awatkins@gbafoundation.org
Internet: http://www.gbafoundation.org/grant.htm
Sponsor: Greater Bridgeport Area Foundation
211 State Street, 3rd Floor
Bridgeport, CT 06604

Greater Cincinnati Foundation Priority and Small Projects/Capacity-Building Grants **1651**

Grants are awarded on a quarterly basis and support projects addressing community needs and priorities in six areas: arts and culture; community progress; education; environment; health; and human services. The Foundation looks for applicants that are established and fiscally sound with strong governance and a demonstrated organizational capacity/track record. Application information is available online. Nonprofits seeking grants of up to $20,000 can get a decision in eight weeks or less; all other grants above $20,000 will be awarded twice a year.
Requirements: The Foundation awards grants to qualified 501(c)3 nonprofit organizations in eight counties: Butler, Clermont, Hamilton, and Warren, Ohio; Boone, Kenton and Campbell, Kentucky; and Dearborn, Indiana.
Restrictions: Funds are not available for: individuals; units of government or government agencies; religious organizations for religious purposes; ongoing operating expenses of nonprofit organizations; annual fund raising drives, event sponsorship or underwriting; stand-alone books, films or videos unless part of a more comprehensive program activity; stand-alone travel expenses for conferences or educational purposes unless part of a more comprehensive program activity; regular operating costs or capital projects for individual public, private or parochial schools, universities, hospitals, nursing or retirement homes; endowments; scholarships; loans; scholarly or medical research; partisan political advocacy; debt retirement or funding of an activity after it is completed.
Geographic Focus: Indiana; Kentucky; Ohio
Amount of Grant: $10,000-$100,000 range
Contact: Kay Pennington, Community Investment Coordinator; (513) 241-2880; fax: (513) 852-6886; email: penningtonk@greatercincinnatifdn.org
Internet: http://www.greatercincinnatifdn.org/page10004265.cfm
Sponsor: Greater Cincinnati Foundation
200 West Fourth Street
Cincinnati, OH 45202

Greater Green Bay Community Foundation Grants **1652**

The Foundation provides assistance to worthy charities serving the people of Brown, Kewaunee, and Oconto counties, Wisconsin. The Foundation's areas of interest are: arts and culture; community development; cultural and ethnic diversity; health and human services; historic preservation; education; and the environment. The Foundation also awards special funds to projects that address issues involved with Alzheimer's Disease, Diabetes, and Hospice. Applicants should share their ideas with the Foundation before completing a formal application. Application information is available online.
Requirements: Eligible recipients meet the following criteria: are tax exempt and have 501(c)3 status; primarily serve residents of Brown, Oconto, and Kewaunee counties; and operate, choose a governing board, and provide services without discrimination.
Restrictions: Funding is not available for: annual or capital campaigns; projects that promote any religious belief; individuals; debt retirement; lobbying; activities that occur prior to the awarding of the grant; efforts substantially serving people outside of Brown, Kewaunee, and Oconto counties.
Geographic Focus: Wisconsin
Samples: Children's Museum of Green Bay (Green Bay, WI)—for the "Pets are People Too" Exhibit, $7,000.; Greater Green Bay YMCA (Green Bay, WI)—for Swim Smart & Family Nights, $3,367.
Amount of Grant: $1,000-$10,000
Date(s) Application is Due: Jan 15; Apr 15; Jul 15; Oct 15
Contact: Lora Warner, Program Officer, (920) 432-0800; fax: (920) 432-5577; email: lora@ggbcf.org
Internet: http://www.ggbcf.org
Sponsor: Greater Green Bay Community Foundation
301 West Walnut Street, Suite 350
Green Bay, WI 54303

Greater Milwaukee Foundation Grants **1653**

The Foundation places its highest funding priority on supporting creative efforts to address issues of poverty in the community, particularly grants focused on education, employment, and strengthening children, youth and families. Lower priority is given to projects that do not meet the above criteria and/or do not address issues of persistent poverty. In addition, the Foundation places special emphasis on programs that accomplish the following: improving understanding among people of different backgrounds through support of efforts addressing issues of racial, cultural and economic diversity; and strengthening the voluntary sector by supporting efforts to enhance the management capacities of nonprofit organizations, promote philanthropy, and encourage civic involvement and community service. Application information is available online.
Requirements: Grants are made only to nonprofit organizations exempt from federal taxation under Section 501(c)3 of the Internal Revenue Code and, on occasion, to governmental agencies. Geographically, funding is limited to projects that will significantly improve the lives of people living in Milwaukee, Waukesha, Ozaukee and Washington counties. Applying organizations will be required to provide evidence of an active, engaged board of directors, sound financial management and the capability to carry out the proposed projects.
Restrictions: Grants for ongoing operational costs or to individuals are not eligible for support from the Foundation's discretionary funds. The Foundation does not provide support for debt reduction, sectarian religious purposes, medical or scientific research, fund drives for sustaining support or organizations that are discriminatory in their practices.
Geographic Focus: Wisconsin
Samples: Foster Care Youth Independence Center of Wisconsin Inc., $15,000—to create a treatment foster care services program in conjunction with the state that would place foster children ages 13 to 18 in private foster care instead of group foster homes. Participating foster care children would receive independent living skills training as part of the program (2009); Bread of Healing Clinic, $25,000—to expand access to medications for uninsured people in Milwaukee through its MedShare program. The program provides medications at low or no cost to the 14 free clinics that make up the Free Clinic Collaborative (2009); Children's Hospital and Health System Foundation Inc., $100,000—grant to be paid over three years, to open a full-service dental clinic at the Next Door Foundation (2009).
Contact: Fran Kowalkiewicz; (414) 272-5805; fax: (414) 272-6235; email: fkowalkiewicz@greatermilwaukeefoundation.org or info@greatermilwaukeefoundation.org
Internet: http://www.greatermilwaukeefoundation.org/grant_seekers/
Sponsor: Greater Milwaukee Foundation
101 West Pleasant Street, Suite 210
Milwaukee, WI 53212

Greater New Orleans Foundation Grants **1654**

The Greater New Orleans Foundation is the community foundation serving the 13-parish region of metropolitan New Orleans. Funding is Focused on: housing, workforce development, education, rural and regional initiatives, healthcare, and arts and culture
Requirements: Nonprofits serving metropolitan New Orleans area are eligible to apply.

Restrictions: The Foundation does not fund the ongoing operational expenses of an established not-for-profit organization.
Geographic Focus: Louisiana
Samples: The Bayou District Foundation,$500,000—to purchase individual lots and vacant homes in St. Bernard (2009); Greater New Orleans Afterschool Partnership, $2,500—to fund a government transperancy project (2009); The Urban Conservancy, $20,000—to implement continuity planning for New Orleans' local businesses (2009).
Contact: Dr. Albert Ruesga, President; (504) 598-4663; fax: (504) 598-4676; email: albert@gnof.org or info@gnof.org
Internet: http://www.gnof.org/nonprofits/
Sponsor: Greater New Orleans Foundation
1055 Saint Charles Avenue, Suite 100
New Orleans, LA 70130

Greater Saint Louis Community Foundation Grants 1655

The Foundation makes grants annually in the broad areas of the arts, community development, education, environment, health, human services and religion. The Foundation administers its discretionary grant program through a periodic series of initiatives related to four areas of interest: a multi-year, issue-focused initiative; capacity building for nonprofits; knowledge development and dissemination related to current community issues; and knowledge development and dissemination related to philanthropy and volunteerism. Organizations interested in learning more about the Foundation's discretionary grant program are encouraged to contact the Director of Community Investment.
Requirements: While the Foundation predominately supports St. Louis area nonprofits, grants are also made to national and international charities.
Geographic Focus: Illinois
Contact: Dwight D. Canning, Vice President; (314) 588-8200, ext. 139; fax: (314) 588-8088; email: dcanning@gstlcf.org
Internet: http://www.stlcf.org/page11503.cfm
Sponsor: Greater Saint Louis Community Foundation
319 North Fourth Street, Suite 300
Saint Louis, MO 63102

Greater Tacoma Community Foundation Grants 1656

The Foundation invests in the community through grants to vital nonprofit agencies in Pierce County. While grants are made across all fields, principal funding areas include: arts and culture; civics; education; the environment; health; and human services. The Foundation also makes capital, equipment, project and operating support grants. Application information is available online.
Requirements: Eligible applicants must meet the following criteria: attest to non-discrimination on the basis of race, sex, age, national origin, religion, physical or mental handicap, veteran status or sexual orientation; provide a service primarily for residents of Pierce County; qualify as tax-exempt under section 501(c)3 of the IRS Code; and apply no more than once a year for any one governing or umbrella organization.
Restrictions: Grants will not be made for: fundraising events or fundraising feasibility projects; individuals; religious organizations for sacramental/theological purposes; production of books, videos, films, or other publications; annual campaign appeals; travel; political or lobbying activities; endowments; debt reduction; events or programs that occur prior to the board of directors decision/notification dates.
Geographic Focus: Washington
Samples: Kids in Distressed Situations (New York, NY)—to provide donated products to low-income children and families in Tacoma and Pierce County, WA, through the Emergency Food Network, $25,000.
Contact: Rose Lincoln Hamilton, President & CEO; (253) 383-5622; fax: (253) 272-8099; email: rlincoln@gtcf.org
Internet: http://www.tacomafoundation.org
Sponsor: Greater Tacoma Community Foundation
950 Pacific Avenue, Suite 1220
Tacoma, WA 98402

Greater Tacoma Community Foundation Ryan Alan Hade Endowment Fund 1657

The Fund is to provide support and care to children who have been through traumatic experiences of abuse and disfigurement. The Foundation is looking for nonprofit partners who serve abused or disfigured children in the Greater Tacoma area to continue or implement programming that will ease these children's lives. Interested applicants should submit a one page letter of intent. LOI information is available online.
Requirements: Nonprofit organizations in the Greater Tacoma area are eligible to apply.
Geographic Focus: Washington
Contact: Kristen Corning, Community Programs Coordinator; (253) 383-5622; email: kcorning@gtcf.org
Internet: http://www.tacomafoundation.org/newsarticle.cfm?articleid=126285&ptsidebaroptid=0&returnto=page19554.cfm&returntoname=Apply%20for%20a%20Grant&siteid=1735&pageid=19538&sidepageid=19554&banner1img=banner%5F1%2EJPG&banner2img=banner%5F2%2EJPG&bannerbg=banner
Sponsor: Greater Tacoma Community Foundation
P.O. Box 1995
Tacoma, WA 98401-1995

Greater Worcester Community Foundation Discretionary Grants 1658

Grants are made to nonprofit organizations to build healthy and vibrant communities. Several large field-of-interest funds are also included in this process, providing support for culture and the arts, academic achievement for disadvantaged youth, progressive education, conservation, homelessness and affordable housing, and health and wellness for women and children. These grants enable us to be responsive to community needs and priorities.
Requirements: The Foundation considers applications only from nonprofit, tax-exempt organizations for activities serving the people of the Central Massachusetts region. Organizations not incorporated as tax-exempt may apply through an established organization that agrees to provide fiscal oversight.
Geographic Focus: Massachusetts
Amount of Grant: $3,000-$25,000 range; $5,000-$15,000 average
Date(s) Application is Due: Mar 15; Sep 15
Contact: Pamela B. Kane; (508) 755-0980; email: pkane@greaterworcester.org
Internet: http://www.greaterworcester.org/grants/disc-grants.htm
Sponsor: Greater Worcester Community Foundation
370 Main Street, Suite 650
Worcester, MA 01608

Greater Worcester Community Foundation Jeppson Memorial Fund for Brookfield Grants 1659

The Fund provides money to civic and community projects that help improve the lives of residents and enrich the cultural environment. The Fund provides support for: cultural or artistic performances; public seminars; festivals or exhibitions; services that help frail or vulnerable citizens, or that contribute to public health and safety; opportunities for educational enrichment; youth involvement in recreation, sports and the arts; and projects that foster community awareness and connections among different groups. Application information is available online.
Requirements: Any nonprofit or civic organization that serves the residents of Brookfield may apply.
Restrictions: Grant funds may not be used for expenses already incurred by the applicant. Fund awards are not intended to replace municipal funds.
Geographic Focus: Massachusetts
Date(s) Application is Due: Jul 15
Contact: Pamela B. Kane; (508) 755-0980; email: pkane@greaterworcester.org
Internet: http://www.greaterworcester.org/grants/Jeppson.htm
Sponsor: Greater Worcester Community Foundation
370 Main Street, Suite 650
Worcester, MA 01608-1738

Green Bay Packers Foundation Grants 1660

The Green Bay Packers organization has enjoyed tremendous fan support through its long and storied history. To give back to the community, the team created the Green Bay Packers Foundation in December 1986. The Foundation assists in a wide variety of activities and programs that benefit education, civic affairs, health services, human services and youth-related programs.
Requirements: 501(c)3 nonprofit organizations in Wisconsin may apply for grant support.
Restrictions: No substantial part of the activities of the organization shall involve carrying on propaganda, or otherwise intervening in any political campaign on behalf of any candidate for public office.
Geographic Focus: Wisconsin
Samples: Packers Scholarship Program, $15,000—$7,500 to Scholarships, Inc., for distribution to students in four-year colleges and $7,500 to Northeast Wisconsin Technical College for distribution to students in two-year associate degree or apprenticeship trades programs (2008); Cooks for Room at the Inn, Green Bay, WI, $2,000—New Community Shelter (2008); Hometown Huddle Program, Green Bay, WI, $5,000—to provide a new playground for the city's Beaumont Elementary School Park (2008).
Contact: Margaret Meyers, Grant Coordinator; (920) 569-7315; fax: (920) 569-7309; email: meyersm@packers.com
Internet: http://www.packers.com/community/packers_foundation
Sponsor: Green Bay Packers Foundation
P.O. Box 10628
Green Bay, WI 54307-0628

Green Foundation Grants 1661

The Foundation's resources are focused on the four specific areas of arts, education, medical/scientific research and special projects. Preferential attention will be given to institutions exhibiting the following positive factors: a history of achievement, good management, and a stable financial condition; significant programs with the promise of making a measurable impact; programs that are self-sustaining and will not necessitate continued dependence on the Foundation. Interested applicants must complete the Foundation's online eligibility questionnaire. Information is available online.
Requirements: 501(c)3 nonprofits (as per the IRS Service Code of 1986) are eligible. Most grantmaking is limited to institutions that serve the Los Angeles community; however the Foundation will consider requests beyond this geographic boundary for those institutions with the potential to impact communities statewide or nationally.
Restrictions: The Foundation does not provide funds for: those with net assets or fund balances of less than $100,000; multi-year commitments; annual meetings, conferences, and/or seminars; religious programs; capital campaigns; direct mail campaigns; conduit institutions, unified funds, fiscal agents, or institutions using grant funds from donors to support other institutions or individuals; private foundations; individuals.
Samples: American Heart Association, $15,000 (2009); New Village Charter School, $25,000 (2009); CA Science Center, $15,000 (2009).
Amount of Grant: $1,000-$150,000 range

Contact: Kylie Wright, Program Director, (626) 793-6200, ext. 1; fax: (626) 793-6201; email: kylies@ligf.org
Internet: http://ligf.org/index.html
Sponsor: Green Foundation
547 South Marengo Avenue
Pasadena, CA 91101

Greene County Foundation Grants **1662**
The Greene County Foundations mission is to work with charitably minded individuals and organizations to strengthen Greene County, Indiana, now and for generations to come. The Foundation administers several funding opportunities. Eligibility, criteria, and supplemental requirements are different for each grant. Contact foundation directly to begin application process.
Geographic Focus: Indiana
Contact: Kerry Conway, Executive Director; (812) 659-3142 or (812) 659-3144; fax: (812) 659-3142; email: gcfound@yahoo.com
Internet: http://www.greenecountyfoundation.org/funds_available.php
Sponsor: Greene County Foundation
RR #2, Box 38X
Bloomfield, IN 47424

Greenfield Foundation of Maine Grants **1663**
The Foundation, established in 1999, offers funding primarily in the form of ongoing general operating support. Focus areas include: federated giving programs; health care; the environment; wildlife; and animal welfare. The geographic focus is primarily in Maine, with an initial approach by Letter of Interest (LOI) and no specific application forms. There are no annual deadlines, and individual grants average $500.
Requirements: Grantees must be 501(C)(3) organizations with a sound track record.
Restrictions: No grants to individuals.
Geographic Focus: Maine
Samples: Maine Audubon Society, $50 (2006); Animal Refuge League, $1,000 (2006).
Amount of Grant: $50 - $1,000 range
Contact: Margaret Cary Curran; (207) 781-5360
Sponsor: Greenfield Foundation
2 Lady Cove
Falmouth, ME 04105-1956

Greenspun Family Foundation Grants **1664**
The foundation awards grants to eligible Nevada organizations in its areas of interest, including cancer research, children's services, higher education, the physically and mentally disabled, and religious welfare programs that provide for the homeless. There are no application forms or deadlines. Submit a letter of request.
Requirements: Nevada nonprofit organizations are eligible. Preference is given to requests from the Las Vegas area.
Geographic Focus: Nevada
Samples: Nevada Cancer Institute (Las Vegas, NV)—for organizational support, $25 million (2005); Nevada Cancer Institute (Las Vegas, NV)—to support cancer-related education, research, and treatment, $5 million (2004).
Contact: Grants Administrator
Sponsor: Greenspun Family Foundation
901 N Green Valley Pkwy, Suite 210
Henderson, NV 89074

Greenwall Foundation Bioethics Grants **1665**
The Foundation provides funding for physicians, lawyers, philosophers, theologians and other professionals to address micro and macro issues in bioethics, providing guidance for those engaged in decision-making at the bedside as well as those responsible for shaping institutional and public policy. The Foundation is especially interested in the work of junior investigators and pilot projects that may lead to NIH support, and it is prepared to address issues regarded by some as sensitive or potentially controversial.
Restrictions: The Foundation is not normally interested in proposals to support equipment purchase, facility construction or renovation, or general operating expenses, and will not normally consider grants to private foundations, endowment funds, or individual applicants.
Amount of Grant: $5000-$50,000 average
Date(s) Application is Due: Feb 1; Aug 1
Contact: Sam Teigen, Grants Administrator; (212) 679-7266; fax: (212) 679-7269; email: steigen@greenwall.org
Internet: http://www.greenwall.org/guidebio.htm
Sponsor: Greenwall Foundation
420 Lexington Avenue, Suite 2500
New York, NY 10170

Gregory B. Davis Foundation Grants **1666**
The Foundation's mission is to enhance the lives of youth and their families through the development and support of health related and educational programs and initiatives. More specifically, GBDF will support healthy life choices and well-being for rural and medically challenged families, caregivers, and youth affected by HIV/AIDS, Alzheimer's Disease, and other debilitating illnesses and those with limited academic and life skills opportunities. There are no specific deadlines, and applicants should forward an entire proposal.
Amount of Grant: $500-$2,000 range
Contact: Edna Davis-Brown, CEO; (301) 593-0644; email: GBDF@gbdf.org
Internet: http://www.gbdf.org/programs.html
Sponsor: Gregory B. Davis Foundation
11404 December Way, Suite 403
Silver Springs, MD 20904-3623

Gregory Family Foundation Grants (Florida) **1667**
The Foundation, established in 1999, offers support to cancer research and prevention, Christian churches and agencies, and hospitals. Funding most often comes in the form of a donation for general operations. The Foundation's geographic restrictions are New York and Florida. A formal application form is required, which should include: a copy of most recent annual report, audited financial statement, or 990; a detailed description of project; and amount of funding requested. There are no specific deadlines.
Requirements: Applicants should be a 501(c)3 located in Florida or New York.
Geographic Focus: Florida; New York
Samples: St. Ambrose Church, Boca Raton, Florida, $1,150—for general operations (2006); Christ Child Society of Boca Raton, Boca Raton, Florida, $800—for general operations (2006).
Amount of Grant: $2,000 maximum
Contact: Dale M. Gregory, President; (561) 362-9868; email: gregory1@bellsouth.net
Sponsor: Gregory Family Foundation, Inc.
101 Plaza Reale S., Apt. 618
Boca Raton, FL 33432-4849

Gregory L. Gibson Charitable Foundation Grants **1668**
The Foundation, established in Terre Haute, Indiana, in 2005, is interested in programs that support children, youth, and families. Its primary areas of interest include: community service programs; education; health care and health care access; hospice care; technology; and youth sports. The specific type of support is for general operations. There are no specific deadlines with which to adhere, and applicants should forward a submission letter.
Requirements: 501(c)3 organizations situated in, or serving the community of, Terre Haute, Indiana, are eligible to apply.
Geographic Focus: Indiana
Amount of Grant: $30,000 maximum
Contact: c/o Cary Sparks, First Financial Bank; (812) 238-6234; fax: (812) 238-6184; email: csparks@first-online.com;; Gregory L. Gibson, President; (812) 466-1233
Sponsor: Gregory L. Gibson Charitable Foundation
3200 E. Haythorne Avenue
Terre Haute, IN 47805-2108

Griffin Family Foundation Grants **1669**
The Foundation, established in 1999, is primarily interested in supporting non-profit organizations in the state of New York. Fields of interest include: Catholic agencies and churches; education; health care clinics and centers; and hospitals. Funding most often comes in the form of general operating support. There are no particular forms, and applicants should submit a copy of the current year's organizational budget and/or the specific project budget.
Requirements: Applicants should have 501(c)3 status with the IRS.
Geographic Focus: New York
Amount of Grant: $20,000 maximum
Contact: William E. Griffin, President; (914) 961-1300; fax: (914) 961-9385
Sponsor: Griffin Family Foundation
51 Pondfield Road
Bronxville, NY 10708-3703

Griffin Foundation Grants **1670**
The Foundation, established in 1991, serves non-profit organizations in Fort Collins, Colorado, and Laramie, Wyoming. Its major fields of interest include: the arts; health care; higher education; performing arts; orchestras; and substance abuse service programs. Funding most often comes in the forms of building construction, renovation, and scholarships. Applicants should request an application form, and submit a detailed description of the project and budget needed.
Geographic Focus: Colorado; Wyoming
Contact: David L. Wood, President; (970) 482-3030; fax: (970) 484-6648; email: carol.wood@thegriffinfoundation.org
Internet: http://www.thegriffinfoundation.org/index.shtml
Sponsor: Griffin Foundation
303 W. Prospect Road
Fort Collins, CO 80526-2003

Grotto Foundation Project Grants **1671**
The foundation is interested in local programs in Minnesota that improve education and promote economic, physical, and social well-being, particularly programs focusing on children and youth, ethnic groups, immigrants and refugees, gays and lesbians, and the economically disadvantaged. Grants support new, innovative projects with special consideration given to programs that show potential to continue after the grant period. General operating grants also are awarded. Application procedures are available on the Web site.
Requirements: Minnesota 501(c)3 nonprofits may submit grant applications.
Restrictions: Policy precludes grants being awarded for capital fund projects, travel, publication of books or manuscripts, undergraduate research projects, or grants to individuals.
Geographic Focus: Minnesota

Samples: W. Harry Davis Leadership Institute (Minneapolis, MN)—for the African American Youth Leadership Training Initiative, $4500.; Girl Scout Council of Saint Croix Valley (MN)—for a volleyball program for Asian American girls, $3000.; Mankato State U (MN)—for a dental health program for Native Americans, $2467.
Amount of Grant: $10,000 maximum
Date(s) Application is Due: Jan 15; Mar 15; Jul 15; Nov 15
Contact: Sarah Marquardt, Grants Manager, (763) 277-3434; fax: (763) 277-3444; email: info@grottofoundation.org
Internet: http://www.grottofoundation.org
Sponsor: Grotto Foundation
5323 Lakeland Ave N, Suite 100
Minneapolis, MN 55429-3115

Gruber Foundation International Prizes **1672**

The Peter and Patricia Gruber Foundation honors and encourages educational excellence, social justice and scientific achievements that better the human condition. The Peter and Patricia Gruber Foundation is a private, United States-based philanthropic organization established in 1993 under the 501(c)3 section of U.S. Corporate Law. It is funded entirely by Peter and Patricia Gruber, who serve as its Chairman and President, respectively. The Foundation is headquartered in St. Thomas, United States Virgin Islands, and maintains a small branch office in New York City. A major focus of the Foundation's philanthropy is its International Prize Program, created to recognize excellence in science and humanities by highlighting five fields that create a better world: Cosmology, Genetics, Neuroscience, Justice, and Women's Rights. Each Prize is given annually, and carries an unrestricted cash award of $500,000 and a gold medal. Independent advisory boards comprised of experts from each field review and select a prize recipient at annual selection meetings held for each discipline. Only fully completed nominations are considered, and the Chair of each Selection Advisory Board screens the nominations, presenting to the Board only those of sufficient caliber. The Selection Advisory Board alone is responsible for the choice of recipient, making its decision from among officially nominated candidates following discussion and deliberation. The Peter and Patricia Gruber Foundation awards its international prizes to recipients only after following a process designed to ensure complete independence and integrity in selecting, as worthy of international recognition, scientific and human rights achievements at the highest levels.
Requirements: Only candidates who have been officially nominated on a fully completed nomination form will be considered for a Peter and Patricia Gruber Foundation International Prize. Additional guidelines and nomination forms are available on line.
Samples: Gruber Cosmology Prize was won by Astronomers Wendy Freedman, Robert Kennicutt, and Jeremy Mould, they led the Hubble Space Telescope Key Project on the Extragalactic Distance Scale, a painstaking ten-year-long effort that resolved the decades-long dispute about the value of the Hubble constant, one of the most important measurements in astronomy. The project's findings have not only effectively determined the age of the universe (about 14 billion years), but have also enabled scientists to more accurately investigate other profound questions about the birth, evolution, and composition of the universe (2009); Gruber Justice Prize was shared by the European Roma Rights Centre and Bryan Stevenson, the executive director of Equal Rights Initiative. Through recourse to litigation, consultation, and other approaches available within the justice and political systems, Bryan Stevenson and the European Roma Rights Centre have courageously helped members of oppressed groups gain access to equal justice (2009);
Amount of Grant: $500,000 plus a gold medal
Date(s) Application is Due: Dec 15
Contact: Bernetia Akin, Foundation Contact; (340) 775-8035 or (340) 775-8014; fax (340) 775 8040; email: info@gruberprizes.org
Internet: http://www.petergruberfoundation.org/GruberPrizes/GruberPrizes.php
Sponsor: The Peter and Patricia Gruber Foundation
6000 Estate Charlotte Amalie, Suite 4
St. Thomas, U.S.VI 00802

Grundy Foundation Grants **1673**

The foundation awards capital grants to eligible Pennsylvania nonprofit organizations in its areas of interest, including children and youth, culture, health care and hospitals, elderly, disabled, and historic preservation. Projects are generally funded for one year and often on a one-time basis. Potential applicants should submit a letter that describes the organization, project or activity, and funds requested.
Requirements: Pennsylvania 501(c)3 organizations in Bucks County are eligible.
Restrictions: Grants are not made to support operating expenses, political or religious organizations, or individuals.
Geographic Focus: Pennsylvania
Samples: Bristol Riverside Theater (Bristol, PA)—for the performance season.; Behanna (Southampton, PA)—for renovations to Swigart House.
Amount of Grant: $1000-$75,000 range
Contact: Roland Johnson, Executive Director, (215) 788-5460; fax: (215) 788-0915; email: grundyf@voicenet.com
Sponsor: Grundy Foundation
P.O. Box 701, 680 Radcliffe Street
Bristol, PA 19007

Guidant Foundation Grants **1674**

The foundation supports charitable and educational programs that lead to improved quality of life for patients who are at risk or suffer from cardiovascular disease. The foundation awards grants in the areas of education, healthcare, and community/social services in Guidant communities and to leading healthcare institutions that provide educational services. Preference will be given to programs that develop a patient-support program, using the Internet, to increase patient awareness of advances in the treatment of cardiovascular disease. There are no application deadlines. Application is available online.
Requirements: 501(c)3 organizations are eligible.
Samples: Cardiovascular Learning Partnership (Atlanta, GA); Denver Health Medical Ctr's Cardiovascular Risk Reduction Program (CO).
Amount of Grant: $12 million total; $500,000 average
Contact: Pat Kuhl, (317) 971-2272; fax: (317) 971-2118; email: pkuhl@guidant.com
Internet: http://www.guidant.com/foundation/index.shtml
Sponsor: Guidant Foundation
111 Monument Cir, Suite 2900
Indianapolis, IN 46244-2159

Guitar Center Music Foundation Grants **1675**

The Guitar Center Music Foundation makes the gift of music available to people across the country by providing funding and resources for music programs. Grants are awarded to music academies, schools, local music programs and national music programs across America. Awards are made in the following categories: In-school music classes, in which the students make music; After-school music programs that are not run by the school; and, Music therapy programs, in which the participants make the music. The intent of the program must be music instruction, not music appreciation or entertainment, and the participants/students cannot be professional or career musicians. The grant committee reviews all applications three times yearly, and grant awards range from $500 to $5,000 in value.
Requirements: Applications are accepted online throughout the year from 501(c)3 or governmental organizations. Qualifying applicants are established, ongoing and sustainable music programs in the United States, which provide music instruction for people of any age who would not otherwise have the opportunity to make music. Almost all of the grants awarded are traditional instruments and the equipment necessary to play them. In specific instances, microphones and PA systems have also been awarded. In order to be eligible for a grant, the instruments and/or equipment must stay in the program for the life of the instrument/equipment and must be played/used by the participants.
Restrictions: Requests that are specifically ineligible are: (a) General operating expenses, including rent, utilities, supplies, travel expenses, etc.; (b) Items or funds to benefit individuals, including scholarships, stipends or salaries; (c) Seed money; (d) Event sponsorship; (e) Music production equipment and/or expenses; (f) Recording studio equipment and/or expenses, including those used for educational purposes; (g) Instrument repairs; (h) Uniforms; (i) Sheet music.
Geographic Focus: Alabama; Alaska; Arizona; Arkansas; California; Colorado; Connecticut; Delaware; District of Columbia; Florida; Georgia; Hawaii; Idaho; Illinois; Indiana; Iowa; Kansas; Kentucky; Louisiana; Maine; Maryland; Massachusetts; Michigan; Minnesota; Mississippi; Missouri; Montana; Nebraska; Nevada; New Hampshire; New Jersey; New Mexico; New York; North Carolina; North Dakota; Ohio; Oklahoma; Oregon; Pennsylvania; Puerto Rico; Rhode Island; South Carolina; South Dakota; Southwest; Tennessee; Texas; Utah; Vermont; Virginia; Washington; West Virginia; Wisconsin; Wyoming
Samples: Music in Schools Today - provides therapeutic percussion, world music and movement classes to the most underserved and at-risk youth, in Bay Area Schools and community centers.; Hijos de la Musica Latina - Non-profit music program that empowers talented Latino youth that are primarily financially, economically and emotionally at-risk, who have a certified talent and gift for Latin music.; Conejo Valley Youth Orchestras - serves an ethnically diverse group of families, with no students being turned away due to socio-economic status or ability, and continues to grow as the demand for music programs continues. The Creative Arts Program at Dana-Farber Cancer Institute Program - offers adult oncology patients and their families the opportunity to receive free music lessons that are especially helpful during difficult times of their treatment. Guitars in the Classroom - provides affordable music instruction in guitar, singing and song leading to educators in 20 states reaching over 3,000 educators and 200,000 students annually.
Amount of Grant: $500 - $5,000
Contact: Larry E. Thomas, Chairman; (818) 735-8800, ext. 2112; fax: (818) 735-7518; email: info@guitarcentermusicfoundation.org
Internet: http://www.guitarcentermusicfoundation.org/grants/index.cfm?sec=overview
Sponsor: Guitar Center Music Foundation
5795 Lindero Canyon Road
Westlake Village, CA 91362

Gulf Coast Community Foundation Grants **1676**

The Foundation is a public charity dedicated to the progressive development of the Mississippi Gulf Coast. Its primary mission is to increase philanthropy to worthy causes by providing donor services, grants and leadership for problem solving. The Foundation carries out donor wishes by making grants in the areas of health and human services, education, arts and culture, historic preservation, and neighborhood enrichment. Grant application and additional guidelines are available online at: http://www.gulfcoastfoundation.org/guidelines.html.
Requirements: Applicants must be non-profit, tax-exempt organizations that are involved in enhancing the quality of life for citizens of South Mississippi. Organizations that have not been recognized as tax-exempt by the IRS may apply if they have a fiscal agent relationship with a 501(c)3 nonprofit organization.
Restrictions: Grants do not support: capital, operating endowment fund drives; political activities; individuals; or religious activities.

Geographic Focus: Mississippi
Contact: Rose Dellenger. Grants Manager, (228) 897-4841; fax: (228) 897-4843; email: rdellenger@mgccf.org
Internet: http://www.gulfcoastfoundation.org/grants.html
Sponsor: Gulf Coast Community Foundation
P.O. Box 984
Gulfport, MS 39503

Gulf Coast Community of Venice Foundation Grants 1677

The Foundation funds grants and programs that are designed to contribute significantly to improving the quality of life for citizens in the communities it serves. Foundation funding is organized around these key areas: arts and culture; civic affairs and the environment; education; health; and human/social services. Application information is available online.
Requirements: The Foundation makes the majority of its grants to nonprofit organizations. In addition, some grants from these funds may be made to government agencies, but not to individuals. Awards will be directed to projects that serve persons living in southern Sarasota County, all of Englewood, Boca Grande, and environs. Nonprofit organizations applying for a grant from these funds may be headquartered outside this geographic area.
Restrictions: Funding is not available for endowments or endowed university chairs, debt reduction, basic scientific research, make loans, sponsor events, or fund travel.
Geographic Focus: Florida
Contact: Mark Pritchett, Vice President for Community Investment, (941) 486-4600; fax: (941) 486-4699; email: info@gulfcoastcf.org
Internet: http://www.gulfcoastcf.org/page27356.cfm
Sponsor: Gulf Coast Community of Venice Foundation
601 Tamiami Trail South
Venice, FL 34285

Guy's and St. Thomas' Charity Grants 1678

The Charity's grants program supports both small (under 20,000 British pounds) and large (between 20,000 and 1 million British pounds) projects under three themes: staff benefits and development; clinical and service innovation; and buildings and the environment. Applications for grants under 20,000 British pounds are considered by the Small Grants Committee, and grants over 20,000 British pounds are assessed by the New Services and Innovations Committee. The small grants deadline dates are: August, 14; September, 25; October 16. Deadline dates for the large grants are: December, 1; March, 6; June, 5; September, 4; November, 20.
Requirements: The Charity only considers applications from anyone working in one of the four NHS Trusts in Lambeth or Southwark, although there are some restrictions for mental health staff.
Samples: Julie Brown, Midwifery Practice Leader for Parent Education, 5,000 pounds (2007); Dr. Danielle Harari, Consultant Physician in Elderly Medicine, 20,000 pounds (2007); Improving dermatology training for primary care professionals, NHS Foundation Trust, 254,000 pounds (2007).
Amount of Grant: 1,000,000 British pounds
Date(s) Application is Due: Aug 14; Sep 25; Oct 16; Dec 1; Mar 6; Jun 5; Sep 4; Nov 20
Contact: Anne Rigby, Grants Manager; 020 7188 1227; email: anne.rigby@gsttcharity.org.uk
Internet: http://www.gsttcharity.org.uk/grants/index.html
Sponsor: Guy's and St. Thomas' Charity
Freepost Lon 15724
London, England SE1 9YA England

H & R Foundation Grants 1679

The Foundation prefers to support projects and programs that strive for excellence, improve service for clients and strengthen the organization. A major emphasis is placed on support of activities that serve underserved, low-income persons living in Jackson, Clay, and Platte counties in Missouri, and Wyandotte and Johnson counties in Kansas.
Requirements: Grants are made only to organizations that are tax-exempt from federal income taxation pursuant to Section 501(c)3 and that are not classified as private foundations within the code.
Restrictions: Except in the most unusual circumstances, the Foundation does not make grants to: organizations that knowingly discriminate on the basis of race, color, religion, gender, national origin, sexual orientation, age, disability, marital status, or status as a veteran; organizations that are not in compliance with laws and regulations that govern them; individuals or businesses; publications; projects for which the Foundation must exercise expenditure responsibility; single-disease causes; travel or conferences; historic preservation; telethons, dinners, advertising, sponsorships, or other special events; animal-related causes; sports-related causes.
Geographic Focus: Kansas; Missouri
Samples: Greater Kansas City Community Foundation, Kansas City, MO, $200,000 (2006); Scholarship America, Saint Peter, MN, $178,845 (2006); Genesis School, Kansas City, MO, $18,495 (2006);
Date(s) Application is Due: Feb 26; Apr 30; Jul 30; Oct 15
Contact: David Miles, President; (816)854-4372 or (816) 854-4361; fax: (816) 854-8025; email: davmiles@hrblock.com
Internet: http://www.blockfoundation.org/nonprofit_organizations/faqs.html
Sponsor: The H & R Foundation
One H&R Bloack Way
Kansas City, MO 64105

H. Schaffer Foundation Grants 1680

The foundation awards grants to nonprofit organizations in New York in the fields of higher education, hospitals and health care, human services, international relief, theater, aging centers and services, federated giving programs, and Jewish agencies and temples. Eligible activites include recreation, children and youth, services, and general charitable giving. There are no application forms or deadlines.
Requirements: Nonprofit organizations in New York, with an emphasis on Schenectady, are eligible.
Geographic Focus: New York
Amount of Grant: $1000-$250,000 average
Contact: Sonya Stall, President; (518) 580-0188
Sponsor: H. Schaffer Foundation
2 Claire Pass
Saratoga Springs, NY 12307

H.A. and Mary K. Chapman Charitable Trust Grants 1681

Grants are provided to support nonprofit organizations involved in a wide variety of charitable purposes, including education, medical research, health and human services, arts and culture, civic and community, and nature and wildlife. Priority is given to: funding projects or programs that will serve a documented need and have a significant impact on the community; financial support of the organization management and board of directors, individuals of the general community affected by the program or project, and other private foundations; sound financial planning for maintenance and continuation of the project or program after the initial funding is complete; projects or programs that potentially benefit a significant segment of people; applicants with committed volunteers and staff leadership. Application information is available online.
Requirements: 501(c)3 nonprofits in Oklahoma, are eligible. Priority will normally be given to Tulsa and surrounding counties and eastern Oklahoma. Depending on the availability of funds, Arkansas and Texas may also be eligible for funding for Colleges and Universities.
Restrictions: Grants are not made for the following purposes: to be passed-through to another organization that is not a 501(c)3 public charity or a governmental entity; to attempt to influence legislation or the outcome of any election, or to political campaigns. Grant requests for the following purposes are not favored: endowments; deficit financing and debt retirement; projects or programs for which the Chapman Trusts would be the sole source of financial support; travel, conferences, conventions, group meetings, or seminars, camp programs and other seasonal activities; religious programs of religious organizations; project or program planning; start-up ventures are not excluded, but organizations with a proven strategy and results are preferred; purposes normally funded by taxation or governmental agencies; requests made less than nine months from the declination of a previous request by an applicant, or within nine months of the last payment made on a grant made to an applicant; requests for more than one project.
Geographic Focus: Arkansas; Oklahoma; Texas
Samples: Oklahoma Methodist Manor (Tulsa, OK)—$100,000.; Bishop Kelly High School (Tulsa, OK)—$75,000.; Oklahoma Baptist Homes for Children (Tulsa, OK)—$50,000.
Contact: Jerry Dickman or Donne Pitman, (918) 496-7882; Fax (918) 496-7887; jerry@chapmantrusts.com
Internet: http://www.chapmantrusts.org/grants_programs.html
Sponsor: H.A. and Mary K. Chapman Charitable Trust
6100 South Yale, Suite 1816
Tulsa, OK 74136

H.J. Heinz Company Foundation Grants 1682

The Foundation is committed to promoting the health and nutritional needs of children and families. Priority is given to programs in communities where Heinz operates with a special focus given to southwestern Pennsylvania. The Foundation proactively donates funds to develop and strengthen organizations that are dedicated to nutrition and nutritional education, youth services and education, diversity, healthy children and families, and quality of life. Application information is available online.
Requirements: Nonprofits in company-operating areas are eligible. Contact program staff for company locations.
Restrictions: The Foundation will not provide grants to individuals nor make multi-year pledges except for major capital or grant campaigns. Generally, the Foundation does not make loans and does not provide grants for individuals, equipment, conferences, travel, general scholarships, religious programs, political campaigns, and unsolicited research projects.
Geographic Focus: Pennsylvania
Samples: North Side Leadership Conference (Pittsburgh, PA)—to provide employment and education programs for local residents, $2 million.; Civic Light Opera (Pittsburgh, PA)—for the Millenium Creche, $10,000.; Mon Valley Initiative (Pittsburgh, PA)—for operating support, $25,000.
Contact: Program Director, (412) 456-5773; fax: (412) 442-3227; email: heinz.foundation@hjheinz.com
Internet: http://www.heinz.com/foundation.aspx
Sponsor: H.J. Heinz Company Foundation
P.O. Box 57
Pittsburgh, PA 15230-0057

H.R. Lissner Award 1683

This award has been established in honor of H.R. Lissner for his pioneering contributions in biomechanical research. The award is bestowed annually for outstanding accomplishments in the area of bioengineering in the form of: significant research

contributions; development of new methods of measuring; design of new equipment and instrumentation; educational impact in the training of bioengineers; or service to the bioengineering community and/or the ASME Bioengineering Division.
Samples: Steven Goldstein—award recipient, $1000 (2005); John Tarbell—award recipient, $1000 (2004).
Amount of Grant: $1000 honorarium and expense supplement
Date(s) Application is Due: Jan 1
Contact: Honors and Awards Department, (212) 705-7735; fax: (212) 705-7739
Internet: http://www.asme.org/honors/ms71/list.html
Sponsor: American Society of Mechanical Engineers
345 E 47th Street
New York, NY 10017-2392

Hackett Foundation Grants **1684**
The Foundation is limited by its giving to the funding of grants for supplies and equipment. Grants are primarily given, but not limited to, Catholic Missions. The primary focus of the Foundation is to provide assistance to those Catholic Organizations which promote the Health, Welfare, Education and Independence of individuals. Application information is available online.
Restrictions: Grants to individuals, scholarships, endowments and fellowships will not be considered. Grants will not be given to supporting organizations having a 509(a)(3) status. Grants will not be used as reimbursement for previously purchased items. Grants are not given for salaries, administrative expenses or matching funds. Grants will not be considered for demonstration projects and/or capital campaigns. Grants will not be provided for non-U.S. based organizations or for taxes or shipping and handling charges.
Geographic Focus: New Jersey; New York; Pennsylvania
Samples: School of the Holy Childhood (Rochester, NY)—to purchase a copier, printers, and power generators for this organization that provides education, training, and employment to developmentally disabled children and adults, $14,000 (2004).
Amount of Grant: $1,000-$20,000
Contact: Maggie Hackett, Grants Manager, (908) 238-9444
Internet: http://fdncenter.org/grantmaker/hackett
Sponsor: Hackett Foundation
P.O. Box 693
Pittstown, NJ 08867

Hagedorn Fund Grants **1685**
The fund supports religious and charitable organizations. Funding interests include: health (including cancer, HIV/AIDS, blindness), gardens, social services, youth, education, senior services and housing and community development. Interested applicants should submit a letter of proposal. Funding decisions are made by December 31st.
Requirements: New York nonprofit organizations are eligible.
Restrictions: No grants are made to individuals or private foundations or for matching gifts or loans.
Geographic Focus: New York
Amount of Grant: $1000-$75,000 range
Date(s) Application is Due: Sep 15
Contact: Erin K. Hogan, c/o JPMorgan Private Bank, Philanthropic Services, (212) 464-2443
Internet: http://fdncenter.org/grantmaker/hagedorn
Sponsor: Hagedorn Fund
345 Park Avenue, 4th Floor, NY1-N040
New York, NY 10154

Hall-Perrine Foundation Grants **1686**
The foundation awards grants to nonprofit organizations in Cedar Rapids and Linn County in its areas of interest, including education (private liberal arts colleges), health care, libraries, social services, and youth.
Requirements: Iowa nonprofit organizations in Cedar Rapids and Linn County are eligible.
Restrictions: Grants do not support religious organizations or elementary/secondary schools.
Geographic Focus: Iowa
Samples: Coe College (Cedar Rapids, IA)—to renovate Stuart Hall, the college's oldest building, in order to expand classroom space and incorporate new technologies, $900,000 (2004); Community Health Free Clinic (Cedar Rapids, IA)—to construct a facility at which volunteers will provide health-care services to low-income people, $1.44 million (2003).
Amount of Grant: $20,000-$100,000
Contact: Grants Administrator, (319) 362-9079
Sponsor: Hall-Perrine Foundation
115 Third St SE, Suite 803
Cedar Rapids, IA 52401-1222

Halliburton Foundation Grants **1687**
The foundation supports education at all levels and charitable organizations in the following ways: matching U.S.- based employee donations on a two-for-one basis up to $20,000 annually per employee for accredited junior colleges, colleges, and universities; matching U.S.-based employee donations to accredited elementary and secondary schools on a two-for-one basis up to $500 annually per employee; making direct donations to U.S.-based elementary and secondary schools and colleges and universities; and recognizing and supporting active U.S.-based employee volunteerism with direct donations through the Halliburton Volunteer Incentive Program. The corporate giving program makes donations to tax-exempt nonprofit organizations dedicated to education, health/welfare, civic issues, and arts and culture. The board meets quarterly. There are no application deadlines or forms.
Geographic Focus: Southwest; Texas
Amount of Grant: $250-$20,000 average
Contact: Margaret Carriere, (713) 676-3717; email: fhoufoundation@halliburton.com
Internet: http://www.halliburton.com/about/community.jsp
Sponsor: Halliburton Foundation
4100 Clinton Drive, Building 1, 7th Floor
Houston, TX 77020

Hallmark Corporate Foundation Grants **1688**
The mission of the Foundation is to help create communities where: all children have the chance to grow up as healthy, productive and caring persons; vibrant arts and cultural experiences enrich the lives of all citizens; there is a strong infrastructure of basic institutions and services, especially for persons in need; and all citizens feel a responsibility to serve their community. Interested applicants should submit an initial letter of contact. There is no application form. Submission information is located online.
Requirements: Eligible applicants should have: charitable status through a 501(c)3; a strong statement of organizational mission; and strong organizational leadership with a capacity to accomplish what is being proposed. The Foundation supports organizations based in and serving citizens of the following communities: Kansas City metropolitan area; Center, Texas; Columbus, Georgia; Enfield, Connecticut; Lawrence, Kansas; Leavenworth, Kansas; Liberty, Missouri; Metamora, Illinois; Topeka, Kansas.
Restrictions: Funding is not available for: individuals for any purpose, including travel, starting a business or paying back loans; religious organizations unless they can demonstrate that services are provided to the community-at-large and separated from religious purposes; fraternal, international and veterans organizations; sports teams and athletic organizations; individual youth clubs, troops, groups or school classrooms; social clubs; disease-specific organizations whose local chapters primarily raise funds for national research; past operating deficits; endowment or foundation funds; conferences; scholarly or health-related research; scholarship funds.
Geographic Focus: Connecticut; Georgia; Illinois; Kansas; Missouri; Texas
Contact: Community Development Manager, (816) 545-6906
Internet: http://www.hallmark.com/webapp/wcs/stores/servlet/article|10001|10051|/HallmarkSite/AboutHallmark/SupportingOurCommunity/VOLUNTEER_SUPP.O.RT
Sponsor: Hallmark Corporate Foundation
Mail Drop 323, P.O. Box 419580
Kansas City, MO 64141-6580

Hamlet Trust Grants **1689**
The trust awards grants in support of self-help initiatives for people with long-term mental health problems in Central and Eastern Europe and the countries of the New Independent States.
Amount of Grant: $1000-$10,000
Contact: Grants Administrator, +44 (0) 20 7247 8666; fax: +44 (0) 20 7247 1984; email: office@hamlettrust.plus.com
Internet: http://www.hamlet-trust.org.uk
Sponsor: Hamlet Trust
Norvin House, 45-55 Commercial Street
London E1 6BD United Kingdom

Hancock County Community Foundation Grants **1690**
The Hancock County Community Foundation has been working to enhance the quality of life in Hancock County, Indiana since 1992. The Community Foundation has established an annual grant program that is available on a competitive basis to incorporated, 501(c)3 organizations serving Hancock County. Each grant program has its own criteria used to evaluate applications. The foundation welcome and encourage contact from organizations that are considering applying for a grant and are happy to clarify and respond to questions concerning policies, guidelines, or application procedures.
Requirements: Annual grant programs begin with a community announcement in which nonprofits are asked to submit a Letter of Intent. Upon review, the invitation to apply for a grant will be made to qualifying organizations. Proposals will be reviewed and compared with other proposals received. Those proposals which best meet our criteria are selected for funding.
Restrictions: The Community Foundation has established an annual grant program that is available on a competitive basis to incorporated, 501(c)3 organizations serving Hancock County.
Geographic Focus: Indiana
Contact: Rachel Strong, Program Officer; (317) 462-8870 ext. 226; email: rstrong@hccf.cc.
Internet: http://www.hccf.cc/granttypes.asp
Sponsor: Hancock County Community Foundation
312 Main Street
Greenfield, IN 46140

Hanna Andersson Children's Foundation Grants **1691**
The Foundation awards grants or gifts to nonprofit programs that create sustainable improvements in the lives of vulnerable children ages birth to ten. Focus is on children who are at-risk due to poverty, child abuse and neglect, domestic violence, homelessness, exposure to substance abuse, physical disabilities or mental health issues. Three criteria

are used for grant and gift allocations: building healthy lives for child; promoting children's participation and empowerment; and supporting not-for-profit coalitions and public policy efforts that support children. The Foundation is not accepting unsolicited proposals at this time.
Requirements: 501(c)3 tax-exempt organizations in areas where the company has a presence are eligible to apply.
Restrictions: The foundation does not fund auctions, capital expenditures, individuals or scholarships, religious activities, or groups that discriminate in the hiring of staff or provision of services due to race, religion, national origin or sexual orientation.
Contact: Director, (503) 242-0920; fax: (503) 222-0544
Internet: http://www.hannafoundation.org/apply/apply.html
Sponsor: Hanna Andersson Childrens Foundation
1010 N.W. Flanders
Portland, OR 97209

Hannaford Charitable Foundation Grants 1692
The foundation awards grants to nonprofit organizations in its areas of interest, including arts and culture, education, environment, children and youth, community development, neighborhoods, and United Way organizations. Types of support include general operating support, capital campaigns, scholarship funds, and exchange programs. There are no application forms or deadlines.
Requirements: Nonprofit organizations are eligible, with preference given to requests in Maine and New Hampshire.
Geographic Focus: Maine; Massachusetts; New Hampshire; New York; Vermont
Amount of Grant: $1000-$10,000 average
Contact: Grants Administrator, c/o Scholarship America, Inc., (507) 931-1682
Internet: http://www.hannaford.com/Contents/Our_Company/Community/index.shtml
Sponsor: Hannaford Charitable Foundation
P.O. Box 1000
Portland, ME 04104

Harden Foundation Grants 1693
The goals of the foundation are to improve the well-being of youth, strengthen families, prevent inappropriate institutionalization of individuals, improve the quality of life through the arts, encourage humane treatment of animals, and improve coordination of social and community services in Monterey County, with emphasis on the Salinas Valley, areas. The foundation supports one-time capital projects, special initiatives, and general operating support.
Requirements: 501(C)3 organizations who provide services or programs in Monterey County, California are eligible to submit grant proposals.
Restrictions: The foundation does not fund sectarian religious programs, educational projects (except agriculture-related requests), endowments, annual events, conferences, or fund-raising events.
Geographic Focus: California
Samples: Boys and Girls Clubs of Monterey County (Seaside, CA)—for youth center at Salinas Sports Complex, $400,000. Kinship Center (Monterey, CA)—for capital campaign for new building in Salinas, $100,000. American Red Cross (Monterey, CA)—to upgrade equipment, purchase disaster supplies, and translate and print training materials for educational purposes, $35,000.
Amount of Grant: $100,000 maximum
Date(s) Application is Due: Mar 1; Sep 1
Contact: Joseph Grainger, Executive Director, (831) 442-3004; fax: (831) 443-1429; email: jgrainger@hardenfoundation.org
Internet: http://www.hardenfoundation.org
Sponsor: Harden Foundation
P.O. Box 779
Salinas, CA 93902

Harley Davidson Foundation Grants 1694
The mission of the Foundation is to support communities with funding and employee volunteerism. The Foundation reaches out to build healthy, thriving communities by placing an emphasis on education, community revitalization, arts and culture, health, and the environment. The Foundation targets areas of greatest need among under-served populations to enhance the quality of life in their communities. The Foundation also supports selected national causes, including veterans initiatives. In making granting decisions, the Foundation looks closely for the following detail: the proposal's relevance to the Foundation's areas of interest; the proposal's clarity in stating the expected project or program outcomes and the strategy for achieving them; the extent to which the strategy involves a collaborative approach to solving a problem or issue affecting the targeted groups or organizations. The program you are nominating should focus on one of the Foundation's funding priorities: education (core curriculum, academic enhancers), community revitalization, job enablers, neighborhood, social services, arts & culture, health, environment. The Common Application Form is located on the company website.
Requirements: 501(c)3 or 170(c) organizations serving metro Milwaukee, Wauwatosa, Franklin, Menomonee Falls or Tomahawk, Wisconson; York, Pennsylvania; Talladega, Alabama; or Kansas City, Missouri are eligible.
Restrictions: The Foundation does not make grants to individuals, political causes or candidates, operating or endowment funds; athletic teams, or religious organizations (unless engaged in a major project benefiting the greater community). The Foundation does not fund conferences or capital campaigns.
Geographic Focus: Alabama; Missouri; Pennsylvania; Wisconsin
Date(s) Application is Due: Jan 23; May 22; Oct 24
Contact: Mary Anne Martiny, Secretary; (414) 343-4001; Fax (414) 343-4254; email: ma.martiny@harley-davidson.com
Internet: http://www.harley-davidson.com/CO/FOU/en/foundation.asp?locale=en_U.S.&bmLocale=en_U.S.
Sponsor: Harley Davidson Foundation
P.O. Box 653
Milwaukee, WI 53201

Harold Alfond Foundation Grants 1695
The foundation awards grants to eligible organizations in its areas of interest, including secondary education, higher education, medical research, health care, and general charities. Grants support: education—public and private colleges and universities, as well as private secondary schools, to fund athletically oriented capital projects and scholarship endowments; medical research—individual research projects are considered when sponsored by a recognized medical research center; health—community support for capital campaigns and endowment funds; and general charities—community organizations that support youth, the arts, persons with disabilities, underprivileged, substance abuse rehabilitation, and annual fund drives of national organizations focusing on the above areas. There are no application deadlines or forms.
Restrictions: Grants are not made to individuals.
Geographic Focus: Florida; Maine
Samples: MaineGeneral Medical Center, Waterville, ME, $2,000,000— for Cancer Center (2007); Thomas College, Waterville, ME, $715,493—for Field House Project (2007).
Amount of Grant: $2,000,000 maximum
Contact: Gregory Powell, c/o Dexter Enterprises; (207) 828-7999
Sponsor: Harold Alfond Foundation
Two Monument Square
Portland, ME 04101-4093

Harold Amos Medical Faculty Development Program 1696
This program offers four-year, postdoctoral research fellowships to minority physicians who have demonstrated superior academic and clinical skills and who are committed to careers in academic medicine. The program seeks to increase the number of minority faculty physician scientists who can achieve senior rank in academic medicine and who will encourage and foster the development of succeeding classes of minority physicians. Applications are accepted from African American, Mexican American, Native American, and mainland Puerto Rican physicians. (Mainland Puerto Ricans are those who have completed at least their postsecondary education on the mainland.) Fellows will pursue biomedical research, clinical investigation, or health services research. Participants will conduct research in association with senior faculty members at academic centers.
Requirements: Eligible to apply are minority physicians who are U.S. citizens at the time of application, have excelled in their postsecondary education within the United States, are now completing or will have completed formal clinical training, and are committed to academic careers.
Samples: Baylor College of Medicine and U of Utah's School of Medicine (UT)—for awards through the Minority Medical Faculty Development Program, $365,400 each.; U of Medicine and Dentistry of New Jersey (NJ)—for programs to help minorities and disadvantaged people pursue careers in healthcare, $200,953.; U of North Carolina at Chapel Hill (NC)—for faculty development programs for minority medical faculty members, $365,400.; New York U (NY)—for faculty development programs for minority medical faculty members, $365,400.
Amount of Grant: $65,000 stipend per year plus $26,350 for research support
Date(s) Application is Due: Mar 23
Contact: National Program Office, (301) 565-4080; email: amfdp@starpower.net
Internet: http://www.amfdp.org/applicat.htm
Sponsor: Robert Wood Johnson Foundation
P.O. Box 2316, Rt 1 and College Rd E
Princeton, NJ 08543-2316

Harold and Arlene Schnitzer CARE Foundation Grants 1697
The Foundation's principal purpose is to assist with Jewish, cultural, youth, education, medical, social service, and community activities. Foundation focus is on proposals for projects that enhance the quality of life in Oregon and Southwest Washington. The Foundation funds grant requests for operating expenses, special projects, matching grants, multiple-year grants and capital campaigns as well as for purchase of specific items. There is no formal application form. Interested applicants may contact the Foundation for guidelines.
Requirements: Nonprofit organizations in Oregon and Washington are eligible. Organizations located in Portland are given first funding priority. Approximately 90% of grant funds stay in the Portland metropolitan area.
Restrictions: The Foundation does not provide funds for individuals, non tax-exempt organizations, other private foundations or political groups.
Geographic Focus: Oregon; Washington
Samples: Mittleman Jewish Community Center, Portland, OR, $400,000—for operating support (2007); Oregon Health and Science University Foundation, Portland, OR, $5,500,000— for Diabetes Center (2007).
Amount of Grant: $1,000-$5,000,000 range
Date(s) Application is Due: Feb 28; May 31; Aug 31; Nov 30
Contact: Barbara Hall, Vice President: (503) 973-0286; fax: (503) 450-0810
Sponsor: Harold and Arlene Schnitzer Foundation
P.O. Box 2708
Portland, OR 97208-2708

Harold Simmons Foundation Grants 1698

The foundation awards grants to Texas nonprofit organizations, with emphasis on social services, religion, health, the arts, and youth. Grants also support community programs and projects, child development, and adult basic education/literacy programs. The foundation also supports international development and relief efforts in Third World countries. Grants are awarded for general operating support, annual campaigns, capital campaigns, building construction/renovation, continuing support, seed money, and program development. Application forms are not required, and there are no deadline dates.

Requirements: Dallas, TX, nonprofits are eligible.

Restrictions: Grants are not awarded to support individuals or for endowment funds or loans.

Geographic Focus: Texas

Samples: Children's Medical Ctr Dallas (TX)—to establish a hospital within the medical center devoted to the needs of child cardiac patients, $5 million (2005); U of Texas Southwestern Medical Ctr (Dallas)—to enhance the Simmons Comprehensive Cancer Center, including supporting the work of its newly recruited director, $15.4 million (2005).

Contact: Lisa Simmons Epstein, President, (972) 233-2134

Sponsor: Harold Simmons Foundation
5430 LBJ Freeway, Suite 1700
Dallas, TX 75240-2697

Harris and Eliza Kempner Fund Grants 1699

The foundation provides grants primarily in the Galveston, TX, area to qualifying organizations in the broad areas of the arts, historic preservation, community development, education, health, and human services. The foundation gives preference to requests for seed money, operating funds, small capital needs, and special projects partnering with other funding sources. Application information is available online.

Requirements: Grants are made primarily to Texas residents.

Restrictions: Funding is not available for: fund-raising benefits; direct mail solicitations; grants to individuals; and grants to non-U.S.A based organizations.

Geographic Focus: Texas

Samples: U of Texas Medical Branch (Galveston, TX)—for its fundraising campaign to support programs to improve access to care; healtcare education; and research on infectious diseases, vaccines, and chronic diseases, $1 million (2003).

Date(s) Application is Due: Mar 15; Oct 15

Contact: Grants Manager, (409) 762-1603; fax: (409) 762-5435; email: information@kempnerfund.org

Internet: http://www.kempnerfund.org/app/programs.html

Sponsor: Harris and Eliza Kempner Fund
2201 Market Street, Suite 601
Galveston, TX 77550-1529

Harrison County Community Foundation Grants 1700

The foundation awards grants to eligible Indiana nonprofit organizations in its areas of interest, including arts and culture, community projects, education, environment, animal protection, health and safety, historical preservation, human services, and recreation. The foundation also awards mini grants to support small projects outside of the regular semiannual grant cycles. Mini grants support unexpected costs such as emergency equipment repairs or purchases, special event support, or other non-routine, nonrecurring expenses. Grants to religious organizations are limited to projects that benefit the community at large, preserve a historical site (typically 100 years or older), or respond to an immediate health or safety related problem. Each spring, the foundation provides funds to each of the county's four high schools for scholarships. Scholarship recipients are selected by the individual high school scholarship selection committee, who also determine the amounts awarded.

Requirements: Nonprofit agencies providing services to residents of Harrison County, IN, are eligible to apply. 501(c)3 tax-exempt organizations and schools, religious organizations, and local governmental units are eligible. All graduating high school seniors in Harrison County are eligible for scholarships.

Restrictions: The foundation does not award grants to purchase real estate that has not been identified and an offer accepted; political activities or those designed to influence legislation; individuals (except scholarships); travel associated with a school-sponsored event; or religious organizations for the purpose of furthering that religion. Traditional equipment, routine maintenance, or facility improvements will not be funded.

Geographic Focus: Indiana

Date(s) Application is Due: Jan 15; Jul 15

Contact: Grants Administrator; (812) 738-6668; fax: (812) 738-6864; email: staff@hccfindiana.org

Internet: http://www.hccfindiana.org

Sponsor: Harrison County Community Foundation
P.O. Box 279, 1523 Foundation Way
Corydon, IN 47112

Harry A. and Margaret D. Towsley Foundation Grants 1701

The foundation awards grants to Michigan organizations in its areas of interest, including environment, medical and preschool education, social services, continuing education, and research in the health sciences. Types of support include annual campaigns, building construction and renovation, capital campaigns, continuing support, employee matching gifts, endowments, general operating support, matching/challenge support, professorships, program development, research, and seed grants. There are no application forms; submit a letter of inquiry between January and the listed application deadline.

Restrictions: Grants are not awarded to individuals or for travel, scholarships, fellowships, conferences, books, publications, films, tapes, audio-visual or communication media, or loans.

Geographic Focus: Michigan

Samples: U of Michigan at Ann Arbor, School of Music ((MI)—to construct a theater and performing-arts center, $1.5 million (2005); Nature Conservancy, Michigan Chapter (Lansing, MI)—for the Northern Great Lakes Forest Project, which will protect 271,000 acres across eight counties in Michigan's Upper Peninsula and link more than 2.5 million acres of protected federal, state, and natural areas, $2 million (2005).

Date(s) Application is Due: Mar 31

Contact: Lynn White, President, (989) 837-1100; fax: (989) 837-3240

Sponsor: Harry A. and Margaret D. Towsley Foundation
P.O. Box 349, 140 Ashman Street
Midland, MI 48640

Harry and Grace Steele Foundation Grants 1702

The foundation's giving emphasizes higher and secondary education including scholarship funds, the fine arts, population control, hospitals and clinics, religion, and youth agencies. Types of support include building funds, endowment funds, scholarship funds, matching funds, continuing support, general purposes, special projects, and equipment grants. Grants are made primarily to California organizations. Application guidelines may be requested; there is no deadline date.

Requirements: IRS 501(c)3 tax-exempt organizations in Orange County, CA, are eligible.

Restrictions: Grants are not made to individuals.

Geographic Focus: California

Samples: Borrego Community Health Society (Borrego Springs, CA)—for general support, $1 million, (2003); Traveler's Aid Society (Garden Grove, CA)—for an additional case worker, $50,000.; Canine Companions for Independence (Rancho Santa Fe, CA)—for training of working dogs, $12,000.; Chapman U—for renovation of the biotechnology laboratory, $200,000.

Amount of Grant: $100,000-$250,000 range

Contact: Audrey Burnand, (949) 631-0418

Sponsor: Harry and Grace Steele Foundation
441 Old Newport Boulevard, Suite 301
Newport Beach, CA 92663

Harry Bramhall Gilbert Charitable Trust Grants 1703

The Harry Bramhall Gilbert Charitable Trust supports tax-exempt organizations that contribute to the health, education, and cultural life of the Tidewater, Virginia region. The Trust currently and substantially funds nonprofits based in the cities of Norfolk, Chesapeake, and Virginia Beach, Virginia. To apply, submit a letter to the Trust (no application form is required) containing the following information: copy of IRS Determination Letter; copy of most recent annual report/audited financial statement/990; listing of board of directors, trustees, officers and other key people and their affiliations; detailed description of project and amount of funding requested. Include two copies.

Requirements: Virginia nonprofit organizations based in the cities of Norfolk, Chesapeake, and Virginia Beach are eligible.

Restrictions: No support for religious or political organizations. No grants to individuals.

Geographic Focus: Virginia

Samples: Chesapeake Public Library Foundation, Chesapeake, VA, $5,000—for additions to collections of books, magazines, newspapers, computers, and software at Central Library (2008); University of Virginia, Charlottesville, VA, $100,000—for merit scholarships for undergraduate students in their fourth-year at UVA meeting certain criteria, who have graduated from Public High School of City of Chesapeake, VA (2008); Virginia Symphony, Norfolk, VA, $25,000—for general support and the Virginia Symphony Endowment Fund (2008).

Amount of Grant: $2,500 -$100,000 range

Date(s) Application is Due: Sep 30

Contact: Stuart D. Glasser, Treasurer; (757) 204-4858; email: sdglasser@cox.net

Internet: http://fdncenter.org/grantmaker/gilbert

Sponsor: Harry Bramhall Gilbert Charitable Trust
316 Scone Castle Loop
Chesapeake, VA 23322

Harry Frank Guggenheim Foundation Research Grants 1704

The foundation invites proposals for natural and social science research that may increase understanding of the causes, manifestations, and control of human violence and aggression. Grants are awarded for one-year support of postdoctoral research. Issues of particular interest are violence and aggression in children, the relationship between drugs and violence, violence in families, techniques for controlling aggression and violence, and political and religious violence. Types of support include salaries, employee benefits, research assistants, supplies, equipment, fieldwork, and technical assistance. Funded programs average two years in duration.

Requirements: The grants are intended to fund individual investigators, not institutional programs.

Restrictions: Funds are not for studies directed toward requirements for the doctoral degree, institutional overhead, nor for conference support.

Amount of Grant: $15,000-$30,000 for one or two years

Date(s) Application is Due: Aug 1

Contact: Program Officer, (646) 428-0971; fax: (646) 428-0981; email: hfgacf@aol.com

Internet: http://www.hfg.org/rg/guidelines.htm
Sponsor: Harry Frank Guggenheim Foundation
25 W 53rd Street
New York, NY 10019-5401

Harry Kramer Memorial Fund Grants **1705**

The Harry Kramer Memorial Fund, established in 1982, supports Jewish organizations in the United States and Israel, involved with the care of the sick or aged, education, and religious organizations. Giving primarily in the southern Florida area. Areas of interest include: aging, centers/services; arts; disasters, 9/11/01; higher education; human services; international terrorism; Jewish federated giving programs; disabled individuals.
Requirements: There are no specific deadlines with which to adhere. Contact the Foundation for further application information and guidelines.
Restrictions: No grants to individuals, or for operating budgets or continuing support.
Geographic Focus: Alabama; Alaska; Arizona; Arkansas; California; Colorado; Connecticut; Delaware; District of Columbia; Florida; Georgia; Guam; Hawaii; Idaho; Illinois; Indiana; Iowa; Kansas; Kentucky; Louisiana; Maine; Maryland; Massachusetts; Michigan; Minnesota; Mississippi; Missouri; Montana; Nebraska; Nevada; New England; New Hampshire; New Jersey; New Mexico; New York; North Carolina; North Dakota; Ohio; Oklahoma; Oregon; Pacific Northwest; Pennsylvania; Puerto Rico; Rhode Island; South Carolina; South Dakota; Tennessee; Texas; U.S. Virgin Islands; Utah; Vermont; Virginia; Washington; West; West Virginia; Wisconsin; WyomingIsrael
Samples: Jewish Museum of Florida, Miami Beach, FL, $15,000 (2006); PEF Israel Endowment Funds, New York, NY, $5,000 (2006); American Friends of Israel Elwyn, Philadelphia, PA, $10,000 (2006);
Amount of Grant: $1,800-$15,000 range
Contact: Leslie J. August, Wachovia Bank, N.A. Trustee; (305) 789-4645;
Sponsor: Harry Kramer Memorial Fund c/o Wachovia Bank, N.A.
100 North Main Street., 13th Floor
Winston-Salem, NC 27150-0001

Harry S. Black and Allon Fuller Fund **1706**

The Harry S. Black & Allon Fuller Fund was established in 1930 to support quality health care and human services programming for underserved populations. The grantmaking focus is in the following areas: Health Care—the Fund supports access to health care; health education; health/wellness promotion and disease prevention; and health policy analysis and advocacy. Emphasis will be placed on programs serving low-income communities; Physical Disabilities—the Fund supports access programs for physically disabled individuals; disability policy analysis and advocacy; workforce development programs; and programs that improve quality of life for the disabled. Grant requests for general operating support or program/project support are strongly encouraged. The Fund has biannual deadlines of April 1 and October 1. Grant decisions for the April 1 deadline will be made by June 30. Grant decisions for the October 1 deadline will be made by December 31.
Requirements: Nonprofit organizations must be geographically located within the city limits of New York City or Chicago to be eligible to apply.
Restrictions: In general, grant requests for endowment campaigns, capital projects, or research will not be considered.
Geographic Focus: Illinois; New York
Amount of Grant: $5,000-$20,000
Date(s) Application is Due: Apr 1; Oct 1
Contact: Christine O'Donnell, c/o Bank of America; (646) 855-1011; email: christine.l.o'donnell@baml.com
Internet: https://www.bankofamerica.com/philanthropic/fn_search.action
Sponsor: Harry S. Black and Allon Fuller Fund
One Bryant Park, NY1-100-28-05
New York, NY 10036

Harry Shwachman Clinical Investigator Award **1707**

This three-year award provides the opportunity for clinically trained physicians to develop into independent biomedical research investigators who have active involvement in cystic fibrosis-related areas. It is also intended to facilitate the transition from postdoctoral training to a career in academic medicine. Applications are due the first Wednesday in September.
Requirements: U.S. citizenship or permanent resident status is required.
Amount of Grant: $70,000 maximum per year plus $15,000 for supplies
Date(s) Application is Due: Sep 1
Contact: Office of Grants Management, (301) 951-4422; fax: (301) 951-6378; email: grants@cff.org
Internet: http://www.cff.org/research/cystic_fibrosis_foundation_grants/research_grants
Sponsor: Cystic Fibrosis Foundation
6931 Arlington Road, 2nd Floor
Bethesda, MD 20814

Harry Sudakoff Foundation Grants **1708**

The Foundation, established in 1956, offers funding primarily in the forms of ongoing support and capital campaigns. Focus areas include: federated giving programs; higher education; and human/social services. Of particular interest are the performing arts, including dance, music, and theater. The geographic focus is Sarasota, Florida, with an initial approach by Letter of Interest. Though there are no specific application forms, the annual deadline for application is August 15, with final notification by November 1st.
Requirements: Grantees must be 501(C)(3) organizations with a sound track record.
Restrictions: Generally the Foundation will not provide grants for: endowments, deficit financing, debt reduction, or ordinary operating expenses; conferences, seminars, workshops, travel, surveys, advertising, fund-raising costs or research; annual giving campaigns; individuals; or projects that have already been completed.
Geographic Focus: Florida
Samples: Mental Health Community Centers, Sarasota, Florida—to provide a 15-passenger van for support programs at Prospect House, $30,000 (2006); Suncoast Communities Blood Bank, Sarasota, Florida, $72,500 (2006).
Amount of Grant: $46,875 average
Date(s) Application is Due: Aug 15
Contact: Janet L Dickens, Asst. V. P., Bank of America; (941) 952-2826; fax: (941) 952-2768; email: janet.dickens@ustrust.com
Sponsor: The Harry Sudakoff Foundation
c/o Janet Lynn Dickens, Bank of America, 1605 Main Street
Sarasota, FL 34236-5840 34236-5840

Hartford Aging and Health Program Awards **1709**

The foundation's two principal programs are Health Care Cost and Quality and Aging and Health. The Health Care Cost and Quality program supports the community health management initiative, health care quality measures, and reducing inappropriate health care services. The Aging and Health program supports strengthening physicians' knowledge of geriatrics, reducing medication problems of the elderly, and demonstrating integrated financing and service delivery for comprehensive geriatric services. Types of support include operating budgets, continuing support, projects/programs, research, publications, and conferences and seminars. The foundation also welcomes inquiries regarding projects that may not fit these specific interests but would further its broad goal of improving health care in America. Types of support include general operations, continuing support, projects/programs, research, publications, and conferences and seminars. Applications are accepted at any time and are reviewed four times each year when the board meets.
Requirements: U.S. health, education, and social service organizations may apply.
Restrictions: Requests will be denied for general research or for projects lasting more than three years.
Contact: Corinne Rieder, Executive Director, (212) 832-7788; fax: (212) 593-4913; email: mail@jhartfound.com
Internet: http://www.jhartfound.org
Sponsor: John A. Hartford Foundation
55 E 59th Street, 16th Floor
New York, NY 10022-1178

Hartford Courant Foundation Grants **1710**

The Foundation established in 1950, supports organizations involved with education, the arts, community development, health and social services, with an emphasis on programs benefiting children, youth and families. Grants in the area of the arts will be made only for outreach or education programs for children or families. Grants may be awarded in support of program, capital and operating expenses, for seed money and as challenge or matching grants. The Hartford Courant Foundation serves: Andover, Avon, Bloomfield, Bolton, Canton, East Granby, East Hartford, East Windsor, Ellington, Enfield, Farmington, Glastonbury, Granby, Hartford, Hebron, Manchester, Marlborough, Middletown, New Britain, Newington, Rocky Hill, Simsbury, Somers, South Windsor, Suffield, Tolland, Vernon, West Hartford, Wethersfield, Windsor, and Windsor Locks.
Requirements: An organization wishing to apply for a grant from The Hartford Courant Foundation must be: within the Foundations service areas; a non-profit organization; submit its request using a Hartford Courant Foundation application form, available on the Foundations website; include supporting documentation.
Restrictions: The Hartford Courant Foundation's policies do not allow funding of: organizations which are not tax exempt under IRS Code section 501(c)3; organizations which have the IRS Private Foundation designation; individuals; endowment funds; religious institutions, other than for their provision of non-sectarian community services; capital projects related to the arts; performances, conferences, trips, one-time events; annual campaigns.
Geographic Focus: Connecticut
Date(s) Application is Due: Dec 15; Mar 15; Jun 15; Sep 15
Contact: Kate Miller, Executive Director; (860) 241-6472 fax: (860) 520-6988; email: kmiller@hcfdn.org
Internet: http://www.hcfdn.org/application/guidelines.htm
Sponsor: The Hartford Courant Foundation
285 Broad Street
Hartford, CT 06115

Hartford Foundation Regular Grants **1711**

The Foundation awards grants for a broad range of purposes to a wide variety of nonprofit organizations in social services, health, education, early childhood and youth services, arts and culture, housing and neighborhood development, and other charitable fields. These grants: enhance or strengthen existing activities; provide start-up for organizations and new programs; provide support for capital improvements. Interested applicants are encouraged to phone a program contact to discuss their project before beginning the application process.
Requirements: Nonprofit organizations in the following Connecticut towns are eligible to apply for funding: Andover, Avon, Bloomfield, Bolton, Canton, East Granby, East Hartford, East Windsor, Ellington, Enfield, Farmington, Glastonbury, Granby,

Hartford, Hebron, Manchester, Marlborough, Newington, Rocky Hill, Simsbury, Somers, South Windsor, Suffield, West Hartford, Wethersfield, Windsor, Windsor Locks, Tolland, and Vernon. Proposals for statewide programs may be considered when there is a substantial benefit to residents of these communities.
Restrictions: The Foundation does not make grants from its unrestricted funds for: sectarian or religious activities; grants directly to individuals; grants to private foundations; endowments or memorials; direct or grass-roots lobbying efforts; conferences; research; or informational activities on topics that are primarily national or international in perspective. In addition, the Foundation generally does not make grants for: federal, state, or municipal agencies or departments supported by taxation; sponsorship of or support for one-time events; liquidation of obligations incurred at a previous date; or sustaining support for recurring operating expenses.
Geographic Focus: Connecticut
Samples: Town of Farmington, Farmington, CT, $19,749 - for construction of a tower and zip line at the youth center and for the Farmington High School's McDonough School Math and Literacy Tutoring Program (2007); The ARC of the Farmington Valley, Inc., Canton, CT, $375,000 - for remodeling, code compliance, and upgrades to the Alleluia property (2007).
Amount of Grant: $500,000 maximum
Contact: Cheryl L. Gerrish, Grants Manager; (860) 548-1888; fax: (860) 524-8346; email: gerrish@hfpg.org or hfpg@hfpg.org
Internet: http://www.hfpg.org/GrantmakingPrograms/Overview/tabid/163/Default.aspx
Sponsor: Hartford Foundation
10 Columbus Boulevard, 8th Floor
Hartford, CT 06106

Hartford Geriatrics Health Outcomes Research Scholars Program **1712**
This program supports physician-scientists committed to improving the health care of older adults during the critical transition from junior faculty to independent researcher. Outcomes research is defined as the study of functional status, impairments, perceptions, social opportunities, and health services utilization that are influenced by disease, injury, treatment, or health policy, including etiology, diagnosis, and intervention. Research must be focused on older adults and may address clinical strategies and effectiveness, innovative outcomes measures, and quality of life. Scholars must have a research sponsor who should have a strong background in training and outcomes research, as well as expertise and interest in the outcomes research that is being proposed. Guidelines and an application request form are available online.
Requirements: The applicant must be a U.S. citizen or permanent resident; be sponsored at a U.S. allopathic or osteopathic institution by a full-time faculty member; have an MD or DO degree; hold a full-time faculty appointment at the level of assistant professor for no longer than two years at the time the grant becomes effective; demonstrate the motivation and ability to devote at least 75 percent of his or her time to conduct outcomes research related to improving the care of older adults with the goal of devoting his/her research career to this area; be a geriatrician or geriatric psychiatrist who has completed all of the requirements to be eligible to sit for a Certificate of Added Qualifications by the time the award commences (July 1), or a general internist (or family physician, neurologist, or subspecialist of internal medicine) who is pursuing a career devoted to aging research and who has completed all the requirements to be eligible to sit for board certification in his/her discipline; and have at least two years of training with one year of clinical experience at an accredited U.S. institution, and one year of research training at a U.S. academic institution.
Amount of Grant: $75,000 per year for two years
Date(s) Application is Due: Jan 15
Contact: Funding Administrator, (800) 247-8779 or (212) 308-1414; fax: (212) 832-8646; email: sreinthaler@americangeriatrics.org
Internet: http://www.healthinaging.org/research
Sponsor: American Geriatrics Society Foundation for Health in Aging
350 Fifth Avenue, Suite 801
New York, NY 10118

Harvest Foundation Grants **1713**
Formed by the sale of Memorial Health Systems, the foundation is managing an endowment to invest in programs and initiatives that will address local challenges in the areas of health, education, and welfare in Martinsville/Henry County. The foundation is committed to honoring the legacy of Memorial Hospital by emphasizing prevention, safety and access to health care; by facilitating opportunities for local citizens to help their community reach its potential; and by improving the learning environment for citizenship, academic, and vocational preparedness. Application and guidelines are available online.
Requirements: To be eligible for consideration, an organization must: be located within, or have its program focused within Martinsville and/or Henry County; have a letter from the IRS stating its 501c3 status; and propose a project within one of the Foundation's three interest areas of health, education or welfare.
Restrictions: The foundation does not fund organizations that discriminate based upon race, creed, gender, or sexual orientation; scholarships, fellowships, or grants to individuals; sectarian religious activities, political lobbying, or legislative activities; profit-making businesses; emergency needs or extremely time sensitive requests; or direct replacement of discontinued government support.
Geographic Focus: Virginia
Samples: Dan River Basin Association, $8,000— to enhance the Uptown Spur Trail (2009); Boy Scouts of America, Blue Ridge Mountains Council, $45,300—to launch the Scoutreach Program aimed at recruiting underserved boys in Martinsville/Henry County to join the Boy Scouts (2009); MARC Workshop, Inc., $241,900—funding paid over 3 years to start-up a mobile employment program for disabled adults, creating competitive, minimum wage jobs for special education students graduating out of the public school system (2009).
Contact: Allyson Rothrock, Executive Director; (276) 632-3329; fax: (276) 632-1878; email: arothrock@theharvestfoundation.org
Internet: http://www.theharvestfoundation.org/page.cfm/topic/strategic-map
Sponsor: Harvest Foundation
P.O. Box 5183, 1 Ellsworth Street
Martinsville, VA 24115

Hasbro Children's Fund **1714**
The mission of the Fund is to assist children triumphing over critical life obstacles as well as bringing the joy of play into their lives. Through the Fund's initiatives, the mission is achieved by supporting programs which provide terminal and seriously ill children respite and access to play, educational programs for children at risk, and basics for children in need. Interested applicants are asked to submit a letter of inquiry through the online system.
Requirements: Applications are accepted from nonprofit organizations around the world.
Restrictions: Funding is not available for: religious organizations; individuals; cash free grants; research; political organizations; scholarships; travel stipends; loans; endowments; goodwill advertising; sponsorship of recreational activities; fundraisers; auctions; and schools.
Geographic Focus: Massachusetts; Rhode Island; Washington
Amount of Grant: $1,000-$10,000
Date(s) Application is Due: Jun 1
Contact: Grants Administrator, email: HCFinfo@hasbro.com
Internet: http://www.hasbro.org/default.cfm?page=grantmaking
Sponsor: Hasbro Children's Fund
1027 Newport Avenue
Pawtucket, RI 02862-1059

Hastings Center International Visiting Scholars Program **1715**
This program responds to the growing interest in comparative bioethics and to the number of foreign scholars and medical professionals interested in the center's work—examining critical ethical issues in medicine, the life sciences, and the professions. The program is designed for advanced scholars and practitioners who have made or will make significant contributions to bioethics in their own countries. International scholars usually stay two weeks to six weeks, dividing their time between their own research and ongoing activities at the center. There is a modest stipend for foreign citizens who require financial assistance. Applications are due four to six months in advance of proposed stay.
Amount of Grant: $500-$1500
Contact: Daniel Callahan, Director, International Programs, (845) 424-4040 ext 222; fax: (845) 424-4545; email: callahand@thehastingscenter.org
Internet: http://www.thehastingscenter.org/visitors/visitorsint.asp
Sponsor: Hastings Center
Rte 9D, 21 Malcolm Gordon Road
Garrison, NY 10524-5555

Hawaii Community Foundation Health Education and Research Grants **1716**
The program provides support from three distinct funds: Tobacco Prevention & Control Trust Fund; the Leahi Fund Research Fund; and the Medical Research Program. Funding will be provided for medical education and research in the fields of: cancer; heart disease; lung disease and research. Priority is given to projects that: demonstrate a foreseeable benefit to the people of Hawaii; support new investigators in Hawaii; and support collaborative efforts. Proposal submission information is available online.
Requirements: To be eligible for consideration an organization must be a 501(c)3 organization or a unit of government. The Principal Investigator must be based in Hawaii and conducting the research in Hawaii.
Geographic Focus: Hawaii
Amount of Grant: $25,000-$50,000
Date(s) Application is Due: Feb 27; Jul 17; Aug 14; Sep 10
Contact: Christel Wuerfel, Philanthropic Services Assistant; (808) 537-6333 or (888) 731-3863; email: cwuerfel@hcf-hawaii.org or jsmith@hcf-hawaii.org
Internet: http://www.hawaiicommunityfoundation.org/index.php?id=71&categoryID=23
Sponsor: Hawaii Community Foundation
1164 Bishop Street, Suite 800
Honolulu, HI 96813

Hawaii Community Foundation Reverend Takie Okumura Family Grants **1717**
The Fund was established by members of the Okumura family to continue the charitable work of Reverend Okumura focusing on the healthy development of Hawaii's young children and youth. Proposals will be accepted in the following areas of focus: youth (ages 6-20 years old) and young children (ages birth to 5 years old). Priorities will be given to programs which: develop the ability to think critically; understand and appreciate one's own culture and those of others; develop the ability to settle differences peacefully; strengthen the early care and education community system. Proposal submission information is available online.
Requirements: Hawai'i organizations that are tax exempt, including nonprofit organizations, 501(c)3 organizations, religious organizations that are exempt from taxation, or units of government are eligible to apply.

Restrictions: Funding is not available for: major capitol projects; endowments; or on-going or general operating costs.
Geographic Focus: Hawaii
Amount of Grant: $5,000-$15,000
Date(s) Application is Due: Aug 5
Contact: Christel Wuerfel, Philanthropic Services Assistant; (808) 537-6333 or (888) 731-3863; email: cwuerfel@hcf-hawaii.org
Internet: http://www.hawaiicommunityfoundation.org/index.php?id=71&category ID=24
Sponsor: Hawaii Community Foundation
1164 Bishop Street, Suite 800
Honolulu, HI 96813

Hawaii Community Foundation West Hawaii Fund Grants **1718**
The West Hawaii Fund was established at the Hawaii Community Foundation in 1992 by a group of concerned citizens for the purpose of accepting charitable gifts for the benefit of the people and communities of West Hawaii, from North Kohala to Hawaiian Ocean View Estates. Today, the Fund continues to grow through additional contributions and planned gifts from donors in the community to respond to current and emerging needs and improve the quality of life for the residents of West Hawaii. The strongest proposals will be those that meet the following criteria: proposal articulates how the proposed project will benefit the West Hawaii community; proposal clearly describes how the project will be implemented and how these particular activities will address critical issues in the West Hawaii community; there are clearly stated outcomes and a plan for measuring and reporting results; project demonstrates collaboration among different sectors of the community; project budget is realistic, relates to project narrative and is reasonable in cost.
Requirements: 501(c)3 organizations - Grant awards will range up to $10,000 Community organizations not designated as 501(c)3 organizations – Grant awards will range up to $2,000 To be eligible for grants of more than $2,000, organization must be designated 501(c)3 or have a 501(c)3 fiscal sponsor
Restrictions: Projects not likely to be funded: projects that do not benefit the residents of West Hawaii; funds for endowments or for the benefit of specific individuals; out-of-state travel expenses; start-up costs of a new organization.
Geographic Focus: Hawaii
Amount of Grant: $2,000-$10,000 range
Date(s) Application is Due: Oct 1
Contact: Diane Chadwick, Fund Director; (808) 885-2174; fax: (808) 885-1857; email: dchadwick@hcf-hawaii.org
Internet: http://www.hawaiicommunityfoundation.org/index.php?id=71&category ID=22
Sponsor: Hawaii Community Foundation
1164 Bishop Street, Suite 800
Honolulu, HI 96813

Hawn Foundation Grants **1719**
The foundation awards grants to Texas arts, education, health care, hospitals, medical research, and social services organizations. Preference will be given to requests from organizations in Dallas, TX.
Restrictions: The Foundation does not award scholarships or fellowships.
Geographic Focus: Texas
Amount of Grant: $1000-$200,000 average range
Date(s) Application is Due: Jun 1
Contact: Joe Hawn Jr., (214) 696-6595; fax: (214) 696-6596
Sponsor: Hawn Foundation
5949 Sherry Lane, Suite 775
Dallas, TX 75225-8043

Hazel Corbin/Maternity Center Association Grant for Evidence-Based Midwifery Care **1720**
The fund provides stipends for students accredited by the American College of Nurse Midwives and accepted in post-RN education programs for nurse-midwifery ending in certification eligibility. Post-RN programs are eight to 12 months in duration, and master's programs usually are from 12 to 24 months. Applicants must write for application forms, enclosing evidence of program acceptance and complete details of the program. Applications are accepted at any time; awards are made as funds permit.
Requirements: Applicants must be registered nurses who are preparing for nurse-midwifery certification in the United States. Students must have a license to practice nursing in a state of the United States and must already have been accepted in an approved nurse-midwifery basic or refresher program at a U.S. school.
Amount of Grant: $4500
Date(s) Application is Due: Apr 30
Contact: Hazel Corbin Grant, (240) 485-1800; fax: (240) 485-1818
Internet: http://www.midwife.org/foundation/award-corbin.cfm
Sponsor: A.C.N.M. Foundation
8403 Colesville Road, Suite 1550
Silver Spring, MD 20910

HCA Foundation Grants **1721**
The Foundation is committed to the care and improvement of human life. Grants are made in the areas of health and well being, childhood and youth development, and the arts. Preference will be given to requests from organizations where an HCA employee volunteers or serves on the board. Application information is available online.
Requirements: 501(c)3 nonprofit organizations are eligible. Because the foundation focuses its giving in Middle Tennessee, all requests outside of the Nashville area should be submitted to the closest HCA facility location or division office.
Restrictions: Funding is not available for: individuals or their projects; private foundations; political activities; advertising or sponsorships of events; social events or similar fund-raising activities. The Foundation does not ordinarily support: organizations in their first three years of operation and organizations involved in research, sports, environmental, wildlife, civic and international affairs. The Foundation does not accept proposals from individual churches or schools, but will support broad faith-based initiatives consistent with our mission and guidelines.
Geographic Focus: Tennessee
Samples: American National Red Cross (Washington, DC)—for relief efforts in South Asia and Africa, $1 million (2005).
Date(s) Application is Due: Dec 8; Mar 16; Jun 22; Sep 14
Contact: Lois Abrams, Grants Manager, (615) 344-2390; fax: (615) 344-5722; lois.abrams@hcahealthcare.com
Internet: http://www.hcacaring.org
Sponsor: HCA Foundation
One Park Plaza, Building 1 - 4th Floor East
Nashville, TN 37203

Health Canada National Seniors Independence Program Grants **1722**
The program is intended to provide financial assistance to Canadian seniors for projects that contribute to improving their health, well-being, and independence and to enhancing their quality of life. Particular attention will be given to projects that address the needs of women seniors, seniors living in rural and remote areas, and seniors who are less advantaged due to life circumstances. The program will provide funds for projects that support action leading to a new or improved resource or organization; test the value or feasibility of new program models; improve the quality and availability of information on particular subjects; and/or develop and strengthen the knowledge, skills, and abilities of seniors or people working with seniors. Groups and organizations interested in submitting an application should contact the appropriate regional office where program representatives are available to meet with groups to discuss their ideas and assist in the preparation of an application. Lists of regional offices are available from the national office.
Requirements: Proposals may be submitted by voluntary, nongovernmental, nonprofit groups and organizations; these may include health or social service agencies, higher educational institutions, professional associations, and other parapublic organizations.
Restrictions: Individuals, for-profit groups, and government departments are not eligible for funding.
Contact: Stephanie Wilson, (613) 954-8549; fax: (613) 954-7363; email: Stephanie_Wilson@hc-sc.gc.ca
Internet: http://www.hc-sc.gc.ca
Sponsor: Health Canada
Postal locator 1912
Ottawa, ON K1A 1B4 Canada

Health Care Financing Research, Demonstrations, and Evaluations Grants **1723**
Project grants (including cooperative agreements) are awarded to support analyses, experiments, demonstrations, and pilot projects in efforts to resolve major health care financing issues or to develop innovative methods for the administration of Medicare and Medicaid. HCFA has identified priority areas for the current fiscal year, including access and quality of care, coordinated care systems, provider payment, health care systems reform and financing, program evaluation and analysis, service delivery systems, and subacute and long-term care. Awardees are required to share in the cost of projects; normally, the minimum cost-sharing requirement is 5 percent of total project costs. Projects are generally funded on a 12-month basis, with support beyond the first year contingent upon acceptable evidence of satisfactory progress, continuing program relevance, and availability of funds. Applications may be submitted at any time.
Requirements: Grants or cooperative agreements may be made to private or public and nonprofit or for-profit agencies/organizations.
Amount of Grant: $25,000-$1 million; $235,000 average
Contact: Judy Norris, (410)786-5130; email: jnorris1@cms.hhs.gov
Internet: http://www.cms.hhs.gov/contracts
Sponsor: Health Care Financing Administration
7500 Security Boulevard
Baltimore, MD 21244-1850

Health Foundation of Greater Cincinnati Grants **1724**
The foundation awards grants to programs and activities that improve health in Cincinnati and 20 surrounding counties in Ohio, Kentucky, and Indiana. Health is broadly defined to include social, behavioral, environmental, and other dimensions beyond the absence of illness. Grant making is focused on strengthening primary care providers to the poor; school-based child health interventions in K-8 school settings; substance abuse; and severe mental illness. Grants also are awarded in response to requests from organizations seeking funds to support a broad range of health-related needs in the community. The Health Foundation of Greater Cincinnati considers projects for funding in three ways: through Requests for Proposals (RFPs), through invitations to submit proposals, and through grantee-initiated requests. In any case, proposals are considered using the same eligibility requirements and proposal evaluation criteria. For more information about the types of proposals, see the Foundations website or call the Grant Manager.

Requirements: 501(c)3 nonprofits in Adams, Brown, Butler, Clermont, Clington, Hamilton, Highland, and Warren Counties in Ohio; Boone, Bracken, Campbell, Gallatin, Grant, Kenton, and Pendleton Counties in Kentucky; and Dearborn, Franklin, Ohio, Ripley, and Switzerland Counties in Indiana are eligible.
Restrictions: The foundation does not normally fund capital campaigns, annual fundraising campaigns, endowments, event sponsorships, clinical research, scholarships, routine operational costs, or direct financial subsidy of health services to individuals or groups.
Geographic Focus: Indiana; Kentucky; Ohio
Contact: Shelly Stolarczyk-George, Grants Manager, (513) 458-6619; fax: (513) 458-6610; email: sstolarczyk@healthfoundation.org
Internet: http://www.healthfoundation.org/grants
Sponsor: Health Foundation of Greater Cincinnati
3805 Edwards Road, Suite 500
Cincinnati, OH 45209-1948

Health Foundation of Greater Indianapolis Grants 1725
The foundation promotes health care for children, youth, and families in Marion County, IN, and seven contiguous Indiana counties. Programs of interest include school-based health, adolescent health, and HIV/AIDS Grants also are awarded to support the development of health careers and to promote cooperative effort between health professionals. Types of support include general operations, building/renovations, equipment, program/project development, conferences and seminars, seed money, technical assistance, and matching funds. Prior to submitting a proposal, contact Stephen L. Everett, Vice President of Programs, to determine if your program and proposal matches The Health Foundation of Greater Indianapolis' funding priorities and application guidelines.
Requirements: Grants are awarded to neighborhood-based service centers in Indiana's Marion County and the seven contiguous counties of Boone, Hamilton, Hancock, Hendricks, Johnson, Morgan and Shelby. Applicants must be a 501 (c)(3) group, organization or agency that provides health-related programs or services.
Restrictions: Grants will not be provided for: individuals; sectarian religious organizations; research projects; purchase of advertising or tickets to events; production and design of educational materials already available; endowments; short or long term loans or payment of financial obligations.
Geographic Focus: Indiana
Samples: Indiana AIDS Fund (Indianapolis, IN)—for a fundraising event for HIV/AIDS organizations, $25,000 (2005); Indianapolis Medical Society Foundation (IN)—for a project designed to improve access to health care for low-income, uninsured Indianapolis residents, $40,000 (2005); Little Red Door Cancer Agency (Indianapolis, IN)—to provide baskets filled with personal-care items to people with cancer, $15,000 (2005); Damien Ctr (Indianapolis, IN)—to implement its HIV Care Network, $50,000 (2005).
Amount of Grant: $10,000-$100,000 average
Contact: Stephen Everett, Program Officer; (317) 630-1805; fax: (317) 630-1806; email: severett@thfgi.org
Internet: http://www.thfgi.org
Sponsor: Health Foundation of Greater Indianapolis, Inc.
429 East Vermont Street, Suite 300
Indianapolis, IN 46202

Health Foundation of Southern Florida Responsive Grants 1726
The foundation awards Responsive Grants through two grant cycles per year. With exceptions, the foundation focuses on providing one to three year grants that do not exceed $300,000 annually. The majority of grants are funded in the $50,000 to $150,000 range over one or two years. Funding is provided in four categories: Project Planning; Health Services; Organizational Capacity Building and Health System/Health Policy Development.
Requirements: Though the foundation welcomes proposal applications anytime, the applications are reviewed on a semi-annual basis. Applicant organizations must be tax-exempt nonprofit under section 501(c)3 of the Internal Revenue Code or a local or state governmental agency. The project must serve exclusively the residents of Broward, Miami-Dade and/or Monroe counties. Initially, a preliminary proposal is required (see the sponsor's website for specific details). If approved, the sponsor will then invite a full proposal. Download the sponsor's grant guide from the website.
Restrictions: The foundation does not fund: Biomedical research or other research that will not impact local residents within the immediate future (1-3 years) or that does not have a direct application to implementing a community-driven health intervention; Capital campaigns of over $1 million (versus grants toward specific health-related equipment or the 'build out' of a specific health-focused space); Secondary and tertiary services (versus preventive and primary medical, oral and behavioral health care services); Health promotion and/or health care with a high per capita cost (this figure will vary depending upon the type of intervention, but over $1,000 per person/year cost may be a rule of thumb); Service expansion or new projects without viable sustainability (unable to reach sustainability without the foundation's resources within a four-year period).
Geographic Focus: Florida
Amount of Grant: $300,000 maximum
Date(s) Application is Due: Mar 13; Apr 24
Contact: Eliane Morales; (305) 374-7200; fax: (305) 374-7003; email: emorales@hfsf.org
Internet: http://www.hfsf.org/ORIGHTML/responsive.html
Sponsor: Health Foundation of Southern Florida
2 South Biscayne Boulevard
Miami, FL 33131

Health Management Scholarships and Grants for Minorities 1727
This financial assistance program provides scholarships and grants to ethnic minority students for graduate study in health care administration/management. Annual tuition scholarships and grants are made to outstanding students in health services management and related programs. Grants are provided to cover the costs of books, tutorial assistance, and other nontuition educational aids. Students are eligible to receive a combination of awards during the same time period.
Requirements: To be eligible, applicants must be members of an ethnic minority group; must be U.S. citizens or have permanent resident status (birth certificate, green card, or current passport); they must be college juniors, seniors or graduate students; they must be health care administration/management majors; they must have a strong academic background (2.5 GPA on a 4.0 scale); and they must have strong extracurricular and community service activities.
Amount of Grant: $2500 scholarship, $500 grant
Contact: Program Contact, (800) 233-0996 or (312) 422-2680; fax: (312) 422-4566
Internet: http://www.diversityconnection.org/diversityconnection_app/career-center/internships/Standard-Internship-page.jsp?fl=S4
Sponsor: Institute for Diversity in Health Management
1 N Franklin, 30th Floor
Chicago, IL 60606

Healthcare Foundation for Orange County Grants 1728
The foundation's mission is to improve the health of the neediest and most underserved residents of Orange County, with particular emphasis on central Orange County. The foundation will address ways of improving the health of residents by advancing access to health information, prevention, and basic health care. Grantmaking is divided among initiatives that support nonprofit hospital working with community-based organizations (Partners for Health); grants directly to community-based organizations (Healthy Orange County); and increased understanding of community needs, and collaborative granting strategies (coalition projects.)
Requirements: California 501(c)3 nonprofit organizations in Orange County that administer health services consistent with the foundation's goals of providing aid to uninsured, poor families are eligible. Eighty-two percent of support goes to or through qualified nonprofit hospitals. Government agencies also are eligible.
Restrictions: Grants generally are not awarded for annual fund drives, building campaigns, major equipment, or biomedical research. Activities that exclusively benefit the members of a religious or fraternal organization are not funded.
Geographic Focus: California
Amount of Grant: $10,000 maximum
Contact: William B. Stannard, Chairman of the Board; (714) 245-1650; fax: (714) 245-1653; email: dflander@hfoc.org
Internet: http://www.hfoc.org/giving/
Sponsor: Healthcare Foundation for Orange County
1450 N Tustin Avenue, Suite 103
Santa Ana, CA 92705-8641

Healthcare Foundation of New Jersey Grants 1729
The Foundation's funding priorities are the vulnerable populations of the greater Newark New Jersey community; the emergent health needs of serving at-risk individuals and families in the MetroWest Jewish community; and clinical research/medical education initiatives that significantly and directly impact these populations. The Foundation seeks grant proposals that promise innovation and change or a significant enhancement of services. Proposals are accepted on a rolling basis throughout the calendar year.
Requirements: Nonprofit organizations in the Greater Newark area are eligible to apply. The Foundation suggests that application documents be submitted electronically.
Restrictions: Grants are made only to private nonprofit organizations that have tax-exempt status under Section 501(c)3 of the Internal Revenue Code and that are not private foundations. The Foundation does not make grants to individuals or government agencies. The Foundation does not typically fund the following: organizations outside of Essex, Morris or Union County, New Jersey; programs not related to health care; direct support of an individual's healthcare needs; fundraising events or endowment campaigns; advertising campaigns; lobbying; or scholarships.
Geographic Focus: New Jersey
Contact: Program Contact, (973) 921-1210; fax: (973) 921-1274; email: info@hfnj.org
Internet: http://www.hfnj.org
Sponsor: Healthcare Foundation of New Jersey
60 East Willow Street, 2nd Floor
Millburn, NJ 07041

Hearst Foundation and William Randolph Hearst Foundation Grants Program 1730
Within a general policy of assisting institutions with providing access and opportunity to underrepresented, low-income, and minority populations, the foundation directors have established priority areas of interest, including education, health, social services, and culture. Organizations in the private sector are favored over those receiving primary support from tax dollars; organizations serving larger geographic areas are generally favored over those of a neighborhood or narrow community nature. Proposals may be submitted throughout the year; board meetings on grant decisions are held in March, June, September, and December. Only fully documented appeals will be considered. As a general policy, meetings are arranged between foundation staff and applicant only if serious consideration of the appeal is anticipated. Programs headquartered east of the Mississippi River should mail appeals to the Hearst Foundations at the New York address. Those west of the Mississippi River should mail requests to Hearst Foundations, 90 New Montgomery Street, San Francisco, CA 94105; (415) 543-0400.

Requirements: Grants are made only to tax-exempt organizations that are not private foundations.
Restrictions: Funding is not available for: individuals; loans and program-related investments; multi-year grants; start-up or seed funding; equipment of any kind, including computers and transportation; publishing projects; radio, film, television or other media-related projects; conferences, workshops or seminars; public policy research; special events, tickets, tables or advertising for fundraising events.
Contact: Mayra Cedeno, Grants Manager, (212) 586-5404; fax: (212) 586-1917
Internet: http://www.hearstfdn.org
Sponsor: Hearst Foundation
300 West 57th Street, 26th Floor
New York, NY 10019-3741

Heart Rhythm Society Fellowships 1731
Fellowships and research grants are available for projects pertaining to cardiac pacing and/or cardiac electrophysiology. All awards are made for one year, renewable in competition. Also available are traveling fellowships, for a one- to three-month duration, to enable a researcher to observe research at other institutions or attend seminars and conferences. One traveling Canadian fellowship is offered; the applicant must be a Canadian citizen or must train at a site in Canada. Annual deadline dates may vary; contact program staff for exact dates.
Requirements: Fellowships are open to applicants who have a doctor of medicine, philosophy, osteopathy, science, or equivalent training or experience in the field of biomedical engineering. Applicants must be citizens or permanent residents of a North American country and include cardiac pacing or cardiac electrophysiology as a central part of his/her long-range career goals.
Amount of Grant: $40,000 for fellowships, $6000 for traveling fellowships, $6000 for traveling Canadian fellowship
Date(s) Application is Due: Sep 15
Contact: Stephanie Mascetta, (508) 647-0100 ext 3046; fax: (508) 647-0124; email: fellowship@HRSonline.org
Internet: http://www.hrsonline.org/society_in_action/fellowships/default.asp
Sponsor: Heart Rhythm Society
Six Strathmore Road
Natick, MA 01760-2499

Heckscher Foundation for Children Grants 1732
The Foundation's mission is to promote the welfare of children, primarily in New York City. The Foundation funds organizations serving youth in the fields of education, family services, job training, health, arts and recreation. The Foundation's giving takes the form of program support, capacity-building, capital projects and general operating support. Interested applicants should submit a letter of inquiry. LOI instructions are available online.
Requirements: New York City 501(c)3 nonprofit organizations are eligible.
Restrictions: Funding is not available for annual appeals, endowments, fundraising events or political efforts.
Geographic Focus: New York
Contact: Virginia Sloane, President, (212) 744-0190; fax: (212) 744-2761
Internet: http://fdncenter.org/grantmaker/heckscher
Sponsor: Heckscher Foundation for Children
123 East 70th Street
New York, NY 10021

Hedco Foundation Grants 1733
The foundation awards grants domestically and internationally to nonprofit organizations in its areas of interest, including education at all levels; health care, including hospitals and health organizations; and organizations serving children and youth. Types of support include building construction/renovation and equipment acquisition. Past grants have supported biomedical research, but research grants generally are not awarded. There are no application deadlines or forms. An audited financial statement and IRS tax-exemption letter must accompany all proposals.
Requirements: 501(c)3 nonprofit organizations are eligible.
Restrictions: Grants do not support individuals or requests for general operating support, publications, special projects, or loans.
Geographic Focus: California
Samples: U of Oregon, College of Education (Eugene, OR)—to construct an education complex, $10 million (2004).
Amount of Grant: $5000-$75,000 average
Contact: Grants Administrator, (925) 242-0257
Sponsor: Hedco Foundation
P.O. Box 1980
San Ramon, CA 94583

HEI Grants 1734
The institute awards research grants for scientific information about the health effects of motor vehicle emissions on the environment and on human health.
Amount of Grant: $70,000-$300,000
Contact: Daniel Greenbaum, President, (617) 886-9330 ext 311; fax: (617) 886-9335; email: dgreenbaum@healtheffects.org
Internet: http://www.healtheffects.org/funding.htm
Sponsor: Health Effects Institute
120 Second Avenue
Boston, MA 02129-4533

Heineman Foundation for Research, Education, Charitable and Scientific Purposes 1735
The purpose of the Heineman Foundation is to provide seed money to start-up projects and new projects within existing organizations for a maximum of three to five years. Preference will be given to organizations that we have not previously funded. The average range of our donations is $20,000.00 to $50,000.00, per annum. An organization must have 501(c)3 status and upload copies of corresponding IRS documents to the online application form in order for the application to be considered. The Foundation's general areas of interest are the following (in no particular order): programs that enable economically challenged women to enter and remain in the workplace; on site day care centers for women in the workplace; job training programs for women; language and leadership skills for women; environmental research that will help prevent, reduce and/or eliminate water degradation; music as education and preserver of culture; research into prevention of and treatment for childhood illnesses; programs that enable youth to think, create and communicate effectively; and programs that support and promote high achievement in music, science, and literature. Applications/proposals must be submitted online no later than September 1st.
Amount of Grant: $20,000-$50,000 range
Date(s) Application is Due: Sep 1
Contact: Simon Rose, President; c/o Brown Brothers Harriman Trust; (212) 493-8000; email: info@heinemanfoundation.org
Internet: http://www.heinemanfoundation.org/guidelines
Sponsor: Heineman Foundation
140 Broadway
New York, NY 10005-1108

Heiser Leprosy and Tuberculosis Research Postdoctoral Fellowships 1736
The program fosters research on leprosy and tuberculosis by supporting the research training of a limited number of young biomedical scientists interested in the field. The program is designed to encourage national and international cooperation and research interchange in the study of the diseases. A maximum of two years of support will be provided to successful applicants at stipend levels adjusted according to U.S. government guidelines for geographical location at which the training is to take place. There are no application forms. Application may be made either by the individual seeking training or by the head of a laboratory engaged in research related to leprosy. In the latter case, the head of the laboratory must name the prospective fellow in the application.
Requirements: Biomedical scientists with either the PhD or MD degree are eligible for these fellowships. Applicants should be at the beginning or in an early phase of their postdoctoral training and interested in obtaining research training in a basic science field directly related to the study of leprosy. There are no citizenship requirements.
Amount of Grant: $35,000 maximum stipend per year; $2000 training allowance; $1500 maximum for health insurance
Date(s) Application is Due: Mar 1
Contact: Len McNally, Director, (212) 686-0010 ext 556; email: lm@nyct-cfi.org
Sponsor: Heiser Program for Research in Leprosy and Tuberculosis
c/o The New York Community Trust , 909 Third Avenue
New York, NY 10022

Heiser Leprosy Research Grants 1737
The grants provide support to laboratories involved in leprosy research training. Proposals of high scientific caliber related to leprosy will be considered. Seed grants may be requested for new projects or facilities that show promise of support from other sources within one year. Leprosy postdoctoral research fellowships and tuberculosis postdoctoral research fellowships also are awarded. There are no application forms. Applicants should submit proposals and budgets along with curriculum vita and relevant bibliographies of participating scientists.
Requirements: Senior investigators who are experienced in leprosy and tuberculosis research and associated with laboratories providing training opportunities in these areas are eligible.
Restrictions: Grants do not support clinical trials, salaries of personnel, or more than 10 percent of institutional overhead.
Amount of Grant: $35,000 maximum
Date(s) Application is Due: Mar 1
Contact: Len McNally, Director, (212) 686-0010 ext 556; email: lm@nyct-cfi.org
Sponsor: Heiser Program for Research in Leprosy and Tuberculosis
c/o The New York Community Trust, 909 Third Avenue
New York, NY 10022

Helen Bader Foundation Grants 1738
The foundation supports innovative pilot projects and programs that are research based, have strong evaluation components, and involve community collaboration. The foundation's primary focus areas are Alzheimer's disease and dementia, early childhood development in Israel, education, economic development, and Jewish life and learning. Modest grants are awarded to support neighborhood renewal and youth development in Milwaukee's Sankofa area. Grants will be awarded primarily in the Delaware River Valley and in particular Milwaukee, WI, with the exception of the Alzheimer's disease and dementia program, which accepts applications from organizations nationwide. International grants are made for projects conducted in Israel. The foundation often funds multiple-year projects but rarely for a period of more than three years. Preliminary proposals must be received by the listed application deadline dates. If the foundation is interested in exploring the grant request further, a member of the program staff will contact the applicant to arrange a meeting or site visit. Applications are available on the Web site.

Requirements: Grants are awarded for projects consistent with one or more of the Helen Bader Foundation's program areas. Grants are given only to U.S. organizations which are tax exempt under Section 501(c)3 of the Internal Revenue Code or to government entities. Grants will only be approved for foreign entities which meet specific charitable status requirements.
Restrictions: The Foundation does not provide direct support for individuals, such as individual scholarships.
Geographic Focus: Wisconsin
Samples: Donors Forum of Wisconsin, Inc., Milwaukee, WI, $45,000—this grant dupports the Donors Forum of Wisconsin's organization of the Milwaukee Area Workforce Funding Alliance, which includes private and public funders that seek to maximize outcomes for low-income families (2009); Aging & Disability Resource Center of Portage County, Stevens Point, WI, $7,000—this grant supports the Aging and Disability Resource Center of Portage County's instituting the Project Lifesaver Program, providing equipment and training to quickly located persons with dementia (2009).
Amount of Grant: $10,000-$100,000 average
Date(s) Application is Due: Feb 24; Mar 24
Contact: Tamara Hogans, Grants Manager; (414) 224-6464; fax: (414) 224-1441; email: tammy@@hbf.org
Internet: http://www.hbf.org/apply.htm
Sponsor: Helen Bader Foundation
233 North Water Street, 4th Floor
Milwaukee, WI 53202

Helen Hay Whitney Foundation Postdoctoral Research Fellowships **1739**
The program provides three-year fellowships for beginning postdoctoral training in basic biomedical research. The program is intended for individuals planning careers in biological or medical research to receive financial support of sufficient duration to help further their professional careers. It is expected that fellowship training will be obtained in an academic setting. The foundation will not consider applicants who plan tenure of the fellowship in the laboratory in which they have already received extensive predoctoral or postdoctoral training; the aim of the fellowship is to broaden postdoctoral training and experience. Applications are available online.
Requirements: Residents of the United States, Canada, and Mexico who are in the final stages of obtaining the MD, PhD, or equivalent degree and are seeking beginning postdoctocral training in basic biomedical research are eligible.
Restrictions: Applications from established scientists or advanced fellows will not be considered. Applicants who have already had one year of postdoctoral laboratory training by the listed deadline date will not be considered.
Amount of Grant: $41,000 for first year, $42,500 for second year, and $44,000 for the third year, plus $2500 to the fellow's laboratory to help defray research expenses
Date(s) Application is Due: Jul 15
Contact: Grants Administrator, (845) 639-6799; fax: (845) 639-6798 or (646) 304-7133; email: hhwf@earthlink.net
Internet: http://www.hhwf.org/HTMLSrc/ResearchFellowships.html
Sponsor: Helen Hay Whitney Foundation
20 Squadron Boulevard, Suite 630
New York, NY 10956

Helen K. and Arthur E. Johnson Foundation Grants **1740**
The foundation makes grants to a wide variety of nonprofit organizations in an attempt to solve community problems and enrich the quality of life in Colorado in the following areas: education, youth, health, community and social services, civic and cultural, and senior citizens. Requests are welcomed throughout the year. However, to be considered at the next board meeting, complete written proposals must be received by the listed application deadline dates. Proposal submission information is available online.
Requirements: IRS 501(c)3 organizations serving Colorado residents may apply.
Restrictions: Funding is not available for: loans or fund endowments; individuals; conferences; scholarships to individuals; multiple year grants; fundraising dinners or special events. The Foundation does not support organizations whose primary purpose is to influence (directly or indirectly) the legislative or judicial process in any manner or for any cause. In addition, the Foundation will not consider grant requests that pass through the nominal grant recipient to another organization.
Geographic Focus: Colorado
Samples: Little Sisters of the Poor (Denver, CO)—for heating and air conditioning system, $250,000.; Educare Colorado (Denver, CO)—for program support, $100,000.
Date(s) Application is Due: Jan 1; Apr 1; Jul 1; Oct 1
Contact: John H. Alexander, Jr., President, (800) 232-9931 or (303) 861-4127; fax: (303) 861-0607; email: info@johnsonfoundation.org
Internet: http://www.johnsonfoundation.org
Sponsor: Helen K. and Arthur E. Johnson Foundation
1700 Broadway, Suite 1100
Denver, CO 80290-1718

Helen McWilliam Memorial Scholarship **1741**
This scholarship is open to full-time graduate students at the University of Calgary interested in pursuing careers in school psychology. Recipients will be selected on the basis of academic excellence, skill in the handling of children referred for testing or guidance, and evidence of interest and ability in the area of school psychology. The award will be based on grades and observations by faculty members of academic and practical work. Annual deadline dates may vary; contact program staff for exact dates.
Requirements: Applicants must be full-time graduate students enrolled in the school psychology program of the Department of Educational Psychology at the master's or doctoral level. Applications should be made at the end of the first academic year.
Amount of Grant: $C2000
Contact: Program Contact, Faculty of Graduate Studies, (403) 220-5690; email: cbusch@acs.ucalgary.ca or ucawards@ucalgary.ca
Internet: http://www.grad.ucalgary.ca/funding/internal_scholarships/lev_4/mcwilliam.htm
Sponsor: University of Calgary
2500 University Dr NW, Earth Sciences Building
Calgary, AB T2N 1N4 Canada

Helen Steiner Rice Foundation Grants **1742**
The Foundation awards grants to worthy charitable programs that assist the needy and the elderly. Essential objectives for grant consideration are: basic necessities and human needs for the poor and elderly; preference for meeting the immediate needs of the poor; and innovative approaches. Organizations in the Greater Cincinnati area should use the contact information for Cincinnati. Organizations in Lorain County should *Contact:* Linda Weaver, Community Foundation Center of Lorain County, (440) 277-0142, Ext. 23. Application forms and instructions are available online.
Requirements: Nonprofit organizations in the greater Cincinnati area and Lorain, OH, may submit grant applications.
Restrictions: Funding is not available for building or endowment programs, direct gifts to individuals, or capital fund drives.
Geographic Focus: Ohio
Samples: Wesley Hall (Cincinnati, OH)—for a program for disadvantaged elderly, $35,000.; Interfaith Hospitality Network (Cincinnati, OH)—for its transportation program, $12,500.; YWCA of Cincinnati (Cincinnati, OH)—to support a school-readiness program for disadvantaged families, $10,000.
Date(s) Application is Due: Jul 1
Contact: James D. Huizenga or Mary LeRoy, (513) 241-2880; fax: (513) 768-6122; email: huizengai@greatercincinnatifdn.org
Internet: http://www.helensteinerrice.com/grants.html
Sponsor: Helen Steiner Rice Foundation
200 West Fourth Street
Cincinnati, OH 45202-2602

Helena Rubinstein Foundation Grants **1743**
The Foundation supports programs in education, community services, arts/arts in education, and health with emphasis on projects which benefit women and children. Grants are primarily targeted to organizations in New York City. Although general operating grants are made, the Foundation prefers to support specific programs. Grant proposals are accepted throughout the year. There is no formal application form; however, the New York Common Application Form may be used. Organizations seeking funds are asked not to make telephone inquiries, but to submit a brief letter outlining the project.
Requirements: U.S. nonprofit organizations are eligible.
Restrictions: Support is not offered to individuals, or for film or video projects. Grants are rarely made to endowment funds and capital campaigns. The foundation does not make loans and cannot provide emergency funds. Funding of new proposals is limited by ongoing commitments and fiscal constraints.
Geographic Focus: New York
Samples: New York City Outward Bound Ctr (NY)—for programs to help high school students develop self-esteem, self-reliance, social responsibility, and improved academic performance, $10,000.; Goodwill Industries of Greater New York (NY)—to support the capital campaign, $10,000.; Winston Preparatory School (NY)—salary support for a vocational guidance counselor, $5000.
Contact: Diane Moss, President, (212) 750-7310
Internet: http://www.helenarubinsteinfdn.org/guide.html
Sponsor: Helena Rubinstein Foundation
477 Madison Avenue, 7th Floor
New York, NY 10022-5802

Hendrick Foundation for Children Grants **1744**
The foundation supports programs designed to provide health, medical, social welfare, and educational services to benefit children with illness, disease, injury, pain, disability, incapacity, or other disadvantages; and improve quality of life for children with life-threatening or chronic injuries, illness, and disabilities. It is also contemplated that the Foundation will honor grants to other charitable and educational organizations sponsoring programs which are community oriented and focus on improving the quality of life of children with life-threatening or chronic injuries, illnesses and disabilities. All requests shall be given careful and thorough consideration by the Hendrick Foundation for Children Grant Committee. Grant awards will be determined on the merits of the organization, its objectives and mission. All grant requests should be submitted in writing on the organization's letterhead
Amount of Grant: $3,500 to $250,000 range
Contact: Charles V. Ricks, President; (704) 568-5550
Internet: http://www.thehendrickfoundation.org/grants.html
Sponsor: Hendrick Foundation for Children
P.O. Box 240070
Charlotte, NC 28224-0070

Henrietta Tower Wurts Memorial Foundation Grants 1745

The Foundation supports organizations which are engaged in helping or caring for people in need, or alleviating the conditions under which they live, primarily for the elderly, women, family and child welfare services. Giving is limited to Philadelphia, Pennsylvania.

Requirements: Non-profits in Philadelphia, Pennsylvania are eligible. The initial approach should be a letter requesting an application form from the Foundation.

Restrictions: No grants to individuals, or for endowment funds, scholarships, fellowships, or matching gifts; no loans. Organizations or programs serving disadvantaged youth and the elderly in Philadelphia, Pennsylvania must have an annual budget of less than 3 million.

Geographic Focus: Pennsylvania

Samples: Empowerment Group, Philadelphia, PA, $7,000 (2007); Juvenile Law Center, Philadelphia, PA, $5,000 (2007); Supportive Older Womens Network, Philadelphia, PA, $4,000 (2007);

Amount of Grant: $1,000-$7,000 range

Date(s) Application is Due: Feb 1; May 1; Sep 1

Contact: Andrew Swinney, President; 215) 563-6417

Sponsor: Henrietta Tower Wurts Memorial Foundation
1234 Market Street, Suite 1800
Philadelphia, PA 19107-3704

Henry and Ruth Blaustein Rosenberg Foundation Grants 1746

The foundation's mission is to improve the human condition through promoting life-long educational opportunities, research advances, and a spectrum of cultural programming. Grants are awarded in four general program areas: education and adult self-sufficiency, including literacy training that enhances individual effectiveness in the family, community, and workplace; arts and culture, particularly local outreach programs that target youth and seek to diversify audiences; health, with a focus on clinical programs that improve the prevention and treatment of specific diseases (currently, breast cancer, diabetes, multiple sclerosis, and kidney disease); and youth development, particulary after-school programs that provide recreation, educational enrichment, and leadership development. Organizations seeking funding should submit a letter of intent or a short proposal outlining the purpose, activities, and budget of the program(s) in need of support, as well as the qualifications of the organization to carry out the proposed activities. Proposals should include a plan for evaluating the impact of the program. Generally, grant decisions are made within six months of proposal submission.

Requirements: 501(c)3 tax-exempt charitable organizations located in and/or primarily serving the metropolitan Baltimore area are eligible.

Restrictions: The foundation does not make grants to individuals; accept unsolicited research proposals; or make grants to local projects located outside the metropolitan Baltimore area.

Geographic Focus: Maryland

Contact: Lara A. Hall, Program Officer: Educational Opportunity, Health and Mental Health; (410) 347-7204; Brenda Bodenheimer Zlatin, Program Officer: Jewish Life, Israel, Human Rights; (410) 347-7207; email: info@blaufund.org

Internet: http://www.blaufund.org/foundations/henryandruth_f.html

Sponsor: Henry and Ruth Blaustein Rosenberg Foundation
P.O. Box 238, 10 E Baltimore Street, Suite 1111
Baltimore, MD 21202-0238

Henry County Community Foundation Grants 1747

As a community foundation, the Henry County Community Foundation addresses the broad needs in Henry County, Indiana which include, but are not limited to, the following five categories: health and medical; social services; education; cultural affairs and civic affairs. All requests for grants are reviewed by the Henry County Community Foundation's Grants Committee, which is made up of members of the Board of Directors and several outside advisers. Reviews and recommendations are then presented to the full Board of Directors at its regularly scheduled meetings in April and October, at which time all final grant decisions are made. However, the Board reserves the right to consider individual requests at any regularly scheduled meeting, if deemed necessary. The Henry County Community Foundation's grant program will emphasize change-oriented and focused types of grants to achieve certain objectives such as becoming more efficient, increasing fund-raising capabilities, delivering better products, etc.

Requirements: Applications from organizations whose programs benefit the residents of Henry County will be accepted only from organizations who attend the spring or fall grant workshops held at the Henry County Community Foundation office. The Spring Grant Workshop is March 11th. The Fall Grant Workshop is August 12th. Organizations must be a 501c (3) tax-exempt or be sponsored by a 501c (3) tax-exempt organization. Grants will also be accepted from school and government entities.

Restrictions: Restrictions for use of grant money: grant money will not be awarded to cover operating cost; no grants will be made solely to individuals; generally, grants will not be made to enable individuals or groups of individuals to attend seminars or take trips except where there are special circumstances which will benefit the community; no grants will be made specifically for sectarian religious purposes but can be made to religious organizations for general community programs. No grants will be made exclusively for endowment purposes of recipient organizations; generally, no grant proposals will be considered which have been proposed by individuals or organizations that are not charitable organizations; generally, grants will not be made for programs and/or equipment which were committed to prior to the submission of grant application.

Geographic Focus: Indiana

Date(s) Application is Due: Mar 31; Aug 28

Contact: Jerry Schaeffer, Executive Director; (765) 529-2235; fax: (765) 529-2284; email: jerry@henrycountycf.org

Internet: http://www.henrycountycf.org/index.php?submenu=Grants&src=gendocs&ref=Grants&category=Grants

Sponsor: Henry County Community Foundation
700 South Memorial Drive, P.O. Box 6006
New Castle, IN 47362

Henry J. Kaiser Family Foundation Grants 1748

The foundation concentrates giving in the following areas: U.S. government's role in health, health of low-income and minority groups with major emphasis on HIV/AIDS policy, reproductive health policy, and health system innovation and reform in California. The foundation also operates a major program to improve health and health care and promote social justice in South Africa. Grants are awarded for one to three years and support a range of activities, including policy analysis, applied research to define and measure public health problems, demonstration and pilot projects, and communications activities that help sharpen health care debates and improve quality of health information. Prospective applicants should submit a preliminary letter (two to three pages in length) that briefly describes the proposed project, along with an estimate of the total budget and the amount requested from the foundation. There are no deadlines and no application forms. Inquiries for projects in South Africa may be addressed to Dr. Michael Sinclair, Senior Vice President, The Henry J. Kaiser Family Foundation, 1450 G St NW, Suite 250, Washington, DC 20005, (202) 347-5270, fax: (202) 347-5274.

Requirements: Grants in response to unsolicited proposals are made only to governmental agencies and to private organizations with IRS 501(c)3 tax-exempt status.

Restrictions: The foundation does not award grants to individuals. Support is not given to ongoing general operating expenses, indirect costs, capital campaigns, annual appeals or other fundraising events, construction, purchase or renovation of facilities, or equipment purchases.

Amount of Grant: $1000-$500,000 typically

Contact: Renee Wells, Grants Manager, (415) 854-9400; fax: (415) 854-4800; email: rwells@kff.org

Internet: http://www.kff.org

Sponsor: Henry J. Kaiser Family Foundation
2400 Sand Hill Road
Menlo Park, CA 94025

Henry J. Kaiser Family Foundation Media Fellowships 1749

The purpose of the fellowship is to help journalists and commentators do the best possible job of keeping the public informed about health issues at this critical time in the evolution of the health care system. The goal of the fellowship is to provide a highly flexible range of opportunities tailored to each fellow's interests; help journalists improve the quality of the work they do; provide time to research specific topics; and deepen participants' commitment to becoming specialists in health reporting. Fellows may want to participate in the fellowship program on a part-time basis and continue writing or reporting during their fellowship. Fellows are encouraged to do reporting based on their fellowship research and to experiment with different media or forms of writing. Most fellows work from home, or base themselves at a local academic or research institution. There is no obligation to pursue academic coursework, although that is an option open to all fellows. There is no application form. Guidelines are available online.

Requirements: Fellowships will be awarded to U.S. journalists interested in U.S. health policy issues.

Amount of Grant: $50,000 maximum for nine-month fellowship

Date(s) Application is Due: Mar 16

Contact: Penny Duckham, Executive Director, (650) 234-9220; fax: (650) 854-4800; email: pduckham@kff.org

Internet: http://www.kff.org/about/mediafellowships.cfm

Sponsor: Henry J. Kaiser Family Foundation
2400 Sand Hill Road
Menlo Park, CA 94025

Hereditary Disease Foundation John J. Wasmuth Postdoctoral Fellowships 1750

Support is offered for research projects that contribute to identifying and understanding the basic defect of Huntington's disease. Areas of interest include trinucleotide expansions, animal models, gene therapy, neurobiology and development of the basal ganglia, cell survival and death, and intercellular signaling in striatal neurons. Awards may be renewed for a third year. To receive an application, submit a letter of intent. Letter of intent forms may be submitted electronically via the Web site.

Amount of Grant: $37,000-$56,000 stipend, plus $8,000 for supplies

Date(s) Application is Due: Feb 15; Jun 15; Oct 15

Contact: Dr. Carl D. Johnson; (212) 928-2121; fax: (212) 928-2172; email: carljohnson@hdfoundation.org

Internet: http://www.hdfoundation.org/funding/postdoct.php

Sponsor: Hereditary Disease Foundation
3960 Broadway, 6th Floor
New York, NY 10032

Hereditary Disease Foundation Lieberman Award 1751

The Hereditary Disease Foundation announces a special Lieberman Award, to catalyze innovative proposals leading to the treatment and cure of Huntington's disease. A Lieberman Award can be funded for two years for up to $75,000 per year. Areas of interest include trinucleotide expansions, animal models, gene therapy, neurobiology

and development of the basal ganglia, cell survival and death, and intercellular signaling in striatal neurons.
Amount of Grant: $75,000 per year for up to 2 years
Contact: Dr. Carl D. Johnson; (212) 928-2121; fax: (212) 928-2172; email: carljohnson@hdfoundation.org
Internet: http://www.hdfoundation.org/funding/lieberman.php
Sponsor: Hereditary Disease Foundation
3960 Broadway, 6th Floor
New York, NY 10032

Hereditary Disease Foundation Research Grants 1752
The focus of the Hereditary Disease Foundation is on Huntington's disease. Support will be for research projects that contribute to identifying and understanding the basic defect in Huntington's disease. Grants are usually for one year, with the possibility of renewal for up to three years. Areas of interest include trinucleotide expansions, animal models, gene therapy, neurobiology and development of the basal ganglia, cell survival and death, and intercellular signaling in striatal neurons. In addition to its regular grants, the foundation also offers the Lieberman Award for innovative proposals accelerating the discovery of a treatment and cure of Huntington's disease. Grants that receive funding are considered seed money. If the project shows promise, it is hoped that other institutions will fund it thereafter. To obtain an application, submit a one-page letter of intent. Letter of intent forms may be submitted electronically via the Web site.
Samples: Dr. Andrew Dwork, Columbia U—for research entitled Ultrastructural Immunohistochemistry of Cortical Biopsies in HD.; Dr. Nansheng Chen, U of British Columbia—for research entitled Regulation of NMDA Receptor Function by Mutant Huntington in Neostriatal Neurons.; Dr. Chris Huang, Massachusetts General Hospital—for research entitled Anti-Huntington Aggregation Agents as Potential Therapeutics for Huntingtons Disease.; Dr. Lucius Passani, Massachusetts General Hospital—for research entitled Evaluation of HYPA/FBP-11, HYPB and HYPC as Candidates for Involvement in HD Pathogenesis.
Amount of Grant: $50,000 maximum
Date(s) Application is Due: Feb 15; Jun 15; Oct 15
Contact: Dr. Carl D. Johnson; (212) 928-2121; fax: (212) 928-2172; email: carljohnson@hdfoundation.org
Internet: http://www.hdfoundation.org/funding/grants.php
Sponsor: Hereditary Disease Foundation
3960 Broadway, 6th Floor
New York, NY 10032

Herman Goldman Foundation Grants 1753
The foundation's broad purpose is to enhance the quality of life in the areas of health, education, social justice, and the arts. Applications submitted by organizations sponsoring projects that will benefit those in need will be considered. With few exceptions, grant making is confined to the New York metropolitan area. A written proposal should include the specific funds requested, a thorough description of existing or intended activities and their expected impact, additional sources of funding on hand as well as those anticipated, and the prospects for the project's continuance and the support envisioned at the expiration of the requested grant. Where possible, a budget should be submitted. The board meets monthly. Grants are considered in April, July, and November. Proposals are due the middle of the month preceding the board meeting.
Requirements: Applicant organizations must submit a copy of the IRS determination letter.
Restrictions: Grants to individuals will not be considered.
Geographic Focus: New York
Samples: Boca Raton Community Hospital (Boca Raton, FL)—to support construction of an urgent care center, $20,000.; New York U School of Medicine—to support Medical Ctr scholarships, $20,000.; American Civil Liberties Union Foundation—to continue support of the Children's Rights Project, $10,000.; Dramatic Risks—to support the development of exemplary projects in the performing arts, theatrical writing, and the arts in education, $5000.
Amount of Grant: $5000-$25,000 average
Contact: Richard Baron, Executive Director, (212) 797-9090
Sponsor: Herman Goldman Foundation
61 Broadway, 18th Floor
New York, NY 10006

Hershey Company Grants 1754
The Hershey Company remains committed to supporting the communities in which it operates and to society in general. Cash and product contributions are made to support a variety of worthy causes and non-profit organizations which support Education, Health & Human Services, Civic & Community initiatives, Arts & Culture and the Environment. Particular emphasis is placed upon causes that support kids and kids at risk. The Hershey Company has plants in the following areas: Hilo, HI; Robinson, IL; Hazleton, PA; Hershey, PA; Lancaster, PA; Memphis, TN; Stuarts Draft, VA; Sao Roque, Brazil; Guadalajara, Mexico; Monterrey, Mexico; Mumbai, India; Shanghai, China. Organizations located in communities in which The Hershey Company has manufacturing operations should direct requests for funding to the management of The Hershey Company facility in their area, see the Hershey website for additional guidelines and contact information.
Requirements: Nonprofit organizations are eligible. Preference is given to nonprofits in corporate-operating locations. All requests must be submitted in writing.
Restrictions: The following are ineligible for funding: organizations without an Internal Revenue Code 501(c)3 non-profit, tax-exempt status; individuals; organizations outside the immediate areas of The Hershey Company's manufacturing facilities, with the exception of national and state-wide organizations whose programs complement Hershey's funding priorities; political campaigns, political or lobbying organizations, or those supporting the candidacy of a particular individual; churches or religious organizations, including seminaries, Bible colleges and theological institutions; fraternal organizations; labor organizations; member agencies of United Way. Exception: requests for capital campaign funding will be considered; affiliate organizations of the Cultural Enrichment Fund in Central Pennsylvania. Exception: requests for capital campaign funding will be considered.
Geographic Focus: Hawaii; Illinois; Pennsylvania; Tennessee; VirginiaBrazil; China; Mexico
Contact: Grants Administrator, (800) 468-1714, fax: (717) 534-6550
Internet: http://www.thehersheycompany.com/about/responsibility.asp
Sponsor: Hershey Company
Community Relations, P.O. Box 810, 100 Crystal A Drive
Hershey, PA 17033-0810

HHK Employment Grants 1755
The majority of the foundation's grants are directed toward increasing employment opportunities for people with physical disabilities. Grants are awarded to organizations that work toward improving the employment and career advancement of people with physical disabilities living in New Jersey. Areas of interest include programs that focus on transition to work for youth and adults; transportation to and from work; workplace accommodations—overcoming barriers to employment, such as access to assistive technology, providing accessible facilities and services, employee education on disabilities; equipment and training programs focusing on workplace preparation and vocational training; supported employment programs; mentoring; school-based enterprises; work-based learning; alternative work solution, such as telecommuting; and employment strategies to support disability recruitment, hiring practices, placement, and retention. Types of support include project/program funds and general operating funds. Grants are awarded for one year. Preference is given to organizations seeking matching funds and that collaborate with other organizations or entities. Guidelines are available online.
Requirements: 501(c)3 tax-exempt organizations are eligible.
Restrictions: The foundation does not support grants to individuals; grants to underwrite fundraising events, such as benefits, dinners, or theater events, ticket purchases, or advertising; endowment campaigns; scholarship funds; deficit reduction or loans; or international causes.
Geographic Focus: New Jersey
Samples: Brain Injury Assoc of New Jersey (Edison, NJ)—for training, technical assistance, and resources for people with brain injuries, $49,980 (2005); Cheshire Home (Florham Park, NJ)—for salary support of a teacher for GED and job preparation and computer-skills training, $12,000 (2005); Employment Horizon (Cedar Knolls, NJ)—for salary support of a driver to transport people with disabilities to work centers in their community, $10,000 (2005).
Amount of Grant: $20,000-$50,000 typically
Contact: Elaine Katz, Director of Development, (973) 324-8367; fax: (973) 324-8373; email: ekatz@hhkfdn.org
Internet: http://www.hhkfdn.org
Sponsor: Henry H. Kessler Foundation
300 Executive Drive, Suite 150
West Orange, NJ 07052

HHMI Biomedical Research Grants for International Scientists in Canada and Latin America 1756
HHMI's International Research Scholars Program provides five-year grants to support promising basic biomedical research scientists working in Canada and Latin America. Eligible epidemiology research includes that directed toward an understanding of disease distribution in populations or of associations that may suggest causality or preventive strategies.
Requirements: The supported research must be conducted in one of the following eight eligible countries: Argentina, Brazil, Canada, Chile, Mexico, Peru, Uruguay, or Venezuela. Applicants must hold a full-time appointment or have a pending full-time appointment at a nonprofit scientific research organization in any one of the eight eligible countries.
Restrictions: Clinical trials and research on health education, health care delivery, or health services are not eligible fields.
Amount of Grant: $50,000-$100,000
Date(s) Application is Due: Sep 14
Contact: Jill G. Conley, Ph.D., Program Director; (301) 215-8873; fax: (301) 215-8888; email: canlatam@hhmi.org
Internet: http://www.hhmi.org/grants/individuals/canlatam.html
Sponsor: Howard Hughes Medical Institute
4000 Jones Bridge Road
Chevy Chase, MD 20815-6789

HHMI Biomedical Research Grants for International Scientists in the Baltics, Central and Eastern Europe, Russia, and Ukraine 1757
The Program will award five-year grants to support promising basic biomedical research scientists working in the Baltics, Central and Eastern Europe, Russia, and Ukraine. Eligible epidemiology research includes that directed toward an understanding of disease distribution in populations or of associations that may suggest causality or preventive strategies. Allowable expense categories include salaries and stipends for award recipients,

graduate students, postdoctoral fellows, and technicians, equipment and supplies, travel, and publication costs. Up to 10 percent of the grant may be used to pay for indirect costs (including administrative costs) of the scientist's institution.
Requirements: The supported research must be conducted in one of the following eligible countries: Bulgaria, Croatia, Czech Republic, Estonia, Hungary, Latvia, Lithuania, Poland, Romania, Russia, Slovak Republic, Slovenia, or Ukraine.
Restrictions: Researchers may not be citizens or permanent residents of the United States. Grant funds may not be used for laboratory renovations.
Amount of Grant: $50,000-$100,000 per year up to five years
Date(s) Application is Due: Nov 17
Contact: Jill G. Conley, Ph.D., Program Director; (301) 215-8873; fax: (301) 215-8888; email: bceeru@hhmi.org
Internet: http://www.hhmi.org/grants/individuals/bceeru.html
Sponsor: Howard Hughes Medical Institute
4000 Jones Bridge Road
Chevy Chase, MD 20815-6789

HHMI Biomedical Research Grants for International Scientists: Infectious Diseases and Parasitology 1758
The Program provides five-year grants to support promising basic biomedical research scientists working in the fields of infectious diseases and parasitology. The Institute seeks to build the strongest foundation of scientific knowledge and capability by creating a global network of scientists who make important contributions outside the U.S. research community. It support these leaders in their home countries to facilitate the application and dissemination of their knowledge and to strengthen research environments and educational opportunities.
Requirements: Applicants must hold a full-time appointment or have a pending appointment at a nonprofit scientific research organization in any country other than the United States and the United Kingdom. Researchers may not be citizens or permanent residents of the United States.
Restrictions: Only scientists working in the research areas specified in the program announcement are eligible to apply for grant support. The Program does not consider unsolicited grant proposals or award grants for clinical trials and research on health education, health-care delivery, or health services.
Amount of Grant: $50,000-$100,000 per year up to five years
Date(s) Application is Due: Sep 15
Contact: Jill G. Conley, Ph.D., Program Director; (301) 215-8873; fax: (301) 215-8888; email: parasite@hhmi.org
Internet: http://www.hhmi.org/grants/individuals/idap.html
Sponsor: Howard Hughes Medical Institute
4000 Jones Bridge Road
Chevy Chase, MD 20815-6789

HHMI Grants and Fellowships Programs 1759
The institute administers a grants program that focuses on improving science education from preschool through postdoctoral training, enhancing the science literacy of the general public, and supporting the research of biomedical scientists in selected foreign countries. Currently, grants are administered through five programs: an international program that supports biomedical scientists outside the United States and provides funding for selected courses and workshops; a precollege science-education program that offers grants for educational activities to science museums, botanical and zoological gardens, etc.; a biomedical-research program that supports medical schools and research organizations; a graduate science-education program that provides fellowships for graduate students, medical students, and physicians, and supports special courses; and a biological-sciences education program that awards grants to selected undergraduate institutions..
Contact: Jill G. Conley, Ph.D., Program Director; (301) 215-8873; fax: (301) 215-8888; email: grantswww@hhmi.org
Internet: http://www.hhmi.org/grants
Sponsor: Howard Hughes Medical Institute
4000 Jones Bridge Road
Chevy Chase, MD 20815-6789

HHMI International Research Scholars Program 1760
This five year grant program supports non-U.S. biomedical scientists, scientific meetings for grant-supported scientists, and other international educational activities. Grants are awarded to promising biomedical scientists who have made significant contributions to fundamental research. Application information is available online.
Requirements: To be considered, individuals must hold a full-time academic or research appointment at a university, medical school, or other nonprofit scientific institution. They are not permitted to have major administrative responsibilities.
Contact: Jill G. Conley, Ph.D., Program Director; (301) 215-8873; fax: (301) 215-8888
Internet: http://www.hhmi.org/grants/for_grantees/
Sponsor: Howard Hughes Medical Institute
4000 Jones Bridge Road
Chevy Chase, MD 20815/6789

HHMI Med into Grad Initiative Grants 1761
HHMI will award grants to institutions to improve the understanding of medicine and pathobiology by scientists conducting biomedical research. Grants will be used to modify existing graduate training or initiate new programs to develop a cadre of Ph.D. researchers who understand pathophysiology and are committed to working at the interface of the basic sciences and clinical medicine. Applications will be accepted from any university in the United States that offers Ph.D.-level training in an appropriate science or engineering discipline. It is expected that as much as $10 million will be awarded in this competition. Awards will range from $400,000 to $1 million, and the grant funds will be allocated over four consecutive years.
Requirements: U.S. institutions that grant PhD degrees in the appropriate science and engineering disciplines are eligible to apply.
Amount of Grant: $400,000-$1 million
Date(s) Application is Due: Apr 27
Contact: Maryrose Franko, Senior Program Officer; (800) 448-4882, ext. 8880; fax: (301) 215-8888; email: medintograd@hhmi.org
Internet: http://www.hhmi.org/grants/institutions/medintograd.html
Sponsor: Howard Hughes Medical Institute
4000 Jones Bridge Road
Chevy Chase, MD 20815-6789

HHMI Physician-Scientist Early Career Award 1762
Through this competitive grant initiative, HHMI awards five-year grants to selected alumni of the HHMI-NIH Research Scholars Program and the HHMI Research Training Fellowships for Medical Students Program to support these individuals as they begin careers as independent physician-scientists. The award provides $375,000 over a five-year period for direct research costs.
Requirements: Only alumni of the HHMI-NIH Research Scholars Program and the HHMI Research Training Fellowship for Medical Students Program who have received an M.D., M.D./Ph.D., D.D.S, or equivalent degree are eligible to apply.
Restrictions: The funds may not be used for the salary of the awardee or institutional indirect costs.
Amount of Grant: $375,000 over a five-year period
Contact: Office of Grants and Special Programs; (800) 448-4882, ext. 8889 or (800) 424-9924; fax: (301) 215-8888; email: earlycareer@hhmi.org
Internet: http://www.hhmi.org/grants/individuals/earlycareer.html
Sponsor: Howard Hughes Medical Institute
4000 Jones Bridge Road
Chevy Chase, MD 20815-6789

HHMI Research Training Fellowships 1763
Medical fellowships are intended to strengthen and expand the nation's pool of medically trained researchers. These fellowships provide funds to help meet fellows' research-related expenses and education costs during the research training period. Fellowships are awarded annually to provide support for one year of full-time training in fundamental biomedical, clinical, translational, or applied research. The fellowship includes a stipend, a research allowance to meet research-related expenses, and a fellow's allowance to be used on behalf of the fellow for health care, tuition and fees, and other research-related expenses. Application information is available online.
Requirements: Fellowships are awarded to students enrolled in medical and dental programs in the U.S.
Date(s) Application is Due: Jan 11
Contact: Program Officer; (301) 215-8500 or (800) 424-9924; fax: (301) 215-8888; email: medfellows@hhmi.org
Internet: http://www.hhmi.org/grants/individuals/medfellows.html
Sponsor: Howard Hughes Medical Institute
4000 Jones Bridge Road
Chevy Chase, MD 20815-6789

HHMI-NIBIB Interfaces Initiative Grants 1764
HHMI and the National Institute of Biomedical Imaging and Bioengineering have formed a partnership to support biomedical research institutions in developing graduate-level research training programs in emerging interdisciplinary fields. The primary goal of this initiative is to train a cadre of PhD scientists who possess the knowledge and skills to conduct interdisciplinary research at the interface between the biomedical sciences and the physical science, computational, engineering, or mathematical disciplines. These fields may include, but are not limited to, chemistry, imaging, science, materials science, nanotechnology, and physics. Another goal is to reduce barriers to interdisciplinary graduate science education. Proposals should reflect the unique educational and scientific capabilities and strengths of the applicant institution(s) as well as address the specific goals of the initiative. The initiative consists of two phases: Phase I supports the establishment of new interdisciplinary training programs; Phase II will sustain the training programs through their critical years. Registration letters of intent to apply are due by January 20, with the proposal submission deadline June 15.
Requirements: All U.S. institutions that grant PhD degrees in appropriate science or engineering disciplines are eligible to apply. Collaborative programs between two or more institutions are acceptable.
Amount of Grant: $1 million maximum for three years
Date(s) Application is Due: Jan 20; Jun 15
Contact: Maryrose Franko, Senior Program Officer; (800) 448-4882, ext. 8880; fax: (301) 215-8888; email: interdisc@hhmi.org
Internet: http://www.hhmi.org/grants/institutions/nibib.html
Sponsor: Howard Hughes Medical Institute
4000 Jones Bridge Road
Chevy Chase, MD 20815-6789

HHMI-NIH Cloister Research Scholars Program 1765
The goal of this program, a joint venture of HHMI and NIH, is to expand the pool of medically trained researchers by encouraging medical students to pursue research

careers. The program provides support for an intensive nine months to one year of full-time research, with a possible one-year extension, at NIH in Bethesda, MD. Most students enter after their second year of medical school. The Cloister, a residential facility for scholars, is available on the NIH campus. The research project is selected upon arrival at NIH, after a round of laboratory visits. Application forms may be downloaded from the Web site or requested from the program officer.
Requirements: Applicant must be in good standing at a medical or dental school in the U.S. or Puerto Rico and must receive permission from the school to participate in the program. The school does not have to be a major academic medical center or research-oriented school.
Restrictions: Enrollees in an M.D./Ph.D. or D.D.S./Ph.D. program are not eligible.
Amount of Grant: $17,800 annual salary
Date(s) Application is Due: Jan 10
Contact: Office of Grants and Special Programs; (800) 424-9924 or (301) 215-8873; fax: (301) 215-8888; email: research_scholars@hhmi.org
Internet: http://www.hhmi.org/research/cloister/program.html
Sponsor: Howard Hughes Medical Institute
4000 Jones Bridge Road
Chevy Chase, MD 20815-6789

HHMI/EMBO Start-up Grants for Central Europe **1766**
The program encourages young scientists to obtain independent faculty positions in select countries that have ongoing HHMI and EMBO science programs. Applications are encouraged from scientists to set up their first independent laboratories in a Central European EMBC member state (Croatia, Czech Republic, Estonia, Hungary, Poland, and Slovenia). Application forms should be completed by the individual scientist and the receiving institute. It is expected that the institute make the applicant an offer that goes beyond that of a position and laboratory space. HHMI will contribute $50,000, while the participating member state must provide the remaining $25,000. Application and guidelines are available online.
Requirements: Eligible scientists should have an excellent publication record; have a maximum of 10 years postdoctoral experience; be negotiating a position at an institute/university in Central Europe by the date of the application; and be located outside Central Europe at the time of application.
Amount of Grant: $75,000 per year for three years
Date(s) Application is Due: Aug 1
Contact: Grants Administrator, (301) 215-8500
Internet: http://www.embo.org/projects/yip/embo_hhmi_startup_grants.html
Sponsor: Howard Hughes Medical Institute
4000 Jones Bridge Road
Chevy Chase, MD 20815-6789

HHS Children's Hospitals Graduate Medical Education Payment Program **1767**
The program provides funds to freestanding children's hospitals to support the training of pediatric and other residents in graduate medical education (GME) programs. This program compensates for the disparity in the level of federal funding for teaching hospitals for pediatrics versus other types of hospitals.
Requirements: To be eligible, a children's hospital must meet all of the following criteria: participates in an approved graduate medical education (GME) program; has a Medicare provider agreement; is excluded from the Medicare inpatient prospective payment system (PPS) under section 1886(d)(1)(B)(iii) of the Social Security Act, and its accompanying regulations; and ss a freestanding hospital.
Amount of Grant: $40 million total
Date(s) Application is Due: May 1; Aug 1
Contact: Kara Castellow, (301) 443-1058; email: kcastellow@hrsa.gov
Internet: http://bhpr.hrsa.gov/childrenshospitalgme/default.htm
Sponsor: Department of Health and Human Services
5600 Fishers Ln, Parklawn Building, Room 9A-05
Rockville, MD 20857

High Meadow Foundation Grants **1768**
The foundation grants funds in support of the performing arts, especially theater and music, and other cultural organizations. Organizations supported are usually located in Berkshire County, MA. Types of support include continuing support, annual campaigns, capital campaigns, building construction/renovation, equipment acquisition, emergency funds, program development, employee-related scholarships, and matching funds. Applications are accepted at any time. Forms are not necessary; a letter outlining the proposed project should include budget and administrative information.
Requirements: Western Massachusetts 501(c)3 tax-exempt organizations in Berkshire County are eligible.
Geographic Focus: Massachusetts
Samples: Massachusetts Museum of Contemporary Art, North Adams, MA, $100,000 (2007); Berkshire Theater Festival, Stockbridge, MA, $60,000 (2007); Lenox Library Association, Lenox, MA, $10,000 (2007);
Contact: Jane Fitzpatrick; (413) 298-5565 or (413) 243-1474; fax: (413) 298-4058
Sponsor: High Meadow Foundation
30 Main Street
Stockbridge, MA 01262

Highmark Corporate Giving Grants **1769**
The Foundation awards grants in the following categories: health; human services; community; education; and arts and culture. Support is expressed in cash grants, sponsorships and in-kind gifts to non-profit organizations. There are no maximum or minimum limits; however, awards to programs and services are granted based on importance to the Foundation's business, social mission and corporate citizen objectives, as well as the initiative's proposed impact. Interested applicants should submit a brief proposal. For additional information or proposal submission, applicants should contact the Community Affairs department in their county of residence. Contact information by county is available online.
Requirements: The Foundation awards grants to nonprofit organizations that are defined as tax exempt under section 501(c)3 of the Internal Revenue Code and as public charities under section 509(a) of that code.
Restrictions: Proposals are not accepted for: multiple-year grants; capital campaigns; individual causes; seed money or start-up organizations; endowment funds; political causes or campaigns; fraternal or civic groups; religious programming; organizations that discriminate on the basis of race, religion, sex, disability or national origin.
Geographic Focus: Pennsylvania
Contact: Mary Ann Papale, (412) 544-4032; email: mary.papale@highmark.com
Internet: https://www.highmark.com/hmk2/community/corpgiving/index.shtml
Sponsor: Highmark Inc
120 Fifth Avenue, FAP 2585
Pittsburgh, PA 15222

Highmark Healthy High 5 **1770**
This program is designed to support schools in the effort to introduce programs that will ultimately create healthier, more successful students. Schools or school districts are invited to submit proposals for innovative programming to improve nutrition education, nutrition services, or increase opportunities for physical activity or education. The School Challenge grant application packet is available online.
Requirements: All schools within the Foundation's 49-county, Pennsylvania service region are eligible to apply. All schools that apply must participate in the PANA Keystone Healthy Zone Program and complete the KHZ Assessment.
Geographic Focus: Pennsylvania
Date(s) Application is Due: Apr 14
Contact: Yvonne Cook, (412) 544-7000; email: yvonne.cook@highmark.com
Internet: https://www.highmark.com/hmk2/community/hmfoundation/index.shtml
Sponsor: Highmark Inc.
120 Fifth Avenue, Suite 2112
Pittsburgh, PA 15222-3099

Highmark Physician eHealth Collaborative Grants **1771**
The program was created to encourage the adoption of health information technology used at the point of care to improve patient safety, quality of care, and cost efficiency for people in western and central Pennsylvania. Physicians may apply to receive grants, which must be used to acquire and use electronic technology systems such as a personal computer, a PDA, or electronic tablet or digital pen to generate and transmit electronically prescriptions to pharmacies. The collaborative will pay up to 75 percent of the cost for a physician's office to acquire, install, and implement the electronic technology system, with the physician's practice to pay the remaining balance. Physicians must apply online.
Requirements: Physicians must be licensed to practice medicine in Pennsylvania and must be a licensed prescriber.
Geographic Focus: Pennsylvania
Amount of Grant: $7000 maximum per physician
Contact: eHealth Grants Administrator, email: info@highmarkehealth.org
Internet: http://www.highmarkehealth.org
Sponsor: Pittsburgh Foundation
1 PPG Pl, 30th Floor
Pittsburgh, PA 15222-5401

Hilda and Preston Davis Foundation Grants **1772**
The Foundation provides funds to charitable organizations whose programs advance the development of all areas of the lives of children and young adults. The Foundation places special emphasis on, and channels most of its financial resources toward, those organizations whose attention is concentrated on eating disorders and education for the underprivileged. Grants may range from $10,000 up to $100,000. In unique circumstances, the Foundation does consider a more significant grant for a program having a major impact in one or more of its areas of interest.
Requirements: 501(c)3 tax-exempt organizations are eligible.
Restrictions: The foundation generally will not provide grants to: non-501(c)3 tax-exempt organizations; individuals; general fundraising drives; endowments; government agencies; or organizations that subsist mainly on third-party funding and have demonstrated no ability or expended little effort to attract private funding.
Amount of Grant: $10,000-$100,000
Contact: Grants Administrator; (203) 629-8552; fax: (203) 547-6112; email: davis@fsllc.net or info@fsllc.net
Internet: http://www.hpdavis.org/application.htm
Sponsor: Hilda and Preston Davis Foundation
640 West Putnam Avenue, 3rd Floor
Greenwich, CT 06830

Hill Crest Foundation Grants **1773**
The foundation awards grants to Alabama nonprofits in its areas of interest, including health, the elderly, arts and culture, community development, higher education, and youth. Types of support include general operating support, capital campaigns, building construction/renovation, equipment acquisition, endowment funds, program

development, professorships, publication, seed money, scholarship funds, research, technical assistance, and matching funds. There are no application forms or deadlines.
Requirements: Alabama nonprofit organizations may apply.
Geographic Focus: Alabama
Amount of Grant: $5000-$50,000 average
Contact: Charles Terry, Senior Chair, (205) 425-5800
Sponsor: Hill Crest Foundation
P.O. Box 530507
Mountain Brook, AL 35253

Hill Foundation Grants **1774**
The foundation awards grants mainly for special health care projects, higher education, equipment funds, and services for the elderly, disabled children, and cultural programs, primarily in Colorado. Some support is provided to social service agencies. Types of support include program development, scholarship funds, and matching funds. There are no application deadlines.
Requirements: Giving primarily in CO and WY.
Restrictions: Grants are not made to individuals nor for capital improvements. The foundation does not make multiyear commitments.
Geographic Focus: Colorado; Wyoming
Amount of Grant: $1000-$45,000 range
Contact: Grants Administrator, c/o Wells Fargo Bank, N.A., (720) 947-6820
Sponsor: Hill Foundation
1740 Broadway, MC 7300-483
Denver, CO 80274

Hillman Foundation Grants **1775**
The foundation provides grants to nonprofit organizations in the city of Pittsburgh and the southwestern Pennsylvania region for programs and projects designed to improve the quality of life in the area. The foundation's areas of interest include community affairs, social services, culture and the arts, education at all levels, and youth services including medical and health. Grants range widely in size and are allocated for large and small capital projects, endowment, new and expanding programs, and on a limited basis, operating support. Applications should include an annual budget of the organization, project information, and evidence of tax-exempt status. Application information is available online.
Requirements: The Foundation considers requests only from organizations classified as tax-exempt under Section 501(c)3 of the U.S. Internal Revenue Code and designated as public charities under Section 509(a).
Restrictions: Grants are not made to individuals, organizations located outside of the United States, for travel expenses for groups, or in support of events, sponsorships and meetings such as conferences, institutes and seminars.
Geographic Focus: Pennsylvania
Samples: Strong Women, Strong Girls, INc., $10,000—towards program for at-risk and low-income girls (2009); Greater Pittsburgh Community Food Bank, $65,000—toward food pantry and outreach program (2009); Carnegie Institute/Museum of Natural History, $50,000—towards purchase of bournonite, amazonite, smoky quarts and rhodochrosite mineral specimens (2009).
Contact: David K. Roger, President; (412) 338-3466; fax: (412) 338-3463; email: foundation@hillmanfo.com
Internet: http://www.hillmanfdn.org/grantprograms.html
Sponsor: Hillman Foundation
330 Grant Street, Suite 2000
Pittsburgh, PA 15219

Hillsdale County Community Foundation Healthy Senior/Healthy Youth Grants **1776**
The Healthy Senior/Healthy Youth Fund provides grants to smoking cessation and prevention programs for young people (under 18) and seniors (over 65) in Hillsdale County. Organizations interested in applying are strongly encouraged to discuss their project with the Executive Director prior to submitting an application. If the project meets the basic eligibility criteria and is consistent with the Foundation's program interests, a formal application will be sent to the applicant. The Grantmaking Committee meets twice a year to review funding requests.
Requirements: The Foundation welcomes applications from the Hillsdale County area or outside Hillsdale County, Michigan, if a significant number of the people to be served reside within Hillsdale County. Applicants shall be tax exempt according to Section 501(c)3 of the Internal Revenue Code.
Geographic Focus: Michigan
Date(s) Application is Due: Nov 1; May 1
Contact: Sharon Bisher, Executive Director, (517) 439-5101; fax: (517) 439-5109; email: s.bisher@abouthccf.org
Internet: http://www.abouthccf.org/funds.asp
Sponsor: Hillsdale County Community Foundation
2 South Howell Street, P.O. Box 276
Hillsdale, MI 49242

Hillsdale County Community General Adult Foundation Grants **1777**
General Adult Foundation grant making is made from the Foundation's named unrestricted endowment funds. These grants focus on improving the quality of life for the citizens of Hillsdale County. Eligible projects generally fall within these categories: education, fine arts, social services, community development, recreation, environmental issues, health and wellness, and improvement in the physical, mental, and moral conditions of Hillsdale County residents. The Foundation aims to support creative approaches to community needs and problems that benefit the widest possible range of people.
Requirements: The Foundation requires applicants to call and discuss their project with the Executive Director prior to submitting the application. Applications from the Hillsdale County area or outside Hillsdale County, Michigan are welcome, if a significant number of the people to be served reside within Hillsdale County. Applicants shall be tax exempt according to Section 501(c)3 of the Internal Revenue Code.
Restrictions: The current objectives of the Foundation do not allow grants for: religious or sectarian purposes; individuals; legislative or political purposes; loans; capital campaigns; routine maintenance, including office equipment; administrative costs for maintaining the present operation of an organization, including, but not limited to, staff salaries, wages, and benefits; basic education materials including state mandated/benchmark core curriculum supplies and resources.
Geographic Focus: Michigan
Samples: Hillsdale Arts Chorale, Hillsdale, MI, $7,500—to underwrite the 2007 Messiah Christmas Concert (2007); Montgomery Fire and Rescue Department, Montgomery, MI, $4,200—to purchase a Self-Contained Breathing Apparatus (2007); Mrs. Stock's Park, Hillsdale, MI, $4,000—to assist in funding costs associated with the 2007 summer festival musical performances (2007).
Date(s) Application is Due: Nov 1; May 1
Contact: Sharon Bisher, Executive Director; (517) 439-5101; fax: (517) 439-5109; email: s.bisher@abouthccf.org
Internet: http://www.abouthccf.org/grants.asp
Sponsor: Hillsdale County Community Foundation
2 South Howell Street, P.O. Box 276
Hillsdale, MI 49242

Hillsdale Fund Grants **1778**
The fund awards grants to nonprofit organizations in its areas of interest, including arts and culture, education, health care, social services delivery, and religion. Call for meeting dates and application materials.
Requirements: Tax-exempt organizations are eligible.
Restrictions: Grants do not support indirect costs or overhead; routine, recurring operating expenses; conferences and seminars; travel and study; or individuals.
Geographic Focus: North Carolina
Samples: College of the Atlantic, Bar Harbor, ME, $50,000 (2006); Rocky Mountain Field Institute, Colorado Springs, CO, $10,000 (2006); Piedmont Environmental Council, Warrenton, VA, $30,000 (2006).
Amount of Grant: $3000-$50,000 average
Contact: Edward Doolan, Grants Administrator, (336) 274-5471
Sponsor: Hillsdale Fund
P.O. Box 20124
Greensboro, NC 27420-0124

Hilton Head Island Foundation Grants **1779**
The Foundation exists to enhance the quality of life for individuals living and/or working in Southern Beaufort County (Hilton Head Island, Daufuskie Island, Bluffton, Okatie). Grantmaking is in the broad areas of: arts, education, and community development. The Board meets three times per year. Application information is available online.
Requirements: To be eligible for funding, an applicant must be: a nonprofit agency with a tax-exempt status under section 501(c)3 of the Internal Revenue code, or eligible to be classified as such, but are not classified as a private foundation; serve the people who live and/or work in the Hilton Head Island area community.
Restrictions: Funding is not available for: sectarian or religious activities; political activities or organizations; grants directly to individuals; endowments; annual fundraising campaigns; special events or fundraisers; scholarships for students in grades K-12.
Geographic Focus: South Carolina
Samples: Hilton Head Island Recreation Assoc (SC)—to support the association???s expanded development and marketing program, $20,000 (2002); Low Country Institute (SC)—to fund the Adopt-A-Watershed citizen-led watershed monitoring effort, $25,000 (2002); Lowcountry Community Development Corp (SC)—for expansion of the corporation's programs, $35,000 (2002); Michael C. Riley Elementary School (SC)—to fund the 100 Book Challenge, which includes instructor training and books for the school, $45,000. Seahawk Theater Guild - $3,749 to purchase a portable sound system for the organization.
Date(s) Application is Due: Apr 1; Aug 1; Dec 1
Contact: Program Contact, (843) 681-9100
Internet: http://www.cf-lowcountry.org/page25039.cfm
Sponsor: Community Foundation of the Lowcountry
P.O. Box 23019, 4 Northridge Drive, Suite A
Hilton Head Island, SC 29925

Hilton Hotels Corporate Giving Program Grants **1780**
The Foundation's giving interests are focused in the areas of K-12 education programs, healthcare programs, youth programs, civic affairs and public policy. The Foundation supports selected organizations with a national constituency or those that are located in communities where the company has a corporate office or a major operating presence. There are no deadlines. Application information is available online.
Requirements: 501(c)3 tax-exempt organizations are eligible.
Restrictions: Funding is not available for: individuals; for-profit entities; local/regional/national sports teams; religious organizations; organizations requesting funds to cover operating deficits; agencies whose majority support comes from the public sector; capital campaigns or endowments; hospitals; private schools/pre-schools/day care facilities/

public schools outside geographic giving area; film or video projects; promotional merchandise; multi-year requests; conferences, tours or one-time special events.
Contact: Grants Administrator, (310) 278-4321
Internet: http://www.hiltonworldwide.com/en/ww/company_info/philanthropy_citizenship.jhtml
Sponsor: Hilton Hotels Corporation
9336 Civic Center Drive
Beverly Hills, CA 90210

Hirtzel Memorial Foundation Grants **1781**
The foundation awards grants to eligible organizations in New York and Pennsylvania in its areas of interest, including medical research and health care; community and neighborhood improvement; higher education; and social and human services. Types of support include building construction and renovation, capital campaigns, scholarships, equipment acquisition, general operating support, research, and scholarships. There are no application deadlines; contact the office for appropriate forms.
Requirements: New York nonprofit organizations in Ripley, Chautauqua County, and Pennsylvania nonprofit organizations in North East, Erie County, are eligible.
Geographic Focus: New York; Pennsylvania
Samples: Mercyhurst College (Erie, PA)—to establish the Institute on Aging and Geriatric Health, $1 million.
Amount of Grant: $750-$250,000 range
Contact: Laurie Moritz, Grants Administrator, c/o Mellon Financial Corporation, (412) 234-0023
Sponsor: Orris C. Hirtzel and Beatrice Dewey Hirtzel Memorial Foundation
P.O. Box 185
Pittsburgh, PA 15230

HIV/AIDS Research Training Fellowship **1782**
This program supports the training of researchers in HIV/AIDS research. The goals of the program are: to increase the number of ethnic minority research scientists studying HIV/AIDS issues among ethnic minority populations; to increase the availability and quality of ethnic minority research training; and to increase the knowledge on issues related to ethnic minority HIV/AIDS prevention and treatment. Fellowships are awarded for one academic year and are renewable for two additional years. Students specializing in such research areas as HIV prevention, AIDS treatment adherence, provider education, or psychoneuroimmunology are encouraged to apply. Students of any specialty in psychology will be considered if they plan careers in HIV/AIDS research.
Requirements: An applicant must be a U.S. citizen or resident with a permanent visa; a member of an ethnic minority group including, but not limited to, African American, Alaskan Native, American Indian, Asian American, Hispanic, Pacific Islander, and Puerto Rican, and/or demonstrate commitment to a career in psychology with a specialty in HIV/AIDS research related to ethnic minority populations; and enrolled full-time in a doctoral degree program in psychology at the time the fellowship is awarded.
Amount of Grant: $9600 approximately
Date(s) Application is Due: Jan 15
Contact: Dr. James Jones, (202) 336-6127; fax: (202) 336-6012; email: mfp@apa.org
Internet: http://www.apa.org/mfp/hprogram.html
Sponsor: American Psychological Association
750 First St NE
Washington, DC 20002-4242

Hoblitzelle Foundation Grants **1783**
The Hoblitzelle Foundation was established by Karl and Esther Hoblitzelle in 1942. Grants made by the Directors are usually focused on specific, non-recurring needs of the educational, social service, medical, cultural, and civic organizations in Texas, particularly in the Dallas area. The Board meets three times per year. It is preferred that the initial approach be through a brief narrative letter describing the project for which funds are asked. Guidelines are available online.
Requirements: Nonprofit organizations in the State of Texas, primarily within the Dallas Metroplex, are eligible to apply.
Restrictions: No grants are made for religious purposes or to individuals. No grants are made outside the State of Texas. Contributions are not made toward operating budgets, debt retirement, research, media productions or publications, scholarships or endowments. The Foundation makes no loans.
Geographic Focus: Texas
Samples: Dallas Arboretum, Texas Discovery Gardens, Dallas, TX—natural resources/environment grant (2009); Dallas Services, Dallas TX—handicapped/disabled grant (2009); Museum of Biblical Art, Dallas, TX—cultural grant (2010); Phoenix House, Dallas, TX-substance abuse grant (2010); Dallas Public Library, Dallas, TX—civic project grant (2010); Baylor Health Care System Foundation, Dallas, TX—medicine & health care grant (2010).
Date(s) Application is Due: Dec 15; Apr 15; Aug 15
Contact: Paul W. Harris, President; (214) 373-0462; email: pharris@hoblitzelle.org
Internet: http://www.hoblitzelle.org/
Sponsor: Hoblitzelle Foundation
5956 Sherry Lane, Suite 901
Dallas, TX 75225

Hogg Foundation for Mental Health Grants **1784**
The Foundation accomplishes its mission through the funding of external and internal projects in strategically selected areas. The Foundation operates major initiatives in three priority areas: integrated health care, cultural competence, and workforce development. Funds available through the Foundation's major initiatives and projects are distributed through a Request for Proposals (RFP) process. The Foundation does not accept unsolicited grant proposals on any topic. To be notified of future RFP opportunities, send an email message including your name, affiliation, and mailing address to: HoggCommunications@austin.utexas.edu.
Geographic Focus: Texas
Samples: People's Community Clinic, Austin, TX, $275,200—paid over three years, this grant was awarded to People's Community Clinic (PCC) in Austin to treat adults with various mental health problems in partnership with Austin Travis County Mental Health Mental Retardation Center.; Texas Children's Pediatric Associates, Houston, TX, $306,500—paid over three years, this grant will benefit children with attention-deficit hyperactivity disorder in its Ripley clinic, located in Houston's East End.
Contact: Program Contact, (888) 404-4336 or (512) 471-5041; fax: (512) 471-9608; email: Hogg-Grants@austin.utexas.edu
Internet: http://www.hogg.utexas.edu/funding_grantmaking.html
Sponsor: Hogg Foundation for Mental Health
University of Texas at Austin, P. O. Box 7998
Austin, TX 78713-7998

Hoglund Foundation Grants **1785**
The foundation supports nonprofits working in the areas of education, health science and services, social services, and children's health and development. Grants are made primarily in Dallas, and Houston, Texas, with a limited number of grants awarded outside of this area. Types of support include project support, capital support, and general operating support. Application guidelines are available on the foundation's Web site.
Requirements: To be eligible for consideration, an organization must provide proof that they have received a determination letter from the Internal Revenue Service indicating that it is a tax exempt organization as described in Section 501(c)3 of the Internal Revenue Code of 1986 and is treated as other than a private foundation as within the meaning of Section 509(a) of the Code. An organization may also qualify under Section 170(c)(1) if the grant requested is to be used exclusively for public purposes as described in the Code.
Restrictions: Grants are not made to individuals.
Geographic Focus: Texas
Samples: University of Virginia Fund, Charlottesville, VA, $33,000-Global Scholarship Fund (2008); Vickery Meadow Learning Center, Dallas, TX, $10,000—Family Literacy program (2008); Victims Outreach, Dallas, TX, $5,000—program services for victims of crime & violence (2008); Reasoning Mind, Inc., Houston, TX, $250,000—program expansion and general operating support (2008).
Amount of Grant: $1000-$200,000 average
Date(s) Application is Due: Mar 15; Jul 15; Nov 15
Contact: Kelly Compton, Executive Director; (214) 987-3605; fax: (214) 363-6507; email: info@hoglundfoundation.org
Internet: http://www.hoglundfoundation.org/grants.html
Sponsor: Hoglund Foundation
5910 North Central Expressway, Suite 255
Dallas, TX 75206

Holland/Zeeland Community Foundation Grants **1786**
This Foundation funds programs and projects that focus on the arts and culture, education, environmental issues, health and human services, youth, seniors, community and economic development, affordable housing, and others that enhance the well-being of all citizens in the community. Proposals that help organizations deliver services more effectively, enhance cooperation and collaboration, address emerging needs or try new approaches, positively impact a large number of people for the resources invested, or focus on prevention receive priority consideration. The Foundation generally awards grants one-time only for a specific program or project. To apply, first call to discuss the project and confirm it meets the Foundation guidelines.
Requirements: Qualifying organizations include nonprofits that are tax-exempt under Section 501(c)3, schools, municipalities, and other governmental entities that serve a charitable purpose in the greater Holland and Zeeland area.
Restrictions: Funding is not available for the following: requests in excess of $15,000; annual fund-raising drives; services which are commonly recognized as government or school obligations (however the foundation does consider applications from schools for pilot projects and innovative programs); endowments, loans, taxes or debt reduction; conference speakers, fieldtrips, travel or tours, for individuals or groups; religious programs that advocate specific religious doctrines or do not serve the broader community.
Geographic Focus: Michigan
Samples: Macatawa Greenway Partnership, $5,000—Trailhead Kiosk: to design, fabricate and install a prototype kiosk along Zuidema bike path; to explore, test and develop potential uses for an efficiently designed trailhead/obelisk (2007); Holland Free Health Clinic, $15,000— pilot program providing free or low cost diabetic supplies and education on the proper use of supplies (2007); Tulipanes Latino Art & Film Festival, Inc., $5,000— to fund programs including purchase and rental of films and productions and live performances by local and regional artists (2007).
Date(s) Application is Due: Jan 18; Jun 7; Sep 20
Contact: Janet DeYoung, Executive Director; (616) 396-6590; fax: (616) 396-3573; email: janet@cfhz.org or nfo@cfhz.org
Internet: http://cfhz.org/files/2010Funding_Guidelines.pdf
Sponsor: Community Foundation of the Holland/Zeeland Area
70 West 8th Street, Suite 100
Holland, MI 49423

Home Building Industry Disaster Relief Fund 1787

The Home Building Industry Disaster Relief Fund (HBIDRF) makes funds available for direct contribution to other recognized charities aiming to meet similar primary needs as the HBIDRF – shelter, health care, education. The board welcomes recommendations of charitable organizations that are actively working in your region to rebuild communities. Guidelines and application form are available at the website.

Requirements: Charities can include corporations, funds, or foundations organized and operated exclusively for charitable, scientific, or educational purposes. These charitable organizations may be involved in making direct contributions to adversely impacted individuals through established process, or with coordinated building projects such as one-day builds, blitzes, etc. Other entities that could be eligible to receive funds might include vocational training programs, temporary shelters or clinics and educational ventures intended to help the local home building industry recover from disastrous events. To apply for funding, contact your local home builders association to determine if any partnering opportunities are available at this time.

Restrictions: The fund does not make assistance available directly to individuals.

Contact: Jerry Howard, Executive Officer; (800) 368-5242; fax: (202) 266-8400

Internet: http://www.nahb.org/generic.aspx?sectionID=842

Sponsor: Home Building Industry Disaster Relief Fund
1201 15th Street, NW
Washington, DC 20005-2800

HomeBanc Foundation Grants 1788

Giving primarily in Florida and Georgia, the HomeBanc Foundation also, gives to national organizations. The Foundation has three main goals: provide support to cancer related causes through funding education, advocacy, and research; support the American dream of homeownership for those who might not reach it on their own; and provide college funding to students who strive to achieve their goals through education beyond high school. Scholarship forms are available online. Send a Letter of Inquiry to the Foundation, unsolicited applications are not excepted. The Foundation will contact you if your proposal fits their criteria.

Requirements: Nonprofit organizations providing services in Georgia and Florida are eligible.

Geographic Focus: Florida; Georgia

Contact: Amanda Albertelli, GrantsManager; (404) 497-1000; email: aalbertelli@homebanc.com

Sponsor: HomeBanc Foundation
2002 Summit Boulevard, Suite 100
Atlanta, GA 30319-1497

Homer Foundation Grants 1789

The Foundation seeks to fund innovative, creative projects that have a high likelihood of success and will have a long-term, positive impact on the community. Funding is available for arts and culture, community development, youth programs, education, health care, scholarships and the environment. Application information is available online.

Requirements: 501(c)3 nonprofit organizations and other qualified nonprofit entities located in the southwestern portion of the Kenai Peninsula, from Ninilchik south and including the communities across Kachemak Bay, are eligible. An individual who applies must be a resident of the region as described above, who will spend the funds on projects completed within this region. Projects taking place outside of this region, but by a resident, will be considered on the merit of the project and how it could benefit the community.

Geographic Focus: Alaska

Amount of Grant: $4,000

Contact: Joy Steward, Director, (907) 235-0541; fax: (907) 235-0542; email: jsteward@homerfund.org

Internet: http://www.homerfund.org/grantmaking.html

Sponsor: Homer Foundation
P.O. Box 2600
Homer, AK 99603

Honda of America Manufacturing Foundation Grants 1790

The Foundation supports community outreach in Ohio. Each year, the Foundation funds various community projects throughout the state. This involvement helps build the community where it does business and where its associates live. The Foundation supports programs and organizations in the areas of education, arts and culture, civic and community, health and human services, and the environment. It places its priorities on the development of programs, and not supporting annual operating budgets.

Requirements: Priority consideration will be given for projects within the West Central Ohio area, including: Allen, Auglaize, Champaign, Clark, Darke, Delaware, Franklin, Hardin, Logan, Madison, Marion, Mercer, Miami, Shelby and Union counties. In addition, Honda considers projects on a case-by-case basis outside this area if the projects are Ohio-based and reflect its priorities of interest.

Restrictions: Honda of America does not make grants to: individuals; religious or political groups; organizations which are not tax-exempt under the U.S. Internal Revenue Code paragraph 501(c)3; or programs outside the state of Ohio. Generally, the Foundation does not provide contributions in support of: conferences or workshops; seminars or pageants; field trips, extra-curricular school activities or sports teams; fraternal or veterans organizations; national health organizations; courtesy advertisements, lobbying organizations, memberships or legal advocacy; staff salaries; or pilot programs.

Geographic Focus: Ohio

Date(s) Application is Due: Mar 31; Jun 30; Sep 30; Dec 31

Contact: Ms. Ginny Milburn, Administrative Coordinator, Corporate Affairs; (937) 645-8792; fax: (937) 645-8787; email: ginny_milburn@ham.honda.com

Internet: http://www.ohio.honda.com/community/giving.cfm

Sponsor: Honda of America Manufacturing Foundation
24000 Honda Parkway
Marysville, OH 43040

Honeywell Foundation Grants 1791

The foundation awards grants to nonprofits in communities where company plants are located. Areas of interest include education, community funds, health, aging, human services, youth agencies, cultural programs, and international exchange programs. Types of support include general operating support, continuing support, annual campaigns, building/renovation, equipment acquisition, employee matching gifts, and fellowship and scholarship aid to colleges and universities that are major sources of future employees.

Requirements: Nonprofit organizations in company-operating areas are eligible. Areas include Arizona, Florida, Illinois, Minnesota, and New Mexico.

Restrictions: Grants do not support individuals, church-related programs, special interest groups (such as labor or veterans) unless activity benefits entire community, political organizations, or for international organizations.

Geographic Focus: Arizona; Florida; Illinois; Minnesota; New Mexico

Amount of Grant: $1000-$25,000 average

Contact: Andre Lewis, Vice President and Executive Director, (973) 455-5876; fax: (612) 951-0433

Internet: http://www.honeywell.com/about/foundation.html

Sponsor: Honeywell Foundation
101 Columbia Road
Morristown, NJ 07962

Horace A. Kimball and S. Ella Kimball Foundation Grants 1792

The Kimball Foundation makes grants almost exclusively to Rhode Island operatives (charities) or those benefitting Rhode Island residents and causes. Although, the Foundation considers gifts to all areas in the state, greater emphasis is placed on South County. Areas of interest for the Foundation are: human services, the environment, and health care.

Requirements: The Foundation will consider any organization which has proper 501(c)3 and 509(a) I.R.S. tax classification status. Application form and guidelines available on foundation Web site. Application form required. Applicants should submit the following: copy of IRS Determination Letter; brief history of organization and description of its mission; copy of most recent annual report/audited financial statement/990.

Restrictions: No support for religious organizations. No grants to individuals, or for feasibility studies, capital projects or multi-year commitments.

Geographic Focus: Rhode Island

Samples: Rhode Island Philharmonic Orchestra, East Providence, RI, $25,000 (2007); Westerly School Department, Westerly, RI, $10,000 (2007); South County Hospital Healthcare System, Wakefield, RI, $25,000 (2007);

Amount of Grant: $1,000-$50,000 range

Date(s) Application is Due: None, but preferably by July 15

Contact: Thomas F. Black III, President; fax: (401) 364-3565;

Internet: http://www.hkimballfoundation.org/index2.htm

Sponsor: The Horace A. Kimball and S. Ella Kimball Foundation
130 Woodville Road
Hope Valley, RI 02832

Horizon Foundation for New Jersey Grants 1793

The Foundation's purpose is to promote health, well-being, and quality of life in New Jersey communities. Foundation goals are to improve health by promoting quality health care programs and access and to enhance arts and cultural opportunities. Application information is available online. Only electronic grant applications will be accepted. Application are accepted between January 1 and September 31.

Requirements: 501(c)3 tax-exempt organizations in New Jersey communities located in and served by Horizon Blue Cross Blue Shield of New Jersey are eligible.

Restrictions: Funding is not available for: capital campaigns; endowments; hospitals or hospital foundations; individuals; political causes; political candidates; political organizations; political campaigns.

Geographic Focus: New Jersey

Samples: ChoiceOne Pregnancy & Sexual Health Resource Centers, Lawrenceville, NJ, $25,000—to support the Sexually Transmitted Diseases Education and Prevention component of its "Straight Talk" Program (2008); Family Guidance Center, Hamilton, NJ, $15.000—to support its Behavioral Health Services-Depression Recovery Program (2008); American Repertory Ballet, New Brunswick, HJ, $7,500—to support the Dance Power Program (2008).

Amount of Grant: $10,000-$50,000

Contact: Michele Berry; email: Foundation_Info@horizonblue.com

Internet: http://www.horizon-bcbsnj.com/foundation/about/funding.html?WT.svl=leftnav

Sponsor: Horizon Foundation for New Jersey
Three Penn Plaza East, PP-15V
Newark, NJ 07105-2200

Horizons Community Issues Grants 1794

Grants support program activities or projects serving lesbian, gay, bisexual, and transgender (LGBT) people of all ages in designated California counties focusing on the following issue areas: arts and culture; advocacy, awareness, and civil rights; children,

youth, and families; and community and social services. Application information is available online.
Requirements: To be eligible, an organization must: be a nonprofit, 501(c)3 organization, or provide documentation that the organization is sponsored under a fiscal agent umbrella that has 501(c)3 status. Organizations or programs must request support for one or more of the following counties: Alameda; Contra; Costa; Marin; Napa; San Francisco; San Mateo; Santa Clara; Solano; Sonoma.
Restrictions: The following are not eligible for support: costs incurred prior to the date of the grant award; government agencies; capital support, including construction and renovation; fundraising or event sponsorship; individuals; Non-LGBT organizations with budget over $1 million.
Geographic Focus: California
Amount of Grant: $10,000-$20,000 range
Contact: Jewelle Gomez, Program Officer; (415) 398-2333, ext. 116; email: jgomez@horizonsfoundation.org
Internet: http://www.horizonsfoundation.org/page/organizations/ci
Sponsor: Horizons Foundation
870 Market Street, Suite 728
San Francisco, CA 94102

Hormel Foods Charitable Trust Grants **1795**
The Charitable Trust was established to benefit various organizations and projects that emphasize education, hunger and quality-of-life initiatives in and around Hormel Foods plant communities. The Program operates as a compliment to its foundation, making charitable contributions to nonprofit organizations directly. Support is given primarily in areas of company operations. Fields of interest include: disaster and preparedness services; education; general charitable giving; and health care. Types of support include: scholarships; matching gifts; general operations; and sponsorships. The Public Relations Department handles giving. Annual donations to a single organization typically do not exceed $15,000. A contributions committee reviews all written requests. Applicants should submit a detailed description of the project and amount of funding requested. The board meets once each month.
Requirements: Only organizations classified as 501(c)3 are eligible for support. Applicants should be located in or serve the communities of: Aurora, Illinois; Austin, Minnesota; Algona, Iowa; Alma, Kansas; Atlanta, Georgia; Beloit, Wisconsin; Chino, California; Fort Dodge, Iowa; Fremont, Nebraska; Knoxville, Iowa; Lathrop, California; Mendota Heights, Minnesota; New Berlin, Wisconsin; Osceola, Iowa; Rochelle, Illinois; Stockton, California; Turlock, California; and Wichita, Kansas.
Restrictions: Giving is primarily limited to areas of company operations.
Geographic Focus: California; Georgia; Illinois; Iowa; Kansas; Minnesota; Nebraska; Wisconsin
Contact: Julie H. Craven, Director of Public Relations; (507) 437-5345; email: media@hormel.com
Internet: http://www.hormelfoods.com/responsibility/philanthropy/default.aspx
Sponsor: Hormel Foods Charitable Trust
1 Hormel Place
Austin, MN 55912-3680

Hormel Foundation Grants **1796**
The Foundation, established in 1941, is a non-profit organization dedicated to supporting higher education, health care and research, social services, and community programs located in or serving the city of Austin, Minnesota. Applications for grants must be presented to the Foundation in writing. They should be as brief as appropriate to present the necessary facts about the applying organization and the project for which the grant is being sought. An application form is required, and must be received by the Foundation office by September 1st of each year.
Requirements: Only 501(c)3 organizations in Minnesota should apply.
Geographic Focus: Minnesota
Date(s) Application is Due: Sep 1
Contact: R.L. Knowlton, Chairperson; (507) 437-9800; fax: (507) 434-6731
Internet: http://www.thehormelfoundation.com/requirements.asp
Sponsor: Hormel Foundation
301 North Main Street
Austin, MN 55912-3498

Houston Endowment Grants **1797**
The Endowment supports nonprofit organizations and educational institutions that improve life for the people of the greater Houston area. The Foundation funds programs in the arts, community enhancement, education, health, human services, the environment and neighborhood development. Requests for funding are accepted throughout the year. Further application information is available online.
Requirements: Nonprofit organizations that are recognized as charitable organizations by the Internal Revenue Code are eligible to apply. Funds are provided primarily to Harris County and contiguous counties. Grants seldom are given outside of Texas and never are made outside of the United States.
Restrictions: The Endowment does not select scholarship recipients or make direct scholarship awards to individuals. Inquiries about scholarship assistance should be made to financial aid offices at colleges and universities. Funding is not available for other grant-making organizations or to charities operated by service clubs. Funds are not available for religious activities; the purchase of uniform, equipment or trips for school-related organizations or sports teams; honoraria for speakers and panelists; fund-raising activities and galas; and memorials for individuals. The Foundation does not make loans or grants to individuals.
Geographic Focus: Texas
Amount of Grant: $2,500-$1 million
Contact: Harriet W. Garland, Grant Manager; (713) 238-8100; fax: (713) 238-8101; email: info@houstonendowment.org
Internet: http://www.houstonendowment.org/grants/grants_apply.htm
Sponsor: Houston Endowment
600 Travis, Suite 6400
Houston, TX 77002-3000

Howard and Bush Foundation Grants **1798**
The foundation's funding is limited to Rensselaer County, NY. with an emphasis on arts and culture, education, civic and urban affairs, legal services, including a women's bar association, and social service and health programs that benefit the areas resident. Requests for equipment acquisition, programs development, matching funds, building/renovation and seed money will receive consideration. There are no deadline dates, funding guidelines are sent upon request. Contact staff prior to submitting a proposal. The board meets twice a year, in April and October. Notification of proposal acceptance will be within 14 days, following the board meeting.
Requirements: Nonprofit organizations benefiting Rensselaer County, NY, and its residents may request grant support.
Restrictions: Grants are not awarded to colleges, schools, churches, or individuals or for endowment purposes, operating budgets, or deficit financing. Generally no support for government or largely tax-supported agencies, or churches not connected with the founders.
Geographic Focus: New York
Samples: Friends of Barker Park, $5,000— for park improvements (2008); East Side Neighborhood Association, $5,000—for security system/modify heating system (2008); Whitney M. Young Jr. Foundation, $10,000—for Troy oral health expansion project (2008).
Amount of Grant: $750-$75,000 range
Contact: Deborah Byers, Program Contact, (518) 271-1134; email: dogclover@aol.com
Sponsor: Howard and Bush Foundation
2 Belle Avenue
Troy, NY 12180

Howe Foundation of North Carolina Grants **1799**
The Howe Foundation, established in 1966, supports organizations involved with arts and culture, education, human services, Christianity, and mentally disabled individuals. Giving limited to the Belmont, North Carolina area.
Requirements: No application form required, submit your proposal to: P.O. Box 749, Belmont, NC 28012.
Restrictions: No grants to individuals.
Geographic Focus: North Carolina
Amount of Grant: $200-$144,000 range
Contact: Henry Howe, Treasure; (704) 825-5372;
Sponsor: The Howe Foundation, Inc.
P.O. Box 227
Belmont, NC 28012-0227

HRB Clinical Research Training Fellowships **1800**
These fellowships are designed to enable medical and dental graduates at any stage in their career to gain specialized clinical research training in a biomedical field in Ireland. Awards are available for up to two years. Fellowships are tenable only in institutions approved of by the board, such as teaching hospitals, universities and research institutes in Ireland. Applications are available on the Web site.
Requirements: Applicants should be graduates in medicine or dentistry from post-registration up to and including senior registrar or equivalent academic level. Applicants should be EU citizens or be graduates from outside the EU with permanent Irish resident status.
Amount of Grant: IR@L46,909-IR@L56,066
Date(s) Application is Due: Sep 16
Contact: Patricia Cranley, Research Grants Officer, (353) 1 6761176 ext 120; fax: (353) 1 6611856; email: pcranley@hrb.ie
Internet: http://www.hrb.ie/display_content.php?page_id=95
Sponsor: Health Research Board
73 Lower Baggot Street
Dublin 2 Ireland

HRB Health Services Research Fellowships **1801**
Fellowships provide an opportunity to graduates with appropriate experience to undertake health services research in Ireland. Research may be interdisciplinary in nature and may involve clinical, epidemiological, public health, statistics, health economics, social science, operational, and management disciplines. Awards are available for up to three years. Application forms are available on the Web site.
Requirements: To be eligible, candidates must hold a primary degree in a discipline relevant to health services research; have acquired appropriate postgraduate experience in the field of health services research; have support from an approved academic department or center; have obtained the prior approval of a head of department for the research study being proposed; be European Union citizens or be graduates from outside the European Union with permanent Irish resident status.
Amount of Grant: IR@L41,902; IR@L43,319; IR@L44,727
Date(s) Application is Due: Oct 14

Contact: Patricia Cranley, Research Grants Officer, (353) 1 6761176 ext 120; fax: (353) 1 6611856; email: pcranley@hrb.ie
Internet: http://www.hrb.ie/display_content.php?page_id=96
Sponsor: Health Research Board
73 Lower Baggot Street
Dublin 2 Ireland

HRB Postdoctoral Research Fellowships 1802
Fellowships enable researchers with a PhD, MD, or equivalent research experience to develop research careers at an advanced level in medicine, dentistry, health-related biological sciences, or epidemiology in Ireland. Awards are available for up to three years. Applications are available on the Web site.
Requirements: Applicants must have a PhD or MD in a related biomedical science field or have submitted a thesis for such at the time of application, or have equivalent research experience. Applicants should not have more than five years postdoctoral experience at the time of application and be European Union citizens or be graduates from outside the European Union with permanent Irish resident status. Applications should be made by the prospective fellow with the support of the head of an appropriate sponsoring laboratory in the Republic of Ireland.
Amount of Grant: IR@L41,902; IR@L43,319; IR@L44,727
Date(s) Application is Due: Oct 7
Contact: Patricia Cranley, Research Grants Officer, (353) 1 6761176 ext 120; fax: (01) 6611856; email: pcranley@hrb.ie
Internet: http://www.hrb.ie/display_content.php?page_id=97
Sponsor: Health Research Board
73 Lower Baggot Street
Dublin 2 Ireland

HRSA Eliminating Disparities in Perinatal Health Grants 1803
The purpose of this program is to enhance a community's capacity to address significant disparities in several perinatal health indicators, with an emphasis on infant mortality rates.
Requirements: Public and private nonprofit community-based organizations are eligible to apply.
Restrictions: Entities that are currently receiving a Healthy Start implementation grant are not eligible to apply.
Amount of Grant: $100,000-$2.3 million; $782,971 average
Contact: Director, Division of Perinatal Systems and Women's Health, (301) 443-0543
Internet: http://www.hrsa.gov
Sponsor: Health Resources and Services Administration
5600 Fishers Ln, Parklawn Building
Rockville, MD 20857

HRSA Emergency Medical Services for Children Grants 1804
State and accredited medical schools may be eligible for grants to support projects that expand and improve emergency medical services for children who need treatment for trauma or critical care. It is expected that maximum distribution of projects among the states will be made and that priority will be given to projects targeted toward populations with special needs, including Native Americans, minorities, and the disabled.
Requirements: States and accredited schools of medicine are eligible to apply.
Amount of Grant: $700,000 average
Date(s) Application is Due: May 7
Contact: Dan Kavanaugh, (301) 443-1321; email: dkavanaugh@hrsa.gov
Internet: http://www.hrsa.gov/grants/preview/mch.htm#hrsa05057
Sponsor: Health Resources and Services Administration
5600 Fishers Ln, Parklawn Building
Rockville, MD 20857

HRSA Geriatric Education Centers 1805
The purpose of this program is to develop geriatric education centers to support development of collaborative arrangements involving several health professions schools and healthcare facilities. Geriatric centers facilitate the training of health professional faculty, students, and practitioners in the diagnosis, treatment, and prevention of disease, disability, and other health problems of the aged. Projects must improve training of health professionals; develop and disseminate curricula relating to treatment; support training and retraining of faculty and continuing education of health professionals who provide geriatric care; and provide students with clinical training in geriatrics in nursing homes, hospitals, ambulatory care centers, and senior centers. HRSA-05-077
Requirements: Accredited health professions schools, physicians assistants training programs, allied health schools, and nursing schools are eligible to apply.
Amount of Grant: $200,000 average
Date(s) Application is Due: Mar 1
Contact: Donna Nash, Grants Managment Specialist, (301) 443-6960; fax: (301) 443-6343; email: dnash@hrsa.gov
Internet: http://www.hrsa.gov/grants/preview/guidanceprofessions/hrsa05077.htm
Sponsor: Health Resources and Services Administration
5600 Fishers Ln, Room 11A-05
Rockville, MD 20857

HRSA Hansen's Disease National Ambulatory Care Program Grants 1806
Grants are provided for screening and testing of contacts of patients diagnosed with Hansen's disease and for ambulatory care and treatment services to any person diagnosed with Hansen's disease who needs and requests care and treatment for that disease. Grants may be used for the cost of providing diagnostic treatment services to patients and contacts of patients diagnosed with Hansen's disease. Contact the office for deadline dates.
Requirements: Existing health care facilities are eligible to apply.
Amount of Grant: $35,000-$375,000
Contact: Office of Grants Management, Bureau of Primary Health Care, (800) 642-2477; fax: (225) 756-3760
Internet: http://bphc.hrsa.gov/nhdp/AMBULATORY_CARE_MAIN_PAGE.htm
Sponsor: Health Resources and Services Administration
4350 East-West Hwy
Bethesda, MD 20814

HRSA Health Professions Scholarships for Disadvantaged Students 1807
The program makes funds available for grants to schools of medicine; osteopathic medicine; dentistry; optometry; pharmacy; podiatric medicine; veterinary medicine; nursing (associate, diploma, baccalaureate, and graduate degree); public health; chiropractic; allied health (baccalaureate or graduate degree programs of dental hygiene, medical laboratory technology, occupational therapy, physical therapy, radiologic technology, speech pathology, audiology, and registered dietitians); graduate programs in behavioral and mental health practice (includes clinical psychology, clinical social work, professional counseling, or marriage and family therapy); and programs providing training of physician assistants for the purpose of assisting such schools in providing scholarships to individuals from disadvantaged backgrounds who are enrolled (or accepted for enrollment) as full-time students in the schools. Notice of awards is issued to the schools, which, in turn, select and issue the awards to the eligible students. Consultation and technical assistance is provided to institutions wishing to apply. Annual deadline dates may vary; contact the office to confirm exact dates.
Requirements: Accredited public or private nonprofit schools of medicine, nursing, osteopathic medicine, dentistry, pharmacy, podiatric medicine, optometry, veterinary medicine, public or allied health, or schools offering graduate programs in clinical psychology are eligible.
Amount of Grant: $727-$650,000; $102,468 average
Contact: Andrea Stampone, Bureau of Health Professions, (301) 443-4776
Internet: http://bhpr.hrsa.gov/dsa/sds.htm
Sponsor: Health Resources and Services Administration
5600 Fishers Ln, Parklawn Building
Rockville, MD 20857

HRSA Nurse Anesthetist Traineeships Program 1808
Grants are awarded to eligible institutions to provide financial support through traineeships for licensed registered nurses enrolled as full-time students beyond the twelfth month of study in a master's nurse anesthesia program. HRSA-05-062
Requirements: Eligible applicants are schools of nursing, academic health centers, and other public or private nonprofit entities which provide registered nurses with full-time anesthetist master's education and have evidence of earned accreditation status from the American Association of Nurse Anesthetists (AANA) Council on Accreditation of Nurse Anesthesia Education Programs.
Amount of Grant: $7100 average
Date(s) Application is Due: Nov 18
Contact: Karen Breeden, Division of Nursing, Bureau of Health Professions, (301) 443-6333; fax: (301) 443-8586; email: kbreeden@hrsa.gov
Internet: http://www.hrsa.gov/grants/preview/professions.htm#hrsa05062
Sponsor: Health Resources and Services Administration
5600 Fishers Ln, Parklawn Building
Rockville, MD 20857

HRSA Nursing Education Opportunities for the Disadvantaged Project Grants 1809
This program is intended to provide financial assistance to eligible schools of nursing and other applicants to meet the costs of special projects to increase nursing education opportunities for individuals from disadvantaged backgrounds. Funds may be used for salaries of personnel specifically employed for the project; consultant fees; supplies and equipment necessary to conduct the project; essential travel expenses; and other expenses related to the project. Indirect administrative costs are allowed, limited to 8 percent of direct costs. Grants may be made for up to three-year project periods and may be renewed competitively for an additional two years.
Requirements: Public and nonprofit private schools of nursing and other public or nonprofit private entities are eligible.
Amount of Grant: $58,800-$518,600; $255,100 average
Contact: Dr. Janice Young, Division of Nursing, Bureau of Health Professions, (301) 443-6193
Internet: http://bhpr.hrsa.gov/dsa/sds.htm
Sponsor: Health Resources and Services Administration
5600 Fishers Ln, Parklawn Building
Rockville, MD 20857

HRSA Physician Assistant Training 1810
Grants are awarded for projects for the training of physician assistants and for the training of individuals who will teach in programs to provide such training. A project supported must meet the following definition of a training program for physician assistants as defined under Section 799B of the Public Health Service Act: has as its objective the education of individuals who will, upon completion of their studies in the program, be qualified to provide primary care under the supervision of a physician; extends for at least one academic year and consists of supervised clinical practice and at

least four months (in the aggregate) of classroom instruction directed toward preparing students to deliver health care; has an enrollment of not less than eight students; and trains students in primary care, disease prevention, health promotion, geriatric medicine, and home health care. The program assists schools to meet the costs of projects to plan, develop, and operate or maintain programs for the training of physician assistants and for the training of individuals who will teach in programs to provide such training. Programs must develop and use methods designed to encourage graduates of the program to work in health professional shortage areas. Programs also must develop and use methods for placing graduates in positions for which they have been trained.
Requirements: Public or nonprofit private hospitals, schools of medicine or osteopathic medicine, or public or private nonprofit entities are eligible to apply. Eligible physician assistant programs are those that are either accredited by the American Medical Association's Committee on Allied Health Education and Accreditation (AMA-CAHEA) or its successor organization, the Commission on Accreditation of Allied Health Education Programs (CAAHEP).
Amount of Grant: $13,487-$257,297; $120,076 average
Contact: Ellie Grant, (301) 443-5404; email: egrant@hrsa.gov
Internet: http://www.hrsa.gov
Sponsor: Health Resources and Services Administration
5600 Fishers Ln, Parklawn Building
Rockville, MD 20857

HRSA Ryan White HIV Early Intervention Services Grants **1811**
To increase the capacity of entities that provide comprehensive primary care services to persons with Human Immunodeficiency Virus (HIV) infection, or who are at-risk of infection, and to offer more early intervention services. The services will include increased counseling and testing, partner involvement in risk reduction, transmission prevention, appropriate primary care diagnostic and treatment services, and, as needed, case-management to ensure that individual service needs are met. A planning and capacity building program provides assistance to organizations wishing to develop a new or expanded HIV program, particularly in rural and underserved areas and communities of color. HRSA-05-020
Requirements: Eligible for grants are public and private nonprofit entities, including migrant and community health centers, health care for the homeless grantees, family planning grantees, comprehensive hemophilia diagnostic and treatment centers, federally qualified health centers, and other groups that currently provide primary care services to people at risk for HIV.
Restrictions: Grant funds may not support construction, in-patient care, residential care, or cash payments to service recipients.
Amount of Grant: $150,000 maximum for three year period
Date(s) Application is Due: Mar 1
Contact: Dr. Jose Morales, (301) 443-0493; email: jmorales@hrsa.gov
Internet: http://www.hrsa.gov/grants/preview/hivaids.htm#hrsa05020
Sponsor: Health Resources and Services Administration
5600 Fishers Lane
Rockville, MD 20857

Huber Foundation Grants **1812**
The Foundation focuses its grants program on three specific aspects of reproductive rights: keeping abortion safe, legal, and preferably increasingly rare; contraceptive choice and availability; and relevant education. The Foundation's major interest lies in funding organizations that will impact these issues on a national level. There is no formal application procedure. A letter describing the project, a budget for the project, and proof of tax-exempt status is required. Though the Foundation board meets four times annually, there are no fixed deadline dates.
Requirements: U.S. nonprofits, including advocacy groups, hospitals, legal defense groups, family planning agencies, educational organizations, universities, and women's groups may submit grant applications.
Restrictions: The foundation does not encourage proposals for projects that are local or regional in scope. It will not consider grants to individuals, foreign organizations, capital campaigns, scholarships, endowment funds, research, international projects, or film productions.
Samples: Planned Parenthood Federation of America (New York, NY)—for general support and Responsible Choices Campaign, $700,000.; Feminist Majority Foundation (Arlington, VA)—for the National Clinic Access Project, $100,000.; Planned Parenthood of Northern New England (Williston, VT)—for general support, $90,000.
Amount of Grant: $10,000-$100,000 average
Contact: Lorraine Barnhart, Executive Director; (732) 933-7700
Sponsor: Huber Foundation
P.O. Box 277
Rumson, NJ 07760-0277

Hudson Webber Foundation Grants **1813**
The purpose of the Foundation is to improve the vitality and quality of life of the metropolitan Detroit community. The Foundation concentrates its giving primarily within the City of Detroit and has a particular interest in the revitalization of the urban core because this area is a focus for community activity and pride and is of critical importance to the vitality of the entire metropolitan community. The Foundation presently concentrates its efforts and resources in support of projects within five program missions: Detroit Physical Revitalization; Economic Development; The Arts; Safe Community; and the Detroit Medical Center. A brief letter signed by a senior officer of the requesting organization is the preferred form of application. Information for completing the letter of request are available online.
Requirements: The foundation concentrates its giving within Detroit.
Geographic Focus: Michigan
Samples: Habitat for Humanity - Metro Detroit, Inc., Detroit, MI, $150,000—Partnership to Build Capacity (2007); Detroit Renaissance Foundation, Inc., Detroit, MI, $100,000—Business Attraction Program (2007); Detroit Science Center, Inc., Detroit, MI, $10,000—General program support (2007); Michigan Community Service Commission, Detroit, MI, $75,000—Winning Futures Program-Mentor Michigan (2007); Harper Hospital, Detroit, MI, $200,000—Renal Transplant Unit (2007).
Contact: Katy Locker, Program Director; (313) 963-7777; fax: (313) 963-2818; email: HWF@hudson-webber.org
Internet: http://www.hudson-webber.org/HowToApply_Instructions.html
Sponsor: Hudson Webber Foundation
333 West Fort Street, Suite 1310
Detroit, MI 48226-3134

Hugh J. Andersen Foundation Grants **1814**
The mission of the Hugh J. Andersen Foundation is to give back to our community through focused efforts that foster inclusivity, promote equality, and lead to increased human independence, self sufficiency and dignity. To fulfill this mission, the Foundation acts as a grantmaker, innovator, and convener. The Foundation's primary geographic area of focus is the St. Croix Valley: Washington County in Minnesota and Pierce, Polk and St. Croix Counties in Wisconsin. Secondarily, there is an interest in St. Paul, Minnesota. From time to time the Foundation may consider programs in other parts of the Metro Area and Greater Minnesota. Please contact the Program Director prior to submitting a proposal to determine if the program might be of interest to the Foundation. The Board generally considers requests in June, September, December and February. Faxed or emailed applications will not be considered.
Requirements: The Hugh J. Andersen Foundation awards grants only to qualified charitable organizations that are designated as tax exempt under Internal Revenue Service Code 501(c)3 and are not classified as private foundations.
Restrictions: The Hugh J. Andersen Foundation: does not make loans, and does not provide grants or scholarships to individuals; does not provide grants for lobbying activities, fundraising dinners and events, or travel; will generally not consider the following types of organizations and programs for funding: agencies/divisions/councils/programs that have counterparts in St. Paul or the St. Croix Valley; arts organizations exclusively focused on music, dance or visual arts; athletic teams; business/economics education; child care centers; civic action groups; debt or after the fact situations; immigration/refugee issues and programs; independent media productions; political/voter education; private or alternative schools; religious institutions. In addition, the Foundation: will generally not fund the entire project budget, but prefers to be part of an effort supported by a number of sources; considers major endowment and capital requests for funding to be a low priority; does not provide funding through fiscal agents; considers letters of inquiry. Letters of inquiry are reviewed at the Foundation's next board meeting. If the board determines that the request falls within its guidelines and interests, a full proposal will be requested from the applicant for review at the following board meeting.
Geographic Focus: Minnesota; Wisconsin
Date(s) Application is Due: Mar 15; Jun 15; Aug 15; Nov 15;
Contact: Brad Kruse, Program Director; (651) 275-4489 or (888) 439-9508; fax: (651) 439-9480; email: hjafdn@srinc.biz
Internet: https://www.srinc.biz/hja/documents/HJAGuidelines09-10.pdf
Sponsor: Hugh J. Andersen Foundation
White Pine Building, 342 Fifth Avenue North
Bayport, MN 55003

Huie-Dellmon Trust Grants **1815**
The trust awards grants to Louisiana nonprofits in its areas of interest, including hospitals, higher and secondary education, libraries, and Protestant churches and organizations. Types of support include general operating support, capital campaigns, building construction/renovation, equipment acquisition, program development, scholarship funds, research, and matching funds. There are no application forms or deadlines.
Requirements: Central Louisiana nonprofit organizations are eligible.
Geographic Focus: Louisiana
Samples: Christus Cabrini Foundation, Alexandria, LA, $100,000 (2008); Calvary Baptist Church, Alexandria, LA, $12,500 (2008); Rapides Parish Library, Alexandria, LA, $30,000 (2008).
Amount of Grant: $1,000-$100,000 average
Contact: Richard Crowell Jr., Trustee, (318) 748-8141
Sponsor: Huie-Dellmon Trust
P.O. Box 330
Alexandria, LA 71309-0330

Human Growth Foundation Small Grants **1816**
The foundation awards grants for investigation of human growth and its disorders, with special consideration given for the chondrodystrophies. Special consideration will be given to new investigators and ideas new to the field. Postdoctoral research dealing with all aspects of normal and abnormal human growth and development including, but not limited to, the areas of biological, psychological, educational, and diet and nutrition will be considered. Up to three grants will be awarded. A synopsis of the research results is required to be submitted the following year. An NIH-type biographical sketch and two-page letter of intent should be sent by May 15; full applications are due by September 1.
Restrictions: No portion of the grant can be used for administrative overhead.
Amount of Grant: $7500-$10,000

Date(s) Application is Due: May 15; Sep 1
Contact: Program Contact, (800) 451-6434 or (516) 671-4041; fax: (516) 671-4055; email: hgf1@hgfound.org
Internet: http://www.hgfound.org/smallgrants.html
Sponsor: Human Growth Foundation
997 Glen Cove Avenue
Glen Head, NY 11545

Human Source Foundation Grants **1817**
The foundation provides assistance and financial support for programs involved with botany, higher education, and human services, with grants coming in the form of general operating funds. Giving is restricted to the State of Texas, primarily in Denton and Fort Worth counties. There are no specific deadlines or application forms with which to adhere, and applicants should begin by forwarding a letter of request.
Requirements: 501(c)3 tax-exempt organizations serving Texas, primarily Denton and Fort Worth counties, are eligible to apply.
Geographic Focus: Texas
Contact: c/o Mary G. Palko; (817) 926-2799; fax: (817) 926-5202; email: mary@ftw.com or mpalko@compuserve.com or info@pauseforpeace.org
Sponsor: Human Source Foundation
P.O. Box 100423, 2409 Winton Terrace West
Fort Worth, TX 76185-0423

Humana Foundation Grants **1818**
The foundation was established to promote worthwhile organizations that improve the health and welfare of communities in its headquarters region of Louisville, KY. It supports nonprofit institutions primarily in the areas of domestic and international health, education, and civic and cultural development. Religious organizations are eligible for project-specific support (e.g., social services outreach) or funds for an accredited, church-affiliated educational institution. Grants also are awarded in Humana market areas outside of the headquarters region. Application information is available online.
Requirements: Applicant organizations must be 501(c)3 tax-exempt located in communities where Humana has a meaningful presence.
Restrictions: Grants are not given to organizations for seed money. The foundation does not contribute to social, labor, political, veterans, or fraternal organizations. Funds cannot be used solely to support an organization's salary expenses or other administrative costs. The foundation does not support lobbying efforts or political action committees.
Geographic Focus: Arizona; Colorado; Florida; Georgia; Illinois; Indiana; Kansas; Kentucky; Louisiana; Michigan; Ohio; Tennessee; Texas; Utah; Wisconsin
Samples: Odyssey House, Louisiana, KY, $100,000--offers services and support systems through a behavioral healthcare facility with an emphasis on addiction treatment (2008); The Warrick Dunn Foundation, Tampa Bay, FL, $100,000—provides opportunities for economically disadvantaged single parents and children who have demonstrated a commitment to achieve financial independence and stability (2008).
Date(s) Application is Due: Jan 15; Jun 15
Contact: Foundation Office, (502) 580-4140; fax: (502) 580-1256; email: HumanaFoundation@humana.com
Internet: http://www.humanafoundation.org/philanthropy/
Sponsor: Humana Foundation
500 West Main Street, Suite 208
Louisville, KY 40202

Humboldt Area Foundation Technical Assistance Program (TAP) Grants **1819**
TAP is a small award program which provides nonprofits with one-on-one technical assistance in a variety of forms: consultants, training workshops, self-pace manuals, software, or any other form identified by applicants. TAP awards typically range from $500 to $2,000. Funds must be used to improve the organization, its leadership or operations, as a whole; not on programs or projects of the agency. Areas of assistance may include: strategic planning, financial management, operational assessments, board development, program assessments, personnel issues, collaborations, and fundraising. TAP applications and information are confidential and will not affect other potential Humboldt Area Foundation grant funding. TAP grant applications are accepted on the first of each month and grants that are awarded are paid directly to a consultant to cover the costs of their consulting services.
Restrictions: TAP will not pay for grant writing, programmatic development or for duties that are typically handled by staff (e.g. data entry). Organizations less than a year old and government entities are not eligible for TAP funds.
Geographic Focus: California
Amount of Grant: $500-$2,000
Date(s) Application is Due: Jan 1; Feb 1; Mar 1; Apr 1; May 1; Jun 1; Jul 1; Aug 1; Sep 1; Oct 1; Nov 1; Dec 1
Contact: Peter Pennekamp, Executive Director; (707) 442-2993, ext. 304; fax: (707) 442-3811; email: peterp@hafoundation.org
Internet: http://www.hafoundation.org/index.php?option=content&task=view&id=74
Sponsor: Humboldt Area Foundation
373 Indianola Road
Bayside, CA 95524

Hunter's Hope Foundation Grants **1820**
Hunter's Hope funds projects directly related to Krabbe disease or other leukodystrophies. Eligible studies may investigate new treatment approaches, or study basic mechanisms related to these diseases. Areas of relevant research include, among others, gene therapy, myelin development, neurodegeneration and transplantation, developmental neurobiology, and molecular biology. Applications are accepted in three project categories: postdoctoral fellowships provide stipend support for individuals who are within five years of receiving their terminal degree (MD, DVM, PhD, or equivalent degree). Fellows will be working with senior investigators within their sponsoring institution. Fellowships are awarded for two years. Pilot studies are one-year projects designed to test new concepts or ideas and can serve as a source of preliminary data for future studies. Major research grants provide support to senior investigators conducting major research studies. Projects may be funded for one to three years. Applications are reviewed twice annually.
Amount of Grant: $100,000 maximum major research grants; $40,000-$60,000 postdoctoral fellowships; $30,000 maximum pilot studies
Date(s) Application is Due: Apr 15; Sep 15
Contact: Executive Director, (877) 984-4673 or (716) 667-1200; fax: (716) 667-1212; email: info@huntershope.org
Internet: http://www.huntershope.org/research/default.asp
Sponsor: Hunter's Hope Foundation
P.O. Box 643
Orchard Park, NY 14127

Huntington Beach Police Officers Foundation Grants **1821**
The Foundation provides funds to various schools and community youth activities, benefits to spouses or children of police officers killed in the line of duty, and medical assistance to children of police officers in need of help. Giving is limited to Huntington Beach, California. There are no specific grant application forms or deadlines with which to adhere. Applicants should contact the Foundation office directly.
Requirements: Support is given only to groups situated in the Huntington Beach, California, region.
Geographic Focus: California
Contact: Kreg Muller, President; (714) 842-8851; fax: (714) 847-0064; email: hbpof@hbpoa.org
Internet: http://www.hbpoa.org/foundation/hbpof.htm
Sponsor: Huntington Beach Police Officers Foundation
20422 Beach Boulevard, Suite 450
Huntington Beach, CA 92648-8301

Huntington Clinical Foundation Grants **1822**
The Foundation, established in 1986, supports health care programs and access, higher education, and medical research. Grant amounts range from approximately $4,000 to $8,000, with some larger amounts available. There are no specific applications or deadlines with which to adhere. The Board meets quarterly, and applicants should forward a detailed description of the project and amount of funding requested.
Requirements: Giving is limited to the Huntington, West Virginia, region.
Geographic Focus: West Virginia
Samples: Hospice of Huntington, Huntington, West Virginia, $5,000—for construction of a new hospice facility (2006); Joan C. Edwards School of Medicine, Huntington, West Virginia, $9,000—for purchase of a video imaging system (2006).
Amount of Grant: $4,000-$8,000 range
Contact: Dr. J. David Daniels, President; (304) 529-4217; fax: (304) 523-6051
Sponsor: Huntington Clinical Foundation
P.O. Box 117
Huntington, WV 25706-0117

Huntington County Community Foundation Grants **1823**
The Foundation funds charitable projects that will make a positive impact on Huntington County and its people. The Foundation is particularly interested in ideas that shed new light on local needs and provide innovative, long term solutions. Grant areas to be considered include, but are not limited to: arts and culture; education; recreation; health and human services; environment and nature; civic affairs; safety; community development; and capital funding and/or start up expenses, preferably matching or last dollar funding.
Requirements: The applicant must be a charitable or not for profit entity exempt from taxation. The proposed grant must qualify for tax exempt funding under federal law. All Information in a grant application is public.
Restrictions: Grants will not be awarded to fund: operational or ongoing recurring (within 60 months) cost of the program; political projects or campaigns; or projects of applicants, or project owners, with taxing authority (e.g. school corporations; units of government).
Geographic Focus: Indiana
Samples: Andrews Elementary School, Andrews, Indiana, $19,072—to fund one half of 2nd through 5th grade playground (2008); Huntington College Foundation, Huntington, Indiana, $18,000—for scholarships for Huntington County residents (2008).
Amount of Grant: $20,000 maximum
Date(s) Application is Due: Apr 21; Oct 20
Contact: Marcia McClelland, Executive Director; (260) 356-8878; fax: (260) 356-0921; email: hccf@onlyinternet.net
Internet: http://www.hccfoundation.com/grants.htm
Sponsor: Huntington County Community Foundation
356 West Park Drive, P.O. Box 5037
Huntington, IN 46750

Huntington National Bank Community Affairs Grants **1824**
The corporation supports a variety of community focused initiatives that benefit children, education, economic development, health, social service housing, and the arts in each community of its banking offices. A letter of request (one to two pages) can serve as an

initial application for both single- and multi-year contributions. The letter should include a brief statement about the organization, its history, objectives, and goals; purpose of the project; visibility for Huntington as a participant in the project; list of officers and directors; target population(s) to be served by contribution; and annual organization budget, total project budget, amount requested, list of other contributors, and amounts of funds anticipated or committed.
Requirements: Tax-exempt organizations in Ohio, Kentucky, Indiana, Michigan, and West Virginia may apply.
Restrictions: Community donations may not be used for political campaigns involving individuals or issues; religious, ethnic, military, fraternal, or labor groups; individuals; organizations outside of the corporate market area; or organizations without IRS 501(c)3 tax-exempt status.
Geographic Focus: Indiana; Kentucky; Michigan; Ohio; West Virginia
Amount of Grant: $1,000-$10,000 average
Contact: Elfi Di Bella, Community Affairs Director; (614) 480-4483; fax: (614) 480-4973; email: elfi.dibella@huntington.com
Internet: http://www.huntington.com/us/HNB3150.htm
Sponsor: Huntington Bancshares Inc
41 South High Street, Huntington Center 3413
Columbus, OH 43215

Huntington's Disease Society of America Research Fellowships **1825**
Fellowships are designed to assist promising young postdoctoral investigators in the early stages of their careers who are engaged in research at the basic and clinical levels relating to the cause and treatment of Huntington's disease. The amount of the award will depend upon the policy of the sponsoring accredited medical school or university and the training and experience of the applicant. Fellowships are awarded for one year with the possibility of renewal. Application forms and requested information on curriculum vita, publications, research proposal, sponsorship, and other sources of funding are provided by the society.
Requirements: All applicants must have an MD or PhD degree or the equivalent and work must in some way be related to Huntington's disease. There is no citizenship requirement.
Amount of Grant: $80,000 maximum over two years
Contact: Robert Graze, Grants Administrator; (212) 242-1968 or (800) 345-4372, ext. 227; email: rgraze@hdsa.org
Internet: http://www.hdsa.org/research/grant-applications.html
Sponsor: Huntington's Disease Society of America
505 Eighth Avenue, Suite 902
New York, NY 10018

Huntington's Disease Society of America Research Grants **1826**
The Society awards research grants for one year for support of basic or clinical research related to Huntington's disease. Grant awards are provided as seed monies for new or innovative research projects in the hope that they will develop sufficiently to attract funding from other sources. Application forms are provided by the society and generally follow the format of NIH grant applications.
Requirements: Applicants may be doctorate or graduate students or equivalent professionals. There is no citizenship requirement.
Samples: Dr. Robert Ferante, Bedford VA Medical Ctr (Bedford, MA)—for research on mechanisms of neurodegeneration in Huntington's Disease, $35,000.; Dr. James Bibb, Rockefeller U (New York, NY)—for research on phosphohuntington, $35,000.
Amount of Grant: $100,000 maximum over two years
Contact: Robert Graze, Grants Administrator; (212) 242-1968 or (800) 345-4372, ext. 227; email: rgraze@hdsa.org
Internet: http://www.hdsa.org/research/grant-applications.html
Sponsor: Huntington's Disease Society of America
505 Eighth Avenue, Suite 902
New York, NY 10018

Hut Foundation Grants **1827**
Since 1998, the Hut Foundation has been funding nonprofits primarily in the states of California and Virginia, in the following areas of interest: arts; children/youth services; community/economic development; education; health care; youth development. Unsolicited requests for funds are not accepted, therefore initial contact should be through a Letter of Inquiry. If the proposal follows the Foundations guidelines, the applicant will be invited to submit an application.
Requirements: Must be a 501(c)3 nonprofit.
Restrictions: No grants to individuals.
Geographic Focus: California; Virginia
Amount of Grant: $5000-$10,000
Contact: Marcus Guerrero, Foundation Representative; (415) 834-2464; email: hutfoundation@gmail.com
Sponsor: Hut Foundation
19 Sutter Street
San Francisco, CA 94104

Hutton Foundation Grants **1828**
The foundation awards grants throughout Santa Barbara County, California to nonprofit organizations in its areas of interest, including education, arts and culture, health and human services, and civic and community development. Preference is given to efforts that promise to bring about major change, build leadership and institutional capacity, and achieve lasting results. Types of support include standard, program related investments, marketing, media, and endowment grants. An application form is available online.
Requirements: California nonprofit organizations headquartered in Santa Barbara county are eligible to apply.
Restrictions: Funding is not available to individuals or organizations that discriminate on the basis of age, gender, race, ethnicity, sexual orientation, disability, national origin, political affiliation or religious belief.
Geographic Focus: California
Contact: Arlene R. Craig, Vice President; (805) 957-4740; fax: (805) 957-4743; email: info@huttonfoundation.org
Internet: Arlene R. Craig, Vice President;
Sponsor: Hutton Foundation
26 West Anapamu Street, 4th Floor
Santa Barbara, CA 93101

i2 Foundation Grants **1829**
The foundation promotes advancements in education, technology, environmental practices, medicine, and economic opportunity through programs improving the quality of life and creating a better society. Although the foundation's main priority is the development and education of youth, proposals related to a wide array of issues are accepted, including illiteracy, youth violence, early childhood development, poverty, improved healthcare, and scientific research. All future grant cycles are currently postponed and new proposals are not being accepted.
Requirements: Nonprofit organizations closely aligned with the foundation's goals are eligible.
Restrictions: Individuals, religious institutions, political organizations, and government entities are ineligible.
Samples: Ctr for Nonprofit Management—to launch the center's Nonprofit Technology program in Texas.; CARE—for its Horn of Africa Emergency Relief Program in Kenya.; Orphan Foundation of America—to fund 15 to 20 postsecondary education scholarships for orphans and foster youth in the United States.; Project Hope—to help expand the maternal and child health programs in Haiti, Dominican Republic, Guatemala, Nicaragua, Peru, Malawi, and Uzbekistan.
Amount of Grant: $5000-$50,000
Contact: Grants Administrator, (469) 357-4200; fax: (469) 357-7777; email: Melis_Jones@i2.com
Internet: http://www.i2.com/company/i2foundation/index.cfm
Sponsor: i2 Foundation
One i2 Pl, 11701 Luna Road
Dallas, TX 75234

IAFF Burn Foundation Research Grants **1830**
The IAFF Burn Foundation Research Grant Program continues to lead to new knowledge and innovative approaches to the prevention and treatment of the physical and psychological problems that impair the quality of life for a burn patient. Research grant proposals are accepted annually and awards are distributed during the American Burn Association Annual Meeting. Topics of interest include by are not limited to pain management, physical and psychological rehabilitation, and wound healing and scarring, especially in children. Clinical projects are recommended. The foundation's Board of Medical Advisors oversees the selection process, reviewing each of the submissions. While all of candidates are deserving, only seven to ten grants are chosen and submitted to the IAFF Burn Foundation for consideration. Typically, five to seven are funded.
Requirements: The foundation welcomes research grant applications from members of the American Burn Association. The areas of funded research fall into three categories: (1) Quality of Life - This area of research is the most common, focusing on issues such as pain management, nutrition, and physical and psychological rehabilitation. The major focus in this area is the care of burned children. (2) Burn Prevention - Research in this area is especially important in shaping prevention programs. (3) Basic Science - Research grants funded in this category surround nutrition, wound healing and scar formation. No animal studies are funded. The required application and detailed guidelines can be found at the sponsor's website.
Restrictions: No animal studies are funded. The grant does not include indirect costs.
Geographic Focus: Alabama; Alaska; Arizona; Arkansas; California; Colorado; Connecticut; Delaware; District of Columbia; Florida; Georgia; Hawaii; Idaho; Illinois; Indiana; Iowa; Kansas; Kentucky; Louisiana; Maine; Maryland; Massachusetts; Michigan; Minnesota; Mississippi; Missouri; Montana; Nebraska; Nevada; New Hampshire; New Jersey; New Mexico; New York; North Carolina; North Dakota; Ohio; Oklahoma; Oregon; Pennsylvania; Rhode Island; South Carolina; South Dakota; Tennessee; Texas; Utah; Vermont; Virginia; Washington; West Virginia; Wisconsin; WyomingCanada
Amount of Grant: $25,000
Contact: Patrick Morrison, Director, IAFF Burn Foundation; (202) 824-8620; fax: (202) 637-0839; email: burnfoundation@iaff.org
Internet: http://burn.iaff.org/grants.shtml
Sponsor: International Association of Fire Fighters (IAFF)
1750 New York Avenue, NW
Washington, DC 20006

IARC Expertise Transfer Fellowship **1831**
The Fellowship is intended to enable an established investigator to spend normally from six to twelve months in an appropriate host institute in a low- to medium-resource country in order to transfer knowledge and expertise in a research area relevant for the host country and related to epidemiology, biostatistics, environmental chemical

carcinogenesis, cancer etiology and prevention, infection and cancer, molecular cell biology, molecular genetics, molecular pathology and mechanisms of carcinogenesis. Applications should include a proposed collaborative research project, specifying the link to IARC's on-going activities and a letter of support from the host lab giving details of feasibility and anticipated benefit to the receiving institute. Priority will be given to projects directly linked to IARC's on-going research program, involving at least one contact at IARC. There will be an annual remuneration of up to $70,000, which will take into account the on-going salary of the Fellow. This amount may include limited support for the project. The cost of travel will also be met.
Requirements: Applicants should be established cancer researchers actively engaged in the field with appropriate scientific or medical qualifications and an excellent publications' record. They must also belong to the staff of a university or a research institution.
Amount of Grant: $70,000 maximum
Date(s) Application is Due: Nov 30
Contact: Dr. Paolo Boffetta; +33-(0)472-73-84-48; fax: +33 (0)472-73-80-80; email: fel@iarc.fr or vsa@iarc.fr
Internet: http://www.iarc.fr/en/education-training/expertisetransfer.php
Sponsor: International Agency for Research on Cancer
150 cours Albert-Thomas
Lyon Cedex 08 69372 France

IARC Postdoctoral Fellowships for Training in Cancer Research 1832
Applications for training fellowships are invited from junior scientists from low- or medium-resource countries wishing to complete their training in those aspects of cancer research related to coordinate and conduct both epidemiological and laboratory research into the causes of cancer. Disciplines covered include: epidemiology, biostatistics, environmental chemical carcinogenesis, cancer etiology and prevention, infection and cancer, molecular cell biology, molecular genetics, molecular pathology and mechanisms of carcinogenesis, with emphasis on interdisciplinary projects. The fellowship is for a period of one year, with the possibility of an extension for a second year subject to satisfactory appraisal.
Requirements: Candidates should have spent less than five years abroad (including doctoral studies) and have finished their doctoral degree within five years of the closing date for application or be in the final phase of completing their doctoral degree (M.D. or Ph.D.). They must provide evidence of their ability to return to their home country and keep working in cancer research. The working languages at IARC are English and French. Candidates must be proficient in English at a level sufficient for scientific communication.
Restrictions: Candidates already working as a postdoctoral fellow at the Agency at the time of application or who have had any contractual relationship with IARC during the 6 months preceding the application deadline or who have already spent more than one year at IARC cannot be considered.
Amount of Grant: 32,000 Euros
Date(s) Application is Due: Nov 30
Contact: Dr. Paolo Boffetta; +33-(0)472-73-84-48; fax: +33-(0)472-73-80-80; email: fel@iarc.fr
Internet: http://www.iarc.fr/en/education-training/postdoc.php
Sponsor: International Agency for Research on Cancer
150 cours Albert-Thomas
Lyon Cedex 08 69372 France

IARC Visiting Scientist Award for Senior Scientists 1833
The IARC is offering this Award for a qualified and experienced investigator with recent publications in international peer-reviewed scientific journals who wishes to spend from six to twelve months at the IARC working on a collaborative project in a research area related to the Agency's programs: epidemiology, biostatistics, environmental chemical carcinogenesis, cancer etiology and prevention, infection and cancer, molecular cell biology, molecular genetics, molecular pathology and mechanisms of carcinogenesis. There will be an annual remuneration of up to $80,000, which will take into account the on-going salary of the visiting scientist plus the cost of travel.
Requirements: Applicants must belong to the staff of a university or a research institution and should provide written assurance of a post to return to at the end of the period of award.
Amount of Grant: $80,000 maximum
Date(s) Application is Due: Nov 30
Contact: Dr. Paolo Boffetta; +33-(0)472-73-84-48; fax: +33-(0)472-73-80-80; email: vsa@iarc.fr
Internet: http://www.iarc.fr/en/education-training/vsa.php
Sponsor: International Agency for Research on Cancer
150 cours Albert-Thomas
Lyon Cedex 08 69372 France

IATA Research Grants 1834
In order to enhance the National Athletic Trainer's Association's (NATA) Research and Education Foundation, the Illinois Athletic Trainers' Association has provided limited funding for athletic training related research in the state of Illinois. Grant monies from the IATA are awarded for projects concerning research in the domains relevant to athletic training within the state of Illinois. Grant applications will be reviewed and monies will be awarded during the Spring and Fall IATA BOD meetings.
Requirements: Applicants must be Certified/Licensed, members in good standing not only with the NATA but also the IATA. Applications must be submitted 3 months prior to the beginning of the research study, and the research must be relevant to the profession of athletic training within the state of Illinois. All applications will be analyzed bi-annually and as stated above must be submitted prior to the beginning of the project. Please note that there is limited funding for these awards, and you may be turned down due to lack of funding.
Restrictions: There will be no awards granted for recovery of cost involved with research that has already been initiated.
Geographic Focus: Illinois
Contact: Contact your Regional Representative
Internet: http://www.illinoisathletictrainers.org/Researchgrts.htm
Sponsor: Illinois Athletic Trainers' Association (IATA)
Wheaton North High School, 701 Thomas Road
Wheaton, IL 60187

IATA Scholarships 1835
Two scholarships of $1,000, three scholarships of $500, and two scholarships of $250 are available from the Illinois Athletic Trainers' Association (IATA). They are available on an annual basis but do not have to be awarded annually, depending on the applicant's qualifications. Scholarships will be awarded by the Vice-President at the IATA State Meeting Awards Luncheon. Certificates will be awarded to the scholarship recipient and their sponsoring Athletic Trainer, or in the case of the offspring scholarship, the parental member of the IATA.
Requirements: All applicants must have a grade point average of 'B,' or its equivalent, or above. All undergraduate and graduate applicants must be a member of the IATA. Applicants for the continuing education scholarship must be a licensed member of the IATA for one year prior to application. The offspring applicant does not need to be a member. Application forms are available from the IATA Vice President. Application requests must be written and will be included in the applicant's application packet. Recipients will be selected based on academic achievement, letters of recommendation and the applicant's autobiographical sketch.
Restrictions: If a committee member is a scholarship applicant, he/she will recuse from the evaluation process. The President-elect or Past-president will gather the committee evaluations.
Geographic Focus: Illinois
Amount of Grant: $250 - $1,000
Date(s) Application is Due: Aug 1
Contact: Mike Overturf, ATC, IATA Vice-President; (630) 575-6212; fax: (630) 575-7412; email: moverturf@athletico.com
Internet: http://www.illinoisathletictrainers.org/Scholarinfo.htm
Sponsor: Illinois Athletic Trainers' Association (IATA)
Wheaton North High School, 701 Thomas Road
Wheaton, IL 60187

Ida Alice Ryan Charitable Trust Grants 1836
The trust awards single-year grants for capital projects to eligible Georgia nonprofit organizations. Grants support programs of the Catholic Church and a wide variety of community causes including health organizations, legal aid societies, youth groups, educational programs, museums, and social services. Application and guidelines are available online.
Requirements: 501(c)3 tax-exempt organizations in the Atlanta area are eligible.
Geographic Focus: Georgia
Samples: Agnes Scott College (GA)—$25,000 (2003); Georgia Assoc for Pastoral Care (GA)—$10,000 (2003); Make-A-Wish Foundation (GA)—$5000 (2003).
Date(s) Application is Due: Feb 1; Aug 1
Contact: Alice Sheets, c/o Wachovia Bank; email: grantinquiriesga@wachovia.com
Internet: http://www.wachovia.com/corp_inst/charitable_services/0,,4269_3301,00.html
Sponsor: Ida Alice Ryan Charitable Trust
3414 Peachtree Road, 5th Floor, MC GA8023
Atlanta, GA 30326

Idaho Community Foundation Eastern Region Competitive Grants 1837
The mission of the Foundation is to enrich life's quality throughout Idaho. Grants are awarded through the regional grant cycle for a wide range of organizations and for a wide range of projects consistent with that mission. Grants are made to fund activities, services, and projects of established organizations, as well as to provide assistance for new organizations to fill unmet and/or emerging community needs. Grant areas include: arts and culture; education; emergency services; libraries; natural sciences; health; recreation; social services; and public projects. Application information is available online.
Requirements: Nonprofit entities in Idaho are eligible to apply.
Restrictions: Funding is not available for: projects which replace school district responsibilities to students or that fund state or federally mandated programs; projects which are considered operating expenses or salaries normally paid by a school district; computer hardware used solely for pre-K through 12th grade educational purposes; religious organizations for the sole purpose of furthering that religion; political activities or those designed to influence legislation; national organizations; or grants that directly benefit a donor to ICF or a donor's family.
Geographic Focus: Idaho
Amount of Grant: $5,000
Date(s) Application is Due: Apr 1
Contact: Grants Administrator, (208) 342-3535; fax: (208) 342-3577; email: grants@idcomfdn.org
Internet: http://www.idcomfdn.org/pages/grant_regional_guidelines.htm
Sponsor: Idaho Community Foundation
P.O. Box 8143
Boise, ID 83707

Idaho Power Company Corporate Contributions 1838

The company awards grants in company operating territories in its areas of interest, including arts and culture, civic and community, education, and health and human services. Types of support include building construction/renovation, capital campaigns, continuing support, equipment, general operating support, matching gifts, scholarships, and sponsorships. The corporate contribution request form is available online. There are no application deadlines.
Requirements: Nonprofit organizations in southern Idaho and eastern Oregon are eligible.
Restrictions: Grants do not support: individuals; loans or investments; churches or religious organizations for purposes of religious advocacy; tickets for contests, raffles, or other prize-oriented activities; organizations that discriminate for any reason, including race, color, religion, creed, age, sex, or national origin; individual school programs or projects with limited participation; fraternal or labor organizations; unrestricted operating funds; special occasion good-will advertising.
Geographic Focus: Idaho; Oregon
Contact: Corporate Contributions, (208) 388-2200
Internet: http://www.idahopower.com/aboutus/community/corporateContributions.htm
Sponsor: Idaho Power Company
P.O. Box 70
Boise, ID 83707

Ignacio Martin-Baro Fund for Mental Health and Human Rights Grants 1839

The organization supports children's programs in health and mental health and is a resource for advocacy, education, prevention, service, and action research. The fund has a strong preference for projects that are developing innovative and progressive ways to deal with the mental health consequences of violence and political repression. Applicants should understand that the foundation does not view mental health and human rights as issues that can be addressed separately, but are seeking to fund activities that explore the links between them. Groups with budgets under $25,000 receive priority consideration. The listed application deadline applies to letters of interest; full proposals are by invitation.
Amount of Grant: $7000 maximum
Date(s) Application is Due: Sep 1
Contact: Grants Administrator, (617) 469-7454; fax: (617) 469-3379; email: apply@martinbarofund.org
Internet: http://www.martinbarofund.org/contact/applying.htm
Sponsor: Ignacio Mart'n-Bar' Fund for Mental Health and Human Rights
P.O. Box 2122
Jamaica Plain, MA 02130

IHS Native American and Alaskan Native Health Research Centers 1840

The purpose of this program is to establish centers that would encourage research on diseases that affect Native American populations and other health issues of importance to tribes and tribal organizations. Funds may be used to reduce health disparities that affect Native Americans and Alaskan Natives, train scientists and health professionals, help encouraging partnerships among health organizations, and for health research. A letter of intent is requested by October 1; full application is due by December 12. Annual deadline dates may vary; contact program staff for exact dates. RFA: GM-00-007
Requirements: Federally recognized tribes, tribal consortia, and nonprofit Indian health organizations are eligible to apply.
Amount of Grant: $27,000-$300,000; $115,000 average
Date(s) Application is Due: Oct 1; Dec 12
Contact: Lois Hodge, Grants Management Officer, (301) 443-5204
Internet: http://www.ihs.gov
Sponsor: Indian Health Service
12300 Twinbrook Plz
Rockville, MD 29852

Ildaura Murillo-Rohde Scholarships 1841

The association awards these scholarships for tuition to outstanding Hispanic associate, diploma, baccalaureate, or graduate students. Recipients will be selected on the basis of potential to graduate, current academic standing in an accredited school of nursing (minimum 3.0 GPA), potential for contribution to the profession, and financial need. The amount awarded each year depends on the availability of funds.
Requirements: An applicant must be currently enrolled in an accredited school of nursing and be a U.S. citizen or legal resident of the United States, Puerto Rico, or the U.S. territories. Applicant must be a member of the association.
Date(s) Application is Due: Apr 30
Contact: Scholarships, (202) 387-2477; fax: (202) 483-7183; email: info@thehispanicnurses.org
Internet: http://www.thehispanicnurses.org
Sponsor: National Association of Hispanic Nurses
1501 16th St NW
Washington, DC 20036

Illinois Children's Healthcare Foundation Grants 1842

The foundation's mission is to improve the health of Illinois children. The foundation focuses its giving on four areas: improving the oral health of underserved children; increasing the incidence of developmental screening in young children and subsequent referrals for treatment; providing Illinois children access to high-quality healthcare services; and, supporting the social/emotional development of children. The listed application deadline is for letters of intent; full proposals are by invitation. Guidelines and RFP are available online.
Requirements: Any 501(c)3 organization determined to be a public charity under section 509(a)1, 2, or 3 of the IRS code or government entity described in section 170(c)1 or 511(a)2(B) is eligible. Proposed activities must serve Illinois children.
Amount of Grant: $50,000-$500,000 range
Date(s) Application is Due: Apr 18
Contact: Susan Kerr, President, (630) 655-2873; fax: (630) 655-4725; email: susankerr@ilchf.org
Internet: http://www.ilchf.org/HOME.asp
Sponsor: Illinois Children's Healthcare Foundation
15 Spinning Wheel Road, Suite 228
Hinsdale, IL 60521

Impact 100 Grants 1843

Impact 100 empowers women to dramatically improve lives by collectively funding significant grants that make a lasting impact in the Greater Cincinnati and Northern Kentucky community. During the first few two months of the year, non-profit organizations in the ten-county Greater Cincinnati/Northern Kentucky area region are encouraged to submit grant applications to Impact 100. The Grant Review Committees of Impact 100 review the applications and conduct site visits to narrow their choices. At the end of the review process, a finalist is chosen by each of the five committees (Education, Health & Wellness, Environment/Preservation & Recreation, Culture and Family). These five finalists present their grant requests at the Annual Awards Celebration. After the finalist presentations, each member casts a vote (or has sent an absentee vote in advance). The votes are immediately tabulated, and the Impact 100 grants are awarded at the end of the evening.
Requirements: Applications that are programmatic, endowment, capital, start-up, or research-oriented are excepted. Applications from non-profit organizations headquartered in any of the following counties are available to apply: Ohio - Adams, Brown, Butler, Clermont, Hamilton, Warren; Kentucky - Boone, Campbell, Kenton; Indiana - Dearborn. Every applying agency must have 501(c)3 status with the IRS.
Restrictions: The following types of applications are not available for funding: operating; partisan; individual churches; indigent care subsidy; travel; loans; or for individuals.
Geographic Focus: Indiana; Kentucky; Ohio
Amount of Grant: $100,000
Date(s) Application is Due: Mar 1
Contact: Luann Scherer, Grant Review Coordinaor; (513) 624-9509; email: Grants@Impact100.org
Internet: http://impact100.org/Grant/Default.aspx
Sponsor: Impact 100, Inc
PMB314 2692 Madison Road NI
Cincinnati, OH 45208-1320

Implant Dentistry Research and Education Foundation Grants 1844

The objective of the grant is to encourage new investigators by providing seed or start-up funding for promising research projects. Grants support basic research and education relating to dental implants. Areas include, but are not limited to, biology, biochemistry, biomechanics, biomaterials, and molecular biology. Grants are awarded after thorough review by an independent scientific advisory board. Grant applications are available upon request.
Requirements: The principal investigator or coprincipal investigator must hold an appropriate terminal degree. A dental resident or PhD candidate may apply if the appropriate department or division chair provides a letter confirming he/she is coming on staff the year a project is funded.
Amount of Grant: $20,000-$25,000
Date(s) Application is Due: Jan 1
Contact: Craig Johnson, Executive Director, IDREF, (800) 442-0525 or (973) 783-6300; fax: (973) 783-1175; email: icoi@dentalimplants.com
Internet: http://www.dentalimplants.com
Sponsor: Implant Dentistry Research and Education Foundation
248 Lorraine Avenue, #3
Upper Montclair, NJ 07043-1454

Inasmuch Foundation Grants 1845

The foundation was established for charitable, scientific, and educational projects primarily in Oklahoma; however, select projects in Colorado Springs, CO, also are supported. The foundation consistently provides funding and support to educational, health and human service, cultural, artistic, historical, and environmental concerns. This funding is not available to individuals, but is available to formal organizations seeking capital and support for existing programs that meet the emerging needs of the community. In order to initiate a proposal, submit a one-page letter of inquiry by the listed application deadlines. Application information is available online.
Restrictions: The foundation generally does not fund endowments or scholarships.
Geographic Focus: Colorado; Oklahoma
Samples: Colorado College (Colorado Springs, CO)—to construct a facility for arts education and performances, $4 million (2004).
Date(s) Application is Due: Feb 15; Aug 15
Contact: Program Contact, (405) 604-5292
Internet: http://www.inasmuchfoundation.org/application.html
Sponsor: Inasmuch Foundation
210 Park Avenue, Suite 3150
Oklahoma City, OK 73102

Independence Blue Cross Charitable Medical Care Grants 1846

The Independence Blue Cross (IBC) Charitable Medical Care Grant Program awards financial and programmatic grant support to nonprofit, privately funded health clinics that provide free or nominal-fee care to the uninsured and medically underserved communities in Bucks, Chester, Delaware, Montgomery, and Philadelphia counties. See website for grant application.

Requirements: To be eligible for a grant through this program, an applicant must meet the following criteria: the mission of the requesting organization aligns with IBC's Social Mission and its funding priorities; the requesting clinic is a privately funded entity. (Note: A clinic may receive federal funding as part of its revenues.); clinic grantee provides direct medical care for free or for a nominal fee to uninsured and/or underinsured residents of southeastern Pennsylvania; all grantees must be located in Bucks, Chester, Delaware, Montgomery, or Philadelphia counties; organizations must be classified as tax-exempt nonprofit under Section 501(c)3 of the IRS code.

Restrictions: Funding is unavailable to: individuals; private foundations; fund-raising events; conferences or seminars; political causes, candidates, organizations, or campaigns; sports teams; endowments; social organizations; religious groups for religious purposes; organizations that do not meet IBC's Social Mission.

Geographic Focus: Pennsylvania

Amount of Grant: $10,000 - $100,000 range

Contact: Courtney Smith, Social Mission Program Analyst; (215) 241-4862; fax: (215) 241-3543; email: courtney.smith@ibx.com

Internet: http://www.ibx.com/social_mission/medical_grants/index.html

Sponsor: Independence Blue Cross
1901 Market Street, 28th floor
Philadelphia, PA 19103

Independence Blue Cross Nurse Scholars Program 1847

This program was created to address the severe threat posed by the current nursing shortage to the quality and cost of health care in southeastern Pennsylvania. The program provides financial assistance to aspiring nurse educators and undergraduate nursing students. It also includes summer internship programs for nursing students and funding for faculty positions at area nursing schools. Application information can be located at the Pennsylvania Higher Education Foundation Web site.

Geographic Focus: Pennsylvania

Samples: Nursing programs in southeastern Pennsylvania (PA)—to establish a scholarship program for graduate students pursuing careers as nursing instructors, $1.74 million over three years (2004); Pennsylvania Higher Education Fdn (Harrisburg, PA)—for a scholarship program for undergraduate nursing students, $750,000 (2004).

Contact: Nurse Scholars Program, (800) 377-4502

Internet: http://www.ibx.com/social_mission/nurse_scholars/index.html

Sponsor: Independence Blue Cross
1901 Market Street
Philadelphia, PA 19103-1480

Independence Blue Cross Nursing Internships 1848

The Independence Blue Cross (IBC) Nursing Internship Program is an integral part of IBC's Nurse Scholars Program and supports the IBC Social Mission commitment to address the nursing shortage and overall health care crisis in the southeastern Pennsylvania region. The IBC Nursing Internship Program is open to undergraduate nursing students who have completed at least one clinical rotation and who attend one of the 31 accredited nursing programs (see website for a complete listing of the participating nursing programs) supported by the IBC Nurse Scholars Program. Two unique student nursing internship opportunities are offered through this program. One is for nursing students who would like to gain experience at IBC in a health care/insurance administration setting; the other is for nursing students interested in exploring the field of public health by interning on site at a community health center clinic.

Requirements: Each program is open to undergraduate nursing students who have completed at least one clinical rotation and who attend an accredited nursing program in southeastern Pennsylvania supported by the IBC Nurse Scholars program. Applications are available on the IBC website. If you are selected to participate, you must be available for the entire ten week internship program beginning June 8 through August 14.

Geographic Focus: Pennsylvania

Date(s) Application is Due: Mar 31

Contact: Courtney Smith, Social Mission Program Analyst; (215) 241-4862; fax: (215) 241-3543; email: courtney.smith@ibx.com

Internet: http://www.ibx.com/social_mission/nurse_scholars/nursing_internship/index.html

Sponsor: Independence Blue Cross
1901 Market Street, 28th floor
Philadelphia, PA 19103

Independence Community Foundation Community Quality of Life Grant 1849

The Foundation makes grants to organizations that engage in community-based efforts that support important institutions or causes. Generally, the grants support: disease awareness and prevention; food pantries; neighborhood greening and graffiti removal; and counseling support for vulnerable populations. Interested applicants should submit an initial letter of inquiry. Application information is available online.

Requirements: Program or project grants are made on a competitive basis to nonprofit organizations located within New York City, Nassau, Suffolk and Westchester counties in New York, and Essex, Bergen, Union, Hudson, Middlesex, Ocean, and Monmouth counties in New Jersey.

Restrictions: The Foundation does not fund: individuals; political contributions; funding for religious purposes; purchase tickets for dinners, golf outings, or similar fundraising events.

Geographic Focus: New Jersey; New York

Date(s) Application is Due: Mar 30; Sep 30

Contact: Program Contact, (718) 722-2300; fax: (718) 722-5757; email: inquiries@icfny.org

Internet: http://www.icfny.org/comm_quality.html

Sponsor: Independence Community Foundation
182 Atlantic Avenue
Brooklyn, NY 11201

Indiana 21st Century Research and Technology Fund Awards 1850

The Indiana 21st Century Research and Technology Fund of the Indiana Economic Development Corporation (IEDC) is open to proposals from all public and private entities for technology-based commercialization activities encompassing science/technology creation, innovation, and transfer intended to have commercial impacts. The fund intends to increase the numbers, and rates of development, of new and expanding technology-based companies by funding promising opportunities that, in some cases, the financial markets might find too risky. The Fund makes awards in two broad categories: Science and Technology Commercialization and Centers of Excellence. In addition, the Fund provides cost-share on behalf of Federal proposals submitted by Indiana-based entities. Generally awards are made in multiples of $50,000 up to $2,000,000. Support for awards in excess of $2,000,000 will be rare.

Requirements: The IEDC defines a technology-based company as one that is involved in transferring advanced technology into products, developing technologies with the near-term intention of creating products, or using new or advanced technologies in its design, development, and/or manufacturing of products. The Fund emphasizes the creation of academic-sector - commercial-sector partnerships. In making awards, the Fund expects significant leverage from the partners involved in the projects. Important: before applying, contact Fund staff (email preferred) to discuss your interest in submitting a proposal and to discuss your technology and commercialization goals. While not a review criterion, the fund encourages the inclusion of interns from any academic institution, or participating commercial sector partner, in order to increase project-related involvement of students at all levels.

Restrictions: Only direct costs will be supported. Institutions will not be provided indirect (overhead) cost support. Entities with previous Fund awards that are not current with regard to financial or technical reporting requirements will be disqualified from making new submissions to the Fund. Resubmissions of previously declined proposals will be considered only if substantive changes have been made to the proposal. Fund staff will determine whether to review resubmissions.

Geographic Focus: Indiana

Samples: 2K Corporation: $400,000 - Commercialization of a Neutron Based Explosives Detection Device (Car Bomb Detection). Arxan Technologies, Inc.: $1,944,096 - Protecting Critical IP in the 21st Century: Advancing Anti-Tamper Technologies. BioVitesse Inc.: $1,300,000 - Rapid Detection and Identification of Live Bacteria. CIS LLC: $1,075,000 - Commercialization of Satellite Radio for Cell Phone Applications.

Amount of Grant: $500,000 - $2,000,000

Contact: Brooke Pyne, Director; (812) 384-3078; email: bpyne@iedc.in.gov;; Carla Phelps, Financial Manager; (317) 233- 4336; email: cphelps@21fund.org

Internet: http://www.21fund.org/

Sponsor: Indiana Economic Development Corporation
One North Capitol Avenue, Suite 900
Indianapolis, IN 46204

Indiana AIDS Fund Grants 1851

Two grant programs are available to Indiana organizations that provide HIV/AIDS advocacy, prevention and direct care services. The Direct Emergency Financial Assistance Fund gives grants to agencies and organizations specifically to help HIV/AIDS patients access emergency financial help for housing, transportation, food, and/or medical care. The Indiana AIDS Fund gives prevention grants in November each year to agencies and organizations that provide persons living with HIV/AIDS direct care services, health education and risk-reduction programs and counseling, testing, and referral programs. Proposal information is available online.

Requirements: Any Indiana-based non-profit 501(c)3 group, organization or agency that provides HIV/AIDS-related programs or services to local constituencies is eligible to apply for grants from the Indiana AIDS Fund. The applicant must function without discrimination or segregation because of race, gender, age, religion, national origin, sexual orientation, disability, military or marital status, in hiring, termination, assignment and promotion of staff, selection of board members or provision of service.

Restrictions: The fund will not make the following types of grants: to individuals; for sectarian religious purposes; to purchase advertising or tickets to events; to support research; for the purpose of deficit reduction; to produce currently available educational materials; to fund endowments; for short- or long-term loans; for multiple-year program funding; for mass media campaigns; for capacity building; or for services not directly related to primary or secondary prevention.

Geographic Focus: Indiana

Contact: Grants Administrator, (317) 630-1805; email: severett@thfgi.org

Internet: http://www.indianaaidsfund.org/index.cfm?navigationid=1844

Sponsor: Indiana AIDS Fund
429 East Vermont Street, Suite 300
Indianapolis, IN 46202

Indiana Minority Teacher/Special Services Scholarships 1852

The Minority Teacher Scholarship was created by the 1988 Indiana General Assembly to address the critical shortage of Black and Hispanic teachers in Indiana. In 1990 the Indiana General Assembly amended the Minority program to include the field of Special Education, and in 1991 the fields of Occupational and Physical Therapy were added. The maximum annual scholarship is $1,000. However, if a minority student applicant demonstrates financial need he/she may be eligible to receive up to $4,000 annually. Colleges will determine the actual amount when reviewing a scholar's financial aid package.

Requirements: To be eligible you must be: 1. A minority student (defined as Black or Hispanic) seeking a teaching certification; or a student seeking a Special Education teaching certification; or a student seeking an Occupational or Physical Therapy certification. 2. An Indiana resident and an U.S. Citizen. 3. Admitted to an eligible institution as a full time student or already attending as a full time student. 4. Pursuing or intend to pursue a course of study that would enable the student upon graduation to teach in an accredited elementary or secondary school in Indiana. 5. Complete and file the Free Application for Federal Student Aid (FAFSA). 6. Not be in default on a State or Federally-funded Student loan. 7. Meet all minimum criteria established by the Commission. In addition, students who are already enrolled in college, must have a Grade Point Average (GPA) of at least 2.0 on a scale of 4.0 or the equivalent, or meet the minimum GPA requirements established at the college for its school of education, if it is higher. Scholars must agree to: 1. Pursue a program which leads to either a teaching or Occupational or Physical Therapy Certification. 2. Complete the Teacher or Occupational or Physical Therapy certification program within six (6) years from the time the first scholarship is received. 3. Teach on a full time basis in an accredited Indiana elementary or secondary school; or, 4. Practice in the field of Occupational or Physical Therapy in an accredited school, vocational rehabilitation center, community mental retardation or other developmental disabilities center, for 3 years out of the first 5 years after certification. Colleges are responsible for making the actual awards. Financial need may be considered but it is not a requirement to apply. Preference will be given to minority students and students enrolling in college for the first time. Applications should be submitted to the Office of Financial Aid at the school where the applicant plans to attend.

Restrictions: Scholarships are non-transferable between universities. Those who fail to fulfill the terms of their scholarship agreements must reimburse the State of Indiana.

Geographic Focus: Indiana

Amount of Grant: up to $4,000

Contact: Ada Sparkman, External Operations Coordinator; (317) 232-2350; email: asparkman@ssaci.in.gov

Internet: http://www.in.gov/ssaci/2342.htm

Sponsor: State Student Assistance Commission of Indiana (SSACI)
150 W. Market Street, Suite 500
Indianapolis, IN 46204

Indiana Nursing Scholarships 1853

The Nursing Scholarship Fund was created by the 1990 Indiana General Assembly to encourage and promote qualified individuals to pursue a nursing career in Indiana. The scholarship can only be applied towards tuition and fees. Colleges will determine the actual award amount when developing a scholar's financial aid package. The maximum annual scholarship is $5,000. However, the amount of the scholarship may be affected by the level of other tuition specific grants and scholarships aid received by an applicant.

Requirements: To be eligible students must: 1) Be admitted to an approved institution of higher learning as a full time (12 hours or more) or part time (6-11 hours) nursing student; 2) Be an Indiana resident and an U.S. citizen; 3) Agree in writing to work as a nurse in an Indiana health care setting for at least the first two (2) years following graduation; 4) Demonstrate a financial need for the scholarship; 5) Have a minimum Grade Point Average (GPA) of at least 2.0 on a scale of 4.0 or the equivalent, or meet the minimum GPA requirements established for the college's nursing program if it is higher; 6) Not be in default on a state or federally sponsored student loan; 7) Complete and file the Free Application for Federal Student Aid (FAFSA); 8) Meet all other minimum criteria established by the Commission. In order to renew the scholarship, Scholars must: 1) Maintain the cumulative GPA required by the college for admission to its nursing program, or; 2) Maintain a GPA of at least 2.0 on a scale of 4.0 or the equivalent if there is no minimum at the college; and, 3) Reapply each year. Applications should be submitted to the Office of Financial Aid where the applicant plans to attend. Applications should not be submitted to SSACI. Colleges will make the award decisions. For a list of colleges and universities participating in the program, go to http://www.in.gov/ssaci/2368.htm.

Geographic Focus: Indiana

Amount of Grant: up to $5,000

Date(s) Application is Due: Mar 10

Contact: Ada Sparkman, External Operations Coordinator; (317) 232-2350; email: asparkman@ssaci.in.gov

Internet: http://www.in.gov/ssaci/2343.htm

Sponsor: State Student Assistance Commission of Indiana (SSACI)
150 W. Market Street, Suite 500
Indianapolis, IN 46204

Infinity Foundation Grants 1854

The foundation awards grants in a broad array of areas including charitable, scientific, religious, educational, and holistic healing activities by organizations and public agencies that work to better the lives of people. Grants also support individuals' research and development of educational materials to improve the authenticity of the portrayal of Indic traditions in the educational system. Proposed projects could result in one or more of the following: books, curriculum development, articles, conferences, CD-Roms, digital slide shows, Internet presentations, and audio/video materials. Topics covered may include philosophy, history, religion, science, art, and sociology, as they pertain to the educational curricula on Indic traditions. Proposals should be submitted by email.

Requirements: Grantee may be a scholar, teacher, visionary, or spiritual leader whose work in the designated topics would be enhanced by a foundation grant.

Contact: Rajiv Malhotra, Founder and President; (609) 683-0548; fax: (609) 683-0478; email: rm.infinity@gmail.com

Internet: http://www.infinityfoundation.com/callforgrantproposals.htm

Sponsor: Infinity Foundation
66 Witherspoon Street, Suite 400
Princeton, NJ 08542

Innovative Technology Development Award Program 1855

The center annually funds biotechnology research projects that promise development of commercializable technologies. In this way, the center aims to further establish and strengthen ties between academic scientists and industry. Grants are for one year, with a continuation seed grant offered for the second and third year if necessary. Proposals are evaluated based on the quality of the science, the commercial potential, and how the project might impact New York state economy. Applications are posted on the Web site or are available by fax or mail.

Requirements: Faculty at any New York state research institution may apply.

Geographic Focus: New York

Samples: Roswell Park Cancer Institute—for DNA damage kits, in collaboration with Zeptogen Corp, $78,000.; Dept of Pathology, SUNY (Brooklyn, NY)—for rational design and testing of new anticancer agents, $32,000.

Amount of Grant: $40,000-$80,000

Contact: Dr. Anil Dhundale, Director of Scientific Affairs, (516) 632-8521; fax: (516) 632-8577; email: anil.dhundale@sunysb.edu

Internet: http://www.biotech.sunysb.edu/techDev/ITD/index.html

Sponsor: Center for Biotechnology
Psychology A Building, 3rd Fl, SUNY Stony Brook
Stony Brook, NY 11794-5208

Institute for Agriculture and Trade Policy Food and Society Fellowships 1856

The IATP Food and Society Fellows Program provides fellowships to professionals in food and agriculture from across North America, enabling them to use mass media channels to inform and shape the public agenda. The goal of the program is to create sustainable food systems that promote good health, vibrant communities, environmental stewardship, worker justice and accessibility for all. Fellows come from many disciplines: chefs, farmers, nutritionists, activists, public health professionals, fishers, policy experts and academics. Together they form an interdisciplinary team that works to: use communication to influence the issues that reach the public agenda, thereby creating policy changes at the personal, organizational and public policy levels that advance sustainable food and farming systems; increase the mass media communications on issues around sustainable food and farming systems that produce healthy, green, fair and affordable foods; raise the profile of the fellows as food system experts among media and policymakers; and build capacity, leadership, and cohesiveness in a group of experts who collaborate and communicate using mass media channels to bring sustainable food system issues to the public agenda.

Requirements: Applicants should be U.S. residents actively involved in a professional career that involves two or more of the following: agriculture, health promotion, youth development, food production, and/or policy analysis.

Contact: Mark Muller, Director; (612) 870-3420; fax: (612) 870-4846; email: mmuller@iatp.org

Internet: http://www.foodandsocietyfellows.org/about/page/about-us

Sponsor: Institute for Agriculture and Trade Policy
2105 First Avenue South
Minneapolis, MN 55404

Institute of Human Values in Health Care Interdisciplinary Fellowships 1857

The program is designed to provide non-clinical professionals who work in health related fields (e.g., law, government, economics, sociology, philosophy, journalism, religion, and history) with first-hand exposure to and involvement with intensive inpatient and ambulatory care of the critically ill within a major academic medical center. The fellowship runs from January through May.

Requirements: Professionals who are active and established in their fields and can devote full time to the program for five months may submit fellowship applications. Postdoctoral candidates also will be considered.

Amount of Grant: $7500

Date(s) Application is Due: Sep 15

Contact: Dr. Robert Sade, (843) 792-5278; fax: (843) 792-8286; email: sader@musc.edu

Internet: http://www.values.musc.edu/news/if_announcement.htm

Sponsor: Medical University of South Carolina
P.O. Box 250612, 96 Jonathan Lucas Street, Suite 409
Charleston, SC 29425

International Cancer Technology Transfer Fellowships 1858

The fellowships are funded by a group of cancer institutes, leagues, societies, associations, foundations, and governmental agencies in North America, Europe, and Australia. The aims of the awards are threefold: to facilitate rapid international transfer of cancer research and clinical technology; exchange knowledge and enhance skills in basic,

clinical, behavioral, and epidemiological areas of cancer research and in cancer control and prevention; and acquire up-to-date clinical management, diagnostic, and therapeutic expertise. Applications are particularly encouraged for projects in the fields of cancer control and prevention, epidemiology and cancer registration, public education, and behavioral sciences. The short-term fellowships permit successful candidates to spend up to three months at a suitable host institute abroad. They are particularly aimed at investigators and clinicians working in places where such teaching is not yet available and where the necessary facilities exist to apply and disseminate the new skills upon return. Applications may be submitted at any time, and funding decisions are generally communicated to candidates within 60 days of receipt of a complete application.
Requirements: Qualified cancer investigators should be at the early stages in their careers; clinicians should be well established in their oncology practice. Experts from any country who have been invited to teach specialized skills abroad also may apply.
Amount of Grant: $3000 average
Contact: International Cancer Research Program, (4122) 809 18 40; fax: (41-22) 809 18 10; email: fellows@uicc.org
Internet: http://fellows.uicc.org/fell4icr.shtml
Sponsor: International Union against Cancer
3, rue de Conseil-General
Geneva 1205 Switzerland

International College of Surgeons Grants and Scholarships **1859**
The ICS makes grants and scholarships available to surgeons who wish to enhance their surgical skills through postgraduate training. Applicants are responsible for making their own arrangements for the program of study; must clearly indicate the place of study, with whom they will be studying, and acceptance by the institution and surgeon for the course of study as defined; and must indicate what it is they expect to achieve upon completion of the study program (e.g. learn a particular procedure, etc.). Guidelines are available online. No formal application form is required.
Requirements: Applicants must have graduated from an accredited medical school, completed their residency, and be licensed to practice surgery in their home country (documentation of licensure must be provided). Applicants need not be ICS fellows.
Contact: Max Downham, Executive Director, (312) 787-6274; fax: (312) 787-9289; email: max@icsglobal.org
Internet: http://www.icsglobal.org/RandS/index.asp
Sponsor: International College of Surgeons
1516 N Lake Shore Drive
Chicago, IL 60610-1694

International Essential Tremor Foundation Grants **1860**
The foundation awards grants for clinical or basic research specific to essential tremor. Data to be derived should lead to grant proposals to governmental or other sources of funds. Two grants are available in the current year. Under exceptional circumstances, funding may be allowed for a second year as a competing renewal. No more than one award can be given to an individual investigator per year. Funding begins in June or July.
Requirements: Grants are awarded to MDs and/or PhDs.
Amount of Grant: $20,000 per year
Contact: Catherine Rice, (888) 387-3667 or (913) 341-3880; fax: (913) 341-1296; email: crice@essentialtremor.org
Internet: http://www.essentialtremor.org/research/index.php
Sponsor: International Essential Tremor Foundation
P.O. Box 14005
Lenexa, KS 66285-4005

International Fellowships in Medical Education **1861**
The program provides opportunities for faculty from schools of medicine outside the United States to study aspects of medical education in the United States that have the potential to improve medical education in their home country institutions. Mentoring will be provided by preceptors in U.S. basic and clinical science departments, medical education departments, and health system institutions. Eligible study areas include educational methodology, curriculum design, evaluation systems, medical school governance, development of basic and clinical science departments, and the design and operation of health care and public health system programs linked to medical education. Fellows may concurrently pursue collaborative research interests with U.S. basic science faculty or observe some clinical activity with clinical faculty. Fellowship allowance generally includes a monthly stipend, round-trip economy-class air fare for the fellow, and travel to one scientific meeting in the United States. Programs may range from six months to one year. The interactive, web-based application is now available online; paper applications are no longer accepted.
Requirements: Candidates must reside and work in their home countries at the time of application; have a graduate or professional degree in medicine or in a basic medical science; have not less than three years of work experience in their chosen field in the home country; hold an academic appointment as a faculty member in a school of medicine; have the ability to communicate effectively in English; have the endorsement of a home country medical school or organization; and have a position to return to in the home country medical school or organization.
Restrictions: Fellowships are not provided for programs in basic or clinical research; degree-granting educational programs that require acceptance to an institution and tuition payments; tuition grants for short-term courses; specialty training in residency programs, or solely for training in clinical procedures.
Amount of Grant: $2400 monthly stipend
Contact: Grants Administrator, (215) 386-5900; fax: (215) 386-9196; email: info@ecfmg.org
Internet: http://www.ecfmg.org/about.html
Sponsor: Educational Commission for Foreign Medical Graduates
3624 Market Street
Philadelphia, PA 19104-2685

International Oncology Nursing Fellowships **1862**
The fellowships are funded by the Oncology Nursing Society and provide an opportunity for qualified nurses to augment their professional knowledge and experience through short-term observerships at a renowned comprehensive cancer center in Australia, North America, or the United Kingdom. A project description must provide full details of the particular cancer nursing skills that the candidate wishes to observe. It should elaborate on the treatment and nursing facilities at the home institute and how the newly acquired knowledge and techniques would be used and disseminated to other nursing staff upon return. Projects need the approval of the candidate's home and host supervisors. The maximum fellowship duration is three months; stipend support is for one month only. The program also contributes to the least expensive international two-way airfare or other appropriate form of transport. Financial support is not provided for dependents.
Requirements: English-speaking registered nurses who are actively engaged in the management of cancer patients in their home institutes and who come from developing or Eastern European countries are eligible, as are established oncology nurses from any country who wish to disseminate their skills in these regions.
Amount of Grant: $2800 average
Date(s) Application is Due: Nov 1
Contact: International Cancer Research Program, (41-22) 809 18 40; fax: (41-22) 809 18 10; email: fellows@uicc.org
Internet: http://fellows.uicc.org/fell5ion.shtml
Sponsor: International Union against Cancer
3, rue de Conseil-General
Geneva 1205 Switzerland

International Spinal Research Trust Grants **1863**
The trust awards grants worldwide for research into the treatment of paralysis caused by spinal cord injury. Grants also are available for the purchase of relevant equipment.
Contact: John Cavanagh, Head of Research, 01483 898786; fax: 01483 898763; email: research@spinal-research.org or john@spinal-research.org
Internet: http://www.spinal-research.org/display_section.asp?section=researchers
Sponsor: International Spinal Research Trust
Station Road, Bramley
Guildford GU5 0AZ United Kingdgom

IOM Gustav O. Lienhard Award **1864**
The award recognizes creative or pioneering efforts that have appreciably improved personal health services, rather than on contributions to the science base of healthcare. Award recipients are selected on the basis of achievement in the area of personal health services; and achievement of national scope. Additional selection criteria include innovative, creative, and pioneering achievement; unique contributions by the nominee to that achievement; positive change over a sustained period not simply for the potential for such change through the nominee's achievement; a qualitative and quantitative impact; and success in overcoming barriers, based on resources available. The recipient must attend the ceremony to receive the award. Complete nomination guidelines and procedures are available online.
Requirements: Any individual or group may submit a nomination. Nominees are not considered on the basis of education or profession.
Amount of Grant: $25,000
Date(s) Application is Due: Apr 30
Contact: Susanne Stoiber, (202) 334-2177; fax: (202) 334-1412; email: lienhard@nas.edu
Internet: http://www.iom.edu/lienhard
Sponsor: Institute of Medicine
500 Fifth Street NW
Washington, DC 20001

Ireland Family Foundation Grants **1865**
Established in 2000, the Ireland Family Foundation givings primarily in North Carolina with some funding available in California. The Foundations supports non-profit organizations involved with autism research, human services and education.
Requirements: The initial approach should be in the form of a letter, followed up with a proposal containing : a copy of IRS Determination Letter; a detailed description of project and amount of funding requested.
Restrictions: No grants to individuals.
Geographic Focus: California; North Carolina
Samples: ARC of Orange County, Chapel Hill, NC., $35,000 (2005);
Amount of Grant: $10,000-$60,000 range
Contact: Lori Ireland, President; (919) 932-3556;
Sponsor: Ireland Family Foundation
1434 Arboretum Drive
Chapel Hill, NC 27517-9161

Irvin Stern Foundation Grants **1866**
The Foundation awards grants to nonprofits primarily in the following areas: human services; civic affairs; and Jewish welfare. Other grant requests should be in the Foundation's other areas of interest which include: aiding the underserved, poor, and disadvantaged; improving the quality of life in urban communities; and enhancing

Jewish community, education and spirituality. Interested applicants may submit an online letter of inquiry or applications may be mailed to the Foundation office.
Requirements: The Foundation makes grants to tax-exempt organizations.
Restrictions: The Foundation does not contribute to endowments, capital campaigns, capital construction projects, and academic or medical research programs of any kind.
Contact: Christine Flood, Grants Administrator; email: christine@irvinstern.org
Internet: http://www.irvinstern.org/guidelines.html
Sponsor: Irvin Stern Foundation
25 West Hubbard Street, 4th Floor
Chicago, IL 60610

Irving S. Gilmore Foundation Grants **1867**
The Irving S. Gilmore Foundation endeavors to develop and to enrich the Greater Kalamazoo community of Michigan and, its residents by supporting the work of nonprofit organizations. The Foundation's funding priorities are: health and well-being; arts; human services; education; community development; culture and humanities. Organizations that are first time Foundation applicants or have not received Foundation funding since 2007 must contact the Foundation at least four weeks prior to an applicable submission deadline.
Requirements: The Foundation supports Kalamazoo County projects, programs, and purposes carried out by charitable institutions, primarily public charities and governmental entities.
Restrictions: Grants are not made to individuals.
Geographic Focus: Michigan
Samples: Michigan Festival of Sacred Music—Operational Support (2008); Hospice Care of Southwest Michigan—Capital Campaign (2008); Volunteer Services of Greater Kalamazoo— BoardConnect Program (2008).
Date(s) Application is Due: Jan 4; Mar 1; May 3; Jul 1; Sep 1; Nov 1
Contact: Janice C. Elliott, Vice President of Administrations; (269) 342-6411; fax: (269) 342-6465;
Internet: http://www.isgilmorefoundation.org/communityinvolvement.htm
Sponsor: Irving S. Gilmore Foundation
136 East Michigan Avenue, Suite 900
Kalamazoo, MI 49007-3912

Isabel Allende Foundation Esperanza Grants **1868**
The Foundation is guided by a vision of a world in which women have achieved social and economic justice. The vision includes empowerment of women and girls and protection of women and children. The Foundation feels that the way to achieve empowerment is: reproductive self-determination; health care; and education. Application information is available online.
Requirements: 501(c)3 organizations (and equivalent international organizations) are eligible to apply. Priority is given to programs in San Francisco Bay Area and Chile.
Restrictions: The foundation does not fund capital campaigns, individual trips or tours, conferences, or events; and projects that benefit political, religious, and/or military organizations. Individuals are not eligible to receive grants and should not apply.
Geographic Focus: California
Amount of Grant: $1,000-$5,000
Date(s) Application is Due: Jan 1; Apr 1; Jul 1; Oct 1
Contact: Lori Barra, Executive Director; (415) 289-0992; fax: (415) 289-1154; email: lori@isabelallendefoundation.org
Internet: http://www.isabelallendefoundation.org/iaf.php?l=en&p=application
Sponsor: Isabel Allende Foundation
116 Caledonia Street
Sausalito, CA 94965

Ittleson Foundation AIDS Grants **1869**
In regards to AIDS, the foundation is particularly interested in new model, pilot, and demonstration efforts: addressing the needs of underserved at-risk populations and especially those programs recognizing the overlap between such programs; responding to the challenges facing community-based AIDS service organizations and those organizations addressing systemic change; providing meaningful school-based sex education; making treatment information accessible, available and easily understandable to those in need of it; or, addressing the psycho-social needs of those infected and affected by AIDS, especially adolescents.
Requirements: Tax-exempt organizations may apply.
Restrictions: The foundation generally does not provide funds for capital building projects, endowments, grants to individuals, scholarships or internships (except as part of a program), direct service programs (especially outside New York City), projects that are local in focus and unlikely to be replicated, continuing or general support, projects and organizations that are international in scope or purpose, or biomedical research.
Samples: AIDS Alliance for Children Youth and Family, Washington, DC, $5,000—to transform the National Consumer Leadership Corps Training Program into one that can be replicated by local AIDS organizations around the nation (2008); Cesar E. Chavez Institute, New York, NY, $40,000—one-time grant to develop new family interventions and a new family-related model of care to reduce risk for HIV and mental health problems in lesbian, gay, bisexual and transgender (LGBT) youth (2008).
Date(s) Application is Due: Sep 1
Contact: Anthony C. Wood, Executive Director; (212) 794-2008; fax: (212) 794-0351
Internet: http://www.ittlesonfoundation.org/aids.html
Sponsor: Ittleson Foundation
15 E. 67th Street, 5th Floor
New York, NY 10021

Ittleson Foundation Mental Health Grants **1870**
For this program, the foundation is interested in innovative, pilot, model and demonstration projects that are: fighting the stigma associated with mental illness and working to change the public's negative perception of people who have mental illness; utilizing new knowledge and current technological advances to improve programs and services for people who have mental illness; bringing the full benefits of this new knowledge and technology to those who presently do not have access to them; or, advancing preventative mental health efforts, especially those targeted to youth and adolescents, with a special focus on strategies that involve parents, teachers, and others in close contact with these populations.
Requirements: Tax-exempt organizations may apply.
Restrictions: The foundation generally does not provide funds for capital building projects, endowments, grants to individuals, scholarships or internships (except as part of a program), direct service programs (especially outside New York City), projects that are local in focus and unlikely to be replicated, continuing or general support, projects and organizations that are international in scope or purpose, or biomedical research.
Samples: Active Minds, Inc., Washington, DC, $10,000—to dramatically expand the network of chapters on college campuses (2008); Partnership with Children, New York, NY, $50,000—one-time grant to develop the Center for Capacity Building to enable the dissemination of the successful counseling and prevention care program for inner-city boys and girls, "Open Heart-Open Mind" to over 100 schools by 2012 (2008).
Date(s) Application is Due: Sep 1
Contact: Anthony C. Wood, Executive Director; (212) 794-2008; fax: (212) 794-0351
Internet: http://www.ittlesonfoundation.org/mental.html
Sponsor: Ittleson Foundation
15 E. 67th Street, 5th Floor
New York, NY 10021

IWMF Public Health Fellowship **1871**
The goals of the fellowship are to offer women newspaper editors and radio producers the opportunity to enhance their ability to cover public health issues, build their journalism skills, and learn first-hand about standards and practices in the U.S. media. The six-month fellowship includes four months in the United States and two months in the fellows' home countries, where the fellows will implement a public health reporting project. Each applicant must clearly identify and describe a public health reporting project that she will focus on when she returns to her home country for that segment of the fellowship. Those demonstrating original approaches to covering HIV/AIDS will be given top consideration. The fellowship includes application costs for a U.S. visa; round-trip economy airfare from the fellows' home countries to Washington, DC; round-trip economy airfare from Washington, DC, to the fellowship site and health insurance; and a fixed stipend to cover lodging, meals, and ground transportation during the U.S. segment of the fellowship. For the home country segment, a fixed stipend will be provided to support the fellow and cover all costs associated with implementing her project. Application and guidelines are available online.
Requirements: The fellowship is open to women journalists who are working in one of the following countries: Asia (China and Indonesia), West Africa (Benin, Burkina Faso, Cameroon, Cape Verde, Chad, Gambia, Ghana, Guinea, Guinea Bissau, Ivory Coast, Liberia, Mali, Mauritania, Niger, Nigeria, Senegal, Sierra Leone, and Togo), and Southern Africa (Angola, Botswana, Lesotho, Malawi, Mozambique, Namibia, Swaziland, Zambia, and Zimbabwe). A successful applicant will be dedicated to a career in journalism and have five or more years of full-time experience in the profession, with at least three of those years having been focused on public health journalism. She must be currently working as a newspaper editor or radio producer and show a strong commitment to sharing knowledge and skills with colleagues upon returning home. The fellow must also have excellent written and spoken English skills.
Date(s) Application is Due: Apr 15
Contact: Fellowship Administrator, (202) 496-1992; fax: (202) 496-1977; email: fellowship@iwmf.org
Internet: http://iwmf.org/programs/8702
Sponsor: International Women's Media Foundation
1625 K St NW, Suite 1275
Washington, DC 20006

J. Walton Bissell Foundation Grants **1872**
The foundation's yearly giving programs are available primarily in the Connecticut River Valley and focus on higher and secondary education, hospitals, youth agencies, care of the aged, aid to the blind, and encouragement of the arts. Brief letters describing projects to be funded, history and current status of requesting organization, and amount desired will be reviewed as received. Organizations interested in applying should apply at least three months before funding is needed. Requests should be submitted three months before funding is needed.
Requirements: Grants are awarded to 501(c)3 charitable organizations in Connecticut, Massachusetts, New Hampshire, and Vermont that are not private foundations.
Restrictions: Grants are not awarded to support campaigns or endowment funding, nor are they awarded to individuals.
Geographic Focus: Connecticut; Massachusetts; New Hampshire; Vermont
Amount of Grant: $1500-$20,000 range
Contact: J.D. Anthony Jr., President, (860) 275-0136; fax: (860) 275-0343
Sponsor: J. Walton Bissell Foundation
P.O. Box 370067
Hartford, CT 06137

J.B. Reynolds Foundation Grants **1873**

The foundation makes grants in the local Kansas City, MO, area, up to a 150-mile radius of the city. Grants are awarded for building and equipment, community development, medical research, social welfare, and the arts and humanities. Some support is given to colleges and universities. Additional types of support include general operating support, continuing support, annual campaigns, endowment funds, publications, and research. The board meets in April and December of each year to consider letters of requests, and only invited proposals are reviewed. All grants are awarded in December.

Requirements: 501(c)3 organizations in the Kansas City, MO, area may submit applications.

Geographic Focus: Missouri

Amount of Grant: \$5,000-\$50,000 range

Contact: Richard L. Finn, Secretary-Treasurer; (816) 753-7000; fax: (816) 753-1354

Sponsor: J.B. Reynolds Foundation
P.O. Box 219139
Kansas City, MO 64141-6139

J.C. Penney Company Grants **1874**

The corporate contributions program awards grants to 501(c)3 nonprofit organizations in the company's areas of interest, including improvement of K- through 12th-grade education through curriculum-based after school care, with a priority on JCPenney Afterschool; support/promotion of associate (employee) volunteerism, primarily through the James Cash Penney Awards for Community Service; and United Way (most of JCPenney's support for health and welfare issues is contributed through local United Ways). Funding for other types of programs and projects is limited. Funding is concentrated on projects and organizations that serve a broad sector of the community; national projects that have a multiplier effect by benefiting local organizations across the country; nonprofits offering direct services; and projects with proven track records. Proposals are accepted year-round. There is no formal grant application. Interested applicants should submit a brief letter of inquiry.

Requirements: JCPenney only considers grants to tax-exempt organizations with 501(c)3 status or organizations that are a political subdivision of the state as described 170(c)1 of the IRS.

Restrictions: JCPenney refrains from or limits support of: individuals (including family reunions); individual student exchange/travel programs; membership organizations, unless the project benefits the entire community; religious organizations, unless the project benefits the entire community; journal or program advertising; fundraising dinners, luncheons or other types of benefits; merchandise donations; door prizes, gift certificates, or other giveaways; conferences and seminars; capital campaigns and multiyear pledges; international projects except in countries with corporate business locations; pilot projects; film and video projects; research projects; scholarships, except at colleges and universities with which the company has a recruiting relationship; higher education institutions, unless the company has a business or recruiting relationship; individual K-12 schools, unless the company has a business partnership with the school (including proms, graduations, PTOs and PTAs); or donations of returned, damaged or excess merchandise. JCPenney does not offer a matching gifts program at this time.

Contact: Jeannette M. Siegel, Community Relations and Contributions Manager; (972) 431-1349; fax: (972) 431-1355; email: jsiegel@jcpenney.com

Internet: http://www.jcpenney.net/about/social_resp/community/default.aspx

Sponsor: J.C. Penney Company Inc
P.O. Box 10001
Dallas, TX 75301-8101

J.E. and L.E. Mabee Foundation Grants **1875**

The purpose of the Foundation is to aid Christian religious organizations, charitable organizations, institutions of higher learning, hospitals and other organizations of a general charitable nature. The Foundation favors organizations that combine sound character and stability with progressiveness and purpose. There is no formal application procedure. Proposal submission information is available online.

Requirements: Nonprofit, tax exempt, and not tax- supported organizations in Arkansas, Kansas, Missouri, New Mexico, Oklahoma, and Texas are eligible.

Restrictions: The foundation does not generally favor grants for deficit financing and debt retirement (except a construction contract that was executed prior to the time of application); operating or program funds or annual fundraising campaigns (except Junior Achievement and United Way in Tulsa, OK, and Midland, TX); reserve purposes or for projects likely to be long delayed; endowments; governmental owned or operated institutions and/or facilities (such as state universities and municipal parks and libraries); educational institutions below the college level; furnishing or equipment (except major medical equipment); or churches.

Geographic Focus: Arkansas; Kansas; Missouri; New Mexico; Oklahoma; Texas

Contact: Thomas R. Brett, Director; (918) 584-4286;

Internet: http://www.mabeefoundation.com/policies.htm

Sponsor: J.E. and L.E. Mabee Foundation
Mid-Continent Tower, 401 South Boston Avenue, Suite 3001
Tulsa, OK 74103-4017

J.L. Bedsole Foundation Grants **1876**

The Foundation considers requests that most closely match its overall mission: to improve the quality of life for the citizens of Southwest Alabama and to strengthen the communities in which they live. The Foundation will consider only those grant applications that meet several of the following guidelines. The project addresses needs in at least one of the following areas: education, arts and culture, health and human services and economic development; potential for permanent, enduring benefits that will provide value to the community and the residents of Southwest Alabama; diverse groups are collaborating on the project to achieve common goals; the organization and the project clearly demonstrate sound fiscal management and accountability; the organization attracts multiple sources of support for the project; the project addresses underserved segments of the population, the economically disadvantaged or citizens of rural communities. The Foundation offers a scholarship program as well, see: http://www.jlbedsolefoundation.org/default.asp?ID=7 for details and guidelines.

Requirements: Nonprofit organizations in Mobile, Baldwin, Clarke, Monroe and Washington County, Alabama are eligible to apply.

Restrictions: The Foundation will not support the following: grants that support political activities or attempts to influence action on specific legislation; multiple year pledges nor make grants beyond the current year; grants to endowment funds of other organizations; grants are not made directly to individuals; grants are not made to organizations, programs or projects outside of the State of Alabama.

Geographic Focus: Alabama

Contact: Christopher L. Lee, Executive Director; (251) 432-3369; fax: (251) 432-1134; email: chrislee@jlbedsolefoundation.org

Internet: http://www.jlbedsolefoundation.org/default.asp?ID=6

Sponsor: J.L. Bedsole Foundation
P.O. Box 1137
Mobile, AL 36633

J.M. Long Foundation Grants **1877**

The Foundation is focused on providing support to organizations involved with health care, education, and conservation in the communities of Northern California and Hawaii. Preference will be given for new, innovative projects, which can be completed with the Foundation contribution. Applications for new grant requests are given by invitation only. In order to receive an invitation, an organization will need to submit to the Foundation a single page Request for Invitation letter using organization letterhead. This Request for Invitation letter should describe the organization's objective and the specific project for which the grant would be used. The applicant should be sure to include an estimated amount for the grant, as well as contact information including email address if available.

Requirements: Hawaiin and Northern California nonprofits are eligible to apply.

Restrictions: Please note that grants will not be made: for the support of solely religious, sacramental or theological functions; in support of political bodies or campaigns; to individuals or foreign organizations; for loans; for purposes of memorializing an individual, although donations may be made to memorial funds as a means of achieving other purposes; for covering operating deficits; to organizations not qualifying as either a federal tax-exempt non-profit private organization or a qualifying public organization; to supporting organizations with a 509(a)(3) designation.

Geographic Focus: California; Hawaii

Samples: California State Parks Foundation, Kentfield, CA - Park Education Legacy Program (2009); Children's Discovery Center, Honolulu, HI - Ready, Set, Grow Program (2009); The Creek, A Middle School Youth Center, Walnut Creek, CA - Start up Funding (2009).

Amount of Grant: \$1000-\$50,000 average

Contact: Brenda Kauten, Grants Administrator; (925) 935-4138; fax: (925) 935-2092

Internet: http://www.jmlongfoundation.org/Grants.html

Sponsor: J.M. Long Foundation
P.O. Box 3827
Walnut Creek, CA 94598-2827

J.W. Kieckhefer Foundation Grants **1878**

The foundation awards grants to support medical research; hospice; health; family planning; disabled; social services; higher, medical, and other education; youth; child welfare; conservation; community funds; public policy; and cultural programs. The grants are awarded for operating budgets, continuing support, annual campaigns, emergency funds, building funds, equipment, land acquisition, endowment funds, matching funds, research, publications, conferences and seminars, and special projects. Applications should be submitted between May and November. The board meets in November and December to consider requests.

Restrictions: Grants are not awarded to individuals or for seed money, deficit financing, scholarships, or demonstration projects.

Amount of Grant: \$350-\$100,000 range

Contact: John Kieckhefer or Eugene Polk, Trustees, (928) 445-4010

Sponsor: J.W. Kieckhefer Foundation
P.O. Box 1151, 116 E Gurley Street
Prescott, AZ 86302

Jackson County Community Foundation Unrestricted Grants **1879**

The Foundation awards grants to nonprofit organizations covering a full range of charitable activity such as health and human services, education, economic/community development, arts and culture, and environmental quality and protection. All grants are evaluated on a competitive basis and priority is given to those projects that show potential for providing maximum benefit to community members. Application information is available online.

Requirements: The Foundation makes grants to Jackson County, Michigan nonprofit, tax-exempt organizations.

Restrictions: While the Foundation remains flexible in trying to address the needs of the community, it do not make grants to individuals (except scholarships), programs that advocate specific religions, or services which are standard government or school

obligations. Applications from organizations not serving Jackson County are not accepted.
Geographic Focus: Michigan
Samples: Smiles on Wheels Preventative Dental Health Care Project, $5,000—to purchase dental supplies and equipment (2009); Jackson School of the Arts, $10,000—Operational support (2009); Center for Family Health, $30,000—Jackson High Teen Health Center (2009).
Amount of Grant: $3,000-$50,000 range
Date(s) Application is Due: Jan 15; May 15; Sep 15
Contact: Diane McDonald, Grant & Scholarship Coordinator; (517) 787-1321; fax: (517) 787-4333; email: jcf@jacksoncf.org
Internet: http://www.jacksoncf.org/grants.html
Sponsor: Jackson County Community Foundation
One Jackson Square, 100 East Michigan Avenue, Suite 308
Jackson, MI 49201-1406

Jackson Laboratory Postdoctoral Research Training Program **1880**
Fellowships are intended for postdoctoral associateships at Jackson Laboratory allowing the fellows to participate in research into gene regulation, developmental genetics, hematology and immunology, and other fields of mammalian biology, with the purpose of the recipient receiving research training under the guidance of experienced researchers. The fellowships are awarded for one year, renewable for up to two years. Applications are accepted at any time.
Requirements: Recent recipients of doctoral degrees in medicine, veterinary medicine, and the biological sciences are eligible to apply. Applicants may be of any nationality.
Contact: Suzanne Serreze, Manager, Sponsored Training Programs, (207) 288-6420; fax: (207) 288-6079; email: sbs@jax.org
Internet: http://www.jax.org/education/postdoc.html
Sponsor: Jackson Laboratory
600 Main Street
Bar Harbor, ME 04609-1500

Jacob and Hilda Blaustein Foundation Grants **1881**
The Foundation promotes social justice and human rights through its five program areas: Jewish life; strengthening Israeli democracy; health and mental health; educational opportunity; and human rights. Support is provided to organizations in the United States and abroad, with a preference to the Baltimore, Maryland area. The Foundation supports organizations that promote systemic change; involve constituents in planning and decision-making; encourage volunteer and professional development; and engage in ongoing program evaluation. Additional guidelines and application information is available online.
Requirements: Nonprofit organizations are eligible to apply.
Restrictions: Support is unavailable for the following: individuals; scholarships to individuals; unsolicited proposals for academic, scientific, or medical research.; direct mail; annual giving; membership campaigns; fundraising; commemorative events.
Geographic Focus: Maryland
Samples: The Foundation for Jewish Campus Life, Washington, DC, $150,000—support offered over a two year period, for Tzedek Hillel, a program that promotes social justice activities among Jewish college students across the country, and support for the Tzedek Leadership Mission to Israel (2007); Fund for Educational Excellence, Baltimore, MD, $250,000—support for over five years, for the implementation of a reform plan for Baltimore's neighborhood high schools (2008); Mental Disability Rights International, Washington, DC, $70,000—support paid over two years, to promote the human rights of people with mental disabilities worldwide (2008).
Contact: Betsy Ringel, Executive Director; (410) 347-7103; fax: (410) 347-7210; email: info@blaufund.org
Internet: http://www.blaufund.org/foundations/jacobandhilda_f.html
Sponsor: Jacob and Hilda Blaustein Foundation
10 East Baltimore Street, Suite 1111
Baltimore, MD 21202

Jacob and Valeria Langeloth Foundation Grants **1882**
The Foundation's grantmaking program is centered on the concepts of health and well-being. The Foundation's purpose is to promote and support effective and creative programs, practices and policies related to healing from illness, accident, physical, social or emotional trauma and to extend the availability of programs that promote healing to underserved populations. The Foundation is particularly interested in funding programs that address the health of individuals who, because of barriers to difficulty accessing care. Preference is given in the areas of: caregivers and; correctional health care.
Requirements: 501(c)3 organizations that promote physical and emotional healing, especially to underserved populations, such as: community-based organizations, health care providers and research institutions in the state of New York are eligible to apply.
Restrictions: The Foundation will not consider proposals for annual or capital campaigns, for building or renovation projects, for budgetary relief, or preventive medicine. The Foundation does not support projects that focus on children or end-of-life issues. Neither will the Foundation make grants to individuals or for sectarian or religious purposes, or for political activities or lobbying. The Foundation will not fund any organization that discriminates on the basis of age, gender, national origin, race, or sexual preference.
Geographic Focus: New York
Samples: AARP Foundation, Washington, DC, $261,000— for professional partners supporting family caregivers (2008); Foundation for Quality Care, Albany, NY, $171,000—for geriatric nursing assistants career development program (2008); New York Academy of Medicine, New York, NY, $200,000— for Prison Health Reentry initiative (2008).
Date(s) Application is Due: Feb 1; Aug 1
Contact: Scott Moyer, President; (212) 687-1133; fax: (212) 681-2628; email: smoyer@langeloth.org
Internet: http://www.langeloth.org/apply.php
Sponsor: Jacob and Valeria Langeloth Foundation
521 Fifth Avenue, Suite 1612
New York, NY 10175-1699

Jacob G. Schmidlapp Trust Grants **1883**
The trust supports tax-exempt organizations in the greater Cincinnati, OH, area. The trust supports charitable or educational purposes; for relief in sickness, suffering, and distress; for the care of young children, the aged, or the helpless; and for the promotion of education to improve living conditions. Support is offered in the form of: endowments; equipment; land acquisition; program development; technical assistance; and seed money grants. An organization interested in submitting a grant proposal should initially contact the Foundation office via a letter of inquiry, an application form is required for proposals. Proposals are reviewed quarterly, March, June, September and, December.
Requirements: Nonprofits in the greater Cincinnati, Ohio area receive the majority of funding, however giving is also available in the surrounding states of Indiana, Kentucky and Michigan.
Restrictions: No support for religious or political purposes. No grants to individuals; no loans.
Geographic Focus: Indiana; Kentucky; Michigan; Ohio
Samples: Jewish Community Center, Cincinnati, OH, $500,000— for capital support (2007); Spectrum Health Foundation, Grand Rapids, MI, $100,000— for capital support (2007); Children Inc., Covington, KY, $100,000— for project/program support (2007); Xavier University, Cincinnati, OH, $250,000—for scholarship (2007).
Amount of Grant: $2,000-$500,000 range
Date(s) Application is Due: Feb 1; May 1; Aug 1; Nov 1
Contact: Heidi B. Jark, Manager, Charitable and Planned Giving Services, c/o Fifth Third Bank; (513) 534-4397
Internet: https://www.53.com:443/wps/portal/personal
Sponsor: Jacob G. Schmidlapp Trust
38 Fountain Square Plaza, MD 1090CA
Cincinnati, OH 45263-0001

James A. and Faith Knight Foundation Grants **1884**
Primarily serving Jackson and Washtenaw counties, Michigan, the Foundation is dedicated to improving communities by providing grant support to qualified nonprofit organizations including, but not limited to, those that address the needs of women and girls, animals and the natural world, and internal capacity. In general, the foundation supports organizations that believe in good nonprofit practices including sound financial management, developed governance practices, and clarity of mission. Attention to gender, diversity, and outcomes are important. Giving is primarily for human services, including a neighborhood center, women's organizations, and family services; support also for nonprofit management, the United Way, housing, the arts, education, and environmental conservation. Fields of interest include: adult education and literacy; basic skills; GED; arts; environment and natural resources; family services; housing development; human services; nonprofit management; and women's services. There are two annual deadlines, and initial approach should be by letter.
Requirements: Giving is limited to Michigan, with emphasis on Jackson and Washenaw counties.
Restrictions: No support is offered for religious or political organizations. No grants to individuals, or for conferences or special events, or for annual campaigns.
Geographic Focus: Michigan
Samples: Center for the Childbearing Year, Ann Arbor, Michigan, $23,000—to increase capacity of the Doulas Care program, with targeted emphasis to improve maternal/infant health outcomes and develop a health career pathway for women (2007); Dahlem Conservancy, Jackson, Michigan, $18,000—to purchase a van to initiate outreach programs (2007).
Date(s) Application is Due: Jan 28; Sep 16
Contact: Margaret A. Talburtt Ph.D., Exec. Director; (734) 769-5653; fax: (734) 769-8383; email: peg@KnightFoundationMi.org or info@knightfoundationmi.org
Internet: http://www.knightfoundationmi.org/guidelines.htm
Sponsor: James A. and Faith Knight Foundation
180 Little Lake Drive, Suite 6B
Ann Arbor, MI 48103-6219

James Ford Bell Foundation Grants **1885**
The Foundation supports organizations primarily in Minnesota. Emphasis is on cultural programs, support is also available for wildlife preservation and conservation, youth agencies, the environment, education, health and human services. A high priority is given to projects with historical connections to the Bell Family. The Trustees meet in the Spring and Fall. Contact the Foundation prior to sending in a proposal. Unsolicited requests for funds are not accepted.
Requirements: Nonprofit organizations in Minnesota are eligible to apply.
Restrictions: No grants are made directly to individuals, nor for scholarships, fellowships, or political campaigns. No funding is available to units of local government. The Foundation does not respond to requests for memberships, annual appeals, or special events and fundraisers.
Geographic Focus: Minnesota

Samples: University of Minnesota Foundation, Minneapolis, MN, $3,000,000 - for general operating support (2007); Minneapolis College of Art and Design, Minneapolis, MN, $1,020,000 - for general operating support (2007); Minnesota Environmental Partnership, Saint Paul, MN, $58,000 - for general operating support (2007).
Contact: Ellen George, C.O.O.; (612) 377-8400; fax: (612) 377-8407; email: ellen@fpadvisors.com
Internet: http://www.fpadvisors.com/jamesfordbell/jamesfordbell.htm
Sponsor: James Ford Bell Foundation
1818 Oliver Avenue South
Minneapolis, MN 55405-2208

James G.K. McClure Educational and Development Fund Grants 1886
The fund devotes most of its resources to an ongoing scholarship program for the students of western North Carolina. When funds are available, the trustees make grants to organizations in the region, primarily those that enhance the lives of the rural citizens of the area. The trustees look favorably on requests from institutions helping to improve the lives of the people within its geographic area. Hospitals, colleges, libraries, and various schools are common recipients. The trustees meet twice each year, usually in May and October.
Requirements: Applicants must be residents of the following counties: Allegheny, Ashe, Avery, Buncombe, Burke, Caldwell, Cherokee, Clay, Graham, Haywood, Henderson, Jackson, Macon, Madison, McDowell, Mitchell, Polk, Rutherford, Swain, Transylvania, Watauga, and Yancey.
Restrictions: No student may apply for a scholarship unless he or she resides in one of the specified counties, and no grant money will be made to organizations outside this district.
Geographic Focus: North Carolina
Amount of Grant: $1000-$5000 typically
Contact: John Curtis Ager, Executive Director; (704) 628-2114; email: jager@ioa.com
Sponsor: James G.K. McClure Educational and Development Fund
John Agner c/o Sugar Hollow Farm, 11 Sugar Hollow Lane
Fairview, NC 28730

James Graham Brown Foundation Grants 1887
The James Graham Brown Foundation fosters the well-being, quality of life, and image of Louisville and Kentucky by actively supporting and funding projects in the fields of education, economic development, health and social services, culture and humanities (excluding performing arts) with an emphasis on community-wide capital campaigns. The Board meets six times annually and determinations are made at the meetings. Funds are dispersed semi-annually.
Requirements: To begin the process of applying, submit a Pre-Grant Request form, available at: http://www.jgbf.org/Home/Deadlines/tabid/74/Default.aspx. If request if accepted, a Formal Application form will be provided to you from the Foundation. Formal Applications must be submitted by the following deadline dates: March 16, Social Services requests; May 12, Culture and Civic requests; July 7, Education requests. Only organizations that have obtained a tax-exempt designation under Section 501(c)3 of the I.R.S. code may apply. The Foundation grants are limited to the Louisville metropolitan area and the state of Kentucky. Campaigns outside the Jefferson County and Louisville metropolitan area must show evidence of significant local community support before being considered by the foundation for funding.
Restrictions: The Foundation does not support the following: organizations outside of the state of Kentucky; those related either directly or indirectly to the performing arts; requests from religious organizations for religious purposes (including theological seminaries); requests from individuals; requests from political entities; requests from national organizations, even if for local projects.
Geographic Focus: Kentucky
Samples: Centre College, $1,000,000 - toward an endowed scholarship fund to be known as the Joe McDowell Rodes Scholarship (2007); Kentucky Christian College, $300,000 - toward the construction of a School of Nursing facility (2007); American Red Cross, Louisville Area Chapter, $750,000 - toward community readiness campaign (2007);
Date(s) Application is Due: Mar 16; May 12; Jul 7
Contact: Dodie McKenzie, Grants Director; (502) 896-2440 or (866) 896-5423; fax: (502) 896-1774; email: grants@jgbf.org
Internet: http://www.jgbf.org
Sponsor: James Graham Brown Foundation
4350 Brownsboro Road, Suite 200
Louisville, KY 40207

James H. Cummings Foundation Grants 1888
The Foundation, gives exclusively for charitable purposes in advancing medical science, research, and education in selected cities in the U.S. and Canada, and for charitable work among underprivileged boys and girls, and aged and infirm persons in designated areas. Priority is given to medical proposals. The funding is limited to: Toronto, Ontario; Canada; Hendersonville, North Carolina and; Buffalo, New York. Grants are available, in the following types of support: building/renovation; capital campaigns; equipment; land acquisition; matching/challenge support; research and seed money.
Requirements: The giving program is limited to the vicinity of the cities of Buffalo, NY; Hendersonville, NC; and Toronto, ON, Canada.
Restrictions: No support for national health organizations. Grants are not awarded to individuals, nor for: loans, annual campaigns, program support, endowment funds, operating budgets, emergency funds, deficit financing, scholarships, fellowships, publications, conferences, or continuing support.
Geographic Focus: New York; North CarolinaCanada
Samples: Child and Family Services Conners Children's Ctr (Buffalo, NY)—to renovate this center that provides residential care for severely disturbed boys between the ages of six and 14, $100,000.; YMCA of Henderson and Henderson County (NC)—program support, $62,500.; Margaret R. Pardee Hospital (NC)—capital support, $100,000.
Amount of Grant: $2000-$250,000 range
Contact: William McFarland, Executive Director; (716) 874-0040; fax: (716) 874-0040; email: cummings.foundation@verizon.net
Sponsor: James H. Cummings Foundation
1807 Elmwood Avenue, Room 112
Buffalo, NY 14207

James Hervey Johnson Charitable Educational Trust Grants 1889
The goal of the trust is to expose religion as against reason, publicize nontheistic views of religion, and publicize James Hervey Johnson's views on health, which are centered primarily in vegetarianism, natural hygiene, and alternative medicine. Interested applicants should contact the Foundation prior to submitting a proposal. The Foundation requires an application form and, will provide guidelines. There are no geographic restrictions, but preference is given to requests from San Diego County, CA.
Requirements: 501(c)3 nonprofits that have been in existence for at least two years are eligible.
Samples: Institute for the Study of the Religious Right—for a Web site that provides information on how the religious right threatens separation of church and state, $9300.; Action on Smoking and Health—for a letter-writing contest on why the U.S. president should proceed with plans to toughen anti-smoking regulations, $7000.; American Natural Hygiene Society—for a new desktop publishing system for producing publications advocating natural hygiene, $8622.
Amount of Grant: $5000-$100,000 range
Date(s) Application is Due: Jun 30;
Contact: Kevin V. Munnelly, Treasurer; fax: (619) 297-9036; email: promotions@home.com
Sponsor: James Hervey Johnson Charitable Educational Trust
P.O. Box 16160
San Diego, CA 92176-6160

James J. and Angelia M. Harris Foundation Grants 1890
The foundation's primary areas of interested include: higher and other education, health services and hospitals, social services, youth, Christian organizations and, Presbyterian churches. Types of support include: annual campaigns, building construction/renovation, capital campaigns, challenge/matching grants, program development, seed money and, scholarship funds. There are no application deadlines or forms. The board meets in May and November to consider requests. Letters of inquiry are due in April and October.
Requirements: Nonprofit organizations in Clarke County, GA, and Mecklenburg County, NC, are eligible.
Geographic Focus: Georgia; North Carolina
Amount of Grant: $1,000-$100,000 range
Contact: Sherri Harrell, Grants Administrator; (704) 364-6046
Sponsor: James J. and Angelia M. Harris Foundation
P.O. Box 220427
Charlotte, NC 28222-0427

James M. Collins Foundation Grants 1891
The foundation awards grants to Texas nonprofit organizations in its areas of interest, including: arts, economic development, health organizations, association, higher education, human services, museums, Salvation Army, secondary school/education. Types of support include research grants, program support, and social services. There are no application deadlines or forms.
Requirements: Texas nonprofit organizations are eligible.
Restrictions: Individuals are not eligible.
Geographic Focus: Texas
Samples: Smithsonian Institution, Washington, DC, $50,475 (2004); Wellesley College, Wellesley, MA, $200,250 (2004); Dallas Museum of Art, Dallas, TX, $17,950 (2004).
Contact: Dorothy Dann Collins Torbert, President; (214) 691-2032;
Sponsor: James M. Collins Foundation
8115 Preston Road, Suite 680
Dallas, TX 75225

James M. Cox Foundation of Georgia Grants 1892
The Foundation awards grants in Cox Enterprises communities in its areas of interest, including journalism, visual and performing arts, child development, education, healthcare, environment, wildlife, and community and family services. Types of support include building construction/renovation, capital campaigns, and program development. There are no application forms or deadlines. Interested applicants should send a request to the Foundation outlining project needs and goals.
Requirements: Nonprofits in Cox Enterprises communities are eligible.
Samples: Colorado State U (Fort Collins, CO)—to endow a chair within the Animal Cancer Center, $3 million.
Contact: Leigh Ann Launius, Assistant Secretary; (678) 645-0929; fax: (678) 645-1708
Internet: http://media.corporate-ir.net/media_files/IROL/76/76341/reports/AR_2003/community.html
Sponsor: James M. Cox Foundation of Georgia, Inc
6205 Peachtree Dunwoody Road
Atlanta, GA 30328

James McKeen Cattell Fund Fellowships 1893
The nonrenewable fellowships advance the science of psychology and its useful applications by enabling faculty members to take a full year sabbatical leave for independent study and research. Annual deadline dates may vary; contact program staff for exact dates.
Requirements: Eligibility is limited to residents of North America. The fellowships are intended for tenured faculty of a psychology department who are eligible for sabbatical leave. Matching institutions' support required.
Amount of Grant: $32,000 maximum
Date(s) Application is Due: Dec 1
Contact: Dr. Christina Williams, Program Contact; email: williams@psych.duke.edu
Internet: http://www.cattell.duke.edu
Sponsor: James McKeen Cattell Fund
9 Flowers Drive, Box 90086, Duke University, Department of Psychological and Brain Sciences
Durham, NC 27708-0086

James R. Dougherty Jr. Foundation Grants 1894
The James R. Dougherty, Jr. Foundation, established in 1950, gives to organizations primarily in Texas. Areas of interest include: family services, domestic violence, human services and women. Support is offered in the form of: annual campaigns, building/renovation, capital campaigns, continuing support, curriculum development, endowments, equipment, general/operating support, income development, management development/capacity building, matching/challenge support, program development, program evaluation, research, scholarship funds, seed money and, technical assistance grants. The board meets twice a year, in the Spring and Fall. No application form is required, contact the Foundation, before submitting a proposal.
Requirements: Nonprofit organizations in Texas are eligible to apply.
Geographic Focus: Texas
Date(s) Application is Due: Mar 1; Sep 1
Contact: Daren Wilder, Grants Administrator, (512) 358-3560
Sponsor: James R. Dougherty Jr. Foundation
P.O. Box 640
Beeville, TX 78104-0640

James S. Copley Foundation Grants 1895
The foundation serves as the philanthropic arm of The Copley Press, Inc., publishers of the Copley newspapers. The foundation offers support in the form of: scholarship funds; capital campaigns; equipment; employee matching gifts; endowments; equipment; building and; renovation grants. Funding organizations involved with arts and culture, education, animals and wildlife, health, recreation, and human services. Giving primarily in areas of company operations in California, Illinois and Ohio.
Requirements: 501(c)3 tax-exempt organizations in the circulation areas of company newspapers/operations are eligible to apply. These areas include: California, Illinois and Ohio.
Restrictions: Ineligible funding opportunities include: religious, fraternal, or athletic organizations, government agencies, local chapters of national organizations, public elementary, secondary schools, public broadcasting systems, individuals, research, publications, conferences, general operating support, large campaigns and loans.
Geographic Focus: California; Illinois; Ohio
Date(s) Application is Due: Jan 2
Contact: Foundation Administrator, (858) 454-0411 Ext. 7671
Sponsor: James S. Copley Foundation
P.O. Box 1530
La Jolla, CA 92038-1530

James S. McDonnell Foundation Brain Cancer Research Collaborative Activity Awards 1896
The Foundation offers Collaborative Activity Awards to initiate interdisciplinary discussions on problems or issues, to help launch interdisciplinary research networks, or to fund communities of researchers/practitioners dedicated to developing new methods, tools, and applications of basic research to applied problems. All proposals submitted to the foundation must clearly link the experimental models and questions to human disease. Proposals primarily intending to characterize basic mechanisms of growth and development that may plausibly but are not yet known to be contributory to human brain cancer are not encouraged. Proposals testing molecules as possible treatment interventions should consider including tests designed to uncover unintended biological effects of such molecules that would disqualify future clinical usefulness. The Foundation is particularly interested in supporting novel research that will generate new knowledge leading to increased rates of survival and improve functional recovery for individuals with brain cancer.
Restrictions: The Foundation does not fund: undergraduate tuition, stipends, scholarships, fellowships, research or travel expenses, or other educational expenses; graduate or postdoctoral stipends, scholarships, fellowships, research or travel expenses, or other educational expenses (exceptions include requests that qualify as allowable budget items as part of specific Research Award applications); expenses tied to projects whose explicit goal is the publication of a book or other bound volume (although publication of a book or special issue of a journal may be one goal or outcome of work funded by the Foundation); expenses tied to the establishment or day-to-day running of a journal or small press; scientific meetings or workshops other than those JSMF puts together or which are affiliated with Collaborative Activity Awards; ongoing operational support for university-based centers, programs, or institutes; professional society meetings or specific sessions at such meetings; charitable functions, museum exhibitions, or similar causes or events; or charitable donations to individuals and organizations.
Contact: Cheryl Washington, Grants Manager; (314) 721-1532; fax: (314) 721-7421; email: washington@jmsf.org or info@jmsf.org
Internet: http://www.jsmf.org/programs/bc/index.htm
Sponsor: James S. McDonnell Foundation
1034 S. Brentwood Boulevard, Suite 1850
Saint Louis, MO 63117

James S. McDonnell Foundation Complex Systems Collaborative Activity Awards 1897
The Foundation offers Collaborative Activity Awards to initiate interdisciplinary discussions on problems or issues, to help launch interdisciplinary research networks, or to fund communities of researchers/practitioners dedicated to developing new methods, tools, and applications of basic research to applied problems. The Program supports scholarship and research directed toward the development of theoretical and mathematical tools that can be applied to the study of complex, nonlinear systems. It is anticipated that research funded in this program will address issues in fields such as biology, biodiversity, climate, demography, epidemiology, technological change, economic Complex Systems development, governance, or computation. While the program's emphasis is on the development and application of theoretical models used in these research fields and not on particular fields per se, JSMF is particularly interested in projects attempting to apply complex systems approaches to real world problems. Proposals attempting to apply tools and models to problems where such approaches are not yet considered usual or mainstream (for example, differentiating normal physiology from disease) are encouraged.
Restrictions: The Foundation does not fund: undergraduate tuition, stipends, scholarships, fellowships, research or travel expenses, or other educational expenses; graduate or postdoctoral stipends, scholarships, fellowships, research or travel expenses, or other educational expenses (exceptions include requests that qualify as allowable budget items as part of specific Research Award applications); expenses tied to projects whose explicit goal is the publication of a book or other bound volume (although publication of a book or special issue of a journal may be one goal or outcome of work funded by the Foundation); expenses tied to the establishment or day-to-day running of a journal or small press; scientific meetings or workshops other than those JSMF puts together or which are affiliated with Collaborative Activity Awards; ongoing operational support for university-based centers, programs, or institutes; professional society meetings or specific sessions at such meetings; charitable functions, museum exhibitions, or similar causes or events; or charitable donations to individuals and organizations.
Contact: Cheryl Washington, Grants Manager; (314) 721-1532; fax: (314) 721-7421; email: washington@jmsf.org or info@jmsf.org
Internet: http://www.jsmf.org/programs/cs/index.htm
Sponsor: James S. McDonnell Foundation
1034 S. Brentwood Boulevard, Suite 1850
Saint Louis, MO 63117

James S. McDonnell Foundation Research Grants 1898
The Awards are designed to support research projects with a high probability of generating new knowledge and insights. Projects submitted for funding consideration should be at an early, even preliminary stage of development that intend to break new ground or to challenge commonly-held assumptions. Projects submitted should be sufficiently novel, cross-disciplinary, or heterodox so that they have a strong likelihood of influencing the development of new ways of thinking about important problems. Awards provide adequate, flexible funding over a sufficient time period to allow investigators to pursue and develop innovative directions to their research programs. Funds can be expended over a minimum of 3 years or a maximum of 6 years. Smaller amounts of money expended over shorter amounts of time may be requested to help investigators pursue pilot projects or test the feasibility of an experimental approach. The applicant can apply the grant funds towards any research-based expense, including travel, equipment, and supplies. Funds can be used to support collaborative projects. A percentage of the funds can also be used to support small workshops organized by the applicant where the goal of the workshop is to gather expertise in support of the research objective.
Requirements: Applications for grants are considered only from 501(c)3 organizations which are not private foundations. Applications from foreign organizations will be considered only if they provide written legal opinion that they qualify as tax-exempt under these sections of the U.S. IRS code or if a qualifying American organization is authorized to receive funds for them under this code. Individuals also are eligible.
Amount of Grant: $450,000 maximum
Contact: Cheryl Washington, Grants Manager; (314) 721-1532; fax: (314) 721-7421; email: washington@jmsf.org or info@jmsf.org
Internet: http://www.jsmf.org/apply/research/index.htm
Sponsor: James S. McDonnell Foundation
1034 S. Brentwood Boulevard, Suite 1850
Saint Louis, MO 63117

James S. McDonnell Foundation Scholar Awards 1899
The Awards program derives from and is consistent with the foundation's commitment to supporting high quality research and scholarship leading to the generation of new knowledge and its responsible application. Currently, the Awards are only available in the Brain, Mind & Behavior program area, and provide largely unrestricted funding over a sufficient time period to allow investigators to pursue and develop new directions to their research programs.
Requirements: Applications must be sponsored by a nonprofit institution as defined by Section 501(c)3 of the United States Internal Revenue Tax Code. Eligible Scholar Award nominees must have completed all doctoral, postdoctoral, or fellowship training

and hold an independent research position. Nominees in the earlier career stages are encouraged.
Restrictions: Researchers with current grant support from JSMF are not eligible to apply for a Scholar Award until all prior JSMF grant funds have been fully expended and a final grant report has been received and approved by the foundation office.
Amount of Grant: $600,000 to be expended over 6 years
Contact: Cheryl Washington, Grants Manager; (314) 721-1532; fax: (314) 721-7421; email: washington@jmsf.org or info@jmsf.org
Internet: http://www.jsmf.org/apply/scholar/index.htm
Sponsor: James S. McDonnell Foundation
1034 S. Brentwood Boulevard, Suite 1850
Saint Louis, MO 63117

James S. McDonnell Foundation Understanding Human Cognition Awards **1900**
The long-standing interest of the James S. McDonnell Foundation on human mind/brain is reflected in changes made to the 2008 RFA, including the explicit emphasis on understanding human cognition. The program is intended to help investigators pursue experiments designed to answer well-articulated questions. JSMF Scholar Awards support research studying how neural systems are linked to and support cognitive functions and how cognitive systems are related to an organism's (preferably human) observable behavior. Studies with model organisms should justify why such models were selected and how data obtained from models advances our understanding of human cognition. Proposals proposing to use functional imaging to identify the "neural correlates" of cognitive or behavioral tasks (for example, mapping the parts of the brain that "light up" when different groups of subjects play chess, solve physics problems, or choose apples over oranges) are not funded through this program. In general, JSMF and its expert advisors have taken an unfavorable view of projects attempting too wide a leap in a single bound. Functional imaging studies using poorly characterized tasks as proxies for complex behavioral issues involving empathy, moral judgments, or social decision-making are generally not appropriate responses to this call for proposals. In past competitions, proposals structured along such lines were eliminated from funding consideration early in the review process.
Requirements: Aspects of proposals appropriate to the JSMF UHC program would include, but are not limited to: characterizing the cognitive operations involved in performing a task; studying how the brain identifies, extracts and uses relevant information from complicated environments; examining how manipulations and/or perturbations at one spatial or temporal scale are meaningful at finer or coarser levels of organization (e.g. does a synaptic change account for a change in network function and vice versa?); re-examining "common wisdom" assumptions (such as the existence of critical periods in human learning); evaluating the usefulness of methodologies or improving the usefulness of methodologies commonly used in mind/brain research; applying approaches and knowledge from cognitive psychology or cognitive science to important problems in education, training, or rehabilitation; taking a comparative, evolutionary approach to characterizing the uniqueness of the human brain and of human cognition.
Restrictions: The Foundation does not fund: undergraduate tuition, stipends, scholarships, fellowships, research or travel expenses, or other educational expenses; graduate or postdoctoral stipends, scholarships, fellowships, research or travel expenses, or other educational expenses (exceptions include requests that qualify as allowable budget items as part of specific Research Award applications); expenses tied to projects whose explicit goal is the publication of a book or other bound volume (although publication of a book or special issue of a journal may be one goal or outcome of work funded by the Foundation); expenses tied to the establishment or day-to-day running of a journal or small press; scientific meetings or workshops other than those JSMF puts together or which are affiliated with Collaborative Activity Awards; ongoing operational support for university-based centers, programs, or institutes; professional society meetings or specific sessions at such meetings; charitable functions, museum exhibitions, or similar causes or events; or charitable donations to individuals and organizations.
Contact: Cheryl Washington, Grants Manager; (314) 721-1532; fax: (314) 721-7421; email: washington@jmsf.org or info@jmsf.org
Internet: http://www.jsmf.org/programs/uhc/index.htm
Sponsor: James S. McDonnell Foundation
1034 S. Brentwood Boulevard, Suite 1850
Saint Louis, MO 63117

Jane Beattie Memorial Scholarship **1901**
The purpose of the fund is to provide scholarships to subsidize travel to the U.S. for purposes of scholarly activity by a foreign scholar in the area of judgment and decision research, broadly defined. Attendance at the annual SJDM meetings is one example of an activity that would be appropriate for support, but by no means the only one. In most years, the Fund awards one or two scholarships in amounts of $400 - $700 each.
Requirements: Applicants should be scholars living and working in a country other than the U.S. who will use the award to help pay for travel to the U.S. for scholarly activities associated with research in judgment and decision making. It is anticipated that most awards will be granted to faculty or graduate students at colleges and universities, especially recent and soon-to-be Ph.D.'s, but others will also be considered. The required application form can be downloaded from: http://gsbwww.uchicago.edu/fac/joshua.klayman/more/BeattieForm.rtf
Restrictions: U.S. Scholars are not eligible to apply.
Amount of Grant: $400 - $700
Date(s) Application is Due: Jul 26
Contact: Joshua Klayman; University of Chicago Graduate School of Business; fax: (773) 834-9134; email: joshk@uchicago.edu
Internet: http://www.sjdm.org/content/beattie-award
Sponsor: Society for Judgment and Decision Making
c/o Bud Fennema, College of Business, Florida State University, P.O. Box 3061110
Tallahassee, FL 32306-1110

Jane Bradley Pettit Foundation Grants **1902**
The Foundation awards grants to initiate and sustain projects in the Greater Milwaukee community, with a focus on programs and projects that serve low-income and disadvantaged individuals, women, children, and the elderly. Grants are awarded to charitable organizations that address these concerns through arts and culture, community and social development, education and health. Initial application should be in the form of a letter of Intent. Application information is available online.
Requirements: Milwaukee-area charitable organizations are eligible.
Geographic Focus: Wisconsin
Date(s) Application is Due: Jan 15; May 15; Sep 15
Contact: Cheryll C. Whiteside, Assistant Director; (414) 227-1266; email: whiteside@cf-law.com
Internet: http://www.jbpf.org/guidelines/index.html
Sponsor: Jane Bradley Pettit Foundation
660 East Mason Street, Fourth Floor
Milwaukee, WI 53202

Jane Coffin Childs Memorial Fund for Medical Research Fellowships **1903**
The fellowships are for furthering of research into the causes, origins, and treatment of cancer. The major effort of the fund, at this time, is directed toward the support of a fellowship program for the training of young men and women at the postdoctoral level for independent research in the same field. Stipend, child dependency allowance, travel for fellow and family, and an institutional allowance are provided. Fellowships are awarded for two to three years.
Requirements: Applicants should not have more than one year of postdoctoral experience. They must either hold the MD degree or PhD degree in the field in which they propose to study. Applicants may be citizens of any country, but awards for foreign nationals will be made only for study in the United States. American citizens may hold fellowships either in the United States or in a foreign country.
Amount of Grant: $41,000 first year, $42,000 second year, $44,000 third year; plus $1500 research allowance per year
Date(s) Application is Due: Feb 1
Contact: Kim Roberts, Administrative Director, (203) 785-4612; fax: (203) 785-3301; email: info@jccfund.org
Internet: http://www.jccfund.org
Sponsor: Jane Coffin Childs Memorial Fund for Medical Research
P.O. Box 208000, 333 Cedar Street
New Haven, CT 06520

Jane's Trust Grants **1904**
The Jane's Trust has particular interest in organizations and projects which primarily benefit underserved populations and disadvantaged communities. Jane's Trust will support grants for general operating purposes, as well, as it's Fields of Interest, which are: arts and culture, education, the environment, health and welfare. The Trust will make grants in the states of Florida, with a preference for southwest and central Florida; Massachusetts, with a preference for greater Boston and eastern Massachusetts; and in the northern New England states of Maine, New Hampshire and Vermont. Preference will be given to organizations located in those states for projects which will primarily provide benefits within those states. The application process begins by submitting of a concept paper. Guidelines are available at the Trusts website.
Requirements: 501(c)3 tax-exempt organizations in Florida, Maine, Massachusetts, New Hampshire, and Vermont are eligible.
Restrictions: Jane's Trust will not support: loans to charitable organizations; attempts to influence legislation; requests from individuals. Please note: Jane's Trust will normally not support public entities, such as municipalities, municipal departments, or public schools directly, but will entertain applications from tax-exempt fiscal agents or partners for collaborative projects with municipalities or schools. This does not apply to public colleges and universities.
Geographic Focus: Florida; Maine; Massachusetts; New Hampshire; Vermont
Samples: Good Shepherd Food-Bank, Auburn, ME, $30,000—for operating support, payable over one year for agency matching funds project to provide for local food pantries and agencies across Maine (2008); Boca Grande Health Clinic Foundation, Inc., Boca Grande, FL, $150,000—capital support in the amount of $100,000 for the renovation of the Boca Grande Health Clinic Annex, $50,000 in endowment support, for the Boca Grande Health Clinic (2008); The Conservation Fund, Arlington, VA, $100,000—capital support for protection of the Three Sisters Springs in Crystal River, Florida, a wintering manatee habitat (2008); Kimball Union Academy, Meriden, NH, $150,000—capital support, payable over two years for construction and renovation of school campus (2008); Vermont Symphony Orchestra, Burlington, VT, $100,000—endowment support for Symphony Kids education programs (2008).
Amount of Grant: $50,000-$1,000,000
Date(s) Application is Due: Jan 25; Jul 15
Contact: Susan Fish, Grants Administrator; (617) 227-7940, ext. 775; fax: (617) 227-0781; email: sfish@hembar.com
Internet: http://www.hembar.com/selectsrv/janes/index.html
Sponsor: Hemenway and Barnes LLP
60 State Street
Boston, MA 02109-1899

Janirve Foundation Grants 1905

The Janirve Foundation, established in 1954, givings primarily to colleges and universities in western North Carolina. However, the Foundation also supports organizations involved with: children and youth services; community/economic development; environment; environment, natural resources; environment, plant conservation; family services; health organizations, association; higher education; hospitals (general); housing/shelter, development; human services.

Requirements: Applicants should contact Asheville, North Carolina, office for application procedures. Proposals from colleges and universities are considered only in the front quarter. Application form required. Applicants should submit the following: copy of IRS Determination Letter; detailed description of project and amount of funding requested; listing of additional sources and amount of support; how project's results will be evaluated or measured; how project will be sustained once grant support is completed; copy of current year's organizational budget and/or project budget; copy of most recent annual report/audited financial statement/990; listing of board of directors, trustees, officers and other key people and their affiliations; signature and title of chief executive officer; five copies of the proposal.

Restrictions: No support for public and private elementary schools, or churches and religious programs. No grants to individuals (except for scholarships), or generally for operating budgets, endowments or for research programs, publication of books or printed material, theatrical productions, videos, radio or television programs; no loans.

Geographic Focus: North Carolina

Amount of Grant: $10,000-$750,000 range

Date(s) Application is Due: Mar 1; Jun 1; Sep 1; Dec 1

Contact: E. Charles Dyson, Chairman; (828) 258-1877; fax: (828) 258-1837; email: janirve@charterinternet.com

Sponsor: Janirve Foundation
1 North Pack Square, Suite 416
Asheville, NC 28801-3409

Japan Heart Foundation Grants 1906

The foundation awards grants in Japan to individuals, organizations, and research institutes for research projects in the area of heart and blood vessel diseases.

Requirements: Research institutes for research in the area of heart and blood vessel diseases, individuals, and organizations in Japan are eligible to apply.

Contact: Grants Administrator, 81-3-3201-0810; fax: 81-3-3213-3920; email: info@jhf.or.jp

Internet: http://www.jhf.or.jp

Sponsor: Japan Heart Foundation
835-A, New Kokusai Bldg,3-4-1, Marunouchi
Chiyoda-ku, Tokyo 100-0005 Japan

Jasper Foundation Jasper County Grants 1907

The purpose of the Foundations is to assist donors in creating a source of assets to meet the ongoing and changing charitable needs and interests of the people living in all of our Jasper and Newton County, Indiana communities. As a Foundation, special emphasis is placed on programs that enrich the quality of life of our community in five distinct areas: arts and culture; preservation of historic and cultural resources; education; health; and social concerns. Applications and guidelines may be obtained from the Foundation office or at the foundations website.

Requirements: The Jasper Foundation welcomes grant applications from non-profit organizations whose programs benefit the residents of Jasper County. Favored grant requests will generally reflect the following characteristics: projects which propose practical solutions to community needs; projects which promote cooperation among existing agencies without duplicating services; projects that will become self-sustaining without requiring on-going Foundation funds.

Restrictions: Grants are not normally made for budget deficits or sectarian religious activities.

Geographic Focus: Indiana

Samples: Jasper County Historical Society - funds to refurbish the interior of the building, $1,500 (2008); Portage Township Education Foundation – funds for financial support for the students from Jasper County, $1,500 (2008); Pathway Family Center – funds to provide a comprehensive range of substance abuse prevention and intervention services to adolescents in the context of their family, $7,000 (2008);

Date(s) Application is Due: Apr 1; Oct 1

Contact: Linda Reiners, Executive Director; (219) 866-5899; fax: (219) 866-0555

Internet: http://www.jasperfdn.org/grants.htm

Sponsor: Jasper Foundation, Inc.
301 N. Van Rensselaer Street / P.O. Box 295
Rensslear, IN 47978

Jasper Foundation Newton County Grants 1908

The purpose of the Foundations is to assist donors in creating a source of assets to meet the ongoing and changing charitable needs and interests of the people living in all of our Jasper and Newton County, Indiana communities. The Newton County Community Foundation welcomes grant applications from non-profit organizations whose programs benefit the residents of Newton County. Grant applications are available in the Foundation office or online at the foundations website.

Requirements: Favored grant requests will generally reflect the following characteristics: projects which propose practical solutions to community needs; projects which promote cooperation among existing agencies without duplicating services; projects that will become self-sustaining without requiring on-going Foundation funds; grants are not normally made for budget deficits or sectarian religious activities. No restrictions are placed on gifts to these funds, allowing the Board of Directors to address community needs.

Geographic Focus: Indiana

Samples: Morocco Lions Club, $1,500 - funding for improvement of the Morocco Lions Club den and kitchen, purchase of stove and commercial coffee maker (2008); Newton/Jasper Community Band, $3,000 - funds to help purchase a tuba that will enable the tuba section to function on a higher level (2008)

Date(s) Application is Due: Apr 1; Oct 1

Contact: Linda Reiners, Executive Director; (219) 866-5899; fax: (219) 866-0555

Internet: http://www.jasperfdn.org/newtgrants.htm

Sponsor: Jasper Foundation, Inc.
301 N. Van Rensselaer Street / P.O. Box 295
Rensslear, IN 47978

Jay and Rose Phillips Family Foundation Grants 1909

The Jay and Rose Phillips Family Foundation has five funding priorities that guide it's grant making: strengthening families; supporting training and education for lifelong success; improving health and wellness; promoting independence and inclusion for people with disabilities and the elderly; and fostering good relations and civic participation. These funding priorities are the combined product of responding to community needs, the legacy of our founders and the current passions and interests of it's Trustees. Across all of these funding priorities, the Foundation place's a high value on supporting efforts that serve the most vulnerable in the community and those with the least access to resources. The Foundation has three program grant rounds each year with deadlines of March 15, July 15 and November 15. All proposals be submitted electronically using an online proposal submission process. The online submission deadline is 11:59 p.m. on the deadline date. The Foundation accepts requests for capital grants once per year through an online Letter of Inquiry (LOI) process. LOI's must be submitted by 11:59 p.m. on January 8.

Requirements: The Foundation awards grants only to organizations which are tax-exempt and publicly supported under Section 501(c)3 of the Internal Revenue Service Code. Grants are awarded primarily in the Twin Cities metropolitan area. Unsolicited proposals are not accepted from organizations located outside of Minnesota.

Restrictions: The foundation does not make grants in support of individuals, for political campaigns, or for lobbying efforts to influence legislation.

Geographic Focus: Minnesota

Samples: Washburn Center for Children, Minneapolis, MN, $40,000—expansion of the school-based mental health services program (2009); Child Care WORKS, Minneapolis, MN, $25,000—support for the Child Care Quality Initiative (2009); Urban Boatbuilders Inc., St. Paul, MN, $20,000—start-up support for the Youth Work Experience Intern Project (2009).

Amount of Grant: $10,000-$100,000 range

Date(s) Application is Due: Jan 8; Mar 15; Jul 15; Nov 15

Contact: Dana Jensen, Grants Manager; (612) 623-1652 or (612) 623-1654; fax: (612) 623-1653; email: djensen@phillipsfnd.org

Internet: http://www.phillipsfnd.org/index.asp?page_seq=15

Sponsor: Jay and Rose Phillips Family Foundation
East Bridge Building, 10 Second Street, N.E., Suite 200
Minneapolis, MN 55413

JDF Career Development Awards 1910

The program awards grants to applicants who have demonstrated superior scholarship and show the greatest promise for future achievement in diabetes research, including either clinically relevant research or basic research. The research plan should be suitable for a five-year project, and awardees must spend at least 75 percent of time and effort on the research project during the period of the award. Research may be conducted at foreign and domestic, for-profit and nonprofit, and public and private organizations such as universities, colleges, hospitals, laboratories, units of state and local governments, and eligible agencies of the federal government. Letters of reference are due two weeks before the application deadline, which are July 15 and January 16.

Requirements: Candidates must have the doctoral degree or the equivalent from an accredited institution, with three to seven years of total professional postdoctoral clinical and/or research experience by the projected start of the award period. Candidate's institution must be a university, medical school, or comparable institution with strong, well-established research and training programs in the chosen area. Research may be conducted at foreign and domestic, for-profit and nonprofit, public and private laboratories; units of state and local governments; and eligible agencies of the federal government.

Restrictions: Individuals holding academic positions of associate professor or professor at the time of the award are not eligible.

Amount of Grant: $150,000 per year

Date(s) Application is Due: Jan 16; Jul 15

Contact: Grant Administrator, (212) 479-7565; fax: (212) 785-9595; email: fellowships@jdrf.org

Internet: http://www.jdrf.org/index.cfm?page_id=103291

Sponsor: Juvenile Diabetes Foundation International
120 Wall Street, 19th Floor
New York, NY 10005-4001

Jean and Louis Dreyfus Foundation Grants 1911

The Jean and Louis Dreyfus Foundation was established in 1979 from the estate of Louis Dreyfus, a music publisher, and that of his wife, Jean. The mission of the Foundation is to enhance the quality of life of New Yorkers, particularly the aging and disadvantaged.

The Foundation disburses grants mainly within the five boroughs of New York City, and supports programs in the arts, health and social services (including youth agencies, women, and the elderly), and education (including literacy). Support is given for program development and matching funds. Application forms are not required. The board meets each year in the spring and in the fall. Initial inquiries should consist of a one or two page letter describing the organization and outlining the project in question. The January 15th and July 15th deadlines are for Letters of Intent.
Requirements: New York City nonprofits are eligible.
Restrictions: Grants are never made to individuals.
Geographic Focus: New York
Date(s) Application is Due: Jan 15; Jul 15
Contact: essica Keuskamp, Program Director; (212) 599-1931; fax: (212) 599-2956; email: jldreyfusfdtn@hotmail.com
Internet: http://foundationcenter.org/grantmaker/dreyfus/guide.html
Sponsor: Jean and Louis Dreyfus Foundation
420 Lexington Avenue, Suite 626
New York, NY 10170

Jeanne Humphrey Block Dissertation Award **1912**
The grant assists dissertation research on the psychological development of women and girls for a doctoral student who is a woman. Proposals should focus on the sex and gender differences or some other developmental issue of particular concern to women or girls. Priority will be given to projects that draw on or contribute to the resources of the Murray Research Center. Research concerned with the life experiences of racially and ethnically diverse populations within the United States is encouraged.
Requirements: Any female student currently enrolled in a doctoral program in a relevant field is eligible to apply. Dissertation proposals must be approved by an advisor or committee before the grant application is submitted.
Amount of Grant: $5000 maximum
Date(s) Application is Due: Apr 1
Contact: Grants Program Administrator, Jeanne Humphrey Block Dissertation Awards Program, (617) 495-8140; fax: (617) 496-3993; email: mrc@radcliffe.com
Internet: http://www.murray.harvard.edu/mra/index.jsp
Sponsor: Radcliffe College Henry A. Murray Research Center
10 Garden Street
Cambridge, MA 02138

Jeffress Research Grants **1913**
The trust supports research in chemical, medical, or other scientific fields through grants to nonprofit educational, charitable, scientific, literary, and research institutions in the Commonwealth of Virginia. Types of support include assistantships, fellowships, research grants, and program grants. Grants are awarded for one year, with possible renewal for two additional years. The deadline for receipt of applications for consideration at the May meeting is March 1; for the November meeting, September 1.
Requirements: Tax-exempt institutions are eligible.
Geographic Focus: Virginia
Amount of Grant: $30,000 maximum first year; $10,000 maximum renewal per year for two years
Date(s) Application is Due: Mar 1; Sep 1
Contact: Dr. Richard Brandt, Advisor, Bank of America , Jeffress Memorial Trust, (804) 788-3698; fax: (804) 788-2700
Internet: http://www.wm.edu/grants/OPPS/jeffress.htm
Sponsor: Jeffress Memorial Trust
P.O. Box 26688
Richmond, VA 23261-6688

JELD-WEN Foundation Grants **1914**
The Foundation seeks to improve the quality of life in company-operating areas and awards grants in the areas of capital campaigns, education, youth activities, community development, health and medical, and arts and humanities. Types of support include building construction/renovation, equipment, general operating support, land acquisition, matching/challenge support, program development, scholarship funds, and seed money. Prescreening and application information are available online.
Requirements: Nonprofit organizations in the Foundation's area of operations.
Samples: Knox Community Hospital, Mt. Vernon, OH, $500,000—grant to help build an outpatient cancer treatment center (2008); Crater Lake Science and Learning Center, Crater Lake, OR, $500,000—to help build the Science and Learning Center at Crater lake National Park (2008); Yakima Valley Museum, Yakima, WA, $250,000—to upgrade and improve the museum facility (2008).
Amount of Grant: $1000-$1,000,000
Contact: JELD-WEN Foundation Headquarters, (503) 478-4478; fax: (503) 478-4474
Internet: http://www.jeld-wenfoundation.org/
Sponsor: Jeld-Wen Foundation
200 SW Market Street, Suite 550
Portland, OR 97201

Jenkins Foundation: Improving the Health of Greater Richmond Grants **1915**
The foundation is committed to expanding access to community-based services through programs and organizations that have the potential to make a significant impact on the quality of health, especially for the youth in its local area.
Requirements: The current areas of focus are: Expanding access to health care services for the uninsured and underserved; Substance abuse prevention services that promote healthy lifestyles and increase availability of services; Violence prevention services that promote safe and healthy environments for children and their families and work toward the elimination of violence in the local communities; In addition, the foundation is committed to the long-term viability of the organizations it supports, and will consider capacity building grants that strengthen an agency's ability to better serve its clients. The foundation will also consider a limited number of proposals outside the above stated focus areas.
Restrictions: Proposals will be accepted from charitable organizations, which serve the residents of the City of Richmond and the counties of Chesterfield, Hanover, Henrico, Goochland, and Powhatan.
Geographic Focus: Virginia
Amount of Grant: up to $50,000
Date(s) Application is Due: May 5; Nov 5
Contact: Elaine Summerfield, Program Officer; (804) 330-7400; fax: (804) 330-5992; email: esummerfield@tcfrichmond.org
Internet: http://www.tcfrichmond.org/Page2954.cfm#Jenkins
Sponsor: Community Foundation Serving Richmond and Central Virginia
7501 Boulders View Drive, Suite 110
Richmond, VA 23225

Jennings County Community Foundation Grants **1916**
The foundation seeks to serve philanthropic and charitable needs in Jennings County, Indiana, by offering endowment services, grant making, scholarships, donor estate and planned gift services to individuals and qualified organizations serving the community of Jennings County, Indiana. The foundations field of interest include: arts; community/economic development; education; health care; human services.
Requirements: Submit 6 copies of the grant proposal; funding is given primarily in the in the Jennings County, Indiana area; contact foundation office for more details
Restrictions: No grants to individuals (except for scholarships)
Geographic Focus: Indiana
Date(s) Application is Due: Mar 1; Sep 1
Contact: Jean Hahn, Executive Director; (812) 346-5553; fax: (812) 346-5553; email: jcff@comcast.net
Internet: http://www.jenningsfoundation.net/index.html
Sponsor: Jennings County Community Foundation, Inc.
265 East Main Street
North Vernon, IN 47265-1510

Jerome and Mildred Paddock Foundation Grants **1917**
The Foundation was established in 1967 to benefit disadvantaged children and elderly populations. Primarily, the foundation is interested in funding programming needs that will improve the quality of life of those less fortunate. Field of interest include: aging; children and youth services; programs for economically disadvantaged; health care support; and human/social services. Though giving is focused in and around Sarasota, the foundation does extend funding beyond Florida. The deadline is January 10th, with final notification by March 15th.
Restrictions: No grants to individuals, or for endowments, debt reduction, operating expenses, conferences or seminars, workshops, travel, surveys, advertising, research, fund raising or for annual campaigns or capital campaigns.
Samples: Florida Studio Theatre, Sarasota, Florida, $10,000—to partially fund the VIP Performing Arts Program for special needs youth (2008); Shodair Childrens Hospital, Helena, Montana, $30,000—to purchase a Coulter automated cell counter (2008); Samaritan Counseling Services, Ann Arbor, Michigan, $10,000—to assist low income, under-insured and uninsured clients (2008).
Amount of Grant: $15,000 average
Date(s) Application is Due: Jan 10
Contact: Joan Greenwood, Charitable Associate, Wachovia Bank, N.A.: (941) 361-5803; email: joan.greenwood@wachovia.com
Sponsor: Jerome and Mildred Paddock Foundation
Wachovia Bank, N.A., P.O. Box 267
Sarasota, FL 34230

Jessie B. Cox Charitable Trust Grants **1918**
The Trust is dedicated to improving the environment and the quality of life for people living in the six New England States. To achieve its goals, the Trust pursues initiatives in three key fields of interest: education: early learning, out-of-school time; environment: habitat conservation, concentrating on fresh and marine water protection; health: access to health care. In all of these funding areas, the Trust is mindful of its special status as one of the few funders with an interest in all six of the New England states. Applications for funding are reviewed in light of the important issues of the region. The Grants Committee meets twice per year to award grants, in April and October. The Trust has a two-step system of application, beginning with a concept paper and progressing to a full grant proposal. Concept papers are due on March 15 and September 15. Applicants who have submitted a concept paper and been asked to submit a complete proposal must do so by July 1 (March applicants) or January 5 (September applicants).
Requirements: All grant applicants are asked to demonstrate a plan for measuring their success. This plan should identify benchmarks against which progress towards identified goals can be measured. Grantees must report on their progress within a year of receiving support and on project completion, with reference to the initial benchmarks.
Restrictions: The Cox Trust does not normally support: general operating support and ongoing maintenance; buildings, equipment or land acquisition; endowments, scholarship funds, or fundraising activities; grant requests of under $50,000; projects for which the Trust is the sole or predominant source of support; programs for which the public sector

normally assumes funding responsibility; core educational programs of public, private, parochial, or charter schools; requests from individuals; sectarian religious activity.
Geographic Focus: Connecticut; Maine; Massachusetts; New England; New Hampshire; Rhode Island; Vermont
Date(s) Application is Due: Mar 15; Sep 15; Jul 1; Jan 5
Contact: Kirstie David, Program Manager; (617) 391-3081; email: kdavid@gmafoundations.com
Internet: http://www.jbcoxtrust.org/?page_id=28
Sponsor: Jessie B. Cox Charitable Trust
c/o GMA Foundations, 77 Summer Street, 8th Floor
Boston, MA 02110-1006

Jessie Ball Dupont Fund Grants **1919**

The fund is a national foundation having a special, though not exclusive, interest in issues affecting the South. Grants awarded include competitive grants—program grants, institutional development, and capacity building; and feasibility grants—smaller grants that enable institutions to carefully explore and develop new concepts and programs. Areas of interest include six focus areas: strengthening the independent sector; organizing and nurturing philanthropy; building assets of people, families, and communities; building the capacity of eligible organizations; stimulating community problem solving; and helping people hold their communities accountable. The fund supports four initiatives: the religion initiative, the nonprofit initiative, the small liberal arts colleges initiative, and the independent schools initiative. Types of support include general operating support, building construction/renovation, equipment acquisition, program development, seed money grants, publication, consulting services, professorships, curriculum development, matching funds, and technical assistance. Grants are awarded generally for one year. The trustees meet in January, March, May, July, September, and November to consider requests.
Requirements: Applying organizations must have received a contribution from Mrs. DuPont between the five-year period of January 1, 1960, and December 31, 1964.
Samples: Jacksonville Symphony Assoc (FL)—to implement a strategic marketing program, $50,000 (2005); Historical Society of Delaware (Wilmington, DE)—to hire a consultant to lead a community-based strategic-planning process, $52,690 (2005); Episcopal Diocese of Southern Ohio (Cincinnati, OH)—to support a partnership with Scioto Christian Ministries to conduct a needs-assessment in Ohio's Scioto County, $28,000 (2005); U of Richmond (VA)—to support the creation of an Internet-based resource center that will serve community organizations in the Northern Neck region of Virginia, $219,975 (2005).
Amount of Grant: $2000-$5000 range for feasibility grants
Contact: Geana Potter, Grants Manager; (904) 353-0890 or (800) 252-3452; fax: (904) 353-3870; email: contactus@dupontfund.org
Internet: http://www.dupontfund.org
Sponsor: Jessie Ball Dupont Fund
One Independent Drive, Suite 1400
Jacksonville, FL 32202-0511

Jessie Smith Noyes Foundation Grants **1920**

The foundation is committed to preventing damage to the natural systems upon which all life depends and to strengthening individuals and institutions committed to protecting natural systems and ensuring a sustainable society. The foundation makes grants primarily in the interrelated areas of environment and reproductive rights. The program components include toxics, sustainable agriculture (both with emphasis on southern and Rocky Mountain states), and U.S. reproductive rights. In addition, a few grants are made in four areas of special concern: sustainable communities, U.S. environmental justice, strengthening the U.S. nonprofit sector, and environmental issues in the metropolitan New York region. Letters of inquiry are received at any time; proposals will be requested from the foundation after review.
Requirements: 501(c)3 tax-exempt organizations are eligible.
Restrictions: Normally, the foundation will not consider requests for direct service, endowments, loans or scholarships to individuals, capital construction funds, conferences, media events, production of media and TV programming, or general fund-raising drives. General research projects are not funded per se.
Samples: Northwest Women's Law Ctr (Seattle, WA)—for its contributions to the field of reproductive-health care and rights in Alaska, Idaho, Montana, Oregon, and Washington State, $100,000 (2005).
Contact: Millie Buchanan, Program Officer, (212) 684-6577; fax: (212) 689-6549; email: noyes@noyes.org
Internet: http://www.noyes.org
Sponsor: Jessie Smith Noyes Foundation
6 E 39th Street, 12th Floor
New York, NY 10016-0112

Jewish Community Foundation of Greater Los Angeles Grants **1921**

The community foundation exists to assist social service agencies in meeting the needs of the Jewish community and the Los Angeles community at large. Major giving categories include community grants, Israel grants, comprehensive development grant projects, and restricted (special purposes) grants. Areas of interest include community and health services, education, social services, arts, and culture. Types of support include awards, building construction/renovation, challenge/matching grants, conferences and seminars, development grants, endowments, internships, program development grants, and seed money grants. Grants are made for a one- or two-year period and are not renewable.
Geographic Focus: California
Amount of Grant: $45 million total
Contact: Grants Administrator, (323) 761-8700; fax: (323) 761-8720; email: info@jewishfoundationla.org
Internet: http://www.jewishfoundationla.org/home1.html
Sponsor: Jewish Community Foundation
6505 Wilshire Boulevard, Suite 1200
Los Angeles, CA 90048

Jewish Foundation for Education of Women Scholarships for Emigres in the Health Professions **1922**

Scholarships are awarded to women emigres from the former Soviet Union for graduate and undergraduate education in medicine, dentistry, nursing, or pharmacy. Approximately 48 scholarships are awarded. Applications are available in late October.
Requirements: Eligible to apply are women who are emigres from the former Soviet Union, live within a 50-mile radius of New York City, and demonstrate financial need.
Restrictions: Pre-medical students are not eligible. Applications submitted directly from students are not accepted.
Geographic Focus: New York
Samples: Jewish Foundation for Education of Women (New York, NY)—to administer scholarships for emigres from the New Independent States who are enrolled in occupational therapy, physical therapy, or physician's assistant programs, $300,000 over three years.
Amount of Grant: $5000
Date(s) Application is Due: Jun 1
Contact: Marge Goldwater, Executive Director, (212) 288-3931; fax: (212) 288-5798; email: FdnScholar@aol.com
Internet: http://www.jfew.org/programs.html#HP
Sponsor: Jewish Foundation for Education of Women
135 East 64th Street
New York, NY 10021

Jewish Fund Grants **1923**

The fund awards grants to sustain, enrich, and address the overall health care needs of both the Jewish community and general community in the metropolitan Detroit area. Funding priorities include programs that address priorities and program initiatives of the DMC/Sinai Hospital; the health care needs of vulnerable/at- risk populations in the general community; and efforts to further positive relationships between the Jewish community and the Detroit community. The fund gives priority to requests for start-up or short-term operating support; new programs within a defined period that address a critical need; and geographical priority to the metropolitan Detroit area of Wayne, Oakland, and Macomb counties. Preference will be given to proposals that can be funded and replicated by others; have a specific plan for continuation funding beyond the grant period; include a financial or in-kind contribution from the organization; involve collaboration with others; and have a well-defined outcome-based evaluation plan. The fund generally will not support a project for more than three years. The first step in the application process is to submit a letter of intent in March or September. Obtain an application packet containing complete guidelines from the office.
Requirements: Michigan 501(c)3 nonprofit organizations that serve the Jewish and/or Detroit communities are eligible.
Geographic Focus: Michigan
Samples: Detroit Institute for Children (Detroit, MI)—to subsidize services for disadvantaged children with special needs, $100,000 (2005); Jewish Community Council (Bloomfield Hills, MI) and Kids Kicking Cancer (Detroit, MI)—to develop a program that uses the martial arts to empower Detroit Public School students to overcome adversity, $300,000 jointly over three years (2005); City Connect (Detroit, MI)—for efforts to increase financial support from the federal government and foundations for the City of Detroit and nonprofit groups in the Detroit area, $20,000 (2005); Arthritis Foundation of Michigan (Southfield, MI)—to develop a comprehensive arthritis education and management program for Jews in the Detroit area, $50,000 (2005).
Contact: Jodee Fishman Raines, Director, The Jewish Fund, (248) 203-1487; fax: (248) 645-7879; email: raines@jfmd.org
Sponsor: Jewish Fund
6735 Telegraph Road
Bloomfield, MI 48303-2030

Jewish Women's Foundation of New York Grants **1924**

The foundation provides support for unmet social, economic, and health needs of Jewish females in the New York metropolitan area and beyond. Strategic grants support cutting-edge projects that address Jewish education, training, and culture—projects related to education, training of educators, leadership development, ethics, spirituality, arts, sports, etc.; mental and physical health—projects involving genetics, self-esteem, violence prevention, issues concerning the end of life, and other areas that relate to women's health as a quality of life; and economic empowerment—projects that give women more independence, knowledge, competency, and responsibility for their economic situations. Grant requests may address innovative programs, services, and/or research. The projects primary target group must be Jewish females. The foundation expects to award three to four grants. The listed deadline is for concept letters; full proposals are by invitation.
Requirements: 501(c)3 tax-exempt organizations in the New York metropolitan area (the five boroughs of New York City, Long Island and/or Westchester) are eligible.
Restrictions: The foundation will not provide grants for scholarships, equipment, capital campaigns, or ongoing support for existing programs.
Geographic Focus: New York
Samples: Jewish Orthodox Feminist Alliance (New York, NY)—to create a gender-sensitive curriculum for use in Jewish Orthodox day schools, $20,000 (2004); Jewish

Outreach Institute (New York, NY)—to develop a program for women who are new to Judaism, $20,000 (2004); Sharsheret (New York, NY)—for a symposium on breast-cancer genetics and Jewish women, $10,000 (2004); Women's Electoral Power (Tel Aviv, Israel)—for workshops for women seeking public office in Israel, $10,000 (2004).
Amount of Grant: $25,000 maximum
Date(s) Application is Due: Sep 30
Contact: Sherri Greenbach, Executive Director, (212) 836-1478; fax: (212) 836-1831
Internet: http://www.jewishwomenny.org
Sponsor: Jewish Women's Foundation of New York
130 E 59th Street, Room 563
New York, NY 10022

Jim Moran Foundation Grants 1925

The mission of the foundation is to improve the quality of life for the youth and families of Florida through the support of innovative programs and opportunities that meet the ever-changing needs of the community. The foundation's funding focuses include: education; literacy; meaningful after school programs; equitable access to technology; and domestic and child abuse intervention. Organizations interested in receiving a grant should submit a letter of inquiry of no more than two typewritten pages to include a proposal summary, proposal budget, project timeline, and anticipated outcomes. Full applications are by invitation.
Requirements: 501(c)3 tax-exempt organizations are eligible. Additionally, the organization must be appropriately recognized by state statutes, laws and regulations that govern tax exempt organizations.
Restrictions: The foundation generally will not consider requests for administrative/overhead costs, sponsorships, or capital campaigns.
Geographic Focus: Florida
Samples: Children's Home Society of Florida (Fort Lauderdale, FL)—for the Reading Enhancement and Development Program, $6387.; Gateway Community Outreach (Deerfield Beach, FL)—to underwrite a portion of the purchase of food staples provided to families in Gateway's 90-day program, $10,000.; Literacy Coalition of Broward County (FL)—for a pediatric literacy program that encourages parents to read to their children on a daily basis, $20,000.; Migrant Assoc of South Florida (FL)—to fund after-school education and tutoring for children of migrant workers in the Boynton Beach school district, as well as program supplies and field trip transportation for these students in K-5, $40,000.
Contact: Grants Administrator, (954) 429-2122; fax: (954) 429-2699; email: information@jimmoranfoundation.org
Internet: http://www.jimmoranfoundation.org/grants_guidelines.asp
Sponsor: Jim Moran Foundation
100 Jim Moran Boulevard
Deerfield Beach, FL 33442

JM Foundation Grants 1926

The foundation awards grants to eligible nonprofit organizations in its areas of interest, including education and research that fosters market-based policy solutions; developing state and national organizations that promote free enterprise, entrepreneurship, and private initiative; and identifying and educating young leaders. Types of support include internships, matching/challenge grants, program grants, publication, research grants, seed grants, and technical assistance. The foundation's board of directors meets bi-annually, usually in May and October. There are no formal proposal deadlines. Inquiries and proposals are processed on an ongoing basis.
Requirements: Public charities, including 501(c)3, 509(a)1, and 170(b)1(a)(vi) nonprofit organizations, that shares the foundation's priority interests is invited to submit a proposal.
Restrictions: Grants do not support individuals, the arts, government agencies, public schools, and international agencies; or requests for operating expenses, annual fundraising campaigns, capital campaigns, equipment, endowment funds, and loans.
Samples: Acton Institute, Grand Rapids, Michigan, $20,000—in support of the Effective Compassion Initiative (2007); Center of the American Experiment, Minneapolis, Minnesota, $40,000—for Intellectual Takeout (2007); National Taxpayers Union Foundation, Alexandria, Virginia, $25,000—toward the National Taxpayers Conference (2007).
Amount of Grant: $5,000-$100,000 range
Contact: Carl Helstrom, Executive Director; (212) 687-7735; fax: (212) 697-5495
Internet: http://foundationcenter.org/grantmaker/jm/guide_jm.html
Sponsor: JM Foundation
654 Madison Avenue, Suite 1605
New York, NY 10065

Joe W. and Dorothy Dorsett Brown Foundation Grants 1927

The foundation awards grants to nonprofit organizations in Louisiana and the Gulf Coast of Mississippi. Areas of interest include medical research; housing for the homeless; support for organizations who care for the sick, hungry or helpless; religious and educational institutions; and organizations and groups concerned with improving the local community. Types of support include operating budgets, research, and student aid. The foundation also supports Service Learning, a learn-by-doing approach to the curriculum. Students receive practical, hands-on experience in the subject matter studied by meeting identified community needs through active participation. The listed deadline date is for Service Learning grants.
Requirements: Louisiana and Mississippi nonprofit organizations, with a focus on South Louisiana, the New Orleans area, and the Mississippi Gulf Coast, are eligible. Service Learning grant applications are available yearly to sixth through 12th grades in the following parishes: Orleans, Jefferson, Plaquemines, Saint Bernard, Saint Charles, Tangipahoa, Saint James, Saint John, Saint Tammany, and Washington.
Geographic Focus: Louisiana; Mississippi
Amount of Grant: $5000-$25,000 average
Date(s) Application is Due: Sep 30
Contact: Beth Buscher, (504) 834-3433; email: BethBuscher@thebrownfoundation.org
Internet: http://www.thebrownfoundation.org
Sponsor: Joe W. and Dorothy Dorsett Brown Foundation
320 Hammond Hwy, Suite 500
Metairie, LA 70005

John Ben Snow Memorial Trust Grants 1928

The mission of the Foundation is to make grants within specific focus areas to enhance the quality of life in Central and Northern New York State. Historically, the Foundation has made grants in the following program areas: arts and culture, community development, education, environment, historic preservation, and journalism. The Foundation responds to the ever-changing needs of various segments of the population, especially to the needs of young people and people who are disadvantaged either physically or economically. It is the Foundation's general policy to give preference to proposals seeking funds for new or enhanced programs, one-time, short-term grants to sustain a program until funding is stabilized, matching grants used to encourage the participation of other donors, and last dollars towards a capital campaign. There are no minimums or maximum grant amounts; however, most grants range from $5,000 to $15,000.
Requirements: Giving is primarily focused in Maryland, Nevada, and central New York.
Restrictions: The Foundation will not accept proposals from individuals or for-profit organizations. Additionally, the Foundation does not encourage proposals from religious organizations or proposals for endowments, contingency funding, or debt reduction.
Amount of Grant: $5,000-$25,000 average
Date(s) Application is Due: Apr 1
Contact: Jonathan L. Snow; (315) 471-5256; fax: (315) 471-5256
Internet: http://www.johnbensnow.com/jbsmt
Sponsor: John Ben Snow Memorial Trust
50 Presidential Plaza, Suite 106
Syracuse, NY 13202

John Deere Foundation Grants 1929

The foundation invests in programs in education, health/human services, community improvement, arts and culture. Types of support include annual campaigns, building construction/renovation, continuing support, fellowships, general operating support, scholarship funds, and seed money grants. Foundation interest also includes support for Third World development through U.S.-based nonprofits with international building funds, research grants, general operating purposes, and continuing support. There are no application deadlines.
Requirements: Nonprofit organizations in communities with major John Deere operating units, and employee presence are eligible. Eligible U.S. locations are: Augusta, GA; Quad City Region, IL; Des Moines, IA, Dubuque, IA, Iowa Quad Cities, IA, Ottumwa, IA, Waterloo, IA, Coffeyville, KS, Lenexa, KS, Thibodaux, LA, Springfield, MO, Cary, NC, Fuquay-Varina, NC, Fargo, ND, Greeneville, TN, Madison, WI, Horicon, WI. Exceptions include: accredited colleges and universities; organizations focused on international development initiatives related to John Deere Solutions for World Hunger initiative. Because John Deere dealerships are owned and operated independently, their communities are not included in this geographic scope. Also eligible to apply are organizations and institutions of national or international scope that reflect the foundation's concerns.
Restrictions: Funds are not available for the following organizations or purposes: individual initiatives, including scholarships; sports teams, racing teams, athletic endeavors or scholarships designated for athletes; faith-based organizations for sectarian purposes; political candidates, campaigns or organizations; private clubs, fraternities or sororities; other foundations for purposes of building endowment; tax-supported entities.
Geographic Focus: Georgia; Illinois; Iowa; Kansas; Louisiana; Missouri; North Carolina; Tennessee; WisconsinBrazil; Canada; Eastern Europe
Contact: Amy Nimmer Director, Corporate Citizenship Center of Excellence; (309) 765-8000;
Internet: http://www.deere.com/en_U.S./globalcitizenship/socialinvestment/index.html
Sponsor: John Deere Foundation
1 John Deere Place
Moline, IL 61265-8098

John Edward Fowler Memorial Foundation Grants 1930

The foundation makes grants to qualified charitable organizations providing grassroots programs for people in need in the Washington, DC, metropolitan area. Preference is given to programs that address the issues of homelessness, hunger, at-risk children and youth (pre-school through high school), adult literacy, free medical care (prenatal to seniors), seniors aging in place, job training and placement. Types of support include general operating support, building construction/renovation, equipment acquisition, program development, and matching funds. The foundation is interested in supporting smaller, well-managed nonprofit organizations that have innovative ideas about how to help people help themselves. Contact the office for application forms. There are no application deadlines.
Requirements: Organizations in Washington, DC, and its close Maryland and Virginia suburbs are eligible.

Restrictions: Grants are not made outside the metropolitan Washington, DC, area, or to/for national health organizations; government agencies; medical research; public school districts; individuals; or arts (except for intensive arts-in-education programs that directly benefit at-risk children and youth).
Geographic Focus: District of Columbia; Maryland; Virginia
Samples: Carpenter's Shelter, Alexandria, VA, $20,000 - housing with intensive supportive services for homeless adults and children (2008); Bucknell University, Lewisburg, PA , $10,000 - general support (2008); All Souls' Episcopal Church, Mechanicsville VA, $15,000 - Orphans Program of the Maseno Mission in Kenya (2008).
Amount of Grant: $5000-$10,000 typically; $20,000 minimum for long-time grantees
Contact: Suzanne Martin, Grant Consultant: (301) 654-2700;
Internet: http://fdncenter.org/grantmaker/fowler/about.html
Sponsor: John Edward Fowler Memorial Foundation
4340 East-West Highway, Suite 206
Bethesda, MD 20814

John G. Duncan Trust Grants **1931**
The trust awards grants in the following areas of interest: arts; education; health care; human services; religion; and support: building/renovation; capital campaigns; emergency funds; equipment; program development; seed money; and research. Contact the foundation, for the application guidelines and application form.
Requirements: IRS 501(c)3 organizations in Colorado are eligible.
Restrictions: No support for other grantmaking organizations, individuals, endowments, or for general operating expenses.
Geographic Focus: Colorado
Amount of Grant: $1,000-$10,000 range
Date(s) Application is Due: Jan 31; Apr 30; Jul 31; Oct 31
Contact: Jason Craig, c/o Wells Fargo Bank, N.A.; (720) 947-6820
Sponsor: John G. Duncan Trust
1740 Broadway, MAC C7300-483
Denver, CO 80274-0001

John G. Martin Foundation Grants **1932**
The foundation awards grants to eligible Connecticut nonprofit organizations in the areas of education at all levels. Grants may be considered in other areas. Preferential consideration will be given to proposals whose benefits include assistance to the aging and elderly or assistance to youth and adolescents. The foundation is interested in the long-term stabilization and advancement of effective organizations specializing in these areas of interest. Types of support include building construction/renovation, capital campaigns, and matching/challenge grants.
Requirements: Nonprofit organizations serving the Hartford, CT, area may submit applications.
Geographic Focus: Connecticut
Samples: Northwest Catholic High School, West Hartford, CT, $20,000 (2007); West Hartford Public Library, West Hartford, CT, $30,000 (2007); Northwest Catholic High School, West Hartford, CT, $20,000 (2007);
Amount of Grant: $10,000-$65,000 range
Contact: Frank Loehmann, President; (860) 677-4574; fax: (860) 674-1490; email: frank@resmgtcorp.com
Sponsor: John G. Martin Foundation
2 Batterson Park Road
Farmington, CT 06032-2553

John H. and Wilhelmina D. Harland Charitable Foundation Grants **1933**
The foundation, offers support for: youth services, community services, cultural programs, education, and health. The focus is local rather than regional or national, and priority is given to institutions in metropolitan Atlanta, Georgia. Grants support: building/renovation; capital campaigns; equipment; general/operating support; matching/challenge support; and scholarship funds. The Foundation prefers a telephone call as opposed to a letter of inquiry for the initial approach.
Requirements: Grant support is available to nonprofit organizations in Georgia, with emphasis on the metropolitan Atlanta area.
Restrictions: Grants are not awarded to individuals.
Geographic Focus: Georgia
Amount of Grant: $4000-$250,000 range
Date(s) Application is Due: Mar 1; Sep 1
Contact: Jane Hardesty, Executive Director; (404) 264-9912
Sponsor: John H. and Wilhelmina D. Harland Charitable Foundation
2 Piedmont Court, Suite 106
Atlanta, GA 30305-1567

John H. Wellons Foundation Grants **1934**
Established in 1950, the John H. Wellons Foundation, is a private foundation. The foundation's support is limited to the Dunn, North Carolina, area. The foundation awards student loans to local area residents, provides housing for the elderly and/or handicapped, and contributes to charitable organizations. There are no specific deadlines with which to adhere. Contact the Foundation for further application information and guidelines.
Geographic Focus: North Carolina
Contact: John H. Wellons, President; (910) 892-0436;
Sponsor: John H. Wellons Foundation, Inc.
P.O. Box 1254
Dunn, NC 28335-1254

John I. Smith Charities Grants **1935**
The foundation supports nonprofit organizations, primarily in South Carolina. With its areas of interest, including: the visual and performing arts, higher education, medical education, theological education, literacy education and basic skills, Christian agencies and churches, child welfare, and programs for the disabled. Grants support general operations, capital campaigns, endowment funds, scholarship funds, and emergency funds. Application forms are not required. The board meets on a quarterly basis. Mail applications to: P.O. Box 1687, Greer, SC 29652
Requirements: Nonprofit organizations in South Carolina are eligible to apply.
Geographic Focus: South Carolina
Samples: Furman University, Greenville, SC, $100,000 (2007); Alliance for Quality Education, Greenville, SC, $27,000 (2007); Columbia Theological Seminary, Decatur, GA, $200,000 (2007).
Amount of Grant: $2500-$200,000 range
Contact: Jefferson Smith, President; (864) 879-2455;
Sponsor: John I. Smith Charities Inc
P.O. Box 40200, FL9-100-10-19
Jacksonville, FL 32203-0200

John J. Leidy Foundation Grants **1936**
The John J. Leidy Foundation was established in 1957. The foundation gives primarily in the metropolitan Baltimore, Maryland, area. Funding is available to people with disabilities, education, health, social services, and Jewish organizations in the form of, scholarship funds, building/renovation, equipment, general/operating support, and program development grants.
Requirements: Maryland non-profits are eligible to apply.
Restrictions: No grants to individuals.
Geographic Focus: Maryland
Contact: Robert L. Pierson, President; (410) 821-3006; email: Leidyfd@attglobal.net
Sponsor: John J. Leidy Foundation
c/o Pierson & Pierson 305 W. Chesapeake Avenue, Suite 308
Towson, MD 21204-4440

John Jewett and Helen Chandler Garland Foundation Grants **1937**
Established in 1959, the John Jewett & Helen Chandler Garland Foundation gives primarily in California, with emphasis on southern California. The foundations area of interest include: the arts, education, health care, children and social services. There are no application deadlines.
Requirements: California nonprofit organizations are eligible.
Restrictions: No telephone inquiries excepted, submit a letter of inquiry as your initial approach.
Geographic Focus: California
Samples: Huntington Library, Friends of the, San Marino, CA, $800,000 - for general support and educational programs at Botanical Center (2004); Marlborough School, Los Angeles, CA, $25,000 - for general support and minority scholarships (2004); Boys and Girls Clubs of Pasadena, Pasadena, CA, $110,000 - for general support and to make swimming pool accessible year-round (2004).
Amount of Grant: $2,500 - $610,000 range
Contact: Lisa M. Hausler, Manager;
Sponsor: John Jewett & Helen Chandler Garland Foundation
P.O. Box 550
Pasadena, CA 91102-0550

John Lord Knight Foundation Grants **1938**
The Foundation, established in 1957, provides funding for program in the Lucas County, Ohio, region and throughout Florida. Its areas of interest include: cancer research; Christian agencies and churches; education; elementary education; federated giving programs; hospitals; human services; public libraries; and youth services. There are no specific deadlines, and applicants should submit a detailed description of project and amount of funding requested to the listed contact person in care of KeyBank.
Geographic Focus: Florida; Ohio
Contact: Erwin Diener, Trust Officer, KeyBank; (419) 259-8372
Sponsor: John Lord Knight Foundation
Three Seagate, P.O. Box 10099
Toledo, OH 43699-0099

John M. Lloyd Foundation Grants **1939**
The foundation has the following funding objectives: to increase funding from public and private sectors to address the HIV/AIDS pandemic, both globally and domestically; to improve domestic and international policies (universal protection of human rights to issues concerning HIV/AIDS, access to HIV/AIDS healthcare and treatment, and access to accurate information about HIV/AIDS); to amplify global awareness of HIV/AIDS and to facilitate broad-based change in attitudes to reduce stigma and change behavior; and to develop the leadership of organizations that fight HIV/AIDS, as well as to foster collaborations among those organizations and leaders. Projects that have promise of making a significant impact and those that are new and innovative receive preference. The listed application deadlines are for concept letters; full proposals are by invitation. Organizations may submit only one concept letter per year.
Requirements: 501(c)3 tax-exempt organizations are eligible. Grants are made to locally focused projects in California, U.S.-based projects with a national or global scope, and international projects.
Restrictions: In general, the foundation does not make contributions more than once per calendar year to any single organization; more than three consecutive years to any single

project; to annual campaigns; to operating budgets of established organizations; to capital expenditures (physical plant, equipment, endowment); to indirect costs; to individuals; to locally focused projects in the United States with the exception of locally focused projects in California; for health care or service provision; or for general support
Amount of Grant: $20,000 maximum
Date(s) Application is Due: Aug 15; Dec 15
Contact: Melanie Havelin, Executive Director; (310) 622-1050; fax: (310) 622-1070; email: Mhavelin@johnmlloyd.org
Internet: http://www.johnmlloyd.org/grant_programs.html
Sponsor: John M. Lloyd Foundation
11777 San Vicente Boulevard, Suite 745
Los Angeles, CA 90049

John Merck Fund Grants **1940**
The foundation fosters innovative advocacy and problem solving in the fields of Developmental Disabilities, Environment, Reproductive Health, Human Rights and Job Opportunities. Its objective is to act as a catalyst, supporting organizations that can effect constructive and measurable change in each of these areas.
Requirements: The foundation actively seeks out projects and programs that may merit support, then requests grant applications on behalf of those it finds most promising. It does not encourage the submission of unsolicited proposals. However, organizations interested in obtaining support for work they do in one of the foundation's areas of interest are welcome to send a brief letter of inquiry. The foundation favors: outstanding individuals working on promising projects in organizations that may have difficulty attracting funds; pilot projects with potential for widespread application; advocacy, including litigation, capable of setting or protecting important precedents; smaller organizations, start-ups included; one-year grant requests (though multi-year grants of up to three years occasionally are made); matching-grant opportunities, particularly to help broaden support for fledgling initiatives.
Restrictions: The foundation does not provide grants for: endowment or capital-fund projects; large organizations with well-established funding sources (except those that need help launching promising new projects for which funding is not readily available); general support (except in the case of small organizations whose entire mission coincides with one of foundation's areas of interest); individuals (except if his or her project is sponsored by a domestic or foreign educational, scientific or charitable organization).
Geographic Focus: Alabama; Alaska; Arizona; Arkansas; California; Colorado; Connecticut; Delaware; District of Columbia; Florida; Georgia; Hawaii; Idaho; Illinois; Indiana; Iowa; Kansas; Kentucky; Louisiana; Maine; Maryland; Massachusetts; Michigan; Midwest; Minnesota; Mississippi; Missouri; Montana; Nebraska; Nevada; New England; New Hampshire; New Jersey; New Mexico; New York; North Carolina; North Dakota; Northeast; Northwest; Ohio; Oklahoma; Oregon; Pacific Northwest; Pennsylvania; Rhode Island; South; South Carolina; South Dakota; Southwest; Tennessee; Texas; Utah; Vermont; Virginia; Washington; West; West Virginia; Wisconsin; Wyoming
Contact: Ruth G. Hennig, Executive Director; (617) 556-4120; fax: (617) 556-4130; email: info@jmfund.org
Internet: http://www.jmfund.org/program.html
Sponsor: John Merck Fund
47 Winter Street, 7th Floor
Boston, MA 02108

John Merck Scholars Awards **1941**
Scholars are chosen from the ranks of the most promising assistant professors currently working, or planning to work, in neurobiological and cognitive sciences relating to the biology of mental disability and developmental disabilities, including developmental studies of cognition, perception, language, reading, learning and motor performance. The foundation will accept one application for a neurobiologist and one for a cognitive scientist from major universities and other research centers. Scholars will receive $75,000 per year for a four-year period, subject to an annual review of research progress. The sponsoring institution is responsible for fiscal management.
Requirements: The foundation will fund the most promising young researchers whose work illuminates neurodevelopmental disorders from the perspectives of (i) synapse formation and synaptic plasticity; (ii) learning and memory, and synaptic plasticity; (iii) perception, cognition and behavior; (iv) neurogenesis and pattern formation; and (v) genetics and early development. Also encouraged are proposals that (i) investigate the possible role of environmental chemicals in the origins of developmental disabilities, or that (ii) aim to distinguish subgroups within accepted diagnostic categories through the use of sophisticated behavioral and neuroimaging tests of perception, cognition, and emotions based on concepts from modern cognitive neuroscience. In all cases, they seek proposals from young scientists conducting research that is of the highest quality and that has the greatest chance of increasing understanding of neurodevelopmental disorders. Applicants must have the following: Academic rank in a university or medical school, or equivalent standing in a research institute or medical center; A record of research in areas relating to the foundation's interest in the underlying causes of developmental disabilities; Not more than four years of experience in an independent faculty position; Evidence of a commitment to a career in neuroscience or cognitive science. Request application forms by mail, email or phone.
Restrictions: Applicants may not: hold tenured positions or their equivalents; apply in more than two rounds of competition; apply for continued postdoctoral support. Holding other fellowships concurrently with the John Merck Scholars Award is discouraged. Prior approval by the foundation for an overlapping fellowship is required and will be given only in unusual circumstances.
Amount of Grant: $75,000 per year for a four-year period
Date(s) Application is Due: Sep 15
Contact: Jason Bentsman, Staff Assistant; (617) 556-4120; fax: (617) 556-4130; email: j bentsman@jmfund.org
Internet: http://www.jmfund.org/jm_scholars_program.html
Sponsor: John Merck Fund
2 Oliver Street, 8th Floor
Boston, MA 02108

John P. McGovern Foundation Grants **1942**
The John P. McGovern Foundation, established in 1961, supports the charitable interests of the donor to support the activities of established nonprofit organizations, which are of importance to human welfare with special focus on children and family health education and promotion, treatment and disease prevention. The Foundation gives primarily in Texas with an emphasis on the Houston area, but also provides funding in the Southwest region as well. The types of support offered are: building/renovation; conferences/seminars; continuing support; curriculum development; emergency funds; endowments; general/operating support; matching/challenge support; professorships; publication; research; and scholarship funds.
Requirements: Non-profits in Texas are eligible to apply.
Geographic Focus: Texas
Samples: University of Texas Health Science Center, Houston, TX. $1,500,000 - for John P. McGovern, MD, Center for Health, Humanities, and Human Spirit/Certificate Program Endowment Fund (2007); Community Family Centers, Houston, TX. $200,000- for John P. McGovern Community Sports and Recreation Building (2007); Salvation Army of Houston, Houston, TX. $150,000 - for general operating fund (2007).
Amount of Grant: $10,000 - $100,000 range
Date(s) Application is Due: Aug 31
Contact: Kathrine G. McGovern, President; (713) 661-4808; fax: (713) 661-3031
Sponsor: John P. McGovern Foundation
2211 Norfolk Street, Suite 900
Houston, TX 77098-4044

John P. Murphy Foundation Grants **1943**
The Foundation awards grants primarily in Cuyahoga County, Ohio, and its immediately adjacent counties. Areas of interest include education—college level, and primary and secondary education to improve educational programs benefiting low income and minority students, most often in Cleveland public schools; arts and culture; social services; community—community activities, agencies, and events; health—institutions and organizations such as hospitals, clinic, and nursing homes; and religion. Grants to national or regional institutions with broad public support will be made only for start-up programs where time is a factor or where the proposal addresses a specific local community need. Guidelines are available online.
Requirements: Ohio organizations properly classified by the IRS as being eligible to receive grants may apply. Each applicant must file its most recent IRS letter of classification with each proposal. National or regional institutions with broad public support may submit proposals that address a specific local community need.
Restrictions: No grants will be made to endowment funds or for scholarships.
Geographic Focus: Ohio
Amount of Grant: $5,000-$75,000 average
Contact: Allan J. Zambie, Executive Vice President; (216) 623-4770 or 623-4771; fax: (216) 623-4773
Internet: http://fdncenter.org/grantmaker/jpmurphy/interest.html
Sponsor: John P. Murphy Foundation
50 Public Square, Suite 924
Cleveland, OH 44113-2203

John R. Oishei Foundation Grants **1944**
The foundation's primary mission is to support medical research and care and education, as well as cultural and social needs existing in the Buffalo Niagara region. The foundation favors creative programs that attempt to advance from the status quo, are strategically sound, and are strongly focused on excellence. Programs that provide opportunities for foundation support to be leveraged into greater support from other sources will be especially favored. The foundation generally does not fund operating expenses, though occasional exceptions may be made for organizations that address basic human needs. Requests for capital funds will not be considered unless they are an integral part of an otherwise eligible proposal. Contact the foundation to discuss eligibility before submitting an application. Grant applications are accepted throughout the year.
Requirements: It is the general policy of the foundation to confine its support to activities located in the Buffalo, NY, metropolitan region.
Restrictions: Grants do not support endowments; capital requests (buildings or equipment); deficit funding or loans; individual scholarships or fellowships (except within specific foundation programs); travel, conferences, seminars, or workshops; fundraising events; or 509(a) private foundations.
Geographic Focus: New York
Amount of Grant: $13 million total; $100,000-$200,000 average
Contact: Blythe T. Merrill Senior Program Officer; (716) 856-9490, ext. 3; fax: (716) 856-9493; email: btmerrill@oisheifdt.org
Internet: http://www.oisheifdt.org/Home/Fund/WhatWeFundOverview
Sponsor: John R. Oishei Foundation
1 HSBC Center, Suite 3650
Buffalo, NY 14203-2805

John S. Dunn Research Foundation Grants and Chairs **1945**
Established in 1985, the foundation funding area is limited to the Texas, providing support to health and medical-related organizations, especially hospitals; support also for cancer, other medical research, and freestanding clinics.
Requirements: Grants are made to nonprofit organizations within Texas having 501(c)3 tax-exempt status.
Restrictions: No grants to individuals, or for multi-year or seed money grants.
Geographic Focus: Texas
Samples: Gulf Coast Consortia, Houston, TX, $1,180,000 - to support drug discovery program (2007); University of Texas M.D. Anderson Cancer Center, Houston, TX, $650,000 - to fund radiological sciences and metabolic lab (2007); Memorial Hermann Healthcare System, Houston, TX, $250,000 - to support life flight services to patients without insurance (2007).
Amount of Grant: $10,000-$100,000 average
Contact: Dr. Lloyd Gregory, Vice President; (713) 626-0368; fax: (713) 626-3866
Sponsor: John S. Dunn Research Foundation
3355 West Alabama street, Suite 720
Houston, TX 77098-1718

John Stauffer Charitable Trust Grants **1946**
The trust awards grants to California higher education institutions and hospitals. Types of support include building construction/renovation, challenge/matching funds, endowments, equipment acquisition, fellowships, professorships, and scholarship funds. There are no application forms or deadlines.
Requirements: California nonprofits are eligible.
Geographic Focus: California
Samples: California Institute of Technology, Pasadena, CA, $500,000 - for construction of research lab in new chemistry building (2008); Loma Linda University, Loma Linda, CA, $250,000 - for classroom for emergency personnel (2008); Occidental College, Los Angeles, CA, $159,320 - for endowment for summer research (2008).
Amount of Grant: $100,000-$500,000 average
Contact: H. Jess Senecal, Treasurer: (626) 793-9400; fax: (626) 793-5900; email: jess@lagerlof.com
Sponsor: John Stauffer Charitable Trust
301 N Lake Avenue, 10th Floor
Pasadena, CA 91101-4108

John W. Alden Trust Grants **1947**
The trust awards grants to Massachusetts nonprofit organizations in its areas of interest, including education and therapy for children who are blind, disabled, retarded, or mentally or physically ill. Grants will normally be made for specific projects rather than general operating purposes. There are no application deadlines. Grant applications should be submitted on-line at www.cybergrants.com/alden. Detailed instructions on the web page will guide you through the process. All questions should be directed to the grants coordinator.
Requirements: Eastern Massachusetts 501(c)3 tax-exempt organizations are eligible.
Restrictions: Grants are not made to individuals.
Geographic Focus: Massachusetts
Samples: Hospice of the North Shore, Inc., $6,000 - Music Therapy Program (2007); - University of Massachusetts Foundation Inc., $12,000 - NERCVE Assistive Technology Center (2007); Franciscan Hospital for Children, $13,000 - aquatic aerobic conditioning program (2007).
Amount of Grant: $15,000 maximum
Date(s) Application is Due: Jan 15; Apr 15; Jul 15; Oct 15
Contact: Susan Monahan, Grants Coordinator; (617) 951-1108; fax: (617) 542-7437; email: smonahan@rackemann.com
Internet: http://www.cybergrants.com/alden
Sponsor: John W. Alden Trust
160 Federal Street, 13th Floor
Boston, MA 02110-1700

John W. and Anna H. Hanes Foundation Grants **1948**
The trust awards grants, primarily for the arts, to nonprofit organizations in North Carolina. Other interests that are funded are children and youth services; education; environment; health care; historic preservation; and human services. Types of support include annual and capital campaigns; building and renovation; emergency funds; endowments and seed money; equipment and land acquisition; matching and challenge support; and program development. The board meets in January, April, July, and October; application forms are required.
Requirements: 501(c)3 North Carolina nonprofit organizations are eligible.
Restrictions: Giving is limited to North Carolina, with emphasis on Forsyth County. No grants are made to individuals, or for operating expenses.
Geographic Focus: North Carolina
Samples: Winston-Salem State University, Winston-Salem, NC, $83,333 (2007); Yadkin Arts Council, Yadkinville, NC, $33,333 (2007); Salem Academy and College, Winston-Salem, NC, $100,000 (2007).
Amount of Grant: $1000-$200,000
Date(s) Application is Due: Mar 15; Jun 15; Sep 15; Dec 15
Contact: Christopher Spaugh, Vice President, Wachovia Bank NA; (336) 732-5991
Sponsor: John W. and Anna H Hanes Foundation c/o Wachovia Bank N.A.
1525 West WT Harris Boulevard
Charlotte, NC 28288-5709

John W. Anderson Foundation Grants **1949**
The John W. Anderson Foundation is an independent foundation established in 1967, in Indiana. The trust was established by John W. Anderson, a manufacturing executive and inventor. Mr. Anderson was president of the Anderson Company. The foundation givings primarily to organizations serving youth; higher educational institutions; community funds; scientific or medical research for the purpose of alleviating suffering; care of needy, crippled or orphaned children; care of needy persons who are sick, aged or helpless; improving the health, and quality of life of all persons; human services; and the arts and humanities. The Foundations gives primarily in Lake and Porter counties in Indiana.
Requirements: Applicants should submit the following: signature and title of chief executive officer; copy of IRS Determination Letter; brief history of organization and description of its mission; copy of most recent annual report/audited financial statement/990; listing of board of directors, trustees, officers and other key people and their affiliations; detailed description of project and amount of funding requested; copy of current year's organizational budget and/or project budget.
Restrictions: Applications sent by fax not considered. Application form not required. An organization may submit a request once in a 12-month period. No support for elementary and secondary schools, or for business or any for-profit organization, or for supporting organizations classified 509(a)3. No grants to individuals, or for endowments, multi-year grants, fund raising events, advertising, seed money, deficit financing; no loans.
Geographic Focus: Indiana
Amount of Grant: $5,000 -$50,000
Date(s) Application is Due: Jan. 20; Mar. 20; May 20; Jul. 20; Sep. 20; Nov. 20
Contact: William N. Vinovich, Vice-Chair; (219) 462-4611
Sponsor: John W. Anderson Foundation
402 Wall Street
Valparaiso, IN 46383-2562

Johns Manville Fund Grants **1950**
The Johns Manville Fund, Inc. gives primarily in areas of company operations in Denver, Colorado, Etowah, Tennessee, and in Canada. The Fund offers support in the areas of: the arts; education; health care; human services; youth services and the American Red Cross. The grants are offered in the form of employee-related scholarships, employee volunteer services, general/operating support, and program development. Contact the Johns Manville Fund, Inc. for a Informational brochure, including application guidelines.
Requirements: Non-profits operating in Denver, Colarado, Etowah, Tennessee, and in Canada are eligible.
Restrictions: No support for religious organizations not of direct benefit to the entire community, hospitals, or non-special needs private educational organizations. No grants for special events.
Geographic Focus: Colorado; TennesseeCanada
Amount of Grant: $1,000 - $27,000 range
Contact: Community Relations Manager; (303) 978-3863; fax: (303) 978-2108
Internet: http://www.jm.com/corporate/careers/1241.htm
Sponsor: Johns Manville Fund
717 17th Street
Denver, CO 80202-3330

Johnson & Johnson Community Health Care Program Grants **1951**
The program provides support for community public health initiatives impacting access and delivery of quality health care services for medically underserved populations, with emphasis on women and children (including infants and adolescents). Additional consideration will be given to programs focusing on the education and prevention of diabetes, obesity, and cardiovascular disease. Grants also will assist organizations in developing a broad-based public and private support network by extending public recognition of their efforts. Second-year continuation grants also are available.
Requirements: Grants are awarded to community/public health care organizations/agencies in Alabama (all areas); Arkansas (all areas); Boston, Massachusetts; Florida (all areas); New Jersey (all areas); Ohio (all areas); San Diego, California; and San Francisco, California.
Restrictions: Proposals from foundations, universities, and political advocacy groups will not be considered.
Geographic Focus: Alabama; Arkansas; California; Florida; Massachusetts; New Jersey; Ohio
Amount of Grant: $150,000 two-year grant
Date(s) Application is Due: Oct 17
Contact: Sierra Veale, Johns Hopkins Bloomberg School of Public Health; (443) 287-5138; fax: (410) 510-1974; email: jandj@jhsph.edu
Internet: http://www.jhsph.edu/johnsonandjohnson/index.html
Sponsor: Johnson & Johnson
615 N Wolfe Street, Room W1100
Baltimore, MD 21205

Johnson & Johnson Corporate Contributions Grants **1952**
Johnson & Johnson and its many operating companies support community-based programs that improve health and well-being. The Company works with community-based partners that have the greatest insight into the needs of local populations and the strategies that stand the greatest chances of success. Giving focuses on: saving and improving the lives of women and children; building on the skills of people who serve community health needs, primarily through education; and preventing diseases and reducing stigma and disability in underserved communities where we have a high potential for impact.

Requirements: Grants are awarded to nonprofit and tax-exempt local, national, and international organizations and institutions.
Restrictions: Grants are not awarded to individuals, for deficit funding, capital or endowment funds, demonstration projects, or publications.
Contact: Michael J. Bzdak, Director of Corporate Contributions; (732) 524-3061; fax: (732) 524-3300;; Shaun Mickus; (732) 524-2086; email: smickus@corus.jnj.com
Internet: http://www.jnj.com/connect/caring/corporate-giving/
Sponsor: Johnson & Johnson
1 Johnson & Johnson Plaza
New Brunswick, NJ 08933-0001

Johnson and Johnson / SAH Arts and Healing Grants **1953**
Johnson & Johnson and the Society for the Arts in Healthcare have provided program funding to 117 organizations in the U.S. and Canada. In 2008, the grant structure was updated to a three-year grant period with a focus on existing programs. This new structure promotes the evaluation and replication of promising models in order to strengthen and expand the arts in healthcare field.
Requirements: To be eligible for consideration, grant applicants must be: a current member of Society for the Arts in Healthcare; located in the U.S. or Canada (partners may be international); a non-profit organization with federal tax exempt status and organized and operated for charitable purposes or a governmental agency (state or local, including education or institutions). Note: U.S. based non-profit organization applicants must be tax exempt under section 501(c)3 of IRS Code; Canada based applicants must be a registered Canadian charity; and able to show a demonstrated ability to work effectively in partnership with other organizations. To be eligible for consideration, proposed programs must: utilize a model that has documented positive impact; and be designed with proposed outcomes, which show initial impact. Program goals should be specific, measurable, attainable, realistic and timely; and Be sustainable based on existing resources and organizational capacity (adequate staffing, funding, space, etc.).
Restrictions: Individuals are ineligible to apply for scholarships or other forms of assistance. Members of the Society for the Arts in Healthcare board of directors, advisory board, or staff are ineligible to apply or partner with any applicant for the purposes of this grant.
Date(s) Application is Due: Oct 15; Jan 13
Contact: Anita Boles; (202) 299-9770; fax: (202) 299-9887; email: mail@thesah.org
Internet: http://www.thesah.org/template/page.cfm?page_id=15
Sponsor: Society for the Arts in Healthcare
2437 15th St NW, B South
Washington, DC 20009

Johnson Controls Foundation Grants **1954**
The foundation makes charitable contributions to nonprofit organizations, primarily in communities where Johnson Controls has a presence. Extra consideration will be given to organizations or institutions in which Johnson Controls employees are involved and are contributing their time and/or funds.
Requirements: In evaluating requests for funds, the Advisory Board has developed policies and guidelines for giving in the following categories: (a) Health & Social Service - includes financial assistance to federated drives, e.g., United Way, hospitals, youth agencies and other health and human service agencies. Ordinarily, operating support of health and social service agencies is reserved for Johnson Controls communities, and generally directed through contributions to United Way. (b) Education - made to public and private higher educational institutions, adult education programs, and education related organizations, including those which seek to increase public knowledge of economics. Included in this area is the funding of a scholarship program for children of employees of Johnson Controls, Inc. Grants are not usually given to public or private pre-schools, elementary, or secondary institutions, but are limited to colleges and universities. (c) Culture and the Arts - contributions to visual, performing, and literary arts, public radio and television, libraries, museums, and other related cultural activities. Priority will be extended to those serving communities in which Johnson Controls employees live and work, and to those in which these employees are involved with their time and/or funds. (d) Civic Activities - includes assistance to programs in the areas of justice and law, community and neighborhood improvements, the environment, civil rights and equal opportunity, citizenship and safety. Requests to finance office equipment and computer systems do not have a high priority. There is no formal application procedure. Proposals are accepted and reviewed throughout the year. Guidelines are available online.
Restrictions: In general, no grants will be made to any political campaign or organization; any municipal, state, federal agency, or department, or to any organization established to influence legislation; any private individual for support of personal needs; any sectarian institutions or programs whose services are limited to members of any one religious group or whose funds are used primarily for the propagation of a religion; for testimonial dinners, fund raising events, tickets to benefits, shows, or advertising; to provide monies for travel or tours, seminars and conferences or for publication of books and magazines or media productions; for specific medical or scientific research projects; foreign-based institutions nor to institutions or organizations for use outside of the United States; fraternal orders or veteran groups; private foundations or to endowment funds. The foundation does not donate equipment, products or labor.
Amount of Grant: $500-$40,000 average
Contact: Charles A. Harvey; Vice President, Diversity and Public Affairs; (414) 524-1200 or (414) 524-2296;
Internet: http://www.johnsoncontrols.com/publish/us/en/about/diversity_and_public/community_relations/johnson_controls_foundation.html
Sponsor: Johnson Controls Foundation
5757 North Green Bay Avenue, P.O. Box 591
Milwaukee, WI 53201

Johnson County Community Foundation Grants **1955**
The Community Foundation seeks to meet the challenges of the Johnson County, Indiana community as a whole. Special attention is given to requests that increase the capacity of not-for-profit organizations to serve the community and requests that demonstrate community support and in-kind investment. The foundation generally supports three kinds of requests: projects of service to the general community and pilot projects; seed money to enable projects to demonstrate their potential or enhance services; emergency funding for community needs.
Requirements: The grants committee will be only accepting applications this year from area organizations that plan to meet a specific need in the area of Health and Human Services. Applicants should submit a letter of inquiry (2-3 pages), also include a copy of your 501(c)3 Letter of Determination. Letters of inquiry should include: a brief statement of the organization's purpose and goals; a brief description of the project, the need and the target population it addresses; short- and long-term outcomes anticipated and plans for assessing achievements; grant amount needed; a statement about the total agency budget and the project budget; a statement about other funding sources for the agency and/or project, specifying both committed and projected sources of support. The staff will review the letter of inquiry to determine if the proposed effort fits within the community foundation's grant program. If so, you will receive a call or letter from a staff member requesting additional information or a full proposal for our next Grant Cycle deadline. The community foundation supports organizations that are tax exempt under Section 501(c)3 of the Internal Revenue Service Code and are not classified as private foundations under Section 509(a) of the Code. In selected cases, it may consider support for projects sponsored by governmental entities.
Restrictions: The Community Foundation does not: take multi-year commitments; support services commonly regarded as the responsibility of government; provide support for political or partisan purposes or for programs in which religious teachings are an integral part; consider more than one proposal from the same organization within a 12-month period; provide discretionary grant support to an organization's ongoing operating budget, building funds, capital campaigns, or endowments; fund raising events and functions; make grants to individuals except for scholarship or special award funds; fund existing obligations or to replenish resources (deficit funding) for such purposes.
Geographic Focus: Indiana
Date(s) Application is Due: Mar 6; Sep 4
Contact: Kim Minton, Programs Director; (317) 738-2213; fax: (317) 738-9113; email: kimm@jccf.org
Internet: http://www.jccf.org/index.asp?p=37
Sponsor: Johnson County Community Foundation Inc.
398 South Main, P.O. Box 217
Franklin, IN 46131-2311

Johnson F. Hammond Memorial Scholarship **1956**
The annual scholarship will be awarded to a medical student of high moral character and outstanding academic achievement with a demonstrated interest and involvement in medical journalism. The scholarship recipient will be selected from among nominees proposed by the deans of AMA approved medical schools, with financial need not being a consideration. Each school may propose one student.
Amount of Grant: $3000
Date(s) Application is Due: Feb 13
Contact: Dina Lindenberg, Program Officer, (312) 464-4193; fax: (312) 464-5973; email: dina.lindenberg@ama-assn.org or amafoundation@ama-assn.org
Internet: http://www.ama-assn.org/ama/pub/category/14772.html
Sponsor: American Medical Association Foundation
515 N State Street
Chicago, IL 60610

Joseph Alexander Foundation Grants **1957**
Established in 1960 in New York, the Foundation supports primarily the New York New York region. Offering support for: higher education, health organizations and medical research, particularly optic nerve research, social services, and Jewish organizations.
Requirements: Nonprofit organizations are eligible to apply.
Restrictions: Grants are not made to individuals.
Geographic Focus: New York
Samples: Bar-Ilan University in Israel, New York, NY, $50,000 (2007); Center for Jewish History, New York, NY, $15,000 (2007); Autism Speaks, New York, NY, $25,000 (2007).
Amount of Grant: $1000-$100,000 range
Contact: Robert Weintraub, President, (212) 355-3688
Sponsor: Joseph Alexander Foundation
110 East 59th Street
New York, NY 10022-1304

Joseph and Luella Abell Charitable Trust Scholarships **1958**
Established in 2003, this Trust (in the care of the Jackson County Bank) offers scholarship awards to individuals that are nursing school students or graduate students of ministry throughout Indiana. The funding, which ranges from $1,000 to $5,000 annually, can be used to defray tuition expenses, books, housing, and other costs associated with attending college. An application form can be secured by contacted the Jackson County Bank, and the annual deadline is April 1st.
Requirements: Only students enrolled in a nursing program or ministry in Indiana may apply.
Geographic Focus: Indiana
Amount of Grant: $1,000-$5,000 range

Date(s) Application is Due: Apr 1
Contact: George F. Spray, Vice-President; (812) 522-3607
Sponsor: Joseph and Luella Abell Charitable Trust
c/o Jackson County Bank, P.O. Box 1001
Seymour, IN 47274-1001

Joseph Collins Foundation Grants **1959**
These grants enable men and women whose own resources are inadequate to attend accredited medical schools of their own choice that offer the MD degree. Consideration will include scholastic record; interest in cultural pursuits; intention to specialize in neurology, psychiatry, or general medicine; moral character; age; and geographical proximity (applicants within 200 miles of the medical school preferred). These awards are tenable at any accredited medical school east of the Mississippi River for one year, and renewable at the discretion of the foundation. Applications should be obtained from appropriate medical school authorities; applications are sent to the school, not to students. The school nominates one student per school year; however, trustees act favorably or unfavorably in their sole discretion. Student must interact with the financial aid officer at his/her school. Request applications in January.
Requirements: Grants are open to anyone attending an accredited medical school in states east of or contiguous to the Mississippi River and who intends to specialize in neurology, psychiatry, or general practice. Applicants must have satisfactorily completed the first year of medical school. Awards are not made to premedical or postgraduate medical students.
Amount of Grant: $10,000 maximum
Date(s) Application is Due: Mar 1
Contact: Jack H. Nusbaum, Chairman; (212) 728-8060; fax: (212) 728-9060; email: jnusbaum@willkie.com
Sponsor: Joseph Collins Foundation
c/o Willkie Farr & Gallagher LLP, 787 Seventh Avenue, Room 3950
New York, NY 10019-7099

Joseph Drown Foundation Grants **1960**
The foundation makes contributions in the areas of education; community, health and social services; and arts and humanities. It supports programs dealing with such issues as the high school drop-out rate, teen pregnancy, lack of sufficient health care, substance abuse, and violence. Types of support include general operating support, program development, seed money, scholarship funds, and matching funds. Most grant making is limited to programs or organizations in California. Requests are considered each year at March, June, September, and December meetings. The foundation makes grants for both operating support and program support but does not make multiyear commitments. No special application form is required. Proposal should include a letter with information about the organization and the project, a copy of 501(c)3 determination letter, a budget for the organization and the project, the most recent audited financial statements, a copy of the most recent IRS Form 990, and a list of the current board of directors. Any additional materials, such as an annual report, may be attached. Questions should be directed to the program director; proposals should be sent to the foundation president.
Requirements: California 501(c)3 organizations may apply.
Restrictions: The foundation does not provide funds to individuals, endowments, capital campaigns, or annual funds. The foundation does not underwrite annual meetings, conferences, or special events, nor does it fund religious programs or purchase tickets to fund-raising events.
Geographic Focus: California
Samples: The Henry Mancini Institute, Los Angeles, CA, $15,000 - for support of the Community Outreach Initiative.; The Museum of Tolerance, Los Angeles, CA, $50,000 - for Tolerance Youth Education programs.; Friends of the Semel Institute for Neuroscience, Los Angeles, CA, $40,000 - for a postdoctoral fellowship.; Los Angeles Leadership Academy, Los Angeles, CA, $30,000 - for a literacy coordinator and development director in initial year of operation.
Amount of Grant: $10,000-$100,000
Date(s) Application is Due: Jan 15; Apr 15; Jul 15; Oct 15
Contact: Alyssa Eichelberger, Program Administrator; (310) 277-4488, ext. 100; fax: (310) 277-4573; email: alyssa@jdrown.org
Internet: http://www.jdrown.org
Sponsor: Joseph Drown Foundation
1999 Avenue of the Stars, Suite 1930
Los Angeles, CA 90067

Joseph H. and Florence A. Roblee Foundation Grants **1961**
The foundation awards grants to enable organizations to promote change by addressing significant social issues in order to improve the quality of life and help fulfill the potential of individuals. The foundation arises out of a Christian framework, and values ecumenical endeavors. The foundation particularly supports programs which work to break down cultural, racial, and ethnic barriers. Organizations and churches are encouraged to collaborate in achieving positive change through advocacy, prevention, and systemic improvements.
Requirements: Giving limited to nonprofit organizations in the greater bi-state St. Louis region, and Miami/Dade, FL. Contact Foundation for additional guidelines.
Restrictions: Support is not given to individuals or for annual campaigns, research, or loans.
Geographic Focus: Florida; Illinois; Missouri
Amount of Grant: $1000-$30,000 average
Date(s) Application is Due: Jan 15; Jun 15
Contact: Peggy Thomas, Bank of America, N.A.; (314) 466-1304; email: kathydc@robleefoundation.org.
Sponsor: Joseph H. and Florence A. Roblee Foundation
P.O. Box 14737, MO2-100-07-19
Saint Louis, MO 63178-4737

Joseph P. Kennedy Jr. Foundation Grants **1962**
The foundation concentrates its funding in the area of mental retardation. Grants providing seed funding are offered to encourage new methods of service and support for people with mental retardation and their families.
Requirements: Nonprofit organizations may apply.
Restrictions: The foundation will not support capital costs or costs of equipment for projects, nor will it pay for ongoing support or operations of existing programs. Individuals are not eligible.
Samples: George Washington U (Washington, DC)—for the Ctr for the Study and Advancement of Disability Policy, $200,000.
Contact: Program Contact, (202) 393-1250; fax: (202) 824-0351; email: eidelman@jpkf.org or info@jpkf.org
Internet: http://www.jpkf.org/JPKF_Info/GRANT.HTML
Sponsor: Joseph P. Kennedy Jr. Foundation
1133 19th Street NW, 12th Floor
Washington, DC 20036-3604

Josephine G. Russell Trust Grants **1963**
The purpose of the trust is for the care, healing, and nursing of the sick and injured, the relief and aid of the poor, the training and education of the young, and any other manner of social service in the city of Lawrence, Massachusetts.
Requirements: Massachusetts nonprofit organizations serving the greater Lawrence metropolitan area are eligible.
Geographic Focus: Massachusetts
Amount of Grant: $40,000 max.
Date(s) Application is Due: Jan 31
Contact: Clifford Elias, Treasurer; (978) 500-3171
Sponsor: Josephine G. Russell Trust
59 Lucerne Drive
Andover, MA 01810-1719

Josephine Goodyear Foundation Grants **1964**
The foundation makes grants in the greater Buffalo, NY, area for programs and projects benefiting indigent women and children, particularly with their physical needs. Grants also support hospitals, child welfare organizations, youth agencies, and community funds. Types of support include capital campaigns, building construction/renovation, equipment acquisition, land acquisition, emergency funds, program development, seed grants, research, employee matching gifts, and matching funds. Applicants are requested to submit a two-page proposal including the purpose of the organization, a description of the project/program or need, budget, other sources of funding, and an IRS determination letter.
Requirements: IRS 501(c)3 tax-exempt organizations serving the greater Buffalo, NY, area are eligible.
Restrictions: Grants are not awarded in support of individuals, continuing support, annual campaigns, deficit financing, endowment funds, scholarships, fellowships, or loans.
Geographic Focus: New York
Amount of Grant: $500-$30,000 average
Date(s) Application is Due: Apr 15; Aug 15
Contact: E.W. Dann Stevens, President, (716) 566-1465; fax: (716) 846-1236; email: ewdstevens@hiscockbarclay.com
Internet: http://www.cfgb.org/index.php/affiliates-and-initiatives/josephine-goodyear-foundation/97-josephine-goodyear-grants
Sponsor: Josephine Goodyear Foundation
3 Fountain Plaza, Suite 1100, M & T Center
Buffalo, NY 14203

Josephine S. Gumbiner Foundation Grants **1965**
The charitable foundation functions for the benefit of women and children in the Long Beach area. The funder supports a wide array of programs, such as the arts; day care; education health care intervention, prevention, and direct services; housing; and recreation. Organizations are not be eligible for funding more than once in any 12-month period. As a general rule, the foundation will not grant funding to any organization for more than three consecutive years. The two-step application process begins with requesting a letter of intent questionnaire, which should be requested through email. Full applications are by invitation. There are no application deadlines. The board meets three or four times each year.
Requirements: Southern California nonprofit organizations are eligible.
Restrictions: Grants do not support political campaigns, lobbying efforts, programs that supplant tradition schooling, pass-through organizations, or groups with endowments greater than $5 million.
Geographic Focus: California
Samples: Children's Dental, CA, $20,000 - I.V. Sedation for L.B. Children Program (2009); Children Today, Long Beach, CA, $15,000 - LCSW Support (2009); Helpline Youth Counseling, Norwalk, CA, $15,000 - L.B. Gang Prevention Program (2009).
Amount of Grant: $5000-$50,000; $10,000 average
Contact: Grants Administrator, (562) 437-2882; fax: (562) 437-4212; email: julie@jsgf.org

Internet: http://www.jsgf.org/
Sponsor: Josephine S. Gumbiner Foundation
333 West Broadway., Suite 302
Long Beach, CA 90802

Josiah Macy Jr. Foundation Grants **1966**

The foundation awards grants to improve the education of physicians and other health care professionals. Grant making focuses on improving medical and health professionals' education in the context of the changing health care system, increasing the number of minority physicians, boosting teamwork between health care professionals, and using educational strategies to increase care for under-served populations. Current initiatives cover the fields of pediatric residency, inter-professional curriculum, improved clinical training, increasing diversity among health care professions, Macy Scholars program, women's health in medical curricula, women in medicine, and funding for a New York post-baccalaureate program. Applications may be submitted at any time. A preliminary letter of inquiry is useful in assisting the foundation staff in determining whether submission of a full proposal is appropriate.
Requirements: Grants are made to colleges, universities, and other 501(c)3 nonprofit organizations for activities within established program areas. Grant proposals, addressed to the president, should include the name of the sponsoring agency or institution; description of the project; names and qualifications of the person who will be responsible for the project; expected cost and duration of the project including an itemized budget; documents substantiating the tax-exempt status of the sponsoring institution; and a letter of endorsement from the sponsoring institution.
Restrictions: Grants are not awarded to individuals or for general undesignated support or for construction/renovation projects.
Amount of Grant: $5 million per year total
Contact: George E. Thibault, President; (212) 486-2424; fax: (212) 644-0765; email: jmacyinfo@josiahmacy
Internet: http://www.josiahmacyfoundation.org/index.php?section=grant_guidelines
Sponsor: Josiah Macy Jr. Foundation
44 East 64th Street
New York, NY 10021

Josiah W. and Bessie H. Kline Foundation Grants **1967**

The foundation was established for charitable, scientific, literary, and educational purposes. The objectives for its grantmaking activities are to aid blind or incapacitated persons or crippled children. Grants are made to Pennsylvania colleges and universities and to hospitals, to institutions for crippled children, or to any other benevolent or charitable institution. Generally, grants are made to such institutions that are located in south-central Pennsylvania. Grants also are made for scientific and medical research. Types of support include continuing support, annual campaigns, capital campaigns, equipment acquisition, building/renovation, curriculum development, scholarship funds, matching funds, research, and emergency funds. The foundation does not have an application form. Instead, a letter of request must be submitted with the following information: a description of the need and purpose of the applicant organization, a project budget, amount requested from the foundation and the dates of the need, and a copy of the 501(c)3 tax-exemption letter. Requests may be submitted at any time. The board generally meets in March and November to consider requests.
Requirements: 501(c)3 organizations serving south-central Pennsylvania communities are eligible.
Restrictions: The foundation does not make loans and does not make grants to individuals or to normal operational phases of established programs, endowments, campaigns or national organizations, or religious programs.
Geographic Focus: Pennsylvania
Amount of Grant: $500-$150,000 range
Contact: John Obrock, Grant Administrator; (717) 561-0820 or (717) 561-4373; fax: (717) 561-0826
Sponsor: Josiah W. and Bessie H. Kline Foundation
515 S 29th Street
Harrisburg, PA 17104

Journal Gazette Foundation Grants **1968**

The foundation awards grants to northeastern Indiana nonprofit organizations in its areas of interest, including community funds, education, higher education, health organizations and hospitals, social services, Christian agencies and churches, and youth. Types of support include general operations and capital campaigns. There are no application deadlines; the board meets quarterly.
Requirements: Indiana nonprofit organizations are eligible. Preference is given to requests from northeastern Indiana.
Restrictions: Grants are not made to individuals.
Geographic Focus: Indiana
Samples: Lincoln Museum (Fort Wayne, Indiana)—for operating support, $6000.
Amount of Grant: $25-$112,000 range
Contact: Jerry Fox, (260) 424-5257
Sponsor: Journal Gazette Foundation
701 S Clinton
Fort Wayne, IN 46802-1883

Joyce Foundation Grants **1969**

The foundation's program areas are education, employment, environment, gun violence, money and politics, and culture. Grantmaking is focused on initiatives that promise to have an impact on the Great Lakes region, specifically the states of Illinois, Indiana, Michigan, Minnesota, Ohio, and Wisconsin. A limited number of environment grants are made to organizations in Canada. Education grantmaking focuses on Chicago, Cleveland, and Milwaukee. Culture grants are primarily focused on the Chicago metropolitan area. The foundation is committed to improving public policy through its grant program. Public policy grants provide general operating support or fund educational advocacy such as nonpartisan research, technical assistance, or examinations of broad social issues. Grant applicants are encouraged to describe the nature of advocacy activities in their grant applications and reports, so the foundation can ensure that it is in compliance with federal tax laws. Guidelines are available online.
Requirements: Applications should be made only by organizations in the Great Lakes region that can demonstrate their tax-exempt status and that can supply complete financial information and permit the results of a grant to be audited.
Restrictions: The foundation generally does not support capital projects, endowment campaigns, religious activities, direct services, or scholarships.
Geographic Focus: Illinois; Indiana; Iowa; Michigan; Minnesota; Ohio; Wisconsin Canada
Amount of Grant: $20,000-$100,000 average
Date(s) Application is Due: Apr 15; Aug 16; Dec 12
Contact: Veronica Salter, Grants Manager, (312) 782-2464; fax: (312) 782-4160; email: info@joycefdn.org
Internet: http://www.joycefdn.org/seekingagrant/seekingmain-fs.html
Sponsor: Joyce Foundation
70 W Madison, Suite 2750
Chicago, IL 60602

Judith and Jean Pape Adams Charitable Foundation ALS Grants **1970**

The Foundation was established in 2004 as a private foundation and is involved in making distributions to charitable organizations on an annual basis. It encompasses two areas of support: organizations and agencies predominantly in Tulsa County, Oklahoma, and national Amyotrophic Lateral Sclerosis (ALS) research. For the latter, the Foundation encourages research that is collaborative, innovative and aggressive. These initiatives may fill gaps not currently being investigated and may involve novel approaches. The research must be of high scientific merit in finding a cure for ALS. Proposals may be longer than two pages. A lay summary is also required. Applications are reviewed by an Advisory Committee comprised of scientific researchers, neurologists and others who have had close relationships with friends and family members afflicted with ALS. The Committee makes funding recommendations to the Trustees.
Requirements: Public agencies and organizations that are classified as a charitable organization described in Section 501(c)3 of the Internal Revenue Code and as a public charity under Section 509(a) of the Internal Revenue Code may apply.
Restrictions: Support groups, education and medical equipment are not supported.
Date(s) Application is Due: Aug 15
Contact: Marcia Y. Manhart, Executive Director; (830) 997-7347; fax: (830) 997-9888; email: mmanhart@jjpafoundation.com
Internet: http://www.jjpafoundation.com/guidelines.html
Sponsor: Judith and Jean Pape Adams Charitable Foundation
105 South Cherry Street
Fredericksburg, TX 78624

Julia Temple Davis Brown Foundation Grants **1971**

The Foundation, established in 1969, is interested in supporting children and youth programs. Because of the limited size of the trust, and limited income available for distribution, the general policy has been to give fewer, but more meaningful grants, rather than spreading the income in smaller amounts to more organizations. The priority has been to the education of youth, from pre-school through high school, with emphasis on the lower age youngsters. Most recently, the Distribution Committee revised the grant emphasis to continue the focus on youth, but to stress youth programs relating to culture and arts, and the environment.
Requirements: Only 501(c)3 organization serving Hawaii are eligible to apply.
Geographic Focus: Hawaii
Samples: Children's Discovery Center, Honolulu, Hawaii, $5,000—for a school group discovery visit program (2007); Hawaii Youth Opera Chorus, Honolulu, Hawaii, $4,000—for scholarships for young choral singers (2007); Reading is Fundamental, Honolulu, Hawaii, $3,000—for implementation of a reading motivation program (2007).
Date(s) Application is Due: Apr 1
Contact: Paula Boyce, AVP & Grants Administration Officer; (808) 538-4945 or (808) 538-4540; fax: (808) 538-4006; email: pboyce@boh.com
Sponsor: Julia Temple Davis Brown Foundation
Foundation Administration #758, P.O. Box 3170, Dept. 715
Honolulu, HI 96802-3170

June Allyson Foundation Research Fellowships **1972**

The purpose of this program is to identify potential future academic leaders and to stimulate their development through the support of research fellowships. The fellowship award is to be used to provide research training and experience for a candidate who exhibits significant evidence of talent and dedication to research. It is expected that the fellow will remain at the same institution for the entire funded period and present his/her research findings at the annual AUGS meeting the year after the fellowship has ended. A full written report will be due one year after the fellowship ends.
Requirements: Grant applicants must have an MD degree and demonstrate that grant proposals are part of ongoing programs representing a serious commitment to reducing or eliminating incontinence and/or its associated problems. The applicant's personal

long-term career goals should include a significant emphasis on incontinence research, treatment, education, etc.
Amount of Grant: $24,000 maximum plus a $2000 allowance for travel
Date(s) Application is Due: Feb 28
Contact: Grant Administrator, AUGS/June Allyson Foundation, (202) 367-1167; fax: (202) 367-2167; email: info@augs.org
Internet: http://www.augs.org/i4a/pages/index.cfm?pageid=229
Sponsor: June Allyson Foundation
2025 M St NW, Suite 800
Washington, DC 20036

K and F Baxter Family Foundation Grants **1973**
The foundation focuses on the special educational challenges encountered by multiracial children; policy recommendations in support of revised school curricula that will be more supportive of multiracial children without sacrificing either basic skills training or appropriate performance standards; and developing, by means of policy studies and analysis, a realistic template for education reform focused on the student rather than the school. In addition, the foundation will consider funding worthwhile projects in the arts, health care, and other areas related to education. Guidelines are available online.
Requirements: Biracial children grants are awarded to nonprofit organizations nationwide. Education grants are limited to schools in California Unified School Districts, including Berkeley, Los Angeles, Oakland, West Contra Costa Counties.
Amount of Grant: $90-$150,000
Date(s) Application is Due: Feb 1; Aug 1
Contact: Stacey Bell, Executive Director, (510) 524-8145; fax: (510) 524-4101; email: kfbaxterfound@aol.com
Internet: http://www.kfbaxterfoundation.com
Sponsor: K and F Baxter Family Foundation
P.O. Box 13053
Berkeley, CA 94712-4053

K. M. Hunter Charitable Foundation Social Welfare Grants **1974**
The Foundation provides a number of major grants to social and health services programs in Ontario. In addition, a series of smaller grants are given to organizations, including housing shelters and hospices for the sick. The Foundation requests that applicants make all contacts through its web site. There are no specific applications or deadlines, and the Board meets two or three times annually to make its funding decisions.
Requirements: Grants are made to registered charitable organizations based in Ontario, with the exception of grants that support AIDS in Africa.
Contact: Sarah Hunter, Vice President
Internet: http://www.kmhunterfoundation.ca/
Sponsor: K. M. Hunter Charitable Foundation
P.O. Box 38, Station E
Toronto, Ontario M6H 4E1 Canada

K21 Health Foundation Cancer Care Fund Grants **1975**
The Kosciusko County Cancer Care Fund, administered by K21 Health Foundation, provides assistance to financially-eligible residents of Kosciusko County who are suffering from cancer. The purpose of the fund is to relieve some of the financial strain that often accompanies that dreaded diagnosis. The assistance provided includes but is not limited to items such as rent or mortgage payments, utilities, insurance, food, car payments, and prescription medications.
Requirements: Eligibility Requirements for Assistance: documented resident of Kosciusko County; verified cancer diagnosis within the last three months; can demonstrate a financial need; completion of the required application (contact the CCF Director for application).
Geographic Focus: Indiana
Contact: Clare Sessa, CCF Director; (574) 372-3500; email: csessa@hcfkc.org
Internet: http://www.k21foundation.org/cancer-care-fund/index.cfm
Sponsor: K21 Health Foundation
2170 North Pointe Drive, P.O. Box 1810
Warsaw, IN 46582

K21 Health Foundation Grants **1976**
K21 Health Foundation exists for the benefit of Kosciusko County, Indiana citizens to ensure health care services are provided, and to advance prevention and healthy lifestyles. This will be accomplished by identifying health needs in our community, and maintaining an endowment so funding is available, through investments and grants, for those needs. Organizations are strongly encouraged to review K21's mission statement as that is the primary tool used to evaluate each application. When submitting an application, organizations must clearly explain how K21's mission will be advanced by supporting the project, program, or service, and the intended benefit(s) to residents of Kosciusko County.
Requirements: To qualify for a grant from K21, your organization must meet the following requirements: must be a non-profit agency with verified IRS tax-exempt status, or a governmental agency; must be in good standing with the Indiana Secretary of State as indicated in a Business Entity Report; your Bylaws must require term limits for Directors and a rotating board is strongly encouraged.
Restrictions: To qualify for a grant from K21, your request must meet the following requirements: the project, program, or service for which you are seeking funding must benefit residents of Kosciusko County; the project, program, or service for which you are seeking funding should provide direct health services or advance prevention and healthy life solutions.
Geographic Focus: Indiana
Date(s) Application is Due: Feb1; May 1; Aug 1; Nov 1
Contact: Holly Swoverland, Grant Coordinator: (574)-269-5188 ext 102; fax: (574) 269-5193
Internet: http://www.k21foundation.org/apply-for-grant/index.cfm
Sponsor: K21 Health Foundation
2170 North Pointe Drive, P.O. Box 1810
Warsaw, IN 46582

Kahuku Community Fund **1977**
The Kahuku Community Fund was established by the Estate of James Campbell in 2005 "to be used for charitable and community purposes within the geographic district of Kahuku, bounded by Turtle Bay and Malaekahana." Preference is given to projects that address educational opportunities; recreational opportunities; economic sufficiency; social conditions; health care; strategic action plan around future development of the Kahuku community; housing opportunities; cultural arts, practices and values of the Ko'olauloa moku. Grant range is between $1,000 to $25,000 with an average of $10,000.
Requirements: Nonprofit, 501(c)3 organizations, schools, units of government, neighborhood groups or projects are eligible to apply. Community organizations without 501(c)3 status are eligible to apply for a grant up to $5,000, provided the activities to be supported are charitable. To be eligible for a grant of more than $5,000, a group must be a tax-exempt 501(c)3 organization or have a 501(c)3 fiscal sponsor. Program or project must benefit the Kahuku community.
Restrictions: Projects not likely to be funded: costs relating to establishing a new 501((c)(3) organization; general operating support, although up to 10% for indirect costs will be considered; funds for an endowment; funds for the benefit of specific individuals; except for emergency assistance through a 501(c)3 organization; full personnel costs (staffing costs are less likely to be funded) of a project or program; major capital improvements, although minor capital improvements required to implement a project may be considered; travel out of state.
Geographic Focus: Hawaii
Amount of Grant: $1,000-$25,000
Date(s) Application is Due: Jan 19
Contact: Amy Luersen, (808) 566-5550 or (888) 731-3863; email: aluersen@hawaiicommunityfoundation.org
Internet: http://www.hawaiicommunityfoundation.org/index.php?id=71&categoryID=22
Sponsor: Hawaii Community Foundation
Attention: Kahuku Community Fund, 1164 Bishop Street, Suite 800
Honolulu, HI 96813

Kaiser Permanente Cares for Communities Grants **1978**
Kaiser Permanente partners with nonprofit organizations to improve the health of its members and the communities it serves. The company's four-pronged approach to improve community health includes: increasing access to coverage and care for vulnerable populations, including children and adults who are ineligible for existing state or private programs due to family income or immigration status, and community-based clinics; evidence-based medicine—successful practices in managing chronic diseases such as diabetes, asthma, depression, and heart failure; education of health care professionals and consumers—graduate medical education programs and nursing scholarships, partnerships with national consumer organizations, and educational theater programs; and national public health policy. Application and guidelines are available online.
Requirements: 501(c)3 nonprofit organizations that have national reach are eligible. Organizations must be nonpartisan and nondenominational.
Samples: Institute for Healthcare Improvement (Boston, MA)—for a scholarship endowment to enable health care professionals to participate in the institute's health-care-improvement programs, including conferences and training courses, $8 million (2005); Doctors Without Borders (New York, NY)—to assist tsunami-relief efforts, $500,000 (2005); American National Red Cross (Washington, DC) and Operation U.S.A (Los Angeles, CA)—to assist tsunami-relief efforts, $250,000 each (2005); Archdiocesan Health Care Network (Washington, DC)—to increase the number of volunteers who provide specialty care to low-income, uninsured people, $15,000 (2004).
Amount of Grant: $343 million total
Contact: Community Relations, (510) 271-5685; fax: (510) 271-6493
Internet: http://www.kaiserpermanentejobs.org/aboutus/community.asp
Sponsor: Kaiser Permanente
1 Kaiser Plz, 21B
Oakland, CA 94612

Kalamazoo Foundation Grants **1979**
The foundation awards unrestricted grants in four priority areas: individuals and families, economic development, education and learning, and community engagement and youth development. Types of support include general operating support, capital campaigns, building construction/renovation, equipment acquisition, emergency funds, program development, seed grants, scholarship funds, technical assistance, employee matching gifts, and matching funds. The period for grant support is normally one year. Guidelines and application are available online.
Requirements: Kalamazoo, MI, organizations recognized (or in the process of applying for recognition) under IRS code 501(c)3 are encouraged to contact foundation staff before submitting a request to determine eligibility.

Restrictions: Generally, the foundation does not provide funding for debt retirement, endowments, individuals, travel for individuals or groups, religious organizations for religious purposes, meetings, conferences, publications, films, or television and radio programming.
Geographic Focus: Michigan
Samples: Interfaith Strategy for Advocacy and Action in the Community (Kalamazoo, MI)—for a voter-registration and community-engagement project, $40,000 (2005); Catholic Family Services (Kalamazoo, MI)—for the Kalamazoo Caring Network's Read Me a Story program, which promotes reading skills and literacy among teenage parents and their children, $25,297 (2005); Michiana Addictions and Prevention Services (Kalamazoo, MI)—to support the merger of this substance-abuse-treatment center with the Guidance Clinic in Kalamazoo, $100,000 (2005); Kalamazoo College (MI)—for a postgraduate fellowship position at the Mary Jane Underwood Stryker Institute for Service Learning, $45,000 (2005).
Contact: Contact, (269) 381-4416; fax: (269) 381-3146; email: info@kalfound.org
Internet: http://www.kalfound.org/page8490.cfm
Sponsor: Kalamazoo Foundation
151 S Rose Street
Kalamazoo, MI 49007

Kansas Health Foundation Grants **1980**
The foundation provides grants to Kansas organizations that share its mission to improve the quality of health in the state. Through solicited requests for proposals, the foundation proactively works as a partner with others in the state on programs that address the greatest health needs and achieve the most positive results. Grants are made in five primary categories, including primary care education, rural health, health promotion and disease prevention, public health, and health policy and research. At times, the foundation may respond to unsolicited proposals that are consistent with current programs. Types of support include fellowships, general operating budgets, special projects, and technical assistance. The foundation also awards recognition grants to honor Kansas grassroots organizations doing innovative work to improve the health of the people of the state.
Requirements: Kansas 501(c)3 nonprofit organizations are eligible.
Restrictions: The foundation does not support clinical or medical research; contributions to capital campaigns; organizations that practice discrimination by race, color, creed, sex, age or national origin; operating deficits or retirement of debt; endowment programs; construction projects or real estate acquisitions; political projects of any kind; and vehicles, such as vans or buses, or emergency medical services equipment.
Geographic Focus: Kansas
Samples: Kansas Health Foundation Leadership Ctr (Wichita, KS)—to establish this center, which will help develop leaders who can spearhead efforts to improve the health of all Kansans, $30 million (2005); Wichita State U, Elliott School of Communication (KS)—to endow a professorship in strategic communication, $2 million (2005).
Date(s) Application is Due: Mar 15; Sep 15
Contact: Grants Manager, (800) 373-7681 or (316) 262-7676; fax: (316) 262-2044; email: info@khf.org
Internet: http://www.kansashealth.org/grants/recognition_grants.jsp
Sponsor: Kansas Health Foundation
309 E Douglas
Wichita, KS 67202-3405

Kate B. Reynolds Charitable Trust Health Care Grants **1981**
The Trust responds to health care and wellness needs and invests in solutions that improve the quality of health for financially needy residents throughout North Carolina. The Health Care Division seeks impact through two program areas: providing treatment and supporting prevention. The trust requires advanced consultation by phone or in writing. Application materials are available online, but applications are not accepted electronically.
Requirements: Nonprofit 501(c)3 organizations in North Carolina are eligible.
Restrictions: Grants are not awarded to individuals.
Geographic Focus: North Carolina
Amount of Grant: $20,000-$200,000 average
Date(s) Application is Due: Mar 15; Sep 15
Contact: John H. Frank, Director Health Care Division; (336) 397-5502 or (866) 551-0690; fax: (336) 723-7765; email: john@kbr.org
Internet: http://www.kbr.org/health-care-division-fund.cfm
Sponsor: Kate B. Reynolds Charitable Trust
128 Reynolda Village
Winston-Salem, NC 27106

Katharine Matthies Foundation Grants **1982**
The foundation awards grants to eligible Connecticut nonprofit organizations in its areas of interest, including arts and culture, civic and public affairs, community development, elderly, elementary/secondary education, environment, ethnic organizations, job training, health care, housing, humanities, religion, social services, women, and youth. Types of support include general operating support, land acquisition, multiyear support, project development, and seed money. Contact the office for application forms.
Requirements: Connecticut 501(c)3 nonprofit organizations serving Seymour, Ansonia, Derby, Oxford, Shelton, and Beacon Falls are eligible. Preference is given to requests from Seymour.
Restrictions: Grants do not support advertising, advocacy organizations, colleges and universities, individuals, international organizations, political organizations, special events, or state and local government agencies.
Geographic Focus: Connecticut
Samples: City of Ansonia, Fiduciary for Omicron Chapter of Delta Kappa Gamma Society International (CT)—to provide scholarships to girls from the Lower Naugatuck high schools, $4000.; City of Ansonia (CT)—to purchase a mass disaster alarm system, $9000 (2003); Birmingham Group Health Services (CT)—to support the Valley Substance Abuse Action Council program, $54,420 (2003).
Date(s) Application is Due: May 1
Contact: Program Contact, (860) 952-7405 or (860) 952-7403
Internet: http://electronicvalley.org/matthies/index.html
Sponsor: Katharine Matthies Foundation
777 Main Street, CT EH 40222B
Hartford, CT 06115

Katherine John Murphy Foundation Grants **1983**
The foundation awards grants to Georgia tax-exempt organizations in its areas of interest, including arts and culture, child welfare, health care, higher education, hospitals, youth, and zoos. Types of support include annual campaigns, building construction/renovation, capital campaigns, continuing support, general operating support, seed grants, and project development. Grants are awarded primarily in Atlanta. Submit a letter of request.
Requirements: Organizations in Atlanta, GA are eligible to apply.
Restrictions: No grants to individuals, or for research, or matching gifts.
Geographic Focus: Georgia
Amount of Grant: $250-$50,000 average range
Date(s) Application is Due: Mar 30; Jun 30; Sep 30; Dec 15
Contact: Brenda Rambeau, (404) 589-8090; email: info@murphyfoundation.org
Internet: http://www.kjmurphyfoundation.org
Sponsor: Katherine John Murphy Foundation
50 Hurt Plaza, Suite 1210
Atlanta, GA 30303

Kathryne Beynon Foundation Grants **1984**
The foundation awards grants to eligible California nonprofit organizations in its areas of interest, including child welfare, substance abuse rehabilitation, and education. Types of support include general operating support, building construction/renovation, endowment funds, and scholarship funds.
Requirements: 501(c)3 southern California tax-exempt organizations are eligible. Preference is given to requests from Pasadena.
Geographic Focus: California
Amount of Grant: $500-$50,000 range
Contact: Mary Ellen Lubow, (626) 584-8800
Sponsor: Kathryne Beynon Foundation
199 S Los Robles Avenue, Suite 711
Pasadena, CA 91101-2460

Kavli Foundation Research Grants **1985**
The Kavli Foundation supports research in the areas of astrophysics, nanoscience, neuroscience, and theoretical physics – three scientific frontiers that promise great discoveries in the 21st century and beyond. This mission is implemented through an international program of research institutes, professorships, symposia and workshops, as well as prizes in the fields of astrophysics, nanoscience, and neuroscience. Dedicated to advancing science for the benefit of humanity and promoting increased public understanding and support for scientists and their work, the Foundation also makes available materials on these sciences at no cost to educational institutions.
Contact: Grants Administrator; (805) 983-6000; fax: (805) 988-4800
Internet: http://www.kavlifoundation.org/areasofscience/
Sponsor: Kavli Foundation
1801 Solar Drive, Suite 250
Oxnard, CA 93031

Kelvin and Eleanor Smith Foundation Grants **1986**
The foundation awards grants to Ohio nonprofits in its areas of interest, including nonsectarian education, the performing and visual arts, health care, and environmental conservation and protection. Types of support include general operating support, continuing support, annual campaigns, capital campaigns, building construction/renovation, and equipment acquisition. There are no required application forms or deadlines.
Requirements: Nonprofit organizations in the greater Cleveland, OH, area are eligible.
Restrictions: Grants are not made in support of individuals or for endowment funds, scholarships, fellowships, matching gifts, or loans.
Geographic Focus: Ohio
Samples: Case Western Reserve University, Kelvin Smith Library (Cleveland, OH)—for capital campaign, $200,000.; Cleveland Museum of Art (Cleveland, OH)—for annual fund, $125,000.
Amount of Grant: $3000-$150,000 average
Contact: Carol Zett, Grants Manager, (216) 591-9111; fax: (216) 591-9557
Sponsor: Kelvin and Eleanor Smith Foundation
30195 Chagrin Boulevard, Suite 275
Cleveland, OH 44124

Ken W. Davis Foundation Grants **1987**
The foundation awards grants in company-operating areas to support charities that directly provide for human welfare, basic needs, and quality of life—food, shelter, clothing, healthcare, disabilities, and childcare. Recipients may be asked to submit a

post-grant evaluation of the project or program. Requests must be in writing and are reviewed and approved throughout the year. Submit requests as early as possible before October 31, the end of the foundation's fiscal year.
Requirements: Texas nonprofit organizations in Midland-Odessa and Forth Worth are eligible.
Restrictions: The foundation does not support religious organizations for religious purposes; activities in support of social political causes; organizations that receive a substantial amount of federal and/or state funding; or organizations (other than the United Way) that receive wide public support.
Geographic Focus: Texas
Contact: Alan Tucker Davis, (817) 332-4081; fax: (817) 332-4095; email: akd@kwdf.org
Internet: http://fdncenter.org/grantmaker/davis/proposal.html
Sponsor: Ken W. Davis Foundation
P.O. Box 3419
Fort Worth, TX 76113-3419

Kendrick Foundation Grants **1988**
Kendrick Foundation, Inc., was created to support health-related programs in Morgan County, Indiana. Support includes making grants to health-related organizations and charities, which may include community health care programs, hospice programs, health care education and training, and tax-exempt medical and health programs. Prior to submitting a grant application, a Letter of Intent must be submitted. Letters of Intent are available for download for a limited amount of time during the opening of the grant cycle. Letters of Intent for the spring grant cycle must be physically received in the office of the Community Foundation of Morgan County, Inc. by March 14, no later than 4 p.m., with invited applications due April 14. Letters of Intent for the fall grant cycle must be physically received in the office of the Community Foundation of Morgan County, Inc. by October 14, no later than 4 p.m., with invited applications due November 14.
Requirements: The Kendrick Foundation will only accept full grant applications from those organizations serving Morgan County, Indiana, which were approved through a Letter of Intent.
Geographic Focus: Indiana
Date(s) Application is Due: Mar 14; Apr 14; Oct 14; Nov 14
Contact: Tom Zoss, Executive Director; (317) 831-1232 or (877) 822-6958; fax: (317) 831-2854; email: tzoss@cfmconline.org
Internet: http://www.cfmconline.org/kendrick/Grants/tabid/129/Default.aspx
Sponsor: Kendrick Foundation, Inc.
250 North Monroe Street
Mooresville, IN 46158

Kenneth T. and Eileen L. Norris Foundation Grants **1989**
The foundation supports Los Angeles County nonprofits in the areas of medicine—to improve access to health care, increase knowledge through research, and provide facilities for those activities to take place; youth—to provide constructive activities, positive role models, and opportunities for disadvantaged, disabled, and misguided children; community—to support law enforcement agencies, good citizenship, and environmental conservation; arts and culture—to support museums, symphony orchestras, and dance and theater companies; and education and science—to focus on private education, especially secondary and college levels. Types of support include general operating support, continuing support, building construction/renovation, equipment acquisition, endowment funds, program development, professorships, scholarship funds, research, and matching funds. Education/science projects are due between May 1 and June 30; youth requests are due between February 15 and March 31; community and cultural (the arts) requests are due between December 1 and January 31; and medicine proposals are due between May 1 and June 30.
Requirements: Grants are awarded to organizations in southern California.
Geographic Focus: California
Samples: Los Angeles Regional Foodbank (Los Angeles, CA)—for general operating support, $10,000.
Amount of Grant: $5000-$25,000 average
Date(s) Application is Due: Jan 31; Mar 31; Jun 30
Contact: Ronald Barnes, Executive Director, (562) 435-8444; fax: (562) 436-0584; email: grants@ktn.org
Internet: http://www.norrisfoundation.org/grant_funding.html
Sponsor: Kenneth T. and Eileen L. Norris Foundation
11 Golden Shore, Suite 450
Long Beach, CA 90802

Kenny's Kids Grants **1990**
The foundation awards grants to U.S. nonprofits in company-operating locations with a focus on programs that improve life for children and young adults. The primary target of grants is giving support to organizations which seek to give youth greater opportunities outside of the classroom to learn and grow, to teach them skills that will enable them to thrive in a technology-oriented society, and to offer them the guidance and attention necessary to develop such skills. Also consideration for youth-oriented organizations and other organizations that promote the welfare of youth, such as those that offer hope and encouragement to the sick and terminally ill, protect those who have suffered from abuse, and offer after-school programs for the underprivileged. There are no application deadlines. Allow eight to 12 weeks for proposal review.
Requirements: Nonprofits in company operating areas of Illinois are eligible.
Restrictions: No support for private foundations, schools (public or private), or corporations. Grants are not made to individuals, or for political campaigns, film, video, or audio productions.
Geographic Focus: Illinois
Amount of Grant: $573,902 total
Contact: Nicholas Pontikes, President
Sponsor: Kenny's Kids
1212 W Lill Street
Chicago, IL 60614

Kettering Family Foundation Grants **1991**
The Kettering Family Foundation (KFF) is a family grant-making organization that supports both Trustee-endorsed and unsolicited proposals that meet specific criteria. Unsolicited requests will be reviewed only one time per KFF fiscal year (ending December 31) from the same requesting organization and/or program. The following categories are of interest to KFF Trustees: cultural and arts; education; environment; medical health; and social/human services. A request summary (letter of interest) is required (by January 31 and July 31) and, if interested, trustees will ask for a full proposal.
Requirements: 501(c)3 tax-exempt organizations are eligible.
Restrictions: Requests for funding for the following areas are not generally approved unless endorsed by a trustee: capital construction; foreign-based or foreign- purpose organizations; religious organizations for religious purposes; individual public elementary or secondary schools or public school districts; local chapters of national organizations; grants, loans, scholarships, fellowships, or memberships; multiyear grants; travel expenses; community drives, event sponsorships; or conduit organizations.
Date(s) Application is Due: Jan 31; Mar 1; Jul 31; Sep 1
Contact: Charles F. Kettering, III, President; (303) 756-7664; email: info@ketteringfamilyfoundation.org
Internet: http://www.ketteringfamilyfoundation.org/main.html
Sponsor: Kettering Family Foundation
2833 S. Colorado Boulevard
Denver, CO 80222

Kettering Fund Grants **1992**
The mission of the Kettering Fund is to support scientific, medical, social and educational studies and research conducted by nonprofit, charitable organizations that are located and/or provide service in Ohio. The Distribution Committee meets on a semi-annual basis to make funding decisions, generally in May and November. The committee will consider support for the following purposes: capital needs (such as the purchase of land, new construction, renovations and equipment); seed grants for new organizations or programs; project support; endowments; research; and scholarship funds.
Requirements: 501(c)3 nonprofit organizations that provide services in or are located in Ohio may apply.
Restrictions: The fund does not support: religious organizations for religious purposes; activities of specific individuals; public elementary or secondary schools; loans; travel; deficit reduction; benefit events; or efforts to carry on propaganda or otherwise attempt to influence legislation.
Geographic Focus: Ohio
Samples: Kettering U (Flint, MI)—to support the Kettering Scholars Program, which awards scholarships to Ohio residents, $2.3 million.
Amount of Grant: $5,000-$200,000 range
Contact: Judith M. Thompson, Executive Director; (973) 228-1021; fax (973) 228-2399; email: info@ketteringfund.org
Internet: http://www.ketteringfund.org/main.html
Sponsor: Kettering Fund
1480 Kettering Tower
Dayton, OH 45423

Kevin P. and Sydney B. Knight Family Foundation Grants **1993**
The Foundation, established in 1997 by the founders of Knight Transportation of Phoenix, Arizona, is focused on the greater Phoenix area. Giving programs are aimed at: children and youth; Catholic agencies and churches; athletics/sports activities (particularly baseball); education; health care; and Mormon affiliated groups. Primary types of support include: community development, general research, and youth programs. There are no specific deadlines or application forms, and initial approach should be by letter.
Restrictions: Funding is restricted primarily to 501(c)3 organization located in Phoenix, Arizona.
Geographic Focus: Arizona
Samples: Leukemia and Lymphoma Society, Phoenix, Arizona, $1,000 (2006); St. Mary's Food Bank, Phoenix, Arizona, $200 (2006); ATA Scholarship Fund, Phoenix, Arizona, $1,500 (2006).
Amount of Grant: $1,000-$2,000 average
Contact: Kevin P. Knight, President; (602) 269-2000; fax: (602) 269-8409
Sponsor: Kevin P. and Sydney B. Knight Family Foundation
5601 W. Buckeye Road
Phoenix, AZ 85043-4603

Key Foundation Grants **1994**
The foundation's objective is to improve the quality of life and economic vibrancy of the places where KeyCorp customers, employees, and shareholders live and work. The foundation supports programs that enhance economic independence in support of two strategic thrusts: financial education and workforce initiatives. To a lesser degree, the foundation will continue to support organizations that enhance quality-of-life in Key communities in the Eastern, Midwestern, and Western United States; and greater Cleveland, OH area. The foundation recognizes the importance of diversity

and, accordingly, will make contributions to organizations that demonstrate a sincere commitment to individual diversity. Guidelines and application are available online.
Requirements: 501(c)3 tax-exempt organizations are eligible.
Restrictions: The foundation does not contribute to individuals, lobbying or political organizations, veteran or fraternal groups, or organizations that discriminate in any way with national equal opportunity policies. The foundation also does not buy journal advertisements or memberships.
Samples: Cleveland Museum of Art (OH)—to support programs that explore how diversity and inclusion influence the arts, to establish the KeyBank Summer Arts Internship Program, and to develop a bilingual distance-learning program that will focus on the art of the ancient Americans, $1.5 million (2005); Cleveland Institute of Music (OH)—for a distance-learning program designed to boost academic and professional development among students and educators, $25,000 (2005); Cuyahoga Community College (Cleveland, OH)—for a new center that will work to facilitate business and economic growth across northeastern Ohio, $1 million over three years (2005).
Contact: Grants Administrator, (216) 689-5458; fax: (216) 689-3865; email: key_foundation@keybank.com
Internet: http://www.key.com/community
Sponsor: Key Foundation
127 Public Sq, 7th Floor
Cleveland, OH 33113-1306

KeySpan Foundation Grants **1995**
The foundation awards grants to eligible nonprofit organizations in its areas of interest, including health and human services; education—K-12 classroom education, scholarships and university partnerships for the underserved, skills training; environment—sustainability of natural resources, educate youth about their connection to the environment, and preserve open spaces for the future; community development; and the arts. Proposals are accepted and reviewed on a first come/first served basis through October. The foundation's board of directors meets on a quarterly basis to review requests and authorize grants.
Requirements: New Hampshire, Massachusetts, and New York nonprofit organizations are eligible.
Restrictions: The foundation does not support religious or political groups, capital or endowment campaigns, advertisements, tables or tickets at dinners, and groups whose combined administrative, management, or fundraising expenses exceed 30 percent of the operating budget.
Geographic Focus: Massachusetts; New England; New Hampshire; New York
Amount of Grant: $5000-$25,000 average
Date(s) Application is Due: Oct 31
Contact: Robert Keller, Executive Director, (516) 545-5147
Internet: http://www.keyspanenergy.com/corpinfo/community/foundation_all.jsp
Sponsor: KeySpan Foundation
175 E Old Country Road
Hicksville, NY 11801

KFC Allied Health Research Grants **1996**
The foundation supports research into the incidence and cure of kidney and urinary tract disease, patient services, and public education. Preference will be given to allied health personnel undertaking research related to the kidney and urinary tract and to a new research project not supported by any other agency. Applications from investigators in related specialty areas also are considered. Types of support include capital grants, fellowships, general operating grants, program development grants, scholarships, and travel assistance. One- and two-year renewable grants are awarded.
Requirements: Application is open to individuals affiliated with Canadian universities for research conducted within Canada.
Restrictions: Grants will not be awarded for equipment only.
Amount of Grant: $C50,000 maximum
Date(s) Application is Due: Oct 15
Contact: Manager, National Research Programs, (514) 369-4806 ext 223 or (800) 361-7494 ext. 223; email: research@kidney.ca
Internet: http://www.kidney.ca/english/research/allied-funding-03.htm
Sponsor: Kidney Foundation of Canada
5165 Rue Sherbrooke Street, Suite 300
Montreal, QC H4A 1T6 Canada

KFC Biomedical Fellowships **1997**
Fellowships support full-time, postdoctoral research training in the renal and urinary tract field for training in Canada or abroad. The award amount is determined by level of experience and the holding of MD, DDS, DVM, and/or PhD degrees. Fellows are expected to devote 12 consecutive months and 80 percent of their time toward fulfilling the objectives of the fellowship. Awards are applied for through the National Office of the Kidney Foundation. Obtain application forms.
Requirements: Applicants must be Canadian citizens or landed immigrants and apply through a university department or affiliated institution.
Amount of Grant: $C45,000
Date(s) Application is Due: Oct 15
Contact: Manager, National Research Programs, (514) 369-4806 ext 225 or (800) 361-7494 ext 225; email: research@kidney.ca
Internet: http://www.kidney.ca/english/research/biomed-funding-03.htm
Sponsor: Kidney Foundation of Canada
5165 Rue Sherbrooke Street, Suite 300
Montreal, QC H4A 1T6 Canada

KFC Biomedical Research Grants **1998**
The program fosters and encourages research about the kidney and urinary tract and the understanding of kidney diseases. Types of support include general operating grants, research grants, materials and supplies, and travel assistance. One- and two-year renewable grants are offered.
Requirements: Canadian citizens or landed immigrants may apply. Research must be conducted in Canada by individuals holding staff appointments at Canadian universities or academic institutions.
Restrictions: Requests for equipment only are denied.
Amount of Grant: $C50,000 maximum
Date(s) Application is Due: Oct 15
Contact: Manager, National Research Programs, (514) 369-4806 ext 225 or (800) 361-7494 ext 225; fax: (514) 369-2472; email: research@kidney.ca
Internet: http://www.kidney.ca/english/research/biomed-funding-03.htm
Sponsor: Kidney Foundation of Canada
5165 Rue Sherbrooke Street, Suite 300
Montreal, PQ H4A 1T6 Canada

KFC Nephrology and Urology Scholarships **1999**
Nephrology and urology scholarships provide salary support for up to two years of an initial faculty appointment at an approved medical school in Canada. Successful applicants must use the scholarship within three years of the date of their first appointment as assistant professor and must commit to spending 75 percent or more time in research.
Amount of Grant: $C45,000 per year for two years
Date(s) Application is Due: Oct 15
Contact: Manager, National Research Programs, (514) 369-4806 ext 225 or (800) 361-7494 ext 225; fax: (514) 369-2472; email: research@kidney.ca
Internet: http://www.kidney.ca/english/research/biomed-funding-03.htm#bio-scholar
Sponsor: Kidney Foundation of Canada
5165 Rue Sherbrooke Street, Suite 300
Montreal, QC H4A 1T6 Canada

KFF Barbara Jordan Health Policy Scholars Program **2000**
The program brings talented African American, Latino, American Indian/Alaska Native, and Asian/Pacific Islander college seniors and recent graduates to Washington, DC, where they are placed in Congressional offices and learn about health policy. Through the nine-week program (May 23 through July 28), scholars gain knowledge about federal legislative procedure and health policy issues, while further developing their critical thinking and leadership skills. Scholars also participate in seminars and site visits to augment their knowledge of health care issues, and write and present a health policy research memo. Scholars receive a stipend upon completion of the program; a daily expense allowance for meals and local transportation; transportation/airfare to and from Washington, DC; and lodging at Howard University in Washington, DC. Application and guidelines are available online.
Requirements: Eligible candidates must be U.S. citizens who will be seniors or recent graduates of an accredited U.S. college or university in the fall. Successful applicants will show evidence of academic achievement and will demonstrate the following: be a member of a population that is adversely affected by racial or ethnic disparities in health; and have experience working in or with programs that address health disparities (e.g., local health departments, community health centers, inner city/rural hospitals, or organizations that conduct research on or develop policy related to health or health care disparities) or have done previous academic work (e.g., taken courses, written papers, or participate in research projects) related to health disparities.
Restrictions: Currently enrolled law, medical, and graduate students are not eligible to apply.
Amount of Grant: $7000 approximately, including $1500 stipend
Date(s) Application is Due: Jan 9
Contact: Grants Administrator, (650) 854-9400; fax: (650) 854-4800
Internet: http://www.kff.org/about/jordanscholars.cfm
Sponsor: Henry J. Kaiser Family Foundation
2400 Sand Hill Road
Menlo Park, CA 94025

Kimberly-Clark Community Grants **2001**
The corporation contributes significant philanthropic resources to organizations and programs that provide vital information, resources, and services that strengthen today's families; involve parents and others in activities that help children grow physically, mentally, and socially; and develop creative, caring options to cope with the issues facing our older relatives. Kimberly-Clark limits its charitable contributions to organizations serving communities where employees live and work. The corporation also supports YMCA of the U.S.A, UNICEF, United Way, and disaster- relief efforts. Send requests in corporate-operating cities to the site manager's attention. All decisions are made locally, not at the corporate level. Guidelines are available online.
Requirements: Nonprofit organizations in Kimberly-Clark communities are eligible, including Alabama (Mobile), Arkansas (Conway, Maumelle), California (Escondido, Fullerton), Connecticut (New Milford), Georgia (LaGrange, Roswell), Idaho (Pocatello), Kentucky (Owensboro), Michigan (Munising), Mississippi (Corinth, Hattiesburg), North Carolina (Hendersonville, Lexington), Ohio (Piqua), Oklahoma (Jenks), Pennsylvania (Chester), South Carolina (Beech Island), Tennessee (Knoxville, Loudon), Texas (Dallas, Del Rio, Fort Worth, Paris, San Antonio), Utah (Draper, Ogden), Washington (Everett), and Wisconsin (Marinette, Neenah, Whiting).

Restrictions: As a general rule, no unsolicited requests for national or international programs will be considered.
Geographic Focus: Alabama; Arkansas; California; Connecticut; Georgia; Idaho; Kentucky; Michigan; Mississippi; North Carolina; Ohio; Oklahoma; Pennsylvania; South Carolina; Tennessee; Texas; Utah; Washington; Wisconsin
Samples: UNICEF (New York, NY)—to assist tsunami-relief efforts, $500,000 (2005); YMCA of the U.S.A (Chicago, IL)—to redistribute to 42 YMCAs nationwide for programs designed to strengthen families, $420,000 (2004).
Contact: Corporate Contributions, (888) 525-8388
Internet: http://www.kimberly-clark.com/aboutus/contrib_program.asp
Sponsor: Kimberly-Clark Corporation
P.O. Box 2020, Dept INT
Neenah, WI 54957-2020

Kimmel Scholar Award **2002**
The foundation seeks to improve the basic understanding of cancer biology and to develop new cancer treatment and prevention methods. Grants support programs of accomplished young cancer researchers that emphasize basic cancer research, rapid translation of basic science concepts into potential therapeutic applications, and clinical research with novel or innovative treatment strategies. Up to 10 awards are made each year. Additional grants are awarded to physicians engaged in translational science. Application and guidelines are available online.
Requirements: Applicants must hold an MD, PhD, or equivalent graduate degree. Researchers who have achieved the equivalent rank of assistant professor on or after July 2001. Physicians who have both clinical and research responsibility are eligible if appointed on or after July 2000. Research must be conducted at U.S. nonprofit organizations.
Samples: Sheil Steart, Washington U (Saint Louis, MO)—for research on cancer, $200,000 over two years (2004); Brian Schaefer, Uniformed Services U of the Health Sciences (Bethesda, MD)—for research on cancer, $200,000 over two years (2004).
Amount of Grant: $100,000 per year for two years
Date(s) Application is Due: Dec 6
Contact: Gary Cohen, (443) 849-3729; fax: (443) 849-3719; email: gcohen@gbmc.org
Internet: http://www.kimmel.org/About41.html
Sponsor: Sidney Kimmel Foundation for Cancer Research
6569 N Charles Street, Suite 201
Baltimore, MD 21204

King Pharmaceuticals Corporate Contributions Grants **2003**
King awards quality-of-life grants in its Tennessee operating communities. Areas of interest include community programs—human health and welfare, with a focus on unmet needs of the community and serving the needs of the disadvantaged; education—innovation in the classroom, quality education for disadvantaged, drug and alcohol education, and youth development activities focused on building leadership and social skills and on preparing young people for the workforce; cultural arts—visual and performing arts organizations, museums, and other organizations with effective outreach programs that broaden cultural experiences for the general public; ministry—broad-based ministry programs that focus on the moral, ethical, and spiritual dimensions of everyday life; athletic programs—health and fitness, teambuilding, and longevity; and economic development—job creation, business development, and community investment. There are no application deadlines.
Requirements: Tennessee nonprofit organizations are eligible.
Geographic Focus: Tennessee
Contact: Corporate Contributions, (800) 776-3637 or (423) 989-8000
Internet: http://www.kingpharm.com/public_relations.htm
Sponsor: King Pharmaceuticals Inc
501 Fifth Street
Bristol, TN 37620

Kiwanis International Foundation Grants **2004**
The foundation supports nonprofits worldwide for programs and activities that meet the needs of young children. Past grants have supported a bloodmobile playground, Reading is Fundamental project, lifetime learning, and an effort to provide pediatric trauma kits. Applicants should contact the local chapter for additional information.
Requirements: U.S. and international nonprofits are eligible.
Restrictions: The foundation does not award grants for capital improvements or programs for more than three years.
Amount of Grant: $50,000 maximum
Date(s) Application is Due: Apr 15; Jul 15; Nov 15
Contact: Program Contact, (800) 549-2647; fax: (317) 879-0204; email: foundation@kiwanis.org
Internet: http://kif.kiwanis.org/kif/grants/grants.asp
Sponsor: Kiwanis International Foundation
3636 Woodview Trace
Indianapolis, IN 46268

Klingenstein Neuroscience Fellowships **2005**
The purpose of the fellowships is to support, in the early stages of their careers, young investigators engaged in basic or clinical research that may lead to a better understanding of epilepsy. Several areas within the neurosciences are of particular interest: cellular and molecular neuroscience, neural systems, and clinical research. Up to 10 fellows will be appointed. While U.S. citizenship is not a requirement, it is expected that candidates will be permanent residents of the United States and that their research will be carried out in U.S. institutions. The award may be used for salary support, research assistants, equipment, or for activities that promote the scientific advancement of the fellow. Payments will be made to the investigator's institution. Holding an award from another foundation concurrently with a Klingenstein award requires the approval of the advisory committee.
Requirements: Investigators must hold the PhD and/or MD degrees and have completed all research training, including postdoctoral training. The candidate should be an independent investigator, holding a tenure-track academic rank (but not yet tenured) in a university or medical school, or the equivalent standing in a research institute or medical center.
Amount of Grant: $150,000 over three years
Date(s) Application is Due: Dec 9
Contact: John Klingenstein, President, (212) 492-6181; fax: (212) 492-7007
Internet: http://www.klingfund.org
Sponsor: Esther A. and Joseph Klingenstein Fund
787 7th Avenue, 6th Floor
New York, NY 10019

Kluge Center David B. Larson Fellowship in Health and Spirituality **2006**
The Library of Congress invites qualified scholars to apply for a postdoctoral fellowship in the field of health and spirituality. It seeks to encourage the pursuit of scholarly excellence in the scientific study of the relation of religiousness and spirituality to physical, mental, and social health. The fellowship provides an opportunity for a period of six to 12 months of concentrated use of the collections of the Library of Congress, through full-time residency in the Library's John W. Kluge Center. If necessary, special arrangements may be made with the National Library of Medicine for access to its materials as well. Applicants must submit a formal application packet, including an application form, a two-page curriculum vita that should indicate major prior scholarship, a one-paragraph project summary, a bibliography of basic sources, a research proposal of no more than 1500 words, and three letters of reference (in English) from people who have read the research proposal.
Requirements: Applicants must by U.S. citizens or permanent residents and must possess a doctoral degree (PhD, MD, ScD, DrPH, DSW, PPsy, DST, ThD, and JD) awarded by the deadline date.
Amount of Grant: $4,200 per month for up to twelve months
Date(s) Application is Due: Apr 17
Contact: Larson Fellowships, (202) 707-3302; fax: (202) 707-3595; email: scholarly@loc.gov
Internet: http://www.loc.gov/loc/kluge/fellowships/larson.html
Sponsor: Library of Congress
101 Independence Avenue, SE
Washington, DC 20540-4860

Knight Family Charitable and Educational Foundation Grants **2007**
The Foundation operates in Michigan, and funding is reserved for elementary and secondary education, religious agencies, and community health and human service programs. Giving is primarily reserved for Michigan-based non-profit organizations. There are no specific deadlines or application forms to adhere to, and final approval is given approximately two months after submission.
Requirements: Applicants should be 501(c)3 organizations based in Michigan.
Amount of Grant: $500-$10,000 range
Contact: N.J. Glasser, Secretary-Treasurer; (517) 547-6131
Sponsor: Knight Family Foundation
215 North Talbot Street
Addison, MI 49220-9698

Knight Public Health Journalism Fellowships at CDC **2008**
The fellowships offer midcareer journalists a chance to break away from the day-to-day rigors of journalism to explore public health in-depth for a period of three months. Housed at CDC in Atlanta, with funding from the John S. and James L. Knight Foundation, the fellowships are a multi-faceted experience in research, field practice, and instruction. This year six Knight Fellows will train with CDC's Epidemic Intelligence Service officers, investigate a disease outbreak, work closely with other CDC scientists, attend seminars and Grand Rounds, and see how public health work is carried out by local and state authorities. Knight fellows receive a stipend to cover modest living expenses. Program guidelines are available online.
Requirements: Journalists with a track record of accomplishment, a minimum of five years of reporting experience, and a desire to strengthen the reporting of public health are invited to apply.
Date(s) Application is Due: Mar 15
Contact: Fellowship Administrator, (888) 880-4232 or (404) 653-0790; fax: (404) 653-0330
Internet: http://www.cdcfoundation.org/pages.html?page=296
Sponsor: Centers for Disease Control Foundation
50 Hurt Plz, Suite 765
Atlanta, GA 30303

Knox County Community Foundation Grants **2009**
Founded in 1996, the Knox County Community Foundation is a nonprofit, public charity created by and for the people of Knox County, Indiana. The foundation helps, nonprofits fulfill their missions by, strengthening their ability to meet community needs through grants that assist charitable programs, address community issues, support community agencies, launch community initiatives, and support leadership development. Grant

proposals are accepted once each year according to the grant cycle. Proposal requirements may change from year to year; therefore, grant seekers are advised to contact the foundation or see the foundations website, prior to beginning the grant application process. Grants are normally given as one-time support of a project but may be considered for additional support for expansions or outgrowths of an initial project. At the start of each cycle, a notice is mailed to nonprofit organizations that have applied for grants in the past, have received grants in the past, or have otherwise requested notification of the start of each cycle. The grant cycle runs from January through May each year. Proposals will be accepted from January through the March deadline. All organizations that have submitted grant proposals will be notified of the outcome of the grants committee's deliberation in writing no later than June 1.
Requirements: The Foundation welcomes proposals from nonprofit organizations that are deemed tax-exempt under sections 501(c)3 and 509(a) of the Internal Revenue Code and from governmental agencies serving the county. Proposals from nonprofit organizations not classified as a 501(c)3 public charity may be considered provided the project is charitable and supports a community need. Proposals submitted by an entity under the auspices of another agency must include a written statement signed by the agency's board president on behalf of the board of directors agreeing to act as the entity's fiscal sponsor, to receive grant monies if awarded, and to oversee the proposed project. Program areas considered for funding are: arts and culture; community development; education; health; human services; other civic endeavors, such as the environment, recreation, and youth development.
Restrictions: Project areas not considered for funding are: religious organizations for religious purposes; political parties or campaigns; endowment creation or debt reduction; operating costs; capital campaigns; annual appeals or membership contributions; travel requests for groups or individuals such as bands, sports teams, or classes. A six-month progress report and a final report at project completion are required by organizations whose proposals are approved for funding. Instructions and appropriate forms will be provided at the time the grant is awarded.
Geographic Focus: Indiana
Samples: Indiana Military Museum, $1,500 - for Website Development and Deployment Project (2008); Walnut Grove United Methodist Church, $2,000 - to support their Back To School Mall Project (2008); Freelandville Community Home, $5,000 - for Ambulance Bay Project (2008);
Date(s) Application is Due: 5 p.m. on the first Wednesday of March.
Contact: Kathy Rinsch; (812) 886-0093; email: kathy@knoxcountyfoundation.org
Internet: http://www.knoxcountyfoundation.org/disc-grants-program
Sponsor: Knox County Community Foundation
20 North Third Street, Suite 301 P.O. Box 273
Vincennes, IN 47591

Komen Greater NYC Clinical Trials Enrollment Grants **2010**
The Greater New York City Affiliate of Susan G. Komen for the Cure (Komen Greater NYC) fulfills its mission of eradicating breast cancer as a life-threatening disease, in part, by offering grants to enhance the capacity of National Cancer Institute- and Department of Defense-approved breast cancer clinical research conducted in the Komen Greater NYC area to increase the number of women enrolled in breast cancer clinical research studies. Komen Greater NYC seeks to fund projects that implement evidence-based strategies to overcome barriers to enrollment in breast cancer clinical research. Collaborative projects between institutions and community-based organizations are encouraged.
Requirements: To apply, the organization must be: a not-for-profit organization (a charitable or educational tax-exempt organization), a government agency, or an Indian tribe; conducting National Cancer Institute (NCI) or Department of Defense (DOD) approved breast cancer clinical research (this includes studies through the Clinical Trials Cooperative Group Program including but not limited to ACOSOG, ECOG, SWOG, NSABP, ACRIN, and RTOG; and located in the Komen Greater NYC service area, which includes the five boroughs of New York City, Long Island, Westchester County, and Rockland County.
Geographic Focus: New York
Amount of Grant: $200,000 over two years
Date(s) Application is Due: Oct 9
Contact: Mary Haviland, Esq. Director of Grants and Public Policy; (212) 560-9590, ext. 230; email: mhaviland@komennyc.org
Internet: http://www.komennyc.org/site/PageServer?pagename=grants_clinicaltrials
Sponsor: Susan G. Komen for the Cure Foundation
341 West 38th Street, 10th Floor
New York, NY 10018-2918

Komen Greater NYC Community Breast Health Grants **2011**
The mission of Komen Greater NYC is to eradicate breast cancer as a life-threatening disease by advancing research, education, screening, and treatment. The Greater New York City Affiliate is, therefore, soliciting applications from non-profit organizations that have current or planned breast health programs within the five boroughs of New York City, Long Island, Westchester County, and Rockland County. The purpose of the Community Breast Health Grants Program (formerly known as Screening, Treatment, and Education Program- STEP) is to support community-based programs that provide the medically under-served with access to breast health education, screening coordination, diagnostic, treatment, and support services.
Requirements: Applicant organizations must be: a not-for-profit organization (a charitable or educational tax-exempt organization), a government agency, or an Indian tribe; located in the Komen Greater NYC service area, which includes the five boroughs of New York City, Long Island, Westchester County, and Rockland County; and a current or planned provider of breast health services.
Geographic Focus: New York
Amount of Grant: $100,000 maximum
Date(s) Application is Due: Oct 9
Contact: Mary Haviland, Esq. Director of Grants and Public Policy; (212) 560-9590, ext. 230; email: mhaviland@komennyc.org
Internet: http://www.komennyc.org/site/PageServer?pagename=grants_breasthealth grants
Sponsor: Susan G. Komen for the Cure Foundation
341 West 38th Street, 10th Floor
New York, NY 10018-2918

Komen Greater NYC Conference Grants **2012**
Komen Greater NYC provides grants to non-profit organizations to support educational conferences, symposiums or meetings. To be considered for funding, events must be specific to breast health or help further the body of knowledge related to breast cancer research, education, screening, diagnosis, treatment and/or support. Grants are considered three times per year, in May, August, and January. Awards will not exceed $5,000. Award notifications are generally made within 6 weeks after receipt of the application.
Requirements: To apply, the organization must be: a not-for-profit organization (a charitable or educational tax-exempt organization), a government agency, or an Indian tribe; conducting National Cancer Institute (NCI) or Department of Defense (DOD) approved breast cancer clinical research (this includes studies through the Clinical Trials Cooperative Group Program including but not limited to ACOSOG, ECOG, SWOG, NSABP, ACRIN, and RTOG; and located in the Komen Greater NYC service area, which includes the five boroughs of New York City, Long Island, Westchester County, and Rockland County.
Geographic Focus: New York
Amount of Grant: $5,000 maximum
Date(s) Application is Due: May 14; Jul 25; Dec 1
Contact: Cara Thunder, Grants Program Associate; (212) 461-6185; cthunder@komennyc.org
Internet: http://www.komennyc.org/site/PageServer?pagename=grants_conference
Sponsor: Susan G. Komen for the Cure Foundation
341 West 38th Street, 10th Floor
New York, NY 10018-2918

Komen Greater NYC Small Grants Program **2013**
Komen Greater NYC is currently offering small grants up to $5,000 to support small and pilot projects in breast health, organize conferences, and travel scholarships. Small Grant Applications are accepted three times a year. The deadlines are announced on the Komen Greater NYC website at: www.komennyc.org/grants. Requests for support of travel scholarships, conferences, or other events must be received at least 3 months prior to the event. Award notifications are generally made within 6 weeks after receipt of the application.
Requirements: Applicants and institutions must conform to the following eligibility criteria to be considered for funding: 1) Applicants must ensure that all past and current Komen-funded grants or awards are up-to-date and in compliance with Komen requirements; 2) Institutions must be located in or providing services to one or more of the following locations: the five boroughs of New York City; Long Island (Suffolk and Nassau Counties); Westchester County; Rockland County; 3) Project must be specific to breast health and/or breast cancer; 4) the applicant must be a non-profit organization with federal tax exemption. Individuals may not receive grants; 5) Small Grant applicants are restricted to a maximum combined award of $5,000 per Komen Greater NYC grant year (April through March), per program for any type of Small Grant- Travel, Conference and/or Small Grant; 6) current Grantees are eligible to apply for small grants.
Geographic Focus: New York
Amount of Grant: $5,000
Contact: Cara Thunder, Grants Program Associate; (212) 461-6185; email: cthunder@komennyc.org.
Internet: http://www.komennyc.org/site/PageServer?pagename=grants_small_grants_program
Sponsor: Susan G. Komen for the Cure Foundation
341 West 38th Street, 10th Floor
New York, NY 10018-2918

Kosair Charities Grants **2014**
In 1923, a committee of members from Louisville's Kosair Shrine Temple, doctors, lawyers, and community leaders formed Kosair Charities. The mission was to provide the highest quality health care possible for children who had nowhere else to turn. Since conception, Kosair Charities has became the largest charity in the history of the region that provides for the medical care of children. All of this is possible thanks to the generous support of individuals and companies. Kosair Charities receives no assistance from United Way, the Crusade for Children, or any governmental entity. Annual grants are awarded in the early summer of each year and applications are due by May 1.
Requirements: Grants are only made to those non-profit agencies and organizations whose program falls within the above stated mission. Two grant requests applications are available for download on the Kosair Charities website in amounts of $1,500 or less and $1,500 or more. With each completed application, attach the following: Copy of IRS determination letter; current year's budget; income and expense statement last two years; copy of last completed audit; copy of roster of Board of Directors; descriptive literature on

agency and its services; if the proposal is for an existing or continuing program, submit latest self-evaluation of program; if the proposal is for one that Kosair Charities has funded in the past, demonstrate use of Kosaid Charities Supported Agency Logo and public acknowledgements; detailed proposal budget; original grant application plus five copies for a total of six copies of all requested information.
Restrictions: Grants are available throughout Kentucky and the southern Indiana region. Grants are made for one year only and do not represent any future commitment on the part of Kosair Charities. Grant recipients are required to use the Kosair Charities Supported Agency logo on all printed and electronic materials and media used by their agency.
Geographic Focus: Indiana; Kentucky
Date(s) Application is Due: May 1
Contact: Jo Barrett, Vice President, Programs & Special Events; (502) 637-7696 / (888) 454-3752; email: jbarrett@kosair.org
Internet: http://www.kosair.org/grants.html
Sponsor: Kosair Charities
982 Eastern Parkway, P.O. Box 37370
Louisville, KY 40233-7370

Kosciusko County Community Foundation Grants **2015**
The Kosciusko County Community Foundation serves Kosciusko County, Indiana and the communities thereof. The Foundations favors activities that: reach abroad segment of the community, especially those citizens whose needs are not being met by existing services that are normally expected to be provided by private rather then government sources; request seed money to realize innovative opportunities to meet needs in the community; stimulate and encourage additional funding; promote cooperation and avoid duplication; help make charitable organization more effective and efficient and better able to be self sustaining. Grant seekers are strongly encouraged to call the Foundation to discuss a grant proposal before submitting a formal application. Application can be obtained at the Foundations office or the Foundations website.
Requirements: Completed applications must be submitted by deadline date with the required attachments: if your organization is a 501(c)3, attach a copy of your IRS Determination letter (1 copy); attach a list of names and addresses of your board of directors and staff (1 copy); attach a copy of your organization's operating budget and a copy of your program/project budget, if applicable (6 copies); complete copies of this application, plus the original. Do not copy any of the attachments such as letters of reference, news articles, brochures, etc.
Geographic Focus: Indiana
Date(s) Application is Due: Jan 15; May 15; Sep 15
Contact: Stephanie Overbey, Communication & Program Director; (574) 267-1901; fax: (574) 268-9780; email: stephanie@kcfoundation.org
Internet: http://www.kcfoundation.org/grants.html
Sponsor: Kosciusko County Community Foundation, Inc.
102 East Market Street
Warsaw, IN 46580

Kraft Cares International Grants **2016**
The company's program for international corporate contributions, has several priority areas for grantmaking. The primary focus area for international giving is the worldwide fight to end hunger. The corporation provides financial support, product donations, meal service, enhanced food delivery systems, nutrition programs, and food security initiatives. Additional funding areas include culture, with particular focus on expanding access to the visual arts and dance to underserved populations; domestic violence, with particular focus on providing food-related support, clothing, shelter, or counseling; AIDS, with particular focus on providing food-related services; and education, with particular focus on helping adults attain literacy competency and supporting at-risk children and adolescents.
Requirements: Funding must be made through a U.S. 501(c)3 organization or qualify as a 501(c)3 equivalent. Program requests must be submitted to a Kraft Foods national or regional office, and address a community need in that market.
Amount of Grant: $10,000-$50,000
Contact: Corporate Contributions Specialist, (847) 646-3332; fax: (847) 646-5241; email: localgrants@kraft.com
Internet: http://www.kraftcares@kraft.com
Sponsor: Kraft Foods Inc
3 Lakes Drive
Northfield, IL 60093

Kraft Cares U.S. Grants **2017**
The corporation's main focus of giving is on hunger, healthy lifestyles, and access to the arts. Grants are awarded to programs that provide direct service to individuals and communities in need. The corporation usually makes grants for specific projects with measurable results, rather than for general operating support, and looks for programs that can be potentially replicated in other communities. A limited number of smaller grants are provided annually to organizations in the areas of conservation and the environment, general education, civic and community involvement, and human services. All requests for applications and guidelines must be made in writing.
Requirements: Organizations with 501(c)3 tax-exempt status are eligible.
Restrictions: Grants do not fund general operating support; operating support for colleges/universities; operating support for high schools or elementary schools; scholarships; endowments; amateur athletic teams; fraternal, veteran, or labor organizations; named charities of foundations; support for specific research or services related to diseases or medical conditions; political campaigns; religious organizations that serve only their denomination; special events (fund-raisers); capital campaigns; travel funds; political or lobbying organizations or those supporting the candidacy of a particular individual; benefit tickets or courtesy advertising; or product donations other than to Second Harvest food banks.
Samples: Art Institute of Chicago, $50,000; Bay Area Food Bank, $48,500; Bienvenidos Children's Center, Inc., $25,000; Catholic Charities Centro Mater Child Care Ctr, $45,000 (all 2005).
Amount of Grant: $10,000-$45,000 typically
Contact: Corporate Contributions Specialist, (847) 646-3332; fax: (847) 646-5241; email: localgrants@kraft.com
Internet: http://www.kraftcares@kraft.com
Sponsor: Kraft Foods Inc
3 Lakes Drive
Northfield, IL 60093

L. A. Hollinger Respiratory Therapy and Nursing Scholarships **2018**
The intent of this scholarship is to promote his strong commitment to education with the emphasis on continually improving the quality of patient care and ensuring the continued preparation of future nurses and respiratory therapists to meet that objective. The scholarship is awarded to those who are currently pursuing a Nursing or Respiratory Therapy undergraduate or graduate degree. All applications must be submitted or postmarked by May 15th.
Requirements: All applicants must have a cumulative GPA of 2.5. All nursing applicants must be a recipient of a Trinity Lutheran Hospital School of Nursing Alumnae Scholarship for the current year. Respiratory Therapy applicants must be enrolled in the Respiratory Therapy program at either Johnson County Community College or the University of Kansas.
Date(s) Application is Due: May 15
Contact: Becky Schaid, Executive Director; (816) 276-7515 or (816) 276-7555; fax: (816) 926-2261; email: becky@btllf.org
Internet: http://www.btllf.org/funding.html
Sponsor: Baptist-Trinity Lutheran Legacy Foundation
6601 Rockhill Road
Kansas City, MO 64131

L. W. Pierce Family Foundation Grants **2019**
Established in 1997, The Foundation supports organizations involved with health, social, and educational services in the areas of alcohol and drug abuse, hospice care and children's welfare. Giving is limited to the Vero Beach, FL and Philadelphia, PA areas.
Requirements: Non-profits in the Vero Beach, FL and Philadelphia, PA areas are eligible.
Restrictions: No grants to individuals.
Geographic Focus: Florida; Pennsylvania
Samples: Homeless Family Center, Vero Beach, FL, $50,000 (2006); Senior Resource Association, Vero Beach, FL, $20,000 (2006); Thomas Jefferson University, Philadelphia, PA, $20,000 (2006);
Amount of Grant: $1,000-$50,000 range
Date(s) Application is Due: Mar 1
Contact: Constance Buckley, President; (610) 862-2105; fax: (610) 862-2120;
Sponsor: The L. W. Pierce Family Foundation
8 Tower Bridge, Suite 1060, 161 Washington Street
Conshohocken, PA 19428-2060

LaGrange County Community Foundation Grants **2020**
The general policy of the foundation is to make grants for innovative and creative projects and programs that are responsive to changing community needs in the areas of, but not restricted to; arts and culture, community development, education, environment, health and human services, recreation and youth development.
Requirements: Non-profit organizations, schools and qualifying government agencies serving the citizens of LaGrange County are invited to apply for a grant through the foundation's application process.
Restrictions: The foundation does not make grants to individuals, except in the form of academic scholarships. Grants are generally given one-time only for specific purposes and will typically not be awarded to provide annual operating expenses or support. Nor will a grant be awarded to replenish funds previously expended. Grants are made with the understanding that the foundation has no obligation or commitment to provide additional support to the grantee. Grants may not be used for any political campaign, or to support attempts to influence legislature of any government body other than through making available the results of nonpartisan analysis, study and research.
Geographic Focus: Indiana
Contact: Grants Administrator, (260) 463-4363; fax: (260) 463-4856; email: lccf@lccf.net
Internet: http://www.lccf.net/grants.html
Sponsor: LaGrange County Community Foundation
109 E. Central Avenue, Suite 3
LaGrange, IN 46761

Lalor Foundation Postdoctoral Research Grants **2021**
Grants are awarded to institutions for basic postdoctoral research in mammalian reproductive physiology and biochemistry yielding improved methods of contraception, termination of pregnancy, and/or sterilization. Funds may be used to cover fellowship stipends, institution overhead, and laboratory and miscellaneous expenses. Less money is awarded for projects requiring less than one year.

Requirements: Applications must come from tax-exempt institutions; individuals nominated must have training and experience at least equal to the PhD, or MD level. People who have held the doctoral degree less than five years are preferred.
Amount of Grant: $35,000 maximum
Date(s) Application is Due: Jan 13
Contact: Pamela Labonte Maksy, (617) 426-7080 ext 314; fax (617) 426-5441; email: pmaksy@grantsmanagement.com
Internet: http://www.lalorfound.org/guidelines.html
Sponsor: Lalor Foundation
77 Summer Street
Boston, MA 02110-1006

LAM Foundation Established Investigator Awards **2022**

The award supports research directly related to lymphangioleiomyomatosis (LAM) and is targeted at established investigators who focus on the abnormal proliferation of smooth muscle that occurs in the disease. Awards provide a maximum of $50,000 per year, renewable for up to two additional years. The structure and terms of this award are identical to the LAM Fellowship Award except that with the LAM Established Award, faculty level investigators are eligible to receive funding for technician support and supplies.
Requirements: U.S. citizens and foreign nationals with appropriate immigrant visa status are eligible. At the time of application, an applicant must hold a doctoral degree and faculty appointment at the level of assistant or associate professor and be undertaking a project related to LAM.
Date(s) Application is Due: Apr 15; Sep 15
Contact: Francis X. McCormack, MD, Director; (513) 558-4831; fax: (513) 558-4858; email: frank.mccormack@uc.edu
Internet: http://www.thelamfoundation.org/research1/research-funding.html&searched=Awards&highlight=ajaxSearch_highlight+ajaxSearch_highlight1
Sponsor: LAM (Lymphangioleiomyomatosis) Foundation
MSB Room 6053 231 Albert Sabin Way
Cincinnati, OH 45267-0564

LAM Foundation Pilot Project Awards **2023**

Pilot project awards are granted for one year to enable investigators to gather sufficient preliminary data for more substantial LAM funding. Funding is intended to support faculty-level investigators, or postdoctoral-level investigators who will be performing LAM research in the laboratory of an established scientist who is an expert in areas that are directly pertinent to LAM. Letters of intent (LOI) are required prior to submission of grant proposals to the LAM Foundation. Application materials and details are available online.
Requirements: Applications are accepted from investigators of all nationalities who have MDs or PhDs, but candidates must possess visas that allow for completion of the proposed project in the original laboratory.
Amount of Grant: $25,000 maximum
Date(s) Application is Due: Apr 15; Sep 15
Contact: Francis X. McCormack, MD, Director; (513) 558-4831; fax: (513) 558-4858; email: frank.mccormack@uc.edu
Internet: http://www.thelamfoundation.org/research1/research-funding.html&searched=Awards&highlight=ajaxSearch_highlight+ajaxSearch_highlight1
Sponsor: LAM (Lymphangioleiomyomatosis) Foundation
MSB Room 6053 231 Albert Sabin Way
Cincinnati, OH 45267-0564

LAM Foundation Research Grants **2024**

The program provides seed money to investigators seeking to understand the abnormal smooth muscle proliferation that occurs in lymphangioleiomyomatosis (LAM). The grant supports clinical, laboratory, epidemiological, or any other kind of research that directly relates to LAM. Grants are subject to annual review and may be granted for up to two years. Scientists who which to apply for LAM Foundation funding must submit a Letter of Intent (LOI). Letters of Intent must reach The LAM Foundation by July 30th.
Requirements: U.S. citizens and foreign nationals with appropriate immigrant visa status are eligible. At the time of application, an applicant must hold a doctoral degree and faculty appointment with an academic institution and have completed two years of research training.
Restrictions: Residents, interns, postdoctoral fellows, students enrolled in degree-granting programs, and established investigators are ineligible.
Amount of Grant: $40,000 maximum per year
Date(s) Application is Due: Sep 15
Contact: Francis X. McCormack, MD, Director; (513) 558-4831; fax: (513) 558-4858; email: frank.mccormack@uc.edu
Internet: http://www.thelamfoundation.org/research1/research-funding.html&searched=Awards&highlight=ajaxSearch_highlight+ajaxSearch_highlight1
Sponsor: LAM (Lymphangioleiomyomatosis) Foundation
MSB Room 6053 231 Albert Sabin Way
Cincinnati, OH 45267-0564

Lance Armstrong Foundation Community Grants **2025**

The foundation awards grants through its community program to nonprofit organizations in support of community-centered, cancer survivorship initiatives that serve the needs identified by the National Action Plan for Cancer Survivorship. Two types of grants will be awarded. One-year planning grants will be considered in two areas: practical issues of cancer survivorship, and outreach to underserved populations. This grant will support the development of a design for the proposed project and a complete plan for its implementation (and evaluation). One-year evaluation grants, awarded in the amount of up to 10 percent of the total project budget, will be considered in five areas: cancer pain, palliative and end-of-life care; physical activity and nutrition; survivorship education; survivorship support; and practical issues of cancer survivorship. The applicant should already have a well-developed design for the project and a complete plan for both its implementation and its impact and effectiveness evaluation. This grant will support the evaluation of the project. The listed deadline is for receipt of applications, accepted only through the online application system. Only the first 100 applications submitted after 9:00 am on August, 29th, will be accepted. Guidelines are available online.
Requirements: Applicants must be U.S. nonprofit organizations, classified as other than a private foundation under the IRS code. Eligible programs include any programmatic project (such as service delivery or education) that fits the guidelines described in the current RFP. For evaluation grants, eligibility includes projects that are finished with implementation, in the midst of implementation, or about to begin implementation—with funding for implementation already secured.
Restrictions: Ineligible programs include nonprogrammatic projects (such as an advertising campaign or a fundraising event or campaign), and other projects that do not fit the guidelines described in the RFP. For evaluation grants, ineligibility includes projects that have not yet been implemented and do not already have funding secured for implementation.
Samples: U of Alabama, School of Public Health (Birmingham, AL)—to provide support services to people with cancer and to cancer survivors, $150,000 (2005); New York U School of Medicine, NYU Cancer Institute (NY)—for education programs to help people deal with the emotional, physical, and practical challenges of cancer, $20,000 (2005).
Amount of Grant: $10,000 maximum planning grants; $10,000 maximum evaluation grants
Date(s) Application is Due: Sep 9
Contact: Grants Administrator, (512) 236-8820; fax: (512) 236-8482
Internet: http://www.livestrong.org/site/c.jvKZLbMRIsG/b.739141/k.9A5A/Community_Program_RFP__Fall.htm
Sponsor: Lance Armstrong Foundation
P O Box 161150
Austin, TX 78716-1150

Lance Armstrong Foundation Research Grants **2026**

The foundation funds and disseminates research that builds on the body of knowledge and services focused on improving the quality of life for cancer survivors across physical, emotional, and practical challenges. The research program also supports research focused on testicular cancer. The foundation funds research that is not readily fundable from traditional sources and that encourages and supports the efforts of both young and established investigators. Young investigators are defined as within eight years of completing a terminal degree or within five years of initiating independent research within a mentored laboratory, while general research awards support new research projects initiated by established investigators. Proposals are accepted from all countries. The listed application deadline is for letters of intent; full RFPs are available online.
Amount of Grant: $50,000 maximum young investigator research awards; $75,000 maximum research awards
Date(s) Application is Due: May 13
Contact: Amy Nunn, Grants Coordinator, (512) 236-8820 ext 181; email: amy.nunn@laf.org or research.grants@laf.org
Internet: http://www.livestrong.org/site/c.jvKZLbMRIsG/b.739079/k.9EDA/Research_Grants.htm
Sponsor: Lance Armstrong Foundation
P.O. Box 161150
Austin, TX 78716-1150

Land O'Lakes Foundation Mid-Atlantic Grants Program **2027**

The grassroots program serves Land O'Lakes dairy communities in the states of Maryland, New Jersey, New York, Pennsylvania, and Virginia, and works to improve quality of life by supporting valuable projects and charitable endeavors in the region. The foundation awards grants to projects that best address the following areas: hunger relief, youth and education, rural leadership, civic improvements, soil and water preservation, and arts and culture. Application procedures are available online.
Requirements: 501(c)3 community organizations serving Land O'Lakes dairy communities in Maryland, New Jersey, New York, Pennsylvania, and Virginia are eligible.
Restrictions: Grants will not be awarded for the following purposes: scholarship funds, gifts or fund raisers for individuals, or non-public church use.
Geographic Focus: Maryland; New Jersey; New York; Pennsylvania; Virginia
Amount of Grant: $500-$5000
Contact: Bonnie Bassett, Executive Director, (651) 481-2222; fax: (651) 481-2000; email: Bbbass@landolakes.com or MLAtkins-Sakry@landolakes.com
Internet: http://www.foundation.landolakes.com/mida_desc.asp
Sponsor: Land O'Lakes Foundation
P.O. Box 64150
Saint Paul, MN 55164-0150

Landon Foundation-AACR Innovator Award for International Collaboration **2028**

This Award will support highly meritorious research that is being conducted collaboratively by investigators in different countries around the world. The goals of the program are to: promote international cancer research collaboration as an effective means to accelerate

progress against cancer; provide the support necessary to sustain and enhance highly meritorious international cancer research collaborations; foster interactions between and among cancer scientists and disseminate the scientific knowledge gained from international collaboration; and contribute to a global impact against cancer. The Award of $100,000 will be provided to the recipients' institutions in the form of a two-year grant to support the collaborative research project, and may be used for such purposes including, but not limited to: direct research expenses attributable to the proposed research, which may include the salary of research assistants or technicians; expenses for travel to the institutions of the collaborators relevant to the research project; expenses for training in new techniques that will benefit the research project, such as training received through a scholar exchange/visiting professor program; and expenses related to the presentation of research data at scientific meetings or through other means that will contribute to the dissemination of the scientific knowledge gained.
Requirements: Two or more independent researchers who working within an established international cancer research collaboration involving institutes in multiple countries may apply. Proposals to initiate a collaborative project will not be accepted. The co-investigators may be affiliated with any institution involved in cancer research, cancer medicine, or cancer-related biomedical science anywhere in the world. There is no limit to the number of co-investigators within each of the collaborating institutes. There are no national or residency status restrictions. Applicants need not be members of the AACR. Applications must be completed online using the proposalCENTRAL website, with one paper copy submitted to the AACR office. Online applications must be completed by 12:00 noon (United States Eastern Daylight Time) on November 20. The paper copy with original signatures and all supporting documents must be postmarked no later than November 25.
Restrictions: Scientific investigators or health professionals who are funded by the tobacco industry for any project, or whose named mentors in the case of mentored grants are funded by the tobacco industry for any project, may not apply and will not be eligible for AACR grants.
Amount of Grant: two-year grant $100,000 ($50,000 per year)
Date(s) Application is Due: Nov 20; Nov 25
Contact: Hanna Hopfinger, Grants Program Assistant; (267) 646-0665; fax: (215) 440-9372; email: hanna.hopfinger@aacr.org
Internet: http://www.aacr.org/home/scientists/research-funding—fellowships/landon-aacr-innovator-award-for-international-collaboration.aspx
Sponsor: American Association for Cancer Research
615 Chestnut Street, 17th Floor
Philadelphia, PA 19106-4404

Landon Foundation-AACR Innovator Award for Cancer Prevention Research **2029**
This Award was established and first given in 2008 to recognize the outstanding achievement of an early career Assistant Professor, and to provide support for cancer prevention research of significant scientific merit in any discipline across the continuum of research. The goals of the program are to: encourage younger investigators to pursue cancer prevention research of significant scientific merit; provide the support necessary to sustain and enhance highly meritorious cancer prevention research; foster interactions between and among cancer scientists and disseminate the scientific knowledge about cancer prevention research; and contribute to a global impact against cancer. A two-year grant of $100,000 ($50,000 per year) will be provided to the recipient's institution to support direct research expenses; salary and benefits; and attendance at the AACR Annual Meeting, Cancer Prevention Conference, or other AACR meeting relevant to cancer prevention for the purpose of participating in scholarly exchange.
Requirements: Candidates must be scientists at the level of Assistant Professor who completed postdoctoral studies or clinical fellowships on or after July 1. Candidates cannot be tenured or under consideration for tenured academic positions at the time of application. A candidate whose title is not Assistant Professor but who believes that he or she meets the eligibility requirements for this Award must attach a letter from the institution's dean certifying that the position held is equivalent to Assistant Professor. Both AACR members and nonmembers are eligible to apply. However, nonmembers must submit a satisfactory application for AACR Active membership on or before October 31. Applications must be submitted by 12:00 noon (United States Eastern Daylight Time) on November 20, using the proposalCENTRAL website at http://proposalcentral.altum.com. One paper copy with original signatures and all supporting documents must be mailed to the AACR office, and be postmarked no later then November 25.
Restrictions: Employees or subcontractors of a national government or private industry are not eligible for this grant.
Amount of Grant: two-year grant $100,000 ($50,000 per year)
Date(s) Application is Due: Nov 20; Nov 25
Contact: Julia Laurence, Program Assistant; (267) 646-0655; fax: (215) 440-9372; email: julia.laurence@aacr.org or awards@aacr.org
Internet: http://www.aacr.org/home/scientists/research-funding—fellowships/landon-aacr-innovator-award-for-cancer-prevention-research.aspx
Sponsor: American Association for Cancer Research
615 Chestnut Street, 17th Floor
Philadelphia, PA 19106-4404

Lands' End Corporate Giving Program **2030**
The corporation awards grants to nonprofits for youth and family services programs. The small grants program is nationwide but the large grants program is limited to certain areas. The company concentrates its large grant awards in Illinois, Iowa, Minnesota, New York, and Wisconsin, in communities where it has operations; however, applications are encouraged from all regions of the country. Areas of interest include education, community development, environment, health, and human services. Application guidelines may be obtained by contacting the company's Web site.
Requirements: U.S. nonprofits are eligible.
Restrictions: The foundation does not consider grants for organizations without nonprofit status; individuals; political organizations, campaigns, or candidates for public office; lobbying groups; advertising in programs, bulletins, yearbooks, or brochures; testimonial/awards dinners; endowments; loans; religious groups for religious purposes; pageants; purchasing of land; salaries; administrative costs; international programs; research programs; or general operating expenses.
Amount of Grant: $100 for small grants; $5000-$10,000 for large grants
Contact: Corporate Contributions, (608) 935-6776 or (608) 935-6728; fax: (608) 935-6432; email: donate@landsend.com
Internet: http://www.landsend.com/cd/fp/help/0,,1_36877_36883_37029_,00.html?sid=6562024422599131030
Sponsor: Lands' End
2 Lands' End Lane
Dodgeville, WI 53595

Larry L. Hillblom Foundation Grants **2031**
The mission of the foundation is to provide philanthropic support exclusively for charitable, religious, scientific, literary, and educational purposes. Primarily, the foundation will support medical research, including basic scientific research, clinical research, and research related to patient self-care and management. Medical research priorities include the areas of diabetes mellitus, diseases associated with aging, and children's physical and neurological diseases. Specific grants include building/institute grants, start-up research grants, network grants, fellowships, endowed chairs, and clinical research grants.
Samples: U of California (Oakland, CA)—to endow a chair in geriatric medicine at the U of California, San Diego, in La Jolla, $2 million (2003); U of California at San Francisco (CA)—to create a center for research on the basic biology of aging, and to support research on diabetes, eye disorders, and neurodegenerative diseases, $12 million.
Amount of Grant: $250,000-$10 million over 7 years
Date(s) Application is Due: Jan 14
Contact: Grants Administrator, (707) 762-6691; fax: (707) 762-6694; email: som@llhf.org
Internet: http://www.llhf.org
Sponsor: Larry L. Hillblom Foundation
755 Baywood Drive, Suite 180
Petaluma, CA 94954

Laura B. Vogler Foundation Grants **2032**
The foundation supports innovative programs and projects in New York City and Long Island in the areas of education, health care, and social services. The foundation is particularly interested in organizations that serve and support children, the elderly, and the disadvantaged. Types of support include general operating support, program development, research grants, and seed money grants. Grants provide one-time, nonrenewable support.
Requirements: Nonprofit organizations in New York City and Long Island, NY, may submit proposals.
Restrictions: Grants are not awarded to support building or endowment funds, annual fund-raising campaigns, or matching gifts.
Geographic Focus: New York
Samples: Shield Institute (NY)—for a joint activities program for preschoolers and the elderly, $2500.; Mercy Ctr Ministries Inc (NY)—to support three shelters for homeless young women and parenting teens, $3500.
Amount of Grant: $1000-$5000
Date(s) Application is Due: Mar 1; Jul 1; Nov 1
Contact: Lawrence D'Amato, President, (718) 423-3000; fax: (718) 631-4808
Internet: http://fdncenter.org/grantmaker/vogler
Sponsor: Laura B. Vogler Foundation
P.O. Box 610508
Bayside, NY 11361-0508

Lavelle Fund for the Blind Grants **2033**
The fund is dedicated to supporting programs that promote the spiritual, moral, intellectual, and physical development of blind and low-vision people of all ages, together with programs that help people avoid vision loss. Priority is given to agencies that concentrate on serving the New York City metropolitan area. The fund gives preference to program creation, expansion, or improvement. (General operating support is rarely provided.) Capital support is generally awarded only in connection with specific program support needs. Application guidelines are available online.
Requirements: 501(c)3 tax-exempt organizations are eligible.
Restrictions: The fund does not make grants to: individuals; medical research programs; conferences or media events (unless they are an integral part of a broader program of direct service); efforts to influence legislation or elections; or organizations seeking support for deficit reduction or emergency funding.
Samples: Cancer Care (New York, NY)—to create a financial-assistance and support program for people with ocular cancers, $122,750 over 18 months (2004); Catholic Near East Welfare Assoc (New York, NY)—for projects at five Palestinian schools for the blind or at vision-rehabilitation groups in the Jerusalem area and the West Bank and Gaza, $209,316 over three years (2004); International Trachoma Initiative (New York, NY)—for a program that will provide sight-saving surgeries in Mali and Niger, two countries with extremely high rates of trachoma, $300,000 Over two years (2004);

Recording for the Blind and Dyslexic (Princeton, NJ)—to create 300 digitally recorded textbooks on mathematics, science, and technology, $320,000 over two years (2004).
Contact: Andrew Fisher, Executive Director, (212) 668-9801; fax: (212) 668-9803; email: afisher@lavellefund.org
Internet: http://fdncenter.org/grantmaker/lavellefund
Sponsor: Lavelle Fund for the Blind
80 Maiden Ln, Suite 1207
New York, NY 10038

Lawrence Foundation Grants **2034**
The foundation awards grants to nonprofit organizations that address the following areas of interest: education (U.S. headquartered organizations for programs in the United States), environment (U.S. headquartered organizations operating programs in the United States or elsewhere in the world), health (U.S. headquartered organizations operating programs in the United States with national scope or specific programs in the Los Angeles area), disaster relief (U.S. headquartered organizations responding to disasters in the United States or elsewhere in the world on an occasional basis), and other (U.S. headquartered organizations operating programs in the United States or elsewhere in the world). Grant amounts vary. The duration of grants will be typically for a single year. Letters of intent are due by the listed deadlines; full proposals are by invitation.
Requirements: Nonprofit organizations that qualify for 501(c)3 public charity status and public schools and libraries are eligible for contributions or grants.
Restrictions: For-profit businesses are not eligible. The foundation does not typically make grants for the following purposes: computers or software; audio or video equipment; designing and producing videos, kiosks, or promotional material; music programs or musical instruments; gardening programs or equipment; physical education programs or equipment; recreational programs; theater arts or performance arts programs or equipment; hospice or old age home programs; religious organizations; religious or charter schools; individuals for any purpose; international organizations that do not have a qualified domestic 501(c)3 representative; political lobbying activities or other political purposes; private foundations; dinners, balls, or other ticketed events; or purposes outside of the foundation's funding priorities.
Amount of Grant: $500-$100,000 average
Date(s) Application is Due: Feb 1; Aug 1
Contact: Lori Mitchell, Executive Director; (310) 451-1567; fax: (310) 451-7580; email: info@thelawrencefoundation.org
Internet: http://www.thelawrencefoundation.org/grant/index.html
Sponsor: Lawrence Foundation
530 Wilshire Boulevard, Suite 207
Santa Monica, CA 90401

Lawrence S. Huntington Fund Grants **2035**
The Foundation, established in 1997 by its namesake, Lawrence J. Huntington, is dedicated to supporting a historical seaport, as well as for environmental conservation, hospitals and human service programs. Mr. Huntington, who serves as the Chairman of St. Luke's Roosevelt Hospital, Chairman of the Woods Hole Research Center, and Vice Chairman of the Board of the South Street Seaport Museum, is primarily interested in preserving the environment and historical landmarks. There are no specific applications or deadlines with which to adhere, and applicants should approach the Foundation in writing.
Requirements: Giving is primarily restricted to the states of New York and Massachusetts, as well as the District of Columbia.
Geographic Focus: New York
Samples: Woods Hole Research Center, Falmouth, Massachusetts, $78,000 (2006); New York Law School, New York, New York, $15,000 (2006).
Amount of Grant: $80,000 maximum
Contact: Lawrence S. Huntington, Director; (212) 717-8633 or (212) 486-2424
Sponsor: Lawrence S. Huntington Fund
46 E. 70th Street, 4th Floor
New York, NY 10021-4928

Layne Beachley Aim For The Stars Foundation Grants **2036**
The Layne Beachley Aim for the Stars Foundation was created to inspire girls and women across Australia to dream and achieve. The Foundation hopes to prevent girls and women alike from having to go through adversity and to encourage, motivate and provide for all aspiring women. Encompassing academic, sport, cultural and community pursuits, Aim for the Stars offers ambitious and dedicated females an opportunity to receive financial and moral support to help them achieve their goals. Support will give them the opportunity to maintain a determined focus on their goal, to achieve their dreams earlier in life and allow them to further their ambitions and aim for the stars. Grants will be awarded, at the discretion of the Foundation, to deserving applicants who meet the criteria and best demonstrate their aspirations to further their educational and/or personal development. Females who aim to achieve their ultimate goal in their field of choice, 12 years of age and above, are eligible to apply.
Requirements: Applicants must be citizens of Australia, a minimum of 12 years old, and female.
Samples: Gabrielle King, Maclean NSW—Sailing (2009); Tayla Walsh—Waterpolo (2009); Nicole Parks, Jindabyne NSW—Mogul Skiing (2009); Anabelle Smith—Diving (2009); Caitlin Gilliman—Soccer (2009); Georgia Gibbs, Dardanup, WA—Rowing (2009); Jessica Brown—Ballet (2009); Samantha Balaton-Chrimes, Wantirna Sth, Victoria—African Studies (2009); Emma—Speed Skating (2009); Julie—Speed Skating (2009); Tatiana—Speed Skating (2009); Melissa Caldecutt—Speed Skating (2009); Bianca Hertel—Rodeo Riding (2009); Bernadette Branca, Meadow Hts, Victoria—Taekwondo (2009).
Amount of Grant: $1,500-$6,000
Date(s) Application is Due: Nov 15
Contact: Program Coordinator; (042) 260-0733; email: info@aimforthestars.com.au
Internet: http://www.aimforthestars.com.au/WhoCanApply/ApplicationChecklist/tabid/1854/language/en-U.S./Default.aspx
Sponsor: Layne Beachley Aim For The Stars Foundation
P.O. Box 666
Forestville, Australia NSW 2087 Australia

Leadership in Education in Neurodevelopmental Disabilities Postdoctoral Fellowships **2037**
Munroe-Meyer Institute, an administrative unit of the Nebraska Medical Center, offers postdoctoral fellowships supported by the Maternal and Child Health Bureau of the Health Resources and Services Administration. Fellowships are available in administration, nursing, nutrition, occupational therapy, pediatrics, physical therapy, psychology, social work, and speech language pathology. The program provides interdisciplinary training for careers and leadership roles in developmental disabilities and children with special needs. The applicant is encouraged to contact the home department director prior to submitting materials to determine if applicant interest is in line with department mission, goals, and objectives. The recruitment/selection committee meets every two weeks, beginning in January, to review materials. Applicants offered an interview will be scheduled to provide a scholarly presentation to the personnel and students within the institute.
Amount of Grant: $18,600 minimum
Contact: Patricia Gromak, Munroe-Meyer Institute, (800) 656-3937 or (402) 559-6402; fax: (402) 559-5737
Internet: http://www.unmc.edu/dept/mmi/index.cfm?L2_ID=60&L1_ID=17&CONREF=14
Sponsor: University of Nebraska Medical Center
985450 Nebraska Medical Ctr
Omaha, NE 68198-5450

Leahi Fund Grants **2038**
The purpose of the Fund is to support programs of research and education in, and the prevention of, pulmonary disease. Highest priority will be given to: research and education with foreseeable clinical application to pulmonary problems that exist in Hawai'i; scientific research in the prevention or treatment of pulmonary diseases and infirmities. Preference will be given to supporting new investigators and to new areas of investigation for established researchers. Application information is available online.
Requirements: Research grants can only be approved for individuals affiliated with tax-exempt organizations classified by the Internal Revenue Services as 501(c)3 type, or with units of government.
Restrictions: Funding is not available for: salary for the principal investigator; patient care; travel; major equipment purchases; printing or publication costs.
Geographic Focus: Hawaii
Amount of Grant: $30,000
Date(s) Application is Due: June 21
Contact: Christel Wuerfel, Philanthropic Services Assistant; (808) 537-6333 or (888) 731-3863; email: cwuerfel@hcf-hawaii.org
Internet: http://www.hawaiicommunityfoundation.org/index.php?id=71&categoryID=23
Sponsor: Hawaii Community Foundation
1164 Bishop Street, Suite 800
Honolulu, HI 96813

Learning and Behavioral Disorders Research Grants **2039**
The foundation's purpose is to provide funds for research and dissemination of research information which targets the proving, diagnosing, or treating of biologically-based disordered behavior. Areas of special interest include nutrition, food and chemical intolerance, neurometrics, neurochemistry, and genetics. Studies ascertaining validity of innovative biomedical therapies are especially encouraged. Initial contact from parties interested in funding an appropriate research project should be by letter which briefly explains the proposed project and states approximate cost. A researcher need not have a doctoral degree to apply.
Amount of Grant: $1000-$50,000
Contact: John Wacker, President, (214) 373-3308; fax: (214) 373-3308
Sponsor: Wacker Foundation
10848 Strait Lane
Dallas, TX 75229

Legacy Foundation Grants **2040**
Legacy Foundation Inc., Lake County, Indiana's Community Foundation, seeks and accepts endowments from public and private sources and distributes the income for community enhancing projects and other charitable purposes. The foundation is dedicated to improving the quality of life in Lake County, Indiana.
Requirements: The Legacy Foundation will make grants to non-profit organizations that implement projects with the potential to make a difference in the quality of life of a substantial number of residents of Lake County, Indiana.
Restrictions: In general the foundation does not support: general operating expenses; endowment campaigns; annual campaigns; fund raising events; travel grants; grants for individual schools or sponsorship of sports teams; previously incurred debt or retroactive

funding for current projects; other grant making organizations; individuals (except designated scholarship funds) & independent scholarly research projects; religious or sectarian programs; political parties or campaigns
Geographic Focus: Indiana
Samples: Charter School of the Dunes, IN — K-6 Guided Reading Project, $6,735.00 (2007); YWCA of the Gary, IN — George Uzelac Young Artists Program, $2,200.00 (2007)
Amount of Grant: $1,000 - $25,000 range
Date(s) Application is Due: Mar 1; May 1; Sep 1; Nov 1
Contact: Grant Coordinator; (219) 736-1880; fax: (219) 736-1940; email: info@legacyfoundationlakeco.org
Internet: http://www.legacyfoundationlakeco.org/grantpages/grantguidelines/index.htm
Sponsor: Legacy Foundation, Inc.
1000 East 80th Place, South Tower 302
Merrillville, IN 46410

Leland McSpadden Memorial Fund for Medical and Scientific Research Grants 2041
The fund invites research proposals aimed at achieving a better understanding of the metabolic basis of Lowe syndrome and/or developing a better understanding and better treatments for the major complications of Lowe syndrome, a genetic disorder that affects boys. Grants are awarded for one year with possible renewal for a second year.
Requirements: The program invites applications from researchers of all types, including but not limited to universities, hospitals, and other nonprofit research organizations.
Restrictions: The grant may not be used as salary for the principal investigator, for honoraria for consultants, for the purchase of standard, nonconsumable laboratory equipment, to purchase services from other research laboratories, or for overhead or indirect costs.
Amount of Grant: $25,000
Date(s) Application is Due: Oct 15
Contact: Mary Tietz, President, (612) 770-8438; email: info@lowesyndrome.org
Internet: http://www.lowesyndrome.org/Research/index.html
Sponsor: Lowe Syndrome Association
18919 Voss Road
Dallas, TX 75287

Lemelson-MIT Lifetime Achievement Award 2042
The award recognizes outstanding individuals whose pioneering spirit and demonstrated inventiveness throughout their careers has improved our society and inspired others. Candidates are living role models in the fields of science, engineering, medicine, and technology. They are U.S. citizens or permanent residents. Candidates are suggested to the program by the inventor community and other national leaders in science and technology. The winner is selected by the Lemelson-MIT board and notified via telephone by the director. Annual deadline dates may vary; contact program staff for exact dates.
Samples: Dr. Ruth Rogan Benerito—for her patented processes in textiles for easy-care cotton and her lifelong commitment to education.
Amount of Grant: $100,000 prize
Contact: Lemelson-MIT Program Office, (617) 253-3352 or (617) 253-3490; email: idudek@mit.edu
Internet: http://web.mit.edu/invent/a-lifetime.html
Sponsor: Massachusetts Institute of Technology
77 Massachusetts Avenue, Building E60-215
Cambridge, MA 02139-4307

Leo Goodwin Foundation Grants 2043
The foundation awards general operating grants, primarily in Florida, in the areas of cancer research, child welfare, education, hospitals, mental health, and youth. There are no application forms.
Requirements: Nonprofit organizations are eligible.
Restrictions: Individuals are not eligible.
Geographic Focus: Florida
Amount of Grant: $1000-$80,000 range
Date(s) Application is Due: Oct 31
Contact: Helen Furia, Secretary-Treasurer, (954) 491-2000
Sponsor: Leo Goodwin Foundation
800 Corporate Drive, Suite 510
Fort Lauderdale, FL 33334-3621

Leonard and Helen R. Stulman Charitable Foundation Grants 2044
The Leonard and Helen R. Stulman Charitable Foundation supports work in four areas of interest. Ninety five percent (95%) of funding from The Foundation is reserved for programs in greater Baltimore and the State of Maryland. The foundation will make a limited number of new grants each year to projects that address one or more of the following: research as to causes and treatment of mental illness and services for people with mental illness and their families; initiatives for an older adult and aging population and programs for geriatric medicine; programs engaged in health care treatment and prevention as well as those involved in medical research; and higher educational institutions. To apply to the Foundation for funding, applicants should submit a two-page letter of inquiry, with basic background on your organization, the identified needs your project proposes to address, an overview of the proposed project, and the amount you intend to request.
Requirements: Organizations (or their fiscal agents) that qualify as public charities under section 501(c)3 of the Internal Revenue Code and do not discriminate on the basis of race, creed, national origin, color, physical handicap, gender or sexual orientation are eligible to apply.
Amount of Grant: $50,000 average
Contact: Cathy Brill, Program Officer; (410) 332-4171; fax: (410) 837-4701; email: cathybrill@comcast.net
Internet: http://www.bcf.org/ourgrants/ourgrantsdetail.aspx?grid=4
Sponsor: Leonard and Helen R. Stulman Charitable Foundation
2 East Read Street, 9th Floor
Baltimore, MD 21202

Leonsis Foundation Grants 2045
The foundation creates opportunities for children that enable them to reach their highest potential; partners with and supports organizations with the creativity, skill, and dedication to help children overcome obstacles and achieve their goals; primarily focuses on innovative programs that expand horizons and create opportunity for children under the age of 18; and is particularly interested in educational and mentoring programs that incorporate computer internet technology. The foundation also has a strong interest in the health and well-being of all children. Unsolicited proposals are not accepted; submit a letter of inquiry. There are no deadline dates.
Geographic Focus: District of Columbia; Maryland; Virginia
Amount of Grant: $1000 average
Contact: Grants Administrator, (202) 266-2298; fax: (202) 347-5580; email: leonsisfdn@aol.com
Internet: http://www.leonsisfoundation.org
Sponsor: Leonsis Foundation
401 Ninth St NW, Suite 750
Washington, DC 20004

Lesbian Health Fund Grants 2046
The fund supports research into lesbian health, including research with the following goals: determination or rates and risk factors for cancers and other diseases among lesbians; issues of access to medical care for lesbians; study of mental health concerns of lesbians and their families; definition and investigation of lesbian family issues; and methodologic exploration of diversity in the lesbian population. Recently funded projects have included the first-ever longitudinal study of lesbian mothers; a survey of lesbian health curricula in U.S. internal medicine residencies; and an effort to develop the phone-survey method as a way of identifying lesbians missed by other survey approaches. Applications are available online.
Restrictions: Grants are not awarded for completed research or for projects in progress.
Amount of Grant: $500-$10,000
Date(s) Application is Due: May 1; Oct 1
Contact: Program Manager, (415) 255-4547; fax: (415) 255-4784; email: info@glma.org
Internet: http://www.glma.org/programs/lhf/index.shtml
Sponsor: Lesbian Health Fund
459 Fulton Street, Suite 107
San Francisco, CA 94102

Lester E. Yeager Charitable Trust B Grants 2047
Established in 1989 in Kentucky, the Lester E. Yeager Charitable Trust B is an independent foundation. Funding is limited to areas of southern Indiana that are adjacent to Kentucky with emphasis on Daviess and Henderson counties in Indiana. The Trust gives primarily for health and human services. Contact Trust coordinator for additional information and to request an application form.
Requirements: Application form required. Applicants should submit the following: detailed description of project and amount of funding requested; additional materials/documentation; one page cover letter with application; four copies of proposal.
Restrictions: No grants are available to individuals. Grant recipients are expected to file a report when project is completed.
Geographic Focus: Indiana; Kentucky
Amount of Grant: $800 - $13,000 range
Contact: Trust Coordinator; (270) 686-8254;
Sponsor: Lester E. Yeager Charitable Trust B
P.O. Box 964
Owensboro, KY 42302-0964

Lester Ray Fleming Scholarships 2048
The North Carolina Governor's Institute on Alcohol and Substance Abuse, Inc. has established scholarships for North Carolina community college students in memory of Lester Ray Fleming, son of Eugene and Mary Fleming and father of Tristan and Curtis. Mr. Fleming was an employee of the Institute at the time of his death in August 2005. It is the hope that these scholarships will benefit and prepare students to educate and serve others in their communities. Those selected will not only receive a $250.00 scholarship but may have the opportunity to attend other venues sponsored by the Institute free of charge where they will gain valuable insight meeting leading researchers, policymakers, and administrators in the field. Scholarship recipients may also have the opportunity to participate in a project at the discretion of the Governor's Institute.
Requirements: Applications can be downloaded from the website.
Geographic Focus: North Carolina
Amount of Grant: $250
Date(s) Application is Due: Mar 19

Contact: Larry Woodard, M.H.S.A., CSAC; (919) 256-7412; fax: (919) 990-9518; email: lwoodard1@mindspring.com
Internet: http://www.governorsinstitute.org/index.php?option=com_content&task=view&id=103&Itemid=66
Sponsor: North Carolina Governor's Institute on Alcohol and Substance Abuse
1730 Varsity Drive, Suite 105
Raleigh, NC 27606

Lettie Pate Whitehead Foundation Grants **2049**
Annual grants are made to accredited educational institutions in the nine specified states in the southeast to fund scholarships for the education of women. The grantee institutions award scholarships on the basis of need to Christian women who reside in one of the named states. Thousands of women receive financial assistance each year in individual amounts determined by the recipient institutions. While most scholarships go toward undergraduate higher education, the foundation maintains a special interest in health education. A significant number of its scholarship grants support education in the medical, nursing, and allied health care fields.
Requirements: Grants are awarded to institutions in Alabama, Florida, Georgia, Louisiana, Mississippi, North Carolina, South Carolina, Tennessee, and Virginia.
Geographic Focus: Alabama; Florida; Georgia; Louisiana; Mississippi; North Carolina; South; South Carolina; Tennessee; Virginia
Contact: Program Contact, (404) 522-6755; fax: (404) 522-7026; email: fdns@woodruff.org
Internet: http://www.lpwhitehead.org
Sponsor: Lettie Pate Whitehead Foundation
50 Hurt Plz, Suite 1200
Atlanta, GA 30303

Leukaemia Research Fund Grants **2050**
The fund was founded to encourage, promote, and assist research into the leukemias, Hodgkin's disease, and other related conditions. The fund supports clinical fellowships and research projects at hospitals and university medical centers throughout the United Kingdom.
Amount of Grant: ?67,866
Contact: Grants Administrator, (020) 7405 0101; fax: (020) 7405 3139; email: info@lrf.org.uk
Internet: http://www.lrf.org.uk/en/1/science.html
Sponsor: Leukaemia Research Fund
43 Great Ormond Street
London WC1N 3JJ United Kingdom

Leukemia and Lymphoma Society Research Grants **2051**
The society's research program is based on the belief that all scientifically sound approaches toward a cure or control of leukemia, lymphoma, and myeloma should be encouraged on a worldwide basis. Basic laboratory research and its application to a clinical setting are supported.
Samples: Baylor College of Medicine, Ctr for Cell and Gene Therapy (TX)—for blood-cancer research, through the Specialized Center of Research grant program, $5 million over five years; To be divided among 32 research projects—to develop new treatments for leukemia, lymphoma, and myeloma, through the Translational Research Program, $11.3 million; Fred Hutchinson Cancer Research Ctr (Seattle, WA)—to support the work of Irwin Bernstein to develop less toxic and more effective immune-based therapies for treating advanced leukemia and lymphoma, $7 million.
Contact: Grants Administrator, (914) 949-5213; fax: (914) 949-6691
Internet: http://www.leukemia-lymphoma.org/all_page?item_id=7427
Sponsor: Leukemia and Lymphoma Society
1311 Mamaroneck Avenue
White Plains, NY 10605

Lewis Preston Fund for Girls Education Grants **2052**
The fund supports women's groups that advance the human rights of women and girls. Grants support women's groups based outside the United States by providing small, flexible, and timely grants for operating and project expenses. Grantees address issues that include but are not limited to building peace and ending gender-based violence; advancing health and sexual and reproductive rights; expanding civic and political participation; ensuring economic and environmental justice; increasing access to education; and fostering social change philanthropy. In addition urgent requests for support to organize or participate in local, regional, or international meetings and conferences will be considered outside of the normal grant cycle. These types of requests must come from organizations, not individuals, and must be received at least eight weeks before the event. Funds for these types of grants are limited.
Requirements: The applicant group must be based in a country outside the United States; demonstrate a strong commitment to women's equality and human rights that is clearly reflected in its activities; be a group of women working together; and be governed, directed, and led by women.
Restrictions: Grants do not support individuals; scholarships; academic research; groups based and working primarily or only in the United States; international organizations proposing projects with local partners; groups without a strong women's rights focus; groups headed and managed by men, or without women in the majority of leadership positions; groups whose sole purpose is to generate income or to provide charity to individuals; or political parties or election campaigns.
Amount of Grant: $500-$20,000
Contact: Executive Assistant, (415) 202-7640; fax: (415) 202-8604; email: proposals@globalfundforwomen.org
Internet: http://www.globalfundforwomen.org/1work/programs/preston.html
Sponsor: Global Fund for Women
1375 Sutter Street, Suite 400
San Francisco, CA 94109

Liberty Bank Foundation Grants **2053**
The foundation's charitable giving is focused primarily on organizations that provide meaningful programs and activities that benefit people within Liberty Bank's market area. Of particular interest are programs and activities that provide assistance and opportunities to improve the quality of life for people of low income, especially families in crisis or at-risk. Top priorities for funding include community and economic development—affordable housing for low/moderate-income individuals and families, community and neighborhood capacity-building, and community services targeted to low/moderate-income individuals; education—programs that address the needs of low/moderate-income individuals; health care and human services—outreach and educational programs on health issues, quality child care, homeless shelters and services, services for victims of domestic violence, and transitional housing assistance; and arts and culture—programs that increase access to arts and culture for people of low income who might not otherwise be able to participate in them. Grants generally support specific programs rather than capital projects, equipment, or general operating expenses. Organizations that have received funding in two consecutive calendar years should refrain from reapplying for one calendar year. Contact the office to discuss the project prior to applying. Guideline and application are available online.
Requirements: 501(c)3 tax-exempt organizations are eligible.
Restrictions: Individuals, fraternal groups, and organizations that are not open to the general public are ineligible. Grants do not support annual funds of colleges, universities or hospitals; trips, tours, or conferences; scientific or medical research; deficit spending or debt liquidation; lobbying or otherwise influencing the outcome of the legislative or electoral process; religious groups, except for nonsectarian programs; or endowments or other foundations.
Samples: Windham InterFaith Ministry—to support the Rooming House rent fund, $2500.; Children's Home—to support the summer jobs program, $3000.; Hospice of Southeastern Connecticut—to support the Live Alone program, $5000.
Amount of Grant: $250 minimum
Date(s) Application is Due: Mar 31; Jun 30; Sep 30; Dec 31
Contact: Grants Administrator, (860) 704-2181; email: smurphy@liberty-bank.com
Internet: http://www.liberty-bank.com/liberty_foundation.asp
Sponsor: Liberty Bank Foundation
P.O. Box 1212
Middletown, CT 06457

Life Sciences Research Foundation Postdoctoral Fellowships **2054**
Each year approximately 12-15 postdoctoral fellowships are awarded in the medical and life sciences to provide training and support of the highest quality young scientists in the best research environments. Research must be performed at nonprofit institutions. The fellowships are awarded for three-year periods. Send a self-addressed envelope for information and an application, or visit the Web site.
Requirements: Applicant must have an MD, PhD, or equivalent degree. Persons working on a second postdoctoral are eligible only if they are transferring to a different supervisor's laboratory and embarking on a new project not connected to their previous research. All U.S. citizens are eligible with no geographic restrictions. Foreign applicants will be eligible for study in U.S. laboratories only.
Restrictions: Candidate must not hold a faculty/permanent appointment. The LSRF does not award an institutional allowance for overhead.
Amount of Grant: $51,000 maximum per year
Date(s) Application is Due: Oct 1
Contact: Susan DiRenzo, Assistant Director, (609) 258-3551; email: sdirenzo@molbio.princeton.edu
Internet: http://www.lsrf.org/geninfo.htm
Sponsor: Life Sciences Research Foundation
c/o Lewis Thomas Laboratory, Princeton University, Washington Road
Princeton, NJ 08544

Liliane Foundation Grants **2055**
The foundation was founded to provide aid for disabled children in developing countries in Africa, Asia, and Central and South America. Grants are awarded to individuals in the field of medical and social rehabilitation.
Contact: G.B. Dollevoet, Manager, 31-73-511-90-29; fax: 31-73-511-73-54; email: liliane@euronet.nl
Internet: http://www.lilianefonds.nl
Sponsor: Liliane Foundation
St Catharinastraat 1, P.O.B 75
Vlijmen 5250 AB The Netherlands

Lillian S. Wells Foundation Grants **2056**
The Lillian S. Wells Foundation established in 1976, primarily supports the Fort Lauderdale, Florida, and Chicago, Illinois regions with funding interests that include: medical research, with emphasis on brain cancer research, women's health, substance abuse, and at-risk youth. Additional funding for education and the arts. Contact the Foundation for an application form, the Board meets quarterly in January, April, July, and October.

Requirements: Nonprofit organizations in Chicago, Illinois and Fort Lauderdale, Florida area are eligible to apply.
Geographic Focus: Florida; Illinois
Amount of Grant: $1,000 - $1,900,000 range
Date(s) Application is Due: Mar 15; Jun 15; Sep 15; Dec 15
Contact: Patricia F. Mulvaney, Executive Director; email: patricia.mulvaney@thewellsfamily.net
Sponsor: Lillian S. Wells Foundation
600 Sagamore Road
Fort Lauderdale, FL 33301-2215

Lillian Sholtis Brunner Summer Fellowships for Historical Research in Nursing 2057
These summer fellowships for historical research in nursing are offered by the Center for the Study of the History of Nursing in the School of Nursing at the University of Pennsylvania. Selection of the scholars will be based on evidence of preparation and/or productivity in historical research related to nursing. It is expected that the research and new materials produced by Brunner scholars will help ensure the growth of scholarly work focused on the history of nursing. The fellowship will support up to eight weeks of residential study and use of the center's collections. The application should be sent via email to either Patricia D'Antonio, PhD, RN, FAAN (dantonio@nursing.upenn.edu) or Barbra Mann Wall, PhD, RN (wallbm@nursing.upenn.edu).
Amount of Grant: $2,500
Date(s) Application is Due: Dec 31
Contact: Dr. Karen Buhler-Wilkerson, Director; (215) 898-4725; fax: (215) 573-2168; email: karenwil@nursing.upenn.edu
Internet: http://www.nursing.upenn.edu/history/Pages/Brunner_Fellowship.aspx
Sponsor: University of Pennsylvania
School of Nursing, 418 Curie Boulevard
Philadelphia, PA 19104-6020

Lincoln Financial Group Foundation Grants 2058
As one of the country's premier financial services organizations, Lincoln Financial Group is committed to providing its customers with the life insurance, retirement and investment products and services they need to maintain their quality of life. As a concerned corporate citizen, the company's foundation has sustained a strategic philanthropic program to improve the quality of life in the communities where employees live and work. These communities include: Chicago, Illinois; Concord, New Hampshire; Fort Wayne, Indiana; Greensboro, North Carolina; Hartford, Connecticut; Omaha, Nebraska; Philadelphia, Pennsylvania.
Requirements: The Lincoln Financial Foundation welcomes grant applications from organizations that meet our geographic, strategic focus, and eligibility guidelines. Local Charitable Contribution Committees meet and review grant applications. Only nonprofit organizations that have a 501(c)3 designation from the Internal Revenue Service are eligible to apply for funding. To apply for a grant, complete the Lincoln Financial Foundation application by using the online form and submitting it electronically. Grant submission deadlines are: Arts and Culture grants applications must be received by January 15; Education/Workforce Development grant applications must be received by April 21; Human Services grant applications must be received by July 21. Applications are reviewed by the local contribution committees within three to four months after the cycle deadline. Notification will be given soon after decisions are rendered.
Restrictions: Qualified organizations are eligible for one grant per calendar year. In general, the Lincoln Foundation will not award grants to: individuals; religious organizations; public or private elementary or secondary schools or school foundations; hospitals or hospital foundations; fraternal, political, or war veteran organizations; general operating support; capital funding; endowments.
Geographic Focus: Connecticut; Illinois; Indiana; Nebraska; New Hampshire; North Carolina; PennsylvaniaUnited Kingdom
Amount of Grant: $5000-$75,000 average
Date(s) Application is Due: Jan 15; Apr 21; Jul 21
Contact: Jean Vrabel, Program Officer; (260) 455-3868; fax: (260) 455-4004; email: Jean.Vrabel@LFG.com
Internet: http://www.lfg.com/LincolnPageServer?LFGPage=/lfg/lfgclient/abt/fingrp/hta/index.html
Sponsor: Lincoln Financial Group Foundation
P.O. Box 7863, 1300 S Clinton Street
Fort Wayne, IN 46802

Lindbergh Grants Program 2059
Grants are awarded to individuals whose proposed projects represent a significant contribution toward the achievement of a better balance between technology and our human and natural environment. Nine to 10 grants are awarded each year. The current funding program is interested in increasing representation in the following areas: aviation/aerospace; agriculture; arts and humanities; biomedical research; conservation of natural resources; exploration; health and population sciences; intercultural communication; oceanography; water resources management; waste disposal management; wildlife preservation; and adaptive technology. Grant application can be obtained by writing the fund; enclose a self-addressed, stamped envelope with request. The Web site contains additional information.
Requirements: Grants are international in scope and open to citizens of all countries. Letters of request, proposals, endorser reports, and required progress and final reports must be submitted in English. The fund welcomes candidates who may or may not be affiliated with academic or nonprofit institutions. Grants are made to individuals, not to affiliated institutions for institutional programs. Note: When sending any materials by fax, seven hard copies via mail or delivery are requested. The deadline for grant applications is the second Thursday of June in the year preceding the awarding of funds.
Restrictions: The fund does not provide support for overhead costs of organizations, tuition, scholarships, fellowships, or travel related to such.
Samples: Dr. Ernest Diedrich, Saint John's College (Collegeville, MN)—for Balancing Energy Consumption with Resource Conservation: A Wind Power Study for Central Minnesota, an Educational Model for the World.;Dr. Ping Liu, Eastern Illinois U (Charleston, IL)—for Analysis of Recycled Plastic Composites to Aid in the Development and Design of Recycled Plastic Products.;Dr. Vivian Charles McAlister, Dalhousie U (Halifax, Nova Scotia)—for Use of Human Response to Parasites to Improve Organ Transplant Survival.;Dr. Carl Wulfman, U of the Pacific (Stockton, CA)—for Clean Energy into Clean Energy: Toward a New Method of Using Sunlight to Produce Electricity.
Amount of Grant: $10,580 maximum
Date(s) Application is Due: Jun 9
Contact: Grants Coordinator, (763) 576-1596; fax: (763) 576-1664; email: info@lindberghfoundation.org
Internet: http://www.lindberghfoundation.org/grants
Sponsor: Charles A. and Anne Morrow Lindbergh Foundation
2150 Third Ave N, Suite 310
Anoka, MN 55303-2200

Little Life Foundation Grants 2060
The Little-Life Foundation is a 501c3 charitable organization founded in 2002 whose primary purpose is to support medical care and research for increasing the survival rates of prematurely born babies. Saint Barnabas Medical Center, where more than 7,500 babies are born each year, will be the primary beneficiary of the Foundation's efforts.
Geographic Focus: New Jersey
Amount of Grant: $66,200 total giving
Contact: Richard P. Rizzuto, Director; (973) 277-2329; fax: 973-401-9799
Internet: http://www.littlelifefoundation.org/
Sponsor: Little Life Foundation
P.O. Box 765
New Vernon, NJ 07976-0765

Littlefield-AACR Grants in Metastatic Colon Cancer Research 2061
The grants will provide support for innovative cancer research projects designed to accelerate the discovery and development of new agents to treat metastatic colon cancer and/or for pre-clinical research with direct therapeutic intent. Special emphasis will be placed on research that holds promise for leading to individualized therapeutic options for treatment in the near future or for developing promising new cancer therapeutics for metastatic colon cancer, which will translate into clinical applications within a one- to two-year period.
Requirements: The prizes are open to all cancer researchers who are affiliated with any institution involved in cancer research, cancer medicine, or cancer-related biomedical science anywhere in the world. Such institutions include those in academia, industry, or government. Candidates must be active researchers and have a record of recent publications.
Amount of Grant: $500,000-$1,000,000
Date(s) Application is Due: Feb 1
Contact: Julia Laurence, Staff Assistant; (215) 440-9300, ext. 102 or (267) 646-0655; fax: (215) 440-9372; email: laurence@aacr.org
Internet: http://www.aacr.org/home/scientists/research-funding—training-grants/research-funding/littlefield-aacr-grants-for-metastatic-colon-cancer-research.aspx
Sponsor: Littlefield 2000 Trust and the American Association for Cancer Research
615 Chestnut Street, 17th Floor
Philadelphia, PA 19106-4404

Lockheed Martin Philanthropic Grants 2062
The corporation awards grants to enhance the quality of life in communities where Lockheed Martin employees live and work. Areas of funding interest include K-16 math and science education—the primary focus, regional and national programs; culture—programs and activities that are accessible to employees and, whenever possible, incorporate an educational component; civic and public interest—local activities that directly benefit employees and quality of life in the community; health and human services; health care providers that provide services directly to employees and local chapters of national health organizations, and the United Way; and voluntarism—programs in which employees actively participate. Applications must be submitted in writing. There are no application deadlines. Organizations outside of Maryland and the District of Columbia should locate the nearest facility; a listing of where to apply is online.
Requirements: 501(c)3 tax-exempt organizations in Lockheed communities are eligible.
Restrictions: Grants are generally not made to: organizations that discriminate by race, creed, gender, sexual orientation, age, religion, disability, or national origin; home-based child care/educational services; individuals (as for business start-ups or scholarships); religious organizations for religious purposes; professional associations, labor organizations, fraternal organizations, social clubs or social events sponsored by social clubs; athletic groups; or advertising in souvenir booklets, yearbooks, or journals unrelated to Lockheed Martin's business interests.
Samples: Phillips Collection (Washington, DC)—for arts exhibitions, $1.5 million over five years (2005); Yellowstone Park Foundation (Bozeman, MT)—to design and build permanent interpretive exhibits for the new visitor-education center at Old Faithful

that describe the relationship between astrobiology and Yellowstone National Park's geothermal features, $200,000 (2005).
Amount of Grant: $8.7 million total
Contact: David Phillips, Manager of Corporate Philanthropy, (301) 897-6292; fax: (301) 897-6485; email: david.e.phillips@lmco.com
Internet: http://www.lockheedmartin.com/wms/findPage.do?dsp=fec&ci=13019&sc=400
Sponsor: Lockheed Martin
6801 Rockledge Drive
Bethesda, MD 20817

Long Island Community Foundation Grants **2063**
The foundation awards grants to eligible New York nonprofit organizations in the following program areas: community building—to address serious issues, break down barriers between groups of people, and foster a sense of community in the area; program start-up in response to critical community needs; organizational development—strengthen or restructure public awareness of the nonprofit's work; arts funding; and field of interest grants, including but not limited to women, music, the poor, maternal and child health, seniors, teenagers suffering from emotional difficulties, innovative classroom projects, and the environment. Projects are preferred that accomplish specific tasks, solve problems, address needs of the disadvantaged, help a large number of people, and use community resources.
Requirements: New York nonprofit organizations are eligible.
Restrictions: Grants do not support requests for ongoing operations, equipment purchase, capital or construction costs, or research.
Geographic Focus: New York
Samples: Adelphi U (Garden City, NY)—for a program in corporate social responsibility, through the Horace and Amy Hagedorn Fund, $1 million (2003).
Amount of Grant: $2500-$15,000
Date(s) Application is Due: Jan 12; May 6; Sep 7
Contact: Grants Administrator, (516) 681-5085
Internet: http://www.licf.org/grants
Sponsor: Long Island Community Foundation
1740 Old Jericho Turnpike
Jericho, NY 11753

Lotus 88 Foundation for Women and Children Grants **2064**
The foundation's mission is to promote the empowerment of women and children through supporting their economic, emotional, and spiritual development. The foundation's focus area is American Indian Country. Grants are awarded in Indian Country for two strategic purposes: revitalizing the council tipis as spiritual, cultural, and service centers; and providing the basic needs through community building. Community building grants are intended to promote and support community building in Indian Country to improve basic living conditions and to encourage a more positive future. Tipi project grants are made to help tribal women living on reservation or off reservation in building community. Grants support cultural and social services, tribal gatherings, educational programs, healing and purification ceremonies, and retreats. Each proposal should identify the specific needs and uses for the tipi and should identify a nonprofit program partner working in the tribal area who will work with the foundation on the project. Guidelines and application are available online.
Requirements: Projects in American Indian communities are eligible.
Contact: Patricia Stout, President, (415) 296-3887; fax: (415) 623-2778; email: benita@lotus88.org
Internet: http://www.lotus88.org
Sponsor: Lotus 88 Foundation for Women and Children
388 Market Street, Suite 400
San Francisco, CA 94111

Louis Calder Foundation Grants **2065**
The foundation supports projects that benefit the children and youth of New York City in the areas of health, welfare, religion, environment, and education. General operating grants, project/program grants, challenge/matching grants, and scholarships are awarded. The foundation's small grants program awards one-time grants to organizations whose programming and budgets would ordinarily fall outside of funding parameters. Small grants are designed to increase the recipient organization's visibility enabling it to attract new potential funding sources.
Requirements: Nonprofit organizations serving the New York City area and its residents are eligible. Typical recipients include schools, hospitals and other medical agencies, youth groups, human service agencies, museums, libraries, and arts groups.
Restrictions: Awards to performing arts groups or private colleges are by invitation only.
Geographic Focus: New York
Samples: Saint John's U (Jamaica, NY)—to endow a scholarship fund, $333,000 challenge grant.; Canisius College (Buffalo, NY)—for scholarships for New York City students who demonstrate academic promise and acute financial need, $250,000 challenge grant.; Citizens Advice Bureau (New York, NY)—for support to implement a whole language-based after-school program for South Bronx children, $25,000.
Amount of Grant: $5000-$250,000 typically; $5000 maximum small grants
Contact: Holly Nuechterlein, Program Manager, (203) 966-8925; fax: (203) 966-5785; email: admin@calderfdn.org
Internet: http://www.louiscalderfdn.org
Sponsor: Louis Calder Foundation
175 Elm Street
New Canaan, CT 06840

Louis R. Cappelli Foundation Grants **2066**
The foundation awards grants to eligible New York nonprofit organizations in its areas of interest, including arts—educational programs for at-risk children and youth in the visual and performing arts, art history, and public libraries; education—programs addressing at-risk children and youth; and health—programs that provide innovative, high-quality health education or organized sports programs serving at-risk children and youth. All requests must be in writing; phone and fax requests are not accepted.
Requirements: New York 501(c)3 tax-exempt organizations located in Sullivan or Westchester Counties are eligible.
Geographic Focus: New York
Date(s) Application is Due: Jun 18
Contact: Executive Director, (914) 769-6500; fax: (914) 747-9268; email: jfevola@cappelli-inc.com
Internet: http://www.cappelli-inc.com/lrc.html
Sponsor: Louis R. Cappelli Foundation
115 Stevens Avenue
Valhalla, NY 10595

Lowe Foundation Grants **2067**
The foundation awards grants to organizations in Texas, primarily for programs that support the critical needs of women and children. The arts and higher education also receive support. Grants are awarded to support capital campaigns, building construction/renovation, and general operations. The board meets in April of each year. The December 1 deadline listed is for pre-proposals, with full proposals by request due December 31.
Requirements: 501(c)3 organizations in Texas may apply for grant support.
Geographic Focus: Texas
Samples: U of Texas Southwestern Medical Ctr at Dallas (Dallas, TX)—to endow a professorship in pediatric critical care, $100,000.
Amount of Grant: $5000-$225,000 range
Date(s) Application is Due: Dec 1; Dec 31
Contact: Clayton Maebius, Trustee; (512) 322-0041; fax: (512) 322-0061; email: info@thelowefoundation.org
Internet: http://www.thelowefoundation.org/guidelines.htm
Sponsor: Lowe Foundation
1005 Congress Avenue, Suite 895
Austin, TX 78701

Lowell Area Community Fund Grants **2068**
The fund awards grants to organizations that assist in fulfilling its mission: to assure community cooperation and participation that supports a healthy, dynamic community. The fund places an emphasis on broad educational initiatives, but also supports initiatives in the areas of arts and culture, community development, environment, health, human services, and recreation. Application and guidelines are available online. Grant applications are accepted three times a year on the third Friday of April, August and December.
Requirements: 501(c)3 tax-exempt organizations are eligible.
Restrictions: The fund generally does not support: political projects, or those that are primarily cause-related; individuals; religious organizations for religious purposes; or profit-making activities.
Amount of Grant: $10,000 maximum
Date(s) Application is Due: Apr 21; Aug 18; Dec 15
Contact: Kate Luckert, (616) 454-1751 ext 117; email: kluckert@grfoundation.org
Internet: http://www.grfoundation.org/lowell.php
Sponsor: Lowell Area Community Fund
161 Ottawa, Suite 209-C
Grand Rapids MI 49503

Lowell Berry Foundation Grants **2069**
The foundation was established with the primary purpose of assisting in strengthening Christian ministry at the local church level. The small number of new grants is restricted to programs in California's Contra Costa and northern Alameda Counties. A proposal for a Christian program should be submitted to the attention of Charles Branagh, president. A proposal for a social service program should be submitted to Barbara Corneille, director. Types of support include conferences and seminars, general operating support, project support, and scholarship funds. The funding cycle runs on a calendar-year basis with committee and board meetings held quarterly. Proposals are received and reviewed continuously throughout the year.
Requirements: 501(c)3 tax-exempt organizations in California may apply.
Restrictions: Grants do not support advertising, advocacy orgnizations, individuals, international organizations, political organizations, local and state government agencies, building funds, capital funds, equipment acquisition, or seed money requests.
Geographic Focus: California
Amount of Grant: $2000-$25,000 average
Contact: Katherine Sanders, Office Manager, (925) 284-4427; fax: (925) 284-4332
Sponsor: Lowell Berry Foundation
3685 Mt Diablo Boulevard, Suite 269
Lafayette, CA 94549

LRF New Investigator Leukemia Research Grants **2070**
The foundation supports leukemia-related research in a broad sense, including such areas as biochemistry, microbiology, virology, molecular biology, genetics, and immunology. Projects related to significant aspects of leukemia, lymphoma, or myelodysplasia also are considered. The goal of the program is to support new investigators; preference will

be given to applicants proposing new lines of investigation. Types of support include research grants and postdoctoral fellowships. Grants and fellowships are for a one-year period and may be renewable for a second year. Annual deadline dates may vary; contact program staff for exact dates.
Requirements: Grants are restricted to researchers who are within five years of the end of their training or of their first independent faculty appointment at the time of the proposed starting date of the grant.
Restrictions: The funds may not be used for salary support of the principal investigator.
Samples: Dr. Curt Horvath, Mount Sinai School of Medicine (New York, NY)—for research to determine how the STAT:IRF complexes function to mediate interferon biological responses, $50,000.; Dr. Alona Weiss, Massachusetts General Hospital (Boston, MA)—for research to further understand the mechanisms and processes involved in normal gene regulation and to contribute to understanding of the causes of diseases, such as leukemia, where these mechanisms fail to function, $25,000.
Amount of Grant: $75,000
Date(s) Application is Due: Feb 15
Contact: Kelli Fitzgerald, Grant Manager, (847) 424-0600; fax: (847) 424-0606; email: Kelli@LRFMail.org
Internet: http://www.leukemia-research.org/phd/application.asp
Sponsor: Leukemia Research Foundation
2700 Patriot Boulevard, Suite 100
Glenview, IL 60026-8021

LRF Physician-Scientist Postdoctoral Fellowships 2071
The foundation awards physician-scientist postdoctoral fellowships to help physicians prepare for independent careers in research of leukemia and related disorders and obtain significant research results. Fellowships support two years of research. Annual deadline dates may vary; contact program staff for exact dates.
Requirements: Fellows (MD, DO, DVM, or equivalent) not yet established as independent investigators are eligible.
Amount of Grant: $30,000 per year
Date(s) Application is Due: Feb 15
Contact: Kelli Fitzgerald, Medical Grants Administrator, (847) 424-0600; fax: (847) 424-0606; email: Kelli@LRFMail.org
Internet: http://www.leukemia-research.org/phd/application.asp
Sponsor: Leukemia Research Foundation
2700 Patriot B;vd, Suite 100
Glenview, IL 60026-8021

LRF Postdoctoral Fellowships 2072
The program awards postdoctoral fellowship support for trainees who wish to work in a research area related to leukemia and related disorders. Fellowships are awarded for two years. Annual deadlines dates may vary; contact program staff for exact dates.
Requirements: Fellows (MD or PhD) with up to three years of training (excluding medical residency) prior to receiving the fellowship are eligible.
Amount of Grant: $30,000 maximum per year
Date(s) Application is Due: Feb 15
Contact: Kelli Fitzgerald, (847) 424-0600; fax: (847) 424-0606; email: Kelli@LRFMail.org
Internet: http://www.leukemia-research.org/phd/application.asp
Sponsor: Leukemia Research Foundation
2700 Patriot Boulevard, Suite 100
Glenview, IL 60026-8021

LSA Fellowships 2073
Fellows of the Leukemia Society are promising investigators with no or minimal prior postdoctoral experience working in fields relevant to leukemia. They will have had less than two years of postdoctoral research training at the time of review. Fellows are encouraged to embark on academic careers involving clinical or fundamental research in leukemia, Hodgkin's disease, the lymphomas, and multiple myeloma. Fellowships are awarded for three years and are nonrenewable; however, an application may be made for a special fellowship in the third year of the fellowship award. The preliminary, two-page application must meet the September application deadline; complete applications must be received by the October date.
Requirements: Applicant must hold a PhD, MD, or equivalent degree at the time a grant is to become effective. There are no restrictions as to citizenship, age, race, sex, or creed.
Restrictions: An award will not be made to an individual with full institutional salary support; applicants must demonstrate lack of or minimal/limited salary support as per institutional policies. Awards are payable to the academic institution on behalf of the investigator.
Amount of Grant: $50,000 (stipend $47,000 + $3000 institutional overhead) per year for three years
Date(s) Application is Due: Sep 15; Oct 1
Contact: Director of Research Administration, (914) 821-8843; fax: (914) 821-8946; email: researchprograms@leukemia-lymphoma.org
Internet: http://www.leukemia-lymphoma.org/all_page?item_id=11618
Sponsor: Leukemia Society of America
1311 Mamaroneck Avenue
White Plains, NY 10605

LSA Scholar Award for Clinical Research 2074
Applicants for this award have demonstrated their ability to design and conduct original research on leukemia, lymphoma, and myeloma. They are expected to hold an independent faculty-level or equivalent position for a period of not less than three years and to have obtained substantial research support from a national agency. This program is designed as a career development award and is not intended for the support of well-established or senior investigators. The award runs for five years; however, annual renewal is required and is based on a yearly noncompetitive progress report review.
Amount of Grant: $110,000 ($105,000 + $5000 institutional overhead) per year for five years
Date(s) Application is Due: Sep 15; Oct 1
Contact: Director of Research Administration, (914) 821-8843; fax: (914) 821-8946; email: researchprograms@lls.org
Internet: http://www.leukemia-lymphoma.org/all_page?item_id=11618
Sponsor: Leukemia Society of America
1311 Mamaroneck Avenue
White Plains, NY 10605

LSA Scholar Awards 2075
This is a career development award for highly qualified scholars who have demonstrated over a five-year period the ability to conduct original research on leukemia, Hodgkin's disease, the lymphomas, and multiple myeloma. Recipients are expected to hold independent faculty-level or equivalent positions and will usually have successfully competed for research grant support for their work. The program has been designed to aid the individual rather than the project and to encourage continued investigation while ensuring the investigator an income. The applicant should have shown the capacity for sustained, original investigation in abnormal cell growth as it relates to leukemia, lymphoma, and myeloma and must desire an investigative career in the field of leukemia, lymphoma, and myeloma. Awards are usually given to individuals in the clinical or basic science departments of universities or associated research institutions. Scholarships are awarded for terms of five years and are nonrenewable. Preliminary, two-page applications must meet the September deadline; complete applications must meet the October deadline.
Requirements: Applicant must hold a PhD, MD, or equivalent degree at the time the grant is to become effective. There are no restrictions as to citizenship, age, race, sex, or creed.
Restrictions: An award will not be made to an individual with full institutional salary support; applicants must demonstrate lack of or minimal/limited salary support as per institutional policies. All awards must be payable to an academic institution.
Amount of Grant: $110,000 ($105,000 + $5000 institutional overhead) per year for five years
Date(s) Application is Due: Sep 15; Oct 1
Contact: Director of Research Administration, (914) 821-8843; fax: (914) 821-8946; email: researchprograms@lls.org
Internet: http://www.leukemia-lymphoma.org/all_page?item_id=11618
Sponsor: Leukemia Society of America
1311 Mamaroneck Avenue
White Plains, NY 10605

LSA Special Fellowships 2076
Special Fellows of the Leukemia Society are scientists who have completed more basic training and education in the field than are required for a fellow but less than is necessary for a scholar. A special fellow has had at least two years of postdoctoral training at the time of review but does not yet hold an independent position and relies on the sponsor for research support. Investigators applying must be willing to dedicate their careers to research bearing on a cure or control of leukemia, Hodgkin's disease, the lymphomas, or multiple myeloma. The special fellowships are awarded for a period of three years and are nonrenewable; however, an application may be made for a scholarship in the third year of the special fellowship award. Proposed research projects must be related directly to the field of leukemia, lymphomas, and myeloma. Preliminary, two-page applications must meet the September deadline; complete applications must meet the October deadline.
Requirements: Applicant should hold a PhD, MD, or equivalent degree at the time a grant is to become effective. There are no restrictions as to citizenship, age, race, sex, or creed.
Restrictions: An award will not be made to an individual with full institutional salary support; applicants must demonstrate lack of or minimal/limited salary support as per institutional policies. Award must be payable to an academic institution.
Amount of Grant: $60,000 ($ 56,000 + $ 4,000 institutional overhead) per year for three years
Date(s) Application is Due: Sep 15; Oct 1
Contact: Director of Research Administration, (914) 821-8843; fax: (914) 821-8946; email: researchprograms@lls.org
Internet: http://www.leukemia-lymphoma.org/all_page?item_id=11618
Sponsor: Leukemia Society of America
1311 Mamaroneck Avenue
White Plains, NY 10605

LSA Specialized Center of Research Grants 2077
The purpose of the program is to increase the cure rate of or prevent leukemia, Hodgkin's and non-Hodgkin's lymphoma, and myeloma in order to foster interdisciplinary and synergistic research. The proposed center should be interdisciplinary, cohesive, and sharply focused and should be composed of at least three relevant scientific projects capable of interacting. The research may be fundamental or applied or an integrated combination of the two approaches. Basic research tied to a related translational research project is encouraged but not mandatory. The most promising ideas and the likelihood of a significant impact on the morbidity and mortality of these diseases will be viewed

favorably regardless of the particular approach. The center grant will also support scientific core laboratories required by the component research programs. Preliminary applications are due November 1; full applications are due March 15. Annual deadlines may vary; contact program staff for exact dates.
Requirements: Applications may be submitted by individuals holding an MD, PhD, or equivalent, working in domestic or foreign nonprofit organizations, such as universities, colleges, hospitals, or laboratories. Applications may be multi-institutional in nature. Applicants need not be U.S. citizens.
Amount of Grant: $1.25 million maximum
Date(s) Application is Due: Mar 15; Nov 1
Contact: Director of Research Administration, (914) 821-8843; fax: (914) 821-8946; email: researchprograms@lls.org
Internet: http://www.leukemia.org/all_page?item_id=11627
Sponsor: Leukemia Society of America
1311 Mamaroneck Avenue
White Plains, NY 10605

LSA Translational Research Program Grants **2078**
The society sponsors research toward a cure or control of leukemia, lymphoma, and myeloma. Grants fund research that shows high promise for translating basic biomedical knowledge to prevention or new treatments and, ultimately, to prolong and enhance life. The goal of the program is to accelerate transfer of findings from the laboratory to clinical application. A renewal of the grant may be funded for an additional two years if it includes an approved clinical trial. A principal intent of the program is to permit the acquisition of sufficient data to apply to an appropriate agency or sponsor for sustained support. Guidelines and sample application are available online.
Requirements: Applications may be submitted by individuals holding an MD or PhD, or equivalent degree, working in domestic or foreign nonprofit organizations, such as universities, colleges, hospitals, laboratories, units of state and local governments, or eligible agencies of the federal government.
Amount of Grant: $200,000 maximum
Date(s) Application is Due: Mar 1
Contact: Director of Research Administration, (914) 821-8843; fax: (914) 821-8946; email: researchprograms@lls.org
Internet: http://www.leukemia-lymphoma.org/all_page?item_id=11620
Sponsor: Leukemia and Lymphoma Society of America
1311 Mamaroneck Avenue
White Plains, NY 10605

Lubbock Area Foundation Grants **2079**
The Lubbock Area Foundation is a nonprofit community foundation that manages a pool of charitable endowment funds, the income from which is used to benefit the South Plains community through grants to nonprofit organizations, educational programs and scholarships. Funding priorities are: art and culture; social services; civic and community; education; social services; health and human services. Grants may be made for start-up funding, general operating support, program support and demonstration programs. Typical grant awards range from $500 - $2,500 with $5,000 as the maximum from the unrestricted funds. Grant application and additional guidelines are available on the Foundation's website.
Requirements: The Foundation restricts its support to organizations in Lubbock and the surrounding South Plains area which are 501(c)3 or the government equivalent.
Restrictions: The Foundation does not make grants to individuals, for political purposes, to retire indebtedness or for payment of interest or taxes.
Geographic Focus: Texas
Samples: Louise Hopkins Underwood Center for the Arts Clay Studio, Lubbock, TX, $8,500—Firehouse Theatre and Marketing Staff Salaries (2009); The Haven Animal Care Shelter, Lubbock, TX—$8,000— funding for veterinary care for animals (2009); Lubbock Children's Health Clinic, Lubbock, TX, $3,600—Pharmacy Assistance Program (2009).
Amount of Grant: $500-$5,000 range
Date(s) Application is Due: Jan 1; Mar 1; May 1; Jul 1; Sep 1; Nov 1
Contact: Kathleen Stocco, Executive Director; (806) 762-8061; fax: (806) 762-8551
Internet: http://www.lubbockareafoundation.org/grant.shtml
Sponsor: Lubbock Area Foundation
1655 Main Street, Suite 202
Lubbock, TX 79401

Lubrizol Foundation Grants Program **2080**
The foundation supports education, youth, health care, human services, the arts, environment, and civic affairs in Lubrizol Corporation operating locations. Funding in education supports higher education scholarships, fellowships in chemistry and chemical and mechanical engineering, adult basic education and literacy, and secondary education. Capital and operating grants are made to colleges and universities and also to private elementary and secondary schools. Health and human services grants support united campaigns and grants to hospitals and organizations providing clothing, rehabilitation, and hospice care. Civic and cultural affairs grants support the performing arts, museums, parks and nature centers, public broadcasting stations, and community special interest groups. Youth activities promoting leadership, citizenship, and recreation also are considered. The foundation operates a matching gift program, which matches gifts up to $5000 per year from Lubrizol Corporation employees on a one-to-one basis. Gifts can support education institutions and other community nonprofit organizations. Applications are accepted at any time.
Requirements: Tax-exempt Ohio and Texas organizations are eligible to apply.
Restrictions: Funds are not awarded directly to individuals or to endowments.
Geographic Focus: Ohio; Texas
Samples: Purdue U—to expand the Lubrizol HP Process Systems Engineering Laboratory, $15,000.; Cleveland Institute of Art—for a scholarship, $4000.
Amount of Grant: $1500-$30,000 average
Contact: Karen Lerchbacher, (440) 347-1797; fax: (440) 347-1858; email: kal@lubrizol.com
Internet: http://corporate.lubrizol.com/Foundation/default.asp
Sponsor: Lubrizol Corporation
29400 Lakeland Boulevard, 053A
Wickliffe, OH 44092

Lucile Horton Howe and Mitchell B. Howe Foundation Grants **2081**
The foundation supports youth organizations, social services, medical research, hospitals, religion, child welfare, drug abuse, education, and family services. Types of support include continuing support, general operating funds, and research. Requests from qualified organizations must be received prior to the second Tuesday of March for the grant year. There is only one consideration meeting a year.
Requirements: Only nonprofit organizations in the Prox-Pasadena area and the San Gabriel Valley of California are eligible. A brief letter and a copy of the organizations 501(c)3 form are the requirements for application.
Restrictions: No restricted grants will be funded by the foundation.
Geographic Focus: California
Amount of Grant: $1,000-$300,000 range
Date(s) Application is Due: Feb 28
Contact: Mitchell B. Howe, Jr., President; (626) 792-2771; email: lhmbhowefoun@earthlink.net
Sponsor: Lucile Horton Howe and Mitchell B. Howe Foundation
180 South Lake Avenue
Pasadena, CA 91101-4932

Lucy Gooding Charitable Foundation Trust **2082**
The trust awards grants to eligible Florida nonprofit organizations in its areas of interest, including child welfare, disabled children, disadvantaged people, homelessness, and hospices. Types of support include building construction/renovation, capital campaigns, equipment and land acquisition, general operating support, seed grants, and United Way. Contact the office for required application form.
Requirements: Florida 501(c)3 nonprofit organizations serving the Jacksonville area are eligible.
Geographic Focus: Florida
Samples: Wolfson Children's Hospital (Jacksonville, FL)—to establish a pediatric neurosurgery center, $5 million (2005); Community Foundation in Jacksonville (FL)—to endow a fund to support organizations that serve children or provide relief services, with an emphasis on Florida's Clay and Duval Counties, $25 million (2004).
Amount of Grant: $2500-$25 million range
Date(s) Application is Due: Sep 30
Contact: Bonnie Smith, Trustee, (904) 786-4796; fax: (904) 786-4796; email: bhsmith@bellsouth.net
Sponsor: Lucy Gooding Charitable Foundation Trust
P.O. Box 37349
Jacksonville, FL 32236-7349

Lucy Gooding Charitable Foundation Trust Grants **2083**
The Foundation, established in 1988, supports organizations involved with children and youth, services, education, human services, residential/custodial care, hospices, economically disadvantaged, people with disabilities, and homelessness. The Foundation gives primarily in the five county area surrounding Jacksonville, Florida.
Requirements: Funding preference is for organizations in the five county area surrounding Jacksonville, FL with projects helping children.
Restrictions: No support for private foundations, religious organizations, or for adults-only services, and individuals.
Geographic Focus: Florida
Samples: Baptist Medical Center, Jacksonville, FL, $1,000,000 - for Pediatric Neurosurgical Center (2006); Bridge of Northeast Florida, Jacksonville, FL, $60,000 - for youth services for disadvantaged (2006); United Way of Northeast Florida, Jacksonville, FL, $450,000 - for establishment of full service site in local school (2006);
Amount of Grant: $5,000 - $1,000,000 range
Date(s) Application is Due: Sep 30
Contact: Bonnie H. Smith, Treasurer; (904) 786-4796; fax: (904) 786-4796; email: bhsmith@bellsouth.net
Sponsor: The Lucy Gooding Charitable Foundation Trust
P.O. Box 37349
Jacksonville, FL 32236-7349

Ludwick Family Foundation Grants **2084**
The foundation is a California nonprofit public benefit corporation established exclusively for charitable, scientific, literary, and educational purposes. The foundation tends to fund tangible types of items that will remain with and can be used repeatedly by the organization.
Requirements: Eligible applicants include U.S. or U.S.-based international organizations, 501(c)3 nonprofit public charities, and government agencies (any level). All grants are to be used exclusively for charitable, public benefit purposes.

Restrictions: The foundation does not grant requests for salaries, general operating expenses, scholarships, endowment funds, fundraising events or capital campaigns, feasibility studies, consulting fees, or advertising. The foundation will no longer accept any unsolicited requests for research or from public/private schools (K-12), universities/colleges, child daycare/development centers, hospitals, or libraries.
Samples: AbilityFirst (Pasadena, CA)—to purchase an American Disabilities Act accessible van to enable the transportation of people who are disabled (2003); Alaska Public Radio Network (AK)—to purchase recorder kits and professional stereo headphones to enable reports of news, current affairs, and cultural information for Alaska's Native People (2003).
Amount of Grant: $5000-$50,000 typically for one year
Date(s) Application is Due: Mar 31; Aug 31
Contact: Deanna Monaghan, (626) 852-0092; fax: (626) 852-0776; email: ludwickfndn@ludwick.org
Internet: http://www.ludwick.org
Sponsor: Ludwick Family Foundation
P.O. Box 1796
Glendora, CA 91740

Lupus Foundation of America Research Grants 2085
Grants are awarded annually to encourage research in lupus erythematosus. It is the foundation's hope that this investment in research will produce new information that may directly lead to much larger projects and substantially increased funding from other sources, particularly the National Institutes of Health, in the future. Grants are awarded for up to two years.
Requirements: Awards are for junior investigators only (assistant professors or below, if in academic medicine). Teachers and aides at teaching centers, hospitals, and colleges are eligible.
Restrictions: First-year fellows are not eligible.
Amount of Grant: $125,000 per year
Date(s) Application is Due: Feb 15
Contact: Grants Coordinator, (202) 349-1155; fax: (202) 349-1156; email: lupusinfo@aol.com
Internet: http://www.lupus.org/research/grantproginfo.html
Sponsor: Lupus Foundation of America
2000 L Street, NW, Suite 710
Washington, DC 20036-4916

Lustgarten Foundation for Pancreatic Cancer Research Grants 2086
The foundation aims to make rapid advances in the battle against pancreatic cancer through a combination of cutting-edge technology and novel ideas. Grants can be submitted in one of three areas: novel technologies for pancreatic cancer genetics; screening for the early detection of pancreatic cancer; and novel therapies in pancreatic cancer. Proposals that exhibit leveraging of institutional resources and the attainment of major new programs are encouraged. This initiative encourages, but does not require, the development of integrative and collaborative teams of investigators from within a single institution or among several institutions. Letters of intent must be received on or before 5:00 p.m. Eastern Time on July 31, with full applications due no later than 5:00 p.m. Eastern Time on August 18. Grants will be awarded for a one-year period for a maximum amount of $100,000, of which no more than 10% can be used for indirect costs.
Requirements: Applications will be accepted from individual investigators as well as collaborating investigators. Applicants must have an MD or a PhD degree to become principal investigators. Eligible organizations include nonprofit organizations; public or private institutions, such as universities, colleges, hospitals, and laboratories; and domestic or foreign institutions/organizations.
Samples: Johns Hopkins University, Allison Klein, Ph.D. - Identification of Pancreatic Cancer Susceptibility Genes (2009); University of Michigan Medical School, Chandan Kumar, Ph.D. - Discovery of Recurrent Gene Fusions in Pancreatic Cancer using High-Throughput Sequencing (2009); Johns Hopkins University School of Medicine, Joshua Mendell, M.D., Ph.D. - Ras-regulated microRNAs in Pancreatic Cancer (2009).
Amount of Grant: $100,000 maximum per year
Contact: Kerri Kaplan, Executive Director; (516) 803-2304 or (866) 789-1000; fax: (516) 803-2303; email: kkaplan@cablevision.com or lsasso@cablevision.com
Internet: http://www.lustgarten.org/Page.aspx?pid=666
Sponsor: Lustgarten Foundation for Pancreatic Cancer Research
1111 Stewart Avenue
Bethpage, NY 11714

Lymphoma Research Foundation Fellowships 2087
Two-year fellowships uniquely permit the uninterrupted development of promising leads and help attract the nation's best scientific talent to careers in lymphoma. Its emphasis upon translational as well as purely basic research assures that breakthroughs are quickly transformed into viable treatment options.
Amount of Grant: $45,000 and $50,000 salary support for year one and year two, respectively; $5000 annual research budget
Date(s) Application is Due: Sep 9
Contact: Director of Medical and Scientific Outreach, (212) 349-2910; fax: (212) 349-2886; email: researchgrants@lymphoma.org
Internet: http://www.lymphoma.org/site/pp.asp?c=bfIKIVMIG&b=38480
Sponsor: Lymphoma Research Foundation
111 Broadway, 19th Floor
New York, NY 10016

Lymphoma Research Foundation Grants 2088
The foundation supports high-quality research that results in safer, more effective treatments and a cure for lymphoma. Applications are accepted for two programs. Fellowship research grants support young investigators (third-year fellows) pursuing careers in lymphoma research. Lymphoma-specific projects submitted by individuals associated with accredited academic institutions, JCAHO-accredited research hospitals, and other research organizations that have national or international reputations for excellence will be considered. Junior faculty research grants support researchers at the assistant or associate professor level. Mantle cell research projects also are funded at both levels.
Samples: U Hospital Grosshadern (Germany)—for research on mantle-cell lymphoma, a rare form of blood cancer, $890,000 (2004); U of Texas MD Anderson Medical Ctr (Houston, TX)—for research on mantle-cell lymphoma, a rare form of blood cancer, $2.4 million (2003).
Amount of Grant: $45,000 maximum fellowships; $75,000 maximum junior faculty research grants
Date(s) Application is Due: Sep 15
Contact: Grants Administrator, (212) 349-2910 or (800) 235-6848; email: ResearchGrants@lymphoma.org
Internet: http://www.lymphoma.org/site/pp.asp?c=bfIKIVMIG&b=36878
Sponsor: Lymphoma Research Foundation
8800 Venice Boulevard, Suite 207
Los Angeles, CA 90034

Lynde and Harry Bradley Foundation Grants 2089
The foundation aims to encourage projects that focus on cultivating a renewed, healthier, and more vigorous sense of citizenship among the American people and among peoples of other nations. Projects likely to be supported will generally treat free people as self-governing, personally responsible citizens, not as victims or clients; aim to restore the intellectual and cultural legitimacy of common sense, the wisdom of experience, everyday morality, and personal character; seek to reinvigorate and re-empower the traditional, local institutions—families, schools, churches, and neighborhoods—that provide training in and room for the exercise of genuine citizenship, that pass on everyday morality to the next generation, and that cultivate personal character; and encourage decentralization of power and accountability away from centralized, bureaucratic, national institutions back to states, localities, and revitalized mediating structures. Eligible projects may address any arena of public life—economics, politics, culture, or civil society; the problem of citizenship at home or abroad; Milwaukee and Wisconsin community and state projects that aim to improve the life of the community through increasing cultural and educational opportunities, grassroots economic development, and social and health services; the resuscitation of citizenship in the economic, political, cultural, or social realms; policy research and writing about approaches encouraging that resuscitation; academic research and writing that explore the intellectual roots of citizenship; and popular writing and media projects that illustrate for a broader public audience the themes of citizenship. The foundation supports programs that research the needs of gifted children and techniques of providing education for students with superior skills and/or intelligence; research programs investigating how learning occurs in gifted children; and demonstration programs of instruction.
Requirements: Tax-exempt and nonprofit organizations should prepare a letter of inquiry presenting a concise description of the project, its objectives and significance, and the qualifications of the organizations and individuals involved. If the project appears to fall within the foundation's mandate, a brochure with detailed proposal requirements will be sent to the applicant.
Restrictions: The foundation favors projects that are normally not financed by public funds and will consider requests from religious organizations that are not denominational in character. Grants without significant importance to the foundation's areas of interest will only under special conditions be considered for endowment or deficit financing proposals. Grants will not be made to individuals, for overhead costs, or for fund-raising counsel.
Amount of Grant: $25,000-$250,000
Date(s) Application is Due: Feb 1; May 1; Aug 1, Nov 1
Contact: Daniel Schmidt, Vice President; (414) 291-9915; fax: (414) 291-9991
Internet: http://www.bradleyfdn.org/app.html
Sponsor: Lynde and Harry Bradley Foundation
1241 North Franklin Place
Milwaukee, WI 53202-2901

Lynde and Harry Bradley Foundation Prizes: Bradley Prizes 2090
The Bradley Prizes formally recognize individuals of extraordinary talent and dedication who have made contributions of excellence in areas consistent with The Lynde and Harry Bradley Foundation's mission. Up to four Prizes of $250,000 each are awarded annually to innovative thinkers and practitioners whose achievements strengthen the legacy of the Bradley brothers and the ideas to which they were committed. Each year, Bradley Prize nominations are solicited from a national panel of more than 100 prominent individuals involved in academia, public-policy research, journalism, civic affairs, and the arts. All nominees are carefully evaluated by a distinguished selection committee that makes recommendations to the Foundation's Board of Directors, which selects them. The Prize winners are then honored at a celebratory awards ceremony.
Amount of Grant: $250,000 each
Contact: Daniel Schmidt, Vice President; (414) 291-9915; fax: (414) 291-9991
Internet: http://www.bradleyfdn.org/bradley_prizes.asp
Sponsor: Lynde and Harry Bradley Foundation
1241 North Franklin Place
Milwaukee, WI 53202-2901

M-A-C AIDS Fund Grants 2091

The fund makes grants to registered charitable, nonprofit organizations that provide basic needs, such as food, clothing, housing, or shelter (short-term or transitional); direct services related to health care; social services, transportation (for medical visits, outpatient visits, and other social services); health-related recreational activities; and programs that bring HIV/AIDS education, awareness, and prevention to public attention. Proposals are reviewed quarterly and must arrive at least one month prior to the quarterly review date. Application guidelines and required format are available online.

Requirements: Grants are awarded to tax exempt, non-profit organizations that are 501(c) (3) and directly associated with HIV/AIDS. A minimum of 80% of the total organization's budget must be is directed to program.

Restrictions: Grants will not fund: individuals; lobbying activities; ongoing general operating expenses or existing deficits; endowments, unless they provide a direct service to PWA's; capital costs; conferences, summits, briefings, PSA's; or research. With the exception of North American based charities, the Fund does not accept unsolicited international grant proposals.

Amount of Grant: $5,000 - $25,000

Internet: http://www.macaidsfund.org/support/givingguidelines.html

Sponsor: M-A-C AIDS Fund
130 Prince Street, 2nd Floor
New York, NY 10012

M. Bastian Family Foundation Grants 2092

The foundation supports nonprofit organizations in its areas of interest, including music, the arts, higher education, health care and health organizations, religion (Christian and Latter-day Saints), social services, and wildlife conservation. Types of support include general operating support and scholarship funds. Contact the office for application forms. There are no application deadlines.

Requirements: Funding focus is primarily in Utah.

Restrictions: Grants are not made to individuals.

Samples: Brigham Young U (Provo, UT)—for scholarship endowment, $200,000.; Pediatric AIDS Foundation (Los Angeles, CA)—for general support, $20,000.; American Diabetes Assoc (Alexandra, VA)—for research, $100,000.

Amount of Grant: $2000-$200,000 range

Contact: McKay Matthews, Program Contact, (801) 225-2455

Sponsor: M. Bastian Family Foundation
51 W Center Street, Suite 305
Orem, UT 84057

M.B. and Edna Zale Foundation Grants 2093

The M.B. & Edna Zale Foundation honors the tradition of its founders through grants that stimulate change. To accomplish this mission, the Foundation acts as a catalyst for collaboration and makes grants in communities where the Directors live or have an interest. Grants are made primarily in the communities of Dallas (Dallas County) and Houston (Harris County), Texas; Boca Raton, Florida; Portland, Oregon; and New York, including Long Island. The Foundation has an interest in four areas of funding: community services; health; education; Jewish heritage.

Requirements: 501(c)3 nonprofits organizations in the communities of Dallas (Dallas County) and Houston (Harris County), Texas; Boca Raton, Florida; Portland, Oregon; and New York, including Long Island are eligible. Contact the Foundation for further application information and guidelines.

Restrictions: The Foundation does not ordinarily provide: major support for the arts; grants to individuals; scholarships and fellowships to individuals (except through colleges and universities).

Geographic Focus: Florida; New York; Oregon; Texas

Amount of Grant: $2000-$100,000 average

Contact: Leonard Krasnow, President; (214) 855-0627; fax: (972) 726-7252; email: mail@zalefoundation.org

Sponsor: M.B. and Edna Zale Foundation
6360 LBJ Highway, Suite 205
Dallas, TX 75240

M.E. Raker Foundation Grants 2094

The foundation was established in 1984, serving the Allen County, Indiana area. Areas of interest include: children/youth, services; education; environment; natural resources; health care; historic preservation/historical societies; human services people with disabilities. Support is offered in the following areas: building/renovation; general/operating support; matching/challenge support; Program development. No support for the arts or to individuals.

Requirements: Indiana nonprofit organizations are eligible. Emphasis is given to requests from Fort Wayne. Send a letter requesting an application to the foundation office. Application form required for grant proposals.

Geographic Focus: Indiana

Amount of Grant: $5000-$40,000 average range

Contact: Jennifer Pickard, Grants Coordinator; (260) 436-2182

Sponsor: M.E. Raker Foundation, Inc.
6207 Constitution Drive
Fort Wayne, IN 46804-1517

M.J. Murdock Charitable Trust Grants 2095

The trust supports nonprofit organizations in the Pacific Northwest. Grantmaking priorities include health and human services—mental health services, early-childhood and youth programs, economic and cultural development, support for the disabled, and disaster relief; education—projects that emphasize innovative learning techniques both in and outside the classroom (e.g., educational programs at museums, nonprofit organizations, schools, universities, and zoos); scientific research in the natural sciences that emphasizes new knowledge or trains students in research techniques; and arts and culture. Prospective applicants should submit a letter of inquiry; guidelines are available on the Web site. A positive response to the letter of inquiry will include an application packet and directions for its completion.

Requirements: Pacific Northwest 501(c)3 tax-exempt organizations in Alaska, Idaho, Montana, Oregon, and Washington State are eligible.

Restrictions: The charitable trust does not support ongoing operations, debt reduction, general fund drives, annual appeals, or emergency funds.

Geographic Focus: Alaska; Idaho; Montana; Oregon; Pacific Northwest; Washington

Samples: Pacific Northwest Research Institute (Seattle, WA)—to purchase equipment for research on the subcellular mechanisms of disease, with a focus on diabetes, $67,500 (2004); Northwest Children's Theater and School (Portland, OR)—to develop a fundraising department, $115,000 over three years (2004); Seattle's Union Gospel Mission (WA)—to repair a shelter that was damaged by an earthquake, $50,000 challenge grant.; NetCorps (Eugene, OR)—to provide technology support to nonprofit organizations in rural Oregon, $90,000 partial challenge grant over three years.

Amount of Grant: $22.8 million total

Contact: Dr. John Van Zytveld, Senior Program Officer, (360) 694-8415

Internet: http://www.murdock-trust.org

Sponsor: M.J. Murdock Charitable Trust
P.O. Box 1618
Vancouver, WA 98668

Mabel H. Flory Charitable Trust Grants 2096

The Mabel H. Flory Charitable Trust was established in 1979 and funds organizations primarily in Washington, DC., and Baltimore, MD. Support is available for research designed to develop new cures and methods of treatment: for children with hearing and sight problems; arthritis in both children and adults; and aphasia related problems.

Requirements: Your initial approach should be in the form of a letter, prior to the deadline date. Mail letter to the following address: c/o BB&T Co. of Virginia, Attn.: Trustee, 6400 Arlington Boulevard, Falls Church, VA, 22042.

Restrictions: No grants to individuals.

Geographic Focus: District of Columbia; Maryland

Date(s) Application is Due: Aug 31

Contact: BB&T Co. Trustee; (703) 531-2053;

Sponsor: Mabel H. Flory Charitable Trust c/o BB&T Co. of Virginia
P.O. Box 2907
Wilson, NC 27894-2907

Mabel Y. Hughes Charitable Trust Grants 2097

The trust awards grants to Denver-area nonprofit organizations in its areas of interest, including community funds, cultural programs, education, health, hospitals, museums, social services, and youth. Types of support include operating support, continuing support, annual campaigns, seed money, emergency funds, building funds, equipment acquisition, endowment funds, research grants, and special projects.

Requirements: Colorado nonprofit organizations are eligible.

Restrictions: Grants do not support conferences, individuals, or ticket purchases for benefits.

Geographic Focus: Colorado

Amount of Grant: $5000-$60,000 range

Contact: Judy Dowling, c/o Wells Fargo Bank, (720) 947-6725

Sponsor: Mabel Y. Hughes Charitable Trust
1740 Broadway, MC 7300 #483
Denver, CO 80274

Madison County Community Foundation Grants 2098

Founded in 1992 by a core of local leaders, the Madison County Community Foundation today is a stable, trustworthy and permanent partner in efforts to sustain and improve our community. With assets at $14 million and growing, the Foundation annually returns hundreds of thousands of dollars to Madison County, Indiana in the form of grants and scholarships. The foundations mission remains constant: to enhance the quality of life of citizens of Madison County by attracting charitable gifts, making philanthropic grants, providing responsible financial stewardship and community leadership.

Requirements: Funding opportunities are limited primarily to Madison County, Indiana area. Contact the foundation office before submitting a proposal.

Geographic Focus: Indiana

Contact: Holly A. Chaille, Development Officer; (765) 644-0002 fax; (765) 644-3392; email: hachaille@madisonccf.org

Internet: http://www.madisonccf.org/grants.html

Sponsor: Madison County Community Foundation, Inc.
33 West 10th Street, Suite 600, P.O. Box 1056
Anderson, IN 46015-1056

Maine Community Foundation Grants 2099

The foundation awards a wide variety of grants. The community building program focuses on proposals that build on community assets and resources and support/promote sustainable, healthy community networks. The goal of the organizational capacity building grant program is to strengthen the impact of Maine-based nonprofit organizations by improving their organizational capacity. The foundation considers requests for equipment purchases or operating expenses, especially if the group is in

the start-up stage. The foundation has several fields of interest and donor-advised funds that make grants within specific interest areas. Several funds make grants to individuals for professional development and special projects (i.e., gay, lesbian, and transgender community, environmental conservation, and arts); there also is a scholarship program. Recent grants have support affordable housing, the arts, economic and community development, education, environment, health, social capital, and youth. Grant sizes, deadlines, and priorities vary for each fund. The board meets quarterly to consider requests. Application deadlines and guidelines are available online.
Requirements: Maine 501(c)3 nonprofit organizations are eligible.
Restrictions: Support is not given to religious organizations for religious purposes; individuals, except scholarship funds; or for endowment funds, equipment, or annual campaigns for regular operations. Grants rarely are made to support capital campaigns.
Geographic Focus: Maine
Samples: College of the Atlantic (Bar Harbor, ME)—for the Cummings Scholarship Fund, to support students from the western mountain area of Maine to attend the college, $10,000.
Amount of Grant: $5,300 average community building grants; $20,000 maximum organizational capacity building grant
Contact: Bethany Murray, Competitive Grants Associate; (877) 700-6800; fax (207) 667-0447; email: bmurray@mainecf.org or info@mainecf.org
Internet: http://www.mainecf.org/html/grants/available/index.html
Sponsor: Maine Community Foundation
245 East Main Street
Ellsworth, ME 04605

Manuel D. and Rhoda Mayerson Foundation Grants **2100**
The foundation awards grants to eligible nonprofit organizations in its areas of interest, including children and youth, people with disabilities, arts and culture, higher education, housing and homelessness, and Jewish life and culture. Types of support include building construction/renovation, conferences and seminars, matching/challenge grants, seed grants, and technical assistance. The board meets quarterly.
Requirements: Nonprofit organizations are eligible. Preference is given to requests from the Cincinnati area.
Restrictions: Individuals are ineligible.
Amount of Grant: $1000-$30,000 average
Contact: Program Contact, (513) 621-7500; fax: (513) 621-2864; email: info@mayersonfoundation.org
Internet: http://www.mayersonfoundation.org
Sponsor: Manuel D. and Rhoda Mayerson Foundation
312 Walnut Street, Suite 3600
Cincinnati, OH 45202

MAP International Medical Fellowships **2101**
The MAP International Medical Fellowship encourages lifelong involvement in global health issues by providing selected medical students firsthand exposure in a Christian context to the health, social and cultural characteristics of a developing world community. MAP International, through a grant from the founders of Reader's Digest, DeWitt and Lila Wallace, sponsors fourth year medical students by funding travel arrangements for medical students to their chosen destination. The field experience must be designed to provide the student exposure to community health in a Christian context. Students select a mission agency or hospital that has an outreach among the poor in a rural or urban setting. Students must spend at least eight weeks in the field (six weeks for residents and interns). The fellowship provides 100 percent of the approved round trip airfare to one destination. In most instances, students pay room and board as well as any in-country travel expenses. To obtain an application, check with the dean of your school or the Student Affairs Office. Applications are sent to all medical schools annually. You may also download the application in PDF or Microsoft Word format on the Map International website.
Requirements: Fourth-year medical students, residents and interns are eligible. Applications should be submitted during the academic year prior to travel.
Date(s) Application is Due: Mar 1
Contact: Margaret Stevenson, Medical Fellowship Coordinator; (404) 880-0540; fax: (912) 265-6170; email: mstevenson@map.org
Internet: http://www.map.org/site/PageServer?pagename=what_Medical_Fellowship
Sponsor: Map International
4700 Glynco Parkway
Brunswick, GA 31525-6800

MAPFRE Foundation for Medicine Grants **2102**
The foundation operates nationally and internationally in the fields of education, medicine and health, science and technology, and social welfare. Types of support include research grants, grants to individuals and organizations, scholarships, fellowships, and prizes.
Contact: Grants Administrator, 34-1-6265704; fax: 34-1-6265825; email: infofmm@mapfremedicina.es
Internet: http://www.mapfre.com/pmapfre/paraguas_mapfre/en/06/0608.shtml
Sponsor: MAPFRE Foundation for Medicine
Carretera de Pozuelo a Majadahonda s/n
Madrid 28220 Spain

Marcia and Otto Koehler Foundation Grants **2103**
Grants are made to support arts and culture, medical, education, and social organizations in San Antonio, Texas. Proposals must demonstrate leadership in effecting positive change; encourage collaborative effort; serve large and diverse sectors of the population; and demonstrate vision, effectiveness, and good fiscal management. Types of support include general operating support, building construction/renovation, and research. Grants are made for one time only. Applicants must send a letter of request for application by March 1 to receive an application.
Requirements: Grants are awarded only to organizations in Bexar County, Texas.
Restrictions: Grants will not be made to individuals or to support other foundations or endowments; salaries; operating deficits; political organizations; or churches, synagogues, or parishes.
Geographic Focus: Texas
Samples: Centro Alameda (San Antonio, TX)—to restore a marquee, canopy, and facade, $30,000.; McNay Art Museum (San Antonio, TX)—to sponsor an art exhibit, $50,000.
Amount of Grant: $2,500-$50,000 range
Date(s) Application is Due: Jun 1
Contact: Thomas K. Killion, Senior Vice President, Bank of America; (210) 270-5422; fax: (210) 270-5520; email: thomas.k.killion@ustrust.com
Sponsor: Marcia and Otto Koehler Foundation
P.O. Box 121
San Antonio, TX 78291-0121

Margaret L. Wendt Foundation Grants **2104**
The foundation awards grants to eligible New York nonprofit organizations in its areas of interest, including education, the arts, social services, churches and religious organizations, health associations, public interest organizations, and youth agencies. There are no application deadlines or forms. The board meets quarterly
Requirements: Western New York nonprofit organizations are eligible. Giving is primarily in Buffalo.
Restrictions: Grants are not awarded to individuals, including scholarships.
Geographic Focus: New York
Samples: D'Youville College (Buffalo, NY)—for its chiropractic program, including equipping a computerized diagnostic-imaging classroom and an off-campus community-based clinic, $350,000 (2005).
Contact: Grants Administrator, (716) 855-2146
Sponsor: Margaret L. Wendt Foundation
40 Fountain Plaza, Suite 277
Buffalo, NY 14202

Margaret T. Morris Foundation Grants **2105**
The foundation awards grants, primarily in Arizona, in its areas of interest, including arts and culture, children and youth, higher education. family, environment and animal welfare, social services, mental health, medical research, marine sciences, music, and hospice. Types of support include general operating costs, building construction/renovation, scholarship funds, deficit financing, endowments, land acquisition, and program development. Proposals are accepted between May and November, and the board meets in August and December.
Restrictions: No support for religious organizations. Grants are not made to individuals.
Geographic Focus: Arizona
Amount of Grant: $350-$100,000 range
Contact: Eugene Polk, Trustee
Sponsor: Margaret T. Morris Foundation
P.O. Box 592
Prescott, AZ 86302

Margoes Foundation Grants **2106**
The foundation awards grants to California nonprofits in its areas of interest, including cardiac research, rehabilitation of mentally ill patients, and scholarships for minority students and for Asian and African nationals studying in the United States. Types of funding include general operating support, continuing support, program development, fellowships, scholarship funds, research, and matching funds. There are no application forms. Applicants should call or submit a preliminary letter prior to submitting a full proposal.
Requirements: California nonprofits are eligible, with preference given to the San Francisco Bay area.
Restrictions: Grants are not awarded to agencies supported by federated campaigns or to individuals.
Geographic Focus: California
Samples: Community Music Center (San Francisco, CA)—for financial aid, $10,000.; U of the Pacific (Stockton, CA)—to increase minority enrollment in the predentistry undergraduate programs, $20,000 over two years.; Fred Finch Youth Ctr (Oakland, CA)—for salary support of a part-time counselor for a transitional independent living program for older adolescents and young adults with severe emotional problems, $15,000.
Amount of Grant: $10,000-$20,000 average
Date(s) Application is Due: Apr 1; Oct 1
Contact: John Blum, Principal Manager, (415) 981-2966; fax: (415) 981-5218; email: margoesfdn@aol.com
Sponsor: Margoes Foundation
57 Post Street, Suite 510
San Francisco, CA 94104

Marijuana Policy Project Grants **2107**

The program supports efforts that promote the legalization and regulation of marijuana. Projects may encompass any aspect of marijuana-law reform, such as: ballot initiatives, grassroots organizing, litigating for the right to use marijuana for religious purposes, lobbying the American Medical Association, marijuana research, and revising the definition of marijuana abuse and dependence in the American Psychiatric Association's Diagnostic and Statistical Manual. Submit letters of inquiry; full proposals are by invitation.

Requirements: Preference is given to 501(c)3 tax-exempt organizations, but such status is not an eligibility requirement.

Restrictions: The grants program does not fund political parties or candidates for office, state ballot initiatives, or hemp-related projects.

Amount of Grant: $60,000 maximum

Date(s) Application is Due: Jan 2; May 1; Sep 1

Contact: Stephanie Vogel, (202) 462-5747 ext 104; fax: (202) 232-0442; email: stephanie@mpp.org

Internet: http://www.mpp.org/grants/index.html

Sponsor: Marijuana Policy Project
P.O. Box 77492
Washington, DC 20013

Marine Biological Laboratory Summer Research Fellowships **2108**

Each year a number of summer research support opportunities for young investigators are awarded for studies and research to be carried out at the Marine Biological Laboratory (MBL) at Woods Hole, MA. The Robert Dale Allen Fellowship supports research in cell motility and cytoarchitecture; and the Frederik B. Bang Fellowship funds research on marine invertebrate immunology, pathology, infectious diseases, and molecular biology. The M.G.F. Fuortes Fellowship sponsors research in the neurosciences, and the Stephen W. Kuffler Fellowship supports research in neurobiology. The H. Burr Steinbach Fellowship funds research in cell biology and physiology. In addition, the Porter Fellowships for Minority Students/Investigators are offered for research in the field of physiology with senior investigators at the MBL. The MBL Summer Fellowships are offered to investigators to conduct independent or collaborative research in any area. Awarded funds may be used to pay laboratory rental fees, housing costs, travel to and from Woods Hole, and appropriate personal expenses. Notification of selection of fellows is made by March 1.

Requirements: Postdoctoral students, instructors, and assistant professors may apply for these fellowships.

Date(s) Application is Due: Jan 15

Contact: Fellowship Coordinator, Office of Research Administration and Education, (508) 289-7441; fax: (508) 289-1924; email: skaufman@mbl.edu

Internet: http://www.mbl.edu/research/summer/fellowships.html

Sponsor: Marine Biological Laboratory
7 MBL Street
Woods Hole, MA 02543

Marion I. and Henry J. Knott Foundation Grants Program **2109**

Grants are awarded to organizations located in areas served by the Archdiocese of Baltimore for projects in private and nonsectarian private school elementary and secondary education, cultural arts and humanities, human and social services, Roman Catholicism, and health. Programs and projects that will be funded include endowment funds, capital and building campaigns, operating expenses, matching funds, equipment, seed money, and new or ongoing program support. All grant requests must be discussed with the foundation's executive director at least one month before submission. Requests should be submitted by a one-page letter; full proposals are by invitation. Deadlines listed are for letters of inquiry.

Requirements: Funding is limited to 501(c)3 organizations serving Baltimore City and the following counties in Maryland: Allegheny, Anne Arundel, Baltimore, Carroll, Frederick, Garrett, Harford, Howard, and Washington.

Restrictions: The following will not be funded: organizations that have not been in operation for at least one year, scholarships, public education/public sector agencies, pro-choice activities, individuals, annual giving, political activities, one-time only events/seminars/workshops, legal services, environment, medical research, day care centers, endowment funds for arts/humanities, national/local chapters for specific diseases, agencies that redistribute grant funds to other nonprofits, or government agencies that form 501(c)3 nonprofits to fund public sector projects.

Geographic Focus: Maryland

Amount of Grant: $20,000-$35,000 average

Date(s) Application is Due: Jun 1; Dec 1

Contact: Program Contact, (410) 235-7068; fax: (410) 889-2577; email: knott@knottfoundation.org

Internet: http://knottfoundation.org

Sponsor: Marion I. and Henry J. Knott Foundation
3904 Hickory Avenue
Baltimore, MD 21211-1834

Marion Park Deaver and Harry Gilbert Deaver Foundation Grants **2110**

The mission of the foundation is to promote education, with major emphasis on financial support to parochial and private schools for facilities, scholarships, computing and network capability, technical support for the use of computers in education, development and presentation of a course for teachers in the use of network for education, and the Deaver Foundation Award for Excellence in Teaching. Other areas designated for financial assistance are religion, science, health, environment, literacy arts, and the indigent. The geographic areas for grants are Florida, Wisconsin, and Minnesota. There are no application forms or deadlines.

Requirements: Florida, Minnesota, and Wisconsin nonprofit organizations are eligible.

Geographic Focus: Florida; Minnesota; Wisconsin

Samples: SpanishNet College (Boynton Beach, FL)—to offer Spanish-language classes to U.S. teachers and other school employees and to nurses and other health-care providers, beginning in Forsyth County, NC, $225,000 (2005).

Contact: Grants Administrator, c/o Wachovia Bank

Internet: http://www.deaverfoundation.org/AboutTheDeaverFoundation.htm

Sponsor: Marion Park Deaver and Harry Gilbert Deaver Foundation
975 S Federal Hwy
Boca Raton, FL 33432

Marjorie C. Adams Charitable Trust Grants **2111**

The Foundation, established in New York in 1987, is administered by the JP Morgan Chase Bank of Newark and supports the care and treatment of deaf and blind people, research into the causes and the treatment of deafness and blindness, and K-12 education. Types of support for these programs include: building and renovation projects, capital campaigns, and endowments. There are no specific application forms required or deadlines with which to adhere.

Geographic Focus: Maryland; New York

Samples: League for the Hard of Hearing, New York, New York, $95,000 (2007); Foundation for Fighting Blindness, Owings Mills, Maryland, $102,000—for an endowment (2007).

Amount of Grant: $150,000 maximum

Contact: Frank Lemma, VP of JP Morgan Chase Bank; (212) 464-2439

Sponsor: Marjorie C. Adams Charitable Trust
345 Park Avenue
New York, NY 10154

Mark and Catherine Winkler Foundation Grants **2112**

The foundation awards grants in its areas of interest, including children and youth, community development, education/higher education, environmental conservation/programs, health care/surgery, human services, and social sciences. Types of support include annual campaigns, building construction/renovation, capital campaigns and endowments, challenge/matching grants, conferences and seminars, equipment acquisition, fellowships, general operating support, professorships, program development, research, and seed grants. There are no application deadlines. The board meets in November to consider requests.

Requirements: Nonprofit organizations are eligible.

Samples: Centre College of Kentucky (Danville, KY)—for program support, $500,000.; Colorado College (Colorado Springs, CO)—to create a professorship and to add a new junior faculty position in the psychology department, $1.5 million.

Amount of Grant: $700-$1 million range

Contact: Lynne Ball, Assistant Treasurer, (703) 998-0400

Sponsor: Mark and Catherine Winkler Foundation
4900 Seminary Road, Suite 900
Alexandria, VA 22311

Marriott Foundation for People with Disabilities Bridges Program Grants **2113**

Bridges works with young people exiting special education, and with local employers, to develop mutually beneficial job placements. The program focuses on the following ideas: to consistently establish successful employment opportunity, the business needs of the employer must take precedence; rather than preoccupation with what people can't do we must focus on their skills and interests; until the talents of all citizens are fully incorporated and utilized, communities will be less than they could be.

Requirements: Nonprofits in Marriott locations are eligible, including Montgomery County, MD; Atlanta, GA; Chicago, IL; Los Angeles, and San Francisco, CA; Philadelphia, PA; and Washington, DC.

Geographic Focus: California; District of Columbia; Georgia; Illinois; Maryland; Pennsylvania

Contact: Michael D'Ovidio, (301) 562-9146 ext 21; TTY: (301) 562-9150; fax: (301) 562-9149

Internet: http://www.marriottfoundation.org

Sponsor: Marriott Foundation for People with Disabilities
8720 Georgia Avenue, Suite 801
Silver Spring, MD 20910

Mars Foundation Grants **2114**

The foundation awards grants to eligible nonprofit organizations primarily within the Washington, DC, metropolitan area, including Virginia, Maryland, and the District of Columbia. Areas of support include arts and culture, animal/wildlife, civic and community, education, environment, health and human services, and historic preservation. Types of support include capital grants, challenge grants, general operating grants, and project grants. Grants are awarded once a year. Requests must be submitted on the foundation's application form.

Requirements: U.S. 501(c)3 nonprofit organizations are eligible.

Samples: Colonial Williamsburg (Williamsburg, VA)—for new 17th- and 18th-century costumes for the casts of the Cry Witch! program, $25,000.

Amount of Grant: $1000-$100,000 range

Date(s) Application is Due: Oct 15

Contact: Grants Administrator, (703) 821-4900; fax: (703) 448-9678

Internet: http://www.mars.com

Sponsor: Mars Foundation
6885 Elm Street
McLean, VA 22101

Marshall Field's Community Grants **2115**
The program awards grants in Marshall Field's communities to nonprofit organizations in its areas of interest, including education—early childhood reading, and youth leadership development; arts and culture—accessibility to the arts, and education through the arts; and health and welfare—children and family wellness, AIDS, and cancer (awareness, research, and treatment). Proposals are considered for both new and ongoing programs. Contact program staff for eligibility. Guidelines and application are available online. Annual deadline dates may vary; contact program staff for exact dates.
Requirements: 501(c)3 nonprofit organizations and units of government, including schools, in operating communities are eligible.
Restrictions: Grants do not support individuals; programs and organizations outside of Marshall Field's operating communities; foundations, endowment fund drives, or capital campaigns; places of worship devoted solely to religious instruction; treatment programs (i.e., substance abuse); athletic teams or events; fundraiser or gala events; advocacy or research groups; or educational institutions for regular instructional programs.
Amount of Grant: $5000 maximum
Date(s) Application is Due: Apr 30
Contact: Community Grants, (800) 634-3537 or (612) 375-2300; email: Fields_Gives@marshallfields.com
Internet: http://www.fields.com/common/comm_grants.jsp
Sponsor: Marshall Field's Corporation
700 On the Mall, MS-859
Minneapolis, MN 55402

Mary Allen Lindsey Branan Foundation Grants **2116**
Income of the trust is to be distributed at least annually to 501(c)3 organizations for the relief of suffering and for charitable purposes—e.g., for the victims of floods, disasters, for the care of the sick, feeble, helpless, and orphans. However, grants are awarded exclusively at the discretion of the Board of Trustees. There are no geographic restrictions on distributions, but it has been the practice of the trustee to make grants within the state of Georgia.
Samples: Moving in the Spirit (GA)—$10,000.; Georgia Health Decisions (GA)—$10,000.; Stepping Stones Educational Therapy Ctr (GA)—$25,000.; Cool Girls (GA)—$5,000.
Contact: Lydia Whitman, c/o Wachovia Bank, (404) 332-6677; email: grantinquiriesga@wachovia.com
Internet: http://www.wachovia.com/corp_inst/charitable_services/0,,3297,00.html
Sponsor: Mary Allen Lindsey Branan Foundation
3414 Peachtree Road, 5th Fl, MC GA8023
Atlanta, GA 30326

Mary Baker Eddy Library Summer Research Fellowships **2117**
The library awards fellowships to scholars and other researchers for research in its collections in the fields of women's history, spirituality and health, religious studies, 19th-century history, and journalism—themes for which the library's collections hold special relevance and value. Consideration will be given to applicants with outstanding writing skills, evidence of having previous publications, and a definite plan for disseminating the research through publication, lecturing, etc. Fellowship recipients are expected to be in regular and continuous use of the collections at the library in Boston during the period of the fellowship (between June 13 and September 2). Fellows are responsible for making their own arrangements for housing in the Boston area. Application and guidelines are available online.
Requirements: Fellowships are open to doctoral and postdoctoral scholars, faculty members, and independent researchers.
Amount of Grant: $700 per scholar week
Date(s) Application is Due: Feb 13
Contact: Fellowships Administrator, (617) 450-7206; email: fellowships@marybakereddylibrary.org
Internet: http://www.marybakereddylibrary.org/programs/fellowshipapplications.jhtml
Sponsor: Mary Baker Eddy Library
200 Massachusetts Avenue
Boston, MA 02115

Mary Black Foundation Grants **2118**
The foundation makes grants to nonprofit organizations in the Spartanburg County, South Carolina, region in its areas of interest, including early childhood development, and active living. Grants support projects in preventive health care, community health and wellness, and education. The community health fund is a small grantmaking resource that allows the foundation to respond to grant applications outside of the active living and early childhood development priority areas, but still within the foundation's mission of improving health and wellness in Spartanburg County. Guidelines and applications are available on the foundation's Web site.
Requirements: Nonprofit organizations in Spartanburg County, SC are eligible.
Restrictions: The foundation does not accept applications from individuals or general fundraising solicitations.
Geographic Focus: South Carolina
Samples: Health Resource Ctr (Spartanburg, SC)—to publish and distribute Parent Talk, a newsletter on child rearing, $15,000.; Senior Ctrs of Spartanburg County (SC)—for a home-repair program for elderly people, $28,000.; Healthy Spartanburg (SC)—for general operating support, $25,000.; Stop the Violence Collaboration of Spartanburg (SC)—to hold a series of violence-prevention institutes for seventh and eighth graders, $25,000.
Date(s) Application is Due: Mar 15; Jun 15; Sep 15; Dec 15
Contact: Program Contact, (864) 573-9500; fax: (864) 573-5805; email: info@maryblackfoundation.org
Internet: http://www.maryblackfoundation.org/application.html
Sponsor: Mary Black Foundation
945 E Main Street
Spartanburg, SC 29302

Mary Ingraham Bunting Institute Biomedical Research Fellowships **2119**
Funded by the Burroughs Wellcome Fund, the fellowships support women scientists in all fields of biomedical research. Two awards will be made in the current year. Fellows may compete for a second year of funding. Fellowships provide office or studio space, auditing privileges, and access to libraries and most other resources of Radcliffe College and Harvard University. Residence in the Boston area and participation in the institute community are required during the fellowship appointment.
Requirements: Women scientists who are U.S. citizens or permanent residents and have held a doctorate (MD or PhD) degree for at least two years prior to appointment are eligible.
Amount of Grant: $55,000 maximum for one year with plus research expenses
Date(s) Application is Due: Oct 1
Contact: Fellowship Coordinator, (617) 496-1324; email: fellowships@radcliffe.edu
Internet: http://www.radcliffe.edu/fellowships/index.php
Sponsor: Bunting Institute of Radcliffe College
34 Concord Avenue
Cambridge, MA 02138

Mary Kay Ash Charitable Foundation Grants **2120**
The foundation, whose mission is to enrich women's lives around the world, supports research grants to help find a cure for cancers affecting women (breast, cervical, ovarian, and uterine). It also funds U.S. women's shelters and offers financial support to organizations that raise awareness and address the problem of violence against women. Proposals may be submitted at any time.
Requirements: Cancer research grants are awarded to accredited U.S. medical schools and schools of public health. Shelters must be U.S. tax-exempt entities.
Samples: U of Texas Southwestern Medical Ctr (Dallas, TX)—to create a professorship in dermatology, $1 million (2005).
Contact: Grants Administrator, (877) 652-2737
Internet: http://www.mkacf.org
Sponsor: Mary Kay Ash Charitable Foundation
P.O. Box 799044
Dallas, TX 75379-9044

Mary Owen Borden Foundation Grants **2121**
The foundation supports programs that address the needs of economically disadvantaged youth and their families. This includes needs such as health, family planning, education, counseling, childcare, substance abuse, and delinquency. Other areas of interest for the foundation include affordable housing, conservation, environment, and the arts.
Requirements: New Jersey nonprofits in Monmouth and Mercer Counties are eligible.
Geographic Focus: New Jersey
Samples: Young Scholars' Institute (Trenton, NJ)—to support after-school, Saturday, and summer programs for more than 200 students (K-12), $18,500.; Union Industrial Home (Trenton, NJ)—to provide residential care for young unwed mothers and their children, and support a program for young fathers, $14,000.; Peace Action Education Fund (Princeton, NJ)—to provide conflict resolution training to Trenton youth, $12,500.
Amount of Grant: $14,000 average; $25,000 maximum
Date(s) Application is Due: Mar 15; Sep 15
Contact: Quinn McKean, Executive Director, (732) 741-4645; fax: (732) 741-2542; email: qmckean@aol.com
Internet: http://fdncenter.org/grantmaker/borden/guide.html
Sponsor: Mary Owen Borden Foundation
4 Blackpoint Horseshoe
Rumson, NJ 07760

Mary S. and David C. Corbin Foundation Grants **2122**
The foundation gives primary consideration to the city of Akron and Summit County, OH, charitable organizations and/or local chapters of national charities located in Akron and Summit County, OH, although extremely worthy causes outside of this preferred area may be considered. Areas of interest include arts and culture, civic and community, education, health care, housing, social services, medical research, and youth. Types of support include building construction/renovation, equipment acquisition, seed grants, research, and matching funds. There are no application forms. The foundation meets at least semiannually to consider requests. Only written applications will be considered. Guidelines are available online.
Requirements: Only residents of Ohio may apply.
Restrictions: Telephone and personal interviews are discouraged unless requested by the foundation. Grants are not made to individuals.
Geographic Focus: Ohio
Samples: U of Akron (OH)—for a common area, $800,000.; Children's Hospital Medical Ctr of Akron (OH)—for burn research, $236,000.
Amount of Grant: $882,500 total

Date(s) Application is Due: Mar 1; Sep 1
Contact: Contact, (330) 762-6427; fax: (330) 762-6428; email: corbin@nls.net
Internet: http://fdncenter.org/grantmaker/corbin
Sponsor: Mary S. and David C. Corbin Foundation
159 S Main Street, Room 910
Akron, OH 44308

Mass Youth Against Tobacco Mini-Grants **2123**
The Mass Youth Against Tobacco grants program is intended to support youth-led tobacco prevention initiatives. Recently, mini-grant categories were developed through a close collaboration between youth and adults. Three categories of application are available: Youth Create Change—strengthening policies for healthier communities; Role Models, Take Action; and Taking Back Our Communities—taking on big tobacco. Between 20 and 25 projects will be funded, ranging from $8,000 to $15,000. See the web site for details.
Restrictions: Monies awarded through the grant cannot be spent on lobbying (calls for action and/or direct support of state legislation) for a specific bill or for direct attacks on the tobacco companies or their employees. Youth groups and their sponsors cannot receive funding nor have an affiliation or contractual relationship with any tobacco company, its affiliates, subsidiaries or its parent company. Funds cannot be used for cessation programs or starting new youth groups or programs.
Geographic Focus: Massachusetts
Amount of Grant: $8,000-$15,000
Date(s) Application is Due: Sep 15
Contact: Brittany Chen, Project Associate; (617) 279-2240, ext. 324 or (617) 451-0049; fax: (617) 451-0062; email: bchen@tmfnet.org
Internet: http://www.makesmokinghistory.org/myat/mini_grants.htm
Sponsor: Medical Foundation
95 Berkeley Street, Suite 208
Boston, MA 02116

Massage Therapy Foundation Community Service Grants **2124**
The Foundation Community Service grants are awarded to organizations that seek to provide massage therapy to communities or groups who currently have little or no access to such services. This program is designed to promote working partnerships between the massage therapy profession and community-based organizations. It benefits the recipient, the massage therapist, and the sponsoring organization by building stronger relationships between these parties. The Community Service deadline is April 1, annually. The normal award for 12 months is $500-$5000 and must be used in the specific time period for which it has been awarded.
Requirements: These grants are available for organizations or affiliates of organizations that have been in existence for at least one year in the respective state or province; are tax-exempt under schedule 501(c)3 in the U.S., non-profit charitable organization in other countries; currently provide some therapeutic or other service programs to the community; and have designated a qualified staff member to oversee the program.
Amount of Grant: $500-$5,000
Date(s) Application is Due: Apr 1
Contact: Alison Pittas, Manager of Research and Grants; (847) 869-5019, ext 167 or (847) 905-1667; fax: (847) 864-1178; email: apittas@massagetherapyfoundation.org
Internet: http://www.massagetherapyfoundation.org/grants_community.html
Sponsor: Massage Therapy Foundation
500 Davis Street, Suite 900
Evanston, IL 60201

Massage Therapy Foundation Practitioner Case Report Contest **2125**
The Foundation has chosen to encourage the writing of case reports to provide an opportunity for massage therapists and bodyworkers to develop research skills and enhance their ability to provide knowledge-based massage to the public. This contest is intended to enhance professional development skills of the practitioner: writing case reports help develop communication skills, critical thinking skills, and could contribute to future research and clinical practice. Cash and publication recognition will be awarded to practitioners submitting the top reports.
Requirements: The Foundation requires that HIPAA guidelines for confidentiality are followed.
Samples: Erika Larson—for Massage Therapy Effects in a Long-Time Prosthetic User with Fibular Hemimelia (2008); Glenda Keller—for The effects of massage therapy in treatment of chronic plantar fasciitis (2008); Robin B. Anderson—for Reduction and Stabilization in Parkinson-related Peripheral Edema with Therapeutic Massage (2008).
Date(s) Application is Due: Oct 8
Contact: Alison Pittas, Manager of Research and Grants; (847) 869-5019, ext 167 or (847) 905-1667; fax: (847) 864-1178; email: apittas@massagetherapyfoundation.org
Internet: http://www.massagetherapyfoundation.org/practitionercontest.html
Sponsor: Massage Therapy Foundation
500 Davis Street, Suite 900
Evanston, IL 60201

Massage Therapy Foundation Research Grants **2126**
One of the primary purposes of the Foundation is to fund solid research studies investigating the many beneficial applications of massage therapy. Foundation research grants are awarded to individuals or teams conducting studies that promise to advance our understanding of specific therapeutic applications of massage, public perceptions of and attitudes toward massage therapy, and the role of massage therapy in health care delivery. The Research Grant deadline is normally March 1 annually (or the following Monday if this falls on a weekend). The normal award for 12 months is $1,000 to $30,000, and must be used in the specific time period for which it has been awarded. This grant supports high quality, independent research that contributes to the basic science of massage therapy application, including applied research investigating massage therapy as a health/mental health treatment and/or prevention modality.
Requirements: Research Grants are available to investigators who: have experience in the relevant field of research; are presently associated with, or have secured the cooperation of a university, independent research organization, health center, or other institution qualified and willing to function as a Sponsoring Organization for the purpose of this project; or new investigators without prior research experience must document support from an experience investigator willing to act as a collaborator.
Restrictions: Research Grants will not be awarded to spouses, domestic partners, children, descendant, spouses of descendants or any other individual related to any officers or trustees of the Massage Therapy Foundation, or to members of the Research Proposal Review Committee.
Amount of Grant: $30,000 maximum
Date(s) Application is Due: Mar 1
Contact: Alison Pittas, Manager of Research and Grants; (847) 869-5019, ext 167 or (847) 905-1667; fax: (847) 864-1178; email: apittas@massagetherapyfoundation.org
Internet: http://www.massagetherapyfoundation.org/grants_research.html
Sponsor: Massage Therapy Foundation
500 Davis Street, Suite 900
Evanston, IL 60201

Massage Therapy Research Grants **2127**
This grant supports high quality, independent research that contributes to the basic science of massage therapy application, including applied research investigating massage therapy as a health/mental health treatment and/or prevention modality. Research grants are awarded to individuals or teams conducting studies that promise to advance understanding of specific therapeutic applications of massage, public perceptions of and attitudes toward massage therapy, and the role of massage therapy in health care delivery.
Requirements: The grant is available to investigators who have experience in the relevant field of research, and are presently associated with or have secured the cooperation of a university, independent research organization, or other institution qualified and willing to function as a sponsoring organization for the purpose of this project.
Samples: Steve Keir, Duke University, $20,000—for Feasibility Study of Massage Therapy within a Brain Tumor Setting (2008); Jennifer Rosen, MD, Boston Medical Center, $20,000—for Pilot RCT of Cancer Patients Undergoing Port-a-Catheter Placement (2008).
Amount of Grant: $1,000-$30,000
Date(s) Application is Due: Mar 1
Contact: Alison Pittas; (847) 869-5019, ext. 167; fax: (847) 864-1178; email: apittas@massagetherapyfoundation.org
Internet: http://www.massagetherapyfoundation.org/grants_research.html
Sponsor: Massage Therapy Foundation
500 Davis Street, Suite 900
Evanston, IL 60201

Matilda R. Wilson Fund Grants **2128**
The fund awards grants, primarily in southeast Michigan, in support of the arts, youth agencies, higher education, hospitals, and social services. Types of support include building construction/renovation, endowments, equipment acquisition, general operating support, matching/challenge grants, program development, research, and scholarship funds. There are no application forms; initial approach should be a letter of request. The board considers requests at quarterly board meetings, in January, June, September, and December.
Requirements: Michigan tax-exempt organizations are eligible.
Restrictions: Grants are not made to individuals.
Geographic Focus: Michigan
Samples: Oakland U (MI)—to repair and restore Meadow Brook Hall, the former home of the university's founder, Matilda Dodge Wilson, $7 million (2004).
Amount of Grant: $10,000-$100,000 average
Contact: David Larsen, Grants Administrator, (313) 259-7777; fax: (313) 393-7579; email: roosterveen@bodmanllp.com
Sponsor: Matilda R. Wilson Fund
100 Renaissance Center, 34th Floor
Detroit, MI 48243

Matsumae International Foundation Grants **2129**
The foundation operates worldwide in the fields of medicine/health and science/technology. Fields of study such as natural science, engineering, and medicine are given first priority. Types of support include grants, scholarships, and fellowships, tenable for three to six months. Awards include a monthly stipend; lump sum on arrival to assist with the cost of lodging, travel expense, etc.; round-trip travel; and insurance.
Requirements: Applicants must apply from outside Japan, be under the age of 40, and be postdoctoral researchers or have a minimum of two years of research experience after receipt of a master's degree. Study in the areas of natural science, engineering, and medicine receive priority.
Amount of Grant: @Y200,000 monthly stipend; @Y300,000 lump sum on arrival
Date(s) Application is Due: Jul 31

Contact: Grants Administrator, 81-3-3214-7611; fax: 81-3-3301-7601; email: contact@matsumae-if.org
Internet: http://www.mars.dti.ne.jp/~mif
Sponsor: Matsumae International Foundation
4-14-46, Kamiogi
Suginami-ku, Tokyo 167-0043 Japan

Mattel Children's Foundation Grants 2130

Charitable organizations that demonstrate that they directly serve children in need may be eligible for grants of $5,000 up to $20,000. Such organizations must have a mission that focuses on the direct service of children ages zero to 12 years. Applicants or programs must show creative and/or innovative methods to address locally defined need directly impacting children, and must be aligned with Mattel's philanthropic priorities: Learnin—increasing access to education for underserved children and in particular, innovative strategies to promote and address literacy; health—supporting the physical health and well-being of children, with particular emphasis on promoting healthy, active lifestyles; and Girl Empowerment—promoting self-esteem in young girls, up to age 12. Organizations may submit under a fiscal agent as long as the program has been in existence for at least two years.
Requirements: Applicants must be a 501(c)3 Public Charity organizations. If an organization is a project under a fiscal sponsor, that sponsor must have a valid tax exemption status. Organizations must serve children in communities within the U.S. Organizations must not discriminate against a person or a group on the basis of age, political affiliation, race, national origin, ethnicity, gender, disability, sexual orientation or religious beliefs. Organizations must have an annual operating budget of less than $1,000,000.
Restrictions: Organizations may not be affiliated in any way with national organizations, regardless of whether funds are received from the national entity. Examples of organizations that are ineligible to apply include Boys & Girls Clubs, United Ways, YMCA's, and disease-affiliated organizations such as the American Heart Association.
Amount of Grant: $5,000-$20,000
Contact: Grants Administrator, (310) 252-2000; fax: (310) 252-2180; email: foundation@mattel.com
Internet: http://corporate.mattel.com/about-us/philanthropy/programs.aspx
Sponsor: Mattel Children's Foundation
333 Continental Boulevard, M1-1418
El Segundo, CA 90245-5012

Mattel International Grants Program 2131

The corporation and its foundation award grants to charitable organizations that directly serve children in need. Funding priorities include international organizations or programs that creatively address a defined need directly impacting children in need, and international organizations or programs that align with Mattel's philanthropic priorities, including health—supporting the physical and mental health and well-being of children, and increasing access to health care services for children in need; education—increasing access to education, promoting literacy to children in need, and resources that promote after-school educational achievement; and girls empowerment—promoting self-esteem of girls and increasing access to education, health, and community resources for girls. Types of support include program-specific grants—funding for new programs or expansion of existing programs; and core operating support—support of organizations to sustain their programs. Applications must be submitted online. Applications will not be accepted by fax or mail. Submit questions via email.
Requirements: Organizations must serve children in non-U.S. communities; and must not discriminate against a person or a group on the basis of age, political affiliation, race, national origin, ethnicity, gender, disability, sexual orientation, or religious belief. Pilot projects and new organizations may be considered as long as all eligibility criteria are met; however, preference will be given to organizations that have at least two years of experience. Preference is given to organizations that have an annual operating budget of less than $1 million and are not affiliated with a national organization.
Restrictions: The program does not not fund capital funding for physical property purchase, renovation, or developments; individuals; political parties, candidates, or partisan political organizations; labor organizations, fraternal organizations, athletic clubs, or social clubs; sectarian or denominational religious organizations, except for programs that are available to anyone, broadly promoted, and free from religious orientation; schools and school districts; fundraising events (e.g., dinners, tournaments); advertising or marketing sponsorships; or research overhead and/or indirect costs (including fiscal sponsor fees) that exceed 15 percent of the direct project costs.
Amount of Grant: $5000-$25,000 typically
Contact: Grants Administrator, (310) 252-2000; fax: (310) 252-2180; email: foundation@mattel.com
Internet: http://corporate.mattel.com/about-us/philanthropy/internationalgrants.aspx
Sponsor: Mattel Children's Foundation
333 Continental Boulevard, M1-1418
El Segundo, CA 90245-5012

Max A. Adler Charitable Foundation Grants 2132

The foundation awards grants to eligible New York nonprofit organizations serving the greater Rochester area in its areas of interest, including arts, children and youth services, Jewish services, health care, higher education, and social services. Types of support include building construction/renovation, capital campaigns, general operating support, and program development. There are no application forms or deadlines.
Requirements: New York 501(c)3 nonprofit organizations serving the greater Rochester area are eligible.
Geographic Focus: New York
Samples: Nazareth College (Rochester, NY)—for its capital campaign to expand the size of its campus, $50,000 (2003).
Amount of Grant: $1000-$25,000 average
Contact: David Gray, President, (585) 232-7290; fax: (585) 232-7260
Sponsor: Max A. Adler Charitable Foundation
1010 Times Sq Building
Rochester, NY 14614

Max and Victoria Dreyfus Foundation Grants 2133

The Foundation awards grants for: museums; cultural, performing, and visual arts programs, schools; hospitals, educational and skills training projects and programs for youth, seniors, and the disabled. Areas of interest include arts, education, health care, hospitals, social services, and medical research. Submit an inquiry letter (three-page maximum) that describes the nonprofit organization, its annual operating budget, the project to be funded, and the project budget; include proof of tax-exempt status.
Requirements: U.S. nonprofit organizations are eligible.
Restrictions: Foreign charitable organizations and individuals are ineligible.
Amount of Grant: $5,000-$20,000 average
Date(s) Application is Due: Mar 10; Jul 10; Nov 10
Contact: John W. Hager; (202) 337-3300; fax: (202) 337-4925
Sponsor: Max and Victoria Dreyfus Foundation
2233 Wisconsin Avenue, NW, Suite 414
Washington, DC 20007-4122

Max Bell Foundation Grants 2134

The foundation focuses its grant making on innovative projects having substantial impact within the areas of health, Canada and the Asian Pacific, and veterinary sciences and education. Under health care, the foundation directs its support to the areas of health education and preventive health care. It is also interested in assisting health care professionals to update their education on a continuing basis. The foundation also supports research intended to build a better understanding of the Asian Pacific area on the part of Canadian policymakers and businesspeople and assists Canadian scholars to build ties to their Asian counterparts. Also funded are major programs at centers of Asian research in Canadian universities. Within the field of veterinary sciences and education, the foundation seeks to provide broad-based support, although it has developed a particular interest in equine research. Applications are reviewed three times annually, eight weeks before the board meets (usually in May September, and November).
Requirements: Funding is restricted to registered Canadian charities. Applicants should submit a brief letter describing the project for which they are seeking funds, an estimated budget, and the organization's charitable gift registration number. If the letter proves of interest to the foundation, a more detailed proposal will be invited.
Restrictions: Support will not be provided for capital projects or building campaigns; continuing operating expenses, funds to cover budget deficits, general fund-raising drives, or annual charitable appeals; academic or sabbatical leaves, internships, bursaries or scholarships; conferences, seminars or workshops, equipment purchases, publication costs, or travel costs.
Samples: AboutFace (Toronto, Ontario)—to provide support to children with facial disfigurements and their families, $C100,000.; U of Toronto (Toronto, Ontario)—to develop a summer study program on the campus of the U of Hong Kong, $C105,000.; U of Guelph (Guelph, Ontario)—to explore the biological and physical attributes of the Great Lakes and consider the continuing impact of humans upon them, $C205,000.
Amount of Grant: $C20,000-$C25,000 average
Contact: Alida White, Administrator, (403) 215-7310; fax: (403) 215-7319; email: apply@maxbell.org
Internet: http://www.maxbell.org
Sponsor: Max Bell Foundation
639 Fifth Ave SW, Suite 1230
Calgary, AB T2P OM9 Canada

Maxon Charitable Foundation Grants 2135

The Maxon Charitable Foundation is a company-sponsored foundation that was established in 1987 in Indiana. The foundation supports hospitals and organizations involved with higher education, natural resources, recreation, human services, community development, and Christianity and awards college scholarships to individuals in the Muncie, Indiana area.
Requirements: Contact the Foundation's office prior to the initial proposal, the office will provide you with the proper Application form.
Geographic Focus: Indiana
Amount of Grant: $500 - $5,000 range
Contact: Jeffrey R. Lang, Secretary; (765) 284-3304;
Sponsor: Maxon Charitable Foundation, Inc.
201 East 18th Street
Muncie, IN 47302-4124

Maxtor Corporate Contributions Grants 2136

Maxtor supports charitable, nonprofit organizations whose programs improve the quality of life through education, health and human services, community services, and cultural endeavors. This program is designed to help eligible organizations in northern California, Massachusetts, and Colorado. Types of support include cash grants, Maxtor products, community service projects, and used equipment or in-kind services.

Requirements: 501(c)3 nonprofits serving northern California, Massachusetts, and Colorado are eligible.
Restrictions: Maxtor does not provide support to organizations without 501(c)3 status; individuals in personal programs; religious activities; school activities such as sporting events, bands, etc.; individual scholarships; team, groups, races, or -athons; travel expenses; or political activities.
Geographic Focus: California; Colorado; Massachusetts
Contact: Program Contact, (408) 894-5000; email: PR@Maxtor.com
Internet: http://www.maxtor.com/en/about/corporate/contributions.htm
Sponsor: Maxtor Corporation
500 McCarthy Boulevard
Milpitas, CA 95035

May and Stanley Smith Trust Grants 2137
The trust awards grants to nonprofit organizations in its areas of interest, including children and youth, people with disabilities, the economically disadvantaged, education, the elderly, social services, and the visually impaired. Types of support include general operating grants and scholarship funds. Grants are awarded primarily in North America, with emphasis on the San Francisco Bay area, and Canada. Applications are accepted from January 1 through the listed deadline date; grants are considered beginning in April.
Restrictions: Grants are not made to individuals.
Amount of Grant: $500-$6000 average
Date(s) Application is Due: Sep 30
Contact: Dale Matheny, (415) 391-0292
Sponsor: May and Stanley Smith Trust
720 Market Street, Suite 250
San Francisco, CA 94102

May Department Stores Charitable Contribution Grants 2138
The company has a long-standing commitment to responsible citizenship and to supporting its operating communities. The foundation contributes to worthy organizations that strive to improve the quality of life for customers, associates, and neighbors. Charitable contributions are concentrated in four areas: health and welfare, including the United Way; education; culture and the arts; and civic causes.
Requirements: Nonprofit organizations in May operating areas are eligible.
Samples: Cathedral of San Fernando (San Antonio, TX)—$10,000 (2004); Jazz at Lincoln Ctr (New York, NY)—$5000 (2004); Legacy Health System (Portland, OR)—$13,700 (2004); Crossroads School (Saint Louis, MO)—$5300 (2004).
Amount of Grant: $15.8 million total
Contact: Deidre Burke, Corporate Communications, (314) 342-6299; fax (314) 342-4461; email: mayfoundation@may-co.com
Internet: http://www2.mayco.com/common/com_index.jsp
Sponsor: May Department Stores Company Foundation
611 Olive Street
Saint Louis, MO 63101

Mayday Fund Grants 2139
The mission of the fund involves one purpose: the reduction of the physical and psychological toll of pain and its consequences. The fund particularly invites projects that will improve public policy to make it more hospitable to the better treatment of pain and that involve multidisciplinary teams including physicians, nurses, pharmacists, and administrators working to introduce routine assessment, documentation, and treatment of pain in hospital settings. Mayday also continues to have special interest in projects that relieve children's pain, involve primary care, and improve the treatment of pain in home care or other settings where a person is in pain after being discharged from a medical institution. There are no deadlines.
Requirements: Grants are made only to public charity organizations, officially recognized as such by the IRS.
Restrictions: Grants generally will not be made for endowments, capital projects, equipment, general operating expenses, ongoing activities, annual fund-raising drives, or in support of international or non-U.S. activities and institutions. Grants are not made to individuals.
Samples: U of Rochester Medical School (Rochester, NY)—to enhance pediatric anesthesiology services, $27,564.; Triumph Over Pain Foundation (Chicago, IL)—for start-up and operating expenses, $10,000.; Saint Mary's Hospital for Children (Bayside, NY)—to develop a pain-management program for children with special health care needs, $150,000.
Amount of Grant: $30,000-$50,000 average
Contact: Christina Spellman, Executive Director, (212) 649-5800; fax: (212) 649-5801; email: inquiry@maydayfund.org
Internet: http://www.painandhealth.org/mayday/mayday-home.html
Sponsor: Mayday Fund
136 W 21st Street, 6th Floor
New York, NY 10011

Mayo Foundation Multidisciplinary Training in Digestive Diseases Research Grants 2140
Postdoctoral fellowships in gastroenterological research are available for two or more years. Faculty members employ a multidisciplinary approach using biochemical, cell/molecular biological, immunological, physiological, and electrophysiological techniques. Applicants may focus on clinical and/or basic studies. A curriculum vita and the names of three references should be submitted to the program director.
Requirements: Applicant should have an MD or PhD degree and must be a U.S. citizen or have permanent visa status.
Contact: Dr. N.F. LaRusso, Program Director, (507) 284-1000
Internet: http://mayoresearch.mayo.edu/mayo/research/traininggrants
Sponsor: Mayo Foundation
200 First St SW
Rochester, MN 55905

McCarthy Family Foundation Grants 2141
The foundation is currently considering grants in four major areas: K-12 science education—to foster increased study of science and to promote further scientific study and careers by qualified students; HIV/AIDS—research (to determine the pathogenesis of HIV and AIDS and related diseases, and to develop new experimental therapies), and education and support (to provide support to HIV-positive individuals and public education regarding the disease); assistance to homeless people—to help with basic needs and support to improve opportunity for independence, health, and self-esteem (including youth and adult education); and child abuse prevention—for child abuse prevention programs and to provide necessary services for victims of child abuse and their families.
Requirements: Proposals will only be accepted for programs within San Diego County.
Restrictions: The foundation does not consider grants for individuals, scholarship funds, or sectarian religious activities. Normally the foundation does not consider requests for general fundraising drives. It does not make grants intended directly or indirectly to support political candidates or to influence legislation.
Geographic Focus: California
Samples: Shelter Partnership (Los Angeles, CA)—for a resource bank, $5000.; KPBS-TV (San Diego, CA)—for the San Diego Night Sky documentary, $25,000.
Amount of Grant: $5000-$15,000 generally
Date(s) Application is Due: Mar 15; Sep 15
Contact: Program Contact, fax: (858) 485-0172; email: mail@mccarthyfamilyfdn.org
Internet: http://www.mccarthyfamilyfdn.org
Sponsor: McCarthy Family Foundation
P.O. Box 27389
San Diego, CA 92198-1389

McCombs Foundation Grants 2142
The foundation makes grants to Texas nonprofit charitable, philanthropic, educational, and benevolent organizations. Areas of interest include arts, education and higher education, historic preservation, medical research, philanthropy, recreation and sports, youth services, and voluntarism. There are no application deadlines or forms.
Requirements: Texas nonprofit organizations are eligible.
Geographic Focus: Texas
Contact: Grants Administrator, (210) 821-6523
Internet: http://www.redmccombs.net/philanthropy.html
Sponsor: McCombs Foundation
755 E Mulberry, Suite 600
San Antonio, TX 78212

McGregor Fund Grants 2143
The fund makes grants to organizations in the following areas: human services—emphasis on activities in southeastern Michigan addressing emergency needs in housing, food, clothing, and other direct aid; education—early child education and development, colleges and universities in the Detroit metropolitan area, liberal arts colleges and universities in Michigan and Ohio; arts and culture in southeastern Michigan; health care—improving access to primary care for underserved populations in Detroit; and public benefit—civic and community organizations that improve the quality of life in southeastern Michigan. Types of support include project support, operating support, special projects, and capital support. Grant decisions are made by the board of trustees four times annually, in February, May, September, and November. Grant requests may be submitted at any time, but requests may take up to three months for staff review. Application guidelines are available online.
Requirements: Organizations in the metropolitan Detroit, MI area, are eligible. Requests will be considered from organizations located elsewhere for programs or projects that significantly benefit the metropolitan Detroit area (city of Detroit and Wayne, Oakland, and Macomb Counties).
Restrictions: The fund discourages proposals for student scholarships, travel, seminars, conferences, workshops, film or video projects, as well as disease-specific organizations and their local affiliates.
Geographic Focus: Michigan
Amount of Grant: $25,000-$50,000 average
Contact: C. David Campbell, President, (313) 963-3495; fax: (313) 963-3512; email: info@mcgregfund.org
Internet: http://www.mcgregorfund.org/guideline.html
Sponsor: McGregor Fund
333 W Fort Street, Suite 2090
Detroit, MI 48226

McInerny Foundation Grants 2144
The foundation awards grants to Hawaii nonprofit organizations in its areas of interest, including arts and culture, education, environment, health care, youth services, and social services. Types of support include general operating support, continuing support, building construction/renovation, equipment acquisition, program development, seed money, scholarship funds, and matching funds. The July 1 deadline is for capital funds;

the November 15 deadline date is for scholarship funds. All other requests are accepted at any time.
Requirements: Hawaii nonprofit organizations are eligible.
Restrictions: Grants are not awarded in support of religious institutions, individuals, endowment funds, deficit financing, or research.
Geographic Focus: Hawaii
Samples: National Tropical Botanical Garden, Kalaheo, HI, $75,000—capital campaign for construction of Botanical Garden Research Center (2007); Boys and Girls Club of Hawaii, Honolulu, HI, $50,000—for RALLY Project at Central Middle School (2007); Honolulu Symphony Society, Honolulu, HI, $40,000-for youth music education program season (2007).
Amount of Grant: $3,000-$250,000 range
Date(s) Application is Due: Jul 1; Nov 15
Contact: Paula Boyce, c/o Bank of Hawaii, (808) 538-4944; fax: (808) 538-4006; email: pboyce@boh.com
Sponsor: McInerny Foundation
P.O. Box 3170 - Dept. 758
Honolulu, HI 96802-3170

McKesson Foundation Grants **2145**

The foundation seeks to enhance the health and quality of life in communities where McKesson HBOC operates and its employees live. Emphasis is focused on youth, especially health services for underserved populations, educational enrichment, the environment, recreation, and youth development activities. The foundation also funds emergency services for children and families, and a variety of social, educational and cultural programs. For culture and the arts, support is given primarily to organizations that reach out to youth and other populations that do not have easy access to such programs. Grants are made for specific projects and programs, and general operating support will be considered in some circumstances. Grants are awarded for one to three years. The Foundation does not accept uninvited applications. Initial approach should be to contact the Foundation directly.
Requirements: 501(c)3 tax-exempt organizations are eligible.
Restrictions: Grants are not made to endowment campaigns, individuals or individual scholarships, religious organizations for religious purposes, political causes or campaigns, advertising in charitable publications, research studies or health organizations concentrating on one disease.
Samples: LA Theater Work (CA)—for a project that creates hands-on performing arts and literary workshops aimed at finding a positive outlet for the aggression of 3000 at-risk and incarcerated youths, $7500.; Massachusetts Coalition for School-Based Health Ctrs (MA)—to hire a coordinator and to continue providing school-based health care, $125,000 over three years.
Amount of Grant: $5,000-$25,000 typically
Contact: Marcia Argyris, Foundation President; (415) 983-8673 or (415) 983-8300; fax: (415) 983-7590; email: marcia.argyris@mckesson.com or community.relations@mckesson.com
Internet: http://www.mckesson.com/en_us/McKesson.com/About%2BUs/Corporate%2BCitizenship/McKesson%2BFoundation.html
Sponsor: McKesson Foundation
1 Post Street, 32nd Floor
San Francisco, CA 94104-5203

McKnight Foundation Grants **2146**

The foundation awards grants to eligible nonprofit organizations in support of efforts to strengthen communities, families, and individuals, particularly those in need. Grants contribute to the arts, encourage preservation of the natural environment, and promote research in selected fields. Types of support include planning, project, and operating support. Application deadlines are for letters of inquiry; full proposals are by invitation.
Requirements: Eligible applicants must be tax-exempt, nonprofit organizations in Minnesota that are not private foundations.
Restrictions: Examples of areas not supported by grants include mental health or disabilities, except for services to enhance parents' capacity to nurture their children; chemical dependency treatment; services for seniors; and health. In addition to these program areas, grants do not support scholarships or other types of assistance for individuals; attendance at or travel to conferences or costs related to conferences; travel, except when related to other McKnight support of an organization; scientific research outside established McKnight research programs; endowments, except in rare cases; or activities that have a specific religious purpose.
Samples: Greater Metropolitan Housing Corp of the Twin Cities (Minneapolis, MN)—for general operating support, $400,000 over two years (2005); Loft (Minneapolis, MN)—for a literary-arts center, and for a national magazine for readers and writers, $160,000 (2005); Resource Inc (Minneapolis, MN)—for a program that trains and supports low-income mothers to help them advance in their jobs, $200,000 (2005); Midwest Environmental Advocates (Madison, WI)—for a campaign to implement and enforce the Clean Water Act, $80,000 (2005).
Amount of Grant: $23 million total annually; $5000-$500,000 typically
Date(s) Application is Due: Jan 15; Apr 15; Jul 15; Oct 15
Contact: Stephanie Duffy, Grants Administration Manager, (612) 333-4220; fax: (612) 332-3833; email: info@mcknight.org
Internet: http://www.mcknight.org
Sponsor: McKnight Foundation
710 S Second Street, Suite 400
Minneapolis, MN 55401

McLean Contributionship Grants **2147**

The program awards grants primarily in Pennsylvania in its areas of interest, including aging, children and youth, education, environment, health care, historic preservation, hospitals, libraries, medical research, museums, nursing homes, performing arts, and youth services. Types of support include building construction/renovation, capital campaigns, conferences and seminars, endowments, equipment, internships, program development, publication, scholarship funds, and seed grants. Applicants can apply using the Delaware Valley Grantmakers Common Grant Application. The board meets quarterly to review requests.
Restrictions: The contributionship does not fund the costs or expenses of existing staff allocated to a project it is asked to support.
Samples: Wistar Institute of Anatomy and Biology (Philadelphia, PA)—to purchase a new tissue processor, $28,000.; Lankenau Hospital Foundation (Wynnewood, PA)—for renovation of the emergency room, $100,000.
Amount of Grant: $2000-$100,000
Contact: Sandra McLean, Executive Director, (610) 527-6330; fax: (610) 527-9733
Internet: http://fdncenter.org/grantmaker/mclean
Sponsor: McLean Contributionship
945 Haverford Road, Suite A
Bryn Mawr, PA 19010-3814

McMillen Foundation Grants **2148**

The McMillen Foundation was incorporated in 1947 and serves the Fort Wayne and Allen Counties of Indiana. Fields of interest include: children/youth services; community/economic development; education; health care; health organizations, association; recreation.
Requirements: The foundation requires no application form and proposals may be submitted at anytime. Applicants should submit the following: copy of IRS Determination Letter; brief history of organization and description of its mission; copy of most recent annual report/audited financial statement/990; listing of board of directors, trustees, officers and other key people and their affiliations; detailed description of project and amount of funding requested; copy of current year's organizational budget and/or project budget; listing of additional sources and amount of support; one copy of the proposal.
Restrictions: Giving limited to Fort Wayne and Allen County, Indiana. No support for churches or religious groups. No grants to individuals.
Geographic Focus: Indiana
Samples: Girl Scouts of the U.S.A., Fort Wayne, IN, $300,000 (2006); Junior Achievement of Northern Indiana, Fort Wayne, IN, $50,000 (2006); Fort Wayne Park Foundation, Fort Wayne, IN, $100,000 (2006).
Amount of Grant: $4,000 - $400,000 range
Contact: Dorothy J. Robinson, Secretary; (260) 484-8631; fax: (260) 484-2141;
Sponsor: McMillen Foundation , Inc.
6610 Mutual Drive
Fort Wayne, IN 46825-4236

McMurry Foundation Grants **2149**

The foundation was established to have a significant and beneficial impact on the communities within Wyoming with special emphasis in Natrona County. Areas of interest include education, religion, children and advocacy for children, health and human services, the arts and humanities, and a favorable business environment. The foundation invests in innovative ventures as well as established community programs that have the potential to make a lasting difference. Funds provide seed money to start new programs; general funds to expand or improve services offered by established agencies; and organizational support, such as strategic planning, increasing management capacity, and board development. Priority will be given to promote strengthening the capacity of nonprofit organizations to do their work, leveraging the dollars of the McMurry Foundation, collaboration and efficient use of nonprofit resources, and addressing the causes or prevention of community problems.
Requirements: Wyoming 501(c)3 nonprofit organizations and organizations who have applied and anticipate receiving such status are eligible.
Restrictions: Grants designated to influence legislation or elect public officials are rejected.
Samples: U of Wyoming (Laramie, WY)—to help renovate the College of Education facility, $250,000 (2005).
Date(s) Application is Due: Jan 15; Apr 15; Jul 15; Oct 15
Contact: Trudi McMurry, Director, fax: (307) 234-4631; email: trudie@mcmurry.net
Internet: https://online.foundationsource.com/public/home/mcmurryfoundation
Sponsor: McMurry Foundation
P.O. Box 2016
Casper, WY 82602-2016

MDA Development Grant **2150**

The association will consider an application for a research grant from a candidate who may be a member of a research team in the laboratory of a senior investigator under whose guidance the applicant will be given flexibility to conduct a neuromuscular disease research project. Awards are for one to three years. Applications must be requested by the listed application deadlines. Guidelines are available online.
Requirements: An applicant must hold a Doctor of Medicine, Doctor of Philosophy, Doctor of Science or equivalent degree; be a professional member at an appropriate institution; be qualified to conduct a program of original research; have an acceptable research plan for a specific disease in MDA's program; have access to institutional resources necessary to conduct the proposed research project; and have eighteen months of postdoctoral research laboratory training at the time of application.

Amount of Grant: $45,000 maximum per year
Date(s) Application is Due: Jun 15; Dec 15
Contact: Grants Program Manager, (520) 529-2000; fax: (520) 529-5454; email: grants@mdausa.org
Internet: http://www.mdausa.org/research/guidelines.html#developmentGrant
Sponsor: Muscular Dystrophy Association
3300 E Sunrise Drive
Tucson, AZ 85718

MDA Neuromuscular Disease Research Grants **2151**
The association supports research into 40 diseases of the neuromuscular system to identify the causes of and effective treatments for the muscular dystrophies and related diseases, which include spinal muscular atrophies and motor neuron diseases, peripheral neuropathies, inflammatory myopathies, metabolic myopathies, and diseases of the neuromuscular junction. Awards cover periods of up to three years. The listed deadlines are for requesting applications.
Requirements: Applicants must be professionals or faculty members at appropriate educational, medical, or research institutions and qualified to conduct and supervise programs of original research; must have access to institutional resources necessary to conduct the proposed research project; and must have the MD, PhD, DSc, or equivalent degree. Preliminary letter requesting an application is required and must include name and address of institution(s) where the research is to be conducted, the specific aim of the proposed research, statement of relevance to the purposes of MDA, and a statement on whether human subjects or tissues will be used.
Samples: Dr. J. Edwin Blalock, U of Alabama (Birmingham, AL)—for research on diagnosis and immunotherapy of myasthenia gravis, $100,000 over two years.; Dr. Terrone Rosenberry, Case Western Reserve U (Cleveland, OH)—for research on catalytic sites and subunity assembly of acetylcholinesterase, $51,500.
Date(s) Application is Due: Jun 15; Dec 15
Contact: Grants Manager, (520) 529-2000; fax: (520) 529-5454; email: grants@mdausa.org
Internet: http://www.mdausa.org/research/guidelines.html
Sponsor: Muscular Dystrophy Association
3300 E Sunrise Drive
Tucson, AZ 85718

MDBD Basic Research Grants **2152**
Grants are awarded to qualified U.S. institutions to support medical and scientific research in the field of birth defects. Research supported by the foundation on the etiology of birth defects takes three main directions. The first supports investigation of the hereditary influences of birth defects. Requests may be to investigate the structure and function of chromosomes, their subunits, genes, and their supporting substructures. The second investigates environmental effects ranging from obvious factors such as drugs, radiation, infections, and malnutrition to more subtle influences such as cytoplasmic influences. The third is the interaction between heredity and environment such as enzymatic feedback and an individual's resistance to disease. Applications will be sent to those whose abstracts are considered relevant to this program. Abstracts must be received with a postmark on or before the listed application deadline date.
Requirements: A request for a new grant should be initiated by a 300-word abstract to the director of grants administration from the principal investigator of the proposed research program. This letter of inquiry, containing a brief protocol of the study, must be submitted before an application form will be provided. Letters of intent may be submitted online at http://researchgrants.modimes.org/LOI.
Samples: Dr. Mary Porter, U of Minnesota (Minneapolis, MN)—for the research study Molecular and Genetic Analyses of the Mechanisms of Flagellar Motility, $37,001.; Dr. John Tamkun, U of California (Santa Cruz, CA)—for the research study Regulators of Homeotic Gene Expression in Drosophilia, $52,242.
Amount of Grant: $25,000 average
Date(s) Application is Due: Apr 30
Contact: Vice President for Research, (914) 997-4555; fax: (914) 997-4560; email: researchgrants@marchofdimes.com
Internet: http://www.marchofdimes.com/professionals/685_2160.asp
Sponsor: March of Dimes Birth Defects Foundation
1275 Mamaroneck Avenue
White Plains, NY 10605

MDBD Research Grants and Basil O'Connor Starter Scholar Award Program **2153**
The program is designed for young scientists at the level of instructor or assistant professor who are embarking on their independent research careers. Both awards support research on birth defects. Grants do not include the recipients' salaries, but provide support for technical help and supplies. Programs may be approved for two years only. Each potential applicant must submit a letter of nomination written by the chair of the department, director of the institute, dean, or other senior person; brief abstract of the proposed research; and curriculum vita. Candidates meeting the criteria of the program will receive application forms. Annual deadline dates may vary; contact program staff for exact dates.
Restrictions: Applicants may not submit simultaneously any other applications for March of Dimes research programs.
Samples: Dr. Anne Calof, U of Iowa (Iowa City, IA)—for the research study Strategies for Identifying Genes that Regulate Neurogenesis in Mammals, $30,000.; Dr. Piero Rinaldo, Yale U (New Haven, CT)—for research on sudden infant death syndrome, $10,000.
Amount of Grant: $75,000 maximum
Date(s) Application is Due: Mar 19
Contact: Grants Administrator, (914) 997-4564 or (888) 663-4637; fax: (914) 997-4560; email: researchgrants@marchofdimes.com
Internet: http://www.marchofdimes.com/professionals/691_1452.asp
Sponsor: March of Dimes Birth Defects Foundation
1275 Mamaroneck Avenue
White Plains, NY 10605

MDBD Research Prize in Developmental Biology **2154**
The prize is awarded to investigators whose research has profoundly advanced the science that underlines understanding of birth defects. Nomination form and guidelines are available online.
Amount of Grant: $250,000
Date(s) Application is Due: Sep 15
Contact: Dr. Michael Katz, (914) 997-4555 or (888) 663-4637; fax: (914) 997-4560; email: mkatz@marchofdimes.com
Internet: http://www.marchofdimes.com/professionals/691_1442.asp
Sponsor: March of Dimes Birth Defects Foundation
1275 Mamaroneck Avenue
White Plains, NY 10605

MDBDF Agnes Higgins Award **2155**
The award recognizes distinguished achievement in research, education, or clinical services in the field of maternal-fetal nutrition. In addition to an honorarium, winners are honored at a presentation and reception at the American Public Health Association Annual Meeting in the year of their award. The award is made every two years. Nominations are invited in even-numbered years.
Requirements: Candidates have been widely involved in maternal-fetal nutrition through teaching, research, or clinical practice for at least five years; shown a demonstrable effect in raising the quality of maternal-fetal nutritional care through scholarly pursuits, research, education, or practice; and demonstrated the ability to apply maternal-fetal nutritional standards of practice or facilitate their implementation by others.
Amount of Grant: $3000
Date(s) Application is Due: Mar 1
Contact: Grants Administrator, (914) 997-4564 or (888) 663-4637; fax: (914) 997-4560; email: ResearchGrants@modimes.org
Internet: http://www.marchofdimes.com/professionals/685_1370.asp
Sponsor: March of Dimes Birth Defects Foundation
1275 Mamaroneck Avenue
White Plains, NY 10605

Mead Johnson Nutritionals Charitable Giving Grants **2156**
Mead Johnson Nutritionals considers requests for charitable giving from a broad range of charitable organizations. Requests for charitable giving must be made in connection with a general fund raising effort by the charitable entity, rather than a request directed only to Mead Johnson Nutritionals. In addition, the request for a contribution must come from the organization itself and not from an individual physician, pharmacist, or health care professional who is not an employee of the charity. Applicants should allow at least three months for the processing of a funding request. Grant applications submitted less than three months prior to an event may be rejected due to insufficient time to process the application. Organizations outside the U.S. that wish to request a charitable gift should refer to Mead Johnson contact information within their country or call the charitable giving department at (812) 429-7800.
Requirements: Charitable giving is permitted if the recipient is a tax-exempt organization under Section 501(c)3 of the Internal Revenue Code.
Restrictions: As with grants, charitable giving may not be tied, in any way, to past, present, or future prescribing, purchasing, or recommending (including formulary recommendations) of any product.
Contact: Grants Administrator, (812) 429-7831; fax: (812) 647-8674; email: meadjohnson.grants1@bms.com
Internet: http://www.mjn.com/app/iwp/MJN/Content2.do?dm=mj&id=/MJN_Home2/mjnBtnSocialResponsibility2/mjnBtnCharitableGivingApplication&iwpst=B2C&ls=0&csred=1&r=3435833953
Sponsor: Mead Johnson Nutritionals
2400 West Lloyd Expressway
Evansville, IN 47721-0001

Mead Johnson Nutritionals Evansville-Area Organizations Grants **2157**
Evansville area non-profit organizations of all varieties may submit charitable giving applications throughout the year. However, if a request exceeds $1,000 it is highly recommended that the applicant submit an application between June 1 and August 31 in the year prior to when the funds are needed. Requests greater than $1,000 are generally reviewed as a group, one time a year. If approved, funding will be awarded in the following year. Requests greater than $1,000 received after August 31 might not be considered and the applicant might be asked to reapply the following year.
Requirements: Evansville area 501(c)3 designated organizations are eligible to apply.
Geographic Focus: Indiana
Date(s) Application is Due: Aug 31
Contact: Grants Administrator, (812) 429-7831; fax: (812) 647-8674; email: meadjohnson.grants1@bms.com
Internet: http://www.mjn.com/app/iwp/MJN/Content2.do?dm=mj&id=/MJN_Home2/mjnBtnSocialResponsibility2/mjnBtnCharitableGivingApplication&iwpst=B2C&ls=0&csred=1&r=3435833953#app

Sponsor: Mead Johnson Nutritionals
2400 West Lloyd Expressway
Evansville, IN 47721-0001

Mead Johnson Nutritionals Medical Education Grants 2158

Mead Johnson Nutritionals has established a Grant program to support medical education and philanthropic initiatives. The program will consider supporting Independent Medical Education (IME) programs and activities designed to enhance the professional skills and knowledge of health care professionals involved in pediatrics, when the program is independently developed and conducted by a qualified medical education provider. Supported programs must be objective, balanced, and scientifically rigorous. Health care provider educational programming can be given for: medical education programs; scientific conferences; creation of health care publications; and other educational and scientific activities. In addition to the U.S. Medical Education Grants, Mead Johnson also funds International Medical Education Grants. Organizations outside the U.S. that wish to request an Independent Medical Education (IME) grant should refer to Mead Johnson contact information within their country or contact Mead Johnson at meadjohnson.grants1@bms.com.
Requirements: Eligible recipients for medical education grants include: academic medical centers; accredited medical education companies; community health centers; hospitals; managed care organizations; medical/professional societies; medical universities; patient advocacy groups; pharmacies; and similar entities.
Restrictions: Grants may not be tied, in any way, to past, present, or future prescribing, purchasing, or recommending (including formulary recommendations) of any product.
Contact: Grants Administrator, (812) 429-7831; fax: (812) 647-8674; email: meadjohnson.grants1@bms.com
Internet: http://www.mjn.com/app/iwp/MJN/Content2.do?dm=mj&id=/MJN_Home2/mjnBtnSocialResponsibility2/mjnBtnMedicalEducationApplications&iwpst=B2C&ls=0&csred=1&r=3435836001
Sponsor: Mead Johnson Nutritionals
2400 West Lloyd Expressway
Evansville, IN 47721-0001

Mead Johnson Nutritionals Scholarships 2159

Mead Johnson Nutritionals provides scholarship grants to medical students, residents, fellows, and other healthcare professionals in training to attend classes and major educational or scientific meetings of a national medical or professional association. The selection of the individuals to receive such support and the grant application must be made by the institution at which they are being trained or the organization hosting the event. Allow at least three months for the processing of your funding application. Independent Medical Education (IME) grant applications submitted less than three months prior to an event may be rejected, due to insufficient time to process the application.
Requirements: Eligible recipients for such grants: academic medical centers; hospitals; medical/professional societies; and medical universities.
Contact: Grants Administrator, (812) 429-7831; fax: (812) 647-8674; email: meadjohnson.grants1@bms.com
Internet: http://www.mjn.com/app/iwp/MJN/Content2.do?dm=mj&id=/MJN_Home2/mjnBtnSocialResponsibility2/mjnBtnMedicalEducationApplications/MedScholarships&iwpst=B2C&ls=0&csred=1&r=3435836794
Sponsor: Mead Johnson Nutritionals
2400 West Lloyd Expressway
Evansville, IN 47721-0001

Mead Witter Foundation Grants 2160

The foundation awards grants to nonprofits in company operating locations, primarily in central and northern Wisconsin. Local community programs are funded, focusing on education, including scholarships in higher education and direct contributions to colleges and universities. Grants also are made to support the arts, health care, human services, youth organizations, environmental programs, and Christian and Roman Catholic organizations for nonreligious purposes. Types of support include general operating support, continuing support, annual campaigns, capital campaigns, building construction/renovation, equipment acquisition, endowment funds, professorships, seed grants, scholarship funds, and employee-matching gifts. The board meets twice annually to consider requests. Full proposal is by invitation only.
Requirements: Wisconsin 501(c)3 organizations may apply.
Restrictions: The foundation does not support religious, athletic, or fraternal groups, except when these groups provide needed special services to the community at large; direct grants or scholarships to individuals; community foundations; or flow-through organizations that redispense funds to other charitable causes.
Geographic Focus: Wisconsin
Amount of Grant: $25,000-$1.8 million range
Contact: Susan Feith, President, (715) 424-3004; fax: (715) 424-1314
Sponsor: Mead Witter Foundation, Inc.
P.O. Box 39
Wisconsin Rapids, WI 54495-0039

Meadows Foundation Grants 2161

Grants are made in five areas of interest: arts and culture, human services, health, education, and civic and public affairs. The foundation looks for innovative, well-planned projects that promote better human relationships and a sense of community. Projects should show the ability to continue and expand after the grant period. Funds support programs, projects, capital projects, general operations, seed grants, equipment acquisition, matching funds, scholarship funds, professorships, internships, fellowships, research, publications, conferences and seminars, and consulting services. The foundation tries to give at least one-half of the grants each year to organizations not previously receiving foundation support. Requests not exceeding $25,000 should be submitted between June 1 and August 31 to be eligible for a special review program.
Requirements: Grants are made to qualified organizations in Texas or programs benefiting Texas residents.
Restrictions: Grants are not made to individuals or for church or seminary construction, annual fund-raising events or drives, biomedical research, out-of-state performances or competition expenses, or professional conferences and symposia.
Geographic Focus: Texas
Amount of Grant: $10,000-$1 million
Contact: Program Contact, (800) 826-9431 or (214) 826-9431; fax: (214) 827-7042; email: grants@mfi.org
Internet: http://www.mfi.org
Sponsor: Meadows Foundation of Texas
3003 Swiss Avenue
Dallas, TX 75204-6090

Measey Foundation Medical Education Grants 2162

The purpose of this grant program is to support and advance the medical education of physicians. Grants are made to medical schools in the immediate Philadelphia, PA, area that will determine eligible recipients. Types of support include fellowships, professorships, and scholarship funds. Grantmaking decisions are made at the quarterly meetings held in March, June, September, and December each year; grant requests should be received at least two weeks prior to the meetings.
Restrictions: Individuals are ineligible.
Geographic Focus: Pennsylvania
Samples: Thomas Jefferson U, Jefferson Medical College (Philadelphia, PA)—to endow a professorship in surgery, $1 million.
Amount of Grant: $15,000-$400,000 average
Contact: James Brennan, Manager and Counsel, (610) 566-5800
Sponsor: Benjamin and Mary Siddons Measey Foundation
P.O. Box 258
Media, PA 19063

Medicaid Infrastructure Grant Program to Support Employment of People with Disabilities 2163

This program is designed to help states support the competitive employment of persons with disabilities by facilitating improvements to states' Medicaid programs. Request applications from Judith Norris,(410)786-5130 or jnorris@cms.hhs.gov.
Requirements: Single state Medicaid agencies and other state agencies in partnership with the single agency are eligible to apply.
Amount of Grant: $500,000 minimum
Date(s) Application is Due: Jul 31
Contact: Jeremy Silanskis, Project Manager, (410) 786-6126; email: jsilanskis@cms.hhs.gov
Internet: http://cms.hhs.gov/twwiia/infrastr.asp
Sponsor: Health Care Financing Administration
7500 Security Boulevard
Baltimore, MD 21244-1850

Medicaid/SCHIP Eligibility Pilots 2164

HCFA is soliciting project proposals from state Medicaid agencies and agencies administering the State Children's Health Insurance Program (SCHIP). The purpose of this project is to identify new and effective ways to simplify the application and enrollment process by piloting and evaluating innovative efforts on a small scale.
Requirements: State Medicaid or SCHIP agencies are eligible to apply. These agencies can collaborate with each other, advocates, schools, community-based organizations, consumers, provider organizations, and other entities.
Amount of Grant: $80,000 maximum
Contact: Candice Hall, (410) 786-4453; email: chall2@hcfa.gov
Internet: http://www.cms.hhs.gov/schip/sho-letters/ch62600.asp
Sponsor: Health Care Financing Administration
7500 Security Boulevard
Baltimore, MD 21244-1850

Medical/Nursing Education, Research, and Health Care Exchanges with Taiwan 2165

This organization provides for the exchange of medical and scientific knowledge and fosters cooperation between health scientists in Taiwan and the United States in biomedical teaching, research, and health care. Three separate programs are sponsored. The fellowship program assists Republic of China graduates or postgraduates to study and do research in the United States. The visiting specialists program provides for U.S. health specialists to teach and lecture in medical schools in Taiwan. The nursing program recruits and sponsors U.S. nurses for positions in Taiwan and places and sponsors nurses from Taiwan in U.S. institutions. In Taiwan, contact Executive Director, Room 9001, 212 Chung Hsiao Tung Lu, Section IV, Taipei, Taiwan 10646, Republic of China, 02-721-6511 ext 367, fax: 02-751-6639.
Requirements: Program recruitment is primarily by invitation.
Contact: Annie Kang, c/o New York Academy of Medicine, (212) 860-1990
Sponsor: American Bureau for Medical Advancement in China
1216 Fifth Avenue, Room 585
New York, NY 10029

MedImmune Charitable Grants **2166**

The program supports educational and charitable activities that ultimately improve patient healthcare and further understanding of disease states and treatment options within the community. While the sponsor will consider initiatives in many areas, priority is given to those in the following areas of interest: (a) health and science education for young people; (b) influenza; (c) immunology; (d) pediatric infectious disease; (e) pediatric respiratory disease.

Requirements: Eligible programs include: (a) Community outreach designed to increase public awareness (e.g, fundraising walk or run, nonprofit community hospital or hospital foundation, etc.); (b) Fellowships; (c) Independent educational/scientific programs, accredited and non-accredited; (d) Medical or Scientific education for Healthcare Professionals; (e) Scholarships; or, (f) Academic Chair Endowments. Applications must be completed online at https://web.medimmune.com/corporategrants/, and must be submitted at least 6 weeks prior to the program date or event.

Restrictions: Applications will not be considered from: (1) individuals, physicians, or physician practices; (2) retroactive support; (3) exhibit or display booths at conventions/ conferences; (4) textbooks; (5) operating expenses; (6) fraternal, social, leisure, labor or political organizations; (7) corporate foundations; (8) public or private schools or scholarship funds, except where a grant is specific to a science education initiative.

Contact: Grants Office; (866) 396-6235; email: corporatefunding@medimmune.com

Internet: http://www.medimmune.com/culture_grants.aspx

Sponsor: MedImmune, Inc.
One MedImmune Way
Gaithersburg, MD 20878

Medtronic Foundation Fitness and Nutrition Grants **2167**

The program supports exemplary school fitness and nutrition programs and encourages new and innovative ways to promote physical activity and good nutrition before, during, and after school. Funds are intended to add to, not replace, school funds already set aside for fitness and nutrition initiatives. Priority is given to schools that serve socio-economically disadvantaged students. Grants supporting existing fitness or nutrition programs in school are intended to help public and private K-12 schools reach the next level as they plan or implement an existing plan to serve their students better. Grants for new and innovative ways to promote physical fitness and nutrition programs will also be made to schools demonstrating measurable efforts to improve health of their students.

Requirements: Grants are only available in Minnesota 's seven country metropolitan area. Schools and parent organizations affiliated with schools are encouraged to apply.

Geographic Focus: Minnesota

Amount of Grant: $5000 maximum

Date(s) Application is Due: Dec 15

Contact: Grants Administrator, (763) 514-4000; fax: (763) 514-4879

Internet: http://www.medtronic.com/foundation/programs_fan_guidelines.html

Sponsor: Medtronic Foundation
710 Medtronic Pkwy
Minneapolis, MN 55432-5604

Medtronic Foundation Full Life Patient Partnership—Heart Rescue Grants **2168**

The program funds organizations and government agencies that provide community-based education, training, and awareness programs related to sudden cardiac death and the use of automatic external defibrillators.

Requirements: National and local nonprofit organizations and government agencies that provide education, training, and awareness programs related to sudden cardiac death, early defibrillation, and early intervention are eligible.

Restrictions: The foundation does not support individuals, including scholarships for individuals; religious groups for religious purposes; fund-raising events or activities, social events or goodwill advertising; reimbursable health treatment or scientific research; general support of educational institutions; long-term counseling or personal development; lobbying, political, or fraternal activities; or programs that receive support from United Way of the Minneapolis area.

Amount of Grant: $5000-$50,000 average

Date(s) Application is Due: Oct 15

Contact: Penny Hunt, Executive Director, (763) 505-2646; fax: (763) 505-2648

Internet: http://www.medtronic.com/foundation/about_news.html

Sponsor: Medtronic Foundation
710 Medtronic Pkwy, LC110
Minneapolis, MN 55432-5604

Medtronic Foundation Health Care Grants **2169**

The foundation supports health education programs that work to help people develop and maintain active, healthy lives. Grants support programs and projects that work to prevent or reduce the effects of disabling and chronic disease, serve children and/or older adults, and provide low-income people with nonreimbursed, preventive health services. Also supported are education programs for service providers that build multicultural understanding; programs that address the relationship between physical, mental, and chemical health; and science and technology for grades K-12. Types of support include continuing support, annual campaigns, seed grants, matching funds, scholarship funds, fellowships, special projects, and employee matching gifts. The foundation discourages requests for general operating support, equipment, capital projects, endowments, and multiyear commitments. Within the Twin Cities area, grants of $5000 or less are generally reviewed within 60 days of receipt of application. Grants over $5000 must meet listed deadlines for review. Outside the Twin Cities area, grants of up to $10,000 are made within three months of receipt of the application. Contact the foundation for deadlines for grants over $10,000. Application forms are available on the Web site.

Requirements: Proposals are considered from nonprofit, tax-exempt organizations, largely from the communities in which the company has operations (Tempe, AZ; Anaheim, Irvine, and San Diego, CA; Parker, CO; Milaca and Minneapolis, MN; Danvers, MA; and Humacao and Villalba, PR).

Restrictions: The foundation does not awards grants to religious or political political groups or for fund-raising events, general support of educational institutions, long-term counseling, or personal development.

Geographic Focus: Minnesota

Samples: Beth Israel Deaconess Medical Ctr (Boston, MA), Scripps Ctr for Integrative Medicine (La Jolla, CA), and Stanford Ctr for Research in Disease Prevention/The Stanford Heart Network (Palo Alto, CA)—to develop integrated acute- and chronic-care models for chronically ill patients that emphasize patient-centered care, $2.4 million divided over three years.

Amount of Grant: $1000-$50,000 average

Date(s) Application is Due: Jan 15; Jul 15; Oct 15

Contact: Deb Anderson, Grants Administrator, (763) 514-4000; fax: (763) 505-2648

Internet: http://www.medtronic.com/foundation

Sponsor: Medtronic Foundation
710 Medtronic Pkwy NE, MS LC110
Minneapolis, MN 55432-5604

Melanoma Research Foundation Grants **2170**

The grant supports promising medical research that will further the goal of developing an effective treatment and possible cure of malignant melanoma, while encouraging a new generation of scientists and clinicians to join in this mission. The program is directed primarily at young independent investigators, e.g., untenured assistant professors and the equivalent who have not yet established strong federal funding, who are working at U.S. institutions. In addition, emphasis will be placed on projects that explore innovative approaches to understanding melanoma and its treatment. Both basic and clinical research projects will be considered. Awards will be announced by December, to commence by January 1 of the following year. Complete guidelines are available online.

Requirements: Researchers who are either U.S. permanent residents or citizens, and hold a PhD or MD degree, and a title equivalent to assistant professor, or have at least four years of postdoctoral experience are eligible to apply. Applicants should have evidence indicating strong departmental or institutional support and commitment, and be within eight years of receiving their advanced degree. The proposed research must be conducted in a nonprofit research organization, medical organization, or educational institution located in the United States.

Amount of Grant: $50,000 per year for two years

Date(s) Application is Due: Jul 1

Contact: Grants Program Director, (800) 673-1290; fax: (732) 821-5955; email: research@melanoma.org

Internet: http://www.melanoma.org

Sponsor: Melanoma Research Foundation
24 Old Georgetown Road
Princeton, NJ 08540

Mental Retardation Distinguished Research Award **2171**

The award recognizes an individual or individuals whose research has had a significant impact on the prevention or amelioration of mental retardation. The recipient will receive, in addition to the monetary award, an expense-paid trip to speak at the luncheon of the national convention. The location of the convention varies; the date of the convention is usually in the fall. Nominations must be received by the listed application deadline. Annual deadline dates may vary; contact program staff for exact dates.

Amount of Grant: $1000

Date(s) Application is Due: May 15

Contact: Dr. Sharon Davis, (301) 565-5456; fax: (301) 565-3843; email: davis@the arc.org or info@thearc.org

Internet: http://thearc.org

Sponsor: The Arc
1010 Wayne Avenue, Suite 650
Silver Spring, MD 20910

Mericos Foundation Grants **2172**

The foundation awards grants to organizations based in Santa Barbara, CA, in support of the arts, medical research, child development and the elderly, and education at all levels. Types of support include program/project support, building/renovations, equipment, endowment funds, fellowships, and matching funds. Grants are usually initiated by the foundation.

Requirements: Organizations in California are eligible to apply.

Restrictions: Grants are not made to individuals.

Geographic Focus: California

Samples: Laguna Cottages for Seniors (Santa Barbara, CA)—to refurbish apartments, $11,000.; Goleta Boys and Girls Club (Goleta, CA)—for renovations, $150,000 challenge grant.; U of California at Santa Barbara (CA)—for a program that matches high school students with mentors who are attending graduate school, $100,000 challenge grant.; Girl Scouts of Tres Condades (Santa Barbara, CA)—for technology upgrades for the Stay Safe project, $25,000.

Amount of Grant: $5000-$380,000 range

Contact: Linda Blinkenberg, Secretary, (626) 441-5188; fax (626) 441-3672

Sponsor: Mericos Foundation
625 S Fair Oaks Avenue, Suite 360
South Pasadena, CA 91030-2630

Meriden Foundation Grants 2173

The foundation awards grants to eligible Connecticut nonprofit organizations in its areas of interest, including arts, children and youth, civic affairs, Christian organizations and churches, health organizations and hospitals, higher education, public libraries, and social services. Types of support include annual campaigns, general operating support, scholarships, and social services delivery. There are no application deadlines.
Requirements: Connecticut nonprofit organizations in the Meriden-Wallingford area are eligible.
Geographic Focus: Connecticut
Samples: Childrens Medical Ctr of Connecticut (Hartford, CT)—for general operating support, $21,540.; Yale U, School of Law (New Haven, CT)—to support the annual fund, $43,080.; Gaylord Hospital (Wallingford, CT)—for general support, $21,540.
Amount of Grant: $175-$10,000 range
Contact: Jeffrey Otis, c/o Webster Trust Co, (203) 782-4531
Sponsor: Meriden Foundation
Michaels Building, Webster Plz
Waterbury, CT 06702

Mesothelioma Applied Research Foundation Grants 2174

The program seeks to stimulate translational research for the treatment of pleural or peritoneal mesothelioma. Grants support projects that apply cutting-edge general cancer research concepts specifically to mesothelioma, and translate directly to improved mesothelioma treatment. Eligible projects may relate to either benchwork research or clinical research, must not be presently funded or pending review, and may be conducted through any not-for-profit academic, medical, or research institution, in the United States or abroad. Grants are awarded for 12 months, renewable for 12 more months.
Requirements: The investigator must be affiliated with a nonprofit academic, medical, or research institution.
Amount of Grant: $50,000 per year for two years
Date(s) Application is Due: Aug 15
Contact: Danele Mangone, Grants Director; (805) 563-8400, 7273; fax: (805) 563-8411; email: dmangone@curemeso.org
Internet: http://www.curemeso.org/site/c.kkLUJ7MPKtH/b.4097447/k.E6A3/Mesothelioma_Research_Grants__Call_for_Applications.htm
Sponsor: Mesothelioma Applied Research Foundation
P.O. Box 91840, 3944 State Street, Suite 340
Santa Barbara, CA 93105

Metro Health Foundation Grants 2175

The foundation awards grants in southeastern Michigan in its areas of interest, including children and youth, disabled, elderly, health associations, homeless, and women. Types of support include challenge grants, equipment acquisition, general operating support, project development, scholarship funds, seed grants, and federated giving. Obtain application materials from the office; the board meets in April and October.
Requirements: Nonprofit organizations in the metropolitan tri-county Detroit, MI, area are eligible to apply.
Restrictions: Grants do not support advertising, advocacy organizations, athletic groups, individuals, international organizations, political organizations, special events, benefit dinners, or state or local government agencies.
Geographic Focus: Michigan
Amount of Grant: $1000-$25,000 average
Date(s) Application is Due: Feb 1; Aug 1
Contact: Theresa Sondys, Program Contact, (313) 965-4220; fax: (313) 965-3626; email: metrohealthfdn@aol.com
Sponsor: Metro Health Foundation
333 W Fort Street, Suite 1370
Detroit, MI 48226-3134

Metrowest Community Health Care Foundation Grants 2176

The foundation seeks to improve the health status of the MetroWest community and awards grants to support of youth and elders initiatives. The youth initiative provides grants to support new, innovative, or expanded programs and services that deal with child and adolescent health issues that include injuries and violence; child abuse; oral health care; asthma; depression and suicide; alcohol and substance abuse; access to health services; and health promotion and disease prevention. The elders initiative invites proposals that offer new, innovative, or expanded models for improving access by the elderly to medical and ancillary services, home health, and social services. Proposals also are invited that promote health and wellness services and mental health, alcohol, and substance abuse services to elders. Proposals must show a clear community need and demonstrated collaboration and/or partnership among community organizations in response to this need. Types of grants include but are not limited to project or program support, capacity building, community education, research and evaluation, and demonstration or pilot projects. The foundation will consider proposals for up to three years of funding, with funding beyond the first year contingent upon careful review.
Requirements: 501(c)3 tax-exempt organizations and organizations recognized as an instrumentality of state/local government in the following Massachusetts communities are eligible: Ashland, Bellingham, Dover, Framingham, Franklin, Holliston, Hopedale, Hopkinton, Hudson, Marlborough, Medfield, Medway, Mendon, Milford, Millis, Natick, Needham, Norfolk, Northborough, Sherborn, Southborough, Sudbury, Wayland, Wellesley, and Westborough.
Restrictions: Grants do not support individuals (except for scholarships—see guidelines online), capital fund drives, fundraising drives, retirement of debt or operating deficits, projects that directly influence legislation, political activities or candidates for public office, programs that are customarily operated by hospitals in Massachusetts, and programs that are outside the service area.
Geographic Focus: Massachusetts
Samples: Hemenway School PTO (Framingham, MA)—for fitness and exercise programs for disabled students, $15,000 (2005); Autism Alliance of MetroWest (Natick, MA)—for organizational development, $24,000 (2005); Natick Senior Ctr (Natick, MA)—to continue its taxi-voucher program, which assists elderly people in getting to and from medical appointments, $22,970 (2005); Screening for Mental Health (Wellesley, MA)—to develop a middle-school curriculum on suicide prevention, $186,311 (2005).
Amount of Grant: $50,000 average
Contact: Cathy Glover, Grants Administrator, (508) 879-7625; fax: (508) 879-7628; email: cglover@mchcf.org or info@mchcf.org
Internet: http://www.mchcf.org
Sponsor: Metrowest Community Health Care Foundation
161 Worcester Road, Suite 202
Framingham, MA 01701

Meyer Foundation Grants 2177

Meyer awards grants to nonprofit organizations that serve the people and communities of Greater Washington. The foundation values community-based organizations that work in concert with members of the community. Programs conducted by national organizations that operate in and with cooperation of the local community also will be considered. Grants fall under the following broad program areas: arts, heritage, and culture; community service—i.e., homelessness, domestic violence, immigrant communities, community building, hunger, and more; education—children and youth, and more; health and mental health; law and justice; neighborhood development and housing—civic engagement, advocacy, and more; management assistance; and nonprofit sector leadership. Eligible candidates are required to first submit a letter of inquiry. Listed deadlines are for letters of inquiry. Guidelines are available online.
Requirements: 501(c)3 nonprofit organizations organized and operated for charitable purposes are eligible. Meyer grantees must be located within and primarily serving the Washington, DC region (which includes Washington, DC; Maryland; and Virginia).
Restrictions: The foundation generally does not fund individuals, either through scholarships or other forms of financial assistance; scientific or medical research; programs that promote religious doctrine; special events or conferences; or endowments.
Amount of Grant: $1500-$50,000
Date(s) Application is Due: Feb 10; Jun 9; Oct 2
Contact: Program Contact, (202) 483-8294; fax: (202) 328-6850; email: meyer@meyerfdn.org
Internet: http://www.meyerfoundation.org
Sponsor: Meyer Foundation
1400 16th St NW, Suite 360
Washington, DC 20036

Meyer Memorial Trust Emergency Grants 2178

Emergency Grants provide expedited consideration of true emergencies. MMT's emergency fund is intended for sudden, unanticipated and unavoidable challenges that, if not addressed immediately, could threaten an organization's stability and/or ability to achieve its mission. Examples of Emergency Grants might include assistance for recovery from fire, flood, and other acts of nature. It is not intended to address failure of an organization to comply with legal requirements or problems that can be attributed to organizational neglect or failure to plan for likely contingencies, such as the breakdown of aging equipment.
Requirements: Grants are awarded to 501(c)3 nonprofit organizations in Oregon and Clark County, Washington.
Restrictions: Meyer does not fund general administrative overhead or indirect rate allocations.
Geographic Focus: Oregon; Washington
Contact: Barbara Gibbs, Grants Director; (503) 228-5512; email: barbara@mmt.org
Internet: http://www.mmt.org/grants_programs/
Sponsor: Meyer Memorial Trust
425 NW 10th Avenue, Suite 400
Portland, OR 97209

Meyer Memorial Trust Grassroots Grants 2179

Grassroots Grants enable smaller organizations, often without development departments, to compete for MMT grants. While organizations with budgets up to $2 million may apply for Grassroots Grants, historically, 70% of small grants have gone to organizations with budgets of $250,000 or less. Grants of $1,000 to $25,000 are awarded for projects with budgets of up to $150,000. Grassroots Grants fund programs, outreach, equipment, facility expansions or repairs, strategic planning, website development, and more. Decisions on Grassroots Grants are made by trustees at the program meetings in February, June and October.
Requirements: Grants are awarded to 501(c)3 nonprofit organizations in Oregon and Clark County, Washington.
Restrictions: Meyer does not fund general administrative overhead or indirect rate allocations.
Geographic Focus: Oregon; Washington
Samples: Assistance League of Klamath Basin, Klamath Falls, Oregon, $14,547—for safety improvements to its resale and consignment shop (2008); Central Oregon Environmental Center, Bend, Oregon, $24,750—to support a merger with reSource to strengthen environmental work in the region (2008).
Amount of Grant: $1,000-$25,000

Date(s) Application is Due: Mar 15; Jul 15; Oct 15
Contact: Barbara Gibbs, Grants Director; (503) 228-5512; email: barbara@mmt.org
Internet: http://www.mmt.org/grants_programs/
Sponsor: Meyer Memorial Trust
425 NW 10th Avenue, Suite 400
Portland, OR 97209

Meyer Memorial Trust Operating Funds Grants **2180**
MMT has launched an Operating Funds grant program to help small- and mid-sized organizations that have been hit particularly hard by the current economic crisis. The purpose of this initiative is organizational stability. Organizations for which a cash infusion is not critical to stability, but wish to request funds to maintain or expand current programming, should continue to apply for support through MMT's Responsive and Grassroots Grant programs, as usual. Applications will be accepted beginning September 1. Application deadline is October 1. Awards announcement is anticipated in December. Applications will be accepted through MMT's Responsive Grant inquiry process.
Requirements: Any 501(c)3 nonprofit organizations the operates in Oregon and Clark County, Washington is eligible to apply.
Restrictions: Meyers does not support the following: direct grants, scholarships, or loans to individuals; endowments; general fund drives, annual appeals, special events, or sponsorships; elimination of operating deficits; projects of sectarian or religious organizations that principally benefit their own members or adherents; direct replacement funding for activities previously supported by federal, state, or local public sources; acquisition of land for conservation purposes (except through Program Related Investments); hospital capital construction projects (except through Program Related Investments); animal welfare organizations (both domestic and wild animals); projects that primarily benefit students of a single K-12 school, unless the school is an independent alternative school primarily serving low-income and/or special needs populations; MMT funds cannot be earmarked for purposes of influencing legislation, and the grantee cannot expend any part of the grant in a way that violates its tax-exempt status.
Geographic Focus: Oregon; Washington
Amount of Grant: $50,000 maximum
Date(s) Application is Due: Oct 1
Contact: Barbara Gibbs, Grants Director; (503) 228-5512; email: barbara@mmt.org
Internet: http://www.mmt.org/grants_programs/
Sponsor: Meyer Memorial Trust
425 NW 10th Avenue, Suite 400
Portland, OR 97209

Meyer Memorial Trust Responsive Grants **2181**
Responsive Grants are awarded in the areas of social services, health, affordable housing, community development, conservation and environment, public affairs and social benefit, arts and culture, and education. They generally range from $30,000 to $500,000; grant periods are from one to three years in length. General purpose grants are given for a wide variety of projects in many fields of activity including program expansions, capacity building, capital projects, and start-ups. Final decisions on Responsive Grants proposals are made by trustees at program meetings every month except January, April and August. Final decisions on proposals for capital projects requesting more than $200,000 are made in May and November. Applicants should time their Initial Inquiry submission at least six months before they hope to have a final decision from MMT.
Requirements: General purpose and small grants are awarded to 501(c)3 nonprofit organizations in Oregon and Clark County, Washington.
Restrictions: Meyer does not fund general administrative overhead or indirect rate allocations.
Geographic Focus: Oregon; Washington
Samples: Confederated Tribes of Warm Springs, Warm Springs, Oregon, $150,000—to help construct a building to co-locate the newspaper office and KWSO radio station (2008); Oregon Ballet Theatre, Portland, Oregon, $200,000—for two years of operating support (2008); South Lane Mental Health Services Cottage Grove, Oregon, $150,000—to purchase and renovate a building as a mental health clinic (2008).
Amount of Grant: $30,000-$500,000 average
Contact: Barbara Gibbs, Grants Director; (503) 228-5512; email: barbara@mmt.org
Internet: http://www.mmt.org/grants_programs/
Sponsor: Meyer Memorial Trust
425 NW 10th Avenue, Suite 400
Portland, OR 97209

MfA Newton Fellowships **2182**
The fellowships are available to mathematically sophisticated individuals who are interested in using their talents to make a difference in the lives of young people. The program seeks college graduates and mid-career professionals who can demonstrate a strong interest in teaching, have a bachelor's degree with substantial coursework in mathematics, and are willing to commit to a five-year program that includes one year of full-time graduate study and four years of teaching mathematics in New York City high schools. Fellows receive a stipend, full tuition to master's in education program, mentoring and coaching, and professional development. Applicants are required to take the ETS Praxis II Math subject tests. Application and guidelines are available online.
Requirements: U.S. citizens and permanent residents are eligible.
Restrictions: Individuals who are currently teaching, are certified to teach, or have completed an education degree program are not eligible.
Geographic Focus: New York
Amount of Grant: $90,000 over five years
Date(s) Application is Due: Feb 10
Contact: Fellowship Administrator, (212) 206-0053; fax: (212) 206-1622; email: info@mathforamerica.org
Internet: http://www.mathforamerica.org
Sponsor: Math for America
101 Fifth Avenue, 5th Floor
New York, NY 10003

MGFA Post-Doctoral Research Fellowships **2183**
The Myasthenia Gravis Foundation of America, Inc. announces a competitive twelve-month post-doctoral research fellowship for clinical or basic research pertinent to myasthenia gravis or related neuromuscular disorders. Research may be concerned with neuromuscular transmission, immunology, molecular or cell biology of the neuromuscular synapse, or the etiology/pathology or diagnosis of myasthenia gravis. See the Foundations website for application and, additional guidelines.
Requirements: The applicant must be: a permanent resident of the United States or Canada who has been accepted to work in the laboratory of an established investigator at an institution in the United States, Canada or abroad deemed appropriate by the Medical/Scientific Advisory Board of the Myasthenia Gravis Foundation of America, Inc.; or a foreign national who has been accepted to work in the laboratory of an established investigator at an institution in the United States or Canada deemed appropriate by the Medical/Scientific Advisory Board of the Myasthenia Gravis Foundation of America.
Amount of Grant: $50,000 maximum
Date(s) Application is Due: Oct 1
Contact: Tor Holtan, Chief Executive; (800) 541-5454 or (212) 297-2156; fax: (212) 370-9047; email: Tor.Holtan@myasthenia.org or mgfa@myasthenia.org
Internet: http://www.myasthenia.org/hp_fellowships.cfm#nursing
Sponsor: Myasthenia Gravis Foundation of America
355 Lexington Avenue, 15th Floor
New York, NY 10017

MGFA Student Fellowships **2184**
These fellowships are awarded annually to current medical students or graduate students interested in the scientific basis of myasthenia gravis or related neuromuscular conditions, serving both to further scientific inquiries into the nature of these disorders and to encourage more research. The stipend is up to $5,000. See the Foundation's website for application form and guidelines.
Requirements: The fellowships are awarded to current medical students or graduate students. Briefly describe, in abstract form, the question that you propose to study, its association to myasthenia gravis or related neuromuscular conditions, and how you will approach the project. Applicants and sponsoring institutions must comply with policies governing the protection of human subjects, the humane care of laboratory animals and the inclusion of minorities in study populations.
Amount of Grant: $5,000
Date(s) Application is Due: Mar 31
Contact: Tor Holtan, Chief Executive; (800) 541-5454 or (212) 297-2156; fax: (212) 370-9047; email: Tor.Holtan@myasthenia.org or mgfa@myasthenia.org
Internet: http://www.myasthenia.org/hp_fellowships.cfm#nursing
Sponsor: Myasthenia Gravis Foundation of America
355 Lexington Avenue, 15th Floor
New York, NY 10017

MHRC Graduate Studentships **2185**
A limited number of studentships are offered to qualified graduate students who are undertaking full-time master's or doctoral programs. Studentships are awarded on a competitive basis. Each candidate must arrange to have three individuals send supporting letters directly to the council. Studentships are initially awarded for a 12-month period and may be renewed. The maximum period of support by the council is two years for individuals enrolled in a master's program, three years for individuals holding a master's degree enrolled in a PhD program, and five years for individuals proceeding directly to a PhD from an honor's BS, BA, or equivalent degree. Recipients should begin their award period by July 1 at the earliest and September 1 at the latest.
Restrictions: In each competition a maximum of one studentship will be awarded per supervisor. Individuals who hold a faculty position are not eligible for graduate studentship awards.
Contact: Program Contact, (204) 775-1096; fax: (204) 786-5401; email: mhrc@cc.umanitoba.ca
Internet: http://www.umanitoba.ca/academic_support/MHRC/PROGRAMS.HTM#contents
Sponsor: Manitoba Health Research Council
770 Bannatyne Avenue
Winnipeg, MB R3E 0W3 Canada

MHRC Operating Grants **2186**
Grants in aid of research are designed to defray the normal direct costs of research including, among others, personnel costs, supplies and expendable materials, experimental animals, equipment costing less than $C5000, computer costs, and publication costs. Up to five percent of the operating grant may be used for travel related to the investigator's research program. Grants are normally awarded for one year. The council gives priority to new investigators and new projects. The starting date for successful grants is July 1.
Requirements: Normally only investigators holding academic appointments or equivalent in the province of Manitoba are eligible to apply. Investigators who do not hold academic

appointments should consult with the council to establish their eligibility before applying.
Restrictions: Individuals holding continuing operating grants from the council are not eligible to apply for other operating grants that would become effective during the tenure of their present grants. Expenditures for student and postdoctoral salaries will not be considered on operating grants.
Amount of Grant: $C100,000 maximum for one year
Contact: Program Contact, (204) 775-1096; fax: (204) 786-5401; email: mhrc@cc.umanitoba.ca
Internet: http://www.umanitoba.ca/academic_support/MHRC/PROGRAMS.HTM#contents
Sponsor: Manitoba Health Research Council
770 Bannatyne Avenue
Winnipeg, MB R3E 0W3 Canada

MHRC Postdoctoral Research Fellowships **2187**
A limited number of fellowships are available to qualified candidates with doctoral degrees whose prior postdoctoral research training shall normally not exceed five years. Fellowships are awarded on a competitive basis and will carry the same monetary value as postdoctoral salaries on the council's operating grants. Only individuals licensed to practice in the province will be eligible for the stipend scale for professional degree holders; all others will receive the PhD stipend. Fellowships are awarded for a 12-month period and may be renewed for one additional year by reapplication and competitive review. Starting dates are between July 1 and September 1.
Requirements: Holders of professional doctoral degrees (MD, DDS, DVM) who will be registered as full-time master's or doctoral students may apply for either a postdoctoral fellowship or a graduate studentship; however, they are eligible for consideration in only one of these two categories and must indicate clearly for which category they wish to be considered. Each candidate must arrange to have three individuals send supporting letters to the council.
Restrictions: In each competition a maximum of one postdoctoral fellowship will be awarded per supervisor. Individuals who hold a faculty position are not eligible for postdoctoral fellowship awards.
Contact: Program Contact, (204) 775-1096; fax: (204) 786-5401; email: mhrc@cc.umanitoba.ca
Internet: http://www.umanitoba.ca/academic_support/MHRC/PROGRAMS.HTM#contents
Sponsor: Manitoba Health Research Council
770 Bannatyne Avenue
Winnipeg, MB R3E 0W3 Canada

Miami County Community Foundation Operation Round Up Grants **2188**
Miami-Cass REMC established this fund with the Northern Indiana Community Foundation in December 2003. Operation Round Up is a national program that allows participating electric cooperatives to partner with their members to provide charitable giving funds in their local community. The concept is simple; each month the total amount of the participating member's bill is rounded up to the nearest dollar and those extra pennies go into the fund designated for distribution to those in need in the area. This fund raising program is completely voluntary. A seven person, volunteer Advisory Board has been created to oversee the designation of funds and ensure that grants are handled wisely. The Miami County Community Foundation holds the funds until the quarterly distribution. Approximately 80% of the Miami-Cass REMC membership participates in Operation Round Up. What may only seem like pennies a month adds up quickly. Collectively approximately $26,000.00 annually could be raised to support local organizations.
Requirements: Applications are available at the Miami-Cass REMC office, the Northern Indiana Community Foundation office and are available to download from the Northern Indiana Community Foundation website.
Restrictions: Operation Round Up funds will not be used for paying utility bills, funding political or private interests.
Geographic Focus: Indiana
Date(s) Application is Due: Mar 31; Jun 30; Sep 30; Dec 31
Contact: Mary Alexander, Associate Director; (765) 475-2859, (877) 432-6423; fax: (765) 472-7378; email: miami@nicf.org
Internet: http://www.nicf.org/miami/grantapplications.html
Sponsor: Miami County Community Foundation
13 East Main Street
Peru, IN 46970

Michael and Susan Dell Foundation Grants **2189**
The mission of the foundation is to encourage and inspire children to reach their greatest potential. The foundation proactively seeks out opportunities to support or develop programs that address five essential areas: children's health—access to affordable health care and insurance; education—improve study and college readiness skills, enable tutoring by licensed teachers, and guide parents and students through the college application process and financial aid process (including the grants and scholarships process); safety—foster care, residential treatment for neglected or abused children, law enforcement, agency child abduction programs, and sexual or domestic violence abuse counseling; youth development—affordable and enriching after school programs to protect and educate children; and early childhood care—increase the quality and reliability of child care. The foundation does not accept unsolicited proposals. Preliminary grant requests may be submitted via the foundation's online form; full application is by invitation. The foundation also sponsors the Dell Scholars Program, which strives to make the dream of a college education possible for a number of underserved youth, especially lower-income students who have experienced obstacles and hardships. Candidates for this particular scholarship are evaluated based on their individual determination to succeed and their demonstrated ability to overcome obstacles and challenges, not on academic record alone.
Requirements: Texas nonprofit organizations are eligible.
Geographic Focus: Texas
Contact: Janet Mountain, Executive Director
Internet: http://www.msdf.org
Sponsor: Michael and Susan Dell Foundation
P.O. Box 163867
Austin, TX 78716-3867

Michael J. Fox Foundation Clinical Discovery Grants **2190**
The goal of this program is to encourage translational research by stimulating well-designed clinical research projects focused on potentially high-impact approaches to the field of Parkinson's disease. Through the program, researchers will be invited to submit grant applications to conduct new or novel clinical research in humans relevant to the cure, cause, prevention, or improved treatment of Parkinson's disease and its complications. The program will support a variety of innovative research studies that are directly related to patients or patient populations affected by the disease. Appliciants may request a project period of up to three years. The foundation employs an expedited, abbreviated granting mechanism to accelerate discoveries and hopefully translate findings to Parkinson's disease patients more quickly. A mandatory letter of intent is due on the listed application deadline; full applications are by invitation.
Requirements: Both U.S. and non-U.S. organizations are eligible. Applications may be submitted by public and private nonprofit entities, units of state and local governments, eligible agencies of the federal government, and for- profit entities. Collaborative efforts are welcome.
Restrictions: Postdoctoral students or fellows are not eligible to apply as principal investigators.
Amount of Grant: $200,000 maximum per year
Date(s) Application is Due: Nov 21
Contact: Grants Administrator, email: research@michaeljfox.org
Internet: http://www.michaeljfox.org/research/index.php
Sponsor: Michael J. Fox Foundation for Parkinson's Research
P.O. Box 4777, Grand Central Sta
New York, NY 10163

Michael J. Fox Foundation for Parkinson's Research LEAPS Program **2191**
Investigators are invited to apply for funding through a novel mechanism called LEAPS (Linked Efforts to Accelerate Parkinson's Solutions). LEAPS are multi-year, potentially multi-million dollar grant awards for collaborative, milestone-driven efforts to address questions that will have significant practical impact on the understanding and treatment of Parkinson's disease. LEAPS grants are goal-oriented and focused on answering a broad research question, one whose answer would represent a major, practical step forward in Parkinson's disease—a solution to a Parkinson's problem. Examples of such questions could be categorized under broad aims of: repairing the PD brain; slowing or halting the progression of PD; preventing or controlling levodopa-induced dyskinesias; and identifying the cause of PD. LEAPS are not intended to be conventional research grants. LEAPS investigators will be asked to interact regularly with foundation staff and advisors to discuss elements of the project, research directions, progress against stated milestones, and possible ways (other than through additional financial resources) the foundation may offer support or assistance. The RFP and preproposal cover sheet are available online.
Requirements: Applications may be submitted by U.S. and non-U.S. entities; public and private nonprofit entities, such as universities, colleges, hospitals, laboratories, units of state and local governments, and eligible agencies of the federal government; and for-profit entities.
Restrictions: Postdoctoral students or fellows are not eligible to apply as coordinating or principal investigators.
Date(s) Application is Due: Apr 29
Contact: Grants Administrator, (800) 708-7644
Internet: http://www.michaeljfox.org
Sponsor: Michael J. Fox Foundation for Parkinson's Research
P.O. Box 4777
New York, NY 10163

Michael J. Fox Foundation Parkinson's Cell Line Research Grants **2192**
Researchers are invited to submit investigator-initiated proposals using embryonic stem cells targeted at achieving optimized transplantation materials and protocols promoting graft survival, stability of dopaminergic phenotype, and long-term functional recovery in animal models of Parkinson's disease. The intent is to use the acquired knowledge to develop cell replacement therapy for PD patients. Work in animal or human cell lines is acceptable; however, a primary focus on human cell lines is required, and research on human embryonic stem cells is considered appropriate. Mandatory letters of intent are due August 9. Guidelines are available online.
Requirements: Investigators with scientific interests and demonstrated success in the development, culture, and manipulation of individual cell lines are invited to apply.
Samples: Ernest Arenas of the Karolinska Institute (Stockholm Sweden), Jun Takahashi of the Kyoto U Graduate School of Medicine (Japan), Xuejun Wen of Clemson U (SC), and Su-Chung Zhang of the U of Wisconsin (Madison, WI)—for stem-cell research related to finding a cure for Parkinson's disease, $1 million divided (2005).

Date(s) Application is Due: Aug 9; Sep 20
Contact: Grants Administrator, (800) 708-7644; email: research@michaeljfox.org
Internet: http://www.michaeljfox.org/research/fundingopps.php?id=9
Sponsor: Michael J. Fox Foundation for Parkinson's Research
P.O. Box 4777, Grand Central Sta
New York, NY 10163

Michigan Psychoanalytic Institute and Society SATA Grants **2193**
The purpose of this grant is to partly sponsor one or more trainees in the mental health field in order for them to attend a national meeting of the American Psychoanalytic Association. The winter meeting of the American is held in New York City and the spring meeting is held in different cities. To apply for a partial scholarship, applicants should send a two-paragraph statement telling us about their background, interest in psychoanalytic thinking, and why he/she would like to attend a meeting of the American Psychoanalytic Association.
Contact: Kathleen Kunkel, Administrative Director; (248) 851-3380 ext. 2 or (248) 865-1164; fax: (248) 851-1806
Internet: http://www.mpi-mps.org/joomla/index.php?option=com_content&task=view&id=32&Itemid=109
Sponsor: Michigan Psychoanalytic Institute and Society
32841 Middlebelt Road, Suite 411
Farmington Hills, MI 48334

Michigan Psychoanalytic Institute and Society Scholarships **2194**
The Continuing Education Division of the Michigan Psychoanalytic Institute offers two Programs, one in Ann Arbor and one in Farmington Hills. The Program is a one-year, clinically-based program which meets once weekly. The program is designed to introduce and further develop an understanding of psychoanalytic principles as applied to psychotherapy with adults, children, and adolescents. Participants meet as a class on a weekly basis with instructors from the faculty of the Michigan Psychoanalytic Institute. Each instructor teaches a 5-6 week segment. Instructors present clinical material to illustrate a psychoanalytic approach to clinical work. Discussion of the case material is utilized to examine psychoanalytic concepts and clinical technique as applied to psychoanalytic psychotherapy. Half of the clinical material presented during the year is from work with adult patients. The other half of the year, child analysts present and discuss clinical material from the treatment of children, adolescents, and their parents. The Scholarship application must be submitted by June 30.
Requirements: The Fellowship Programs are ideally suited for mental health clinicians who are in practice, recently graduated, or in training in their respective fields (psychiatry, psychology, social work, counseling, or nursing). It is also useful as preparation for clinicians who are considering more extensive training in psychoanalytic psychotherapy or psychoanalysis in the future.
Date(s) Application is Due: Jun 30
Contact: Jean Lewis, Program Director; (248) 851-3380; fax: (248) 851-1806; email: jlewis@mpi-mpi.org
Internet: http://www.mpi-mps.org/joomla/index.php?option=com_content&task=view&id=62&Itemid=216
Sponsor: Michigan Psychoanalytic Institute and Society
32841 Middlebelt Road, Suite 411
Farmington Hills, MI 48334

Microsoft Research Cell Phone as a Platform for Healthcare Grants **2195**
Microsoft Research will support selected academic research with the goal of advancing the state-of-the-art in smart cell phones for health care applications. Successful projects must seek to increase the capacity of cell phone-based health care solutions in under-served rural and urban communities. They must also take into consideration the social context of application deployment. Topics to consider include: medical applications that are relevant, worldwide, for smart mobile phones (application and Web-enabled) in rural, and urban, communities; and appropriate services and infrastructures needed to provide affordable and accessible health care services. The total amount available under this request for proposals (RFP) is $1,000,000. Microsoft Research anticipates making approximately 10-12 awards averaging $80,000, with a maximum of $100,000 for any single award. Awards are made for the purpose of seed-funding larger initiatives, proofs of concept, or demonstrations of feasibility. It is important to understand that funding will continue after the first year only in exceptional circumstances, and that the principal investigators should therefore make every effort to leverage Microsoft Research funds as one component of a diverse funding base in a larger or longer-running project.
Requirements: All qualifying institutions are eligible without regard for geographic location. The proposing institution must be either: an accredited degree-granting college or university (or international equivalent) with non-profit status and awarding degrees at the baccalaureate level or above; or a research institution with non-profit status.
Restrictions: For all awards, payment of indirect costs (overhead) is not permitted.
Amount of Grant: $100,000 maximum
Date(s) Application is Due: Oct 29
Contact: Rick Rashid, Senior Vice President; (800) 642-7676; fax: (425) 936-7329; email: erpinq@microsoft.com
Internet: http://research.microsoft.com/en-us/um/redmond/about/collaboration/awards/cellphone-healthcare_awards.aspx
Sponsor: Microsoft Research
One Microsoft Way
Redmond, WA 98052-6399

Middlesex Savings Charitable Foundation Grants **2196**
The foundation supports eligible Massachusetts nonprofit organizations, services and programs in a wide variety of fields, including education, health and welfare, arts and culture, and community development. Philanthropic programs include: educational opportunities—organizations that provide unique educational opportunities to children and adults; capacity building—organizational-capacity building of local nonprofits; and community development—projects and programs whose primary goal is to improve the lives of low- and moderate-income families and individuals throughout the foundation's communities. Guidelines and application are available online.
Requirements: Eastern Massachusetts 501(c)3 tax-exempt organizations serving one or more communities served by Middlesex Savings Bank, including Acton, Ashland, Ayer, Bedford, Bellingham, Berlin, Bolton, Boxborough, Carlisle, Chelmsford, Concord, Dover, Dunstable, Framingham, Franklin, Groton, Harvard, Holliston, Hopedale, Hopkinton, Hudson, Lexington, Lincoln, Littleton, Marlborough, Maynard, Medfield, Medway, Milford, Millis, Natick, Needham, Newton, Norfolk, Northborough, Pepperell, Sherborn, Shirley, Southborough, Stow, Sudbury, Townsend, Tyngsborough, Upton, Walpole, Waltham, Wayland, Wellesley, Westborough, Westford, and Weston, are eligible.
Restrictions: The foundation will not fund political or sectarian activities.
Geographic Focus: Massachusetts
Amount of Grant: $15,000 maximum
Date(s) Application is Due: May 15; Aug 30
Contact: Dana Neshe, (508) 652-4503; email: dneshe@middlesexbank.com
Internet: http://www.middlesexbank.com/mscf/index.asp
Sponsor: Middlesex Savings Charitable Foundation
P.O. Box 358, 6 Main Street
Natick, MA 01760

Miguel Aleman Foundation Grants **2197**
The foundation operates in Mexico in the fields of conservation and the environment, the arts and humanities, economic development, education, international affairs, medicine and health, science and technology, and social welfare. Types of support include research, grants to organizations, and prizes.
Contact: Fernando Castro y Castro, Director, 52-5-250-65-76; fax: 52-5-250-10-43; email: 103503.1144@compuserve.com
Internet: http://www.miguelaleman.org.mx
Sponsor: Miguel Aleman Foundation
Ruben Dario 187
Col Chapultepec Morales 11570 Mexico

Milagro Foundation Grants **2198**
Started by musician Carlos Santana and his wife Deborah, the foundation supports educational efforts that help youths live healthy, literate, and culturally enriched lives. Priority is helping at-risk and vulnerable populations acquire the skills to succeed in life. The foundation is especially interested in arts education. Unsolicited completed applications are not accepted. Preliminary letters of inquiry are accepted at any time. The board meets in February, June, and October.
Requirements: Nonprofit organizations are eligible. In order of priority, the foundation has an interest in helping children in San Rafael, the remainder of California, the United States, and other nations in which Carlos Santana performs.
Samples: Friends of School of the Arts Foundation (San Francisco, CA)—to repair and replace instruments for the school orchestra and jazz bands at this public high school that serves artistic and creatively talented youths, $15,000.; Huckleberry Youth Programs (San Rafael, CA)—to provide teenagers with health-education services, including information n HIV prevention, drug and alcohol abuse, and pregnancy prevention, $10,000.; Jeanette Prandi Children's Ctr (San Rafael, CA)—to provide medical services to child victims of sexual assault, $12,000.
Amount of Grant: $2,500-$5,000 average
Contact: Grants Administrator; (415) 460-9939; fax: (415) 460-6802; email: info@milagrofoundation.org or apply@milagrofoundation.org
Internet: http://www.milagrofoundation.org/apply.asp
Sponsor: Milagro Foundation
P.O. Box 9125
San Rafael, CA 94912-9125

Miles of Hope Breast Cancer Foundation Grants **2199**
The Fund provides programs and support services for women and families in the Hudson Valley, New York, affected by breast cancer. All funds raised for the Foundation are used in the Hudson Valley. The Miles of Hope Breast Cancer Foundation is currently offering grants for projects in the areas of breast health and breast cancer education, outreach, screening, treatment and support projects.
Requirements: Services must be provided in the eight counties served by the Miles of Hope Breast Cancer Foundation, which include: Columbia, Dutchess, Greene, Orange, Putnam, Rockland, Westchester and Ulster.
Restrictions: Project must be specific to breast health and/or breast cancer. Applicants must be a U.S. nonprofit (federally tax-exempt) organization. Nonprofit organizations, known educational institutions (i.e. college or university), government agencies, and Indian tribes are eligible. Equipment costs, if applicable, may not exceed 30% of direct costs and should be used exclusively on this project. Salaries, if requested, are for personnel related to this project only and not the general work of the employee. Funds will not be awarded to capital campaigns
Geographic Focus: New York

Contact: Program Administrator, (845) 527-6884 or (845) 264-2005; email: info@milesofhopebcf.org
Internet: http://www.milesofhopebcf.org/funds.html#grants
Sponsor: Miles of Hope Breast Cancer Foundation
P.O. Box 405
La Grangeville, NY 12540

Milheim Foundation Cancer Research Grants **2200**
Project grants provide support for research work for the prevention, treatment, and cure of cancer. In addition to a written proposal and completed application form, at least one letter of recommendation and one curriculum vita must be submitted. The grants are awarded for one year; renewal is possible but not encouraged.
Requirements: Organizations that are incorporated as nonprofit and operate within the continental limits of the United States are eligible. PI must hold MD, PhD, or the equivalent.
Restrictions: Grants do not support travel or presentation of papers, overhead expenses or support and maintenance of hospitals, salaries of academic personnel, or individuals.
Amount of Grant: $10,000-$22,000
Date(s) Application is Due: Mar 15
Contact: Barbara Cole, c/o U.S. Bank PFS/Trust, (303) 316-5945 or (303) 316-5948; fax: (303) 388-9387; email: jnelson@foundation.sdsu.edu
Sponsor: Milheim Foundation for Cancer Research
200 University Boulevard
Denver, CO 80206

Military Ex-Prisoners of War Foundation Grants **2201**
The Military Ex-Prisoners of War Foundation was founded primarily to assist Military Ex-P.O.W Veterans, and to fund their National Educational Scholarship Program for qualified heirs. The mission of the Military Ex-Prisoners of War Foundation is to support educational programs designed to inform Americans about the P.O.W experience; offer scholarships to children and grandchildren of former P.O.Ws and other such activities as may be approved by the Foundation's board of directors.
Requirements: Children, grandchildren, and great-grandchildren of former prisoners-of-war (P.O.Ws) who served after December 7, 1941 are eligible to apply. Applicants must include the following: completed application (available at the Foundations website); short autobiographical statement (not to exceed one typed page); Transcript requirements: copy of official transcripts of high school grades including SAT/ACT test scores, official transcripts of college grades; two letters of recommendation, one must be from a present/former teacher; short essay, limited to 1,000 words, on the impact of WWII on society today; statement about your grandparent's experience as a prisoner of war, 1,000 words or less. Completed applications should be mailed to: Dorris Livingstone, Recording Secretary, Military Ex-Prisoners of War Foundation, 1561 Glen Hollow Lane South, Dunedin, FL 34698. If you have any questions, email your inquiry to: Dorris2001@aol.com with "Foundation Scholarship Application/Question" typed into the Subject line.
Restrictions: No support for individuals not related to former prisoners of war, religious, political causes, or for organizations.
Amount of Grant: $2,000
Date(s) Application is Due: Apr 1
Contact: F. Paul Dallas, President; (910) 867-2775; fax: (910) 867-0339; email: threatt273@aol.com
Internet: http://www.militarypowfoundation.org/072409-scholarships.html
Sponsor: Military Ex-Prisoners of War Foundation
916 Bingham Drive
Fayetteville NC 27803

Military Medical Research and Development Grants **2202**
The objective of the program is to reduce illness and injury acquired by U.S. military personnel on the battlefield through basic and applied medical research executed largely through grants and contracts with civilian educational and research institutions. The maximum period acceptable for a research proposal is five years. Preproposals are encouraged prior to submission of a formal application. There are no overall deadline dates for applications. Individual research areas may initiate deadlines, which will be communicated upon review of the preproposal.
Requirements: Applicant must be a public, nonprofit organization; other public organization; private nonprofit organization; specialized group; or quasi-public nonprofit organization.
Samples: Characterization and Utilization of Opioid-Like Hibernation Factors, $621,000.; Analysis of Investigational Drugs in Biological Fluids, Method Development and Routine Assay, $2.4 million.; Studies of Altered Response to Infection Induced by Severe Injury, $1.1 million; and Mechanisms of Cutaneous Vesication, $862,000.
Amount of Grant: $100,000-$5 million; $650,000 average
Contact: Craig Lebo, U.S. Army Medical Research Acquisitions, (301) 619-2036
Internet: https://mrmc-www.army.mil/mrdindex.asp
Sponsor: U.S. Army Medical Research and Material Command
SCRD-RMA-RC, Fort Detrick
Frederick, MD 21702-5014

Millipore Foundation Grants **2203**
The foundation supports nonprofit organizations in company operating communities in five main areas: education and research, social services, culture, health care, and public policy. Types of support include general operating support, employee matching gifts, and employee-related scholarships. Applications are accepted throughout the year.
Requirements: 501(c)3 tax-exempt organizations are eligible.
Amount of Grant: $2500-$5000 average
Contact: Charleen Johnson, Executive Director, (978) 715-1268; fax: (978) 715-1385; email: Charleen_Johnson@millipore.com
Internet: http://www.millipore.com/corporate/milliporefoundation.nsf/foundationhome
Sponsor: Millipore Foundation
290 Concord Road
Billerica, MA 01821-7037

Millipore/Charles P. Schaufus Parenteral-Processing Technology Grant **2204**
The grant is intended to stimulate research in parenteral processing through the support of a graduate student. Parenteral processing includes the investigation of aspects in bulk manufacture of parenteral drugs, such as fermentation and scale-up; intermediate steps, such as crystallization and purification; equipment surfaces, such as their contribution to particulate matter and their resistance to corrosion; and computer-assisted manufacture, such as software and its validation. Emphasis of this research is to be on parenteral processing. The grant is for up to three years and includes cash and equipment each year. Applications are available on the Web site.
Requirements: Applicants must be associated with U.S. 501(c)3 and 509(a)(1)(2) or (3) tax-exempt organizations.
Samples: Dr. Bhogi Sheth, U of Tennessee (Memphis, TN)—three-year parenteral research grant recipient, $10,000 in cash and $10,000 in Millipore equipment.
Amount of Grant: $22,500 for one year; $22,500 in equipment
Date(s) Application is Due: Sep 15
Contact: Deanna Morton, c/o Morton Communications/Infinitech, (516) 829-5501; fax: (516) 829-1008; email: DeeMorton@aol.com
Internet: http://www.pdafoundation.org/grant_offerings.html
Sponsor: Parenteral Drug Association Foundation for Pharmaceutical Sciences
111 Great Neck Road, Suite 308
Great Neck, NY 11021

Milton Wexler Postdoctoral Fellowships **2205**
Support will be for research projects that contribute to identifying and understanding the basic defect of Huntington's disease. Areas of interest include trinucleotide expansions, animal models, gene therapy, neurobiology and development of the basal ganglia, cell survival and death, and intercellular signaling in striatal neurons. Awards may be renewed for a third year. To receive an application, submit a letter of intent. Letter of intent forms may be submitted electronically at any time via the Web site.
Amount of Grant: $43,000 starting salary, $12,000 for supplies, and $2000 travel allowances for two years
Date(s) Application is Due: Feb 15; Jun 15; Oct 15
Contact: Dr. Carl Johnson, (310) 458-4183; fax: (310) 458-3937; email: carljohnson@hdfoundation.org
Internet: http://www.hdfoundation.org/fundinga.htm
Sponsor: Hereditary Disease Foundation
3960 Broadway, 6th Floor
New York, NY 10032

Minneapolis Foundation Community Grants **2206**
The foundation awards grants throughout Minnesota. Eligible activities include policy and systems change work in the following areas: affordable housing; economic opportunity; educational achievement; and the health and well-being of children, youth, and families. The foundation also focuses on systems and policy work that addresses the intersection of issues, such as housing and health. Types of support include program/project support, operating support, capital support (limited to the seven-county metro area); and some multiyear grants. Proposals are accepted throughout the year.
Requirements: 501(c)3 nonprofit organizations located in the seven-county metropolitan area of Minneapolis and Saint Paul may apply.
Restrictions: The foundation does not fund individuals, organizations/activities outside of Minnesota, conference registration fees, memberships, direct religious activities, political organizations or candidates, direct fundraising activities, telephone solicitations, courtesy advertising, or financial deficits.
Geographic Focus: Minnesota
Date(s) Application is Due: Mar 15; Sep 15
Contact: Paul Verrette, Senior Grants Administrator; (612) 672-3836; email: pverrette@mplsfoundation.org
Internet: http://www.mplsfoundation.org/grants/guidelines.htm
Sponsor: Minneapolis Foundation
800 IDS Center, 80 South Eighth Street
Minneapolis, MN 55402

Minority Doctoral Fellowships in Science and Engineering **2207**
The university accepts applications from members of minority groups for doctoral fellowships in the life sciences, physical sciences, and engineering. Contact the program director for detailed information on application and amounts of fellowships offered. Annual deadline dates may vary; contact program staff for exact dates. Contact program staff for program availability.
Requirements: Citizens or permanent residents of the United States who are African American, Hispanic, or Native American may apply. The recipient must have an earned baccalaurate degree and be accepted for admission to a doctoral program in the fields of life sciences, physical sciences, engineering, or mathematics at a participating Illinois institution. Upon completion, recipients must agree to seek and accept a full-time faculty appointment at an Illinois institution of higher learning for a period equal to the number of years of the award.

Amount of Grant: $1100 monthly stipend
Date(s) Application is Due: Jan 23
Contact: Karen Jennings, Graduate School, (618) 453-4555; fax: (618) 453-4562; email: kjenning@siu.edu or gaoffice@siu.edu
Internet: http://www.siu.edu/gradschl/doctoral_fellowship.htm
Sponsor: Southern Illinois University at Carbondale
Graduate School, Woody Hall B130
Carbondale, IL 62901-4716

Miriam and Peter Haas Fund Grants **2208**
The fund, which limits grant making to the San Francisco Bay area of California, supports nonprofit organizations in the areas of education, early childhood education and development (ages two to five), family services, arts, humanities, health, social services, public affairs, and the environment. Types of support include operating budgets, capital campaigns, equipment acquisition, continuing support, deficit financing funds, building challenge/matching grants, equipment acquisition, special projects, and technical assistance. There are no application deadlines.
Requirements: Nonprofit organizations in the San Francisco Bay area of California may submit grant requests.
Restrictions: Individuals are not eligible.
Geographic Focus: California
Samples: Child Development Policy Institute Education Fund (CA)—for general operating support, $25,000.; Ctr for the Arts, Yerba Buena Gardens (CA)—to support educational and marketing efforts, $100,000.; Performing Arts Workshop (CA)—to train a core group of artists to teach creative movements in San Francisco preschools, $10,000.
Amount of Grant: $5000-$50,000 average
Contact: David Thesell, Grants Manager, (415) 296-9249; fax: (415) 296-8842; email: dThesell@mphf.org
Sponsor: Miriam and Peter Haas Fund
201 Filbert Street, 5th Floor
San Francisco, CA 94133

MLA Ida and George Eliot Prize **2209**
The prize is presented annually for a work published in the preceding calendar year that has been judged most effective in furthering medical librarianship. The recipient receives a cash award and a certificate at the association's annual meeting. The recipient will be notified in February.
Requirements: Nominations are accepted from the membership at large, and should include a complete bibliographic citation, a copy of the nominee's work whenever possible, and any other pertinent information regarding the availability, content, and impact of the work.
Samples: Robert M. Braude, PhD (New York, NY) for his article, The Organization of the Digital Library.; Valerie Florence, PhD (Rochester, NY) for her article, Educating Physicians to Use the Digital Library.; Mark E. Frisse, MD (St. Louis, MO) for his article Informatics and Medical Libraries: Changing Needs and Changing Roles.
Contact: Lisa Fried, Program Contact, (312) 419-9094 ext 28; fax: (312) 419-8950; email: info@mlahq.org
Internet: http://www.mlanet.org/awards/honors/eliot.html
Sponsor: Medical Library Association
65 E Wacker Pl, Suite 1900
Chicago, IL 60601-7298

MLA Lois Ann Colaianni Award for Excellence and Achievement in Hospital Librarianship **2210**
The award is a general award for outstanding contributions to hospital librarianship as demonstrated by excellence and achievement in service, advocacy, leadership, publications, presentations, teaching, research, technology, administration, special projects, or any combination of these areas. The award is generally aimed at the midcareer hospital librarian but is not restricted to midcareer. Nominating petitions are available from the awards committee chair or from MLA headquarters.
Requirements: Nominees must be members of the MLA and be hospital librarians who have worked in a hospital library for at least five years preceding the award.
Contact: Lisa Fried, (312) 419-9094 ext 28; fax: (312) 419-8950; email: mlapd2@mlahq.org
Internet: http://www.mlanet.org/awards/honors/colaianni.html
Sponsor: Medical Library Association
65 E Wacker Pl, Suite 1900
Chicago, IL 60601-7298

MMRF Research Grants **2211**
The foundation's mission is to accelerate a cure for multiple myeloma. The program supports three categories of research grants. Fellows awards support researchers entering the field of multiple myeloma working under the direction of a research sponsor (March 1 deadline). Senior research awards support investigators with an interest in myeloma who have been working in cancer research for a minimum of five years (May 2 deadline). Collaborative programs grants support multidisciplinary research in multiple myeloma. Cohesive and synergistic grant proposals that involve several research projects across one or more scientific core laboratories are sought (preliminary deadline for submitting a Collaborative Program Grant application is June 15, final application deadline is September 15).
Samples: Johns Hopkins U (Baltimore, MD)—for research on immunotherapy of myeloma at the Sidney Kimmel Comprehensive Cancer Ctr, $1.5 million (2004).
Amount of Grant: $50,000 fellows awards; $100,000 senior research awards; $1.5 million collaborative program grants
Contact: Jill Shook, Grants Administrator, (203) 972-1250; fax: (203) 972-1259; email: shookj@themmrf.org
Internet: http://www.multiplemyeloma.org/research
Sponsor: Multiple Myeloma Research Foundation
3 Forest Street
New Canaan, CT 06840

MNI Jeanne Timmins Fellowships **2212**
The institute offers annual postdoctoral fellowships to support research and study in neurology, neurosurgery, or neuroscience for a period of one year at the institute. One renewal is possible. An application form may be requested in writing. Successful applicants will be notified by letter.
Requirements: Candidates must have MD or PhD degrees; those with MDs will ordinarily have completed clinical studies in neurology or neurosurgery.
Amount of Grant: $C25,000 maximum
Date(s) Application is Due: Oct 31
Contact: Assistant to the Director, (514) 398-1903; fax: (514) 398-8248; email: john@mni.lan.mcgill.ca
Internet: http://www.mni.mcgill.ca/MNIfellowships.html
Sponsor: Montreal Neurological Institute
3801 University Street, Room 636
Montreal, PQ H3A 2B4 Canada

Monfort Family Foundation Grants **2213**
The foundation awards general operating grants to Colorado nonprofit organizations in its areas of interest, including education, health and medical research, arts and culture, agriculture, and general charitable giving. Application forms must be obtained.
Requirements: Colorado nonprofits, primarily in Weld County, are eligible.
Restrictions: Grants are not made to individuals.
Geographic Focus: Colorado
Samples: U of Northern Colorado, College of Business Administration (Greeley, CO)—to bring nationally prominent business leaders to campus to teach; to create a technology center; and to establish an entrepreneurship institute, a lecture series, and an instruction-improvement fund, $10.5 million.
Amount of Grant: $5000-$100,000 average range
Date(s) Application is Due: May 1; Oct 1
Contact: Dave Evans, Program Contact, (970) 454-1357
Sponsor: Monfort Family Foundation
Box 337300
Greeley, CO 80633

Montgomery County Community Foundation Grants **2214**
The Montgomery County Community Foundation (MCCF) builds bridges to support the future of Montgomery County. Since its founding, MCCF has granted well over $8 million dollars to the Montgomery County Community. Large grants have been awarded to the Crawfordsville District Public Library, Boys and Girls Club, the Economic Development Committee, the Christian Nursing Service, MUFFY, the Montgomery County Historical Society, the Montgomery County Cultural Foundation, the Family Crisis Shelter, the Youth Service Bureau, and many, many more. Generally, if a proposal makes sense, if it is good for Montgomery County, and if funds are available, MCCF is interested in reviewing a proposal for funding. A properly completed grant application must be received in the MCCF office by noon on June 30th.
Requirements: Grant applications will be accepted from any new or existing nonprofit organization in Montgomery County. These organizations must be a tax-exempt organization whose purposes are described in Section 501(c) of the Internal Revenue Service Code. Grant applications will also be accepted from the three Montgomery County school corporations.
Geographic Focus: Indiana
Amount of Grant: $50,000 maximum
Date(s) Application is Due: Jun 30
Contact: Ann Malott, Executive Director; (765) 362-1267; email: ann@mccf-in.org
Internet: http://www.mccf-in.org/
Sponsor: Montgomery County Community Foundation
118 East Main Street, P.O. Box 334
Crawfordsville, IN 47933

MONY Foundation Grants **2215**
The foundation awards grants in its areas of interest, including after-school community service and volunteer programs for youth, New York, NY; meeting the essential after-school needs of children and teens at risk, Syracuse, NY; and meeting the essential needs of minority children nationwide (with local MONY sales office). Types of support include employee matching gifts, employee-related scholarships, general operating support, in-kind gifts, matching/challenge support, and program development. Contact headquarters or local office by mail to obtain guidelines.
Restrictions: Grants do not support private foundations; fully participating members of the United Way; religious, fraternal, athletic, social, or veterans' organizations; individuals; capital fund drives; endowments; or deficit financing.
Amount of Grant: $1500-$10,000 average
Contact: Grants Administrator, (212) 708-2468; fax: (212) 708-2001; email: lynn_stekas@mony.com
Internet: http://www.mony.com

Sponsor: MONY Foundation
1740 Broadway, Mail Drop 10-36
New York, NY 10019

Morgan Adams Foundation Grants **2216**

The Morgan Adams Foundation supports laboratory and clinical research in the area of pediatric cancer, with an emphasis on cancers of the brain and spine. The Foundation's particular interest is to provide seed and bridge grants for viable investigations not yet ripe enough for total funding by larger organizations. Additionally, the Foundation is able to partially fund translational studies, experimental therapeutics studies and/or Phase I and II clinical trials on a case by case basis. The Foundation is seeking out projects that are highly collaborative and/or multi-institutional in nature, hoping to facilitate through the strategic placement of funding, more rapid trials development in order to get the best possible treatment options into circulation with the greatest expediency possible. Through careful consideration and placement of its funding, the Foundation encourages and supports research intended to improve treatment effectiveness, improve treatment outcomes and improve the quality of life for children battling cancer.
Contact: Joan Slaughter, Executive Director; (303) 758-2130; fax: (303) 758-2134; email: joan@morganadamsfoundation.org or info@morganadamsfoundation.org
Internet: http://www.morganadamsfoundation.org/fundsBecomeHope.html
Sponsor: Morgan Adams Foundation
5303 E. Evans Avenue, Suite 202
Denver, CO 80222

Morris and Gwendolyn Cafritz Foundation Grants **2217**

The Morris & Gwendolyn Cafritz Foundation supports IRS-registered, tax-exempt, 501(c)3 organizations with a public charity status of 509(a)(1) or 509(a)(2) only. These organizations must serve residents in the District of Columbia, Prince George's and Montgomery Counties in Maryland, Arlington and Fairfax Counties, and the cities of Alexandria and Falls Church in Virginia. Grants are made in four program areas: Arts and Humanities, Community Services, Education and Health.
Requirements: Nonprofits serving residents in the District of Columbia, Prince George's and Montgomery Counties in Maryland, Arlington and Fairfax Counties, and the cities of Alexandria and Falls Church in Virginia may apply.
Restrictions: The Foundation does not generally fund the following projects: capital campaigns; endowments; multi-year grants; special events or tables for special events. Please also note, the Foundation does not fund: organizations that do not have 501(c)3 tax-exempt status with the IRS; private foundations; public charities with a non-private foundation status of 509(a)(3); individuals; organizations whose missions fall outside the Foundations funding priorities; organizations serving residents outside the Washington, DC metropolitan area.
Geographic Focus: District of Columbia; Maryland; Virginia
Samples: Theater Downtown, Washington, DC, $200,000 - for Staging Our Future Campaign (2008); Prince Georges Child Resource Center, Largo, MD, $25,000 - for Family Literacy Program (2008); Spanish Catholic Center, Washington, DC, $75,000 - for oral health treatment and education for low-income, uninsured immigrants (2008);
Date(s) Application is Due: Mar 1; Jul 1; Nov 1
Contact: Rose Ann Cleveland, Executive Director; (202) 223-3100; fax: (202) 296-7567; email: info@cafritzfoundation.org
Internet: http://www.cafritzfoundation.org/Applicant/app_guidelines.asp
Sponsor: Morris and Gwendolyn Cafritz Foundation
1825 K Sreet North West, Suite 1400
Washington, DC 20006

Morton K. and Jane Blaustein Foundation Grants **2218**

The foundation makes grants in the United States and abroad. Support is provided in the program areas of educational opportunity—to improve educational opportunities for underserved K-12 children, with preference given to initiatives in Baltimore and New York City; health and mental health—to improve health and mental health care for underserved people, with preference given to programs in Baltimore and New York City; and human rights—to advance fundamental human rights both in the United States and abroad, with preference given to grassroots efforts.
Requirements: Education and human services organizations in Maryland and New York are eligible to apply.
Restrictions: No support for fundraising events, or direct mail solicitations. Grants are not made to individuals.
Geographic Focus: Maryland; New York
Samples: Johns Hopkins U (Baltimore, MD)—for a fellowship endowment at the School of Nursing, $1 million (2005).
Contact: Grants Administrator, (410) 347-7205; email: info@blaufund.org
Internet: http://www.blaufund.org/foundations/mortonandjane_f.html
Sponsor: Morton K. and Jane Blaustein Foundation
10 E Baltimore Street, Suite 1111
Baltimore, MD 21202

Moses Cone-Wesley Long Community Health Foundation Grants **2219**

The foundation awards grants to eligible North Carolina organizations and programs in its areas of interest, including access to necessary health services, with particular emphasis on eliminating the barriers often encountered by persons in need; or wellness, with particular attention to physical activity, nutrition/obesity, substance abuse (including tobacco use prevention/cessation), responsible sexual behavior (especially the prevention of HIV/AIDS, STDs, and adolescent pregnancy), mental health, and injury prevention. Grants are awarded through the community health improvement fund ($50,000 maximum), direct foundation grants ($50,000 minimum), and special funding initiatives. In addition, the foundation funds organizational development and technical assistance projects that help communities build the capacity to help themselves improve the health of those in their communities. Funding priorities will be reviewed annually, and change is expected to occur periodically every three to five years. Applications and guidelines are available online.
Requirements: North Carolina nonprofit organizations, government agencies, schools, academic and research institutions, and collaborative consortia serving Greensboro, Winston-Salem, and High Point are eligible.
Geographic Focus: North Carolina
Samples: Nonprofit groups in the metropolitan Greensboro, NC, area (NC)—to support activities related to healthcare access, health promotion, injury prevention, mental health, physical activity and nutrition, responsible sexual behavior, and substance abuse treatment and prevention, $2 million (2005); Twenty-four nonprofit groups and government agencies (Greensboro, NC)—to support activities related to health-care access, health promotion, injury prevention, mental health, physical activity and nutrition, responsible sexual behavior, and substance-abuse treatment and prevention, $3.194 million (2004).
Contact: Program Director, (336) 832-9555; fax: (336) 832-9559; email: antonia.reaves@mosescone.com
Internet: http://www.mcwlhealthfoundation.org
Sponsor: Moses Cone-Wesley Long Community Health Foundation
P.O. Box 4426, 721 Green Valley Road, Suite 102
Greensboro, NC 27404-4426

Mount Zion Health Fund Grants **2220**

The fund provides grants predominantly in the San Francisco Bay area to nonprofit organizations in its areas of interest, including UCSF at Mount Zion and its affiliates, the Institute on Aging, and the Bay Area Jewish community. MZHF will consider proposals for grants for up to three years in duration. For multiyear grants, grant distributions will be contingent upon annual review of the grantee's progress toward defined expectations. There are no deadlines for submission. Applicants will generally receive a response within three months after submitting a complete proposal.
Requirements: California 501(c)3 tax-exempt organizations and organizations with 501(c)3 fiscal sponsors are eligible.
Restrictions: Grants are not awarded to support the personal benefit of individuals; endowments, annual appeals, membership drives, and fundraising events; or the reducation of operating deficits.
Geographic Focus: California
Samples: Bay Area Jewish Healing Ctr (San Francisco, CA)—for Jewish spiritual care, outreach, and education, $145,000 (2004); Homeless Prenatal Program (San Francisco, CA)—to provide care to homeless pregnant women and mothers, $15,000 (2004); Jewish Home (San Francisco, CA)—for general support of this geriatric center, $100,000 (2004); Life Tapes Project (San Francisco, CA)—to produce videotaped interviews designed to help relatives of people diagnosed with cancer, $40,000 (2004).
Amount of Grant: $5000-$100,000 generally
Date(s) Application is Due: Feb 15; Sep 15
Contact: Grants Administrator, (415) 750-4100; fax: (415) 495-6635; email: information@mzhf.org
Internet: http://sandbox.sfjcf.org/mountzion/grantapp
Sponsor: Mount Zion Health Fund
P.O. Box 194065
San Francisco, CA 94119-4065

MRC Career Establishment Grants **2221**

Career establishment grants provide research support for scientists and clinicians newly appointed to academic posts in medical schools, teaching hospitals, and universities who are at an early stage in the development of their research career and who can show that they have the potential to become the research team leaders of the future. A career establishment grant is intended to help award holders to establish themselves as independent scientists capable of winning support in open competition by the time the grant ends.
Requirements: An applicant must be in an established academic post in a university, medical school, teaching hospital, or similar institution; have a PhD or DPhil (for scientifically qualified applicants) or an MD (for medically qualified applicants); have at least three years postdoctoral research experience; be planning to make a long-term career in biomedical or health-related research; and make their initial application for a career establishment grant within the first three years of appointment to their first established academic post.
Restrictions: Scientists who do not hold an established academic appointment are not eligible to apply. Grants are not intended for researchers whose career in research is already well established, as demonstrated by their publication track record and their success in winning research funding.
Samples: Dr. C.R. Byrne, School of Biological Science, U of Manchester—for research on the relationship between fetal skin patterning and epidermal differentiation, @ L310,000.; Dr. S.L. Dickson, Physiological Laboratory, U of Cambridge—for research on hypothalamic circuits involved in body weight homeostasis, @L276,000.; Dr. S.J. Talbot, Department of Medical Microbiology, U of Edinburgh—for research on characterization of HHV-8 latency associated genes and the development of an animal model for studying tumorigenesis, @L476,000.
Contact: Michele Michalczuk, Research Management Group, 020 7636 5422; fax: 020 7436 6179; email: michele.michalczuk@headoffice.mrc.ac.uk

Internet: http://www.mrc.ac.uk/index/funding/funding-specific_schemes/funding-revised_grant_schemes.htm
Sponsor: Medical Research Council
20 Park Crescent
London W1B 1AL England

Ms. Foundation for Women Grants Program 2222
The foundation funds in the areas of economic security; health and safety; and girls, young women and leadership. It also supports organizing and public policy advocacy work that cuts across these issue areas. Guidelines are available on the Web site.
Requirements: Applicants must be tax-exempt groups and organizations. Applications, in five pages or less, should describe the organization or group; project for which funds are requested and why the organization is particularly suited to carry it out; community affected; general budget and project budget with specific amount being requested; other funding sources, presently and in the past; references; and a copy of IRS letter of determination of tax exemption. The foundation does not accept or reply to unsolicited requests that are not sent in response to an RFP.
Restrictions: Grants do not support cultural or media projects, publications, individuals, scholarships, university-based research, state agencies, religious institutions, or international programs.
Samples: Asian Immigrant Woman Advocates (Oakland, CA)—for general operating support, through its Public Voices, Public Policy—Realizing the Power of Women of Color grant program, $75,000 (2005); White House Project/Women's Leadership Fund (New York, NY)—to help more women become political leaders in the United States, $1 million (2004).
Contact: Program Contact, (212) 742-2300; fax: (212) 742-1653; email: info@ms.foundation.org
Internet: http://www.ms.foundation.org/wmspage.cfm?parm1=5
Sponsor: Ms. Foundation for Women
120 Wall Street, 33rd Floor
New York, NY 10005

Ms. Foundation Women and AIDS Fund Grants 2223
The Women and AIDS Fund supports and builds the capacity of community-based, peer-focused organizations led by women with HIV/AIDS. Proposals will be considered for efforts that seek to enhance organizational capacity around: advocacy programs that provide leadership training and skills building for HIV-positive women to increase their participation at the planning and decision-making level; advocacy programs that increase the understanding around the unique issues facing HIV-infected women to the general public and seek ways to enlist HIV-positive women to take action in seeking redress; and expanding HIV-positive women's access to currently available resources, such as clinical trials, new medications, and funding, that have often overlooked or underutilized women. Three-year general operating and project specific grants are awarded. Annual deadline dates may vary; contact program staff for exact dates.
Requirements: Grants are awarded to nonprofit groups working in the United States and Puerto Rico. The leadership of the specific project must be substantially made up of women with HIV/AIDS. Priority will be given to independent, women-focused organizations and programs.
Restrictions: Start-up projects in organizations that have no track record in women and AIDS will not be considered. The fund does not support videos, stand-alone conferences, individuals, scholarships, fundraising events, university-based research, or government agencies.
Amount of Grant: $10,000 per year
Contact: Grants Administrator, (212) 742-2300; fax: (212) 742-1653; email: info@ms.foundation.org
Internet: http://www.ms.foundation.org/wmspage.cfm?parm1=5
Sponsor: Ms. Foundation for Women
120 Wall Street, 33rd Floor
New York, NY 10005

MSSC Career Development Awards 2224
The awards further research into the cause, prevention, treatment, and cure of multiple sclerosis. Awards are intended to support independent research by the young, beginning researcher who holds a doctoral degree and intends to work full time at a Canadian school of medicine on research relevant to multiple sclerosis. Awards are normally made for three years with possible renewal.
Date(s) Application is Due: Oct 1
Contact: Jackie Munroe, Research Grants Manager, (416) 967-3001; fax: (416) 967-3040; email: jackie.munroe@mssociety.ca or info@mssoc.ca
Internet: http://www.mssociety.ca/en/research/researchfunding.htm
Sponsor: Multiple Sclerosis Society of Canada
175 Bloor St E, Suite 700, N Tower
Toronto, ON M4W 3R8 Canada

MSSC Postdoctoral Fellowships 2225
The fellowships further research into the cause, prevention, treatment, and cure of multiple sclerosis. These fellowships are intended for qualified scientists who have MDs or PhDs and intend to pursue further training in research related to multiple sclerosis. Fellowships are awarded for one year, renewable for up to three years if progress is deemed satisfactory.
Date(s) Application is Due: Oct 1
Contact: Jackie Munroe, Research Grants Manager, (416) 967-3001; fax: (416) 922-7538; email: jackie.munroe@mssociety.ca or info@mssoc.ca
Internet: http://www.mssociety.ca/en/research/researchfunding.htm
Sponsor: Multiple Sclerosis Society of Canada
175 Bloor St E, Suite 700, N Tower
Toronto, ON M4W 3R8 Canada

MSSC Research Grants 2226
The grants further independent research into the cause, prevention, treatment, and cure of multiple sclerosis. Research grants are awarded for projects covering a one- to three-year period. Research must be conducted in or under the authority of an institution approved by the society. Grants are to be used to cover research costs, including funding of equipment up to $C5000.
Samples: Drs. Albert Aguayo and Garth Bray, McGill U—for Neuron-Glia Interactions: Experimental Manipulation of Trophic Factors in Demyelination, $88,100.; Dr. Luanne Metz, U of Calgary—for The Cost of Multiple Sclerosis, $5050.
Date(s) Application is Due: Oct 1
Contact: Jackie Munroe, Research Grants Manager, (416) 967-3001; fax: (416) 922-7538; email: jackie.munroe@mssociety.ca or info@mssoc.ca
Internet: http://www.mssociety.ca/en/research/researchfunding.htm
Sponsor: Multiple Sclerosis Society of Canada
175 Bloor St E, Suite 700, N Tower
Toronto, ON M4W 3R8 Canada

MSSC Research Studentships 2227
Studentships are for doctoral candidates who require further training. The awards offer candidates an opportunity to acquire this training in specialized areas related to research into the cause, prevention, treatment, and/or cure of multiple sclerosis. Awards are for a maximum period of four years, renewable annually.
Date(s) Application is Due: Oct 1
Contact: Jackie Munroe, Research Grants Manager, (416) 967-3001; fax: (416) 922-7538; email: jackie.munroe@mssociety.ca or info@mssoc.ca
Internet: http://www.mssociety.ca/en/research/researchfunding.htm
Sponsor: Multiple Sclerosis Society of Canada
175 Bloor St E, Suite 700, N Tower
Toronto, ON M4W 3R8 Canada

Multiple Sclerosis Foundation Brighter Tomorrow Grants 2228
The goal of the grant is provide individuals with MS with goods or services (valued at up to $1000.00 per recipient) to improve their quality of life by enhancing safety, self-sufficiency, comfort, or well-being. Recipients have used the grant to purchase wheelchairs, walkers, eye glasses, computers, appliances, furniture, therapeutic equipment, hobby supplies, and for care repairs and various home modifications.
Requirements: To qualify, a person must be 18 years of age or older and diagnosed with MS, or the parent of a minor child diagnosed with MS, and be a permanent U.S. resident. They must not have any other means of fulfilling the need they express.
Amount of Grant: $1,000
Date(s) Application is Due: Oct 10
Contact: Program Services Department; (888) 673-6287 or (954) 776-6805; fax: (954) 351-0630; email: support@msfocus.org
Internet: http://www.msfocus.org/Brighter-Tomorrow-Grant.aspx
Sponsor: Multiple Sclerosis Foundation
6350 North Andrews Avenue
Fort Lauderdale, FL 33309-2130

Musculoskeletal Rehabilitation Fellowships 2229
The fellowship provides a unique opportunity for specialized training in clinical, education, and research aspects of musculoskeletal rehabilitation. Resources at the clinic are vast and include a multispecialty spine center, sports medicine center, biomechanics department, hand center, arthritis clinic, pain clinic, and orthopedic and general musculoskeletal rehabilitation. Fellows will have the opportunity to assist in medical coverage of sporting events in southeastern Minnesota to gain musculoskeletal management skills. Multiple educational opportunities are available, including the teaching of medical students and residents. Dedicated research time can be allotted with faculty mentorship and integrated use of other departments. Appointments and application deadlines vary each year.
Requirements: Candidate must have successfully completed an accredited residency program in physical medicine and rehabilitation and be board eligible or board certified.
Date(s) Application is Due: Aug 30
Contact: Cindy Weber, (507) 284-2946; fax: (507) 284-3431; email: pmreduc@mayo.edu
Internet: http://www.mayo.edu/msgme/physmed-musculo-rch.html
Sponsor: Mayo Clinic
200 First St SW
Rochester, MN 55905

NAF Fellowships 2230
The foundation supports new and innovative studies that are relevant to the cause, pathogenesis, or treatment of the hereditary or sporadic ataxias. Postdoctoral fellowship awards serve as a bridge from postdoctoral positions to junior faculty positions. The award will permit individuals to spend an additional third year in a postdoctoral position and increase chances to establish an independent ataxia research program. Letters of Intent should arrive by August 15, with full proposals due by September 15. Application and guidelines are available online.

Requirements: Applicants should have completed at least one year of postdoctoral training, but not more than two at the time of application, and should have shown a commitment to research in the field of ataxia.
Restrictions: Indirect costs are not allowed.
Amount of Grant: $35,000 average
Date(s) Application is Due: Aug 15; Sep 15
Contact: Administrator; (763) 553-0020; fax: (763) 553-0167; email: naf@ataxia.org
Internet: http://www.ataxia.org/research/ataxia-research-grants.aspx
Sponsor: National Ataxia Foundation
2600 Fernbrook Lane, Suite 119
Minneapolis, MN 55447-4752

NAF Kyle Bryant Translational Research Award **2231**
The Friedreich's Ataxia Research Alliance (FARA) and the National Ataxia Foundation (NAF) invite proposals, under a competitive Request for Applications (RFA) process, to award a grant focusing on pre-clinical investigations that will facilitate clinical trials for Friedreich's Ataxia. Funding will be for one year. The total award is limited to $120,000 (direct costs only). The Foundation is requesting that applicants submit Letters of Intent by July 15, and full applications by July 31.
Requirements: Each application must include a project objectives and lay summary that will be used as FARA and NAF wishes and should not contain confidential information. The other parts of the grant application are considered confidential and will only be released to review committee, FARA and NAF staff and Board of Directors. Applications will be accepted from for-profit organizations, non-profit organizations, public or private institutions, and foreign institutions.
Amount of Grant: $120,000 maximum in direct costs
Date(s) Application is Due: Jul 15; Jul 31
Contact: Jennifer Farmer, Grant Manager; (610) 246-9017; email: jen.farmer@cureFA.org;; Susan Hagen; email: (763) 553-0020; susan@ataxia.org
Internet: http://www.ataxia.org/research/ataxia-research-grants.aspx
Sponsor: National Ataxia Foundation
2600 Fernbrook Lane, Suite 119
Minneapolis, MN 55447-4752

NAF Research Grants **2232**
NAF research grants are for new and innovative studies that are relevant to the cause, pathogenesis or treatment of the hereditary or sporadic ataxias. Due to the larger availability of funding for Ataxia-Telangiectasia (A-T), those research proposals will receive a lower priority. However, a higher ranking will be given to those Ataxia-Telangiectasia research studies which lend themselves to an overall better understanding of the ataxia process. Research grants are offered primarily as seed monies to assist investigators in the early or pilot phase of their studies and as additional support for ongoing investigations on demonstration of need. It is hoped that these studies will be further developed to attract future funding from other sources. Grants are awarded for one year only. If funding for a second year is desired then another grant application should be submitted for that funding period. The average funds granted will be up to $15,000, but funding may be considered for up to $30,000 for projects deserving special consideration.
Restrictions: Indirect costs will not be funded.
Amount of Grant: $5,000-$15,000 average; $30,000 for special projects
Date(s) Application is Due: Aug 15
Contact: Administrator; (763) 553-0020; fax: (763) 553-0167; email: naf@ataxia.org
Internet: http://www.ataxia.org/research/ataxia-research-grants.aspx
Sponsor: National Ataxia Foundation
2600 Fernbrook Lane, Suite 119
Minneapolis, MN 55447-4752

NAF Young Investigator Awards **2233**
The purpose of this award is to encourage young clinical and scientific investigators to pursue a career in the field of ataxia research. It is the foundation's hope that ataxia research will be invigorated by the work of young, talented individuals supported by stable multi-year funding. This award will be made to the sponsoring institution and will be used as salary support or for direct research expenses. The sponsoring institution must agree in writing to the following provision: a clinical investigator (MD) must be free to allocate a minimum of half time for a project; a non-clinician investigator (PhD) must allocate a minimum of three-fourths time for the project. Periodic progress reports will be required. Applicants are asked to submit a brief email with the intentions to apply for NAF funding, including a full title of the research proposal, on or before August 1. Deadline for full application is September 1.
Requirements: Candidates must have attained the MD or PhD degree, and have an appointment as a junior faculty member. Clinicians must have finished their residency no more than five years prior to applying, and investigators must have completed their postdoctoral training no more than five years prior to applying.
Restrictions: Individuals at the associate professor level are not eligible. Awards are for direct costs only, not for indirect costs or institutional overhead.
Amount of Grant: $50,000 per year for two years
Date(s) Application is Due: Aug 1; Sep 1
Contact: Administrator; (763) 553-0020; fax: (763) 553-0167; email: naf@ataxia.org
Internet: http://www.ataxia.org/research/ataxia-research-grants.aspx
Sponsor: National Ataxia Foundation
2600 Fernbrook Lane, Suite 119
Minneapolis, MN 55447-4752

Nancy R. Gelman Foundation Breast Cancer Seed Grants **2234**
The program awards seed grants to fund projects aimed at improving outcomes for women with breast cancer. Proposed projects must: demonstrate a need for start-up, interim, or supplemental funding for a one-year period beginning April 1; not already be funded by other sources (projects that represent a clear new initiative extending beyond the scope of a currently funded project are permissible); and prospectively state an objective outcome measure that will be used to gauge project success. Types of projects seed grants might fund include: a mentored summer fellowship for a medical student to work in a laboratory, gaining experience in basic research on breast cancer mechanisms or therapies; community-based efforts to promote breast cancer awareness and early detection among populations at increased risk; development of information materials to encourage appropriate screening and to help guide newly diagnosed patients, or those whose cancer has recurred, through the challenging maze of treatment options; fledgling research studies to pave the way for further advances in breast cancer therapy; quality initiatives in cancer or emergency department nursing units to improve care for patients with breast cancer; and a summer research project studying end-of-life care for breast cancer patients and making recommendations to hospitals and hospice organizations to improve care. The application and guidelines are available online.
Amount of Grant: $1,500 maximum
Date(s) Application is Due: Aug 5
Contact: Michael Gelman, President; (206) 441-7225; email: michael@nrgf.org or grants@nrgf.org
Internet: http://www.nrgf.org/grants.html
Sponsor: Nancy R. Gelman Foundation
1133 Broadway, Suite 706
New York, NY 10010

NAPNAP Foundation Elaine Gelman Scholarship **2235**
The purpose of this annual scholarship is to support the education of a nurse practitioner student who demonstrates the ability to articulate and follow through an innovative solution through clinical competence, academic achievement and involvement in political activism relating to a pediatric health care issue. Preference is given to applicants in an accredited PNP program or those with interest or experience in health policy or advocacy. The recipient will receive an award up to $1000 if all criteria are met. The recipient will be recognized in The Pediatric Nurse Practitioner newsletter and again at the Annual NAPNAP Conference Awards Breakfast.
Requirements: Applicant must be a full or part time NP Student enrolled in an accredited NP program with an expected graduation date of two years or less. Applicants must submit two (2) letters of support from professional colleagues addressing the applicant's clinical competence, academic achievement and involvement in political activism relating to health care issues.
Amount of Grant: $1,000 maximum
Date(s) Application is Due: Jun 30
Contact: Dolores Jones, Director; (856) 857-9700; fax (856) 857-1600; email: djones@napnap.org or info@napnap.org
Internet: http://www.napnap.org/PNPResources/research/AvailGrantsScholarships.aspx
Sponsor: National Association of Pediatric Nurse Associates and Practitioners
20 Brace Road, Suite 200
Cherry Hill, NJ 08034-2634

NAPNAP Foundation Graduate Student Research Grant **2236**
The program supports research by graduate students currently enrolled in a pediatric nurse practitioner program. The purposes of the award are to: encourage graduate students to participate in the research process; and stimulate interest in research regarding children and their families. The recipient of the award will be invited to participate at the research presentation session at the annual conference in the spring following the award. Application and guidelines are available online.
Requirements: The graduate student must be a current member of NAPNAP.
Samples: Cathy Woodward—for Routine Chest Radiographs Post Chest Tube Removal in Children, $1,000 (2006-07); Sheri Vlam—for ADHD Assessment Methods Used by APRNs, $500 (2003-04); Jacqueline Rychnovsky—for A Pediatric Perspective of Maternal Fatigue Across the First Ten Weeks Postpartum, $1,000 (2002-03).
Amount of Grant: $1,000
Date(s) Application is Due: Apr 1
Contact: Dolores Jones, Director; (856) 857-9700; fax (856) 857-1600; email: djones@napnap.org or info@napnap.org
Internet: http://www.napnap.org/PNPResources/research/AvailGrantsScholarships.aspx
Sponsor: National Association of Pediatric Nurse Associates and Practitioners
20 Brace Road, Suite 200
Cherry Hill, NJ 08034-2633

NAPNAP Foundation Innovative Health Care Small Grant **2237**
The Innovative Health Care Small Grant Program is designed to encourage NAPNAP members and chapters to develop and implement innovative, feasible, and cost-effective programs to improve children's health services. These projects are intended to improve the accessibility of health services to underserved children and those in need of health care; enhance family education regarding the importance of health care maintenance and preventive care; increase utilization rates for children without services or who are underserved; and encourage providers to pursue new mechanisms in delivery of health services to children in need. Guidelines are available online.
Requirements: Each application must be submitted by a national NAPNAP member (or group of members) or by a NAPNAP chapter; represent a local initiative that is community-based, family-centered, and culturally appropriate; describe the project's

target population; offer innovative or improved access to health education and/or health care services for children; clearly state project goal; define measurable objectives of the project and identify those activities that lead to their achievement; develop a simple evaluation mechanism reflecting extent to which goal and objectives have been achieved; and include a budget for the project (monies may not be used for salary, consultation, or gifts).
Amount of Grant: $4,000 maximum
Date(s) Application is Due: Sep 15
Contact: Dolores Jones, Director; (856) 857-9700; fax (856) 857-1600; email: djones@napnap.org or info@napnap.org
Internet: http://www.napnap.org/PNPResources/research/AvailGrantsScholarships.aspx
Sponsor: National Association of Pediatric Nurse Associates and Practitioners
20 Brace Road, Suite 200
Cherry Hill, NJ 08034-2633

NAPNAP Foundation McNeil Grant-in-Aid **2238**
The purpose of the NAPNAP Foundation is to support nursing research and clinical practice efforts that contribute to the improvement of the quality of life for children and their families. Through the generosity of grants from the McNeil Consumer Healthcare Division of McNeil-PPC, Inc., the NAPNAP Foundation offers up to $5,000 for members and one student to attend the annual conference.
Amount of Grant: $5,000
Date(s) Application is Due: Oct 4
Contact: Dolores Jones, Director; (856) 857-9700; fax (856) 857-1600; email: djones@napnap.org or info@napnap.org
Internet: http://www.napnap.org/PNPResources/research/AvailGrantsScholarships.aspx
Sponsor: National Association of Pediatric Nurse Associates and Practitioners
20 Brace Road, Suite 200
Cherry Hill, NJ 08034-2633

NAPNAP Foundation McNeil PNP Scholarships **2239**
NAPNAP will award two annual McNeil Scholarships to students enrolled in pediatric nurse practitioner programs. Scholarships for each academic year are awarded for both the fall and spring semesters/quarters. Individuals who are enrolled in a program within the current academic year will be reviewed. Students who begin a program in January may also apply the following May if clinical course work will continue into the next academic year. Scholarship recipients will be determined by NAPNAP and notified within two months of the application deadline. The recipients will be formally recognized at NAPNAP's annual conference. Airfare and conference registration fees will be paid by NAPNAP. Instructions and application are available online.
Requirements: Applicant must be a registered nurse with at least three years previous work experience in pediatrics; have documented acceptance at a recognized PNP program; have no previous formal pediatric nurse practitioner education; demonstrate financial need, based on submission of information regarding resources; and state rationale for seeking PNP education that is consistent with NAPNAP's mission statement. In addition, students must maintain the following: full-time status (nine or more credit hours/semester) while in PNP program; GPA of 3.0 or higher; NAPNAP membership; provide NAPNAP with ongoing accounts regarding student status, as requested.
Amount of Grant: $1,500 scholarship
Date(s) Application is Due: Apr 30
Contact: Dolores Jones, Director; (856) 857-9700; fax (856) 857-1600; email: djones@napnap.org or info@napnap.org
Internet: http://www.napnap.org/index.cfm?page=13&sec=102
Sponsor: National Association of Pediatric Nurse Associates and Practitioners
20 Brace Road, Suite 200
Cherry Hill, NJ 08034-2634

NAPNAP Foundation McNeil Rural and Underserved Scholarships **2240**
Through the support of McNeil Consumer Healthcare Division of McNeil-PPC, Inc., NAPNAP members can apply for the McNeil Rural & Underserved Scholarship. This scholarship of up to $10,000 will cover a full academic year for a PNP student who will provide primary care to children and families in rural areas after graduating. The deadline for applications is June 15.
Requirements: To be eligible for the scholarship, applicants must meet the following criteria: plan on practicing in a rural or under served geographical region for the first two years after PNP education completed; be a registered nurse who has completed at least 2 semesters or quarters as defined by the university; show documented acceptance at a recognized Master's Degree program; have no previous formal pediatric nurse practitioner education; demonstrate financial need, based on submission of information regarding resources; and state rational for seeking PNP education that is consistent with NAPNAP's mission statement. In addition, students must maintain the following: full-time status (9 or more credit hours/semester) while in PNP program; G.P.A. of 3.0 or higher; NAPNAP membership; and provide NAPNAP with ongoing accounts regarding student status.
Amount of Grant: $10,000
Date(s) Application is Due: Jun 15
Contact: Dolores Jones, Director; (856) 857-9700; fax (856) 857-1600; email: djones@napnap.org or info@napnap.org
Internet: http://www.napnap.org/PNPResources/research/AvailGrantsScholarships.aspx
Sponsor: National Association of Pediatric Nurse Associates and Practitioners
20 Brace Road, Suite 200
Cherry Hill, NJ 08034-2634

NAPNAP Foundation Nursing Research Grants **2241**
The foundation supports nursing research efforts that contribute to the improvement of the quality of life for children and their families. The foundation is primarily interested in the following areas of research: impact of nurse practitioner role in healthcare delivery; development/implementation of innovative methods for delivery of health care services in the areas of school health, community health, behavior and development, adolescent health, and chronic disease management; health care problems of children and their families; advanced nursing practice problems and issues; exploratory/evaluative research of PNP education and credentialing; and educational programs and materials for healthcare providers and/or children and families. Up to two grants will be awarded annually.
Amount of Grant: $2,500
Date(s) Application is Due: Apr 1
Contact: Dolores Jones, Director; (856) 857-9700; fax (856) 857-1600; email: djones@napnap.org or info@napnap.org
Internet: http://www.napnap.org/index.cfm?page=13&sec=102
Sponsor: National Association of Pediatric Nurse Associates and Practitioners
20 Brace Road, Suite 200
Cherry Hill, NJ 08034-2633

NAPNAP Foundation Reckitt Benckiser Student Scholarship **2242**
Through a grant from Reckitt Benckiser Inc., the NAPNAP Foundation will award two grants of $1,600 to a Pediatric Nurse Practitioner Student to allow for attendance at the NAPNAP Annual Meeting in April. The postmark deadline for applications is November 2. The grant recipient will be determined by the NAPNAP Foundation and the recipient will be formally recognized at NAPNAP's Annual Conference.
Requirements: To be eligible for the grant, applicants must meet the following criteria: be a registered nurse and a graduate student who has completed at least 1 semester of graduate studies in a Pediatric Nurse Practitioner Program; provide documentation from the PNP Program Coordinator/Director that the student is enrolled in a recognized program of study leading to completion of qualifications for education and practice as a PNP; and be a member of NAPNAP.
Amount of Grant: $1,600
Date(s) Application is Due: Nov 2
Contact: Dolores Jones, Director; (856) 857-9700; fax (856) 857-1600; email: djones@napnap.org or info@napnap.org
Internet: http://www.napnap.org/PNPResources/research/AvailGrantsScholarships.aspx
Sponsor: National Association of Pediatric Nurse Associates and Practitioners
20 Brace Road, Suite 200
Cherry Hill, NJ 08034-2634

NAPNAP Foundation Shourd Parks Immunization Project Small Grants **2243**
The NAPNAP Foundation is pleased to offer the Shourd-Parks Immunization Project Small Grant, as part of a national effort to improve health care for infants through young adults. Biennially, a $500 grant will be awarded to a NAPNAP member or chapter. To keep grant activities consistent with the goals of NAPNAP and the NAPNAP Foundation, grant applications should focus on improving health care in the area of child, adolescent and/or young adult immunizations. Four copies of the proposal and the application should be mailed to the NAPNAP National Office and postmarked no later than September 15.
Requirements: Each NAPNAP Foundation application should meet at least one of the following: 1) Improve access to immunizations for children and/or adolescents in any health care setting. 2) Strengthen existing or new health education programs in the area of immunizations. 3) Strengthen existing or new methods in the delivery of immunizations. 4) Incorporates NAPNAP's and NAPNAP Foundation priorities. Each application must meet these specific requirements: 1) Be submitted by a national NAPNAP member (or group of members) or by a NAPNAP Chapter. 2) Describe the project's target population. 3) Clearly state the project purpose, goal(s) or aim(s). 4) Define one measurable outcome for the project. 5) Develop an evaluation mechanism for the one outcome. 6) Include a brief budget.
Amount of Grant: $500
Date(s) Application is Due: Sep 15
Contact: Dolores Jones, Director; (856) 857-9700; fax (856) 857-1600; email: djones@napnap.org or info@napnap.org
Internet: http://www.napnap.org/PNPResources/research/AvailGrantsScholarships.aspx
Sponsor: National Association of Pediatric Nurse Associates and Practitioners
20 Brace Road, Suite 200
Cherry Hill, NJ 08034-2633

NAPNAP Foundation Wyeth Pediatric Immunization Grant **2244**
These grants will give NAPNAP members the opportunity to develop innovative programs to enhance the immunization rates in their communities. Examples of the ways in which a grant could be used include: parent education/awareness activities or materials; provider education workshops on current vaccines topics and true contra-indications to vaccinating; development of clinic policies to prevent missed opportunities; strategies for immunization registries; community outreach endeavors to assess and eliminate barriers to immunizations translation services for diverse communities; and evaluation research on effectiveness of vaccine programs to increase immunization rates. Two grants of $2,500 each and one grant of $7,500 are available.
Requirements: NAPNAP members are eligible to apply.
Amount of Grant: $2,500-$7,500
Date(s) Application is Due: Dec 15

Contact: Dolores Jones, Director; (856) 857-9700; fax (856) 857-1600; email: djones@napnap.org or info@napnap.org
Internet: http://www.napnap.org/PNPResources/research/AvailGrantsScholarships.aspx
Sponsor: National Association of Pediatric Nurse Associates and Practitioners
20 Brace Road, Suite 200
Cherry Hill, NJ 08034-2633

Narcolepsy Network Seed Grants **2245**
The network supports medical/scientific research of narcolepsy and awards seed/pilot grants in the following categories: tissue banks—facilitation of acquisition, storage, or utilization of tissue; subjects—addition of subjects with narcolepsy to an ongoing or recently completed study of some other condition; food—as regards understanding of short-term adverse effects in cataplectic-narcoleptic persons of some aspect of food consumption; and comorbidities—the sesarch for coexsisting structural or physiological alterations in persons with narcolepsy, which along with alterations in sleep reflect narcolepsy susceptibility gene(s). The network anticipates awarding one grant in each category. Complete application information is available online. Annual deadline dates may vary; contact program staff for exact dates.
Requirements: 501(c)3 tax-exempt organizations are eligible. A principal investigator with the MD, PhD, or DO degree must originate or be responsible for the projectt.
Amount of Grant: $8000
Date(s) Application is Due: Sep 15
Contact: Grants Administrator, (401) 667-2523; fax: (401) 633-6567; email: narnet@narcolepsynetwork.org
Internet: http://www.narcolepsynetwork.org
Sponsor: Narcolepsy Network
P.O. Box 294
Pleasantville, NY 10570

NARSAD Distinguished Investigator Award **2246**
The award supports established scientists who maintain peer-reviewed competitively funded scientific programs. This program is intended to stimulate new approaches and projects from senior investigators, rather than extending current work of established investigators. Research must be relevant to schizophrenia; major affective disorders; or other serious mental illnesses, including bipolar disease, borderline disorders with depression or suicide, or research with children. Applicants must demonstrate that, without new funds, the proposed work is not feasible.
Requirements: The researcher must be at the full professor academic rank (or equivalent), maintain a laboratory, and be affiliated with a university or research institution.
Amount of Grant: $100,000 maximum
Date(s) Application is Due: May 15
Contact: Audra Moran, Director, Research Grants Program, (800) 829-8289 or (516) 829-5576; email: amoran@narsad.org
Internet: http://www.narsad.org/research/apply
Sponsor: National Alliance for Research on Schizophrenia and Depression
60 Cutter Mill Road, Suite 404
Great Neck, NY 11021

NARSAD Independent Investigator Award **2247**
The program provides up to two years of support to enable the scientist at the academic level of associate professor or equivalent, who has won national competitive support as a principal investigator, to facilitate innovative research opportunities. Research must be relevant to schizophrenia, major affective disorders, or other serious mental illnesses, including bipolar disease, borderline disorders with depression or suicide, and research with children. The award is not renewable; applicants may reapply for a second award immediately following the completion of the first award, pending they have fulfilled all requirements for the first award. A maximum of two NARSAD Independent Investigator Awards may be received.
Requirements: The researcher must be at the associate professor academic rank (or equivalent), have received national competitive support as a principal investigator, and be affiliated with a university or research institution.
Amount of Grant: $50,000 maximum per year; up to $100,000 for two years
Date(s) Application is Due: Mar 6
Contact: Audra Moran, (800) 829-8289 or (516) 829-5576; fax: (516) 487-6930; email: amoran@narsad.org or grants@narsad.org
Internet: http://www.narsad.org/research/apply/independent
Sponsor: National Alliance for Research on Schizophrenia and Depression
60 Cutter Mill Road, Suite 404
Great Neck, NY 11021

National 4-H Healthy Lifestyles Grants **2248**
The program is designed to help communities create educational programs and public awareness that will confront the climbing trends of obesity. The council, with funding from Kraft Foods, offers local grants to develop or expand innovative and fun programs that partner youth ages five to 12 with adults to reverse these trends. Applicants must have demonstrated interest and experience in dealing with the issues of obesity, fitness, nutrition, and healthy lifestyles. Grants are intended for direct programmatic activities only. Download application online.
Restrictions: Grants do not support indirect costs/overhead (e.g., rent, utilities).
Amount of Grant: $7500
Date(s) Application is Due: Jan 14
Contact: Grants Administrator, (301) 961-2800; fax: (301) 961-2894; email: info@fourhcouncil.edu
Internet: http://www.fourhcouncil.edu/GrantsHealthyLifestyles.aspx
Sponsor: National 4-H Council
7100 Connecticut Avenue
Chevy Chase, MD 20815

National Blood Foundation Research Grant Program **2249**
Research grants support investigator-initiated original research in blood banking and transfusion medicine. Projects dealing with all aspects of blood banking, including transfusion sciences, blood banking administration, and education will be considered. Priority will be given to the following areas: transfusion medicine and immunology, hematology, immunohematology, infectious diseases, and medicine administration. Preference will be given to innovative new projects; applications from junior and less well-established investigators are encouraged. Grants will be awarded for periods of one or two years. Applications are available on the Web site.
Requirements: Preference is given to new investigators in the field. There is a $150 application fee.
Amount of Grant: $65,000 maximum
Date(s) Application is Due: Dec 13
Contact: Program Contact, (301) 215-6552; fax: (301) 907-6895; email: nbf@aabb.org
Internet: http://www.aabb.org/about_the_aabb/nbf/nbf2.htm#3
Sponsor: National Blood Foundation
8101 Glenbrook Road
Bethesda, MD 20814-2749

National City Corporation Contributions Grants **2250**
National City has been providing diversified financial services to its customers for more than 150 years. Its success depends on the prosperity and development of the communities in which it has a presence. As a conscientious corporate citizen, National City recognizes its responsibility to its communities in which we live, learn, and work. Its objective is to support organizations that enhance educational, economic, and cultural priorities of its local communities and to provide for the health and welfare of all citizens. Such support may be in the form of cash donations, in-kind gifts or services, and employee volunteers. To accomplish its goal and to be responsive to local community needs and priorities, each affiliate bank receives and acts upon grant requests from organizations located only in the respective area in the states of Ohio, Pennsylvania, Michigan, Illinois, Indiana, Kentucky and Missouri. National City seeks to maximize the benefits of its contributions by giving to entities which have widespread corporate, foundation and community support.
Requirements: Requests for contributions must be in writing and should include: copy of letter from IRS granting tax-exempt not-for-profit 501(C)(3) status; statement of purpose; history of the organization; listing of current board members, showing an active and responsible governing body serving without compensation, holding regular meetings and exercising administrative control; description of program activities and goals; complete budget for the project or period; detailed annual budget translating program plans into financial terms, showing that current fund raising is directed to a wide base in the community; annual audit prepared by a certified accountant showing all revenues and expenditures in reasonable detail; any other information that will aid the Charitable Contributions Committee in making its decision. Each state has it's own Public Affairs office (which is dedicated to grant proposals) see website for the address of the office in your area.
Restrictions: Grant requests available to organizations located only in the respective area in the states of Ohio, Pennsylvania, Michigan, Illinois, Indiana, Kentucky and Missouri. Requests will be acted upon on a quarterly basis following the receipt of all necessary information.
Geographic Focus: Illinois; Indiana; Kentucky; Michigan; Missouri; Ohio; Pennsylvania
Contact: Joanne Clark, Senior Vice President; (216) 222-2000; fax: (216) 222-2670; email: joanne.clark@nationalcity.com
Internet: https://www.nationalcity.com/about-us/community/community-relations/pages/charitable-giving.asp
Sponsor: National City Corporation
1900 E. 9th Street, LOC-2157
Cleveland, OH 44114-3484

National Dairy Promotion and Research Board Scholarships **2251**
Scholarships are awarded annually to up to 19 students enrolled in college/university programs that emphasize dairy food science, technology, or marketing. Scholarships are awarded based upon outstanding academic achievement; a commitment to a career in a dairy food-related discipline; and demonstrated leadership, initiative, and integrity. Application forms are available on the Web site.
Requirements: Applications must be accompanied by an official transcript of all completed university credits and a letter of recommendation from a faculty member familiar with the applicant's scholastic performance. Sophomore, junior, and/or senior undergraduate students enrolled in college/university programs that emphasize dairy and majoring in communications, public relations, journalism, marketing, business, economics, nutrition, food science or ag education are eligible to apply.
Amount of Grant: $1500
Date(s) Application is Due: May 31
Contact: Scholarship Administrator, (847) 803-2000 ext 255 or (800) 853-2479
Internet: http://www.dairycheckoff.com/DairyCheckoff/about/scholarship.htm
Sponsor: National Dairy Council
10255 W Higgins Road, Suite 900
Rosemont, IL 60018-5616

National Emergency Medicine Association Grants 2252

The association supports projects that foster the development and delivery of quality emergency services, with special emphasis given to heart attack and stroke. Proposals should address education or direct services to victims. Also to receive consideration are childrens' emergency issues and projects teaching good parenting skills. Programs must be related to health and emergency issues and prevention or diminishing of trauma events. Types of support include capital, program development, research, and training grants. Applications are accepted on an ongoing basis.

Samples: Beebe Medical Ctr (Lewes, DE)—to improve its trauma care services for people in southern Delaware, $83,778.; National Stroke Assoc (Englewood, CO)—to update a publication that educates emergency room physicians about emergency evaluation and treatment of stroke victims, $17,000.

Contact: Grants Administrator, (410) 494-0300; fax: (410) 494-0725; email: info@nemahealth.org

Internet: http://www.nemahealth.org/organization/grants.htm

Sponsor: National Emergency Medicine Association
306 W Joppa Road
Baltimore, MD 21204

National Headache Foundation Research Grants 2253

The National Headache Foundation is interested in research protocols that are objectively sound and whose results can, when published in the medical literature, contribute to the better understanding and treatment of headache and pain. Grants may be used for the purchasing of supplies needed for the study (chemical or pharmacological reagents, laboratory animals, tissue culture materials. forms, etc.) and for costs related to the recruiting of patients, data analysis, interpreting or reading results, etc. Applications are available online, and are due by December 1.

Requirements: Funds for a research project approved by the National Headache Foundation are awarded to the individual who is the principal investigator of the study. The funds are sent to the institution that employs the PI but designated for the PI and the approved study.

Restrictions: Grants from the NHF will not cover costs including overhead, salaries (payment for technicians, others collecting data, administrative services, etc.), purchasing of equipment, rent or other indirect expenses.

Date(s) Application is Due: Dec 1

Contact: Carolyn Smith, Executive Assistant; (312) 274-2652 or (312) 274-2650; fax: (312) 640-9049; email: info@headaches.org

Internet: http://www.headaches.org/For_Professionals/Research_Grants

Sponsor: National Headache Foundation
820 N. Orleans, Suite 217
Chicago, IL 60610-3132

National Headache Foundation Seymour Diamond Clinical Fellowship in Headache Education 2254

The one-year fellowship is intended to encourage, provide for, and engage physicians in the clinical management of headache patients. The program is an individualized hands-on approach at a headache clinic mutually selected by the committee and the applicant. The objectives are to develop competence in the management of common and complex headache problems, to publish a research paper keyed to the treatment of headache, and to prepare the applicant for a career in treating headache patients. The participating institution will be a specialized facility dedicated primarily to headache management, with facilities for inpatient and outpatient treatment. Up to 80 percent of the fellow's time will be clinical, 20 percent study/research.

Requirements: Applicant will be a graduate of an approved U.S. medical school and be four years or more postgraduate.

Amount of Grant: $40,000 stipend

Date(s) Application is Due: Feb 1

Contact: Fellowship Selection Committee; (312) 274-2650; fax: (312) 640-9049; email: info@headaches.org

Internet: http://www.headaches.org/For_Professionals/Fellowship_Grants

Sponsor: National Headache Foundation
820 N. Orleans, Suite 217
Chicago, IL 60610-3132

National Heart Foundation of New Zealand Grants 2255

The foundation is dedicated to the reduction of premature death and disability from heart and circulatory disease, including stroke. Types of support include research project grants, training fellowships enabling New Zealand cardiology trainees to study abroad, senior fellowships, and a chair in cardiovascular studies.

Contact: Program Contact, (09) 571 9191; fax: (09) 571 9190; email: info@nhf.org.nz

Internet: http://www.nhf.org.nz/index.asp?PageID=2145820407

Sponsor: National Heart Foundation of New Zealand
P.O. Box 17160
Greenlane, Auckland 1130 New Zealand

National Lottery Community Fund Grants 2256

The organization operates in the United Kingdom and internationally and awards grants to charitable, benevolent, and philanthropic organizations. The organization particularly wants to support projects that help people who face disadvantage that is severe, long-term, difficult to tackle, or who face a combination of needs. Grants support projects that try to prevent or reduce, as far as possible, future disadvantage.

Contact: Gerald Oppenheim, Director, 44-020-7-747-5299; fax: 44-020-7-747-5214; email: enquiries.res@biglotteryfund.org.uk

Internet: http://www.community-fund.org.uk/about-us/our-grants-programmes/index.html

Sponsor: National Lottery Community Fund
Saint Vincent House, 16 Suffolk Street
London SW1Y 4NL United Kingdom

National MPS Society Grants 2257

The society awards research grants and fellowships to qualified individuals to promote medical research in the fields of mucopolyssaccharidosis (MPS) and mucolipidosis (ML). The program supports MPS (I, II, III IV, V, and VI) research, ML II/III research, and general MPS research. Grants and fellowships are awarded for a two-year period. Application forms and guidelines are available online.

Requirements: Qualified medical researchers are eligible.

Samples: Mount Sinai School of Medicine (New York, NY)—to support the work of Caleogera Simanaro, for medical research on bone and joint diseases in mucopolysaccharide diseases, $100,000 (2005); Iowa State U (IA)—to support the work of Matthew Ellinwood, for medical research on Sanfilippo syndrome, a genetic disease that prevents the normal degeneration of cells and progressively complicates cognitive and physical function, $60,000 (2005).

Amount of Grant: $30,000 per year

Date(s) Application is Due: May 1

Contact: Barbara Wedehase, Executive Director, (207) 947-1445; fax: (207) 990-3074; email: barbara@mpssociety.org

Internet: http://www.mpssociety.org/grants.html

Sponsor: National MPS Society
P.O. Box 736
Bangor, ME 04402-0736

National Patient Safety Foundation Patient Safety Research Grants 2258

NPSF seeks to stimulate new, innovative projects directed toward enhancing patient safety in the United States. Its objective is to promote studies leading to prevention of human errors, system errors, and any forms of preventable injuries in health care and the adverse consequences to patients that may result. In the first stage of a two-stage application process, letters of intent (LOIs) are solicited for research and development that is broadly related to identifying the causes of preventable injuries and errors and/or developing prevention strategies and methods to implement them. From these LOIs, a subset will be selected for preparation of a more detailed proposal. Highest priority is given to investigations that apply to a broad spectrum of problems and patients and that are clearly relevant to patient safety. Priority is also given to projects with the promise of improved methods of patient safety with a defined and direct path to implementation into health care. Areas of research include, but are not limited to: identifying, reporting on, analyzing, or otherwise assisting in the understanding of the causes of preventable injuries in health care; enhancing understanding of the impact of the changes in health care on the system, on human error, and on safety; developing methods for avoiding preventable injuries; assessing the cost effectiveness of techniques designed to increase patient safety; and developing educational tools and/or training materials designed to alter behaviors to prevent errors and increase safety. Innovation and creativity are strongly encouraged, as are cross-disciplinary research teams. Priority will be given to topics that do not have other available sources for funding. LOIs are due July 1; full applications are due December 2.

Requirements: Awards are made to a sponsoring institution, not to individuals or to departments. Any official member of a nonprofit institution in the United States may apply. Only one person should be listed as the principal investigator. All coinvestigators, collaborators, and consultants should be listed on the LOI.

Amount of Grant: $100,000 maximum for up to two years

Date(s) Application is Due: Jul 1; Dec 2

Contact: Contact, (703) 506-3280; fax: (703) 506-3266; email: info@npsf.org.

Internet: http://www.npsf.org/html/research

Sponsor: American Medical Association Foundation
8405 Greensboro Drive, Suite 800
McLean, VA 22102

National Psoriasis Foundation Research Grants 2259

The foundation will award up to five $50,000 one year pilot project grants to support advancement of both basic and clinical research into the cause and cure of psoriasis and psoriatic arthritis. The purpose of pilot project grants is to provide support for innovative early stage ideas. These grants are designed to allow the investigator to determine whether their idea is worth pursuing and then to secure longer-term funding.

Requirements: Applicants should use their NIH biographical sketches. Download the required application form from the website.

Amount of Grant: up to $50,000

Date(s) Application is Due: Oct 20

Contact: Bruce F. Bebo, Jr., Ph.D.; Director of Research and Medical Programs; (503) 244-7404 or (800) 723-9166; email: research@psoriasis.org

Internet: http://www.psoriasis.org/research/grants/index.php

Sponsor: National Psoriasis Foundation
6600 SW 92nd Avenue, Suite 300
Portland, OR 97223-7195

National Sleep Foundation Pickwick Postdoctoral Fellowship 2260

The fellowships enable young researchers to devote full-time professional effort to research related to the study of sleep or sleep disorders. Fellows receive funding for one or two years. The second year of support is dependent upon satisfactory progress in the

first year. Applicants must conduct research in recognized U.S. or Canadian programs of study or laboratories with strong mentorship in the appropriate area. Fellowships are available for basic, applied, or clinical research. Minorities are encouraged to apply.
Requirements: Candidates must hold either an MD, DVM, PhD, or DO degree in which the degree or subsequent training has been completed within the past five years.
Restrictions: Individuals in a faculty position or who have received an NIH grant are ineligible.
Amount of Grant: $45,048 maximum per year; $5500 maximum benefit allowance
Date(s) Application is Due: Dec 1
Contact: Jessica Steinitz, (202) 347-3471 ext 209; fax: (202) 347-3472; email: jsteinitz@sleepfoundation.org
Internet: http://www.sleepfoundation.org/nsfalert/index.php?id=31&secid=159#item159
Sponsor: National Sleep Foundation
1522 K St NW, Suite 500
Washington, DC 20005

National Starch and Chemical Foundation Grants 2261
The foundation supports nonprofits in company-operating locations in the areas of higher education, children's services, and hospitals. Types of support include general operating support, continuing support, employee-related scholarships, and employee matching gifts. There are no application guidelines. Applicants are asked to submit a written proposal.
Requirements: Nonprofits in company operating areas such as Georgia, Illinois, Indiana, Missouri, North Carolina, New Jersey, Pennsylvania, South Carolina, and Tennessee may apply.
Geographic Focus: Georgia; Illinois; Indiana; Missouri; New Jersey; North Carolina; Pennsylvania; South Carolina; Tennessee
Amount of Grant: $500-$10,000 average
Contact: Carmen Ortiz, (908) 685-5201; email: carmen.ortiz@nstarch.com
Internet: http://news.nationalstarch.com/NewsStory.asp?newsItemId=214
Sponsor: National Starch and Chemical Foundation
10 Finderne Avenue
Bridgewater, NJ 08807

National Student Nurses' Association Foundation Scholarships 2262
Scholarships are based on academic achievement, financial need, and involvement in nursing student organizations and community activities related to health care. Regular scholarships are open to all nursing students; career mobility scholarships are open to licensed practical nurses enrolled in programs leading to licensure as a registered nurse and to registered nurses enrolled in baccalaureate programs in nursing. Specialty scholarships have additional criteria set by the sponsors. Applicants submit one application and are considered for all scholarships for which they are eligible.
Requirements: Students currently enrolled in state-approved schools of nursing or pre-nursing programs in baccalaureate, diploma, generic doctorate, and generic master's programs are eligible. Applications must be accompanied by a $10 processing fee.
Restrictions: Graduating high school seniors are not eligible. Funds are not available for graduate study, unless it is for a first degree in nursing.
Amount of Grant: $1000-$2500
Date(s) Application is Due: Jan 20
Contact: Diane Mancino, Executive Director, (718) 210-0705; fax: (718) 210-0710; email: diane@nsna.org
Internet: http://www.nsna.org/foundation/index.asp
Sponsor: National Student Nurses' Association Foundation
45 Main Street, Suite 606
Brooklyn, NY 11201

NBME Stemmler Medical Education Research Fund Grants 2263
The purpose of the fund is to provide support for research or development of innovative evaluation methodology or techniques with the potential to advance assessment in medical education or practice, at eligible medical schools. Collaborative investigations within or among institutions are eligible, particularly as they strengthen the likelihood of the project's contribution and success. Proposed projects may request up to two years of support. Applicants for both new proposals and competing renewals may request up to $150,000 of NBME funding support for a project period of up to two years.
Requirements: Medical schools accredited by the Liaison Committee on Medical Education or the American Osteopathic Association are eligible.
Amount of Grant: $150,000 maximum for two years
Date(s) Application is Due: Oct 3
Contact: Officer of Research Support; (215) 590-9657; fax: (215) 590-9488; email: stemmlerfund@nbme.org
Internet: http://www.nbme.org/research/stemmler/index.html
Sponsor: National Board of Medical Examiners
3750 Market Street
Philadelphia, PA 19104

NBNA Lauranne Sams Scholarships 2264
NBNA awards undergraduate and graduate nursing scholarships primarily to African Americans enrolled at any level in a nursing program. Each chapter must submit completed NBNA scholarship application forms filled out by each candidate it recommends. Scholarship winners are notified by July 1, and the awards are presented at the annual August conference.
Requirements: Candidate must be enrolled in a nursing program (AD, BSN, or LPN/LVN) and be in good scholastic standing at the time of application. Applications must be accompanied by two letters of recommendation (one from the school of nursing and one from the local chapter). Letters from the school of nursing and a nurse in the area will suffice for candidates who have no local chapter in the area.
Amount of Grant: $500-$2000 range
Date(s) Application is Due: Apr 15
Contact: Scholarships Administrator, (800) 575-6298 or (301) 589-3200; fax: (301) 589-3223; email: NBNA@erols.com
Internet: http://www.nbna.org/scholarship.htm
Sponsor: National Black Nurses Association
8630 Fenton Street, Suite 330
Silver Spring, MD 20910-3803

NCCAM Exploratory Developmental Grants for Complementary and Alternative Medicine (CAM) Studies of Humans 2265
The National Center for Complementary and Alternative Medicine (NCCAM), the National Cancer Institute (NCI), the National Institute on Aging (NIA), and the Office of Dietary Supplements (ODS) invites high quality exploratory/developmental research grant applications of humans in all domains of complementary and alternative medicine (CAM), in order to obtain preliminary data that can be used as a foundation for a larger clinical study. NCCAM groups CAM practices into four domains: biologically-based practices; energy medicine; manipulative and body-based therapies, and mind-body medicine. In addition, NCCAM funds studies of whole medical systems that employ practices drawn from the four domains. The total project period for an application submitted in response to this funding opportunity may not exceed three years. Direct costs are limited to $400,000 over a three-year period, with no more than $250,000 in direct costs allowed in any single year.
Requirements: The following organizations and institutions may apply: public/state controlled institutions of higher education; private institutions of higher education; Hispanic-serving institutions; historically Black colleges and universities (HBCUs); tribally controlled colleges and universities (TCCUs); Alaska native and native Hawaiian serving institutions; nonprofits with 501(c)3 IRS status; nonprofits without 501(c)3 IRS status; small businesses; for-profit organizations; State governments; regional organizations; U.S. territories or possessions; Indian/Native American tribal governments; Indian/Native American tribally designated organizations; county governments; city or township governments; special district governments; independent school districts; public housing authorities/Indian housing authorities; eligible agencies of the Federal government; and faith-based or community based organizations.
Amount of Grant: $250,000 maximum for single entity; $400,000 maximum for 3-year project
Date(s) Application is Due: Feb 16; Jun 16; Oct 16
Contact: April Bower; (301) 451-3560; fax: (301) 480-3621; email: bowera@mail.nih.gov
Internet: http://grants.nih.gov/grants/guide/pa-files/PAR-08-135.html#SectionVII
Sponsor: National Center for Complementary and Alternative Medicine (NCCAM)
6707 Democracy Boulevard, Suite 401
Bethesda, MD 20892

NCCAM Ruth L. Kirschstein National Research Service Awards for Postdoctoral Training in Complementary and Alternative Medicine 2266
The National Center for Complementary and Alternative Medicine (NCCAM) awards individual postdoctoral research training fellowships to promising applicants with the desire and potential to become productive, independent investigators in the field of complementary and alternative medicine (CAM) research. The primary objective of this funding opportunity is to help ensure that diverse pools of highly trained scientists will be available in adequate numbers and in appropriate research areas to carry out the Nation's biomedical, behavioral, and clinical CAM research agendas. Applicants may come from a range of career backgrounds, including biomedical research, conventional allopathic medicine, or CAM healing practices. The number of awards and the total amount of funding that NCCAM expects to award through this announcement will depend on the scientific merit of applications received, relevance to NCCAM's program priorities, and the availability of funds.
Requirements: Eligible organizations include for-profit and non-profit organizations, public or private institutions such as universities, colleges, hospitals and laboratories, units of State and local governments, eligible agencies and labs of the Federal government including NIH intramural labs, and domestic or foreign institutions/organizations. Applicant fellows must be citizens or non-citizen nationals of the United States, or have been lawfully admitted to the United States for permanent residence and have in their possession an Alien Registration Receipt Card.
Restrictions: Individuals on temporary or student visas are not eligible.
Date(s) Application is Due: Apr 8; Aug 8; Dec 8
Contact: Nancy J. Pearson; (301) 594-0519; fax: (301) 480-3621; email: pearsonn@mail.nih.gov
Internet: http://grants.nih.gov/grants/guide/pa-files/PAR-07-319.html
Sponsor: National Center for Complementary and Alternative Medicine (NCCAM)
6707 Democracy Boulevard, Suite 401, MSC 5475
Bethesda, MD 20892-5475

NCCAM Translational Tools for Clinical Studies of CAM Interventions Grants 2267
This Funding Opportunity Announcement (FOA) issued by the National Center for Complementary and Alternative Medicine (NCCAM) of the National Institutes of Health (NIH) encourages investigator(s)-initiated applications that propose to develop, enhance, and validate translational tools to facilitate rigorous study of complementary and alternative medicine (CAM) approaches that are in wide use by the public. Multidisciplinary studies and collaboration among investigators with expertise in

appropriate disciplines are encouraged. NCCAM intends to award up to $3 million (total costs) per year, to support approximately 4 to 6 new grants. A maximum of $300,000 (direct costs) per year may be requested and the total project period for an application submitted in response to this FOA will be five years.
Requirements: The following organizations and institutions are eligible to apply: individuals; public/state controlled institutions of higher education; private institutions of higher education; Hispanic-serving institutions; historically Black colleges and universities (HBCUs); tribally controlled colleges and universities (TCCUs); Alaska Native and Native Hawaiian serving institutions; nonprofits with 501(c)3 IRS status; nonprofits without 501(c)3 IRS status; for-profit organizations; state governments; Indian/Native American tribal governments (federally recognized); Indian/Native American tribally designated organizations; county governments; city or township governments; special district governments; independent school districts; public housing authorities/Indian housing authorities; U.S. territory or possession; Indian/Native American tribal governments (other than federally recognized); regional organizations; non-domestic (non-U.S.) entities (foreign organizations); other eligible agencies of the federal government; and faith-based or community-based organizations.
Amount of Grant: $300,000 per year
Date(s) Application is Due: Jul 17
Contact: Dr. Partap S. Khalsa, Division of Extramural Research; (301) 594-3462; fax: (301) 480-1587; email: khalsap@mail.nih.gov
Internet: http://grants.nih.gov/grants/guide/rfa-files/RFA-AT-09-002.html
Sponsor: National Center for Complementary and Alternative Medicine (NCCAM)
6707 Democracy Boulevard, Suite 401
Bethesda, MD 20892-5475

NCI Academic-Industrial Partnerships for Development and Validation of In Vivo Imaging Systems and Methods for Cancer Investigations 2268

The overall goal of this Funding Opportunity Announcement (FOA) is to accelerate the transition of in vivo spectroscopic and imaging systems and methods into cancer research, clinical trials, and/or clinical practice. A related goal is to advance new technologies and methods for animal imaging. To promote these goals, the Cancer Imaging Program (CIP) of the National Cancer Institute (NCI) solicits applications from multi-institutional research partnerships formed by academic, industrial, and other investigators. The partners will establish an inter-disciplinary, multi-institutional research team for the purpose of developing imaging technology that is applicable to cancer research involving human subjects and/or animal models. The academic-industrial partnerships must be dedicated to the complete research and development cycle, culminating in the product prototype stage. The partnership model is expected to more readily overcome various barriers to the development of new imaging devices and technologies faced by either academia or industry working alone.
Requirements: Eligible institutions include: public and state controlled institutions of higher education; private institutions of higher education; nonprofits with 501(c)3 IRS status (other than institutions of higher education); nonprofits without 501(c)3 IRS status (other than institutions of higher education); small businesses; for-profit organizations (other than small businesses); state governments; U.S. territories or possessions; non-domestic (non-U.S.) entities (foreign organizations); and eligible agencies of the federal government.
Date(s) Application is Due: Feb 5; Jun 5; Oct 5
Contact: Guoying Liu, Ph.D.; (301) 496-9531; fax: (301) 480-3507; email: guoyingl@mail.nih.gov
Internet: http://grants.nih.gov/grants/guide/pa-files/PAR-07-214.html
Sponsor: National Cancer Institute (NCI)
6130 Executive Plaza, EPN Suite 6000, MSC 7412
Bethesda, MD 20892-7412

NCI Application and Use of Transformative Emerging Technologies in Cancer Research 2269

This Funding Opportunity Announcement (FOA) solicits grant applications proposing exploratory research projects on evaluating the performance of emerging molecular and cellular analysis technologies utilizing an appropriate cancer-relevant biological system. Technologies proposed for evaluation may have broad applicability but must ultimately be suitable for cancer-relevant analyses such as the detection (at various molecular and cellular levels) of cancer-related characteristics and/or structural and/or functional alterations. Letters of intent are requested by January 23, April 27, and August 30; full proposal deadlines are February 23, May 27, and September 30. Annual deadline dates may vary; contact program staff for exact dates.
Requirements: Eligible institutions include: public and state controlled institutions of higher education; private institutions of higher education; nonprofits with 501(c)3 IRS status (other than institutions of higher education); nonprofits without 501(c)3 IRS status (other than institutions of higher education); small businesses; for-profit organizations (other than small businesses); state governments; U.S. territories or possessions; non-domestic (non-U.S.) entities (foreign organizations); and eligible agencies of the federal government.
Amount of Grant: $275,000 maximum request per two-year period
Date(s) Application is Due: Jan 23; Feb 23; Apr 27; May 27; Aug 30; Sep 30
Contact: Richard Aragon, Ph.D.; (301) 496-1550; fax: (301) 496-7807; email: raragon@mail.nih.gov
Internet: http://grants.nih.gov/grants/guide/rfa-files/RFA-CA-09-006.html
Sponsor: National Cancer Institute
Building 31, Room 10A52, MSC 2580
Bethesda, MD 20892-2580

NCI Application of Metabolomics for Translational and Biological Grants 2270

The purpose of this Funding Opportunity Announcement (FOA), sponsored by multiple NIH Institutes/Centers (ICs), is to promote the use of metabolomic technologies in translational research in human health and disease for the purposes of enabling and improving disease detection, diagnosis, risk assessment, prognosis, and prediction of therapeutic responses. In addition to this overall goal, specific scopes and objectives of the participating ICs are presented below. Using the NIH Research Project Grant (R01) funding mechanism, this FOA focuses on well developed projects supported by preliminary data.
Requirements: Application can be made by the following institutions and organizations: public and state controlled institutions of higher education; private institutions of higher education; small businesses; for-profit organizations (other than small businesses); and non-domestic (non-U.S.) entities (foreign organizations).
Date(s) Application is Due: Feb 5; Feb 16; Jun 5; Jun 16; Oct 5; Oct 16
Contact: Padma Maruvada, Ph.D.; (301) 496-3893; fax: (301) 402-8990; email: maruvadp@mail.nih.gov
Internet: http://grants.nih.gov/grants/guide/pa-files/PA-07-301.html
Sponsor: National Cancer Institute (NCI)
6130 Executive Boulevard, EPN Suite 3144, MSC 7362
Bethesda, MD 20892-7362

NCI Basic Cancer Research in Cancer Health Disparities Grants 2271

Through this Funding Opportunity Announcement (FOA), the Center to Reduce Cancer Health Disparities (CRCHD) and the Division of Cancer Biology (DCB), at the National Cancer Institute (NCI), invite cooperative agreement research (U01) grant applications from investigators interested in conducting basic research studies into the causes and mechanisms of cancer health disparities. These awards will support pilot and feasibility studies, development and testing of new methodologies, secondary data analyses, and innovative mechanistic studies that investigate biological/genetic bases of cancer health disparities. This FOA is also designed to aid and facilitate the growth of a nationwide cohort of scientists with a high level of basic research expertise in cancer health disparities research who can develop resources and tools, such as biospecimens, cell lines and methods that are necessary to conduct basic research in cancer health disparities. The total project period for an application submitted in response to this funding opportunity may not exceed five years. Direct costs are limited to $250,000/year and may not exceed 5 years.
Requirements: The following organizations and institutions are eligible to apply: public/state controlled institutions of higher education; private institutions of higher education; Hispanic-serving institutions; historically Black colleges and universities (HBCUs); tribally controlled colleges and universities (TCCUs); Alaska Native and Native Hawaiian serving institutions; nonprofits with 501(c)3 IRS status; nonprofits without 501(c)3 IRS status; small businesses; for-profit organizations; state governments; Indian/Native American tribal governments (federally recognized); Indian/Native American tribally designated organizations; U.S. territories or possessions; Indian/Native American tribal governments (other than federally recognized); regional organizations; eligible agencies of the federal government; and units of local governments.
Amount of Grant: $250,000 per year for up to 5 years
Date(s) Application is Due: Jun 23; Nov 23
Contact: Phillip J. Daschner; (301) 496-1951; fax: (301) 496-2025; email: PD93U@nih.gov;; Kenneth C. Chu; (301) 435-9213; fax: (301) 435-9225; email: kc10d@nih.gov
Internet: http://grants.nih.gov/grants/guide/pa-files/PAR-09-161.html
Sponsor: National Cancer Institute (NCI)
Executive Plaza North (EPN), Room 5014, 6130 Executive Boulevard, MSC 7344
Bethesda, MD 20892-7344

NCI Diet, Epigenetic Events, and Cancer Prevention Grants 2272

The purpose of this Funding Opportunity Announcement (FOA) is to promote innovative preclinical and clinical research to determine how diet and dietary factors, including dietary supplements, impact epigenetic processes involved in cancer prevention. Although much evidence exists that dietary components are linked to cancer prevention, the specific nutrients and sites of action remain elusive. Diet, in fact, has been implicated in many of the pathways of cancer, including apoptosis, cell cycle control, differentiation, inflammation, angiogenesis, DNA repair, and carcinogen metabolism. These are also processes that are likely regulated by epigenetic events to impact gene function and chromatin stability. Thus, research supported by this initiative could address one of the following issues: How bioactive food components regulate epigenetic events for cancer prevention, how bioactive food components might alter aberrant epigenetic patterns or events and restore gene function, and how these components might circumvent or compensate for genes and pathways that are altered by epigenetic events. Another important aim of this FOA is to encourage collaborations between nutrition scientists and experts in epigenetics to study bioactive food components with cancer-preventative properties and to examine key epigenetic events in cancer processes (e.g., carcinogen metabolism, cell division, differentiation, and apoptosis) in order to begin to establish linkages between epigenetic events and patterns, and tumor incidences/behaviors. NIDDK is particularly interested in receiving applications that address normal and neoplastic conditions focusing on the impact of epigenetics on cell division, differentiation, and/or apoptosis in the gastrointestinal (GI) tract and related organs. It is also expected that each application demonstrate experience in nutrition and cancer prevention as well as in epigenetic research. Because the nature and scope of the proposed research will vary from application to application, it is anticipated that the size and duration of each award will also vary.
Requirements: Application can be made by the following institutions and organizations: public/state controlled institutions of higher education; private institutions of higher

education; nonprofits with 501(c)3 IRS status (other than institutions of higher education); nonprofits without 501(c)3 IRS status (other than institutions of higher education); small businesses; for-profit organizations (other than small businesses); state governments; U.S. territories or possessions; Indian/Native American tribal governments (federally recognized); Indian/Native American tribal governments (other than Federally recognized); Indian/Native American tribally designated organizations; non-domestic (non-U.S.) entities (foreign organizations); Hispanic-serving institutions; historically Black colleges and universities (HBCUs); tribally controlled colleges and universities (TCCUs); Alaska Native and Native Hawaiian serving institutions; regional organization; eligible agencies of the Federal government; and faith-based or community based organizations.
Date(s) Application is Due: Feb 5; Jun 5; Oct 5
Contact: Sharon Ross, Ph.D.; (301) 594-7547; fax: (301) 480-3925; email: rosssha@mail.nih.gov;; Vishnudutt Purohit, Ph.D.; (301) 443-2689; fax: (301) 594-0673; email: vpurohit@mail.nih.gov
Internet: http://grants.nih.gov/grants/guide/pa-files/PA-07-175.html
Sponsor: National Cancer Institute (NCI)
6130 Executive Boulevard, EPN Suite 3157, MSC 7328
Bethesda, MD 20892-7328

NCI Engineered Isogenic Cell Lines with Relevant Cancer Targets Grants 2273
This PA encourages the small business community to develop isogenic cell lines in which functions of a molecular activity or pathway found in human tumors can be analyzed in pair-wise fashion. Such cell lines could be used for drug screening with the intent of identification of compounds that influence the action of the identified target. The end result of the PA-supported projects would be a series of genetically engineered screening models that the small businesses could market directly or utilize in a license agreement or other type of collaboration. PAR-98-068 may be obtained through the NIH grant line (301-402-2221), the NIH Web site, mail, and email.
Contact: Dr. George Johnson, Division of Cancer Treatment and Diagnosis, (301) 496-8783; fax: (301) 402-5200; email: gj16m@nih.gov; Toby Friedberg, Division of Extramural Activities, (301) 496-3428; fax: (301) 402-0275; email: friedbet&7dea.nci.nih.gov
Internet: http://www.grants.nih.gov/grants/guide/pa-files/PAR-98-068.html
Sponsor: National Cancer Institute
6130 Executive Boulevard, Executive Plz N
Bethesda, MD 20892

NCI Exploratory Grants for Behavioral Research in Cancer Control 2274
This FOA will support innovative pilot projects or feasibility studies, which will facilitate the growth of research science in the cancer control continuum from a behavioral perspective. This FOA includes and incorporates the research interests of the Behavioral Research program, the Office of Cancer Survivorship, and the Community Oncology and Prevention Trials Research Group. This FOA is appropriate for testing timely interventions in pilot studies for feasibility or using rigorous qualitative research methods to assess the potential efficacy of an intervention. It is also appropriate for the psychometric evaluation of new measures or culturally appropriate ones to be adapted for use in populations where measures have not yet been developed or validated. This FOA encourages applications that include small cross-disciplinary teams of investigators who bring perspectives from the behavioral and social sciences, as well as other fields of public health.
Requirements: Eligible institutions and agencies include: public/state controlled institutions of higher education; private institutions of higher education; nonprofits with 501(c)3 IRS status (other than institutions of higher education); nonprofits without 501(c)3 IRS status (other than institutions of higher education); small businesses; for-profit organizations (other than small businesses); state governments; U.S. territories or possessions; regional organizations; non-domestic (non-U.S.) entities (foreign organizations); eligible agencies of the federal government; and units of local governments.
Amount of Grant: $275,000 maximum request per two-year period
Date(s) Application is Due: Feb 16; Jun 16; Oct 16
Contact: Sabra F. Woolley, Ph.D.; (301) 435-4589; fax: (301) 594-0673; email: woolleys@mail.nih.gov;; Barbara C. Sorkin, Ph.D.; (301) 594-8018; email: sorkinb@mail.nih.gov
Internet: http://grants.nih.gov/grants/guide/pa-files/PA-09-130.html
Sponsor: National Cancer Institute (NCI)
6130 Executive Boulevard, Room 4084, MSC 7365
Bethesda, MD 20850-7365

NCI Improving Diet and Physical Activity Assessment Grants 2275
This Funding Opportunity Announcement (FOA) is aimed at advancing the quality of measurements of dietary intake and physical activity pertinent to cancer and/or other pathologies through support of research on improved instruments, technologies, and/or statistical/analytical techniques. Studies proposed in the grant applications should be aimed at optimizing the combined use of objective and self-report measures of physical activity and/or dietary intake for testing in both general and diverse populations. Applicants responding to this FOA, which uses the R01 grant mechanism, should have already tested and validated new approaches and have obtained feasibility data in the context of cancer or other relevant diseases. Because the nature and scope of the proposed research will vary from application to application, it is anticipated that the size and duration of each award will also vary.
Requirements: Application can be made by the following institutions and organizations: public/state controlled institutions of higher education; private institutions of higher education; nonprofits with 501(c)3 IRS status (other than institutions of higher education); nonprofits without 501(c)3 IRS status (other than institutions of higher education); small businesses; for-profit organizations (other than small businesses); state governments; U.S. territories or possessions; Indian/Native American tribal governments (federally recognized); Indian/Native American tribal governments (other than Federally recognized); Indian/Native American tribally designated organizations; non-domestic (non-U.S.) entities (foreign organizations); Hispanic-serving institutions; historically Black colleges and universities (HBCUs); tribally controlled colleges and universities (TCCUs); Alaska Native and Native Hawaiian serving institutions; regional organization; eligible agencies of the Federal government; and faith-based or community based organizations.
Restrictions: Applicants without sufficiently extensive preliminary data or those who wish to explore the utility of new untested dietary or physical activity assessment methods in pilot studies are advised to consider submitting applications under the parallel FOA, PAR-06-103, which uses the Exploratory/Developmental Grant (R21) award mechanism.
Date(s) Application is Due: Feb 5; Jun 5; Oct 5
Contact: Amy Subar, Ph.D.; (301) 594-0831; fax: (301) 435-3710; email: subara@mail.nih.gov;; Richard Troiano, Ph.D.; (301) 435-6822; fax: (301) 435-3710; email: troianor@mail.nih.gov
Internet: http://grants.nih.gov/grants/guide/pa-files/PAR-09-225.html
Sponsor: National Cancer Institute (NCI)
6130 Executive Boulevard, EPN Room 4005, MSC 7344
Bethesda, MD 20892-7344

NCI Mentored Career Development Award to Promote Diversity 2276
This mechanism establishes a pathway of recruiting, training, and retaining underrepresented investigators in research fields that address problems pertinent to the biology, etiology, pathogenesis, prevention, diagnosis, control, and treatment of human cancer and who can conduct independent competitive cancer research programs. The Mentored Career Development Award to Promote Diversity (K01) provides support for a sustained period of protected time for intensive research career development under the guidance of an experienced mentor, or sponsor, in the biomedical, behavioral or clinical sciences leading to research independence. The expectation is that through this sustained period of research career development and training, awardees will launch independent research careers and become competitive for new research project grant funding.
Requirements: The following organizations and institutions may apply: for-profit and non-profit organizations; public or private institutions, such as universities, colleges, hospitals, and laboratories; and domestic institutions.
Restrictions: Foreign institutions and organizations are not eligible to apply.
Amount of Grant: $75,000 salary plus fringe benefits
Date(s) Application is Due: Feb 12; Mar 12; Jun 12; Jul 12; Oct 12; Nov 12
Contact: Belinda Locke; (301) 496-7344; fax: (301) 402-4551; email: Lockeb@mail.nih.gov
Internet: http://grants.nih.gov/grants/guide/pa-files/PAR-06-220.html
Sponsor: National Cancer Institute (NCI)
6116 Executive Boulevard, Suite 7031, MSC 8350
Bethesda, MD 20892-8350

NCI Ruth L. Kirschstein National Research Service Award Institutional Research Training Grants 2277
The National Institutes of Health (NIH) will award Ruth L. Kirschstein National Research Service Award (NRSA) Institutional Research Training Grants (T32) to eligible institutions as the primary means of supporting predoctoral and postdoctoral research training to help ensure that a diverse and highly trained workforce is available to assume leadership roles related to the Nation's biomedical, behavioral and clinical research agenda. The primary objective of the T32 program is to prepare qualified individuals for careers that have a significant impact on the health-related research needs of the Nation. This program supports predoctoral, postdoctoral and short term research training programs at domestic institutions of higher education with the T32 funding mechanism. Stipends are provided as a subsistence allowance for trainees to help defray living expenses during the research training experience and are based on a 12-month appointment period.
Requirements: The following organizations are eligible to apply: public/state controlled institutions of higher education; private institutions of higher education; nonprofits with 501(c)3 IRS status (other than institutions of higher education); nonprofits without 501(c)3 IRS status (other than institutions of higher education); for-profit organizations (other than small businesses); state governments; U.S. territories or possessions; Indian/Native American tribal governments (Federally recognized); Hispanic-serving institutions; historically Black colleges and universities (HBCUs); tribally controlled colleges and universities (TCCUs); Alaska Natives and Native Hawaiians serving institutions; regional organizations; eligible agencies of the federal government; faith-based or community based organizations.
Date(s) Application is Due: Apr 8; Aug 8; Dec 8
Contact: Crystal Wolfrey; (301) 496-8634; (301) 496-8601; email: wolfreyc@mail.nih.gov
Internet: http://grants.nih.gov/grants/guide/pa-files/PA-08-226.html
Sponsor: National Cancer Institute (NCI)
6120 Executive Boulevard, Room 243, MSC 7150
Bethesda, MD 20892-7150

NCI Stages of Breast Development: Normal to Metastatic Disease Grants 2278
The National Cancer Institute (NCI), National Institute of Child Health and Human Development (NICHD), National Institute of Diabetes and Digestive and Kidney Diseases (NIDDK), National Institute on Aging (NIA), and National Institute of Environmental Health Sciences (NIEHS) invite investigator-initiated research grant applications to study the molecular, cellular, endocrine, and other physiological

influences on the development and maturation of the normal mammary gland and alterations involved in early malignant and metastatic breast cancer. Multi-disciplinary collaborations, for example between cell biologists, molecular endocrinologists, bioengineers, geneticists, and mammary pathologists, are encouraged. Appropriate studies include, but are not limited to, documenting the role of dynamic hormonal influences and determining the role of cell growth, apoptosis, and differentiation in mammary gland maturation; integrating knowledge of cell signaling in breast tissue with whole organ biology; developing models of breast differentiation; and studies focusing on the characteristics of breast tumor physiology particularly in relation to metastasis. It is expected that a complete understanding of mammary gland development will form critical underpinnings for continued advances in detecting, preventing and treating breast cancer.
Requirements: Applications may be submitted by domestic and foreign, for-profit and non-profit organizations, public and private, such as universities, colleges, hospitals, laboratories, units of State or local governments, and eligible agencies of the Federal government.
Amount of Grant: $250,000 maximum per year
Date(s) Application is Due: Feb 5; Jun 5; Oct 5
Contact: Padma Maruvada, Ph.D.; (301) 496-3893; fax: (301) 402-8990; email: maruvadp@mail.nih.gov
Internet: http://grants.nih.gov/grants/guide/pa-files/PA-99-162.html
Sponsor: National Cancer Institute (NCI)
6130 Executive Boulevard, EPN Suite 3144, MSC 7362
Bethesda, MD 20892-7362

NCI Technologies and Software to Support Integrative Cancer Biology Research (SBIR) Grants 2279
This Funding Opportunity Announcement (FOA), issued by the National Cancer Institute (NCI), invites Small Business Innovation Research (SBIR) grant applications from small business concerns (SBCs) that propose the development of commercial software tools, computational/mathematical methods, and technologies that will enable integrative cancer biology research. Integrative cancer biology focuses on understanding cancer as a complex biological system by utilizing both computational and experimental biology to integrate heterogeneous data sources and ultimately to generate predictive computational models of cancer processes. Phase I applications may request up to 2 years of support with total costs of up to $300,000 for the duration of the award (not to exceed $200,000 total costs in any one year). Budgetary requests of Phase II applications will conform to standard SBIR guidelines (up to $750,000 total costs for up to two years).
Requirements: Only United States small business concerns (SBCs) are eligible to submit SBIR applications.
Amount of Grant: $300,000 maximum for Phase 1; $750,000 maximum for Phase 2
Date(s) Application is Due: Apr 5; Aug 5; Dec 5
Contact: Greg Evans, Ph.D.; (301) 594-8807; fax: (301) 480-4082; email: evansgl@mail.nih.gov
Internet: http://grants.nih.gov/grants/guide/pa-files/PA-09-188.html
Sponsor: National Cancer Institute (NCI)
Building 31, Room 10A19, 31 Center Drive, MSC 2580
Bethesda, MD 20892-2580

NCI/NIDA Transdisciplinary Tobacco Use Research Centers Grants 2280
Transdisciplinary tobacco use research centers (TTURCs) are expected to conduct research that will lead to major scientific advances in knowledge of tobacco use, nicotine addiction, prevention and treatment interventions, and the translation of this knowledge into practice. There are several overarching goals: increase the number of investigators from relevant disciplines who focus on the study of tobacco use as part of transdisciplinary teams; generate basic research evidence to improve understanding of the etiology and natural history of tobacco use; produce evidence-based tobacco use interventions that can translate to the community and specific understudied or underserved populations; increase the number of evidence-based interventions that are novel, including the development, testing and dissemination of innovative behavioral treatments and prevention strategies based upon findings from basic research; train transdisciplinary investigators capable of conducting cutting-edge tobacco use research; and to increase the number of peer-reviewed publications in the area of tobacco use, nicotine addiction, and treatment. RFA-CA-04-012
Requirements: Applications may be submitted by public and private, domestic, for-profit and nonprofit organizations, units of state and local governments, and eligible agencies of the federal government. Domestic applications with foreign components are permitted. To be considered, applicant organizations must have: (1) an established investigator as a strong principal investigator who can oversee and conduct planning activities, provide direction to the TTURC, ensure a transdisciplinary research emphasis, and build a career development program; full institutional commitment from the applicant institution; clearly delineated and formally confirmed, subcontracted, collaborative scientific arrangements with scientists from other institutions, including foreign institutions, may be included.
Contact: Crystal Wolfrey, Grants Administration Branch, NCI, (301) 496-8634; email: crystal.wolfrey@nih.gov
Internet: http://grants1.nih.gov/grants/guide/rfa-files/RFA-CA-04-012.html
Sponsor: National Cancer Institute
6130 Executive Boulevard, Executive Plz N
Rockville, MD 20852

NCIC Canadian Breast Cancer Research Initiative Grants 2281
The initiative is a broad alliance of partners, comprising the Canadian Cancer Society, Health Canada through the National Health Research and Development Program, the Medical Research Council, the National Cancer Institute of Canada, the Breast Cancer International Centre, the Canadian Breast Cancer Foundation, and the Canadian Breast Cancer Network. The grants provide research support for up to three years to individuals formally affiliated with Canadian universities or other recognized Canadian institutions. Proposals must clearly state their relevance to the problem of breast cancer. Grantees are required to submit annual progress reports. Obtain application form 801 from the institute.
Restrictions: Applications may not be submitted in duplicate to sponsoring agencies. Applications for support of infrastructure will not be accepted.
Contact: Dr. Pascale Macgregor, Research Program Director, (416) 596-6598 ext 360; fax; (416) 596-1714; email: pfmacgregor@cbcf.org
Internet: http://www.breast.cancer.ca/cbcra_research_program
Sponsor: National Cancer Institute of Canada
10 Alcorn Avenue, Suite 200
Toronto, ON M4V 3B1 Canada

NCIC Canadian Cancer Society Research Grants 2282
The grants are intended to stimulate Canadian investigators in the design and execution of clinical and psychosocial/behavioral research in cancer and in the exploration of all the areas of the basic sciences having relevance to cancer. Grants for research will be awarded to projects deemed worthy of support, provided that the basic equipment and research facilities are available in the institution concerned and that it will provide the necessary administrative services. Such awards will be granted for the purchase and maintenance of animals, for expendable supplies, minor items of equipment, payment of graduate students and other assistants, and for research travel. Researchers focusing on breast cancer are strongly encouraged to submit applications to the Canadian Breast Cancer Research Initiative.
Requirements: A researcher who is designated as the principal investigator must be based in, or formally affiliated with (but not necessarily receive salary support from), a Canadian host institution such as a university, research institute, or healthcare agency.
Restrictions: Funds may not be used for personal salary support of the grantee.
Samples: Ralph Durand, British Columbia Cancer Research Centre—for a three-year project beginning in 1998 entitled Modifying Tumour Physiology to Improve Response to Radiation, $C149,544 per year.; Christopher Overall, U of British Columbia—for a three-year project beginning in 1998 entitled Cellular Activation of Human Gelatinase A, $C121,500 per year.; Heather Sutherland, U of British Columbia—for a three-year project beginning in 1998 entitled Purification and Characterization of Human Acute Myeloid Leukemia Stem Cells, $C97,600 per year.; Kevin Kane, U of Alberta—for a three year project beginning in 1998 entitled Ly-49 Interactions with Class I Major Histocompatibility Complex Molecules, $C95,390 per year.
Amount of Grant: $C300,000 maximum per year
Date(s) Application is Due: Oct 17
Contact: Director of Research Programs, (416) 961-7223; fax: (416) 961-4189; email: research@cancer.ca
Internet: http://www.ncic.cancer.ca/ncic/internet/standard/0,3621,84658243_85805597__langId-en,00.html
Sponsor: National Cancer Institute of Canada
10 Alcorn Avenue, Suite 200
Toronto, ON M4V 3B1 Canada

NCIC Canadian Cancer Society Travel Award for Senior Level PhD Students 2283
The purpose of this program is to provide financial assistance to senior-level PhD or MD/PhD students by helping to defray the travel costs associated with making a scientific presentation at a conference, symposium, or other appropriate professional gathering. The travel award will be made to defray actual costs of travel, registration, accommodation, etc. Three competitions are held annually. Conference dates for which funding is being requested must occur within six months of the competition deadline. Individuals may receive this award only once. A maximum of one award per supervisor will be given in the current calendar year. Applications must be completed using form 405/96. Letters announcing the results of eligible applications will be issued approximately one month following the deadline date.
Requirements: Applicants must be students enrolled in a PhD or MD/PhD program at a Canadian institution and be in their final phase of study. Candidates must be attending a conference for the purpose of presenting data (paper or poster presentation) from a cancer-related project on a first-author basis. It is not a requirement that the student and/or the supervisor be supported by an NCIC grant.
Amount of Grant: $C1500 maximum
Date(s) Application is Due: Apr 1; Sep 1; Dec 1
Contact: Contact, (416) 961-7223; fax: (416) 961-4189; email: research@cancer.ca
Internet: http://www.ncic.cancer.ca/ncic/internet/standard/0,3621,84658243_85813951_91005239_langId-en,00.html
Sponsor: National Cancer Institute of Canada
10 Alcorn Avenue, Suite 200
Toronto, ON M4V 3B1 Canada

NCIC Equipment Grants 2284
The grants provide for the purchase of items of permanent equipment necessary for research projects supported by the institute, if such equipment is not otherwise available. Application for minor items of apparatus and equipment with a total cost for each item of less than $C10,000 should be included as part of the application for the research grant.

Application for funds to purchase each item with a total cost of less than $C100,000 but more than $C5000 may be made either as part of an application for a grant for research or as a separate request if the applicant is the recipient of a continuing award. For items of specialized major equipment having a value of $C100,000 or more, the institute may have to contemplate alternative approaches to funding; therefore, a prior consultation with the institute is required.
Amount of Grant: $C75,000 maximum
Date(s) Application is Due: Oct 17
Contact: Grants Administrator, (416) 961-7223; fax: (416) 961-4189; email: research@cancer.ca
Internet: http://www.ncic.cancer.ca/ncic/internet/standard/0,3621,84658243_85808828__langId-en,00.html
Sponsor: National Cancer Institute of Canada
10 Alcorn Avenue, Suite 200
Toronto, ON M4V 3B1 Canada

NCIC Terry Fox Postdoctoral Research Fellowships **2285**
Fellowships are designed to provide training in cancer research for outstanding candidates who plan careers in Canada in this field of investigation. Post-MD fellowships are made to provide support for specialized training in the research aspects of the broad field of oncology (including epidemiology, medical statistics, clinical trials, and other forms of biomedical research). Initial tenure of a fellowship will normally be two years. One or more years of additional support may be available to individuals who demonstrate a serious commitment to cancer research, e.g., by registration in a degree program. Post-MD fellows may wish to maintain their clinical skills by means of service to the host institution during the period of the award. Such activities are acceptable provided the service is directly related to the cancer-oriented plan of the fellow and neither exceeds 10 working hours per week nor adversely affects the quantity or quality of the research training.
Requirements: Candidates must be graduates of universities recognized by NCIC and must be accepted for postdoctoral training in the field of cancer research in an academic environment also recognized by NCIC.
Restrictions: In general, applicants will not be eligible for funding beyond five years of postdoctoral training.
Amount of Grant: $C35,000-$C47,500 per year based on number of years of postdoctoral experience; Plus for up to $C1,200 per year to use towards the cost of attending and/or travelling to scientific meetings or conferences
Date(s) Application is Due: Feb 1
Contact: Director of Research Programs, (416) 961-7223; fax: (416) 961-4189; email: research@cancer.ca
Internet: http://www.ncic.cancer.ca/ncic/internet/standard/0,3621,84658243_85811512_90904221_langId-en,00.html
Sponsor: National Cancer Institute of Canada
10 Alcorn Avenue, Suite 200
Toronto, ON M4V 3B1 Canada

NCIC Terry Fox Research Studentships **2286**
Research studentships provide training to PhD students in cancer research and are offered to outstanding individuals who plan a career in cancer research in Canada. Awards are made for up to a maximum of four years and are not renewable. Research studentship award recipients must devote full time to the research and training program during the tenure of the studentship. If the supervisor considers a certain amount of teaching to be part of the training, such teaching and duties must be limited to not more than 10 hours per week. At the completion of each award year, a letter summarizing the progress to date, signed by the research student and the research supervisor, must be submitted to the institute.
Requirements: Applicants must be residents of Canada and be enrolled in a PhD program at a Canadian institution at the time of application. Candidates must have completed at least two years of research training at the graduate level or have equivalent research experience.
Amount of Grant: $C21,500; Plus up to $C1200 per year to use towards the cost of attending and/or travelling to scientific meetings or conferences
Contact: Michael Wosnick, Executive Director, (416) 934-5672; fax: (416) 961-4189; email: mwosnick@cancer.ca
Internet: http://www.ncic.cancer.ca/ncic/internet/standard/0,3621,84658243_85813949_90911828_langId-en,00.html
Sponsor: National Cancer Institute of Canada
10 Alcorn Avenue, Suite 200
Toronto, ON M4V 3B1 Canada

NCRR Networks and Pathways Collaborative Research Projects Grants **2287**
This announcement solicits applications for research project grants that will leverage and complement the ongoing technology development being pursued in the National Technology Centers for Networks and Pathways (TCNPs), a program of the NIH Roadmap for Medical Research. These collaborative projects should focus either on addressing a challenging biological problem using the technology developed in one or more of the TCNPs, or on the development of technology that will complement that which is being developed in the centers. Applicants may request support for their own work as well as supplemental support for components pursued in the participating TCNP. While the nature and scope of these applications will vary, it is anticipated that the annual direct costs for these projects will typically range from $150,000 to $250,000.
Requirements: Application can be made by the following institutions and organizations: public/state controlled institutions of higher education; private institutions of higher education; nonprofits with 501(c)3 IRS status (other than institutions of higher education); nonprofits without 501(c)3 IRS status (other than institutions of higher education); small businesses; for-profit organizations (other than small businesses); state governments; U.S. territories or possessions; non-domestic (non-U.S.) entities (foreign organizations); historically Black colleges and universities (HBCUs); Tribally controlled colleges and universities (TCCUs); and other eligible agencies of the Federal government.
Amount of Grant: $150,000 to $250,000 range
Date(s) Application is Due: Feb 5; Jun 5; Oct 5
Contact: Douglas M. Sheeley, Sc.D.; (301) 594-9762; email: sheeleyd@mail.nih.gov;; David M. Balshaw, Ph.D.; (919) 541-2448; email: balshaw@niehs.nih.gov
Internet: http://grants.nih.gov/grants/guide/pa-files/PA-07-266.html
Sponsor: National Center for Research Resources (NCRR)
6701 Democracy Boulevard, MSC 4874
Bethesda, MD 20892-4874

NCRR Novel Approaches to Enhance Animal Stem Cell Research **2288**
The purpose of this funding opportunity announcement (FOA) is to encourage the submission of applications for research to enhance animal stem cells as model biological systems. Innovative approaches to isolate, characterize and identify toti-potent and multi-potent stem cells from nonhuman biomedical research animal models, as well as to generate reagents and techniques to characterize and separate those stem cells from other cell types is encouraged.
Requirements: The following organizations and institutions may apply: public/state controlled institutions of higher education; private institutions of higher education; Hispanic-serving institutions; historically Black colleges and universities (HBCUs); tribally controlled colleges and universities (TCCUs); Alaska Native and Native Hawaiian serving institutions; nonprofits with 501(c)3 IRS status (other than institution of higher education); nonprofits without 501(c)3 IRS status (other than institution of higher education); non-domestic (non-U.S.) entities (foreign organizations); small businesses; for-profit organizations (other than small businesses).
Restrictions: Studies involving human subjects are not allowed.
Date(s) Application is Due: Feb 5; Jun 5; Oct 5
Contact: John D. Harding, PhD; (301) 435-0744; fax: (301) 480-3819; email: hardingj@mail.nih.gov;; Donald Blair, Ph.D.; (301) 496-7028; fax: (301) 402-1037; email: blaird@mail.nih.gov
Internet: http://grants.nih.gov/grants/guide/pa-files/PA-07-303.html
Sponsor: National Center for Research Resources (NCRR)
6701 Democracy Boulevard, Room 950, MSC 4874
Bethesda, MD 20892-4874

NEDA/AED Charron Family Research Grant **2289**
Committed to promoting study into the causes, cures and prevention of eating disorders, NEDA first established the Research Grants Program in 2002 in partnership with the Academy for Eating Disorders (AED). The aim of these grants is to expand eating disorders research while drawing promising new scientists into the field. In 2004 Shelley Charron-Bahniuk died from complications of her eating disorder while she was in recovery. The Charron Family Research Grant was created as a direct result of this illness that impacted both her immediate and extended family.
Requirements: Individuals working in the field of eating disorders who have completed their training, and have the doctorate degree or beyond are eligible.
Amount of Grant: $10,000
Contact: Dee Christoff, Development Director; (206) 382-3587, ext. 15; fax: (206) 829-8501; email: info@nationaleatingdisorders.org
Internet: http://www.nationaleatingdisorders.org/p.asp?WebPage_ID=712
Sponsor: National Eating Disorders Association / Academy for Eating Disorders
603 Stewart Street, Suite 803
Seattle, WA 98101

NEDA/AED Joan Wismer Research Grant **2290**
Committed to promoting study into the causes, cures and prevention of eating disorders, NEDA first established the Research Grants Program in 2002 in partnership with the Academy for Eating Disorders (AED). The aim of these grants is to expand eating disorders research while drawing promising new scientists into the field.
Requirements: Individuals working in the field of eating disorders who have completed their training, and have the doctorate degree or beyond are eligible.
Amount of Grant: $10,000
Contact: Dee Christoff, Development Director; (206) 382-3587, ext. 15; fax: (206) 829-8501; email: info@nationaleatingdisorders.org
Internet: http://www.nationaleatingdisorders.org/p.asp?WebPage_ID=818
Sponsor: National Eating Disorders Association / Academy for Eating Disorders
603 Stewart Street, Suite 803
Seattle, WA 98101

NEDA/AED Tampa Bay Eating Disorders Task Force Award **2291**
The National Eating Disorders Association sponsors a small grants program to support research in the areas of eating disorders etiology, prevention, and treatment. Through the grants, the organization seeks to expand innovative eating disorders research while supporting investigators in the early stages of their careers in the eating disorders field. Support can be included for: salary for technicians, research assistants and other ancillary personnel; laboratory, radiological and pharmaceutical costs in clinical research projects; rating instruments and questionnaires; equipment and supplies; acquisition and maintenance of laboratory animals; subject payment; and advertising.

Requirements: Any junior investigator worldwide who works in the field of eating disorders and has completed their terminal graduate level degree and training is eligible.
Restrictions: Trainees (e.g. students, grad students, residents) are not eligible and investigators must be within seven years following the end of their training. Individuals who previously served or currently serve as a principal investigator on a substantial externally funded grant (e.g. RO1, RO3, or K award in the U.S.) are ineligible. Funds cannot be used for the following purposes: salary support for residents, fellows or other trainees; faculty or investigator salary; secretarial salary and benefits; tuition for residents, graduate students or post-doctoral fellows; publication costs or purchase of reprints or books; room and board for clinical subjects; studies that are also sponsored by pharmaceutical firms; computers; or travel.
Amount of Grant: $10,000
Contact: Dee Christoff, Development Director; (206) 382-3587, ext. 15; fax: (206) 829-8501; email: info@nationaleatingdisorders.org
Internet: http://www.nationaleatingdisorders.org/p.asp?WebPage_ID=816
Sponsor: National Eating Disorders Association / Academy for Eating Disorders
603 Stewart Street, Suite 803
Seattle, WA 98101

NEI Clinical Study Planning Grant 2292
This program provides support for the development of a comprehensive research protocol for a large-scale clinical trial or epidemiologic study. This grant provides early peer review of the proposed clinical study in terms of its rationale, design, organizational structure, and implementation plan. The planning grant is used to support the development of a detailed MOP and may include preliminary studies to refine study procedures or to document recruitment potential. PAR-05-115
Requirements: Applications may be submitted by domestic for-profit and nonprofit organizations, both public and private; units of state and local governments; and eligible agencies of the federal government; domestic and foreign institutions.
Restrictions: Foreign institutions are not eligible.
Amount of Grant: $150,000 maximum for two years
Internet: http://grants.nih.gov/grants/guide/pa-files/PAR-05-115.html
Sponsor: National Eye Institute
5635 Fishers Lane, Suite 1300, MSC 9300
Bethesda, MD 20892-9300

NEI Clinical Vision Research Development Award 2293
This award is intended to strengthen interactions among clinicians, biostatisticians, epidemiologists, statistical geneticists, and other clinical trial specialists to facilitate the design and conduct of clinical research projects, such as the development of coordinating center capabilities. The intent of this projects is to advance the understanding, prevention, or clinical management of visual system disorders. A number of experienced investigators and research groups are needed to provide leadership in the design and implementation of such clinical vision research projects. Therefore, NEI wishes to help institutions with NEI-funded investigators augment staff expertise and acquire the resources necessary to enhance their clinical vision research programs. PA: PAR-00-050
Requirements: Applications may be submitted by domestic for-profit and non-profit organizations, public and private, such as universities, colleges, hospitals, laboratories, units of State and local governments, and eligible agencies of the Federal government.
Restrictions: Foreign institutions and institutions having current or past NEI Core Grant for Vision Research (P30) support for a biostatistics module are not eligible to apply.
Amount of Grant: $100,000 maximum
Contact: Mary Frances Cotch, (301) 496-5983; fax: (301) 402-0528; email: mfcotch@nei.nih.gov or deverett@nei.nih.gov
Internet: http://grants.nih.gov/grants/guide/pa-files/PAR-00-050.html
Sponsor: National Eye Institute
6120 Executive Boulevard, MSC 7164
Bethesda, MD 20892-7164

NEI Innovative Patient Outreach Programs And Ocular Screening Technologies To Improve Detection Of Diabetic Retinopathy Grants 2294
This Funding Opportunity Announcement (FOA) solicits Small Business Innovation Research (SBIR) grant applications from small business concerns (SBCs) that propose to 1) develop educational outreach programs to create a greater awareness of the blinding consequences of diabetes; and, 2) develop tools and systems to be used for increasing patient access to eye exams for detecting Diabetic Retinopathy (DR). This FOA will utilize the SBIR (R43/R44) grant mechanisms for Phase I, Phase II, and Fast-Track applications. The estimated amount of funds available for support of 2-4 projects awarded as a result of this announcement is $2 million for this fiscal year.
Requirements: Only United States small business concerns (SBCs) are eligible to submit SBIR applications. A small business concern is one that, at the time of award of Phase I and Phase II, meets all of the criteria listed. Any individual(s) with the skills, knowledge, and resources necessary to carry out the proposed research as the PD/PI is invited to work with his/her organization to develop an application for support. Individuals from underrepresented racial and ethnic groups as well as individuals with disabilities are always encouraged to apply for NIH support. See website for details.
Amount of Grant: $2,000,000
Date(s) Application is Due: Mar 23, Dec 23
Contact: Jerome Wujek, (301) 451-2020; fax: (301) 402-0528; email: wujekjer@nei.nih.gov
Internet: http://grants.nih.gov/grants/guide/rfa-files/RFA-EY-09-001.html
Sponsor: National Eye Institute
5635 Fishers Lane, Suite 1300
Bethesda, MD 20892-9300

NEI Mentored Clinical Scientist Development Program Award (K12) 2295
The NEI Mentored Clinician Scientist Development Award (K12) is an award to an educational institution or professional organization to facilitate and support career development experiences which lead clinician scientists to research independence. It is expected that scholars appointed to the program will subsequently apply for their own individual research support. The program should be designed to accommodate candidates with varying levels of research experience who require an individualized career development program ranging from two to five years. Applications for this award should propose a structured, phased development plan overseen by a Program Director and a Program Advisory Committee. A designated period of didactic training should be followed by a period of supervised research experience. Candidates should be exposed to both research that is typically undertaken with a few investigators and to research approaches that require a multidisciplinary team to address complex research questions as appropriate. It is expected that at the end of the career development period, appointees will transition successfully into positions as independent investigators. This award provides five years of potentially renewable support. The subsequent continuation will depend in part on the progress made by the Scholars in achieving independent research support. Renewal applications must contain a progress report documenting the accomplishments and current career activities of former Scholars. PA# PAR-09-083
Requirements: The following organizations and institutions are eligible to apply: public/state controlled institutions of higher education; private institutions of higher education; hispanic-serving Institutions; historically black colleges and universities; tribally controlled colleges and universities; Alaska Native and Native Hawaiian serving institutions; nonprofits with 501(c)3 IRS Status (other than institutions of higher education); nonprofits without 501(c)3 IRS Status (other than institutions of higher education). Any individual with the skills, knowledge, and resources necessary to carry out the proposed research is invited to work with his/her institution to develop an application for support. Individuals from underrepresented racial and ethnic groups as well as individuals with disabilities are always encouraged to apply for NIH support.
Restrictions: Foreign institutions are not eligible to apply.
Amount of Grant: $1,125,000
Date(s) Application is Due: May 13
Contact: Neeraj Agarwal, (301) 451-2020; fax: (301) 402-0528; email: agarwalnee@nei.nih.gov
Internet: http://grants.nih.gov/grants/guide/pa-files/PAR-09-083.html
Sponsor: National Eye Institute
5635 Fishers Lane, Suite 1300
Bethesda, MD 20892-9300

NEI Research Grant For Secondary Data Analysis Grants 2296
The NEI Research Grant for Secondary Data Analysis (R21) program is designed to provide investigators with the support necessary to conduct secondary data analyses utilizing existing database resources. Applications may be related to, but must be distinct from, the specific aims of the original data collection. The total project period for an application submitted in response to this funding opportunity may not exceed two years. Direct costs are limited to $275,000 over an R21 two-year period, with no more than $200,000 in direct costs allowed in any single year. PA # PAR-06-326
Requirements: Eligible organizations: for-profit and non-profit organizations; public and private institutions (such as universities, colleges, hospitals, and laboratories); units of state and local governments; eligible agencies of the federal government; units of state; local tribal governments; domestic and foreign institutions. Eligible Project Directors/Principal Investigators (PD/PIs): any individual with the skills, knowledge, and resources necessary to carry out the proposed research. Individuals from underrepresented racial and ethnic groups as well as individuals with disabilities are always encouraged to apply for NIH support.
Amount of Grant: $275,000 over a two year period
Date(s) Application is Due: May 8
Contact: Natalie Kurinij, (301) 451-2020; fax: (301) 402-0528; email: kurinijn@mail.nih.gov
Internet: http://grants.nih.gov/grants/guide/pa-files/PAR-06-326.html
Sponsor: National Eye Institute
5635 Fishers Lane, Suite 1300, MSC 9300
Bethesda, MD 20892-9300

NEI Ruth L. Kirschstein National Research Service Award Short-Term Institutional Research Training Grants 2297
The National Institutes of Health (NIH) will award Ruth L. Kirschstein National Research Service Award (NRSA) Short-Term Institutional Research Training Grants (T35) to eligible institutions to develop or enhance research training opportunities for individuals interested in careers in biomedical, behavioral and clinical research. Many of the NIH Institutes and Centers (ICs) use this grant mechanism exclusively to support intensive, short-term research training experiences for students in health professional schools during the summer. In addition, the Short-Term Institutional Research Training Grant may be used to support other types of predoctoral and postdoctoral training in focused, often emerging scientific areas relevant to the mission of the funding IC. The proposed training must be in either basic, behavioral or clinical research aspects of the health-related sciences. This program is intended to encourage graduate and/or health professional students to pursue research careers by exposure to and short-term involvement in the health- related sciences. The training should be of sufficient depth to enable the trainees, upon completion of the program, to have a thorough exposure to the principles underlying the conduct of research. PA # PA-08-227
Requirements: The following organizations/institutions are eligible to apply: public/state controlled institutions of higher education; private institutions of higher

education; hispanic-serving institutions; historically black colleges and universities (HBCUs); tribally controlled colleges and universities (TCCUs); Alaska Native and Native Hawaiian serving institutions; nonprofits with 501(c)3 IRS Status (Other than Institutions of Higher Education); nonprofits without 501(c)3 IRS Status (Other than institutions of higher education); indian/native american tribal governments (federally recognized); indian/native american tribally designated organizations; U.S. Territory or possession; indian/native american tribal governments (other than federally recognized); faith-based or community-based organizations. Only domestic, non-profit, private or public institutions may apply for grants to support National Research Service Award (NRSA) short-term research training programs. Foreign institutions are not eligible to apply. The applicant institution must have a strong and high quality research program in the area(s) proposed for the research training and must have the requisite staff and facilities on site to conduct the proposed research training program. Any individual with the skills, knowledge, and resources necessary to organize and implement a high-quality research training program is invited to work with their institution to develop an application for support. Individuals from underrepresented racial and ethnic groups, individuals with disabilities, and individuals from disadvantaged backgrounds are always encouraged to apply for NIH support.
Restrictions: Foreign institutions are not eligible to apply.
Date(s) Application is Due: Sep 8
Contact: Neeraj Agarwal, (301) 451-2020; fax: (301) 402-0528; email: agarwalnee@mail.nih.gov
Internet: http://grants.nih.gov/grants/guide/pa-files/PA-08-227.html
Sponsor: National Eye Institute
5635 Fishers Lane, Suite 1300
Rockville, MD 20892-9300

NEI Scholars Program **2298**
This program provides an opportunity for outstanding individuals to obtain laboratory or clinical research training within NEI intramural environment and to facilitate the successful transition to continue their research career at an extramural institution as independent vision researchers. This is accomplished by first providing individuals with the necessary resources to receive high quality research training for three to four years at NEI. This is followed by providing extramural funding to support the research program for two years at the extramural institution to which NEI scholar is recruited. It is anticipated that NEI scholars will subsequently compete for independent funding to continue their research. During the intramural phase, the scholar is expected to spend full time on research. During the extramural phase, the scholar must spend a minimum of 75 percent of a full-time professional effort conducting research and engaging in research career development activities for the two years of the award. Applicants are encouraged to contact NEI extramural staff regarding their eligibility for this award and NEI intramural laboratory scientist regarding sponsorship information, prior to submitting an application. PA: PAR-98-107
Requirements: Individuals must have a research or health professional doctoral level degree or its equivalent and must have demonstrated the potential for a highly productive research career during predoctoral training and the immediate postdoctoral period, if applicable. Individuals at NEI or other NIH intramural laboratories who meet the eligibility requirements are eligible to apply. Before submitting an application for the program, the candidate must identify an individual in the NEI Division of Intramural Research who will serve as the sponsor and will be committed to supervise the training and research project. The sponsor must be an active investigator in the area of the proposed research and have research training experience and resources needed to support the NEI scholar.
Restrictions: Individuals who have had more than five years of postdoctoral research training at the time of application are not eligible to apply; however, clinical training does not count against the five years. Former principal investigators on NIH research project grants R01; SBIR/STTR awards R43, R44/R41, R42; subprojects of program project grants P01; center grants P30, P50; K08, K23, K24, or the equivalent are not eligible.
Amount of Grant: $175,000 maximum per year or $350,000 for two years
Date(s) Application is Due: Feb 1; Jun 1; Oct 1
Contact: Dr. Maria Giovanni, Division of Extramural Research, (301) 496-0484; fax: (301) 402-0528; email: myg@nei.nih.gov
Internet: http://www.grants.nih.gov/grants/guide/pa-files/PAR-98-107.html
Sponsor: National Eye Institute
9000 Rockville Pike, Building 31
Bethesda, MD 20892

NEI Translational Research Program On Therapy For Visual Disorders **2299**
This program continues support of collaborative, multidisciplinary research programs focused on new therapeutic approaches to restore or prevent the loss of function due to visual system diseases and disorders. The rapid and efficient translation of laboratory research findings into clinical development requires a comprehensive and highly integrated approach involving collaborative teams of scientists and clinicians with expertise in multiple disciplines. Such a collaborative approach would be particularly appropriate for research focused on pathways that will likely be targeted by biological intervention, such as gene therapy, cell-based therapy, pharmacological approaches, or development of appropriate delivery systems. The intention of this program is to make resources available to scientists from several disciplines to form research teams to address scientific and technical questions that would be beyond the capabilities of any one research group. It is anticipated that applications funded under this program will lead to therapies that can be tested in a clinical trial.
Requirements: Eligible Institutions, you may submit an application (s) if your organization has any of the following characteristics: for-profit organizations; non-profit organizations; public or private institutions, such as universities, colleges, hospitals, and laboratories; units of State government; units of local government; eligible agencies of the Federal government; domestic Institutions Foreign components to domestic applications will be allowed if the foreign component provides significant scientific input that is critical to the program and for which there is no similar resource in the United States. Eligible Individuals: any individual with the skills, knowledge, and resources necessary to carry out the proposed research is invited to work with their institution to develop an application for support. Individuals from underrepresented racial and ethnic groups as well as individuals with disabilities are always encouraged to apply for NIH programs.
Amount of Grant: $2 million maximum
Contact: Peter Dudley, (301) 451-2020; fax: (301) 402-0528; email: pad@nei.nih.gov
Internet: http://grants.nih.gov/grants/guide/pa-files/PAR-05-110.html
Sponsor: National Eye Institute
5635 Fishers Lane, Suite 1300, MSC 9300
Bethesda, MD 20892

NEI Vision Research Core Grants **2300**
The primary objective of Core Grants for Vision Research is to provide groups of investigators who have achieved independent National Eye Institute (NEI) funding with additional, shared support to enhance their own and their institution's capability for conducting vision research. Secondary objectives of this program include facilitating collaborative studies and attracting other scientists to research on the visual system.
Requirements: Institutions applying for a Core Grant must hold, on the receipt date, a minimum of eight NEI research project grants (R01), Bioengineering Research Partnership Grants (R24), Mentored Clinical Scientist Development Awards (K08), Mentored Patient-Oriented Research Career Development Award (K23), or Midcareer Investigator Award in Patient-Oriented Research (K24), including any noncompeting extensions of these awards made with or without additional funds. No other mechanisms or source of research support will be considered in determining eligibility. Only one Core Grant will be made to any single applicant organization. For multicampus institutions, no more than one Core Grant will be made to each campus. Joint applications may be submitted by investigators at neighboring, independent institutions.
Amount of Grant: $2,000,000 - $2,500,000 range over a five-year period
Date(s) Application is Due: Sep 25
Contact: Hemin Chin, (301) 451-2020; fax: (301) 402-0528; email: hemin@nei.nih.gov
Internet: http://www.nei.nih.gov/funding/p30.asp
Sponsor: National Eye Institute
5635 Fishers Lane, Suite 1300 MSC 9300
Bethesda, MD 20892-9300

Nelda C. and H.J. Lutcher Stark Foundation Grants **2301**
The foundation awards grants in its areas of interest, including education, health and social services, medical and dental, community enrichment, arts and culture. Giving is primarily in Texas, with preference to programs that directly impact Southeast Texas and limited giving in Southwest Louisiana. There are no application forms. Submit a letter of proposal containing the following information: description of the project signed by the president or CEO; brief history, description, programs, and mission of the organization; project time line; specific amount requested; list of other funding sources and amounts; list of board of directors and occupations; form 990 for most recent year-end; most recent audited financial statements or organization prepared statements; and current copy of IRS determination letter certifying tax-exempt status. Guidelines are available online. All grants from the third quarter of 2008 and for 2009 have been suspended due to recovery efforts in which the Foundation must engage for its own operations as a result of damages from Hurricane Ike, together with the negative impact of the downturn in financial markets on the Foundation's corpus, the Stark Foundation will continue the prior suspension of the grant-making aspect of its operations through the entirety of Year 2009. Therefore, the Stark Foundation will not accept any grant applications for Year 2009, nor will be able to consider any grant applications that may be submitted notwithstanding this suspension.
Requirements: To be eligible for a grant, an organization must: be exempt from taxation under Section 501(c)3 of the Internal Revenue Code; not be a private foundation within the meaning of Section 509(a) of the Code. No grants are made for endowment purposes, to individuals, or to supporting organizations as described in Section 509(a)(3) of the Internal Revenue Code.
Samples: Lamar State College, Orange, Texas $128,269 - Funding to establish a regional EMT training program in cooperation with Acadian Ambulance Service (2007); Texas Energy Museum, Beaumont, Texas $2,500 - Matching funds for an interactive science exhibit (2007); Orange Community Band, Orange, Texas $12,340 - equipment and program support (2007); Orange County Historical Commission, Orange, Texas $2,800 - matching funds to capture in digital format and place on-line the large collection of historical photographs belonging to the Historical Commission (2007); The Conservation Fund, Austin, Texas $375,000 - funding for purchase of strategic conservation lands in Orange County, Texas for donation to the Big Thicket National Preserve for permanent protection (2007);
Date(s) Application is Due: Mar 1; Jun 1; Oct 1
Contact: Grant Department
Internet: http://www.starkfoundation.org/Grants/Grant-Guidelines.aspx
Sponsor: Nelda C. and H.J. Lutcher Stark Foundation
P.O. Box 909
Orange, TX 77631-0909

Nell Warren Elkin and William Simpson Elkin Foundation 2302

The foundation awards grants to charitable organizations in its areas of interest, including universities, cancer clinics, specific disease associations, religious groups, and Bible studies. Application form and guidelines are available online.

Requirements: Nonprofit, charitable organizations are eligible.

Amount of Grant: $2000-$10,000 average

Date(s) Application is Due: Feb 28; Jul 31

Contact: Dale Welch, c/o SunTrust Bank, Atlanta, (404) 724-3773; email: rs.foundationinfo@suntrust.com

Internet: http://www.elkinfoundation.org

Sponsor: Nell Warren Elkin and William Simpson Elkin Foundation
P.O. Box 4655, MC 221
Atlanta, GA 30302

New Jersey Osteopathic Education Foundation Scholarships 2303

Approximately five scholarships are awarded each year to deserving students entering their first year in an osteopathic college. They must be residents of New Jersey and have completed four years of pre-medical education. Selection of awardees is based on undergraduate academic achievement, financial need, motivation, and professional promise as an osteopathic physician.

Requirements: Student must be a resident of the state of New Jersey, must be osteopathically oriented, and must be a student member of the American Osteopathic Association and the New Jersey Association of Osteopathic Physicians and Surgeons throughout his/her medical education. Applicants should have a B average or a 3.0 grade point average or better on a 4.0 scale and be in the upper 25 percent in class standing. The required forms can be downloaded from the sponsor's website.

Geographic Focus: New Jersey

Amount of Grant: $5000 minimum

Date(s) Application is Due: Apr 30

Contact: Robert Bowen, NJAOPS Executive Director; (732) 940-9000; fax: (732) 940-8899; email: njaops@njosteo.com

Internet: http://www.njosteo.com/displaycommon.cfm?an=1&subarticlenbr=68

Sponsor: New Jersey Osteopathic Education Foundation
One Distribution Way, Suite 201
Monmouth Junction, NJ 08852-3001

New York Life Foundation Grants 2304

The foundation awards grants to nonprofit organizations in its areas of interest. Periodically, the foundation selects an area of special priority. The current focus, Nurturing the Children, directs the majority of the foundation's resources toward organizations, programs, and services aimed at helping young people. This initiative specifically focuses on safe places to learn and grow; educational enhancement; and mentoring. The foundation has initiated a new grant award program for nonprofit organizations based in New York City. Youth In Action recognizes innovative Nurturing the Children programs that engage youth in planning, coordinating and/or helping to provide services.

Requirements: Nonprofit 501(c)3 organizations may submit grant requests. The foundation funds projects in New York City, where New York Life's Home Office is located. The foundation also considers multi-site projects implemented by national organizations. These projects must serve two or more of the following: Atlanta; Cleveland; Clinton/Hunterdon County, New Jersey; Dallas; Kansas City; Minneapolis; New York City; Parsippany/Morris County, New Jersey; Tampa; and Westchester County, New York.

Restrictions: The foundation does not support sectarian or religious organizations or activities; fraternal, social, professional, athletic, or veterans groups; seminars or conferences; preschool, primary, or secondary education; endowments; memorials; basic or applied research; capital campaigns; or fund-raising activities.

Date(s) Application is Due: Dec 1

Contact: Program Contact, (212) 576-7341; fax: (212) 576-6220; email: NYLFoundation@newyorklife.com

Internet: http://www.newyorklife.com/foundation/index.html

Sponsor: New York Life Foundation
51 Madison Avenue, Room 1600
New York, NY 10010-1655

New York University Steinhardt School of Education Fellowships 2305

The program awards fellowships for doctoral study in the field of education. Named fellowships include Founders Fellowships, Phyllis and Gerald LeBoff Fellowship in Media Ecology, and the Steinhardt Fellowship in Education and Jewish Studies. Fellowships provide up to three years of full-tuition support and annual stipends. Faculty in relevant disciplines are also invited to nominate qualified students for these awards for doctoral study in education, applied psychology, health, nursing, art, music, and media studies.

Requirements: Successful candidates are expected to have a history of collaborative and scholarly work with faculty, strong academic records, and an ability to draw on the resources of their program's faculty at the university.

Amount of Grant: $10,000-$18,000 per year

Date(s) Application is Due: Jan 15

Contact: Grants Administrator, Office of Graduate Admissions, School of Education, (800) 771-4698 ext K28 or (212) 998-5030; email: ed.gradadmissions@nyu.edu

Internet: http://www.education.nyu.edu

Sponsor: New York University
82 Washington Square E, 2nd Floor
New York, NY 10003-6680

Newman's Own Inc Grants 2306

The corporate giving program awards general support grants to a broad array of charitable and educational causes, including children and youth, health, education, elderly, environment, the arts, handicapped, literacy, substance abuse education, programs for the needy (i.e., housing and food). More than 600 grants are made annually. Funding levels vary each year based on after-tax profits. Actor and company president, Paul L. Newman, reviews each proposal and selects the groups and organizations to receive contributions. He is interested in organizations outside of the charity mainstream that help those who often cannot help themselves. Social service agencies in Australia and Canada also receive support. Early submission of proposals is encouraged. Faxed or emailed proposals are not accepted.

Requirements: IRS 501(c)3 nonprofits are eligible for grant support.

Restrictions: Paul Newman and the Newman's Own Foundation do not support individual donations and scholarships.

Amount of Grant: $2,000-$15,000 typically

Contact: Paul L. Newman; c/o Newman's Own

Internet: http://www.newmansownfoundation.org/giving/

Sponsor: Newman's Own Inc
246 Post Road East
Westport, CT 06880-3615

NFID Advanced Vaccinology Course Travel Grant 2307

These grants are intended to assist recent postdoctoral graduates who have a demonstrated interest in a career in vaccinology. This program provides participants with a comprehensive overview of vaccinology, from immunology to the social, economic, political, and ethical issues of vaccination. Practical approaches to the implementation of effective vaccination programs suitable for particular population groups will be discussed. To be eligible for this award the applicant must have made separate application to the course. Further information about the course can be obtained from: Betty Dodet, Fondation Merieux, 17, rue Bourgelat, BP 2021, Lyon Cedex 02, France. Annual deadline dates vary; contact program staff for exact dates. Note: Please do not contact NFID for information about the course. Contact the listed contact person.

Requirements: Individuals who are U.S. citizens who reside in the United States at the time of the course and who are within three years of obtaining a doctoral degree, or in the case of physicians, within two years of completing specialty training or a subspecialty fellowship, are eligible to apply. Candidates must have a demonstrated commitment to vaccinology as a career, and must be conducting research or working in a recognized and accredited U.S. institution of higher learning or in a governmental agency.

Amount of Grant: $4000

Date(s) Application is Due: Nov 14

Contact: Betty Dodet, Fondation Merieux; fax: (33-4) 72 40 79 50; email: betty.dodet@fond-merieux.org

Internet: http://www.nfid.org/fellow/grantsfellow.pdf

Sponsor: National Foundation for Infectious Diseases
4733 Bethesda Avenue, Suite 750
Bethesda, MD 20814

NFID Colin L. Powell Minority Postdoctoral Fellowship in Tropical Disease Research 2308

The program, sponsored by NFID and GlaxoSmithKline, invites applications from qualified minority researchers to become specialists and investigators in the field of tropical diseases. The one-year fellowship includes a stipend, $3000 of which may be used for travel and supplies. Fellowships commence on or about July 1, with notification on or about April 15. Annual deadline dates may vary; contact program staff for exact dates.

Requirements: The applicant must hold a doctorate from a recognized U.S. university and be a U.S. citizen or permanent resident or spouse of a U.S. citizen or permanent resident.

Amount of Grant: $30,000 stipend

Date(s) Application is Due: Jan 6

Contact: Senior Executive Director, (301) 656-0003; fax: (301) 907-0878; email: info@nfid.org

Internet: http://www.nfid.org/fellow/grantsfellow.pdf

Sponsor: National Foundation for Infectious Diseases
4733 Bethesda Avenue, Suite 750
Bethesda, MD 20814

NFID John P. Utz Medical Mycology Postdoctoral Fellowship 2309

The fellowship is intended to encourage and assist a qualified physician to become a specialist and investigator in medical mycology. Selection criteria for the one-year fellowship will include, but not be limited to, the applicant's record of scholarship performance and professional qualifications; scientific merit of the clinical research project proposed; and validity of research rationale and adequacy of facilities available to the applicant, host department, and host institution. The recipient will be required to submit two single-spaced, one-page progress reports during his/her year of clinical research. One report will be due after six months and the second after 12 months or upon completion of the fellowship year. Notification of award will be made on or about April 15.

Requirements: The applicant must be a physician who is a U.S. citizen. He/she must demonstrate aptitude and accomplishment in research and must confirm arrangements for conduct of the proposed research in a recognized host laboratory. A letter from the chairperson of the department of infectious diseases expressing a willingness to assume responsibility for training the applicant must accompany the application.

Restrictions: The fellowship may not be awarded if the applicant has received or will receive a major fellowship, research grant, or traineeship from the federal government or another foundation in excess of the amount of this award.
Amount of Grant: $40,000 stipend which includes $1000 for travel and supplies
Date(s) Application is Due: Jan 6
Contact: Senior Executive Director, (301) 656-0003; fax: (301) 907-0878; email: info@nfid.org
Internet: http://nfid.org/fellow/grantsfellow.pdf
Sponsor: National Foundation for Infectious Diseases
4733 Bethesda Avenue, Suite 750
Bethesda, MD 20814-5278

NFID New Investigator Matching Grants **2310**
Matching grants are intended to assist new investigators who are beginning their research. The proposal must be based on research relevant to infectious diseases, microbiology, clinical medicine, epidemiology, nursing, etc. Priority will be given to applications proposing research on HIV and AIDS; tuberculosis, influenza, and other respiratory diseases; hospital-acquired and opportunistic infections; viral hepatitis; gastrointestinal, diarrheal, and food-borne diseases; sexually transmitted diseases; antibiotic resistance; tropical, travelers', and parasitic diseases; diseases transferred from animals to humans; and new and reemerging infectious diseases. Each application must be accompanied by an agreement from the applicant's sponsoring institution to match the award with equal funds.
Requirements: A new investigator is defined as an individual with full-time junior faculty (instructor or assistant professor) status at a recognized and accredited institution of higher learning. Priority will be given to those who do not have research grants and whose studies represent pilot work with intent to further develop their research.
Samples: Dr. Nancy Connell, UMDNJ/New Jersey Medical School (NJ)—to support experiments to study the cell wall and membranes of mycobacteria, $2000.; Dr. Christine Wanke, Harvard U Medical School (MA)—to support research on E. coli in adult patients infected with HIV with chronic diarrhea, $2000.
Amount of Grant: $2000
Date(s) Application is Due: Feb 14
Contact: Senior Executive Director, (301) 656-0003; fax: (301) 907-0878; email: info@nfid.org
Internet: http://www.nfid.org/fellow/grantsfellow.pdf
Sponsor: National Foundation for Infectious Diseases
4733 Bethesda Avenue, Suite 750
Bethesda, MD 20814

NFID Nosocomial Infection Research and Training Postdoctoral Fellowship **2311**
The fellowship is intended to encourage and assist a qualified physician researcher to become a specialist and investigator in the field of nosocomial infections. Priority will be given to the study of gram positive nosocomial infections. Each application must be accompanied by a letter from the host laboratory and signed by the laboratory director or appropriate department chairperson indicating a willingness to accept the applicant and to provide guidance, research space, and necessary research equipment. Overhead to the sponsoring institution will not be paid. One thousand dollars of the stipend may be used for travel and supplies.
Requirements: The applicant must be a physician and a citizen of the United States. He/she must demonstrate aptitude and accomplishment in research and must confirm arrangements for conduct of the proposed research in a recognized host laboratory. An applicant with no grant support will receive priority consideration.
Restrictions: Applicants receiving or to be awarded grants in the same academic year in excess of the amount of this award are ineligible.
Amount of Grant: $40,000 total
Date(s) Application is Due: Jan 6
Contact: Senior Executive Director, (301) 656-0003; fax: (301) 907-0878; email: info@nfid.org
Internet: http://nfid.org/fellow/grantsfellow.pdf
Sponsor: National Foundation for Infectious Diseases
4733 Bethesda Avenue, Suite 750
Bethesda, MD 20814-5278

NFID Postdoctoral Fellowships in Emerging Infectious Diseases **2312**
This one-year fellowship is intended to encourage and assist a qualified physician to become a recognized authority on emerging infectious diseases and epidemiology. The fellow will be assigned to the National Center for Infectious Diseases, CDC, in Atlanta, GA, and will participate in analysis and reporting of the national burden of infectious diseases and potential threats of emerging infectious diseases.
Requirements: The applicant must be a physician who is a U.S. citizen who preferably will have completed an infectious diseases fellowship.
Restrictions: The fellowship may not be awarded if the applicant has received or will receive a major fellowship, research grant, or traineeship from the federal government or another foundation in excess of $20,000.
Amount of Grant: $50,000 stipend
Date(s) Application is Due: Jan 6
Contact: Executive Director, (301) 656-0003; fax: (301) 907-0878; email: info@nfid.org
Internet: http://nfid.org/fellow/grantsfellow.pdf
Sponsor: National Foundation for Infectious Diseases
4733 Bethesda Avenue, Suite 750
Bethesda, MD 20814

NFX Patient-Oriented Research Grants **2313**
The foundation supports a broad range of research endeavors that will lead to better recognition, treatment, and an eventual cure of children and adults with fragile X syndrome. The following forms of investigation are potentially appropriate for the current round of funding: educational or therapy interventions, medical treatment interventions, studies of family support and counseling, and diagnostic and reproductive studies. Basic research and patient-oriented research grants are awarded on a six-month alternating cycle. The January deadline is for basic science and clinical research applications. Applications should be submitted both as email attachments and as hard-copy documents.
Requirements: The program is open to all investigators with demonstrated ability to carry out research on fragile X syndrome.
Amount of Grant: $35,000 maximum for junior investigators; $50,000 maximum for senior investigators
Date(s) Application is Due: Jan 31
Contact: Grants Administrator, (800) 688-8765 or (925) 938-9300; fax: (925) 938-9315; email: NATLFX@FragileX.org
Internet: http://www.fragilex.org/html/request_for_application.htm
Sponsor: National Fragile X Foundation
P.O. Box 190488
San Francisco, CA 94119

NFX Summer Research Fellowships **2314**
The foundation awards summer research fellowships in the area of fragile X syndrome. Proposals should be no longer than four pages, and should describe the research project in depth and the specific roles and activities of the summer fellow and the mentor. The curriculum vitas of the mentor and the fellow should be included as an addendum. Guidelines are available online.
Requirements: The fellow can be either an undergraduate or graduate student, and the mentor should be experienced in research concerning fragile X syndrome.
Amount of Grant: $2500
Date(s) Application is Due: Apr 17
Contact: Grants Administrator, (800) 688-8765 or (925) 938-9300; fax: (925) 938-9315; email: NATLFX@FragileX.org
Internet: http://www.fragilex.org/html/request_for_application.htm
Sponsor: National Fragile X Foundation
P.O. Box 190488
San Francisco, CA 94119

NHGRI Mentored Research Scientist Development Award **2315**
These awards are intended to foster the career development of individuals with expertise in scientific disciplines that would further technological developments critical to the success of the Human Genome Project and the understanding of the genetic basis of diseases. Up to three scientists may be selected and appointed to this program by the grantee institutions. Up to the Federal salary cap, plus fringe benefits, is available. Up to $20,000 of research support per year is also available.
Requirements: Eligibility is limited to individuals with degrees in computer sciences, mathematics, chemistry, engineering, physics, and closely related scientific disciplines, such as bioinformatics, computational biology, statistics, biomathematics, bioengineering. Applications will be accepted from domestic, nonfederal organizations of higher education that have strong, well-established research and training programs. The following organizations and institutions may apply: public/state controlled institutions of higher education; private institutions of higher education; Hispanic-serving institutions; historically Black colleges and universities (HBCUs); tribally controlled colleges and universities (TCCUs); Alaska native and native Hawaiian serving institutions; nonprofits with 501(c)3 IRS status; nonprofits without 501(c)3 IRS status; small businesses; for-profit organizations; State governments; regional organizations; U.S. territories or possessions; Indian/Native American tribal governments; Indian/Native American tribally designated organizations; eligible agencies of the Federal government; and faith-based or community based organizations.
Date(s) Application is Due: Feb 12; Mar 12; Jun 12; Jul 12; Oct 12; Nov 12
Contact: Bettie J. Graham; (301) 496-7531; email: bettie_graham@nih.gov
Internet: http://grants.nih.gov/grants/guide/pa-files/PAR-98-062.html
Sponsor: National Human Genome Research Institute (NHGRI)
5635 Fishers Lane, Suite 4076
Rockville, MD 20852

NHLBI Airway Smooth Muscle Function and Targeted Therapeutics in Human Asthma Grants **2316**
The purpose of this funding opportunity announcement, issued by the NHLBI, NIH, is to solicit Research Project Grant applications from institutions and organizations that propose to investigate the complex role of airway smooth muscle (ASM) functions in the development of human asthma and identify novel therapeutic targets. Budgets for direct costs of up to $350,000 per year (exclusive of indirect costs associated with consortia) and a project duration of up to four years may be requested for a maximum of $1,400,000 direct costs over a four-year project period. Letters of Intent should be received by December 8, and full proposals are due by January 6.
Requirements: The following organizations and institutions are eligible to apply: public/state controlled institutions of higher education; private institutions of higher education; Hispanic-serving institutions; historically Black colleges and universities (HBCUs); tribally controlled colleges and universities (TCCUs); Alaska Native and Native Hawaiian serving institutions; nonprofits with 501(c)3 IRS status; nonprofits without 501(c)3 IRS status; for-profit organizations; state governments; Indian/Native American tribal governments (federally recognized); Indian/Native American tribally designated

organizations; county governments; city or township governments; special district governments; independent school districts; public housing authorities/Indian housing authorities; U.S. territory or possession; Indian/Native American tribal governments (other than federally recognized); regional organizations; non-domestic (non-U.S.) entities (foreign organizations); other eligible agencies of the federal government; and faith-based or community-based organizations.
Amount of Grant: $350,000 per year maximum
Date(s) Application is Due: Dec 8; Jan 6
Contact: Susan Banks-Schlegel, Ph.D.; (301) 435-0202; fax: (301) 480-3557; email: Schleges@nhlbi.nih.gov;; Dorothy Gail, Ph.D.; (301) 435-0222; fax: (301) 480-3557; email: Gaild@nhlbi.nih.gov
Internet: http://grants1.nih.gov/grants/guide/rfa-files/RFA-HL-09-007.html
Sponsor: National Heart, Lung, and Blood Institute (NHLBI)
6701 Rockledge Drive
Bethesda, MD 20892-7952

NHLBI Ancillary Studies in Clinical Trials **2317**
The purpose of this Funding Opportunity Announcement (FOA) is to solicit research grant applications to conduct time-sensitive ancillary studies related to heart, lung, and blood diseases and sleep disorders in conjunction with ongoing NIH- or non-NIH-supported clinical trials. An applicant may request a project period of up to four years and a budget for direct costs up to $250,000 (10 modules) per year. Dates for Letters of Intent are: December 30, April 29, and August 31. Respective due dates fot full applications are: January 30, May 29, and September 30.
Requirements: The following organizations and institutions are eligible to apply: individuals; public/state controlled institutions of higher education; private institutions of higher education; Hispanic-serving institutions; historically Black colleges and universities (HBCUs); tribally controlled colleges and universities (TCCUs); Alaska Native and Native Hawaiian serving institutions; nonprofits with 501(c)3 IRS status; nonprofits without 501(c)3 IRS status; for-profit organizations; state governments; Indian/Native American tribal governments (federally recognized); Indian/Native American tribally designated organizations; county governments; city or township governments; special district governments; independent school districts; public housing authorities/Indian housing authorities; U.S. territory or possession; Indian/Native American tribal governments (other than federally recognized); regional organizations; non-domestic (non-U.S.) entities (foreign organizations); other eligible agencies of the federal government; and faith-based or community-based organizations.
Amount of Grant: $250,000 per year for up to 4 years
Date(s) Application is Due: Jan 30; May 29; Sep 30
Contact: Gail Weinmann, M.D.; (301) 435-0233; fax: (301) 480-3547; email: weinmang@nhlbi.nih.gov;; Peter Kaufmann, Ph.D.; (301) 435-0422; fax: (301) 480-1773; email: kaufmannp@nhlbi.nih.gov
Internet: http://grants.nih.gov/grants/guide/rfa-files/RFA-HL-09-001.html
Sponsor: National Heart, Lung, and Blood Institute
6701 Rockledge Drive, Room 10188
Bethesda, MD 20892-7952

NHLBI Bioengineering and Obesity Grants **2318**
The purpose of this FOA is to solicit applications to develop and validate new and innovative engineering approaches to address clinical problems related to energy balance, intake, and expenditure. Novel sensors, devices, imaging, and other technologies, including technologies to detect biochemical markers of energy balance are expected to be developed and evaluated by collaborating engineers, physical scientists, mathematicians, and scientists from other relevant disciplines with expertise in obesity and nutrition. Basic and applied scientific applications with rigorous hypothesis-testing designs or for design-directed research are encouraged. The goal is to increase the number of useful technologies and tools available to scientists to facilitate their research in energy balance and health. Eventually these research tools should facilitate therapeutic advances and behavioral changes to address such problems as weight control and obesity.
Requirements: The following organizations and institutions are eligible to apply: public/state controlled institutions of higher education; private institutions of higher education; Hispanic-serving institutions; historically Black colleges and universities (HBCUs); tribally controlled colleges and universities (TCCUs); Alaska Native and Native Hawaiian serving institutions; nonprofits with 501(c)3 IRS status; nonprofits without 501(c)3 IRS status; for-profit organizations; state governments; Indian/Native American tribal governments (federally recognized); Indian/Native American tribally designated organizations; county governments; city or township governments; special district governments; independent school districts; public housing authorities/Indian housing authorities; U.S. territory or possession; Indian/Native American tribal governments (other than federally recognized); regional organizations; non-domestic (non-U.S.) entities (foreign organizations); other eligible agencies of the federal government; and faith-based or community-based organizations.
Date(s) Application is Due: Feb 5; Jun 5; Oct 5
Contact: Abby G. Ershow; (301) 435-0550; fax: (301) 480-1338; email: ErshowA@mail.nih.gov;; J. Timothy Baldwin; (301) 435-0513; fax: (301) 480-1335; email: BaldwinT@mail.nih.gov
Internet: http://grants.nih.gov/grants/guide/pa-files/PA-07-354.html
Sponsor: National Heart, Lung, and Blood Institute (NHLBI)
6701 Rockledge Drive, Suite, MSC 7956
Bethesda, MD 20892-7956

NHLBI Bioengineering Approaches to Energy Balance and Obesity Grants for SBIR **2319**
This funding opportunity will develop and validate new and innovative bioengineering technology to address clinical problems related to energy balance, intake, and expenditure. Novel sensors, devices, imaging, and other approaches are expected to be developed and evaluated by collaborating engineers, physical scientists, and scientists from other relevant disciplines with expertise in obesity and nutrition. The goal is to increase the number of useful technologies and tools available to scientists to facilitate their research in energy balance and health. Eventually these research tools should facilitate therapeutic advances and behavioral changes to address such problems as weight control and obesity. Because the nature and scope of the proposed research will vary from application to application, it is anticipated that the size and duration of each award will also vary. The total amount awarded and the number of awards will depend upon the mechanism numbers, quality, duration, and costs of the applications received.
Requirements: Only United States small business concerns (SBCs) are eligible to submit SBIR applications.
Date(s) Application is Due: Apr 5; Aug 5; Dec 5
Contact: Abby G. Ershow; (301) 435-0550; fax: (301) 480-1338; email: ErshowA@mail.nih.gov;; J. Timothy Baldwin; (301) 435-0513; fax: (301) 480-1335; email: BaldwinT@mail.nih.gov
Internet: http://grants.nih.gov/grants/guide/pa-files/PA-07-435.html
Sponsor: National Heart, Lung, and Blood Institute (NHLBI)
Two Rockledge Center, Suite 9152, MSC 7956, 6701 Rockledge Drive
Bethesda, MD 20892-7956

NHLBI Bioengineering Approaches to Energy Balance and Obesity Grants for STTR **2320**
This funding opportunity will develop and validate new and innovative bioengineering technology to address clinical problems related to energy balance, intake, and expenditure. Novel sensors, devices, imaging, and other approaches are expected to be developed and evaluated by collaborating engineers, physical scientists, and scientists from other relevant disciplines with expertise in obesity and nutrition. The goal is to increase the number of useful technologies and tools available to scientists to facilitate their research in energy balance and health. Eventually these research tools should facilitate therapeutic advances and behavioral changes to address such problems as weight control and obesity. Because the nature and scope of the proposed research will vary from application to application, it is anticipated that the size and duration of each award will also vary. The total amount awarded and the number of awards will depend upon the mechanism numbers, quality, duration, and costs of the applications received.
Requirements: Only United States small business concerns (SBCs) are eligible to submit STTR applications.
Date(s) Application is Due: Apr 5; Aug 5; Dec 5
Contact: Abby G. Ershow; (301) 435-0550; fax: (301) 480-1338; email: ErshowA@mail.nih.gov;; J. Timothy Baldwin; (301) 435-0513; fax: (301) 480-1335; email: BaldwinT@mail.nih.gov
Internet: http://grants.nih.gov/grants/guide/pa-files/PA-07-436.html
Sponsor: National Heart, Lung, and Blood Institute (NHLBI)
Two Rockledge Center, Suite 9152, MSC 7956, 6701 Rockledge Drive
Bethesda, MD 20892-7956

NHLBI Biomedical Research Training Program for Individuals from Underrepresented Groups **2321**
The NHLBI established the Biomedical Research Training Program for Individuals from Underrepresented Groups (BRTPUG) to offer opportunities for underrepresented post-baccalaureate individuals, undergraduate, and graduate students to receive training in fundamental biomedical sciences and clinical research disciplines. The purpose of the program is to enhance career opportunities in biomedical and behavioral research, including clinical and laboratory medicine, epidemiology, and biostatistics as applied to the etiology and treatment of heart, blood vessel, lung, and blood diseases. BRTPUG offers each participant the opportunity to work closely with leading research scientists in the Division of Intramural Research and extramural scientists in the Division of Prevention and Population Sciences. The program provides students with hands-on training in a research environment, which will prepare them to continue their studies and advance their careers in clinical and basic research. The trainee's appointment is a one-time appointment of 6 (2 summers) to 24 months over a 2 year period beginning the summer of selection. Each trainee is assigned to a mentor who is responsible for designing a carefully planned training program. For placements beginning in June of the calendar year or summer opportunities, NHLBI strongly encourages applicants to submit your application by January 15. For Post-Baccalaureate 1-2 year research internships beginning in July-September of the calendar year, applications should be submitted by March 1.
Requirements: Underrepresented post-baccalaureate individuals, and undergraduate and graduate students planning to pursue advanced degrees in the biomedical and behavioral sciences and meeting all other program criteria are eligible. Applicants must have a cumulative grade point average (GPA) or science course GPA of 3.3 or better on a 4.0 scale, or 4.3 or better on a 5.0 scale, and be U.S. citizens or permanent residents.
Date(s) Application is Due: Jan 15; Mar 1
Contact: Helena O. Mishoe, PhD; (301) 451-5081; fax: (301) 480-0862; email: mishoeh@nhlbi.nih.gov
Internet: http://www.nhlbi.nih.gov/funding/training/redbook/undbrtum.htm
Sponsor: National Heart, Lung, and Blood Institute (NHLBI)
6701 Rockledge Drive, Room 8188
Bethesda, MD 20892-7913

NHLBI Blood Diseases and Resources Research Grants 2322

To foster research for the prevention, improved diagnosis, and treatment of non-malignant blood diseases such as Coolie's anemia, sickle cell disease, hemophilia, hemochromatosis, and disorders of hemostasis and thrombosis; to support research on hematopoietic stem cell biology and transplantation and on the use of transplantation to treat blood diseases; and to promote research in transfusion medicine for improving the availability, safety, and use of blood and blood products; and to develop new scientists for blood disease and resources research. Grants may support salaries, equipment, supplies, travel, and patient hospitalization as required to perform the research effort. National Research Service Awards (NRSAs) are made directly to individuals for research training in specified biomedical shortage areas. Grants may be made to institutions to enable them to make NRSAs to individuals selected by them.

Requirements: Any nonprofit organization engaged in biomedical research and institutions (or companies) organized for profit may apply for grants, with the exception of NRSAs. An individual may apply for a NRSA or, in some cases, may qualify for a research grant if adequate facilities in which to perform the research are available. SBIR grants can be awarded only to domestic small businesses (entities that are independently owned and operated for profit, are not dominant in the field in which research is proposed, and have no more than 500 employees).

Restrictions: Restrictions or limitations are imposed against the use of funds for entertainment, foreign travel, general-purpose equipment, alterations and renovations, and other items not regularly required for the performance of research.

Amount of Grant: $67,988-$2.9 million; $470,787 average

Date(s) Application is Due: Feb 1; Jun 1; Oct 1

Contact: Director, Division of Blood Diseases and Resources; (301) 435-0080; Suzanne White, Grants Management Officer, (301) 435-0144

Internet: http://www.federalgrantswire.com/blood-diseases-and-resources-research.html

Sponsor: National Heart, Lung, and Blood Institute
6701 Rockledge Drive
Bethesda, MD 20892

NHLBI Cardiac Development Consortium Grants 2323

The National Heart, Lung, and Blood Institute (NHLBI) and the Canadian Institutes of Health Research (CIHR) invite applications to participate in a new NHLBI Cardiac Development Consortium, a cooperative investigative group that will drive an integrated approach to the investigation of cardiovascular development. The purpose of this initiative is to support basic collaborative research leading to a comprehensive understanding of the regulatory networks controlling cardiovascular development. The consortium will consist of up to four Research Centers, scientific Cores as necessary, and a Steering Committee. Research Center applicants will propose projects that will select key regulatory pathways, identify the components of the pathways and targets, and rapidly disseminate data to the scientific community. The Research Centers will collaborate to maximize interoperability of the data. This Consortium is part of a new NHLBI translational program in pediatric cardiovascular disease, which includes the companion NHLBI Pediatric Cardiac Genomics Consortium and Administrative Coordinating Center. These consortia will interact with each other and the NHLBI Pediatric Heart Network to encourage translation of results from basic science to clinical research, and to provide clinical input on pressing needs for basic research. Maximum allowable direct costs for the research centers are $160,000 in the Year 1 planning phase, and up to $1,070,000 per year in years two through six. Letters of Intent should be received by January 6, and full proposals are due by February 6.

Requirements: The following organizations and institutions are eligible to apply: public/state controlled institutions of higher education; private institutions of higher education; Hispanic-serving institutions; historically Black colleges and universities (HBCUs); tribally controlled colleges and universities (TCCUs); Alaska Native and Native Hawaiian serving institutions; nonprofits with 501(c)3 IRS status; nonprofits without 501(c)3 IRS status; small businesses; for-profit organizations; state governments; and non-domestic (non-U.S.) entities in North America.

Amount of Grant: $160,000 maximum in the Year 1 planning phase; $1,070,000 maximum per year in years 2-6

Date(s) Application is Due: Jan 6; Feb 6

Contact: Charlene Schramm; (301) 435-0510; email: SchrammC@nhlbi.nih.gov

Internet: http://grants.nih.gov/grants/guide/rfa-files/RFA-HL-09-002.html

Sponsor: National Heart, Lung, and Blood Institute (NHLBI)
Rockledge 2, Room 8100, 6701 Rockledge Drive, MSC 7940
Bethesda, MD 20892

NHLBI Cardiac Translational Research Implementation Program Grants 2324

The National Heart, Lung, and Blood Institute (NHLBI) solicits Stage 1 exploratory planning (P20) applications to the Cardiac Translational Research Implementation Program (C-TRIP). The overall objective of the entire two-staged C-TRIP is to accelerate translation of promising new therapeutic interventions derived from fundamental research discoveries for the treatment and prevention of heart failure or arrhythmias through the planning and execution of well-designed clinical trials to demonstrate safety and efficacy. Stage 1 exploratory planning (P20) applications will support the planning and development of Stage 2 specialized center (P50) applications that support the conduct of the safety and efficacy trials recommended for support following a second phase of peer review. Subsequent Stage 2 (P50) applications for the conduct of the clinical trials planned and developed during Stage 1 will be solicited at a later time. The to-be-released solicitation for Stage 2 specialized center (P50) applications will be limited to successful Stage 1 applicants. Stage 2 (P50) applications will be anticipated 18 months following the initial award of Stage 1 applications. Support during Stage 2 of C-TRIP is expected to provide up to $1,515,000 direct costs per year for up to five years. During this period, applicants may request no more than $500,000 per year in direct costs for a maximum of $1,000,000 direct costs.

Requirements: The following organizations and institutions are eligible to apply: individuals; public/state controlled institutions of higher education; private institutions of higher education; Hispanic-serving institutions; historically Black colleges and universities (HBCUs); tribally controlled colleges and universities (TCCUs); Alaska Native and Native Hawaiian serving institutions; nonprofits with 501(c)3 IRS status; nonprofits without 501(c)3 IRS status; for-profit organizations; state governments; Indian/Native American tribal governments (federally recognized); Indian/Native American tribally designated organizations; county governments; city or township governments; special district governments; independent school districts; public housing authorities/Indian housing authorities; U.S. territory or possession; Indian/Native American tribal governments (other than federally recognized); regional organizations; non-domestic (non-U.S.) entities (foreign organizations); other eligible agencies of the federal government; and faith-based or community-based organizations.

Amount of Grant: $500,000

Date(s) Application is Due: Apr 28; May 28

Contact: David A. Lathrop, Ph.D.; (301) 435-0507; fax: (301) 451-5458; email: lathropd@nhlbi.nih.gov

Internet: http://grants.nih.gov/grants/guide/rfa-files/RFA-HL-10-001.html

Sponsor: National Heart, Lung, and Blood Institute
6701 Rockledge Drive, MSC 7956
Bethesda, MD 20892-7956

NHLBI Career Enhancement Awards for Stem Cell Research 2325

The Career Enhancement Award for Stem Cell Research enables investigators to acquire new research capabilities in the use of human or animal embryonic, adult, or cord blood stem cells. Candidates must have a clinical or research doctoral degree and be actively engaged in research of interest to the NHLBI. Candidates must meet the NIH career development requirements. Actual salary is based on candidate's full-time, 12-month institutional salary, and the level of effort requested. Most recently, for mid-career and senior investigators, the maximum allowable salary was $186,600 for full-time effort. For junior faculty, maximum allowable salary was $75,000. Salary adjustments are announced in the NIH Guide. Up to $50,000 per year is allowed for research expenses, tuition, technical support, personnel consultant fees for mentor, and travel.

Requirements: Investigators at U.S. institutions with current or previous independent research support are eligible.

Amount of Grant: $200,000 maximum

Date(s) Application is Due: Feb 12; Mar 12; Jun 12; Jul 12; Oct 12; Nov 12

Contact: Traci Heath Mondoro, Ph.D.; (301) 435-0052; fax: (301) 480-1060; email: mondorot@nhlbi.nih.gov

Internet: http://www.nhlbi.nih.gov/funding/training/redbook/k18est-junior.htm

Sponsor: National Heart, Lung, and Blood Institute (NHLBI)
Two Rockledge Center, Room 9174, 6701 Rockledge Drive, MSC 7950
Bethesda, MD 20892-7950

NHLBI Career Transition Award 2326

The goal of the program is to provide highly qualified new investigators with an opportunity to receive research and research training experience in the NHLBI Division of Intramural Research and then to provide them with bridge funding to facilitate the transition of their research programs to extramural institutions. Total direct costs for the extramural phase cannot exceed $150,000 including fringe benefits per year in direct costs or $300,000 for the two-year period.

Requirements: The candidate must have a research or a health-professional doctorate, or its equivalent, and must have completed at least three and no more than five years of postdoctoral training, during which the potential for highly productive basic or clinical research was demonstrated.

Restrictions: Individuals on temporary or student visas are not eligible.

Amount of Grant: $150,000 total for intramural phase; $300,000 total direct costs for extramural phase

Date(s) Application is Due: Feb 5; Jun 5; Oct 5

Contact: Herbert M. Geller; (301) 451-9440; fax: (301) 594-8133; email: direducation@nhlbi.nih.gov

Internet: http://grants.nih.gov/grants/guide/pa-files/PAR-07-317.html#SectionVII

Sponsor: National Heart, Lung, and Blood Institute
10 Center Drive, Room 2N242, MSC 1754
Bethesda, MD 20892-1754

NHLBI Characterizing the Blood Stem Cell Niche Grants 2327

This FOA issued by the National Heart, Lung, and Blood Institute, National Institutes of Health, solicits Research Project Grant applications in a specific area of stem cell research, the blood stem cell niche, an area critical to advancing stem cell biology and its applications to cellular therapeutics including hematopoietic stem cell transplantation. This FOA is being initiated to foster collaborative research projects and insightful approaches to dissect the cellular components and factors involved in the hematopoietic stem cell niche. Development of conditional genetic knock-out models to test the role of factors in specific cell lineages and imaging technology to facilitate following stem cell engraftment in the niche in vivo are integral to this initiative. An individual research grant application may not request more than $250,000 direct cost a year unless collaborative in vivo cell imaging studies are included, in which case up to $350,000 direct cost may be requested in a year. An applicant may request a project period of up to 4 years. Letters of Intent should be received by December 8, and full proposals are due by January 6.

Requirements: The following organizations and institutions are eligible to apply: public/state controlled institutions of higher education; private institutions of higher education; Hispanic-serving institutions; historically Black colleges and universities (HBCUs); tribally controlled colleges and universities (TCCUs); Alaska Native and Native Hawaiian serving institutions; nonprofits with 501(c)3 IRS status; nonprofits without 501(c)3 IRS status; for-profit organizations; state governments; Indian/Native American tribal governments (federally recognized); Indian/Native American tribally designated organizations; county governments; city or township governments; special district governments; independent school districts; public housing authorities/Indian housing authorities; U.S. territory or possession; Indian/Native American tribal governments (other than federally recognized); regional organizations; non-domestic (non-U.S.) entities (foreign organizations); other eligible agencies of the federal government; and faith-based or community-based organizations.
Amount of Grant: $250,000 maximum for single entity; $350,000 maximum for collaboratives
Date(s) Application is Due: Dec 8; Jan 6
Contact: John Thomas, Ph.D.; (301) 435-0065; fax: (301) 451-5453; email: ThomasJ@NHLBI.NIH.Gov
Internet: http://grants.nih.gov/grants/guide/rfa-files/RFA-HL-09-010.html
Sponsor: National Heart, Lung, and Blood Institute (NHLBI)
Rockledge II, Suite 9030, 6701 Rockledge Drive
Bethesda, MD 20892-7950

NHLBI Childhood Obesity Prevention and Treatment Research Consortium Grants 2328

The goal of this Funding Opportunity Announcement (FOA) is to fund randomized trials testing intervention approaches to prevent excess weight gain in non-overweight youth and in those already overweight, and/or to reduce weight in obese and severely obese youth. The whole program is designed to promote collaboration, coordination and exchange of scientific information among institutions, and partnerships with local, state and national agencies. The ultimate goal is to improve children's health by preventing obesity-related morbidity and mortality from cardiovascular and other chronic diseases. Letters of Intent are due by September 8, with full proposals received by October 6.
Requirements: The following organizations and institutions are eligible to apply: individuals; public/state controlled institutions of higher education; private institutions of higher education; Hispanic-serving institutions; historically Black colleges and universities (HBCUs); tribally controlled colleges and universities (TCCUs); Alaska Native and Native Hawaiian serving institutions; nonprofits with 501(c)3 IRS status; nonprofits without 501(c)3 IRS status; for-profit organizations; state governments; Indian/Native American tribal governments (federally recognized); Indian/Native American tribally designated organizations; county governments; city or township governments; special district governments; independent school districts; public housing authorities/Indian housing authorities; U.S. territory or possession; Indian/Native American tribal governments (other than federally recognized); regional organizations; non-domestic (non-U.S.) entities (foreign organizations); other eligible agencies of the federal government; and faith-based or community-based organizations.
Amount of Grant: $700,000 in years 1 and 2; $1,500,000 per year in years 3-6; $700,000 in year 7
Date(s) Application is Due: Sep 8; Oct 6
Contact: Charlotte A. Pratt, Program Director; (301) 435-0382; fax: (301) 480-5158; email: prattc@nhlbi.nih.gov;; Terry T-K Huang, Director, Obesity Research Strategic Core; (301) 594-1846; fax: (301) 480-9791; email: huangter@mail.nih.gov
Internet: http://grants.nih.gov/grants/guide/rfa-files/RFA-HL-10-004.html
Sponsor: National Heart, Lung, and Blood Institute (NHLBI)
6701 Rockledge Drive, MSC 7936, Room 10018
Bethesda, MD 20892

NHLBI Childhood Obesity Prevention and Treatment Research Coordinating Unit Grants 2329

This funding opportunity announcement (FOA) invites applications from eligible institutions to participate as the Research Coordinating Unit (RCU) for the childhood obesity prevention and treatment research consortium, which runs in parallel to this FOA. Applicants for the clinical trial will conduct randomized controlled trials that are innovative and that would test innovative interventions to prevent overweight and obesity in youth and to treat existing overweight, obesity and severe obesity in youth. The participating organizations intend to award up to $5.25 million over seven years under this FOA. It is anticipated that one Research Coordinating Unit (RCU) award will be made. Budgets for direct costs of up to $500,000 per year and a project duration of up to seven years may be requested for a maximum of $3.5 million direct costs over a seven year project period. Letters of Intent are due by September 8, with full proposals received by October 6.
Requirements: The following organizations and institutions are eligible to apply: individuals; public/state controlled institutions of higher education; private institutions of higher education; Hispanic-serving institutions; historically Black colleges and universities (HBCUs); tribally controlled colleges and universities (TCCUs); Alaska Native and Native Hawaiian serving institutions; nonprofits with 501(c)3 IRS status; nonprofits without 501(c)3 IRS status; for-profit organizations; state governments; Indian/Native American tribal governments (federally recognized); Indian/Native American tribally designated organizations; county governments; city or township governments; special district governments; independent school districts; public housing authorities/Indian housing authorities; U.S. territory or possession; Indian/Native American tribal governments (other than federally recognized); regional organizations; non-domestic (non-U.S.) entities (foreign organizations); other eligible agencies of the federal government; and faith-based or community-based organizations.
Amount of Grant: $500,000 per year for 7 years
Date(s) Application is Due: Sep 8; Oct 6
Contact: Charlotte A. Pratt, Program Director; (301) 435-0382; fax: (301) 480-5158; email: prattc@nhlbi.nih.gov
Internet: http://grants.nih.gov/grants/guide/rfa-files/RFA-HL-10-005.html
Sponsor: National Heart, Lung, and Blood Institute (NHLBI)
6701 Rockledge Drive, MSC 7936, Room 10018
Bethesda, MD 20892

NHLBI Circadian-Coupled Cellular Function in Heart, Lung, and Blood Tissue Grants 2330

The purpose of this FOA is to stimulate Phase I translation (T1) of fundamental genome-based circadian biology to improve our understanding of heart, lung, and blood disease pathogenesis in non-neural tissues. For the purpose of this initiative, T1 research starts after gene discovery and has as its goal the development of molecular models with application to an improved understanding of human health and disease pathogenesis, predictive testing for disease susceptibility, prognostic testing, or the selection of therapeutic strategies. Budget for direct costs up to $325,000 per year for project duration of up to four years may be requested. Letters of Intent should be received by December 8, and full proposals are due by January 6.
Requirements: The following organizations and institutions are eligible to apply: public/state controlled institutions of higher education; private institutions of higher education; Hispanic-serving institutions; historically Black colleges and universities (HBCUs); tribally controlled colleges and universities (TCCUs); Alaska Native and Native Hawaiian serving institutions; nonprofits with 501(c)3 IRS status; nonprofits without 501(c)3 IRS status; for-profit organizations; state governments; Indian/Native American tribal governments (federally recognized); Indian/Native American tribally designated organizations; county governments; city or township governments; special district governments; independent school districts; public housing authorities/Indian housing authorities; U.S. territory or possession; Indian/Native American tribal governments (other than federally recognized); regional organizations; non-domestic (non-U.S.) entities (foreign organizations); other eligible agencies of the federal government; and faith-based or community-based organizations.
Amount of Grant: $325,000 per year maximum
Date(s) Application is Due: Dec 8; Jan 6
Contact: Aaron Laposky, Ph.D.; (301) 435-0199; fax: (301) 480-3451; email: laposkya@nhlbi.nih.gov
Internet: http://grants.nih.gov/grants/guide/rfa-files/RFA-HL-09-012.html
Sponsor: National Heart, Lung, and Blood Institute (NHLBI)
6701 Rockledge Dr. MSC 7952
Bethesda, MD 20892-7952

NHLBI Clinical Centers for the NHLBI Asthma Network Grants 2331

The purpose of this funding opportunity, issued by NHLBI, NIH, is to invite applications to participate in the NHLBI Asthma Network (AsthmaNet), a clinical research network that will develop and conduct multiple clinical trials to address the most important asthma management questions and new treatment approaches in pediatric and adult populations. AsthmaNet is designed to promote cooperation and coordination, facilitate scientific exchange, provides training opportunities, and leverage resources. AsthmaNet will include multiple Clinical Centers and one Data Coordinating Center. The protocols will include clinical trials to evaluate and/or compare existing or new therapeutic approaches to asthma management as well as a limited number of proof-of-concept studies to advance the development of novel therapies and studies that investigate the mechanistic bases for interventions examined in AsthmaNet. Letters of Intent should be received by December 30, and full proposals are due by January 30.
Requirements: The following organizations and institutions are eligible to apply: public/state controlled institutions of higher education; private institutions of higher education; Hispanic-serving institutions; historically Black colleges and universities (HBCUs); tribally controlled colleges and universities (TCCUs); Alaska Native and Native Hawaiian serving institutions; nonprofits with 501(c)3 IRS status; nonprofits without 501(c)3 IRS status; for-profit organizations; state governments; Indian/Native American tribal governments (federally recognized); Indian/Native American tribally designated organizations; county governments; city or township governments; special district governments; independent school districts; public housing authorities/Indian housing authorities; U.S. territory or possession; Indian/Native American tribal governments (other than federally recognized); regional organizations; non-domestic (non-U.S.) entities (foreign organizations); other eligible agencies of the federal government; and faith-based or community-based organizations.
Date(s) Application is Due: Dec 30; Jan 30
Contact: Virginia S. Taggart; (301) 435-0202; email: taggartv@nhlbi.nih.gov;; Robert Smith, Ph.D.; (301) 435-0202; email: smithra3@nhlbi.nih.gov
Internet: http://grants.nih.gov/grants/guide/rfa-files/RFA-HL-08-010.html
Sponsor: National Heart, Lung, and Blood Institute (NHLBI)
6701 Rockledge Drive
Bethesda, MD 20892-7952

NHLBI Developmental Origins of Altered Lung Physiology and Immune Function Grants 2332

This FOA issued by the NHLBI, National Institutes of Health, solicits Research Project Grant applications from institutions and organizations that propose to perform research that will enhance the understanding of how the pre- and postnatal environments affect

the interplay of the lung and immune system during development resulting in sustained changes in lung physiology and immune function that compromise respiratory health and outcomes. Budgets for direct costs of up to $350,000 per year (exclusive of indirect costs associated with consortia) and a project duration of up to five years may be requested for a maximum of $1,750,000 direct costs over a five-year project period. Letters of Intent should be received by September 19, and full proposals are due by October 21.
Requirements: The following organizations and institutions are eligible to apply: public/state controlled institutions of higher education; private institutions of higher education; Hispanic-serving institutions; historically Black colleges and universities (HBCUs); tribally controlled colleges and universities (TCCUs); Alaska Native and Native Hawaiian serving institutions; nonprofits with 501(c)3 IRS status; nonprofits without 501(c)3 IRS status; for-profit organizations; state governments; Indian/Native American tribal governments (federally recognized); Indian/Native American tribally designated organizations; county governments; city or township governments; special district governments; independent school districts; public housing authorities/Indian housing authorities; U.S. territory or possession; Indian/Native American tribal governments (other than federally recognized); regional organizations; non-domestic (non-U.S.) entities (foreign organizations); other eligible agencies of the federal government; and faith-based or community-based organizations.
Amount of Grant: $350,000 per year maximum
Date(s) Application is Due: Sep 19; Oct 21
Contact: Patricia Noel, Ph.D.; (301) 435-0202; email: noelp@nhlbi.nih.gov
Internet: http://grants.nih.gov/grants/guide/rfa-files/RFA-HL-08-009.html
Sponsor: National Heart, Lung, and Blood Institute (NHLBI)
6701 Rockledge Drive
Bethesda, MD 20892-7952

NHLBI Elucidating Nature's Solutions to Heart, Lung, and Blood Diseases and Sleep Disorder Processes Research Grants 2333

This Funding Opportunity Announcement (FOA) issued by the National Heart, Lung, and Blood Institute (NHLBI), National Institutes of Health (NIH), solicits grant applications proposing studies that elucidate the natural molecular and cellular adaptations of mammalian species to extreme environmental conditions that would rapidly evoke life-threatening cardiovascular or respiratory responses in other species, including humans. Extreme environmental conditions may include food scarcity, limited access to oxygen, or temperature extremes. The overall objective of the funding opportunity is to identify new targets for therapeutic interventions to treat and prevent heart, blood, and lung diseases and sleep disorders. There are no set aside specific dollars for this funding opportunity, and the amount of each award will be limited to $250,000 in direct costs for up to four years. Check the website for various deadlines.
Requirements: The following organizations and institutions are eligible to apply: individuals; public/state controlled institutions of higher education; private institutions of higher education; Hispanic-serving institutions; historically Black colleges and universities (HBCUs); tribally controlled colleges and universities (TCCUs); Alaska Native and Native Hawaiian serving institutions; nonprofits with 501(c)3 IRS status; nonprofits without 501(c)3 IRS status; for-profit organizations; state governments; Indian/Native American tribal governments (federally recognized); Indian/Native American tribally designated organizations; county governments; city or township governments; special district governments; independent school districts; public housing authorities/Indian housing authorities; U.S. territory or possession; Indian/Native American tribal governments (other than federally recognized); regional organizations; non-domestic (non-U.S.) entities (foreign organizations); other eligible agencies of the federal government; and faith-based or community-based organizations.
Restrictions: This FOA will not support the examination of animal models that simply mimic the progression of human cardiovascular and respiratory diseases.
Amount of Grant: $250,000 in direct costs for up to four years
Date(s) Application is Due: Jan 16; May 15
Contact: David Lathrop; (301) 435-0504; fax: (301) 451-5458; email: LathropD@nhlbi.nih.gov;; David Reiter, Grants Operations Branch; (301) 480-3310; email: reiterd@nhlbi.nih.gov
Internet: http://grants.nih.gov/grants/guide/pa-files/PAR-07-102.html
Sponsor: National Heart, Lung, and Blood Institute
6701 Rockledge Drive, MSC 7940
Bethesda, MD 20892-7940

NHLBI Exploratory Studies in the Neurobiology of Pain in Sickle Cell Disease 2334

The goal of this initiative is to foster novel basic and translational research of the neurobiology of pain in sickle cell disease. Priority will be given to the application of investigational techniques that have been utilized in other pain syndromes in both human and nonhuman studies. A multidisciplinary collaboration, between neurobiologists, clinical specialists in pain, and hematologists will be necessary to maximize the research effort.
Requirements: The following organizations and institutions are eligible to apply: public/state controlled institutions of higher education; private institutions of higher education; Hispanic-serving institutions; historically Black colleges and universities (HBCUs); tribally controlled colleges and universities (TCCUs); Alaska Native and Native Hawaiian serving institutions; nonprofits with 501(c)3 IRS status; nonprofits without 501(c)3 IRS status; for-profit organizations; state governments; Indian/Native American tribal governments (federally recognized); Indian/Native American tribally designated organizations; county governments; city or township governments; special district governments; independent school districts; public housing authorities/Indian housing authorities; U.S. territory or possession; Indian/Native American tribal governments (other than federally recognized); regional organizations; non-domestic (non-U.S.) entities (foreign organizations); other eligible agencies of the federal government; and faith-based or community-based organizations.
Amount of Grant: $300,000 per year maximum
Date(s) Application is Due: Jan 5; Feb 3
Contact: Harvey Luksenburg, M.D.; (301) 435-0050; fax: (301) 480-0868; email: luksenburgh@mail.nih.gov
Internet: http://grants.nih.gov/grants/guide/rfa-files/RFA-HL-09-008.html
Sponsor: National Heart, Lung, and Blood Institute (NHLBI)
6701 Rockledge Drive, MSC 7950
Bethesda, MD 20892-7950

NHLBI Hyperglycemic Exacerbation of Ischemia/Reperfusion Injury after Ischemic Insult Grants 2335

This funding opportunity announcement (FOA) will stimulate a focus on the causal relationship between hyperglycemia and impaired cardioprotection in a cohesive, integrated manner. The concept of this initiative evolved from a survey of the grant portfolio in ischemic heart disease and from the literature and consultation with investigators in the scientific community. Appropriate topics for investigation under this FOA include but are not limited to the following: to elucidate mechanisms of acute hyperglycemic exacerbation of myocardial ischemic injury following an ischemic insult to identify new therapeutic targets; to examine the relationship between severity of hyperglycemia and increases in myocardial infarct size mediated by hyperglycemia-induced impairment of cardioprotective signal transduction; to determine the role of inflammatory cells and oxidative stress in the hyperglycemic exacerbation of myocardial injury in infarction; to examine the interaction of metabolic and sex specific hormonal effects on endothelial and coronary microvascular function with acute hyperglycemia; to elucidate the specific mechanisms by which hyperglycemia affects glucose and lipid metabolism in the myocardium; and to study the pathogenesis of cardiovascular disease during acute hyperglycemia in suitable animal models.
Requirements: The following organizations and institutions are eligible to apply: individuals; public/state controlled institutions of higher education; private institutions of higher education; Hispanic-serving institutions; historically Black colleges and universities (HBCUs); tribally controlled colleges and universities (TCCUs); Alaska Native and Native Hawaiian serving institutions; nonprofits with 501(c)3 IRS status; nonprofits without 501(c)3 IRS status; for-profit organizations; state governments; Indian/Native American tribal governments (federally recognized); Indian/Native American tribally designated organizations; county governments; city or township governments; special district governments; independent school districts; public housing authorities/Indian housing authorities; U.S. territory or possession; Indian/Native American tribal governments (other than federally recognized); regional organizations; non-domestic (non-U.S.) entities (foreign organizations); other eligible agencies of the federal government; and faith-based or community-based organizations.
Date(s) Application is Due: Feb 5; Jun 5; Oct 5
Contact: Isabella Liang, Ph.D.; (301) 435-0504; fax: (301) 451-5458; email: Liangi@mail.nih.gov
Internet: http://grants.nih.gov/grants/guide/pa-files/PA-07-323.html
Sponsor: National Heart, Lung, and Blood Institute (NHLBI)
6701 Rockledge Drive, MSC 7940
Bethesda, MD 20892-7940

NHLBI Hypersensitivity Pneumonitis – Grants for Early Identification and Mechanisms of Disease 2336

The objectives of this funding opportunity announcement (FOA) are to investigate basic mechanisms and early clinical identification of hypersensitivity pneumonitis (HP) interstitial lung disease, in order to elucidate how chronic disease progresses and how it can evolve into either interstitial fibrosis or airway obstructive disease.
Requirements: The following organizations and institutions are eligible to apply: individuals; public/state controlled institutions of higher education; private institutions of higher education; Hispanic-serving institutions; historically Black colleges and universities (HBCUs); tribally controlled colleges and universities (TCCUs); Alaska Native and Native Hawaiian serving institutions; nonprofits with 501(c)3 IRS status; nonprofits without 501(c)3 IRS status; for-profit organizations; state governments; Indian/Native American tribal governments (federally recognized); Indian/Native American tribally designated organizations; county governments; city or township governments; special district governments; independent school districts; public housing authorities/Indian housing authorities; U.S. territory or possession; Indian/Native American tribal governments (other than federally recognized); regional organizations; non-domestic (non-U.S.) entities (foreign organizations); other eligible agencies of the federal government; and faith-based or community-based organizations.
Date(s) Application is Due: Feb 5; Jun 5; Oct 5
Contact: Herbert Y. Reynolds, M.D.; (301) 435-0222; fax: (301) 480-3557; email: Reynoldh@nhlbi.nih.gov
Internet: http://grants.nih.gov/grants/guide/pa-files/PA-07-300.html
Sponsor: National Heart, Lung, and Blood Institute (NHLBI)
6701 Rockledge Drive, 2 Rockledge Center, Suite 10042
Bethesda, MD 20892-7952

NHLBI Immunomodulatory, Inflammatory, and Vasoregulatory Properties of Transfused Red Blood Cell Units as a Function of Preparation and Storage 2337

The goal of this Funding Opportunity Announcement (FOA) in blood banking and transfusion medicine is to solicit novel basic and translational research projects which will identify the molecular and cellular changes that occur during red blood cell unit preparation and storage; and evaluate the immunomodulatory, inflammatory, and

vasoactive effects of storage lesion elements from red blood cell units on the blood vessel wall, host cells, and tissue oxygenation. Only research applications involving human red blood cell units (and their components) suitable for transfusion in the U.S. and that are collected and stored according to methods approved by the U.S. FDA will be considered responsive to this FOA. Applications are encouraged that propose collaborations between investigators from different disciplines such as hematology, blood banking, transfusion medicine, immunology, cell biology, rheology, nanotechnologies, molecular biology, and other relevant disciplines. This program will promote interactions and resource sharing among the award recipients to maximize their research efforts. Letters of Intent should be received by April 21 (1st cycle) or December 19 (2nd cycle), and full proposals are due by either May 21 (1st cycle) or January 21 (2nd cycle).
Requirements: The following organizations and institutions are eligible to apply: public/state controlled institutions of higher education; private institutions of higher education; Hispanic-serving institutions; historically Black colleges and universities (HBCUs); tribally controlled colleges and universities (TCCUs); Alaska Native and Native Hawaiian serving institutions; nonprofits with 501(c)3 IRS status; nonprofits without 501(c)3 IRS status; small businesses; for-profit organizations; state governments; Indian/Native American tribal governments; Indian/Native American tribally designated organizations; and U.S. territories or possessions.
Date(s) Application is Due: Apr 21; May 21; Dec 19; Jan 21
Contact: Simone Glynn, M.D.; (301) 435-0065; email: glynnsa@nhlbi.nih.gov
Internet: http://grants.nih.gov/grants/guide/rfa-files/RFA-HL-08-005.html
Sponsor: National Heart, Lung, and Blood Institute (NHLBI)
Rockledge II, Room 9142, 6701 Rockledge Drive
Bethesda, MD 20892-7950

NHLBI Improving Heart Failure Disease Management Grants **2338**
The purpose of this initiative is to stimulate innovative research to address inadequately answered questions about disease management in clinical practice for chronic heart failure (HF). The broader goal is to identify and improve, better implement, and disseminate clinically effective disease management tools into clinical practice to reduce HF morbidity and mortality and improve patient outcomes. Because the nature and scope of the proposed research will vary from application to application, it is anticipated that the size and duration of each award will also vary. The total amount awarded and the number of awards will depend upon the mechanism numbers, quality, duration, and costs of the applications received.
Requirements: The following organizations and institutions are eligible to apply: individuals; public/state controlled institutions of higher education; private institutions of higher education; Hispanic-serving institutions; historically Black colleges and universities (HBCUs); tribally controlled colleges and universities (TCCUs); Alaska Native and Native Hawaiian serving institutions; nonprofits with 501(c)3 IRS status; nonprofits without 501(c)3 IRS status; for-profit organizations; state governments; Indian/Native American tribal governments (federally recognized); Indian/Native American tribally designated organizations; county governments; city or township governments; special district governments; independent school districts; public housing authorities/Indian housing authorities; U.S. territory or possession; Indian/Native American tribal governments (other than federally recognized); regional organizations; non-domestic (non-U.S.) entities (foreign organizations); other eligible agencies of the federal government; and faith-based or community-based organizations.
Date(s) Application is Due: Feb 5; Jun 5; Oct 5
Contact: Lawton S. Cooper, M.D., M.P.H.; (301) 435-0419; fax: (301) 480-1773; email: CooperLS@nhlbi.nih.gov;; Patrice Desvigne-Nickens, M.D.; (301) 435-0504; fax: (301) 480-1336; email: DesvignP@mail.nih.gov
Internet: http://grants.nih.gov/grants/guide/pa-files/PA-07-355.html
Sponsor: National Heart, Lung, and Blood Institute
6701 Rockledge Drive, Room 10108, MSC 7936
Bethesda, MD 20892-7936

NHLBI Independent Scientist Award **2339**
The award is a special salary-only grant designed to provide protected time for newly independent scientists who currently have non-research obligations such as heavy teaching loads, clinical work, committee assignments, service, and administrative duties that prevent them from having a period of intensive research focus. The award is targeted to persons with doctoral degrees who have completed their research training, have independent peer-reviewed research support, and who need a period of protected research time in order to foster their research career development. New applications are due February 12, June 12, and October 12, while renewal applications are due March 12, July 12, and November 12. Up to $75,000 per year plus fringe benefits is available. No other research development support funds are provided.
Requirements: The following organizations and institutions are eligible to apply: public/state controlled institutions of higher education; private institutions of higher education; nonprofits with 501(c)3 IRS status; nonprofits without 501(c)3 IRS status; small businesses; for-profit organizations; State governments; U.S. territories or possessions; Indian/Native American tribal governments (Federally recognized and other than Federally recognized); Indian/Native American tribally designated organizations; Hispanic-serving institutions; historically Black colleges and universities (HBCUs); tribally controlled colleges and universities (TCCUs); Alaska Native and Native Hawaiian serving institutions; regional organizations; and faith-based or community based organizations.
Restrictions: The award is not intended for investigators who already have full time to perform research, or have substantial publication records or considerable research support indicating that they are well established in their fields. Foreign institutions are not eligible to apply.
Amount of Grant: $75,000 per year maximum, plus fringe benefits
Date(s) Application is Due: Feb 12; Mar 12; Jun 12; Jul 12; Oct 12; Nov 12
Contact: Traci Heath Mondoro, Ph.D.; (301) 435-0052; fax: (301) 480-1060; email: mondorot@nhlbi.nih.gov
Internet: http://grants.nih.gov/grants/guide/pa-files/PA-09-038.html
Sponsor: National Heart, Lung, and Blood Institute (NHLBI)
6701 Rockledge Drive, MSC 7950
Bethesda, MD 20892-7950

NHLBI Individual Postdoctoral National Research Service Awards **2340**
This program offers health scientists the opportunity to receive full-time research training for up to 3 years in areas that reflect the national need for biomedical, clinical and behavioral research in cardiovascular, pulmonary, hematologic, and sleep disorders.
Requirements: When the fellowship begins, the applicant must have received a doctoral degree and have arranged to work with a sponsor affiliated with an institution that has the staff and facilities needed for the proposed training. Applicants must be U.S. citizens, noncitizen nationals, or legal permanent residents of the U.S. Training can be conducted abroad if the site provides opportunities that are not available in this country.
Restrictions: These grants are not intended for study leading to the M.D., D.O., D.D.S., or equivalent professional degrees, nor do they support residency training. One month of payback for each month of training, up to a maximum of 12 months, is required. This requirement can be fulfilled by teaching or research (a minimum of 20 hours per week) on a continuous basis beginning within 2 years after support ends.
Date(s) Application is Due: Apr 8; Aug; Dec 8
Contact: Sandra Colombini Hatch, M.D.; (301) 435-0222; fax: (301) 480-3557; email: Hatchs@nhlbi.nih.gov;; Hannah H. Peavy, M.D.; (301) 435-0222; fax: (301) 480-3557; email: peavyh@nhlbi.nih.gov
Internet: http://www.nhlbi.nih.gov/funding/training/redbook/phdf32.htm
Sponsor: National Heart, Lung, and Blood Institute
Two Rockledge Center, Room 10162, 6701 Rockledge Drive, MSC 7952
Bethesda, MD 20892-7952

NHLBI Individual Predoctoral Fellowships to Promote Diversity in Health-Related Research **2341**
This program encourages students from underrepresented racial and ethnic groups, individuals with disabilities, and individuals from disadvantaged backgrounds to seek graduate degrees in the biomedical and behavioral sciences to help increase the number of well-trained scientists from underrepresented groups. The fellowship provides up to 5 years of support for research training leading to the Ph.D. or equivalent research degree, the combined M.D./Ph.D. degree, or other combined degrees in the biomedical or behavioral sciences.
Requirements: At the time of appointment, students must be U.S. citizens, noncitizen nationals, or lawfully admitted to the U.S. for permanent residence. Individuals on temporary or student visas are not eligible. Individuals with disabilities, or from racial and ethnic groups, or individuals from disadvantaged backgrounds pursuing advanced degrees in the biomedical and behavioral sciences are eligible.
Date(s) Application is Due: Apr 13; Aug 13; Dec 13
Contact: Ann Rothgeb; (301) 435-0202; fax: (301) 480-3557; email: rothgeba@mail.nih.gov
Internet: http://www.nhlbi.nih.gov/funding/training/redbook/gradf31.htm
Sponsor: National Heart, Lung, and Blood Institute
Two Rockledge Center, Room 10158, 6701 Rockledge Drive, MSC 7952
Bethesda, MD 20892-7952

NHLBI Integrating Lung Genetics and Genomics in Human Populations Grants **2342**
The purpose of this Funding Opportunity Announcement (FOA) is to stimulate innovative approaches to merge genetic and genomic techniques to find genes associated with human complex traits for lung disease. Because the nature and scope of the proposed research will vary from application to application, it is anticipated that the size and duration of each award will also vary. The total amount awarded and the number of awards will depend upon the mechanism numbers, quality, duration, and costs of the applications received.
Requirements: The following organizations and institutions are eligible to apply: individuals; public/state controlled institutions of higher education; private institutions of higher education; Hispanic-serving institutions; historically Black colleges and universities (HBCUs); tribally controlled colleges and universities (TCCUs); Alaska Native and Native Hawaiian serving institutions; nonprofits with 501(c)3 IRS status; nonprofits without 501(c)3 IRS status; for-profit organizations; state governments; Indian/Native American tribal governments (federally recognized); Indian/Native American tribally designated organizations; county governments; city or township governments; special district governments; independent school districts; public housing authorities/Indian housing authorities; U.S. territory or possession; Indian/Native American tribal governments (other than federally recognized); regional organizations; non-domestic (non-U.S.) entities (foreign organizations); other eligible agencies of the federal government; and faith-based or community-based organizations.
Date(s) Application is Due: Feb 5; Jun 5; Oct 5
Contact: Susan Banks-Schlegel, Ph.D.; (301) 435-0202; fax: (301) 480-3557; email: Schleges@nhlbi.nih.gov;; Dorothy Gail, Ph.D.; (301) 435-0222; fax: (301) 480-3557; email: Gaild@nhlbi.nih.gov
Internet: http://grants.nih.gov/grants/guide/pa-files/PA-07-135.html
Sponsor: National Heart, Lung, and Blood Institute
Two Rockledge Center, Suite 10018, 6701 Rockledge Drive
Bethesda, MD 20892-7952

NHLBI Intramural Research Training Awards 2343

The Office of Education of the Division of Intramural Research coordinates and assists the training program and provides administrative support and resources for all research training activities within the Division. Programs are available within the Laboratories and Branches within the Division to provide specialized research training for high school students, college students, graduate and medical students, postdoctoral fellows and medical residents and fellows. The Office of Education provides assistance to applicants at each of these levels. NHLBI is committed to improving the representation of underrepresented groups, including minorities, women, and scientists with disabilities in the mainstream of basic and clinical research.

Contact: Herbert M. Geller; (301) 451-9440; fax: (301) 594-8133; email: direducation@nhlbi.nih.gov

Internet: http://www.training.nih.gov/student/pre-irta/previewpostbac.asp

Sponsor: National Heart, Lung, and Blood Institute (NHLBI)
Building 10, Room 2N242, 10 Center Drive MSC 1754
Bethesda, MD 20892-1754

NHLBI Investigator Initiated Multi-Site Clinical Trials 2344

The purpose of this Funding Opportunity Announcement is to provide a vehicle for submitting grant applications for investigator-initiated multi-site Phase II or Phase III randomized, controlled clinical trials. The trials may address any research question related to the mission and goals of NHLBI and may test clinical or behavioral interventions. The trials may randomize at the individual (patient) level or at a group or cluster level (e.g., randomization of clinics, schools, worksites, etc.).

Requirements: The following organizations and institutions are eligible to apply: public/state controlled institutions of higher education; private institutions of higher education; Hispanic-serving institutions; historically Black colleges and universities (HBCUs); tribally controlled colleges and universities (TCCUs); Alaska Native and Native Hawaiian serving institutions; nonprofits with 501(c)3 IRS status; nonprofits without 501(c)3 IRS status; for-profit organizations; state governments; Indian/Native American tribal governments (federally recognized); Indian/Native American tribally designated organizations; county governments; city or township governments; special district governments; independent school districts; public housing authorities/Indian housing authorities; U.S. territory or possession; Indian/Native American tribal governments (other than federally recognized); regional organizations; non-domestic (non-U.S.) entities (foreign organizations); other eligible agencies of the federal government; and faith-based or community-based organizations.

Restrictions: This Funding Opportunity Announcement is not intended for support of single-center studies or multi-center observational studies that are not testing an intervention. Foreign institutions are not eligible to apply.

Date(s) Application is Due: Feb 5; Jun 5; Oct 5

Contact: David Gordon; (301) 435-0564; fax: (301) 480-7971; email: gordond@nhlbi.nih.gov

Internet: http://grants.nih.gov/grants/guide/pa-files/PAR-07-373.html

Sponsor: National Heart, Lung, and Blood Institute (NHLBI)
6701 Rockledge Drive, MSC 7940
Bethesda, MD 20892-7940

NHLBI Lymphatic Biology in Health and Disease Grants 2345

This Funding Opportunity Announcement (FOA) issued by the National Heart, Lung, and Blood Institute (NHLBI) solicits Research Project Grant (R01) applications from qualified researchers to investigate the biology of the lymphatic system and potential new therapeutic implications. The purpose of this program announcement is to stimulate research on the biology of the lymphatic system at all biologic levels: molecular, cellular, tissue, organ, and whole body levels. Further, it includes research on innovations for identifying and intervening in lymphatic diseases across all age groups and disease states. Individuals with the skills, knowledge, and resources necessary to carry out the proposed research are invited to work with their institution/organization to develop an application for support. Individuals from underrepresented racial and ethnic groups as well as individuals with disabilities are always encouraged to apply for NIH support. Letters of Intent are due on August 17, while full ptoposals must arrive by September 18.

Requirements: The following organizations and institutions are eligible to apply: public/state controlled institutions of higher education; private institutions of higher education; Hispanic-serving institutions; historically Black colleges and universities (HBCUs); tribally controlled colleges and universities (TCCUs); Alaska Native and Native Hawaiian serving institutions; nonprofits with 501(c)3 IRS status; nonprofits without 501(c)3 IRS status; for-profit organizations; state governments; Indian/Native American tribal governments (federally recognized); Indian/Native American tribally designated organizations; county governments; city or township governments; special district governments; independent school districts; public housing authorities/Indian housing authorities; U.S. territory or possession; Indian/Native American tribal governments (other than federally recognized); regional organizations; non-domestic (non-U.S.) entities (foreign organizations); other eligible agencies of the federal government; and faith-based or community-based organizations.

Restrictions: Foreign institutions are not eligible to apply.

Date(s) Application is Due: Aug 17; Sep 18

Contact: Stephen Goldman, Ph.D.; (301) 435-0560; fax: (301) 480-7971; email: goldmans@nhlbi.nih.gov;; A. Tyl Hewitt, Ph.D.; (301) 496-5541; fax: (301) 480-0303; email: th119v@nih.gov

Internet: http://grants.nih.gov/grants/guide/pa-files/PAR-07-420.html

Sponsor: National Heart, Lung, and Blood Institute (NHLBI)
6701 Rockledge Drive, Rockledge II, Room 8108
Bethesda, MD 20892-7940

NHLBI Mentored Career Award For Faculty At Minority Institutions 2346

The NHLBI Mentored Career Award for Faculty at Minority Institutions is a three-to-five-year non-renewable career development award made to faculty at a minority institution. The candidates are faculty members at a minority institution, must have research experience (length of time may vary), and be committed to developing into independent biomedical investigators in research areas relevant to the mission of the NHLBI (i.e, cardiovascular, pulmonary, hematologic, or sleep disorders research). The award will enable suitable faculty members holding doctoral degrees, such as the Ph.D., M.D., D.O., D.V.M., or an equivalent degree, to undertake special study and supervised research under a mentor who is an accomplished investigator in the research area proposed and has experience in developing independent investigators. Letters of Intent are due on June 21, while full proposals are due by July 19.

Requirements: Minority scientists and physicians with limited research experience needing guided coursework and supervised laboratory experiences, as well as minority faculty needing only an intensive research experience under the guidance of an established scientist, are eligible to apply. At the time of award, it is required that at least two years have elapsed since the receipt of the doctoral degree and that the candidate have at least one year of prior documented research experience.

Restrictions: Current or past principal investigators of an NIH grant or its equivalent, including the Clinical Investigator Award, Physician Scientist Award, Clinical Investigator Development Award, or Mentored Clinical Scientist Development Award are not eligible for the Mentored Research Scientist Development Award for Minority Faculty. Similarly, individuals serving as responsible investigators or project leaders on large grants, such as a Program Project Grant, are not eligible for the Mentored Research Scientist Development Award for Minority Faculty.

Amount of Grant: $1.2 million total

Date(s) Application is Due: Jun 21; Jul 19

Contact: Traci Heath Mondoro, Ph.D.; (301) 435-0052; fax: (301) 480-1060; email: mondorot@nhlbi.nih.gov

Internet: http://grants.nih.gov/grants/guide/rfa-files/RFA-HL-05-016.html#SectionVII

Sponsor: National Heart, Lung, and Blood Institute
6701 Rockledge Drive, MSC 7950
Bethesda, MD 20892-0052

NHLBI Mentored Career Award for Faculty at Minority Institutions 2347

This program provides research support to faculty members at minority institutions who have the potential to conduct high quality research in the areas of cardiovascular, pulmonary, hematologic, or sleep disorders. Important NHLBI program goals are to enhance the minority institution's science infrastructure by developing the research career and teaching skills of the candidate. All faculty members at domestic institutions with student enrollment drawn substantially from minority racial and ethnic groups (such as African Americans/Blacks, Hispanics, American Indians, Alaska Natives, Native Hawaiians, and non-Asian Pacific Islanders) currently underrepresented in biomedical and behavioral research are eligible. Up to $75,000 per year is available for salary, plus fringe benefits, and up to $36,000 for research development support.

Requirements: Candidates for this award must be minority school faculty members who: are U.S. citizens, noncitizen nationals, or permanent residents by the time of the award; have a doctoral degree or equivalent in a biomedical or behavioral science at least two years prior to the award; and wish to receive specialized training in cardiovascular, pulmonary, hematologic, or sleep disorders research. Each candidate must identify and complete arrangements with a mentor (at the same institution or at a collaborating research center) who is recognized as an accomplished investigator in the proposed research area and who will provide guidance for the candidate's career development and research plan.

Amount of Grant: $75,000 per year for salary; $36,000 maximum for research development

Date(s) Application is Due: Aug 15

Contact: Traci Heath Mondoro, Ph.D.; (301) 435-0052; fax: (301) 480-1060; email: mondorot@nhlbi.nih.gov

Internet: http://www.nhlbi.nih.gov/funding/training/redbook/newrek01.htm

Sponsor: National Heart, Lung, and Blood Institute (NHLBI)
Two Rockledge Center, Room 9174, 6701 Rockledge Drive, MSC 7950
Bethesda, MD 20892-7950

NHLBI Mentored Career Development Award to Promote Faculty Diversity/Re-Entry in Biomedical Research 2348

This award is offered to encourage underrepresented faculty members at U.S. institutions to enhance their research skills in areas of interest to the NHLBI and to increase the number of highly trained investigators from diverse backgrounds or who have experienced an interruption in their research careers. It is geared toward individuals whose basic and clinical research interests are grounded in the advanced methods and experimental approaches needed to solve problems related to cardiovascular, pulmonary, hematological, and sleep disorders research. Salary support up to $75,000 per year plus fringe benefits is available, with research support up to $30,000 per year.

Requirements: Faculty members who have been determined by the grantee institution to be underrepresented on faculty in biomedical and behavioral research on a national or institutional basis, such as individuals from racial and ethnic minority groups, individuals with disabilities, individuals from disadvantaged backgrounds or individuals who have experienced an interruption in their research careers are eligible.

Amount of Grant: $105,000 maximum

Date(s) Application is Due: Aug 15

Contact: Lorraine M. Silsbee; (301) 435-0709; fax: (301) 480-1667; email: Lorraine_Silsbee@nih.gov

Internet: http://www.nhlbi.nih.gov/funding/training/redbook/newsck01.htm
Sponsor: National Heart, Lung, and Blood Institute (NHLBI)
Two Rockledge Center, Room 10018, 6701 Rockledge Drive, MSC 7936
Bethesda, MD 20892-7936

NHLBI Mentored Clinical Scientist Research Career Development Awards 2349
This award enables candidates holding professional degrees (e.g., M.D., D.O., D.V.M., or equivalent degrees) to undertake 3 to 5 years of special study and supervised research with the goal of becoming independent investigators. The award also allows awardees to pursue a research career development program suited to their experience and capabilities under a mentor who is competent to provide guidance in the chosen research area. Institutions may submit applications on behalf of candidates who hold professional degrees. At least 2 years must have elapsed since the health professional degree was granted. Candidates can have varying levels of clinical training and research experience. New applications are due February 12, June 12, and October 12, while resubmitted applications are due March 12, July 12, and November 12. Up to $75,000 per year plus fringe benefits is available, and up to $25,000 per year for research support for new awards.
Requirements: All candidates must be U.S. citizens, non-citizen nationals, or legal permanent residents of the U.S. Persons with temporary or student visas are not eligible. The grantee institution must have a strong, well-established research and research training program in the chosen area, accomplished faculty in the basic and clinical sciences, and a commitment to the candidate's research development. The proposed program should include an appropriate mentor.
Amount of Grant: $100,000 maximum
Date(s) Application is Due: Feb 12; Mar 12; Jun 12; Jul 12; Oct 12; Nov 12
Contact: Lorraine M. Silsbee; (301) 435-0709; fax: (301) 480-1667; email: Lorraine_Silsbee@nih.gov
Internet: http://www.nhlbi.nih.gov/funding/training/redbook/newrek08.htm
Sponsor: National Heart, Lung, and Blood Institute (NHLBI)
6701 Rockledge Drive, MSC 7936, Two Rockledge Center, Room 10202
Bethesda, MD 20892-7936

NHLBI Mentored Patient-Oriented Research Career Development Awards 2350
This award supports the career development of investigators who are committed to patient-oriented research. It provides support for supervised study and research for clinically trained professionals who have the potential to develop into productive, clinical investigators focusing on patient-oriented research. This program provides research development opportunities for clinicians with varying levels of research experience. Support is provided for a minimum of 3 years and a maximum of 5 years. Up to $75,000 per year in salary, plus fringe benefits, is available. In addition, $30,000 for research development support per year is available (with sufficient justification up to $50,000 per year can be requested). New applications are due February 12, June 12, and October 12, while resubmitted applications are due March 12, July 12, and November 12.
Requirements: All candidates must be U.S. citizens, noncitizen nationals, or legal permanent residents of the U.S. Candidates must have an M.D., D.D.S., D.M.D., D.O., D.C., Pharm.D. or the Ph.D. or other doctoral degrees in disciplines such as clinical psychology, nursing, clinical genetics, and rehabilitation, or equivalent degree from an accredited domestic or foreign institution at the time of application. Certification by an authorized individual at the degree-granting institution that all degree requirements have been met is acceptable. Candidates must have completed their clinical training, including specialty and, if applicable, subspecialty training prior to receiving an award.
Restrictions: Persons with temporary or student visas are not eligible.
Amount of Grant: $125,000 maximum
Date(s) Application is Due: Feb 12; Mar 12; Jun 12; Jul 12; Oct 12; Nov 12
Contact: Ann Rothgeb; (301) 435-0202; fax: (301) 480-3557; email: rothgeba@mail.nih.gov
Internet: http://www.nhlbi.nih.gov/funding/training/redbook/newk23.htm
Sponsor: National Heart, Lung, and Blood Institute (NHLBI)
Two Rockledge Center, Room 10158, 6701 Rockledge Drive, MSC 7952
Bethesda, MD 20892-7952

NHLBI Mentored Quantitative Research Career Development Awards 2351
The goal of this program is to foster interdisciplinary collaboration in biomedical and behavioral research by supporting supervised research experiences for scientists with quantitative and engineering backgrounds. This award provides research and career development opportunities for scientists and engineers with little or no biomedical or behavioral research experience who are committed to establishing themselves in careers as independent biomedical or behavioral investigators. Examples of quantitative scientific and technical backgrounds outside of biology and medicine considered appropriate for this award include, but are not limited to: mathematics, statistics, computer science, informatics, physics, chemistry, and engineering. This mechanism is intended for research-oriented investigators from the postdoctoral level to the level of senior faculty. Institutions may submit applications on behalf of candidates who hold an advanced degree in a quantitative area of science or engineering. Up to $75,000 per year plus fringe benefits and up to $40,000 per year for research development support is available. New applications are due February 12, June 12, and October 12, while resubmitted applications are due March 12, July 12, and November 12.
Requirements: All candidates must be U.S. citizens, noncitizen nationals, or legal permanent residents of the U.S. The grantee institution must have a strong, well-established research and research training program in the chosen area, accomplished faculty in the basic and clinical sciences, and a commitment to the candidate's research development. The proposed program should include an appropriate mentor.
Amount of Grant: $115,000 maximum
Date(s) Application is Due: Feb 12; Mar 12; Jun 12; Jul 12; Oct 12; Nov 12
Contact: Michael Commarato, Ph.D.; (301) 435-0535; fax: (301) 480-7971; email: CommaraM@nhlbi.nih.gov
Internet: http://www.nhlbi.nih.gov/funding/training/redbook/newk25.htm
Sponsor: National Heart, Lung, and Blood Institute (NHLBI)
Two Rockledge Center, Room 8140, 6701 Rockledge Drive, MSC 7940
Bethesda, MD 20892-7940

NHLBI Microbiome of the Lung and Respiratory Tract in HIV-Infected Individuals and HIV-Uninfected Controls 2352
The National Heart, Lung, and Blood Institute (NHLBI) solicits grant applications under this Funding Opportunity Announcement (FOA) to characterize the microbiome of the lung (the airways and airspaces below the glottis and the lung parenchyma) alone or in combination with the nasal and/or oropharyngeal cavities in HIV-infected individuals and matched HIV-uninfected controls, including normal healthy controls, using molecular techniques to identify bacteria and if possible other organisms, e.g., viruses, cell-wall deficient organisms, protozoa, and fungi. Investigators should use high-throughput technology platforms to create a data set of sufficient quality and depth to allow analysis of how changes of microbiota relate to HIV lung disease progression/complications. These data will be used to examine the impact of changes in the respiratory microbiome on the pathogenesis and progression of HIV disease, on HIV-related respiratory complications, and the effects of anti-HIV therapies. The NHLBI also invites applications for four Clinical/Sequencing research sites and one supporting Data Coordinating Center (DCC). Each application for a clinical/sequencing research site should propose approaches to characterize the lung microbiome and applicants are encouraged to include at least one hypothesis-driven mechanistic aim. Direct costs up to $525,000 per year for project duration of up to five years may be requested. Letters of Intent are due by February 25, with full proposals to be received by March 25.
Requirements: The following organizations and institutions are eligible to apply: individuals; public/state controlled institutions of higher education; private institutions of higher education; Hispanic-serving institutions; historically Black colleges and universities (HBCUs); tribally controlled colleges and universities (TCCUs); Alaska Native and Native Hawaiian serving institutions; nonprofits with 501(c)3 IRS status; nonprofits without 501(c)3 IRS status; for-profit organizations; state governments; Indian/Native American tribal governments (federally recognized); Indian/Native American tribally designated organizations; county governments; city or township governments; special district governments; independent school districts; public housing authorities/Indian housing authorities; U.S. territory or possession; Indian/Native American tribal governments (other than federally recognized); regional organizations; non-domestic (non-U.S.) entities (foreign organizations); other eligible agencies of the federal government; and faith-based or community-based organizations.
Amount of Grant: $525,000 maximum per year for up to 5 years
Date(s) Application is Due: Feb 25; Mar 25
Contact: Sandra Colombini Hatch, M.D.; (301) 435-0222; fax: (301) 480-3557; email: Hatchs@nhlbi.nih.gov;; Hannah H. Peavy, M.D.; (301) 435-0222; fax: (301) 480-3557; email: peavyh@nhlbi.nih.gov
Internet: http://grants.nih.gov/grants/guide/rfa-files/RFA-HL-09-006.html
Sponsor: National Heart, Lung, and Blood Institute (NHLBI)
6701 Rockledge Dr. MSC 7952
Bethesda, MD 20892-7952

NHLBI Midcareer Investigator Award in Patient-Oriented Research 2353
This award provides support for established clinicians within 15 years of their specialty training to further their research and mentoring of outstanding patient-oriented investigators. It will enable them to expand their potential for significant contributions to their field, and to act as mentors for beginning clinical researchers. This award provides protected time to enable the clinician to carry out these activities. The salary that may be requested and awarded is 25% to 50% of the recipient's institutional salary, exclusive of fringe benefits, up to the maximum allowable annual salary rate in effect at the time of award. New applications are due February 12, June 12, and October 12, while resubmitted applications are due March 12, July 12, and November 12.
Requirements: Patient-oriented investigators at U.S. institutions with independent research support are eligible.
Date(s) Application is Due: Feb 12; Mar 12; Jun 12; Jul 12; Oct 12; Nov 12
Contact: Sandra Colombini Hatch, M.D.; (301) 435-0222; fax: (301) 480-3557; email: Hatchs@nhlbi.nih.gov;; Hannah H. Peavy, M.D.; (301) 435-0222; fax: (301) 480-3557; email: peavyh@nhlbi.nih.gov
Internet: http://www.nhlbi.nih.gov/funding/training/redbook/estk24.htm
Sponsor: National Heart, Lung, and Blood Institute (NHLBI)
Two Rockledge Center, 6701 Rockledge Drive, MSC 7952
Bethesda, MD 20892-7952

NHLBI Minority Institution Research Scientist Development Award 2354
This program provides research support to faculty members at minority institutions who have the interest and potential to conduct high quality research in the areas of cardiovascular, pulmonary, hematologic, or sleep disorders. Important goals are to enhance the institution's science programs and to assist in the acquisition of hands-on research opportunities for minority students at the applicant's institution. Annual deadline dates may vary; contact the program office for exact dates.
Requirements: The institution must be a domestic medical or non-medical college, university, or equivalent school in which students of underrepresented minority ethnic groups including African Americans, Hispanics, American Indians, Alaska Natives, and

Pacific Islanders compose a majority (more than 50 percent) of the school's enrollment. It must have ongoing staff and facilities required for the proposed program.
Amount of Grant: $400,000 maximum
Date(s) Application is Due: Jul 21; Sep 12
Contact: Joyce Creamer, Division of Blood Diseases and Resources; (301) 435-0064; fax: (301) 480-0867; email: CreamerJ@gwgate.nhlbi.nih.gov
Internet: http://www.grants.nih.gov/grants/guide/rfa-files/RFA-HL-00-017.html
Sponsor: National Heart, Lung, and Blood Institute
6701 Rockledge Drive, MSC 7952
Bethesda, MD 20892-7952

NHLBI Minority Institutional Research Training Program Grants **2355**
The NHLBI's Minority Institutional Research Training Program is a Ruth L. Kirschstein National Research Service Award Program intended to support training of predoctoral and health professional students and individuals in postdoctoral training at minority schools having the potential to develop meritorious training programs in cardiovascular, pulmonary, hematologic, and sleep disorders. Predoctoral and health professional students and individuals in postdoctoral training in minority schools need further opportunities to develop biomedical and behavioral research skills. The NHLBI Minority Institutional Research Training Program is designed to attract students in their developmental stages; to increase their awareness of cardiovascular, pulmonary, hematologic, and sleep disorders research; and to encourage them to pursue research career opportunities in these areas. Trainee appointments will be determined by the institution and carried out in a manner that will include the recruitment of racial and ethnic minorities, individuals from disadvantaged backgrounds, individuals with disabilities, and women into heart, lung, blood, and sleep disorders scientific research areas. Letters of Intent are due on July 15, with full proposals due by August 15.
Requirements: The institution must be a domestic medical or non-medical college, university, or equivalent school in which students from underrepresented minority groups including African Americans, Hispanics, American Indians, Alaska Natives, and Pacific Islanders compose a majority or a significant proportion of the school enrollment. The individual to be trained must be a citizen of the United States, a noncitizen national, or have been lawfully admitted to the United States for permanent residence at the time of appointment for training, and have a baccalaureate degree. Trainees must be training at the post-baccalaureate level (i.e., predoctoral level) in a relevant biomedical or behavioral science and have made a strong commitment to completing a doctoral degree, be enrolled in a minority health professional school, or have a doctoral degree or equivalent in a biomedical or behavioral science. The program may not support studies leading to a health professional degree.
Amount of Grant: $250,000 total
Date(s) Application is Due: Jul 15; Aug 15
Contact: Sandra Colombini Hatch, M.D.; (301) 435-0222; fax: (301) 480-3557; email: Hatchs@nhlbi.nih.gov;; Hannah H. Peavy, M.D.; (301) 435-0222; fax: (301) 480-3557; email: peavyh@nhlbi.nih.gov
Internet: http://grants.nih.gov/grants/guide/rfa-files/RFA-HL-08-017.html
Sponsor: National Heart, Lung, and Blood Institute
Two Rockledge Center, Suite 10162, MSC 7952, 6701 Rockledge Drive
Bethesda, MD 20892-7952

NHLBI Multidisciplinary Translational Research in Critical Care Grants **2356**
The purpose of this funding opportunity is to promote multidisciplinary translational research that will improve the treatment, diagnosis, and outcome of patients with critical illness and increase the understanding of fundamental processes causing critical illness in humans of all ages. The research team must include scientists from at least two medical or surgical specialties with direct relevance to critical care. Individuals with the skills, knowledge, and resources necessary to carry out the proposed research are invited to work with their institution/organization to develop an application for support.
Requirements: The following organizations and institutions are eligible to apply: individuals; public/state controlled institutions of higher education; private institutions of higher education; Hispanic-serving institutions; historically Black colleges and universities (HBCUs); tribally controlled colleges and universities (TCCUs); Alaska Native and Native Hawaiian serving institutions; nonprofits with 501(c)3 IRS status; nonprofits without 501(c)3 IRS status; for-profit organizations; state governments; Indian/Native American tribal governments (federally recognized); Indian/Native American tribally designated organizations; county governments; city or township governments; special district governments; independent school districts; public housing authorities/Indian housing authorities; U.S. territory or possession; Indian/Native American tribal governments (other than federally recognized); regional organizations; non-domestic (non-U.S.) entities (foreign organizations); other eligible agencies of the federal government; and faith-based or community-based organizations.
Date(s) Application is Due: Feb 5; Jun 5; Oct 5
Contact: Andrea L Harabin, Ph.D.; (301) 435-0222; email: harabin@nih.gov;; Basil Eldadah, M.D., Ph.D.; (301) 496-4996; email: eldadahb@mail.nih.gov
Internet: http://grants.nih.gov/grants/guide/pa-files/PA-07-233.html
Sponsor: National Heart, Lung, and Blood Institute
6701 Rockledge Drive, MSC 7952
Bethesda, MD 20892-7952

NHLBI National Research Service Award Programs in Cardiovascular Epidemiology and Biostatistics **2357**
This program enables research institutions to support pre- and post-doctoral training in areas of particular interest to the Institute and to prepare individuals for careers in biomedical and behavioral research. The cardiovascular epidemiology and biostatistics research training programs offer opportunities in the fields of epidemiology of cardiovascular diseases and statistical analysis. Trainees are selected through review procedures established by the program director at the grantee institution. Attention is given to recruiting individuals from minority groups that are under-represented nationally in the biomedical sciences (African Americans, Hispanics, Native Americans, Alaskan Natives, and Pacific Islanders).
Requirements: Students must be U.S. citizens, noncitizen nationals, or legal permanent U.S. residents. Trainees must have received a baccalaureate degree and must be training at the postbaccalauareate level in a program leading to a PhD, ScD, or equivalent degree.
Restrictions: These awards do not support study leading to the MD, DDS, or other similar professional degrees, nor do they support residency training. Persons on temporary or student visas are not eligible.
Date(s) Application is Due: Apr 5; Aug 5; Dec 5
Contact: Lorraine M. Silsbee; (301) 435-0709; fax: (301) 480-1667; email: Lorraine_Silsbee@nih.gov
Internet: http://www.nhlbi.nih.gov/funding/training/epi-bio/nrsa.htm
Sponsor: National Heart, Lung, and Blood Institute
6701 Rockledge Drive
Bethesda, MD 20892-7934

NHLBI National Research Service Awards for Senior Fellowships **2358**
This program enables experienced scientists to change the direction of their research careers, broaden their scientific background, acquire new research capabilities, or enlarge their command of an allied research field. Selection is by national competition. All experienced scientists interested in changing the direction of their careers are eligible to apply.
Requirements: When the fellowship begins, an applicant must have received the Ph.D., M.D., D.O., D.D.S., D.V.M., O.D., D.P.M., Sc.D., D.Eng., DNSc., or equivalent degree. The applicant also must have at least 7 subsequent years of relevant postdoctoral research or professional training, and must have a sponsor affiliated with a public or private institution with appropriate facilities for the proposed training.
Restrictions: One month of payback for each month of training, up to a maximum of 12 months, is required. This requirement can be fulfilled by teaching or research (a minimum of 20 hours per week) on a continuous basis beginning within 2 years after support ends.
Date(s) Application is Due: Apr 8; Aug; Dec 8
Contact: Charlotte A. Pratt, Program Director; (301) 435-0382; fax: (301) 480-5158; email: prattc@nhlbi.nih.gov
Internet: http://www.nhlbi.nih.gov/funding/training/redbook/estf33.htm
Sponsor: National Heart, Lung, and Blood Institute (NHLBI)
Two Rockledge Center, Room 10118, 6701 Rockledge Drive, MSC 7936
Bethesda, MD 20892-7936

NHLBI New Approaches to Arrhythmia Detection and Treatment Grants for SBIR **2359**
The purpose of this initiative is to improve our ability to detect, treat and prevent cardiac arrhythmias using new or improved methods, tools, and technologies. Applications are invited for the development and significant improvements of innovative monitoring tools, diagnostic methods, and therapeutic approaches for arrhythmia detection, treatment and prevention.
Requirements: Only United States small business concerns (SBCs) are eligible to submit SBIR applications.
Date(s) Application is Due: Apr 5; Aug 5; Dec 5
Contact: Bishow B. Adhikari, Ph.D.; (301) 435-0507; fax: (301) 480-7971; email: AdhikarB@NHLBI.NIH.GOV;; David A. Lathrop, Ph.D.; (301) 435-0507; fax: (301) 451-5458; email: LathropD@NHLBI.NIH.GOV
Internet: http://grants.nih.gov/grants/guide/pa-files/PA-07-032.html
Sponsor: National Heart, Lung, and Blood Institute (NHLBI)
Rockledge Two, Room 9192, 6701 Rockledge Drive
Bethesda, MD 20892

NHLBI New Approaches to Arrhythmia Detection and Treatment Grants for STTR **2360**
The purpose of this initiative is to improve our ability to detect, treat and prevent cardiac arrhythmias using new or improved methods, tools, and technologies. Applications are invited for the development and significant improvements of innovative monitoring tools, diagnostic methods, and therapeutic approaches for arrhythmia detection, treatment and prevention.
Requirements: Only United States small business concerns (SBCs) are eligible to submit STTR applications.
Date(s) Application is Due: Apr 5; Aug 5; Dec 5
Contact: Bishow B. Adhikari, Ph.D.; (301) 435-0507; fax: (301) 480-7971; email: AdhikarB@NHLBI.NIH.GOV;; David A. Lathrop, Ph.D.; (301) 435-0507; fax: (301) 451-5458; email: LathropD@NHLBI.NIH.GOV
Internet: http://grants.nih.gov/grants/guide/pa-files/PA-07-031.html
Sponsor: National Heart, Lung, and Blood Institute (NHLBI)
Rockledge Two, Room 9192, 6701 Rockledge Drive
Bethesda, MD 20892

NHLBI Nutrition and Diet in the Causation, Prevention, and Management of Heart Failure Research Grants **2361**
The purpose of this Funding Opportunity Announcement (FOA) is to encourage submission of investigator-initiated research applications on the role of nutrition and diet in the causation, prevention, and treatment of cardiomyopathies and heart failure.

Basic, translational, and applied interdisciplinary research applications with rigorous hypothesis-testing designs for projects in animals or humans are of interest. The overall goal is to develop a satisfactory science base for preventive approaches in high-risk individuals and for rational nutritional management of patients in various stages of heart failure.
Requirements: The following groups are eligible to apply: for-profit organizations on-profit organizations; public or private institutions, such as universities, colleges, hospitals, and laboratories; units of State government; units of local government; eligible agencies of the Federal government; foreign institutions; domestic institutions; faith-based or community-based organizations; units of State tribal government; and units of local Tribal government.
Amount of Grant: $200,000 maximum annually
Date(s) Application is Due: Feb 16; Jun 16; Oct 16
Contact: Abby G. Ershow; (301) 435-0550; fax: (301) 480-1338; email: ErshowA@mail.nih.gov
Internet: http://grants.nih.gov/grants/guide/pa-files/PA-06-136.html
Sponsor: National Heart, Lung, and Blood Institute (NHLBI)
6701 Rockledge Drive, Suite, MSC 7956
Bethesda, MD 20892-7956

NHLBI Pathogenesis And Treatment Of Lymphedema And Lymphatic Diseases Grants **2362**
The purpose of this Funding Opportunity Announcement (FOA) is to stimulate research on the lymphatic system, to characterize its function on the molecular, cellular, tissue, organ, and intact organism levels and pathophysiologic mechanisms that cause disease, to develop new methods for imaging and/or quantitating lymph flow, and to discover new therapeutic interventions, including nursing, complementary and alternative treatments. The scope of this research includes developmental biology and genetics of the lymphatic system to identify and characterize processes important for its organization and regulation. Such knowledge will help to improve early diagnosis of affected individuals, the choice and timing of treatment, and genetic counseling. Research is also needed on disorders of skin and subcutaneous tissue due to chronic lymphedema, and lymphedema which results from cancers or cancer treatment, with a goal to develop better therapies.
Requirements: The following organizations and institutions are eligible to apply: public/state controlled institutions of higher education; private institutions of higher education; Hispanic-serving institutions; historically Black colleges and universities (HBCUs); tribally controlled colleges and universities (TCCUs); Alaska Native and Native Hawaiian serving institutions; nonprofits with 501(c)3 IRS status; nonprofits without 501(c)3 IRS status; for-profit organizations; state governments; Indian/Native American tribal governments (federally recognized); Indian/Native American tribally designated organizations; non-domestic (non-U.S.) entities (foreign organizations); Hispanic-serving institutions; and regional organization.
Date(s) Application is Due: Feb 5; Jun 5; Oct 5
Contact: Henry Chang, M.D.; (301) 435-0067; fax: (301) 480-1060; email: changh@nih.gov;; Stephen S. Goldman, Ph.D.; (301) 435-0565; fax: (301) 480-2849; email: goldmans@nih.gov
Internet: http://grants.nih.gov/grants/guide/pa-files/PA-07-165.html
Sponsor: National Heart, Lung, and Blood Institute (NHLBI)
6701 Rockledge Drive, MSC 7950
Bethesda, MD 20892-7950

NHLBI Pathway to Independence Award **2363**
The Pathway to Independence (PI) Award is designed to facilitate a timely transition from a mentored postdoctoral research position to a stable independent research position with independent NIH or other independent research support at an earlier stage than is currently the norm. The PI award will provide up to 5 years of support consisting of two phases. The initial phase will provide 1-2 years of mentored support for postdoctoral research scientists. This phase will be followed by up to 3 years of independent support contingent on securing an independent tenure-track or equivalent research position. A typical successful candidate will have an impressive record of research productivity and publications, and will have identified a unique research direction to pursue after the mentored phase of the award. Domestic for-profit or non-profit institutions and organizations, or public or private institutions, such as universities, colleges, hospitals and laboratories, eligible agencies of the federal government, and NIH intramural laboratories are eligible (all institution and organization types listed above are eligible for both the mentored and independent phase, with one exception: ineligible agencies of the Federal government, such as the NIH intramural program, are eligible only for the mentored phase). For the Mentored Phase, salary up to $75,000 plus fringe benefits per year is available, with up to $25,000 additional per year for support (F&A costs will be provided at 8% of modified direct costs). During the Independent investigator phase, total cost may not exceed $249,000 per year. New applications are due February 12, June 12, and October 12, while resubmitted applications are due March 12, July 12, and November 12.
Requirements: At the time of application submission (or resubmission) candidates for this award must have earned a terminal clinical or research doctorate (including Ph.D., M.D., D. O., D.C., N.D., D.D.S., D.V.M., Sc.D., D.N.S., Pharm. D., or equivalent doctoral degree, or a combined clinical and research doctoral degree); and have no more than 5 years (60 months) of research experience since completing the requirements of the doctoral degree (resubmissions must also comply with this requirement).
Restrictions: Foreign institutions are not eligible.
Amount of Grant: $100,000 maximum for mentored phase; $249,000 for Independent Investigator phase
Date(s) Application is Due: Feb 12; Mar 12; Jun 12; Jul 12; Oct 12; Nov 12
Contact: Herbert Geller, Ph.D.; (301) 451-9440; fax: (301) 594-8133; email: direducation@nhlbi.nih.gov
Internet: http://www.nhlbi.nih.gov/funding/training/redbook/phdk99r00.htm
Sponsor: National Heart, Lung, and Blood Institute (NHLBI)
Building 10, Room 2N242, 10 Center Drive, MSC 1754
Bethesda, MD 20892-1754

NHLBI Pediatric Cardiac Genomics Consortium Grants **2364**
The purpose of this initiative is to support collaborative genetic and genomic research leading to a comprehensive understanding of the causes and outcomes of congenital heart disease in the human population. The Consortium will consist of up to 6 Research Centers, Cores, and a Steering Committee. Research Center applicants will propose detailed investigation of the genetics and genomics of one or more human cardiac malformations, with the goal of identifying genetic influences on outcome, as well as causative genes. Individual Research Centers will collaborate in recruitment of individuals with congenital heart disease and their families for all Research Center projects. Maximum allowable direct costs for the Research Centers per year are $160,000 in Year 1, and $535,000 per year in years 2-6. Letters of Intent should be received by January 6, and full proposals are due by February 6.
Requirements: The following organizations and institutions are eligible to apply: public/state controlled institutions of higher education; private institutions of higher education; Hispanic-serving institutions; historically Black colleges and universities (HBCUs); tribally controlled colleges and universities (TCCUs); Alaska Native and Native Hawaiian serving institutions; nonprofits with 501(c)3 IRS status; nonprofits without 501(c)3 IRS status; for-profit organizations; small businesses; state governments; non-domestic (non-U.S.) entities in North America; and other eligible agencies of the Federal Government.
Amount of Grant: $160,000 maximum in year 1 planning; $535,000 in years 2-6
Date(s) Application is Due: Jan 6; Feb 6
Contact: Gail D. Pearson; (301) 435-0510; email: pearsong@mail.nih.gov
Internet: http://grants.nih.gov/grants/guide/rfa-files/RFA-HL-09-003.html
Sponsor: National Heart, Lung, and Blood Institute (NHLBI)
6701 Rockledge Drive, Room 8104
Bethesda, MD 20892

NHLBI Phase II Clinical Trials of Novel Therapies for Lung Diseases **2365**
The purpose of this FOA is to solicit research grant applications to conduct Phase II clinical therapeutic trials that have the potential to advance development of novel therapies for a lung disease or a cardiopulmonary disorder of sleep. Each application will propose one Phase II interventional trial that will most likely use physiological or biochemical rather than clinical endpoints along with at least one smaller basic ancillary research study that is tightly related to the clinical question. Although definitive Phase III trials will not be supported, the proposed studies must provide proof of concept for a novel intervention that has high potential for modifying current treatments and could be disease modifying.
Requirements: The following organizations and institutions are eligible to apply: public/state controlled institutions of higher education; private institutions of higher education; Hispanic-serving institutions; historically Black colleges and universities (HBCUs); tribally controlled colleges and universities (TCCUs); Alaska Native and Native Hawaiian serving institutions; nonprofits with 501(c)3 IRS status; nonprofits without 501(c)3 IRS status; for-profit organizations; state governments; Indian/Native American tribal governments (federally recognized); Indian/Native American tribally designated organizations; county governments; city or township governments; special district governments; independent school districts; public housing authorities/Indian housing authorities; U.S. territories or possessions; Indian/Native American tribal governments (other than federally recognized); regional organizations; non-domestic (non-U.S.) entities (foreign organizations); other eligible agencies of the federal government; and faith-based or community-based organizations.
Amount of Grant: $800,000 maximum 1st year; $1,515,000 maximum 2nd and 3rd year
Date(s) Application is Due: May 18; Jun 18; Dec 30; Jan 29; Aug 15; Sep 15
Contact: Andrea L. Harabin, Ph.D.; (301) 435-0222; email: harabina@nhlbi.nih.gov
Internet: http://grants.nih.gov/grants/guide/rfa-files/RFA-HL-10-003.html
Sponsor: National Heart, Lung and Blood Institute (NHLBI)
6701 Rockledge Drive
Bethesda, MD 20892-7952

NHLBI Prematurity and Respiratory Outcomes Program (PROP) Grants **2366**
This RFA intends to fill the need for understanding the underlying pathophysiology by supporting the investigation of the molecular mechanisms that contribute to acute and chronic respiratory morbidity of the premature infant. The well phenotyped populations developed in this program will significantly increase the chance of studying groups with common pathophysiology and lay the groundwork for novel biomarker discovery. The program will use the cooperative agreement mechanism and require multidisciplinary expertise including neonatologists/pulmonologists, and physiological, molecular, biological, or bioinformatics scientists. Participating sites will plan and coordinate their own research and will develop and implement shared protocols for respiratory phenotyping and respiratory outcomes of the premature infant NICU graduate. Letters of Intent should be received by May 4, and full proposals are due by June 2 each year.
Requirements: The following organizations and institutions are eligible to apply: public/state controlled institutions of higher education; private institutions of higher education; Hispanic-serving institutions; historically Black colleges and universities (HBCUs); tribally controlled colleges and universities (TCCUs); Alaska Native and Native Hawaiian serving institutions; nonprofits with 501(c)3 IRS status; nonprofits without

501(c)3 IRS status; for-profit organizations; state governments; Indian/Native American tribal governments (federally recognized); Indian/Native American tribally designated organizations; county governments; city or township governments; special district governments; independent school districts; public housing authorities/Indian housing authorities; U.S. territories or possessions; Indian/Native American tribal governments (other than federally recognized); regional organizations; non-domestic (non-U.S.) entities (foreign organizations); other eligible agencies of the federal government; and faith-based or community-based organizations.
Amount of Grant: $150,000 maximum in year 1; $350,000 maximum in years 2-5.
Date(s) Application is Due: May 4; Jun 2
Contact: Carol J. Blaisdell, M.D.; (301) 435-0222; email: blaisdellcj@nhlbi.nih.gov
Internet: http://grants.nih.gov/grants/guide/rfa-files/RFA-HL-10-007.html
Sponsor: National Heart, Lung, and Blood Institute (NHLBI)
6701 Rockledge Drive
Bethesda, MD 20892

NHLBI Progenitor Cell Biology Consortium Administrative Coordinating Center Grants 2367

The goal of the Consortium is to identify and characterize progenitor cell lineages, to direct the differentiation of stem and progenitor cells to desired cell fates, and to develop new strategies to address the unique challenges presented by the transplantation of these cells. The Consortium will assemble multiple independent research projects, each with a multi-disciplinary team of Principal Investigators, core research support facilities, and skills development components to establish synergistic virtual hubs focused on progenitor cell biology. The total project period for an application submitted in response to this FOA is 7 years. Maximum allowable direct costs are $600,000 per year for ACC operations. Letters of Intent are dur by April 1, while full applications should arrive by May 1.
Requirements: The following organizations and institutions are eligible to apply: public/state controlled institutions of higher education; private institutions of higher education; Hispanic-serving institutions; historically Black colleges and universities (HBCUs); tribally controlled colleges and universities (TCCUs); Alaska Native and Native Hawaiian serving institutions; nonprofits with 501(c)3 IRS status; nonprofits without 501(c)3 IRS status; small businesses; for-profit organizations; and state governments.
Amount of Grant: $600,000 per year maximum for 7 years
Date(s) Application is Due: Apr 1; May 1
Contact: Denis Buxton, Ph.D.; (301) 435-0513; email: Buxtond@nhlbi.nih.gov;; Carol J. Blaisdell, M.D.; (301) 435-0222; email: blaisdellcj@nhlbi.nih.gov
Internet: http://grants.nih.gov/grants/guide/rfa-files/RFA-HL-09-005.html
Sponsor: National Heart, Lung, and Blood Institute (NHLBI)
Rockledge 2, Room 8216, 6701 Rockledge Drive, MSC 7940
Bethesda, MD 20892

NHLBI Progenitor Cell Biology Consortium Research Hubs 2368

The National Heart, Lung, and Blood Institute (NHLBI) invites applications to participate in the NHLBI Progenitor Cell Biology Consortium. The goal of the Consortium is to identify and characterize progenitor cell lineages, to direct the differentiation of stem and progenitor cells to desired cell fates, and to develop new strategies to address the unique challenges presented by the transplantation of these cells. The Consortium will assemble clusters of synergistic research projects, each with a multi-disciplinary team of Principal Investigators, to establish virtual Research Hubs focused on progenitor cell biology. The Consortium will also contain core research support facilities and skills development components. The expected direct cost amount for the Consortium awards will be up to $750,000 per year. Letters of Intent are due by April 1, with full proposals received by May 1.
Requirements: The following organizations and institutions are eligible to apply: public/state controlled institutions of higher education; private institutions of higher education; Hispanic-serving institutions; historically Black colleges and universities (HBCUs); tribally controlled colleges and universities (TCCUs); Alaska Native and Native Hawaiian serving institutions; nonprofits with 501(c)3 IRS status; nonprofits without 501(c)3 IRS status; small businesses; for-profit organizations; and state governments.
Amount of Grant: $750,000 per year
Date(s) Application is Due: Apr 1; May 1
Contact: Denis Buxton, Ph.D.; (301) 435-0513; email: Buxtond@nhlbi.nih.gov;; Carol J. Blaisdell, M.D.; (301) 435-0222; email: blaisdellcj@nhlbi.nih.gov
Internet: http://grants.nih.gov/grants/guide/rfa-files/RFA-HL-09-004.html
Sponsor: National Heart, Lung, and Blood Institute (NHLBI)
Rockledge 2, Room 8216, 6701 Rockledge Drive, MSC 7940
Bethesda, MD 20892

NHLBI Protein Interactions Governing Membrane Transport in Pulmonary Health and Disease Grants 2369

This Funding Opportunity Announcement (FOA) issued by the National Heart, Lung, and Blood Institute, National Institutes of Health (NIH), solicits research grant applications to delineate the protein interactions and pathways governing membrane trafficking pathways operative in pulmonary health and disease and develop novel therapeutic interventions. Because the nature and scope of the proposed research will vary from application to application, it is anticipated that the size and duration of each award will also vary. The total amount awarded and the number of awards will depend upon the mechanism numbers, quality, duration, and costs of the applications received.
Requirements: The following organizations and institutions are eligible to apply: public/state controlled institutions of higher education; private institutions of higher education; Hispanic-serving institutions; historically Black colleges and universities (HBCUs); tribally controlled colleges and universities (TCCUs); Alaska Native and Native Hawaiian serving institutions; nonprofits with 501(c)3 IRS status; nonprofits without 501(c)3 IRS status; for-profit organizations; state governments; Indian/Native American tribal governments (federally recognized); Indian/Native American tribally designated organizations; county governments; city or township governments; special district governments; independent school districts; public housing authorities/Indian housing authorities; U.S. territory or possession; Indian/Native American tribal governments (other than federally recognized); regional organizations; non-domestic (non-U.S.) entities (foreign organizations); other eligible agencies of the federal government; and faith-based or community-based organizations.
Date(s) Application is Due: Feb 5; Jun 5; Oct 5
Contact: Susan Banks-Schlegel, Ph.D.; (301) 435-0202; fax: (301) 480-3557; email: Schleges@nhlbi.nih.gov;; Dorothy Gail, Ph.D.; (301) 435-0222; fax: (301) 480-3557; email: Gaild@nhlbi.nih.gov
Internet: http://grants.nih.gov/grants/guide/pa-files/PA-07-137.html
Sponsor: National Heart, Lung, and Blood Institute (NHLBI)
Two Rockledge Center, Suite 10018, 6701 Rockledge Drive
Bethesda, MD 20892-7952

NHLBI Research Demonstration and Dissemination Grants 2370

The purpose of this Funding Opportunity Announcement (FOA) is to encourage the scientific community to conduct Demonstration and Dissemination (D&D) studies to test the effectiveness of interventions in children, adolescents, and/or adults to: promote healthful behaviors; reduce risk factors for heart, lung, and blood diseases, and sleep disorders; improve the prevention or management of heart, lung, and blood diseases, and sleep disorders, including the delivery of health care services; and enhance understanding of the processes of intervention implementation and diffusion, or sustainability in a defined population, or defined clinical or community setting. The total project period for an application submitted in response to this funding opportunity may not exceed 5 years. Direct costs are limited to less than $500,000 in any single year, unless pre-approval is obtained from the Institute.
Requirements: The following organizations and institutions are eligible to apply: public/state controlled institutions of higher education; private institutions of higher education; Hispanic-serving institutions; historically Black colleges and universities (HBCUs); tribally controlled colleges and universities (TCCUs); Alaska Native and Native Hawaiian serving institutions; nonprofits with 501(c)3 IRS status; nonprofits without 501(c)3 IRS status; for-profit organizations; state governments; Indian/Native American tribal governments (federally recognized); Indian/Native American tribally designated organizations; county governments; city or township governments; special district governments; independent school districts; public housing authorities/Indian housing authorities; U.S. territory or possession; Indian/Native American tribal governments (other than federally recognized); regional organizations; non-domestic (non-U.S.) entities (foreign organizations); other eligible agencies of the federal government; and faith-based or community-based organizations.
Amount of Grant: $500,000 per year maximum for 5 years
Date(s) Application is Due: Jan 25; May 25; Sep 25
Contact: Charlotte Pratt, Ph.D.; (301) 435-0382; fax: (301) 480-5158; email: PrattC@nhlbi.nih.gov
Internet: http://grants.nih.gov/grants/guide/pa-files/PA-07-017.html
Sponsor: National Heart, Lung, and Blood Institute (NHLBI)
6701 Rockledge Drive, MSC 7936, Room 8134
Bethesda, MD 20892

NHLBI Research Grants on the Relationship Between Hypertension and Inflammation 2371

This Funding Opportunity Announcement (FOA) solicits grant applications that propose the study of the sequence of events in which the vascular inflammatory state contributes to the development and maintenance of hypertension. Ample evidence suggests that inflammation may play a role in the pathogenesis of hypertension or that it may characterize a functional state of the vessel wall as a consequence of high blood pressure. Angiotensin II (Ang II), a widely recognized vasoconstrictor and anti-natriuretic involved in blood pressure regulation, also acts as a pro-inflammatory factor in the cardiovascular system. Ang II stimulates the expression of several inflammatory cytokines, which in turn affect blood pressure. A potential linkage between Ang II and immuno-cytokines is their shared ability to induce the level of reactive oxygen species (ROS), which serve as second messengers for many intracellular signaling pathways. The production of ROS not only decreases bioavailability of nitric oxide (NO), a vasodilator, but also initiates the functional and morphological alterations, such as remodeling, in the vascular wall that accompany the hypertensive state over time. This FOA would provide an opportunity to bring focus on the potential causal relationship between hypertension and inflammation in a cohesive, integrated manner. A new understanding of hypertension and inflammation would provide novel opportunities to prevent and treat the disease.
Requirements: The following organizations and institutions are eligible to apply: public/state controlled institutions of higher education; private institutions of higher education; Hispanic-serving institutions; historically Black colleges and universities (HBCUs); tribally controlled colleges and universities (TCCUs); Alaska Native and Native Hawaiian serving institutions; nonprofits with 501(c)3 IRS status; nonprofits without 501(c)3 IRS status; for-profit organizations; state governments; Indian/Native American tribal governments (federally recognized); Indian/Native American tribally designated organizations; county governments; city or township governments; special district governments; independent school districts; public housing authorities/Indian housing

authorities; U.S. territory or possession; Indian/Native American tribal governments (other than federally recognized); regional organizations; non-domestic (non-U.S.) entities (foreign organizations); other eligible agencies of the federal government; and faith-based or community-based organizations.
Date(s) Application is Due: Feb 5; Jun 5; Oct 5
Contact: Eser Tolunay, Ph.D.; (301) 435-0560; email: tolunaye@nhlbi.nih.gov
Internet: http://grants.nih.gov/grants/guide/pa-files/PA-07-138.html
Sponsor: National Heart, Lung, and Blood Institute (NHLBI)
6701 Rockledge Drive
Bethesda, MD 20892

NHLBI Research on the Role of Cardiomyocyte Mitochondria in Heart Disease: An Integrated Approach 2372

The National Heart, Lung, and Blood Institute (NHLBI) invites applications for collaborative research projects to develop an integrated understanding of cardiomyocyte mitochondria and its contributions to myocardial adaptations and heart disease progression by combining functional data with information derived from powerful new technologies. Budgets for direct costs of up to $500,000 per year and a project duration of up to four years may be requested for a maximum of $2,000,000 direct costs over a four-year project period. Because the nature and scope of the proposed research will vary from application to application, it is anticipated that the size and duration of each award will also vary.
Requirements: The following organizations and institutions are eligible to apply: individuals; public/state controlled institutions of higher education; private institutions of higher education; Hispanic-serving institutions; historically Black colleges and universities (HBCUs); tribally controlled colleges and universities (TCCUs); Alaska Native and Native Hawaiian serving institutions; nonprofits with 501(c)3 IRS status; nonprofits without 501(c)3 IRS status; for-profit organizations; state governments; Indian/Native American tribal governments (federally recognized); Indian/Native American tribally designated organizations; county governments; city or township governments; special district governments; independent school districts; public housing authorities/Indian housing authorities; U.S. territory or possession; Indian/Native American tribal governments (other than federally recognized); regional organizations; non-domestic (non-U.S.) entities (foreign organizations); other eligible agencies of the federal government; and faith-based or community-based organizations.
Amount of Grant: $500,000 direct costs per year for no more than four years
Date(s) Application is Due: Apr 20; May 19
Contact: Isabella Liang, Ph.D.; (301) 435-0504; fax: (301) 451-5458; email: Liangi@mail.nih.gov
Internet: http://grants.nih.gov/grants/guide/rfa-files/RFA-HL-10-002.html
Sponsor: National Heart, Lung, and Blood Institute (NHLBI)
Two Rockledge Center, Room 8178, 6701 Rockledge Drive, MSC 7956
Bethesda, MD 20892-7956

NHLBI Research Supplements to Promote Diversity in Health-Related Research (Postdoctoral Individuals/New Independent Researchers) 2373

Supplement enables principal investigators with eligible NHLBI research grants to include recently appointed junior faculty from underrepresented racial and ethnic groups and individuals with disabilities in their projects. Nationally, underrepresented groups in biomedical research careers include but are not limited to, African Americans, Hispanic Americans, American Indians/Alaska Natives, Native Hawaiians and Pacific Islanders. The research proposed for the investigator must be a logical extension of the parent grant. The investigator must be given opportunities to interact with other individuals on the grant, to contribute intellectually to the study, and to enhance his or her research skills and knowledge. Funds may be requested to make changes or adjustments in the laboratory setting that will enable the investigator with disabilities to perform the essential functions associated with his or her research project. Accommodation requests must be reasonable in relationship to the direct costs of the parent grant. There is no application receipt date. However, awards are generally made four times per year (December, March, June, and September). Principal Investigators are encouraged to synchronize the supplement requested start date with the parent grant budget period start date. A maximum of $75,000 per year in salary is available (plus fringe benefits), and a maximum of $10,000 per year for supplies and travel.
Requirements: All principal investigators at U.S. institutions with eligible NHLBI research grants are eligible to apply.
Amount of Grant: $85,000 maximum
Contact: Helena O. Mishoe, PhD; (301) 451-5081; fax: (301) 480-0862; email: mishoeh@nhlbi.nih.gov
Internet: http://www.nhlbi.nih.gov/funding/training/redbook/newmirs.htm
Sponsor: National Heart, Lung, and Blood Institute (NHLBI)
6701 Rockledge Drive, Room 8188
Bethesda, MD 20892-7913

NHLBI Research Supplements to Promote Diversity in Health-Related Research for Established Investigators Who Become Disabled 2374

This supplement enables principal investigators with eligible NHLBI research grants who become disabled to obtain additional support to continue their research. Funds may be requested to make changes or adjustments in the laboratory setting that will enable the disabled investigator to perform the essential functions associated with his or her research project and/or to hire an assistant. Accommodation requests must be reasonable in relationship to the direct costs of the parent grant. Applications can be submitted at any time, but no later than 3 months before the last 2 years remaining on the NHLBI research grant. Applicants may request support for special equipment, an assistant, or other modifications to facilitate reasonable accommodation to a disabling injury or illness that has occurred during the current project period.
Requirements: All principal investigators at U.S. institutions with eligible NHLBI research grants who become disabled are eligible to apply.
Contact: Helena O. Mishoe, PhD; (301) 451-5081; fax: (301) 480-0862; email: mishoeh@nhlbi.nih.gov
Internet: http://www.nhlbi.nih.gov/funding/training/redbook/estdissu.htm
Sponsor: National Heart, Lung, and Blood Institute (NHLBI)
6701 Rockledge Drive, Room 8188
Bethesda, MD 20892-7913

NHLBI Research Supplements to Promote Diversity in Health-Related Research for Graduate Research Assistants 2375

This supplement enables principal investigators with eligible NHLBI research grants to include graduate students in their projects. Priority is given to applications requesting support for students with disabilities and/or from underrepresented racial and ethnic groups. The research activity proposed for the student must be part of the approved research for the parent grant or a logical extension. The student must be given opportunities to interact with other individuals on the grant and to contribute intellectually to the study. Applications can be submitted at any time, but no later than 3 months before the last 2 years remaining on the NHLBI research grant. Stipends include: salary (including fringe benefits) up to a maximum of $26,000 per year; and a maximum of $4,000 a year for supplies, travel (up to $1,000 for travel to scientific meetings), and other.
Requirements: All principal investigators at U.S. institutions with eligible NHLBI research grants who wish to offer research experiences to students with disabilities and/or students from underrepresented racial and ethnic groups who are pursuing a masters or doctoral degree in one of the biomedical or behavioral sciences or enrolled in a master's degree program in nursing are eligible to apply.
Amount of Grant: $30,000 maximum
Contact: Helena O. Mishoe, PhD; (301) 451-5081; fax: (301) 480-0862; email: mishoeh@nhlbi.nih.gov
Internet: http://www.nhlbi.nih.gov/funding/training/redbook/gradsup.htm
Sponsor: National Heart, Lung, and Blood Institute
6701 Rockledge Drive, Room 8188
Bethesda, MD 20892-7913

NHLBI Research Supplements to Promote Diversity in Health-Related Research for Individuals in Postdoctoral Training 2376

This supplement enables principal investigators with eligible NHLBI research grants to include postdoctoral individuals from underrepresented racial and ethnic groups and individuals with disabilities in their projects. Nationally, underrepresented groups in biomedical research careers include but are not limited to African Americans, Hispanic Americans, American Indians/Alaska Natives, Native Hawaiians and Pacific Islanders. The research proposed for the individual must be a logical extension of the parent grant. The individual must be given opportunities to interact with other researchers on the grant, to contribute intellectually to the study, and to enhance his or her research skills and knowledge. Funds may be requested to make changes or adjustments in the laboratory setting that will enable the investigator with disabilities to perform the essential functions associated with his or her research project. Accommodation requests must be reasonable in relationship to the direct costs of the parent grant. There is no application receipt date. However, awards are generally made four times per year (December, March, June, and September). Principal Investigators are encouraged to synchronize the supplement requested start date with the parent grant budget period start date. Up to $40,000 per year is provided for salary and fringe benefits, plus up to $10,000 per year for supplies, travel, and other.
Requirements: The individual may be affiliated with the principal investigator's institution or another institution. Supplements are available for long-term research support for individuals with a postdoctoral degree. A minimum of two years and a maximum of four years full-time research effort (at least 40 hours a week) is required.
Restrictions: Normally, funding will not be provided for postdoctoral individuals to work with their former predoctoral mentors. If the postdoctoral mentor is the individual's predoctoral mentor, a justification for continued mentorship must be provided. Cumulative Postdoctoral research experience must not exceed 6 years.
Amount of Grant: $50,000 maximum
Contact: Helena O. Mishoe, PhD; (301) 451-5081; fax: (301) 480-0862; email: mishoeh@nhlbi.nih.gov
Internet: http://www.nhlbi.nih.gov/funding/training/redbook/phdressu.htm
Sponsor: National Heart, Lung, and Blood Institute
6701 Rockledge Drive, Room 8188
Bethesda, MD 20892-7913

NHLBI Research Supplements to Promote Diversity in Health-Related Research for Undergraduate Students 2377

This supplement enables principal investigators with eligible NHLBI research grants to include undergraduate students in their projects. Priority is given to applications requesting support for students with disabilities and/or from underrepresented racial and ethnic groups. The research proposed for the student must be part of the approved research for the parent grant or a logical extension. The student must be given opportunities to interact with other individuals on the study, to contribute intellectually, and to enhance his or her research skills and knowledge. The program is designed to support undergraduate students who are interested in biomedical or behavioral research and who will devote at least 2 years (two 3-month periods) to the program. Support should

be requested for at least 3 months during any 1 year. Applications can be submitted any time, but no later than 3 months before the last 2 years remaining on the NHLBI research grant. Stipend include: $10 per hour for salary; and supplies, travel (up to $1,000 for travel to scientific meeting(s) or between home/school and worksite), and other up to $2,400.
Requirements: All principal investigators at U.S. institutions with eligible NHLBI research grants are eligible.
Contact: Helena O. Mishoe, PhD; (301) 451-5081; fax: (301) 480-0862; email: mishoeh@nhlbi.nih.gov
Internet: http://www.nhlbi.nih.gov/funding/training/redbook/undersup.htm
Sponsor: National Heart, Lung, and Blood Institute
6701 Rockledge Drive, Room 8188
Bethesda, MD 20892-7913

NHLBI Right Heart Function in Health and Chronic Lung Diseases Grants 2378
This program will promote research on cellular, molecular and physiological determinants of right ventricular function in health, and function/ dysfunction in association with chronic lung diseases. The goal is to encourage research which concentrates on building a foundation of basic knowledge of right ventricular physiology and the basic molecular and biomechanical factors contributing to right ventricular dysfunction associated with pulmonary diseases. This knowledge base will be used in determining the best methods of preventing, diagnosing and treating right heart failure. This FOA seeks to fill the current gaps that exist in our understanding of the right heart and how right heart function affects lung function in both health and disease. The emphasis on interaction of the heart and the lung during chronic lung disease in this program is intended to promote collaboration between the heart and lung research communities.
Requirements: The following organizations and institutions are eligible to apply: public/state controlled institutions of higher education; private institutions of higher education; Hispanic-serving institutions; historically Black colleges and universities (HBCUs); tribally controlled colleges and universities (TCCUs); Alaska Native and Native Hawaiian serving institutions; nonprofits with 501(c)3 IRS status; nonprofits without 501(c)3 IRS status; for-profit organizations; state governments; Indian/Native American tribal governments (federally recognized); Indian/Native American tribally designated organizations; county governments; city or township governments; special district governments; independent school districts; public housing authorities/Indian housing authorities; U.S. territory or possession; Indian/Native American tribal governments (other than federally recognized); regional organizations; non-domestic (non-U.S.) entities (foreign organizations); other eligible agencies of the federal government; and faith-based or community-based organizations.
Date(s) Application is Due: Feb 5; Jun 5; Oct 5
Contact: Elizabeth M. Denholm, Ph.D.; (301) 435-0222; fax: (301) 480-3557; email: denholme@mail.nih.gov
Internet: http://grants.nih.gov/grants/guide/pa-files/PA-07-043.html
Sponsor: National Heart, Lung, and Blood Institute (NHLBI)
6701 Rockledge Drive, MSC 7952
Bethesda, MD 20892-7952

NHLBI Ruth L. Kirschstein National Research Service Award (NRSA) Institutional Research Training Grants 2379
This award enables research institutions to support predoctoral research training in specific areas and fields of shortage. Selection of institutions is by national competition; trainees are selected through local review procedures established by the program director at the grantee institution. Institutional grants are renewable, through competition, for up to 5 years. The NHLBI will accept all types of competing T32 applications (new, renewal/competing continuation, resubmission/amended) until January 25. Only resubmission/amended T32 applications will be accepted until September 25.
Requirements: Trainees are required to pursue their research training full-time, and trainees in clinical areas are expected to confine their clinical duties to those that are part of their research training. Trainees must be U.S. citizens, noncitizen nationals, or legal permanent residents of the U.S. Persons on temporary or student visas are not eligible.
Date(s) Application is Due: Jan 25; Sep 25
Contact: Michael Commarato, Ph.D.; (301) 435-0535; fax: (301) 480-7971; email: CommaraM@nhlbi.nih.gov
Internet: http://www.nhlbi.nih.gov/funding/training/redbook/gradt32.htm
Sponsor: National Heart, Lung, and Blood Institute
Two Rockledge Center, 6701 Rockledge Drive, Room 8140, MSC 7940
Bethesda, MD 20892-7940

NHLBI Ruth L. Kirschstein National Research Service Award Short-Term Institutional Research Training Grants 2380
This program provides funds to research institutions to make awards to individuals in health professional schools for research opportunities that would not be available through their regular course of study. Awards are made to training institutions by national competition. The applicant institution may request the proportion of the NIH standard annual NRSA Training Related Expenses to help defray other costs of the short-term training experience, such as research supplies, tuition, fees, certain types of travel, and other expenses. Amounts for TRE are $4,200 annually ($350/month) for each predoctoral trainee and $7,850 annually ($654/month) for each postdoctoral trainee. Health insurance is an allowable expense that may be charged to the Trainee Related Expenses budget category but only to the extent that the same health insurance fees are charged to non-Federally students and postdoctoral individuals.
Requirements: Trainees are selected by the grantee institution and must be U.S. citizens, noncitizen nationals, or legal permanent residents of the U.S. Trainees should have successfully completed at least 1 semester at an accredited school of medicine, optometry, osteopathy, dentistry, veterinary medicine, pharmacy, or public health before entering the program. The award cannot be used to support courses that are required for the M.D., D.O., D.D.S., D.V.M., or similar professional degrees.
Date(s) Application is Due: Jan 25
Contact: Charlotte Pratt, Ph.D.; (301) 435-0382; fax: (301) 480-5158; email: PrattC@nhlbi.nih.gov
Internet: http://www.nhlbi.nih.gov/funding/training/redbook/gradt35.htm
Sponsor: National Heart, Lung, and Blood Institute (NHLBI)
6701 Rockledge Drive, MSC 7936
Bethesda, MD 20892-7936

NHLBI Ruth L. Kirschstein National Research Service Awards for Individual Predoctoral MD/PhD Fellows 2381
The National Heart, Lung, and Blood Institute (NHLBI) provides Ruth L. Kirschstein National Research Service Awards (Kirschstein-NRSA) to individuals for combined MD/PhD fellowship training. The NHLBI awards this Kirschstein-NRSA individual fellowship to promising applicants with the potential to become productive, independent, highly trained physician-scientists, including patient-oriented physician-scientists in its scientific mission area. The Institute plans, conducts, fosters, and supports an integrated and coordinated program of basic research, clinical investigations and trials, observational studies, and demonstration and education projects. Research is related to the causes, prevention, diagnosis, and treatment of heart, blood vessel, lung, and blood diseases; and sleep disorders. The NIH will reimburse 60 percent of the cost of tuition up to $21,000.
Requirements: Applications may be submitted by: for-profit organizations; non-profit organizations; public or private institutions, such as universities, colleges, hospitals, and laboratories; eligible agencies of the Federal government; and domestic Institutions
Date(s) Application is Due: Apr 8; Aug 8; Dec 8
Contact: Jane D. Scott, Sc.D., M.S.N.; (301) 435-0535; fax: (301) 480-7404; email: scottj2@nhlbi.nih.gov
Internet: http://grants.nih.gov/grants/guide/pa-files/PA-08-021.html
Sponsor: National Heart, Lung, and Blood Institute
6701 Rockledge Drive, MSC 7940
Bethesda, MD 20892-7940

NHLBI Sarcoidosis: Research Grants into the Cause of Multi-Organ Disease and Clinical Strategies for Therapy 2382
The purpose of this Funding Opportunity Announcement (FOA) is to stimulate research on the etiology and management of sarcoidosis, an immune–mediated granulomatous inflammatory disorder. Studies supported by this FOA would include investigations to find the etiology(ies) and related host factors that might enhance susceptibility to sarcoidosis, especially development of symptomatic multi-organ disease that has a propensity to involve critical organs (such as lungs, heart, eyes, central/peripheral nervous system, liver, kidneys and other abdominal viscera) that create serious illness. Study of the still problematic management and the biological, behavioral, or psychosocial burden on individuals, families, and community is encouraged. Moreover, there is interest for approaches to risk reduction, psychological coping, and management of complications and side effects of treatment. Because the nature and scope of the proposed research will vary from application to application, it is anticipated that the size and duration of each award will also vary. The total amount awarded and the number of awards will depend upon the mechanism numbers, quality, duration, and costs of the applications received.
Requirements: The following organizations and institutions are eligible to apply: public/state controlled institutions of higher education; private institutions of higher education; Hispanic-serving institutions; historically Black colleges and universities (HBCUs); tribally controlled colleges and universities (TCCUs); Alaska Native and Native Hawaiian serving institutions; nonprofits with 501(c)3 IRS status; nonprofits without 501(c)3 IRS status; for-profit organizations; state governments; Indian/Native American tribal governments (federally recognized); Indian/Native American tribally designated organizations; county governments; city or township governments; special district governments; independent school districts; public housing authorities/Indian housing authorities; U.S. territory or possession; Indian/Native American tribal governments (other than federally recognized); regional organizations; non-domestic (non-U.S.) entities (foreign organizations); other eligible agencies of the federal government; and faith-based or community-based organizations.
Date(s) Application is Due: Feb 5; Jun 5; Oct 5
Contact: Herbert Y. Reynolds, M.D.; (301) 435-0222; fax: (301) 480-3557; email: Reynoldh@nhlbi.nih.gov
Internet: http://grants.nih.gov/grants/guide/pa-files/PA-07-136.html
Sponsor: National Heart, Lung, and Blood Institute (NHLBI)
Two Rockledge Center, Suite 10018, 6701 Rockledge Drive, MSC 7952
Bethesda, MD 20892-7952

NHLBI Short-Term Research Education Program to Increase Diversity in Health-Related Research 2383
This FOA issued by the National Heart, Lung, and Blood Institute, National Institutes of Health, solicits Research Education (R25) applications from institutions/organizations to promote diversity in undergraduate and health professional student populations by providing short-term research education support to stimulate career development in cardiovascular, pulmonary, hematologic, and sleep disorders research. The overall goal of the program is to provide research opportunities for individuals from disadvantaged backgrounds, racial and ethnic minorities, and others who are underrepresented

in biomedical and behavioral research (e.g., individuals with disabilities), that will significantly contribute to a diverse research workforce in the future. The estimated funds (total costs) available for the first year of support for the entire program are expected to be $850,000. Up to eight new awards are anticipated, depending on the number of student participants requested and the availability of funds.
Requirements: The following organizations and institutions are eligible to apply: domestic institutions; non-profit organizations; public/state controlled institutions of higher education; private institutions of higher education; nonprofits with 501(c)3 IRS status; for-profit organizations (other than small businesses); state governments; county governments; city or township governments; special district governments; and faith-based or community-based organizations.
Restrictions: Applications from foreign institutions will not be accepted. Individuals on temporary or student visas and individuals holding PhD, MD, DVM, or equivalent doctoral degrees in the health sciences are not eligible.
Amount of Grant: $850,000 total
Date(s) Application is Due: Jul 15; Aug 15
Contact: Dr. Michael Commarato; (301) 435-0530; fax: (301) 480-1454; email: michael_commarato@nih.gov
Internet: http://grants.nih.gov/grants/guide/rfa-files/RFA-HL-08-016.html
Sponsor: National Heart, Lung, and Blood Institute
6701 Rockledge Drive, MSC 7940
Bethesda, MD 20892-7924

NHLBI Stress Management Interventions to Reduce Risk of Coronary Artery Disease 2384

The purpose of this program announcement is to encourage applications that evaluate the efficacy of stress management interventions on intermediate outcomes purported to be in the biological or behavioral mechanistic pathway through which mental stress (MS) is thought to influence major adverse cardiac events (MACE) in patients with confirmed coronary artery disease (CAD). These include subclinical measures of atherosclerosis, measures of cardiac or endothelial function, or measures such as cardiovascular reactivity or neurohumoral response to a provocative mental stress test. The ultimate goal is to determine whether stress management interventions can slow progression of CAD or reduce MACE and, if so, to translate effective stress management interventions to clinical practice.
Requirements: The following organizations and institutions are eligible to apply: individuals; public/state controlled institutions of higher education; private institutions of higher education; Hispanic-serving institutions; historically Black colleges and universities (HBCUs); tribally controlled colleges and universities (TCCUs); Alaska Native and Native Hawaiian serving institutions; nonprofits with 501(c)3 IRS status; nonprofits without 501(c)3 IRS status; for-profit organizations; state governments; Indian/Native American tribal governments (federally recognized); Indian/Native American tribally designated organizations; county governments; city or township governments; special district governments; independent school districts; public housing authorities/Indian housing authorities; U.S. territory or possession; Indian/Native American tribal governments (other than federally recognized); regional organizations; non-domestic (non-U.S.) entities (foreign organizations); other eligible agencies of the federal government; and faith-based or community-based organizations.
Date(s) Application is Due: Feb 5; Jun 5; Oct 5
Contact: Peter G. Kaufmann, Ph.D.; (301) 435-2467; fax: (301) 480-1773; email: KaufmannP@mail.nih.gov;; Cristina Rabadan-Diehl, Ph.D.; (301) 435-0550; fax: (301) 480-2858
Internet: http://grants.nih.gov/grants/guide/pa-files/PA-07-322.html
Sponsor: National Heart, Lung, and Blood Institute (NHLBI)
6701 Rockledge Drive, Room 8118, MSC 7936
Bethesda, MD 20892-7936

NHLBI Summer Institute for Training in Biostatistics II 2385

The National Heart, Lung, and Blood Institute (NHLBI) and the National Center for Research Resources (NCRR) invite applications for grants to develop, conduct, and evaluate summer courses in the basic principles and methods of biostatistics as employed in biomedical research. The courses would introduce participants to the field of biostatistics for the purpose of attracting new students into the field. The course will attract students from the entire U.S.A and will cover the fundamental concepts of probability, statistical reasoning and inferential methods motivated, in part, by examples that include data collected in studies of heart, lung, blood, and sleep disorders. The course will be taught during the summer, with appropriate modifications or refinements following each of the first two summers' sessions. Programs may choose an area of emphasis, such as clinical trials, statistical genetics, bioinformatics or epidemiology or take a general approach. Recent college graduates as well as advanced undergraduates should be eligible to participate provided they have not participated in SIBS previously. Direct costs are limited to $248,000 per year for a three-year period. Letters of Intent should be received by December 5, and full proposals are due by January 6.
Requirements: The following organizations and institutions are eligible to apply: public/state controlled institutions of higher education; private institutions of higher education; Hispanic-serving institutions; historically Black colleges and universities (HBCUs); tribally controlled colleges and universities (TCCUs); Alaska Native and Native Hawaiian serving institutions; nonprofits with 501(c)3 IRS status; nonprofits without 501(c)3 IRS status; for-profit organizations; state governments; Indian/Native American tribal governments (federally recognized); Indian/Native American tribally designated organizations; county governments; city or township governments; special district governments; independent school districts; public housing authorities/Indian housing authorities; U.S. territory or possession; Indian/Native American tribal governments (other than federally recognized); regional organizations; non-domestic (non-U.S.) entities (foreign organizations); other eligible agencies of the federal government; and faith-based or community-based organizations.
Amount of Grant: $248,000 maximum per year for a three-year period
Date(s) Application is Due: Dec 5; Jan 6
Contact: Song Yang; (301) 435-0431; fax: (301) 480-1862; email: yangso@nhlbi.nih.gov
Internet: http://grants.nih.gov/grants/guide/rfa-files/RFA-HL-09-009.html
Sponsor: National Heart, Lung, and Blood Institute (NHLBI)
6701 Rockledge Drive, Room 9210
Bethesda, MD 20892

NHLBI Summer Internship Program in Biomedical Research 2386

The goal of the Summer Internship Program in Biomedical Research at NHLBI is to expose students to research investigation in a highly enriched environment that is devoted exclusively to biomedical research and training. The Program is open to high school and college, graduate or Medical and Dental Students. Participants join a research laboratory for a minimum of ten weeks between June and August and conduct research in selected areas of investigation under the guidance of an NHLBI intramural research scientist. To augment the training experience, students participate in a Seminar Series at the NHLBI, as well as the National Institutes of Health Summer Seminar Series and Summer Research Program Poster Day. While applications may be filed between Nov. 15 and March 1, early applications are encouraged.
Requirements: Applicants must be either U.S. citizens or permanent residents and be currently enrolled full-time in high school, college, professional or graduate school with a minimum GPA of 3.0 on a 4.0 scale. College graduates are eligible for the summer between graduation and beginning either graduate or professional school. High school students should be at least 16 years of age prior to June 1. Applications must be submitted online using the link for provided for Summer Internship Applicants.
Date(s) Application is Due: Mar 1
Contact: Llewellyn, Jessica, MBA, Program Coordinator; (301) 451-9440; fax: (301) 594-8133; email: llewellj@mail.nih.gov or direducation@nhlbi.nih.gov
Internet: http://dir.nhlbi.nih.gov/oe/summerprogs.asp
Sponsor: National Heart, Lung, and Blood Institute (NHLBI)
6701 Rockledge Drive, Building 10, Room 2N242
Bethesda, MD 20892-1754

NHLBI Targeted Approaches to Weight Control for Young Adults Grants 2387

The National Heart, Lung, and Blood Institute (NHLBI) of the National Institutes of Health (NIH) invites applications for cooperative agreements (U01) to conduct two-phase clinical research studies to develop, refine, and test innovative behavioral and/or environmental approaches for weight control in young adults at high risk for weight gain. Weight control interventions can address weight loss, prevention of weight gain, or prevention of excessive weight gain during pregnancy. The first phase will consist of formative research to refine the proposed intervention, recruitment, retention, and adherence strategies targeted to young adults. The second phase will consist of a randomized controlled trial to test the efficacy of the intervention. For the purpose of this FOA, young adults are defined as 18-35 years of age. The maximum award for the research component will be approximately $3,000,000 in direct costs, including direct costs of up to $500,000 for the first year, $650,000 for the second year, $650,000 for the third year, $650,000 for the fourth year, and $550,000 for the fifth year. Letters of Intent should be received by September 10, and full proposals are due by October 10.
Requirements: The following organizations and institutions are eligible to apply: public/state controlled institutions of higher education; private institutions of higher education; Hispanic-serving institutions; historically Black colleges and universities (HBCUs); tribally controlled colleges and universities (TCCUs); Alaska Native and Native Hawaiian serving institutions; nonprofits with 501(c)3 IRS status; nonprofits without 501(c)3 IRS status; for-profit organizations; Indian/Native American tribal governments; Indian/Native American Tribally Designated Organizations; eligible agencies of the federal government; faith-based or community-based organizations; and regional organizations.
Amount of Grant: $500,000-$650,000 maximum
Date(s) Application is Due: Sep 10; Oct 10
Contact: Catherine (Cay) Loria, Ph.D.; (301) 435-0702; fax: (301) 480-5158; email: loriac@nhlbi.nih.gov
Internet: http://grants.nih.gov/grants/guide/rfa-files/RFA-HL-08-007.html
Sponsor: National Heart, Lung, and Blood Institute (NHLBI)
6701 Rockledge Drive, Suite 10118, MSC 7936
Bethesda, MD 20892-7936

NHLBI Targeting Calcium Regulatory Molecules for Arrhythmia Prevention Grants 2388

The purpose of this Funding Opportunity Announcement (FOA) is to stimulate the development of therapeutic strategies for cardiac arrhythmias that target Ca2+ handling and Ca2+ signaling molecules. The overall goal is to exploit present knowledge of Ca2+ regulatory molecules and the role they play in arrhythmogenesis to develop novel therapeutic targets. Critical components of successful responses to this program announcement are: preclinical or early clinical testing of promising new therapeutic strategies to terminate and prevent cardiac arrhythmias in established models of human arrhythmogenic disease; and the feasibility to move positive findings to Phase I or II clinical trials. Grantees must budget for and attend two Project Director/Principal Investigator (PD/PI) meetings in Bethesda, MD, usually scheduled during the second and fourth year of the award.

Requirements: The following organizations and institutions are eligible to apply: public/state controlled institutions of higher education; private institutions of higher education; Hispanic-serving institutions; historically Black colleges and universities (HBCUs); tribally controlled colleges and universities (TCCUs); Alaska Native and Native Hawaiian serving institutions; nonprofits with 501(c)3 IRS status; nonprofits without 501(c)3 IRS status; for-profit organizations; state governments; Indian/Native American tribal governments (federally recognized); Indian/Native American tribally designated organizations; county governments; city or township governments; special district governments; independent school districts; public housing authorities/Indian housing authorities; U.S. territory or possession; Indian/Native American tribal governments (other than federally recognized); regional organizations; non-domestic (non-U.S.) entities (foreign organizations); other eligible agencies of the federal government; and faith-based or community-based organizations.
Date(s) Application is Due: Feb 5; Jun 5; Oct 5
Contact: Dennis A. Przywara, Ph.D.; (301) 435-0506; fax: (301) 480-1454; email: przywarad@nhlbi.nih.gov
Internet: http://grants.nih.gov/grants/guide/pa-files/PA-07-101.html
Sponsor: National Heart, Lung, and Blood Institute (NHLBI)
6701 Rockledge Drive, Room 9186, MSC 7940
Bethesda, MD 20892-7940

NHLBI Transfusion-Related Acute Lung Injury Basic Research Grants 2389
This Funding Opportunity Announcement (FOA) issued by the National Heart, Lung, and Blood Institute (NHLBI), National Institutes of Health, solicits Research Project Grant (R01) applications from institutions/organizations that propose to study the mechanisms responsible for acute lung injury after blood transfusion and stimulate the development of strategies to improve the prevention, diagnosis, and treatment of the disorder for the four million transfusion recipients per year in the U.S. who may be at risk for developing Transfusion-Related Acute Lung Injury (TRALI).
Requirements: The following organizations and institutions are eligible to apply: individuals; public/state controlled institutions of higher education; private institutions of higher education; nonprofits with 501(c)3 IRS status; nonprofits without 501(c)3 IRS status; small businesses; for-profit organizations; and non-domestic (non-U.S.) entities.
Date(s) Application is Due: Feb 5; Jun 5; Oct 5
Contact: Traci Heath Mondoro, Ph.D.; (301) 435-0052; fax: (301) 480-1060; email: mondorot@nhlbi.nih.gov
Internet: http://grants.nih.gov/grants/guide/pa-files/PA-07-385.html
Sponsor: National Heart, Lung, and Blood Institute
6701 Rockledge Drive, MSC 7950
Bethesda, MD 20892-0052

NHLBI Translating Basic Behavioral and Social Science Discoveries into Interventions to Reduce Obesity: Centers for Behavioral Intervention Development Grants 2390
This FOA solicits cooperative agreement (U01) applications from institutions/organizations that propose to translate findings from basic research on human behavior into more effective clinical, community, and population interventions to reduce obesity and improve obesity-related behaviors. This FOA will support Centers for Behavioral Intervention Development (CBIDs) in which interdisciplinary teams of basic and applied behavioral and social science researchers develop and refine novel interventions to reduce obesity and alter obesity-related health behaviors (e.g., diet, physical activity). The interventions to be developed include any of a wide range of strategies aimed at promoting weight loss and/or preventing weight gain. Interventions can be targeted to the individual, family, social network, community, environmental, clinical or population level, or combinations of these, and to any age group. Investigators at each CBID will conduct several types of studies during the funding period, including laboratory experimental studies, formative research, early phase trials and pilot/feasibility studies, in order to create promising new avenues for reducing obesity and improving obesity-related behaviors. The maximum award for the research component will be approximately $3,750,000 in direct costs across five years, with a limit of $750,000 in direct cost for any single year. Letters of Intent should be received by December 16, and full proposals are due by January 13.
Requirements: The following organizations and institutions are eligible to apply: public/state controlled institutions of higher education; private institutions of higher education; Hispanic-serving institutions; historically Black colleges and universities (HBCUs); tribally controlled colleges and universities (TCCUs); Alaska Native and Native Hawaiian serving institutions; nonprofits with 501(c)3 IRS status; nonprofits without 501(c)3 IRS status; for-profit organizations; state governments; Indian/Native American tribal governments (federally recognized); Indian/Native American tribally designated organizations; county governments; city or township governments; special district governments; independent school districts; public housing authorities/Indian housing authorities; U.S. territory or possession; Indian/Native American tribal governments (other than federally recognized); regional organizations; non-domestic (non-U.S.) entities (foreign organizations); other eligible agencies of the federal government; and faith-based or community-based organizations.
Amount of Grant: $750,000 maximum per year
Date(s) Application is Due: Dec 16; Jan 13
Contact: Susan M. Czajkowski, Ph.D.; (301) 435-0406; fax: (301) 480-1773; email: czajkows@mail.nih.gov
Internet: http://grants.nih.gov/grants/guide/rfa-files/RFA-HL-08-013.html
Sponsor: National Heart, Lung, and Blood Institute (NHLBI)
6701 Rockledge Drive, Suite 10118, MSC 7936
Bethesda, MD 20892-7936

NHLBI Translational Programs in Lung Diseases 2391
The purpose of this program is to encourage interdisciplinary approaches to lung translational research, allowing for potentially high-impact research, which will translate basic observations to applied clinical research. An application to NHLBI requires a minimum of three interrelated research projects that focus a number of scientific disciplines on investigations of a complex biomedical theme or research question. Applicants will be required to propose research that will become progressively more clinical and translational during the life of the program project, and they are expected to assemble interactive, multidisciplinary teams that have the combined expertise to formulate a plan for successful translation. Research teams are not required to have prior collaborative experience but must be able to demonstrate an integrated, practical approach that will result in the effective progression of mechanistic/basic concepts toward application in the clinic. This program allows for a maximum of two 5-year awards (a new application and one competing renewal). There are two application cycles. Letters of Intent should be received by April 25 and August 25 (respectively), and full proposals are due by May 25 and September 25 (respectively).
Requirements: The following organizations and institutions are eligible to apply: public/state controlled institutions of higher education; private institutions of higher education; Hispanic-serving institutions; historically Black colleges and universities (HBCUs); tribally controlled colleges and universities (TCCUs); Alaska Native and Native Hawaiian serving institutions; nonprofits with 501(c)3 IRS status; nonprofits without 501(c)3 IRS status; for-profit organizations; state governments; Indian/Native American tribal governments (federally recognized); Indian/Native American tribally designated organizations; county governments; city or township governments; special district governments; independent school districts; public housing authorities/Indian housing authorities; U.S. territories or possessions; Indian/Native American tribal governments (other than federally recognized); regional organizations; non-domestic (non-U.S.) entities (foreign organizations); other eligible agencies of the federal government; and faith-based or community-based organizations.
Date(s) Application is Due: Apr 25; May 25; Aug 25; Sep 25
Contact: Patricia Noel, Ph.D.; (301) 435-0202; email: noelp@nhlbi.nih.gov
Internet: http://grants.nih.gov/grants/guide/pa-files/PAR-09-185.html
Sponsor: National Heart, Lung and Blood Institute (NHLBI)
6701 Rockledge Drive
Bethesda, MD 20892-7952

NIA Aging Research Dissertation Awards to Increase Diversity 2392
This Funding Opportunity Announcement (FOA) issued by the National Institute on Aging (NIA) of the National Institutes of Health (NIH) publicizes the re-issuance of an FOA that publicizes the availability of dissertation awards in aging research to increase the diversity of the research-on-aging workforce. These awards are available to all qualified Predoctoral students in accredited research doctoral programs in the United States (including Puerto Rico and other U.S. territories or possessions).
Requirements: Public or private institutions, such as universities, colleges, hospitals, and laboratories, that offer accredited research doctoral programs may submit an application.
Restrictions: Domestic institutions only are eligible.
Amount of Grant: $50,000 average
Date(s) Application is Due: Feb 16; Jun 16; Oct 16
Contact: Michael-David A.R.R. Kerns; (301) 402-7713; fax: (301) 402-2945; email: michael-david.kerns@nih.hhs.gov
Internet: http://grants.nih.gov/grants/guide/pa-files/PAR-08-250.html
Sponsor: National Institute on Aging (NIA)
7201 Wisconsin Avenue, Suite 2C-218
Bethesda, MD 20814

NIA Aging, Oxidative Stress and Cell Death Grants 2393
The purpose of this Program Announcement is to encourage the submission of applications to support research on the relationship between oxidative stress and apoptosis, and how these biological processes are involved in aging and/or change with age. Although the National Institute of General Medical Sciences is not participating in this program announcement, that Institute continues to be interested in receiving applications on basic mechanisms of programmed cell death and oxidative stress when these applications do not focus on aging mechanisms. Modular Grant applications will request direct costs in $25,000 modules, up to a total direct cost request of $250,000 per year.
Requirements: The following organizations and institutions may apply: public/state controlled institutions of higher education; private institutions of higher education; Hispanic-serving institutions; historically Black colleges and universities (HBCUs); tribally controlled colleges and universities (TCCUs); Alaska native and native Hawaiian serving institutions; nonprofits with 501(c)3 IRS status; nonprofits without 501(c)3 IRS status; small businesses; for-profit organizations; State governments; regional organizations; U.S. territories or possessions; Indian/Native American tribal governments; Indian/Native American tribally designated organizations; county governments; city or township governments; special district governments; independent school districts; public housing authorities/Indian housing authorities; eligible agencies of the Federal government; and faith-based or community based organizations.
Amount of Grant: $250,000 maximum per year
Date(s) Application is Due: Feb 5; Jun 5; Oct 5
Contact: Chyren Hunter, Ph.D.; (301) 496-9322; fax: (301) 402-0528; email: Hunterc@nia.nih.gov
Internet: http://grants.nih.gov/grants/guide/pa-files/PA-00-081.html
Sponsor: National Institute on Aging (NIA)
7201 Wisconsin Avenue, MSC 9205, Gateway Building, Room 2C218
Bethesda, MD 20892-9205

NIA AIDS and Aging: Behavioral Sciences Prevention Research Grants 2394

NIA, NIMH, and NINR invite qualified researchers to submit applications to investigate prevention issues relevant to AIDS in middle-aged and older populations. This announcement solicits AIDS prevention research proposals to study primary prevention of disease transmission as well as secondary and tertiary prevention of negative behavioral and social consequences of HIV/AIDS for persons with AIDS, their families, and communities. Thus, the primary goals are to identify social and behavioral factors associated with HIV transmission and disease progression in later life; examine behavioral and social consequences of HIV infection/AIDS across the life course; develop and evaluate age-appropriate behavioral and social interventions for preventing AIDS in middle-aged and older adults and/or ameliorating problems associated with older adult caregiver responsibilities and burdens; explore health care issues surrounding AIDS care; and strengthen existing research and evaluation methods.

Requirements: Applications may be submitted by domestic and foreign for-profit and non-profit organizations, public and private, such as universities, colleges, hospitals, laboratories, units of State and local governments, and eligible agencies of the Federal government. Applications may be submitted by single institutions or by a consortia of institutions.

Date(s) Application is Due: Feb 5; Feb 16; Jun 5; Jun 16; Oct 5; Oct 16

Contact: Ying Tian, M.D.; (301) 496-6761; fax: (301) 402-1784; email: tiany@nia.nih.gov;; John W. Kusek, Ph.D.; (301) 594-7735; fax: (301) 480-3510; email: kusekj@extra.niddk.nih.gov

Internet: http://www.grants.nih.gov/grants/guide/pa-files/PA-97-069.html

Sponsor: National Institute on Aging (NIA)
7201 Wisconsin Avenue, Gateway Building, Suite 3C-307
Bethesda, MD 20892-9205

NIA Alzheimer's Disease Core Centers Grants 2395

The National Institute on Aging (NIA) invites applications from qualified institutions for support of Alzheimer's Disease Core Centers (ADCCs). These centers are designed to support and conduct research on Alzheimer's disease (AD), to serve as shared research resources that will facilitate research in AD and related disorders, distinguish them from the processes of normal brain aging and mild cognitive impairment (MCI), provide a platform for training, develop novel techniques and methodologies, and translate these research findings into better diagnostic, prevention and treatment strategies. New applications should request a project period of five years and a budget for direct costs of up to $750,000 per year. Competing renewal applications may request direct costs for all cores (both required and optional), and the other listed functions, i.e., satellites and pilot grants at a level not exceeding the combined direct costs of all funded activities awarded during the final year of the present funding period plus a 3% increase, or $750,000 per year, whichever is larger. Letters of Intent should arrive by the April 6 deadline, with full proposals due by May 5

Requirements: The following organizations and institutions are eligible to apply: public/state controlled institutions of higher education; private institutions of higher education; Hispanic-serving institutions; historically Black colleges and universities (HBCUs); tribally controlled colleges and universities (TCCUs); Alaska Native and Native Hawaiian serving institutions; nonprofits with 501(c)3 IRS status (other than institutions of higher education); and nonprofits without 501(c)3 IRS status (other than institutions of higher education).

Restrictions: At the time of award, the applicant institution cannot have another Alzheimer's Disease Center funded by the NIA.

Amount of Grant: $750,000 per year for five years

Date(s) Application is Due: Apr 6; May 5

Contact: Creighton H. Phelps, (301) 496-9350; fax: (301) 496-1494; email: phelpsc@nia.nih.gov

Internet: http://grants.nih.gov/grants/guide/rfa-files/RFA-AG-10-001.html

Sponsor: National Institute on Aging (NIA)
7201 Wisconsin Avenue, Suite 350
Bethesda, MD 20892-9205

NIA Alzheimer's Disease Drug Development Program Grants 2396

The NIA and other NIH Institutes currently support research projects for the study of the epidemiology, etiology, diagnosis, and treatment of Alzheimer's disease (AD). Investigators in all relevant scientific disciplines and organizations are invited to develop and pre-clinically test compounds which can slow the disease progression, reverse the disease process, or delay the onset of or prevent AD, mild cognitive impairment (MCI), or age-related cognitive decline.

Requirements: The following organizations and institutions may apply: public/state controlled institutions of higher education; private institutions of higher education; nonprofits with 501(c)3 IRS status; nonprofits without 501(c)3 IRS status; small businesses; for-profit organizations; State governments; and non-domestic (non-U.S.) entities.

Amount of Grant: $300,000-$800,000 annually in direct costs

Date(s) Application is Due: Jan 2; Feb 2; Sep 1; Oct

Contact: Suzana Petanceska, Ph.D.; (301) 496-9350; fax: (301) 496-1494; email: petanceskas@nia.nih.gov

Internet: http://grants.nih.gov/grants/guide/pa-files/PAR-08-266.html

Sponsor: National Institute on Aging (NIA)
7201 Wisconsin Avenue, Suite 350, MSC 9205
Bethesda, MD 20892-9205

NIA Alzheimer's Disease Pilot Clinical Trials 2397

The objective of the Alzheimer's Disease Pilot Clinical Trials initiative is to improve the quality of clinical research designed to evaluate interventions for the prevention and treatment of Alzheimer's disease (AD), mild cognitive impairment (MCI), and age-associated cognitive decline by stimulating applications for pilot clinical trials to test interventions aimed at delaying the onset of or preventing AD, MCI, and age-associated cognitive decline; slowing, halting, or, if possible, reversing the progressive decline in cognitive function; and modifying the cognitive and behavioral symptoms in AD and MCI. The goal is not to duplicate or compete with pharmaceutical companies but to encourage, complement, and accelerate the process of testing new, innovative, and effective treatments. The pilot research project application should directly address how it will inform and advance the design of a subsequent full-scale clinical trial. The application should also address the intrinsic scientific merit of the pilot trial itself. The application may include the following: studies to refine the intervention strategy (e.g. drug dosage, duration, delivery system; behavioral intensity and duration); studies to define and refine the target population and ensure adequate enrollment, protocol adherence and subject retention; collection of preliminary data for establishing measures of clinical efficacy including clinical/neuropsychological/behavioral measures, neuroimaging measures, and other biological measures in blood and cerebrospinal fluid; assessment of efficacy (including primary and secondary outcome and assessment measures for both patients and caregivers); and studies of safety.

Requirements: The following organizations and institutions may apply: public/state controlled institutions of higher education; private institutions of higher education; Hispanic-serving institutions; historically Black colleges and universities (HBCUs); tribally controlled colleges and universities (TCCUs); Alaska native and native Hawaiian serving institutions; nonprofits with 501(c)3 IRS status; nonprofits without 501(c)3 IRS status; small businesses; for-profit organizations; State governments; regional organizations; U.S. territories or possessions; Indian/Native American tribal governments; Indian/Native American tribally designated organizations; county governments; city or township governments; special district governments; independent school districts; public housing authorities/Indian housing authorities; eligible agencies of the Federal government; and faith-based or community based organizations.

Amount of Grant: $450,000 per year for up to 3 years

Date(s) Application is Due: Feb 5; Jun 5; Oct 5

Contact: Laurie M. Ryan, PhD; (301) 496-9350; fax: (301) 496-1494; email: ryanl@nia.nih.gov;; April Bower, RN; (301) 451-3560; fax: (301) 480-3621; email: bowera@mail.nih.gov

Internet: http://grants.nih.gov/grants/guide/pa-files/PAR-08-062.html

Sponsor: National Institute on Aging (NIA)
7201 Wisconsin Avenue, Suite 350, MSC 9205
Bethesda, MD 20892-9205

NIA Alzheimer's Disease Research Centers Grants 2398

The National Institute on Aging (NIA) invites applications from qualified institutions for support of Alzheimer's Disease Research Centers (ADRCs). These centers are designed to support and conduct research on Alzheimer's disease (AD), to serve as shared research resources that will facilitate research in AD and related disorders, distinguish them from the processes of normal brain aging and mild cognitive impairment (MCI), provide a platform for training, develop novel techniques and methodologies, and translate these research findings into better diagnostic, prevention and treatment strategies. New applications should request a project period of five years and a budget for direct costs of up to $1 million per year. Letters of Intent are due by April 6 annually, with full applications received by May 5.

Requirements: The following organizations and institutions are eligible to apply: public/state controlled institutions of higher education; private institutions of higher education; Hispanic-serving institutions; historically Black colleges and universities (HBCUs); tribally controlled colleges and universities (TCCUs); Alaska native and native Hawaiian serving institutions; nonprofits with 501(c)3 IRS status (other than institutions of higher education); and nonprofits without 501(c)3 IRS status (other than institutions of higher education).

Amount of Grant: $1 million maximum per year for five years

Date(s) Application is Due: Apr 5; May 6

Contact: Creighton H. Phelps, Ph.D.; (301) 496-9350; fax: (301) 496-1494; email: phelpsc@nia.nih.gov

Internet: http://grants.nih.gov/grants/guide/rfa-files/RFA-AG-10-002.html

Sponsor: National Institute on Aging (NIA)
7201 Wisconsin Avenue, Suite 350
Bethesda, MD 20892-9205

NIA Archiving and Development of Socialbehavioral Datasets in Aging Related Studies Grants 2399

This Funding Opportunity Announcement (FOA), issued by the National Institute on Aging (NIA) is seeking small grant applications to stimulate and facilitate data archiving and development related to cognitive psychology, behavioral interventions in the context of randomized controlled trials (RCTs), demography, economics, epidemiology, behavioral genetics and other behavioral research on aging for secondary analysis.

Requirements: The following organizations and institutions may apply: public/state controlled institutions of higher education; private institutions of higher education; Hispanic-serving institutions; historically Black colleges and universities (HBCUs); tribally controlled colleges and universities (TCCUs); Alaska native and native Hawaiian serving institutions; nonprofits with 501(c)3 IRS status; nonprofits without 501(c)3 IRS status; small businesses; for-profit organizations; State governments; regional organizations; U.S. territories or possessions; Indian/Native American tribal governments; Indian/Native American tribally designated organizations; county governments; city or township governments; special district governments; independent school districts; public housing authorities/Indian housing authorities; eligible agencies of the Federal government; and faith-based or community based organizations.

Amount of Grant: $100,000 maximum over two years
Date(s) Application is Due: Feb 16; Jun 16; Oct 16
Contact: Partha Bhattacharyya, Ph.D.; (301) 496-3136; fax: (301) 402-0051; email: bhattacharyyap@mail.nih.gov
Internet: http://grants.nih.gov/grants/guide/pa-files/PA-08-252.html
Sponsor: National Institute on Aging (NIA)
7201 Wisconsin Avenue, Gateway 533
Bethesda, MD 20892

NIA Awards to Support Research on the Biology of Aging in Invertebrates Grants **2400**

This Funding Opportunity Announcement (FOA) issued by the National Institute on Aging (NIA), National Institutes of Health, invites applications that propose the identification and development of new invertebrate models for use in biomedical research that is highly relevant to the biology of aging. Applications should focus on the identification, development and characterization of new invertebrate models that have short lifespans. Invertebrate models with tractable genetics and genome sequence available or in progress, negligible or induced senescence, and tissue regeneration in adults are of particular interest to NIA. Examples of invertebrate models of interest include, but are not limited to planaria, hydra, rotifers, and tunicates. These invertebrate models are currently not well developed for aging research. Within the scope of this FOA, invertebrate models other than those mentioned above currently used by the biomedical research community, but not yet fully developed or realized for aging research, will be considered responsive to this FOA. In particular, applications that focus on the characterization of these novel models for aging research utilizing molecular, genetic, cellular or physiological tools and approaches to identify genes involved in longevity, senescence and cellular pathways in tissue homeostasis during aging are encouraged. Letters of Intent are due by September 30, with final applications due by October 30.
Requirements: The following organizations and institutions are eligible to apply for support: public/state controlled institutions of higher education; private institutions of higher education; Hispanic-serving institutions; historically Black colleges and universities (HBCUs); tribally controlled colleges and universities (TCCUs); Alaska Native and Native Hawaiian serving institutions; nonprofits with 501(c)3 IRS status (other than institutions of higher education); nonprofits without 501(c)3 IRS status (other than institutions of higher education); Indian/Native American tribal governments (federally recognized); Indian/Native American tribally designated organizations; U.S. territories or possessions; and eligible agencies of the federal government.
Amount of Grant: $250,000 maximum
Date(s) Application is Due: Sep 30; Oct 30
Contact: Anna M. McCormick, Ph.D.; (301) 496-6402; email: mccormia@nia.nih.gov
Internet: http://grants.nih.gov/grants/guide/rfa-files/RFA-AG-10-004.html
Sponsor: National Institute on Aging (NIA)
Gateway Building, Suite 2C231, 7201 Wisconsin Avenue
Bethesda, MD 20892-9205

NIA Behavioral and Social Research Grants on Disasters and Health **2401**

The purpose of this FOA is to stimulate research in the behavioral and social sciences on the consequences of natural and man-made disasters for the health of children, the elderly, and vulnerable groups, with an ultimate goal of preventing and mitigating harmful consequences and health disparities. Disasters include severe weather-related events, earthquakes, large-scale attacks on civilian populations, technological catastrophes or perceived catastrophes, and influenza pandemics. For the elderly and for children and youth, the health outcomes of greatest interest include mortality, disability and resilience, severe distress and clinically significant morbidity (as opposed to mild or transient symptoms and dysphoria), and economic hardship sufficient to harm health. For children and youth, long-term effects on development are also of interest.
Requirements: The following organizations and institutions may apply: for-profit organizations; non-profit organizations; public or private institutions, such as universities, colleges, hospitals, and laboratories; units of State government; units of Local government; units of State Tribal government; units of Local Tribal government; eligible agencies of the Federal government; foreign institutions; domestic institutions; faith-based or community-based organizations; Indian/Native American tribal governments (federally recognized); Indian/Native American tribal governments (other than federally recognized); and Indian/Native American tribally designated organizations.
Date(s) Application is Due: Feb 16; Jun 16; Oct 16
Contact: John G. Haaga, Ph.D.; (301) 496-3131; email: HaagaJ@mail.nih.gov;; Rebecca L. Clark, Ph.D.; (301) 496-1175; email: rclark@mail.nih.gov
Internet: http://grants.nih.gov/grants/guide/pa-files/PA-06-452.html
Sponsor: National Institute on Aging (NIA)
7201 Wisconsin Avenue, Gateway Building, Room 533
Bethesda, MD 20892-9205

NIA Bioenergetics, Fatigability, and Activity Limitations in Aging **2402**

This FOA encourages Research Project Grant applications proposing to study bioenergetic factors underlying increased fatigability and activity limitations in aging. Increased fatigability is a significant cause of restricted physical and cognitive activity in older adults. Alterations in bioenergetics - the production and utilization of energy, and the regulation of these processes - may contribute significantly to increased fatigability. This FOA encourages applications that propose to: elucidate specific alterations in bioenergetics related to increased fatigability and activity limitations; develop and evaluate improved measures of fatigability related to bioenergetics; and evaluate interventions for increased fatigability and activity limitations that target alterations in bioenergetics and lead to improved quality of life.
Requirements: The following organizations and institutions may apply: public/state controlled institutions of higher education; private institutions of higher education; Hispanic-serving institutions; historically Black colleges and universities (HBCUs); tribally controlled colleges and universities (TCCUs); Alaska native and native Hawaiian serving institutions; nonprofits with 501(c)3 IRS status; nonprofits without 501(c)3 IRS status; small businesses; for-profit organizations; State governments; regional organizations; U.S. territories or possessions; Indian/Native American tribal governments; Indian/Native American tribally designated organizations; county governments; city or township governments; special district governments; independent school districts; public housing authorities/Indian housing authorities; eligible agencies of the Federal government; and faith-based or community based organizations.
Date(s) Application is Due: Feb 5; Feb 16; Jun 5; Jun 16; Oct 5; Oct 16
Contact: Basil Eldadah; (301) 496-6761; fax: (301) 402-1784; email: eldadahb@nia.nih.gov;; Cheryl L. McDonald; (301) 435-0560; fax: (301) 480-2858; email: mcdonalc@nhlbi.nih.gov
Internet: http://grants.nih.gov/grants/guide/pa-files/PA-09-190.html
Sponsor: National Institute on Aging (NIA)
7201 Wisconsin Avenue, 3C-307
Bethesda, MD 20892-9205

NIA Diversity in Medication Use and Outcomes in Aging Populations Grants **2403**

The National Institute on Aging (NIA) in collaboration with the National Center for Complementary and Alternative Medicine, the Office of Research on Minority Health and the Office of Research on Women"s Health invites qualified researchers to submit applications to investigate issues relevant to medication use and outcomes among older people. This program announcement solicits both basic and applied research proposals to investigate the multiple factors that influence medication use by the elderly. Goals of this announcement are to: identify the epidemiological, psychosocial, health care and clinical factors associated with medication use by older people, including the use of unconventional medical products; assess social, behavioral, psychological and cognitive factors that play a role in older people's understanding of and adherence to medication regimens; determine the role of medical and pharmaceutical professionals in facilitating or hindering proper use of prescribed and over-the-counter medications and unconventional medications including herbs and dietary supplements; refine methodologies to link these factors to medical or psychosocial outcomes; investigate interventions to improve medication adherence; and increase our understanding of biological factors which contribute to therapeutic outcomes in the use of medications by the elderly.
Requirements: Applications may be submitted by foreign and domestic for-profit and non-profit organizations, public and private, such as universities, colleges, hospitals, laboratories, units of state and local governments, and eligible agencies of the Federal government.
Contact: Laurie M. Ryan, PhD; (301) 496-9350; fax: (301) 496-1494; email: ryanl@nia.nih.gov;; April Bower, RN; (301) 451-3560; fax: (301) 480-3621; email: bowera@mail.nih.gov
Internet: http://grants.nih.gov/grants/guide/pa-files/PA-99-097.html
Sponsor: National Institute on Aging (NIA)
7201 Wisconsin Avenue, Suite 350, MSC 9205
Bethesda, MD 20892-9205

NIA Effects of Gene-Social Environment Interplay on Health and Behavior in Later Life Grants **2404**

The National Institute on Aging (NIA) invites applications for the development of multidisciplinary collaborations among existing longitudinal twin and family studies, with a focus on social and behavioral factors associated with aging outcomes. This FOA is intended to lay the foundation for future studies of the role of gene-environment interplay in accounting for links between social experiences and physical health, functionality, and psychological well-being in midlife and older age. Of particular interest are applications that can embed this foundation within a lifespan perspective. Applicants are encouraged to use this FOA as a starting point for: developing collaborations among existing data sets; harmonizing social phenotypes across a number of twin and family studies; conducting analyses aimed at further refining social phenotypes for genetic analysis; using animal models of gene-social environment interplay to inform work using twin studies; and/or establishing preliminary data on the feasibility of genetic/genomic approaches that could be applied to questions of how social experiences are biologically embedded and influence middle and later life outcomes. Use of existing data is strongly encouraged; funds from this award are not intended for new data collection, but a small percentage of funds may be used for adding modules to ongoing data collection efforts to augment phenotypic or genetic data. NIA expects to make 1-2 awards totaling $750,000 total costs in the first year, and $3,750,000 in total costs over the 5 year project period. Direct costs are expected to range from $200,000 -$500,000 in the first year. Letters of Intent are due by October 9, with final applications due by November 9.
Requirements: The following organizations and institutions may apply: public/state controlled institutions of higher education; private institutions of higher education; Hispanic-serving institutions; historically Black colleges and universities (HBCUs); tribally controlled colleges and universities (TCCUs); Alaska native and native Hawaiian serving institutions; nonprofits with 501(c)3 IRS status; nonprofits without 501(c)3 IRS status; small businesses; for-profit organizations; State governments; regional organizations; U.S. territories or possessions; Indian/Native American tribal governments; Indian/Native American tribally designated organizations; county governments; city or township governments; special district governments; independent school districts; public housing authorities/Indian housing authorities; eligible agencies of the Federal government; and faith-based or community based organizations.
Amount of Grant: $200,000-$500,000 in the first year

Date(s) Application is Due: Oct 9; Nov 9
Contact: Erica L. Spotts, Ph.D.; (301) 451-4503; fax: (301) 402-0051; email: spottse@mail.nih.gov
Internet: http://grants.nih.gov/grants/guide/rfa-files/RFA-AG-10-006.html
Sponsor: National Institute on Aging (NIA)
7201 Wisconsin Avenue, Suite 533
Bethesda, MD 20892-9201

NIA Factors Affecting Cognitive Function in Adults with Down Syndrome Grants **2405**

The purpose of this solicitation is to encourage investigator initiated research to focus on various factors that maximize and maintain cognitive function in adults (>21 years of age) with Down syndrome. This solicitation encourages applications from investigators from very diverse backgrounds and interdisciplinary and transdisciplinary proposals, as well as those that involve systematic longitudinal study rather than study of samples of convenience. These studies could serve to form an evidence base that will inform not only health care management and treatment, but also issues such as quality of life, access to services, education, and ultimately affect public policy. This solicitation encourages applications that would inform several areas of inquiry: the natural history of medical and mental health issues in adults with Down syndrome, their incidence and onset; health disparities that occur, and their prevention or effective treatment; the development of better diagnostic tools to assess functional and cognitive impairment in adults with Down syndrome; improved quality of life measures; community-based interventions that improve individual educational, occupational, and social outcomes; the impact of early entry to services, type of intervention, and/or family history on quality of life for adults with Down Syndrome; and the impact of family structure and ancestry on critical life transitions, co-occurring conditions, and developmental changes of adults with Down syndrome through longitudinal studies rather than studies of samples of convenience. The requested budget is limited to $500,000 total costs per year for a maximum of five years. Letters of Intent are due by May 29, and full applications should arrive by June 30.
Requirements: The following organizations and institutions are eligible to apply: public/state controlled institutions of higher education; private institutions of higher education; nonprofits with 501(c)3 IRS status (other than institutions of higher education); nonprofits without 501(c)3 IRS status (other than institutions of higher education); for-profit organizations (other than small businesses); State governments; county governments; eligible agencies of the Federal government; and faith-based or community-based organizations.
Restrictions: Foreign institutions may not submit applications, but collaborators at foreign institutions are allowed.
Amount of Grant: $500,000 maximum per year for up to five years
Date(s) Application is Due: May 29; Jun 30
Contact: Mary Lou Oster-Granite; (301) 435-6866; fax: (301) 496-3791; email: mo96o@nih.gov
Internet: http://grants.nih.gov/grants/guide/rfa-files/RFA-HD-09-028.html
Sponsor: Eunice Kennedy Shriver National Institute of Child Health and Human Development (NICHD) / National Institute on Aging (NIA)
6100 Executive Boulevard, Room 4B05L, MSC 7510
Bethesda, MD 20892-7510

NIA Grants for Alzheimer's Disease Drug Discovery **2406**

The objective of this solicitation is to stimulate preclinical research in the discovery, design, development and testing of novel compounds aimed at slowing, halting, or, if possible, reversing the progressive decline in cognitive function and modifying the behavioral symptoms in Alzheimer's disease as well as delaying the onset of or preventing AD. This initiative is intended to stimulate basic research and development efforts. The goal is not to duplicate or compete with pharmaceutical companies but to encourage, complement, and accelerate the process of discovering new, innovative, and effective compounds for the prevention and treatment of the cognitive impairment and behavioral symptoms associated with Alzheimer's disease. The development of compounds for ameliorating, modifying, or improving potential aberrations in neuronal cellular communication mechanisms is encouraged. These compounds should be designed to affect fundamental processes such as the neuronal dysfunction, death, and loss of connectivity associated with the disease by targeting molecules and mechanisms such as neurotransmitters, neuromodulators, and neurotrophins; receptors and ion channels; second and third messenger systems; all facets of relevant amyloid precursor protein, amyloid beta protein, and tau neurobiology; protein synthesis, aggregation, and degradation; energy utilization; and oxidative, immunological, and inflammatory mechanisms.
Requirements: The following organizations are eligible to apply: for-profit organizations; non-profit organizations; public or private institutions, such as universities, colleges, hospitals, and laboratories; units of State government; units of local government; eligible agencies of the Federal government; foreign institutions; and domestic institutions.
Amount of Grant: $200,000 maximum per year; $275,000 maximum per two-year cycle
Date(s) Application is Due: Feb 16; Jun 16; Oct 16
Contact: Neil S. Buckholtz, Ph.D.; (301) 496-9350; fax: (301) 496-1494; email: Buckholn@nia.nih.gov
Internet: http://grants.nih.gov/grants/guide/pa-files/PAS-06-261.html
Sponsor: National Institute on Aging (NIA)
7201 Wisconsin Avenue, Suite 350, MSC 9205
Bethesda, MD 20892-9205

NIA Harmonization of Longitudinal Cross-National Surveys of Aging Grants **2407**

The National Institute on Aging (NIA) will provide support through the R21 mechanism to facilitate the ex-ante and ex-post harmonization of international longitudinal surveys of aging populations to the Health and Retirement Study to maximize cross-national comparability of data. Facilitation will include, but is not limited to, meetings, pilots, and the development of methods to improve cross-national comparability of international aging surveys to the Health and Retirement Study and existing international data files that are harmonized with the HRS: the English Longitudinal Study on Ageing (ELSA); and the Survey of Health, Ageing, and Retirement in Europe (SHARE).
Requirements: The following organizations and institutions may apply: public/state controlled institutions of higher education; private institutions of higher education; nonprofits with 501(c)3 IRS status; nonprofits without 501(c)3 IRS status; for-profit organizations; State governments; and non-domestic (non-U.S.) entities (foreign organizations).
Amount of Grant: $200,000 maximum per year; $275,000 maximum per two-year cycle
Date(s) Application is Due: Feb 16; Jun 16; Oct 16
Contact: John W. R. Phillips, Ph.D.; (301) 496-3138; fax: (301) 402-0051; email: phillipj@mail.nih.gov
Internet: http://grants.nih.gov/grants/guide/pa-files/PAS-07-387.html
Sponsor: National Institute on Aging (NIA)
7201 Wisconsin Avenue, Gateway Building, Room 533
Bethesda, MD 20892

NIA Health Behaviors and Aging Grants **2408**

The National Institute on Aging (NIA) invites qualified researchers to submit applications for research and research training on those health-related behaviors and attitudes of older adults, their families, and significant others, that can affect health and functioning as people grow older. Studies are sought that extend scientific understanding of how older adults health behaviors and attitudes develop under varying social conditions; how they relate to health promotion and disease prevention, care and treatment of disease, rehabilitation or death; and how they can be modified as relevant new scientific knowledge is developed.
Requirements: Applications may be submitted by foreign and domestic, for-profit and non-profit organizations, public and private, such as universities, colleges, hospitals, laboratories, units of State and local governments, and eligible agencies of the Federal government. Applications from minority individuals and women are encouraged.
Amount of Grant: $150,000 maximum per year
Date(s) Application is Due: Feb 5; Jun 5; Oct 5
Contact: Chyren Hunter, Ph.D.; (301) 496-9322; fax: (301) 402-0528; email: Hunterc@nia.nih.gov
Internet: http://grants.nih.gov/grants/guide/pa-files/PA-93-064.html
Sponsor: National Institute on Aging (NIA)
7201 Wisconsin Avenue, MSC 9205, Gateway Building, Room 2C218
Bethesda, MD 20892-9205

NIA Healthy Aging through Behavioral Economic Analyses of Situations Grants **2409**

The National Institute on Aging (NIA), National Institutes of Health, solicits Research Project Grant applications that propose to translate basic findings from Behavioral Economics into behavior change interventions targeting health behaviors associated with chronic health conditions of mid-life and older age. Applications should propose small pilot clinical trials or demonstration projects, ideally based on collaborations between individuals with expertise in behavioral economics and psychologists, psychiatrists, clinicians, or others with expertise in aging or implementing behavioral interventions. Depending on the availability of funding, the NIA expects to make 4 or 5 awards totaling $1,250,000 total costs in the first year, and $3,750,000 over the 3 year project period. The direct cost amount for each individual award will be no greater than $525,000 in total for three years, and no more than $175,000 in any year. Letters of Intent are due by October 2, with final applications due by November 2.
Requirements: The following organizations and institutions may apply: public/state controlled institutions of higher education; private institutions of higher education; Hispanic-serving institutions; historically Black colleges and universities (HBCUs); tribally controlled colleges and universities (TCCUs); Alaska native and native Hawaiian serving institutions; nonprofits with 501(c)3 IRS status; nonprofits without 501(c)3 IRS status; small businesses; for-profit organizations; State governments; regional organizations; U.S. territories or possessions; Indian/Native American tribal governments; Indian/Native American tribally designated organizations; county governments; city or township governments; special district governments; independent school districts; public housing authorities/Indian housing authorities; eligible agencies of the Federal government; and faith-based or community based organizations.
Amount of Grant: $525,000 maximum for three years; $175,000 maximum per year
Date(s) Application is Due: Oct 2; Nov 2
Contact: Dr. Jonathan W. King; (301) 402-4156; fax: (301) 402-0051; email: kingjo@nia.nih.gov
Internet: http://grants.nih.gov/grants/guide/rfa-files/RFA-AG-10-008.html
Sponsor: National Institute on Aging (NIA)
7201 Wisconsin Avenue, Room 533
Bethesda, MD 20892-9205

NIA Higher-Order Cognitive Functioning and Aging Grants **2410**

The National Institute on Aging (NIA) invites qualified researchers to submit new applications for research projects that focus on adulthood and aging related changes in the higher-order processes and strategies required for judgment, decision-making, reasoning, problem-solving, and processing complex information. As in earlier periods of life older adults continue to make decisions related to everyday life, but with advanced age, new, and sometimes even more complex, decision-making is required of them. Recent research indicates that age-related limitations in cognitive processing resources

(e.g., speed and working memory) may impact decision-making. Research also indicates that some older adults experience growth in specific areas of cognitive functioning (e.g., expertise, semantic knowledge, emotional regulation) and continue to use adaptive intelligence, demonstrating multi-directionality in adult cognitive change. It is generally recognized that research on higher-order processing is underdeveloped in the field of aging. Research proposals are needed that examine the actual processes that are engaged when older adults make important decisions, how these processes change with age and context, and what environmental supports, interventions, and training may be necessary for optimal functioning. Research may investigate either individual or collaborative, or social processes. Modular Grant applications will request direct costs in $25,000 modules, up to a total direct cost request of $250,000 per year.
Requirements: Applications may be submitted by foreign and domestic, for-profit and non-profit, public and private organizations such as universities, colleges, hospitals, laboratories, units of State and local governments, and eligible agencies of the Federal government. Racial/ethnic minority individuals, women, and persons with disabilities are encouraged to apply as principal investigators.
Amount of Grant: $250,000 maximum per year
Date(s) Application is Due: Feb 16; Jun 16; Oct 16
Contact: Chyren Hunter, Ph.D.; (301) 496-9322; fax: (301) 402-0528; email: Hunterc@nia.nih.gov
Internet: http://grants.nih.gov/grants/guide/pa-files/PA-00-052.html
Sponsor: National Institute on Aging (NIA)
7201 Wisconsin Avenue, MSC 9205, Gateway Building, Room 2C218
Bethesda, MD 20892-9205

NIA Human Biospecimen Resources for Aging Research Grants 2411
The purpose of this announcement is to disseminate information about available human biospecimen resources for age-related studies, and promote independent use of existing human biospecimen resources through collaborative and other arrangements with the studies that collect biospecimens. Websites for the participating studies are accessed via the Virtual Repository. NIA is interested in aging-related research that integrates biomarker analyses with the study of normal aging, age-associated diseases, and behavioral and psychosocial data. Budgets for direct costs of up to $50,000 per year and a project duration of up to two years may be requested for a maximum of $100,000 direct costs over a two-year project period.
Requirements: The following organizations and institutions may apply: for-profit organizations; non-profit organizations; public or private institutions, such as universities, colleges, hospitals, and laboratories; units of State government; units of Local government; units of State Tribal government; units of Local Tribal government; eligible agencies of the Federal government; foreign institutions; domestic institutions; faith-based or community-based organizations; Indian/Native American tribal governments (federally recognized); Indian/Native American tribal governments (other than federally recognized); and Indian/Native American tribally designated organizations.
Amount of Grant: $50,000 maximum per year for up to 2 years
Date(s) Application is Due: Feb 16; Jun 16; Oct 16
Contact: Nancy L. Nadon, Ph.D.; (301) 402-7744; fax: (301) 402-0010; email: nadonn@nia.nih.gov
Internet: http://grants.nih.gov/grants/guide/pa-files/PA-06-443.html
Sponsor: National Institute on Aging (NIA)
7201 Wisconsin Avenue, GW 2C231
Bethesda, MD 20892

NIA Independent Scientist Award 2412
The award is a special salary-only grant designed to provide protected time for newly independent scientists who currently have non-research obligations such as heavy teaching loads, clinical work, committee assignments, service, and administrative duties that prevent them from having a period of intensive research focus. The award is targeted to persons with doctoral degrees who have completed their research training, have independent peer-reviewed research support, and who need a period of protected research time in order to foster their research career development. New applications are due February 12, June 12, and October 12, while renewal applications are due March 12, July 12, and November 12. Up to 75% per year of base salary plus fringe benefits is available. No other research development support funds are provided.
Requirements: The following organizations and institutions are eligible to apply: public/state controlled institutions of higher education; private institutions of higher education; nonprofits with 501(c)3 IRS status; nonprofits without 501(c)3 IRS status; small businesses; for-profit organizations; State governments; U.S. territories or possessions; Indian/Native American tribal governments (Federally recognized and other than Federally recognized); Indian/Native American tribally designated organizations; Hispanic-serving institutions; historically Black colleges and universities (HBCUs); tribally controlled colleges and universities (TCCUs); Alaska Native and Native Hawaiian serving institutions; regional organizations; and faith-based or community based organizations. The candidate must have a doctoral degree and peer-reviewed, independent research support at the time the award is made. The candidate must spend a minimum of 75 percent effort conducting research during the period of the award.
Restrictions: The award is not intended for investigators who already have full time to perform research, or have substantial publication records or considerable research support indicating that they are well established in their fields. Foreign institutions are not eligible to apply.
Date(s) Application is Due: Feb 12; Mar 12; Jun 12; Jul 12; Oct 12; Nov 12
Contact: Chyren Hunter, Ph.D.; (301) 496-9322; fax: (301) 402-0528; email: Hunterc@nia.nih.gov
Internet: http://grants.nih.gov/grants/guide/pa-files/PA-09-038.html
Sponsor: National Institute on Aging (NIA)
7201 Wisconsin Avenue, MSC 9205, Gateway Building, Room 2C218
Bethesda, MD 20892-9205

NIA Malnutrition in Older Persons Research Grants 2413
NIA continues to encourage research on the full spectrum of issues related to the causes, prevention, and treatment as well as sociobehavioral and economic aspects related to malnutrition in older persons. Support for this program will be through the research project grant and mentored research scientist development award. Applications will compete for available funds on the basis of scientific merit with all other applications assigned to the institute.
Requirements: Applications may be submitted by foreign and domestic, for-profit and non-profit organizations, public and private, such as universities, colleges, hospitals, laboratories, unit of State and local governments, and eligible agencies of the Federal government. Applications from minority individuals and women are encouraged.
Date(s) Application is Due: Feb 12; Mar 12; Jun 12; Jul 12; Oct 12; Nov 12
Contact: Chyren Hunter, Ph.D.; (301) 496-9322; fax: (301) 402-0528; email: Hunterc@nia.nih.gov
Internet: http://grants.nih.gov/grants/guide/pa-files/PA-94-088.html
Sponsor: National Institute on Aging (NIA)
7201 Wisconsin Avenue, Gateway 533
Bethesda, MD 20892

NIA Mechanisms Underlying the Links between Psychosocial Stress, Aging, the Brain and the Body Grants 2414
This FOA encourages multidisciplinary and interdisciplinary research to elucidate the mechanistic links between psychosocial stress and health in aging, as well as how the aging process and age-related diseases affect the responses to psychosocial stressors. Generally, research should be focused on: aging and how neural mechanisms respond to psychosocial stress and affect other body systems; characterizing the behavioral, psychological and social mechanisms and pathways involved in transducing psychosocial stressors into health outcomes; how stressors modulate physiological process underlying life-span, immune mechanisms, and metabolism; and how psychosocial stress contributes to the development or progression of geriatric syndromes, chronic medical conditions, and disabilities in later life. Research is strongly encouraged that aims to identify appropriate targets for intervention, at any level of analysis, from societal to molecular. Research spanning multiple levels of analysis is particularly encouraged.
Requirements: The following organizations and institutions are eligible to apply: public/state controlled institutions of higher education; private institutions of higher education; Hispanic-serving institutions; historically Black colleges and universities (HBCUs); tribally controlled colleges and universities (TCCUs); Alaska native and native Hawaiian serving institutions; nonprofits with 501(c)3 IRS status (other than institutions of higher education); nonprofits without 501(c)3 IRS status (other than institutions of higher education); small businesses; for-profit organizations (other than small businesses); state governments; Indian/Native American tribal governments (federally recognized); Indian/Native American tribally designated organizations; county governments; city or township governments; special district governments; independent school districts; public housing authorities/Indian housing authorities; U.S. territories or possessions; Indian/native American tribal governments (other than federally recognized); regional organizations; and non-domestic (non-U.S.) entities (foreign organizations).
Restrictions: Research focused on oxidative stress or on environmental or physical stressors of a non-psychosocial nature is not appropriate for this FOA.
Date(s) Application is Due: Mar 5; Jul 5; Nov 5
Contact: Suzana S. Petanceska, Ph.D.; (301) 496-9350; fax: (301) 496-1494; email: petanceskas@mail.nih.gov
Internet: http://grants.nih.gov/grants/guide/pa-files/PA-09-216.html
Sponsor: National Institute on Aging (NIA)
Gateway Building, Suite 350 7201, Wisconsin Avenue, MSC 9205
Bethesda, MD 20892-9205

NIA Mechanisms, Measurement, and Management of Pain in Aging: from Molecular to Clinical 2415
This FOA encourages Research Project Grant applications from institutions and organizations that propose to: study biological, neurobiological, psychosocial, and clinical mechanisms and processes by which aging and/or age-related diseases affect the experience of pain; examine biological, neurobiological, psychosocial, and clinical factors that impact pain experience and prevalence in older people; evaluate existing pain assessment and/or management approaches in older adults; or develop new assessment methods and/or management strategies for pain with particular attention to the needs of older adults. Studies involving animal models or human subjects are appropriate under this program announcement.
Requirements: The following organizations and institutions may apply: public/state controlled institutions of higher education; private institutions of higher education; Hispanic-serving institutions; historically Black colleges and universities (HBCUs); tribally controlled colleges and universities (TCCUs); Alaska native and native Hawaiian serving institutions; nonprofits with 501(c)3 IRS status; nonprofits without 501(c)3 IRS status; small businesses; for-profit organizations; State governments; regional organizations; U.S. territories or possessions; Indian/Native American tribal governments; Indian/Native American tribally designated organizations; county governments; city or township governments; special district governments; independent school districts; public housing authorities/Indian housing authorities; eligible agencies of the Federal government; and faith-based or community based organizations.
Date(s) Application is Due: Feb 5; Feb 16; Jun 5; Jun 16; Oct 5; Oct 16

Contact: Wen G. Chen, Ph.D.; (301) 496-9350; fax: (301) 496-1494; email: chenw@nia.nih.gov;; Basil Eldadah; (301) 496-6761; fax: (301) 402-1784; email: eldadahb@nia.nih.gov
Internet: http://grants.nih.gov/grants/guide/pa-files/PA-09-193.html
Sponsor: National Institute on Aging (NIA)
7201 Wisconsin Avenue, Gateway Building, Suite 350
Bethesda, MD 20892

NIA Medical Management of Older Patients with HIV/AIDS Grants **2416**
The National Institute on Aging (NIA), the National Institute of Allergy and Infectious Diseases (NIAID), the Center for Mental Health Research on AIDS of the National Institute of Mental Health (NIMH), and the National Institute of Nursing Research (NINR), invite Research Project Grant applications addressing clinical and translational health issues in the diagnosis and/or management of HIV infection and its consequences in older persons. The goal of this funding opportunity is to improve medical outcomes, functional status and quality of life in older patients with HIV/AIDS through improved understanding of interactions among aging processes, HIV viral infection, treatment effects and toxicities, and multiple morbidities commonly occurring in older persons.
Requirements: The following organizations and institutions may apply: public/state controlled institutions of higher education; private institutions of higher education; Hispanic-serving institutions; historically Black colleges and universities (HBCUs); tribally controlled colleges and universities (TCCUs); Alaska native and native Hawaiian serving institutions; nonprofits with 501(c)3 IRS status; nonprofits without 501(c)3 IRS status; small businesses; for-profit organizations; State governments; regional organizations; U.S. territories or possessions; Indian/Native American tribal governments; Indian/Native American tribally designated organizations; county governments; city or township governments; special district governments; independent school districts; public housing authorities/Indian housing authorities; eligible agencies of the Federal government; and faith-based or community based organizations.
Date(s) Application is Due: May 7; Sep 7; Jan 7
Contact: Susan G. Nayfield, M.D.; (301) 496-6761; fax: (301) 402-1784; email: nayfiels@nia.nih.gov
Internet: http://grants.nih.gov/grants/guide/pa-files/PA-09-017.html
Sponsor: National Institute on Aging (NIA)
7201 Wisconsin Avenue, Gateway Building, Suite 3C-307
Bethesda, MD 20892-9205

NIA Mentored Clinical Scientist Research Career Development Awards **2417**
The overall objective of the NIH Research Career Development Award program is to prepare qualified individuals for careers that have a significant impact on the health-related research needs of the Nation. The objective of the NIH Mentored Clinical Scientist Research Career Development Award (K08) program is to support didactic study and mentored research for individuals with clinical doctoral degrees (e.g., M.D., D.D.S., D.M.D., D.O., D.C., O.D., N.D., D.V.M., Pharm.D., or Ph.D. in clinical disciplines). The purpose of this Funding Opportunity Announcement (FOA) is to continue the long-standing NIH support of the K08 program. This award provides support and protected time for an intensive, mentored research career development experience in biomedical or behavioral research, including translational research. For the purpose of this award, translational research is defined as application of basic research discoveries toward the diagnosis, management, and prevention of human disease.
Requirements: The following organizations and institutions may apply: public/state controlled institutions of higher education; private institutions of higher education; Hispanic-serving institutions; historically Black colleges and universities (HBCUs); tribally controlled colleges and universities (TCCUs); Alaska native and native Hawaiian serving institutions; nonprofits with 501(c)3 IRS status; nonprofits without 501(c)3 IRS status; small businesses; for-profit organizations; State governments; regional organizations; U.S. territories or possessions; Indian/Native American tribal governments; Indian/Native American tribally designated organizations; county governments; city or township governments; special district governments; independent school districts; public housing authorities/Indian housing authorities; eligible agencies of the Federal government; and faith-based or community based organizations.
Restrictions: Individuals on temporary or student visas and organizations described in section 501(c)4 of the Internal Revenue Code that engage in lobbying are not eligible.
Amount of Grant: $100,000 maximum
Date(s) Application is Due: Feb 12; Mar 12; Jun 12; Jul 12; Oct 12; Nov 12
Contact: Chyren Hunter, Ph.D.; (301) 496-9322; fax: (301) 402-0528; email: Hunterc@nia.nih.gov
Internet: http://grants.nih.gov/grants/guide/pa-files/PA-09-042.html
Sponsor: National Institute on Aging (NIA)
7201 Wisconsin Avenue, MSC 9205, Gateway Building, Room 2C218
Bethesda, MD 20892-9205

NIA Mentored Research Scientist Development Award **2418**
The award is for research scientists who have established careers in biomedical, behavioral, or social research and wish to change career direction toward aging research; for more junior researchers with training in aging research who need additional periods of mentored research experience prior to becoming fully independent; or for researchers with training and experience in some aspect of aging research who wish to gain complementary training to expand their research interests in aging. The primary purpose of the program is to provide support and protected time (three, four, or five years) for an intensive, supervised career development experience in the biomedical, behavioral, or clinical sciences leading to research independence.
Requirements: The candidate must have a research or health-professional doctorate or its equivalent and must have demonstrated the capacity or potential for highly productive independent research in the period after the doctorate. The candidate must identify a mentor with extensive research experience and must spend a minimum of 75 percent of full-time professional effort conducting research for the period of the award. The following organizations and institutions may apply: public/state controlled institutions of higher education; private institutions of higher education; Hispanic-serving institutions; historically Black colleges and universities (HBCUs); tribally controlled colleges and universities (TCCUs); Alaska native and native Hawaiian serving institutions; nonprofits with 501(c)3 IRS status; nonprofits without 501(c)3 IRS status; small businesses; for-profit organizations; State governments; regional organizations; U.S. territories or possessions; Indian/Native American tribal governments; Indian/Native American tribally designated organizations; eligible agencies of the Federal government; and faith-based or community based organizations.
Amount of Grant: $75,000 salary plus fringe benefits
Date(s) Application is Due: Feb 12; Mar 12; Jun 12; Jul 12; Oct 12; Nov 12
Contact: Chyren Hunter, Ph.D.; (301) 496-9322; fax: (301) 402-0528; email: Hunterc@nia.nih.gov
Internet: http://grants.nih.gov/grants/guide/pa-files/PAR-09-060.html
Sponsor: National Institute on Aging (NIA)
7201 Wisconsin Avenue, MSC 9205, Gateway Building, Room 2C218
Bethesda, MD 20892-9205

NIA Minority Dissertation Research Grants in Aging **2419**
Small grants to support doctoral dissertation research will be available for underrepresented minority doctoral candidates. Grant support is designed to aid the research of such investigators and to encourage underrepresented minority individuals from a variety of academic disciplines and programs to conduct research related to aging. It is anticipated that a total of five to six new applications will be funded in each year. The maximum budget request should be limited to $25,000 in direct costs for the initial budget period. No more than $30,000 in total direct costs will be provided across the two year period.
Requirements: This research initiative is to provide underrepresented minority students assistance to complete their dissertation research on an aging-related topic and thereby increase their representation in aging research.
Amount of Grant: $25,000 maximum per year; $30,000 maximum for 2-year period
Date(s) Application is Due: Mar 15; Nov 15
Contact: Laurie M. Ryan, PhD; (301) 496-9350; fax: (301) 496-1494; email: ryanl@nia.nih.gov;; April Bower, RN; (301) 451-3560; fax: (301) 480-3621; email: bowera@mail.nih.gov
Internet: http://grants.nih.gov/grants/guide/pa-files/PAR-98-110.html
Sponsor: National Institute on Aging (NIA)
7201 Wisconsin Avenue, Suite 350, MSC 9205
Bethesda, MD 20892-9205

NIA Multicenter Study on Exceptional Survival in Families: The Long Life Family Study (LLFS) Grants **2420**
This limited competition FOA is to continue the Long Life Family Study (LLFS). The LLFS was designed to determine the degree and patterns of familial transmission and aggregation of exceptional longevity and healthy survival to advanced age as characterized by a variety of phenotypic measures, with a further goal of also understanding potential genetic factors that contribute to exceptional survival. Five awards, to four study centers and one data management and coordinating center, were made in response to RFA-AG-03-004.
Date(s) Application is Due: Aug 30; Sep 30
Contact: Winifred K. Rossi; (301) 496-3836; fax: (301) 402-1784; email: winnie_rossi@nih.gov
Internet: http://grants.nih.gov/grants/guide/rfa-files/RFA-AG-10-005.html
Sponsor: National Institute on Aging (NIA)
7201 Wisconsin Avenue, Room 3C307
Bethesda, MD 20892-9205

NIA Nathan Shock Centers of Excellence in Basic Biology of Aging Grants **2421**
The NIA invites applications for support of centers, known as Nathan Shock Centers of Excellence in Basic Biology of Aging. These center grants will provide funding for research and training activities related to basic biology of aging. They are intended for institutions with a substantial investment in and commitment to aging research, but they are not intended to directly support clinical research or clinical trials. The goal of this program is to enhance the ability of institutions with well-developed research programs in basic research on aging to utilize state-of-the-art research resources to provide the strongest environment for the conduct of research on aging. Thus, this RFA is intended to enhance the quality of research in the basic biology of aging, facilitate the planning and coordination of aging research activities, provide support and a suitable environment for investigators new to aging research to acquire research skills and experience at institutions that have demonstrated commitment to, and expertise in, basic biology of aging research, and to develop potential regional and/or national resource centers. Annual deadline dates may vary.
Requirements: Applications may be submitted by domestic nonprofit organizations and institutions, state and local governments and their agencies, and authorized federal institutions. The applicant institution must currently support a minimum of 15 peer-reviewed, externally funded research projects on aging to be eligible. In the case of currently funded program projects (P01s), or similar multiproject research grants, each

research project will be deemed to be a separate project. (Core components do not qualify.)
Date(s) Application is Due: Apr 16; May 20
Contact: Dr. Huber Warner, Ph.D., Associate Director; (301) 496-4996; fax: (301) 402-0010; email: warnerh@nia.nih.gov
Internet: http://grants.nih.gov/grants/guide/rfa-files/RFA-AG-04-010.html
Sponsor: National Institute on Aging
7201 Wisconsin Avenue, Gateway Building, Suite 2C231
Bethesda, MD 20892-9205

NIA NRSAs—Individual Postdoctoral Fellowships **2422**
The fellowships support training for basic and clinical research on aging and the problems of the aging and the aged. The training should be directed toward long-term involvement in research in aging and gerontology. The institute will accept proposals in the behavioral and social sciences related to aging and in the biological and biomedical sciences related to aging. Support may be requested for up to three years. PA: PA-03-067
Requirements: Applicants must be citizens of the United States or permanent resident aliens who have received doctoral degrees before the beginning date of the fellowship.
Amount of Grant: $26,256-$41,268
Date(s) Application is Due: Apr 5; Aug 5; Dec 5
Contact: Dr. Robin Barr, Extramural Affairs, (301) 496-9322; fax: (301) 402-2945; email: rb42h@nih.gov
Internet: http://grants.nih.gov/grants/guide/pa-files/PA-03-067.html
Sponsor: National Institute on Aging
6701 Rockledge Drive, Room 1040, MSC 7710
Bethesda, MD 20892-7710

NIA NRSAs—Institutional Training Awards **2423**
NIA will award new and competing renewal NRSA (NRSA) Institutional Training Grants (T32) to eligible institutions to develop or enhance research training opportunities for individuals, selected by the institution, who are training for careers in specified areas of aging research. The purpose of this announcement is to help ensure a broad cadre of researchers trained in the content and methods of aging research and in the major biomedical, behavioral, and social areas of research most closely related to their field of study within aging. NIA supports both predoctoral and postdoctoral training in aging. The institute also supports short-term research training for students in health-professional programs as part of an overall T32 program. The NIA has a single receipt date each year for applications. PA: PA-00-057
Requirements: Applicant must be a citizen or noncitizen national of the United States or must have been lawfully admitted for permanent residence. Predoctoral trainees must have received a baccalaureate degree by the beginning date of their NRSA appointment, and must be training at the postbaccalaureate level and enrolled in a program leading to a PhD in science or in an equivalent research doctoral degree program. Postdoctoral trainees must have received, as of the beginning date of the NRSA appointment, a PhD, MD, or comparable doctoral degree from an accredited domestic or foreign institution. To be eligible for short-term predoctoral research training positions, health-professional students must have completed at least one quarter in a program leading to a clinical doctorate prior to participating in the program.
Contact: Dr. Robin Barr, Extramural Affairs, (301) 496-9322; fax: (301) 402-2945; email: rb42h@nih.gov
Internet: http://grants.nih.gov/grants/guide/pa-files/PA-00-057.html
Sponsor: National Institute on Aging
7201 Wisconsin Avenue, Gateway Building
Bethesda, MD 20892

NIA Paul Beeson Career Development Awards in Aging **2424**
The program will foster the independent research careers of clinically trained investigators whose research will enhance the health and quality of life of Americans, particularly older people. The aims of the program are to encourage and assist the development of future leaders in the field of aging by supporting junior and midcareer faculty members to gain additional research training as needed and to establish independent programs in aging research; deepen the commitment of research institutions to academic research in aging and to translating research outcomes to geriatric medicine by involving mentor and recipient in establishing and advancing the recipient's career in aging research; expand medical research on aging broadly defined as including the biology of aging, maintenance of health and independence in old age, diseases and disabilities of old age and issues in their clinical management, and systems of care for the elderly. Project periods of three, four, or five years are supported. A letter of intent is requested but not required by October 24. Program information and guidelines are available online.
Requirements: Eligible institutions are for-profit or nonprofit, public or private, units of state and local governments, and eligible agencies of the federal government. Individuals eligible to become principal investigators have a clinical doctoral degree (e.g., MD, DO, DDS) or its equivalent. At the time of award, applicants must be U.S. citizens or noncitizen nationals, or have been lawfully admitted to the United States for permanent residence.
Restrictions: Foreign institutions are not eligible to apply. Ineligible individuals include current and former principal investigators on NIH research projects, FIRST Awards, sub-projects of program project, or center grants. Individuals on temporary or student visas are not eligible.
Amount of Grant: $200,000 maximum per year
Date(s) Application is Due: Nov 23
Contact: Office of Extramural Affairs, (301) 496-9322; fax: (301) 402-2945; email: BarrR@nia.nih.gov
Internet: http://grants1.nih.gov/grants/guide/rfa-files/RFA-AG-06-005.html
Sponsor: National Institutes of Health
7201 Wisconsin Avenue, Room 2C218, MSC 9205
Bethesda, MD 20892-9205

NIA Pilot Research Grant Program **2425**
NIA is seeking small grant applications in specific areas to stimulate and facilitate the entry of promising new investigators into aging research or encourage established investigators to enter new targeted, high-priority areas in this research field. This small grant program provides support for pilot research that is likely to lead to subsequent individual research project grants and/or a significant advancement of aging research. Annual deadline dates may vary; contact program staff for exact dates.
Requirements: Applications may be submitted by domestic for-profit and nonprofit organizations, both public or private; units of state and local governments; and eligible agencies of the federal government. The program supports new and established investigators. For a new investigator to be eligible, the individual should be in the first five years of his or her independent research career. If the applicant is in the final stages of training it is permissible to apply for an R03, but no award will be made to individuals who are still in training or fellowship status at the time of award. For an established investigator to be eligible, the individual must propose research that is unrelated to a currently funded research project in which the investigator participates.
Restrictions: Foreign organizations and institutions are not eligible.
Amount of Grant: $50,000 maximum direct costs for one year
Contact: Dr. David Finkelstein, Biology of Aging Program; (301) 496-6402; fax: (301) 402-0010; email: BAPquery@extramur.nia.nih.gov
Internet: http://grants.nih.gov/grants/guide/pa-files/PA-99-049.html
Sponsor: National Institute on Aging (NIA)
7201 Wisconsin Avenue, Gateway Building, Suite 2C231, MSC 9205
Bethesda, MD 20892

NIA Postdoctoral Training in Research on Aging in Canada **2426**
The objective of the National Research Service Award (NRSA) F32 program is to provide support to promising postdoctoral applicants who have the potential to become productive and successful independent research investigators in scientific health-related fields relevant to the missions of the participating NIH Institutes and Centers (ICs). A primary purpose of this initiative is to offer training in research on aging that exposes developing American postdoctoral investigators to diverse combinations of expertise and resources singularly available in Canada through the Canadian Institutes of Health-Institute on Aging (CIHR-IA), combinations that also take into account the unique cultural and ethnic composition of Canada and its aging population.
Requirements: Applicants must choose Canadian institutions and mentors selected by CIHR-IA. These institutions and mentors can be located through the CIHR Funding Database. Any individual with the skills, knowledge, and resources necessary to carry out the proposed research training is invited to work with his/her sponsor and institution to develop an application for support. Individuals from underrepresented racial and ethnic groups as well as individuals with disabilities are always encouraged to apply for NIH support.
Restrictions: Candidates for the postdoctoral fellowship award must be citizens or non-citizen nationals of the United States, or must have been lawfully admitted to the United States for Permanent Residence.
Date(s) Application is Due: Apr 8; Aug 8; Dec 8
Contact: Michael-David A.R.R. Kerns; (301) 402-7713; fax: (301) 402-2945; email: michael-david.kerns@nih.hhs.gov
Internet: http://grants.nih.gov/grants/guide/pa-files/PA-06-469.html
Sponsor: National Institute on Aging (NIA)
7201 Wisconsin Avenue, Suite 2C-218
Bethesda, MD 20892 -9205

NIA Promoting Careers in Aging and Health Disparities Research Grants **2427**
The Mentored Research Scientist Development Award provides support for a sustained period of protected time for intensive research career development under the guidance of an experienced mentor, or sponsor, in the biomedical, behavioral or clinical sciences leading to research independence. The expectation is that through this sustained period of research career development and training, awardees will launch independent research careers and become competitive for new research project grant funding.
Requirements: The following organizations and institutions may apply: public/state controlled institutions of higher education; private institutions of higher education; Hispanic-serving institutions; historically Black colleges and universities (HBCUs); tribally controlled colleges and universities (TCCUs); Alaska native and native Hawaiian serving institutions; nonprofits with 501(c)3 IRS status; nonprofits without 501(c)3 IRS status; small businesses; for-profit organizations; State governments; regional organizations; U.S. territories or possessions; Indian/Native American tribal governments; Indian/Native American tribally designated organizations; county governments; city or township governments; special district governments; independent school districts; public housing authorities/Indian housing authorities; eligible agencies of the Federal government; and faith-based or community based organizations.
Amount of Grant: $150,000 dollars per year for a project period of up to 3-5 years
Date(s) Application is Due: Feb 12; Jun 12; Oct 12
Contact: Dr. J. Taylor Harden; (301) 496-0765; fax: (301) 496-2525; email: Taylor_Harden@nih.gov
Internet: http://grants.nih.gov/grants/guide/pa-files/PAR-09-136.html
Sponsor: National Institute on Aging (NIA)
31 Center Drive
Bethesda, MD 20892-2292

NIA Prostate Cancer Aging, Race, and Ethnicity Research Grants **2428**

NIA invites research project grant applications to expand the understanding of biological and clinical factors leading to the development, progression, and treatment of prostate cancer in aging men. The increased risk of prostate cancer with advancing age and its prominence in older-aged men are well-known characteristics of this tumor. The unusually high incidence and mortality rates of prostate cancer for older white and black American men and, by contrast, the much lower rates in men of Hispanic and Asian descent, provide the need for research that emphasizes the role of race and ethnic factors, as well as age, in early diagnosis, management, and etiology of this malignancy. The purpose of this RFA is to support research that will provide information leading to better prevention, diagnosis, prognosis, and treatment of prostate cancer in the age range in which prostate cancer most frequently occurs in the diverse population groups at risk (i.e., in men 65 years and older). Proposals to address the issues indicated above may be focused on genetic and environmental risk factors, pre-malignant changes, tumorigenesis, detection of localized and advanced disease, prognostic indicators, disease progression, and response to treatment. Studies to evaluate or refine the ability of existing diagnostic, screening, or follow-up methods of persons of different age, race, and ethnicity are also responsive to this RFA. The PA, which describes the research objectives, application procedures, review considerations, and award criteria may be obtained electronically through the NIH grant line (301-402-2221), the NIH Web site, and by mail and email. RFA: AG-02-003

Contact: Dr. Rosemary Yancik, Geriatrics Program, (301) 496-5278; fax: (301) 496-2793; email: YancikR@31.nia.nih.gov

Internet: http://grants2.nih.gov/grants/guide/rfa-files/RFA-AG-02-003.html

Sponsor: National Institute on Aging
7201 Wisconsin Avenue, Gateway Building
Bethesda, MD 20892

NIA Renal Function and Chronic Kidney Disease in Aging Grants **2429**

This Funding Opportunity Announcement (FOA) issued by the National Institute on Aging (NIA) and the National Institute of Diabetes and Digestive and Kidney Diseases (NIDDK), National Institutes of Health, invites applications that propose basic, clinical, and translational research on chronic kidney disease (CKD) and its consequences in aging and in older persons. Applications should focus on: biology and pathophysiology of CKD in animal models; etiology and pathophysiology of CKD in the elderly; epidemiology and risk factors for the development of CKD with advancing age; and/or diagnosis, medical management and clinical outcomes of CKD in this population. Research supported by this initiative should enhance knowledge of CKD and its consequences in the elderly and provide evidence-based guidance in the diagnosis, prevention, and treatment of CKD in older persons.

Requirements: The following organizations and institutions may apply: public/state controlled institutions of higher education; private institutions of higher education; Hispanic-serving institutions; historically Black colleges and universities (HBCUs); tribally controlled colleges and universities (TCCUs); Alaska native and native Hawaiian serving institutions; nonprofits with 501(c)3 IRS status; nonprofits without 501(c)3 IRS status; small businesses; for-profit organizations; State governments; regional organizations; U.S. territories or possessions; Indian/Native American tribal governments; Indian/Native American tribally designated organizations; county governments; city or township governments; special district governments; independent school districts; public housing authorities/Indian housing authorities; eligible agencies of the Federal government; and faith-based or community based organizations.

Date(s) Application is Due: Feb 5; Feb 16; Jun 5; Jun 16; Oct 5; Oct 16

Contact: Susan G. Nayfield; (301) 496-6761; fax: (301) 402-1784; email: nayfiels@mail.nih.gov;; John W. Kusek, Ph.D.; (301) 594-7735; fax: (301) 480-3510; email: kusekj@extra.niddk.nih.gov

Internet: http://grants.nih.gov/grants/guide/pa-files/PA-09-165.html

Sponsor: National Institute on Aging (NIA)
7201 Wisconsin Avenue, Gateway Building, Suite 3C-307
Bethesda, MD 20892-9205

NIA Research Grants on Chemical Senses: Neurotransmitters and Neuromodulators **2430**

NIDCD and NIA sponsor research grants that support research fundamental to understanding the neurochemistry of pathways in the olfactory and gustatory systems throughout the life span. This research includes the identification and characterization of the neurotransmitters, neuromodulators, receptors, and secondary messengers throughout the chemosensory systems. More information may be obtained by mail and email, or through the NIH grant line (301-402-2221), and the NIH Web site.

Requirements: Applications may be submitted by domestic and foreign, for-profit and non-profit organizations, public and private, such as universities, colleges, hospitals, laboratories, units of state and local governments, and eligible agencies of the federal government.

Contact: Dr. Judy Finkelstein, (301) 496-9350; fax: (301) 496-1494; email: FinkelsJ@gw.nia.nih.gov

Internet: http://www.grants.nih.gov/grants/guide/pa-files/PA-96-035.html

Sponsor: National Institute on Aging
7201 Wisconsin Avenue, Gateway Building
Bethesda, MD 20892

NIA Role of Apolipoprotein E, Lipoprotein Receptors and CNS Lipid Homeostasis in Brain Aging and Alzheimer's Disease **2431**

This FOA encourages multidisciplinary and interdisciplinary research to elucidate how Apolipoprotein E, lipoprotein receptors and CNS lipid homeostasis influence brain aging and the transition to neurodegeneration in Alzheimer's disease (AD). The ultimate goal is to gain an in depth understanding of the mechanisms by which the Apolipoprotein E e4 allele confers increased AD risk for the purpose of advancing the overall search for efficacious AD treatments and Apolipoprotein E e4-directed therapeutics in particular. To this end we encourage research spanning multiple levels of analysis in multiple species (from mice to man). Studies aimed at identifying new therapeutic targets for the treatment of AD and other age-related neurodegenerative conditions associated with lipid neurobiology are strongly encouraged. Also of great interest are projects that aim to use lipidomics, various types of imaging and other cutting edge technologies to identify and develop early biomarkers of neurodegeneration associated lipid dyshomeostasis. The estimated amount of funds available to support projects under this FOA is $2,500,000.

Requirements: The following organizations and institutions are eligible to apply: public/state controlled institutions of higher education; private institutions of higher education; Hispanic-serving institutions; historically Black colleges and universities (HBCUs); tribally controlled colleges and universities (TCCUs); Alaska native and native Hawaiian serving institutions; nonprofits with 501(c)3 IRS status (other than institutions of higher education); nonprofits without 501(c)3 IRS status (other than institutions of higher education); small businesses; for-profit organizations (other than small businesses); state governments; Indian/Native American tribal governments (federally recognized); Indian/Native American tribally designated organizations; county governments; city or township governments; special district governments; independent school districts; public housing authorities/Indian housing authorities; U.S. territories or possessions; Indian/native American tribal governments (other than federally recognized); regional organizations; and non-domestic (non-U.S.) entities (foreign organizations).

Date(s) Application is Due: Mar 5; Jul 5; Nov 5

Contact: Suzana S. Petanceska, Ph.D.; (301) 496-9350; fax: (301) 496-1494; email: petanceskas@mail.nih.gov

Internet: http://grants.nih.gov/grants/guide/pa-files/PA-09-217.html

Sponsor: National Institute on Aging (NIA)
7201 Wisconsin Avenue, Suite 350
Bethesda, MD 20892-9205

NIA Role of Nuclear Receptors in Tissue and Organismal Aging Grants **2432**

This Funding Opportunity Announcement (FOA) solicits grant applications proposing to conduct research into underlying biologic mechanisms involving nuclear receptors, their co-regulators and intracellular signaling systems in the process of aging and the connections of the aging process with pathophysiology in middle- and old-age. The focus of the proposed research must be on processes of aging and/or age-related changes, i.e., research proposed in applications responding to this FOA must have clear relevance to aging. Potential topic areas of interest to the NIA include, but are not limited to, the following: age-changes in levels, sensitivity, and gene expression activation profiles of NRs and co-regulators, and their effects on processes of aging (e.g., age-changes in tissue function, inflammation, glucose and lipid metabolism, adipogenesis, muscle, and brain function) and connections with disease processes for diseases common in older individuals; modification of lifespan in model organisms (e.g., the NR homologue DAF-12 in the insulin-IGF-like pathway in the nematode, and mammalian homologues) and the health-protecting, life-extending effects of caloric restriction or other life-span altering genetic mutations or transgenic models in mammalian organisms; and age-changes in steroid metabolism or in tissue sensitivity and/or response to exogenous sex steroid (or tissue-selective sex steroid receptor modulators) therapy in middle- and old-age.

Requirements: The following organizations and institutions may apply: public/state controlled institutions of higher education; private institutions of higher education; Hispanic-serving institutions; historically Black colleges and universities (HBCUs); tribally controlled colleges and universities (TCCUs); Alaska native and native Hawaiian serving institutions; nonprofits with 501(c)3 IRS status; nonprofits without 501(c)3 IRS status; small businesses; for-profit organizations; State governments; regional organizations; U.S. territories or possessions; Indian/Native American tribal governments; Indian/Native American tribally designated organizations; eligible agencies of the Federal government; and faith-based or community based organizations.

Date(s) Application is Due: Feb 5; Jun 5; Oct 5

Contact: Jill Carrington, Ph.D.; (301) 496-6402; fax: (301) 402-0010; email: carringj@mail.nih.gov;; Ronald Margolis, Ph.D.; (301) 594-8819; fax: (301) 435-6047; email: rm76f@nih.gov

Internet: http://grants.nih.gov/grants/guide/pa-files/PAS-07-267.html

Sponsor: National Institute on Aging (NIA)
Gateway Building, Suite 2C231, 7201 Wisconsin Avenue
Bethesda, MD 20892-9205

NIA Significance of Sarcopenia in Old Age Grants **2433**

NIA and NIAMS invite research project applications to elucidate the metabolic/physiological and functional consequences of sarcopenia in old age. Sarcopenia is defined as the loss of skeletal muscle mass, quality, and strength. More information may be obtained by mail and email, or through the NIH grant line (301-402-2221) and the NIH Web site. PA: PA-96-038

Requirements: Applications may be submitted by foreign and domestic, for-profit and nonprofit organizations, both public and private; units of state and local governments; and eligible agencies of the federal government.

Contact: Dr. Chhanda Dutta, Geriatrics Program, (301) 496-6761; fax: (301) 402-1784; email: DuttaC@gw.nia.nih.gov

Internet: http://www.grants.nih.gov/grants/guide/pa-files/PA-96-038.html

Sponsor: National Institute on Aging
7201 Wisconsin Avenue, Gateway Building
Bethesda, MD 20892

NIA Sociobehavorial Data Analysis and Archiving in Aging 2434

NIA) is seeking small grant (R03) applications to stimulate and facilitate data archiving and secondary analyses of data related to caregiving, cognition, demography, economics, epidemiology, behavioral genetics and other behavioral research on aging; provide support for preliminary projects using secondary analysis that could lead to subsequent applications for other research project grant award mechanisms; provide support for rapid analyses of new databases and experimental modules for purposes such as informing the design and content of future study waves; provide support for the development, enhancement and assembly of new databases from existing data; and provide support for pilot research on under-utilized databases. PA: PA-04-123

Requirements: Applications may be submitted by domestic for-profit and nonprofit organizations, public and private, such as universities, colleges, hospitals, laboratories, units of state and local governments, and eligible agencies of the federal government.

Restrictions: Foreign organizations and institutions are not eligible.

Amount of Grant: $850,000 maximum

Contact: Linda Whipp, Grants and Contracts Management Office, (301) 496-1472; fax: (301) 402-3672; email: lw17m@nih.gov

Internet: http://grants.nih.gov/grants/guide/pa-files/PA-04-123.html

Sponsor: National Institute on Aging
7201 Wisconsin Avenue, Gateway Building
Bethesda, MD 20892

NIA Support of Scientific Meetings as Cooperative Agreements 2435

The purpose of the program announcement is to inform the scientific community that the National Institute on Aging (NIA) will now support scientific meetings as cooperative agreements in addition to the current practice of supporting them through the traditional grant mechanism. This program provides guidelines for when it is appropriate to request support of a meeting as a cooperative agreement and explains procedures for preparing and submitting such applications. The Principal Investigator will have the primary authority and responsibility to define objectives and approaches; plan, publicize, and conduct the scientific meeting; and publish the results of the meeting.

Requirements: Applications may be submitted by U.S. institutions, including scientific or professional societies eligible to receive grants from Public Health Service (PHS) agencies. In the case of an international conference, the U.S. representative organization of an established international scientific or professional society is the eligible applicant.

Restrictions: Foreign institutions are not eligible.

Contact: Chyren Hunter, Ph.D.; (301) 496-9322; fax: (301) 402-0528; email: Hunterc@nia.nih.gov

Internet: http://grants.nih.gov/grants/guide/pa-files/PA-00-128.html

Sponsor: National Institute on Aging (NIA)
Gateway Building, Room 2C218, 7201 Wisconsin Avenue, MSC 9205
Bethesda, MD 20892-9205

NIA Symptom Management for Chronic Neurological Conditions Grants 2436

NINR, NIA, NICHD, NIDCD, and NINDS are interested in facilitating investigator-initiated research designed to deal with symptoms associated with chronic neurological conditions including stroke, epilepsy, brain and spinal cord injury, multiple sclerosis, and Parkinson's disease. The overall goals are to manage symptoms effectively, to prevent secondary effects of the condition when possible, to maximize the health potential, and to improve the health-related quality of life for patients, care givers, and families. The mechanism of support is the research project grant (R01). PA-98-030 may be obtained through the NIH grant line (301-402-2221), the NIH Web site, mail, and email.

Requirements: Applications may be submitted by domestic and foreign for-profit and nonprofit organizations, public or private.

Contact: Dr. Judith Finkelstein, Sensory/Motor Disorders of Aging Program, (301) 496-9350; fax: (301) 496-1494; email: jf119k@nih.gov; Joseph Ellis, Grants Management Officer, (301) 496-1472; fax: (301) 402-3672; email: ellisj@exmur.nia.nih.gov

Internet: http://www.grants.nih.gov/grants/guide/pa-files/PA-98-030.html

Sponsor: National Institute on Aging
7201 Wisconsin Avenue, Gateway Building
Bethesda, MD 20892

NIA Thyroid in Aging Grants 2437

The purpose of this funding opportunity announcement (FOA) is to encourage submission of investigator-initiated research applications on the thyroid in aging. This FOA is intended to promote basic, translational, and clinical studies leading to increased understanding of the physiology of the aging thyroid and improved diagnosis and management of thyroid disease in the elderly.

Requirements: The following organizations and institutions may apply: public/state controlled institutions of higher education; private institutions of higher education; Hispanic-serving institutions; nonprofits with 501(c)3 IRS status; nonprofits without 501(c)3 IRS status; small businesses; for-profit organizations; State governments; regional organizations; U.S. territories or possessions; Indian/Native American tribal governments; Indian/Native American tribally designated organizations; non-domestic (non-U.S.) entities (foreign organizations); Hispanic-serving institutions; historically Black colleges and universities (HBCUs); tribally controlled colleges and universities (TCCUs); Alaska native and native Hawaiian serving institutions; and regional organizations.

Date(s) Application is Due: Feb 5; Feb 16; Jun 5; Jun 16; Oct 5; Oct 16

Contact: Basil A. Eldadah, MD; (301) 496-6761; fax: (301) 402-1784; email: eldadahb@nia.nih.gov;; Nancy J. Emenaker, PhD; (301) 496-0116; fax: (301) 480-3925; email: emenaken@mail.nih.gov

Internet: http://grants.nih.gov/grants/guide/pa-files/PA-08-037.html

Sponsor: National Institute on Aging (NIA)
7201 Wisconsin Avenue, Gateway Building, Suite 3C-307
Bethesda, MD 20892-9205

NIA Transdisciplinary Research on Fatigue and Fatigability in Aging Grants 2438

The purpose of this Funding Opportunity Announcement (FOA) is to encourage submission of research applications on fatigue and fatigability in aging. This FOA is intended to promote research studies employing transdisciplinary approaches that could lead to increased understanding of mechanisms contributing to, assessment of, or potential interventions for, increased fatigue or fatigability in older persons. Both animal models and humans are appropriate for study under this FOA.

Requirements: The following organizations and institutions may apply: public/state controlled institutions of higher education; private institutions of higher education; Hispanic-serving institutions; historically Black colleges and universities (HBCUs); tribally controlled colleges and universities (TCCUs); Alaska native and native Hawaiian serving institutions; nonprofits with 501(c)3 IRS status; nonprofits without 501(c)3 IRS status; small businesses; for-profit organizations; State governments; regional organizations; U.S. territories or possessions; Indian/Native American tribal governments; Indian/Native American tribally designated organizations; county governments; city or township governments; special district governments; independent school districts; public housing authorities/Indian housing authorities; eligible agencies of the Federal government; and faith-based or community based organizations.

Date(s) Application is Due: Feb 5; Feb 16; Jun 5; Jun 16; Oct 5; Oct 16

Contact: Basil A. Eldadah, MD; (301) 496-6761; fax: (301) 402-1784; email: eldadahb@nia.nih.gov;; Kathleen Jett, PhD; (301) 594-2154; fax: (301) 480-8260; email: jettk@mail.nih.gov

Internet: http://grants.nih.gov/grants/guide/pa-files/PA-08-161.html

Sponsor: National Institute on Aging (NIA)
7201 Wisconsin Avenue, Suite 3C307
Bethesda, MD 20892-9205

NIA Translational Research at the Aging/Cancer Interface (TRACI) Grants 2439

The purpose of this Funding Opportunity Announcement (FOA) is to enhance translational research in the overlapping areas of human aging and cancer by: integrating knowledge of basic processes in cancer biology and aging into clinical care of older patients with cancer (bench to bedside); and exploring clinical observations from the patient care setting at more basic and molecular levels (bedside to bench). Ultimately, information from the research supported by this initiative should lead to further improvements in prevention, diagnosis and disease management, improving the health and well-being of elderly patients at risk for, or diagnosed with, cancer and decreasing the functional impairment and morbidity associated with cancer in this population.

Requirements: The following organizations and institutions may apply: public/state controlled institutions of higher education; private institutions of higher education; Hispanic-serving institutions; historically Black colleges and universities (HBCUs); tribally controlled colleges and universities (TCCUs); Alaska native and native Hawaiian serving institutions; nonprofits with 501(c)3 IRS status; nonprofits without 501(c)3 IRS status; small businesses; for-profit organizations; State governments; regional organizations; U.S. territories or possessions; Indian/Native American tribal governments; Indian/Native American tribally designated organizations; county governments; city or township governments; special district governments; independent school districts; public housing authorities/Indian housing authorities; eligible agencies of the Federal government; and faith-based or community based organizations.

Date(s) Application is Due: Feb 5; Feb 16; Jun 5; Jun 16; Oct 5; Oct 16

Contact: Susan G. Nayfield, M.D.; (301) 496-6761; fax: (301) 402-1784; email: nayfiels@nia.nih.gov

Internet: http://grants.nih.gov/grants/guide/pa-files/PA-08-230.html

Sponsor: National Institute on Aging (NIA)
7201 Wisconsin Avenue, Gateway Building, Suite 3C-307
Bethesda, MD 20892-9205

NIA Vulnerable Dendrites and Synapses in Aging and Alzheimer's Disease Grants 2440

The purpose of this initiative is to solicit research proposals that will investigate the factors regulating synaptic plasticity and dysfunction with a particular emphasis on the age-dependent changes in the functions of dendrites, spines and synapses of key cell types in regions of brain that are selectively vulnerable in certain neurodegenerative disorders such as AD, or with aging using, for example, in vitro and in vivo models.

Requirements: The following organizations and institutions may apply: public/state controlled institutions of higher education; private institutions of higher education; Hispanic-serving institutions; historically Black colleges and universities (HBCUs); tribally controlled colleges and universities (TCCUs); Alaska native and native Hawaiian serving institutions; nonprofits with 501(c)3 IRS status; nonprofits without 501(c)3 IRS status; small businesses; for-profit organizations; State governments; regional organizations; U.S. territories or possessions; Indian/Native American tribal governments; Indian/Native American tribally designated organizations; county governments; city or township governments; special district governments; independent school districts; public housing authorities/Indian housing authorities; eligible agencies of the Federal government; and faith-based or community based organizations.

Date(s) Application is Due: Feb 5; Jun 5; Oct 5

Contact: D. Stephen Snyder; (301) 496-9350; fax; (301) 496-1494; email: ss82f@nih.gov

Internet: http://grants.nih.gov/grants/guide/pa-files/PA-09-061.html

Sponsor: National Institute on Aging (NIA)
7201 Wisconsin Avenue, Gateway Building, Room 350
Bethesda, MD 20892-9205

NIA/NIEHS Biomedical Epidemiologic and Intervention Studies Planning Grants 2441

This program provides grant support for planning and protocol development of biomedical epidemiologic and intervention studies in research areas supported by NIA's geriatrics program. PA: PA-99-145

Requirements: Applications may be submitted by foreign and domestic for-profit and nonprofit organizations, both public and private; units of state and local governments; and eligible agencies of the federal government.

Amount of Grant: $150,000 maximum

Contact: Dr. Evan Hadley, Associate Director, NIA; fax: (301) 402-1784; email: HadleyE@exmur.nia.nih.gov; Dr. Gwen Collman, Program Administrator, Environmental and Molecular Epidemiology, NIEHS, (301) 541-4980; fax: (919) 541-4937; email: Collman@niehs.nih.go

Internet: http://grants.nih.gov/grants/guide/pa-files/PA-99-145.html

Sponsor: National Institute on Aging
7201 Wisconsin Avenue
Bethesda, MD 20892

NIAAA Hepatitis C Infection and Alcoholic Liver Disease 2442

NIAAA invites basic and clinical research grant applications that focus on the synergistic interactions between alcohol consumption and hepatitis C virus (HCV) infection to produce chronic liver disease. This announcement solicits grant applications for research that elucidate mechanism(s) in the development and progression of liver disease in a setting of combined alcohol use and HCV infection. Studies that focus on cellular and molecular mechanisms of viral pathogenesis, immune responses and liver disease, in the context of gender, race, and age are encouraged. Development of animal models and in vitro experimental systems to study the interactive effects of alcohol exposure and HCV pathogenesis are highly encouraged. Annual deadline dates may vary; contact program staff for exact dates. PA: PAS-99-155

Requirements: Applications may be submitted by domestic and foreign, for-profit and nonprofit organizations, both public and private; units of state and local governments; and eligible agencies of the federal government.

Amount of Grant: $2 million total

Contact: Thomas Kresina, Division of Basic Research, (301) 443-6537; fax: (301) 594-0673; email: tk13v@nih.gov; Raye Litten, Division of Clinical and Prevention Research, (301) 443-0796; fax: (301) 443-8774; email: rlitten@willco.niaa.nih.gov

Internet: http://grants.nih.gov/grants/guide/pa-files/PAS-99-155.html

Sponsor: National Institute on Alcohol Abuse and Alcoholism
6000 Executive Boulevard
Bethesda, MD 20892

NIAAA Independent Scientist Award 2443

The award is a special salary-only grant designed to provide protected time for newly independent scientists who currently have non-research obligations such as heavy teaching loads, clinical work, committee assignments, service, and administrative duties that prevent them from having a period of intensive research focus. The award is targeted to persons with doctoral degrees who have completed their research training, have independent peer-reviewed research support, and who need a period of protected research time in order to foster their research career development. New applications are due February 12, June 12, and October 12, while renewal applications are due March 12, July 12, and November 12. Up to 75% per year of base salary plus fringe benefits is available. Research support is not provided in most cases. Individuals engaged in predominantly theoretical work, such as modeling or computer simulation, may request up to $25,000 per year for research expenses.

Requirements: The following organizations and institutions are eligible to apply: public/state controlled institutions of higher education; private institutions of higher education; nonprofits with 501(c)3 IRS status; nonprofits without 501(c)3 IRS status; small businesses; for-profit organizations; State governments; U.S. territories or possessions; Indian/Native American tribal governments (Federally recognized and other than Federally recognized); Indian/Native American tribally designated organizations; Hispanic-serving institutions; historically Black colleges and universities (HBCUs); tribally controlled colleges and universities (TCCUs); Alaska Native and Native Hawaiian serving institutions; regional organizations; and faith-based or community based organizations. The candidate must have a doctoral degree and peer-reviewed, independent research support at the time the award is made. The candidate must spend a minimum of 75 percent effort conducting research during the period of the award.

Restrictions: The award is not intended for investigators who already have full time to perform research, or have substantial publication records or considerable research support indicating that they are well established in their fields. Foreign institutions are not eligible to apply.

Amount of Grant: $100,000 maximum

Date(s) Application is Due: Feb 12; Mar 12; Jun 12; Jul 12; Oct 12; Nov 12

Contact: Michael Hilton, Ph.D.; (301) 402- 9402; email: mhilton@mail.nih.gov

Internet: http://grants.nih.gov/grants/guide/pa-files/PA-09-038.html

Sponsor: National Institute on Alcohol Abuse and Alcoholism (NIAAA)
5635 Fishers Lane
Bethesda, MD 20892-9304

NIAAA Mechanisms of Alcohol and Drug-Induced Pancreatitis Grants 2444

This Funding Opportunity Announcement (FOA) issued by the National Institute on Alcohol Abuse and Alcoholism (NIAAA), the National Institute of Diabetes and Digestive and Kidney Diseases (NIDDK), and the National Institute on Drug Abuse (NIDA), National Institutes of Health (NIH), solicits grant applications from institutions/organizations that propose to investigate the underlying molecular, biochemical, and cellular mechanisms by which long-term alcohol ingestion and drugs lead to the development of pancreatitis. Research is also encouraged to understand the role of various predisposing factors, including substance abuse, that make the pancreas susceptible to alcoholic injury. Understanding the mechanisms as well as the role of predisposing factors may help in developing strategies for the prevention or treatment of the disease. Because the nature and scope of the proposed research will vary from application to application, it is anticipated that the size and duration of each award will also vary.

Requirements: Application can be made by the following institutions and organizations: public/state controlled institutions of higher education; private institutions of higher education; nonprofits with 501(c)3 IRS status (other than institutions of higher education); nonprofits without 501(c)3 IRS status (other than institutions of higher education); small businesses; for-profit organizations (other than small businesses); state governments; U.S. territories or possessions; Indian/Native American tribal governments (federally recognized); Indian/Native American tribal governments (other than Federally recognized); Indian/Native American tribally designated organizations; non-domestic (non-U.S.) entities (foreign organizations); Hispanic-serving institutions; historically Black colleges and universities (HBCUs); tribally controlled colleges and universities (TCCUs); Alaska Native and Native Hawaiian serving institutions; regional organization; eligible agencies of the Federal government; and faith-based or community based organizations.

Date(s) Application is Due: Feb 5; Jun 5; Oct 5

Contact: Vishnudutt Purohit, Ph.D.; (301) 443-2689; fax: (301) 443-0673; email: vpurohit@mail.nih.gov

Internet: http://grants.nih.gov/grants/guide/pa-files/PA-07-067.html

Sponsor: National Institute on Alcohol Abuse and Alcoholism (NIAAA)
5635 Fishers Lane, Room 2035, MSC 9304
Bethesda, MD 20892-9304

NIAAA Mechanisms of Alcohol-Induced Hepatic Fibrosis Research Grants 2445

The Division of Basic Research of NIAAA invites grant applications that focus on the developmental mechanisms of hepatic fibrosis that occur in alcohol-induced liver disease. PA: PA-99-110

Requirements: Applications may be submitted by domestic and foreign, for-profit and nonprofit organizations, public and private. Applicants requesting $500,000 or more in direct costs for any year must contact program staff before submitting the application.

Amount of Grant: $50,000 maximum direct costs per year

Contact: Dr. Vishnudutt Purohit, Division of Basic Research, (301) 443-2689; email: vpurohit@willco.niaaa.nih.gov; Dr. Leslie Isaki, Division of Basic Research, (301) 594-6228; fax: (301) 594-0673; email: lisaki@willco.niaaa.nih.gov

Internet: http://www.grants.nih.gov/grants/guide/pa-files/PA-99-110.html

Sponsor: National Institute on Alcohol Abuse and Alcoholism
6000 Executive Boulevard, Willco Building
Bethesda, MD 20892

NIAAA Mentored Clinical Scientist Research Career Development Awards 2446

This award enables candidates holding professional degrees (e.g., M.D., D.O., D.V.M., or equivalent degrees) to undertake 3 to 5 years of special study and supervised research with the goal of becoming independent investigators. The award also allows awardees to pursue a research career development program suited to their experience and capabilities under a mentor who is competent to provide guidance in the chosen research area. Institutions may submit applications on behalf of candidates who hold professional degrees. At least 2 years must have elapsed since the health professional degree was granted. Candidates can have varying levels of clinical training and research experience. New applications are due February 12, June 12, and October 12, while resubmitted applications are due March 12, July 12, and November 12. Up to Up to 75 percent of base salary plus fringe benefits is available, and up to $50,000 per year for research support for new awards.

Requirements: All candidates must be U.S. citizens, non-citizen nationals, or legal permanent residents of the U.S. Persons with temporary or student visas are not eligible. The grantee institution must have a strong, well-established research and research training program in the chosen area, accomplished faculty in the basic and clinical sciences, and a commitment to the candidate's research development. The proposed program should include an appropriate mentor.

Amount of Grant: $100,000 average

Date(s) Application is Due: Feb 12; Mar 12; Jun 12; Jul 12; Oct 12; Nov 12

Contact: Judith A. Arroyo, Ph.D.; (301) 402-0717; fax: (301) 443-6077; email: jarroyo@mail.nih.gov

Internet: http://grants.nih.gov/grants/guide/pa-files/pa-06-512.html

Sponsor: National Institute on Alcohol Abuse and Alcoholism (NIAAA)
5635 Fishers Lane, Room 2079
Bethesda, MD 20892 -9304

NIAAA Peptide Regulation of Alcohol Intake 2447

The purpose of this program is to identify peptides and their receptors that regulate alcohol consumption, ultimately leading to an understanding of their mechanism(s) of action. Although not exclusive, several areas have potential for further investigation including the hypothalamic-pituitary-adrenal axis, opioid peptides, the renin-angiotensin system, plus the group of peptides regulating food intake and energy balance, exemplified by leptin and neuropeptide Y. The goal of this initiative is to elucidate the role of peptides in pathological alcohol consumption, suggesting novel pharmacotherapeutic approaches for alcoholism. Annual deadlines may vary; contact program staff for exact dates. PA: PAS-99-156

Requirements: Applications may be submitted by domestic and foreign, for-profit and nonprofit organizations, both public and private; units of state and local governments; and eligible agencies of the federal government.
Amount of Grant: $2 million total
Contact: Jules Selden, Division of Basic Research, (301) 443-2678; fax: (301) 594-0673; email: jselden@willco.niaaa.nih.gov
Internet: http://grants.nih.gov/grants/guide/pa-files/PAS-99-156.html
Sponsor: National Institute on Alcohol Abuse and Alcoholism
6000 Executive Boulevard
Bethesda, MD 20892

NIAAA Secondary Analysis of Existing Health Services Data Sets Grants 2448
The NIAAA is soliciting exploratory/developmental research grant applications (R21) to support the secondary analysis of existing data sets relevant to developing a knowledge base to improve the delivery of services for alcohol-related problems, including both treatment and preventive interventions. Research objectives of this PA include, but are not limited to, five major areas: determining the effects of financing and reimbursement mechanisms on alcohol-related healthcare program availability, accessibility, delivery, organization, content, quality, and outcomes; assessing sources of variation in access to and utilization of treatment and prevention interventions for alcohol-related problems; identifying organizational and managerial factors that influence the delivery of treatment and prevention services for alcohol-related problems, either within or across regions, populations, and settings; evaluating the cost, cost-effectiveness, cost-benefit, and cost-utility of alcohol-related treatment and prevention services; and identifying and assessing the effectiveness and outcomes of alcohol-related treatment and preventive services. PA: PA-00-100
Requirements: Applications may be submitted by foreign and domestic, for-profit and nonprofit organizations, both public and private; units of state and local governments; and eligible agencies of the federal government.
Amount of Grant: $100,000 maximum in direct costs per year for two years
Contact: Dr. Harold Perl, Division of Clinical and Prevention Research, (301) 443-0788; fax: (301) 443-8774; email: hperl@willco.niaaa.nih.gov
Internet: http://grants.nih.gov/grants/guide/pa-files/PA-00-100.html
Sponsor: National Institute on Alcohol Abuse and Alcoholism
6000 Executive Boulevard, Willco Building
Bethesda, MD 20892

NIAID Allergy, Immunology, and Transplantation Program Research Grants 2449
This program concerns the immune system as it functions in the maintenance of health and as it malfunctions in the production of disease. Because of this dual focus, the program encompasses both basic research (immunology) and clinical research (allergic and immunologic diseases). Basic research is supported under immunobiology and immunochemistry to provide the information necessary for understanding immune system structure and function and under genetics and transplantation biology, directed more specifically at the histocompatibility antigens and their role in graft rejection, autoimmunity, immune responsiveness, and a variety of diseases. Clinical research is supported under asthma and allergic diseases, directed at determining the cause and improving the diagnosis, prevention, and treatment of a variety of common allergic diseases, and under immunologic diseases covering disorders of the human immune system and their underlying pathophysiologic inflammation and immunopathologic mechanisms and consequences. Clinical aspects of transplantation and genetic predisposition to disease are supported under genetics and transplantation biology. The small instrumentation program supports the purchase of relatively low-cost pieces of research equipment that generally are not funded in research project grants and that do not qualify for support under the NIH larger shared instrumentation program.
Requirements: Universities, colleges, hospitals, laboratories, and other public or private nonprofit domestic institutions, including state and local units of government, and individuals are eligible for grant support of research by a named principal investigator or a research career development candidate. Also, for-profit organizations are eligible.
Amount of Grant: $9.24 million-$4.72 million; $373,726 average
Date(s) Application is Due: Feb 1; Jun 1; Oct 1
Contact: Dr. John McGowan, Acting Director, Division of Extramural Activities, (301) 496-7291; Mary Kirker, Grants Management Officer, (301) 496-7075; email: mk35h@nih.gov
Internet: http://12.46.245.173/pls/portal30/CATALOG.PROGRAM_TEXT_RPT.show
Sponsor: National Institute of Allergy and Infectious Diseases
6003 Executive Boulevard, Solar Building
Bethesda, MD 20892

NIAID Allergy, Immunology, Transplantation, Infectious Diseases, and AIDS NRSAs—Individual 2450
NRSAs are offered to increase the number of biomedical investigators who are conducting high-quality research in the areas of allergy, immunology, transplantation, infectious diseases, and AIDS. Predoctoral fellowships for minority and disabled students provide up to five years of support. NRSA postdoctoral fellowships provide support for up to three years. NRSA senior fellowships provide support for two years. Deadlines for postdoctoral and senior fellowships are April 5, August 5, and December 5. Annual deadline dates may vary; contact program, staff for exact dates.
Requirements: Awards are given only to U.S. citizens and noncitizen nationals. Minority predoctoral fellowships are available to underrepresented minority students (African Americans, Hispanic, Native Americans, and Pacific Islanders) or scientists with disabilities who will be entering a PhD program. Postdoctoral fellowship applicants must have a doctoral degree (PhD, MD, DVM, DDS, OD, etc.). Senior fellowship applicants should plan to do research that will provide training the candidate does not have and will become an asset to her or his academic career.
Amount of Grant: $7586-$743,606; $113,228 average
Date(s) Application is Due: Apr 5; Aug 5; Dec 5
Contact: Mary Kirker, Grants Management Officer, (301) 496-7075
Internet: http://12.46.245.173/pls/portal30/CATALOG.PROGRAM_TEXT_RPT.show
Sponsor: National Institute of Allergy and Infectious Diseases
6003 Executive Boulevard, Solar Building
Bethesda, MD 20892

NIAID Challenge Grants: Joint Ventures in Biomedicine and Biotechnology 2451
The purpose of this initiative is to support research and development efforts whose outcomes could significantly reduce the impact of infectious diseases nationally and worldwide. NIAID has identified areas of high importance where it believes successful product research and development combined with existing infrastructures and federal challenge grant funding could significantly impact a major health or medical problem. Applications in response to this RFA for challenge grants are limited to these areas: Medicines for Malaria; Medicines for Tuberculosis; Vaccines for Influenza; Vaccines for Emerging and Resistant Infections; and Therapeutics for Emerging and Resistant Infections. Awards will be made in two Phases: Phase I awards will be short-term (two month), small dollar ($25,000) research grants for development of detailed plans for implementation of research and development efforts (i.e., a Phase II grant application); and Phase II awards will be cooperative agreement awards to those Phase I awardees whose research plans present the best opportunities, based on peer review and potential public health significance, for products that will benefit the public health. Annual deadline dates may vary; contact program staff for exact dates. RFA: AI-00-010
Requirements: Applications may be submitted by domestic for-profit and nonprofit organizations such as biotechnology, bioengineering and pharmaceutical companies with collaborators as necessary from universities, colleges, hospitals, and laboratories.
Restrictions: Phase I applications must directly address one or more of the research topics listed. Only Phase I awardees will be eligible for Phase II awards.
Amount of Grant: $20 million total for Phases I and II
Contact: Program Officer; email: niaidchallenge@niaid.nih.gov
Internet: http://grants.nih.gov/grants/guide/rfa-files/RFA-AI-00-010.html
Sponsor: National Institute of Allergy and Infectious Diseases
6700-B Rockledge Drive
Bethesda, MD 20892

NIAID Enhancing Vaccine-Elicited Protective Immunity in Malaria Research Grants 2452
NIAID invites applications for research project (R01) grants to conduct innovative research to advance fundamental understanding of eliciting optimal protective immune responses with candidate malaria vaccines. As part of its Malaria Vaccine Development Plan, NIAID seeks to identify and validate methods and strategies for improved antigen delivery, processing, and presentation or enhancement of protective immunity with existing candidate antigens. Identification, characterization, and evaluation of new candidate vaccines, especially combination vaccines based on a rational strategy for antigen inclusion, are also encouraged. Because many of the poorest nations of the world are afflicted with malaria, to be effective any intervention must be inexpensive, cost-effective, and relatively easy to administer and maintain. Annual deadline dates may vary; contact program staff for exact dates. RFA: AI-99-006
Requirements: Applications may be submitted by domestic and foreign for-profit and nonprofit organizations and public and private institutions.
Amount of Grant: $250,000 maximum per year
Contact: Dr. B.F. Hall, Division of Microbiology and Infectious Diseases, (301) 496-2544; fax: (301) 402-0659; email: bh24q@nih.gov
Internet: http://www.grants.nih.gov/grants/guide/rfa-files/RFA-AI-99-006.html
Sponsor: National Institute of Allergy and Infectious Diseases
6003 Executive Boulevard, Solar Building
Bethesda, MD 20892

NIAID HIV Prevention Trial Units Grants 2453
NIAID invites applications for HIV Prevention Trial Units (HPTUs), which will be integral parts of an HIV Prevention Trials Network (HPTN) designed to carry out a comprehensive scientific agenda on HIV prevention strategies. The HPTN will conduct domestic and international research on promising biomedical and behavioral strategies for the prevention of HIV transmission among adult, pediatric, and adolescent populations. Modalities of interventions may include, but are not limited to, antiretroviral drugs, microbicides, behavioral approaches, barrier and other contraceptive/STD prevention methods, vaccines (in perinatal settings), chemoprophylaxis, treatment of sexually transmitted diseases, and combined approaches. The HPTUs will contribute to the HPTN research agenda; conduct/participate in Phase I, II, and/or III prevention intervention clinical trials domestically and/or internationally; and expand for multiple prevention efficacy trials. Potential applicants should refer to the following Web site for further information on this initiative: http://www.niaid.nih.gov/daids/vtn-ptn. Annual deadline dates may vary; contact program staff for exact dates. RFA: AI-99-010
Requirements: Applications may be submitted by domestic and foreign for-profit and nonprofit organizations, public and private institutions, and eligible agencies of the federal government.
Contact: Rodney Hoff, Division of AIDS, (301) 496-6177; fax: (301) 402-3684; email: rh25v@nih.gov

Internet: http://www.grants.nih.gov/grants/guide/rfa-files/RFA-AI-99-010.html
Sponsor: National Institute of Allergy and Infectious Diseases
6003 Executive Boulevard, Solar Building
Bethesda, MD 20892

NIAID HIV Vaccine Clinical Trial Units Grants 2454

The Division of AIDS (DAIDS) of NIAID solicits applications for HIV Vaccine Trial Clinical Units (HVTUs) that are integral parts of an HIV Vaccine Trials Network (HVTN) designed to carry out a comprehensive scientific agenda on HIV vaccines. The HVTUs will contribute to the HVTN research agenda, participate in domestic and international Phase I and II clinical trials of candidate HIV vaccines, and participate in domestic and international Phase III efficacy trials of HIV vaccines. Potential applicants should refer to the following Web site for further information on this initiative: http://www.niaid.nih.gov/daids/vtn-ptn. In addition to the HVTN, NIAID supports the creation of the HIV Prevention Trials Network (HPTN) to perform Phase I, II, and III trials of other prevention strategies to prevent HIV-1 transmission, domestically and internationally. Clinical trials of vaccines focused on questions around maternal-infant transmission will be conducted within the HPTN in collaboration with the HVTN and, when desirable, the Pediatric AIDS Clinical Trials Network. Sites funded under the HPTN may serve as effective venues for the eventual implementation of larger HIV vaccine trials; therefore, linkages between HPTN and HVTN, in addition to other scientific organizations, are strongly encouraged. Annual deadline dates may vary; contact program staff for exact dates. RFA: AI-99-009
Requirements: Applications may be submitted by domestic and foreign for-profit and nonprofit organizations, public and private institutions, and eligible agencies of the federal government.
Contact: Dr. Jorge Flores, Division of AIDS, (301) 435-3578; fax: (301) 402-3684; email: jf30t@nih.gov
Internet: http://www.grants.nih.gov/grants/guide/rfa-files/RFA-AI-99-009.html
Sponsor: National Institute of Allergy and Infectious Diseases
6003 Executive Boulevard, Solar Building
Bethesda, MD 20892

NIAID HIV Vaccine Research and Design—Program Project Grants 2455

NIAID invites applications for research aimed at obtaining an efficacious vaccine against HIV or AIDS. NIAID supports all stages of AIDS vaccine research and development—from basic research to iterative product development through clinical trials. Applications may target any area of AIDS vaccine research. These areas include, but are not limited to, HIV antigen processing, correlates of immunity, animal model development, DNA vaccination, studies of the structure of HIV immunogens, development of virus and bacterial vaccine vectors, studies of existing vaccine cohorts, studies targeting initial infection (dendritic cells), and extensive modeling of vaccine concepts in macaques or chimps, etc. Clinical studies involving humans would not be considered appropriate for this announcement.
Requirements: Applications may be submitted by domestic and foreign, for-profit and nonprofit organizations, public and private.
Date(s) Application is Due: Jun 10; Nov 10
Contact: Dr. Michael Pensiero, Division of AIDS, (301) 435-3749; fax: (301) 402-3684; email: mpensiero@niaid.nih.gov
Internet: http://grants.nih.gov/grants/guide/pa-files/PAR-00-093.html
Sponsor: National Institute of Allergy and Infectious Diseases
6003 Executive Boulevard, Solar Building
Bethesda, MD 20892

NIAID Independent Scientist Award 2456

The award is a special salary-only grant designed to provide protected time for newly independent scientists who currently have non-research obligations such as heavy teaching loads, clinical work, committee assignments, service, and administrative duties that prevent them from having a period of intensive research focus. The award is targeted to persons with doctoral degrees who have completed their research training, have independent peer-reviewed research support, and who need a period of protected research time in order to foster their research career development. New applications are due February 12, June 12, and October 12, while renewal applications are due March 12, July 12, and November 12. Up to $75,000 plus fringe benefits per year is available. Additional research is not generally provided.
Requirements: The following organizations and institutions are eligible to apply: public/state controlled institutions of higher education; private institutions of higher education; nonprofits with 501(c)3 IRS status; nonprofits without 501(c)3 IRS status; small businesses; for-profit organizations; State governments; U.S. territories or possessions; Indian/Native American tribal governments (Federally recognized and other than Federally recognized); Indian/Native American tribally designated organizations; Hispanic-serving institutions; historically Black colleges and universities (HBCUs); tribally controlled colleges and universities (TCCUs); Alaska Native and Native Hawaiian serving institutions; regional organizations; and faith-based or community based organizations. The candidate must have a doctoral degree and peer-reviewed, independent research support at the time the award is made. The candidate must spend a minimum of 75 percent effort conducting research during the period of the award.
Restrictions: The award is not intended for investigators who already have full time to perform research, or have substantial publication records or considerable research support indicating that they are well established in their fields. Foreign institutions are not eligible to apply.
Amount of Grant: $75,000 plus fringe benefits
Date(s) Application is Due: Feb 12; Mar 12; Jun 12; Jul 12; Oct 12; Nov 12
Contact: Milton J. Hernandez, Ph.D.; (301) 496-3775; email: mh35c@nih.gov
Internet: http://grants.nih.gov/grants/guide/pa-files/PA-09-038.html
Sponsor: National Institute of Allergy and Infectious Diseases (NIAID)
6700B Rockledge Drive, Room 2149
Bethesda, MD 20886

NIAID Integrated Preclinical/Clinical AIDS Vaccine Development Grants 2457

NIAID invites applications for research aimed at obtaining a safe and efficacious vaccine against HIV or AIDS. The overall goal of this program is to support multidisciplinary research that will lead to a safe and protective AIDS vaccine. As such, IPCAVD applications must include human clinical studies within the term of the award. Applicants must address the following issues in their application regarding human studies: design of the clinical trial, plans for recruitment, enrollment, education and follow-up of clinical subjects, including attention to the possibility of social harms and discrimination arising from vaccine- induced positive screening tests that may be interpreted incorrectly as HIV infection, plus documentation of compliance with all applicable federal (FDA), state and local laws and regulations governing clinical research. Annual deadlines may vary; contact program staff for exact dates. PA: PAR-00-072
Requirements: Applications may be submitted by domestic for-profit and nonprofit organizations, both public and private; units of state and local governments; and eligible agencies of the federal government.
Contact: Dr. Michael Pensiero, Division of AIDS, (301)-435-3749; fax: (301) 402-3684; email: mpensiero@niaid.nih.gov
Internet: http://grants.nih.gov/grants/guide/pa-files/PAR-00-072.html
Sponsor: National Institute of Allergy and Infectious Diseases
6003 Executive Boulevard, Solar Building
Bethesda, MD 20892

NIAID Laboratory Methods to Assess Responses to HIV Vaccine Candidates Research Grants 2458

NIAID invites applications to conduct innovative research to develop and improve technologies for evaluation of immune responses to HIV vaccines and to expand the range and scope of immune functions currently measured in vaccine trials. This PA intends to complement the scope of vaccine research carried out in human volunteers and animals receiving experimental HIV/SIV vaccines in prophylactic and/or therapeutic trials funded through other programs. Development of new techniques that detect and quantitate changes in innate (nonspecific) and HIV-specific responses will be fostered. Research may include comparative analysis of samples acquired from individuals infected with HIV or who have been exposed to, but not infected with, HIV. Studies in animals, particularly primates that have received SIV/SHIV vaccines, are also encouraged. Applications to develop reagents (including non-clade B based materials), to adapt assays to field conditions and to improve on cell cryopreservation methods are also appropriate. The PA is not intended to directly support the conduct of human or animal clinical trials. Contact the program office for deadline dates. PA: PA-99-044
Requirements: Applications may be submitted by domestic and foreign, for-profit and nonprofit organizations, public and private.
Contact: Dr. Jorge Flores, Division of AIDS, (301) 435-3758; fax: (301) 402-3684; email: jf30t@nih.gov
Internet: http://www.grants.nih.gov/grants/guide/pa-files/PA-99-044.html
Sponsor: National Institute of Allergy and Infectious Diseases
6003 Executive Boulevard, Solar Building
Bethesda, MD 20892

NIAID Microbiology and Infectious Diseases Research Grants and Contracts 2459

This program supports research with the broad aim of improving health by controlling diseases caused by infectious or parasitic agents. Investigator-originated and grant-supported research focuses on all aspects of microbiology, with particular emphasis on human pathogens. Projects range from studies of microbial physiology and antigenic structure to collaborative trials of experimental drugs and vaccines. NIAID also supports studies on the mechanisms of resistance to antibiotics as well as research dealing with epidemiologic observations in hospitalized patients or community populations. Program project grants and research contracts are used to fund selected projects of high institute relevance in the branches covering molecular microbiology; bacteriology, mycobacteriology, and mycology; virology; and parasitology.
Requirements: Universities, colleges, hospitals, laboratories, and other public or private nonprofit domestic institutions, including state and local units of government, are eligible. Individuals are eligible to make application for grant support of research by a named principal investigator or a research career development candidate.
Amount of Grant: $2000-$18.07 million; $389,416 average
Date(s) Application is Due: Feb 1; Jun 1; Oct 1
Contact: Dr. John McGowan, Acting Director, Division of Extramural Activities, (301) 496-7291; Mary Kirker, Grants Management Officer, (301) 496-7075
Internet: http://12.46.245.173/pls/portal30/CATALOG.PROGRAM_TEXT_RPT.show
Sponsor: National Institute of Allergy and Infectious Diseases
6003 Executive Boulevard, Solar Building
Bethesda, MD 20892

NIAID Pediatric Clinical Trials Program for AIDS 2460

The purpose of this RFA is to solicit applications from institutions interested in establishing cooperative clinical trials groups to plan and direct pediatric therapeutics and prevention research. The awardees will have the capacity and expertise to conduct all phases of clinical trials involving children, adolescents, and pregnant women with all stages of infection. Studies focus on high priority research questions on the treatment and

pathogenesis of HIV disease and its sequelae. The scope of activities ranges from studies requiring in-depth laboratory support to research in long-term clinical outcomes. Annual deadline dates may vary: contact program staff for exact dates. RFA: AI-00-015
Requirements: Applications may be submitted by domestic for-profit and nonprofit organizations, both public and private; units of state and local governments; and eligible agencies of the federal government.
Restrictions: Foreign institutions are not eligible to apply as primary grantees; however, foreign institutions may participate as part of a domestic application.
Amount of Grant: $36 million total
Contact: Dr. Frederick Batzold, Division of AIDS, (301) 402-0143; fax: (301) 480-4582; email: fb10c@nih.gov
Internet: http://grants.nih.gov/grants/guide/rfa-files/RFA-AI-00-015.html
Sponsor: National Institute of Allergy and Infectious Diseases
6700-B Rockledge Drive
Bethesda, MD 20892-7624

NIAID Preparedness against Illegitimate Use of Bacterial Pathogens 2461
The purpose of this program is to support basic research on molecular and genetic aspects of pathogenesis of, and host immune/defense responses to, the following bacterial pathogens: Bacillus anthracis, Yersinia pestis, Francisella tularensis, Coxiella burnetii, or Brucella species. It is hoped that research from funded projects will be used to devise appropriate defense strategies that can be implemented shortly before or soon after bioterrorist acts. Annual deadline dates may vary; contact program staff for exact dates. RFA: AI-01-002
Requirements: Applications may be submitted by domestic for-profit and nonprofit organizations, both public and private; units of state and local governments; and eligible agencies of the federal government.
Amount of Grant: $1.5 million total
Contact: Dr. Phillip Baker, Division of Microbiology and Infectious Diseases, (301) 435-2855; fax: (301) 402-2508; email: pb26o@nih.gov
Internet: http://grants.nih.gov/grants/guide/rfa-files/RFA-AI-01-002.html
Sponsor: National Institute of Allergy and Infectious Diseases
6700-B Rockledge Drive
Bethesda, MD 20892

NIAID Research Scholar Development Award 2462
NIAID invites applications from outstanding intramural and extramural postdoctoral fellows for the Research Scholar Development Award (RSDA). The RSDA provides support for postdoctoral fellows who are moving to assistant professor positions in academic institutions. The purpose of the RSDA is to ease the transition to an academic position by enabling the awardee to focus on the establishment of his or her research laboratory prior to submitting applications for grant support.
Requirements: The candidate must have a health professional doctoral degree and have demonstrated the capacity for highly productive, independent postdoctoral research in her or his chosen field prior to applying for this award.
Contact: Dr. Milton Hernandez, Division of Extramural Activities, (301) 496-3775; fax: (301) 402-0369; email: mh35c@nih.gov; Barbara Huffman, Division of Extramural Activities, (301) 496-3821; fax: (301) 402-0369; email: bh23g@nih.gov
Internet: http://www.grants.nih.gov/grants/guide/pa-files/PAR-98-072.html
Sponsor: National Institute of Allergy and Infectious Diseases
6003 Executive Boulevard, Solar Building
Bethesda, MD 20892

NIAID Small Business Innovation Research Advanced Technology Grants 2463
This PA invites grant applications for Small Business Innovation Research (SBIR) projects with award duration and amounts greater than those routinely allowed under the SBIR program. This PA provides examples of advanced technology areas in which NIAID will entertain SBIR applications and provides NIAID's interpretation and clarification of instructions relating to total cost, dates of project period, and page limitations for these applications. Information may be obtained through the NIH grant line (301-402-2221), the NIH Web site, mail, and email. PA: PA-04-127
Date(s) Application is Due: Apr 1; Aug 1; Dec 1
Contact: Gregory Milman, Division of Extramural Activities, (301) 496-8666; fax: (301) 402-0369; email: gm16s@nih.gov
Internet: http://grants.nih.gov/grants/guide/pa-files/PA-04-127.html
Sponsor: National Institute of Allergy and Infectious Diseases
6003 Executive Boulevard, Solar Building
Bethesda, MD 20892

NIAID Statistical Methods in HIV and AIDS Research Grants 2464
NIAID and NIMH invite applications for the development of original statistical methods to advance the understanding, treatment, and prevention of HIV and AIDS. Traditional research project grant (R01) applications may be submitted in response to this PA. PA-98-054 may be obtained through the NIH grant line (301-402-2221), the NIH Web site, mail, and email.
Requirements: Applications may be submitted by domestic and foreign, for-profit and nonprofit organizations, public or private.
Contact: Dr. Jeffrey Albert, Division of AIDS, (301) 435-3752; fax: (301) 480-5703; email: ja24o@nih.gov; Mary Ledford, Grants Management, (301) 402-6446; fax: (301) 480-3780; email: m128g@nih.gov
Internet: http://www.grants.nih.gov/grants/guide/pa-files/PA-98-054.html
Sponsor: National Institute of Allergy and Infectious Diseases
6003 Executive Boulevard, Solar Building
Bethesda, MD 20892

NIAID Therapeutics Research on AIDS-Associated Opportunistic Infections 2465
The goal of this program is the discovery of agents for treatment of AIDS-associated opportunistic infections. Given present advances in molecular biology, the principal objectives of the program are to stimulate original and innovative preclinical research to identify and characterize new, pathogen-specific molecular targets and to develop promising therapeutic approaches based on new targets. Program announcement is available on the Web site along with an addendum (http://grants2.nih.gov/grants/guide/notice-files/NOT-AI-00-001.html). PA: PA-99-124
Requirements: Applications may be submitted by domestic and foreign, for-profit and nonprofit organizations, both public and private; units of state and local governments; and eligible agencies of the federal government. Racial/ethnic minority individuals, women, and persons with disabilities are encouraged to apply.
Amount of Grant: $25,000-$250,000 R01 modules; $50,000 R03 modules
Contact: Dr. Chris Lambros, (301) 435-3769; fax: (301) 402-3171; email: clambros@niaid.nih.gov
Internet: http://www.grants.nih.gov/grants/guide/pa-files/PA-99-124.html
Sponsor: National Institute of Allergy and Infectious Diseases
6003 Executive Boulevard, Solar Building
Bethesda, MD 20892

NIAMS Clinical Trial Planning Grants 2466
The goal of this program is to provide support for planning activities critical for the successful implementation of clinical trials in areas of interest to NIAMS. In addition, the grant is intended to allow for early peer review of the rationale and design for complex or large-scale clinical trials and studies in those areas that are in the NIAMS mission; provide support for the development of a detailed clinical trial research plan, including a manual of operations and procedures, as a means of decreasing the long start-up time often needed for initiating large trials after award; and provide support to refine critical components of a clinical trial protocol, such as outcome measures, recruitment strategies, inclusion and exclusion criteria, etc. Annual deadline dates may vary; contact program staff for exact dates. RFA: AR-00-010
Requirements: Applications may be submitted by domestic for-profit and nonprofit organizations, both public and private; units of state and local governments; and eligible agencies of the federal government.
Amount of Grant: $500,000 total
Contact: Dr. Joan McGowan, Bone Diseases, (301) 594-5055; fax: (301) 480-4543; email: Joan_Mcgowan@nih.gov; Dr. Alan Moshell, Skin Diseases, (301) 594-5017; fax: (301) 480-4543; email: Alan_N_Moshell@nih.gov
Internet: http://grants.nih.gov/grants/guide/rfa-files/RFA-AR-00-010.html
Sponsor: National Institute of Arthritis and Musculoskeletal and Skin Diseases
45 Center Drive
Bethesda, MD 20892

NIAMS Collaborative Arthritis and Musculoskeletal and Skin Diseases Science Award 2467
The objective of the Collaborative Arthritis and Musculoskeletal and Skin Diseases Science Award (CAMSSA) program is to develop and promote competitive scientific research programs in areas within the mission of the National Institute of Arthritis and Musculoskeletal and Skin Diseases at institutions with substantial minority enrollment. The CAMSSA program is designed to encourage collaborative investigations among scientists at institutions with substantial minority enrollment with grantees from research-intensive institutions who have grant support to conduct research in arthritis, musculoskeletal diseases or skin diseases. The nature of the collaborations will include joint research efforts, specialized training in research techniques, and participation in research seminars. The CAMSSA program should develop and expand scientific opportunities among the participating institutions for research in arthritis, musculoskeletal diseases or skin diseases. PAR 04-003
Requirements: Applicant institution must be an institution with substantial minority enrollment that may be a non-Federal, public or private nonprofit institution located in the United States, its possessions or territories. The collaborating institution must also be a non-Federal, public or private nonprofit institution located in the United States, its possessions or territories. Individuals are eligible to become principal investigators. Applicant investigator must have a doctoral degree in a basic or clinical science area, and have completed one or more years of postdoctoral research experience and must be a full-time employee of the applicant institution.
Amount of Grant: $750,000 maximum direct costs
Date(s) Application is Due: Feb 1; Jun 1; Oct 1
Contact: Melinda Nelson, Chief Grants Management Officer, (301) 594-3535; fax: (301) 480-5450; email: nelsonm@mail.nih.gov
Internet: http://grants2.nih.gov/grants/guide/pa-files/PAR-04-003.html
Sponsor: National Institute of Arthritis and Musculoskeletal and Skin Diseases
Building 31, Room 4C02, 31 Center Dr MSC 2350
Bethesda, MD 20892-2350

NIAMS Core Centers for Musculoskeletal Disorders Grants 2468
NIAMS invites applications for research core centers in musculoskeletal disorders. The centers will provide the resources for a number of established, currently funded investigators, often from different disciplines, to adopt a multidisciplinary approach to common research problems in musculoskeletal disorders and to ensure greater productivity than from each of the separate projects. Annual deadline dates may vary; contact program staff for exact dates. RFA: AR-98-004

Requirements: Applications may be submitted by domestic for-profit and nonprofit organizations, public or private.
Restrictions: Foreign institutions are not eligible for center grants.
Amount of Grant: $400,000 maximum
Contact: Dr. Julia Freeman, Centers Program, (301) 594-5052; fax: (301) 480-4543; email: Julia_B_Freeman@nih.gov
Internet: http://grants.nih.gov/grants/guide/rfa-files/RFA-AR-98-004.html
Sponsor: National Institute of Arthritis and Musculoskeletal and Skin Diseases
45 Center Drive, Natcher Building
Bethesda, MD 20892

NIAMS Exploratory Developmental Grants for Multidisciplinary Clinical Studies of Sarcopenia 2469
NIAMS, with NIA, invites exploratory developmental research grant (R21) applications for multidisciplinary clinical studies on the mechanisms underlying the physical functional consequences of sarcopenia in older persons. This exploratory grants program is intended to facilitate new collaborative efforts in the development of novel scientific hypotheses on the causes of changes in skeletal muscle morphology and/or metabolism that lead to physical disabilities in old age, by providing research support for the appropriate pilot/feasibility studies to refine these hypotheses. Multidisciplinary approaches may include collaborations among various types of clinical research expertise or between basic and clinical researchers, with or without previous aging research experience.
Contact: Dr. Richard Lymn, Muscle Biology and Musculoskeletal Fitness Program Director, (301) 594-5128; fax: (301) 480-4543; email: lymnr@ep.niams.nih.gov
Internet: http://www.grants.nih.gov/grants/guide/pa-files/PA-97-060.html
Sponsor: National Institute of Arthritis and Musculoskeletal and Skin Diseases
45 Center Drive, Natcher Building
Bethesda, MD 20892

NIAMS High Risk Arthritis and Musculoskeletal and Skin Diseases Research 2470
This program seeks to broaden the base of inquiry in fundamental biomedical, biobehavioral, and biomedical technology research by encouraging research projects that involve a high degree of innovation and novelty. It supports research in rheumatic diseases; cartilage biology and diseases; bone biology and diseases (e.g., osteoporosis, Paget's disease); skin biology and skin diseases; autoimmune diseases (e.g., lupus); connective tissue diseases; musculoskeletal diseases, injuries, and disorders; muscle biology and diseases (e.g., muscular dystrophy); exercise physiology and musculoskeletal fitness; sports injuries; occupational diseases and injuries; and orthopedics and bioengineering. Annual deadline dates may vary; contact program staff for exact dates.
Requirements: Applications may be submitted by domestic for-profit and nonprofit organizations, both public and private; units of state and local governments; and eligible agencies of the federal government.
Amount of Grant: $50,000 maximum
Contact: Dr. Bernadette Tyree, Cartilage and Connective Tissue, (301) 594-5032; email: bt16w@nih.gov; Dr. Elizabeth Gretz, Rheumatic Diseases, (301) 594-5032; email: gretze@mail.nih.gov; Dr. Deborah Ader, Behavioral and Prevention Research, (301) 594-5032; e-m
Internet: http://grants.nih.gov/grants/guide/rfa-files/RFA-AR-01-004.html
Sponsor: National Institute of Arthritis and Musculoskeletal and Skin Diseases
45 Center Drive, Natcher Building
Bethesda, MD 20892

NIAMS Low-Back Pain and Common Spinal Disorders Research Grants 2471
The program is sponsored by NIAMS, NICHD, NINDS, and NIOSH at the CDC. This initiative invites applications directed to the study of the pathogenesis, epidemiology, prevention, and treatment of three common causes of low-back pain: herniated nucleus pulposus, spinal stenosis, and idiopathic low-back pain. The support mechanism for grants in this area will be the individual investigator-initiated research grant (R01). PA-97-058 may be obtained electronically through the NIH grant line (301-402-2221), the NIH Web site, and by mail and email.
Contact: Dr. James Panagis, Orthopaedics Program, (301) 594-5055; fax: (301) 480-4543; email: panagisj@ep.niams.nih.gov
Internet: http://www.grants.nih.gov/grants/guide/pa-files/PA-97-058.html
Sponsor: National Institute of Arthritis and Musculoskeletal and Skin Diseases
45 Center Drive, Natcher Building
Bethesda, MD 20892

NIAMS Mechanisms of Chondroprotection Research Grants 2472
Approximately six to eight awards will be made for research on mechanisms of chondroprotection. Applications may be for individual research projects or for exploratory/development grants. The objective of the exploratory/developmental mechanism is to encourage applications from individuals who are interested in testing innovative or conceptually creative ideas that are scientifically sound and may advance our understanding of chondroprotective mechanisms. Research should be specifically targeted towards identification and evaluation of chondroprotective agents to prevent cartilage destruction and/or facilitate its repair in such conditions as rheumatoid arthritis, juvenile rheumatoid arthritis, and osteoarthritis, where there is a decline in the structural integrity of the articular cartilage. This request for applications is for basic and applied research projects, but not epidemiological treatment projects. Annual deadline dates may vary; contact program staff for exact dates. RFA: AR-99-004
Requirements: Applications may be submitted by domestic and foreign public and private for-profit and nonprofit organizations, including universities, colleges, hospitals, laboratories, units of state and local government, and eligible agencies of the federal government.
Amount of Grant: $1.5 million total
Contact: Dr. Bernadette Tyree, Cartilage and Connective Tissue Program, or Dr. Susana Serrate-Sztein, Arthritis Branch, (301) 594-5032; fax: (301) 480-4543; email: tyreeb@ep.niams.nih.gov or szteins@ep.niams.nih.gov
Internet: http://www.grants.nih.gov/grants/guide/rfa-files/RFA-AR-99-004.html
Sponsor: National Institute of Arthritis and Musculoskeletal and Skin Diseases
45 Center Drive, Natcher Building
Bethesda, MD 20892

NIAMS Molecular Pathogenesis and New Interventions in Scleroderma 2473
The goal of this RFA is to foster developmental and traditional research projects to advance understanding of the pathogenesis of scleroderma and to promote the design, development, and pilot testing of hypothesis-driven innovative therapeutic approaches. Annual deadline dates may vary; contact program staff for exact dates. RFA: AR-00-007
Requirements: Applications may be submitted by domestic for-profit and nonprofit organizations, both public and private; units of state and local governments; and eligible agencies of the federal government.
Restrictions: Foreign institutions are not eligible to apply for these grants, however, applicants may collaborate, through consultation or contractual agreements, with investigators at foreign institutions.
Amount of Grant: $1.5 million total
Contact: Dr. Susana Serrate-Sztein, Rheumatic Diseases Branch, (301) 594-5032; fax: (301) 480-4543; email: szteins@mail.nih.gov
Internet: http://grants.nih.gov/grants/guide/rfa-files/RFA-AR-00-007.html
Sponsor: National Institute of Arthritis and Musculoskeletal and Skin Diseases
45 Center Drive
Bethesda, MD 20892

NIAMS Pathogenesis and Therapy of the Muscular Dystrophies Research Grants 2474
NINDS and NIAMS encourage investigator-initiated research grant applications to study the pathogenesis and therapy of the various forms of muscular dystrophy in children and adults. Responses to this PA may include studies in appropriate animal models or preclinical or clinical studies in patients with facioscapulohumeral dystrophy (FSH), limb-girdle muscular dystrophy (LGMD), myotonic dystrophy, congenital muscular dystrophy (CMD), Emery-Dreifuss muscular dystrophy (EMD), Duchenne muscular dystrophy (DMD), Becker muscular dystrophy (BMD), or other forms of muscular dystrophy. Support mechanisms for grants are research project grant (R01) and program project grant (P01). PA-98-044 may be obtained through the NIH grant line (301-402-2221), the NIH Web site, mail, and email.
Requirements: Applications may be submitted by domestic and foreign, for-profit and nonprofit organizations, public or private.
Contact: Dr. Richard Lymn, Muscle Biology Program, (301) 594-4128; fax: (301) 480-4543; email: r128b@nih.gov; Sally Nichols, Grants Management Officer, (301) 594-3535; fax: (301) 480-5450; email: nicholss@ep.niams.nih.gov
Internet: http://www.grants.nih.gov/grants/guide/pa-files/PA-98-044.html
Sponsor: National Institute of Arthritis and Musculoskeletal and Skin Diseases
45 Center Drive, Natcher Building
Bethesda, MD 20892

NIAMS Repetitive Motion Disorders Research Grants 2475
The program is sponsored by NIAMS, NICHD, NINDS, and NIOSH at the CDC. This initiative invites applications directed to the study of the pathogenesis, epidemiology, prevention, and treatment of repetitive motion disorders. The support mechanism for grants in this area will be the individual investigator-initiated research grant (R01). PA-97-059 may be obtained electronically through the NIH grant line (301-402-2221), the NIH Web site, and by mail and email.
Contact: Dr. James Panagis, Orthopaedics Program, (301) 594-5055; fax: (301) 480-4543; email: panagisj@ep.niams.nih.gov
Internet: http://www.grants.nih.gov/grants/guide/pa-files/PA-97-059.html
Sponsor: National Institute of Arthritis and Musculoskeletal and Skin Diseases
45 Center Drive, Natcher Building
Bethesda, MD 20892

NIAMS Research on Musculoskeletal Fitness and Sports Medicine Grants 2476
NIAMS and NINR invite investigator-initiated research grant applications to study a broad range of basic and clinical topics related to musculoskeletal fitness, exercise physiology, and sports medicine. The National Center for Medical Rehabilitation Research of NICHD encourages applications for both basic and clinical studies of musculoskeletal fitness and exercise physiology of persons with physical disabilities. The principal investigator and participating investigators will plan, direct, and perform the research. Applicants for program project grants are requested to contact NIAMS representative as early as possible in the planning stages. NINR will support individual research project grants. PA-97-025 may be obtained electronically through the NIH grant line (301-402-2221), the NIH Web site, and by mail and email.
Contact: Dr. Richard Lymn, Muscle Biology and Musculoskeletal Fitness Program Director, (301) 594-5128; fax: (301) 480-4543; email: lymnr@ep.niams.nih.gov
Internet: http://www.grants.nih.gov/grants/guide/pa-files/PA-97-025.html
Sponsor: National Institute of Arthritis and Musculoskeletal and Skin Diseases
45 Center Drive, Natcher Building
Bethesda, MD 20892

NIAMS Significance of Sarcopenia in Old Age Grants **2477**

NIA and NIAMS invite research project applications to elucidate the metabolic/physiological and functional consequences of sarcopenia in old age. Sarcopenia is defined as the loss of skeletal muscle mass, quality, and strength. More information may be obtained by mail and email, or through the NIH grant line (301-402-2221) or the NIH Web site.
Amount of Grant: $10,000-$1.5 million; $239,000 average
Date(s) Application is Due: Feb 1; Jun 1; Oct 1
Contact: Dr. S. Hausman, Director, Extramural Program, (301) 594-2463; Sally Nichols, Grants Management Officer, Extramural Program, (301) 594-3535
Internet: http://www.grants.nih.gov/grants/guide/pa-files/PA-96-038.html
Sponsor: National Institute of Arthritis and Musculoskeletal and Skin Diseases
45 Center Drive, Natcher Building
Bethesda, MD 20892

NIAMS Skin Diseases Research Core Centers Grants **2478**

NIAMS is accepting applications for research core centers in skin diseases. The centers will provide the resources for a number of established, currently funded investigators, often from different disciplines, to adopt a multidisciplinary approach to common research problems in skin diseases and to ensure greater productivity through interaction among the investigators of individually funded research projects. New research directions are encouraged through a pilot and feasibility component. Broad advances in skin disease research can be effectively fostered by research core centers. Examples of advances include, but are not limited to, stratum corneum—biochemistry, structure, function; epidermis—differentiation, keratinization, cellular constituents; dermal-epidermal junction—structure, functions, diseases; skin and an immunological organ; and autoimmune skin diseases.
Requirements: Applications may be submitted by domestic for-profit and nonprofit organizations, both public and private; units of state and local governments; and eligible agencies of the federal government. An established clinical and basic research program in skin diseases must be present.
Restrictions: Foreign institutions are not eligible for center grants.
Amount of Grant: $400,000 maximum
Contact: Dr. Julia Freeman, Centers Program, Extramural Program, (301) 594-5052; fax: (301) 480-4543; email: Julia_B_Freeman@nih.gov
Internet: http://grants.nih.gov/grants/guide/rfa-files/RFA-AR-99-009.html
Sponsor: National Institute of Arthritis and Musculoskeletal and Skin Diseases
45 Center Drive, Natcher Building
Bethesda, MD 20892

NIAMS Specialized Centers of Research in Osteoarthritis and Systemic Lupus Erythematosus **2479**

NIAMS invites applications for specialized centers of research in osteoarthritis and systemic lupus erythematosus. These centers should foster a coordinated research effort that strongly emphasizes basic disciplines but also involves significant interaction between basic research and clinical investigations. Annual deadline dates may vary; contact program staff for exact dates. RFA: AR-01-005
Requirements: Applications may be submitted by domestic for-profit and nonprofit organizations, both public and private; units of state and local governments; and eligible agencies of the federal government.
Amount of Grant: $750,000 maximum
Contact: Dr. Julia Freeman, Centers Program, (301) 594-5052; fax: (301) 480-4543; email: Julia_B_Freeman@nih.gov; Melinda Nelson, Grants Management Officer, (301) 594-3535; fax: (301) 480-5450; email: nelsonm@exchange.nih.gov
Internet: http://grants.nih.gov/grants/guide/rfa-files/RFA-AR-01-005.html
Sponsor: National Institute of Arthritis and Musculoskeletal and Skin Diseases
45 Center Drive, Natcher Building
Bethesda, MD 20892

NIAMS Specialized Centers of Research in Osteoporosis, Rheumatoid Arthritis, and Scleroderma **2480**

NIAMS invites applications for specialized centers of research in the following disease areas: osteoporosis, rheumatoid arthritis, and scleroderma. A center should foster a coordinated research effort that strongly emphasizes basic disciplines but also involves significant interaction between basic research and clinical investigations. More information may be obtained by mail and email or through the NIH grant line (301-402-2221), and the NIH Web site.
Requirements: Domestic for-profit and nonprofit organizations, both public and private; units of state and local governments; and eligible agencies of the federal government may apply.
Amount of Grant: $750,000 maximum
Contact: Dr. Julia Freeman, Centers Program, (301) 594-5052; fax: (301) 480-4543; email: freemanj@ep.niams.nih.gov; Sally Nichols, Grants Management Officer, (301) 594-3535; fax: (301) 480-5450; email: nicholss@exchange.nih.gov
Internet: http://grants.nih.gov/grants/guide/rfa-files/RFA-AR-98-001.html
Sponsor: National Institute of Arthritis and Musculoskeletal and Skin Diseases
45 Center Drive, Natcher Building
Bethesda, MD 20892

NIAMS/NICHD Deep Infections of Total Joint Replacements **2481**

This PA seeks to stimulate the receipt of a broad range of basic science and clinical studies to better understand the pathophysiology, diagnosis, and treatment of deep infections around total joint replacement implants. PA: PA-00-014
Requirements: Applications may be submitted by domestic and foreign, for-profit and nonprofit organizations, both public and private; units of state and local governments; and eligible agencies of the federal government.
Contact: Dr. James Panagis, Director, Orthopaedics Program, NIAMS, (301) 594-5055; fax: (301) 480-4543; email: jp149d@nih.gov; Dr. Ralph Nitkin, NICHD, (301) 402-2242; fax: (301) 402-0832; email: rn21e@nih.gov
Internet: http://grants.nih.gov/grants/guide/pa-files/PA-00-014.html
Sponsor: National Institute of Arthritis and Musculoskeletal and Skin Diseases
6500 Center Drive, Natcher Building
Bethesda, MD 20892

NICHD Central Nervous System Effects of HIV Infection: Neurobiological, Neurovirological, and Neurobehavioral Studies Grants **2482**

NIMH, NINDS, NIAAA, and NIDA, invites applications for support of research focused on determining the pathogenic mechanisms involved in Human Immunodeficiency Virus (HIV)-1 associated neurobehavioral and neurological dysfunction in domestic and international settings. The objective of this cooperative effort is to foster investigations that will provide the foundation for the rapid development of therapeutic interventions to prevent and treat the effects of HIV-1 on the central nervous system (CNS). Applications ranging from basic research to clinical diagnosis and treatment are of interest. Multidisciplinary research teams and collaborative alliances are encouraged but not required. Applications will be accepted under PHS receipt dates for AIDS applications. PA: PA-04-154
Requirements: Applications may be submitted by domestic and foreign, for-profit and nonprofit organizations, both public and private; units of state and local governments; and eligible agencies of the federal government.
Amount of Grant: $375,000 maximum
Contact: Dr. Jeymohan Joseph, (301) 443-3012; fax: (301) 443-9719; email: jjeymoha@mail.nih.gov
Internet: http://grants.nih.gov/grants/guide/pa-files/PA-04-154.html
Sponsor: National Institute of Child Health and Human Development
6100 Executive Boulevard
Bethesda, MD 20892

NICHD Clinical Trial Planning Grants for Pediatric Rehabilitation **2483**

The purpose of this grant is to provide support for the organization of an effective research group and development of elements essential for a successful clinical trial. Applications may address the development of activities relevant to such elements as plans for recruitment of patients, experimental design and protocols, testing of procedures, data management, analysis techniques, facilities, administrative procedures, and collaborative arrangements. Detailed information regarding the rationale for the clinical trial based on preclinical and preliminary clinical research must be included in the application. Annual deadline dates may change; contact program staff for exact dates. RFA: HD-01-006
Requirements: Applications may be submitted by foreign and domestic, for-profit and nonprofit organizations, both public and private; units of state and local governments; and eligible agencies of the federal government.
Restrictions: Clinical trial planning support is for new projects and may not be used to supplement research projects already being supported or to provide interim support of projects under review.
Amount of Grant: $75,000 maximum
Contact: Dr. Beth Ansel, Director, Clinical Practices Research Program, (301) 402-2242; fax: (301) 402-0832; email: Beth_Ansel@nih.gov
Internet: http://grants.nih.gov/grants/guide/rfa-files/RFA-HD-01-006.html
Sponsor: National Institute of Child Health and Human Development
6100 Executive Boulevard
Bethesda, MD 20892

NICHD Cooperative Specialized Infertility Research Centers **2484**

The objective of this program is to expedite the development of new approaches for the diagnosis and treatment of human male or female infertility. Annual deadline dates may vary; contact program staff for exact dates. RFA: HD-01-001
Requirements: Applications may be submitted by domestic for-profit and nonprofit organizations, both public and private; units of state and local governments; and eligible agencies of the federal government.
Amount of Grant: $3 million total
Contact: Dr. Louis DePaolo, Reproductive Sciences Branch, (301) 435-6970; fax: (301) 496-0962; email: ld38p@nih.gov
Internet: http://grants.nih.gov/grants/guide/rfa-files/RFA-HD-01-001.html
Sponsor: National Institute of Child Health and Human Development
6100 Executive Boulevard
Bethesda, MD 20892

NICHD Innovative Therapies and Clinical Studies for Screenable Disorders Grants **2485**

This Funding Opportunity Announcement (FOA) issued by the National Institute of Child Health and Human Development (NICHD), the National Institute on Deafness and Other Communication Disorders (NIDCD), and the National Institute of Diabetes and Digestive and Kidney Diseases (NIDDK), National Institutes of Health (NIH), solicit applications for research relevant to the basic understanding and development of therapeutic interventions for currently screened conditions and high priority genetic conditions for which screening could be possible in the near future. Because the nature and scope of the proposed research will vary from application to application, it is anticipated that the size and duration of each award will also vary. The total amount awarded and the number of awards will depend upon the numbers, quality, duration, and costs of the applications received.

Requirements: Application can be made by the following institutions and organizations: public/state controlled institutions of higher education; private institutions of higher education; nonprofits with 501(c)3 IRS status (other than institutions of higher education); nonprofits without 501(c)3 IRS status (other than institutions of higher education); small businesses; for-profit organizations (other than small businesses); state governments; U.S. territories or possessions; Indian/Native American tribal governments (federally recognized); Indian/Native American tribal governments (other than Federally recognized); Indian/Native American tribally designated organizations; non-domestic (non-U.S.) entities (foreign organizations); Hispanic-serving institutions; historically Black colleges and universities (HBCUs); tribally controlled colleges and universities (TCCUs); Alaska Native and Native Hawaiian serving institutions; regional organization; eligible agencies of the Federal government; and faith-based or community based organizations.

Date(s) Application is Due: Feb 5; Mar 5; Jun 5; Jul 5; Oct 5; Nov 5

Contact: Gilian Engelson; (301) 451-2137; fax: (301) 451-5512; email: engelsong@mail.nih.gov

Internet: http://grants.nih.gov/grants/guide/pa-files/PAR-07-184.html

Sponsor: National Institute of Child Health and Human Development (NICHD)
6100 Executive Boulevard, Room 4A05E, MSC 7510
Bethesda, MD 20892-7510

NICHD Low-Back Pain and Common Spinal Disorders Research Grants **2486**

The program is sponsored by NIAMS, NICHD, NINDS, and NIOSH at the CDC. This initiative invites applications directed to the study of the pathogenesis, epidemiology, prevention, and treatment of three common causes of low-back pain: herniated nucleus pulposus, spinal stenosis, and idiopathic low-back pain. The support mechanism for grants in this area will be the individual investigator-initiated research grant (R01). Information may be obtained electronically through the NIH grant line (301-402-2221), the NIH Web site, and by mail and email. PA-97-058

Requirements: Applications may be submitted by foreign and domestic, for-profit and nonprofit organizations, both public and private; units of state and local governments; and eligible agencies of the federal government.

Restrictions: Foreign institutions or organizations in foreign countries are not eligible.

Contact: Dr. Stephen Tuel, National Center for Medical and Rehabilitation Research, (301) 402-2242; fax: (301) 402-0832; email: tuels@hd01.nichd.nih.gov

Internet: http://www.grants.nih.gov/grants/guide/pa-files/PA-97-058.html

Sponsor: National Institute of Child Health and Human Development
6100 Executive Boulevard
Bethesda, MD 20892

NICHD Medical Rehabilitation Research **2487**

This program announcement invites qualified researchers to submit grant applications for research on restoring, replacing, or enhancing the function of adults and children with disabilities. Medical rehabilitation research is directed towards restoration and improvement of functional capability lost as a consequence of injury, disease, or congenital disorders. The mission of the NCMRR is to increase the effectiveness of medical rehabilitation practices through research on improving functional mobility; promoting behavioral adaptation to functional losses; assessing the efficacy and outcomes of medical rehabilitation therapies and practices; developing improved assistive technology; understanding whole body system responses to physical impairments and functional changes; developing more precise methods to measure impairments, disabilities, and societal and functional limitations; and training research scientists in the field of medical rehabilitation.

Requirements: Applications for research project grants (R01) may be submitted by domestic and foreign, for-profit and nonprofit organizations, both public and private; units of state or local governments; and eligible agencies of the federal government.

Contact: Dr. Louis Quatrano, Behavioral Sciences and Rehabilitation Engineering Program, (301) 402-2242; email: lq2n@nih.gov

Internet: http://www.grants.nih.gov/grants/guide/pa-files/PA-99-041.html

Sponsor: National Institute of Child Health and Human Development
6100 Executive Boulevard
Rockville, MD 20852

NICHD NRSAs—Individual **2488**

The program offers health scientists with doctoral degrees the opportunity to receive full-time research training in areas that reflect the national need for biomedical and behavioral research on specific programs of mothers and children and population and reproductive research. Areas of concentration include pregnancy and infancy, developmental biology and nutrition, learning and behavior, mental retardation, fertility-infertility, fertility regulation, nutrition and reproduction, social and behavioral aspects of reproduction, and population change. These fellowships may not be used for study leading to an MD, DO, DDS, or similar degree, or for the support of residency training. Awardees are subject to the payback provisions of the NRSA by which one year of research or teaching, or acceptable combination thereof, is required for each year of support, except for the first 12 months, which are free of the payback obligation.

Requirements: Universities, colleges, medical, dental, and nursing schools and schools of public health, laboratories, hospitals, state and local health departments, other for-profit public or private institutions, and individuals may apply for research grants. NRSA support is provided for academic and research training only, in health and health-related areas that are periodically specified by the NIH. SBIR grants can be awarded only to domestic small businesses. STTR grants can be awarded only to domestic small business concerns that partner with research institutions in cooperative research and development.

Date(s) Application is Due: Apr 5; Aug 5; Dec 5

Contact: NICHD Office of Program & Public Liaison, (301) 496-0536 or (301) 435-3447

Internet: http://www.nichd.nih.gov/funding/funding.htm

Sponsor: National Institute of Child Health and Human Development
Building 31 Room 2A32, MSC 2425, 31 Center Drive
Bethesda, MD 20892-2425

NICHD NRSAs—Institutional **2489**

Awards provide opportunities for research training in the biological and/or behavioral science aspects of child health and human development. Primary concern in awarding institution awards will be given to multidisciplinary or interdisciplinary programs that cannot be provided through individual fellowships. Although major concern is for postdoctoral training, predoctoral training will be considered where a special case for support can be justified. In the Center for Research for Mothers and Children, areas covered include pregnancy and infancy, developmental biology and nutrition, learning and behavior, and mental retardation. In the Center for Population Research, areas covered include fertility-infertility, fertility regulation, nutrition and reproduction, social and behavioral aspects of reproduction, and population change. The training program director at the grantee institution will be responsible for the selection and appointment of trainees and for the overall direction of the program. These grants are not made for study leading to the MD, DDS, DVM, or other similar health professional degrees. Trainees are subject to the payback provisions of the NRSA by which one year of research or teaching, or acceptable combination thereof, is required for each year of support, except for the first 12 months, which are free of payback obligation.

Requirements: Universities; colleges; medical, dental, and nursing schools and schools of public health; laboratories; hospitals; state and local health departments; other for-profit public or private institutions; and individuals may apply for research grants. NRSA support is provided for academic and research training only, in health and health-related areas that are periodically specified by the National Institutes of Health. SBIR grants can be awarded only to domestic small businesses. STTR grants can be awarded only to domestic small business concerns that partner with research institutions in cooperative research and development.

Date(s) Application is Due: May 10

Contact: NICHD Office of Program & Public Liaison, (301) 496-0536 or (301) 435-3447

Internet: http://www.nichd.nih.gov/funding/funding.htm

Sponsor: National Institute of Child Health and Human Development
Building 31 Room 2A32, MSC 2425, 31 Center Drive
Bethesda, MD 20892-2425

NICHD Population Research Grants **2490**

The objective of the program is to seek solutions to the fundamental problems of the reproductive processes; to strive to develop and evaluate safer and more effective contraceptives; and to understand how population structure and change affect the health and well-being of individuals and society. The Center for Population Research supports biomedical research in the reproductive sciences, clinical and epidemiological studies of contraceptives and the risk of sexually transmitted diseases (STDs) including HIV, and behavioral and demographic studies on population processes and structure. Mechanisms are projects grants, small business innovation research (SBIR) grants, small business technology transfer (STIR) grants, and individual fellowships (NRSAs).

Requirements: Project grants: Universities, colleges, medical, dental, and nursing schools, and schools of public health; laboratories, hospitals, state and local health departments, and other nonprofit or for-profit public or private institutions; and individuals. NRSAs: Individuals with a professional or scientific degree are eligible (MD, PhD, DDS, DO, DVM, ScD, DEng, or equivalent domestic or foreign degree). SBIR and STIR grants can be awarded only to domestic small businesses (entities that are independently owned and operated for profit, are not dominant in the field in which research is proposed, and have no more than 500 employees).

Amount of Grant: $50,000-$5 million range; $318,200 average

Date(s) Application is Due: Feb 1; Jun 1; Oct 1

Contact: Dr. Florence Haseltine, Director, Center for Population Research, (301) 496-1101; fax: (301) 496-0962; email: haseltif@mail.nih.gov

Internet: http://www.nichd.nih.gov/cpr

Sponsor: National Institute of Child Health and Human Development
6100 Executive Boulevard, Executive Building
Bethesda, MD 20892

NICHD Repetitive Motion Disorders Research Grants **2491**

The program is sponsored by NIAMS, NICHD, NINDS, and NIOSH at the CDC. This initiative invites applications directed to the study of the pathogenesis, epidemiology, prevention, and treatment of repetitive motion disorders. The support mechanism for grants in this area will be the individual investigator-initiated research grant (R01). Information may be obtained electronically through the NIH grant line (301-402-2221), the NIH Web site, and by mail and email. PA-97-059

Requirements: Applications may be submitted by foreign and domestic, for-profit and nonprofit organizations, both public and private; units of state and local governments; and eligible agencies of the federal government.

Restrictions: Foreign institutions or organizations in foreign countries are not eligible.

Contact: Dr. Stephen Tuel, National Center for Medical and Rehabilitation Research, (301) 402-2242; fax: (301) 402-0832; email: tuels@hd01.nichd.nih.gov

Internet: http://www.grants.nih.gov/grants/guide/pa-files/PA-97-059.html

Sponsor: National Institute of Child Health and Human Development
6100 Executive Boulevard, Executive Building
Bethesda, MD 20892

NICHD Research on Musculoskeletal Fitness and Sports Medicine Grants 2492

NIAMS and NINR invite investigator-initiated research grant applications to study a broad range of basic and clinical topics related to musculoskeletal fitness, exercise physiology, and sports medicine. The National Center for Medical Rehabilitation Research of NICHD encourages applications for both basic and clinical studies of musculoskeletal fitness and exercise physiology of persons with physical disabilities. PA: PA-97-025

Requirements: Applications may be submitted by domestic and foreign, for-profit organizations, both public and private; units of state or local governments; and eligible agencies of the federal government.

Contact: Dr. Danuta Krotoski, National Center for Medical Rehabilitation Research, (301) 402-2242; email: krotoskd@hd01.nichd.nih.gov

Internet: http://www.grants.nih.gov/grants/guide/pa-files/PA-97-025.html

Sponsor: National Institute of Child Health and Human Development
6100 Executive Boulevard
Bethesda, MD 20892

NICHD Ruth L. Kirschstein National Research Service Award Institutiona Predoctoral Training Program in Systems Biology of Developmental Biology & Birth Defects 2493 1

The objective of this NRSA T32 program is to provide research training to predoctoral students interested in establishing research careers that use systems biology approaches to study developmental biology and the formation of structural birth defects. Stipends are provided as a subsistence allowance to help defray trainees' living expenses during the research training experience. Funds are provided to offset the cost of tuition and fees. The NIH provides 60% of the combined requested costs, up to $16,000 annually per Ph.D. student, and up to $21,000 annually for students in formal programs leading to combined professional and Ph.D. degrees. Letters of Intent are due by April 25, with full applications due May 25.

Requirements: The following organizations are eligible to apply: public/state controlled institutions of higher education; private institutions of higher education; nonprofits with 501(c)3 IRS status (other than institutions of higher education); nonprofits without 501(c)3 IRS status (other than institutions of higher education); for-profit organizations (other than small businesses); state governments; U.S. territories or possessions; Indian/Native American tribal governments (Federally recognized); Hispanic-serving institutions; historically Black colleges and universities (HBCUs); tribally controlled colleges and universities (TCCUs); Alaska Natives and Native Hawaiians serving institutions; regional organizations; eligible agencies of the federal government; faith-based or community based organizations.

Date(s) Application is Due: Apr 25; May 25

Contact: James Coulombe, Ph.D.; (301) 496-5541; fax: (301) 480-0303; email: coulombej@mail.nih.gov

Internet: http://grants.nih.gov/grants/guide/pa-files/PAR-08-054.html

Sponsor: National Institute of Child Health and Human Development (NICHD)
6100 Executive Boulevard, 4B01 MSC 7510
Bethesda, MD 20892-7510

NICHD Small Grants Program 2494

Applications for these small grants may be submitted by new or more established investigators for support of research in any scientific area relevant to the institute's programs in the Center for Population Research, the Center for Research for Mothers and Children, or the National Center for Medical Rehabilitation Research. Although proposals may involve a wide variety of biomedical, biobehavioral, or clinical disciplines, relevance to the mission of NICHD must be clear. Deadline dates are February 1, June 1, or October 1 for new applications; March 1, or July 1, or November 1 for revised applications. Additional information may be obtained by mail and email, or through the NIH grant line (301-402-2221), and the NIH Web site. PA: PAR-99-126

Requirements: Applications may be submitted by domestic, for-profit and nonprofit organizations, both public and private; units of state and local governments; and eligible agencies of the federal government.

Restrictions: Foreign institutions and organizations are not eligible.

Amount of Grant: $50,000 for one year; $100,000 for two years

Date(s) Application is Due: Feb 1; Jun 1; Oct 1

Contact: Program Contact, (301) 435-0714; email: grantsinfo@nih.gov

Internet: http://grants.nih.gov/grants/guide/pa-files/PAR-99-126.html

Sponsor: National Institute of Child Health and Human Development
6100 Executive Boulevard, Executive Building
Bethesda, MD 20892

NICHD Socioeconomic Status and Health Across the Life Course 2495

NHLBI, NIA, NICHD, NIEHS, and NIMH seek research grant applications on the cumulative and contemporaneous relationships between socioeconomic status (SES) and physical and mental health and functioning over the life course and across generations. Given that the relationships between SES and physical and mental health, morbidity, disability, and mortality have been long and extensively documented, additional studies aimed at merely describing or demonstrating these relationships are outside the scope of this program announcement. Encouraged are studies relating to appropriate conceptualization and measurement of SES over the life course, across generations, and in various population groups; specification of the processes through which SES influences cumulatively and contemporaneously physical and mental health, disability, morbidity, and mortality outcomes over the life course, and how these outcomes, in turn, impact on SES; the relationship between SES and physical and mental health, disability, morbidity, and mortality over the life course in various population groups. PA: PA-98-098

Requirements: Applications may be submitted by public and private, foreign and domestic for-profit and nonprofit organizations, and eligible agencies of the federal government.

Contact: Dr. Rose Maria Li, Center for Population Research, (301) 496-1174; fax: (301) 496-0962; email: Rose_Li@nih.gov

Internet: http://www.grants.nih.gov/grants/guide/pa-files/PA-98-098.html

Sponsor: National Institute of Child Health and Human Development
6100 Executive Boulevard
Bethesda, MD 20892

NICHD Symptom Management for Chronic Neurological Conditions Research Grants 2496

NINR, NIA, NICHD, NIDCD, and NINDS are interested in facilitating investigator-initiated research designed to deal with symptoms associated with chronic neurological conditions including stroke, epilepsy, brain and spinal cord injury, multiple sclerosis, and Parkinson's disease. The overall goals are to manage symptoms effectively, to prevent secondary effects of the condition when possible, to maximize the health potential, and to improve the health-related quality of life for patients, caregivers, and families. The mechanism of support is the research project grant (R01). Information may be obtained through the NIH grant line (301-402-2221), the NIH Web site, mail, and email. PA-98-030

Requirements: Research applications may be submitted by domestic and foreign, for-profit and nonprofit organizations, both public and private; units of state and local governments; and eligible agencies of the federal government.

Contact: Dr. Louis Quatrano, National Center for Medical Rehabilitation Research, (301) 402-2242; fax: (301) 402-0832; email: LQ2N@nih.gov; Mary Ellen Colvin, Grants Management Branch, (301) 496-1303; fax: (301) 402-0915; email: MC113B@nih.gov

Internet: http://www.grants.nih.gov/grants/guide/pa-files/PA-98-030.html

Sponsor: National Institute of Child Health and Human Development
6100 Executive Boulevard, Executive Building
Bethesda, MD 20892

Nicholas H. Noyes Jr. Memorial Foundation Grants 2497

The foundation awards grants to eligible Indiana nonprofit organizations in its areas of interest, including arts and culture, education from early childhood through higher education, disadvantaged, museums, social services, health, hospitals, family services, performing arts, and youth. Types of support include general operating support, endowment funds, and scholarship funds.

Requirements: Proposals are welcomed, and encouraged, to be submitted at any time after January 1st for the first funding cycle or after June 1st for the final funding cycle. Submit the following with your proposal: thirteen copies of the complete grant application (available at the foundations website or office) including attachments (i.e. applicable budget(s) as required). You may recreate the application form for ease in completing, but please limit your response to the space provided and use a minimum font of 12. It is also require that you use both sides of the paper i.e. side one is page 1 with page 2 on the flip-side etc.; one copy of your organization's 501(c)3 tax determination letter from the IRS; one copy of your organization's most recent audited financial statement for all organizations requesting $25,000 or more.

Restrictions: Organizations may apply only one time in any calendar year. The Foundation does not make grants to individuals. The principle geographic region served by the Noyes Foundation is the greater Indianapolis area. If you intend to request a grant in excess of $50,000, please contact the Foundation's Program Officer before submitting your grant request.

Geographic Focus: Indiana

Amount of Grant: $150,000 maximum

Date(s) Application is Due: Feb 1; Aug 29

Contact: Kelly Mills, Executive Administrator; (317) 844-8009; fax: (317) 844-8099; email: kmills@noyesfoundation.org

Internet: http://www.noyesfoundation.org

Sponsor: Nicholas H. Noyes Jr. Memorial Foundation
1950 E Greyhound Pass, No 18
Carmel, IN 46033-7730

NIDA Behavioral Science Track Awards for Rapid Transition 2498

NIDA invites newly independent investigators to submit applications for small-scale, exploratory (i.e., pilot) research projects related to NIDA's behavioral sciences mission. The award (B/START-NIDA) provides rapid review and funding decisions of applications. Experimentally based research applications are encouraged across a wide variety of behavioral factors in drug abuse, including neurocognitive, cognitive, and perceptual processes; psychosocial; and more broadly motivational, social, and community factors in drug abuse. Given the role that drug abuse plays in HIV/AIDS transmission, studies applying basic behavioral science models and methods to address this issue are especially encouraged. More information may be obtained by mail and email or through the NIH grant line (301-402-2221), and the NIH Web site. PAR-03-146

Amount of Grant: $50,000 maximum

Contact: Gary Fleming, Grants Management Branch, (301) 443-6710

Internet: http://grants2.nih.gov/grants/guide/pa-files/PAR-03-146.html

Sponsor: National Institute on Drug Abuse
5600 Fishers Ln, Parklawn Building
Rockville, MD 20857

NIDA Behavioral Therapies Development Program Grants 2499

The purpose of the program is to reaffirm NIDA's continued and ongoing commitment to a major program of research on behavioral therapies for drug abuse and dependence. The term behavioral therapy is used here in a broad sense and includes various forms of psychotherapy, behavior therapy, cognitive therapy, family therapy, skills training, counseling, and other rehabilitative therapies. Behavioral therapy research has been conceptualized, for the purposes of this initiative, to consist of three stages. Stage I, or early therapy development, involves research on the development, refinement, and pilot testing of behavioral interventions. Stage I includes research aimed at translating basic behavioral and cognitive research into novel behavioral therapies. Stage II involves the efficacy testing of therapies that show promise and includes research on the hypothesized mechanisms through which these therapies may have their effect. Stage III is research aimed at determining if and how efficacious behavioral therapies may be transported to community settings, including primary care sites. Stage III includes research examining methods of training therapists and counselors to administer new behavioral therapies. PA: PA-03-066

Requirements: Applications may be submitted by domestic and foreign, for-profit and nonprofit organizations, both public and private; units of state and local government; and eligible agencies of the federal government.

Amount of Grant: $100,000 maximum per year

Contact: Gary Fleming, NIDA, Grants Management Branch, (301) 443-6710; fax: (301) 594-6849; email: GF6S@NIH.GOV

Internet: http://grants2.nih.gov/grants/guide/pa-files/PA-03-066.html

Sponsor: National Institute on Drug Abuse
6001 Executive Boulevard, Executive Building
Bethesda, MD 20892

NIDA Clinical Research Education Programs in Drug Abuse and Addiction 2500

Grants support educational programs developing the research skills of investigators who wish to focus on clinical, prevention, health services, or treatment issues in drug abuse; or developing a cadre of clinical drug abuse experts proficient in the use of research findings (for example, in public health, behavioral science, or medicine) to develop or implement early detection, diagnosis, treatment, or prevention interventions. This latter category would also include applications of health services research findings. Programs that address both of these aims are particularly desired. NIDA will grant awards to eligible institutions to develop or enhance research training opportunities for individuals, selected by the institution, who are training for careers as researchers, as clinicians (broadly defined), or (ideally) as a combination of the two. Educational partnerships between research institutions and drug abuse treatment organizations are highly encouraged in order to broaden research training and educational opportunities and as a result, increase the number of well-trained clinical and health services researchers in the field. Contact program staff for deadline dates. PA: PAR-04-054

Requirements: Applications may be submitted by domestic, for-profit and nonprofit organizations, both public and private; units of state and local governments; and eligible agencies of the federal government; All students must be U.S. citizens, nationals, or lawfully admitted permanent residents of the United States. Predoctoral students must have an MS, MSW, or equivalent degree in biostatistics, nursing, psychology, or other social sciences as a prerequisite to pursuing a doctorate degree.

Restrictions: This award will not support a master's degree for a predoctoral student.

Amount of Grant: $350,000 maximum

Contact: Gary Fleming, Chief, Grants Management Officer, (301) 443-6710; fax: (301) 594-6847; email: gf6s@nih.gov

Internet: http://grants.nih.gov/grants/guide/pa-files/PAR-04-054.html

Sponsor: National Institute on Drug Abuse
6101 Executive Boulevard, Suite 242, MSC 8403
Bethesda, MD 20892-8403

NIDA Cutting-Edge Basic Research Awards (CEBRA) 2501

The goal of this program is to foster highly innovative or conceptually creative research that advances our understanding of drug abuse and addiction and how to prevent and treat them. It is specifically designed to support research that is high-risk and potentially high-impact and that is underrepresented or not included in NIDA's current portfolio. The program is aimed at experienced drug abuse research investigators who wish to develop or adapt new methods or techniques and at new investigators or scientists with expertise in fields other than drug abuse who wish to establish new programs in drug abuse research. PA: PAR-01-047

Requirements: Applications may be submitted by domestic and foreign, for-profit and nonprofit organizations, both public and private; units of state and local governments; and eligible agencies of the federal government.

Restrictions: Amended R21 applications for CEBRA will not be accepted.

Amount of Grant: $1 million total; $100,000 maximum for Stage I awards

Contact: Dr. Rebekah Rasooly, (301) 443-6300; fax: (301) 594-6043; email: rr185i@nih.gov

Internet: http://grants.nih.gov/grants/guide/pa-files/PAR-01-047.html

Sponsor: National Institute on Drug Abuse
6001 Executive Boulevard
Bethesda, MD 20892

NIDA Drug Abuse Dissertation Research: Epidemiology, Prevention, Treatment, Services, and Women and Gender Differences 2502

NIDA announces the availability of small grants (R03) to support drug abuse doctoral dissertation research in epidemiology, prevention, treatment, services, and women and sex/gender differences, areas in which there is a significant need for new investigators. Grant support is designed to encourage doctoral candidates from a variety of academic disciplines and programs to conduct research in these areas of interest to NIDA. It is hoped that this program will ultimately facilitate the entry of promising new investigators into the field of drug abuse research. PA: PAR-05-083

Requirements: The applicant investigator must be enrolled in an accredited doctoral degree program in the behavioral, biomedical, or social sciences and must be conducting or intending to conduct research in one of the areas specified. The applicant must be a registered doctoral candidate student. All requirements for the doctoral degree other than the dissertation and clinical internship, if applicable, must be completed by the time of the award. This information and the approval of the dissertation topic by a named committee must be verified in a letter of certification from the thesis chairperson and submitted with the grant application. The applicant institution administering the grant on behalf of the proposed applicant must be domestic. Applications may be submitted by any public or private nonprofit university, college, or professional school. The doctoral candidate must be a citizen or noncitizen national of the United States or hold a permanent residence visa.

Restrictions: An applicant who receives support for dissertation research under a grant from NIDA may not hold concurrently another federally sponsored fellowship or similar Federal award, such as a National Research Service Award (NRSA) that provides a stipend or otherwise duplicates provisions of this grant program.

Contact: Gary Fleming, (301) 443-6710; fax: (301) 594-6849; email: gfleming@nida.nih.gov

Internet: http://grants.nih.gov/grants/guide/pa-files/PAR-05-083.html

Sponsor: National Institute on Drug Abuse
5600 Fishers Ln, Parklawn Building
Rockville, MD 20857

NIDA Drug Addiction Neuroscience Research Grants 2503

The intent of this program announcement is to continue to encourage investigator interest in the wide range of neuroscience research relevant to drug abuse, drug dependence, and drug addiction supported by NIDA. The research relevant to this announcement does not involve human subjects; for information about the neuroscience research program involving human subjects, contact Dr. Joseph Frascella, (301) 443-4877, jf80t@nih.gov. The scientific understanding gained by this research is anticipated ultimately to be applicable to improved treatment and prevention of drug abuse and drug addiction, and their consequences. The specific research topics emphasized in this program announcement are animal models to study the neurobiology of addiction; vulnerability to drug addiction; neuroadaptation and neurotoxicity; developmental neurobiology; drugs and learning, memory, and cognition; pain and analgesia; drug effects on sensory and perceptual systems; drugs of abuse; sleep and circadian rhythms; neuropsychopharmacology of drugs of abuse; and central nervous system (CNS) interaction with other systems. Contact the program officer for deadline dates. PA: PA-02-085

Requirements: Applications may be submitted by public and private, domestic and foreign, for-profit and nonprofit organizations, units of state and local governments, and eligible agencies of the federal government. Racial/ethnic minority individuals, women, and persons with disabilities are encouraged to apply as principal investigators.

Contact: Dr. Roger Brown, Division of Basic Research, (301) 443-1887; fax: (301) 594-6043; email: rb99w@nih.gov

Internet: http://grants2.nih.gov/grants/guide/pa-files/PA-02-085.html

Sponsor: National Institute on Drug Abuse
6100 Executive Boulevard, Executive Building
Rockville, MD 20892

NIDA HIV Drug Therapy for HIV Users: Access, Adherence, Effectiveness 2504

NIDA invites applications for research on access, adherence, and effectiveness relevant to the treatment of drug users with HIV. This initiative supports research on a broad range of HIV care-related issues, including, but not limited to, access issues related to receipt of HIV-related treatment and outreach strategies to improve access; factors influencing initiation of HIV treatment and long-term adherence to HIV treatment regimens; and the development of intervention strategies to improve use of and adherence to complex medical regimens in a variety of settings. Annual deadline dates may vary; contact program staff for exact dates. RFA: DA-00-007

Requirements: Applications may be submitted by domestic and foreign for-profit and nonprofit organizations, both public and private; units of state and local governments; and eligible agencies of the federal government.

Amount of Grant: $3 million total

Contact: Dr. Elizabeth Lambert, (301) 402-1933; fax: (301) 443-4100; email: el46i@nih.gov

Internet: http://grants.nih.gov/grants/guide/rfa-files/RFA-DA-00-007.html

Sponsor: National Institute on Drug Abuse
5600 Fishers Ln, Parklawn Building
Rockville, MD 20857

NIDA International Studies on Drug Abuse and HIV/AIDS 2505

This program invites applications for international, cross-disciplinary research on HIV/AIDS, other blood-borne infections [i.e., hepatitis B virus (HBV), hepatitis C virus (HCV)], tuberculosis (TB), and comorbid conditions and consequences in injecting and noninjecting drug users, their sexual partners, and their children. This RFA is intended to build on lessons learned in developed countries in response to the intertwined epidemics of drug abuse and the spread of HIV/AIDS and other infectious diseases. It seeks to foster cross-national and international research collaborations that, through both independent research and the recruitment, training, and mentoring of new, multi-disciplinary researchers, lead to the development, adaptation, replication, and evaluation of effective interventions and approaches to slow or reverse the spread of HIV and other infections in vulnerable drug-using populations. Annual deadline dates may vary; contact program staff for exact dates. RFA: DA-01-006

Requirements: Applications may be submitted by domestic and foreign for-profit and nonprofit organizations, both public and private; units of state and local governments; and eligible agencies of the federal government.

Amount of Grant: $1.5 million total

Contact: Helen Cesari, Center on AIDS and Other Medical Consequences of Drug Abuse, (301) 402-1918; fax: (301) 443-4100; email: hc30x@nih.gov

Internet: http://grants.nih.gov/grants/guide/rfa-files/RFA-DA-01-006.html

Sponsor: National Institute on Drug Abuse
6001 Executive Boulevard
Bethesda, MD 20892

NIDA Medications Development for Cannabis-Related Disorder **2506**

This program seeks grant applications focusing on the identification, evaluation, and development of safe and effective pharmacological treatments for cannabis-related disorders (CRDs), such as cannabis abuse or dependence, and cannabis-induced disorders (e.g., intoxication, delirium, psychotic disorder, and anxiety disorder), and their comorbidity with other medical and psychiatric disorders (e.g., depression), with special interest in the treatment of children and adolescents. Cannabis use includes marijuana, hashish, and other tetrahydrocannabinol (THC) containing substances. This RFA will support clinical trials to test potential medications in humans, and the preclinical development of new chemical entities (NCEs) for advancement to the clinical development stage. Applications may focus on the pharmacotherapy of cannabis abuse and they may target one or various CRDs or clinical manifestations of the disorders. Annual deadline dates may vary; contact program staff for exact dates. RFA-DA-04-014

Requirements: Applications may be submitted by domestic and foreign, for-profit and nonprofit organizations, both public and private; units of state and local governments; and eligible agencies of the federal government.

Contact: Gary Fleming, Grants Management Branch, (301) 443-6710; fax: (301) 594-6847; email: gf6s@nih.gov

Internet: http://www.grants.nih.gov/grants/guide/rfa-files/RFA-DA-04-014.html

Sponsor: National Institute on Drug Abuse
6101 Executive Boulevard
Bethesda, MD 20892-8403

NIDA Mentored Clinical Scientist Research Career Development Awards **2507**

The overall objective of the NIH Research Career Development Award program is to prepare qualified individuals for careers that have a significant impact on the health-related research needs of the Nation. The objective of the NIH Mentored Clinical Scientist Research Career Development Award (K08) program is to support didactic study and mentored research for individuals with clinical doctoral degrees (e.g., M.D., D.D.S., D.M.D., D.O., D.C., O.D., N.D., D.V.M., Pharm.D., or Ph.D. in clinical disciplines). The purpose of this Funding Opportunity Announcement (FOA) is to continue the long-standing NIH support of the K08 program. This award provides support and protected time for an intensive, mentored research career development experience in biomedical or behavioral research, including translational research. For the purpose of this award, translational research is defined as application of basic research discoveries toward the diagnosis, management, and prevention of human disease.

Requirements: The following organizations and institutions may apply: public/state controlled institutions of higher education; private institutions of higher education; Hispanic-serving institutions; historically Black colleges and universities (HBCUs); tribally controlled colleges and universities (TCCUs); Alaska native and native Hawaiian serving institutions; nonprofits with 501(c)3 IRS status; nonprofits without 501(c)3 IRS status; small businesses; for-profit organizations; State governments; regional organizations; U.S. territories or possessions; Indian/Native American tribal governments; Indian/Native American tribally designated organizations; county governments; city or township governments; special district governments; independent school districts; public housing authorities/Indian housing authorities; eligible agencies of the Federal government; and faith-based or community based organizations.

Amount of Grant: $90,000 salary maximum per yer plus fringe benefits; $50,000 for research support

Date(s) Application is Due: Feb 12; Mar 12; Jun 12; Jul 12; Oct 12; Nov 12

Contact: Mimi M. Ghim, Ph.D.; (301) 443-6071; email: ghimm@mail.nih.gov;; Carol Alderson; (301) 594-5614; email: ca10h@nih.gov

Internet: http://grants.nih.gov/grants/guide/pa-files/PA-09-042.html#SectionIII

Sponsor: National Institute on Drug Abuse (NIDA)
6001 Executive Boulevard, Room 5232, MSC 9591
Bethesda, MD 20892

NIDA Microarray-Based Research on Drug Abuse **2508**

With this announcement, NIDA plans to develop a strong, multidisciplinary basic research program—drawing from neuroscience, genetics, behavioral science, bioengineering, and computational biology—aimed at adapting and applying microarray techniques to the general problem of drug abuse. Eventually, it is anticipated that the identification of genes and gene products that may underlie the process of addiction will provide new targets for the development of new medications and therapies for drug abuse. Annual deadline dates may vary; contact program staff for exact dates. RFA: DA-00-003

Requirements: Applications may be submitted by domestic and foreign, for-profit and nonprofit organizations, both public and private; units of state and local governments; and eligible agencies of the federal government.

Amount of Grant: $2 million total

Contact: Dr. Rebekah Rasooly, (301) 443-6300; fax: (301) 594-6043; email: rr185i@nih.gov

Internet: http://grants.nih.gov/grants/guide/rfa-files/RFA-DA-00-003.html

Sponsor: National Institute on Drug Abuse
6001 Executive Boulevard
Bethesda, MD 20892

NIDA Minority Institutions Drug Abuse Research Development Grants **2509**

In its efforts to broaden and strengthen drug abuse research in minority institutions, NIDA is initiating MIDARP. Grants will be provided to develop the capacity of minority institutions and their faculty, staff, and students to conduct rigorous drug abuse research in all areas of research supported by NIDA including neuroscience, behavioral, clinical, social science, public health, biological, HIV/AIDS, and health services areas. In addition, this PA seeks to broaden the scientific knowledge base in drug abuse in those areas where minority institutions may have particular interest, knowledge, and commitment. Awards under this PA will use the R24 grant mechanism. Applicants are responsible for the planning, direction, and execution of the proposed projects. The total project period for applications submitted in response to this PA may not exceed five years. PAR-98-001 may be obtained electronically through the NIH Web site, email, and by mail.

Requirements: An applicant institution must be a public or private nonprofit university, four-year college, or other institution with a traditionally high (more than 50 percent) minority student enrollment; an institution with a substantial enrollment of minority students, which provides evidence of efforts to recruit into scientific careers members of ethnic or racial groups who have been found to be underrepresented in biomedical and behavioral research; or a Native American tribe that, in conjunction with one or more institutions of higher learning, offers undergraduate and graduate degrees in ADM disciplines.

Contact: Dr. Lula Beatty, Special Populations Office, (301) 443-0441; fax: (301) 480-8179; email: lb75x@nih.gov; Dr. Pushpa Thadani, Division of Basic Research, (301) 443-6300; fax: (301) 443-6043; email: pt24e@nih.gov; Dr. C. Jamie Biswas, Medications Develop

Internet: http://www.grants.nih.gov/grants/guide/pa-files/PAR-98-001.html

Sponsor: National Institute on Drug Abuse
5600 Fishers Ln, Parklawn Building
Rockville, MD 20857

NIDA National Drug Abuse Treatment Clinical Trials Network **2510**

NIDA invites cooperative agreement applications from established clinical investigators to participate in the National Drug Abuse Treatment Clinical Trials Network (CTN). Awardees will conduct and participate in coordinated multisite clinical trials of behavioral, pharmacological, and combined behavioral/pharmacological therapies for drug abuse and addiction, and conduct research on practices, i.e., studies of factors that impact upon successful adoption of new treatments. The overall goal of the program is to improve the quality of drug abuse treatment throughout the nation, thereby reducing the prevalence, morbidity, and mortality of drug abuse and addiction. Some of the program objectives include supporting studies of behavioral, pharmacological, and combined behavioral and pharmacological treatment interventions of established efficacy in rigorous, multisite clinical trials to determine effectiveness across a broad range of treatment settings and patient populations; encouraging research on the translation of science-based, effective treatment interventions into clinical practice by establishing effectiveness in community-based treatment programs and by determining effective strategies for transporting effective treatments; furthering the development of effective treatments by integrating behavioral, pharmacological, and practice research; investigating the impact of advances in treatment research on community-level treatment practices; and ensuring that treatment research in drug abuse and addiction meets the needs of the wider community, including minorities, women, children, and underserved populations. The complete RFA is available on the Web site. Annual deadline dates may vary; contact a program officer for exact dates. RFA: DA-00-002

Requirements: Applications may be submitted by domestic for-profit and nonprofit organizations, both private and public. Principal investigators should be able to document a substantial history of managing complex research initiatives in clinical sites and have an extensive publication record in clinical research.

Restrictions: Foreign applicants are not eligible, and domestic applications may not include a foreign site.

Amount of Grant: $11 million total

Contact: Dr. Jack Blaine, Division of Clinical and Services Research, (301) 443-0107; fax: (301) 443-8674; email: jb167n@nih.gov; Dr. Betty Tai, Medications Development Division, (301) 443-2397; fax: (301) 443-2599; email: bt26r@nih.gov

Internet: http://grants.nih.gov/grants/guide/rfa-files/RFA-DA-00-002.html

Sponsor: National Institute on Drug Abuse
6001 Executive Boulevard, Executive Building
Bethesda, MD 20892

NIDA Neurobiological and Behavioral Research on Nicotine and Tobacco Products **2511**

The purpose of this PA is to expand the basic science knowledge base on the neurobiological and behavioral effects of nicotine and associated tobacco chemicals, as part of continuing efforts to explain and prevent their use and to develop effective treatments for nicotine addiction. This PA encourages research on any aspect of the effects of nicotine and other tobacco components, using neurobiological, behavioral, or other methods in humans, animals, or in vitro systems, that seeks to explain nicotine use, addiction, or other

effects in humans. This PA solicits research in two general categories, neurobiology and behavioral sciences. Neurobiological, cognitive, behavioral, and social processes, methods, and models are all relevant to this announcement. For both neurobiological and behavioral studies, approaches are encouraged that consider differences in gender, race, ethnicity, and age or developmental stage. PA: PA-00-045
Requirements: Applications may be submitted by domestic and foreign, for-profit and nonprofit organizations, both public and private; units of state and local governments; and eligible agencies of the federal government.
Contact: Dr. Thomas Aigner, Neurobiological Studies, (301) 443-6975; fax: (301) 594-6043; email: ta17r@nih.gov; Dr. Jaylan Turkkan, Cognitive or Behavioral Studies, (301) 443-1263; fax: (301)-594-6043; email: jt58t@nih.gov
Internet: http://grants.nih.gov/grants/guide/pa-files/PA-00-045.html
Sponsor: National Institute on Drug Abuse
6001 Executive Boulevard
Bethesda, MD 20892

NIDA Origins and Pathways to Drug Abuse Research Grants **2512**
The main goal of this PA is to stimulate innovative investigations that enhance our understanding of: drug use patterns and trends within and across populations; interplay of social interactions, social environment, structural context with individual behavioral characteristics and genetic vulnerability; the phenotypic heterogeneity of drug abuse; causal mechanisms leading to onset, maintenance, and remittance of drug abuse, as well as protective mechanisms that reduce the risk of drug abuse; and drug abuse over the life course, including developmental processes that influence drug use trajectories and behavioral, health, and social consequences of drug abuse. In addition, research is encouraged to develop methodologies to improve the accuracy, efficiency, scope, timeliness, and analytic yield of drug abuse epidemiologic data. PA: PA-04-100
Requirements: Applications may be submitted by foreign and domestic, for-profit and nonprofit organizations, both public and private; units of state or local governments; and eligible agencies of the federal government.
Restrictions: Foreign institutions are not eligible for program project or centers (P-Series) awards.
Contact: Gary Fleming, Grants Management, (301) 443-6710; fax: (301) 594-6849; email: gfleming@nida.nih.gov
Internet: http://grants.nih.gov/grants/guide/pa-files/PA-04-100.html
Sponsor: National Institute on Drug Abuse
6001 Executive Boulevard
Bethesda, MD 20892

NIDA Pilot and Feasibility Studies in Preparation for Drug Abuse Prevention Trials **2513**
This FOA for R34 applications seeks to support: pilot and/or feasibility testing of new, revised, or adapted preventive intervention approaches targeting the initiation of drug use, the progression to abuse or dependence, and the acquisition or transmission of HIV infection among diverse populations and settings; and pre-trial feasibility testing for prevention services and systems research.
Requirements: The following organizations and institutions may apply: public/state controlled institutions of higher education; private institutions of higher education; Hispanic-serving institutions; historically Black colleges and universities (HBCUs); tribally controlled colleges and universities (TCCUs); Alaska native and native Hawaiian serving institutions; nonprofits with 501(c)3 IRS status; nonprofits without 501(c)3 IRS status; small businesses; for-profit organizations; State governments; regional organizations; U.S. territories or possessions; Indian/Native American tribal governments; Indian/Native American tribally designated organizations; county governments; city or township governments; special district governments; independent school districts; public housing authorities/Indian housing authorities; eligible agencies of the Federal government; and faith-based or community based organizations.
Restrictions: The NIDA R34 mechanism does not support the development of intervention protocols, manuals, or the standardization of protocols.
Amount of Grant: $225,000 annually; $450,00 maximum for three years
Date(s) Application is Due: Feb 16; Jun 16; Oct 16
Contact: Aleta Meyer, Ph.D.; (301) 402-1725; fax: (301) 443-2636; email: meyera2@nida.nih.gov
Internet: http://grants.nih.gov/grants/guide/pa-files/PA-09-146.html
Sponsor: National Institute on Drug Abuse (NIDA)
6001 Executive Boulevard, Room 5170
Bethesda, MD 20892

NIDA Role of Limbic System and Brain Ontogeny in Drug Abuse Research Grants **2514**
This initiative is designed to support basic research into the fundamental mechanisms of development of the midbrain and basal forebrain structures that mediate the euphoric properties of drugs as well as understanding how drugs of abuse affect the cellular and molecular mechanism underlying nervous system development. In the past, vertebrate model systems (such as chick, frog, mouse, and zebrafish) and invertebrate systems (such as Drosophila and C. Elegans) have provided insights into mechanisms of development and are also likely to provide new information about the formation and specification of the limbic system. Approaches using these or other model systems both in vitro and in vivo are applicable to this PA. PA-02-015 may be obtained through the NIH grant line (301-402-2221), the NIH Web site, mail, and email.
Requirements: Applications may be submitted by foreign and domestic for-profit and nonprofit organizations, public or private.
Amount of Grant: $90,000 maximum direct costs per year
Contact: Dr. Jonathan Pollock, Division of Basic Research, (301) 443-6300; fax: (301) 594-6043; email: jp183r@nih.gov; Gary Fleming, Grants Management Branch, (301) 443-6710; fax: (301) 594-6847; email: gf6s@nih.gov
Internet: http://grants2.nih.gov/grants/guide/pa-files/PA-02-015.html
Sponsor: National Institute on Drug Abuse
5600 Fishers Ln, Parklawn Building
Rockville, MD 20857

NIDA Senior Scientist Award **2515**
The Senior Scientist Award provides support to outstanding scientists who have demonstrated sustained, high levels of productivity and whose expertise, research accomplishments, and contributions to the field have been and will continue to be critical to the mission of the particular NIH center or institute. The award provides salary support for award periods of five years. Contact the program office for more information.
Requirements: The candidate must be a senior scientist and a recognized leader in the field with a distinguished record of original contributions, must have long-term support from a funding institute or center, and must have peer-reviewed grant support at the time of the award. Applications may be submitted on behalf of candidates by domestic, nonfederal organizations, both public or private; or other institutions. Candidates must be U.S. citizens, noncitizen nationals, or permanent residents.
Amount of Grant: $1000-$1.235 million; $190,000 average
Date(s) Application is Due: Feb 1; Jun 1; Oct 1
Contact: Dr. Timothy Condon, Office of Science Policy, Education, and Legislation, (301) 443-6072; fax: (301) 443-6277; email: tc52x@nih.gov; Dr. Charles Sharp, Division of Basic Research, (301) 443-1887; fax: (301) 594-6043; email: cs107m@nih.gov
Internet: http://www.grants.nih.gov/grants/guide/pa-files/PA-95-051.html
Sponsor: National Institute on Drug Abuse
5600 Fishers Ln, Parklawn Building
Rockville, MD 20857

NIDA Transition from Drug Abuse to Drug Addiction **2516**
The intent of this program is to stimulate research on the processes and mechanisms underlying the transition from drug use to drug addiction from a wide variety of academic disciplines and approaches. Research from epidemiologic, basic, and clinical disciplines, including research on other transitional states with relevance to addiction, will be supported under this program. Annual deadline dates may vary; contact program staff for exact dates.
Requirements: Applications may be submitted by domestic, for-profit and nonprofit organizations, both public and private; units of state and local governments; and eligible agencies of the federal government.
Amount of Grant: $400,000 maximum
Contact: Dr. Steven Gust, (301) 443-6480; fax: (301) 443-9127; email: sgust@mail.nih.gov
Internet: http://grants.nih.gov/grants/guide/rfa-files/RFA-DA-01-004.html
Sponsor: National Institute on Drug Abuse
6001 Executive Boulevard
Bethesda, MD 20892

NIDCD Clinical Trial Planning Grant **2517**
NIDCD provides funding to those who are seeking to improve health by supporting well-executed clinical trials in its mission areas of hearing, balance, smell, taste, voice, speech, and language. Investigators who submit applications for large-scale clinical trials for consideration are expected to provide detailed information regarding the study rationale, design, protocols and procedures, analytical techniques, facilities and environment, administrative procedures, and collaborative arrangements. PA: PAR-02-158
Requirements: Applications may be submitted by domestic for-profit and nonprofit organizations, both public and private; units of state and local governments; and eligible agencies of the federal government.
Restrictions: Foreign organizations are not eligible to apply.
Amount of Grant: $75,000 maximum
Contact: A. Julianna Gulya, Chief, Clinical Trials Branch, (301) 435-4085; fax: (301) 402-6251; email: julie_gulya@nih.gov
Internet: http://grants2.nih.gov/grants/guide/pa-files/PAR-02-158.html
Sponsor: National Institute on Deafness and Other Communication Disorders
6120 Executive Boulevard
Bethesda, MD 20892

NIDCD Communicative Competence of Users of Augmentative and Alternative Communication Systems Research Grants **2518**
Awards are given for the support of research studies on issues related to the communicative competence of users of augmentative and alternative communication (AAC) systems. Such studies promise to lead to a better understanding of the impact of AAC on the development of or restoration of communicative competence of individuals with severe communication difficulties commonly seen in association with developmental or acquired disorders such as brain injury and other diseases or disorders affecting the oral motor system. It will also define the ways in which augmentative and alternative strategies can influence all phases of communication development and activity. Findings from these studies will direct the establishment and refinement of tools and intervention strategies enabling the development or recovery of communicative function.
Amount of Grant: $72,486-$458,342; $200,000 average
Date(s) Application is Due: Feb 1; Jun 1; Oct 1
Contact: Sara Stone, Grants Management, (301) 402-0909
Internet: http://www.grants.nih.gov/grants/guide/pa-files/PA-96-032.html

Sponsor: National Institute on Deafness and Other Communication Disorders
6120 Executive Boulevard, Executive Plaza S
Bethesda, MD 20892

NIDCD Exploratory Research: Feasibility Pilot Studies Grants **2519**
The NIDCD invites applications for exploratory, initial feasibility pilot studies focused on hearing, balance, smell, taste, voice, speech, and language, the organization's scientific mission areas. Exploratory research involves initial feasibility pilot studies in which the technological, methodological, or theoretical approach to a problem lacks sufficient preliminary/baseline data and a body of peer-reviewed publications, but whose successful outcome would make a significant contribution to a scientific area or field. It is anticipated that most applications will be submitted by investigators with ongoing research programs who wish to change the focus of their current research effort or move into a new area of research within the communication sciences but need additional funds to complete initial pilot studies. The NIDCD encourages applications from investigators conducting research outside the communication sciences who possess expertise with methodological or technological approaches which have not been typically applied to but which would greatly promote scientific progress within the communication sciences. Annual deadline dates may vary; contact program staff for exact dates. PA: PAR-01-103
Requirements: Applications may be submitted by domestic for-profit and nonprofit organizations, both public and private; units of state or local governments; and eligible agencies of the federal government.
Contact: Dr. Amy Donahue, Hearing, (301) 402-3458; email: amy_donahue@nih.gov; Dr. Lynn Luethke, Hearing, (301) 402-3461; email: lynn_huerta@nih.gov; Dr. Daniel Sklare, Balance/Vestibular, (301) 496-1804; email: daniel_sklare@nih.gov
Internet: http://grants2.nih.gov/grants/guide/pa-files/PAR-01-103.html
Sponsor: National Institute on Deafness and Other Communication Disorders
6120 Executive Boulevard, Executive Plaza S
Bethesda, MD 20892

NIDCD Exploratory/Developmental Research Grants **2520**
NIDCD invites grant applications from basic and clinical investigators who are interested in pursuing high-risk/high-impact (HR/HI) research focused on hearing, balance, smell, taste, voice, speech, or language related to the specific mission of the institute. HR/HI research involves pilot/feasibility studies in which the technological, methodological, or theoretical approach to the problem lacks a traditional historical basis or pilot data, but which could have a major impact on a scientific area or field. Additional information may be obtained electronically through the NIH grant line (301-402-2221), and by mail and email from the program contact listed. Annual deadline dates may vary; contact program staff for exact dates. PA: PAR-96-073
Amount of Grant: $72,486-$458,342; $200,000 average
Date(s) Application is Due: Feb 1; Jun 1; Oct 1
Contact: Sharon Hunt, Grants Management, (301) 402-0909
Internet: http://www.grants.nih.gov/grants/guide/pa-files/PAR-96-073.html
Sponsor: National Institute on Deafness and Other Communication Disorders
6120 Executive Boulevard, Executive Plaza S
Bethesda, MD 20892

NIDCD Health Promotion and Disease Prevention: Health Communication, Development, and Dissemination **2521**
The purpose of this RFA is to encourage the submission of research grant applications that create, develop, and evaluate health communication information. Projects should be based in current health communication theory and directed to address important problems of disease prevention, health promotion, and improved understanding of the basis for human communication disorders through public information. Annual deadline dates may vary; contact program staff for exact dates. RFA: DC-00-003
Requirements: Applications may be submitted by domestic and foreign, for-profit and nonprofit organizations, both public and private; units of state and local governments; and eligible agencies of the federal government.
Amount of Grant: $600,000 total
Contact: Dr. Amy Donahue, (301) 402-3458; fax: (301) 402-6251; email: Amy_Donahue@nih.gov
Internet: http://grants.nih.gov/grants/guide/rfa-files/RFA-DC-00-003.html
Sponsor: National Institute on Deafness and Other Communication Disorders
6120 Executive Boulevard, Executive Plaza S
Bethesda, MD 20892

NIDCD Mentored Clinical Scientist Research Career Development Award **2522**
This award enables candidates holding professional degrees (e.g., M.D., D.O., D.V.M., or equivalent degrees) to undertake 3 to 5 years of special study and supervised research with the goal of becoming independent investigators. The award also allows awardees to pursue a research career development program suited to their experience and capabilities under a mentor who is competent to provide guidance in the chosen research area. Institutions may submit applications on behalf of candidates who hold professional degrees. At least 2 years must have elapsed since the health professional degree was granted. Candidates can have varying levels of clinical training and research experience. New applications are due February 12, June 12, and October 12, while resubmitted applications are due March 12, July 12, and November 12. Up to $105,000 per year plus fringe benefits is available, and up to $85,000 per year for research support for new awards.
Requirements: A candidate must have a clinical degree or its equivalent, must have initiated postgraduate clinical training, must identify a mentor with extensive research experience, and must be willing to spend a minimum of 75 percent of full-time professional effort conducting research. Applications may be submitted on behalf of candidates by domestic, nonfederal organizations, public or private, such as medical, dental, or nursing schools or other institutions of higher education. Candidates must be U.S. citizens, noncitizen nationals, or permanent residents.
Amount of Grant: $185,000 maximum
Date(s) Application is Due: Feb 12; Mar 12; Jun 12; Jul 12; Oct 12; Nov 12
Contact: Dr. Daniel Sklare; (301) 496-1804; fax: (301) 402-6251; email: sklared@nidcd.nih.gov
Internet: http://grants.nih.gov/grants/guide/pa-files/pa-06-512.html
Sponsor: National Institute on Deafness and Other Communication Disorders (NIDCD)
6120 Executive Blvd. , MSC-7180
Bethesda, MD 20892-7180

NIDCD Mentored Research Scientist Development Award **2523**
The NIDCD utilizes the K01 Program for the retooling and transition of junior- and midcareer-level scientists and clinicians (generally below the rank of full professor, or the equivalent in nonacademic settings) into two research domains: translational research, i.e., the application of basic research discoveries toward advancing the diagnosis, management and prevention of deafness and other communication disorders; and clinical research. Junior-level clinically-trained individuals should apply for the Mentored Clinical Scientist Development Award or the Mentored Patient-Oriented Research Career Development Award, as appropriate.
Requirements: The candidate must have a research or health-professional doctorate or its equivalent, and must have demonstrated the capacity or potential for highly productive independent research in the period after the doctorate. The candidate must identify a mentor with extensive research experience, and must be willing to spend a minimum of 75 percent of full-time professional effort conducting research and research career development activities for the period of the award. Applications may be submitted on behalf of candidates by domestic, public or private, nonfederal organizations. Candidates must be U.S. citizens or noncitizen nationals.
Amount of Grant: $105,000 maximum salary per year plus fringe benefits; $50,000 per year for research support
Date(s) Application is Due: Feb 12; Mar 12; Jun 12; Jul 12; Oct 12; Nov 12
Contact: Daniel A. Sklare; (301) 496-1804; email: sklared@nidcd.nih.gov
Internet: http://www.grants.nih.gov/grants/guide/pa-files/PAR-99-027.html
Sponsor: National Institute on Deafness and Other Communication Disorders (NIDCD)
6120 Executive Blvd. , MSC-7180, Executive Plaza South, Room 400C
Bethesda, MD 20892-7180

NIDCD Minority Dissertation Research Grants in Human Communication **2524**
NIDCD invites applications for small grants to support doctoral dissertation research in human communication for doctoral candidates who are members of racial and ethnic minority groups that are under-represented in biomedical and behavioral research. The goals of this program are to aid the research of new minority investigators and to encourage minority individuals from a variety of academic disciplines and programs to conduct research in hearing, balance, smell, taste, voice, speech, and language. These grants are not eligible for competitive renewal. Annual deadline dates may vary; contact the program office for exact dates. More information may be obtained by mail and email, or through the NIH grant line (301-402-2221) and the NIH Web site. RFA: DC-00-001
Requirements: Candidates for this award must be graduate students in good standing and must be identified by the grantee institution as a member of an ethnic or racial group that is underrepresented in biomedical or behavioral research.
Amount of Grant: $36,000 maximum direct costs for up to two years, $30,000 maximum direct costs for any one year
Contact: Daniel Sklare, Division of Extramural Research, (301) 496-1804; fax: (301) 402-6251; email: daniel_sklare@nih.gov
Internet: http://grants2.nih.gov/grants/guide/rfa-files/RFA-DC-00-001.html
Sponsor: National Institute on Deafness and Other Communication Disorders
6120 Executive Boulevard, Executive Plaza S
Bethesda, MD 20892

NIDCD Molecular and Cellular Pathology of the Human Auditory and Vestibular Systems Grants **2525**
These grants support cellular biologic, molecular biologic, and molecular genetic studies of newly acquired and archival human temporal bones and associated brain tissues of individuals who had well-documented evidence of disorders of hearing and/or balance before death. It is believed that studies of this kind can lead to a better understanding of the pathogenesis and pathophysiology of disorders of the human auditory and vestibular systems. Further information may be obtained by mail and email or through the NIH grant line (301-402-2221), and the NIH Web site. Annual deadline dates may vary; contact program staff for exact dates. RFA: DC-96-005
Requirements: Applications may be submitted by domestic and foreign for-profit and non-profit organizations, public and private; and eligible agencies of the federal government.
Amount of Grant: $72,486-$458,342; $200,000 average
Contact: Sharon Hunt, Grants Management, (301) 402-0909
Internet: http://www.grants.nih.gov/grants/guide/rfa-files/RFA-DC-96-005.html
Sponsor: National Institute on Deafness and Other Communication Disorders
6120 Executive Boulevard, Executive Plaza S
Bethesda, MD 20892

NIDCD Neurobiology and Genetics of Autism Grants **2526**

NICHD and NIDCD fund grants for research that will elucidate the biological basis of autism and contribute to the discovery of a biological and/or diagnostic marker for autism. The purpose of these grants is to provide support for collaborative, multidisciplinary, and methodologically rigorous programs of research that will use advanced techniques in the biological and behavioral sciences to study the diagnosis, biological etiology, pathophysiology, and developmental course of autism. Annual deadline dates may vary; contact program staff for exact dates. More information may be obtained by mail and email, or through the NIH grant line (301-402-2221), and the NIH Web site. RFA: HD-96-004

Amount of Grant: $36,000-$2.3 million; $282,409 average
Date(s) Application is Due: Feb 1; Jun 1; Oct 1
Contact: Marie Bristol, Center for Research for Mothers and Children, (301) 496-1383; fax: (301) 496-3791; email: BRISTOLM@HD01.NICHD.NIH.GOV
Internet: http://www.grants.nih.gov/grants/guide/rfa-files/RFA-HD-96-004.html
Sponsor: National Institute on Deafness and Other Communication Disorders
6120 Executive Boulevard, Executive Plaza S
Bethesda, MD 20892

NIDCD Physiologic and Molecular Bases of Tinnitus Research Grants **2527**

Three to five exploratory/developmental grants will be awarded to support research addressing the physiologic and molecular bases of tinnitus. The goal is to stimulate research on pathologic processes in the auditory system that produce tinnitus. More information may be obtained by mail and email, or through the NIH grant line (301-402-2221), and the NIH Web site. Annual deadline dates vary; contact program staff for exact dates. RFA: DC-96-003

Amount of Grant: $72,486-$458,342; $200,000 average
Contact: Sharon Hunt, Grants Management, (301) 402-0909
Internet: http://www.grants.nih.gov/grants/guide/rfa-files/RFA-DC-96-003.html
Sponsor: National Institute on Deafness and Other Communication Disorders
6120 Executive Boulevard, Executive Plaza S
Bethesda, MD 20892

NIDCD Program for Postdoctoral Research Training in Clinical Trials **2528**

Grants support programs of postdoctoral research training in the design and conduct of clinical trials for individuals trained in the clinical disciplines of human communications. The purpose of this initiative is to foster the development of trained professionals into independent investigators capable of conducting clinical trials of the efficacy of treatment for diseases and disorders affecting hearing, balance, smell, taste, voice, speech, or language. More information may be obtained by mail and email, or through the NIH grant line (301-402-2221), and the NIH Web site. Annual deadline dates may vary; contact program staff for exact dates. PA: PA-96-024

Amount of Grant: $72,486-$458,342; $200,000 average
Date(s) Application is Due: Feb 1; Jun 1; Oct 1
Contact: Daniel Sklare, Division of Human Communication, (301) 496-1804; fax: (301) 402-6251; email: daniel_sklare@nih.gov; Sharon Hunt, Grants Management, (301) 402-0909
Internet: http://www.grants.nih.gov/grants/guide/pa-files/PA-96-024.html
Sponsor: National Institute on Deafness and Other Communication Disorders
6120 Executive Boulevard, Executive Plaza S
Bethesda, MD 20892

NIDCD Research Core Centers **2529**

NIDCD invites grant applications for research core centers. The overall goal of a core center is to promote a cooperative interaction among basic science and/or clinical investigators in a manner that will enrich the effectiveness of ongoing research and promote new research directions. Grants support centralized resources and facilities shared by investigators with existing research projects. A letter of intent is requested by April 1, August 1, and December 1; full application is due by February 1, June 1, and October 1. Annual deadline dates may vary; contact program staff for exact dates.

Requirements: Applications may be submitted by domestic for-profit and nonprofit organizations, both public and private; units of state or local governments; and eligible agencies of the federal government.
Restrictions: Foreign organizations or organizations in foreign countries are not eligible; subcontracts to foreign organizations are not allowed.
Date(s) Application is Due: Feb 1; Apr 1; Jun 1; Aug 1; Oct 1; Dec 1
Contact: Amy Donahue, (301) 402-3458; fax: (301) 402-6251; email: amy_donahue@nih.gov
Internet: http://grants.nih.gov/grants/guide/pa-files/PA-01-011.html
Sponsor: National Institute on Deafness and Other Communication Disorders
6120 Executive Boulevard, Executive Plaza S
Bethesda, MD 20892

NIDCD Research Grants on Chemical Senses: Neurotransmitters and Neuromodulators **2530**

NIDCD and NIA sponsor research grants that support research fundamental to understanding the neurochemistry of pathways in the olfactory and gustatory systems throughout the lifespan. This research includes the identification and characterization of the neurotransmitters, neuromodulators, receptors, and secondary messengers throughout the chemosensory systems. More information may be obtained by mail and email, or through the NIH grant line (301-402-2221), and the NIH Web site. Annual deadline dates may vary; contact program staff for exact dates. PA: PA-96-035

Amount of Grant: $72,486-$458,342; $200,000 average
Date(s) Application is Due: Feb 1; Jun 1; Oct 1
Contact: Program Contact, Division of Human Communication, (301) 496-5061; Sara Stone, Grants Management, (301) 402-0909
Internet: http://www.grants.nih.gov/grants/guide/pa-files/PA-96-035.html
Sponsor: National Institute on Deafness and Other Communication Disorders
6120 Executive Boulevard, Executive Plaza S
Bethesda, MD 20892

NIDCD Small Grants Program **2531**

NIDCD provides support for pilot research that is likely to lead to subsequent application for individual research project grants or first independent research support and transition grants. The research must be focused on one or more of the areas within the biomedical and behavioral scientific mission of NIDCD: hearing, balance, smell, taste, voice, speech, or language. Applicants may request support for up to two years, nonrenewable. For additional information, investigators are encouraged to contact NIDCD staff responsible for grants in the investigator's particular area of interest. PA: PAR-99-018

Requirements: This program is designed solely to support basic and clinical scientists with limited research experience who are at the beginning stages of their research careers. Former recipients of federally funded Training or Career Development awards are eligible for this program.
Restrictions: Current and previous principal investigators of NIH research grants or other federal funding agencies are ineligible.
Amount of Grant: $35,000 maximum per year
Contact: Dr. Beth Ansel, Voice/Speech, (301) 402-3461; fax: (301) 402-6251; email: Beth_Ansel@nih.gov; Dr. Chyren Hunter, Hearing, (301) 402-3461; email: Chyren_Hunter@nih.gov; Dr. Daniel Sklare, Balance/Vestibular, (301) 496-1804; email: Daniel_Sklare@nih.g
Internet: http://www.grants.nih.gov/grants/guide/pa-files/PAR-99-018.html
Sponsor: National Institute on Deafness and Other Communication Disorders
6120 Executive Boulevard, Executive Plaza S
Bethesda, MD 20892

NIDCD Symptom Management for Chronic Neurological Conditions Research Grants **2532**

NINR, NIA, NICHD, NIDCD, and NINDS are interested in facilitating investigator-initiated research designed to deal with symptoms associated with chronic neurological conditions including stroke, epilepsy, brain and spinal cord injury, multiple sclerosis, and Parkinson's disease. The overall goals are to manage symptoms effectively, to prevent secondary effects of the condition when possible, to maximize the health potential, and to improve the health-related quality of life for patients, caregivers, and families. The mechanism of support is the research project grant (R01). PA-98-030 may be obtained through the NIH grant line (301-402-2221), the NIH Web site, mail, and email.

Requirements: Applications may be submitted by domestic and foreign for-profit and nonprofit organizations, public or private.
Contact: Dr. Beth Ansel, Division of Human Communication, (301) 402-3461; fax: (301) 402-6251; email: Beth_Ansel@nih.gov
Internet: http://www.grants.nih.gov/grants/guide/pa-files/PA-98-030.html
Sponsor: National Institute on Deafness and Other Communication Disorders
6120 Executive Boulevard, Executive Plaza S
Bethesda, MD 20892

NIDCR Clinical Trial Pilot Grant **2533**

The goal of this program is to identify effective preventive, diagnostic, and treatment approaches to craniofacial, oral and dental diseases, and disorders that will improve health by supporting well-executed clinical trials and to support pilot studies to obtain preliminary data necessary to address preliminary design and methodological issues for clinical trials. PA: PAR-99-158

Requirements: Applications may be submitted by foreign and domestic, for-profit and nonprofit organizations, both public and private; units of state and local governments; and eligible agencies of the federal government.
Amount of Grant: $250,000 maximum for enrollment centers; $350,000 maximum for coordinating centers
Contact: Dr. Ann Sandberg, Division of Extramural Research, (301) 594-2419; email: Ann.Sandberg@nih.gov
Internet: http://grants.nih.gov/grants/guide/pa-files/PAR-99-158.html
Sponsor: National Institute of Dental and Craniofacial Research
45 Center Drive
Bethesda, MD 20892

NIDCR Clinical Trial Planning Grant **2534**

The goal of this program is to identify effective preventive, diagnostic, and treatment approaches to craniofacial, oral and dental diseases, and disorders that will improve health by supporting well-executed clinical trials. PA: PAR-03-042

Requirements: Applications may be submitted by domestic and foreign, for-profit and nonprofit organizations, both public and private; units of state and local governments; and eligible agencies of the federal government.
Amount of Grant: $250,000 maximum
Contact: Dr. Bruce Pihlstrom, Acting Director, Division of Clinical Research and Health Promotion, (301) 594-4830; fax: (301) 480-8322; email: bruce.Pihlstrom@nih.gov
Internet: http://grants.nih.gov/grants/guide/pa-files/PAR-03-042.html
Sponsor: National Institute of Dental and Craniofacial Research
45 Center Drive
Bethesda, MD 20892

NIDCR HIV/AIDS Associated Oral Viral Infections 2535

NIDCR invites new and experienced scientists to submit research grant applications for basic, behavioral, epidemiological, or clinical investigations to study the pathogenesis, infectivity, transmission, reactivation, and pathotropic spread of viral infections in the oral cavity of the immunocompromised host. This RFA is intended to solicit a broad range of research proposals on oral opportunistic infections with viruses, including human herpes virus, Epstein Barr virus, cytomegalovirus varicella-zoster virus, and human papillomavirus in HIV-infected/AIDS individuals. The institute encourages collaborative projects that bring together investigators from all relevant scientific disciplines including microbiology, immunology, biochemistry, and pathology interested in studying viral infections of the oral cavity. Applications that include collaboration with foreign scientists conducting unique research on this topic are also encouraged. The goal of this RFA is to increase our understanding of how virulence, infection, and host response is modified in the immune compromised patient to allow infection, activation, or reactivation of opportunistic pathogens. This understanding can lead to improved diagnosis, prevention, and treatment strategies, for the various opportunistic pathogens. Annual deadline dates may vary; contact program staff for exact dates. RFA: DE-00-002

Requirements: Applications may be submitted by domestic and foreign, for-profit and nonprofit organizations, both public and private; units of state and local governments; and eligible agencies of the federal government. Although an application must be submitted from a single institution, collaborative arrangements with other institutions are encouraged.

Amount of Grant: $200,000 maximum; $225,000 maximum for collaborative agreements

Contact: Dr. Denise Anne Russo, Infectious Diseases and Immunity, (301) 594-2617; fax: (301) 480-8318; email: Denise.Russo@nih.gov

Internet: http://grants.nih.gov/grants/guide/rfa-files/RFA-DE-00-002.html

Sponsor: National Institute of Dental and Craniofacial Research
45 Center Drive
Bethesda, MD 20892

NIDCR International Collaborative Oral Health Research Planning Grant 2536

The objective of this scientific program is to promote research that will advance understanding of the underlying causes of craniofacial dysmorphologies such as ectodermal dysplasia, enamel dysplasia, cleft lip and palate, and osteogenesis imperfecta. International collaboration in relevant areas such as genetic research, epidemiology, genetic registries, and treatment modalities can help speed progress toward the goal of improved prevention, diagnosis, and treatment by combining scientific talents from different countries to focus on selected populations at high risk. An international approach that includes all disciplines relevant to specific craniofacial anomalies might dramatically enhance the possibility of resolving the many complex issues surrounding these malformations. PA: PAR-00-012

Requirements: Applications may be submitted by foreign and domestic, for-profit and nonprofit organizations, both public and private; units of state and local governments; and eligible agencies of the federal government.

Amount of Grant: $75,000 maximum

Contact: Dr. Judy Small, Craniofacial Anomalies and Injuries Branch, (301) 594-2425; Dr. Dennis Mangan, Infectious Diseases Branch, (301) 594-2421; Dr. Ann Sandberg, Neoplastic Diseases Branch, (301) 594-2419

Internet: http://grants.nih.gov/grants/guide/pa-files/PAR-00-012.html

Sponsor: National Institute of Dental and Craniofacial Research
45 Center Drive, Natcher Building
Bethesda, MD 20892

NIDCR Oral Microbiology/Immunology of Type 1 Diabetes 2537

The purpose of this program is to encourage submission of applications for two-year exploratory grants that will broaden research on the oral microbiology and immunology of Type 1 diabetes. In particular, research is needed on the oral microflora, cytokines, and antibodies in the subgingival crevice. Annual deadline dates may vary; contact program staff for exact dates. RFA: DE-01-001

Requirements: Applications may be submitted by domestic and foreign, for-profit and nonprofit organizations, both public and private; units of state and local governments; and eligible agencies of the federal government.

Amount of Grant: $100,000 maximum

Contact: Dr. Dennis Mangan, Infectious Diseases and Immunity Branch, (301) 594-2421; fax: (301) 480-8318; email: Dennis.Mangan@nih.gov

Internet: http://grants.nih.gov/grants/guide/rfa-files/RFA-DE-01-001.html

Sponsor: National Institute of Dental and Craniofacial Research
45 Center Drive, Natcher Building
Bethesda, MD 20892

NIDCR Priorities in Behavioral Research in Cancer Prevention and Control Grants 2538

NCI and NIDCR invite researchers to submit research project grant (R01) applications that address behavioral research issues in cancer prevention and control. The PA addresses recommendations made by a special Behavioral Research in Cancer Prevention and Control Working Group in 1996 that consisted of leading national experts whose role was to identify behavioral research needs in cancer prevention and control during the coming years. PA-97-055 may be obtained electronically through the NIH grant line (301-402-2221), the Web site, and by mail and email.

Contact: Dr. Patricia Bryant, Behavior, Health Promotion, and Environment Program, (301) 594-2095; email: bryantp@de45.nidr.nih.gov

Internet: http://grants.nih.gov/grants/guide/pa-files/PA-97-055.html

Sponsor: National Institute of Dental and Craniofacial Research
45 Center Drive, Natcher Building
Bethesda, MD 20892

NIDDK Advances in Polycystic Kidney Disease Grants 2539

The National Institute of Diabetes and Digestive and Kidney Diseases (NIDDK) through its Division of Kidney, Urologic and Hematologic Diseases (DKUHD) invites experienced and new investigators to submit research grant applications to pursue basic and applied investigations in order to better understand the etiology and pathogenesis of Polycystic Kidney Disease (PKD), in both its autosomal dominant and autosomal recessive forms. Such applications may examine the genetic determinants, and cellular and molecular mechanisms, which disrupt normal kidney function; mechanisms of cyst formation and growth; development of experimental model systems; development of markers of disease progression; and the identification of innovative therapeutic interventions and gene targeted strategies to prevent progressive renal insufficiency due to this disorder. The intent of this funding opportunity is to intensify investigator-initiated research, to attract new investigators to the field, and to increase interdisciplinary research. The ultimate aim is to facilitate PKD-related research studies, which will provide the basis for new therapeutic approaches.

Requirements: The following organizations may apply: for-profit organizations; non-profit organizations; public or private institutions, such as universities, colleges, hospitals, and laboratories; units of State government; units of local government; eligible agencies of the Federal government; foreign institutions; domestic institutions; and faith-based or community-based organizations.

Date(s) Application is Due: Feb 5; Jun 5; Oct 5

Contact: Catherine M. Meyers, M.D.; (301) 594-7717; fax: (301) 480-3510; email: cm420i@nih.gov

Internet: http://grants.nih.gov/grants/guide/pa-files/PA-06-158.html

Sponsor: National Institute of Diabetes and Digestive and Kidney Diseases (NIDDK)
6707 Democracy Boulevard, Room 641
Bethesda, MD 20892-5458

NIDDK Ancillary Studies of Kidney Disease Accessing Information from Clinical Trials, Epidemiological Studies, and Databases Grants 2540

The National Institute of Diabetes and Digestive and Kidney Diseases (NIDDK) invites investigator-initiated research project applications for ancillary studies to ongoing or completed clinical trials and epidemiological studies of kidney disease as well as clinical trials and epidemiological studies for other diseases or populations that lend themselves to the study of kidney disease. These studies may range from new analyses of existing datasets of completed studies to additional collection of data and biological specimens in ongoing investigations. The goal of these studies should be to extend our understanding of the risk factors for developing kidney disease and their associated co-morbid illnesses such as malnutrition and cardiovascular disease, factors associated with rapid decline in kidney function among persons with chronic kidney disease, and the impact of these diseases on quality of life and mental and physical functioning. Studies of biomarkers for patients with acute renal failure and other kidney diseases, for example, are also appropriate topics for further investigation. Studies ancillary to both government and non-government supported clinical trials and epidemiological studies are encouraged. Analysis of large public access databases and other databases is also encouraged.

Requirements: The following organizations and institutions may apply: public/state controlled institutions of higher education; private institutions of higher education; Hispanic-serving institutions; historically Black colleges and universities (HBCUs); tribally controlled colleges and universities (TCCUs); Alaska native and native Hawaiian serving institutions; nonprofits with 501(c)3 IRS status; nonprofits without 501(c)3 IRS status; small businesses; for-profit organizations; State governments; regional organizations; U.S. territories or possessions; Indian/Native American tribal governments; Indian/Native American tribally designated organizations; eligible agencies of the Federal government; and faith-based or community based organizations.

Date(s) Application is Due: Feb 5; Jun 5; Oct 5

Contact: John W. Kusek; (301) 594-7735; fax: (301) 480-3510; email: jk61x@nih.gov

Internet: http://grants.nih.gov/grants/guide/pa-files/PA-07-050.html

Sponsor: National Institute of Diabetes and Digestive and Kidney Diseases (NIDDK)
6707 Democracy Boulevard, Room 617
Bethesda, MD 20892-5458

NIDDK Ancillary Studies to Major Ongoing NIDDK and NHLBI Clinical Research Studies 2541

This Funding Opportunity Announcement (FOA) solicits grant applications from qualified investigators to conduct ancillary studies of selected ongoing major clinical research studies, including clinical trials, epidemiological studies and disease databases, supported by the National Institute of Diabetes and Digestive and Kidney Diseases and the National Heart, Lung, and Blood Institute, National Institutes of Health (NIH). The objective is to introduce NIDDK-oriented ancillary studies into either NIDDK or NHLBI-funded parent studies, or NHLBI-oriented ancillary studies into NIDDK-funded parent studies.

Requirements: The following organizations and institutions may apply: public/state controlled institutions of higher education; private institutions of higher education; Hispanic-serving institutions; historically Black colleges and universities (HBCUs); tribally controlled colleges and universities (TCCUs); Alaska native and native Hawaiian serving institutions; nonprofits with 501(c)3 IRS status; nonprofits without 501(c)3 IRS status; small businesses; for-profit organizations; State governments; regional organizations; U.S. territories or possessions; Indian/Native American tribal

governments; Indian/Native American tribally designated organizations; eligible agencies of the Federal government; and faith-based or community based organizations.
Date(s) Application is Due: Feb 5; Jun 5; Oct 5
Contact: John W. Kusek; (301) 594-7735; fax: (301) 480-3510; email: jk61x@nih.gov
Internet: http://grants.nih.gov/grants/guide/pa-files/PAR-07-024.html
Sponsor: National Institute of Diabetes and Digestive and Kidney Diseases (NIDDK)
Two Democracy Plaza, Room 617, 6707 Democracy Boulevard
Bethesda, MD 20892-5458

NIDDK Basic and Clinical Studies of Congenital Urinary Tract Obstruction Grants 2542

The purpose of this funding opportunity is to address the numerous scientific and clinical uncertainties related to the development, treatment and prognosis of congenital obstructive uropathy, by encouraging and facilitating research in diverse areas. These areas include: the development of objective prognostic markers; the genetic determinants of this congenital disorder; the development of reliable animal models of the disorder; and, evaluation of the long-term effectiveness of various treatment strategies. Because the nature and scope of the proposed research will vary from application to application, it is anticipated that the size and duration of each award will also vary. The total amount awarded and the number of awards will depend upon the mechanism numbers, quality, duration, and costs of the applications received.
Requirements: The following organizations and institutions may apply: public/state controlled institutions of higher education; private institutions of higher education; Hispanic-serving institutions; historically Black colleges and universities (HBCUs); tribally controlled colleges and universities (TCCUs); Alaska native and native Hawaiian serving institutions; nonprofits with 501(c)3 IRS status; nonprofits without 501(c)3 IRS status; small businesses; for-profit organizations; State governments; regional organizations; U.S. territories or possessions; Indian/Native American tribal governments; Indian/Native American tribally designated organizations; eligible agencies of the Federal government; and faith-based or community based organizations.
Date(s) Application is Due: Feb 5; Jun 5; Oct 5
Contact: Marva Moxey-Mims, M.D.; (301) 594-7717; fax: (301) 480-3510; email: mm726k@nih.gov
Internet: http://grants.nih.gov/grants/guide/pa-files/PA-07-059.html
Sponsor: National Institute of Diabetes and Digestive and Kidney Diseases (NIDDK)
6707 Democracy Boulevard, Room 639
Bethesda, MD 20892-5458

NIDDK Basic Research Grants in the Bladder and Lower Urinary Tract 2543

This funding opportunity encourages basic cellular, molecular, developmental and genetic research relevant to the bladder and lower urinary tract. Basic research studies that address age and gender differences in bladder and lower urinary tract function are also encouraged. New and established investigators from related fields of study are encouraged to apply their expertise to these problem areas. Investigators with diverse basic science and clinical backgrounds are encouraged to develop collaborative research relationships. Discoveries resulting from these studies may serve as the basis for the development of new agents, techniques, and strategies for detecting, preventing, and treating diseases of the bladder and lower urinary tract, as well as dealing with bladder complications resulting from other diseases, such as diabetes.
Requirements: Application can be made by the following institutions and organizations: for-profit organizations; non-profit organizations; public or private institutions (such as universities, colleges, hospitals, and laboratories); units of State government; units of local government; eligible agencies of the Federal government; foreign institutions; and domestic institutions.
Date(s) Application is Due: Feb 5; Jun 5; Oct 5
Contact: Chris Mullins; (301) 594-7717; fax: (301) 480-3510; email: cm419z@nih.gov
Internet: http://grants.nih.gov/grants/guide/pa-files/PA-06-254.html
Sponsor: National Institute of Diabetes and Digestive and Kidney Diseases (NIDDK)
6707 Democracy Boulevard, Room 637
Bethesda, MD 20892-5458

NIDDK Calcium Oxalate Stone Diseases Grants 2544

The purpose of this Funding Opportunity Announcement (FOA) is to increase investigator interest in research into the genetics and heritability of oxalate regulation and the oxalate stone diseases, and to develop new treatments for the disorder. This initiative solicits research as well as pilot and feasibility studies that utilize new and innovative approaches to study the diagnosis, treatment and prevention of these disorders. Because the nature and scope of the proposed research will vary from application to application, it is anticipated that the size and duration of each award will also vary. The total amount awarded and the number of awards will depend upon the mechanism numbers, quality, duration, and costs of the applications received.
Requirements: The following organizations and institutions may apply: public/state controlled institutions of higher education; private institutions of higher education; Hispanic-serving institutions; historically Black colleges and universities (HBCUs); tribally controlled colleges and universities (TCCUs); Alaska native and native Hawaiian serving institutions; nonprofits with 501(c)3 IRS status; nonprofits without 501(c)3 IRS status; small businesses; for-profit organizations; State governments; regional organizations; U.S. territories or possessions; Indian/Native American tribal governments; Indian/Native American tribally designated organizations; eligible agencies of the Federal government; and faith-based or community based organizations.
Date(s) Application is Due: Feb 5; Jun 5; Oct 5
Contact: Rebekah S. Rasooly, Ph.D.; (301) 594-6007; fax: (301) 480-3510; email: rr185i@nih.gov
Internet: http://grants.nih.gov/grants/guide/pa-files/PA-07-051.html
Sponsor: National Institute of Diabetes and Digestive and Kidney Diseases (NIDDK)
6707 Democracy Boulevard, Room 643
Bethesda, MD 20892-5458

NIDDK Cell-Specific Delineation of Prostate and Genitourinary Development 2545

This RFA is intended to encourage the development of new research tools and methods to study the development and biology of the prostate and genitourinary tract. Strategies to be supported include systematic assessment of gene expression in specific cell types in the developing prostate and genitourinary tract; methods to tag individual cell types for purification, analysis, and characterization; tools to manipulate gene expression in vivo in individual cell types; and development of clinically relevant cell lines. The major goal of this initiative is to ensure that research tools are available so that a broad range of innovative methods can be applied to studying prostate development. Annual deadline dates may vary; contact program staff for exact dates.
Requirements: Application can be made by the following institutions and organizations: public/state controlled institutions of higher education; private institutions of higher education; nonprofits with 501(c)3 IRS status (other than institutions of higher education); nonprofits without 501(c)3 IRS status (other than institutions of higher education); small businesses; for-profit organizations (other than small businesses); state governments; U.S. territories or possessions; Indian/Native American tribal governments (federally recognized); Indian/Native American tribal governments (other than Federally recognized); Indian/Native American tribally designated organizations; non-domestic (non-U.S.) entities (foreign organizations); Hispanic-serving institutions; historically Black colleges and universities (HBCUs); tribally controlled colleges and universities (TCCUs); Alaska Native and Native Hawaiian serving institutions; regional organization; eligible agencies of the Federal government; and faith-based or community based organizations.
Amount of Grant: $350,000 maximum for RO1 grants; $100,000 maximum for R21 grants
Date(s) Application is Due: Feb 5; Mar 5; Jun 5; Jul 5; Oct 5; Nov 5
Contact: Dr. Robert Star; (301) 594-7715; fax: (301) 480-3510; email: StarR@extra.niddk.nih.gov; Dr. Michael McClure, Organs and Systems Toxicology, (919) 541-5327; fax: (919) 541-5064; email: mm461n@nih.gov
Internet: http://grants.nih.gov/grants/guide/rfa-files/RFA-DK-00-015.html
Sponsor: National Institute of Diabetes and Digestive and Kidney Diseases (NIDDK)
Room 9A-35, 31 Center Drive, MSC 2560
Bethesda, MD 20892-2560

NIDDK Co-Activators and Co-Repressors in Gene Expression Grants 2546

This initiative stems from an NIDDK workshop in molecular endocrinology and is designed to stimulate research that addresses the fundamental underlying mechanisms by which nuclear accessory proteins mediate signaling through hormone receptors at the level of the regulation of gene expression. Staff contact prior to submission is highly recommended.
Requirements: Applications may be submitted by domestic and foreign, for-profit and nonprofit organizations, both public and private; units of state and local governments; and eligible agencies of the federal government.
Amount of Grant: $100,000 maximum per year R21 grants, $250,000 maximum per year modular R01 grants
Date(s) Application is Due: Feb 16; Jun 16; Oct 16
Contact: Dr. Ronald Margolis; (301) 594-8819; fax: (301) 435-6047; email: rm76f@nih.gov
Internet: http://grants.nih.gov/grants/guide/pa-files/PA-99-111.html
Sponsor: National Institutes of Health
6707 Democracy Boulevard, Building 2DEM, Room 693
Bethesda, MD 20892

NIDDK Collaborative Interdisciplinary Team Science in Diabetes, Endocrinology and Metabolic Diseases Grants 2547

The purpose of the Collaborative Interdisciplinary Team Science Program described in this announcement is to provide support to enable strong investigative teams to do inter- and/or trans-disciplinary research on a complex problem in biomedical science relevant to Diabetes, Endocrinology and Metabolic Diseases. It is anticipated that 1-3 projects will be funded per year, but because the nature and scope of the proposed research will vary from application to application, it is anticipated that the size and duration of each award will also vary. The total amount awarded and the number of awards will depend upon the quality, duration, and costs of the applications received, as well as on the availability of funds.
Requirements: The following organizations and institutions are eligible to apply: public/state controlled institutions of higher education; private institutions of higher education; Hispanic-serving institutions; historically Black colleges and universities (HBCUs); tribally controlled colleges and universities (TCCUs); Alaska Native and Native Hawaiian serving institutions; and non-domestic (non-U.S.) entities (foreign organizations).
Date(s) Application is Due: Feb 24; Mar 24
Contact: Karen Salomon; (301) 594-7733; fax: (301) 435-6047; email: ks495c@nih.gov
Internet: http://grants.nih.gov/grants/guide/pa-files/PAR-08-182.html
Sponsor: National Institute of Diabetes and Digestive and Kidney Diseases (NIDDK)
6707 Democracy Boulevard, Room 687
Bethesda, MD 20892-5460

NIDDK Development of Assays for High-Throughput Drug Screening Grants 2548
The overall goal of the Molecular Libraries Initiative, part of the NIH Roadmap for Medical Research, is to offer public sector researchers opportunities to screen small molecules with the high-throughput chemical screening (HTS) methods commonly used by the private sector to develop therapeutic agents. The purpose of this FOA is to support the development of innovative assays that may ultimately be adapted for automated screening. The assay should aim to identify new tools for basic research or promising new avenues for therapeutics development, especially in areas related to the missions of the participating institutes. Awards issued under this FOA are contingent upon the availability of funds and the submission of a sufficient number of meritorious applications. The total amount awarded and the number of awards will depend upon the quality and costs of the applications received.
Requirements: The following organizations and institutions may apply: public/state controlled institutions of higher education; private institutions of higher education; Hispanic-serving institutions; historically Black colleges and universities (HBCUs); tribally controlled colleges and universities (TCCUs); Alaska native and native Hawaiian serving institutions; nonprofits with 501(c)3 IRS status; nonprofits without 501(c)3 IRS status; small businesses; for-profit organizations; State governments; regional organizations; U.S. territories or possessions; Indian/Native American tribal governments; Indian/Native American tribally designated organizations; eligible agencies of the Federal government; and faith-based or community based organizations.
Date(s) Application is Due: Feb 5; Jun 5; Oct 5
Contact: Laura K. Moen; (301) 594-4748; fax: (301) 480-3510; email: lm232f@nih.gov
Internet: http://grants.nih.gov/grants/guide/pa-files/PA-07-320.html
Sponsor: National Institute of Diabetes and Digestive and Kidney Diseases (NIDDK)
6707 Democracy Boulevard, Room 623
Bethesda, MD 20892-5458

NIDDK Development of Disease Biomarkers Grants 2549
The goal of this Funding Opportunity Announcement (FOA) is to validate biomarkers for well-defined human diseases of liver, kidney, urological tract, digestive and hematologic systems, and endocrine and metabolic disorders, diabetes and its complications, and obesity, for which there are no or very few biomarkers, or for which standard biomarkers are currently prohibitively invasive or expensive. New biomarkers will stimulate bench to bedside translation by providing measures of the biological effects of potential new treatments. The ideal biomarker can be measured in a minimally invasive way, can be measured repeatedly over time, identifies early stages of disease, is indicative of disease prognosis, and correlates well with progression and response to therapy. Especially of interest would be studies designed to test the validity of candidate biomarkers or new technologies to monitor candidate biomarkers in patient tissue samples or small groups of well-characterized patients. For biomarkers already validated in human subjects, the larger effort might be to establish a reliable assay prior to pursuing larger patient studies. Priority will be given to those projects with high promise for improving clinical care in the relatively near future. Studies of potential biomarkers conducted in animal models of disease, and extended prospective clinical trials for marker validation against hard clinical endpoints, are outside the scope of this initiative. Because the nature and scope of the proposed research will vary from application to application, it is anticipated that the size and duration of each award will also vary.
Requirements: Application can be made by the following institutions and organizations: public/state controlled institutions of higher education; private institutions of higher education; nonprofits with 501(c)3 IRS status (other than institutions of higher education); nonprofits without 501(c)3 IRS status (other than institutions of higher education); small businesses; for-profit organizations (other than small businesses); state governments; U.S. territories or possessions; Indian/Native American tribal governments (federally recognized); Indian/Native American tribal governments (other than Federally recognized); Indian/Native American tribally designated organizations; non-domestic (non-U.S.) entities (foreign organizations); Hispanic-serving institutions; historically Black colleges and universities (HBCUs); tribally controlled colleges and universities (TCCUs); Alaska Native and Native Hawaiian serving institutions; regional organization; eligible agencies of the Federal government; and faith-based or community based organizations.
Date(s) Application is Due: Feb 5; Jun 5; Oct 5
Contact: Maren R. Laughlin, Ph.D.; (301) 594-8802; fax: (301) 480-0475; email: ml33q@nih.gov
Internet: http://grants.nih.gov/grants/guide/pa-files/PA-07-052.html
Sponsor: National Institute of Diabetes and Digestive and Kidney Diseases (NIDDK)
6707 Democracy Boulevard, Room 787
Bethesda, MD 20892-5460

NIDDK Developmental Biology and Regeneration of the Liver Grants 2550
The purpose of this FOA is to invite qualified scientific investigators to submit applications on liver development and regeneration to fully define the molecular and cellular mechanisms underlying these processes in health and disease and to apply these findings to developing improved therapies for liver disease. Because the nature and scope of the proposed research will vary from application to application, it is anticipated that the size and duration of each award will also vary. The total amount awarded and the number of awards will depend upon the mechanism numbers, quality, duration, and costs of the applications received.
Requirements: The following organizations and institutions may apply: public/state controlled institutions of higher education; private institutions of higher education; Hispanic-serving institutions; historically Black colleges and universities (HBCUs); tribally controlled colleges and universities (TCCUs); Alaska native and native Hawaiian serving institutions; nonprofits with 501(c)3 IRS status; nonprofits without 501(c)3 IRS status; small businesses; for-profit organizations; State governments; regional organizations; U.S. territories or possessions; Indian/Native American tribal governments; Indian/Native American tribally designated organizations; eligible agencies of the Federal government; and faith-based or community based organizations.
Date(s) Application is Due: Feb 5; Jun 5; Oct 5
Contact: Jose Serrano; (301) 594-8871; fax: (301) 480-8300; email: js362q@nih.gov;; Samir Zakhari, Ph.D.; (301) 4 43-0799; fax: (301) 594-0673; email: szakhari@mail.nih.gov
Internet: http://grants.nih.gov/grants/guide/pa-files/PA-07-026.html
Sponsor: National Institute of Diabetes and Digestive and Kidney Diseases (NIDDK)
6707 Democracy Boulevard, Room 657
Bethesda, MD 20892-5450

NIDDK Diabetes Research Centers 2551
The mission of the Diabetes Centers is to serve as a key component of the NIDDK-supported research effort to develop new therapies and improve the health of Americans with, or at risk for, diabetes and related endocrine and metabolic disorders. The Centers promote new discoveries and enhance scientific progress through support of cutting-edge basic and clinical research related to the etiology and complications of diabetes, with the goal of rapidly translating research findings into novel strategies for the prevention, treatment and cure of diabetes and related conditions. This Funding Opportunity Announcement (FOA) solicits new and competing continuation applications for Diabetes Endocrinology Research Centers (DERCs) and Diabetes Research and Training Centers (DRTCs). Both types of Centers are designed to support and enhance the national research effort in diabetes and related endocrine and metabolic diseases. DERCs support three primary research-related activities: biomedical research cores, a Pilot and Feasibility (P&F) program, and an Enrichment program. DRTCs possess all elements of a DERC, with additional dedicated core services and P&F awards to support research in diabetes prevention and control. All activities pursued by Diabetes Centers are designed to enhance the efficiency, productivity, effectiveness and multidisciplinary nature of research in Diabetes Center topic areas.
Requirements: The following organizations and institutions are eligible to apply: public/state controlled institutions of higher education; private institutions of higher education; Hispanic-serving institutions; historically Black colleges and universities (HBCUs); tribally controlled colleges and universities (TCCUs); Alaska Native and Native Hawaiian serving institutions; nonprofits with 501(c)3 IRS status (other than institutions of higher education); nonprofits without 501(c)3 IRS status (other than institutions of higher education); for-profit organizations (other than small businesses); and state governments.
Date(s) Application is Due: Jun 22; Jul 15
Contact: James F. Hyde, Ph.D.; (301) 594-7692; fax: (301) 480-3503; email: jh486z@nih.gov
Internet: http://grants.nih.gov/grants/guide/rfa-files/RFA-DK-08-008.html
Sponsor: National Institute of Diabetes and Digestive and Kidney Diseases (NIDDK)
6707 Democracy Boulevard, Room 789
Bethesda, MD 20892-5460

NIDDK Diabetes, Endocrinology, and Metabolic Diseases NRSAs—Individual 2552
Individual National Research Service Awards (NRSAs) are given only at the postdoctoral level for research training in diabetes, endocrine, or metabolic diseases. To receive one, an individual must submit an application that describes a specific research project, which is guided and sponsored by a specific preceptor at a particular institution. The award may be for up to 36 months of training and consists of a stipend and an allowance to help meet expenses incurred during the course of fellowship.
Requirements: All awardees must be citizens or have been admitted to the United States for permanent residence. Individuals and public and private institutions, nonprofit and for-profit, that propose to establish, expand, and improve research activities in health sciences and related fields may apply for research grants. Individuals must be nominated and sponsored by public or nonprofit private institutions having staff and facilities appropriate to the proposed research training programs. SBIR grants can be awarded only to domestic small businesses. STTR grants can be awarded only to domestic small business concerns that partner with research institutions in cooperative research and development.
Amount of Grant: $16,600-$2.09 million; $180,100 average
Date(s) Application is Due: Apr 5; Aug 5; Dec 5
Contact: Dr. Judith Fradkin, Director; (301) 496-7348
Internet: http://grants.nih.gov/grants/guide/pa-files/PA-07-107.html
Sponsor: National Institute of Diabetes and Digestive and Kidney Diseases
45 Center Drive, Natcher Building
Bethesda, MD 20892-2560

NIDDK Diet Composition and Energy Balance Grants 2553
The goal of this funding opportunity announcement (FOA) is to invite Research Project Grant applications investigating the role of diet composition in energy balance, including studies in both animals and humans. Both short and longer-term studies are encouraged, ranging from basic studies investigating the impact of micro-or macronutrient composition on appetite, metabolism, and energy expenditure through clinical studies evaluating the efficacy of diets differing in micro- or macronutrient composition, absorption, dietary variety, or energy density for weight loss or weight maintenance. Because the nature and scope of the proposed research will vary from application to application, it is anticipated that the size and duration of each award will also vary. The total amount awarded and the number of awards will depend upon the mechanism numbers, quality, duration, and costs of the applications received.

Requirements: The following organizations and institutions may apply: public/state controlled institutions of higher education; private institutions of higher education; Hispanic-serving institutions; historically Black colleges and universities (HBCUs); tribally controlled colleges and universities (TCCUs); Alaska native and native Hawaiian serving institutions; nonprofits with 501(c)3 IRS status; nonprofits without 501(c)3 IRS status; small businesses; for-profit organizations; State governments; regional organizations; U.S. territories or possessions; Indian/Native American tribal governments; Indian/Native American tribally designated organizations; eligible agencies of the Federal government; and faith-based or community based organizations.
Date(s) Application is Due: Feb 5; Jun 5; Oct 5
Contact: Susan Z. Yanovski, M.D.; (301) 594-8882; fax: (301) 480-8300; email: sy29f@nih.gov
Internet: http://grants.nih.gov/grants/guide/pa-files/PA-07-218.html
Sponsor: National Institute of Diabetes and Digestive and Kidney Diseases (NIDDK)
6707 Democracy Boulevard, Room 665
Bethesda, MD 20892-5450

NIDDK Education Program Grants **2554**
This funding opportunity announcement (FOA) solicits Research Education grant applications from applicant organizations that propose to create educational opportunities to attract undergraduate students, graduate students, and postdoctoral fellows to careers in areas of biomedical or behavioral research of particular interest to the NIDDK while fostering the career development of these students and fellows. The NIDDK is especially interested in attracting students and postdoctoral fellows from scientific disciplines underrepresented in disease-oriented biomedical research such as engineering, informatics, computer science, and computational sciences, to encourage them to apply their expertise to research relevant to diabetes and other endocrine and metabolic diseases, digestive and liver diseases, nutrition, obesity research and prevention, and kidney, urologic and hematologic diseases. The total project period for an application submitted in response to this funding opportunity may not exceed five years. Direct costs are limited to $100,000 per year.
Requirements: The following organizations and institutions may apply: public/state controlled institutions of higher education; private institutions of higher education; Hispanic-serving institutions; historically Black colleges and universities (HBCUs); tribally controlled colleges and universities (TCCUs); Alaska native and native Hawaiian serving institutions; nonprofits with 501(c)3 IRS status; nonprofits without 501(c)3 IRS status; and Indian/Native American tribally designated organizations.
Amount of Grant: $100,000 maximum per year
Date(s) Application is Due: Jan 25; May 25; Sep 25
Contact: James F. Hyde, Ph.D.; (301) 594-7692; fax: (301) 480-3503; email: jh486z@nih.gov
Internet: http://grants.nih.gov/grants/guide/pa-files/PAR-06-554.html
Sponsor: National Institute of Diabetes and Digestive and Kidney Diseases (NIDDK)
6707 Democracy Boulevard, Room 785
Bethesda, MD 20892-5460

NIDDK Endoscopic Clinical Research Grants In Pancreatic & Biliary Diseases **2555**
These small grants (R03) may be used as planning grants for full-scale multi-center clinical trials or for pilot studies that could lead to full-scale multi-center clinical trials designed to provide evidence for or against changes in the current standard of care. Pilot epidemiological studies are encouraged that could lead to more extended research that would provide evidence for or against changes in health policy, especially as related to disease and cancer prevention. It is expected that these R03 grants will serve as a basis for planning future multi-center research project grant applications (R01) or cooperative agreement (U01) awards. New and experienced investigators in relevant fields and disciplines may apply for these small grants. Investigators are encouraged to take advantage of recent endoscopic and laboratory developments. In addition, the small grant is a good mechanism for new and experienced investigators to become better equipped to perform clinical and epidemiological research. A project period of up to two years and a budget for direct costs of up to two $25,000 modules or $50,000 per year may be requested.
Requirements: The following organizations and institutions may apply: for-profit organizations; non-profit organizations; public or private institutions, such as universities, colleges, hospitals, and laboratories; units of State government; units of local government; eligible agencies of the Federal government; domestic institutions; and foreign institutions.
Date(s) Application is Due: Feb 16; Jun 16; Oct 16
Contact: Frank Hamilton M.D.; (301) 594-8877; fax: (301) 480-8300; email: fh14e@nih.gov;; Jose Serrano M.D., Ph.D.; (301) 594-8871; fax: (301) 480-8300; email: js362q@nih.gov
Internet: http://grants.nih.gov/grants/guide/pa-files/PAR-06-171.html
Sponsor: National Institute of Diabetes and Digestive and Kidney Diseases (NIDDK)
6707 Democracy Boulevard, Room 669
Bethesda, MD 20892-5450

NIDDK Enhancing Zebrafish Research with Research Tools and Techniques **2556**
This FOA encourages investigator-initiated applications designed to exploit the power of the zebrafish as a vertebrate model for biomedical and behavioral research. Applications proposing to develop new research tools or techniques that are of high priority to the zebrafish community and that will advance the detection and characterization of genes, pathways, and phenotypes of interest in development and aging, organ formation, neural processes, behavior, sensory processing, physiological processes, and disease processes are welcome. Budgets for direct costs under $500,000 (direct costs) per year and a project duration of up to five years may be requested. Letters of Intent should arrive by August 17, with full proposals due by September 17.
Requirements: The following organizations and institutions may apply: public/state controlled institutions of higher education; private institutions of higher education; Hispanic-serving institutions; historically Black colleges and universities (HBCUs); tribally controlled colleges and universities (TCCUs); Alaska native and native Hawaiian serving institutions; nonprofits with 501(c)3 IRS status; nonprofits without 501(c)3 IRS status; small businesses; for-profit organizations; State governments; regional organizations; U.S. territories or possessions; Indian/Native American tribal governments; Indian/Native American tribally designated organizations; eligible agencies of the Federal government; and faith-based or community based organizations.
Date(s) Application is Due: Aug 17; Sep 17
Contact: Dr. Rebekah S. Rasooly; (301) 594-6007; fax: (301) 480-3510; email: rr185i@nih.gov
Internet: http://grants.nih.gov/grants/guide/pa-files/PAR-08-139.html
Sponsor: National Institute of Diabetes and Digestive and Kidney Diseases (NIDDK)
6707 Democracy Boulevard, MSC 5458
Bethesda, MD 20892-5458

NIDDK Erythroid Lineage Molecular Toolbox Grants **2557**
The ultimate goals of this Funding Opportunity Announcement (FOA) will be to use erythroid cells at different stages of development and differentiation to assemble the complete collection of genes expressed, describe how they are expressed and elucidate physical parameters, including subcellular localization of the proteins translated during erythropoiesis. These reagents may then be used to discover the structure-function relationships that exist in erythroid cells with possible application to other cell types. Because the nature and scope of the proposed research will vary from application to application, it is anticipated that the size and duration of each award will also vary.
Requirements: Application can be made by the following institutions and organizations: public/state controlled institutions of higher education; private institutions of higher education; nonprofits with 501(c)3 IRS status (other than institutions of higher education); nonprofits without 501(c)3 IRS status (other than institutions of higher education); small businesses; for-profit organizations (other than small businesses); state governments; U.S. territories or possessions; Indian/Native American tribal governments (federally recognized); Indian/Native American tribal governments (other than Federally recognized); Indian/Native American tribally designated organizations; non-domestic (non-U.S.) entities (foreign organizations); Hispanic-serving institutions; historically Black colleges and universities (HBCUs); tribally controlled colleges and universities (TCCUs); Alaska Native and Native Hawaiian serving institutions; regional organization; eligible agencies of the Federal government; and faith-based or community based organizations.
Date(s) Application is Due: Feb 5; Jun 5; Oct 5
Contact: Terry Rogers Bishop, Ph.D.; (301) 594-7726; email: tb232j@nih.gov
Internet: http://grants.nih.gov/grants/guide/pa-files/PA-07-011.html
Sponsor: National Institute of Diabetes and Digestive and Kidney Diseases (NIDDK)
6707 Democracy Boulevard, Room 619
Bethesda, MD 20892-5458

NIDDK Erythropoiesis: Components and Mechanisms Grants **2558**
This FOA issued by the National Institute of Diabetes and Digestive and Kidney Diseases (NIDDK) the National Institute of Aging (NIA), and the National Heart, Lung, and Blood Institute (NHLBI), National Institutes of Health, encourages investigator-initiated R01 applications that propose hypothesis-driven research using erythroid cells. The aim of this program is to support research efforts towards a complete description of the molecular and cellular components of erythropoiesis and how these components contribute to erythropoiesis. Components include genes that are expressed (transcriptome) in erythroid cells, either during development or during differentiation, and the proteins (proteome) that are translated in erythroid cells, especially with post-translational modifications or subcellular localizations that are unique to erythroid cells. A long range goal of this program is to generate a concise description of erythropoiesis that unifies genetics, molecular processes and cytokine determinants in the erythroid lineages so that new therapeutics may be developed to measure and combat anemia. Budgets for direct costs of up to $500,000 per year and a project duration of up to five years may be requested.
Requirements: The following organizations and institutions may apply: public/state controlled institutions of higher education; private institutions of higher education; Hispanic-serving institutions; historically Black colleges and universities (HBCUs); tribally controlled colleges and universities (TCCUs); Alaska native and native Hawaiian serving institutions; nonprofits with 501(c)3 IRS status; nonprofits without 501(c)3 IRS status; small businesses; for-profit organizations; State governments; regional organizations; U.S. territories or possessions; Indian/Native American tribal governments; Indian/Native American tribally designated organizations; county governments; city or township governments; special district governments; independent school districts; public housing authorities/Indian housing authorities; eligible agencies of the Federal government; and faith-based or community based organizations.
Amount of Grant: $500,000 maximum per year for five years
Date(s) Application is Due: Feb 5; Jun 5; Oct 5
Contact: Terry Rogers Bishop, Ph.D.; (301) 594-7726; email: tb232j@nih.gov
Internet: http://grants.nih.gov/grants/guide/pa-files/PA-09-255.html
Sponsor: National Institute of Diabetes and Digestive and Kidney Diseases (NIDDK)
6707 Democracy Boulevard, Room 619
Bethesda, MD 20892-5458

NIDDK Exploratory/Developmental Clinical Research Grants in Obesity 2559

The goal of this initiative is to encourage exploratory/developmental clinical research that will accelerate the development of effective interventions for prevention or treatment of overweight or obesity in adults and/or children. The goal of this mechanism is to provide flexibility for initiating exploratory, short-term studies, thus allowing new ideas to be investigated in a more expeditious manner without stringent requirements for preliminary data. Such support is needed to encourage investigators to pursue new approaches, underdeveloped topics, or more creative avenues for research including new partnerships. Epidemiological research with a goal of informing translational/clinical research on prevention or treatment of obesity or overweight in adults and/or children is encouraged. The emphasis is thus on the development of exploratory clinical studies, pilot and feasibility studies, or small randomized clinical trials that will provide preliminary data for intervention and epidemiological studies that will inform translational/clinical research.
Requirements: The following organizations and institutions may apply: public/state controlled institutions of higher education; private institutions of higher education; Hispanic-serving institutions; historically Black colleges and universities (HBCUs); tribally controlled colleges and universities (TCCUs); Alaska native and native Hawaiian serving institutions; nonprofits with 501(c)3 IRS status; nonprofits without 501(c)3 IRS status; small businesses; for-profit organizations; State governments; regional organizations; U.S. territories or possessions; Indian/Native American tribal governments; Indian/Native American tribally designated organizations; eligible agencies of the Federal government; and faith-based or community based organizations.
Amount of Grant: $200,000 in direct costs allowed in any single year; $275,000 for the combined two-year award
Date(s) Application is Due: Feb 16; Jun 16; Oct 16
Contact: Carolyn W. Miles, Ph.D.; (301)451-3759; fax: (301) 480-8300; email: cm294e@nih.gov
Internet: http://grants.nih.gov/grants/guide/pa-files/PA-09-124.html
Sponsor: National Institute of Diabetes and Digestive and Kidney Diseases (NIDDK)
6707 Democracy Boulevard, Room 665
Bethesda, MD 20817

NIDDK Grants for Basic Research in Glomerular Diseases 2560

This FOA invites applications from investigators with diverse scientific interests to apply their expertise in basic research to enhance the understanding of the pathogenesis of the various primary or secondary forms of glomerular disease. Recent observations regarding intrinsic glomerular cell biology, particularly in the podocyte, have provided exciting new insights into potential pathogenic mechanisms of human glomerular disease. Although both immune and nonimmune mechanisms of glomerular injury have been studied previously, experimental models of disease and recent techniques that provide tools for molecular and proteomic profiling show great promise for identifying glomerular disease biomarkers. Despite these recent advances, additional basic studies are needed to facilitate a better understanding of glomerular disease pathogenesis and ultimately impact on the treatment of human glomerulopathies. It is anticipated that applications submitted in response to this FOA could address a number of different aspects concerning the pathogenesis, natural history, therapy pre-emption or prevention of the various morphologic forms of experimental glomerular disease.
Requirements: The following organizations and institutions may apply: public/state controlled institutions of higher education; private institutions of higher education; Hispanic-serving institutions; historically Black colleges and universities (HBCUs); tribally controlled colleges and universities (TCCUs); Alaska native and native Hawaiian serving institutions; nonprofits with 501(c)3 IRS status; nonprofits without 501(c)3 IRS status; small businesses; for-profit organizations; State governments; regional organizations; U.S. territories or possessions; Indian/Native American tribal governments; Indian/Native American tribally designated organizations; eligible agencies of the Federal government; and faith-based or community based organizations.
Date(s) Application is Due: Feb 5; Jun 5; Oct 5
Contact: Marva Moxey-Mims, M.D.; (301) 594-7717; fax: (301) 480-3510; email: mm726k@nih.gov
Internet: http://grants.nih.gov/grants/guide/pa-files/PA-07-367.html
Sponsor: National Institute of Diabetes and Digestive and Kidney Diseases (NIDDK)
6707 Democracy Boulevard, Room 639
Bethesda, MD 20892-5458

NIDDK Identifying and Reducing Diabetes and Obesity Related Health Disparities within Healthcare Systems 2561

This FOA requests applications designed to identify or address factors or barriers that result in disparate outcomes within a healthcare system. All applications should measure the impact of identified factors or interventions on health outcomes. Research is sought that examines at least one of the following factors in a healthcare system and/or the interaction between these factors; healthcare professionals, healthcare organizations, and the patients and communities they serve.
Requirements: The following organizations and institutions may apply: public/state controlled institutions of higher education; private institutions of higher education; Hispanic-serving institutions; historically Black colleges and universities (HBCUs); tribally controlled colleges and universities (TCCUs); Alaska native and native Hawaiian serving institutions; nonprofits with 501(c)3 IRS status; nonprofits without 501(c)3 IRS status; small businesses; for-profit organizations; State governments; regional organizations; U.S. territories or possessions; Indian/Native American tribal governments; Indian/Native American tribally designated organizations; eligible agencies of the Federal government; and faith-based or community based organizations.
Date(s) Application is Due: Feb 5; Jun 5; Oct 5
Contact: Christine Hunter; (301) 594-4728; fax: (301) 480-3503; fax: ch514c@.nih.gov
Internet: http://grants.nih.gov/grants/guide/pa-files/PA-07-388.html
Sponsor: National Institute of Diabetes and Digestive and Kidney Diseases (NIDDK)
6707 Democracy Boulevard, Room 605
Bethesda, MD 20892-5460

NIDDK Insulin Signaling and Receptor Cross Talk Grants 2562

This Funding Opportunity Announcement (FOA) solicits investigator-initiated research projects that will define the mechanistic basis of crosstalk between the insulin receptor signaling pathway and other signaling pathways, with the goal of defining how insulin action is influenced by the complex microenvironment found in insulin responsive tissues.
Requirements: The following organizations and institutions may apply: public/state controlled institutions of higher education; private institutions of higher education; Hispanic-serving institutions; historically Black colleges and universities (HBCUs); tribally controlled colleges and universities (TCCUs); Alaska native and native Hawaiian serving institutions; nonprofits with 501(c)3 IRS status; nonprofits without 501(c)3 IRS status; small businesses; for-profit organizations; State governments; regional organizations; U.S. territories or possessions; Indian/Native American tribal governments; Indian/Native American tribally designated organizations; eligible agencies of the Federal government; and faith-based or community based organizations.
Date(s) Application is Due: Feb 5; Jun 5; Oct 5
Contact: Kristin Abraham, Ph.D.; (301) 451-8048; fax: (301) 480-3503; email: ka136s@nih.gov
Internet: http://grants.nih.gov/grants/guide/pa-files/PA-07-058.html
Sponsor: National Institute of Diabetes and Digestive and Kidney Diseases (NIDDK)
6707 Democracy Boulevard, Room 795
Bethesda, MD 20892-5460

NIDDK Intestinal Failure, Short Gut Syndrome and Small Bowel Transplantation Grants 2563

The National Institute of Diabetes and Digestive and Kidney Diseases (NIDDK) seeks grant applications to study the pathogenesis, natural history, treatment and complications of intestinal failure and its therapies, including parenteral nutrition and small bowel transplantation. The overall objective of this funding opportunity is to encourage basic and clinical research into intestinal failure, short gut syndrome and intestinal transplantation. Because the nature and scope of the proposed research will vary from application to application, it is anticipated that the size and duration of each award will also vary.
Requirements: Application can be made by the following institutions and organizations: public/state controlled institutions of higher education; private institutions of higher education; nonprofits with 501(c)3 IRS status (other than institutions of higher education); nonprofits without 501(c)3 IRS status (other than institutions of higher education); small businesses; for-profit organizations (other than small businesses); state governments; U.S. territories or possessions; Indian/Native American tribal governments (federally recognized); Indian/Native American tribal governments (other than Federally recognized); Indian/Native American tribally designated organizations; non-domestic (non-U.S.) entities (foreign organizations); Hispanic-serving institutions; historically Black colleges and universities (HBCUs); tribally controlled colleges and universities (TCCUs); Alaska Native and Native Hawaiian serving institutions; regional organization; eligible agencies of the Federal government; and faith-based or community based organizations.
Date(s) Application is Due: Feb 5; Jun 5; Oct 5
Contact: Dr. Michael K. May; (301) 594-8884; fax: (301) 480-8300; email: mm102i@nih.gov
Internet: http://grants.nih.gov/grants/guide/pa-files/PA-07-010.html
Sponsor: National Institute of Diabetes and Digestive and Kidney Diseases (NIDDK)
6707 Democracy Boulevard, Room 663, MSC 5450
Bethesda, MD 20892-5450

NIDDK Intestinal Stem Cell Consortium Grants 2564

This FOA invites new applications to participate in the Intestinal Stem Cell Consortium (ISCC). The goals of this initiative are: to establish a network of individual research projects and a Coordinating Center focused on research on stem cells of the small intestine; to isolate, culture, characterize, functionally validate, and compare stem cell populations from the small intestine epithelium in vivo and in vitro; to share data, biomaterials, models, reagents, resources and methods between projects in the ISCC; and make these publicly available through a web site to be developed by the Coordinating Center. The objective of support for this consortium is to accelerate research on stem cells of the intestinal epithelium in order to facilitate understanding of the biology and function of the intestine and aid development of therapies for intestinal diseases and conditions where damage and replacement of this epithelium are important components. Direct costs are limited to $250,000 per year for a maximum five-year period for research projects and $350,000 per year for a maximum five-year period for the Coordinating Center.
Requirements: Application can be made by the following institutions and organizations: public/state controlled institutions of higher education; private institutions of higher education; nonprofits with 501(c)3 IRS status (other than institutions of higher education); nonprofits without 501(c)3 IRS status (other than institutions of higher education); small businesses; for-profit organizations (other than small businesses); state governments; U.S. territories or possessions; Indian/Native American tribal governments (federally recognized); Indian/Native American tribal governments (other than Federally recognized); Indian/Native American tribally designated organizations; non-domestic (non-U.S.) entities (foreign organizations); Hispanic-serving institutions;

historically Black colleges and universities (HBCUs); tribally controlled colleges and universities (TCCUs); Alaska Native and Native Hawaiian serving institutions; regional organization; eligible agencies of the Federal government; and faith-based or community based organizations.
Amount of Grant: $250,000 maximum per year for five years
Date(s) Application is Due: Mar 18
Contact: Jill Carrington, Ph.D.; (301) 496-6402; fax: (301) 402-0010; email: carringj@mail.nih.gov;; Ronald Margolis, Ph.D.; (301) 594-8819; fax: (301) 435-6047; email: rm76f@nih.gov
Internet: http://grants.nih.gov/grants/guide/rfa-files/RFA-DK-08-010.html
Sponsor: National Institute of Diabetes and Digestive and Kidney Diseases (NIDDK)
Democracy 2, Room 661, 6707 Democracy Boulevard, MSC 5450
Bethesda, MD 20892

NIDDK Mentored Research Scientist Development Award **2565**
The overall objective of the NIH Research Career Development Award program is to prepare qualified individuals for careers that have a significant impact on the health-related research needs of the Nation. The objective of the NIDDK Mentored Research Scientist Development Award (K01) is to provide support for a sustained period of protected time for intensive research career development under the guidance of an experienced mentor, or sponsor, in the biomedical, behavioral or clinical sciences leading to research independence, thereby ensuring a future cadre of well-trained Ph.D. scientists working in research areas supported by NIDDK. The expectation is that through this sustained period of research career development and training, awardees will launch independent research careers and become competitive for new research project grant (R01) funding. By providing support for the critical transition period between postdoctoral training and independent R01 funding for non-clinical investigators, the NIDDK hopes to foster the careers of these investigators who are vital for the future excellence of the NIDDK research endeavor. Applicants must justify the need for a period of mentored research experience and provide a convincing case that the proposed period of support will substantially enhance their careers as independent investigators.
Requirements: The following organizations and institutions may apply: public/state controlled institutions of higher education; private institutions of higher education; Hispanic-serving institutions; historically Black colleges and universities (HBCUs); tribally controlled colleges and universities (TCCUs); Alaska native and native Hawaiian serving institutions; nonprofits with 501(c)3 IRS status; nonprofits without 501(c)3 IRS status; small businesses; for-profit organizations; State governments; regional organizations; U.S. territories or possessions; Indian/Native American tribal governments; Indian/Native American tribally designated organizations; eligible agencies of the Federal government; and faith-based or community based organizations.
Date(s) Application is Due: Mar 12; Jul 12; Nov 12
Contact: James F. Hyde, Ph.D.; (301) 594-7692; fax: (301) 480-3503; email: jh486z@nih.gov
Internet: http://grants.nih.gov/grants/guide/pa-files/PAR-09-060.html
Sponsor: National Institute of Diabetes and Digestive and Kidney Diseases (NIDDK)
6707 Democracy Boulevard, Room 789
Bethesda, MD 20892-5460

NIDDK Multi-Center Clinical Study Cooperative Agreements **2566**
This PAR provides for grant applications for investigator-initiated, multi-center clinical studies. NIDDK supports investigator-initiated, multi-center clinical studies through a two-part process that includes an implementation planning (U34) grant. Beginning with the receipt date, NIDDK will accept, peer review, and consider for funding applications for investigator-initiated, multi-center clinical studies only from NIDDK Multi-Center Clinical Study Implementation Planning (U34) grant awardees. Because the nature and scope of the proposed research will vary from application to application, it is anticipated that the size and duration of each award will also vary. The total amount awarded and the number of awards will depend upon the mechanism numbers, quality, duration, and costs of the applications received.
Requirements: The following organizations and institutions may apply: public/state controlled institutions of higher education; private institutions of higher education; Hispanic-serving institutions; historically Black colleges and universities (HBCUs); tribally controlled colleges and universities (TCCUs); Alaska native and native Hawaiian serving institutions; nonprofits with 501(c)3 IRS status; nonprofits without 501(c)3 IRS status; small businesses; for-profit organizations; State governments; regional organizations; U.S. territories or possessions; Indian/Native American tribal governments; Indian/Native American tribally designated organizations; eligible agencies of the Federal government; and faith-based or community based organizations.
Date(s) Application is Due: Feb 5; Jun 5; Oct 5
Contact: Catherine Meyers, M.D.; (301) 451-4901; fax: (301) 480-3510; email: meyersc@mail.nih.gov
Internet: http://grants.nih.gov/grants/guide/pa-files/PAR-08-058.html
Sponsor: National Institute of Diabetes and Digestive and Kidney Diseases (NIDDK)
Two Democracy Plaza, Room 641, 6707 Democracy Boulevard
Bethesda, MD 20892-5458

NIDDK Multi-Center Clinical Study Implementation Planning Grants **2567**
NIDDK supports investigator-initiated, multi-center clinical studies through a two-part process that includes an implementation planning grant. The planning grant is designed to: permit early peer review of the rationale for the proposed clinical study; permit assessment of the design/protocol of the proposed study; provide support for the development of a complete study protocol and associated documents including a manual of operations; and support the development of other essential elements required for the conduct of a clinical study. Completion of the required products of a U34 grant is a prerequisite for submission of a multi-center clinical study cooperative agreement application, which will support the actual conduct of the study. Because the nature and scope of the proposed research will vary from application to application, it is anticipated that the size and duration of each award will also vary. The total project period for an application submitted in response to this funding opportunity may not exceed two years. Applicants may request up to $250,000 in direct costs per year.
Requirements: The following organizations and institutions may apply: public/state controlled institutions of higher education; private institutions of higher education; Hispanic-serving institutions; historically Black colleges and universities (HBCUs); tribally controlled colleges and universities (TCCUs); Alaska native and native Hawaiian serving institutions; nonprofits with 501(c)3 IRS status; nonprofits without 501(c)3 IRS status; small businesses; for-profit organizations; State governments; regional organizations; U.S. territories or possessions; Indian/Native American tribal governments; Indian/Native American tribally designated organizations; eligible agencies of the Federal government; and faith-based or community based organizations.
Date(s) Application is Due: Jun 23; Mar 18
Contact: Catherine Meyers, M.D.; (301) 451-4901; fax: (301) 480-3510; email: meyersc@mail.nih.gov
Internet: http://grants.nih.gov/grants/guide/pa-files/PAR-08-057.html
Sponsor: National Institute of Diabetes and Digestive and Kidney Diseases (NIDDK)
Two Democracy Plaza, Room 641, 6707 Democracy Boulevard
Bethesda, MD 20892-5458

NIDDK Neurobiology of Diabetic Complications Grants **2568**
NIDDK invites investigator-initiated research grant applications to study the mechanisms by which diabetes results in painful and disabling neuropathies and other neurological complications and to apply this information to the development of interventions to prevent, limit, or reverse these complications. The intent of this RFA is to attract basic neuroscientists to the study of diabetic neuropathy and neurobiology relevant to diabetes, and enhance interdisciplinary approaches to research in this area. Annual deadline dates may vary; contact the appropriate NIH institute for exact dates. Letters of intent are due by March 24, with full applications due by April 25 each year.
Requirements: Applications may be submitted by domestic and foreign, for-profit and nonprofit organizations, both public and private; units of state and local governments; and eligible agencies of the federal government.
Amount of Grant: $3 million total
Date(s) Application is Due: Mar 24; Apr 25
Contact: Dr. Barbara Linder; (301) 594-0021; fax: (301) 480-3503; email: bl99n@nih.gov;; Dr. Paul Nichols; (301) 496-9964; fax: (301) 402-2060; email: pn13w@nih.gov
Internet: http://grants.nih.gov/grants/guide/rfa-files/RFA-NS-00-002.html
Sponsor: National Institute of Diabetes and Digestive and Kidney Diseases (NIDDK)
45 Center Drive, MSC 6600
Bethesda, MD 20892-6600

NIDDK Neuroimaging in Obesity Research Grants **2569**
This FOA issued by the National Institute of Diabetes and Digestive and Kidney Diseases, the National Institute on Drug Abuse, and the National Institute of Biomedical Imaging and Bioengineering, of the National Institutes of Health, solicits Research Project Grant (R01) applications from institutions/ organizations that propose to use neuroimaging approaches in obesity research in human subjects and animal models. Many areas of the brain interact or communicate with other organs to control eating behavior, physical activity and energy metabolism, and functional neuroimaging holds enormous promise for expanding our understanding of how food intake and energy expenditure are mismatched in a setting of abundantly available nutrients, leading to excessive fat storage. The total amount of funding that the ICs expect to award through this announcement is up to $4.5 Million, to fund approximately 9-15 awards. The duration and requested direct costs will vary depending on the scope of the proposed research, but cannot exceed 5 years and $500,000 per year. Letters of intent are due by February 18, with full applications due by 5:00 p.m. on March 18.
Requirements: Application can be made by the following institutions and organizations: public/state controlled institutions of higher education; private institutions of higher education; nonprofits with 501(c)3 IRS status (other than institutions of higher education); nonprofits without 501(c)3 IRS status (other than institutions of higher education); small businesses; for-profit organizations (other than small businesses); state governments; U.S. territories or possessions; Indian/Native American tribal governments (federally recognized); Indian/Native American tribal governments (other than Federally recognized); Indian/Native American tribally designated organizations; non-domestic (non-U.S.) entities (foreign organizations); Hispanic-serving institutions; historically Black colleges and universities (HBCUs); tribally controlled colleges and universities (TCCUs); Alaska Native and Native Hawaiian serving institutions; regional organization; eligible agencies of the Federal government; and faith-based or community based organizations.
Amount of Grant: $500,000 maximum in direct costs per year, for up to 5 years
Date(s) Application is Due: Feb 18; Mar 18
Contact: Maren R. Laughlin, Ph.D.; (301) 594-8802; fax: (301) 480-0475; email: ml33q@nih.gov
Internet: http://grants.nih.gov/grants/guide/rfa-files/RFA-DK-08-009.html
Sponsor: National Institute of Diabetes and Digestive and Kidney Diseases (NIDDK)
6707 Democracy Boulevard Room 787, MSC 5460
Bethesda, MD 20892-5460

NIDDK New Technologies for Liver Disease SBIR 2570

The purpose of this Funding Opportunity Announcement (FOA) is to solicit Small Business Innovation Research (SBIR) grant applications from small business concerns (SBCs) that propose to develop resources, research tools, instrumentations, biomarkers, devices, drugs or new and innovative approaches to diagnosis, monitoring, management, treatment and prevention of liver diseases. Areas of interest include development of reliable and practical means of diagnosis of liver diseases; biomarkers for disease activity and stage; noninvasive tests for inflammation, fibrosis and fat in the liver; and drugs, complementary and alternative modalities, biologics or molecular reagents for the therapy or prevention of liver diseases. The goal of this announcement is to enlist members of the small business research community in advancing means of diagnosis, treatment and prevention of liver disease and facilitate the goals outlined in the trans-NIH Action Plan for Liver Disease Research.

Requirements: Only United States small business concerns (SBCs) are eligible to submit SBIR applications.

Amount of Grant: $100,000 maximum for Phase 1; $750,000 maximum for Phase 2

Date(s) Application is Due: Apr 5; Aug 5; Dec 5

Contact: Christine L. Densmore, M.S.; (301) 402-8714; fax: (301) 480-8300; email: cd121z@nih.gov

Internet: http://grants.nih.gov/grants/guide/pa-files/PA-09-095.html

Sponsor: National Institute of Diabetes and Digestive and Kidney Diseases (NIDDK)
6707 Democracy Boulevard, Room 649
Bethesda, MD 20892-5450

NIDDK New Technologies for Liver Disease STTR 2571

The objective of this FOA is to encourage and enable scientists at small businesses to develop and evaluate new technologies, drugs, devices, and approaches to diagnosis, management, and prevention of liver disease. Development of new technologies as well as application of existing technologies may be proposed. Studies may include use of animal models or human participants or both. If appropriate, plans for manufacturing and clinical evaluation of developed technologies, drugs, devices and innovative approaches should be included in the application. However, clinical trials beyond Phase I studies will not be considered appropriate to this announcement.

Requirements: Only United States small business concerns (SBCs) are eligible to submit STTR applications.

Amount of Grant: $100,000 maximum for Phase 1; $750,000 maximum for Phase 2

Date(s) Application is Due: Apr 5; Aug 5; Dec 5

Contact: Christine L. Densmore, M.S.; (301) 402-8714; fax: (301) 480-8300; email: cd121z@nih.gov

Internet: http://grants.nih.gov/grants/guide/pa-files/PA-09-094.html

Sponsor: National Institute of Diabetes and Digestive and Kidney Diseases (NIDDK)
6707 Democracy Boulevard, Room 649
Bethesda, MD 20892-5450

NIDDK Non-Invasive Methods for Diagnosis and Progression of Diabetes, Kidney, Urological, Hematological and Digestive Diseases 2572

This funding opportunity is a call for the application of imaging and other non- or minimally-invasive technologies to detect, characterize, diagnose, identify persons with predisposition to, or monitor treatment of diseases of interest to the National Institute of Diabetes and Digestive and Kidney Diseases. Also needed are new, robust surrogate markers for clinical trial endpoints, and new ways to characterize normal and pathological tissues in vivo. Diseases of interest include type 1 and 2 diabetes, obesity, and kidney, liver, urologic, hematologic, digestive, endocrine and metabolic diseases and their complications. Applicable techniques include molecular imaging and functional imaging approaches, imaging methods with high spatial, chemical or time resolution, and new spectroscopic or sensor array technologies for monitoring metabolic or physiological events.

Requirements: The following organizations and institutions may apply: for-profit organizations; non-profit organizations; public or private institutions, such as universities, colleges, hospitals, and laboratories; units of State government; units of local government; eligible agencies of the Federal government; foreign institutions; domestic institutions; and faith-based or community-based organizations.

Date(s) Application is Due: Feb 5; Jun 5; Oct 5

Contact: Maren R. Laughlin, Ph.D.; (301) 594-8802; fax: (301) 480-0475; email: ml33q@nih.gov

Internet: http://grants.nih.gov/grants/guide/pa-files/PA-06-143.html

Sponsor: National Institute of Diabetes and Digestive and Kidney Diseases (NIDDK)
6707 Democracy Boulevard, Room 787
Bethesda, MD 20892-5460

NIDDK Pancreatic Development and Regeneration Grants: Toward Cellula Therapies for Diabetes 2573 r

This Funding Opportunity Announcement (FOA) is intended to promote basic research in pancreatic development, stem cell biology and regeneration that will provide the foundation for the rationale design of future cell replacement therapies for diabetes. Appropriate topics for investigation include, but are not limited to: prospective isolation, purification and characterization of pancreatic stem/progenitor cells; identification of the signals, signaling pathway components and transcriptional factors that could direct the formation of pancreatic endoderm and progenitors, islet cell differentiation, morphogenesis, growth, function and survival in vitro; use of existing NIH-approved human ES cell lines or mouse embryonic cells, pancreatic stem cells, non-pancreatic adult stem cells such as those from liver or gut, human amniotic cells or bone marrow-derived cells to efficiently generate endoderm, pancreatic progenitor cells, or differentiated beta cells in culture; development of methods and reagents to assess quantitatively, the survival, migration, fate and function of transplanted animal or human pancreatic progenitors and their progeny in the living animal; determination of the factors important for beta cell regeneration and designing strategies to foster regeneration; development of new animal models that can used to identify exogenous or endogenous factors that might promote beta cell regeneration or neogenesis; characterization the lineage of cells that may contribute or participate in beta cell regeneration by genetic marking; and development of assays to screen chemical libraries for modifiers of beta cell regeneration, differentiation, and or expansion.

Requirements: The following organizations and institutions may apply: public/state controlled institutions of higher education; private institutions of higher education; Hispanic-serving institutions; historically Black colleges and universities (HBCUs); tribally controlled colleges and universities (TCCUs); Alaska native and native Hawaiian serving institutions; nonprofits with 501(c)3 IRS status; nonprofits without 501(c)3 IRS status; small businesses; for-profit organizations; State governments; regional organizations; U.S. territories or possessions; Indian/Native American tribal governments; Indian/Native American tribally designated organizations; eligible agencies of the Federal government; and faith-based or community based organizations.

Date(s) Application is Due: Feb 5; Jun 5; Oct 5

Contact: Sheryl M. Sato, Ph.D.; (301) 594-8811; fax: (301) 480-0475; email: ss68z@nih.gov

Internet: http://grants.nih.gov/grants/guide/pa-files/PA-07-056.html

Sponsor: National Institute of Diabetes and Digestive and Kidney Diseases (NIDDK)
2 Democracy Plaza, Room 790, 6707 Democracy Boulevard
Bethesda, MD 20892-5460

NIDDK Pilot and Feasibility Clinical Research Grants in Diabetes, Endocrine and Metabolic Diseases 2574

The goal of this initiative is to encourage exploratory/developmental clinical research related to the prevention or treatment of diabetes, obesity and endocrine and genetic metabolic diseases. The Pilot and Feasibility Clinical Research Grants Program is designed to allow initiation of exploratory, short-term clinical studies, so that new ideas may be investigated without stringent requirements for preliminary data. Such support can be used by experienced investigators, as well as new investigators, to pursue new approaches and investigate underdeveloped research areas. The short-term studies should focus on research questions that are likely to have high clinical impact. They can include testing a new prevention strategy, a new intervention, or unique combinations of therapies. A high priority is the use of such studies to help stimulate the translation of promising research developments from the laboratory into clinical practice in diabetes, endocrine diseases and genetic metabolic diseases, including cystic fibrosis.

Requirements: The following organizations and institutions may apply: public/state controlled institutions of higher education; private institutions of higher education; Hispanic-serving institutions; historically Black colleges and universities (HBCUs); tribally controlled colleges and universities (TCCUs); Alaska native and native Hawaiian serving institutions; nonprofits with 501(c)3 IRS status; nonprofits without 501(c)3 IRS status; small businesses; for-profit organizations; State governments; regional organizations; U.S. territories or possessions; Indian/Native American tribal governments; Indian/Native American tribally designated organizations; eligible agencies of the Federal government; and faith-based or community based organizations.

Amount of Grant: $200,000 in direct costs allowed in any single year; $275,000 for the combined two-year award

Date(s) Application is Due: Feb 16; Jun 16; Oct 16

Contact: Karen Salomon; (301) 594-7733; fax: (301) 435-6047; email: ks495c@nih.gov

Internet: http://grants.nih.gov/grants/guide/pa-files/PA-09-133.html

Sponsor: National Institute of Diabetes and Digestive and Kidney Diseases (NIDDK)
6707 Democracy Boulevard, Democracy 2, Room 687
Bethesda, MD 20892-5460

NIDDK Pilot and Feasibility Clinical Research Grants in Kidney or Urologic Diseases 2575

This funding opportunity announcement (FOA) is a re-issuance of PAR-06-113 and specifically encourages the submission of applications for small scale or pilot and feasibility clinical and translational research studies, including epidemiological studies or clinical trials related to kidney or urologic disease research that address important clinical and translational questions and are potentially of high impact. It is anticipated that some applications for pilot and feasibility studies may lead to full-scale clinical studies including evaluation of diagnostic strategies, epidemiologic studies, or trials in the diagnosis, prevention, or treatment of kidney or urologic diseases. These grants may be used to plan, evaluate the feasibility, or implement clinical trials that assess pharmacological, dietary, surgical, or behavioral interventions for the prevention or treatment of kidney or urologic disease. Small scale or pilot epidemiological studies are also encouraged.

Requirements: The following organizations and institutions may apply: public/state controlled institutions of higher education; private institutions of higher education; Hispanic-serving institutions; historically Black colleges and universities (HBCUs); tribally controlled colleges and universities (TCCUs); Alaska native and native Hawaiian serving institutions; nonprofits with 501(c)3 IRS status; nonprofits without 501(c)3 IRS status; small businesses; for-profit organizations; State governments; regional organizations; U.S. territories or possessions; Indian/Native American tribal governments; Indian/Native American tribally designated organizations; eligible agencies of the Federal government; and faith-based or community based organizations.

Amount of Grant: $200,000 in direct costs allowed in any single year; $275,000 for the combined two-year award

Date(s) Application is Due: Feb 16; Jun 16; Oct 16
Contact: Catherine M. Meyers, M.D.; (301) 594-7717; fax: (301) 480-3510; email: cm420i@nih.gov
Internet: http://grants.nih.gov/grants/guide/pa-files/PAR-09-077.html
Sponsor: National Institute of Diabetes and Digestive and Kidney Diseases (NIDDK)
6707 Democracy Boulevard, Room 641
Bethesda, MD 20892-5458

NIDDK Pilot and Feasibility Clinical Research Studies in Digestive Diseases and Nutrition 2576

The goal of this pilot and feasibility mechanism is to provide flexibility for initiating preliminary, short-term clinical studies, thus allowing new ideas to be investigated in a more expeditious manner without stringent requirements for preliminary data. Such support is needed to encourage experienced investigators as well as new investigators to pursue new approaches, underdeveloped topics, or more creative avenues of research. If successful, these awards should lead to significant scientific advances in digestive disease research and should facilitate translation into clinical practice to improve patient outcomes.
Requirements: The following organizations and institutions are eligible to apply: public/state controlled institutions of higher education; private institutions of higher education; Hispanic-serving institutions; historically Black colleges and universities (HBCUs); tribally controlled colleges and universities (TCCUs); Alaska Native and Native Hawaiian serving institutions; nonprofits with 501(c)3 IRS status (other than institutions of higher education); nonprofits without 501(c)3 IRS status (other than institutions of higher education); small businesses; for-profit organizations (other than small businesses); state governments; Indian/Native American tribal governments (federally recognized); Indian/Native American tribally designated organizations; county governments; city or township governments; special district governments; independent school districts; public housing authorities; Indian housing authorities; U.S. territory or possession; Indian/Native American tribal governments (other than federally recognized); regional organizations; non-domestic (non-U.S.) entities (foreign organizations); other eligible agencies of the federal government; and faith-based or community-based organizations.
Date(s) Application is Due: Feb 16; Jun 16; Oct 16
Contact: Mary Evans, Ph.D.; (301) 594-4578; fax: (301) 480-8300; email: me189d@nih.gov
Internet: http://grants.nih.gov/grants/guide/pa-files/PA-09-151.html
Sponsor: National Institute of Diabetes and Digestive and Kidney Diseases (NIDDK)
6707 Democracy Boulevard, Room 681
Bethesda, MD 20892-5450

NIDDK Planning Grants For Translational Research For The Prevention And Control Of Diabetes And Obesity 2577

The National Institute of Diabetes and Digestive and Kidney Diseases (NIDDK) seeks to develop cost effective and sustainable interventions, that can be adopted in real world settings, for the prevention and control of diabetes and obesity. Research should be based on interventions already proven efficacious in clinical trials to prevent and reverse obesity and type 2 diabetes, to improve care of type 1 and type 2 diabetes and to prevent or delay its complications. The interventions proposed under this solicitation should have the potential to be widely disseminated to clinical practice, individuals and communities at risk. Relevant topics include: methods to improve health care delivery to patients with or at risk of diabetes; to enhance diabetes self management; methods to develop strategies to promote healthy lifestyles to reduce the risk of diabetes; and methods to promote lifestyle change that will prevent or reverse overweight and obesity, and 5) new cost effective ways to identify people with pre-diabetes and undiagnosed diabetes. This FOA will use the National Institutes of Health (NIH) clinical trial planning grant (R34) award mechanism, which will provide up to $150,000 in direct costs per year.
Requirements: Applications may be submitted by: for-profit organizations; non-profit organizations; public or private institutions, such as universities, colleges, hospitals, and laboratories; units of State government; units of local government; eligible agencies of the Federal government; domestic institutions; faith-based or community-based organizations; Indian/Native American tribal governments; and Indian/Native American tribally designated organizations.
Amount of Grant: $150,000 maximum per year
Date(s) Application is Due: Feb 16; Jun 16; Oct 16
Contact: Sanford Garfield; (301) 594-8803; fax: (301) 480-3503; email: sg50o@nih.gov
Internet: http://grants.nih.gov/grants/guide/pa-files/PAR-06-358.html
Sponsor: National Institute of Diabetes and Digestive and Kidney Diseases
6707 Democracy Boulevard, Room 685
Bethesda, MD 20892-5460

NIDDK Proteomics: Diabetes, Obesity, And Endocrine, Digestive, Kidney, Urologic, And Hematologic Diseases 2578

This Funding Opportunity Announcement (FOA) issued by the National Institute of Diabetes and Digestive and Kidney Diseases (NIDDK), National Institutes of Health (NIH), solicits projects that advance research to identify and quantitate protein expression patterns, post-translational modification of proteins, and protein-protein interactions on cells, tissues, organ systems relevant to diabetes, obesity, endocrine and metabolic diseases, nutritional function and diseases of the alimentary tract, exocrine pancreas, liver, kidney, bladder and prostate and normal biological processes related to the function of these systems. The development and improvement of innovative proteomic technologies is also encouraged through their application to relevant biological questions related to the pathophysiology of endocrine glands, gastrointestinal tract, liver and kidney, bladder and prostate.
Requirements: The following organizations and institutions may apply: public/state controlled institutions of higher education; private institutions of higher education; Hispanic-serving institutions; historically Black colleges and universities (HBCUs); tribally controlled colleges and universities (TCCUs); Alaska native and native Hawaiian serving institutions; nonprofits with 501(c)3 IRS status; nonprofits without 501(c)3 IRS status; small businesses; for-profit organizations; State governments; regional organizations; U.S. territories or possessions; Indian/Native American tribal governments; Indian/Native American tribally designated organizations; eligible agencies of the Federal government; and faith-based or community based organizations.
Date(s) Application is Due: Feb 5; Jun 5; Oct 5
Contact: Salvatore Sechi; (301) 594-8814; fax: (301) 480-2688; email: ss24q@nih.gov
Internet: http://grants.nih.gov/grants/guide/pa-files/PA-07-016.html
Sponsor: National Institute of Diabetes and Digestive and Kidney Diseases (NIDDK)
6707 Democracy Blvd. Room 611
Bethesda, MD 20892-5460

NIDDK Race/Ethnic Disparities in the Incidence of Diabetes Complications 2579

This PA solicits research to investigate differences among contemporary populations in the United States, categorized by race-ethnicity and other factors, in risk factors for complications of diabetes and in rates of these complications; and the extent to which factors, including inherent metabolic and genetic variations, medical care, socioeconomic status, and behavioral factors, account for these differences. PA: PA-02-165
Requirements: Applications may be submitted by domestic for-profit and nonprofit organizations, both public and private; units of state and local governments; and eligible agencies of the federal government.
Contact: Dr. Kristin Abraham, (301) 451-8048; fax: (301) 480-3503; email: ka136s@nih.gov
Internet: http://grants2.nih.gov/grants/guide/pa-files/PA-02-165.html
Sponsor: National Institute of Diabetes and Digestive and Kidney Diseases
45 Center Drive, Natcher Building
Bethesda, MD 20892

NIDDK Research Grants for Studies of Hepatitis C in the Setting of Renal Disease 2580

It is the intent of this Funding Opportunity Announcement (FOA) to invite applications from investigators with diverse scientific interests, who wish to apply their expertise into basic and applied research to enhance the understanding of the pathogenesis, natural history, therapy,and prevention of hepatitis C in the setting of renal disease or renal transplantation. Because the nature and scope of the proposed research will vary from application to application, it is anticipated that the size and duration of each award will also vary. The total amount awarded and the number of awards will depend upon the mechanism numbers, quality, duration, and costs of the applications received.
Requirements: The following organizations and institutions may apply: public/state controlled institutions of higher education; private institutions of higher education; Hispanic-serving institutions; historically Black colleges and universities (HBCUs); tribally controlled colleges and universities (TCCUs); Alaska native and native Hawaiian serving institutions; nonprofits with 501(c)3 IRS status; nonprofits without 501(c)3 IRS status; small businesses; for-profit organizations; State governments; regional organizations; U.S. territories or possessions; Indian/Native American tribal governments; Indian/Native American tribally designated organizations; eligible agencies of the Federal government; and faith-based or community based organizations.
Date(s) Application is Due: Feb 5; Jun 5; Oct 5
Contact: Catherine M. Meyers, M.D.; (301) 594-7717; fax: (301) 480-3510; email: cm420i@nih.gov
Internet: http://grants.nih.gov/grants/guide/pa-files/PA-07-015.html
Sponsor: National Institute of Diabetes and Digestive and Kidney Diseases (NIDDK)
6707 Democracy Boulevard, Room 641
Bethesda, MD 20892-5458

NIDDK Research Grants on Improving Health Care for Obese Patients 2581

This funding opportunity announcement (FOA) solicits Research Project Grant applications from institutions and organizations that propose to conduct research to determine the barriers to optimal health care for obese patients, and to test innovations or modifications in care delivery to improve health outcomes for obese patients independent of weight loss. Awards issued under this FOA are contingent upon the availability of funds and the submission of a sufficient number of meritorious applications. Applications can be renewed by competing for additional project periods.
Requirements: The following organizations and institutions may apply: public/state controlled institutions of higher education; private institutions of higher education; Hispanic-serving institutions; historically Black colleges and universities (HBCUs); tribally controlled colleges and universities (TCCUs); Alaska native and native Hawaiian serving institutions; nonprofits with 501(c)3 IRS status; nonprofits without 501(c)3 IRS status; small businesses; for-profit organizations; State governments; regional organizations; U.S. territories or possessions; Indian/Native American tribal governments; Indian/Native American tribally designated organizations; eligible agencies of the Federal government; and faith-based or community based organizations.
Date(s) Application is Due: Feb 5; Jun 5; Oct 5
Contact: Susan Z. Yanovski; (301) 594-8882; fax: (301) 480-8300; email: sy29f@nih.gov
Internet: http://grants.nih.gov/grants/guide/pa-files/PA-07-013.html
Sponsor: National Institute of Diabetes and Digestive and Kidney Diseases (NIDDK)
6707 Democracy Boulevard, Room 675
Bethesda, MD 20892-5450

NIDDK Role of Gastrointestinal Surgical Procedures in Amelioration of Obesity-Related Insulin Resistance and Diabetes Independent of Weight Loss 2582

This Funding Opportunity Announcement (FOA) issued by the National Institute of Diabetes and Digestive and Kidney Diseases, National Institutes of Health encourages Research Project Grant (R01) applications from institutions and organizations that propose to explain the underlying mechanism(s) by which various gastrointestinal surgical procedures ameliorate obesity-related insulin resistance and diabetes independent of the resultant weight loss. Awards issued under this FOA are contingent upon the availability of funds and the submission of a sufficient number of meritorious applications.
Requirements: The following organizations and institutions may apply: public/state controlled institutions of higher education; private institutions of higher education; Hispanic-serving institutions; historically Black colleges and universities (HBCUs); tribally controlled colleges and universities (TCCUs); Alaska native and native Hawaiian serving institutions; nonprofits with 501(c)3 IRS status; nonprofits without 501(c)3 IRS status; small businesses; for-profit organizations; State governments; regional organizations; U.S. territories or possessions; Indian/Native American tribal governments; Indian/Native American tribally designated organizations; eligible agencies of the Federal government; and faith-based or community based organizations.
Date(s) Application is Due: Feb 5; Jun 5; Oct 5
Contact: Carolyn W. Miles, Ph.D.; (301)451-3759; fax: (301) 480-8300; email: cm294e@nih.gov
Internet: http://grants.nih.gov/grants/guide/pa-files/PA-08-014.html
Sponsor: National Institute of Diabetes and Digestive and Kidney Diseases (NIDDK)
6707 Democracy Boulevard, Room 665
Bethesda, MD 20892-5450

NIDDK Secondary Analyses in Obesity, Diabetes and Digestive and Kidney Diseases Grants 2583

The specific objectives of this announcement on Secondary Analyses In Obesity, Diabetes, Digestive and Kidney Diseases are to support the following: secondary analyses of data related to the epidemiology of disease areas of NIDDK; important and/or innovative hypotheses explored through analysis of existing data sets; secondary analyses designed to inform and support subsequent applications for individual research awards; rapid analyses of new databases and experimental modules to inform the design and content of future studies; the archiving of datasets to be made publicly available for research purposes related to disease areas of NIDDK, including both epidemiological studies and multi-center clinical trials. Research that employs analytic techniques that demonstrate or promote methodological advances in patient oriented and epidemiologic research is also of interest. International comparative analyses are encouraged. Applications that are innovative and high risk with the likelihood for high impact are especially encouraged.
Requirements: The following organizations and institutions may apply: public/state controlled institutions of higher education; private institutions of higher education; Hispanic-serving institutions; historically Black colleges and universities (HBCUs); tribally controlled colleges and universities (TCCUs); Alaska native and native Hawaiian serving institutions; nonprofits with 501(c)3 IRS status; nonprofits without 501(c)3 IRS status; small businesses; for-profit organizations; State governments; regional organizations; U.S. territories or possessions; Indian/Native American tribal governments; Indian/Native American tribally designated organizations; eligible agencies of the Federal government; and faith-based or community based organizations.
Amount of Grant: $200,000 in direct costs allowed in any single year; $275,000 for the combined two-year award
Date(s) Application is Due: Feb 16; Jun 16; Oct 16
Contact: James E. Everhart, MD, MPH; (301) 594-8878; fax: (301) 480-8300; email: je17g@nih.gov
Internet: http://grants.nih.gov/grants/guide/pa-files/PA-09-131.html
Sponsor: National Institute of Diabetes and Digestive and Kidney Diseases (NIDDK)
6707 Democracy Boulevard, Room 655
Bethesda, MD 20892-5450

NIDDK Seeding Collaborative Interdisciplinary Team Science in Diabetes, Endocrinology and Metabolic Diseases Grants 2584

The purpose of the Seeding Collaborative Interdisciplinary Team Science Program described in this announcement is to provide initial support to enable strong new investigative teams to form, and to foster preliminary research activities. It is anticipated that research teams receiving seeding support under this program will be well positioned to compete for funds through the parent NIDDK Collaborative Interdisciplinary Research Program in Diabetes, Endocrinology and Metabolic Diseases solicitation. It is anticipated that 5-10 projects will be funded, but because the nature and scope of the proposed research will vary from application to application, it is anticipated that the size and duration of each award will also vary. Budgets for direct costs of up to $300,000 per year with a project duration of up to one year may be requested.
Requirements: The following organizations and institutions are eligible to apply: public/state controlled institutions of higher education; private institutions of higher education; Hispanic-serving institutions; historically Black colleges and universities (HBCUs); tribally controlled colleges and universities (TCCUs); Alaska Native and Native Hawaiian serving institutions; and non-domestic (non-U.S.) entities (foreign organizations).
Amount of Grant: $375,000 maximum
Date(s) Application is Due: Jan 25; May 25; Sep 25
Contact: Karen Salomon; (301) 594-7733; fax: (301) 435-6047; email: ks495c@nih.gov
Internet: http://grants.nih.gov/grants/guide/pa-files/PAR-08-181.html
Sponsor: National Institute of Diabetes and Digestive and Kidney Diseases (NIDDK)
6707 Democracy Boulevard, Room 687
Bethesda, MD 20892-5460

NIDDK Silvio O. Conte Digestive Diseases Research Core Centers Grants 2585

The objective of the Silvio O. Conte Digestive Diseases Research Core Centers is to bring together, on a cooperative basis, basic science and clinical investigators to enhance the effectiveness of their research related to digestive and/or liver diseases and their complications. A core center must be an identifiable unit within a single university medical center or a consortium of cooperating institutions, including an affiliated university. An existing program of excellence in biomedical research in the area of digestive and/or liver diseases is a prerequisite for applying. This research must be in the form of NIH research projects, program projects, or other peer-reviewed research that is already funded at the time of submission of a center grant application. Close cooperation, communication, and collaboration among all involved personnel of various professional disciplines are the ultimate objectives.
Requirements: The following organizations and institutions are eligible to apply: public/state controlled institutions of higher education; private institutions of higher education; nonprofits with 501(c)3 IRS status (other than institutions of higher education); nonprofits without 501(c)3 IRS status (other than institutions of higher education); and for-profit organizations (other than small businesses).
Amount of Grant: $750,000 per year for five years
Date(s) Application is Due: Oct 12; Nov 9
Contact: Judith Podskalny; (301) 594-8876; fax: (301) 480-8300; email: jp53s@nih.gov
Internet: http://grants.nih.gov/grants/guide/rfa-files/RFA-DK-09-005.html
Sponsor: National Institute of Diabetes and Digestive and Kidney Diseases (NIDDK)
6707 Democracy Boulevard, MSC 5450
Bethesda , MD 20892

NIDDK Small Business Innovation Research to Develop New Therapeutics and Monitoring Technologies for Type 1 Diabetes (T1D)—Towards an Artificial Pancreas (SBIR) 2586

A promising therapeutic option for the treatment of diabetes is a system (termed an artificial pancreas or closed-loop) that can mimic normal pancreatic beta cell function thereby restoring normal metabolic homeostasis without causing hypoglycemia. The design of any system capable of achieving this goal is complex and raises scientific, clinical and regulatory challenges. This FOA solicits Small Business Innovation Research (SBIR) grant applications from small business concerns (SBCs) for funding to perform research leading to the development of innovative technologies that may advance progress toward integrated long term glucose regulated insulin delivery system (artificial pancreas). Letters of Intent are due by March 16, with full proposals to be received by April 15.
Requirements: Only United States small business concerns (SBCs) are eligible to submit SBIR applications.
Amount of Grant: $500,000 maximum for phase I; $1,000,000 maximum for phase II
Date(s) Application is Due: Mar 16; Apr 15
Contact: Dr. Guillermo Arreaza; (301) 594-4724; fax: (301) 480-3503; email: ga96b@nih.gov
Internet: http://grants.nih.gov/grants/guide/rfa-files/RFA-DK-09-001.html
Sponsor: National Institute of Diabetes and Digestive and Kidney Diseases (NIDDK)
6707 Democracy Boulevard, Room 6101
Bethesda, MD 20892

NIDDK Small Grant Program for K08/K23 Recipients 2587

The NIDDK invites recipients of its K08/K23 awards to apply for grant support during the final two years of their awards through the NIDDK Small Grant Program. This additional support will enable K awardees to either expand their current research objectives or to branch out to a closely related pilot study, thus demonstrating their growth as investigators and their independence. This should facilitate the transition to fully independent investigator status. The added grant support in the latter years of an award is expected to have the following benefits: increased fiscal independence for the K08/K23 award recipient as a precursor to complete independence; an opportunity for the recipient to generate additional publications and data to form the basis for an R01 application; an opportunity for a Scientific Review Group (SRG) to evaluate accomplishments made during the first two years of the K08/K23 award; an opportunity for the applicant to provide more detailed research plans for the last two years of the K award; and an opportunity for the applicant to demonstrate additional success in the peer review process during the course of their K08/K23 award. A project period of up to two years and a budget for direct costs of up to two $25,000 modules or $50,000 per year may be requested.
Requirements: This award is available only to those currently holding the K08 award from NIDDK. Details of the K08 award are given in NIH Program Announcement PA-00-003. Applications may be submitted on behalf of candidates by domestic non-federal nonprofit organizations, public or private.
Amount of Grant: $50,000 per year for two years
Date(s) Application is Due: Feb 16; Jun 16; Oct 16
Contact: Dr. James Hyde, Ph.D.; (301) 594-7692; fax: (301) 480-0475; email: jh486z@nih.gov;; Dr. Judith Podskalny, Ph.D.; (301) 594-8876; fax: (301) 480-8300; email: jp53s@nih.gov
Internet: http://grants.nih.gov/grants/guide/pa-files/PAR-06-172.html
Sponsor: National Institute of Diabetes and Digestive and Kidney Diseases
6707 Democracy Boulevard, Room 786
Bethesda, MD 20892-5460

NIDDK Small Grants for Underrepresented Minority Scientists in Diabetes and Digestive and Kidney Diseases 2588

The goal of this program is to enable the applicant to accept a tenure-earning position, gain additional research experience and obtain preliminary data on which to base a subsequent research grant application in an area of diabetes, endocrinology, metabolism,

digestive diseases, and nutrition, kidney, urology, or hematology. Annual deadline dates may vary; contact program staff for exact dates.
Requirements: Awards will be limited to minority citizens or non-citizen nationals of the United States or to individuals who have been lawfully admitted for permanent residence at the time of application. Applicants must also have a doctoral degree.
Restrictions: Applicants may not hold, nor apply concurrently for any other PHS research project grant at the time of this application.
Amount of Grant: $250,000 maximum
Date(s) Application is Due: Mar 22
Contact: Dr. Charles H. Rodgers; (301) 594-7717; email: rodgersc@extra.niddk.nih.gov
Internet: http://grants.nih.gov/grants/guide/rfa-files/RFA-DK-00-007.html
Sponsor: National Institute of Diabetes and Digestive and Kidney Diseases (NIDDK)
45 Center Drive, Room 6AS 19J, MSC 6600
Bethesda, MD 20892-6600

NIDDK Traditional Conference Grants 2589
Conference Grants are awarded to institutions and organizations (not individuals) to provide partial support for international or domestic meetings, conferences, and workshops to coordinate, exchange, and disseminate research information. NIDDK is especially interested in conference grants used to cover travel expenses for young and minority investigators, although meeting publications, salaries, consultant services, equipment rental, and supplies may be requested. Indirect costs normally are not allowed.
Requirements: Applicants must submit a letter of intent to apply at least 8 weeks before the application receipt date. This letter should include the names of the organizing committee, a preliminary agenda, a list of accepted or invited speakers, a proposed budget and other planned sources of funding, and a description of how the conference will address each of the above criteria.
Contact: Dr. M. Ken May, Nutrient Metabolism Program Director; (301) 594-8884; fax: (301) 480-8300; email: maym@mail.nih.gov
Internet: http://www2.niddk.nih.gov/Funding/Grants/ApplicantGuidelines/ConferenceSupport.htm
Sponsor: National Institute of Diabetes and Digestive and Kidney Diseases (NIDDK)
Building 2DEM, Room 663, 6707 Democracy Boulevard
Bethesda, MD 20892-1754

NIDDK Training in Clinical Investigation in Kidney and Urology Grants 2590
The Division of Kidney, Urology, and Hematology (DKUH) has long been interested in stimulating more training in clinical research methods in programs related to nephrology and urology. At the same time, there is a dearth of clinicians that have advanced training in clinical trial methodology. The purpose of this program announcement is to encourage applications for new training programs and to encourage program directors of existing Institutional Training Grants supported by DKUH to collaborate with schools of public health and departments of epidemiology, statistics, and biostatistics to offer didactic and practical training in clinical research methodologies. The goal of this program announcement is to increase the number of well-trained investigators who are capable of conceiving, designing, conducting, analyzing, and presenting the results of clinical research in areas pertaining to nephrology or urology.
Requirements: For new training programs, only domestic, nonprofit, private or public institutions may apply. The applicant institution must have the staff and facilities required for the proposed program. The research training program director at the institution will be responsible for the selection and appointment of trainees to receive National Research Service Award (NRSA) support and for the overall direction of the program.
Restrictions: Positions on NRSA institutional grants may not be used for study leading to the MD, DDS or other clinical health professional degrees except when those studies are a part of a formal combined research degree program such as the MD/PhD. Similarly, trainees may not accept NRSA support for studies which are a part of residency training leading to a medical specialty or subspecialty except when the residency program credits a period of full-time, postdoctoral research training toward board certification and the trainee intends to pursue a research career.
Amount of Grant: $2000 maximum for tuition and fees plus 60 percent of costs exceeding that amount
Date(s) Application is Due: Mar 10
Contact: Dr. Charles Rodgers; (301) 594-7717; fax: (301) 480-3510; email: rodgersc@extra.niddk.nih.gov
Internet: http://grants.nih.gov/grants/guide/pa-files/PAR-99-012.html
Sponsor: National Institute of Diabetes and Digestive and Kidney Diseases
45 Center Drive, MSC 6600
Bethesda, MD 20892-6600

NIDDK Translational Research for the Prevention and Control of Diabetes and Obesity 2591
The National Institute of Diabetes and Digestive and Kidney Diseases (NIDDK), the National Institute of Nursing Research and the Office of Behavior and Social Sciences Research seek to develop cost effective and sustainable interventions that can be adopted in real world settings, for the prevention and control of diabetes and obesity. Research should be based on interventions already proven efficacious in clinical trials to prevent and reverse obesity and type 2 diabetes, to improve care of type 1 and type 2 diabetes and to prevent or delay its complications. The interventions proposed under this solicitation should have the potential to be widely disseminated to clinical practice, individuals and communities at risk. Relevant topics include: methods to improve health care delivery to patients with or at risk of diabetes; strategies to enhance diabetes self management; methods to develop strategies to promote healthy lifestyles to reduce the risk of diabetes; methods to promote lifestyle change that will prevent or reverse overweight and obesity; and new cost effective ways to identify people with pre-diabetes and undiagnosed diabetes.
Requirements: The following organizations and institutions may apply: public/state controlled institutions of higher education; private institutions of higher education; Hispanic-serving institutions; historically Black colleges and universities (HBCUs); tribally controlled colleges and universities (TCCUs); Alaska native and native Hawaiian serving institutions; nonprofits with 501(c)3 IRS status; nonprofits without 501(c)3 IRS status; small businesses; for-profit organizations; State governments; regional organizations; U.S. territories or possessions; Indian/Native American tribal governments; Indian/Native American tribally designated organizations; eligible agencies of the Federal government; and faith-based or community based organizations.
Date(s) Application is Due: Jan 25; May 25; Sep 25
Contact: Sanford Garfield; (301) 594-8803; fax: (301) 480-3503; email: sg50o@nih.gov
Internet: http://grants.nih.gov/grants/guide/pa-files/PAR-06-532.html
Sponsor: National Institute of Diabetes and Digestive and Kidney Diseases (NIDDK)
6707 Democracy Boulevard, Room 685
Bethesda, MD 20892-5460

NIDDK Transmission of Human Immunodeficiency Virus (HIV) In Semen 2592
The National Institute of Diabetes and Digestive and Kidney Diseases (NIDDK) through its Division of Kidney, Urologic and Hematologic Diseases (DKUHD) and the National Institute of Child Health and Human Development, Center for Population Research invite investigators to submit research grant applications that will increase the basic and clinical knowledge of the biology of HIV in semen. Direct exposure to semen of HIV seropositive men is a major route for transmission of HIV type I. This Funding Opportunity Announcement (FOA) focuses on studies that will elucidate the factors that determine HIV shedding in the male genital tract. This includes studies that elucidate the infectivity of HIV in semen fractions, the effect of antiretroviral therapy on HIV infectivity in semen fractions, the relationship between the immunobiology of the male genital tract and HIV replication and infectivity, and factors such as genital tract inflammation which influence HIV transmission through semen. Of particular interest are studies of the anatomic sites of virus infected cells and virus production in the male genital tract. The intent of this Funding opportunity is to encourage investigator-initiated research, to attract new investigators to the field, and to increase interdisciplinary research to enhance the scope and effectiveness of research in this area. Because the nature and scope of the proposed research will vary from application to application, it is anticipated that the size and duration of each award will also vary. The total amount awarded and the number of awards will depend upon the mechanism numbers, quality, duration, and costs of the applications received.
Requirements: The following organizations and institutions are eligible to apply: public/state controlled institutions of higher education; private institutions of higher education; Hispanic-serving institutions; historically Black colleges and universities (HBCUs); tribally controlled colleges and universities (TCCUs); Alaska Native and Native Hawaiian serving institutions; nonprofits with 501(c)3 IRS status (other than institutions of higher education); nonprofits without 501(c)3 IRS status (other than institutions of higher education); small businesses; for-profit organizations (other than small businesses); state governments; Indian/Native American tribal governments (federally recognized); Indian/Native American tribally designated organizations; county governments; city or township governments; special district governments; independent school districts; public housing authorities; Indian housing authorities; U.S. territory or possession; Indian/Native American tribal governments (other than federally recognized); regional organizations; non-domestic (non-U.S.) entities (foreign organizations); other eligible agencies of the federal government; and faith-based or community-based organizations.
Date(s) Application is Due: Feb 5; Jun 5; Oct 5
Contact: Leroy M. Nyberg, Jr.; (301) 594-7717; email: ln10f@nih.gov
Internet: http://grants.nih.gov/grants/guide/pa-files/PA-07-044.html
Sponsor: National Institute of Diabetes and Digestive and Kidney Diseases (NIDDK)
6707 Democracy Boulevard, Room 627
Bethesda, MD 20892

NIDDK Type 2 Diabetes in the Pediatric Population Research Grants 2593
NIDDK and NICHD invite investigator-initiated research grant applications to study the epidemiology, natural history, pathophysiology, prevention, and treatment of type 2 diabetes in children in the United States. Type 2 diabetes has traditionally been viewed as a disease of adults. More recently, however, it has become apparent that an increasing number of cases of type 2 diabetes are being reported in children. New hypothesis-driven studies are needed to describe the epidemiology, refine the diagnosis, define the metabolic abnormalities, and formulate treatment options for type 2 diabetes in children. Annual deadline dates may vary; contact program staff for exact dates.
Requirements: Applications may be submitted by domestic for-profit and nonprofit organizations, both public and private; units of state and local governments; and eligible agencies of the federal government.
Contact: Dr. Barbara Linder; (301) 594-0021; fax: (301) 480-3503; email: linderb@mail.nih.gov;; Dr. Gilman Grave; (301) 496-5593; fax: (301) 480-9791
Internet: http://www2.niddk.nih.gov/Research/ScientificAreas/Diabetes/Type2Diabetes/DM2K.htm
Sponsor: National Institute of Diabetes and Digestive and Kidney Diseases (NIDDK)
Building 2DEM, Room 699, 6707 Democracy Boulevard
Bethesda, MD 20892

NIDRR Field-Initiated Projects 2594
The goals of this project include: developing methods and technologies that maximize the integration of individuals with disabilities into society; employment and family

environments; and improving the effectiveness of services authorized under the Rehabilitation Act. Applicants who receive awards under this program may carry out either research or development activities, and applications for each type of project will be reviewed separately. The applicant is responsible for indicating which type of project is being proposed. Projects may last up to three years. Annual deadline dates may vary; contact program staff for exact dates.
Requirements: Proposals will be accepted from any public or private agency or organization.
Contact: Donna Nangle; (202) 245-7462; fax: (202) 245-7323; email: Donna.Nangle@ed.gov
Internet: http://www.ed.gov/fund/grant/apply/nidrr/index.html
Sponsor: National Institute on Disability and Rehabilitation Research
550 12th Street SW, 6th Floor, Switzer Building
Washington, DC 20202-6510

NIEHS Applied Toxicological Research and Testing Grants **2595**
A small number of grants are supported to further the primary aims of the program to determine the toxicity and health hazards of chemicals by the best means available and to develop and validate better test methods. Toward the latter objective, the conventional two-year bioassays previously used to detect and assess carcinogenesis alone have been modified to assess other toxic responses in the same animals. Chemicals of interest are selected on the basis of recommendations from public and private sources including state and local government agencies, colleges and universities, trade unions, and industry. Testing priorities are established by an executive committee made up of personnel from key federal regulatory and research agencies. Testing of selected chemicals has been broadened and improved with new quality assessment standards, expanded screening for effects in various organs, on fertility and fetal development, and on distribution, metabolism, and excretion of the chemicals. Program emphases include development of reliable test methods, improvement of existing bioassay systems, and development of model test systems for xenobiotics.
Requirements: A university, college, hospital, state or local government, nonprofit research institution, or for-profit organization may submit an application and receive a grant for support or research by a named principal investigator.
Amount of Grant: $141,500-$1.6 million; $332,897 average
Date(s) Application is Due: Feb 1; Jun 1; Oct 1
Contact: Dr. William Suk, (919) 541-0797; email: suk@niehs.nih.gov
Internet: http://12.46.245.173/pls/portal30/CATALOG.PROGRAM_TEXT_RPT.show
Sponsor: National Institute of Environmental Health Sciences
P.O. Box 12233
Research Triangle Park, NC 27709

NIEHS Biological Response to Environmental Health Hazards Research Grants **2596**
The aim of this program is to develop a better understanding of the mechanisms of injury and disease caused by environmental factors. Research focuses on perturbations by chemical and physical agents at the molecular, cellular, tissue, and organ levels. This is a broad area of inquiry that integrates the traditional disciplines of anatomy, physiology, cell biology, endocrinology, genetics, biochemistry, and reproduction. Problem areas include, but are not limited to, neurological and behavioral disorders, respiratory diseases, cardiovascular disease, biochemical and endocrine disturbances, kidney dysfunction, carcinogenesis, mutagenesis, reproductive disorders, and birth defects.
Requirements: A university, college, hospital, state or local government, nonprofit research institution, or for-profit organization may submit an application and receive a grant for support of research by a named principal investigator.
Amount of Grant: $38,500-$2.03 million; $350,490 average
Date(s) Application is Due: Feb 1; Jun 1; Oct 1
Contact: Dr. William Suk, Director, Office of Program Development, (919) 541-0797; email: suk@niehs.nih.gov
Internet: http://12.46.245.173/pls/portal30/CATALOG.PROGRAM_TEXT_RPT.show
Sponsor: National Institute of Environmental Health Sciences
P.O. Box 12233
Research Triangle Park, NC 27709

NIEHS Carcinogenicity of Drinking Water Disinfection By-Products **2597**
NIEHS, in collaboration with EPA, is conducting short-term and long-term toxicity studies of the disinfection by-products found in drinking water, on traditional rodent models with additional studies in genetically modified (transgenic) mice. Emphasis should be on whether lower concentrations, which may not cause cancer in rodents, can be either expected to pose a human health hazard or may be considered of minimal risk for the human population, including sensitive subpopulations. Annual deadline dates may vary; contact program staff for exact dates. RFA: ES-99-007
Requirements: Applications may be submitted by domestic, for-profit and nonprofit organizations, public and private, such as universities, colleges, hospitals, laboratories, units of state or local governments and eligible agencies of the federal government.
Restrictions: Foreign institutions and organizations are not eligible.
Amount of Grant: $450,000 total
Contact: Dr. Jerrold Heindel, (919) 541-0781; fax: (919) 541-5064; email: heindelj@niehs.nih.gov
Internet: http://grants.nih.gov/grants/guide/rfa-files/RFA-ES-99-007.html
Sponsor: National Institute of Environmental Health Sciences
P.O. Box 12233
Research Triangle Park, NC 27709

NIEHS Environmental Justice: Partnerships for Communication **2598**
The purpose of this program is to strengthen the NIEHS effort that supports research aimed at achieving environmental equity for socioeconomically disadvantaged and medically underserved populations in the United States. One goal of the institute is to stimulate investigative efforts that attempt to address questions related to the influence of economic and social factors on the health status of individuals exposed to environmental toxicants. The main objective of this announcement is to establish a new model for linking members of a community who are directly affected by adverse environmental conditions with researchers and health care providers. The mechanism of support for this program will be the NIH Education Grant. The total project period for applications submitted in response to the announcement may not exceed four years, and projects are not renewable. Annual deadline dates may vary; contact the program office for exact dates. RFA: ES-99-005
Requirements: Applications may be submitted by domestic for-profit, nonprofit, public, and private institutions.
Amount of Grant: $200,000 maximum per year
Contact: Dr. Frederick Tyson, Chemical Exposures and Molecular Biology Branch, (919) 541-0176; fax: (919) 541-4937; email: tyson2@niehs.nih.gov
Internet: http://www.grants.nih.gov/grants/guide/rfa-files/RFA-ES-99-005.html
Sponsor: National Institute of Environmental Health Sciences
P.O. Box 12233
Research Triangle Park, NC 27709

NIEHS Hazardous Materials Worker Health and Safety Training Grants **2599**
This FOA issued by the National Institute of Environmental Health Sciences (NIEHS) invites applications for cooperative agreements to support the development of model programs for the training and education of workers engaged in activities related to hazardous materials and waste generation, removal, containment, transportation and emergency response. The major objective of this solicitation is to prevent work-related harm by assisting in the training of workers in how best to protect themselves and their communities from exposure to hazardous materials encountered during hazardous waste operations, hazardous materials transportation, environmental restoration of contaminated facilities or chemical emergency response. A variety of sites, such as those involved with chemical waste clean up and remedial action and transportation-related chemical emergency response may pose severe health and safety concerns to workers and the surrounding communities. These sites contain a multiplicity of hazardous substances, sometimes unknown substances, and often the site is uncontrolled. A major goal of the Worker Education and Training Program (WETP) is to provide assistance to organizations in developing their institutional competency to provide appropriate model training and education programs. The total project period for an application submitted in response to this funding opportunity must be 5 years. A new applicant may request a budget for direct costs of up to $700,000 for the first year. Letters of Intent (LOIs) are due by October 23, with full proposals due by November 23.
Requirements: The following organizations and institutions are eligible to apply: public/state controlled institutions of higher education; private institutions of higher education; Hispanic-serving institutions; historically Black colleges and universities (HBCUs); tribally controlled colleges and universities (TCCUs); Alaska Native and Native Hawaiian serving institutions; and nonprofits with 501(c)3 IRS status (other than institutions of higher education).
Amount of Grant: $700,000 maximum for the first year
Date(s) Application is Due: Oct 23; Nov 23
Contact: Joseph Hughes, Director; (919) 541-0217; fax: (919) 541-0462; email: hughes3@niehs.nih.gov
Internet: http://grants.nih.gov/grants/guide/rfa-files/RFA-ES-09-004.html
Sponsor: National Institute of Environmental Health Sciences (NIEHS)
Keystone Building, Room 3039, P.O. Box 12233, MD K3-14
Research Triangle Park, NC 27709-2233

NIEHS Hazmat Training at Doe Nuclear Weapons Complex Grants **2600**
The National Institute of Environmental Health Sciences (NIEHS) invites applications for cooperative agreements to support the development of model programs for the training and education of workers engaged in activities related to hazardous materials and waste generation, removal, containment, transportation and emergency response within the Department of Energy (DOE) Nuclear Weapons Complex. The major objective of this solicitation is to prevent work related harm by assisting in the training and education of workers in the DOE nuclear weapons complex. Safety and health training will transmit skills and knowledge to workers in how best to protect themselves and their communities from exposure to hazardous materials encountered during hazardous waste operations, facility decommissioning and decontamination, hazardous materials transportation, environmental restoration of contaminated facilities or chemical emergency response. The total project period for an application submitted in response to this funding opportunity must be 5 years. A new applicant may request a budget for direct costs of up to $700,000 for the first year. Letters of Intent (LOIs) are due by October 23, with full proposals due by November 23.
Requirements: The following organizations and institutions are eligible to apply: public/state controlled institutions of higher education; private institutions of higher education; Hispanic-serving institutions; historically Black colleges and universities (HBCUs); tribally controlled colleges and universities (TCCUs); Alaska Native and Native Hawaiian serving institutions; and nonprofits with 501(c)3 IRS status (other than institutions of higher education).
Amount of Grant: $700,000 maximum for the first year
Date(s) Application is Due: Oct 23; Nov 23

Contact: Joseph Hughes, Director; (919) 541-0217; fax: (919) 541-0462; email: hughes3@niehs.nih.gov
Internet: http://grants.nih.gov/grants/guide/rfa-files/RFA-ES-09-003.html
Sponsor: National Institute of Environmental Health Sciences (NIEHS)
Keystone Building, Room 3039, P.O. Box 12233, MD K3-14
Research Triangle Park, NC 27709-2233

NIEHS Independent Scientist Award **2601**
The award is a special salary-only grant designed to provide protected time for newly independent scientists who currently have non-research obligations such as heavy teaching loads, clinical work, committee assignments, service, and administrative duties that prevent them from having a period of intensive research focus. The award is targeted to persons with doctoral degrees who have completed their research training, have independent peer-reviewed research support, and who need a period of protected research time in order to foster their research career development. Strong preference is given to candidates with active research project grant support from the NIEHS. New applications are due February 12, June 12, and October 12, while renewal applications are due March 12, July 12, and November 12. Up to $75,000 per year of base salary plus fringe benefits is available. Research support of up to $25,000 is provided in some cases. Individuals engaged in predominantly theoretical work, such as modeling or computer simulation, may request up to $25,000 per year for research expenses.
Requirements: The following organizations and institutions are eligible to apply: public/state controlled institutions of higher education; private institutions of higher education; nonprofits with 501(c)3 IRS status; nonprofits without 501(c)3 IRS status; small businesses; for-profit organizations; State governments; U.S. territories or possessions; Indian/Native American tribal governments (Federally recognized and other than Federally recognized); Indian/Native American tribally designated organizations; Hispanic-serving institutions; historically Black colleges and universities (HBCUs); tribally controlled colleges and universities (TCCUs); Alaska Native and Native Hawaiian serving institutions; regional organizations; and faith-based or community based organizations. The candidate must have a doctoral degree and peer-reviewed, independent research support at the time the award is made. The candidate must spend a minimum of 75 percent effort conducting research during the period of the award.
Restrictions: The award is not intended for investigators who already have full time to perform research, or have substantial publication records or considerable research support indicating that they are well established in their fields. Foreign institutions are not eligible to apply.
Contact: Carol Shreffler; (919) 541-1445; fax: (919) 541-5064; email: shreffl1@niehs.nih.gov
Internet: http://grants.nih.gov/grants/guide/pa-files/PA-09-038.html
Sponsor: National Institute of Environmental Health Sciences (NIEHS)
P.O. Box 12233
Research Triangle Park, NC 27709

NIEHS Mentored Clinical Scientist Research Career Development Awards **2602**
This award enables candidates holding professional degrees (e.g., M.D., D.O., D.V.M., or equivalent degrees) to undertake 3 to 5 years of special study and supervised research with the goal of becoming independent investigators. The award also allows awardees to pursue a research career development program suited to their experience and capabilities under a mentor who is competent to provide guidance in the chosen research area. Institutions may submit applications on behalf of candidates who hold professional degrees. At least 2 years must have elapsed since the health professional degree was granted. Candidates can have varying levels of clinical training and research experience. New applications are due February 12, June 12, and October 12, while resubmitted applications are due March 12, July 12, and November 12. Up to $75,000 per year plus fringe benefits is available, and up to $25,000 per year for research support for new awards.
Requirements: All candidates must be U.S. citizens, non-citizen nationals, or legal permanent residents of the U.S. Persons with temporary or student visas are not eligible. The grantee institution must have a strong, well-established research and research training program in the chosen area, accomplished faculty in the basic and clinical sciences, and a commitment to the candidate's research development. The proposed program should include an appropriate mentor.
Amount of Grant: $100,000 maximum
Date(s) Application is Due: Feb 12; Mar 12; Jun 12; Jul 12; Oct 12; Nov 12
Contact: Dr. Carol Shreffler; (919) 541-1445; fax: (919) 541-5064; email: shreffl1@niehs.nih.gov
Internet: http://grants.nih.gov/grants/guide/contacts/pa-06-512_contacts.htm
Sponsor: National Institute of Environmental Health Sciences (NIEHS)
P.O. Box 12233
Research Triangle Park, NC 27709

NIEHS Mentored Research Scientist Development Award **2603**
The MRSDA is for a research scientist who needs an additional period of sponsored research experience as a way to gain expertise in a research area new to the candidate or in an area that would demonstrably enhance the candidate's scientific career. Research projects proposed in response to this Announcement will be expected to have a defined impact on the environmental health sciences and be directly responsive to the mission of the NIEHS, which is distinguished from that of other Institutes by its focus on research programs seeking to link the effects of environmental exposures to the cause, mechanisms, moderation, or prevention of a human disease or disorder or relevant pathophysiologic process. Applications must include as part of the justification the specific human disease, dysfunction, pathophysiologic condition, or relevant human biologic process altered, and the specific environmentally relevant toxicant. Examples of environmentally relevant toxicants include industrial chemicals or manufacturing byproducts, metals, pesticides, herbicides, air pollutants and other inhaled toxicants, particulates or fibers, fungal, bacterial, or biologically derived toxins. Agents considered non-responsive to this announcement include, but are not limited to: alcohol, chemotherapeutic agents, radiation which is not the result of an ambient environmental exposure, drugs of abuse, and infectious or parasitic agents. Ecologic, biomonitoring, biotransformation or biodegradation studies are also not responsive. Applicants must demonstrate a significant career shift or career enhancement activity which will achieve research independence upon completion of the program. Preference will be given to candidates whose mentor has NEIHS research grant support.
Requirements: The candidate must have a research or health-professional doctorate or its equivalent and must have demonstrated the capacity or potential for highly productive independent research in the period after the doctorate. The candidate must identify a mentor with extensive research experience and must spend a minimum of 75 percent of full-time professional effort conducting research for the period of the award. Applications may be submitted on behalf of candidates by domestic, nonfederal organizations, public or private, such as medical, dental, or nursing schools or other institutions of higher education. Candidates must be U.S. citizens, noncitizen nationals, or permanent residents.
Amount of Grant: $75,000 plus fringe benefits
Date(s) Application is Due: Feb 12; Mar 12; Jun 12; Jul 12; Oct 12; Nov 12
Contact: Carol Shreffler; (919) 541-1445; fax: (919) 541-5064; email: shreffl@niehs.nih.gov
Internet: http://grants.nih.gov/grants/guide/pa-files/PA-09-040.html
Sponsor: National Institute of Environmental Health Sciences (NIEHS)
P.O. Box 12233
Research Triangle Park, NC 27709

NIEHS SBIR E-Learning for HAZMAT and Emergency Response Grants **2604**
This funding opportunity announcement (FOA) solicits Small Business Innovation Research (SBIR) grant applications from small business concerns (SBCs) that propose to further the development of Advanced Technology Training (ATT) Products for the health and safety training of hazardous materials (HAZMAT) workers, emergency responders, and skilled support personnel. These products would complement the goals and objectives of the Worker Education and Training Program (WETP). The major objective of the NIEHS/WETP is to prevent work related harm by assisting in the training of workers in how best to protect themselves and their communities from exposure to hazardous materials. There is a need to ensure that learning and training technologies are further developed, field tested and applied to real world situations. It is the intent of this solicitation to support the development of products to support e-collaboration, e-teaching, e-certification, and e-learning in safety and health training for workers engaged in hazardous materials response. A new applicant may request a budget for direct costs of up to $300,000 for the first year. Letters of Intent (LOIs) are not required, and full proposals are due by August 3.
Requirements: Only United States small business concerns (SBCs) are eligible to submit SBIR applications. A small business concern is one that, at the time of award of SBIR Phase I and Phase II, meets all of the following criteria: is organized for profit, with a place of business located in the United States, which operates primarily within the United States or which makes a significant contribution to the United States economy through payment of taxes or use of American products, materials or labor; is in the legal form of an individual proprietorship, partnership, limited liability company, corporation, joint venture, association, trust or cooperative, except that where the form is a joint venture, there can be no more than 49 percent participation by foreign business entities in the joint venture; is at least 51 percent owned and controlled by one or more individuals who are citizens of, or permanent resident aliens in, the United States, or it must be a for-profit business concern that is at least 51% owned and controlled by another for-profit business concern that is at least 51% owned and controlled by one or more individuals who are citizens of, or permanent resident aliens in, the United States, except in the case of a joint venture, where each entity to the venture must be 51 percent owned and controlled by one or more individuals who are citizens of, or permanent resident aliens in, the United States; and; has, including its affiliates, not more than 500 employees.
Amount of Grant: $300,000 for first fiscal year
Date(s) Application is Due: Aug 3
Contact: Ted Outwater; (919) 541-2972; fax: (919) 541-0462; email: outwater@niehs.nih.gov
Internet: http://grants.nih.gov/grants/guide/rfa-files/RFA-ES-09-006.html
Sponsor: National Institute of Environmental Health Sciences (NIEHS)
P.O. Box 12233, MD: K3-14
Research Triangle Park, NC 27709-2233

NIEHS Small Business Innovation Research (SBIR) Program Grants **2605**
The focus of these grants is on understanding how chemical and physical agents cause pathological changes in molecules, cells, tissues, and organs and become manifested as respiratory disease; neurological, behavioral, and developmental abnormalities; cancer; and other disorders. By understanding the relationship between environmental exposures and the subsequent development of disease or biological injury, human health may be protected. SBIR program objectives are to stimulate technological innovation, use small businesses to meet federal research and development needs, increase private sector commercialization of innovations derived from federal research and development, and foster and encourage participation by minority and disadvantaged persons in technological innovation. Phase I awards, generally for six months, establish the technical merit and feasibility of proposed research efforts that may lead to commercial products or processes. Phase II awards are for the continuation of research initiated in Phase I.

Requirements: SBIR grants can be awarded only to domestic small businesses (entities that are independently owned and operated for profit, are not dominant in the field in which research is proposed, and have no more than 500 employees). Primary employment (more than one-half) of the principal investigator must be with the small business at the time of award and during the conducting of the proposed research. In both Phase I and II, the research must be performed in the United States.
Amount of Grant: $100,000 Phase I grants; $750,000 maximum Phase II grants
Date(s) Application is Due: Apr 15; Aug 15; Dec 15
Contact: Jo Anne Goodnight, SBIR/STTR, (301) 435-2688; fax: (301) 480-0146; email: jg128w@nih.gov or sbir@od.nih.gov
Internet: http://grants.nih.gov/grants/funding/sbir.htm#sbir
Sponsor: National Institute of Environmental Health Sciences
P.O. Box 12233
Research Triangle Park, NC 27709

NIEHS Structure-Function Relationships of Environmentally Relevant Genetic Variants Research Grants 2606
The objective of this RFA is to encourage multidisciplinary projects to identify and characterize the gene products coded by allelic variants of environmental responsive genes. NIEHS is the principal funding agency that supports this RFA and NIA is the cosponsor. Data generated from the studies will allow for rapid developments of innovative approaches to elucidate the mechanisms of the xenobiotic-induced molecular alterations in specific target cells and organs. Collaborative research efforts between investigators in environmental health sciences and in molecular and structural biology, and/or molecular modeling disciplines are especially encouraged. The major research objectives for this RFA include: biochemical and structural biological studies of the proteins coded by the allelic variants of candidate genes; evaluation of the functional significance of single nucleotide polymorphisms or other allelic variations in candidate genes and their regulatory regions; characterization of the molecular mechanisms controlling temporal and cellular regulation of expression of the allelic variants of a specific class of genes; functional genomic studies to assess the expression patterns and functions of these classes of environmental responsive genes at the organ/tissue/cell levels; and studies on protein-protein interactions. RFA: ES-98-007
Requirements: Applications may be submitted by domestic and foreign, for-profit and nonprofit organizations, both public and private; units of state or local governments; and eligible agencies of the federal government. Applications from minority individuals and women are encouraged.
Amount of Grant: $3.5 million
Contact: Dr. Jose Velazquez, Division of Extramural Research and Training, (919) 541-4998; fax: (919) 541-4937; email: velazqu1@niehs.nih.gov
Internet: http://www.grants.nih.gov/grants/guide/rfa-files/RFA-ES-98-007.html
Sponsor: National Institute of Environmental Health Sciences
P.O. Box 12233
Research Triangle Park, NC 27709

NIEHS Superfund Hazardous Substances Basic Research and Education Grants 2607
Grants support a wide range of research to address the broad public health concerns arising from the release of hazardous chemical wastes and other hazardous substances into the environment from waste-disposal sites. The primary objective is to expand the base of scientific knowledge needed for adequate assessment of exposure and health risks from environmental contamination, reduction in the amount and toxicity of hazardous substances, and ultimately to prevent adverse human health effects. Grants fund university-based research programs to develop advanced techniques for the detection, assessment, and evaluation of the effects of hazardous substances on human health; methods to assess the risks to human health presented by hazardous substances; methods and technologies to detect hazardous substances in the environment; and basic biological, chemical, and physical methods to reduce the amount and toxicity of hazardous substances. Advanced or graduate training should be integrated into the second year of the multidisciplinary research program to provide for training in environmental and occupational health and safety and the engineering aspects of hazardous wastes control, and graduate training in the geosciences including hydrogeology, geological engineering, geophysics, geochemistry, and related fields. Contact the program office for deadline dates. RFA: ES-99-001
Requirements: An accredited institution of higher education may submit an application and receive a grant for support of research by a named principal investigator. Subcontracts may be made with public and private organizations including generators of hazardous wastes; persons involved in the detection, assessment, evaluation, and treatment of hazardous substances; owners and operators of facilities at which hazardous substances are located; and state and local governments. Strong biomedical research is a requisite of this program. A minimum of three approved biomedical projects is required for funding.
Restrictions: Single-project applications will not be accepted. This program is not intended to support individual research project grants.
Amount of Grant: $182,787$3.81 million; $1.31 million average
Contact: Dr. William Suk, Director, Superfund Hazardous Substance Basic Research and Training Program, (919) 541-0797; fax: (919) 541-2843; email: suk@niehs.nih.gov; Dorothy Duke, Grants Management Officer, Division of Extramural Research and Training, (919) 541
Internet: http://www.grants.nih.gov/grants/guide/rfa-files/RFA-ES-99-001.html
Sponsor: National Institute of Environmental Health Sciences
P.O. Box 12233
Research Triangle Park, NC 27709

NIEHS/NINDS Role of the Environment in Parkinson's Disease 2608
The objective of this program is to stimulate research on the relative roles of environmental, endogenous neurochemical and modifying genetic factors in the cause of Parkinson's disease. Annual deadline dates may vary; contact program staff for exact dates.
Requirements: Applications may be submitted by domestic and foreign, for-profit and nonprofit organizations, public and private, such as universities, colleges, hospitals, laboratories, units of state and local governments, and agencies of the federal government.
Amount of Grant: $4 million total
Contact: Dr. Annette Kirshner, Division of Extramural Research and Training, (919) 541-0488; fax: (919) 541-5064; email: kirshner@niehs.nih.gov; Dr. Eugene Oliver, Division of Stroke, Trauma and Neurodegenerative Disorders, (301) 496-5680; fax: (301) 480-1080
Internet: http://grants.nih.gov/grants/guide/rfa-files/RFA-ES-00-002.html
Sponsor: National Institute of Environmental Health Sciences
P.O. Box 12233
Research Triangle Park, NC 27709

NIGMS Exploratory Studies for High Risk/High Impact Research Grants 2609
This program attempts to broaden the base of inquiry in fundamental biomedical research by encouraging applications for research projects that involve an especially high degree of innovation and novelty, such that their potential for highly significant outcomes may be difficult to judge by the standard criteria used in evaluating R01 proposals. Research projects proposed under this program may lack preliminary data establishing feasibility, but should present the opportunity for conceptual or technological breakthroughs. PA-03-100 may be obtained electronically through the NIH grant line (301-402-2221), the NIH Web site, and by mail and email.
Amount of Grant: $275,000 maximum for two years
Contact: Joe Ellis, Grants Management Officer, (301) 594-5135; fax: (301) 480-1969; email: ellisj@nigms.nih.gov; Dr. James Cassatt, Division of Cell Biology and Biophysics, (301) 594-0828; fax: (301) 480-2004; email: cassattj@nigms.nih.gov
Internet: http://grants2.nih.gov/grants/guide/pa-files/PA-03-100.html
Sponsor: National Institute of General Medical Sciences
45 Center Drive, Natcher Building
Bethesda, MD 20892

NIGMS Fellowships in Quantitative Biology 2610
The NIGMS encourages applications for individual postdoctoral and senior fellowships from highly qualified individuals with doctoral training in both the traditional quantitative disciplines (such as mathematics, physics, engineering, and computer science) and biology. NIGMS supports individual postdoctoral and senior fellowships in those areas covered by its research grant portfolio. These areas include biomedical engineering, cell biology, molecular biophysics, genetics and developmental biology, pharmacology, physiology, especially burn and trauma research, and biological chemistry. PA 98-082
Requirements: Individuals must be citizens or noncitizen nationals of the United States, or have been lawfully admitted to the United States for permanent residence (i.e., possess a currently valid Alien Registration Receipt Card I-551, or other legal verification of such status) at the time of application. Applicants for individual postdoctoral fellowships must have completed all of the requirements for the doctoral degree by the time of award. Applicants for senior fellowships must have had at least seven years of relevant research or professional experience beyond the doctoral degree. In addition, a significant amount of retraining is required for senior fellowship applicants. Applications from women, underrepresented minorities, and individuals with disabilities are especially encouraged.
Restrictions: Individuals on temporary or student visas are not eligible.
Amount of Grant: $21,000-$33,012 stipend; $4000 allowance per 12-month period for sponsoring institutions (nonfederal and nonprofit organizations)
Date(s) Application is Due: Apr 5; Aug 5; Dec 5
Contact: Dr. James Cassatt, Division of Cell Biology and Biophysics, (301) 594-0828; fax: (301) 402-2004; email: cassattj@nigms.nih.gov; Dr. James Anderson, Division of Genetics and Developmental Biology, (301) 594-0943; fax: (301) 480-2228
Internet: http://www.grants.nih.gov/grants/guide/pa-files/PA-98-082.html
Sponsor: National Institute of General Medical Sciences
45 Center Drive, Natcher Building
Bethesda, MD 20892

NIGMS Individual Postdoctoral NRSA Fellowships in Clinical Pharmacology 2611
Fellowships support high-quality physicians seeking research training in the field of clinical pharmacology. These fellowships are intended to support up to three years of advanced training to individuals with the MD degree to qualify them to perform basic laboratory and/or clinical investigations of the effects and mechanisms of drug actions in humans, in the scientific areas consistent with the mission of NIGMS. One goal of this initiative is to promote high-quality clinical pharmacology research training at academic health centers. Therefore, a special feature of this award is to encourage applicants at institutions with a General Clinical Research Center (GCRC) supported by the NCRR to submit a letter of endorsement from the director of the training institution's GCRC. The intent is to promote interaction between the applicant and the staff and director of the GCRC, expose the applicant to the extensive resources and rich research environment of the GCRC, and raise the visibility of this important area of translational research within the institution. PA: PA-99-078
Requirements: The candidate must have an MD degree or its equivalent and must meet the criteria for the NIH National Research Service Awards for Individual Postdoctoral Fellows (F32) described in program announcement PA-99-025, available on the Web site at http://www.nih.gov/grants/guide/pa-files/PA-99-025.htm l.

Contact: Dr. Alison Cole, Division of Pharmacology, Physiology, and Biological Chemistry, (301) 594-1826; fax: (301) 480-2802; email: colea@nigms.nih.gov
Internet: http://www.grants.nih.gov/grants/guide/pa-files/PA-99-078.html
Sponsor: National Institute of General Medical Sciences
45 Center Drive, Natcher Building
Bethesda, MD 20892

NIGMS Initiative for Minority Students: Bridges to the Baccalaureate Degree 2612
NIGMS and the Office of Research on Minority Health (ORMH) reannounce two research initiatives directed at increasing the number of underrepresented minorities entering careers in biomedical research. The programs target two different underrepresented minority student populations: those in colleges and universities offering only master of science (MS) degree programs in biomedically-related sciences and those in two-year junior or community colleges. These have been identified as two key transition points for students considering careers in biomedical research. This RFA solicits new applications for a partnership program involving two-year colleges awarding the associate's degree and institutions awarding the baccalaureate degree. Annual deadline dates may change; contact program staff for exact dates. RFA: GM-01-002
Requirements: Applications may be submitted by domestic, private or public, educational institutions and state or local systems of higher education.
Amount of Grant: $600,000 maximum
Contact: Dr. Irene Eckstrand, (301) 594-5402; fax: (301) 480-2228; email: eckstrai@nigms.nih.gov
Internet: http://grants.nih.gov/grants/guide/rfa-files/RFA-GM-01-002.html
Sponsor: National Institute of General Medical Sciences
45 Center Drive, Natcher Building
Bethesda, MD 20892

NIGMS Initiative for Minority Students: Bridges to the Doctoral Degree 2613
The program develops partnerships between educational institutions to support underrepresented minorities in the transition to doctoral programs. Besides reflecting the plans and priorities of the individual institutions, the partnership must address the needs of the minority graduate students. Support activities the institutions may implement include, but are not limited to, enhancing the curriculum of the master's institution; establishing a mentor program for master's students with faculty at the doctoral institution; enabling and encouraging students from either institution to take classes at the other institution; and providing research opportunities for master's students at the doctoral institution or in private industrial laboratories. Annual deadline dates may vary; contact program staff for exact dates. RFA: GM-01-003
Requirements: Partnerships involve a minimum of two educational institutions. One institution must have a significant enrollment of underrepresented minorities, and the highest postgraduate degree offered in the related sciences must be the master's degree. The other participating institution must be a research university and offer doctoral degrees in biomedical relevant areas. Applications also may represent several institutions within a single state, with one institution designated as the applicant institution.
Amount of Grant: $20 million total
Contact: Dr. Irene Eckstrand, (301) 594-5402; fax: (301) 480-2228; email: eckstrai@nigms.nih.gov
Internet: http://grants.nih.gov/grants/guide/rfa-files/RFA-GM-01-003.html
Sponsor: National Institute of General Medical Sciences
45 Center Drive, Natcher Building
Bethesda, MD 20892

NIGMS Institutional Research and Academic Career Development Award 2614
The goal of this program is to prepare qualified individuals for careers that significantly impact the nation's research agenda. The objectives of this initiative are: to enhance research-oriented teaching at minority serving institutions (MSIs); to increase the research and other skills needed by developing scientists to conduct high quality research in an academic environment; and to promote linkages between research-intensive institutions and MSIs that can lead to further collaborations in research and teaching; and to increase the number of well-qualified underrepresented minority students entering competitive careers in biomedical research. Grant funds may be used to support the following expenses: salary/wages and benefits for a full-time, 12-month staff appointment; tuition, fees, and books; research expenses; supplies; travel to one training or scientific meeting per year; and statistical services. PAR-98-085.
Requirements: An application must be submitted on behalf of a consortium of domestic private or public educational institutions; the applicant institution should be the primary site of the postdoctoral research experience. An institution may not submit more than one application. A consortium must include one or more partners that are MSIs. Candidates appointed under this program award must be U.S. citizens or noncitizen nationals, or have been lawfully admitted for permanent residence and possess Alien Registration Receipt Cards (I-151 or I-551) or some other verification of legal status as permanent residents. Postdoctoral candidates must have received, as of the beginning date of the appointment to the program, the PhD, MD, or comparable doctoral degree from an accredited domestic or foreign institution.
Restrictions: Individuals on temporary or student visas are not eligible.
Contact: Dr. Clifton Poodry, Division of Minority Opportunities in Research, (301) 594-3900; fax: (301) 480-2753; email: poodryc@nigms.nih.gov
Internet: http://www.grants.nih.gov/grants/guide/pa-files/PAR-98-085.html
Sponsor: National Institute of General Medical Sciences
45 Center Drive, Natcher Building
Bethesda, MD 20892

NIGMS Integrative and Collaborative Approaches to Research Grants 2615
The purpose of this PA is to encourage collaborative and integrative approaches to research on multifaceted biological problems. While the traditional R01 research project grant remains the backbone of NIH and NIGMS support for biomedical science, individual R01 grants may be inadequate to support larger efforts that require collaborative approaches. In some cases, individual investigators with existing R01 or R37 support, or other sources of independent funding, will need to attract and coordinate expertise in different disciplines and approaches and may also require access to specialized resources, such as computational facilities, high-throughput technologies, and equipment. In order to provide a new mechanism to support such collaborative and interactive activities, this initiative will use the R24 consortium grant mechanism, designed for groups of currently funded investigators. This PA also strongly encourages consideration of existing and previously announced mechanisms whenever appropriate, to enhance collaborative and integrative approaches to research problems. These include administrative supplements to NIGMS-funded research grants, competitive supplements to NIGMS-funded research grants, individual R01 grants containing a consortium arrangement for a collaborative component, program project (P01) and center (P50) grants, and Interactive Research Project Grants (IRPG). PA: PA-00-099
Requirements: Applications may be submitted by domestic and foreign, for-profit and nonprofit organizations, both public and private; units of state and local governments; and eligible agencies of the federal government.
Amount of Grant: $300,000 maximum direct costs per year
Contact: Dr. Marion Zatz, Division of Genetics and Developmental Biology, (301) 594-0943; fax: (301) 480-2228; email: zatzm@nigms.nih.gov
Internet: http://grants.nih.gov/grants/guide/pa-files/PA-00-099.html
Sponsor: National Institute of General Medical Sciences
45 Center Drive, Natcher Building
Bethesda, MD 20892

NIGMS Large-Scale Collaborative Project Awards 2616
The purpose of this program is to enable the solution of major problems in biomedical research and to facilitate the next evolutionary stage of integrative biomedical science. The intention is to make resources available for independently funded scientists to form research teams to solve a complex biological problem that would be beyond the means of any one research group, and that is of central importance to biomedical science and to the mission of NIGMS. It is expected that the participating investigators will already hold externally peer reviewed and funded research grants in the area of the proposal, and, in general, support of new individual research projects will not be a part of these large-scale project awards. A high level of resources may be requested to allow participating investigators to extend their research efforts to form a consortium to approach a research problem of overarching importance in a comprehensive and highly integrated fashion. Grants for this initiative will be awarded in two phases. The purpose of the Phase I award is to provide resources for detailed planning to applicants who have demonstrated the selection of an appropriate complex biological problem, an innovative plan, and appropriate commitments to its solution from participating investigators and institutions. Phase I applicants will submit an overview of the proposed large-scale project for peer review. Successful Phase I applicants will receive a $25,000 (direct costs) planning grant, and those applicants who receive awards will be eligible to submit a more extensively planned and detailed application for a Phase II award to support the large-scale project itself. Annual deadline dates may vary; contact program staff for exact dates. RFA: GM-02-007
Requirements: Applications may be submitted by domestic, nonprofit organizations, both public and private; units of state and local governments; and eligible agencies of the federal government. Multi-institutional applications are encouraged. A collaborative project may include participating investigators from foreign and/or for-profit organizations. Participation by industry is also encouraged.
Contact: Dr. Michael Rogers, Division of Pharmacology, Physiology, and Biological Chemistry, (301) 594-3827; fax: (301) 480-2802; email: rogersm@nigms.nih.gov; Dr. James Cassatt, Division of Cell Biology and Biophysics, (301) 594-0828; fax: (301) 480-2004; e-mai
Internet: http://grants2.nih.gov/grants/guide/rfa-files/RFA-GM-02-007.html
Sponsor: National Institute of General Medical Sciences
45 Center Drive, Natcher Building
Bethesda, MD 20892

NIGMS MARC Undergraduate Student Training in Academic Research 2617
The Minority Access to Research Careers (MARC) Program Branch of the Division of Minority Opportunity in Research of NIGMS provides research training opportunities that target students and faculty from minority groups who are underrepresented in the biomedical sciences, including mathematics. As part of its ongoing commitment to the development of prospective underrepresented minority researchers and the enhancement of their training environment, the MARC Program provides support directed at underrepresented minority students to improve their preparation for graduate training in the biomedical sciences. PA: PAR-02-033
Requirements: Only domestic, nonprofit, private or public institutions which offer the baccalaureate degree and in which student enrollments are drawn substantially from ethnic minority groups that are underrepresented in the biomedical sciences, including mathematics, may apply. Only one grant per eligible institution will be awarded. The program is open to qualified undergraduate honors students majoring in the sciences with expressed interest in careers in biomedical research and intentions to pursue graduate education leading to the PhD, MD/PhD or other combined professional degree/PhD.
Contact: Dr. Adolphus Toliver, Division of Minority Opportunities in Research, (301) 594-3900; fax: (301) 480-2753; email: tolivera@nigms.nih.gov

Internet: http://grants2.nih.gov/grants/guide/pa-files/PAR-02-033.html
Sponsor: National Institute of General Medical Sciences
45 Center Drive, Natcher Building
Bethesda, MD 20892

NIGMS Mentored Clinical Scientist Research Career Development Awards **2618**
This award enables candidates holding professional degrees (e.g., M.D., D.O., D.V.M., or equivalent degrees) to undertake 3 to 5 years of special study and supervised research with the goal of becoming independent investigators. The award also allows awardees to pursue a research career development program suited to their experience and capabilities under a mentor who is competent to provide guidance in the chosen research area. Institutions may submit applications on behalf of candidates who hold professional degrees. At least 2 years must have elapsed since the health professional degree was granted. Candidates can have varying levels of clinical training and research experience. New applications are due February 12, June 12, and October 12, while resubmitted applications are due March 12, July 12, and November 12. Up to $75,000 per year plus fringe benefits is available, and up to $20,000 per year for research support for new awards.
Requirements: The candidate must have an MD degree or its equivalent, must have completed postgraduate clinical training and have secured a faculty appointment in an appropriate research-intensive environment, must identify a mentor with extensive research experience, and must be willing to spend a minimum of 75 percent of full-time professional effort conducting research and research career development. Applications may be submitted on behalf of candidates by domestic, nonfederal organizations, public or private, such as medical schools. Minorities and women are encouraged to apply. Candidates must be U.S. citizens or noncitizen nationals, or must have been lawfully admitted for permanent residence and possess Alien Registration Receipt Card (I-551) or some other verification of legal admission as permanent residents.
Restrictions: Former principal investigators on NIH research project (R01), sub-projects of program project (P01), or center grants (P50), or the equivalent, are not eligible. A candidate for the award may not concurrently apply for any other PHS award that duplicates the provisions of this award nor have another application pending award. K08 recipients are encouraged to apply for independent research grant support during the period of this award. The K08 recipient would be allowed to maintain the award if other PHS support is procured, as long as the new support does not interfere with the ability to meet the MCSDA requirements.
Amount of Grant: $95,000 salary per year maximum
Date(s) Application is Due: Feb 12; Mar 12; Jun 12; Jul 12; Oct 12; Nov 12
Contact: Dr. Alison Cole, Anesthesiology Program; (301) 594-1826; fax: (301) 480-2802; email: colea@nigms.nih.gov
Internet: http://www.grants.nih.gov/grants/guide/pa-files/PAR-98-084.html
Sponsor: National Institute of General Medical Sciences (NIGMS)
45 Center Drive, Natcher Building, Room 2AS-49, MSC6200
Bethesda, MD 20892-6200

NIGMS Minority Access to Research Careers Ancillary Training Activities Grants **2619**
The MARC program provides research training opportunities for students and faculty from minority groups underrepresented in the biomedical and behavioral sciences relevant to biomedicine, including mathematics and engineering. Under the ancillary training initiative, the program provides support for ancillary research training activities that are harmonious with its overall objective of increasing the number of underrepresented minorities who participate fully in the biomedical enterprise of this country. Program-related scientific meetings, conferences, technical assistance workshops, and other ancillary training activities will be funded. Funds may be used for salaries, equipment, supplies, travel expenses, per diem costs, conference services, publication costs, registration fees, and speaker fees. Grant amounts are variable, based on the nature and scope of proposed activities. A letter of intent is requested by January 1, May 1, and September 1; full application is due February 1, June 1, and October 1. Annual deadline dates may vary; contact program officer for exact dates. PA: PAR-99-091
Requirements: Applications may be submitted by U.S. institutions, including scientific or professional societies, eligible to receive grants from the Department of Health and Human Services.
Restrictions: Foreign organizations are not eligible.
Date(s) Application is Due: Jan 1; Feb 1; May 1; Jun 1; Sep 1; Oct 1
Contact: Dr. Hinda Zlotnick, MARC Program Director, (301) 594-3900; fax: (301) 480-2573; email: hindaz@nigms.nih.gov
Internet: http://www.grants.nih.gov/grants/guide/pa-files/PAR-99-091.html
Sponsor: National Institute of General Medical Sciences
45 Center Drive, Natcher Building
Bethesda, MD 20892

NIGMS Minority Access to Research Careers (MARC) Program **2620**
The program's goals are to increase the number and capabilities of scientists from underrepresented minority groups who are engaged in biomedical research and to strengthen science curricula and student research opportunities at institutions with substantial minority enrollments in order to prepare minority students for research careers. The program offers postdoctoral and predoctoral fellowships, and undergraduate student training. PA: PAR-03-140
Requirements: Applications are accepted from domestic private and public universities, and research institutions or centers with graduate programs that offer a solid research environment as evidenced by a high level of faculty involvement in biomedical and/or behavioral research. To be eligible for participation in the program as a PREP scholar, individuals from underrepresented minority groups must have graduated with a baccalaureate degree in a biomedically relevant science from an accredited U.S. college or university no more than 36 months prior to the date of submission of the application. PREP scholars must be U.S. citizens or permanent residents.
Restrictions: An applicant institution may submit only one application for this program announcement.
Contact: Dr. Adolphus Toliver, Chief, MARC Branch, (301) 594-3900; fax: (301) 480-8506; email: rm63f@nih.gov
Internet: http://grants.nih.gov/grants/guide/pa-files/PAR-03-140.html
Sponsor: National Institute of General Medical Sciences
45 Center Drive, Natcher Building
Bethesda, MD 20892

NIGMS Molecular Pharmacology of Anesthetic Action Research Grants **2621**
NIGMS invites applications for the study of the molecular mechanisms of action of general and local anesthetics. The objective of this program is to encourage the submission of applications from individuals who have been trained either in basic or clinical research and who possess experience in research disciplines that are pertinent to answering questions germane to the understanding of anesthetic action such as the neurosciences, the pharmacological sciences, biophysics, biochemistry, and cell biology. Presumably, a wide variety of approaches and model systems could be employed to study anesthetic action at the molecular level. These model systems would include, but are not limited to, artificial membranes; ion channels, receptors, and other macromolecules in reconstituted membranes; electrophysiological measurements and biochemical determinations in isolated whole membrane systems; studies of whole cell responses to anesthetics; and actions of anesthetics on integrated systems such as brain slices and the spinal cord. Additionally, experimental designs utilizing recombinant DNA and molecular biological techniques, immunological approaches, and biophysical procedures whose aims are to elucidate structural features of anesthetic interactions with components of biological systems would also be of interest. There are no limits to the types of approaches that may be proposed to answer questions relevant to anesthetic action, so long as those approaches emphasize clarification of molecular aspects of anesthetic pharmacodynamics. Ideally, the ultimate goal of this research would be to develop hypotheses that might explain the relationship between molecular actions and physiological effects of general and local anesthetics. Additional information may be obtained by mail and email or through the NIH grant line (301-402-2221) or the NIH Web site. PA: PA-96-026
Requirements: Research project awards can be made to any public or private, for-profit or nonprofit university, college, hospital, laboratory, or other institution, including state and local units of government, qualifying small businesses, and individuals. SBIR grants can be awarded only to domestic small businesses. STTR grants can be awarded only to domestic small business concerns that partner with research institutions in cooperative research and development.
Date(s) Application is Due: Feb 1; Jun 1; Oct 1
Contact: Dr. Alison Cole, (301) 594-1826; fax: (301) 480-2802; email: colea@gm1.nigms.nih.gov
Internet: http://www.grants.nih.gov/grants/guide/pa-files/PA-96-026.html
Sponsor: National Institute of General Medical Sciences
45 Center Drive, Natcher Building
Bethesda, MD 20892

NIGMS MORE Faculty Development Awards **2622**
The MORE program provides support for eligible faculty to spend a summer or one academic term every year for two to five years in full-time research in a research-intensive laboratory. Contact the program office for deadline dates. PA: PAR-95-048
Date(s) Application is Due: Feb 1; Jun 1; Oct 1
Contact: Dr. Adolphus Toliver, Predoctoral NRSA Awards, (301) 594-3900; Carol Tippery, Grants Management Officer, (301) 594-5135
Internet: http://grants.nih.gov/grants/guide/pa-files/PAR-95-048.html
Sponsor: National Institute of General Medical Sciences
45 Center Drive, Natcher Building
Bethesda, MD 20892

NIGMS Pharmacogenomics Research Network Grants **2623**
The purpose of this funding opportunity announcement is to allow new and renewal applications for research groups to compete to become part of the Pharmacogenomics Research Network (PGRN), and to create network resources that serve the entire PGRN. The PGRN is a consortium of interdisciplinary groups with a core mission to conduct research into understanding the genetic basis of variable drug responses, both therapeutic and adverse. The scientific objectives of the research network include definition of the pressing problems for safe and effective use of medications, establishment of truly cross-disciplinary research groups, application of the most appropriate genetic and genomic methods to important sample collections, discovery and replication studies that identify variation in critical genes and biological pathways, elucidation of the functional consequences of genetic variation for the drugs being studied, and understanding the clinical implications of genotyping to predict drug responses. The expected direct costs amount for each individual research group award is $1 to $1.5 million per year, and for each add-on network resource is $0.1 to $0.5 million per year. Letters of Intent are due by May 2, with full proposals received by June 2.
Requirements: The following organizations and institutions are eligible to apply: public/state controlled institutions of higher education; private institutions of higher education; Hispanic-serving institutions; historically Black colleges and universities (HBCUs); nonprofits with 501(c)3 IRS status (other than institutions of higher education); nonprofits without 501(c)3 IRS status (other than institutions of higher education); small businesses; and for-profit organizations (other than small businesses).

Date(s) Application is Due: May 2; Jun 2
Contact: Rochelle M. Long, PhD; (301) 594-3827; email: rochelle.long@nih.gov;; Richard A. Anderson, MD, PhD; (301) 594-0943; email: andersor@nigms.nih.gov
Internet: http://grants.nih.gov/grants/guide/rfa-files/RFA-GM-10-001.html
Sponsor: National Institute of General Medical Sciences (NIGMS)
45 Center Drive, Building 45
Bethesda, MD 20892

NIGMS Pilot Projects for the Protein Structure Initiative **2624**
This program funds research centers that serve as pilots to examine the best approach for developing subsequent integrated, large-scale research networks in structural genomics. This is part of the institute's Protein Structure Initiative (PSI), whose goal is the understanding of protein structural families, structural folds, and the relationship of structure and function. These research centers should include all the constituent tasks of structural genomics and should test strategies for large-scale high throughput structure determination by X-ray crystallography and/or NMR. A letter of intent is requested by November 3; full application is due February 12. Annual deadline dates may vary; contact program staff for exact dates. RFA: GM-00-006
Requirements: Applications may be submitted by domestic for-profit and nonprofit organizations, both public and private; units of state and local governments; and eligible agencies of the federal government.
Restrictions: Foreign institutions are not eligible for research center grants.
Amount of Grant: $3 million maximum
Date(s) Application is Due: Feb 12; Nov 3
Contact: Dr. John Norvell, Division of Cell Biology and Biophysics, (301) 594-0533; fax: (301) 480-2004; email: norvellj@nigms.nih.gov
Internet: http://grants.nih.gov/grants/guide/rfa-files/RFA-GM-00-006.html
Sponsor: National Institute of General Medical Sciences
45 Center Drive
Bethesda, MD 20892

NIGMS Predoctoral Training in Bioinformatics and Computation Biology Grants **2625**
The purpose of this program is to develop a mechanism to train a cadre of scientists whose primary professional identification and disciplinary affiliation is bioinformatics or computational biology. For the purpose of this announcement, bioinformatics and computational biology are defined broadly to include the use of theory, computer implementation, and application to the full spectrum of basic research in the biomedical sciences. The terms thus include analysis of molecular sequence and structure, molecular function, cellular function, physiology, genomics, and genetics, as well as computational modeling of complex phenomena such as neural circuits and equilibrium phenomena, population biology, theoretical and mathematical biology, and the analysis of complex systems. The goal of this program is to train PhD students in the background theory, computational implementation, and biological application of information sciences (including computer science, statistics, mathematics and others), and to use this training to study problems relevant to biomedical research. PA: PAR-99-146
Requirements: Applications may be submitted by domestic public and private institutions with established programs leading to a PhD degree.
Amount of Grant: $14,688 annual stipend, $1500 total direct support costs, $300 per year for travel
Contact: Dr. James Cassatt, Director, Division of Cell Biology and Biophysics, (301) 594-0828; fax: (301) 402-2004; email: cassattj@nigms.nih.gov; Dr. Marion Zatz, Division of Genetics and Developmental Biology, (301) 594-0943; fax: (301) 480-2228; email: zatzm
Internet: http://grants.nih.gov/grants/guide/pa-files/PAR-99-146.html
Sponsor: National Institute of General Medical Sciences
45 Center Drive, Natcher Building
Bethesda, MD 20892

NIGMS Quantitative Approaches to the Analysis of Complex Biological Systems **2626**
The purpose of this program announcement is to advertise NIGMS and NIMH interest in supporting research projects that develop quantitative approaches to describe, analyze, and predict the behavior of complex biological systems, especially those requiring the integration of potentially large amounts of molecular, biochemical, cell biological, and physiological data. Such studies, adapted to the analysis of complex systems in humans, will ultimately have an impact on the treatment of human disorders and disease. These projects are expected to require the participation of individuals with diverse expertise and therefore to be of a collaborative and cross disciplinary nature. Additional information for this program may be obtained by phone, fax, email, or the Internet. PA: PA-98-077
Requirements: Applications may be submitted by foreign and domestic, for-profit and nonprofit organizations, both public and private. Racial/ethnic minority individuals, women, and persons with disabilities are encouraged to apply.
Restrictions: Foreign institutions are not eligible for program project (P01) grants.
Contact: Dr. James Cassatt, Division of Cell Biology and Biophysics, (301) 594-0828; fax: (301) 480-2004; email: czj@cu.nih.gov; Dr. Judith Greenberg, Division of Genetics and Developmental Biology, (301) 594-0943; fax: (301) 480-2228; email: greenbej@nigms.ni
Internet: http://www.grants.nih.gov/grants/guide/pa-files/PA-98-077.html
Sponsor: National Institute of General Medical Sciences
45 Center Drive, Natcher Building
Bethesda, MD 20892

NIGMS Ruth L. Kirschstein National Research Service Awards for Individual Predoctoral Fellows in PharmD/PhD Grants **2627**
NIGMS is committed to increasing the number of pharmacy students who wish to pursue doctoral research in the pharmaceutical sciences. It recognizes that current career paths for Doctor of Pharmacy graduates have reduced the number of individuals who pursue academic research training. NIGMS's intent in issuing this Funding Opportunity Announcement (FOA) is to provide individual research training fellowships to promising predoctoral applicants who are enrolled in PharmD/PhD programs in Schools of Pharmacy who desire to become productive and successful independent investigators whose research meets the mission of NIGMS. This fellowship program will provide support for the dissertation stage of predoctoral students enrolled in joint PharmD/PhD programs. It is expected that the length of time for an award will be 3 years or less
Requirements: The following organizations and institutions are eligible to apply: for-profit organizations; non-profit organizations; domestic institutions; public or private institutions, such as universities, colleges, and hospitals; units of State and local governments; eligible agencies of the Federal government.
Restrictions: Individuals on temporary or student visas are not eligible.
Date(s) Application is Due: Apr 8; Aug 8; Dec 8
Contact: Richard Okita, Ph.D.; (301) 594-3827; fax: (301) 480-2802; email: okitar@nigms.nih.gov
Internet: http://grants.nih.gov/grants/guide/pa-files/PA-09-029.html
Sponsor: National Institute of General Medical Sciences (NIGMS)
45 Center Drive, 2AS.49A, MSC 6200
Bethesda, MD 20892-6200

NIGMS Short Courses on Mathematical and Statistical Tools for the Study of Complex Phenotypes and Complex Systems **2628**
The purpose of this program is to provide support for short courses or workshops to assist scientists in preparing for research on complex phenotypes and complex systems. This program announcement solicits applications for education grants (R25), which provide for one to five years of support for short courses. Support is limited to courses that are highly focused and that reach a wide audience of scientists. The program announcement is not intended for university course or curriculum development. A variety of approaches will be considered. The nature of the activity, the needs of the target community, and the course goals should determine the instructional approach. These might include new approaches, such as Web-based instruction, or more traditional approaches, such as summer workshops or on-site instruction. PA: PA-98-083
Requirements: Applications may be submitted by domestic nonprofit and for-profit organizations, public and private.
Restrictions: Foreign organizations are not eligible.
Contact: Dr. Irene Anne Eckstrand, (301) 594-0943; fax: (301) 480-2228; email: Irene_Eckstrand@nih.gov
Internet: http://www.grants.nih.gov/grants/guide/pa-files/PA-98-083.html
Sponsor: National Institute of General Medical Sciences
45 Center Drive, Natcher Building
Bethesda, MD 20892

NIGMS Short Courses on Mathematical, Statistical, and Computational Tools for Studying Biological Systems **2629**
The goal of this FOA is to prepare researchers at all professional levels for multidisciplinary research on complex biological systems and phenotypes by improving integration of mathematical, statistical, and computational approaches into biological and/or behavioral research. Progress in contemporary biological and behavioral disciplines depends heavily on investigators who are skilled in the use of mathematics, computation, and statistics (collectively referred to as quantitative methods). This FOA issued by the National Institute of General Medical Sciences, the National Center for Complementary and Alternative Medicine, the National Institute on Aging and the National Institute of Mental Health encourages applications for Research Education Grants (R25) from institutions and organizations to conduct workshops and short courses to improve integration of mathematical, statistical, and computational approaches into biological and/or behavioral research. Support will be limited to activities that reach a wide audience of researchers.
Requirements: Application can be made by the following institutions and organizations: public/state controlled institutions of higher education; private institutions of higher education; nonprofits with 501(c)3 IRS status (other than institutions of higher education); nonprofits without 501(c)3 IRS status (other than institutions of higher education); small businesses; for-profit organizations (other than small businesses); state governments; U.S. territories or possessions; Indian/Native American tribal governments (federally recognized); Indian/Native American tribal governments (other than Federally recognized); Indian/Native American tribally designated organizations; non-domestic (non-U.S.) entities (foreign organizations); Hispanic-serving institutions; historically Black colleges and universities (HBCUs); tribally controlled colleges and universities (TCCUs); Alaska Native and Native Hawaiian serving institutions; regional organization; eligible agencies of the Federal government; and faith-based or community based organizations.
Restrictions: The program announcement is not intended for university course or curriculum development.
Amount of Grant: $200,000 maximum annually
Date(s) Application is Due: Jan 25; May 25; Sep 25
Contact: Matthew E. Portnoy, Ph.D.; (301) 594-0943; fax: (301) 480-2228; email: mportnoy@nigms.nih.gov
Internet: http://grants.nih.gov/grants/guide/pa-files/PA-09-002.html
Sponsor: National Institute of General Medical Sciences (NIGMS)
Building 45, 2AS.25P, 45 Center Drive
Bethesda, MD 20892-6200

NIGMS Supplements for the Study of Complex Biological Systems 2630

The purpose of this initiative is to support new quantitative approaches to the study of complex, fundamental biological processes by encouraging nontraditional collaborations across disciplinary lines. NIGMS will provide supplements to existing NIGMS grants to support the salary and expenses of collaborating investigators such as physicists, engineers, mathematicians, and other experts with quantitative skills relevant to the analysis of complex systems. It is expected that the collaboration will result in new directions for the parent project, or new research projects that will compete for independent funding. PA-98-024 may be obtained through the NIH grant line (301-402-2221), the NIH Web site, mail, and email.

Requirements: Applications may be submitted by foreign, domestic, for-profit and nonprofit organizations, public or private.

Contact: Dr. James Cassatt, Division of Cell Biology and Biophysics, (301) 594-0828; fax: (301) 480-2004; email: czj@cu.nih.gov; Dr. Judith Greenberg, Division of Genetics and Developmental Biology, (301) 594-0943; fax: (301) 480-2228; email: greenbej@nigms.ni

Internet: http://www.grants.nih.gov/grants/guide/pa-files/PA-98-024.html

Sponsor: National Institute of General Medical Sciences
45 Center Drive, Natcher Building
Bethesda, MD 20892

NIGMS Support of Competitive Research (SCORE) Pilot Project Awards 2631

The objective of the SCORE program is to foster the development of faculty at minority serving institutions (MSIs) in order to increase their research competitiveness and promote their transition to non-SCORE external sources of funding. This objective is expected to translate into an increase in the number of individuals from groups underrepresented in biomedical and behavioral research professionally engaged in these areas of research, and an enhancement of an institution's research base. SCORE SC grants are offered to eligible MSIs. For the purposes of this program, eligible MSIs are those with more than 50% student enrollment of individuals from groups underrepresented in biomedical and behavioral research. The SC2 awards may not exceed $300,000 (direct costs) for the entire length of the award which may be one to three years maximum.

Requirements: Eligible applicants include: public or private post secondary educational institution, such as a university or college awarding associate, undergraduate or graduate degrees located in the United States of America or its territories including Puerto Rico, Guam and Virgin Islands with more than 50 percent student enrollment from groups underrepresented in the biomedical and behavioral sciences (such as African American, Hispanic American, Native American, Alaska Natives or natives of the U.S. Pacific Islands); an Indian tribe that has a recognized governing body and that performs substantial governmental functions, or an Alaska Regional Corporation (ARC), as defined in the Alaska Native Claims Settlement Act (43 U.S.C. 1601 et. Seq.); or an institution that has a significantly high student enrollment from groups underrepresented in the biomedical or behavioral sciences but less than 50% (if the Secretary of the Department of Health and Human Services, through the MBRS Chief, determines that the institution has demonstrated special commitment to the retention and graduation of students from groups underrepresented in the biomedical and behavioral sciences and to the hiring and retention of science faculty from underrepresented groups).

Restrictions: Foreign institutions are not eligible to apply.

Amount of Grant: $50,000 to $100,000 maximum

Date(s) Application is Due: Jan 25; May 25; Sep 25

Contact: Hinda Zlotnik, Ph.D.; (301) 594-3900; fax: (301) 480-2753; email: zlotnikh@nigms.nih.gov

Internet: http://grants.nih.gov/grants/guide/pa-files/PAR-08-027.html

Sponsor: National Institute of General Medical Sciences (NIGMS)
45 Center Drive, Room 2AS.37, MSC 6200
Bethesda, MD 20892-6200

NIGMS Support of Competitive Research Research Advancement Awards 2632

The objective of the SCORE program is to foster the development of faculty at minority serving institutions (MSIs) in order to increase their research competitiveness and promote their transition to non-SCORE external sources of funding. This objective is expected to translate into an increase in the number of individuals from groups underrepresented in biomedical and behavioral research professionally engaged in these areas of research, and an enhancement of an institution's research base. SCORE SC grants are offered to eligible MSIs. For the purposes of this program, eligible MSIs are those with more than 50% student enrollment of individuals from groups underrepresented in biomedical and behavioral research. The anticipated amount of individual SC1 awards is expected to range between $125,000 to $250,000 maximum direct costs per year.

Requirements: Eligible applicants include: public or private post secondary educational institution, such as a university or college awarding associate, undergraduate or graduate degrees located in the United States of America or its territories including Puerto Rico, Guam and Virgin Islands with more than 50 percent student enrollment from groups underrepresented in the biomedical and behavioral sciences (such as African American, Hispanic American, Native American, Alaska Natives or natives of the U.S. Pacific Islands); an Indian tribe that has a recognized governing body and that performs substantial governmental functions, or an Alaska Regional Corporation (ARC), as defined in the Alaska Native Claims Settlement Act (43 U.S.C. 1601 et. Seq.); or an institution that has a significantly high student enrollment from groups underrepresented in the biomedical or behavioral sciences but less than 50% (if the Secretary of the Department of Health and Human Services, through the MBRS Chief, determines that the institution has demonstrated special commitment to the retention and graduation of students from groups underrepresented in the biomedical and behavioral sciences and to the hiring and retention of science faculty from underrepresented groups).

Restrictions: Foreign institutions are not eligible to apply.

Amount of Grant: $125,000-$250,000

Date(s) Application is Due: Jan 25; May 25; Sep 25

Contact: Hinda Zlotnik, Ph.D.; (301) 594-3900; fax: (301) 480-2753; email: zlotnikh@nigms.nih.gov

Internet: http://grants1.nih.gov/grants/guide/pa-files/PAR-08-026.html

Sponsor: National Institute of General Medical Sciences (NIGMS)
45 Center Drive, Room 2AS.37, MSC 6200
Bethesda, MD 20892-6200

NIGMS/NIDCR Evolution of Infectious Diseases Research Grants 2633

The goal of this joint NIGMS/NIDCR request for applications is to encourage development of a predictive science of infectious diseases by applying the perspectives, theories, and methods of population and evolutionary biology to important issues of disease emergence, prevention, and treatment. To achieve this goal, this RFA seeks collaborations between two major groups of scientists: those with expertise in population and evolutionary biology and molecular phylogenetics, including mathematical modeling and complexity theory; and infectious disease experts such as clinicians, epidemiologists, immunologists, microbiologists, veterinarians, or plant pathologists. PA: PA-99-147

Requirements: Applications may be submitted by domestic and foreign, for-profit and nonprofit organizations, units of state and local governments, and eligible agencies of the federal government.

Restrictions: Foreign institutions are not eligible for program project grants.

Amount of Grant: $250,000 total for direct costs per year

Contact: Dr. Irene Anne Eckstrand, Division of Genetics and Developmental Biology, (301) 594-0943; fax: (301) 480-2228; email: Irene_Eckstrand@nih.gov

Internet: http://grants2.nih.gov/grants/guide/pa-files/PA-99-147.html

Sponsor: National Institute of General Medical Sciences
45 Center Drive, Natcher Building
Bethesda, MD 20892

NIH Academic Career Awards 2634

The awards support individuals interested in introducing or improving curriculum in a particular scientific field as a means of enhancing the educational or research capacity at the grantee institution. The award supports two types of activities. Development—support for more junior candidates who are interested in developing academic and research expertise in particular fields as a way to increase the overall pool of individuals capable of research or teaching in the identified area. Leadership—supports more senior individuals with acknowledged scientific expertise and leadership skills who are interested in improving the curricula and enhancing the research capacity within an academic institution. Inquiries may be directed to program staff at the appropriate NIH institute: Dr. Robin Barr, Office of Extramural Affairs, (301) 496-9322, NIA, 7201 Wisconsin Avenue, Bethesda, MD 20892; Dr. Ernestine Vanderveen, Division of Basic Research, (301) 443-1273, NIAAA, 6000 Executive Boulevard, Bethesda, MD 20892; Dr. Richard Lymn, Extramural Programs, (301) 594-5128, NIAMS, Natcher Building, Bethesda, MD 20892; Dr. John Schneider, (301) 496-8580, NCI, Executive Plaza North, Bethesda, MD 20892; Dr. Annette Kirshner, (919) 541-0488, NIEHS, P.O. Box 12233, Research Triangle Park, NC 27709; and Dr. George Niederehe, (301) 443-3264, NIMH, 5600 Fishers Ln, Rockville, MD 20857. Annual deadline dates may vary; contact program staff for exact dates. PA: PA-95-052

Requirements: Candidate for this award must have a clinical or doctoral degree. Candidate for the development award must demonstrate the potential to develop into an excellent academician and must be able to identify a mentor who is an expert in the research field of interest. Candidate must also be able to devote 75 percent of full-time professional effort to the research program. For the leadership award, candidate must have sufficient clinical training, research, or teaching experience in the academic area of interest to implement a program of curriculum development within the applicant institution; must have an academic appointment at a level sufficient to exert an influence on the coordination of research, teaching, and clinical practice in an emerging field; and must be able to devote at least 25 percent effort to the program.

Date(s) Application is Due: Feb 1; Jun 1; Oct 1

Contact: Program Officer

Internet: http://www.grants.nih.gov/grants/guide/pa-files/PA-95-052.html

Sponsor: National Institutes of Health
6701 Rockledge Drive
Bethesda, MD 20892

NIH Academic Research Enhancement Awards (AREA) 2635

NIH makes a special effort to stimulate research in educational institutions that provide baccalaureate training for a significant number of the nation's research scientists but that historically have not been major recipients of NIH support. The AREA funds are intended to support new research projects or expand ongoing research activities proposed by faculty members of these institutions in areas related to the health sciences. Funding decisions will be based on the proposed research project's scientific merit and relevance to NIH programs and the institution's contribution to the undergraduate preparation of doctoral-level health professionals. Annual deadline dates vary; contact program staff for exact dates. PA: PA-99-062

Requirements: All health professional schools/colleges and other academic components of domestic institutions offering baccalaureate or advanced degrees in the sciences related to health are eligible to apply.

Restrictions: Applicant principal investigators must not have active research grant support from either NIH or ADAMHA at the applicant institution at the time of award of an AREA grant; may not submit a regular NIH or ADAMHA research grant application

for essentially the same project as a pending AREA application; are expected to conduct the majority of their research at their own institutions, although limited access to special facilities or equipment other institutions is permitted; and may not be awarded more than one AREA grant at a time nor be awarded a second AREA grant to continue research initiated under the first AREA grant.
Amount of Grant: $150,000 maximum in direct costs
Date(s) Application is Due: May 7; Jun 25; Sep 7
Contact: Denise Russo, Ph.D., Office of Extramural Research; (301) 451-7972; fax: (301) 480-0146; email: drussol@mail.nih.gov
Internet: http://grants.nih.gov/grants/guide/pa-files/PA-06-042.html
Sponsor: National Institutes of Health
6705 Rockledge Drive, Rockledge I Building, Room 3524
Bethesda, MD 20892

NIH Alzheimer's Disease Clinical Trial Planning Grant **2636**
NIA, NIMH, and NINDS invite qualified investigators to submit research grant applications for clinical trial planning grants directed toward the drug treatment of the cognitive and behavioral symptoms of Alzheimer's disease (AD). The purpose of the grant is to allow for early peer review of the rationale and design for Alzheimer's disease clinical drug trials and to provide support for the development of a detailed clinical trial research plan, including a manual of operations and procedures. Note: There is a companion program announcement available for Alzheimer's Disease Pilot Clinical Trials (PA-99-038). Inquiries may be directed to program staff at the appropriate NIH institute: Dr. Neil Buckholtz, (301) 496-9350, Neuroscience and Neuropsychology of Aging Program, NIA, 7201 Wisconsin Avenue, Bethesda, MD 20892; Dr. Eugene Oliver, (301) 496-5680, Division of Stroke, Trauma, and Neurodegenerative Disorders, NINDS, 7550 Wisconsin Avenue, Bethesda, MD 20892; Dr. George Niederehe, (301) 443-1185, NIMH, 5600 Fishers Ln, Rockville, MD 20857. PA: PA-99-039
Requirements: Applications may be submitted by foreign and domestic, for-profit and nonprofit organizations, both public and private.
Restrictions: The award cannot be renewed.
Amount of Grant: $150,000 maximum direct costs for one year
Contact: Program Officer
Internet: http://www.grants.nih.gov/grants/guide/pa-files/PA-99-039.html
Sponsor: National Institutes of Health
6701 Rockledge Drive
Bethesda, MD 20892

NIH Autism and Autism Spectrum Disorders Research **2637**
The purpose of this program announcement is to encourage grant applications for the support of research designed to elucidate the diagnosis, epidemiology, etiology, genetics, treatment, and optimal means of service delivery in relation to autistic disorder (autism) and autism spectrum disorders. Inquiries may be directed to program staff at the appropriate NIH institute: Dr. Judith Rumsey, (301) 443-9264, NIMH, 5600 Fishers Ln, Rockville, MD 20857; Dr. Marie Bristol, (301) 496-1383, NICHD, 6100 Executive Boulevard, Bethesda, MD 20892; Dr. Judith Cooper, (301) 496-5061, NIDCD, Executive Plaza South, Bethesda, MD 20892; and Dr. Giovanna Spinella, (301) 496-5821, NINDS, 7550 Wisconsin Avenue, Bethesda, MD 20892. PA: PA-98-108
Requirements: Applications may be submitted by foreign and domestic, for-profit organizations, both public and private; units of state and local governments; and eligible agencies of the federal government.
Restrictions: Foreign institutions are not eligible to apply.
Contact: Program Officer
Internet: http://www.grants.nih.gov/grants/guide/pa-files/PA-98-108.html
Sponsor: National Institutes of Health
6701 Rockledge Drive
Bethesda, MD 20892

NIH Biobehavioral Pain Research Grants **2638**
The purpose of this PA is to inform the scientific community of the interests of the various institutes at the NIH and to stimulate and foster a wide range of basic and clinical studies on pain as they relate to the missions of these institutes. Applicants are encouraged to study individual differences in pain responses which may be due to factors such as genetic differences, endocrine activity, neural activity, immune function, psychological state, disability state, age, gender, and cultural background. Research is also needed in areas such as understanding the neuroanatomical pathways and the neurophysiological mechanisms in pain. The pain experience needs to be examined at all levels of research including the gene, molecule, cell, organ, and individual with the goal of developing biobehavioral interventions to manage or prevent pain. Inquiries may be directed to the appropriate NIH institute: Dr. Martha Hare, (301) 451-3874, Office of Extramural Programs, NINR, 6701 Democracy Boulevard, Room 710, Bethesda, MD 20892; Dr. Patricia Bryant, (301) 594-2095, Division of Extramural Research, NIDCR, Building 45, Bethesda, MD 20892; Dr. Judith Finkelstein, (301) 496-9350, Neuroscience and Neuropsychology of Aging Program, NIA, 7201 Wisconsin Avenue, Bethesda, MD 20892; Dr. Deborah Ader, (301) 594-5032, Behavior and Prevention Research Program Director, NIAMS, Building 45, Bethesda, MD 20892; Dr. Louis Quatrano, (301) 402-4221, Behavioral Sciences and Rehabilitation Engineering, NICHD, 6100 Executive Boulevard, Bethesda MD 20892; Dr. David Thomas, (301) 443-6975, Behavioral Neurobiology Research Branch, NIDA, 5600 Fishers Ln, Rockville, MD 20857; Dr. Peter Muehrer, (301) 443-4708, Prevention, Early Intervention, and Epidemiology Research Branch, NIMH, 5600 Fishers Ln, Rockville, MD 20857; Dr. Linda Porter, (301) 496-9964, Systems and Cognitive Neuroscience, NINDS, 6001 Executive Boulevard, Bethesda, MD 20892; and Dr. Nancy Pearson, (301) 594-0519, NCCAM, 6707 Democracy Boulevard, Bethesda, MD 20892. PA: PA-03-152
Requirements: Applications may be submitted by foreign and domestic, for-profit and nonprofit, both public and private organizations; units of state and local governments; and eligible agencies of the federal government.
Contact: Program Officer
Internet: http://grants2.nih.gov/grants/guide/pa-files/PA-03-152.html
Sponsor: National Institutes of Health
6701 Rockledge Drive
Bethesda, MD 20892

NIH Biobehavioral Research for Effective Sleep **2639**
The goal of this program announcement is to stimulate clinical and applied research on behavioral, psychosocial, and physiological consequences of acute and chronic partial sleep deprivation in either chronically ill or healthy individuals and to develop environmental, clinical management, and other interventions with the potential to reduce sleep disturbances and significantly improve the health of large numbers of people. Although sleep disorders are a cause of sleep loss in affected individuals, the questions to be addressed under this solicitation should focus on causes and consequences of sleep deprivation, apart from any sleep pathology. Inquiries may be directed to program staff at the appropriate NIH institute.
Requirements: Applications may be submitted by domestic and foreign, for-profit and non-profit organizations, public and private, such as universities, colleges, hospitals, laboratories, units of State and local governments, and eligible agencies of the Federal government. Racial/ethnic minority individuals, women, and persons with disabilities are encouraged to apply as Principal Investigators.
Amount of Grant: $250,000 maximum per year
Date(s) Application is Due: Feb 16; Jun 16; Oct 16
Contact: Susan Grove, Program Officer; (301) 435-0714; email: sg16d@nih.gov or grantsinfo@od.nih.gov
Internet: http://grants.nih.gov/grants/guide/pa-files/PA-00-046.html
Sponsor: National Institutes of Health (NIH)
6701 Rockledge Drive
Bethesda, MD 20892

NIH Bioengineering Nanotechnology Initiative **2640**
NIH invites grant applications for projects on nanotechnologies useful to biomedicine. Nanotechnology is defined as the creation of functional materials, devices, and systems through control of matter at the scale of one to 100 nanometers, and the exploitation of novel properties and phenomena at the same scale. Inquiries may be directed to program staff at the appropriate NIH institute. See web site for listing of program staff. PA: PA-02-125
Amount of Grant: $400,000 maximum
Date(s) Application is Due: Apr 1; Aug 1; Dec 1
Contact: Program Officer
Internet: http://grants2.nih.gov/grants/guide/pa-files/PA-02-125.html
Sponsor: National Institutes of Health
6701 Rockledge Drive
Bethesda, MD 20892

NIH Biology, Development, and Progression of Malignant Prostate Disease Research Grants **2641**
Investigator-initiated research grants will be made to examine a range of fundamental biological issues considered critical for progress in defeating prostate cancer. The purpose of funding is to encourage new projects focusing on the biology that underlies the development and progression of malignant prostatic disease. Multidisciplinary collaborations between basic and clinical scientists in projects ranging from exploratory basic biology studies to disease progression in appropriate biological systems or models are encouraged.
Requirements: Applications may be submitted by foreign or domestic for-profit and nonprofit organizations, both public and private; units of state and local government; and eligible agencies of the federal government.
Amount of Grant: $250,000 maximum per year
Date(s) Application is Due: Feb 5; Feb 16; Jun 5; Jun 16; Oct 5; Oct 16
Contact: Frank Bellino, Ph.D.; (301) 496-6402; fax: (301) 402-0010; email: fb12a@nih.gov
Internet: http://grants.nih.gov/grants/guide/pa-files/PA-99-081.html
Sponsor: National Institutes of Health (NIH)
Gateway Building, Suite 2C231
Bethesda, MD 20892

NIH Biomedical Research on the International Space Station **2642**
The National Institutes of Health (NIH) and the National Aeronautics and Space Administration (NASA) are cooperating to facilitate biomedical research in space for better understanding of human physiology and human health on Earth. Applications to this FOA should propose innovative biomedical research on the molecular or cellular level that is directly relevant to the NIH mission and can be carried out on the ISS. Awards made through this FOA will initially support milestone-driven, ground based preparatory studies (UH2 ground feasibility phase), with possible rapid transition to the second, ISS-based research phase (UH3 ISS experimental phase). The ground feasibility phase (UH2) will allow investigators to focus on ground-based preparatory work to meet scientific milestones and technical requirements leading to the ISS experimental phase (UH3). The UH3 phase will include preparing the experiments for launch, conducting

them on the ISS, and the subsequent data analyses on Earth. UH3s will be awarded after administrative review of the eligible UH2s that have met the scientific milestones and feasibility requirements necessary to conduct research on the ISS. Applicants should contact individuals at the specific departments listed on the web site. Letters of Intent are due by August 31, and full applications should arrive by September 30.
Requirements: The UH2/UH3 application must be submitted as a single application, and applicants should note specific instructions for each phase in this FOA. The following organizations and institutions may apply: public/state controlled institutions of higher education; private institutions of higher education; Hispanic-serving institutions; historically Black colleges and universities (HBCUs); tribally controlled colleges and universities (TCCUs); Alaska native and native Hawaiian serving institutions; nonprofits with 501(c)3 IRS status; nonprofits without 501(c)3 IRS status; small businesses; for-profit organizations; State governments; regional organizations; U.S. territories or possessions; Indian/Native American tribal governments; Indian/Native American tribally designated organizations; county governments; city or township governments; special district governments; independent school districts; public housing authorities/ Indian housing authorities; eligible agencies of the Federal government; and faith-based or community based organizations.
Amount of Grant: $300,000 in direct costs per year
Date(s) Application is Due: Aug 31; Sep 30
Contact: Susan Grove, Program Officer; (301) 435-0714; email: sg16d@nih.gov or grantsinfo@od.nih.gov
Internet: http://grants.nih.gov/grants/guide/pa-files/PAR-09-120.html
Sponsor: National Institutes of Health (NIH)
6701 Rockledge Drive
Bethesda, MD 20892-0052

NIH Bone and the Hematopoietic and Immune Systems Research Grants 2643
The participating institutes seek investigator-initiated projects that have the potential to illuminate functional interactions between bone and the hematopoietic and immune systems. Recent observations underscore the linkage between endochondral bone formation and the establishment of hematopoietic marrow, and suggest that interactions between bone, marrow, and the immune system persist in the mature skeleton. Marrow stromal cells include the precursors of the osteochondrogenic lineage, exert important influences on osteoclastogenesis and lymphopoiesis, and mediate the effects of some systemic factors on bone turnover. Recent evidence indicates that hematopoietic cells can influence the differentiation of osteogenic cells, and suggests that mature lymphocytes can influence osteoclastic and osteoblastic functions. In order to explore the mechanisms that underlie these interactions, the participating institutes support outstanding projects that have the potential to either clarify the importance of specific cell types and effector molecules or identify previously unrecognized cellular and molecular agents that influence bone physiology. Collaborations among bone biologists, hematologists, and immunologists, and between basic scientists and clinical investigators, are particularly encouraged. Inquiries may be directed to the staff at the appropriate NIH institute: Dr. William Sharrock, Musculoskeletal Diseases Branch, NIAMS, 45 Center Drive, Bethesda, MD 20892; Dr. Frank Bellino, (301) 496-6402, Biology of Aging Program, NIA, Gateway Building, Bethesda, MD 20892; Dr. Kenneth Gruber, (301) 584-4836, Chronic and Disabling Diseases Branch, NIDCR, 45 Center Drive, Bethesda, MD 20892; and Dr. Charles Peterson, (301) 435-0050, Division of Blood Diseases and Resources, NHLBI, 6701 Rockledge Drive, Bethesda, MD 20892. PA: PA-99-085
Requirements: Applications may be submitted by domestic and foreign, for-profit and nonprofit, public and private organizations, units of state and local governments, and eligible agencies of the federal government.
Restrictions: Foreign institutions are not eligible for program project grant support.
Amount of Grant: $250,000 maximum per year
Contact: Frank Bellino, Ph.D.; (301) 496-6402; fax: (301) 402-0010; email: fb12a@ nih.gov
Internet: http://grants.nih.gov/grants/guide/pa-files/PA-99-085.html
Sponsor: National Institutes of Health (NIH)
Gateway Building, Suite 2C231
Bethesda, MD 20892

NIH Building Interdisciplinary Research Careers in Women's Health Grants 2644
The NIH Office of Research on Women's Health (ORWH) and its cosponsors invite institutional career development award applications for Building Interdisciplinary Research Careers in Women's Health (BIRCWH) Career Development Programs, hereafter termed Programs. Programs will support mentored research career development of junior faculty members, known as BIRCWH Scholars, who have recently completed clinical training or postdoctoral fellowships, and who will be engaged in interdisciplinary basic, translational, behavioral, clinical, and/or health services research relevant to women's health or sex/gender factors. Direct costs are limited to $500,000 total costs for a five-year period. Letters of Intent are due by September 23, with final applications due by October 22.
Requirements: The following organizations and institutions are eligible to apply for support: public/state controlled institutions of higher education; private institutions of higher education; Hispanic-serving institutions; historically Black colleges and universities (HBCUs); tribally controlled colleges and universities (TCCUs); Alaska Native and Native Hawaiian serving institutions; nonprofits with 501(c)3 IRS status (other than institutions of higher education); nonprofits without 501(c)3 IRS status (other than institutions of higher education); Indian/Native American tribal governments (federally recognized); Indian/Native American tribally designated organizations; U.S. territories or possessions; and eligible agencies of the federal government.
Amount of Grant: $500,000 maximum for a five-year period
Date(s) Application is Due: Sep 23; Oct 22
Contact: Joan Davis Nagel; (301) 496-9186; fax: (301) 402-1798; email: joandav@mail.nih.gov
Internet: http://grants.nih.gov/grants/guide/rfa-files/RFA-OD-09-006.html
Sponsor: National Institutes of Health (NIH)
6707 Democracy Boulevard, Suite 400
Bethesda, MD 20892

NIH Cancer Surveillance Using Health Claims-Based Data System Grants 2645
Three institutes of the NIH invite investigator-initiated grant applications for research to investigate the utility of health claims information as a reporting source for assessing the national cancer burden. Health claims include secondary data sources, for example fee-for-service insurance bills, managed care encounter data, and discharge summaries. Responses to this program announcement would initiate mechanisms to expand understanding of the capability of and methods needed to use claims data for cancer surveillance as well as applying these findings to the claims data in order to assess all aspects of cancer surveillance, such as cancer screening, incidence, treatment, and outcomes. The NIDCR's specific interests focus on health claims-based data as related to oral and pharyngeal cancers or the oral complications of cancer therapies. Inquiries may be directed to the program contact at the appropriate NIH institute: Dr. Joan Warren, (301) 496-5184, Applied Research Branch, NCI, Executive Plaza N, Bethesda, MD 20892; Dr. Patricia Bryant, (301) 594-2095, Division of Extramural Research, NIDCR, 45 Center Drive, Bethesda, MD 20892; and Dr. Bernard Friedman, (301) 594-6819, AHCPR, 2101 E Jefferson Street, Rockville, MD 20852. Annual deadline dates vary; contact program staff for exact dates. PA: PA-04-012
Requirements: Applications may be submitted by public and private, foreign and domestic, for-profit and nonprofit organizations.
Contact: Crystal Wolfrey, Grants Administration Branch, (301) 496-8634; fax: (301) 496-8601; email: wolfreyc@il.nih.gov
Internet: http://grants2.nih.gov/grants/guide/pa-files/PA-04-012.html
Sponsor: National Institutes of Health
6701 Rockledge Drive
Bethesda, MD 20892

NIH Career Development Awards: Child Abuse and Neglect Research 2646
The five sponsoring institutes invite applications in response to this announcement for the career development of investigators who have made a commitment to focus their research endeavors on child abuse and neglect through research career enhancement to conduct high-quality, multidisciplinary, clinically relevant research on basic biological, behavioral, and social aspects of child and adolescent abuse and neglect. While the focus of the career development program is on child abuse and neglect in human populations, the award may include complementary, appropriate laboratory and animal research related to the child abuse and neglect research proposed in the application. Inquiries may be directed to program staff at the appropriate NIH institute: Dr. Malcolm Gordon, (301) 443-4709, NIMH, 6001 Executive Boulevard, Bethesda, MD 20892; Dr. Cheryl A. Boyce, (301) 443-0848, NIMH, 6001 Executive Boulevard, Bethesda, MD 20892; Dr. Joseph S. Drage, (301) 496-4188, NINDS, 6001 Executive Boulevard, Suite 3309, Bethesda, MD 20892; Dr. G. Reid Lyon, (301) 496-9849, NICHD, Building 6100, Room 4B05, MSC 7510, Bethesda, MD 20892; Dr. Coryl Jones, (301) 443-6637, NIDA, 6001 Executive Boulevard, Room 5169, MSC 9589, Bethesda, MD 20892; and Dr. Susan Martin, (301) 443-8767, NIAAA, 6000 Executive Boulevard, Suite 505, Rockville, MD 20892. PA: PA-99-133
Requirements: Prospective candidates should contact the program staff most relevant to the applicant's research interests to ascertain the conditions of the award supported by each institute.
Date(s) Application is Due: Feb 1; Jun 1; Oct 1
Contact: Program Officer
Internet: http://grants.nih.gov/grants/guide/pa-files/PA-99-133.html
Sponsor: National Institutes of Health
6701 Rockledge Drive, Room 1040
Bethesda, MD 20892

NIH Centers for AIDS Research (CFARs) 2647
Participating institutes of NIH invite applications for center core grants (P30) to support Centers for AIDS Research (CFARs). CFAR cores provide infrastructure and promote basic, clinical, behavioral and translational AIDS research activities at institutions that receive significant AIDS funding from multiple NIH institutes or centers. CFARs foster synergy and improve coordination of research, support emerging research opportunities, and promote economy of scale through resources shared by multiple independent laboratories. Inquiries may be directed to program staff at the appropriate NIH institute; see web site for staff listings. PA: PAR-03-089
Requirements: Applications may be submitted by domestic for-profit and nonprofit organizations, both public and private; units of state or local government; and eligible agencies of the federal government.
Restrictions: Foreign institutions are not eligible to apply.
Date(s) Application is Due: Jun 16
Contact: Lori Zimand, Program Contact, (301) 451-4580; fax; (301) 493-0597; email: lz36k@nih.gov
Internet: http://grants2.nih.gov/grants/guide/pa-files/PAR-03-089.html
Sponsor: National Institutes of Health
6701 Rockledge Drive
Bethesda, MD 20892

NIH Centers for Dietary Supplements Research: Botanicals 2648

Applications are invited to establish specialized research centers to investigate the biological effects of botanicals including, but not limited to, botanicals available as dietary supplements. The creation of such centers is needed to advance the quality and quantity of scientific information on botanicals and to promote further research in this area. The major goal of this RFA is to foster interdisciplinary research to develop systematic evaluation of the safety and efficacy of botanicals. General inquiries may be directed to Dr. Christine Swanson, (301) 435-2920, Office of Dietary Supplements, NIH, Building 31, Bethesda, MD 20892. Programmatic inquiries may be directed to the staff at the appropriate NIH institute: Dr. Joshua Rosenthal, (301) 496-2516, Biodiversity Program, FIC, 31 Center Drive, Bethesda, MD 20892; Dr. Carolyn Clifford, (301) 496-8573, Division of Cancer Prevention, NCI, Executive Plaza N, Bethesda, MD 20892; Dr. Neal West, (301) 402-5867, NCCAM, Building 31, Bethesda, MD 20892; Dr. Momtaz Wassef, (301) 435-0550, Vascular Research Program, NHLBI, 6701 Rockledge Drive, Bethesda, MD 20892; Dr. Peter Preusch, (301) 594-5938, Pharmacology, Physiology, and Biological Chemistry Division, NIGMS, 45 Center Drive, Bethesda, MD 20892; Dr. Michael Ken May, (301) 594-8884, Division of Digestive Diseases and Nutrition, NIDDK, 45 Center Drive, Bethesda, MD 20892; Dr. Pamela Starke-Reed, (301) 496-6402, Office of Nutrition, NIA, 7201 Wisconsin Avenue, Bethesda, MD 20892; Dr. Jag Khalsa, (301) 443-1801, Center on AIDS and Other Medical Consequences of Drug Abuse, NIDA, 6001 Executive Building, Bethesda, MD 20892; Dr. Michael McClure, (919) 541-5327, Division of Extramural Research and Training, NIEHS, 111 TW Alexander Drive, Building 401, Research Triangle Park, NC 27709; and Dr. Kay Anderson, Research Program Director, (301) 402-1770, ORWH, 1 Center Drive, Bethesda, MD 20892. Annual deadline dates may vary; contact program staff for exact dates. RFA: OD-00-004

Requirements: Applications may be submitted by domestic for-profit and nonprofit organizations, both public and private; units of state and local governments; and eligible agencies of the federal government. Foreign organizations may participate if they are components of domestic U.S. organizations or via contractual or consortium agreements with domestic U.S. organizations.

Amount of Grant: $1.5 million maximum for up to five years

Contact: Program Officer

Internet: http://grants.nih.gov/grants/guide/rfa-files/RFA-OD-00-004.html

Sponsor: National Institutes of Health
6701 Rockledge Drive
Bethesda, MD 20892

NIH Clinical Bioethics Postdoctoral Fellowships 2649

The Department of Clinical Bioethics of the Warren Grant Magnuson Clinical Center, NIH, offers a limited number of postdoctoral fellowship positions in bioethics. Fellows will participate in the activities and the intellectual life of the department and study ethical issues related to conduct of research, clinical practice, and health policy. Fellows will conduct their research under the guidance of senior faculty, participate in weekly bioethics seminars, case conferences, ethics consultations, and IRB deliberations, and have access to multiple educational opportunities at the NIH. Fellowships are two years in length, and stipends are based on the applicant's previous experience and the current U.S. government schedule. Guidelines are available online.

Requirements: Applicants should have a PhD, MD, JD, or other advanced degree in a relevant field. Fellows will be selected on the basis of their previous academic or professional achievements, commitment to scholarship, and the contribution they are likely to make in the field of bioethics. No prior experience in bioethics is necessary.

Date(s) Application is Due: Dec 30

Contact: Becky Chen, Department of Clinical Bioethics, (301) 496-2429; fax: (301) 496-0760; email: bioethics-inquiries@mail.nih.gov

Internet: http://www.bioethics.nih.gov/opportunities/post-doc.html

Sponsor: National Institutes of Health
10 Center Drive, Building 10, Room 1C118
Bethesda, MD 20892-1156

NIH Clinical Bioethics Predoctoral Fellowships 2650

The Department of Clinical Bioethics of the Warren Grant Magnuson Clinical Center, NIH, supports a limited number of predoctoral fellowship positions in bioethics. Fellows will participate in the activities and intellectual life of the department, and study ethical issues related to the conduct of research, clinical practice, and health policy. Fellows will conduct their research under the guidance of the senior faculty, participate in weekly bioethics seminars, case conferences, ethics consultations, and IRB deliberations, and have access to multiple educational opportunities at NIH. Fellowships are two years in length. Stipends are based on the current U.S. government schedule. Application guidelines are available online.

Requirements: Applicants should have an undergraduate degree and should be planning postgraduate work. Fellows will be selected on the basis of their previous academic achievements, commitment to scholarship, and the contribution they are likely to make in the field of bioethics. No prior experience in bioethics is necessary.

Date(s) Application is Due: Jan 15

Contact: Program Contact, Department of Clinical Bioethics, (301) 496-2429; fax: (301) 496-0760; email: bioethics-inquiries@mail.nih.gov

Internet: http://www.bioethics.nih.gov/opportunities/pre-doc.html

Sponsor: National Institutes of Health
10 Center Drive, Building 10, Room 1C118
Bethesda, MD 20892-1156

NIH Collaborations for Advanced Strategies in Complication of HIV Infection 2651

NIDA, NIAAA, NIDDK, and NIMH invite applicants to expand the clinical knowledge of the complications of HIV by expediting the translation of promising innovative preclinical findings into clinical research applications. The focus of the program is to support focused collaborative research between preclinical and clinical scientists to test, refine, and improve diagnostic, pathogenic, or therapeutic concepts. It anticipates such research will lead to innovative approaches for the prevention and management of complications causing significant morbidity or mortality in HIV infected persons, including the recently recognized metabolic complications, coincident pathogens such as hepatitis C virus, and the opportunistic pathogens. Inquiries may be directed to program staff at the appropriate NIH institute: Dr. Barbara Laughon, (301) 402-2304, NIAID, 6700 B Rockledge Drive, Bethesda, MD 20892; Dr. Jag Khalsa, Health Scientist Administrator, (301) 443-1801, NIDA, 6001 Executive Boulevard, Bethesda, MD 20892; Dr. Thomas Kresina, Chief, Biomedical Research Branch, (301) 443-6537, NIAAA, 6000 Executive Boulevard, Bethesda, MD 20892; Dr. Philip Smith, Senior Advisor, (301) 594-8816, NIDDK, 45 Center Drive, Bethesda, MD 20892; and Dr. Dianne Rausch, (301) 443-7281, NIMH, 6001 Executive Boulevard, Bethesda, MD 20892. Annual deadline dates vary; contact program staff for exact dates.

Requirements: Applications may be submitted by domestic and foreign, for-profit and nonprofit organizations, both public and private; units of state and local governments; and eligible agencies of the federal government.

Contact: Program Officer

Internet: http://grants.nih.gov/grants/guide/pa-files/PA-00-048.html

Sponsor: National Institutes of Health
6701 Rockledge Drive
Bethesda, MD 20892

NIH Complementary and Alternative Medicine Postdoctoral Training Grants 2652

The Office of Alternative Medicine funds individual postdoctoral training awards using the National Research Service Award (NRSA) mechanism. The purpose is to provide a cadre of investigators capable of conducting systematic studies on safety, efficacy, cost effectiveness, or mechanisms of action of unconventional methods for treating major diseases and promoting well-being. This training is expected to attract postdoctoral candidates who are in the early stages of their careers. They will have obtained expertise in conventional research methodology and some familiarity with/or interest in alternative medical procedures. Prospective trainees will be expected to form alliances with established researchers to provide mutual learning experiences. Individuals may request up to three years of aggregate NRSA support at the postdoctoral level. Written and telephone inquiries are invited. PA: PA-01-088

Requirements: U.S. citizens or noncitizen nationals may apply if, prior to beginning the award, they have received the PhD, MD, DO, DDS, DVM, OD, DPM, ScD, D.Eng, DrPH, DNS, DPharm, or equivalent doctoral degree from an accredited domestic or foreign institution. Before submitting an application, the applicant must arrange for appointment to an appropriate accredited university, hospital, or other institution with facilities including staff for postdoctoral training. The candidate should be accepted by a sponsor who will actively supervise the training. The sponsor should have research experience in clinical medicine and/or basic preclinical research along with an involvement in the evaluation of alternative medicine. The sponsor should be qualified to supervise in the application of rigorous study design to the assessment of individual alternative therapies.

Amount of Grant: $28,260-$44,412 depending on years of experience

Date(s) Application is Due: Apr 5; Aug 5; Dec 5

Contact: Dr. Nancy Pearson, (301) 594-0519; fax: (301) 480-3621; email: pearsonn@mail.nih.gov

Internet: http://grants2.nih.gov/grants/guide/pa-files/PA-01-088.html

Sponsor: National Institutes of Health
6120 Executive Boulevard, Executive Plaza S
Rockville, MD 20892-9904

NIH Demographic Research on Sexual Behaviors Related to HIV 2653

NICHD, NIDR and NIMH invite qualified researchers to submit applications to study the social and behavioral aspects of the transmission of HIV through sexual intercourse, including oral sexual practices. Inquiries may be directed to program staff at the appropriate NIH institute: Dr. Susan Newcomer, (301) 496-1174, NICHD, 6100 Executive Boulevard, Bethesda, MD 20892; Dr. Willo Pequegnat, (301) 443-6100, NIMH, Parklawn Building, 5600 Fishers Ln, Rockville, MD 20857. Annual deadline dates may vary; contact program staff for exact dates. PAS-00-136

Requirements: Applications may be submitted by domestic for-profit and nonprofit organizations, both public and private; units of state and local governments; and eligible agencies of the federal government.

Amount of Grant: $2.7 million total

Contact: Program Officer

Internet: http://grants2.nih.gov/grants/guide/pa-files/PAS-00-136.html

Sponsor: National Institutes of Health
6701 Rockledge Drive
Bethesda, MD 20892

NIH Dietary Supplement Research Centers: Botanicals Grants 2654

ODS, NCCAM and NCI invite new and renewal applications to support research centers which will: promote collaborative integrated interdisciplinary study of botanicals, particularly those found as ingredients in dietary supplements; and conduct research of high potential for being translated into practical benefits for human health. This initiative is intended to advance the spectrum of botanical research activities, ranging from plant

identification and characterization to early phase clinical studies. Preclinical research that will inform future clinical studies is encouraged as the primary research focus of this program. ODS has a particular interest in botanicals as part of health care for conditions relating to health maintenance or primary prevention. NCCAM is interested in the study of botanicals broadly used by the American public. The NCI Division of Cancer Prevention is interested in supporting research focused on mechanisms by which botanically derived bioactive food components might influence cancer risk and tumor behavior. An applicant may request a project period of up to five years; an annual budget in direct costs up to $1.0 million.
Requirements: The following organizations and institutions are eligible to apply: individuals; public/state controlled institutions of higher education; private institutions of higher education; Hispanic-serving institutions; historically Black colleges and universities (HBCUs); tribally controlled colleges and universities (TCCUs); Alaska Native and Native Hawaiian serving institutions; nonprofits with 501(c)3 IRS status; nonprofits without 501(c)3 IRS status; for-profit organizations; state governments; Indian/Native American tribal governments (federally recognized); Indian/Native American tribally designated organizations; county governments; city or township governments; special district governments; independent school districts; public housing authorities/Indian housing authorities; U.S. territory or possession; Indian/Native American tribal governments (other than federally recognized); regional organizations; non-domestic (non-U.S.) entities (foreign organizations); other eligible agencies of the federal government; and faith-based or community-based organizations.
Amount of Grant: $1,000,000 per year
Date(s) Application is Due: Dec 3
Contact: Christine A. Swanson, Ph.D., Director, Botanical Research Centers Program; (301) 435-2920; fax: (301) 480-1845; email: Swansonc@od.nih.gov
Internet: http://grants.nih.gov/grants/guide/pa-files/PAR-09-091.html
Sponsor: National Institutes of Health (NIH)
6100 Executive Boulevard, Room 3B01, MSC 7517
Bethesda, MD 20892

NIH Earth-Based Research Relevant to the Space Environment 2655
The purpose of this Program Announcement (PA) is to stimulate ground-based research on basic, applied, and clinical biomedical and behavioral problems that are relevant to human space flight or that could use the space environment as a laboratory. Although none of the research supported under this initiative would be conducted in space, it is anticipated that it would form a basis for future competitively reviewed studies which could be conducted on the International Space Station, or other space flight opportunities, by skilled on-board specialists. Modular Grant applications will request direct costs in $25,000 modules, up to a total direct cost request of $250,000 per year.
Requirements: The following organizations and institutions may apply: public/state controlled institutions of higher education; private institutions of higher education; Hispanic-serving institutions; historically Black colleges and universities (HBCUs); tribally controlled colleges and universities (TCCUs); Alaska native and native Hawaiian serving institutions; nonprofits with 501(c)3 IRS status; nonprofits without 501(c)3 IRS status; small businesses; for-profit organizations; State governments; regional organizations; U.S. territories or possessions; Indian/Native American tribal governments; Indian/Native American tribally designated organizations; county governments; city or township governments; special district governments; independent school districts; public housing authorities/Indian housing authorities; eligible agencies of the Federal government; and faith-based or community based organizations.
Amount of Grant: $250,000 maximum per year
Date(s) Application is Due: Feb 5; Jun 5; Oct 5
Contact: Susan Grove, Program Officer; (301) 435-0714; email: sg16d@nih.gov or grantsinfo@od.nih.gov
Internet: http://grants.nih.gov/grants/guide/pa-files/PA-00-088.html
Sponsor: National Institutes of Health (NIH)
6701 Rockledge Drive
Bethesda, MD 20892

NIH Ecology of Infectious Diseases 2656
NIH, NSF, NASA, U.S.GS, and the Agricultural Research Service (ARS) invite applications for the establishment of research programs to elucidate the underlying mechanisms that govern the relationships between anthropogenic environmental changes and the transmission dynamics of infectious diseases. This RFA calls for the development of interdisciplinary research programs on the ecology of infectious diseases in the context of anthropogenic environmental changes such as biodiversity loss, habitat transformation, environmental contamination, climate change, and other influences. The focus of this RFA is on discovery of basic ecological and biological mechanisms and development of predictive models for the emergence and transmission of diseases in humans and other animals, and ultimately the development of strategies to prevent or control them. Annual deadline dates may vary; contact program staff for exact dates. RFA: TW-00-002
Requirements: Applications may be submitted by domestic and foreign, for-profit and nonprofit organizations, both public and private (including domestic institutions with foreign collaborators); units of state and local governments; and eligible agencies of the federal government.
Amount of Grant: $4 million total
Contact: Program Officer
Internet: http://grants.nih.gov/grants/guide/rfa-files/RFA-TW-00-002.html
Sponsor: National Institutes of Health
6701 Rockledge Drive
Bethesda, MD 20892

NIH Economic Studies in Cancer Prevention, Screening, and Care 2657
NCI and AHCPR invite investigator-initiated grant applications for research directed at increasing the knowledge base in the area of the economic aspects of cancer prevention, screening, and care. The goal of this program announcement is to generate new economic knowledge that will promote the optimal design of cancer prevention and control trial studies and interventions and will facilitate the formulation of effective health care policy related to cancer prevention and control. NIDCR has an interest in economic and health services studies as these relate specifically to oral and pharyngeal cancers and health care policies related to prevention and control of oral cancers. This initiative requests research applications on new methods development, the synthesis and extension of existing methods, and innovative data gathering strategies. Applications that propose to implement actual data collection on a pilot or full-scale basis as well as analytical studies that use existing data and methodology will be entertained. PA: PA-04-017
Requirements: Foreign and domestic, for-profit and nonprofit organizations, both public and private; units of state and local governments; and eligible agencies of the federal government may apply.
Contact: Crystal Wolfrey, Grants Administration Branch, NCI, (301) 496-8634; fax: (301) 496-4801; email: wolfreyc@mail.nih.gov
Internet: http://grants1.nih.gov/grants/guide/pa-files/PA-04-017.html
Sponsor: National Institutes of Health
6701 Rockledge Drive
Bethesda, MD 20892

NIH Endocrine Disruptors: Epidemiologic Approaches Grants 2658
Through this program NIOSH, EPA, NIEHS, and NCI support research on the relationship between exposure to endocrine disruptors and adverse health effects in humans, particularly reproductive and developmental, with a focus on epidemiologic approaches. Synthetic chemicals released in the workplace and environment collectively called endocrine disruptors (EDs) or endocrine disrupting chemicals (EDCs) are thought to interfere with one or more aspects of the normal endocrine functions that are responsible for the maintenance of homeostasis and the regulation of developmental processes. The cooperating agencies support research that examines human health consequences of exposure to physical and chemical toxicants in the environment and in occupational settings as well as the underlying mechanisms involved in environmentally related disease and dysfunction. Research applications are sought that will investigate the relationships between exposure to endocrine disruptors and adverse health effects, particularly reproductive/developmental effects in humans. Annual deadline dates may vary; contact program staff for exact dates. Inquiries may be directed to program staff at the appropriate institute: Michael Galvin, Research Grants Program, (404) 639-3343, NIOSH, 1600 Clifton Rd NE, Atlanta, GA 30333; David Reese, (202) 564-6919, EPA, 1200 Pennsylvania Ave NW, Washington, DC 20460; Kumiko Iwamoto, (301) 435-4911, NCI, 6130 Executive Boulevard, Bethesda, MD 20892; and Gwen Collman, (919) 541-4980, NIEHS, P.O. Box 12233, MD EC-21, Research Triangle Park, NC 27709.
Requirements: Applications may be submitted by domestic and foreign, public and private nonprofit and for-profit organizations, and by governments and their agencies; state and local governments or their bona fide agents; and federally recognized Indian tribal governments, Indian tribes, or Indian tribal organizations.
Amount of Grant: $6 million total
Contact: Program Officer
Internet: http://www.grants.nih.gov/grants/guide/rfa-files/RFA-OH-01-001.html
Sponsor: National Institutes of Health
6701 Rockledge Drive
Bethesda, MD 20892

NIH Enhancing Adherence to Diabetes Self-Management Behaviors 2659
This PA solicits applications for investigator-initiated research related to sociocultural, environmental, and behavioral mechanisms and biological/technological factors that contribute to successful and ongoing self-management in diabetes. Self-management is defined as client strategies and behaviors that contribute to blood glucose normalization, improved health, and prevention or reduction of complications. It is broader than adherence to specific regimen components and incorporates deliberate problem solving and decision-making processes. Applications are encouraged for both type 1 and type 2 diabetes; representative and minority populations; and all age groups. Inquiries may be directed to program staff at the appropriate NIH institute. Modular Grant applications will request direct costs in $25,000 modules, up to a total direct cost request of $250,000 per year.
Requirements: Applications may be submitted by domestic and foreign, for-profit and non-profit organizations, public and private, such as universities, colleges, hospitals, laboratories, units of State and local governments, and eligible agencies of the Federal government. Racial/ethnic minority individuals, women, and persons with disabilities are encouraged to apply as principal investigators.
Amount of Grant: $250,000 maximum
Date(s) Application is Due: Feb 16; Jun 16; Oct 16
Contact: Susan Grove, Program Officer; (301) 435-0714; email: sg16d@nih.gov or grantsinfo@od.nih.gov
Internet: http://grants.nih.gov/grants/guide/pa-files/PA-00-049.html
Sponsor: National Institutes of Health (NIH)
6701 Rockledge Drive
Bethesda, MD 20892

NIH Epidemiological and Behavioral Research in Oral Health 2660
This program seeks to stimulate epidemiological and behavioral research to improve oral health or increase the understanding of the determinants of oral health. It supports studies that expand and enhance the integration of population-based, genetic, social,

and behavioral research. Specific research activities highlighted in the strategic plan include, but are not limited to, furthering the understanding of how genetic, behavioral, and environmental factors interact to contribute to disease susceptibility or resistance; assessing and bridging gaps in the knowledge, opinions, and practices of the public, educators, and health care professionals about oral diseases and their prevention; identifying risk factors and markers for the progression of disease to oral, dental, and craniofacial diseases and disorders; improving oral health literacy; and developing more effective strategies to encourage the appropriate and timely adoption of research findings into clinical practice. PA Number: PA-04-022
Requirements: Applications may be submitted by domestic and foreign, for-profit and nonprofit organizations, both public and private; units of state and local governments; and eligible agencies of the federal government.
Contact: Mary Daley, Grants Management Branch, (301) 594-4808; (301) 480-3562; email: daleym@mail.nih.gov
Internet: http://www.grants.nih.gov/grants/guide/pa-files/PA-04-022.html
Sponsor: National Institutes of Health
6701 Rockledge Drive
Bethesda, MD 20892

NIH Ethical Issues in Human Studies Research Grants **2661**
NIH and CDC invite research grant applications (R01) for support to conduct research on ethical issues that arise with research involving human participants. Grants may be requested in $25,000 direct cost modules. Annual deadline dates may vary; contact program staff for exact dates. PA: PA-02-103
Requirements: Applications may be submitted by any domestic and foreign, for-profit and nonprofit, public and private organizations; units of state and local governments; and eligible agencies of the federal government. Applicants are encouraged to visit the Web sites of the participating institutes and centers to learn more about their specific interests.
Restrictions: The PA does not solicit essays, editorials, literature or historical reviews of science, conferences, or speculative, theoretical, or policy analyses.
Amount of Grant: $250,000 maximum per year
Date(s) Application is Due: Feb 1; Jun 1; Oct 1
Contact: Dr. Della Hann, Program Contact, (301) 402-2725; email: hannd@od.nih.gov
Internet: http://grants2.nih.gov/grants/guide/pa-files/PA-02-103.html
Sponsor: National Institutes of Health
6701 Rockledge Drive
Bethesda, MD 20892

NIH Exceptional, Unconventional Research Enabling Knowledge Acceleration (EUREKA) Grants **2662**
The purpose of the EUREKA (Exceptional Unconventional Research Enabling Knowledge Acceleration) initiative is to foster exceptionally innovative research that, if successful, will have an unusually high impact on the areas of science that are germane to the mission of one or more of the participating NIH Institutes. Before submitting an application, it is extremely important to verify that the proposed research is of interest to at least one of the NIH Institutes that is participating in the EUREKA FOA, since applications that are not germane to the mission of one or more of the participating Institutes will be withdrawn without review.
Requirements: The following organizations and institutions are eligible to apply: public/state controlled institutions of higher education; private institutions of higher education; Hispanic-serving institutions; historically Black colleges and universities (HBCUs); tribally controlled colleges and universities (TCCUs); Alaska Native and Native Hawaiian serving institutions; nonprofits with 501(c)3 IRS status (other than institutions of higher education); nonprofits without 501(c)3 IRS status (other than institutions of higher education); small businesses; for-profit organizations (other than small businesses); non-domestic (non-U.S.) entities (foreign organizations).
Restrictions: EUREKA is for new projects, not for continuation of existing projects. Nor is EUREKA for support of pilot projects, i.e., projects of limited scope that are designed primarily to generate data that will enable the PI to seek other funding opportunities.
Amount of Grant: $800,000 maximum in direct costs
Date(s) Application is Due: Nov 24
Contact: Laurie Tompkins, Ph.D.; (301) 594-0943; fax: (301) 480-2228; email: tompkinL@nigms.nih.gov;; Judy Mietz, Ph.D.; (301) 496-9326; fax: (301) 496-1224; email: mietzj@mail.nih.gov
Internet: http://grants.nih.gov/grants/guide/rfa-files/RFA-GM-10-009.html
Sponsor: National Institutes of Health (NIH)
45 Center Drive, MSC 6200
Bethesda, MD 20892-6200

NIH Exploratory Centers for Alternative Medicine Research Grants **2663**
The objective of the program is to develop exploratory centers for the purpose of investigating and validating alternative therapies. These centers will support new interdisciplinary programs involving experienced investigators from conventional medicine with clinicians and investigators from alternative medicine and should provide clinical/scientific/technical assistance to alternative medicine clinicians who may have potentially useful accumulations of patient data that could be evaluated for treatment outcome. It will be important that the research faculty at these centers have expertise in broad areas such as biostatistics, computer processing, data management, and protocol design. Additionally, through a peer review process that will be established by the centers, small prospective pilot studies will be started. Program areas to be developed and evaluated can include nutrition, diet, and lifestyle/behavioral health changes; mind/body control therapies; traditional and ethnomedicine therapies; structural manipulations and energetic therapies; pharmacological and biological therapies; and bioelectromagnetic therapies. Annual deadline dates vary; contact program staff for exact dates. RFA: OD-94-004
Requirements: Applications may be submitted by domestic for-profit, nonprofit, public, and private organizations.
Amount of Grant: $30,000 planning grants, $20,000-$30,000 training grants, $350,000 cooperative agreements, $115,000 investigator-initiated grants
Contact: Dr. John Spencer, Office of Alternative Medicine, (301) 402-2466; fax: (301) 402-4741
Internet: http://www.grants.nih.gov/grants/guide/rfa-files/RFA-OD-94-004.html
Sponsor: National Institutes of Health
6120 Executive Boulevard, Executive Plaza S
Rockville, MD 20892

NIH Exploratory Innovations in Biomedical Computational Science and Technology (BISTI) Grants **2664**
The NIH is interested in promoting research and developments in computational science and technology that will support rapid progress in areas of scientific opportunity in biomedical research. As defined here, biomedical computing or biomedical information science and technology includes database design, graphical interfaces, querying approaches, data retrieval, data visualization and manipulation, data integration through the development of integrated analytical tools, and tools for electronic collaboration, as well as computational and mathematical research including the development of structural, functional, integrative, and analytical models and simulations. This particular FOA is intended to support exploratory biomedical informatics and computational biology research - applications should be innovative, with high risk/high impact in new areas that are lacking preliminary data or development. Because the nature and scope of the proposed research will vary from application to application, it is anticipated that the size and duration of each award will also vary.
Requirements: Application can be made by the following institutions and organizations: for-profit organizations; non-profit organizations; public or private institutions (such as universities, colleges, hospitals, and laboratories); units of state government; units of local government; eligible agencies of the Federal government; foreign institutions; domestic institutions; faith-based or community-based organizations; Indian/Native American tribal governments (federally recognized); Indian/Native American tribal governments (other than federally recognized); and Indian/Native American tribally designated organizations.
Date(s) Application is Due: Feb 16; Jun 16; Oct 16
Contact: Peter Lyster, Ph.D.; (301) 451-6446; email: lysterp@mail.nih.gov
Internet: http://grants.nih.gov/grants/guide/pa-files/PAR-06-411.html
Sponsor: National Institutes of Health (NIH)
45 Center Drive, Room 2AS.55k, MSC 6200
Bethesda, MD 20892-6200

NIH Exploratory/Development Grants for Mental Health Intervention Research **2665**
NIMH is requesting research grant applications to develop somatic, pharmacologic, psychosocial, or combination interventions for the prevention, rehabilitation, treatment, and/or management of mental disorders and emotional or behavioral problems; research the co-occurrence of mental, physical, and substance abuse problems and the functional consequences of these problems across the life span; and to perform preliminary tests of feasibility, acceptability, and efficacy/effectiveness of interventions. PA-03-078
Requirements: Applications may be submitted by domestic and foreign, for-profit and nonprofit organizations, both public and private; units of state and local governments; and eligible agencies of the federal government.
Amount of Grant: $125,000 average
Contact: Joy Knipple, Grants Management Branch, National Institute of Mental Health, (301) 443-8811; fax: (301) 443-6885; email: jk173@nih.gov
Internet: http://grants.nih.gov/grants/guide/pa-files/PAR-03-078.html
Sponsor: National Institute of Mental Health
6701 Rockledge Drive, Room 1040, MSC 7710
Bethesda, MD 20892

NIH Exploratory/Developmental Research Grant **2666**
The Exploratory/Developmental Grant (R21) mechanism is intended to encourage exploratory and developmental research projects by providing support for the early and conceptual stages of these projects. These studies may involve considerable risk but may lead to a breakthrough in a particular area, or to the development of novel techniques, agents, methodologies, models, or applications that could have a major impact on a field of biomedical, behavioral, or clinical research.
Requirements: Eligible organizations: for profit organizations; non-profit organizations; public or private institutions, such as universities, colleges, hospitals and laboratories; units of state government; units of local government; eligible institutions of the federal government; domestic institutions; foreign institutions; faith-based or community-based organizations; units of state tribal government; and units of local tribal government. Eligible Project Directors/Principal Investigators: any individual with the skills, knowledge and resources necessary to carry out the proposed research, is invited to work with his/her institution to develop an application for support; individuals from underrepresented racial and ethnic groups; individuals with disabilities
Amount of Grant: $275,000 over the two years of the R21 award
Date(s) Application is Due: Feb 16, Jun 16, Oct 16
Contact: Ellen S. Liberman, Ph.D., (301) 451-2020; email: esl@nei.nih.gov

Internet: http://grants.nih.gov/grants/guide/pa-files/PA-06-181.html
Sponsor: National Eye Institute
5635 Fishers Lane, Suite 1300
Bethesda, MD 20892-9300

NIH Fine Mapping and Function of Genes for Type 1 Diabetes Grants 2667

The purpose of this initiative is to bring together investigators with experience in genetics, immunology, and biochemistry to perform fine mapping of the loci discovered and study the function of the genes being identified and to identify the mechanisms by which newly discovered genes predispose to T1D. This would lead to elucidation of the mechanisms whereby changes in the function or regulation of these genes are likely to provide crucial new insights into disease pathogenesis. The discovery of the genes would be relevant to developing a predictive strategy for individuals who may develop diabetes. In the future, genetic testing may lead to personalized treatment regimens by identifying the most appropriate class of drugs for particular patients. Total funding available for this five year program is $20 million to fund 4-10 applications, contingent upon the availability of funds and the submission of a sufficient number of meritorious applications. The maximum direct costs are $5 million that can be spent on a project period of up to 5 years. Letters of Intent are due by February 27, with final applications due by March 30. The office strongly urges communication from applicants via email.
Requirements: The following organizations and institutions are eligible to apply: public/state controlled institutions of higher education; private institutions of higher education; Hispanic-serving institutions; historically Black colleges and universities (HBCUs); tribally controlled colleges and universities (TCCUs); Alaska Native and Native Hawaiian serving institutions; nonprofits with 501(c)3 IRS status (other than institutions of higher education); nonprofits without 501(c)3 IRS status (other than institutions of higher education); small businesses; for-profit organizations (other than small businesses); non-domestic (non-U.S.) entities (foreign organizations); and other eligible agencies of the federal government.
Amount of Grant: $1,500,000-$5,000,000 over five years
Date(s) Application is Due: Feb 27; Mar 30
Contact: Beena Akolkar, PhD.; (301) 594-8812; email: ba92i@nih.gov
Internet: http://grants.nih.gov/grants/guide/rfa-files/rfa-dk-08-006.html
Sponsor: National Institutes of Health (NIH)
6707 Democracy Boulevard, Room 6105
Bethesda, MD 20892-5460

NIH Genetic Architecture of Complex Phenotypes 2668

The purpose of this initiative is to support new studies on the architecture of complex phenotypes, including research using human and model systems as well as research using theoretical approaches.The studies targeted by this program announcement are expected to expand our understanding of the roles of genetic and environmental variation and their interactions in causing phenotypic variation in populations; increase the quantity and quality of population-based data; lead to the development of mathematical and statistical tools for analyzing measured genotype data; lead to improvements in study design; and create biologically relevant models for understanding the origins, roles, and implications of genetic variation in causing variation in phenotypes. This program announcement encourages efforts including organization of DNA sequence variation in populations and subpopulations with the goal of understanding the causal forces that shape that organization; studies of the relationship of genotypic and phenotypic variation; data analysis; research on study design, including comparisons of different strategies for studying complex phenotypes; development of statistical and analytical tools; and construction of meaningful tests of relationships between genotypic and phenotypic data. Further information for this program is available on the Web site. Inquiries may be directed to program staff at the appropriate NIH institute; Dr. Irene Anne Eckstrand, (301) 594-0943, NIGMS, 45 Center Drive, Bethesda, MD 20892; Dr. Jose Velazquez, (919) 541-4998, NIEHS, P.O. Box 12233, Research Triangle Park, NC 27709; Dr. William Sharrock, (301) 594-5055, NIAMS, 45 Center Drive, Bethesda, MD 20892; Dr. Evan Hadley, (301) 435-3048, NIA, 7201 Wisconsin Avenue, Bethesda, MD 20892; Dr. Steven Moldin, (301) 443-2037, NIMH, 5600 Fishers Ln, Rockville, MD 20857; Dr. Harold Gordon, (301) 443-4877, NIDA, 5600 Fishers Ln, Rockville, MD 20857; Dr. Robert Karp, (301) 443-4223, NIAAA, 6000 Executive Boulevard, Bethesda, MD 20892; Dr. Ralph Nitkin, (301) 496-1383, NICHD, 6100 Executive Boulevard, Bethesda, MD 20892; Dr. Lisa Brooks, (301) 496-7531, NHGRI, 38 Library Drive, Bethesda, MD 20892; and Dr. Cashell Jaquish, (301) 435-0447, NHLBI, 6701 Rockledge Drive, Bethesda, MD 20892. PA: PA-02-110
Requirements: Applications may be submitted by domestic and foreign, for-profit and nonprofit organizations, both public and private. Racial/ethnic minority individuals, women, and persons with disabilities are encouraged to apply.
Restrictions: Foreign institutions are not eligible for program projects (P01) grants.
Contact: Program Officer
Internet: http://grants2.nih.gov/grants/guide/pa-files/PA-02-110.html
Sponsor: National Institutes of Health
6701 Rockledge Drive
Bethesda, MD 20892

NIH Genetic Susceptibility and Variability of Human Malformations Research Grants 2669

NICHD, NIDCR, NIEHS, and EPA invite research grant applications to study the genetic susceptibility and mechanisms of human congenital malformations including research on the contribution of potential genetic and environmental factors, identified at the molecular level, to the etiology, distribution, and prevention of disease within families and across populations. The research conducted as a result of this RFA will provide the direction and focus for future initiatives to dissect the molecular and genetic mechanisms underlying specific human malformations. The current initiative is designed to encourage collaborative, interdisciplinary, and innovative studies that integrate the latest advances in developmental genetics, functional genomics, epidemiology, and high throughput biotechnology with the new mathematical, methodological, and statistical tools for analyzing and evaluating data related to the etiology and distribution of birth defects in populations. The primary objective of this initiative is to develop and use integrated multidisciplinary approaches to obtain information that will enhance our knowledge of and provide a basis for future initiatives focusing on the basic mechanisms and etiologies of human malformations. This RFA is part of a larger birth defects program which will include an upcoming initiative related to fundamental developmental mechanisms underlying the formation of structural anomalies. Inquiries may be directed to the staff at the appropriate institute/organization: Dr. Deborah Henken, (301) 496-5541, Center for Research for Mothers and Children, NICHD, Executive Building, 6100 Executive Boulevard, Bethesda, MD 20892; Dr. Judy Small, (301) 594-2425, Craniofacial Anomalies and Injury Branch, NIDCR, Building 45, Bethesda, MD 20892; Dr. Gwen Collman, (919) 541-4980, Chemical Exposures and Molecular Biology Branch, Division of Extramural Research and Training, NIEHS, P.O. Box 12233 Research Triangle Park, NC 27709; and Dr. Chris Saint, (202) 564-6909, National Center for Environmental Research & Quality Assurance, EPA, 1300 Pennsylvania Avenue, Washington, DC 20004. Annual deadline dates may vary; contact program staff for exact dates. RFA: HD-99-002
Requirements: Applications may be submitted by domestic and foreign, for-profit and nonprofit, public and private organizations; units of state and local governments; and eligible agencies of the federal government.
Restrictions: Applications limited to descriptive or traditional epidemiological approaches will be considered nonresponsive. The EPA will not be able to consider applications from for-profit organizations or federal agencies.
Amount of Grant: $700,000 maximum
Contact: Program Officer
Internet: http://www.grants.nih.gov/grants/guide/rfa-files/RFA-HD-99-002.html
Sponsor: National Institutes of Health
6701 Rockledge Drive
Bethesda, MD 20892

NIH Genetics of Neurobehavioral Disorders in Existing Samples Grants 2670

The purpose of the program is to encourage applications for multidisciplinary, collaborative genetic research projects, employing state-of-the-art diagnostic procedures and analytic methods, to integrate different pedigree data sets that have already been collected for the study of a given neurobehavioral disorder. Applications will implement the assembling of data from multiple research groups for combined analysis, and will focus on one of the following: attention-deficit hyperactivity disorder, bipolar disorder or other related mood disorders, recurrent early-onset depression, eating disorders, obsessive-compulsive disorder or other anxiety disorders, panic disorder, schizophrenia or other psychotic disorders, personality disorders, or Tourette's syndrome. The creation and analysis of clinically well-characterized samples of sufficient size for linkage analyses and for linkage disequilibrium mapping studies in genetically isolated populations studied previously may be facilitated by the establishment of international consortia. Full collaborations between American scientists and scientists at international institutions are encouraged, when scientifically appropriate. In these cases, awards may be made to international institutions or to domestic applications that include international components. Inquiries may be directed to program staff at the appropriate NIH institute: Dr. Steven Moldin, Division of Neuroscience and Basic Behavioral Science, NIMH, (301) 443-2037, 6001 Executive Boulevard, Bethesda, MD 20892; Dr. Lisa Freund, Child Development and Behavior Branch, NICHD, (301) 435-6879, Building 6100, 9000 Rockville Pike, Bethesda, MD 20892. Annual deadline dates may vary; contact program staff for exact dates. PA: PAR-99-120
Requirements: Applications may be submitted by domestic, for-profit and nonprofit organizations, both public and private; units of state and local governments; and eligible agencies of the federal government.
Amount of Grant: $250,000 maximum per year
Date(s) Application is Due: Feb 1; Jun 1; Oct 1
Contact: Program Officer
Internet: http://www.grants.nih.gov/grants/guide/pa-files/PA-99-120.html
Sponsor: National Institutes of Health
6701 Rockledge Drive
Bethesda, MD 20892

NIH Health Promotion Among Racial and Ethnic Minority Males 2671

This Funding Opportunity Announcement solicits Exploratory/Developmental grant applications from applicants that propose to stimulate and expand research in the health of minority men. Specifically, this initiative is intended to: enhance our understanding of the numerous factors (e.g., sociodemographic, community, societal, personal) influencing the health promoting behaviors of racial and ethnic minority males and their sub-populations across the life cycle; and solicit applications focusing on the development and testing of culturally and linguistically appropriate health-promoting interventions designed to reduce health disparities among racially and ethnically diverse males and their sub-populations age 21 and older. The total project period for an application submitted in response to this funding opportunity may not exceed two years. Direct costs are limited to $275,000 over an R21 two-year period, with no more than $200,000 in direct costs allowed in any single year.
Requirements: Application can be made by the following institutions and organizations: public/state controlled institutions of higher education; private institutions of higher

education; nonprofits with 501(c)3 IRS status (other than institutions of higher education); nonprofits without 501(c)3 IRS status (other than institutions of higher education); small businesses; for-profit organizations (other than small businesses); state governments; U.S. territories or possessions; Indian/Native American tribal governments (federally recognized); Indian/Native American tribal governments (other than Federally recognized); Indian/Native American tribally designated organizations; non-domestic (non-U.S.) entities (foreign organizations); Hispanic-serving institutions; historically Black colleges and universities (HBCUs); tribally controlled colleges and universities (TCCUs); Alaska Native and Native Hawaiian serving institutions; regional organization; eligible agencies of the Federal government; and faith-based or community based organizations.
Amount of Grant: $200,000 maximum per year; $275,000 maximum per two-year cycle
Date(s) Application is Due: Feb 16; Jun 16; Oct 16
Contact: Dr. Charlotte Pratt, Program Director; (301) 435-0382; fax: (301) 480-5158; email: prattc@nhlbi.nih.gov
Internet: http://grants.nih.gov/grants/guide/pa-files/PA-07-421.html
Sponsor: National Institutes of Health (NIH)
6701 Rockledge Drive, Suite 10118, MSC 7936
Bethesda, MD 20892-7936

NIH Human Brain Project (Neuroinformatics) Phase I & II **2672**
The purpose of this initiative is to encourage and support investigator- initiated research on neuroscience informatics (neuroinformatics). This research will lead to the development of new web based databases, analytical tools, and knowledge management systems to foster sharing of data for all domains of neuroscience research. This program combines neuroscience and informatics (neuroinformatics) research to develop and apply advanced tools and approaches essential for efficient understanding of the structure, function and development in health and disorders of the nervous system, from the genetic to whole systems level. Annual deadline dates may vary; contact program staff for exact dates.
Requirements: Applications may be submitted by domestic and foreign, for-profit and nonprofit organizations, both public and private; units of state and local governments; and eligible agencies of the federal government.
Restrictions: Foreign institutions are not eligible to apply.
Date(s) Application is Due: Jan 21; May 20; Sep 22
Contact: Stephen Koslow, Office on Neuroinformatics, NIMH, (301) 443-1815; fax: (301) 443-1867; email: koz@helix.nih.gov
Internet: http://grants2.nih.gov/grants/guide/pa-files/PAR-03-035.html
Sponsor: National Institutes of Health
6701 Rockledge Drive, Room 1040
Bethesda, MD 20892

NIH Human Connectome Project Grants **2673**
This Funding Opportunity Announcement is issued as an initiative of the NIH Blueprint for Neuroscience Research. The Neuroscience Blueprint is a collaborative framework through which 16 NIH Institutes, Centers and Offices jointly support neuroscience-related research, with the aim of accelerating discoveries and reducing the burden of nervous system disorders. The overall purpose of this five year Human Connectome Project (HCP) is to develop and share knowledge about the structural and functional connectivity of the human brain. This purpose will be pursued through the following specific efforts: existing, but cutting-edge, non-invasive imaging technologies will be optimized and combined to acquire structural and functional in vivo data about axonal projections and neural connections from brains of hundreds of healthy adults. Demographic data and data regarding sensory, motor, cognitive, emotional, and social function will also be collected for each subject, as will DNA samples and blood (to establish cell lines). Models to better understand and use these data will be developed. Connectivity patterns will be linked to existing architectonic data. Data and models will be made available to the research community immediately via a user-friendly system to include tools to query, organize, visualize and analyze data. Outreach activities will be conducted to engage and educate the research community about the imaging tools, data, models, and informatics tools. After five years, these specific efforts are expected to deliver: a set of integrated, non-invasive imaging tools to obtain connectivity data from humans in vivo; a high quality and well characterized, quantitative set of human connectivity data linked to behavioral and genetic data as well as to general, existing architectonic data, and associated models, from up to hundreds of healthy adult female and male subjects; and rapid, user-friendly dissemination of connectivity data, models, and tools to the research community via outreach activities and an informatics platform. Letters of Intent are due by October 24, with final applications due by November 24.
Requirements: The following organizations and institutions are eligible to apply for support: public/state controlled institutions of higher education; private institutions of higher education; Hispanic-serving institutions; historically Black colleges and universities (HBCUs); tribally controlled colleges and universities (TCCUs); Alaska Native and Native Hawaiian serving institutions; nonprofits with 501(c)3 IRS status (other than institutions of higher education); nonprofits without 501(c)3 IRS status (other than institutions of higher education); Indian/Native American tribal governments (federally recognized); Indian/Native American tribally designated organizations; U.S. territories or possessions; and eligible agencies of the federal government.
Amount of Grant: $6 million maximum per year for five years
Date(s) Application is Due: Oct 24; Nov 24
Contact: Michael F. Huerta, Ph.D.; (301) 443-1815; fax: (301) 443-1731; email: mhuertl@mail.nih.gov
Internet: http://grants.nih.gov/grants/guide/rfa-files/RFA-MH-10-020.html
Sponsor: National Institutes of Health (NIH)
6001 Executive Boulevard, Room 7202, MSC 9645
Bethesda, MD 20892-9645

NIH Human Models and Markers of Skeletal Aging Grants **2674**
NIA, NIAMS, NIDR, and NIDDK invite research grant applications to develop or refine models and markers using human bone, bone marrow, or bone cell constituents that more accurately reflect those age-related and/or pathophysiological processes occurring within the mature human skeleton that lead to osteoporosis and other age-related skeletal diseases. It is expected that improved human models and markers of age-related changes in skeletal tissue structure and function will enhance the accuracy and reliability of diagnostic and prognostic capabilities and serve to expedite the development of more effective, targeted preventative, and therapeutic strategies. Annual deadlines vary; contact program staff for exact dates. Additional information may be obtained by mail and email, or through the NIH grant line (301-402-2221), and the NIH Web site. PA: PA-96-022
Requirements: Applications may be submitted by domestic and foreign, for-profit and nonprofit organizations, both public and private; units of state and local governments; and eligible agencies of the federal government.
Date(s) Application is Due: Feb 1; Jun 1; Oct 1
Contact: Dr. Richard Sprott, Biology of Aging, (301) 496-4996; Dr. Evan Hadley, Geriatrics and Clinical Research, (301) 496-6761
Internet: http://www.grants.nih.gov/grants/guide/pa-files/PA-96-022.html
Sponsor: National Institutes of Health
6701 Rockledge Drive
Bethesda, MD 20892

NIH Hyperaccelerated Award/Mechanisms in Immunomodulation Trials **2675**
NIAID, NIA, NIAMS, NIDCR, NIDDK, and NINDS invite investigator-initiated research applications for mechanistic studies in clinical trials of: immunomodulatory interventions for immune system mediated diseases, including, but not limited to: asthma and allergic diseases; graft failure in solid organ, cell, tissue and stem cell transplantation; and chronic inflammatory, autoimmune, and immunodeficiency diseases; and preventative and therapeutic, vaccines for non-HIV/AIDS infectious diseases, including NIAID Category A, B, and C agents of bioterrorism and emerging/re-emerging infectious diseases. Applications will be accepted monthly on the ninth of each month; a letter of intent is due one month prior to application receipt date. RFA: AI-01-001
Requirements: Applications may be submitted by domestic and foreign, for-profit and nonprofit organizations, both public and private; units of state and local governments; and eligible agencies of the federal government.
Amount of Grant: $2 million total
Contact: Ann White-Devine, NIAID, (301) 402-5601; fax: (301) 480-3780; email: ad22x@nih.gov
Internet: http://grants.nih.gov/grants/guide/rfa-files/RFA-AI-01-001.html
Sponsor: National Institutes of Health
6701 Rockledge Drive
Bethesda, MD 20892

NIH Impact of HAART on HIV/CNS Disease **2676**
This RFA solicits applications to study the effects of HAART on HIV/CNS disease with respect to the clinical, neurological, neuropsychological, virological, immunological, and neuropathological response to the drugs. This solicitation also includes studies to develop drug formulations with improved ability to cross the blood-brain barrier, studies to develop improved methods of delivering drugs to the CNS, and the interaction of anti-retrovirals with psychotropic drugs. Annual deadline dates vary; contact program staff for exact dates. Inquiries may be directed to program staff at the appropriate NIH institute: Dr. Dianne Rausch, (301) 443-7281, NIMH, 6001 Executive Boulevard, Bethesda, MD 20892; Dr. A.P. Kerza-Kwiatecki, (301) 496-1431, NINDS, 6001 Executive Boulevard, Bethesda, MD 20892; and Dr. Thomas Johnson, (301) 402-3461, NIDCD, 6120 Executive Boulevard, Bethesda, MD 20892. RFA: MH-00-003
Requirements: Applications may be submitted by domestic and foreign, for-profit and nonprofit organizations, both public and private; units of state and local governments; and eligible agencies of the federal government.
Amount of Grant: $3.4 million total
Contact: Program Officer
Internet: http://grants.nih.gov/grants/guide/rfa-files/RFA-MH-00-003.html
Sponsor: National Institutes of Health
6701 Rockledge Drive
Bethesda, MD 20892

NIH Independent Scientist Award **2677**
The award is a special salary-only grant designed to provide protected time for newly independent scientists who currently have non-research obligations such as heavy teaching loads, clinical work, committee assignments, service, and administrative duties that prevent them from having a period of intensive research focus. The award is targeted to persons with doctoral degrees who have completed their research training, have independent peer-reviewed research support, and who need a period of protected research time in order to foster their research career development. New applications are due February 12, June 12, and October 12, while renewal applications are due March 12, July 12, and November 12.
Requirements: The following organizations and institutions are eligible to apply: public/state controlled institutions of higher education; private institutions of higher education; nonprofits with 501(c)3 IRS status; nonprofits without 501(c)3 IRS status; small businesses; for-profit organizations; State governments; U.S. territories or possessions; Indian/Native American tribal governments (Federally recognized and other than Federally recognized); Indian/Native American tribally designated organizations; Hispanic-serving institutions; historically Black colleges and universities (HBCUs);

tribally controlled colleges and universities (TCCUs); Alaska Native and Native Hawaiian serving institutions; regional organizations; and faith-based or community based organizations. The candidate must have a doctoral degree and peer-reviewed, independent research support at the time the award is made. The candidate must spend a minimum of 75 percent effort conducting research during the period of the award.
Restrictions: The award is not intended for investigators who already have full time to perform research, or have substantial publication records or considerable research support indicating that they are well established in their fields. Foreign institutions are not eligible to apply.
Amount of Grant: \$75,000-\$100,000 average
Date(s) Application is Due: Feb 12; Mar 12; Jun 12; Jul 12; Oct 12; Nov 12
Contact: Susan Grove, Program Officer; (301) 435-0714; email: sg16d@nih.gov or grantsinfo@od.nih.gov
Internet: http://grants.nih.gov/grants/guide/contacts/PA-09-038_contacts.html
Sponsor: National Institutes of Health (NIH)
6701 Rockledge Drive
Bethesda, MD 20892

NIH Individual Postdoctoral Fellowships in Genomics and Related ELSI Topics 2678
The purpose of these fellowships is to train scientists who will have the multidisciplinary skills that will enable them to engage in research to accomplish the short- and long-term objectives of the HGP and similar genomic projects and to take full advantage of the resulting genomic data and resources to solve biomedical and bioethical problems. Broad areas of research that are relevant include genomic analysis (including technology development) and the ethical, legal, and social implications of human genetics research. The goal of the fellowship program in the area of genomic analysis and technology is to train highly skilled scientists who will use the expertise gained to develop research programs in the mapping and sequencing of the human genome and the genomes of other organisms, in sequence variation, in the analysis and interpretation of the resulting data, and in the development of biological, medical, or biotechnological applications based on the data, or in the development of technologies to support any of this research. Inquiries may be directed to program staff at the appropriate NIH institute: Dr. Bettie Graham, (301) 496-7531, Division of Extramural Research, NHGRI, Building 38A, Bethesda, MD 20892; Dr. Lisa Begg, (301) 496-8580, Office of Centers, Training and Resources, NCI, 6130 Executive Boulevard, Bethesda, MD 20892; Dr. Carol Shreffler, (919) 541-1445, Division of Extramural Research and Training, NIEHS, P.O. Box 12233, Research Triangle Park, NC 27709; Dr. Laurie Tompkins, (301) 594-0943, NIGMS, Building 45, Bethesda, MD 20892; and Dr. Hilary Sigmon, (301) 594-5970, Nursing Fellowships in Genetics, NINR, Building 45, Bethesda, MD 20815.
Requirements: Individuals must meet the criteria for the NIH National Research Service Awards for Individual Postdoctoral Fellows (F32) described in program announcement PA-99-025, available in the NIH Guide for Grants and Contracts. By the time of award, individuals must be citizens or noncitizen nationals of the United States, or have been lawfully admitted to the United States for permanent residence. Before an NRSA award can be activated, the individual must have received a doctoral degree or its equivalent to be eligible for an individual postdoctoral fellowship (F32). To be eligible for a senior fellowship (F33), individuals must have received a doctoral degree and must have had at least seven subsequent years of relevant research or professional experience.
Restrictions: Individuals on temporary or student visas are not eligible.
Amount of Grant: \$26,256-\$41,268 depending on experience
Date(s) Application is Due: Apr 5; Aug 5; Dec 5
Contact: Program Officer
Internet: http://www.grants.nih.gov/grants/guide/pa-files/PA-99-122.html
Sponsor: National Institutes of Health
6701 Rockledge Drive
Bethesda, MD 20892

NIH Innovations in Biomedical Computational Science and Technology Grants 2679
The NIH is interested in promoting research and developments in computational science and technology that will support rapid progress in areas of scientific opportunity in biomedical research. As defined here, biomedical computing or biomedical information science and technology includes database design, graphical interfaces, querying approaches, data retrieval, data visualization and manipulation, data integration through the development of integrated analytical tools, and tools for electronic collaboration, as well as computational and mathematical research including the development of structural, functional, integrative, and analytical models and simulations. Because the nature and scope of the proposed research will vary from application to application, it is anticipated that the size and duration of each award will also vary.
Requirements: Application can be made by the following institutions and organizations: for-profit organizations; non-profit organizations; public or private institutions (such as universities, colleges, hospitals, and laboratories); units of state government; units of local government; eligible agencies of the Federal government; foreign institutions; domestic institutions; faith-based or community-based organizations; Indian/Native American tribal governments (federally recognized); Indian/Native American tribal governments (other than federally recognized); and Indian/Native American tribally designated organizations.
Amount of Grant: \$500,000 maximum per year
Date(s) Application is Due: Feb 5; Jun 5; Oct 5
Contact: Peter Lyster, Ph.D.; (301) 451-6446; email: lysterp@mail.nih.gov
Internet: http://grants.nih.gov/grants/guide/pa-files/PAR-09-218.html
Sponsor: National Institutes of Health (NIH)
45 Center Drive, Room 2AS.55k, MSC 6200
Bethesda, MD 20892-6200

NIH Innovations in Biomedical Computational Science and Technology Initiative Grants for SBIR 2680
This funding opportunity announcement (FOA) solicits Small Business Innovation Research (SBIR) grant applications from small business concerns (SBCs) that propose innovative research in biomedical computational science and technology to promote the progress of biomedical research. There exists an expanding need to speed the progress of biomedical research through the power of computing to manage and analyze data and to model biological processes. The NIH is interested in promoting research and developments in biomedical computational science and technology that will support rapid progress in areas of scientific opportunity in biomedical research. As defined here biomedical computing or biomedical information science and technology includes database design, graphical interfaces, querying approaches, data retrieval, data visualization and manipulation, data integration through the development of integrated analytical tools, and tools for electronic collaboration, as well as computational research including the development of structural, functional, integrative, and analytical models and simulations.
Requirements: Only United States small business concerns (SBCs) are eligible to submit SBIR applications.
Amount of Grant: \$150,000 maximum per year in phase 1; \$750,000 maximum per year in phase 2
Date(s) Application is Due: Apr 5; Aug 5; Dec 5
Contact: Peter Lyster, Ph.D.; (301) 451-6446; email: lysterp@mail.nih.gov
Internet: http://grants.nih.gov/grants/guide/pa-files/PAR-07-160.html
Sponsor: National Institutes of Health (NIH)
45 Center Drive, Room 2AS.55k, MSC 6200
Bethesda, MD 20892-6200

NIH Innovations in Biomedical Computational Science and Technology Initiative Grants for STTR 2681
This funding opportunity announcement (FOA) solicits Small Business Technology Transfer (STTR) grant applications from small business concerns (SBCs) that propose innovative research in biomedical computational science and technology to promote the progress of biomedical research. There exists an expanding need to speed the progress of biomedical research through the power of computing to manage and analyze data and to model biological processes. The NIH is interested in promoting research and developments in biomedical computational science and technology that will support rapid progress in areas of scientific opportunity in biomedical research. As defined here biomedical computing or biomedical information science and technology includes database design, graphical interfaces, querying approaches, data retrieval, data visualization and manipulation, data integration through the development of integrated analytical tools, and tools for electronic collaboration, as well as computational research including the development of structural, functional, integrative, and analytical models and simulations.
Requirements: Only United States small business concerns (SBCs) are eligible to submit STTR applications.
Amount of Grant: \$150,000 maximum per year in phase 1; \$750,000 maximum per year in phase 2
Date(s) Application is Due: Apr 5; Aug 5; Dec 5
Contact: Peter Lyster, Ph.D.; (301) 451-6446; email: lysterp@mail.nih.gov
Internet: http://grants.nih.gov/grants/guide/pa-files/PAR-07-161.html
Sponsor: National Institutes of Health (NIH)
45 Center Drive, Room 2AS.55k, MSC 6200
Bethesda, MD 20892-6200

NIH Investigator-Initiated Interactive Research Project Grants 2682
This program provides support for formal, investigator-initiated, collaborative relationships. An IRPG group could be used constructively to support collaborative efforts to accelerate the development of fundamental knowledge and/or enhance the clinical application of that knowledge. The IRPG program may provide an effective means to fund applications for focused clinical research and related, correlative laboratory studies. Annual deadline dates may vary; contact program staff for exact dates.
Requirements: Applications may be submitted by foreign and domestic, for-profit and nonprofit organizations, both public and private; state and local governments; and eligible agencies of the federal government.
Date(s) Application is Due: Feb 15; Jun 15; Oct 15
Contact: Division of Research Grants, (301) 435-0715
Internet: http://www.grants.nih.gov/grants/guide/pa-files/PA-96-001.html
Sponsor: National Institutes of Health
6701 Rockledge Drive
Bethesda, MD 20892

NIH Low Birthweight in Minority Populations Research Grants 2683
This PA solicits research to expand our understanding of the underlying mechanisms that contribute to the ethnic variations in low birth weight (LBW) and strategies for prevention. The goals of this PA are the development of innovative strategies to prevent LBW in minority populations and to expand our understanding of how psychosocial and environmental factors affect or interact with the biologic mechanisms that influence pregnancy outcomes. Inquiries may be directed to the program staff at the appropriate NIH institute: Dr. Cara Krulewitch, (301) 594-2542, Division of Extramural Activities, NINR, Building 45, Bethesda, MD 20892; Dr. Dennis Mangan, (301) 594-2421, Division of Extramural Research, NIDCR, 45 Center Drive, Bethesda, MD 20892; Dr. Gwen Collman, (919) 541-4980, Division of Extramural Research and Training, NIEHS, Box 12233 Research Triangle Park, NC 27709; and Dr. Jonelle Rowe, (301)

496-5575, Center for Research for Mothers and Children, NICHD, 6100 Executive Boulevard, Rockville, MD 20852. PA: PA-99-045
Requirements: Applications may be submitted by foreign and domestic for-profit and nonprofit organizations, public and private.
Contact: Program Officer
Internet: http://www.grants.nih.gov/grants/guide/pa-files/PA-99-045.html
Sponsor: National Institutes of Health
6701 Rockledge Drive
Bethesda, MD 20892

NIH Mechanisms of Orofacial Pain: Anatomy, Genomics, and Proteomics 2684
NINDS and NIDCR invite applications to stimulate and support innovative, interdisciplinary research studies to elucidate the molecular mechanisms underlying orofacial pain, particularly the discovery of proteins and protein networks critical to processing nociceptive information. The purpose of this RFA is to encourage the use of genomic and proteomic approaches and imaging techniques to clarify the molecular events involved in acute orofacial pain, the transition from unrelieved acute pain to chronic pain (i.e. neuroplasticity), neuronal hyperexcitability as manifested by hyperalgesia and allodynia, and chronic orofacial pain disorders of an inflammatory and neuropathic origin. This improved understanding could lead to new therapeutic interventions to effectively treat chronic pain conditions. A letter of intent is requested by April 19; full proposal is due May 14. Annual deadline dates may vary; contact program staff for exact dates. RFA: RFA-DE-05-004
Requirements: Applications may be submitted by domestic and foreign, for-profit and nonprofit organizations, both public and private; units of state and local governments; and eligible agencies of the federal government.
Amount of Grant: $250,000 maximum
Date(s) Application is Due: Apr 19; May 14
Contact: Mary Daley, Chief Grants Management Officer, (301) 594-4808; fax: (301) 480-3562; email: daleym@mail.nih.gov
Internet: http://www.grants.nih.gov/grants/guide/rfa-files/RFA-DE-05-004.html
Sponsor: National Institutes of Health
45 Center Drive, Building 45, Room 4AN-44F
Bethesda, MD 20892-6402

NIH Mechanisms Underlying Individual Variations in Drug Responses 2685
The purpose of this program announcement is to stimulate research into identifying the critical candidate proteins and/or genes that play essential roles in determining individual variations in drug responses. The study of pharmacogenetic/pharmacogenomic variation presents opportunities to a wide range of researchers, working at levels ranging from the most molecular to the most clinical, in the fields of pharmacology, genetics, genomics, medicine, epidemiology, statistics, and computer science. Although NIGMS is leading the initiative, a number of other institutes of NIH are participating, and they are particularly interested in studies in the following areas: NCI—drug response proteins and/or genes involved in cancer, genetic/molecular epidemiologic studies of polymorphisms associated with cancer, and studies of nicotine susceptibility; NHLBI—drug response proteins and/or genes involved in cardiovascular, pulmonary, and hematologic systems; NICHD—development of drug response proteins and/or genes in children; NIEHS—drug response proteins and/or genes affected by environmental exposure; NIMH—drug response proteins and/or genes involved in the treatment of mental disorders and cognitive disorders; NIA—drug response proteins and/or genes involved in susceptibility to adverse drug reactions and drug-drug interactions in older persons; NIAAA—drug response proteins and/or genes that mediate the effects of alcohol and/or drugs that modify alcohol's effects. Applicants may contact the appropriate institute for information: Dr. Kumiko Iwamoto, (301) 496-9600, Division of Cancer Control and Population Sciences, NCI, Executive Plaza N, Rockville, MD 20852; Dr. Mary Wolpert, (301) 496-8783, Division of Cancer Treatment and Diagnosis, NCI, Executive Plaza N, Rockville, MD 20852; Dr. Peter Savage, (301) 435-0421, Division of Epidemiology and Clinical Applications, NHLBI, 2 Rockledge Center, Bethesda, MD 20817; Dr. George Giacoia, (301) 496-5589, Endocrinology, Nutrition and Growth Branch, NICHD, Building 62, Bethesda, MD 20892; Dr. Jose Velazquez, (919) 542-4998, Division of Extramural Research and Training, NIEHS, P.O. Box 12233, Research Triangle Park, NC 27709; Dr. Linda Brady, (301) 443-9875, Division of Basic and Clinical Science Research, NIMH, Parklawn Building, Rockville, MD 20857; Dr. Stanley Slater, (301) 496-6761, Geriatrics Program, NIA, Gateway Building, Bethesda, MD 20892; or Dr. Samir Zakhari, (301) 443-0799, Division of Basic Research, Willco Building, NIAAA, Bethesda, MD 20892. PA: PA-99-016
Requirements: Applications may be submitted by domestic and foreign, for-profit and nonprofit organizations, units of state and local governments, and eligible agencies of the federal government
Contact: Program Officer
Internet: http://www.grants.nih.gov/grants/guide/pa-files/PA-99-016.html
Sponsor: National Institutes of Health
45 Center Drive, Natcher Building
Bethesda, MD 20892

NIH Mechanisms Underlying Secondary Conditions in Mobility Disorders 2686
Primary disabling conditions are often associated with secondary conditions that further inhibit full participation, cause additional negative health consequences, and dramatically increase the burden of the disorder. Treatment or prevention of such secondary conditions (e.g., spasticity, pain, ulceration, infection, weakness and limited motion) will help to create a more enabling environment for persons with limited mobility, so that functioning of the whole person is enhanced. To accomplish these goals, additional research is required to investigate the underlying mechanisms that exacerbate secondary conditions in mobility disorders. Inquiries may be directed to program staff at the appropriate NIH institute: Dr. Mary Ellen Cheung, (301) 402-2242, NICHD, 6100 Executive Boulevard, Bethesda, MD 20892; Dr. Chhanda Dutta, (301) 435-3048, NIA, 7201 Wisconsin Avenue, Bethesda, MD 20892; Dr. James Panagis, (301) 594-5055, NIAMS, 45 Center Drive, Bethesda, MD 20892; Dr. Sanford Garfield, (301) 594-8803, NIDDK, 45 Center Drive, Bethesda, MD 20892; Dr. Scott Somers, (301) 594-5560, NIGMS, 45 Center Drive, Bethesda, MD 20892; and Dr. Karin Helmers, Program Director, (301) 594-2177, NINR, Building 45, Bethesda, MD 20892. Annual deadline dates vary; contact program staff for exact dates. PA: PA-99-096
Requirements: Applications may be submitted by domestic and foreign, for-profit and nonprofit organizations, both public and private; units of state or local governments; and eligible agencies of the federal government.
Amount of Grant: $250,000 maximum per year
Contact: Program Officer
Internet: http://www.grants.nih.gov/grants/guide/pa-files/PA-99-096.html
Sponsor: National Institutes of Health
6701 Rockledge Drive
Bethesda, MD 20892

NIH Mentored Clinical Scientist Development Award 2687
This award enables candidates holding professional degrees (e.g., M.D., D.O., D.V.M., or equivalent degrees) to undertake 3 to 5 years of special study and supervised research with the goal of becoming independent investigators. The award also allows awardees to pursue a research career development program suited to their experience and capabilities under a mentor who is competent to provide guidance in the chosen research area. Institutions may submit applications on behalf of candidates who hold professional degrees. At least 2 years must have elapsed since the health professional degree was granted. Candidates can have varying levels of clinical training and research experience. New applications are due February 12, June 12, and October 12, while resubmitted applications are due March 12, July 12, and November 12.
Requirements: All candidates must be U.S. citizens, non-citizen nationals, or legal permanent residents of the U.S. Persons with temporary or student visas are not eligible. The grantee institution must have a strong, well-established research and research training program in the chosen area, accomplished faculty in the basic and clinical sciences, and a commitment to the candidate's research development. The proposed program should include an appropriate mentor.
Date(s) Application is Due: Feb 12; Mar 12; Jun 12; Jul 12; Oct 12; Nov 12
Contact: Susan Grove, Program Officer; (301) 435-0714; email: sg16d@nih.gov or grantsinfo@od.nih.gov
Internet: http://grants.nih.gov/grants/guide/pa-files/pa-06-512.html
Sponsor: National Institutes of Health
6701 Rockledge Drive
Bethesda, MD 20892

NIH Mentored Patient-Oriented Research Career Development Award 2688
The purpose of this program is to support the career development of investigators who have made a commitment to focus their research endeavors on patient-oriented research. This mechanism provides support for three to five years of supervised study and research for clinically trained professionals who have the potential to develop into productive, clinical investigators focusing on patient-oriented research. Inquiries may be directed to program staff at the appropriate NIH institute. See the following web page for specific contact information: http://grants.nih.gov/grants/guide/contacts/PA-09-043_contacts.html
Requirements: Applicants must have a clinical doctoral degree or its equivalent and must have completed their clinical training, specialty and, if applicable, sub-specialty training prior to receiving an award. However, candidates may submit an application prior to the completion of clinical training. Candidates must identify a mentor with extensive research experience, and must be willing to spend a minimum of 75 percent of full-time professional effort conducting research career development and clinical research.
Restrictions: Current and former principal investigators on NIH research project (R01), FIRST Awards (R29), comparable career development awards (K01, K07, or K08), sub-projects of program project (P01) or center grants (P50), and the equivalent are not eligible for funding under this grant.
Contact: Susan Grove, Program Officer; (301) 435-0714; email: sg16d@nih.gov or grantsinfo@od.nih.gov
Internet: http://grants.nih.gov/grants/guide/pa-files/PA-09-043.html#SectionVII
Sponsor: National Institutes of Health (NIH)
6701 Rockledge Drive
Bethesda, MD 20892

NIH Mentored Research Scientist Development Awards 2689
The overall objective of the NIH Research Career Development Award program is to prepare qualified individuals for careers that have a significant impact on the health-related research needs of the Nation. The objective of the NIH Mentored Research Scientist Development Award is to provide support for a sustained period of protected time for intensive research career development under the guidance of an experienced mentor, or sponsor, in the biomedical, behavioral or clinical sciences leading to research independence. The expectation is that through this sustained period of research career development and training, awardees will launch independent research careers and become competitive for new research project grant funding. Inquiries should be directed to program staff at the appropriate NIH institute. See the website for specific contact information.

Requirements: Applications may be submitted, on behalf of candidates, by domestic, non-federal organizations, public or private, such as medical, dental, or nursing schools or other institutions of higher education. Candidates must be U.S. citizens or non-citizen nationals, or must have been lawfully admitted for permanent residence by the time of award. Candidates must have a research or a health-professional doctorate or its equivalent; have demonstrated the capacity or potential for highly productive independent research in the period after the doctorate; must identify a mentor with extensive research experience; and must be willing to spend a minimum of 75 percent of full-time professional effort conducting research and research career development during the entire award period.
Restrictions: Individuals on temporary or student visas are not eligible for this award.
Amount of Grant: $75,000-$100,000 average
Date(s) Application is Due: Feb 12; Mar 12; Jun 12; Jul 12; Oct 12; Nov 12
Contact: Susan Grove, Program Officer; (301) 435-0714; email: sg16d@nih.gov or grantsinfo@od.nih.gov
Internet: http://grants.nih.gov/grants/guide/pa-files/PA-09-040.html
Sponsor: National Institutes of Health (NIH)
6701 Rockledge Drive
Bethesda, MD 20892

NIH Midcareer Investigator Award in Mouse Pathobiology Research Grants 2690
The purpose of the program is to provide support for established pathobiologists to allow them protected time to devote to mouse pathobiology research and to act as mentors for beginning investigators. The target candidates are outstanding scientists engaged in pathobiology research who are within 15 years of their specialty training, who can demonstrate the need for a period of intensive research focus as a means of enhancing their research careers, and who are committed to mentoring the next generation of mouse pathobiologists. The award is intended to relieve mouse pathobiologists from time consuming service obligations and administrative responsibilities, thereby increasing the opportunities for their own research and for mentoring. Direct inquiries regarding programmatic issues to: Dr. Franziska Grieder, Comparative Medicine Area, (301) 435-0744, NCRR, 6705 Rockledge Drive, Bethesda, MD 20892. Inquiries regarding research and training related to age-related pathology may be directed to: Dr. Huber Warner, (301) 496-6402, Biology of Aging Program, NIA, Gateway Building, Bethesda, MD 20892. PA: PAR-01-064
Requirements: Most candidates for this award will have a Doctor of Veterinary Medicine degree (or equivalent) from an institution recognized by the American Veterinary Medical Association (AVMA). In addition, individuals holding other clinical (such as the MD) or research (such as the PhD) degree(s) may apply for the award if they have been certified or have demonstrated the necessary expertise to perform high quality, funded research in mouse pathobiology. Candidates must have completed their specialty or research training within 15 years of submitting the application, and there is no age limit for candidates. In exceptional circumstances, the period of eligibility may be extended if it can be demonstrated that candidates had an interruption in their career progression due to family or personal circumstances. Applications may be submitted on behalf of candidates by domestic, nonfederal organizations, public or private. At the time of award, candidates must be U.S. citizens or noncitizen nationals.
Restrictions: Individuals on temporary visas are not eligible.
Contact: Program Officer
Internet: http://grants.nih.gov/grants/guide/pa-files/PAR-01-064.html
Sponsor: National Institutes of Health
6701 Rockledge Drive
Bethesda, MD 20892

NIH Molecular Epidemiology of Prostate Carcinogenesis Grants 2691
NCI, NIDDK, and NIEHS invite investigator-initiated research grant applications of molecular epidemiologic studies for understanding prostate cancer development and progression. The purpose of this initiative is to stimulate development and application of biological markers of prostate cancer risk and tumor aggressiveness in developing strategies for prostate cancer prevention and control. Of special interest are studies of markers to elucidate multiethnic differences in prostate cancer susceptibility. Interdisciplinary collaborations, which may include multicenter study sites as well as joint effort between NIH/NCI intramural and extramural scientists, are encouraged. These collaborations may include utilization of shared laboratory and specimen resources whenever possible. Investigations in understudied populations and in populations of contrasting risk, including those who are residing outside of the United States, are strongly encouraged. This PA invites a range of interdisciplinary investigations, including molecular epidemiologic, family, or population-based studies of prostate cancer, utilizing available or new/novel biomarkers (e.g., biochemical, molecular, cellular, genetic) and sources of specimens (e.g., prostate tissue, prostatic fluid, blood components) whenever possible. Annual deadline dates vary; contact program staff for exact dates. PA: PA-00-080
Requirements: Applications may be submitted by foreign and domestic, for-profit and nonprofit organizations, public and private.
Contact: Dr. Kumiko Iwamoto, Division of Cancer Control and Population Sciences, NCI (Executive Plaza N, Bethesda, MD 20892), (301) 435-4911; fax: (301) 402-4279; email: ki6n@nih.gov; Dr. Leroy Nyberg, Urology Program, NIDDK (Natcher Building, Bethesda, MD 20892), (
Internet: http://grants2.nih.gov/grants/guide/pa-files/PA-00-080.html
Sponsor: National Institutes of Health
6701 Rockledge Drive
Bethesda, MD 20892

NIH Mouse Mutagenesis and Phenotyping: Developmental Defects Research Grants 2692
Funds will be awarded to establish a facility for large-scale mutagenesis and phenotyping of developmental defects in the laboratory mouse. The immediate objective of the facility is to produce and characterize mouse strains harboring mutations that affect normal developmental processes. Ultimately, the mutant mice produced are expected to help elucidate the basic cellular, molecular, and genetic mechanisms that direct embryonic and post-embryonic growth and function, as well as yield insights into the mechanisms of human disease. It is anticipated that this facility will devise and perform efficient genome-wide mutagenesis, devise and perform high-throughput phenotyping to screen for mutations that disrupt normal developmental processes, and devise and perform detailed characterization of mutants that display defects in development. Mutant mice, protocols, assays, assessment criteria, and other materials and information generated in projects will be made available to the wider biomedical community. The activities of this facility will be coordinated with the facility(s) established in response to RFA MH-99-007, Mouse Mutagenesis and Phenotyping: Nervous System and Behavior. Inquiries may be directed to program staff at the appropriate NIH institute: Dr. Steven Klein, (301) 496-5541, Developmental Biology, Genetics and Teratology Branch, NICHD, 6100 Executive Boulevard, Rockville, MD 20852; Dr. Judith Greenberg, (301) 594-0943, Division of Genetics and Developmental Biology, NIGMS, Building 45, Bethesda, MD 20892; Dr. Huber Warner, (301) 496-6402, Biology of Aging Program, NIA, Gateway Building, Bethesda, MD 20892; Dr. William Sharrock, (301) 594-5055, Musculoskeletal Diseases Branch, NIAMS, Building 45, Bethesda, MD 20892; Dr. Judy Small, (301) 594-2425, Inherited Craniofacial Diseases and Injury Program, NIDCR, Building 45, Bethesda, MD 20892; Dr. Josie Briggs, (301) 496-6325, Division of Kidney, Urology and Hemotology, NIDDK, Building 31, 31 Center Drive, Bethesda, MD 20892; Dr. John Fakunding, (301) 435-0544, Heart Research Program, Division of Heart and Vascular Disease, NHLBI, 6701 Rockledge Drive, Bethesda, MD 20892. A letter of intent is requested by August 2; full application is due October 14. Annual deadline dates may vary; contact program staff for exact dates. RFA: HD-99-007
Requirements: Applications may be submitted by domestic public and private for-profit and nonprofit organizations such as universities, colleges, hospitals, laboratories, units of state and local government, and eligible agencies of the federal government.
Restrictions: Foreign institutions are not eligible to apply.
Amount of Grant: $2.8 million approximate total funding available
Date(s) Application is Due: Aug 2; Oct 14
Contact: Diane Watson, Grants Management Branch, National Institute of Child Health and Human Development, (301) 496-5001; fax: (301) 402-0915; email: watsond@exchange.nih.gov
Internet: http://www.grants.nih.gov/grants/guide/rfa-files/RFA-HD-99-007.html
Sponsor: National Institutes of Health
6701 Rockledge Drive
Bethesda, MD 20892

NIH Mouse Mutagenesis and Phenotyping: Nervous System and Behavior Research Grants 2693
Funds will be awarded to establish facilities for large-scale mutagenesis and phenotyping of nervous system functions and complex behaviors in the laboratory mouse. Neuroscience-focused mutagenesis and phenotyping facilities established are expected to serve as a national resource by producing a bank of mouse strains that harbor a wide range of mutations affecting murine nervous system function and behavior. Data and biomaterials produced in projects supported will be made widely available to the scientific community. Projects may be funded for up to five years. Inquiries may be directed to program staff at the appropriate NIH institute: Dr. Hemin Chin, (301) 443-1706, Division of Neuroscience and Basic Behavioral Science, NIMH, 6001 Executive Boulevard, Bethesda, MD 20892; Dr. Jonathan Pollock, (301) 435-1309, Division of Basic Research, NIDA, 6001 Executive Boulevard, Bethesda, MD 20892; Dr. Robert Karp, (301) 443-4223, Division of Basic Research, NIAAA, 6000 Executive Boulevard, Bethesda, MD 20892; Dr.Bradley Wise, (301) 496-9350, Neuroscience and Neuropsychology of Aging Program, NIA, 7201 Wisconsin Avenue, Bethesda, MD 20892; Dr. Maria Giovanni, (301) 496-0484, Fundamental Retinal Processes, NEI, 6120 Executive Boulevard, Bethesda, MD 20892; Dr. Gabrielle Leblanc, (301) 496-5745, Division of Fundamental Neuroscience and Developmental Disorders, NINDS, 6001 Executive Boulevard, Bethesda, MD 20892; Dr. Rochelle Small, (301) 402-3464, Division of Human Communication, NIDCD, 6120 Executive Boulevard, Bethesda, MD 20892. A letter of intent is requested by August 2; full application is due October 14. Annual deadline dates vary; contact program staff for exact dates. RFA: MH-99-007
Requirements: Applications may be submitted by domestic public and private for-profit and nonprofit organizations such as universities, colleges, hospitals, laboratories, units of state and local government, and eligible agencies of the federal government.
Restrictions: Foreign institutions are not eligible.
Amount of Grant: $5.5 million total approximately
Date(s) Application is Due: Aug 2; Oct 14
Contact: Robert Barnie, (301) 443-4116; fax: (301) 443-0501; email: rb245s@nih.gov
Internet: http://www.grants.nih.gov/grants/guide/rfa-files/RFA-MH-99-007.html
Sponsor: National Institutes of Health
6701 Rockledge Drive
Bethesda, MD 20892

NIH Multidisciplinary Approach for Research on Oral Complications of HIV Infection 2694
This initiative is designed to encourage multidisciplinary research on the oral complications of HIV infection and their prevention that crosses several academic

disciplines (e.g., virology, immunology, cell biology, pathology, epidemiology, biochemistry, pharmacology, medical imaging, etc.) It is anticipated that this research will increase the knowledge of the basic mechanisms involved in the pathogenesis of the oral disorders associated with AIDS and that it will identify novel strategies for prevention, treatment, and diagnosis of the oral manifestations of AIDS. A letter of intent is due by August 17; full applications are due September 14. Annual deadline dates may vary; contact program staff for exact dates. RFA Number: RFA-DE-05-003
Requirements: Applications may be submitted by domestic and foreign, for-profit and nonprofit organizations, both public and private; units of state and local governments; and eligible agencies of the federal government.
Amount of Grant: $1.1 million maximum per year
Date(s) Application is Due: Aug 17; Sep 14
Contact: Mary Daley, Grants Management Branch, NIDCR, (301) 594-4808; fax: (301) 480-3562; email: md74u@nih.gov
Internet: http://www.grants.nih.gov/grants/guide/rfa-files/RFA-DE-05-003.html
Sponsor: National Institutes of Health
Building 45, Room 4AN-44F
Bethesda, MD 20892-6402

NIH National Centers for Neurofibromatosis Research **2695**
NINDS and NIDCD invite qualified investigators to submit grant applications for the establishment of National Centers for Neurofibromatosis Research. Recent discoveries have created important opportunities for basic, translational, and clinical research on the neurofibromatoses. The purpose of this Program Announcement (PA) is to encourage the formation and development of research centers that can capitalize on these opportunities, and ultimately develop therapeutic interventions for neurofibromatosis patients. These centers are intended to provide focused expertise and resources, and establish a multi-disciplinary environment that will accelerate research progress. PA Number: PAR-04-018
Requirements: Applications may be submitted by domestic and foreign, for-profit and nonprofit organizations, both public and private; units of state and local governments; and eligible agencies of the federal government.
Contact: Kathleen Howe, Grants Management Branch, NINDS, (301) 496-9231; fax: (301) 402-0219; email: kh52x@nih.gov; Sara Stone, Division of Extramural Activities, NIDCD, (301) 402-0909; fax: (301) 402-1758; email: stones@nidcd.nih.gov
Internet: http://grants1.nih.gov/grants/guide/pa-files/PAR-04-018.html
Sponsor: National Institutes of Health
6701 Rockledge Drive, Room 1040, MSC 7710
Bethesda, MD 20892-7710

NIH National Occupational Research Agenda Grants **2696**
The purpose of the grants program is to develop knowledge that can be used in preventing occupational diseases and injuries and to better understand their underlying pathophysiology. The following types of research projects will be supported: causal research to identify and investigate the relationships between hazardous working conditions and associated occupational diseases and injury; the nature and magnitude of special risk factors experienced by older and/or minority workers; methods research to develop more sensitive means of evaluating hazards at work sites; and evaluations of the effectiveness of prevention and intervention programs, including new approaches or combinations of techniques such as control technologies, personal protective equipment, and changes in work organization factors which have been developed and implemented in workplaces. Inquiries may be directed to program staff at the appropriate NIH institute: Dr. Roy Fleming, (404) 639-3343, Research Grants, NIOSH, 1600 Clifton Rd NE, Atlanta, GA 30333; Dr. Kumiko Iwamoto, (301) 435-4911, Epidemiology and Genetics Research, NCI, 6130 Executive Boulevard, Bethesda, MD 20892; Dr. Gail Weinmann, (301) 435-0202, Division of Lung Diseases, NHLBI, 6701 Rockledge Drive, Bethesda, MD 20892; Dr. Sidney Stahl, (301) 402-4156, Behavioral and Social Research, NIA, 7201 Wisconsin Avenue, Bethesda, MD 20892; Dr. Amy Donhaue, (301) 402-3458, Hearing and Balance/Vestibular Sciences, NIDCD, 6120 Executive Boulevard, Bethesda, MD 20892; Dr. Gwen Collman, (919) 541-4980, Division of Extramural Research and Training, NIEHS, P.O. Box 12233, Research Triangle Park, NC 27709. Awards will be made for projects lasting one to three years. Annual deadline dates may vary; contact program staff for exact dates. RFA: OH-99-002
Requirements: Applications may be submitted by domestic and foreign public and private nonprofit and for-profit organizations; state and local governments or their bona fide agents; and federally recognized Indian tribal governments, Indian tribes, or Indian tribal organizations.
Restrictions: Any organization involved in lobbying activities is not eligible.
Amount of Grant: $250,000 maximum per year
Contact: Program Officer
Internet: http://www.grants.nih.gov/grants/guide/rfa-files/RFA-OH-99-002.html
Sponsor: National Institutes of Health
6701 Rockledge Drive
Bethesda, MD 20892

NIH National Research Service Awards—Senior Fellows **2697**
This program awards senior fellowships to experienced scientists who wish to make major changes in the direction of their research careers or who wish to broaden their scientific background by acquiring new research capabilities. These awards will enable individuals with at least seven years of research experience beyond the doctorate, and who have progressed to the stage of independent investigator, to take time from regular professional responsibilities for the purpose of receiving training to increase their scientific capabilities. In most cases, this award is used to support sabbatical experiences for established independent scientists. This program is not designed for postdoctoral- level investigators seeking to prove their research potential prior to independence. Inquiries may be directed to program staff at the appropriate NIH institute: Dr. Robin Barr, (301) 496-9322, NIA; Dr. Ernestine Vanderveen, (301) 443-2530, NIAAA; Dr. Milton Hernandez, (301) 496-3775, NIAID; Dr. Richard Lymn, (301) 594-5128, NIAMS; Dr. Lisa Begg, (301) 496-8580, NCI; Dr. Steven Klein, (301) 496-5541, NICHD, Dr. Daniel Sklare, (301) 496-1804, NIDCD; Dr. James Lipton, (301) 594-2618, NIDR; Dr. Judith Podskalny, (301) 594-8876, NIDDK; Dr. Carol Shreffler, (919) 541-1445, NIEHS; Dr. Chyren Hunter, (301) 496-5301, NEI; Dr. John Norvell, (301) 594-0533, NIGMS; Dr. Sarah Knox, (301) 435-0409, NHLBI; Dr. Henry Khachaturian, (301) 496-4188, NINDS; Dr. Nell Armstrong, (301) 594-5973, NINR; Dr. Bettie Graham, (301) 496-7531, NCHGR; Dr. David Wilde, (301) 435-0799, NCRR; and Dr. Neal West, (301) 402-5867, NCCAM. Annual deadline dates may vary; contact program staff for exact dates. PA: PA-00-131
Requirements: Applicants must have at least seven years of postdoctoral research or professional experience in the field. By the time of award, individuals must be citizens or noncitizen nationals of the United States or have been lawfully admitted to the United States for permanent residence. The sponsoring institution may be private (profit or nonprofit) or public.
Date(s) Application is Due: Apr 5; Aug 5; Dec 5
Contact: Program Officer; email: grantsinfo@nih.gov
Internet: http://grants.nih.gov/grants/guide/pa-files/PA-00-131.html
Sponsor: National Institutes of Health
6701 Rockledge Drive
Bethesda, MD 20892

NIH New Directions in Pain Research Grants **2698**
This program encourages investigator-initiated research project grant applications to study mechanisms underlying analgesic response and pain to advance the development of novel pain interventions, treatments, and management strategies. The purpose of this PA is to inform the scientific community of broad, shared interests in pain research encompassing the various components of the NIH, and to stimulate and foster a wide range of basic, translational, and patient-oriented clinical studies on pain. Applications are particularly encouraged to study pain throughout the lifespan from the perspectives of molecular genetics, transcriptional controls, signal transduction, including cellular/molecular mechanisms, innovative imaging technologies, plasticity, and from hormonal or gender influences. The pain experience needs to be examined at all levels of analysis from the gene, molecule, cell, tissue, and organ, to the individual, family, and community, with the ultimate goal of developing new insights into pain intervention, treatment, and management. Inquiries may be directed to program staff at the appropriate NIH institute: Dr. Cheryl Kitt, (301) 496-1431, Division of Convulsive, Infectious, and Immune Disorders, NINDS, Federal Building, Bethesda, MD 20892; Dr. Patricia Bryant, (301) 594-2095, Temporomandibular Joint Disorders and Neuropathies and Neurodegenerative Diseases, NIDRC, 45 Center Drive, Bethesda, MD 20892; Claudette Varricchio, (301) 496-8541, Division of Cancer Prevention, NCI, 6130 Executive Boulevard, Bethesda, MD, 20892; Dr. Judith Finkelstein, (301) 496-9350, Neuroscience and Neuropsychology of Aging Programs, NIA, 7201 Wisconsin Avenue, Bethesda, MD, 20892; Dr. John Killen, (301) 496-0545, Division of Acquired Immunodeficiency Syndrome, NIAID, 6003 Executive Boulevard, Rockville, MD 20892; Dr. James Panagis, (301) 594-5055, Orthopedics Program, NIAMS, 45 Center Drive, Bethesda, MD 20892; Dr. Rochelle Small, Division of Human Communication, (301) 402-3464, NIDCD, 6120 Executive Boulevard, Bethesda, MD 20892; Dr. David Thomas, (301) 443-4975, Division of Basic Research, NIDA, 5600 Fishers Ln, Rockville, MD 20857; Dr. Alison Cole, (301) 594-1826, Division of Pharmacology, Physiology, and Biological Chemistry, NIGMS, 45 Center Drive, Bethesda, MD 20892; Dr. Mary Leveck, (301) 594-5963, Program Director, NINR, Building 45, Bethesda, MD 20892; and Joyce Rudick, (301) 402-1770, Office of Research on Women's Health, NIH, Building 1, Bethesda, MD 20892. PA: PA-98-102
Requirements: Applications may be submitted by foreign and domestic, for-profit and nonprofit organizations, public and private.
Contact: Program Officer
Internet: http://www.grants.nih.gov/grants/guide/pa-files/PA-98-102.html
Sponsor: National Institutes of Health
9000 Rockville Pike
Bethesda, MD 20892

NIH Nonhuman Primate Immune Tolerance Cooperative Study Group Grants **2699**
NIAID and NIDDK invite applications from single institutions or consortia of institutions to participate in a multi-center, cooperative research program to evaluate existing and new tolerance induction treatment regimens and to elucidate the underlying mechanisms of the induction, maintenance and/or loss of tolerance in nonhuman primate models of kidney and islet transplantation. The goals of this research program are to evaluate further the safety, toxicity, and efficacy of existing tolerance induction regimens; define the underlying mechanisms of action of the therapeutic approaches under investigation; and develop and validate immune and/or surrogate markers of the induction, maintenance, and loss of tolerance, graft function, graft acceptance, and graft survival. The deadline for Letters of Intent is August 22, with full applications due September 22.
Requirements: Applications may be submitted by domestic for-profit and nonprofit organizations and public and private institutions.
Restrictions: Foreign institutions are not eligible to apply. This RFA will not support: studies in animal models other than non-human primates; human studies or trials; xenotransplantation; preliminary development of a non-human primate transplantation

model; studies to improve the isolation, preservation, or supply of organs, tissues or cells; hematopoietic stem cell transplantation, unless in the context of kidney or islet transplantation (i.e. bone marrow chimerism experiments); heart or lung transplantation models; or studies of non-immunological side effects of an immuno-modulatory agent.
Amount of Grant: $6.7 million approximate total
Date(s) Application is Due: Aug 22; Sep 22
Contact: Kristy Kraemer, Ph.D., Division of Allergy, Immunology and Transplantation; (301) 496-5598; fax: (301) 480-0693; email: kkraemer@niaid.nih.gov
Internet: http://grants.nih.gov/grants/guide/rfa-files/RFA-AI-06-018.html
Sponsor: National Institutes of Health
6610 Rockledge Drive, Room 3043, MSC-6601
Bethesda, MD 20892

NIH NRSAs for Individual Predoctoral Fellowships 2700
The awards are provided to individuals for research training in specified areas of biomedical and behavioral research to help ensure that highly trained scientists will be available in adequate numbers and in appropriate research areas and fields to meet the nation's mental health, drug abuse, alcohol abuse, and alcoholism research needs. As such, this program is intended to provide a mechanism to train future generations of outstanding scientists committed to pursuing a career in mental health, drug abuse, and/or alcohol abuse and alcoholism research. Inquiries may be directed to program staff at the appropriate NIH institute: Dr. Henry Khachaturian, (301) 443-4335, NIMH, 5600 Fishers Ln, Rockville, MD 20857; Dr. Cindy Miner, (301) 443-6071, NIDA, 5600 Fishers Ln, Rockville, MD 20850; and Dr. Tina Vanderveen, (301) 443-2531, NIAAA, 6000 Executive Boulevard, Bethesda, MD 20892. Annual deadline dates vary; contact program staff for exact dates. PA: PA-00-125
Requirements: Applicants must be citizens or non-citizen nationals of the United States, or have been lawfully admitted to the United States for permanent residence and have in their possession an Alien Registration Receipt Card at the time of award. Applicants must have received, as of the activation date of the award, a baccalaureate degree and must be enrolled in a program leading to a research doctorate such as the PhD or DSc, or a combined clinical and research degree such as MD/PhD, by the proposed fellowship activation date.
Contact: Program Officer
Internet: http://grants.nih.gov/grants/guide/pa-files/PA-00-125.html
Sponsor: National Institutes of Health
6701 Rockledge Drive
Bethesda, MD 20892

NIH NRSAs Predoctoral Fellowship Awards for Students with Disabilities 2701
The intent of this program is to encourage students with disabilities to seek graduate degrees and thus further the goal of increasing the number of scientists with disabilities who are prepared to pursue careers in biomedical and behavioral research. Inquiries may be directed to program staff at the appropriate NIH institute: Dr. Robin Barr, (301) 496-9322, NIA; Dr. Ernestine Vanderveen, (301) 443-1273, NIAAA; Dr. Milton Hernandez, (301) 496-7291, NIAID; Dr. Richard Lymn, (301) 594-5128, NIAMS; Dr. John Schneider, (301) 496-8580, NCI; Hildegard Topper, (301) 496-0104, NICHD; Dr. Daniel Sklare, (301) 496-1804, NIDCD; Dr. James Lipton, (301) 594-2618, NIDR; Dr. Ronald Margolis, (301) 594-8819, NIDDK; Dr. Charles Sharp, (301) 443-1887, NIDA; Dr. Michael Galvin Jr., (919) 541-7825, NIEHS; and Dr. Maria Giovanni, (301) 496-0484, NEI. Annual deadline dates may vary; contact program staff for exact dates. PA: PA-95-028
Requirements: Applicants must be citizens or non-citizen nationals of the United States, or have been lawfully admitted to the United States for permanent residence.
Restrictions: Individuals on temporary or student visas are not eligible.
Amount of Grant: $10,008 annual stipend plus a $2000 institutional allowance
Contact: Program Officer
Internet: http://www.grants.nih.gov/grants/guide/pa-files/PA-95-028.html
Sponsor: National Institutes of Health
6701 Rockledge Drive
Bethesda, MD 20892

NIH Pathological Gambling: Basic, Clinical, and Services Research Grants 2702
NIMH, NIAAA, and NIDA invite investigator-initiated research relevant to their programs that will advance basic, clinical, and services research concerning pathological gambling, as well as enable more effective clinical assessment, prevention, and treatment. This program announcement encourages research that builds on extant research findings concerning pathological gambling and research that expands the breadth and depth of scientific knowledge through increased involvement of various disciplines, e.g., epidemiology; genetics; neuroscience; developmental psychopathology; and behavioral, cognitive, and social science. Multidisciplinary research is especially encouraged. Major questions include factors that predispose for pathological gambling and that distinguish types of pathological gamblers; models for explaining pathological gambling, e.g., social learning, addiction, impulse dyscontrol; developmental pathways and course; gender, age, and sociocultural factors; mechanisms involved in onset, continuation, and cessation; efficacious clinical interventions for the prevention of onset, for treatment, and for prevention and management of relapse; effectiveness of interventions in general use; and effects of the organization and financing of services. Inquiries may be directed to the appropriate NIH institute: Dr. James Breiling, (301) 443-3527, Division of Mental Disorders, Behavior, and AIDS Research, NIMH, 5600 Fishers Ln, Rockville, MD 20857; Darryl Bertolucci, (301) 443-4898, Epidemiology Branch, NIAAA, 6000 Executive Boulevard, Bethesda, MD 20892; and Dr. Meyer Glantz, Division of Epidemiology and Prevention Research, NIDA, 5600 Fishers Ln, Rockville, MD 20857. Annual deadline dates may vary; contact program staff for exact dates. PA: PA-98-106
Requirements: Applications may be submitted by public and private, foreign and domestic, for-profit and nonprofit organizations.
Date(s) Application is Due: Oct 19; Nov 16
Contact: Program Officer
Internet: http://grants.nih.gov/grants/guide/pa-files/PA-98-106.html
Sponsor: National Institutes of Health
6003 Executive Boulevard
Bethesda, MD 20892

NIH Predoctoral Fellowship Awards for Minority Students 2703
These fellowships are for well-qualified students from minority groups found to be underrepresented in the biomedical and behavioral sciences in the United States. The intent of this program is to encourage students from minority groups that are underrepresented in the biomedical and behavioral sciences to seek graduate degrees and thus further the goal of increasing the number of minority scientists who are prepared to pursue careers in biomedical and behavioral research. Inquiries may be directed to program staff at the appropriate NIH institute: Dr. Robin Barr, (301) 496-9322, NIA; Dr. Ernestine Vanderveen, (301) 443-1273, NIAAA; Dr. Milton Hernandez, (301) 496-7291, NIAID; Dr. Richard Lymn, (301) 594-5128, NIAMS; Dr. John Schneider, (301) 496-8580, NCI; Hildegard Topper, (301) 496-0104, NICHD; Dr. Daniel Sklare, (301) 496-1804, NIDCD; Dr. James Lipton, (301) 594-2618, NIDR; Dr. Ronald Margolis, (301) 594-8819, NIDDK; Dr. Charles Sharp, (301) 443-1887, NIDA; Dr. Michael Galvin Jr., (919) 541-7825, NIEHS; and Dr. Maria Giovanni, (301) 496-0484, NEI. Annual deadline dates may vary; contact program staff for exact dates. PA: PA-95-029
Requirements: Applicants must be citizens or non-citizen nationals of the United States, or have been lawfully admitted to the United States for permanent residence
Restrictions: Individuals on temporary or student visas are not eligible.
Amount of Grant: $10,008 annual stipend plus a $2000 institutional allowance
Contact: Program Officer
Internet: http://www.grants.nih.gov/grants/guide/pa-files/PA-95-029.html
Sponsor: National Institutes of Health
6701 Rockledge Drive
Bethesda, MD 20892

NIH Protein Structure Initiative (Structural Genomics) Research Grants 2704
The purpose of this PA is to encourage research on the development of methodology and technology underpinning the emerging field of structural genomics, whose goal is the understanding of protein structural families, structural folds, and the relation of structure and function. Projects related to high throughput structure determination by x-ray crystallography and/or NMR, as well as those addressing other constituent tasks of structural genomics, are relevant to this PA. Inquiries may be directed to the staff at the appropriate NIH institute: Dr. John Norvell, (301) 594-0533, Division of Cell Biology and Biophysics, NIGMS, 45 Center Drive, Bethesda, MD 20892; Dr. Abraham Levy, (301) 435-0755, Biomedical Technology, NCRR, 6705 Rockledge Drive, Bethesda, MD 20892; and Dr. Jose Velazquez, (919) 541-4998, Division of Extramural Research and Training, NIEHS, P.O. Box 12233, Research Triangle Park, NC 27709. Annual deadlne dates vary; contact program staff for exact dates. PA: PA-99-116
Requirements: Applications may be submitted by domestic and foreign, for-profit and nonprofit organizations, public and private.
Restrictions: Foreign institutions are not eligible for program project (P01) grants.
Date(s) Application is Due: Feb 1; Jun 1; Oct 1
Contact: Program Officer
Internet: http://www.grants.nih.gov/grants/guide/pa-files/PA-99-116.html
Sponsor: National Institutes of Health
6701 Rockledge Drive
Bethesda, MD 20892

NIH Protein Structure Initiative (Structural Genomics)—SBIR/STTR Grants 2705
The purpose of this SBIR/STTR program announcement is to encourage research on the development of methodology and technology underpinning the emerging field of structural genomics, whose goal is the understanding of protein structural families, structural folds, and the relation of structure and function. Projects related to high-throughput structure determination by x-ray crystallography and/or NMR, as well as those addressing other constituent tasks of structural genomics, are relevant to this
Requirements: Any small business concern, independently owned and operated by U.S. citizens or lawfully admitted permanent resident aliens, which is located in the United States and is organized for profit, may apply.
Date(s) Application is Due: Apr 1; Aug 1; Dec 1
Contact: Dr. John Norvell, Division of Cell Biology and Biophysics, (301) 594-0533; fax: (301) 480-2004; email: norvellj@nigms.nih.gov
Internet: http://grants2.nih.gov/grants/guide/pa-files/PA-99-117.html
Sponsor: National Institutes of Health
6701 Rockledge Drive
Bethesda, MD 20892

NIH Receptors and Signaling in Bone in Health and Disease 2706
The objective of this initiative is to elicit grant submissions that focus on systemic hormones, local growth factors, and bone-active cytokines, their receptors and mechanisms of signaling in bone. While the primary focus is on basic research, the long-term emphasis is on identifying mechanisms or processes related to hormone action with potential applicability as targets for therapeutic agents that may have efficacy in

the treatment of diseases that adversely affect bone, such as osteoporosis and primary hyperparathyroidism. Modular Grant applications will request direct costs in $25,000 modules, up to a total direct cost request of $250,000 per year.
Requirements: Applications may be submitted by domestic and foreign for-profit and nonprofit organizations, public and private, such as universities, colleges, hospitals, laboratories, units of State and local governments, and eligible agencies of the Federal Government. Racial/ethnic minority individuals, women, and persons with disabilities are encouraged to apply as principal investigators.
Amount of Grant: $250,000 maximum per year
Date(s) Application is Due: Feb 5; Jun 5; Oct 5
Contact: Susan Grove, Program Officer; (301) 435-0714; email: sg16d@nih.gov or grantsinfo@od.nih.gov
Internet: http://grants.nih.gov/grants/guide/pa-files/PA-00-017.html
Sponsor: National Institutes of Health (NIH)
6701 Rockledge Drive
Bethesda, MD 20892

NIH Recovery Act Limited Competition: Academic Research Enhancement Awards 2707

The purpose of the Academic Research Enhancement Award (AREA) program is to stimulate research in educational institutions that provide baccalaureate or advanced degrees for a significant number of the Nation's research scientists, but that have not been major recipients of NIH support. These AREA grants create opportunities for scientists and institutions otherwise unlikely to participate extensively in NIH programs, to contribute to the Nation's biomedical and behavioral research effort. AREA grants are intended to support small-scale health-related research projects proposed by faculty members of eligible, domestic institutions. The requested budget is limited to $300,000 total costs for the entire three-year project (maximum time period). Applicants should contact individuals at the specific departments listed on the web site. No Letters of Intent are necessary, though full applications should arrive by September 24.
Requirements: The following institutions and organizations may apply: public/state controlled institutions of higher education; private institutions of higher education; Hispanic-serving institutions; historically Black colleges and universities (HBCUs); tribally controlled colleges and universities (TCCUs); Alaska Native and Native Hawaiian serving institutions; public or private institutions and components of institutions defined below as health professional schools or colleges; and other academic components.
Restrictions: Foreign organizations/institutions are not permitted as the applicant organization.
Amount of Grant: $300,000 maximum total direct costs for a three-year period
Date(s) Application is Due: Sep 24
Contact: Susan Grove, Program Officer; (301) 435-0714; email: sg16d@nih.gov or grantsinfo@od.nih.gov
Internet: http://grants.nih.gov/grants/guide/rfa-files/RFA-OD-09-007.html
Sponsor: National Institutes of Health (NIH)
6701 Rockledge Drive
Bethesda, MD 20892

NIH Recovery Act Limited Competition: Biomedical Research, Development, and Growth to Spur the Acceleration of New Technologies (BRDG-SPAN) Pilot Program Grants 2708

This Funding Opportunity Announcement (FOA), supported by funds provided to the NIH under the American Recovery & Reinvestment Act of 2009 (Recovery Act or ARRA), Public Law 111-5, solicits grant applications for a new initiative called Biomedical Research, Development, and Growth to Spur the Acceleration of New Technologies (BRDG-SPAN) Pilot Program. The purpose of this pilot program is to address the funding gap between promising research and development (R&D) and transitioning to the market — often called the Valley of Death — by contributing to the critical funding needed by applicants to pursue the next appropriate milestone(s) toward ultimate commercialization; i.e., to carry out later stage research activities necessary to that end. This program aims to accelerate the transition of research innovations and technologies toward the development of products or services that will improve human health, help advance the mission of NIH and its Institutes and Centers (ICs), and create significant value and economic stimulus. This program also aims to foster partnerships among a variety of research and development (R&D) collaborators working toward these aims. The requested budget is limited to $1 million total costs per year for a maximum of three years. Applicants should contact individuals at the specific departments listed on the web site. Letters of Intent are due by August 3, and full applications should arrive by September 1.
Requirements: The applicant United States institution and organization must be located in the 50 states, territories and possessions of the U.S., Commonwealth of Puerto Rico, Trust Territory of the Pacific Islands, or District of Columbia.
Restrictions: Foreign organizations/institutions are not permitted as the applicant organization.
Amount of Grant: $1,000,000 total costs per year over three years
Date(s) Application is Due: Aug 3; Sep 1
Contact: Susan Grove, Program Officer; (301) 435-0714; email: sg16d@nih.gov or grantsinfo@od.nih.gov
Internet: http://grants.nih.gov/grants/guide/rfa-files/RFA-OD-09-008.html
Sponsor: National Institutes of Health (NIH)
6701 Rockledge Drive
Bethesda, MD 20892

NIH Recovery Act Limited Competition: Building Sustainable Community-Linked Infrastructure to Enable Health Science Research 2709

Applications are invited from domestic (United States) institutions/organizations proposing to develop or expand needed infrastructures that will fundamentally transform collaboration and communication between academic health centers and local communities. Such collaborative infrastructures are essential to advance the health science research enterprise while ensuring that important research findings are effectively disseminated and implemented to improve public health and advance health care delivery. The primary intent is to fund projects to develop infrastructure for productive and sustainable academic-community research partnerships that can be leveraged in the future for efficiently conducting research that includes and is relevant to affected communities, and through which research findings can be disseminated in a manner that maximizes impact on public health. It is expected that each grantee will be able to leverage this Recovery Act funding into future research grants using the infrastructure partnership between itself and the participating community. Letters of Intent are due by November 12, with final applications due by December 11.
Requirements: The following organizations and institutions may apply: public/state controlled institutions of higher education; private institutions of higher education; Hispanic-serving institutions; historically Black colleges and universities (HBCUs); tribally controlled colleges and universities (TCCUs); Alaska native and native Hawaiian serving institutions; nonprofits with 501(c)3 IRS status; nonprofits without 501(c)3 IRS status; small businesses; for-profit organizations; State governments; regional organizations; U.S. territories or possessions; Indian/Native American tribal governments; Indian/Native American tribally designated organizations; county governments; city or township governments; special district governments; independent school districts; public housing authorities/Indian housing authorities; eligible agencies of the Federal government; and faith-based or community based organizations.
Restrictions: This RFA is not intended to fund research or evaluation projects, clinical trials, or public health campaigns. Foreign organizations/institutions are not permitted as the applicant organization.
Date(s) Application is Due: Nov 12; Dec 11
Contact: Dr. Suzanne Heurtin-Roberts; (301) 402-2277; email: sheurtin@mail.nih.gov
Internet: http://grants.nih.gov/grants/guide/rfa-files/RFA-OD-09-010.html
Sponsor: National Institutes of Health (NIH)
1 Center Drive, Room B3-11
Bethesda, MD 20892

NIH Recovery Act Limited Competition: Small Business Catalyst Awards for Accelerating Innovative Research Grants 2710

This NIH Funding Opportunity Announcement, supported by funds provided to the NIH under the American Recovery and Reinvestment Act of 2009 (Recovery Act or ARRA), Public Law 111-5, invites grant applications from small business concerns that propose to accelerate innovation through high risk, high reward research and development (R&D) that has commercial potential and is relevant to the mission of the NIH. The Small Business Catalyst Award is further expected to support entrepreneurs of exceptional creativity, drawn from scientific and technological environments beyond NIH, who propose pioneering and possibly transformative approaches to addressing major biomedical or behavioral challenges with the potential for downstream commercial development. The Small Business Catalyst Award for Accelerating Innovative Research funding opportunity seeks to encourage fresh research perspectives and approaches to serve the mission of NIH. In particular, applications from small business concerns without a history of NIH Small Business Innovation Research (SBIR) or Small Business Technology Transfer (STTR) support may receive funding priority. Solicited are applications for support for projects that have the potential to generate high impact results (e.g., products, processes or services) and/or innovative research applications, research tools, techniques, devices, inventions, or methodologies. The outcomes of the research supported should have potential to lead to products that will improve public health and create significant value and economic stimulus. This FOA solicits early-stage ideas that promise to lead to major leaps forward in capabilities important to serving the mission of NIH rather than incremental improvements of existing technologies. In accord with the funding priority of this initiative to attract applicants without a history of SBIR/STTR support from NIH, the focus of the projects solicited by this FOA is on early stage technology development. Budget requests are limited to $200,000 total costs for a maximum project period of one year. Applicants should contact individuals at the specific departments listed on the web site. Letters of Intent are due by August 3, and full applications should arrive by September 1.
Requirements: Only United States small business concerns (SBCs) are eligible to submit SBIR applications. A small business concern is one that, at the time of award of SBIR Phase I and Phase II, meets all of the following criteria: is organized for profit, with a place of business located in the United States, which operates primarily within the United States or which makes a significant contribution to the United States economy through payment of taxes or use of American products, materials or labor; is in the legal form of an individual proprietorship, partnership, limited liability company, corporation, joint venture, association, trust or cooperative, except that where the form is a joint venture, there can be no more than 49 percent participation by foreign business entities in the joint venture; is at least 51 percent owned and controlled by one or more individuals who are citizens of, or permanent resident aliens in, the United States, or it must be a for-profit business concern that is at least 51% owned and controlled by another for-profit business concern that is at least 51% owned and controlled by one or more individuals who are citizens of, or permanent resident aliens in, the United States, except in the case of a joint venture, where each entity to the venture must be 51 percent owned and controlled by one or more individuals who are citizens of, or permanent resident aliens in, the United States; and has, including its affiliates, not more than 500 employees.

Amount of Grant: $200,000 over a one-year period
Date(s) Application is Due: Aug 3; Sep 1
Contact: Susan Grove, Program Officer; (301) 435-0714; email: sg16d@nih.gov or grantsinfo@od.nih.gov
Internet: http://grants.nih.gov/grants/guide/rfa-files/RFA-OD-09-009.html
Sponsor: National Institutes of Health (NIH)
6701 Rockledge Drive
Bethesda, MD 20892

NIH Recovery Act Limited Competition: Supporting New Faculty Recruitment to Enhance Research Resources through Biomedical Research Core Centers Grants 2711

This initiative, which is supported by funds provided to the NIH under the Recovery Act, is designed to provide the necessary resources for U.S. academic institutions/organizations to enhance their biomedical research efforts through the development of Biomedical Research Core Centers. For this announcement, Biomedical Core Centers are defined as a community of multidisciplinary researchers focusing on areas of biomedical research relevant to NIH, such as centers, departments, programs, and/or trans-departmental collaborations or consortia. These Core Centers are designed to provide scientific and programmatic support for promising research faculty and their areas of research. The NIH invites applications that include plans to recruit and hire investigators to conduct biomedical research in all scientific disciplines, including the field of bioethics. Applicants should contact individuals at the specific departments listed on the web site. Letters of Intent are due by April 29, and full applications should arrive by May 29.
Requirements: The following institutions and organizations may apply: public/state controlled institutions of higher education; private institutions of higher education; Hispanic-serving institutions; historically Black colleges and universities (HBCUs); tribally controlled colleges and universities (TCCUs); Alaska Native and Native Hawaiian serving institutions; nonprofits with 501(c)3 IRS status (other than institutions of higher education); nonprofits without 501(c)3 IRS status (other than institutions of higher education); and Indian/Native American tribally designated organizations .
Restrictions: Foreign organizations/institutions are not permitted to apply.
Date(s) Application is Due: Apr 29; May 29
Contact: Susan Grove, Program Officer; (301) 435-0714; email: sg16d@nih.gov or grantsinfo@od.nih.gov
Internet: http://grants.nih.gov/grants/guide/rfa-files/RFA-OD-09-005.html
Sponsor: National Institutes of Health (NIH)
6701 Rockledge Drive
Bethesda, MD 20892

NIH Research On Ethical Issues In Human Subjects Research 2712

The purpose of this funding opportunity announcement is to solicit research addressing the ethical challenges of human subjects research in order to optimize the protection of human subjects and enhance the ethical conduct of human subjects research. The research design for studies on ethical issues in human subjects research should be appropriate to the nature of the project(s) proposed and the disciplines involved. Given the conceptual and methodological complexity of many of these research questions, interdisciplinary and collaborative projects are encouraged, particularly those involving clinical researchers, ethicists, and behavioral/social scientists.
Requirements: The following organizations and institutions may apply: public/state controlled institutions of higher education; private institutions of higher education; nonprofits with 501(c)3 IRS status (other than institution of higher education); nonprofits without 501(c)3 IRS status (other than institution of higher education); small businesses; for-profit organizations (other than small business); State governments; U.S. territories or possessions; Indian/Native American tribal governments (Federally recognized); Indian/Native American tribal governments (other than Federally recognized); Indian/Native American tribally designated organizations; non-domestic (non-U.S.) entities (foreign organization); eligible agencies of the Federal government; and faith-based or community based organizations.
Date(s) Application is Due: Feb 5; Jun 5; Oct 5
Contact: Kim Witherspoon; (301) 496-8866; fax: (301) 480-4663; email: withersk@ctep.nci.nih.gov;; Ellen M. Werner, Ph.D.; (301) 435-0050; fax: (301) 480-0868; email: wernere@nhlbi.nih.gov
Internet: http://grants.nih.gov/grants/guide/pa-files/PA-07-277.html
Sponsor: National Institutes of Health (NIH)
6130 Executive Blvd. (EPN), Room 7009, MSC 7432
Bethesda, MD 20892-7432

NIH Research on Sleep and Sleep Disorders 2713

This Funding Opportunity Announcement (FOA) solicits grant applications proposing research to advance biomedical knowledge related to sleep or sleep disorders, improve understanding of the neurobiology or functions of sleep over the life-span, enhance timely diagnosis and effective treatment for individuals affected by sleep-related disorders, or implement and evaluate innovative community-based public health education and intervention programs. Because the nature and scope of the proposed research will vary from application to application, it is anticipated that the size and duration of each award will also vary. The total amount awarded and the number of awards will depend upon the mechanism numbers, quality, duration, and costs of the applications received.
Requirements: The following organizations and institutions may apply: public/state controlled institutions of higher education; private institutions of higher education; nonprofits with 501(c)3 IRS status; nonprofits without 501(c)3 IRS status; small businesses; State governments; non-domestic (non-U.S.) entities (foreign organizations); eligible agencies of the Federal government; and faith-based or community based organizations.
Date(s) Application is Due: Feb 5; Jun 5; Oct 5
Contact: Susan Grove, Program Officer; (301) 435-0714; email: sg16d@nih.gov or grantsinfo@od.nih.gov
Internet: http://grants.nih.gov/grants/guide/pa-files/pa-07-140.html
Sponsor: National Institutes of Health (NIH)
6701 Rockledge Drive
Bethesda, MD 20892

NIH Research Project Grants 2714

The Research Project Grant (R01) is an award to support a discrete, specified, circumscribed project to be performed by named Project Directors/Principal Investigators (PDs/PIs) in areas representing the investigators' specific interests and competencies, based on the mission of the NIH. The R01 is the original and historically the oldest grant mechanism used by the NIH to support health-related research and development. The NIH awards R01 grants to institutions/organizations of all types. This mechanism allows the PDs/PIs to define the scientific focus or objective of the research based on particular areas of interest and competence. Although the PDs/PIs write the grant application and are responsible for conducting and supervising the research, the actual applicant is the research institution/organization. Research grant applications are assigned to an NIH IC based on receipt and referral guidelines and many applications are assigned to multiple ICs with related research interests. Each IC maintains a Web site with funding opportunities and areas of interest. Contact with an IC representative may help focus the research plan based on an understanding of the mission of the IC. For specific information about the mission of each NIH IC, see http://www.nih.gov/icd, which provides a brief summary of the research interests in each IC and access to individual IC home pages.
Requirements: The following organizations and institutions may apply: public/state controlled institutions of higher education; private institutions of higher education; Hispanic-serving institutions; historically Black colleges and universities (HBCUs); tribally controlled colleges and universities (TCCUs); Alaska native and native Hawaiian serving institutions; nonprofits with 501(c)3 IRS status; nonprofits without 501(c)3 IRS status; small businesses; for-profit organizations; State governments; regional organizations; U.S. territories or possessions; Indian/Native American tribal governments; Indian/Native American tribally designated organizations; eligible agencies of the Federal government; and faith-based or community based organizations.
Date(s) Application is Due: Feb 5; Jun 5; Oct 5
Contact: Visit the web site for departmental contact information
Internet: http://grants.nih.gov/grants/guide/pa-files/PA-07-070.html
Sponsor: National Institutes of Health (NIH)
6100 Executive Boulevard
Bethesda, MD 20892

NIH Rett Syndrome: Genetics, Pathophysiology, and Biomarkers Research Grants 2715

The Mental Retardation and Developmental Disabilities (MRDD) Branch and the Center for Research for Mothers and Children (CRMC) of NICHD and the Division of Fundamental Neuroscience and Developmental Disorders (DFNDD) of NINDS invite research grant applications that address the genetics, pathophysiological mechanisms, and the development of biomarkers for Rett syndrome. Areas of interest include developmental neurobiology, pathophysiology, genetics, epidemiology, structure-function correlations, and clinical studies that have a direct link to Rett syndrome. Specific funds will be set aside to support investigator-initiated applications responsive to this grant solicitation. PA: PAS-99-037
Requirements: Applications may be submitted by domestic, for-profit and nonprofit organizations, both public and private; units of state or local governments; and eligible agencies of the federal government.
Amount of Grant: $1.5 million total
Contact: Dr. Mary Lou Oster-Granite, NICHD, 6100 Executive Boulevard, Bethesda, MD 20892; (301) 496-1383; fax: (301) 496-3791; email: mo96o@nih.gov; Dr. Giovanna Spinella, NINDS, (301) 496-5821; (301) 402-1501;email: gs41b@nih.gov
Internet: http://www.grants.nih.gov/grants/guide/pa-files/PAS-99-037.html
Sponsor: National Institutes of Health
6701 Rockledge Drive
Bethesda, MD 20892

NIH Role of Microglia in Normal and Abnormal Immune Responses of the Nervous System 2716

NINDS, NIMH, NCRR, NIDCD, and NIDA invite applications to promote research into the role of microglia in the initiation and expansion of autoimmune processes of the central nervous system (CNS) and the resulting injury to CNS components. The intent of this PA is to intensify interest and investigator-initiated research to attract new investigators to this field and to mobilize interdisciplinary approaches. Inquiries may be directed to program staff at the appropriate NIH institute: Dr. A.P. Kerza-Kwiatecki, Neural Environment Team, (301) 496-1431, NINDS, 6001 Executive Boulevard, Bethesda, MD 20892; Dr. John Strandberg, Comparative Medicine, (301) 435-0744, NCRR, 1 Rockledge Ctr, Bethesda, MD 20892; Dr. Dianne Rausch, (301) 443-7281, NIMH, 6001 Executive Boulevard, Bethesda, MD 20892; Dr. Thomas Johnson, Program Officer, (301) 402-3461, NIDCD, 6120 Executive Boulevard, Bethesda, MD 20892; and Dr. Charles William Sharp, Division of Basic Research, (301) 443-1887, NIDA, 6001 Executive Boulevard, Bethesda, MD 20892. PA: PA-00-029
Requirements: Applications may be submitted by foreign and domestic, for-profit and nonprofit organizations, both public and private; units of state and local governments; and eligible agencies of the federal government.
Contact: Program Officer

Internet: http://grants.nih.gov/grants/guide/pa-files/PA-00-029.html
Sponsor: National Institutes of Health
6701 Rockledge Drive
Bethesda, MD 20892

NIH Roybal Centers for Translational Research on Aging 2717
The long-range objectives of the Roybal Centers are to improve the health, quality of life, and productivity of middle-aged and older people, through: facilitating the translation from the basic behavioral and social sciences (including human factors) to practical outcomes, including new technologies, for the benefit of the aged, and if possible also stimulating new "use-inspired" basic research in the behavioral and social sciences. A letter of intent is due by December 22; full application is due January 22. Annual deadline dates mayb vary; contact program staff for exact dates. RFA Number:
Requirements: An Edward R. Roybal Center Grant (P30) requires relevant pre-existing research activity at the institution. Any individual with the skills, knowledge, and resources necessary to carry out the proposed research is invited to work with their institution to develop an application for support.
Restrictions: Foreign organizations are not eligible to apply for P30 grants.
Amount of Grant: $360,000 maximum allowable annual costs
Date(s) Application is Due: Jan 22; Dec 22
Contact: Jean Richelsen, Grants and Contracts Management Office, (301) 496-1472; email: richelsj@nia.nih.gov
Internet: http://grants1.nih.gov/grants/guide/rfa-files/RFA-AG-04-007.html
Sponsor: National Institutes of Health
6701 Rockledge Drive, Room 1040, MSC 7701
Bethesda, MD 20892-7710

NIH Ruth L. Kirschstein National Research Service Awards (NRSA) for Individual Senior Fellows 2718
The objective of the National Research Service Award (NRSA) F33 program is to provide senior fellowship support to experienced scientists who wish to make major changes in the direction of their research careers or who wish to broaden their scientific background by acquiring new research capabilities as independent research investigators in scientific health-related fields relevant to the missions of the participating NIH Institutes and Centers (ICs). Senior fellowship applicants for the F33 award must include a research training proposal that offers an opportunity for individuals to broaden their scientific background or to extend their potential for research in health-related areas as independent researchers. These awards will enable individuals with at least seven years of research experience beyond the doctorate, and who have progressed to the stage of independent investigator, to take time from regular professional responsibilities for the purpose of receiving training to increase their scientific capabilities. In most cases, this award is used to support sabbatical experiences for established independent scientists seeking support for retraining or additional career development.
Requirements: The following organizations are eligible to apply: for-profit organizations; non-profit organizations; public or private institutions, such as universities, colleges, hospitals, and laboratories; eligible agencies and labs of the Federal government, including NIH intramural labs; domestic institutions; and foreign institutions.
Restrictions: This program is not designed for postdoctoral level investigators seeking to enhance their research experience prior to independence.
Date(s) Application is Due: Apr 8; Aug 8; Dec 8
Contact: Nancy Lohrey; (301) 496-8580; fax: (301) 402-4472; email: lohreyn@mail.nih.gov
Internet: http://grants.nih.gov/grants/guide/pa-files/PA-07-172.html
Sponsor: National Institutes of Health (NIH)
6116 Executive Boulevard, Suite 7019, MSC 8346
Bethesda, MD 20892-8346

NIH Ruth L. Kirschstein National Research Service Awards for Individual Postdoctoral Fellows 2719
The purpose of the National Research Service Award Act (NRSA) is to help ensure that diverse pools of highly trained scientists will be available in adequate numbers and in appropriate research areas to carry out the Nation's biomedical, behavioral and clinical research agendas. The National Institutes of Health (NIH) awards individual postdoctoral fellowships (F32) to promising applicants who have the potential to become productive, independent investigators in fields related to the mission of participating NIH Institutes and Centers. The proposed postdoctoral training must be within the broad scope of biomedical, behavioral, or clinical research or other specific disciplines relevant to the research mission of the participating NIH Institutes and Centers. The proposed training must offer an opportunity to enhance the fellow's understanding of the health-related sciences and extend his/her potential for a productive research career.
Requirements: Applicant organizations must have any of the following characteristics: for-profit organizations; non-profit organizations; public or private institutions, such as universities, colleges, hospitals, and laboratories; units of State and local governments; eligible agencies and labs of the Federal government including NIH intramural labs; domestic institutions; and foreign institutions.
Date(s) Application is Due: Apr 8; Aug 8; Dec 8
Contact: Walter Schaffer; (301) 435-2687; fax: (301) 480-0146; email: ws11q@nih.gov
Internet: http://grants.nih.gov/grants/guide/pa-files/PA-06-373.html
Sponsor: National Institutes of Health (NIH)
45 Center Drive, Natcher Building
Bethesda, MD 20892

NIH Ruth L. Kirschstein National Research Service Awards for Individual Predoctoral Fellows 2720
The objective of this funding opportunity announcement is to help ensure that highly trained scientists will be available in adequate numbers and in appropriate research areas to carry out the Nation's biomedical, behavioral, and clinical research agenda. The participating Institutes of the National Institutes of Health (NIH) provide individual predoctoral research training fellowship awards to promising doctoral candidates who have the potential to become productive, independent investigators in research fields relevant to the missions of these participating NIH Institutes and Centers. Each participating NIH Institute has a unique scientific purview and different program goals and initiatives that evolve over time. Prior to preparing an application, it is critical that all applicants consult the appropriate Institute website for details of research areas supported by that Institute. Applicants should also contact the appropriate Institute scientific/research contact to obtain current information about specific program priorities and policies.
Requirements: The following organizations are eligible to apply: for-profit organizations; non-profit organizations; public or private institutions, such as universities, colleges, hospitals, and laboratories; eligible agencies and labs of the Federal government, including NIH intramural labs; domestic institutions; and foreign institutions.
Date(s) Application is Due: Apr 8; Aug 8; Dec 8
Contact: Michael-David Kerns; (301) 496-9322; email: kernsmd@mail.nih.gov;; Dennis Twombly; (301) 443-9334; fax: (301) 443-1650; email: dtwombly@mail.nih.gov
Internet: http://grants.nih.gov/grants/guide/pa-files/PA-07-002.html
Sponsor: National Institutes of Health (NIH)
6120 Executive Boulevard
Bethesda, MD 20892-7180

NIH Ruth L. Kirschstein National Research Service Awards for Individual Predoctoral Fellowships to Promote Diversity in Health-Related Research 2721
The purpose of the F31 predoctoral fellowship to promote diversity in health-related research is to provide up to five years of support for research training leading to the PhD or equivalent research degree, the combined MD/PhD degree; or another formally combined professional degree and research doctoral degree in biomedical, behavioral, health services, or clinical sciences. These fellowships will enhance the diversity of the biomedical, behavioral, health services, and clinical research labor force in the United States by providing opportunities for academic institutions to identify and recruit students from diverse population groups to seek graduate degrees in health-related research and apply for this fellowship. The goal of this program is to increase the number of scientists from diverse population groups who are prepared to pursue careers in biomedical, behavioral, social, clinical, or health services research.
Requirements: The following organizations and institutions are eligible to apply: public/state controlled institutions of higher education; private institutions of higher education; Hispanic-serving institutions; historically Black colleges and universities (HBCUs); tribally controlled colleges and universities (TCCUs); Alaska Native and Native Hawaiian serving institutions; nonprofits with 501(c)3 IRS status (other than institutions of higher education); nonprofits without 501(c)3 IRS status (other than institutions of higher education); for-profit organizations (other than small businesses); non-domestic (non-U.S.) entities (foreign organizations); and other eligible agencies of the Federal Government.
Date(s) Application is Due: Apr 8; Aug 8; Dec 8
Contact: Susan Grove, Program Officer; (301) 435-0714; email: sg16d@nih.gov or grantsinfo@od.nih.gov
Internet: http://grants.nih.gov/grants/guide/pa-files/PA-09-209.html
Sponsor: National Institutes of Health (NIH)
6701 Rockledge Drive
Bethesda, MD 20892

NIH Ruth L. Kirschstein National Research Service Awards for Individual Predoctoral MD/PhD and Other Dual Doctoral Degree Fellows 2722
The purpose of the Ruth L. Kirschstein National Research Service Awards (Kirschstein-NRSA) is to provide support to individuals for combined MD/PhD and other dual doctoral degree training (e.g. DO/PhD, DDS/PhD, AuD/PhD). The participating Institutes award this Kirschstein-NRSA individual fellowship to qualified applicants with the potential to become productive, independent, highly trained physician-scientists and other clinician-scientists, including patient-oriented researchers in their scientific mission areas. This funding opportunity supports individual predoctoral F30 fellowships with the expectation that these training opportunities will increase the number of future investigators with both clinical knowledge and skills in basic, translational or clinical research.
Requirements: The following organizations and institutions are eligible to apply: public/state controlled institutions of higher education; private institutions of higher education; Hispanic-serving institutions; historically Black colleges and universities (HBCUs); tribally controlled colleges and universities (TCCUs); Alaska Native and Native Hawaiian serving institutions; nonprofits with 501(c)3 IRS status (other than institutions of higher education); nonprofits without 501(c)3 IRS status (other than institutions of higher education); for-profit organizations (other than small businesses); and other eligible agencies of the Federal Government.
Restrictions: Non-domestic (non-U.S.) entities (foreign organizations) are not eligible to apply.
Date(s) Application is Due: Apr 8; Aug 8; Dec 8
Contact: Nancy C. Lohrey; (301) 496-8580; fax: (301) 402-4472; email: lohreyn@mail.nih.gov
Internet: http://grants.nih.gov/grants/guide/pa-files/PA-09-207.html
Sponsor: National Institutes of Health (NIH)
6116 Executive Boulevard, Suite 7019, MSC 8346
Bethesda, MD 20892-8346

NIH Sarcoidosis: Research into the Cause of Multi-Organ Disease and Clinical Strategies for Therapy Grants 2723

The purpose of this Funding Opportunity Announcement (FOA) is to stimulate research on the etiology and management of sarcoidosis, an immune–mediated granulomatous inflammatory disorder. Studies supported by this FOA would include investigations to find the etiology(ies) and related host factors that might enhance susceptibility to sarcoidosis, especially development of symptomatic multi-organ disease that has a propensity to involve critical organs (such as lungs, heart, eyes, central/peripheral nervous system, liver, kidneys and other abdominal viscera) that create serious illness. Study of the still problematic management and the biological, behavioral, or psychosocial burden on individuals, families, and community is encouraged. Moreover, there is interest for approaches to risk reduction, psychological coping, and management of complications and side effects of treatment.

Requirements: The following organizations and institutions may apply: public/state controlled institutions of higher education; private institutions of higher education; Hispanic-serving institutions; historically Black colleges and universities (HBCUs); tribally controlled colleges and universities (TCCUs); Alaska native and native Hawaiian serving institutions; nonprofits with 501(c)3 IRS status; nonprofits without 501(c)3 IRS status; small businesses; for-profit organizations; State governments; regional organizations; U.S. territories or possessions; Indian/Native American tribal governments; Indian/Native American tribally designated organizations; eligible agencies of the Federal government; and faith-based or community based organizations.

Date(s) Application is Due: Feb 5; Jun 5; Oct 5

Contact: Herbert Y. Reynolds, M.D.; (301) 435-0222; fax: (301) 480-3557; email: Reynoldh@nhlbi.nih.gov

Internet: http://grants.nih.gov/grants/guide/pa-files/PA-07-136.html

Sponsor: National Institutes of Health (NIH)
Two Rockledge Center, Suite 10018, 6701 Rockledge Drive, MSC 7952
Bethesda, MD 20892-7952

NIH SBIR/STTR Study and Control of Microbial Biofilms Research Grants 2724

Several NIH institutes invite research grant applications to conduct studies on microbial biofilms leading to improved strategies and technologies to diagnose, prevent, and treat biofilm-associated infectious diseases. Inquiries may be directed to the staff at the appropriate NIH institute: Dr. Joyce Reese, (301) 594-2088, Division of Extramural Research, NIDCR, Building 45, Bethesda, MD 20892; Dr. Stephen Heyse, (301) 496-7728, Division of Microbiology and Infectious Diseases, NIAID, Solar Building, Bethesda, MD 20892; Dr. Kenneth Gruber, (301) 402-3458, Division of Human Communication, NIDCD, 6120 Executive Boulevard, Bethesda, MD 20892; Dr. James Panagis, (301) 594-5055, Orthopedics Program, NIAMS, 45 Center Drive, 4500 Bethesda, MD 20892; Dr. Scott Somers, (301) 594-5560, Division of Pharmacology, Physiology, and Biological Chemistry, NIGMS, 45 Center Drive, Bethesda, MD 20892; Dr. Susan Banks-Schlegel, (301) 435-0202, Airway Biology and Disease Program, NHLBI, 6701 Rockledge Drive, 7952 Bethesda, MD 20892; Dr. Lawrence Agodoa, (301) 594-7717, Division of Kidney, Urologic, and Hematologic Diseases, NIDDK, 45 Center Drive, Bethesda, MD 20892; Dr. Eugene Hayunga, (301) 402-1770, Office of Research on Women's Health, Building 1, Bethesda, MD 20892; Dr. Louis Quatrano, (301) 402-2242, National Center for Medical Rehabilitation Research, NICHD, 6100 Executive Boulevard, Rockville, MD 20852; Dr. Hilary Sigmon, (301) 594-5970, Division of Extramural Activities, NINR, 45 Center Drive, Bethesda, MD 20892; and Dr. William Heetderks, (301) 496-1447, Division of Stroke, Trauma, and Neurodegenerative Disorders, NINDS, Federal Building, Bethesda, MD 20892. Contact program staff for availability. PA: PA 99-084

Date(s) Application is Due: Apr 1; Aug 1; Dec 1

Contact: Program Officer

Internet: http://www.grants.nih.gov/grants/guide/pa-files/PA-99-084.html

Sponsor: National Institutes of Health
6701 Rockledge Drive
Bethesda, MD 20892

NIH School-based Interventions to Prevent Obesity 2725

This Funding Opportunity Announcement (FOA) encourages the formation of partnerships between academic institutions and school systems in order to develop and implement controlled, school-based intervention strategies designed to reduce the prevalence of obesity in childhood. This FOA also encourages evaluative comparisons of different intervention strategies, as well as the use of methods to detect synergistic interactions between different types of interventions. Because the nature and scope of the proposed research will vary from application to application, it is anticipated that the size and duration of each award will also vary. The total amount awarded and the number of awards will depend upon the mechanism numbers, quality, duration, and costs of the applications received.

Requirements: The following organizations and institutions may apply: public/state controlled institutions of higher education; private institutions of higher education; Hispanic-serving institutions; historically Black colleges and universities (HBCUs); tribally controlled colleges and universities (TCCUs); Alaska native and native Hawaiian serving institutions; nonprofits with 501(c)3 IRS status; nonprofits without 501(c)3 IRS status; small businesses; for-profit organizations; State governments; regional organizations; U.S. territories or possessions; Indian/Native American tribal governments; Indian/Native American tribally designated organizations; eligible agencies of the Federal government; and faith-based or community based organizations.

Date(s) Application is Due: Feb 5; Jun 5; Oct 5

Contact: Gilman Grave, M.D.; (301) 496-5593; fax: (301) 480-9791; email: graveg@mail.nih.gov

Internet: http://grants.nih.gov/grants/guide/pa-files/PA-07-180.html

Sponsor: National Institutes of Health (NIH)
6100 Executive Boulevard, 4B-11, MSC 7510
Bethesda, MD 20892-7510

NIH Self-Management Strategies Across Chronic Diseases Grants 2726

The purpose of this Program Announcement (PA) is to solicit applications to expand research on established self-management interventions to multiple chronic diseases across the life-course. Interventions aimed at chronic disease self-management are numerous and many are well described in the literature. They are often presented as specific to a particular chronic disease. This PA encourages applicants to investigate the applicability of effective self-management interventions to a broader spectrum of chronic diseases. Chronic disease, for this announcement, is defined as illnesses that are prolonged, are rarely cured completely, and require self-management behaviors by affected individuals and/or their caretakers. Modular Grant applications will request direct costs in $25,000 modules, up to a total direct cost request of $250,000 per year.

Requirements: The following organizations and institutions may apply: public/state controlled institutions of higher education; private institutions of higher education; Hispanic-serving institutions; historically Black colleges and universities (HBCUs); tribally controlled colleges and universities (TCCUs); Alaska native and native Hawaiian serving institutions; nonprofits with 501(c)3 IRS status; nonprofits without 501(c)3 IRS status; small businesses; for-profit organizations; State governments; regional organizations; U.S. territories or possessions; Indian/Native American tribal governments; Indian/Native American tribally designated organizations; county governments; city or township governments; special district governments; independent school districts; public housing authorities/Indian housing authorities; eligible agencies of the Federal government; and faith-based or community based organizations.

Amount of Grant: $250,000 maximum per year

Date(s) Application is Due: Feb 5; Jun 5; Oct 5

Contact: Susan Grove, Program Officer; (301) 435-0714; email: sg16d@nih.gov or grantsinfo@od.nih.gov

Internet: http://grants.nih.gov/grants/guide/pa-files/PA-00-109.html

Sponsor: National Institutes of Health (NIH)
6701 Rockledge Drive
Bethesda, MD 20892

NIH Senior Scientist Award 2727

This award provides stability of support to outstanding scientists who have demonstrated a sustained, high level of productivity and whose expertise, research accomplishments, and contributions to the field have been and will continue to be critical to the mission of the particular NIH center or institute. The award provides salary support for award periods of up to five years as a means of enhancing the individual recipient's skills and dedication to his/her area of research. It permits NIH institutes and centers to identify and support exceptionally talented investigators who are well established in their field of research. Inquiries may be directed to program staff at the appropriate NIH institute: Dr. Ernestine Vanderveen, (301) 443-2531, NIAAA; Dr. Lester Gorelic, (301) 496-8580, NCI; Dr. Andrea Baruchin, (301) 443-6071, NIDA; Dr. Henry Khachaturian, (301) 443-4335, NIMH; and Dr. Neal West, (301) 402-5867, NCCAM. PA: PA-00-021

Requirements: Applications may be submitted on behalf of candidates by domestic, nonfederal organizations, public or private, such as medical, dental, or nursing schools or other institutions of higher education. At the time of award, candidates must be citizens or noncitizen nationals of the United States or must have been lawfully admitted for permanent residence. The candidate must be a senior scientist and a recognized leader in the field with a distinguished record of original contributions; must have a record of support from a funding institute or center; and must have peer-reviewed grant support at the time of the award to be eligible.

Restrictions: Individuals on temporary or student visas are not eligible.

Contact: Program Officer

Internet: http://grants.nih.gov/grants/guide/pa-files/PA-00-021.html

Sponsor: National Institutes of Health
6701 Rockledge Drive
Bethesda, MD 20892

NIH Small Business Innovation Research (SBIR): Animal Models of HCV Infection Research Grants 2728

This is a multi-institute solicitation targeting the development/identification of one or more small animal models of hepatitis C infection and disease progression including acute and chronic states, fibrosis/cirrhosis, and liver tumor development—not necessarily all in the same model. Identification of a small, inexpensive, reproducible, well-defined, and nonendangered mammalian animal model for hepatitis C research is critical to the progress of exploration of this pathogen. Such a model is needed to study the pathogenesis, immunology, natural history, and viral replication of hepatitis C, as well as to act as a model for the testing of new therapies and vaccine candidates. This RFA invites grant applications for SBIR projects with award duration and amounts greater than those routinely allowed under the SBIR program. Inquiries may be directed to the appropriate NIH institute: Dr. Leslye Johnson, (301) 496-7051, Division of Microbiology and Infectious Diseases, NIAID, 6003 Executive Boulevard, Bethesda, MD 20892; Dr. John Cole III, (301) 496-1718, Division of Cancer Biology, NCI, Executive Plaza N, Bethesda, MD 20892; Dr. Raymond O'Neil, (301) 435-0744, Comparative Medicine, NCRR, 6701 Rockledge Drive, Bethesda, MD 20892; and Dr. Thomas Kresina, (301) 443-6537, Biomedical Research Branch, NIAAA, 6000 Executive Boulevard, Bethesda, MD 20892. Annual deadline dates may vary; contact program staff for exact dates. RFA: AI-00-008

Requirements: Any small business, independently owned and operated by U.S. citizens or permanent resident aliens may apply. Such a business must be organized for profit, cannot be dominant in its field of expertise, and must have its principal place of business in the United States. Including any affiliates, the company can be the employer of no more than 500 people. Full eligibility details may be found in the NIH Omnibus Solicitation.
Amount of Grant: $3.2 million
Contact: Program Officer
Internet: http://grants.nih.gov/grants/guide/rfa-files/RFA-AI-00-008.html
Sponsor: National Institutes of Health
6701 Rockledge Drive
Bethesda, MD 20892

NIH Solicitation of Assays for High Throughput Screening (HTS) in the Molecular Libraries Probe Production Centers Network (MLPCN) 2729

he NIH Molecular Libraries Roadmap Initiative wishes to encourage HTS assay applications from investigators who have the interest and capability to work with the Molecular Libraries Probe Production Centers Network (MLPCN) for chemical probe development. This Funding Opportunity Announcement (FOA) promotes discovery and development of new chemical probes as research tools for use by scientists in both the public and private sectors to advance the understanding of biological functions and disease mechanisms. This initiative is one of the integrated components of the NIH Molecular Libraries Roadmap initiative that offers biomedical researchers access to large-scale automated high throughput screening (HTS) centers in the MLPCN, diverse compound libraries in the Small Molecule Repository (MLSMR) and information on biological activities of small molecules in the PubChem BioAssay public database. Letters of Intent (LOIs) are due on December 4, April 4, and August 3 respectively. Full application must be received by January 4, May 4, and September 3 respectively.
Requirements: The following organizations and institutions are eligible to apply: public/state controlled institutions of higher education; private institutions of higher education; Hispanic-serving institutions; historically Black colleges and universities (HBCUs); tribally controlled colleges and universities (TCCUs); Alaska native and native Hawaiian serving institutions; nonprofits with 501(c)3 IRS status (other than institutions of higher education); nonprofits without 501(c)3 IRS status (other than institutions of higher education); small businesses; for-profit organizations (other than small businesses); state governments; Indian/Native American tribal governments (federally recognized); Indian/Native American tribally designated organizations; county governments; city or township governments; special district governments; independent school districts; public housing authorities/Indian housing authorities; U.S. territories or possessions; Indian/native American tribal governments (other than federally recognized); regional organizations; non-domestic (non-U.S.) entities (foreign organizations); eligible agencies of the federal government; and faith-based or community-based organizations.
Amount of Grant: $50,000 maximum
Date(s) Application is Due: Jan 4; May 4; Sep 3
Contact: Yong Yao, Ph.D.; (301) 443-6102; email: yyao@mail.nih.gov
Internet: http://grants.nih.gov/grants/guide/pa-files/PAR-09-129.html#SectionIII
Sponsor: National Institutes of Health (NIH)
6001 Executive Boulevard, Room 7175, MSC 9641
Bethesda, MD 20892-9641

NIH Structural Biology of Membrane Proteins Grants 2730

This PA solicits applications to develop research and methods to enhance the rate of membrane protein structure determination and to determine specific membrane protein structures. Innovative methods for expression, oligomerization, solubilization, stabilization, purification, characterization, crystallization, isotopic labeling, and structure determination of unique and biologically significant membrane proteins by x-ray diffraction, nuclear magnetic resonance (NMR), electron microscopic, mass spectrometry, and other biophysical techniques are encouraged. Projects that will lead in the near term to determining the structures of biologically important membrane proteins are also encouraged.
Requirements: Applicant organizations must be: for-profit organizations; non-profit organizations; public or private institutions, such as universities, colleges, hospitals, and laboratories; units of State government; units of local government; eligible agencies of the Federal government; foreign institutions; domestic institutions; faith-based agencies; or community-based organizations.
Date(s) Application is Due: Feb 5; Jun 5; Oct 5
Contact: Peter C. Preusch, Ph.D.; (301) 594-3827; email: preuschp@nigms.nih.gov;; Jean Chin, Ph.D.; (301) 594-0828; email: chinj@nigms.nih.gov
Internet: http://grants.nih.gov/grants/guide/pa-files/PA-06-119.html
Sponsor: National Institutes of Health (NIH)
Building 45, 2AS.55E 45 Center Drive, MSC 6200
Bethesda, MD 20892

NIH Studies of Ethical, Legal, and Social Implications of Research into Human Genetic Variation Grants 2731

The program solicits projects that examine the ethical, legal, and social implications of the study of human DNA sequence variation. Of particular interest are studies that explore how research on human genetic variation can be conducted in an ethically and culturally sensitive way; how the information that results from this research will interact with current concepts of race and ethnicity; how cultural and socioeconomic factors influence the interpretation and use of this information; and how this information may influence access to and use of genetic health services by various groups. The study of sequence variation and the exploration of related ethical, legal, and social issues have been identified as two of the new five-year goals of the U.S. Human Genome Project and will be of continuing interest to the NHGRI program over the next several years. Inquiries may be directed to program staff at the appropriate NIH institute: Jean Cahill, Division of Extramural Research, NHGRI, (301) 402-1733, 38 Library Drive, Bethesda, MD 20892; Sherry Dennison, Grants Management Branch, NIDCD, (301) 402-0909, 6120 Executive Boulevard, Bethesda, MD 20892; David Mineo, Division of Extramural Research and Training, NIEHS, (919) 541-1373, P.O. Box 12233, T.W. Alexander Drive, E Campus, Research Triangle Park, NC 27709; Antoinette Holland, Grants Administration Branch, NIGMS, (301) 594-5132, Building 45, Bethesda, MD 20892. Annual deadline dates vary; contact program staff for exact dates. RFA: HG-99-002
Requirements: Applications may be submitted by domestic and foreign, for-profit and nonprofit, public and private organizations; units of state and local governments; and eligible agencies of the federal government.
Amount of Grant: $2 million per year for up to three years
Contact: Program Officer
Internet: http://www.grants.nih.gov/grants/guide/rfa-files/RFA-HG-99-002.html
Sponsor: National Institutes of Health
6701 Rockledge Drive
Bethesda, MD 20892

NIH Summer Internship Program in Biomedical Research 2732

Summer programs at the National Institutes of Health (NIH) provide an opportunity to spend a summer working side-by-side with some of the leading scientists in the world, in an environment devoted exclusively to biomedical research. The NIH consists of the 240-bed Mark O. Hatfield Clinical Research Center and more than 1,200 laboratories located on the main campus in Bethesda, Maryland, as well as in Baltimore and Frederick, Maryland; Research Triangle Park, North Carolina; Phoenix, Arizona; Hamilton, Momtana; and Detroit, Michigan. Awards cover a minimum of eight weeks, with students generally arriving at the NIH in May or June. The stipends for trainees are adjusted yearly, with supplements for prior experience. Prospective candidates must apply online. The application is available from mid-November to March 1.
Requirements: The Summer Internship Program is for students who will be sixteen years of age or older at the time they begin the program and who are currently enrolled at least half-time in high school or an accredited U.S. college or university. Students who have been accepted into a college or university program may also apply.
Restrictions: To be eligible, candidates must be U.S. citizens or permanent residents.
Amount of Grant: $1,700 - $3,100 per month
Date(s) Application is Due: Mar 1
Contact: Arnetta Courtney; (301) 827-3724; email: arnetta.courtney@fda.hhs.gov
Internet: http://www.training.nih.gov/student/sip/info.asp
Sponsor: National Institutes of Health (NIH)
Building 31, Room 9A06, 31 Center Drive, MSC 2560
Bethesda, MD 20892-2560

NIH Supplements to Promote Reentry into Biomedical and Behavioral Research Careers 2733

NIH provides administrative supplements to research grants to support individuals with high potential to reenter an active research career after taking time off to care for children or parents or to attend to other family responsibilities. This program will provide administrative supplements to existing NIH research grants for the purpose of supporting full-time or part-time research by these individuals in a program geared to bring their existing research skills and knowledge up to date. For more information, contact the program officer at the appropriate institute. PA: PA-99-106
Requirements: Candidates must have a doctoral degree, such as MD, DDS, PhD, OD, DVM, or equivalent; at least two years of postdoctoral research experience; and must have had sufficient prior research experience to have qualified for a faculty appointment at the assistant professor or equivalent level at the time of their leaving active research.
Restrictions: Candidates who have begun the reentry process through a fellowship, traineeship, or similar mechanism are not eligible.
Amount of Grant: $40,000 maximum
Contact: NIAAA, (301) 443-2531; NIA, (301) 496-9322; NIAID, (301) 496-8697; NIAMS, (301) 594-5052; NCI, (301) 496-7344; NICHD, (301) 496-1848; NIDCD, (301) 496-5061; NIDR, (301) 594-2089; NIDDK, (301) 594-8842; NIDA, (301) 443-0441; NIEHS, (919) 541-7723
Internet: http://www.grants.nih.gov/grants/guide/pa-files/PA-99-106.html
Sponsor: National Institutes of Health
6701 Rockledge Drive
Bethesda, MD 20892

NIH Targeting Research Gaps in HIV Therapeutics Research Grants 2734

NIAID, NIDDK, and NIMH invite applications to conduct applied studies in specific gap areas identified in current HIV therapeutics. Study areas include new delivery or formulation methods to enhance the clinical potential of anti-HIV drugs (FDA-approved or those undergoing clinical testing) in infected adults and children; validating new viral and cellular targets for HIV inhibition and for developing new drugs (or developing new agents against existing targets); and defining and validating the role of innate (nonacquired) immune responses in susceptibility to HIV infection, modulation of disease progression, and their potential use in therapeutic application in infected adults and children. Studies targeted in this PA should generate preclinical proof-of-concept on the therapeutic feasibility of the specific target or approach, and engage in applied preclinical studies. When relevant, applications with clinical studies (e.g., evaluating a drug delivery method) will be considered. Inquiries regarding eligibility and research scope may contact Dr. Nava Sarver, (301) 496-2970, Division of AIDS, NIAID, 6003 Executive Boulevard, Bethesda, MD 20892, email: ns18p@nih.gov. Inquiries regarding

other programmatic issues may contact Dr. Dianne Rausch, (301) 443-7281, Office of AIDS Research, NIMH, 6001 Executive Boulevard, Bethesda, MD 20892; or Dr. Philip Smith, (301) 594-8816, Division of Diabetes, Endocrinology, and Metabolic Diseases, NIDDK, 45 Center Drive, Bethesda, MD 20892. PA-99-067
Requirements: Applications may be submitted by domestic and foreign for-profit and nonprofit organizations, both public and private; units of state and local governments; and eligible agencies of the federal government.
Contact: Program Officer
Internet: http://www.grants.nih.gov/grants/guide/pa-files/PA-99-067.html
Sponsor: National Institutes of Health
6701 Rockledge Drive
Bethesda, MD 20892

NIH Technologies to Improve the Utility of Animal Models Research Grants 2735
This PA encourages the small business community to develop technologies, reagents, and equipment to improve the utility of animal models for biomedical research. The results of projects supported under this PA are expected to be improvement of laboratory animal welfare, improved long-term maintenance and preservation of laboratory animal models, and improved technologies for generation of animal models of human diseases. Cost-effective methods, reagents, and equipment to improve animal health and to characterize, culture, and preserve biomedically important organisms are critical needs for biomedical research. Reagents to diagnose and control laboratory animal diseases, including those of aquatic animals, are needed. Equipment and techniques for cost-effective husbandry of animal models in controlled environments are needed for a variety of aquatic and nonaquatic laboratory animals. Improved technologies for the cryopreservation of embryos and gametes are needed for several scientific and economic reasons. Projects supported under the PA are to be directed along one or more of these objectives. This PA must be read in conjunction with the Omnibus Solicitations for SBIR and STTR applications (available on the Web site). Inquiries may be directed to the staff at the appropriate NIH institute: Director, Comparative Medicine, (301) 435-0744, NCRR, 6705 Rockledge Drive, Bethesda, MD 20892; Jo Anne Goodnight, (301) 496-5307, Division of Cancer Biology, NCI, Executive Plaza N, Bethesda, MD 20892; Dr. Christine Kelley, (301) 435-0565, Division of Heart and Vascular Diseases, NHLBI, 2 Rockledge Center, Bethesda, MD 20892; Dr. Joyce Reese, (301) 594-2088, Division of Extramural Research, NIDCR, Building 45, Bethesda, MD 20892; and Dr. Michael Galvin Jr., (910) 541-7825, Division of Extramural Research and Training, NIEHS, P.O. Box 12233, Research Triangle Park, NC 27709. PA: PA-99-048
Requirements: Any small business, independently owned by U.S. citizens and located in the United States, may apply.
Contact: Program Officer
Internet: http://www.grants.nih.gov/grants/guide/pa-files/PA-99-048.html
Sponsor: National Institutes of Health
6701 Rockledge Drive
Bethesda, MD 20892

NIH Transitional Career Development Award in Women's Health Research 2736
This award is designed to support career development experiences leading to independence for clinical investigators interested in patient-oriented or population-based research related to women's health. The career development program will provide an opportunity for investigators to develop solid clinical research skills during two years of study and research within the environment of the NIH Intramural Research Programs (IRP). The award will also include a follow-on two-year period of salary and research support at an academic institution of the candidate's choice. This period of extramural support will facilitate the transition to independence as a clinical researcher specializing in research issues related to women's health. Inquiries may be directed to program staff at the appropriate NIH institute: Dr. Robin Barr, (301) 496-9322, NIA, 7201 Wisconsin Avenue, Bethesda, MD 20892; Dr. Milton Hernandez, (301) 496-7291, NIAID, Solar Building, Bethesda, MD 20892; Dr. Richard Lymn, (301) 594-5128, NIAMS, Building 45, Bethesda, MD 20892; Dr. Lester Gorelic, (301) 496-8580, NCI, Executive Plaza N, Bethesda, MD 20892; Dr. Donna Vogel, (301) 496-6515, NICHD, Building 6100, Bethesda, MD 20892; Dr. James Lipton, (301) 594-2618, Natcher Building, Bethesda, MD 20892; Dr. Cora Lee Wetherington, (301) 443-1263, NIDA, 6001 Executive Boulevard, Bethesda, MD 20892; Dr. Carol Shreffler, (919) 541-5064, NIEHS, P.O. Box 12233, Research Triangle Park, NC 27709; and Dr. Beth Schucker, (301) 435-0535, NHLBI, 6701 Rockledge Drive, Bethesda, MD 20892. PA: OD-00-003
Requirements: Individuals must have a health-professional doctoral degree or its equivalent and must be able to demonstrate the potential for highly productive patient-oriented research. Candidates should possess aptitudes for independent, patient-oriented, or population-based research (e.g. epidemiology, behavior, or disease prevention) and should be able to demonstrate a commitment to the study of diseases that occur in women. Candidates must be U.S. citizens or noncitizen nationals, or must have been lawfully admitted for permanent residence and possess an Alien Registration Card.
Restrictions: Individuals on temporary or student visas are not eligible to apply.
Contact: Program Officer
Internet: http://grants.nih.gov/grants/guide/rfa-files/RFA-OD-00-003.html
Sponsor: National Institutes of Health
6701 Rockledge Drive
Bethesda, MD 20892

NIH Undergraduate Scholarships 2737
The program offers competitive one-year scholarships to students from disadvantaged backgrounds who are committed to careers in biomedical, behavioral, and social science health-related research. Scholarships support tuition, educational expenses, and reasonable living expenses. Recipients may reapply for additional years (not to exceed four scholarship years).The program is designed to improve access to education leading to research careers for those who have had fewer opportunities than others, and to provide an incentive for exceptional scholars to pursue research careers at the NIH. For each full or partial scholarship year, the recipient will incur two types of service obligation: 10-week summer laboratory experience; and employment at the NIH after graduation. Guidelines are available online.
Requirements: The applicant must be a U.S. citizen, national, or qualified noncitizen; enrolled or accepted for enrollment as a full-time student for the academic year at an accredited undergraduate institution; from a disadvantaged background; and must have a grade point average of 3.5 (on a 4.0 scale) or be within the top 5 percent of his or her class.
Amount of Grant: $20,000 maximum per year
Date(s) Application is Due: Feb 28
Contact: Office of Loan Repayment and Scholarship, (800) 528-7689; fax: (301) 480-3123; email: ugsp@nih.gov
Internet: http://ugsp.info.nih.gov/exesumfaq.htm
Sponsor: National Institutes of Health
2 Center Drive, MSC 0230
Bethesda, MD 20892-0230

NIH Urinary Incontinence Treatment Network 2738
NIDDK and NICHD invite cooperative agreement applications for investigators to design and implement a multicenter, prospective cohort study to clarify the benefits of the different surgical interventions for treatment of patients with urinary incontinence. This study will assess the long-term outcomes of the most commonly utilized surgical interventions to correct urinary incontinence in adult women and the utilization of concomitant medical and behavioral therapy. These cooperative agreements will support a collaborative network of continence treatment centers and a biostatistical coordinating center that will prospectively assess the outcomes of different surgical interventions for the treatment of urinary incontinence in women over a three- to four-year period. This group of investigators will develop standardized diagnostic and outcome measures that can be applied uniformly to all of the different surgical cohorts to be evaluated by this initiative. This includes the establishment of diagnostic entry criteria, identification of clinically and patient relevant outcomes, and the development of questionnaires to measure quality of life and other patient-reported factors. Inquiries may be directed to program staff at the appropriate NIH institute: Dr. John Kusek, Program Director, (301) 594-7717, NIDDK, 45 Center Drive, Bethesda, MD 20892; and Dr. Trent MacKay, (301) 435-6972, NICHD, 6100 Executive Boulevard, Bethesda, MD 20892. Annual deadline dates may vary; contact program staff for exact dates. RFA: DK-99-001
Requirements: Applications may be submitted by domestic, for-profit and nonprofit institutions, both public and private organizations; units of state and local government; and eligible agencies of the federal government. Racial/ethnic minorities, women, and persons with disabilities are encouraged to apply.
Restrictions: Foreign institutions are not eligible to apply.
Amount of Grant: $250,000-$750,000
Contact: Program Officer
Internet: http://www.grants.nih.gov/grants/guide/rfa-files/RFA-DK-99-001.html
Sponsor: National Institutes of Health
6701 Rockledge Drive
Bethesda, MD 20892

NIH Xenobiotics and Cell Death/Injury in Neurodegenerative Disease Research Grants 2739
The objective of this program announcement is to stimulate research on the relative roles of environmental, endogenous, neurochemical, and genetic factors in the cause of neurodegenerative diseases (e.g., Parkinson's disease, Alzheimer's disease, and amyotrophic lateral sclerosis). Attempts are needed to understand the contribution of environmental exposure, endogenous susceptibility factors, and increasing age in the etiopathology of neurodegenerative disease and will require a concurrent advancement and refinement of methodologies and sciences. Of particular significance may be those approaches that can be used across species from lower animals to humans. Such approaches permit a precise characterization in animal models of alterations arising from defined environmental exposures which can serve as a cogent guide to underlying cellular and molecular mechanisms. The results of these investigations should help clarify the part xenobiotics play in the etiology of these diseases. Applications that are collaborations between basic and clinical neuroscientists and/or are interdisciplinary in nature are encouraged. Inquiries may be directed to the staff of the appropriate NIH institute: Dr. Annette Kirshner, (919) 541-0488, Division of Extramural Research and Training, NIEHS, Research Triangle Park, NC 27709; Dr. Eugene Oliver, (301) 496-5680, Division of Stroke, Trauma, and Neurodegenerative Disorders, NINDS, 7550 Wisconsin Avenue, Bethesda, MD 20892; Dr. Bradley Wise, (301) 496-9350, Neuroscience and Neuropsychology of Aging Program, NIA, 7201 Wisconsin Avenue, Bethesda, MD 20892; and Dr. Linda Brady, Preclinical and Clinical, Therapeutics Research Branch, NIMH, 5600 Fishers Ln, Rockville, MD 20857. PA: PAS-99-054
Requirements: Applications may be submitted by domestic and foreign, for-profit and nonprofit organizations, public and private.
Amount of Grant: $2 million total per year
Contact: Program Officer
Internet: http://www.grants.nih.gov/grants/guide/pa-files/PAS-99-054.html
Sponsor: National Institutes of Health
6701 Rockledge Drive
Bethesda, MD 20892

NIH Zebrafish as an Animal Model for Development and Disease Research Grants 2740

The purpose of this PA is to solicit applications as part of an NIH initiative to increase support of the zebrafish as an animal model for research. The goals of this PA are to encourage new and innovative research and approaches using the zebrafish to identify the genes and elucidate the molecular and genetic mechanisms responsible for normal and defective development and disease. The mechanism of support for this PA will be the investigator-initiated research project grant (R01) award. Applications from new investigators are particularly encouraged. Inquiries may be directed to program staff at the appropriate NIH institute: Dr. Deborah Henken, (301) 496-5541, NICHD; Dr. David Badman, (301) 594-7717, NIDDK; Dr. Grace Shen, (301) 435-5226, NCI; Dr. Jill Carrington, (301) 435-0776, NCRR; Dr. Maria Giovanni, (301) 496-0484, NEI; Dr. Carol Letendre, (301) 435-0080, NHLBI; Dr. Adam Felsenfeld, (301) 496-7531, NHGRI; Dr. Bradley Wise, (301) 496-9350, NIA; Dr. Robert Karp, (301) 443-2239, NIAAA; Dr. Vicki Seyfert, (301) 496-7551, NIAID; Dr. Richard Lymn, (301) 594-5130, NIAMS; and Dr. Chyren Hunter, (301) 402-3461, NIDCD. PA: PA-01-095

Requirements: Applications may be submitted by domestic and foreign, for-profit and nonprofit organizations, public or private. The total project period for an application submitted in response to this PA may not exceed five years.

Contact: Program Officer

Internet: http://grants.nih.gov/grants/guide/pa-files/PA-01-095.html

Sponsor: National Institutes of Health
6705 Rockledge Drive
Bethesda, MD 20892

NIH/EPA Mechanistic-Based Cancer Risk Assessment Methods Research Grants 2741

This RFA solicits studies that focus on the development of cancer risk assessment methods and practices. Emphasis should be on the development of new methods and practices that reduce the uncertainties associated with cancer risk assessment, especially uncertainties that are encountered in extrapolating from animal species to humans. Studies that propose refinement, validation, or invalidation of existing methods and practices are also acceptable if they will result in a significant reduction in uncertainty. Methods of development can be based on in vitro and/or in vivo animal model systems, in vitro human cell model systems, and exploratory epidemiologic approaches. Short-term, mechanistic-based methods that can be used to augment long-term bioassays are also encouraged. A clear and unambiguous demonstration of mechanistic commonality with humans is a requirement of any method based on animal model systems. Inquiries may be directed to the staff at the appropriate organization/institute: Dr. Roy Fleming, Director, (404) 639-3343, Research Grants Program, National Institute for Occupational Safety and Health, CDC, 1600 Clifton Rd NE, Building 1, Atlanta, GA 30333; Dr. David Reese, (202) 564-6919, National Center for Environmental Research and Quality Assurance, EPA, 401 M St SW, Washington, DC 20460; and Dr. Kumiko Iwamoto, Epidemiology and Genetics Research Program, NCI, 6130 Executive Boulevard, Bethesda, MD 20892. Annual deadline dates may vary; contact program staff for exact dates.

Requirements: Applications may be submitted by domestic and foreign, public and private, nonprofit and for-profit organizations; governments and their agencies; and federally recognized Indian tribal governments, Indian tribes, or Indian tribal organizations.

Amount of Grant: $250,000 maximum average

Contact: Program Officer

Internet: http://www.grants.nih.gov/grants/guide/rfa-files/RFA-OH-99-003.html

Sponsor: National Institutes of Health
6701 Rockledge Drive
Bethesda, MD 20892

NIHCM Foundation Health Care Print Journalism Awards 2742

To encourage outstanding work from journalists furthering innovation in health care policy and management, The National Institute for Health Care Management Research and Educational Foundation (NIHCM Foundation) recognizes excellence in health care reporting and writing on the financing and delivery of health care and the impact of health care policy with two $10,000 awards. NIHCM Foundation awards prizes to the winning entry in the following two categories, Health Care Article or Series from General Circulation Publications and Health Care Article or Series from Trade Publications. The award prize will be presented to the winner at a dinner in Washington, DC in May.

Requirements: Articles must originally have been published during calendar year 2009. Entries will be accepted from all staff reporters and editors, as well as freelance writers for articles that appeared in a General Circulation or Trade Publication. Online articles will be accepted if produced and disseminated originally on the web in affiliation with a General Circulation or Trade Publication. Articles should be timely and produce new insights into health care financing and delivery or health care policy.

Amount of Grant: $10,000

Date(s) Application is Due: FEB 26

Contact: Nancy Chockley, President and CEO; (202) 296-4426; fax: (202) 296-4319; email: nihcm@nihem.org

Internet: http://nihcm.org/awards/journalism

Sponsor: National Institute for Health Care Management Foundation
1225 19th Street, NW, Suite 710
Washington, DC 20036

NIHCM Foundation Health Care Research Awards 2743

To encourage outstanding work from researchers furthering innovation in health care policy and management, the National Institute for Health Care Management (NIHCM) Research and Educational Foundation recognizes excellence in original and creative research with a $10,000 award. Selection criteria for the award includes the originality and creativity of the research. Impact that the research may have in advancing the public policy debate, improving health care delivery, management and the relevance to one or more of the subject areas. The award will be presented to the winner at a dinner in Washington, DC in May.

Requirements: Articles must have been published in a peer-reviewed journal or similar quality publication during calendar year 2009. Applications are encouraged from authors in diverse fields, including economics, health policy, political science, public health, etc. and from individuals in non-academic settings, such as research firms and policy organizations. All research articles must address some aspect of health care financing, delivery, organization or the implementation of health care policy.

Amount of Grant: $10,000 prize

Date(s) Application is Due: Feb 26

Contact: Nancy Chockley, President and CEO; (202) 296-4426; fax: (202) 296-4319; email: nihcm@nihem.org

Internet: http://nihcm.org/awards/research

Sponsor: National Institute for Health Care Management Foundation
1225 19th Street, NW, Suite 710
Washington, DC 20036

NIHCM Foundation Health Care Television and Radio Journalism Awards 2744

The Third Annual NIHCM Foundation Health Care Television and Radio Journalism Award recognizes excellence in television and radio reporting on health care issues and policy. Selection criteria will include, new insights generated by the reporting, impact on health care policy and quality of writing and production. A $10,000 prize will be presented to the winner at a dinner in Washington, DC in May.

Requirements: Entries must originally have aired during calendar year 2009. Entries will be accepted from staff employees of national or local news organizations, nationally-distributed cable programs, or from freelance journalists who have produced reports disseminated by same. Online stories will be accepted if produced for and disseminated originally on the web in affiliation with a television or radio news organization. Material repurposed from other media will not be accepted.

Amount of Grant: $10,000

Date(s) Application is Due: Feb 26

Contact: Nancy Chockley, President and CEO; (202) 296-4426; fax: (202) 296-4319; email: nihcm@nihem.org

Internet: http://nihcm.org/awards/televison_and_radio_journalism

Sponsor: National Institute for Health Care Management Foundation
1225 19th Street, NW, Suite 710
Washington, DC 20036

NIMH AIDS and Aging: Behavioral Sciences Prevention Research Grants 2745

NIA, NIMH, and NINR invite qualified researchers to submit applications to investigate prevention issues relevant to AIDS in middle-aged and older populations. This announcement solicits AIDS prevention research proposals to study primary prevention of disease transmission as well as secondary and tertiary prevention of negative behavioral and social consequences of HIV/AIDS for persons with AIDS, their families, and communities. Thus, the primary goals are to identify social and behavioral factors associated with HIV transmission and disease progression in later life; examine behavioral and social consequences of HIV infection/AIDS across the life course; develop and evaluate age-appropriate behavioral and social interventions for preventing AIDS in middle-aged and older adults and/or ameliorating problems associated with older adult caregiver responsibilities and burdens; explore health care issues surrounding AIDS care; and strengthen existing research and evaluation methods.

Requirements: Applications may be submitted by domestic and foreign for-profit and non-profit organizations, public and private, such as universities, colleges, hospitals, laboratories, units of State and local governments, and eligible agencies of the Federal government. Applications may be submitted by single institutions or by a consortia of institutions.

Date(s) Application is Due: Feb 5; Feb 16; Jun 5; Jun 16; Oct 5; Oct 16

Contact: Dr. Willo Pequegnat; (301) 443-6100; fax: (301) 443-9719; email: wpequegn@nih.gov

Internet: http://www.grants.nih.gov/grants/guide/pa-files/PA-97-069.html

Sponsor: National Institute of Mental Health (NIMH)
5600 Fishers Lane, Parklawn Building, Room 18-101
Rockville, MD 20857

NIMH Basic and Translational Research in Emotion Grants 2746

This Funding Opportunity Announcement encourages Research Project Grant applications to expand basic and translational research on the processes and mechanisms involved in the experience, expression, and regulation of emotion. The study of emotion encompasses a wide range of physiological, psychological, social, cognitive, and developmental phenomena. Emotional processes can be studied in human or animal subjects. Important objects of study include, but are not limited to: central and peripheral nervous system activity in the origins, expression, regulation and modulation of emotion; the contribution of emotional and motivational systems to cognitive faculties such as perception, attention, learning, and memory; investigations of overt behaviors, interpersonal relationships, communication and decision making; and the environmental circumstances and experiences that evoke and modulate different emotions.

Requirements: The following organizations and institutions may apply: public/state controlled institutions of higher education; private institutions of higher education; Hispanic-serving institutions; historically Black colleges and universities (HBCUs); tribally controlled colleges and universities (TCCUs); Alaska native and native

Hawaiian serving institutions; nonprofits with 501(c)3 IRS status; nonprofits without 501(c)3 IRS status; small businesses; for-profit organizations; State governments; regional organizations; U.S. territories or possessions; Indian/Native American tribal governments; Indian/Native American tribally designated organizations; county governments; city or township governments; special district governments; independent school districts; public housing authorities/Indian housing authorities; eligible agencies of the Federal government; and faith-based or community based organizations.
Date(s) Application is Due: Feb 5; Jun 5; Oct 5
Contact: Janine Simmons; (301) 443-6652; fax: (301) 402-4740; email: simmonsj@mail.nih.gov;; Wendy Nelson; (301) 435 4590; fax: (301) 435 7547; email: nelsonw@mail.nih.gov
Internet: http://grants.nih.gov/grants/guide/pa-files/PA-09-137.html
Sponsor: National Institute of Mental Health (NIMH)
6001 Executive Boulevard, Room 7179, MSC 9637
Bethesda, MD 20892-9637

NIMH Behavior Genetics in Adulthood and Old Age Research Grants **2747**
NIA and NIMH invite qualified researchers to submit research grant applications on behavior genetics in adulthood and old age. The goal of this PA is to further scientific knowledge about the relative contributions of hereditary and environmental factors in the health, well-being, and quality of life of adults (age 21 and over) and older persons. This PA encourages research that will address one or more of the following: behavior genetics and cognitive functioning/intellectual ability and behavior genetics and personality.
Requirements: Applications may be submitted by foreign and domestic for-profit and nonprofit organizations, public or private.
Contact: Dr. Marilyn Miller, National Institute on Aging,(301) 496-9350; fax: (301) 496-1494; email: Millerm@nia.nih.gov
Internet: http://www.grants.nih.gov/grants/guide/pa-files/PAS-03-128.html
Sponsor: National Institute of Mental Health
5600 Fishers Ln, Parklawn Building
Rockville, MD 20857

NIMH Career Opportunities in Research (COR) Education and Training Honors High School Research Education Grant **2748**
This program encourages applications for training activities designed to stimulate interest among minority youth in research careers in biomedical and behavioral sciences relevant to mental health. This program is specifically designed to increase the participation of groups that are underrepresented in biomedical and behavioral sciences, including African Americans, Hispanics, Native Indians and Alaska Natives, and Asians/Pacific Islanders. The program is intended to support activities that allow hands-on experiences in research or science education and encourage high school students to make the choice of a research career in a mental health-related field. PA: PAR-01-009
Requirements: Applicant institutions must have a currently funded NIMH Career Opportunities in Research Education and Training Program Honors Undergraduate Research Training Grant. Such institutions are baccalaureate granting, four-year domestic, public or private, nonprofit colleges, universities, or health professional schools with at least 50 percent minority students.
Restrictions: Foreign organizations are not eligible to apply.
Amount of Grant: $25,000-$35,000
Date(s) Application is Due: May 10
Contact: Dr. Carolyn Strete, Office for Special Populations, (301) 443-2847; fax: (301) 443-8552; email: cstrete@nih.gov
Internet: http://grants.nih.gov/grants/guide/pa-files/PAR-01-009.html
Sponsor: National Institute of Mental Health
6001 Executive Boulevard
Bethesda, MD 20892

NIMH Career Opportunities in Research (COR) Education and Training Honors Undergraduate Research Training Grant **2749**
This program is intended to strengthen research and research training experiences of undergraduate minority students in scientific disciplines related to mental health. It is directed specifically to four-year colleges and universities that serve substantial numbers of students of one or more racial/ethnic minority groups, including African Americans, Hispanics, Native Americans and Alaska Natives, and Asians/Pacific Islanders. An applicant institution must propose a two-year COR Honors Undergraduate program for which six to 10 highly talented third-and fourth-year undergraduate students are selected. Proposed training programs should provide students with special research training experiences designed to improve their qualifications for entry into advanced research career training programs leading to doctoral-level or MD research career degrees. PA: PAR-01-008
Requirements: Applicant institutions must be four-year public or private, nonprofit colleges, universities, or heath professional schools with at least 50 percent racial/ethnic minority students; and be able to develop the faculty and institutional facilities in order to provide a suitable research environment and high-quality research training in areas relevant to mental health.
Restrictions: Foreign organizations are not eligible to apply.
Amount of Grant: $300,000 total
Contact: Robert Mays, Office for Special Populations, (301) 443-3017; fax: (301) 443-8022; email: rmays@mail.nih.gov
Internet: http://grants.nih.gov/grants/guide/pa-files/PAR-01-008.html
Sponsor: National Institute of Mental Health
6001 Executive Boulevard
Bethesda, MD 20892

NIMH Centers for AIDS Research (CFARs) **2750**
NIMH is interested in establishing AIDS research centers to provide support for coordinated, multidisciplinary research programs on the mental health and drug abuse aspects of AIDS, ARC, and HTLV-III infection. AIDS research centers support may be requested for up to five years. The overall aims of the center must be clearly defined for the requested period of support. Areas of future development should be indicated and justified. Annual deadline dates may vary; contact program staff for exact dates. PA: PAR-03-089
Contact: Dr. Dianne Rausch, (301) 443-7281; fax: (301) 443-9719; email: dr89b@nih.gov
Internet: http://grants2.nih.gov/grants/guide/pa-files/PAR-03-089.html
Sponsor: National Institute of Mental Health
5600 Fishers Ln, Parklawn Building
Rockville, MD 20857

NIMH Central Nervous System Effects of HIV Infection: Neurobiological, Neurovirological, and Neurobehavioral Studies Grants **2751**
NIMH, with NINDS, NICHD, and NIDA, invites applications for support of research on the role of HIV in the central nervous system and its consequent effects on behavior. Applicants may request up to five years of support. Applications will be accepted under PHS receipt dates for AIDS applications. Potential applicants should contact the AIDS coordinator. PA: PA-04-154
Contact: Brian Albertini, NIMH Grants Management Branch, (301) 443-0004; fax: (301) 443-0219; email: albertib2@mail.nih.gov
Internet: http://grants.nih.gov/grants/guide/pa-files/PA-04-154.html
Sponsor: National Institute of Mental Health
5600 Fishers Ln, Parklawn Building
Rockville, MD 20857

NIMH Collaborative R01s for Clinical Studies of Mental Disorders **2752**
NIMH invites applications for collaborative research efforts on clinical studies of mental disorders (CSMD), including schizophrenia, mood disorders, anxiety disorders, and other severe mental illnesses. This PA provides guidelines for the conceptualization, preparation, review, and administration of collaborative CSMD applications submitted to the NIMH. PA-01-123 may be obtained through the NIH grant line (301-402-2221), the NIH Web site, mail, and email.
Requirements: This mechanism requires more than one applicant organization, although multiple campuses of a single institution are also eligible. Applications may be submitted by domestic and foreign, for-profit and nonprofit organizations, public and private.
Contact: Dr. Barry Lebowitz, Division of Services and Intervention Research, (301) 443-1185; fax: (301) 443-4045; email: blebowit@nih.gov; Diana Trunnell, Grants Management Branch, (301) 443-2805; fax: (301) 443-6885; email: Diana_Trunnell@nih.gov
Internet: http://grants2.nih.gov/grants/guide/pa-files/PA-01-123.html
Sponsor: National Institute of Mental Health
5600 Fishers Ln, Parklawn Building
Rockville, MD 20857

NIMH Core Support Program for Mental Health/AIDS Research Grants **2753**
The purpose of this program is to provide a mechanism to facilitate currently funded investigators in improving and expanding research infrastructure, including administrative coordination, subject recruitment, equipment, laboratories, statistical analysis, and database management. A letter of intent is requested by December 1; full application is due by January 2. Annual deadline dates may vary; contact program staff for exact dates.
Requirements: Applications may be submitted by domestic, for-profit and nonprofit organizations, both public and private; units of state and local governments; and eligible agencies of the federal government.
Amount of Grant: $2 million total
Date(s) Application is Due: Jan 2; Dec 1
Contact: Dr. Dianne Rausch, Office of AIDS Research, (301) 443-7281; fax: (301) 443-9719; email: dr89b@nih.gov
Internet: http://grants.nih.gov/grants/guide/pa-files/PAR-03-142.html
Sponsor: National Institute of Mental Health
6001 Executive Boulevard
Bethesda, MD 20892

NIMH Curriculum Development Award in Neuroinformatics Research and Analysis **2754**
The purpose of this program is to encourage and support applications from individuals, with the requisite scientific expertise and leadership, for the development of courses and curricula designed to train interdisciplinary neuroinformatics scientists at U.S. educational institutions. The field of neuroinformatics combines neuroscience research with informatics research developed from the computer sciences, mathematics, physics, engineering or closely related sciences. It is anticipated that these courses or curricula would be useful to students and scientists who wish: to develop new conceptual approaches to basic and/or clinical neuroscientific research and analysis; or to acquire, store, retrieve, organize, manage, analyze, visualize, manipulate, integrate, synthesize, disseminate, and share data about the brain and behavior. Development of courses at the graduate and undergraduate level is encouraged. As part of this program, awardees will be expected to develop and implement the courses or curricula in their institution. It is expected that such courses and curricula will be models that could be transferable to other institutions in whole or in part.
Requirements: The principal investigator must be engaged in neuroscience research or research in computer science, mathematics, physics, engineering, or a related informatics

field. Collaborator(s) who will contribute to the interdisciplinary nature of the courses or curricula must be identified. The principal investigator must be willing to spend at least 20 percent of full-time professional effort on course(s) and curricula development during the period of the award. The principal investigator must also identify appropriate researcher(s) who will agree to collaborate on the development of course(s) and curricula.
Date(s) Application is Due: Feb 16; Jun 16; Oct 16
Contact: Stephen H. Koslow; (301) 443-1815; fax: (301) 443-1867; email: koz@helix.nih.gov
Internet: http://grants.nih.gov/grants/guide/pa-files/PAR-99-135.html
Sponsor: National Institute of Mental Health (NIMH)
6001 Executive Boulevard, Room 6167, MSC 9613
Bethesda, MD 20892

NIMH Early Detection of HIV Grants 2755
NIMH offers funds to conduct research on ways to promote early detection of HIV, and the impact of these findings on prevention. Research should look at new strategies to increase HIV testing and communication of test results to at-risk individuals, as well as develop innovative prevention strategies associated with emerging technologies in the early detection of HIV. A letter of intent is requested by February 10; full proposal is due March 10. Annual deadline dates may vary; contact program staff for exact dates. RFA: MH-00-008
Requirements: Public and private nonprofits may apply.
Amount of Grant: $1 million total
Date(s) Application is Due: Feb 10; Mar 10
Contact: Louis Steinberg, (301) 443-6100; fax: (301) 443-9719; email: lsteinbe@nih.gov
Internet: http://grants.nih.gov/grants/guide/rfa-files/RFA-MH-00-008.html
Sponsor: National Institute of Mental Health
5600 Fishers Ln, Parklawn Building
Rockville, MD 20857

NIMH Early Identification and Treatment of Mental Disorders in Children and Adolescents Grants 2756
This program supports research on early identification and treatment of mental disorders in children and adolescents. In particular, this announcement intends to encourage research on disorders such as schizophrenia, schizoaffective disorder, bipolar disorder, major depression, obsessive-compulsive disorder, and anorexia nervosa, alone or comorbid with other common mental or substance abuse disorders. PA: PA-00-094
Requirements: Applications may be submitted by domestic for-profit and nonprofit organizations, both public and private; units of state or local governments; and eligible agencies of the federal government.
Amount of Grant: $125,000; $250,000
Contact: Rebecca Claycamp, Grants Management Officer, (301) 443-2811
Internet: http://www.nimh.nih.gov/researchfunding/grants.cfm
Sponsor: National Institute of Mental Health
6001 Executive Boulevard
Bethesda, MD 20892

NIMH HIV/AIDS, Severe Mental Illness, and Homelessness Research Grants 2757
This PA is sponsored by the NIMH to stimulate investigator-initiated research that targets persons with severe mental illness (SMI) either before or after HIV infection and to expand HIV-related research to homeless persons. It solicits studies on the SMI population and/or homeless persons with special attention to the development, implementation, and evaluation of effective HIV-prevention interventions and their dissemination and translation to the community and public health service organizations. also solicit studies on the SMI population and/or homeless persons that propose improved methodologies to study descriptive/analytic epidemiology of HIV infection and epidemiology of the behavior associated with risk and the spread of HIV infection. An important objective of this PA is to encourage integration both across and within the different research areas by establishing multidisciplinary research teams and collaborative alliances. PA: PA-04-024
Requirements: Applications may be submitted by domestic and foreign, for-profit and nonprofit organizations, both public and private; units of state and local governments; and eligible agencies of the federal government.
Contact: Dr. David Stoff, (301) 443-4625; fax: (301) 443-9719; email: dstoff@nih.gov; Brian Albertini, (301) 443-0004; fax: (301) 443-6885; email: albertib2@mail.nih.gov
Internet: http://www.grants.nih.gov/grants/guide/pa-files/PA-04-024.html
Sponsor: National Institute of Mental Health
6701 Rockledge Drive
Bethesda, MD 20817

NIMH Informed Consent in Research Grants 2758
This program invites applications for a three-year research grant to stimulate investigations into the informed consent process in scientific research involving human participants. The grant is being offered because voluntary informed consent is the defining aspect of interactions between researchers and participants and is integral to the conduct of scientific research. One of the goals of this project is to bring together perspectives of different agencies, because various areas of research reflect a diversity of issues relating to informed consent. The focus of the program will be to document the degree of understanding achieved by research participants regarding the identity of the sponsoring federal agency or agencies; the purposes for which the research is being conducted; the comprehension of a study's methods and procedures; the relative risks and benefits of deciding to consent or refuse participation; the confidentiality and any exceptions to confidentiality; the implications of withdrawal from a study; and the planned and other possible use of the data. The goal of the present initiative is to develop and test alternative strategies for obtaining informed consent in diverse populations and to determine optimal ways to obtain informed consent for research participation. Additional information may be obtained electronically through the NIH grant line (301-402-2221), the NIH Web site, and by mail and email from the program contact listed. Annual deadline dates may vary; contact program, staff for exact dates. RFA: OD-97-001
Requirements: Applications may be submitted by any domestic or foreign, for-profit or nonprofit organizations, both public or private; units of state and local governments; or eligible agencies of the federal government.
Contact: Dr. John Hsiao, Chief, Special Projects Research Program, (301) 443-1185; fax: (301) 594-6784; email: jhsiao@heilix.nih.gov or jh23f@nih.gov
Internet: http://www.grants.nih.gov/grants/guide/rfa-files/RFA-OD-97-001.html
Sponsor: National Institute of Mental Health
5600 Fishers Ln, Parklawn Building
Rockville, MD 20857

NIMH Interdisciplinary Behavioral Science Centers for Mental Health 2759
The purpose of these centers is to support collaborative, hypothesis-driven basic research activities that will extend the most cutting-edge theories and approaches in basic behavioral science to incorporate current approaches in neuroscience. A letter of intent is requested by January 18; full application is due February 18. Annual deadline dates may vary; contact program staff for exact dates. PA: PAR-04-004
Requirements: Applications may be submitted by domestic, for-profit and nonprofit organizations, both public and private; units of state and local governments; and eligible agencies of the federal government.
Amount of Grant: $1.5 million maximum for full-scale centers; $600,000 maximum for start-up centers
Date(s) Application is Due: Jan 18; Feb 18
Contact: Dr. Mary Ellen Oliveri, (301) 443-3942; fax: (301) 443-9876; email: moliveri@nih.gov
Internet: http://grants.nih.gov/grants/guide/pa-files/PAR-04-004.html
Sponsor: National Institute of Mental Health
6001 Executive Boulevard, Room 7220, MSC 9651
Bethesda, MD 20892-9651

NIMH Interventions Infrastructure Program Research Grants 2760
NIMH is seeking to expand the capacity of the field to support state-of-the-art public health-oriented studies in the treatment, rehabilitation, and prevention of mental disorders in children, adolescents, and in mid- and late-life adults. The Interventions Infrastructure Program (IIP) encourages the expansion of intervention research collaborations between academic health centers and health care provider organizations that are oriented to community care, and have access to large, stable, and diverse patient populations. The purpose of the IIP is to provide the infrastructure for the support of research that has sufficient power to define standards of appropriate and cost-effective care for the diverse populations of patients with mental disorders seen in all health care settings. Applications are accepted annually. Annual deadline date may vary; contact program staff for exact dates. PA: PAR-04-015
Requirements: Applications may be submitted by domestic, for-profit and nonprofit organizations, public and private.
Restrictions: This program is nonrenewable.
Amount of Grant: $250,000 maximum, plus negotiated indirect costs, up to five years
Date(s) Application is Due: Jun 1
Contact: Dr. Junius Gonzales, NIMH, (301) 443-3364; fax: (301) 443-4045; email: jgonzale@mail.nih.gov
Internet: http://grants2.nih.gov/grants/guide/pa-files/PAR-04-015.html
Sponsor: National Institute of Mental Health
6001 Executive Boulevard
Bethesda, MD 20892

NIMH Jointly Sponsored Ruth L. Kirschstein National Research Service Award Institutional Predoctoral Training Program in the Neurosciences 2761
The Jointly Sponsored NIH Predoctoral Training Program in the Neurosciences supports broad and fundamental, early-stage graduate research training in the neurosciences via institutional NRSA research training grants (T32) at domestic institutions of higher education. Trainees are supported during years 1 and 2 of their graduate training when they are typically not committed to a dissertation laboratory. The primary objective is to prepare qualified individuals for careers in neuroscience that have a significant impact on the health-related research needs of the Nation. Because the nature and scope of the proposed research training will vary from application to application, it is anticipated that the size and duration of each award will also vary. The total amount awarded and the number of awards will depend upon the number, quality, duration, and costs of the applications received.
Requirements: The following organizations are eligible to apply: non-profit organizations; public or private institutions, such as universities, colleges, hospitals, and laboratories; and domestic institutions.
Date(s) Application is Due: Apr 25; May 25
Contact: Lindsey Grandison, Ph.D.; (301) 443-0606; fax: (301) 443-1650; email: lgrandis@mail.nih.gov
Internet: http://grants.nih.gov/grants/guide/pa-files/PAR-08-101.html
Sponsor: National Institute of Mental Health (NIMH)
5635 Fishers Lane, MSC 9304
Bethesda, MD 20892-9304

NIMH Mental Health Dissemination Research Grants 2762
NIMH invites applications for studies addressing factors influencing the dissemination of mental health research knowledge across mental health service settings. The purpose of this announcement is to stimulate research on the array of influences, and their interaction, that beneficially or adversely affect the adoption of valid mental health research findings into clinical practice; and to promote the development of a sound knowledge base on the effectiveness of knowledge dissemination interventions. PA: PA-02-131
Requirements: Applications may be submitted by domestic and foreign, for-profit and nonprofit organizations, public and private.
Restrictions: Foreign institutions are not eligible for small (R03) awards.
Contact: Dr. David Chambers, Division of Services and Intervention Research, (301) 443-3747; fax: (301) 443-4045; email: dchamber@mail.nih.gov; Joy Knipple, Grants Management Branch, (301) 443-8811; fax: (301) 443-6885; email: jk173r@nih.gov
Internet: http://grants2.nih.gov/grants/guide/pa-files/PA-02-131.html
Sponsor: National Institute of Mental Health
6001 Executive Boulevard
Bethesda, MD 20892

NIMH Minority Research Infrastructure Support Program Grants 2763
The purpose of this program is to increase the capacity of minority institutions and their faculty to conduct rigorous mental health-relevant research. The intent of the research infrastructure program is to strengthen the research environments of minority institutions through grant support to develop and/or expand existing capacities for conducting behavioral and neuroscience research in all fields related to mental health. The program provides for two types of activities: institutional development support to strengthen the institutional infrastructure and enhance the capability of individual faculty members to undertake mental health-related research; and individual investigator research support for developing research scientists to conduct small grant research activities that can lead to successful applications for funding under regular research grant mechanisms. PA: PAR-01-029
Requirements: Applications may be submitted by domestic for-profit and nonprofit organizations, public and private; units of state and local governments; and eligible agencies of state and local government.
Amount of Grant: $400,000 maximum
Date(s) Application is Due: Jun 1
Contact: Dr. Robert Mays Jr., Office for Special Populations, (301) 443-3017; fax: (301) 443-8022; email: rmays@mail.nih.gov
Internet: http://grants.nih.gov/grants/guide/pa-files/PAR-01-029.html
Sponsor: National Institute of Mental Health
5600 Fishers Ln, Parklawn Building
Rockville, MD 20857

NIMH National Research Service Awards (NRSA)—Individual 2764
A National Research Service Award to an individual supports research training experiences in mental health areas of biomedical and behavioral research. The NIMH research objective is to increase the knowledge of, and improve research methods on, mental and behavioral disorders; to generate information regarding basic biological and behavioral processes underlying these disorders and the maintenance of mental health; and to improve mental health services. PA: PA-99-025
Requirements: Applicants must be citizens or noncitizen nationals of the United States. Predoctoral applicants must have completed two or more years of graduate work and be enrolled in a doctoral degree program by the proposed activation date of the fellowship. Postdoctoral applicants must have received a doctoral or equivalent degree as of the proposed activation date, or submit certification by an authorized official of the degree-granting institution that all requirements have been met.
Amount of Grant: $14,688 predoctoral stipend; $26,256-$41-268 postdoctoral stipend
Date(s) Application is Due: Apr 5; Aug 5; Dec 5
Contact: Dr. Robin Barr, (301) 443-2530; email: rb42h@nih.gov
Internet: http://www.grants.nih.gov/grants/guide/pa-files/PA-99-025.html
Sponsor: National Institute of Mental Health
5600 Fishers Ln, Parklawn Building
Rockville, MD 20857

NIMH New Minority Faculty Scientist Development Award 2765
The purpose of this program is to enable new minority faculty members to have the necessary time and assistance early in their academic careers to initiate a program of research and to help them to become outstanding independent investigators in mental health research. PA: PAR-99-169
Requirements: Applications may be submitted on behalf of the proposed candidate by domestic, nonprofit, public and private universities, colleges, and professional schools that are engaged in mental health research. The candidate must be a citizen or non-citizen national of the United States or hold a permanent residence visa. Candidates for this award must be new, non-tenured minority faculty in their first or second faculty position who have earned a doctoral degree (PhD, MD, DSc, etc.) by the time the award is made.
Contact: Henry Khachaturian, Office of Science Policy and Program Planning, (301) 443-4335; fax: (301) 443-3225; email: hkhachat@mail.nih.gov
Internet: http://grants.nih.gov/grants/guide/pa-files/PAR-99-169.html
Sponsor: National Institute for Mental Health
6001 Executive Boulevard
Bethesda, MD 20892

NIMH Pilot Effectiveness Trials for Mental Disorders Grants 2766
The purpose of the program is to obtain needed preliminary data and to conduct studies to support subsequent effectiveness trials of interventions for mental disorders of children and adults. This is part of a series of four program announcements making up a broad-scale public health-oriented intervention research program. Projects may be funded for up to three years. Annual deadline dates may vary; contact program staff for exact dates. PA: PAR-03-078
Requirements: Applications may be submitted by domestic, for-profit and nonprofit organizations, both public and private; units of state and local governments; and eligible agencies of the federal government.
Amount of Grant: $125,000 maximum per year
Date(s) Application is Due: Feb 1; Jun 1; Oct 1
Contact: Dr. Barry Lebowitz, Adult and Geriatric Division, (301) 443-1419; fax: (301) 594-6784; email: blebowit@mail.nih.gov; Joy Knipple, Grants Management Division, (301) 443-8811; fax: (301) 443-6885; email: jk173@nih.gov
Internet: http://www.grants.nih.gov/grants/guide/pa-files/PAR-03-078.html
Sponsor: National Institute of Mental Health
6001 Executive Boulevard
Bethesda, MD 20892

NIMH Quantitative Approaches to the Analysis of Complex Biological Systems 2767
The purpose of this program announcement is to advertise the interest of NIGMS and NIMH in supporting research projects that develop quantitative approaches to describe, analyze, and predict the behavior of complex biological systems, especially those requiring the integration of potentially large amounts of molecular, biochemical, cell biological, and physiological data. These projects are expected to require the participation of individuals with diverse expertise and therefore to be of a collaborative and cross-disciplinary nature. NIMH expresses particular interest in studies using mathematical, computational, or theoretical approaches to understanding the fundamental biological mechanisms underlying behavior. PA: PA-98-077
Requirements: Applications may be submitted by foreign and domestic, for-profit and nonprofit organizations, both public and private. Racial/ethnic minority individuals, women, and persons with disabilities are encouraged to apply.
Restrictions: Foreign institutions are not eligible for program project (P01) grants.
Contact: Dr. Dennis Glanzman, Division of Basic and Clinical Neuroscience Research, (301) 443-1576; fax: (301) 443-4822; email: glanzman@helix.nih.gov; Diana Trunnell, Grants Management Branch, (301) 443-2805; fax: (301) 433-6885; email: Diana_Trunnel@nih.gov
Internet: http://www.grants.nih.gov/grants/guide/pa-files/PA-98-077.html
Sponsor: National Institute of Mental Health
5600 Fishers Ln, Parklawn Building
Rockville, MD 20857

NIMH Risk Factors for Psychopathology Using Existing Data Sets Grants 2768
The program encourages extensive and innovative use of existing data sets to study the development of psychopathology or resilience in order to guide the development of prevention and early intervention strategies. The aims of the program are to mine the full potential of public use and other extant data sets to increase our knowledge of risk and protective factors for the development of psychopathology or resilience in community-based and clinical populations, and to encourage applications from new investigators to examine these research areas using state-of-the-art data analytic procedures. NIMH encourages proposals to conduct analyses using mental health research data that is in public-use format or that is privately held by a principal investigator. Annual deadline dates may vary; contact program staff for exact dates. PA: PA-03-044
Requirements: Applications may be submitted by domestic and foreign, for-profit and nonprofit organizations, both public and private; units of state and local governments; and eligible agencies of the federal government.
Restrictions: Foreign institutions are not eligible for NIMH R03 (small grant) awards.
Amount of Grant: $250,000 maximum
Date(s) Application is Due: Feb 1; Jun 1; Oct 1
Contact: Karen Bourdon, (301) 443-5944; fax: (301) 480-4415; email: kbourdon@nih.gov
Internet: http://www.grants.nih.gov/grants/guide/pa-files/PA-03-044.html
Sponsor: National Institute of Mental Health
6701 Executive Boulevard
Bethesda, MD 20892

NIMH Short Courses in Neuroinformatics 2769
The purpose of this program is to encourage and support short-term research for the development of short courses, seminars, and workshops on interdisciplinary neuroinformatics education . This short-term training will be provided to scientists seeking to combine knowledge about the various subdisciplines of neuroscience and behavioral science research with expertise in informatics research. It is anticipated that these short courses will allow the participants to acquire new conceptual approaches to basic neuroscience research and analyses; and learn to develop unique strategies for acquiring, storing, retrieving, organizing, managing, analyzing, visualizing, manipulating, integrating, synthesizing, disseminating, and sharing data about the brain and behavior.
Requirements: Any nonprofit or for-profit organization engaged in health-related education or research and located in the United States, its possessions, or territories is eligible to apply.
Amount of Grant: $150,000 maximum
Date(s) Application is Due: Feb 16; Jun 16; Oct 16

Contact: Stephen H. Koslow; (301) 443-1815; fax: (301) 443-1867; email: koz@helix.nih.gov
Internet: http://grants.nih.gov/grants/guide/pa-files/PAR-99-137.html
Sponsor: National Institute of Mental Health (NIMH)
6001 Executive Boulevard, Room 6167, MSC 9613
Bethesda, MD 20892

NIMH Short Courses on Mathematical and Statistical Tools for the Study of Complex Phenotypes and Complex Systems **2770**
The purpose of this program announcement is to provide support for short courses or workshops to assist scientists in preparing for research on complex phenotypes and complex systems. This program announcement solicits applications for education grants (R25), which provide for one to five years of support for short courses. Support is limited to courses that are highly focused and that reach a wide audience of scientists. The program announcement is not intended for university course or curriculum development. A variety of approaches will be considered. The nature of the activity, the needs of the target community, and the course goals should determine the instructional approach. These might include new approaches, such as Web-based instruction, or more traditional approaches, such as summer workshops or on-site instruction. PA: PA-98-083
Requirements: Applications may be submitted by domestic nonprofit and for-profit organizations, both public and private.
Restrictions: Foreign organizations are not eligible.
Contact: Dr. Walter Goldschmidts, Division of Basic and Clinical Neurosciences Research, (301) 443-3563; fax: (301) 443-1731; email: wg8u@nih.gov
Internet: http://www.grants.nih.gov/grants/guide/pa-files/PA-98-083.html
Sponsor: National Institute of Mental Health
5600 Fishers Ln, Parklawn Building
Rockville, MD 20857

NIMH Silvio O. Conte Centers for Neuroscience Research Grants **2771**
NIMH invites research grant applications for centers. The primary goal of this initiative is to encourage investigators representing a variety of disciplines and/or approaches to bring to the field of mental health research the full range of expertise and advanced technologies available in the basic sciences. Centers for the feasibility of neuroscience research, centers for neuroscience research, and centers for the neuroscience of mental disorders will be represented. The letter of intent receipt date is July 1, and the application receipt date is October 20. PAR-02-122 may be obtained through the NIH grant line (301-402-2221), the NIH Web site, mail, and email.
Requirements: Applications may be submitted by domestic, for-profit and nonprofit organizations, public or private.
Contact: Carol Robinson, Grants Management Branch, (301) 443-3858; fax: (301) 443-6885; email: crobinso@mail.nih.gov
Internet: http://grants2.nih.gov/grants/guide/pa-files/PAR-02-122.html
Sponsor: National Institute of Mental Health
5600 Fishers Ln, Parklawn Building
Rockville, MD 20857

NIMH Socioeconomic Status and Health Across the Life Course **2772**
NHLBI, NIA, NICHD, NIEHS, and NIMH seek research grant applications on the cumulative and contemporaneous relationships between socioeconomic status (SES) and physical and mental health and functioning over the life course and across generations. Given that the relationships between SES and physical and mental health, morbidity, disability, and mortality have been long and extensively documented, additional studies aimed at merely describing or demonstrating these relationships are outside the scope of this program announcement. Encouraged are studies relating to appropriate conceptualization and measurement of SES over the life course, across generations, and in various population groups; specification of the processes through which SES influences cumulatively and contemporaneously physical and mental health, disability, morbidity, and mortality outcomes over the life course, and how these outcomes, in turn, impact on SES; and the relationship between SES and physical and mental health, disability, morbidity, and mortality over the life course in various population groups. PA: PA-98-098
Requirements: Applications may be submitted by public and private, foreign and domestic for-profit and nonprofit organizations, and eligible agencies of the federal government.
Contact: Dr. Emeline Otey, Division of Mental Disorders, Behavioral Research, and AIDS, (301) 443-9400; fax: (301) 443-9876; email: eotey@nih.gov
Internet: http://www.grants.nih.gov/grants/guide/pa-files/PA-98-098.html
Sponsor: National Institute of Mental Health
5600 Fishers Lane
Rockville, MD 20857

NIMH Supplements for Underrepresented Minorities **2773**
NIMH recognizes the need to increase the number of underrepresented minority scientists participating in mental health research. Therefore, funds are made available for administrative supplements designed to provide a continuum of support for underrepresented minority scientists and students. These supplements may support research experience for minority undergraduate students, graduate research assistants, and minority investigators. The aim of these programs is to attract and encourage these minority individuals to pursue biomedical and behavioral research careers in areas within the mission of NIMH by providing supplemental funding to ongoing research grants. The minority individual must be given the opportunity to interact with individuals on the parent grant, to contribute intellectually to the research, and to enhance her/his research skills and knowledge regarding the particular area of biomedical or behavioral science. Applications are accepted at any time. Copies of the specific guidelines may be obtained upon request. PA: PA-99-104
Requirements: Any principal investigator at a domestic institution holding an active ADAMHA grant that has a minimum of two years of research support remaining at the time of a requested supplemental award is eligible. In making requests, the grantee institution, on behalf of the principal investigator of the parent grant and in cooperation with the minority individual, should submit the request for supplemental funds directly to the project officer for the parent grant.
Contact: Deputy Associate Director for Special Populations, (301) 443-2847; fax: (301) 443-8552; email: sr14j@nih.gov
Internet: http://grants.nih.gov/grants/guide/pa-files/PA-99-104.html
Sponsor: National Institute of Mental Health
5600 Fishers Ln, Parklawn Building
Rockville, MD 20857

NIMH Therapeutic Effectiveness Protocol Development Program Grants **2774**
The program is directed toward the development of infrastructure and resources for investigation of effectiveness of therapeutic interventions through support of protocol design. This program has been developed in response to a recommendation of the Clinical Treatment and Services Research Workgroup of the National Advisory Mental Health Council. The program will support effectiveness trial development that will lead to large-scale studies focusing on diseases and populations of major public health significance that are consistent with the mission of NIMH. This is part of a series of four program announcements. Projects may receive funding for up to three years. Annual deadline dates may vary; contact program staff for exact dates. PA: PAR-03-078
Requirements: Applications may be submitted by domestic, for-profit and nonprofit organizations, both public and private; units of state and local governments; and eligible agencies of the federal government.
Amount of Grant: $125,000 maximum per year
Date(s) Application is Due: Feb 1; Jun 1; Oct 1
Contact: Dr. Linda Street, Division of Services and Intervention Research, (301) 443-0651; fax: (301) 594-6784; email: Lstreet@nih.gov; Joy Knipple, Grants Management Branch, (301) 443-8811; fax: (301) 443-6885; email: jk173@nih.gov
Internet: http://www.grants.nih.gov/grants/guide/pa-files/PAR-03-078.html
Sponsor: National Institute of Mental Health
6001 Executive Boulevard
Bethesda, MD 20892

NIMH/NIDA Children's Services Program Grants **2775**
The purpose of this program is to encourage research grant applications on services delivered to children, adolescents, and their families. Conducting the proposed research at one of the Children's Services Program sites (either existing sites or graduated sites) is a prerequisite for funding under this PA. This PA encourages studies of the effectiveness of treatments or services delivered at these sites, the nature and impact of routine clinical practice, and factors related to successful implementation of treatments or services. PA: PA-04-019
Requirements: Applications may be submitted by domestic and foreign, for-profit and nonprofit organizations, both public and private; units of state and local governments; and eligible agencies of the federal government.
Restrictions: Research grant funds may not be used to operate treatment, rehabilitation, or service programs.
Amount of Grant: $25,000-$250,000
Contact: Dr. Heather Ringeisen, Chief, Child and Adolescent Services Research Program, (301) 496-7227; fax: (301) 443-4045; email: hringeis@mail.nih.gov
Internet: http://grants.nih.gov/grants/guide/pa-files/PA-04-019.html
Sponsor: National Institute of Mental Health
6001 Executive Boulevard
Bethesda, MD 20892

Nina Mason Pulliam Charitable Trust Grants **2776**
The Nina Mason Pulliam Charitable Trust provides grants that focus on the areas of service Nina Pulliam supported during her lifetime: helping people in need; protecting animals and nature; enriching community life. The Trust awards grants for program projects and capital needs, and provides application opportunities three times during the calendar year. The Trust prefers to disperse funds as a one-year grant, but will consider projects of up to three years.
Requirements: Primary consideration is given to 501(c)3 charitable organizations that serve metropolitan Indianapolis and Phoenix. Secondary consideration is given to the states of Indiana and Arizona. National organizations whose programs benefit these priority areas and/or benefit society as a whole are occasionally considered.
Restrictions: Grants are not awarded for international purposes or academic research, Grants are not awarded to individuals, sectarian organizations for religious purposes, or to non-operating private foundations except in extraordinary circumstances.
Geographic Focus: Arizona; Indiana
Samples: Chrysalis Academy of Life and Learning, $75,000 for a residential program to develop self-sufficiency among young men ages 18-24 (2006); Indiana Legal Services, to continue a project that helps individuals avoid losing their homes in inner-city Indianapolis neighborhoods because of abusive lending practices, $35,000 (2005); Camptown, Inc., to send 100 underprivileged youths on wilderness trips, $28,000 (2005); St. Francis Healthcare Foun dation, Inc., $35,000 to hire an additional social worker to serve residents in the Garfield Park area (2006).
Date(s) Application is Due: Jan 4; May 4; Sep 4
Contact: David Hillman or Lee Ann Hoy; (317) 231-6075; fax: (317) 231-9208

Internet: http://www.ninapulliamtrust.org
Sponsor: Nina Mason Pulliam Charitable Trust
135 N Pennsylvania Street, Suite 1200
Indianapolis, IN 46204

NINDS Central Nervous System Effects of HIV Infection: Neurobiological, Neurovirological, and Neurobehavioral Studies Grants 2777
NINDS, with NIMH, NICHD, and NIDA, invites applications for support of research on the role of the HIV virus in the central nervous system and its consequent effects on behavior. Applicants may request up to five years of support. Applications will be accepted under PHS receipt dates for AIDS applications. PA: PA-04-154
Requirements: Any public, private, nonprofit, or for-profit institution is eligible to apply for research grants. For-profit institutions are not eligible for institutional NRSAs but are eligible for individual NRSAs. SBIR grants can be awarded only to domestic small businesses. STTR grants can be awarded only to domestic small business concerns that partner with a research institution in cooperative research and development.
Date(s) Application is Due: Feb 1; Jun 1; Oct 1
Contact: Dr. Jeymohan Joseph, Chief, HIV Neurovirology, (301) 443-3012; fax: (301) 443-9719; email: jjeymoha@mail.nih.gov
Internet: http://grants.nih.gov/grants/guide/pa-files/PA-04-154.html
Sponsor: National Institute of Neurological Disorders and Stroke
6701 Rockledge Drive, Room 1040, MSC 7710
Bethesda, MD 20892-7710

NINDS Cerebral Radiobiology and Neuroimaging of Brain Tumors Research Grants 2778
This program supports research that will increase our knowledge of the genetic, molecular, cellular, and physiological mechanisms of radiation-induced cell injury and recovery, and the sensitizing and protective mechanisms in the central nervous system under radiation treatment conditions for brain tumors. The intent of this program announcement is to encourage investigator-initiated applications to study tumor and normal brain cell injury and repair mechanisms induced by brain tumor radiotherapy including stereotactic radiosurgery procedures such as the Gamma Knife, altered fractionation and/or radioenhancing agents, using state-of-the-art neurobiological and neuroimaging approaches. An applicant planning to submit a new (Type 1) investigator-initiated grant application requesting $500,000 or more in direct costs for any year is advised that he or she must contact the program staff before submitting the application.
Requirements: Applications may be submitted by domestic and foreign, for-profit and nonprofit organizations, both public and private; units of state and local governments; and eligible agencies of the federal government.
Restrictions: Foreign institutions are not eligible for P01 grants.
Contact: Dr. Thomas Jacobs, Division of Stroke, Trauma, and Neurodegenerative Disorders, (301) 496-4226; fax: (301) 480-1080; email: TJ12G@nih.gov
Internet: http://www.grants.nih.gov/grants/guide/pa-files/PA-98-094.html
Sponsor: National Institute of Neurological Disorders and Stroke
6001 Executive Boulevard, Suite 2209
Bethesda, MD 20892

NINDS Low-Back Pain and Common Spinal Disorders Research Grants 2779
The program is sponsored by NIAMS, NICHD, NINDS, and NIOSH at CDC. This initiative invites applications directed to the study of the pathogenesis, epidemiology, prevention, and treatment of three common causes of low-back pain: herniated nucleus pulposus, spinal stenosis, and idiopathic low-back pain. The support mechanism for grants in this area will be the individual investigator-initiated research grant (R01). PA-97-058 may be obtained electronically through the NIH grant line (301-402-2221), the NIH Web site, and by mail and email.
Requirements: Applications may be submitted by foreign and domestic, for-profit and nonprofit organizations, both public and private; units of state and local governments; and eligible agencies of the federal government.
Restrictions: Foreign institutions or organizations in foreign countries are not eligible for First Independent Research Support and Transition (R29) awards.
Contact: Dr. Mary Ellen Cheung, Division of Stroke, Trauma, and Neurodegenerative Disorders, (301) 496-4226; fax: (301) 480-1080; email: mm108w@nih.gov
Internet: http://www.grants.nih.gov/grants/guide/pa-files/PA-97-058.html
Sponsor: National Institute of Neurological Disorders and Stroke
6001 Executive Boulevard, Suite 2209
Bethesda, MD 20892

NINDS Optimization of Small Molecule Probes for the Nervous System (SBIR) Grants 2780
This Funding Opportunity Announcement (FOA) encourages Small Business Innovation Research (SBIR) grant applications from small business concerns (SBCs) that propose to develop new small molecule probes for investigating biological function in the nervous system via the application of advanced medicinal chemistry and the biological testing of compounds. Eligible SBCs will have identified probe candidates via screening of small molecule collections, using in vitro assays of biological activity developed to interrogate these collections, and be able to show that the structural features of these small molecules are related to their biological activity. Applications should nominate small molecule probe candidates from distinct structural series for the further, iterative design and testing of analogues in structure-activity relationship studies, using in vitro assays of biological function adapted to the medium throughput screening requirements of this work. These studies should have the goal of developing a small molecule probe possessing the attributes (eg: affinity, selectivity, activity) required for its use in future pharmacological studies proposed by the SBC. Applicants are strongly encouraged to utilize publicly available cheminformatic capabilities for the acquisition of compounds, and semi-custom synthesis of analogues.
Requirements: Only United States small business concerns (SBCs) are eligible to submit SBIR applications.
Amount of Grant: $150,000 maximum per year
Date(s) Application is Due: Apr 5; Aug 5; Dec 5
Contact: Mark Scheideler, Ph.D.; (301) 496-1779; fax: (301) 402-1501; email: scheidelerm@ninds.nih.gov
Internet: http://grants.nih.gov/grants/guide/pa-files/PAR-09-260.html
Sponsor: National Institute of Neurological Disorders and Stroke (NINDS)
6001 Executive Boulevard, NSC 2107
Bethesda, MD 20892-9527

NINDS Optimization of Small Molecule Probes for the Nervous System (STTR) Grants 2781
This Funding Opportunity Announcement (FOA) encourages Small Business Technology Transfer (STTR) grant applications from small business concerns (SBCs) that propose to develop new small molecule probes for investigating biological function in the nervous system via the application of advanced medicinal chemistry and the biological testing of compounds. Eligible SBCs will have identified probe candidates via screening of small molecule collections, using in vitro assays of biological activity developed to interrogate these collections, and be able to show that the structural features of these small molecules are related to their biological activity. Applications should nominate small molecule probe candidates from distinct structural series for the further, iterative design and testing of analogues in structure-activity relationship studies, using in vitro assays of biological function adapted to the medium throughput screening requirements of this work. These studies should have the goal of developing a small molecule probe possessing the attributes (eg: affinity, selectivity, activity) required for its use in future pharmacological studies proposed by the SBC. Applicants are strongly encouraged to utilize publicly available cheminformatic capabilities for the acquisition of compounds, and semi-custom synthesis of analogues, which is required of these studies.
Requirements: Only United States small business concerns (SBCs) are eligible to submit STTR applications.
Amount of Grant: $150,000 maximum per year
Date(s) Application is Due: Apr 5; Aug 5; Dec 5
Contact: Mark Scheideler, Ph.D.; (301) 496-1779; fax: (301) 402-1501; email: scheidelerm@ninds.nih.gov
Internet: http://grants.nih.gov/grants/guide/pa-files/PAR-09-260.html
Sponsor: National Institute of Neurological Disorders and Stroke (NINDS)
6001 Executive Boulevard, NSC 2107
Bethesda, MD 20892-9527

NINDS Optimization of Small Molecule Probes for the Nervous System Grants 2782
This FOA issued by participating institutes of the National Institutes of Health, encourages research grant applications from institutions/ organizations that propose to develop new small molecule probes for investigating biological function in the nervous system via the application of advanced medicinal chemistry and the biological testing of compounds. Eligible investigators will have identified probe candidates via screening of small molecule collections, using in vitro assays of biological activity developed to interrogate these collections, and be able to show that the structural features of these small molecules are related to their biological activity. Proposals should nominate small molecule probe candidates from distinct structural series for the further, iterative design and testing of analogues in structure-activity relationship studies, using in vitro assays of biological function adapted to the medium throughput screening requirements of this work. These studies should have the goal of developing a small molecule probe possessing the attributes (eg: affinity, selectivity, activity) required for its use in future pharmacological studies proposed by the investigator. Applicants are strongly encouraged to utilize publicly available cheminformatic capabilities for the acquisition of compounds, and semi-custom synthesis of analogues.
Requirements: The following organizations and institutions are eligible to apply: public/state controlled institutions of higher education; private institutions of higher education; Hispanic-serving institutions; historically Black colleges and universities (HBCUs); tribally controlled colleges and universities (TCCUs); Alaska native and native Hawaiian serving institutions; nonprofits with 501(c)3 IRS status (other than institutions of higher education); nonprofits without 501(c)3 IRS status (other than institutions of higher education); small businesses; for-profit organizations (other than small businesses); state governments; Indian/Native American tribal governments (federally recognized); Indian/Native American tribally designated organizations; county governments; city or township governments; special district governments; independent school districts; public housing authorities/Indian housing authorities; U.S. territories or possessions; Indian/native American tribal governments (other than federally recognized); regional organizations; non-domestic (non-U.S.) entities (foreign organizations); eligible agencies of the federal government; and faith-based or community-based organizations.
Amount of Grant: $150,000 maximum per year
Date(s) Application is Due: Feb 16; Jun 16; Oct 16
Contact: Mark Scheideler, Ph.D.; (301) 496-1779; fax: (301) 402-1501; email: scheidelerm@ninds.nih.gov
Internet: http://grants.nih.gov/grants/guide/pa-files/PAR-09-251.html
Sponsor: National Institute of Neurological Disorders and Stroke (NINDS)
6001 Executive Boulevard, NSC 2107
Bethesda, MD 20892-9527

NINDS Pathogenesis and Therapy of the Muscular Dystrophies Research Grants 2783

NINDS and NIAMS encourage investigator-initiated research grant applications to study the pathogenesis and therapy of the various forms of muscular dystrophy in children and adults. Responses to this PA may include studies in appropriate animal models or preclinical or clinical studies in patients with facioscapulohumeral dystrophy (FSH), limb-girdle muscular dystrophy (LGMD), myotonic dystrophy, congenital muscular dystrophy (CMD), Emery-Dreifuss muscular dystrophy (EMD), Duchenne muscular dystrophy (DMD), Becker muscular dystrophy (BMD), or other forms of muscular dystrophy. Support mechanisms for grants are research project grant (R01) and program project grant (P01). Information may be obtained through the NIH grant line (301-402-2221), the NIH Web site, mail, and email. PA: PA-98-044
Requirements: Applications may be submitted by domestic and foreign, for-profit and nonprofit organizations, both public and private; units of state and local governments; and eligible agencies of the federal government.
Contact: Dr. Paul Nichols, Division of Convulsive, Infectious, and Immune Disorders, (301) 496-1431; fax: (301) 402-2060; email: pn13w@nih.gov; Dawn Richardson, Grants Management Branch, (301) 496-9231; fax: (301) 402-0219; email: r128b@nih.gov
Internet: http://www.grants.nih.gov/grants/guide/pa-files/PA-98-044.html
Sponsor: National Institute of Neurological Disorders and Stroke
6001 Executive Boulevard, Suite 2209
Bethesda, MD 20892

NINDS Repetitive Motion Disorders Research Grants 2784

The program is sponsored by NIAMS, NICHD, NINDS, and NIOSH at CDC. This initiative invites applications directed to the study of the pathogenesis, epidemiology, prevention, and treatment of repetitive motion disorders. The support mechanism for grants in this area will be the individual investigator-initiated research grant (R01). PA-97-059 may be obtained electronically through the NIH grant line (301-402-2221), the NIH Web site, and by mail and email.
Requirements: Applications may be submitted by foreign and domestic, for-profit and nonprofit organizations, both public and private; units of state and local governments; and eligible agencies of the federal government.
Restrictions: Foreign institutions or organizations in foreign countries are not eligible for First Independent Research Support and Transition (FIRST) (R29) awards.
Contact: Dr. Paul Nichols, (301) 496-1431; fax: (301) 402-2060; email: pn13w@nih.gov
Internet: http://www.grants.nih.gov/grants/guide/pa-files/PA-97-059.html
Sponsor: National Institute of Neurological Disorders and Stroke
6001 Executive Boulevard, Suite 2209
Bethesda, MD 20892

NINDS Specialized Neuroscience Research Programs (SNRP) on Health Disparity: HIV and the Nervous System 2785

The purpose of this program is to augment and strengthen the research capabilities of faculty, students, and fellows at minority institutions by supporting the development of new, and/or the enhancement of ongoing basic and clinical neuro-AIDS related research projects and programs. Applicants planning to submit an investigator-initiated new, competing continuation, competing supplement, or any amended/revised version of the preceding grant application types requesting $500,000 or more in direct costs for any year are advised that he or she must contact institute program staff before submitting the application. Annual deadline dates may vary; contact program staff for exact dates.
Requirements: Applications will only be accepted from domestic, public or private, nonprofit, academic institutions that offer PhD, MD, and/or equivalent health professional degrees, at which more than 50 percent of the students enrolled are from ethnic or racial minority groups. Each applicant institution must identify a collaborating institution that can be a domestic federal or nonfederal, public or private, nonprofit organization. The principal investigator, who serves as SNRP director, must be a U.S. citizen, permanent resident, or noncitizen national.
Amount of Grant: $1 million maximum
Contact: Dr. Joana Rosario, Office of Special Programs in Neuroscience, (301) 496-5489; fax: (301) 594-5929; email: jr69z@nih.gov; Dr. A.P. Kerza-Kwiatecki, (301) 496-1431; fax: (301) 402-4020; email: ak45w@nih.gov
Internet: http://grants.nih.gov/grants/guide/rfa-files/RFA-NS-01-009.html
Sponsor: National Institute of Neurological Disorders and Stroke
6001 Executive Boulevard, Suite 2209
Bethesda, MD 20892

NINDS Support of Scientific Meetings as Cooperative Agreements 2786

The purpose of the program announcement is to inform the scientific community that the National Institute of Neurological Disorders and Stroke (NINDS) will now support scientific meetings as cooperative agreements in addition to the current practice of supporting them through the traditional grant mechanism. This program provides guidelines for when it is appropriate to request support of a meeting as a cooperative agreement and explains procedures for preparing and submitting such applications. The Principal Investigator will have the primary authority and responsibility to define objectives and approaches; plan, publicize, and conduct the scientific meeting; and publish the results of the meeting.
Requirements: Applications may be submitted by U.S. institutions, including scientific or professional societies eligible to receive grants from Public Health Service (PHS) agencies. In the case of an international conference, the U.S. representative organization of an established international scientific or professional society is the eligible applicant.
Restrictions: Foreign institutions are not eligible.
Contact: Danilo A. Tagle, Ph.D.; (301) 496-5745; fax: (301) 402-2060; email: tagled@ninds.nih.gov
Internet: http://grants.nih.gov/grants/guide/notice-files/NOT-NS-02-003.html
Sponsor: National Institute of Neurological Disorders and Stroke (NINDS)
6001 Executive Boulevard, Neuroscience Center, Room 2114
Bethesda, MD 20892-9525

NINDS Symptom Management for Chronic Neurological Conditions Research Grants 2787

NINR, NIA, NICHD, NIDCD, and NINDS are interested in facilitating investigator-initiated research designed to deal with symptoms associated with chronic neurological conditions including stroke, epilepsy, brain and spinal cord injury, multiple sclerosis, and Parkinson's disease. The overall goals are to manage symptoms effectively, to prevent secondary effects of the condition when possible, to maximize the health potential, and to improve the health-related quality of life for patients, care givers, and families. The mechanism of support is the research project grant (R01). More information may be obtained through the NIH grant line (301-402-2221), the NIH Web site, mail, and email. PA: PA-98-030
Requirements: Research applications may be submitted by domestic and foreign, for-profit and nonprofit organizations, both public and private; units of state and local governments; and eligible agencies of the federal government.
Contact: Dr. Mary Ellen Cheung, Division of Stroke, Trauma, and Neurodegenerative Disorders, (301) 496-4226; fax: (301) 480-1080; email: MM108W@nih.gov; Gladys Melendez-Bohler, Grants Management Branch, (301) 496-9231; fax: (301) 402-0219; email: GB13Y@nih.gov
Internet: http://www.grants.nih.gov/grants/guide/pa-files/PA-98-030.html
Sponsor: National Institute of Neurological Disorders and Stroke
6001 Executive Boulevard, Suite 2209
Bethesda, MD 20892

NINR Acute and Chronic Care During Mechanical Ventilation Research Grants 2788

NINR seeks research applications for investigator-initiated research to improve the clinical management and care delivery of patients who require mechanical ventilation. For the purpose of this program announcement, the time course of mechanical ventilation is defined as beginning with endotracheal or tracheal tube intubation, maintenance of full and/or partial ventilatory support, discontinuation of mechanical ventilation via weaning techniques, and concluding with care of patients who require chronic mechanical ventilation. Two different, but related, types of basic science and/or clinical research on acute and/or chronic mechanical ventilation are encouraged: studies examining the effects of physiological, environmental, and/or psychological approaches to facilitate the care of patients during any phase of mechanical ventilation, and studies directed toward examining the physical and psychological ramifications of technology dependency on patients and their families/significant others. Priority research areas include optimum ways to deliver patient care during mechanical ventilatory support; ethical issues related to initiation, maintenance, and withdrawal of life support technology; emotional support and communication during mechanical ventilation; methods of optimally managing the artificial airway; impact of care on family dynamics; and decision making regarding withdrawal of ventilatory support. Research is also needed to describe and intervene with care-giving resources, family functioning, and quality of life for patients on mechanical ventilation particularly chronically ill children and adults being maintained on home ventilators; optimum methods and techniques to deliver nursing care while critically ill patients receive mechanical ventilation; and determine optimal measures for promoting recovery as patients move through levels of care in acute, intermediate, and long-term care. This PA covers a wide range of topics relevant to clinical management and clinical problem solving issues for patients who require mechanical ventilation.
Requirements: Applications may be submitted by public and private, domestic and foreign, for-profit and nonprofit organizations; units of state and local governments; and eligible agencies of the federal government.
Restrictions: The total project period for an application may not exceed five years.
Date(s) Application is Due: Feb 5; Feb 16; Jun 5; Jun 16; Oct 5; Oct 16
Contact: Josephine Boyington; (301) 594-2542; fax: (301) 480-8260; email: boyingtonje@mail.nih.gov
Internet: http://grants.nih.gov/grants/guide/pa-files/PA-99-003.html
Sponsor: National Institute of Nursing Research (NINR)
6701 Democracy Boulevard, Suite 710, Room 715
Bethesda, MD 20892-4870

NINR Aging Women and Breast Cancer Grants 2789

NINR, NCI, and NIA are supporting grants that focus on the unique problems of older women with breast cancer. Their purpose is to inform the scientific community of the interests of NIA and NCI and to expand the knowledge base on breast cancer in older women through studies in the fields of biology, clinical medicine, epidemiology, and the behavioral and social sciences. More information may be obtained by mail and email or through the NIH grant line (301-402-2221), and the NIH Web site. PA: PA-00-001
Requirements: Foreign and domestic for-profit and nonprofit organizations, both public and private; units of state and local governments; and eligible agencies of the federal government are eligible to apply.
Amount of Grant: $29,175-$627,861; $272,777 average
Date(s) Application is Due: Feb 1; Jun 1; Oct 1
Contact: Dr. Janice Phillips, Program Director, (301) 594-6152; fax: (301) 480-8260; email: Janice_Phillips@nih.gov
Internet: http://grants.nih.gov/grants/guide/pa-files/PA-00-001.html
Sponsor: National Institute of Nursing Research
45 Center Drive, Natcher Building
Bethesda, MD 20892

NINR AIDS and Aging: Behavioral Sciences Prevention Research Grants 2790
NIA, NIMH, and NINR invite qualified researchers to submit applications to investigate prevention issues relevant to AIDS in middle-aged and older populations. This announcement solicits AIDS prevention research proposals to study primary prevention of disease transmission as well as secondary and tertiary prevention of negative behavioral and social consequences of HIV/AIDS for persons with AIDS, their families, and communities. Thus, the primary goals are to identify social and behavioral factors associated with HIV transmission and disease progression in later life; examine behavioral and social consequences of HIV infection/AIDS across the life course; develop and evaluate age-appropriate behavioral and social interventions for preventing AIDS in middle-aged and older adults and/or ameliorating problems associated with older adult caregiver responsibilities and burdens; explore health care issues surrounding AIDS care; and strengthen existing research and evaluation methods.
Requirements: Applications may be submitted by domestic and foreign for-profit and non-profit organizations, public and private, such as universities, colleges, hospitals, laboratories, units of State and local governments, and eligible agencies of the Federal government. Applications may be submitted by single institutions or by a consortia of institutions.
Date(s) Application is Due: Feb 5; Feb 16; Jun 5; Jun 16; Oct 5; Oct 16
Contact: Josephine Boyington; (301) 594-2542; fax: (301) 480-8260; email: boyingtonje@mail.nih.gov
Internet: http://www.grants.nih.gov/grants/guide/pa-files/PA-97-069.html
Sponsor: National Institute of Nursing Research (NINR)
6701 Democracy Boulevard, Suite 710, Room 715
Bethesda, MD 20892-4870

NINR Career Transition Award 2791
The overall goal of this program is to support outstanding individuals to obtain a research training experience at the NIH in the intramural research laboratories and to facilitate their successful transition to an extramural environment as independent researchers. Annual deadline dates may vary; contact program staff for exact dates.
Requirements: Registered Nurses (RN) who are recent recipients of a doctoral degree or its equivalent and who have demonstrated the potential for a highly productive research career are eligible to apply.
Amount of Grant: $125,000 maximum
Contact: Hilary Sigmon, NINR, (301) 594-5970; fax: (301) 480-8260; email: hilary_sigmon@nih.gov
Internet: http://www.grants.nih.gov/grants/guide/rfa-files/RFA-NR-01-003.html
Sponsor: National Institute of Nursing Research
Building 45
Bethesda, MD 20892

NINR Chronic Illness Self-Management in Children and Adolescents Grants 2792
The purpose of this Funding Opportunity Announcement (FOA) issued by the NINR, NICHD, NIDDK, NCI, and the ODS is to solicit research to improve self-management and quality of life in children and adolescents with chronic illnesses. Biobehavioral studies of children within the context of family and family-community dynamics are encouraged. Children with a chronic disease and their families have a long-term responsibility for self-management. The child with the illness will have a life-long responsibility to maintain and promote health and prevent complications. Research related to sociocultural, environmental, and behavioral mechanisms as well as biological/technological factors that contribute to successful and ongoing self-management of particular chronic illnesses in children is encouraged. Because the nature and scope of the proposed research will vary from application to application, it is anticipated that the size and duration of each award will also vary.
Requirements: Application can be made by the following institutions and organizations: public/state controlled institutions of higher education; private institutions of higher education; nonprofits with 501(c)3 IRS status (other than institutions of higher education); nonprofits without 501(c)3 IRS status (other than institutions of higher education); small businesses; for-profit organizations (other than small businesses); state governments; U.S. territories or possessions; Indian/Native American tribal governments (federally recognized); Indian/Native American tribal governments (other than Federally recognized); Indian/Native American tribally designated organizations; non-domestic (non-U.S.) entities (foreign organizations); Hispanic-serving institutions; historically Black colleges and universities (HBCUs); tribally controlled colleges and universities (TCCUs); Alaska Native and Native Hawaiian serving institutions; regional organization; eligible agencies of the Federal government; and faith-based or community based organizations.
Restrictions: This FOA is restricted to studies of chronic illnesses in children and adolescents ages 8 to 21 grouped by developmental stages according to the discretion of the investigator. Studies of chronic mental illness or serious cognitive disability are beyond the scope of this FOA.
Date(s) Application is Due: Feb 5; Jun 5; Oct 5
Contact: Dr. Linda S. Weglicki, PhD; (301) 594-6908; fax: (301) 480-8260; email: weglickils@mail.nih.gov
Internet: http://grants.nih.gov/grants/guide/pa-files/PA-07-097.html
Sponsor: National Institute of Nursing Research (NINR)
6701 Democracy Boulevard, Suite 710, One Democracy Plaza
Bethesda, MD 20892-4870

NINR Clinical Interventions for Managing the Symptoms of Stroke Grants 2793
NINR, NINDS, NIA, NIDCD, and NICHD seek research applications that address effective nonpharmacological approaches to managing the initial events and subsequent symptoms of a stroke. This research would focus on reducing the impairments, preventing secondary complications, and improving the functional independence and the quality of life for the individual following a stroke. Research areas that need to be explored include, but are not limited to: techniques to improve assessment during the initial stroke event and at each stage of recovery to guide nonpharmacologic treatment decisions and monitor patient progress; interventions to manage common symptoms, such as dysphagia, aphasia, bowel and bladder problems, sensorimotor deficits, depression, cognitive and perceptual deficits as well as difficulties in nutrition, hydration, skin integrity, and sleep; strategies to determine optimal timing, intensity, and duration of nonpharmacologic treatments; methods to prevent secondary complications, improve function, and address the sequelae of common comorbid conditions; strategies to promote self-care in both activities of daily living and instrumental activities of daily living and to enhance or maintain health promotion activities; measures to enhance family caregiving during all stages of recovery; methods to improve care during transition from one setting to another and care in specialized nurse managed units; and studies on the extent to which age and pre-existing conditions, such as specific diseases, sensory, motor, and cognitive declines, influence treatment outcome and management after stroke.
Requirements: Applications may be submitted by domestic and foreign, for-profit and nonprofit organizations, public and private.
Amount of Grant: $250,000 maximum per year
Contact: Karin F. Helmers; (301) 594-2177; fax: (301) 480-8260; email: karin_helmers@nih.gov
Internet: http://www.grants.nih.gov/grants/guide/pa-files/PA-99-088.html
Sponsor: National Institute of Nursing Research (NINR)
6701 Rockledge Drive, Building 45, Room 3AN-12
Bethesda, MD 20892

NINR Clinical Trials: Collaborations for Nursing Research 2794
NINR invites nurse investigators to participate in an initiative that capitalizes on the substantial NIH resource of available study populations in clinical trials from the unique perspective of nursing research and special expertise of nurse researchers. The purpose of this RFA is to link substudies posed by nurse researchers to currently funded clinical research studies, or to link substudies by non-nurse researchers with ongoing clinical studies where nurse researchers are the principal investigators. Collaborations and consortia promoting the cross-fertilization of ideas are encouraged. The rationale for this RFA is that substudies are cost effective ways to stimulate ongoing research while capitalizing on resources expended on a parent clinical trial. Nurse researchers are to collaborate with non-nurse PIs and/or the steering committees on currently funded clinical trials where resources can be accessed to answer a clinical question or solve a nursing problem. Likewise, non-nurse researchers in various fields are encouraged to collaborate with an NIH-funded nurse researcher to access a study population in a scientific field of their choice. Annual deadline dates may vary; contact program staff for exact dates. RFA: NR-01-004
Requirements: Registered nurses with doctoral preparation who pose a research question from her/his ongoing program of research that can be answered by accessing a currently funded clinical trial, or, a non-nurse doctorally prepared scientist who seeks to answer a clinical question or solve a nursing problem using the clinical study resources where the PI is a nurse researcher are eligible to apply. Applications may be submitted by domestic and foreign for-profit and nonprofit organizations, both public and private; units of state or local governments; and eligible agencies of the federal government.
Amount of Grant: $1.5 million total
Contact: Dr. Hilary Sigmon, Program Director, (301) 594-5970; fax: (301) 480-8260; email: Hilary_Sigmon@nih.gov
Internet: http://www.grants.nih.gov/grants/guide/rfa-files/RFA-NR-01-004.html
Sponsor: National Institute of Nursing Research
45 Center Drive, Natcher Building
Bethesda, MD 20892

NINR Diabetes Self-Management in Minority Populations Grants 2795
This Program Announcement (PA) solicits applications for investigator-initiated research related to sociocultural, environmental, and behavioral mechanisms and biological/technological factors that contribute to successful and ongoing self-management of diabetes in minority populations. Applications that expand accepted intervention strategies in majority populations to minority populations are encouraged. Testing new interventions designed to promote self-management in minority diabetes populations will also be responsive to the PA. Self-management is defined as client strategies and behaviors that contribute to blood glucose normalization, improved health, and prevention or reduction of complications. The concept is broader than adherence to specific regimen components and incorporates deliberate problem solving and decision making processes. Applications are encouraged for both type 1 and type 2 diabetes and all age groups. Modular Grant applications will request direct costs in $25,000 modules, up to a total direct cost request of $250,000 per year.
Requirements: Applications may be submitted by domestic and foreign, for-profit and non-profit organizations, public and private, such as universities, colleges, hospitals, laboratories, units of State and local governments, and eligible agencies of the Federal government. Racial/ethnic minority individuals, women, and persons with disabilities are encouraged to apply as principal investigators.
Amount of Grant: $250,000 maximum per year
Date(s) Application is Due: Feb 5; Jun 5; Oct 5
Contact: Dr. Karen Huss, Ph.D.; (301) 594-5970; fax: (301) 451-5649; email: husk@mail.nih.gov
Internet: http://grants.nih.gov/grants/guide/pa-files/PA-00-113.html
Sponsor: National Institute of Nursing Research (NINR)
6701 Democracy Boulevard, Room 710
Bethesda, MD 20892-4870

NINR Management of Symptoms at the End of Life Grants 2796

NINR, NCI, NIAID, NIMH, and the Office of Alternative Medicine, NIH, seek research grant applications concerning the clinical management of symptoms and syndromes that are associated with life-limiting illness, such as pain, dyspnea, delirium, cachexia, nausea, fatigue, and depression. The purpose of this initiative is to stimulate research that will lead to improved quality of life for those at the end of life and decreased distress for their caregivers.

Requirements: Applications may be submitted by domestic and foreign, for-profit and nonprofit organizations, public and private.

Contact: Dr. June Lunney, Division of Extramural Activities, (301) 594-6908; fax: (301) 480-8260; email: Lunneyj@ninr.nih.gov; Jeff Carow, Grants Management Branch, (301) 496-7800 ext 250; fax: (301) 496-8601; email: Jeff_Carow@nih.gov

Internet: http://grants.nih.gov/grants/guide/pa-files/PA-98-019.html

Sponsor: National Institute of Nursing Research
6300 Center Drive
Bethesda, MD 20892

NINR Mechanisms, Models, Measurement, & Management in Pain Research Grants 2797

The purpose of this Funding Opportunity Announcement (FOA), Mechanisms, Models, Measurement, and Management in Pain Research, is to inform the scientific community of the pain research interests of the various Institutes and Centers (ICs) at the National Institutes of Health (NIH) and to stimulate and foster a wide range of basic, clinical, and translational studies on pain as they relate to the missions of these ICs. New advances are needed in every area of pain research, from the micro perspective of molecular sciences to the macro perspective of behavioral and social sciences. Although great strides have been made in some areas, such as the identification of neural pathways of pain, the experience of pain and the challenge of treatment have remained uniquely individual and unsolved. Furthermore, our understanding of how and why individuals transition to a chronic pain state after an acute insult is limited. Research to address these issues conducted by interdisciplinary and multidisciplinary research teams is strongly encouraged, as is research from underrepresented, minority, disabled, or female investigators.

Requirements: The following organizations and institutions are eligible to apply: public/state controlled institutions of higher education; private institutions of higher education; Hispanic-serving institutions; historically Black colleges and universities (HBCUs); tribally controlled colleges and universities (TCCUs); Alaska native and native Hawaiian serving institutions; nonprofits with 501(c)3 IRS status (other than institutions of higher education); nonprofits without 501(c)3 IRS status (other than institutions of higher education); small businesses; for-profit organizations (other than small businesses); state governments; Indian/Native American tribal governments (federally recognized); Indian/Native American tribally designated organizations; county governments; city or township governments; special district governments; independent school districts; public housing authorities/Indian housing authorities; U.S. territories or possessions; Indian/native American tribal governments (other than federally recognized); regional organizations; non-domestic (non-U.S.) entities (foreign organizations); eligible agencies of the federal government; and faith-based or community-based organizations.

Amount of Grant: $200,000 maximum annually; $275,000 maximum per two-year period

Date(s) Application is Due: Feb 16; Jun 16; Oct 16

Contact: Dr. Susan Marden; (301) 496-9623; fax: (301) 480-8260; email: mardens@mail.nih.gov

Internet: http://grants.nih.gov/grants/guide/pa-files/PA-10-007.html

Sponsor: National Institute of Nursing Research (NINR)
6701 Democracy Boulevard, Suite 710, One Democracy Plaza
Bethesda, MD 20892-4870

NINR Mentored Research Scientist Development Award 2798

The objective of the NIH Mentored Research Scientist Development Award is to provide support for a sustained period of protected time for intensive research career development under the guidance of an experienced mentor, or sponsor, in the biomedical, behavioral or clinical sciences leading to research independence. The expectation is that through this sustained period of research career development and training, awardees will launch independent research careers and become competitive for new research project grant funding. NINR encourages mentored research scientist development in areas of symptom management, pulmonary, critical care, trauma, reproductive health, end-of-life and palliative care. NINR limits the length of the K01 award to a 3-year period and generally considers career development applications only from doctorally prepared applicants who will advance the science of nursing.

Requirements: The candidate must have a research or health-professional doctorate or its equivalent and must have demonstrated the capacity or potential for highly productive independent research in the period after the doctorate. The candidate must identify a mentor with extensive research experience and must spend a minimum of 75 percent of full-time professional effort conducting research for the period of the award. Applications may be submitted on behalf of candidates by domestic, nonfederal organizations, public or private, such as medical, dental, or nursing schools or other institutions of higher education. Candidates must be U.S. citizens, noncitizen nationals, or permanent residents.

Amount of Grant: $50,000 maximum salary plus fringe benefits

Date(s) Application is Due: Feb 12; Mar 12; Jun 12; Jul 12; Oct 12; Nov 12

Contact: David Banks; (301) 496-9558; fax: (301) 480-8260; email: banksd@mail.nih.gov

Internet: http://grants.nih.gov/grants/guide/pa-files/PA-09-040.html

Sponsor: National Institute of Nursing Research (NINR)
6701 Democracy Boulevard, Suite 710, One Democracy Plaza
Bethesda, MD 20892-4870

NINR Nursing National Research Service Awards (NRSA)—Individuals 2799

NRSAs are given to increase the opportunities for qualified nurses to engage in full-time graduate study and research training; to prepare professional nurses to conduct independent research, collaborate in interdisciplinary research, and stimulate and guide others in nursing research; to promote the availability and utilization of nurses with research training in nursing and/or the basic sciences to function as faculty in schools of nursing at undergraduate and graduate levels; and to prepare nurses to conduct scientific inquiry in disciplines that have significance for nursing theory and practice.

Requirements: Applicant must be a registered professional nurse with either a baccalaureate and/or a master's degree in nursing, must be a U.S. citizen or lawfully admitted for permanent residence. Applicants for postdoctoral study must have received PhD, DN, ScD, or equivalent prior to beginning date of proposed fellowship.

Restrictions: Those on temporary or student visas are ineligible.

Date(s) Application is Due: Apr 5; Aug 5; Dec 5

Contact: Dr. Nell Armstrong, (301) 594-5973; email: armstrongn@nih.gov

Internet: http://grants.nih.gov/grants/guide/pa-files/PA-03-067.html

Sponsor: National Institute of Nursing Research
45 Center Drive, Natcher Building
Bethesda, MD 20892

NINR Nursing Research Exploratory Center Grants 2800

NINR invites applications for exploratory center grants in key clinical and basic areas of nursing research that establish a scientific basis for the care of individuals across the life span. NINR seeks to increase the numbers of research-intensive schools of nursing through this program. These grants augment the research resources in schools of nursing by facilitating the growth of infrastructure to centralize resources and facilities in a specific area of inquiry that has a beginning base of research funding. Annual deadline dates may vary; contact program staff for exact dates. RFA: NR-01-001

Requirements: Applications may be submitted by domestic, for-profit and nonprofit organizations both public and private; units of state and local governments; and eligible agencies of the federal government.

Restrictions: Foreign institutions are not eligible for the center program grants.

Contact: Carole Hudgings, (301) 594-5976; fax: (301) 480-8260; email: carole_hudgings@nih.gov

Internet: http://grants.nih.gov/grants/guide/rfa-files/RFA-NR-01-001.html

Sponsor: National Institute of Nursing Research
45 Center Drive, Natcher Building
Bethesda, MD 20892

NINR Opportunities in Genetics and Nursing Research Grants 2801

The purpose of the PA is to integrate genetics and nursing research. Currently PHS-funded investigators with at least two years remaining on an NIH-funded research project grant (R01) are eligible. Nurse researchers are encouraged to collaborate with an ethicist, geneticist, molecular biologist, or an equivalent professional trained in genetic research. Likewise, PHS-funded genetic researchers in fields of ethics, genetics, molecular biology, or equivalent fields are encouraged to collaborate with a nurse researcher. Collaborations and consortia promoting the cross-fertilization of ideas are welcome. In such cases, each participant's contribution should be identified and well-integrated into the overall design. PA-97-047 may be obtained electronically through the NIH grant line (301-402-2221), the NIH Web site, and by mail and email.

Contact: Dr. Hilary Sigmon, Division of Extramural Activities, (301) 594-5970; fax: (301) 480-8260; email: hsigmon@ep.ninr.nih.gov

Internet: http://www.grants.nih.gov/grants/guide/pa-files/PA-97-047.html

Sponsor: National Institute of Nursing Research
45 Center Drive, Natcher Building
Bethesda, MD 20892

NINR Quality of Life for Individuals at the End of Life Grants 2802

The National Institute of Nursing Research (NINR) and 6 other ICs seek research grant applications that will generate scientific knowledge to improve the quality of life for individuals who are facing end-of-life issues and for their families. Research applications may include basic, clinical or care delivery studies focused on management of physical and psychological symptoms, patient-provider and patient-family communication, ethics and clinical decision-making, caregiver support, or the context of care delivery for those facing life-limiting illnesses. In a broad sense the purpose of this program announcement is to enhance the quality of life remaining for individuals who are nearing the end of their lives. Modular Grant applications will request direct costs in $25,000 modules, up to a total direct cost request of $250,000 per year.

Requirements: Applications may be submitted by domestic and foreign, for-profit and non-profit organizations, public and private, such as universities, colleges, hospitals, laboratories, units of State and local governments, and eligible agencies of the Federal government. Racial/ethnic minority individuals, women, and persons with disabilities are encouraged to apply as principal investigators.

Amount of Grant: $250,000 maximum per year

Date(s) Application is Due: Feb 5; Jun 5; Oct 5

Contact: Nancy C. Lohrey; (301) 496-8580; fax: (301) 402-4472; email: lohreyn@mail.nih.gov

Internet: http://grants.nih.gov/grants/guide/pa-files/PA-00-127.html

Sponsor: National Institute of Nursing Research (NINR)
6116 Executive Boulevard, Suite 7019, MSC 8346
Bethesda, MD 20892-8346

NINR Research on Musculoskeletal Fitness and Sports Medicine Grants 2803

NIAMS and NINR invite investigator-initiated research grant applications to study a broad range of basic and clinical topics related to musculoskeletal fitness, exercise physiology, and sports medicine. The National Center for Medical Rehabilitation Research of NICHD encourages applications for both basic and clinical studies of musculoskeletal fitness and exercise physiology of persons with physical disabilities. The principal investigator and participating investigators will plan, direct, and perform the research. Applicants for program project grants are requested to contact the NIAMS representative as early as possible in the planning stages. PA-97-025 may be obtained electronically through the NIH grant line (301-402-2221), the NIH Web site, and by mail and email.
Contact: Dr. Hilary Sigmon, Division of Extramural Activities, (301) 594-5970; fax: (301) 480-8260; email: hsigmon@ep.ninr.nih.gov
Internet: http://www.grants.nih.gov/grants/guide/pa-files/PA-97-025.html
Sponsor: National Institute of Nursing Research
45 Center Drive, Natcher Building
Bethesda, MD 20892

NINR Ruth L. Kirschstein National Research Service Award (NRSA) for Individual Predoctoral Fellows in Nursing Research 2804

This grant program will provide predoctoral training support for doctoral students. The applicant must propose a research training program and dissertation research that is consistent with the scientific mission of the NINR. Research topics and skills that will serve as a foundation for an ongoing program of research are of particular interest. The research training experience must enhance the applicant's conceptualization of research problems and research skills, under the guidance and supervision of a committed mentor who is an active and established investigator in the area of the applicant's proposed research. The research training program should be carried out in a research environment that includes appropriate human and technical resources and is demonstrably committed to the research training of the applicant in the program he/she proposes in the application. Up to five years of aggregate NRSA support may be provided. Fellowship awardees are required to pursue their research training on a full-time basis, devoting at least 40 hours per week to the training program.
Requirements: The following organizations are eligible to apply: for-profit organizations; non-profit organizations; public or private institutions, such as universities, colleges, hospitals, and laboratories; and domestic institutions.
Date(s) Application is Due: Apr 8; Aug 8; Dec 8
Contact: David Banks, Ph.D.; (301) 496-9558; fax: (301) 480-8260; email: banksd@mail.nih.gov
Internet: http://grants.nih.gov/grants/guide/pa-files/PAR-09-227.html
Sponsor: National Institute of Nursing Research (NINR)
6701 Democracy Boulevard, Suite 710, One Democracy Plaza
Bethesda, MD 20892-4870

NINR Symptom Management for Chronic Neurological Conditions Research Grants 2805

NINR, NIA, NICHD, NIDCD, and NINDS are interested in facilitating investigator-initiated research designed to deal with symptoms associated with chronic neurological conditions, including stroke, epilepsy, brain and spinal cord injury, multiple sclerosis, and Parkinson's disease. The overall goals are to manage symptoms effectively, to prevent secondary effects of the condition when possible, to maximize the health potential, and to improve the health-related quality of life for patients, care givers, and families. The mechanism of support is the research project grant (R01). PA-98-030 may be obtained through the NIH grant line (301-402-2221), the NIH Web site, mail, and email.
Requirements: Applications may be submitted by domestic and foreign for-profit and nonprofit organizations, public or private.
Contact: Dr. Mary Leveck, Scientific Program Administrator, (301) 594-5963; fax: (301) 480-8260; email: mary_leveck@nih.gov; Jeff Carow, Grants Management Officer, (301) 594-6869; fax: (301) 480-8260; email: jcarow@ep.ninr.nih.gov
Internet: http://grants.nih.gov/grants/guide/pa-files/PA-98-030.html
Sponsor: National Institute of Nursing Research
45 Center Drive, Natcher Building
Bethesda, MD 20892

NINR/NHGRI Nursing and Genetics Research Individual Postdoctoral and Senior Fellowships 2806

NINR and NHGRI announce the availability of long- and short-term support for individual postdoctoral and senior fellowships to scientists who are seeking training that will enable them to investigate the clinical implications of human genetics research. The three-fold purpose of this initiative is to incorporate genetic research into programs of research and research training for nurse scientists; integrate nursing research with research training programs for genetic scientists; and provide opportunities for addressing the ethical, legal, and social implications of genetic research training. PA-97-039 may be obtained electronically through the NIH grant line (301-402-2221), the NIH Web site, and by mail and email.
Contact: Dr. Hilary Sigmon, Scientific Program Administrator, (301) 594-5970; fax: (301) 480-8260; email: hsigmon@ep.ninr.nih.gov; Dr. Elizabeth Thomson, NHGRI, (301) 402-4997; fax: (301) 402-083; email: Elizabeth_Thomson@nih.gov
Internet: http://grants.nih.gov/grants/guide/pa-files/PA-97-039.html
Sponsor: National Institute of Nursing Research
45 Center Drive, Natcher Building
Bethesda, MD 20892

NIOSH Occupational Safety and Health Research and Demonstration Grants 2807

This program aims to increase knowledge about the underlying characteristics of occupational safety and health problems to prevent occupational diseases and injuries. Research projects supported include causal research to identify and investigate relationships between hazardous working conditions and associated occupational diseases and injuries; methods research to develop more sensitive means of evaluating hazards at work sites, as well as methods for measuring early markers of adverse health effects and injuries; control research to develop new protective equipment, engineering control technology, and work practices to reduce the risks of occupational hazards; and demonstrations to evaluate the technical feasibility or application of a new or improved occupational safety and health procedure, method, technique, or system. Funds support career development, small grants, and competing renewal and revised applications.
Requirements: Eligible applicants include for-profit and nonprofit organizations, universities, colleges, research institutions, and other public and private organizations, including state and local governments, and small minority- and/or women-owned businesses.
Samples: Epidemiologic Study of Isocyanate Asthma in Autobody Shops—to assess the impact of isocyanate exposures on the development of adult asthma and to assess potential biomarkers for exposure to isocyanates, and genetic markers of susceptibility to isocyanate-induced asthma.; Trunk Stability and Spinal Load during MMH Lifting—to use biomechanical modeling to quantify spinal loads and musculoskeletal behavior in response to unstable events.; Electrostatic Sampling of Airborne Microorganisms—to use electrostatic mechanisms to collect the airborne microorganisms.
Amount of Grant: $30,000-$400,000; $220,000 average
Date(s) Application is Due: Mar 1; Jul 1; Nov 1
Contact: Susan Board, Office of Extramural Programs, (404) 498-2512; fax: (404) 498-2517; email: sboard@cdc.gov
Internet: http://grants.nih.gov/grants/guide/pa-files/PA-04-038.html
Sponsor: National Institute for Occupational Safety and Health
1600 Clifton Rd NE
Atlanta, GA 30333

NIOSH Repetitive Motion Disorders Research Grants 2808

The program is sponsored by NIAMS, NICHD, NINDS, and NIOSH at CDC. This initiative invites applications directed to the study of the pathogenesis, epidemiology, prevention, and treatment of repetitive motion disorders. PA-97-059 may be obtained electronically through the NIH grant line (301-402-2221), the NIH Web site, and by mail and email.
Contact: Roy Fleming, Grants Management Branch, (404) 639-2810; fax: (404) 639-2196; email: rmf2@cdc.gov
Internet: http://www.grants.nih.gov/grants/guide/pa-files/PA-97-059.html
Sponsor: National Institute for Occupational Safety and Health
1600 Clifton Rd NE
Atlanta, GA 30333

NKF Clinical Scientist Awards 2809

The award supports investigators who have demonstrated outstanding clinical or basic research potential to promote their continued success as independent investigators. Scientists are expected to devote a minimum of 75 percent of their time to research. This undertaking includes the establishment of a new Study Section which will review all proposals involving clinical research for all funding mechanisms, based on the following definition from the Nathan Report, which describes three categories of clinical research: Patient-Oriented Research, defined as research conducted with human subjects (or on material of human origin such as tissues, specimens and cognitive phenomena) for which an investigator (or colleague) directly interacts with human subjects in either an outpatient or inpatient setting; Epidemiologic and Biobehavioral Studies; and Outcomes Research and Health Services Research. Applications must be submitted electronically no later than November 30.
Requirements: Applicants must be citizens or permanent residents of the United States at the time of application. Applicants must hold an M.D. or equivalent domestic or foreign degree and must be full-time staff members of a department within an institution in the United States at the time of the award. Applicants will generally have at least five, but not more than 10 years of postdoctoral research experience in nephrology by the beginning of the award date.
Amount of Grant: $50,000 per year
Date(s) Application is Due: Nov 30
Contact: Emily B. Newell, Scientific Communications Director; (212) 889-2210, ext. 288 or (800) 622-9010; fax: (212) 689-9261; email: emilyn@kidney.org or research@kidney.org
Internet: http://www.kidney.org/professionals/research/index.cfm
Sponsor: National Kidney Foundation
30 East 33rd Street
New York, NY 10016

NKF Franklin McDonald/Fresenius Medical Care Clinical Research Grants 2810

The National Kidney Foundation is soliciting applications for the annual Franklin McDonald/Fresenius Medical Care Clinical Research Grant. Applicants should be able to spend a minimum of 50% of their time conducting research and 25% of effort in the direct care of maintenance dialysis patients and/or in teaching medical students, residents or nephrology fellows the pathophysiology and treatment of CKD, ESRD, or maintenance dialysis. Proposals are due on December 1.
Requirements: Applicants must hold a full-time faculty appointment at a university or an equivalent position as a scientist on the staff of a research organization.
Date(s) Application is Due: Dec 1

Contact: Emily B. Newell, Scientific Director; (212) 889-2210, ext. 288 or (800) 622-9010; fax: (212) 689-9261; email: emilyn@kidney.org or research@kidney.org
Internet: http://www.kidney.org/professionals/research/index.cfm
Sponsor: National Kidney Foundation
30 East 33rd Street
New York, NY 10016

NKF Professional Councils Research Grants **2811**

The purpose of the CNNT Research Grants Program is to further knowledge of nursing and technician issues in the management of kidney failure. The grants may cover basic or applied research on nursing and technical issues in the area of kidney failure; early intervention and treatment of chronic kidney disease; development and evaluation of education programs to enhance patient/family understanding of kidney failure treatment; demonstration projects related to kidney failure and rehabilitation. Letter of intent due on October 15, and full proposals must be received by December 1.
Requirements: Applicants must hold a regular membership in CNNT, a minimum of two years work experience as a nephrology nurse or technician, residence in the U.S. or its territories, written approval from the department head or facility director at the institution/facility where the research is to be conducted, and have prior research training or evidence of support from an individual with research experience.
Restrictions: Project support and stipend not to exceed 20% of requested amount; consultant fees not to exceed 15% of total requested funds.
Amount of Grant: $20,000 maximum
Date(s) Application is Due: Oct 15; Dec 1
Contact: Beverly Sneed, Grant Contact; (214) 514-3846 or (800) 622-9010; fax: (212) 689-9261; email: bevyann1@sbcglobal.net or research@kidney.org
Internet: http://www.kidney.org/professionals/research/profcouncil.cfm
Sponsor: National Kidney Foundation
30 East 33rd Street
New York, NY 10016

NKF Research Fellowships **2812**

The purpose of National Kidney Foundation (NKF) Research Fellowships is: to foster training of young and new investigators with the potential of making contributions to the understanding and cure of kidney diseases; to foster, through training fellows, kidney-related research that is of high merit; and to encourage high quality applicants who want to make a career change into academic Nephrology. The fellowships are open to qualified investigators of any nationality who are interested in a career in kidney research and who will not have had more than four and one-half years of research training prior to the commencement of the award. The one-year awards may be renewed.
Requirements: Applicants must have completed no more than 4.5 years of post-doctoral research training (after receipt of M.D., Ph.D, D.O., or equivalent degree) at time of the activation of the award. For those applying for a second year (competitive renewal), applicants must have completed no more than 5.5 years of post-doctoral training.
Restrictions: Anyone who has ever held a faculty appointment at the level of Assistant Professor is ineligible.
Amount of Grant: $50,000 per year for a maximum of two years
Date(s) Application is Due: Nov 30
Contact: Emily B. Newell, Director; (212) 889-2210, ext. 288 or (800) 622-9010; fax: (212) 689-9261; email: emilyn@kidney.org or research@kidney.org
Internet: http://www.kidney.org/professionals/research/awards.cfm
Sponsor: National Kidney Foundation
30 East 33rd Street
New York, NY 10016

NKF Young Investigator Grants **2813**

The purpose of this program is to support research in the fields of nephrology, urology, and related disciplines by junior faculty now starting their investigative work, who are often hampered in their progress by difficulty in obtaining suitable financial support for their research during the formative periods of their careers. The applicant's research and career goals must be directed to the study of normal or abnormal kidney function or of diseases of the kidney or urinary tract.
Requirements: Applicants must have completed research fellowship training in nephrology, urology or closely related field prior to the start of the grant award, intend to pursue directly related research, and hold a full-time appointment to a faculty position at a university or an equivalent position as a scientist on the staff of a research oriented institution for no more than four years at the start of the award. Recipients typically hold an appointment as Assistant Professor.
Amount of Grant: $50,000 maximum
Date(s) Application is Due: Nov 30
Contact: Emily B. Newell, Scientific Communications Director; (212) 889-2210, ext. 288 or (800) 622-9010; fax: (212) 689-9261; email: emilyn@kidney.org or research@kidney.org
Internet: http://www.kidney.org/professionals/research/awards.cfm
Sponsor: National Kidney Foundation
30 East 33rd Street
New York, NY 10016

NLM Academic Research Enhancement Awards (AREA) **2814**

The purpose of the Academic Research Enhancement Award (AREA) program is to stimulate research in educational institutions that provide baccalaureate or advanced degrees for a significant number of the Nation's research scientists, but that have not been major recipients of support. NLM's participation is confined to applications that address research in biomedical informatics and bioinformatics. Only electronic applications are accepted. Deadlines for new applications are February 25, June 25 and October 25 each year.
Date(s) Application is Due: Feb 25; Jun 25; Oct 25
Contact: Dr. Hua-Chuan Sim, Clinical and Public Health Informatics; (301) 594-5983; fax: (301) 402-1384; email: simh@mail.nih.gov
Internet: http://www.nlm.nih.gov/ep/area.html
Sponsor: National Library of Medicine
6705 Rockledge Drive, Suite 301
Bethesda, MD 20892

NLM Exceptional, Unconventional Research Grants Enabling Knowledge Acceleration **2815**

This RFA is for exceptionally innovative research on novel hypotheses or difficult problems, solutions to which would have an extremely high impact on biomedical or biobehavioral research that is germane to the mission of the National Library of Medicine. The RFA supports new projects, not continuation of projects that have already been initiated. For the EUREKA program, NLM seeks innovative applications in the following two discovery science areas: integrated discovery mining for biology and medicine; and integrated hypothesis testing for biology and medicine. Only electronic applications are accepted. The deadline for Letter of Intent is September 29, and the deadline for new applications is October 28.
Restrictions: This grant does not support pilot projects, i.e., projects of limited scope that are designed primarily to generate data that will enable the PI to seek other funding opportunities.
Date(s) Application is Due: Sep 29; Oct 28
Contact: Dr. Valerie Florance; (301) 594-5983; fax: (301) 402-1384; email: florancev@mail.nih.gov
Internet: http://www.nlm.nih.gov/ep/eureka.html
Sponsor: National Library of Medicine
6705 Rockledge Drive, Suite 301
Bethesda, MD 20892

NLM Exploratory/Developmental Grants **2816**

The purpose of this program is to support for early stage conceptual work and feasibility tests in biomedical informatics and bioinformatics. These studies may involve considerable risk but may lead to a breakthrough in a particular area, or to the development of novel techniques or approaches that could have major impact on a field of biomedical, behavioral, or clinical research. Preliminary data are not required, but applicants are urged to provide milestones by which progress on the project can be measured. Only electronic applications are accepted. Deadlines for new applications are February 16, June 16 and October 16 each year. Deadlines for revised applications are March 16, July 16 and November 16 each year.
Date(s) Application is Due: Feb 16; Mar 16; Jun 16; Jul 16; Oct 16; Nov 16
Contact: Dr. Hua-Chuan Sim, Clinical and Public Health Informatics; (301) 594-5983; fax: (301) 402-1384; email: simh@mail.nih.gov;; Dr. Jane Ye, Bioinformatics and Computational Biology; (301) 594-5983; fax: (301) 402-1384; email: yej@mail.nih.gov
Internet: http://www.nlm.nih.gov/ep/GrantExDev.html
Sponsor: National Library of Medicine
6705 Rockledge Drive, Suite 301
Bethesda, MD 20892

NLM Express Research Grants in Biomedical Informatics and Bioinformatics **2817**

The purpose of the program is to provide support for rigorous scientific research in biomedical informatics and bioinformatics. NLM Express Research Grant applications are limited to a 15-page research plan and to a modular budget. The scope of interests is outlined in the funding opportunity announcement. Investigators whose needs are not met by this announcement can also apply through the NIH Parent R01 (PA 07-070), with a cover letter requesting assignment to NLM. Those who do so should use PAR 08-080 as a source of guidance about NLM's research grant priorities and scope of interest. Deadlines for new applications are February 5, June 5 and October 5 each year. Deadlines for revised applications are March 5, July 5 and November 5 each year.
Date(s) Application is Due: Feb 5; Mar 5; Jun 5; Jul 5; Oct 5; Nov 5
Contact: Dr. Hua-Chuan Sim, Clinical and Public Health Informatics; (301) 594-5983; fax: (301) 402-1384; email: simh@mail.nih.gov;; Dr. Jane Ye, Bioinformatics and Computational Biology; (301) 594-5983; fax: (301) 402-1384; email: yej@mail.nih.gov
Internet: http://www.nlm.nih.gov/ep/GrantResearch.html
Sponsor: National Library of Medicine
6705 Rockledge Drive, Suite 301
Bethesda, MD 20892

NLM Grants for Scholarly Works in Biomedicine and Health **2818**

Small grants are awarded for up to three years to provide short-term assistance for the preparation of book-length manuscripts and, in some cases, the publication of important scientific information needed by U.S. health professionals. Grants are awarded for major critical reviews and analyses of current developments in important areas of the health sciences, historical studies, works about health sciences informatics, librarianship, and certain kinds of secondary information and literature tools in the health sciences. Publication may be in formats other than print-on-paper (e.g., electronic, film, etc.), and may involve new and innovative ways of organizing and presenting information. Only electronic applications are accepted.
Requirements: Grants may be made to public or private, nonprofit institutions on behalf of a principal investigator; or to unaffiliated individuals to support salaries, consultant fees, equipment and supplies, travel, and other justified costs.

Restrictions: The program does not support textbooks, the production of curriculum materials, the initial reporting of original biomedical scientific research findings, proceedings of annual meetings, projects highly likely to have substantial commercial sales (best-seller type publications), or projects of local interest only. The program does not provide support for the free distribution of publications resulting from grants.
Amount of Grant: $50,000 maximum direct annual costs for up to three years
Date(s) Application is Due: Feb 2
Contact: Dr. Hua-Chuan Sim, Clinical and Public Health Informatics; (301) 594-5983; fax: (301) 402-1384; email: simh@mail.nih.gov
Internet: http://www.nlm.nih.gov/ep/GrantPubs.html
Sponsor: National Library of Medicine
6705 Rockledge Drive, Suite 301
Bethesda, MD 20892

NLM Informatics Conference Grants **2819**
The purpose of the program is to provide support for scientific meetings, conferences, and workshops that are relevant to scientific development in biomedical informatics, bioinformatics, computational biology, and information sciences. The typical award is $10,000 per year in direct costs. The maximum amount that can be requested for a single year is $20,000 in direct costs. Only electronic applications are accepted.
Restrictions: NLM will not support the annual meeting for an organization.
Amount of Grant: $20,000 maximum
Date(s) Application is Due: Apr 12; Aug 12; Dec 12
Contact: Dr. Hua-Chuan Sim, Clinical and Public Health Informatics; (301) 594-5983; fax: (301) 402-1384; email: simh@mail.nih.gov;; Dr. Jane Ye, Bioinformatics and Computational Biology; (301) 594-5983; fax: (301) 402-1384; email: yej@mail.nih.gov
Internet: http://www.nlm.nih.gov/ep/GrantConf.html
Sponsor: National Library of Medicine
6705 Rockledge Drive, Suite 301
Bethesda, MD 20892

NLM Internet Connection for Medical Institutions Grants **2820**
NLM encourages the development of a communications infrastructure to promote the rapid interchange of medical information nationally and throughout the world. Internet access provides health professionals engaged in education, research, clinical care, and administration with a means of accessing remote databases and libraries, transferring files and images, and interacting with colleagues throughout the world. To accelerate the pace with which health-related institutions become part of the electronic information web, NLM offers grants to support Internet connections. Funds may be used for the purchase and installation of a gateway system and associated connection hardware. Funds may also be used to defray the cost of installation and leasing of communication circuits to connect the network. Annual deadline dates may vary; contact the program office for exact dates.
Requirements: Domestic public and private nonprofit institutions working in health sciences administration, education research, and/or clinical care services can apply for these grants. Groups that are health-related institutions are also encouraged to apply.
Amount of Grant: $30,000 maximum for a single institution; $50,000 maximum for a group of institutions
Contact: Dr. Hua-Chuan Sim, Clinical and Public Health Informatics; (301) 594-5983; fax: (301) 402-1384; email: simh@mail.nih.gov;; Dr. Jane Ye, Bioinformatics and Computational Biology; (301) 594-5983; fax: (301) 402-1384; email: yej@mail.nih.gov
Internet: http://grants.nih.gov/grants/guide/rfa-files/RFA-LM-00-001.html
Sponsor: National Library of Medicine
8600 Rockville Pike, Building 38A
Bethesda, MD 20894

NLM Limited Competition for Continuation of Biomedical Informatics Bioinformatics Resource Grants **2821**
This limited competition funding opportunity announcement (FOA) solicits competitive renewal applications from investigators currently supported under PAR-04-142, NLM Resource Grant in Biomedical Informatics/Bioinformatics (P41) or its predecessors. NLM's Biomedical Informatics/Bioinformatics Resource Grant program provides support for five (5) resource centers that support activities, databases or software tools that advance research or practice in the biomedical sciences, clinical medicine or health services research. Direct costs for the first year may not exceed 5% above the current award of the active year of NLM funding at the time of application, or a maximum of $500,000, whichever is smaller. Applicants may include cost-of-living increases of up to 3% per year for direct costs in future years. The deadline for Letters of Intent is July 28, while the deadline for Renewal Applications is August 27.
Date(s) Application is Due: Jul 28; Aug 27
Contact: Dr. Valerie Florance; (301) 594-5983; fax: (301) 402-1384; email: florancev@mail.nih.gov
Internet: http://www.nlm.nih.gov/ep/grantp41.html
Sponsor: National Library of Medicine
6705 Rockledge Drive, Suite 301
Bethesda, MD 20892

NLM Manufacturing Processes of Medical, Dental, and Biological Technologies (SBIR) Grants **2822**
NLM is encouraging eligible United States small business concerns to submit SBIR and STTR Phase I, Phase II, and Fast-Track grant applications whose biomedical research is related to advanced processing, manufacturing processes, equipment and systems, and manufacturing workforce skills and protection. Only electronic applications are accepted.
Date(s) Application is Due: Apr 5; Aug 5; Dec 5
Contact: Dr. Jane Ye, Bioinformatics and Computational Biology; (301) 594-5983; fax: (301) 402-1384; email: yej@mail.nih.gov
Internet: http://www.nlm.nih.gov/ep/grantsbmanu.html
Sponsor: National Library of Medicine
6705 Rockledge Drive, Suite 301
Bethesda, MD 20892

NLM New Technologies for Liver Disease Grants **2823**
The goal of this announcement is to enlist members of the small business research community in advancing means of diagnosis, treatment and prevention of liver disease and facilitate the goals outlined in the trans-NIH Action Plan for Liver Disease Research. Annual deadline dates are April 5, August 5 and December 5.
Date(s) Application is Due: Apr 5; Aug 5; Dec 5
Contact: Dr. Jane Ye, Bioinformatics and Computational Biology; (301) 594-5983; fax: (301) 402-1384; email: yej@mail.nih.gov
Internet: http://www.nlm.nih.gov/ep/grantsbliver.html
Sponsor: National Library of Medicine
6705 Rockledge Drive, Suite 301
Bethesda, MD 20892

NLM Predictive Multiscale Models of the Physiome in Health and Disease Grants **2824**
The goal of this funding opportunity announcement (FOA) is to move the field of biomedical computational modeling forward through the development of more realistic and predictive models of health and disease. NIH recognizes the need for sophisticated, predictive, computational models of development and disease that encompass multiple biological scales. These models may be designed to uncover biological mechanisms or to make predictions about clinical outcome and may draw on a variety of data sources including relevant clinical data. Ultimately the models and the information derived from their use will enable researchers and clinicians to better understand, prevent, diagnose and treat the diseases or aberrations in normal development. Specifically this FOA solicits the development of predictive multiscale models of health and disease states that must include higher scales of the physiome. The specific objectives are to develop multiscale models that are physiologically mechanistic and biomedically relevant, to bring together modeling and biomedical expertise to collaborate on building models, to validate and test models with standard datasets, and to develop models that can be explicitly shared with other modelers.
Date(s) Application is Due: Jan 14; May 14; Sep 15
Contact: Dr. Jane Ye, Bioinformatics and Computational Biology; (301) 594-5983; fax: (301) 402-1384; email: yej@mail.nih.gov
Internet: http://www.nlm.nih.gov/ep/predictive.html
Sponsor: National Library of Medicine
6705 Rockledge Drive, Suite 301
Bethesda, MD 20892

NLM Research Project Grants **2825**
The primary purpose of this program is to provide support for rigorous scientific research in biomedical informatics and bioinformatics. Medical informatics is an interdisciplinary field that combines health sciences specialty areas with the information and computer sciences, computational linguistics, and decision theory, among others. NLM's program emphasizes knowledge issues without restriction as to specific categorical diseases. Proposed research must be clearly health relevant. Areas of interest include knowledge representation, more effective human-machine interfaces, and more efficient information storage and retrieval. The cognitive aspects of information-related behaviors are of particular interest. This area includes problems of medical decision analysis, medical decision support systems, and retrieval from image databases. Deadlines for new applications are February 5, June 5 and October 5 each year. Deadlines for revised applications are March 5, July 5 and November 5 each year.
Requirements: Institutions or organizations with research capabilities in the health information fields or in medical informatics are eligible to apply.
Amount of Grant: $25,000-$2 million; $225,000 average
Date(s) Application is Due: Feb 5; Mar 5; Jun 5; Jul 5; Oct 5; Nov 5
Contact: Dr. Hua-Chuan Sim, Clinical and Public Health Informatics; (301) 594-5983; fax: (301) 402-1384; email: simh@mail.nih.gov;; Dr. Jane Ye, Bioinformatics and Computational Biology; (301) 594-5983; fax: (301) 402-1384; email: yej@mail.nih.gov
Internet: http://www.nlm.nih.gov/ep/GrantResearchParent.html
Sponsor: National Library of Medicine
6705 Rockledge Drive, Suite 301
Bethesda, MD 20892

NLM Research Supplements to Promote Reentry in Health-Related Research **2826**
Principal Investigators holding NIH research grants of the specified types (see announcement) can apply for administrative supplements to support individuals with high potential to reenter an active research career after taking time off to care for children or attend to other family responsibilities. It is anticipated that at the completion of the supplement, the reentry scientist will be in a position to apply for a career development award, a research award, or some other form of independent research support. The grantee institution must submit the application for supplemental funds directly to the awarding component that supports the parent grant. The application must not be submitted to the NIH Center for Scientific Review.
Contact: Dr. Hua-Chuan Sim, Clinical and Public Health Informatics; (301) 594-5983; fax: (301) 402-1384; email: simh@mail.nih.gov

Internet: http://www.nlm.nih.gov/ep/grantsupreentry.html
Sponsor: National Library of Medicine
6705 Rockledge Drive, Suite 301
Bethesda, MD 20892

NLM Understanding and Promoting Health Literacy Research Grants **2827**
The goal of these Program Announcements (Understanding and Promoting Health Literacy Research Grants and Understanding and Promoting Health Literacy Small Project Grants) is to increase scientific understanding of the nature of health literacy and its relationship to healthy behaviors, illness prevention and treatment, chronic disease management, health disparities, risk assessment of environmental factors, and health outcomes including mental and oral health.
Date(s) Application is Due: Jan 25; May 25
Contact: Dr. Hua-Chuan Sim, Clinical and Public Health Informatics; (301) 594-5983; fax: (301) 402-1384; email: simh@mail.nih.gov
Internet: http://www.nlm.nih.gov/ep/healthlit.html
Sponsor: National Library of Medicine
8600 Rockville Pike
Bethesda, MD 20894

NMF Aura E. Severinghaus Award **2828**
One award is presented annually to an underrepresented minority (African American, Mexican American, mainland Puerto Rican, or Native American) student attending Columbia University's College of Physicians and Surgeons in recognition of outstanding academic achievement, leadership, and community service. A committee of faculty and administrators at the college selects the student most deserving of this award and presents the candidate's dossier to NMF for final approval.
Requirements: This award is open only to underrepresented minority students enrolled in their senior year at the College of Physicians and Surgeons at Columbia University.
Geographic Focus: New York
Amount of Grant: $2,000
Contact: Programs Department; (212) 483-8880; fax: (212) 483-8897; email: nmf1@nmfonline.org
Internet: http://www.nmfonline.org/index.html
Sponsor: National Medical Fellowships Inc
5 Hanover Square
New York, NY 10004

NMF Franklin C. McLean Award **2829**
One award is presented annually to a senior underrepresented minority (African American, Mexican American, mainland Puerto Rican, and Native American) student enrolled in an accredited U.S. medical school in recognition of outstanding academic achievement, leadership, and community service. Annual deadline dates may vary; contact program staff for exact dates.
Requirements: Candidates must be nominated by medical school deans. Nominations are requested in June. Schools are required to submit letters of recommendation and official academic transcripts for each candidate.
Amount of Grant: $3,000
Contact: Programs Department; (212) 483-8880; fax: (212) 483-8897; email: nmf1@nmfonline.org
Internet: http://www.nmf-online.org/Programs/MeritAwards/McLean/Overview.htm
Sponsor: National Medical Fellowships, Inc.
5 Hanover Square
New York, NY 10004

NMF General Electric Medical Scholars Fellowships **2830**
The sponsor has established a partnership with General Electric (GE) to provide need-based scholarship support to historically underrepresented minority medical students, and to allow them to engage in clinical work in underserved communities. The program also offers eligible students an opportunity to complete a two-month elective in Ghana, West Africa focusing on areas of critical need such as HIV/AIDS, diabetes, tuberculosis, heart disease, cancer and infant mortality. Five fellowships are awarded annually. Students will be matched with a mentor for the period of the program. Travel, hosing and a stipend will be provided for students.
Requirements: Students must be nominated by their medical school deans. Eligible candidates must be underrepresented minority students enrolled in their fourth year in an accredited U.S. medical school. Candidates must demonstrate outstanding academic achievement, leadership, and potential for community-based work or initiation of innovative projects in school or community. Additionally, candidates must also demonstrate potential for distinguished contributions to medicine. Complete application requirements can be found at the sponsor's website.
Contact: Dr. Stephen Keith, President and COO of Panacea Pharmaceuticals, Inc.; (240) 243-8000; fax: (240) 465-0450
Internet: http://www.nmfonline.org/index.html
Sponsor: National Medical Fellowships, Inc.
5 Hanover Square
New York, NY 10004

NMF Henry G. Halladay Awards **2831**
Five supplemental scholarships are presented annually to African American men who have been accepted into the first-year classes of accredited U.S. medical schools and who have overcome significant obstacles to obtain a medical education. Staff members review NMF first-year general scholarship applicants and select five students who, on the basis of recommendations, personal statements, and financial need, are most deserving of these awards. Annual deadline dates may vary; contact program staff for exact dates.
Requirements: Applicants must have been accepted to AAMC or AOA-accredited U.S. medical schools for study leading to MD or DO degrees.
Amount of Grant: $760
Contact: Programs Department; (212) 483-8880; fax: (212) 239-9718; email: nmf2@nmfonline.org
Internet: http://www.nmfonline.org/index.html
Sponsor: National Medical Fellowships, Inc.
5 Hanover Square
New York, NY 10004

NMF Hugh J. Andersen Memorial Scholarship **2832**
This scholarship program was established by the family of the late Hugh J. Andersen. Need-based merit scholarships are annually presented to Minnesota residents enrolled in any accredited U.S. medical school or students attending medical schools in Minnesota. Up to 5 scholarships of $2,500 are presented annually.
Requirements: Eligible candidates must be underrepresented minority students enrolled beyond their first year in an accredited U.S. medical school. Candidates must demonstrate outstanding academic achievement as indicated in academic transcripts, faculty evaluations, by receipt of special academic honors, fellowships, awards or induction into national medical honor societies, leadership (as indicated by active participation in community-based work or initiation of innovative projects in school or community), and potential for distinguished contributions to medicine as indicated by participation in research, publications or unique clerkships. Students must also provide documented proof of financial need. Students must be nominated by medical school deans. Schools are required to submit letters of recommendations and official academic transcripts. Applicants must submit scholarship applications and include documented proof of financial need. See the sponsor's website for the required application form and further instructions.
Geographic Focus: Minnesota
Amount of Grant: $2,500 stipend
Contact: Programs Department, (212) 714-0933; fax: (212) 239-9718; email: nmf1@nmfonline.org
Internet: http://www.nmfonline.org/index.html
Sponsor: National Medical Fellowships, Inc.
5 Hanover Square
New York, NY 10004

NMF Irving Graef Memorial Scholarship **2833**
This two-year scholarship is presented annually to a third-year student and recognizes outstanding academic achievement, leadership, and community service. The scholarship is renewable in the fourth year if the award recipient continues in good academic standing. The scholarship is open only to rising third-year minority medical students who received NMF financial assistance during their second year. One new scholarship is awarded each year. Annual deadline date may vary; contact program staff for exact dates.
Requirements: Students must be nominated by medical school deans. Schools are required to submit letters of recommendation as well as official academic transcripts. Candidates must demonstrate outstanding academic achievement, submit the scholarship application (excluding proof of financial need), personal essay and current cirriculum vitae.
Amount of Grant: $2,000
Contact: Programs Department; (212) 483-8880; email: nmf1@nmfonline.org
Internet: http://www.nmfonline.org/index.html
Sponsor: National Medical Fellowships, Inc.
5 Hanover Square
New York, NY 10004

NMF Mary Ball Carrera Scholarship **2834**
This need-based merit scholarship is annually presented to a Native American woman enrolled in any accredited U.S. medical school and recognizes outstanding academic achievement, leadership and community services. Recipients receive a one-time award of $2,500. Scholarships are granted on the basis of financial need as determined by the student's total resources (including parental and spousal support), education costs, and receipt of other scholarships and grants.
Requirements: Eligible candidates must be first- or second-year medical students. Students must provide proof of admission by an accredited medical school. Applicants must demonstrate financial need and submit a current financial aid award letter.
Restrictions: All applicants must reside within the 50 U.S.A. states and provide proof of citizenship.
Amount of Grant: $2,500
Contact: Programs Department; (212) 483-8880; email: nmf1@nmfonline.org
Internet: http://www.nmfonline.org/index.html
Sponsor: National Medical Fellowships, Inc.
5 Hanover Square
New York, NY 10004

NMF Metropolitan Life Foundation Awards Program for Academic Excellence in Medicine **2835**
Need-based scholarships are awarded annually to third- and fourth-year underrepresented minority medical students who have demonstrated academic achievement and leadership. Applicants must attend medical schools or have legal residence in cities, designated each year; contact office for current eligible area. Nominations are requested in August. Annual deadline dates may vary; contact program staff for exact dates.

Requirements: Students must be nominated by medical school deans. Schools are required to submit letters of recommendation as well as official academic transcripts. Candidates are required to submit scholarship applications including personal statements and verification of financial need.
Amount of Grant: $4,000
Contact: Programs Department; (212) 483-8880; fax: (212) 483-8897; email: nmf1@nmfonline.org
Internet: http://www.nmfonline.org/index.html
Sponsor: National Medical Fellowships, Inc.
5 Hanover Square
New York, NY 10004

NMF National Medical Association Awards for Medical Journalism **2836**
In general, these awards recognize academic achievement, leadership, and potential for distinguished contributions to medicine. Specifically, these awards recognize demonstrated skills in journalism. Deadlines vary - contact the sponsor for dates.
Requirements: Eligibility is limited to African-American medical students. Each medical school may submit up to two nominations. Candidates must be in the third or fourth year of medical school and must have published articles and photographs in, or been writers, editors, photographers on the staffs of: medical school newspapers; medical students' journals; recognized professional journals; or, other accredited scientific journal. Students who have written, produced or directed health-related films, commercials or videos are also encouraged to submit their applications and samples of their work. Applicants must also submit samples of their journalistic work (articles, photographs, audio tapes, video tapes, etc.) for review by the selection committee. Entries must have been published or produced within the last three years.
Amount of Grant: $2,500
Contact: Programs Department; (212) 483-8880; fax: (212) 239-9718; email: nmf2@nmfonline.org
Internet: http://www.nmfonline.org/index.html
Sponsor: National Medical Fellowships, Inc.
5 Hanover Square
New York, NY 10004

NMF National Medical Association Emerging Scholar Awards **2837**
The National Medical Association and NMF sponsor need-based award programs that recognize and reward African American medical students for special achievements, academic excellence, leadership, and potential for outstanding contributions to medicine. The NMA Emerging Scholar Awards are presented to current first, second, and third-year medical students.
Requirements: Eligibility for these awards is limited to African-American medical students. Each school may submit two nominations. Applicants must demonstrate and document financial need. Deadlines vary - contact the sponsor for specific dates.
Amount of Grant: $2,250
Contact: Programs Department; (212) 483-8880; email: nmf1@nmfonline.org
Internet: http://www.nmfonline.org/index.html
Sponsor: National Medical Fellowships, Inc.
5 Hanover Square
New York, NY 10004

NMF National Medical Association Patti LaBelle Award **2838**
This award is one of the highest honors presented to students by the National Medical Association. It recognizes academic achievement, leadership and potential for distinguished contributions to medicine. This award is presented to current first-, second-, and third-year medical students with demonstrated financial need.
Requirements: Eligibility is limited to African-American medical students. Application materials must include a letter of recommendation that fully discusses the candidate's academic performance, extracurricular activities and other qualifications; a complete scholarship application form; an essay of at least 500 words discussing the applicant's motivation for a career in medicine and plans over the next ten years; and, an official academic transcript.
Amount of Grant: $5,000
Contact: Programs Department; (212) 483-8880; fax: (212) 483-8897; email: nmf1@nmfonline.org
Internet: http://www.nmfonline.org/index.html
Sponsor: National Medical Fellowships, Inc.
5 Hanover Square
New York, NY 10004

NMF Need-Based Scholarships **2839**
The program provides financial assistance to United States citizens from groups currently underrepresetned in the medical profession; specifically, African-Americans, Mexican-Americans, Native Americans, Alaska Natives, Native Hawaiians, and mainland Puerto Ricans who permanently reside within the 50 U.S. states. These awards are offered to first- and second-year medical students. Scholarships are granted on the basis of financial need as determined by the student's total resources (including parental and spousal support), cost of education, and receipt of other scholarships and grants. Awards have ranged from $500 to $10,000.
Requirements: Applicants must be U.S. citizens by the application deadline and must have been accepted to AAMC or AOA-accredited U.S. medical schools for study leading to M.D. or D.O. degrees. The application form and FAQs can be found at the sponsor's website. Applicants must demonstrate and document financial need by submitted complete copies of their parents', spouse's and their own most recent 1040, 1040A or 1040EZ tax forms. All nontaxable income (e.g. AFDC, ADC, Social Security benefits, etc.) must also be documented by the appropriate agency. Applicants with neither taxable nor nontaxable income must provide verification of means of support. All parental financial data must be submitted in order to evaluate dependent status.
Amount of Grant: $500 -$10,000
Date(s) Application is Due: Aug 31
Contact: Programs Department; (212) 483-8880 ext 304; fax: (212) 483-8897; email: NMF1@NMFonline.org or info@NMFonline.org
Internet: http://www.nmfonline.org/programs.html
Sponsor: National Medical Fellowships, Inc.
5 Hanover Square
New York, NY 10004

NMF Ralph W. Ellison Prize **2840**
The prize is presented to a graduating underrepresented medical student who has demonstrated outstanding academic achievement, leadership, and potential to make significant contributions to medicine. One prize is presented each year (nonrenewable) and includes a certificate of merit and a stipend. Annual deadline date may vary; contact program staff for exact dates.
Requirements: African-Americans, mainland Puerto Ricans, Mexican-Americans, Native Hawaiians, Alaska Natives, and American Indians who are U.S. citizens attending M.D. degree-granting institutions accredited by the Liaison Committee on Medical Education of the Association of American Medical Colleges, or in D.O. degree-granting colleges of osteopathic medicine accredited by the Bureau of Professional Education of the American Osteopathic Association are eligible.
Amount of Grant: $500
Contact: Programs Department; (212) 483-8880; fax: (212) 483-8897; email: nmf1@nmfonline.org
Internet: http://www.nmfonline.org/index.html
Sponsor: National Medical Fellowships, Inc.
5 Hanover Square
New York, NY 10004

NMF William and Charlotte Cadbury Award **2841**
This award is presented annually to a senior, underrepresented student enrolled in an accredited U.S. medical school. Candidates must demonstrate outstanding academic achievement, leadership, and community service. A certificate of merit is included in the award. Annual deadline dates may vary; contact program staff for exact dates.
Requirements: Students must be nominated by medical school deans. Schools are required to submit letters of recommendation and official academic transcripts for each candidate. Competition is open to senior, underrepresented minority students enrolled in accredited U.S. medical schools. Candidates must demonstrate outstanding academic achievement and leadership.
Amount of Grant: $2,000
Contact: Programs Department; (212) 483-8880; fax: (212) 483-8897; email: nmf1@nmfonline.org
Internet: http://www.nmfonline.org/index.html
Sponsor: National Medical Fellowships, Inc.
5 Hanover Square
New York, NY 10004

NMSS Daniel Haughton Senior Faculty Awards **2842**
The award is granted to established investigators seeking support for specialized training in a field which they are not currently expert, inasmuch as such training will enhance their capacity to conduct research related to multiple sclerosis. Awards may be used for sabbatical support.
Date(s) Application is Due: Feb 13
Contact: Dr. Timothy Coetzee, Director, Research Training Programs, (212) 476-0478; email: timothy.coetzee@nmss.org
Internet: http://www.nationalmssociety.org/Research-srfaculty.asp
Sponsor: National Multiple Sclerosis Society
733 Third Avenue
New York, NY 10017

NMSS Harry Weaver Neuroscience Scholar Awards **2843**
These junior faculty awards provide higher support for qualified candidates who have concluded their research training and begun academic careers as independent investigators in areas of the neurosciences related to multiple sclerosis. The awards are designed to provide salary and grant support for a five-year period, thus permitting the awardee to establish competence in his/her chosen research area. Candidates may request up to 75 percent annual salary support, not to exceed $50,000 in the first year of the award, with a 5 percent annual increase in each of the remaining four years. Research support of $25,000 may be requested in the first year and up to $35,000 in the last year.
Requirements: Candidate must hold the MD, PhD, or equivalent with no more than five years of independent research experience and must have been offered a position equivalent to assistant professor at an approved institution.
Date(s) Application is Due: Feb 1
Contact: Timothy Coetzee, Director, Research Training Programs, (212) 476-0478; email: timothy.coetzee@nmss.org
Internet: http://www.nationalmssociety.org/Research-jrfaculty.asp
Sponsor: National Multiple Sclerosis Society
733 Third Avenue
New York, NY 10017-3288

NMSS Research Grants 2844
Grants are awarded for fundamental or applied research in scientific areas pertinent to multiple sclerosis. Grants are available for clinical or nonclinical studies, providing they show a reasonable relevance to the society's interests. Annual deadline dates may vary; contact program staff for exact dates.
Requirements: Qualified investigators affiliated with appropriate institutions are eligible to apply. Institutions are the official recipients of the grants.
Amount of Grant: $35,568-$51,036
Date(s) Application is Due: Feb 1; Aug 3
Contact: Dr. Patricia O'Looney, Research Programs Department, (212) 476-0413; fax: (212) 986-7981; email: patricia.olooney@nmss.org
Internet: http://www.nationalmssociety.org/Research-Grants.asp
Sponsor: National Multiple Sclerosis Society
733 Third Avenue
New York, NY 10017-3288

NMSS Scholarships 2845
The society awards unrestricted scholarships to defray expenses related to post-high school education. Decisions are based on financial need, an academic record that shows the applicant is able to succeed in his or her chosen area, and on a personal essay discussing the impact of multiple sclerosis (MS) on the applicant's life.
Requirements: Application is open to high school seniors who have MS; high school seniors who have a parent or guardian with MS; and adults with MS who have never enrolled in a postsecondary institution.
Amount of Grant: $2000-$3000
Date(s) Application is Due: Mar 1
Contact: c/o Scholarship America, (800) 344-4467 or (510) 268-0572; email: info@msconnection.org
Internet: http://www.nationalmssociety.org/can/event/event_detail.asp?e=8108#scholarship
Sponsor: National Multiple Sclerosis Society
P.O. Box 297, 1505 Riverview Road
Saint Peter, MN 56082 56082

NMSS Sylvia Lawry Physician Fellowships 2846
The society welcomes applications for support of physicians for training in key elements associated with conducting multiple sclerosis clinical trials. The purpose of this award is to help maintain and foster high quality clinical trials in multiple sclerosis and to ensure that there is a continuing pool of physicians who are trained in this area. In this program the individual with an MD or equivalent medical degree will acquire formal training, under the tutelage of an established investigator, in key elements associated with conducting clinical trials in MS. Annual deadline dates may vary; contact program staff for exact dates.
Requirements: Individuals must have received the MD or equivalent medical degree from an accredited institution and must be licensed to practice medicine in the United States.
Amount of Grant: $40,000 maximum
Date(s) Application is Due: Feb 1
Contact: Dr. Timothy Coetzee, Research Programs Department, (212) 476-0478; email: timothy.coetzee@nmss.org
Internet: http://www.nationalmssociety.org/Research-physfellow.asp
Sponsor: National Multiple Sclerosis Society
733 Third Avenue
New York, NY 10017-3288

NNEDVF/Altria Doors of Hope Program 2847
The goal of this initiative is to strengthen the safety net available to survivors of domestic violence through the provision of grant awards that support organizational excellence, innovation, and leadership in the provision of shelter and legal advocacy services. Direct service grants are awarded to domestic violence service providers for shelter services and advocacy/legal services. There is a two stage application process; stage one consists of registration online, which includes key questions that will be used to determine which applicants will be invited to apply for stage two. For the current funding year, grantmaking will be by invitation only. Applicants will be contacted if they are eligible to apply. Additional assistance and information is provided at www.nnedv.org.
Requirements: Eligible organizations must have a primary mission which includes the provision of direct services to survivors of domestic violence; provide shelter and/or legal advocacy services to survivors of domestic violence; be a U.S. based non-profit, non-governmental, tax-exempt organization; have been in operation for a minimum of three years with an organization budget greater than or equal to $250,000; and have nondiscrimination policies that include ethnicity, race, religious creed, national origin, disability, sexual orientation, marital status, age, and gender.
Restrictions: Applications will only be accepted through the online RFP.
Samples: Hmong American Friendship Association (Milwaukee, WI)—to provide group facilitators, education groups in the workplace, and domestic violence training for Hmong elders, $24,000.
Amount of Grant: $10,000-$50,000
Contact: Grants Administrator, (202) 543-5566; fax: (202) 543-5626; email: altriadoorsofhope@nnedv.org
Internet: http://www.altria.com/responsibility/4_9_1_1_2_1_domviolprograms.asp
Sponsor: National Network to End Domestic Violence Fund
660 Pennsylvania Ave SE, Suite 303
Washington, DC 20003

Noble County Community Foundation Grants 2848
The Noble County Community Foundation helps build an enduring source of charitable assets to meet the changing needs of the people in Noble County, Indiana. The general policy of the Foundation and Community Initiatives is to make grants for innovative, creative projects and programs responsive to changing community needs in the areas of health and human services, education, arts, and culture and civic affairs. The funding from the Foundation and Community Initiatives is not limited to these areas and grant seekers are encouraged to respond to emerging community needs. The Noble County Community Foundation, Inc. and it's supporting organization, Community Initiatives, Inc. are offering four grant cycles per year. Grants will be considered in April, June, August, and December. Applicants may telephone or submit a letter of intent briefly describing the project before submitting a proposal in order to find out if their ideas are potentially fundable by the Foundation.
Requirements: The Foundation considers only not-for-profit projects that: promote cooperation among organizations without duplicating services; promote volunteer involvement; demonstrate practical approaches to current community issues; enhance or improve an organization's self-sufficiency and effectiveness; emphasize prevention. In addition, the Foundation is inclined to give favorable consideration to projects that: affect a broad segment of the population; are pilot programs clearly replicable in their design; have reasonable prospects for future support; serve people whose needs are not being met by existing services and which encourage independence; move the community to a higher cultural awareness.
Restrictions: Discretionary funds generally will not be used to support: routine operating support for ongoing programs and multi-year funding; research; uniforms and performance apparel. Discretionary funds will not be used under any circumstances to support: deficit spending; political purposes; annual fund campaigns; lobbying; organizations whose primary function is to allocate funds to other charitable organizations or projects; projects that don't serve residents of Noble County; travel; augmenting endowments; underwriting for fund raising events; loans.
Geographic Focus: Indiana
Date(s) Application is Due: Mar 2; May 2; Jul 2; Nov 2
Contact: NCCF Office; (260) 894-3335; email: nccf@ligtel.com
Internet: http://www.noblecounty.org/NCCF/grants.html
Sponsor: Noble County Community Foundation, Inc.
1599 Lincolnway South
Ligonier, IN 46767

NORD Orphan Diseases Research Grants 2849
The program provides seed money in small grants to academic scientists studying new treatments or diagnostics for rare diseases. One-year clinical-research projects should focus on the early detection, diagnosis, or treatment of one of the following disorders: adenoid cystic carcinoma, alveolar capillary dysplasia, Cat Eye Syndrome, Ehlers-Danlos Syndrome, erythromelalgia, giant hypertrophic gastritis, and olivopontocerebellar atrophy or closely related diseases. The clinical researchers supported by the research grants provide preliminary data indicating that a treatment (drug, device, or medical food) may be safe and effective when used for a larger number of patients. Researchers can then use the preliminary data to apply for larger multiyear government grants or to attract a commercial sponsor who will manufacture an orphan product and get it approved for marketing by the U.S. Food and Drug Administration.
Requirements: Individuals who have earned an MD or MD/PhD in the past 10 years are eligible.
Samples: Dr. Cynthia Jackson and Dr. Douglas Gnepp, Rhode Island Hospital (RI)—to focus on the identification of genes as potentially new prognostic markers, as well as to study their contribution to the development of adenoid cystic carcinoma.; Dr. Eli Chang, Doheny Eye Institute, Keck School of Medicine of the U of Southern California (CA)—to research the establishment of an animal model for adenoid cystic carcinoma of the lacrimal gland, which may lead to the development of new and improved treatment modalities.
Contact: Grants Administrator, (203) 744-0100; fax: (203) 798-2291; email: orphan@rarediseases.org
Internet: http://www.rarediseases.org/research/requests
Sponsor: National Organization for Rare Disorders
55 Kenosia Avenue
Danbury, CT 06813-1968

NORD Roscoe Brady Lysosomal Storage Disease Fellowships 2850
The fellowships assist physicians who desire to establish careers in lysosomal storage diseases (LSDs) clinical medicine. Clinical research funded by the fellowships will be collaborative, involve multidisciplinary teams, and focus on genetics, new treatments and diagnostics, and/or epidemiology of LSDs in general, or for a specific LSD. The program's primary goal is to develop and support clinicians beginning their medical career that will specialize and focus on research, treatment, and coordination of multidisciplinary care for people suffering with LSDs. The research will be conducted in the United States, countries of the European Union, Canada, Australia, New Zealand, Brazil, Argentina, Chile, South Africa, Japan, or Israel, and where supervision of grant administration is possible. Complete guidelines and application are available online.
Requirements: Applicants should have earned the degree(s) of MD or MD/PhD within the past 10 years.
Amount of Grant: $50,000-$70,000
Date(s) Application is Due: Apr 13
Contact: Fellowships Administrator, (203) 744-0100 or (800) 999-6673 (voicemail only);TDD: (203) 797-9590; fax: (203)798-2291; email: orphan@rarediseases.org
Internet: http://www.rarediseases.org/research/roscoe

Sponsor: National Organization for Rare Disorders
55 Kenosia Avenue
Danbury, CT 06813-1968

Nordson Corporation Foundation Grants 2851
The corporate foundation awards grants to nonprofit organizations in geographic areas where Nordson facilities and employees are located: Cuyahoga and Lorain counties in Ohio; the Greater Atlanta, Georgia area; California, Rhode Island and Southeastern Massachusetts. The foundation provides a source of stable funding for community programs and projects in the areas of education, human welfare, civic, and arts and culture. Educational support is generally limited to improving elementary and secondary schools and certain programs for public and private higher education. Human welfare grants focus on children and youth. The foundation considers other funding areas, including urban affairs, volunteerism, public policy, health and health organizations, and literacy. Grants are awarded for general operating support, continuing support, annual campaigns, capital campaigns, building construction/renovation, equipment acquisition, emergency funds, seed money, scholarship funds, employee matching gifts, and technical assistance. The board meets four times each year. Deadlines vary by state; contact program staff for appropriate deadlines. Application forms are available on the website and may only be submitted online.
Requirements: Private, nonprofit organizations in California, Georgia, Ohio, Rhode Island, and southeastern Massachusetts may apply.
Restrictions: Funding is not provided for organizations whose services are not provided within the foundation's geographic areas of interest; direct grants or scholarships to individuals; organizations not eligible for tax-deductible support; organizations not exempt under Section 501(c)3 of the Internal Revenue Code; political causes, candidates, organizations or campaigns; organizations that discriminate on the basis of race, sex, or religion; or special occasion, goodwill advertising, i.e., journals or dinner programs.
Geographic Focus: California; Georgia; Massachusetts; Ohio; Rhode Island
Samples: Ctr for Leadership in Education (Lorain, OH)—for general operating support, $250,000.; Salvation Army of Lorain (Lorain, OH)—for the capital campaign, $50,000.; Neighborhood House Assoc of Lorain County (Lorain, OH)—for rejuvenation of the Cityview Ctr, $39,625.
Amount of Grant: $1.5 million total
Date(s) Application is Due: Feb 15; May 15; Aug 15; Nov 15
Contact: Cecilia H. Render, Director; (440) 892-1580, ext. 5172; email: crender@nordson.com
Internet: http://www.nordson.com/Corporate/Community/Foundation
Sponsor: Nordson Corporation Foundation
28601 Clemens Road
Westlake, OH 44145-1119

North Carolina Biotechnology Center Event Sponsorship Grants 2852
This popular Biotechnology Center grant promotes and supports events advancing the understanding or application of biotechnology to benefit North Carolina. Events must promote information sharing and personal interaction focused on biotechnology research, education, or business. The highest amount awarded is $3,000. Awards typically cover costs such as speaker fees, travel expenses, event-site rental and publicity.
Requirements: All award money is disbursed directly to the applicant's organization. The money must be used solely to support the event outlined in this application.
Restrictions: This sponsorship does not provide money either to promote a specific product to benefit a few companies or individuals. This sponsorship does not cover food or refreshments for event attendees.
Geographic Focus: North Carolina
Amount of Grant: $3,000 maximum
Contact: Ginny DeLuca; (919) 549-8842; fax: (919) 549-9710; email: virginia_deluca@ncbiotech.org
Internet: http://www.ncbiotech.org/services_and_programs/grants_and_loans/biotechnology_event_sponsorship/index.html
Sponsor: North Carolina Biotechnology Center
P.O. Box, 13547, 15 T.W. Alexander Drive
Research Triangle Park, NC 27709-3547

North Carolina Biotechnology Center Grantsmanship Training Grants 2853
The Grantsmanship Training Grant (GTG) program is a one-time funding opportunity that provides financial support for grant writing training activities for faculty and staff of North Carolina colleges and universities and other non-profits who are involved in research or programs related to the life sciences. Funds can be requested to support a variety of grantsmanship training activities, including workshops and other training events. The following individuals and groups would be eligible for training support under the GTG program: academic faculty members who seek funding related to life science research or life science-related economic development; research administration staff affiliated with departments or institutions that regularly submit proposals in life science research or life science-related economic development; and staff of non-profit organizations involved in activities related to biotechnology or the life sciences. A maximum of $5,000 may be requested based on the type of training activity proposed.
Requirements: Proposed programs and activities must clearly relate to biotechnology research, development, commercialization, education, or training. Priority will be giving to proposals requesting support for innovative programs or activities in biotechnology. Applicants are required to contribute a cash match equaling the requested amount (dollar-for-dollar).
Restrictions: Awards are not made to individuals.
Geographic Focus: North Carolina
Amount of Grant: $5,000 maximum
Contact: Deborah De, Program Manager; (919) 549-8845; fax: (919) 549-9710; email: deborah_de@ncbiotech.org
Internet: http://www.ncbiotech.org/gtg/
Sponsor: North Carolina Biotechnology Center
P.O. Box, 13547, 15 T.W. Alexander Drive
Research Triangle Park, NC 27709-3547

North Carolina Biotechnology Center Meeting Grants 2854
This grant promotes and supports national and international meetings which advance the understanding or application of biotechnology and focus national and international attention on the North Carolina scientific community. Meetings must promote information sharing and personal interaction focused on biotechnology research, education, or business. The highest amount awarded is $10,000. Awards typically cover costs such as speaker fees, travel expenses, event-site rental and publicity.
Requirements: All award money is given to the applicant's organization. The money must be used solely to support the event outlined in this application.
Restrictions: This sponsorship does not provide money either to promote a specific product to benefit a few companies or individuals. This sponsorship does not cover food or refreshments for event attendees.
Geographic Focus: North Carolina
Amount of Grant: $10,000 maximum
Contact: Ginny DeLuca; (919) 549-8842; fax: (919) 549-9710; email: virginia_deluca@ncbiotech.org
Internet: http://www.ncbiotech.org/services_and_programs/grants_and_loans/BiotechnologyMeetingGrant.html
Sponsor: North Carolina Biotechnology Center
P.O. Box, 13547, 15 T.W. Alexander Drive
Research Triangle Park, NC 27709-3547

North Carolina Biotechnology Center Regional Development Grants 2855
The goal of the Regional Development Grant Program (PDF) is to build capacity through collaborative projects, providing a foundational resource for biotechnology development in the community that was not there previously and that the community could not have achieved without Biotechnology Center funding. Preproposals are required: cycle 1 preproposals are due no later than January 28, while cycle 2 preproposals should be received by August 20. The deadlines for final proposals are April 1 (cycle 1) and October 15 (cycle 2).
Requirements: Proposed programs and activities must clearly relate to biotechnology research, development, commercialization, education, or training. Priority will be giving to proposals requesting support for innovative programs or activities in biotechnology. Only North Carolina academic institutions, non profit research organizations, or businesses may apply.
Restrictions: Awards are not made to individuals.
Geographic Focus: North Carolina
Amount of Grant: $75,000 maximum
Date(s) Application is Due: Jan 28; Apr 1; Aug 20; Oct 15
Contact: Deborah De, Program Manager; (919) 549-8845; fax: (919) 549-9710; email: deborah_de@ncbiotech.org
Internet: http://www.ncbiotech.org/services_and_programs/grants_and_loans/regional_development/index.html
Sponsor: North Carolina Biotechnology Center
P.O. Box, 13547, 15 T.W. Alexander Drive
Research Triangle Park, NC 27709-3547

North Carolina Biotechnology Center Technology Enhancement Grants 2856
The Technology Enhancement Grant (TEG) Program provides funding to North Carolina Universities or other research institutions in the state through their respective technology transfer offices. Under this program, awards of up to $50,000 are available to fund research studies determined to be critical to enhancing the university's licensing position for specified technologies with commercial opportunity. Eligible technologies are those for which intellectual property rights are assigned to the university or institution and have not been committeed through license, option or letter-of-intent to license to any third party commercial interest at the time of award. Funds are intended to support an approved research project designed to yield a significant technical milestone in the evolution of a technology from basic science to licensable commercial product or service. Examples of such projects include proof-of-concept, validation, lead identification and optimization using a proprietary platform technology, etc. Due to legal constraints, funds provided under the TEG program can only be used to offset direct costs associated with the project.
Requirements: Technology transfer offices associated with any North Carolina university or not-for-profit research institution are eligible and encouraged to apply.
Restrictions: Prohibited charges include (but are not limited to): purchase or lease of real estate, building construction or renovations; salaries for administrative personnel; overhead or indirect costs; and atenting costs.
Geographic Focus: North Carolina
Amount of Grant: $50,000 maximum
Contact: Dr. Rob Lindberg; (919) 541-9366; fax: (919) 549-9710; email: rob_lindberg@ncbiotech.org
Internet: http://www.ncbiotech.org/services_and_programs/grants_and_loans/technology_enhancement/index.html
Sponsor: North Carolina Biotechnology Center
P.O. Box, 13547, 15 T.W. Alexander Drive
Research Triangle Park, NC 27709-3547

North Carolina Biotechnology Centers of Innovation Grants 2857

The Centers of Innovation Program is bringing together North Carolina's best scientific and technical minds in the life sciences. This program is designed to focus the state's efforts in biotechnology research, development and commercialization in targeted industrial sectors important to economic development and job creation. The North Carolina Biotechnology Center (NCBC) will work with university researchers, technology transfer offices, industrial partners, non-profit stake holders as well as regional and state-wide community leaders to establish nine Centers of Innovation (COI). Initial Centers of Innovation will complement efforts already under way in the state to align academic and industrial resources. The Phase I award is a 12-month $100,000 planning grant that will allow the development of a business plan and organization plan. The Phase II award is funding for the implementation of the business plan. Only invited applicants may apply. Potential applicants will need to demonstrate that they have established a cohesive academic-industry consortium in order to receive an invitation to submit an application.
Geographic Focus: North Carolina
Amount of Grant: $100,000 maximum (phase I); $2,400,000 maximum (phase II)
Contact: Mary Beth Thomas, Ph.D.; (919) 541-9366; fax: (919) 549-9710; email: marybeth_thomas@ncbiotech.org
Internet: http://www.ncbiotech.org/services_and_programs/COI/index.html
Sponsor: North Carolina Biotechnology Center
P.O. Box, 13547, 15 T.W. Alexander Drive
Research Triangle Park, NC 27709-3547

North Carolina Community Development Grants 2858

The foundation supports nonprofit organizations in North Carolina to enrich the quality of life in the state, with special concern for rural regions and Cabarrus County. Grants are awarded primarily for healthcare, higher education, and community service. Other more limited areas of interest are arts, culture, historic preservation, religion, and the environment. Grants generally will be awarded for capital improvements, challenge opportunities, or special purposes rather than for operating purposes. Grant requests are considered on a quarterly basis.
Requirements: IRS 501(c)3 organizations serving North Carolina communities are eligible. Churches and governmental agencies also may apply.
Restrictions: Normally, the foundation does not make multiyear grants or frequent grants to the same organization (except for select, historic relationships); or provide operating funds, start-up funding, or lead gifts. The foundation does not make grants to individuals, to endowment funds, for loans, or for scholarships or fellowships.
Geographic Focus: North Carolina
Samples: Lenoir-Rhyne College (Hickory, NC)—for equipment and technology upgrades, $156,000 (2003); Mars Hill College (Mars Hill, NC)—to purchase two boilers and a fire-alarm system, $150,000.
Amount of Grant: $10,000-$30,000 average
Date(s) Application is Due: Jan 5; Apr 5; Jul 5; Oct 5
Contact: Frank Davis, Executive Director, (704) 786-8216; fax: (704) 785-2051
Internet: http://www.thecannonfoundationinc.org/guidelines.asp
Sponsor: Cannon Foundation
P.O. Box 548
Concord, NC 28026-0548

North Carolina Community Foundation Grants 2859

The community foundation exists to meet the needs of nonprofit organizations and improve the lives of citizens of North Carolina counties, including Allegheny, Caldwell, Cherokee, Clay, Craven, Eastern Bank of Cherokee Indians, Franklin Community, Franklin, Graham, Harnett, Haywood, Jackson, Johnston, Madison, Montgomery, Moore, Pender, Pitt, Randolph, Rockingham, Swain, Wake, Watauga, and Wilkes. Support is available for programs that enrich the quality of life in the areas of civic affairs, education, health, religion, social services, arts, and the conservation and preservation of environmental, historical preservation, and cultural resources. Grants will be awarded to support programs and projects, endowments, conferences and seminars, and consulting services. Grants are awarded in local communities; use the "Affiliate Webpage" link to contact the office serving your area.
Requirements: Nonprofit organizations throughout North Carolina are eligible to apply.
Geographic Focus: North Carolina
Contact: Jennifer Tolle Whiteside, President; (800) 201-9533 or (919) 828-4387; fax: (919) 828-5495; email: jtwhiteside@nccommunityfoundation.org
Internet: http://nccommunityfoundation.org/05_grants_available.php
Sponsor: North Carolina Community Foundation
4601 Six Forks Road, Suite 524
Raleigh, NC 27609

North Carolina GlaxoSmithKline Foundation Grants 2860

The foundation supports activities primarily in North Carolina that help meet the needs of today's society and future generations by funding programs that emphasize the understanding and application of health, science, and mathematics at all educational and professional levels. Although providing seed funds for new and worthwhile educational programs is the foundation's primary focus, requests for funding of ongoing projects will also receive consideration. Types of support include operating budgets, professorships, and conferences and seminars. Proposals may be submitted for either one-year or multi-year funding with a maximum of five years' duration. The foundation's board of directors meets four times a year to consider and award grants. Completed applications must be received by the listed deadline dates. If the stated deadline falls on a weekend or holiday, the next business day serves as the official deadline. All applicants will be notified of the board's decisions within 15 days of the board meeting.
Requirements: The foundation makes grants only to North Carolina 501(c)3 tax-exempt organizations and institutions or to governmental agencies.
Restrictions: Grants are not made to individuals for construction or restoration projects, or for international programs unless specifically exempted by the board. Funds are not ordinarily provided to programs that benefit a limited geographic region.
Geographic Focus: North Carolina
Samples: North Carolina Center for Public Policy Research, $446,000 (2006); The Carolina Ballet, Healthier Living Through the Arts, $650,000 (2006); Prevent Blindness North Carolina, $100,000 (2006).
Amount of Grant: $25,000-$1,000,000 average
Date(s) Application is Due: Jan 1; Apr 1; Jul 1; Oct 1
Contact: Marilyn Foote-Hudson, Executive Director; (919) 483-2140; fax: (919) 315-3015; email: community.partnership@gsk.com
Internet: http://us.gsk.com/html/community/community-grants-foundation.html
Sponsor: North Carolina GlaxoSmithKline Foundation
Five Moore Drive, P.O. Box 13398
Research Triangle Park, NC 27709

North Central Health Services Grants 2861

North Central Health Services (NCHS) was created in 1984 to serve as the parent company of a family of corporations which included Lafayette Home Hospital, Home Hospital Foundation, and Service Frontiers Incorporated. Today, NCHS is a medical services company whose primary purpose is to operate an ambulatory surgery center, where sterilization services are made available to the Greater Lafayette community. NCHS also is a grant making organization providing primarily capital grants to 501(c)3 organizations serving the citizens of Benton, Carroll, Clinton, Fountain, Montgomery, Tippecanoe, Warren, and White counties in Indiana. Grants are awarded to organizations for projects that relate to Health, and Healthy Communities. NCHS prefers to fund projects that have a significant potential for positive impact on the community. NCHS encourages collaboration among agencies and organizations that efficiently utilize resources, and provide services that are not duplicative of existing programs. NCHS provides grants that will: advance technology and scientific development in health care; develop and promote community health education; provide direct, individual social welfare and human service; promote a Healthy Community; improve the quality of life for all the communities people.
Requirements: The first step for an organization to apply for a grant is to submit a written letter of inquiry. This letter should include a concise description of the organization, a statement of the problem or need being addressed, and an explanation of the project, estimated total costs, and the amount being requested from NCHS. The letter should be addressed to: North Central Health Services, Inc., Attn: Rita Smith, Program Director, P.O. Box 528, Lafayette, In. 47902. Upon receipt of the letter of inquiry, initial review will determine whether or not the request meets the funding focus and priorities of NCHS. You will be promptly notified in writing of the initial determination, and informed of application opportunities.
Restrictions: Beginning in 2008, NCHS implemented the following grant categories and cycles. Grant requests and cycles: letter of inquiry requesting funds in excess of $250,000, accepted May 1 to August 15 of each calendar year. If approved, funding would be available for distribution after January 1 of the following year; letter of inquiry requesting funds of $100,000 to $250,000 will be accepted throughout the calendar year. If approved, funding would generally be available for distribution within 90 days of board approval; letter of inquiry requesting funds of $25,000 to $100,000 will be accepted throughout the calendar year. If approved, funding would generally be available within 60 days of board approval; letter of inquiry requesting funds of less than $25,000 will be accepted throughout the calendar year. If approved, funding would generally be available within 60 days of approval.
Geographic Focus: Indiana
Samples: Lauramie Township EMS - Purchase Zoll E series AED to update equipment for EMS basic life support ambulance service, $8,693.00 (2009); St. Elizabeth Regional Health - Gifts for hospitalized children, $4,155.00 (2009); Indiana Regular Baptist Youth Camp, Inc. - Build a new Health Center for Twin Lakes Camp & Conference Center, $150,000.00 (2008).
Contact: Rita Smith, Program Director; (765) 423-1604
Internet: http://www.nchsi.com/grantmaking.cfm
Sponsor: North Central Health Services, Inc.
201 Main Street, Suite 606, P.O. Box 528
Lafayette, IN 47902

North Georgia Community Foundation Grants 2862

The foundation serves Banks, Dawson, Fannin, Forsyth, Franklin, Habersham, Hall, Hart, Jackson, Lumpkin, Rabun, Stephens, Towns, Union, and White counties. The foundation looks favorably at efforts which promise to affect a broad constituency in its service area. The foundation is interested in those organizations which can demonstrate that they have planned their projects in light of overall community need, and that similar projects by other organizations do not duplicate the proposed services. A request which asks the foundation to provide a portion of the support for a project generally will receive greater priority than one which looks to it as the single funding source. The foundation is especially interested in leveraging additional income from other sources.
Requirements: Grants are made only to Georgia nonprofit tax-exempt organizations in the counties listed for charitable purposes, unless donor-advised funds are designated to qualifying entities outside the foundation's area of emphasis.

Restrictions: Funding is not generally provided for annual fund campaigns, lobbying, operating support other than start-up, or to individuals.
Geographic Focus: Georgia
Amount of Grant: $3000 maximum
Contact: Program Officer, (770) 535-7880; fax: (770) 503-0439; email: info@ngcf.org
Internet: http://www.ngcf.org/main.asp
Sponsor: North Georgia Community Foundation
615F Oak Street, Suite 1300
Gainesville, GA 30501

Northeast Utilities Foundation Grants **2863**
The foundation supports community efforts to improve education, social and economic conditions, and protect the quality of the environment. Areas of focus include education, civic and community, human services, environment, and culture and arts. Grant requests are evaluated using criteria such as organizational and financial management, program objectives, diverse number of people who will benefit, existing service, funding sources and stability, organizational history, and measures of success. The board meets in February, April, August, and November.
Restrictions: Grants do not support individuals; corporations that do not qualify as charitable organizations according to IRS codes; private foundations; projects benefiting limited groups—religious, fraternal, political; athletic outings; reducing or eliminating a preexisting debt; or health care issues or organizations.
Geographic Focus: Connecticut; Massachusetts; New Hampshire; Northeast
Samples: Saint Joseph College, West Hartford, CT, $500,000 — to reconfigure two science laboratories, and to establish the Fresh Water Institute.
Date(s) Application is Due: Jan 10; Apr 11; Jul 11; Oct 10
Contact: Patricia McCullough
President, Executive Director; (888) 682-4639 or (860) 665-5822; fax: (860) 721-4331; email: NUFoundation@NU.com
Internet: http://northeastutilitiesfoundation.org/what/index.html
Sponsor: Northeast Utilities Foundation
P.O. Box 270
Hartford, CT 06141-0270

Northern New York Community Foundation Grants **2864**
The foundation is looking for innovative programs that address problems to be solved, or opportunities to be seized, in the northern New York area. Grants are made only for capital items and for seed money for new agencies, or new projects by established agencies.
Requirements: Grants are made to nonprofit, tax-exempt organizations in or serving Jefferson and/or Lewis counties in New York State. Governmental units are also eligible provided that the purpose of the grant goes beyond the expected limits of government service. The foundation does not make grants to churches and religious organizations except in cases where projects clearly benefit the entire community. Applicants should contact the office to provide a brief summary of the project and needs. The applicant will be notified of grant award or denial by letter after the board of directors meets, which is generally one month following application deadline dates. Grant requests under $5,000 may be approved at the committee level. Larger grant requests are referred to the board of directors with a committee recommendation.
Restrictions: Individuals are ineligible. The foundation does not fund operations or pay off deficits.
Geographic Focus: New York
Samples: 4th Qtr 2008: The Handweaving Museum and Arts Center - $35,000 to help fund a new Director of Development position.; Northern Area Health Education Center (NAHEC) - $3,575 for student internships in technical fields.; Ogdensburg Command Performances - $7,000 to match a Land Trust Alliance grant to develop a Point Peninsula conservation plan.; Pendragon Theatre - $2,784 for three Shakespeare performances at Jefferson Community College.; Trinity Episcopal Church, Watertown - $2,500 for a Trinity Concert Series performance of Handel's Messiah.; Watertown Housing Authority - $5,000 to help fund a new playground for East Hills and Meadowbrook family housing projects.; American Red Cross of Northern New York - $5,306 for access to donor management software.
Date(s) Application is Due: Jan 30; Apr 24; Aug 28; Oct 23
Contact: Alex Velto, Executive Director; (315) 782-7110; fax: (315) 782-0047; email: info@nnycf.org
Internet: http://www.nnycf.org/grantguidelines.asp?mm=5
Sponsor: Northern New York Community Foundation
120 Washington Street, Suite 400
Watertown, NY 13601

Northern Trust Company Charitable Trust and Corporate Giving Program **2865**
Contributions from the Charitable Trust support program, general operating, capital, or endowment priorities. Grants usually are confined to programs and agencies that focus on advancing the well-being of disadvantaged women and children, and people with disabilities. Priority is given to programs or agencies that serve the following Chicago neighborhoods: Chatham, Englewood, Humboldt Park, Logan Square, Loop, Washington Park, and West Town. Applications, including all material specified in the checklist must be received in the Community Affairs office before 5:00 pm on the deadline date. Deadlines for requests for funding are determined by area of service, as follows: social welfare—January 13 and August 12, education-'May 13; and arts and culture—May 13.
Requirements: Nonprofit organizations in Illinois are eligible. A proposal should include a short cover letter, an operating budget for the current year, a copy of the agency's most recent audited financial statement, a list of members of the agency's governing board, a list of Chicago-based corporate and foundation contributors and amounts each has contributed in the last calendar year, and a letter from the IRS indicating tax-exempt status.
Geographic Focus: Illinois
Samples: Parents United for Responsible Education (Chicago, IL)—for operating support, $5000.; Chicago Reporter (Chicago, IL)—for operating support, $3000.
Amount of Grant: $2500-$5000 typically
Date(s) Application is Due: Jan 13; May 13; Aug 12
Contact: Dawn McGovern, Program Contact, (312) 444-4059
Internet: http://www.northerntrust.com/aboutus/community/charitable/index.html
Sponsor: Northern Trust Company
50 S LaSalle Street, Suite L-7
Chicago, IL 60675

Northrop Grumman Corporation Grants **2866**
Northrop's concentrated giving program is designed to ensure that each recipient organization can accomplish its mission on an expanded basis or undertake specific projects or programs that otherwise would be unfeasible. Areas of interest include youth programs; community access to health services; career and employment counseling; precollege education; human services; environmental, civic, and cultural; and United Way of Greater Los Angeles. Contribution guidelines are available online.
Requirements: Organizations applying must be tax-exempt under 501(c)3.
Restrictions: The foundation does not make grants to religious organizations, political groups, fraternal organizations, individuals, fundraising events, campus student organizations, athletic teams, choirs, bands, advertising or underwriting expenses, capital campaigns, or endowment funds.
Samples: U of Central Florida, College of Optics and Photonics (Orlando, FL)—for use in its work on a semiconductor-manufacturing process called extreme ultraviolet lithography, $22 million approximately in equipment and intellectual property (2004); U.S. Naval Academy Foundation (Annapolis, MD)—for the Ctr for the Study of Professional Military Ethics, $1 million (2004); People Assisting the Homeless (Los Angeles, CA)—to improve social services and other resources that can help homeless people become self-sufficient, $1 million over 10 years (2003).
Amount of Grant: $8.4 million total
Date(s) Application is Due: Dec 31
Contact: Corporate Director of Diversity, EEO & Contributions, (310) 553-6262; email: Community_Relations@northgrum.com
Internet: http://www.northgrum.com/com_rel/guidelines.html
Sponsor: Northrop Grumman Corporation
1840 Century Park E, 131/CC
Los Angeles, CA 90067

Northrop Grumman Newport News Grants **2867**
The shipbuilder makes grants in Virginia and nationally in the areas of education, arts and humanities, civic and community affairs, and health and human services. Education grants have been awarded to K-12 schools, youth-oriented nonprofits, and higher education. Science and engineering programs for minority students are of special interest. There are no application deadlines; proposals are reviewed at quarterly meetings, in March, June, September, and December.
Requirements: Nonprofit organizations, including schools, are eligible.
Samples: Hampton U (VA)—for engineering programs, $300,000.; Christopher Newport U (VA)—for a new performing arts center, $250,000.; People to People (VA)—for ongoing support to improve race relations, $250,000.
Contact: Brenda Roth, Community Relations, (757) 380-3011; email: brenda.roth@ngc.com
Internet: http://www.nn.northropgrumman.com/about/community.html
Sponsor: Northrop Grumman Newport News
4101 Washington Avenue
Newport News, VA 23607

Northwest Airlines KidCares Medical Travel Assistance **2868**
The program provides air travel to children age 18 and younger who are unable to receive treatment in their home area. The KidCares program is fueled by generous mileage donations of Northwest's WorldPerks members. Availability of the program is based on that donated WorldPerks mileage, and consideration of each request is based on the guidelines below. Each application received must be evaluated on a case-by-case basis.
Requirements: Guidelines are as follows: (1) Only one round-trip per family is permitted. (2) A letter from the child's physician must accompany the application, stating: (a) patient's diagnosis; (b) confirmation of the need for travel; (c) the patient has medical clearance for air travel; (d) dates of appointments/surgery; and (e) length of stay. (3) The patient must be 18 years old or younger at the time the travel request is made. (4) The medical treatment for which the child is traveling must be unavailable in the child's home location. (5) KidCares travel can only be provided by Northwest Airlines or one of its airline partners. (6) Families demonstrating financial need are given priority consideration for KidCares travel. (7) One adult companion may accompany the child on KidCares travel at no additional cost. Applications may be found on Northwest's Web site, nwa.com at the following location http://www.nwa.com/corpinfo/aircares/about/KidCares_Application.pdf. You may also call (612) 726-4206 and leave detailed information regarding where the application should be sent and to whom.
Restrictions: KidCares travel is not available to families with insurance coverage that covers the cost of travel for medical treatment. KidCares travel is not eligible for Northwest Airlines WorldPerks bonus mileage credit. KidCares travel is not provided

to St. Jude Children's Research Hospital, which is covered by a separate Northwest Airlines travel program.
Contact: Community Relations; (612) 726-4206; fax: (612) 726-3942; email: aircares@nwa.com
Internet: http://www.nwa.com/corpinfo/aircares/feature/
Sponsor: Northwest Airlines, Inc.
2700 Lone Oak Parkway, Department A1300
St. Paul, MN 55121

Northwest Minnesota Foundation Women's Fund Grants **2869**
Formed in 1997 as a tax exempt charitable component of the Northwest Minnesota Foundation (NMF), the Women's Fund serves as a catalyst for improving the quality of life for women and girls by promoting ideas and supporting programs for the continued strengthening and empowerment of all women. The Women's Fund will consider grant requests of up to $2,500 addressing one or more of the following areas meeting the needs of females: cultural interactions; economic development; education; healthcare; and housing.
Requirements: Minnesota counties served by NMF are Beltrami, Clearwater, Hubbard, Kittson, Lake of the Woods, Mahnomen, Marshall, Norman, Pennington, Polk, Red Lake, and Roseau.
Geographic Focus: Minnesota
Amount of Grant: $2,500 maximum
Date(s) Application is Due: May 1
Contact: Jim Steenerson; (218) 759-2057; fax: (218) 759-2328; email: jims@nwmf.org or nwmf@nwmf.org;; Lisa Peterson; (800) 659-7859; email: lisap@nwmf.org
Internet: http://www.nwmf.org/prog_grant_aproc.php
Sponsor: Northwest Minnesota Foundation
4225 Technology Drive NW
Bemidji, MN 56601

Northwestern Mutual Foundation Grants **2870**
The people of Northwestern Mutual have a long history of community involvement. To carry out its corporate contributions program, Northwestern Mutual created a private foundation, The Northwestern Mutual Foundation. The Northwestern Mutual Foundation focuses its funding in Milwaukee, where the company is headquartered. Therefore, applying for a grant from the Northwestern Mutual Foundation is limited to Milwaukee-area nonprofit organizations with programs centered on Education, Health & Human Services or Arts & Culture.
Requirements: Northwestern Mutual Foundation does not accept unsolicited grant requests. Groups new to the Foundation are asked to submit a written letter of intent, describing the organization, funding request, and provide information about the program for which you are seeking support. The Foundations team will review your letter of intent and, if they are interested in learning more about your project, you will receive an application form. Groups that have an active relationship with the Foundation and currently receive funding are allowed to apply annually for support. Once an organization submits an application, the review process takes about 90 days. The Foundation review's Milwaukee-area grants on a monthly basis.
Restrictions: Milwaukee-area nonprofits are eligible to apply. The Foundation defines the Milwaukee-area as Milwaukee County, with limited programmatic grants in Waukesha, Racine and Ozaukee Counties.
Geographic Focus: Wisconsin
Samples: Boys and Girls Clubs of Greater Milwaukee, Milwaukee, WI, $800,000 (2008); United Performing Arts Fund, Milwaukee, WI, $605,000 (2008); Scholarship America, Saint Peter, MN, $205,425 (2008);
Amount of Grant: $10,000- $800,000 range
Contact: Edward J. Zore President and CEO; (414) 271-1444;
Internet: http://www.nmfn.com/tn/aboutus—fd_intro
Sponsor: Northwestern Mutual Foundation
720 East Wisconsin Avenue
Milwaukee, WI 53202-4797

Northwood University/Alden B. Dow Creativity Center Summer Residency **2871**
The program provides a 10-week residency at the university from mid-June through mid-August to allow each successful applicant to pursue innovative ideas having the potential for impact in his or her field. Project ideas must be specific with accomplishable goals for the 10-week period. Selection is based on newness and uniqueness of idea. Fellows are expected to be capable of independent research on their proposed projects. From education and literature to health care and chemistry, physics, engineering, and architecture and the arts, no creative area will be overlooked when a project idea may result in a significant advancement. Foreign citizens are also invited, provided they can communicate in written and spoken English. Project budgets are approved on an individual basis; however, ideas involving heavy developmental costs are discouraged. The grant includes travel within the United States (foreign applicants must provide transportation to the United States), room and board, and a stipend for personal expenses and/or project materials. Application fee is $10; forms and instructional brochures are available upon request.
Amount of Grant: $750 stipend
Date(s) Application is Due: Dec 31
Contact: Dr. Grover Proctor, Jr, Executive Director, (989) 837-4478; fax: (989) 837-4468; email: creativity@northwood.edu
Internet: http://www.northwood.edu/abd
Sponsor: Northwood University
4000 Whiting Drive
Midland, MI 48640-2398

Norwin S. and Elizabeth N. Bean Foundation Grants **2872**
The Norwin S. and Elizabeth N. Bean Foundation was established in 1967 as a general purpose foundation to serve the communities of Manchester and Amherst and, consistent with the wishes of the founders, grants are made in the fields of arts and humanities, education, environment, health, human services, and public/society benefit.
Requirements: Applications are accepted from nonprofit 501(c)3 organizations and municipal and public agencies serving the communities of Manchester and Amherst, New Hampshire. Priority consideration is given to organizations operating primarily in those two communities. However, the Foundation will consider applications from statewide or regional organizations which provide a substantial and documented level of service to Manchester and Amherst.
Restrictions: The foundation does not make grants to individuals or provide scholarship aid.
Geographic Focus: New Hampshire
Date(s) Application is Due: Dec 1; Apr 1; Sep 1
Contact: Kathleen Cook, Grant Manager; (603) 493-7257; email: KCook@BeanFoundation.org
Internet: http://www.beanfoundation.org/grants/bean-foundation-grant/application-criteria.aspx
Sponsor: Norwin S. and Elizabeth N. Bean Foundation
40 Stark Street
Manchester, NH 03301

NSERC Brockhouse Canada Prize for Interdisciplinary Research in Science and Engineering Grant **2873**
The Brockhouse Canada Prize for Interdisciplinary Research in Science and Engineering recognizes outstanding Canadian teams of researchers from different disciplines who have combined their expertise to produce achievements of outstanding international significance in the natural sciences and engineering. The prize, accompanied by a team research grant of $250,000, reflects NSERC's commitment to supporting Canadian research through strategic investments in people, discovery and innovation. The grant supports the direct costs of university-based research and/or the enhancement of research facilities. The grant may be distributed in one lump sum or up to five instalments, depending on the needs of the recipients.
Requirements: Research teams nominated for the Brockhouse Canada Prize must have at least two members who are independent researchers, one of whom must hold an NSERC grant. The team can be part of an international effort, but the majority of the nominated team members must be employed at a Canadian university or public or private organization. NSERC recognizes that teams may change between the time of the specific research achievements and the time of nomination. Nominations will be accepted when changes have occurred but only as long as the core of the team remains intact. Contributions must be primarily in the natural sciences and engineering, and of an interdisciplinary and collaborative nature.
Restrictions: Any Canadian citizen may nominate a research team for the Brockhouse Canada Prize. Self nominations will not be accepted. Current NSERC Council members cannot be nominated. Since the prize is for interdisciplinary research, nominators should consult NSERC's Guidelines for the Preparation and Review of Applications in Interdisciplinary Research. Nominators should also consult NSERC's Guidelines for the Preparation and Review of Applications in Engineering and the Applied Sciences. See website for deadline & hyper links to above mentioned guidelines.
Amount of Grant: $250,000
Date(s) Application is Due: Jun 1
Contact: (613) 995-5829; fax: (613) 992-5337; email: brockhouse@nserc-crsng.gc.ca
Internet: http://www.nserc-crsng.gc.ca/Prizes-Prix/Brockhouse-Brockhouse/Index-Index_eng.asp
Sponsor: Natural Sciences and Engineering Research Council of Canada
350 Albert Street
Ottawa, Ontario K1A 1H5 Canada

NSF Alan T. Waterman Award **2874**
The annual award recognizes an outstanding young researcher in any field of science or engineering supported by the National Science Foundation. In addition to a medal, the awardee receives a grant of $500,000 over a three year period for scientific research or advanced study in the mathematical, physical, biological, engineering, social, or other sciences at the institution of the recipient's choice.
Requirements: Candidates must be U.S. citizens, normally 35 years of age or younger, or not more than seven years beyond receipt of the PhD degree by December 31 of the year nominated. Candidates should have demonstrated exceptional individual achievements in scientific or engineering research of sufficient quality to place them at the forefront of their peers. Criteria include originality, innovation, and significant impact on the field.
Samples: David Charbonneau, Professor of Astronomy, Harvard University (2009); Terence Tao, Professor of Mathematics, University of California, Los Angeles (2008); Peidong Yang, Associate Professor of Chemistry, University of California, Berkeley (2007).
Amount of Grant: $500,000 over a three-year period
Date(s) Application is Due: Dec 31
Contact: Mayra N. Montrose, Program Contact; (703) 292-8040; fax: (703) 292-9040; email: mmontros@nsf
Internet: http://www.nsf.gov/od/waterman/waterman.jsp
Sponsor: National Science Foundation
4201 Wilson Boulevard
Arlington, VA 22230

NSF Animal Developmental Mechanisms Grants 2875
Animal Developmental Systems programmatic area supports research that seeks to understand the processes that result in the complex phenotype of animals. Because different organisms may be more amenable to certain approaches than others, analyses of development in a wide range of different species are encouraged. The Developmental Systems Cluster is also particularly interested in understanding how emergent properties result in the development of complex phenotypes and lead to the evolution of developmental mechanisms. Proposals may be submitted at any time; however, receipt by target dates will ensure review at the regular panel meeting. Full proposals should be submitted via the FastLane system at NSF or Grants.gov.
Requirements: The most frequent recipients of support are academic institutions and nonprofit research groups. In special circumstances, grants also are awarded to other types of institutions and to individuals.
Date(s) Application is Due: Jan 12; Jul 12
Contact: James Deshler, Program Director; (703) 292-8417; email: jdeshler@nsf.gov
Internet: http://www.nsf.gov/funding/pgm_summ.jsp?pims_id=501087
Sponsor: National Science Foundation
4201 Wilson Boulevard
Arlington, VA 22230

NSF Behavioral Neurosciences Research Grants 2876
This program focuses on the neural regulation of behavioral events ranging from simple movements to complex adaptive and interactive responses. Major activities are sensorimotor integration, biological rhythms, and cognitive functions such as attention, spatial representation, and learning and memory. Approaches that use novel techniques to study behavior within an evolutionary and ecological context are encouraged. Proposals may be submitted at any time. For review within six months, proposals should be submitted in line with the listed target dates for applications.
Requirements: The most frequent recipients of support are academic institutions and nonprofit research groups. In special circumstances, grants also are awarded to other types of institutions and to individuals.
Date(s) Application is Due: Jan 12; Jul 12
Contact: Judith Verbeke, Acting Division Director, (703) 292-8420; fax: (703) 292-9153; email: jverbeke@nsf.gov
Internet: http://www.nsf.gov/pubs/progdesc/1998/bio/ibn/1191.htm
Sponsor: National Science Foundation
4201 Wilson Boulevard
Arlington, VA 22230

NSF BIO Minority Postdoctoral Research Fellowships 2877
These fellowships seek to provide opportunities for recent minority doctoral scientists to obtain additional training, to gain research experience under the sponsorship of established scientists, and to broaden their scientific horizons beyond their research experiences during their undergraduate or graduate training. They are further designed to assist new scientists to direct their research efforts across traditional disciplinary lines and to avail themselves of unique research resources, sites, and facilities, including foreign locations. Fellows must affiliate with an appropriate research institution and are expected to devote themselves full time to the fellowship activities for the duration of the fellowship. At the conclusion of the fellowship, a fellow who accepts a tenure-track appointment at a U.S. institution eligible to receive NSF funds may apply for a research starter grant. Application materials are available on request. The deadline for FastLane submission of new postdoctoral fellowships is 5 p.m. local time on the first Monday in December each year. NSF 00-139
Requirements: Applicants must be U.S. nationals from underrepresented minority groups. Graduate students who will complete the PhD within one year or have completed it within the previous four years and who have not completed more than two years of postdoctoral support are eligible to apply.
Amount of Grant: $1.8 million total
Date(s) Application is Due: Dec 5
Contact: Carter Kimsey, Program Officer, (703) 292-8470; email: ckimsey@nsf.gov
Internet: http://www.nsf.gov/pubs/2001/nsf00139/nsf00139.txt
Sponsor: National Science Foundation
4201 Wilson Boulevard
Arlington, VA 22230

NSF Biological Physics (BP) 2878
The program supports projects in which the analytical and experimental tools of physics are applied to the study of problems originating in the living world. Both experimental and theoretical projects will be considered, although the main focus of the program is in the experimental area. Of particular interest are projects in which new experimental approaches are brought to bear on a well-identified problem. These approaches should at the same time have the potential for broad applicability to a set of similar problems, thereby adding to the set of tools the scientist has for addressing biological problems in general. While the problems under study must be important to advancing understanding of the living world in a meaningful way, particular emphasis will be placed on those projects in which the lessons learned from the application serve to foster new concepts and ideas that expand the intellectual basis of physics. The program funds individual investigators, although collaborative proposals between physicists and biologists are welcome.
Requirements: Unrestricted (i.e., open to any type of entity)
Samples: Trustees of Boston University - ($195,000) Electronic Recognition of Gene Regulatory Proteins Bound to DNA; University of California-Berkeley - ($300,000) In vitro and in vivo Single Molecular Experiments of Biological Systems; University of Illinois at Chicago - ($180,000) Study of the Dynamics of Protein-DNA Interactions to Probe Site-Specific Recognition; University of California-Davis - ($135,000) Computational study of DNA repair enzyme photolyase.
Amount of Grant: $135,000 - $500,000
Date(s) Application is Due: Jul 31
Contact: C. D. Caldwell, dcaldwel@nsf.gov, (703) 292-7371; James M. Olsen, jolsen@nsf.gov, (703) 292-7388; Ramona Winkelbauer, winkelb@nsf.gov, (703) 292-7390
Internet: http://nsf.gov/funding/pgm_summ.jsp?pims_id=6673&org=NSF&sel_org=NSF&from=fund
Sponsor: National Science Foundation
4201 Wilson Boulevard
Arlington, VA 22230

NSF Biomedical Engineering and Engineering Healthcare Grants 2879
The mission of the Biomedical Engineering and Engineering Healthcare cluster is to provide opportunities to develop novel ideas into projects that integrate engineering and life science principles in solving biomedical problems that serve humanity. The cluster focuses on high impact transforming technologies for deriving information from cells, tissues, organs, and organ systems, extraction of useful information from complex biomedical signals, new approaches to the design of structures and materials for eventual medical use, biophotonics, and new methods of controlling living systems. This cluster is also directed toward the characterization, restoration, and/or substitution of normal functions in humans.
Contact: Marcia Rawlings, Information Technology Specialist; (703) 292-7956; fax: (703) 292-9013; email: mrawling@nsf.gov
Internet: http://www.nsf.gov/funding/pgm_summ.jsp?pims_id=501032
Sponsor: National Science Foundation
4201 Wilson Boulevard
Arlington, VA 22230

NSF Biomolecular Systems Cluster Grants 2880
The Biomolecular Systems Cluster emphasizes the structure, function, dynamics, interactions, and interconversions of biological molecules. The context for such studies can range from investigations of individual macromolecules to the large-scale integration of metabolic and energetic processes. Research supported by this cluster includes development of cutting-edge technologies integrating theoretical, computational, and experimental approaches to the study of biological molecules and their functional complexes; mechanistic studies of the regulation and catalysis of enzymes and RNA, and higher-order characterization of the biochemical processes by which all organisms acquire, transform, and utilize energy from substrates. This cluster emphasizes the importance of multi-disciplinary research carried out at the interfaces of biology, physics, chemistry, mathematics and computer science, and engineering.
Requirements: Standard NSF Grant Proposal Guidelines apply (see http://www.nsf.gov/publications/pub_summ.jsp?ods_key=gpg).
Date(s) Application is Due: Jan 12; Jul 12
Contact: Kamal Shukla, Program Director; (703) 292-7131; email: kshukla@nsf.gov
Internet: http://www.nsf.gov/funding/pgm_summ.jsp?pims_id=12771
Sponsor: National Science Foundation
4201 Wilson Boulevard
Arlington, VA 22230

NSF Cell Systems Cluster Grants 2881
The Cellular Systems Cluster, one of three thematic areas within the Division of Molecular and Cellular Biosciences, supports research, across all taxa, into the structure and organization of cells and the dynamics of cellular processes. The Cellular Systems cluster is interested not only in traditional areas of cell biology (such as the organization, function, and dynamics of membranes, organelles and other subcellular compartments, and intracellular and transmembrane signal transduction mechanisms and cell-cell signaling processes) but also in the development of quantitative, theory-driven approaches to cell biology that integrate experimental studies at the molecular genetic, biochemical, biophysical, transcriptomic and proteomic levels. Network theory (e.g., as applied to signal transduction) and molecular dynamic modeling (e.g., as applied to the structure/function relationships of cellular structures) are also of particular interest.
Requirements: While proposals using approaches and model systems traditional in the field of cell biology are welcome, studies focused on novel, unique approaches and on non-traditional model organisms are encouraged.
Date(s) Application is Due: Jan 12; Jul 12
Contact: Gregory Warr, Program Director; (703) 292-8284; email: gwarr@nsf.gov;; LaJoyce Debro, Program Director: (703) 292-7135; email: ldebro@nsf.gov
Internet: http://www.nsf.gov/funding/pgm_summ.jsp?pims_id=12772
Sponsor: National Science Foundation (NSF)
4201 Wilson Boulevard
Arlington, VA 22230

NSF Chemical, Biochemical, and Biotechnology Systems Research Grants 2882
The Chemical, Biochemical, and Biotechnology cluster deals with problems involved in the processing and manufacture of products of economic importance by effectively utilizing chemical resources and renewable resources of biological origin, often with the aid of bioinformatics originating from genomic and proteomic information. This cluster supports fundamental and applied research on catalytic processes and understanding the kinetics and mechanisms of pertinent reactions. Research in control, optimization, and process modeling are also supported. Chemical and Biological Separations, Biochemical Engineering, Biotechnology, Catalysis and Biocatalysis, and Process and Reaction Engineering are funded as part of this activity.

Amount of Grant: $400,000 maximum
Contact: Marcia Rawlings, Information Technology Specialist; (703) 292-7956; fax: (703) 292-9013; email: mrawling@nsf.gov
Internet: http://www.nsf.gov/funding/pgm_summ.jsp?pims_id=13481
Sponsor: National Science Foundation
4201 Wilson Boulevard, Room 565
Arlington, VA 22230

NSF Chemistry Research Experiences for Undergraduates (REU) **2883**

The program supports active research participation by undergraduate students in any of the areas of research funded by the National Science Foundation. The NSF Division of Chemistry funds about 20-25 REU Sites a year (depending on the availability of funds) as part of the NSF-wide REU activity. Projects involve students in meaningful ways in ongoing research programs or in research projects specifically designed for the program. Two mechanisms are featured for support of student research: (1) REU Sites are based on independent proposals to initiate and conduct projects that engage a number of students in research. REU Sites may be based in a single discipline or academic department, or on interdisciplinary or multi-department research opportunities with a coherent intellectual theme. Proposals with an international dimension are welcome. A partnership with the Department of Defense supports REU Sites in DoD-relevant research areas. (2) REU Supplements may be requested for ongoing NSF-funded research projects or may be included as a component of proposals for new or renewal NSF grants or cooperative agreements.
Requirements: For REU Site proposals, a single individual should be designated as the Principal Investigator. This individual will be responsible for overseeing all aspects of the award. However, one additional person may be designated as Co-Principal Investigator, if developing and operating the REU Site would involve such shared responsibility. Other anticipated research supervisors should be listed as Non-Co-PI Senior Personnel. Undergraduate student participants in either Sites or Supplements must be citizens or permanent residents of the United States or its possessions. An undergraduate student is a student who is enrolled in a degree program (part-time or full-time) leading to a baccalaureate or associate degree. Students who are transferring from one college or university to another and are enrolled at neither institution during the intervening summer may participate. High school graduates who have been accepted at an undergraduate institution but who have not yet started their undergraduate study are also eligible to participate. Students who have received their bachelor's degrees and are no longer enrolled as undergraduates are generally not eligible to participate. For REU Sites, a significant fraction of the student participants should come from outside the host institution or organization. Some NSF directorates encourage inclusion in the REU program of K-12 teachers of science, technology, engineering, and mathematics. Please contact the appropriate disciplinary program officer for guidance.
Restrictions: Students may not apply to NSF to participate in REU activities. Students apply directly to REU Sites and should consult the directory of active REU Sites.
Contact: Wilfredo Colon, Program Director; (703) 292-8171; fax: (703) 292-9061; email: wcolon@nsf.gov
Internet: http://www.nsf.gov/funding/pgm_summ.jsp?pims_id=503210
Sponsor: National Science Foundation
4201 Wilson Boulevard
Arlington, VA 22230

NSF Doctoral Dissertation Improvement Grants in the Directorate for Biological Sciences (DDIG) **2884**

This program awards grants in selected areas of the biological sciences. These grants provide partial support of doctoral dissertation research to improve the overall quality of research. Allowed are costs for doctoral candidates to participate in scientific meetings, to conduct research in specialized facilities or field settings, and to expand an existing body of dissertation research. NSF 08-564.
Requirements: U.S. institutions and organizations that are eligible for awards from the National Science Foundation, including colleges, universities, and other nonprofit research organizations such as botanical gardens, marine and freshwater institutes, and natural history museums may submit proposals. See Chapter I, Section E of the NSF Grant Proposal Guide (GPG) for specific definitions of these categories of proposers. The NSF encourages collaborations with scientists at foreign organizations; however, primary support for any foreign participants' activities must be secured through their own national sources. A student must have advanced to candidacy for a Ph.D. degree before the submission deadline to be eligible to submit a proposal. A statement that the student has advanced to candidacy for a Ph.D., signed and dated by the department chairperson, graduate dean, or similar administrative official is required. The proposal must be submitted through regular organizational channels by the dissertation advisor(s) on behalf of a graduate student who is at the point of initiating or is already conducting dissertation research. The student must be enrolled at a U.S. institution, but need not be a U.S. citizen. Organizations should limit applications to outstanding dissertation proposals with unusual financial requirements that cannot be met otherwise. Preference may be given to projects that are underway and for which feasibility is demonstrated.
Restrictions: Indirect costs not allowed.
Amount of Grant: up to $15,000
Date(s) Application is Due: Nov 20
Contact: DEB Program Officer, (703) 292-8480, ddig-deb@nsf.gov; IOS Program Officer, (703) 292-8423, ddig-ios@nsf.gov
Internet: http://www.nsf.gov/funding/pgm_summ.jsp?pims_id=5234&org=BIO&sel_org=BIO&from=fund
Sponsor: National Science Foundation
4201 Wilson Boulevard
Arlington, VA 22230

NSF Emerging Frontiers in Research and Innovation (EFRI) Grants **2885**

The Directorate for Engineering at the National Science Foundation has established the Office of Emerging Frontiers in Research and Innovation (EFRI) to serve a critical role in focusing on important emerging areas in a timely manner. The EFRI Office is launching a new funding opportunity for interdisciplinary teams of researchers to embark on rapidly advancing frontiers of fundamental engineering research. For this program, they will consider proposals that aim to investigate emerging frontiers in the following two specific research areas: (1) BioSensing & BioActuation: Interface of Living and Engineered Systems (BSBA), and (2) Hydrocarbons from Biomass (HyBi). EFRI seeks proposals with transformative ideas that represent an opportunity for a significant shift in fundamental engineering knowledge with a strong potential for long term impact on national needs or a grand challenge. It is anticipated that 11 or more standard grants will be made (4-year awards).
Requirements: Proposals may be submitted by a single organization or a group of organizations consisting of a lead organization in partnership with one or more partner organizations. Only U.S. academic institutions with significant research and degree-granting education programs in disciplines normally supported by NSF are eligible to be the lead organization. Principal investigators are encouraged to form synergistic collaborations among researchers and with private and public sector organizations, government laboratories, and scientists and engineers at foreign organizations where appropriate, though no NSF funds will be provided to those organizations. Submission of Letters of Intent is required, due by October 14. Submission of Preliminary Proposals is required, due by December 2. Full proposals will be due by April 30. Each project team may receive support of up to a total of $500,000 per year for up to four years, pending the availability of funds. It is not expected that all awards will receive the maximum amount; the size of awards will depend upon the type of research program proposed. See the website for the detailed solicitation, which includes guidelines, requirements, and application instructions.
Restrictions: The principal investigator and co-principal investigators may participate in one proposal submitted to this program.
Amount of Grant: up to $500,000 per year
Date(s) Application is Due: Oct 14; Dec 2; Apr 30
Contact: Sohi Rastegar, Director, Office of Emerging Frontiers in Research and Innovation (EFRI); (703) 292-8305; email: srastega@nsf.gov
Internet: http://www.nsf.gov/funding/pgm_summ.jsp?pims_id=13708
Sponsor: National Science Foundation
4201 Wilson Boulevard
Arlington, VA 22230

NSF Genes and Genome Systems Cluster Grants **2886**

Grants support studies on genomes and genetic mechanisms in all organisms, whether prokaryote, eukaryote, phage, or virus. Proposals on the structure, maintenance, expression, transfer, and stability of genetic information in DNA, RNA, and proteins and how those processes are regulated are appropriate. Areas of interest include genome organization, molecular and cellular evolution, replication, recombination, repair, and vertical and lateral transmission of heritable information. Of equal interest are the processes that mediate and regulate gene expression, such as chromatin structure, epigenetic phenomena, transcription, RNA processing, editing and degradation, and translation. The use of innovative in vivo and/or in vitro approaches, including biochemical, physiological, genetic, genomic, and/or computational methods, is encouraged, as is research at the interfaces of biology, physics, chemistry, mathematics and computer science, and engineering.
Requirements: Standard NSF Grant Proposal Guidelines apply (see http://www.nsf.gov/publications/pub_summ.jsp?ods_key=gpg).
Date(s) Application is Due: Jan 12; Jul 12
Contact: Patrick P. Dennis, Program Director; (703) 292-7145; fax: (703) 292-9061; email: pdennis@nsf.gov
Internet: http://www.nsf.gov/funding/pgm_summ.jsp?pims_id=12780
Sponsor: National Science Foundation
4201 Wilson Boulevard
Arlington, VA 22230

NSF Grant Opportunities for Academic Liaison with Industry (GOALI) **2887**

Grant Opportunities for Academic Liaison with Industry (GOALI) promotes university-industry partnerships by making project funds or fellowships/traineeships available to support an eclectic mix of industry-university linkages. Special interest is focused on affording the opportunity for: faculty, postdoctoral fellows, and students to conduct research and gain experience in an industrial setting; industrial scientists and engineers to bring industry's perspective and integrative skills to academe; and interdisciplinary university-industry teams to conduct research projects. This solicitation targets high-risk/high-gain research with a focus on fundamental research, new approaches to solving generic problems, development of innovative collaborative industry-university educational programs, and direct transfer of new knowledge between academe and industry. GOALI seeks to fund transformative research that lies beyond that which industry would normally fund.
Contact: Donald Senich, Program Director; (703) 292-7082; fax: (703) 292-9056; email: dsenich@nsf.gov
Internet: http://www.nsf.gov/funding/pgm_summ.jsp?pims_id=13706
Sponsor: National Science Foundation
4201 Wilson Boulevard
Arlington, VA 22230

NSF Instrument Development for Biological Research (IDBR) 2888

The IDBR program provides support for development of the following: (1) New instrumentation that addresses emerging biological research needs with the capacity to transform biological research; (2) Novel instrument configurations (hybrids, etc.) that demonstrably address a fundamental biological research challenge; (3) Instrumentation that leverages advances in micro- and nano-fabrication and device design to provide new capabilities in measurement and observation of biological phenomena; (4) Concept and proof-of-concept of novel instruments for biological research; (5) New instruments that provide new capabilities for detection, measurement, and/or observation of biological phenomena, or that greatly extend currently achievable sensitivity, accuracy or resolution; (6) Sensors that meet emerging biological research needs and that have the potential to transform biological research at any level of organization (7) Data acquisition and analysis tools that, through the development of novel devices/instruments, meet biological research needs. The program is not limited to the above mentioned activities. Any proposal that is designed to meet the goals of the Program will be considered. Proposals must, in all cases, demonstrate a strong connection to biological research needs through, for example, collaboration with biological researchers as well as demonstrate that the need for the instrumentation is firmly based on biological research drivers. NSF Program Solicitation 08-566.

Requirements: The program encourages proposals which conduct collaborative and planning activities such as workshops and the development of virtual organization frameworks. Those activities which promote interactions between the instrument development community and biological researchers as well as innovative networking strategies that foster research collaborations or enable new instrument development directions are especially encouraged. Activities which increase participation of colleagues at smaller institutions, minority-serving institutions, community colleges, and K-12 students and teachers are also recommended. Recognizing that the development and use of novel instrumentation have become increasingly integral to activities supported by all BIO programs, the IDBR program will place a higher priority on proposals that create novel instrumentation that enables biological research in a new and potentially transformative way and that serves a broad user community. Check the NSF Grant Proposal Guide (GPG) available electronically on the NSF website at: http://www.nsf.gov/publications/pub_summ.jsp?ods_key=gpg for other general eligibility guidelines.

Restrictions: The program does not support research or technique development activities, except to the extent these are required as part of the development of the new or improved instrument, or for the testing of its utility. Projects emphasizing the development of new research techniques should be addressed to an appropriate research program. The anticipated uses of the instrumentation to be developed or improved should include areas of research that fall within the scope of the Directorate for Biological Sciences (see BIO Home Page at http://www.nsf.gov/bio). Projects aimed at instrumentation whose primary use will be in studies of the etiology, diagnosis or treatment of physical or mental disease, abnormality, or malfunction in human beings or animals, is not supported by IDBR. Similarly, the development or testing of drugs or of instruments whose primary application is in pharmaceutical chemistry are not eligible for support. Such projects should be addressed to an appropriate program in another NSF Directorate or to another agency. Projects in which the main portion of the instrument development activity will be subcontracted to a Federally Funded Research and Development Center (FFRDC) or a commercial (for profit) organization are also not eligible for support by IDBR, and should be addressed to an appropriate NSF program or to another agency.

Date(s) Application is Due: Aug 28

Contact: Robyn Hannigan, Program Director; (703) 292-8470; fax: (703) 292-9063; email: dbiiid@nsf.gov

Internet: http://www.nsf.gov/publications/pub_summ.jsp?ods_key=nsf08566&org=NSF

Sponsor: National Science Foundation
4201 Wilson Boulevard
Arlington, VA 22230

NSF Major Research Instrumentation Program (MRI) Grants 2889

The MRI program assists in the acquisition or development of major research instrumentation that is, in general, too costly for support through other NSF programs. This program seeks to improve the quality and expand the scope of research and research training in science and engineering, and to foster the integration of research and education by providing instrumentation for research-intensive learning environments. For proposals over $2 million, requests must be for the acquisition of a single instrument. For proposals requesting $2 million or less, investigators may seek support for instrument development or for acquisition of a single instrument, a large system of instruments, or multiple instruments that share a common or specific research focus. Submission of Letters of Intent is required (only for acquisition requests between $2 million and $4 million).

Requirements: Proposals may only be submitted by the following: (1) U.S. colleges, universities and organizations of higher education located in the U.S., its territories and possessions; (2) U.S. independent research museums located in the U.S., its territories and possessions; (3) U.S. independent nonprofit research organizations located in the U.S., its territories and possessions, including consortia whose members consist only of organizations described in items (1) and (2). (Requests for instrumentation that will be located at a Federally Funded Research and Development Center (FFRDC) must be submitted as consortium proposals. This is the only mechanism by which instrumentation, whether purchased or developed, can be placed at an FFRDC.); (4) U.S. small businesses located in the U.S., its territories and possessions are eligible for instrument development support as private sector partners with submitting organizations; they may not submit proposals as a lead organization. The deadline is the fourth Thursday in January. Proposers are required to prepare and submit all proposals for this program solicitation through use of the NSF FastLane system.

Restrictions: The MRI program will NOT support proposal requests for: Computer networks used for general-purposes; General laboratory equipment or assorted instruments that do not share a common or specific research or research training focus; Instrumentation used primarily for standard science and engineering courses; Renovation or modernization of research facilities, fixed equipment, or facilities such as research vessels, airplanes, large telescopes, and supercomputing centers. The term 'research facilities' refers to the bricks-and-mortar physical plant in which sponsored or unsponsored research activities (including research training) take place, including related infrastructure, systems (e.g., HVAC and power systems, toxic waste removal systems), and fixed equipment. The term 'fixed equipment' refers to the permanent components of a research facility that are integral (i.e., built in, rather than affixed) to the facility (e.g., clean rooms, fume hoods, elevators, laboratory casework); their removal would affect the integrity or basic operation of the facility.

Amount of Grant: up to $4,000,000

Date(s) Application is Due: Jan 22

Contact: Joan M. Frye, (703) 292-8040, email: jfrye@nsf.gov; Randy Phelps, (703) 292-8040, email: rphelps@nsf.gov

Internet: http://nsf.gov/funding/pgm_summ.jsp?pims_id=5260

Sponsor: National Science Foundation
4201 Wilson Boulevard
Arlington, VA 22230

NSF Perception, Action & Cognition Research Grants 2890

This program supports research on perception, action and cognition including the development of these capacities. Emphasis is on research strongly grounded in theory. Research topics include vision, audition, haptics, attention, memory, reasoning, written and spoken discourse, motor control, and developmental issues in all topic areas. The program encompasses a wide range of theoretical perspectives, such as symbolic computation, connectionism, ecological, nonlinear dynamics, and complex systems, and a variety of methodologies including both experimental studies and modeling. Research involving acquired or developmental deficits is appropriate if the results speak to basic issues of perception, action, and cognition.

Amount of Grant: $1100-$4.9 million range; $85,000 average

Date(s) Application is Due: Feb 1; Aug 1

Contact: Vincent R. Brown, Program Director; (703) 292-7305; email: vrbrown@nsf.gov;; Betty K. Tuller, Program Director; (703) 292-7238; email: btuller@nsf.gov

Internet: http://www.nsf.gov/funding/pgm_summ.jsp?pims_id=5686

Sponsor: National Science Foundation (NSF)
4201 Wilson Boulevard
Arlington, VA 22230

NSF Postdoctoral Research Fellowships in Biology (PRFB) 2891

The Directorate for Biological Sciences (BIO) awards Postdoctoral Research Fellowships in Biology to recent recipients of the doctoral degree for research and training in selected areas of biology supported by BIO to encourage independence early in their research careers and to permit them to pursue their research and training goals in the most appropriate research locations regardless of the availability of funding for the Fellows at that site. The fellowships are also designed to provide active mentoring of the Fellows by the sponsoring scientists who will benefit from having additional members in their research groups. The research and training plan of each fellowship must address important scientific questions in contemporary biology within the scope of the BIO Directorate and the specific guidelines in this fellowship program solicitation. Because the fellowships are offered only to postdoctoral scientists early in their careers, doctoral advisors are encouraged to discuss the availability of BIO fellowships with their graduate students early in their doctoral programs. Fellowships are awards to individuals, not institutions, and are administered by the Fellows. Fellowship stipends are being adjusted on a yearly basis.

Requirements: Only individuals may apply. NSF postdoctoral fellowships are awards to individuals, and applications are submitted directly by applicants to NSF. However, applications must include sponsoring scientists' statements and the applicants must affiliate with institutions (e.g., colleges and universities, and privately-sponsored nonprofit institutes and museums, government agencies and laboratories, and, under special conditions, for-profit organizations) anywhere in the world. Applicants must: (1) be U.S. citizens (or nationals) or legally admitted permanent residents of the United States (i.e., have a 'green card') at the time of application; (2) earn or plan to earn the doctoral degree in a scientific or engineering field prior to the requested start date of the fellowship; (3) either currently be a graduate student or, at the deadline date, have served in a position requiring the doctoral degree for no more than 12 full time months since earning the degree. There is a one time exception to this criterion for Biological Informatics in November, 2007 only, as described below; (4) must present a research and training plan that falls within the purview of BIO and includes the required information for the specific competition as described below; (5) select a host institution and sponsoring scientist different from the doctoral degree and current position or provide compelling justification for why such a change is not being proposed; (6) not have received Federal funding of more than $20,000 as PI or co-PI (except graduate fellowships and doctoral dissertation improvement grants); (7) not have submitted concurrently the same project to another NSF program; (8) not be a named participant on any other proposal submitted to NSF, including regular research proposals, concurrent with the fellowship application, regardless of who is the named principal investigator; AND (9) meet other limitations on eligibility imposed within the specific competitive areas, if any. There is no limit on the number of applicants that an institution may host. For now, submission can only be made using NSF's FastLane system, given that Grants.gov does not support all required forms. Applications are due the first Monday in November by 5 p.m. proposer's local time.

Amount of Grant: $60,000 - $66,000 per year

Date(s) Application is Due: Nov
Contact: Carter Kimsey, Program Manager, Broadening Participation, (703) 292-8470, email: ckimsey@nsf.gov; Peter McCartney, Program Director, Informatics, (703) 292-8470, email: pmccartn@nsf.gov
Internet: http://www.nsf.gov/publications/pub_summ.jsp?ods_key=nsf07580&org=BIO
Sponsor: National Science Foundation
4201 Wilson Boulevard
Arlington, VA 22230

NSF Presidential Early Career Awards for Scientists and Engineers Grants 2892
Each year NSF selects nominees for the Presidential Early Career Awards for Scientists and Engineers (PECASE) from among the most meritorious new CAREER awardees. Selection for this award is based on two important criteria: innovative research at the frontiers of science and technology that is relevant to the mission of the sponsoring organization or agency, and community service demonstrated through scientific leadership, education or community outreach. These awards foster innovative developments in science and technology, increase awareness of careers in science and engineering, give recognition to the scientific missions of the participating agencies, enhance connections between fundamental research and national goals, and highlight the importance of science and technology for the Nation's future. Individuals cannot apply for PECASE. These awards are initiated by the participating federal agencies. At NSF, up to twenty nominees for this award are selected each year from among the PECASE-eligible CAREER awardees who are most likely to become the leaders of academic research and education in the twenty-first century. The White House Office of Science and Technology Policy makes the final selection and announcement of the awardees.
Requirements: Applicant must be employed at an institution in the United States, its territories or possessions, or Puerto Rico, that awards a baccalaureate or advanced degree in a field supported by NSF; be in their first or second full-time tenure-track academic appointment and have begun the first tenure-track or appointment (at any institution) on or after October 1, 1996, and before October 1, 2001; not be tenured or have held tenure on or before October 1, 2001; and not be a previous recipient of a CAREER or PECASE award. Contact program officer for exact requirements.
Restrictions: No salary support for other Senior Personnel is permitted, in either the primary budget or in any sub awards.
Amount of Grant: $400,000 - $500,000 for a 5-yr period
Date(s) Application is Due: Jul 21; Jul 22; Jul 23
Contact: Elizabeth L. Rom, Program Director; (703) 292-7709; fax: (703) 292-9085; email: elrom@nsf.gov;; Donald Elthon; (703) 292-8580; fax: (703) 292-9085; email: delthon@nsf.gov
Internet: http://www.nsf.gov/funding/pgm_summ.jsp?pims_id=5262
Sponsor: National Science Foundation
4201 Wilson Boulevard
Arlington, VA 22230

NSF Small Business Innovation Research (SBIR) Grants 2893
The Small Business Innovation Research (SBIR) Program stimulates technological innovation in the private sector by strengthening the role of small business concerns in meeting Federal research and development needs, increasing the commercial application of federally supported research results, and fostering and encouraging participation by socially and economically disadvantaged and women-owned small businesses.
Requirements: Eligible to apply are small business firms—those organized for profit, individually owned or operated, not dominant in the field in which they are bidding, and with an average of no more than 500 employees in all affiliated firms. In addition, the primary employment of the principal investigator must be with the small business firm at the time of the award.
Samples: Inrad Inc (Northvale, NJ)—Growth of potassium iodate single crystals for nonlinear applications (Phase I SBIR), $65,000.; Metcal Inc (Menlo Park, CA)—Computer design of a new class of magnetic alloys (Phase I SBIR), $65,000.
Amount of Grant: $5000-$4 million; $119,000 average
Contact: Gregory T. Baxter, Program Director; (703) 292-7795; fax: (703) 292-9057; email: gbaxter@nsf.gov
Internet: http://www.nsf.gov/funding/pgm_summ.jsp?pims_id=503361
Sponsor: National Science Foundation
4201 Wilson Boulevard
Arlington, VA 22230

NSF Social Psychology Research Grants 2894
Grants support laboratory and field research in all areas of human social behavior, including attitude formation and change, social cognition, personality processes, interpersonal relations and group processes, the self, emotion, social comparison and social influence, the social psychology of health, and the psychophysiological correlates of social behavior. This program also supports research on social development over the human life span. Proposals are accepted at any time; target dates indicate the approximate time of review panel meetings. PD 98-1332
Date(s) Application is Due: Jan 15; Jul 15
Contact: Amber Story, Program Director, (703) 292-7249; email: astory@nsf.gov
Internet: http://www.nsf.gov/funding/pgm_summ.jsp?pims_id=5712
Sponsor: National Science Foundation
4201 Wilson Boulevard
Arlington, VA 22230

NSF Systematic Biology and Biodiversity Inventories Grants 2895
The Systematic Biology and Biodiversity Inventories Cluster supports research in taxonomy and systematics that contributes to: 1) using phylogenetic methods to understand the evolution of life in time and space, 2) discovery, description, and cataloguing global species diversity, and 3) organizing information from the above in efficiently retrievable forms that best meet the needs of science and society. The Systematic Biology and Biodiversity Inventories Cluster funds projects within the two Programs, Systematic Biology and Biodiversity Inventories, in addition to the PEET and PBI solicitations listed below. In addition, the cluster participates in AToL and other related funding opportunities. The SBBI Cluster continues to encourage and support studies that seek to synthesize available and new species-level taxonomic information in the context of providing revisionary treatments and predictive classifications for particular groups of organisms. NSF PD 047374.
Requirements: The most frequent recipients are academic institutions and nonprofit research groups. In special circumstances, grants also are awarded to other types of institutions and to individuals. Standard NSF Grant Proposal Guidelines apply (see http://www.nsf.gov/publications/pub_summ.jsp?ods_key=gpg).
Date(s) Application is Due: Jan 9; Jul 9
Contact: Maureen Kearney, Program Director; (703) 292-7187; email: mkearney@nsf.gov
Internet: http://www.nsf.gov/publications/pub_summ.jsp?ods_key=pd047374&org=NSF
Sponsor: National Science Foundation
4201 Wilson Boulevard
Arlington, VA 22230

NSF Undergraduate Research and Mentoring in the Biological Sciences 2896
This program will fund projects that have strong research and mentoring activities designed to prepare students for successful entry into graduate programs. URM will support projects involving the recruitment, retention and development of undergraduate students, especially those from underrepresented groups, for the purpose of preparing them for graduate study in the biological sciences. Proposed projects are expected to create a URM program that will actively engage students in interesting and exciting research ideas, provide hands-on research experience, and develop their academic skills. URM will enable institutions to create innovative programs that will increase the number and diversity of students who enter graduate research programs in the biological sciences. URM will support well-defined research and mentoring activities that will enable students, especially underrepresented minorities, to become independent thinkers and effective communicators, as well as professional development activities that will expose students to exciting careers in biology. Students are expected to be recruited early in their academic career. The project should frame all student activities around an effective mentoring strategy. Factors that are known to increase the likelihood of success for students to enter, and complete, graduate research programs should be emphasized. Approximately $4,000,000 will be available for this program, subject to the availability of funds. Under the solicitation, requests may be submitted for funding amounts up to a total of $1,000,000 for up to 5 years. However, funding beyond the first year is contingent upon satisfactory progress in the program. The program expects to make at least eight awards, depending upon the quality of submissions and the availability of funds.
Requirements: Preliminary Proposals (deadline: Sep. 18) are required prior to submitting a Full Proposal (deadline: Mar. 4). Proposals may only be submitted by academic institutions located in the United States. Collaborative Proposals from two or more institutions are allowed. The proposing institution is expected to foster an enriched and intellectually stimulating research and educational environment. URM proposals should involve year-round mentoring and include a major emphasis on direct student participation in research leading to publishable data. URM projects may be based in a single discipline or academic department, or on interdisciplinary or multi-department research opportunities. A proposal should reflect the unique combination of the proposing organization's interests and capabilities and those of any partnering organizations. Partnerships between minority-serving institutions, especially Historically Black Colleges and Universities (HBCU), Tribal Colleges and Universities (TCU), and Hispanic-Serving Institutions (HSI), community colleges, and research intensive institutions are encouraged, if such partnerships will result in a diverse pool of qualified participants as well as an enriched research environment for the students. Undergraduate student participants supported with NSF funds must be citizens or permanent residents of the United States or its possessions. An undergraduate student is one who is enrolled in a degree program (part-time or full-time) leading to a baccalaureate or associates degree. High school graduates who have not yet enrolled, and students who have received their bachelor's degrees and are no longer enrolled as undergraduates, are not eligible.
Restrictions: All collaborative proposals submitted as separate submissions from multiple organizations must be submitted via the NSF FastLane system.
Samples: University of Arkansas (AR) $149,233 - RIG: Biophysical Characterization of Cdc42Hs Forms Associated with Cell Transformation; University of Montana (MT) $170,382 - Collaborative UMEB: Training American Indians in Environmental Biology; Salish Kootenai College (MT) $132,715 - Collaborative UMEB: Training American Indians in Environmental Biology; University of Maryland Eastern Shore (MD) $150,000 - Discovery of Novel Transcription Factor III Proteins in Trypanosomes
Amount of Grant: $1,000,000 maximum
Date(s) Application is Due: Sep 18; Mar 4
Contact: URM Program Director; phone: (703) 292-8470; email: biourm@nsf.gov
Internet: http://www.nsf.gov/funding/pgm_summ.jsp?pims_id=500036
Sponsor: National Science Foundation
4201 Wilson Boulevard
Arlington, VA 22230

NSF-NIST Interaction in Chemistry, Materials Research, Molecular Biosciences, Bioengineering, and Chemical Engineering 2897

This program is intended to facilitate interactions between faculty and students supported by the National Science Foundation (NSF) and scientists at the National Institute of Standards and Technology's (NIST) Chemical Science and Technology Laboratory (CSTL) and Materials Science and Engineering Laboratory (MSEL), including the NIST Center for Neutron Research (NCNR). Chemistry, materials research, molecular biology, bioengineering, and chemical engineering are centralized at NIST in these laboratories. Support may be requested for supplements to existing NSF awards to provide the opportunity for faculty and students to participate in research at NIST facilities. Support may be requested as supplements to existing NSF awards for travel expenses and per diem associated with work at these NIST laboratories for faculty, students and other personnel associated with the NSF/NIST activity. It is estimated that 10-20 supplements will be made annually, up to $20,000 each.
Requirements: Support may be requested only by organizations that have currently active awards in any of the participating NSF Divisions, viz. the Division of Bioengineering and Environmental Systems (BES), the Division of Chemical and Transport Systems (CTS), the Division of Chemistry (CHE), the Division of Materials Research (DMR), and the Division of Molecular and Cellular Biosciences (MCB). Only faculty who are principal investigators on current NSF awards from BES, CHE, CTS, DMR, or MCB are eligible to apply for supplements. Standard NSF Grant Proposal Guidelines apply (see http://www.nsf.gov/publications/pub_summ.jsp?ods_key=gpg).
Restrictions: Indirect costs (F&A) are not allowed.
Amount of Grant: up to $20,000
Contact: Dr. William F. Koch, Deputy Director, (301) 975-8301, fax: (301) 975-3845, william.koch@nist.gov; Dr. Stephen W. .Freiman, Deputy Director; (301) 975-5658, fax: (301) 975-5012, stephen.freiman@nist.gov
Internet: http://www.nsf.gov/publications/pub_summ.jsp?ods_key=nsf03568
Sponsor: National Science Foundation
4201 Wilson Boulevard
Arlington, VA 22230

Nuffield Foundation Africa Program Grants 2898

The Commission for Africa highlighted the importance of strengthening Africa's science capacity, recommending that donors develop incentives for research and development in health that meet Africa's needs, and increase funding to African-led research. With that in mind, the Foundation has recently replaced its Commonwealth Program with Africa Program grants, which aims to improve services in health, education and civil justice in Southern and Eastern Africa through the development of the expertise and experience of practitioners and policy makers.
Contact: Sarah Lock; 44-171-631-0566; fax: 44-171-323-4877; email: africaprogram@nuffieldfoundation.org
Internet: http://www.nuffieldfoundation.org/go/grants/commonwealth/page_100.html
Sponsor: Nuffield Foundation
28 Bedford Square
London WC1B 3JS United Kingdom

Nuffield Foundation Children and Families Grants 2899

The foundation was founded for the advancement of health through medical research and teaching and for the care of the elderly through scientific research and education. The Children and Families program supports work to help ensure that the legal and institutional framework is best adapted to meet the needs of children and families. At present, particular interests include (but are not limited to): work that links education and child development, either in the case of adolescent mental health or younger children; work that considers policies relevant to child welfare in a broader institutional context: parents' paid working patterns; childcare and early years provision; work that considers especially the well-being of children growing up in adverse conditions, and what institutional responses may be appropriate; work in family law, including cohabitation, child contact, child support; and work in child protection and placement (adoption and fostering) but only when it raises significant issues. Where a proposal is for a research study, Trustees are interested in the dispassionate examination of evidence. It notes that evidence is likely to be different in different cases, for different types of children and families, and are more likely to support work that takes this approach.
Requirements: Usually grants are made only to United Kingdom organizations, and support work that will be mainly based in the United Kingdom, although the Trustees welcome proposals for collaborative projects involving partners in European or Commonwealth countries.
Restrictions: The Foundation does not make grants for the running costs of voluntary bodies but will consider making a contribution to voluntary sector overheads on funded projects.
Samples: Gillian Douglas, Cardiff Law School—for Attitudes towards the law of inheritance in the context of changing family structures, 193,542 GBP (2009); Ingrid Schoon, Department of Quantitative Social Sciences, Institute of Education, 152,771 GBP (2009).
Amount of Grant: 5,000-150,000 GBP
Date(s) Application is Due: Jan 8; May 7; Sep 3
Contact: Sharon Witherspoon; 44-171-631-0566; fax: 44-171-323-4877; email: sfwpa@nuffieldfoundation.org or info@nuffieldfoundation.org
Internet: http://www.nuffieldfoundation.org/go/grants/cplfj/page_30.html
Sponsor: Nuffield Foundation
28 Bedford Square
London WC1B 3JS United Kingdom

Nuffield Foundation Law and Society Grants 2900

The foundation was founded for the advancement of health through medical research and teaching and for the care of the elderly through scientific research and education. The Foundation has long had an interest in the area of law. Its current objectives in this area are: to promote developments in the legal system that will improve its accessibility to all people; to promote wider access to legal services and advice and a better understanding of the obstacles to access to justice; to fund research and promote developments in alternative dispute resolution; to help promote a greater knowledge of the rights and duties of the individual, including those of the European citizen; to examine the implications of new human rights' obligations on civil (not criminal) justice; and to help promote a greater public understanding of the role of law in society and of the legal system.
Requirements: Usually grants are made only to United Kingdom organizations, and support work that will be mainly based in the United Kingdom, although the Trustees welcome proposals for collaborative projects involving partners in European or Commonwealth countries.
Samples: Jo Shaw, School of Law, University of Edinburgh—for Friction and overlap between EU free movement rules and immigration law in the United Kingdom, 65,171 GBP (2009); Nigel Blackwood, Forensic Mental Health Science, King's College London, 193,398 GBP, (2008).
Amount of Grant: 5,000-150,000 GBP
Date(s) Application is Due: Jan 8; May 7; Sep 3
Contact: Sharon Witherspoon; 44-171-631-0566; fax: 44-171-323-4877; email: sfwpa@nuffieldfoundation.org or info@nuffieldfoundation.org
Internet: http://www.nuffieldfoundation.org/go/grants/accesstojustice/page_57.html
Sponsor: Nuffield Foundation
28 Bedford Square
London WC1B 3JS United Kingdom

Nuffield Foundation Oliver Bird Rheumatism Program Grants 2901

The Fund will offer grants to up to five United Kingdom Higher Education Institutions where students of outstanding potential will be recruited into doctoral training. The institutions will provide multidisciplinary environments for researching problems in rheumatic disease, and be able to develop both the students' awareness of the broader context of these diseases and the professional skills required of future scientists. For each studentship the grant will provide: a stipend of not less than 13,500GBP per annum plus United Kingdom fees; research expenses at a rate of 8,000GBP per annum; and a meeting and travel allowance of 1,000GBP per annum. In addition the Fund will provide a grant to each institution of 25,000GBP over the five years of the program to support such activities as: meetings within the Collaborative Center to promote the field and assist the recruitment and training of doctoral students; the hosting of a program meeting to be attended by all program participants from the other Collaborative Centers; and occasional bursaries for interested undergraduates to work alongside the doctoral students and potential supervisors or to attend meetings in the Collaborative Centers.
Amount of Grant: 27,500GBP per year for four years
Date(s) Application is Due: Feb 28
Contact: Vicki Hughes; 44-171-631-0566; fax: 44-171-323-4877; email: oliverbird@nuffieldfoundation.org
Internet: http://www.nuffieldfoundation.org/go/grants/oliverbird/page_86.html
Sponsor: Nuffield Foundation
28 Bedford Square
London WC1B 3JS United Kingdom

Nuffield Foundation Open Door Grants 2902

The Foundation keeps an open door to proposals of exceptional merit for research projects or practical innovations that lie outside our main program areas, but that meet Trustees' wider interests. These must have some bearing on the Foundation's widest charitable object. Particular interest is given to projects which identify change or interventions which will have a practical implications for policy or practice, or that will improve the quality of research evidence in areas of public debate. Through the Open Door, the Foundation may also identify emerging areas that justify more sustained attention.
Requirements: Usually grants are made only to United Kingdom organizations, and support work that will be mainly based in the United Kingdom, although the Trustees welcome proposals for collaborative projects involving partners in European or Commonwealth countries.
Samples: Dr Alex Bryson, National Institute of Economic & Social Research—for British Workplaces in the shadow of recession, 219,167 GBP (2009); Colin Aitken, School of Mathematics, University of Edinburgh, 75,869 GBP (2009).
Amount of Grant: 5,000-150,000 GBP
Date(s) Application is Due: Jan 8; May 7; Sep 3
Contact: Sharon Witherspoon; 44-171-631-0566; fax: 44-171-323-4877; email: sfwpa@nuffieldfoundation.org or info@nuffieldfoundation.org
Internet: http://www.nuffieldfoundation.org/go/grants/opendoor/page_115.html
Sponsor: Nuffield Foundation
28 Bedford Square
London WC1B 3JS United Kingdom

Nuffield Foundation Small Grants 2903

Most recently, the Foundation has decided that it will no longer try to fund across the full range of all social sciences, but will focus on work that more closely matches the wider interests of the Foundation. As a consequence, the budgetary ceiling for individual grants will be raised from the current maximum of 12,000GBP.
Amount of Grant: 12,000GBP
Date(s) Application is Due: Jul 17

Contact: Sarah Lock; 44-171-631-0566; fax: 44-171-323-4877; email: smallgrants@nuffieldfoundation.org
Internet: http://www.nuffieldfoundation.org/go/grants/smallgrants/page_123.html
Sponsor: Nuffield Foundation
28 Bedford Square
London WC1B 3JS United Kingdom

NWHF Community-Based Participatory Research Grants **2904**
The Northwest Health Foundation supports community-based participatory research as a tool to generate meaningful information about community health and build the capacity of groups united by common challenges to organize and advocate for change. The RFP will seek to support community-based participatory research (CBPR) projects that: build community capacity for policy advocacy; and apply research findings to support policy change that improves community health.
Requirements: 501(c)3 educational institutions and governmental entities are eligible. Generally speaking, foundation programs serve the entire state of Oregon, and the following Washington counties: Clark, Cowlitz, Pacific, Skamania, and Wahkiakum. Specific programs and funds may have additional geographic restrictions. Applying organizations must sign a statement of nondiscrimination in leadership, staffing, and services.
Restrictions: Support will not be considered for basic operations, or for salaries or other expenses associated with ongoing programs.
Geographic Focus: Oregon; Washington
Date(s) Application is Due: Sep 8
Contact: Judith Woodruff, Program Director; (503) 220-1955; fax: (503) 220-1355; email: judith@nwhf.org;; Chris Kabel, Program Officer; (503) 220-1955; fax: (503) 220-1355; email: ckabel@nwhf.org
Internet: http://www.nwhf.org/index.php?/apply/cbpr
Sponsor: Northwest Health Foundation / Robert Wood Johnson Foundation
221 NW Second Avenue, Suite 300
Portland, OR 97209

NWHF Health Advocacy Small Grants **2905**
Awards of up to $10,000 will be available for 15-20 projects dedicated to one of the following areas: grassroots organizing; coalition building; communications; and policy analysis. For example, organizations may request funds to develop communications materials or enhance their Web site, dedicate staff time to keep abreast of health-reform related activity in Salem during the legislative session, or build their organizational capacity to develop a coalition focused on health reform. In addition to grant dollars, organizations can apply for approximately two days of technical assistance from the Consumer Voices for Coverage team in one or more of the areas listed above.
Requirements: 501(c)3 educational institutions and governmental entities are eligible. Generally speaking, foundation programs serve the entire state of Oregon, and the following Washington counties: Clark, Cowlitz, Pacific, Skamania, and Wahkiakum. Specific programs and funds may have additional geographic restrictions. Applying organizations must sign a statement of nondiscrimination in leadership, staffing, and services.
Restrictions: Support will not be considered for basic operations, or for salaries or other expenses associated with ongoing programs.
Geographic Focus: Northwest
Amount of Grant: $10,000 maximum
Date(s) Application is Due: Feb 4
Contact: Chris DeMars, Program Officer; (971) 230-1292 or (503) 220-1955; email: cdemars@nwhf.org
Internet: http://www.nwhf.org/index.php?/apply/access
Sponsor: Northwest Health Foundation
221 NW Second Avenue, Suite 300
Portland, OR 97209

NWHF Kaiser Permanente Community Fund Grants **2906**
The Kaiser Permanente Community Fund (KPCF) at Northwest Health Foundation was established in late 2004 to advance the health of the communities served by Kaiser Permanente Northwest. The Fund intends to achieve this goal by addressing those factors in the social, policy, and physical environment that impact community health. Often referred to as the social determinants of health, these factors have been shown to play a major role in the development of health disparities based on race, ethnicity, and socio-economic status.
Requirements: To be eligible to apply for a grant from the Community Fund, the service area of your project must fall within the geographic region roughly spanning from Longview, Washington to Salem, Oregon and portions of the Willamette Valley.
Geographic Focus: Oregon; Washington
Date(s) Application is Due: Jul 2
Contact: Judith Woodruff, Program Director; (503) 220-1955; fax: (503) 220-1355; email: judith@nwhf.org;; Chris Kabel, Program Officer; (503) 220-1955; fax: (503) 220-1355; email: ckabel@nwhf.org
Internet: http://www.nwhf.org/index.php?/apply/kaiser
Sponsor: Northwest Health Foundation
221 NW Second Avenue, Suite 300
Portland, OR 97209

NWHF Mark O. Hatfield Research Fellowship **2907**
The Mark O. Hatfield Research Fellowship Program was established in 2005 to honor the legacy of Senator Mark O. Hatfield, founding Board Chairman of the Northwest Health Foundation (NWHF). The purpose of the Fellowship program is to advance the research career of health practitioners who serve communities in Oregon and southwest Washington. The fellowship is open to health professionals from a variety of disciplines who wish to launch, renew, or expand their research activities in biomedical, applied, or translational research. A secondary purpose is to increase the intellectual resources of research-based institutions. One two-year fellowship of up to $150,000 will be awarded. Funds will be distributed to the fellow's sponsoring institution in two annual disbursements of half of the amount awarded.
Requirements: Eligible candidates must: be a clinical, allied health, public health, or social service provider (early-career researchers specializing in translational research are also encouraged to apply); possess (or be in the process of completing) a doctoral degree or equivalent in an appropriate field related to medicine, nursing, health care, public health, or biomedical sciences; obtain sponsorship from a research-based institution that can act as fiscal manager of the award; and demonstrate a commitment to communities in Oregon and southwest Washington.
Amount of Grant: $150,000 maximum
Date(s) Application is Due: Mar 16
Contact: R. David Rebanal, Officer; (503) 220-1955; email: drebanal@nwhf.org
Internet: http://www.nwhf.org/index.php?/apply/hatfield
Sponsor: Northwest Health Foundation
221 NW Second Avenue, Suite 300
Portland, OR 97209

NWHF Partners Investing in Nursing's Future Grants **2908**
Partners Investing in Nursing's Future is a collaborative initiative of the RWJ Foundation and Northwest Health Foundation that will address nursing issues at the local level through funding partnerships with community and regional foundations. The goal of this initiative is to enable local foundations to act as catalysts in developing the comprehensive strategies that are vital to establishing a stable, adequate nursing workforce. Grants support the capacity, involvement, and leadership of local foundations to advance nursing workforce solutions in their communities. Local foundations must match funds with at least $1 for every $1 provided by the program. Proposals must be submitted online. Guidelines are available online. Letters of Intent are due by October 2, and invited proposals are due on December 19.
Requirements: U.S. local or regional private, family, or community foundations are eligible. Eligible foundations are those classified under IRS codes as 501(c)3 tax exempt, a nonexempt charitable trust treated as a private foundation under 4947(a)1, or organizations claiming status as a private operating foundation under 4942(j)3 or 5. Government entities, corporations, or corporate grantmakers may participate in funding collaboratives but may not serve as the applicant organization.
Amount of Grant: $250,000 maximum
Date(s) Application is Due: Oct 2; Dec 19
Contact: Judith Woodruff, Director; (503) 220-1955; fax: (503) 220-1355; email: judith@nwhf.org;; Chris Kabel; (503) 220-1955; fax: (503) 220-1355; email: ckabel@nwhf.org
Internet: http://www.partnersinnursing.org/grants.html
Sponsor: Northwest Health Foundation / Robert Wood Johnson Foundation
221 NW Second Avenue, Suite 300
Portland, OR 97209

NYAM Brock Lecture, Award and Visiting Professorship in Pediatrics **2909**
The New York Academy of Medicine invites pediatric program directors from New York area medical schools and medical centers to nominate candidates for the annual fall Millie and Richard Brock Lecture, Award and Visiting Professorship in Pediatrics. The Brock Lecture, Award and Visiting Professorship in Pediatrics was established by Millie and Richard Brock in 1995 on the 100th anniversary of The Academy's Section on Pediatrics to sponsor a nationally recognized leader in pediatrics to engage in a one to two day visiting professorship at a New York-area pediatrics training program, to deliver the annual Brock Lecture, and to receive the Brock Award for distinguished contributions to pediatrics. The one to two day visiting professorship to a New York area pediatric training program should be part of a program which include a grand rounds lecture as well as teaching interactions with medical students, pediatric residents, fellows, and members of the attending staff. The Brock Lecture held at the Academy must address issues concerned with providing care for underserved children. Suggested topics for discussion include, but are not restricted to: childhood nutrition, HIV and AIDS, substance abuse, child abuse, asthma, violence, and environmental issues such as lead poisoning. The Brock program includes an honorarium of $1,000 and all expenses for travel, lodging, and meals. Letters of nomination, including an outline of the proposed plan for the visit and the topic for the Brock Lecture, as well as the curriculum vitae of the nominee, should be forwarded via email to: brock@nyam.org.
Samples: Mark W. Kline, MD, Professor of Pediatrics and Chief of Retrovirology at the Baylor College of Medicine and Texas Children's Hospital, Academy Lecture: "Pediatric AIDS: Worlds Apart", Visiting Professorship: Weill Cornell Medical Center (2009); Glenn Flores, MD, Professor of Pediatrics and Public Health, Director of General Pediatrics, the Judith and Charles Ginsburg Chair in Pediatrics, and the Director of the Academic General Pediatrics Fellowship at University of Texas Southwestern and Children's Medical Center Dallas, Academy Lecture: "Racial and Ethnic Disparities in U.S. Children's Health and Healthcare: How We Can Level the Playing Field", Visiting Professorship: New York University School of Medicine (2008).
Amount of Grant: $1,000 honorarium and expenses
Date(s) Application is Due: Mar 1
Contact: Coordinator, (212) 822-7204; fax: (212) 822-7338; email: brock@nyam.org
Internet: https://www.nyam.org/grants/brock.shtml
Sponsor: New York Academy of Medicine
1216 Fifth Avenue
New York, NY 10029-5202

NYAM Charles A. Elsberg Fellowship 2910
The Fellowship in Neurological Surgery was established to support research training in the specialty of neurological surgery for individuals who have completed, or will shortly complete, accredited residency training in neurological surgery, and who intend to use research training for continued development of academic careers in this field. The Elsberg Fellowship program seeks to support individuals in supervised programs that will develop the candidate's capacity to perform independent clinical or laboratory research.
Requirements: Candidates who have, or will have completed an accredited neurological surgery residency program by June 30, and whose career direction suggests eligibility for subsequent research support are invited to apply. In general, applicants are expected to be at the start of their academic careers, having completed their residency training within the past year or two. Candidates must be board certified or eligible for certification by the beginning of the grant period. The proposed research must be conducted at an institution located in the United States under the mentorship of a senior researcher.
Samples: Aaron S. Dumont, MD, University of Virginia School of Medicine (2008-09); Ziv Williams, MD, Massachusetts General HospitalJason (2007-08); H. Huang, MD, University of Rochester School of Medicine and Dentistry (2006-07).
Amount of Grant: $50,000
Contact: Program Administrator, (212) 822-7204; fax: (212) 822-7338; email: elsberg@nyam.org
Internet: http://www.nyam.org/grants/elsberg.shtml
Sponsor: New York Academy of Medicine
1216 Fifth Avenue
New York, NY 10029-5202

NYAM David E. Rogers Fellowships 2911
The Fellowship is meant to enrich the educational experiences of medical and dental students through projects that bear on medicine and dentistry as social enterprises, such as enterprises devoted to the capacity of these professions in any and all of their expressions to serve human needs. Particularly, the focus is on the needs of underserved or disadvantaged patients or populations. The content of the Fellowship might include clinical investigation, health policy analysis, activities linking biomedicine, the social infrastructure and human need, or community activities.
Requirements: Available to first-year medical and dental students for support of projects to be executed during the summer between the first and second years of medical or dental school.
Samples: Abdulrahman Mohamed El-Sayed, University of Michigan Medical School (2008); Patricia Kuan-Pei Foo, Stanford University School of Medicine (2008); Christina Marie Hupman, Medical College of Georgia (2008).
Amount of Grant: $3,500
Contact: Office of Medical and Academic Affairs; (212) 822-7204; fax: (212) 996-7338; email: rogers@nyam.org
Internet: http://www.nyam.org/grants/rogers.shtml
Sponsor: New York Academy of Medicine
1216 Fifth Avenue
New York, NY 10029-5202

NYAM Edward N. Gibbs Memorial Lecture and Award in Nephrology 2912
The New York Academy of Medicine seeks nominations of physician scientists who have dedicated their careers to advances in nephrology or are presently making cutting-edge discoveries in the field. The distinguished recipient of this honor will present his or her research at a lecture before a broad audience of scientists and clinicians, to be held at The New York Academy of Medicine in the fall. The award recipient will receive the Edward N. Gibbs Memorial Medal and an honorarium of $7,500; all travel expenses associated with the lecture will be paid by the Edward N. Gibbs Memorial Endowment. It is expected that the manuscript from this lecture will be submitted to a scholarly journal for publication.
Requirements: Candidates must hold an MD degree and be citizens of the United States to be considered for this award.
Samples: Maurice B. Burg, MD, National Institutes of Health (2008); Franklin H. Epstein, MD, Harvard Medical School (2006); Gerhard H. Giebisch, MD, Yale University School of Medicine (2004).
Amount of Grant: $7,500 honorarium
Date(s) Application is Due: Mar 1
Contact: Program Coordinator, (212) 822-7204; fax: (212) 822-7338; email: gibbs@nyam.org
Internet: https://www.nyam.org/grants/gibbs.shtml
Sponsor: New York Academy of Medicine
1216 Fifth Avenue
New York, NY 10029-5202

NYAM Edwin Beer Research Fellowship 2913
The Edwin Beer Research Fellowship seeks to increase the number of investigators in urology and urology-related fields by providing transitional funding in support of research conducted by qualified candidates. The program provides two-year grants of up to $80,000 for research projects commencing July of the award year. The grants are made to the awardees' institutions for the direct support of their salary and research activities. Fellows are required to devote at least fifty percent of their time to the research funded by the program.
Requirements: Candidates must hold an MD, PhD, or equivalent degree and are expected to conduct research in a supervised program in the United States. Applicants should have completed residency and fellowship or postdoctoral training, having demonstrated their ability to perform and direct research, and should currently be under the mentorship of a senior researcher. Fellowships are awarded to qualified candidates who are at a stage of transition prior to receiving major independent funding. Because the program seeks to increase the number of investigators in urology and urology-related fields, applicants must have a direct association with the department of urology at their sponsoring institution. Candidates are not required to be United States citizens; however, non-citizen applicants are required to provide assurances of employment eligibility to perform the proposed research.
Samples: David C. Miller, MD, University of Michigan Medical School (2009); Aria F. Olumi, MD, Massachusetts General Hospital (2009); Jayoung Kim, PhD, Harvard Medical School (2008).
Amount of Grant: $80,000 maximum
Date(s) Application is Due: Feb 2
Contact: Office of Medical and Academic Affairs; (212) 822-7204; fax: (212) 822-7338; email: beer@nyam.org
Internet: http://www.nyam.org/grants/beer.shtml
Sponsor: New York Academy of Medicine
1216 Fifth Avenue
New York, NY 10029-5202

NYAM Ferdinand C. Valentine Fellowship 2914
The Fellowship offers one-year, $50,000 fellowships in support of research by individuals who have completed, or will shortly complete, residency training acceptable to the American Board of Urology, and who intend to pursue academic research careers in urology.
Requirements: Fellows must commit no less than fifty percent of their time to the supported research and preference is given to investigators conducting their research at institutions in the greater New York area.
Restrictions: Indirect costs and fringe benefits will not be paid.
Samples: Gerald J. Wang, MD, New York Presbyterian Hospital, Weill Cornell Medical Center (2009-10); Maurico Davalos, MD, New York Medical College (2008-09); Gerald Y. Tan, MD, Weill Medical College of Cornell University (2009-09).
Amount of Grant: $50,000
Date(s) Application is Due: Feb 2
Contact: Program Administrator, (212) 822-7204; fax: (212) 822-7338; email: valentine@nyam.org
Internet: http://www.nyam.org/grants/valentine.shtml
Sponsor: New York Academy of Medicine
1216 Fifth Avenue
New York, NY 10029-5202

NYAM Lewis Rudin Glaucoma Grants 2915
This $50,000 prize is awarded for the most outstanding scholarly article on glaucoma published in a peer-reviewed journal during the previous calendar year. Nominations are solicited from leaders of the ophthalmologic community and reviewed in the spring of the award year. One prize winner is recommended for ratification by the Academy's Board of Trustees by the Lewis Rudin Glaucoma Prize Selection Committee, a group of nationally recognized experts in glaucoma research chaired by David H. Abramson, MD of Memorial Sloan-Kettering Cancer Center and Weill Medical College of Cornell University. The winner is announced in July of the award year.
Requirements: Nominees for this award must be the first or last author of the published work and must hold primary responsibility for the research. Authors may nominate themselves but may not submit multiple articles and must choose only one article to submit for consideration by the committee. All authors of the article receive recognition, however the monetary prize is granted solely to the primary researcher specified in the nomination. Copies of the published article must accompany the completed nomination form.
Samples: Oscar A. Candia, MD, Mount Sinai School of Medicine (2009); Claude Burgoyne, MD, Devers Eye Institute (2008); John Danias, MD, PhD, Mount Sinai School of Medicine (2007); Cynthia Lee Grosskreutz, MD, PhD, Harvard Medical School and Massachusetts Eye and Ear Infirmary (2006).
Amount of Grant: $50,000
Date(s) Application is Due: May 1
Contact: Program Coordinator, (212) 822-7204; fax: (212) 822-7338; email: rudinglaucoma@nyam.org
Internet: https://www.nyam.org/grants/rudin.shtml
Sponsor: New York Academy of Medicine
1216 Fifth Avenue
New York, NY 10029-5202

NYAM Mary and David Hoar Fellowship 2916
The Mary and David Hoar Fund was established to promote research in the prevention and treatment of hip fractures. The Fund provides a two-year grant of $100,000 to support pilot programs in clinical, epidemiologic and health services research in the following areas related to hip fractures: clinical care and treatment; prevention; rehabilitation; and model program development.
Requirements: Candidates must hold an MD, PhD, or equivalent degree and are expected to conduct research in a supervised program in the greater New York area. Preferential consideration will be given to new investigators for whom this award is likely to provide interim support pending future funding, or to more senior investigators who are making a change in career or research direction for whom this award will facilitate the transition. Candidates are not required to be United States citizens; however, non-citizen applicants are required to provide assurances, such as permanent resident status, of legal eligibility for employment to perform the proposed research throughout the award period, regardless of the disposition of this or any other pending grants.

Samples: Amanda S. Carmel, Weill Medical College of Cornell University (2008-10); Marcella D. Walker, Columbia University College of Physicians and Surgeons (2007-09); Knox H. Todd, Beth Israel Medical Center (2006-08).
Amount of Grant: $100,000
Contact: Administrator, (212) 822-7204; fax: (212) 822-7338; email: hoar@nyam.org
Internet: http://www.nyam.org/grants/hoar.shtml
Sponsor: New York Academy of Medicine
1216 Fifth Avenue
New York, NY 10029-5202

NYAM Student Essay Grants **2917**
The New York Academy of Medicine invites entries for the New York Academy of Medicine Student Essay Prize, awarded to the best unpublished essay by a graduate student in a medical, public health, pharmacy, or nursing program in the United States. Essays should address topics in the history of public health or medicine as they relate to urban health issues; social or environmental factors in the health of urban populations, institutional histories, or specific diseases may be considered. The winner will receive $500, and the winning essay will receive expedited review for possible publication in the Journal of Urban Health. Honorable Mention prizes may also be awarded at the discretion of the Prize Committee.
Requirements: The contest is open to students in accredited professional degree programs in medicine, nursing, pharmacy, and public health. The writer must have been a student at the time the essay was written.
Amount of Grant: $500
Contact: Program Coordinator, (212) 822-7314; fax: (212) 822-7338; email: historyessay@nyam.org
Internet: https://www.nyam.org/grants/studentessay.shtml
Sponsor: New York Academy of Medicine
1216 Fifth Avenue
New York, NY 10029-5202

NYC Managed Care Consumer Assistance Workshop Re-Design Grants **2918**
The New York City Managed Care Consumer Assistance Program (NYC MCCAP), a program of the Community Service Society of NY invites you to submit a proposal for the workshop re-design project. We are seeking individuals or agencies that have interest and knowledge around training, organizational structuring and curriculum development expertise. The goal of the workshop project is to create a more flexible workshop structure that can be easily adapted to different trainers, audiences and settings ranging from busy hospitals and clinics to classrooms and health fairs.
Requirements: 501(c)3 social service agencies with a history of providing education and counseling for low-income communities, immigrants, and populations with special health care needs are encouraged to apply.
Date(s) Application is Due: May 21
Contact: Priya Mendon; (212) 614-5400; fax: (212) 614-5305; email: pmendon@cssny.org or mccap@cssny.org
Internet: http://www.nycmccap.org/newsitems.html#rfp
Sponsor: Community Service Society of New York
105 East 22nd Street, 8th Floor
New York, NY 10010

NYCT AIDS/HIV Grants **2919**
The Trust supports projects that strengthen preventive health care, improve access to services, promote the efficient use of health resources, and develop the skills and independence of people with special needs. The goal of this program is to address the complex social, medical, and legal problems of people with HIV. Since this issue cuts across a number of program areas, projects may fall within a number of funding categories. A limited amount of support is available specifically for policy research and advocacy efforts that: increase public understanding of AIDS and HIV infection; improve the funding and delivery of services; and improve coordination among service organizations. The grant review process takes from two to six months. Grants range from $5,000 to $100,000; an average grant is around $60,000.
Requirements: Grants are made primarily to nonprofit organizations located in the five boroughs of New York City. Grants for programs outside the area are generally from funds designated for specific charities or have been made at the suggestion of donors.
Restrictions: The trust does not make grants to individuals, offer general or capital funding, endowments, building construction/renovation, deficit financing, films, or religion.
Geographic Focus: New York
Amount of Grant: $5,000-$100,000
Date(s) Application is Due: Sep 14
Contact: Joyce M. Bove, Senior Vice President; (212) 686-0010, ext. 552; fax: (212) 534-8528; email: info@nycommunitytrust.org or grants@nycommunitytrust.org
Internet: http://www.nycommunitytrust.org/HowtoApply/RequestsforProposals/NewYorkCityAIDSFund/tabid/408/Default.aspx
Sponsor: New York Community Trust
909 Third Avenue, 22nd Floor
New York, NY 10022

NYCT Biomedical Research Grants **2920**
The Trust supports projects that strengthen preventive health care, improve access to services, promote the efficient use of health resources, and develop the skills and independence of people with special needs. The Trust provides funding for biomedical research projects in four areas: blood diseases, cancer, leprosy and tuberculosis. Grants for these projects are awarded in response to requests for proposals.
Requirements: Grants are made primarily to colleges, universities, and research organizations located in the five boroughs of New York City. Grants for programs outside the area are generally from funds designated for specific charities or have been made at the suggestion of donors.
Restrictions: The trust does not make grants to individuals, offer general or capital funding, endowments, building construction/renovation, deficit financing, films, or religion.
Geographic Focus: New York
Amount of Grant: $5,000-$100,000
Contact: Joyce M. Bove, Senior Vice President; (212) 686-0010, ext. 552; fax: (212) 534-8528; email: info@nycommunitytrust.org or grants@nycommunitytrust.org
Internet: http://www.nycommunitytrust.org/ForGrantSeekers/GrantmakingGuidelines/HealthandPeoplewithSpecialNeeds/tabid/207/Default.aspx
Sponsor: New York Community Trust
909 Third Avenue, 22nd Floor
New York, NY 10022

NYCT Blindness and Visual Disabilities Grants **2921**
The Trust supports projects that strengthen preventive health care, improve access to services, promote the efficient use of health resources, and develop the skills and independence of people with special needs. The goals of this program are to support program innovation and reform and eliminate service gaps. Specifically, grants are made to projects that: improve services to those people with visual disabilities who are presently underserved, such as the elderly, minorities, people with multiple disabilities, people in institutions, and youth in transition from school to work (projects need not be limited to direct service, and may include advocacy and organizational improvement); involve people with visual disabilities more fully in community activities; expand programs that identify people with vision problems at an early stage and link them with appropriate resources; empower persons with visual disabilities by enabling them to participate in planning programs that affect them; and support research in the prevention and treatment of blindness (this may include clinical, epidemiological, and applied studies). The grant review process takes from two to six months. Grants range from $5,000 to $100,000; an average grant is around $60,000.
Requirements: Grants are made primarily to nonprofit organizations located in the five boroughs of New York City. Grants for programs outside the area are generally from funds designated for specific charities or have been made at the suggestion of donors.
Restrictions: The trust does not make grants to individuals, offer general or capital funding, endowments, building construction/renovation, deficit financing, films, or religion.
Geographic Focus: New York
Amount of Grant: $5,000-$100,000
Contact: Joyce M. Bove, Senior Vice President; (212) 686-0010, ext. 552; fax: (212) 534-8528; email: info@nycommunitytrust.org or grants@nycommunitytrust.org
Internet: http://www.nycommunitytrust.org/ForGrantSeekers/GrantmakingGuidelines/HealthandPeoplewithSpecialNeeds/tabid/207/Default.aspx
Sponsor: New York Community Trust
909 Third Avenue, 22nd Floor
New York, NY 10022

NYCT Blood Disease Research Grants **2922**
The New York Community Trust is a charitable foundation concerned with the needs of the Greater New York area. The NYCT has a special fund to be used in support of research in the field of blood diseases. A panel of recognized hematologists will convene to review proposals solicited from the major medical research institutions on a competitive basis. It is estimated that about $700,000 will be available this year to support such research projects. A total of no more than two projects may be submitted from any one organization. Basic laboratory research. Candidates may apply for support totaling $100,000 for up to 2 years, but funds for any one project year may not exceed $50,000. Second-year funding is contingent upon submission of a satisfactory progress report at the end of the first year. Research that may have application to New York City residents is of particular interest to The Trust. Young investigators will be given special consideration.
Requirements: Proposals are due no later than 5:00 p.m. on September 25th. Additional guidelines and forms are available online at the NYCT website.
Geographic Focus: New York
Amount of Grant: $100,000 over two years
Date(s) Application is Due: Sep 25
Contact: Joyce M. Bove, Senior Vice President; (212) 686-0010, ext. 552; fax: (212) 534-8528; email: info@nycommunitytrust.org or grants@nycommunitytrust.org
Internet: http://www.nycommunitytrust.org/BloodDiseaseResearch/tabid/504/Default.aspx
Sponsor: New York Community Trust
909 Third Avenue, 22nd Floor
New York, NY 10022

NYCT Children and Youth with Disabilities Grants **2923**
The Trust supports projects that strengthen preventive health care, improve access to services, promote the efficient use of health resources, and develop the skills and independence of people with special needs. The goals of this program are to stimulate policymakers and service providers to improve existing services for children with disabilities and to encourage a service approach that emphasizes independence and the development of full potential. Specifically, grants are made to projects that: foster integration into community life, independent living, and improved self-image; improve early identification of disability, encourage early intervention, and increase access to early

childhood education; provide comprehensive treatment, planning, and referral programs for children and their families; and assess needs, develop policy, and advocate to improve the delivery and coordination of services. The grant review process takes from two to six months. Grants range from $5,000 to $100,000; an average grant is around $60,000.
Requirements: Grants are made primarily to nonprofit organizations located in the five boroughs of New York City. Grants for programs outside the area are generally from funds designated for specific charities or have been made at the suggestion of donors.
Restrictions: The trust does not make grants to individuals, offer general or capital funding, endowments, building construction/renovation, deficit financing, films, or religion.
Geographic Focus: New York
Amount of Grant: $5,000-$100,000
Contact: Joyce M. Bove, Senior Vice President; (212) 686-0010, ext. 552; fax: (212) 534-8528; email: info@nycommunitytrust.org or grants@nycommunitytrust.org
Internet: http://www.nycommunitytrust.org/ForGrantSeekers/GrantmakingGuidelines/HealthandPeoplewithSpecialNeeds/tabid/207/Default.aspx
Sponsor: New York Community Trust
909 Third Avenue, 22nd Floor
New York, NY 10022

NYCT Girls and Young Women Grants **2924**
The Trust works in partnership with government and private agencies to develop the strengths of families and young people; to improve their living and working conditions; to improve family and child welfare services; and to advance social work practice. The goal of this Program is to improve conditions and opportunities for those who are poor and disadvantaged, particularly minorities and young, single mothers. Specifically, the program funds projects that: prepare girls and young women for economic self-sufficiency by providing the economic and personal support necessary to gain access to jobs and promoting innovative ways to include indigent and vulnerable young women in the workplace; and reduce the effects of health and social problems that threaten the lives and well-being of girls and young women through direct services and policy and advocacy efforts. Particular emphasis is placed on projects addressing the issues of teen pregnancy, homelessness, and AIDS. The grant review process takes from two to six months. Grants range from $5,000 to $100,000; an average grant is around $60,000.
Requirements: Grants are made primarily to nonprofit organizations located in the five boroughs of New York City. Grants for programs outside the area are generally from funds designated for specific charities or have been made at the suggestion of donors.
Restrictions: The trust does not make grants to individuals, offer general or capital funding, endowments, building construction/renovation, deficit financing, films, or religion.
Geographic Focus: New York
Amount of Grant: $5000-$100,000
Contact: Joyce M. Bove, Senior Vice President; (212) 686-0010, ext. 552; fax: (212) 534-8528; email: info@nycommunitytrust.org or grants@nycommunitytrust.org
Internet: http://www.nycommunitytrust.org/ForGrantSeekers/GrantmakingGuidelines/ChildrenYouthandFamilies/tabid/205/Default.aspx
Sponsor: New York Community Trust
909 Third Avenue, 22nd Floor
New York, NY 10022

NYCT Grants for the Elderly **2925**
The Trust supports projects that strengthen preventive health care, improve access to services, promote the efficient use of health resources, and develop the skills and independence of people with special needs. The goals of this program are to enable elderly people to remain active in their communities and to meet the basic needs of those who are vulnerable and dependent. Resources are primarily targeted toward the most underserved elderly and those whose needs are most acute, including members of racial and ethnic minorities, the poor, and those with chronic illnesses or mental or functional disabilities. Specifically, grants are made to projects that: increase the number of elderly who are able to participate in community activities, particularly those involving contact with young people; enable the elderly to assume a leadership role in planning, influencing, or changing the programs that serve them; improve the management, capacity, and resources of government and voluntary agencies serving the elderly, and encourage collaboration among agencies; and assess need, develop policy, and advocate to improve the delivery and coordination of services. The grant review process takes from two to six months. Grants range from $5,000 to $100,000; an average grant is around $60,000.
Requirements: Grants are made primarily to nonprofit organizations located in the five boroughs of New York City. Grants for programs outside the area are generally from funds designated for specific charities or have been made at the suggestion of donors.
Restrictions: The trust does not make grants to individuals, offer general or capital funding, endowments, building construction/renovation, deficit financing, films, or religion.
Geographic Focus: New York
Amount of Grant: $5,000-$100,000
Contact: Joyce M. Bove, Senior Vice President; (212) 686-0010, ext. 552; fax: (212) 534-8528; email: info@nycommunitytrust.org or grants@nycommunitytrust.org
Internet: http://www.nycommunitytrust.org/ForGrantSeekers/GrantmakingGuidelines/HealthandPeoplewithSpecialNeeds/tabid/207/Default.aspx
Sponsor: New York Community Trust
909 Third Avenue, 22nd Floor
New York, NY 10022

NYCT Health Services, Systems, and Policies Grants **2926**
The Trust supports projects that strengthen preventive health care, improve access to services, promote the efficient use of health resources, and develop the skills and independence of people with special needs. The primary goal of this program is to improve the effectiveness, responsiveness, and equity of health care in New York City. Specifically, the program makes grants: for services, policy research, advocacy, and technical assistance that promote the accessibility of basic health services, especially in minority and immigrant communities; to strengthen health service providers, especially those serving the city's poorest residents; and to promote healthy lifestyles. The grant review process takes from two to six months. Grants range from $5,000 to $100,000; an average grant is around $60,000.
Requirements: Grants are made primarily to nonprofit organizations located in the five boroughs of New York City. Grants for programs outside the area are generally from funds designated for specific charities or have been made at the suggestion of donors.
Restrictions: The trust does not make grants to individuals, offer general or capital funding, endowments, building construction/renovation, deficit financing, films, or religion.
Geographic Focus: New York
Amount of Grant: $5,000-$100,000
Contact: Joyce M. Bove, Senior Vice President; (212) 686-0010, ext. 552; fax: (212) 534-8528; email: info@nycommunitytrust.org or grants@nycommunitytrust.org
Internet: http://www.nycommunitytrust.org/ForGrantSeekers/GrantmakingGuidelines/HealthandPeoplewithSpecialNeeds/tabid/207/Default.aspx
Sponsor: New York Community Trust
909 Third Avenue, 22nd Floor
New York, NY 10022

NYCT Mental Health and Mental Retardation Grants **2927**
The Trust supports projects that strengthen preventive health care, improve access to services, promote the efficient use of health resources, and develop the skills and independence of people with special needs. The goals of this program are to foster the independence of people with mental illness and mental retardation, and to encourage a community-based system of care. Specifically, grants are made to projects that: improve the quality and availability of community housing and services for people with chronic mental illnesses; improve and expand the delivery of mental health services to children and adolescents, especially those that stress the early identification and remediation of problems; strengthen advocacy groups that promote reimbursement practices and allocation of mental health resources that correspond to community needs; and direct the attention of service providers, policy makers, and the general public to the mental health concerns of racial and ethnic minorities. The grant review process takes from two to six months. Grants range from $5,000 to $100,000; an average grant is around $60,000.
Requirements: Grants are made primarily to nonprofit organizations located in the five boroughs of New York City. Grants for programs outside the area are generally from funds designated for specific charities or have been made at the suggestion of donors.
Restrictions: The trust does not make grants to individuals, offer general or capital funding, endowments, building construction/renovation, deficit financing, films, or religion.
Geographic Focus: New York
Amount of Grant: $5,000-$100,000
Contact: Joyce M. Bove, Senior Vice President; (212) 686-0010, ext. 552; fax: (212) 534-8528; email: info@nycommunitytrust.org or grants@nycommunitytrust.org
Internet: http://www.nycommunitytrust.org/ForGrantSeekers/GrantmakingGuidelines/HealthandPeoplewithSpecialNeeds/tabid/207/Default.aspx
Sponsor: New York Community Trust
909 Third Avenue, 22nd Floor
New York, NY 10022

NYCT Substance Abuse Grants **2928**
The Trust works in partnership with government and private agencies to develop the strengths of families and young people; to improve their living and working conditions; to improve family and child welfare services; and to advance social work practice. The goal of this program is to address the treatment needs of the most under-served, with a focus on women, ex-offenders, and adolescents. Specifically, grants are made to projects that: promote coordinated drug treatment, particularly between treatment providers and other systems such as mental health and child welfare; expand treatment by building the capacity of mid-sized drug treatment programs. We will help groups strengthen and increase existing services and develop new capacity to accommodate people not being treated; and promote strategies that reduce or prevent substance abuse among elders. The grant review process takes from two to six months. Grants range from $5,000 to $100,000; an average grant is around $60,000.
Requirements: Grants are made primarily to nonprofit organizations located in the five boroughs of New York City. Grants for programs outside the area are generally from funds designated for specific charities or have been made at the suggestion of donors.
Restrictions: The trust does not make grants to individuals, offer general or capital funding, endowments, building construction/renovation, deficit financing, films, or religion.
Geographic Focus: New York
Amount of Grant: $5,000-$100,000
Contact: Joyce M. Bove, Senior Vice President; (212) 686-0010, ext. 552; fax: (212) 534-8528; email: info@nycommunitytrust.org or grants@nycommunitytrust.org
Internet: http://www.nycommunitytrust.org/ForGrantSeekers/GrantmakingGuidelines/ChildrenYouthandFamilies/tabid/205/Default.aspx
Sponsor: New York Community Trust
909 Third Avenue, 22nd Floor
New York, NY 10022

NYCT Technical Assistance Grants **2929**
The Trust focuses on relieving New York's chronic shortage of affordable housing, strengthening the local economy, and protecting the environment. It supports community-based agencies working on these issues at the neighborhood level, and

government and nonprofit institutions developing strategies for the City as a whole. The goal of this program is to improve the management capacity of nonprofits and strengthen the nonprofit sector. Specifically, The Trust provides grants: up to $10,000 to current and prospective grantees to hire consultants to help with specific management needs; to advance public and nonprofit service by developing skills and expertise of professionals in the field; and to support service and umbrella organizations providing technical assistance to groups of nonprofits. The grant review process takes from two to six months. Grants range from $5,000 to $100,000; an average grant is around $60,000.
Requirements: Grants are made primarily to nonprofit organizations located in the five boroughs of New York City. Grants for programs outside the area are generally from funds designated for specific charities or have been made at the suggestion of donors.
Restrictions: The trust does not make grants to individuals, offer general or capital funding, endowments, building construction/renovation, deficit financing, films, or religion.
Geographic Focus: New York
Amount of Grant: $5,000-$100,000
Contact: Joyce M. Bove, Senior Vice President; (212) 686-0010, ext. 552; fax: (212) 534-8528; email: info@nycommunitytrust.org or grants@nycommunitytrust.org
Internet: http://www.nycommunitytrust.org/ForGrantSeekers/GrantmakingGuidelines/CommunityDevelopmentandtheEnvironment/tabid/204/Default.aspx
Sponsor: New York Community Trust
909 Third Avenue, 22nd Floor
New York, NY 10022

Oakland Fund for Children and Youth Grants **2930**
Grants support Oakland, CA, nonprofit organizations in two categories. The general grants program awards grants to organizations serving children and youth ages 0-20 in four priority areas: support for children's success in school, child health and wellness, healthy transitions to adulthood, and youth empowerment. The Community Promotions Program for Service Organizations and the Youth Violence/Drug Prevention Program award grants to organizations providing parent/caregiver support services, youth drug prevention services, or work to prevent youth violence. Annual deadline dates may vary; contact program staff for exact date.
Requirements: Oakland, CA, nonprofit organizations serving children and youth are eligible.
Geographic Focus: California
Amount of Grant: $20,000-$250,000 range
Date(s) Application is Due: Jan 6
Contact: Ayako Miyashita, Grant Coordinator, (510) 238-4913; fax: (510) 238-4971; email: amiyashita@oaklandnet.com
Internet: http://www.ofcy.org
Sponsor: East Bay Community Foundation, Oakland Fund for Children and Youth
150 Frank H Ogawa Plz, Suite 4216
Oakland, CA 94612

Obsessive-Compulsive Foundation Research Awards **2931**
The foundation invites proposals for research projects on any aspect of obsessive-compulsive disorders. Applicants should submit a proposal limited to five pages and a budget. The foundation will request more detailed proposals following initial review.
Amount of Grant: $39,000-$49,000
Contact: Jeannette Cole, (888) 302-6662 or (203) 401-2069; fax: (203) 315-2196; email: cole@ocfoundation.org
Internet: http://www.ocfoundation.org/ocf1140a.htm
Sponsor: Obsessive-Compulsive Foundation
337 Notch Hill Road
North Branford, CT 06471

OBSSR Behavioral and Social Science Research on Understanding and Reducing Health Disparities Grants **2932**
The purpose of this program is to encourage behavioral and social science research on the causes and solutions to health and disabilities disparities in the U. S. population. Health disparities between, on the one hand, racial/ethnic populations, lower socioeconomic classes, and rural residents and, on the other hand, the overall U.S. population are major public health concerns. Emphasis is placed on research in and among three broad areas of action: public policy; health care; and disease/disability prevention. Particular attention is given to reducing health gaps among groups. Proposals that utilize an interdisciplinary approach, investigate multiple levels of analysis, incorporate a life-course perspective, and/or employ innovative methods such as system science or community-based participatory research are particularly encouraged. The NIH anticipates supporting 20 to 30 awards. Because the nature and scope of the proposed research will vary from application to application, it is anticipated that the size and duration of each award will also vary.
Requirements: Application can be made by the following institutions and organizations: public/state controlled institutions of higher education; private institutions of higher education; nonprofits with 501(c)3 IRS status (other than institutions of higher education); nonprofits without 501(c)3 IRS status (other than institutions of higher education); small businesses; for-profit organizations (other than small businesses); state governments; U.S. territories or possessions; Indian/Native American tribal governments (federally recognized); Indian/Native American tribal governments (other than Federally recognized); Indian/Native American tribally designated organizations; non-domestic (non-U.S.) entities (foreign organizations); Hispanic-serving institutions; historically Black colleges and universities (HBCUs); tribally controlled colleges and universities (TCCUs); Alaska Native and Native Hawaiian serving institutions; regional organization; eligible agencies of the Federal government; and faith-based or community based organizations.
Date(s) Application is Due: Feb 5; Jun 5; Oct 5
Contact: Ronald P. Abeles, Ph.D.; (301) 496-7859; fax: (301) 435-8779; email: abeles@nih.gov
Internet: http://grants.nih.gov/grants/guide/pa-files/PAR-07-379.html
Sponsor: Office of Behavioral and Social Sciences Research (OBSSR)
31 Center Drive, Building 31, Room B1C19
Bethesda, MD 20892-2027

OceanFirst Foundation Grants **2933**
The foundation awards two types of grants (small and major) to nonprofit organizations in OceanFirst Bank's service area and its neighboring communities for programs that expand home ownership opportunities and provide access to affordable rental housing; support youth development programs to improve life options through education and work skills; support community organizations that contribute to the quality of life; and support nonprofit medical facilities. There are no application deadlines; requests are considered in the first, second, and fourth quarters of the year.
Requirements: New Jersey nonprofit organizations serving Middlesex, Monmouth, and Ocean Counties are eligible.
Geographic Focus: New Jersey
Amount of Grant: $3500 maximum for small grants; $3500 minimum for major grants
Contact: Katherine Durante, Executive Director, (732) 341-4676; fax: (732) 473-9641; email: kdurante@oceanfirstfdn.org
Internet: http://www.oceanfirstfdn.org
Sponsor: OceanFirst Foundation
1415 Hooper Avenue, Suite 304
Toms River, NJ 08753

Oceanside Charitable Foundation Grants **2934**
The Oceanside Charitable Foundation will focus on supporting projects that inspire and strengthen Civil Society in its communities; in particular, projects that foster community participation, consensus-building and collective problem solving in the field of children and youth programs. The Oceanside Charitable Foundation will fund Civil Society projects for school-aged (K-12) children and youth that are managed by non-profit organizations or government agencies.
Requirements: Projects for which funding is requested must serve children and/or youth in the geographical limits of the City of Oceanside.
Restrictions: The Oceanside Charitable Foundation does not make grants for: annual campaigns and fund raising events for non-specific purposes; capital campaigns for buildings or facilities; stipends for attendance at conferences; endowments or chairs; for-profit organizations or enterprises; individuals unaffiliated with a qualified fiscal sponsor; projects that promote religious or political doctrine; research projects (medical or otherwise); scholarships; or existing obligations or debt.
Geographic Focus: California
Date(s) Application is Due: Dec 18
Contact: Kerry Helmer; (619) 814-1384; email: kerry@sdfoundation.org;; Trudy Amstrong, Regional Manager; (619) 814-1384; email: trudy@sdfoundation.org
Internet: http://www.endowoceanside.org/grants.html
Sponsor: Oceanside Charitable Foundation / San Diego Foundation
2508 Historic Decatur Road, Suite 200
San Diego, CA 92106

Office Depot Corporation Community Grants **2935**
The corporate giving program awards grants to nonprofit organizations aligned with Office Depot's mission to directly impact the health, education, and welfare of children. Office Depot supports nonprofit organizations at the local level with donations of products, contributions of funds, and efforts to encourage employees and customers to become involved. To request a monetary donation, provide a brief description of the organization, the federal tax-ID number, an explanation of what is being requested, and the rationale based on Office Depot's charitable giving guidelines. The request should be submitted on organization letterhead and sent to the office.
Requirements: 501(c)3 nonprofit organizations are eligible.
Restrictions: Grants do not support individuals, advertising, athletic teams or events, fashion shows, project graduation, capital campaigns, individual or group travel, political causes, film/video projects, or nonprofit organizations that spend more than 25 percent of their revenue on management overhead and fundraising expenses.
Contact: Melissa Perlman, Public Relations; (561) 438-0704; email: Melissa.Perlman@officedepot.com
Internet: http://www.community.officedepot.com/local.asp
Sponsor: Office Depot Corporation
2200 Old Germantown Road
Delray Beach, FL 33445

Office Depot Foundation Grants **2936**
Everywhere Office Depot conducts business, its belief in the fundamental importance of corporate citizenship is readily apparent. The Foundation's funding focus includes: making a difference in children's lives—to support activities that serve, teach and inspire children, youth and families; building communities—to support civic organizations and activities that serve the needs of our community; and disaster relief—to support disaster relief efforts of recognized national, regional and local agencies, and to provide disaster relief to Office Depot associates who have experienced catastrophic loss. The Foundation will consider proposals from organizations related to disaster relief and recovery throughout the year.
Requirements: 501(c)3 nonprofit organizations are eligible.

Restrictions: Office Depot does not contribute to individuals and does not make donations in return for advertising. In addition, grants do not support athletic teams or events; fashion shows; project graduation; capital campaigns; individual or group travel; political causes; film/video projects; or nonprofit organizations that spend more than 25 percent of their revenue on management overhead and fundraising expenses.
Amount of Grant: $250-$10,000 range
Date(s) Application is Due: Jun 30
Contact: Brian Levine, Public Relations; (561) 438-2895; email: brian.levine@officedepot.com
Internet: http://www.community.officedepot.com/odfoundation.asp
Sponsor: Office Depot Foundation
2200 Old Germantown Road
Delray Beach, FL 33445

Ogden Codman Trust Grants 2937
The trust awards grants to eligible Massachusetts nonprofit organizations in its areas of interest, including environmental conservation, historic preservation, cultural activities, health care, and social services. Grants support special programs intended to improve the quality of life. Matching funds are sometimes requested
Requirements: Lincoln, MA, nonprofit organizations are eligible to apply.
Restrictions: General operating grants are rarely awarded.
Samples: Campaign for Drumlin Farm, Lincoln, MA, $25,000 (2007); Lincoln Public Schools, Lincoln, MA, $25,000 (2006).
Contact: Susan Monahan, Grants Coordinator; email: smonahan@rackemann.com
Sponsor: Ogden Codman Trust
160 Federal Street, 13th Floor
Boston, MA 02110-1700

Ohio County Community Foundation Grants 2938
Established in 1998, the Ohio County Community Foundation is charged with assisting donors in building, managing and distributing a lasting source of charitable funds for the good of Ohio County. The Community Foundation currently offers services that include endowment creation, scholarship administration and charitable gift funds. Currently, there are two annual grant cycles, with deadlines on April 15 and October 15 respectively.
Requirements: Grants will be made only to organizations whose programs benefit the residents of Ohio County.
Restrictions: No grants will be made solely to individuals but can be made for the benefit of certain individuals for such purposes as scholarships and special programs through educational institutions and other sponsoring recipient organizations. Generally grants will not be made to enable individuals or groups of individuals to take trips except where there are special circumstances which will benefit the larger community.
Geographic Focus: Indiana
Amount of Grant: $3,000 maximum
Date(s) Application is Due: Apr 15; Oct 15
Contact: Stephanie Scott, Program Coordinator; (812) 438-9401: fax: (812) 438-9488; email: sscott@occfrisingsun.com
Internet: http://www.occfrisingsun.com/grants.html
Sponsor: Ohio County Community Foundation
591 Smart Drive, P.O. Box 170
Rising Sun, IN 47040

Ohio County Community Foundation Mini-Grants 2939
Established in 1998, the Ohio County Community Foundation is charged with assisting donors in building, managing and distributing a lasting source of charitable funds for the good of Ohio County. The Ohio County Community Foundation will seek and accept mini-grant applications from area non-profit organizations whose programs benefit the residents of Ohio County. Each mini-application will be reviewed after submission by the Program Coordinator to ensure the application is complete and the organization is eligible to make application.
Requirements: Grants will be made only to organizations whose programs benefit the residents of Ohio County.
Restrictions: No grants will be made solely to individuals but can be made for the benefit of certain individuals for such purposes as scholarships and special programs through educational institutions and other sponsoring recipient organizations. Generally grants will not be made to enable individuals or groups of individuals to take trips except where there are special circumstances which will benefit the larger community.
Geographic Focus: Indiana
Amount of Grant: $100 maximum
Contact: Stephanie Scott, Program Coordinator; (812) 438-9401: fax: (812) 438-9488; email: sscott@occfrisingsun.com
Internet: http://www.occfrisingsun.com/grants.html
Sponsor: Ohio County Community Foundation
591 Smart Drive, P.O. Box 170
Rising Sun, IN 47040

Ohio Learning Network Grants 2940
The network funds programs to help Ohioans increase work-related knowledge and skills through college credits; assist faculty in teaching using emerging technologies; and better understand the role of technology in learning. Grants support emerging needs, learning communities, distance learning research, partnership grants, and technology initiatives/innovations.
Geographic Focus: Ohio
Amount of Grant: $100,000 maximum
Contact: Judith M. Leach, Assistant Director; (614)485-6738 or (614) 995-3240; email: jleach@oln.org
Internet: http://www.oln.org/about_oln/grants.php
Sponsor: Ohio Learning Network
35 E. Chestnut Street, 8th Floor
Columbus, OH 43215-2541

Oleonda Jameson Trust Grants 2941
The trust awards grants to New Hampshire nonprofit organizations in its areas of interest, including arts/culture, community foundations, children and youth, health care, housing, social sciences, human services, federated giving programs and, social services. Types of support include capital campaigns, building construction/renovation, equipment acquisition, emergency funds, and scholarship funds. There are no application forms or deadlines. The board meets in March, June, September, and December.
Requirements: New Hampshire nonprofit organizations are eligible. Requests from Concord nonprofits receive preference.
Restrictions: Grants do not support endowments or general operating expenses.
Geographic Focus: New Hampshire
Samples: New Hampshire Charitable Foundation, Concord, NH, $25,000 (2007); Riverbend Community Mental Health, Concord, NH, $15,000 (2007); Arts in Reach, Dover, NH, $7,500 (2007).
Amount of Grant: $1000-$60,000 range
Contact: McLane Graf Raulerson & Middleton Professional Association, (603) 226-0400;
Sponsor: Oleonda Jameson Trust
c/o McLane Graf Raulerson & Middleton, 11 South Main Street, Suite 500
Concord, NH 03301-4945

Olfactory Research Fund Grants 2942
The fund sponsors innovative scientific research in the olfactory arts and sciences. Grants promote the study of olfaction and also support educational and outreach programs about the sense of smell. The fund is especially interested in supporting research that integrates the study of olfaction with current issues in developmental, perceptual, social and cognitive psychology, and related disciplines. The fund is currently seeking proposals for research that focuses on the influence of olfaction in the mental and physical aspects of performance. Contact organization for submission deadlines.
Requirements: Applicants must have a doctoral degree.
Restrictions: Generally, the following types of research are ineligible for support: studies not directly related to olfaction and/or the human reaction to odors; studies exclusively on animal olfaction without direct relevance to humans; or invasive human studies.
Contact: Theresa Molnar, Executive Administrator, (212) 725-2755; fax: (212) 779-9072; email: tmolnar@senseofsmell.org or info@senseofsmell.org
Internet: http://www.senseofsmell.org/resources/research.php
Sponsor: Olfactory Research Fund
145 E 32nd Street
New York, NY 10016

Olin Corporation Charitable Trust Grants 2943
The charitable trust supports nonprofits in company-operating areas. Grants focus on three priority categories: education, with a science and technology emphasis; programs that include Olin employees as volunteers and that impact communities in which Olin employees work and live; and conservation, environmental education, and environmental research. Types of support include general operating budgets, continuing support, annual campaigns, seed money, emergency funds, building funds, equipment, land acquisition, special projects, research, publications, conferences and seminars, internships, scholarship funds, employee-related scholarships, fellowships, and employee matching gifts. U.S.-based nonprofits with an international focus are supported primarily through matching gifts. There are no application deadlines. Applicants should submit a letter of request. The board meets in January to consider requests.
Requirements: Support is directed primarily to communities where Olin has a major employee presence.
Restrictions: Grants are not awarded to individuals or for endowments.
Samples: Thirteen communities in Olin operating areas—for education programs, with a focus on computer technology and science education, $242,137 divided.
Amount of Grant: $50-$50,000
Contact: Program Contact, (314) 480-1400
Internet: http://www.olin.com/about/charitable.asp
Sponsor: Olin Corporation Charitable Trust
190 Carondelet Plz, Suite 1530
Clayton, MO 63105-3443

OneSight Research Foundation Block Grants 2944
Formerly known as the Pearle Vision Foundation, the OneSight Research Foundation is dedicated to sight preservation through research and education. A significant portion of their grant dollars will be awarded to fund research and treatment for diabetic eye diseases, hoping to find a cure for diabetic retinopathy, the number one cause of adult blindness in the United States.
Requirements: U.S. 501(c)3 nonprofits are eligible for grant support. Requests for funding should cover a period of time not to exceed one year. Exceptions to this policy will be considered on an individual basis.
Restrictions: Grants will not be considered for endowments or operating expenses.

Samples: Retina Foundation of the Southwest (Dallas, TX)—to equip and furnish a new visual-testing laboratory at the Morchower Pediatric Eye Research Laboratory, $16,342.; Lighthouse International (New York, NY)—to study a new reading method for people with macular degeneration and other diseases that result in central-vision loss, $10,000.; New Eyes for the Needy (Short Hills, NV)—for eyeglass vouchers to serve individuals nationwide, $25,000.
Amount of Grant: $5,000-$50,000
Date(s) Application is Due: Jun 30; Dec 31
Contact: Trina Parasiliti, Administrator; (972) 277-6191; fax: (972) 277-6414; email: tparasil@onesight.org
Internet: http://www.onesight.org/northamerica/na/
Sponsor: OneSight Research Foundation
2465 Joe Field Road
Dallas, TX 75229

OneStar Foundation AmeriCorps Grants **2945**
OneStar NSC seeks to fund programs that engage members to address health, public safety, homeland security, education, or human service needs in Texas communities. Funds support the state priority grant, professional corps grant, and education award grant. AmeriCorps education awards for members who successfully complete their full term of service will also be supported. Guidelines are available online.
Requirements: Local or statewide nonprofit organizations, state and local units of government, and institutions of higher education are eligible.
Contact: Grants Administrator; (512) 287-2000; fax: (512) 473-8228 or (512) 287-2039; email: onestar@onestarfoundation.org
Internet: http://www.onestarfoundation.org/page/americorpstexas
Sponsor: OneStar Foundation
816 Congress, Stuite 900
Austin, TX 78701

ONF Career Development Awards **2946**
The awards support the career development of professional nurses in the field of oncology nursing. The awards allow attendance in an educational program focusing on clinical ethics that will further the nurse's professional goals and potential to contribute to oncology nursing. This award is not intended to supplement tuition in a graduate degree program. Preference will be given to applicants who are seeking beginning level knowledge in clinical ethics.
Requirements: All applicants must be registered nurses or nurse administrators actively involved in some aspect of cancer patient care, education, or research.
Amount of Grant: $1000
Contact: ONS Foundation Office, (412) 859-6100 ext 8503; email: customer.service@ons.org or member@ons.org
Internet: http://www.ons.org/awards/foundawards/ethics.shtml
Sponsor: Oncology Nursing Foundation
125 Enterprise Drive
Pittsburgh, PA 15275-1214

ONF Small Grants Program **2947**
These grant awards are designed to support oncology nursing research conducted by beginning and experienced researchers. The majority of the small grants are for general investigator-initiated oncology topics. Funding preference is given to research that addresses the ONS Research Priorities and Research Agenda. A letter of intent is requested by October 1; full proposal is due November 1. Annual deadline dates may vary; contact program staff for exact dates.
Requirements: The principal investigator must be actively involved in some aspect of cancer patient care, education, or research. Funding preference is given to projects that involve nurses in the design and conduct of the research activity and that promote oncology nursing theory and a scientific basis for practice.
Samples: Kimberly Kahn, U of Virginia Health Science Ctr (Charlottesville, VA)—nursing education research grant, The Informed Consent Process in Oncology Clinical Trials, $7500.; Dr. June Eilers, U of Nebraska Medical Ctr (Omaha, NE)—research grant, Longitudinal Study of the Impact of BMT on Family Members, $5000.
Amount of Grant: $10,000
Date(s) Application is Due: Oct 1; Nov 1
Contact: Grants Administrator, email: research@ons.org
Internet: http://www.ons.org/awards/foundawards/smallGrants.shtml
Sponsor: Oncology Nursing Foundation
125 Enterprise Drive, RIDC Park W
Pittsburgh, PA 15275-1214

ONR Human Performance Division Research Grants **2948**
The mission of the Human Performance S&T Division is to direct, plan, foster and encourage Science and Technology in cognitive science, computational neuroscience, bio-inspired systems, social/organizational science, manpower & personnel, training, human factors, decision making and human systems integration as related to Naval needs. Major goals include: to sustain warfighter performance and enhanced decision making in all environments through training technologies, manpower management, and human systems integration; to create options for future (perhaps unanticipated) naval decisions, based upon fundamental understanding of the cognitive and neurosciences; to support integrated interdisciplinary research programs; and to cultivate transition of findings to government and commercial funding of applied research, advanced technology development, small business and acquisition projects. Submission of the Research Proposal should always be preceded by submission of a Preproposal and a discussion of that Preproposal with the assigned Program Officer.
Requirements: Grants are awarded to academic, industrial, and nonprofit organizations, with strong emphasis on university research.
Restrictions: New grants or contracts are typically started near the beginning of the fiscal year (October 1). New proposals for the next fiscal year should be submitted no later than June 1, unless otherwise directed by the BAA. Competitive renewals should be submitted no later than six months prior to the award termination date after contacting the Program Officer. Conference proposals should be submitted at least four months prior to the conference.
Amount of Grant: $70,000-$150,000 per year
Contact: Dr. John F. Tangney; (703) 696-4501 or (703) 588-2427; fax: (703) 696-5940; email: john.f.tangney@navy.mil
Internet: http://www.onr.navy.mil/sci_tech/34/341/
Sponsor: Office of Naval Research
875 North Randolph Street, Suite 1425
Arlington, VA 22203-1995

ONS Major Research Grants **2949**
Applications are invited for research proposals which focus on increasing understanding of and management of understudied symptoms and/or symptom clusters in diverse populations and across settings. Priority will be given to proposals that address management of symptoms and/or symptom clusters that include dermatologic problems in cancer patients. Examples of symptom clusters include dermatitis, pain, and sleep/wake disturbances or fatigue, depression, and sleep/wake disturbances. Other symptom clusters and symptoms will be considered. Justification must be provided for selecting the cluster and/or the rationale for the research needed for the symptom. Membership in ONS is not required.
Requirements: The principal investigator must be actively involved in some aspect of cancer patient care, education, or research.
Amount of Grant: $50,000
Contact: Research, (412) 859-6298; fax: (877) 369-5497; email: research@ons.org
Internet: http://www.ons.org/awards/foundawards
Sponsor: Oncology Nursing Society
125 Enterprise Drive
Pittsburgh, PA 15275-1214

ONS Scholarships **2950**
Nursing scholarships are awarded each year to enable registered nurses to continue their education in the area of oncology nursing. Each year, undergraduate scholarships, graduate scholarships, and doctoral scholarships are awarded. In addition Congress Scholarships (December 1 deadline) may be applied toward registration, travel to and from Congress, and per diem Congress expenses. Guidelines are available online.
Requirements: An applicant must have a current license to practice as a registered nurse and be enrolled in (or accepted in) a nursing-degree program in an NLN-accredited school of nursing.
Amount of Grant: $2000 undergraduate, $3000 master's, $3000-$5000 doctoral; $1000 Congress Scholarship
Date(s) Application is Due: Feb 1
Contact: Research Team, (412) 859-6100; email: foundation@ons.org
Internet: http://www.ons.org
Sponsor: Oncology Nursing Society
125 Enterprise Drive
Pittsburgh, PA 15275-1214

Oracle Corporate Contributions Grants **2951**
The corporation awards grants for medical research in the areas of cancer, AIDS, and neuroscience; endangered animal protection; environmental protection, specifically for education and preservation of important open space; and K-12 education, with emphasis on mathematics, science, and technology programs. Grants are awarded in February and August.
Requirements: Nonprofits nationwide and in operating communities are eligible.
Restrictions: Grants generally do not support fundraising benefits, charitable dinners, sporting events, and marketing brochures. The corporation does not award multiyear grants and rarely approves funds for more than three consecutive years.
Samples: United Negro College Fund (Fairfax, VA)—to strengthen the technical capacities of its 39 member institutions, $10 million, including cash donation, scholarships, internships, and curricular training, certification, and technology resources.
Contact: Corporate Giving, (650) 506-7000
Internet: http://www.oracle.com/corporate/giving/community/index.html?giveform.html
Sponsor: Oracle Corporation
500 Oracle Pkwy, MS 50P11
Redwood City, CA 94065

Ordean Foundation Grants **2952**
The Foundation, established in 1933, supports organizations involved with alcoholism, children/youth, services, crime/violence prevention, youth, education, family services, food services, health care, homeless, human services, housing/shelter, human services, medical care, rehabilitation, mental health/crisis services, substance abuse, services, YM/YWCAs & YM/YWHAs, aging, disabilities, economically disadvantaged. Grants will be awarded for up to three years. Applications are reviewed on an ongoing basis; the deadline is the 15th of each month.

Requirements: Non-profits in the Duluth and contiguous cities and townships in St. Louis County, Minnesota are eligible. The Foundation accepts the Minnesota Common Grant Application Form.
Restrictions: No support for direct religious purposes, or for political campaigns or lobbying activities. No grants to individuals (directly), or for endowment funds, travel, conferences, seminars or workshops, telephone solicitations, benefits, dinners, research, including biomedical research, deficit financing, national fund raising campaigns, or to supplant government funding.
Geographic Focus: Minnesota
Amount of Grant: $1,000-$290,000 range
Contact: Stephen A. Mangan, Executive Director; (218) 726-4785; fax: (218) 726-4848; email: ordean@computerpro.com
Sponsor: Ordean Foundation
501 Ordean Building
Duluth, MN 55802-4725

OREF Educational Awards **2953**
The awards support continuing medical education programs and other projects of relevance to orthopedic surgeons of all ages developed in conjunction with a national, recognized organization. Types of support include conferences and seminars, visiting scholars, and program grants. Honorariums support visiting scholars for lectureships; program grants vary in amount.
Requirements: Departments and state orthopedic societies may apply for honorariums. Orthopedic departments and regional and national specialty societies may apply for special symposia, conferences, and workshops.
Amount of Grant: $25,000 maximum
Date(s) Application is Due: Oct 3
Contact: Jean Maguire, VP Grants, (847) 698-9980; fax: (847) 698-7806
Internet: http://www.oref.org/rga/rga.html#educational
Sponsor: Orthopaedic Research and Education Foundation
6300 N River Road, Suite 700
Rosemont, IL 60018

OREF Orthopedic Career Development Awards **2954**
Career development awards are granted to candidates who have demonstrated a commitment to scientific research as well as excellence in clinical training in the field of orthopedic surgery. Program requirements specify that recipients spend a minimum of 20 percent of a five-day week on the research project. A minimum of 50 percent of grant funds may be used for the candidate's salary. Applications must note budget requirements. Awards for up to two years, conditional upon annual review, will be considered. The grant period each year runs from July 1 through June 30 following the year of application. Recipients will be notified by letter after the annual board meeting held in the first quarter of each year.
Requirements: Candidates must have completed a residency in orthopaedic surgery and demonstrated a sustained interest in research and excellence in clinical training. Letters of nomination and support must offer convincing evidence of the candidate's potential to develop as an investigator.
Restrictions: Recipients of current or past NIH RO1 grants are ineligible.
Amount of Grant: $75,000 maximum per year for three years
Date(s) Application is Due: Oct 3
Contact: Jean McGuire, Vice President of Grants, (847) 698-9980; fax: (847) 698-7806; email: mcguire@oref.org
Internet: http://www.oref.org/rga/rga.html#career
Sponsor: Orthopaedic Research and Education Foundation
6300 N River Road, Suite 700
Rosemont, IL 60018

OREF Orthopedic Resident Research Awards **2955**
Applications will be considered for one year of laboratory or clinical research by orthopedic surgery residents in approved orthopedic programs at U.S. medical centers. The objective of these awards is to encourage young investigators by providing funding for research projects that would not ordinarily be funded. Grants provide funds for supplies and expenses but not for a resident's salary. The foundation will notify each applicant by letter after the annual meeting of the board, held in the first quarter of each year.
Requirements: The principal investigator must be an orthopedic surgery resident in an approved U.S. or Canadian orthopedic program.
Amount of Grant: $15,000 maximum for one year
Date(s) Application is Due: Oct 3
Contact: Jean McGuire, Vice President of Grants, (847) 698-9980; fax: (847) 698-7806; email: mcguire@oref.org
Internet: http://www.oref.org/rga/rga.html#resident
Sponsor: Orthopaedic Research and Education Foundation
6300 N River Road, Suite 700
Rosemont, IL 60018

OREF Prospective Clinical Research Proposal Grants **2956**
The objective of these grants is to provide funding for promising prospective clinical research projects in areas of high clinical importance in orthopedic surgery. Subject to available funds, at least four applications will be considered each year for funding up to three years, conditional on annual review. Annual deadline dates may vary; contact program staff for exact dates.
Requirements: The principal or coprincipal investigator must be a suitably qualified orthopedic surgeon working at a U.S. institution. Investigators with an MD, PhD, or DVM degree may serve with the orthopedic surgeon.
Amount of Grant: $50,000 maximum per year for up to three years
Date(s) Application is Due: Oct 3
Contact: Jean McGuire, Vice President of Grants, (847) 698-9980; fax: (847) 698-7806; email: mcguire@oref.org
Internet: http://www.oref.org/rga/rga.html#prospective
Sponsor: Orthopaedic Research and Education Foundation
6300 N River Road, Suite 700
Rosemont, IL 60018

OREF Research Grants **2957**
The objective of the program is to encourage research into the causes, cure, and prevention of orthopedic-related injuries, illness, and conditions, and to encourage research by new investigators in the field of orthopedic musculoskeletal surgery. Grants provide seed and start-up funding for promising research projects for no more than two years, conditional upon annual review. Grant period runs from July 1st through June 30th for two years. Successful applicants will be notified by letter after the annual board meeting, which is held in the first quarter of each year.
Requirements: The principal or coprincipal investigator must be an orthopedic surgeon at a U.S. or Canadian institution. In addition, the candidate must have adequate protected time to accomplish the proposed grant within a 24-month time period.
Restrictions: Recipients of current or past NIH RO1 grants are ineligible.
Amount of Grant: $50,000 per year for up to two years
Date(s) Application is Due: Oct 3
Contact: Jean McGuire, Vice President of Grants, (847) 698-9980; fax: (847) 698-7806; email: mcguire@oref.org
Internet: http://www.oref.org/rga/rga.html#research
Sponsor: Orthopaedic Research and Education Foundation
6300 N River Road, Suite 700
Rosemont, IL 60018

OREF/AAOS Clinical Research Training Fellowship **2958**
The goal of this program is to encourage the development of a cadre of orthopaedic surgeons who have the research skills necessary to undertake and manage various types of health services and outcomes research. The candidate is encouraged to earn a public health degree. Candidates who have completed an accredited North American orthopedic residency and are recommended by their department chairs may apply.
Requirements: Applicants must have completed an orthopedic residency at an accredited North American institution and be recommended by their department chairs.
Amount of Grant: $70,000 per year
Date(s) Application is Due: Oct 3
Contact: Jean McGuire, Vice President, (847) 698-9980; email: mcguire@oref.org
Internet: http://www.oref.org/rga/rga.html#aaos
Sponsor: Orthopaedic Research and Education Foundation
6300 N River Road, Suite 700
Rosemont, IL 60018

Orentreich Foundation for the Advancement of Science Grants **2959**
Occasional and limited grants are made for joint or collaborative biomedical research, usually initiated by OFAS, with emphasis in dermatology, aging, endocrinology, and serum markers for human diseases. The amount of the grants varies with joint interest and need. Unsolicited applications may be submitted at any time.
Requirements: Applicants must be at or above postgraduate level in science or medicine at accredited universities and research institutions in the United States. There is no restriction on citizenship. Submit an outline of proposed program, curriculum vita of principal investigator, and estimated budget.
Amount of Grant: $50,000 total
Contact: Dr. Rozlyn Krajcik, fax: (914) 265-4210; email: ofas@orentreich.org
Internet: http://www.orentreich.org/research.htm
Sponsor: Orentreich Foundation for the Advancement of Science Inc
Cold Spring-on-Hudson
New York, NY 10516

ORISE Postgraduate Research Participation at the Agency for Toxic Substances and Disease Registry **2960**
An interagency agreement between DOE and ATSDR enables ORISE to provide opportunities and support for research in exposure and disease registries, health investigations, public health assessments, toxicological profiles, emergency response, and health education. The one-year, renewable grants are tenable at the ATSDR in Atlanta, GA. Stipends are based on research area and degree, and include reimbursement for inbound travel and moving. Applications are accepted at any time.
Requirements: Applicants should have completed graduate degree requirements within the last three years; others are considered on a case-by-case basis.
Date(s) Application is Due: Feb 1
Contact: Linda McCamant, Group Manager, (865) 576-9361; email: mccamanl@orau.gov; Tasha Powell, Program Specialist, (865) 574-3911; email: powellt@orau.gov
Internet: http://www.orau.gov/orise/edu/ATSDR/gi-gugsrp.htm
Sponsor: Oak Ridge Institute for Science and Education
P.O. Box 117
Oak Ridge, TN 37831-0117

ORISE Postgraduate Research Participation at the National Center for Toxicological Research 2961

An interagency agreement between DOE and FDA enables ORISE to administer this program, which provides opportunities and support for research in biological effects of potentially toxic chemicals and deriving solutions to problems in toxicology that have a major impact on human health and the environment. The program is tenable at the NCTR in Jefferson, AR. Stipends are based on research area and degree. Applications are accepted at any time for the one-year, renewable grants. Applications for summer appointments due March 1.
Requirements: Candidates should have completed graduate degree requirements within the last three years; others are considered on a case-by-case basis.
Contact: Linda McCamant, Group Manager, (865) 576-1089; email: mccamanl@orau.gov; Tasha Powell, Program Specialist, (865) 574-3911; email: powellt@orau.gov
Internet: http://www.orau.gov/orise/edu/FDA/gi-gugNCTR.htm
Sponsor: Oak Ridge Institute for Science and Education
P.O. Box 117
Oak Ridge, TN 37831-0117

ORISE Postgraduate Research Program at the Center for Devices and Radiological Health 2962

These one-year renewable grants provide opportunities and support for research concerning medical devices and radiation emissions from electronic products. This is an interagency agreement between the DOE and FDA, with the positions located at the Center for Devices and Radiological Health in Rockville, MD. Stipends are based on research area and degree and include limited reimbursement for inbound travel and moving.
Requirements: Applicants must have completed bachelor's or graduate degree within last three years; others are considered on a case-by-case basis.
Contact: Linda McCamant, Project Manager, (865) 576-1089; email: mccamanL@orau.gov; Sherry Edwards, Program Specialist, (865) 576-7385; email: warrens@orau.gov
Internet: http://www.orau.gov/orise/edu/FDA/gi-rgpdCDRH.htm
Sponsor: Oak Ridge Institute for Science and Education
P.O. Box 117
Oak Ridge, TN 37831-0117

Oscar Rennebohm Foundation Grants 2963

The foundation awards grants to nonprofit organizations in the Madison, WI area. Areas of interest, include: higher education, the arts, environmental conservation, health and social service agencies. Types of support include building construction/renovation, equipment acquisition, and research. There are no application forms or deadlines.
Geographic Focus: Wisconsin
Contact: Grants Administrator, (608) 274-5991
Sponsor: Oscar Rennebohm Foundation
P.O. Box 5187
Madison, WI 53705

OSI Access to Essential Medicines Grants 2964

The project supports efforts to increase access to essential medicines to developing countries and marginalized populations. Work has focused on three key areas: transparency and monitoring of the pharmaceutical industry; procurement mechanisms; and intellectual property. The project promotes civil society engagement with these issues and actively supports a civil society platform around the WHO Working Group on innovation for neglected diseases. The project works closely with OSI's palliative care and harm reduction initiatives. In an effort to strengthen needed capacity, the OSI programs are seeking applications from qualified organizations interested in receiving institutional support for their work on access to essential medicines. Grants for up to $75,000, renewable for up to three years, will be awarded to local NGOs with a mandate and demonstrated capacity to advance policy and civil society engagement related to access to medicines in Brazil, India, Kenya, Malaysia, South Africa, and Thailand. If requested, technical assistance will be offered throughout the length of the grant period. OSI may further sponsor seminars and meetings for grantees to share lessons learned. Applicants will be notified of final selection results no later than September 14th.
Requirements: Legally registered NGOs based in one of the following countries should apply: Brazil, India, Kenya, Malaysia, South Africa, and Thailand.
Amount of Grant: $75,000, renewable for up to three years
Date(s) Application is Due: Jul 16
Contact: Jane Li; (212) 548-0600; fax: (646) 557-2550; email: jli@sorosny.org
Internet: http://www.soros.org/initiatives/health/news/access_20070608
Sponsor: Open Society Institute
400 West 59th Street, 3rd Floor
New York, NY 10019

OSI European Commission Internships for Young Roma Graduates 2965

The European Commission, in cooperation with the OSI, offers internships for young Roma university graduates from all new EU member states (excluding Cyprus and Malta), Croatia, Macedonia, Serbia (including Kosovo), and Montenegro. The training periods involve work experience in one of the Commission's departments. The primary aims of the program are: to give Roma interns a general idea of the objectives and problems of European integration; to provide them with practical knowledge of the working of Commission departments; to enable them to acquire personal experience by means of contacts made in the course of their everyday work; and to enable them to further and put into practice the knowledge they have acquired during their studies or professional careers. This is a five-month internship, with a starting date of October 1. The grant covers: travel expenses to and from Brussels/Luxembourg (using the cheapest available means of transportation, actual cost being counted by OSI up to a maximum of 600 euro); and accommodation, subsistence, and health and accident insurance: 6,000 euro (1,200 euro per month).
Requirements: Nationals from all new EU member states (excluding Cyprus and Malta), Croatia, Macedonia, Serbia, including Kosovo, and Montenegro, who are of Roma origin may apply. Applications from women are encouraged. Preference will be given to candidates with proven experience in civil society work. Working knowledge of at least English or French is required, as is ability to draft reports in one of these languages. Minimum computer literacy is also required. The age limit for interns is minimum 25.
Restrictions: Candidates must have completed a course of university education and obtained a full degree or its equivalent by the closing date for applications.
Amount of Grant: 6,600 euro, including travel
Date(s) Application is Due: Jul 15
Contact: Bernard Rorke, Director; +36-1-327-3100; fax: +36-1-327-3101; email: brorke@osi.hu or rpp@osi.hu
Internet: http://www.soros.org/initiatives/roma/focus/internship/grants/internship
Sponsor: Open Society Institute
Oktober 6. ut. 12
Budapest H-1051 Hungary

OSI Harm Reduction and Drug Use Grants 2966

Founded in 1995, the International Harm Reduction Development Program (IHRD) works to reduce HIV and other harms related to injecting drug use, and to press for policies that reduce stigmatization of illicit drug users and protect their human rights. IHRD, which has supported more than 200 programs in Central and Eastern Europe, the former Soviet Union, and Asia, bases its activities on the philosophy that people unable or unwilling to abstain from drug use can make positive changes to protect their health and that of their families and communities. Since 2001, IHRD has prioritized advocacy to expand availability of needle exchange, opiate substitution treatment, and treatment for HIV; to reform discriminatory policies and practices; and to increase the political participation of people who use drugs and those living with HIV.
Contact: Janna Ataiants, Program Coordinator; (212) 548-0600; fax: (212) 548-4679; email: jataiants@sorosny.org
Internet: http://www.soros.org/initiatives/health/focus/ihrd/about
Sponsor: Open Society Institute
400 West 59th Street, 3rd Floor
New York, NY 10019

OSI Indonesia Project Grants 2967

In concert with the Tifa Foundation, OSI facilitates grants and operational programs through the Indonesia Project, which focuses on access to justice, media, local government capacity building, and public health. The Project accepts proposals for programs taking place in Indonesia in the following areas: access to justice; media; local government capacity building; and public health. Concept papers are accepted on a rolling basis. Papers should be 2–3 pages in length and give a detailed summary of project objectives and activities. Organizations whose concept papers fall within the Project funding priorities will be invited to submit complete proposals in accordance with project guidelines.
Restrictions: The program cannot fund the follow types of projects: unsolicited research projects, conference proposals, and organizational newsletters; social welfare projects, including health care, schools, orphanages, and provision of social services; cultural projects, including those related to cultural heritage and preservation, museums, literature, and fine and performing arts unless directly connected to the protection and promotion of civil and political rights; environmental projects unless directly connected to the protection and promotion of civil and political rights; development projects (i.e., construction of buildings, well digging); micro-finance and loans; or grants to individuals.
Contact: Sumaya Regal; +27 21 683 3489; fax: +27 21 683 3550; email: sumaya@ct.org.za
Internet: http://www.soros.org/initiatives/bpsai/focus_areas/indonesia
Sponsor: Open Society Institute
400 W. 59th Street, 3rd Floor
New York, NY 10019

OSI Integrating Health and Legal Services Grants 2968

The Law and Health Initiative supports the integration of legal and paralegal advocacy into community-based health services, both to increase access to justice and ensure comprehensive care for vulnerable groups. The aim is to ensure access to timely, effective, and affordable legal assistance for underserved populations such as women and girls, people who use drugs, sex workers, LGBT persons, and people living with HIV and other terminal illnesses. LAHI welcomes letters of intent from organizations seeking support for projects in one of five focus areas: Integrating Health and Legal Services; Human Rights in Patient Care; HIV/AIDS and Human Rights; Law and Health Capacity Development; and Legal Strategies in Health Monitoring.
Requirements: Geographically, LAHI limits its support to Central and Eastern Europe and the former Soviet Union, sub-Saharan Africa, and China and Southeast Asia.
Contact: Francoise Girard; (212) 548-0600; fax: (212) 548-4679; email: fgirard@sorosny.org
Internet: http://www.soros.org/initiatives/health/focus/law/focus_areas/integrating/guidelines
Sponsor: Open Society Institute
400 W. 59th Street, 3rd Floor
New York, NY 10019

OSI Mental Health Grants 2969
The Public Health Program's Mental Health Initiative provides grants to projects that stimulate the reform of national health, social welfare, education, and employment policies. The initiative also provides technical assistance and training in substantive areas to its grantees. Many grantees provide high-quality, community-based services which demonstrate that people with mental disabilities can live in their communities when they receive appropriate support.
Contact: Francoise Girard; (212) 548-0600; fax: (212) 548-4679; email: fgirard@sorosny.org
Internet: http://www.soros.org/initiatives/health/focus/mhi/focus_areas
Sponsor: Open Society Institute
400 W. 59th Street, 3rd Floor
New York, NY 10019

OSI Palliative Cancer Care Grants 2970
OSI's International Palliative Care Initiative supports organizations in resource-limited countries to integrate palliative care into national health care plans and policies, budgets, delivery systems, and professional and public education. The initiative also supports efforts to ensure that essential medications for pain relief are available to all patients who need them. This International Palliative Care Initiative funding program provides a two-year grant to a cancer center or general hospital with a focused oncology program, to support the salary of a clinical palliative care physician to develop a palliative care program.
Contact: Mary Callaway, Project Director; (212) 548-0600; fax: (212) 548-4679; email: mcallaway@sorosny.org
Internet: http://www.soros.org/initiatives/health/focus/ipci/grants/cancer
Sponsor: Open Society Institute
400 W. 59th Street, 3rd Floor
New York, NY 10019

OSI Supplementary Grant Program: Burma 2971
The Supplementary Grant Program–Burma (SGPB) was established in 1994 to address the needs of Burmese students, both inside and outside of the country, whose college education was disrupted due to political instability in Burma. The program provides supplemental financial assistance to Burmese students enrolled in academic programs at accredited colleges and universities leading to a degree. For individuals who are studying or intend to study in the United States, Canada, Europe and Australia, only those studying in the humanities and social sciences are eligible to apply—with preference given to graduate study in the following fields: Public Health, Social Policy, Social Work, Education, Environmental Policy, Public Policy, Public Administration, Economic Policy, and Law. The March 15 deadline is for students studying in India, Asia and Australia. The May 15 deadline is for students studying in Europe and North America.
Requirements: Applicants must be between the ages of 18-40, must be accepted into a full-time study program, must already have partial support, and must intend to return to Burma.
Restrictions: Requests for support in the following fields are ineligible: Business Administration/Management Training, Computer Science, Finance/Banking/Marketing, Engineering, Hard & Natural Sciences (Physics, Biology, Chemistry, etc.), Mathematics, Medical Science, Fine and Performing Arts.
Date(s) Application is Due: Mar 15; May 15
Contact: Maureen Aung-Thwin, Director; (212) 548-0632; fax: (212) 548-4655; email: maungthwin@sorosny.org
Internet: http://www.soros.org/initiatives/scholarship/focus_areas/supplementary_burma
Sponsor: Open Society Institute
400 W. 59th Street, 3rd Floor
New York, NY 10019

OSI-Baltimore Special Opportunities Program Grants 2972
The Special Opportunities Program allows OSI–Baltimore to make occasional grants outside its usual target areas that further its mission. For example, a grant to Your Public Radio Corporation helped develop a local news department and underwrite Just Words, a new weekly show that highlights justice issues relevant to the region. In addition, the Association of Baltimore Area Grantmakers received support for its Neighborhood Indicators Alliance, an information system that helps community groups access data about their neighborhoods and use it to improve local policy making. There are no specific deadlines or guidelines.
Geographic Focus: Maryland
Samples: Association of Baltimore Area Grantmakers, Baltimore, MD, $11,000—to provide general support (2008); Megaphone Project Inc., Baltimore, MD, $10,000— to provide general support during a leadership transition (2008).
Contact: Diana Morris, Director; (410) 234-1091, ext. 205; fax: (410) 234-2816; email: dmorris@sorosny.org
Internet: http://www.soros.org/initiatives/baltimore/focus_areas/special_opportunities
Sponsor: Open Society Institute
201 North Charles Street, Suite 1300
Baltimore, MD 21201

OSI-Baltimore Tackling Drug Addiction Grants 2973
The initiative aims to increase the access of uninsured drug-dependent citizens to comprehensive services that respond to their individual needs. To achieve this objective, the Program is helping Baltimore City to develop a sustainable, high-quality treatment system that uses research-based clinical practices and that benefits from inter-agency coordination. The initiative also seeks to demonstrate to policymakers and the general public that sound treatment practices and policies will save lives, reduce crime, rebuild families and communities, and use public funds wisely. Grants seek to fund three major priorities: to make available drug treatment that integrates services targeting poverty-related barriers to self-sufficiency; to engage more drug-dependent citizens in the treatment system by supporting aggressive outreach efforts and by removing barriers to treatment entry; and to promote a comprehensive, high-quality public treatment system by supporting infrastructure development and advocacy and public education efforts.
Requirements: Baltimore area non-profit and for-profit entities may apply.
Geographic Focus: Maryland
Contact: Robert Schwartz; (410) 234-1091, ext. 207; fax: (410) 234-2816; email: rschwartz@sorosny.org
Internet: http://www.soros.org/initiatives/baltimore/focus_areas/drug_addiction/guidelines
Sponsor: Open Society Institute
201 North Charles Street, Suite 1300
Baltimore, MD 21201

Osserman-Sosin Postdoctoral Myasthenia Gravis Research Fellowships 2974
These postdoctoral fellowships are intended to provide some support to physicians, PhD scientists, and allied health professionals for conducting research into myasthenia gravis (MG) or related conditions. Clinical investigations as well as laboratory studies concerned with research on MG and with underlying mechanisms of neuromuscular transmission and the pathogenesis of myasthenia gravis are supported. A qualified candidate desiring training in MG-related research first finds a scientist with an established research program who will agree to supervise her/his training and the basic or clinical research to be carried out. The number of fellowships awarded per year is dependent on the amount of funds available.
Requirements: applicant must be a permanent resident of the United States or Canada who has been accepted to work in the laboratory of an established investigator at an institution in the United States, Canada, or abroad; or a foreign national who has been accepted to work in the laboratory of an established investigator a an institution in the United States or Canada.
Samples: Dr. Marika Falcone, U of Arizona—to study the role of B-lymphocytes as antigen-presenting cells in the induction of the pathogenic T-cell responses against nicotinic acetylcholine receptor, $30,000.; Dr. Brian Hare, Harvard Medical School—to study the solution structure determination of a single chain T-cell receptor and design of T-cell ligands with therapeutic potential, $30,000.; Drs. Anthony Auerbach and Claudio Grosman, State U of New York at Buffalo—to study binding, gating, and desensitization of the acetylcholine receptor channel.
Amount of Grant: $50,000 maximum
Date(s) Application is Due: Oct 1
Contact: Fellowships Administrator, (651) 917-6256 or (800) 541-5454; fax: (651) 917-1835; email: mgfa@myasthenia.org
Internet: http://www.myasthenia.org/research/MGFA_PostDoctoralFellowship.pdf
Sponsor: Myasthenia Gravis Foundation of America
1821 University Ave W, Suite S256
St. Paul, MN 55104

Osteogenesis Imperfecta Foundation Research Grants 2975
Funding is available for fellowships for young investigators working to develop expertise in osteogenesis imperfecta (OI) research or seed grants for either basic or clinical studies with relevance to OI. Michael Geisman Research Fellowships provide support for investigator's salary and for supplies. (Second year funding may be available.) Seed grants may be funded for one year. (Grants do not support indirect costs or principal investigator salaries.) Clinical Seed Grants may be funded for two years. (Grants do not support indirect costs or principal investigator salaries.)
Amount of Grant: $50,000 per year Michael Geisman Research Fellowships; $60,000 maximum seed grants; $120,000 clinical seed grants for two years
Date(s) Application is Due: Nov 1
Contact: Research Department, (301) 947-0083; fax: (301) 947-0456; email: bonelink@oif.org
Internet: http://www.oif.org/site/PageServer?pagename=OIFGrantApp
Sponsor: Osteogenesis Imperfecta Foundation
804 W Diamond Avenue, Suite 210
Gaithersburg, MD 20878

Oticon Focus on People Awards 2976
The national awards program honors individuals with mild, moderate, or severe hearing loss who demonstrate through their accomplishments that hearing loss does not limit a person's ability to make a difference in his/her family, community, and the world. The awards program aims to change outdated stereotypes of what it means to have a hearing loss—stereotypes that often prevent people from seeking professional help. This year, awards are offered in five categories: youth, for children ages five to 12; student, for young people ages 13 to 25 who are full-time students; adults, for those over the age of 18; advocacy, for individuals of all ages who are actively involved in advocacy or support efforts for the hard-of-hearing and deaf community; and practitioner, a special award for hearing care professionals who are currently in practice. First-place category winners will receive an award and a $1,000 donation by Oticon to a not-for-profit cause of their choice. Guidelines and a nomination form are available online.
Requirements: Anyone may nominate themselves or another with a hearing loss.
Amount of Grant: $1000 first-place award, $500 second-place award, $250 third-place award
Contact: Program Contact, (732) 560-1220; fax: (732) 560-0029

Internet: http://www.oticon.dk/eprise/main/Oticon/U.S._en/SEC_Professionals/FocusOnPeopleAwards/_index
Sponsor: Oticon Corporation
29 Schoolhouse Road
Somerset, NJ 08873

Otto Bremer Foundation Grants **2977**
The foundation concentrates its grantmaking activity in communities served by Bremer-affiliated banks and provides financial assistance to nonprofit organizations whose work contributes to the well-being of these towns. The foundation looks to support programs that promote civil and political rights, including freedom of assembly, speech, and religion; economic and social rights, including the right to education, food, health care, and shelter; and cultural and environmental rights, including the right to live in a clean environment and participate in the cultural and political events of one's community. Types of support include program development, operating support, capital (including building and equipment), matching or challenge grants, and internships. Applications are accepted throughout the year. Most grants are given for a one-year period, although some multiyear grants are awarded. The foundation encourages initial telephone or written inquiries concerning its interest in a particular project. Applicants are also encouraged to contact foundation staff for assistance in the development of a proposal.
Requirements: Private nonprofit or public 501(c)3 tax-exempt organizations whose beneficiaries are residents of Minnesota, North Dakota, or Wisconsin with priority given to those communities or regions served by Bremer affiliates.
Restrictions: Requests for the following types of projects are discouraged: annual fund drives; benefit events; camps; commercial and business development; K-12 education; medical research; sporting activities; building endowments other than for the development of community foundations; capital requests for hospitals and nursing homes; theatrical productions, including motion pictures, books, and other artistic or media projects; municipal and government services; or historical preservation, museums, and interpretive centers.
Geographic Focus: Minnesota; North Dakota; Wisconsin
Amount of Grant: $552-$259,235; $20,455 average
Contact: Danielle Cheslog, Grants Manager; (651) 312-3717 or (651) 227-8036; fax: (651) 312-3665; email: danielle@ottobremer.org or obf@ottobremer.org
Sponsor: Otto Bremer Foundation
445 Minnesota Stret, Suite 2250
Saint Paul, MN 55101-2107

OUT Fund for Lesbian and Gay Liberation Grants **2978**
The organization is dedicated to a range of social justice, race, class, gender, and sexuality issues and supports radical organization projects to build community among lesbians, gay men, bisexuals, and transgender people. Proposals are sought that originate in marginalized communities like the poor, young, old, or disabled; serve rural areas; develop long-term coalitions in and out of diverse communities; organize antiracism efforts; foster organization through cultural projects; and focus on HIV health policy, prevention, and education efforts. Proposals that identify and target multi-issues, such as race, class, gender, and poverty, are preferred.
Requirements: 501(c)3 tax-exempt organizations and organizations with a 501(c)3 fiscal sponsor are eligible. 501(c)4 lobbying organizations may be eligible under very specific circumstances.
Contact: Grants Administrator, (212) 529-5300; fax: (212) 982-9272; email: info@fex.org
Internet: http://www.fex.org/grantmaking.shtml
Sponsor: Funding Exchange
666 Broadway, Suite 500
New York, NY 10012

Owen County Community Foundation Grants **2979**
The Owen County Community Foundation was established in 1996 and serves the Owen County, Indiána area. The Foundation connects donors with the causes they care about. The foundation provides support for organizations involved with arts and culture, education, animal welfare, health care, human services, and community development.
Requirements: A letter of intent is required prior to submitting a grant request. The letter of intent must be submitted before June 1, 4:00 pm and must be: one page in length; include name, address, and phone number of organization; include name and title of contact person; include mission statement of agency/organization; list project description; list anticipated results. A copy of tax-exempt verification must accompany the letter of intent as well. You will be contacted approximately one month after the deadline as to whether or not to submit a full proposal. A full proposal should include the following: grant application and agreement page (available at the foundation office or the foundations website); organizations background, including history, mission statement, number of staff, and number of persons served by agency or program; proposed program, please indicate desired outcomes; program methods; evaluation; funding the program; timetable; project budget; agency budget; governing organization; financial statement and balance sheet; tax exempt status; audit, with the original proposal only, provide one copy of your organization's most recently completed audit. Mail or hand deliver an original signed and completed grant proposal, along with eight copies with no permanent binding to the Owen Community Foundation office no later then September 15, 4:00 pm. The Board will contact you in late October with it's funding decision and grant checks will be presented in November.
Restrictions: Giving limited to Owen County, Indiana. No grants for endowments, deficit funding, conferences, publications, films, television, or radio programs, travel, annual appeals, religious purposes or membership contributions.
Geographic Focus: Indiana
Date(s) Application is Due: Jun 1; Sep 15
Contact: Maggie Burton, Program Manager; (812) 829-1725; fax: (812) 829-9958; email: maggie@owencountycf.org
Internet: http://www.owencountycf.org/Grants.asp
Sponsor: Owen County Community Foundation, Inc.
201 W. Morgan Street, Suite 202, P.O. Box 503
Spencer, IN 47460

Oxalosis and Hyperoxaluria Foundation Grants **2980**
Grants are awarded for research on hyperoxaluria, the presence of excess oxalic acid or oxalates in the urine, and the related conditions oxalosis and calcium-oxalate kidney stones. The foundation seeks to fund grants that will increase the understanding of hyperoxaluria and oxalosis and improve the clinical management and treatment of these two orphan diseases. Investigation into alternative methods of treatment that will alleviate the need for transplantation therapy are encouraged. Applications for up to two years of support will be considered. These funds may be used for salaries for technical assistance, special equipment, animals, supplies, and travel. Other organizations that have been approached about supporting the same project should be identified.
Requirements: Applicants must hold an MD, PhD, or equivalent degree by the time the funding period begins.
Amount of Grant: $160,000 maximum
Date(s) Application is Due: Oct 15
Contact: Program Contact, (212) 777-0470; fax: (212) 777-0471; email: execdirector@ohf.org
Internet: http://www.ohf.org/prof_application.html
Sponsor: Oxalosis and Hyperoxaluria Foundation
201 E 19th Street, 12E
New York, NY 10003

PacifiCare Foundation Grants **2981**
The foundation's mission is to improve the quality of life for residents of areas where PacifiCare Health Systems does business. The foundation's focus areas are child/youth, including child care, youth activity programs, at-risk youth, and counseling programs; education, including school programs that promote self-esteem, encourage academic achievement and the development of specific skills, literacy programs, training programs, and programs that improve the effectiveness of the educational system; health, including prevention, health education, access to health care, and improved quality of health care of targeted populations; human/social services, including housing, shelters, education, protection, community development, crime prevention, food, transportation, and other social services for targeted populations; and senior, including social services, nutrition, education, volunteer, and and adult day care. Preference will be given to proposals for specific projects. Requests for operating costs will be considered if the request is very specific and clearly defined. Seed grant requests also receive consideration. Organizations funded by the foundation are welcome to reapply annually. Guidelines and foundation application forms are available on the foundation's Web site.
Requirements: IRS 501(c)3 nonprofit organizations serving residents of PacifiCare regions in Arizona, California, Colorado, Nevada, Oklahoma, Oregon, Texas, and Washington are eligible.
Restrictions: The foundation will not consider grants for arts/cultural programs, associations, annual campaigns, associations—professional/technical, capital campaigns, challenge/matching grants, hosting/supporting conferences, individual support, private foundations, programs that promote religious doctrine, research, scholarships, or sponsorship of special events.
Geographic Focus: Arizona; California; Colorado; Nevada; Oklahoma; Oregon; Texas; Washington
Samples: Casa de Esperanza (Green Valley, AZ)—to provide intergenerational community programming for children and the elderly, $10,000.; Escape Family Resource Ctr (Houston, TX)—for a school-based child abuse prevention and family support program, $10,000.
Amount of Grant: $2000-$10,000 range
Date(s) Application is Due: Jan 1; Jul 1
Contact: Riva Gebel, Director, (714) 825-5233
Internet: http://www.pacificare.com/commonPortal/application?origin=hnav_bar.jsp&event=bea.portal.framework.internal.portlet.event&pageid=ContentDisplay&portletid=contentdisplay&wfevent=link.viewarticle&navnode=Foundation.1
Sponsor: PacifiCare Foundation
P O Box 25186
Santa Ana, CA 92799

PacifiCorp Foundation for Learning Grants **2982**
The foundation awards grants to eligible nonprofit organizations in four broad areas, including educational and research institutions, both public and private, from early childhood through university level; youth organizations; cultural enrichment organizations dedicated to the performing arts, the visual arts, historic preservation, cross-cultural education, and other such activities; and health and human services organizations, including chemical dependency treatment and prevention programs, senior citizen centers, runaway youth services, and domestic violence treatment and prevention programs. Deadline for education organizations is March 15; for civic, community, and organizations not covered in other categories, June 15; for culture and arts organizations, September 15; for health, welfare, and social service organizations, December 15. Guidelines and application are available online.

Requirements: 501(c)3 community organizations in Idaho, Oregon, Utah, California, Washington, and Wyoming are eligible.
Restrictions: Organizations and activities not eligible for foundation support include religious groups for religious purposes; political organizations, ballot measure campaigns, or candidates for public office; organizations that discriminate against individuals on the basis of creed, color, sex, age, national origin, or veteran status; individuals; contributions to or memberships in chambers of commerce, service clubs, taxpayer associations, and other similar bodies; or any non-charitable purpose. As a general rule, the foundation also will not support establishment or support of endowments; coverage of operating deficits; capital campaigns; conferences, conventions, and events; projects that do not have a bearing on communities within the six-state region served by PacifiCorp subsidiaries or communities served by PacifiCorp Power Marketing.
Geographic Focus: California; Idaho; Oregon; Utah; Washington; Wyoming
Amount of Grant: $1000-$10,000 average
Date(s) Application is Due: Mar 15; Jun 15; Sep 15; Dec 15
Contact: Grants Manager, (503) 813-7257; fax: (503) 813-5272; email: pacificorpfoundation@pacificorp.com
Internet: http://www.pacificorpfoundation.org/Article/Article25110.html
Sponsor: PacifiCorp Foundation for Learning
825 NE Multnomah, Suite 2000
Portland, OR 97232-4116

PAHO-ASM International Professorship for Latin America 2983
The program provides funding support to an ASM member from the U.S. who is scientifically recognized in his/her area to teach a hands-on, highly interactive short course in the area of antimicrobial resistance at an institution of higher learning in Bolivia, Colombia, Costa Rica, Dominican Republic, Ecuador, El Salvador, Guatemala, Honduras, Nicaragua, Panama, Paraguay, or Peru. One Teaching Professorship offered per program year.
Requirements: The application must be made jointly between a hosting institution and the visiting professor. Eligibility for Host Institution: institution with graduate students enrolled in a masters, doctoral or equivalent program, post-doctoral fellows or residents, and teaching faculty; institution where at least 12 students will be enrolled full-time in the short course; commitment to maximizing use of the course, as demonstrated by the applicability of the course's contents to existing programs at the institution or to the field of research of the Research Professor. demonstrated commitment to international collaborations and partnerships; demonstrated commitment to advancing the microbiological sciences through interactions with professional organizations; institutions in developed nations, as defined by the UN high HDI group, are ineligible. Eligibility for Visiting Teaching Professor: scientifically recognized their area of microbiological expertise; actively engaged in teaching at the post-secondary level; commitment to international collaborations and partnerships; must be an ASM member during the term of the Professorship. Preference will be given to: applicants who will be able to make maximal use of the course, as demonstrated either by the applicability of the course's contents to existing programs at the host institution or to the field of research of the visiting Professor; applications that demonstrate a commitment to building an ongoing institutional relationship. It is strongly recommended that the course include a hands-on component, such as a wet lab or other practical activity.
Amount of Grant: $4,000
Date(s) Application is Due: Apr 15; Oct 15
Contact: International Professorship Program, (202) 942-9368; fax: (202) 942-9328; email: international@asmusa.org
Internet: http://www.asm.org/International/index.asp?bid=57785
Sponsor: American Society for Microbiology
1752 N Street NW
Washington, DC 20036-2804

PAHO/WHO Fellowships 2984
Fellowship is a specially tailored training activity for an individual or a group with the purpose of fulfilling specific learning objectives. Fellowships may be of short or long duration and take place in a training institution or in the field inside or outside of the fellow's country. Each of the six regional WHO offices share responsibility for management and administration of the fellowship program within its region: regional office for Europe in Copenhagen, Denmark; regional office for Eastern Mediterranean in Alexandria, Egypt; regional office for the Western Pacific in Manila, the Philippines; regional office for Africa in Brazzaville, Congo; regional office for South-East Asia in New Delhi, India; and regional office for the Americas in Washington, DC. The Pan American Health Organization (PAHO) serves as the Regional WHO Office for all of the Americas.
Requirements: Fellowships are open to nationals of member states of the PAHO who are public health workers in all fields, especially deans or faculty members of schools of public health, medicine, dentistry, engineering, veterinary medicine, and nursing. Individual must be recommended by his/her own government and return to his/her home country for at least three years service on completion of studies. Contact program staff for specific eligibility.
Restrictions: Candidates normally should not be more than 55 years of age.
Contact: Regional Office for the Americas, Pan American Health Organization, (202) 974-3000; fax: (202) 974-3663; email: postmaster@paho.org
Internet: http://www.paho.org/English/HSP/HSR/fellowships.htm
Sponsor: Pan American Health Organization
525 23rd St NW
Washington, DC 20037

Pajaro Valley Community Health Grants 2985
The trust awards responsive grants to eligible nonprofit organizations in its areas of interest, including oral health—community-based projects devoted to dental disease prevention and oral health education efforts; farm workers and their families—programs addressing a wide range of health issues affecting farm workers and their families (proposals are welcome for health education services and increased access and linkage to existing services or medical benefits); and children and youth ages six to 21/making healthy life choices—programs dealing with a variety of issues related to youth making healthy life choices (i.e., Hepatitis C prevention, support services for teen parents, substance abuse prevention, violence prevention, cultural and after-school activities that build self-esteem, and prevention of obesity and reducing sedentary lifestyles). Types of support include operating support, capacity building and infrastructure, and funding for new or expanded services. Guidelines are available online.
Requirements: California 501(c)3 organizations, organizations with 501(c)3 fiscal sponsors, and school-based health programs in the primary service area consisting of zip codes 95076, 95019, and 95004, in the communities of Watsonville, Pajaro, Freedom, and Aromas are eligible.
Geographic Focus: California
Samples: Ctr for Community Advocacy (Watsonville, CA)—to expand the Promotores de Salud program to include indigenous Mexican farm workers, $15,000 (2003); Family Services Assoc of the Pajaro Valley (Watsonville, CA)—to explain and provide mental-health services to farmworker families, $10,000 (2003); Salud Para la Gente (Watsonville, CA)—to develop and expand its dental-services program, $30,000 (2003); Pajaro Valley Prevention and Student Assistance (Watsonville, CA)—for a school-based violence-prevention and conflict-resolution program, $15,000 (2003).
Amount of Grant: $5000-$30,000
Date(s) Application is Due: Feb 3
Contact: Kathleen McCarthy, Program and Grants Manager, (831) 761-5695; fax: (831) 763-6084; email: grants@pvhealthtrust.org
Internet: http://www.pvhealthtrust.org/html/grants.html
Sponsor: Pajaro Valley Community Health Trust
85 Nielson Street
Watsonville, CA 95076

Palm Beach and Martin Counties Grants 2986
The community foundation supports nonprofit organizations serving Florida's Palm Beach and Martin Counties in eight program areas: arts and culture, education, environment, health, human services, community development, the conservation and preservation of historical and cultural resources, and human and race relations. Guidelines and forms are available online.
Requirements: Florida organizations based in and serving Palm Beach and Martin Counties are eligible to apply.
Restrictions: Proposals will not be funded for routine operating expenses, endowments, building campaigns, computers, fund-raising events, celebration functions, feasibility studies, religious organizations for religious purposes, or recurring requests for the same purpose.
Geographic Focus: Florida
Samples: Pleasant City Family Reunion Committee (West Palm Beach, FL)—to support artists and instructors who work with disadvantaged youths, $15,000 (2003); TAB Development Corp (West Palm Beach, FL)—for classes and training courses for first-time homebuyers, $15,000 (2003); FAI/FIU Joint Ctr for Environmental and Urban Problems (Jupiter, FL)—to integrate economic, environmental, and social concerns in community design, $15,000 (2003); Florida Resource Ctr for Women and Children (Riviera Beach, FL)—for salary and program expenses of an antiviolence program for teenagers, $25,000 (2003).
Amount of Grant: $25,000 maximum
Contact: Linda Raybin, Program Contact, (561) 659-6800; fax: (561) 832-6542; email: lraybin@cfpdmc.org
Internet: http://www.cfpbmc.org/grant/Guidelines.asp
Sponsor: Community Foundation for Palm Beach and Martin Counties
700 S Dixie Hwy, Suite 200
West Palm Beach, FL 33401

Pancreatic Cancer Action Network-AACR Fellowship 2987
The Pancreatic Cancer Action Network-AACR Fellowship represents a joint effort to attract young scientist to careers in pancreatic cancer research. The Fellowship is open to Postdoctoral Fellows and Clinical Research Fellows working at an academic, medical, or research institution who will be in the 1st, 2nd, or 3rd year of their postdoctoral training at the start of the grant term on July 1. The Fellowship provides a one-year grant of $45,000 to support the salary and benefits of the Fellow while working on a mentored pancreatic cancer research project. A partial amount of funds, up to 25% of the total grant, may be designated for direct research support. The research proposed for funding may be basic, translational, clinical or epidemiological in nature and must have direct application and relevance to pancreatic cancer. It is anticipated that one Fellowship will be funded. AACR requires applicants submit both an online and a paper application. The online application must be submitted by 12:00 noon (United Sates Eastern Time) on October 28, using the proposalCENTRAL website at http://proposalcentral.altum.com. The paper copy with original signatures and all required documents must be postmarked and sent no later then October 30.
Requirements: Applicants must have acquired a doctoral degree (including Ph.D., M.D., D.O., D.C., N.D., D.D.S., D.V.M., Sc.D., D.N.S., Pharm.D., or equivalent doctoral degree, or a combined clinical and research doctoral degree) in a related field and may not currently be candidate for another degree. Applicants must be in the 1st, 2nd, or 3rd

year of Postdoctoral or Clinical Research Fellowship at an academic, medical, or research institution within the United States at the start of the Fellowship term on July 1.
Restrictions: Scientific investigators or health professionals who are funded by the tobacco industry for any project, or whose named mentors in the case of mentored grants are funded by the tobacco industry for any project, may not apply and will not be eligible for AACR grants.
Amount of Grant: $45,000
Date(s) Application is Due: Oct 28; Oct 30
Contact: Hanna Hopfinger, Grants Program Assistant; (267) 646-0665; fax: (215) 440-9372; email: hanna.hopfinger@aacr.org
Internet: http://www.aacr.org/home/scientists/research-funding—fellowships/postdoctoral-fellowships.aspx
Sponsor: American Association for Cancer Research
615 Chestnut Street, 17th Floor
Philadelphia, PA 19106-4404

Pancreatic Cancer Action Network-AACR Pathway to Leadership Grants 2988
The Pancreatic Cancer Action Network-AACR Pathway to Leadership Grant represents a joint effort to ensure the future leadership of pancreatic cancer research by supporting outstanding early career investigators beginning in their postdoctoral research positions and continuing through their successful transition to independence. Applicants must be in the first five years of their postdoctoral or clinical research fellowships at the time of application and not already have a full-time tenure track assistant professor position (or equivalent). The Pathway to Leadership Grant will provide up to five years of support, for a total of $600,000, consisting of two phases. The initial Mentored Phase lasts up up two years, during which time recipients will receive $75,000 per year and are expected to work closely with mentors to develop their research. During the subsequent three years, recipients are expected to be independent research positions and will be funded at $150,000 per year. AACR requires applicants to submit both an online and a paper application. Online applications must be completed by 12:00 noon (United States Eastern Daylight Time) on October 28, using the proposalCENTRAL website. The paper copy with original signatures and all supporting documents must be postmarked and sent no later than October 30.
Requirements: Applicants must be in mentored training positions at an academic, medical, or research institution within the United States. There are no citizenship requirements. The applicant institution will be the mentored phase institution. Employees or subcontractors of a government entity or for-profit private industry are not eligible. Exceptions may apply if an applicant holds a full-time position at a Veterans' Hospital or national laboratory in the U.S. Contact AACR before submitting an application to determine your eligibility. Applicants must be Postdoctoral or Clinical Research Fellows who completed all doctoral degree requirements no more then five years prior to the start of the grant term.
Amount of Grant: $600,000
Date(s) Application is Due: Oct 28; Oct 30
Contact: Elizabeth Martin, Program Assistant; (267) 646-0664; fax: (215) 440-9372; email: grants@aacr.org
Internet: http://www.aacr.org/home/scientists/research-funding—fellowships/postdoctoral-fellowships.aspx
Sponsor: American Association for Cancer Research
615 Chestnut Street, 17th Floor
Philadelphia, PA 19106-4404

Parker B. Francis Fellowships in Pulmonary Research 2989
Grants are awarded to institutions for the purpose of providing stipends, fringe benefits, and modest travel expenses in support of qualified post-doctoral fellows or newly appointed assistant professors. Award recipients will thereby be enabled to devote the major part of their professional effort to research related to pulmonary disease and lung biology. Sponsorship of the fellow by an established investigator is required. There can be only two fellows in a department at any one time. Only one application will be accepted from a department annually. Fellowships are awarded for three years.
Requirements: Fellows must be U.S. or Canadian citizens, or intend to make permanent residence in the United States or Canada, must hold doctoral degrees, and must be sponsored by established investigators. Foreign nationals must document intent to become permanent residents or citizens of North America.
Samples: Dr. Zissis Chroneos, Pediatrics, Children's Hospital Medical Ctr—for research entitled Cloning of the SP-A Receptor Gene.; Dr. Emily DiMango, Medicine, Columbia U—for research entitled Signal Transduction of Inflammation in Cystic Fibrosis.; Dr. Michael DuVall, Anesthesiology, U of Alabama, Birmingham—for research entitled Effects of Reactive Nitrogen Species on C1-secretion in Airway Epithelium.
Amount of Grant: $44,000 first year, $46,000 second year, $48,000 third year; plus $1500 maximum for travel and fringe benefits
Date(s) Application is Due: Oct 17
Contact: Dr. Joseph Brain, Director of the Fellowship Program, (617) 432-4099; fax: (617) 277-2382; email: brain@hsph.harvard.edu
Internet: http://www.francisfellowships.org
Sponsor: Francis Families Foundation
Harvard School of Public Health, Room 1411, Building 1
Boston, MA 02115

Partners for Youth with Disabilities Grants 2990
Proposals are invited from faith-based and community-based organizations throughout the country to start up, sustain, or expand mentoring programs for youth with disabilities. Mentoring programs must promote positive employment and transition outcomes for youth with disabilities. Priorities include: depending on qualifications, one grant will be reserved for a Massachusetts-based organization; mentoring activities must serve youth with disabilities between the ages of 16 and 24; mentoring activities may include one-to-one mentoring between adults and youth with disabilities, one-to-one e-mentoring between adults and youth with disabilities, or group mentoring programs for youth with disabilities. Guidelines are available online.
Requirements: To be eligible, the primary applicant: must be a community- or faith-based organization that has social services as a major part of its mission; is headquartered in the local community to which it provides social services; has a social services budget of $300,000 or less, excluding salaries and expenses, or has six or fewer full-time equivalent employees; is 501(c)3 tax exempt; and is located in the United States.
Amount of Grant: $5000-$25,000
Contact: Genelle Campbell, PYD National Mentoring Director, (617) 556-4075 ext 28; fax: (617) 556-4074; email: gcampbell@pyd.org
Internet: http://www.pyd.org/mentoring_programs/mentor_match.htm
Sponsor: Partners for Youth with Disabilities
95 Berkeley Street, Suite 109
Boston, MA 02116

Partnership for Cures Charles E. Culpeper Scholarships in Medical Science 2991
The program awards scholarships in medical science to support the career development of academic physicians. In direct costs, $100,000 per year to the sponsoring institution will be committed for up to three consecutive years. It is expected that a significant portion of the award will be used as a contribution to the Scholar's salary. Up to $50,000 (plus fringe benefits) of this sum may be used for this purpose; the rest for support of research including personnel and some travel costs. Eight percent will be added to each award for indirect costs. All scientific research relevant to human health is eligible for consideration.
Requirements: Candidates must: be U.S. citizens or aliens who have been granted permanent U.S. residence (proof required); hold the M.D. degree from a U.S. medical school or the equivalent of an M.D. degree from an educational institution equivalent to a United States medical school; and be judged worthy of support by virtue of the quality of their research proposals and their potential for successful careers in academic medicine. Applicants must have at least one year of post-doctoral clinical training.
Restrictions: Individuals who have achieved a rank above assistant professor are ineligible for this program, and an awardee who is promoted above the rank of assistant professor before the initiation of the scholarship will be ineligible to receive the award.
Amount of Grant: $108,000 per year for three years
Date(s) Application is Due: Aug 16
Contact: Dr. Bruce E. Bloom; (312) 696-1366; fax: (312) 263-0939; email: Bruce@4cures.org
Internet: http://www.4cures.org/home/culpeper_scholar_program_research
Sponsor: Partnership for Cures
70 West Madison Street, Suite 1500
Chicago, IL 60602

Partnership for Cures Two Years To Cures Grants 2992
The Initiative is intended to bring researchers, funders and institutions together to produce better treatments and cures for patients with disease right now. The Program works to quickly bring together: breakthrough scientific discoveries about diseases and treatments; FDA approved drugs and other medical therapies (Eastern and Western) with new potential uses; research teams at top institutions ready to proceed with urgency and focus; and independent validation, compressed time lines, and financial leverage. Projects must be able to create a direct patient impact in 24 months from the date of initiation of the project. Budgets can range from $35,000 to $500,000. The Program is accepting research projects in any catastrophic disease, but has special interest in the following diseases: lupus, Crohns disease, MS, ALS, protein intolerances in children, ischemic colitis, autism, type I diabetes, lung cancer, osteosarcoma, Fragile X syndrome, Jewish genetic diseases, and Parkinsons disease. There is no deadline for submissions, but funders are looking for projects right now.
Requirements: Each project must come with a minimum of 30% matching funds. Those funds can come from the institution itself, from government or other public funders, or from individuals, foundations or other private funders.
Restrictions: No more than 10% of the budget can be allocated to overhead, travel and publications.
Amount of Grant: $35,000 to $500,000
Contact: Dr. Bruce E. Bloom; (312) 696-1366; fax: (312) 263-0939; email: Bruce@4cures.org
Internet: http://www.4cures.org/home/funding_opportunities
Sponsor: Partnership for Cures
70 West Madison Street, Suite 1500
Chicago, IL 60602

Partnership for Pediatric Epilepsy Research Grants 2993
This program stimulates epilepsy research by providing funding for investigators in the early stages of their careers. Seed grants are awarded to clinical investigators or basic scientists for support of biological or behavioral research which will advance the understanding, treatment, and prevention of epilepsy. All research must be conducted in the United States. The partnership is a consortium of professional organizations and individuals with the common objective of researching treatments and cures to pediatric epilepsy.
Requirements: Proposals are invited from investigators who hold an advanced degree (MD or PhD) and have completed all research training. Investigators may be based at corporations as well as academic/university settings.

Amount of Grant: $100,000 maximum for two years
Date(s) Application is Due: Sep 1
Contact: Grants Administrator, (301) 459-3700; fax: (301) 577-2684; email: grants@efa.org
Internet: http://www.epilepsyfoundation.org/research/grants.cfm
Sponsor: Partnership for Pediatric Epilepsy
4351 Garden City Drive
Landover, MD 20785

Pasadena Foundation Average Grants **2994**
The community foundation serves the greater Pasadena, CA, area and awards grants for capital improvements to agencies serving children, the elderly, and the disabled. Fields of interest include child development, the elderly, disabled, youth, drug abuse, family planning, education, arts and the humanities, mental health, community development, and the environment. Challenge/matching grants also are awarded. The deadline is the first business day in March.
Restrictions: Schools, religious institutions, and political organizations are ineligible.
Geographic Focus: California
Samples: Women at Work—for the acquisition of three computer systems, $6000.; Pasadena Boys Choir—to purchase concert uniforms, $5725.; All Saints Children's Ctr—to purchase cots and floor coverings, $2610.
Amount of Grant: $8000 maximum
Contact: Program Contact, (626) 796-2097; fax: (626) 583-4738; email: pcfstaff@pasadenacf.org
Internet: http://www.pasadenacf.org/grant_reg.htm
Sponsor: Pasadena Foundation
260 S Los Robles Avenue, #119
Pasadena, CA 91101

Paso del Norte Health Foundation Grants **2995**
The foundation offers support to nonprofits serving West Texas and Southern New Mexico, with limited funding to provide health and wellness to the underserved. The foundation issues RFPs to request proposals in target areas, such as health and nutrition and exercise and health. Eligible groups must serve low-income areas. Contact the foundation with ideas on a particular project.
Requirements: Nonprofits serving West Texas and Southern New Mexico are eligible.
Geographic Focus: Texas
Samples: Texas Tech U Health Sciences Ctr (El Paso, TX)—for scholarships and loans for medical students who choose to practice in El Paso, contingent on Texas Legislative approval of a four-year medical school in El Paso, $1.25 million over five years.
Contact: Eric Hutson, Program Officer, (915) 544-7636 ext 20; fax (915) 544-7713; email ehutson@pdnhf.org
Internet: http://www.pdnhf.org
Sponsor: Paso del Norte Health Foundation
1100 N Stanton Street, Suite 510
El Paso, TX 79902

Patron Saints Foundation Grants **2996**
The foundation awards one-year grants to California nonprofit organizations to improve health care in the West San Gabriel Valley. Areas of interest include medical care and medical research. Types of support include capital grants, matching gifts, project grants, research grants, and seed money grants. Applications must be postmarked by the first Friday in March and October.
Requirements: California 501(c)3 tax-exempt organizations serving the West San Gabriel Valley are eligible.
Geographic Focus: California
Amount of Grant: $3500-$15,000 range
Contact: Program Contact, (626) 564-0444; fax: (626) 564-0444; email: patronsaintsfdn@sbcglobal.net
Internet: http://www.patronsaintsfoundation.org
Sponsor: Patron Saints Foundation
260 S Los Robles Avenue, Suite 201
Pasadena, CA 91101

Paul and Mary Haas Foundation Contributions and Student Scholarships **2997**
Grants are given to tax-exempt organizations in six areas: civic and charitable, education (including adult basic education, adult/family literacy training, curriculum development, and vocational programs), health, religion, the arts, and college scholarships. Funding is generally seed money for innovative services in the Corpus Christi, TX, area. Creative, innovative, and exploratory projects are encouraged, with less interest in building projects and areas covered by normal budgets. Additional types of support include general operating support, equipment acquisition, program development, conferences and seminars, and scholarship funds and scholarships to individuals. Requests for support are normally reviewed on a year-round basis in the order in which they are received. All grants are made for one year and are not automatically renewed. Applications for scholarships are due in August at the beginning of senior high school year; application for other grants are accepted at any time.
Requirements: Grants are made to Texas organizations with 501(c)3 status. Initial inquiries should be made in the form of a one- to two-page written proposal.
Geographic Focus: Texas
Samples: Corpus Christi Neighborhood Ctrs (TX)—for general operating support, $5000.
Amount of Grant: $35-$250,000 average
Contact: Karen Wesson, Administrative Director, (361) 887-6955; fax: (361) 883-5992; email: haasfdn@aol.com
Sponsor: Paul and Mary Haas Foundation
P.O. Box 2928
Corpus Christi, TX 78403

Paul Balint Charitable Trust Grants **2998**
The trust operates in the United Kingdom and internationally and awards grants to nonprofit charities in the fields of Jewish charities, medicine, disability, with a specific interest in aging and elderly and improving the daily lives of those with disabilities.
Contact: Andrew Balint, 020 7624 2098
Sponsor: Paul Balint Charitable Trust
C/O 26 Church Crescent
London N20 0JP United Kingdom

Paul E. and Klare N. Reinhold Foundation Grants **2999**
The foundation makes grants in Clay County, Florida, for projects in health, religion, children and youth, music appreciation and education, art appreciation and education, and public improvement. Types of support include building construction/renovation, capital campaigns, emergency funds, equipment, land acquisition, matching/challenge grants, operating grants, and seed money grants. Details are available on the Web site.
Requirements: 501(c)3 tax-exempt organizations in Florida's Clay County are eligible.
Restrictions: Grants do not support advertising for fund-raising campaigns, tickets, debt reduction, endowments, attempts to influence legislation, or basic operating costs.
Geographic Focus: Florida
Samples: Clay County Habitat For Humanity, Inc (FL)—to supplement a Capacity Building Grant to help pay the Executive Director's salary, $20,000.; Alzheimer's Assoc (FL)—to support Caregiver Education By enhancing the resource library, $3000.; Christ Episcopal Church Building Fund (FL)—dedication of family/gathering room in honor of Thomas E. Camp, III, $50,000.; Keystone Heights Elementary School (FL)—for additional supplies for Project Playground, $500.
Amount of Grant: $10,000 maximum
Contact: Contact, (904) 269-5857; fax: (904) 269-8382; email: lhoke@reinhold.net
Internet: http://www.reinhold.org/html/guidelines.htm
Sponsor: Paul E. and Klare N. Reinhold Foundation
1845 Town Center Boulevard, Suite 105
Orange Park, FL 32003

Paul G. Allen Family Foundation Grants **3000**
The single foundation, created through the consolidation of Allen's six previous foundations (The Allen Foundation for the Arts, The Paul G. Allen Charitable Foundation, The Paul G. Allen Foundation for Medical Research, The Paul G. Allen Forest Protection Foundation, The Allen Foundation for Music, and The Paul G. Allen Virtual Education Foundation), will continue to focus on the Allen family's philanthropic interests in the areas of arts and culture, youth engagement, community development and social change, and scientific and technological innovation. The Arts and Culture Program fosters creativity and promotes critical thinking by helping strong arts organizations become sustainable and supporting projects that feature innovative and diverse artistic forms. The Youth Engagement Program improves the way young people learn by supporting organizations that use innovative teaching strategies and provide opportunities for children to address issues relevant to their lives. The Community Development and Social Change Program promotes individual and community development by supporting initiatives and organizations that provide access to resources and opportunities. The Scientific and Technological Innovation Program advances promising scientific and technology research that has the potential to enhance understanding and stewardship of the world in which we live. Organizations may only receive one grant per year. Organizations must not have any delinquent final reports due to any of the Paul G. Allen Foundations for previous grants. Grantseekers are encouraged to apply through the online application process, where basic organizational and project information will be requested. Guidelines are available online.
Requirements: 501(c)3 tax-exempt organizations, status from the Internal Revenue government entities, and IRS-recognized tribes are eligible. Eligible organizations must be located in, or serving populations of, the Pacific Northwest, which includes Alaska, Idaho, Montana, Oregon, and Washington.
Restrictions: In general, the foundation will not consider requests for general fund drives, annual appeals, or federated campaigns; special events or sponsorships; direct grants, scholarships, or loans for the benefit of specific individuals; projects of organizations whose policies or practices discriminate on the basis of race, ethnic origin, sex, creed, or sexual orientation; contributions to sectarian or religious organizations whose principle activity is for the benefit of their own members or adherents; loans or debt retirement; projects that will benefit the students of a single school; general operating support for ongoing activities; or projects not aligned with the foundation's specified program areas. 509(a) private foundations are ineligible.
Geographic Focus: Alaska; Idaho; Montana; Northwest; Oregon; Pacific Northwest; Washington
Date(s) Application is Due: Mar 31; Sep 30
Contact: Grants Administrator, (206) 342-2030; fax: (206) 342-3030; email: info@pgafamilyfoundation.org
Internet: http://www.pgafamilyfoundation.org
Sponsor: Paul G. Allen Family Foundation
505 Fifth Ave S, Suite 900
Seattle, WA 98104

Paul G. Duke Foundation Grants 3001

The Foundation is primarily interested in supporting projects for children, young adults, and the family. Grants are generally made in the fields of the arts, education, health, and social services. The Foundation will also consider making challenge grants for worthwhile projects to encourage matching gifts or additional funding from other donors. Requests may be for general, capital, or specific project support, including seed money for innovative programs. The Foundation accepts proposals twice per year, and support is generally given for one year.

Requirements: Nonprofit organizations having recognition under Section 501(c)3 of the Internal Revenue Code are eligible for grants.

Restrictions: The Foundation generally does not make grants for transportation, computer hardware or software, and research or treatment for specific diseases. The Foundation does not award grants to individuals. Generally, grants are not made for religious purposes, budget deficits, or projects that are normally the responsibility of a public agency.

Geographic Focus: Ohio

Date(s) Application is Due: Apr 1; Aug 1

Contact: Tami Durrence; (614) 251-4000; fax: (614) 251-4009; email: mail@supportingfoundations.org

Internet: http://www.columbusfoundation.org/paul_g_duke.aspx

Sponsor: Paul G. Duke Foundation
1234 East Broad Street
Columbus, OH 43205-1453

Paul Marks Prizes for Cancer Research 3002

The prizes recognize outstanding young investigators who have made significant contributions to increase the understanding of cancer or improve the treatment of the disease through basic or clinical research. The winners will present their work at the center, be honored at a dinner, and share a cash award of $150,000. Nomination packets must include a letter from the nominator outlining the significance of the accomplishments for which the candidate should be recognized; a one-page scientific biography of the candidate; a list of up to eight of the candidate's significant published papers with a brief (fewer than 100 words) explanation of the importance of each one; and the candidate's curriculum vita. Up to three supporting letters may also be submitted. Annual deadline date may vary; contact program staff for exact dates.

Requirements: Nominees are required to be age 45 or younger at the time of submission.

Amount of Grant: $150,000

Date(s) Application is Due: Apr 29

Contact: Paizhe Pressley, Program Contact, (212) 639-6561; email: presslep@mskcc.org

Internet: http://www.mskcc.org/mskcc/html/53983.cfm

Sponsor: Memorial Sloan-Kettering Cancer Center
1275 York Avenue
New York, NY 10021

Paul Ogle Foundation Grants 3003

The Paul Ogle Foundation, Inc., was incorporated as an Indiana non-profit corporation in 1979 and is qualified under the IRS 501(c)3 as a private foundation. The Foundation's founder and original benefactor was Paul W. Ogle, who lived in Clark County, Indiana. The Foundation is headquartered in Jeffersonville, Indiana, and provides grants to deserving IRS 501(c)3 organizations in Clark, Floyd, Harrison, Switzerland, Scott, and Washington Counties in Indiana and Jefferson County, Kentucky. The Board of Directors has established guidelines for programs which they will consider for grant funding of capital projects and endowments.

Requirements: First read guidelines prior to contacting the foundations office, then send a letter of intent to the office. The letter should be typed on your institutions letterhead and should not exceed for typewritten pages in length. It should contain the following information about the proposed project: a brief description of the need that will be addressed by the proposal; a statement of the project's principal objectives; how the need will be met; the total estimated project budget and other sources of support that may be forthcoming, including a list of donors and amounts; the staff that will carry out the project and their qualifications; a timetable for the project; brief background on the organization; list of board members; the name of the primary contact person for follow-up; copy of IRS 501(c)3 exemption letter. Based on review of your letter of intent, the foundation may request a full proposal. If a proposal is requested, you will be provided with a grant form along with specific instructions. All projects are funded only on the authorization of the Foundation's Board of Director, this may take up to six months. Formal written communications from the foundation is the ONLY way you will be advised of a favorable funding decision.

Restrictions: Grants are not made to: private foundations; religious organizations for religious purposes; individuals; primary or secondary schools; political entities; national organizations, even if for local projects; annual operating support or debt reduction.

Geographic Focus: Indiana; Kentucky

Contact: Robert W. Lanum, Chair; fax: (812) 284-5519; email: klanum@ogle-fdn.org

Internet: http://www.ogle-fdn.org/Guidelines.htm

Sponsor: Paul Ogle Foundation, Inc.
321 East Court Avenue, P.O. Box 845
Jeffersonville, IN 47131

Payless ShoeSource Foundation Grants 3004

The foundation is dedicated to improving the quality of life in the communities where its corporate associates and customers live. Grants support programs that achieve measurable results in these communities (50 U.S. states, Puerto Rico, Guam, Saipan, the U.S. Virgin Islands, Canada, Central America, the Caribbean, and South America). There are no application deadlines. Submit requests in writing at least 60 days prior to when the grant is needed. Small requests (under $5000) are considered monthly; large requests (more than $5000) are reviewed quarterly. Guidelines are available online.

Requirements: 501(c)3 tax-exempt organizations are eligible.

Restrictions: Grants do not support religious or political organizations or individuals.

Contact: Grants Administrator, (877) 452-7500

Internet: http://www.payless.com/en-U.S./Corporate/Foundation/Foundation.htm

Sponsor: Payless ShoeSource Foundation
3231 SE 6th Avenue
Topeka, KS 66607

PDF International Research Grants 3005

The International Research Grants Program (IRGP) is designed to promote innovative research that has a high potential to significantly advance the knowledge of Parkinson's disease (PD) but little likelihood of securing funding through more traditional sources. By supporting novel, "high risk/high reward" research, the goal of the IRGP is to enable investigators to demonstrate the feasibility of their ideas while generating preliminary data necessary for the support of future funding. At its core, research supported by the IRGP must be directly relevant to the treatment and/or understanding of Parkinson's disease. Successful IRGP projects are: novel research hypotheses of Parkinson's disease; inventive in terms of methodology or approach; and clinical, preclinical, or basic research proposals that will directly impact Parkinson's disease or its treatment. IRGP awards will now reach a maximum of $75,000 per year for two years (compared to the previous maximum of $50,000 per year for one year of research), subject to review of first year progress. Research grants are now also eligible for an additional ten percent in indirect costs. All applications must be submitted online through the PDF website; no paper copies will be accepted. Visit grants.pdf.org, after Monday, November 2, to create an account, see more detailed instructions and submit your application. The deadline for submission of grant applications will be 11:59 PM EST on Tuesday, February 2.

Requirements: The IRGP is open to applicants both nationally and internationally and basic, translational and clinical research proposals are eligible for support. All applicants must possess a Ph.D. or a M.D. (or equivalent). Preference will be given to scientists who are at an early stage in their professional careers.

Restrictions: Investigators who receive funding from PDF may not receive funding for other projects supported by PDF during the same year, nor receive funding from other foundations or institutions for the same project during that year.

Amount of Grant: $75,000 per year for two years

Date(s) Application is Due: Feb 2

Contact: Robin Anthony Elliott, Executive Director; (212) 923-4700; fax: (212) 923-4778; email: info@pdf.org

Internet: http://www.pdf.org/en/grant_funding_irg#focus

Sponsor: Parkinson's Disease Foundation
1359 Broadway, Suite 1509
New York, NY 10018

PDF Postdoctoral Fellowships for Basic Scientists 3006

The Postdoctoral Fellowships for Basic Scientists are one-year fellowships for young scientists, fresh from their Ph.D. training, to study at major research institutions. The programs grants funding in the amount of $40,000 for one year as well as a research allowance of $5,000 to be used at the discretion of the Fellow, with approval of the sponsor/mentor, to pay for such items as books, training courses, travel costs (up to $2,000) or a computer. There is no provision for the deduction of postdoctoral taxes, institutional overhead or fees. However, if the Fellow submits a written request, $3,000 of the research allowance may be used to defray the cost of premiums for health insurance. Fellows may competitively reapply for continued funding after their first year for a total of three years of support. In these instances, a progress report of the current research would be due along with the new application. All applications must be submitted online through the PDF website; no paper copies will be accepted. The deadline for submission of grant applications will be 11:59 PM ET on Tuesday, February 2. Visit grants.pdf.org after Monday, November 2, to create an account, see more detailed instructions and submit your application. Final grant decisions are expected by mid-May.

Requirements: The applicant must have completed a Ph.D. or M.D. and must identify a research mentor who will serve as mentor for the fellow and supervisor of the research.

Amount of Grant: $45,000

Date(s) Application is Due: Feb 2

Contact: Robin Anthony Elliott, Executive Director; (212) 923-4700; fax: (212) 923-4778; email: info@pdf.org

Internet: http://www.pdf.org/en/grant_funding_fellow#pdflabres

Sponsor: Parkinson's Disease Foundation
1359 Broadway, Suite 1509
New York, NY 10018

PDF Postdoctoral Fellowships for Neurologists 3007

For young clinicians who have completed their neurology residency and are seeking clinical research experience, PDF offers the Postdoctoral Fellowships for Neurologists, one-year awards in the amount of $55,000. A research allowance of $5,000 may be used at the discretion of the Fellow, with approval of the mentor, to pay for such items as books, training courses, travel costs (up to $2,000) or a computer. There is no provision for the deduction of postdoctoral taxes, institutional overhead or fees. However, if the Fellow submits a written request, $3,000 of the research allowance may be used to defray the cost of premiums for health insurance. Fellows may competitively reapply for continued funding after their first year for a total of three years of support. In these instances, a progress report of the current research would be due along with the new application. All

applications must be submitted online through the PDF website; no paper copies will be accepted. The deadline for submission of grant applications will be 11:59 PM EST on Tuesday, February 2. Visit grants.pdf.org, after Monday, November 2, to create an account, see more detailed instructions and submit your application. Final decisions are expected by mid-May.
Requirements: Applicants seeking a Postdoctoral Fellowship for Neurologists must have an M.D. and be completing or have completed a neurology residency.
Restrictions: Applicants may not have their own lab.
Amount of Grant: $55,000
Date(s) Application is Due: Feb 2
Contact: Robin Anthony Elliott, Executive Director; (212) 923-4700; fax: (212) 923-4778; email: info@pdf.org
Internet: http://www.pdf.org/en/grant_funding_fellow#pdflabres
Sponsor: Parkinson's Disease Foundation
1359 Broadway, Suite 1509
New York, NY 10018

PDF Summer Fellowships 3008
PDF's Summer Fellowship Program is used to support students – from advanced undergraduates to graduate and medical students – in their pursuit of Parkinson's-related summer research projects. The goal of the Summer Fellowship is to cultivate an early interest in Fellows into the cause(s) and possible treatments for Parkinson's disease. Fellows work under the close supervision of a sponsor who is an expert in the Parkinson's community and oversees the project. Typically, summer fellowships are offered for 10 weeks of laboratory work with an award of $3,000. The application period for Summer Student Fellowships will open on Monday, November 2, apply by 11:59 PM ET on Friday, January 15.
Requirements: Undergraduate students, graduate students and medical students are all eligible for summer fellowships. Each applicant must identify a mentor, with whom he or she will conduct the proposed project.
Amount of Grant: $3,000
Date(s) Application is Due: Jan 15
Contact: Robin Anthony Elliott, Executive Director; (212) 923-4700; fax: (212) 923-4778; email: info@pdf.org
Internet: http://www.pdf.org/en/grant_funding_fellow#pdflabres
Sponsor: Parkinson's Disease Foundation
1359 Broadway, Suite 1509
New York, NY 10018

PDF-AANF Clinician-Scientist Development Awards 3009
The Parkinson's Disease Foundation (PDF) and the American Academy of Neurology Foundation (AANF) collaborated in 2007 to create the Clinician Scientist Development Award to support our mutual interest in training outstanding residency-level clinicians in the field of Parkinson's disease. Successful applicants will receive a three-year award of $85,000. This award supports three years of research training in an environment where talented young clinicians address problems in Parkinson's disease with the most current scientific tools. It is expected that upon completion of the program, participants will be committed to a research or combined clinical/research career in PD and will be in line to direct robust research programs relevant to PD. This award is given every three years. It will be offered again until 2011.
Requirements: Eligibility & Guidelines: applicants must hold an M.D., D.O., or equivalent clinical degree from an accredited institution; applicants must have completed residency training but be less than seven years from completion of residency when funding begins; there is no citizenship requirement; however, the individual applying for the award must be licensed to practice medicine in the United States at the time of application; may only submit one application per department. The department is considered to be the one at which the applicant's training and research program will occur; each applicant must agree to a phone interview with a member of the PDF-AANF Advisory Committee, if necessary, during the application review period.
Amount of Grant: $85,000 over three years
Contact: Robin Anthony Elliott, Executive Director; (212) 923-4700; fax: (212) 923-4778; email: info@pdf.org;; Terry Heinz, Grants Administrator; (651) 695-2746; email: theinz@aan.com
Internet: http://www.pdf.org/en/grant_funding_fellow#pdflabres
Sponsor: Parkinson's Disease Foundation
1359 Broadway, Suite 1509
New York, NY 10018

Peabody Foundation Grants 3010
The giving program of this foundation consists of grants primarily to provide care, treatment, rehabilitation, education, and assistance to children and for medical research relating to disabled children. The majority of recipient organizations will be located in the Boston, MA, area. Proposals may be submitted at any time and are reviewed in the spring.
Restrictions: Grants are not made to individuals.
Geographic Focus: Massachusetts
Amount of Grant: $3000-$275,000
Date(s) Application is Due: Feb 1
Contact: William Tripp III, c/o Choate, Hall & Stewart, (617) 523-2700
Sponsor: Peabody Foundation
53 State Street, Exchange Pl
Boston, MA 02109-2804

Peacock Foundation Grants 3011
Established by Henry B. Peacock, Jr. in 1947, the mission of Peacock Foundation, Inc. is to enhance and promote the good health and well being of children, families, and underprivileged persons in Southeast Florida, through contributions, gifts, and grants to eligible nonprofit organizations. The priorities of Peacock Foundation, Inc. include: making grants to human services providers that promote youth development, assist abused or neglected children, women, and the elderly, and seek to reduce abuse, prevent homelessness, and end hunger in our community; supporting educational programs in the arts and the environment, as well as special education for disabled persons; contributing to medical research, health care organizations, and hospitals.
Requirements: All applicants must be IRS recognized 501(c)3 public charities classified as not a private foundation, registered with the Department of Agriculture to solicit funds in Florida, when applicable, and located in and/or of significant benefit to residents to the Southeast Florida counties of Miami-Dade, Broward, or Monroe. In order for a proposal to be considered for funding, the applicant first must send a brief letter of inquiry. See Foundations website for letter of inquiry guidelines: http://www.peacockfoundationinc.org/review_progress.html.
Restrictions: Peacock Foundation, Inc. does not fund: capital campaigns, construction, or renovation projects; deficit financing or debt reduction; conferences or festivals; fundraising events or advertising; special events or athletic events; individuals; lobbying to influence legislation; religious organizations, unless engaged in a significant project benefiting the entire community.
Geographic Focus: Florida
Contact: Joelle Allen, Executive Director; (305) 373-1386
Internet: http://www.peacockfoundationinc.org/eligibility.html
Sponsor: Peacock Foundation, Inc.
100 South East Second Street, Suite 2370
Miami, FL 33131

Pediatric Brain Tumor Research Grants 3012
The foundation awards grants in the area of basic pediatric brain tumor research. The laboratory-based, hypothesis driven project should demonstrate the potential to advance basic scientific research in brain tumors. Funds may be used for start-up projects or as supplementary funding. Guidelines and application are available online.
Requirements: Grant applications will be accepted from institutions in the United States, Canada, and Australia.
Amount of Grant: $50,000 per year
Date(s) Application is Due: Sep 30
Contact: Dianne Traynor, Grants Administrator, (800) 253-6530 or (828) 665-6891; fax: (828) 665-6894; email: dtraynor@pbtfus.org
Internet: http://www.pbtfus.org/grants/grntfund.htm
Sponsor: Pediatric Brain Tumor Foundation of the United States
302 Ridgefield Ct
Asheville, NC 28806

Pediatric Cancer Research Foundation Grants 3013
The foundation focuses its efforts on improving the care, quality of life, and survival rate of children with malignant diseases. One-year grants support laboratory research that translates into immediate treatment for children with cancer. The foundation funds research that brings innovative approaches to the treatment, diagnosis, or prevention of pediatric cancer. Applications proposing novel approaches to the prevention, management, or cure of pediatric cancer are sought. Proposals should be based on molecular, cellular, or integrated systems and be conceptually innovative. The application should have a clear plan for study and future clinical use of the facutal data obtained.
Requirements: Applications may be submitted by individuals holding a MD, PhD, or equivalent degree working in domestic nonprofit organizations such as universities, colleges, hospitals, or laboratories.
Samples: Columbmia U, College of Physicians and Surgeons, Division of Pediatric Oncology (New York, NY) and New York-Presbyterian Children's Hospital (New York, NY)—to establish a state-of-the-art laboratory for research on pediatric cancer, $3 million jointly over three years.
Amount of Grant: $25,000-$100,000
Date(s) Application is Due: Sep 30
Contact: Grants Administrator, (949) 859-6312; fax: (949) 859-6323; email: admin@pcrf-kids.com
Internet: http://www.pcrf-kids.com
Sponsor: Pediatric Cancer Research Foundation
9272 Jeronimo Road, Suite A-107A
Irvine, CA 92618

Perkins Charitable Foundation Grants 3014
The Perkins Charitable Foundation Trust was established in 1950, by members of the Perkins family. The Foundation gives primarily for education, the arts, environmental conservation, animals, wildlife, health and medical care, and children, youth and social services. They offer funding on a national basis, with some emphasis on Ohio and Vermont.
Requirements: Contact the Foundation's office by letter or phone prior to your proposal. No Application form is required.
Restrictions: No grants to individuals.
Contact: Marilyn Best, Secretary; (216) 621-0465;
Sponsor: The Perkins Charitable Foundation
1030 Hanna Building, 1422 Euclid Avenue
Cleveland, OH 44115-2001

Perpetual Trust for Charitable Giving Grants 3015

The Foundation, established in 1957, supports organizations involved with education, health care, and family services. Giving is limited to Massachusetts. Contact the Foundation for further application information and guidelines.

Requirements: Must be a non-profit in Massachusetts to be eligible.

Restrictions: No grants to individuals.

Geographic Focus: Massachusetts

Samples: Boston Urban Youth Foundation, Boston, MA, $20,000 (2004); Pine Street Inn, Boston, MA, $30,000 - for program support (2004); Education Resources Institute, Boston, MA, $35,000 - for CKP program (2004);

Amount of Grant: $1,000-$50,000 range

Date(s) Application is Due: Sep 1

Contact: Kerry Sullivan. Director, Bank of America, N.A. Foundation & Philanthropic Services; (617) 4334-4846; email: kerry.h.sullivan@bankofamerica.com

Sponsor: Perpetual Trust for Charitable Giving
100 Federal Street, MA5-100-16-01
Boston, MA 02110

Perry County Community Foundation Grants 3016

The Perry County Community Foundation is a nonprofit, public charity created by and for the people of Perry County, Indiana. We connect donors with the causes they care about. The Foundation will accept grant proposals from all charitable organizations seeking funding; however, special attention will be given to projects that promote healthy living and that offer training and/or support to potential small business entrepreneurship. The foundation considers proposals for grants on a yearly cycle which begins each July. At the start of each cycle, a notice is mailed to nonprofit organizations that have applied for grants in the past, have received grants in the past, or have otherwise requested notification of the start of each cycle. The foundations grant cycle runs from July through November each year. Proposals will be accepted from July through the September deadline. Proposals submitted after the September deadline (date varies, contact foundation office for current deadline) will not be considered. The grants committee will make its recommendations on funding to the Foundation's Board of Trustees, which will make final funding recommendations to the board of directors of the Community Foundation Alliance (our governing body). All organizations that have submitted grant proposals will be notified of the outcome of the grants committee's deliberation in writing no later than December 1.

Requirements: The foundation welcomes proposals from nonprofit organizations that are deemed tax-exempt under sections 501(c)3 and 509(a) of the Internal Revenue Code and from governmental agencies serving the county. Proposals from nonprofit organizations not classified as a 501(c)3 public charity may be considered provided the project is charitable and supports a community need. Proposals submitted by an entity under the auspices of another agency must include a written statement signed by the agency's board president on behalf of the board of directors agreeing to act as the entity's fiscal sponsor, to receive grant monies if awarded, and to oversee the proposed project.

Restrictions: Project areas NOT considered for funding: religious organizations for religious purposes; political parties or campaigns; endowment creation or debt reduction; operating costs; capital campaigns; annual appeals or membership contributions; travel requests for groups or individuals such as bands, sports teams, or classes. A six-month progress report and a final report at project completion are required by organizations whose proposals are approved for funding. Instructions and appropriate forms will be provided at the time the grant is awarded.

Geographic Focus: Indiana

Contact: Sally Houzanme; (812) 547-3176; email: sallyh@perrycommunityfoundation.org

Internet: http://www.perrycommunityfoundation.org/disc-grants-program

Sponsor: Perry County Community Foundation, inc.
601 Main Street, Suite B, P.O. Box 13
Tell City, IN 47586

Pet Care Trust Sue Busch Memorial Award 3017

Incorporated in Washington, D.C. in 1990, The Pet Care Trust is a non-profit, charitable, public foundation. The purpose of The Pet Care Trust is to help promote public understanding regarding the value of and right to enjoy companion animals, to enhance knowledge about companion animals through research and education, and to promote professionalism among members of the companion animal community. The Pet Care Trust invites you submit a letter of recommendation for a graduating veterinary technician student who has been selected by your faculty as having a keen interest in companion animals (dogs, cats, small pet mammals, birds, reptiles, amphibians or pond and aquarium fish) as well as dedicating time to community service related to animals while maintaining a high academic standard. Please include instances relating to the above mentioned criteria. If selected, the student you have recommended will receive one of three $500 Sue Busch Memorial Awards for the year. Our goal is not only to bring recognition to a fine student but recognition as well to the institution instrumental in educating that student. Please submit your recommendations on or before Feb 1 You will be notified on or before April 30 in order for the Check and Certificate to be presented at your graduation ceremony.

Amount of Grant: $500

Date(s) Application is Due: Feb 1

Contact: Steve Hellem, Executive Director; (202) 530-5910; email: shellem@navista.net

Internet: http://www.petcaretrust.org/i4a/pages/index.cfm?pageid=3297

Sponsor: Pet Care Trust
1155 Fifteenth Street, NW, Suite 500
Washington, DC 20005 20005

Peter and Elizabeth C. Tower Foundation Community Grants 3018

The foundation makes grants to community organizations serving children, adolescents, and families affected by psychological disorders, developmental disabilities, and substance abuse. Priority is given to projects that focus on prevention or early intervention projects, especially those targeted towards at'risk youth; overcoming the stigma of mental illness; improve public awareness of effective treatment; introduce effective treatment modalities; identify individuals in the target group and link them to appropriate services; focus on delivery of state'of'the'art treatment; and focus on capacity'building—projects that enhance organizational self'sufficiency or service delivery. Priority is given to projects where the incremental costs, i.e., the costs that are new to the organization as a result of the proposed project, are a substantial portion of the grant request. Multiyear grants are encouraged. Preference is given to projects that benefit 100 or more individuals. The funding year is November through October. Letters of intent are due on the listed application deadlines; full proposals are by invitation. Guidelines are available online.

Requirements: 501(c)3 nonprofit organizations operating in Massachusetts—Martha's Vineyard and the North Shore area, as defined by the area of Essex County east of I-95; and New York State— Erie and Niagara Counties are eligible.

Restrictions: The foundation does not fund capital campaigns or programs/projects that may be used for the private benefit of any grant recipient or affiliated person; attempt to influence legislation; attempt to influence or intervene in any political campaign.

Geographic Focus: Massachusetts; New York

Samples: Lake Shore Behavioral Health (Buffalo, NY)—for child-rearing and children's services at a residential drug-treatment facility for women and their children, $88,925 over three years (2004); People Inc (Buffalo, NY)—to help families manage severe behavioral problems, $60,000 over two years (2004); Vista Vocational and Life Skills (Westbrook, CT)—to develop new communication materials about employment opportunities, $16,000 (2004).

Amount of Grant: $25,000-$75,000

Date(s) Application is Due: Apr 12

Contact: Glenda Cadwallader, Executive Director, (716) 689-0370; fax: (716) 689-3716; email: info@thetowerfoundation.com

Internet: http://thetowerfoundation.com/grant_guidelines/community_grant_guidelines.asp

Sponsor: Peter and Elizabeth C. Tower Foundation
90B John Muir Drive, Suite 100
Amherst, NY 14228-1148

Pew Charitable Trusts Biomedical Research Grants 3019

Pew invests in an array of programs related to science that are aimed at improving the quality of scientific research as well as making data widely available. These projects are working toward solutions to environmental, health and safety dilemmas. Pew also has a decades-long commitment to support groundbreaking research by biomedical researchers early in their careers. All of these initiatives are part of our broader effort to study and promote nonpartisan policy solutions for pressing and emerging problems affecting the American public and the global community. Pew's experts partner with leading authorities in science, the environment and associated fields to conduct research and advance fact-based solutions to compelling problems. Pew targets the frontiers of scientific knowledge where it can make a difference.

Requirements: Grants are made only to colleges and universities, as well as 501(c)3 tax-exempt organizations that are not private foundations.

Restrictions: Grants are not made to individuals or for endowments, capital campaigns, unsolicited construction requests, debt reduction, or scholarships or fellowships that are not part of a program initiated by the Trusts.

Contact: Susan A. Magill, Managing Director; (202) 552-2129 or (202) 552-2000; fax: (202) 552-2299; email: smagill@pewtrusts.org or info@pewtrusts.com

Internet: http://www.pewtrusts.org/our_work_category.aspx?id=336

Sponsor: Pew Charitable Trusts
2005 Market Street, Suite 1700
Philadelphia, PA 19103-7077

Pew Charitable Trusts Children and Youth Grants 3020

The Pew Charitable Trusts seeks to study and promote nonpartisan policy solutions for pressing and emerging problems that affect the next generation. Pew supports initiatives, grounded in research and evidence, that aim to help children and youth become active, contributing members of society both in Philadelphia and around the country. At the national level, Pew supports efforts to prevent children from languishing in foster care without safe, permanent families. Pew works to provide access to high-quality preschool for all three- and four-year-olds, and supports a public health initiative that seeks to reduce young people's exposure to alcohol advertising. Locally, the Pew Fund for Health and Human Services in Philadelphia offers operating and project-specific support to a number of nonprofits that aid youth in the city and four nearby counties.

Requirements: Grants are made only to 501(c)3 tax-exempt organizations that are not private foundations.

Restrictions: Grants are not made to individuals or for endowments, capital campaigns, unsolicited construction requests, debt reduction, or scholarships or fellowships that are not part of a program initiated by the Trusts.

Contact: Susan A. Magill, Managing Director; (202) 552-2129 or (202) 552-2000; fax: (202) 552-2299; email: smagill@pewtrusts.org or info@pewtrusts.com

Internet: http://www.pewtrusts.org/our_work_category.aspx?id=4

Sponsor: Pew Charitable Trusts
2005 Market Street, Suite 1700
Philadelphia, PA 19103-7077

Pew Scholars in the Biomedical Sciences 3021

This program is designed to support young investigators of outstanding promise in the basic and clinical sciences relevant to the advancement of human health. The funding of the awards is provided by The Pew Charitable Trusts. The award is intended to provide assured support, during their earlier years, for junior members of the faculty as they establish their laboratories. It is hoped that the assurance provided through the program will encourage successful applicants to be more venturesome in their research and future applications for support than would otherwise be likely. ALL applicants must be nominated by their institution and complete the online application.
Requirements: The program is open to individuals with a doctorate in medicine, other health related professions, or biomedical sciences. Candidates must hold full- time appointments at the rank of assistant professor or independent researcher on the faculty of the sponsoring institution.
Restrictions: A biomedical scholar cannot apply on his/her own for this scholarship but must apply through a selected institution.
Samples: U of California at San Francisco (CA)—for the Pew Scholars Program in the Biomedical Sciences, $3.6 million over four years (2004).
Amount of Grant: $60,000 per year
Date(s) Application is Due: Nov 1
Contact: Leslie Tucker, Program Officer, (215) 575-4850; email: shans@pewtrusts.com or info@pewtrust.com
Internet: http://futurehealth.ucsf.edu/biomed/scholdes.html
Sponsor: Pew Charitable Trusts
2005 Market Street, Suite 1700
Philadelphia, PA 19103-7077

PeyBack Foundation Grants 3022

The foundation was established by NFL quarterback Peyton Manning with the purpose of promoting the future success of disadvantaged youth by assisting programs that provide leadership and growth opportunities for children at risk (ages 6-18). The nature of the programs and their immediate long-term benefit shall be guiding considerations in funding grants. Although the foundation does not have a dollar limit on grant requests, most grant amounts range between $1,500 and $10,000.
Requirements: Due to the close association of Peyton Manning with the Indiana, Tennessee and the New Orleans Metropolitan area, programs and projects related to the youth in these areas are of primary concern to the foundation. Proposals will be only considered from organizations that have tax-exempt status under Section 501(c)3 of the Internal Revenue Code. A proposal asking to consider providing a portion of the support for a project will generally receive greater preference than one seeking exclusive funding. Download the required application form at the website.
Restrictions: The following are not areas that the PeyBack Foundation supports: organizations without 501(c)3 tax-exempt status – will immediately be eliminated; Fundraising and sponsorship events (e.g., golf tournaments, telethons, banquets); Groups outside of Indiana, Tennessee and New Orleans, LA; Projects/groups benefiting an individual or just a few persons; Building/renovating expenses of any kind; To defray meeting, conferences, workshops or seminars expenses; Payment of travel of individuals or groups; Re-granting organizations; Post-event fundraising; Multi-year gifts.
Geographic Focus: Indiana; Louisiana; Tennessee
Samples: Boy Scouts of America, Indianapolis, IN, $10,000 (2009); Start the Adventure in Reading, New Orleans, LA, $10,000 (2009); Eighteenth Avenue Family Enrichment Center, Nashville, TN, $8,000 (2009).
Amount of Grant: $1,500 - $10,000
Date(s) Application is Due: Feb 1
Contact: Elizabeth Ellis, Executive Director; (877) 873-9225; email: PeyBack@PeytonManning.com
Internet: http://www.peytonmanning.com/Peyback/GrantGuidelines.html
Sponsor: PeyBack Foundation
6325 North Guilford, Suite 201
Indianapolis, IN 46220

Pezcoller Foundation-AACR International Award for Cancer Research 3023

The Award for Cancer Research was established in 1997 to annually recognize a scientist: who has made a major scientific discovery in basic cancer research OR who has made significant contributions to translational cancer research; who continues to be active in cancer research and has a record of recent, noteworthy publications; and whose ongoing work holds promise for continued substantive contributions to progress in the field of cancer. More than one scientist may be co-nominated and selected to share the Award when their investigations are closely related in subject matter and have resulted in work that is worthy of the Award. The Award consists of an unrestricted grant of Euro 75,000 and a commemorative plaque.
Requirements: Eligible candidates are cancer researchers affiliated with institutions in academia, industry, or government that are involved in cancer research, cancer medicine, or cancer-related biomedical science anywhere in the world.
Restrictions: Institutions or organizations are not eligible for the Award.
Amount of Grant: Euro 75,000
Date(s) Application is Due: Sep 15
Contact: Monique P. Eversley, Staff Associate; (267) 646-0576 or (215) 440-9300, ext. 1400; fax: (215) 440-9372; email: monique.eversley@aacr.org or awards@aacr.org
Internet: http://www.aacr.org/home/scientists/scientific-achievement-awards/pezcoller-aacr-international-award.aspx
Sponsor: Pezcoller Foundation / American Association for Cancer Research
615 Chestnut Street, 17th Floor
Philadelphia, PA 19106-4404

Pfizer Foundation Epilepsy Scholarship Award 3024

The scholarship honors 16 outstanding students who have overcome the challenges of epilepsy, been successful in school, done well in activities out of the classroom, and shown the ability to make the most out of college or graduate school. Experts in education and medicine will choose the winners. Information and application are available online.
Requirements: An applicant must be under a doctor's care for epilepsy; a high school senior who has applied to college; a freshman, sophomore, or junior in college; or a college senior who has applied to graduate school.
Amount of Grant: $3000
Date(s) Application is Due: Mar 1
Contact: Pfizer Epilepsy Scholarship, (800) 292-7373; email: Scholarship@edencomgroup.com
Internet: http://www.epilepsy-scholarship.com
Sponsor: Eden Communications Group
515 Valley Street, Suite 200
Maplewood, NJ 07040

Pfizer Foundation Grants 3025

The foundation's charitable giving programs provide grants through targeted initiatives focused primarily on health care and science education. Areas of interest include: global health—health literacy programs to improve the ability of low-income, low-literate populations to effectively comprehend and act on health information; HIV/AIDS—programs to provide Pfizer's antifungal medicine (Diflucan) to low-income HIV/AIDS patients in the world's least developed countries where the disease is most prevalent, the training of health-care workers in opportunistic infections related to HIV, and health-promotion programs that target those at high-risk of HIV infection living in countries where Pfizer is donating Diflucan; international trachoma initiative—programs to provide Pfizer's key antibiotic (Zithromax) to countries implementing public-health programs to combat trachoma, including community-based initiatives to provide surgery, antibiotics, promotion of clean faces, and education about the disease; disaster relief—requests for product donations following floods, earthquakes, droughts, wars, and other disasters domestically and abroad; K-12 science education—partnerships between Pfizer sites and local schools, with an emphasis on training teachers, developing curriculum, constructing science labs, and support of exhibits and educational outreach programs at science-rich institutions across the country; and community and cultural—programs in Pfizer communities, with a particular focus in the New York City for a range of organizations that address urgent community needs, seek long-term solutions to community issues, and strengthen the cultural vitality of diverse communities.
Requirements: Nonprofit 501(c)3 organizations and schools are eligible.
Restrictions: The following types of organizations or activities are excluded from support: fundraising events or activities such as telethons, walkathons, and races; specific performances or concerts; sporting events; endowment campaigns; building fund drives and capital campaigns (except science lab renovations in partner schools and universities); film, video, television, or radio projects (except as part of a health literacy program); requests for loans or debt retirement; trips, tours, or cultural exchange programs; conferences, seminars, briefing programs, and similar activities (except in instances where the event evolves from Pfizer programs in health care and science education); organizations already supported through United Way contributions; operating expenses of United Way local agencies (except through annual United Way campaigns); grants to individuals; political causes or candidates; anti-business organizations; or organizations that practice discrimination or limit membership on the basis of race, creed, gender, age, sexual preference, or national origin.
Contact: Grants Administrator, (800) 733-4717 or (212) 573-2323
Internet: http://www.pfizer.com/subsites/philanthropy/caring/index.html
Sponsor: Pfizer Inc
235 E 42nd Street
New York, NY 10017-5755

Pfizer Foundation Health Literacy Grant Program 3026

The program invites applications for research to advance the understanding of health literacy and for an intervention that overcomes problems associated with low levels of health literacy. Examples of proposed projects include developing new measures or new ways of looking at the causes or impact of health literacy; developing programs that demonstrate improved health literacy; or creating policy initiatives that promote improved health outcomes. Proposals for community-based research and interventions are encouraged.
Requirements: Applications are encouraged from investigators in diverse fields such as health literacy, adult education, health economics, medicine, nursing, pharmacy, public health, anthropology, health policy, social work, management sciences, and ethics.
Amount of Grant: $65,000 per year
Contact: Programs Administrator, (212) 733-4250
Internet: http://www.pfizerhealthliteracy.com/partnerships_awards.html
Sponsor: Pfizer Foundation
235 E 42nd Street
New York, NY 10017-5755

Pfizer/AAFP Foundation Visiting Professorship Program in Family Medicine 3027

This program is designed to bring educational benefits to U.S. medical schools, teaching hospitals, and community hospitals. Recipient institutions may select and invite prominent physician scientists for three days of teaching and interaction with the faculty, students, residents, research fellows, and physicians involved in family medicine at the medical center. During the visit, the guest faculty may give lectures and participate in rounds, seminars, and conferences. Awards are intended to cover the Visiting Professor's

honorarium, travel expenses, and other direct expenses incurred by the host institution in conducting program activities. Amounts allotted for each item are at the discretion of the host institution.
Requirements: This program is open to any family medicine department within a U.S. medical school or any accredited family medicine residency program. Applications from community-based programs are encouraged. Each hospital may submit only one application. Submissions must originate from the Chair of the Family Medicine Department or the Residency Director.
Restrictions: Only one visit per year per visiting professor will be funded.
Amount of Grant: $7,500
Date(s) Application is Due: Mar 28
Contact: Susie Morantz, Senior Program Manager; (800) 274-2237 ext. 4470; fax: (913) 906-6095; email: smorantz@aafp.org;; Perry A. Pugno, Medical Education Director; (800) 274-2237 ext. 6700; email: ppugno@aafp.org
Internet: http://www.aafpfoundation.org/x500.xml
Sponsor: American Academy of Family Physicians (AAFP) Foundation
11400 Tomahawk Creek Parkway, Suite 440
Leawood, KS 66211-2672

Pharmacia-ASPET Award for Experimental Therapeutics **3028**
The Pharmacia-ASPET Award in Experimental Therapeutics is given annually to recognize and stimulate outstanding research in pharmacology and experimental therapeutics—basic laboratory or clinical research that has had, or potentially will have, a major impact on the pharmacological treatment of disease. The winner will receive a $2,500 honorarium, a plaque, hotel and economy airfare for the winner and spouse to the award ceremony at the ASPET annual meeting.
Requirements: Nominations must be made by ASPET members; however, the nominee need not be a member. No restrictions exist as to age or institutional affiliation of nominee.
Amount of Grant: $2,500
Date(s) Application is Due: Sep 15
Contact: Christine Carrico, Ph.D., Executive Officer; (301) 634-7060; fax: (301) 634-7061; email: ccarrico@aspet.org or info@aspet.org
Internet: http://www.aspet.org/public/awards/exp_ther_award.html
Sponsor: Pfizer / American Society for Pharmacology and Experimental Therapeutics
9650 Rockville Pike
Bethesda, MD 20814-3995

Philadelphia Foundation Organizational Effectiveness Grants **3029**
Organizational Effectiveness Grants are designed to strengthen and improve the business and operational practices of nonprofit organizations in Bucks, Chester, Delaware, Montgomery and Philadelphia counties. As in business, these practices are critical to the success of nonprofits' ability to lead, adapt, manage and effectively operate their organizations. These core competencies are critical to nonprofits at all stages of development and size for the effective delivery of services, implementation of best practices, utilization of data to drive decision-making and the ability to adapt to new demands, risks and opportunities. new applications for General Operating Support or Organizational Effectiveness cannot be accepted until January 1st.
Requirements: IRS 501(c)3 tax-exempt organizations located in Bucks, Chester, Delaware, Montgomery, and Philadelphia Counties of Pennsylvania are eligible.
Restrictions: Grants are rarely made to affiliates of national or international organizations, government agencies, organizations not located in Southeastern Pennsylvania, organizations with budgets of more than $1.5 million, private schools, or umbrella-funding organizations. Requests usually are denied for capital campaigns, conferences, deficit financing, endowments, publications, research projects, tours, and trips. Individuals are ineligible.
Geographic Focus: Pennsylvania
Amount of Grant: $3,000-$30,000 range
Contact: Libby Walsh, Program Associate; (215) 563-6417; fax: (215) 563-6882; email: lwalsh@philafound.org or oeapplications@philafound.org
Internet: https://www.philafound.org/ForNonprofits/DiscretionaryGrantmaking/OrganizationalEffectiveness/tabid/238/Default.aspx
Sponsor: Philadelphia Foundation
1234 Market Street, Suite 1800
Philadelphia, PA 19107

Phoenix Suns Charities Grants **3030**
The Phoenix Suns Charities awards general operating grants, project grants, challenge grants, and capital building grants to Arizona nonprofit organizations. Specific areas of grantmaking interest include arts and cultural programs focusing on children; education primarily focusing on pre-K-12; health care education for youth; museums and science centers and science projects for youth; and social services focusing on children and family issues. Recipients of the Playmaker Award may use funds for building projects.
Requirements: Arizona 501(c)3 organizations, primarily in Maricopa County, may apply.
Geographic Focus: Arizona
Amount of Grant: $1000-$10,000 average; $500,000 total
Date(s) Application is Due: Apr 30
Contact: Thomas Ambrose, Executive Director, (602) 379-7767; fax: (602) 530-2251
Internet: http://www.nba.com/suns/news/charities_index.html
Sponsor: Phoenix Suns
201 E Jefferson
Phoenix, AZ 85004

PhRMA Foundation Health Outcomes Post Doctoral Fellowships **3031**
The program provides stipend support for individuals engaged in a research training program that will create or extend their credentials in health outcomes. The intent of this program is to support post doctoral career development activities of individuals prepared (or preparing) to engage in research that will strengthen representation of health outcomes in schools of pharmacy, medicine, nursing and public health. To accomplish these goals, support will be provided for a two-year period to selected individuals who are beginning careers in health outcomes research and who give promise of outstanding development as researchers. The award, consisting of a $40,000 annual stipend, is made to the institution on behalf of the fellow. The award is intended solely as a stipend and may not be used otherwise.
Requirements: Eligible applicants include well-trained graduates from Pharm. D., M.D., and Ph.D. programs who seek to further develop and refine their research skills through formal postdoctoral training. They must also have a firm commitment from an accredited U.S. university and be a U.S. citizen or permanent resident. The application must include a research plan written by the applicant, the mentor's research record, and a description of how the mentored experience will enhance the applicant's career development in health outcomes research. The sponsor (mentor) of the post doctoral program must describe how the goals of the research training program will be accomplished and provide assurance that key collaborating mentors endorse and are willing to support the training plan.
Restrictions: Applications, however good, which do not meet the aims of the program will be disapproved.
Amount of Grant: $40,000
Contact: Eileen M. Cannon, Executive Director; (202) 572-7756; fax: (202) 572-7799; email: info@phrmafoundation.org
Internet: http://www.phrmafoundation.org/awards/outcomes/postdoc.php
Sponsor: Pharmaceutical Research and Manufacturers of America (PhRMA) Foundation
950 F Street, N.W., Suite 300
Washington, DC 20004

PhRMA Foundation Health Outcomes Pre-Doctoral Fellowships **3032**
To provide some assistance in this training sequence, the PhRMA Foundation program aims at supporting promising students during their thesis research. The program provides a stipend and funds to cover costs incidental to the training. Applications will be accepted for a minimum of one year and a maximum of two years. The program is designed for candidates who expect to complete the requirements for the Ph.D. in the field of health outcomes in two years or less from the time the fellowship begins. The program assumes that the fellows will devote full-time (including summers) to their research. The award is made to the university on behalf of the fellow. The fellowship provides a stipend of $20,000 a year payable monthly for a minimum of one year and a maximum of two years. Of the $20,000 awarded annually, $500 a year may be used for incidentals directly associated with the thesis research preparation (e.g., secretarial help, artwork, books, travel, etc.). The second year of a fellowship is contingent upon certification by the thesis advisor that satisfactory progress is being achieved.
Requirements: The fellowship program of pre-doctoral support is designed to assist full-time, in-residence Ph.D. candidates in the fields of health outcomes who are enrolled in U.S. schools of medicine, pharmacy, dentistry or schools of public health. The program seeks to support advanced students who will have completed the bulk of their pre-thesis requirements (two years of study) and are starting their thesis research by the time the award is activated. Students just starting in graduate school should not apply. A candidate enrolled in an M.D./Ph.D. program should not be taking required clinical course work or clerkships during the tenure of the fellowship. Before an individual is eligible to apply for a PhRMA Foundation award, the applicant must first have a firm commitment from a U.S. university. Applications must be submitted by an accredited U.S. school, and all applicants must be U.S. citizens or permanent residents.
Restrictions: The fellowship may not be used as a supplement to funds from other fellowships, traineeships or assistantships. The focus of the program is to assist in the pre doctoral training of the candidate. It should not be viewed as a program to fund a research project. An individual may not simultaneously hold or interrupt any other fellowship providing stipend support during the PhRMA Foundation fellowship.
Amount of Grant: $20,000
Contact: Eileen M. Cannon, Executive Director; (202) 572-7756; fax: (202) 572-7799; email: info@phrmafoundation.org
Internet: http://www.phrmafoundation.org/awards/outcomes/predoc.php
Sponsor: Pharmaceutical Research and Manufacturers of America (PhRMA) Foundation
950 F Street, N.W., Suite 300
Washington, DC 20004

PhRMA Foundation Health Outcomes Research Starter Grants **3033**
The purpose of the program is to offer financial support to individuals beginning their independent research careers at the faculty level. The program provides a research grant of $30,000 per year for up to two years. This program supports individuals beginning independent research careers in academia who do not have other substantial sources of research.
Requirements: Those holding the academic rank of instructor or assistant professor and investigators at the doctoral level with equivalent positions are eligible to apply, providing their proposed research is neither directly nor indirectly subsidized to any significant degree by an extramural support mechanism. The program is not intended for those in postdoctoral training programs. However, individuals in postdoctoral training scheduled to conclude and who will hold an academic appointment by January 1 may apply. Applicants must be sponsored by the department or unit within which the

proposed research is to be undertaken. The grant is made to the university on behalf of the applicant and with the understanding that the university will administer the funds. Schools of medicine, pharmacy, public health, nursing, dentistry and schools of other areas where appropriate are eligible for this award. Applications must be submitted by an accredited school in the U.S., and all applicants must be U.S. citizens or permanent residents. Before an individual is eligible to apply for a PhRMA Foundation award, the applicant must first have a firm commitment from a U.S. university.
Restrictions: This program is not offered as a means to augment substantially funded research efforts. It is intended to offer support for researchers who are starting their independent research efforts. This award is granted in part based on need. If an individual currently has or is guaranteed substantial funding, they should not apply.
Amount of Grant: $30,000
Contact: Eileen M. Cannon, Executive Director; (202) 572-7756; fax: (202) 572-7799; email: info@phrmafoundation.org
Internet: http://www.phrmafoundation.org/awards/outcomes/starter.php
Sponsor: Pharmaceutical Research and Manufacturers of America (PhRMA) Foundation
950 F Street, N.W., Suite 300
Washington, DC 20004

PhRMA Foundation Health Outcomes Sabbatical Fellowships **3034**
The fellowship provides stipend support for individuals engaged in a multidisciplinary research training program that will create or extend their credentials in health outcomes. The program enables faculty with active research programs to work outside of their home institution for periods of six months to one year to learn new skills or develop new collaborations that will enhance their research and research training capabilities in health outcomes. The applicant and mentor of the program must describe how the multidisciplinary goals of the research experiential program will be accomplished and provide assurance that key collaborating mentors endorse and are willing to support the plan. Matching funds must be provided by the home institution. Awards may be activated beginning January 1 or on the first day of any month thereafter, up to and including December 1. Guidelines and application are available online.
Requirements: Eligible applicants must (1) hold a PhD, Pharm.D., M.D. or Sc.D. degree in a field of study logically or functionally related to the proposed post doctoral activities, (2) hold a faculty appointment that imparts eligibility for a sabbatical leave from their home institution, (3) have institutional approval of a sabbatical plan that includes partial salary that matches the PhRMA stipend, (4) hold an endorsement from a mentor who agrees to sponsor the applicant's visiting scientist activity, and (5) be a U.S. citizen or permanent resident. Matching funds must be provided by the home institution.
Restrictions: The program provides no other subsidies (travel, tuition, fringe benefit costs, etc.), and indirect costs to the institution are not provided.
Amount of Grant: $40,000
Contact: Eileen M. Cannon, Executive Director; (202) 572-7756; fax: (202) 572-7799; email: info@phrmafoundation.org
Internet: http://www.phrmafoundation.org/awards/outcomes/sabbatical.php
Sponsor: Pharmaceutical Research and Manufacturers of America (PhRMA) Foundation
950 F Street, N.W., Suite 300
Washington, DC 20004

PhRMA Foundation Informatics Sabbatical Fellowships **3035**
The fellowship supports individuals engaged in a multidisciplinary research training program that will create or extend their credentials in informatics. The program enables faculty with active research programs to work outside of their home institution for periods of six months to one year to learn new skills or develop new collaborations that will enhance their research and research training capabilities in informatics. Applicants are expected to engage in research that supports career development of scientists engaged in computational and experimental research to integrate cutting edge information technology with advanced biological, chemical, and pharmacological sciences in the fields of genetics, genomics, and proteomics biological pathways. Emphasis will be placed on the development of new informatics technologies that demonstrate the translation of genomic data into an elucidation and understanding of biological and disease processes. The applicant and mentor of the program must describe how the multidisciplinary goals of the research experiential program will be accomplished and provide assurance that key collaborating mentors endorse and are willing to support the plan. The award provides up to $40,000 stipend support for mid-career scientists to engage in an academic year or calendar year experiential program intended to redirect their core research focus to an area of emerging importance to pharmaceutical research and development.
Requirements: Eligible applicants must hold a PhD or MD degree in a field of study logically or functionally related to the proposed postdoctoral activities; hold a faculty appointment that imparts eligibility for a sabbatical leave from their home institution; have institutional approval of a sabbatical plan that includes partial salary that matches the PhRMA stipend; and be a U.S. citizen or permanent resident. Preference will be given to those individuals whose research combines novel computational methods with experimental validation. Emphasis will be placed on the development of new informatics technologies that demonstrate the translation of genomic data into an elucidation and understanding of biological and disease processes. Matching funds must be provided by the home institution.
Restrictions: The program provides no other subsidies (travel, tuition, fringe benefit costs, etc.), and indirect costs to the institution are not provided.
Amount of Grant: $40,000
Contact: Eileen M. Cannon, Executive Director; (202) 572-7756; fax: (202) 572-7799; email: info@phrmafoundation.org
Internet: http://www.phrmafoundation.org/awards/informatics/sabbatical.php
Sponsor: Pharmaceutical Research and Manufacturers of America (PhRMA) Foundation
950 F Street, N.W., Suite 300
Washington, DC 20004

PhRMA Foundation Informatics Post Doctoral Fellowships **3036**
The postdoctoral program provides stipend support for individuals engaged in a multidisciplinary research training program that will create or extend their credentials in informatics. The intent of this program is to support postdoctoral career development activities of individuals preparing to engage in research that will bridge the gap between experimental and computational approaches in genomic and biomedical studies. It is anticipated that this research training will be accomplished in academic and/or industrial laboratory settings where multidisciplinary teams are organized to address problems that span the range of biological complexity rather than focus on the application of single technologies. The award, consisting of a $40,000 annual stipend, is made to the institution on behalf of the fellow. The award is intended solely as a stipend and may not be used otherwise.
Requirements: Eligible applicants must either hold a PhD degree in a field of study logically or functionally related to the proposed postdoctoral activities, or expect to receive the PhD before activating the award. They must also have a firm commitment from an accredited U.S. university and be a U.S. citizen or permanent resident. The sponsor (mentor) of the postdoctoral program must describe how the multidisciplinary goals of the research training program will be accomplished and provide assurance that key collaborating mentors endorse and are willing to support the training plan.
Restrictions: The program provides no other subsidies (travel, tuition, fringe benefit costs, etc.) and indirect costs to the institution are not provided. The second year of this award is contingent upon a progress report approved by the Foundation and submission of a financial report.
Amount of Grant: $40,000
Contact: Eileen M. Cannon, Executive Director; (202) 572-7756; fax: (202) 572-7799; email: info@phrmafoundation.org
Internet: http://www.phrmafoundation.org/awards/informatics/postdoc.php
Sponsor: Pharmaceutical Research and Manufacturers of America (PhRMA) Foundation
950 F Street, N.W., Suite 300
Washington, DC 20004

PhRMA Foundation Informatics Pre Doctoral Fellowships **3037**
The program is designed for candidates who expect to complete the requirements for the Ph.D. in the fields of informatics in two years or less from the time the fellowship begins. It aims at supporting promising students during their thesis research. The award is made to the university on behalf of the fellow. The fellowship provides a stipend of $20,000 a year payable monthly for a minimum of one year and a maximum of two years. Of the $20,000 awarded annually, up to $500 a year may be used for incidentals directly associated with the thesis research preparation (e.g., secretarial help, artwork, books, travel, etc.). Applications will be accepted for a minimum of one year and a maximum of two years. The program assumes that the fellows will devote full-time (including summers) to their research.
Requirements: The fellowship program of pre doctoral support is designed to assist full-time, in-residence Ph.D. candidates in the fields of informatics who are enrolled in U.S.A schools of medicine, pharmacy, dentistry or veterinary medicine. The program supports full-time advanced students who will have completed the bulk of their pre-thesis requirements (at least two years of study) and are engaged in thesis research as Ph.D. Candidates by the time the award is activated. Students just starting in graduate school should not apply. Highest priority will be given to applications who support the goal of the Informatics Programs. The goal of the program is to promote the use of informatics in an integrative approach to the understanding of biological and disease processes. Informatics awards will support career development of scientists engaged in computational and experimental research to integrate cutting-edge information technology with advanced biological, chemical, and pharmacological sciences. Applications must be submitted by an accredited U.S. school, and all applicants must be U.S. citizens or permanent residents.
Restrictions: The fellowship may not be used to supplement funds from other fellowships, traineeships or assistantships, unless necessary to make stipend levels compliant with institutional policy. The focus of the program is to assist in the predoctoral training of the candidate. It should not be viewed as a program to fund a research project. Indirect costs are not provided to the institution and PhRMA Foundation grant funds may not be used for this purpose.
Amount of Grant: $20,000
Contact: Eileen M. Cannon, Executive Director; (202) 572-7756; fax: (202) 572-7799; email: info@phrmafoundation.org
Internet: http://www.phrmafoundation.org/awards/informatics/predoc.php
Sponsor: Pharmaceutical Research and Manufacturers of America (PhRMA) Foundation
950 F Street, N.W., Suite 300
Washington, DC 20004

PhRMA Foundation Informatics Research Starter Grants **3038**
This program supports individuals beginning independent research careers in academia who do not have other substantial sources of research. The areas of interest within this program consists of research that supports career development of scientists engaged in computational and experimental research to integrate cutting edge-edge information

technology with advanced biological, chemical, and pharmacological sciences in: Genetics (Molecular, Medical-human, Pharmaco, Population); Genomics (Function, Structural, Toxico, Pharmaco, Comparative); Proteomics; Biological pathways. The program provides a research grant of $30,000 per year for up to two years. The 'starter' aspect of the program strives to assist those individuals who are establishing careers as independent investigators in the field of informatics. The program is not offered as a means to augment an ongoing research effort or is the grant intended to be used for any direct effort to obtain further extramural funding. The funds are to be used to conduct the proposed research.
Requirements: Those holding the academic rank of instructor or assistant professor and investigators at the doctoral level with equivalent positions are eligible to apply for these research starter grants, providing their proposed research is neither directly nor indirectly subsidized to any significant degree by an extramural support mechanism. The program is not intended for those in postdoctoral training programs. However, individuals in postdoctoral training scheduled to conclude and who will hold an academic appointment by January 1 may apply. Applicants must be sponsored by the department or unit in which the proposed research is to be undertaken. The grant is made to the university on behalf of the applicant and with the understanding that the university will administer the funds. Applications must be submitted by an accredited U.S. school, and all applicants must be U.S. citizens or permanent residents.
Restrictions: Research projects that extend or develop the proprietary value of specific drug products are not acceptable in this program. This exclusion does not preclude research in which specific drug products are used to test hypotheses that have a general applicability. The funds may not be used for salary support of the grantee, but may be used to support technical assistance. No more than $500 a year may be used for travel to professional meetings by the grantee. Indirect costs are not provided to the institution, and grant funds may not be used for this purpose.
Amount of Grant: $30,000
Contact: Eileen M. Cannon, Executive Director; (202) 572-7756; fax: (202) 572-7799; email: info@phrmafoundation.org
Internet: http://www.phrmafoundation.org/awards/informatics/starter.php
Sponsor: Pharmaceutical Research and Manufacturers of America (PhRMA) Foundation
950 F Street, N.W., Suite 300
Washington, DC 20004

PhRMA Foundation Paul Calabresi Medical Student Research Fellowship 3039
The fellowship is offered to medical or dental students who have substantial interests in research and teaching careers in pharmacology - clinical pharmacology and who are willing to spend full-time in a specific research effort within a pharmacology or clinical pharmacology unit. Fellowships are available for a minimum period of three months or any period of time up to 24 months. The commitment must be full-time. The student may undertake this investigative effort at his/her own school or at another institution. Requests for a fellowship are to be submitted online by the appropriate representative of the school or university. The fellowship is made to the institution on behalf of the student and the institution must agree to administer the funds. The program offers funding of up to $1,500 per month. It is expected that the funds will be distributed to the fellow in regular payments over the period of the fellowship by the recipient school. The funds may be used towards the stipend, tuition or affiliated fees for the fellow. Fellowships are available for a minimum period of six months or any period of time up to 24 months. However, if the student's award period is 24 months, the maximum stipend is still $18,000.
Requirements: A candidate must be enrolled in a U.S. medical/dental school and have finished at least one year of the school curriculum. Priority consideration will be given to those candidates who project strong commitments to careers in the field of clinical pharmacology. The applicant must be sponsored by the pharmacology or clinical pharmacology program in which the investigative project is to be undertaken. The sponsoring unit must have a demonstrated commitment to training in the fields of pharmacology or clinical pharmacology. Applications must be submitted by an accredited U.S. school, and all applicants must be U.S. citizens or permanent residents.
Restrictions: There are no indirect costs provided to the institution nor may any of the funds be used for this purpose. Once an individual has received a Medical Student Fellowship, that individual may not reapply.
Amount of Grant: up to $18,000
Contact: Eileen M. Cannon, Executive Director; (202) 572-7756; fax: (202) 572-7799; email: info@phrmafoundation.org
Internet: http://www.phrmafoundation.org/awards/clinical/medstudent.php
Sponsor: Pharmaceutical Research and Manufacturers of America (PhRMA) Foundation
950 F Street, N.W., Suite 300
Washington, DC 20004

PhRMA Foundation Pharmaceutics Postdoctoral Fellowships 3040
The purpose of the fellowships is to encourage graduates from PhD programs in pharmaceutics to continue to refine their research skills through formal postdoctoral training. Applicants should indicate a strong determination to continue their research careers in pharmaceutics following completion of the fellowship. Applications will be accepted for postdoctoral research training extending over a minimum of one year and a maximum of two years. Each fellowship carries an annual stipend of $40,000 which can be supplemented by the sponsor and/or his/her institution.
Requirements: To be eligible, applicants must either hold a PhD degree in pharmaceutics from a school of pharmacy accredited by the American Council on Pharmaceutical Education or expect to receive such a degree before activating the fellowship. The mentor of the fellow must be in an accredited school of pharmacy. Alternatively, a student with a Ph.D. from a school of pharmacy may use the fellowship to study with a mentor in any science or engineering department. An equally important aspect of eligibility is that suitable facilities for the necessary training and research must be available to the applicant. The program with which the applicant is, or will be, associated must provide an environment where the applicant's potential can be developed to the fullest extent possible.
Restrictions: The award is intended solely as a stipend and may not be used otherwise. If necessary, the institution may supplement the award to a level that is consistent with other postdoctoral fellowships it currently offers. Research projects that extend or develop the proprietary value of specific drug products are not acceptable in this program. The program provides no other subsidies (travel, tuition, fringe benefit costs, etc.) and indirect costs to the institution are not provided.
Amount of Grant: $40,000
Contact: Eileen M. Cannon, Executive Director; (202) 572-7756; fax: (202) 572-7799; email: info@phrmafoundation.org
Internet: http://www.phrmafoundation.org/awards/pharmaceutics/postdoc.php
Sponsor: Pharmaceutical Research and Manufacturers of America (PhRMA) Foundation
950 F Street, N.W., Suite 300
Washington, DC 20004

PhRMA Foundation Pharmaceutics Pre Doctoral Fellowships 3041
To encourage the entry of more qualified individuals into this area, the program aims at supporting promising students during their thesis research by providing assistance in the form of stipend and funds to cover costs incidental to the training. Applications will be accepted for a minimum of one year and a maximum of two years. The program is designed for applicants who expect to complete the requirements for the Ph.D. in pharmaceutics in two years or less from the time the fellowship begins. For the purposes of this program, pharmaceutics includes basic pharmaceutics, biopharmaceutics and pharmaceutical technology. The fundamental aspects of pharmacokinetics are not included since these are covered by PhRMA Foundation awards in pharmacology and toxicology.
Requirements: To be eligible, applicants must hold a B.S., M.S., or Pharm.D. degree in pharmacy or a related area such as chemistry or biology from an accredited school in the U.S. A candidate enrolled in a Pharm.D./Ph.D. program should not be taking required clinical course work or clinical clerkships during the tenure of the fellowship. Also, before an individual is eligible to apply for a PhRMA Foundation award, the applicant must first have a firm commitment from a U.S. university, and must be a U.S. citizen or permanent resident. The program assumes that the fellows will devote full-time (including summers) to their research. The fellowship may not be used as a supplement to funds from other fellowships or assistantships. However, this does not preclude institutions supplementing a fellowship with their own funds in order to bring the stipend within the normal range of the institution.
Restrictions: Research projects which extend or develop the proprietary value of specific drug products are not acceptable in this program. This exclusion does not preclude research in which specific drug products are used to test hypotheses which have a general applicability. Applications, however good, which do not meet the aims of the program will be disapproved.
Contact: Eileen M. Cannon, Executive Director; (202) 572-7756; fax: (202) 572-7799; email: info@phrmafoundation.org
Internet: http://www.phrmafoundation.org/awards/pharmaceutics/predoc.php
Sponsor: Pharmaceutical Research and Manufacturers of America (PhRMA) Foundation
950 F Street, N.W., Suite 300
Washington, DC 20004

PhRMA Foundation Pharmaceutics Research Starter Grants 3042
The purpose of the starter grants is to offer financial support to individuals beginning their independent research careers at the faculty level. The areas of interest within this program are research efforts in the fields of pharmaceutics. The program provides a research grant of $30,000 per year for up to two years. For the purposes of this program, pharmaceutics includes basic pharmaceutics, biopharmaceutics, pharmaceutical technology and pharmaceutical biotechnology. The fundamental aspects of pharmacokinetics are not included since they are covered by PhRMA Foundation programs in pharmacology and toxicology. The 'starter' aspect of the program strives to assist those individuals who are establishing careers as independent investigators in the fields listed above.
Requirements: Those holding the academic, tenure track, rank of instructor or assistant professor and investigators at the doctoral level with equivalent positions are eligible to apply for these research starter grants, providing their proposed research is neither directly nor indirectly subsidized to any significant degree by an extramural support mechanism. It is anticipated that this research experience will occur in an academic and/or industrial laboratory setting. Applications must be submitted by a school of pharmacy accredited by the American Council on Pharmaceutical Education, and all applicants must be U.S. citizens or permanent residents. The grant is made to the university on behalf of the applicant and with the understanding that the university will administer the funds. Only schools of pharmacy are eligible for this award.
Restrictions: The program is not offered as a means to augment an ongoing research effort. Nor is the grant intended to be used for any direct effort to obtain further extramural funding. The funds are to be used to conduct the proposed research. The funds may not be used for salary support of the grantee, but may be used to support technical assistance. No more than $500 a year may be used for travel to professional meetings by the grantee. Indirect costs are not provided to the institution, and grant funds may not be used for this purpose.
Amount of Grant: $30,000

Contact: Eileen M. Cannon, Executive Director; (202) 572-7756; fax: (202) 572-7799; email: info@phrmafoundation.org
Internet: http://www.phrmafoundation.org/awards/pharmaceutics/starter.php
Sponsor: Pharmaceutical Research and Manufacturers of America (PhRMA) Foundation
950 F Street, N.W., Suite 300
Washington, DC 20004

PhRMA Foundation Pharmaceutics Sabbatical Fellowships **3043**
The purpose of this program is to enable faculty with active research programs to work outside of their home institution for periods of 6 months to one year to learn new skills or develop new collaborations that will enhance their research and research training capabilities in pharmaceutics. For the purposes of this program, pharmaceutics includes basic pharmaceutics, biopharmaceutics, pharmaceutical technology and pharmaceutical biotechnology. The fundamental aspects of pharmacokinetics are not included since they are covered by PhRMA Foundation programs in pharmacology and toxicology. It is anticipated that this research experience will occur in an academic and/or industrial laboratory setting. The award provides up to $40,000 stipend support for mid-career scientists to engage in an academic year or calendar year experiential program intended to redirect their core research focus to an area of emerging importance to pharmaceutical research and development.
Requirements: Eligible applicants must hold a PhD degree in pharmaceutics from a School of Pharmacy accredited by the American Council on Pharmaceutical Education; hold a faculty appointment that imparts eligibility for a sabbatical leave from their home institution; have institutional approval of a sabbatical plan that includes partial salary that matches the PhRMA stipend; hold an endorsement from a mentor who agrees to sponsor the applicants visiting scientist activity; and be a U.S. citizen or permanent resident. The applicant and mentor of the program must describe how the multidisciplinary goals of the research experiential program will be accomplished and provide assurance that key collaborating mentors endorse and are willing to support the plan. Matching funds must be provided by the home institution.
Restrictions: The program provides no other subsidies (travel, tuition, fringe benefit costs, etc.) and indirect costs to the institution are not provided.
Amount of Grant: $40,000
Contact: Eileen M. Cannon, Executive Director; (202) 572-7756; fax: (202) 572-7799; email: info@phrmafoundation.org
Internet: http://www.phrmafoundation.org/awards/pharmaceutics/sabbatical.php
Sponsor: Pharmaceutical Research and Manufacturers of America (PhRMA) Foundation
950 F Street, N.W., Suite 300
Washington, DC 20004

PhRMA Foundation Pharmacology/Toxicology Post Doctoral Fellowships **3044**
The postdoctoral program provides stipend support for individuals engaged in a multidisciplinary research training program that will create or extend their credentials in pharmacology or toxicology. The intent of this program is to support postdoctoral career development activities of individuals prepared (or preparing) to engage in research that integrates information on molecular or cellular mechanisms of action with information on the effect of an agent in the intact organism. It is anticipated that this research training will be accomplished in academic and/or industrial laboratory settings where multidisciplinary teams are organized to integrate informatics, molecular, cell, and systems biology with pharmacology/toxicology research. Funding is for up to 2 years but not beyond the 3rd year of the existing Post Doc.
Requirements: Eligible applicants must either hold a PhD degree or appropriate terminal research doctorate in a field of study logically or functionally related to the proposed post doctoral activities; or expect to receive the PhD before activating the award. They must also have a firm commitment from an accredited U.S. university and be a U.S. citizen or permanent resident. The sponsor (mentor) must describe how the multidisciplinary goals of the research training program will be accomplished and provide assurance that key collaborating mentors endorse and are willing to support the training plan. The award, consisting of a $40,000 annual stipend, is made to the institution on behalf of the fellow. The award is intended solely as a stipend and may not be used otherwise. If necessary, the institution may supplement the award to a level that is consistent with other postdoctoral fellowships it currently offers.
Restrictions: The program provides no other subsidies (travel, tuition, fringe benefit costs, etc.) and indirect costs to the institution are not provided. The second year of this award is contingent upon a progress report approved by the foundation and submission of a financial report.
Amount of Grant: $40,000
Contact: Eileen M. Cannon, Executive Director; (202) 572-7756; fax: (202) 572-7799; email: info@phrmafoundation.org
Internet: http://www.phrmafoundation.org/awards/pharmacology/postdoc.php
Sponsor: Pharmaceutical Research and Manufacturers of America (PhRMA) Foundation
950 F Street, N.W., Suite 300
Washington, DC 20004

PhRMA Foundation Pharmacology/Toxicology Pre Doctoral Fellowships **3045**
The program is designed for candidates who expect to complete the requirements for the Ph.D. in the fields of pharmacology or toxicology in two years or less from the time the fellowship begins. The award is made to the university on behalf of the fellow. The fellowship provides a stipend of $20,000 a year payable monthly for a minimum of one year and a maximum of two years. Of the $20,000 awarded annually, up to $500 a year may be used for incidentals directly associated with the thesis research preparation (e.g., secretarial help, artwork, books, travel, etc.). Awards may be activated beginning January 1 or on the first day of any month thereafter, up to and including August 1. The second year of a fellowship is contingent upon certification by the thesis advisor that satisfactory progress is being achieved.
Requirements: The fellowship program of pre doctoral support is designed to assist full-time, in-residence Ph.D. candidates in the fields of pharmacology or toxicology who are enrolled in U.S.A schools of medicine, pharmacy, dentistry or veterinary medicine. The program supports full-time advanced students who will have completed the bulk of their pre-thesis requirements (at least two years of study) and are engaged in thesis research as Ph.D. Candidates by the time the award is activated. Students just starting in graduate school should not apply. In the field of pharmacology or toxicology, highest priority will be given to applications for research that attempts to integrate information on the mechanism of action of a drug or chemical at a molecular or cellular level with the drug's effects in the intact laboratory animal or human, encompassing the potential influences of biochemical, physiological or behavioral systems. The pharmacology/toxicology research and teaching mission of the unit awarding the degree must be apparent as a core mission component on their web site. Applications must be submitted by an accredited U.S. school, and all applicants must be U.S. citizens or permanent residents. The program assumes that the fellows will devote full-time (including summers) to their research. The PhRMA Foundation fellowship may not be used to supplement funds from other fellowships, traineeships or assistantships, unless necessary to make stipend levels compliant with institutional policy. The focus of the program is to assist in the predoctoral training of the candidate. It should not be viewed as a program to fund a research project.
Restrictions: A candidate enrolled in an M.D./Ph.D. program should not be taking required clinical course work or clerkships during the tenure of the fellowship. The foundation will accept only one application per academic institution. Exceptions may be considered for institutions with multiple campuses. Indirect costs are not provided to the institution and PhRMA Foundation grant funds may not be used for this purpose.
Amount of Grant: $20,000
Contact: Eileen M. Cannon, Executive Director; (202) 572-7756; fax: (202) 572-7799; email: info@phrmafoundation.org
Internet: http://www.phrmafoundation.org/awards/pharmacology/predoc.php
Sponsor: Pharmaceutical Research and Manufacturers of America (PhRMA) Foundation
950 F Street, N.W., Suite 300
Washington, DC 20004

PhRMA Foundation Pharmacology/Toxicology Research Starter Grants **3046**
The purpose of the program is to offer financial support to individuals beginning their independent research careers at the faculty level. The areas of interest within this program are research efforts in the fields of pharmacology and drug toxicology. The program provides a research grant of $30,000 per year for up to two years. The 'starter' aspect of the program strives to assist those individuals who are establishing careers as independent investigators in the fields listed above. The program is not offered as a means to augment an ongoing research effort. The funds are to be used to conduct the proposed research. This program supports individuals beginning independent research careers in academia who do not have other substantial sources of research. Applicants will be judged on the scientific merit of the proposed research, and on the degree of financial need.
Requirements: Those holding the academic rank of instructor or assistant professor and investigators at the doctoral level with equivalent positions are eligible to apply for these research starter grants, providing their proposed research is neither directly nor indirectly subsidized to any significant degree by a competitive extramural grant. The program is not intended for those in postdoctoral training programs. However, individuals in postdoctoral training scheduled to conclude and who will hold an academic appointment by January 1 may apply. Applicants must be sponsored by the department or unit in which the proposed research is to be undertaken. The sponsoring unit must have responsibility for pharmacology/toxicology teaching and research as part of its core mission. If the pharmacology/toxicology mission is not apparent on the sponsoring unit's web site, the sponsor letter must describe how the academic appointment will support the applicant's career development in pharmacology/toxicology. The grant is made to the university on behalf of the applicant, with the understanding that the university will administer the funds. Schools of medicine (human or veterinary), pharmacy and dentistry are eligible for this award. In the field of pharmacology or toxicology, highest priority will be given to applications for research that attempts to integrate information on the mechanism of action of a drug or chemical at a molecular or cellular level with the drug's effects in the intact laboratory animal or human, encompassing the potential influences of biochemical, physiological or behavioral systems. Applications must be submitted by an accredited U.S. school, and all applicants must be U.S. citizens or permanent residents.
Restrictions: Research projects that extend or develop the proprietary value of specific drug products are not acceptable in this program. This exclusion does not preclude research in which specific drug products are used to test hypotheses that have a general applicability. The funds may not be used for salary support of the grantee, but may be used to support technical assistance. No more than $500 a year may be used for travel to professional meetings by the grantee. Indirect costs are not provided to the institution, and grant funds may not be used for this purpose. Applicants holding multi-year national competitive awards or grants supporting their independent research will not be considered. If a national competitive grant is obtained after the application has been submitted, the Foundation must be so informed.
Amount of Grant: $30,000
Contact: Eileen M. Cannon, Executive Director; (202) 572-7756; fax: (202) 572-7799; email: info@phrmafoundation.org

Internet: http://www.phrmafoundation.org/awards/pharmacology/starter.php
Sponsor: Pharmaceutical Research and Manufacturers of America (PhRMA) Foundation
950 F Street, N.W., Suite 300
Washington, DC 20004

PhRMA Foundation Pharmacology/Toxicology Sabbatical Fellowships **3047**

This program provides stipend funding to enable faculty members at all levels with active research programs an opportunity to work at other institutions for periods of six months to one year to learn new skills or develop new collaborations that will enhance their research and research training activities in pharmacology/toxicology. Applicants are expected to engage in multidisciplinary research that integrates information on molecular or cellular mechanisms of action with information on the effect of an agent in the intact organism. It is anticipated that this research experience will occur in academic and/or industrial laboratory settings as part of a multidisciplinary team organized to integrate informatics, molecular, cell, and systems biology with pharmacology/toxicology research. The award provides up to $40,000 stipend support for mid-career scientists to engage in an academic year or calendar year experiential program intended to redirect their core research focus to an area of emerging importance to pharmaceutical research and development.
Requirements: Eligible applicants must hold a PhD degree or appropriate terminal doctorate and record of research accomplishment in a field of study logically or functionally related to the proposed post doctoral activities; hold a faculty appointment that imparts eligibility for a sabbatical leave from their home institution; have institutional approval of a sabbatical plan that includes partial salary that matches the PhRMA stipend; hold an endorsement from a mentor who agrees to sponsor the applicants visiting scientist activity; and be a U.S. citizen or permanent resident. The applicant and mentor of the program must describe how the multidisciplinary goals of the research experiential program will be accomplished and provide assurance that key collaborating mentors endorse and are willing to support the plan. Matching funds must be provided through the university.
Restrictions: The program provides no other subsidies (travel, tuition, fringe benefit costs, etc.) and indirect costs to the institution are not provided.
Amount of Grant: $40,000
Contact: Eileen M. Cannon, Executive Director; (202) 572-7756; fax: (202) 572-7799; email: info@phrmafoundation.org
Internet: http://www.phrmafoundation.org/awards/pharmacology/sabbatical.php
Sponsor: Pharmaceutical Research and Manufacturers of America (PhRMA) Foundation
950 F Street, N.W., Suite 300
Washington, DC 20004

Piedmont Natural Gas Grants **3048**

Piedmont Natural Gas supports programs and activities that benefit its customers and employees. Corporate contributions are primarily awarded to nonprofit organizations in the following categories: health and human services—United Way; hospitals and medical centers; health and human service organizations—youth agencies, and senior citizens programs; education—higher education, community colleges, education-related organizations, drop-out prevention programs, foundations that achieve progressive and far-reaching change in education, and public/private education partnerships; culture and the arts—arts funds or councils; museums or cultural centers, visual and performing arts organizations, and public libraries; civic and community—housing, environment and ecology, community development, zoos and parks, economic development, employment, and job training; and other—public television and radio, and public policy research organizations. There are no application deadlines.
Requirements: 501(c)3 tax-exempt organizations in company-operating areas in North Carolina, South Carolina, and Tennessee are welcome.
Restrictions: As a general rule, grants do not support individuals, non-501(c)3 organizations; pre-college level private schools except through employee matching gifts; travel and conferences; third-party professional fund-raising organizations; controversial social causes; fraternal and veterans organizations or private clubs; religious organizations with programs limited to or expressly for their membership only; agencies already receiving corporate support through United Way or a united arts drive, with the exception of approved capital campaigns; or athletic events and programs.
Geographic Focus: North Carolina; South Carolina; Tennessee
Contact: Administrator, (704) 364-3120; email: contributions@piedmontng.com
Internet: http://www.piedmontng.com/eprise/main/piedmontng/itc/guidelinesPolicies/guidelinesPolicies_main
Sponsor: Piedmont Natural Gas Corporation
P.O. Box 33068, 1915 Rexford Road
Charlotte, NC 28233

Pike County Community Foundation Grants **3049**

Founded in 1998, the Pike County Community Foundation is a charitable organization formed to strengthen the Pike County, Indiana community by awarding grants to local nonprofits, by bringing individuals together to address community needs, and by offering personalized charitable gift planning services to our donors. The foundation considers proposals for grants on a yearly cycle which begins each July. At the start of each cycle, a notice is mailed to nonprofit organizations that have applied for grants in the past, have received grants in the past, or have otherwise requested notification of the start of each cycle. The foundations grant cycle runs from July through November each year. Proposals will be accepted from July through the September deadline. Proposals submitted after the September deadline (date varies, contact foundation office for current deadline) will not be considered. The grants committee will make its recommendations on funding to the Foundation's Board of Trustees, which will make final funding recommendations to the board of directors of the Community Foundation Alliance (our governing body). All organizations that have submitted grant proposals will be notified of the outcome of the grants committee's deliberation in writing no later than December 1.
Requirements: The Foundation welcomes proposals from nonprofit organizations that are deemed tax-exempt under sections 501(c)3 and 509(a) of the Internal Revenue Code and from governmental agencies serving Pike County. Proposals from nonprofit organizations not classified as a 501(c)3 public charity may be considered provided the project is charitable and supports a community need. Proposals submitted by an entity under the auspices of another agency must include a written statement signed by the agency's board president on behalf of the board of directors agreeing to act as the entity's fiscal sponsor, to receive grant monies if awarded, and to oversee the proposed project.
Restrictions: Project areas NOT considered for funding: religious organizations for religious purposes; political parties or campaigns; endowment creation or debt reduction; operating costs; capital campaigns; annual appeals or membership contributions; travel requests for groups or individuals such as bands, sports teams, or classes. A six-month progress report and a final report at project completion are required by organizations whose proposals are approved for funding. Instructions and appropriate forms will be provided at the time the grant is awarded.
Geographic Focus: Indiana
Samples: Evansville Philharmonic Orchestra - for Pike County third through fifth grade students to participate in the youth concert program, $300.00.; Petersburg Ministerial Fellowship - to purchase clothing for the "Clothe-a-Child" program, $2,000.00.; Tri-Cap - to assist with emergency financial assistance for families in need, $918.00.
Contact: Tom Dooley, Director; (812) 354-6797; fax: (812) 354-6797; email: tom@pikecommunityfoundation.org
Internet: http://www.pikecommunityfoundation.org/grantmaking
Sponsor: Pike County Community Foundation
714 Main Street, P.O. Box 587
Petersburg, IN 47567

Pinellas County Grants **3050**

The Pinellas Community Foundation was established in 1969, it distributes grants twice annually to a wide variety of non-profit agencies, organizations and programs that enhance and support the quality of life in Pinellas County, Florida. Areas of interest are: art, culture, health care, environment, community development, employment opportunities, the underserved, and social services.
Requirements: Eligibility: a non-profit, 501(c)3; be headquartered in Pinellas County; provide social services to people in Pinellas County; not have a large endowment or fund raising staff; provide recent audited financial statements. For Grant Applications call Pinellas Community Foundation: (727)531-0058.
Geographic Focus: Florida
Date(s) Application is Due: Jun 15; Oct 1
Contact: Julie Scales, Executive Director; (727) 531-0058; fax: (727) 531-0053; email: info@pinellasccf.org
Internet: http://www.pinellasccf.org/pinellas-community-foundation-pcf-clearwater-fl-our-grants-programs.htm
Sponsor: Pinellas County Community Foundation
5200 East Bay Drive, Suite 202
Clearwater, FL 33764

Pioneer Hi-Bred Community Grants **3051**

The international corporation supports community-based projects in the areas of agriculture, education, farm safety, and the environment. Priority consideration is given to projects located in Pioneer facility communities or rural agricultural regions and to organizations with active Pioneer management/employee participation and company-related expertise and interest. Types of support include capital grants, general operating grants, program development grants, and seed money grants. The company accepts proposals from nonprofit organizations nationwide but favors programs in its operating communities. Pioneer prefers to make direct contributions to organizations, rather than sponsorships, ticket or table purchases. This allows more funding to go directly toward the non-profit organization; however, we are willing to consider sponsorships when Pioneer employees are actively involved with the organization. The employee must present the request to Community Investment at least one month in advance. Due to the number of non-profit events held annually, there is a $1,000 maximum contribution level per event per year. The company favors proposals that demonstrate cooperation with other community-based programs, broad-based funding, community need, and positive results. Grant proposals are reviewed on a quarterly basis.
Requirements: Nonprofit organizations are eligible. All requests should be directed to the Pioneer Hi-Bred office within the local area. Otherwise, send to the contact listed. Pioneer does not respond favorably to verbal requests.
Restrictions: Grants are not made to individuals, religious or political organizations that promote a particular doctrine, elected officials, company marketing or advertising, or organizations where there is a conflict of interest with Pioneer Hi-Bred.
Amount of Grant: $250-$1,000 average; $5,000 maximum
Contact: Grants Administrator; (800) 247-6803, ext. 3915; fax: (515) 334-4415; email: community.investment@pioneer.com
Internet: http://www.pioneer.com/web/site/portal/menuitem.bb020a6d93d9d318bc0c0a03d10093a0/
Sponsor: Pioneer Hi-Bred International, Inc.
6900 NW 62nd Avenue, P.O. Box 246
Johnston, IA 50131

Pioneer Hi-Bred Society Fellowships 3052

The Pioneer Hi-Bred Society Fellowship is designed to contribute to agricultural research and education by providing financial support for outstanding students studying for graduate level degrees in plant breeding. Leading societies that support plant improvement graduate programs in crops of interest to Pioneer have been selected by the Fellowship Sub-committee. The institutions are responsible for student selection and administering the program. Funded societies include: Agronomic Science Foundation; American Phytopathological Society; American Society of Plant Biologists; the Consultative Group on International Agricultural Research (CGIAR); and the Entomological Foundation.

Requirements: Pioneer prefers this grant to be used solely to fund a student(s) progressing towards a graduate degree in plant breeding from the funded institution. No university overhead will be paid from these funds.

Contact: David Harwood; (515) 270-3200 or (800) 247-6803, ext. 3915; fax: (515) 334-4415; email: David.Harwood@pioneer.com

Internet: http://www.pioneer.com/web/site/portal/menuitem.07196fe7964ae318bc0c0a03d10093a0/

Sponsor: Pioneer Hi-Bred International, Inc.
6900 NW 62nd Avenue, P.O. Box 246
Johnston, IA 50131

Piper Jaffray Companies Building Strong Communities Grants 3053

The foundation supports organizations and programs that enhance the lives of people living and working in communities in which the company has offices. Of primary interest is support for organizations that increase opportunities for individuals to improve their lives and help themselves. Highest priority is given to family stability programs (including housing, family violence, responsible parenting), early childhood development, job training/career development, youth development, and adult education services. The foundation will also consider requests from organizations that work to increase citizen understanding or involvement in civic affairs or that enhance the artistic and cultural life of the community. Requests for general operating support from proven nonprofit organizations will be considered. Requests for project and capital support will be considered on a very selective basis. Support for higher education and K-12 public and private schools is provided primarily through the company gift-matching program. Contact the foundation for deadline dates.

Requirements: IRS 501(c)3 organizations located in the Minneapolis/Saint Paul metropolitan area should submit requests directly to the foundation. Organizations located outside the Minneapolis/Saint Paul metropolitan area should submit requests to the nearest Piper Jaffray office for forwarding to the foundation.

Restrictions: Requests will not be considered from newly formed nonprofit organizations; individuals; teams; religious, political, veterans, or fraternal organizations; or organizations working to treat or eliminate specific diseases. Support is not available for basic or applied research, travel, event sponsorship, benefits or tickets, or to eliminate an organization's operating deficit.

Geographic Focus: Arizona; Arkansas; California; Colorado; Idaho; Illinois; Iowa; Kansas; Kentucky; Minnesota; Missouri; Montana; Nebraska; Nevada; North Dakota; Ohio; Oregon; South Dakota; Tennessee; Utah; Washington; Wisconsin; Wyoming

Samples: Abbott Northwestern Hospital Park House (Minneapolis, MN)—for capital support.; CARE Foundation (Plymouth, MN)—for general operating support.; United Way of the Minneapolis Area (Minneapolis, MN)—for operating support.

Amount of Grant: $1000-$5000 average

Date(s) Application is Due: Mar 31; Jul 15; Oct 1

Contact: Kris Kewitsch, Director of Community Relations, (612) 303-5515; fax: (612) 342-6085; email: kristin.k.kewitsch@pjc.com or communityrelations@pjc.com

Internet: http://www.piperjaffray.com/info3.aspx?id=220

Sponsor: Piper Jaffray Companies Foundation
800 Nicollet Mall, Suite 800
Minneapolis, MN 55402

Pittsburgh Foundation Community Fund Grants 3054

The Pittsburgh Foundation, established in 1945, is the 14th largest community foundation in the county. The foundation awards grants to organizations operating primarily in the Pittsburgh area and Allegheny County, PA. The Foundation supports five targeted areas of impact: education; economic development; families, children and youth; health care; arts.

Requirements: Grants in the five targeted areas for impact are awarded to nonprofit organizations that are defined as tax-exempt under Section 501(c)3 of the Internal Revenue Code and are located within Allegheny County, or can demonstrate that a significant majority of their population served is from Allegheny County.

Geographic Focus: Pennsylvania

Amount of Grant: $30,000-$150,000 typically

Contact: Jane Downing, Senior Program Officer; (412) 391-5122; fax: (412) 391-7259; email: downingj@pghfdn.org

Internet: http://www.pittsburghfoundation.org/page8894.cfm

Sponsor: The Pittsburgh Foundation
5 PPG Place, Suite 250
Pittsburgh, PA 15222-5414

Pittsburgh Foundation Medical Research Grants 3055

Through the generosity of individuals and families who have established medical research funds with The Pittsburgh Foundation, the Foundation provides support for this cutting edge research. Based on the donors' fields of interest, the Foundation provides grants for the following: Richard S. Caliguiri Fund - for research in the field of amyloidosis; The Walter L. Copeland Fund - for cranial research (disease of the brain/neurological disease), to be conducted within the Department of Neurological Surgery at the University of Pittsburgh; John F. and Nancy A. Emmerling Fund - for research in the field of neuropsychobiology (with emphasis on biochemistry) of mental disorders, with the goal of discovering the causes and cure, of amelioration, of mental disorders. The principal investigator must have full time status at the University of Pittsburgh; Albert B. Ferguson, M.D. Orthopaedic Fund - for orthopaedic research; GLBT Health and Wellness Fund - to assess the incidence, cause or cure of certain diseases (i.e., cancer, heart disease, diabetes, arthritis, AIDS and Alzheimer's disease) in the Gay, Lesbian, Bisexual and Transgender (GLBT) community; Medical Research Funding - for research in the field of cancer, heart disease, arthritis, diabetes, multiple sclerosis and geriatric diseases (with focuses particularly on Alzheimer's disease and other related diseases of the elderly).

Requirements: Pennsylvania not-for-profit institutions with 501(c)3 tax-exempt status are invited to apply for funding. Support is given to investigators in Allegheny County with a proven record of performance in the area under investigation. Guidelines and applications vary, see: http://www.pittsburghfoundation.org/page32428.cfm for a complete listing of each grant.

Geographic Focus: Pennsylvania

Contact: Judy Powell, Support; (412) 394-4294; email: powellj@pghfdn.org

Internet: http://www.pittsburghfoundation.org/page32428.cfm

Sponsor: Pittsburgh Foundation
5 PPG Place, Suite 250
Pittsburgh, PA 15222-5414

PKD Foundation Lillian Kaplan International Prize for the Advancement in the Understanding of Polycystic Kidney Disease 3056

The prize is a joint venture between the foundation and the International Society of Nephrology. The winning nominee of the initial award received the prize in Berlin; it has been awarded every other year since. Each award consists of a monetary award, a framed certificate with an appropriate citation, and a designated sculpture to clinicians and scientists who have made outstanding discoveries in basic science or who have made outstanding clinical contributions to the care of individuals. This is the largest cash prize for a clinical medical specialty in the world signaling the prestige and importance it carries. PKD experts from both organizations judge nominations.

Requirements: Awards are made to residents of any country without restriction to gender, race, religion, creed, or nationality. Nomination letters should describe the key role of the nominee(s) in a biomedical advance relevant to PKD and should be accompanied by a full curriculum vita with a complete mailing address and at least two supporting letters that detail a major discovery or sustained advance. If two individuals are nominated to share the prize, the reasons for why the prize would be shared must be clearly delineated.

Samples: Dr. Corinne Antignac, Necker Hospital, Paris, France, $50,000 (2009); Dr. Lisa Guay-Woodford, University of Alabama at Birmingham, $50,000 (2009); Dr. Friedhelm Hildebrandt, University of Michigan, $50,000 (2009).

Amount of Grant: $50,000

Date(s) Application is Due: Feb 1

Contact: Dan Lara, Government Relations Manager; (816) 268-8480; fax: (816) 931-8655; email: larad@pkdcure.org or pkdcure@pkdcure.org

Internet: http://www.pkdcure.org

Sponsor: PKD Foundation
9221 Ward Parkway, Suite 400
Kansas City, MO 64114-3367

PKD Foundation Research Grants 3057

The PKD Foundation, established in 1982 by Joseph H. Bruening and Jared J. Grantham, leads the fight against polycistic kidney disease through vital research funding and patient education. Annually, the PKD Foundation funds more than $4.2 million in vital PKD research. Most recently, clinical trials in cardiovascular health, Rapamycin, Somatostatin, Tolvaptan, and more have offered help and hope to the 12.5 million worldwide with the disease.

Amount of Grant: $25,000-$1,000,000

Contact: Dan Lara, Government Relations Manager; (816) 268-8480; fax: (816) 931-8655; email: larad@pkdcure.org or pkdcure@pkdcure.org

Internet: http://www.pkdcure.org/Research/tabid/82/Default.aspx

Sponsor: PKD Foundation
9221 Ward Parkway, Suite 400
Kansas City, MO 64114-3367

Plastic Surgery Educational Foundation Basic Research Grants 3058

The Plastic Surgery Educational Foundation and the American Society for Aesthetic Plastic Surgery offer annual research grants to provide seed money to U.S. and Canadian surgeons for research projects in the field of plastic and reconstructive surgery. Nonmembers of PSEF must submit a letter of sponsorship from a foundation member.

Requirements: Applicant must be a plastic surgeon, MD, or PhD working in plastic surgery.

Samples: Dr. James Anthony, U of California (San Francisco, CA)—for research on wound cytokine levels, $4600. Dr. Steven Buchman, U of Michigan (MI)—for research on cranial suture closure, $4998. Dr. James Doyle, U of Massachusetts Medical Ctr (MA)—for research questioning IL-10 as an immunosuppressive factor in chronic wound fluid, $5000.

Amount of Grant: $5,000

Date(s) Application is Due: Jan 17

Contact: Carol V. Wargo, Director of Corporate Relations; (847) 228-3358 or (847) 228-9900; fax: (847) 228-9131 or (847) 228-0628; email: cvw@plasticsurgery.org or cschmieden@plasticsurgery.org
Internet: http://www.plasticsurgery.org/medical_professionals/research/Grant-Applications.cfm
Sponsor: Plastic Surgery Educational Foundation
444 E. Algonquin Road
Arlington Heights, IL 60005

Plastic Surgery Educational Foundation Research Fellowship Grants **3059**
The Research Fellowship Grants are awarded for the purpose of encouraging research and academic career development in Plastic Surgery. The PSEF Research Fellowship is for training in any area of Plastic Surgery and is designed for those who wish to supplement one year of clinical training for a research experience. The PSEF/KCI Wound Care Research Fellowship is open to plastic surgery residents and recent plastic surgery resident graduates focusing on a project in wound care management.
Samples: Dr. Emmanuella Joseph (Boston, MA)—senior award winner for clinical research, $3000. Dr. Jayesh Panchal (Oklahoma City, OK)—junior award winner for clinical research, $3000. Dr. W.P. Andrew Leww (Boston, MA)—senior award winner for basic science, $3000. Dr. Vaishali Doolabh (Saint Louis, MO)—junior award winner for basic science, $3000.
Contact: Carol V. Wargo, Director of Corporate Relations; (847) 228-3358 or (847) 228-9900; fax: (847) 228-9131 or (847) 228-0628; email: cvw@plasticsurgery.org or cschmieden@plasticsurgery.org
Internet: http://www.plasticsurgery.org/medical_professionals/research/Grant-Applications.cfm
Sponsor: Plastic Surgery Educational Foundation
444 E. Algonquin Road
Arlington Heights, IL 60005

Plastic Surgery Educational Foundation/AAO-HNSF Combined Grant **3060**
The PSEF/AAO-HNSF Combined Grant is designed to promote interdisciplinary research by encouraging a collaborative research effort between the specialties of Plastic Surgery and Otolaryngology. Recipients of this grant must demonstrate a potential for excellence in research and training and a commitment to an academic research career in either Plastic Surgery or Otolaryngology.
Requirements: Applicants must have demonstrated a potential for excellence in research and teaching and serious commitment to an academic research career in otolaryngology or plastic surgery. Priority will be given to senior residents, fellows or faculty who have completed residencies or fellowships within four years of the application receipt date.
Amount of Grant: $20,000 maximum
Date(s) Application is Due: Dec 15
Contact: Carol V. Wargo, Director of Corporate Relations; (847) 228-3358 or (847) 228-9900; fax: (847) 228-9131 or (847) 228-0628; email: cvw@plasticsurgery.org or cschmieden@plasticsurgery.org
Internet: http://www.plasticsurgery.org/medical_professionals/research/Grant-Applications.cfm
Sponsor: Plastic Surgery Educational Foundation
444 E. Algonquin Road
Arlington Heights, IL 60005

Plough Foundation Grants **3061**
The foundation awards grants to nonprofit organizations in Shelby County, Tennessee, (emphasis on Memphis) for charitable purposes that will benefit the greatest number of people in the state. Areas of interest include early childhood and elementary education, crime, health care, economic development, social service agencies, housing and homelessness, and the arts. Types of support include building/renovation, capital campaigns, endowments, equipment, land acquisition, management development/capacity building, matching/challenge support, professorships, program-related investments/loans, program development, program evaluation, and seed money. Applicants should submit a brief letter of three pages or less explaining the specific project for which funds are needed and the results anticipated if the project is funded. Organizations whose projects are within the focus area will be invited to submit full proposals. The board meets in February, May, August, and November to review requests.
Requirements: Nonprofit organizations in Shelby County, TN, with particular emphasis on Memphis, may submit letters of request.
Restrictions: Funding requests are denied for annual operating expenses, individuals, and projects outside the Memphis, TN, area.
Geographic Focus: Tennessee
Amount of Grant: $1,000-$1,250,000
Date(s) Application is Due: Jan 10; Apr 10; Jul 10; Oct 10
Contact: Scott McCormick, Executive Director; fax: (901) 529-4063; email: mail@plough.org
Sponsor: Plough Foundation
62 North Main Street, Suite 201
Memphis, TN 38103

Plum Creek Foundation Grants **3062**
The corporate foundation awards grants to improve the quality of life in company operating areas. The foundation supports human services for children, at-risk youth, seniors, low-income, and abused individuals; education, particularly public and private colleges; youth organizations; hospitals, equipment, and medical programs; arts and cultural organizations; environmental education and conservation efforts; and civic affairs such as crime prevention, parks, and community development. Applications are reviewed quarterly. Application materials are available on the Web site.
Requirements: Nonprofit organizations in Alabama, Arkansas, Florida, Georgia, Idaho, Louisiana, Maine, Mississippi, Montana, North Carolina, Oklahoma, Oregon, Pennsylvania, South Carolina, Texas, Virginia, Washington, West Virginia, and Wisconsin are eligible.
Geographic Focus: Alabama; Arkansas; Florida; Georgia; Idaho; Louisiana; Maine; Mississippi; Montana; North Carolina; Oklahoma; Oregon; Pennsylvania; South Carolina; Texas; Virginia; Washington; West Virginia; Wisconsin
Amount of Grant: $1000-$10,000
Contact: Foundation Administrator, (206) 467-3600; fax: (206) 467-3799; email: foundation@plumcreek.com
Internet: http://www.plumcreek.com/community/default.php
Sponsor: Plum Creek Foundation
999 Third Avenue, Suite 4300
Seattle, WA 98104-4096

PMI Foundation Grants **3063**
The foundation awards grants nationally, with emphasis on California, to a wide range of organizations with the goal of expanding homeownership. The foundation also contributes generously to deserving causes and charities in the areas of arts, education, health organizations, human services, and youth services. There are no application deadlines. Submit an IRS determination letter, along with a description of the project and the amount of funding requested.
Requirements: Nonprofit organizations are eligible.
Amount of Grant: $50-$750,000 range
Contact: Laura Kinney, (800) 288-1970; email: pmi.contactus@pmigroup.com
Internet: http://www.pmigroup.com//careers/culture_c4_foundation.html
Sponsor: PMI Foundation
3003 Oak Road
Walnut Creek, CA 94597

PNC Charitable Trust and Foundation Grants **3064**
The PNC Charitable Trust Grant Review Committee serves over thirty perpetual charitable trusts and private foundations for which PNC is trustee. PNC's mission is to implement the legacies set forth by the individual donors who established these trust relationships with PNC. The Committee distributes grants from these charitable trusts to worthy 501c3 non-profit organizations at local and regional levels. In accordance with the provisions of the trust agreements, the Committee funds grant requests that demonstrate a capacity and commitment to charitable service and enhance the quality of life for the people and their communities.
Requirements: Before developing and submitting a full grant proposal, PNC asks that you follow these steps when applying to the Charitable Trust Grant Review Committee: Call PNC or submit a letter of inquiry. Provide a brief overview of your organization and description of your proposed project; If PNC believe's there is a potential fit between your proposed project our donors' intent and availability of funds, PNC will then invite you to submit a full grant proposal. PNC require's the use of the common grant application format that is accepted by many foundations. See PNC's website for more information. PNC's grantmaking priorities: organizations that are direct providers of services, with projects and programs that meet our donors' intent; programs in communities where donors lived and/or engaged in their grantmaking activities; currently these areas are Greater Cincinnati, Greater Philadelphia, Greater Pittsburgh, Central Pennsylvania, Washington DC, Steubenville, Ohio, and Hardin and Jefferson Counties, Kentucky; applicant demonstrates a capacity to meet the request's stated objectives; and those objectives are clearly articulated and measurable; the critical nature of the need being addressed by the proposed program; organizations with strong leadership, diversified income streams, and long-term sustainability that have demonstrated efficiencies in delivering their services. Other Considerations: PNC seeks to support projects and programs that: reflect the core social mission of the applicant's organization; address a need in the community and for which there is a demonstrated demand; have broad impact, or benefit under served populations; have measurable outcomes and a plan for documenting results; have detailed project budgets and demonstrate effective financial accountability; involve collaboration with other organizations; are of longer duration than events, conferences, or seminars; complements rather than duplicates the work of other non-profit organizations.
Restrictions: Multi-year pledges are rarely made; PNC grants are one-time events and not pledges of continued support. Size of grants depends on the fit with donors' intent, availability of funds, breadth of organizations represented in the grant proposal mix, and the project's social impact. PNC will not provide grants for: organizations that discriminate based on race, color, creed, gender, or national origin; individuals or private foundations; for-profit organizations; fraternal, political, advocacy or labor organizations; event sponsorships; general operating costs.
Geographic Focus: Delaware; Indiana; Kentucky; Maryland; New Jersey; Ohio; Pennsylvania; Washington
Date(s) Application is Due: Feb 1; May 1; Aug 1; Oct 1
Contact: Eva T. Blum, Chairperson; (412) 762-2748; fax: (412) 705-3584; email eva.blum@pnc.com
Internet: https://www.pnc.com/webapp/sec/Solutions.do?siteArea=/PNC/Home/Corporate+and+Institutional/Non-profits+and+Government+Institutions/Charitable+Trust+Grants
Sponsor: The PNC Foundation
One PNC Plaza, 249 5th Avenue, P1-P.O.PP-20-1
Pittsburgh, PA 15222

Polaroid Fund Grants Program 3065

The foundation supports nonprofit organizations whose work benefits Massachusetts communities where Polaroid operates, in particular Boston, Cambridge, Greater New Bedford, and Waltham. Within the community, the foundation invests its resources where it can make the greatest difference in helping disadvantaged children and adults to develop skills and competencies that enable them to create full and self-sufficient lives for themselves and others. Priorities include basic adult education, literacy, English as a second or other language, job training, and life skills. Types of support include matching funds, employee matching gifts, employee-related scholarships, seed money, emergency funds, scholarship funds, exchange programs, fellowships, general operating budgets, annual campaigns, capital campaigns, continuing support, equipment, loans, publications, and special projects. The foundation supports new and promising, as well as established programs. Proposals are accepted only during the months of November through July. Letters of inquiry are reviewed at any time.

Requirements: The foundation supports nonprofit organizations whose work benefits Massachusetts communities where Polaroid operates, in particular Boston, Cambridge, Greater New Bedford, and Waltham. Requests for funding should be submitted on organizational letterhead and should include a grant application, brief history of the program, description of the population served, outline of the program or project for which support is requested, annual budget for the specific project, latest audited financial statement, and a copy of the IRS tax-exemption letter. In lieu of this information, Polaroid will accept the AGM common proposal format. A request for Polaroid photographic equipment should be submitted in letter form on organizational letterhead and include an outline of the program, description of the population served, specific account of the role instant photography will play in the program, and a general statement regarding how much equipment is required. An IRS letter is not required. Organizations that qualify will be contacted directly by staff personnel.

Restrictions: The foundation does not make contributions for research or for purchasing advertisements, tables or tickets at dinners, or other functions; does not provide cameras or film for any fund-raising activities, nor for prizes, raffles, photo booths, fairs, conferences, or similar activities; and does not usually make more than one grant to an organization in any calendar year. Grants are not made to individuals.

Geographic Focus: Massachusetts

Samples: Community Economic Development Ctr of Southeastern Massachusetts (New Bedford, MA)—to maintain ongoing functioning of the computer centers and to introduce new training programs, $15,000.; Nemasket Group (Fairhaven, MA)—for a school-to-work program for students with severe disabilities, $20,000.

Amount of Grant: $10,000-$25,000 average

Date(s) Application is Due: Jun 15

Contact: Corey Davis, Grants Manager, (617) 338-2521; fax: (617) 338-1606; email: cld@tbf.org

Internet: http://www.polaroid.com/company_info/fund.jsp

Sponsor: Polaroid Fund
75 Arlington Street
Boston, MA 02116

Polk Bros. Foundation Grants 3066

The primary focus of the Foundation is programs that work with populations of need, particularly children, youth, and families—in underserved Chicago communities. Very few awards are made to organizations located outside the city of Chicago. Grants are made for both new and ongoing initiatives in four program areas: social service, education, culture and health care. In all areas, proposals should address increased access to services and improvement of the quality of life for area residents. Grants are seldom made for capital support.

Requirements: Illinois 501(c)3 nonprofit organizations are eligible. Preference is given to requests from Chicago. An organization that has not previously received a grant from the Foundation should first call the Foundation office or complete the pre-application form available on the Foundation website. The Foundation will then mail an application form or contact the organization with further questions.

Restrictions: The Polk Bros. Foundation will not support: organizations that devote a substantial portion of their activities to attempting to influence legislation or to participating in campaigns on behalf of candidates for public office; religious institutions seeking support for programs whose participants are restricted by religious affiliation or whose services promote a particular creed; purchase of dinner or raffle tickets or advertising in dinner programs; medical, scientific, or academic research; grants to individuals; tax-generating entities (municipalities, school districts, etc.) for services within their normal responsibilities. The Foundation will not consider more than one request from an organization or its affiliates in a 12-month period, nor will it generally fund more than eight percent of an organization's operating budget.

Geographic Focus: Illinois

Samples: Chicago High School for the Arts, $750,000 - general operating (2009); Advocate Illinois Masonic Medical Center, $90,000 - school-based health centers at Amundsen and Lake View High Schools (2009); Albany Park Theater Project, $80,000 - youth development through theater program (2009); America Scores Chicago, $25,000 - salary support for the education and soccer directors (2009);

Amount of Grant: $15,000 maximum small grants

Contact: Suzanne Doombos Kerbow, Asst. Director; (312) 527-4684; fax: (312) 527-4681; email: questions@polkbrosfdn.org

Internet: http://www.polkbrosfdn.org/guidelines.htm

Sponsor: Polk Bros. Foundation
20 West Kinzie Street, Suite 1110
Chicago, IL 60611

Portland General Electric Foundation Grants 3067

Portland General Electric is committed to improving the quality of life for all Oregonians. Priorities for the company's foundation are to support the concept and development of healthy families, focus resources on projects that explore and demonstrate productive and effective ways to promote a quality environment across Oregon, promote activities that highlight and celebrate cultural diversity and support for minority initiatives, and place resources in the educational system that maintain and/or strengthen the quality of education in Oregon to ensure a competent work force and prepare future leaders. Employee Volunteer grants allow an employee to apply for a $500 grant for a nonprofit organization in which he or she is actively involved. Types of support include awards, development grants, product donations, program grants, scholarships, seed money grants, and technical assistance. Applications are accepted at any time throughout the year. However, the review and approval process may take up to 90 days; be sure to apply at least three months before funds are needed.

Requirements: 501(c)3 nonprofits in Oregon are eligible.

Restrictions: The foundation does not fund: bridge grants, debt retirement or operational deficits; endowment funds; general fund drives or annual appeals; political entities, ballot measure campaigns or candidates for political office; organizations that discriminate against individuals on the basis of creed, color, gender, sexual orientation, age, religion or national origin; fraternal, sectarian and religious organizations; individuals; travel expenses; conferences, symposiums, festivals, events, team sponsorships or user fees; salaries of employees, with the exception of costs relating directly to the funded project; or capital requests that include building improvements, equipment purchases or anything considered an asset of the organization.

Geographic Focus: Oregon

Contact: Alice Chang, Contributions Coordinator, (503) 464-7618; fax: (503) 464-2929; email: Alice.Chang@pgn.com

Internet: http://www.pgefoundation.org/eligibility.html

Sponsor: Portland General Electric Foundation
121 SW Salmon Street, One World Trade Ctr, 3rd Floor
Portland, OR 97204

Posey Community Foundation Grants 3068

The Posey County Community Foundation is a nonprofit, public charity created by and for the people of Posey County, Indiana. The Foundation connects donors with the causes they care about. The Foundations discretionary grants program accepts grant proposals once a year according to the grant cycle. Proposal requirements may change from year to year; therefore, grant seekers are advised to visit The Foundations website prior to beginning the grant application process. Grants are normally given as one time support of a project but may be considered for additional support for expansions or outgrowths of an initial project. The Foundation considers proposals for grants on a yearly cycle which begins each January. At the start of each cycle, a notice is mailed or emailed to nonprofit organizations that have applied for grants in the past, have received grants in the past, or have otherwise requested notification of the start of each cycle. The requirements and instructions provided here are to be considered current and accurate only for the duration of the Foundation's grant cycle, which runs from January through May each year. Proposals will be accepted from January through the March deadline. Proposals submitted after the March deadline will not be considered. Contact the Foundations office for current deadlines.

Requirements: The Foundation welcomes proposals from nonprofit organizations that are deemed tax-exempt under sections 501(c)3 and 509(a) of the Internal Revenue Code and from governmental agencies serving the county. Proposals from nonprofit organizations not classified as a 501(c)3 public charity may be considered provided the project is charitable and supports a community need. Proposals submitted by an entity under the auspices of another agency must include a written statement signed by the agency's board president on behalf of the board of directors agreeing to act as the entity's fiscal sponsor, to receive grant monies if awarded, and to oversee the proposed project. Required Documents: Cover Sheet (see "Online Forms" at the Foundations website); Narrative addressing the following (two to four pages): project summary; funding; implementation; evaluation. Supporting Documents: The following documents are to be attached to the Cover Sheet and Narrative described above. It is important to provide ALL requested attachments and that they be labeled in the following manner: Attachment 1: Project Budget Worksheet (see website "Online Forms" page); Attachment 2: Mission statement and nondiscrimination policy; Attachment 3: Statement of qualifications of project personnel; Attachment 4: Current board roster with professional affiliations; Attachment 5: Copy of IRS determination letter establishing 501(c)3 and 509(a) status (and fiscal sponsor agreement letter, if applicable); Attachment 6: Organization's current annual operating budget; Attachment 7: Most recent financial statement (monthly, quarterly, etc.); Attachment 8: Most recent audited financial statement or completed IRS Form 990 (if available). The original and thirteen copies of the proposal must be postmarked or delivered to the Foundation office no later than 4:30 p.m. on the first Tuesday of March. Use 8 1/2 by 11 inch paper. Attach all required documents using paperclips or binder clips only (no binders or folders).

Restrictions: Project areas NOT considered for funding: religious organizations for religious purposes; political parties or campaigns; endowment creation or debt reduction; operating costs (costs that keep the organization running and the doors open, i.e., general computer software or hardware, staff salary, general office supplies or equipment, utilities, etc.); capital campaigns (Large capital projects that may take several years to complete where there is no defined area for use of the grant); annual appeals or membership contributions; travel requests for groups or individuals such as bands, sports teams, or classes. A six month progress report and a final report at project completion are required by organizations whose proposals are approved for funding. Instructions and appropriate forms will be provided at the time the grant is awarded.

Geographic Focus: Indiana
Samples: Cynthiana Area Recreation & Environmental, Inc. - to purchase wood mulch for under the playground structure at the town park, $350.00.; Mt. Vernon Band Boosters - to purchase four Euphonia for the Mt. Vernon High School Band, $2,800.00.; Posey County Sheriff Department - to purchase a narcotics dog and provide handler training, $10,000.
Contact: Julie Eickhoff, Director; (812) 838-0288; fax:(812) 838-8009; email: julie@poseycommunityfoundation.org
Internet: http://www.poseycommunityfoundation.org/disc-grants
Sponsor: Posey Community Foundation
402 Main Street, P.O. Box 746
Mt. Vernon, IN 47620

Posey Community Foundation Womens Fund Grants **3069**
The Posey County Community Foundation is a nonprofit, public charity created by and for the people of Posey County, Indiana. The Foundation connects donors with the causes they care about. The Women's Fund of Posey County grant program is used to make yearly grants to support a variety of projects or programs serving women and girls in Posey County, Indiana such as programs that prevent domestic violence, secure family supporting jobs, promote health and education, and develop confidence. The programs or projects for which funding is being requested must address the needs and opportunities which support the Fund's mission of providing opportunities, encouragement, knowledge and hope to our community's women and girls. Grant proposals are accepted once each year according to the grant cycle. Proposal requirements may change from year to year; therefore, grant seekers are advised to contact the Foundations office or visit the Foundations website prior to beginning the grant application process. Grants are normally given as one time support of a project but may be considered for additional support for expansions or outgrowths of an initial project. The Foundation considers proposals for grants on a yearly cycle which begins each June. At the start of each cycle, a notice is mailed to nonprofit organizations that have applied for grants in the past, have received grants in the past, or have otherwise requested notification of the start of each cycle, which runs from June through October each year. Proposals will be accepted from June through the July deadline. Proposals submitted after the July deadline will not be considered, contact the Foundation office for current deadline dates.
Requirements: The Women's Fund of Posey County welcomes proposals from non-profit organizations that are tax-exempt under sections 501(c)3 and 509(a) of the Internal Revenue Code and from governmental agencies serving Posey County women and girls. Proposals from other non-profit organizations to carry out charitable projects or activities that address issues facing women and girls in Posey County may be accepted. Proposals submitted by an entity under the auspices of another agency must include a written statement signed by the agency's board president on behalf of the board of directors agreeing to act as the entity's fiscal sponsor, to receive grant monies if awarded, and to oversee the proposed project. When submitting a grant proposal, include the following: cover sheet; narrative; project summary; funding; implementation; evaluation. The following documents are to be attached to the cover sheet and narrative. It is important to provide ALL requested attachments and that they be labeled in the following manner: attachment 1: project budget worksheet; attachment 2: mission statement and nondiscrimination policy; attachment 3: statement of qualifications of project personnel; attachment 4: current board roster with professional affiliations; attachment 5: copy of IRS determination letter establishing 501(c)3 and 509(a) status (and fiscal sponsor agreement letter, if applicable); attachment 6: organization's current annual operating budget; attachment 7: most recent financial statement (monthly, quarterly, etc.); attachment 8: most recent audited financial statement or completed IRS Form 990 (if available). The cover sheet form and the project budget worksheet form are provided on the Foundations website. When submitting the proposal send the original and fifteen copies. The proposal must be postmarked or delivered to the Foundation office no later than 4:30 p.m. on the fourth Tuesday in July. Use 8 1/2 by 11 inch paper. Attach all required documents using paperclips or binder clips only (no binders or folders).
Restrictions: If the grant proposal is approved, the organization is required to submit a six-month progress report and a final report at project completion. Appropriate forms will be provided.
Geographic Focus: Indiana
Samples: Posey County Steps Ahead Council, Family Matters - to purchase ten portable cribs, $1,190.00 (2008); Willow Tree of Posey County - for materials used in community outreach projects, $1,211.00 (2007); Farmersville Elementary School, Girl Power Program - which focuses on self-esteem, nutrition, careers, manners and community service-for fifth-grade girls, $1,120.00 (2007); Posey County Council on Aging - to support Tai Chi classes for aging women at Poseyville and Mt. Vernon Senior centers to help them maintain good physical and mental health, $2,350.00 (2008).
Contact: Julie Eickhoff, Director; (812) 838-0288; fax:(812) 838-8009; email: julie@poseycommunityfoundation.org
Internet: http://www.poseycommunityfoundation.org/wf-grantmaking
Sponsor: Posey Community Foundation
402 Main Street, P.O. Box 746
Mt. Vernon, IN 47620

Postdoctoral Research Fellowships in Gerontological Public Health **3070**
The Center for Research on Health and Aging (CRHA) at the university offers postdoctoral fellowships in gerontological public health. These are two- to three-year appointments sponsored by the National Institute on Aging. This program focuses on developing research skills through mentoring, a comprehensive curriculum, hands-on research experience, presentations and publications, and opportunities for grantsmanship. The goal of the program is to foster and hone the research skills of future faculty and academic researchers in health and aging. This is an integrated multidisciplinary program with academic faculty and researchers in public health, gerontology, geriatrics, epidemiology, biostatistics, psychology, sociology, disability and human development, medicine and occupational therapy. Each postdoc fellow will be matched with a mentor from the Training Program Core Faculty. This primary mentor will work with the fellow to guide and collaborate on research projects. The fellowship includes a salary, with reimbursement for health insurance and yearly travel support. Additional financial support is also available. All fellows will have office space, a computer, phone, and access to university resources through the CRHA. Applications are accepted at any time for open positions. Guidelines are available online.
Requirements: Candidates should have received (or be very close to receiving) a doctoral degree in public health, gerontology, sociology, medicine, disability studies, or a related discipline.
Amount of Grant: $35,568 per year
Contact: Dr. Thomas Prohaska, Center for Research on Health and Aging, (312) 413-9830; fax: (312) 413-9835; email: prohaska@uic.edu
Internet: http://www.uic.edu/depts/ovcr/hrpc/centers/fellow_gphpost.html
Sponsor: University of Illinois at Chicago
1747 W Roosevelt Road
Chicago, IL 60608

Pott Foundation Grants **3071**
Established in 1963 by Herman T. Pott, The Pott Foundation is a non-profit organization supporting children, education and health and human services. Most of the grant recipients are located in Herman Pott's adopted city of St. Louis, Missouri. The Foundation distributes approximately $1.5 million annually to over 100 charities.
Requirements: Non-profit 501(c)3 organization are eligible to apply in Missouri. Mail grant applications to: The Pott Foundation, C/O U.S. Bank, N.A., The Private Client Reserve, Attn: Carol Eaves, Mail Loc: SL-MO-CTCS, 10 North Hanley, Clayton, MO 63105.
Geographic Focus: Missouri
Date(s) Application is Due: Apr 1
Contact: Carol Eaves, U.S. Bank, N.A.; (314) 418-8317;
Sponsor: The Pott Foundation
10 North Hanley
Clayton, MO 63105

Potts Memorial Foundation Grants **3072**
The Potts Memorial Foundation is a private foundation, incorporated in 1922 in New York. The Foundation gives on a national and international basis. The foundation was established to provide for the care, treatment, and rehabilitation of persons afflicted with tuberculosis; support for tuberculosis eradication, including fellowship programs for physicians. Grants given for tuberculosis and related disorders.
Requirements: Application form not required, Applicants should submit a detailed description of project and amount of funding requested. Proposal must be submitted via mail.
Restrictions: No grants to individuals, or for endowment funds or matching gifts; no loans.
Samples: Johns Hopkins University, Baltimore, Maryland, $41,800 (2007); Columbia Memorial Hospital, Hudson, New York, $20,000 (2007);
Amount of Grant: $15,000 - $45,000 range
Date(s) Application is Due: Apr 15; Sep 15
Contact: Charles Inman, Secretary, (518) 828-3365
Sponsor: Potts Memorial Foundation
444 Warren Street
Hudson, NY 12534-2415

Powell Foundation Grants **3073**
The foundation's current emphasis is in the field of education in the broadest sense. Other areas of interest continue to be community service projects focused on the needs of children, the disadvantaged, the urban environment, and the visual and performing arts, especially in the greater Houston area. Special consideration will be given to those requests addressing critical and/or basic needs and/or having timing of the essence. Guidelines are available online.
Requirements: Texas tax-exempt organizations serving Harris, Walker, and Travis counties are eligible.
Restrictions: Normally, the foundation will not consider requests for building funds or grant commitments extending into successive calendar years. The foundation does not support grants to religious organizations for religious purposes; testimonial dinners, fundraising events, or advertising; other private foundations; past operating deficits or debt retirement; or individuals. Normally, the foundation will not consider requests for building funds or grant commitments extending into successive calendar years.
Geographic Focus: Texas
Samples: U of Texas at Austin (TX)—to establish an endowment for the UTeach program, which trains students to become mathematics and science teachers, $1 million.
Amount of Grant: $5000-$10,000 average
Contact: Caroline Sabin, Executive Director, (713) 523-7557; fax: (713) 523-7553; email: info@powellfoundation.org
Internet: http://www.powellfoundation.org/powellguide.htm
Sponsor: Powell Foundation
2121 San Felipe, Suite 110
Houston, TX 77019-5600

Premera CARES Grants 3074

Premera CARES supports nonprofit organizations and programs that address prevention and treatment of major diseases and health conditions that have a large impact on the residents in corporate communities including: diabetes; heart disease, stroke, heart attack, and hypertension; cancer (especially breast and colon cancer); children's health (especially immunizations, well baby checks, and routine preventive care); behavioral health; smoking cessation; osteoporosis; and special regional community health needs. Application and guidelines are available online.
Requirements: Application is open to Washington, Alaska, and Oregon 501(c)3 organizations, government agencies, and public schools or school districts (if the contribution is made for exclusively public purposes).
Restrictions: Premera CARES does not make charitable grants to religious organizations for religious purposes; for-profit organizations; organizations that discriminate against individuals based on gender, race, religion, ethnicity, sexual orientation, etc.; or individuals.
Geographic Focus: Alaska; Oregon; Washington
Contact: Juna Sexton, (907) 677-2414
Internet: https://www.premera.com/stellent/groups/public/documents/xcpproject/ak_premera_cares_giving_guidel.asp
Sponsor: Premera Blue Cross Blue Shield of Alaska
2550 Denali Street, Suite 1404
Anchorage, AK 99503

Presbyterian Health Foundation Bridge, Seed and Equipment Grants 3075

The primary objective of bridge grants is to provide funding of limited duration to enhance faculty competitiveness for national extramural funding. The seed grant program provides start-up funding for young investigators or for investigators launching into a new research direction. The equipment grants program provides the funding for laboratory equipment needed to advance research.
Requirements: Oklahoma nonprofit organizations are eligible. Submit a letter of application. Applications are due the last week in March, June, September, and December.
Restrictions: Grants are not made to individuals, private foundations, for-profit organizations or for operating funds of organizations.
Geographic Focus: Oklahoma
Samples: U of Oklahoma Health Sciences Ctr (OK)—for research on genetics, $1.2 million over two years (2003),; U of Oklahoma Health Sciences Ctr (OK)—to build the Stanton L. Young Research Center, $5 million (2003).
Amount of Grant: $25,000-$250,000 average
Contact: Michael D. Anderson, Ph.D., President, (405) 319-8150; fax: (405) 319-8168; email: manderson@phfokc.com
Internet: http://www.phfokc.com/bridge.htm
Sponsor: Presbyterian Health Foundation
655 Research Park Way, Suite 500
Oklahoma City, OK 73104-3603

Presbyterian Patient Assistance Program 3076

The goal program is to be able to provide temporary assistance in times of urgent and emergency need to patients and clinical clients and their immediate families. Funding can be used to assist with temporary medication, food, utility and housing assistance, and/or clinically-related travel. Costs, expenses and other related expenses are sometimes covered by these funds.
Requirements: Requests for funding come to the foundation via their Chaplains, social workers, case workers, and other related individuals. Each case is evaluated on an individual basis and applicants must be able to provide documentation that verifies the needs for which assistance is requested. Those having the most devastating direct impact on an patient will take precedence.
Contact: Program Coordinator, (505) 724-6580
Internet: http://www.phs.org/foundation/assistance.shtml
Sponsor: Presbyterian Healthcare Foundation
P.O. Box 26666
Albuquerque, NM 87125-6666

Priddy Foundation Grants 3077

The foundation makes grants in three geographic areas: in Texas within a 120 mile radius of Wichita Falls, in Oklahoma within a 75 mile radius of Wichita Falls, and, to a limited degree, in the Dallas/Fort Worth area. Requests for grants outside the above geographic area should provide statewide benefit. Primary grant categories include arts and culture, community enhancement, education, health, human services, and youth programs. The application process consists of a brief preliminary grant application for the purpose of policy screening. Full proposals are by request. Deadlines listed are for preliminary applications.
Requirements: 501(c)3 Texas and Oklahoma nonprofit organizations are eligible.
Restrictions: The foundation does not normally provide funding for the following: annual operating budgets on an ongoing basis, research, endowments, lobbying activities, churches or church denominations with the limited exception of certain Presbyterian-sponsored organizations, individuals, or individual scholarships.
Geographic Focus: Oklahoma; Texas
Samples: U of North Texas (TX)—to provide fellowships to students devoted to becoming leaders in the arts and music, $2.5 million over five years (2005).
Amount of Grant: $6 million total
Date(s) Application is Due: Feb 1; Aug 1
Contact: Debbie White, Grants Director, (940) 723-8720; fax: (940) 723-8656; email: debbiecw@priddyfdn.org
Internet: http://www.priddyfdn.org
Sponsor: Priddy Foundation
807 Eighth Street, Suite 1010
Wichita Falls, TX 76301-3310

Pride Foundation Grants and Scholarships 3078

The community foundation works to strengthen the lesbian, gay, transgender, and bisexual community primarily in Washington state and extending to the four neighboring states of Alaska, Idaho, Montana, and Oregon. The foundation will strive to balance funds awarded to projects in education and advocacy, AIDS education and support, arts and recreation, youth and family services, lesbian health, and other health and human services. Types of support include endowments, general operating grants, program grants, scholarships, and seed money grants. The listed application deadlines are January 13, for scholarships; and January 20, for grants. Guidelines are available online.
Requirements: IRS 501(c)3 tax-exempt organizations or organizations affiliated with tax-exempt organizations are eligible. Applicants must use foundation-supplied application form.
Geographic Focus: Alaska; Idaho; Montana; Oregon; Pacific Northwest; Washington
Samples: 25 nonprofit organizations in Alaska, Idaho, Oregon, and Washington State—for programs to benefit gay men and lesbians, including youth and family services, AIDS education, the arts, recreation, and women's health, $101,699 divided.
Amount of Grant: $5000 maximum
Date(s) Application is Due: Jan 13; Jan 20
Contact: Jeff Hedgepeth, Grants Manager, (800) 735-7287 or (206) 323-3318; fax: (206) 323-1017; email: grants@pridefoundation.org; Randy Brians, Scholarships Manager, (800) 735-7287 or (206) 323-3318; fax: (206) 323-1017; email: scholarships@pridefoundation.or
Internet: http://www.pridefoundation.org
Sponsor: Pride Foundation
1122 E Pike, Suite 1001
Seattle, WA 98122-3934

Prince Charitable Trusts Chicago Grants 3079

The trusts awards grants to eligible Chicago nonprofit organizations in its areas of interest: arts and culture, education, environment, health, and social services.
Requirements: The Trusts Chicago program only funds organizations within the city limits of Chicago (with the exception of grants made through the MacArthur Fund for Arts and Culture at Prince). The Trusts make grants only to charitable organizations that are exempt from federal income tax under Section 501(c)3 of the Internal Revenue Code and are classified as public charities under Sections 509(a)(1) or 509(a)(2). All grant applications must include a Prince Charitable Trusts cover sheet, see the Trusts website, http://foundationcenter.org/grantmaker/prince/chi_app.html for proper form and additional guidelines.
Restrictions: The Trusts do not fund projects that promote or proselytize any religion. While the Trusts do fund the projects of faith-based organizations, those projects must be secular in nature. The Trusts do not fund organizations that discriminate on the basis of ethnicity, race, color, creed, religion, gender, national origin, age, disability, marital status, sexual orientation, gender identity, or any veteran's status.
Geographic Focus: Illinois
Date(s) Application is Due: Jan 13; May 1; Jun 1
Contact: Sharon Robison, Grants Manager; (312) 419-8700; fax: (312) 419-8558; email: srobison@prince-trusts.org
Internet: http://www.fdncenter.org/grantmaker/prince/chicago.html
Sponsor: Prince Charitable Trusts
303 West Madison Street, Suite 1900
Chicago, IL 60606

Prince Charitable Trusts District of Columbia Grants 3080

The trusts awards grants to eligible Washington D.C. nonprofit organizations in its areas of interest: arts and culture, community, environment, health, emergency services, youth and provide a limited number of capital grants each year.
Requirements: The Trusts make grants only to charitable organizations that are exempt from federal income tax under Section 501(c)3 of the Internal Revenue Code and are classified as public charities under Sections 509(a)(1) or 509(a)(2). Electronic proposals are preferred. Attachments may be mailed separately. Proposals should include the Prince Charitable Trust Grant Application Cover Sheet and the Common Grant Application Format of Washington Grantmakers. These forms and additional guidelines may be obtained at the Trusts website, http://foundationcenter.org/grantmaker/prince/dc_app.html.
Restrictions: The Trusts do not make grants to individuals, nor does it fund projects that promote or proselytize any religion. While the Trusts do fund the projects of faith-based organizations, those projects must be secular in nature.
Geographic Focus: District of Columbia
Amount of Grant: $10,000-$30,000 average
Date(s) Application is Due: Feb 1; Sep 1; Aug 10;
Contact: Kristin Pauly, Managing Director; (202) 728-0646; fax: (202) 466-4726; email: kpauly@princetrusts.org
Internet: http://www.fdncenter.org/grantmaker/prince/dc_interest.html
Sponsor: Prince Charitable Trusts
816 Connecticut Avenue, NW
Washington, DC 20006

Princeton Area Community Foundation Greater Mercer Grants 3081

The Greater Mercer Grants Program is a competitive program for projects benefiting residents of Mercer County, New Jersey, and the immediately adjoining areas of surrounding counties. There are three distinct categories. In addressing the needs of low-income individuals and families (Category 1), grants up to $15,000 are made to nonprofit organizations only. In support of community organizing in low-income neighborhoods (Category 2), grants of $500 to $20,000 are made to 501(c)3 nonprofit organizations, neighborhood associations, and groups of residents forming a neighborhood association to work on a project. And in support of building community within and among municipalities (Category 3), grants generally range from $10,000 to $35,000, but may be as much as $50,000, made to nonprofit organizations only.
Requirements: Nonprofit organizations that have tax-exempt status under Section 501(c)3 of the Internal Revenue Code are eligible. They must be registered with the State of New Jersey as a charity, unless they are religious organizations, or schools that file their curricula with the Department of Education and are exempt from the provisions of the New Jersey Charitable Registration and Investigation Act.
Restrictions: Nonprofits may submit one application per calendar year in each category, for a maximum of three. Neighborhood associations or groups of residents who will form a neighborhood association may apply only once annually for a Community Organizing in Low-Income Neighborhoods grant.
Geographic Focus: New Jersey
Samples: Trenton Film Society, $15,000— expansion of Year-Round Trenton Film Society Programming (2008); Rescue Mission of Trenton, $10,000—job training program for Rescue Mission residents (2008); Womanspace, $10,000— Womanspace Non-Denominational Chaplaincy Program to provide faith-based resources to victims of domestic violence and sexual assault to "meet the victim where they are at" if that meeting point is their faith (2008).
Amount of Grant: $500-$35,000 range
Contact: Deborah Thomas, Director of Grants & Programs; (609) 219-1800; fax: (609) 219-1850; email: daubert-thomas@pacf.org
Internet: http://www.pacf.org/grants/polCalendarEvent.cfm?Program_Code=12
Sponsor: Princeton Area Community Foundation
15 Princess Road
Lawrenceville, NJ 08648

Principal Financial Group Foundation Grants 3082

The foundation addresses concerns in the areas of health and human services, education, arts and culture, environment, and recreation and tourism. The primary objective is to support, through charitable contributions, selected nonprofit organizations primarily located in the greater Des Moines, IA, area. The foundation also will consider requests from organizations located in areas where the corporation has offices, including Des Moines, Mason City and Cedar Falls, IA; Grand Island, NE; Spokane, WA; Wilmington, DE; Appleton, WI; and Phoenix, AZ. The objectives, priorities, and programs seek to reflect the needs and concerns of communities in which the corporation operates. Support is given for annual campaigns, building funds, capital campaigns, continuing support, employee matching gifts, in-kind gifts, performances and exhibitions, conferences and workshops, adult basic education, vocational programs, operating budgets, internships, demonstration grants, matching grants, and seed grants. Contribution requests are considered on a quarterly basis, in accordance with the following schedule: health and human services, March 1; education, June 1; arts and culture, September 1; and environment, recreation, and tourism, December 1.
Requirements: 501(c)3 tax-exempt organizations in company operating locations may apply.
Restrictions: Proposals for athletic groups, conferences, endowments, fellowships, festivals, fraternal organizations, health care facility fund drives, libraries, or religious groups are denied.
Geographic Focus: Delaware; Iowa; Nebraska; Washington
Amount of Grant: $1000-$50,000 average
Date(s) Application is Due: Mar 1; Jun 1; Sep 1; Dec 1
Contact: Laura Sauser, Community Investment Consultant, (515) 247-7227; fax: (515) 246-5475
Internet: http://www.principal.com/about/giving/grant.htm
Sponsor: Principal Financial Group Foundation Inc
711 High Street
Des Moines, IA 50392-0150

Procter and Gamble Fund Grants 3083

The fund supports nonprofit organizations in company-operating locations in the areas of education, health and social services, civic projects, cultural organizations, disaster relief, and environmental efforts. Grants are awarded to education initiatives in local communities, such as teacher training efforts, with a focus on economic teaching; and other efforts by public policy, research, and economic education organizations. Employee voluntarism is prevalent in many K-12 initiatives. Most health and human services funding supports the United Way. The Salvation Army, Red Cross, hospitals, food banks, and other social service organizations receive support. Community support is awarded through grants that bolster economic growth and enrichment, including support for a youth jobs program, libraries, zoos, and local chambers of commerce. Support is awarded to a variety of arts organizations, including theater, dance, music, and visual arts. Major environmental groups also receive support. Grant Application Cycles are July 1 through September 30 and December 1 through February 28, grant requests are only accepted during those times.
Requirements: 501(c)3 organizations in communities where Procter and Gamble Company manufacturing plants are located are eligible.
Amount of Grant: $25 million total
Contact: Brenda Ratliff, Administrator, Corporate Philanthropy; (513) 945-8454; fax: (513) 945-5211; email: pgfund.im@pg.com
Internet: http://www.pg.com/company/our_commitment/grant_application_guidelines.shtml
Sponsor: Procter and Gamble Fund
P.O. Box 599
Cincinnati, OH 45201

Progress Energy Foundation Grants 3084

The foundation partners with nonprofits in Florida, North Carolina, and South Carolina to improve the lives of Progress Energy's customers. Grants focus on education, the environment, economic development and employee involvement. Education grants support K-12 teacher quality, math and science, and principal and superintendent leadership development (February 1 deadline); and scholarships to institutions of higher education that support the company's recruiting strategy (November 1 deadline). Environment grants support projects that protect or improve water quality through the restoration, enhancement, and preservation of riparian lands (August 1 deadline). Economic Development grants support major community initiatives that support the company's economic development plans (May 1 deadline). Employee Involvement grants provide funding for nonprofits selected for the Employee Giving Campaign or programs in which there is substantial employee involvement. Nonprofit organizations providing services to Progress Energy customers in the focus areas are encouraged to contact a contributions specialist to discuss funding opportunities.
Requirements: Tax-exempt organizations in Florida and North and South Carolina may apply.
Geographic Focus: Florida; North Carolina; South Carolina
Samples: Western North Carolina Economic Development Commission (Fletcher, NC)—general operating support (2004); Cary Academy (Carey, NC)—funding for a summer technology course for K-12 teachers (2004); U of Florida (Gainesville, FL)—for College of Engineering scholarships, and lab renovation (2004); Wilmington Children's Museum (NC)—funding for science education area in new museum facility (2004).
Amount of Grant: $9.7 million total; $10,000-$100,000 average
Date(s) Application is Due: Feb 1; May 1; Aug 1; Nov 1
Contact: Deborah Shipley, Florida, (727) 820-5348; Merrilee Jacobson, North Carolina/South Carolina, (919) 546-6441
Internet: http://www.progress-energy.com/community
Sponsor: Progress Energy Foundation
P.O. Box 2591
Raleigh, NC 27602-1551

Prospect Burma Scholarships 3085

By funding education for young Burmese, Prospect Burma seeks to help create a cadre of Burmese who will be competent to run the country once democracy returns. Its aim is to educate those who will bring their knowledge and skills back to Burma for its future development. Preference is given to applicants studying one of the following subjects: Agriculture; Civil Society; Development; Ecology/Conservation; Economics; Education/Teacher Training; Engineering; Human Rights; Nursing; Public Administration; Public Health; or Science subjects. Preference is also given to students at educational institutions in South-East Asia or South Asia.
Requirements: You may qualify for an award if you are of Burmese origin and have been accepted for, or enrolled in a degree course at an accredited college or university, and are: accepted for and/or enrolled in a first degree (undergraduate) course at a college or university; already studying, or accepted for, a Master's degree course; or a postgraduate student who has already started on a Doctorate, or has a confirmed offer of a place to read for a Doctorate.
Restrictions: The Program does not contribute to international travel, computer equipment or debts. Furthermore, it does not make a contribution to the costs of dependants (spouses, partners, children).
Date(s) Application is Due: Mar 31
Contact: Shona Kirkwood, Education Project Coordinator; email: bpeoshona@gmail.com; Ian C Sloane, Executive Director, (44) (0) 207 371 0887; email: scholarships@prospectburma.org
Internet: http://www.prospectburma.org/index.php?option=com_content&task=category&sectionid=5&id=18&Itemid=39
Sponsor: Prospect Burma
Rivermead Court, Ranelagh Gardens
London SW6 3SF England

Prostate Cancer Foundation Research Grants 3086

The heart of the Prostate Cancer Foundation's effort to to find better treatments and a cure for recurrent prostate cancer is its research awards programs. Each year, the PCF invests millions of dollars in research projects that have the greatest potential to advance the fight against prostate cancer. The PCF's research awards program has three components: Competitive Awards, Special Awards and Donor-Directed Awards. The foundation favors research applications focused on translational and clinical programs with potential for near term benefit for patients with recurrent prostate cancer. The listed application deadline is for competitive awards. Application guidelines and form are available online.
Requirements: Applications from individuals with or without institutional affiliations will be considered.

Restrictions: For-profit organizations or government agencies are not eligible for consideration.
Amount of Grant: $25,000-$100,000
Date(s) Application is Due: Dec 2
Contact: Grants Administrator, (310) 570-4700; fax: (310) 570-4701
Internet: http://www.prostatecancerfoundation.org/site/pp.asp?c=itIWK2OSG&b=68790
Sponsor: Prostate Cancer Foundation
1250 Fourth Street, Suite 360
Santa Monica, CA 90401

Prudential Foundation Grants **3087**

The foundation's areas of interest are ready-to-learn programs, ready-to-work programs, and ready-to-live programs. Grants support programs in the areas of business and economic research; education; health; public affairs; conservation and ecology; cultural activities; urban and community affairs; research and professional training in long-term health care and family care; job creation, employment of the elderly, and welfare-to-work programs; building and equipment needs; programs for children and youth; and assistance to minorities. Types of support include operating support, continuing support, annual campaigns, seed money, matching funds and employee matching gifts, consulting services, technical assistance, employee-related scholarships, research, capital campaigns, conferences and seminars, and projects/programs. The foundation is especially interested in proposals that anticipate and address potential major problems. Funds are targeted to areas where Prudential has a strong presence. Applicant should make initial contact with a brief letter to determine whether a more detailed proposal would be acceptable. Applications are available on the web site.
Requirements: Tax-exempt nonprofit organizations are eligible. Priority in order of preference goes to programs in Newark and surrounding communities; Los Angeles, CA; Jacksonville, FL; Atlanta, GA: Minneapolis, MN; Philadelphia, PA; and Houston, TX. Third priority are national programs that can be implemented or replicated in the above cities.
Geographic Focus: Arizona; California; Florida; Georgia; Minnesota; New Jersey; Pennsylvania; Texas
Samples: National Governors Assoc (Washington, DC)—for efforts to create and implement ways to improve high school-graduation and college-preparedness rates in 13 states, $1 million; For relief efforts in South Asia and Africa, $1 million.
Amount of Grant: $27.6 million total
Contact: Foundation Director; (973) 802-4791; email: community.resources@prudential.com
Internet: http://www.prudential.com/view/page/public/12154
Sponsor: Prudential Foundation
751 Broad Street, 15th Floor
Newark, NJ 07102-3777

PSG Mentored Clinical Research Awards **3088**

The Mentored Clinical Research Award (MCRA) for new investigators is funded by a grant from the Parkinson's Disease Foundation (PDF) to the Parkinson Study Group (PSG). The PDF has partnered with the PSG to encourage the professional and scientific development of young investigators on their path to independence. To this end, this grant will support a new investigator for a one year project in patient oriented research in Parkinson's disease or other parkinsonian disorders under the mentorship of an experienced investigator. The training should lead a junior investigator to gain skills in clinical research. The research plan should address unmet needs of people living with PD, have the potential for broad application among the PD community, and lead to advances in clinically relevant treatment options. An award of $75,000 will be available this year. An electronic copy of the proposal in Microsoft Word or pdf-format must be received by the PSG on or before Friday, March 26. Applications should be sent by email to: Roseanna.Battista@ctcc.rochester.edu with a cover note that includes the candidate's name and the title of proposal. The candidate's proposal should be formatted according to the guidelines indicated in the "toolkit" available on the PSG website http://www.parkinson-study- group.org/PSGToolkit.asp. Applicants will be notified of the results of these reviews by May 21.
Requirements: Appropriate applicants for the MCRA are clinicians and scientists who are within 5 years of having completed formal training (this includes PhD professionals working in the field of Parkinson's disease). Fellows may apply. See website for additional guidelines.
Amount of Grant: $75,000
Date(s) Application is Due: Mar 26
Contact: Karl Kieburtz, PSG Chair; email: karl.kieburtz@ctcc.rochester.edu;; Roseanna Battista, PSG Mentoring Committee Administrator; roseanna.battista@ctcc.rochester.edu
Internet: http://www.parkinson-study-group.org/Resources/PSG%20SRC%20Mentored%20Clinical%20Research%20Award%20RFP%202010-2011%20FINAL.pdf
Sponsor: Parkinson Study Group
c/o Karl Kieburtz, MD, MPH, University of Rochester, 1351 Mt. Hope Avenue, Suite 223
New York, NY 14620

Public Welfare Foundation Grants **3089**

Grants are awarded primarily to grassroots organizations in the United States and abroad, with emphasis on the environment, disadvantaged elderly and youth, population and reproductive health, economic development, welfare reform, health, human rights and global security, criminal justice, and community development. Programs must serve low-income populations, with preference to short-term needs. Types of support include matching funds, operating budgets, seed money, continuing support, and special projects. Grant guidelines are available upon request. Proposal with cover letter should be addressed to the Steering Committee at the address listed.
Requirements: Nonprofit organizations and, in certain cases, organizations without 501(c)3 status, may apply for grant support. Eligible exceptions are listed in the guidelines (available upon request).
Restrictions: Grants will not be made to individuals or for religious purposes, building funds, capital improvements, endowments, scholarships, graduate work, foreign study, conferences, seminars, publications, research, workshops, consulting services, annual campaigns, or deficit financing.
Samples: Fair Housing Agency of Alabama (Mobile, AL)—to provide temporary and long-term housing and other support to people in Mobile, AL, left homeless by Hurricane Katrina, $10,000 (2005); Louisiana Bucket Brigade (Baton Rouge, LA)—to train people to monitor environmental pollution in their neighborhoods, $25,000 (2005); Share Foundation (San Francisco, CA)—to provide relief and support for reconstruction efforts in El Salvador following Hurricane Stan, $25,000 (2005); Environmental Support Ctr (Washington, DC)—to provide small grants to environmental justice groups in the Gulf Coast region that are struggling to reestablish their programs in the wake of recent hurricanes, $75,000 (2005).
Amount of Grant: $25,000-$50,000 average
Contact: Grants Administrator, (202) 965-1800; fax: (202) 265-8851; email: reviewcommittee@publicwelfare.org
Internet: http://www.publicwelfare.org/about/about.asp
Sponsor: Public Welfare Foundation
1200 U St NW
Washington, DC 20009

Puerto Rico Community Foundation Grants **3090**

The foundation seeks to contribute to the achievement of a healthier economy and enhance the quality of life in Puerto Rico. Grants are awarded in the areas of economic development, education, the elderly, community development, science and technological innovation, health (including AIDS programs and drug and alcohol abuse), arts and cultural activities (including dance and fine arts), criminal justice, agriculture, animal welfare, and civic affairs. Types of support include general operating support, emergency funds, conferences and seminars, professorships, publications, research, technical assistance, consulting services, and matching funds. There are no application deadlines; the board meets in March, June, September, and December to consider requests.
Requirements: Grants are awarded to nonprofits in Puerto Rico.
Restrictions: The foundation does not make grants to support individuals, annual campaigns, seed money, endowments, deficit financing, scholarships, or building funds.
Geographic Focus: Puerto Rico
Samples: La Fondita de Jesus (PR)—for development of a housing project for homeless people, $20,000.; Taller de Arte y Cultura (Adjuntas, PR)—for computer equipment, $5000.
Amount of Grant: $1.45 million total
Contact: Administrator, (787) 721-1037; fax: (787) 721-1673; email: fcpr@fcpr.org
Internet: http://www.fcpr.org/english/solicitadonativo.htm
Sponsor: Puerto Rico Community Foundation
P.O. Box 70362
San Juan 00936-8362
Puerto Rico

Pulaski County Community Foundation Grants **3091**

The Pulaski County Community Foundation was established in 1994 and serves the citizens of Pulaski County, Indiana. The Pulaski County Community Foundation welcomes grant requests from any nonprofit organization in Pulaski County. The Foundation also invites applications to help fund new organizations who seek to meet demonstrated needs or to benefit the community through creative and innovative projects and programs. Grants are made only to organizations that serve the Pulaski County area. Grant seekers may call the Foundation office to speak with a staff member prior to writing a grant proposal. This will allow the applicant to explain the nature of the grant request and obtain an application.
Requirements: The Foundation will generally favor grant requests which: impact a substantial number of people in our community; propose practical solutions to current problems or address a current community interest; examine and address underlying causes of local needs; encourage cooperation and elimination of duplicate services; build the capacity of the applying organization; are from established agencies tax exempt under Section 501 (c)(3) of the IRS Code.
Restrictions: As a general rule, the Foundation does not make grants from its discretionary funds for the following: ongoing operating expenses or annual fund raising drives; existing obligations, debt reduction or building campaigns; individuals or travel expenses; loans or endowments; political purposes. Grantees are required to complete a Final Report (program and financial) detailing how the grant funds were spent.
Geographic Focus: Indiana
Date(s) Application is Due: Mar 18
Contact: Wendy Rose, Executive Director; (574) 946-0906; fax: (574) 946-0971; email: wrose@pulaskionline.org
Internet: http://pccf.pulaskionline.org/content/view/47/66/
Sponsor: Pulaski County Community Foundation, Inc.
127 E. Pearl Street, P.O. Box 407
Winamac, IN 46996

Pulte Homes Corporate Contributions **3092**
The charitable giving program is committed to addressing the life challenges facing individuals and families by partnering with organizations that have a significant positive impact on the future of society. Pulte's focus is in four primary categories: housing—funds are allocated for this category through 2006; education—major capital improvements or professorship endowments to improve programs targeted toward the residential homebuilding industry at U.S. universities; environmental—sustainable conservation projects or major initiatives to improve the environment; and health and human services. In the health and human services category, requests for funds benefiting the metropolitan Detroit area will be considered at the listed office location. Requests for funds for other geographic areas should be forwarded to the local Pulte market office. Guidelines and application are available online.
Requirements: 501(c)3 tax-exempt organizations are eligible.
Restrictions: Grants do not support individuals (except for residential homebuilding-industry scholarships); organizations that discriminate on the basis of race, religion, ethnicity, sexual preference, or other unlawful classification; or religious, fraternal, or veterans' organizations unless they benefit the community at large. Appeals for unrestricted funds or for organizations that distribute funds to other charities will not be considered.
Amount of Grant: $50,000 minimum education grant; $25,000 minimum environmental grant
Contact: Charitable Giving Administrator, (248) 433-4534
Internet: http://www.pulte.com/about_us/contributions_missionstatement.asp?ss={4F1CC3DE-CDDA-4CA2-BBE7-800009464021}
Sponsor: Pulte Homes Corporation
100 Bloomfield Hills Pkwy, Suite 300
Bloomfield Hills, MI 48304

Putnam County Community Foundation Grants **3093**
The Putnam County Community Foundation is a nonprofit public charity established in 1985 to administer funds, award grants and provide leadership, enriching the quality of life and strengthening community in Putnam County. The Community Foundation administers more than 174 funds for donors supporting a variety of charitable activities. Three types of grants offered include: community grants, non-profit endowment building grants, and youth philanthropy grants. Types of support include: building renovation; consulting services; income development; matching/challenge support; program-related investments/loans; program development; scholarship funds; seed money; and technical assistance. The first funding cycle has a preliminary grant application due date of February 1, with full grants due by March 9; the second funding cycle has a preliminary grant application due date of August 1, with full grants due by September 9.
Requirements: A final report is due at the time of project completion. Unless other arrangements are made, it is expected that projects will be completed within one year of the grant award.
Restrictions: In general, grants from the Community Grants Program will not be awarded for the following: individuals; ongoing operational expenses (salaries, rent, and utilities); projects that do not serve Putnam County citizens; projects normally fully funded by units of government; projects to build or fund an endowment; religious activities or programs that appear to serve one denomination and not the community at large; political organizations or campaigns; national and state-wide fund raising projects; projects that could be considered discriminatory; projects operated by for-profit companies; or projects requesting retroactive funding.
Geographic Focus: Indiana
Date(s) Application is Due: Feb 1; Mar 9; Aug 1; Sep 9
Contact: M. Elaine Peck, Executive Director; (765) 653-4978; fax: (765) 653-6385; email: epeck@pcfoundation.org or info@pcfountation.org
Internet: http://www.pcfoundation.org/grant_what_we_fund.html
Sponsor: Putnam County Community Foundation
2 South Jackson Street, P.O. Box 514
Greencastle, IN 46135

Quality Health Foundation Grants **3094**
The foundation's focus is on programs that demonstrate improved health care delivery, quality, and outcomes from a consumer's perspective. Priority areas include improved treatment through the use of best practices; improved access to health care services; and improved communication of health knowledge. Types of projects might include promotion of healthy lifestyles and quality of life; promotion of culturally and linguistically appropriate care; promotion of consumer-centered care and decision-making; improvements in dissemination of health-related information; promotion of patient safety; promotion of best practices; and programs that reach underserved populations (rural, homeless, uninsured, etc.). The foundation supports projects of many types, including service demonstrations and rapid cycle change projects that have the potential to produce high impacts on health outcomes. Grants are awarded annually, for a one-year timeframe. Projects may apply each year for continued funding.
Requirements: Applicants must be from Maryland or the District of Columbia, where Delmarva is the Quality Improvement Organization (QIO) for the area. All organizations must be committed to improving the health of individuals at the community level. Examples of organizations that may apply for funding include faith-based, nonprofit, government, hospital/provider, and educational.
Restrictions: The foundation will not fund reimbursable direct patient-care services; individuals; ongoing operating expenses; capital expenses; lobbying; fundraising activities; or conferences (unless associated with an approved grant).
Geographic Focus: District of Columbia; Maryland
Amount of Grant: $50,000 maximum
Date(s) Application is Due: Jan 15
Contact: Mariana Lesher, (410) 763-6227; email: lesherm@dfmc.org
Internet: http://www.qualityhealthfoundation.org/html/How_to.html
Sponsor: Delmarva Foundation
9240 Centreville Road
Easton, MD 21601

Quantum Corporation Snap Server Grants **3095**
The Snap Server Donation program focuses its charitable efforts on increasing access to storage technology by supporting organizations in the areas of human services and civic development. Quantum makes grants of storage appliances to nonprofit organizations worldwide. Its goal is to help bring the benefits of storage technology to people and their communities, to provide support to the communities in which its employees live, and to support its employees by taking an active role in their community. Snap Server donations are focused on youth organizations, local community programs, science and technology organizations, and humanitarian causes.
Geographic Focus: California
Contact: Sean Lamb, Manager of Public Relations; (408) 879-8776; fax: (408) 371-1783; email: sean.lamb@quantum.com
Internet: http://www.quantum.com
Sponsor: Quantum Corporation
2001 Logic Drive
San Jose, CA 95035

Quantum Foundation Grants **3096**
The foundation makes grants to approved charitable organizations, as well as state and local governmental entities, serving Palm Beach County, Florida, in the areas of health—improving access to insurance, health care, and prevention programs and reforming the health care delivery system; education—early childhood development, along with academic and career achievement for K-12 students; and community betterment (by invitation only)—promoting diversity, helping special needs populations, reducing family violence, and reducing child abuse and neglect. Types of support include capital grants, challenge/matching grants, program development grants, and seed money grants. Submit concept papers before full proposals.
Requirements: Nonprofits serving West Palm Beach, Florida, are eligible.
Geographic Focus: Florida
Contact: Christine Koehn, Ph.D., Vice President for Programs; (561) 832-7497; fax: (561) 832-5794; email: chrisk@quantumfnd.org
Internet: http://www.quantumfnd.org
Sponsor: Quantum Foundation
2701 North Australian Avenue, Suite 200
West Palm Bach, FL 33407

Questar Corporate Contributions Grants **3097**
The corporation funds health and social services in the West, including some parts of Colorado, Oklahoma, Utah, and Wyoming. Grants have been awarded to hospitals, especially to build emergency rooms; substance abuse prevention programs, especially in the schools; child abuse prevention programs; and HIV/AIDS prevention and care. Questar determines the size of the grants based on the number of its employees in its facilities in the area, as well as how many other organizations of the same type it has funded nearby. Requests should be submitted in writing and describe the problem, outline the project, and state the amount sought. Applications are accepted at any time.
Requirements: Nonprofits in the West are eligible.
Geographic Focus: Colorado; Oklahoma; Utah; West; Wyoming
Amount of Grant: $5000 maximum small grants; $10,000-$20,000 large grants
Contact: Jan Bates, Questar Community Affairs; (801) 324-5132 or (801) 324-5202; email: Jan.Bates@Questar.com
Internet: http://www.questar.com/about_us/community/contributions.html
Sponsor: Questar Corporation
P.O. Box 45433, Mailstop QB 811 or 180 East 100 South
Salt Lake City, UT 84145-0433

R.C. Baker Foundation Grants **3098**
The foundation makes grants to U.S. nonprofit organizations for projects and programs that support social services for youth and the elderly, crime prevention, education, religion (Christian, Episcopal, Friends, Jewish, Methodist, and Presbyterian), scientific research, culture, and health. Support will be provided for fellowships and scholarships, general operating grants, challenge/matching grants, emergency funds, building funds, equipment, continuing support, annual campaigns, capital campaigns, renovation projects, and special projects. Submit cover letter with proposal. The board meets in June and November to consider requests.
Requirements: Nonprofit organizations are eligible. $25,000 to
Geographic Focus: West
Samples: Anaheim Memorial Medical Center, Anaheim, CA - $40,000 (2006); Harvey Mudd College, Claremont, CA - $25,000 (2006);
Amount of Grant: $1000-$280,000 average
Date(s) Application is Due: May 1; Oct 1
Contact: Frank Scott, Chairman, (714) 750-8987
Sponsor: R.C. Baker Foundation
P.O. Box 6150
Orange, CA 92863-6150

RACGP Cardiovascular Research Grants in General Practice **3099**
Individual grants of up to $25,000 will be offered for a period of one year to fund projects investigating various aspects of cardiovascular disease including hypertension, stroke, lipid disorder, health promotion and lifestyle changes. The Cardiovascular Research Grants (CVRGs) in General Practice are a joint initiative of the RACGP and the Australian Association of Academic General Practice (AAAGP).
Requirements: To be eligible for the Cardiovascular Research Grants, the chief investigator must be a GP or GP registrar who is a member of the RACGP or the AAAGP. New and emerging researchers are particularly encouraged to apply.
Restrictions: Unless otherwise indicated, Grants must be used in the year for which they are awarded. Grants will be paid only to incorporated bodies that have an ABN and ACN and not to individuals. By applying for a Grant each applicant will be taken to have consented to permit the RACGP to publicise their name, institution, and title of their research project.
Amount of Grant: $25,000 maximum
Date(s) Application is Due: May 8
Contact: Samantha Fernandes, Research and Grants Program Administrator, phone: 03-8699-0496; fax: 03-8699-0400; email: research@racgp.org.au
Internet: http://www.racgp.org.au/researchfoundation/awards/cvrg
Sponsor: Royal Australian College of General Practitioners
College House, 1 Palmerston Crescent
South Melbourne VIC 3205 Australia

RACGP National Asthma Council Research Award **3100**
The Award is awarded annually by the National Asthma Council to the best presenter of an asthma related abstract or poster at the RACGP Annual Scientific Convention. The award is to the value of $500 and is presented at the closing ceremony.
Requirements: To be eligible for the award, an individual must be: a GP or GP registrar; a member of the RACGP; in the early stages of their research career; presenting an asthma-related paper or poster at the RACGP Annual Scientific Conference, and; a major contributor to the research study being presented.
Restrictions: By applying each applicant will be taken to have consented to permit RACGP to publicise their name, their institution, and the title of their research project.
Amount of Grant: $500
Date(s) Application is Due: Sep 1
Contact: Samantha Fernandes, Research and Grants Program Administrator, phone: 03-8699-0496; fax: 03-8699-0400; email: research@racgp.org.au
Internet: http://www.racgp.org.au/researchfoundation/awards/nac
Sponsor: Royal Australian College of General Practitioners
College House, 1 Palmerston Crescent
South Melbourne VIC 3205 Australia

RACGP Vicki Kotsirilos Integrative Medicine Grants **3101**
The Vicki Kotsirilos Integrative Medicine Grant is to encourage research that assists the integration of safe and ethical forms of natural and complementary medicines or therapies into mainstream general practice. The Grant is designed to encourage research that assists the integration of safe and ethical forms of natural and complementary medicines or therapies into mainstream general practice. A Grant of up $5,000 is offered to applicants conducting general practice research in the following areas: clinical research that contributes to the knowledge base concerning the efficacy of natural and complementary medicines or therapies; any project that supports research in behavioural and lifestyle factors impacting on health eg. diet, exercise, stress management, and; research that contributes to the efficient dissemination of the evidence regarding integrative medicine.
Requirements: Applicants must be: a General Practitioner or General Practice Registrar, and; a member of the RACGP.
Restrictions: Unless otherwise indicated, the Grant must be used in the year for which it is awarded. The Grant will be paid only to incorporated bodies that have an ABN and ACN and not to individuals. By applying for the Grant each applicant will be taken to have consented to permit the RACGP to publicise their name, institution, and title of their research project.
Amount of Grant: $5,000
Date(s) Application is Due: May 8
Contact: Samantha Fernandes, Research and Grants Program Administrator, phone: 03-8699-0496; fax: 03-8699-0400; email: research@racgp.org.au
Internet: http://www.racgp.org.au/researchfoundation/awards/kotsirilos
Sponsor: Royal Australian College of General Practitioners
College House, 1 Palmerston Crescent
South Melbourne VIC 3205 Australia

Rainbow Endowment Grants **3102**
Once a year, the Rainbow Endowment invites non-profit organizations having a national impact on the LGBT community to submit a request for funding. The proposals are reviewed by the Endowment's Grant Committee, which makes funding recommendations to the Board of Directors. The endowment supports national efforts to encourage positive physical and mental health; promote increased visibility; and advance full participation and access to social, cultural, and civic life for the gay and lesbian community. The Endowment seeks to support LGBT organizations whose efforts are national in scope in the areas of health and community. Priority is given to efforts that have practical implications or applications. In the area of health, grants are made to promote awareness of gay and lesbian mental and physical health issues among consumers and health care providers; to advocate for and develop public policy for equal health care treatment or equal access to health care treatment; and to advocate for and develop public policy to prevent further HIV/AIDS infection and to improve the lives of people with HIV/AIDS. In the area of community, grants are made to protect lesbian and gay rights; promote coalitions that work to strengthen advocacy efforts to improve conditions for lesbians and gays; and to develop policies that benefit lesbian and gay youth and the children of lesbian and gay families. Proposals can be submitted at anytime; however, they are reviewed only once per year. The deadline is the third Friday in May.
Requirements: U.S. nonprofit 501(c)3 organizations are eligible to apply.
Restrictions: The endowment does not support direct services, state or local projects, government agencies, individuals, regularly held meetings, fund-raising events, K-12 schools, religious purposes, endowments, or capital projects. Organizations may not apply more than once each calendar year.
Amount of Grant: $5,000-$20,000 range
Contact: Jean E. Bochnowski, Executive Director; (215) 241-7280; fax: (215) 241-7278; email: jeb35@aol.com or endowment@rainbowcard.com
Internet: http://www.rainbowendowment.org/what.html
Sponsor: Rainbow Endowment
1501 Cherry Street
Philadelphia, PA 19102-1403

Rainbow Fund Grants **3103**
The Trust was established in 1954 in Georgia. Giving is primarily focused on theological education and other Christian endeavors. Support is also offered for substance abuse treatment and music education through mentoring high school students and conservatory musicians. There are no specific guidelines or application forms, and potential applicants are advised to contact the office directly.
Requirements: Eligible applicants from Florida, Georgia, Kentucky, Mississippi, and Texas can apply.
Geographic Focus: Florida; Georgia; Kentucky; Mississippi; Texas
Samples: Wesley Biblical Center, Jackson, Mississippi, $2,000,000—for theology instruction (2007); Champions for Life, Duncanville, Texas, $50,000—for prison ministry (2007).
Amount of Grant: $25,000-$2,000,000
Contact: Burton S. Luce, Manager; (954) 764-7724; fax: (954) 764-3603; email: lluce@drmail.com
Sponsor: Rainbow Fund
2408 Sunrise Key Boulevard
Fort Lauderdale, FL 33304

Rajiv Gandhi Foundation Grants **3104**
The foundation conducts activities in India in the areas of the arts and humanities, conservation and the environment, economic affairs, education, international affairs, law and human rights, medicine and health, science and technology, and social welfare. Main projects are concerned with literacy and primary education, empowering women and children, aid for the disabled, health care services in rural and poor urban areas, and decentralized government. Types of support include research grants to institutions and scholarships, fellowships, and prizes to individuals.
Contact: Jawahar Bhawan, Director; (091-11) 23755117 or (091-11) 23312456; fax: (091-11) 23755119; email: info@rgfindia.com
Internet: http://www.rgfindia.com
Sponsor: Rajiv Gandhi Foundation
Dr. Rajendra Prasad Road
New Delhi 110 001
India

Ralph F. Hirschmann Award in Peptide Chemistry **3105**
This award, supported by Merck Research Laboratories, is given annually to recognize and encourage outstanding achievements in the chemistry, biochemistry, and biophysics of peptides. The award is granted without regard to age or nationality of the recipient. The award consists of $5,000 and a certificate. Up to $2,500 for travel expenses to the meeting at which the award will be presented will be reimbursed.
Requirements: Any individual, except a member of the award committee, may submit one nomination or seconding letter for each award in any given year. Nominating documents consist of a letter of not more than 1000 words containing an evaluation of the nominee's accomplishments and a specific identification of the work to be recognized, a biographical sketch including date of birth, and a list of publications and patents authored by the nominee.
Restrictions: Self-nominations are not accepted.
Samples: Morten P. Meldal—award winner, $5,000 (2009); William F. DeGrado—award winner, $5,000 (2008); Samuel H. Gellman—award winner, $5,000 (2007).
Amount of Grant: $5,000 and reimbursement of travel expenses to award meeting
Date(s) Application is Due: Nov 1
Contact: Felicia Dixon, Awards Administrator; (800) 227-5558 or (202) 872-4408; fax: (202) 776-8008; email: f_dixon@acs.org or awards@acs.org
Internet: http://portal.acs.org/portal/acs/corg/content?_nfpb=true&_pageLabel=PP_ARTICLEMAIN&node_id=1319&content_id=CTP_004547&use_sec=true&sec_url_var=region1
Sponsor: American Chemical Society
1155 Sixteenth Street, NW
Washington, DC 20036

Ralphs Food 4 Less Foundation Grants **3106**
The foundation supports nonprofits primarily in areas of company operations in southern California, from Santa Barbara to San Diego, for programs and activities to improve the well-being of youth through education, recreation, and health-related programs; expand

cultural awareness and appreciation of the arts; strengthen neighborhoods; and assist communities in the aftermath of local disasters. Types of support include special projects and general operating expenses. There are no application deadlines. Applicants should submit a letter of application.
Requirements: To be eligible, your organization must be: a 501(3) tax exempt nonprofit; located in Southern California; working in one of the focus areas. Requests for funding must arrive eight (8) weeks prior to the event date or date of need.
Restrictions: Funding is not available to: individuals; capital campaigns; travel expenses; projects of sectarian or religious organizations whose principal benefit is for their own members or adherents; organizations that discriminate on the basis of sex, race, religion, sexual orientation or national origin; third party giving.
Geographic Focus: California
Samples: Los Angeles Rescue Mission, Los Angeles, CA - $10,000 (2008); Community Environmental Council, Santa Barbara, CA - to support its annual Earth Day Festival $1,250 (2009); The Museum of Tolerance (MOT), Los Angeles, CA - to fund the MOT's student programs $10,000 (2008);
Contact: Michelle Williams, Executive Director; (310) 884-6205 or (310) 900-3522
Internet: http://www.ralphs.com/corpnewsinfo_charitablegiving_art5.htm
Sponsor: Ralph's-Food 4 Less Foundation
P.O. Box 54143
Los Angeles, CA 90054

Raskob Foundation for Catholic Activities Grants 3107
The foundation supports Roman Catholic church organizations and missionary activities worldwide. Grants support elementary and secondary education, community action and development, missionary activities, ministries (including youth and parish), health care, social concerns, AIDS victims, finance and development, and relief services. Types of support include operating budgets, seed money, emergency funds, equipment, land acquisition, conferences and seminars, program-related investments, renovation projects, special projects, and matching funds. Deadlines are June 8 and August 8 for the fall meeting; and December 8 and February 8 for the spring meeting.
Requirements: Roman Catholic organizations listed in the Kenedy Directory of Official Catholic Organizations may apply.
Amount of Grant: $5000-$15,000 typically
Date(s) Application is Due: Feb 8; Aug 8
Contact: Maureen Horner, Grants Management, (302) 655-4440; fax: (302) 655-3223
Internet: http://www.rfca.org/grantinfo.htm
Sponsor: Raskob Foundation for Catholic Activities
P.O. Box 4019
Wilmington, DE 19807

Rasmuson Foundation Grants 3108
The Rasmuson Foundation supports non-profit organizations which strive to improve the quality of life for people throughout the state of Alaska. By assisting these groups which address basic needs, special circumstances, the arts and education, the Rasmuson Foundation contributes to healthy, enriched and productive lives for Alaskans of all ages. Types of support include capital grants and challenge/matching grants. Tier 1 and tier 2 grants are awarded. An application cover sheet is available on the Web site.
Requirements: Alaskan organizations that have received 501(c)3 status from the Internal Revenue Service and are classified as not a private foundation under section 509(a) of the Code, units of government, and federally-recognized tribes. Please note, for religious organizations, only projects with a broad community impact are considered. For units of government and tribes, only projects with a broad community impact beyond traditional government functions are considered.
Restrictions: The Foundation will not support: general operations, administrative, indirect, or overhead costs, deficits or debt reduction, endowments, scholarships, fund-raising events or sponsorships, K-12 education reimbursement for items already purchased, electronic health records and other emerging technologies.
Geographic Focus: Alaska
Samples: City of Ambler, Ambler, AK, $16,640 - Community center renovation to repair and rebuild the foundation and entryway (2008); Abused Women's Aid in Crisis, Anchorage, AK, $24,497 - Paint the interior and exterior of Harmony House Transitional Living facility (2008); Delta/Greely School District, Delta Junction, AK, $300,000 - Challenge grant to match federal, state, school district, and private funds for construction of a trades training facility (2009).
Contact: Barbara Bach, Director of Grant Management; (907) 297-2825 or (907) 297-2700; fax: (907) 297-2770; email: bbach@rasmuson.org
Internet: http://www.rasmuson.org
Sponsor: Rasmuson Foundation
301 W Northern Lights Boulevard, Suite 400
Anchorage, AK 99503

Rathmann Family Foundation Grants 3109
The foundation's main funding areas are education, with priority given to science and math; the arts; children and youth health organizations; and preservation of the environment. Types of support include general operating support, continuing support, capital campaigns, equipment acquisition, endowment funds, program development, conferences and seminars, seed grants, curriculum development, fellowships, internships, scholarship funds, research, and matching funds.
Requirements: Grants are awarded to organizations in the San Francisco Bay, CA area; Annapolis, MD; Seattle, WA; Philadelphia, PA: and metropolitan Minneapolis/Saint Paul, MN.
Restrictions: Grants are not awarded to/for private foundations; religious organizations for religious activities; civil rights; social action; advocacy organizations; fraternal groups; political purposes; mental health counseling; individuals; or fundraisers, media events, public relations, annual appeals, or propaganda.
Geographic Focus: California; Maryland; Minnesota; Pennsylvania; Washington
Samples: U of Washington, School of Medicine (Seattle, WA)—to endow a chair in patient-centered clinical education, $1.5 million.
Amount of Grant: $1000-$100,000 average
Contact: Rick Rathmann, (410) 349-2376; fax: (410) 349-2377
Sponsor: Rathmann Family Foundation
1290 Bay Dale Drive, PMB No 352
Arnold, MD 21012

Raymond John Wean Foundation Grants 3110
The foundation awards grants to children's nonprofits in northeast Ohio and southwest Pennsylvania in the areas of education and human services. In education, the foundation supports programs helping teachers and schools prepare students for life and work, especially projects improving educational opportunities, standards, performance, and achievement. In the human services category, the foundation prefers programs strengthening families, providing opportunities for at-risk youth, and helping disadvantaged people. The foundation also is interested in improving healthcare access.
Requirements: Nonprofit organizations serving northeast Ohio and southwest Pennsylvania are eligible.
Geographic Focus: Ohio; Pennsylvania
Amount of Grant: $1,000-$5,000 average
Date(s) Application is Due: Mar 1; Jun 1; Sep 1; Dec 1
Contact: Grants Administrator; (330) 394-5600; fax: (330) 394-5601; email: info@rjweanfoundation.org
Internet: http://www.rjweanfoundation.org
Sponsor: Raymond John Wean Foundation
108 Main Avenue, South West, Suite 1005
Warren, OH 44481-1058

Rayonier Foundation Grants 3111
The foundation awards grants to eligible nonprofit organizations in its areas of interest, including children and youth, community development, disadvantaged (economically), education, engineering, environmental programs, families, health care and hospitals, libraries, minorities, performing arts, recreation science, social services, technology, and volunteerism. Types of support include annual campaigns, building construction/renovation, continuing support, employee matching gifts, employee-related scholarships, endowments, equipment acquisition, general operating support, matching/challenge grants, performing arts, program development, recreation, science, research grants, scholarship funds, and seed grants.
Requirements: Nonprofit organizations in Florida, Georgia, and Washington are eligible.
Geographic Focus: Florida; Georgia; Washington
Samples: United Way of Clallam County, Port Angeles, WA - $4,243 (2006); Florida Community College at Jacksonville Foundation, Jacksonville, FL - $25,000 (2006); University of Virginia, Charlottesville, VA - $7,500 (2006);
Amount of Grant: $250 - $25,000 range
Contact: Charles H. Hood, President; (904) 357-9100; fax: (904) 357-9101; email: info@rayonier.com
Sponsor: Rayonier Foundation
50 North Laura Street, Stuite 1900
Jacksonville, FL 32202

RCPSC Balfour M. Mount Visiting Professorship in Palliative Medicine 3112
The Royal College of Physicians and Surgeons of Canada, in collaboration with the Robert Pope Foundation of Nova Scotia, has established this professorship in order to bring to the health science faculties in Canada the most distinguished international lecturers in the palliative care community to engage in discussion about, and to lecture on, the physical, psycho-social and spiritual needs of patients requiring palliative care. The professorship is meant to facilitate the work of the multidisciplinary team that contributes to palliative care expertise in the community and university being visited. The professor will be appointed in alternate years and will visit the health science faculties of at least two universities in Canada. Using a variety of teaching tools, the professor will bring to the host faculties knowledge and research related to the physical, psycho-social, and spiritual needs of patients requiring palliative care.
Contact: Ines Martin; (800) 668-3740, ext. 212 or (613) 730-6212; fax (613) 730-2410; email: imartin@rcpsc.edu
Internet: http://rcpsc.medical.org/awards/bmm-palliative_e.php
Sponsor: Royal College of Physicians and Surgeons of Canada
774 Echo Drive
Ottawa, ON K1S 5N8 Canada

RCPSC Canadian Research Awards for Specialty Residents 3113
The purpose of the awards is to provide national recognition for original work by postgraduate trainees. Any original work in the field of clinical investigation, in the basic sciences relating to medicine or surgery, in medical education, or in medical ethics, is acceptable. Work described in manuscripts published or submitted for publication during the 12 months preceding January 31 is acceptable, providing the other conditions are fulfilled. The manuscripts must be received no later than January 29, at 5 p.m. The

recipients will receive a certificate that bears the logo or crest of the three participating organizations together with a check for $2,000. The prizes are presented at the Royal College Annual Conference.
Requirements: The candidate must be a resident (postgraduate trainee registered with a university office of postgraduate education) and enrolled in a residency program accredited by the Royal College. Those certified in a primary specialty but continuing their residency towards a subspecialty in an approved residency program are also eligible. The work must have been done mainly in Canada. Residents who have not previously won this award in either category are eligible.
Amount of Grant: $2,000
Date(s) Application is Due: Jan 29
Contact: Ines Martin; (800) 668-3740, ext. 212 or (613) 730-6212; fax (613) 730-2410; email: imartin@rcpsc.edu
Internet: http://rcpsc.medical.org/awards/residents_e.php
Sponsor: Royal College of Physicians and Surgeons of Canada
774 Echo Drive
Ottawa, ON K1S 5N8 Canada

RCPSC Detweiler Traveling Fellowships **3114**
Fellowships are made to improve the quality of medical and surgical practice in Canada. The fellowships will enable the recipients to visit medical centers in Canada or abroad to study or gain experience in the use or application of new knowledge or techniques in their fields or to further the pursuit of a fundamental or clinical research problem. Five or more fellowships offered annually to a maximum of $21,000 will be reserved for junior applicants. Two additional fellowships offered annually will be reserved for senior applicants: one will be granted to a Fellow who has held Royal College certification for five years or more and has been in private practice for at least three years, and one will be granted to a Fellow who has held Royal College certification for five years or more and has been in academic practice for at least three years. Each award will be to a maximum of $10,500.
Requirements: Applicants must be Fellows of the Royal College in good standing, or residents in the final year of their training who will be admitted to Fellowship in the Royal College prior to December 31st.
Restrictions: Travel fellowships will not be awarded retroactively.
Amount of Grant: $1,750 per month to a maximum of 12 months (up to $21,000)
Date(s) Application is Due: Sep 30
Contact: Allison Shaw, Awards and Grants Section; (800) 668-3740, ext. 355 or (613) 730-8177; fax: (613) 730-2410; email: awards@rcpsc.edu
Internet: http://rcpsc.medical.org/awards/detweiler_e.php
Sponsor: Royal College of Physicians and Surgeons of Canada
774 Echo Drive
Ottawa, ON K1S 5N8 Canada

RCPSC Duncan Graham Award **3115**
One of the notable and outstanding awards that The Royal College of Physicians and Surgeons of Canada may bestow upon an individual is the Duncan Graham Award. The Duncan Graham Award was introduced in 1969 in honor of the late Dr. Duncan Graham, for many years a professor of medicine at the University of Toronto. The Award is conferred upon any individual, whether physician or not, in recognition of outstanding lifelong contribution to medical education. The award is in the amount of $1,000 accompanied by a suitably engraved memento. It is usually conferred each year at the Convocation of the Royal College Annual Meeting. Nominations are solicited from the Deans of the Faculties of medicine. The Awards Committee of the Royal College selects the recipient of the Duncan Graham Award. At its discretion, the Awards Committee may add to the list of nominations.
Amount of Grant: $1,000 accompanied by a suitably engraved memento
Date(s) Application is Due: Sep 30
Contact: Ines Martin; (800) 668-3740 ext. 212 or (613) 730-6212; fax (613) 730-2410; email: imartin@rcpsc.edu
Internet: http://rcpsc.medical.org/awards/duncan-graham_e.php
Sponsor: Royal College of Physicians and Surgeons of Canada
774 Echo Drive
Ottawa, ON K1S 5N8 Canada

RCPSC Events, Speakers and Visiting Professors Grants **3116**
The purpose of the grant is to help defray the cost of special events, speakers, and visiting professors. Events must be primarily organized for Fellows and residents of the RCPSC. The RACs represent the following regions of Canada: Region 1—British Columbia, Alberta, Yukon Territory, and Northwest Territories; Region 2—Saskatchewan and Manitoba; Region 3—Ontario and Nunavut; Region 4—Quebec; and Region 5—New Brunswick, Nova Scotia, Prince Edward Island, and Newfoundland and Labrador. Up to $1,200 is available in regions 1, 2, 3 and 5, and up to $1,000 is available in region 4.
Restrictions: No consideration given to applications submitted or received after the event. The application must be submitted by a Fellow of the RCPSC in good standing.
Amount of Grant: $1,200 maximum
Contact: Allison Shaw, Awards and Grants Section; (800) 668-3740, ext. 355 or (613) 730-8177; fax: (613) 730-2410; email: awards@rcpsc.edu
Internet: http://rcpsc.medical.org/awards/cme_e.php
Sponsor: Royal College of Physicians and Surgeons of Canada
774 Echo Drive
Ottawa, ON K1S 5N8 Canada

RCPSC Faculty Development Grants **3117**
The objective of the grant is to support the creation, promotion, and evaluation of, and/or research on, new and innovative methods of faculty development to foster the training of quality teachers. Proposals to create new and innovative faculty development programs must, at a minimum, contain an evaluative component in order to be considered. Innovative pilot research projects focused on faculty development will also be considered. Although not a requirement, applicants are encouraged to seek matching funds from the participating university. Preference will be given to projects that are generic, practical, applicable to postgraduate medical education, and relevant to the defined objective of the grant.
Requirements: Applicants must be members of a Canadian faculty of medicine involved in teaching and/or educational research. It is not necessary to be a Fellow of the RCPSC or a physician.
Restrictions: Budgets should not include salary, honoraria, travel, accommodation or meals for investigators; however, a maximum of $500 may be requested to defray the costs for travel, accommodation, meals or conference registration for investigators to disseminate the project findings. Ineligible costs include tuition fees, capital equipment costs (e.g. computer hardware, office equipment), overhead costs, university or other organization administrative fees.
Amount of Grant: $5,000 maximum
Date(s) Application is Due: Mar 2
Contact: Allison Shaw, Awards and Grants Section; (800) 668-3740, ext. 355 or (613) 730-8177; fax: (613) 730-2410; email: awards@rcpsc.edu
Internet: http://rcpsc.medical.org/awards/faculty_e.php
Sponsor: Royal College of Physicians and Surgeons of Canada
774 Echo Drive
Ottawa, ON K1S 5N8 Canada

RCPSC International Traveling Fellowship **3118**
The objective of the fellowship is to enable fellows residing outside of Canada to study in a Canadian medical center in order to acquire a new knowledge and skills applicable to clinical practice, undertake clinical research, or to enable fellows residing in Canada to practice and teach in a less developed country. The fellowship is applicable for visits of six to 12 months duration. Visits may be broken into separate time blocks but must be completed within two years. An amount equivalent to 75% of the award will be given at the beginning of the fellowship and the remainder upon receipt of the final report at the end of the fellowship. The fellowship may be used to supplement financial assistance granted from other sources.
Requirements: Applicants must be Fellows of the Royal College in good standing, or residents in the final year of their training who will be admitted to Fellowship in the Royal College prior to December 31.
Amount of Grant: $1,750 per month to a maximum of 12 months (up to $21,000)
Date(s) Application is Due: Sep 30
Contact: Allison Shaw, Awards and Grants Section; (800) 668-3740, ext. 355 or (613) 730-8177; fax: (613) 730-2410; email: awards@rcpsc.edu
Internet: http://rcpsc.medical.org/awards/international_e.php
Sponsor: Royal College of Physicians and Surgeons of Canada
774 Echo Drive
Ottawa, ON K1S 5N8 Canada

RCPSC James H. Graham Award of Merit **3119**
In 1987, the Council of The Royal College of Physicians and Surgeons of Canada recommended that an award of merit be given to a person whose outstanding achievements reflect the aims and objectives of the Royal College. This person need not be a physician. The Awards Committee will be the selection committee for the award of merit. The selection committee will receive nominations (with curriculum vitae) from the RCPSC Council (limit of two), and the Regional Advisory Committees (one per RAC). The presentation for the award of merit will be made at the Annual Meeting of the Royal College. The winner will receive a suitably engraved memento. The travel and maintenance expenses of the award winner and spouse will be paid in accordance with Royal College guidelines.
Samples: Dr. Robert Y. McMurty, London, Canada (2009); Dr. Paul M. O'Byrne, Ancaster, Canada (2008); Dr. Eldon R. Smith, Calgary, Canada (2007).
Date(s) Application is Due: Sep 30
Contact: Ines Martin; (800) 668-3740 ext. 212 or (613) 730-6212; fax (613) 730-2410; email: imartin@rcpsc.edu
Internet: http://rcpsc.medical.org/awards/james-graham_e.php
Sponsor: Royal College of Physicians and Surgeons of Canada
774 Echo Drive
Ottawa, ON K1S 5N8 Canada

RCPSC Janes Visiting Professorship in Surgery **3120**
The purpose of this visiting professorship is to stimulate and increase an interest in the latest developments in surgery and surgical techniques. The visiting professor, preferably a Canadian surgeon of national stature, spends up to one week visiting one to three medical schools according to a mutually agreed schedule. The professor participates in undergraduate and postgraduate teaching and in the exchange of ideas with practicing surgeons, residents and students. The professorship is supported by a grant of $7,000 and is usually selected every second year.
Amount of Grant: $7,000
Date(s) Application is Due: Sep 30
Contact: Ines Martin; (800) 668-3740, ext. 212 or (613) 730-6212; fax (613) 730-2410; email: imartin@rcpsc.edu

Internet: http://rcpsc.medical.org/awards/janes-surgery_e.php
Sponsor: Royal College of Physicians and Surgeons of Canada
774 Echo Drive
Ottawa, ON K1S 5N8 Canada

RCPSC Kilborn Memorial Visiting Professorship 3121

The Royal College of Physicians and Surgeons of Canada, in collaboration with the Kilborn Memorial Fund, has established a visiting professorship to West China Centre of Medical Sciences (WCCMS), formerly West China University of Medical Sciences (WCUMS), to honour the contributions made by members of the Kilborn family to the founding and development of the faculty of medicine and health sciences at WCCMS in Chengdu, Sichuan, China. The purpose of the visiting professorship is to enable Canadian specialists to visit WCCMS for a predetermined time (e.g., 2–4 weeks), and to contribute to the education of students and the professional development of the faculty of the school of medical sciences and/or related health sciences in the discipline identified by the host center.
Contact: Ines Martin; (800) 668-3740, ext. 212 or (613) 730-6212; fax (613) 730-2410; email: imartin@rcpsc.edu
Internet: http://rcpsc.medical.org/awards/kilborn_e.php
Sponsor: Royal College of Physicians and Surgeons of Canada
774 Echo Drive
Ottawa, ON K1S 5N8 Canada

RCPSC KJR Wightman Award for Scholarship in Ethics 3122

The Royal College of Physicians and Surgeons of Canada awards a prize for the best scholarly paper presented by a resident registered in a postgraduate program accredited by the Royal College. Papers arising from a clinical case, addressing ethical issues pertinent to the CanMEDS roles (medical expert, communicator, collaborator, manager, health advocate, scholar, professional), or on the topic of equity in any aspect relevant to the work of the College are welcome. The recipient will receive $1,000 as well as a certificate. The award will be presented during the Convocation Ceremony at the Annual Conference. The travel expenses of the recipient and guest to the Annual Conference will be paid in accordance with Royal College guidelines.
Requirements: Submissions for the award must be accompanied by a curriculum vitae and submitted electronically. The manuscript must be between 2500 and 5000 words, excluding the bibliography.
Samples: Dr. Michel Shamy, University of Toronto, Toronto, Ontario—Narrative, Argument and Evidence: An Ethical Justification for the Use of Suggestion in the Treatment of Psychogenic Illness (2008); Dr. Trevor Langhan, Calgary, Alberta—Simulation training for emergency medicine procedural skills: Should we move away from practicing on people? (2007).
Amount of Grant: $1,000 as well as a certificate
Date(s) Application is Due: Apr 30
Contact: Ines Martin; (800) 668-3740 ext. 212 or (613) 730-6212; fax (613) 730-2410; email: imartin@rcpsc.edu
Internet: http://rcpsc.medical.org/awards/wightman_e.php
Sponsor: Royal College of Physicians and Surgeons of Canada
774 Echo Drive
Ottawa, ON K1S 5N8 Canada

RCPSC McLaughlin-Gallie Visiting Professorship 3123

The Royal College of Physicians and Surgeons of Canada established the McLaughlin-Gallie Visiting Professorship in 1960. The professorship commemorates the outstanding contributions to surgical science of Dr. William Edward Gallie of Toronto. McLaughlin-Gallie Visiting Professors may be selected from any country in the world and may represent any branch of medicine. They spend up to one week at each of two Canadian faculties of medicine. They participate in undergraduate and postgraduate teaching, and in the exchange of ideas with the staff, the researchers and the undergraduate and postgraduate students.
Amount of Grant: $10,000
Contact: Ines Martin; (800) 668-3740, ext. 212 or (613) 730-6212; fax (613) 730-2410; email: imartin@rcpsc.edu
Internet: http://rcpsc.medical.org/awards/mclaughlin-gallie_e.php
Sponsor: Royal College of Physicians and Surgeons of Canada
774 Echo Drive
Ottawa, ON K1S 5N8 Canada

RCPSC Medical Education Research Grants 3124

The primary objective of the grant is to support quality research in Canada relevant to the field of postgraduate medical education or continuing professional development. Applications may be individual or joint, involving one or more departments, disciplines, or faculties of medicine. It is not necessary to be a Fellow of the RCPSC or a physician; however, a Fellow of the Royal College must contribute to the research project. The following areas of research are encouraged: curriculum design and implementation; instructional methods; assessment; program evaluation; continuing education; professional development; and faculty development.
Requirements: Applicants must be involved in teaching and/or medical education research in Canada. Applications must meet contemporary standards of educational research, which include the relevance of the research question, the quality of the research design, ethical review of the submission, accountability for funds received, and the ability to complete the project during the funding period. One or more grants, of up to $25,000 per year of study, will be awarded annually.
Restrictions: Ineligible costs include tuition fees, capital equipment costs (e.g. computer hardware, office equipment), overhead costs, university or other organization administrative fees.
Amount of Grant: $25,000 maximum per year of study
Date(s) Application is Due: Mar 2
Contact: Allison Shaw, Awards and Grants Section; (800) 668-3740, ext. 355 or (613) 730-8177; fax: (613) 730-2410; email: awards@rcpsc.edu
Internet: http://rcpsc.medical.org/awards/MERG_e.php
Sponsor: Royal College of Physicians and Surgeons of Canada
774 Echo Drive
Ottawa, ON K1S 5N8 Canada

RCPSC Medical Education Traveling Fellowships 3125

The objective of the fellowship is to enable the recipient to acquire knowledge and expertise in the field of medical education. Upon completion, the recipient will be able to use education principles to develop educational programs and proceed to the evaluation of learning experiences at the undergraduate, postgraduate, or continuing education level. Fellowships are applicable for visits of six to 12 months duration. Up to 75 percent of the fellowship stipend will be given at the beginning of the fellowship and the remainder upon receipt of the final report at the end of the fellowship. The fellowship may be used to supplement financial assistance granted from other sources.
Requirements: Applicants must be Fellows of the Royal College in good standing, or residents in the final year of their training who will be admitted to Fellowship in the Royal College prior to December 31st.
Amount of Grant: $2,500 per month to a maximum of $21,000
Date(s) Application is Due: Sep 30
Contact: Allison Shaw, Awards and Grants Section; (800) 668-3740, ext. 355 or (613) 730-8177; fax: (613) 730-2410; email: awards@rcpsc.edu
Internet: http://rcpsc.medical.org/awards/medical_e.php
Sponsor: Royal College of Physicians and Surgeons of Canada
774 Echo Drive
Ottawa, ON K1S 5N8 Canada

RCPSC National Specialty Society Annual Meeting Grants 3126

The National Specialty Society Annual Meeting Grants program was established to assist Royal College Fellows in their professional development activities by providing some financial support to national forums on specialty medicine. Funding can support: the speaker of the Royal College of Physicians and Surgeons of Canada; and postgraduate coursework at the time of the national specialty society's annual meeting. Up to $1,200 including expenses and honorarium.
Requirements: The national specialty society must be duly constituted and must represent a specialty or a sub-specialty recognized by the Royal College. Consideration may also given to multidisciplinary societies if a large percentage of its members are Fellows of the Royal College. The application form must be submitted by a Fellow of the Royal College at least eight (8) weeks before the society's annual meeting.
Amount of Grant: $1,200 maximum
Contact: Allison Shaw, Awards and Grants Section; (800) 668-3740, ext. 355 or (613) 730-8177; fax: (613) 730-2410; email: awards@rcpsc.edu
Internet: http://rcpsc.medical.org/awards/nssgrant_e.php
Sponsor: Royal College of Physicians and Surgeons of Canada
774 Echo Drive
Ottawa, ON K1S 5N8 Canada

RCPSC Royal College Fellowship for Studies in Medical Education 3127

The goal of this fellowship is to increase the number and quality of professionally trained medical educators in Canada by providing training in the science of medical education to selected promising candidates. The program is to help specialists acquire knowledge and skills in the field of medical education in order to develop educational programs and evaluation methods that apply to any phase of the continuum of medical education. This fellowship funding is for one year. Applicants may reapply for one additional year of funding; however, repeat or renewal applications will be considered on a competitive basis with all other applications received in the same year, and will require an outline of the progress of the previous year's work.
Requirements: Applicants must register in a Masters or PhD level university program leading to a degree in Education, or a subject field/program of study closely related to medical education. The candidate must be registered and attending university as a full time or part time student, either within Canada or abroad. Applicants must be Canadian citizens or permanent residents who, are Fellows of the Royal College in good standing or residents who, at the time of the application, are registered in a program accredited by the Royal College.
Amount of Grant: $45,000 for residents and Fellows per year of study
Date(s) Application is Due: Sep 30
Contact: Allison Shaw, Awards and Grants Section; (800) 668-3740, ext. 355 or (613) 730-8177; fax: (613) 730-2410; email: awards@rcpsc.edu
Internet: http://rcpsc.medical.org/awards/fellow_e.php
Sponsor: Royal College of Physicians and Surgeons of Canada
774 Echo Drive
Ottawa, ON K1S 5N8 Canada

RCPSC Royal College Medal Award in Medicine 3128

The Royal College of Physicians and Surgeons of Canada offers annually a competition for the RCPSC Medal in Medicine. This award provides national recognition for original work by a clinical investigator who has completed his/her training within the past 10

years. Any original work in clinical investigation or in the basic sciences relating to medicine is acceptable. The deadline for receipt of the manuscript is November 28, at 5 p.m. The recipient will receive a gold medal and $5,000.
Requirements: The candidate must be a Fellow of the Royal College and the work must have been done mainly in Canada. Only applicants who have not previously won the Medal are eligible.
Restrictions: Work which is directed or overseen by a supervisor such as in a graduate or post-doctoral training program is not eligible.
Amount of Grant: $5,000
Date(s) Application is Due: Nov 30
Contact: Ines Martin; (800) 668-3740 ext. 212 or (613) 730-6212; fax (613) 730-2410; email: imartin@rcpsc.edu
Internet: http://rcpsc.medical.org/awards/medals_e.php
Sponsor: Royal College of Physicians and Surgeons of Canada
774 Echo Drive
Ottawa, ON K1S 5N8 Canada

RCPSC Royal College Medal Award in Surgery 3129
The Royal College of Physicians and Surgeons of Canada offers annually a competition for the RCPSC Medal in Surgery. This award provides national recognition for original work by a clinical investigator who has completed his/her training within the past 10 years. Any original work in clinical investigation or in the basic sciences relating to surgery is acceptable. The deadline for receipt of the manuscript is November 30, at 5 p.m. The recipient will receive a gold medal and $5,000.
Requirements: The candidate must be a Fellow of the Royal College and the work must have been done mainly in Canada. Only applicants who have not previously won the Medal are eligible.
Restrictions: Work which is directed or overseen by a supervisor such as in a graduate or post-doctoral training program is not eligible.
Samples: Dr. Mohit Bhandari, FRCSC, Burlington, Ontario, $5,000 - Trial of Reamed and Unreamed Intramedullary Nailing of Tibial Shaft Fractures (2009); D Robert Nam, Toronto, Ontario, $5,000 - Expression of the TMPRSS2:ERG fusion gene predicts cancer recurrence after surgery for localized prostate cancer (2008); Dr. Marc Ruel, Ottawa, Canada, $5,000 - Comparative effects of mesenchymal progenitor cells, endothelial progenitor cells or their combination on myocardial infarct regeneration and cardiac function (2007).
Amount of Grant: $5,000
Date(s) Application is Due: Nov 30
Contact: Ines Martin; (800) 668-3740 ext. 212 or (613) 730-6212; fax (613) 730-2410; email: imartin@rcpsc.edu
Internet: http://rcpsc.medical.org/awards/medals_e.php
Sponsor: Royal College of Physicians and Surgeons of Canada
774 Echo Drive
Ottawa, ON K1S 5N8 Canada

RCPSC Royal College Visiting Professorships in Medical Research 3130
The intent of this grant is to provide medical students and residents with the opportunity to meet established researchers from other centers in order to promote medical research as a career choice. It is intended that the visiting professor have the opportunity to interact with both undergraduate medical students and residents through rounds and other teaching sessions, and that the visit not be department-specific. Such interaction will provide the visiting professor with opportunities to expound on the challenges and rewards of a career in medical research. A $3,000 grant is available for each medical faculty.
Amount of Grant: $3,000
Date(s) Application is Due: Sep 30
Contact: Ines Martin; (800) 668-3740, ext. 212 or (613) 730-6212; fax (613) 730-2410; email: imartin@rcpsc.edu
Internet: http://rcpsc.medical.org/awards/visiting-medresearch_e.php
Sponsor: Royal College of Physicians and Surgeons of Canada
774 Echo Drive
Ottawa, ON K1S 5N8 Canada

RCPSC Teasdale-Corti Humanitarian Award 3131
The purpose of the Teasdale-Corti Humanitarian Award is to acknowledge and celebrate Canadian physicians who, while providing health care or emergency medical services, go beyond the accepted norms of routine practice, which may include exposure to personal risk. The recipient's action will exemplify altruism and integrity, courage and perseverance in the alleviation of human suffering. The award may be bestowed upon Canadian physicians whose current practice reflects the above description or upon those who have made such a contribution in the past. The Award will be open to Canadian physicians worldwide. Nominations will be widely solicited and may be submitted by any Fellow of the Royal College. The recipient will be presented with a suitably engraved memento that will be presented at the Royal College Annual Conference or other suitable venue. The travel and maintenance expenses of the award winner and companion will be paid in accordance with Royal College guidelines. The Royal College may make a donation to the relief organization with which the recipient is affiliated.
Date(s) Application is Due: Sep 30
Contact: Ines Martin; (800) 668-3740 or (613) 730-6212; fax (613) 730-2410; email: imartin@rcpsc.edu
Internet: http://rcpsc.medical.org/awards/index.php
Sponsor: Royal College of Physicians and Surgeons of Canada
774 Echo Drive
Ottawa, ON K1S 5N8 Canada

RCPSC Traineeships 3132
These Traineeships are provided for periods of personalized professional development (to learn a skill, surgical procedure or expand an area of competence). Applications should be received at least eight (8) weeks before the start of the traineeship. Up to $3,000 is available per applicant.
Restrictions: Applications are restricted to Fellows of the RCPSC in good standing.
Amount of Grant: $3,000 maximum
Contact: Allison Shaw, Awards and Grants Section; (800) 668-3740, ext. 355 or (613) 730-8177; fax: (613) 730-2410; email: awards@rcpsc.edu
Internet: http://rcpsc.medical.org/awards/traineeships_e.php
Sponsor: Royal College of Physicians and Surgeons of Canada
774 Echo Drive
Ottawa, ON K1S 5N8 Canada

RCPSC Walter C. MacKenzie Fellowship in Surgery 3133
The fellowship will enable the recipient to visit one or more centers to acquire surgical research or clinical surgical training. Knowledge gained should have a direct application to the recipient's clinical surgical practice. One or more fellowship are offered annually, depending on budget. Tenable for visits of two weeks to 12 months duration; visits may be broken into separate time blocks but must be completed within two years. An amount equivalent to 75% of the award will be given at the beginning of the fellowship, and the remainder upon receipt of a final report at the end of the fellowship. The fellowship may be used to supplement financial assistance granted from other sources.
Requirements: Applications are accepted from practicing surgeons who are fellows of the Royal College in good standing at the time of application and who reside in Canada. Practicing surgeons are those who have spent at least 50 percent of their professional time in active clinical surgery over the last five years.
Amount of Grant: $5,000 per month (up to $15,000 prorated)
Date(s) Application is Due: Sep 30
Contact: Allison Shaw, Awards and Grants Section; (800) 668-3740, ext. 355 or (613) 730-8177; fax: (613) 730-2410; email: awards@rcpsc.edu
Internet: http://rcpsc.medical.org/awards/mackenzie_e.php
Sponsor: Royal College of Physicians and Surgeons of Canada
774 Echo Drive
Ottawa, ON K1S 5N8 Canada

RCPSC Wightman Visiting Professorship in Medicine 3134
The Wightman Visiting Professor participates in undergraduate and postgraduate teaching and in discussions with peers, both in internal medicine and in the professor's particular area of academic interest. The visiting professor spends one or two weeks visiting two or three Canadian faculties of medicine. The Professorship is supported by a grant of $7,000.
Amount of Grant: $7,000
Date(s) Application is Due: Sep 30
Contact: Ines Martin; (800) 668-3740, ext. 212 or (613) 730-6212; fax (613) 730-2410; email: imartin@rcpsc.edu
Internet: http://rcpsc.medical.org/awards/visiting-wightman_e.php
Sponsor: Royal College of Physicians and Surgeons of Canada
774 Echo Drive
Ottawa, ON K1S 5N8 Canada

RCPSC/AMS CanMEDs Research and Development Grants 3135
The primary objective of the grant is to support research, development, and/or implementation of projects to enhance specialty education in the promotion of the key roles for specialists as defined by CanMEDS. Applications may be individual or joint, involving one or more departments, disciplines, or faculties of medicine. It is not necessary to be a Fellow of the RCPSC or a physician; however, a Fellow of the Royal College must contribute to the project. Eligible projects may include faculty development, course development and/or medical education research that both apply and promote the CanMEDS roles. Budgets may include requests to defray the costs for travel, accommodation and meals for investigators to disseminate the project findings. One or more grants of up to $25,000 will be awarded each year.
Requirements: Applicants must be involved in teaching and/or medical education research in Canada. Applications that include research must meet contemporary standards of educational research, which include the relevance of the research question, the quality of the research design, ethical review of the submission, accountability for funds received, and the ability to complete the project during the funding period. Applications that include project development must include an evaluative component assessing the impact of the project.
Restrictions: Budgets should not include salary or honoraria for investigators. Ineligible costs include tuition fees, capital equipment costs (e.g. computer hardware, office equipment), overhead costs, university or other organization administrative fees.
Amount of Grant: $25,000 maximum
Date(s) Application is Due: Mar 2
Contact: Allison Shaw, Awards and Grants Section; (800) 668-3740, ext. 355 or (613) 730-8177; fax: (613) 730-2410; email: awards@rcpsc.edu
Internet: http://rcpsc.medical.org/awards/ams_e.php
Sponsor: Royal College of Physicians and Surgeons of Canada
774 Echo Drive
Ottawa, ON K1S 5N8 Canada

RCPSC/AMS Donald Richards Wilson Award 3136
The Royal College of Physicians and Surgeons of Canada, in collaboration with Associated Medical Services, Inc. has established an award to honour and acknowledge

the contribution of Dr. Donald R. Wilson (President, RCPSC, 1988-1990) to medical education. This award will be given annually to a medical educator (not necessarily a Fellow) or an identified leader of a team, program, or department who has demonstrated excellence in integrating the CanMEDS roles into a Royal College or other health related training programs. Nominations will be received from Deans, Department or program heads, peers, or trainees. The successful applicant(s) will receive an award of $2,000 and a suitably engraved recognition.
Restrictions: Self-applications are ineligible.
Amount of Grant: $2,000
Date(s) Application is Due: Apr 30
Contact: Ines Martin; (800) 668-3740, ext. 212 or (613) 730-6212; fax (613) 730-2410; email: imartin@rcpsc.edu
Internet: http://rcpsc.medical.org/awards/wilson_e.php
Sponsor: Royal College of Physicians and Surgeons of Canada
774 Echo Drive
Ottawa, ON K1S 5N8 Canada

Reader's Digest Partners for Sight Foundation Grants **3137**
The foundation awards grants to nonprofit organizations that serve the blind and visually impaired. Multiyear grants and smaller one-year grants are made to organizations that work on the local level. The listed deadline is for preliminary applications for multiyear grants; preliminary applications for one-year grants may be submitted at anytime. Grants are awarded every three years.
Requirements: 501(c)3 nonprofit organizations are eligible.
Amount of Grant: $1 million maximum for multiyear grants
Date(s) Application is Due: Sep 15
Contact: Dianna Kelly-Naghizadeh, (914) 244-5830 or (800) 877-5293; fax: (914) 244-7481; email: PartnersForSight@rd.com
Internet: http://www.rd.com/corporate/rd_fundblind.html
Sponsor: Reader's Digest Partners for Sight Foundation
Reader's Digest Road
Pleasantville, NY 10570-7000

Regence Foundation Access to Health Care Grants **3138**
Grants in this category support the health care safety-net and insurance access programs, including efforts to: increase access to health and medical care for low-income, uninsured or underinsured individuals; provide a medical home to those who would otherwise go without; improve medical outcomes; and help eligible individuals and families navigate the process of accessing available health insurance coverage.
Requirements: The Foundation funds: organizations that are nonprofit and tax-exempt under 501(c)3 of the Internal Revenue Service Code (IRC) and defined as a public charity under 509(a) 1, 2, or 3 (types I, II, or a functionally integrated type III); organizations that serve residents of Idaho, Oregon, Washington and/or Utah; accredited schools or universities; units of government and public agencies; and programs and services that align with our mission and program areas.
Restrictions: The Foundation does not fund: capital construction; award dinners, athletic events, competitions, special events or tournaments; conferences or seminars; religious organizations for religious purposes; political causes, candidates, organizations or campaigns; grants to individuals; grants to 509(a)3, type III supporting organizations that are not functionally integrated; or grants to organizations that are not doing significant work in Idaho, Oregon, Washington and/or Utah.
Geographic Focus: Idaho; Oregon; Utah; Washington
Amount of Grant: $50,000-$115,000
Contact: Monique Barton, Executive Director; (503) 276-1965; email: mxbarto@regence.com or RegenceFoundation@regence.com
Internet: http://www.regencefoundation.org/programs/transformation.html
Sponsor: Regence Foundation
100 SW Market Street, MS E-8T
Portland, OR 97201

Regence Foundation Health Care Community Awareness and Engagement Grants **3139**
At the core of this program area is a laser-focus on increasing the accessibility and usability of information for consumers to make informed health care decisions. Grants in this category support efforts that encourage consumers to seek information about the value and quality of their health care, and develop tools to access that information, such as: community collaborative pilot projects; campaigns promoting consumer education and engagement; and research on consumer use of health care information.
Requirements: The Foundation funds: organizations that are nonprofit and tax-exempt under 501(c)3 of the Internal Revenue Service Code (IRC) and defined as a public charity under 509(a) 1, 2, or 3 (types I, II, or a functionally integrated type III); organizations that serve residents of Idaho, Oregon, Washington and/or Utah; accredited schools or universities; units of government and public agencies; and programs and services that align with our mission and program areas.
Restrictions: The Foundation does not fund: capital construction; award dinners, athletic events, competitions, special events or tournaments; conferences or seminars; religious organizations for religious purposes; political causes, candidates, organizations or campaigns; grants to individuals; grants to 509(a)3, type III supporting organizations that are not functionally integrated; or grants to organizations that are not doing significant work in Idaho, Oregon, Washington and/or Utah.
Geographic Focus: Idaho; Oregon; Utah; Washington
Amount of Grant: $45,000-$150,000
Contact: Monique Barton, Executive Director; (503) 276-1965; email: mxbarto@regence.com or RegenceFoundation@regence.com
Internet: http://www.regencefoundation.org/programs/transparency.html
Sponsor: Regence Foundation
100 SW Market Street, MS E-8T
Portland, OR 97201

Regence Foundation Health Care Connections Grants **3140**
Grants in this category support general health programs that are innovative and solve community-identified problems, including efforts to: manage chronic conditions; make healthy lifestyle choices; and serve a target population whose health care needs may be unmet and/or who may be experiencing health disparities.
Requirements: The Foundation funds: organizations that are nonprofit and tax-exempt under 501(c)3 of the Internal Revenue Service Code (IRC) and defined as a public charity under 509(a) 1, 2, or 3 (types I, II, or a functionally integrated type III); organizations that serve residents of Idaho, Oregon, Washington and/or Utah; accredited schools or universities; units of government and public agencies; and programs and services that align with our mission and program areas.
Restrictions: The Foundation does not fund: capital construction; award dinners, athletic events, competitions, special events or tournaments; conferences or seminars; religious organizations for religious purposes; political causes, candidates, organizations or campaigns; grants to individuals; grants to 509(a)3, type III supporting organizations that are not functionally integrated; or grants to organizations that are not doing significant work in Idaho, Oregon, Washington and/or Utah.
Geographic Focus: Idaho; Oregon; Utah; Washington
Amount of Grant: $15,000-$50,000
Contact: Monique Barton, Executive Director; (503) 276-1965; email: mxbarto@regence.com or RegenceFoundation@regence.com
Internet: http://www.regencefoundation.org/programs/transformation.html
Sponsor: Regence Foundation
100 SW Market Street, MS E-8T
Portland, OR 97201

Regence Foundation Improving End-of-Life Grants **3141**
The Regence Foundation works to transform health care and address core problems in our health care system with innovative solutions. The Foundation supports a transformational health care system where consumers partner with their physicians and other providers to make health care decisions based on what's valuable to them — such as end-of-life decisions — just as they do when making other economic decisions.
Requirements: The Foundation funds: organizations that are nonprofit and tax-exempt under 501(c)3 of the Internal Revenue Service Code (IRC) and defined as a public charity under 509(a) 1, 2, or 3 (types I, II, or a functionally integrated type III); organizations that serve residents of Idaho, Oregon, Washington and/or Utah; accredited schools or universities; units of government and public agencies; and programs and services that align with our mission and program areas.
Restrictions: The Foundation does not fund: capital construction; award dinners, athletic events, competitions, special events or tournaments; conferences or seminars; religious organizations for religious purposes; political causes, candidates, organizations or campaigns; grants to individuals; grants to 509(a)3, type III supporting organizations that are not functionally integrated; or grants to organizations that are not doing significant work in Idaho, Oregon, Washington and/or Utah.
Geographic Focus: Idaho; Oregon; Utah; Washington
Contact: Monique Barton, Executive Director; (503) 276-1965; email: mxbarto@regence.com or RegenceFoundation@regence.com
Internet: http://www.regencefoundation.org/programs/endOfLife.html
Sponsor: Regence Foundation
100 SW Market Street, MS E-8T
Portland, OR 97201

Regence Foundation Tools and Technology Grants **3142**
At the core of this program area is a laser-focus on increasing the accessibility and usability of information for consumers to make informed health care decisions. Grants in this category support innovative technology solutions that work to overcome practical barriers and improve the quality and safety of health care. Projects might include: multi-stakeholder technology collaborations; not-for-profit technology initiatives that include providers in development and testing; research on the usage and effects of technology collaborations in health care; and approaches that address patients who receive services from multiple providers across the spectrum.
Requirements: The Foundation funds: organizations that are nonprofit and tax-exempt under 501(c)3 of the Internal Revenue Service Code (IRC) and defined as a public charity under 509(a) 1, 2, or 3 (types I, II, or a functionally integrated type III); organizations that serve residents of Idaho, Oregon, Washington and/or Utah; accredited schools or universities; units of government and public agencies; and programs and services that align with our mission and program areas.
Restrictions: The Foundation does not fund: capital construction; award dinners, athletic events, competitions, special events or tournaments; conferences or seminars; religious organizations for religious purposes; political causes, candidates, organizations or campaigns; grants to individuals; grants to 509(a)3, type III supporting organizations that are not functionally integrated; or grants to organizations that are not doing significant work in Idaho, Oregon, Washington and/or Utah.
Geographic Focus: Idaho; Oregon; Utah; Washington
Contact: Monique Barton, Executive Director; (503) 276-1965; email: mxbarto@regence.com or RegenceFoundation@regence.com

Internet: http://www.regencefoundation.org/programs/transparency.html
Sponsor: Regence Foundation
100 SW Market Street, MS E-8T
Portland, OR 97201

Regenstrief Geriatrics Fellowship 3143
The Department of Medicine and the Division of General Internal Medicine and Geriatrics offer a 2-year fellowship in Geriatric Medicine (with an optional third year). Residents who have completed three years of training in internal medicine or family practice and who are board eligible or board certified may apply for the fellowship. Fellows will be trained in clinical geriatrics, research, teaching, and/or administration in preparation for a successful career in academic geriatric medicine. Formal instruction will be provided by a structured curriculum with goals and objectives that will be met by clinical experiences in a variety of settings, didactic seminars to augment the clinical experiences, and seminars in research, teaching and administration. For further information on the Geriatric Fellowship contact the Program Director.
Contact: Glenda Westmorland, Program Director: (317) 630-6906; fax: (317) 630-2667; email: GWestmorland@regenstrief.org
Internet: http://www.regenstrief.org/training/geriatrics-fellowship-program
Sponsor: Regenstrief Institute
410 West 10th Street, Suite 2000
Indianapolis, IN 46202-3012

Regenstrief General Internal Medicine - General Pediatrics Fellowships 3144
The Regenstrief Institute and the Division of General Internal Medicine offers a 2-year research oriented fellowship (with an optional third year) to prepare physicians for academic careers in general internal medicine and general pediatrics. Fellows receive formal didactic training through classes and seminars taught by faculty from both the Institute as well as Indiana University.
Requirements: Candidates for the Fellowship must hold the M.D. or equivalent degree, and must be U.S. citizens or permanent residents. Minority applicants are encouraged to apply.
Contact: Kurt Kroenke, Program Director: (317) 630-7447; fax: (317) 630-6611; email: KKroenke@regenstrief.org
Internet: http://www.regenstrief.org/training/general-internal-medicine-pediatric-research-fellowship-program
Sponsor: Regenstrief Institute
410 West 10th Street, Suite 2000
Indianapolis, IN 46202-3012

Regenstrief Master Of Science In Clinical Research/CITE Program 3145
Indiana University has received funding from the National Institute of Health through a K-30 grant to develop and implement the Clinical Investigation and Translational Education (CITE) program. The purpose of this program is to prepare health care professionals for a career in clinical research. Following completion of the program, graduates can embark on a career in clinical research with the skills necessary to successfully compete for grant funding, conduct and analyze research findings, and publish their work in scientific journals. By participating in the program, CITE trainees will complete a two-year formal clinical research curriculum, at the end of which they will receive a Master of Science in Clinical Research degree. The program is designed for participants that already have or are in training for a doctoral degree (e.g., MD, PhD, DNS, DDS, DPT).
Requirements: Most participants will already have a doctoral degree (e.g., MD, PhD, DNS, DDS, or DPT) or be in training for a doctoral degree. Potential applicants include, but are not limited to, the following: fellows or other health care professional trainees who have substantial protected time for clinical research; junior faculty who have career awards or support from their division or department head for participation in the CITE program; other faculty who previously have focused on basic research or other academic activities but now are committed to pursuing a career in clinical research CITE constitutes the formal didactic requirements for certain types of federal training grants (such as K-23's) and other career awards. Individuals in these programs would be expected to participate in CITE unless they were enrolled in some other type of formal degree program.
Contact: Kurt Kroenke, Program Director: (317) 630-7447; fax: (317) 630-6611; email: KKroenke@regenstrief.org
Internet: https://www.indianactsi.org/cite/citeapplication
Sponsor: Regenstrief Institute
1050 Wishard Boulevard, RG-6
Indianapolis, IN 46202-2872

Rehab Therapy Foundation Grants 3146
The foundation awards grants to North Carolina nonprofit organizations. Areas of priority include organizations that serve children with developmental disabilities and their families; and impact inadequately insured or underserved children with developmental disabilities and their families. Grant applications are available year round at the Foundations website however, applications will only be accepted once a year beginning in January and must be received by February 28th. Award recipients will be notified by mail on or about May 15th.
Requirements: Applicant must be a nonprofit 501(c)3 organization or public school in North Carolina.
Restrictions: Proposals benefiting religious organizations, university level education, research, events, individuals, trusts, or political causes will not be funded.
Geographic Focus: North Carolina
Amount of Grant: $50,000 total
Date(s) Application is Due: Feb 28
Contact: Kimberly D. Reilly, Wachovia Philanthropic Services; email: info@rehabtherapyfoundation.org
Internet: http://www.rehabtherapyfoundation.org/grant.htm
Sponsor: Rehab Therapy Foundation, Inc.
150 Fayetteville Street, Seventh Floor
Raleigh, NC 27602

Rehabilitation Nursing Foundation Research Grants 3147
The Foundation makes available research grants totaling $44,500. RNF offers funding of up to $30,000 for rehabilitation nursing research which is awarded in the form of multiple grants. A New Investigator Award, offered to encourage nurses who are novice researchers, will be awarded for up to $10,000. Up to two grants from the remaining amount will be awarded to recipients, who will be designated RNF Research Fellows. Research proposals that address clinical practice or educational or administrative dimensions of rehabilitation nursing are accepted. Quantitative and qualitative research projects will be reviewed. Funding may be awarded in the form of multiple grants. The Research Grant Committee reviews proposals once a year. Proposals must be postmarked by February 1. Grant recipients will be notified in September, and funding begins January of the following year for the selected proposals.
Requirements: The principal investigator for the research project must be a registered nurse who is active in rehabilitation or who demonstrates interest in and significant contributions to rehabilitation nursing. Membership in the Association of Rehabilitation Nurses is not required. Graduate student researchers are eligible for funding.
Samples: Maryann Abendroth, Research Title: Understanding Caregivers' Decision Process When Choosing to Institutionalize a Relative with Parkinson's Disease (2008); Cheryl Gies, Research Title: Web-based Psychosocial Assessment for Caregivers of Persons with Dementia: A Feasibility Study (2008); Susan Newman, Research Title: Community Integration after Spinal Cord Injury: Identifying Barriers and Facilitators through Photovoice (2007).
Amount of Grant: $44,500 maximum
Date(s) Application is Due: Feb 1
Contact: Director; (847) 375-4710 or (800) 229-7530; email: info@rehabnurse.org
Internet: http://www.rehabnurse.org/research/researchgrants.html
Sponsor: Rehabilitation Nursing Foundation
4700 W. Lake Avenue
Glenview, IL 60025-1485

Rehabilitation Nursing Foundation Scholarships 3148
ARN offers financial assistance in the form of two distinct types of scholarships: a $1,000 award to nurses working toward a Bachelor of Science in Nursing (BSN) degree; and the Mary Ann Mikulic Scholarship, which covers one full tuition to the Professional Rehabilitation Nursing Course. Each award has a deadline of June 1.
Requirements: The BSN Scholarship eligibility requirements include: membership and involvement in ARN; enrollment in a Bachelor of Science in Nursing (BSN) program in good standing and successful completion of at least one course; current practice in rehabilitation nursing; and a minimum of 2 years experience in rehabilitation nursing. The Mary Ann Mikulic Scholarship eligibility requirements include: being a registered nurse with a current license; currently practicing in the specialty of rehabilitation nursing; and the ability to meet all other financial responsibilities incurred by participating in the course.
Amount of Grant: $1,000
Date(s) Application is Due: Jun 1
Contact: Gayle Elliott; (847) 375-4710 or (800) 229-7530; email: gelliott@connect2amc.com
Internet: http://www.rehabnurse.org/awards/allscholar.html
Sponsor: Rehabilitation Nursing Foundation
4700 W. Lake Avenue
Glenview, IL 60025-1485

Religion and Health: Effects, Mechanisms, and Interpretation RFP 3149
The Center seeks proposals to elucidate how religious involvement (religious attendance, worship, altruistic and caring activities) influences individual and community health. The goals of this research program are to: quantitatively document effects on health (where health is broadly defined); clarify the biological, social, psychological mechanisms involved; and interpret what the findings mean for individual, congregational, and community health through trans-disciplinary collaboration and deliberation. This RFP focuses on research that examines the contribution of context and caring as part of the mechanism that accounts for the effects of religion on health, in particular the effects of membership and practices within a faith community. Letters of Intent are due July 15. Thirty finalists will be invited to submit full proposals; seven $200,000 grants will be awarded to outstanding research proposals. Finalists will be selected by Aug 5, with full proposals due by November 1, and awards announced on January 1.
Amount of Grant: $200,000
Date(s) Application is Due: Jul 15
Contact: Catherine Craver, Assistant Director; (919) 660-7578; fax: (919) 684-8569; email: catherine.craver@duke.edu
Internet: http://www.dukespiritualityandhealth.org/proposals/
Sponsor: Center for Spirituality, Theology and Health at Duke University Medical Center
Box 3825, Duke University Medical Center
Durham, NC 27710

Retirement Research Foundation General Program Grants 3150

The Retirement Research Foundation, based in Chicago, was established in the 1950s and endowed in 1978 by the late John D. MacArthur. The Foundation is devoted solely to serving the needs of older persons in the U.S. and enhancing their quality of life. The Foundation supports a range of programs and special initiatives designed to: improve access to and quality of community-based and residential health and long-term care; promote economic security for all older adults by strengthening social insurance, pension, and personal savings programs; and support adequate training of, and compensation for, those already working directly with older persons and their families to bring higher quality of care to larger numbers of older adults. The Foundation's historic interest in innovative projects continues. RRF also has a strong interest in projects that implement or adapt proven models that address clearly identified needs and gaps. Requests for support of projects focusing on advocacy, research, or education and training will be considered from anywhere in the United States. Direct service requests will be considered only from organizations in these seven states: Illinois, Indiana, Iowa, Kentucky, Missouri, Wisconsin, and Florida.

Requirements: The Retirement Research Foundation does not use a standard application form, proposals for funds should include the following elements: cover page; Summary; project significance; statement of objectives; description of methodology; dissemination; budget and timetable; plans for continued support; list of personnel; applicant organization; tax exempt status. Application submission must include: the signature of the chief executive officer of the applicant organization; the proposal and attachments must be submitted in triplicate; only one copy of the annual report and financial/audit are needed.

Restrictions: Funding for vans is limited to applicants from Illinois and Florida. Funding is not generally available for: biomedical research; computer equipment; conferences, publications or travel unless they are components of other larger Foundation-funded projects; construction of facilities; dissertation research; endowment or developmental campaigns; general operating expenses of established organizations; grants or scholarships to individuals; production of films and videos; projects of governmental organizations except for state universities, area agencies on aging, and programs of the Veterans Administration; projects outside the United States

Samples: Alivio Medical Center, Chicago, Illinois $255,000 - three-year grant to design and implement a chronic disease self-management program for seniors (2008); Family Caregiver Alliance, San Francisco, California $148,650 - An 18-month grant to facilitate advocacy around state and federal policies designed to assist caregivers through organization and dissemination of policy and resources (2008); Organization of New City, Chicago, Illinois $150,000 - Three-year grant to help low-income elderly families cope with safety, utility, and housing issues (2008);

Date(s) Application is Due: Feb1; May 1; Aug 1;

Contact: Irene Frye, Executive Director; (773) 714-8080; fax: (773) 714-8089; email: info@rrf.org

Internet: http://www.rrf.org/generalProgram.htm

Sponsor: The Retirement Research Foundation
8765 West Higgins Road, Suite 430
Chicago, IL 60631-4170

Rett Syndrome Research Foundation Grants 3151

The foundation (RSRF) awards research grants and postdoctoral fellowships for international biomedical research for the treatment and cure of Rett Syndrome. Relevant disciplines include but are not limited to developmental biology, molecular biology, genetics, biochemistry, cellular physiology, neurology, immunology, pharmacology, gastroenterology, orthopedics, and experimental neurotherapeutics. Treatment-related research is especially encouraged. RSRF seeks to encourage research that encompasses innovative approaches and techniques that will lead to NIH and other funding sources. The foundation is committed to funding senior investigators as well as junior, provided they have a supportive environment. Teams working together from different disciplines, institutions as well as industry are encouraged to apply. Grants are made for technical support, supplies, equipment, and relevant travel. No salary support is provided for the Principal Investigator. Indirect costs of up to 10 percent of direct costs may be included. Letters of intent must be received by the listed application deadline; full proposals are by invitation. Guidelines are available online.

Amount of Grant: $50,000 maximum per year ($40,000 salary plus $10,000 of expendables)

Date(s) Application is Due: Jan 31

Contact: Monica Coenraads, Director of Research, (203) 445-9233; fax: (203) 445-9234; email: monica@rsrf.org

Internet: http://www.rsrf.org/researchers/4.7.1.html

Sponsor: Rett Syndrome Research Foundation
4600 Devitt Drive
Cincinnati, OH 45246

Reynolds and Reynolds Associate Foundation Grants 3152

Reynolds has a long-standing reputation as a leading corporate citizen within the communities where it has a large presence. The company encourages its associates to roll up their sleeves and get involved in organizations they believe in, and in which they often are involved personally. The mission of The Foundation is to provide a vehicle for Dayton associates to improve health and human services in the local communities. Since 1956, the Foundation has provided financial support to area health and human service agencies throughout an eight-county area. Focus areas include: health and human services with emphasis on domestic violence and child abuse; youth-at-risk; hunger; issues of the elderly; homelessness; literacy; and life-threatening illnesses.

Requirements: Giving is limited to the eight-county region in and around Dayton, Ohio.

Restrictions: There is no support available for non 501(c)3 organizations, sectarian organizations with a predominately religious purpose, fraternal or veterans' organizations, individual primary or secondary schools (except for occasional special projects), or tax-supported universities and colleges (except for occasional special projects) No grants are offered to individuals, or for endowments, courtesy advertising, fund raising events, deficit or debt retirement, or capital campaigns.

Geographic Focus: Ohio

Samples: Dayton Fund for Home Rehab, $2,500 - care for the Elderly, Homelessness, Youth at Risk (2008); Project READ, $4,000 - Literacy, Youth at Risk (2008); A Special Wish Foundation, $3,500 - Life Threatening Illness (2008).

Amount of Grant: $500-$5,000 average; $40,000 maximum

Date(s) Application is Due: Jan 7; Mar 11; Jun 10; Sep 9

Contact: Alice Davisson, Treasurer; (937) 485-4409 or (937) 485-8138; email: alice_davisson@reyrey.com

Internet: http://www.reyrey.com/company/community/associate_foundation.asp

Sponsor: Reynolds and Reynolds Associate Foundation
P.O. Box 2608
Dayton, OH 45401-2608

RGK Foundation Grants 3153

RGK Foundation awards grants in the broad areas of Education, Community, and Medicine/Health. The foundation's primary interests within Education include programs that focus on formal K-12 education (particularly mathematics, science and reading), teacher development, literacy, and higher education. Within Community, the foundation supports a broad range of human services, community improvement, abuse prevention, and youth development programs. Human service programs of particular interest to the foundation include children and family services, early childhood development, and parenting education. The foundation supports a variety of Community Improvement programs including those that enhance non-profit management and promote philanthropy and voluntarism. Youth development programs supported by the foundation typically include after-school educational enrichment programs that supplement and enhance formal education systems to increase the chances for successful outcomes in school and life. The foundation is also interested in programs that attract female and minority students into the fields of mathematics, science, and technology. The foundation's current interests in the area of Medicine/Health include programs that promote the health and well-being of children, programs that promote access to health services, and Foundation-initiated programs focusing on ALS.

Requirements: Although there are no geographic restrictions to the foundation's grantmaking program, the foundation no longer accepts unsolicited requests for international agencies or programs. All applicants must complete an electronic Letter of Inquiry from the Web site as the first step. RGK Foundation will entertain one electronic Letter of Inquiry (LOI) per organization in a twelve-month period. While the foundation occasionally awards grants for operating expenses, capital campaigns, endowments, and international projects, such grants are infrequent and usually initiated by the foundation. Grants are made only to nonprofit organizations certified as tax exempt under Sections 501(c)3 or 170(c) of the IRS code. Hospitals, educational institutions, and governmental institutions meeting these requirements are eligible to apply.

Restrictions: The foundation refrains from funding annual funds, galas or other special-event fundraising activities; debt reduction; emergency or disaster relief efforts; dissertations or student research projects; indirect/administrative costs; sectarian religious activities, political lobbying, or legislative activities; institutions that discriminate on the basis of race, creed, gender, or sexual orientation in policy or in practice; or loans, scholarships, fellowships, or grants to individuals; unsolicited requests for international organizations or programs or for ALS research projects.

Samples: 2008: COMMUNITY - Ark House Foundation (Richardson, TX) to provide low cost, temporary housing for patients and their families while undergoing long-term medical treatment in the Dallas area.; Rider University (Lawrenceville, NJ) to expand the Minding Our Business after-school and summer entrepreneurship program serving 6th-8th grade students in Trenton public schools.; YWCA of Greater Atlanta (Atlanta, GA) expansion of Teen Girls in Technology Program to middle school girls at Title One schools. EDUCATION - BookSpring (Austin, TX) to build regional alliance's capacity following merger with Reading is Fundamental of Austin.; Generations Incorporated (Boston, MA) to expand the Classroom Literacy program using older adults as literacy aids in Boston Public elementary schools.; The Field Museum (Chicago, IL) to improve curriculum in Chicago Public Schools as part of the High School Transformation Project.; MEDICINE/HEALTH - Ambulatory Surgery Access Coalition (San Francisco, CA) to provide essential outpatient surgery to uninsured through a volunteer network.; Marathon Kids (Austin, TX) to enhance national program capacity through technology upgrades for the website.; Travis County Medical Society Foundation (Austin, TX) support program and ongoing enhancements for Project Access that will add dental services and Bilingual Patient Service Coordinator.

Amount of Grant: $1000-$25,000 average

Contact: Suzanne Haffey, Grants Associate; (512) 474-9298; fax (512) 474-7281; email: shaffey@rgkfoundation.org

Internet: http://www.rgkfoundation.org/public/guidelines

Sponsor: RGK Foundation
1301 West 25th Street, Suite 300
Austin, TX 78705-4236

Rhode Island Foundation Grants 3154

The foundation seeks to promote philanthropic activities that will improve the living conditions and well-being of the inhabitants of Rhode Island. Grants for capital and operating purposes principally to agencies working in the fields of education, health

care, the arts and cultural affairs, youth, the aged, social services, urban affairs, historic preservation, and the environment.
Requirements: Rhode Island nonprofits organizations may apply. See Foundations website for additional guidelines.
Restrictions: The foundation does not make grants for endowments, research, religious groups for religious purposes, hospital equipment, capital needs of health organizations, or to educational institutions for general operating expenses.
Geographic Focus: Rhode Island
Samples: Ocean State Action Fund, Cranston, RI, $50,000 - for continued funding for grassroots organizing, coalition work, and public communications in support of affordable, quality health care for all Rhode Islanders (2008); Community Housing Land Trust of Rhode Island, Providence, RI, $50,000 - for new program targeting foreclosed properties or those close to being foreclosed upon (2008); Sakonnet Preservation Association, Little Compton, RI, $25,000 - for three-community partnership to preserve drinking water quality and open space in Newport County (2008);
Contact: Owen Heleen, Vice President for Grant Programs; (401) 427-4009 or (401) 274-4564; fax: (401) 331-8085; email: oheleen@rifoundation.org
Internet: http://www.rifoundation.org/Nonprofits/GrantOpportunities/tabid/175/Default.aspx
Sponsor: Rhode Island Foundation
One Union Station
Providence, RI 02903

Rice Foundation Grants **3155**
The foundation awards grants to Illinois nonprofit organizations in its areas of interest, including civic affairs, higher education, hospitals, libraries, medical education, and youth programs. Project and operating support are available. There are no application forms or deadlines.
Requirements: Applicants should submit a proposal with directly to the Foundation including the following: statement of problem project will address; copy of IRS Determination Letter; brief history of organization and description of its mission; detailed description of project and amount of funding requested.
Geographic Focus: Illinois
Samples: John G. Shedd Aquarium, Chicago, IL $1,000,000 - for general support (2005); Northwestern University, Evanston, IL $386,700 - for general support (2005); Big Shoulders Fund, Chicago, IL $30,000 - for general support (2005);
Amount of Grant: $25,000-$1,000,000 average
Contact: Peter Nolan, President; (847) 581-9999
Sponsor: Daniel F. and Ada L. Rice Foundation
8600 Gross Point Road
Skokie, IL 60077-2151

Rich Foundation Grants **3156**
The foundation awards grants to nonprofit organizations in Atlanta, GA, to support community funds, performing arts, cultural programs, higher education, social services, homeless, youth, hospitals, heart disease, theater, and AIDS. Types of support include annual campaigns, building funds, continuing support, equipment acquisition, operating budgets, technical assistance, and research. Contact the office for application forms. The board meets quarterly to review requests.
Requirements: Nonprofit organizations in the Atlanta, GA, area are eligible for grant support.
Geographic Focus: Georgia
Amount of Grant: $5000-$100,000 average
Date(s) Application is Due: Mar 15; Jun 15; Sep 15; Dec 15
Contact: Anne Poland Berg, Grant Consultant, (404) 262-2266
Sponsor: Rich Foundation
11 Piedmont Ctr, Suite 204
Atlanta, GA 30305

Richard and Helen DeVos Foundation Grants **3157**
The foundation supports nonprofit organizations primarily in western Michigan and central Florida in its areas of interest, including religious agencies and churches and education and outreach, social services, the arts, public policy, and health care. Types of support include general operating support, continuing support, annual campaigns, capital campaigns, building construction/renovation, program development, seed grants, and matching funds.
Requirements: Application forms are not required. Applicants should submit the following: copy of IRS Determination Letter; copy of current year's organizational budget and/or project budget. The Board meets every 3 months, submit your proposal two weeks prior to the review (contact Foundation for deadline dates). Mail applications to: 126 Ottawa Avenue, N.W., Suite 500, Grand Rapids, MI 49503
Restrictions: No grants to individuals.
Geographic Focus: Florida; Michigan
Samples: Michigan State University, East Lansing, Michigan, $5,000,000 - For general support, payable over 1 year (2007)); Salvation Army of West Palm Beach, West Palm Beach, Florida, $50,000 - For general support, payable over 1 year (2007);
Amount of Grant: $300 - $5,000,000 range
Contact: Ginny Vander Hart, Foundation Director; (616) 643-4700; fax: (616) 774-0116; email: virginiav@rdvcorp.com
Sponsor: Richard and Helen DeVos Foundation Grants
P.O. Box 230257
Grand Rapids, MI 49523-0257

Richard and Rhoda Goldman Fund Grants **3158**
The fund is interested in supporting programs that will have a significant positive impact in an array of fields, including culture, the environment, population, Jewish affairs, violence prevention, children and youth, the elderly, and social and human services. Types of support include general operating support, continuing support, capital campaigns, program development, and seed money. Funds will be allocated primarily in the San Francisco Bay area of California and to organizations benefiting this area. There are no application deadlines.
Requirements: Nonprofit organizations serving primarily the San Francisco Bay area of California are eligible.
Restrictions: The fund does not accept applications for research or award grants or scholarships for individuals, conferences, documentary films, or fund-raisers. Unsolicited proposals for support of arts organizations or institutions of primary, secondary, or higher education will not be accepted.
Geographic Focus: California
Samples: San Francisco Beautification (CA)—for efforts to increase green schoolyards, $10,000 (2005); American Jewish Joint Distribution Committee (New York, NY)—for relief efforts following the earthquake and tsunamis that struck Southeast Asia in 2004, $30,000 (2005); United States Public Interest Research Group Education Fund (Washington, DC)—for efforts to increase attention to the role of hard money in federal political campaigns, $20,000 (2005); Community Awareness and Treatment Services (San Francisco, CA)—for support of this 24-hour shelter and transitional-housing program for women, $25,000 (2005).
Amount of Grant: $1000-$500,000
Contact: Sam Salkin, Executive Director, (415) 345-6300; fax: (415) 345-9686; email: info@goldmanfund.org
Internet: http://www.goldmanfund.org
Sponsor: Richard and Rhoda Goldman Fund
P.O. Box 29924, 211 Lincoln Boulevard
San Francisco, CA 94129

Richard and Susan Smith Family Foundation Grants **3159**
The foundation awards grants to Massachusetts nonprofit organizations in its areas of interest, including arts and culture, children and youth, disadvantaged (economically), education (early childhood, elementary, and higher), minorities, biomedical research, health care and social services delivery. Types of support include annual campaigns, building construction/renovation, capital campaigns, curriculum development, general operating grants, program/project support, seed grants, and service delivery programs. There are no application forms.
Requirements: Massachusetts nonprofit organizations serving the greater Boston area are eligible.
Restrictions: Grants do not support political activities; religious activities; individuals; or requests for deficit financing or endowment funds.
Geographic Focus: Massachusetts
Samples: Compassionate Care ALS, West Falmouth, MA $25,000 - for the purchase of a cargo van to transport adaptive equipment to and from patient homes (2009); United Teen Equality Center, Lowell, MA $944,780 - funding provides violence prevention, youth development, education and community organizing programs for the youth center, the grant is payable over 5 years (2009);
Amount of Grant: $5000-$238,000 range
Date(s) Application is Due: Mar 15; Aug 15
Contact: David Ford, Executive Director; (617) 278-5200; fax: (617) 278-5250; email: dford@smithfamilyfoundation.net
Internet: http://www.smithfamilyfoundation.net
Sponsor: Richard and Susan Smith Family Foundation
1280 Boylston Street, Suite 100
Chestnut Hill, MA 02467

Richard E. Griffin Family Foundation Grants **3160**
The Foundation, established in 1997, is dedicated to supporting higher education, human and social services, and federated giving programs. Funding most often comes in the form of general operating support. Though there are no specific application forms or deadlines with which to adhere, applicants should make an initial approach by letter outlining the project and budgetary need.
Samples: Nantucket Historical Association, Nantucket, Massachusetts, $36,000—for general operations (2006); Massachusetts College of Pharmacy and Health Sciences, Boston, Massachusetts, $55,000—for general operations (2006).
Amount of Grant: $1,000-$100,000
Contact: Gregory J. Englund, Foundation Contact; (617) 439-6779 or (617) 292-4602; fax: (617) 439-6920; email: GJEnglund@EnglundLawFirm.com;; Richard E. Griffin; (603) 472-4652
Sponsor: Richard E. Griffin Family Foundation
75 Federal Street, Suite 413
Boston, MA 02110-1904

Richard King Mellon Foundation Grants **3161**
On a national basis, the foundation makes grants to acquire and preserve key tracts of land in danger of being lost to urban growth and environmentally insensitive development. Mellon gives to nonprofits in Pittsburgh and throughout southwestern Pennsylvania to improve human services, education, medical care, civic affairs, and cultural activities. Types of support include capital grants, challenge/matching grants, general operating grants, project grants, and seed money grants. Application and guidelines are available online.

Requirements: Projects originating in Pittsburgh and southwestern Pennsylvania are given special priority.
Restrictions: Grants are not made to individuals. The foundation does not consider requests for individuals or organizations that pass funds to other agencies or projects outside of the United States.
Geographic Focus: Pennsylvania
Samples: Saint Vincent College (LaTrobe, PA)—for a business and conference center, $5 million (2005); Westminster College (New Wilmington, PA)—to renovate an academic and administration building, $300,000 (2005); Carnegie Museums of Pittsburgh (PA)—to renovate and expand dinosaur exhibits at the Carnegie Museum of Natural History, $3 million (2005); Direct Relief International (Santa Barbara, CA)—to assist tsunami-relief efforts, $500,000 (2005).
Amount of Grant: $74.1 million total
Contact: Michael Watson, Vice President, (412) 392-2800; fax: (412) 392-2837
Internet: http://fdncenter.org/grantmaker/rkmellon
Sponsor: Richard King Mellon Foundation
500 Grant Street, Suite 4106
Pittsburgh, PA 15219-2502

Richard M. Fairbanks Foundation Grants **3162**
The Richard M. Fairbanks Foundation, Inc. was established in 1986 by Richard M. Fairbanks, founder and owner of Fairbanks Communications. An independent private foundation granting funds to qualifying nonprofit organizations, programs, and projects in the greater Indianapolis, Indiana area. Exceptions to this geographic limitation are normally made only for organizations historically supported by the Fairbanks family or for national disasters. If you are interested in learning if your organization and project/program matches the Richard M. Fairbanks Foundation's areas of interest and funding guidelines, you may contact the foundation by telephone, email or brief written letter of inquiry. Please note that the Fairbanks Foundation does not accept unsolicited proposals.
Requirements: The Foundation: makes grants only to tax exempt public charities as defined in Sections 501(c)3 & 509(a)(1)(2)(3) of the Internal Revenue Code, except as prohibited for 509(a)(3) Type III organizations; will not consider requests for loans and grants to individuals; does not make grants or give support to conferences, seminars, media events, or workshops unless they are an integral part of a broader program; ordinarily considers grant requests only from organizations located in Greater Indianapolis, Indiana.
Geographic Focus: Indiana
Samples: Prevent Blindness Indiana - in support of General Operations, $15,000 (2008); Indiana University School of Nursing - in support of School of Nursing Learning Consortium for Faculty Development in Simulation Technology, $167,887 (2008).
Contact: Claire Fiddian-Green, Grants Officer; (317) 663-4189 or (317) 846-7111; fax: (317) 844-0167; email: Fiddiangreen@rmfairbanksfoundation.org
Internet: http://www.rmfairbanksfoundation.org/default.asp?p=3
Sponsor: Richard M. Fairbanks Foundation, Inc.
9292 North Meridian Street, Suite 304
Indianapolis, IN 46260

Richard P. Covert Scholarship **3163**
Two scholarships are awarded annually, one each at the undergraduate and graduate levels, in the field of health care information and management systems. Funding is provided by HIMSS. Completed application form, available from the society, must be accompanied by relevant transcripts, a technical paper and/or an essay, and a faculty recommendation. Annual deadline dates may vary; contact the program office for exact dates.
Requirements: Applicant must be at least a junior when the scholarship is awarded and must be a student member of HIMSS. Previous winners are not eligible, although an undergraduate winner is eligible if pursuing a graduate degree.
Amount of Grant: $5000
Date(s) Application is Due: Oct 31
Contact: John Page, Executive Director, HIMSS Scholarship Committee, (312) 644-4467; fax: (312) 664-6143; email: jpage@himss.org
Internet: http://www.himss.org/ASP/scholarship_ms.asp
Sponsor: Healthcare Information and Management Systems Society
230 E Ohio Street, Suite 500
Chicago, IL 60611-3269

Richmond Eye and Ear Fund Grants **3164**
The fund is committed to serving the city of Richmond, Colonial Heights, Hopewell and Petersburg, and the counties of Chesterfield, Hanover, Henrico, Goochland, New Kent, Charles City, Lancaster, Northumberland, Richmond, Westmoreland and Powhatan in the fields of ophthalmology, otolaryngology, and oral maxillofacial surgery for qualified organizations. Grantmaking focuses on underserved, uninsured, or medically indigent children and adults in need of ophthalmological (eye), otolaryngological (ear, nose, and throat), and/or oral maxillofacial services (conditions, defects, injuries, and aesthetic aspects of the mouth, teeth, and jaws); improving access and outreach as it relates to the stated services mentioned; and healthcare education/preventive care consistent with purposes of this fund. Guidelines are available online. The Fund???s grantmaking focuses on: Underserved, uninsured or medically indigent children and adults in need of ophthalmological (eye), otolaryngological (ear, nose and throat), and/or oral maxillofacial services (conditions, defects, injuries, and aesthetic aspects of the mouth, teeth, and jaws). Improving Access and Outreach as it relates to the services mentioned above. Healthcare Education/preventive care consistent with purposes of this fund.
Requirements: Proposals will be accepted from charitable organizations, which serve the residents of the focus area.
Geographic Focus: Virginia
Amount of Grant: $50,000 maximum
Date(s) Application is Due: May 5; Nov 5
Contact: Elaine Summerfield, Program Officer; (804) 330-7400; fax: (804) 330-5992; email: esummerfield@tcfrichmond.org
Internet: http://www.tcfrichmond.org/Page2954.cfm#ear
Sponsor: The Community Foundation
7501 Boulders View Drive, Suite 110
Richmond, VA 23225

Riley Foundation Grants **3165**
The foundation's purpose is to make grants, distributions, and/or loans to charitable and governmental organizations for charitable purposes and to provide financial resources and assistance for community wide projects and programs in health care; education; and the betterment of cultural, environmental, and economic conditions for the people of Meridian and Lauderdale County, Mississippi. Applications are reviewed at quarterly meetings in January, April, July, and October and must be in by noon on the listed deadline days.
Requirements: Mississippi governmental agencies and 501(c)3 organizations that are not private foundations as defined under Section 509(a) are eligible.
Restrictions: Best of Both Worlds Addiction Center, Inc. $75,000 - Operating Support (2009); Meridian Community College $5,000 - Lucile Reisman Rosenbaum Memorial Scholarship Endowmen (2009);
Geographic Focus: Mississippi
Samples: Care Lodge Domestic Violence Shelter, Inc (MS)—to renovate the kitchen and add a bathroom, $33,975.; City of Meridian (MS)—to support a feasibility study for a proposed downtown hotel development, $12,000.; Meridian Little Theatre (MS)—to purchase 60 student season tickets $2100.; Montgomery Institute (MS)—to support the Regional Leadership Institute, $325,000.
Amount of Grant: $2000-$300,000 typically
Date(s) Application is Due: Feb 15; May 15; Aug 15; Nov 15
Contact: Becky Lewis, (601) 481-1430; fax: (601) 481-1434; email: info@rileyfoundation.org
Internet: http://www.rileyfoundation.org/guide.htm?46,10
Sponsor: Riley Foundation
4518 Poplar Springs Drive
Meridian, MS 39305

Ripley County Community Foundation Grants **3166**
The Ripley County Community Foundation, Inc. was formed in February 1997. The effort to create the Foundation was a result of the vision of a group of philanthropic minded Ripley County residents who wanted to improve the quality of life for Ripley County, Indiana residents. Organizations seeking grants from the Ripley County Community Foundation must file an "Intent to Apply" form before preparing a complete grant application. This process will allow the Foundation to review and determine if the grant request meets Ripley County Community Foundation guidelines and/or whether the grant is likely to be funded. This "Intent to Apply" form must be received at the Foundation's office no later then 4:00 PM on August 14th. A grant application will be mailed within two weeks if you are eligible to apply. Grant applications must be received at the Foundation's office no later then 4:00 PM on September 11th. If you have any questions, call the Foundations office.
Requirements: Grant applicants must qualify as exempt organizations under Internal Revenue Code Section 501(c), or be sponsored by such organizations, or qualify as governmental or educational entities or possess similar attributes per IRS Code Section 509(a). Grants will be made only to organizations that have a responsible fiscal agent and adequate accounting procedures.
Restrictions: No grants will be made: solely to individuals; to defray travel or lodging expenses to enable individuals or groups to attend seminars or take trips; exclusively for endowment purposes of recipient organizations; for programs which will have been completed and funded prior to the Ripley County Community Foundation publicized date for grant decisions; to repay acquisition costs for equipment already purchased or paid for; for acquisition of weapons, firearms or destructive devices as defines in the Indiana Code under IC 35-41-1-8 or IC 35-47.5-2-4; specifically for sectarian religious purposes, but can be made to religious organizations for general community programs, or to preserve an historical site; organizations who have been awarded prior grants must have complied with all reporting requirements and be in good standing before submitting another grant application. Non-compliance will result in exclusion from future granting; to attempt to influence legislation or to intervene in any political campaign on behalf of any candidate for public office. Ripley County Community Foundation reserves the right to refuse any and all grant applications. Grant recipients and fiscal agents will sign and abide by the respective conditions as set forth in the foundation's " Grant Award Agreements" and "Grant Report Forms".
Geographic Focus: Indiana
Samples: Morris Fireman's Assoc. - self-contained breathing apparatus, $4,500 (2008); SEICHN, Inc. - Breast Health Screening, $4,600 (2008); American Legion Post 337 - chairs and cart, $1,115 (2008).
Contact: Jane Deiwert Program Officer; (877) 234-5220 or (812) 933-1098; fax: (812) 933-0096; email: jdeiwert@rccfonline.org
Internet: http://www.rccfonline.org/grants.asp
Sponsor: Ripley County Community Foundation, Inc.
132 South Main Street
Batesville, IN 47006

Robert and Joan Dircks Foundation Grants 3167
The foundation supports non-profit organizations that enrich and improve the quality of life for individuals primarily located in the New Jersey area. The focus is to encourage innovative programs and projects that benefit and improve the lives of children and individuals who are physically mentally or economically disadvantaged.
Requirements: Submit your inquiry online, using the Grant Request Information form provided on the Robert and Joan Dircks Foundation website: http://www.dircksfoundation.org/application2.asp
Restrictions: The Robert and Joan Dircks Foundation does not award grants for political or lobbying activities, environmental or cultural projects, capital or annual campaigns, endowments, operating budgets, deficit or debt reduction, loans or housing projects. Also, grants are not made to programs of national or international scope.
Geographic Focus: Northeast
Amount of Grant: $1000-$15,000 range
Contact: Grants Administrator; email: grants@dircksfoundation.org
Internet: http://www.dircksfoundation.org/guidelines.html
Sponsor: Robert and Joan Dircks Foundation
P.O. Box 6
Mountain Lakes, NJ 07046

Robert and Polly Dunn Foundation Grants 3168
The foundation awards grants in the U.S. Southeast, with emphasis on the Atlanta, GA, area, for projects in the area of youth, child development, and higher education. Types of support include capital campaigns, general operating support, and scholarship funds. There are no application forms. The board meets in June and December to consider requests.
Restrictions: Grants do not support individuals and not awarded to support endowment funds, loans, or program-related investments
Geographic Focus: Georgia
Amount of Grant: $587,925 total
Date(s) Application is Due: Apr 30; Sep 30
Contact: Karen Wilbanks, Executive Director, (404) 816-2883; fax: (404) 816-2883
Sponsor: Robert and Polly Dunn Foundation
P.O. Box 723194
Atlanta, GA 31139

Robert B McMillen Foundation Grants 3169
The Robert B McMillen Foundation is a non-profit charitable foundation. The Foundation offers funding in the states of Washington and Alaska. The two areas of intent are: medical and social enhancement. Fifty percent of the annual funding is earmarked for medical research. The Foundation will consider making grants to non-profit organizations involved in researching cardiology, lipid and organ transplants. Twenty-five percent of annual giving is earmarked for social areas including, but not limited to, Goodwill, Salvation Army & United Way. Preference is given to organizations and/or programs that use art as the vehicle to impact communities and change individual lives.
Requirements: The Foundation does not accept uninvited medical or social proposals. Contact the Foundations office for information on, how to be invited to make a medical or social proposal to the McMillen Foundation.
Restrictions: The Foundation do not make grants to: religious, fraternal or other organizations primarily benefiting their own members; other private foundations nor political organizations; for-profit entities; other than scholarships, the foundation will not make multi-year grants.
Geographic Focus: Alaska; Washington
Samples: Seattle Children's Hospital – Pediatric Heart Failure, Organ Transplantation and Neovascularization (2008); ArtsEd Washington – PAL Program and Arts Partners Project (2008); Seattle Goodwill – General Support (2008).
Contact: Cassandra Town, President; (425) 313-5711; fax: (425) 313-8955; email: cassandra@mcmillenfoundation.org
Internet: http://www.mcmillenfoundation.org/mission.htm
Sponsor: Robert B McMillen Foundation
55 1st Place NW, Suite 2, P.O. Box 1523
Issaquah, WA 98027

Robert E. and Evelyn McKee Foundation Grants 3170
The foundation awards grants in the following categories: civic, cultural, and religion; education and scholarships; hospitals; medical and medical research; welfare, rehabilitation, and mental health; United Way; and youth activities. Grants awarded for scholarships are made to a few selected high schools and universities, who select scholarship recipients. Religious contributions are basically limited to the local Episcopal churches. The majority of funding is made to local charitable organizations or through local affiliates of national or statewide organizations.
Requirements: 501(c)3 tax-exempt organizations are eligible.
Restrictions: Funding is not available to organizations outside the United States or those limited by race or ethnic origin. The foundation refrains from awarding grants for endowments or deficit financing. Grants are not made to other foundations, except for a local community foundation.
Geographic Focus: Texas
Samples: Saint Francis on the Hill Episcopal Church (El Paso, TX)—$1000 (2003); U of Texas at El Paso (TX)—for Department of Engineering scholarships, $8000 (2003); Texas Tech U Health Sciences Ctr (El Paso, TX)—for the University Breast Care Center, $3000.; Special Olympics, Area 19 (El Paso, TX)— $1000 (2003).
Amount of Grant: $1000-$10,000
Date(s) Application is Due: Dec 15
Contact: Grants Administrator, (915) 581-4025; fax: (915) 833-3714; email: mckeefoundation@directway.com
Internet: http://www.mckeefoundation.org
Sponsor: Robert E. and Evelyn McKee Foundation
5835 Cromo Drive, Suite 1
El Paso, TX 79912

Robert F. Stoico / FIRSTFED Charitable Foundation Grants 3171
The foundation was established to support the local communities of southeastern Massahusetts and Rhode Island. The foundation's main areas of interest are affordable housing, economic/job development, educational programs, arts and cultural programs that benefit the public or the traditionally underserved, and accessible health care for all. Small grants (under $2501) are reviewed throughout the year on a rolling basis. Large grant requests are reviewed four times a year (in April, July, October and January). Application and guidelines are available online.
Requirements: Massachusetts and Rhode Island 501(c)3 nonprofit organizations in the counties where FIRSTFED America Bancorp had business involvement are eligible.
Restrictions: The foundation does not support sports programs, political organizations, individual schools, individuals, or organizations that are not classified 501(c)3.
Geographic Focus: Massachusetts; Rhode Island
Samples: Thomas Chew Memorial Boys and Girls Club (Fall River, MA)—for its capital campaign, $1 million (2005).
Contact: Stacie Charbonneau, Manager, (508) 235-1368; fax: (508) 235-1854; email: info@stoicofirstfed.org
Internet: http://www.stoicofirstfed.org/apply.htm
Sponsor: Robert F. Stoico / FIRSTFED Charitable Foundation
P.O. Box 438
Swansea, MA 02777

Robert P. & Clara I. Milton Fund for Senior Housing 3172
The purpose of this fund is to support innovative programs focusing on issues related to senior housing. Given the fund's significant resources, projects will be considered that look to make a meaningful impact while promoting dignity, independence and quality of life. Taking into consideration the evolving needs of an aging population, this fund strives to make St. Joseph County a regional model for senior housing by acting as a catalyst through the funding of innovative approaches. Senior housing may range from institutional care to in-home care, as well as the various ancillary services related to this issue. Special consideration will be given to projects that serve the most vulnerable of the aging population.
Requirements: 501(c)3 organizations operating in St. Joseph County and not-for-profit educational institutions and other public agencies (agencies of the state, county or local government) in St. Joseph County. The priorities for funding include Education/Training; Home & Community Based Services; Programs/Projects Serving Vulnerable Seniors, and; Public Policy Issues.
Restrictions: Annual appeals or membership contributions, grants to individuals directly or special event underwriting will not be funded.
Geographic Focus: Indiana
Samples: REAL Services for a consumer directed homemaker pilot program; South Bend Heritage Foundation for enhanced security at the Robertson's apartment building; Alzheimer's Services of Northern Indiana to rehab part of the Milton Adult Day Services Center; Health in Hospital to implement a restaurant style dining program in its facility.
Date(s) Application is Due: May 1; Nov 1
Contact: Malissa Ayala, Program Officer; (574) 232-0041; fax: (574) 233-1906; email: malissa@cfsjc.org
Internet: http://www.cfsjc.org/initiatives/senior/milton_grants.html
Sponsor: Community Foundation of St. Joseph County
205 West Jefferson Boulevard, P.O. Box 837
South Bend, IN 46624

Robert Sterling Clark Foundation Reproductive Rights and Health Grants 3173
The objective of the Foundation's work in this field is to protect and expand women's access to reproductive health services in the belief that the ability to control one's fertility and prevent unintended pregnancy is fundamental to the advancement of women's opportunities. The strategy employed by the Foundation to achieve this objective is to support policy analysis, advocacy, litigation, research, message development, and/or organizing aimed at: promoting the implementation of laws, policies and practices that will enable all women to have access to comprehensive reproductive health information and services, including emergency contraception and abortion; challenging laws and legal decisions that undermine reproductive rights and developing legal theory in support of these rights; mobilizing an informed grassroots constituency; developing new pro-choice messages, based on current opinion research, that resonate with a broad public; informing the development of judicial selection criteria that will produce non-ideological courts; and promoting the use of comprehensive sexuality education curricula in the schools.
Requirements: The Foundation makes support available to national and regional organizations working on these issues.
Amount of Grant: $1,000-$200,000
Contact: Margaret C. Ayers, Executive Director; (212) 288-8900; fax: (212) 288-1033; email: rcsf@rsclark.org
Internet: http://www.rsclark.org/index.php?page=reproductive-right-and-health
Sponsor: Robert Sterling Clark Foundation
135 East 64th Street
New York, NY 10065-7045

Robin Hood Foundation Grants 3174

The foundation's mission is to end poverty in New York City. Grants are awarded in the areas of early childhood—child development, comprehensive healthcare, parenting skills, and school preparation; education—public education reform; after-school programs—academic tutoring linked with healthcare, sex education, counseling, and job training; job training—job-traning and -placement for people with histories of substance abuse, crime, and homelessness; and basic survival initiatives—issues such as hunger, AIDS, domestic violence, and inadequate housing.
Geographic Focus: New York
Amount of Grant: $50 million total
Contact: Karen Moody, Grants Manager, (212) 227-6601; fax: (212) 227-6698; email: grants@robinhood.org
Internet: http:/www.robinhood.org
Sponsor: Robin Hood Foundation
826 Broadway, 9th Floor
New York, NY 10003

Robins Foundation Grants 3175

The foundation awards grants to nonprofit organizations in the Richmond, VA, area. Areas of interest include general grants—including cultural, charitable, scientific, environmental, and educational programs, and at-risk youth; and early childhood/quality improvement grants— for organizations that devote a major portion of their resources to young children and their families. The goal is to help improve the quality of services by providing funding for accreditation, staff training, facilities improvements, and similar initiatives. The foundation seeks projects that meet well-defined community needs, use effective approaches that build on proven programs, develop models with potential for wider application, foster self-reliance and/or end dependency, and focus on prevention as well as treatment. Types of support include capital grants and endowments.
Requirements: 501(c)3 organizations based in Virginia are eligible. Organizations based in Virginia that have or support programs outside Virginia or the United States also are eligible.
Restrictions: In general, the foundation does not make grants to support annual operating funds or budgets, special events or fundraising benefits, or religious purposes unless they are otherwise compatible with the objectives of the foundation.
Geographic Focus: Virginia
Amount of Grant: $5.1 million total; $10,000-$100,000
Contact: William Roberts Jr., Executive Director; (804) 697-6917; fax: (804) 697-6797; email: wlrjr@robins-foundation.org
Internet: http://www.robins-foundation.org
Sponsor: Robins Foundation
P.O. Box 1124, Capitol Station
Richmond, VA 23218-1124

Rochester Area Community Foundation Grants 3176

The foundation seeks to improve the quality of life in the community and awards grants in the areas of child development, education, the environment, arts and cultural programs, health services, community development, and social services and general charitable giving. Types of support include general operating support, building construction/renovation, equipment acquisition, program development, conferences and seminars, publication, seed grants, scholarship funds, technical assistance, consulting services, and scholarships to individuals. There are no application deadlines. The board meets in January, February, March, May, June, July, October, and November.
Requirements: Nonprofits in Monroe, Livingston, Ontario, Orleans, Genessee, and Wayne Counties, NY, are eligible.
Restrictions: Grants do not support partisan political organizations or religious projects, individuals, annual campaigns, deficit financing, land acquisition, endowments, or emergency funds.
Geographic Focus: New York
Samples: Heritage Christian Services, $5,000—to support the annual Sheep Shearing Festival at Springdale Farm (2009); Step by Step of Rochester, $12,000—to support the merger of Step by Step and Samaritan Women. Both organizations provide support to incarcerated women and their children (2009); Arts & Cultural Council for Greater Rochester, $42,500—for Community Arts Grants, which are administered by the Arts & Cultural Council, have a capacity-building focus, and are aimed at smaller arts organizations (2009); Lifespan of Greater Rochester, $10,000—for a financial management program which trains volunteers to provide in-home assistance with bill paying, budgeting, government benefits (such as Medicare and Medicaid), and other financial tasks for physically and/or mentally frail older adults (2009).
Contact: Marlene Cole, Administrative Assistant; (585) 341-4333; fax: (585) 271-4292; email: mcole@racf.org
Internet: http://www.racf.org/page10000903.cfm
Sponsor: Rochester Area Community Foundation
500 East Avenue
Rochester, NY 14607-1912

Rochester Area Foundation Grants 3177

The foundation makes grants in the fields of arts and culture, community development, education, human services and recreation in the greater Rochester, Minnesota area.
Requirements: Organizations must be one of the following to be eligible to receive grant funding: a tax-exempt 501(c)3 organization, a government unit (city, township, county), or a government-created organization such as a public agency. Download the required pre-application form from the website. If your pre-application is approved, you will be notified and asked to submit a full application to the foundation.
Geographic Focus: Minnesota
Samples: Rochester Public Library, $7,500—matching grant for an online tutoring program available to all students with a library card (2009); Children's Dental Health Services, $8,000—for dental equipment required to meet growing demand for services (2009); Child Care Resource & Referral, $5,300—for a new van for transporting participants of income-eligible services (2009).
Amount of Grant: $1,000 - $25,000
Date(s) Application is Due: Jan 2; May 1; Sep 1
Contact: Steve Thornton, Executive Director; (507) 424-2400 or (507) 424-3755, ext. 102; fax: (507) 282-4938; email: Steve@RochesterArea.org
Internet: http://www.rochesterarea.org/grant-resources/index.html
Sponsor: Rochester Area Foundation
400 South Broadway, Suite 300
Rochester, MN 55904

Rockefeller Archive Center Research Grants 3178

The foundation awards grants for travel and research at the Rockefeller Archive Center, which contains records of the Rockefeller Foundation, Rockefeller University, and other affiliated philanthropic organizations and individuals. The center also will award grants to support research on the history of basic medical research, the life of the Nobel laureate Paul Ehrlich, and on postcolonial studies.
Requirements: Scholarly reseearchers, particularly students preparing dissertations, are eligible.
Restrictions: The Archive Center's programs do not support research at other institutions, and they do not provide general tuition support.
Contact: Camilla Harris, Grants Administrator; (914) 366-6311 or (914) 631-4505; fax: (914) 631-6017; email: charris@rockarch.org or archive@rockarch.org
Internet: http://www.rockarch.org/grants/
Sponsor: Rockefeller Foundation
15 Dayton Avenue
Sleepy Hollow, NY 10591-1598

Rockefeller Brothers Fund Peace and Security Grants 3179

The Fund's Peace and Security Program focuses on two factors that may be key to advancing or undermining global problem solving: the content and style of U.S. global engagement in the face of new perils and opportunities; and the strength and quality of relationships between Muslim and Western societies. In addition, peace and security is a theme that may be identified for attention in one or more of the Fund's pivotal places. Two specific goals have emerged: to advance U.S. policies and behaviors that reflect a broadly shared vision of constructive, cooperative, principled, farsighted, and effective global engagement; and to reduce the divisive and destabilizing tensions that exist between much of the Islamic world and the West, particularly the United States, and to increase the potential for collaboration among Muslim and Western societies on behalf of a better, safer world.
Requirements: A prospective grantee in the United States or foreign counterpart must be either a tax-exempt organization or an organization seeking support for a project that would qualify as educational or charitable.
Restrictions: The fund does not make grants to individuals, nor does it as a general rule support research, graduate study, or the writing of books or dissertations by individuals.
Amount of Grant: $25,000-$300,000; $75,000 average
Contact: Benjamin Shute, Jr.; (212) 812-4200; fax: (212) 812-4299; email: info@rbf.org
Internet: http://www.rbf.org/programs/
Sponsor: Rockefeller Brothers Fund
437 Madison Avenue, 37th Floor
New York, NY 10022-7001

Rockefeller Brothers Fund Pivotal Places Grants: South Africa 3180

The Fund will support human advancement through its work to improve basic education and to meet the developmental needs of orphans and vulnerable children. In addition, the RBF is exploring linkages between HIV/AIDS and the Fund's other substantive concerns: democratic practice, sustainable development, and peace and security. While the Fund recognizes the critical importance of HIV/AIDS education, prevention, and treatment, many other donors are active in these fields. The RBF seeks to complement these efforts by contributing to the development of integrated responses to the broad societal impacts of the pandemic. Specifically, the Fund seeks to: improve the quality and accessibility of basic education for children in the areas of early childhood development and primary learning; assist orphans and vulnerable children in achieving their full potentials individuals and as members of society; and strengthen understanding of the linkages between HIV/AIDS and democratic practice, sustainable development, and peace and security issues in South Africa, and to promote integrated responses to the broad societal impacts of the HIV/AIDS pandemic.
Requirements: A prospective grantee in the United States or foreign counterpart must be either a tax-exempt organization or an organization seeking support for a project that would qualify as educational or charitable.
Restrictions: The fund does not make grants to individuals, nor does it as a general rule support research, graduate study, or the writing of books or dissertations.
Contact: Nancy L. Muirhead, Program Director; (212) 812-4200; fax: (212) 812-4299; email: nmuirhead@rbf.org or info@rbf.org
Internet: http://www.rbf.org/programs/
Sponsor: Rockefeller Brothers Fund
437 Madison Avenue, 37th Floor
New York, NY 10022-7001

Rockefeller Foundation Grants 3181

The foundation provides grants to institutions and individuals seeking to improve the lives of poor people with a focus on the issues and region where the foundation works. The foundation works globally but provides the majority of its grants to organizations whose work is focused in Southern and Eastern Africa, Southeast Asia, and North America through programs that address agriculture, health, employment, housing, education, arts and culture, and global policy. The foundation also operates special programs, including a conference and study program at its Bellagio Center, the Program Venture Experiment, and the Philanthropy Workshop.

Requirements: Nonprofit organizations are eligible.

Restrictions: The foundation does not give or lend money for personal aid to individuals, support attempts to influence legislation, or, except in rare cases, provide general institutional support, fund endowments, or contribute to building and operating funds.

Samples: Criterion Ventures, Haddam, CT—toward the start-up costs of a new mission-driven venture that will provide healthcare financial services to groups of American workers who are struggling with the negative economic and health impacts of paying cash for health services, $500,000 (2009); Water and Sanitation for the Urban Poor, London, England—toward the costs of building the capacity of community and local service groups and of testing innovative water and sanitation delivery systems in Gatwekera, Nairobi and the surrounding municipality to provide sustainable, equitable and affordable water and sanitation services, $249,900 (2009)

Contact: Grants Administrator; (212) 869-8500; fax: (212) 764-3468

Internet: http://www.rockfound.org/grants/grants.shtml

Sponsor: Rockefeller Foundation
420 Fifth Avenue
New York, NY 10018-2729

Rockwell Collins Charitable Contributions 3182

The corporation has identified two distinct funding priorities, and special consideration will be given to proposals that integrate these issues: education and youth development, with emphasis in math, science and engineering; and culture and the arts, with emphasis on youth educational programs. Rockwell Collins also contributes to health, human services, and civic organizations. Special consideration is given to qualifying organizations where employees volunteer; however, the majority of gifts to these organizations are made through Rockwell Collins United Way corporate contributions or employee campaigns.

Requirements: Applying organizations must be tax exempt under the federal code; able to provide current full, certified, audited financial statements; and not be private foundations. Non-U.S. organizations must provide nongovernmental organization (NGO) documentation.

Restrictions: Funding will not be considered for general endowments, deficit reduction, grants to individuals, federated campaigns, religious organizations for religious purposes, or fraternal or social organizations.

Amount of Grant: $5000 maximum

Contact: Cindy Dietz, Manager Community Relations, (319) 295-7444; fax: (319) 295-9374; email: communityrelations@rockwellcollins.com

Internet: http://www.rockwellcollins.com/about/community/index.html

Sponsor: Rockwell Collins Corporation
400 Collins Rd NE
Cedar Rapids, IA 52498-0001

Rockwell International Corporate Trust Grants Program 3183

Grants are awarded in the areas of education and youth development, with emphasis in math, science, and engineering; and culture and the arts, with emphasis on youth educational programs. Rockwell also contributes to health, human services, and civic organizations and also gives special consideration to qualifying organizations in which employees are involved as volunteers. Types of support include capital grants, challenge/matching grants, conferences and seminars, development grants, endowments, research grants, scholarship funds, and general operating grants. Awards include single-year, multiple-year, and provisional continuing support of specific programs. Applicants should submit full, detailed proposals. Proposals are accepted at any time. At the Web site, click on About Us, then Corporate Citizenship, and then Rockwell Automation Corporation Trust.

Restrictions: Organizations are not eligible if they have not received a permanent, tax-exempt ruling determination from the federal government; if they cannot provide current full, certified, audited financial statements; or if they are private foundations. Funding will not be considered for the following purposes: general endowments, deficit reduction, grants to individuals, federated campaigns, organizations or projects outside the United States, religious organizations for religious purposes, or fraternal or social organizations.

Amount of Grant: $1000-$50,000 average

Contact: Rockwell International Corporation General Information; (562) 797-3311

Internet: http://www.rockwell.com

Sponsor: Rockwell International Corporate Trust
1201 S Second Street
Milwaukee, WI 53204

Roeher Institute Research Grants 3184

The institute, through the support of the Scottish Rite Charitable Foundation of Canada, offers research grants to associates, associations, and agencies in a broad range of fields relating to human services and intellectual disability. The renewable grants are offered for one year. Research projects must be under the direction of the Roeher Institute academic associates or other university faculty or under researchers approved by the Roeher Institute. Areas constituting research priorities for the Roeher Institute are issues affecting people with intellectual disabilities; integration of people who have an intellectual disability into society; prevention, early identification, and minimization of disabling conditions; and strategies for social change that improve the quality of life of persons with intellectual disabilities. Applicants are asked to submit a summary of their research project, budget, and financial requirements.

Requirements: Applications are invited from university faculty, department heads, supervisors, Roeher Institute associates, and/or consultants.

Amount of Grant: $C10,000 maximum

Contact: Cameron Crawford, President; (416) 661-9611; fax: (416) 661-5701; email: cameronc@roeher.ca or cameronc@worldchat.com

Internet: http://www.roeher.ca/english/about/about.htm

Sponsor: Roeher Institute
4700 Keele Street, York University, Kinsmen Building
North York, ON M3J 1P3 Canada

Rohm and Haas Company Grants 3185

The company awards grants in five key philanthropic categories: education, environment, civic and community, health and human services, and arts and culture. Education grants support programs linking education in science, technology, and math to workplace and career opportunities; and educational enrichment for students, particularly in the areas of math, science, technology, and the environment either during or after school hours (including weekends, summer, and other times when school is not in session). Environment grants support after-school programs that build environmental awareness and understanding; sustainability programs that educate and promote development that meets the needs of the present society without compromising the ability of future generations to meet their own needs; pollution prevention and waste management, environmental conservation and biodiversity, and energy and water conservation; and community beautification. Civic and community grants support regional efforts that build local competitiveness and strengthen the economic and social base in Rohm and Haas host communities; programs that cut across multiple giving categories and/or that impact key stakeholders in Rohm and Haas communities; and programs that focus on volunteerism. Health and human services grants support public safety awareness; disaster preparedness; structured youth development such as leadership training; and structured youth activities and recreation. Arts and culture grants support organizational capacity building in the form of plan implementation—technology implementation and/or enhancement, communications and marketing, outreach and audience development, financial management and fundraising, board development, strategic development, professional development, and educational program development. Application and guidelines are available online.

Requirements: Eligible national and international organizations include performing and visual arts, humanities and historical societies, and museums. Preference is given to requests from Chicago, IL, and the greater Philadelphia area.

Restrictions: Grants are not awarded to individuals or for fundraising, advertising, or testimonials.

Amount of Grant: $250-$50,000

Contact: Alexandra Samuels, (215) 592-3644; fax: (215) 592-6808; email: alexandra_samuels@rohmhaas.com

Internet: http://www.rohmhaas.com/community/giving/guidelines/guidelines.html

Sponsor: Rohm and Haas Company
100 Independence Mall W
Philadelphia, PA 19106-2399

Rollin M. Gerstacker Foundation Grants Program 3186

The primary purpose of the foundation is to furnish financial aid to charities of all types supported by Mr. and Mrs. R.M. Gerstacker during their lifetimes. These charities are concentrated in Michigan and Ohio. The foundation's areas of interest include churches, community development, education, environment, health care, music and arts, research, social services, and youth, and grants are also awarded for services to the elderly and the emotionally disturbed. Some funds are designated for cultural programs and for colleges. Applications are accepted at any time.

Restrictions: Grants are not awarded to individuals, or for scholarships or fellowships

Geographic Focus: Michigan; Ohio

Samples: Alma College (MI)—to construct and maintain a residence hall, $1 million (2005); Nature Conservancy, Michigan Chapter (Lansing, MI)—for the Northern Great Lakes Forest Project, which will protect 271,000 acres across eight counties in Michigan's Upper Peninsula and link more than 2.5 million acres of protected federal, state, and natural areas, $800,000 (2005).

Date(s) Application is Due: Apr 15; Aug 15; Nov 15

Contact: E.N. Brandt, Vice President, (989) 631-6097; fax: (989) 832-8842

Sponsor: Rollin M. Gerstacker Foundation
P.O. Box 1945
Midland, MI 48641-1945

Rosalinde and Arthur Gilbert Foundation/AFAR New Investigator Awards in Alzheimer's Disease 3187

The major goal of this program is to support important research in areas in which more scientific investigation is needed to improve the prevention, diagnosis, and treatment of Alzheimer's Disease. The program will also serve to encourage junior investigators in the United States and Israel to pursue research and academic careers in the neurosciences, and Alzheimer's disease in particular. Projects in basic and translational research related to Alzheimer's disease (AD) that are clinically relevant, will be considered. Examples of

promising areas of research include, but are not limited to: basic mechanisms of aging in the central nervous system; genetics of AD; neuroimaging and precursors of AD; cellular and Molecular pathways of AD; biological Markers of AD; exercise and dietary factors; neurogenesis and AD; impact of environmental agents in CNS aging and early AD; inflammation; cardiovascular and cerebrovascular factors; drug discovery. It is anticipated that 5 grants of up to $75,000 each will be awarded. Applicants may propose to use the award over the course of one or two years as justified by the proposed research. Funds may not be requested for overhead or indirect costs. Funding will begin July 1.
Requirements: The applicant must be an independent investigator with assigned independent space and must have received a junior faculty appointment (instructor, assistant professor or equivalent) no sooner then July 1st. The proposed research must be conducted at any type of not-for-profit setting in the United States or Israel. Five criteria are used to determine the merit of an application: qualifications of the applicant; quality of the proposed research; relevance of the proposal to how mechanisms of aging may lead to AD; excellence of the research environment; likelihood that the project will advance the applicant's career in basic research on the mechanisms of aging and AD. All candidates must submit applications endorsed by their institution. The deadline for receipt of applications and supporting materials from candidates based in the U.S. is December 16th, at 5:00 p.m. EST. The deadline for receipt of applications and supporting materials from candidates based in Israel is December 30th. See website for instruction sheet and application for complete application procedures. Incomplete applications cannot be considered.
Restrictions: The Gilbert/AFAR Research Grant Program does not provide support for: Postdoctoral fellows in the laboratory of a senior investigator; investigators who have already received major extramural funding for research on Alzheimer's disease and/or aging (such as an R01 grant); Senior faculty, i.e. at the rank of Associate Professor level or higher; NIH Intramural program employees. Applicants cannot apply for the AFAR Research Grant Program or Glenn/AFAR BIG Program.
Amount of Grant: $75,000
Date(s) Application is Due: Dec 16 U.S.A; Dec 30 Israel
Contact: Grants Manager; (212) 703-9977 or (888) 582-2327; fax: (212) 997-0330; email: grants@afar.org or info@afar.org
Internet: http://afar.org/Gilbert.html
Sponsor: American Federation for Aging Research
55 West 39th Street, 16th Floor
New York, NY 10018

Rosalynn Carter Institute Georgia Caregiver of the Year Awards **3188**
To honor their work and to focus public attention on the contributions of caregivers throughout the State of Georgia, the Rosalynn Carter Institute on Caregiving in cooperation with the Georgia CARE-NETS initiated the Georgia Caregiver of the Year Awards in 2007. Awardess are presented with a gilded rose and a check for $1,000.
Requirements: Nominees must be caregivers from the State of Georgia.
Geographic Focus: Georgia
Amount of Grant: $1,000
Contact: Laura Bauer Granberry, Director; (229) 931-2034; fax: (229) 931-2663; email: lbgran@gsw.edu
Internet: http://www.rosalynncarter.org/caregiver2/
Sponsor: Rosalynn Carter Institute for Caregiving
800 GSW Drive
Americus, GA 31709-4379

Rosalynn Carter Institute John and Betty Pope Fellowships **3189**
The John and Betty Pope Fellowship in Caregiving is a unique program of the Rosalynn Carter Institute for Caregiving at Georgia Southwestern State University. The fellowship provides financial support for outstanding individuals pursuing training and careers in fields related to caregiving, and provides a structure and course of study intended to prepare them for leadership in the field. The certificate program of study includes courses in psychology, nursing, sociology and special education taken over up to four years of study at GSW.
Requirements: Award of Pope Fellowships is currently limited to students pursuing a degree program at Georgia Southwestern State University and who are or will be enrolled in the Caregiver Specialist Certificate at GSW. Applicants must have a grade point average of 3.0 as well as an established interest in academic study related to caregiving or a record of outstanding professional or informal caregiving. In addition, Pope Fellows must: enroll for minimum of 12 credit hours each semester (undergraduate) or 9 credit hours (graduate) for a full award; attend Pope Fellowship orientation and other required meetings; and make steady progress in fulfilling requirements of the Caregiver Specialist Certificate.
Amount of Grant: $6000 per year graduate Pope fellows; $3000 per year undergraduate Pope fellows; $3000 per year graduate scholarships; $1500 per year undergraduate scholarships
Date(s) Application is Due: Feb 15
Contact: Leisa Easom, Pope Fellowship Director; (229) 928-1234; fax: (229) 931-2663; email: leasom@gsw.edu or rci@canes.gsw.edu
Internet: http://www.rosalynncarter.org/PopeFellowship/
Sponsor: Georgia Southwestern State University
800 GSW Drive
Americus, GA 31709-4379

Rosalynn Carter Institute Mattie J. T. Stepanek Caregiving Scholarships **3190**
The Mattie Stepanek Caregiving Scholarship was created in memory of renowned poet and peacemaker Mattie J.T. Stepanek. The purpose of the Scholarship is to provide financial assistance to family, professional, or paraprofessional caregivers who are seeking training or education in specific skills, procedures and strategies that lead to more effective care, while also protecting the health and well-being of the caregiver.
Contact: Laura Bauer Granberry, Director; (229) 931-2034; fax: (229) 931-2663; email: lbgran@gsw.edu
Internet: http://www.rosalynncarter.org/08mattie/
Sponsor: Rosalynn Carter Institute for Caregiving
800 GSW Drive
Americus, GA 31709-4379

Roy and Christine Sturgis Trust Grants **3191**
The Roy and Christine Sturgis Charitable and Educational Trust established in 1981, supports organizations involved with arts, education, engineering/technology, food services, health care, the economically disadvantaged, health organizations, associations for homeless human services, hospitals, social services, homelessness, libraries/library science, medical research, institute, and science. Giving is primarily centered in the states of Arkansas and Texas. Contact the Foundation for further application information and guidelines.
Restrictions: No grants to individuals or for seminars; no loans.
Geographic Focus: Arkansas; Texas
Amount of Grant: $15,000 - $700,000 range
Date(s) Application is Due: Dec 31
Contact: Daniel J. Kelly Vice President,Trustee, (214) 209-1965; email: dan.kelly@nationsbank.com
Sponsor: Roy and Christine Sturgis Charitable and Educational Trust
P.O. Box 830241
Dallas, TX 75283-0241

Roy J. Carver Charitable Trust Medical and Science Research Grants **3192**
The trust supports Iowa and western Illinois nonprofit organizations and projects in the area of medical and scientific research. The goal of the program in medical and scientific research is to provide support for innovative investigation that may hold great promise for advancing scientific knowledge and improving human health. In this context, the Trust has recognized a variety of university-based scientific endeavors, most notably in the fields of medicine, engineering and the natural sciences. Although grants are occasionally awarded to address institutional capital needs, the focus of this program area is typically on the work of specific laboratories, often emphasizing multidisciplinary approaches and the development of untried, inherently risky research directions. Applicants are encouraged to contact staff prior to the development of a proposal. The board considers requests at quarterly meetings in January, April, July, and October. Approved grant payments are made semiannually in April and October.
Requirements: Grants are made to 501(c)3 tax-exempt scientific organizations in Iowa and western Illinois.
Restrictions: The trust does not support annual campaigns or ongoing operations, direct grants to individuals, religious activities, organizations without 501(c)3 status, fund-raising benefits or program advertising, or political parties or candidates.
Geographic Focus: Illinois; Iowa
Samples: Iowa State University, Ames IA—A study of high-intensity ultrasound technology for clinical applications, $166,458 (2006); University of Illinois, Urbana, IL—Enhance bioinformatics & mass spectrometry resources, $1,804,293 (2006); University of Iowa Foundation, Iowa City, IA—Continuing support for program, endowment and capital needs at the Carver College of Medicine, $6,104,365 (2006).
Amount of Grant: $10,000-$150,000 average
Date(s) Application is Due: Feb 15; May 15; Aug 15; Nov 15
Contact: Dr. Troy Ross, Executive Administrator; (563) 263-4010; fax: (563) 263-1547; email: info@carvertrust.org
Internet: https://www.carvertrust.org/index.php?page=56
Sponsor: Roy J. Carver Charitable Trust
202 Iowa Avenue
Muscatine, IA 52761-3733

RRF General Program Grants **3193**
The program funds service, education, research, and advocacy projects. The foundation is particularly interested in innovative projects that have the potential to change practice, policy, or delivery systems. The foundation's programs seek to improve the availability and quality of community-based and institutional long-term care programs; expand opportunities for older persons to play meaningful roles in society; support selected basic, applied, and policy research into the causes and solutions of significant problems of the aged; and increase the number of professionals and paraprofessionals adequately prepared to serve the elderly. Proposals fall into three general categories: research, model projects and service, and education and training. Guidelines are available online.
Requirements: Direct service projects that seek to improve the availability and quality of community-based and institutional long-term care programs; expand opportunities for older persons to play meaningful roles in society; support selected applied and policy research into the causes and solutions of significant problems of the aged; increase the number of professionals and paraprofessionals adequately prepared to serve the elderly.
Restrictions: The foundation will only consider proposals from applicants in Illinois, Indiana, Iowa, Kentucky, Missouri, Wisconsin, and Florida. Priority is given to nonprofit organizations serving the Chicago metropolitan area.
Geographic Focus: Florida; Illinois; Indiana; Iowa; Kentucky; Missouri; Wisconsin
Amount of Grant: $15 million total
Date(s) Application is Due: Feb 1; May 1; Aug 1
Contact: Marilyn Hennessy, President; (773) 714-8080; fax: (773) 714-8089; email: info@rrf.org

Internet: http://www.rrf.org/generalProgram.htm
Sponsor: Retirement Research Foundation
8765 W. Higgins Road, Suite 430
Chicago, IL 60631-4170

RRF Organizational Capacity Building Grants **3194**

The foundation provides grants for capacity-building activities that will help a nonprofit organization improve its management or governance to better serve the elderly. The following are examples of activities that will be supported but are not meant to exclude other ideas: planning (strategic, business, and financial plans) to steer an organization through changes; organizational assessments to identify problem areas that need to be strengthened; evaluation to develop outcome measures and determine progress in order to strengthen accountability to constituents and funding sources; public relations, communications, and marketing to increase awareness and utilization of services; financial management and resource development to improve financial systems, explore revenue options, and develop a stronger funding base; human resources management to enhance professional development, do team building, and improve the working environment; information systems management to identify and incorporate technology to improve efficiency; restructuring and building relations among organizations to strengthen service delivery, reduce costs, share resources, develop joint evaluations, or achieve other benefits; and board assessment, recruitment, training and structuring to strengthen the governance of the organization. All organizations that receive a grant are eligible for additional funding over the course of the grant, to be used flexibly for technical assistance opportunities that arise during the course of the grant. These may include seminars, workshops, short-term courses, publications, or other training opportunities related to organizational capacity building.
Requirements: For an organization to be eligible, it must meet the following criteria: be a nonprofit organization, but not a unit of government; be located in Cook, DuPage Kane, Kendall, Lake, or McHenry County, IL; provide services to the elderly; and intentionally give a high priority to the elderly.
Restrictions: The foundation will not fund building, renovation or capital improvements; emergency needs; deficits; or one-time events that do not build long-term capacity, i.e. fundraising events or one-time conferences.
Geographic Focus: Illinois
Amount of Grant: \$30,000 - \$75,000
Date(s) Application is Due: Feb 1; May 1; Aug 1
Contact: Mary O'Donnell, Coordinator; (773) 714-8080; email: info@rrf.org
Internet: http://www.rrf.org/organizationalCapacityBuildingProgram.htm
Sponsor: Retirement Research Foundation
8765 W. Higgins Road, Suite 430
Chicago, IL 60631-4170

RSC Abbyann D. Lynch Medal in Bioethics **3195**

The award was created to honour bioethicist and Past-President of AMS, Professor Abbyann D. Lynch, C.M., Ph.D., for her substantial achievements and support of biomedical ethics in Canada. Its purpose is to raise the profile of ethics in medicine and science by honouring leading Canadian exponents in these fields and bring recognition to their work. The bronze medal and a cash amount of \$2,000 are offered every year if there is a suitable candidate.
Requirements: The medal is awarded for a major contribution in bioethics by a Canadian. The contribution may be a book, a report, a scholarly article, a monograph or series of articles, which will normally be published in the two years preceding the nomination. Candidates shall be Canadian citizens or persons having permanent resident status, and who have lived in Canada during the three years preceding the date of nomination. Nominations shall be made by three persons with the initiator being a Fellow of the Society. The form for nomination can be downloaded from the sponsor's website.
Restrictions: Self-nomination for an award is not permitted.
Samples: 2007 - Eike-Henner W. Kluge; 2006 - Christine Overall; 2005 - Jocelyn Downie; 2003 - Hubert Doucet.
Amount of Grant: \$2,000 CAN
Date(s) Application is Due: Dec 1
Contact: Erin Hearty, Officer, Fellowship & Awards; (613) 991-6990; fax: (613) 991-6996; email: fellowship@rsc-src.ca
Internet: http://www.rsc.ca/index.php?page_id=61&lang_id=1&award_id=16
Sponsor: Royal Society of Canada
170 Waller Street
Ottawa, ON K1N 9B9 Canada

RSC Jason A. Hannah Medal **3196**

The Jason A. Hannah Medal was established in 1976 by RSC with the assistance of Associated Medical Services Incorporated, through its Hannah Institute for the History of Medicine. The medal was established to honor the late President and Managing Director of AMS Inc., Dr. Jason A. Hannah, and to bring recognition to the work of Canadian research in the history of medicine. The award is normally made for a book published in the two years preceding its nomination. The bronze medal and a cash amount are offered every year if there is a suitable nomination.
Requirements: The medal is awarded for an important Canadian publication in the history of medicine. In this context, the word 'Canadian' refers to the citizenship or residence of the author, or to a content clearly relevant to Canadian medicine and health care. Nominations shall be made by three persons with the initiator being a Fellow of the Society.
Samples: (2007) Michael Bliss, 'Harvey Cushing: A Life in Surgery'. (2006) James Opp, 'Home, Work, and Play: Situating Canadian Social History, 1840-1980'. (2005) David and Rosemary R. Gagan, 'or Patients of Moderate Means: A Social History of the Voluntary Public General Hospital in Canada, 1890-1950'. (2004) F. J. Paul Hackett, 'A Very Remarkable Sickness: Disease and Epidemics in the Petit Nord, 1670-1846'.
Amount of Grant: \$1,500 CAN
Date(s) Application is Due: Mar 1
Contact: Erin Hearty, Officer, Fellowship & Awards; (613) 991-6990; fax: (613) 991-6996; email: fellowship@rsc-src.ca
Internet: http://www.rsc.ca/index.php?page_id=61&lang_id=1&award_id=14
Sponsor: Royal Society of Canada
170 Waller Street
Ottawa, ON K1N 9B9 Canada

RSC McLaughlin Medal **3197**

This medal and cash award are given annually for important research of sustained excellence in any branch of medical sciences. Nominations must be received by the listed application deadline.
Requirements: Candidates are to be Canadian citizens or persons who have been Canadian residents for the five years prior to award date. Nominations must be made by three persons, with the initiator being a fellow of the society, and consist of citation of not more than 250 words stating concisely why the nominee should be considered, curriculum vita, list of publications, and detailed appraisal of nominee's work. The nomination dossier will remain valid for three years from the year of first nomination.
Restrictions: Self-nomination for an award is not permitted.
Amount of Grant: \$2,500 CAN
Date(s) Application is Due: Dec 1
Contact: Erin Hearty, Officer, Fellowship & Awards; (613) 991-6990; fax: (613) 991-6996; email: fellowship@rsc-src.ca
Internet: http://www.rsc.ca/index.php?page_id=61&lang_id=1&award_id=17
Sponsor: Royal Society of Canada
170 Waller Street
Ottawa, ON K1N 9B9 Canada

RSC McNeil Medal for the Public Awareness of Science **3198**

The McNeil Medal for the Public Awareness of Science was established in 1991 through McNeil Consumer Healthcare. It is intended to highlight the important role that science plays within our society and to encourage the communication of science to students and the public. The bronze medal and a cash amount are awarded every year if there is a suitable candidate.
Requirements: The medal is awarded to a candidate who has demonstrated outstanding ability to promote and communicate science to students and the public within Canada (the term public is defined in its broadest sense). Candidates shall be Canadian citizens or persons having permanent resident status, and who have lived in Canada during the three years preceding the date of nomination. Nominations shall be made by three persons with the initiator being a Fellow of the Society.
Restrictions: Self-nomination for an award is not permitted.
Samples: (2007) Mary Anne White - Her contributions have been made through helping establish an interactive science center, newspaper columns, encyclopedia contributions and science booklets, and through public lectures, innovative courses, radio, television, and many public venues, including libraries, shopping malls, and Parliament Hill. (2006) Reginald Harry Mitchell - In the area of awareness of science, his principal audience is young people and his Chemistry 'magic show', experienced by more than 30,000 BC students to date, is legendary.
Amount of Grant: \$1,500 CAN
Date(s) Application is Due: Dec 1
Contact: Erin Hearty, Officer, Fellowship & Awards; (613) 991-6990; fax: (613) 991-6996; email: fellowship@rsc-src.ca
Internet: http://www.rsc.ca/index.php?page_id=61&lang_id=1&award_id=18
Sponsor: Royal Society of Canada
170 Waller Street
Ottawa, ON K1N 9B9 Canada

RSC Thomas W. Eadie Medal **3199**

The medal is awarded annually in recognition of major contributions to any field through engineering or applied science, with preference given to those having an impact on communications, in particular the development of the Internet. Nominations must be received by the listed application deadline. The award includes a bronze medal and a cash amount.
Requirements: Candidates are to be Canadian citizens or persons who have been Canadian residents for the five years prior to award date. Nominations must be made by three persons, with the initiator being a fellow of the society, and consist of citation of not more than 250 words stating concisely why the nominee should be considered, curriculum vita, list of publications, and detailed appraisal of nominee's work. The nomination dossier will remain valid for five years from the year of first nomination.
Restrictions: Self-nomination for an award is not permitted.
Samples: 2007 - Hussein T. Mouftah; 2006 - Alberto Leon-Garcia; 2005 - Norman C. Beaulieu; 2004 - Vijay K. Bhargava; 2003 - Morrel P. Bachynski.
Amount of Grant: \$3000 CAN
Date(s) Application is Due: Dec 1
Contact: Erin Hearty, Officer, Fellowship & Awards; (613) 991-6990; fax: (613) 991-6996; email: fellowship@rsc-src.ca
Internet: http://www.rsc.ca/index.php?page_id=61&lang_id=1&award_id=5
Sponsor: Royal Society of Canada
170 Waller Street
Ottawa, ON K1N 9B9 Canada

Rush County Community Foundation Grants 3200

The Rush County Community Foundation, is a nonprofit public charity established in 1991 to serve donors, award grants and scholarships, and provide leadership to enrich and enhance the quality of life in Rush County, Indiana. The Rush County Community Foundation now holds over 130 funds, and have permanent endowment assets of over $6.5 million. As a public foundation, it helps donors provide grant making dollars for not-for-profit organizations that serve Rush County citizens. For additional information contact the Foundations office.

Requirements: Funding opportunities must serve the Rush County citzens.
Geographic Focus: Indiana
Date(s) Application is Due: Feb 15; Jun 15; Oct 15
Contact: Garry Cooley, Executive Director; (765) 938-1177; fax: (765) 938-1719; email: rccf@verizon.net
Internet: http://www.rushcountyfoundation.org/funds.php
Sponsor: Rush County Community Foundation, Inc
117 North Main Street
Rushville, IN 46173

Russell Berrie Foundation Grants 3201

The foundation supports nonprofit organizations primarily in Israel and the New York and New Jersey metropolitan areas. Grants are awarded for education (colleges and universities, Jewish education, divinity schools, parochial elementary and secondary schools, and religious higher education), health care (hospitals and respite homes), international programs (development programs, ministries, and missions), religious organizations (religious welfare, synagogues, and temples), social issues, and youth welfare. Types of support include capital support and general operating support. Applicants should submit a brief letter of inquiry and include a description of the program and the organization, including a financial statement. There are no application deadlines.

Requirements: Christian, Jewish, and Roman Catholic organizations in New York, New Jersey, and Israel are eligible.
Geographic Focus: New Jersey; New YorkIsrael
Samples: Pave the Way Foundation (New York, NY)—for unrestricted support of this organization that promotes good will and reconciliation between different religions, $100,000 (2005); American Technion Society (New York, NY)—to establish a nanotechnology institute at the Technion-Israel Institute of Technology, in Haifa, $26 million (2005).
Amount of Grant: $5000-$20,000 typically
Contact: Susan Strunk, Administrative Director, (201) 928-1880
Internet: http://www.russberrie.com/foundation.html
Sponsor: Russell Berrie Foundation
300 Frank Burr Boulevard, Building E, 7th Floor
Teaneck, NJ 07666-6704

Ruth Eleanor Bamberger and John Ernest Bamberger Memorial Foundation Grants 3202

The Foundation is dedicated to fulfilling the Founders' desires to help people reach their individual potential. The Foundation assists people of all ages, but especially children and young people through educational opportunities and scholarships, supporting crisis care and protective services, dental aid, after school programs, etc.

Requirements: Only residents of Utah may apply.
Restrictions: Grants and scholarships are given only to organizations, not individuals.
Geographic Focus: Utah
Amount of Grant: $1000-$20,000 range
Date(s) Application is Due: Mar 16; Sep 28
Contact: Eleanor Roser, Treasurer; (801) 364-2045; email: bambergermemfdn@qwestoffice.net
Internet: http://www.ruthandjohnbambergermemorialfdn.org/
Sponsor: Ruth Eleanor Bamberger and John Ernest Bamberger Memorial Foundation
136 S Main, Suite 418
Salt Lake City, UT 84101-1690

Ruth H. and Warren A. Ellsworth Foundation Grants 3203

The foundation awards grants to nonprofits in Massachusetts in support of the arts, children and youth, community development, education and higher education, and health care and hospitals. Types of support include general operating support, continuing support, annual campaigns, building construction/renovation, equipment acquisition, emergency funds, and seed grants. There are no application forms.

Requirements: Nonprofits in the Worcester, MA, area are eligible.
Restrictions: Grants are not awarded to individuals or for endowment funds, scholarships, fellowships, research, publications, conferences, matching gifts, or loans.
Geographic Focus: Massachusetts
Samples: Bancroft School, Worcester, MA, $125,000 (2006); UMass Memorial Foundation, Worcester, MA, $50,000 (2006);
Amount of Grant: $500-$100,000 average
Contact: Sumner Tilton Jr., Trustee; (508) 798-8621
Sponsor: Ruth H. and Warren A. Ellsworth Foundation
370 Main Street, 12th Floor, Suite 1250
Worcester, MA 01608-1723

Ruth Mott Foundation Grants 3204

The community is invited to submit grant requests for the program areas of arts—culture, music, theater, dance, media, graphics, photography, storytelling, and crafts; beautification—enhance neighborhoods and quality of life in the greater Flint area; and health promotion—healthy and active lifestyles and environments such as physical activity, proper nutrition, responsible sexual behavior, and overall well-being. Types of support include special projects, capacity building (planning, technical assistance, and resource development), evaluation, and general purposes. Priority is given to requests that bring diverse segments of the community together to share ideas and common interests and to respectfully address and resolve differences; enable the engagement of citizens in civic life, community service and leadership; ensure that all stakeholders are informed and involved in decisions affecting them; promote life-long learning and involvement; share and celebrate community members' unique talents, histories, cultures, and contributions; and benefit low-income segments of the community and reduce social, economic, and racial disparities. Concept papers may be submitted at any time throughout the year; full proposals are by invitation.

Requirements: Michigan nonprofit organizations are eligible. Preference is given to requests from Flint, MI.
Amount of Grant: $6.5 million total
Contact: Grants Administrator, (810)233-0170
Internet: http://www.ruthmottfoundation.org
Sponsor: Ruth Mott Foundation
111 E Court Street, Suite 3C
Flint, MI 48502-1649

RWJF Bridging the Gap: Research Informing Practice and Policy for Healthy Youth Behavior 3205

RWJF has developed three integrated strategies to reverse the childhood obesity epidemic: evidence, action and advocacy. The Bridging the Gap: Research Informing Practice and Policy for Healthy Youth Behavior program is intended to improve understanding of school, community, state and national policies and environmental factors affecting youth diet, physical activity, obesity, and tobacco, alcohol and drug use, and to evaluate the effectiveness of interventions to prevent youth obesity and tobacco use.

Requirements: Eligible applicants for research grants are scholars associated with educational institutions, research organizations, health care providers or other public or nonprofit organizations. Preference will be given to public entities or nonprofit organizations tax exempt under Section 501(c)3 of the Internal Revenue Code. Applicants may be independent of or associated with organizations currently receiving grants. All proposals must be submitted only through the RWJF Grantmaking Online system.
Contact: C. Tracy Orleans; (609) 627-5962 or (877) 843-7953; email: cto@rwjf.org
Internet: http://www.rwjf.org/grants/npo.jsp?FUND_ID=55100
Sponsor: Robert Wood Johnson Foundation
College Road East and Route 1, P.O. Box 2316
Princeton, NJ 08543-2316

RWJF Changes in Health Care Financing and Organization Grants 3206

The program supports policy analysis, research, evaluation and demonstration projects that provide policy leaders timely information on health care policy and financing issues. Supported projects include: examining significant issues and interventions related to health care financing and organization and their effects on health care costs, quality and access; and exploring or testing major new ways to finance and organize health care that have the potential to improve access to more affordable and higher quality health services. The grant period is 12 or fewer months for small grants and 12 or more months for large grants. There are no application deadlines. Program information and the online application process are available online.

Requirements: Researchers, as well as practitioners and public and private policy-makers working with researchers, are eligible to apply. Projects may be initiated from within many disciplines, including health services research, economics, sociology, political science, public policy, public health, public administration, law and business administration. Multidisciplinary teams and researchers who are just beginning their careers—perhaps teaming with a more senior researcher to develop the analytic approach—are especially encouraged to apply. Preference will be given to applicants that are public agencies or are tax-exempt under Section 501(c)3 of the Internal Revenue Code and are not private foundations as defined under Section 509(a). Proposals for this program must be submitted through the RWJF Grantmaking Online system.
Restrictions: Grant funds may not be used to subsidize individuals for the cost of health care, to construct or renovate facilities, for lobbying, or as a substitute for funds currently being used to support similar activities.
Amount of Grant: $100,000 maximum small grants; $100,000 minimum large grants
Contact: Program Officer; (202) 292-6700; fax: (202) 292-6800; email: hcfo@academyhealth.org
Internet: http://www.rwjf.org/applications/solicited/cfp.jsp?ID=19274
Sponsor: Robert Wood Johnson Foundation
College Road East and Route 1, P.O. Box 2316
Princeton, NJ 08543-2316

RWJF Clinical Scholars Program Grants 3207

The program fosters the development of leaders who will transform U.S. health and health care. These future leaders will be equipped to work with communities and to conduct innovative research as a result of the didactic and experiential learning they receive at each of four chosen training sites (University of California, Los Angeles; University of Michigan; University of Pennsylvania; and Yale University). The program's focus emphasizes community-based research and leadership training. The goal of the program is the integration of scholars' clinical training with skills in program development and research methodology to help them find solutions for issues in public policy, community health, and health services research. The program offers graduate-level study and research as part of a university-based postresidency training program.

Up to 29 scholars will be selected for appointments beginning the following year. Under the program, the universities provide Scholars with their stipends and health insurance. Stipends currently range from $49,000 to $51,500 per year, depending on the training site. Limited financial support is also available at each university for expenses associated with Scholars' research, including travel.
Requirements: To be eligible, physicians must be U.S. citizens; be committed to a career consonant with the program's purposes and priorities; be highly regarded by those responsible for their clinical training; and plan to complete the clinical requirements of their residency/fellowship training by the date of entry into the program (except for surgeons). Scholars may not hold appointments as sub-specialty fellows during their tenure in the program.
Amount of Grant: $49,000 - $51,500 per year
Date(s) Application is Due: Feb 15
Contact: Desmond Kimo Runyan, Program Director; (919) 843-8261; fax: (650) 566-2340; email: drunyan@med.unc.edu or rwjcsp_admin@med.unc.edu
Internet: http://rwjcsp.unc.edu/
Sponsor: Robert Wood Johnson Foundation
333 MacNider Hall
Chapel Hill, NC 27599-7105

RWJF Community Health Leaders Awards **3208**
Each year, the program honors ten outstanding individuals who overcome daunting odds to expand access to health care and social services to underserved and isolated populations in communities across the United States. Awards include a personal stipend and a grant for program enhancement. Potential nominators must submit a letter of intent; if a letter of intent is approved, a packet is sent to the nominator. For more information, contact the program office.
Requirements: Candidates must be residents of the United States, be affiliated with a 501(c)3 tax-exempt organization, have a five- to 15-year record of work in the community-health field, have experience as a direct provider of health-care services or be involved in the improvement of health-care access and delivery, demonstrate a full-time commitment to working with needy people, and have received no significant national recognition.
Restrictions: Nominations are not accepted from development and public relations departments or professional grant writers. Self-nominations are not accepted.
Amount of Grant: $125,000
Date(s) Application is Due: Oct 15
Contact: Helen Dundas, Health Care Group; (609) 627-5947 or (609) 627-5809; fax: (609) 419-8347; email: hdundas@rwjf.org
Internet: http://www.rwjf.org/applications/solicited/cfp.jsp?ID=20902
Sponsor: Robert Wood Johnson Foundation
College Road East and Route 1, P.O. Box 2316
Princeton, NJ 08543-2316

RWJF Evaluating Innovations in Nursing Education Grants **3209**
Evaluating Innovations in Nursing Education (EIN) will support evaluations of interventions that expand teaching capacity or promote faculty recruitment and retention in nursing schools. The program aims to increase the number of nursing school graduates by evaluating strategies that address the nurse faculty shortage. An important activity of the program will be disseminating successful strategies so they can be replicated in other nursing education settings.
Requirements: Nursing schools or health care organizations who will act as the applicant institution and subcontract to the evaluation team are eligible. Preference will be given to applicant organizations that are tax-exempt under Section 501(c)3 of the Internal Revenue Code and are not private foundations as defined under Section 509(a). The Robert Wood Johnson Foundation makes grants to organizations in the United States and its territories only.
Amount of Grant: $300,000 maximum
Date(s) Application is Due: Nov 24
Contact: Director; (732) 932-4670; email: info@evaluatinginnovationsinnursing.org
Internet: http://www.evaluatinginnovationsinnursing.org/
Sponsor: Robert Wood Johnson Foundation
College Road East and Route 1, P.O. Box 2316
Princeton, NJ 08543-2316

RWJF Executive Nurse Fellowships **3210**
This program is an advanced leadership program for nurses in senior executive roles who are aspiring to lead and shape the U.S. health care system of the future. The three-year fellowships are intended to offer participating nurses the experiences, insights, competencies, and skills necessary to achieve or advance in executive leadership positions in a health care system undergoing unprecedented change. Each Fellow's individual learning activities are supported by a leadership development account of $15,000 ($7,000 in year one, $4,000 in year two, and $4,000 in year three). These funds support self-directed learning activities, independent study, and access to an electronic communications network. The program office also will provide matching support for the Fellow's leadership project of $20,000 over the first two years of the program ($10,000 in year one and $10,000 in year two). The Fellow's employing organization must match the project resources of $20,000 dollar for dollar, either in cash or in-kind. Applications must be submitted online.
Requirements: Nurses in executive roles in the fields of health services, public and community health, or nursing education who possess a strong professional record reflecting positions of increasing leadership responsibility are eligible.
Samples: Jeannette Andrews, PhD, APRN, BC-Chair and Associate Professor, Biobehavioral Nursing Medical College of Georgia (Augusta, GA); Kim Hoover, PhD, RN-Associate Dean for Research and Evaluation, School of Nursing, University of Mississippi Medical Center (Jackson, MS); Susan Bakewell-Sachs, PhD, RN, APRN, BC-Dean and Professor, School of Nursing, Health & Exercise Science, The College of New Jersey (Ewing, NJ); Jill Briggs, RN, MS, MPH-Manager, Community and Family Health Division, Minnesota Department of Health (St. Paul, MN)
Amount of Grant: $15,000
Date(s) Application is Due: Feb 1
Contact: Maryjoan D. Ladden, Program Officer; (415) 502-4770; fax: (415) 502-4992; email: maryd@thecenter.ucsf.edu
Internet: http://futurehealth.ucsf.edu/Public/Leadership-Programs/Home.aspx?pid=34
Sponsor: Robert Wood Johnson Foundation
College Road East and Route 1, P.O. Box 2316
Princeton, NJ 08543-2316

RWJF Finding Answers: Disparities Research for Change Grants **3211**
The program was created to support rigorous evaluations of practical and replicable solutions designed to reduce and eliminate disease specific racial and ethnic health care disparities. It seeks to improve the quality of health care provided to patients affected by racial and ethnic disparities by: Granting funds to discover and evaluate practical and replicable solutions designed to reduce and eliminate disease specific racial and ethnic health care disparities; Focusing on interventions aimed at health care delivery for one or more of the following health concerns: cardiovascular disease, depression, or diabetes; Conducting systematic reviews of the literature regarding racial and ethnic health care disparities interventions; and Disseminating results from these research efforts and systematic reviews to encourage health care systems to address racial and ethnic gaps in care.
Requirements: For-profit organizations are eligible to apply, however preference will be given to applicants that are public agencies or are tax-exempt under Section 501(c) (3) of the Internal Revenue Code and are not private foundations as defined under Section 509(a). Proposals must focus on innovative interventions that reduce racial and ethnic disparities in the treatment of cardiovascular disease, depression, and diabetes. There are no age restrictions for the target populations of the interventions proposed for evaluation using program funds. Although there are no restrictions on the age of target populations, proposals targeting pediatric and geriatric populations are encouraged. Applications are accepted in two phases. The first phase is a brief proposal submission open to all interested research teams. The second phase is a full proposal submission and will be accepted by invitation only. All applications, both the brief and full proposals, must be submitted through the Robert Wood Johnson Foundation's Grantmaking Online system.
Restrictions: Individuals are not eligible to apply. Stand-alone prevention interventions such as tobacco cessation or exercise programs are not eligible unless they are one part of a larger, more comprehensive, intervention. The program will only directly fund health care delivery institutions. However, eligible institutions may partner/sub-contract with academic or research groups.
Amount of Grant: $100,000 - $275,000
Contact: Marshall H. Chin, Director; (866) 344-9800 or (773) 702-4769; email: mchin@medicine.bsd.uchicago.edu
Internet: http://www.solvingdisparities.org/
Sponsor: Robert Wood Johnson Foundation
College Road East and Route 1, P.O. Box 2316
Princeton, NJ 08543-2316

RWJF Generalist Physician Faculty Scholars **3212**
This national career development program is designed to develop leaders in primary care academics by providing funding for junior faculty research. Each year the program provides $300,000 for 15 junior faculty members in family medicine, internal medicine and general pediatrics, to conduct four-year research projects nationwide. Under the program, the scholars, sponsored by their medical schools, receive support to enhance their research productivity, develop innovative mentoring programs for medical students, and participate in the design and implementation of primary education initiatives. The program coordinates several activities including an annual meeting for the scholars to present their research findings and conference calls for the scholars to discuss professional issues.
Requirements: Accredited colleges and universities within the United States are eligible to apply.
Samples: Dartmouth Medical School Center for the Evaluative Clinical Sciences, $240,906.; University of California, San Francisco, School of Medicine, $300,000.; University of Colorado at Denver and Health Sciences Center, $299,980.; Mount Sinai School of Medicine of New York University, $300,000.; University of Pennsylvania School of Medicine, $299,993.
Amount of Grant: $300,000 maximum
Contact: Cynthia D. Mulrow; (210) 877-2275; email: mulrowc@uthscsa.edu
Internet: http://www.rwjf.org/applications/solicited/npo.jsp?FUND_ID=55121
Sponsor: Robert Wood Johnson Foundation
College Road East and Route 1, P.O. Box 2316
Princeton, NJ 08543-2316

RWJF Harold Amos Medical Faculty Development Scholars **3213**
The Harold Amos Medical Faculty Development Program supports basic/biomedical, clinical, and health services/epidemiology research. The purpose of the AMFDP award is to facilitate the transition of the newly-trained clinician who wishes to develop into an independent investigator. A completed application consists of two parts: the completion of the online proposal process, and submission of other (paper) supporting documents.

Requirements: To be eligible, applicants must be physicians from historically disadvantaged backgrounds (ethnic, financial, or educational) who are U.S. citizens or permanent residents at the time of application deadline; have excelled in their education; are now completing or have completed their formal clinical training; are prepared to devote four consecutive years to research; are committed to pursuing academic careers; and are committed to improving the health status of the underserved, decreasing health disparities, or serving as role models for students and faculty from historically disadvantaged backgrounds Preference will be given to physicians who have recently completed their formal clinical training. In order to pursue the advanced research training required by this program, applicants must identify faculty mentors with whom a research plan will be developed. The mentor's experience in the supervision of trainees and the adequacy of the mentor's research environment and support will be strongly considered. Deadline for receipt of completed online applications - March 23. Deadline for postmark of all supporting documents and hard copies - March 24. Complete guidelines and application instructions are available at the website.
Amount of Grant: $104,140
Date(s) Application is Due: Mar 23; Mar 24
Contact: Nina Ardery, Program Deputy Director; (301) 565-4080 or (317) 278-0500; fax: (301) 565-4088; email: nardery@erols.com or amfdp@starpower.net
Internet: http://www.amfdp.org/applicat.htm
Sponsor: Robert Wood Johnson Foundation
College Road East and Route 1, P.O. Box 2316
Princeton, NJ 08543-2316

RWJF Health & Society Scholars **3214**
The program is a two-year fellowship designed to build the nation's capacity for research, leadership, and action to address the broad range of factors affecting health. The goal of the program is to improve health by training scholars to rigorously investigate the connections between biological, behavioral, environmental, economic, and social determinants of health; and develop, evaluate, and disseminate knowledge and interventions based on integration of these determinants. Each year the program will enable up to 18 outstanding individuals who have completed doctoral training to engage in an intensive two-year program at one of six nationally prominent universities. Applications and guidelines are available online.
Requirements: Individuals must apply only through the foundation's online system (http://www.hsscholars.org). To be eligible, scholars must have completed doctoral training by the time of entry into the program (August or September) in one of a variety of fields including, but not limited, to the behavioral and social sciences, the biological and natural sciences, health professions, public policy, public health, history and ethics; have significant research experience; clearly connect their research interests to substantive population health concerns; and be citizens or permanent residents of the United States or its territories. Applications from candidates with diverse backgrounds are encouraged.
Restrictions: Individuals placed in the program must be willing to relocate to the institution designated during the match process for the duration of the two-year program.
Amount of Grant: $89,000 plus health insurance
Date(s) Application is Due: Oct 2
Contact: Pamela G. Russo, Program Officer; (212) 419-3566; fax: (212) 419-3569; email: hss@nyam.org
Internet: http://www.healthandsocietyscholars.org
Sponsor: Robert Wood Johnson Foundation
College Road East and Route 1, P.O. Box 2316
Princeton, NJ 08543-2316

RWJF Health Care Costs: Research to Inform Policy Grants **3215**
The Robert Wood Johnson Foundation, through its Changes in Health Care Financing and Organization (HCFO) initiative, is issuing a special topic solicitation for proposals to conduct research and analyses on the complex causes and potential solutions to rising health care costs. The solicitation seeks research contributing to an evidence base that defines and addresses the problem of rising health care costs, and how it relates to health insurance coverage. Research should focus on identifying sources of continued cost growth, examining promising cost control efforts, and exploring the relationship between health care costs and health insurance. The research questions are broken down into four major categories (Cost Controls, Affordability, Pricing, and Cost Estimates). The questions are not an exhaustive list, but have been identified among the priorities for the foundation. However, these should not be viewed as prescriptive.
Requirements: Researchers should have a demonstrated track record in health services research, economics, financing, or public policy. Junior researchers may apply as the principal investigator. However, to be competitive, the proposal must provide evidence that there is sufficient senior research oversight and support. All applicants are required to submit a brief proposal.
Restrictions: Grants are not available for ongoing general operating expenses or existing deficits; endowment or capital costs, including construction, renovation, or equipment purchases; basic biomedical research; conferences, symposia, publications, or media projects, unless they are clearly related to the foundation's goals; research on unapproved drug therapies or devices; international programs and institutions; or direct support to individuals.
Contact: Bonnie J. Austin, Deputy Director; (202) 292-6700; fax: (202) 292-6800; email: Bonnie.Austin@academyhealth.org or hcfo@academyhealth.org
Internet: http://www.hcfo.net/grants.htm
Sponsor: Robert Wood Johnson Foundation
College Road East and Route 1, P.O. Box 2316
Princeton, NJ 08543-2316

RWJF Health Impact Project Grants **3216**
The Health Impact Project, a collaboration of the Robert Wood Johnson Foundation and The Pew Charitable Trusts, encourages the use of health impact assessment (HIA) to help decision-makers better assess proposed policies, projects and programs with respect to their impact on health, in order that they may avoid adverse health consequences and costs and improve health. The foundations are issuing this call for proposals to demonstrate the effectiveness of HIAs and promote their incorporation into local, state, tribal and federal decision-making. Grants will range from $25,000 to $150,000 and must be completed within 24 months. Proposals for more than $150,000 may be considered under rare and exceptional circumstances.
Requirements: Eligible applicant organizations include: state, tribal or local agencies; tax-exempt educational institutions; or publicly supported charitable organizations that are exempt from federal income tax as an organization described by Section 501(c)3 of the Code. Applicant organizations must be located in the United States or its territories at the time of application.
Amount of Grant: $25,000-$150,000 range
Contact: Program Director; (202) 540-6012; email: healthimpactproject@pewtrusts.org
Internet: http://www.rwjf.org/applications/solicited/cfp.jsp?ID=20921
Sponsor: Robert Wood Johnson Foundation
College Road East and Route 1, P.O. Box 2316
Princeton, NJ 08543-2316

RWJF Health Policy Fellowships **3217**
The purpose of this fellowship is to give outstanding mid-career health professionals in academic and community-based settings an opportunity to learn more about the legislative process through direct participation. Fellows actively contribute to the formulation of national health policies and accelerate their careers as leaders in health policy. Up to six grants of up to $165,000 each will be made. Each fellow will receive up to $94,000 for the Washington stay in salary plus fringe benefits or fellowship stipend. Fellows will receive an additional allowance for relocation subject to limitations provided in detail on the program's Web site. November 13 is the deadline for receipt of applications submitted online, with January 29 the deadline for receipt of full proposals.
Requirements: Applicants may have backgrounds in the following disciplines: allied health professions; biomedical sciences; dentistry; economics or other social sciences; health services organization and administration; medicine; nursing; public health; or social and behavioral health. Applicants must be U.S. citizens or have permanent residency status at the time of application. Potential applicants must obtain documented sponsorship from an eligible institution to support their application. Nonprofit health care organizations and academic centers are eligible sponsors. Eligible institutions may sponsor more than one candidate, but no more than one individual will be selected from any one sponsoring organization.
Restrictions: No additional direct costs (such as laptops or PDAs) or indirect costs are paid for during the first year of this program.
Amount of Grant: $165,000 maximum over three years
Date(s) Application is Due: Nov 13; Jan 29
Contact: Marie Michnich, Director; (202) 334-1506; fax: (202) 334-3862; email: mmichnich@nas.edu
Internet: http://www.rwjf.org/applications/solicited/cfp.jsp?ID=20904
Sponsor: Robert Wood Johnson Foundation
College Road East and Route 1, P.O. Box 2316
Princeton, NJ 08543-2316

RWJF Healthy Eating Research Grants **3218**
Healthy Eating Research is a national program that will support research to identify, analyze, and evaluate environmental and policy strategies that can promote healthy eating among children and prevent childhood obesity. Special emphasis will be given to research projects that benefit children in the low-income and racial/ethnic populations at highest risk for obesity. The program will fund two types of research grants: studies to identify and/or evaluate promising school food environment and policy changes (12- to 18-month awards up to $100,000 each, and 18- to 36-month awards up to $400,000 each); and analyses of macro-level policy or system determinants of school food environments and policies (12- to 18-month awards up to $75,000 each). Applications must be submitted through the online process.
Requirements: Preference will be given to those applicants that may be either public entities or nonprofit organizations that are tax-exempt under Section 501(c)3 of the Internal Revenue Code. Applicant organizations must be based in the United States or U.S. Territories. The focus of this program is the United States; studies of policies in other countries will be considered only to the extent that they may directly inform U.S. policy. The experience and qualifications of the research team is one of the primary criteria for proposal review. A doctorate or terminal degree is preferred for the principal investigator. Deadline for receipt of brief proposals - February 13. Select applicants will be invited to submit full proposals. Deadline for receipt of full proposals - May 23.
Restrictions: This program does not fund demonstration projects. The foundation does not award grants to private individuals or applicants from outside the U.S. or U.S. Territories. No faxed, emailed or mailed proposals will be accepted.
Amount of Grant: $400,000 maximum
Contact: Kathy Kosiak, Research Coordinator; (800) 578-8636; fax: (612) 624-9328; email: healthyeating@umn.edu
Internet: http://www.healthyeatingresearch.org/
Sponsor: Robert Wood Johnson Foundation
College Road East and Route 1, P.O. Box 2316
Princeton, NJ 08543-2316

RWJF Interdisciplinary Nursing Quality Research Initiative 3219

The initiative awards two-year grants to support the generation, dissemination, and translation of research to improve the contributions of nursing to the quality of hospital care. It will support interdisciplinary teams of nurse scholars and scholars from other disciplines to address gaps in knowledge about the relationship between nursing and health care quality. Topic areas include: identifying, developing, and testing new measures to advance quality nursing research; and testing the effects of implementing the nursing-sensitive performance measures endorsed by the National Quality Forum. Investigator-initiated ideas that are consistent with the broader set of program goals also will be considered. The two-phase application process begins with online submittal of a brief proposal dur by December 4; full proposals are by invitation, and are due by April 9. Guidelines are available online.

Requirements: Teams of researchers who are U.S. citizens or permanent residents are eligible. Each team must have at least one nursing researcher and at least one researcher from another discipline. Preference will be given to 501(c)3 applicants that are not 509(a) private foundations.

Amount of Grant: $300,000 maximum over two years

Date(s) Application is Due: Dec 4; Apr 9

Contact: Lori A. Melichar, Grants Administrator; (301) 571-8161 or (800) 978-8309; email: INQRIhelpdesk@constellagroup.com

Internet: http://www.inqri.org

Sponsor: Robert Wood Johnson Foundation
College Road East and Route 1, P.O. Box 2316
Princeton, NJ 08543-2316

RWJF Investigator Awards in Health Policy Research 3220

The program supports researchers whose cross-cutting and innovative ideas promise to contribute meaningfully to improving health and health policy in America. Each year, the program awards 24- to 36-month grants of up to $335,000 to highly qualified individuals to fund approximately 10 research projects that have national policy relevance. The program funds projects with a broader scope than traditional NIH or NSF grants. Data-driven health services research focusing on a narrowly defined research question is not appropriate for this program, nor are pilot projects that are designed to evaluate clinical care in a specific geographic area or to demonstrate service delivery programs or financing strategies.

Requirements: Individuals in the United States who are affiliated either with a U.S.-based educational institution or a 501(c)3 tax-exempt organization are eligible. Applications are welcomed from investigators in fields such as anthropology, business, demography, economics, engineering, ethics, genetics, health and social policy, history, journalism, law, medicine, nursing, political science, psychology, public health, science policy, social work, sociology and others. The program seeks a diverse group of applicants including minorities, researchers early in their careers, and individuals in nonacademic settings. Key Dates: Deadline for receipt of letters of intent - March 28; Applicants will be notified by mail if they have been selected to submit a full proposal. Deadline for receipt of full proposals - July 27.

Restrictions: Past awardees and teams of more than two researchers are not eligible.

Samples: Michael D. Cohen, Ph.D. - Handoffs in Hospitals: Research for the Design of Better Practices; Julie Fairman, Ph.D., FAAN, R.N. - Practice Politics: History of Nursing 1975 to the Present; Joseph J. Fins, M.D. - Minds Apart: Severe Brain Injury and Health Policy; Dominick L. Frosch, Ph.D., Jose A. Pagan, Ph.D. - Direct-to-Consumer Advertising: Do Television Pharmaceutical Ads Prompt More Than Just Prescription Requests?

Amount of Grant: up to $335,000

Date(s) Application is Due: Mar 28; Jul 27

Contact: Cynthia Church, Program Administrator; (732) 932-3817; fax: (732) 932-3819; email: depdir@ifh.rutgers.edu

Internet: http://www.investigatorawards.org

Sponsor: Robert Wood Johnson Foundation
College Road East and Route 1, P.O. Box 2316
Princeton, NJ 08543-2316

RWJF Jobs to Careers: Promoting Work-Based Learning for Quality Care Research Grants 3221

The program will support partnerships to advance and reward the skill and career development of incumbent (currently employed) workers providing care and services on the front lines of our health and health care systems. The program seeks to develop and redesign systems that support and institutionalize learning and career advancement and test new models of work-based learning. The research grants will support applied research to inform these efforts. Research funded through this program will complement and supplement learnings from the Jobs to Careers' implementation grants, which will fund partnerships of health and health care employers and educational institutions to promote the program's objectives. Grant funds may be used for project staff salaries, consultant fees, data collection and analysis, meetings, supplies, project-related travel, and other direct project expenses, including a limited amount of equipment essential to the project.

Requirements: Eligible applicants for research grants through Jobs to Careers are scholars associated with educational institutions, research organizations, health care providers or other public or nonprofit organizations. Preference will be given to public entities or nonprofit organizations tax exempt under Section 501(c)3 of the Internal Revenue Code. Applicants may be independent of or associated with organizations currently receiving Jobs to Careers implementation grants. All proposals must be submitted only through the RWJF Grantmaking Online system.

Restrictions: Grant funds may not be used to subsidize individuals for the costs of their health care, to support clinical trials of unapproved drugs or devices, to construct or renovate facilities, for lobbying, or as a substitute for funds currently being used to support similar activities.

Amount of Grant: up to $200,000

Date(s) Application is Due: Jun 19

Contact: Maria Kniesler Flynn, Director; (617) 728-4446; email: mflynn@jff.org

Internet: http://www.jobs2careers.org

Sponsor: Robert Wood Johnson Foundation
College Road East and Route 1, P.O. Box 2316
Princeton, NJ 08543-2316

RWJF Ladder to Leadership: Developing the Next Generation of Community Health Leaders Fellowships 3222

Ladder to Leadership: Developing the Next Generation of Community Health Leaders is a collaborative initiative of the Robert Wood Johnson Foundation (RWJF) and the Center for Creative Leadership. The initiative aims to enhance the leadership capacity of community-based nonprofit health organizations serving vulnerable populations. RWJF is committed to leadership development and improving the health of all Americans, particularly those in the most vulnerable communities—where people are often economically disadvantaged and have limited educational opportunities and inadequate access to health services. The program will be delivered in nine priority communities on a staggered schedule over the next four years. Each phase of the three-part curriculum includes a mixture of face-to-face training sessions, individualized executive coaching and mentoring, and team project work—all anchored within the context of the communities in which these leaders live and work to maximize the application and impact of the program concepts.

Requirements: Only one applicant from each organization will be considered. Qualified applicants must: be an early- to mid-career professional with one to five years of supervisory experience; be an employee of a community-based, health or health-related nonprofit or government organization that serves vulnerable populations; work in one of the priority communities targeted by the initiative; commit to a 16-month leadership development initiative and curriculum; have the support of their organization's executive director or senior leader and their board of directors; and be a citizen or permanent resident of the United States or its territories at the time of application.

Restrictions: Up to 30 fellows will be selected to participate in the program in each of nine targeted communities across the United States: Central New York; Cleveland, Ohio; Birmingham, Alabama; Albuquerque, New Mexico; Eastern North Carolina; Portland, Oregon; Mid-South Region (Western Tennessee, Eastern Arkansas and Northern Mississippi); New Jersey (specific site/region to be determined); and Starr County, Texas.

Contact: Christy Schaefer, Project Manager; (336) 286-4595; email: schaeferc@ccl.org or info@laddertoleadership.org

Internet: http://www.rwjf.org/applications/solicited/cfp.jsp?ID=20281

Sponsor: Robert Wood Johnson Foundation
College Road East and Route 1, P.O. Box 2316
Princeton, NJ 08543-2316

RWJF Local Funding Partnerships Program Grants 3223

The foundation awards matching grants to establish funding partnerships with local grantmakers in support of innovative, community-based projects that focus on the health and health care of underserved and at-risk populations. Priority will be given to projects that involve cooperation among public- and private-sector service providers; have other financial sponsors; include continuation of the proposed innovation after support expires; and have local government support. Grants are awarded for 36 to 48 months and must be matched one-to-one. Grant funds may be used for project staff salaries, consultant fees, data collection and analysis, meetings, supplies, project-related travel, and other direct project expenses, including a limited amount of equipment deemed essential to the project. The full RFP is available online.

Requirements: Applicants may be either 501(c)3 public entities or nonprofit organizations and not classified as a private foundation under Section 509(a).

Restrictions: In-kind services and money to pay for capital costs or renovation may not be used to match funds.

Samples: Northern Virginia Community College Educational Foundation (VA)—for community-based efforts to reduce health disparities, as part of the Local Initiative Funding Partners Program, $500,000.

Amount of Grant: $50,000-$200,000 average

Contact: Leticia Peguero, Deputy Director; (609) 275-4128; email: lpeguero@localfundingpartnerships.org

Internet: http://www.rwjf.org/applications/solicited/cfp.jsp?ID=20781

Sponsor: Robert Wood Johnson Foundation
College Road East and Route 1, P.O. Box 2316
Princeton, NJ 08543-2316

RWJF New Careers in Nursing Scholarships 3224

The Robert Wood Johnson Foundation New Careers in Nursing is a scholarship program to help alleviate the nursing shortage and increase the diversity of nursing professionals. Through grants to schools of nursing, the program will provide scholarships to college graduates with degrees in other fields who are enrolled in accelerated baccalaureate and master's degree nursing programs. A school of nursing may apply for between five and 30 scholarships per year to be awarded to students from underrepresented groups in nursing or disadvantaged backgrounds. Up to 400 scholarship awards will be made during this funding cycle. The deadline for receipt of applications and supporting documents submitted online is December 15.

Requirements: To be eligible, applicant institutions must: offer an entry-level accelerated baccalaureate nursing program or master's nursing program for non-nursing college graduates; and be accredited by a nursing accrediting agency recognized by the U.S. Department of Education.

Contact: Vernell DeWitty, Ph.D.; (202) 463-6930; email: vdewitty@aacn.nche.edu

Internet: http://www.rwjf.org/applications/solicited/cfp.jsp?ID=20905

Sponsor: Robert Wood Johnson Foundation
College Road East and Route 1, P.O. Box 2316
Princeton, NJ 08543-2316

RWJF New Jersey Health Initiatives Grants **3225**

The program funds grants that promote the development of innovative, community-based health services in New Jersey. Special emphasis is placed on projects that improve access to primary health care, address the complex service needs of people with chronic health conditions, and reduce substance abuse. Grant funds may be used for staff salaries, project-related travel, data processing, supplies, a limited amount of equipment, and other expenses essential to the project. The primary emphasis of the program is the demonstration of new service delivery approaches, although a limited amount of funding will be available for planning, feasibility, and program development. The program will also support a small number of health services research or evaluation projects in the goal areas.

Requirements: Public entities or IRS 501(c)3 organizations located in New Jersey are eligible for funding. Applicants are asked to propose projects that respond to one of the following RWJF interest areas: Addiction Prevention & Treatment; Childhood Obesity; or Vulnerable Populations. Projects must address all of the following: Reach people who are not served by traditional health and social services; Focus on meeting the needs of individuals and families, touching their lives directly; Address the lack of policy, financing and service integration among state and local agencies that creates barriers to helping people.

Restrictions: Private 509(a) foundations are not eligible. Grant funds may not be used for capital costs (including construction, renovation, and most equipment purchases), to support ongoing general operating expenses or existing deficits, or to substitute for funds currently supporting similar services. No hard-copy brief or full proposals will be accepted.

Geographic Focus: New Jersey

Amount of Grant: $50,000-$300,000

Date(s) Application is Due: Jan 15

Contact: Gretchen Hartling, Program Co-Director; Rutgers, The State University of New Jersey; Institute for Health, Health Care Policy and Aging Research; 323 Cooper Street; Camden, NJ 08102-1519; (856) 225-6733; fax: (856) 225-6736; email: info@njhi.org

Internet: http://www.njhi.org

Sponsor: Robert Wood Johnson Foundation
College Road East and Route 1, P.O. Box 2316
Princeton, NJ 08543-2316

RWJF Partners Investing in Nursing's Future Grants **3226**

The program is a collaborative initiative of the Robert Wood Johnson Foundation (RWJF) and the Northwest Health Foundation (NWHF), with the intention of addressing nursing issues at the community level through funding partnerships with local and regional foundations. Up to 10 awards of up to $250,000 each will be made for projects lasting up to 24 months. Local foundations, with other partners (such as state workforce investment boards, hospital and long-term-care associations, foundations and other funding sources) will match these awards with at least $1 for every $2 provided by the program. Funding will be commensurate with the size and scope of the proposed activity and the foundation's experience with nursing issues. Funding is not intended to support the continuation of ongoing projects, but it may support new programs led by foundations that are already working in the field of nursing. October 29 is the deadline for receipt of brief proposals, and January 5 is the deadline for receipt of invited full proposals.

Requirements: Eligible institutions include local or regional private, family or community foundations and public charities. Eligible foundations are those classified as tax-exempt under Section 501(c)3 as a public charity or private foundation, a nonexempt charitable trust treated as a private foundation under Section 4947(a)(1), or organizations that claim status as private operating foundations under Section 4942(j)(3) or (5) of the Internal Revenue Code. Government entities, corporate grantmakers and others may participate as part of funding collaboratives; however, they may not serve as the applicant institution. All proposals to this program must address one or more of these topics: (1) Diversity; (2) Educational Infrastructure and Faculty Development; (3) Public Health; (4) Long-Term Care; and/or (5) Mid-Level Management. Proposals for planning as well as implementation projects will be considered. Deadline for receipt of brief proposals - November 9. Deadline for receipt of invited full proposals - February 1.

Restrictions: This program accepts only proposals submitted through the RWJF Grantmaking Online system at http://grantmaking.rwjf.org/pin2.

Amount of Grant: up to $250,000

Date(s) Application is Due: Oct 29; Jan 5

Contact: Judith L. Woodruff, J.D., Program Director; (971) 230-0093; email: judith@nwhf.org

Internet: http://www.rwjf.org/applications/solicited/cfp.jsp?ID=20903

Sponsor: Robert Wood Johnson Foundation
College Road East and Route 1, P.O. Box 2316
Princeton, NJ 08543-2316

RWJF Pioneer Portfolio Grants **3227**

The program aims to support novel, high-return ideas that may have far-reaching impact on people's health, the quality of care they receive and the systems through which that care is provided. It seeks ideas not only from the mainstream of health and health care but also looks to sources outside of these fields for innovations that might have transformative impact. Several projects apply approaches from diverse sectors such as finance, design and entertainment to forge new solutions in health and health care arenas.

Requirements: Preference is given to public agencies, public charities or are tax-exempt under section 501(c)3 of the Internal Revenue Code. Organizations must be located in the United States or one of its territories.

Restrictions: The organization does not fund any of the following: Ongoing general operating expenses or existing deficits; Endowment or capital costs; Basic biomedical research; Research on drug therapies or devices; International programs; Direct support of individuals; Lobbying of any kind. Additionally, RWJF no longer funds projects in the following areas: End-of-life care; Long-term care; Specific chronic conditions (that are not part of the strategies of other Program Areas); Physical activity for adults age 50 or older.

Samples: Ramanan Laxminaryan, Extending the Cure: Laxminaryan is reframing how we fight drug-resistant diseases by suggesting we manage antibiotics as a shared societal resource. Working with regulatory, health, pharmaceutical and economic experts, he is building evidence and consensus around incentive-based policy alternatives to ensure a vital pipeline of effective antibiotics and combat 'superbugs' that cannot be eliminated with existing drugs.; Project HealthDesign: A national program that supports interdisciplinary teams to look beyond stand-alone personal health records (PHR) to design next-generation PHR systems that empower patients to better manage their health and health care.; Influenza Prediction Markets: University of Iowa business school professors teamed up with an infectious disease expert to test whether the Iowa Electronic Markets—prediction markets that aggregate information and are best known for predicting election and film box office results—can target where influenza may strike in advance.; Myelin Repair Foundation (MRF): MRF's innovative research model provides the infrastructure for five scientific teams—spread across different university labs in the U.S. and Canada—to work virtually toward treatment breakthroughs for patients suffering from multiple sclerosis.

Contact: Chinwe Onyekere, Program Officer; (609) 627-7504 or (888) 631-9989; email: conyeke@rwjf.org

Internet: http://www.rwjf.org/pioneer/submission.jsp

Sponsor: Robert Wood Johnson Foundation
College Road East and Route 1, P.O. Box 2316
Princeton, NJ 08543-2316

RWJF Pipeline, Profession and Practice: Community-Based Dental Education Grants **3228**

Three national foundations provide grants to dental schools in the United States under the Pipeline, Profession & Practice: Community-Based Dental Education (Dental Pipeline) program, including: the Robert Wood Johnson Foundation (RWJF); the California Endowment; and W.K. Kellogg Foundation. The primary purposes of the Program is to assist dental schools in: increase services provided to vulnerable populations through dental school-community-based collaborations; train graduates with the cultural knowledge and communication skills they need to treat racially and ethically diverse patients; increase student body diversity; and graduate more dentists who choose to practice in communities-in-need.

Contact: Judith S. Stavisky, Senior Program Director; (888) 631-9989; fax: (609) 627-6401; email: JStavis@rwjf.org

Internet: http://www.dentalpipeline.org/

Sponsor: Robert Wood Johnson Foundation
P.O. Box 2316, College Road East and Route 1
Princeton NJ 08543

RWJF Scholars in Health Policy Research Fellowships **3229**

The program is a two-year fellowship targeted to outstanding new PhDs in economics, political science, and sociology to advance their involvement in health policy research. Each year, the program enables up to 12 individuals to spend two years at one of three nationally prominent universities—Harvard University, the University of California at Berkeley (in collaboration with the University of California at San Francisco), and the University of Michigan. Those selected as scholars will have access to the full range of university resources, including libraries, computers, databases and research support, and will receive stipends from their university of $80,000 for the first year and $83,000 for the second year. Application and guidelines are available online.

Requirements: Applicants must be U.S. citizens or permanent residents at the time of application and have received a doctoral degree after January 2002 but no later than July 15, 2007. Applicants must have received a doctoral degree in economics, political science, or sociology. Preference will be given to applicants who have not previously worked in the areas of health or health policy research.

Amount of Grant: $89,000

Date(s) Application is Due: Oct 21

Contact: Coordinator; (617) 353-9220; fax: (617) 353-9227; email: rwjf@bu.edu

Internet: http://www.rwjf.org/applications/solicited/cfp.jsp?ID=20841

Sponsor: Robert Wood Johnson Foundation
College Road East and Route 1, P.O. Box 2316
Princeton, NJ 08543-2316

RWJF State Coverage Initiatives Grants **3230**

These grants are designed to support states in the early stages of planning coverage expansions and those states that have decided on a new coverage expansion mechanism

and seek assistance designing and implementing the program. Both policy planning and demonstration grants are available. Specific new grant opportunities are occasionally announced on the sponsor's web site, however, states may submit project ideas at any time. The program offers primarily two types of grants: policy planning and demonstration grants. Policy planning grants are small, fast-track grants for up to $150,000 to support states in the early stages of the planning process toward expanding coverage. Grantees have used the funds to conduct health insurance surveys, analyze private market options, model specific strategies, hold policy summits, and bring together a consortium of stakeholders. Large demonstration grants of up to $1.5 million are awarded to states that have selected a coverage expansion mechanism and seek assistance in designing and implementing the coverage expansion programs. These grants have helped states to make substantial progress toward a sizable coverage objective, such as expanding eligibility to all children in a state or implementing public-private initiatives for the working uninsured. In certain circumstances, the foundation will provide special grants, such as implementation grants to assist in the successful implementation of a new coverage program.
Requirements: State organizations are eligible to apply. Contact sponsor for specific guidelines and application information.
Amount of Grant: up to $1.5 million
Contact: Isabel Friedenzohn; (202) 292-6726; email: isabel.friedenzohn@academyhealth.org
Internet: http://www.statecoverage.net
Sponsor: Robert Wood Johnson Foundation
College Road East and Route 1, P.O. Box 2316
Princeton, NJ 08543-2316

RWJF Summer Medical and Dental Education Program (SMDEP) 3231
The program was originally established as the Minority Medical Education Program (MMEP) with the aim of increasing the number of highly qualified medical school applicants from minority groups that were underrepresented in medicine—primarily African Americans, Hispanics, and American Indians. In 2003, the program changed its name to the Summer Medical Education Program (SMEP), reflecting the inclusion of students representing a wide range of economic, cultural, racial, and ethnic diversity, also expanding to include pre-dental students who face challenges similar to those of pre-medical students. The program is a free (full tuition, housing, and meals) six-week summer medical and dental school preparatory program that offers eligible students intensive and personalized medical and dental school preparation. Stipends are designed to support scholars throughout the six weeks at SMDEP. Each program site determines the amount given based on local factors such as cost of living, whether or not meals or travel are included, etc. Even though amounts vary among program sites, the stipend allowance given to each scholar is adequate to support them with their day-to-day living expenses during the six weeks attending the program.
Requirements: To be eligible for the program, an applicant must be currently enrolled as a freshman or sophomore in college; have a minimum overall GPA of 3.0, with 2.75 in the sciences; and be a U.S. citizen or hold a permanent resident visa. Other factors considered in the admissions process include whether an applicant has a combined verbal and math SAT score of at least 950 or ACT score of at least 20; comes from a group that is racially/ethnically underrepresented in medicine and dentistry (as defined independently by each program site); comes from an economically or educationally disadvantaged background; has demonstrated interest in issues affecting underserved populations; has local and/or regional residency; and submits a strong personal statement and strong letters of recommendation.
Restrictions: Former participants are not eligible to apply.
Date(s) Application is Due: Mar 1
Contact: Charles Terrell; (202) 828-0584; email: cterrell@aamc.org
Internet: http://www.smdep.org
Sponsor: Robert Wood Johnson Foundation
College Road East and Route 1, P.O. Box 2316
Princeton, NJ 08543-2316

RWJF Vulnerable Populations Portfolio Grants 3232
Programs within the Vulnerable Populations Portfolio have four elements in common: they offer an opportunity to improve health by taking a fresh approach to a long standing problem; they address poor health status in the context of other factors like housing, education and poverty; they make fundamental changes in how services are organized and delivered; and they address the lack of policy, financing, or service integration among local service providers and state and federal agencies. While RWJF awards most of its grants in response to calls for proposals, it also award grants in response to unsolicited proposals in the Vulnerable Populations Portfolio.
Requirements: Preference is given to public agencies, public charities or are tax-exempt under section 501(c)3 of the Internal Revenue Code. Organizations must be located in the United States or one of its territories. Guidelines and application information is available at the website.
Restrictions: This program will not provide funding for efforts that do not incorporate the social factors that drive health status as part of their proposed model. Additionally, the program does not fund documentaries, research, programs that address a single medical condition, or provide core support for free or safety net clinics, disease management models, or well-tested models whose effectiveness have already been established and that have been widely disseminated.
Contact: Thomas Andruszewski; (888) 631-9989; email: tandrus@rwjf.org
Internet: http://www.rwjf.org/programareas/approach.jsp?pid=1144
Sponsor: Robert Wood Johnson Foundation
College Road East and Route 1, P.O. Box 2316
Princeton, NJ 08543-2316

RWJF Young Epidemiology Scholars (YES) Competition 3233
The competition for original student research is designed to inspire talented students to investigate the many behavioral, biological, environmental and social factors that affect health and, based upon this knowledge, to identify ways to improve the health of the public. The competition awards up to 120 college scholarships each year to high school juniors and seniors who conduct outstanding research projects that apply epidemiological methods of analysis to a health-related issue.
Requirements: The student competition is open to high-school juniors and seniors who are citizens or permanent residents of the United States and enrolled in a high school in the United States, Puerto Rico, Guam, U.S. Virgin Islands American Samoa, Wake and, Midway Islands or the Marianas. Home-schooled students are also eligible. To enter the competition, you must register online and upload a written report of your research project. Reports sent via email, fax or mail will not be accepted.
Restrictions: Only one project per student will be accepted. Team projects are not eligible. If you are a previous national finalist or scholarship winner, you may not submit the same topic as a previous year unless you have significantly advanced your research (e.g., adding substantive new data, analysis or other material).
Amount of Grant: up to $50,000
Date(s) Application is Due: Feb 1
Contact: YES Program Coordinator; The College Board; 11911 Freedom Drive, Suite 300; Reston VA 20190; (800) 626-9795, ext. 5849; fax: (703) 707-5599; email: yes@collegeboard.org
Internet: http://www.collegeboard.com/yes
Sponsor: Robert Wood Johnson Foundation
College Road East and Route 1, P.O. Box 2316
Princeton, NJ 08543-2316

Ryan Gibson Foundation Grants 3234
The Foundation welcomes any and all research grant requests from around the country. The main focus is on blood related cancers. Applicants should submit a one to two page proposal with the following information: description of the procedure and or drug that is to be tested/developed, and what the desired/expected result will be; some background on the researcher and the facility that will be used (past projects success and or failures should be included); and a budget of anticipated costs. Mail all requests to the following address: The Ryan Gibson Foundation, Attn: Research Proposal, 18111 Preston Road, Suite 650, Dallas, TX 75252
Amount of Grant: $50,000 average
Contact: National Director, (214) 987-0008; fax: (214) 365-9293; email: mail@trgf.org
Internet: http://www.trgf.org/grants.shtml
Sponsor: Ryan Gibson Foundation
5910 North Central Expressway, Suite 770
Dallas, TX 75206

S. Livingston Mather Charitable Trust Grants 3235
The S. Livingston Mather Charitable Trust was established in 1953 in Ohio by Cleveland-Cliffs vice-president Samuel Livingston Mather. The Trust's primary areas of interest include cultural programs, education, child welfare, and social services. Support is also available for youth programs, the environment, and natural resources. Giving is primarily restricted to the northeastern Ohio area. Applicants should contact the Trust prior to submitting an application.
Requirements: Unsolicited requests for funds not accepted, contact the Trust before sending a proposal.
Restrictions: No support is available for: endowments; science; medical research programs; in areas appropriately supported by the government and/or the United Way; individuals; or deficit financing.
Geographic Focus: Ohio
Samples: Cleveland Museum of Art, Cleveland, OH, $20,000.; Cuyahoga Valley Countryside Conservancy, Peninsula, OH, $7,500.
Amount of Grant: $100 - $100,000 range
Contact: Janet W. Havener, Director, c/o Glenmede Trust Company; (215) 419-6000; fax: (215) 419-6790
Sponsor: The S. Livingston Mather Charitable Trust
1 Corporate Exchange, 25825 Science Park Drive, Suite 110
Beachwood, OH 44122

S. Mark Taper Foundation Grants 3236
The S. Mark Taper Foundation, founded in 1989, is a private family foundation dedicated to enhancing the quality of people's lives by supporting nonprofit organizations and their work in the Los Angeles, Long Beach, Santa Ana, California communities. Areas of interest are broad and include but are not limited to education, the environment, independent living for the disabled, abused women, immigrant health care, children, hunger, housing, AIDS, teenage pregnancy prevention, job creation and economic revitalization, individuals with visual impairments, and the arts. Types of support include capital grants, challenge/matching grants, general operating grants, research grants, program/project grants, seed money grants, and scholarships. Grants are made generally for one year.
Requirements: 501(c)3 nonprofit organizations in California are eligible for grant support. Application forms are required therefore your initial approach should be a Letter of Inquiry containing one copy of the proposal and the following: brief history of organization and description of its mission; copy of most recent annual report/audited financial statement/990; detailed description of project and amount of funding requested; list of source(s) of last three years of funding for the specific project (if any) and, the organization.

Geographic Focus: California
Samples: Korean Health Education Information and Research Center, Los Angeles, CA - $500,000 (2006); Santa Clarita Child and Family Development Center, Santa Clarita, CA - $100,000 (2006); Los Angeles Unified School District Education Foundation, Los Angeles, CA - $200,000 (2006);
Amount of Grant: $5,000 - $500,000 range
Date(s) Application is Due: Dec 1 - Feb 28
Contact: Raymond Reister, Executive Director; (310) 476-5413; fax: (310) 471-4993; email: rreisler@smtfoundation.org or info@smtfoundation.org
Internet: http://www.smtfoundation.org/
Sponsor: S. Mark Taper Foundation
12011 San Vicente Boulavard, Suite 400
Los Angeles, CA 90049

S.H. Cowell Foundation Grants **3237**
The foundation awards grants for a wide variety of causes to nonprofit organizations in northern California. Projects of interest include those that support children, youth, and families; education; housing; alcohol abuse prevention; religious organizations, education, and welfare; school-to-work employment training; population and environment; family planning; and conventional arms control. Applicants are encouraged to obtain most of their operating and project funding from other sources. Matching and challenge grants will be awarded under appropriate circumstances. The foundation prefers to award grants for one-time capital needs or for specific projects that are time-definite in nature and likely to become self-sufficient within several years. The application process should begin with a phone call. If interested, the foundation will request a short letter and then a formal proposal.
Requirements: Grants are made only to 501(c)3 tax-exempt organizations primarily in northern California.
Restrictions: The foundation does not normally make grants to individuals, for start-up of new organizations, for academic or other research, for general support, for annual fund-raising, to governmental agencies, to churches for religious support, to hospitals for medical research or treatment, for conferences, for media projects, or for political lobbying.
Geographic Focus: California
Samples: Adventure Risk Challenge, Truckee, CA, $25,000 - to launch year-round expansion of the Adventure Risk Challenge (ARC) summer program (2008); Boys & Girls Clubs of the North Valley Chico, CA, $500,000 - to launch a Boys & Girls Club in South Oroville (2008); East Bay Asian Local Development Corporation Oakland, CA, $375,000 - to complete the budget to install a park at Lion Creek Crossings (2008);
Amount of Grant: $500,000 maximum; $20,000-$100,000 average
Contact: Susan Vandiver, Program Contact; (415) 397-0285; fax: (415) 986-6786; email: info@shcowell.org
Internet: http://www.shcowell.org/grant/grant.php
Sponsor: S.H. Cowell Foundation
120 Montgomery Street, Suite 2570
San Francisco, CA 94104

SAG Motion Picture Players Welfare Fund Grants **3238**
The Motion Picture Players Welfare Fund (MPPWF) is an emergency financial assistance fund of the Screen Actors Guild New York region designed to assist eligible members who are struggling with a financial, personal or medical crisis. The Screen Actors Guild contracts with The Actors Fund to administer the MPPWF as well as provide an array of services to meet each members needs. Services include counseling and referrals for personal, family or work-related problems. Linkage to community resources for legal services, elder care, entitlement benefits or childcare. Workshops are offered on locating affordable housing, financial education as well as health insurance options. Financial assistance is available for rent, utilities, mental health and medical care as well as other basic living expenses. Grants are approved on a case–by-case basis based on need.
Requirements: All SAG members should feel free to call The Actors Fund for information, referrals and access to our social services. To be eligible for financial assistance from MPPWF you must be: living in the New York Tri-State area; a SAG member for at least six dues periods; a member in good standing at the time of application or be vested for pension purposes; and, able to document a need for emergency financial assistance.
Geographic Focus: New York
Contact: Actors Fund Intake Unit; (212) 221-7300, ext. 119
Internet: http://new.actorsfund.org/services/Partner_Programs/Motion_Picture_Players/index_html
Sponsor: Screen Actors Guild (SAG)
360 Madison Avenue, 12th Floor
New York, NY 10017

Saint Luke's Foundation Grants **3239**
The foundation exists to improve the health and well being of individuals and families living in Greater Cleveland. Proposals are invited for activities intended to enhance community involvement and ownership; promote healthy behaviors and life styles by education and outreach programs aimed at increasing the capacity of individuals and families to protect and improve their own health; increase and improve health care by improving access to affordable, high-quality, comprehensive, culturally competent and appropriate health care; educate health care professionals to increase their capacity in serving the health and health care needs of inner-city residents; and increase knowledge by furthering research on: the determinants of health; innovative systems, strategies, and collaborations designed to improve health and well being in the community; and the underlying causes of diseases and disabilities particularly prevalent in the communities.
Requirements: 501(c)3 tax-exempt organizations and governmental units/agencies are eligible. The grant application is a 3 step process: step 1: Letter of Inquiry; step 2: site visit; step 3: proposal submission. See website for detailed description of each step. The deadlines posted are for the Letter of Inquiry.
Restrictions: The Foundation does not fund: individuals; religious organizations for religious or evangelical purposes; projects outside Greater Cleveland that do not directly benefit Cleveland residents; fundraising events; endowment funds; biomedical research; debt retirement; lobbying.
Geographic Focus: Ohio
Date(s) Application is Due: Jan 5; Apr 1; Jul 1; Aug 1; Oct 1
Contact: Peg Butler, Grants Manager; (216) 431-8010; fax: (216) 431-8015; email: pbutler@saintlukesfoundation.org
Internet: http://www.saintlukesfoundation.org/grants/community-grants.html
Sponsor: Saint Luke's Foundation of Cleveland, Ohio
4208 Prospect Avenue
Cleveland, OH 44103

Saint Luke's Health Initiatives Grants **3240**
The trust was established for the purpose of addressing critical health needs in Maricopa County, AZ. Community grants support innovative approaches that address community health from a broad perspective, including funding for such projects as professional education and training, public education/advocacy demonstration projects, program planning and expansion, and equipment to address the health needs of populations that are considered underserved and vulnerable. Community grants are awarded for up to two years. Bridge grants support small, emerging organizations or new programs of larger organizations that have infrastructure or developmental needs. Grants support strategic planning, technical training, purchasing equipment, or convening discussion groups on community health issues. Bridge grants are awarded for one year. Inquiries are encouraged prior to proposal submission.
Requirements: To be eligible for a community partnership grant, a prospective organization must: demonstrate tax-exempt status under Section 501(c)3 of the Internal Revenue Service Code or be recognized as an instrumentality of state/local government; be located in Arizona. Preference is given to organizations within Maricopa County, although a statewide program with impact on Maricopa County will be considered.
Restrictions: The trust does not fund individuals, participate in large capital campaigns or endowment drives, provide grants for ongoing annual operating support, or fund projects of sectarian or religious organizations.
Geographic Focus: Arizona
Samples: Maricopa Council on Youth, Sports and Physical Activity, Phoenix, AZ, $23,000 - creation of an interactive map and resource directory to document healthy food accessibility (2009); The Centers for Habilitation, Pheonix, AZ, $12,000 - development of a family support group: "J.O.E.," Just Our Experiences (2009);
Amount of Grant: $10,000-$100,000 to community groups over two years or less; bridge grants up to $10,000
Date(s) Application is Due: Feb 12; Aug 14
Contact: Jane Pearson, Associate Director, Programs; (602) 385-6500; fax: (602) 385-6510; email: Jane.Pearson@slhi.org or info@slhi.org
Internet: http://www.slhi.org/community_grants/how_to_apply.shtml
Sponsor: Saint Luke's Health Initiatives
2929 North Central Avenue, Suite 1550
Phoenix, AZ 85012

Salem Foundation Charitable Trust Grants **3241**
The Foundation provides funding for a large variety of community based programs that serve the greater Salem area. In partnership with donors, the Foundation supports nonprofit and other community organizations with funds for health and human services, affordable housing, early childhood development, community arts, culture and other important areas of need. Grant making decisions are made by the Distribution Committee, comprised of five Salem area residents.
Requirements: Must be a community-based organization that serves the greater Salem region. Grants may be made only to organizations which have received appropriate determination letters from the Internal Revenue Service that they are exempt under the Internal Revenue Code.
Geographic Focus: Oregon
Samples: Camerata Musica—to support 2007-2008 concerts at the Salem Public Library (2007); Family Building Blocks—for staff members to attend National Conference on Child Abuse and Neglect (2007); Lord & Schryver Conservancy—Garden rehabilitation at Historic Deepwood Estate (2007).
Date(s) Application is Due: May 1; Dec 1
Contact: Trustee of the Salem Foundation, (503) 363-3136; email: salemfoundation@pioneertrustbank.com
Internet: http://www.pioneertrustbank.com/salemfoundation/index.html
Sponsor: Salem Foundation Charitable Trust
109 Commercial Street NE, P.O. Box 2305
Salem, OR 97308

Salem Foundation Grants **3242**
The primary purpose of the Foundation is support of higher education, cultural activities, health services, hospital building funds, and Christian giving. Its fields of interest include: arts; Christian agencies and churches; the disabled; education (secondary and higher); the environment; family services; federated giving programs; health care (particularly heart and circulatory disease research); hospitals; human services; museums; and Protestant federated giving programs. Types of support include: annual campaigns,

building/renovation projects, capital campaigns, general operating support, and program development. There is no formal application process and no deadlines. Please contact via letter.
Restrictions: Giving primarily in Florida, Maine and Minnesota. No grants to individuals.
Geographic Focus: Florida; Maine; Minnesota
Amount of Grant: $10,000 maximum
Contact: Robert S. Parish, President, (952) 476-6292
Sponsor: Salem Foundation, Inc.
2181 Springwood Road
Wayzata, MN 55391-2254

Salisbury Community Foundation Grants 3243
The foundation was created to address the needs of the Salisbury, NC, community and its residents. Nonprofit organizations may apply for project support in the categories of arts, education, environment, historic preservation, human services, health and medical research, public and civic affairs, religion, the elderly, and youth services. Applications are accepted throughout the year.
Requirements: Tax-exempt, charitable organizations in Salisbury, NC, and Rowan county are eligible.
Geographic Focus: North Carolina
Samples: American Symphony Orchestra—to support the arts, $2000.; Brevard College—to support education, $48,200.; NC Coastal Federation—to support environmental programs, $5000.
Amount of Grant: $10,000 average
Date(s) Application is Due: Jan 31; Apr 30; Jul 31; Oct 31
Contact: McCray Benson, Assistant Secretary, (704) 973-4559; fax: (704) 973-4946; email: mvbenson@fftc.org
Internet: http://www.fftc.org/affiliates/community/nc/salisbury
Sponsor: Salisbury Community Foundation
217 S Tryon Street
Charlotte, NC 28202

SAMHSA Campus Suicide Prevention Grants 3244
The purpose of this program is to facilitate a comprehensive approach to preventing suicide in institutions of higher education. This program is designed to assist colleges and universities in their efforts to prevent suicide attempts and completions and to enhance services for students with mental and behavioral health problems, such as depression and substance abuse, which put them at risk for suicide and suicide attempts. Applications are due by November 25.
Requirements: Eligibility for SAMHSA's Campus Suicide Prevention Grant program is limited to institutions of higher education. Applicants from both public and private institutions may apply, including State universities, private four-year colleges and universities (including those with religious affiliations), Minority Serving Institutions of higher learning, and community colleges.
Amount of Grant: $100,000 per year for three years
Date(s) Application is Due: Nov 25
Contact: Scott J. Salvatore, Center for Mental Health Services; (240) 276-1866; email: Scott.Salvatore@samhsa.hhs.gov;; Gwendolyn Simpson, Division of Grants Management; (240) 276-1408; email: gwendolyn.simpson@samhsa.hhs.gov
Internet: http://www.samhsa.gov/Grants/2009/sm_09_001.aspx
Sponsor: Substance Abuse and Mental Health Services Administration
1 Choke Cherry Road, Room 7-1085
Rockville, MD 20857

SAMHSA Child Mental Health Initiative (CMHI) Grants 3245
The purpose of this program is to support States, political subdivisions within States, the District of Columbia, Territories, Native American Tribes and tribal organizations, in developing integrated home and community-based services and supports for children and youth with serious emotional disturbances and their families by encouraging the development and expansion of effective and enduring systems of care. Applications are due by January 15.
Requirements: Eligibility for this program is statutorily limited to public entities such as: state governments; Indian or tribal organizations (as defined in Section 4[b] and Section 4[c] of the Indian Self-Determination and Education Assistance Act); governmental units within political subdivisions of a State, such as a county, city or town; District of Columbia government; and Commonwealth of Puerto Rico, Northern Mariana Islands, Virgin Islands, American Samoa and Trust Territory of the Pacific Islands (now Palau, Micronesia and the Marshall Islands).
Restrictions: Proposed budgets cannot exceed the allowable amount in total costs (direct and indirect) in any year of the proposed project. Annual continuation awards will depend on the availability of funds, grantee progress in meeting project goals and objectives, timely submission of required data and reports and compliance with all terms and conditions of award.
Amount of Grant: $1,000,000 maximum first year
Date(s) Application is Due: Jan 15
Contact: Diane L. Sondheimer, Deputy Chief; (240) 276-1980; fax: (240) 276-1930; email: diane.sondheimer@samhsa.hhs.gov;; Gwendolyn Simpson, Division of Grants Management; (240) 276-1408; email: gwendolyn.simpson@samhsa.hhs.gov
Internet: http://www.samhsa.gov/Grants/2009/sm_09_002.aspx
Sponsor: Substance Abuse and Mental Health Services Administration
1 Choke Cherry Road, Room 7-1085
Rockville, MD 20857

SAMHSA Conference Grants 3246
The purpose of the Conference Grant program is to disseminate knowledge about practices within the mental health services and substance abuse prevention and treatment fields and to integrate that knowledge into real-world practice as effectively and efficiently as possible. The maximum Conference Grant award is $50,000 for a 12-month project period. Only direct costs will be funded under this program. Applications are due on the recurring dates of March 31 and September 30 each year.
Requirements: Applications may be submitted by public and domestic private nonprofit and for-profit entities.
Amount of Grant: $50,000 maximum
Date(s) Application is Due: Mar 31; Sep 30
Contact: David Morrissette; (240) 276-1960; email: david.morrissette@samhsa.hhs.gov;; Gwendolyn Simpson, Division of Grants Management; (240) 276-1408; email: gwendolyn.simpson@samhsa.hhs.gov
Internet: http://www.samhsa.gov/Grants/2008/OA_08_002cmhs.aspx
Sponsor: Substance Abuse and Mental Health Services Administration
1 Choke Cherry Road, Room 7-1085
Rockville, MD 20857

SAMHSA Drug Free Communities Support Program Grants 3247
This Program is a collaborative initiative sponsored by ONDCP in partnership with SAMHSA in order to achieve two major goals: establish and strengthen collaboration among communities, private nonprofit agencies, and Federal, State, local, and tribal governments to support the efforts of community coalitions to prevent and reduce substance abuse among youth; and reduce substance abuse among youth and, over time, among adults by addressing the factors in a community that increase the risk of substance abuse and promoting the factors that minimize the risk of substance abuse. Substances include, but are not limited to, narcotics, depressants, stimulants, hallucinogens, cannabis, inhalants, alcohol, and tobacco, where their use is prohibited by Federal, State, or local law.
Requirements: DFC grant funds are intended to support eligible community-based coalitions.
Amount of Grant: $125,000 per year for up to five years
Date(s) Application is Due: Mar 30
Contact: Dan Fletcher; (240) 276-1270; email: dfcnew2009@samhsa.hhs.gov;; Barbara Orlando; (240) 276-1422; email: barbara.orlando@samhsa.hhs.gov
Internet: http://www.samhsa.gov/grants/2009/sp_09_002.aspx
Sponsor: Substance Abuse and Mental Health Services Administration
1 Choke Cherry Road, Room 7-1085
Rockville, MD 20857

SAMHSA Strategic Prevention Framework State Incentive Grants 3248
The purpose of the SPF SIG program is to provide funding to States, Federally recognized Tribes and U.S. Territories in order to: prevent the onset and reduce the progression of substance abuse, including childhood and underage drinking; reduce substance abuse-related problems; and build prevention capacity and infrastructure at the State, tribal, territorial and community-levels. Applications are due by November 7.
Requirements: Eligible applicants are the immediate Office of the Chief Executive (e.g., Governor) in the States, U.S. Territories or District of Columbia; and Federally recognized Tribes. The Chief Executive of the State, Territory, or District of Columbia; or of the Federally recognized Tribe must sign the application.
Amount of Grant: $2.3 million per year maximum
Date(s) Application is Due: Nove 7
Contact: Mike Lowther, Division Director; (240) 276-2581; email: mike.lowther@samhsa.hhs.gov;; Edna Frazier, Division of Grants Management; (240) 276-1405; email: edna.frazier@samhsa.hhs.gov
Internet: http://www.samhsa.gov/Grants/2009/sp_09_001.aspx
Sponsor: Substance Abuse and Mental Health Services Administration
1 Choke Cherry Road, Room 7-1085
Rockville, MD 20857

Samuel Freeman Charitable Trust Grants 3249
The trust has broad funding interests in supporting U.S. charitable, scientific, literary, and education programs. The trust awards grants to support cancer research and treatment; the preservation, exhibition, and operation of historical railway equipment; and secondary schools and universities. Types of support include general operating support, continuing support, annual campaigns, and seed money. There are no application deadlines; proposals are reviewed throughout the year.
Requirements: U.S. nonprofit organizations may apply.
Amount of Grant: $1000-$150,000 average
Contact: Linda Franciscovich, U.S. Trust Company, (212) 852-3683; fax: (212) 852-3377
Sponsor: Samuel Freeman Charitable Trust
114 W 47th Street
New York, NY 10036-1532

Samuel Roberts Noble Foundation Grants Program 3250
The foundation is engaged in basic plant biology research as well as agricultural research, consultation, and development. Grants are made in a number of areas, with primary focus on capital funding for higher education and on health research and delivery systems. Requests are initiated with a letter describing the organization and the project for which funds are requested. Applications are provided if the request is in a current area of interest. Public affairs requests are initiated with a two-page summary of the

organization and the project. Applications must be submitted a month preceding a Trustee meeting. Requests may not be submitted by fax.
Requirements: Generally, grants are geographically limited to the southwestern United States, with primary emphasis in Oklahoma. Matching funds are required.
Amount of Grant: \$5 million-\$12 million total approximately
Date(s) Application is Due: Mar 1; Jun 1; Sep 1; Dec 1
Contact: Donna Windel, (580) 223-5810 ext 6245; fax: (580) 221-7362; email: dkwindel@nobel.org
Internet: http://www.noble.org/Admin/Granting/grGuides.html
Sponsor: Samuel Roberts Noble Foundation
P.O. Box 2180
Ardmore, OK 73402

Samuel S. Johnson Foundation Grants **3251**
The Samuel S. Johnson Foundation was incorporated in 1948 and supports organizations primarily in Oregon and Clark County, Washington region. The Foundation gives to: formal education programs leading to an R.N. status or baccalaureate or higher college/university degree in nursing; vocational education programs targeting high school drop-outs and high school grads who are not able to pursue junior college or higher formal education and which offer them job-specific technical training, mentoring or coaching; emergency food assistance programs; rural mobile health screening/care projects benefiting the uninsured medically needy; environmental programs, coastal & marine ecosystems, sustainable agriculture and communities.
Requirements: Grants are awarded to non-profit organizations in Oregon and Clark County, Washington. Contact the Foundation for current focus and guidelines with a phone call before submitting a proposal. No Application form is required, however you must include the following in your proposal: copy of IRS Determination Letter; brief history of organization and description of its mission; copy of most recent annual report/audited financial statement/990; listing of board of directors, trustees, officers and other key people and their affiliations; detailed description of project and amount of funding requested; contact person; copy of current year's organizational budget and/or project budget; listing of additional sources and amount of support. Include one copy of the proposal. The board meets twice a year, in May and October, with no deadline date for the submitting of proposals. If your proposal is accepted, you will receive notification within 2 - 3 weeks after the board meets.
Restrictions: No support for foreign organizations. No grants or scholarships to individuals, or for leadership training or staff development, campaigns to retire debt, annual campaigns, deficit financing, construction, sole underwriting of major proposals or projects, demolition or endowments.
Geographic Focus: Oregon; Washington
Amount of Grant: \$400-\$100,000 range
Contact: Mary A. Krenowicz, Secretary/Treasurer; (541) 548-8104; fax: (541) 548-2014; email: mary@tssjf.org
Sponsor: The Samuel S. Johnson Foundation
P.O. Box 356
Redmond, OR 97756-0079

Samueli Foundation Health Grants **3252**
The Foundation considers grants to agencies, primarily in Orange County, California, that serve the community, and whose programs meet the guidelines listed. Grants are usually approved for a defined period of time, but may be paid over a multi-year period. In the area of Health, its goals are to: support programs promoting alternative and integrative medicine; and utilize creative and innovative approaches to education, prevention, treatment and research of disease and illness.
Requirements: 501(c)3 tax-exempt organizations are eligible.
Restrictions: The foundation does not fund umbrella fund raising organizations, political campaigns, or grants to individuals.
Amount of Grant: \$1,000-\$50,000 average
Date(s) Application is Due: Nov 24
Contact: Maggie Sherer, Grants Administrator; (949) 760-4400; fax: (949) 759-5707; email: Info@samueli.org
Internet: http://www.samueli.org/health.aspx
Sponsor: Samueli Foundation
2101 East Coast Highway, 3rd Floor
Corona del Mar, CA 92625

Samueli Institute Scientific Research Grants **3253**
The Institute operates in conjunction with the Uniformed Services University of Health Sciences and Universitatsklinikum Freiburg Institute. Its mission is is to transform health care through the scientific exploration of healing. The Institute is one of an elite group of organizations in the nation with a track record in complementary and integrative medicine, healing relationships and military medical research. The major purpose of funding is to investigate healing processes and their application in promoting health and wellness, preventing illness, and treating disease. Researchers should respond to Requests for Applications or Program Announcements.
Amount of Grant: \$2,000-\$600,000 range
Contact: Matt Fritts; (703) 299-4800; email: mfritts@SamueliInstitute.org
Internet: http://www.siib.org/funding/investigator-home/218-SIIB.html
Sponsor: Samueli Institute
1737 King Street, Suite 600
Alexandria, VA 22314

San Antonio Area Foundation Grants **3254**
Grants are usually awarded in the areas of health care and biomedical research, community and social services, arts and culture, education (early childhood education, higher education, medical schools, nursing schools, adult basic education and literacy), and animal services. Types of support include operating budgets, continuing support, annual campaigns, seed grants, emergency funds, equipment acquisition, matching funds, scholarship funds, research, lectureships, professorships, and building renovations. Applicants must submit a letter of intent to apply; if the letter is approved, the foundation will send a request for a proposal to the applicant. The foundation only reviews full proposals from applicants whose letters of intent have been approved. If asked to submit a proposal, the applicant will be sent an application package with a letter of notification in early February.
Requirements: Grants are made to organizations in the San Antonio, Texas, area.
Geographic Focus: Texas
Amount of Grant: \$250-\$250,000 average
Date(s) Application is Due: Nov 15
Contact: Lydia R. Saldana, Program Officer; (210) 228-3753 or (210) 225-2243; fax: (210) 225-1980; email: lsaldana@saafdn.org or info@saafdn.org
Internet: http://www.saafdn.org/NetCommunity/Page.aspx?pid=254
Sponsor: San Antonio Area Foundation
110 Broadway Street, Suite 230
San Antonio, TX 78205-1948

San Diego Foundation for Change Grants **3255**
The foundation seeks funding proposals from grassroots community organizations who work to achieve social, economic, and environmental justice in San Diego County. Foundation concerns cover the range of progressive social issues, including: ending discrimination in any form; halting environmental pollution; promoting peace; expanding immigrant rights; improving San Diego's neighborhoods and workplaces; working toward racial equality; fighting for women's rights; developing youth projects; addressing domestic violence; and preventing violence in the community. Priority goes to projects with limited access to other sources of funding. In addition to the general funds, the foundation has the following special grants: the Danzig Award; and the James Mitsuo Cua Award. Organizations submitting a general application will be considered for these special grants with no additional application necessary. Letters of Intent are due on February 5, while full proposals are due by April 2.
Requirements: California nonprofit organizations in San Diego are eligible.
Restrictions: Grants do not support social or human service organizations that do not have a strong community organizing component; individual efforts; national or statewide projects unless there is a strong local focus; direct union organizing; private businesses or profit-making organizations; or electoral campaigns or candidates.
Date(s) Application is Due: Feb 5; Apr 2
Contact: John Fanestil, Executive Director; (619) 692-0527; fax: (619) 255-3640; email: john@foundation4change.org or info@foundation4change.org
Internet: http://www.foundation4change.org/forapplicants.php
Sponsor: San Diego Foundation for Change
3758 30th Street
San Diego, CA 92104

San Diego Foundation Health & Human Services Grants **3256**
The San Diego Foundation's Health and Human Services Working Group was established with the vision to improve the health, well-being and self-sufficiency of individuals, families and communities in the San Diego region. The Health and Human Services Working Group's research, investigation and grant awards to date indicate that families who are vulnerable to episodic homelessness benefit from financial education that leads to budget management, traditional banking relationships, reduction of debt improved credit, and increased savings. This initiative will support financial education and asset building programs of community-based organizations that serve the residents of the San Diego region.
Requirements: To be eligible, organizations must be providing services in San Diego County. The organizations must have a 501(c)3 IRS tax exempt status. An organization may serve as a fiscal sponsor for a charitable organization that does not have a 501(c)3 status if a cooperative relationship between the two can clearly be demonstrated. The fiscal sponsor must be willing to administer the grant if awarded.
Restrictions: Generally, the Foundation does not make grants for: organizations that have previously received funding from the Foundation but have not submitted required final reports; major building/capital campaigns; scholarships; endowments; for-profit organizations; projects that promote religious doctrine; individuals; organizations outside San Diego County; marketing and/or promotional materials (annual reports, brochures, video productions); re-granting dollars to other nonprofit organizations or individuals; short-term, annual or one time events, including festivals, performances and conferences; travel outside of the San Diego region, or; existing obligations or debt.
Geographic Focus: California
Amount of Grant: \$30,000
Date(s) Application is Due: Jan 16
Contact: Kerri Favela; (619) 235-2300, ext. 1329; email: kerri@sdfoundation.org;; Shelley Lyford, Research & Development Manager; (619) 235-2300; email: Shelley@sdfoundation.org
Internet: http://www.sdfoundation.org/communityimpact/cycle2006.html#ac
Sponsor: San Diego Foundation
2508 Historic Decatur Road, Suite 200
San Diego, CA 92106

San Diego Foundation Paradise Valley Hospital Community Fund Grants 3257

The Foundation has created a joint process managed by the San Diego Foundation and Alliance Healthcare Foundation for the distribution of funds to tax-exempt community-based health and social service organizations. Grant making decisions and oversight of funded projects will be provided by an advisory committee comprised of diverse individuals representing stakeholders in the PVH service area, as well as members of The San Diego Foundation's Health & Human Services Working Group.
Requirements: To be eligible, organizations must be providing services in San Diego County. The organizations must have a 501(c)3 IRS tax exempt status. An organization may serve as a fiscal sponsor for a charitable organization that does not have a 501(c)3 status if a cooperative relationship between the two can clearly be demonstrated. The fiscal sponsor must be willing to administer the grant if awarded.
Geographic Focus: California
Contact: Anahid Brakke, Director of Health & Human Services; (619) 235-2300; email: anahid@sdfoundation.org
Internet: http://www.sdfoundation.org/communityimpact/healthservices/pvhfund.html
Sponsor: San Diego Foundation
2508 Historic Decatur Road, Suite 200
San Diego, CA 92106

San Diego HIV Funding Collaborative (SDHFC) Grants 3258

The mission of the Collaborative is to raise, leverage and collaboratively allocate private funds to reduce the impact of HIV in the San Diego region. Donations are pooled and re-granted to local service organizations to help people affected by HIV/AIDS. Funds from the local community are used to make grants to local organizations and assist grantees with technical support. All grant applicants must start by submitting a Letter of Intent.
Requirements: The Foundation does not fund projects and programs outside San Diego and Imperial Counties.
Restrictions: The Foundation does not fund: research; lobbying; underwriting of medical expenses; general operating expenses we deem to be excessive; construction or renovation; the purchase of costly equipment; development activities, such as fund raising events, capital campaigns or annual fund drives; projects or proposals from individuals; or organizations that do not have 501(c)3 status.
Geographic Focus: California
Contact: Hamse Warfa, Program Officer; (858) 614-4892 or (858) 874-3788; fax: (858) 874-3656; email: hwarfa@alliancehf.org
Internet: http://www.alliancehf.org/sdhiv/who_we_are.html
Sponsor: Alliance Healthcare Foundation
9325 Sky Park Court, Suite 350
San Diego, CA 92123

San Diego Women's Foundation Grants 3259

The San Diego Women's Foundation (SDWF) strengthens and improves women's capacities to engage in significant philanthropy in the San Diego region. The foundation chooses one focus area of grant making each year. Its primary focus areas include: education, arts and culture, environment, employment and economic development, civil society, and health and human services. Check the web site each September for that year's focus guidelines.
Requirements: Only 501(c)3 organization within San Diego County should apply.
Geographic Focus: California
Samples: AjA Project in Community Heights, $40,000; Eveoke Dance Theater: Young Artists Program, $28,000; La Jolla Playhouse: Enriching Children's Lives Through Theater, $17,000.
Amount of Grant: $25,000 minimum
Date(s) Application is Due: Dec 6
Contact: Tracy Johnson, Director; (619) 814-1374 or (619) 235-2300; fax: (619) 239-1710; email: tracy@sdfoundation.org
Internet: http://www.sdwomensfoundation.org/
Sponsor: San Diego Women's Foundation
2508 Historic Decatur Road, Suite. 200
San Diego, CA 92106

San Francisco Foundation Community Health Grants 3260

The San Francisco Foundation welcomes unsolicited applications twice a year. The Community Health Program works to expand access to health services and promote health prevention in the five counties we serve. Community Health's efforts focus on improving health on a community level and providing the social supports for communities to improve health. The Bay Area counties included are: Martin, Contra Costa, San Francisco, Alameda and San Mateo.
Requirements: Grants are made to nonprofit organizations in Alameda, Contra Costa, Marin, San Francisco, and San Mateo Counties of California.
Restrictions: The foundation generally does not fund projects outside the Bay Area community; long-term operating support; medical, academic, or scientific research; religious activities (religious institutions may apply for nonsectarian programs); direct assistance to individuals; or conferences or one-time events.
Geographic Focus: California
Samples: California Pan-Ethnic Health Network, Oakland, CA—to provide core operating support for public policy work and building relationships with primary constituents, $50,000 (2008);Latina Breast Cancer Agency, San Francisco, CA—to perform a needs and community assessment around the California Every Women Counts Cancer Detection Program, $25,000 (2008).
Amount of Grant: $15,000-$80,000
Date(s) Application is Due: Jan 16; Jul 1
Contact: Denise Martin, Program Officer; (415) 733-8569: email: dkm@sff.org
Internet: http://www.sff.org/programs/community-health
Sponsor: San Francisco Foundation
225 Bush Street, Suite 500
San Francisco, CA 94104-4224

San Francisco Foundation Disability Rights Advocate Fund Emergency Grants 3261

The program awards emergency grants to positively impact large populations of people with disabilities in the Bay Area and northern California. Grants are available to organizations to assist mobilizing people with disabilities to act upon time-sensitive and urgent matters affecting the disability community. For example, funds may be used to cover the transportation and/or personal assistant costs associated with a community mobilization effort. Requests are accepted throughout the year; decisions are made, based on availability of funds, within four to six weeks of submission. Requests should be submitted via electronic mail. Guidelines are available online.
Requirements: Organizations located in the Bay Area and northern California are eligible.
Geographic Focus: California
Amount of Grant: $10,000
Contact: Denise Martin, Community Health Program Officer; (415) 733-8500; email: dkm@sff.org
Internet: http://www.sff.org
Sponsor: San Francisco Foundation
225 Bush Street, Suite 500
San Francisco, CA 94104

Sandler Program for Asthma Research Grants 3262

The mission of the foundation is to develop important new pathways of investigation in basic research regarding asthma. The program, which is open to investigators from all fields, particularly encourages applications from investigators not currently studying asthma. Innovation and risk are strongly encouraged. The program especially (but not exclusively) seeks applications in the following areas: development of new animal models for asthma; studies in humans or of human materials (excluding clinical trials); genetics of asthma; and technology development relevant to asthma. Three-year senior investigator awards and three-year junior investigator awards will be made. Awards to junior investigators are intended to support investigators who have demonstrated exceptional early accomplishment as independent investigators, permitting the expansion of their work into the field of asthma; they are not start-up funds. The proposed work should be directed toward uncovering basic mechanisms in the pathogenesis of asthma.
Requirements: Senior investigators will have well-established research programs and an international reputation for their research. They will usually hold a full-time academic appointment as professor, tenured associate professor, or the equivalent. Junior investigators will have already established an independent research program. They will usually hold a full-time academic appointment as an assistant professor, early associate professor, or the equivalent. Investigators may apply from any U.S. or Canadian nonprofit organization that can and will provide the necessary facilities and infrastructure for the research, and that will assure compliance with guidelines for animal and human studies established by the U.S. Department of Health and Human Services. Applicants from Canadian institutions must also provide evidence that the institution has been designated as a public charity by the U.S. Internal Revenue Service.
Samples: Robinna G. Lorenz, M.D., Ph.D., University of Alabama at Birmingham (2006); Boris Reizis, Ph.D., Columbia University (2006); John B. Wallingford, Ph.D., University of Texas at Austin (2006).
Amount of Grant: $250,000 per year senior investigator award; $150,000 per year junior investigator award
Date(s) Application is Due: Feb 8
Contact: William E. Seaman, Program Director, (415) 514-0730; fax: (415) 514-0734; email: seamanb@sandlerresearch.org
Internet: http://www.sandlerresearch.org
Sponsor: Sandler Foundation
Box 0509, UCSF
San Francisco, CA 94143-0509

Sarah Scaife Foundation Grants Program 3263

Approximately 80 percent of the annual grants are made to public policy programs that address major domestic and international issues. There are no geographic restrictions. Other grants are made in the fields of education and culture, health and medicine, scientific research, public affairs, and recreation and equipment in all geographic areas, but primarily in western Pennsylvania. Types of support include general operating support, continuing support, program development, conferences and seminars, publication, seed grants, fellowships, research, and matching funds. Applications are accepted at any time. Foundation staff considers requests in February, May, September, and November.
Restrictions: Grants are not made to individuals or to national organizations for general fund-raising purposes.
Samples: U of Pittsburgh (Pittsburgh, PA)—to construct facilities for the planned Pittsburgh Institute for Neurodegenerative Diseases, $5.4 million.
Amount of Grant: $25,000-$200,000 average
Contact: Michael Gleba, Vice President of Programs, (412) 392-2900
Internet: http://www.scaife.com/sarah.html
Sponsor: Sarah Scaife Foundation
1 Oxford Ctr, 301 Grant Street, Suite 3900
Pittsburgh, PA 15219

Sarasota Memorial Healthcare Foundation Grants 3264

The Foundation is an organization with the mission to improve the delivery of health care in the Sarasota area through the acquisition and utilization of philanthropic funds. Although the Foundation primarily supports Sarasota Memorial Health Care System, it also awards grants to other area nonprofit organizations to meet the community's changing health care needs. Grants totaling more than $32,000,000 have been provided since the Foundation's establishment in 1976. Current fields of interest include: health care; medical care; and community health systems.
Requirements: Health care programs and organization in the Sarasota, Florida, region are eligible to apply.
Geographic Focus: Florida
Contact: Alexandra Quarles, President: (941) 917-1286; email: alex-quarles@smh.com
Internet: http://www.smhf.org
Sponsor: Sarasota Memorial Healthcare Foundation
1515 S. Osprey Avenue, Suite B4
Sarasota, FL 34239

Sasco Foundation Grants 3265

The Foundation focus of support is on the arts, education, the environment, health, and human services. Although the main geographic areas are limited to Connecticut, Maine, and New York, the Foundation also occasionally supports programs of national importance. There are no deadlines and no formal applications. Please contact the Foundation for further details.
Requirements: Must be a 501(c)3 organization. Grants are not given to individuals.
Geographic Focus: Connecticut; Maine; New York
Contact: c/o Uwe Linder, J.P. Morgan Private Bank, (800) 576-6209
Sponsor: Sasco Foundation
345 Park Avenue, 6th Floor
New York, NY 10154-1002

Savoy Foundation Post-Doctoral and Clinical Research Fellowships 3266

Fellowships of the Savoy Foundation are available to Canadian researchers and to foreign nationals or for projects conducted in Canada. Post-doctoral and clinical research fellowships of $30,000 will be awarded to scientists or medical specialists (Ph.D. or M.D.) wishing to carry out a full time research project in the field of epilepsy. The grant will be for one (1) year, but will be renewable, exceptionally, once upon request. As a rule, the modalities of attribution and amounts awarded will be similar to those of governmental funding agencies (MRC or FRSQ). The fellow with the highest mark will received the prestigious Steriade-Savoy award of an additional $1,500.
Restrictions: Fellows funded by the Savoy Foundation must not cumulate two major awards.
Amount of Grant: $30,000
Date(s) Application is Due: Jan 15
Contact: Fellowship Coordinator; (450) 358-9779; fax: (450) 346-1045; email: epilepsy@savoy-foundation.ca
Internet: http://www.savoy-foundation.ca/eng/mission/defaut.htm
Sponsor: Savoy Foundation
230 Foch Street
St Jean Sur Richelieu, Quebec J3B 6B2

Savoy Foundation Research Grants 3267

A small number of research grants are available each year to clinicians and/or established scientists working on epilepsy or related subjects. These grants will be attributed for the following purposes: launching of a new research project, preliminary studies in preparation of a more substantial request to be addressed to another agency, continuation or completion of a project, sharing of expenses, or a limited project not requiring funding in excess of the limit. As a rule, these grants are not renewable. Contact the foundation for application forms.
Requirements: Research grants are available to Canadian citizens or for projects conducted in Canada.
Amount of Grant: $25,000
Date(s) Application is Due: Jan 15
Contact: Grants Administrator; (450) 358-9779; fax: (450) 346-1045; email: epilepsy@savoy-foundation.ca
Internet: http://www.savoy-foundation.ca/eng/mission/defaut.htm
Sponsor: Savoy Foundation
230 Foch Street
St Jean Sur Richelieu, Quebec J3B 6B2 Canada

Savoy Foundation Studentships 3268

Studentships of the Savoy Foundation are available to Canadian researchers and to foreign nationals or for projects conducted in Canada. Studentships will be awarded to meritorious applicants wishing to acquire training and pursue research in a biomedical discipline, the health sciences or social sciences related to epilepsy. These studentships last one year, but will be renewable three times, upon request, for a maximum duration of four years. The stipend will be $15,000 per year. The student with the highest mark will receive the prestigious Van Gelder-Savoy award of an additional $1,500. An annual sum of $1,000 will be allocated to the laboratory or institution as additional support for the research project.
Requirements: To be eligible, the candidate must have a good university record (B. Sc., M.D. or equivalent diploma) and have ensured that a qualified researcher affiliated to a university and/or hospital, will supervise his/her work. Concomitant registration in a graduate program (M. Sc. or Ph. D.) is encouraged.
Restrictions: Students funded by the Savoy Foundation must not cumulate two studentship awards.
Amount of Grant: $15,000
Date(s) Application is Due: Jan 15
Contact: Caroline Savoy, (450) 358-9779; fax: (450) 346-1045; email: epileps@savoy-foundation.ca
Internet: http://www.savoy-foundation.ca/eng/mission/defaut.htm
Sponsor: Savoy Foundation
230 Foch
St Jean Sur Richelieu, Quebec J3B 2B2 Canada

Schering-Plough Foundation Community Initiatives Grants 3269

The Schering-Plough Foundation, a non-profit membership corporation established in 1955, is dedicated to working with the citizens of our communities to help them realize their full potential and enhance their quality of life. Support for community development takes many forms and allows the Foundation to reach out to numerous, highly diverse groups within its communities. The Foundation continues to support organizations that promote culture and the arts, environmental issues, legal services, etc. and are always seeking out new and innovative ways to serve the citizens of its communities.
Requirements: The Foundation considers requests from tax-exempt, 501(c)3 non-profit organizations located in the United States, or its possessions, whose goals and activities fall within its stated objectives and areas of interest. All requests for funding must be made online. National organizations are eligible to apply.
Restrictions: Grants are not made to individuals.
Amount of Grant: $5,000-$200,000 range
Contact: Christine Fahey, Assistant Secretary; (908) 298-7232; fax: (908) 298-7349
Internet: http://www.schering-plough.com/company/foundation.aspx
Sponsor: Schering-Plough Foundation
2000 Galloping Hill Road
Kennilworth, NJ 07033-0530

Schering-Plough Foundation Health Grants 3270

The Schering-Plough Foundation, a non-profit membership corporation established in 1955, is dedicated to working with the citizens of our communities to help them realize their full potential and enhance their quality of life. The Foundation's interest in improving the health and well-being of its communities remains a top priority and is reflected in the numerous initiatives that have been developed to benefit these communities. The Foundation invests in the future of those communities by building meaningful partnerships that enhance the quality of life. Currently, the Foundation is involved in several partnerships that seek to expand the quality and availability of health care in its underserved communities.
Requirements: The Foundation considers requests from tax-exempt, 501(c)3 non-profit organizations located in the United States, or its possessions, whose goals and activities fall within its stated objectives and areas of interest. All requests for funding must be made online. National organizations are eligible to apply.
Restrictions: Grants are not made to individuals.
Samples: New Jersey Institute of Technology (Newark, NJ)—to enhance its master's degree program in pharmaceutical engineering, $250,000.
Amount of Grant: $5,000-$200,000 range
Contact: Christine Fahey, Assistant Secretary; (908) 298-7232; fax: (908) 298-7349
Internet: http://www.schering-plough.com/company/foundation.aspx
Sponsor: Schering-Plough Foundation
2000 Galloping Hill Road
Kennilworth, NJ 07033-0530

Schurz Communications Foundation Grants 3271

The Schurz Communications Foundation, Inc. is a company sponsored foundation which was incorporated in 1940. The Foundations donors are: Schurz Communications, Incorporated; South Bend Tribune Corporation; WSBT, Incorporated. The Foundation supports community service clubs and organizations involved with arts and culture, higher education, youth development and disabled people.
Requirements: Giving is limited to the South Bend Indiana area.
Geographic Focus: Indiana
Samples: Studebaker National Museum, South Bend, IN - $25,000 (2006); Boys and Girls Club of Saint Joseph County, South Bend, IN - $10,000 (2006); United Way of Saint Joseph County, South Bend, IN - $40,000 (2006);
Amount of Grant: $1,000 - $40,000 range
Contact: David C. Ray, President: (574) 235-6241;
Sponsor: Schurz Communications Foundation, Inc.
225 West Colfax Avenue
South Bend, IN 46624

Scientific Communities Initiative Grants 3272

The coalition is awarding grants to digital ventures offering information in the areas of science, technology, and medicine (STM). The purpose of the grants is to stimulate and accelerate the creation of new university-based information communities serving users in key STM fields. Proposed projects should offer strategic alternatives to inefficiencies in the current, traditional scientific communication process. Projects should provide increased responsiveness to the needs of scientists—as authors and information users—and to libraries by offering an effective new electronic venue for publication of research; aggregating content/links needed by targeted users in sufficient breadth and mass; addressing important objectives of universities and colleges; delivering convenient, efficient access to this information in a Web environment optimized to the needs of

scientists in the target discipline; and fostering a more open and competitive marketplace in which academe exercises an increased role in assuring broad dissemination of research. Partnerships and collaborations among universities and professional societies are encouraged. Letters of intent must meet the listed application deadline; full applications will be requested.
Amount of Grant: $100,000 minimum; $500,000 total
Contact: Heather Joseph, (202) 296-2296; email: sparc@arl.org
Internet: http://www.arl.org/sparc/core/index.asp?page=f17
Sponsor: Scholarly Publishing and Academic Resources Coalition
21 Dupont Circle, Suite 800
Washington, DC 20036

Scott County Community Foundation Grants **3273**
In order to fulfill most effectively its philanthropic responsibilities within the limits of its resources, the Scott County Community Foundation's grant program will emphasize focused and effective types of grants. The Scott County Community Foundation currently has one grants cycle per year. Applications are typically accepted in the summer and recipients are announced in early fall. The broad purpose of the Scott County Community Foundation is to improve the quality of life of the residents of Scott County, Indiana. Grant funding will focus on the encouragement of programs that enhance cooperating and collaboration among institutions within our community. Foundation funds ordinarily are not given to agencies for the purpose of meeting routine budgets. Funding will focus on effectiveness of special non-recurring projects which enrich health, education, cultural or recreational situations in Scott County. However, special consideration will be given to agencies that partner with other organizations to complete a unified project.
Requirements: The grant policies are: grants will be made only to organizations whose programs benefit the residents of Scott County; grants from the Scott County Community Foundation must meet legal and tax requirements as to the purpose and may be made only to charitable organizations and/or cause; grantees may be required to attend an interview by the Grants Committee; grantees must submit a final grant evaluation report; the Grantee will not be allowed to participate in any future Grant Cycles until the final report is on file in the Foundation office; grant money must be used for the specific purpose as stated in the line item budget provided in the grant application; any changes in purpose must be requested in writing and approved by the Foundation prior to any changes being made; any portion of the amount granted which is not used for the purpose of the grant will be repaid; grants will only be made to organizations, that as required by law make equal opportunities available to all persons without regard to race, age, color, religion, national origin, disability, citizenship status, or any other category protected under state or local law; after evaluation, the Grants Committee makes recommendations to the Board of Directors, which makes all funding decisions; applicants must submit 10 hole-punched copies of the application.
Restrictions: The Foundation does not typically fund: on going operational expenses; existing obligations; services primarily supported by tax dollars or responsibility of a public agency; individuals or travel expenses; multi-year grants or repeat funding; advocacy or political purposes; religious or sectarian purposes; loans or endowments.
Geographic Focus: Indiana
Contact: L.L. Lowry, Executive Director; (812) 752-2057; fax: (812) 752-9257; email: info@scottcountyfoundation.org
Internet: http://www.scottcountyfoundation.org/grants.htm
Sponsor: Scott County Community Foundation
60 North Main Street, P.O. Box 25
Scottsburg, IN 47170

Seabury Foundation Grants **3274**
In general, The Seabury Foundation makes one-time, special project grants, rather than general operating support. Areas of interest of the Foundation include: Arts, Culture and Humanities; Human Capacity-building; Health; Education; Conservation and Environment; Children, Youth and Families. On occasion, the Foundation may invite grant renewal requests for up to two consecutive succeeding years. After that period, the Foundation will not consider a request for funding from that organization until a minimum of two full years have passed since the final grant was awarded. Please note that all grants awarded are within the City of Chicago with the exception of projects personally sponsored by family members.
Requirements: Chicago, IL, nonprofit organizations are eligible. Initial contact should be through a Letter of Inquiry, letters need only be 1-2 pages in length. Deadline dates for Letter of Inquiry are: September 15; January 15; June 15. If after reviewing the Letter of Inquiry, if your organization is invited to submit a full proposal, the deadline dates are: November 1; March 1; August 1.
Restrictions: The Seabury Foundation do not entertain grants in support of gala events, annual fundraising events, or annual fundraising drives.
Geographic Focus: Illinois
Date(s) Application is Due: Jan 15; June 15; Sep 15; Mar 1; Aug 1; Nov 1;
Contact: Boyd McDowell III, Director; (312) 587-7146; fax: (312) 587-7332; email: bmcdowell@seaburyfoundation.org
Internet: http://www.seaburyfoundation.org/apply.htm
Sponsor: Seabury Foundation
1111 North Wells Street, Suite 503
Chicago, IL 60610-7633

Searle Scholars Program Grants **3275**
The program's aim is to identify junior faculty members who have demonstrated a potential for doing innovative research in the biomedical sciences. Approximately 15 scholars are selected each year to receive the award. Scholars will receive a grant to support their research over the next three years. Application forms are distributed through invited institutions.
Requirements: Applicants will be expected to be pursuing independent research careers in biochemistry, cell biology, genetics, immunology, neuroscience, pharmacology, related areas in chemistry, medicine, and the biological sciences. Candidates should be in their first or second year at the assistant professor level. This appointment must be a tenure-track position and must be in an academic department of an invited, degree-granting institution. Potential applicants whose institutions do not have tenure-track appointments should consult with the scientific director of the program prior to preparing an application.
Restrictions: Applications from any institution not invited to participate will not be considered. No more than two applications will be accepted from any one institution.
Amount of Grant: $80,000 per year for three years
Date(s) Application is Due: Sep 30
Contact: Mary Tarpey, Program Contact, (847) 714-1702; fax: (847) 714-1716; email: mary.tarpey@kinshipcorp.com
Internet: http://www.searlescholars.net/apply
Sponsor: Searle Scholars Program
400 Skokie Boulevard, Suite 300
Northbrook, IL 60062

Seattle Foundation Grants **3276**
The Foundation considers grant proposals from tax-exempt nonprofit organizations serving King County, Washington residents. Grants are awarded through a number of programs and Foundation funds, the targeted area of interest are : basic needs, the environment, the economy, education, arts and culture, neighborhoods and communities, and health and wellness. See the Foundations website for a application form.
Requirements: Nonprofit organizations serving King County, Washington residents maintaining a tax-exempt status under Section 501(c)3 of the IRS may apply.
Geographic Focus: Washington
Contact: Jared Watson Vice President, Program & Donor Services; (206) 515-2114 or (206) 622-2294; fax: (206) 622-7673; email: grantmaking@seattlefoundation.org
Internet: http://www.seattlefoundation.org/page29609.cfm
Sponsor: The Seattle Foundation
1200 Fifth Avenue, Suite 1300
Seattle, WA 98101-3151

Self Foundation Grants **3277**
The Self Family Foundation primarily serves the Greenwood, South Carolina and surrounding counties. The Self Family Foundation will consider requests from other regions of South Carolina, if they have statewide impact. The Foundation supports non-profit organizations in the following areas of interest: Education - enhancing children's school readiness and ability to achieve educational goals with success; working together with schools, families, youth-serving organizations and other community organizations to support the intellectual and social development of young people; Arts, Culture & History - increasing awareness of and access to activities that broaden the horizons and knowledge of all residents, within Greenwood, South Carolina; Civic & Community - improving neighborhood resources and community attitudes and services, emphasizing the utilization of existing facilities, skills and talents to create a stronger, more unified community through collaboration with organizations, businesses, public institutions and residents; Health and Human Services - promoting individual and community wellness, prevention and literacy.
Requirements: IRS 501(c)3 tax-exempt or 509(a) nonprofit organizations in South Carolina are eligible. Letters of Inquiry or requests for information may be emailed to: application@selffoundation.org or mailed to Foundation. Contact Foundation Program Officer by email or phone prior to submitting proposal. All applicants must have the financial potential to sustain the project on a continuing basis after any funding is approved.
Restrictions: No grants to individuals and no loans available.
Geographic Focus: South Carolina
Amount of Grant: $1500-$50,000
Date(s) Application is Due: Feb 15; May 15; Aug 15; Nov 15
Contact: (864) 953-2441 or (864) 941-4036; fax: (864) 941- 4091; email: info@selffoundation.org
Internet: http://www.selffoundation.org/grantmaking4.htm
Sponsor: Self Family Foundation
P.O. Box 1017
Greenwood, SC 29648-1017

Seneca Foods Foundation Grants **3278**
The Seneca Foods Foundation was established in 1988 in New York and is sponsored by the Seneca Foods Corporation. The foundation supports fire departments and organizations involved with education, health, Down Syndrome, agriculture and food, recreation, and youth. Funding is primarily in areas of company processing facilities, with emphasis on New York.
Requirements: Nonprofit organizations in Seneca Foods operating locations are eligible. Contact foundation for application form.
Restrictions: Grants are not made to individuals.
Contact: Kraig H. Kayser, President; (315) 926-8100; email: foundation@senecafoods.com
Sponsor: Seneca Foods Corporation
3736 South Main Street
Marion, NY 14505-9751

Sexually Transmitted Diseases Postdoctoral Fellowships 3279

The ASHA Research Fund fellowships program is intended to expand the number of trained scientists working in the field of sexually transmissible diseases research by providing postdoctoral candidates with the opportunity to spend two years in a challenging, stimulating, and instructive STD research environment under the sponsorship of an established researcher. Applications for research training relative to any aspect of the sexually transmissible diseases are welcome. ASHA has supported projects in chancroid, human papilloma virus (HPV), group B streptococcal infection, herpes, gonorrhea, chlamydia, HIV, pelvic inflammatory disease (PID), and syphilis. In funding HIV-related research, ASHA gives priority to researchers exploring the relationship between HIV and other STDs. Although applications covering fellowship training in basic investigations are not discouraged, it is the intent of this program to focus on research of short- or medium-term duration. Requests for applications are usually issued in May of odd-numbered years, with an application deadline of October 15, and the award being given the following spring for a fellowship period commencing on July 1.

Requirements: Applications are requested from MDs, PhDs, DSc who will be conducting two-year research projects under the sponsorship of established STD investigators. Applicants are required to study at established U.S. institutions.

Restrictions: ASHA fellowships may not be used in support of faculty positions unless approved by ASHA's management. Current ASHA fellows are not eligible to apply for other ASHA fellowships.

Amount of Grant: $35,500 first year; $36,000 second year

Date(s) Application is Due: Nov 15

Contact: Grant Administrator; (919) 361-8400; fax: (919) 361-8425

Internet: http://www.ashastd.org/programs/arf.html

Sponsor: American Social Health Association
P.O. Box 13827
Research Triangle Park, NC 27709

Shaw's Supermarkets Donations 3280

Shaw's focuses its support on not-for-profit 501(c)3 organizations that help create healthy, thriving communities. Shaw's provides financial support, volunteer support and in-kind product donations to organizations that benefit communities in areas where they operate, and meet the following focus areas: (1) Hunger Relief - Ending hunger in the stores' local communities via both product and financial support to hunger-relief organizations. (2) Nutrition Education - support for organizations that educate and promote healthy lifestyles and nutrition by emphasizing disease management and prevention through diet. (3) Environmental Stewardship - environmental stewardship and sustainable operations and that will continually work to use energy more efficiently and reduce waste. Shaw's supports local efforts towards sustainability. (4) Community Connections - select local events that build strong communities by broadly engaging community pride and spirit.

Requirements: 501(c)3 tax-exempt organizations in Connecticut, Maine, Massachusetts, New Hampshire, Rhode Island, and Vermont are eligible. If the grant request involves an event, the request should be sent at least 8 weeks prior to event date. Download the application form from the website.

Restrictions: Shaw's will generally not support: individuals; travel or research expenses; fees for participation in competitive programs; veteran, fraternal or labor organizations; lobbying, political or religious programs; or, organizations that are not tax-exempt.

Geographic Focus: Connecticut; Maine; Massachusetts; New Hampshire; Rhode Island; Vermont

Contact: Donation Committee; email: shaws.donations@shaws.com

Internet: http://www.shaws.com/pages/community/donationRequests.php

Sponsor: Shaw's Supermarkets, Inc.
P.O. Box 600
East Bridgewater, MA 02333

Shell Oil Company Foundation Grants 3281

Shell makes monetary grants to nonprofit organizations within the U.S. Priority consideration will be given to organizations in or near communities where Shell Oil Company or its affiliates in the United States have a major presence. Shell Oil Company and the Shell Oil Company Foundation will consider charitable contributions to eligible nonprofit organizations for select programs that fall within our focused areas of contributions: health and welfare; community outreach; workforce development / education and; environment. There are no deadline dates for submitting a proposal, proposals are reviewed on a regular basis.

Requirements: Nonprofit organizations in company operating locations are eligible.

Restrictions: Shell Oil Company and the Shell Oil Company Foundation will not consider contributions for the following purposes: individuals; private Foundations; non-profit organizations without a current 501(c)3 exempt status; conferences or symposia; endowment funds; fraternal and labor organizations; capital campaigns; conferences, workshops, or seminars not directly related to Shell business interests; religious organizations that do not serve the general public on a non-denominational basis; organizations located in or benefiting nations other than U.S. and its territories; organizational operating expenses.

Amount of Grant: $10,000-$50,000 average

Contact: A.H. Myres, Vice President, (713) 241-3616; fax: (713) 241-3329; email: socfoundation@shellus.com

Internet: http://www.shell.us/home/content/usa/responsible_energy/shell_in_the_society/giving_back/grant/grant_request_060208.html

Sponsor: Shell Oil Company Foundation
One Shell Plaza, 910 Louisiana, Suite 4478A
Houston, TX 77002

Sheltering Arms Fund Grants 3282

The purpose of the fund is to complement and extend Sheltering Arms Hospital's mission by funding health related initiatives that serve uninsured and underinsured adults who are experiencing physical or cognitive disabilities or who are at risk for developing functional limitations. Emphasis will be placed on responding to the needs of individuals with a Rehab Impairment Category diagnosis as defined by the Centers for Medicaid and Medicare (CMS)

Requirements: Proposals will be accepted from charitable organizations, which serve the residents of the metropolitan Richmond and Central Virginia. Proposed programs should align with the goals of the fund: Improve access to health and related support services such as Primary Care, Specialty clinics (Diabetes, Podiatry, Dental, Women's Health, etc.), and Nutritional Support; Increase functional independence (Home care, Day care, Transportation, Use of assistive devices and technology, Facility renovations to improve handicapped access); Promote disability prevention for at risk populations through education and/or public health initiatives.

Geographic Focus: Virginia

Amount of Grant: up to $100,000

Date(s) Application is Due: May 5

Contact: Susan Hallett, Program Officer; (804) 330-7400; fax: (804) 330-5992; email: shallett@tcfrichmond.org

Internet: http://www.tcfrichmond.org/page2954.cfm#SAF

Sponsor: Community Foundation Serving Richmond and Central Virginia
7501 Boulders View Drive, Suite 110
Richmond, VA 23225

SHF Reach—Connecting Communities and Youth for a Healthy Future Grants 3283

The foundation supports the healthy development of youth in the California Capital Region. The program awards one-year grants to improve the quality of youth programs or increase the number of youth that participate in quality programs. Examples of projects that will be considered include design or testing of new youth development program components, including the purchase of curriculum; training of staff on cultural competency, youth development best practices, and program improvement; purchasing of computers to add a skills-building component for youth; evaluation planning and implementation to measure the program's effectiveness; computer support to develop better systems of outcomes measurement; improving current program design and effectiveness by engaging youth in focus groups; expansion of programs or adding new sites; developing more or better community/school partnerships; marketing and outreach to youth; transportation of youth to and from programs; incentives to participate; and fund development research and proposal writing to sustain existing programs. Attendance at a proposers' conference is highly encouraged, though not required to apply for a grant. Application and guidelines are available online.

Requirements: The program will fund applicants that are 501(c)3 tax-exempt; have or wish to add a youth-serving program, primarily focused on youth age 10 to 15; reflect in the proposal an understanding of and commitment to youth development principles and practices; engage or plan to engage youth in projects, programs, and the organization's leadership and decision-making; and serve youth in the California Capital Region (the organization's office may be located outside of this region), which includes an area encompassing all of Sacramento County and parts of the surrounding counties bounded by the Sacramento County line in the south, Jackson (Amador County) in the southeast, Pollock Pines (El Dorado County) in the east, Grass Valley (Nevada County) in the northeast, Marysville/Yuba City (Yuba and Sutter counties) in the north, Winters (Yolo County) in the west, and Fairfield (Solano County) in the southwest.

Restrictions: Grants are not intended for general operating or ongoing service support.

Geographic Focus: California

Amount of Grant: $10,000 maximum

Date(s) Application is Due: Jan 15; Apr 15; Sep 15

Contact: Grants Administrator, (916) 922-4755; fax: (916) 922-4024; email: info@sierrahealth.org

Internet: http://www.sierrahealth.org/programs/reach/program_improvemnt_grants.html

Sponsor: Sierra Health Foundation
1321 Garden Hwy
Sacramento, CA 95833

Sid W. Richardson Foundation Grants 3284

Grants are provided to tax-exempt organizations in Texas in the areas of education (museums, learning centers, day schools, K-12 schools, higher education institutions, and business and economic education), health (medical schools, organ donor registries, hospitals, disease prevention, health science centers, and nursing associations), arts (arts councils, visual and performing arts festivals, museums, ballet, symphony orchestra, and arts education programs), and human services (boys' and girls' clubs, united funds, the elderly, crime prevention, the disabled, housing opportunities, food programs, and drug and alcohol abuse prevention); specific goals within these larger areas change periodically. Types of support include operating budgets, seed grants, building construction funds, equipment acquisition, endowment funds, research, publications, conferences and seminars, matching funds, continuing support, and projects/programs. Award amounts vary depending on proposed projects.

Requirements: Proposals must cover programs and projects within Texas.

Restrictions: Grants are not made to individuals.

Geographic Focus: Texas

Samples: All Saints Episcopal School (Fort Worth, TX)—for its capital campaign, $1 million (2005).

Amount of Grant: $10,000-$100,000 typically

Date(s) Application is Due: Jan 15
Contact: Valleau Wilkie Jr., Executive Director, (817) 336-0494; fax: (817) 332-2176
Internet: http://www.sidrichardson.org/GrantInfo.html
Sponsor: Sid W. Richardson Foundation
309 Main Street
Fort Worth, TX 76102

Siebert Lutheran Foundation Grants **3285**
Specific areas of interest vary from time to time. At present, the Foundation is supportive of the following: Clergy and lay education and training, community development and outreach, health ministry, evangelism and youth. Grants are occasionally made to provide seed money or start-up costs for a program or project. In such instances, the participation of other donors is desired. Grants are made only to Lutheran organizations exempt under Section 501(c)3 of the Internal Revenue Code and are generally awarded for a one-year period.
Requirements: The Foundation utilizes an on-line grant application. Potential grant applicants, who represent Wisconsin congregations or Wisconsin recognized service organizations in the Lutheran church, may complete the Foundation's formal, online, letter of inquiry. A telephone call is not necessary prior to completing the letter of inquiry for Lutheran organizations in Wisconsin. If your organization does not meet the above criteria and you would like to discuss possible funding, contact the Foundation office (262-754-9160).
Restrictions: The Foundation does not approve grants for the following: endowment funds, fellowships and scholarships, trusts, and other grant-making foundations. Grants are generally not made to churches for capital or operating expenses. No grants are made outside the United States.
Geographic Focus: Wisconsin
Date(s) Application is Due: Mar 1; Jun 1; Sep 1; Dec 1
Contact: Deborah Engel, Administrative Assistant; (262) 754-9160; fax: (262) 754-9162; email: contactus@Siebertfoundation.org
Internet: http://www.siebertfoundation.org/grants.htm
Sponsor: Siebert Lutheran Foundation
300 North Corporate Drive, Suite 200
Brookfield, WI 53045

Sigrid Juselius Foundation Grants **3286**
The Sigrid Juselius Foundation, offers funding for domestic medical research. To enable established foreign medical researchers to work in a Finnish institution for 1-12 months, the Foundation also offers grants to nationals of other countries. Resources are allocated to senior and post doc researchers. The grants cover all disciplines of medical science. The grants can cover personal expenses (living costs) and travel.
Requirements: The Foundation does not award direct grants to foreign medical research. A foreign scientist interested in coming over to Finland has to get in touch with a Finnish scientist of his particular field, and the application should be made on the part of the Finnish host together with the proposed visiting researcher. A electronic application is available on the Sigrid Juselius Foundation website.
Restrictions: The funds are not available for studies or doctoral theses.
Date(s) Application is Due: Apr 15; Sep 15
Contact: Funding Officer; 358 20 710 9082 or 358 20 710 9083; fax: 358 20 710 9089
Internet: http://www.sigridjuselius.fi/index.php?page_id=48
Sponsor: Sigrid Juselius Foundation
Aleksanterinkatu 48 B
Helsinki FI-00100 Finland

Simmons Foundation Grants **3287**
The foundation awards grants to Maine nonprofits in its areas of interest, including arts, higher education, family services, health care, food services, health organizations, human services, children and youth, services and women. Types of support include general operating support, building construction/renovation, equipment acquisition, and scholarship funds.
Requirements: There are no application forms or deadlines however your initial approach should be in the form of a letter. Applicants should submit the following: detailed description of project and amount of funding requested; brief history of organization and description of its mission; descriptive literature about organization; copy of IRS Determination Letter.
Geographic Focus: Maine
Contact: Suzanne McGuffey; Treasurer, (207) 774-2635
Sponsor: Simmons Foundation
1 Canal Plaza
Portland, ME 04101-4098

Simone and Cino del Duca Grand Prix Awards **3288**
The Simone and Cino del Duca Foundation of the Institut de France awards each year a scientific Grand Prix based on the recommendations of a jury of members of the Institut de France. The amount of the Grand Prix will be 364,000 euros: 250,000 euros to finance the work of the award-winning group, 50,000 euros awarded to the director of the research group, and an additional 64,000 euros towards hiring one or more French or foreign postdoctoral researchers to be selected by the group director.
Requirements: The Grand Prix will reward an internationally recognized French or European mathematician proposing an ambitious research project based on the collective work of a group under his/her direction. The proposal should describe the scientific objectives and the means that will be used to implement the project (duration of the project, invitations, meetings, seminars, etc.).
Amount of Grant: 364,000 EU
Date(s) Application is Due: Jan 25
Contact: Grants Administrator; 01 47 66 01 21; fax: 01 46 22 45 02; email: fondation-del-duca@institut-de-france.fr
Internet: http://www.enseignementsup-recherche.gouv.fr/cid23192/call-for-applications-for-the-grand-prix-scientifique-simone-and-cino-del-duca-2009.html
Sponsor: Institut de France
23, quai Conti
Paris 75270 France

Simple Advise Education Center Grants **3289**
The Simple Advise Education Center supports organizations, centers & services, primarily in North Carolina. Giving to improve the quality of life of citizens with developmental disabilities.
Requirements: There are no specific deadlines with which to adhere. Contact the Foundation for further application information and guidelines.
Geographic Focus: North Carolina
Contact: Barbara J. Spigner, Director; (800) 677-7306
Sponsor: Simple Advise Education Center, Inc. c/o BJ Hills and Assoc., Inc.
P.O. Box 758
Fayetteville, NC 28302-0758

Simpson Fund Grants **3290**
The fund serves a broad range of organizations in its operating communities that address key community needs such as education, health services, economic development, the arts, and more. Simpson also provides support to environmental and conservation projects, such as environmental education, habitat restoration, research relevant to the timber industry, as well as other projects that impact the timber business. The fund makes an extra effort to support organizations of interest to, or recommended by, Simpson employees. Support is generally committed for one year at a time. Capital projects are given priority over requests for contributions to operating funds. The fund supports the United Way in all of its operating communities. Guidelines are available online.
Requirements: Contributions are limited to Simpson communities: Washington—Pierce, Mason, Thurston and Grays Harbor Counties; Oregon—Lincoln and Tillamook Counties; and California—Del Norte and Humboldt Counties.
Geographic Focus: California; Oregon; Washington
Amount of Grant: $1000-$10,000
Contact: Grants Administrator, (206) 224-5198; email: cmusgra@simpson.com
Internet: http://www.simpson.com/communitycontribute.cfm
Sponsor: Simpson Fund
1301 Fifth Avenue, Suite 2800
Seattle, WA 98101-2613

Sir Dorabji Tata Trust Grants for NGOs or Voluntary Organizations **3291**
Thoughtful and committed programs initiated by organizations in priority areas are considered for financial support. The Trust draws on the expertise of its staff and specialist consultants who travel widely, study project proposals and keep abreast of developments in each of the sectors (see below).
Requirements: The trust limits its funding to projects within India. This program focuses on specific sectors for its funding: Management of Natural Resources; Livelihood; Education; Health; and Social Development Initiatives. While no specific format is prescribed, applications should preferably include: (a) description of the proposed project with clearly articulated objectives, plans/programs or activities, and mechanisms for impact assessment; (b) profile of the project holder (qualifications, achievements, experience) and a brief background of the core team; (c) Registration Certificates of the organization and Income-tax Exemption Certificates; (d) The financial audited statements of the last three years and Annual Reports.
Contact: R.M. Lala, Director; +91 (22) 6665-8282; fax: +91 (22) 2204-5427 / + 91 (22) 2282 6092; email: sdtt@sdtatatrust.com
Internet: http://www.dorabjitatatrust.org/ngo/ngo_grants.asp
Sponsor: Sir Dorabji Tata Trust
Bombay House, 24 Homi Mody Street
Mumbai 400 001 India

Sir Dorabji Tata Trust Individual Medical Grants **3292**
The Sir Dorabji Tata Trust provides individual medical grants to needy and deserving patients for medical and surgical care. The maximum disbursement for an individual patient is Rs 100,000, covering expenses incurred towards costs of major surgeries like neurosurgery, cardiac surgery, skin graft surgery for burns, cancer, kidney transplant and others. The grants are also available to patients who are physically handicapped. Though the quantum offered is modest and small, the grants bring much-needed financial relief to the patients and their families. The thrust is to help poor patients from government and municipal hospitals. Individual medical grants are one-time grants.
Requirements: The Trust gives priority to cases within Mumbai in view of the difficulties in assessing cases outside Mumbai. To apply for a medical grant from the Sir Dorabji Tata Trust, you are required to visit the Trust Office at Mulla House, 3rd Floor, 51 M.G. Road, Mumbai 400001 between 3:00 pm to 5:00 pm from Monday to Friday, and pick up the application form. Please ensure that you have all the following documents: (a) Doctor's Certificate; (b) Discharge Certificate; (c) Income Certificate; (d) Copies of Hospital/Medical Bills; (e) Proof of Residence i.e. Ration Card or any other document; (e) Recommendation Letter from Medical Social Worker from a general, municipal or government hospital; (f) Employers Reimbursement; (g) Medical Insurance. The

completed forms should be submitted in person to the Trust Office along with the required documents within a month of collecting the form.
Restrictions: Limited to India.
Amount of Grant: 100,000 Rs maximum
Contact: R.M. Lala, Director; +91 (22) 6665-8282; fax: +91 (22) 2204-5427 / + 91 (22) 2282 6092; email: sdtt@sdtatatrust.com
Internet: http://www.dorabjitatatrust.org/ind_grants/ind_img.asp
Sponsor: Sir Dorabji Tata Trust
Bombay House, 24 Homi Mody Street
Mumbai 400 001 India

Sir Halley Stewart Trust Grants **3293**
The trust awards grants worldwide to organizations and individuals in the areas of medical research, social and education, and religion. Medical research grants focus on problems of the elderly, preventing disability in children, tropical diseases, and Crohn's disease. In the education and social category, grants support research and innovative development projects that attempt to prevent and resolve conflicts, promote reconciliation, and increase understanding within families and across racial, cultural, class, religious, and professional divides. Religion grants advance Christianity and include theological training, teaching in the United Kingdom about Christianity, encouragement of specific groups of people (e.g., the elderly, people with disability, students in higher education, etc.) to explore their spiritual needs and strengths, communicating the Christian message through the media, projects that attempt to help disadvantaged people, etc. Applications will not be accepted by fax or email.
Requirements: Nonprofit organizations worldwide are eligible.
Restrictions: Grants do not support general appeals of any kind; personal education fees or fees for taught courses—unless connected with research that falls within current priority areas; educational or 'GAP' year travel projects for young people; purchase, erection, or conversion of buildings; capital costs; running costs of established organizations; or university overhead charges.
Amount of Grant: @L875,000 total
Contact: Sue West, Administrator, 44-1954-260707
Internet: http://www.sirhalleystewart.org
Sponsor: Sir Halley Stewart Trust
22 Earith Road
Willingham, Cambridge CB4 5LS United Kingdom

Siragusa Foundation Health Services & Medical Research Grants **3294**
The Siragusa Foundation, established in 1950 by Ross D. Siragusa, is a private family foundation that is committed to honoring its founder by sustaining and developing Chicago's extraordinary nonprofit resources. The Foundation's Health Services and Medical Research Program is balanced between medical research organizations, which are concerned with scientific inquiry and the exploration of treatment methods, and health service organizations, which provide direct social and clinical care. The Foundation primarily funds fellowships, single-disease research programs and clinical treatment services. The Foundation believes it is critical to fund research efforts, health support services, patient care services and treatment, and advocacy programs for both adults and youth, all of which are highly complementary to each other.
Requirements: Nonprofit 501(c)3 organization in Chicago are eligible to apply. Before submitting a formal proposal to the Foundation, prospective applicants should submit a two-page letter of inquiry outlining the background of the organization and the proposed project. The letter of inquiry should describe succinctly the project for which funding is requested, including how it relates to the Foundation's interests, the target audience, the estimated budget and request amount. After reviewing the letter of inquiry, the Foundation may or may not request a formal proposal.
Restrictions: The Foundation limits potential grantees from applying for funds to once per calendar year. The Foundation does not accept unsolicited proposals from outside the Chicago area and does not support individuals or political advocacy. The foundation typically does not support capital expenditures or endowments.
Geographic Focus: Illinois
Samples: Arthritis Foundation, Greater Chicago Chapter, Chicago, Illinois, $5,000 (2008); Children's Memorial Foundation, Chicago, Illinois, $215,000 (2008); Rehabilitation Institute of Chicago, Chicago, Illinois, $16,666 (2008).
Contact: Kristen M. Buerster, Adminstrative Assistant/ Grants Administrator; (312) 755-0064; fax: (312) 755-0069
Internet: http://www.siragusa.org/pages/program_areas/13.php
Sponsor: Siragusa Foundation
One East Wacker Drive, Suite 2910
Chicago, IL 60601

Sisters of Mercy of North Carolina Foundation Grants **3295**
The foundation provides grants to tax-exempt health care, educational, and social service organizations that assist women, children, the elderly, and the poor to improve the quality of their lives. Types of support include start-up grants for new organizations or programs, ongoing operating expenses for individual organizations, program or project expenses, building renovation, and equipment acquisition. Preference will be given to organizations whose efforts are collaborative, ecumenical, and multicultural. Particular attention will be given to organizations that serve the unserved or underserved. Annual deadline dates may vary; contact program staff for exact dates.
Requirements: Tax-exempt health care, education, and social service organizations in North and South Carolina are eligible to apply.
Restrictions: The foundation does not ordinarily support projects, programs, or organizations that serve a limited audience; biomedical or clinical research; units of the federal government; political activities; publication of newsletters, magazines, books and the production of videos; conferences and travel; endowment funds; capital fundraising campaigns; annual giving campaigns; or social events or similar fundraising activities.
Geographic Focus: North Carolina; South Carolina
Samples: Greater Carolinas Chapter of the American Red Cross (Charlotte, NC)—to provide free transportation to and from medical appointments, $50,000 (2004).
Amount of Grant: $25,000 - $150,000 range
Date(s) Application is Due: Apr 1; Aug 1; Dec 1
Contact: Grants Administrator, (704) 366-0087; fax: (704) 366-8850; email: contact@somncfdn.org
Internet: http://www.somncfdn.org/grantseekers.html
Sponsor: Sisters of Mercy of North Carolina Foundation
2115 Rexford Road, Suite 401
Charlotte, NC 28211

Sisters of Saint Joseph Charitable Fund Grants **3296**
The charitable fund awards community support grants to nonprofits in West Virginia and Ohio counties in three areas: Healthy Communities grants support efforts to mobilize resources and citizen energy for communitywide health promotion, environmental protection, and local development; Healthy Families funding goes to efforts to provide children and youth with sustained, caring adult relationships that will encourage responsible behavior and positive self-identity; Healthy Senior Citizens grants support efforts to engage the elderly in the community by promoting wellness and preventive health care, independent living, voluntary service, and growth through learning. Community Initiative grants support grassroots community-based groups that are addressing health and human service needs directly affecting their local areas. The listed application deadline dates are for one-page letters of inquiry. If interested, the fund will send an application packet. Annual deadline dates may vary; contact program staff for exact dates.
Requirements: 501(c)3 tax-exempt organizations in Calhoun, Jackson, Pleasants, Ritchie, Roane, Tyler, Wirt, and Wood counties of West Virginia; and Athens, Meigs, and Washington counties of Ohio may apply for grant support. Eligible volunteer groups, such as neighborhood associations or church outreach communities, must be sponsored by a 501(c)3 organization.
Restrictions: The fund is unable to make grants to organizations without a 501(c)3 designation, whose projects do not benefit residents of the SSJCF service area, or whose projects do not promote health and wellness in the community it serves. Individuals are not eligible. Organizations that promote proselytizing or religious conversion as a goal of their programming or proposal; or Endowment funds.
Geographic Focus: Ohio; West Virginia
Amount of Grant: $18,000 average
Date(s) Application is Due: Jan 9; Jul 12
Contact: Grants Manager, (304) 424-6080; fax (304) 424-6081; email: info@ssjcharitablefund.org
Internet: http://www.ssjcharitablefund.org/grant_program.htm
Sponsor: Sisters of Saint Joseph Charitable Fund
P.O. Box 4440
Parkersburg, WV 26104-4440

Sisters of St. Joseph Healthcare Foundation Grants **3297**
The Sisters of St. Joseph Healthcare Foundation is a non-profit, public benefit corporation, which addresses the needs of the working and indigent poor in: Southern California; San Francisco Bay Area; Humboldt County; Fresno County. The Sisters of St. Joseph Healthcare Foundation funds programs which directly serve the needs of the underserved, especially families and children at risk. The Foundation sponsors or supports long-term efforts which are closely identified with the Sisters of St. Joseph of Orange and their mission of bringing unity and healing where divisiveness and oppression exist. The foundation supports the concept of "Healthy Communities" and desire to fund programs and organizations that: provide direct health-related services; support and transform the individual, social, economic, institutional, and cultural aspects of communities; provide change within larger societal systems to benefit low-income and at-risk populations; and develop the leadership and capacity for self-determination of those served by our funding. The Sisters of St. Joseph Healthcare Foundation is particularly interested in proposals which fall into these funding categories: mental health services; health services; homeless services; violence prevention.
Requirements: Southern California, Humbolt County, Fresno County and San Francisco bay area nonprofits are eligible.
Restrictions: The Foundation does not fund direct support to individuals, annual fund drives, or capital campaigns.
Geographic Focus: California
Samples: Access OC, Irvine, CA $50,000 - to improve access to specialty care for the safety net population (2008); Boys & Girls Clubs, Garden Grove, CA $30,000 - to fund transportation to improve access to healthcare for low-income families (2008); Casa Teresa, Orange, CA $40,000 - to assist homeless pregnant women with services to help them move from a low-income situation to self-sufficiency (2008);
Amount of Grant: $1,000 - $50,000 range
Contact: Sister Regina Fox, SSND, Program Director; (714) 633-8121 ext. 7109; email: rfox@csjorange.org
Sponsor: Sisters of St. Joseph Healthcare Foundation
440 South Batavia Street
Orange, CA 92868-3998

Skin Cancer Foundation Research Grants **3298**

Funding is provided annually for basic research, clinical studies, and educational programs related to skin cancer. The foundation's grants program is intended for pilot projects, which, if successful, can be further developed in order to be eligible for larger grants from other sources. Grants include: The Dr. Patricia Wexler Research Grant Awards (one-year, $10,000 grant for a research project); The Theodore S. Tromovitch Memorial Award (one-year, $5,000 grant for a research project); The Melissa K. Bambino Memorial Award (one-year, $8,000 grant for a research project); The Robert N. Cooke Memorial Award (one-year, $3,000 grant for a research project); Pevonia Botantica Research Award (one-year, $10,000 grant for a research project)
Requirements: Candidates must comply with all directions on the application form (available at the website). All projects are selected on the basis of their applicability to the foundation's mission of reducing the incidence, morbidity and mortality of skin cancer. Research must be conducted at institutions within the U.S. Preference is given to projects that address, at the basic science and clinical level, improved methods of prevention, detection, and treatment of skin cancers.
Restrictions: Overhead or indirect costs are not eligible.
Amount of Grant: $3,000 - $10,000
Date(s) Application is Due: Oct 1
Contact: Grants Administrator; (800) 754-6490; email: info@skincancer.org
Internet: http://www.skincancer.org/research-grants-2010.html
Sponsor: Skin Cancer Foundation
149 Madison Avenue, Suite 901
New York, NY 10016

Smith Family New Investigator Awards **3299**

These awards are made to promote basic research in the areas of AIDS, cancer, cardiovascular disease, diabetes, neuroscience, autism, and related disorders. The program favors innovative research, clearly presented proposals, realistic objectives, qualified personnel, and financial viability. The program will make six to eight two-year awards.
Requirements: Massachusetts medical groups may submit proposals.
Geographic Focus: Massachusetts
Amount of Grant: $100,000 per year
Contact: Grants Advisory Services, (617) 451-0049 ext 702; fax: (617) 423-4619; email: research@tmfnet.org
Internet: http://www.tmfnet.org/grantmake.html
Sponsor: The Medical Foundation
95 Berkeley Street, Suite 201
Boston, MA 02116

Snee Reinhardt Charitable Foundation Grants **3300**

The foundation awards a large variety of grants that have an impact on the social issues that Americans face every day. Recent grantees have included children's museums, universities, health agencies, theaters, schools, hospitals, youth issues, and environmental causes. Precedence is given to organizations situated within or whose activities are concentrated in, first, southwestern Pennsylvania, then northern West Virginia, northern Maryland, the Commonwealth of Pennsylvania and, lastly, the United States. Application and guidelines are available online.
Requirements: 501(c)3 nonprofit organizations are eligible.
Restrictions: Organizations, activities, and/or programs excluded from support include general capital improvement; general operating expenses, including salaries and fringe benefits; chairs or professorships; endowment funding; grants to individuals; political contributions; highly specialized health or medical programs that do not have specific impact on the community; organizations and programs designed to influence legislation or elect candidates to public office; organizations that discriminate by race, color, creed, gender, or national origin; or programs that promote, research, or support the prevention of life, abortion, the practice of euthanasia, or cruelty to animals.
Amount of Grant: $50,000 maximum
Date(s) Application is Due: Apr 15; Aug 15
Contact: Grants Administrator, (412) 390-2690; fax: (412) 390-2686
Internet: http://www.snee-reinhardt.org/index.html
Sponsor: Snee Reinhardt Charitable Foundation
River Park Commons Two, 2425 Sidney Street
Pittsburgh, PA 15203

SNM Molecular Imaging Research Grant For Junior Medical Faculty **3301**

The objective of this program is to provide salary support for one junior faculty member in an academic/research setting to enable them to engage in Molecular Imaging research related to diagnostic or therapeutic applications. The grant will support new, innovative pilot projects in any area of molecular imaging research. The grant may supplement other funds, but not duplicate other support.
Requirements: Applicant Eligibility: applicants must have MD degree (or equivalent) and have completed a residency and be certified in their specialty; applicants must be practicing in an academic/research setting as a faculty member in the United States; applicants must be within 5 years of their initial faculty appointment with an academic rank of instructor or assistant professor (or equivalent); applicants must provide a detailed proposal of the proposed research activity; applicants must not have received grant/contract amounts totaling $50,000.00 or more in a single calendar year as the principle investigator; preference will be given to individuals who have demonstrated great potential for a research career in the field of molecular imaging; multidisciplinary projects are encouraged; only one application per faculty member is accepted per grant; no grantee may receive more than one SNM research grant in any one year. Likewise no other research grant request or continuation will be considered until a satisfactory summary of an earlier grant is received; applicants are required to be a SNM member at the time of application.
Restrictions: The grant will not pay institutional overhead costs or indirect costs
Amount of Grant: $100,000 over two years
Date(s) Application is Due: Jan 20
Contact: Nicole Kern, SNM Program Manager; (703) 652-6795 ext. 1255; fax: (703) 708-9015; email: nkern@snm.org
Internet: http://interactive.snm.org/index.cfm?PageID=7252
Sponsor: Society of Nuclear Medicine
1850 Samuel Morse Drive
Reston, VA 20190

SNM PDEF Mickey Williams Minority Student Scholarships **3302**

This scholarship supports minority students pursuing a two or four year degree in nuclear medicine. It honors the memory of Mickey Williams, a past SNMTS President who immigrated to the United States from Jamaica.
Requirements: To be eligible for the PDEF Mickey Williams Minority Student Scholarship, candidates must: be of African American, Native American, Hispanic American, Asian American or Pacific Islander decent [Eligible Native Americans include American Indian, Eskimo, Hawaiian and Samoan]; hold current U.S. residency status of U.S. citizen, U.S. national, or U.S. permanent resident; be currently enrolled in or accepted into an entry-level nuclear medicine technology program at the time of application; Award is open to students in associate and baccalaureate level programs only; demonstrate financial need; have maintained a cumulative grade point average of 2.5 or better on a four-point scale, with evidence of high academic performance. See SNM website for application.
Restrictions: Individuals with a visitor, student, or G-series visa are not eligible. Individuals with previous certificates or degrees in nuclear medicine sciences are ineligible.
Amount of Grant: $5,000
Date(s) Application is Due: Jan 15
Contact: Nicole Kern, SNM Program Manager; (703) 652-6795 ext. 1255; fax: (703) 708-9015; email: nkern@snm.org
Internet: http://interactive.snm.org/index.cfm?PageID=2682&RPID=2259
Sponsor: Society of Nuclear Medicine
1850 Samuel Morse Drive
Reston, VA 20910

SNM Pilot Research Grants **3303**

The pilot research grants are designed to help basic or clinical scientists in the early stages of their career conduct research that may lead to further funding. The Mitzi and William Blahd, MD Pilot Research Grant is awarded to the applicant with the highest-ranked proposal. Preference will be given to individuals who have demonstrated great potential for a research career in the field of nuclear medicine/molecular imaging.
Requirements: Applicant Eligibility: basic or clinical scientists employed by academic and research-oriented organizations in North America are eligible; applicants must not be no more than five years post training.
Amount of Grant: $25,000
Date(s) Application is Due: Feb 20
Contact: Nicole Mitchell, Program Manager; (703) 652-6795; email: nkern@snm.org
Internet: http://interactive.snm.org/index.cfm?PageID=2255
Sponsor: Society of Nuclear Medicine
1850 Samuel Morse Drive
Reston, VA 20190

SNM Pilot Research Grants in Nuclear Medicine/Molecular Imaging **3304**

The pilot research grants are designed to help basic or clinical scientists in the early stages of their career conduct research that may lead to further funding.
Requirements: Applicant Eligibility: basic or clinical scientists employed by academic and research-oriented organizations in North America are eligible; applicants must be no more than five years post training; applicant must not have served as the principal investigator of a peer-reviewed grant for more than $50,000 in a single calendar year; preference will be given to individuals who have demonstrated great potential for a research career in the field of nuclear medicine/molecular imaging.
Restrictions: The grant will not pay salaries, institutional overhead costs or indirect costs. Funds may supplement other funds, but not duplicate other support. Grants will be limited to a time span of one year. No grantee may receive more than one grant in any one year.
Amount of Grant: $25,000
Date(s) Application is Due: Feb 20
Contact: Nicole Kern, SNM Program Manager; (703) 652-6795 ext. 1255; fax: (703) 708-9015; email: nkern@snm.org
Internet: http://interactive.snm.org/index.cfm?PageID=2255
Sponsor: Society of Nuclear Medicine
1850 Samuel Morse Drive
Reston, VA 20190

SNM Postdoctoral Molecular Imaging Scholar Grants **3305**

The postdoctoral program will support a two-year research endeavor that promotes integration of molecular imaging into the career of the trainee. The funds maybe used for new, innovative pilot projects in any area of molecular imaging research. The grant may supplement other funds, but not duplicate other support. A summary report and an accounting of funds will be requested at the halfway point and upon completion of the research project. Grantees are expected to submit results of the research as an abstract

for presentation at the SNM Annual Meeting and/or as a scientific manuscript to the Journal of Nuclear Medicine. A final report is due within 60 days after completion of the research project.
Requirements: Applicant Eligibility: MD, MD/PhD, and PhD applicants are eligible; applicants from any country may apply; applicants must hold a full-time position in an educational institution when the award starts; applicants must have completed all basic training and be no more than 2 years post training; applicants must not have served as a principal investigator on peer-reviewed grants totaling $50,000 or more in a single calendar year; preference will be given to individuals who have demonstrated great potential for a research career in the field of molecular imaging; only one application per trainee is accepted; no grantee may receive more than one SNM research grant in any one year. Likewise no other research grant request or continuation will be considered until a satisfactory summary of an earlier grant is received.
Restrictions: Grant extensions are not often allowed, but will be reviewed and decided upon by the SNM Grants and Awards Committee if requested. The grant will not pay institutional overhead costs or indirect costs.
Amount of Grant: $60,000 over two years
Date(s) Application is Due: Jan 20
Contact: Nicole Kern, SNM Program Manager; (703) 652-6795 ext. 1255; fax: (703) 708-9015; email: nkern@snm.org
Internet: http://interactive.snm.org/index.cfm?PageID=7252
Sponsor: Society of Nuclear Medicine
1850 Samuel Morse Drive
Reston, VA 20190

SNM Student Fellowship Awards **3306**
The SNM Student Fellowships are designed to stimulate interest in molecular imaging/nuclear medicine by supporting their full-time participation in clinical and basic research activities for three months (or less). These Fellowships are made possible by support of the Education and Research Foundation for SNM.
Requirements: Candidates from any country may apply. Students must be enrolled in a medical, pharmacy or graduate school, or be an undergraduate student demonstrating outstanding competence in nuclear medicine and/or molecular imaging research. Fellowship must be carried out during a three-month that starts no earlier then March and completed no later then December 31st.
Amount of Grant: $3000
Date(s) Application is Due: Jan 23
Contact: Nicole Kern, SNM Program Manager; (703) 652-6795, ext. 1255; fax: (703) 708-9015; email: nkern@snm.org
Internet: http://interactive.snm.org/index.cfm?PageID=2254
Sponsor: Society of Nuclear Medicine
1850 Samuel Morse Drive
Reston, VA 20190

SNM Tetalman Memorial Young Investigator Awards **3307**
Established by the family and friends of Dr. Tetalman, this award honors the work of a young investigator who is pursuing a career in nuclear medicine. It is named in memory of a highly respected and productive clinician and researcher, Mark Tetalman, M.D., whose career was cut tragically short. The award is based on a submitted paper supporting current research efforts and accomplishments, teaching, clinical service and administration. Service to the Society and a commitment to academic nuclear medicine will also be considered.
Requirements: Applicants must be 36 years old or younger as of July 1 of the application year and must have obtained certification in Nuclear Medicine or Nuclear Radiology or have completed a PhD program within the last seven years. Complete applications must be must be received, not simply post-marked by November 14th. One original unstapled copy of the completed application must be sent to: SNM Development Office, Attention: SNM Committee on Awards
Amount of Grant: $2500
Date(s) Application is Due: Nov 14
Contact: Nicole Kern, SNM Program Manager; (703) 652-6795 ext. 1255; fax: (703) 708-9015; email: nkern@snm.org
Internet: http://interactive.snm.org/index.cfm?PageID=2253
Sponsor: Society of Nuclear Medicine
1850 Samuel Morse Drive
Reston, VA 20190

SNM/ Covidien Seed Grant in Molecular Imaging/Nuclear Medicine Research **3308**
The Society of Nuclear Medicine is pleased to offer the SNM/Covidien Seed Grant in Nuclear Medicine Research. This grant is designed to assist researchers in conducting new and innovative pilot projects that have potential for future support from foundations, corporations or government agencies.
Requirements: Applicant Eligibility: basic or clinical scientists employed by academic and research-oriented organizations; applicants from any country may apply; applicants must hold a full-time faculty position in an educational institution when the award period begins; applicants must have completed all advanced training and be no more than five years post training; applicants must not have served as a principal investigator on peer-reviewed grants totaling $50,000 or more in a single calendar year; preference will be given to individuals who have demonstrated great potential for a research career in the field of nuclear medicine/molecular imaging.
Restrictions: No grantee may receive more than one SNM research grant in any one year. The grant will not pay institutional overhead costs or indirect costs. No salary support for principal investigator or co-principal investigators. Grants will be limited to a time span of one year; no extensions are allowed
Amount of Grant: $25,000
Date(s) Application is Due: Feb 20
Contact: Nicole Kern, SNM Program Manager; (703) 652-6795 ext. 1255; fax: (703) 708-9015; email: nkern@snm.org
Internet: http://interactive.snm.org/index.cfm?PageID=2255
Sponsor: Society of Nuclear Medicine
1850 Samuel Morse Drive
Reston, VA 20910

SNMTS Clinical Advancement Scholarships **3309**
The SNMTS Clinical Advancement Scholarships serve to support technologists who are pursuing clinical advancement through didactic educational programs. Ten (10) $500 scholarships will be awarded. Scholarship application form is available on the SNM website.
Requirements: To be eligible for the SNMTS Clinical Advancement Scholarship, candidates must: be a member of the SNMTS; demonstrate financial need; be currently enrolled in a didactic educational program(s) (ex. CT, DEXA, physics, statistics) which is/are college credit eligible; complete the said class or program. It is not required that class/program completion results in a degree.
Amount of Grant: $500
Date(s) Application is Due: May 1
Contact: Nicole Kern, SNM Program Manager; (703) 652-6795 ext. 1255; fax: (703) 708-9015; email: nkern@snm.org
Internet: http://interactive.snm.org/index.cfm?PageID=7270&RPID=2259
Sponsor: Society of Nuclear Medicine Technologist Section
1850 Samuel Morse Drive
Reston, VA 20910

SNMTS Outstanding Educator Awards **3310**
The purpose of this award to is to recognize a SNMTS member who has significantly contributed to providing knowledge that advances and promotes the field of nuclear medicine technology through outstanding work in education. The winner will receive $750 along with a plaque to be presented at the SNM Annual Meeting.
Requirements: Eligible candidates include teachers but also educators in the non-traditional sense such as industry and clinical professionals. Evidence of their outstanding work must be shown in the following required supporting documentation: Curriculum Vitae, including listing of publications, presentations, programs, awards and honors; one letter of support from recent student/graduate (within 5 years) or participant in program; one letter of support from current program director or supervisor; one letter of support from a colleague; completed Nomination Form (see website).
Amount of Grant: $750
Date(s) Application is Due: Mar 13
Contact: Nicole Kern, SNM Program Manager; (703) 652-6795 ext. 1255; fax: (703) 708-9015; email: nkern@snm.org
Internet: http://interactive.snm.org/index.cfm?PageID=2256
Sponsor: Society of Nuclear Medicine Technologist Section
1850 Samuel Morse Drive
Reston, VA 20910

SNMTS Outstanding Technologist Awards **3311**
The purpose of this award to is to recognize an SNMTS (SNM Technologist Section) member who has demonstrated outstanding service and dedication to the field of nuclear medicine technology. The winner will receive $750 along with a plaque to be presented at the SNM Annual Meeting.
Requirements: Eligible candidates include SNMTS members in any area of the field of nuclear medicine technology who have exhibited commitment to advancing the field in their workplace and through their involvement with the Society. Nominees must be involved with the Society at the local, regional and/or national level and have at least five years of experience in nuclear medicine technology. Evidence of their outstanding work must be shown in the following required supporting documentation: curriculum vitae- including listing of publications, presentations, programs, awards and honors; one letter of support from current supervisor; one letter of support from a colleague; one letter of support from a colleague who is a member of the SNMTS; completed Nomination Form (see website for application form).
Amount of Grant: $750
Date(s) Application is Due: Mar 13
Contact: Nicole Kern, SNM Program Manager; (703) 652-6795 ext. 1255; fax: (703) 708-9015; email: nkern@snm.org
Internet: http://interactive.snm.org/index.cfm?PageID=2256
Sponsor: Society of Nuclear Medicine
1850 Samuel Morse Drive
Reston, VA 20190

SNMTS Paul Cole Scholarships **3312**
The Paul Cole Scholarship is named in memory of Paul Cole, CNMT, who served as President of the SNM Technologist Section (SNMTS) in 1986 and who was known as a champion of education for technologists. This scholarship is funded by the Education and Research Foundation for the SNM.
Requirements: To be eligible for the Paul Cole Scholarship, candidates must: demonstrate financial need; be enrolled in or accepted into an institution accredited through the Joint Review Committee on Educational Programs in Nuclear Medicine Technology

(JRCNMT). To see if your institution is accredited with JRCNMT, visit their website at www.jrcnmt.org. Award is open to students in associate, baccalaureate, and certificate level programs; have maintained a minimum cumulative GPA of 2.5 or better (on a 4.0 scale) or B average in a nuclear medicine technology core curriculum.
Amount of Grant: $1,000
Date(s) Application is Due: Jan 15
Contact: Nicole Kern, SNM Program Manager; (703) 652-6795 ext. 1255; fax: (703) 708-9015; email: nkern@snm.org
Internet: http://interactive.snm.org/index.cfm?PageID=2681&RPID=2259
Sponsor: Society of Nuclear Medicine Technologist Section
1850 Samuel Morse Drive
Reston, VA 20190

SOBP A.E. Bennett Research Award **3313**
The awards, supported by the A.E. Bennett Neuropsychiatric Research Foundation, are in recognition of basic science and clinical science research in biological psychiatry by young investigators. Candidates must be actively engaged in the research for which the award is sought. Applicants need only write a brief description of their research, submit 2-3 published or submitted papers and arrange for two letters of support (at least one of the letters needs to be from a member of the Society).
Requirements: Submissions are welcomed from laboratory researchers in any country who have not passed their 45th birthday or have not been engaged in research for greater than 10 years following award of their terminal degree or the end of formal clinical/fellowship training, whichever is later by deadline date; candidates need not be current members of the society.
Amount of Grant: $2,000
Date(s) Application is Due: Jan 15
Contact: Maggie Peterson; (904) 953-2842; fax: (904) 953-7117; email: maggie@mayo.edu or sobp@sobp.org
Internet: http://www.sobp.org/i4a/pages/index.cfm?pageID=3379
Sponsor: Society of Biological Psychiatry
4500 San Pablo Road
Jacksonville, FL 32224

SOBP International Travel Fellowships **3314**
The Society offers International Travel Fellowships of up to U.S. $1,500 each to promising young investigators under the age of 35 from less-developed and less well-funded countries of the five IBRO Regions (Africa, Asian/Pacific, Central and Eastern Europe, Latin America, Western Europe) who would benefit from attending the annual meeting of the Society of Biological Psychiatry. This program will provide exposure of the fellowship recipients to the best science the Society has to offer and facilitate the professional contacts that may yield enduring collaborative and collegial relationships.
Requirements: Nominees must be: from a less developed and less well-funded country; and less than 35 years of age.
Amount of Grant: $1,500 maximum
Date(s) Application is Due: Jan 15
Contact: Maggie Peterson; (904) 953-2842; fax: (904) 953-7117; email: maggie@mayo.edu or sobp@sobp.org
Internet: http://www.sobp.org/i4a/pages/index.cfm?pageID=3375
Sponsor: Society of Biological Psychiatry
4500 San Pablo Road, Birdsall 310
Jacksonville, FL 32224

SOBP Travel Fellowships **3315**
The training of a new generation of psychiatric academicians is a major objective of the Society. Participation in professional meetings, where new information is exchanged and contacts are made, can have a critical impact on the career of a developing clinician-scientist. In recognition of the importance of academic exchange, the Society, through an educational grant from Eli Lilly and Company, Forest Laboratories and Elsevier Science, announces the continuation of annual Travel Fellowships. Each Fellowship will provide $1,500 to help defray the cost of attending the Society's Annual Meeting. In addition to the stipend and the opportunity to attend sessions of interest to them, Fellows also receive certificates of excellence and participate in a special ceremony held during the meeting in their honor. To receive the travel award, applicants are expected to attend the entire meeting and be present for the recognition events.
Requirements: For medical graduates, each University Department of Psychiatry in the United States, Canada and Mexico may nominate one candidate for this award. Medical graduates must be in their third, fourth, or fifth year of residency or in a bona fide research training program or sub-specialty training program within four years of leaving a general psychiatry residency training program.
Amount of Grant: $1,500 maximum
Date(s) Application is Due: Jan 15
Contact: Maggie Peterson; (904) 953-2842; fax: (904) 953-7117; email: maggie@mayo.edu or sobp@sobp.org
Internet: http://www.sobp.org/i4a/pages/index.cfm?pageID=3372
Sponsor: Society of Biological Psychiatry
4500 San Pablo Road, Birdsall 310
Jacksonville, FL 32224

SOBP Ziskind-Somerfeld Research Awards **3316**
The Society offers an annual award of $2,500 in either basic or clinical research for the purpose of stimulating investigations in biological psychiatry by senior investigators who are members in good standing of the Society of Biological Psychiatry. The Ziskind-Somerfeld Research Foundation makes this award possible. No submission is required to be considered for this award.
Requirements: Candidates will be at least thirty-five years of age at the time of submission. When more than one investigator is listed as an author on the submitted work, the principal investigators (first and last authors) must be over the age of 45.
Amount of Grant: $2,500
Contact: Maggie Peterson; (904) 953-2842; fax: (904) 953-7117; email: maggie@mayo.edu or sobp@sobp.org
Internet: http://www.sobp.org/i4a/pages/index.cfm?pageID=3380#top
Sponsor: Society of Biological Psychiatry
4500 San Pablo Road, Birdsall 310
Jacksonville, FL 32224

SOCFOC Catholic Ministries Grants **3317**
The Sisters of Charity Foundation of Cleveland belongs to a community of Catholic health and social service organizations inspired to service by the healing ministry of Jesus Christ. As a supporting foundation to the congregation of the Sisters of Charity of St. Augustine, the Foundation gives priority to the ministries of the Sisters of Charity Health System. A limited amount of remaining funds may be available to other Catholic ministries in health and human services in Cuyahoga County. Funding is limited to Invited Proposals.
Requirements: Each proposal to the Foundation must include a completed application form, proposal narrative, budget, and Budget Narrative. The application form and guidelines for the proposal narrative may be found on this website under the specific program area. Eligible organizations are 501(c)3 organizations or governmental agencies or units.
Restrictions: The Foundation does not make grants to individuals.
Geographic Focus: Ohio
Samples: Secretariat for Parish Life & Development, OH, $10,000 .;2008.; St. Vincent Charity Hospital, OH, $151,600 .;2008.;
Amount of Grant: $10,000 - $150,000 range
Contact: Lynn Berner, Program Officer, (216) 241-9300; fax: (216) 241-9345; email: lberner@socfdncleveland.org
Internet: http://www.socfdncleveland.org/RespondingToOurCommunity/CatholicMinistries/tabid/313/Default.aspx
Sponsor: Sisters of Charity Foundation of Cleveland
The Halle Building, Suite 330, 1228 Euclid Avenue
Cleveland, OH 44115-1834

SOCFOC Reducing Health & Educational Disparities in the Central Neighborhood Grants **3318**
The Sisters of Charity Foundation of Cleveland is committed to helping families and individuals overcome the challenges of poverty. In this grant opportunity the Foundation focuses on health, housing and education as key components to building stronger families and stable neighborhoods. The Foundation seeks to reduce both health and educational disparities in the Cuyahoga County.
Requirements: Applicants must be 501(c)3 organizations or governmental units or agencies (such as schools) that primarily serve the Cuyahoga County.
Geographic Focus: Ohio
Samples: Health Disparities/Community Health, OH, $125,000 .;2007.;
Amount of Grant: $20,000 - $75,000 per year, larger for two year period
Date(s) Application is Due: Apr 7
Contact: Ursula Craig, Grants Coordinator, (216) 241-9300; fax: (216) 241-9345; email: ucraig@socfdncleveland.org
Internet: http://www.socfdncleveland.org/sistersofcharity/OurFocusAreas/HealthDisparities/HealthintheCentralNeighborhood/tabid/344/Default.aspx
Sponsor: Sisters of Charity Foundation of Cleveland
The Halle Building, Suite 330, 1228 Euclid Avenue
Cleveland, OH 44115-1834

Society for Biomedical Screening Small Grants **3319**
The society's small grants program will provide start-up funding for research projects with potential to advance the disciplines, technologies, and skills involved in screening and molecular discovery, including the support of graduate or undergraduate training in these areas. The program is intended to support projects that may have an applied focus or those that may involve radically new concepts. Applications are considered without regard to race, religion, national origin, physical handicap, or age of the candidates.
Requirements: Applicants must be employed full time in a college, university, or nonprofit research institute in order to serve as principal investigators.
Date(s) Application is Due: Feb 18
Contact: David Roman, (203) 743-1336; fax: (203) 748-7557; email: droman@sbsonline.org
Internet: http://www.sbsonline.org/awards_grants
Sponsor: Society for Biomedical Screening
36 Tamarack Avenue, #348
Danbury, CT 06811

Society for Imaging Informatics in Medicine (SIIM) Emeritus Mentor Grants **3320**
The mission of SIIM, The Society for Imaging Informatics in Medicine, is to advance computer applications and information technology in medical imaging through education and research. In support of this mission, the SIIM Research and Development Committee offers a $20,000 grant for a retired, or semi-retired, expert in imaging informatics to act as a mentor for a trainee (student, resident, fellow) or junior faculty

member for hypothesis-driven research. Any area of research involving medical imaging informatics is eligible for support, as well as development of new hardware, software, or processes to support electronic imaging practice, education, or research.
Requirements: A senior, experienced investigator jointly applies with a resident, fellow, graduate student, or junior faculty for a SIIM emeritus mentor grant. Preference will be given to projects at SIIM institutions and to projects that contribute to the development of careers of new or prospective researchers. This grant may not be applied for in conjunction with another SIIM grant covering the same subject material.
Amount of Grant: $20,000
Date(s) Application is Due: Aug 3
Contact: Grant Manager; (703) 723-0432; fax: (703) 723-0415; email: grants@siimweb.org or info@siimweb.org
Internet: http://www.scarnet.org/index.cfm?id=63
Sponsor: Society for Imaging Informatics in Medicine (SIIM)
19440 Golf Vista Plaza, Suite 330
Leesburg, VA 20176-8264

Society for Imaging Informatics in Medicine (SIIM) Micro Grants 3321
The mission of SIIM, The Society for Imaging Informatics in Medicine, is to advance computer applications and information technology in medical imaging through education and research. In support of this mission, the SIIM Research and Development Committee offers a $5,000 grant for hypothesis-driven experiments of short duration and high risk. Prior preliminary data is not required. An imaging informatics project that needs resources falls between what a researcher is willing to fund personally or is more than his/her department provides in seed money and what is typically requested in grant applications. Examples include trying unconventional hardware or software in an imaging informatics experiment, trying a particular piece of hardware for a user-interface design, paying for short duration consulting assistance, or paying for an educational course that the researcher needs to enhance a particular study.
Requirements: There are no restrictions on who may apply for the grant. Trainees (residents, fellows, and graduate students) are required to include a letter from a faculty member, acting as an advisor, to show that the applicant's department supports the project. Preference will be given to projects at SIIM institutions and to projects that may yield high value results or provide enough preliminary data to justify additional work and application for traditional grant funding.
Amount of Grant: $5,000
Date(s) Application is Due: Aug 3
Contact: Grant Manager; (703) 723-0432; fax: (703) 723-0415; email: grants@siimweb.org or info@siimweb.org
Internet: http://www.scarnet.org/index.cfm?id=63
Sponsor: Society for Imaging Informatics in Medicine (SIIM)
19440 Golf Vista Plaza, Suite 330
Leesburg, VA 20176-8264

Society for Imaging Informatics in Medicine (SIIM) Research Grants 3322
The mission of SIIM, The Society for Imaging Informatics in Medicine, is to advance computer applications and information technology in medical imaging through education and research. In support of this mission, the SIIM Research and Development Committee offers two $50,000 grants for original research. Any area of research involving medical imaging informatics is eligible for support, as well as development of new hardware, software, or processes to support electronic imaging practice, education, or research.
Requirements: Residents, fellows, graduate students, or faculty may apply for SIIM research grants. Preference will be given to projects at SIIM institutions and to projects that contribute to the development of careers of new or prospective researchers. Residents, fellows, and students must conduct their projects under the guidance of experienced investigators. Grant recipients will not be eligible for concurrent support through other SIIM grants.
Amount of Grant: $50,000
Date(s) Application is Due: Aug 3
Contact: Grant Manager; (703) 723-0432; fax: (703) 723-0415; email: grants@siimweb.org or info@siimweb.org
Internet: http://www.scarnet.org/index.cfm?id=63
Sponsor: Society for Imaging Informatics in Medicine (SIIM)
19440 Golf Vista Plaza, Suite 330
Leesburg, VA 20176-8264

Society for Imaging Informatics in Medicine (SIIM) Small Grant for Product Support Development 3323
The mission of SIIM, The Society for Imaging Informatics in Medicine, is to advance computer applications and information technology in medical imaging through education and research. In support of this mission, the SIIM Research and Development Committee offers a $20,000 grant to support the development of a product or tool for use in the field of imaging informatics. Any area of product or tool development for use in the field of medical imaging informatics is eligible for support (e.g., open source application development, work flow measurement tools, replacement PACS change management tools).
Requirements: Residents, fellows, graduate students, or faculty may apply for product support development grants. Preference will be given to projects at SIIM institutions and to projects that contribute to the development of careers of new or prospective researchers. Residents, fellows, and students must conduct their projects under the guidance of experienced investigators.
Amount of Grant: $20,000
Date(s) Application is Due: Aug 3
Contact: Grant Manager; (703) 723-0432; fax: (703) 723-0415; email: grants@siimweb.org or info@siimweb.org
Internet: http://www.scarnet.org/index.cfm?id=63
Sponsor: Society for Imaging Informatics in Medicine (SIIM)
19440 Golf Vista Plaza, Suite 330
Leesburg, VA 20176-8264

Society for Imaging Informatics in Medicine (SIIM) Small Training Grants 3324
The mission of SIIM, The Society for Imaging Informatics in Medicine, is to advance computer applications and information technology in medical imaging through education and research. In support of this mission, the SIIM Research and Development Committee offers a $20,000 grant targeted at providing training opportunities in the field of imaging informatics for students and imaging informatics professionals. Any area of training within medical imaging informatics is eligible for support. The grant is designed to support hands-on training or experience with a designated mentor or sponsor in the imaging informatics arena. It is not intended to support tuition or other traditional education-related expenses. The period of training must last a minimum of three months and may extend no longer than twelve months.
Requirements: Residents, fellows, graduate students, or faculty members at recognized institutions may apply for SIIM training grants. Preference will be given to training experiences at SIIM institutions and to those that contribute to the careers of new or prospective imaging informatics personnel.
Amount of Grant: $20,000
Date(s) Application is Due: Aug 3
Contact: Grant Manager; (703) 723-0432; fax: (703) 723-0415; email: grants@siimweb.org or info@siimweb.org
Internet: http://www.scarnet.org/index.cfm?id=63
Sponsor: Society for Imaging Informatics in Medicine (SIIM)
19440 Golf Vista Plaza, Suite 330
Leesburg, VA 20176-8264

Society for Investigative Dermatology Career Development Award 3325
The society makes one-year career development awards to encourage trainees in skin-related fields to become skin scientists. Applications will be considered in the following areas: skin biology, skin disease, skin research publishing, and presentation of skin research at a forum. Application forms may be obtained from the Dermatology Foundation, 1563 Maple Avenue, Evanston, IL 60201. Contact program staff to determine availability of awards.
Requirements: Eligible applicants include MDs and PhDs engaged in projects related to the skin and skin diseases.
Amount of Grant: $40,000 per year
Contact: Program Contact, Department of Dermatology, Columbia University, (216) 579-9300; fax: (216) 579-9333; email: sid@sidnet.org
Internet: http://www.sidnet.org
Sponsor: Society for Investigative Dermatology Inc
820 W Superior Avenue, 7th Floor
Cleveland, OH 44113-1800

Society for the Arts in Healthcare Consulting Grants 3326
The Society for the Arts in Healthcare has partnered with the National Endowment for the Arts to provide hundreds of consulting grants to arts and/or health care organizations across the U.S.. Through a roster of over 20 trained arts in health care consultants, these grants assist organizations in utilizing a diverse array of arts media including performing arts, visual arts, literature, film, or design to promote the health and well-being of equally diverse populations. Organizations may apply for up to 20 hours of consulting with an experienced leader in the field. This grant pays for all consultant fees and grantees cover any additional costs such as long-distance phone calls or consultant travel and accommodation. Consultants are available to travel to organizations for site visits or to provide information and support via phone or email. The Consulting Service can assist in: program planning/strategic planning; artist training; fundraising and promotion; community collaborations and effective partnerships; evaluation; and improving health care facility design and environments. Projects can range from specific technical assistance such as designing a job description, creating a survey, feedback on a grant application, or developing guidelines for exhibitions to thinking through a strategic plan for a program. Prospective clients can request the number of hours that would be most appropriate for their needs.
Requirements: Applicant organizations must be based in the United States.
Date(s) Application is Due: Nov 16
Contact: Anita Boles, Executive Director; (202) 299-9770; fax: (202) 299-9887; email: anita@thesah.org
Internet: http://www.thesah.org/template/page.cfm?page_id=466
Sponsor: Society for the Arts in Healthcare (SAH)
2437 15th Street, NW
Washington, DC 20009

Society for the Arts in Healthcare Environmental Arts Research Grant 3327
The American Art Resources and Society for the Arts in Healthcare Environmental Arts Research Grant program offers a cash award sponsored by American Art Resources in Houston, Texas. The program is provided to a Principal Investigator to conduct or supplement Arts in Healthcare research. Selection is made on the merit, innovation and feasibility of the research proposal.
Requirements: Applicant organizations must be based in the United States.

Contact: Anita Boles, Executive Director; (202) 299-9770; fax: (202) 299-9887; email: anita@thesah.org
Internet: http://www.thesah.org/template/page.cfm?page_id=570
Sponsor: Society for the Arts in Healthcare (SAH)
2437 15th Street, NW
Washington, DC 20009

Society of Cosmetic Chemists Allan B. Black Award Sponsored by Presperse 3328
Dedicated to the advancement of cosmetic science, the Society strives to increase and disseminate scientific information through meetings and publications. By promoting research in cosmetic science and industry, and by setting high ethical, professional and educational standards, it strives to improve the qualifications of cosmetic scientists. Its mission is to further the interests and recognition of cosmetic scientists while maintaining the confidence of the public in the cosmetic and toiletries industry. With the Allan B. Black Award, a scroll and honorarium are awarded annually for the Best Paper on make-up technology either presented at an annual meeting, a seminar, or published in the Journal of Cosmetic Science, the Official Journal of the Society of Cosmetic Chemists.
Contact: Theresa Cesario, Executive Director; (212) 668-1500; fax: (212) 668-1504; email: TCesario@SCConline.org
Internet: http://www.scconline.org/website/about_scc/awards_fellowships.shtml
Sponsor: Society of Cosmetic Chemists
120 Wall Street, Suite 2400
New York, NY 10005-4088

Society of Cosmetic Chemists Award Sponsored by McIntyre Group, Ltd. 3329
Dedicated to the advancement of cosmetic science, the Society strives to increase and disseminate scientific information through meetings and publications. By promoting research in cosmetic science and industry, and by setting high ethical, professional and educational standards, it strives to improve the qualifications of cosmetic scientists. Its mission is to further the interests and recognition of cosmetic scientists while maintaining the confidence of the public in the cosmetic and toiletries industry. This award, given in the form of a scroll and honorarium, are awarded for the best paper presented at the Society's Annual Scientific Meeting.
Contact: Theresa Cesario, Executive Director; (212) 668-1500; fax: (212) 668-1504; email: TCesario@SCConline.org
Internet: http://www.scconline.org/website/about_scc/awards_fellowships.shtml
Sponsor: Society of Cosmetic Chemists
120 Wall Street, Suite 2400
New York, NY 10005-4088

Society of Cosmetic Chemists Award Sponsored by The HallStar Company 3330
Dedicated to the advancement of cosmetic science, the Society strives to increase and disseminate scientific information through meetings and publications. By promoting research in cosmetic science and industry, and by setting high ethical, professional and educational standards, it strives to improve the qualifications of cosmetic scientists. Its mission is to further the interests and recognition of cosmetic scientists while maintaining the confidence of the public in the cosmetic and toiletries industry. Offered in the form of a scroll and honorarium, this honor is awarded for the Best Paper that makes the greatest scientific contribution to knowledge in the field of protecting against or ameliorating damage to human skin caused by exposure to UV radiation presented at the Society's Annual Scientific Seminar.
Contact: Theresa Cesario, Executive Director; (212) 668-1500; fax: (212) 668-1504; email: TCesario@SCConline.org
Internet: http://www.scconline.org/website/about_scc/awards_fellowships.shtml
Sponsor: Society of Cosmetic Chemists
120 Wall Street, Suite 2400
New York, NY 10005-4088

Society of Cosmetic Chemists Chapter Best Speaker Award 3331
Dedicated to the advancement of cosmetic science, the Society strives to increase and disseminate scientific information through meetings and publications. By promoting research in cosmetic science and industry, and by setting high ethical, professional and educational standards, it strives to improve the qualifications of cosmetic scientists. Its mission is to further the interests and recognition of cosmetic scientists while maintaining the confidence of the public in the cosmetic and toiletries industry. The Chapter Best Speaker Award is given for the best scientific paper presented before each Chapter during a given calendar year. Recommendations for this award originates with the Chapters and are submitted to the National Office. A scroll and honorarium ($250 for a manuscript submission and $150 for an abstract submission) is provided by National for presentation by the Chapter.
Contact: Theresa Cesario, Executive Director; (212) 668-1500; fax: (212) 668-1504; email: TCesario@SCConline.org
Internet: http://www.scconline.org/website/about_scc/awards_fellowships.shtml
Sponsor: Society of Cosmetic Chemists
120 Wall Street, Suite 2400
New York, NY 10005-4088

Society of Cosmetic Chemists Chapter Merit Award 3332
Dedicated to the advancement of cosmetic science, the Society strives to increase and disseminate scientific information through meetings and publications. By promoting research in cosmetic science and industry, and by setting high ethical, professional and educational standards, it strives to improve the qualifications of cosmetic scientists. Its mission is to further the interests and recognition of cosmetic scientists while maintaining the confidence of the public in the cosmetic and toiletries industry. The Chapter Merit Award is awarded to a Chapter Member for outstanding service, dedication and voluntary services over a period of time. A scroll is provided by National for presentation by the Chapter. Recommendations for this award originates with each Chapter and are submitted to the National Office.
Contact: Theresa Cesario, Executive Director; (212) 668-1500; fax: (212) 668-1504; email: TCesario@SCConline.org
Internet: http://www.scconline.org/website/about_scc/awards_fellowships.shtml
Sponsor: Society of Cosmetic Chemists
120 Wall Street, Suite 2400
New York, NY 10005-4088

Society of Cosmetic Chemists Frontier of Science Award 3333
Dedicated to the advancement of cosmetic science, the Society strives to increase and disseminate scientific information through meetings and publications. By promoting research in cosmetic science and industry, and by setting high ethical, professional and educational standards, it strives to improve the qualifications of cosmetic scientists. Its mission is to further the interests and recognition of cosmetic scientists while maintaining the confidence of the public in the cosmetic and toiletries industry. The Frontier of Science Award is an honorarium given to a speaker who has achieved exceptional national or international stature in the scientific community for delivering a lecture at the Annual Scientific Meeting.
Contact: Theresa Cesario, Executive Director; (212) 668-1500; fax: (212) 668-1504; email: TCesario@SCConline.org
Internet: http://www.scconline.org/website/about_scc/awards_fellowships.shtml
Sponsor: Society of Cosmetic Chemists
120 Wall Street, Suite 2400
New York, NY 10005-4088

Society of Cosmetic Chemists Hans Schaeffer Award 3334
Dedicated to the advancement of cosmetic science, the Society strives to increase and disseminate scientific information through meetings and publications. By promoting research in cosmetic science and industry, and by setting high ethical, professional and educational standards, it strives to improve the qualifications of cosmetic scientists. Its mission is to further the interests and recognition of cosmetic scientists while maintaining the confidence of the public in the cosmetic and toiletries industry. The Hans Schaeffer Award, offered in the form of a scroll and honorarium, are awarded annually for the Most Innovative Paper presented at either an annual meeting or a seminar.
Contact: Theresa Cesario, Executive Director; (212) 668-1500; fax: (212) 668-1504; email: TCesario@SCConline.org
Internet: http://www.scconline.org/website/about_scc/awards_fellowships.shtml
Sponsor: Society of Cosmetic Chemists
120 Wall Street, Suite 2400
New York, NY 10005-4088

Society of Cosmetic Chemists Joseph P. Ciaudelli Award 3335
Dedicated to the advancement of cosmetic science, the Society strives to increase and disseminate scientific information through meetings and publications. By promoting research in cosmetic science and industry, and by setting high ethical, professional and educational standards, it strives to improve the qualifications of cosmetic scientists. Its mission is to further the interests and recognition of cosmetic scientists while maintaining the confidence of the public in the cosmetic and toiletries industry. The Joseph P. Ciaudelli Award, offered in the form of a scroll and honorarium, are bestowed annually for the best article appearing in the Journal of Cosmetic Science on the subject of hair care technology.
Contact: Theresa Cesario, Executive Director; (212) 668-1500; fax: (212) 668-1504; email: TCesario@SCConline.org
Internet: http://www.scconline.org/website/about_scc/awards_fellowships.shtml
Sponsor: Society of Cosmetic Chemists
120 Wall Street, Suite 2400
New York, NY 10005-4088

Society of Cosmetic Chemists Keynote Award Lecture Sponsored by Ruger Chemical Corporation 3336
Dedicated to the advancement of cosmetic science, the Society strives to increase and disseminate scientific information through meetings and publications. By promoting research in cosmetic science and industry, and by setting high ethical, professional and educational standards, it strives to improve the qualifications of cosmetic scientists. Its mission is to further the interests and recognition of cosmetic scientists while maintaining the confidence of the public in the cosmetic and toiletries industry. The Keynote Award is an honorarium given to a speaker who has achieved exceptional national or international stature in the scientific community for delivering a lecture at the Annual Scientific Meeting.
Contact: Theresa Cesario, Executive Director; (212) 668-1500; fax: (212) 668-1504; email: TCesario@SCConline.org
Internet: http://www.scconline.org/website/about_scc/awards_fellowships.shtml
Sponsor: Society of Cosmetic Chemists
120 Wall Street, Suite 2400
New York, NY 10005-4088

Society of Cosmetic Chemists Literature Award 3337
Dedicated to the advancement of cosmetic science, the Society strives to increase and disseminate scientific information through meetings and publications. By promoting

research in cosmetic science and industry, and by setting high ethical, professional and educational standards, it strives to improve the qualifications of cosmetic scientists. Its mission is to further the interests and recognition of cosmetic scientists while maintaining the confidence of the public in the cosmetic and toiletries industry. Through the Literature Award, a scroll and honorarium are presented annually to the author or authors of scientific papers in basic research judged to be an outstanding contribution to cosmetic science and technology.
Contact: Theresa Cesario, Executive Director; (212) 668-1500; fax: (212) 668-1504; email: TCesario@SCConline.org
Internet: http://www.scconline.org/website/about_scc/awards_fellowships.shtml
Sponsor: Society of Cosmetic Chemists
120 Wall Street, Suite 2400
New York, NY 10005-4088

Society of Cosmetic Chemists Maison G. de Navarre Medal **3338**
Dedicated to the advancement of cosmetic science, the Society strives to increase and disseminate scientific information through meetings and publications. By promoting research in cosmetic science and industry, and by setting high ethical, professional and educational standards, it strives to improve the qualifications of cosmetic scientists. Its mission is to further the interests and recognition of cosmetic scientists while maintaining the confidence of the public in the cosmetic and toiletries industry. The Society's highest honor, the Maison G. de Navarre Medal, recognizes individuals for their technical contributions to cosmetic science. The award is presented annually.
Contact: Theresa Cesario, Executive Director; (212) 668-1500; fax: (212) 668-1504; email: TCesario@SCConline.org
Internet: http://www.scconline.org/website/about_scc/awards_fellowships.shtml
Sponsor: Society of Cosmetic Chemists
120 Wall Street, Suite 2400
New York, NY 10005-4088

Society of Cosmetic Chemists Merit Award **3339**
Dedicated to the advancement of cosmetic science, the Society strives to increase and disseminate scientific information through meetings and publications. By promoting research in cosmetic science and industry, and by setting high ethical, professional and educational standards, it strives to improve the qualifications of cosmetic scientists. Its mission is to further the interests and recognition of cosmetic scientists while maintaining the confidence of the public in the cosmetic and toiletries industry. The Merit Award is presented annually for outstanding service and distinguished leadership in Society activities.
Contact: Theresa Cesario, Executive Director; (212) 668-1500; fax: (212) 668-1504; email: TCesario@SCConline.org
Internet: http://www.scconline.org/website/about_scc/awards_fellowships.shtml
Sponsor: Society of Cosmetic Chemists
120 Wall Street, Suite 2400
New York, NY 10005-4088

Society of Cosmetic Chemists Robert A. Kramer Lifetime Service Award **3340**
Dedicated to the advancement of cosmetic science, the Society strives to increase and disseminate scientific information through meetings and publications. By promoting research in cosmetic science and industry, and by setting high ethical, professional and educational standards, it strives to improve the qualifications of cosmetic scientists. Its mission is to further the interests and recognition of cosmetic scientists while maintaining the confidence of the public in the cosmetic and toiletries industry. The Robert A. Kramer Lifetime Service Award, given at the discretion of the Board of Directors, goes to an individual who has given extraordinary service over the course of his or her membership.
Contact: Theresa Cesario, Executive Director; (212) 668-1500; fax: (212) 668-1504; email: TCesario@SCConline.org
Internet: http://www.scconline.org/website/about_scc/awards_fellowships.shtml
Sponsor: Society of Cosmetic Chemists
120 Wall Street, Suite 2400
New York, NY 10005-4088

Society of Cosmetic Chemists Shaw Mudge Award **3341**
Dedicated to the advancement of cosmetic science, the Society strives to increase and disseminate scientific information through meetings and publications. By promoting research in cosmetic science and industry, and by setting high ethical, professional and educational standards, it strives to improve the qualifications of cosmetic scientists. Its mission is to further the interests and recognition of cosmetic scientists while maintaining the confidence of the public in the cosmetic and toiletries industry. The Shaw Mudge Award, given in the form of a scroll and honorarium, are awarded for the best paper presented at the Society's Annual Scientific Seminar.
Contact: Theresa Cesario, Executive Director; (212) 668-1500; fax: (212) 668-1504; email: TCesario@SCConline.org
Internet: http://www.scconline.org/website/about_scc/awards_fellowships.shtml
Sponsor: Society of Cosmetic Chemists
120 Wall Street, Suite 2400
New York, NY 10005-4088

Society of Cosmetic Chemists Student Poster Awards **3342**
Dedicated to the advancement of cosmetic science, the Society strives to increase and disseminate scientific information through meetings and publications. By promoting research in cosmetic science and industry, and by setting high ethical, professional and educational standards, it strives to improve the qualifications of cosmetic scientists. Its mission is to further the interests and recognition of cosmetic scientists while maintaining the confidence of the public in the cosmetic and toiletries industry. The Student Poster Award, sponsored by DD-Chemco, Inc., is given annually in conjunction with the Annual Scientific Seminar. Honorariums are given for first, second, third and fourth place Best Student Poster.
Contact: Theresa Cesario, Executive Director; (212) 668-1500; fax: (212) 668-1504; email: TCesario@SCConline.org
Internet: http://www.scconline.org/website/about_scc/awards_fellowships.shtml
Sponsor: Society of Cosmetic Chemists
120 Wall Street, Suite 2400
New York, NY 10005-4088

Society of Cosmetic Chemists Young Scientist Awards **3343**
The Young Scientist Awards are presented each year to recognize the outstanding achievements of new cosmetic scientists throughout the industry. Each year every manufacturer, supplier or other organization in the personal care industry may select an individual in their employ as a recipient of this award. The criteria for selection is made by the individual company. Information is sent in March of each year and is posted on the SCC Website. The submission deadline is July 1st each year. The awards may be presented at an SCC Chapter Meeting or through an internal corporate presentation. Recipient names are listed in the SCC Winter Newsletter.
Requirements: Recipients be an active member of the Society for at least one year and working in the industry less than 10 years.
Date(s) Application is Due: Jul 1
Contact: Theresa Cesario, Executive Director; (212) 668-1500; fax: (212) 668-1504; email: TCesario@SCConline.org
Internet: http://www.scconline.org/website/about_scc/awards_fellowships.shtml
Sponsor: Society of Cosmetic Chemists
120 Wall Street, Suite 2400
New York, NY 10005-4088

Society of Medical Friends of Wine Research Award **3344**
One award is given biennially for published original research identifying substances in wine; ascertaining the effects of wine components on living cells, tissues, or organs; or indicating appropriate clinical applications of wine in treatment or prevention of disease. Applications are accepted at any time.
Amount of Grant: $2000
Contact: Susan Guerguy, Executive Secretary, (925) 933-9691; fax: (925) 939-5224; email: marq@inreach.com
Internet: http://www.medicalfriendsofwine.org
Sponsor: Society of Medical Friends of Wine
511 Jones Pl
Walnut Creek, CA 94597

Society of Neuroscience Minority Fellowships **3345**
The goal of the program is to increase the diversity of the pool of individuals participating in mental-health related neuroscience research and teaching programs. The program recruits and trains outstanding individuals of traditionally underrepresented racial and ethnic minorities. Training stipends are available for predoctoral (up to three years) and postdoctoral (up to two years) fellowships. The program includes training stipends in accordance with NRSA standard guidelines; travel assistance and registration to attend the annual meeting, in addition to SFN member resources; enrichment programs including funds to participate in activities outside of the fellow's home laboratory; and mentoring opportunities, with a mentor from among SFN memberships. Details and application are available online.
Date(s) Application is Due: Jan 1; Apr 1; Sep 1
Contact: Jessica Pearce, Program Coordinator,(202) 462-6688; fax: (202) 462-9740; email: jessica@sfn.org
Internet: http://www.sfn.org/content/Programs/DiversityinNeuroscience/mnfp/index.html
Sponsor: Society for Neuroscience
11 Dupont Circle NW, Suite 500
Washington, DC 20036

Solo Cup Foundation Grants **3346**
The foundation awards grants to Illinois nonprofit organizations in its areas of interest, including higher education, health, social services, and Christian organizations and churches. Types of support include capital campaigns, general operating support, and scholarship funds. There are no application deadlines or forms.
Requirements: Illinois nonprofit organizations are eligible.
Geographic Focus: Illinois
Samples: La Rashida Children's Hospital (Chicago, IL)—for a capital campaign to modernize and upgrade its inpatient facility, $1 million.; Immaculate Conception Church (Chicago, IL)—for restoration project, $85,000.; Congregation of the Passion (Chicago, IL)—for general support, $50,000.
Amount of Grant: $5000-$85,000
Contact: Robert M. Korzenski, President and CEO; (847) 831-4800; fax: (847) 579-3245; email: info@solocup.com
Sponsor: Solo Cup Foundation
1700 Old Deerfield Road
Highland Park, IL 60035

Sonoco Foundation Grants 3347

The Sonoco Products Company is the company sponsor of the Sonoco Foundation. The foundation was established in 1983, in the state of South Carolina. The foundation supports organizations involved with education, crime and violence prevention, human services, youth, and community development. Giving primarily in areas of company operations, with emphasis on Hartsville, South Carolina.

Requirements: South Carolina nonprofit organizations are eligible to apply for these grants. There is no application form required. Applicants should submit a detailed description of project and amount of funding requested.

Restrictions: The foundation does not support religious, political, or lobbying organizations. Grants aren't available to individuals, or for educational capital funds programs, endowments, trips, or tours.

Geographic Focus: South Carolina

Amount of Grant: $1,000 - $600,000 range

Contact: Joyce Beasley, (800) 377-2692 or (843) 383-7851

Internet: http://www.sonoco.com

Sponsor: Sonoco Foundation
1 North Second Street M.S. A09
Hartsville, SC 29550-3300

Sosland Foundation Grants 3348

The foundation awards grants to nonprofit organizations in the metropolitan bistate Kansas City area. Areas of interest include arts and culture, higher education, health care, Jewish services, and social services. Types of support include program development, building construction/renovation, equipment acquisition, development grants, endowments, general operating grants, and matching gifts. There are no application forms or deadlines. Applicants should send a letter including a description of the program and the organization, a list of board and staff, and proof of tax-exempt status.

Requirements: Metropolitan bistate Kansas City 501(c)3 nonprofit organizations are eligible.

Restrictions: Individuals and publications or conferences are ineligible.

Geographic Focus: Kansas; Missouri

Samples: William Jewell College (Liberty, MO)—to renovate Jewell Hall, $50,000.

Amount of Grant: $1000-$5000 average

Contact: Program Contact, (816) 756-1000; fax: (816) 756-0494

Internet: http://www.soslandfoundation.org

Sponsor: Sosland Foundation
4800 Main Street, Suite 100
Kansas City, MO 64112

South Madison Community Foundation Grants 3349

South Madison Community Foundation, Inc. is a not-for-profit 501(c)3 charitable organization that was established in 1992 to assist donors in meeting their philanthropic interests. It is governed by a professional volunteer Board of Directors, and assisted by volunteer committee members and a dedicated staff. SMCF serves the residents in Adams, Fall Creek, Green, and Stony Creek Townships of Madison County. It was established due to a vision of a handful of community residents who embraced the concept of a community foundation, a unique charitable organization that is funded by a variety of individuals and organizations and governed by a board of community citizens. The Board of Directors of the South Madison Community Foundation, Inc. has developed a procedure for submission and evaluation of grant proposals. Because of time constraints, all proposals must be submitted in writing, no personal presentations are accepted. The Grants Committee makes its recommendation to the Board of Directors who must give final approval for the funding. Applicants are notified within one month of the submission deadline of approval or denial of their request for funding.

Requirements: The priorities of the South Madison Community Foundation, Inc. are: to focus on the prevention of problems rather than the symptoms; to maintain both a proactive focus and an ability to respond to creative ideas from grant seekers; to assist grant seekers to better respond to the changing needs of the South Madison County community; to encourage programs that enhance cooperation and collaboration among institutions within the community; to leverage funds through the use of match and challenge grants; to fund projects that will make a significant improvement in the community. While the Community Foundation remains flexible in attempting to meet community needs, the following items generally will not be funded: operational expenses of existing programs; endowments or deficit funding; funds for redistribution by the grantee; conferences, publication, films, television and radio programs unless integral to the project for which the grant is sought; religious or political purposes; travel for individuals or groups such as bands, sports teams and classes; annual appeals and membership contributions; major capital improvements.

Geographic Focus: Indiana

Samples: Pendleton Historical Museum - matching grant opportunity to be used toward the renovation/remodeling of the 3rd floor attic space, $5000 (2008); Alternatives - to purchase shoes and socks for South Madison residents temporarily residing in the Shelter, $500 (2008); Pendleton Police Department - to purchase First Responder equipment, $634.50 (2008).

Amount of Grant: $150 - $10,000 range

Date(s) Application is Due: Feb 1; Jun 1; Oct 1

Contact: Lisa Floyd, Exec. Director; (765) 778-8444; fax: (765) 778-9144; email: smcfed@verizon.net

Sponsor: South Madison Community Foundation, Inc.
233 South Main Street
Pendleton, IN 46064

Southbury Community Trust Fund 3350

The Fund awards grants in the areas of arts, community and economic development, education, the environment, and health and human services. High priority is given to program development, program implementation, organizational capacity building, and policy change addressing root causes of problems. Interested applicants should complete a letter of inquiry. Information for submission is available online.

Requirements: Organizations with IRS 501(c)3 status serving Southbury are eligible to submit letters of inquiry.

Restrictions: Funding is not available for: religious purposes; political campaigns; annual appeals; building fund/capital, endowment or memorial campaigns; loans or deficit financing; federal, state, or municipal agencies or departments supported by taxation; individuals.

Geographic Focus: Connecticut

Date(s) Application is Due: Jan 15

Contact: Anne Watkins , Director of Programs, (203) 334-7511; fax: (203) 333-4652; email: awatkins@gbafoundation.org

Internet: http://www.gbafoundation.org/grants/apply.asp

Sponsor: Greater Bridgeport Area Foundation
211 State Street, 3rd Floor
Bridgeport, CT 06604

Southwest Florida Community Foundation Competitive Grants 3351

Program/project grants are primarily for new or expanded programs and pilot or demonstration projects, which meet a documented need. Capital grants primarily support the construction, acquisition and renovation of facilities. The foundation offers competitive grants for programs and projects in eight focus areas: animal welfare, arts and culture, community development, conservation and preservation, education, the environment, health, and human services.

Requirements: IRS 501(c)3 tax-exempt organizations undertaking programs to improve the quality of life in Florida's Lee County and contiguous counties, including Charlotte, Collier, Gledes, and Hendry, are eligible. (NOTE: Agencies located in Collier County must also serve one of the other four counties in order to be eligible.) Applicants must employ staff, elect a governing board, and conduct business without discrimination on the basis of race, religion, gender, sexual orientation, age, national origin or disability.

Restrictions: The foundation generally will not fund: Normal operating expenses or existing obligations; Annual campaigns; Endowments; Sectarian purposes (i.e. programs that promote or require a religious doctrine except where designated by a donor); Debt retirement Monetary awards; Professional conferences, sports team travel, class trips, etc.; Individuals; Fraternal organizations, societies, etc.; Political organizations or campaigns; Fund-raising or feasibility studies; Research; or, Re-granting.

Geographic Focus: Florida

Samples: Calusa Nature Center & Planetarium - $26,000.; Fellowship of Christian Athletes - $20,000.; Harry Chapin Food Bank - $20,000.; Literacy Council of Bonita Springs - $15,000.; Take Stock in Children - $13,615.; Vineyards Elementary School - $23,000

Date(s) Application is Due: Jun 19

Contact: Carol McLaughlin, Chief Program Officer; (239) 274-5900 ext. 225; fax: (239) 274-5930; email: cmclaughlin@floridacommunity.com

Internet: http://www.floridacommunity.com/grantseekers/

Sponsor: Southwest Florida Community Foundation
8260 College Parkway, Suite 101
Fort Myers, FL 33919

Southwest Gas Corporation Foundation Grants 3352

The corporate foundation supports nonprofit organizations in its service communities. General support grants and employee matching gifts are made in the areas of education (universities, colleges, and literacy programs) and social services (United Way organizations, youth groups, community service, and volunteer organizations). Additional areas of interest are arts/culture and health. Types of support include general operating grants, projects grants, conferences and seminars, building construction/renovation, capital campaigns, emergency funds, employee matching gifts,research grants, donated equipment, and in-kind services. In southern Arizona, contact Marty Looney, P.O. Box 26500, Tucson, AZ 85726-6500; (520) 794-6416.

Requirements: Nonprofit organizations in Arizona; San Bernardino County, CA; and Nevada may apply.

Geographic Focus: Arizona; California; Nevada

Samples: Phoenix Art Museum (Phoenix, AZ)—for general support, $3000.; Boys and Girls Clubs (Tucson, AZ)—for general support, $1000.; Community Food Bank (Phoenix, AZ)—for general support, $3500.

Amount of Grant: $620,567 total

Contact: Suzanne Farinas; (702) 876-7247; fax: (702) 876-7037

Internet: http://www.swgas.com

Sponsor: Southwest Gas Corporation
P.O. Box 98510
Las Vegas, NV 89193-8510

Southwire Company Grants 3353

The company awards grants to nonprofits located in company-operating communities in Cleburne and Randolph Counties, AL; Mississippi County, AR; Mohave County, AZ; Carroll, Clarke and Oconee, GA; Daviess and Hancock Counties, KY; Oktibeeha County, MS; and Clay County, IL. Corporate community relations supports local community health and development, families in need, at-risk youth, disadvantaged youth, youth education, and religious development. The one-year grants vary in size.

Requests are reviewed monthly. Interested applicants should apply at least 45 days prior to the date funding is needed.
Restrictions: The company does not make contributions to individuals; political, labor, athletic, or social groups; advertising campaigns; or fundraising benefits.
Geographic Focus: Alabama; Arkansas; Georgia; Illinois; Kentucky; Mississippi; Texas; Utah
Contact: Community Relations, (800) 444-1700 or (770) 832-4242; fax: (770) 832-4929; email: gift@southwire.com
Internet: http://www.southwire.com
Sponsor: Southwire Company
1 Southwire Drive
Carrollton, GA 30119

Soy Health Research Program Incentive Awards **3354**
This program supports the development of complete research proposals on the topic of soy and bone health, soy and prostate health, and the dose-response relationship between isoflavone consumption and health and efficacy.
Amount of Grant: $10,000
Date(s) Application is Due: Mar 15
Contact: Steve Veile, Project Manager, (573) 635-3265 or (888) 772-8449; email: stevev@communiqueinc.com or soy@communiqueinc.com
Internet: http://www.talksoy.com/Shrp/default.htm
Sponsor: United SoyBean Board
P.O. Box 237, 512 E Capitol Avenue
Jefferson City, MO 65102

Special Olympics Health Professions Student Grants **3355**
The purpose of this program is to engage health professions students to work with persons with intellectual disabilities as a way of filling in a gap that exists in most health program curricula. The program promotes short-term projects exploring issues that impact the health and well-being of all persons with intellectual disabilities, including, but not limited to, Special Olympics athletes. Projects may include: data collection and analysis on issues impacting persons with intellectual disabilities; measurement of attitudes, opinions and behaviors of health professionals, coaches, family/caregivers and athletes; follow-up assessments of existing programs; or health promotion projects. Projects that involve collaborations with Special Olympics Programs or other CDC grant recipients (e.g., state and local health departments) are encouraged. Special Olympics is not currently prioritizing specific research areas for funding, as the program???s primary goal is to engage health professions students to work with the population of persons with intellectual disabilities. All awards will be made to the institution on behalf of the student grantee. Funding must include all expenses and no indirect costs may be covered by this grant. Applications are accepted year-round. Application and guidelines are available online.
Requirements: Health professions students at the bachelor, master, doctorate and postdoctorate levels from accredited institutions or programs in the United States or other countries are eligible. Fields or disciplines may include, audiology, dentistry, pre-med, medicine, nursing, optometry, physical therapy, podiatry, public health, social work, law, public administration, or other related health areas. All students??? projects will require a faculty advisor.
Amount of Grant: $5,000 maximum
Contact: Darcie Mersereau, Grants Administrator; (202) 628-3600 or (800) 700-8585; fax: (202) 824-0200; email: 2006hastudentgrant@specialolympics.org
Internet: http://info.specialolympics.org/Special%20Olympics%20Public%20Website/English/Initiatives/Research/Health%20Student%20Grants%20Available.htm
Sponsor: Special Olympics
1133 19th Street, NW
Washington, DC 20036-3604

Special People in Need Grants **3356**
The program awards grants to individuals and organizations operating in the fields of education, health, and assistance to people who are disabled, ill, or economically disadvantaged. There are no application deadlines or forms. Applicants should submit a cover letter, which will be reviewed by the grant committee.
Requirements: Nonprofit organizations are eligible.
Amount of Grant: $500 - $5,000
Contact: Gary Kline, (312) 715-5235
Sponsor: Special People in Need Foundation
Citicorp Center, 500 W. Madison Street, Suite 3700
Chicago, IL 60661

Special People in Need Scholarships **3357**
This scholarship is for undergraduate students with disabilities pursuing a postsecondary education. Applicants must demonstrate a strong financial need and a potential to benefit from an education, which might not otherwise be possible. The institution the student is attending must be willing to serve as a sponsor for disbursement.
Requirements: There are no formal deadlines. To be considered send an application with transcripts, letter of acceptance, and agreement from the institution to act as sponsor, letter of recommendation from an educator, financial statements, biographical data, and other relevant information.
Contact: Gary Kline, (312) 715-5235
Sponsor: Special People in Need Foundation
Citicorp Center, 500 W. Madison Street, Suite 3700
Chicago, IL 60661

Spencer County Community Foundation Grants **3358**
The Spencer County Community Foundation is a nonprofit, public charity created by and for the people of Spencer County, Indiana. The Foundation helps nonprofits fulfill their missions by strengthening their ability to meet community needs through grants that assist charitable programs, address community issues, support community agencies, launch community initiatives, and support leadership development. Grant proposals are accepted once each year according to the grant cycle. Grants are normally given as one time support of a project but may be considered for additional support for expansions or outgrowths of an initial project. Proposals will be accepted from January through the March 2 deadline. Grant awards will be presented in June.
Requirements: The Foundation welcomes proposals from nonprofit organizations that are deemed tax exempt under sections 501(c)3 and 509(a) of the Internal Revenue Code and from governmental agencies serving the county. Proposals from nonprofit organizations not classified as a 501(c)3 public charity may be considered provided the project is charitable and supports a community need. Proposals submitted by an entity under the auspices of another agency must include a written statement signed by the agency's board president on behalf of the board of directors agreeing to act as the entity's fiscal sponsor, to receive grant monies if awarded, and to oversee the proposed project.
Restrictions: Project areas not considered for funding: religious organizations for religious purposes; political parties or campaigns; endowment creation or debt reduction; operating costs; capital campaigns; annual appeals or membership contributions; travel requests for groups or individuals such as bands, sports teams, or classes. A six month progress report and a final report at project completion are required by organizations whose proposals are approved for funding. Instructions and appropriate forms will be provided at the time the grant is awarded.
Geographic Focus: Indiana
Samples: Evansville Philharmonic Orchestral Corporation - for Young People's Concerts and classroom materials that help the teachers make the most of the cultural experience with their students, $500 (2008); Friends of Lincoln State Park, Inc. - for a nature center Lincoln Mural, $1000 (2008); Carter Fire District - to install a Weather Alert System for the west side of Dale, $5,108 (2008);
Amount of Grant: $400 - $10,000 range
Date(s) Application is Due: Mar 2
Contact: Barbara Hinton, Director; (812) 649-5724; email: bhinton@spencercommunityfoundation.org
Internet: http://www.spencercommunityfoundation.org/disc-grants
Sponsor: Spencer County Community Foundation
321 Main Street, Suite A, P.O. Box 3
Rockport, IN 47635

Sprague Foundation Grants Program **3359**
Grants are made to hospitals, arts and cultural organizations, civic and community affairs, educational institutions, and health and human service organizations and charities located in New York and Massachusetts. Types of support include general operating support, matching and challenge funds, and program development. The initial approach should be a letter requesting the foundation's guidelines. Grants are awarded at the June and December board meetings.
Requirements: Only residents of New York and Massachusetts may apply.
Restrictions: No grants are provided to individuals, for building funds, or for loans.
Geographic Focus: Massachusetts; New York
Amount of Grant: $1000-$55,000 range
Date(s) Application is Due: Apr 15; Oct 1
Contact: Linda Franciscovich, U.S. Trust Company of New York, fax: (212) 852-3377
Sponsor: Seth Sprague Educational and Charitable Foundation
114 W 47th Street
New York, NY 10036-1532

Springs Close Foundation Grants **3360**
Since it was chartered in 1942, the Springs Close Foundation has contributed over $85 million to a wide variety of charitable and educational causes designed to improve the quality of life and well-being of the people in Chester, Lancaster and York Counties. Support includes, but is not limited to, food, shelter and medical assistance. This temporary change in focus is in response to high levels of unemployment and economic distress in the Foundation's service areas. The Foundation also makes occasional statewide grants in South Carolina. There are three major areas of program interest: Recreation and Environment, Public Education and Early Childhood Development, Community Service and Health
Requirements: Grants are made only to organizations that are tax-exempt under Section 501(c)3 of the Internal Revenue Code. No grants are made to individuals.
Restrictions: The Foundation will only consider grant requests from eligible nonprofit organizations that can effectively deliver emergency and basic support to citizens in Chester and Lancaster counties and a portion of York County.
Geographic Focus: South Carolina
Amount of Grant: $5,000-$50,000 average
Date(s) Application is Due: Mar 1; Oct 1
Contact: Angela McCrae, President; (803) 548-2002; fax: (803) 548-1797
Internet: http://www.thespringsclosefoundation.org/grants.htm
Sponsor: Springs Close Foundation
1826 Second Baxter Crossing
Fort Mill, SC 29708

Square D Foundation Grants 3361

The foundation makes donations for operating support, capital development needs, and special projects to nonprofit organizations in the areas of education, social welfare, arts and cultural and civic affairs, and health. Each year the foundation supports United Way in communities where the company and its domestic subsidiaries have significant operations. Donations are not normally made to organizations already receiving support through United Way. Support of higher education is achieved through scholarships, endowments for faculty and acquisition or expansion of equipment or facilities, unrestricted operating support, and the matching gift program. Submit letters of application between June and August.

Requirements: Giving primarily to 501(c)3 tax-exempt organizations in areas of company operations, with emphasis on: Illinois; Indiana; Iowa; Kentucky; Missouri; Nebraska; North Carolina; Ohio; South Carolina; Tennessee; and Wisconsin.

Restrictions: Grants are not made to religious organizations for religious purposes, political groups and organizations, labor unions and organizations, organizations making requests by telephone, organizations listed by the U.S. attorney general as subversive, or to individuals.

Geographic Focus: Illinois; Indiana; Iowa; Kentucky; Nebraska; North Carolina; Tennessee; Texas; Wisconsin

Amount of Grant: $2.7 million total

Date(s) Application is Due: Aug 31

Contact: Harry Wilson, Secretary, (847) 397-2600

Internet: http://www.squared.com

Sponsor: Square D Foundation
1415 South Roselle Road
Palatine, IL 60067

SRC Medical Research Grants 3362

The Scientific Council for Medicine supports research throughout the discipline of Medical Science, i.e. Medicine, Odontology, Pharmaceutics and Health Sciences. Medical research supported by the Scientific Council ranges from studies at molecular and cell level, and research involving laboratory animal science and patients, to epidemiological studies on groups of human subjects. The Program offers grants for research and junior research positions; grants for research periods for clinical researchers; grants for research stays (sabbaticals) abroad; project research grants (distributed, as a rule, for three years for salary, materials, travel, publication, etc); international postdoctoral fellowships and grants for postdoctoral positions in Sweden; networks; symposium; research equipment; collaboration grant and grant for inviting a visiting scientist.

Contact: Paola Norlin, Research Administrator; +46 (0)8 546 44 311; fax: +46-8-546-44-180; email: paola.norlin@vr.se

Internet: http://www.vr.se/responsibilities/researchfunding/medicine.4.69f66a93108e85f68d48000837.html

Sponsor: Swedish Research Council
Klarabersgviadukten 82
Stockholm, Sweden SE-103 78 Sweden

SSHRC Image, Text, Sound and Technology (ITST) Grants 3363

The program will provide funding for researchers and their graduate students to develop expertise in applying advanced technology through summer institutes, workshops and conferences. The ITST program will help researchers refine their ability to apply digital multimedia technologies to their research on image, text and sound. The overall objectives of the ITST program are to: reflect on, interpret, and analyze new digital media, multimedia, and text-based computing technologies and integrate these into humanities and social sciences research; bring together theorists, experimentalists, and technologists from different disciplines, to share and nurture ideas and methods that challenge research to advance through the use of audio-visual and text-based technologies; and facilitate the creation of national and international networks of, and partnerships among, researchers, industries, governments, and individuals that will promote and sustain social sciences and humanities research and resources worldwide. Up to $50,000 is available for twelve months.

Requirements: Canadian postsecondary institutions are eligible to apply. The summer institute, workshop or conference must be held at the applying institution. Detailed instructions accompany the application form.

Amount of Grant: $50,000 maximum

Date(s) Application is Due: Sep 15

Contact: Garry Pinard, Program Officer; (613) 992-5129; fax: (613) 947-0223; email: garry.pinard@sshrc.ca

Internet: http://www.sshrc.ca/web/apply/program_descriptions/itst/workshops_e.asp

Sponsor: Social Sciences and Humanities Research Council of Canada
350 Albert Street, P.O. Box 1610
Ottawa, ON K1P 6G4 Canada

SSHRC Research/Creation Grants in Fine Arts 3364

The broad purpose of the pilot program is to support and develop excellence in research in artistic disciplines. The program invites artist-researchers affiliated with Canadian postsecondary institutions, within a broad range of disciplines, to apply for research grants of up to three years' duration to support research/creation. Grants are available for programs of research/creation of up to three years. The value of these grants is up to a maximum of $100,000 per year, but totalling not more than $250,000 in a three-year period. SSHRC welcomes both small- and large-scale projects.

Requirements: Only those who fulfill the definition of artist-researcher are eligible to apply to this program. Humanities and social science scholars affiliated with Canadian postsecondary institutions who engage in research/creation are also eligible to apply.

Amount of Grant: $100,000 annually; $250,000 over 3 years

Date(s) Application is Due: Oct 20

Contact: Mathieu Ravignat, Senior Program Officer; (613) 947-3724; fax: (613) 947-0223; email: mathieu.ravignat@sshrc.ca

Internet: http://www.sshrc.ca/web/apply/program_descriptions/fine_arts_e.asp

Sponsor: Social Sciences and Humanities Research Council of Canada
350 Albert Street, P.O. Box 1610
Ottawa, ON K1P 6G4 Canada

SSRC HIV/AIDS and Public Health Policy Research in Africa Fellowships 3365

The program is open to African researchers, policy analysts, program planners and practitioners to support research on health and social policy in Eastern and Southern Africa relating to: political economy of care-giving and HIV/AIDS with particular emphasis on gender analysis; or sexual violence and HIV/AIDS. Two senior fellowships of up to $25,000 and six associate fellowships of up to $10,000 will be awarded. Primary goals are to: increase knowledge and understanding about the implications of HIV/AIDS in Eastern and Southern Africa as it relates to care-giving and sexual violence; improve public health policy responses to the pandemic and increase understanding about the interaction between local and global health systems; and foster collaboration among African institutions, researchers, policy analysts, program planners and practitioners both within and outside of the continent.

Requirements: Fellowships will be awarded to African researchers (master's degree and above) and mid-career policy analysts, program planners and practitioners with at least eight years of field experience. Preference will be given to applicants based in Eastern and Southern Africa. Applications will be reviewed on the basis of their academic quality and rigor; policy relevance; feasibility; potential contribution to the field; and the applicant's professional and research background and achievements.

Amount of Grant: $10,000 for associate fellowships; $25,000 for senior fellowships

Date(s) Application is Due: Jul 15

Contact: Alex de Waal, Program Director; (212) 377-2700, ext. 619; fax: (212) 377-2727; email: dewaal@ssrc.org

Internet: http://www.ssrc.org/programs/hiv-aids-program/

Sponsor: Social Science Research Council
One Pierrepont Plaza, 15th Floor
Brooklyn, NY 11201

SSSS Student Research Grants 3366

The society awards three grants annually for graduate research in areas of human sexuality. The purpose of the research is to advance the knowledge about sexuality. An applicant must send one copy each of a completed application fact sheet (available on the Web site) and a letter from the department chairperson stating student status within the institution and the educational purpose of the research. Also, an applicant must send seven copies each of a 10-page description of the proposed research, a proposed budget for the project, and a 150-word abstract.

Requirements: Students enrolled in a graduate degree-granting program working toward their master's degree or doctorate are eligible to apply, although the research need not be for the thesis.

Amount of Grant: $1000

Date(s) Application is Due: Feb 1; Sep 1

Contact: Program Contact, (610) 530-2483; fax: (610) 530-2485; email: thesociety@inetmail.att.net

Internet: http://www.sexscience.org/awards/index.php?category_id=427

Sponsor: Society for the Scientific Study of Sexuality
P.O. Box 416
Allentown, PA 18105

St. Joseph Community Health Foundation Burn Care and Prevention Grants 3367

The St. Joseph Community Health Foundation, sponsored by the Poor Handmaids of Jesus Christ, exists to steward resources that strengthen, improve, and sustain long-term community health in Allen County, Indiana. The Foundation mission is to invest, and collaborate with other community agencies to improve the physical, mental, and spiritual health of the poor and under served. The Burn Care and Prevention Grants are restricted funds to promote burn prevention education and to help educate health care professionals and first responders to emergency situations to treat severe burns with best care practices available. Grants typically range in size from $500 to $5,000.

Requirements: Applicants should have a demonstrated history of serving poor and powerless populations residing in Allen County. Applicants should be not-for-profit entities classified as 501(c)3 by the Internal Revenue Service. Some government agencies involved in related service areas may be eligible for support. The Foundation will consider requests for program, program-related equipment, staff continuing education, technical assistance and small capital grants. *Restrictions:* Grant applications will not be accepted elimination of deficits, support of political activities, individuals, or projects all ready completed.

Geographic Focus: Indiana

Samples: Allen County Juvenile Firesetters Task Force, $5,000 - Funding for a seminar pertaining to the identification and treatment of juvenile fire setters (2007); Public Safety Foundation of Northeast Indiana, Inc., $50,000 - Partial funding of construction costs for a new classroom/office building in the Safety Village (2007).

Amount of Grant: $500 - $5,000 range

Date(s) Application is Due: Mar 1; Jun 1; Sep 1; Dec 1

Contact: Meg Distler, Executive Director; (260) 969-2001, ext. 201; fax: (260) 969-2004; email: mdistler@sjchf.org

Internet: http://www.stjosephhealthfdn.org/index.php?option=com_content&view=article&id=72&Itemid=71
Sponsor: St. Joseph Community Health Foundation
2826 South Calhoun Street
Fort Wayne, IN 46807

St. Joseph Community Health Foundation Improving Healthcare Access Grants 3368
The St. Joseph Community Health Foundation was established in 1998 when the Poor Handmaids of Jesus Christ sold the St. Joseph Medical Center and reorganized the St. Joseph Community Health Foundation with a significant share of the proceeds. Proceeds from the Foundation's endowment are redistributed as grants typically ranging from $5,000 to $35,000 to advance programs, projects and partnerships that improve the access to quality health care and the health of the poor and powerless of Allen County, Indiana. Typically, only programs that can demonstrate that greater than 51 percent of their clients are very low income with health issues are considered for these grants. The Foundation also considers these values of the Poor Handmaids as a part of its grant review process: respecting and valuing each person; standing with the poor and powerless; using our talents and resources to respond to the emerging needs of society; nurturing leadership in our efforts to bring peace to the world. The Foundation will consider requests for program support, operations, seed monies, program-related equipment, staff continuing education, technical assistance, and matching funds. The Foundation will commit support on an annual basis only. Additional funding will be contingent upon program performance.
Requirements: Applicants should have a demonstrated history of serving poor and powerless populations with medical, dental, mental, and/or spiritual health care and wellness services. Applicants should be not-for-profit entities classified as 501(C)(3) by the Internal Revenue Service. Partnerships between not-for-profits are encouraged. The proposed grant must be operated for the benefit of residents of Allen County, Indiana.
Restrictions: Grant applications will not be accepted for building projects, elimination of deficits, support of political activities, individuals, or projects already completed.
Geographic Focus: Indiana
Amount of Grant: $5,000 - $35,000
Date(s) Application is Due: Mar 1; Sep 1
Contact: Meg Distler, Executive Director; (260) 969-2001, ext. 201; fax: (260) 969-2004; email: mdistler@sjchf.org
Internet: http://www.stjosephhealthfdn.org/index.php?option=com_content&view=article&id=79&Itemid=70
Sponsor: St. Joseph Community Health Foundation
2826 South Calhoun Street
Fort Wayne, IN 46807

St. Joseph Community Health Foundation Pfeiffer Fund Grants 3369
The St. Joseph Community Health Foundation, sponsored by the Poor Handmaids of Jesus Christ, exists to steward resources that strengthen, improve, and sustain long-term community health in Allen County, Indiana. The Foundation mission is to invest, and collaborate with other community agencies to improve the physical, mental, and spiritual health of the poor and under served. The Pfeiffer grants are restricted to health serving organizations for capital improvements or acquiring medical & surgical equipment. These funds have primarily been directed to help local clinics acquire medical equipment. All grants will be made to non-profit agencies, not individuals.
Requirements: Applicants should have a demonstrated history of serving poor and powerless populations residing in Allen County, Indiana. Applicants should be not-for-profit entities classified as 501(c)3 by the Internal Revenue Service. Some government agencies involved in related service areas may be eligible for support. Applications are available on the Foundation's website.
Restrictions: Grant applications will not be accepted for elimination of deficits, support of political activities, individuals, or projects all ready completed.
Geographic Focus: Indiana
Amount of Grant: $500 - $25,000
Date(s) Application is Due: Mar 1; Sep 1
Contact: Meg Distler, Executive Director; (260) 969-2001, ext. 201; fax: (260) 969-2004; email: mdistler@sjchf.org
Internet: http://www.stjosephhealthfdn.org/index.php?option=com_content&view=article&id=106&Itemid=129
Sponsor: St. Joseph Community Health Foundation
2826 South Calhoun Street
Fort Wayne, IN 46807

St. Joseph Community Health Foundation Schneider Fellowships 3370
The late Dr. Louis and Mrs. Anne Schneider understood and valued the importance of well-trained health and wellness care providers in the community. As a result, they established these fellowships to assist local not-for-profit agencies build the capacity of their agencies and staffs to provide quality care to the people of Allen County, Indiana. A preference will be to provide Fellowships that broaden the base of community health knowledge with new skills, services, health and wellness care abilities of health professionals in the community. Agencies may apply to use the Fellowships to either send staff or volunteers to continuing education opportunities, or to bring an expert to the community to provide specialized health and wellness care training for a group of staff, volunteers, and/or community members. The Foundation will commit support on an annual basis only.
Requirements: Applicants should have a demonstrated history of primarily serving poor and powerless populations residing in Allen County. Applicants should be not-for-profit entities classified as 501(c)3 by the Internal Revenue Service. The Foundation will consider requests for program, program-related equipment, staff continuing education, and technical assistance. Grant applications are available at the Foundation's website.
Restrictions: The Foundation will not fund anything destructive of human life. Grant applications will not be accepted for building projects, elimination of deficits, support of political activities, individuals, or projects all ready completed.
Geographic Focus: Indiana
Samples: Children's Autism Center, Inc., $2,000 - Funding to present continuing education workshops to staff, volunteers, and parents (2007); IPFW – Personal & Professional Department, $2,000 - Funding for a keynote speaker to speak at a day-long transcultural healthcare conference in Allen County (2008);
Amount of Grant: $2,000
Date(s) Application is Due: Mar 1; Jun 1; Sep 1; Dec 1
Contact: Meg Distler, Executive Director; (260) 969-2001, ext. 201; fax: (260) 969-2004; email: mdistler@sjchf.org
Internet: http://www.stjosephhealthfdn.org/index.php?option=com_content&view=article&id=105&Itemid=123
Sponsor: St. Joseph Community Health Foundation
2826 South Calhoun Street
Fort Wayne, IN 46807

Stackner Family Foundation Grants 3371
The foundation awards grants concentrated in the Milwaukee metropolitan area for building programs and equipment acquisition, medical research, programs at all levels of education, social welfare, child welfare, and programs that assist the physically disabled. Additional categories of support include general operating support, continuing support, annual campaigns, capital campaigns, and program development. The board meets each year in January, April, July, and October. Application forms are not required.
Requirements: Nonprofit organizations in the greater Milwaukee, WI, area may request grant support.
Geographic Focus: Wisconsin
Samples: Horizon House (Milwaukee, WI)—for an outpatient program, $4000.;Penfield Childrens Ctr (Milwaukee, WI)—for the capital campaign, $10,000.
Amount of Grant: $25-$25,000 range
Date(s) Application is Due: Mar 15; Jun 15; Sep 15; Dec 15
Contact: Paul Tillman, fax: (414) 646-5409; email: Stackner@MSH.com
Sponsor: Stackner Family Foundation
411 E Wisconsin Avenue
Milwaukee, WI 53202-4497

Staglin Family Music Festival NARSAD Schizophrenia Research Award 3372
The award supports an investigator with the MD, PhD, or doctoral degree and postdoctoral training applicable to schizophrenia. The candidate should be at the assistant or associate professor level, and be age 45 or younger. Applications should be sent electronically (as one document) via email. Guidelines are available online.
Requirements: The candidate should be nominated by the dean, department chair, or head of his/her scientific program of the university in which he or she is employed.
Amount of Grant: $250,000
Date(s) Application is Due: Dec 2
Contact: email: grants@narsad.org
Internet: http://www.narsad.org/research/apply
Sponsor: National Alliance for Research on Schizophrenia
60 Cutter Mill Road, Suite 404
Great Neck, NY 11021

Stan and Sandy Checketts Foundation 3373
The foundation's primary focus is on human services and helping individuals defray medical expenses. Applicants should submit a detailed description of the project, along with the amount of funding requested. There are no deadlines, and the primary geographic focus is Utah.
Geographic Focus: Utah
Contact: Stan Checketts, President; (435) 752-1987; Fax (435) 752-1948
Sponsor: S&S Power
350 West 2500 North
Logan, UT 84341

Staney Foundation Treatment Trials for Schizophrenia and Bipolar Disorder 3374
The foundation is interested in supporting studies of compounds not supported by the pharmaceutical industry in the treatment of schizophrenia and bipolar disorder, including novel agents and studies of off-label use of drugs approved for other conditions. Grants are awarded for a maximum of three years, depending on design. Applicant may apply online.
Amount of Grant: $300,000 maximum per year for a period of up to three years
Date(s) Application is Due: Mar 1; Oct 1
Contact: Xiomara Herrera, Grants Administrator, (301) 571-0760 ext 124; fax: (301) 571-0769; email: herrerax@stanleyresearch.org
Internet: http://www.stanleyresearch.org/application
Sponsor: Stanley Foundation
5430 Grosvenor Ln, Suite 200
Bethesda, MD 20814

Stanley Foundation Schizophrenia and Bipolar Disorder Research Grants 3375
The program supports researchers at all levels of development who are already in the field of schizophrenia and bipolar disorder, as well as researchers in other fields of medicine

and biology (e.g., neurology, immunology, biochemistry, and epidemiology) who wish to initiate new research projects in schizophrenia and bipolar disorder. Up to two years of research will be supported.
Amount of Grant: $75,000 per year
Date(s) Application is Due: Mar 1
Contact: Rhoda Marte, (301) 571-0760 ext 118; fax: (301) 571-0769; email: marter@stanleyresearch.org
Internet: http://www.stanleyresearch.org/application
Sponsor: Stanley Foundation
5430 Grosvenor Ln, Suite 200
Bethesda, MD 20814

Stark Community Foundation Women's Fund Grants 3376

The Women's Fund is a permanent endowment to benefit future generations and increase vital funding for programs which advance the economic, educational, physical, emotional, social, artistic, and personal growth of women and to educate and inspire women to become leaders in philanthropy. The interest area of this fund includes nonprofit agencies and their programs or projects that meet the needs of women and children in the Stark County area.
Requirements: The Women's Fund would like to fund grassroots nonprofit organizations, churches, and educational components that have unique projects serving women and/or women and children, and their basic needs for daily living.
Geographic Focus: Ohio
Amount of Grant: $500 - $3,000
Date(s) Application is Due: Mar 5
Contact: Cindy Lazor, Vice President for Program; (330) 454-3426
; fax: (330) 454-5855;
email: cmlazor@starkcf.org
Internet: http://www.starkcf.org/the_womens_fund.asp
Sponsor: Stark Community Foundation
400 Market Avenue North, Suite 200
Canton, OH 44702

Starr Foundation Grants 3377

The foundation awards grants to nonprofit organizations in the areas of education, medicine and health care, human needs, public policy, and culture. Education grants support scholarships for deserving students, groups that offer need-based financial aid, and international-exchange programs. Human needs grants support food programs for the poor, job training, literacy, adequate housing, and programs for the disabled. Medicine and health care grants include capital grants to hospitals, significant research grants, and grants to assist in the provision of health care to underserved communities. Public policy grants support international relations and democratic institutions around the world. Culture grants go to exchange programs and provide services to the elderly and/or disabled. The foundation rarely funds local charities outside of New York City but may fund national organizations that serve communities outside of New York. Types of support include multiyear grants, general operating grants, and capacity-building grants. There are no application deadlines. The board meets throughout the year.
Amount of Grant: $70 million total
Contact: Florence Davis, President, (212) 770-6882; email: florence.davis@starrfdn.org or grants@starrfoundation.org
Internet: http://fdncenter.org/grantmaker/starr
Sponsor: Starr Foundation
70 Pine Street, 14th Floor
New York, NY 10270

Staunton Farm Foundation Grants 3378

The foundation awards grants in the field of mental health in southwestern Pennsylvania. Projects that represent new and different approaches for organizations and ultimately affect patient care are encouraged. Support may be for more than one year, but the project must become self-sustaining following the grant period. Applicants should submit a letter of intent; full proposals are by invitation.
Requirements: Nonprofit organizations in the 10-county area in southwestern Pennsylvania including Washington, Greene, Fayette, Westmoreland, Armstrong, Butler, Lawrence, Beaver, Indiana, and Allegheny are eligible.
Geographic Focus: Pennsylvania
Samples: Squirrel Hill Health Center, Pittsburgh, PA, $172,000 - for Comprehensive Mental Health Care and Collaborative Wellness Program (2006); Hill House Association, Pittsburgh, PA, $77,500 - for Ex-Offenders and Non-Custodial Parents Employment Program (2006); Allegheny County Department of Human Services, Pittsburgh, PA, $69,000 - for Community Reintegration Project (2006);
Date(s) Application is Due: Jun 1; Dec 1
Contact: Joni Schwager, Executive Director; (412) 281-8020; fax: (412) 232-3115; email: jschwager@stauntonfarm.org
Internet: http://www.stauntonfarm.org
Sponsor: Staunton Farm Foundation
650 Smithfield Street, Centre City Tower, Suite 210
Pittsburgh, PA 15222

Steelcase Foundation Grants 3379

The foundation make grants to nonprofit organizations, projects, and programs in corporate communities. Grants are awarded in the areas of human service, health, education, community development, the arts, and the environment. Preference is given to programs designed to improve the quality life for disadvantaged, disabled, young, and elderly people. Matching gifts are made to educational, arts, and environment programs supported by Steelcase employees, retirees, and directors. To obtain a grant application, send a letter on letterhead, signed by the organization's chief executive officer. Include the following items in the letter: description of the organization or project; expected results of the project; amount of grant funds requested; and a copy of 501(c)3 nonprofit certification. Guidelines are available online.
Requirements: The foundation makes grants to IRS-certified nonprofit organizations in areas where Steelcase manufacturing plants are located (Grand Rapids, MI; Fletcher, NC; City of Industry, CA; Athens, AL; Toronto, Canada; and Tijuana, Mexico.)
Restrictions: The foundation does not provide grants to individuals or to organizations that discriminate on the basis of race, religion, sex, disability, or national origin; have received a Steelcase foundation grant within the past 12 months; request support for a conference or seminar; or request support for religious programs (nonsectarian programs for humanitarian purposes are eligible for consideration.)
Geographic Focus: Alabama; California; MichiganCanada; Mexico
Samples: Aquinas College (Grand Rapids, MI)—for its Sustainable Business Program, $1 million (2005).
Amount of Grant: $2000-$673,000 average
Contact: Executive Director, (616) 475-2009; fax (616) 475-2200; email: sbroman@steelcase.com
Internet: http://www.steelcase.com/na/ourcompany.aspx?f=10042&c=10022
Sponsor: Steelcase Foundation
P.O. Box 1967, CH4E
Grand Rapids, MI 49501

Steele-Reese Foundation Grants 3380

The foundation's available income is divided equally for grants to operating charities in southern Appalachia (particularly Kentucky) and in the Northwest (particularly Idaho). In both areas the funds are devoted to education, health, welfare, and the humanities. Types of support include general operating support, equipment, endowment funds, matching funds, professorships, scholarship funds, and capital campaigns. The foundation gives preference to projects that have, among others, the following characteristics: rural, modest in ambition, narrow in function, unglamorous, based on experience, enjoying community financial support, and essential rather than merely desirable. While the foundation considers southern Kentucky and Idaho to be its territories of primary concern, it makes grants to organizations operating throughout southern Appalachia and in Oregon, Montana, and Wyoming.
Requirements: Applicant should submit a letter requesting guidelines. Only residents of Georgia, Idaho, Kentucky, Montana, North Carolina, Texas, and Wyoming are eligible to apply. Personal and telephone inquiries are not encouraged.
Restrictions: The foundation does not make grants to individuals, to community chest or similar drives, for conferences or workshops, for efforts to influence elections or legislation, for planning purposes or experimental projects, for emergencies, or for permanent support except for occasional endowment grants to organizations where stability is critically important.
Geographic Focus: Georgia; Idaho; Kentucky; Montana; North Carolina; Texas; Wyoming
Samples: Frontier Nursing Service, Wendover, KY, $40,000 - to purchase a new phone system for the Mary Breckenridge Hospital (2005); Mountain Home Montana, Missoula, MT, $28,000 - salary support for the director of a teen-mother residency program (2005); West Central Highlands Resource Conservation and Development Council, Emmett, ID, $10,000 - for upgrades and renovations of the Indian Valley Community Hall (2005).
Amount of Grant: $10,000-$50,000 average
Date(s) Application is Due: Mar 1;
Contact: Charles U. Buice; (212) 505-2696; email: charlesbuice@hotmail.com
Internet: http://www.steele-reese.org/what.html
Sponsor: Steele-Reese Foundation
32 Washington Square West
New York, NY 10011

Stephen Bechtel Fund Preventive Healthcare and Selected Research Grants 3381

The Foundation and the Fund believe that preventive health care and research programs can help individuals of all ages increase life expectancy and improve their quality of life. To meet these objectives, the Foundation and the Fund seek to: support selected health care programs that focus on prevention and/or seek to improve the quality and delivery of medical care, particularly for the underserved Bay Area populations; support capital needs of hospitals within the Foundation's and Fund's grantee portfolio; and support selected research related to Alzheimer's Disease or other Board-determined specific research initiatives. The Foundation provides: capital support; operational support; and project support. The Foundation/Fund do not accept unsolicited proposals and do not currently publish annual reports. However, brief letters of intent (not to exceed two pages) that focus on a primary or secondary program area of the Foundation or the Fund and are within their geographic focus areas may be reviewed, with the possibility of being invited to submit a full proposal. Proposals received after October 1st will be reviewed in the next calendar year.
Requirements: The primary geographic focus of the Foundation and the Fund is the San Francisco Bay area.
Restrictions: The Foundation/Fund do not provide endowment funding, international grants, or grants for individuals.
Geographic Focus: California
Amount of Grant: $5,000-$25,000 typically
Date(s) Application is Due: Oct 1

Contact: Program Coordinator; (415) 284-8675; fax: (415) 284-8571; email: sdbjr@sdbjrfoundation.org
Internet: http://www.sdbjrfoundation.org/secondary_program_areas.htm
Sponsor: S. D. Bechtel, Jr. Foundation / Stephen Bechtel Fund
P.O. Box 193809
San Francisco, CA 94119-3809

Stephen S. Chang Award **3382**
This award is given annually to recognize a scientist, technologist, or engineer who has made distinguished accomplishments in basic research, and the knowledge the person thus produced must have been utilized by industries for the improvement or development of products related to lipids. A prospective recipient must agree to be present for acceptance of the award and to deliver an award address at an AOCS annual meeting.
Requirements: Eligibility for nomination shall be demonstrated through high-quality scientific papers, patents, or the marketing of commercial products developed through the nominee's scientific or technological efforts. The award shall be made without regard for national origin, place of residence, race, color, creed, or gender.
Amount of Grant: $6000 approximately
Date(s) Application is Due: Oct 15
Contact: Program Contact, (217) 359-2344; fax: (217) 351-8091; email: membership@aocs.org
Internet: http://www.aocs.org/member/awards/awd-chang.asp
Sponsor: American Oil Chemists' Society
P.O. Box 3489
Champaign, IL 61826-3489

Steuben County Community Foundation Grants **3383**
The Steuben County Community Foundation works to preserve and enhance the lifestyle and assets of Steuben County, Indiana, for current and future generations by providing ongoing assessment and financial support of identified needs through philanthropic giving and endowment building.
Requirements: Prospective applicants are strongly encouraged to discuss their grant requests with Community Foundation staff before beginning the application process. Applications can be obtained on the Foundation's website. The Steuben County Community Foundation encourages projects that: address priority community concerns; encourage more effective use of community resources; test or demonstrate new approaches and techniques in the solution of community problems; are intended to strengthens the management capabilities of agencies, and; promote volunteer participation and citizen involvement in community affairs.
Restrictions: If approved, each grant recipient must sign an agreement that includes the following obligations: public acknowledgment of the Foundation's support; expenditure of the monies as specified in the proposal; return of any unused portion of the grant; completion of an evaluation report; any special conditions as mutually agreed (failure to do so can adversely affect any subsequent requests).
Geographic Focus: Indiana
Date(s) Application is Due: Jan 31; Mar 31; May 31; Jul 31; Sep 30; Nov 30
Contact: Bill Stockberger Grant Administrator; (260) 665-6656; fax: (260) 665-8420
Internet: http://www.steubenfoundation.org/grants/index.html
Sponsor: Steuben County Community Foundation
1701 N. Wayne Street
Angola, IN 46703

Stewart Huston Charitable Trust Grants **3384**
The purpose of the Trust is to provide funds, technical assistance and collaboration on behalf of non-profit organizations engaged exclusively in religious, charitable or educational work; to extend opportunities to deserving needy persons. Giving primarily in the Savannah, GA, area and Coatesville, PA.
Requirements: 501(c)3 nonprofit organizations are eligible.
Restrictions: Grants are not awarded for scholarship support to individuals, endowment purposes, purchases of tickets or advertising for benefit purposes, coverage of continuing operating deficits, or document publication costs. Support is not provided to intermediate or pass-through organizations (other than United Way) that in turn allocate funds to beneficiaries or to fraternal organizations, political parties or candidates, veterans, labor or local civic groups, volunteer fire companies, or groups engaged in influencing legislation.
Geographic Focus: Georgia; Pennsylvania
Amount of Grant: $1000-$15,000 average
Date(s) Application is Due: Jan 15; Mar 1; Sep 1
Contact: Scott Huston, Program Director, (610) 384-2666; fax: (610) 384-3396; email: admin@stewarthuston.org
Internet: http://www.stewarthuston.org
Sponsor: Stewart Huston Charitable Trust
50 South First Avenue
Coatesville, PA 19320

Stroke Association Allied Health Professional Research Bursaries **3385**
The Research Bursary Awards are primarily intended for the purpose of training nurses and therapists, but consideration will be given to other health professionals. These bursaries will be awarded to United Kingdom departments that can demonstrate a track record and current participation in stroke research. The host department will be required to provide appropriate supervision and a research training program suitable for equipping the candidate for a career in stroke research, and to enable them to obtain a post graduate qualification. Bursaries may be taken up on a part-time, pro-rata basis.
Requirements: Research must take place in the United Kingdom.
Samples: Trudi Pelton, University of Birmingham (2008); Holly Robson, University of Manchester (2008); Linda Hammett, St. George's, University of London (2007); Andrea Atzori, University of Southampton (2007); Emma Jones, University of Sheffield (2007).
Amount of Grant: 30,000 Britsh pounds per annum for up to two years (up to a maximum of 60,000 British pounds)
Contact: Research Department, (020) 7566-0345; fax: (020) 7490-2686; textphone: (020) 7251-9096; email: research@stroke.org.uk
Internet: http://www.stroke.org.uk/research/research_we_fund/allied_health_professional_bursaries/index.html
Sponsor: Stroke Association
Stroke House, 240 City Road
London, England EC1V 2PR England

Stroke Association Clinical Fellowships **3386**
Fellowships are awarded to individuals for training in stroke medicine, and are intended to enable a specialist registrar to gain the appropriate clinical experience and accreditation required for a career in the prevention, treatment or rehabilitation of stroke.
Requirements: Applicants are required to nominate a supervisor and training program in a host institution that has been approved for stroke medicine training by the Stroke Medicine Sub-specialty Advisory Committee (SSAC). The funding is not to be taken as part of a one year taught course or for those who have completed the SpR training program and have certification.
Amount of Grant: 40,000 British pounds
Date(s) Application is Due: Jan 6
Contact: Research Department, (020) 7566-0345; fax: (020) 7490-2686; textphone: (020) 7251-9096; email: research@stroke.org.uk
Internet: http://www.stroke.org.uk/research/research_we_fund/fellowships/index.html
Sponsor: Stroke Association
Stroke House, 240 City Road
London, England EC1V 2PR England

Stroke Association Research Project Grants **3387**
Research project grants are awarded to doctors, professors, research fellows, therapists, psychologists and nurses at universities and hospitals across the United Kingdom. Project grants can last for up to three years. The Stroke Association's priorities for funding include research into the prevention, treatment, rehabilitation and long-term care of stroke patients. The majority of funded projects are patient orientated. The Stroke Association has recently undertaken a review of its activities and has developed a new Research and Development Strategy. As a result, applications for Research Project Grants have been revised and new application forms have been developed. All applications for funding by The Stroke Association will now undergo review by a panel of service users in addition to expert peer review. Therefore all applicants will now be required to complete a Project Grant Lay Summary Form, as well as the main Research Project Grant Application Form. Details of the new procedures and forms can be found on online.
Requirements: Research must take place in the United Kingdom.
Restrictions: Applications that are not submitted on the new forms will not be accepted for this application round.
Amount of Grant: 70,000 British pounds per annum for up to three years (up to a maximum of 210,000 British pounds)
Date(s) Application is Due: Feb 5
Contact: Research Department, (020) 7566-0345; fax: (020) 7490-2686; textphone: (020) 7251-9096; email: research@stroke.org.uk
Internet: http://www.stroke.org.uk/research/apply_for_funding/index.html
Sponsor: Stroke Association
Stroke House, 240 City Road
London, England EC1V 2PR England

Strowd Roses Grants **3388**
Strowd Roses, Inc. is a private charitable foundation which was established in 2001 under the will of Mrs. Irene Harrison Strowd of Chapel Hill, North Carolina. The Board of Directors of Strowd Roses, Inc. makes grants to qualified tax-exempt charitable, educational, religious and public organizations that are based in Chapel Hill or Carrboro, or are devoted primarily to benefiting the citizens of those communities. Grants may also be made to individuals engaged in projects designed to enhance the Chapel Hill/Carrboro community. Grants may, at the Board's discretion, include support for operating as well as capital expenditures, seed money and matching grants. Grants to individuals may be used for scholarships or fellowships; to produce a report or similar product; or to improve or enhance a literary, artistic, musical, scientific, teaching or similar capacity, skill or talent which will be used to benefit the life of the community. Particular consideration is given to those projects and purposes which further the interests of Mr. and Mrs. Strowd, including the welfare of children and youth, the enhancement of the environment, and the promotion of a sense of civic duty.
Requirements: Applicants should submit the appropriate application form (see foundations website), along with a proposed budget and evidence of their tax-exempt status (IRS determination letter or comparable documentation) to: Board of Directors, Strowd Roses, Inc., P.O. Box 3558, Chapel Hill, NC, 27515-3558.
Geographic Focus: North Carolina
Amount of Grant: $10,000

Date(s) Application is Due: Jan 31; Apr 30; Jul 31; Oct 31;
Contact: Jennifer Boger, Grant Coordinator; (919) 929-1984; fax: (919) 929-1990; email: jboger@strowdroses.org
Internet: http://www.strowdroses.org/grantApp.htm
Sponsor: Strowd Roses, Inc.
P.O. Box 3558
Chapel Hill, NC 27515-3558

STTI Doris Bloch Research Awards 3389
The purpose of the STTI Doris Bloch Research Awards is to encourage nurses to contribute to the advancement of nursing through research. Allocation of funds is based on the quality of the proposed research, the future promise of the applicant and the applicant's research budget. Applications from novice researchers who have received no other national research funds are encouraged and will receive preference for funding, other aspects being equal. Preference will be given to Sigma Theta Tau International members, other qualifications being equal. Funding is provided by a gift to the honor society's Research Endowment from the Doris Bloch estate.
Requirements: Eligibility Criteria: registered nurse with current license; hold a master's or doctoral degree or be enrolled in a doctoral program; submission of a completed research application package and signed research agreement via on-line submission system; ready to implement research project when funding is received.
Amount of Grant: $5,000 max.
Date(s) Application is Due: Dec 1
Contact: Research Services; (888) 634-7575 or (317) 634-8171; fax: (317) 634-8188; email: research@stti.iupui.edu
Internet: http://www.nursingsociety.org/Research/SmallGrants/Pages/grant_bloch.aspx
Sponsor: Sigma Theta Tau International
550 West North Street
Indianapolis, IN 46202

STTI Emergency Nurses Association Foundation Grant 3390
The ENA Foundation and Sigma Theta Tau International, Inc. (STTI) have combined resources to offer this annual research grant. The ENA Foundation/STTI research grant provides funding for research that will advance the specialized practice of emergency nursing. All relevant research topics will be considered. Priority will be given to research studies relating to the ENA/ENA Foundation research initiatives.
Requirements: Eligibility Criteria: principal investigator must be a registered nurse; team members may be from other disciplines; principal investigator must have a master's degree; submit a completed research application package and signed research agreement; be ready to start, or have already started, the research project. An electronic Research Grant Application is available on the ENA Foundation website. All applications MU.S.T be returned to ENA Foundation.
Restrictions: Application packets submitted to Sigma Theta Tau International will not be reviewed.
Samples: Sarah Lynn Anderson, MSN, PhD., University of Virginia - Changes in Genital Injuries in Women Based on Skin color after Consensual Intercourse (2008);
Amount of Grant: $6000
Date(s) Application is Due: Mar 1
Contact: Department of Research; (847) 460-4119; fax: (847) 460-4005; email: res@ena.org;; Suling Li, Director of Research; (847) 460-4110; email: sli@ena.org
Internet: http://www.nursingsociety.org/Research/SmallGrants/Pages/grant_ena.aspx
Sponsor: Emergency Nurses Association Foundation
915 Lee Street
Des Plaines, IL 60016 -6569

STTI Environment of Elder Care Nursing Research Grants 3391
The Environment of Elder Care Nursing Research Grant co-sponsored by Hill-Rom Company will advance the science of nursing through research focused on critical aspects of elder care including clear lungs, no falls, safe skin, patient comfort and ease-of-use. Applications from novice researchers who have received no other national research funds are encouraged. Preference will be given to Sigma Theta Tau International members, other qualifications being equal. Allocation of funds is based on the quality of the proposed research, the future promise of the applicant, and the applicant's research
Requirements: Eligibility Criteria: registered nurse with a current license; hold at minimum a Master's degree or its equivalent, and/or be enrolled in a Doctoral program; submission of completed research application packet and a signed research agreement via our on-line submission system; ready to implement research project when funding is received; submit to STTI a final report; submit completed abstract to STTI's Virginia Henderson International Nursing Research Library; and submit an abstract for publication to Hill-Rom regarding the research done as a product of the grant, and credit research grant partners in all publications and presentations of the research.
Amount of Grant: $9,000 max.
Date(s) Application is Due: Jul 1
Contact: Research Services; (888) 634-7575 or (317) 634-8171; fax: (317) 634-8188; email: research@stti.iupui.edu
Internet: http://www.nursingsociety.org/Research/SmallGrants/Pages/EnvironmentofCare.aspx
Sponsor: Sigma Theta Tau International
550 West North Street
Indianapolis, IN 46202

STTI Joan K. Stout RN Research Grants 3392
The purpose of the Sigma Theta Tau International/Joan K. Stout, RN, Research Grant is to advance ongoing evidence-based study by nurse researchers on the impact of the practice of simulation education in schools of nursing and clinical care settings. The allocation of funds is based upon a research project that is ready for implementation. The proposed research project should be designed to ensure the ongoing practice of nurse-led simulation in improving quality of care in clinical and/or academic settings with the potential for further funding and ongoing research. Funds provided by interest from a research endowment established at Sigma Theta Tau International Foundation for Nursing, with a donation by the Hugoton Foundation.
Requirements: Eligibility Criteria: registered nurse with current license; have a master's degree, and/or be enrolled in a Doctoral program; submit a completed research application via online submission system; ready to implement research project when funding is received; complete project within one (1) year of funding; submit to STTI a final report; submit completed abstract to STTI's Virginia Henderson International Nursing Research Library.
Amount of Grant: $5,000
Date(s) Application is Due: Jul 1
Contact: Research Services; (888) 634-7575 or (317) 634-8171; fax: (317) 634-8188; email: research@stti.iupui.edu
Internet: http://www.nursingsociety.org/Research/SmallGrants/Pages/JoanKStout.aspx
Sponsor: Sigma Theta Tau International
550 West North Street
Indianapolis, IN 46202

STTI National League for Nursing Grants 3393
Funds for this grant are made possible from a gift from Dr. Diane Billings to Sigma Theta Tau International Foundation for Nursing's research endowment. The purpose of this grant is to support research that advances the science of nursing education and learning through the use of technology in dissemination of knowledge.
Requirements: Eligibility Criteria: preference given to Sigma Theta Tau International and/or National League for Nursing members; grant proposals must advance the science of nursing education through the use of technology in the dissemination of knowledge; registered nurse with current license; hold a master's or doctoral degree or be enrolled in a doctoral program; submit a completed research application package and signed research agreement; ready to implement research project when funding is received. All applications must be submitted via the online submission system (see STTI website)
Amount of Grant: $5,000
Date(s) Application is Due: Jun 1
Contact: Research Services; (888) 634-7575 or (317) 634-8171; fax: (317) 634-8188; email: research@stti.iupui.edu
Internet: http://www.nursingsociety.org/Research/SmallGrants/Pages/grant_nln.aspx
Sponsor: Sigma Theta Tau International
550 West North Street
Indianapolis, IN 46202

STTI Rosemary Berkel Crisp Research Awards 3394
The purpose of the STTI Rosemary Berkel Crisp Research Awards is to support nursing research in the critical areas of women's health, oncology, and pediatrics. The allocation of funds is based upon a research project that is ready for implementation in the area of women's health, oncology, or pediatrics; the quality of the proposed research, future potential of the application, appropriateness of the research budget, and feasibility of time frame. Funds provided by interest from a gift from The Harry L. Crisp, II and Rosemary Berkel Crisp Foundation to the honor society's Research Endowment.
Requirements: Eligibility Criteria: registered nurse with current license; hold a master's or doctoral degree or be enrolled in a doctoral program; submit a completed research application package and signed research agreement via the online submission system; ready to implement research project when funding is received; member of Sigma Theta Tau International; Note: Some preference will be given to applicants residing in Illinois, Missouri, Arkansas, Kentucky, and Tennessee.
Amount of Grant: $5,000 max.
Date(s) Application is Due: Dec 1
Contact: Research Services; (888) 634-7575 or (317) 634-8171; fax: (317) 634-8188; email: research@stti.iupui.edu
Internet: http://www.nursingsociety.org/Research/SmallGrants/Pages/grant_crisp.aspx
Sponsor: Sigma Theta Tau International
550 West North Street
Indianapolis, IN 46202

STTI Small Grants 3395
The purpose of the Sigma Theta Tau International Small Grants is to encourage nurses to contribute to the advancement of nursing through research. Allocation of funds is based on the quality of the proposed research, the future promise of the applicant, and the applicant's research budget. Applications from novice researchers who have received no other national research funds are encouraged and will receive preference for funding, other aspects being equal. Preference will be given to Sigma Theta Tau members, other qualifications being equal.
Requirements: Eligibility Criteria: registered nurse with current license; have a master's or doctoral degree or be enrolled in a doctoral program; submit a completed research application package and signed research agreement via the online submission system; ready to implement research project when funding is received.
Amount of Grant: $5000 maximum

Date(s) Application is Due: Dec 1
Contact: Research Services; (888) 634-7575 or (317) 634-8171; fax: (317) 634-8188; email: research@stti.iupui.edu
Internet: http://www.nursingsociety.org/Research/SmallGrants/Pages/small_grants.aspx
Sponsor: Sigma Theta Tau International
550 West North Street
Indianapolis, IN 46202-2156

STTI Virginia Henderson Clinical Research Grants **3396**
The purpose of the Sigma Theta Tau International Virginia Henderson Clinical Research Grant is to encourage the research career development of clinically based nurses through support of clinically oriented research. Allocation of funds is based on a research project ready for implementation, the quality of the proposed research, the future potential of the applicant, appropriateness of the research budget and feasibility of the time frame. Funds for this biennial grant are provided by interest from the Virginia Henderson Clinical Research Endowment Fund.
Requirements: Eligibility Criteria: registered nurse actively involved in some aspect of health care delivery, education or research in a clinical setting; hold a master's or doctoral degree or be enrolled in a doctoral program; submit a completed research application package and signed research agreement via the online submission system; ready to implement research project when funding is received; member of Sigma Theta Tau International.
Amount of Grant: $5,000 max.
Date(s) Application is Due: Dec 1
Contact: Research Services; (888) 634-7575 or (317) 634-8171; fax: (317) 634-8188; email: research@stti.iupui.edu
Internet: http://www.nursingsociety.org/Research/SmallGrants/Pages/grant_VHL.aspx
Sponsor: Sigma Theta Tau International
550 West North Street
Indianapolis, IN 46202

STTI/ATI Educational Assessment Nursing Research Grants **3397**
The purpose of this grant, co-sponsored by Assessment Technologies Institute (ATI), with the Honor Society of Nursing, Sigma Theta Tau International will support research that encourages the appropriate use of a standardized assessment program in a nursing education curriculum, including, but not limited to: use of formative assessment to drive remediation; use of summative assessment to guide curricular evaluation and revision; timing of assessment administration within a program of study; identification of key markers of at-risk student status.
Requirements: Eligibility Criteria: registered nurse with current license; have a master's or doctoral degree or be enrolled in a doctoral program; submit a completed research application package and signed research agreement via the online submission system; ready to implement research project when funding is received; submit a final report; submit completed abstract to the Virginia Henderson Research Library and credit research grant partners in all publications and presentations of the research.
Amount of Grant: $4,500
Date(s) Application is Due: Jul 1
Contact: Research Services; (888) 634-7575 or (317) 634-8171; fax: (317) 634-8188; email: research@stti.iupui.edu
Internet: http://www.nursingsociety.org/Research/SmallGrants/Pages/STTIATI.aspx
Sponsor: Sigma Theta Tau International
550 West North Street
Indianapolis, IN 46202

STTI/Council for the Advancement of Nursing Science Grants **3398**
The purpose of the Sigma Theta Tau International/The Council for Advancement of Nursing Science research grant is to encourage qualified nurses to improve the health of the world's people through research. Proposals for clinical, educational or historical research, including plans for broadly disseminating the research findings, may be submitted for the grant.
Requirements: Eligibility Criteria: preference given to Sigma Theta Tau International member; hold at minimum a Master's degree or equivalent; submission of completed research application via on-line submission system; ready to implement research project when funding is received; submit a final report; submit completed abstract to Virginia Henderson International Nursing Research Library; submit completed project's abstract for presentation at Sigma Theta Tau or Council for Advancement of Nursing Science research meeting; and credit research grant partners in all publications and presentations of the research.
Amount of Grant: $5,000
Date(s) Application is Due: Jul 1
Contact: Research Services; (888) 634-7575 or (317) 634-8171; fax: (317) 634-8188; email: research@stti.iupui.edu
Internet: http://www.nursingsociety.org/Research/SmallGrants/Pages/CANS.aspx
Sponsor: Sigma Theta Tau International
550 West North Street
Indianapolis, IN 46202

Sulzberger Foundation Grants **3399**
The foundation awards grants to eligible nonprofit organizations in its areas of interest, including arts and culture, education, environmental protection and natural resource conservation, hospitals, and social services delivery. Types of support include annual campaigns, building construction/renovation, endowments, general operating support, multiyear grants, programs and projects, and scholarship funds. There are no application forms or deadlines. Preference is given to requests from New York City and Chatanooga.
Restrictions: Individuals are not eligible. Loans and matching grants are not awarded.
Samples: New York Times Company Foundation (New York, NY)—for the Neediest Cases Fund, $100,000 (2003).
Amount of Grant: $100-$255,000 average
Contact: Marian Heiskell, President, (212) 556-1400
Sponsor: Sulzberger Foundation
229 W 43rd Street, Suite 1031
New York, NY 10036

Sunderland Foundation Grants **3400**
The foundation makes grants annually to publicly supported charitable organizations in its areas of interest, including higher education; churches; youth serving agencies; health facilities; community buildings; museums; civic projects; and and low maintenance, energy efficient housing projects sponsored by qualified tax-exempt organizations. The Foundation generally awards grants to larger, well-established nonprofit organizations. The Sunderland Foundation primarily makes grants in the geographic areas that have connections to the Ash Grove Cement Company. Grants are awarded in Western Missouri, Kansas, Nebraska, Arkansas, and Western Iowa, and to a lesser extent, in Idaho, Oregon, Washington, Utah and Montana.
Requirements: All grant requests should be submitted in writing, and proposals should include the following: a clear description of the project for which funds are being requested, including program goals and objectives, documentation of need and expected outcomes; a brief background on the proposing organization or agency; a detailed expense budget for the project indicating how the funds would be spent and over what time period; an income statement showing other sources of project support, public and/or private, which have been or will be solicited, including a statement of funds that have been received or pledged to date; a financial plan showing how the project will be supported beyond the grant period; the organization's current board of directors and their terms of office; a copy of the organization's most recent 501 (c)(3) tax-exempt ruling from the IRS; the organization's most recent certified audit or audited financial statement, where applicable. Proposals should be submitted by mail to the address listed in the "Sponsoring Organization" catagory. Proposals will also be accepted by email. Send a PDF file to the following address: sunderlandfoundation@ashgrove.com.
Restrictions: The Foundation does not award grants: for annual operating expenses; for programs or endowments; provide sponsorship for special events; to primary and secondary schools are generally not considered; to individuals. No scholarships are available from the Foundation.
Geographic Focus: Arkansas; Idaho; Iowa; Kansas; Missouri; Montana; Nebraska; Oregon; Utah; Washington
Samples: Pleasant Valley Baptist Church, Liberty, MO, $50,000 (2006%2Proxy-Connection: keep-alive Cache-Control: max-age=0; Salvation Army of Greater Kansas City, Kansas City, MO, $50,000 (2006); MD Anderson Cancer Center, Houston, TX, $100,000 (2006); Donnelly College, Kansas City, KS, $25,000 (2006);
Contact: Kent Sunderland, President; (913) 451-8900; email: sunderlandfoundation@ashgrove.com
Internet: http://www.sunderlandfoundation.org
Sponsor: Sunderland Foundation
P.O. Box 25900
Overland Park, KS 66225

Sunflower Foundation Bridge Grants **3401**
Bridge Grant funding is intended to provide core transitional financial support for new or expanded medical, mental, dental and/or public health services that provide primary care or primary prevention services to the uninsured and the underinsured. Funds are available for: salaries, benefits, allowable indirect expenses appropriate to the health care practitioners needed for the program; administrative services (e.g. financial & medical record clerks, clerical staff) resulting from the new or expanded services for which funding is being requested from the Foundation. Applicants must demonstrate a cost share in the project through a cash match of $1 to $1 of the total amount requested. Grants will not exceed $200,000 each and may be for projects up to three years in length.
Requirements: Proposals are invited from private nonprofit or public organizations that have a mission to improve health status or access to quality, affordable health care for Kansans.
Restrictions: The foundation will not fund ongoing general operating expenses or existing deficits; capital, endowment or specific fund-raising campaigns; fund raising events; routine continuing education; travel to conferences not directly related to the project; programs that are not Kansas-based; programs that require additional staff but demonstrate no clear means of sustainability after foundation funding; individual medical care or support; medical equipment; capital equipment (except for allowable technology); political purposes; or support of organizations that practice discrimination. Additional exclusions include: requests for new construction; and facility renovations. Any Safety Net clinic that qualifies for the Dental Hub initiative should contact the Sunflower Foundation program staff prior to application (there may be some restrictions for Dental Bridge Grant funding for organizations eligible for Dental Hub funding).
Geographic Focus: Kansas
Amount of Grant: $200,000 maximum
Date(s) Application is Due: Oct 23

Contact: Cheryl Bean, Grants Manager; (785) 232-3000, ext. 104; email: cbean@sunflowerfoundation.org
Internet: http://www.sunflowerfoundation.org/areas_of_interest-health_care_access.php
Sponsor: Sunflower Foundation: Health Care for Kansans
1200 SW Executive Drive, Suite 100
Topeka, KS 66615-3850

Sunflower Foundation Capacity Building Grants **3402**
The Foundation funds two types of Capacity Building grants: Assessment (grant limit is based on scope of work) —the first step of any effort to build capacity within an organization is an assessment of present capacity to identify what is working well and what needs to be strengthened (the Foundation will fund technical assistance, consulting, and other expenses related to conducting a formal assessment of current organizational capacity); and Implementation ($20,000 grant limit)—the Foundation will fund the implementation of capacity building strategies. Allowable expenses typically include such items as technical assistance/consulting, technology (hardware and/or software), limited equipment (e.g. telephone systems), training and assessment/evaluation.
Requirements: Proposals are invited from private nonprofit or public organizations that have a mission to improve health status or access to quality, affordable health care for Kansans.
Restrictions: The foundation will not fund ongoing general operating expenses or existing deficits; capital, endowment or specific fund-raising campaigns; fund raising events; routine continuing education; travel to conferences not directly related to the project; programs that are not Kansas-based; programs that require additional staff but demonstrate no clear means of sustainability after foundation funding; individual medical care or support; medical equipment; capital equipment (except for allowable technology); political purposes; or support of organizations that practice discrimination. Additional exclusions include: program expenses; existing staff salaries/benefits; Electronic Medical Records (EMR) technology; medical equipment; capital equipment (except for allowable technology); routine continuing education; and travel to conferences not directly related to the project.
Geographic Focus: Kansas
Amount of Grant: $20,000 maximum
Date(s) Application is Due: Jun 19
Contact: Grants Administrator, (785) 232-3000 or (866) 232-3020; email: info@sunflowerfoundation.org
Internet: http://www.sunflowerfoundation.org/flash/request.html
Sponsor: Sunflower Foundation: Health Care for Kansans
1200 SW Executive Drive, Suite 100
Topeka, KS 66615-3850

Sunflower Foundation Walking Trails Grants **3403**
The Foundation is seeking projects that bring together public and private support to construct Walking Trails as a means to increase physical activity among Kansans. Grant funds may be used for Walking Trails building materials only. Walking Trails are generally expected to be at least ???? mile in length. Grants awards will be for one year and will not exceed $15,000. Organizations that are seeking matching funding to secure state or federal grants for larger Trail projects should contact the Foundation before submitting a proposal.
Requirements: Proposals are invited from private nonprofit or public organizations that have a mission to improve health status or access to quality, affordable health care for Kansans. Public access to the Walking Trail is required. Applicants must demonstrate a cost share in the project through a cash match of $1 to $1 of the total amount requested from the Sunflower Foundation.
Restrictions: The foundation will not fund ongoing general operating expenses or existing deficits; capital, endowment or specific fund-raising campaigns; fund raising events; routine continuing education; travel to conferences not directly related to the project; programs that are not Kansas-based; programs that require additional staff but demonstrate no clear means of sustainability after foundation funding; individual medical care or support; medical equipment; capital equipment (except for allowable technology); political purposes; or support of organizations that practice discrimination. Additional exclusions include: requests for physical fitness equipment; and fitness facility dues/membership fees.
Geographic Focus: Kansas
Amount of Grant: $15,000 maximum
Date(s) Application is Due: Jun 29
Contact: Grants Administrator, (785) 232-3000 or (866) 232-3020; email: info@sunflowerfoundation.org
Internet: http://www.sunflowerfoundation.org/flash/request.html
Sponsor: Sunflower Foundation: Health Care for Kansans
1200 SW Executive Drive, Suite 100
Topeka, KS 66615-3850

Sunshine Natural Wellbeing Foundation Grants **3404**
The foundation awards grants to nonprofit organizations for existing or upstart programs relating to alternative treatments and research for asthma, immune disorders, and other similar illnesses, as well as children's educational programs relative to alternative health. Submit a proposal with specific goals, project budget, organization budget, audited financial reports, 501(c)3 letter, IRS 990 for previous year, list of current contributors, and list of board members.
Requirements: 501(c)3 nonprofit organizations are eligible. Giving is primarily made in Florida.
Restrictions: Individuals are not eligible.
Geographic Focus: Florida
Date(s) Application is Due: Sep 1
Contact: Delores Wooldridge, (941) 346-5297
Sponsor: Sunshine Natural Wellbeing Foundation
6547 Midnight Pass Road, Suite 19
Sarasota, FL 34242

Supelco AOCS Research Award **3405**
This award is given annually to a qualified scientist for outstanding original research on fats, oils, lipid chemistry, and/or biochemistry, the results of which have been published in technical papers of high quality. A travel and expense allowance and a plaque are provided. Application materials are available upon request.
Amount of Grant: $8000
Date(s) Application is Due: Nov 1
Contact: Awards Officer, (217) 359-2344; fax: (217) 351-8091; email: membership@aocs.org
Internet: http://www.aocs.org/member/awards/awd-research.asp
Sponsor: American Oil Chemists' Society
P.O. Box 3489
Champaign, IL 61826-3489

Support Our Aging Religious (SOAR) Grants **3406**
Support Our Aging Religious (SOAR) was established to raise national public awareness of the religious retirement crisis, to network concerned laity, and to provide financial resources to religious communities to assist them in the care of their elderly members. Each year the program awards grants to congregations across the country in its areas of interest, including the fields of education, social services, and health care. Grant categories include: building renovations to allow for handicapped accessibility, physical therapy, and medical equipment; and safety needs—fire alarms, sprinklers, hospital beds, and nurse call systems.
Requirements: SOAR welcomes applications from religious institutes that need assistance to provide critically needed items to care for their retired and infirm members.
Restrictions: SOAR is unable to provide: ongoing living expenses of retired religious in assisted living or skilled nursing facilities; major contributions to retirement funds; funds for construction of new buildings; funds for operational expenses; or cosmetic improvements that do not directly relate to the physical well-being of the retired. Proposals which request partial funding for large projects if additional funds have not been obtained cannot be supported.
Samples: Sisters, Servants of the IHM, Monroe, MI — handicapped accessible van (2008); Society of the Sacred Heart, Atherton, CA — backup generator (2008); Conception Abbey, Inc., Conception, Missouri — elevator upgrade (2008).
Amount of Grant: $500-$30,000; $13,252 average
Date(s) Application is Due: Nov 1
Contact: Deborah Hudson Vornbrock, Grants Administrator; (202) 529-7627; fax: (202) 529-7633; email: dvornbrock@soar-usa.org or info@soar-usa.org
Internet: http://www.soar-usa.org/published/index.html
Sponsor: Support Our Aging Religious (SOAR)
900 Varnum Street, NE
Washington, DC 20017-2145

Susan G. Komen Breast Cancer Foundation Basic, Clinical, and Translational Research Grants **3407**
The foundation awards funding for basic, clinical, and translational breast cancer research. Grants offer two years of support for a variety of research projects in such areas as complementary and alternative medicine; detection and diagnosis, prognosis; risk, prevention, and epidemiology; local treatment; psychosocial treatment; systemic treatment; and tumor cell biology. The foundation gives preference to projects that have potential for high impact in their field, may not be considered by other funders, and benefit the medically underserved in communities. Application deadlines are August 1 for electronic submittal of abstracts; August 8 for electronic submittal of applications; and August 15 for hard-copy applications. Information and application forms are posted on the foundation's Web site.
Requirements: A wide range of nonprofits, including research groups and health and human service agencies, are eligible to apply.
Samples: Dr. Eliot Rosen, Long Island Jewish Medical Ctr (NY)—for the study BRCA1 as a Target for Chemoprevention Agents, $249,939 (2003); Dr. Margot Ip, Roswell Park Cancer Institute—for the study Stromal-Vascular Precursors as a Target for Breast Cancer Prevention, $249,987 (2003); Dr. Georgia Chenevix-Trench, Queensland Institute of Medical Research—for the study The role of the ATM Gene in Familial Breast Cancer, $249,300 (2003); Dr. Amanda Spurdle, Queensland Institute of Medical Research—for the study Evaluation of BRCA1 and BRCA2 Unclassified Sequence Variants, $248,250 (2003).
Amount of Grant: $250,000 maximum over two years
Date(s) Application is Due: Aug 1; Aug 8; Aug 15
Contact: Grants Manager, (888) 300-5582; fax: (972) 855-1640; email: grants@komen.org
Internet: http://www.komen.org/intradoc-cgi/idc_cgi_isapi.dll?IdcService=SS_GET_PAGE&nodeId=390
Sponsor: Susan G. Komen Breast Cancer Foundation
5005 LBJ Fwy, Suite 370
Dallas, TX 75244

Susan G. Komen Breast Cancer Foundation Breast Health, Breast Cancer Education, and Outreach Programs Grants **3408**

Grants are made for breast health, breast cancer education, or outreach programs targeting services not otherwise available to the medically under served in Arizona. See website for grant deadline dates.
Requirements: Applicants must be 501(c)3 public charity, educational institute, and/or government agency based in Arizona.
Geographic Focus: Arizona
Contact: (888) 300-5582; fax: (972) 855-1640; email grants@komen.org
Internet: http://www.komen.org/grants
Sponsor: Susan G. Komen Breast Cancer Foundation
5005 LBJ Freeway, Suite 250
Dallas, TX 75244

Susan G. Komen Breast Cancer Foundation Hurricane Relief Grants **3409**

The foundation awards grants to nonprofit institutions and providers of breast health and breast cancer care in areas affected by Hurricanes Katrina and Rita, and to organizations offering patient services in communities responding to the needs of displaced populations. Two types of grants are available. Rebuilding Grants are intended for nonprofit institutions and providers of breast cancer care in areas affected by the hurricanes for rebuilding efforts, including but not limited to, rebuilding facilities, replacing equipment, hiring staff, replacing/buying supplies, retrieving records, locating patients, and reassigning providers. Patient Services Grants are intended to enable nonprofit institutions and providers of breast cancer care in communities responding to displaced populations to maintain breast cancer services. Funding is designed to assist breast cancer care providers with patient treatment needs, including pharmaceutical and medical supplies; transportation of patients to and from treatment; and child care for patients undergoing treatment and patient navigation services. The foundation is unable to provide funds directly to individuals, but is collaborating with organizations like CancerCare to ensure patients' needs are being met. Individuals with breast health needs who were affected by the hurricane can contact the foundation's national toll-free Breast Care Helpline (800-462-9273). Application and guidelines are available online.
Requirements: Nonprofit organizations and providers of breast health and breast cancer care in areas affected by Hurricanes Katrina and Rita, and organizations offering patient services in communities responding to the needs of displaced populations are eligible.
Amount of Grant: $1 million total; $50,000 maximum rebuilding grants; $30,000 maximum patient services grants
Contact: Grants Administrator, (972) 855-1600; fax: (972) 855-1605
Internet: http://www.komen.org/intradoc-cgi/idc_cgi_isapi.dll?IdcService=SS_GET_PAGE&ssDocName=katrina
Sponsor: Susan G. Komen Breast Cancer Foundation
5005 LBJ Freeway, Suite 250
Dallas, TX 75244

Susan G. Komen Breast Cancer Foundation Interdisciplinary Fellowships **3410**

The foundation serves as a catalyst to develop fellowship training for interdisciplinary programs in breast care that will prepare physicians for careers devoted to serving the multispecialty needs of the breast cancer patient; offer an interdisciplinary curriculum integrated into a comprehensive program; and provide special emphasis on enhancing the physician's understanding of the patient with benign and malignant breast disease while developing a better treatment environment for future patients. The program will fund two consecutive one-year fellowships. Guidelines are available online.
Requirements: The host institution must be an accredited medical institution in the United States or similarly recognized non-U.S. institution.
Restrictions: For-profit organizations are not eligible.
Amount of Grant: $35,000 per year
Date(s) Application is Due: Feb 7
Contact: Dianne McDonald, Research Grants Manager, (888) 300-5582; email: grants@komen.org
Internet: http://www.komen.org/intradoc-cgi/idc_cgi_isapi.dll?IdcService=SS_GET_PAGE&nodeId=395
Sponsor: Susan G. Komen Breast Cancer Foundation
5005 LBJ Freeway, Suite 250
Dallas, TX 75244

Susan G. Komen Breast Cancer Foundation Postdoctoral Fellowships **3411**

Postdoctoral fellowships offer three years of support for basic, clinical, or translational cancer research and public health or epidemiology studies. Detailed program-specific eligibility requirements and application information are available directly from the foundation or its Web site. Abstracts submitted electronically are due August 1; applications submitted electronically are due August 8; hard-copy applications are due August 15.
Requirements: The fellowship candidate must be no more than three years post completion of PhD or equivalent or five years post completion of MD or comparable doctoral degree in the clinical health profession. U.S. citizenship or residency is not required.
Samples: Dr. Carolyn Bertozzi, U of California at Berkeley (CA)—fellowship recipient, for Disruption of 4-Epimerase: A Novel Anti-Metastasis Strategy for Breast Cancer, $135,000 (2003); Dr. Christopher Contag, Stanford U—fellowship recipient, for In Vivo Recruitment and Activation of NK-T Cells into Tumors, $135,000 (2003); Dr. Carol Lange, U of Minnesota Cancer Ctr (MN)—fellowship recipient, for Molecular Regulation of Breast Tumor Kinase, $135,000 (2003); Dr. Wayne Marasco, Dana-Farber Cancer Institute—fellowship recipient, for Isolation and Characterization of Human Anti-Human CXCR4 Antibodies for Immunotherapy of Breast Cancer Metastasis, $135,000 (2003).
Amount of Grant: $45,000 per year
Date(s) Application is Due: Aug 1; Aug 8; Aug 15
Contact: Director, Grants and Sponsored Programs, (888) 300-5582; fax: (972) 855-1640; email: grants@komen.org
Internet: http://www.komen.org/intradoc-cgi/idc_cgi_isapi.dll?IdcService=SS_GET_PAGE&nodeId=391
Sponsor: Susan G. Komen Breast Cancer Foundation
5005 LBJ Fwy, Suite 250
Dallas, TX 75244

Susan Mott Webb Charitable Trust Grants **3412**

The trust awards grants to eligible Alabama nonprofit organizations in its areas of interest, including the arts, civic and public affairs, animals/wildlife, community development, education, health care, religion, social services, youth programs and homelessness. Types of support include annual campaigns, building construction/renovation, capital campaigns, continuing support, curriculum development, emergency funds, endowments, equipment, general/operating support, internship funds, program development, publication, and technical assistance. Contact the Foundation for further application information and guidelines.
Requirements: Giving limited to the greater Birmingham, AL, area.
Restrictions: Grants do not support advertising, individuals, international organizations, or political organizations.
Geographic Focus: Alabama
Samples: Alabama Symphonic Association, Birmingham, AL, $40,000 (2006); Crisis Resource Center of Southeast Kansas, Pittsburg, KS, $25,000 (2006);
Amount of Grant: $2000-$100,000 average
Date(s) Application is Due: Apr 1; Oct 1
Contact: Laura Wainwright, Vice President, c/o Regions Bank; (205) 801-0380; fax: (205) 581-7433; email: laura.wainwright@regions.com
Sponsor: Susan Mott Webb Charitable Trust
P.O. Box 11426
Birmingham, AL 35202-1426

Susan Vaughan Foundation Grants **3413**

The Susan Vaughan Foundation established in 1952, supports non-profits involved with: education, particularly to a library; arts; environment, natural resources; higher education; human services. The Foundation gives primarily in Houston and Austin Texas area with support in the form of: annual campaigns; building/renovation; capital campaigns; general/operating support; matching/challenge support.
Requirements: There is no formal application form required, applicant must be a non-profit in the Houston and Austin, Texas region. Initial contact should be made through a Letter of Inquiry.
Geographic Focus: Texas
Amount of Grant: $2,500-$630,000 range
Contact: Jennifer Grosvenor, Grant Coordinator c/o Legacy Trust Co.; (713) 651-8980; email: jgrosvenor@legacytrust.com
Sponsor: The Susan Vaughan Foundation
600 Jefferson Street, Suite 300
Houston, TX 77002-7377

Sybil G. Jacobs Award for Outstanding Use of Tobacco Industry Documents **3414**

The award recognizes a person who has made a significant and well-recognized contribution to the health of the public in the recent past through use of tobacco documents. The award also honors innovation in the use and application of tobacco industry documents to improve the public's health and, where applicable, to further the goals of tobacco prevention and control in order to help build a world where young people reject tobacco and anyone can quit. Those nominated should be individuals who have made a notable impact through innovative use of tobacco industry documents as applied to research, policy, or advocacy.
Requirements: At least one of the following two criteria must be met by the nominated individual: Nominees must have made a remarkable research, policy, or advocacy contribution with the use of tobacco industry documents, and/or; Nominees must have employed innovative, creative approaches to the employment of tobacco industry documents that result in an improvement in the health or public awareness of a community or nation. Nominations may be made by individuals such as colleagues, peers, coworkers, instructors/professors, governments, or CBOs that are qualified to make such a nomination because of their familiarity with the nominee's work and contribution.
Restrictions: Nominees must not have any affiliation with the tobacco industry. Members of the awards committee may not nominate potential recipients, although they may provide written support as part of a nomination package. Employees and directors of the American Legacy Foundation and their relatives are not eligible.
Amount of Grant: $7,500
Date(s) Application is Due: Feb 6
Contact: Virginia Lockmuller, Grant Coordinator; (202) 454-5555; fax: (202) 454-5599; email: awards@americanlegacy.org
Internet: http://www.legacyforhealth.org/awards/
Sponsor: American Legacy Foundation
Legacy Awards, 724 Massachusetts Avenue, NW
Washington, DC 20036

Take Care to Learn: Teaching Clinical Care Management Grants 3415
The program awards grants to primary-care residency and nurse-practitioner programs, as well as managed-care organizations. The goal is to support education programs leading to improving care for patients with asthma or diabetes and make sure trainees have the skills needed to deliver high-quality health care. Ten two-year grants will be awarded.
Requirements: Healthcare institutions are eligible.
Amount of Grant: $300,000 maximum
Contact: Elizabeth March, Deputy Director, (617) 509-9811; fax: (617) 859-8112; email: Elizabeth_March@harvardpilgrim.org
Internet: http://www.pqe.org/programs-takecare.html
Sponsor: Partnerships for Quality Education
133 Brookline Avenue, 6th Floor
Boston, MA 02215

Takemi Program in International Health Research and Advanced Training Fellowships 3416
This midcareer program offers a limited number of fellowship positions for research and advanced training on critical issues of international health, especially those relating to developing countries. This interdisciplinary program has four major objectives: to create better methods for mobilizing and using health resources in both rich and poor countries; to promote cooperative research and comparative analysis of health policies and programs in different countries; to study transnational causes of health conditions such as population migration, disease transmission, and air and water pollution; and to bring together leading health professionals and scholars from many nations for research and training. Fellowship positions cover estimated costs for the program, which includes 10 months in residence at the Harvard School of Public Health.
Requirements: Applicants should have completed graduate degrees and demonstrated potential leadership capacity in their home countries. They are expected to show strong promise and appropriate preparation to enable them to benefit from a period at Harvard. Applicants may come from the disciplines of medicine, law, public health, economics, management, and social sciences. Applicants should submit a curriculum vita and publications list, a proposal of research and writing to be undertaken during the fellowship, and three letters of reference. The proposal should not exceed five typed pages and should include a clear statement of objectives, significance or relevance, data sources, and methodology.
Restrictions: Clinical research will not be funded. Individuals enrolled in degree-granting programs are ineligible.
Contact: Program Coordinator, Takemi Program in International Health, Harvard School of Public Health, (617) 432-0686; fax: (617) 432-1251; email: takemi@hsph.harvard.edu
Internet: http://www.hsph.harvard.edu/takemi
Sponsor: Harvard University
665 Huntington Avenue, Building 1-1207
Boston, MA 02115-6021

Taproot Foundation Capacity-Building Service Grants 3417
The program seeks to strengthen the capacity of strong charitable organizations that provide effective, high-quality programs. Applicant organizations must have a mission that fits in one of four categories: education—organizations that strengthen the public education (pre-K and K-12) system or enhance the educational success of students; environment—organizations that preserve or restore the environment; health—organizations that improve people's physical or emotional health; and social services—organizations that provide social services to those who suffer hardship or who have been unable to participate fully in the social and economic life of the community. The foundation makes grants of high-quality professional services that target capacity-building needs nonprofit organizations, including fundraising, marketing, information technology, and talent management. Each grant is staffed by professionals from the business community who donate their time and expertise to help the community. The grant also includes a project plan with estimated timing based on volunteers donating five hours per week. Guidelines and application are available online.
Requirements: 501(c)3 nonprofit organizations that provide direct benefits primarily or entirely to residents of the five boroughs of New York City (Manhattan, Bronx, Queens, Staten Island, and Brooklyn) and the six counties of the California Bay Area (Alameda, San Francisco, San Mateo, Santa Clara, Marin, and Contra Costa counties) are eligible. The organization must also have its headquarters in one of these areas.
Restrictions: The foundation does not support nonprofits with other than 501(c)3 status, for-profit corporations, or individuals. Service Grants are not expressly intended to support candidates for political office, or to influence legislation. Grants are not awarded to support religious purposes. (Agencies operated by religious organizations that serve secular needs are eligible.)
Geographic Focus: California; New York
Date(s) Application is Due: Mar 1; Jun 1; Sep 15; Dec 1
Contact: Administrator, (415) 359-0226; email: national@taprootfoundation.org
Internet: http://taprootfoundation.org/npo/index.shtml
Sponsor: Taproot Foundation
466 Geary Street, Suite 300
San Francisco, CA 94102

Tellabs Foundation Grants 3418
The foundation awards grants to eligible nonprofit organizations in the following areas: educational programs with a particular focus on local and national programs and curricula for engineering, science, mathematics and technology; health and human services programs for projects involving health and wellness-related, research, education and treatment in the United States (The primary focus is on projects involving hospitals and health care facilities); and environmental programs that encourage the understanding and protection of the environment. Generally, grants are awarded for specific programs rather than for general operating funds or capital projects. The primary focus of the foundation is to support programs in areas in which Tellabs employees live and work. Tellabs Inc and its affiliates also have direct giving programs, including an employee matching gift program, giving to the United Way, and limited direct corporate grants. The board meets quarterly (January, April, July and October); submit proposals at least four weeks before scheduled meetings.
Requirements: Unless invited by the foundation board to submit a full grant proposal, all applicants or programs must first submit a letter of inquiry. There is no set format, but it should be 1-2 pages in length. All grant recipients must be recognized by the IRS as tax exempt, not-for-profit organizations under Section 501(c)3 of the Internal Revenue Code.
Restrictions: The foundation generally will not consider requests from: Organizations which do not have a 501(c)3 status; Political organizations or parties, candidates for political office, and organizations whose primary purpose is to influence legislation; Labor unions or organizations; Local athletic or sports programs; Service organizations raising money for community purposes; Individuals; Travel funds for tours, expeditions, or trips by individuals or groups; Dues or gifts to national or local alumni groups, clubs or fraternities; Institutional memberships or subscription fees for publications; Gifts to individual churches, synagogues or other entities organized exclusively for religious purposes; Donations for benefit events, raffle tickets or fundraising efforts that involve value returned to the donor; Organizations not operating for the benefit of the general public or that have discriminatory practices; Any grantee who receives funds of $50,000 or more shall not be entitled to submit another grant proposal for three years from the date of grant.
Samples: Purdue U (West Lafayette, IN)—to construct a facility for the department of computer sciences, $30,000.
Amount of Grant: $10,000 minimum
Contact: Meredith Hilt, Executive Director; (630) 798-2506; fax: (630) 798-4778; email: meredith.hilt@tellabs.com
Internet: http://www.tellabs.com/about/foundation.shtml
Sponsor: Tellabs Foundation
1415 W. Diehl Road, Mail Stop 10
Naperville, IL 60563

Temple-Inland Foundation Grants 3419
The foundation makes grants to IRS 501(c)3 tax-exempt organizations located in geographic operating areas of Temple-Inland Inc's subsidiary companies. Areas of interest include services for children and youth, Christian churches and organizations, education at all levels, health care and organizations, human services, and arts and culture. Types of support include general operating support, research, employee matching gifts, and employee-related scholarships. Requests should be received two weeks prior to quarterly board meetings. Submit a written request for guidelines and specific application deadlines. The listed deadline date is for scholarships.
Restrictions: Ineligible applicants include fraternal, veterans, political, local social, and service organizations.
Amount of Grant: $1000-$30,000 average
Date(s) Application is Due: Mar 15
Contact: Richard Warner, (936) 829-1721; fax: (936) 829-7727
Internet: http://www.templeinland.com
Sponsor: Temple-Inland Foundation
1300 S Mopac
Austin, TX 78749

Texas Commission on the Arts Arts Respond Project Grants 3420
This program provides project assistance grants on a short-term basis and may include administrative costs directly related to the project. Projects must address one of the following priority areas: education, health and human services, economic development, public safety, criminal justice, natural resources, or agriculture. Organizations that are eligible are: Arts Organizations, Established Arts Organizations, Minority Arts Organizations, Rural Arts Providers.
Requirements: To be eligible for TCA grants, an organization must: be a tax-exempt nonprofit organization as designated by the Internal Revenue Service and/or must be an entity of government; be incorporated in Texas; have fulfilled all its outstanding contractual obligations to the State of Texas (i.e. student loans, child support, taxes, etc.); and comply with regulations pertaining to federal grant recipients including Title VI of the Civil Rights Act of 1964, Section 504 of the Rehabilitation Act of 1973, the Age Discrimination Act of 1975, the Education Amendments of 1972, the Americans with Disabilities Act of 1990, and the Drug Free Workplace Act of 1988.
Geographic Focus: Texas
Amount of Grant: $45,000 maximum
Contact: Director of Programs; (512) 463-5535 or (800) 252-9415; fax: (512) 475-2699; email: front.desk@arts.state.tx.us
Internet: http://www.arts.state.tx.us/index.php?option=com_wrapper&view=wrapper&Itemid=86
Sponsor: Texas Commission on the Arts
P.O. Box 13406
Austin, TX 78711-3406

Thelma Doelger Charitable Trust Grants 3421
The trust awards grants in the San Francisco Bay area to zoos, hospitals, and organizations supporting animal welfare and senior citizens. Grants are awarded for general purposes and to support operating budgets. There are no application deadlines. Application forms are required.

Requirements: Nonprofit organizations in the San Francisco Bay area of northern California may submit grant requests.
Restrictions: Individuals are not eligible.
Geographic Focus: California
Samples: San Francisco Zoo (CA)—for operating support, $100,000.; Marin Humane Society (Novato, CA)—for operating support, $70,000.
Amount of Grant: $2000-$75,000 range
Contact: D. Eugene Richard, Trustee, (650) 755-2333
Sponsor: Thelma Doelger Charitable Trust
950 Daly Boulevard, Suite 300
Daly City, CA 94015-3004

Thomas and Dorothy Leavey Foundation Grants **3422**
Thomas Leavey and partner John C. Tyler began the Farmer's Insurance Company in 1928. The foundation was begun in 1952 by Leavey and his wife, Dorothy. Thomas Leavey died in 1980 and Dorothy actively led the foundation until her death in 1998. Giving primarily in southern California, the Foundation offers support for: hospitals, medical research, higher and secondary education, Catholic church groups; and provides scholarships to children of employees of Farmers Group.
Requirements: The foundation gives primarily in southern California.
Geographic Focus: California
Samples: Childrens Museum of Los Angeles, Lake View Terrace, CA, $250,000 (2007); Santa Clara University, Santa Clara, CA, $2,000,000 (2007); Orthopaedic Hospital, Los Angeles, CA, $100,000 (2007).
Amount of Grant: $10,000-$2,000,000 range
Contact: Kathleen Leavey McCarthy, Chair, (310) 551-9936
Sponsor: Thomas and Dorothy Leavey Foundation
10100 Santa Monica Boulevard, Suite 610
Los Angeles, CA 90067-4110

Thomas C. Ackerman Foundation Grants **3423**
The foundation awards grants to California nonprofits in its areas of interest, including arts and culture, community development, education, and health and human services. Types of support include general operating support, emergency grants, seed grants, scholarship funds, and matching grants. Contact the office for application forms. Deadlines listed are for letters of intent. Annual deadline dates may vary; contact program staff for exact dates.
Requirements: California nonprofits, primarily in San Diego County, are eligible.
Restrictions: The foundation does not award grants to religious organizations for religious purposes; individuals; or for brick-and-mortar projects, conferences, symposia, or human medical or biological research.
Geographic Focus: California
Samples: San Diego Senior Olympics (San Diego, CA)—for Website Online Registration Development, $3500.; San ElderHelp of San Diego (San Diego, CA)—for Shared Housing Program, $10,000.; Museum of Contemporary Art (San Diego, CA)—for the program Off Broadway: Emerging Artists in Downtown San Diego, $7500.
Amount of Grant: $300-$25,000 typically
Date(s) Application is Due: Jan 31; Apr 29; Jul 29; Oct 31
Contact: Program Contact, (619) 699-5411; fax: (619) 232-8311; email: Info@AckermanFoundation.org or pgarcia@luce.com
Internet: http://www.ackermanfoundation.org
Sponsor: Thomas C. Ackerman Foundation
600 W Broadway, Suite 2600
San Diego, CA 92101-3391

Thomas M. and Irene B. Kirbo Charitable Trust Grants **3424**
The trust awards grants to nonprofit organizations in support of religion, hospitals, universities, and youth. The trust supports higher education, libraries, hospitals, youth organizations, and Christian agencies and churches. Applications must be requested.
Requirements: Nonprofit organizations in Florida and Georgia are eligible.
Restrictions: Grants are not made to individuals.
Geographic Focus: Florida; Georgia
Samples: Elon College (Elon College, NC)—for a new library, $150,000.
Amount of Grant: $1000-$125,000 range
Contact: R. Murray Jenks, President, (904) 354-7212
Sponsor: Thomas M. and Irene B. Kirbo Charitable Trust
112 W Adams Street, Suite 1111
Jacksonville, FL 32202

Thompson Charitable Foundation Grants **3425**
Established in 1987, the Foundation supports organizations involved with education, Christian organizations, Autism research, health, human services, youth, including funding for capital and building improvements for human service organizations and educational institutions. Giving is limited to Bell, Clay, Laurel, and Leslie counties, Kentucky; Anderson, Blount, Knox, and Scott counties, Tennessee; and Buchanan and Tazewell counties, Virginia.
Requirements: Nonprofits operating in Bell, Clay, Laurel, and Leslie counties, Kentucky; Anderson, Blount, Knox, and Scott counties, Tennessee; and Buchanan and Tazewell counties, Virginia are eligible to apply. Initial contact should be a letter, no more then 2 pages long. The letter should include: a statement of the problem, the project will address; a detailed description of project, and amount of funding requested.
Restrictions: No support for religious or political organizations, budget deficits or endowments.
Geographic Focus: Kentucky; Tennessee; Virginia
Amount of Grant: $2,000-$500,000
Date(s) Application is Due: Mar 31; Sep 1
Contact: Debbie Black, Exec. Director; (865) 588-0491; fax: (865) 588-4496; email: debbie@cf.org
Sponsor: The Thompson Charitable Foundation
800 South Gay Street, Suite 2021
Knoxville, TN 37929-9710

Thrasher Research Fund Grants **3426**
The fund awards grants in support of research that seeks to improve children's health where insufficient research and investigation have been performed. In particular, the fund supports medical research that seeks to prevent or cure children's critical illnesses, injuries, and disabilities. Projects should be scientifically sound and culturally appropriate; document methods and practices that have sustainable benefits; have specific aims and a well-designed methodology; and evaluate the significance of impact on children's health. The fund normally supports projects no longer than three years. Financial support may be provided for supplies, minor equipment (items less than U.S.$1000), and technical personnel assistance related to a specific fund-sponsored project. The fund requires the principal investigator to submit semiannual project progress and financial reports. The initial application procedure is to submit a five-page prospectus, which should include a brief background statement justifying the proposed project; hypothesis to be tested; specific aims of the project; design and methodology of the proposed project, including evaluation component; time schedule and detailed budget; and investigator(s) curriculum vita (in addition to four-page prospectus). Applicants are encouraged to consult program staff prior to submitting a prospectus.
Restrictions: The fund does not award grants for general operations, construction or renovation of buildings or facilities, loans, scholarships, or the purchase of major equipment. Grants generally are not awarded for conferences, workshops, or symposia. Proposals in the areas of sexually transmitted diseases, abortion or reproductive physiology, and contraceptive technology will not be considered. In addition, proposals involving the use of therapeutically aborted human fetal tissue will not be considered.
Samples: Dr. Rebecca Stoltzfus, Johns Hopkins School of Hygiene and Public Health (Baltimore, MD)—for a study to improve iron status and growth of preschool children in East Africa, $141,529 total.; Paul Calvert, Intermediate Technology (Rugby, England)—for study on environmental health and sanitation for fishing communities, $117,250 total.
Amount of Grant: $100,000-$350,000 average
Contact: Julie Busse, (801) 240-4720; fax: (801) 240-1625; email: BusseJ@thrasherresearch.org
Internet: http://www.thrasherresearch.org
Sponsor: Thrasher Research Fund
15 W South Temple Street, Suite 1650
Salt Lake City, UT 84101

Tides Foundation Syringe Access Fund **3427**
The Syringe Access fund is a collaborative grant making initiative that strives to reduce the risk of HIV infection and other blood-borne pathogens among injection drug users, their sexual partners and children through expanded access to sterile syringes. Grants are awarded to fund expanded access to clean syringes via syringe exchange programs and networking/capacity development among local syringe exchange programs; and coordinated, local/state-level education programs focusing on policies to expand access to sterile syringes, including the decriminalization of syringe exchange programs or the sale of syringes without a prescription. The program also seeks to broaden public support for syringe exchange programs as well as for policies designed to expand access to sterile syringes. The listed application deadline is for letters of intent, which must be submitted via email; proposals are by invitation. Guidelines and letter of intent form are available online.
Requirements: Applications are accepted from all 50 states, the District of Columbia, Native American reservations/tribal land, and Puerto Rico.
Amount of Grant: $50,000 per year for policy work; $25,000 per year for program/direct services
Contact: Tierney Gleason, Syringe Access Fund; (212) 509-4975 or (202) 408-4848 ext. 203; fax: (212) 509-1059; email: syringeaccess@tides.org or saf@aidsfund.org
Internet: http://www.tidesfoundation.org/services-strategies/collective-giving/syringe-access-fund/index.html
Sponsor: Tides Foundation
55 Exchange Place, Suite 402
New York, NY 10005-1965

Tifa Foundation Grants **3428**
The Tifa Foundation has two grant making mechanism. The first, known as Pro-Active Grants, is through a proactive approach in which Tifa assumes an active role in working together with other organizations that correspond with Tifa's mission. The second, known as Open Grants, is through the endorsement of program proposals that conform to Tifa's strategic direction and priority/supporting programs.
Requirements: Grants are awarded to: organizations with proposed program activities that are in accordance with Tifa's vision and mission; organizations that possess unblemished an track record during their involvement with Tifa as well as with other donor institutions; organizations with legal entities; organizations that cooperate with government agencies; and institutions under the control of a particular university.
Restrictions: Grants are not eligible for: individuals, including proposals for scholarships, trips, conferences and others; all government agencies, legislative and judiciary bodies, political parties, military or those with affiliation/direct relationship with

the aforementioned bodies; all organizations with profit-seeking interests; program proposals where the end product or outcome is sold to the public (except upon Tifa's approval); organizations that are still engaged in cooperation with Tifa for the ongoing period except upon prior approval.
Date(s) Application is Due: Jan 15; Jul 15
Contact: Yayasan Tifa; (62) 021 829 2776; fax: (62) 021 837 83648; email: public@tifafoundation.org
Internet: http://www.tifafoundation.org/
Sponsor: Tifa Foundation
Jl. Jaya Mandala II No. 14 E
Menteng Dalam – South Jakarta 12870
Indonesia

Topeka Community Foundation Kansas Blood Services Scholarships **3429**
The Kansas Blood Services Fund with the Topeka Community Foundation provides scholarships for individuals in the medical field of blood banking or a related field. The scholarship can be used to cover expenses related to attending a professional conference or meeting (including conference fees, hotel, meals and transportation).
Requirements: Residents of Nemaha, Riley, Pottawatomie, Jackson, Jefferson, Douglas, Shawnee, Wabaunsee, Osage and Lyon counties in Kansas are eligible to apply.
Geographic Focus: Kansas
Contact: Marsha Pope, Vice President; (785) 272-4804; fax: (785) 272-4644; email: pope@topekacommunityfoundation.org
Internet: http://www.topekacommunityfoundation.org/newsarticle.cfm?articleid=10023450&ptsidebaroptid=0&returnto=page31525.cfm&returntoname=Grant Information&siteid=1897&pageid=31520&sidepageid=31525
Sponsor: Topeka Community Foundation
5431 SW 29th Street, Suite 300
Topeka, KS 66614

Topfer Family Foundation Grants **3430**
The mission of the foundation (TFF) is to fund programs and organizations that connect people to the tools and resources they need to build self-sufficient and fulfilling lives. Programs areas of interest include child abuse prevention and treatment; youth enrichment; job training and support services; children's health; and aging in place. The Topfer family is keenly interested in understanding the unique needs of the communities in which they invest foundation resources. Therefore, contributions are limited to the communities in which the family resides: the greater Austin, TX, and the greater Chicago, IL, metropolitan areas. In Illinois, preference is given to organizations serving Du Page and Cook Counties. Note to Chicago area applicants: The foundation is not accepting unsolicited applications in the Job Training or Children's Health program areas from the Chicago area at this time. Guidelines and application are available online.
Requirements: 501(c)3 nonprofit organizations in Illinois and Texas are eligible.
Restrictions: The foundation does not generally support: grants or loans to individuals; loans to charitable organizations; more than 20 percent of an organization's operating budget; administrative costs; organizations that exclude participants based on race or religion; the purchase of dinner, gala, or raffle tickets; school fundraisers or events (including sports and other extracurricular activities); tax-generating entities (municipalities, school districts, etc.) for services within their normal responsibilities; public or private educational institutions for recurrent operating, administrative, or capital expenses (i.e., acquisition, construction, improvement, and maintenance of buildings and equipment), or scholarships that subsidize existing funding base; academic or scientific research; advertising or marketing efforts; political campaigns or purposes; or any one program more than once a calendar year.
Geographic Focus: Illinois; Texas
Contact: (866) 897-0298 or (512) 329-0009
Internet: http://www.topferfamilyfoundation.org
Sponsor: Topfer Family Foundation
5000 Plaza on the Lake, Suite 170
Austin, TX 78746

Toro Foundation Grants **3431**
The foundation supports nonprofit organizations in corporate operating areas to improve the quality of life for employees and customers. The foundation's primary giving focus is to support organizations that preserve the outdoor environment. The foundation also contributes to programs that enhance education, health and welfare, culture, the arts, and civic projects. Preference is given to requests for program funds over endowment or capital fund requests and to organizations where Toro employees volunteer. Grants are evaluated based on criteria such as mission, employee involvement, geographical area, environmental component, industry relevance, and the presence of United Way funds. Proposals are accepted throughout the years. Guidelines are available online.
Requirements: 501(c)3 tax-exempt organizations in corporate communities are eligible, including Minneapolis/Saint Paul, and Windom, MN; El Cajon, Madera, and Riverside, CA; Oxford, MS; Beatrice, NE; Baraboo, Tomah, and Plymouth, WI; and Abilene, and El Paso, TX.
Restrictions: Grants do not support religious or political activities; general, capital, or endowment support for educational institutions; health treatment, scientific research, or substance abuse treatment programs; travel for individuals or groups; fundraising events or activities, social events, or goodwill advertising, except where Toro employees are participating; individuals or for-profit organizations; or organizations funded by the United Way.
Geographic Focus: California; Minnesota; Mississippi; Nebraska; Texas; Wisconsin
Contact: Administrator, (800) 348-2424 or (952) 887-8870; fax: (952) 887-8258
Internet: http://www.thetorocompany.com/community/foundation.html
Sponsor: Toro Foundation
8111 Lyndale Ave S
Bloomington, MN 55420-1196

Tourette Syndrome Association Post-Doc Fellowships **3432**
The Fellowship program is interested in supporting any research that has the potential to contribute to the understanding of Tourette Syndrome, including genetics, pathogenesis, pathophysiology, clinical treatments and animal model development. Post-doctoral research fellowships of up to $40,000 for one year are awarded. For preliminary screening, a Letter of Intent briefly describing the scientific basis and relevance of the proposed project should be sent to tsadevel@earthlink.net by October 1. The cover page to accompany each letter can be downloaded from the website. Applicants will be notified electronically as to whether or not to proceed with a full grant proposal. If invited to apply for a research grant, detailed instructions will be provided, and full proposals are due by December 9th.
Requirements: Candidates must have a M.D., Ph.D. or equivalent. Previous experience in the field of movement disorders is desirable, but not essential. Applicants may reside outside the United States.
Amount of Grant: $40,000 maximum
Date(s) Application is Due: Oct 1; Dec 9
Contact: Fellowship Administrator; (718) 224-2999, ext. 222; fax: (718) 279-9596; email: grantadministrator@tsa-usa.org
Internet: http://tsa-usa.org/research.html
Sponsor: Tourette Syndrome Association
42-40 Bell Boulevard
Bayside, NY 11361-2820

Tourette Syndrome Association Research Grants **3433**
The Program is interested in receiving applications from any research study that has the potential to contribute to the understanding of Tourette Syndrome, including genetics, pathogenesis, pathophysiology, clinical treatments and animal model development. Research grants of up to $75,000 for one year are awarded. Applicants may apply for a second year of funding, which is reviewed competitively. For preliminary screening, a Letter of Intent briefly describing the scientific basis and relevance of the proposed project should be sent as an email attachment to tsadevel@earthlink.net by October 1st. The cover page to accompany each letter can be downloaded from the website. Applicants will be notified electronically as to whether or not to proceed with a full grant proposal. If invited to apply for a research grant, detailed instructions will be provided, and full proposals are due by December 9th.
Requirements: Candidates must have a M.D., Ph.D. or equivalent. Previous experience in the field of movement disorders is desirable, but not essential. Applicants may reside outside the United States.
Amount of Grant: $75,000
Date(s) Application is Due: Oct 1; Dec 9
Contact: Heather Cowley, Manager; (718) 224-2999, ext. 247; fax: (718) 279-9596; email: Heather.Cowley@tsa-usa.org or grantadministrator@tsa-usa.org
Internet: http://tsa-usa.org/research.html
Sponsor: Tourette Syndrome Association
42-40 Bell Boulevard
Bayside, NY 11361

TRDRP California Research Awards **3434**
This program is focused on research projects that address questions specific to tobacco-related disease or tobacco control issues in California. The awards will provide funding for average annual direct costs of $140,000; $170,000 per year for research involving human subjects. Full indirect costs are paid to eligible institutions. Maximum duration is 3 years. (This is a new TRDRP award mechanism as of 2009.)
Requirements: Principal Investigators from California not-for-profit organizations are eligible for funding. Research undertaken with TRDRP funds must be conducted primarily in California. The Principal Investigator must conduct and supervise the research project directly and in person. Underrepresented racial and ethnic investigators are encouraged to submit applications. To be competitive, proposals must present a compelling justification, including evidence if available, supporting the California-specific criterion. The proposal should be fully developed, scientifically rigorous, and include sound background information, hypothesis, and promising preliminary studies or preliminary data.
Restrictions: All submitted applications will be screened for their direct relevance to tobacco use or tobacco-related disease. Proposed research that is not relevant will not undergo peer review for scientific merit. It is incumbent on the applicant to make a compelling case that the proposed work is directly relevant to the mission of TRDRP.
Geographic Focus: California
Samples: Examples of previously-funded TRDRP grants that addressed California-specific research questions (but not limited to): Diabetes & tobacco exposure in So CA American Indians - Study tobacco use patterns with California Indian tribal members and tribal tobacco control policies.; Environmental contexts of smoking for Southeast Asians - Investigate the relationship between the social environment and smoking among Southeast Asians in California urban areas.; The geography of tobacco related disease in California - Describe the spatial distribution of hospital admitted tobacco-related disease prevalence rates and smoking prevalence in California.
Amount of Grant: $140,000 - $170,000 per year
Date(s) Application is Due: Dec 5

Contact: Kamlesh Asotra, Ph.D., (510) 287-3366, kamlesh.asotra@ucop.edu; M.F. Bowen, Ph.D., (510) 987-9811, mf.bowen@ucop.edu; Phillip Gardiner, Dr.P.H., (510) 987-9853, phillip.gardiner@ucop.edu
Internet: http://www.trdrp.org/fundingopps/callawardmechs.asp#calrchawd
Sponsor: Tobacco-Related Disease Research Program (TRDRP)
University of California—Office of the President, 300 Lakeside Drive, 6th Floor
Oakland, CA 94612-3550

TRDRP Exploratory/Developmental Research Awards **3435**
The purpose of these grants is to gather preliminary data or demonstrate proof-of-principle (i.e., pilot projects), or to conduct a research project within the specified limits of money and time. The ultimate goal of these awards is to provide the foundation for proposals for fully-developed research project awards from other funding programs. Total direct costs of $250,000 for the entire project duration (maximum of 2 years). Indirect costs are paid to eligible institutions.
Requirements: Principal Investigators from California not-for-profit organizations are eligible for funding. Research undertaken with TRDRP funds must be conducted primarily in California. The Principal Investigator must conduct and supervise the research project directly and in person. Underrepresented racial and ethnic investigators are encouraged to submit applications. Although Principal Investigators may submit as many proposals for these awards as they wish for separate projects, no more than one Exploratory/Developmental Research Award will be made to any individual PI in the same year. Only proposals that address one of TRDRP's Primary research area will be eligible and will undergo peer review. Exploratory/Developmental Research Awards are for new projects only; that is, competing renewal applications will not be accepted.
Restrictions: All submitted applications will be screened for their direct relevance to tobacco use or tobacco-related disease. Proposed research that is not relevant will not undergo peer review for scientific merit. It is incumbent on the applicant to make a compelling case that the proposed work is directly relevant to the mission of TRDRP.
Amount of Grant: $250,000
Date(s) Application is Due: Dec 5
Contact: Kamlesh Asotra, Ph.D., (510) 287-3366, kamlesh.asotra@ucop.edu; M.F. Bowen, Ph.D., (510) 987-9811, mf.bowen@ucop.edu; Phillip Gardiner, Dr.P.H., (510) 987-9853, phillip.gardiner@ucop.edu
Internet: http://www.trdrp.org/fundingopps/callawardmechs.asp#explordev
Sponsor: Tobacco-Related Disease Research Program (TRDRP)
University of California—Office of the President, 300 Lakeside Drive, 6th Floor
Oakland, CA 94612-3550

Tri-County Electric People Fund Grants **3436**
The fund awards grants for charitable purposes to benefit people and organizations in the Tri-County Electric service area. Grants are awarded for food, shelter, clothing, health, and other humane needs for programs or services that benefit a significant segment of a community. An organization's financial statements, bylaws, and nonprofit status must be submitted with its application. Individuals or families must submit copies of previous federal income tax forms. The fund has the right to fully audit the use of donations at any time. Guidelines and application are available online.
Requirements: Individuals and organizations in mid-Michigan, including Ionia, Eaton, Ingham, Clinton, Gratiot, Montcalm, Isabella, and Mcosta Counties, are eligible.
Restrictions: No funds shall in any fashion be used to support any candidate for political office or any political purpose. An applicant may not reapply within six months from a previous application.
Geographic Focus: Michigan
Samples: Eaton County Clothing and Furniture Project (MI)—for their back-to-school program, $3000 (2004); EightCAP (Ionia and Montcalm Counties, MI)—for Camp Wah-Wah-Tay-See program expenses, $2000 (2004); Montcalm County family to help with medical expenses, $309.09 (2004); Women's Aid Service (Mount Pleasant, MI)—for replacement windows, $2000 (2004).
Amount of Grant: $10,000 maximum annually to an organization; $2500 maximum annually to a family or individual
Contact: People Fund, (877) 466-3957 (choose option #1); email: tricoenergy@homeworks.org.
Internet: http://www.tricoenergy.com/people_fund1/guidelines.htm
Sponsor: Tri-County Electric People Fund
P.O. Box 503
Portland, MI 48875

Triangle Community Foundation Donor-Advised Grants **3437**
Established in 1983, the Triangle Community Foundation is a nonprofit organization that serves Chatham, Durham, Orange and Wake counties of North Carolina. There's no application process for the donor-advised grants, rather, fundholders advise Foundation staff as to where they would like their grants made. Often, fundholders seek guidance from staff about which nonprofits are doing work matching their charitable interests. For this reason, it is important nonprofits keep members of the Philanthropic Services Team informed about their organizations, including special projects and funding needs. For more information, nonprofit organizations should contact the following staff: Arts, Culture, & Humanites - Lori O'Keefe, lori@trianglecf.org; Community Building - Agnes Vishnevkin, agnes@trianglecf.org; Education & Youth Development - Robyn Fehrman, robyn@trianglecf.org; Health & Human Services - Sandra Rodriguez, sandra@trianglecf.org; Law, Justice, & Public Action - Robyn Fehrman, robyn@trianglecf.org; Natural Resources - Tracy Joseph, tracy@trianglecf.org; Volunteerism & Community Support - Libby Long, libby@trianglecf.org; Religious & Spiritual Development - Tracy Joseph, tracy@trianglecf.org.
Requirements: North Carolina 501(c)3 tax-exempt organizations, government units, and religious congregations planning projects that benefit residents of Chatham, Durham, Orange and Wake counties of North Carolina are eligible.
Geographic Focus: North Carolina
Contact: Lori O'Keefe, Director of Philanthropic Services; (919) 474-8370, ext. 144; fax: (919) 941-9208; email: lori@trianglecf.org
Internet: http://www.trianglecf.org/page33699.cfm
Sponsor: Triangle Community Foundation
324 Blackwell Street, Suite 1220
Durham, NC 27701

Triangle Community Foundation Shaver-Hitchings Scholarship **3438**
The Shaver-Hitchings Scholarship Fund was created in 1990 by Dr. George H. Hitchings and Dr. Joyce Shaver Hitchings to honor and reward individuals with a commitment to helping others in the area of drug and alcohol addiction. The Scholarship is available to any graduate student, physician's assistant, or medical student in the Triangle area who has worked (preferably as a volunteer) to help others with alcoholism, drug abuse and addictive disorder treatment or with preventive education on the subject of addiction. The fund is designed to recognize the recipient for his or her work or volunteer activity and to provide financial aid. Excellent candidates who have demonstrated a commitment to working with others in the area of addictive disorders, especially those who have done so as volunteers, are sought. One Scholarship of $1,500 will be awarded each year. The Scholarship may be applied toward expenses for tuition, required fees, and required books or materials not covered by other financial aid.
Requirements: Applicant must be a resident of Durham, Orange, Wake, or Chatham County.
Restrictions: The Scholarship does not cover living expenses such as room and board, transportation, or childcare.
Geographic Focus: North Carolina
Date(s) Application is Due: Mar 15
Contact: Libby Long Richards, Scholarship Coordinator; (919) 474-8370, ext. 134; fax: (919) 941-9208; email: libby@trianglecf.org
Internet: http://www.trianglecf.org/grants_support/view_scholarships/shaver-hitchings_scholarship/
Sponsor: Triangle Community Foundation
4813 Emperor Boulevard
Durham, NC 27703

Trinity Lutheran School of Nursing Alumnae Scholarships **3439**
The Trinity Lutheran Hospital School of Nursing Alumnae Scholarship fund was established to assist persons who wish to pursue a career in nursing (such as undergraduate, advanced degree, etc.) and need financial assistance. Applications for the scholarship must be received by May 1st. Renewal of the scholarship is possible each year for those who reapply and meet the criteria.
Requirements: Applicants must: be a student currently enrolled in an accredited RN school of nursing or in an accredited higher education nursing program; have completed at least one semester at an accredited school; be a full or part-time student and the course work must be continuous; and have a cumulative GPA of 2.5.
Date(s) Application is Due: May 1
Contact: Becky Schaid, Executive Director; (816) 276-7515 or (816) 276-7555; fax: (816) 926-2261; email: becky@btllf.org
Internet: http://www.btllf.org/funding.html
Sponsor: Baptist-Trinity Lutheran Legacy Foundation
6601 Rockhill Road
Kansas City, MO 64131

Triological Society Research Career Development Awards **3440**
The purpose of this award is to provide support for the research career development of otolaryngologists (head and neck surgeons) who have made a commitment to focus their research endeavors on patient-oriented research, e.g., clinical trials, translational research. Research training supported by this award may be related to any research questions relevant to the specialty of otolaryngology, as long as it is demonstrated that the training will have a direct impact on the applicant's ability to pursue his/her long-range research objectives. Grants can be for one to two years, are non-renewable, and have a $40,000 maximum award limitation. There are approximately six grants awarded annually. Letters of Intent are due by December 15, with full proposals received by January 15 annually.
Requirements: Otolaryngologists-head and neck surgeons who hold full-time, part-time or contributed service medical school faculty appointments and who have made a commitment to focus their research endeavors on patient-oriented research may apply. Applicants must be sponsored by the Chair of his/her division or department and by an official representative of the institution which would administer the award and in whose name the application is formally submitted.
Amount of Grant: $40,000 maximum
Date(s) Application is Due: Dec 15; Jan 15
Contact: Gail Binderup; (402) 346-5500; fax: (402) 346-5300; email: info@triological.org;; Stephanie L. Jones, Assistant Director; (703) 519-1586 or (703) 836-4444; email: sljones@entnet.org
Internet: http://www.triological.org/researchgrants.htm
Sponsor: Triological Society
555 North 30th Street
Omaha, NE 68131

Trull Foundation Grants 3441

The Trull Foundation was established to share God's bounty in Texas and beyond. The Foundation supports organizations involved with: health care, the coastal Texas environment, seniors, child abuse, neglect, farming, ranching, agriculture, birds, hunger, substance abuse, religion, charity, education, improving the quality of life, especially for those living in poor or oppressed conditions, with a special concern for the needs of Palacios and Matagorda County where the Foundation has it's roots.

Requirements: 501(c)3 tax-exempt organizations and departments, agencies, and other services operated within federal, state, or local government agencies and institutions and agencies affiliated with organized religions and religious bodies are eligible. Proposals should be mailed directly to the foundation, faxed or emailed proposals will not be excepted. See foundation's website for additional proposal guidelines and application forms.

Restrictions: The foundation usually will not make long term commitments; make grants for buildings, endowments, or research; repeat grants to the same project longer than three years; or fund operational expenses except during initial years. Any scholarship funds granted are made to institutions and are administered by those institutions. No scholarships or other funds are granted to individuals.

Samples: El Buen Pastor Early Childhood Development Center, Austin, TX, $8,000 - Student Tuition Scholarships (2008); Palmer Drug Abuse Program of Corpus Christi, Inc., Corpus Christi, TX, $7,000 - Reaching out to the Rural Areas of South Texas (2008); Ducks Unlimited, Inc., Memphis, TN, $10,000 - Texas Prairie Wetlands (2008); Louise Independent School District, Louise, TX, $3,000 - TI-83 calculators for students in Grades 9-12 (2008); Blessing Historical Foundation, Blessing, TX, $15,000 - Hotel Restoration (2008);

Amount of Grant: $250-$20,000 range

Contact: E. Gail Purvis, Executive Director; (361) 972-5241; fax: (361) 972-1109; email: gpurvis@trullfoundation.org

Internet: http://www.trullfoundation.org

Sponsor: Trull Foundation
404 Fourth Street
Palacios, TX 77465

TSA Research Grant Awards 3442

The association accepts applications for grants in the following categories: proposals in basic neuroscience specifically relevant to Tourette syndrome (TS); clinical studies related to the etiology, pathophysiology, and treatment of TS; and one postdoctoral fellowship. Relevant scientific fields include animal models, basal ganglia physiology, biochemistry, epidemiology, genetics, molecular biology, neuroanatomy, neuroimaging, neurology, neuropathology, neuropsychology, neurophysiology, pharmacology, psychiatry, and psychology. As a means of preliminary screening to assess the relevance and quality of intended proposals, a letter of intent briefly describing the scientific basis of the proposed project is requested. An approximate level of project funding should be included. Letters of intent must meet the application deadline. All applicants will be promptly informed as to whether to proceed with a final proposal. Deadline listed is for letter of intent.

Requirements: Investigators already studying TS and those currently working in areas of science that can be applied to the problems of TS are invited to apply.

Amount of Grant: $75,000 maximum PhD and MD applicants; $40,000 maximum postdoctoral fellowships

Date(s) Application is Due: Oct 17

Contact: TSA Scientific Advisory Board, (718) 224-2999 ext 222; fax: (718) 279-9596; email: grantadministrator@tsa-usa.org

Internet: http://www.tsa-usa.org

Sponsor: Tourette Syndrome Association
42-40 Bell Boulevard
Bayside, NY 11361-2874

TWS Foundation Grants 3443

The foundation awards grants to eligible nonprofit organizations in its areas of interest, including community development, arts, health care, public policy, research, and human services. Types of support include general operating support and scholarship funds. There are no application forms or deadlines.

Requirements: Nonprofit organizations, primarily in Connecticut, New York, Rhode Island, and Texas, are eligible.

Geographic Focus: Connecticut; New York; Rhode Island; Texas

Samples: National Center for Policy Analysis (Dallas, TX)—$200,000.; Westerly Hospital Foundation (Westerly, RI)—$100,000.; Philharmonic-Symphony Society of New York (New York, NY)—$10,000.

Amount of Grant: $100-$230,000 range

Contact: Thomas Smith, Trustee

Sponsor: TWS Foundation
323 Railroad Avenue
Greenwich, CT 06830-6306

Tylenol Scholarship 3444

The makers of the Tylenol Family of Products will award 170 scholarships in the amounts of $1000 and $5000 for higher education to students who demonstrate leadership in community activities and school activities and who intend to major in areas that will lead to health-related fields. Apply online at the sponsor's website.

Requirements: Application is open to students who will be attending an undergraduate or graduate course of study in the fall at an accredited two- or four-year college, university or vocational-technical school. This includes those students currently enrolled in an undergraduate or graduate course of study and have one or more years of school remaining. Applicants will be judged on leadership qualities and academic performance.

Amount of Grant: $5,000 - $10,000 range

Date(s) Application is Due: May 15

Contact: Scholarship Program Administrators, Inc. (third party); (615) 320-3149

Internet: http://tylenol.com/page.jhtml?id=tylenol/news/subptyschol.inc&s_kwcid=ContentNetwork|1522864193

Sponsor: McNeil Consumer Healthcare
7050 Camp Hill Road
Fort Washington, PA 19034

U.S. Department of Education 21st Century Community Learning Centers 3445

This program supports the creation of community learning centers that provide academic enrichment opportunities for children, particularly students who attend high-poverty and low-performing schools. The program helps students meet state and local student standards in core academic subjects, such as reading and math; offers students a broad array of enrichment activities that can complement their regular academic programs; and offers literacy and other educational services to the families of participating children.

Requirements: Awards are made to State Education Agencies (SEAs). Local education agencies (LEAs) and nonprofit organization may apply to states for subgrants. Formula grants are awarded to State educational agencies, which in turn manage statewide competitions and award grants to eligible entities. For this program, eligible entity means a local educational agency, community-based organization, another public or private entity, or a consortium of two or more of such agencies, organizations, or entities. States must give priority to applications that are jointly submitted by a local educational agency and a community-based organization or other public or private entity. Consistent with this definition of eligible entities, faith-based organizations are eligible to participate in the program. Each eligible entity that receives an award from the state may use the funds to carry out a broad array of before- and after-school activities (including those held during summer recess periods) to advance student achievement. Many states around the country are conducting competitions to award 21st Century Community Learning Center grants. The State Contact List (http://www.ed.gov/programs/21stcclc/contacts.html#state) now includes links to State websites and application due dates.

Contact: Peter Eldridge, Acting Program Contact; (202) 260-2514; fax: (202) 260-8969; email: 21stCCLC@ed.gov or Peter.Eldridge@ed.gov

Internet: http://www.ed.gov/programs/21stcclc/index.html

Sponsor: U.S. Department of Education
400 Maryland Ave. S.W., Room 3E246
Washington, DC 20202-6200

U.S. Department of Education Erma Byrd Scholarships 3446

The Erma Byrd Scholarship Program provides scholarships to individuals pursuing a course of study that will lead to a career in industrial health and safety occupations, including mine safety. This program is designed to increase the skilled workforce in these fields at both the fundamental skills level and the advanced skills level. The program has a service obligation component, requiring recipients of the scholarship to be employed in a career position directly related to industrial health and safety, including mine safety, for a period of one year upon completion of the degree program. The selected areas of study are: mining and mineral engineering, industrial engineering, occupational safety and health technology/technician, quality control technology/technician, industrial safety technology/technician, hazardous materials information systems technology/technician, mining technology/technician, and occupational health and industrial hygiene. Scholarship recipients must begin such employment no more than six months after the completion of their degree program. Average awards will be as follows: $2,500 associate's degree; $5,000 bachelor's degree; $10,000 graduate degree.

Requirements: Applicants must be: U.S. citizen, national, or permanent resident; pursuing a degree in mining and mineral engineering, industrial engineering, occupational safety and health technology/technician, quality control technology/technician, industrial safety technology/technician, hazardous materials information systems technology/technician, mining technology/technician, or occupational health and industrial hygiene; and, within two years of completing an associate's, bachelor's, or graduate degree at an accredited U.S. institution of higher education. As part of your application package, your Social Security Number must be submitted to the U.S. Department of Education via postal mail using the form on page 34 of the application package. For security reasons, DO NOT submit this form via email with the rest of your application.

Amount of Grant: $2,500 - $10,000

Date(s) Application is Due: Jul 31

Contact: Lauren Kennedy; (202) 502-7630; fax: (202) 502-7675; email: ermabyrdprogram@ed.gov

Internet: http://www.ed.gov/programs/ermabyrd/index.html

Sponsor: U.S. Department of Education
1990 K Street, N.W., Room 6121
Washington, DC 20006-8524

U.S. Department of Education Rehabilitation Engineering Research Centers Grants 3447

RERCs support activities that: (1) lead to the development of methods, procedures, and devices that will benefit individuals with disabilities, especially those with the most severe disabilities; or (2) involve technology for the purposes of enhancing opportunities for meeting the needs of and addressing the barriers confronted by individuals with disabilities in all aspects of their lives. Types of activities supported include: the development of technological systems for persons with disabilities; stimulation of the production and distribution of equipment in the private sector; and clinical evaluations

of equipment. Awards are for five years, except that grants to new recipients or to support new or innovative research may be made for fewer than five years.
Requirements: States, Institutions of Higher Education (IHEs), Nonprofit Organizations, public or private agencies – including for-profit agencies, Indian tribes, and tribal organizations may apply. RERCs must be operated by or in collaboration with one or more institutions of higher education or nonprofit organizations.
Amount of Grant: $850,000 – $1,000,000
Date(s) Application is Due: Apr 1; Aug 1
Contact: Donna Nangle; (202) 245-7462; fax: (202) 245-7323; email: donna.nangle@ed.gov
Internet: http://www.ed.gov/programs/rerc/index.html
Sponsor: U.S. Department of Education
OSERS, 400 Maryland Avenue, S.W., Room 6030, PCP
Washington, DC 20202-2700

U.S. Department of Education Rehabilitation Research Training Centers 3448
The RRTCs conduct coordinated and advanced programs of research, training, and information dissemination. Each RRTC has a major program of research in a particular area, such as mental illness, vocational rehabilitation (VR), or independent living, which is specified by the National Institute on Disability and Rehabilitation Research (NIDRR). The RRTCs must serve as centers of national excellence and national or regional resources for providers and individuals with disabilities and their representatives. RRTC awards are for five years, except that grants to new recipients or to support new or innovative research may be made for fewer than five years.
Requirements: Note: Each year, competitions are held in specific areas that determine the types of projects. Eligible applicants include Institutions of Higher Education and Nonprofit Organizations. States, public or private agencies – including for-profit agencies, Indian tribes, and tribal organizations may also apply. Rehabilitation research and training centers must be operated by or in collaboration with: (1) one or more institutions of higher education or (2) one or more providers of rehabilitation or other appropriate services.
Amount of Grant: up to $675,000
Date(s) Application is Due: Aug 21; Aug 22
Contact: Donna Nangle; (202) 245-7462; fax: (202) 245-7323; email: donna.nangle@ed.gov
Internet: http://www.ed.gov/programs/rrtc/index.html
Sponsor: U.S. Department of Education
OSERS, 400 Maryland Avenue, SW, Room 6030, PCP
Washington, DC 20202-2700

U.S. Department of Education Rehabilitation Training—Rehabilitation Continuing Education Programs — Institute on Rehabilitation Issues 3449
The purpose of the Technical Assistance and Dissemination To Improve Services and Results For Children With Disabilities program is to promote academic achievement and to improve results for children with disabilities by providing technical assistance (TA), supporting model demonstration projects, disseminating useful information, and implementing activities that are supported by scientifically based research. The purpose of this priority is to support the establishment and operation of State Technical Assistance Projects To Improve Services and Results for Children Who Are Deaf-Blind (projects). Grants are available to support projects in the District of Columbia; Puerto Rico; and the Virgin Islands.
Requirements: Eligible applicants include: SEAs; LEAs, including public charter schools that are considered LEAs under State law; IHEs; other public agencies; private nonprofit organizations; outlying areas; FAS; Indian tribes or tribal organizations; and for-profit organizations. The projects funded under this competition must make positive efforts to employ and advance in employment qualified individuals with disabilities (see section 606 of IDEA). Applicants and grant recipients funded under this competition must involve individuals with disabilities or parents of individuals with disabilities ages birth through 26 in planning, implementing, and evaluating the projects (see section 682(a)(1)(A) of IDEA).
Restrictions: Funds awarded under this priority may not be used to provide direct early intervention services under Part C of IDEA, or direct special education and related services under Part B of IDEA. The Department will reject an application for a State project that proposes a budget exceeding the funding level for any single budget period of 12 months.
Geographic Focus: District of Columbia; Puerto Rico; U.S. Virgin Islands
Amount of Grant: $30,000 - $65,000
Date(s) Application is Due: Jul 17
Internet: http://www.ed.gov/programs/rsatrain/applicant.html#84264c
Sponsor: U.S. Department of Education
400 Maryland Avenue, SW, Room 5038
Washington, DC 20202-2800

U.S. Department of Education Special Education—National Activities— Parent Information Centers 3450
The purpose of this program is to ensure that parents of children with disabilities receive training and information to help improve results for their children. Awards are made for parent information centers, community parent centers, and for technical assistance to such centers. This program includes the following grants competitions: Community Parent Resource Centers (CFDA 84.328C); Parent Training and Information Centers (CFDA 84.328M); and, Technical Assistance for the Parent Centers (CFDA 84.328R).
Requirements: Nonprofit organizations are eligible to apply. For Parent Training and Information (PTI) Centers (# 84.328M), parent organizations may apply. A parent organization is a private nonprofit organization (other than an institution of higher education [IHE]) that: (a) has a board of directors (1) the majority of whom are parents of children with disabilities ages birth through 26; (2) that includes (i) individuals working in the fields of special education, related services, and early intervention, (ii) individuals with disabilities, and (iii) the parent and professional members of which are broadly representative of the population to be served, including low-income parents of limited English proficient (LEP) children; and (b) has as its mission serving families of children with disabilities who are ages birth through 26, and have the full range of disabilities described in Sec. 602(3) of the Individuals with Disabilities Education Act(IDEA). For Community Parent Resource Centers (CPRC; # 84.328C), local parent organizations may apply (same requirements as listed above for PTI Centers). Additionally, *Community to be served* refers to a community whose members experience significant isolation from available sources of information and support as a result of cultural, economic, linguistic, or other circumstances deemed appropriate by the secretary of education. For Technical Assistance for Parent Training and Information Centers (# 84.328R), state education agencies (SEAs); local education agencies (LEAs); public charter schools that are LEAs under state law; IHEs; other public agencies; private nonprofit organizations; outlying areas (American Samoa, Guam, the Northern Mariana Islands, and the U.S. Virgin Islands); freely associated states; Indian tribes or tribal organizations; and for-profit organizations may apply.
Amount of Grant: $100,000 – $500,000
Date(s) Application is Due: Feb 26; Apr 18
Contact: Lisa Gorove; (202) 245-7357; fax: (202) 245-7617; email: Lisa.Gorove@ed.gov
Internet: http://www.ed.gov/programs/oseppic/index.html
Sponsor: U.S. Department of Education
OSERS, 400 Maryland Avenue, S.W., Room 4056, PCP
Washington, DC 20202-2600

U.S. Department of Education United States-Russia Program: Improving Research and Educational Activities in Higher Education 3451
The program provides grants that demonstrate partnerships between Russian and American institutions of higher education that contribute to the development and promotion of educational opportunities between the two nations, particularly in the areas of mutual foreign language learning and the cooperative study of mathematics and science. Collaborative projects comprised of partnerships of Russian and American universities and colleges will be supported.
Requirements: Institutions of Higher Education (IHEs) or combinations of IHEs and other public and private nonprofit institutions and agencies are eligible to apply. Applicants must select one of three academic discipline as the subject area for their grant proposal: (A) Environmental Science Studies; (B) Biotechnology; or, (C) Any discipline, other than (A) and (B). Applications are invited from institutions of higher education with the capacity to contribute to a collaborative project in the areas listed with a Russian institution. The consortium partners, through promoting the study of and communication in foreign languages, are expected to increase awareness and understanding of the two cultures, and to strengthen the professional and scholarly ties between the two countries. Russian institutions will apply to The Russian Ministry of Education and Science for funding.
Restrictions: Any application that proposes a budget exceeding $150,000 for a single budget period of 12 months will be rejected. The Assistant Secretary for Postsecondary Education may change the maximum amount through a notice published in the Federal Register.
Amount of Grant: $189,000 average
Date(s) Application is Due: Jul 7
Contact: Krish Mathur, Coordinator, U.S.-Russia Program; (202) 502-7512; fax: (202) 502-7877; email: Krish.Mathur@ed.gov
Internet: http://www.ed.gov/programs/fipserussia/index.html
Sponsor: U.S. Department of Education
1990 K Street, N.W., Room 6155
Washington, DC 20006-8544

U.S. Department of Education Vocational Rehabilitation Services Projects for American Indians with Disabilities Grants 3452
The program provides financial assistance for the establishment and operations of vocational rehabilitation (VR) services programs for American Indians with disabilities living on or near a federal or state reservation. The purpose of this program is to assist tribal governments to develop or to increase their capacity to provide a program of vocational rehabilitation services, in a culturally relevant manner, to American Indians with disabilities residing on or near federal or state reservations. The program's goal is to enable these individuals, consistent with their individual strengths, resources, priorities, concerns, abilities, capabilities, and informed choice, to prepare for and engage in gainful employment. Program services are provided under an individualized plan for employment and may include native healing services.
Requirements: The governing body of an Indian tribe or consortia of such governing bodies located on federal and state reservations may apply.
Amount of Grant: $350,000 - $450,000
Date(s) Application is Due: May 5; Jun 12
Contact: Alfreda Reeves (202) 245-7485, email: alfreda.reeves@ed.gov; August Martin (202) 245-7410, email: august.martin@ed.gov
Internet: http://www.ed.gov/programs/vramerind/index.html
Sponsor: U.S. Department of Education
OSERS, 400 Maryland Avenue, S.W., Room 5051, PCP
Washington, DC 20202-6400

U.S. Lacrosse EAD Grants 3453

U.S. Lacrosse is playing a leading role in ongoing research and is committed to educating the national lacrosse community about the life-saving value of having Automatic External Defibrillators (AEDs) available during lacrosse games and practices. In order to achieve that goal, U.S. Lacrosse, the national governing body of the sport, and Cardiac Science, a leading manufacturer of cardiology products, are offering an AED grant program which provides an AED and comprehensive management of AED and CPR training to lacrosse leagues or U.S. Lacrosse chapters.
Requirements: Applicant must be a current member of U.S. Lacrosse. Awarded group must budget $1295 towards the AED Grant Program.
Date(s) Application is Due: Nov 30
Contact: Sarah Newman, Manager of Programs and Grants; (410) 235-6882; fax: (410) 366-6735; email: snewman@uslacrosse.org
Internet: http://www.uslacrosse.org/programs/AEDgrantprogram.phtml
Sponsor: U.S. Lacrosse
113 W. University Parkway
Baltimore, MD 21210

UCLA / RAND Corporation Post-Doctoral Fellowships 3454

The post-doctoral training program is jointly housed in the RAND Health Sciences program and the UCLA School of Public Health. Post-doctoral fellows have the option of pursuing a Masters degree in the UCLA Department of Health Services. The grant covers all tuition and fees, as well as a stipend, which currently ranges from $35,568 to $51,036, depending on the number of years of post-doctoral experience. Travel money is also available for fellows to attend professional meetings.
Requirements: To be eligible, candidates must have obtained a Ph.D., medical degree, or other professional doctoral degree. Awards will last two years. Fellows will be required to attend at least 8 courses at UCLA or RAND, including three courses in health services research methods, two in statistics, and three in health services issue areas. Those pursuing a Masters degree must complete a total of 12 courses. Upon arrival, fellows will align with an ongoing research project at RAND or UCLA. RAND and UCLA have numerous ongoing projects in the health services research area. These fall into several areas, including: access/utilization among the underserved; assessing quality, effectiveness, outcomes; health behaviors; alternative delivery systems; hospital and physician payment; health care cost containment; technology assessment; private health insurance; international comparisons. By the end of the first year, the fellow will identify a research idea and write a proposal. The proposal may be addressed to the principal investigator of an ongoing research project, or to an outside funding agency. By the end of the program, the fellow will prepare an article on research conducted during the fellowship, and submit it to a peer reviewed journal. This can either be done alone, or in collaboration with the research director or other member of the fellow's research team.
Amount of Grant: $35,568 - $51,036
Contact: RAND Health Communications; (310) 393-0411, ext. 7775; email: RAND_Health@rand.org
Internet: http://www.ph.ucla.edu/hs/post_doctoral.html
Sponsor: RAND Corporation
1776 Main Street, P.O. Box 2138
Santa Monica, CA 90407-2138

UICC American Cancer Society International Fellowships for Beginning Investigators 3455

The international fellowships fund 12-month basic or clinical research projects in the areas of epidemiology, prevention, detection, diagnosis, treatment, and psycho-oncology that foster a bidirectional flow of knowledge, experience, expertise, and innovation to and from the United States. Candidates should be in the early stages of their careers. Applications that are geared to the development of specific cancer control measures in developing and central and east European countries are particularly encouraged. Six to eight fellowships, with tenures beginning in April, will be awarded each year.
Requirements: Eligible candidates should hold assistant professorships or similar positions at their home institutes and have, ordinarily, a minimum of two and a maximum of ten years of postdoctoral experience after obtaining their MD or PhD degrees or equivalents.
Restrictions: Candidates who are physically present at the proposed host institute while their applications are under consideration are not eligible for UICC fellowships.
Samples: Paula Ximena Fernandez-Calotti, from Laboratory of Oncohematology Institute of Hematology Research, M.R. Castex, Argentina, to the Department of Biochemistry and Molecular Biology, University of Barcelona, Spain (2007); Nikita A. Makretsov, from the Department of Pathology & Laboratory Medicine, Memorial University of Newfoundland, Canada, to the Department of Oncology Hutchinson / MRC Research Centre, United Kingdom (2007).
Amount of Grant: $45,000
Date(s) Application is Due: Dec 1
Contact: Beate Vought, Fellowships Coordinator; +41 22 809 1843; fax: +41 22 809 1810; email: fellows@uicc.ch
Internet: http://www.uicc.org/index.php?option=com_content&task=view&id=14259&Itemid=182
Sponsor: International Union Against Cancer / American Cancer Society
62, route de Frontenex
Geneva 1207 Switzerland

UICC International Cancer Technology Transfer (ICRETT) Fellowships 3456

The program helps to facilitate rapid international transfer of cancer research techiques and technology and clinical management skills. It is hoped that funding will support the exchange of knowledge and enhance skills in basic, clinical, behavioral, and epidemiological areas of cancer research, in cancer control and prevention (including tobacco control). Participants should acquire appropriate clinical management, diagnostic and therapeutic skills for effective application and use in the home organization upon their return. There are 120 to 150 awards available annually, with applications accepted at any time and notification generally within 60 days of registration.
Requirements: Eligible applicants include appropriately qualified investigators, pathologists, epidemiologists, cancer registrars, behavioral scientists, tobacco control activists, laboratory technicians, clinicians and general practitioners, generally in the early stages of their careers.
Amount of Grant: $3,400
Contact: Beate Vought, Fellowships Coordinator; +41 22 809 1843; fax: +41 22 809 1810; email: fellows@uicc.ch
Internet: http://www.uicc.org/index.php?option=com_content&task=view&id=14262&Itemid=185
Sponsor: International Union Against Cancer
62, route de Frontenex
Geneva 1207 Switzerland

UICC Raisa Gorbachev Memorial International Cancer Fellowships 3457

This award is funded by UICC International Cancer Foundation and enables qualified beginning pathologists to carry out specific research or training project relating to the many fields of oncology, and should be centred on an appropriate training period in modern diagnostic tools in the field of pathology. The Fellowship is conditional on Fellows returning to the home institutes/country at the end of the fellowship period. The original Fellowships cannot be prolonged, or run concurrently with other awards, even those funded by other agencies. They can however, be extended subject to the written approval of home and host supervisors and at no additional cost to UICC i.e. up to a total duration of 3 months. Should return of the Fellow to their home country be delayed past these 3 months, 50 percent of the travel award must be reimbursed to UICC.
Requirements: The candidate must possess the appropriate professional qualifications and experience according to the specifications described on the website and must currently be engaged in cancer research, clinical oncology practice, or cancer society work. To permit effective communication at the host institute, the candidate must have adequate fluency in a common language. The candidate must also be on the staff payroll of a university, research laboratory or institute, hospital, oncology unit to where they will return at the end of a fellowship.
Restrictions: Candidates attached to commercial entities are not eligible. Fellowships cannot be granted to candidates who are already physically present at the proposed host institute whilst their applications are under consideration.
Contact: Beate Vought, Fellowships Coordinator; +41 22 809 1843; fax: +41 22 809 1810; email: fellows@uicc.ch
Internet: http://www.uicc.org/index.php?option=com_content&task=view&id=15956&Itemid=301
Sponsor: International Union Against Cancer
62, route de Frontenex
Geneva 1207 Switzerland

UICC Yamagiwa-Yoshida Memorial International Cancer Study Grants 3458

These study grants enable cancer investigators from any country to establish bilateral research projects abroad that exploit complementary materials or skills, including advanced training in experimental methods or special techniques. There are 14 to 16 three-to six-month grants awarded each year. Selection takes place twice annually, with recipients notified in mid-April and mid-October. Grants should be taken up within six months following notification. Travel awards contribute toward the least expensive international two-way airfare or other appropriate form of transport. Financial support is not provided for dependents. Application materials are available on the Web site.
Requirements: Candidates should have appropriate scientific or medical qualifications and be actively engaged in cancer research.
Samples: Dr. Hakan Akbulut, from Department of Medical Oncology, Cebeci Hospital, Turkey, to Sydney Kimmel Cancer Center, U.S.A (2007); Dr. Gil Ast, from Department of Human Molecular Genetics & Biochemistry, Sackler School of Medicine, Israel, to Department of Biochemistry, School of Medicine, University of Washington, U.S.A (2007).
Amount of Grant: $10,000 average for three months
Date(s) Application is Due: Jan 15; Jul 1
Contact: Beate Vought, Fellowships Coordinator; +41 22 809 1843; fax: +41 22 809 1810; email: fellows@uicc.ch
Internet: http://www.uicc.org/index.php?option=com_content&task=view&id=15958&Itemid=302
Sponsor: International Union Against Cancer
62, route de Frontenex
Geneva 1207 Switzerland

United Kingdom Foundation for the Study of Infant Deaths Grants 3459

The foundation awards grants in England, Wales, and Northern Ireland for research into sudden infant death syndrome. Specific areas of interest include epidemiology, immunology, pathology, statistics, and infection. Graduate researchers of all nationalities are considered.
Amount of Grant: @L100,000 maximum
Date(s) Application is Due: Mar 1
Contact: Secretary-General, 0870 787 0885; fax: 0870 787 0725; email: research@sids.org.uk

Internet: http://www.sids.org.uk/fsid/grants.htm
Sponsor: United Kingdom Foundation for the Study of Infant Deaths
Artillery House, 11-19 Artillery Row
London SW1P 1RT United Kingdom

Union Benevolent Association Grants **3460**

The Union Benevolent Association attempts to distribute its limited resources as widely as is consistent with the needs of its recipients. It tends to select projects that aid large groups of individuals among the disadvantaged. Grants have frequently been given to help support summer camping and educational experiences for inner city youths, to aid programs for the elderly and handicapped, to assist those involved in legal, medical, and social difficulties, to improve the quality of life in deteriorating neighborhoods, and to provide deprived young people with employable skills and artistic and cultural experiences. The Board prefers to make grants for specific projects and, as a rule, does not contribute toward general operating revenues or major building programs. It limits its grants to projects serving the needs of residents of Philadelphia. Preference is given to organizations with budgets of 2 million and below, and which leverage the use of volunteers.
Requirements: The Association makes grants only to 501 (c)(3) non-profit organizations,that work with people in need, within the city of Philadelphia, PA. Submitted proposals must be on the Delaware Valley Grantmakers Common Application Form (available on the Union Benevolent Association website) and be received (not posted) by email AND regular mail on or before 5:00PM on the deadline date.
Restrictions: The Association does not make grants to support capital renovations or to individuals.
Geographic Focus: Pennsylvania
Date(s) Application is Due: Apr 30; Sep 30
Contact: Fernando Chang-Muy, Administrator; (215) 763-7670
; fax: (215) 731-9457; email: info@uba1831.org
Internet: http://www.uba1831.org/grant_guide.html
Sponsor: Union Benevolent Association
1616 Walnut Street, Suite 800
Philadelphia, PA 19103

Union County Community Foundation Grants **3461**

Established in 1989, the Union County Community Foundation is a regional affiliate of Foundation for the Carolinas. The Foundation assists donors in making charitable gifts to the community, provides services for nonprofit organizations to create new or manage existing endowments and makes grants for new projects. Preference will be given to programs that meet the following criteria: serve those who are mentally or physically challenged as a result of visual and/or hearing impairments; provide professional development for Union County public school teachers; or address community needs through innovative approaches (funding available only to programs that cannot be covered by normal budgets of existing charitable agencies). Giving limited for the benefit of Union County, NC.
Requirements: Non-profits in or benefiting the community of Union County, North Carolina are eligible to apply. Contact the Foundation, an application form is required to submit a proposal. Applicants should submit the following: signature and title of chief executive officer; copy of most recent annual report/audited financial statement/990; copy of current year's organizational budget and/or project budget; listing of board of directors, trustees, officers and other key people and their affiliations; copy of IRS Determination Letter.
Restrictions: No grants to individuals, or for capital campaigns, ongoing operating budgets beyond the seed level, publication of books, conferences, or endowment funds.
Geographic Focus: North Carolina
Contact: Karen Coppadge; (704) 973-4559; email: kcoppadge@fftc.org
Sponsor: Union County Community Foundation
217 South Tryon Street
Charlotte, NC 28202-3201

United Cerebral Palsy Research Grants **3462**

The foundation is interested in stimulating and providing funding for pilot studies on research important to the prevention of cerebral palsy and to improvement in the quality of life of persons with disabilities due to cerebral palsy and related developmental disorders. Research grants generally are awarded in support of basic and clinical science pilot studies or for time-limited clinical studies or trials. High priority is given to prevention of prematurity, decrease of perinatal neurologic morbidity, prevention of central nervous system infections of the newborn and to medical, surgical, and bioengineering methods that may improve the functioning of persons with cerebral palsy addressing issues such as impaired mobility, impaired communication skills, swallowing, drooling, and effects of aging on further diminution of function. Funds are awarded initially for a period not to exceed two years and may be renewed for a one- or two-year period, to a total of four years.
Requirements: Grants are awarded to institutions or organizations on behalf of a principal investigator in support of biomedical and bioengineering research in areas that have a significant relationship to cerebral palsy.
Amount of Grant: $50,000 maximum annually
Contact: Medical Director, (202) 973-7140; fax: (202) 776-0414; email: lsmithslade@ucp.org
Internet: http://www.ucp.org/ucp_generaldoc.cfm/1/4/23/23-23/113
Sponsor: United Cerebral Palsy Research and Educational Foundation
1660 L St NW, Suite 700
Washington, DC 20036-5602

United Methodist Church Global AIDS Fund Grants **3463**

This fund represents the commitment of every United Methodist to put a stop to HIV/AIDS in our world. It supports education, prevention, care, and treatment programs for people living with HIV/AIDS. The plan specifies that 25 percent of what each annual conference raises should be used in that conference for AIDS work, either locally or in global projects.
Requirements: Overseas programs fitting the mission of the Global AIDS Fund may apply to receive a grant. The application should propose work in one or more of the following types of activities: (1) Promoting HIV/AIDS awareness and prevention by education and information; (2) Behavior modification; (3) Voluntary testing and counseling; (4) Treatment of persons with AIDS; (5) Home Based Care; (6) Care of orphans and vulnerable children.
Restrictions: This program is only for grants covering primarily United Methodist or Methodist-related projects for up to a one-year period.
Samples: 2008: Mozambique Annual Conference- Communicating against HIV/AIDS newspaper ($10,000); University Church in Toledo, Ohio- HIV/AIDS education for pastors of sub-Saharan Africa, Zambia ($11,850); Helping Children Worldwide, Inc-Mercy Hospital HIV/AIDS Outreach, Sierra Leone ($10,000); Five Points Institute for Pastoral Education, U.S.A- Pastoral Counseling Training, for pastors, health workers and social workers, Bedfordview Methodist Church ($3,000); Jamkhed Comprehensive Rural Health Project, India- Promote HIV/AIDS awareness and prevention education and information ($15,000).
Contact: Linda Bales, email: lbales@umc-gbcs.org; Donna Brandyberry, email: dbrandyberry@umc-gbcs.org
Internet: http://new.gbgm-umc.org/umcor/work/health/hivaids/aids-fund/
Sponsor: United Methodist Church
475 Riverside Drive
New York, NY 10115

United Methodist Church Malaria Control Grants **3464**

United Methodists are joining forces with others to make malaria's grip on the lives of children and adults a part of history. These efforts include the United Methodist Community-Based program that provides education, medication, and mosquito nets to prevent and treat malaria.
Requirements: The application should propose work in one or more of the following types of activities: (1) Promoting Malaria awareness and prevention by education and information; (2) Distribution of Insecticide Treated Bed Nets; (3) Indoor spraying; (4) Testing; (5) Malaria case management; (6) Preventative treatment in pregnant women. Download the required application form at the sponsor's website.
Restrictions: This program is only for United Methodist and Methodist-related projects outside the U.S.
Contact: Dr. Cherian Thomas; Health and Welfare Ministries; (212) 870-3870; email: cthomas@gbgm-umc.org
Internet: http://new.gbgm-umc.org/umcor/work/health/malaria/
Sponsor: United Methodist Church
475 Riverside Drive, Room 330
New York, NY 10115

United Methodist Health Ministry Fund Grants **3465**

Grants are awarded to health care projects proposed by eligible organizations to respond to needs and build on assets of local, regional, and state situations. The Health Fund is targeting three areas for funding: Access to health care; Oral health; and, Healthy nutrition and exercise.
Requirements: Grants can be awarded only to 501(c)3 organizations or governmental entities with projects to benefit the health of Kansas residents. Grants have one or more of the following purposes: (a) Develop new or expanded, sustainable program resources to provide quality services; (b) Change the delivery system to meet demands, improve access/quality, or reduce cost; (c) Test innovative ideas for improved service delivery; (d) Offer public education for improvement of individual and community health care; (e) Provide group opportunities for health care providers to improve critical skills; (f) Develop technical expertise, collaborations, and similar supports for improvement and change in health care service delivery and education. Contact the sponsor before beginning a grant application - the Health Fund will not accept unsolicited and unauthorized applications, and will be automatically rejected them without consideration.
Restrictions: Grants are not awarded to individuals or for individual medical, dental, or other personal care treatment. Generally, capital projects and endowments are not funded. The fund does not provide regular operating expenses of on-going projects. The Health Fund does not fund projects in other U.S. states (outside of Kansas) or foreign nations.
Contact: Virginia Elliott, Vice President for Programs; (620) 662-8586; fax: (620) 662-8597; email: velliot@healthfund.org
Internet: http://www.healthfund.org/funding.php
Sponsor: United Methodist Health Ministry Fund
100 East First Avenue, P.O. Box 1384
Hutchinson, KS 67504-1384

United Technologies Corporation Grants **3466**

The corporation focuses its contributions programs in communities where UTC has major facilities with a substantial employee residence population. In Greater Hartford, UTC supports grants in arts and culture, math and science education, the environment, and human services (through the United Way). Nationally, UTC provides grants to arts organizations and groups engaged in environmental sustainability work. Funding proposals should include a brief letter, the organization's most recent financial statement,

a list of its directors, and IRS tax-exemption documents. UTC has an employee matching gift program limited to degree-granting educational institutions, cultural, and environmental organizations. The corporation, on a limited basis, contributes to capital building funds in support of specific business objectives. General operating grants, program development grants, and work-study programs are additional types of support. UTC Corporate will accept online grant applications throughout the year. UTC business units accept grant applications between March 1 and June 1 of each year.
Requirements: U.S. 501(c)3 tax-exempt organizations and international tax-exempt organizations are eligible.
Restrictions: The corporation will not fund partisan political organizations, individuals, organizations, religious organizations with programs limited to or expressly for their membership, controversial social causes on which there are strong differences of opinion, organizations that are the recipients of federated drives to which the corporation contributes (capital campaigns excluded), and endowment campaigns.
Date(s) Application is Due: Jun 1
Contact: Krista Pilot, Director, (860) 728-7000; fax: (860) 728-7041; email: contribu@corphq.utc.com
Internet: http://www.utc.com/responsibility/social/index.htm
Sponsor: United Technologies Corporation
1 Financial Plaza, MS 503
Hartford, CT 06101

Unity Foundation Of LaPorte County Grants 3467
The Unity Foundation of LaPorte County makes discretionary and field of interest grants to charitable organizations in the area of the arts, education, health and human services, the environment, and the community for the benefit of the citizens of LaPorte County, Indiana. The Unity Foundation of LaPorte County is particularly interested in funding: projects that are not adequately being serviced by existing community resources;start-up costs for new programs; one-time projects or needs; projects that provide leverage for generating other funds and community resources; projects that facilitate cooperation and collaboration between organizations and the communities within LaPorte County, Indiana.
Requirements: Generally, only charitable organizations with a verifiable 501(c)3 IRS status operating or offering programs in LaPorte County, Indiana will be considered for funding.
Restrictions: No grants will be made: to churches for sectarian religious programs; for operating budgets or for basic municipal or educational functions and services; for endowment campaigns or for previously incurred debts; to provide long-term funding. No grants will be made for post-event or after-the-fact situations.
Geographic Focus: Indiana
Date(s) Application is Due: July 15
Contact: Unity Foundation Office; (219) 879-0327 or (888) 898-6489; email: unity@uflc.net
Internet: http://www.grantselect.com/gs/editorial/
Sponsor: Unity Foundation Of LaPorte County, Inc.
619 Franklin Street, P.O. Box 527
Michigan City, IN 46361

University of Calgary Nursing Alumni Scholarship 3468
One scholarship per year is given to a Canadian citizen or landed immigrant of high academic standing who is registered in or admitted to a full-time master's program, who intends to make a career in nursing, and who is a registered member of the University of Calgary Faculty of Nursing Alumni Association. The scholarship may be used for any area or discipline at the master's level related to nursing. Annual deadline dates may vary; contact program staff for exact dates.
Requirements: To be eligible, applicants must be Canadian citizens or landed immigrants; graduate students in a master's program who intend to make a career in nursing; and registered members of the University of Calgary Faculty of Nursing Alumni Association.
Amount of Grant: $C1000
Date(s) Application is Due: Dec 2
Contact: Maria Lavoie, Graduate Scholarship Officer, (403) 220-8483; email: lavoiem@ucalgary.ca or ucawards@ucalgary.ca
Internet: http://www.grad.ucalgary.ca/funding/internal_scholarships/lev_4/nurs_alum_burs.htm
Sponsor: University of Calgary
2500 University Dr NW, Earth Sciences Building, Room 720
Calgary, AB T2N 1N4 Canada

University of California President's Postdoctoral Fellowships 3469
The fellowship, originally designed to encourage applications from minority and women scholars in areas where they were severely underrepresented, is now open to all qualified candidates. The program provides postdoctoral fellowships to qualified persons who intend to pursue academic careers and to enhance their prospects for appointment to faculty positions at the University of California and other institutions of higher education. In addition to financial support, fellowships include mentorship and guidance in areas critical to success in an academic career. Application materials are available upon request.
Requirements: Applicants must be U.S. citizens or permanent residents and must hold a PhD from an accredited university. Applicants are required to have earned their PhD degree by June 30 of the year for which they are applying.
Amount of Grant: $40,000-$50,000 (depending on experience) annual stipend and up to $4000 for research-related expenses
Date(s) Application is Due: Nov 15
Contact: Kim Adkinson, President's Fellowships, (510) 987-9503; fax: (510) 587-6077; email: kim.adkinson@ucop.edu
Internet: http://www.ucop.edu/acadadv/ppfp
Sponsor: University of California Office of the President
1111 Franklin Street, 11th Floor
Oakland, CA 94607-5200

University of Georgia Counseling and Psychological Services Postdoctoral Fellowship 3470
The program is designed to develop advanced skills in the practice of clinical and counseling psychology. The postdoctoral program provides fellows an opportunity to refine and expand experience in the following areas: clinical practice with individuals, couples and groups, assessment, crisis intervention, workshops, and educational programming. Postdoctoral fellows will work in close collaboration with senior staff and will function as professionals with many of the same responsibilities. Fellows attend all case conferences, professional development workshops, and staff meetings. In addition to the stipend, fellows are also eligible for staff benefits, including health and dental insurance, retirement, vacation, sick leave, professional development, exercise facility, library privileges, and licensing preparation time. Guidelines are available online. Annual deadline dates may vary; contact program staff for exact dates.
Requirements: Admission requirements include completion of all professional degree requirements from a regionally accredited institution of higher education or an APA/CPA'accredited program and completion of an APA approved predoctoral internship. Fellow must have received diploma before first day of fellowship or have a letter from Director of Graduate Studies verifying that all degree requirements have been met. Previous counseling center experience is preferred.
Amount of Grant: $25,000 stipend
Date(s) Application is Due: Mar 11
Contact: Dr. Al Clarke, University Health Center, (706) 542-2273; email: aclarke@uhs.uga.edu
Internet: http://www.uhs.uga.edu/CAPS/postdoc/index.html
Sponsor: University of Georgia
University of Georgia Health Ctr
Athens, GA 30602-1755

Until There's a Cure Foundation Grants 3471
The foundation supports HIV/AIDS organizations throughout the United States. Grants focus on four priorities: care and services to meet the immediate needs of people living with HIV/AIDS, prevention education, vaccine development and research, and policy development and research. Types of support include capital campaigns, equipment acquisition, program development, and general operating support.
Requirements: 501(c)3 nonprofit U.S. organizations are eligible for grant support.
Restrictions: The foundation does not make grants for: for walk-a-thons, tournaments, or special events; to organizations with religious affiliations, unless the program is open to the entire community without regard to religious beliefs; for costs already incurred by an organization; or to fund general administration expenses of an organization rather than for specific projects and programs
Samples: AIDS Service Agency of North Carolina (NC)—$9000.; AIDS Task Force Greater Cleveland (Cleveland, OH)—$41,818.; AIDS Walk Atlanta (Atlanta, GA)—$15,000.; Wisconsin AIDS Fund (WI)—$40,000.
Amount of Grant: $1000-$40,000 range; $2500-$4000 average
Date(s) Application is Due: Apr 29
Contact: Grants Administrator, (800) 888-6845 or (650) 332-3200; fax: (650) 332-3210; email: grants@utac.org
Internet: http://www.utac.org
Sponsor: Until There's a Cure Foundation
560 Mountain Home Road
Redwood City, CA 94062

U.S. Airways Community Contributions 3472
U.S. Airways invests in community organizations and initiatives to enhance quality of life in markets served by the airline. The airline's funding priorities include arts and culture, health and human services, and education and environment in the following hub markets and focus cities: Boston, Charlotte, Las Vegas, New York, Philadelphia, Phoenix, Pittsburgh and Washington, DC.
Requirements: Tax exempt organizations in the airline's market areas are eligible to apply. All requests must be submitted in writing on the organization's letterhead 6-8 weeks prior to the event and any print deadlines. All completed proposals will receive a written response within 6-8 weeks from receipt. The Contributions Committee meets bi-weekly to review requests.
Restrictions: Funding will not be considered for: Pass through and start-up organizations; Individuals, including support for specific students, researchers or conference fees; Endowment programs; Foundations which are themselves grant-making entities; Professional associations; Debt-reduction campaigns; Fundraising activities related to individual sponsorship (i.e. walk-a-thons); Service clubs (i.e. Lions, Rotary, Kiwanis); Sports teams, political, labor or fraternal organizations, scouting groups and religious organizations; Organizations or programs funded 50% or more by government sources; Individual schools; district and system-wide education programs will be considered; Capital and building campaigns.
Geographic Focus: Arizona; District of Columbia; Massachusetts; Nevada; New York; North Carolina; Pennsylvania
Contact: Community Relations; email: community.relations@usairways.com

Internet: http://www.usairways.com/awa/content/aboutus/corporategiving/default.aspx
Sponsor: U.S. Airways Inc.
Community Relations Department, 4000 E. Sky Harbor Boulevard
Phoenix, AZ 85034

U.S. Airways Community Foundation Grants 3473

The community foundation supports multi-year capital and building campaigns by 501(c)3 non-profit organizations operating in U.S. Airways' hub markets of Charlotte, Philadelphia and Phoenix. Grant application deadlines are April 1 and October 1 of each year. Grants will be made in late May and November.
Requirements: Grantees must be 501 (c)(3) nonprofit organizations that operate in one of U.S. Airways' hub cities (Charlotte, Philadelphia and Phoenix) and improve the quality and availability of charitable health care; artistic and cultural organizations; education; and/or community services. Support includes multi-year capital and building campaigns only
Restrictions: The foundation will not consider funding for endowment programs; professional associations; debt-reduction campaigns; service clubs (i.e. Lions, Rotary and Kiwanis); political, labor/fraternal or sports organizations; individual schools; general operating support; staff/consultant fees; hardware, software; infrastructure; religious activities.
Geographic Focus: Arizona; North Carolina; Pennsylvania
Date(s) Application is Due: Apr 1; Oct 1
Contact: Julie Coleman, Vice President; (480) 693-3652; email: community.relations@usairways.com
Internet: http://www.usairways.com/awa/content/aboutus/corporategiving/default.aspx
Sponsor: U.S. Airways Community Foundation
4000 E. Sky Harbor Boulevard
Phoenix, AZ 85034

U.S. CRDF Leishmaniasis: Collaborative Research Opportunities in North Africa and the Middle East 3474

The U.S. Civilian Research and Development Foundation (CRDF) is a nonprofit organization authorized by the U.S. Congress and established in 1995 by the National Science Foundation. This unique organization promotes international scientific and technical collaboration through grants, technical resources, and training. CRDF, with funding from the National Institute for Allergy and Infectious Diseases (NIAID), announces a targeted, collaborative grant competition on Leishmaniasis in the North Africa and the Middle East (MENA) Region. This grant competition is a follow-on activity to the June 2009 interdisciplinary research conference in Tunisia sponsored by NIAID that brought together regional and international scientists to discuss research opportunities on sand fly biology, leishmania parasites, immunology, leishmaniasis epidemiology, animal reservoirs, clinical manifestations, genetics, diagnostics, treatment, and prevention of leishmaniasis in North Africa and the Middle East. These follow-on grants will provide up to one- year's support to joint research teams of U.S. and MENA scientists, with the possibility of up to a one year no-cost extension, if justified. CRDF and NIAID anticipate that the research implemented through these awards will lay the foundation for future grant proposals to NIAID and other funding agencies. The average anticipated grant will provide up to $30,000 U.S. dollars for a period of one year. At least 80% of the funds awarded to each project will be used for project-related expenses of the MENA component of the research team, including institutional support. No more than 20% may be used for U.S. team expenses. As part of the grant, the CRDF strongly encourages a member of the MENA team to visit the U.S. team's laboratory, and members of the U.S. team are encouraged to visit the MENA laboratory.
Requirements: Each proposal submitted to the CRDF must have at least one MENA Principal Investigator and at least one U.S. Principal Investigator, who share overall responsibility for the project in their respective countries, coordinating all project participants and institutions. Each proposal must meet each of the following eligibility criteria: 1) Only workshop attendees and their institutions are eligible to apply. 2) Each Principal Investigator must work full-time in a civilian research environment. (U.S. Government Laboratories working on civilian-oriented R&D projects are eligible to apply to this program.) 3) The U.S. Principal Investigator and participants of the U.S. team may be foreign nationals, but must reside in the U.S during the course of the grant award. Graduate students on the U.S. team may be foreign nationals, but they must be enrolled in an accredited degree program at a U.S. institution. A PI from Navy Medical Research Unit 3 (NAMRU3) may serve as either a U.S. or MENA researcher. 4) All projects must be in one of the following subject areas: Sand fly biology; Leishmania Parasites; Immunology; Leishmaniasis Epidemiology; Animal reservoirs; Clinical manifestations, treatment, and prevention of leishmaniasis in North Africa and the Middle East (but not clinical trials involving interventions); Genetics; Diagnostics. 5) Only one proposal will be accepted from a U.S. or MENA PI. 6) All projects must be oriented toward non-military objectives and must be carried out in a civilian research environment. Use of human subjects requires appropriate approvals from all institutions involved including Local Ethics Committee (LEC) and U.S. IBR. Middle East countries: Afghanistan, Behrain, Iran, Iraq, Israel, Jordan, Kyrgyzstan, Kuwait, Lebanon, Oman, Pakistan, Palestine, Qatar, Saudi Arabia, Syria, Tajikistan, Turkey, Turkmenistan, United Arab Emirates, Uzbekistan, Yemen. North African countries: Algeria, Egypt, Libya, Morocco, Sudan, Tunisia, Western Sahara.
Restrictions: No clinical trials involving interventions will be accepted for this competition.
Amount of Grant: up to $30,000
Date(s) Application is Due: Sep 30
Contact: Mr. Stuart Politi, Senior Program Manager; (703) 526-9720; fax: (703) 526-9721; email: cgp@crdf.org
Internet: http://www.crdf.org/funding/funding_show.htm?doc_id=949719
Sponsor: U.S. Civilian Research and Development Foundation
1530 Wilson Boulevard, 3rd Floor
Arlington, VA 22209

U.S. Trust Corporation Foundation Grants 3475

The foundation supports worthy, nonprofit organizations in the communities in which U.S. Trust does business. Funded organizations include cultural and arts institutions and community services organizations that assist low-to moderate-income residents. The corporate contributions committee reviews proposals continuously throughout the year, and meets formally twice per year to award grants. Types of support include general operating support, continuing support, annual campaigns, capital campaigns, building construction/renovation, endowment funds, program development, and matching funds. Preference is given to organizations that demonstrate an ability to solve problems and provide direct services, innovative programs with broad-based community support and community development impact, organizations in which U.S. Trust employees are active, privately supported rather than tax-supported organizations, and programs that encourage self-sufficiency of participants. Proposals are reviewed year round. Proposal deadlines are March 1 for culture and arts grants and September 1 for community services grants.
Requirements: Grant giving is concentrated in the communities in which U.S. Trust does business, and is directed to 501(c)3 nonprofit organizations.
Restrictions: Grants are not made to individuals for education or other purposes; educational, religious, veterans, fraternal, or labor organizations unless engaged in a significant project benefiting the entire community; organizations, projects, or programs outside the United States; political organizations or candidates; organizations requesting support for advertising; organizations supported by umbrella organizations; or organizations with operating budgets of $150,000 or less.
Geographic Focus: California; Connecticut; Delaware; District of Columbia; Florida; Minnesota; New Jersey; New York; North Carolina; Oregon; Pennsylvania; Texas; Virginia
Amount of Grant: $10,000-$30,000 range
Date(s) Application is Due: Mar 1; Sep 1
Contact: Carol Strickland, Chairman of the Corporate Contributions Committee, (212) 852-1330; fax: (212) 852-1341; email: cstrickland@ustrust.com or foundation@ustrust.com
Internet: http://www.ustrust.com/public/ustrust/our_firm/community_contributions?cmsid=P-564113&lvl1=our_firm&lvl2=community_contributions
Sponsor: U.S. Trust Corporation Foundation
114 W 47th Street
New York, NY 10036

U.S.CM HIV/AIDS Prevention Grants 3476

The U.S.CM HIV Prevention Grants Program, in cooperation with the Centers for Disease Control and Prevention, provides financial and technical assistance to local health departments and community-based organizations to implement HIV prevention programs. The goal of this effort is to strengthen the capacity of local service providers to carry out effective HIV/AIDS prevention activities.
Requirements: Grants are awarded on the recommendation of an independent external review panel composed of HIV/AIDS experts drawn from local and state health departments, national organizations, and local community-based organizations.
Contact: Crystal D. Swann Assistant Executive Director, (202) 861-6707; fax: (202) 293-2352; email: cswann@usmayors.org
Internet: http://www.usmayors.org/hivprevention/hiv_prevention_grant.asp
Sponsor: United States Conference of Mayors
1620 Eye Sreet NW
Washington, DC 20006

Vancouver Foundation Grants and Community Initiatives Program 3477

Vancouver Foundation's Grants and Community Initiatives program provides Community Impact Grants in nine fields of interest: Animal Welfare; Arts and Culture; Children, Youth and Families; Education; Environment; Health and Social Development; Health and Medical Research; Youth Homelessness; Youth Philanthropy. The Vancouver Foundation has a two-stage application process. The first stage is a letter of intent. This consists of a brief proposal to determine basic suitability. The second stage is submission of a full grant application by a specific date. The letter of intent may be submitted online. You will be notified, if you are invited to submit a full grant application. The following is a list of deadline dates for the letters of intent and applications. Animal Welfare, Arts and Culture, Children, Youth and Families, Education, Environment, and Health and Social Development grants have a deadline date of: Letter of Intent, June 18, Application, August 6. Youth Homelessness grants: Letter of Intent, August 6, Application, September 24. Youth Philanthropy grants: Letter of Intent, September 17, Application, October 1. Health and Medical Research grants deadline dates are undetermined, at this time.
Requirements: Under our Grants and Community Initiatives program, Vancouver Foundation funds eligible applicants, which include: registered charities and qualified donees under the Income Tax Act; First Nations that may be considered a public body performing a function of government.
Restrictions: The Foundation does not fund the following: 100% of a proposal's costs; an organization's ongoing operational or core expenses; retroactive funding, or for any expenses to be incurred prior to the Foundation's decision date; debt retirement or reserves; mortgage pay-downs; conferences, competitions, symposia, annual events, or travel to/attendance at such events; office equipment and furniture; activities of religious organizations that serve primarily their membership and/or their direct religious purposes, unless the community at large will benefit significantly; sabbatical leaves,

student exchanges; medical facilities or equipment; league-based sports and recreation programs; library acquisitions and construction; school construction; publication of books; academic or dissertation research; research with human subjects; endowment matching grants; capital requests, with the exceptions noted above; activities previously supported through government funding; bursaries, scholarships and awards; school trips, annual events or equipment; grants to individuals or businesses; funding requests if reports on any previous grants are overdue.
Contact: Mark Gifford, Director, Grants and Community Initiatives; (604) 629-5362; email: markg@vancouverfoundation.ca;; Catharine Hume, Grants and Community Initiatives; (604) 629-5361; email: catharineh@vancouverfoundation.ca
Internet: http://www.vancouverfoundation.ca/grants/communityinitiatives.htm
Sponsor: Vancouver Foundation
555 West Hastings Street, Suite 1200
Vancouver, BC V6B 4N6 Canada

Vancouver Foundation Public Health Bursary Package **3478**
With funding from the BC Associated Boards of Health Dr. Ken Benson Memorial Bursary and the Isabel Loucks Foster Public Health Bursary Funds, bursaries are available to qualified students who are or wish to engage in post-graduate study in a field of Public or Community health practice within any recognized discipline. The funds are managed by the Vancouver Foundation and the Bursary funds will be released to a successful applicant(s) annually on the recommendation of the Health Officers' Council. The Health Officers' Council is comprised of the Medical Health Officers and public health physicians of British Columbia. Bursaries in an amount up to $3,000 are available to eligible applicants on a one- time-only basis. Successful candidates will be notified by October 31st.
Requirements: Eligibility for the Isabel Loucks Foster Public Health Bursary Fund: full-time students engaged in post-graduate study in a field of Public/Community Health Practice within an applicable discipline (e.g. nurses, nutritionists, environmental health officers, physicians, etc.); persons must be ordinarily resident in B.C.; persons must have demonstrated excellence in performance and leadership ability; studies may be undertaken at any suitable educational institution either within or outside British Columbia.
Amount of Grant: $3,000
Date(s) Application is Due: Sep 4
Contact: Faye Wightman, President & CEO; (604) 688-2204; fax: (604) 688-4170; email: info@vancouverfoundation.ca
Internet: http://www.vancouverfoundation.ca/grants/specialprograms.htm
Sponsor: Vancouver Foundation
555 West Hastings Street, Suite 1200
Vancouver, BC V6B 4N6 Canada

Vancouver Sun Children's Fund Grants **3479**
In partnership with Vancouver Foundation, the Vancouver Sun Children's Fund provides grants twice yearly to registered charities in British Columbia that directly serve the needs of children and youth (up to18 years) with special challenges. Grants range from $100 to $5,000 and recommendations are made by Vancouver Foundation's Children, Youth and Families Advisory Committee whose members have knowledge and experience in the fields of children's physical, mental and emotional health.
Requirements: Eligible applicants are registered charities and other qualified organizations under the Income Tax Act. They must demonstrate fiscal responsibility and effective management. To apply, submit your Letter of Intent electronically.
Restrictions: Grants are not made to individuals or businesses.
Amount of Grant: $100 - $5,000 range
Contact: Mark Gifford Director, Grants and Community Initiatives; (604) 688-2204; fax: (604) 688-4170; email: markg@vancouverfoundation.ca
Internet: http://www.vancouverfoundation.ca/grants/specialprograms.htm
Sponsor: The Vancouver Sun Children's Fund c/o Vancouver Foundation
Suite 1200, 555 West Hastings Street, Box 12132, Harbour Centre
Vancouver, B C V6B 4N6 Canada

Vanderburgh Community Foundation Grants **3480**
The Vanderburgh Community Foundation is a nonprofit, public charity created by and for the people of Vanderburgh County, Indiana. The Foundation assists nonprofits fulfill their missions by strengthening their ability to meet community needs through grants that assist charitable programs, address community issues, support community agencies, launch community initiatives, and support leadership development. The Foundation's grant cycle will be announced by the end of July.
Requirements: A Letter of Intent is the required first step for submitting funding requests to be considered by the Community Foundation. The Letter of Intent helps in determining whether a funding request qualifies for consideration before the applicant invests time and effort in completing a full grant proposal. The Foundation's office will provide additional information on proposal procedure or you may access the Foundation's website. The Foundation gives primarily to 501(c)3 tax-exempt organizations in Vanderburgh County, Indiana.
Geographic Focus: Indiana
Date(s) Application is Due: $1,000 - $10,000 range
Contact: Barbara Dicken, Director; (812) 422-1245; fax: (812) 429-0840; barb@vcfoundation.org
Internet: http://www.vanderburghcommunityfoundation.org/disc-grants
Sponsor: Vanderburgh Community Foundation
18 Northwest Forth Street, Suite 220
Evansville, IN 47708

Varian Medical Systems Grants **3481**
Varian Medical Systems makes grants, donations, and gifts to nonprofit organizations committed to supporting the provision of information and services involving the prevention, detection, and treatment of cancer. The company also supports education through matching gifts that employees make to nonprofit educational institutions. Applications must be received at least 60 days in advance of the time that the funding is needed. Application and guidelines are available online.
Requirements: Nonprofit organizations are eligible.
Restrictions: The following are ineligible: applications that are in any way associated with planned, current, or past purchases, or the recommendation to purchase, any Varian Medical Systems, Inc, products or services; local chapter programs already supported by Varian at the national level (i.e., National Survivor's Day, Relay for Life); capital campaigns for new buildings and/or major equipment purchases; sporting or entertainment events (i.e., golf); individual requests for personal needs/projects; a-thon fundraisers (i.e., walk-a-thon, telethon); religious or political organizations; or advertising programs (i.e., radio/television).
Contact: Program Contact, (650) 493-4000; fax: (650) 424-6822; email: giving@varian.com
Internet: http://www.varian.com/com/ctz000.html
Sponsor: Varian Medical Systems, Inc
3100 Hansen Wy, MS E-210
Palo Alto, CA 94304

VDH Commonwealth of Virginia Nurse Educator Scholarships **3482**
Scholarships will be provided to full/part-time graduate nursing students who are accepted to or enrolled in a master's or doctoral level nursing program in the Commonwealth of Virginia. The purpose of this program is to increase the number of nursing faculty by providing master's/doctoral students with financial support. Additionally, this program will assist Virginia nursing schools to recruit and retain new nursing faculty, which enables the schools to increase enrollment.
Requirements: Full/part-time master's or doctoral nursing students enrolled or accepted in nursing program in Virginia will be eligible to apply. Students must complete their degree requirements in two years or less. Priority shall be given to master's degree candidates who will teach in community colleges. Applications will be accepted from June 1 through July 31 each calendar year. Complete and submit a Nursing Scholarship Application along with all required materials. Applications will be available online at: http://www.vdh.virginia.gov/healthpolicy/primarycare/incentives/nursing/index.htm
Restrictions: Recipients will be required to give two years of teaching service as a faculty member for every year they receive a scholarship. Recipients who do not take teaching positions at a Virginia nursing program will be required to pay back the scholarship with a 9% interest penalty. Repayment must be paid in full within two years of degree completion. Recipients must begin their teaching service within three months of completing their educational program.
Geographic Focus: Virginia
Amount of Grant: $20,000
Date(s) Application is Due: Jul 31
Contact: Aileen Harris, Health Care Workforce Manager; (804) 864-7436; fax: (804) 864-7440; email: Aileen.Harris@vdh.virginia.gov ...
Internet: http://www.vdh.virginia.gov/healthpolicy/primarycare/incentives/nursing/va_nsp_guidelines.htm
Sponsor: Virginia Department of Health
Post Office Box 2448
Richmond, VA 23218

VDH Emergency Medical Services Training Fund (EMSTF) **3483**
The EMS Training Fund program is designed to provide financial assistance for Virginia Certified EMS providers and Virginia Office of EMS approved Emergency Medical Services courses. These funds shall supplement local support for Emergency Medical Services Courses. The Emergency Medical Services Training Funds are monies available for student expenses related to attending EMS Certification programs, tuition reimbursement, auxiliary programs and continuing education programs whose lessons are based upon or resemble the learning objectives in the United States Department of Transportation's Intermediate-99 and Paramedic curricula and the Enhanced curricula as defined in 12VAC5-31. See website for application.
Requirements: These funds are designed for non-profit entities and individuals participating in Virginia's EMS System.
Geographic Focus: Virginia
Contact: Jackie Hunter, Program Support Technician; (804) 864-7585; email: Jacqueline.Hunter@vdh.virginia.gov
Internet: http://www.vdh.virginia.gov/OEMS/Training/EMSTF.htm
Sponsor: Virginia Department of Health
Post Office Box 2448
Richmond, VA 23218

VDH Rescue Squad Assistance Fund Grants **3484**
The Financial Assistance for Emergency Medical Services Grants Program, known as the Rescue Squad Assistance Fund (RSAF) Grant Program is a multi-million dollar matching grant program for Virginia governmental, non-profit EMS agencies and organizations to provide financial assistance based on a demonstrated need. Items eligible for funding include EMS equipment and vehicles, computers, EMS management programs, courses/classes and projects benefiting the recruitment and retention of EMS members. RSAF is primarily a reimbursement grant that requires the grantee to make the purchase for the awarded item(s) and then submit an invoice for reimbursement.

Requirements: Applicant must be a Virginia non-profit agency/organization or governmental organization involved in emergency medical service (ems); applicant must submit verification of its FIN. Verification can be provided in the following formats: copy of the original letter from the IRS issuing FIN, copy of the latest tax returns (1st page only), statement from the County Administrator or City Manager of the municipality stating that the application is non-profit or a government agency and verifies their FIN; applicant must submit a copy (1st page only) of the most recent Federal Tax Return from the IRS (Form 990); applicant must submit the Virginia Office of EMS Affirmation Page in its entirety including the original signature of the Authorized Agent, the Fiscal Officer (Treasurer) and the Operational Medical Director (OMD). All Grant Applications must be submitted via the Internet. The Affirmation page is due by September 15 with original signatures. Faxed Applications will not be accepted. Submit all grant information to: Office of Emergency Medical Services, Attn: Amanda Davis - Grant Manager, 109 Governor Street, Suite UB-55, Richmond, VA 23219.
Restrictions: Applications submitted with line items less then $500.00 will be disqualified.
Geographic Focus: Virginia
Date(s) Application is Due: Sep 15
Contact: Amanda Davis, Grant Manager: (804) 864-7600; fax: (804) 864-7580
Internet: http://www.vdh.virginia.gov/OEMS/Grants/index.htm
Sponsor: Virginia Department of Health
Post Office Box 2448
Richmond, VA 23218

Vectren Foundation Grants **3485**

The foundation focuses its efforts in four major areas of giving: Education, Arts & Culture, Civic, and Health & Human Services. Priority will be given to those organizations and activities that serve to improve the quality of life in the communities Vectren serves.
Requirements: The only awards grants to organizations exempt from Federal Tax under Section 501(c)3 of the IRS code. The funding request application can be downloaded from the website. Applications should include a copy of your tax-exempt ruling from the IRS; a list of current board members and annual report, if available; and, a current operating and project budget. Applications for contributions to capital fund drives or to purchase equipment should also provide a clear description of the project, including its goals and objectives; and, a financial plan showing how the project will be funded. The plan should include other possible sources of support and funds that have been pledged or received to date.
Restrictions: The foundation will not: support programs, activities or campaigns that advance a specific religious agenda.; make contributions to political, fraternal, labor or veteran's organizations, unless the activity is for direct community involvement; make contributions to issues-oriented organizations; will not award scholarships or grants that benefit individuals (This includes individuals raising funds for charitable purposes, student ambassador programs and sponsorship of individual sports or academic teams.); or, award grants involving travel outside of the Vectren Service Territory.
Geographic Focus: Indiana
Samples: Morgan County Public Library's Youth Art month; Cornerstone Center for the Arts, Arts Adventure program; Lakeview Volunteer Firefighters; United Way Campaigns
Contact: Mark H. Miller, Community Affairs Manager, Vectren Corporation; (812) 491-4176; fax: (812) 491-4078; email: mmiller@vectren.com
Internet: http://www.vectren.com/web/holding/discover/foundation/foundation_i.jsp
Sponsor: Vectren Foundation
One Vectren Square
Evansville, IN 47708

Verizon Foundation Health Care and Accessibility Grants **3486**

The Verizon Foundation invests in projects that provide technology to help under served populations and people with disabilities access information on critical health issues. It also supports innovative technology that helps health care providers increase their efficiency, effectiveness and reach. The Foundation only accepts electronic proposals through its online process, and reviews unsolicited proposals on a continuous calendar year basis from January 1st through October 31st.
Requirements: Proposals will be considered from eligible tax-exempt organizations in certain 501(c)3 subsections as defined by the Internal Revenue Service (IRS). Proposals will also be considered from elementary and secondary schools (public and private) that are registered with the National Center for Education Statistics (NCES). Proposals may also be considered from eligible tax-exempt organizations in the subsection 170(B)(1)(a)(i)—Church, provided that the proposal will benefit a large portion of a community without regard to religious affiliation and does not duplicate the work of other agencies in the community.
Restrictions: The Verizon Foundation does not provide funding for any of the following: individuals; private charity or foundation; organizations not exempt under Section 501(c)3 of the Internal Revenue Code, and not eligible for tax-deductible support; religious organizations, unless the particular program will benefit a large portion of a community without regard to religious affiliation and does not duplicate the work of other agencies in the community; political causes, candidates, organizations or campaigns; organizations that discriminate on the basis of age, color, citizenship, disability, disabled veteran status, gender, race, religion, national origin, marital status, sexual orientation, military service or status or Vietnam-era veteran status; organizations whose primary purpose is to influence legislation; endowments or capital campaigns; film, music, TV, video and media production projects or broadcast program underwriting; research studies, unless related to projects we are already supporting; sports sponsorships; performing arts tours; association memberships; or organizations that have received a grant from the Verizon Foundation in the last three consecutive years - organization may reapply after a one-year hiatus.
Amount of Grant: $5,000-$10,000 average
Contact: Patrick Gaston, President; (800) 360-7955; fax: (908) 630-2660; email: patrick.g.gaston@erizon.com
Internet: http://foundation.verizon.com/core/health.shtml
Sponsor: Verizon Foundation
One Verizon Way
Basking Ridge, NJ 07920

Verizon Foundation Maryland Grants **3487**

The foundation invites applications, in Maryland, to receive financial grants that support education, literacy, health care access, workforce development, and the reduction of domestic violence. Consideration will be given to proposals for programs that provide job training for individuals, including welfare-to-work and school-to-work training programs; and assist people with disabilities in acquiring computer skills through adaptive technology that prepares them to enter the workforce. The Foundation only accepts electronic proposals through its online process, and reviews unsolicited proposals on a continuous calendar year basis from January 1st through October 31st.
Requirements: Proposals will be considered from eligible tax-exempt organizations in certain 501(c)3 subsections as defined by the Internal Revenue Service (IRS). Proposals will also be considered from elementary and secondary schools (public and private) that are registered with the National Center for Education Statistics (NCES). Proposals may also be considered from eligible tax-exempt organizations in the subsection 170(B)(1)(a)(i)—Church, provided that the proposal will benefit a large portion of a community without regard to religious affiliation and does not duplicate the work of other agencies in the community.
Restrictions: The Verizon Foundation does not provide funding for any of the following: individuals; private charity or foundation; organizations not exempt under Section 501(c)3 of the Internal Revenue Code, and not eligible for tax-deductible support; religious organizations, unless the particular program will benefit a large portion of a community without regard to religious affiliation and does not duplicate the work of other agencies in the community; political causes, candidates, organizations or campaigns; organizations that discriminate on the basis of age, color, citizenship, disability, disabled veteran status, gender, race, religion, national origin, marital status, sexual orientation, military service or status or Vietnam-era veteran status; organizations whose primary purpose is to influence legislation; endowments or capital campaigns; film, music, TV, video and media production projects or broadcast program underwriting; research studies, unless related to projects we are already supporting; sports sponsorships; performing arts tours; association memberships; or organizations that have received a grant from the Verizon Foundation in the last three consecutive years - organization may reapply after a one-year hiatus.
Geographic Focus: Maryland
Amount of Grant: $5,000-$10,000 average
Contact: Diane Miles, Director; (410) 393-7450 or (800) 360-7955; fax: (908) 630-2660; email: diane.f.miles@verizon.com
Internet: http://foundation.verizon.com/cybergrants/plsql/vznadmin.vz_www.iyc?x_zip=21202
Sponsor: Verizon Foundation
One East Pratt Street, 10E
Baltimore, MD 21202

Verizon Foundation New York Grants **3488**

The Verizon Foundation—the philanthropic arm of Verizon Communications—supports a variety of programs and events in communities from Buffalo to Brooklyn. As one of the largest corporate contributors in New York, Verizon is proud to have directed more than 6,000 grants totaling more than $14 million to some 2,700 non-profits across the state. Those non-profits include school districts and universities, multicultural groups and hospitals, children's organizations and those assisting the disabled and victims of domestic violence. Through the Foundation, Verizon New York underscores the company's commitment to key funding priorities—combating literacy and domestic violence, empowering communities with technology, bridging the digital divide, creating a skilled work force, and galvanizing employees to volunteer. The Foundation only accepts electronic proposals through its online process, and reviews unsolicited proposals on a continuous calendar year basis from January 1st through October 31st.
Requirements: Proposals will be considered from eligible tax-exempt organizations in certain 501(c)3 subsections as defined by the Internal Revenue Service (IRS). Proposals will also be considered from elementary and secondary schools (public and private) that are registered with the National Center for Education Statistics (NCES). Proposals may also be considered from eligible tax-exempt organizations in the subsection 170(B)(1)(a)(i)—Church, provided that the proposal will benefit a large portion of a community without regard to religious affiliation and does not duplicate the work of other agencies in the community.
Restrictions: The Verizon Foundation does not provide funding for any of the following: individuals; private charity or foundation; organizations not exempt under Section 501(c)3 of the Internal Revenue Code, and not eligible for tax-deductible support; religious organizations, unless the particular program will benefit a large portion of a community without regard to religious affiliation and does not duplicate the work of other agencies in the community; political causes, candidates, organizations or campaigns; organizations that discriminate on the basis of age, color, citizenship, disability, disabled veteran status, gender, race, religion, national origin, marital status, sexual orientation, military service or status or Vietnam-era veteran status; organizations whose primary purpose is to influence legislation; endowments or capital campaigns; film, music, TV, video

and media production projects or broadcast program underwriting; research studies, unless related to projects we are already supporting; sports sponsorships; performing arts tours; association memberships; or organizations that have received a grant from the Verizon Foundation in the last three consecutive years - organization may reapply after a one-year hiatus.
Geographic Focus: New York
Amount of Grant: $5,000-$10,000 average
Contact: Sandy Wilson, Director; (800) 360-7955; fax: (908) 630-2660; email: sandra.c.wilson@verizon.com
Internet: http://foundation.verizon.com/cybergrants/plsql/vznadmin.vz_www.iyc?x_zip=10007
Sponsor: Verizon Foundation
140 West Street, 26 Floor, Room 2621
New York, NY 10007

Verizon Foundation Northeast Region Grants **3489**
The Verizon Foundation is committed to supporting programs and projects that leverage technology to improve basic computer literacy and domestic violence initiatives, seeking organizations that serve the needs of diverse communities, people with disabilities, and the economically and socially challenged. The Foundation only accepts electronic proposals through its online process, and reviews unsolicited proposals on a continuous calendar year basis from January 1st through October 31st.
Requirements: Proposals will be considered from eligible tax-exempt organizations in certain 501(c)3 subsections as defined by the Internal Revenue Service (IRS). Proposals will also be considered from elementary and secondary schools (public and private) that are registered with the National Center for Education Statistics (NCES). Proposals may also be considered from eligible tax-exempt organizations in the subsection 170(B)(1)(a)(i)—Church, provided that the proposal will benefit a large portion of a community without regard to religious affiliation and does not duplicate the work of other agencies in the community.
Restrictions: The Verizon Foundation does not provide funding for any of the following: individuals; private charity or foundation; organizations not exempt under Section 501(c)3 of the Internal Revenue Code, and not eligible for tax-deductible support; religious organizations, unless the particular program will benefit a large portion of a community without regard to religious affiliation and does not duplicate the work of other agencies in the community; political causes, candidates, organizations or campaigns; organizations that discriminate on the basis of age, color, citizenship, disability, disabled veteran status, gender, race, religion, national origin, marital status, sexual orientation, military service or status or Vietnam-era veteran status; organizations whose primary purpose is to influence legislation; endowments or capital campaigns; film, music, TV, video and media production projects or broadcast program underwriting; research studies, unless related to projects we are already supporting; sports sponsorships; performing arts tours; association memberships; or organizations that have received a grant from the Verizon Foundation in the last three consecutive years - organization may reapply after a one-year hiatus.
Geographic Focus: Massachusetts; Rhode Island
Amount of Grant: $5,000-$10,000 average
Contact: Rick Colon, Regional Director; (781) 849-2046; email: richard.b.colon@verizon.com
Internet: http://foundation.verizon.com/cybergrants/plsql/vznadmin.vz_www.iyc?x_zip=02184
Sponsor: Verizon Foundation
125 Lundquist Drive, Room 1730
Braintree, MA 02184

Verizon Foundation Pennsylvania Grants **3490**
Verizon Foundation Pennsylvania is investing in online resources, community-based initiatives and state-wide programs that teach non readers to read and advance the complex skills necessary for educational achievement and job success in the 21st Century. The grants have enabled the recipient organizations to improve basic literacy skills, create new and diverse approaches to technology-based learning, and help domestic violence victims rebuild their lives. The Foundation only accepts electronic proposals through its online process, and reviews unsolicited proposals on a continuous calendar year basis from January 1st through October 31st.
Requirements: Proposals will be considered from eligible tax-exempt organizations in certain 501(c)3 subsections as defined by the Internal Revenue Service (IRS). Proposals will also be considered from elementary and secondary schools (public and private) that are registered with the National Center for Education Statistics (NCES). Proposals may also be considered from eligible tax-exempt organizations in the subsection 170(B)(1)(a)(i)—Church, provided that the proposal will benefit a large portion of a community without regard to religious affiliation and does not duplicate the work of other agencies in the community.
Restrictions: The Verizon Foundation does not provide funding for any of the following: individuals; private charity or foundation; organizations not exempt under Section 501(c)3 of the Internal Revenue Code, and not eligible for tax-deductible support; religious organizations, unless the particular program will benefit a large portion of a community without regard to religious affiliation and does not duplicate the work of other agencies in the community; political causes, candidates, organizations or campaigns; organizations that discriminate on the basis of age, color, citizenship, disability, disabled veteran status, gender, race, religion, national origin, marital status, sexual orientation, military service or status or Vietnam-era veteran status; organizations whose primary purpose is to influence legislation; endowments or capital campaigns; film, music, TV, video and media production projects or broadcast program underwriting; research studies, unless related to projects we are already supporting; sports sponsorships; performing arts tours; association memberships; or organizations that have received a grant from the Verizon Foundation in the last three consecutive years - organization may reapply after a one-year hiatus.
Geographic Focus: Pennsylvania
Amount of Grant: $5,000-$10,000 average
Contact: Denise Loughlin; (215) 466-3351; email: denise.g.loughlin@verizon.com
Internet: http://www22.verizon.com/about/community/pa/community/comm_index.html
Sponsor: Verizon Foundation
3478 Kirkwood Road
Philadelphia, PA 19114

Verizon Foundation Vermont Grants **3491**
The Foundation is committed to supporting programs and projects that leverage technology to improve basic computer literacy and domestic violence initiatives, seeking organizations that serve the needs of diverse communities, people with disabilities, and the economically and socially challenged. Last year, Verizon Foundation donated close to $250,000 to Vermont nonprofit organizations and our employees clocked more than 16,000 volunteer hours to community organizations. The Foundation only accepts electronic proposals through its online process, and reviews unsolicited proposals on a continuous calendar year basis from January 1st through October 31st.
Requirements: Proposals will be considered from eligible tax-exempt organizations in certain 501(c)3 subsections as defined by the Internal Revenue Service (IRS). Proposals will also be considered from elementary and secondary schools (public and private) that are registered with the National Center for Education Statistics (NCES). Proposals may also be considered from eligible tax-exempt organizations in the subsection 170(B)(1)(a)(i)—Church, provided that the proposal will benefit a large portion of a community without regard to religious affiliation and does not duplicate the work of other agencies in the community.
Restrictions: The Verizon Foundation does not provide funding for any of the following: individuals; private charity or foundation; organizations not exempt under Section 501(c)3 of the Internal Revenue Code, and not eligible for tax-deductible support; religious organizations, unless the particular program will benefit a large portion of a community without regard to religious affiliation and does not duplicate the work of other agencies in the community; political causes, candidates, organizations or campaigns; organizations that discriminate on the basis of age, color, citizenship, disability, disabled veteran status, gender, race, religion, national origin, marital status, sexual orientation, military service or status or Vietnam-era veteran status; organizations whose primary purpose is to influence legislation; endowments or capital campaigns; film, music, TV, video and media production projects or broadcast program underwriting; research studies, unless related to projects we are already supporting; sports sponsorships; performing arts tours; association memberships; or organizations that have received a grant from the Verizon Foundation in the last three consecutive years - organization may reapply after a one-year hiatus.
Geographic Focus: Vermont
Amount of Grant: $5,000-$10,000 average
Contact: Stephanie Lee, Regional Director; (617) 743-5440; email: stephanie.s.lee@verizon.com;; Phil Santoro; (617) 743-4760; email: philip.g.santoro@verizon.com
Internet: http://foundation.verizon.com/cybergrants/plsql/vznadmin.vz_www.iyc?x_zip=05403
Sponsor: Verizon Foundation
185 Franklin Street, Room 1702
Boston, MA 02110

Verizon Foundation Virginia Grants **3492**
Verizon Foundation grants have touched and will continue to affect thousands of lives in Virginia. Verizon is committed to investing in the technological, financial, and human resources necessary to build more literate communities that can prosper in the information era, and to foster domestic violence awareness, prevention, and recovery. The Foundation will continue to form strong partnerships with Virginia's non-profit community to achieve its funding priority goals and improve the quality of life for people across the Commonwealth. The Foundation only accepts electronic proposals through its online process, and reviews unsolicited proposals on a continuous calendar year basis from January 1st through October 31st.
Requirements: Proposals will be considered from eligible tax-exempt organizations in certain 501(c)3 subsections as defined by the Internal Revenue Service (IRS). Proposals will also be considered from elementary and secondary schools (public and private) that are registered with the National Center for Education Statistics (NCES). Proposals may also be considered from eligible tax-exempt organizations in the subsection 170(B)(1)(a)(i)—Church, provided that the proposal will benefit a large portion of a community without regard to religious affiliation and does not duplicate the work of other agencies in the community.
Restrictions: The Verizon Foundation does not provide funding for any of the following: individuals; private charity or foundation; organizations not exempt under Section 501(c)3 of the Internal Revenue Code, and not eligible for tax-deductible support; religious organizations, unless the particular program will benefit a large portion of a community without regard to religious affiliation and does not duplicate the work of other agencies in the community; political causes, candidates, organizations or campaigns; organizations that discriminate on the basis of age, color, citizenship, disability, disabled veteran status, gender, race, religion, national origin, marital status, sexual orientation, military service or status or Vietnam-era veteran status; organizations whose primary purpose is to influence legislation; endowments or capital campaigns; film, music, TV, video

and media production projects or broadcast program underwriting; research studies, unless related to projects we are already supporting; sports sponsorships; performing arts tours; association memberships; or organizations that have received a grant from the Verizon Foundation in the last three consecutive years - organization may reapply after a one-year hiatus.
Geographic Focus: Virginia
Amount of Grant: $5,000-$10,000 average
Contact: Stephan Clementi; (804) 772-1673 or (800) 360-7955; fax: 908-630-2660; email: steve.clementi@verizon.com
Internet: http://foundation.verizon.com/cybergrants/plsql/vznadmin.vz_www.iyc?x_zip=24012
Sponsor: Verizon Foundation
703 East Grace Street, 7th Floor
Richmond, VA 23219

Vermont Community Foundation Grants **3493**
The foundation has broad program interests and will consider any project that meets a clearly defined community need in Vermont. Categories of support include, but are not limited to: the arts and humanities; education; the environment; historic resources; health; public affairs and community development; and social services.
Requirements: To be eligible, an organization must: have 501(c)3 tax-exempt status and not be classified as a private foundation; be located in or serve the people of Vermont; and employ staff and provide services without discrimination on the basis of race, religion, sex, age, national origin, disability, or sexual orientation. See Foundations website for additional guidelines, including rolling deadlines, and application forms.
Restrictions: The foundation does not make grants for endowments, annual operating or capital campaigns, religious purposes, individuals, debts, or equipment unless it is an integral part of an otherwise eligible project.
Geographic Focus: Vermont
Amount of Grant: $25,000 maximum
Contact: Peter Espenshade Vice President for Community Philanthropy; (802) 388-3355 ext 248; fax: (802) 388-3398; email: pespenshade@vermontcf.org
Internet: http://www.vermontcf.org/apply/
Sponsor: Vermont Community Foundation
P.O. Box 30, 3 Court Street
Middlebury, VT 05753

VFW Ladies Auxiliary Cancer Research Postdoctoral Fellowships **3494**
The VFW Ladies Auxiliary offers three postdoctoral research fellowships annually so that recipient researchers can devote their full time for one year to the challenge of cancer research. The fellowship is not renewable. The grant is not to be used for lab equipment or supplies; it is a stipend for personal living expenses of the accredited researcher. The application must be filed on appropriate application form and must describe the proposed research project that the nominee will be conducting, including abstract and brief outline of methods, procedures, and significance. The proposed research must be the principal professional responsibility of the recipient during the stated period of the award. The application must be accompanied by a letter of recommendation.
Requirements: Nominees must be U.S. citizens who are qualified in a specific cancer-related specialty and must have earned a doctoral level degree by the time the fellowship is activated (July 1). Colleges and research institutions are invited to nominate researchers; institutions may nominate more than one person.
Amount of Grant: $50,000
Date(s) Application is Due: Mar 1
Contact: Judy Millick, Program Contact, (816) 561-8655; fax: (816) 931-4753; email: jmillick@vfw.org or info@ladiesauxvfw.com
Internet: http://www.ladiesauxvfw.com/cancer%20fellowships.html
Sponsor: Veterans of Foreign Wars Ladies Auxiliary
406 W 34th Street
Kansas City, MO 64111

VHA Health Foundation Grants **3495**
The Foundation has dedicated its resources to create a legacy strategy, which will build on its vision of the last decade by focusing on two critical issues that will significantly improve the delivery of health care: patient safety and disaster relief. Programs submitted for funding consideration must represent a new and innovative approach to hospital emergency preparedness and be beyond the concept stage - ready to test, implement, expand, or diffuse. Innovations should be either transformational (i.e. involve significant change in current operations) and/or disruptive (i.e., have profound impact on services and economics) in nature.
Requirements: Unsolicited inquires may be submitted at any time during the year. The Letter of Inquiry is the required first step in the process. Eligible programs should clearly incorporate four key elements: Innovation, Impact, Replicability and Sustainability. Grants are available to U.S. health care providers, including hospitals, health care systems, clinics, and medical practices with IRS tax-exempt 501(c)3 status. Local partnerships are encouraged to apply, but, since the hospital is the foundation's primary audience, the health care provider must serve as fiduciary agent and play an integral role in the program. An organization may submit multiple inquiries for consideration. Previously funded organizations may apply. Applicants are required to financially invest in the program with cash from any source and/or through in-kind contributions specific to the grant period. The minimum level of the investment is equal to one-half of the funding requested from the foundation.
Restrictions: The foundation will not consider requests for seed money or planning grants; primary research and development of technology; construction or renovation; indirect costs or overhead; endowments; political activities or attempts to influence specific legislation; individual scholarships or tuition assistance; or programs outside the United States.
Samples: MeritCare Health System, Fargo, ND and Medcenter One Health System, Bismarck, ND, $62,500—disaster relief, North Dakota flooding (2009); Arkansas Methodist Medical Center, Paragould, AR, St. Bernard's Regional Medical Center, Jonesboro, AR, and Washington Regional Medical Center, Fayetteville, AR, $170,850—disaster relief, Arkansas winter storm (2009).
Amount of Grant: $100,000-$250,000
Contact: Michael Regier, Senior Vice President; (877) 847-1450 or (972) 830-0422; fax: (972) 830-0332; email: vhahealthfoundation@vha.com
Internet: https://www.vhafoundation.org/portal/server.pt?open=512&objID=1204&PageID=0&cached=true&mode=2&userID=504686
Sponsor: VHA Health Foundation
220 Easr Las Colinas Boulevard
Irving, TX 75039-5500

Viets Medical Student Myasthenia Gravis Research Fellowships **3496**
This fellowship is for the purpose of initiating and furthering the interests of potential investigators from colleges and medical schools in the area of causative or treatment research in myasthenia gravis (MG), including clinical investigations as well as laboratory studies concerned with research on MG, underlying mechanisms of neuromuscular transmission, and the pathogenesis of MG. A qualified candidate desiring training in MG-related research should first find a scientist with an established research program who will agree to supervise her/his training and the research to be carried out. The research can be basic or clinical and conducted in the student's own medical school or in one close to the student's residence. The number of fellowships awarded each year is limited by the amount of funds available. Application guidelines are available online.
Requirements: Submit eight copies of the following: cover letter, summary of the research proposal and its association to Myasthenia Gravis or related neuromuscular conditions, curriculum vita of applicant and sponsoring preceptor, and letter of recommendation from preceptor that indicates acceptance of the candidate and outlines the proposed work plan for the research study.
Amount of Grant: $3000
Date(s) Application is Due: Mar 15
Contact: Fellowships Administrator, (800) 541-5454 or (651) 917-6256; fax: (651) 917-1835; email: mgfa@myasthenia.org
Internet: http://www.myasthenia.org/research
Sponsor: Myasthenia Gravis Foundation
1821 University Ave W, Suite S256
Saint Paul, MN 55104

Viking Children's Fund Grants **3497**
The fund supports the needs of children in Minnesota and the upper Midwest. Grants support research at the University of Minnesota Department of Pediatrics into the major diseases and disorders of childhood; and nonprofits that focus efforts in the areas of health education and family services supporting the well-being of children in the upper Midwest.
Requirements: Nonprofit organizations in Minnesota and the upper Midwest, including Iowa, North Dakota, South Dakota, and Wisconsin, are eligible.
Geographic Focus: Iowa; Minnesota; North Dakota; South Dakota; Wisconsin
Amount of Grant: $500-$5000
Date(s) Application is Due: Apr 1
Contact: Patrick Leopold, Viking Children's Fund Coordinator, (952) 828-6500; email: info@vikings.com
Internet: http://www.vikings.com/commchildfund.html
Sponsor: Minnesota Vikings Football Club
9520 Viking Drive
Eden Prairie, MN 55344

Virginia Department of Health Mary Marshall Nursing Scholarships for Licensed Practical Nurses **3498**
The Mary Marshall Nursing Scholarships for Licensed Practical Nurses are funded by the Virginia General Assembly along with a donation from The Board of Nursing. The scholarship amount is dependent upon amount of scholarship source and the number of qualified applicants. It is important that all applicants fully understand the conditions of accepting a Mary Marshall Nursing Scholarship. These awards are not gifts. Scholarship recipients must agree to engage in full time nursing in Virginia for one month for every $100 received.
Requirements: To be considered for a Mary Marshall Nursing Scholarship, an applicant must meet the following criteria: residency in Virginia for at least one year; acceptance or enrollment as a full-time or part-time student in a practical school of nursing in the state of Virginia; and have submitted a completed application form and a recommendation from the Program Director regarding scholastic attainment and financial need prior to June 30. Applications and guidelines are available online from May 1 to June 30 every year. Applications must be typed, printed and mailed (with original signatures) to the: Virginia Department of Health, Office of Minority Health and Public Health Policy, ATTN: Nursing Scholarship, 109 Governor Street, Suite 1016, East Richmond, Virginia 23219.
Restrictions: The award recipient has 60 days from the date of graduation to obtain his/her license. Full time employment must begin within 90 days of the recipient's license date. Voluntary military service, even if stationed in Virginia, cannot be used to repay scholarship awards.

Geographic Focus: Virginia
Date(s) Application is Due: Jun 30
Contact: Aileen Harris, Health Care Workforce Manager; (804) 864-7436; fax: (804) 864-7440; email: Aileen.Harris@vdh.virginia.gov ...
Internet: http://www.vdh.virginia.gov/healthpolicy/primarycare/incentives/nursing/lpn_guidelines.htm
Sponsor: Virginia Department of Health
Post Office Box 2448
Richmond, VA 23218

Virginia Department of Health Mary Marshall Nursing Scholarships for Registered Nurses 3499
The Mary Marshall Nursing Scholarships are funded by the Virginia General Assembly along with a donation from The Board of Nursing. The scholarship amount is dependent upon amount of scholarship source and the number of qualified applicants. It is important that all applicants fully understand the conditions of accepting a Mary Marshall Nursing Scholarship. These awards are not gifts. Scholarship recipients must agree to engage in full time nursing in Virginia for one month for every $100 received.
Requirements: To be considered for a Mary Marshall Nursing Scholarship, an applicant must meet the following criteria: residency in Virginia for at least one year; acceptance or enrollment as a full time or part time student in a school of nursing in the state of Virginia; demonstration of a cumulative grade point average of at least 3.0 in required courses, not electives; demonstration of financial need, verified by the Financial Aid Office/authorized person at the applicant's nursing school; and have submitted a completed application form and an official grade transcript. Applications and guidelines are available online from May 1 to June 30 every year. Applications must be typed, printed and mailed (with original signatures) to the: Virginia Department of Health, Office of Minority Health and Public Health Policy, ATTN: Nursing Scholarship, 109 Governor Street, Suite 1016, East Richmond, Virginia 23219.
Restrictions: The award recipient has 60 days from the date of graduation to obtain his/her license. Full time employment must begin within 90 days of the recipient's license date. Voluntary military service, even if stationed in Virginia, cannot be used to repay scholarship awards.
Geographic Focus: Virginia
Date(s) Application is Due: June 30
Contact: Aileen Harris, Health Care Workforce Manager; (804) 864-7436; fax: (804) 864-7440; email: Aileen.Harris@vdh.virginia.gov ...
Internet: http://www.vdh.virginia.gov/healthpolicy/primarycare/incentives/nursing/rn_guidelines.htm
Sponsor: Virginia Department of Health
Post Office Box 2448
Richmond, VA 23218

Virginia Department of Health Nurse Practitioner/Nurse Midwife Scholarships 3500
The program awards nurse practitioner/nurse midwife scholarships on a competitive basis. Considerations for award selections include scholastic achievement; character; and stated commitment to postgraduate employment in a medically undeserved area of Virginia, in an employment setting that provides services to persons who are unable to pay for the service and participates in all government-sponsored insurance programs designed to assure access to medical care services for covered persons. Student recipients must agree to engage in full-time practice in a designated medically underserved area for a period of years equal to the number of annual scholarships received. Preference will be given to residents of the commonwealth; minority students; students enrolled in family practice, obstetrics and gynecology, pediatric, adult health, and geriatric nurse practitioner programs; and residents of medically undeserved areas of Virginia, as determined by the board of health, in accordance with the provisions of its regulations for that purpose. The application period for this scholarship is May 1st - June 30th.
Requirements: The applicant must meet the following criteria: residency in Virginia for at least one year; acceptance or enrollment as a full-time student in a nurse practitioner/nurse midwifery program in Virginia or a nurse midwifery program in a nearby state; demonstration of a cumulative grade- point average of at least 3.0 in graduate and/or undergraduate courses; have submitted a completed application form, official grade transcript of graduate and/or undergraduate courses, and a statement of intent to practice as a nurse practitioner/nurse midwife in an undeserved area of Virginia following graduation; submission of two reference letters; and submission of all materials to the Virginia Department of Health, Office of Minority Health and Public Health Policy, ATTN: Nursing Scholarship, 109 Governor Street, Suite 1016, East Richmond, Virginia 23219
Geographic Focus: Virginia
Date(s) Application is Due: June 30
Contact: Aileen Harris, Health Care Workforce Manager; (804) 864-7436; fax: (804) 864-7440; email: Aileen.Harris@vdh.virginia.gov ...
Internet: http://www.vdh.virginia.gov/healthpolicy/primarycare/incentives/nursing/index.htm
Sponsor: Virginia Department of Health
Post Office Box 2448
Richmond, VA 23218

Virginia Tuition Assistance Grants 3501
Grants are awarded to any full-time undergraduate or graduate (including medical or law) student, regardless of financial need, who is a domiciliary resident of Virginia enrolled at an eligible private college or university in Virginia. Completed applications must be submitted to the financial aid office of the institution on, or before, July 31 prior to the fall semester of enrollment. Applications submitted after July 31, but no later than December 1, will be considered for an award only if funds are available.
Requirements: Applicant must be a domiciliary resident of Virginia; enrolled full-time as an undergraduate, graduate, or professional student; and enrolled at an eligible institution pursuing an eligible degree that is not in religious training or theological education.
Geographic Focus: Virginia
Amount of Grant: $2500 undergraduate; $1900 graduate
Date(s) Application is Due: Jul 31; Dec 1
Contact: Elizabeth Waddy, Student Aid Program Specialist, (804) 225-2632 or (804) 225-2600; fax: (804) 225-2604; email: ElizabethWaddy@schev.edu
Internet: http://www.schev.edu/students/factsheetvtag.asp?from=schevs
Sponsor: State Council of Higher Education for Virginia
101 N 14th Street
Richmond, VA 23219

Virginia W. Kettering Foundation Grants 3502
The Virginia W. Kettering Foundation, a private family foundation in Dayton, Ohio, was activated in 2003 when Virginia Kettering passed away at the age of 95. To continue her legacy of confident determination and passionate commitment to the Dayton area, Virginia Kettering directed the stewards of her foundation to support charitable organizations for charitable purposes within Montgomery, Greene, Clark, Miami, Darke, Preble, Butler and Warren Counties.
Requirements: 501(c)3 organizations located in, or that serve, the counties of Montgomery, Greene, Clark, Miami, Darke, Preble, Butler and Warren in Ohio.
Geographic Focus: Ohio
Amount of Grant: $5,000-$50,000 range
Date(s) Application is Due: Mar 1; Sep 1
Contact: Judith M. Thompson, Executive Director; (973) 228-1021; fax (973) 228-2399; email: info@ketteringfund.org
Internet: http://vwketteringfoundation.org/main.html
Sponsor: Virginia W. Kettering Foundation
1480 Kettering Tower
Dayton, OH 45423

Volkswagen of America Corporate Contributions Grants 3503
The corporation accepts proposals broadly from programs servicing needs in healthcare, wellness, children, medical research, education and diversity.
Requirements: There are no specific deadlines, however the review committee does meet quarterly to go over proposals received. The committee considers the type of organization, its mission and the intended use of the funds.
Restrictions: Grants are available to 501(c)3 organizations only.
Amount of Grant: $100,000 total per year; $1000-$2500 average
Contact: Tara Jones, email: tara.jones@vw.com; (248) 754-4693
Sponsor: Volkswagen of America, Inc.
3800 Hamlin Road
Auburn Hills, MI 48326

Vulcan Materials Company Foundation Grants 3504
The company foundation supports nonprofit organizations in company-operating areas. Grants support a broad array of programs and projects in the areas of health and welfare, community and economic development, education (including an employee matching grants program), the environment, law and justice, women and children, arts and humanities, minorities, and literacy. Requests will be considered for support of general operating expenses, capital and annual campaigns, scholarship funds, research, continuing support, and seed money. There are no application deadlines.
Requirements: The foundation awards grants only to public charities and units of government, such as public schools and parks. A public charity is any Section 501(c)3 charitable organization that is not a private foundation because it meets one of the three internal Revenue Code definitions: 509(a)1, 509(a)2 or 509(a)3.
Restrictions: The foundation does not fund individuals; organizations outside the United States; telephone or mass-mail appeals, political organizations; testimonial dinners; sectarian religious activities; organizations which have discriminatory practices; or athletic, labor, fraternal and veterans associations. The Foundation generally will not consider requests from organizations located in communities where Vulcan has no operations, offices or employees.
Geographic Focus: Alabama; Arizona; Arkansas; California; Florida; Georgia; Illinois; Indiana; Iowa; Kansas; Kentucky; Louisiana; Maryland; Mississippi; Missouri; New Mexico; North Carolina; Pennsylvania; South Carolina; Tennessee; Texas; Virginia; Wisconsin
Samples: Auburn U Foundation (Auburn U, AL)—for scholarships and fellowships, $45,000.; Family and Child Services (Birmingham, AL)—for youth programs, $20,000.; Metropolitan Arts Council (Birmingham, AL)—for general support, $79,233.
Amount of Grant: $2.8 million total
Contact: Program Contact, (205) 298-3222; email: giving@vmcmail.com
Internet: http://www.vulcanmaterials.com/social.asp?content=guidelines
Sponsor: Vulcan Materials Company Foundation
P.O. Box 385014
Birmingham, AL 35238-5014

W. C. Griffith Foundation Grants 3505
The W. C. Griffith Foundation was established in 1959 by a donation of William C. Griffith, and Ruth Perry Griffith. The Foundation gives primarily in Indianapolis-Carmel, Indiana area. The Foundation provides support primarily for hospitals, health

associations, medical and cancer research, the arts, including music and museums, community funds and development, higher, secondary, and other education, family planning services, child welfare, the homeless, the environment, libraries, and Christian religious organizations.
Requirements: Applicants should submit the following: detailed description of project and amount of funding requested; 1 Copy of the proposal.
Geographic Focus: Indiana
Samples: Eiteljorg Museum of American Indians and Western Art, Indianapolis, IN, $25,000 (2007); Providence Cristo Rey High School, Indianapolis, IN, $10,000 (2007);
Amount of Grant: $1,000 - $45,000 range
Contact: Trust Coordinator; (317) 693-2504
Sponsor: W. C. Griffith Foundation
101 West Ohio Street, Suite 1450
Indianapolis, IN 46204-1998

W. Clarke Swanson, Jr. Foundation Grants **3506**
The Foundation, established in 1998, is the brain-child of W. Clarke Swanson, Jr., founder of Swanson Vineyards. The Foundation is primarily interested in supporting the arts, education, and health care in California, there is some national giving. The type of funding typically comes in the form of general operating support. Although there is no specific application form required, applicants should submit a detailed description of the project and amount of funding requested.
Samples: Friends of Lincoln Theater, Yountville, California, $172,200 (2007); University of California at San Francisco Foundation, San Francisco, California, $50,000 (2007).
Amount of Grant: $3,000-$250,000 range
Contact: W. Clarke Swanson, Jr., Director; (707) 944-0905, ext. 20; email: clarke@swansonvineyards.com
Sponsor: W. Clarke Swanson, Jr. Foundation
1050 Oakville Cross Road, P.O. Box 148
Oakville, CA 94562

W.K. Kellogg Foundation Healthy Kids Grants **3507**
The Foundation believes that children need nutrition, stimulation, healthy living conditions and access to quality health care. It helps many of them get all four, by funding organizations that improve birth outcomes and first food experiences, create access to healthy foods, improve health services, and educate families and communities about the inter-related factors that determine well-being. The Foundation especially focuses on children who are disadvantaged by multiple societal factors, a disproportionate percentage of whom are children of color.
Requirements: To be eligible for support, your organization or institution, as well as the purpose of the proposed project, must qualify under regulations of the United States Internal Revenue Service. The Kellogg Foundation does not have any submission deadlines. Grant applications are accepted throughout the year and are reviewed at its headquarters in Battle Creek, Michigan, or in its regional office in Mexico.
Restrictions: In general, the Foundation does not provide funding for: operational phases of established programs; capital requests (which includes the construction, purchase, renovation, and/or furnishing of facilities); equipment; conferences and workshops; films, television and/or radio programs; endowments; development campaigns; or research/studies (unless they are an integral part of a larger program budget being considered for funding).
Contact: Deborah A. Rey, Supervisor of Proposal Processing; (269) 969-2133 or (269) 968-1611; fax: (269) 968-0413
Internet: http://www.wkkf.org/what-we-support/healthy-kids.aspx
Sponsor: W.K. Kellogg Foundation
One Michigan Avenue East
Battle Creek, MI 49017-4012

W.K. Kellogg Foundation Secure Families Grants **3508**
The primary needs of the family must be addressed to create pathways out of poverty for children. The Foundation supports programs that increase family stability, foster quality jobs, careers and entrepreneurship, and promote secondary achievement and financial independence. It further supports strategies that increase income, assets, and aspirations of vulnerable children and their families and reduce disparities based on class, gender and race. The Foundation focuses on three areas, each with a direct impact on the ability of families to generate income and accumulate assets: family stability; career ladders; and financial independence.
Requirements: To be eligible for support, your organization or institution, as well as the purpose of the proposed project, must qualify under regulations of the United States Internal Revenue Service. The Kellogg Foundation does not have any submission deadlines. Grant applications are accepted throughout the year and are reviewed at its headquarters in Battle Creek, Michigan, or in its regional office in Mexico.
Restrictions: In general, the Foundation does not provide funding for: operational phases of established programs; capital requests (which includes the construction, purchase, renovation, and/or furnishing of facilities); equipment; conferences and workshops; films, television and/or radio programs; endowments; development campaigns; or research/studies (unless they are an integral part of a larger program budget being considered for funding).
Contact: Deborah A. Rey, Supervisor of Proposal Processing; (269) 969-2133 or (269) 968-1611; fax: (269) 968-0413
Internet: http://www.wkkf.org/what-we-support/secure-families.aspx
Sponsor: W.K. Kellogg Foundation
One Michigan Avenue East
Battle Creek, MI 49017-4012

W.W. Smith Charitable Trust Grants for Medical Research in Cancer, AIDS, and Heart Disease **3509**
Concentration of the grant program in this area is toward basic scientific research that can help uncover and solve some of the mysteries of cancer, heart disease, and AIDS. Types of support include challenge/matching grants, general operating grants, program development grants, research grants, and scholarships. Funding is directed to projects that are new or headed by little-known investigators who are not yet qualified for large government grants. The trust also supports promising research outside the conventional pathways. Grant applications should be submitted no later than June 15 for cancer and AIDS research and no later than September 15 for cardiovascular research. Each application should be accompanied by an audited financial statement for the institution of the researcher. Projects requested should be one to three years in length and should not request funds for equipment alone. A special application form is required.
Requirements: Institutions in the general geographic area of New Jersey, eastern Pennsylvania, and Maryland may submit proposals. Specialized application form and specific guidelines should be obtained from the trust prior to submitting a proposal.
Restrictions: Only 10 percent of indirect costs are allowed on all grant proposals. Funds to support students, fellows, and postdoctoral candidates should be supported by curriculum vita. Applications should be submitted for the work of individual investigators and not for general work of research centers.
Geographic Focus: New Jersey
Samples: Thomas Jefferson U, Jefferson Medical College (Philadelphia, PA)—to endow a chair in cardiac research, $1.5 million.; Coriell Institute for Medical Research—to support cancer research, $165,000.; Fox Chase Cancer Ctr—to support AIDS research, $166,645.
Date(s) Application is Due: Jun 15; Sep 15
Contact: Frances Pemberton, Trust Administrator, (610) 397-1844; fax: (610) 397-1680; email: info@wwsmithcharitabletrust.org
Internet: http://www.wwsmithcharitabletrust.org
Sponsor: W.W. Smith Charitable Trust
200 Four Falls Corporate Center, Suite 300
West Conshohocken, PA 19428

Wabash Valley Community Foundation Grants **3510**
The foundation's mission is to promote community investment for a better tomorrow. Giving primarily for arts and culture, education, human services, community development, and religion. Each year, the Foundation provides grants to charitable organizations for projects that meet the charitable needs in the Wabash Valley. These grants respond to specific community challenges and improve the vitality of the community. The Foundation teaches the area's youth leaders by engaging them in allocating limited resources for them to grant to worthy charitable projects. Deadlines for letters of intent are as follows: Clay County—May 1; Sullivan County—May 1. Vigo County—May 1 and November 15.
Restrictions: Giving is restricted to Clay, Sullivan, and Vigo counties in Indiana. No grants are given for endowments, deficit funding, annual appeals and membership contributions, travel for groups such as bands, sports teams and classes, conferences, publications, films, television, or radio programs (unless integral to the project for which the grant is sought.
Geographic Focus: Indiana
Date(s) Application is Due: Nov 15; May 1
Contact: Beth Tevlin, Executive Director; (812) 232-2234 or (877) 232-2230; fax: (812) 234-4853; email: beth@wvcf.com
Internet: http://www.wvcf.com/wvcf_index3.htm
Sponsor: Wabash Valley Community Foundation
2901 Ohio Boulevard, Suite 153
Terre Haute, IN 47803

Wachovia Foundation Grants **3511**
The foundation awards grants to eligible tax-exempt organizations in four primary areas: education, community and economic development, arts and culture, and health and human services. Its mission is to build strong and vibrant communities, improve the quality of life, and make a positive difference in Wachovia communities. Contributions are coordinated through regional Wachovia Community Affairs offices (list available online), in Florida; Georgia; New Jersey, New York, and Connecticut; North and South Carolina (except for Charlotte); North Carolina'Charlotte); Pennsylvania and Delaware; Virginia, Maryland, and Washington, DC; Wachovia Securities; and national requests. Guidelines and application are available online.
Requirements: Applicant organizations must have a 501(c)3 nonprofit tax-exempt classification, be located or provide service in Wachovia's markets, have broad community support and address specific community needs; and demonstrate fiscal and administrative stability.
Restrictions: Grants are not made to support individuals; travel or conferences; political causes or candidates; organizations whose primary purpose is to influence legislation; religious, veteran, or fraternal organizations for programs limited to specific groups; retirement homes or communities; precollege-level private schools; or organizations already receiving support through United Way or a United Arts drive, except for approved capital campaigns.
Amount of Grant: $5000-$100,000 typically
Contact: Grants Administrator, (704) 374-4085; fax: (704) 374-2484
Internet: http://www.wachovia.com/inside/page/0,,139_414_430,00.html
Sponsor: Wachovia Foundation
301 S College Street, NC0143
Charlotte, NC 28288-0143

Waitt Family Foundation Grants 3512
The Waitt Family Foundation is looking for programs with real potential to improve the lives of people in at-risk populations throughout the world. These programs, supported by the Waitt Helping Hands Fund, will encourage collaboration across various disciplines or related organizations in order to change the way people see themselves, others, and the opportunities before them. The Foundation is interested in programs that foster independence, self-help, and self-reliance, and want people to obtain the skills necessary to better themselves and their communities. Most importantly, the Foundation is looking for projects that create long-term change to help the greatest number of people. There is a $100,000 minimum for all grant requests. Multi-year proposals will be considered.
Requirements: Organizations must have a U.S. tax identification number and be able to provide a current copy of their IRS 501(c)3 determination letter. Only organizations with federal non-profit agency tax status can receive financial support.
Restrictions: The Foundation does not fund the following categories: individuals; for-profit organizations; capital campaigns; endowments; debt reduction; arts; religious organizations; public education institutions; health care organizations or hospitals; or lobbying prohibited by the Internal Revenue Code.
Geographic Focus: California; Iowa; Nebraska; South Dakota
Amount of Grant: $100,000 minimum
Date(s) Application is Due: Feb 1; May 1; Aug 1; Oct 1
Contact: Cherie Jacobson; (858) 551-4400; fax: (858) 551-6871; email: grants@waittfoundation.org
Internet: http://waittfoundation.org/grants/guidelines.html
Sponsor: Waitt Family Foundation
P.O. Box 1948
La Jolla, CA 92038-1948

Wal-Mart Foundation Community Grants 3513
The sponsor encourages its stores to award grants in its four areas of focus: Education, Health, Job Skills Training and Sustainability. All requests for funding must be directed through Wal-Mart Stores, SAM'S CLUBS, Neighborhood Markets and Distribution Centers. Proposals mailed directly to the Wal-Mart Foundation will not be considered.
Requirements: Eligible organizations include 501(c)3 organizations; schools—public, parochial, and private; churches—faith-based organizations that are conducting projects benefiting a broad section of the community; government-funded agencies. Request a grant application by speaking with the facility manager at your local Wal-Mart Stores, Inc. facility.
Restrictions: Grants are not awarded to support annual meetings; capital campaigns; endowments; faith-based organization's projects that benefit primarily or entirely on their members or adherents; film and video projects; individuals; organizations outside of the United States or Puerto Rico; political causes; program advertising; funding for projects used for benefit outside of the local community; or travel.
Amount of Grant: up to $5,000
Contact: Community Involvement Coordinator at the Wal-Mart or Sam's Club location closest to you
Internet: http://walmartstores.com/CommunityGiving/238.aspx
Sponsor: Wal-Mart Foundation
702 SW Eighth Street
Bentonville, AR 72716-8611

Wal-Mart State Giving Program Grants 3514
Through this program, the sponsor awards grants at the state and regional level to support unmet needs that are not directly addressed by any of their current giving programs. The foundation has adopted four areas of focus: Education, Job Skills Training, Environmental Sustainability and Health. The minimum grant size for this program is $5,000.
Requirements: While the sponsor encourages funding requests that align with its four areas of focus – programs that do not align with the four areas of focus will also be given full consideration. (See the sponsor's website for more information on the areas of focus.) Applications will be accepted year-round through the online application system. Applications will be valid only for the Fiscal Year during which they were submitted (February – January). Only organizations with a current tax-exempt status under Section 501(c)3 of the Internal Revenue Code are eligible to request funding. (NOTE: Organizations must be listed in the most current IRS 50 State Master File at the time the grant request is submitted.)
Restrictions: Organizations and Projects that are excluded from funding: (1) Organizations without a valid 501(c)3 tax exemption status; (2) Scholarship programs; (3) Athletic teams or events; (4) Political advocacy groups; (5) Gala and event sponsorships; (6) Association/Chamber memberships; (7) Organizations whose services are limited to its members; (8) Projects that send products or people for relief efforts to a foreign country; (9) Advertising, film or video projects; (10) Program advertising or marketing venues; (11) Children's Miracle Network; (12) General operating expenses; (13) Churches and other faith-based organizations when the proposed grant will only benefit the organization or its members. Examples of such projects include: (a) Youth groups, (b) Purchase of real estate, (c) Mission trips, or (d) Sunday school supplies; (14) Organizations that have received a State Giving Program grant within the current fiscal year; (15) Multi-year commitments - (a) Organizations are to be funded on a year by year basis; (b) Organizations that receive funding must submit additional funding applications in order to be considered for additional funding each year.
Amount of Grant: $5,000 minimum
Date(s) Application is Due: Apr 17; Jun 3; Sep 18; Nov 4
Contact: Grants Administrator; (479) 273-4000
Internet: http://walmartstores.com/CommunityGiving/8168.aspx
Sponsor: Wal-Mart Foundation
702 SW Eighth Street
Bentonville, AR 72716-8611

Wallace H. Coulter Foundation Grants 3515
The foundation awards grants to support research and education in the fields of engineering, medicine, and science. Past grants also have supported humanitarian interests. There are no application deadlines or forms.
Restrictions: Grants do not support religious organizations or individuals.
Samples: Boston U, Biomedical Engineering Dept (MA)—to help advance promising biomedical technologies to the clinical-application phase, $2.9 million (2005).
Amount of Grant: $35,000-$200,000 average
Contact: Wayne Barlin, Vice President, (305) 559-2991; fax: (305) 559-5490; email: wb@whcf.org
Internet: http://www.whcf.org
Sponsor: Wallace H. Coulter Foundation
790 NW 107th Avenue, Suite 215
Miami, FL 33172

Walt Disney Company Foundation Grants 3516
The foundation funds medical and health services, health and welfare of children, youth activities, higher education, community funds, music, and cultural arts in Los Angeles and Orange Counties in California and Orange and Osceola Counties in Florida. Types of support include general operating support, continuing support, annual campaigns, capital campaigns, program development, scholarship funds, fellowships, and employee-related scholarships. Previous grants have supported downtown revitalization in both New York City, where Disney redeveloped an old Times Square theater, and Los Angeles, where support has been given for a new music hall that will be home to the Los Angeles Philharmonic Orchestra.
Requirements: 501(c)3 tax-exempt organizations in California and Florida may apply.
Restrictions: Disney will not make grants for scholarships, religious organizations, building campaigns, start-up campaigns, seed purposes, research, loans, conferences, general fund drives, annual charitable appeals, and political purposes.
Geographic Focus: California; Florida; New York
Amount of Grant: $1000 scholarships
Contact: Tillie Baptie, Executive Director, (818) 560-1006; fax: (818) 563-5271
Internet: http://disney.go.com/disneyhand/contributions/wdcfoundation.html
Sponsor: Walt Disney Company Foundation
500 S Buena Vista Street
Burbank, CA 91521-0987

Walter Nicolai Prize in Biomedical Gerontology 3517
This award is given annually for meritorious research by a graduate or medical student in the area of biomedical gerontology. For purposes of the prize, biomedical gerontology is defined as basic biological or clinical research involving normal aging or age-associated diseases. The research should be oriented toward improving the quality of later life. There is one prize plus awards to the first two runners-up to help enable them to attend the annual meeting of the American Aging Association (AGE). Nomination should include four copies each of the following: six- to 10-page (double-spaced) report of the research with name and departmental affiliations in the format used by the AGE journal, sponsor's letter commenting on the significance of the work, and candidate's curriculum vita with current professional address. The sponsor's letter will serve as the nominating document. The recipient of the prize, as well as the two runners-up, will be notified and the prizes will be presented at the annual meeting.
Requirements: A nomination may be made by any member of a society associated with aging research. The sponsor may reside in the United States, Canada, or Mexico.
Amount of Grant: $500 first prize
Contact: Program Contact, (610) 627-2626; fax: (610) 565-9747; email: ameraging@aol.com
Internet: http://www.americanaging.org
Sponsor: American Aging Association (AGE)
110 Chesley Drive
Media, PA 19063

Warren Alpert Foundation Prize 3518
The annual prize recognizes scientists and researchers from around the world for their contributions to humanity and their breakthroughs in the understanding and curing of major diseases. Many of the world's foremost scientific and medical professionals, working in a variety of disciplines, are nominated by their colleagues for this prestigious honor. Winners are presented with a monetary award at the foundation's annual luncheon. Recipients are selected by the foundation's scientific advisory board, which comprises internationally renowned biomedical scientists.
Samples: David Goeddel, PhD; Sidney Pestka, MD; and Charles Weissmann, MD, PhD—award recipients, for their pioneering work on the purification, characterization, and cloning of human interferon-alpha, $150,000 each (2003).
Amount of Grant: $100,000 award
Contact: Patrick Gilligan, (617) 432-2094; email: patrick_gilligan@hms.harvard.edu
Internet: http://www.hms.harvard.edu/fa/alpertprize
Sponsor: Warren Alpert Foundation
25 Shattuck Street, Room 206
Boston, MA 02115

Warrick County Community Foundation Grants 3519

The Warrick County Community Foundation is a nonprofit, public charity created by and for the people of Warrick County, Indiana. The Foundation helps nonprofits fulfill their missions by strengthening their ability to meet community needs through grants that assist charitable programs, address community issues, support community agencies, launch community initiatives, and support leadership development.

Requirements: The Foundation welcomes proposals from nonprofit organizations that are deemed tax-exempt under sections 501(c)3 and 509(a) of the Internal Revenue Code and from governmental agencies serving the Warrick County. Proposals from nonprofit organizations not classified as a 501(c)3 public charity may be considered provided the project is charitable and supports a community need.

Restrictions: Project areas not considered for funding: religious organizations for religious purposes; political parties or campaigns; endowment creation or debt reduction; operating costs; capital campaigns; annual appeals or membership contributions; travel requests for groups or individuals such as bands, sports teams, or classes.

Geographic Focus: Indiana

Samples: Youth Resources of Southwestern Indiana $1,500 - for the Teen Advisory Council and Youth Make a Difference Grant Program (2008); Lampion Center $1,937 - for the Nurturing Program for Abused Children (2008); Evansville Philharmonic Orchestra $1,500 - for the 2008-2009 Warrick County Youth Concert Series (2008).

Date(s) Application is Due: Sep 1

Contact: Susan Sublett, Director; (812) 897-2030; email: susan@warrickcommunityfoundation.org

Internet: http://www.warrickcommunityfoundation.org/disc-grants

Sponsor: Warrick County Community Foundation
224 West Main Street, P.O. Box 215
Boonville, IN 47601

Washington Post Contributions Program Grants 3520

The contributions program supports qualified nonprofit organizations of the Washington, DC, metropolitan community whose ongoing programs directly benefit those in the community who are in need and that focus on key issues in the areas of education, health and human services, the arts, civic betterment, and community service. Special interest is given to organizations whose programs serve the most needy and least able citizens; seek to fill unmet societal needs or solve long-standing community problems; and address key community issues and concerns in collaborative and imaginative ways. Grants are awarded to support specific programs or for general operating support. Funding rarely is available for capital campaigns. Applications for capital campaigns that meet the Post's general guidelines are held until December and will be funded only if resources are available at the time of review. There are no application forms. Proposals should include a one-page cover sheet; a three- to five-page application letter; supporting documents; list of board of directors and officers; a copy of the most recent annual report; and several relevant articles, reviews, brochures, etc., about the project or organization. Deadlines are the first Tuesday in March, June, September, and December.

Requirements: Organizations that are tax-exempt under section 501(c)3 of the Internal Revenue Code that operate in the Washington, DC, metropolitan area are eligible.

Restrictions: Funding is not available for individuals; national or other organizations whose programs do not directly serve Washington-area needs; religious organizations for religious purposes; fraternal, membership, or veterans organizations or athletic teams, volunteer fire/emergency services, or similar groups; political action or advocacy groups; multiyear grants; challenge grants; third-party fund-raising efforts; conferences; research; or start-up projects. Applications are not accepted.

Contact: Eric Grant, Director, (202) 334-6834; fax: (202) 334-5609

Internet: http://washpost.com/community/charities/contributions.shtml

Sponsor: Washington Post Educational Foundation
1150 15th St NW
Washington, DC 20071

Wasie Foundation Grants 3521

The foundation limits grantmaking activities to organizations in Minnesota and currently makes grants in the areas of higher education, specifically endowed scholarship programs, and the care and treatment of individuals afflicted with schizophrenia. Types of support include equipment acquisition, endowment funds, program development, conferences and seminars, scholarship funds, research, and matching funds. Call or write for application procedures and current deadlines; the foundation encourages phone contact.

Requirements: Organizations in Florida and Minnesota are eligible.

Restrictions: Grant making is limited to the Saint Paul/Minneapolis metropolitan area.

Geographic Focus: Florida; Minnesota

Amount of Grant: $15,000-$200,000 average

Contact: Jan Preble, Program Associate, (612) 455-6880; fax: (612) 455-6888

Sponsor: Wasie Foundation
4999 France Ave S, Suite 250
Minneapolis, MN 55410

Wayne and Gladys Valley Foundation Grants 3522

The foundation awards grants to California nonprofits in its primary areas of interest, including education at all levels, health care and medical research, youth and families, human services, sciences and engineering, and religion. Types of support include general operating support, building construction/renovation, program development, professorships, research, and matching funds. There are no application forms or deadlines. The board meets in February, May, September, and November to consider requests.

Requirements: California nonprofits in Alameda, Contra Costa, and Santa Clara Counties are eligible.

Geographic Focus: California

Samples: U of the Pacific (Stockton, CA)—for its new biological-sciences center, $2.5 million (2005); Santa Clara U (CA)—to construct a new library, $15 million (2004); Dominican U of California (San Rafael, CA)—for a new science and technology center, $2.25 million (2004).

Contact: Michael Desler, Executive Director, (510) 466-6060; fax (510) 466-6067; email: info@wgvalley.org

Sponsor: Wayne and Gladys Valley Foundation
1939 Harrison Street, Suite 510
Oakland, CA 94612-3532

Weatherwax Foundation Grants 3523

The foundation awards grants in Michigan to projects that promote and support education, civic and social programs, culture, science, and the arts, primarily in the greater Jackson area and, to a lesser extent, in the adjacent counties. Types of support include building construction and renovation; matching and challenge grants; general operating grants; program development; scholarships; annual and capital campaigns; and emergency funds. The initial approach is a two-page grant proposal that may be submitted at any time. Granting decisions are made in January, May, and August.

Requirements: Giving primarily in Hillsdale, Lenawee, and Jackson counties, MI.

Restrictions: No grants to individuals; or for computer purchases.

Geographic Focus: Michigan

Samples: Albion College (MI)—for music facility renovation, $125,000.; Michigan Theatre (MI)—for restoration, strategic planning, and executive search, $27,500.; Family Service and Children's Aid (MI)—for general operating support and neighborhood outreach activities, $45,491.

Amount of Grant: $1000-$200,000 average range

Contact: Program Contact, (517) 787-2117; fax: (517) 787-2118

Internet: http://www.lib.msu.edu/harris23/grants/wfbrochu.htm

Sponsor: Weatherwax Foundation
P.O. Box 1111
Jackson, MI 49204

Weingart Foundation Grants 3524

Weingart Foundation makes grants to assist organizations that work in the areas of health, human services, and education. The Foundation gives highest priority to activities that provide greater access to people who are economically disadvantaged and underserved. Of particular interest to the Foundation are applications that specifically address the needs of low-income children and youth, older adults, and people affected by disabilities and homelessness. The Foundation also funds activities that benefit the general community and improve the quality of life for all individuals in Southern California. Weingart Foundation offers the following types of grants: core support; capital; capacity building; program; and a small grant program. See website for a description of each grant type: http://www.weingartfnd.org/default.asp?PID=5

Requirements: An organization that is certified as tax exempt under Section 501(c) (3) of the U.S. Internal Revenue Code and is not a private foundation as defined in section 509(a) of that Code is eligible for consideration. Preference is given to organizations providing services in the following six Southern California counties: Los Angeles, Orange, Riverside, Santa Barbara, San Bernardino, and Ventura.

Restrictions: Grants are not made: for propagandizing, influencing legislation and/or elections, promoting voter registration; for political candidates, political campaigns; for litigation; to institutions limiting their services to persons of a single religious sect or denomination; for social or political issues outside the United States of America; to individuals; to federated appeals or for the collection of funds for redistribution to other nonprofit groups; for conferences, workshops, temporary exhibits, travel, surveys, films or publishing activities; for endowment funds; for contingencies, deficits or debt reduction; for fundraising dinners or events; for research. Grants generally are not approved for: national organizations that do not have local chapters operating in the geographic area of grant focus; projects or programs normally financed by government sources; refugee or religious programs, consumer interest or environmental advocacy; feasibility studies. The Foundation does not fund Section 509(a) (3) Type III non-functionally integrated supporting organizations.

Geographic Focus: California

Samples: National Urban Fellows, $25,000—program support for the Southern California Capacity Building Initiative (2010); Performing Arts Center of Los Angeles, $150,000—core support for Music Center education programs (2010); JWCH Medical Clinic, $900,000— capacity building support to strengthen administrative infrastructure (2010); University of Southern California, $10,000—support for the Los Angeles Leadership Group (2010); Church of Our Saviour, $150,000—core support (2010).

Contact: Grants Administrator, (213) 688-7799; fax: (213) 688-1515; email: info@weingartfnd.org

Internet: http://www.weingartfnd.org

Sponsor: Weingart Foundation
1055 W. Seventh Street, Suite 3050
Los Angeles, CA 90017-2305

Welborn Baptist Foundation Grants 3525

Welborn Baptist Foundation is continuing to make significant grants in its target areas, which include: promotion of healthy adolescent development; improvements to community health status; faith-based initiatives; school based health; promotion of early childhood development; and general opportunity. Types of support include: building renovation; capital campaigns; conferences/seminars; curriculum development; equipment; challenge support; and program development.

Requirements: Giving limited to: Gallatin, Saline, Wabash, Wayne and White counties in Illinous; Dubois, Gibson, Perry, Pike, Posey, Spencer, Vanderburgh, and Warrick counties in Indiana; and Henderson County, Kentucky.
Restrictions: Typically, projects designed to meet urgent human needs such food pantries, soup kitchens, direct shelter services, rental and utility assistance programs and the like are not considered to be mission-critical to the Foundation. No support is available for: basic scientific research; individuals; endowments; annual fund drives; debt service; deficit spending; scholarships; fellowships; general operating costs; venture capital or fund-raising; or loans.
Geographic Focus: Illinois; Indiana; Kentucky
Date(s) Application is Due: Mar 27
Contact: Garz W. Bauer; (812) 437-8260 or (877) 437-8260; fax: (812) 437-8269; email: info@welbornfdn.org
Internet: http://www.welbornfdn.org/page.aspx?PageID=a7a64ca2-e45e-424a-8b09-7212a9ee9cff&ParentPageID=72d50394-86af-45a2-bf89-ae6b403dac17
Sponsor: Welborn Baptist Foundation, Inc.
Twenty-One Southeast Third Street, Suite 610
Evansville, IN 47708

Wellmark Foundation Grants **3526**
The foundation encourages proposals that measurably decrease the number of community members suffering from an acute or chronic disease or improve the health status of community members afflicted with an acute or chronic disease. Priority areas include asthma, diabetes, heart failure and cardiovascular risk factors, major depression, and end-of-life care with an emphasis on pain control. Mini grants award smaller amounts of money available for projects that support one or more of the five priority areas. The listed application deadline is for mini grants.
Requirements: 501(c)3 tax exempt in Iowa or South Dakota are eligible.
Restrictions: 509(a) private foundations and primary contracting entities that have a contractual relationship with Wellmark are ineligible.
Geographic Focus: Iowa; South Dakota
Contact: Grants Administrator, (515) 245-4819; fax: (515) 235-4455; email: WMFoundation@wellmark.com
Internet: http://www.wellmark.com/community/wellmark_foundation/wellmark_foundation.htm
Sponsor: Wellmark Foundation
636 Grand Avenue, Sta 150
Des Moines, IA 50309-2565

Wells County Foundation Grants **3527**
The Wells County Foundation, Inc. is a nonprofit public charity established in 1957 to serve donors, award grants, and provide leadership to improve the Wells County, Indiana area forever. The Foundation gives priority to programs having a positive effect on the Wells County community. Grant making fields of interest include arts and culture, education, economic and community development, health and human services, and other charitable purposes. In general, the Foundation does not award multi-year grants. With the exception of the scholarship funds administered by the Foundation, grants are not made to individuals. Awards are made with the understanding that the Foundation has no obligation or commitment to provide any additional support. The Foundation operates without discrimination as to race, national origin, religion, gender, gender preference, age, or disability or that perceived as a disability in the consideration of grant requests. Likewise, grants will be awarded only to those organizations operating without the aforementioned discriminations. Requests for support of projects presented by religious groups will be considered if a general community need is being met and the project does not promote the teachings or doctrine of a particular church or religious organization.
Requirements: The most efficient way of making initial contact with The Wells County Foundation, Inc. is by a phone call. Be prepared to give a brief description of the purpose for the grant request. Factual information should be provided to enable the Foundation to determine whether the request falls within grant-making guidelines. Grant proposals for programs or projects should include the following, if applicable: Title page - organization's name, address, and telephone number; contact person and title; project/program title and amount requested; date of application. Proposal narrative - issues project/program will address; expectations of project/program; how many will benefit from project/program; role for volunteers in project/program; plan for evaluation of project/program; signed endorsement of the proposal by the organization's Board of Directors. Financial information - Budget for proposed project / program, including income and expense data; minimum of two pricing quotes for equipment requested; listing of other funding sources applied to and / or received for project / program; if applicable, how project / program will be funded in future. Organizational information - brief history of organization, including mission and purpose; list of officers and members of governing board, including addresses and telephone numbers; year-end financial statement or audit; if more than six months since statement or audit, also include most recent financial statement; copy of tax exemption from Internal Revenue Service. If you have any questions in the preparation of your proposal, please call the Foundation office at (260)824-8620.
Restrictions: No grants will be made to any political organization or to support attempts to influence the legislation of any governing body other than through making available to the community at large the results of non-partisan analysis, study and/or research.
Geographic Focus: Indiana
Samples: Wells County Master Gardeners, $5,000 - to provide funding for the Cook-Williamson Memorial Iris Garden (2008); Southern Wells Community Schools, $3,655 - to provide funding for Musical Magic Summer School Enrichment Program (2008); JobWorks, Inc., $10,000 - to provide funding for the Wells County Community GED Tutoring Project (2008).
Date(s) Application is Due: Feb 16; Jun 15; Oct 15
Contact: Tom Stogdill, Grant Committee Chair: (260) 824-8620; fax: (260) 824-3981; email: wellscountyfound@wellscountyfound.org or tstogdill@parlorcity.com
Internet: http://www.wellscountyfound.org/Grants.htm
Sponsor: Wells County Foundation, Inc.
109 North Scott Street
Bluffton, IN 46714

Western Indiana Community Foundation Grants **3528**
The Western Indiana Community Foundation focuses its attention on local needs within the geographical boundaries as set by the Board of Directors (i.e. the school corporation boundaries), with consideration given to the areas of health, charitable service, education, cultural affairs, and community improvement. All endowment funds, which stipulate in the fund agreement the areas to be supported from the income, earned on the fund assets will be honored regardless of location of grant recipient. Primary fields of interest include: health, charitable service, education, cultural affairs, and community improvement. The Foundation is especially interested in learning of plans for: startup costs for new programs; one-time projects or needs; and capital needs beyond an applicant's capabilities and needs. Grant applications may be submitted at anytime throughout the year. Applicants will be notified immediately following the Board of Directors decision.
Requirements: Programs serving the residents of the Fountain County region of western Indiana are eligible to apply.
Restrictions: The Foundation will not consider: grants for individuals except for scholarships; organizations for political or religious purposes; support for regular operating budgets; contributions to endowments; providing for long term funding; post-event situations; or apparel (such as school/sport uniforms).
Geographic Focus: Indiana
Amount of Grant: $10,000 maximum
Contact: Dale White, Executive Director; (765)-793-0702; fax: (765)-793-0703; email: dwhite@wicf-inc.org or info@wicf-inc.org
Internet: http://www.wicf-inc.org/grant_guidelines.asp
Sponsor: Western Indiana Community Foundation
135 S. Stringtown Road, P.O. Box 175
Covington, IN 47932-0175

Western Union Foundation Grants **3529**
The Foundation generally awards grants in the United States and internationally in its areas of interest, including education; and health and human services addressing literacy, health care for the uninsured, nutrition, pre- and postnatal care, childhood immunizations, poverty, language barriers, and cultural adjustment. In order to maximize resources and create a greater impact in communities, the Foundation will not accept unsolicited proposals in 2010. The Foundation will work with its current NGO partners and solicit proposals from NGOs that closely align with the Foundation's education and economic development program areas.
Restrictions: In general grants do not support general operating support, individuals, endowments, special events, capital projects, early childhood education, other post-secondary scholarship programs, deficits or retirement of debt, re-granting agencies, and awards.
Geographic Focus: Colorado; Florida; Nebraska; New York; Texas
Date(s) Application is Due: Mar 1; Jun 1; Dec 1
Contact: Luella Chavez D'Angelo, President; (720) 332-4763 or (720) 332-6606; fax: (720) 332-4772; email: luella.dangelo@westernunion.com
Internet: http://foundation.westernunion.com/ourProgramsDirect.html
Sponsor: Western Union Foundation
12500 East Belford Avenue, Suite 1-I
Englewood, CO 80112

Westinghouse Charitable Giving Grants **3530**
The foundation makes charitable contributions to community priorities primarily where Westinghouse has a presence. Areas of emphasis include education—elementary, secondary, and high school programs that emphasize math and science (some non-fine arts programs); health and welfare—to improve quality of life in the community; and civic and social affairs—to support economic development, environmental quality, and the preservation of public safety. Within each area, the foundation actively encourages programs that meet the needs of special populations, such as the disadvantaged, the young, the elderly, the gifted, people with disabilities, minorities, and women. Because of the foundation's approach to funding in Westinghouse plant locations, all organizations, except colleges and universities, should submit their requests for support to the nearest Westinghouse location. Applications are accepted on an ongoing basis.
Requirements: 501(c)3 tax-exempt organizations are eligible.
Restrictions: The following organizations and activities are ineligible: individuals; political contributions; religious organizations; highly specialized health, medical, or welfare programs; fine arts organizations/programs; organizations that discriminate by race, color, creed, gender, or national origin; hospitals; colleges, universities, and two-year institutions; capital improvement or building projects; medical education; chairs or professorships; liberal arts, fine arts, or similar educational programs; educational research programs, regardless of academic discipline; graduate education; general endowment; equipment purchases at universities; United Way-affiliated agencies; tickets; or memberships.
Samples: Regional Math/Science Collaborative (Pittsburgh, PA)—to support education reform and international economic education, $20,000.; NAACP Benton-Franklin

County Chapter (Pasco, WA)—to encourage academic excellence in the sciences, humanities, and visual and performing arts for African American ninth-12th grade students, $10,000.
Amount of Grant: $5000 maximum
Contact: Program Officer, Contributions and Community Affairs, (412) 374-6824; fax: (412) 642-4874
Internet: http://www.westinghousenuclear.com/E2.asp
Sponsor: Westinghouse Electric Corporation
P.O. Box 355, ECE 575C
Pittsburgh, PA 15230-0355

WHAS Crusade for Children Grants **3531**
The organization, established in Kentucky in 1954, is dedicated to helping the handicapped children of today and to expanding the ability to care for and prevent the handicaps of tomorrow. The crusade supports organizations which serve children suffering from a variety of mental and physical disabilities. WHAS Crusade for Children grants are made to non-profit agencies, schools and hospitals to help children (up to age 18) overcome physical, mental, emotional or medical challenges. Grants are for direct services only, and are made for specific programs or equipment that provide direct benefit to special needs children. Applications are mailed out each year in November and December. All agencies that received a grant this year receive an application for next year. To request an application, a non-profit agency, school or hospital should send a letter (on letterhead signed by the agency director or school superintendent) to the WHAS Crusade for Children at the address listed. The deadline for applications is late January each year.
Requirements: Agencies serving special needs children from Kentucky and southern Indiana are eligible to receive grants. The Crusade must have support from a county before grants can be made to a school, hospital or agency located in that county.
Restrictions: Grants are not made to individuals, and are not considered operating grants.
Geographic Focus: Indiana; Kentucky
Contact: Dawn Lee, President; (502) 582-7706; fax: (502) 582-7712; email: dlee@whas11.com or contact-crusade@whascrusade.org
Internet: http://www.whascrusade.org/grants/
Sponsor: WHAS Crusade for Children
P.O. Box 1100
Louisville, KY 40201-1100

Whitaker International Fellows and Scholars Program **3532**
The Program consists of two branches: Whitaker Fellows and Whitaker Scholars. The goal of both Programs is to assist in the development of professional leaders who are not only superb engineers and scientists, but who also will lead and serve the profession with an international outlook. The term of the Fellow awards will be one academic year (as defined by the academic calendar of the host country). The term of the Scholar awards can be for as little as one academic semester or as long as a full academic year. Awards will typically begin between July 1st and October 1st, but may begin as late as March 31st.
Requirements: U.S. citizens and non-citizen permanent residents may apply. Fellows must have a BS or MS degree in biomedical engineering (or bioengineering, which is considered here synonymous if the program emphasizes biomedical engineering), and they will not have a doctorate at the time they start the grant. The Fellows applicant's most recent degree may not have been obtained more than two years prior to the start of the grant. Scholars must have a either degree in biomedical engineering and a doctorate which may not have been obtained more than two years prior to the start of the grant, or must be advanced PhD candidates who have been admitted to candidacy and who will receive the PhD prior to departure.
Amount of Grant: $15,000 maximum
Date(s) Application is Due: Jan 25
Contact: Vijay Renganathan, Manager; (212) 984-5442; email: whitaker@iie.org
Internet: http://whitakerawards.org/program-overview
Sponsor: Institute of International Education
809 United Nations Plaza
New York, NY 10017

Whitehall Foundation Neurobiology Research Grants **3533**
Through its program of grants and grants in aid, the foundation assists scholarly research in the life sciences. The foundation is currently interested in basic research in invertebrate and vertebrate (excluding clinical) neurobiology, specifically investigations of neural mechanisms involved in sensory, motor, and other complex functions of the whole organism as these relate to behavior. Research grants are available to established scientists of all ages working at accredited institutions and will be awarded for up to three years, with possible renewal on a competitive basis for a maximum of two years. Grants in aid are designed for researchers at the assistant professor level who experience difficulty in competing for research funds because they have not yet become firmly established. Grants in aid will also be made to senior scientists. The foundation's policy is to assist those dynamic areas of basic biological research that are not heavily supported by federal agencies or other foundations with specialized missions. Types of support include personnel (salary support for students and technicians); permanent equipment, materials, and supplies needed to complete the project; travel for research; publication costs; and overhead (no more than 25 percent or supplies). Applicant should initiate the proposal process by submitting a one-page letter written in technical language identifying the nature of the research proposal and indicating whether the request is for a grant or grant in aid. Grant application forms will be sent to those applicants whose proposed project matches the foundation's current funding interests. Deadlines listed are for letters of intent.
Requirements: Accredited U.S. institutions are eligible. The foundation prefers to support scientists at the beginning of their career and those senior scientists who have maintained productivity. The principal investigator must hold no less than the position of assistant professor or the equivalent.
Samples: Daniel Pollen, U of Massachusetts (MA)—for research on the cerebral integration in the primate visual system, $40,000 of three-year grant.; Richard Ivry, U of California (CA)—for research on the role of the cerebellum in temporal processing, $24,000 final payment on three-year grant.; Paul Black, Boston U (Boston, MA)—to support research on brain-immune system interactions, $130,020 final payment on three-year grant.
Amount of Grant: $30,000-$75,000 typically; $30,000 maximum grants in aid
Date(s) Application is Due: Jan 15; Apr 15; Oct 1
Contact: Director, (561) 655-4474; fax (561) 655-4978; email: email@whitehall.org
Internet: http://www.whitehall.org
Sponsor: Whitehall Foundation
P.O. Box 3423
Palm Beach, FL 33480

WHO Foundation General Grants **3534**
The foundation nationally supports grass-roots charities serving the overlooked needs of women and children. Grants are provided to organizations serving women and/or children in the United States and Puerto Rico. Specific projects and programs addressing health, education, and social service needs are the priority. The foundation recognizes the value of new programs created to respond to changing needs and will consider funding projects of an original or pioneering nature within an existing organization. Application and guidelines are available for download at the sponsor's website.
Requirements: 501(c)3 nonprofit organizations in the United States and Puerto Rico are eligible. Organizations must have been incorporated for a minimum of three years prior to application. Preference will be given to organizations with an operating budget of $3 million or less, those not dependent upon government grants, and those with greater organizational program costs than personnel costs. Funding requests must be made using the WHO Foundation application. Electronic and faxed submissions will not be accepted.
Restrictions: The following types of organizations, activities or purposes will not be considered: personal requests, loans or scholarships to individuals.; educational institutions; endowment campaigns; international programs or projects; government agencies; fiscal agents; religious organizations (including young Men's and Women's Christian Association); political causes, candidates, organizations or campaigns; foundations that are grant making institutions; advertising in charitable publications; sports organizations; labor groups; research projects; travel for individuals or groups; conferences, galas, charity balls, sponsorships, seminars, or reunions; capital campaigns; salaries; or building campaigns (i.e. Habitat for Humanity).
Amount of Grant: $5,000-$30,000
Contact: Cindy Turek, Executive Director; (800) 946-4663; fax: (972) 386-8736; email: who@beauticontrol.com
Internet: http://www.whofoundation.org/WHO_FundingCriteria.htm
Sponsor: WHO (Women Helping Others) Foundation
P.O. Box 816029
Dallas, TX 75381-6029

Wilhelm Sander Foundation Grants **3535**
The purpose of the Foundations grants are to support research in the field of human medicine with a focus on cancer research.
Restrictions: The grant is limited to Germany and Switzerland.
Contact: J. Koppenhofer: (089) 544-1870; fax: (089) 544-18720; email: info@sanst.de
Internet: http://www.wilhelm-sander-stiftung.de
Sponsor: Wilhelm Sander Foundation
Goethe route 74
Munich 80336 Germany

Wilkins Family Foundation Grants **3536**
The foundation awards grants to U.S. nonprofit organizations in its areas of interest, including projects, community service organizations, economic development activities, and cultural organizations involved with education and health issues of children 17 years of age and younger. Letters of intent are accepted online; full proposals are by invitation.
Requirements: 501(c)3 tax-exempt organizations are eligible.
Restrictions: The foundation does not make multiyear commitments and prefers to fund causes, rather than management expenses.
Date(s) Application is Due: Feb 1
Contact: Grants Administrator, email: proposals@wilkinsfamilyfoundation.org
Internet: http://fdncenter.org/grantmaker/wilkinsfamily/procedure.html
Sponsor: Wilkins Family Foundation
302 N Rock Road, Suite 200
Wichita, KS 67206-2255

William G. Gilmore Foundation Grants **3537**
The foundation supports nonprofits primarily in the San Francisco Bay Area, CA; some funding also in Pueblo, CO and Portland, OR. Giving primarily for the arts, health, and children, youth, and social services.
Requirements: California, Colorado, and Oregon nonprofits are eligible to apply. Contact the Foundation for additional application information.
Restrictions: No grants to individuals.
Geographic Focus: California; Colorado; Oregon
Samples: YMCA of Pueblo, Pueblo, CO, $50,000 (2006); Queen of the Valley Hospital Foundation, Napa, CA, $50,000 (2006); Pueblo Child Advocacy Center, Pueblo, CO, $5,000 (2006);
Amount of Grant: $1,000-$50,000 range

Contact: Faye Wilson, Executive Director; (415) 546-1400; fax: (415) 391-8732
Sponsor: William G. Gilmore Foundation
120 Montgomery Street, Suite 1880
San Francisco, CA 94104-4317

William G. Kelley Foundation Grants 3538

The foundation's grants are available to help individuals and families overcome physical challenges. Grants are awarded based on physical and financial need. Priority will be given to applicants requesting assistance in the fields of assistive technology or universal design. Interested applicants are invited to send a letter of inquiry to the foundation, at the above address, describing the intended use of the funds, including estimates for materials and labor. Applicants should demonstrate financial need. One project grant will also be available to a nonprofit organization that provides support to individuals with physical challenges. Projects aiming to foster inclusion of people with challenges through accessibility and universal design will be given priority. Grant applications are accepted on a rolling basis. Application and guidelines are available online.
Requirements: Residents and nonprofit organizations of Essex and Middlesex Counties in Massachusetts may apply.
Geographic Focus: Massachusetts
Amount of Grant: $1000 maximum individual grant; $2000 maximum nonprofit organization grant
Contact: Grants Administrator, email: info@williamgkelley.org
Internet: http://www.williamgkelley.org/news_events.htm
Sponsor: William G. Kelley Foundation
1 Marlboro Road
Georgetown, MA 01833

William G. McGowan Charitable Fund Grants 3539

The fund awards grants to eligible nonprofit organizations that are devoted to three specific philanthropic goals: developing the talents and gifts of the very young, especially those who have been disenfranchised by virtue of low income status, inner-city conditions or family situations; funding for selected areas of medical research directed toward finding cures for, or relieving the pain and suffering of, those afflicted with debilitating conditions or diseases; and the McGowan Scholars program, which provides financial assistance to selected college and university students interested in pursuing an undergraduate or graduate degree at a college or university business school accredited by the International Association for Management Education or Association of Collegiate Business Schools and Programs.
Requirements: Nonprofit organizations in the following states and cities are eligible: Chicago, IL; District of Columbia and its Virginia suburbs; metropolitan Kansas City, western New York; and northeast Pennsylvania.
Restrictions: The fund does not support multiyear grants; accept requests online; or fund art or theatrical activities, building funds, church renovation campaigns, or endowments.
Geographic Focus: California; District of Columbia; Illinois; Missouri; New York; Pennsylvania; Virginia
Samples: Rochester Institute of Technology, College of Applied Science (NY)—to construct the Center for Telecommunications, $2 million (2004); U of the Pacific (Stockton, CA)—for a scholarship for a business student, $18,000 (2004); Foundation for the National Archives (Washington, DC)—for the National Archives Experience, which will make important American documents accessible to the public and teach visitors about the value of archives, $5 million (2003).
Amount of Grant: $8.1 million total; $10,000-$100,000 average
Date(s) Application is Due: Jan 2; May 1; Sep 1
Contact: Bernard Goodrich, Executive Director, (301) 320-8570; fax: (301) 320-8627; email: goodric@aol.com or info@mcgowanfund.org
Internet: http://www.mcgowanfund.org/guidelines.html
Sponsor: William G. McGowan Charitable Fund
P.O. Box 40515
Washington, DC 20016-0515

William H. Hannon Foundation Grants 3540

The foundation awards grants to eligible California nonprofit organizations in its areas of interest, including Roman Catholic education (elementary, secondary, and higher); churches; medical research; hospitals; health care and human services, especially for those least able to afford quality care; and needs of the disadvantaged, aged, sick, and the homeless. There are no application deadlines or forms. Applications should be sent at least three weeks before quarterly board meetings, in March, June, September, and December.
Requirements: California nonprofit organizations serving Los Angeles and southern California areas are eligible.
Geographic Focus: California
Contact: Kathleen Hannon Aikenhead, President, (310) 260-2470; fax: (310) 260-9740; email: williamhannonfdn@yahoo.com
Internet: http://www.hannonfoundation.org
Sponsor: William H. Hannon Foundation
729 Montana Avenue, Suite 5
Santa Monica, CA 90403

William T. Grant Foundation Research Grants 3541

The foundation supports research to improve the lives of youth ages 8 to 25 in the United States. This is done primarily by investing in high quality empirical studies. The foundation's Current Research Interests are understanding and improving social settings (i.e., families, schools, peer groups, organizations, programs, etc.), their effects on youth, and the use and influence of scientific evidence. Within these interests, the foundation is interested in descriptive and intervention studies. There are no geographical boundaries for its support of research projects.
Requirements: The grants are limited, without exception, to established tax-exempt, private organizations and institutions. To apply for a major grant, the Principal Investigator must submit a Letter of Inquiry to the grants coordinator briefly describing the project or program and the financial needs. Letters of Inquiry are due on the deadline dates listed. If it is determined that the project falls within the current program interests and priorities, a full proposal will be requested. Full proposal deadlines are four to six months prior to the quarterly board meetings in March and October.
Restrictions: The foundation does not support or make contributions to building funds, fundraising drives, endowment funds, general operating budgets, or scholarships. Grants are made to organizations or institutions, not individuals.
Amount of Grant: $200,000 - $500,000
Date(s) Application is Due: Nov 1; Jan 3; Apr 1
Contact: Nancy Rivera-Torres, Research Grants Coordinator; (212) 752-0071; fax: (212) 752-1398; email: nrivera@wtgrantfdn.org
Internet: http://www.wtgrantfoundation.org/funding_opportunities/research_grants
Sponsor: William T. Grant Foundation
570 Lexington Avenue, 18th Floor
New York, NY 10022-6837

Wilson-Wood Foundation Grants 3542

The Wilson-Wood Foundation established in 1983, supports organizations involved with: adult education; aging, centers/services; children/youth, services; education; health care; housing/shelter, development; human services; nutrition; women, centers/services. Giving is limited to the Manatee-Sarasota, Florida area, for for the underprivileged and the less fortunate in the community.
Requirements: Non-profits in the Manatee-Sarasota, Florida area are eligible to apply. Initial approach should be a phone call to the Foundation prior to submitting a the letter of inquiry (must be received by June 1). There is no application form required. Applicants must submit two copies of the proposal. Application must include the following information: timetable for implementation and evaluation of project; qualifications of key personnel; name, address and phone number of organization; copy of IRS Determination Letter, must be dated within the past 10 years; brief history of organization and description of its mission; copy of most recent annual report/audited financial statement/990; descriptive literature about organization; listing of board of directors, trustees, officers and other key people and their affiliations; detailed description of project and amount of funding requested; copy of current year's organizational budget and/or project budget; listing of additional sources and amount of support.
Restrictions: No support for foreign organizations, supporting organizations, or private foundations. No grants to individuals, or for endowment funds, deficit financing, travel projects, research, fundraising costs, multi-year projects, conferences, emergency funding or start up costs.
Geographic Focus: Florida
Samples: Childrens Academy of Southwest Florida, Bradenton, FL, $30,000 (2007); Meals on Wheels Plus of Manatee, Bradenton, FL, $20,000 (2007); Habitat for Humanity, Venice Area, Venice, FL, $25,000 (2007);
Amount of Grant: $8,000-$30,000 range
Date(s) Application is Due: Jun 1
Contact: Susan Wood, Executive Director; (941) 966-3635
Sponsor: Wilson-Wood Foundation, Inc.
930 Scherer Way
Osprey, FL 34229-6867

Winifred & Harry B. Allen Foundation Grants 3543

Established in 1963 in honor of Harry B. Allen, president of the Belvedere Land Company, and his wife, the Foundation has as its primary fields of interest: animal and wildlife preservation; education; the environmental programs; environmental education; protection of natural resources; health care; health organizations; human services; immigrants/refugees; performing arts; and visual arts. Though giving is centered around Marin County, California, the Foundation has also supported 501(c)3 organizations in Massachusetts, Georgia, New York, and the District of Columbia. Applicants should contact the Foundation in writing, stating the purpose and offering proof of tax exempt status. Though there are no specific deadlines, the Board meets four times annually, including April 15, June 15, September 15, and December 15.
Restrictions: No grants are given to individuals.
Geographic Focus: California; District of Columbia; Georgia; Massachusetts; New York
Samples: Angel Island Association, Tiberton, California, $1,000—for general operating costs (2008); Belvedere Public Library Foundation, Belvedere, California, $5,300—for general operations (2008); Cornell Lab of Ornithology, Ithica, New York, $2,000—for research (2008).
Amount of Grant: $500-$5,000 range
Contact: Howard B. Allen; (415) 435-2439; fax: (415) 435-3166
Sponsor: Winifred & Harry B. Allen Foundation
P.O. Box 380, 83 Beach Road
Belvedere, CA 94920-0380

Winston-Salem Foundation Competitive Grants 3544

The foundation makes competitive grant awards to tax-exempt, nonprofit agencies in the greater Forsyth County, North Carolina, area. Its charitable purposes include: public interest, education and recreation, health, human services, arts and culture, youth,

and older adults. Grants ordinarily are made for proposals that initiate, expand, or improve direct services to people and for endowment purposes under certain conditions. Additional types of support include program development, seed grants, scholarship funds, technical assistance, employee matching gifts, scholarships to individuals, and matching funds. Except in unusual cases, grants will be approved for one year at a time. Potential applicants should contact the office for an appointment to introduce the proposed project.
Requirements: Organizations in Davidson, Davie, Forsyth, Surry, Stokes, Wilkes, and Yadkin counties in North Carolina are eligible to apply.
Restrictions: Grants for major equipment purposes and for capital campaigns in support of local community facilities are of low priority.
Geographic Focus: North Carolina
Amount of Grant: $15,000-$20,000 average
Contact: Brittney Gaspari, Grants Director; (336) 725-2382; fax: (336) 727-0581; email: bgaspari@wsfoundation.org or info@wsfoundation.org
Internet: http://www.wsfoundation.org/grant-seekers/types-of-grants/competitive-grants/
Sponsor: Winston-Salem Foundation
860 W. Fifth Street
Winston-Salem, NC 27101-2506

Winston-Salem Foundation Elkin/Tri-County Grants **3545**
The Funds consist of three component trusts established by Richard T. Chatham, Lucy Hanes Chatham, and citizens of Elkin to benefit the community. Ordinarily, grants are made for projects that initiate, expand or improve direct service to people. Applicants should send a two or three page letter describing the need for the project, its goals and objectives, its cost and the portion of the cost requested.
Requirements: A list of board members is required, as well as organizational and project budgets, and evidence of non-profit 501(c)3 tax-exempt status. The chief board officer must sign the proposal or write an endorsement cover letter.
Restrictions: Grants will be made only to legally recognized non-profit organizations and educational institutions in Wilkes, Surry, and Yadkin Counties. Those that benefit residents of the Elkin-Jonesville-Dobson-Roaring River radius will be of priority interest to the advisory committee. Grants will not be made for on-going operating expenses. Foundation funds will not be granted to supplant tax or government funds for projects or institutions that would ordinarily receive public funding support.
Geographic Focus: North Carolina
Samples: Communities in Schools of Wilkes, $3,500 (2007); Hugh Chatham Memorial Hospital Foundation, $7,000 (2007); Mountain Valley Hospice and Palliative Care, $2,500 (2007).
Amount of Grant: $500-$7,000
Date(s) Application is Due: Jun 15
Contact: Brittney Gaspari, Grants Director; (336) 725-2382; fax: (336) 727-0581; email: bgaspari@wsfoundation.org or info@wsfoundation.org
Internet: http://www.wsfoundation.org/grant-seekers/types-of-grants/elkintri-county-grants/
Sponsor: Winston-Salem Foundation
860 W. Fifth Street
Winston-Salem, NC 27101-2506

Winston-Salem Foundation Stokes County Grants **3546**
The Trust provides grants to non-profit organizations or informal groups in Stokes County for worthy public and charitable purposes with an emphasis on developing leaders and inspiring others. Leadership can be either formal and traditional, or demonstrated in less traditional ways that are creative and innovative, including leading by example. The trust is designed both to work with established organizations and to encourage new initiatives. Special attention will be given to encouraging leadership in certain focus areas: education; arts; environmental protection and recreational use; historical preservation; local government and community services; health; and organizations and issues affecting minorities and low-resource communities.
Requirements: Applicants can be informal groups of people with innovative ideas, including those that might grow into nonprofit organizations; or established organizations with 501(c)3 tax-exempt status. The Advisory Board will also consider letters from small groups of people with good ideas who need guidance about turning them into formal grant proposals in the future.
Restrictions: Grants will not be made for projects or institutions that would ordinarily receive public funding. However, public institutions such as schools or parks may submit proposals for innovative projects for which funds are not ordinarily provided.
Geographic Focus: North Carolina
Amount of Grant: $3,000 maximum
Date(s) Application is Due: Sep 11
Contact: Brittney Gaspari, Grants Director; (336) 725-2382; fax: (336) 727-0581; email: bgaspari@wsfoundation.org or info@wsfoundation.org
Internet: http://www.wsfoundation.org/grant-seekers/types-of-grants/stokes-county-grants/
Sponsor: Winston-Salem Foundation
860 W. Fifth Street
Winston-Salem, NC 27101-2506

Winston-Salem Foundation Victim Assistance Grants **3547**
The fund provides financial assistance to victims of violent crime to help minimize complications from the event. The fund also provides grants for statewide organizations that provide information in a supportive manner to victims of violent crime. Victims of violent crime such as rape or assault are eligible for assistance from the fund. The fund is also available to assist surviving family members of homicide victims and victims of violent crime resulting from domestic violence. The victim can receive monetary support for expenses such as the following: relocation expenses; locks, alarms, or repair of damages from break-ins; clothes, especially for rape victims when clothes are retained as evidence; transportation to counseling visits; lost wages that may be reimbursed to the Fund at a later date by North Carolina Crime Victims Compensation; and help with payment of bills that are late because of the consequences of the crime.
Requirements: Victims should be residents of Forsyth, Davie, or Stokes counties (or the area being served by Family Services, Inc.).
Restrictions: The fund is not for assistance to organizations serving victims (except, as noted in the purpose, for nonprofit statewide organizations that provide information in a supportive manner to victims of violent crime).
Geographic Focus: North Carolina
Contact: Betty Gray Davis; (336) 725-2382; fax: (336) 727-0581; email: bgdavis@wsfoundation.org
Internet: http://www.wsfoundation.org/grant-seekers/types-of-grants/victim-assistance-grants/
Sponsor: Winston-Salem Foundation
860 W. Fifth Street
Winston-Salem, NC 27101-2506

Women of the ELCA Opportunity Scholarships for Lutheran Laywomen **3548**
The purpose of these scholarships is to provide assistance to women studying for a career other than the ordained ministry. The following scholarships are offered: Amelia Kemp Scholarship— for ELCA women of color in undergraduate, graduate, professional, or vocational courses of study; Belmer, Flora Prince Scholarships—for ELCA women studying for ELCA service abroad; Kahler, Vickers/Raup, Emma Wettstein Scholarships—for ELCA women studying for service in health professions associated with ELCA projects abroad; Irene Drinkall Franke, Mary Seeley Knudstrup Scholarships—for ELCA women in graduate courses of study preparing for occupations in Christian service; and Cronk Memorial, First Triennium Board, General, Mehring, Paepke, Piero/Wade/Wade, Edwin, and Edna Robeck Scholarships—for ELCA women in undergraduate, graduate, professional, or vocational courses of study.
Requirements: The applicant must be at least 21 years old, be a U.S. citizen, hold membership in the Evangelical Lutheran Church in America, and have experienced an interruption in education of two or more years since completion of high school. Scholarship funds must be used within the year following the award.
Amount of Grant: $800-$1,000
Contact: Valora Starr, Coordinator; (800) 638-3522 ext. 2741; fax: (773) 380-2419; email: Valora.Starr@elca.org
Internet: http://www.elca.org/Growing-In-Faith/Ministry/Women-of-the-ELCA/Engage-in-action-and-support-one-another-in-our-callings/Scholarships/For-Lutheran-Laywomen.aspx
Sponsor: Evangelical Lutheran Church in America
8765 W. Higgins Road
Chicago, IL 60631-4189

Women's Foundation of California Community Action Fund **3549**
The foundation awards grants to support projects of organizations working to improve the lives of women and girls in California. Requests will only be considered in one of the following issue areas: economic rights and justice; environmental health and justice; and reproductive rights and justice. Types of support include general operating support, project/program-specific grants, and planning grants. Serious consideration will be given to cross-sector collaborations as well as to emerging organizations, especially in rural and non-urban areas. Funding for publications and one-time events will only be considered if they are integrated within a larger strategy for social change.
Requirements: California organizations that work with low-income women and girls are eligible. Priority is given to projects serving women and girls of color; immigrant, undocumented, and refugees women and girls; lesbian, bisexual, transgender, intersex, and questioning women and girls; women and girls with disabilities; women over 50; indigenous women and girls; young and/or single mothers; and women and girls in rural and non-urban communities.
Restrictions: The program does not fund capital improvements, endowments, loans, individuals, debt reduction, expenses that accrued prior to the date of the grant award, or fundraising events.
Geographic Focus: California
Amount of Grant: $25,000 maximum general or program grants; $10,000 maximum planning grants; $35,000 maximum collaborative grants
Date(s) Application is Due: Dec 16
Contact: Grants Administrator, (415) 837-1113; fax: (415) 837-1144
Internet: http://www.womensfoundca.org
Sponsor: Women's Foundation of California
340 Pine Street, Suite 302
San Francisco, CA 94104

Women's Foundation of California Grants **3550**
The Women's Foundation of California envisions a future where communities in California are healthy, safe and economically prosperous. The Foundation achieve's this vision by focusing on women and girls as change agents through their central role in families and communities. The Foundation supports organizations that meet the following objectives: organizations mobilizing communities to change policies and systems; to improve the lives of women and girls; developing the leadership of women and

girls working to change policies and systems and create stronger movements for social justice; promoting the human rights of women and girls in all sectors of society, including economic, political, social, environmental, sexual, cultural and civil rights.
Requirements: The foundation awards grants to: California 501(c)3 nonprofit corporations or California nonprofit groups with a 501(c)3 fiscal sponsor; organization/program prioritize low-income women and girls in California; health and safety: this includes reproductive health and justice, environmental health and justice and gender-based violence; economic prosperity: this includes efforts towards economic security and economic development. Organizations or programs that utilize one or more of the following strategies to bring about measurable and sustainable change: policy advocacy; community organizing; leadership development; media and/or public education; civic participation; participatory action research; youth-led programs and initiatives. Contact the Foundation for further application information and guidelines.
Restrictions: The Women's Foundation of California does not make grants to or for the following: individuals; for-profit organizations or small businesses; start-up loans; capital projects; direct services; fundraising events; shelters; scholarships; capital improvements; endowments; loans; debt reduction; expenses that accrued prior to the date of the grant award. Funding for publications and one-time events such as retreats and conferences will only be considered if they are integrated within a larger strategy for social change.
Geographic Focus: California
Amount of Grant: $10,000 - $40,000 range
Contact: Maya Thornell-Sandifor, Senior Program Officer; (415) 837-1113; fax: (415) 837-1144; email: mayat@womensfoundca.org
Internet: http://www.womensfoundca.org/grantmaking.html
Sponsor: Women's Foundation of California
340 Pine Street, Suite 302
San Francisco, CA 94104

Women's Sports Foundation Grants **3551**
Founded by Billie Jean King in 1974, the Women's Sports Foundation builds on her legacy as a champion athlete, advocate of social justice and agent of change. The Foundation strives for gender equity and to fight discrimination in sports. These grants provide girls and women with educational materials and scholarships, research on leadership development and opportunities to participate in sports and physical activity. Behind every Women's Sports Foundation grant lies one concrete objective: provide girls access to sport and physical activity despite background or financial ability. Grants are awarded to girl-serving organizations who strive to provide diverse, underserved populations of girls ages 8 to 18 with a way to get involved in sport and physical activity. The Women's Sports Foundation awards grants nationwide, but places a strong emphasis on Atlanta, Boston, Chicago and San Antonio metropolitan areas.
Contact: Grants Administrator; (800) 227-3988 or (516) 542-4700; fax: (516) 542-4716; email: Info@WomensSportsFoundation.org
Internet: http://www.womenssportsfoundation.org/Grants-And-Scholarships.aspx
Sponsor: Women's Sports Foundation
1899 Hempstead Turnpike, Suite 400
East Meadow, NY 11554

Woodward Fund Grants **3552**
Grants support nonprofit institutions, corporations, and associations that are located in Georgia or one of its neighboring states and are organized and operated exclusively for religious, educational, and charitable and scientific purposes. Grantmaking focuses on capital projects. The distribution committee makes its decisions based on materials provided in the grant request. The trust does not require a formal application form, but requests a proposal outlining the project or program and containing the following information: project/program description; complete itemized project budget, including project schedule; need for the project; other funding sources, including the amount received from each source; names and qualifications of those conducting the project; objectives and how they will be achieved; a brief description of the applicant organization; method and criteria for project evaluation; list of officers, board of directors, or trustees; copy of the 501(c)3 designation letter; and plans for recognition of the trust in the project. Applicants should not contact committee members personally concerning a proposal or anticipated approach to the fund.
Requirements: 501(c)3 nonprofit organizations in Georgia and its neighboring states are eligible. Government agencies to which contributions by individuals are made deductible from income by IRS laws also are eligible.
Restrictions: Grants are not awarded to individuals or for scholarships or student loans.
Geographic Focus: Alabama; Florida; Georgia; North Carolina; South Carolina; Tennessee
Amount of Grant: $5000-$300,000
Date(s) Application is Due: May 1; Nov 1
Contact: Alice Sheets, c/o Wachovia Bank, NA Trustee, email: grantinquiries8@wachovia.com
Internet: https://www.wachovia.com/charitable_services/woodward_overview.asp
Sponsor: David, Helen, and Marian Woodward Fund
Wachovia Bank, NA Trustee, 3280 Peachtree Road, N.E. Suite 400, MC: G0141-041
Atlanta, GA 30305

WWNFF Dissertation Grants in Women's Health **3553**
Dissertation grants encourage original and significant research on issues related to women's health. This program emphasizes the implications of research for the understanding of women's lives and significance for public policy or treatment. Previous grant recipients have explored such topics as postpartum depression; contraceptive law; sex hormones and ovarian cancer; dietary determinants of morbidity; sex and violence in everyday life; and sexuality on the Internet. Grant funds may be used for expenses connected with the dissertation, including but are not limited to, travel, books, microfilming, taping, and computer services. Ten awards will be made. Guidelines are available online. Annual deadline dates may vary; contact program staff for exact dates.
Requirements: Students in doctoral programs such as nursing, public health, anthropology, history, sociology, psychology, and social work, at graduate schools in the United States are eligible to apply. Candidates must have completed all pre-dissertation requirements by October 24 and expect to complete their dissertations by the summer of next year.
Restrictions: Candidates who are within a few months of completing their work should not apply.
Amount of Grant: $6000
Date(s) Application is Due: Oct 11
Contact: Women's Health Dissertation Fellowships, (609) 452-7007; fax: (609) 452-0066; email: contact@woodrow.org
Internet: http://www.woodrow.org/womens-studies/health/purpose.html
Sponsor: Woodrow Wilson National Fellowship Foundation
P.O. Box 5281
Princeton, NJ 08543-5281

Xoran Technologies Resident Research Grant **3554**
The purpose of this grant is to stimulate original resident research in otolaryngology projects that are well-conceived and scientifically valid, with potential to clarify the role of head and neck computed tomography in diagnosis or treatment. Awards are for one year, are non renewable, and have a $10,000 maximum limit. Generally, a single award is made available annually. Letters of Intent are due on December 15, with full proposals due by January 15.
Requirements: Application is open to residents of an accredited otolaryngolgoy-head and neck surgery training program in the U.S. and Canada for projects that are well-conceived and scientifically valid, with potential to clarify the role of the head and neck computed tomography in diagnosis or treatment.
Amount of Grant: $10,000 maximum total direct costs
Date(s) Application is Due: Dec 15; Jan 15
Contact: Stephanie L. Jones, Assistant Director; (703) 519-1586 or (703) 836-4444; email: sljones@entnet.org
Internet: http://www.entnet.org/EducationAndResearch/coreGrants.cfm
Sponsor: Xoran Technologies, Inc.
One Prince Street
Alexandria, VA 22314-3357

YSA Get Ur Good On Grants **3555**
Get Ur Good On Grants are available for youth-led service initiatives on Global Youth Service Day, April 23-25. Available to children and youth around the world, YSA's Get Ur Good On Grants will award 100 $500 grants to support projects addressing critical community needs such as poverty, education, and environmental sustainability. Grant applications are due February 22. Additional guidelines are available at: www.YSA.org/grants.
Amount of Grant: $500
Date(s) Application is Due: Feb 22
Contact: Megan Brudney, Grants Manager; (202) 296-2992; fax: (202) 296-4030; email: Brudney@ysa.org
Internet: http://www.ysa.org/grants/programs/get-ur-good-grants
Sponsor: Youth Service America
1101 15th Street NW, Suite 200
Washington, DC 20005

YSA UnitedHealth Heroes Service Learning Grants **3556**
UnitedHealthcare and Youth Service America are are offering the UnitedHealth HEROES service-learning grant program for youth-led community education projects in Alabama, Arizona, California, Colorado, Indiana, Maryland, New Jersey, North Carolina, Ohio, Pennsylvania, South Carolina and Tennessee, and in the following specific areas: Florida—selected counties, Illinois—Chicagoland and Peoria, and New York—Long Island, New York City and Syracuse. These grants of up to $1,000 support teachers, service-learning coordinators and students in the health professions to implement service-learning projects around childhood obesity and engage children and youth ages 5 to 25 as volunteers. Semester-long projects that launch in February, and celebrate Global Youth Service Day, are encouraged.
Requirements: Applicants must meet the following requirements: (1) The proposed project must take place in Alabama, Arizona, California, Colorado, Indiana, Maryland, New Jersey, North Carolina, Ohio, Pennsylvania, South Carolina, Tennessee, or in the following specific areas: Florida—selected counties, Illinois—Chicagoland and Peoria, and New York—Long Island, New York City and Syracuse (2) The applicant must be (a) a teacher or service-learning coordinator at a public, private, faith-based, or charter school; or (b) an instructor or service-learning coordinator at an institution of higher education; or (c) student(s) in the health professions; or (d) staff at a community-based, non-profit organization. Projects must be youth-led and are encouraged to take place between February and April. A significant component of the project must take place on or around Global Youth Service Day. This timeline may include significant project planning components. Please check with your school district to make sure your project plans will not conflict with school closings and spring break. Applications must be submitted online via the sponsor's website. Download the guidelines and application information at the website.

Geographic Focus: Alabama; Arizona; California; Colorado; Florida; Illinois; Indiana; Maryland; New Jersey; New York; North Carolina; Ohio; Pennsylvania; South Carolina; Tennessee
Amount of Grant: $1,000 maximum
Date(s) Application is Due: Oct 22
Contact: Megan Brudney, Grants Manager; (202) 296-2992; fax: (202) 296-4030; email: Brudney@ysa.org or healthheroes@ysa.org
Internet: http://www.ysa.org/grants/programs/unitedhealth-heroes
Sponsor: Youth Service America (YSA)
1101 15th Street, Suite 200
Washington DC 20005

Z. Smith Reynolds Foundation Small Grants **3557**

The Z. Smith Reynolds Foundation now offers a Small Grants Process for grant requests of up to $35,000 per year for up to two years. Small grants are made in the areas of community building and economic development, the environment, governance, public policy and civic engagement, pre-collegiate education, and social justice or equity. In addition to funding projects that achieve the goals of each focus area, the foundation has an interest in building the capacity of organizations and in promoting organizational development. New programs, rather than those that are well-established and well-funded, receive priority consideration. Types of support include operating budgets, continuing support, annual campaigns, seed grants, matching funds, projects/programs, conferences and seminars, and technical assistance.
Requirements: The foundation makes grants only to nonprofit, tax-exempt, charitable organizations and institutions in North Carolina.
Restrictions: The foundation does not give priority to: the arts; capital campaigns; computer hardware or software purchases; conferences, seminars, or symposiums; crisis intervention programs; fund raising events; historic preservation; local food banks; or substance abuse treatment programs.
Geographic Focus: North Carolina
Amount of Grant: $35,000 maximum
Date(s) Application is Due: Aug 3
Contact: Leslie Winner, Executive Director; (800) 443-8319, ext. 105 or (336) 725-7541, ext. 105; fax: (336) 725-6069; email: lwinner@zsr.org or info@zsr.org
Internet: http://www.zsr.org/small_grants.htm
Sponsor: Z. Smith Reynolds Foundation
147 South Cherry Street, Suite 200
Winston-Salem, NC 27101-5287

Subject Index

Aboriginal Studies
Vancouver Fndn Grants and Comm Initiatives Program, 3477

Abortion
Huber Fndn Grants, 1812
Lalor Fndn Postdoctoral Research Grants, 2021

Academic Achievement
3M Fndn Grants, 11
Albertson's Charitable Giving Grants, 330
Alice Tweed Tuohy Fndn Grants, 357
AON Fndn Grants, 491
ARCO Fndn Education Grants, 526
Cargill Citizenship Fund-Corp Giving Grants, 865
Carnegie Corp of New York Grants, 879
Clarence E. Heller Charitable Fndn Grants, 1022
Comm Fndn of Santa Cruz County Grants, 1122
Comm Fndn Silicon Valley Grants, 1133
Comm Impact Fund, 1135
CPhA Centennial Award, 1156
Fluor Fndn Grants, 1517
Gamble Fndn Grants, 1582
General Mills Fndn Grants, 1590
Greater Milwaukee Fndn Grants, 1653
Harvest Fndn Grants, 1713
Helena Rubinstein Fndn Grants, 1743
Jane's Trust Grants, 1904
Jessie B. Cox Charitable Trust Grants, 1918
Johnson F. Hammond Memorial Scholarship, 1956
Louis Calder Fndn Grants, 2065
Louis R. Cappelli Fndn Grants, 2066
Lynde and Harry Bradley Fndn Grants, 2089
Lynde and Harry Bradley Fndn Prizes: Bradley Prizes, 2090
Mattel Children's Fndn Grants, 2130
Mattel International Grants, 2131
National Dairy Promotion and Research Board Scholarships, 2251
NIH Academic Career Awards, 2634
NMF Franklin C. McLean Award, 2829
NMF Hugh J. Andersen Memorial Scholarship, 2832
NMF Metropolitan Life Fndn Awards Program for Academic Excellence in Medicine, 2835
NMF National Medical Association Awards for Medical Journalism, 2836
NMF National Medical Association Emerging Scholar Awards, 2837
NMF National Medical Association Patti LaBelle Award, 2838
NMF Ralph W. Ellison Prize, 2840
NMF William and Charlotte Cadbury Award, 2841
PacifiCare Fndn Grants, 2981
Quantum Fndn Grants, 3096
RGK Fndn Grants, 3153
S. Mark Taper Fndn Grants, 3236
Z. Smith Reynolds Fndn Small Grants, 3557

Access
OSI Access to Essential Medicines Grants, 2964

Accidents
Jacob and Valeria Langeloth Fndn Grants, 1882

Accounting
NIGMS MORE Faculty Development Awards, 2622

Acoustics
ASHFndn Research Grant in Speech Science, 583

Addictions
AACAP-NIDA K12 Career Development Awards, 55
American Psychiatric Association Minority Medical Student Summer Externship in Addiction Psychiatry, 445
Boyd Gaming Corp Contributions, 788
Bush Fndn Health & Human Services Grants, 814
Comm Fndn Of Greater Lafayette Grants, 1110
CTCRI Idea Grants, 1170
Griffin Fndn Grants, 1670
Johnson & Johnson Corp Contributions Grants, 1952
NCI/NIDA Transdisciplinary Tobacco Use Research Centers Grants, 2280
NIDA Behavioral Science Track Awards for Rapid Transition, 2498
NIDA Behavioral Therapies Development Grants, 2499
NIDA Cutting-Edge Basic Research Awards, 2501
NIDA Drug Addiction Neuroscience Research Grants, 2503
NIDA Microarray-Based Research on Drug Abuse, 2508
NIDA National Drug Abuse Treatment Clinical Trials Network, 2510
NIDA Neurobiological and Behavioral Research on Nicotine and Tobacco Products, 2511
NIDA Origins and Pathways to Drug Abuse Research Grants, 2512
NIDA Pilot and Feasibility Studies in Preparation for Drug Abuse Prevention Trials, 2513
NIDA Transition from Drug Abuse to Drug Addiction, 2516
NIH Pathological Gambling: Basic, Clinical, and Services Research Grants, 2702
OSI-Baltimore Tackling Drug Addiction Grants, 2973
Rainbow Fund Grants, 3103
TRDRP California Research Awards, 3434
Triangle Comm Fndn Shaver-Hitchings Scholarship, 3438

Adolescent Health
Agnes M. Lindsay Trust Grants, 263
Blowitz-Ridgeway Fndn Grants, 767
CDC School Health Programs to Prevent the Spread of HIV Cooperative Agreements, 928
Crail-Johnson Fndn Grants, 1157
DHHS Emergency Medical Services for Children Program, 1249
DHHS HIV Demonstration Program for Children, Adolescents, and Women, 1262
DHHS Oral Health Promotion Research Across the Lifespan, 1269
EPA Baseline Assessment of Risks of Exposure to Lead Poisoning of Native American Children, 1419
Fairlawn Fndn Grants, 1447
Flinn Fndn Grants Programs, 1511
Fndn for Seacoast Health Grants, 1533
General Service Fndn Reproductive Health and Rights Grants, 1592
Greater Tacoma Comm Fndn Ryan Alan Hade Endowment Fund, 1657
Humana Fndn Grants, 1818
John Edward Fowler Memorial Fndn Grants, 1930
Johnson & Johnson Comm Health Care Grants, 1951
NAPNAP Fndn Shourd Parks Immunization Project Small Grants, 2243
NIAID HIV Prevention Trial Units Grants, 2453
NIAID Pediatric Clinical Trials Program for AIDS, 2460
NINR Chronic Illness Self-Management in Children and Adolescents Grants, 2792
Oakland Fund for Children and Youth Grants, 2930
Partnership for Cures Two Years To Cures Grants, 2992
Robert and Joan Dircks Fndn Grants, 3167

Adolescent Psychiatry
AACAP Child and Adolescent Psychiatry Teaching Scholarships, 31
AACAP Congressional Fellowships, 32
AACAP Educational Outreach Program for Child and Adolescent Psychiatry Residents, 33
AACAP Educational Outreach Program for General Psychiatry Residents, 34
AACAP Elaine Schlosser Lewis Award for Research on Attention-Deficit Disorder, 35
AACAP George Tarjan Award for Contributions in Developmental Disabilities, 36
AACAP Irving Philips Award for Prevention, 37
AACAP Jeanne Spurlock Lecture and Award on Diversity and Culture, 38
AACAP Jeanne Spurlock Minority Medical Student Clinical Fellowship in Child and Adolescent Psychiatry, 39
AACAP Klingenstein Third Generation Fndn Award for Research in Depression or Suicide, 42
AACAP Norbert and Charlotte Rieger Award for Scientific Achievement, 43
AACAP Norbert and Charlotte Rieger Psychodynamic Psychotherapy Award, 44
AACAP Pilot Research Awards, Supported by Eli Lilly and Company, 47
AACAP Rieger Service Program Award for Excellence, 49
AACAP Robert Cancro Academic Leadership Award, 50
AACAP Sidney Berman Award for the School-Based Study and Intervention for Learning Disorders and Mental Ilness, 51
AACAP Simon Wile Leadership in Consultation Award, 52
APF Call for Proposals, 505
APF James H. Scully Jr., M.D., Educational Fund Grants, 508
APF Typical or Troubled School Mental Health Education Grants, 510
Blowitz-Ridgeway Fndn Grants, 767

Adolescent Psychology
Blowitz-Ridgeway Fndn Grants, 767
Greater Tacoma Comm Fndn Ryan Alan Hade Endowment Fund, 1657
NIMH Early Identification and Treatment of Mental Disorders in Children and Adolescents Grants, 2756
NIMH Interventions Infrastructure Program Research Grants, 2760
William T. Grant Fndn Research Grants, 3541

Adolescents
AON Fndn Grants, 491
AT&T Fndn Civic and Comm Service Grants, 658
Comm Fndn for Southeastern Michigan Grants, 1094
Connecticut Comm Fndn Grants, 1141
Dell Fndn Open Grants, 1218
DHHS Comprehensive Comm Mental Health Services Grants for Children with Serious Emotional Disturbances, 1247
FCD Child Development Grants, 1458
Greater Worcester Comm Fndn Discretionary Grants, 1658
Laura B. Vogler Fndn Grants, 2032
Margoes Fndn Grants, 2106
Ms. Fndn for Women Grants, 2222
NIH Career Development Awards: Child Abuse and Neglect Research, 2646
NIMH/NIDA Children's Services Grants, 2775
Oakland Fund for Children and Youth Grants, 2930

Adoption
Abell-Hanger Fndn Grants, 183
DHHS Adolescent Family Life Demonstration Projects, 1243
Taproot Fndn Capacity-Building Service Grants, 3417

Adult and Continuing Education
Ahmanson Fndn Grants, 303
Allen P. and Josephine B. Green Fndn Grants, 361
Allyn Fndn Grants, 365
Arkell Hall Fndn Grants, 534
Arlington Comm Fndn Grants, 536
AT&T Excelerator, 657
Atlanta Fndn Grants, 662
Auburn Fndn Grants, 664
Ball Brothers Fndn Grants, 684
Battle Creek Comm Fndn Grants, 703
Bayer Hemophilia Caregivers Education Award, 707

Benton Comm Fndn Grants, 743
Bernard and Audre Rapoport Fndn Grants, 746
Berrien Comm Fndn Grants, 749
Besser Fndn Grants, 752
Blackford County Comm Fndn Grants, 763
Blue Mountain Comm Fndn Grants, 769
Blue River Comm Fndn Grants, 770
Bodenwein Public Benevolent Fndn Grants, 775
Boettcher Fndn Grants, 778
Booth-Bricker Fund Grants, 780
Boston Fndn Grants, 783
Brown County Comm Fndn Grants, 807
Carl and Lily Pforzheimer Fndn Grants, 868
Carl B. and Florence E. King Fndn Grants, 869
Cass County Comm Fndn Grants, 887
CDC Promoting Prevention in Managed Care Cooperative Agreements, 925
Cemala Fndn Grants, 933
Chicago Board of Trade Fndn Grants, 988
CIGNA Fndn Grants, 1011
Colorado Springs Comm Trust Fund Grants, 1061
Comm Fndn of Bartholomew County Heritage Fund Grants, 1096
Comm Fndn of Bartholomew County James A. Henderson Award for Fund-Raising, 1097
Comm Fndn of Boone County Grants, 1099
Comm Fndn of Central Illinois Grants, 1101
Comm Fndn of Greater Fort Wayne: Comm Endowment & Clarke Endowment Fund Grants, 1108
Connelly Fndn Grants, 1143
Constantin Fndn Grants, 1145
Constellation Energy Group and Baltimore Gas and Electric Corp Contributions, 1146
Coors Brewing Corp Contributions Grants, 1151
Cornerstone Fndn of Northeastern Wisconsin Grants, 1152
Cowles Charitable Trust Grants, 1155
Cruise Industry Charitable Fndn Grants, 1166
Dayton Power and Light Fndn Grants, 1205
DHHS Maternal and Child Health Research and Training Programs Grants, 1264
eBay Fndn Comm Grants, 1363
Emma B. Howe Memorial Fndn Grants, 1415
Evjue Fndn Grants, 1439
Field Fndn of Illinois Grants, 1499
Fisher Fndn Grants, 1508
Frances L. and Edwin L. Cummings Memorial Fund Grants, 1547
G.N. Wilcox Trust Grants, 1581
Goodrich Corp Fndn Grants, 1638
Gulf Coast Comm of Venice Fndn Grants, 1677
Hallmark Corp Fndn Grants, 1688
Harold Simmons Fndn Grants, 1698
Helen Steiner Rice Fndn Grants, 1742
Henry & Ruth Blaustein Rosenberg Fndn Grants, 1746
Howard and Bush Fndn Grants, 1798
James A. and Faith Knight Fndn Grants, 1884
James Ford Bell Fndn Grants, 1885
John H. and Wilhelmina D. Harland Charitable Fndn Grants, 1933
Joseph H. and Florence A. Roblee Fndn Grants, 1961
Liberty Bank Fndn Grants, 2053
Lubrizol Fndn Grants, 2080
Max Bell Fndn Grants, 2134
Middlesex Savings Charitable Fndn Grants, 2196
NBME Stemmler Medical Education Research Fund Grants, 2263
Paul and Mary Haas Fndn Contributions and Student Scholarships, 2997
Perry County Comm Fndn Grants, 3016
Pfizer Fndn Health Literacy Grants, 3026
Pike County Comm Fndn Grants, 3049
Piper Jaffray Companies Building Strong Communities Grants, 3053
Principal Financial Group Fndn Grants, 3082
Pulaski County Comm Fndn Grants, 3091
Richard and Rhoda Goldman Fund Grants, 3158
Samuel S. Johnson Fndn Grants, 3251
San Antonio Area Fndn Grants, 3254
Sisters of Saint Joseph Charitable Fund Grants, 3296
SOCFOC Reducing Health & Educational Disparities in the Central Neighborhood Grants, 3318
Vanderburgh Comm Fndn Grants, 3480
Warrick County Comm Fndn Grants, 3519
Wilson-Wood Fndn Grants, 3542

Adult Basic Education
McCarthy Family Fndn Grants, 2141

Adult Development
George Family Fndn Grants, 1598
NSF Social Psychology Research Grants, 2894

Adults
Carrie E. and Lena V. Glenn Fndn Grants, 882
Charles Delmar Fndn Grants, 963
Mabel H. Flory Charitable Trust Grants, 2096
NHLBI Targeted Approaches to Weight Control for Young Adults Grants, 2387

Advertising
Google Grants Beta, 1640
NCI/NIDA Transdisciplinary Tobacco Use Research Centers Grants, 2280

Africa
Annenberg Fndn Grants, 479
ASM-UNESCO Leadership Grant for International Educators, 626
Atkinson Fndn International Grants, 661
Besser Fndn Grants, 752
Doris Duke Charitable Fndn Operations Research on AIDS Care and Treatment in Africa Grants, 1319
Fulbright Traditional Scholar Program in Sub-Saharan Africa, 1573
Margoes Fndn Grants, 2106
SSRC HIV/AIDS and Public Health Policy Research in Africa Fellowships, 3365

Africa, Northern
Fulbright Traditional Scholar Program in the Near East and North Africa Region, 1575

Africa, Sub-Saharan
Fulbright Traditional Scholar Program in Sub-Saharan Africa, 1573

Africa, Western
NMF General Electric Medical Scholars Fellowships, 2830

African Americans
African American Fund of New Jersey Grants, 260
American Sociological Association Minority Fellowships, 458
Arkansas Comm Fndn Arkansas Black Hall of Fame Grants, 532
ASM Robert D. Watkins Graduate Research Fellowship, 614
Boston Fndn Grants, 783
Charles Delmar Fndn Grants, 963
CMA Fndn Grants, 1042
CMS Historically Black Colleges and Universities Health Services Research Grants, 1044
Coca-Cola Fndn Grants, 1052
Connecticut Comm Fndn Grants, 1141
DHHS AIDS and HIV Epidemiologic Research Studies Grants, 1244
DHHS Maternal and Child Health Projects Grants, 1263
Effie and Wofford Cain Fndn Grants, 1385
FDHN Student Research Fellowships, 1480
Harold Amos Medical Faculty Development Program, 1696
NIA Prostate Cancer Aging, Race, and Ethnicity Research Grants, 2428
NIMH Career Opportunities in Research Education and Training Honors High School Research Education Grant, 2748
NIMH Career Opportunities in Research Education and Training Honors Undergraduate Research Training Grant, 2749
NMF Franklin C. McLean Award, 2829
Philadelphia Fndn Organizational Effectiveness Grants, 3029
Saint Luke's Health Initiatives Grants, 3240
SNM PDEF Mickey Williams Minority Student Scholarships, 3302
Strowd Roses Grants, 3388

African Americans (Student Support)
AMA Fndn Minority Scholars Awards, 395
KFF Barbara Jordan Health Policy Scholarships, 2000
NMF National Medical Association Patti LaBelle Award, 2838

After-School Programs
Boston Globe Fndn Grants, 784
Carnegie Corp of New York Grants, 879
Comm Fndn of Broward Grants, 1100
Comm Fndn of Greenville Hollingsworth Funds Program/Project Grants, 1114
CVS Comm Grants, 1177
Emma B. Howe Memorial Fndn Grants, 1415
Foellinger Fndn Grants, 1519
Fremont Area Comm Fndn Grants, 1561
Ginn Fndn Grants, 1616
Global Fund for Children Grants, 1629
Hanna Andersson Children's Fndn Grants, 1691
Henry & Ruth Blaustein Rosenberg Fndn Grants, 1746
J.C. Penney Company Grants, 1874
Jim Moran Fndn Grants, 1925
Kenny's Kids Grants, 1990
Louis Calder Fndn Grants, 2065
Mattel Children's Fndn Grants, 2130
Mattel International Grants, 2131
Michael and Susan Dell Fndn Grants, 2189
Milagro Fndn Grants, 2198
MONY Fndn Grants, 2215
New York Life Fndn Grants, 2304
Paul G. Allen Family Fndn Grants, 3000
Robin Hood Fndn Grants, 3174
Rohm and Haas Company Grants, 3185
Samuel S. Johnson Fndn Grants, 3251
Southbury Comm Trust Fund, 3350
U.S. Department of Education 21st Century Comm Learning Centers, 3445

Age Discrimination
Allstate Corp Giving Grants, 363
Allstate Corp Hometown Commitment Grants, 364

Aging/Gerontology
AAFCS International Graduate Fellowships, 109
AAFCS National Graduate Fellowships, 110
AAFCS National Undergraduate Scholarships, 111
AARP Fndn Gerontology Graduate Scholarships and Fellowships, 175
Abington Fndn Grants, 184
Administration on Aging Senior Medicare Patrol Project Grants, 236
AFAR CART Fund Grants, 254
AFAR Medical Student Training in Aging Research Program, 255
AFAR Paul Beeson Career Development Awards in Aging Research for the Island of Ireland, 256
AFAR Research Grants, 257
Ahn Family Fndn Grants, 304
American Academy of Nursing Building Academic Geriatric Nursing Capacity Scholarships, 414
American Academy of Nursing Claire M. Fagin Fellowships, 415
American Academy of Nursing Mayday Fund Grants, 416
American Academy of Nursing MBA Scholarships, 417
American Society on Aging Graduate Student Research Award, 455
American Society on Aging Mental Health and Aging Awards, 456

American Society on Aging NOMA Award for Excellence in Multicultural Aging, 457
Andersen Fndn Grants, 471
APSA Congressional Fellowships Health and Aging Policy Fellows Program, 514
Arlington Comm Fndn Grants, 536
ASA Metlife Fndn MindAlert Awards, 545
Austin-Bailey Health and Wellness Fndn Grants, 669
Bender Fndn Grants, 742
Brookdale Fndn Leadership in Aging Fellowships, 805
Carl B. and Florence E. King Fndn Grants, 869
Carl W. and Carrie Mae Joslyn Trust Grants, 873
Catherine Kennedy Home Fndn Grants, 890
CF Roger C. Bone Award for Advances in End-of-Life Care, 941
Charles Delmar Fndn Grants, 963
CHCF Grants, 979
Claude Pepper Fndn Grants, 1032
Clay Fndn Grants, 1034
Comm Fndn of Howard County Grants, 1116
Daniels Fund Grants, 1200
Daphne Seybolt Culpeper Memorial Fndn Grants, 1201
Duke University Postdoctoral Research Fellowships in Aging, 1348
Effie and Wofford Cain Fndn Grants, 1385
Ellison Medical Fndn/AFAR Julie Martin Mid-Career Award in Aging Research, 1403
Ellison Medical Fndn/AFAR Postdoctoral Fellows in Aging Research Program, 1404
Ellison Medical Fndn/AFAR Senior Postdoctoral Fellows Research Program, 1405
Fallon OrNda Comm Health Fund Grants, 1449
FIC Israeli Ministry of Health Postdoctoral Research Fellowships, 1494
Glenn/AFAR Breakthroughs in Gerontology Awards, 1627
Glenn/AFAR Research Grants for Postdoctoral Fellows, 1628
Greater Worcester Comm Fndn Jeppson Memorial Fund for Brookfield Grants, 1659
Harden Fndn Grants, 1693
Harry Kramer Memorial Fund Grants, 1705
Hartford Aging and Health Program Awards, 1709
Hartford Geriatrics Health Outcomes Research Scholars Program, 1712
Hawaii Comm Fndn Health Education and Research Grants, 1716
Helen Steiner Rice Fndn Grants, 1742
Henrietta Tower Wurts Memorial Fndn Grants, 1745
Honeywell Fndn Grants, 1791
Horace A. Kimball and S. Ella Kimball Fndn Grants, 1792
HRSA Geriatric Education Centers, 1805
James H. Cummings Fndn Grants, 1888
Jerome and Mildred Paddock Fndn Grants, 1917
John G. Martin Fndn Grants, 1932
Kavli Fndn Research Grants, 1985
Larry L. Hillblom Fndn Grants, 2031
Leonard and Helen R. Stulman Charitable Fndn Grants, 2044
M.B. and Edna Zale Fndn Grants, 2093
Margaret L. Wendt Fndn Grants, 2104
McLean Contributionship Grants, 2147
NHLBI Independent Scientist Award, 2339
NIA Aging Research Dissertation Awards to Increase Diversity, 2392
NIA Aging, Oxidative Stress and Cell Death Grants, 2393
NIA AIDS and Aging: Behavioral Sciences Prevention Research Grants, 2394
NIA Alzheimer's Disease Core Centers Grants, 2395
NIA Archiving and Development of Socialbehavioral Datasets in Aging Related Studies Grants, 2399
NIA Awards to Support Research on the Biology of Aging in Invertebrates Grants, 2400
NIA Bioenergetics, Fatigability, and Activity Limitations in Aging, 2402
NIA Diversity in Medication Use and Outcomes in Aging Populations Grants, 2403
NIA Effects of Gene-Social Environment Interplay on Health and Behavior in Later Life Grants, 2404
NIA Harmonization of Longitudinal Cross-National Surveys of Aging Grants, 2407
NIA Health Behaviors and Aging Grants, 2408
NIA Healthy Aging through Behavioral Economic Analyses of Situations Grants, 2409
NIA Higher-Order Cognitive Functioning and Aging Grants, 2410
NIA Human Biospecimen Resources for Aging Research Grants, 2411
NIA Independent Scientist Award, 2412
NIA Malnutrition in Older Persons Research Grants, 2413
NIA Mechanisms, Measurement, and Management of Pain in Aging: from Molecular to Clinical, 2415
NIA Medical Management of Older Patients with HIV/AIDS Grants, 2416
NIA Mentored Research Scientist Development Award, 2418
NIA Minority Dissertation Research Grants in Aging, 2419
NIA Multicenter Study on Exceptional Survival in Families: The Long Life Family Study Grants, 2420
NIA Nathan Shock Centers of Excellence in Basic Biology of Aging Grants, 2421
NIA NRSAs—Individual Postdoctoral Fellowships, 2422
NIA NRSAs—Institutional Training Awards, 2423
NIA Paul Beeson Career Development Awards in Aging, 2424
NIA Pilot Research Grant Program, 2425
NIA Postdoctoral Training in Research on Aging in Canada, 2426
NIA Promoting Careers in Aging and Health Disparities Research Grants, 2427
NIA Prostate Cancer Aging, Race, and Ethnicity Research Grants, 2428
NIA Renal Function and Chronic Kidney Disease in Aging Grants, 2429
NIA Role of Apolipoprotein E, Lipoprotein Receptors and CNS Lipid Homeostasis in Brain Aging and Alzheimer's Disease, 2431
NIA Role of Nuclear Receptors in Tissue and Organismal Aging Grants, 2432
NIA Significance of Sarcopenia in Old Age Grants, 2433
NIA Sociobehavorial Data Analysis and Archiving in Aging, 2434
NIA Support of Scientific Meetings as Cooperative Agreements, 2435
NIA Thyroid in Aging Grants, 2437
NIA Transdisciplinary Research on Fatigue and Fatigability in Aging Grants, 2438
NIA Translational Research at the Aging/Cancer Interface Grants, 2439
NIA Vulnerable Dendrites and Synapses in Aging and Alzheimer's Disease Grants, 2440
NIA/NIEHS Biomedical Epidemiologic and Intervention Studies Planning Grants, 2441
NIAAA Hepatitis C Infection and Alcoholic Liver Disease, 2442
NIAMS Significance of Sarcopenia in Old Age Grants, 2477
NIEHS Structure-Function Relationships of Environmentally Relevant Genetic Variants Research Grants, 2606
NIH Human Models and Markers of Skeletal Aging Grants, 2674
NIH Midcareer Investigator Award in Mouse Pathobiology Research Grants, 2690
NIH Pathological Gambling: Basic, Clinical, and Services Research Grants, 2702
NIH Research on Sleep and Sleep Disorders, 2713
NIH Roybal Centers for Translational Research on Aging, 2717
NIH Xenobiotics and Cell Death/Injury in Neurodegenerative Disease Research Grants, 2739
NIMH AIDS and Aging: Behavioral Sciences Prevention Research Grants, 2745
NIMH Behavior Genetics in Adulthood and Old Age Research Grants, 2747
NINR Aging Women and Breast Cancer Grants, 2789
NINR AIDS and Aging: Behavioral Sciences Prevention Research Grants, 2790
NSF Biomedical Engineering and Engineering Healthcare Grants, 2879
Ordean Fndn Grants, 2952
Orentreich Fndn for the Advancement of Science Grants, 2959
Paul Balint Charitable Trust Grants, 2998
Posey Comm Fndn Grants, 3068
Posey Comm Fndn Womens Fund Grants, 3069
Powell Fndn Grants, 3073
Quantum Fndn Grants, 3096
Retirement Research Fndn General Grants, 3150
Rhode Island Fndn Grants, 3154
Rosalinde and Arthur Gilbert Fndn/AFAR New Investigator Awards in Alzheimer's Disease, 3187
S. Mark Taper Fndn Grants, 3236
Steelcase Fndn Grants, 3379
Strowd Roses Grants, 3388
STTI Environment of Elder Care Nursing Research Grants, 3391
United Cerebral Palsy Research Grants, 3462
Walter Nicolai Prize in Biomedical Gerontology, 3517
Wilson-Wood Fndn Grants, 3542

Agribusiness
CLIF Bar Family Fndn Grants, 1040

Agricultural Planning/Policy
American Jewish World Service Grants, 437
Clarence E. Heller Charitable Fndn Grants, 1022
Institute for Agriculture and Trade Policy Food and Society Fellowships, 1856

Agriculture
Agway Fndn Grants, 265
ALSAM Fndn Grants, 369
Canada Graduate Scholarships and NSERC Postgraduate Scholarships, 845
Canada-U.S. Fulbright New Century Scholars, 846
Canada-U.S. Fulbright Senior Specialists Grants, 847
Canadian Friends of Hebrew University Research and Study Grants, 850
CLIF Bar Family Fndn Grants, 1040
Comm Fndn of Grant County Grants, 1104
Fulbright Alumni Initiatives Awards Grants, 1566
Fulbright Distinguished Chairs Grants, 1567
Fulbright New Century Scholars Grants, 1570
Fulbright Specialists Grants, 1571
Fulbright Traditional Scholar Program in Europe and Eurasia, 1572
Fulbright Traditional Scholar Program in Sub-Saharan Africa, 1573
Fulbright Traditional Scholar Program in the East Asia/Pacific Region, 1574
Fulbright Traditional Scholar Program in the Near East and North Africa Region, 1575
Fulbright Traditional Scholar Program in the South and Central Asia Region, 1576
Fulbright Traditional Scholar Program in the Western Hemisphere, 1577
Gamble Fndn Grants, 1582
Institute for Agriculture and Trade Policy Food and Society Fellowships, 1856
John Deere Fndn Grants, 1929
Lindbergh Grants, 2059
Monfort Family Fndn Grants, 2213
NIH Ecology of Infectious Diseases, 2656
Perry County Comm Fndn Grants, 3016
Posey Comm Fndn Grants, 3068
Prospect Burma Scholarships, 3085
Puerto Rico Comm Fndn Grants, 3090
RSC Thomas W. Eadie Medal, 3199
Samuel Roberts Noble Fndn Grants, 3250
Samuel S. Johnson Fndn Grants, 3251
Seneca Foods Fndn Grants, 3278
Trull Fndn Grants, 3441

Agriculture Education
Comm Fndn of Grant County Scholarships, 1105
Dean Foods Comm Involvement Grants, 1209
Posey Comm Fndn Grants, 3068

AIDS
25th Anniversary Fndn Grants, 8
AAAAI Summer Clinical Research Fellowship Medical Student Grants, 27
AAAAI Summer Research Fellowship Medical Student Grants, 28
Abbott Fund Global AIDS Care Grants, 178
Abbott Fund Science and Medical Innovation Grants, 179
AEC Trust Grants, 242
AIDS Vaccine Advocacy Coalition Fund Grants, 315
Alexander Fndn Insurance Continuation Grants, 343
Alexis Gregory Fndn Grants, 349
AMA Fndn Seed Grants for Research, 398
amfAR Fellowships, 462
amfAR Global Initiatives Grants, 463
amfAR Mathilde Krim Fellowships in Basic Biomedical Research, 464
amfAR Public Policy Grants, 465
amfAR Research Grants, 466
Ann and Robert H. Lurie Family Fndn Grants, 475
ASM Merck Irving S. Sigal Memorial Awards, 606
ASM/CCID Fellowships, 627
Assurant Fndn Grants, 654
Atkinson Fndn International Grants, 661
Bernard Van Leer Fndn Grants, 748
Blowitz-Ridgeway Fndn Grants, 767
Bodenwein Public Benevolent Fndn Grants, 775
Boston Fndn Grants, 783
Bristol-Myers Squibb Fndn Global HIV/AIDS Initiative Grants, 796
Bristol-Myers Squibb Fndn Health Disparities Grants, 797
Bristol-Myers Squibb Virology and Oncology M.D. Research Fellowships, 802
Cable Positive's Tony Cox Comm Fund Grants, 827
Campbell Fndn HIV/AIDS Research Grants, 839
CDC Intervention Epidemiologic Research Studies of HIV/AIDS, 915
CDC Prevention Education & Access to Care Services for Persons Infected and Affected by HIV, 922
Charles Delmar Fndn Grants, 963
Chestnut Hill Charitable Fndn, Inc Grants, 987
Children Affected by AIDS Fndn Camp Network Grants, 994
Children Affected by AIDS Fndn Domestic Grants, 995
Children Affected by AIDS Fndn Family Assistance Emergency Fund Grants, 996
Colin Higgins Fndn Grants, 1056
Comer Fndn Grants, 1072
Comm Fndn AIDS Endowment Awards, 1088
Comm Fndn for Southern Arizona Grants, 1095
Comm Fndn of Broward Grants, 1100
Cooper Industries Fndn Grants, 1150
Coors Brewing Corp Contributions Grants, 1151
Cornerstone Fndn of Northeastern Wisconsin Grants, 1152
Cowles Charitable Trust Grants, 1155
Dade Comm Fndn Comm AIDS Partnership Grants, 1184
Dade Comm Fndn Grants, 1185
Dallas Women's Fndn Grants, 1191
Danellie Fndn Grants, 1198
David Geffen Fndn Grants, 1202
DHHS AIDS Project Grants, 1245
DHHS Health Care Systems Cost and Access Research and Development Grants, 1252
DHHS HIV Demonstration Program for Children, Adolescents, and Women, 1262
DHHS Project Grants for Renovation or Construction of Nonacute Health Care Facilities, 1275
Doris Duke Charitable Fndn Clinical Scientist Development Award, 1316
Doris Duke Charitable Fndn Operations Research on AIDS Care and Treatment in Africa Grants, 1319
Duchossois Family Fndn Grants, 1337
Eddie C. and Sylvia Brown Family Fndn Grants, 1367
Elisabeth Severance Prentiss Fndn Grants, 1392
Elizabeth Glaser Pediatric AIDS Fndn International Leadership Awards, 1393
Elizabeth Glaser Pediatric AIDS Fndn Operations Research Grants, 1394
Elizabeth Glaser Pediatric AIDS Fndn Pediatric HIV Vaccine Research Grants, 1395
Elizabeth Glaser Pediatric AIDS Fndn Two-Year International Scholar Award, 1396
Elizabeth Glaser Pediatric AIDS Fndn Two-Year Scholar Awards, 1397
Elizabeth Glaser Scientist Award, 1398
Emily Davie and Joseph S. Kornfeld Fndn Grants, 1414
Ensworth Charitable Fndn Grants, 1416
FAR Fund, 1453
FIC International Cooperative Biodiversity Groups Grants, 1487
FIC/NIH AIDS International Training and Research Program, 1496
Frances L. and Edwin L. Cummings Memorial Fund Grants, 1547
Frank E. and Seba B. Payne Fndn Grants, 1551
Gill Fndn - Gay and Lesbian Fund Grants, 1613
Green Bay Packers Fndn Grants, 1660
Hagedorn Fund Grants, 1685
Hasbro Children's Fund, 1714
Henry J. Kaiser Family Fndn Grants, 1748
HIV/AIDS Research Training Fellowship, 1782
Indiana AIDS Fund Grants, 1851
Ittleson Fndn AIDS Grants, 1869
John M. Lloyd Fndn Grants, 1939
Johnson & Johnson Corp Contributions Grants, 1952
Johnson and Johnson / SAH Arts and Healing Grants, 1953
Kraft Cares International Grants, 2016
M-A-C AIDS Fund Grants, 2091
M. Bastian Family Fndn Grants, 2092
Marshall Field's Comm Grants, 2115
McCarthy Family Fndn Grants, 2141
Ms. Fndn Women and AIDS Fund Grants, 2223
New York Life Fndn Grants, 2304
NFID New Investigator Matching Grants, 2310
NHLBI Blood Diseases and Resources Research Grants, 2322
NIA AIDS and Aging: Behavioral Sciences Prevention Research Grants, 2394
NIA Medical Management of Older Patients with HIV/AIDS Grants, 2416
NIAID Allergy, Immunology, Transplantation, Infectious Diseases, and AIDS NRSAs—Individual, 2450
NIAID HIV Vaccine Clinical Trial Units Grants, 2454
NIAID Integrated Preclinical/Clinical AIDS Vaccine Development Grants, 2457
NIAID Laboratory Methods to Assess Responses to HIV Vaccine Candidates Research Grants, 2458
NIAID Pediatric Clinical Trials Program for AIDS, 2460
NIAID Therapeutics Research on AIDS-Associated Opportunistic Infections, 2465
NICHD Central Nervous System Effects of HIV Infection: Neurobiological, Neurovirological, and Neurobehavioral Studies Grants, 2482
NICHD Population Research Grants, 2490
NIDA Behavioral Science Track Awards for Rapid Transition, 2498
NIDA International Studies on Drug Abuse and HIV/AIDS, 2505
NIDA Minority Institutions Drug Abuse Research Development Program (MIDARP) Grants, 2509
NIDCR HIV/AIDS Associated Oral Viral Infections, 2535
NIDDK Transmission of Human Immunodeficiency Virus In Semen, 2592
NIH Centers for AIDS Research, 2647
NIH Demographic Research on Sexual Behaviors Related to HIV, 2653
NIH Multidisciplinary Approach for Research on Oral Complications of HIV Infection, 2694
NIMH AIDS and Aging: Behavioral Sciences Prevention Research Grants, 2745
NIMH Centers for AIDS Research, 2750
NIMH Central Nervous System Effects of HIV Infection: Neurobiological, Neurovirological, and Neurobehavioral Studies Grants, 2751
NIMH Core Support Program for Mental Health/AIDS Research Grants, 2753
NIMH HIV/AIDS, Severe Mental Illness, and Homelessness Research Grants, 2757
NINDS Central Nervous System Effects of HIV Infection: Neurobiological, Neurovirological, and Neurobehavioral Studies Grants, 2777
NINDS Specialized Neuroscience Research Programs on Health Disparity: HIV and the Nervous System, 2785
NINR AIDS and Aging: Behavioral Sciences Prevention Research Grants, 2790
NYCT AIDS/HIV Grants, 2919
NYCT Girls and Young Women Grants, 2924
Oracle Corp Contributions Grants, 2951
OSI Harm Reduction and Drug Use Grants, 2966
Pfizer Fndn Grants, 3025
Pittsburgh Fndn Medical Research Grants, 3055
Puerto Rico Comm Fndn Grants, 3090
Quantum Corp Snap Server Grants, 3095
Questar Corp Contributions Grants, 3097
Rhode Island Fndn Grants, 3154
Rich Fndn Grants, 3156
Robin Hood Fndn Grants, 3174
Rockefeller Brothers Fund Pivotal Places Grants: South Africa, 3180
S. Mark Taper Fndn Grants, 3236
San Diego HIV Funding Collaborative Grants, 3258
San Francisco Fndn Comm Health Grants, 3260
Smith Family New Investigator Awards, 3299
SSRC HIV/AIDS and Public Health Policy Research in Africa Fellowships, 3365
United Methodist Church Global AIDS Fund Grants, 3463
Until There's a Cure Fndn Grants, 3471
USCM HIV/AIDS Prevention Grants, 3476
W.W. Smith Charitable Trust Grants for Medical Research in Cancer, AIDS, and Heart Disease, 3509

AIDS Counseling
AIDS Vaccine Advocacy Coalition Fund Grants, 315
Ann and Robert H. Lurie Family Fndn Grants, 475
Children Affected by AIDS Fndn Domestic Grants, 995
Comm Fndn AIDS Endowment Awards, 1088
Dade Comm Fndn Comm AIDS Partnership Grants, 1184
DHHS Adolescent Family Life Demonstration Projects, 1243
Eddie C. and Sylvia Brown Family Fndn Grants, 1367
M-A-C AIDS Fund Grants, 2091
NIA Medical Management of Older Patients with HIV/AIDS Grants, 2416
NYCT AIDS/HIV Grants, 2919
OSI Harm Reduction and Drug Use Grants, 2966
Robin Hood Fndn Grants, 3174
Rockefeller Brothers Fund Pivotal Places Grants: South Africa, 3180
San Diego HIV Funding Collaborative Grants, 3258
United Methodist Church Global AIDS Fund Grants, 3463

AIDS Education
Abbott Fund Science and Medical Innovation Grants, 179
African American Fund of New Jersey Grants, 260
AIDS Vaccine Advocacy Coalition Fund Grants, 315
Alexis Gregory Fndn Grants, 349
amfAR Fellowships, 462

amfAR Global Initiatives Grants, 463
amfAR Mathilde Krim Fellowships in Basic Biomedical Research, 464
amfAR Public Policy Grants, 465
amfAR Research Grants, 466
Cable Positive's Tony Cox Comm Fund Grants, 827
CDC Prevention Education & Access to Care Services for Persons Infected and Affected by HIV, 922
CDC School Health Programs to Prevent the Spread of HIV Cooperative Agreements, 928
Colin Higgins Fndn Grants, 1056
Comer Fndn Grants, 1072
Comm Fndn AIDS Endowment Awards, 1088
Dade Comm Fndn Comm AIDS Partnership Grants, 1184
Eddie C. and Sylvia Brown Family Fndn Grants, 1367
Fairlawn Fndn Grants, 1447
FCNY Union Square Awards, 1461
Frances L. and Edwin L. Cummings Memorial Fund Grants, 1547
Gill Fndn - Gay and Lesbian Fund Grants, 1613
Health Fndn of Greater Indianapolis Grants, 1725
Ittleson Fndn AIDS Grants, 1869
M-A-C AIDS Fund Grants, 2091
McCarthy Family Fndn Grants, 2141
Morris and Gwendolyn Cafritz Fndn Grants, 2217
NIH Centers for AIDS Research, 2647
NYCT AIDS/HIV Grants, 2919
OSI Harm Reduction and Drug Use Grants, 2966
Pride Fndn Grants and Scholarships, 3078
Robin Hood Fndn Grants, 3174
Rockefeller Brothers Fund Pivotal Places Grants: South Africa, 3180
San Diego HIV Funding Collaborative Grants, 3258
United Methodist Church Global AIDS Fund Grants, 3463
Until There's a Cure Fndn Grants, 3471
USCM HIV/AIDS Prevention Grants, 3476

AIDS Prevention
Abbott Fund Global AIDS Care Grants, 178
Abbott Fund Science and Medical Innovation Grants, 179
AIDS Vaccine Advocacy Coalition Fund Grants, 315
Alexander Fndn Insurance Continuation Grants, 343
Alexis Gregory Fndn Grants, 349
Cable Positive's Tony Cox Comm Fund Grants, 827
CDC Intervention Epidemiologic Research Studies of HIV/AIDS, 915
CDC Prevention Education & Access to Care Services for Persons Infected and Affected by HIV, 922
CDC School Health Programs to Prevent the Spread of HIV Cooperative Agreements, 928
CDC Technology Translation and Transfer of Effective HIV Behavioral Interventions, 931
Colin Higgins Fndn Grants, 1056
Comm Fndn AIDS Endowment Awards, 1088
Dade Comm Fndn Comm AIDS Partnership Grants, 1184
Eddie C. and Sylvia Brown Family Fndn Grants, 1367
Elizabeth Glaser Pediatric AIDS Fndn Operations Research Grants, 1394
Elizabeth Glaser Pediatric AIDS Fndn Two-Year Scholar Awards, 1397
FCNY Union Square Awards, 1461
Frances L. and Edwin L. Cummings Memorial Fund Grants, 1547
Gates Global HIV/AIDS Vaccine Grants, 1583
HIV/AIDS Research Training Fellowship, 1782
Ittleson Fndn AIDS Grants, 1869
M-A-C AIDS Fund Grants, 2091
Morris and Gwendolyn Cafritz Fndn Grants, 2217
Moses Cone-Wesley Long Comm Health Fndn Grants, 2219
NIA AIDS and Aging: Behavioral Sciences Prevention Research Grants, 2394
NIAID HIV Vaccine Research and Design—Program Project Grants, 2455
NIAID Integrated Preclinical/Clinical AIDS Vaccine Development Grants, 2457
NIAID Statistical Methods in HIV and AIDS Research Grants, 2464
NIDDK Transmission of Human Immunodeficiency Virus In Semen, 2592
NIH Centers for AIDS Research, 2647
NIH Multidisciplinary Approach for Research on Oral Complications of HIV Infection, 2694
NIMH AIDS and Aging: Behavioral Sciences Prevention Research Grants, 2745
NIMH HIV/AIDS, Severe Mental Illness, and Homelessness Research Grants, 2757
NINR AIDS and Aging: Behavioral Sciences Prevention Research Grants, 2790
NYCT AIDS/HIV Grants, 2919
OSI Harm Reduction and Drug Use Grants, 2966
Questar Corp Contributions Grants, 3097
Rainbow Endowment Grants, 3102
Robin Hood Fndn Grants, 3174
Rockefeller Brothers Fund Pivotal Places Grants: South Africa, 3180
San Diego HIV Funding Collaborative Grants, 3258
SSRC HIV/AIDS and Public Health Policy Research in Africa Fellowships, 3365
United Methodist Church Global AIDS Fund Grants, 3463
Until There's a Cure Fndn Grants, 3471
USCM HIV/AIDS Prevention Grants, 3476

Air Pollution
Bullitt Fndn Grants, 809
Carrier Corp Contributions Grants, 884
Colorado Interstate Gas Grants, 1060
San Diego Fndn for Change Grants, 3255
Takemi Program in International Health Research and Advanced Training Fellowships, 3416

Airplanes
Northwest Airlines KidCares Medical Travel Assistance, 2868

Alaskan Natives
AMA Fndn Minority Scholars Awards, 395
ASM Robert D. Watkins Graduate Research Fellowship, 614
CDC Increasing Breast and Cervical Cancer Screening Services for Urban American Indian/Alaska Native Women, 912
DHHS Health Professions Preparatory Scholarship Program for Indians, 1257
DHHS Health Professions Scholarship Program, 1258
FDHN Student Research Fellowships, 1480
IHS Native American and Alaskan Native Health Research Centers, 1840
NHLBI Minority Institutional Research Training Grants, 2355
NIMH Career Opportunities in Research Education and Training Honors High School Research Education Grant, 2748
NIMH Career Opportunities in Research Education and Training Honors Undergraduate Research Training Grant, 2749

Alcohol Education
Coors Brewing Corp Contributions Grants, 1151
Fairlawn Fndn Grants, 1447
King Pharmaceuticals Corp Contributions Grants, 2003
NYCT Girls and Young Women Grants, 2924
NYCT Substance Abuse Grants, 2928

Alcohol/Alcoholism
Adaptec Fndn Grants, 232
African American Fund of New Jersey Grants, 260
Alcohol Misuse and Alcoholism Research Grants, 335
Alliance Healthcare Fndn Grants, 362
AMA Fndn Fund for Better Health Grants, 388
amfAR Fellowships, 462
amfAR Global Initiatives Grants, 463
amfAR Mathilde Krim Fellowships in Basic Biomedical Research, 464
amfAR Public Policy Grants, 465
amfAR Research Grants, 466
Andersen Fndn Grants, 471
Barberton Comm Fndn Grants, 693
Berks County Comm Fndn Grants, 745
Bodman Fndn Grants, 776
Bush Fndn Health & Human Services Grants, 814
Cambridge Comm Fndn Grants, 837
Carlisle Fndn Grants, 874
Carpenter Fndn Grants, 881
Cass County Comm Fndn Grants, 887
Cleo Fndn Grants, 1035
Colorado Springs Comm Trust Fund Grants, 1061
Comm Fndn for Southern Arizona Grants, 1095
Comm Fndn of Broward Grants, 1100
Constantin Fndn Grants, 1145
Coors Brewing Corp Contributions Grants, 1151
D.F. Halton Fndn Grants, 1181
Dallas Women's Fndn Grants, 1191
Daniels Fund Grants, 1200
Dennis and Phyllis Washington Fndn Grants, 1222
DOJ Mental Health and Juvenile Justice, 1304
EIF Comm Grants, 1386
Farmers Insurance Group of Companies Grants, 1455
Fndn for a Healthy Kentucky Grants, 1527
Frances and John L. Loeb Family Fund Grants, 1546
Greater Worcester Comm Fndn Discretionary Grants, 1658
Hasbro Children's Fund, 1714
Health Fndn of Greater Cincinnati Grants, 1724
Johnson & Johnson Corp Contributions Grants, 1952
Joseph Drown Fndn Grants, 1960
Joseph H. and Florence A. Roblee Fndn Grants, 1961
Kalamazoo Fndn Grants, 1979
Kathryne Beynon Fndn Grants, 1984
L. W. Pierce Family Fndn Grants, 2019
Lesbian Health Fund Grants, 2046
Lester Ray Fleming Scholarships, 2048
Margaret L. Wendt Fndn Grants, 2104
Mary Owen Borden Fndn Grants, 2121
Moses Cone-Wesley Long Comm Health Fndn Grants, 2219
Newman's Own Inc Grants, 2306
NIAAA Hepatitis C Infection and Alcoholic Liver Disease, 2442
NIAAA Independent Scientist Award, 2443
NIAAA Mechanisms of Alcohol and Drug-Induced Pancreatitis Grants, 2444
NIAAA Mechanisms of Alcohol-Induced Hepatic Fibrosis Research Grants, 2445
NIAAA Peptide Regulation of Alcohol Intake, 2447
NIAAA Secondary Analysis of Existing Health Services Data Sets Grants, 2448
NIH Exploratory/Development Grants for Mental Health Intervention Research, 2665
NIH NRSAs for Individual Predoctoral Fellowships, 2700
NIH Research on Sleep and Sleep Disorders, 2713
NIMH Early Identification and Treatment of Mental Disorders in Children and Adolescents Grants, 2756
Northern Trust Company Charitable Trust and Corp Giving Program, 2865
NYCT Substance Abuse Grants, 2928
Ordean Fndn Grants, 2952
PacifiCorp Fndn for Learning Grants, 2982
Pajaro Valley Comm Health Grants, 2985
Peter and Elizabeth C. Tower Fndn Comm Grants, 3018
Puerto Rico Comm Fndn Grants, 3090
Quantum Corp Snap Server Grants, 3095
Questar Corp Contributions Grants, 3097
Rayonier Fndn Grants, 3111
RWJF New Jersey Health Initiatives Grants, 3225
S.H. Cowell Fndn Grants, 3237
SAMHSA Conference Grants, 3246
SAMHSA Drug Free Communities Support Grants, 3247
SAMHSA Strategic Prevention Framework State Incentive Grants, 3248
Sid W. Richardson Fndn Grants, 3284

Southbury Comm Trust Fund, 3350
Stewart Huston Charitable Trust Grants, 3384
Triangle Comm Fndn Shaver-Hitchings Scholarship, 3438

Allergy
AAAAI / Schering Allergy/Immunology Fellowship of Excellence Training Awards, 20
AAAAI Allergy, Asthma and Immunology Education and Research Trust Allied Health Travel Grants, 21
AAAAI Allergy, Asthma and Immunology Education and Research Trust Clinical Research Grants, 22
AAAAI Allergy, Asthma and Immunology Education and Research Trust Faculty Development Award, 23
AAAAI Research Award Grants, 25
AAAAI STAR Grants, 26
AAAAI Summer Clinical Research Fellowship Medical Student Grants, 27
AAAAI Summer Research Fellowship Medical Student Grants, 28
Coca-Cola Fndn Grants, 1052
NIAID Allergy, Immunology, and Transplantation Program Research Grants, 2449
NIAID Allergy, Immunology, Transplantation, Infectious Diseases, and AIDS NRSAs—Individual, 2450
NIAID Independent Scientist Award, 2456
NIAID Research Scholar Development Award, 2462
NIAID Small Business Innovation Research Advanced Technology Grants, 2463
NIH Hyperaccelerated Award/Mechanisms in Immunomodulation Trials, 2675

Allied Health Education
AAHPERD-AAHE Barbara A. Cooley Scholarships, 129
AAHPERD-AAHE Delbert Oberteuffer Scholarships, 130
CVS All Kids Can Grants, 1175
CVS Comm Grants, 1177
DHHS Health Careers Opportunity Grants, 1253
DHHS Health Education and Training Centers Project Grants, 1256
DHHS Health Professions Training in Geriatrics Grants, 1259
DHHS Oral Health Promotion Research Across the Lifespan, 1269
Health Fndn of Greater Indianapolis Grants, 1725
HRSA Geriatric Education Centers, 1805
HRSA Health Professions Scholarships for Disadvantaged Students, 1807
HRSA Physician Assistant Training, 1810
J.M. Long Fndn Grants, 1877
James G.K. McClure Educational and Development Fund Grants, 1886
Jewish Fndn for Education of Women Scholarships for Emigres in the Health Professions, 1922
Josiah Macy Jr. Fndn Grants, 1966
Lettie Pate Whitehead Fndn Grants, 2049
Schering-Plough Fndn Health Grants, 3270

Alternative Fuels
Alfred P. Sloan Fndn Research Fellowships, 353

Alternative Medicine
Blowitz-Ridgeway Fndn Grants, 767
Fannie E. Rippel Fndn Grants, 1452
GPP Charles E. Culpeper Fndn Biomedical Pilot Projects Initiative Grants, 1641
James Hervey Johnson Charitable Educational Trust Grants, 1889
NCCAM Exploratory Developmental Grants for Complementary and Alternative Medicine Studies of Humans, 2265
NCCAM Ruth L. Kirschstein National Research Service Awards for Postdoctoral Training in Complementary and Alternative Medicine, 2266
NIH Centers for Dietary Supplements Research: Botanicals, 2648
NIH Complementary and Alternative Medicine Postdoctoral Training Grants, 2652
NIH Exploratory Centers for Alternative Medicine Research Grants, 2663
NINR Management of Symptoms at the End of Life Grants, 2796
NINR Quality of Life for Individuals at the End of Life Grants, 2802
RACGP Vicki Kotsirilos Integrative Medicine Grants, 3101
Sunshine Natural Wellbeing Fndn Grants, 3404
Susan G. Komen Breast Cancer Fndn Basic, Clinical, and Translational Research Grants, 3407
U.S. Department of Education Vocational Rehabilitation Services Projects for American Indians with Disabilities Grants, 3452

Alternative Modes of Education
Chicago Comm Trust Grants, 989
U.S. Department of Education Vocational Rehabilitation Services Projects for American Indians with Disabilities Grants, 3452

Alzheimer's Disease
AHAF Alzheimer's Disease Research Grants, 266
Alzheimer's Association Everyday Technologies for Alzheimer Care Research Grants, 377
Alzheimer's Association Investigator-Initiated Research Grants, 378
Alzheimer's Association Mentored New Investigator Research Grants to Promote Diversity, 379
Alzheimer's Association Molecular Imaging Grants, 380
Alzheimer's Association New Investigator Research Grants, 381
Alzheimer's Association New Investigator Research Grants to Promote Diversity, 382
Alzheimer's Association Senator Mark Hatfield Award, 383
Alzheimer's Association Zenith Fellows Awards, 384
Alzheimer's Association Conference Grants, 385
Balfe Family Fndn Grants, 682
Brookdale Fndn Leadership in Aging Fellowships, 805
F.M. Kirby Fndn Grants, 1443
Fairlawn Fndn Grants, 1447
Fremont Area Comm Fndn Grants, 1561
G.N. Wilcox Trust Grants, 1581
Grand Rapids Area Comm Fndn Grants, 1645
Harden Fndn Grants, 1693
Hawaii Comm Fndn Health Education and Research Grants, 1716
Helen Bader Fndn Grants, 1738
NIA Alzheimer's Disease Core Centers Grants, 2395
NIA Alzheimer's Disease Drug Development Grants, 2396
NIA Alzheimer's Disease Pilot Clinical Trials, 2397
NIA Alzheimer's Disease Research Centers Grants, 2398
NIA Grants for Alzheimer's Disease Drug Discovery, 2406
NIA Role of Apolipoprotein E, Lipoprotein Receptors and CNS Lipid Homeostasis in Brain Aging and Alzheimer's Disease, 2431
NIA Vulnerable Dendrites and Synapses in Aging and Alzheimer's Disease Grants, 2440
NIH Alzheimer's Disease Clinical Trial Planning Grant, 2636
NIH Xenobiotics and Cell Death/Injury in Neurodegenerative Disease Research Grants, 2739
Northwestern Mutual Fndn Grants, 2870
Pittsburgh Fndn Medical Research Grants, 3055
Rosalinde and Arthur Gilbert Fndn/AFAR New Investigator Awards in Alzheimer's Disease, 3187

American Recovery and Reinvestment Act
NIH Recovery Act Limited Competition: Academic Research Enhancement Awards, 2707
NIH Recovery Act Limited Competition: Biomedical Research, Development, and Growth to Spur the Acceleration of New Technologies (BRDG-SPAN) Pilot Grants, 2708
NIH Recovery Act Limited Competition: Small Business Catalyst Awards for Accelerating Innovative Research Grants, 2710
NIH Recovery Act Limited Competition: Supporting New Faculty Recruitment to Enhance Research Resources through Biomedical Research Core Centers Grants, 2711

American Studies
Canada-U.S. Fulbright New Century Scholars Grants, 846
Canada-U.S. Fulbright Senior Specialists Grants, 847
Fulbright Alumni Initiatives Awards Grants, 1566
Fulbright Distinguished Chairs Grants, 1567
Fulbright New Century Scholars Grants, 1570
Fulbright Specialists Grants, 1571
Fulbright Traditional Scholar Program in Europe and Eurasia, 1572
Fulbright Traditional Scholar Program in Sub-Saharan Africa, 1573
Fulbright Traditional Scholar Program in the East Asia/Pacific Region, 1574
Fulbright Traditional Scholar Program in the Near East and North Africa Region, 1575
Fulbright Traditional Scholar Program in the South and Central Asia Region, 1576
Fulbright Traditional Scholar Program in the Western Hemisphere, 1577

Amyotrophic Lateral Sclerosis
NIH Xenobiotics and Cell Death/Injury in Neurodegenerative Disease Research Grants, 2739

Anatomy
Deafness Research Fndn Research Grants, 1208
NIEHS Biological Response to Environmental Health Hazards Research Grants, 2596
PhRMA Fndn Pharmacology/Toxicology Post Doctoral Fellowships, 3044

Anemia
Cooley's Anemia Research Fellowships, 1149

Anesthesiology
AGS Dennis W. Jahnigen Career Development Scholars Awards, 264
Duke University Adult Cardiothoracic Anesthesia and Critical Care Medicine Fellowships, 1340
Duke University Ambulatory and Regional Anesthesia Fellowships, 1341
Duke University Obstetric Anesthesia Fellowships, 1345
Duke University Pediatric Anesthesiology Fellowship, 1347
HRSA Nurse Anesthetist Traineeships Program, 1808
Mayday Fund Grants, 2139
NIGMS Mentored Clinical Scientist Research Career Development Awards, 2618
NIGMS Molecular Pharmacology of Anesthetic Action Research Grants, 2621
Parker B. Francis Fellowships in Pulmonary Research, 2989

Animal Behavior/Ethology
Fyssen Fndn Postdoctoral Study Grants, 1580

Animal Breeding and Facilities, Scientific
NIH Technologies to Improve the Utility of Animal Models Research Grants, 2735

Animal Care
Adam Richter Charitable Trust Grants, 230
Alberto Culver Corp Contributions Grants, 329
Armstrong McDonald Fndn Grants, 537
Batchelor Fndn Grants, 701
Bearemy's Kennel Pals Grants, 728

Benton County Fndn Grants, 744
Champlin Fndns Grants, 960
Charlotte County (FL) Comm Fndn Grants, 973
Comm Fndn of Broward Grants, 1100
Comm Fndn of Madison and Jefferson County Grants and Scholarships, 1117
Comm Fndn of Tampa Bay Grants, 1128
Dade Comm Fndn Grants, 1185
Dean Foods Comm Involvement Grants, 1209
DeRoy Testamentary Fndn Grants, 1239
Fargo-Moorhead Area Fndn Grants, 1454
Gamble Fndn Grants, 1582
Green Bay Packers Fndn Grants, 1660
Greenfield Fndn of Maine Grants, 1663
Harden Fndn Grants, 1693
Jane's Trust Grants, 1904
Lubbock Area Fndn Grants, 2079
Margaret T. Morris Fndn Grants, 2105
Owen County Comm Fndn Grants, 2979
Perkins Charitable Fndn Grants, 3014
Perry County Comm Fndn Grants, 3016
Pet Care Trust Sue Busch Memorial Award, 3017
Puerto Rico Comm Fndn Grants, 3090
San Antonio Area Fndn Grants, 3254
Southwest Florida Comm Fndn Competitive Grants, 3351
Vancouver Fndn Grants and Comm Initiatives Program, 3477
Vanderburgh Comm Fndn Grants, 3480

Animal Development
NIH Mouse Mutagenesis and Phenotyping: Developmental Defects Research Grants, 2692

Animal Diseases/Pathology
ACVIM Fndn Clinical Investigation Grants, 227
DOI Biological Resource Division Brucellosis Program, 1302
NIH Technologies to Improve the Utility of Animal Models Research Grants, 2735

Animal Drugs
DOI Biological Resource Division Brucellosis Program, 1302

Animal Ecology
Greenfield Fndn of Maine Grants, 1663

Animal Research Policy
Alternatives Research and Development Fndn Alternatives in Education Grants, 370
Alternatives Research and Development Fndn Grants, 371
Center for Alternatives to Animal Testing Grants, 934
Ethical Research Grants and Fellowships, 1431
NCRR Novel Approaches to Enhance Animal Stem Cell Research, 2288
NIH Technologies to Improve the Utility of Animal Models Research Grants, 2735
NIH Zebrafish as an Animal Model for Development and Disease Research Grants, 2740
Vancouver Fndn Grants and Comm Initiatives Program, 3477

Animal Rights
Adam Richter Charitable Trust Grants, 230
Andersen Fndn Grants, 471
Ann Jackson Family Fndn Grants, 477
Blue Mountain Comm Fndn Grants, 769
Bodenwein Public Benevolent Fndn Grants, 775
Comm Fndn of Broward Grants, 1100
Comm Fndn of Crawford County Grants and Scholarships, 1103
Frank Stanley Beveridge Fndn Grants, 1553
Harrison County Comm Fndn Grants, 1700
Horace A. Kimball and S. Ella Kimball Fndn Grants, 1792
NIH Technologies to Improve the Utility of Animal Models Research Grants, 2735
Perkins Charitable Fndn Grants, 3014
Rhode Island Fndn Grants, 3154
Thelma Doelger Charitable Trust Grants, 3421
Vancouver Fndn Grants and Comm Initiatives Program, 3477

Animal Science
ACVIM Fndn Clinical Investigation Grants, 227
NSF Animal Developmental Mechanisms Grants, 2875
NSF Cell Systems Cluster Grants, 2881

Animal Welfare
Annenberg Fndn Grants, 479
Arkansas Comm Fndn Grants, 533
Central Okanagan Fndn Grants, 937

Animals as Pets
Bearemy's Kennel Pals Grants, 728
Comm Fndn of Madison and Jefferson County Grants and Scholarships, 1117

Animals for Assistance/Therapy
Bearemy's Kennel Pals Grants, 728
Harry and Grace Steele Fndn Grants, 1702

Anorexia Nervosa
NIMH Early Identification and Treatment of Mental Disorders in Children and Adolescents Grants, 2756

Anthropology
AHFMR Population Health Investigator Awards, 292
Canada-U.S. Fulbright New Century Scholars Grants, 846
Canada-U.S. Fulbright Senior Specialists Grants, 847
EF Behavioral Sciences Student Fellowships, 1379
Fulbright Alumni Initiatives Awards Grants, 1566
Fulbright Distinguished Chairs Grants, 1567
Fulbright New Century Scholars Grants, 1570
Fulbright Specialists Grants, 1571
Fulbright Traditional Scholar Program in Europe and Eurasia, 1572
Fulbright Traditional Scholar Program in Sub-Saharan Africa, 1573
Fulbright Traditional Scholar Program in the East Asia/Pacific Region, 1574
Fulbright Traditional Scholar Program in the Near East and North Africa Region, 1575
Fulbright Traditional Scholar Program in the South and Central Asia Region, 1576
Fulbright Traditional Scholar Program in the Western Hemisphere, 1577
Fyssen Fndn Postdoctoral Study Grants, 1580
Pfizer Fndn Health Literacy Grants, 3026

Antibiotics
NFID New Investigator Matching Grants, 2310
Pfizer Fndn Grants, 3025

Antivirals
Doris Duke Charitable Fndn Operations Research on AIDS Care and Treatment in Africa Grants, 1319

Appalachia
Commission on Religion in Appalachia Grants, 1074

Archaeology
Canada-U.S. Fulbright New Century Scholars Grants, 846
Canada-U.S. Fulbright Senior Specialists Grants, 847
Fulbright Alumni Initiatives Awards Grants, 1566
Fulbright Distinguished Chairs Grants, 1567
Fulbright New Century Scholars Grants, 1570
Fulbright Specialists Grants, 1571
Fulbright Traditional Scholar Program in Europe and Eurasia, 1572
Fulbright Traditional Scholar Program in Sub-Saharan Africa, 1573
Fulbright Traditional Scholar Program in the East Asia/Pacific Region, 1574
Fulbright Traditional Scholar Program in the Near East and North Africa Region, 1575
Fulbright Traditional Scholar Program in the South and Central Asia Region, 1576
Fulbright Traditional Scholar Program in the Western Hemisphere, 1577
Stewart Huston Charitable Trust Grants, 3384

Architecture
Chicago Tribune's Corp Contributions Grants, 991
Denver Fndn Comm Grants, 1227
Northwood University/Alden B. Dow Creativity Center Summer Residency Program, 2871

Archives
Grammy Fndn Grants, 1643

Arrhythmia
NHLBI New Approaches to Arrhythmia Detection and Treatment Grants for SBIR, 2359
NHLBI New Approaches to Arrhythmia Detection and Treatment Grants for STTR, 2360
NHLBI Targeting Calcium Regulatory Molecules for Arrhythmia Prevention Grants, 2388

Art Appreciation
Benton County Fndn Grants, 744
Boyd Gaming Corp Contributions Program, 788
Carl B. and Florence E. King Fndn Grants, 869
Carrier Corp Contributions Grants, 884
Comm Fndn of Madison and Jefferson County Grants and Scholarships, 1117
Honda of America Manufacturing Fndn Grants, 1790
Paul E. and Klare N. Reinhold Fndn Grants, 2999
Perry County Comm Fndn Grants, 3016
Pike County Comm Fndn Grants, 3049
San Diego Women's Fndn Grants, 3259
Vanderburgh Comm Fndn Grants, 3480
Warrick County Comm Fndn Grants, 3519

Art Conservation
Pike County Comm Fndn Grants, 3049

Art Education
2 Depot Square Ipswich Charitable Fndn Grants, 7
3M Fndn Grants, 11
Abbott Fund Comm Vitality Grants, 177
Abell-Hanger Fndn Grants, 183
Ahn Family Fndn Grants, 304
Alaska Airlines Corp Giving Grants, 323
Alaska Airlines Fndn Grants, 324
Angels Baseball Fndn Grants, 473
Annenberg Fndn Grants, 479
Ashland Corp Contributions Grants, 586
Assurant Health Fndn Grants, 655
Benton County Fndn Grants, 744
Boyd Gaming Corp Contributions Program, 788
Carl and Lily Pforzheimer Fndn Grants, 868
Chicago Comm Trust Grants, 989
Connecticut Comm Fndn Grants, 1141
Cooper Industries Fndn Grants, 1150
DAAD Research Stays for University Academics and Scientists, 1183
Eisner Fndn Grants, 1387
Erie Comm Fndn Grants, 1427
Ethel S. Abbott Charitable Fndn Grants, 1430
Ford Motor Company Fund Grants, 1522
Grand Rapids Area Comm Fndn Grants, 1645
Grand Rapids Area Comm Fndn Nashwauk Area Endowment Fund Grants, 1646
Greater Worcester Comm Fndn Discretionary Grants, 1658
Green Fndn Grants, 1661
H & R Fndn Grants, 1679
Herman Goldman Fndn Grants, 1753
Honda of America Manufacturing Fndn Grants, 1790
Horizon Fndn for New Jersey Grants, 1793
Jacob and Hilda Blaustein Fndn Grants, 1881
Jane's Trust Grants, 1904
Jewish Women's Fndn of New York Grants, 1924

Julia Temple Davis Brown Fndn Grants, 1971
Lettie Pate Whitehead Fndn Grants, 2049
Lincoln Financial Group Fndn Grants, 2058
Louis R. Cappelli Fndn Grants, 2066
Lubrizol Fndn Grants, 2080
Marion I. and Henry J. Knott Fndn Grants, 2109
McGregor Fund Grants, 2143
Mead Johnson Nutritionals Evansville-Area Organizations Grants, 2157
Milagro Fndn Grants, 2198
Miriam and Peter Haas Fund Grants, 2208
Morris and Gwendolyn Cafritz Fndn Grants, 2217
North Carolina GlaxoSmithKline Fndn Grants, 2860
OSI-Baltimore Special Opportunities Grants, 2972
Paul E. and Klare N. Reinhold Fndn Grants, 2999
Peacock Fndn Grants, 3011
Pike County Comm Fndn Grants, 3049
Rockwell International Corp Trust Grants, 3183
San Diego Women's Fndn Grants, 3259
Sid W. Richardson Fndn Grants, 3284
Vancouver Fndn Grants and Comm Initiatives Program, 3477
Weatherwax Fndn Grants, 3523
Westinghouse Charitable Giving Grants, 3530

Art History
Louis R. Cappelli Fndn Grants, 2066
Pike County Comm Fndn Grants, 3049

Art in Public Places
Abbott Fund Comm Vitality Grants, 177
Amador Comm Fndn Grants, 409
Boyd Gaming Corp Contributions Program, 788
Grand Rapids Area Comm Fndn Grants, 1645
Grand Rapids Area Comm Fndn Nashwauk Area Endowment Fund Grants, 1646

Art Works/Artifacts
Bank of America Client Fndn Grants, 690

Art, Experimental
Connecticut Comm Fndn Grants, 1141

Arthritis
AF Doctoral Dissertation Award for Arthritis Health Professionals, 253
Arthritis Fndn of Australia Grants, 541
Balfe Family Fndn Grants, 682
Comm Fndn of Broward Grants, 1100
Fairlawn Fndn Grants, 1447
Mabel H. Flory Charitable Trust Grants, 2096
Musculoskeletal Rehabilitation Fellowships, 2229
NIAMS Clinical Trial Planning Grants, 2466
NIAMS Collaborative Arthritis and Musculoskeletal and Skin Diseases Science Award, 2467
NIAMS High Risk Arthritis and Musculoskeletal and Skin Diseases Research, 2470
NIAMS Mechanisms of Chondroprotection Research Grants, 2472
NIAMS Specialized Centers of Research in Osteoarthritis and Systemic Lupus Erythematosus, 2479
NIAMS Specialized Centers of Research in Osteoporosis, Rheumatoid Arthritis, and Scleroderma, 2480
Pittsburgh Fndn Medical Research Grants, 3055

Arts
Abramson Family Fndn Grants, 188
Annenberg Fndn Grants, 479
Assurant Health Fndn Grants, 655
Autodesk Comm Relations Grants, 671
Blanche and Julian Robertson Family Fndn Grants, 765
Carolyn Fndn Grants, 880
Chazen Fndn Grants, 978
CIT Corp Giving Grants, 1014
Columbus Fndn Competitive Grants, 1066
Comm Fndn of Morgan County Grants and Scholarships, 1118
Dale and Edna Walsh Fndn Grants, 1189
Drs. Bruce and Lee Fndn Grants, 1333
DuPage Comm Fndn Grants, 1352
Eastman Chemical Company Fndn Grants, 1362
Elizabeth Morse Genius Charitable Trust Grants, 1400
Fndn for the Carolinas Grants, 1535
GlaxoSmithKline Corp Grants, 1623
Goodyear Tire Grants, 1639
Green Fndn Grants, 1661
Hanna Andersson Children's Fndn Grants, 1691
Harold Alfond Fndn Grants, 1695
Johnson and Johnson / SAH Arts and Healing Grants, 1953
Josephine S. Gumbiner Fndn Grants, 1965
K and F Baxter Family Fndn Grants, 1973
Kraft Cares International Grants, 2016
Lowell Area Comm Fund Grants, 2068
Maine Comm Fndn Grants, 2099
Margaret L. Wendt Fndn Grants, 2104
Matilda R. Wilson Fund Grants, 2128
McCombs Fndn Grants, 2142
McMurry Fndn Grants, 2149
Meyer Fndn Grants, 2177
Middlesex Savings Charitable Fndn Grants, 2196
Oscar Rennebohm Fndn Grants, 2963
PMI Fndn Grants, 3063
Ruth Mott Fndn Grants, 3204
Society for the Arts in Healthcare Consulting Grants, 3326
Steelcase Fndn Grants, 3379

Arts Administration
Alcatel-Lucent Technologies Fndn Grants, 333
Andersen Fndn Grants, 471
Frey Fndn Grants, 1562
J.L. Bedsole Fndn Grants, 1876
Procter and Gamble Fund Grants, 3083
Sid W. Richardson Fndn Grants, 3284

Arts and Culture
AIG American General Corp Grants, 316
John W. and Anna H. Hanes Fndn Grants, 1948
Sosland Fndn Grants, 3348
Sprague Fndn Grants, 3359
Stewart Huston Charitable Trust Grants, 3384
TWS Fndn Grants, 3443
Weatherwax Fndn Grants, 3523

Arts Festivals
Angels Baseball Fndn Grants, 473
Bank of America Charitable Fndn Anchor Institutions Grants, 688
Honda of America Manufacturing Fndn Grants, 1790

Arts, General
2 Depot Square Ipswich Charitable Fndn Grants, 7
3M Fndn Grants, 11
A Friend's Fndn Trust Grants, 13
A. Gary Anderson Family Fndn Grants, 17
Aaron Fndn (Massachusetts) Grants, 174
Abbott Fund Comm Vitality Grants, 177
Achelis and Bodman Fndns Grants, 206
Adam Richter Charitable Trust Grants, 230
Adams County Fndn Grants - Pennsylvania, 231
Adobe Comm Investment Grants, 237
AEC Trust Grants, 242
AEGON Transamerica Fndn Grants, 243
AFG Industries Grants, 259
African American Fund of New Jersey Grants, 260
Agnes Gund Fndn Grants, 262
Ahmanson Fndn Grants, 303
Ahn Family Fndn Grants, 304
Air Products and Chemicals Grants, 319
Alabama Power Fndn Grants, 321
Aladdin Industries Fndn Grants, 322
Alaska Airlines Corp Giving Grants, 323
Alaska Airlines Fndn Grants, 324
Alberto Culver Corp Contributions Grants, 329
Albuquerque Comm Fndn Grants, 331
Alcatel-Lucent Technologies Corp Contributions Grants, 332
Alcatel-Lucent Technologies Fndn Grants, 333
Alcoa Fndn Grants, 334
Alex Brown and Sons Charitable Fndn Grants, 337
Alexander & Baldwin Fndn Hawaiian and Pacific Island Grants, 338
Alexander & Baldwin Fndn Mainland Grants, 339
Alexis Gregory Fndn Grants, 349
Alice Tweed Tuohy Fndn Grants, 357
Allegheny Technologies Charitable Trust, 359
Altman Fndn Health Care Grants, 372
Amador Comm Fndn Grants, 409
Amarillo Area/Harrington Fndns Grants, 410
American Schlafhorst Fndn Grants, 454
Andersen Fndn Grants, 471
Angels Baseball Fndn Grants, 473
Annenberg Fndn Grants, 479
Annie Sinclair Knudsen Memorial Fund/Kaua'i Comm Grants, 480
AON Fndn Grants, 491
AptarGroup Fndn Grants, 522
Arizona Cardinals Grants, 529
Arizona Public Service Corp Giving Grants, 531
Arkansas Comm Fndn Grants, 533
Arlington Comm Fndn Grants, 536
Armstrong McDonald Fndn Grants, 537
ARS Fndn Grants, 538
Assisi Fndn Grants, 653
Atherton Family Fndn Grants, 659
Athwin Fndn Grants, 660
Atlanta Fndn Grants, 662
Audrey and Sydney Irmas Charitable Fndn Grants, 665
Aurora Fndn Grants, 667
Autzen Fndn Grants, 672
Bacon Family Fndn Grants, 679
Bailey Fndn Grants, 680
Ball Brothers Fndn General Grants, 683
Banfi Vintners Fndn Grants, 687
Bank of America Client Fndn Grants, 690
Barberton Comm Fndn Grants, 693
Barker Welfare Fndn Grants, 695
Barnes Group Fndn Grants, 696
Barra Fndn Comm Fund Grants, 698
Barra Fndn Project Grants, 699
Batchelor Fndn Grants, 701
Baton Rouge Area Fndn Grants, 702
Battle Creek Comm Fndn Grants, 703
Batts Fndn Grants, 704
Beazley Fndn Grants, 730
Beckley Area Fndn Grants, 732
Belk Fndn Grants, 739
Benton Comm Fndn Grants, 743
Benton County Fndn Grants, 744
Berks County Comm Fndn Grants, 745
Bernard and Audre Rapoport Fndn Grants, 746
Berrien Comm Fndn Grants, 749
Besser Fndn Grants, 752
Bildner Family Fndn Grants, 755
Binney and Smith Comm Grants, 757
Biogen Corp Giving Grants, 758
Blackford County Comm Fndn Grants, 763
Blanche and Irving Laurie Fndn Grants, 764
Blue Grass Comm Fndn Grants, 768
Blue Mountain Comm Fndn Grants, 769
Blue River Comm Fndn Grants, 770
Bodenwein Public Benevolent Fndn Grants, 775
Boeing Company Contributions Grants, 777
Bonfils-Stanton Fndn Grants, 779
Borkee-Hagley Fndn Grants, 781
Bosque Fndn Grants, 782
Boston Fndn Grants, 783
Boston Globe Fndn Grants, 784
Bradley Turner Fndn Grants, 789
Bridgestone/Firestone Trust Fund Grants, 792
Brook J. Lenfest Fndn Grants, 804
Brown County Comm Fndn Grants, 807
Bruce and Adele Greenfield Fndn Grants, 808
Burlington Industries Fndn Grants, 811
Burlington Northern Santa Fe Fndn Grants, 812
Business Bank of Nevada Comm Grants, 817
Byron W. and Alice L. Lockwood Fndn Grants, 824

C.R. Bard Fndn Grants, 825
C.W. Titus Fndn Grants, 826
Caleb C. and Julia W. Dula Educational and Charitable Fndn Grants, 830
Cambridge Comm Fndn Grants, 837
Canada-U.S. Fulbright New Century Scholars Grants, 846
Canada-U.S. Fulbright Senior Specialists Grants, 847
Canadian Friends of Hebrew University Research and Study Grants, 850
Cardinal Health Fndn Grants, 864
Carl and Eloise Pohlad Family Fndn Grants, 867
Carl B. and Florence E. King Fndn Grants, 869
Carl C. Icahn Fndn Grants, 870
Carpenter Fndn Grants, 881
Carrie E. and Lena V. Glenn Fndn Grants, 882
Cemala Fndn Grants, 933
Central Okanagan Fndn Grants, 937
Cessna Fndn Grants, 938
CFFVR Opportunity Grants, 952
Champlin Fndns Grants, 960
Charles H. Dater Fndn Grants, 966
Charles Lafitte Fndn Grants, 970
Charles M. Bair Family Trust Grants, 972
Charlotte County (FL) Comm Fndn Grants, 973
Chestnut Hill Charitable Fndn, Inc Grants, 987
Chicago Board of Trade Fndn Grants, 988
Chicago Comm Trust Grants, 989
Chiles Fndn Grants, 1003
Christy-Houston Fndn Grants, 1008
Chula Vista Charitable Fndn Grants, 1009
CICF Legacy Fund Comm Fndn Grants, 1010
CIGNA Fndn Grants, 1011
Cinergy Fndn Grants, 1013
Citizens Bank Mid-Atlantic Charitable Fndn Grants, 1015
Clarcor Fndn Grants, 1021
Clark County Comm Fndn Grants, 1028
Claude Worthington Benedum Fndn Grants, 1033
Cleveland Browns Fndn Grants, 1036
CNA Fndn Grants, 1046
Coastal Comm Fndn of South Carolina Grants, 1051
Cockrell Fndn Grants, 1053
Coeta and Donald Barker Fndn Grants, 1054
Collins Fndn Grants, 1058
Columbus Fndn Mary Eleanor Morris Fund Grants, 1069
Comer Fndn Grants, 1072
Comm Fndn Alliance City of Evansville Endowment Fund Grants, 1089
Comm Fndn for Monterey County Grants, 1092
Comm Fndn for Muskegon County Grants, 1093
Comm Fndn for Southeastern Michigan Grants, 1094
Comm Fndn for Southern Arizona Grants, 1095
Comm Fndn of Bartholomew County Heritage Fund Grants, 1096
Comm Fndn of Bartholomew County James A. Henderson Award for Fund-Raising, 1097
Comm Fndn of Bloomington and Monroe County Grants, 1098
Comm Fndn of Boone County Grants, 1099
Comm Fndn of Broward Grants, 1100
Comm Fndn of Central Illinois Grants, 1101
Comm Fndn of Champaign County Grants, 1102
Comm Fndn of Crawford County Grants and Scholarships, 1103
Comm Fndn of Greater Birmingham Grants, 1106
Comm Fndn of Greater Flint Grants, 1107
Comm Fndn of Greater Fort Wayne: Comm Endowment & Clarke Endowment Fund Grants, 1108
Comm Fndn of Greater Greensboro Grants, 1109
Comm Fndn Of Greater Lafayette Grants, 1110
Comm Fndn of Greater New Britain Grants, 1111
Comm Fndn of Greater Tampa Grants, 1112
Comm Fndn of Greenville Comm Enrichment Grants, 1113
Comm Fndn of Greenville Hollingsworth Funds Program/Project Grants, 1114
Comm Fndn of Greenville-Greenville Women Giving Grants, 1115
Comm Fndn of Mount Vernon and Knox County Grants, 1119
Comm Fndn of Randolph County Grants, 1121
Comm Fndn of Santa Cruz County Grants, 1122
Comm Fndn of South Alabama Grants, 1123
Comm Fndn of South Puget Sound Grants, 1124
Comm Fndn of Southeastern Connecticut Grants, 1125
Comm Fndn of Switzerland County Grants, 1127
Comm Fndn of Tampa Bay Grants, 1128
Comm Fndn of the Eastern Shore Comm Needs Grants, 1129
Comm Fndn of the Ozarks Grants, 1130
Comm Fndn of Wabash County Grants, 1131
Comm Fndn of Western North Carolina Grants, 1132
Comm Fndn Silicon Valley Grants, 1133
Comm Impact Fund, 1135
Compass Bank Fndn Grants, 1138
ConAgra Foods Fndn Grants, 1140
Connecticut Comm Fndn Grants, 1141
Connelly Fndn Grants, 1143
ConocoPhillips Fndn Grants, 1144
Constantin Fndn Grants, 1145
Consumers Energy Fndn, 1147
Cooke Fndn Grants, 1148
Cooper Industries Fndn Grants, 1150
Cornerstone Fndn of Northeastern Wisconsin Grants, 1152
Cowles Charitable Trust Grants, 1155
Cranston Fndn Grants, 1158
CSRA Comm Fndn Grants, 1168
CSX Corp Contributions Grants, 1169
Cudd Fndn Grants, 1171
CUNA Mutual Group Fndn, 1174
Cyrus Eaton Fndn Grants, 1178
D.V. and Ida J. McEachern Charitable Trust Grants, 1182
Dade Comm Fndn Grants, 1185
DaimlerChrysler Corp Fund Grants, 1186
Dairy Queen Corp Contributions Grants, 1187
Dana Corp Fndn Grants, 1196
David Geffen Fndn Grants, 1202
Davis Family Fndn Grants, 1204
Daywood Fndn Grants, 1206
Deaconess Comm Fndn Grants, 1207
Dearborn Comm Fndn City of Lawrenceburg Comm Grants, 1210
Dearborn Comm Fndn County Progress Grants, 1211
Delaware Comm Fndn Grants, 1215
Dell Fndn Open Grants, 1218
DeMatteis Family Fndn Grants, 1221
Denver Fndn Comm Grants, 1227
DeRoy Testamentary Fndn Grants, 1239
Donald and Sylvia Robinson Family Fndn Grants, 1310
Dorothy Rider Pool Health Care Grants, 1322
Dorrance Family Fndn Grants, 1323
Dr. Leon Bromberg Charitable Trust Fund Grants, 1328
Dubois County Comm Fndn Grants, 1336
Duke Energy Fndn Grants, 1339
E.L. Wiegand Fndn Grants, 1361
Eberly Fndn Grants, 1364
Eddie C. and Sylvia Brown Family Fndn Grants, 1367
EDS Fndn Grants, 1371
Educational Fndn of America Grants, 1372
Edwin W. and Catherine M. Davis Fndn Grants, 1377
Eisner Fndn Grants, 1387
El Paso Comm Fndn Grants, 1388
El Paso Corp Fndn Grants, 1389
El Pomar Fndn Awards and Grants, 1390
Elkhart County Comm Fndn Grants, 1401
Elsie Lee Garthwaite Memorial Fndn Grants, 1408
Emerson Electric Company Contributions Grants, 1413
Ensworth Charitable Fndn Grants, 1416
Entergy Comm Partnership Grants, 1417
Erie Comm Fndn Grants, 1427
Essex County Comm Fndn Discretionary Fund Grant, 1428
Estee Lauder Grants, 1429
Ethel S. Abbott Charitable Fndn Grants, 1430
Eugene and Agnes E. Meyer Fndn Grants, 1432
Eugene M. Lang Fndn Grants, 1434
Evanston Comm Fndn Grants, 1438
ExxonMobil Grants, 1442
F.M. Kirby Fndn Grants, 1443
Fairfield County Comm Fndn Grants, 1446
Fargo-Moorhead Area Fndn Grants, 1454
Farmers Insurance Group of Companies Grants, 1455
Faye McBeath Fndn Grants, 1456
Fayette County Fndn Grants, 1457
Ferree Fndn Grants, 1486
Fidelity Fndn Grants, 1498
Fifth Third Fndn Grants, 1501
Fireman's Fund Fndn Grants, 1504
Fishman Family Fndn Grants, 1510
Foellinger Fndn Grants, 1519
Fondren Fndn Grants, 1520
Ford Motor Company Fund Grants, 1522
Forrest C. Lattner Fndn Grants, 1523
Frances and John L. Loeb Family Fund Grants, 1546
Francis L. Abreu Charitable Trust Grants, 1549
Frank Stanley Beveridge Fndn Grants, 1553
Franklin County Comm Fndn Grants, 1554
Fred Baldwin Memorial Fndn Grants, 1556
Fred L. Emerson Fndn Grants, 1557
Fremont Area Comm Fndn Grants, 1561
Fuji Film Grants, 1565
Fulbright Alumni Initiatives Awards Grants, 1566
Fulbright Distinguished Chairs Grants, 1567
Fulbright New Century Scholars Grants, 1570
Fulbright Specialists Grants, 1571
Fulbright Traditional Scholar Program in Europe and Eurasia, 1572
Fulbright Traditional Scholar Program in Sub-Saharan Africa, 1573
Fulbright Traditional Scholar Program in the East Asia/Pacific Region, 1574
Fulbright Traditional Scholar Program in the Near East and North Africa Region, 1575
Fulbright Traditional Scholar Program in the South and Central Asia Region, 1576
Fulbright Traditional Scholar Program in the Western Hemisphere, 1577
Fulton County Comm Fndn Grants, 1579
Gebbie Fndn Grants, 1585
GenCorp Fndn Grants, 1587
General Mills Fndn Grants, 1590
General Motors Fndn Grants Support Program, 1591
George Frederick Jewett Fndn Grants, 1599
George Kress Fndn Grants, 1601
George S. and Dolores Dore Eccles Fndn Grants, 1602
Gheens Fndn Grants, 1610
Gibson Fndn Grants, 1612
Gill Fndn - Gay and Lesbian Fund Grants, 1613
Gilroy and Lillian P. Roberts Charitable Fndn Grants, 1614
Ginn Fndn Grants, 1616
Giving Sum Annual Grant, 1619
Gladys Brooks Fndn Grants, 1620
Glendale Comm Fndn Grants, 1626
Halliburton Fndn Grants, 1687
Goodrich Corp Fndn Grants, 1638
Grand Haven Area Comm Fndn Grants, 1644
Grand Rapids Area Comm Fndn Grants, 1645
Grand Rapids Area Comm Fndn Nashwauk Area Endowment Fund Grants, 1646
Greater Cincinnati Fndn Priority and Small Projects/Capacity-Building Grants, 1651
Greater Green Bay Comm Fndn Grants, 1652
Greater Milwaukee Fndn Grants, 1653
Greater New Orleans Fndn Grants, 1654
Greater Saint Louis Comm Fndn Grants, 1655
Greater Tacoma Comm Fndn Grants, 1656
Greater Worcester Comm Fndn Jeppson Memorial Fund for Brookfield Grants, 1659

Greene County Fndn Grants, 1662
Griffin Fndn Grants, 1670
Gulf Coast Comm Fndn Grants, 1676
Gulf Coast Comm of Venice Fndn Grants, 1677
H & R Fndn Grants, 1679
H.A. and Mary K. Chapman Charitable Trust Grants, 1681
H.J. Heinz Company Fndn Grants, 1682
Hallmark Corp Fndn Grants, 1688
Hancock County Comm Fndn Grants, 1690
Hannaford Charitable Fndn Grants, 1692
Harden Fndn Grants, 1693
Harley Davidson Fndn Grants, 1694
Harold and Arlene Schnitzer CARE Fndn Grants, 1697
Harold Simmons Fndn Grants, 1698
Harris and Eliza Kempner Fund Grants, 1699
Harrison County Comm Fndn Grants, 1700
Harry Bramhall Gilbert Charitable Trust Grants, 1703
Harry Kramer Memorial Fund Grants, 1705
Hartford Courant Fndn Grants, 1710
Hartford Fndn Regular Grants, 1711
Hawaii Comm Fndn West Hawaii Fund Grants, 1718
Hawn Fndn Grants, 1719
HCA Fndn Grants, 1721
Heckscher Fndn for Children Grants, 1732
Helena Rubinstein Fndn Grants, 1743
Henrietta Tower Wurts Memorial Fndn Grants, 1745
Henry & Ruth Blaustein Rosenberg Fndn Grants, 1746
Herman Goldman Fndn Grants, 1753
Hershey Company Grants, 1754
High Meadow Fndn Grants, 1768
Hill Crest Fndn Grants, 1773
Hillman Fndn Grants, 1775
Hillsdale County Comm General Adult Fndn Grants, 1777
Hillsdale Fund Grants, 1778
Hilton Head Island Fndn Grants, 1779
Hoglund Fndn Grants, 1785
Holland/Zeeland Comm Fndn Grants, 1786
Honda of America Manufacturing Fndn Grants, 1790
Horace A. Kimball and S. Ella Kimball Fndn Grants, 1792
Horizons Comm Issues Grants, 1794
Houston Endowment Grants, 1797
Howard and Bush Fndn Grants, 1798
Howe Fndn of North Carolina Grants, 1799
Hudson Webber Fndn Grants, 1813
Hugh J. Andersen Fndn Grants, 1814
Humana Fndn Grants, 1818
Huntington County Comm Fndn Grants, 1823
Huntington National Bank Comm Affairs Grants, 1824
Hut Fndn Grants, 1827
Hutton Fndn Grants, 1828
Idaho Comm Fndn Eastern Region Competitive Grants, 1837
Idaho Power Company Corp Contributions, 1838
Inasmuch Fndn Grants, 1845
Irvin Stern Fndn Grants, 1866
Irving S. Gilmore Fndn Grants, 1867
J. Walton Bissell Fndn Grants, 1872
J.B. Reynolds Fndn Grants, 1873
J.M. Long Fndn Grants, 1877
Jackson County Comm Fndn Unrestricted Grants, 1879
Jacob and Hilda Blaustein Fndn Grants, 1881
James A. and Faith Knight Fndn Grants, 1884
James Ford Bell Fndn Grants, 1885
James Graham Brown Fndn Grants, 1887
James M. Collins Fndn Grants, 1891
James S. Copley Fndn Grants, 1895
Jane Bradley Pettit Fndn Grants, 1902
Jane's Trust Grants, 1904
Jasper Fndn Jasper County Grants, 1907
Jasper Fndn Newton County Grants, 1908
Jay and Rose Phillips Family Fndn Grants, 1909
Jean and Louis Dreyfus Fndn Grants, 1911
JELD-WEN Fndn Grants, 1914
Jennings County Comm Fndn Grants, 1916
Jessie Ball Dupont Fund Grants, 1919
Jewish Comm Fndn of Greater Los Angeles Grants, 1921
John Ben Snow Memorial Trust Grants, 1928
John Deere Fndn Grants, 1929
John G. Duncan Trust Grants, 1931
John H. and Wilhelmina D. Harland Charitable Fndn Grants, 1933
John I. Smith Charities Grants, 1935
John J. Leidy Fndn Grants, 1936
John Jewett and Helen Chandler Garland Fndn Grants, 1937
John Lord Knight Fndn Grants, 1938
John P. Murphy Fndn Grants, 1943
John W. Alden Trust Grants, 1947
John W. Anderson Fndn Grants, 1949
Johns Manville Fund Grants, 1950
Johnson Controls Fndn Grants, 1954
Joseph Alexander Fndn Grants, 1957
Joseph Drown Fndn Grants, 1960
Josiah W. and Bessie H. Kline Fndn Grants, 1967
Julia Temple Davis Brown Fndn Grants, 1971
Kahuku Comm Fund, 1977
Katharine Matthies Fndn Grants, 1982
Katherine John Murphy Fndn Grants, 1983
Kenneth T. and Eileen L. Norris Fndn Grants, 1989
Kettering Family Fndn Grants, 1991
KeySpan Fndn Grants, 1995
Kosciusko County Comm Fndn Grants, 2015
Kraft Cares US Grants, 2017
Land O'Lakes Fndn Mid-Atlantic Grants, 2027
Legacy Fndn Grants, 2040
Lester E. Yeager Charitable Trust B Grants, 2047
Liberty Bank Fndn Grants, 2053
Lillian S. Wells Fndn Grants, 2056
Lincoln Financial Group Fndn Grants, 2058
Louis Calder Fndn Grants, 2065
Lowe Fndn Grants, 2067
Lowell Berry Fndn Grants, 2069
Lubbock Area Fndn Grants, 2079
Lubrizol Fndn Grants, 2080
Lucile Horton Howe and Mitchell B. Howe Fndn Grants, 2081
Lucy Gooding Charitable Fndn Trust Grants, 2083
Ludwick Family Fndn Grants, 2084
M. Bastian Family Fndn Grants, 2092
M.J. Murdock Charitable Trust Grants, 2095
Madison County Comm Fndn Grants, 2098
Manuel D. and Rhoda Mayerson Fndn Grants, 2100
Marcia and Otto Koehler Fndn Grants, 2103
Margaret T. Morris Fndn Grants, 2105
Mars Fndn Grants, 2114
Marshall Field's Comm Grants, 2115
Mary Owen Borden Fndn Grants, 2121
Mary S. and David C. Corbin Fndn Grants, 2122
Max A. Adler Charitable Fndn Grants, 2132
Max and Victoria Dreyfus Fndn Grants, 2133
May Department Stores Charitable Contribution Grants, 2138
McGregor Fund Grants, 2143
McInerny Fndn Grants, 2144
McKesson Fndn Grants, 2145
McKnight Fndn Grants, 2146
Mead Johnson Nutritionals Evansville-Area Organizations Grants, 2157
Mead Witter Fndn Grants, 2160
Meadows Fndn Grants, 2161
Mericos Fndn Grants, 2172
Meriden Fndn Grants, 2173
Meyer Memorial Trust Emergency Grants, 2178
Meyer Memorial Trust Grassroots Grants, 2179
Meyer Memorial Trust Operating Funds Grants, 2180
Meyer Memorial Trust Responsive Grants, 2181
Miguel Aleman Fndn Grants, 2197
Miriam and Peter Haas Fund Grants, 2208
Monfort Family Fndn Grants, 2213
Morris and Gwendolyn Cafritz Fndn Grants, 2217
National City Corp Contributions Grants, 2250
Nelda C. and H.J. Lutcher Stark Fndn Grants, 2301
New York Life Fndn Grants, 2304
New York University Steinhardt School of Education Fellowships, 2305
Newman's Own Inc Grants, 2306
Nicholas H. Noyes Jr. Memorial Fndn Grants, 2497
Nina Mason Pulliam Charitable Trust Grants, 2776
Noble County Comm Fndn Grants, 2848
Nordson Corp Fndn Grants, 2851
North Carolina Comm Development Grants, 2858
North Carolina Comm Fndn Grants, 2859
North Georgia Comm Fndn Grants, 2862
Northeast Utilities Fndn Grants, 2863
Northern Trust Company Charitable Trust and Corp Giving Program, 2865
Northrop Grumman Newport News Grants, 2867
Northwestern Mutual Fndn Grants, 2870
Northwood University/Alden B. Dow Creativity Center Summer Residency Program, 2871
Norwin S. and Elizabeth N. Bean Fndn Grants, 2872
Oceanside Charitable Fndn Grants, 2934
Oleonda Jameson Trust Grants, 2941
OSI-Baltimore Special Opportunities Grants, 2972
Owen County Comm Fndn Grants, 2979
PacifiCorp Fndn for Learning Grants, 2982
Palm Beach and Martin Counties Grants, 2986
Paul and Mary Haas Fndn Contributions and Student Scholarships, 2997
Paul G. Allen Family Fndn Grants, 3000
Paul G. Duke Fndn Grants, 3001
Peacock Fndn Grants, 3011
Perpetual Trust for Charitable Giving Grants, 3015
Perry County Comm Fndn Grants, 3016
Phoenix Suns Charities Grants, 3030
Piedmont Natural Gas Grants, 3048
Pike County Comm Fndn Grants, 3049
Pinellas County Grants, 3050
Piper Jaffray Companies Building Strong Communities Grants, 3053
Pittsburgh Fndn Comm Fund Grants, 3054
Plough Fndn Grants, 3061
PNC Charitable Trust and Fndn Grants, 3064
Polk Bros. Fndn Grants, 3066
Portland General Electric Fndn Grants, 3067
Posey Comm Fndn Grants, 3068
Posey Comm Fndn Womens Fund Grants, 3069
Powell Fndn Grants, 3073
Priddy Fndn Grants, 3077
Pride Fndn Grants and Scholarships, 3078
Prince Charitable Trusts Chicago Grants, 3079
Prince Charitable Trusts District of Columbia Grants, 3080
Princeton Area Comm Fndn Greater Mercer Grants, 3081
Principal Financial Group Fndn Grants, 3082
Puerto Rico Comm Fndn Grants, 3090
Pulaski County Comm Fndn Grants, 3091
Putnam County Comm Fndn Grants, 3093
Rajiv Gandhi Fndn Grants, 3104
Ralphs Food 4 Less Fndn Grants, 3106
Rasmuson Fndn Grants, 3108
Rathmann Family Fndn Grants, 3109
Rhode Island Fndn Grants, 3154
Richard and Helen DeVos Fndn Grants, 3157
Richard and Susan Smith Family Fndn Grants, 3159
Ripley County Comm Fndn Grants, 3166
Robert B McMillen Fndn Grants, 3169
Robert F. Stoico / FIRSTFED Charitable Fndn Grants, 3171
Rochester Area Comm Fndn Grants, 3176
Rochester Area Fndn Grants, 3177
Rockwell International Corp Trust Grants, 3183
Rohm and Haas Company Grants, 3185
Rollin M. Gerstacker Fndn Grants, 3186
Roy and Christine Sturgis Trust Grants, 3191
Rush County Comm Fndn Grants, 3200
Ruth H. and Warren A. Ellsworth Fndn Grants, 3203
S. Livingston Mather Charitable Trust Grants, 3235
S. Mark Taper Fndn Grants, 3236
Salem Fndn Charitable Trust Grants, 3241
Salem Fndn Grants, 3242

Salisbury Comm Fndn Grants, 3243
Samuel S. Johnson Fndn Grants, 3251
San Antonio Area Fndn Grants, 3254
Sasco Fndn Grants, 3265
Schering-Plough Fndn Comm Initiatives Grants, 3269
Schurz Communications Fndn Grants, 3271
Scott County Comm Fndn Grants, 3273
Seabury Fndn Grants, 3274
Seattle Fndn Grants, 3276
Self Fndn Grants, 3277
Simmons Fndn Grants, 3287
Simpson Fund Grants, 3290
Society for the Arts in Healthcare Environmental Arts Research Grant, 3327
Sonoco Fndn Grants, 3347
Sosland Fndn Grants, 3348
South Madison Comm Fndn Grants, 3349
Southbury Comm Trust Fund, 3350
Southwest Florida Comm Fndn Competitive Grants, 3351
Southwest Gas Corp Fndn Grants, 3352
Spencer County Comm Fndn Grants, 3358
Square D Fndn Grants, 3361
Stark Comm Fndn Women's Fund Grants, 3376
Steuben County Comm Fndn Grants, 3383
Strowd Roses Grants, 3388
Sulzberger Fndn Grants, 3399
Sunderland Fndn Grants, 3400
Susan Mott Webb Charitable Trust Grants, 3412
Susan Vaughan Fndn Grants, 3413
Thomas C. Ackerman Fndn Grants, 3423
Toro Fndn Grants, 3431
Triangle Comm Fndn Donor-Advised Grants, 3437
Trull Fndn Grants, 3441
Union Benevolent Association Grants, 3460
United Technologies Corp Grants, 3466
Unity Fndn Of LaPorte County Grants, 3467
US Airways Comm Contributions, 3472
US Airways Comm Fndn Grants, 3473
Vancouver Fndn Grants and Comm Initiatives Program, 3477
Vanderburgh Comm Fndn Grants, 3480
Vectren Fndn Grants, 3485
Vermont Comm Fndn Grants, 3493
Virginia W. Kettering Fndn Grants, 3502
Vulcan Materials Company Fndn Grants, 3504
W. C. Griffith Fndn Grants, 3505
W. Clarke Swanson, Jr. Fndn Grants, 3506
Wabash Valley Comm Fndn Grants, 3510
Wachovia Fndn Grants, 3511
Walt Disney Company Fndn Grants, 3516
Warrick County Comm Fndn Grants, 3519
Washington Post Contributions Grants, 3520
Weingart Fndn Grants, 3524
Wells County Fndn Grants, 3527
William G. Gilmore Fndn Grants, 3537
Winston-Salem Fndn Competitive Grants, 3544
Winston-Salem Fndn Stokes County Grants, 3546
YSA Get Ur Good On Grants, 3555

Asia
ASM-UNESCO Leadership Grant for International Educators, 626
Fulbright Traditional Scholar Program in the East Asia/Pacific Region, 1574
Margoes Fndn Grants, 2106
Max Bell Fndn Grants, 2134

Asia, East (Far East)
Fulbright Traditional Scholar Program in the East Asia/Pacific Region, 1574

Asia, Southeast
Fulbright Traditional Scholar Program in the East Asia/Pacific Region, 1574

Asian Americans
American Sociological Association Minority Fellowships, 458
Grotto Fndn Project Grants, 1671
John R. Oishei Fndn Grants, 1944
NIA Prostate Cancer Aging, Race, and Ethnicity Research Grants, 2428
NIMH Career Opportunities in Research Education and Training Honors High School Research Education Grant, 2748
NIMH Career Opportunities in Research Education and Training Honors Undergraduate Research Training Grant, 2749
Philadelphia Fndn Organizational Effectiveness Grants, 3029
SNM PDEF Mickey Williams Minority Student Scholarships, 3302

Asian Arts
E. Rhodes and Leona B. Carpenter Fndn Grants, 1356

Assisted-Living Programs
California Endowment CommunitiesFirst Grants, 833
Jenkins Fndn: Improving the Health of Greater Richmond Grants, 1915
Sheltering Arms Fund Grants, 3282

Assistive Technology
U.S. Department of Education Rehabilitation Engineering Research Centers Grants, 3447

Asthma
AAAAI Allergy, Asthma and Immunology Education and Research Trust Clinical Research Grants, 22
AAAAI Summer Clinical Research Fellowship Medical Student Grants, 27
AAAAI Summer Research Fellowship Medical Student Grants, 28
AAFA Investigator Research Grants, 108
ACAAI Fndn Research Grants, 189
CF Clinical Research Trainee Awards, 940
Fairlawn Fndn Grants, 1447
NHLBI Airway Smooth Muscle Function and Targeted Therapeutics in Human Asthma Grants, 2316
NHLBI Clinical Centers for the NHLBI Asthma Network (AsthmaNet) Grants, 2331
NIH Hyperaccelerated Award/Mechanisms in Immunomodulation Trials, 2675
NIOSH Occupational Safety and Health Research and Demonstration Grants, 2807
Quantum Fndn Grants, 3096
RACGP National Asthma Council Research Award, 3100
Sandler Program for Asthma Research Grants, 3262
Sunshine Natural Wellbeing Fndn Grants, 3404
Take Care to Learn: Teaching Clinical Care Management Grants, 3415
Wellmark Fndn Grants, 3526

Astronomy
Alfred P. Sloan Fndn History of Science and Technology Grants, 352
Canada Graduate Scholarships and NSERC Postgraduate Scholarships, 845
Roy J. Carver Charitable Trust Medical and Science Research Grants, 3192

Astrophysics
Brinson Fndn Grants, 794

At-Risk Youth
Acushnet Fndn Grants, 226
Alliance Healthcare Fndn Grants, 362
AT&T Excelerator, 657
Boston Fndn Grants, 783
Charles Lafitte Fndn Grants, 970
CIT Corp Giving Grants, 1014
Citizens Bank Mid-Atlantic Charitable Fndn Grants, 1015
CMA Fndn Grants, 1042
Columbus Fndn Traditional Grants, 1071
Commonweal Fndn Comm Assistance Grants, 1075
Comm Fndn of Greater Greensboro Grants, 1109
Cruise Industry Charitable Fndn Grants, 1166
Dallas Women's Fndn Grants, 1191
Denver Broncos Charities Fund Grants, 1226
DHHS Maternal and Child Health Projects Grants, 1263
Educational Fndn of America Grants, 1372
EPA Children's Health Protection Grants, 1420
Express Scripts Fndn Grants, 1441
Global Fund for Children Grants, 1629
Greater Tacoma Comm Fndn Ryan Alan Hade Endowment Fund, 1657
Hanna Andersson Children's Fndn Grants, 1691
Hasbro Children's Fund, 1714
Health Fndn of Greater Cincinnati Grants, 1724
Jim Moran Fndn Grants, 1925
John Edward Fowler Memorial Fndn Grants, 1930
Kraft Cares International Grants, 2016
Lillian S. Wells Fndn Grants, 2056
Louis R. Cappelli Fndn Grants, 2066
Mary Owen Borden Fndn Grants, 2121
Mattel Children's Fndn Grants, 2130
Mattel International Grants, 2131
McKesson Fndn Grants, 2145
Milagro Fndn Grants, 2198
MONY Fndn Grants, 2215
New York Life Fndn Grants, 2304
PacifiCorp Fndn for Learning Grants, 2982
Paul G. Allen Family Fndn Grants, 3000
Peter and Elizabeth C. Tower Fndn Comm Grants, 3018
PeyBack Fndn Grants, 3022
Plum Creek Fndn Grants, 3062
Raymond John Wean Fndn Grants, 3110
Robins Fndn Grants, 3175
RWJF Local Funding Partnerships Grants, 3223
Southwire Company Grants, 3353
Stewart Huston Charitable Trust Grants, 3384
Topfer Family Fndn Grants, 3430
W.K. Kellogg Fndn Healthy Kids Grants, 3507
Z. Smith Reynolds Fndn Small Grants, 3557

Attention Deficit Disorder
AACAP Elaine Schlosser Lewis Award for Research on Attention-Deficit Disorder, 35
AACAP Pilot Research Award for Attention-Deficit Disorder, Supported by the Elaine Schlosser Lewis Fund, 45
EF Behavioral Sciences Student Fellowships, 1379
NIH Genetics of Neurobehavioral Disorders in Existing Samples Grants, 2670

Audience Development
Air Products and Chemicals Grants, 319
Connecticut Comm Fndn Grants, 1141
Kraft Cares US Grants, 2017
McKesson Fndn Grants, 2145
Meyer Memorial Trust Emergency Grants, 2178
Meyer Memorial Trust Grassroots Grants, 2179
Meyer Memorial Trust Responsive Grants, 2181

Audiology
ASHA Multicultural Activities Projects Grants, 571
ASHA Students Preparing for Academic & Research Careers Award, 574
ASHFndn Graduate Student International Scholarship, 576
ASHFndn Graduate Student Scholarships for Minority Students, 578
ASHFndn Graduate Student with a Disability Scholarship, 579
ASHFndn New Century Scholars Program Doctoral Scholarships, 580
ASHFndn New Century Scholars Research Grant, 581
ASHFndn Research Grant for New Investigators, 582
ASHFndn Student Research Grants in Audiology, 584
DHHS National Health Service Corps Scholarships Program, 1266
Special Olympics Health Professions Student Grants, 3355

Audiovisual Materials
Vermont Comm Fndn Grants, 3493

Australia
American College of Surgeons Australia and New Zealand Chapter Travelling Fellowships, 423

Autism
CAN Autism Treatment-Related Study Awards, 842
CAN Pilot Research Projects, 843
CAN Young Investigator Awards, 844
FAR Fund, 1453
Horizon Fndn for New Jersey Grants, 1793
Ireland Family Fndn Grants, 1865
NIDCD Neurobiology and Genetics of Autism Grants, 2526
NIH Autism and Autism Spectrum Disorders Research, 2637
NWHF Mark O. Hatfield Research Fellowship, 2907
Partnership for Cures Two Years To Cures Grants, 2992
Smith Family New Investigator Awards, 3299
Thompson Charitable Fndn Grants, 3425

Autoimmunity
Glaucoma Research Pilot Project Grants, 1622
NIAMS High Risk Arthritis and Musculoskeletal and Skin Diseases Research, 2470
NIAMS Skin Diseases Research Core Centers Grants, 2478
NIH Hyperaccelerated Award/Mechanisms in Immunomodulation Trials, 2675
NIH Role of Microglia in Normal and Abnormal Immune Responses of the Nervous System, 2716

Automotive Engineering
ArvinMeritor Grants, 544

Aviation
Lindbergh Grants, 2059

Back Pain
FCER Research Grants and Fellowships, 1460
NIAMS Low-Back Pain and Common Spinal Disorders Research Grants, 2471
NICHD Low-Back Pain and Common Spinal Disorders Research Grants, 2486
NINDS Low-Back Pain and Common Spinal Disorders Research Grants, 2779

Bacteriology
Ethical Research Grants and Fellowships, 1431
NIAID Microbiology and Infectious Diseases Research Grants and Contracts, 2459
NIAID Preparedness against Illegitimate Use of Bacterial Pathogens, 2461

Bangladesh
Fulbright Traditional Scholar Program in the South and Central Asia Region, 1576

Baptist Church
Booth-Bricker Fund Grants, 780
Bosque Fndn Grants, 782
Bradley Turner Fndn Grants, 789
Effie and Wofford Cain Fndn Grants, 1385

Basic Living Expenses
SAG Motion Picture Players Welfare Grants, 3238

Basic Research
Auburn Fndn Grants, 664
Drs. Bruce and Lee Fndn Grants, 1333

Basic Science
AMSSM Fndn Research Grants, 469

Basic Skills Education
Ahmanson Fndn Grants, 303
Allen P. and Josephine B. Green Fndn Grants, 361
Allyn Fndn Grants, 365
Arkell Hall Fndn Grants, 534
Atlanta Fndn Grants, 662
Auburn Fndn Grants, 664
Ball Brothers Fndn Grants, 684
Baptist Comm Ministries Grants, 691
Battle Creek Comm Fndn Grants, 703
Benton Comm Fndn Grants, 743
Berrien Comm Fndn Grants, 749
Blackford County Comm Fndn Grants, 763
Blue Mountain Comm Fndn Grants, 769
Blue River Comm Fndn Grants, 770
Bodenwein Public Benevolent Fndn Grants, 775
Boettcher Fndn Grants, 778
Booth-Bricker Fund Grants, 780
Boston Fndn Grants, 783
Brown County Comm Fndn Grants, 807
Carl and Lily Pforzheimer Fndn Grants, 868
Carl B. and Florence E. King Fndn Grants, 869
Cemala Fndn Grants, 933
Chicago Board of Trade Fndn Grants, 988
CIGNA Fndn Grants, 1011
Colorado Springs Comm Trust Fund Grants, 1061
Comm Fndn of Bartholomew County Heritage Fund Grants, 1096
Comm Fndn of Bartholomew County James A. Henderson Award for Fund-Raising, 1097
Comm Fndn of Boone County Grants, 1099
Comm Fndn of Central Illinois Grants, 1101
Comm Fndn of Greater Fort Wayne: Comm Endowment & Clarke Endowment Fund Grants, 1108
Cornerstone Fndn of Northeastern Wisconsin Grants, 1152
Cowles Charitable Trust Grants, 1155
Cruise Industry Charitable Fndn Grants, 1166
Dayton Power and Light Fndn Grants, 1205
Evjue Fndn Grants, 1439
Field Fndn of Illinois Grants, 1499
Frances L. and Edwin L. Cummings Memorial Fund Grants, 1547
G.N. Wilcox Trust Grants, 1581
Hallmark Corp Fndn Grants, 1688
Harold Simmons Fndn Grants, 1698
Helen Steiner Rice Fndn Grants, 1742
Howard and Bush Fndn Grants, 1798
John H. and Wilhelmina D. Harland Charitable Fndn Grants, 1933
John I. Smith Charities Grants, 1935
Johnson Controls Fndn Grants, 1954
Joseph H. and Florence A. Roblee Fndn Grants, 1961
Lubrizol Fndn Grants, 2080
Paul and Mary Haas Fndn Contributions and Student Scholarships, 2997
Principal Financial Group Fndn Grants, 3082
Richard and Rhoda Goldman Fund Grants, 3158
San Antonio Area Fndn Grants, 3254
U.S. Department of Education Rehabilitation Training—Rehabilitation Continuing Education Programs—Institute on Rehabilitation Issues, 3449
Wilson-Wood Fndn Grants, 3542

Behavioral Medicine
Allen P. and Josephine B. Green Fndn Grants, 361
CDC Technology Translation and Transfer of Effective HIV Behavioral Interventions, 931
International Cancer Technology Transfer Fellowships, 1858
James S. McDonnell Fndn Research Grants, 1898
James S. McDonnell Fndn Scholar Awards, 1899
NCI Stages of Breast Development: Normal to Metastatic Disease Grants, 2278
NCIC Canadian Cancer Society Research Grants, 2282
NEI Ruth L. Kirschstein National Research Service Award Short-Term Institutional Research Training Grants, 2297
NIA AIDS and Aging: Behavioral Sciences Prevention Research Grants, 2394
NIAID HIV Prevention Trial Units Grants, 2453
NICHD Central Nervous System Effects of HIV Infection: Neurobiological, Neurovirological, and Neurobehavioral Studies Grants, 2482
NIDA Behavioral Science Track Awards for Rapid Transition, 2498
NIDA Minority Institutions Drug Abuse Research Development Program (MIDARP) Grants, 2509
NIDA National Drug Abuse Treatment Clinical Trials Network, 2510
NIDCD Neurobiology and Genetics of Autism Grants, 2526
NIDCR HIV/AIDS Associated Oral Viral Infections, 2535
NIDDK Race/Ethnic Disparities in the Incidence of Diabetes Complications, 2579
NIEHS Biological Response to Environmental Health Hazards Research Grants, 2596
NIH Alzheimer's Disease Clinical Trial Planning Grant, 2636
NIH Genetics of Neurobehavioral Disorders in Existing Samples Grants, 2670
NIH NRSAs for Individual Predoctoral Fellowships, 2700
NIH Pathological Gambling: Basic, Clinical, and Services Research Grants, 2702
NIH Research on Sleep and Sleep Disorders, 2713
NIH Ruth L. Kirschstein National Research Service Awards for Individual Postdoctoral Fellows, 2719
NIMH AIDS and Aging: Behavioral Sciences Prevention Research Grants, 2745
NIMH Behavior Genetics in Adulthood and Old Age Research Grants, 2747
NIMH Central Nervous System Effects of HIV Infection: Neurobiological, Neurovirological, and Neurobehavioral Studies Grants, 2751
NIMH Minority Research Infrastructure Support Grants, 2763
NIMH Quantitative Approaches to the Analysis of Complex Biological Systems, 2767
NINDS Central Nervous System Effects of HIV Infection: Neurobiological, Neurovirological, and Neurobehavioral Studies Grants, 2777
NINR Aging Women and Breast Cancer Grants, 2789
NINR AIDS and Aging: Behavioral Sciences Prevention Research Grants, 2790
Premera CARES Grants, 3074

Behavioral Sciences
ACS Research Scholar Grants in Psychosocial and Behavioral and Cancer Control Research, 224
Alzheimer's Association Investigator-Initiated Research Grants, 378
APA Congressional Fellowships, 492
Arizona Diamondbacks Charities Grants, 530
CCFF Fellowships, 893
CCFF Studentships, 897
CCFF Summer Studentship, 898
CDC Injury Control Research Centers Grants, 913
Duke University Postdoctoral Research Fellowships in Aging, 1348
EF Behavioral Sciences Student Fellowships, 1379
FIC International Research Fellowship Program, 1490
FIC International Research Scientist Development Award, 1491
FIC Israeli Ministry of Health Postdoctoral Research Fellowships, 1494
FIC Swedish Medical Research Council Fellowships, 1495
FIC/ORMH Minority International Research Training Grants, 1497
Fyssen Fndn Postdoctoral Study Grants, 1580
Health Fndn of Greater Cincinnati Grants, 1724
James S. McDonnell Fndn Scholar Awards, 1899
James S. McDonnell Fndn Understanding Human Cognition Awards, 1900
NCI Exploratory Grants for Behavioral Research in Cancer Control, 2274
NCI Ruth L. Kirschstein National Research Service Award Institutional Research Training Grants, 2277

NCI/NIDA Transdisciplinary Tobacco Use Research Centers Grants, 2280
NHLBI Short-Term Research Education Program to Increase Diversity in Health-Related Research, 2383
NHLBI Translating Basic Behavioral and Social Science Discoveries into Interventions to Reduce Obesity: Centers for Behavioral Intervention Development Grants, 2390
NIA Alzheimer's Disease Core Centers Grants, 2395
NIA Archiving and Development of Socialbehavioral Datasets in Aging Related Studies Grants, 2399
NIAMS High Risk Arthritis and Musculoskeletal and Skin Diseases Research, 2470
NICHD NRSAs—Institutional, 2489
NICHD Population Research Grants, 2490
NIDA Behavioral Therapies Development Grants, 2499
NIDA Microarray-Based Research on Drug Abuse, 2508
NIDA Neurobiological and Behavioral Research on Nicotine and Tobacco Products, 2511
NIDDK Planning Grants For Translational Research For The Prevention And Control Of Diabetes And Obesity, 2577
NIGMS Minority Access to Research Careers Ancillary Training Activities Grants, 2619
NIGMS Minority Access to Research Careers Program, 2620
NIGMS Ruth L. Kirschstein National Research Service Awards for Individual Predoctoral Fellows in PharmD/PhD Grants, 2627
NIH Biobehavioral Research for Effective Sleep, 2639
NIH Career Development Awards: Child Abuse and Neglect Research, 2646
NIH Enhancing Adherence to Diabetes Self-Management Behaviors, 2659
NIH Exploratory/Developmental Research Grant, 2666
NIH Mentored Research Scientist Development Awards, 2689
NIH Mouse Mutagenesis and Phenotyping: Nervous System and Behavior Research Grants, 2693
NIH NRSAs Predoctoral Fellowship Awards for Students with Disabilities, 2701
NIH Predoctoral Fellowship Awards for Minority Students, 2703
NIH Supplements to Promote Reentry into Biomedical and Behavioral Research Careers, 2733
NIH Transitional Career Development Award in Women's Health Research, 2736
NIMH Career Opportunities in Research Education and Training Honors High School Research Education Grant, 2748
NIMH Interdisciplinary Behavioral Science Centers for Mental Health, 2759
NIMH Short Courses in Neuroinformatics, 2769
NSF Alan T. Waterman Award, 2874
NSF Behavioral Neurosciences Research Grants, 2876
NSF Doctoral Dissertation Improvement Grants in the Directorate for Biological Sciences, 2884
OBSSR Behavioral and Social Science Research on Understanding and Reducing Health Disparities Grants, 2932
Simone and Cino del Duca Grand Prix Awards, 3288
Whitehall Fndn Neurobiology Research Grants, 3533

Behavioral/Experimental Psychology
NIA Behavioral and Social Research Grants on Disasters and Health, 2401

Behavioral/Social Sciences
Mark and Catherine Winkler Fndn Grants, 2112

Beverages, Alcoholic
Adolph Coors Fndn Grants, 238
Alcohol Misuse and Alcoholism Research Grants, 335
NIH Mechanisms Underlying Individual Variations in Drug Responses, 2685
Society of Medical Friends of Wine Research Award, 3344

Beverages, Non-alcoholic
Adolph Coors Fndn Grants, 238

Bioassay
NIEHS Applied Toxicological Research and Testing Grants, 2595
NIH/EPA Mechanistic-Based Cancer Risk Assessment Methods Research Grants, 2741

Biochemical Engineering
NSF Chemical, Biochemical, and Biotechnology Systems Research Grants, 2882

Biochemistry
AHAF National Glaucoma Research Grants, 268
Alfred Bader Award in BioInorganic or BioOrganic Chemistry, 350
Barth Syndrome Fndn Research Grants, 700
Beckman Scholars Grants, 734
Deafness Research Fndn Research Grants, 1208
DOE Medical Applications and Measurement Science Grants, 1301
EF Predoctoral Research Training Fellowship, 1383
Greater Milwaukee Fndn Grants, 1653
Helen Hay Whitney Fndn Postdoctoral Research Fellowships, 1739
Implant Dentistry Research and Education Fndn Grants, 1844
Lalor Fndn Postdoctoral Research Grants, 2021
LRF New Investigator Leukemia Research Grants, 2070
Mayo Fndn Multidisciplinary Training in Digestive Diseases Research Grants, 2140
Millipore Fndn Grants, 2203
NIA Research Grants on Chemical Senses: Neurotransmitters and Neuromodulators, 2430
NIAAA Mechanisms of Alcohol-Induced Hepatic Fibrosis Research Grants, 2445
NIAMS Skin Diseases Research Core Centers Grants, 2478
NIDCD Research Grants on Chemical Senses: Neurotransmitters and Neuromodulators, 2530
NIDCR HIV/AIDS Associated Oral Viral Infections, 2535
NIEHS Biological Response to Environmental Health Hazards Research Grants, 2596
NIEHS Structure-Function Relationships of Environmentally Relevant Genetic Variants Research Grants, 2606
NIGMS Fellowships in Quantitative Biology, 2610
NIGMS Molecular Pharmacology of Anesthetic Action Research Grants, 2621
NIGMS Quantitative Approaches to the Analysis of Complex Biological Systems, 2626
NIH Molecular Epidemiology of Prostate Carcinogenesis Grants, 2691
NIH Multidisciplinary Approach for Research on Oral Complications of HIV Infection, 2694
NIH Ruth L. Kirschstein National Research Service Awards for Individual Postdoctoral Fellows, 2719
NIMH Quantitative Approaches to the Analysis of Complex Biological Systems, 2767
NSF Biomolecular Systems Cluster Grants, 2880
NSF Chemistry Research Experiences for Undergraduates, 2883
NSF Genes and Genome Systems Cluster Grants, 2886
NSF-NIST Interaction in Chemistry, Materials Research, Molecular Biosciences, Bioengineering, and Chemical Engineering, 2897
Pittsburgh Fndn Medical Research Grants, 3055
Ralph F. Hirschmann Award in Peptide Chemistry, 3105
Rett Syndrome Research Fndn Grants, 3151
Searle Scholars Grants, 3275
Sigrid Juselius Fndn Grants, 3286
Supelco AOCS Research Award, 3405
TSA Research Grant Awards, 3442

Biochemistry, Lipids
Stephen S. Chang Award, 3382

Biodiversity
FIC International Cooperative Biodiversity Groups Grants, 1487
James S. McDonnell Fndn Complex Systems Collaborative Activity Awards, 1897
NIH Ecology of Infectious Diseases, 2656
Rohm and Haas Company Grants, 3185

Bioenergetics
NIA Bioenergetics, Fatigability, and Activity Limitations in Aging, 2402

Bioengineering
Food, Pharmaceutical, and Bioengineering Division Award in Chemical Engineering, 1521
GPP Charles E. Culpeper Fndn Biomedical Pilot Projects Initiative Grants, 1641
H.R. Lissner Award, 1683
NHGRI Mentored Research Scientist Development Award, 2315
NHLBI Bioengineering and Obesity Grants, 2318
NHLBI Bioengineering Approaches to Energy Balance and Obesity Grants for SBIR, 2319
NHLBI Bioengineering Approaches to Energy Balance and Obesity Grants for STTR, 2320
NHLBI Individual Postdoctoral National Research Service Awards, 2340
NIA Human Biospecimen Resources for Aging Research Grants, 2411
NIAID Challenge Grants: Joint Ventures in Biomedicine and Biotechnology, 2451
NIAMS High Risk Arthritis and Musculoskeletal and Skin Diseases Research, 2470
NIDA Microarray-Based Research on Drug Abuse, 2508
NIH Bioengineering Nanotechnology Initiative, 2640
NSF Emerging Frontiers in Research and Innovation Grants, 2885
United Cerebral Palsy Research Grants, 3462

Bioethics
NIH Clinical Bioethics Postdoctoral Fellowships, 2649
NIH Clinical Bioethics Predoctoral Fellowships, 2650

Biofeedback
NIH Exploratory Centers for Alternative Medicine Research Grants, 2663

Bioinformatics
NLM Limited Competition for Continuation of Biomedical Informatics/Bioinformatics Resource Grants, 2821

Biological Markers
NCI/NIDA Transdisciplinary Tobacco Use Research Centers Grants, 2280
NIDCD Mentored Research Scientist Development Award, 2523
NIDCD Neurobiology and Genetics of Autism Grants, 2526
NIH Human Models and Markers of Skeletal Aging Grants, 2674
NIH Hyperaccelerated Award/Mechanisms in Immunomodulation Trials, 2675
NIH Molecular Epidemiology of Prostate Carcinogenesis Grants, 2691
NIH Nonhuman Primate Immune Tolerance Cooperative Study Group Grants, 2699
NIH Rett Syndrome: Genetics, Pathophysiology, and Biomarkers Research Grants, 2715
NIOSH Occupational Safety and Health Research and Demonstration Grants, 2807
Orentreich Fndn for the Advancement of Science Grants, 2959

Biological Response Modifiers
Cancer Treatment Research Fndn Clinical Investigation Grants, 861

Biological Sciences

AAAS Science & Technology Policy Fellowships - National Defense & Global Security, 29
Beckman Scholars Grants, 734
Brookdale Fndn Leadership in Aging Fellowships, 805
DOE Environmental Remediation Grants, 1297
Ellison Medical Fndn/AFAR Postdoctoral Fellows in Aging Research Program, 1404
EMBO Installation Grants, 1409
Eppendorf & Science Prize for Neurobiology, 1424
Eppley Fndn Postdoctoral Grants, 1425
Flinn Fndn Grants Programs, 1511
Fndn for Medical Research Grants, 1528
Fyssen Fndn Postdoctoral Study Grants, 1580
HHMI Grants and Fellowships Programs, 1759
HRB Postdoctoral Research Fellowships, 1802
James Ford Bell Fndn Grants, 1885
John Stauffer Charitable Trust Grants, 1946
Minority Doctoral Fellowships in Science and Engineering, 2207
NCI Application of Metabolomics for Translational and Biological Research Grants, 2270
NIDA Minority Institutions Drug Abuse Research Development Program (MIDARP) Grants, 2509
NIDCD Neurobiology and Genetics of Autism Grants, 2526
NLM Manufacturing Processes of Medical, Dental, and Biological Technologies Grants, 2822
NSF Alan T. Waterman Award, 2874
NSF BIO Minority Postdoctoral Research Fellowships, 2877
NSF Doctoral Dissertation Improvement Grants in the Directorate for Biological Sciences, 2884
NSF Instrument Development for Biological Research, 2888
NSF Postdoctoral Research Fellowships in Biology, 2891
NSF Undergraduate Research and Mentoring in the Biological Sciences, 2896
PhRMA Fndn Informatics Sabbatical Fellowships, 3035
PhRMA Fndn Informatics Research Starter Grants, 3038
Richard King Mellon Fndn Grants, 3161
Searle Scholars Grants, 3275
SOBP Ziskind-Somerfeld Research Awards, 3316
Society of Cosmetic Chemists Allan B. Black Award Sponsored by Presperse, 3328
Society of Cosmetic Chemists Award Sponsored by McIntyre Group, Ltd., 3329
Society of Cosmetic Chemists Award Sponsored by The HallStar Company, 3330
Society of Cosmetic Chemists Chapter Best Speaker Award, 3331
Society of Cosmetic Chemists Chapter Merit Award, 3332
Society of Cosmetic Chemists Frontier of Science Award, 3333
Society of Cosmetic Chemists Hans Schaeffer Award, 3334
Society of Cosmetic Chemists Joseph P. Ciaudelli Award, 3335
Society of Cosmetic Chemists Keynote Award Lecture Sponsored by Ruger Chemical Corp, 3336
Society of Cosmetic Chemists Literature Award, 3337
Society of Cosmetic Chemists Maison G. de Navarre Medal, 3338
Society of Cosmetic Chemists Merit Award, 3339
Society of Cosmetic Chemists Robert A. Kramer Lifetime Service Award, 3340
Society of Cosmetic Chemists Shaw Mudge Award, 3341
Society of Cosmetic Chemists Student Poster Awards, 3342
Society of Cosmetic Chemists Young Scientist Awards, 3343

Biology

Alfred P. Sloan Fndn Research Fellowships, 353
American Fndn for Suicide Prevention Grants, 436
Award in Separations Science and Technology, 677
BWF Ad Hoc Grants, 818
BWF Investigators in the Pathogenesis of Infectious Disease, 823
Canada Graduate Scholarships and NSERC Postgraduate Scholarships, 845
Canada-U.S. Fulbright New Century Scholars Grants, 846
Canada-U.S. Fulbright Senior Specialists Grants, 847
CFF Postdoctoral Research Fellowships, 946
Collins Fndn Grants, 1058
DOE Health Effects and Life Sciences Research Grants, 1298
DOE Low Dose Radiation Research Program, 1300
Dr. Sydney Segal Research Grants, 1331
Eppendorf & Science Prize for Neurobiology, 1424
FDHN Funderburg Research Scholar Award in Gastric Biology Related to Cancer, 1471
Fulbright Alumni Initiatives Awards Grants, 1566
Fulbright Distinguished Chairs Grants, 1567
Fulbright New Century Scholars Grants, 1570
Fulbright Specialists Grants, 1571
Fulbright Traditional Scholar Program in Europe and Eurasia, 1572
Fulbright Traditional Scholar Program in Sub-Saharan Africa, 1573
Fulbright Traditional Scholar Program in the East Asia/Pacific Region, 1574
Fulbright Traditional Scholar Program in the Near East and North Africa Region, 1575
Fulbright Traditional Scholar Program in the South and Central Asia Region, 1576
Fulbright Traditional Scholar Program in the Western Hemisphere, 1577
HHMI Grants and Fellowships Programs, 1759
Human Growth Fndn Small Grants, 1816
Implant Dentistry Research and Education Fndn Grants, 1844
Jackson Laboratory Postdoctoral Research Training Program, 1880
James S. McDonnell Fndn Complex Systems Collaborative Activity Awards, 1897
Marion I. and Henry J. Knott Fndn Grants, 2109
NCI Stages of Breast Development: Normal to Metastatic Disease Grants, 2278
NHGRI Mentored Research Scientist Development Award, 2315
NHLBI Progenitor Cell Biology Consortium Administrative Coordinating Center Grants, 2367
NHLBI Progenitor Cell Biology Consortium Research Hubs, 2368
NIA Awards to Support Research on the Biology of Aging in Invertebrates Grants, 2400
NIA Nathan Shock Centers of Excellence in Basic Biology of Aging Grants, 2421
NIDA Microarray-Based Research on Drug Abuse, 2508
NIDDK Developmental Biology and Regeneration of the Liver Grants, 2550
NIGMS Fellowships in Quantitative Biology, 2610
NIGMS Integrative and Collaborative Approaches to Research Grants, 2615
NIGMS Predoctoral Training in Bioinformatics and Computation Biology Grants, 2625
NIGMS Quantitative Approaches to the Analysis of Complex Biological Systems, 2626
NIGMS Supplements for the Study of Complex Biological Systems, 2630
NIH Career Development Awards: Child Abuse and Neglect Research, 2646
NIH Ecology of Infectious Diseases, 2656
NIH Enhancing Adherence to Diabetes Self-Management Behaviors, 2659
NIH Midcareer Investigator Award in Mouse Pathobiology Research Grants, 2690
NIMH Quantitative Approaches to the Analysis of Complex Biological Systems, 2767
NINR Aging Women and Breast Cancer Grants, 2789
North Carolina GlaxoSmithKline Fndn Grants, 2860
NSF Biological Physics (BP), 2878
NSF Postdoctoral Research Fellowships in Biology, 2891
SOBP Ziskind-Somerfeld Research Awards, 3316
US CRDF Leishmaniasis: Collaborative Research Opportunities in North Africa and the Middle East, 3474

Biology Education

Amgen Fndn Grants, 467
NSF Undergraduate Research and Mentoring in the Biological Sciences, 2896

Biology, Behavioral

NIH Ruth L. Kirschstein National Research Service Awards for Individual Predoctoral Fellows, 2720

Biology, Cellular

AAAAI Summer Clinical Research Fellowship Medical Student Grants, 27
AAAAI Summer Research Fellowship Medical Student Grants, 28
AFAR Research Grants, 257
AHAF National Glaucoma Research Grants, 268
Cancer Research UK Fellowships, 858
CFF Postdoctoral Research Fellowships, 946
CFF Research Grants, 947
Eppendorf & Science Prize for Neurobiology, 1424
FDHN Fellowship to Faculty Transition Awards, 1470
Glaucoma Research Pilot Project Grants, 1622
Helen Hay Whitney Fndn Postdoctoral Research Fellowships, 1739
Hereditary Disease Fndn John J. Wasmuth Postdoctoral Fellowships, 1750
Hereditary Disease Fndn Lieberman Award, 1751
Hereditary Disease Fndn Research Grants, 1752
Hunter's Hope Fndn Grants, 1820
IARC Expertise Transfer Fellowship, 1831
IARC Postdoctoral Fellowships for Training in Cancer Research, 1832
IARC Visiting Scientist Award for Senior Scientists, 1833
LSA Scholar Awards, 2075
LSA Translational Research Grants, 2078
Marine Biological Laboratory Summer Research Fellowships, 2108
Mayo Fndn Multidisciplinary Training in Digestive Diseases Research Grants, 2140
MDBD Basic Research Grants, 2152
Milton Wexler Postdoctoral Fellowships, 2205
NCI Engineered Isogenic Cell Lines with Relevant Cancer Targets Research Grants, 2273
NCIC Canadian Cancer Society Research Grants, 2282
NHLBI Progenitor Cell Biology Consortium Administrative Coordinating Center Grants, 2367
NHLBI Progenitor Cell Biology Consortium Research Hubs, 2368
NIA Nathan Shock Centers of Excellence in Basic Biology of Aging Grants, 2421
NIAAA Hepatitis C Infection and Alcoholic Liver Disease, 2442
NIAAA Mechanisms of Alcohol-Induced Hepatic Fibrosis Research Grants, 2445
NIAMS Skin Diseases Research Core Centers Grants, 2478
NIDA Role of Limbic System and Brain Ontogeny in Drug Abuse Research Grants, 2514
NIDCD Molecular and Cellular Pathology of the Human Auditory and Vestibular Systems Grants, 2525
NIDDK Cell-Specific Delineation of Prostate and Genitourinary Development, 2545
NIEHS Biological Response to Environmental Health Hazards Research Grants, 2596
NIGMS Fellowships in Quantitative Biology, 2610
NIGMS Integrative and Collaborative Approaches to Research Grants, 2615
NIGMS Molecular Pharmacology of Anesthetic Action Research Grants, 2621

NIGMS Predoctoral Training in Bioinformatics and Computation Biology Grants, 2625
NIGMS Quantitative Approaches to the Analysis of Complex Biological Systems, 2626
NIH Human Models and Markers of Skeletal Aging Grants, 2674
NIH Molecular Epidemiology of Prostate Carcinogenesis Grants, 2691
NIH Mouse Mutagenesis and Phenotyping: Developmental Defects Research Grants, 2692
NIH New Directions in Pain Research Grants, 2698
NIH Research on Sleep and Sleep Disorders, 2713
NIH Xenobiotics and Cell Death/Injury in Neurodegenerative Disease Research Grants, 2739
NIMH Quantitative Approaches to the Analysis of Complex Biological Systems, 2767
NSF Behavioral Neurosciences Research Grants, 2876
NSF Biomedical Engineering and Engineering Healthcare Grants, 2879
NSF Cell Systems Cluster Grants, 2881
NSF Chemical, Biochemical, and Biotechnology Systems Research Grants, 2882
ONR Human Performance Division Research Grants, 2948
PhRMA Fndn Pharmacology/Toxicology Post Doctoral Fellowships, 3044
PhRMA Fndn Pharmacology/Toxicology Pre Doctoral Fellowships, 3045
PhRMA Fndn Pharmacology/Toxicology Research Starter Grants, 3046
PhRMA Fndn Pharmacology/Toxicology Sabbatical Fellowships, 3047
Searle Scholars Grants, 3275
Simone and Cino del Duca Grand Prix Awards, 3288

Biology, Developmental/Evolutionary
AHAF Alzheimer's Disease Research Grants, 266
Alfred P. Sloan Fndn History of Science and Technology Grants, 352
NIAAA Mechanisms of Alcohol-Induced Hepatic Fibrosis Research Grants, 2445
NICHD NRSAs—Individual, 2488
NICHD NRSAs—Institutional, 2489
NICHD Ruth L. Kirschstein National Research Service Award Institutional Predoctoral Training Program in Systems Biology of Developmental Biology & Birth Defects, 2493
NIGMS Fellowships in Quantitative Biology, 2610
NIGMS Integrative and Collaborative Approaches to Research Grants, 2615
NSF Animal Developmental Mechanisms Grants, 2875
Rett Syndrome Research Fndn Grants, 3151

Biology, Molecular
AAAAI Summer Clinical Research Fellowship Medical Student Grants, 27
AAAAI Summer Research Fellowship Medical Student Grants, 28
AHAF Alzheimer's Disease Research Grants, 266
AHAF National Glaucoma Research Grants, 268
Alfred P. Sloan Fndn History of Science and Technology Grants, 352
Cancer Research UK Fellowships, 858
DOE Health Effects and Life Sciences Research Grants, 1298
DOE Human Genome Program—Ethical, Legal, and Social Implications, 1299
EMBO Installation Grants, 1409
EMBO Long-Term Fellowships, 1410
EMBO Short-Term Fellowships, 1411
Eppendorf & Science Prize for Neurobiology, 1424
FDHN Fellowship to Faculty Transition Awards, 1470
Fndn for Medical Research Grants, 1528
GE & Science Prize for Young Life Scientists, 1584
Glaucoma Research Pilot Project Grants, 1622
Helen Hay Whitney Fndn Postdoctoral Research Fellowships, 1739
IARC Expertise Transfer Fellowship, 1831
IARC Postdoctoral Fellowships for Training in Cancer Research, 1832
IARC Visiting Scientist Award for Senior Scientists, 1833
Implant Dentistry Research and Education Fndn Grants, 1844
LRF New Investigator Leukemia Research Grants, 2070
LSA Translational Research Grants, 2078
Marine Biological Laboratory Summer Research Fellowships, 2108
Mayo Fndn Multidisciplinary Training in Digestive Diseases Research Grants, 2140
MDBD Basic Research Grants, 2152
NCI Academic-Industrial Partnerships for Development and Validation of In Vivo Imaging Systems and Methods for Cancer Investigations, 2268
NCI Application and Use of Transformative Emerging Technologies in Cancer Research, 2269
NCI Engineered Isogenic Cell Lines with Relevant Cancer Targets Research Grants, 2273
NCI/NIDA Transdisciplinary Tobacco Use Research Centers Grants, 2280
NIA Nathan Shock Centers of Excellence in Basic Biology of Aging Grants, 2421
NIAAA Hepatitis C Infection and Alcoholic Liver Disease, 2442
NIAID Preparedness against Illegitimate Use of Bacterial Pathogens, 2461
NIAID Therapeutics Research on AIDS-Associated Opportunistic Infections, 2465
NIDA Role of Limbic System and Brain Ontogeny in Drug Abuse Research Grants, 2514
NIDCD Mentored Research Scientist Development Award, 2523
NIDCD Molecular and Cellular Pathology of the Human Auditory and Vestibular Systems Grants, 2525
NIEHS Biological Response to Environmental Health Hazards Research Grants, 2596
NIEHS Structure-Function Relationships of Environmentally Relevant Genetic Variants Research Grants, 2606
NIGMS Molecular Pharmacology of Anesthetic Action Research Grants, 2621
NIGMS Predoctoral Training in Bioinformatics and Computation Biology Grants, 2625
NIGMS Quantitative Approaches to the Analysis of Complex Biological Systems, 2626
NIH Genetic Susceptibility and Variability of Human Malformations Research Grants, 2669
NIH Mechanisms Underlying Individual Variations in Drug Responses, 2685
NIH Molecular Epidemiology of Prostate Carcinogenesis Grants, 2691
NIH Mouse Mutagenesis and Phenotyping: Developmental Defects Research Grants, 2692
NIH New Directions in Pain Research Grants, 2698
NIH Research on Sleep and Sleep Disorders, 2713
NIH Xenobiotics and Cell Death/Injury in Neurodegenerative Disease Research Grants, 2739
NIMH Quantitative Approaches to the Analysis of Complex Biological Systems, 2767
NINR Opportunities in Genetics and Nursing Research Grants, 2801
NSF Behavioral Neurosciences Research Grants, 2876
NSF Biomolecular Systems Cluster Grants, 2880
NSF Systematic Biology and Biodiversity Inventories Grants, 2895
ONR Human Performance Division Research Grants, 2948
PhRMA Fndn Pharmacology/Toxicology Post Doctoral Fellowships, 3044
PhRMA Fndn Pharmacology/Toxicology Pre Doctoral Fellowships, 3045
PhRMA Fndn Pharmacology/Toxicology Research Starter Grants, 3046
PhRMA Fndn Pharmacology/Toxicology Sabbatical Fellowships, 3047
Rett Syndrome Research Fndn Grants, 3151
Simone and Cino del Duca Grand Prix Awards, 3288
TSA Research Grant Awards, 3442

Biology, Reproductive
Lalor Fndn Postdoctoral Research Grants, 2021
NSF Animal Developmental Mechanisms Grants, 2875

Biology, Structural
DOE Health Effects and Life Sciences Research Grants, 1298
NIEHS Structure-Function Relationships of Environmentally Relevant Genetic Variants Research Grants, 2606
NIH Structural Biology of Membrane Proteins Grants, 2730
NSF Emerging Frontiers in Research and Innovation Grants, 2885

Biology, Systematic
AACR Team Science Award, 89
NICHD Ruth L. Kirschstein National Research Service Award Institutional Predoctoral Training Program in Systems Biology of Developmental Biology & Birth Defects, 2493
NIH Biology, Development, and Progression of Malignant Prostate Disease Research Grants, 2641
NSF Emerging Frontiers in Research and Innovation Grants, 2885
NSF Systematic Biology and Biodiversity Inventories Grants, 2895

Biomarkers
NIDDK Development of Disease Biomarkers Grants, 2549

Biomaterials
Implant Dentistry Research and Education Fndn Grants, 1844

Biomechanics
CDC Injury Prevention and Control Research and State and Comm Based Programs, 914
H.R. Lissner Award, 1683
Implant Dentistry Research and Education Fndn Grants, 1844
Musculoskeletal Rehabilitation Fellowships, 2229
NIOSH Occupational Safety and Health Research and Demonstration Grants, 2807

Biomedical Education
AHFMR Full-Time M.D./Ph.D. Studentships, 277
AHFMR Infrastructure Funding Grants, 283
AHFMR Part-Time Studentships, 289
AHFMR Personnel Funding Grants, 290
AHFMR Scholar Awards, 295
AHFMR Scientist Awards, 296
AHFMR Senior Investigator Awards, 297
AHFMR Senior Scholar Awards, 299
HHMI Biomedical Research Grants for International Scientists in Canada and Latin America, 1756
HHMI Biomedical Research Grants for International Scientists in the Baltics, Central and Eastern Europe, Russia, and Ukraine, 1757
HHMI Biomedical Research Grants for International Scientists: Infectious Diseases and Parasitology, 1758
HHMI Physician-Scientist Early Career Award, 1762
NCI Ruth L. Kirschstein National Research Service Award Institutional Research Training Grants, 2277
NIGMS Minority Access to Research Careers Ancillary Training Activities Grants, 2619
NIH Summer Internship Program in Biomedical Research, 2732
NIH Undergraduate Scholarships, 2737
NIMH Career Opportunities in Research Education and Training Honors High School Research Education Grant, 2748
NYCT Biomedical Research Grants, 2920
Topeka Comm Fndn Kansas Blood Services Scholarships, 3429

Biomedical Engineering
Heart Rhythm Society Fellowships, 1731
NHLBI Individual Postdoctoral National Research Service Awards, 2340
NHLBI Intramural Research Training Awards, 2343
NIGMS Fellowships in Quantitative Biology, 2610
NSF Biomedical Engineering and Engineering Healthcare Grants, 2879
NSF Emerging Frontiers in Research and Innovation Grants, 2885
Whitaker International Fellows and Scholars Program, 3532

Biomedical Programs
Alpha Research Fndn Grants, 367

Biomedical Research
100 Mile Man Fndn Grants, 2
25th Anniversary Fndn Grants, 8
A.O. Smith Comm Grants, 18
AACR Award for Outstanding Achievement in Cancer Research, 67
AACR Team Science Award, 89
AAMC Award for Distinguished Research, 135
Achelis and Bodman Fndns Grants, 206
Adaptec Fndn Grants, 232
AFAR CART Fund Grants, 254
Affymetrix Corp Contributions Grants, 258
AHFMR Clinical Fellowships, 269
AHFMR Clinical Investigator Awards, 270
AHFMR Clinical Investigator Awards, 270
AHFMR Comm Support Grants, 271
AHFMR Dr. Lionel E. McLeod Health Research Scholarship, 272
AHFMR Establishment and Independent Establishment Grants, 273
AHFMR Fast-Track Studentships and Fellowships, 274
AHFMR Forefront Internship Grants, 275
AHFMR Full-Time Fellowships, 276
AHFMR Full-Time M.D./Ph.D. Studentships, 277
AHFMR Full-Time Studentships, 278
AHFMR Health Research Career Renewal Awards, 279
AHFMR Health Research Full-Time Studentships, 280
AHFMR Health Research Fund Grants, 281
AHFMR Heritage Summer Studentships, 282
AHFMR Infrastructure Funding Grants, 283
AHFMR Interdisciplinary Team Grants, 284
AHFMR Major Equipment Grants, 285
AHFMR Medical or Health Scholars Investigator Grants, 286
AHFMR Medical or Health Scientist Awards, 287
AHFMR Part-Time Fellowships, 288
AHFMR Part-Time Studentships, 289
AHFMR Personnel Funding Grants, 290
AHFMR Polaris Awards, 291
AHFMR Proposals for Special Initiatives, 293
AHFMR Research Prize, 294
AHFMR Scholar Awards, 295
AHFMR Scientist Awards, 296
AHFMR Senior Investigator Awards, 297
AHFMR Senior Medical or Health Scholars Investigator Grants, 298
AHFMR Senior Scholar Awards, 299
AHRQ Individual Awards for Postdoctoral Fellows Ruth L. Kirschstein National Research Service Awards, 314
Albany Medical Center Prize in Medicine and Biomedical Research, 325
Albert and Mary Lasker Fndn Awards, 327
Alcoa Fndn Grants, 334
Allyn Fndn Grants, 365
ALSAM Fndn Grants, 369
Amgen Fndn Grants, 467
Annenberg Fndn Grants, 479
Anthony R. Abraham Fndn Grants, 490
APF Disaster Recovery Fund for Psychiatrists, 506
Arizona Cardinals Grants, 529
Armstrong McDonald Fndn Grants, 537
ASCO Improving Cancer Care Grants, 546
ASCO State Affiliate Grants, 547
ASCO Advanced Clinical Research Award in Colorectal Cancer, 548
ASCO Advanced Clinical Research Awards in Breast Cancer, 549
ASCO Advanced Clinical Research Awards in Sarcoma, 550
ASCO Career Development Award, 551
ASCO Comm Oncology Research Grants, 552
ASCO Comparative Effectiveness Research Professorship in Breast Cancer, 553
ASCO Long-Term International Fellowships, 556
ASCO Medical Student Rotation Grants, 557
ASCO Translational Research Professorships, 561
ASCO/UICC International Cancer Technology Transfer (ICRETT) Fellowships, 563
ASM Abbott Laboratories Award in Clinical and Diagnostic Immunology, 587
Australian Academy of Science Grants, 670
Award in Separations Science and Technology, 677
Barth Syndrome Fndn Research Grants, 700
Batchelor Fndn Grants, 701
BCBSNC Fndn Grants, 725
Beckman Coulter Comm Relations Grants, 733
Blue Shield of California Grants, 771
Blum-Kovler Fndn Grants, 772
Bodman Fndn Grants, 776
Booth-Bricker Fund Grants, 780
Bosque Fndn Grants, 782
Bright Family Fndn Grants, 793
Brinson Fndn Grants, 794
Bristol-Myers Squibb Fndn Global HIV/AIDS Initiative Grants, 796
Bristol-Myers Squibb Fndn Health Disparities Grants, 797
Bristol-Myers Squibb Virology and Oncology M.D. Research Fellowships, 802
Brookdale Fndn Leadership in Aging Fellowships, 805
Burden Trust Grants, 810
Bushrod H. Campbell and Adah F. Hall Charity Fund Grants, 816
BWF Clinical Scientist Awards in Translational Research, 821
BWF Institutional Program Unifying Population and Laboratory Based Sciences, 822
Byron W. and Alice L. Lockwood Fndn Grants, 824
Carl C. Icahn Fndn Grants, 870
Carl J. Herzog Fndn Grants, 872
Carrie Estelle Doheny Fndn Grants, 883
Catherine Holmes Wilkins Fndn Grants, 889
CCFF Fellowships, 893
CCFF Studentships, 897
CCFF Summer Studentship, 898
CDC Injury Control Research Centers Grants, 913
Charles Edison Fund Grants, 964
Charles H. Revson Fndn Grants, 969
Charles Lafitte Fndn Grants, 970
Chateaubriand Exact Sciences, Engineering, and Medicine Research Scholarships, 976
Chest Fndn Geriatric Development Research Awards, 984
Chiles Fndn Grants, 1003
Chiron Fndn Comm Grants, 1004
Claude Pepper Fndn Grants, 1032
CMA Fndn Grants, 1042
CMS Research and Demonstration Grants, 1045
Columbus Fndn Competitive Grants, 1066
Comm Fndn of Broward Grants, 1100
Compass Bank Fndn Grants, 1138
Connecticut Health Fndn Health Initiative Grants, 1142
DAAD Research Stays for University Academics and Scientists, 1183
Dana Clinical Hypotheses Program in Brain and Immuno-Imaging Research Grants, 1195
Dana Fndn Science and Health Grants, 1197
DeBakey Medical Fndn Fellowships and Scholarships, 1212
Del E. Webb Fndn Grants, 1213
Delta Air Lines Fndn Grants, 1220
DeMatteis Family Fndn Grants, 1221
Denton A. Cooley Fndn Grants, 1225
DOD Breast Cancer Center of Excellence Award, 1290
DOD Clinical Translational Research Grants, 1291
Donaghue Practical Benefit Initiatives Grants, 1309
Doris Duke Charitable Fndn Clinical Interfaces Award Program, 1314
Doris Duke Charitable Fndn Clinical Research Fellowships for Medical Students, 1315
Doris Duke Charitable Fndn Clinical Scientist Development Award Bridge Grants, 1317
Doris Duke Charitable Fndn Distinguished Clinical Scientist Award Program, 1318
Dorothea Haus Ross Fndn Grants, 1320
Dr. Scholl Fndn Grants, 1329
Duke University Postdoctoral Research Fellowships in Aging, 1348
Edwin S. Webster Fndn Grants, 1376
Effie and Wofford Cain Fndn Grants, 1385
Elisabeth Severance Prentiss Fndn Grants, 1392
Elizabeth Glaser Pediatric AIDS Fndn Two-Year Scholar Awards, 1397
Ellison Medical Fndn/AFAR Postdoctoral Fellows in Aging Research Program, 1404
Emerson Charitable Trust Grants, 1412
Emma B. Howe Memorial Fndn Grants, 1415
Eugene M. Lang Fndn Grants, 1434
Eugene McDermott Fndn Grants, 1435
Fairlawn Fndn Grants, 1447
Feldman Fndn Grants, 1484
FIC International Research Fellowship Program, 1490
FIC Swedish Medical Research Council Fellowships, 1495
FIC/ORMH Minority International Research Training Grants, 1497
Fidelity Fndn Grants, 1498
Fight for Sight Research Grants, 1502
Fishman Family Fndn Grants, 1510
Flinn Fndn Grants Programs, 1511
Forrest C. Lattner Fndn Grants, 1523
Fndn for Psychocultural Research Postdoctoral Fellowships, 1531
Frank Stanley Beveridge Fndn Grants, 1553
Frederick Gardner Cottrell Fndn Grants, 1560
Fritz B. Burns Fndn Grants, 1564
Gates Global HIV/AIDS Vaccine Grants, 1583
Gebbie Fndn Grants, 1585
Gerber Fndn Grants, 1606
Gheens Fndn Grants, 1610
Good Samaritan Inc Grants, 1637
GPP Charles E. Culpeper Fndn Biomedical Pilot Projects Initiative Grants, 1641
Green Fndn Grants, 1661
Greenspun Family Fndn Grants, 1664
H.A. and Mary K. Chapman Charitable Trust Grants, 1681
Harold Amos Medical Faculty Development Program, 1696
Harry A. and Margaret D. Towsley Fndn Grants, 1701
Hawn Fndn Grants, 1719
Healthcare Fndn of New Jersey Grants, 1729
Hearst Fndn and William Randolph Hearst Fndn Grants, 1730
Hedco Fndn Grants, 1733
Helen Hay Whitney Fndn Postdoctoral Research Fellowships, 1739
HHMI Biomedical Research Grants for International Scientists in Canada and Latin America, 1756
HHMI Biomedical Research Grants for International Scientists in the Baltics, Central and Eastern Europe, Russia, and Ukraine, 1757
HHMI Biomedical Research Grants for International Scientists: Infectious Diseases and Parasitology, 1758
HHMI Grants and Fellowships Programs, 1759
HHMI International Research Scholars Program, 1760
HHMI Physician-Scientist Early Career Award, 1762

HHMI Research Training Fellowships, 1763
HHMI-NIBIB Interfaces Initiative Grants, 1764
HHMI-NIH Cloister Research Scholars Program, 1765
Hilda and Preston Davis Fndn Grants, 1772
HomeBanc Fndn Grants, 1788
HRB Postdoctoral Research Fellowships, 1802
i2 Fndn Grants, 1829
IHS Native American and Alaskan Native Health Research Centers, 1840
J.B. Reynolds Fndn Grants, 1873
J.W. Kieckhefer Fndn Grants, 1878
Jackson Laboratory Postdoctoral Research Training Program, 1880
James H. Cummings Fndn Grants, 1888
Jeffress Research Grants, 1913
Joe W. and Dorothy Dorsett Brown Fndn Grants, 1927
John R. Oishei Fndn Grants, 1944
John S. Dunn Research Fndn Grants and Chairs, 1945
Johnson & Johnson Corp Contributions Grants, 1952
Joseph Drown Fndn Grants, 1960
Josiah W. and Bessie H. Kline Fndn Grants, 1967
Kavli Fndn Research Grants, 1985
Kenneth T. and Eileen L. Norris Fndn Grants, 1989
Kettering Fund Grants, 1992
Lance Armstrong Fndn Research Grants, 2026
Larry L. Hillblom Fndn Grants, 2031
Lillian S. Wells Fndn Grants, 2056
Lindbergh Grants, 2059
Lucile Horton Howe and Mitchell B. Howe Fndn Grants, 2081
M.J. Murdock Charitable Trust Grants, 2095
MAPFRE Fndn for Medicine Grants, 2102
Margaret L. Wendt Fndn Grants, 2104
Margaret T. Morris Fndn Grants, 2105
Mark and Catherine Winkler Fndn Grants, 2112
Marshall Field's Comm Grants, 2115
Mary Ingraham Bunting Institute Biomedical Research Fellowships, 2119
Mary S. and David C. Corbin Fndn Grants, 2122
Matsumae International Fndn Grants, 2129
McCarthy Family Fndn Grants, 2141
McCombs Fndn Grants, 2142
McLean Contributionship Grants, 2147
MDBD Research Prize in Developmental Biology, 2154
Medical/Nursing Education, Research, and Health Care Exchanges with Taiwan, 2165
Mericos Fndn Grants, 2172
MHRC Graduate Studentships, 2185
MHRC Operating Grants, 2186
MHRC Postdoctoral Research Fellowships, 2187
Military Medical Research and Development Grants, 2202
MMRF Research Grants, 2211
Monfort Family Fndn Grants, 2213
Mount Zion Health Fund Grants, 2220
MRC Career Establishment Grants, 2221
National Lottery Comm Fund Grants, 2256
National MPS Society Grants, 2257
NCI Ruth L. Kirschstein National Research Service Award Institutional Research Training Grants, 2277
NEI Ruth L. Kirschstein National Research Service Award Short-Term Institutional Research Training Grants, 2297
NHLBI Biomedical Research Training Program for Individuals from Underrepresented Groups, 2321
NHLBI Career Enhancement Awards for Stem Cell Research, 2325
NHLBI Hyperglycemic Exacerbation of Ischemia/ Reperfusion Injury after Ischemic Insult Grants, 2335
NHLBI Independent Scientist Award, 2339
NHLBI Individual Postdoctoral National Research Service Awards, 2340
NHLBI Individual Predoctoral Fellowships to Promote Diversity in Health-Related Research, 2341
NHLBI Intramural Research Training Awards, 2343
NHLBI Investigator Initiated Multi-Site Clinical Trials, 2344
NHLBI Lymphatic Biology in Health and Disease Grants, 2345
NHLBI Mentored Career Award for Faculty at Minority Institutions, 2347
NHLBI Mentored Career Development Award to Promote Faculty Diversity/Re-Entry in Biomedical Research, 2348
NHLBI Mentored Clinical Scientist Research Career Development Awards, 2349
NHLBI Mentored Patient-Oriented Research Career Development Awards, 2350
NHLBI Mentored Quantitative Research Career Development Awards, 2351
NHLBI Midcareer Investigator Award in Patient-Oriented Research, 2353
NHLBI Multidisciplinary Translational Research in Critical Care Grants, 2356
NHLBI National Research Service Awards for Senior Fellowships, 2358
NHLBI Pathway to Independence Award, 2363
NHLBI Research Demonstration and Dissemination Grants, 2370
NHLBI Ruth L. Kirschstein National Research Service Award Institutional Research Training Grants, 2379
NHLBI Ruth L. Kirschstein National Research Service Award Short-Term Institutional Research Training Grants, 2380
NHLBI Short-Term Research Education to Increase Diversity in Health-Related Research, 2383
NHLBI Summer Internship Program in Biomedical Research, 2386
NHLBI Transfusion-Related Acute Lung Injury Basic Research Grants, 2389
NIA Alzheimer's Disease Core Centers Grants, 2395
NIA Independent Scientist Award, 2412
NIA Mentored Clinical Scientist Research Career Development Awards, 2417
NIA Paul Beeson Career Development Awards in Aging, 2424
NIA/NIEHS Biomedical Epidemiologic and Intervention Studies Planning Grants, 2441
NIAAA Independent Scientist Award, 2443
NIAAA Mentored Clinical Scientist Research Career Development Awards, 2446
NIAID Challenge Grants: Joint Ventures in Biomedicine and Biotechnology, 2451
NIAID Independent Scientist Award, 2456
NIDCD Mentored Clinical Scientist Research Career Development Award, 2522
NIDDK Ancillary Studies to Major Ongoing NIDDK and NHLBI Clinical Research Studies, 2541
NIDDK Erythropoiesis: Components and Mechanisms Grants, 2558
NIEHS Hazardous Materials Worker Health and Safety Training Grants, 2599
NIEHS Hazmat Training at Doe Nuclear Weapons Complex Grants, 2600
NIEHS Independent Scientist Award, 2601
NIEHS SBIR E-Learning for HAZMAT and Emergency Response Grants, 2604
NIGMS Exploratory Studies for High Risk/High Impact Research Grants, 2609
NIGMS Initiative for Minority Students: Bridges to the Baccalaureate Degree, 2612
NIGMS Initiative for Minority Students: Bridges to the Doctoral Degree, 2613
NIGMS Institutional Research and Academic Career Development Award, 2614
NIGMS Large-Scale Collaborative Project Awards, 2616
NIGMS MARC Undergraduate Student Training in Academic Research (U-STAR) Program, 2617
NIGMS Minority Access to Research Careers Program, 2620
NIGMS Ruth L. Kirschstein National Research Service Awards for Individual Predoctoral Fellows in PharmD/PhD Grants, 2627
NIH Academic Research Enhancement Awards, 2635
NIH Biomedical Research on the International Space Station, 2642
NIH Earth-Based Research Relevant to the Space Environment, 2655
NIH Exceptional, Unconventional Research Enabling Knowledge Acceleration (EUREKA) Grants, 2662
NIH Exploratory Innovations in Biomedical Computational Science and Technology Grants, 2664
NIH Exploratory/Developmental Research Grant, 2666
NIH Independent Scientist Award, 2677
NIH Innovations in Biomedical Computational Science and Technology Grants, 2679
NIH Innovations in Biomedical Computational Science and Technology Initiative Grants for SBIR, 2680
NIH Innovations in Biomedical Computational Science and Technology Initiative Grants for STTR, 2681
NIH Investigator-Initiated Interactive Research Project Grants, 2682
NIH Mentored Clinical Scientist Development Award, 2687
NIH Mentored Research Scientist Development Awards, 2689
NIH NRSAs for Individual Predoctoral Fellowships, 2700
NIH NRSAs Predoctoral Fellowship Awards for Students with Disabilities, 2701
NIH Predoctoral Fellowship Awards for Minority Students, 2703
NIH Recovery Act Limited Competition: Academic Research Enhancement Awards, 2707
NIH Recovery Act Limited Competition: Biomedical Research, Development, and Growth to Spur the Acceleration of New Technologies (BRDG-SPAN) Pilot Grants, 2708
NIH Recovery Act Limited Competition: Small Business Catalyst Awards for Accelerating Innovative Research Grants, 2710
NIH Recovery Act Limited Competition: Supporting New Faculty Recruitment to Enhance Research Resources through Biomedical Research Core Centers Grants, 2711
NIH Ruth L. Kirschstein National Research Service Awards for Individual Senior Fellows, 2718
NIH Ruth L. Kirschstein National Research Service Awards for Individual Predoctoral Fellows, 2720
NIH Ruth L. Kirschstein National Research Service Awards for Individual Predoctoral Fellowships to Promote Diversity in Health-Related Research, 2721
NIH Ruth L. Kirschstein National Research Service Awards for Individual Predoctoral MD/PhD and Other Dual Doctoral Degree Fellows, 2722
NIH Senior Scientist Award, 2727
NIH Summer Internship Program in Biomedical Research, 2732
NIH Supplements to Promote Reentry into Biomedical and Behavioral Research Careers, 2733
NIH Undergraduate Scholarships, 2737
NIMH Basic and Translational Research in Emotion Grants, 2746
NIMH Supplements for Underrepresented Minorities, 2773
NLM Academic Research Enhancement Awards, 2814
NLM Exceptional, Unconventional Research Grants Enabling Knowledge Acceleration, 2815
NLM Express Research Grants in Biomedical Informatics and Bioinformatics, 2817
NLM Grants for Scholarly Works in Biomedicine and Health, 2818
NLM Internet Connection for Medical Institutions Grants, 2820
NLM Limited Competition for Continuation of Biomedical Informatics/Bioinformatics Resource Grants, 2821

NLM Predictive Multiscale Models of the Physiome in Health and Disease Grants, 2824
NLM Research Supplements to Promote Reentry in Health-Related Research, 2826
NORD Orphan Diseases Research Grants, 2849
NORD Roscoe Brady Lysosomal Storage Disease Fellowships, 2850
NSF Alan T. Waterman Award, 2874
NSF Emerging Frontiers in Research and Innovation Grants, 2885
NSF Instrument Development for Biological Research, 2888
NSF Postdoctoral Research Fellowships in Biology, 2891
Nuffield Fndn Africa Grants, 2898
Nuffield Fndn Law and Society Grants, 2900
Nuffield Fndn Small Grants, 2903
NYCT Biomedical Research Grants, 2920
Orentreich Fndn for the Advancement of Science Grants, 2959
Partnership for Cures Two Years To Cures Grants, 2992
Pasadena Fndn Average Grants, 2994
Patron Saints Fndn Grants, 2996
Peabody Fndn Grants, 3010
Pediatric Cancer Research Fndn Grants, 3013
Pew Charitable Trusts Biomedical Research Grants, 3019
Pew Scholars in the Biomedical Sciences, 3021
PKD Fndn Lillian Kaplan International Prize for the Advancement in the Understanding of Polycystic Kidney Disease, 3056
Presbyterian Health Fndn Bridge, Seed and Equipment Grants, 3075
Rajiv Gandhi Fndn Grants, 3104
RCPSC Detweiler Traveling Fellowships, 3114
Rett Syndrome Research Fndn Grants, 3151
RGK Fndn Grants, 3153
Richard and Susan Smith Family Fndn Grants, 3159
Robert E. and Evelyn McKee Fndn Grants, 3170
Rockefeller Archive Center Research Grants, 3178
Roy J. Carver Charitable Trust Medical and Science Research Grants, 3192
RSC McLaughlin Medal, 3197
RSC Thomas W. Eadie Medal, 3199
Russell Berrie Fndn Grants, 3201
Saint Luke's Fndn Grants, 3239
Salisbury Comm Fndn Grants, 3243
Samuel Roberts Noble Fndn Grants, 3250
San Antonio Area Fndn Grants, 3254
Sarah Scaife Fndn Grants, 3263
Savoy Fndn Studentships, 3268
Schering-Plough Fndn Health Grants, 3270
Scientific Communities Initiative Grants, 3272
Searle Scholars Grants, 3275
Sigrid Juselius Fndn Grants, 3286
Simone and Cino del Duca Grand Prix Awards, 3288
Sir Halley Stewart Trust Grants, 3293
Skin Cancer Fndn Research Grants, 3298
Society for Biomedical Screening Small Grants, 3319
Society of Cosmetic Chemists Allan B. Black Award Sponsored by Presperse, 3328
Society of Cosmetic Chemists Award Sponsored by McIntyre Group, Ltd., 3329
Society of Cosmetic Chemists Award Sponsored by The HallStar Company, 3330
Society of Cosmetic Chemists Chapter Best Speaker Award, 3331
Society of Cosmetic Chemists Chapter Merit Award, 3332
Society of Cosmetic Chemists Frontier of Science Award, 3333
Society of Cosmetic Chemists Hans Schaeffer Award, 3334
Society of Cosmetic Chemists Joseph P. Ciaudelli Award, 3335
Society of Cosmetic Chemists Keynote Award Lecture Sponsored by Ruger Chemical Corp, 3336
Society of Cosmetic Chemists Literature Award, 3337
Society of Cosmetic Chemists Maison G. de Navarre Medal, 3338
Society of Cosmetic Chemists Merit Award, 3339
Society of Cosmetic Chemists Robert A. Kramer Lifetime Service Award, 3340
Society of Cosmetic Chemists Shaw Mudge Award, 3341
Society of Cosmetic Chemists Student Poster Awards, 3342
Society of Cosmetic Chemists Young Scientist Awards, 3343
Starr Fndn Grants, 3377
Takemi Program in International Health Research and Advanced Training Fellowships, 3416
Tellabs Fndn Grants, 3418
Thomas and Dorothy Leavey Fndn Grants, 3422
Tourette Syndrome Association Post-Doc Fellowships, 3432
Tourette Syndrome Association Research Grants, 3433
Wallace H. Coulter Fndn Grants, 3515
Wayne and Gladys Valley Fndn Grants, 3522
Whitehall Fndn Neurobiology Research Grants, 3533
William G. McGowan Charitable Fund Grants, 3539
William H. Hannon Fndn Grants, 3540

Biomedical Research Resources

AHFMR Establishment and Independent Establishment Grants, 273
AHFMR Forefront Internship Grants, 275
AHFMR Polaris Awards, 291
AHFMR Proposals for Special Initiatives, 293
NHLBI Biomedical Research Training Program for Individuals from Underrepresented Groups, 2321
NHLBI Career Enhancement Awards for Stem Cell Research, 2325
NHLBI Individual Postdoctoral National Research Service Awards, 2340
NHLBI Intramural Research Training Awards, 2343
NHLBI Mentored Career Award for Faculty at Minority Institutions, 2347
NHLBI Mentored Career Development Award to Promote Faculty Diversity/Re-Entry in Biomedical Research, 2348
NHLBI Mentored Clinical Scientist Research Career Development Awards, 2349
NHLBI Mentored Patient-Oriented Research Career Development Awards, 2350
NHLBI Mentored Quantitative Research Career Development Awards, 2351
NHLBI Midcareer Investigator Award in Patient-Oriented Research, 2353
NHLBI Research Demonstration and Dissemination Grants, 2370
NHLBI Ruth L. Kirschstein National Research Service Award Institutional Research Training Grants, 2379
NHLBI Ruth L. Kirschstein National Research Service Award Short-Term Institutional Research Training Grants, 2380
NIAAA Mentored Clinical Scientist Research Career Development Awards, 2446
NIDCD Mentored Clinical Scientist Research Career Development Award, 2522
NIGMS Large-Scale Collaborative Project Awards, 2616
NIH Exploratory Innovations in Biomedical Computational Science and Technology Grants, 2664
NIH Innovations in Biomedical Computational Science and Technology Grants, 2679
NIH Innovations in Biomedical Computational Science and Technology Initiative Grants for SBIR, 2680
NIH Innovations in Biomedical Computational Science and Technology Initiative Grants for STTR, 2681
NIH Mentored Clinical Scientist Development Award, 2687
NIH Recovery Act Limited Competition: Supporting New Faculty Recruitment to Enhance Research Resources through Biomedical Research Core Centers Grants, 2711
NLM Academic Research Enhancement Awards, 2814
NLM Limited Competition for Continuation of Biomedical Informatics/Bioinformatics Resource Grants, 2821
NSF Emerging Frontiers in Research and Innovation Grants, 2885
Partnership for Cures Two Years To Cures Grants, 2992
Pew Charitable Trusts Biomedical Research Grants, 3019

Biomedical Research Training

AHFMR Polaris Awards, 291
AHFMR Proposals for Special Initiatives, 293
Harry Shwachman Clinical Investigator Award, 1707
NEI Ruth L. Kirschstein National Research Service Award Short-Term Institutional Research Training Grants, 2297
NHLBI Biomedical Research Training Program for Individuals from Underrepresented Groups, 2321
NHLBI Individual Predoctoral Fellowships to Promote Diversity in Health-Related Research, 2341
NHLBI Intramural Research Training Awards, 2343
NHLBI Minority Institutional Research Training Grants, 2355
NHLBI Ruth L. Kirschstein National Research Service Award Institutional Research Training Grants, 2379
NHLBI Ruth L. Kirschstein National Research Service Award Short-Term Institutional Research Training Grants, 2380
NSF Postdoctoral Research Fellowships in Biology, 2891
PhRMA Fndn Informatics Sabbatical Fellowships, 3035
PhRMA Fndn Pharmaceutics Postdoctoral Fellowships, 3040
PhRMA Fndn Pharmacology/Toxicology Pre Doctoral Fellowships, 3045
Topeka Comm Fndn Kansas Blood Services Scholarships, 3429

Biomedicine

ASPEN C. Richard Fleming Grant, 629
ASPEN Douglas Wilmore Grant, 630
ASPEN Maurice Shils Grant, 633
ASPEN Norman Yoshimura Grant, 634
ASPEN Nutrition Research Grants, 635
Heart Rhythm Society Fellowships, 1731
HHMI-NIBIB Interfaces Initiative Grants, 1764
NIH Earth-Based Research Relevant to the Space Environment, 2655
NIH Exploratory Innovations in Biomedical Computational Science and Technology Grants, 2664
NIH Innovations in Biomedical Computational Science and Technology Grants, 2679
NIH Innovations in Biomedical Computational Science and Technology Initiative Grants for SBIR, 2680
NIH Innovations in Biomedical Computational Science and Technology Initiative Grants for STTR, 2681
NIH Ruth L. Kirschstein National Research Service Awards for Individual Predoctoral Fellows, 2720
NIH Undergraduate Scholarships, 2737
NLM Academic Research Enhancement Awards, 2814
NLM Exceptional, Unconventional Research Grants Enabling Knowledge Acceleration, 2815
NLM Express Research Grants in Biomedical Informatics and Bioinformatics, 2817
NLM Limited Competition for Continuation of Biomedical Informatics/Bioinformatics Resource Grants, 2821
NLM Predictive Multiscale Models of the Physiome in Health and Disease Grants, 2824
NYCT Biomedical Research Grants, 2920
Partnership for Cures Two Years To Cures Grants, 2992

Prudential Fndn Grants, 3087
RSC Abbyann D. Lynch Medal in Bioethics, 3195
Topeka Comm Fndn Kansas Blood Services Scholarships, 3429

Biometry
CDC Minority Health Statistics Dissertation Research Grants, 916
DHHS Public Health Students Traineeships and Other Graduate Public Health Programs, 1277
HRB Health Services Research Fellowships, 1801
NCI Basic Cancer Research in Cancer Health Disparities Grants, 2271
NCIC Terry Fox Postdoc Research Fellowships, 2285
NEI Clinical Vision Research Development Award, 2293
NHLBI National Research Service Award Programs in Cardiovascular Epidemiology and Biostatistics, 2357
NIA Nathan Shock Centers of Excellence in Basic Biology of Aging Grants, 2421
NIGMS Short Courses on Mathematical and Statistical Tools for the Study of Complex Phenotypes and Complex Systems, 2628
NIGMS Short Courses on Mathematical, Statistical, and Computational Tools for Studying Biological Systems, 2629
NIH Exploratory Centers for Alternative Medicine Research Grants, 2663
NIH Genetic Architecture of Complex Phenotypes, 2668
NIH Urinary Incontinence Treatment Network, 2738
NIMH Short Courses on Mathematical and Statistical Tools for the Study of Complex Phenotypes and Complex Systems, 2770

Biophysics
Grass Fndn Marine Biological Laboratory Fellowships, 1648
NIGMS Fellowships in Quantitative Biology, 2610
NIGMS Integrative and Collaborative Approaches to Research Grants, 2615
NIGMS Molecular Pharmacology of Anesthetic Action Research Grants, 2621
NIH Structural Biology of Membrane Proteins Grants, 2730
NSF Biological Physics (BP), 2878
NSF Biomolecular Systems Cluster Grants, 2880
PhRMA Fndn Pharmaceutics Postdoctoral Fellowships, 3040
PhRMA Fndn Pharmaceutics Pre Doctoral Fellowships, 3041

Biostatistics
NHLBI Summer Institute for Training in Biostatistics II, 2385

Biosynthesis
NSF Biomolecular Systems Cluster Grants, 2880

Biotechnology
ASM Promega Biotechnology Research Award, 610
Canada Graduate Scholarships and NSERC Postgraduate Scholarships, 845
Deland Fellowships in Health Care and Society, 1214
Harry and Grace Steele Fndn Grants, 1702
Innovative Technology Development Awards, 1855
Joyce Fndn Grants, 1969
Kavli Fndn Research Grants, 1985
Millipore/Charles P. Schaufus Parenteral-Processing Technology Research Grant, 2204
NHLBI Summer Institute for Training in Biostatistics II, 2385
NIAID Challenge Grants: Joint Ventures in Biomedicine and Biotechnology, 2451
NIAMS High Risk Arthritis and Musculoskeletal and Skin Diseases Research, 2470
NIH Genetic Susceptibility and Variability of Human Malformations Research Grants, 2669
NIH Individual Postdoctoral Fellowships in Genomics and Related ELSI Topics, 2678
NINR Acute and Chronic Care During Mechanical Ventilation Research Grants, 2788
North Carolina Biotechnology Center Event Sponsorship Grants, 2852
North Carolina Biotechnology Center Grantsmanship Training Grants, 2853
North Carolina Biotechnology Center Meeting Grants, 2854
North Carolina Biotechnology Center Regional Development Grants, 2855
North Carolina Biotechnology Center Technology Enhancement Grants, 2856
North Carolina Biotechnology Centers of Innovation Grants, 2857
NSF Biomedical Engineering and Engineering Healthcare Grants, 2879
NSF Chemical, Biochemical, and Biotechnology Systems Research Grants, 2882
NSF Chemistry Research Experiences for Undergraduates, 2883
NSF Emerging Frontiers in Research and Innovation Grants, 2885
ONR Human Performance Division Research Grants, 2948
PhRMA Fndn Pharmaceutics Research Starter Grants, 3042
PhRMA Fndn Pharmaceutics Sabbatical Fellowships, 3043

Bipolar Disorder
AACAP Quest for the Test Bipolar Disorder Pilot Research Award, 48
American Psychiatric Association/AstraZeneca Young Minds in Psychiatry International Awards, 450

Birth/Congenital Defects
DHHS Priority Health Conditions Studies Initiative, 1273
FACES Assistance Grants, 1444
Little Life Fndn Grants, 2060
MDBD Basic Research Grants, 2152
MDBD Research Prize in Developmental Biology, 2154
NICHD Ruth L. Kirschstein National Research Service Award Institutional Predoctoral Training Program in Systems Biology of Developmental Biology & Birth Defects, 2493
NIEHS Biological Response to Environmental Health Hazards Research Grants, 2596
NIH Genetic Susceptibility and Variability of Human Malformations Research Grants, 2669

Bladder
NIDDK Basic Research Grants in the Bladder and Lower Urinary Tract, 2543

Blood
Chiron Fndn Comm Grants, 1004

Blood Coagulation
ACCP Anticoagulation Training Grants, 197
NHLBI Immunomodulatory, Inflammatory, and Vasoregulatory Properties of Transfused Red Blood Cell Units as a Function of Preparation and Storage Grants, 2337

Blood Diseases
Bayer Clinical Scholarship Award, 706
Bayer Hemophilia Caregivers Education Award, 707
Chest Fndn Grant in Venous Thromboembolism, 985
Cooley's Anemia Research Fellowships, 1149
CSL Behring Local Empowerment for Advocacy Development Grants, 1167
Doris Duke Charitable Fndn Clinical Scientist Development Award, 1316
E.D.Thomas Fellowship, 1359
Fairlawn Fndn Grants, 1447
NHLBI Blood Diseases and Resources Research Grants, 2322
NHLBI Career Transition Award, 2326
NHLBI Characterizing the Blood Stem Cell Niche Grants, 2327
NHLBI Circadian-Coupled Cellular Function in Heart, Lung, and Blood Tissue Grants, 2330
NHLBI Elucidating Nature's Solutions to Heart, Lung, and Blood Diseases and Sleep Disorder Processes Research Grants, 2333
NHLBI Immunomodulatory, Inflammatory, and Vasoregulatory Properties of Transfused Red Blood Cell Units as a Function of Preparation and Storage Grants, 2337
NHLBI Mentored Career Award For Faculty At Minority Institutions, 2346
NHLBI Stress Management Interventions to Reduce Risk of Coronary Artery Disease, 2384
NIDDK Grants for Basic Research in Glomerular Diseases, 2560
NYCT Biomedical Research Grants, 2920
NYCT Blood Disease Research Grants, 2922

Blood Disorders
Leukemia and Lymphoma Society Research Grants, 2051

Blood Pressure
Fairlawn Fndn Grants, 1447
NIDDK Grants for Basic Research in Glomerular Diseases, 2560

Bolivia
Fulbright Traditional Scholar Program in the Western Hemisphere, 1577

Bone Disorders
NIAMS High Risk Arthritis and Musculoskeletal and Skin Diseases Research, 2470
NIH Bone and the Hematopoietic and Immune Systems Research Grants, 2643
NIH Human Models and Markers of Skeletal Aging Grants, 2674
NIH Receptors and Signaling in Bone in Health and Disease, 2706
Osteogenesis Imperfecta Fndn Research Grants, 2975

Bone Marrow
Leukemia and Lymphoma Society Research Grants, 2051
MMRF Research Grants, 2211
NIH Bone and the Hematopoietic and Immune Systems Research Grants, 2643
NIH Human Models and Markers of Skeletal Aging Grants, 2674

Botanical Gardens
Auburn Fndn Grants, 664
Bruce and Adele Greenfield Fndn Grants, 808
Ethel S. Abbott Charitable Fndn Grants, 1430
Kelvin and Eleanor Smith Fndn Grants, 1986
Perry County Comm Fndn Grants, 3016
Posey Comm Fndn Grants, 3068
Spencer County Comm Fndn Grants, 3358
Vanderburgh Comm Fndn Grants, 3480
Warrick County Comm Fndn Grants, 3519

Botanicals
NIH Dietary Supplement Research Centers: Botanicals Grants, 2654

Botany
Human Source Fndn Grants, 1817
NIH Centers for Dietary Supplements Research: Botanicals, 2648

Brain
Alzheimer's Association Investigator-Initiated Research Grants, 378
CDC Cooperative Agreement for Continuing Enhanced National Surveillance for Prion Diseases in the United States, 904

Dana Clinical Hypotheses Program in Brain and Immuno-Imaging Research Grants, 1195
Dana Fndn Science and Health Grants, 1197
EF Postdoctoral Research Training Fellowships, 1382
James S. McDonnell Fndn Brain Cancer Research Collaborative Activity Awards, 1896
James S. McDonnell Fndn Research Grants, 1898
James S. McDonnell Fndn Scholar Awards, 1899
James S. McDonnell Fndn Understanding Human Cognition Awards, 1900
NIA Symptom Management for Chronic Neurological Conditions Research Grants, 2436
NICHD Symptom Management for Chronic Neurological Conditions Research Grants, 2496
NIDA Role of Limbic System and Brain Ontogeny in Drug Abuse Research Grants, 2514
NIDCD Communicative Competence of Users of Augmentative and Alternative Communication Systems Research Grants, 2518
NIDCD Symptom Management for Chronic Neurological Conditions Research Grants, 2532
NIGMS Molecular Pharmacology of Anesthetic Action Research Grants, 2621
NIH Human Brain Project (Neuroinformatics) Phase I & II, 2672
NIMH Short Courses in Neuroinformatics, 2769
NINDS Cerebral Radiobiology and Neuroimaging of Brain Tumors Research Grants, 2778
NINDS Symptom Management for Chronic Neurological Conditions Research Grants, 2787
NINR Symptom Management for Chronic Neurological Conditions Research Grants, 2805
Whitehall Fndn Neurobiology Research Grants, 3533

Brain Tumors
Children's Brain Tumor Fndn Research Grants, 998
Goldhirsh Fndn Brain Tumor Research Grants, 1634
James S. McDonnell Fndn Brain Cancer Research Collaborative Activity Awards, 1896
NINDS Cerebral Radiobiology and Neuroimaging of Brain Tumors Research Grants, 2778
Pediatric Brain Tumor Research Grants, 3012

Brazil
Fulbright Traditional Scholar Program in the Western Hemisphere, 1577
OSI Access to Essential Medicines Grants, 2964

Breast Cancer
1 in 9: Long Island Breast Cancer Action Coalition Grants, 1
AACR Outstanding Investigator Award for Breast Cancer Research, 84
ASCO Improving Cancer Care Grants, 546
ASCO Advanced Clinical Research Awards in Breast Cancer, 549
ASCO Career Development Award, 551
ASCO Comparative Effectiveness Research Professorship in Breast Cancer, 553
ASCO Loan Repayment Grants, 555
ASCO Young Investigator Award, 562
ASCO/UICC International Cancer Technology Transfer (ICRETT) Fellowships, 563
Avon Fndn Breast Care Fund Grants, 674
Avon Products Fndn Grants, 675
BCRF Research Grants, 726
BCRF-AACR Grants for Translational Breast Cancer Research, 727
Breast Cancer Fund Grants, 790
CDC Increasing Breast and Cervical Cancer Screening Services for Urban American Indian/ Alaska Native Women, 912
CDC National Breast and Cervical Cancer Early Detection Program, 917
CMA Fndn Grants, 1042
DOD Breast Cancer Center of Excellence Award, 1290
DOD Clinical Translational Research Grants, 1291
DOD Era of Hope Scholar Award, 1292
DOD HBCU/MI Partnership Training Award, 1293
DOD Idea Award for Breast Cancer Research, 1294
DOD Multidisciplinary Postdoctoral Award for Breast Cancer Research, 1295
DOD Predoctoral Traineeship in Breast Cancer Research, 1296
Henry & Ruth Blaustein Rosenberg Fndn Grants, 1746
Komen Greater NYC Clinical Trials Enrollment Grants, 2010
Komen Greater NYC Comm Breast Health Grants, 2011
Komen Greater NYC Conference Grants, 2012
Komen Greater NYC Small Grants, 2013
Lesbian Health Fund Grants, 2046
Mary Kay Ash Charitable Fndn Grants, 2120
Miles of Hope Breast Cancer Fndn Grants, 2199
Nancy R. Gelman Fndn Breast Cancer Seed Grants, 2234
NCI Stages of Breast Development: Normal to Metastatic Disease Grants, 2278
NCIC Canadian Breast Cancer Research Initiative Grants, 2281
NCIC Canadian Cancer Society Research Grants, 2282
NINR Aging Women and Breast Cancer Grants, 2789
Pezcoller Fndn-AACR International Award for Cancer Research, 3023
Premera CARES Grants, 3074
Susan G. Komen Breast Cancer Fndn Basic, Clinical, and Translational Research Grants, 3407
Susan G. Komen Breast Cancer Fndn Breast Health, Breast Cancer Education, and Outreach Programs Grants, 3408
Susan G. Komen Breast Cancer Fndn Hurricane Relief Grants, 3409
Susan G. Komen Breast Cancer Fndn Interdisciplinary Fellowships, 3410

Broadcast Media
AMA-RFS and AMA Fndn Medical Student & Resident/Fellow Elective-Medicine & the Media, 406
American Academy of Nursing Media Awards, 418
Henry J. Kaiser Family Fndn Grants, 1748

Building Grants
Gladys Brooks Fndn Grants, 1620
Home Building Industry Disaster Relief Fund, 1787
Jennings County Comm Fndn Grants, 1916
Paul Ogle Fndn Grants, 3003
Potts Memorial Fndn Grants, 3072
Pulte Homes Corp Contributions, 3092

Buildings, Residential
Pulte Homes Corp Contributions, 3092

Burma
OSI Supplementary Grant Program: Burma, 2971
Prospect Burma Scholarships, 3085

Burns
CDC National Training Information and Exchange Program, 920
IAFF Burn Fndn Research Grants, 1830
John S. Dunn Research Fndn Grants and Chairs, 1945
NIGMS Fellowships in Quantitative Biology, 2610
NIGMS Mentored Clinical Scientist Research Career Development Awards, 2618
St. Joseph Comm Health Fndn Burn Care and Prevention Grants, 3367

Business
Aladdin Industries Fndn Grants, 322
Archer Daniels Midland Fndn Grants, 525
ARCO Fndn Education Grants, 526
AT&T Fndn Civic and Comm Service Grants, 658
Beldon Fund Grants, 738
Boyd Gaming Corp Contributions Program, 788
Castle Rock Fndn Grants, 888
Charles G. Koch Charitable Fndn Grants, 965
Collins C. Diboll Private Fndn Grants, 1057
Deland Fellowships in Health Care and Society, 1214
Duke Energy Fndn Grants, 1339
E.L. Wiegand Fndn Grants, 1361
ExxonMobil Grants, 1442
Ford Motor Company Fund Grants, 1522
Graco Fndn Grants, 1642
John Ben Snow Memorial Trust Grants, 1928
Kenny's Kids Grants, 1990
Lincoln Financial Group Fndn Grants, 2058
Max Bell Fndn Grants, 2134
McMurry Fndn Grants, 2149
New York Life Fndn Grants, 2304
Phoenix Suns Charities Grants, 3030
Procter and Gamble Fund Grants, 3083
Prudential Fndn Grants, 3087
United Technologies Corp Grants, 3466

Business Administration
Advocate HealthCare Post Graduate Administrative Fellowship, 241
American Academy of Nursing Claire M. Fagin Fellowships, 415
American Academy of Nursing Mayday Fund Grants, 416
American Academy of Nursing MBA Scholarships, 417
Canada-U.S. Fulbright New Century Scholars Grants, 846
Canada-U.S. Fulbright Senior Specialists Grants, 847
Cargill Citizenship Fund-Corp Giving Grants, 865
Fulbright Alumni Initiatives Awards Grants, 1566
Fulbright Distinguished Chairs Grants, 1567
Fulbright New Century Scholars Grants, 1570
Fulbright Specialists Grants, 1571
Fulbright Traditional Scholar Program in Europe and Eurasia, 1572
Fulbright Traditional Scholar Program in Sub-Saharan Africa, 1573
Fulbright Traditional Scholar Program in the East Asia/Pacific Region, 1574
Fulbright Traditional Scholar Program in the Near East and North Africa Region, 1575
Fulbright Traditional Scholar Program in the South and Central Asia Region, 1576
Fulbright Traditional Scholar Program in the Western Hemisphere, 1577
William G. McGowan Charitable Fund Grants, 3539

Business Development
Arkansas Comm Fndn Arkansas Black Hall of Fame Grants, 532
Bailey Fndn Grants, 680
Boyd Gaming Corp Contributions Program, 788
Frey Fndn Grants, 1562
General Motors Fndn Grants Support Program, 1591
Grand Haven Area Comm Fndn Grants, 1644
Harold Alfond Fndn Grants, 1695
Helen Bader Fndn Grants, 1738
Humboldt Area Fndn Technical Assistance Program Grants, 1819
Indiana 21st Century Research and Technology Fund Awards, 1850
Northern Trust Company Charitable Trust and Corp Giving Program, 2865
Pulaski County Comm Fndn Grants, 3091
Southbury Comm Trust Fund, 3350
U.S. Department of Education Vocational Rehabilitation Services Projects for American Indians with Disabilities Grants, 3452

Business Education
3M Fndn Grants, 11
Abell-Hanger Fndn Grants, 183
Alcoa Fndn Grants, 334
Allstate Corp Giving Grants, 363
Allstate Corp Hometown Commitment Grants, 364
American Academy of Nursing Claire M. Fagin Fellowships, 415
American Academy of Nursing Mayday Fund Grants, 416
American Academy of Nursing MBA Scholarships, 417
AMI Semiconductors Corp Grants, 468

Benton Comm Fndn Grants, 743
Blackford County Comm Fndn Grants, 763
Blue River Comm Fndn Grants, 770
Boettcher Fndn Grants, 778
Bright Family Fndn Grants, 793
Brown County Comm Fndn Grants, 807
Chazen Fndn Grants, 978
Coca-Cola Fndn Grants, 1052
Comm Fndn of Bartholomew County Heritage Fund Grants, 1096
Comm Fndn of Bartholomew County James A. Henderson Award for Fund-Raising, 1097
Comm Fndn of Boone County Grants, 1099
Comm Fndn of Greater Fort Wayne: Comm Endowment & Clarke Endowment Grants, 1108
Consumers Energy Fndn, 1147
D.F. Halton Fndn Grants, 1181
DaimlerChrysler Corp Fund Grants, 1186
F.M. Kirby Fndn Grants, 1443
FMC Fndn Grants, 1518
GenCorp Fndn Grants, 1587
General Motors Fndn Grants Support Program, 1591
James M. Collins Fndn Grants, 1891
Monfort Family Fndn Grants, 2213
Olin Corp Charitable Trust Grants, 2943
Richard and Helen DeVos Fndn Grants, 3157
Sid W. Richardson Fndn Grants, 3284
Wayne and Gladys Valley Fndn Grants, 3522
William G. McGowan Charitable Fund Grants, 3539

Cable Television
Cable Positive's Tony Cox Comm Fund Grants, 827

Campaign Finance Reform
Joyce Fndn Grants, 1969

Canada
CCFF Scholarships, 895
CCFF Small Conference Grants, 896
CCFF Summer Studentship, 898
CCFF Visiting Scientist Awards, 900
Fulbright Traditional Scholar Program in the Western Hemisphere, 1577
Max Bell Fndn Grants, 2134
NIA Postdoctoral Training in Research on Aging in Canada, 2426
RSC Jason A. Hannah Medal, 3196

Canadian Studies
Canada-U.S. Fulbright New Century Scholars Grants, 846
Canada-U.S. Fulbright Senior Specialists Grants, 847

Cancer
AEGON Transamerica Fndn Grants, 243
Partnership for Cures Two Years To Cures Grants, 2992

Cancer Detection
1 in 9: Long Island Breast Cancer Action Coalition Grants, 1
2COBS Private Charitable Fndn Grants, 9
A/H Fndn Grants, 19
AACR Award for Lifetime Achievement in Cancer Research, 66
AACR Award for Outstanding Achievement in Chemistry in Cancer Research, 68
AACR Brigid G. Leventhal Scholar in Cancer Research Awards, 69
AACR Centennial Postdoctoral Fellowships in Cancer Research, 71
AACR Centennial Pre-doctoral Fellowships in Cancer Research, 72
AACR Fellows Grants, 74
AACR G.H.A. Clowes Memorial Award, 75
AACR Gertrude Elion Cancer Research Award, 76
AACR Henry Shepard Bladder Cancer Research Grants, 77
AACR Joseph H. Burchenal Memorial Award, 78
AACR Kirk A. Landon and Dorothy P. Landon Fndn Prizes, 80
AACR Margaret Foti Award for Leadership and Extraordinary Achievements in Cancer Research, 81
AACR Minority Scholar in Cancer Research Awards, 82
AACR Minority-Serving Institution Faculty Scholar in Cancer Research Awards, 83
AACR Outstanding Investigator Award for Breast Cancer Research, 84
AACR Princess Takamatsu Memorial Lectureship, 85
AACR Team Science Award, 89
AACR-American Cancer Society Award for Research Excellence in Cancer Epidemiology and Prevention, 91
AACR-Colorectal Cancer Coalition Fellows Grant, 92
AACR-FNAB Fellows Grant for Translational Pancreatic Cancer Research, 93
AACR-FNAB Fellows Grant for Translational Pancreatic Cancer Research, 94
AACR-FNAB Fndn Career Development Award for Translational Cancer Research, 95
AACR-Genentech BioOncology Career Development Award for Cancer Research on the HER Family Pathway, 96
AACR-Genentech BioOncology Fellowship for Cancer Research in Angiogenesis, 97
AACR-GlaxoSmithKline Clinical Cancer Research Scholar Awards, 98
AACR-National Brain Tumor Fndn Fellows Grant, 100
AACR-NCI International Investigator Opportunity Grants, 101
AACR-Pancreatic Cancer Action Network Career Development Award for Pancreatic Cancer Research, 102
AACR-Pancreatic Cancer Action Network Innovative Grants, 103
AACR-Prevent Cancer Fndn Award for Excellence in Cancer Prevention Research, 104
AACR-WICR Scholar Awards, 105
ACGT Young Investigator Grants, 205
American-Italian Cancer Fndn Fellowships, 459
Angel Kiss Fndn Grants, 472
Angels Baseball Fndn Grants, 473
Ann and Robert H. Lurie Family Fndn Grants, 475
Avon Fndn Breast Care Fund Grants, 674
Avon Products Fndn Grants, 675
Balfe Family Fndn Grants, 682
Breast Cancer Fund Grants, 790
CDC Cancer Prevention and Control Programs, 903
CDC Increasing Breast and Cervical Cancer Screening Services for Urban American Indian/ Alaska Native Women, 912
CDC National Breast and Cervical Cancer Early Detection Program, 917
Charlotte Geyer Fndn Cancer Research Grants, 974
CMA Fndn Grants, 1042
Coleman Fndn Cancer Care Grants, 1055
Damon Runyon Cancer Fndn Fellowships, 1193
FDHN Funderburg Research Scholar Award in Gastric Biology Related to Cancer, 1471
Fndn of CVPH Chelsea's Rainbow Fund Grants, 1539
General Motors Fndn Grants Support Program, 1591
IARC Expertise Transfer Fellowship, 1831
IARC Postdoctoral Fellowships for Training in Cancer Research, 1832
IARC Visiting Scientist Award for Senior Scientists, 1833
International Cancer Technology Transfer Fellowships, 1858
James S. McDonnell Fndn Brain Cancer Research Collaborative Activity Awards, 1896
Littlefield-AACR Grants in Metastatic Colon Cancer Research, 2061
Lustgarten Fndn for Pancreatic Cancer Research Grants, 2086
Mary Kay Ash Charitable Fndn Grants, 2120
Morgan Adams Fndn Grants, 2216
NCI Diet, Epigenetic Events, and Cancer Prevention Grants, 2272
NIH Biology, Development, and Progression of Malignant Prostate Disease Research Grants, 2641
NIH Economic Studies in Cancer Prevention, Screening, and Care, 2657
NIH Molecular Epidemiology of Prostate Carcinogenesis Grants, 2691
NYCT Biomedical Research Grants, 2920
Paul Marks Prizes for Cancer Research, 3002
Pediatric Cancer Research Fndn Grants, 3013
Pezcoller Fndn-AACR International Award for Cancer Research, 3023
Prostate Cancer Fndn Research Grants, 3086
Ryan Gibson Fndn Grants, 3234
UICC American Cancer Society International Fellowships for Beginning Investigators, 3455
Varian Medical Systems Grants, 3481
W. C. Griffith Fndn Grants, 3505

Cancer Prevention
1 in 9: Long Island Breast Cancer Action Coalition Grants, 1
2COBS Private Charitable Fndn Grants, 9
A/H Fndn Grants, 19
AACR Award for Lifetime Achievement in Cancer Research, 66
AACR Award for Outstanding Achievement in Chemistry in Cancer Research, 68
AACR Brigid G. Leventhal Scholar in Cancer Research Awards, 69
AACR Career Development Awards for Pediatric Cancer Research, 70
AACR Centennial Postdoctoral Fellowships in Cancer Research, 71
AACR Centennial Pre-doctoral Fellowships in Cancer Research, 72
AACR Clinical and Translational Research Fellowships, 73
AACR Fellows Grants, 74
AACR G.H.A. Clowes Memorial Award, 75
AACR Gertrude Elion Cancer Research Award, 76
AACR Henry Shepard Bladder Cancer Research Grants, 77
AACR Joseph H. Burchenal Memorial Award, 78
AACR Judah Folkman Career Development Award for Anti-Angiogenesis Research, 79
AACR Kirk A. Landon and Dorothy P. Landon Fndn Prizes, 80
AACR Margaret Foti Award for Leadership and Extraordinary Achievements in Cancer Research, 81
AACR Minority Scholar in Cancer Research Awards, 82
AACR Minority-Serving Institution Faculty Scholar in Cancer Research Awards, 83
AACR Outstanding Investigator Award for Breast Cancer Research, 84
AACR Princess Takamatsu Memorial Lectureship, 85
AACR Team Science Award, 89
AACR-American Cancer Society Award for Research Excellence in Cancer Epidemiology and Prevention, 91
AACR-Colorectal Cancer Coalition Fellows Grant, 92
AACR-FNAB Fellows Grant for Translational Pancreatic Cancer Research, 93
AACR-FNAB Fellows Grant for Translational Pancreatic Cancer Research, 94
AACR-FNAB Fndn Career Development Award for Translational Cancer Research, 95
AACR-Genentech BioOncology Career Development Award for Cancer Research on the HER Family Pathway, 96
AACR-Genentech BioOncology Fellowship for Cancer Research in Angiogenesis, 97
AACR-GlaxoSmithKline Clinical Cancer Research Scholar Awards, 98
AACR-National Brain Tumor Fndn Fellows Grant, 100

AACR-NCI International Investigator Opportunity Grants, 101
AACR-Pancreatic Cancer Action Network Career Development Award for Pancreatic Cancer Research, 102
AACR-Pancreatic Cancer Action Network Innovative Grants, 103
AACR-Prevent Cancer Fndn Award for Excellence in Cancer Prevention Research, 104
AACR-WICR Scholar Awards, 105
AACR Basic Cancer Research Fellowships , 107
ACGT Young Investigator Grants, 205
American-Italian Cancer Fndn Fellowships, 459
Angel Kiss Fndn Grants, 472
Angels Baseball Fndn Grants, 473
Ann and Robert H. Lurie Family Fndn Grants, 475
ASCO Improving Cancer Care Grants, 546
ASCO State Affiliate Grants, 547
ASCO Advanced Clinical Research Award in Colorectal Cancer, 548
ASCO Advanced Clinical Research Awards in Breast Cancer, 549
ASCO Advanced Clinical Research Awards in Sarcoma, 550
ASCO Comm Oncology Research Grants, 552
ASCO Comparative Effectiveness Research Professorship in Breast Cancer, 553
ASCO Loan Repayment Grants, 555
ASCO Long-Term International Fellowships, 556
ASCO Medical Student Rotation Grants, 557
ASCO Translational Research Professorships, 561
Balfe Family Fndn Grants, 682
Bill and Melinda Gates Fndn Grants, 756
Breast Cancer Fund Grants, 790
CDC Cancer Prevention and Control Programs, 903
CDC Increasing Breast and Cervical Cancer Screening Services for Urban American Indian/ Alaska Native Women, 912
CDC National Breast and Cervical Cancer Early Detection Program, 917
Charlotte Geyer Fndn Cancer Research Grants, 974
Coleman Fndn Cancer Care Grants, 1055
Comm Fndn of Broward Grants, 1100
Cowles Charitable Trust Grants, 1155
Damon Runyon Cancer Fndn Fellowships, 1193
Fairlawn Fndn Grants, 1447
FDHN Funderburg Research Scholar Award in Gastric Biology Related to Cancer, 1471
Fndn of CVPH Chelsea's Rainbow Fund Grants, 1539
Georgia Power Fndn Grants, 1603
Gerber Fndn Grants, 1606
Greenfield Fndn of Maine Grants, 1663
Greenwall Fndn Bioethics Grants, 1665
Gregory Family Fndn Grants (Florida), 1667
IARC Expertise Transfer Fellowship, 1831
IARC Postdoctoral Fellowships for Training in Cancer Research, 1832
IARC Visiting Scientist Award for Senior Scientists, 1833
International Cancer Technology Transfer Fellowships, 1858
James S. McDonnell Fndn Brain Cancer Research Collaborative Activity Awards, 1896
Kimmel Scholar Award, 2002
Landon Fndn-AACR Innovator Award for International Collaboration, 2028
Landon Fndn-AACR Innovator Award for Cancer Prevention Research, 2029
Leukemia & Lymphoma Society Research Grants, 2051
Littlefield-AACR Grants in Metastatic Colon Cancer Research, 2061
Mary Kay Ash Charitable Fndn Grants, 2120
Milheim Fndn Cancer Research Grants, 2200
Morgan Adams Fndn Grants, 2216
NCI Basic Cancer Research in Cancer Health Disparities Grants, 2271
NCI Diet, Epigenetic Events, and Cancer Prevention Grants, 2272
NCI Exploratory Grants for Behavioral Research in Cancer Control, 2274
NIDCR Priorities in Behavioral Research in Cancer Prevention and Control Grants, 2538
NIH Economic Studies in Cancer Prevention, Screening, and Care, 2657
NIH Molecular Epidemiology of Prostate Carcinogenesis Grants, 2691
NYCT Biomedical Research Grants, 2920
OSI Palliative Cancer Care Grants, 2970
Paul Marks Prizes for Cancer Research, 3002
Pediatric Cancer Research Fndn Grants, 3013
Pezcoller Fndn-AACR International Award for Cancer Research, 3023
Prostate Cancer Fndn Research Grants, 3086
Ryan Gibson Fndn Grants, 3234
Susan G. Komen Breast Cancer Fndn Breast Health, Breast Cancer Education, and Outreach Programs Grants, 3408
UICC American Cancer Society International Fellowships for Beginning Investigators, 3455
Varian Medical Systems Grants, 3481
W. C. Griffith Fndn Grants, 3505

Cancer/Carcinogenesis

2COBS Private Charitable Fndn Grants, 9
AACR Award for Lifetime Achievement in Cancer Research, 66
AACR Award for Outstanding Achievement in Cancer Research, 67
AACR Award for Outstanding Achievement in Chemistry in Cancer Research, 68
AACR Career Development Awards for Pediatric Cancer Research, 70
AACR Centennial Postdoctoral Fellowships in Cancer Research, 71
AACR Centennial Pre-doctoral Fellowships in Cancer Research, 72
AACR Clinical and Translational Research Fellowships, 73
AACR Fellows Grants, 74
AACR G.H.A. Clowes Memorial Award, 75
AACR Gertrude Elion Cancer Research Award, 76
AACR Henry Shepard Bladder Cancer Research Grants, 77
AACR Joseph H. Burchenal Memorial Award, 78
AACR Judah Folkman Career Development Award for Anti-Angiogenesis Research, 79
AACR Kirk A. Landon and Dorothy P. Landon Fndn Prizes, 80
AACR Margaret Foti Award for Leadership and Extraordinary Achievements in Cancer Research, 81
AACR Minority Scholar in Cancer Research Awards, 82
AACR Minority-Serving Institution Faculty Scholar in Cancer Research Awards, 83
AACR Outstanding Investigator Award for Breast Cancer Research, 84
AACR Princess Takamatsu Memorial Lectureship, 85
AACR Richard and Hinda Rosenthal Memorial Awards, 86
AACR Team Science Award, 89
AACR-American Cancer Society Award for Research Excellence in Cancer Epidemiology and Prevention, 91
AACR-Colorectal Cancer Coalition Fellows Grant, 92
AACR-FNAB Fellows Grant for Translational Pancreatic Cancer Research, 93
AACR-FNAB Fellows Grant for Translational Pancreatic Cancer Research, 94
AACR-FNAB Fndn Career Development Award for Translational Cancer Research, 95
AACR-Genentech BioOncology Career Development Award for Cancer Research on the HER Family Pathway, 96
AACR-GlaxoSmithKline Clinical Cancer Research Scholar Awards, 98
AACR-Minorities in Cancer Research Jane Cooke Wright Lectureship Awards, 99
AACR-National Brain Tumor Fndn Fellows Grant, 100
AACR-NCI International Investigator Opportunity Grants, 101
AACR-Pancreatic Cancer Action Network Career Development Award for Pancreatic Cancer Research, 102
AACR-Pancreatic Cancer Action Network Innovative Grants, 103
AACR-Prevent Cancer Fndn Award for Excellence in Cancer Prevention Research, 104
AACR-WICR Scholar Awards, 105
AACR-Women in Cancer Research Charlotte Friend Memorial Lectureship Awards, 106
AACR Basic Cancer Research Fellowships , 107
ACGT Investigators Grants, 204
ACGT Young Investigator Grants, 205
ACS Master's Training Grants in Clinical Oncology Social Work, 208
ACS Cancer Control Career Development Awards for Primary Care Physicians, 209
ACS Clinical Research Professor Grants, 210
ACS Doctoral Degree Scholarships in Cancer Nursing, 211
ACS Doctoral Scholarships in Cancer Nursing, 212
ACS Doctoral Training Grants in Oncology Social Work, 213
ACS Graduate Scholarships in Cancer Nursing Practice, 214
ACS Institutional Research Grants, 215
ACS MEN2 Thyroid Cancer Professorship Grants, 216
ACS Mentored Research Scholar Grant in Applied and Clinical Research, 217
ACS Physician Training Awards in Preventive Medicine, 218
ACS Pilot and Exploratory Projects in Palliative Care of Cancer Patients and Their Families Grants, 219
ACS Postdoctoral Fellowships, 220
ACS Research Professor Grants, 221
ACS Research Scholar Grants for Health Services and Health Policy Research, 222
ACS Research Scholar Grants in Basic, Preclinical, Clinical and Epidemiology Research, 223
ACS Research Scholar Grants in Psychosocial and Behavioral and Cancer Control Research, 224
Affymetrix Corp Contributions Grants, 258
AJCC Cancer Staging Grants, 320
Alexander and Margaret Stewart Trust Grants, 340
AMA Fndn Seed Grants for Research, 398
American-Italian Cancer Fndn Fellowships, 459
Andersen Fndn Grants, 471
Angels Baseball Fndn Grants, 473
ArvinMeritor Fndn Health Grants, 543
ASCO Improving Cancer Care Grants, 546
ASCO State Affiliate Grants, 547
ASCO Advanced Clinical Research Award in Colorectal Cancer, 548
ASCO Advanced Clinical Research Awards in Breast Cancer, 549
ASCO Advanced Clinical Research Awards in Sarcoma, 550
ASCO Career Development Award, 551
ASCO Comm Oncology Research Grants, 552
ASCO Comparative Effectiveness Research Professorship in Breast Cancer, 553
ASCO Loan Repayment Grants, 555
ASCO Long-Term International Fellowships, 556
ASCO Medical Student Rotation Grants, 557
ASCO Merit Awards, 558
ASCO Resident Travel Awards, 559
ASCO State Affiliate Grants, 560
ASCO Translational Research Professorships, 561
ASCO Young Investigator Award, 562
ASCO/UICC International Cancer Technology Transfer (ICRETT) Fellowships, 563
Bodenwein Public Benevolent Fndn Grants, 775
Booth-Bricker Fund Grants, 780
Bristol-Myers Squibb Fndn Health Disparities Grants, 797
Cancer Research Postdoctoral Fellowships for Basic and Physician Scientists, 856

Cancer Research Society Fellowships and Grants, 857
Cancer Research UK Fellowships, 858
Cancer Research UK Grants, 859
Cancer Society of New Zealand Grants, 860
Cancer Treatment Research Fndn Clinical Investigation Grants, 861
CDC Cancer Prevention and Control Programs, 903
CDC National Breast and Cervical Cancer Early Detection Program, 917
CF Clinical Research Trainee Awards, 940
Charles Lafitte Fndn Grants, 970
Charlotte Geyer Fndn Cancer Research Grants, 974
Chestnut Hill Charitable Fndn, Inc Grants, 987
Chicago Board of Trade Fndn Grants, 988
Chicago White Metal Charitable Fndn Grants, 992
Children's Medical Research Institute Grants, 1000
Chiron Fndn Comm Grants, 1004
CIIT Postdoctoral Fellowships, 1012
Coleman Fndn Cancer Care Grants, 1055
Comm Fndn of Broward Grants, 1100
Constellation Energy Group and Baltimore Gas and Electric Corp Contributions, 1146
Cooper Industries Fndn Grants, 1150
Coors Brewing Corp Contributions Grants, 1151
CRH Fndn Grants, 1160
CRI Clinical Investigator Award in Cancer Immunology, 1161
CRI Postdoctoral Fellowships, 1162
CRI Prostate Cancer Initiative Grants, 1163
D.F. Halton Fndn Grants, 1181
Damon Runyon Cancer Fndn Fellowships, 1193
Dermatology Research Career Development Awards, 1238
DeRoy Testamentary Fndn Grants, 1239
DHHS Priority Health Conditions Studies Initiative, 1273
DOD Breast Cancer Center of Excellence Award, 1290
DOD Clinical Translational Research Grants, 1291
DOD Era of Hope Scholar Award, 1292
DOD HBCU/MI Partnership Training Award, 1293
DOD Idea Award for Breast Cancer Research, 1294
DOD Multidisciplinary Postdoctoral Award for Breast Cancer Research, 1295
DOD Predoctoral Traineeship in Breast Cancer Research, 1296
Doris Duke Charitable Fndn Clinical Scientist Development Award, 1316
Duchossois Family Fndn Grants, 1337
E.L. Wiegand Fndn Grants, 1361
Educational Fndn of America Grants, 1372
Elizabeth McGraw Fndn Grants, 1399
Elsa U. Pardee Fndn Grants, 1407
Emerson Charitable Trust Grants, 1412
Emma B. Howe Memorial Fndn Grants, 1415
ExxonMobil Grants, 1442
Fannie E. Rippel Fndn Grants, 1452
Farmers Insurance Group of Companies Grants, 1455
FIC International Cooperative Biodiversity Groups Grants, 1487
FIC Israeli Ministry of Health Postdoctoral Research Fellowships, 1494
Fondren Fndn Grants, 1520
Fndn for Medical Research Grants, 1528
General Motors Fndn Grants Support Program, 1591
Georgia Power Fndn Grants, 1603
Greenspun Family Fndn Grants, 1664
Greenwall Fndn Bioethics Grants, 1665
Hagedorn Fund Grants, 1685
Hawaii Comm Fndn Health Education and Research Grants, 1716
Hearst Fndn and William Randolph Hearst Fndn Grants, 1730
HHMI Biomedical Research Grants for International Scientists in Canada and Latin America, 1756
HHMI Biomedical Research Grants for International Scientists in the Baltics, Central and Eastern Europe, Russia, and Ukraine, 1757
HHMI Biomedical Research Grants for International Scientists: Infectious Diseases and Parasitology, 1758
Hillman Fndn Grants, 1775
HomeBanc Fndn Grants, 1788
Horizon Fndn for New Jersey Grants, 1793
IARC Expertise Transfer Fellowship, 1831
IARC Postdoctoral Fellowships for Training in Cancer Research, 1832
IARC Visiting Scientist Award for Senior Scientists, 1833
Innovative Technology Development Awards, 1855
International Cancer Technology Transfer Fellowships, 1858
International Oncology Nursing Fellowships, 1862
James S. McDonnell Fndn Brain Cancer Research Collaborative Activity Awards, 1896
James S. McDonnell Fndn Research Grants, 1898
Jane Coffin Childs Memorial Fund for Medical Research Fellowships, 1903
John S. Dunn Research Fndn Grants and Chairs, 1945
K21 Health Fndn Cancer Care Fund Grants, 1975
Kimmel Scholar Award, 2002
Komen Greater NYC Clinical Trials Enrollment Grants, 2010
Komen Greater NYC Comm Breast Health Grants, 2011
Komen Greater NYC Conference Grants, 2012
Lance Armstrong Fndn Comm Grants, 2025
Lance Armstrong Fndn Research Grants, 2026
Landon Fndn-AACR Innovator Award for International Collaboration, 2028
Landon Fndn-AACR Innovator Award for Cancer Prevention Research, 2029
Leo Goodwin Fndn Grants, 2043
Leukemia and Lymphoma Society Research Grants, 2051
Lillian S. Wells Fndn Grants, 2056
Littlefield-AACR Grants in Metastatic Colon Cancer Research, 2061
Louis R. Cappelli Fndn Grants, 2066
LSA Fellowships, 2073
LSA Scholar Award for Clinical Research, 2074
LSA Scholar Awards, 2075
LSA Special Fellowships, 2076
LSA Specialized Center of Research Grants, 2077
Lustgarten Fndn for Pancreatic Cancer Research Grants, 2086
Lymphoma Research Fndn Grants, 2088
Marshall Field's Comm Grants, 2115
Mary Kay Ash Charitable Fndn Grants, 2120
Melanoma Research Fndn Grants, 2170
Mesothelioma Applied Research Fndn Grants, 2174
Milheim Fndn Cancer Research Grants, 2200
MMRF Research Grants, 2211
NCI Academic-Industrial Partnerships for Development and Validation of In Vivo Imaging Systems and Methods for Cancer Investigations, 2268
NCI Application and Use of Transformative Emerging Technologies in Cancer Research, 2269
NCI Basic Cancer Research in Cancer Health Disparities Grants, 2271
NCI Engineered Isogenic Cell Lines with Relevant Cancer Targets Research Grants, 2273
NCI Exploratory Grants for Behavioral Research in Cancer Control, 2274
NCI Stages of Breast Development: Normal to Metastatic Disease Grants, 2278
NCI Technologies and Software to Support Integrative Cancer Biology Research Grants, 2279
NCIC Canadian Breast Cancer Research Initiative Grants, 2281
NCIC Canadian Cancer Society Research Grants, 2282
NCIC Canadian Cancer Society Travel Award for Senior Level PhD Students, 2283
NCIC Equipment Grants, 2284
NCIC Terry Fox Postdoctoral Research Fellowships, 2285
NCIC Terry Fox Research Studentships, 2286
Nell Warren Elkin and William Simpson Elkin Fndn, 2302
NIA Prostate Cancer Aging, Race, and Ethnicity Research Grants, 2428
NIEHS Applied Toxicological Research and Testing Grants, 2595
NIEHS Biological Response to Environmental Health Hazards Research Grants, 2596
NIEHS Carcinogenicity of Drinking Water Disinfection By-Products, 2597
NIEHS Small Business Innovation Research Grants, 2605
NIH Cancer Surveillance Using Health Claims-Based Data System Grants, 2645
NIH Economic Studies in Cancer Prevention, Screening, and Care, 2657
NIH Mechanisms Underlying Individual Variations in Drug Responses, 2685
NIH Molecular Epidemiology of Prostate Carcinogenesis Grants, 2691
NIH Small Business Innovation Research: Animal Models of HCV Infection Research Grants, 2728
NIH/EPA Mechanistic-Based Cancer Risk Assessment Methods Research Grants, 2741
NINDS Cerebral Radiobiology and Neuroimaging of Brain Tumors Research Grants, 2778
NINR Aging Women and Breast Cancer Grants, 2789
NYCT Biomedical Research Grants, 2920
Oracle Corp Contributions Grants, 2951
OSI Palliative Cancer Care Grants, 2970
Pancreatic Cancer Action Network-AACR Fellowship, 2987
Pancreatic Cancer Action Network-AACR Pathway to Leadership Grants, 2988
Paul Marks Prizes for Cancer Research, 3002
Pediatric Cancer Research Fndn Grants, 3013
Pezcoller Fndn-AACR International Award for Cancer Research, 3023
Pittsburgh Fndn Medical Research Grants, 3055
Premera CARES Grants, 3074
Prostate Cancer Fndn Research Grants, 3086
Russell Berrie Fndn Grants, 3201
Samuel Freeman Charitable Trust Grants, 3249
Skin Cancer Fndn Research Grants, 3298
Smith Family New Investigator Awards, 3299
Susan G. Komen Breast Cancer Fndn Basic, Clinical, and Translational Research Grants, 3407
Susan G. Komen Breast Cancer Fndn Interdisciplinary Fellowships, 3410
Susan G. Komen Breast Cancer Fndn Postdoctoral Fellowships, 3411
Thompson Charitable Fndn Grants, 3425
UICC American Cancer Society International Fellowships for Beginning Investigators, 3455
UICC International Cancer Technology Transfer (ICRETT) Fellowships, 3456
UICC Raisa Gorbachev Memorial International Cancer Fellowships, 3457
UICC Yamagiwa-Yoshida Memorial International Cancer Study Grants, 3458
Varian Medical Systems Grants, 3481
VFW Ladies Auxiliary Cancer Research Postdoctoral Fellowships, 3494
W. C. Griffith Fndn Grants, 3505
W.W. Smith Charitable Trust Grants for Medical Research in Cancer, AIDS, and Heart Disease, 3509
Wilhelm Sander Fndn Grants, 3535
William G. McGowan Charitable Fund Grants, 3539

Carbohydrates

American Chemical Society Claude S. Hudson Awards, 419

Cardiology

Abbott Fund Science and Medical Innovation Grants, 179
ACCP Heart Failure Training Grants, 198
AFAR Research Grants, 257
Duke University Clinical Cardiac Electrophysiology Fellowships, 1342

Duke University Interventional Cardiology Fellowships, 1344
Genentech Corp Charitable Contributions Grants, 1588
Heart Rhythm Society Fellowships, 1731
Joseph Drown Fndn Grants, 1960
Margoes Fndn Grants, 2106
Nell Warren Elkin and William Simpson Elkin Fndn, 2302
NHLBI Ancillary Studies in Clinical Trials, 2317
NHLBI Cardiac Development Consortium Grants, 2323
NHLBI Cardiac Translational Research Implementation Grants, 2324
NHLBI Pediatric Cardiac Genomics Consortium Grants, 2364
NHLBI Research on the Role of Cardiomyocyte Mitochondria in Heart Disease: An Integrated Approach, 2372

Cardiomyocyte Mitochondria
NHLBI Research on the Role of Cardiomyocyte Mitochondria in Heart Disease: An Integrated Approach, 2372

Cardiovascular Diseases
Abbott Fund Science and Medical Innovation Grants, 179
Alcohol Misuse and Alcoholism Research Grants, 335
AMA Fndn Seed Grants for Research, 398
Andersen Fndn Grants, 471
Balfe Family Fndn Grants, 682
C.R. Bard Fndn Grants, 825
Cardiac Arrhythmias Research and Education Fndn Research Grants, 863
CDC Core Capacity Grants, 907
Chest Fndn/LUNGevity Fndn Clinical Research in Lung Cancer Grants, 986
Chestnut Hill Charitable Fndn, Inc Grants, 987
Children's Cardiomyopathy Fndn Research Grants, 1002
Compass Bank Fndn Grants, 1138
CVS All Kids Can Grants, 1175
D.F. Halton Fndn Grants, 1181
DeBakey Medical Fndn Fellowships and Scholarships, 1212
Dietetic Outcomes Research Study Grants, 1285
Doris Duke Charitable Fndn Clinical Scientist Development Award, 1316
Duke University Interventional Cardiology Fellowships, 1344
E.L. Wiegand Fndn Grants, 1361
Educational Fndn of America Grants, 1372
Emma B. Howe Memorial Fndn Grants, 1415
Fannie E. Rippel Fndn Grants, 1452
FIC International Cooperative Biodiversity Groups Grants, 1487
FIC Israeli Ministry of Health Postdoctoral Research Fellowships, 1494
Gerber Fndn Grants, 1606
Guidant Fndn Grants, 1674
Hawaii Comm Fndn Health Education and Research Grants, 1716
Jacob and Valeria Langeloth Fndn Grants, 1882
Japan Heart Fndn Grants, 1906
Johnson & Johnson Comm Health Care Grants, 1951
Lesbian Health Fund Grants, 2046
Medtronic Fndn Full Life Patient Partnership Program—Heart Rescue Grants, 2168
National Emergency Medicine Association Grants, 2252
National Heart Fndn of New Zealand Grants, 2255
Nell Warren Elkin and William Simpson Elkin Fndn, 2302
NHLBI Ancillary Studies in Clinical Trials, 2317
NHLBI Cardiac Development Consortium Grants, 2323
NHLBI Cardiac Translational Research Implementation Grants, 2324
NHLBI Career Transition Award, 2326
NHLBI Elucidating Nature's Solutions to Heart, Lung, and Blood Diseases and Sleep Disorder Processes Research Grants, 2333
NHLBI Improving Heart Failure Disease Management Grants, 2338
NHLBI Mentored Career Award For Faculty At Minority Institutions, 2346
NHLBI Minority Institution Research Scientist Development Award, 2354
NHLBI Minority Institutional Research Training Grants, 2355
NHLBI National Research Service Awards in Cardiovascular Epidemiology and Biostatistics, 2357
NHLBI Research on the Role of Cardiomyocyte Mitochondria in Heart Disease: An Integrated Approach, 2372
NHLBI Short-Term Research Education Program to Increase Diversity in Health-Related Research, 2383
NHLBI Stress Management Interventions to Reduce Risk of Coronary Artery Disease, 2384
NIEHS Biological Response to Environmental Health Hazards Research Grants, 2596
NIH Mechanisms Underlying Individual Variations in Drug Responses, 2685
NIH Research on Sleep and Sleep Disorders, 2713
Premera CARES Grants, 3074
RACGP Cardiovascular Research Grants in General Practice, 3099
Rich Fndn Grants, 3156
Saint Luke's Health Initiatives Grants, 3240
Smith Family New Investigator Awards, 3299
W.W. Smith Charitable Trust Grants for Medical Research in Cancer, AIDS, and Heart Disease, 3509
Wellmark Fndn Grants, 3526

Cardiovascular Health
Anthem Blue Cross and Blue Shield School Nurse Grants, 489

Cardiovascular System
CDC Core Capacity Grants, 907
Chest Fndn/LUNGevity Fndn Clinical Research in Lung Cancer Grants, 986
Children's Cardiomyopathy Fndn Research Grants, 1002
Duke University Interventional Cardiology Fellowships, 1344
NHLBI Cardiac Translational Research Implementation Grants, 2324
Simone and Cino del Duca Grand Prix Awards, 3288

Care Givers
Rosalynn Carter Institute Georgia Caregiver of the Year Awards, 3188

Career Education and Planning
Actors Fund Social Services and Financial Assistance, 225
Adaptec Fndn Grants, 232
AFAR Paul Beeson Career Development Awards in Aging Research for the Island of Ireland, 256
AHNS/AAO-HNSF Surgeon Scientist Combined Award, 307
AHNS/AAO-HNSF Young Investigator Combined Award, 308
AMD Corp Contributions Grants, 411
Chiron Fndn Comm Grants, 1004
Cleveland Browns Fndn Grants, 1036
Comer Fndn Grants, 1072
Comm Fndn of Greater Flint Grants, 1107
DaimlerChrysler Corp Fund Grants, 1186
Ford Motor Company Fund Grants, 1522
Hartford Aging and Health Program Awards, 1709
Highmark Corp Giving Grants, 1769
Lincoln Financial Group Fndn Grants, 2058
McCarthy Family Fndn Grants, 2141
NCI Mentored Career Development Award to Promote Diversity, 2276
NCI/NIDA Transdisciplinary Tobacco Use Research Centers Grants, 2280
NEI Scholars Program, 2298
New York Life Fndn Grants, 2304
NHGRI Mentored Research Scientist Development Award, 2315
NIA Mentored Research Scientist Development Award, 2418
NIEHS Mentored Research Scientist Development Award, 2603
NIGMS Institutional Research and Academic Career Development Award, 2614
NIH Transitional Career Development Award in Women's Health Research, 2736
NIMH Career Opportunities in Research Education and Training Honors High School Research Education Grant, 2748
NIMH Career Opportunities in Research Education and Training Honors Undergraduate Research Training Grant, 2749
NINR Mentored Research Scientist Development Award, 2798
Northrop Grumman Corp Grants, 2866
NSF Presidential Early Career Awards for Scientists and Engineers (PECASE) Grants, 2892
Piper Jaffray Companies Building Strong Communities Grants, 3053
RWJF Summer Medical and Dental Education Program, 3231
U.S. Department of Education 21st Century Comm Learning Centers, 3445

Caries
DHHS Oral Health Promotion Research Across the Lifespan, 1269
NIH Ruth L. Kirschstein National Research Service Awards for Individual Postdoctoral Fellows, 2719

Cataloging and Classification
ASM USFCC/J. Roger Porter Award, 623

Catalysis/Kinetics
ONR Human Performance Division Research Grants, 2948

Catholic Church
Anthony R. Abraham Fndn Grants, 490
Archer Daniels Midland Fndn Grants, 525
Booth-Bricker Fund Grants, 780
Carrie Estelle Doheny Fndn Grants, 883
Charles Delmar Fndn Grants, 963
Collins C. Diboll Private Fndn Grants, 1057
Connelly Fndn Grants, 1143
Eugene B. Casey Fndn Grants, 1433
Hackett Fndn Grants, 1684
Ida Alice Ryan Charitable Trust Grants, 1836
Kevin P. and Sydney B. Knight Family Fndn Grants, 1993
Marion I. and Henry J. Knott Fndn Grants, 2109
Raskob Fndn for Catholic Activities Grants, 3107
Thomas and Dorothy Leavey Fndn Grants, 3422
William H. Hannon Fndn Grants, 3540

Cell Death
NIA Aging, Oxidative Stress and Cell Death Grants, 2393

Central America
Fulbright Traditional Scholar Program in the Western Hemisphere, 1577

Cerebral Palsy
F.M. Kirby Fndn Grants, 1443
United Cerebral Palsy Research Grants, 3462

Chamber Music
Ann Arbor Area Comm Fndn Grants, 476
Clarence E. Heller Charitable Fndn Grants, 1022

Charter Schools
Achelis and Bodman Fndns Grants, 206

Chemical Dynamics
NSF Chemistry Research Experiences for Undergraduates, 2883

Chemical Engineering
Food, Pharmaceutical, and Bioengineering Division Award in Chemical Engineering, 1521
Lubrizol Fndn Grants, 2080
NSF-NIST Interaction in Chemistry, Materials Research, Molecular Biosciences, Bioengineering, and Chemical Engineering, 2897

Chemical Sciences
ExxonMobil Grants, 1442
PhRMA Fndn Informatics Sabbatical Fellows, 3035
PhRMA Fndn Informatics Research Starter Grants, 3038

Chemistry
AACR Award for Outstanding Achievement in Chemistry in Cancer Research, 68
AACR Team Science Award, 89
AHAF Alzheimer's Disease Research Grants, 266
Alfred P. Sloan Fndn Research Fellowships, 353
American Chemical Society Claude S. Hudson Awards, 419
American Chemical Society GCI Pharmaceutical Roundtable Research Grants, 420
Award in Separations Science and Technology, 677
Beckman Scholars Grants, 734
Beckman Young Investigators Grants, 735
BWF Career Awards at the Scientific Interface, 819
Canada Graduate Scholarships and NSERC Postgraduate Scholarships, 845
Canada-U.S. Fulbright New Century Scholars Grants, 846
Canada-U.S. Fulbright Senior Specialists Grants, 847
DOE Environmental Remediation Grants, 1297
FIC International Training and Research in Environmental and Occupational Health, 1493
Frederic Stanley Kipping Award in Silicon Chemistry, 1559
Fulbright Alumni Initiatives Awards Grants, 1566
Fulbright Distinguished Chairs Grants, 1567
Fulbright New Century Scholars Grants, 1570
Fulbright Specialists Grants, 1571
Fulbright Traditional Scholar Program in Europe and Eurasia, 1572
Fulbright Traditional Scholar Program in Sub-Saharan Africa, 1573
Fulbright Traditional Scholar Program in the East Asia/Pacific Region, 1574
Fulbright Traditional Scholar Program in the Near East and North Africa Region, 1575
Fulbright Traditional Scholar Program in the South and Central Asia Region, 1576
Fulbright Traditional Scholar Program in the Western Hemisphere, 1577
HHMI-NIBIB Interfaces Initiative Grants, 1764
Jeffress Research Grants, 1913
John Stauffer Charitable Trust Grants, 1946
Lubrizol Fndn Grants, 2080
Marion I. and Henry J. Knott Fndn Grants, 2109
Millipore Fndn Grants, 2203
NHGRI Mentored Research Scientist Development Award, 2315
North Carolina GlaxoSmithKline Fndn Grants, 2860
Northwood University/Alden B. Dow Creativity Center Summer Residency Program, 2871
NSF Chemistry Research Experiences for Undergraduates, 2883
Ralph F. Hirschmann Award in Peptide Chemistry, 3105
Searle Scholars Grants, 3275
Society of Cosmetic Chemists Allan B. Black Award Sponsored by Presperse, 3328
Society of Cosmetic Chemists Award Sponsored by McIntyre Group, Ltd., 3329
Society of Cosmetic Chemists Award Sponsored by The HallStar Company, 3330
Society of Cosmetic Chemists Chapter Best Speaker Award, 3331
Society of Cosmetic Chemists Chapter Merit Award, 3332
Society of Cosmetic Chemists Frontier of Science Award, 3333
Society of Cosmetic Chemists Hans Schaeffer Award, 3334
Society of Cosmetic Chemists Joseph P. Ciaudelli Award, 3335
Society of Cosmetic Chemists Keynote Award Lecture Sponsored by Ruger Chemical Corp, 3336
Society of Cosmetic Chemists Literature Award, 3337
Society of Cosmetic Chemists Maison G. de Navarre Medal, 3338
Society of Cosmetic Chemists Merit Award, 3339
Society of Cosmetic Chemists Robert A. Kramer Lifetime Service Award, 3340
Society of Cosmetic Chemists Shaw Mudge Award, 3341
Society of Cosmetic Chemists Student Poster Awards, 3342
Society of Cosmetic Chemists Young Scientist Awards, 3343
Supelco AOCS Research Award, 3405

Chemistry Education
FMC Fndn Grants, 1518
North Carolina GlaxoSmithKline Fndn Grants, 2860

Chemistry, Analytical
NSF Chemistry Research Experiences for Undergraduates, 2883

Chemistry, Environmental
Award for Creative Advances in Environmental Science and Technology, 676
NSF Chemistry Research Experiences for Undergraduates, 2883

Chemistry, Inorganic
Alfred Bader Award in BioInorganic or BioOrganic Chemistry, 350
NSF Chemistry Research Experiences for Undergraduates, 2883

Chemistry, Materials
NSF Chemistry Research Experiences for Undergraduates, 2883

Chemistry, Organic
Alfred Bader Award in BioInorganic or BioOrganic Chemistry, 350
NSF Chemistry Research Experiences for Undergraduates, 2883
PhRMA Fndn Pharmaceutics Postdoctoral Fellowships, 3040
PhRMA Fndn Pharmaceutics Pre Doctoral Fellowships, 3041

Chemistry, Physical
NIH Ruth L. Kirschstein National Research Service Awards for Individual Postdoctoral Fellows, 2719
NSF Chemistry Research Experiences for Undergraduates, 2883
PhRMA Fndn Pharmaceutics Postdoctoral Fellowships, 3040
PhRMA Fndn Pharmaceutics Pre Doctoral Fellowships, 3041

Chemistry, Separations
Award in Separations Science and Technology, 677

Chemistry, Surface
NSF Chemistry Research Experiences for Undergraduates, 2883

Chemopreventive Agents
DOD Clinical Translational Research Grants, 1291

Chemotherapy
ASM sanofi-aventis ICAAC Award, 616
DOD Clinical Translational Research Grants, 1291
Elsa U. Pardee Fndn Grants, 1407

Child Abuse
Baxter International Fndn Grants, 705
Burton G. Bettingen Grants, 813
Carl B. and Florence E. King Fndn Grants, 869
Carl C. Icahn Fndn Grants, 870
Charles Lafitte Fndn Grants, 970
Children's Advocacy Center Grants, 997
Children's Trust Fund of Oregon Grants, 1001
ConocoPhillips Fndn Grants, 1144
Dade Comm Fndn Grants, 1185
Delaware Comm Fndn-Youth Philanthropy Board for Kent County, 1216
Detroit Lions Charities Grants, 1241
DHHS Promoting Safe and Stable Families Grants, 1276
Doris and Victor Day Fndn Grants, 1313
Elliot Fndn Inc Grants, 1402
Faye McBeath Fndn Grants, 1456
Global Fund for Children Grants, 1629
Greater Bridgeport Area Fndn Comm Impact Grants, 1650
Greater Tacoma Comm Fndn Ryan Alan Hade Endowment Fund, 1657
Green Bay Packers Fndn Grants, 1660
Hanna Andersson Children's Fndn Grants, 1691
Hasbro Children's Fund, 1714
Hoglund Fndn Grants, 1785
Huie-Dellmon Trust Grants, 1815
Jane Bradley Pettit Fndn Grants, 1902
Jim Moran Fndn Grants, 1925
Kenny's Kids Grants, 1990
McGregor Fund Grants, 2143
Michael and Susan Dell Fndn Grants, 2189
NIH Career Development Awards: Child Abuse and Neglect Research, 2646
PacifiCare Fndn Grants, 2981
Peacock Fndn Grants, 3011
Questar Corp Contributions Grants, 3097
Reynolds and Reynolds Associate Fndn Grants, 3152
Southbury Comm Trust Fund, 3350
Topfer Family Fndn Grants, 3430

Child Care
Alexander and Margaret Stewart Trust Grants, 340

Child Development
Children's Trust Fund of Oregon Grants, 1001

Child Psychiatry
AACAP Beatrix A. Hamburg Award for the Best New Research Poster by a Child and Adolescent Psychiatry Resident, 30
AACAP Child and Adolescent Psychiatry Teaching Scholarships, 31
AACAP Congressional Fellowships, 32
AACAP Educational Outreach Program for Child and Adolescent Psychiatry Residents, 33
AACAP Educational Outreach Program for General Psychiatry Residents, 34
AACAP Elaine Schlosser Lewis Award for Research on Attention-Deficit Disorder, 35
AACAP George Tarjan Award for Contributions in Developmental Disabilities, 36
AACAP Irving Philips Award for Prevention, 37
AACAP Jeanne Spurlock Lecture and Award on Diversity and Culture, 38
AACAP Jeanne Spurlock Minority Medical Student Clinical Fellowship in Child and Adolescent Psychiatry, 39
AACAP Junior Investigator Awards, 41
AACAP Klingenstein Third Generation Fndn Award for Research in Depression or Suicide, 42
AACAP Norbert and Charlotte Rieger Award for Scientific Achievement, 43

AACAP Norbert and Charlotte Rieger Psychodynamic Psychotherapy Award, 44
AACAP Pilot Research Award for Attention-Deficit Disorder, Supported by the Elaine Schlosser Lewis Fund, 45
AACAP Pilot Research Awards, Supported by Eli Lilly and Company, 47
AACAP Quest for the Test Bipolar Disorder Pilot Research Award, 48
AACAP Rieger Service Program Award for Excellence, 49
AACAP Robert Cancro Academic Leadership Award, 50
AACAP Sidney Berman Award for the School-Based Study and Intervention for Learning Disorders and Mental Ilness, 51
AACAP Simon Wile Leadership in Consultation Award, 52
APF Call for Proposals, 505
APF James H. Scully Jr., M.D., Educational Fund Grants, 508
APF Typical or Troubled School Mental Health Education Grants, 510
Greater Tacoma Comm Fndn Ryan Alan Hade Endowment Fund, 1657
WHAS Crusade for Children Grants, 3531

Child Psychology/Development

AON Fndn Grants, 491
Assurant Fndn Grants, 654
Carnegie Corp of New York Grants, 879
Chestnut Hill Charitable Fndn, Inc Grants, 987
Chicago Board of Trade Fndn Grants, 988
Colorado Interstate Gas Grants, 1060
Comm Fndn of Greater New Britain Grants, 1111
Connecticut Comm Fndn Grants, 1141
Constellation Energy Group and Baltimore Gas and Electric Corp Contributions, 1146
CVS All Kids Can Grants, 1175
DHHS Emergency Medical Services for Children Program, 1249
DHHS Neurodevelopmental Test Methods Research Grants, 1268
EF Research and Training Fellowships for Clinicians, 1384
Effie and Wofford Cain Fndn Grants, 1385
Elizabeth Glaser Pediatric AIDS Fndn International Leadership Awards, 1393
Elizabeth Glaser Pediatric AIDS Fndn Operations Research Grants, 1394
Elizabeth Glaser Pediatric AIDS Fndn Two-Year International Scholar Award, 1396
FCD Child Development Grants, 1458
FIC Israeli Ministry of Health Postdoctoral Research Fellowships, 1494
Fndn for Seacoast Health Grants, 1533
George Family Fndn Grants, 1598
Gerber Fndn Grants, 1606
Harold Simmons Fndn Grants, 1698
Helen Bader Fndn Grants, 1738
Henrietta Tower Wurts Memorial Fndn Grants, 1745
Hoglund Fndn Grants, 1785
i2 Fndn Grants, 1829
Jeanne Humphrey Block Dissertation Award, 1912
John Merck Scholars Awards, 1941
Mericos Fndn Grants, 2172
Miriam and Peter Haas Fund Grants, 2208
NICHD Socioeconomic Status and Health Across the Life Course, 2495
NIEHS Small Business Innovation Research Grants, 2605
NIMH Early Identification and Treatment of Mental Disorders in Children and Adolescents Grants, 2756
NIMH Interventions Infrastructure Program Research Grants, 2760
NSF Perception, Action & Cognition Research Grants, 2890
NSF Social Psychology Research Grants, 2894
Pasadena Fndn Average Grants, 2994
Piper Jaffray Companies Building Strong Communities Grants, 3053
Robert and Polly Dunn Fndn Grants, 3168
Salem Fndn Charitable Trust Grants, 3241
Seabury Fndn Grants, 3274
WHAS Crusade for Children Grants, 3531
William T. Grant Fndn Research Grants, 3541

Child Sexual Abuse

ACF Standing Announcement for Unaccompanied Alien Children Grants, 202
Greater Tacoma Comm Fndn Ryan Alan Hade Endowment Fund, 1657
Michael and Susan Dell Fndn Grants, 2189
Reynolds and Reynolds Associate Fndn Grants, 3152

Child Welfare

1104 Fndn Grants, 3
Agnes M. Lindsay Trust Grants, 263
Allen P. and Josephine B. Green Fndn Grants, 361
Alliance Healthcare Fndn Grants, 362
Andersen Fndn Grants, 471
Ann Jackson Family Fndn Grants, 477
Atkinson Fndn International Grants, 661
Blum-Kovler Fndn Grants, 772
Bodenwein Public Benevolent Fndn Grants, 775
Bodman Fndn Grants, 776
Burton G. Bettingen Grants, 813
Caleb C. and Julia W. Dula Educational and Charitable Fndn Grants, 830
Carl B. and Florence E. King Fndn Grants, 869
Carl C. Icahn Fndn Grants, 870
Carls Fndn Grants, 876
Carolyn Fndn Grants, 880
Carrie Estelle Doheny Fndn Grants, 883
Charles Lafitte Fndn Grants, 970
Colonel Stanley R. McNeil Fndn Grants, 1059
Colorado Springs Comm Trust Fund Grants, 1061
Comm Fndn for Greater Buffalo Grants, 1090
Comm Fndn for Muskegon County Grants, 1093
D. W. McMillan Fndn Grants, 1180
Daniels Fund Grants, 1200
Detlef Schrempf Fndn Grants, 1240
DHHS Abandoned Infants Assistance Grants, 1242
DHHS Oral Health Promotion Research Across the Lifespan, 1269
Dorothea Haus Ross Fndn Grants, 1320
Hawaii Comm Fndn Reverend Takie Okumura Family Grants, 1717
Hoblitzelle Fndn Grants, 1783
J.W. Kieckhefer Fndn Grants, 1878
Janirve Fndn Grants, 1905
John H. and Wilhelmina D. Harland Charitable Fndn Grants, 1933
John I. Smith Charities Grants, 1935
Josephine Goodyear Fndn Grants, 1964
Katherine John Murphy Fndn Grants, 1983
Kathryne Beynon Fndn Grants, 1984
Kenny's Kids Grants, 1990
L. W. Pierce Family Fndn Grants, 2019
Leo Goodwin Fndn Grants, 2043
Lucile Horton Howe and Mitchell B. Howe Fndn Grants, 2081
Lucy Gooding Charitable Fndn Trust, 2082
Michael and Susan Dell Fndn Grants, 2189
Nuffield Fndn Children and Families Grants, 2899
Oakland Fund for Children and Youth Grants, 2930
Ruth Eleanor Bamberger and John Ernest Bamberger Memorial Fndn Grants, 3202
W. C. Griffith Fndn Grants, 3505
W.K. Kellogg Fndn Secure Families Grants, 3508
Walt Disney Company Fndn Grants, 3516

Child/Maternal Health

AAP Comm Access To Child Health Advocacy Training Grants, 157
AAP Comm Access to Child Health Planning Grants, 159
AAP Comm Access To Child Health Residency Training Grants, 160
AAP Comm Access To Child Health Resident Grants, 161
AAP Leonard P. Rome Comm Access to Child Health Visiting Professorships, 164
Abbott Fund Access to Health Care Grants, 176
AHRQ Independent Scientist Award, 313
Alcatel-Lucent Technologies Fndn Grants, 333
APF Jeanne Spurlock Congressional Fellowships, 509
Batchelor Fndn Grants, 701
BCBSNC Fndn Grants, 725
Ben B. Cheney Fndn Grants, 741
Bill and Melinda Gates Fndn Grants, 756
Blowitz-Ridgeway Fndn Grants, 767
California Endowment CommunitiesFirst Grants, 833
California Wellness Fndn Work and Health Grants, 834
CFF Research Grants, 947
Charles H. Dater Fndn Grants, 966
Charles H. Hood Fndn Child Health Research Grants, 968
Children Affected by AIDS Fndn Domestic Grants, 995
Children's Brain Tumor Fndn Research Grants, 998
Cleveland Browns Fndn Grants, 1036
Comm Fndn for Greater Buffalo Grants, 1090
Comm Toolbox for Children's Environmental Health Grants, 1137
Connecticut Health Fndn Initiative Grants, 1142
Dallas Women's Fndn Grants, 1191
DHHS Emergency Medical Services for Children Program, 1249
DHHS Health Centers Grants for Residents of Public Housing, 1254
DHHS Healthy Tomorrows Partnership for Children, 1261
DHHS HIV Demonstration Program for Children, Adolescents, and Women, 1262
DHHS Maternal and Child Health Projects Grants, 1263
DHHS Maternal and Child Health Research and Training Programs Grants, 1264
DHHS Public Health Students Traineeships and Other Graduate Public Health Programs, 1277
DHHS Technical and Non-Financial Assistance to Health Centers, 1280
DHHS Universal Newborn Hearing Screening and Intervention, 1282
Edwards Memorial Trust Grants, 1375
El Paso Comm Fndn Grants, 1388
Elizabeth Glaser Pediatric AIDS Fndn International Leadership Awards, 1393
Elizabeth Glaser Pediatric AIDS Fndn Operations Research Grants, 1394
Elizabeth Glaser Pediatric AIDS Fndn Pediatric HIV Vaccine Research Grants, 1395
Elizabeth Glaser Pediatric AIDS Fndn Two-Year International Scholar Award, 1396
EPA Children's Health Protection Grants, 1420
Express Scripts Fndn Grants, 1441
F.M. Kirby Fndn Grants, 1443
Fairlawn Fndn Grants, 1447
Flinn Fndn Grants Programs, 1511
Fndn for Seacoast Health Grants, 1533
Frances and John L. Loeb Family Fund Grants, 1546
Gerber Fndn Grants, 1606
GlaxoSmithKline Corp Grants, 1623
Hanna Andersson Children's Fndn Grants, 1691
Health Fndn of Greater Cincinnati Grants, 1724
Health Fndn of Greater Indianapolis Grants, 1725
Healthcare Fndn of New Jersey Grants, 1729
Hoglund Fndn Grants, 1785
HRSA Eliminating Disparities in Perinatal Health Grants, 1803
HRSA Emergency Medical Services for Children Grants, 1804
i2 Fndn Grants, 1829
Illinois Children's Healthcare Fndn Grants, 1842
Jewish Fund Grants, 1923
Johnson & Johnson Comm Health Care Grants, 1951
Johnson & Johnson Corp Contributions Grants, 1952

Josiah Macy Jr. Fndn Grants, 1966
Kaiser Permanente Cares for Communities Grants, 1978
Kansas Health Fndn Grants, 1980
Ken W. Davis Fndn Grants, 1987
Kiwanis International Fndn Grants, 2004
Larry L. Hillblom Fndn Grants, 2031
Leadership in Education in Neurodevelopmental Disabilities Postdoctoral Fellowships, 2037
Leonsis Fndn Grants, 2045
Long Island Comm Fndn Grants, 2063
Lowe Fndn Grants, 2067
Mary Black Fndn Grants, 2118
Max Bell Fndn Grants, 2134
Mayday Fund Grants, 2139
Medicaid/SCHIP Eligibility Pilots, 2164
Medtronic Fndn Health Care Grants, 2169
Michael and Susan Dell Fndn Grants, 2189
Mount Zion Health Fund Grants, 2220
NAPNAP Fndn Innovative Health Care Small Grant, 2237
NAPNAP Fndn McNeil Grant-in-Aid, 2238
NAPNAP Fndn Nursing Research Grants, 2241
National Emergency Medicine Association Grants, 2252
NIAID HIV Vaccine Clinical Trial Units Grants, 2454
NIAID Pediatric Clinical Trials Program for AIDS, 2460
NICHD NRSAs—Individual, 2488
NICHD NRSAs—Institutional, 2489
NICHD Small Grants, 2494
NICHD Socioeconomic Status and Health Across the Life Course, 2495
NIDA International Studies on Drug Abuse and HIV/AIDS, 2505
NIDA National Drug Abuse Treatment Clinical Trials Network, 2510
NIH Mechanisms Underlying Individual Variations in Drug Responses, 2685
NIH Research on Sleep and Sleep Disorders, 2713
NIH Rett Syndrome: Genetics, Pathophysiology, and Biomarkers Research Grants, 2715
NIH Targeting Research Gaps in HIV Therapeutics Research Grants, 2734
Oakland Fund for Children and Youth Grants, 2930
Pajaro Valley Comm Health Grants, 2985
Pediatric Brain Tumor Research Grants, 3012
Pediatric Cancer Research Fndn Grants, 3013
Premera CARES Grants, 3074
Prince Charitable Trusts Chicago Grants, 3079
Quantum Corp Snap Server Grants, 3095
Quantum Fndn Grants, 3096
RGK Fndn Grants, 3153
Robin Hood Fndn Grants, 3174
Stewart Huston Charitable Trust Grants, 3384
Sunshine Natural Wellbeing Fndn Grants, 3404
Thrasher Research Fund Grants, 3426
Topfer Family Fndn Grants, 3430
Walt Disney Company Fndn Grants, 3516
WHO Fndn General Grants, 3534
Wilkins Family Fndn Grants, 3536

Children (Patients)
Northwest Airlines KidCares Medical Travel Assistance, 2868
NYAM Brock Lecture, Award and Visiting Professorship in Pediatrics, 2909

Children and Youth
1104 Fndn Grants, 3
1976 Fndn Grants, 5
2 Depot Square Ipswich Charitable Fndn Grants, 7
3M Fndn Grants, 11
A Friend's Fndn Trust Grants, 13
AACAP Junior Investigator Awards, 41
AACAP Pilot Research Award for Attention-Deficit Disorder, Supported by the Elaine Schlosser Lewis Fund, 45
AACAP Quest for the Test Bipolar Disorder Pilot Research Award, 48
AACAP-NIDA K12 Career Development Awards, 55
AAP Anne E. Dyson Child Advocacy Awards, 156
Aaron & Cecile Goldman Family Fndn Grants, 171
Aaron Fndn (California) Grants, 173
Abbott Fund Comm Vitality Grants, 177
AcademyHealth Nemours Child Health Services Research Awards, 194
ACE Charitable Fndn Grants, 199
ACF Preferred Communities Grants, 201
ACF Standing Announcement for Unaccompanied Alien Children Grants, 202
ACF Supplemental Services for Recently Arrived Refugees Grants, 203
Achelis and Bodman Fndns Grants, 206
Adaptec Fndn Grants, 232
Administaff Comm Affairs Grants, 235
AEGON Transamerica Fndn Grants, 243
Aetna Fndn Regional Comm Health Grants, 249
Agnes M. Lindsay Trust Grants, 263
Agway Fndn Grants, 265
Alcatel-Lucent Technologies Fndn Grants, 333
Alcohol Misuse and Alcoholism Research Grants, 335
Alice Tweed Tuohy Fndn Grants, 357
Allegis Group Fndn Grants, 360
Alliance Healthcare Fndn Grants, 362
American Academy of Dermatology Camp Discovery Scholarships, 412
American Schlafhorst Fndn Grants, 454
Angels Baseball Fndn Grants, 473
Anheuser-Busch Fndn Grants, 474
Ann and Robert H. Lurie Family Fndn Grants, 475
Annenberg Fndn Grants, 479
Annunziata Sanguinetti Fndn Grants, 481
Anthem Blue Cross and Blue Shield School Nurse Grants, 489
Anthony R. Abraham Fndn Grants, 490
APF Jeanne Spurlock Congressional Fellowships, 509
Arcadia Fndn Grants, 524
Arizona Cardinals Grants, 529
Arizona Diamondbacks Charities Grants, 530
Arizona Public Service Corp Giving Grants, 531
Arlington Comm Fndn Grants, 536
Assurant Fndn Grants, 654
AT&T Fndn Civic and Comm Service Grants, 658
Austin College Leadership Award, 668
Austin-Bailey Health and Wellness Fndn Grants, 669
Avon Products Fndn Grants, 675
Bailey Fndn Grants, 680
Baltimore Washington Center Child Psychotherapy Fellowships, 686
Bank of America Client Fndn Grants, 690
Baptist Comm Ministries Grants, 691
Barberton Comm Fndn Grants, 693
Barker Fndn Grants, 694
Barr Fund Grants, 697
Barth Syndrome Fndn Research Grants, 700
Batchelor Fndn Grants, 701
Batts Fndn Grants, 704
Baxter International Fndn Grants, 705
BCBSM Building Healthy Communities Engaging Elementary Schools and Comm Partners Grants, 713
BCBSM Corp Contributions Grants, 716
Bella Vista Fndn Grants, 740
Bender Fndn Grants, 742
Benton County Fndn Grants, 744
Bernard Van Leer Fndn Grants, 748
Berrien Comm Fndn Grants, 749
Bill and Melinda Gates Fndn Grants, 756
Birmingham Fndn Grants, 760
BJ's Charitable Fndn Grants, 761
Blackford County Comm Fndn Grants, 763
Blanche and Irving Laurie Fndn Grants, 764
Blowitz-Ridgeway Fndn Grants, 767
Bodenwein Public Benevolent Fndn Grants, 775
Booth-Bricker Fund Grants, 780
Borkee-Hagley Fndn Grants, 781
Boston Globe Fndn Grants, 784
Boston Psychoanalytic Society and Institute Fellowship in Child Psychoanalytic Psychotherapy, 786
Bradley Turner Fndn Grants, 789
Brian G. Dyson Fndn Grants, 791
Bright Family Fndn Grants, 793
Bristol-Myers Squibb Fndn Health Education Grants, 798
Burden Trust Grants, 810
Burlington Industries Fndn Grants, 811
Burton G. Bettingen Grants, 813
Cailloux Fndn Grants, 829
Cambridge Comm Fndn Grants, 837
Caring Fndn Grants, 866
Carl B. and Florence E. King Fndn Grants, 869
Carl W. and Carrie Mae Joslyn Trust Grants, 873
Carlisle Fndn Grants, 874
Carlos and Marguerite Mason Trust Grants, 875
Carls Fndn Grants, 876
Carolyn Fndn Grants, 880
Carpenter Fndn Grants, 881
Carrie E. and Lena V. Glenn Fndn Grants, 882
Carrie Estelle Doheny Fndn Grants, 883
Carroll County Comm Fndn Grants, 885
Catherine Holmes Wilkins Fndn Grants, 889
Cemala Fndn Grants, 933
Central Okanagan Fndn Grants, 937
Cessna Fndn Grants, 938
Champ-A Champion Fur Kids Grants, 959
CharityWorks Grants, 961
Charles Delmar Fndn Grants, 963
Charles H. Dater Fndn Grants, 966
Charles Lafitte Fndn Grants, 970
Chestnut Hill Charitable Fndn, Inc Grants, 987
Chicago Board of Trade Fndn Grants, 988
Children Affected by AIDS Fndn Camp Network Grants, 994
Children Affected by AIDS Fndn Domestic Grants, 995
Children Affected by AIDS Fndn Family Assistance Emergency Fund Grants, 996
Children's Trust Fund of Oregon Grants, 1001
Children's Cardiomyopathy Fndn Research Grants, 1002
Chula Vista Charitable Fndn Grants, 1009
CIT Corp Giving Grants, 1014
Citizens Bank Mid-Atlantic Charitable Fndn Grants, 1015
Clark Fndn Grants, 1029
Cleo Fndn Grants, 1035
Cleveland Browns Fndn Grants, 1036
CLIF Bar Family Fndn Grants, 1040
CNCS Foster Grandparent Projects Grants, 1048
Coeta and Donald Barker Fndn Grants, 1054
Columbus Fndn Traditional Grants, 1071
Comer Fndn Grants, 1072
Commonweal Fndn Comm Assistance Grants, 1075
Commonweal Fndn Grants, 1076
Commonwealth Fund Harkness Fellowships in Health Care Policy and Practice, 1079
Comm Fndn for Greater Buffalo Grants, 1090
Comm Fndn for Greater New Haven Grants, 1091
Comm Fndn for Muskegon County Grants, 1093
Comm Fndn for Southeastern Michigan Grants, 1094
Comm Fndn for Southern Arizona Grants, 1095
Comm Fndn of Bloomington and Monroe County Grants, 1098
Comm Fndn of Broward Grants, 1100
Comm Fndn of Grant County Grants, 1104
Comm Fndn of Greater Flint Grants, 1107
Comm Fndn Of Greater Lafayette Grants, 1110
Comm Fndn of Greater New Britain Grants, 1111
Comm Fndn of Greater Tampa Grants, 1112
Comm Fndn of Howard County Grants, 1116
Comm Fndn of Mount Vernon and Knox County Grants, 1119
Comm Fndn of Randolph County Grants, 1121
Comm Fndn of Santa Cruz County Grants, 1122
Comm Fndn of Southeastern Connecticut Grants, 1125
Comm Fndn of Western North Carolina Grants, 1132

Comm Impact Fund, 1135
Compass Bank Fndn Grants, 1138
Comprehensive Health Education Fndn Grants, 1139
ConAgra Foods Fndn Grants, 1140
Crail-Johnson Fndn Grants, 1157
CSRA Comm Fndn Grants, 1168
CSX Corp Contributions Grants, 1169
Cudd Fndn Grants, 1171
CVS Comm Grants, 1177
D. W. McMillan Fndn Grants, 1180
D.V. and Ida J. McEachern Charitable Trust Grants, 1182
Dade Comm Fndn Grants, 1185
Dairy Queen Corp Contributions Grants, 1187
Daisy Marquis Jones Fndn Grants, 1188
Dallas Mavericks Fndn Grants, 1190
Dammann Fund Grants, 1192
Dana Brown Charitable Trust Grants, 1194
Danellie Fndn Grants, 1198
Daphne Seybolt Culpeper Memorial Fndn Grants, 1201
Daywood Fndn Grants, 1206
Deaconess Comm Fndn Grants, 1207
Delaware Comm Fndn-Youth Philanthropy Board for Kent County, 1216
Dell Fndn Healthy Communities, Literate Communities, and Connected Communities Grants, 1217
Dell Fndn Open Grants, 1218
Delta Air Lines Fndn Grants, 1220
Dennis and Phyllis Washington Fndn Grants, 1222
Denver Fndn Comm Grants, 1227
Dept of Ed Safe and Drug-Free Schools and Communities State Grants, 1230
Dept of Ed Special Education—Personnel Development to Improve Services and Results for Children with Disabilities, 1231
Dept of Ed Special Education-National Activities-Technology and Media Services for Individuals with Disabilities, 1234
Detlef Schrempf Fndn Grants, 1240
DHHS Abandoned Infants Assistance Grants, 1242
DHHS Comprehensive Comm Mental Health Services Grants for Children with Serious Emotional Disturbances, 1247
DHHS Emergency Medical Services for Children Program, 1249
DHHS Healthy Tomorrows Partnership for Children, 1261
DHHS Oral Health Promotion Research Across the Lifespan, 1269
Dickson Fndn Grants, 1284
Dole Food Company Charitable Contributions, 1307
Dora Roberts Fndn Grants, 1311
Dorothea Haus Ross Fndn Grants, 1320
Dr. John T. Macdonald Fndn Grants, 1327
Dr. Scholl Fndn Grants, 1329
Duke University Pediatric Anesthesiology Fellowship, 1347
E.L. Wiegand Fndn Grants, 1361
eBay Fndn Comm Grants, 1363
Eckerd Corp Fndn Grants, 1366
Edina Realty Fndn Grants, 1369
Edward S. Moore Fndn Grants, 1374
Edwards Memorial Trust Grants, 1375
Edyth Bush Charitable Fndn Grants, 1378
Eisner Fndn Grants, 1387
El Paso Comm Fndn Grants, 1388
Elizabeth Morse Genius Charitable Trust Grants, 1400
Elliot Fndn Inc Grants, 1402
Elsie Lee Garthwaite Memorial Fndn Grants, 1408
Emma B. Howe Memorial Fndn Grants, 1415
Entergy Comm Partnership Grants, 1417
Entergy Corp Open Grants for Healthy Families, 1418
EPA Baseline Assessment of Risks of Exposure to Lead Poisoning of Native American Children, 1419
EPA Lead Awareness Outreach for Native American Tribes, 1421
Eugene and Agnes E. Meyer Fndn Grants, 1432
Eugene McDermott Fndn Grants, 1435
Evanston Comm Fndn Grants, 1438
Express Scripts Fndn Grants, 1441
Fairfield County Comm Fndn Grants, 1446
Fallon OrNda Comm Health Fund Grants, 1449
FAR Fund, 1453
Fargo-Moorhead Area Fndn Grants, 1454
Faye McBeath Fndn Grants, 1456
Fayette County Fndn Grants, 1457
FCD Child Development Grants, 1458
Federal Express Corp Contributions Program, 1483
Ferree Fndn Grants, 1486
Fireman's Fund Fndn Grants, 1504
Florida BRAIVE Fund of Dade Comm Fndn, 1512
Florida BRAIVE Fund of Gulf Coast Comm Fndn of Venice, 1513
Florida BRAIVE Fund of The Comm Fndn in Jacksonville, 1514
Floyd A. and Kathleen C. Cailloux Fndn Grants, 1516
Foellinger Fndn Grants, 1519
Foster Fndn Grants, 1524
Fndn of CVPH Chelsea's Rainbow Fund Grants, 1539
Fndn of CVPH Roger Senecal Endowment Fund Grants, 1542
Fourjay Fndn Grants, 1544
Frances L. and Edwin L. Cummings Memorial Fund Grants, 1547
Francis L. Abreu Charitable Trust Grants, 1549
Francis T. & Louise T. Nichols Fndn Grants, 1550
Frank E. and Seba B. Payne Fndn Grants, 1551
Frank Stanley Beveridge Fndn Grants, 1553
Fred Baldwin Memorial Fndn Grants, 1556
Fred L. Emerson Fndn Grants, 1557
Freddie Mac Fndn Grants, 1558
Frey Fndn Grants, 1562
Gamble Fndn Grants, 1582
Gebbie Fndn Grants, 1585
General Mills Champions for Healthy Kids Grants, 1589
General Mills Fndn Grants, 1590
George and Ruth Bradford Fndn Grants, 1595
George Kress Fndn Grants, 1601
George S. and Dolores Dore Eccles Fndn Grants, 1602
Gerber Fndn Grants, 1606
Ginn Fndn Grants, 1616
Giving in Action Society Children & Youth with Special Needs Grants, 1617
Global Fund for Children Grants, 1629
Godfrey Fndn Grants, 1631
Golden State Warriors Fndn Grants, 1633
Graco Fndn Grants, 1642
Grammy Fndn Grants, 1643
Grand Haven Area Comm Fndn Grants, 1644
Grand Rapids Area Comm Fndn Grants, 1645
Grand Rapids Area Comm Fndn Nashwauk Area Endowment Fund Grants, 1646
Grand Rapids Comm Fndn Grants, 1647
Greater New Orleans Fndn Grants, 1654
Greater Tacoma Comm Fndn Ryan Alan Hade Endowment Fund, 1657
Greater Worcester Comm Fndn Discretionary Grants, 1658
Greater Worcester Comm Fndn Jeppson Memorial Fund for Brookfield Grants, 1659
Green Bay Packers Fndn Grants, 1660
Greenspun Family Fndn Grants, 1664
Gregory B. Davis Fndn Grants, 1666
Gregory L. Gibson Charitable Fndn Grants, 1668
Grotto Fndn Project Grants, 1671
Grundy Fndn Grants, 1673
H.J. Heinz Company Fndn Grants, 1682
Hagedorn Fund Grants, 1685
Hall-Perrine Fndn Grants, 1686
Hanna Andersson Children's Fndn Grants, 1691
Hannaford Charitable Fndn Grants, 1692
Harold & Arlene Schnitzer CARE Fndn Grants, 1697
Harry Frank Guggenheim Fndn Research Grants, 1704
Hartford Courant Fndn Grants, 1710
Hartford Fndn Regular Grants, 1711
Hasbro Children's Fund, 1714
Hawaii Comm Fndn Reverend Takie Okumura Family Grants, 1717
HCA Fndn Grants, 1721
Heckscher Fndn for Children Grants, 1732
Hedco Fndn Grants, 1733
Heineman Fndn for Research, Education, Charitable and Scientific Purposes, 1735
Helena Rubinstein Fndn Grants, 1743
Hendrick Fndn for Children Grants, 1744
Henrietta Tower Wurts Memorial Fndn Grants, 1745
Henry County Comm Fndn Grants, 1747
Herman Goldman Fndn Grants, 1753
Hershey Company Grants, 1754
Highmark Healthy High 5, 1770
Hilda and Preston Davis Fndn Grants, 1772
Hill Fndn Grants, 1774
Hillman Fndn Grants, 1775
Hillsdale County Comm Fndn Healthy Senior/Healthy Youth Fund Grants, 1776
Hilton Head Island Fndn Grants, 1779
Hoglund Fndn Grants, 1785
Holland/Zeeland Comm Fndn Grants, 1786
Horace A. Kimball and S. Ella Kimball Fndn Grants, 1792
Horizons Comm Issues Grants, 1794
Howard and Bush Fndn Grants, 1798
Hugh J. Andersen Fndn Grants, 1814
Humana Fndn Grants, 1818
Huntington Beach Police Officers Fndn Grants, 1821
Huntington National Bank Comm Affairs Grants, 1824
Hut Fndn Grants, 1827
Hutton Fndn Grants, 1828
Ignacio Martin-Baro Fund for Mental Health and Human Rights Grants, 1839
Illinois Children's Healthcare Fndn Grants, 1842
Impact 100 Grants, 1843
Institute for Agriculture and Trade Policy Food and Society Fellowships, 1856
Irving S. Gilmore Fndn Grants, 1867
Isabel Allende Fndn Esperanza Grants, 1868
J.C. Penney Company Grants, 1874
Jacob and Hilda Blaustein Fndn Grants, 1881
Jacob G. Schmidlapp Trust Grants, 1883
James Ford Bell Fndn Grants, 1885
James H. Cummings Fndn Grants, 1888
James J. and Angelia M. Harris Fndn Grants, 1890
James M. Cox Fndn of Georgia Grants, 1892
James S. Copley Fndn Grants, 1895
Jane Bradley Pettit Fndn Grants, 1902
Janirve Fndn Grants, 1905
Jay and Rose Phillips Family Fndn Grants, 1909
JELD-WEN Fndn Grants, 1914
Jerome and Mildred Paddock Fndn Grants, 1917
Jim Moran Fndn Grants, 1925
JM Fndn Grants, 1926
John Edward Fowler Memorial Fndn Grants, 1930
John Jewett and Helen Chandler Garland Fndn Grants, 1937
John Merck Scholars Awards, 1941
John P. McGovern Fndn Grants, 1942
John W. Alden Trust Grants, 1947
John W. and Anna H. Hanes Fndn Grants, 1948
John W. Anderson Fndn Grants, 1949
Johnson Controls Fndn Grants, 1954
Joseph H. and Florence A. Roblee Fndn Grants, 1961
Josephine G. Russell Trust Grants, 1963
Josephine Goodyear Fndn Grants, 1964
Josephine S. Gumbiner Fndn Grants, 1965
Josiah W. and Bessie H. Kline Fndn Grants, 1967
Julia Temple Davis Brown Fndn Grants, 1971
K and F Baxter Family Fndn Grants, 1973
Kaiser Permanente Cares for Communities Grants, 1978
Ken W. Davis Fndn Grants, 1987
Kenny's Kids Grants, 1990
Kevin P. and Sydney B. Knight Family Fndn Grants, 1993
Kimberly-Clark Comm Grants, 2001
Kiwanis International Fndn Grants, 2004
Kosair Charities Grants, 2014
Kosciusko County Comm Fndn Grants, 2015
Kraft Cares International Grants, 2016

L. W. Pierce Family Fndn Grants, 2019
Land O'Lakes Fndn Mid-Atlantic Grants, 2027
Lands' End Corp Giving Program, 2030
Larry L. Hillblom Fndn Grants, 2031
Laura B. Vogler Fndn Grants, 2032
Layne Beachley Aim For The Stars Fndn Grants, 2036
Legacy Fndn Grants, 2040
Leonsis Fndn Grants, 2045
Liliane Fndn Grants, 2055
Long Island Comm Fndn Grants, 2063
Lotus 88 Fndn for Women and Children Grants, 2064
Louis Calder Fndn Grants, 2065
Louis R. Cappelli Fndn Grants, 2066
Lucile Horton Howe and Mitchell B. Howe Fndn Grants, 2081
Lucy Gooding Charitable Fndn Trust, 2082
Lucy Gooding Charitable Fndn Trust Grants, 2083
Ludwick Family Fndn Grants, 2084
M.E. Raker Fndn Grants, 2094
Mabel H. Flory Charitable Trust Grants, 2096
Manuel D. and Rhoda Mayerson Fndn Grants, 2100
Margaret L. Wendt Fndn Grants, 2104
Margaret T. Morris Fndn Grants, 2105
Mark and Catherine Winkler Fndn Grants, 2112
Marriott Fndn for People with Disabilities Bridges Grants, 2113
Marshall Field's Comm Grants, 2115
Mary Black Fndn Grants, 2118
Mass Youth Against Tobacco Mini-Grants, 2123
Mattel Children's Fndn Grants, 2130
Mattel International Grants, 2131
Max A. Adler Charitable Fndn Grants, 2132
Maxon Charitable Fndn Grants, 2135
Maxtor Corp Contributions Grants, 2136
May and Stanley Smith Trust Grants, 2137
McKesson Fndn Grants, 2145
McKnight Fndn Grants, 2146
McLean Contributionship Grants, 2147
McMillen Fndn Grants, 2148
McMurry Fndn Grants, 2149
Mead Johnson Nutritionals Evansville-Area Organizations Grants, 2157
Meriden Fndn Grants, 2173
Metro Health Fndn Grants, 2175
Metrowest Comm Health Care Fndn Grants, 2176
Meyer Fndn Grants, 2177
Meyer Memorial Trust Emergency Grants, 2178
Meyer Memorial Trust Grassroots Grants, 2179
Meyer Memorial Trust Operating Funds Grants, 2180
Meyer Memorial Trust Responsive Grants, 2181
Michael and Susan Dell Fndn Grants, 2189
Milagro Fndn Grants, 2198
Minneapolis Fndn Comm Grants, 2206
MONY Fndn Grants, 2215
Morgan Adams Fndn Grants, 2216
Morris and Gwendolyn Cafritz Fndn Grants, 2217
NAPNAP Fndn Elaine Gelman Scholarship, 2235
NAPNAP Fndn Graduate Student Research Grant, 2236
NAPNAP Fndn Innovative Health Care Small Grant, 2237
NAPNAP Fndn McNeil Grant-in-Aid, 2238
NAPNAP Fndn McNeil PNP Scholarships, 2239
NAPNAP Fndn McNeil Rural and Underserved Scholarships, 2240
NAPNAP Fndn Nursing Research Grants, 2241
NAPNAP Fndn Reckitt Benckiser Student Scholarship, 2242
NARSAD Distinguished Investigator Award, 2246
NARSAD Independent Investigator Award, 2247
National Starch and Chemical Fndn Grants, 2261
Nelda C. and H.J. Lutcher Stark Fndn Grants, 2301
New York Life Fndn Grants, 2304
Newman's Own Inc Grants, 2306
NHLBI Childhood Obesity Prevention and Treatment Research Consortium Grants, 2328
Nicholas H. Noyes Jr. Memorial Fndn Grants, 2497
NIMH Pilot Effectiveness Trials for Mental Disorders Grants, 2766
NIMH/NIDA Children's Services Grants, 2775
Nina Mason Pulliam Charitable Trust Grants, 2776
NINR Chronic Illness Self-Management in Children and Adolescents Grants, 2792
Nordson Corp Fndn Grants, 2851
North Carolina Comm Development Grants, 2858
Northwest Airlines KidCares Medical Travel Assistance, 2868
Northwestern Mutual Fndn Grants, 2870
Nuffield Fndn Children and Families Grants, 2899
NYCT Children and Youth with Disabilities Grants, 2923
NYCT Girls and Young Women Grants, 2924
NYCT Mental Health and Mental Retardation Grants, 2927
Oakland Fund for Children and Youth Grants, 2930
Oceanside Charitable Fndn Grants, 2934
Office Depot Corp Comm Grants, 2935
Office Depot Fndn Grants, 2936
Ohio County Comm Fndn Grants, 2938
Ohio County Comm Fndn Mini-Grants, 2939
Oleonda Jameson Trust Grants, 2941
Ordean Fndn Grants, 2952
OUT Fund for Lesbian & Gay Liberation Grants, 2978
PacifiCare Fndn Grants, 2981
Pajaro Valley Comm Health Grants, 2985
Partnership for Pediatric Epilepsy Research Grants, 2993
Pasadena Fndn Average Grants, 2994
Paul E. and Klare N. Reinhold Fndn Grants, 2999
Paul G. Allen Family Fndn Grants, 3000
Paul G. Duke Fndn Grants, 3001
Peabody Fndn Grants, 3010
Pediatric Brain Tumor Research Grants, 3012
Pediatric Cancer Research Fndn Grants, 3013
Perkins Charitable Fndn Grants, 3014
Perpetual Trust for Charitable Giving Grants, 3015
Peter and Elizabeth C. Tower Fndn Comm Grants, 3018
Pew Charitable Trusts Children & Youth Grants, 3020
PeyBack Fndn Grants, 3022
Philadelphia Fndn Organizational Effectiveness Grants, 3029
Phoenix Suns Charities Grants, 3030
Pike County Comm Fndn Grants, 3049
Pinellas County Grants, 3050
Pittsburgh Fndn Comm Fund Grants, 3054
Plough Fndn Grants, 3061
Plum Creek Fndn Grants, 3062
Polaroid Fund Grants, 3065
Polk Bros. Fndn Grants, 3066
Posey Comm Fndn Grants, 3068
Posey Comm Fndn Womens Fund Grants, 3069
Pott Fndn Grants, 3071
Prince Charitable Trusts Chicago Grants, 3079
Prudential Fndn Grants, 3087
Public Welfare Fndn Grants, 3089
Pulaski County Comm Fndn Grants, 3091
Putnam County Comm Fndn Grants, 3093
Quantum Fndn Grants, 3096
Rainbow Endowment Grants, 3102
Rajiv Gandhi Fndn Grants, 3104
Rathmann Family Fndn Grants, 3109
Raymond John Wean Fndn Grants, 3110
Rayonier Fndn Grants, 3111
Rehab Therapy Fndn Grants, 3146
Reynolds and Reynolds Associate Fndn Grants, 3152
RGK Fndn Grants, 3153
Rhode Island Fndn Grants, 3154
Richard and Rhoda Goldman Fund Grants, 3158
Richard and Susan Smith Family Fndn Grants, 3159
Richard King Mellon Fndn Grants, 3161
Robert and Joan Dircks Fndn Grants, 3167
Robert B McMillen Fndn Grants, 3169
Robin Hood Fndn Grants, 3174
Robins Fndn Grants, 3175
Rochester Area Comm Fndn Grants, 3176
Rochester Area Fndn Grants, 3177
Rockwell Collins Charitable Contributions, 3182
Rush County Comm Fndn Grants, 3200
Ruth H. and Warren A. Ellsworth Fndn Grants, 3203
RWJF Bridging the Gap: Research Informing Practice & Policy for Healthy Youth Behavior, 3205
RWJF Healthy Eating Research Grants, 3218
RWJF Local Funding Partnerships Grants, 3223
S. Livingston Mather Charitable Trust Grants, 3235
S. Mark Taper Fndn Grants, 3236
S.H. Cowell Fndn Grants, 3237
SAMHSA Child Mental Health Initiative Grants, 3245
SAMHSA Strategic Prevention Framework State Incentive Grants, 3248
Samuel S. Johnson Fndn Grants, 3251
San Diego Fndn for Change Grants, 3255
Schurz Communications Fndn Grants, 3271
Scott County Comm Fndn Grants, 3273
Seabury Fndn Grants, 3274
Seattle Fndn Grants, 3276
Self Fndn Grants, 3277
Seneca Foods Fndn Grants, 3278
SHF Reach—Connecting Communities and Youth for a Healthy Future Grants, 3283
Sid W. Richardson Fndn Grants, 3284
Siebert Lutheran Fndn Grants, 3285
Simmons Fndn Grants, 3287
Sir Halley Stewart Trust Grants, 3293
Sisters of Mercy of North Carolina Fndn Grants, 3295
Sisters of Saint Joseph Charitable Fund Grants, 3296
Sisters of St. Joseph Healthcare Fndn Grants, 3297
Sonoco Fndn Grants, 3347
Southbury Comm Trust Fund, 3350
Spencer County Comm Fndn Grants, 3358
Sprague Fndn Grants, 3359
Stark Comm Fndn Women's Fund Grants, 3376
Steelcase Fndn Grants, 3379
Strowd Roses Grants, 3388
Sunderland Fndn Grants, 3400
Susan Mott Webb Charitable Trust Grants, 3412
Taproot Fndn Capacity-Building Service Grants, 3417
Thompson Charitable Fndn Grants, 3425
Topfer Family Fndn Grants, 3430
Triangle Comm Fndn Donor-Advised Grants, 3437
Trull Fndn Grants, 3441
U.S. Lacrosse EAD Grants, 3453
Union Benevolent Association Grants, 3460
United Methodist Health Ministry Fund Grants, 3465
Vancouver Fndn Grants and Comm Initiatives Program, 3477
Vancouver Sun Children's Fund Grants, 3479
Vanderburgh Comm Fndn Grants, 3480
Viking Children's Fund Grants, 3497
Volkswagen of America Corp Contributions Grants, 3503
Vulcan Materials Company Fndn Grants, 3504
W. C. Griffith Fndn Grants, 3505
W.K. Kellogg Fndn Secure Families Grants, 3508
Wachovia Fndn Grants, 3511
Waitt Family Fndn Grants, 3512
Wal-Mart Fndn Comm Grants, 3513
Warrick County Comm Fndn Grants, 3519
Weingart Fndn Grants, 3524
Western Union Fndn Grants, 3529
Westinghouse Charitable Giving Grants, 3530
WHAS Crusade for Children Grants, 3531
Wilkins Family Fndn Grants, 3536
William G. McGowan Charitable Fund Grants, 3539
William T. Grant Fndn Research Grants, 3541
Wilson-Wood Fndn Grants, 3542
Winston-Salem Fndn Competitive Grants, 3544
Winston-Salem Fndn Elkin/Tri-County Grants, 3545
Women's Fndn of California Grants, 3550
Women's Sports Fndn Grants, 3551
YSA UnitedHealth Heroes Service Learning Grants, 3556
Z. Smith Reynolds Fndn Small Grants, 3557

Children's Museums

Angels Baseball Fndn Grants, 473
Anschutz Family Fndn Grants, 486
Athwin Fndn Grants, 660
Phoenix Suns Charities Grants, 3030

Children's Television
Farmers Insurance Group of Companies Grants, 1455
Chiropractic
DHHS Chiropractic Demonstration Project Grants, 1246
DHHS Health Careers Opportunity Grants, 1253
FCER Chiropractic Research Grants, 1459
FCER Research Grants and Fellowships, 1460

Chromatography
Ethical Research Grants and Fellowships, 1431

Chronic Illness
Aetna Fndn Health Grants in Connecticut, 244
BCBS of Minnesota Healthy Together Grants, 712
CDC Oral Diseases Prevention and Oral Health Promotion Grants, 921
CDC Promoting Prevention in Managed Care Cooperative Agreements, 925
CFF Research Grants, 947
Emma B. Howe Memorial Fndn Grants, 1415
FIC International Research Scientist Development Award, 1491
Gerber Fndn Grants, 1606
Health Fndn of Greater Cincinnati Grants, 1724
Josiah Macy Jr. Fndn Grants, 1966
Kaiser Permanente Cares for Communities Grants, 1978
Kenny's Kids Grants, 1990
Leonard and Helen R. Stulman Charitable Fndn Grants, 2044
Medtronic Fndn Health Care Grants, 2169
NAPNAP Fndn Nursing Research Grants, 2241
NIA Symptom Management for Chronic Neurological Conditions Research Grants, 2436
NICHD Symptom Management for Chronic Neurological Conditions Research Grants, 2496
NIDCD Symptom Management for Chronic Neurological Conditions Research Grants, 2532
NIH Biobehavioral Research for Effective Sleep, 2639
NIH Research on Sleep and Sleep Disorders, 2713
NIH Small Business Innovation Research: Animal Models of HCV Infection Research Grants, 2728
NINDS Symptom Management for Chronic Neurological Conditions Research Grants, 2787
NINR Acute and Chronic Care During Mechanical Ventilation Research Grants, 2788
NINR Chronic Illness Self-Management in Children and Adolescents Grants, 2792
NINR Symptom Management for Chronic Neurological Conditions Research Grants, 2805
NSF Biomedical Engineering and Engineering Healthcare Grants, 2879
RWJF New Jersey Health Initiatives Grants, 3225
Special People in Need Grants, 3356
Wellmark Fndn Grants, 3526

Churches
Abel Fndn Grants, 181
Adam Richter Charitable Trust Grants, 230
Adams County Fndn Grants - Pennsylvania, 231
ALSAM Fndn Grants, 369
Andersen Fndn Grants, 471
Anthony R. Abraham Fndn Grants, 490
Archer Daniels Midland Fndn Grants, 525
Atkinson Fndn International Grants, 661
Booth-Bricker Fund Grants, 780
Bosque Fndn Grants, 782
Boston Fndn Grants, 783
Caddock Fndn Grants, 828
Callaway Fndn Grants, 835
Carnahan-Jackson Fndn Grants, 878
Catherine Kennedy Home Fndn Grants, 890
Champlin Fndns Grants, 960
Chiles Fndn Grants, 1003
Commission on Religion in Appalachia Grants, 1074
Comm Fndn of Champaign County Grants, 1102
Comm Fndn of Greenville Comm Enrichment Grants, 1113
Comm Fndn of Greenville Hollingsworth Funds Program/Project Grants, 1114
Danellie Fndn Grants, 1198
General Mills Fndn Grants, 1590
George Kress Fndn Grants, 1601
Gregory Family Fndn Grants (Florida), 1667
Griffin Family Fndn Grants, 1669
Helen Steiner Rice Fndn Grants, 1742
High Meadow Fndn Grants, 1768
Howe Fndn of North Carolina Grants, 1799
James M. Collins Fndn Grants, 1891
Jessie Ball Dupont Fund Grants, 1919
John H. and Wilhelmina D. Harland Charitable Fndn Grants, 1933
John I. Smith Charities Grants, 1935
Maxon Charitable Fndn Grants, 2135
Perkins Charitable Fndn Grants, 3014
Richard and Helen DeVos Fndn Grants, 3157
Rollin M. Gerstacker Fndn Grants, 3186
Sunderland Fndn Grants, 3400
Support Our Aging Religious Grants, 3406
Susan Mott Webb Charitable Trust Grants, 3412
Temple-Inland Fndn Grants, 3419
Thomas M. and Irene B. Kirbo Charitable Trust Grants, 3424
W. C. Griffith Fndn Grants, 3505
William H. Hannon Fndn Grants, 3540

Circadian Rhythms
NHLBI Circadian-Coupled Cellular Function in Heart, Lung, and Blood Tissue Grants, 2330
NIDA Drug Addiction Neuroscience Research Grants, 2503
NIH Research on Sleep and Sleep Disorders, 2713

Circulatory Disease
Edna G. Kynett Memorial Fndn Grants, 1370

Citizenship
Battle Creek Comm Fndn Grants, 703
Carnegie Corp of New York Grants, 879
Citizens Bank Mid-Atlantic Charitable Fndn Grants, 1015
Greater Bridgeport Area Fndn Comm Impact Grants, 1650
Harvest Fndn Grants, 1713
John Edward Fowler Memorial Fndn Grants, 1930
Kenneth T. and Eileen L. Norris Fndn Grants, 1989
Kraft Cares US Grants, 2017
Lubrizol Fndn Grants, 2080
Piper Jaffray Companies Building Strong Communities Grants, 3053
Richard King Mellon Fndn Grants, 3161

Civic Affairs
A.O. Smith Comm Grants, 18
Abbott Fund Global AIDS Care Grants, 178
Acushnet Fndn Grants, 226
Advanced Micro Devices Comm Affairs Grants, 239
AEGON Transamerica Fndn Grants, 243
AFG Industries Grants, 259
Alabama Power Fndn Grants, 321
Alaska Airlines Corp Giving Grants, 323
Alaska Airlines Fndn Grants, 324
Albert Pick Jr. Fund Grants, 328
Alberto Culver Corp Contributions Grants, 329
Alcatel-Lucent Technologies Fndn Grants, 333
Alcoa Fndn Grants, 334
Alex Brown and Sons Charitable Fndn Grants, 337
Alice Tweed Tuohy Fndn Grants, 357
Allegheny Technologies Charitable Trust, 359
Annenberg Fndn Grants, 479
Arie and Ida Crown Memorial Grants, 528
Arizona Cardinals Grants, 529
Arkansas Comm Fndn Grants, 533
Armstrong McDonald Fndn Grants, 537
ArvinMeritor Grants, 544
Ashland Corp Contributions Grants, 586
Autodesk Comm Relations Grants, 671
Banfi Vintners Fndn Grants, 687
Barker Welfare Fndn Grants, 695
Bechtel Group Fndn Building Positive Comm Relationships Grants, 731
Ben B. Cheney Fndn Grants, 741
Bernard and Audre Rapoport Fndn Grants, 746
Bertha Russ Lytel Fndn Grants, 751
Besser Fndn Grants, 752
Binney and Smith Comm Grants, 757
Blum-Kovler Fndn Grants, 772
Boeing Company Contributions Grants, 777
Boston Globe Fndn Grants, 784
Bridgestone/Firestone Trust Fund Grants, 792
Burlington Industries Fndn Grants, 811
Burlington Northern Santa Fe Fndn Grants, 812
C.R. Bard Fndn Grants, 825
Cailloux Fndn Grants, 829
Cass County Comm Fndn Grants, 887
Central Carolina Comm Fndn Comm Impact Grants, 936
Charles M. Bair Family Trust Grants, 972
Chatlos Fndn Grants, 977
Chesapeake Corp Fndn Grants, 982
Chicago Tribune's Corp Contributions Grants, 991
Chicago White Metal Charitable Fndn Grants, 992
CICF Legacy Fund Comm Fndn Grants, 1010
CIGNA Fndn Grants, 1011
Clarcor Fndn Grants, 1021
CNA Fndn Grants, 1046
Cockrell Fndn Grants, 1053
Colorado Interstate Gas Grants, 1060
Columbus Fndn Mary Eleanor Morris Fund Grants, 1069
Comerica Charitable Fndn Grants, 1073
Comm Fndn for Greater Buffalo Grants, 1090
Comm Fndn for Southeastern Michigan Grants, 1094
Comm Fndn of Greater Greensboro Grants, 1109
Comm Fndn of Howard County Grants, 1116
Comm Fndn of Santa Cruz County Grants, 1122
Comm Fndn of South Alabama Grants, 1123
Comm Fndn of Southeastern Connecticut Grants, 1125
Comm Fndn of St. Joseph County Special Project Challenge Grants, 1126
Comm Impact Fund, 1135
ConAgra Foods Fndn Grants, 1140
Connelly Fndn Grants, 1143
Constellation Energy Group and Baltimore Gas and Electric Corp Contributions, 1146
Consumers Energy Fndn, 1147
Cooper Industries Fndn Grants, 1150
Cranston Fndn Grants, 1158
Cruise Industry Charitable Fndn Grants, 1166
CSRA Comm Fndn Grants, 1168
CSX Corp Contributions Grants, 1169
DaimlerChrysler Corp Fund Grants, 1186
Dana Corp Fndn Grants, 1196
Dayton Power and Light Fndn Grants, 1205
Dell Fndn Open Grants, 1218
Delta Air Lines Fndn Grants, 1220
Denver Fndn Comm Grants, 1227
Detroit Lions Charities Grants, 1241
Dr. Scholl Fndn Grants, 1329
Dunspaugh-Dalton Fndn Grants, 1351
Eastman Chemical Company Fndn Grants, 1362
eBay Fndn Comm Grants, 1363
El Paso Comm Fndn Grants, 1388
El Pomar Fndn Awards and Grants, 1390
Elmer L. and Eleanor J. Andersen Fndn Grants, 1406
Evan and Susan Bayh Fndn Grants, 1437
ExxonMobil Grants, 1442
F.M. Kirby Fndn Grants, 1443
Fargo-Moorhead Area Fndn Grants, 1454
Farmers Insurance Group of Companies Grants, 1455
Faye McBeath Fndn Grants, 1456
Ferree Fndn Grants, 1486
Fifth Third Fndn Grants, 1501
FirstEnergy Fndn Comm Grants, 1505
Floyd A. and Kathleen C. Cailloux Fndn Grants, 1516
Fluor Fndn Grants, 1517
Ford Motor Company Fund Grants, 1522
Fndn for the Carolinas Grants, 1535

Fndn Northwest Grants, 1537
Frey Fndn Grants, 1562
Fulton County Comm Fndn Grants, 1579
GenCorp Fndn Grants, 1587
George F. Baker Trust Grants, 1597
Goodrich Corp Fndn Grants, 1638
Goodyear Tire Grants, 1639
Grand Haven Area Comm Fndn Grants, 1644
Greater Bridgeport Area Fndn Comm Impact Grants, 1650
Greater New Orleans Fndn Grants, 1654
Greater Tacoma Comm Fndn Grants, 1656
Greater Worcester Comm Fndn Discretionary Grants, 1658
Green Bay Packers Fndn Grants, 1660
Gruber Fndn International Prizes, 1672
Gulf Coast Comm Fndn Grants, 1676
H.A. and Mary K. Chapman Charitable Trust Grants, 1681
Halliburton Fndn Grants, 1687
Hallmark Corp Fndn Grants, 1688
Hancock County Comm Fndn Grants, 1690
Helen K. and Arthur E. Johnson Fndn Grants, 1740
Hillman Fndn Grants, 1775
Hilton Hotels Corp Giving Grants, 1780
Hoblitzelle Fndn Grants, 1783
Howard and Bush Fndn Grants, 1798
Hugh J. Andersen Fndn Grants, 1814
Huntington County Comm Fndn Grants, 1823
Hutton Fndn Grants, 1828
J.L. Bedsole Fndn Grants, 1876
John Deere Fndn Grants, 1929
John J. Leidy Fndn Grants, 1936
John Merck Fund Grants, 1940
Johnson Controls Fndn Grants, 1954
Katharine Matthies Fndn Grants, 1982
Kosciusko County Comm Fndn Grants, 2015
Land O'Lakes Fndn Mid-Atlantic Grants, 2027
Legacy Fndn Grants, 2040
Lewis Preston Fund for Girls Education Grants, 2052
Lockheed Martin Philanthropic Grants, 2062
Lubbock Area Fndn Grants, 2079
Lubrizol Fndn Grants, 2080
Lynde and Harry Bradley Fndn Grants, 2089
Lynde and Harry Bradley Fndn Prizes: Bradley Prizes, 2090
Madison County Comm Fndn Grants, 2098
Maine Comm Fndn Grants, 2099
Mars Fndn Grants, 2114
May Department Stores Charitable Contribution Grants, 2138
Meadows Fndn Grants, 2161
Meriden Fndn Grants, 2173
Meyer Fndn Grants, 2177
Morris and Gwendolyn Cafritz Fndn Grants, 2217
Nina Mason Pulliam Charitable Trust Grants, 2776
Noble County Comm Fndn Grants, 2848
Nordson Corp Fndn Grants, 2851
Northern Trust Company Charitable Trust and Corp Giving Program, 2865
Northrop Grumman Newport News Grants, 2867
PacifiCorp Fndn for Learning Grants, 2982
Paul and Mary Haas Fndn Contributions and Student Scholarships, 2997
Paul Ogle Fndn Grants, 3003
Piedmont Natural Gas Grants, 3048
Piper Jaffray Companies Building Strong Communities Grants, 3053
Plum Creek Fndn Grants, 3062
Princeton Area Comm Fndn Greater Mercer Grants, 3081
Procter and Gamble Fund Grants, 3083
Puerto Rico Comm Fndn Grants, 3090
Rainbow Endowment Grants, 3102
RGK Fndn Grants, 3153
Rice Fndn Grants, 3155
Richard and Rhoda Goldman Fund Grants, 3158
Richard King Mellon Fndn Grants, 3161
Rochester Area Comm Fndn Grants, 3176
Rockefeller Brothers Fund Peace and Security Grants, 3179
Rockwell Collins Charitable Contributions, 3182
Rohm and Haas Company Grants, 3185
Salisbury Comm Fndn Grants, 3243
San Diego Women's Fndn Grants, 3259
Shell Oil Company Fndn Grants, 3281
Sosland Fndn Grants, 3348
Spencer County Comm Fndn Grants, 3358
Sprague Fndn Grants, 3359
Square D Fndn Grants, 3361
Stewart Huston Charitable Trust Grants, 3384
Sunderland Fndn Grants, 3400
Toro Fndn Grants, 3431
United Technologies Corp Grants, 3466
Vectren Fndn Grants, 3485
Wachovia Fndn Grants, 3511
Washington Post Contributions Grants, 3520
Weatherwax Fndn Grants, 3523
Wells County Fndn Grants, 3527
Westinghouse Charitable Giving Grants, 3530
Women's Fndn of California Grants, 3550
Z. Smith Reynolds Fndn Small Grants, 3557

Civic Engagement
Rockefeller Brothers Fund Peace and Security Grants, 3179

Civics
Gill Fndn - Gay and Lesbian Fund Grants, 1613
Hershey Company Grants, 1754

Civics Education
ACF Ethnic Comm Self-Help Grants, 200
Richard King Mellon Fndn Grants, 3161

Civil Engineering
NSF-NIST Interaction in Chemistry, Materials Research, Molecular Biosciences, Bioengineering, and Chemical Engineering, 2897

Civil Law
John Merck Fund Grants, 1940
OSI Indonesia Project Grants, 2967

Civil Service
John Merck Fund Grants, 1940

Civil Society
Cowles Charitable Trust Grants, 1155
Prospect Burma Scholarships, 3085

Civil/Human Rights
Allstate Corp Giving Grants, 363
Allstate Corp Hometown Commitment Grants, 364
Assisi Fndn Grants, 653
Blumenthal Fndn Grants, 773
Carrier Corp Contributions Grants, 884
Cass County Comm Fndn Grants, 887
Castle Rock Fndn Grants, 888
Coastal Comm Fndn of South Carolina Grants, 1051
Commission on Religion in Appalachia Grants, 1074
Comm Fndn of Greater Greensboro Grants, 1109
Comm Fndn of Western North Carolina Grants, 1132
Cowles Charitable Trust Grants, 1155
David Geffen Fndn Grants, 1202
Eugene McDermott Fndn Grants, 1435
Fargo-Moorhead Area Fndn Grants, 1454
Frank Stanley Beveridge Fndn Grants, 1553
Gill Fndn - Gay and Lesbian Fund Grants, 1613
Harold Simmons Fndn Grants, 1698
Henry J. Kaiser Family Fndn Grants, 1748
Herman Goldman Fndn Grants, 1753
Horizons Comm Issues Grants, 1794
Ignacio Martin-Baro Fund for Mental Health and Human Rights Grants, 1839
Jacob and Hilda Blaustein Fndn Grants, 1881
John Merck Fund Grants, 1940
Knox County Comm Fndn Grants, 2009
Lewis Preston Fund for Girls Education Grants, 2052
Margaret L. Wendt Fndn Grants, 2104
Minneapolis Fndn Comm Grants, 2206
Morton K. and Jane Blaustein Fndn Grants, 2218
OSI Indonesia Project Grants, 2967
OUT Fund for Lesbian and Gay Liberation Grants, 2978
Philadelphia Fndn Organizational Effectiveness Grants, 3029
Rainbow Endowment Grants, 3102
Rajiv Gandhi Fndn Grants, 3104
Samuel S. Johnson Fndn Grants, 3251
San Diego Fndn for Change Grants, 3255
Sir Dorabji Tata Trust Grants for NGOs or Voluntary Organizations, 3291
Steelcase Fndn Grants, 3379
Tifa Fndn Grants, 3428
Vanderburgh Comm Fndn Grants, 3480
Warrick County Comm Fndn Grants, 3519
Women's Fndn of California Grants, 3550
Z. Smith Reynolds Fndn Small Grants, 3557

Classroom Instruction
Arkema Fndn Science Teachers Program, 535
Coca-Cola Fndn Grants, 1052
Kettering Fund Grants, 1992
KeySpan Fndn Grants, 1995
King Pharmaceuticals Corp Contributions Grants, 2003
Long Island Comm Fndn Grants, 2063
Meyer Memorial Trust Emergency Grants, 2178
Meyer Memorial Trust Grassroots Grants, 2179
Meyer Memorial Trust Responsive Grants, 2181
NSF Presidential Early Career Awards for Scientists and Engineers (PECASE) Grants, 2892
Vectren Fndn Grants, 3485

Climate
James S. McDonnell Fndn Complex Systems Collaborative Activity Awards, 1897

Climatology
Bullitt Fndn Grants, 809
DOE Health Effects and Life Sciences Research Grants, 1298
NIH Ecology of Infectious Diseases, 2656

Clinical Medicine, General
AHFMR Clinical Fellowships, 269
AHFMR Fast-Track Studentships and Fellowships, 274
American College of Surgeons and The Triological Society Clinical Scientist Development Awards, 422
American Philosophical Society Daland Fellowships in Clinical Investigation, 441
CDC Evidence-Based Laboratory Medicine: Quality/Performance Measure Evaluation, 901
CVS All Kids Can Grants, 1175
Doris Duke Charitable Fndn Clinical Interfaces Award Program, 1314
Doris Duke Charitable Fndn Clinical Research Fellowships for Medical Students, 1315
Doris Duke Charitable Fndn Clinical Scientist Development Award Bridge Grants, 1317
Doris Duke Charitable Fndn Distinguished Clinical Scientist Award Program, 1318
EF Research and Training Fellowships for Clinicians, 1384
FIC International Research Scientist Development Award, 1491
FIC International Training and Research in Environmental and Occupational Health, 1493
Fndn for Medical Research Grants, 1528
Harry Shwachman Clinical Investigator Award, 1707
Henry & Ruth Blaustein Rosenberg Fndn Grants, 1746
NCI Ruth L. Kirschstein National Research Service Award Institutional Research Training Grants, 2277
NCI Stages of Breast Development: Normal to Metastatic Disease Grants, 2278
NEI Clinical Vision Research Development Award, 2293

NFID New Investigator Matching Grants, 2310
NHLBI Multidisciplinary Translational Research in Critical Care Grants, 2356
NIA Alzheimer's Disease Core Centers Grants, 2395
NIDA Minority Institutions Drug Abuse Research Development Program (MIDARP) Grants, 2509
NIDA Transition from Drug Abuse to Drug Addiction, 2516
NIDDK Pilot and Feasibility Clinical Research Grants in Kidney or Urologic Diseases, 2575
NIGMS Individual Postdoctoral NRSA Fellowships in Clinical Pharmacology, 2611
NIH Investigator-Initiated Interactive Research Project Grants, 2682
NIH Mentored Research Scientist Development Awards, 2689
NINR Aging Women and Breast Cancer Grants, 2789
NLM Internet Connection for Medical Institutions Grants, 2820
NYAM Mary and David Hoar Fellowship, 2916
PhRMA Fndn Health Outcomes Pre-Doctoral Fellowships, 3032
PhRMA Fndn Paul Calabresi Medical Student Research Fellowship, 3039
Regenstrief Master Of Science In Clinical Research/ CITE Program, 3145
RWJF Clinical Scholars Grants, 3207

Clinical Psychology
DHHS Health Careers Opportunity Grants, 1253
University of Georgia Counseling and Psychological Services Postdoctoral Fellowship, 3470

Clinical Research
AMSSM Fndn Research Grants, 469

Clinical Trials
Alton Ochsner Award, 373
ASCO State Affiliate Grants, 547
ASCO Advanced Clinical Research Award in Colorectal Cancer, 548
ASCO Advanced Clinical Research Awards in Breast Cancer, 549
ASCO Advanced Clinical Research Awards in Sarcoma, 550
ASCO Comm Oncology Research Grants, 552
ASCO Long-Term International Fellowships, 556
ASCO Medical Student Rotation Grants, 557
CDC Evidence-Based Laboratory Medicine: Quality/ Performance Measure Evaluation, 901
CRI Prostate Cancer Initiative Grants, 1163
Dermatology Clinical Career Development Awards, 1235
FDA Orphan Products Clinical Studies Grants, 1462
International Essential Tremor Fndn Grants, 1860
NCIC Terry Fox Postdoctoral Research Fellowships, 2285
NEI Clinical Study Planning Grant, 2292
NEI Clinical Vision Research Development Award, 2293
NHLBI Investigator Initiated Multi-Site Clinical Trials, 2344
NHLBI Mentored Clinical Scientist Research Career Development Awards, 2349
NIAAA Mentored Clinical Scientist Research Career Development Awards, 2446
NIAID HIV Prevention Trial Units Grants, 2453
NIAID HIV Vaccine Clinical Trial Units Grants, 2454
NIAID HIV Vaccine Research and Design—Program Project Grants, 2455
NIAID Pediatric Clinical Trials Program for AIDS, 2460
NIAMS Clinical Trial Planning Grants, 2466
NICHD Clinical Trial Planning Grants for Pediatric Rehabilitation, 2483
NICHD Innovative Therapies and Clinical Studies for Screenable Disorders Grants, 2485
NIDA National Drug Abuse Treatment Clinical Trials Network, 2510
NIDCD Clinical Trial Planning Grant, 2517
NIDCD Mentored Clinical Scientist Research Career Development Award, 2522
NIDCD Program for Postdoctoral Research Training in Clinical Trials, 2528
NIDCR Clinical Trial Pilot Grant, 2533
NIDCR Clinical Trial Planning Grant, 2534
NIDDK Ancillary Studies of Kidney Disease Accessing Information from Clinical Trials, Epidemiological Studies, and Databases Grants, 2540
NIDDK Ancillary Studies to Major Ongoing NIDDK and NHLBI Clinical Research Studies, 2541
NIDDK Basic and Clinical Studies of Congenital Urinary Tract Obstruction Grants, 2542
NIDDK Exploratory/Developmental Clinical Research Grants in Obesity, 2559
NIDDK Multi-Center Clinical Study Cooperative Agreements, 2566
NIGMS Individual Postdoctoral NRSA Fellowships in Clinical Pharmacology, 2611
NIH Alzheimer's Disease Clinical Trial Planning Grant, 2636
NIH Mentored Clinical Scientist Development Award, 2687
NIH Rett Syndrome: Genetics, Pathophysiology, and Biomarkers Research Grants, 2715
NIH Sarcoidosis: Research into the Cause of Multi-Organ Disease and Clinical Strategies for Therapy Grants, 2723
NINR Clinical Trials: Collaborations for Nursing Research, 2794
NKF Franklin McDonald/Fresenius Medical Care Clinical Research Grants, 2810
NMSS Sylvia Lawry Physician Fellowships, 2846
ONF Small Grants, 2947
PDF Postdoctoral Fellowships for Neurologists, 3007
Tourette Syndrome Association Post-Doc Fellowships, 3432
Tourette Syndrome Association Research Grants, 3433

Clinics
Andersen Fndn Grants, 471
Ann Arbor Area Comm Fndn Grants, 476
California Comm Fndn Health Care Grants, 831
CCFF Small Conference Grants, 896
CDC Evaluation of the Use of Rapid Testing For Influenza in Outpatient Medical Settings, 910
E. Rhodes and Leona B. Carpenter Fndn Grants, 1356
Fondren Fndn Grants, 1520
Gladys Brooks Fndn Grants, 1620
Harry and Grace Steele Fndn Grants, 1702
Sheltering Arms Fund Grants, 3282

Cloning of Cells
Parker B. Francis Fellowships in Pulmonary Research, 2989

Coastal Processes
Richard and Rhoda Goldman Fund Grants, 3158

Cognitive Development/Processes
CVS Comm Grants, 1177
DHHS Neurodevelopmental Test Methods Research Grants, 1268
Fyssen Fndn Postdoctoral Study Grants, 1580
Gerber Fndn Grants, 1606
James S. McDonnell Fndn Research Grants, 1898
James S. McDonnell Fndn Scholar Awards, 1899
James S. McDonnell Fndn Understanding Human Cognition Awards, 1900
NIA Factors Affecting Cognitive Function in Adults with Down Syndrome Grants, 2405
NIA Higher-Order Cognitive Functioning and Aging Grants, 2410
NIDA Behavioral Science Track Awards for Rapid Transition, 2498
NIDA Behavioral Therapies Development Grants, 2499
NIDA Drug Addiction Neuroscience Research Grants, 2503
NIDA Neurobiological and Behavioral Research on Nicotine and Tobacco Products, 2511
NIH Alzheimer's Disease Clinical Trial Planning Grant, 2636
NIH Mechanisms Underlying Individual Variations in Drug Responses, 2685
NIH Pathological Gambling: Basic, Clinical, and Services Research Grants, 2702
NIMH Behavior Genetics in Adulthood and Old Age Research Grants, 2747
NLM Research Project Grants, 2825
NSF Perception, Action & Cognition Research Grants, 2890
Olfactory Research Fund Grants, 2942
RCPSC Royal College Fellowship for Studies in Medical Education, 3127

Colitis
Broad Fndn IBD Research Grants, 803
Crohn's Disease and Colitis Research Fellowships, 1164
Crohn's Disease and Ulcerative Colitis Senior Research Grants, 1165
Partnership for Cures Two Years To Cures Grants, 2992

College Students
Alcohol Misuse and Alcoholism Research Grants, 335

College-Preparatory Education
3M Fndn Grants, 11
Florida High School/High Tech Project Grants, 1515
Michael and Susan Dell Fndn Grants, 2189
RWJF Young Epidemiology Scholars Competition, 3233

Columbia
Fulbright Traditional Scholar Program in the Western Hemisphere, 1577

Communication Systems
NIDCD Communicative Competence of Users of Augmentative and Alternative Communication Systems Research Grants, 2518

Communications
AAFCS International Graduate Fellowships, 109
AAFCS National Graduate Fellowships, 110
AAFCS National Undergraduate Scholarships, 111
Abell-Hanger Fndn Grants, 183
AMA-RFS and AMA Fndn Medical Student & Resident/Fellow Elective-Medicine & the Media, 406
ASHFndn New Century Scholars Research Grant, 581
ASM Public Communications Award, 611
AVDF Health Care Grants, 673
Canada Graduate Scholarships and NSERC Postgraduate Scholarships, 845
Canada-U.S. Fulbright New Century Scholars Grants, 846
Canada-U.S. Fulbright Senior Specialists Grants, 847
CDC Promoting Prevention in Managed Care Cooperative Agreements, 925
Chicago Board of Trade Fndn Grants, 988
DOL Occupational Safety and Health—Susan Harwood Training Grants, 1305
EPA Children's Health Protection Grants, 1420
Fulbright Alumni Initiatives Awards Grants, 1566
Fulbright Distinguished Chairs Grants, 1567
Fulbright New Century Scholars Grants, 1570
Fulbright Specialists Grants, 1571
Fulbright Traditional Scholar Program in Europe and Eurasia, 1572
Fulbright Traditional Scholar Program in Sub-Saharan Africa, 1573
Fulbright Traditional Scholar Program in the East Asia/Pacific Region, 1574
Fulbright Traditional Scholar Program in the Near East and North Africa Region, 1575
Fulbright Traditional Scholar Program in the South and Central Asia Region, 1576
Fulbright Traditional Scholar Program in the Western Hemisphere, 1577

Heineman Fndn for Research, Education, Charitable and Scientific Purposes, 1735
Henry J. Kaiser Family Fndn Grants, 1748
Josiah Macy Jr. Fndn Grants, 1966
NCI/NIDA Transdisciplinary Tobacco Use Research Centers Grants, 2280
New York University Steinhardt School of Education Fellowships, 2305
NIDCD Health Promotion and Disease Prevention: Health Communication, Development, and Dissemination, 2521
NLM Internet Connection for Medical Institutions Grants, 2820
NSF Chemistry Research Experiences for Undergraduates, 2883
RSC Thomas W. Eadie Medal, 3199
Scientific Communities Initiative Grants, 3272
Tellabs Fndn Grants, 3418
United Cerebral Palsy Research Grants, 3462

Communicative Disorders, Hearing
ASHA Advancing Academic-Research Careers Award, 569
ASHA Minority Student Leadership Program Awards, 570
ASHA Research Mentoring-Pair Travel Award, 572
ASHA Student Research Travel Award, 573
ASHA Students Preparing for Academic & Research Careers Award, 574
ASHFndn Clinical Research Grants, 575
ASHFndn Graduate Student International Scholarship, 576
ASHFndn Graduate Student Scholarships, 577
ASHFndn Graduate Student Scholarships for Minority Students, 578
ASHFndn Graduate Student with a Disability Scholarship, 579
ASHFndn New Century Scholars Program Doctoral Scholarships, 580
ASHFndn New Century Scholars Research Grant, 581
ASHFndn Research Grant for New Investigators, 582
ASHFndn Student Research Grants in Audiology, 584
Deafness Research Fndn Research Grants, 1208
DHHS Universal Newborn Hearing Screening and Intervention, 1282
NIDCD Exploratory Research: Feasibility Pilot Studies Grants, 2519
NIDCD Exploratory/Developmental Research Grants, 2520
NIDCD Health Promotion and Disease Prevention: Health Communication, Development, and Dissemination, 2521
NIDCD Mentored Clinical Scientist Research Career Development Award, 2522
NIDCD Minority Dissertation Research Grants in Human Communication, 2524
NIDCD Program for Postdoctoral Research Training in Clinical Trials, 2528
NIDCD Research Core Centers, 2529
NIDCD Small Grants, 2531

Communicative Disorders, Speech
ASHA Advancing Academic-Research Careers Award, 569
ASHA Minority Student Leadership Program Awards, 570
ASHA Research Mentoring-Pair Travel Award, 572
ASHA Student Research Travel Award, 573
ASHA Students Preparing for Academic & Research Careers Award, 574
ASHFndn Clinical Research Grants, 575
ASHFndn Graduate Student International Scholarship, 576
ASHFndn Graduate Student Scholarships, 577
ASHFndn Graduate Student Scholarships for Minority Students, 578
ASHFndn Graduate Student with a Disability Scholarship, 579
ASHFndn New Century Scholars Program Doctoral Scholarships, 580
ASHFndn New Century Scholars Research Grant, 581
ASHFndn Research Grant for New Investigators, 582
ASHFndn Research Grant in Speech Science, 583
NIDCD Communicative Competence of Users of Augmentative and Alternative Communication Systems Research Grants, 2518
NIDCD Exploratory Research: Feasibility Pilot Studies Grants, 2519
NIDCD Exploratory/Developmental Research Grants, 2520
NIDCD Health Promotion and Disease Prevention: Health Communication, Development, and Dissemination, 2521
NIDCD Mentored Clinical Scientist Research Career Development Award, 2522
NIDCD Minority Dissertation Research Grants in Human Communication, 2524
NIDCD Program for Postdoctoral Research Training in Clinical Trials, 2528
NIDCD Small Grants, 2531

Community and School Relations
American Express Fndn Comm Service Grants, 435
Bank of America Charitable Fndn National Programs and Partners Grants, 689
DOJ Gang-Free Schools and Communities Intervention Grants, 1303
Evanston Comm Fndn Grants, 1438
Farmers Insurance Group of Companies Grants, 1455
Joe W. and Dorothy Dorsett Brown Fndn Grants, 1927
Mead Johnson Nutritionals Evansville-Area Organizations Grants, 2157
Princeton Area Comm Fndn Greater Mercer Grants, 3081
Self Fndn Grants, 3277
Vancouver Fndn Grants and Comm Initiatives Program, 3477

Community Development
2 Depot Square Ipswich Charitable Fndn Grants, 7
3M Company Health and Human Services Grants, 10
A/H Fndn Grants, 19
AAP Resident Initiative Fund Grants, 167
Abbott Fund Access to Health Care Grants, 176
Abbott Fund Comm Vitality Grants, 177
Able To Serve Grants, 185
ACF Ethnic Comm Self-Help Grants, 200
Adobe Comm Investment Grants, 237
AEC Trust Grants, 242
Agnes M. Lindsay Trust Grants, 263
AIG American General Corp Grants, 316
Air Products and Chemicals Grants, 319
Albert Pick Jr. Fund Grants, 328
Alexander & Baldwin Fndn Hawaiian and Pacific Island Grants, 338
Alexander & Baldwin Fndn Mainland Grants, 339
Alexander Eastman Fndn Grants, 341
Alice Tweed Tuohy Fndn Grants, 357
Allyn Fndn Grants, 365
Altman Fndn Health Care Grants, 372
AMA Fndn Fund for Better Health Grants, 388
AMA Fndn Healthy Communities/Healthy America Grants, 390
AMA Fndn Jack B. McConnell, MD Awards for Excellence in Volunteerism, 391
AMA Fndn Leadership Awards, 394
AMA-MSS Chapter Involvement Grants, 401
AMA-MSS Chapter of the Year Award, 402
Amador Comm Fndn Grants, 409
AMD Corp Contributions Grants, 411
American Express Fndn Comm Service Grants, 435
American Jewish World Service Grants, 437
Angels Baseball Fndn Grants, 473
Anheuser-Busch Fndn Grants, 474
Ann and Robert H. Lurie Family Fndn Grants, 475
Ann Arbor Area Comm Fndn Grants, 476
Annie Sinclair Knudsen Memorial Fund/Kaua'i Comm Grants, 480
Arizona Public Service Corp Giving Grants, 531
Arkansas Comm Fndn Grants, 533
Arlington Comm Fndn Grants, 536
Armstrong McDonald Fndn Grants, 537
ASCO State Affiliate Grants, 547
Autodesk Comm Relations Grants, 671
Bacon Family Fndn Grants, 679
Bailey Fndn Grants, 680
Ball Brothers Fndn General Grants, 683
Ball Brothers Fndn Grants, 684
Bank of America Charitable Fndn National Programs and Partners Grants, 689
Barberton Comm Fndn Grants, 693
Barnes Group Fndn Grants, 696
Baton Rouge Area Fndn Grants, 702
Battle Creek Comm Fndn Grants, 703
Batts Fndn Grants, 704
BCBSM Building Healthy Communities Engaging Elementary Schools & Comm Partners Grants, 713
BCBSM Comm Health Matching Grants, 715
Beazley Fndn Grants, 730
Beckley Area Fndn Grants, 732
Bill and Melinda Gates Fndn Grants, 756
Biogen Corp Giving Grants, 758
Birmingham Fndn Grants, 760
Black River Falls Area Fndn Grants, 762
Blackford County Comm Fndn Grants, 763
Blanche and Julian Robertson Family Fndn Grants, 765
Bodenwein Public Benevolent Fndn Grants, 775
Boeing Company Contributions Grants, 777
Bonfils-Stanton Fndn Grants, 779
Bosque Fndn Grants, 782
Boyd Gaming Corp Contributions Program, 788
Brian G. Dyson Fndn Grants, 791
Bridgestone/Firestone Trust Fund Grants, 792
Burlington Industries Fndn Grants, 811
Business Bank of Nevada Comm Grants, 817
C.R. Bard Fndn Grants, 825
C.W. Titus Fndn Grants, 826
Caleb C. and Julia W. Dula Educational and Charitable Fndn Grants, 830
California Comm Fndn Health Care Grants, 831
California Comm Fndn Human Development Grants, 832
Callaway Fndn Grants, 835
Cambridge Comm Fndn Grants, 837
Caring Fndn Grants, 866
Carl B. and Florence E. King Fndn Grants, 869
Carnahan-Jackson Fndn Grants, 878
Carrie E. and Lena V. Glenn Fndn Grants, 882
Carrier Corp Contributions Grants, 884
Carroll County Comm Fndn Grants, 885
Catherine Kennedy Home Fndn Grants, 890
Catholic Campaign for Human Development Comm Organizing Grants, 891
Central Okanagan Fndn Grants, 937
Cessna Fndn Grants, 938
CFFVR Opportunity Grants, 952
Champlin Fndns Grants, 960
Charles Delmar Fndn Grants, 963
Charles M. and Mary D. Grant Fndn Grants, 971
Charlotte County (FL) Comm Fndn Grants, 973
Chesapeake Corp Fndn Grants, 982
Chicago Comm Trust Grants, 989
Christy-Houston Fndn Grants, 1008
Chula Vista Charitable Fndn Grants, 1009
Cinergy Fndn Grants, 1013
Claude Worthington Benedum Fndn Grants, 1033
CNA Fndn Grants, 1046
Coastal Bend Comm Fndn Grants, 1050
Coeta and Donald Barker Fndn Grants, 1054
Coleman Fndn Cancer Care Grants, 1055
Colorado Springs Comm Trust Fund Grants, 1061
Comerica Charitable Fndn Grants, 1073
Comm Fndn Alliance City of Evansville Endowment Fund Grants, 1089
Comm Fndn for Greater Buffalo Grants, 1090
Comm Fndn for Muskegon County Grants, 1093
Comm Fndn of Bloomington and Monroe County Grants, 1098
Comm Fndn of Champaign County Grants, 1102

Comm Fndn of Crawford County Grants and Scholarships, 1103
Comm Fndn of Grant County Grants, 1104
Comm Fndn of Greater Birmingham Grants, 1106
Comm Fndn of Greater Greensboro Grants, 1109
Comm Fndn Of Greater Lafayette Grants, 1110
Comm Fndn of Greater New Britain Grants, 1111
Comm Fndn of Greater Tampa Grants, 1112
Comm Fndn of Greenville Comm Enrichment Grants, 1113
Comm Fndn of Greenville Hollingsworth Funds Program/Project Grants, 1114
Comm Fndn of Greenville-Greenville Women Giving Grants, 1115
Comm Fndn of Howard County Grants, 1116
Comm Fndn of Madison and Jefferson County Grants and Scholarships, 1117
Comm Fndn of Morgan County Grants and Scholarships, 1118
Comm Fndn of Mount Vernon and Knox County Grants, 1119
Comm Fndn of Muncie and Delaware County Grants, 1120
Comm Fndn of Randolph County Grants, 1121
Comm Fndn of Santa Cruz County Grants, 1122
Comm Fndn of St. Joseph County Special Project Challenge Grants, 1126
Comm Fndn of Switzerland County Grants, 1127
Comm Fndn of Tampa Bay Grants, 1128
Comm Fndn of the Eastern Shore Comm Needs Grants, 1129
Comm Fndn of the Ozarks Grants, 1130
Comm Fndn of Wabash County Grants, 1131
Comm Fndn of Western North Carolina Grants, 1132
Comm Technology Fndn of California Building Communities Through Technology Grants, 1136
Connelly Fndn Grants, 1143
ConocoPhillips Fndn Grants, 1144
Constantin Fndn Grants, 1145
Constellation Energy Group and Baltimore Gas and Electric Corp Contributions, 1146
Cornerstone Fndn of Northeastern Wisconsin Grants, 1152
Crestlea Fndn Grants, 1159
Cruise Industry Charitable Fndn Grants, 1166
CSL Behring Local Empowerment for Advocacy Development Grants, 1167
CSRA Comm Fndn Grants, 1168
CSX Corp Contributions Grants, 1169
CVS All Kids Can Grants, 1175
D. W. McMillan Fndn Grants, 1180
D.F. Halton Fndn Grants, 1181
Dade Comm Fndn Comm AIDS Partnership Grants, 1184
Dade Comm Fndn Grants, 1185
Daisy Marquis Jones Fndn Grants, 1188
Danellie Fndn Grants, 1198
Daviess County Comm Fndn Health Grants, 1203
Daywood Fndn Grants, 1206
Dearborn Comm Fndn City of Lawrenceburg Comm Grants, 1210
Delaware Comm Fndn Grants, 1215
Delta Air Lines Fndn Grants, 1220
Dept of Ed Safe and Drug-Free Schools and Communities State Grants, 1230
DeRoy Testamentary Fndn Grants, 1239
Dole Food Company Charitable Contributions, 1307
Duke Energy Fndn Grants, 1339
Duneland Health Council InCorpd Grants, 1350
Dyson Fndn Mid-Hudson Valley General Operating Support Grants, 1354
Eberly Fndn Grants, 1364
Eddie C. and Sylvia Brown Family Fndn Grants, 1367
Edina Realty Fndn Grants, 1369
Edwin S. Webster Fndn Grants, 1376
Edyth Bush Charitable Fndn Grants, 1378
El Paso Corp Fndn Grants, 1389
El Pomar Fndn Awards and Grants, 1390
Elkhart County Comm Fndn Grants, 1401
Elliot Fndn Inc Grants, 1402
Ensworth Charitable Fndn Grants, 1416
Entergy Comm Partnership Grants, 1417
Entergy Corp Open Grants for Healthy Families, 1418
Ethel S. Abbott Charitable Fndn Grants, 1430
Eugene and Agnes E. Meyer Fndn Grants, 1432
Eugene McDermott Fndn Grants, 1435
Evanston Comm Fndn Grants, 1438
Evjue Fndn Grants, 1439
Fairfield County Comm Fndn Grants, 1446
FAR Fund, 1453
Fayette County Fndn Grants, 1457
Feldman Fndn Grants, 1484
Ferree Fndn Grants, 1486
Fidelity Fndn Grants, 1498
Fifth Third Fndn Grants, 1501
FirstEnergy Fndn Comm Grants, 1505
Fisher Fndn Grants, 1508
Fishman Family Fndn Grants, 1510
Florida BRAIVE Fund of Dade Comm Fndn, 1512
Florida BRAIVE Fund of Gulf Coast Comm Fndn of Venice, 1513
Florida BRAIVE Fund of The Comm Fndn in Jacksonville, 1514
FMC Fndn Grants, 1518
Foellinger Fndn Grants, 1519
Fondren Fndn Grants, 1520
Ford Motor Company Fund Grants, 1522
Foster G. McGaw Prize, 1525
Fndn for the Mid-South Grants, 1536
Fndn Northwest Grants, 1537
Fourjay Fndn Grants, 1544
Frances L. and Edwin L. Cummings Memorial Fund Grants, 1547
Frances W. Emerson Fndn Grants, 1548
Frank Stanley Beveridge Fndn Grants, 1553
Franklin County Comm Fndn Grants, 1554
Fred Baldwin Memorial Fndn Grants, 1556
Freddie Mac Fndn Grants, 1558
Fremont Area Comm Fndn Grants, 1561
Genentech Corp Charitable Contributions Grants, 1588
George Kress Fndn Grants, 1601
Georgiana Goddard Eaton Memorial Fund Grants, 1604
Geraldine R. Dodge Fndn Morris County Grants, 1605
Gertrude and William C. Wardlaw Fund Grants, 1607
Gertrude E. Skelly Charitable Fndn Grants, 1609
Gheens Fndn Grants, 1610
Giant Eagle Fndn Grants, 1611
Ginn Fndn Grants, 1616
Giving Sum Annual Grant, 1619
Gladys Brooks Fndn Grants, 1620
GlaxoSmithKline Corp Grants, 1623
Godfrey Fndn Grants, 1631
Graco Fndn Grants, 1642
Grand Rapids Comm Fndn Grants, 1647
Greater Cincinnati Fndn Priority and Small Projects/ Capacity-Building Grants, 1651
Greater Green Bay Comm Fndn Grants, 1652
Greater Milwaukee Fndn Grants, 1653
Greater New Orleans Fndn Grants, 1654
Greater Saint Louis Comm Fndn Grants, 1655
Greater Worcester Comm Fndn Jeppson Memorial Fund for Brookfield Grants, 1659
Greene County Fndn Grants, 1662
Gregory L. Gibson Charitable Fndn Grants, 1668
Gruber Fndn International Prizes, 1672
Gulf Coast Comm Fndn Grants, 1676
Gulf Coast Comm of Venice Fndn Grants, 1677
H & R Fndn Grants, 1679
Hagedorn Fund Grants, 1685
Hancock County Comm Fndn Grants, 1690
Hannaford Charitable Fndn Grants, 1692
Harley Davidson Fndn Grants, 1694
Harold Alfond Fndn Grants, 1695
Harold and Arlene Schnitzer CARE Fndn Grants, 1697
Harris and Eliza Kempner Fund Grants, 1699
Harry Bramhall Gilbert Charitable Trust Grants, 1703
Harry Kramer Memorial Fund Grants, 1705
Harry S. Black and Allon Fuller Fund, 1706
Hartford Courant Fndn Grants, 1710
Hartford Fndn Regular Grants, 1711
Harvest Fndn Grants, 1713
Hawaii Comm Fndn Reverend Takie Okumura Family Grants, 1717
Hawaii Comm Fndn West Hawaii Fund Grants, 1718
Health Fndn of Greater Cincinnati Grants, 1724
Henrietta Tower Wurts Memorial Fndn Grants, 1745
Henry County Comm Fndn Grants, 1747
Henry County Comm Fndn Grants, 1747
Hershey Company Grants, 1754
High Meadow Fndn Grants, 1768
Highmark Corp Giving Grants, 1769
Hill Crest Fndn Grants, 1773
Hillman Fndn Grants, 1775
Hillsdale County Comm General Adult Fndn Grants, 1777
Hilton Head Island Fndn Grants, 1779
Hirtzel Memorial Fndn Grants, 1781
Hoglund Fndn Grants, 1785
Holland/Zeeland Comm Fndn Grants, 1786
Homer Fndn Grants, 1789
Honda of America Manufacturing Fndn Grants, 1790
Horace A. Kimball and S. Ella Kimball Fndn Grants, 1792
Horizon Fndn for New Jersey Grants, 1793
Hormel Fndn Grants, 1796
Houston Endowment Grants, 1797
Howard and Bush Fndn Grants, 1798
Howe Fndn of North Carolina Grants, 1799
Hudson Webber Fndn Grants, 1813
Hugh J. Andersen Fndn Grants, 1814
Humana Fndn Grants, 1818
Humboldt Area Fndn Technical Assistance Grants, 1819
Huntington Clinical Fndn Grants, 1822
Huntington County Comm Fndn Grants, 1823
Hut Fndn Grants, 1827
Hutton Fndn Grants, 1828
Idaho Comm Fndn Eastern Region Competitive Grants, 1837
Idaho Power Company Corp Contributions, 1838
Impact 100 Grants, 1843
Inasmuch Fndn Grants, 1845
Independence Blue Cross Charitable Medical Care Grants, 1846
Independence Comm Fndn Comm Quality of Life Grant, 1849
Ireland Family Fndn Grants, 1865
Irvin Stern Fndn Grants, 1866
Irving S. Gilmore Fndn Grants, 1867
Isabel Allende Fndn Esperanza Grants, 1868
J.B. Reynolds Fndn Grants, 1873
J.C. Penney Company Grants, 1874
J.E. and L.E. Mabee Fndn Grants, 1875
J.L. Bedsole Fndn Grants, 1876
J.W. Kieckhefer Fndn Grants, 1878
Jackson County Comm Fndn Unrestricted Grants, 1379
Jacob and Hilda Blaustein Fndn Grants, 1881
Jacob G. Schmidlapp Trust Grants, 1883
James A. and Faith Knight Fndn Grants, 1884
James Ford Bell Fndn Grants, 1885
James Graham Brown Fndn Grants, 1887
James J. and Angelia M. Harris Fndn Grants, 1890
James R. Dougherty Jr. Fndn Grants, 1894
James S. Copley Fndn Grants, 1895
Jane Bradley Pettit Fndn Grants, 1902
Janirve Fndn Grants, 1905
Jasper Fndn Jasper County Grants, 1907
Jasper Fndn Newton County Grants, 1908
JELD-WEN Fndn Grants, 1914
Jennings County Comm Fndn Grants, 1916
Joe W. and Dorothy Dorsett Brown Fndn Grants, 1927
John Ben Snow Memorial Trust Grants, 1928
John Deere Fndn Grants, 1929
John G. Duncan Trust Grants, 1931
John H. and Wilhelmina D. Harland Charitable Fndn Grants, 1933
John H. Wellons Fndn Grants, 1934

John Jewett and Helen Chandler Garland Fndn Grants, 1937
John P. McGovern Fndn Grants, 1942
John S. Dunn Research Fndn Grants and Chairs, 1945
John W. Alden Trust Grants, 1947
John W. Anderson Fndn Grants, 1949
Johnson County Comm Fndn Grants, 1955
Josephine G. Russell Trust Grants, 1963
Josephine Goodyear Fndn Grants, 1964
K21 Health Fndn Cancer Care Fund Grants, 1975
K21 Health Fndn Grants, 1976
Kahuku Comm Fund, 1977
Katharine Matthies Fndn Grants, 1982
KeySpan Fndn Grants, 1995
Knox County Comm Fndn Grants, 2009
Kosciusko County Comm Fndn Grants, 2015
L. W. Pierce Family Fndn Grants, 2019
Lands' End Corp Giving Program, 2030
Legacy Fndn Grants, 2040
Liberty Bank Fndn Grants, 2053
Lillian S. Wells Fndn Grants, 2056
Long Island Comm Fndn Grants, 2063
Lotus 88 Fndn for Women and Children Grants, 2064
Lowell Area Comm Fund Grants, 2068
Lowell Berry Fndn Grants, 2069
Lubbock Area Fndn Grants, 2079
Lucy Gooding Charitable Fndn Trust Grants, 2083
M.B. and Edna Zale Fndn Grants, 2093
Mabel Y. Hughes Charitable Trust Grants, 2097
Madison County Comm Fndn Grants, 2098
Maine Comm Fndn Grants, 2099
Margaret L. Wendt Fndn Grants, 2104
Mark and Catherine Winkler Fndn Grants, 2112
Massage Therapy Fndn Comm Service Grants, 2124
Maxon Charitable Fndn Grants, 2135
McKnight Fndn Grants, 2146
McMillen Fndn Grants, 2148
Mead Johnson Nutritionals Evansville-Area Organizations Grants, 2157
Meyer Fndn Grants, 2177
Meyer Memorial Trust Emergency Grants, 2178
Meyer Memorial Trust Grassroots Grants, 2179
Meyer Memorial Trust Operating Funds Grants, 2180
Meyer Memorial Trust Responsive Grants, 2181
Miami County Comm Fndn Operation Round Up Grants, 2188
Middlesex Savings Charitable Fndn Grants, 2196
Montgomery County Comm Fndn Grants, 2214
Morris and Gwendolyn Cafritz Fndn Grants, 2217
National City Corp Contributions Grants, 2250
National Lottery Comm Fund Grants, 2256
Nelda C. and H.J. Lutcher Stark Fndn Grants, 2301
Noble County Comm Fndn Grants, 2848
North Carolina Biotechnology Center Meeting Grants, 2854
North Carolina Biotechnology Center Regional Development Grants, 2855
North Carolina Comm Fndn Grants, 2859
North Central Health Services Grants, 2861
North Georgia Comm Fndn Grants, 2862
Northern New York Comm Fndn Grants, 2864
Northern Trust Company Charitable Trust and Corp Giving Program, 2865
Northwest Minnesota Fndn Women's Fund Grants, 2869
Northwestern Mutual Fndn Grants, 2870
Norwin S. and Elizabeth N. Bean Fndn Grants, 2872
NWHF Comm-Based Participatory Research Grants, 2904
NWHF Kaiser Permanente Comm Fund Grants, 2906
NYCT Girls and Young Women Grants, 2924
NYCT Grants for the Elderly, 2925
NYCT Technical Assistance Grants, 2929
Oceanside Charitable Fndn Grants, 2934
Office Depot Fndn Grants, 2936
Ohio County Comm Fndn Grants, 2938
Ohio County Comm Fndn Mini-Grants, 2939
Oleonda Jameson Trust Grants, 2941
OneStar Fndn AmeriCorps Grants, 2945
Oscar Rennebohm Fndn Grants, 2963
OSI-Baltimore Special Opportunities Grants, 2972
Otto Bremer Fndn Grants, 2977
Owen County Comm Fndn Grants, 2979
PacifiCare Fndn Grants, 2981
Palm Beach and Martin Counties Grants, 2986
Paul G. Allen Family Fndn Grants, 3000
Paul Ogle Fndn Grants, 3003
Peacock Fndn Grants, 3011
Perkins Charitable Fndn Grants, 3014
Perpetual Trust for Charitable Giving Grants, 3015
Perry County Comm Fndn Grants, 3016
Pet Care Trust Sue Busch Memorial Award, 3017
Philadelphia Fndn Organizational Effectiveness Grants, 3029
Piedmont Natural Gas Grants, 3048
Pike County Comm Fndn Grants, 3049
Pinellas County Grants, 3050
Pittsburgh Fndn Comm Fund Grants, 3054
Plough Fndn Grants, 3061
Plum Creek Fndn Grants, 3062
PNC Charitable Trust and Fndn Grants, 3064
Polk Bros. Fndn Grants, 3066
Portland General Electric Fndn Grants, 3067
Posey Comm Fndn Grants, 3068
Posey Comm Fndn Womens Fund Grants, 3069
Pott Fndn Grants, 3071
Priddy Fndn Grants, 3077
Prince Charitable Trusts District of Columbia Grants, 3080
Princeton Area Comm Fndn Greater Mercer Grants, 3081
Public Welfare Fndn Grants, 3089
Puerto Rico Comm Fndn Grants, 3090
Pulaski County Comm Fndn Grants, 3091
Putnam County Comm Fndn Grants, 3093
Quantum Fndn Grants, 3096
Raskob Fndn for Catholic Activities Grants, 3107
Rasmuson Fndn Grants, 3108
Rayonier Fndn Grants, 3111
Regence Fndn Access to Health Care Grants, 3138
Regence Fndn Health Care Comm Awareness and Engagement Grants, 3139
Regence Fndn Health Care Connections Grants, 3140
Regence Fndn Improving End-of-Life Grants, 3141
Regence Fndn Tools and Technology Grants, 3142
Retirement Research Fndn General Grants, 3150
Reynolds and Reynolds Associate Fndn Grants, 3152
Rhode Island Fndn Grants, 3154
Rich Fndn Grants, 3156
Richard M. Fairbanks Fndn Grants, 3162
Ripley County Comm Fndn Grants, 3166
Robert and Joan Dircks Fndn Grants, 3167
Robert B McMillen Fndn Grants, 3169
Rochester Area Comm Fndn Grants, 3176
Rochester Area Fndn Grants, 3177
Rockefeller Fndn Grants, 3181
Rockwell International Corp Trust Grants, 3183
Rollin M. Gerstacker Fndn Grants, 3186
Roy and Christine Sturgis Trust Grants, 3191
Rush County Comm Fndn Grants, 3200
Ruth H. and Warren A. Ellsworth Fndn Grants, 3203
RWJF Ladder to Leadership: Developing the Next Generation of Comm Health Leaders Fellowships, 3222
RWJF Pipeline, Profession and Practice: Comm-Based Dental Education Grants, 3228
RWJF Vulnerable Populations Portfolio Grants, 3232
S. Livingston Mather Charitable Trust Grants, 3235
Samuel S. Johnson Fndn Grants, 3251
San Diego Fndn Paradise Valley Hospital Comm Fund Grants, 3257
San Diego Women's Fndn Grants, 3259
Schering-Plough Fndn Comm Initiatives Grants, 3269
Schurz Communications Fndn Grants, 3271
Scott County Comm Fndn Grants, 3273
Seattle Fndn Grants, 3276
Self Fndn Grants, 3277
Shaw's Supermarkets Donations, 3280
Shell Oil Company Fndn Grants, 3281
Siebert Lutheran Fndn Grants, 3285
Simple Advise Education Center Grants, 3289
Sir Dorabji Tata Trust Grants for NGOs or Voluntary Organizations, 3291
SOCFOC Catholic Ministries Grants, 3317
SOCFOC Reducing Health & Educational Disparities in the Central Neighborhood Grants, 3318
Sonoco Fndn Grants, 3347
South Madison Comm Fndn Grants, 3349
Southbury Comm Trust Fund, 3350
Southwest Florida Comm Fndn Competitive Grants, 3351
Southwest Gas Corp Fndn Grants, 3352
Southwire Company Grants, 3353
Spencer County Comm Fndn Grants, 3358
Sprague Fndn Grants, 3359
Springs Close Fndn Grants, 3360
St. Joseph Comm Health Fndn Improving Healthcare Access Grants, 3368
Stackner Family Fndn Grants, 3371
Steelcase Fndn Grants, 3379
Steuben County Comm Fndn Grants, 3383
Strowd Roses Grants, 3388
Sunderland Fndn Grants, 3400
Susan Mott Webb Charitable Trust Grants, 3412
Susan Vaughan Fndn Grants, 3413
Temple-Inland Fndn Grants, 3419
Thomas and Dorothy Leavey Fndn Grants, 3422
Thomas C. Ackerman Fndn Grants, 3423
Thompson Charitable Fndn Grants, 3425
Triangle Comm Fndn Donor-Advised Grants, 3437
Trull Fndn Grants, 3441
TWS Fndn Grants, 3443
U.S. Department of Education 21st Century Comm Learning Centers, 3445
Union Benevolent Association Grants, 3460
Union County Comm Fndn Grants, 3461
Unity Fndn Of LaPorte County Grants, 3467
USCM HIV/AIDS Prevention Grants, 3476
Vancouver Fndn Grants and Comm Initiatives Program, 3477
Vancouver Sun Children's Fund Grants, 3479
Vanderburgh Comm Fndn Grants, 3480
Vermont Comm Fndn Grants, 3493
Vulcan Materials Company Fndn Grants, 3504
W. C. Griffith Fndn Grants, 3505
W.K. Kellogg Fndn Secure Families Grants, 3508
Wabash Valley Comm Fndn Grants, 3510
Wachovia Fndn Grants, 3511
Warrick County Comm Fndn Grants, 3519
Welborn Baptist Fndn Grants, 3525
Western Indiana Comm Fndn Grants, 3528
William G. Gilmore Fndn Grants, 3537
Wilson-Wood Fndn Grants, 3542
Winston-Salem Fndn Elkin/Tri-County Grants, 3545
Women's Fndn of California Grants, 3550
YSA Get Ur Good On Grants, 3555

Community Outreach Programs

3M Fndn Grants, 11
Able To Serve Grants, 185
AHFMR Comm Support Grants, 271
Allstate Corp Giving Grants, 363
Allstate Corp Hometown Commitment Grants, 364
American Express Fndn Comm Service Grants, 435
Angels Baseball Fndn Grants, 473
APF Helping Hands Grants, 507
Bank of America Charitable Fndn National Programs and Partners Grants, 689
Batchelor Fndn Grants, 701
Bernard and Audre Rapoport Fndn Grants, 746
Boston Fndn Grants, 783
Cable Positive's Tony Cox Comm Fund Grants, 827
California Comm Fndn Human Development Grants, 832
Cambridge Comm Fndn Grants, 837
Caring Fndn Grants, 866
Carl B. and Florence E. King Fndn Grants, 869
Carrie E. and Lena V. Glenn Fndn Grants, 882
Carrier Corp Contributions Grants, 884
Catherine Kennedy Home Fndn Grants, 890

Catholic Campaign for Human Development Comm Organizing Grants, 891
Cessna Fndn Grants, 938
Charles Delmar Fndn Grants, 963
Columbus Fndn Traditional Grants, 1071
Commonweal Fndn Grants, 1076
Comm Fndn of Grant County Grants, 1104
Comm Fndn Of Greater Lafayette Grants, 1110
Comm Fndn of Greater New Britain Grants, 1111
Comm Fndn of Greenville Comm Enrichment Grants, 1113
Comm Fndn of Greenville Hollingsworth Funds Program/Project Grants, 1114
Comm Fndn of Howard County Grants, 1116
Comm Fndn of Madison and Jefferson County Grants and Scholarships, 1117
Comm Fndn of Randolph County Grants, 1121
Comm Fndn of Switzerland County Grants, 1127
Cowles Charitable Trust Grants, 1155
D. W. McMillan Fndn Grants, 1180
Dade Comm Fndn Comm AIDS Partnership Grants, 1184
Danellie Fndn Grants, 1198
Delaware Comm Fndn-Youth Philanthropy Board for Kent County, 1216
DHHS Healthy Tomorrows Partnership for Children, 1261
Edina Realty Fndn Grants, 1369
Eisner Fndn Grants, 1387
EPA Children's Health Protection Grants, 1420
Evan and Susan Bayh Fndn Grants, 1437
Florida BRAIVE Fund of Dade Comm Fndn, 1512
Florida BRAIVE Fund of Gulf Coast Comm Fndn of Venice, 1513
Florida BRAIVE Fund of The Comm Fndn in Jacksonville, 1514
Fndn for the Mid-South Grants, 1536
George Family Fndn Grants, 1598
Georgiana Goddard Eaton Memorial Fund Grants, 1604
Geraldine R. Dodge Fndn Morris County Grants, 1605
Giant Eagle Fndn Grants, 1611
Giving Sum Annual Grant, 1619
Harley Davidson Fndn Grants, 1694
Harry Kramer Memorial Fund Grants, 1705
Hartford Courant Fndn Grants, 1710
Harvest Fndn Grants, 1713
Health Fndn of Greater Cincinnati Grants, 1724
Henrietta Tower Wurts Memorial Fndn Grants, 1745
High Meadow Fndn Grants, 1768
Hilton Head Island Fndn Grants, 1779
Horace A. Kimball and S. Ella Kimball Fndn Grants, 1792
Horizons Comm Issues Grants, 1794
Ireland Family Fndn Grants, 1865
Janirve Fndn Grants, 1905
Jasper Fndn Newton County Grants, 1908
Jennings County Comm Fndn Grants, 1916
John H. Wellons Fndn Grants, 1934
John W. Anderson Fndn Grants, 1949
Johnson County Comm Fndn Grants, 1955
K21 Health Fndn Cancer Care Fund Grants, 1975
K21 Health Fndn Grants, 1976
Kosciusko County Comm Fndn Grants, 2015
L. W. Pierce Family Fndn Grants, 2019
Legacy Fndn Grants, 2040
Lucy Gooding Charitable Fndn Trust Grants, 2083
M.B. and Edna Zale Fndn Grants, 2093
Madison County Comm Fndn Grants, 2098
Maine Comm Fndn Grants, 2099
Maxon Charitable Fndn Grants, 2135
Mead Johnson Nutritionals Evansville-Area Organizations Grants, 2157
MedImmune Charitable Grants, 2166
Meyer Fndn Grants, 2177
Military Ex-Prisoners of War Fndn Grants, 2201
NAPNAP Fndn Wyeth Pediatric Immunization Grant, 2244
NEI Innovative Patient Outreach Programs And Ocular Screening Technologies To Improve Detection Of Diabetic Retinopathy Grants, 2294
NIH Recovery Act Limited Competition: Building Sustainable Comm-Linked Infrastructure to Enable Health Science Research, 2709
NNEDVF/Altria Doors of Hope Program, 2847
North Central Health Services Grants, 2861
Northwestern Mutual Fndn Grants, 2870
NWHF Comm-Based Participatory Research Grants, 2904
OSI-Baltimore Special Opportunities Grants, 2972
Peacock Fndn Grants, 3011
Perpetual Trust for Charitable Giving Grants, 3015
Perry County Comm Fndn Grants, 3016
Pike County Comm Fndn Grants, 3049
Pinellas County Grants, 3050
Plough Fndn Grants, 3061
Polk Bros. Fndn Grants, 3066
Posey Comm Fndn Grants, 3068
Posey Comm Fndn Womens Fund Grants, 3069
Pott Fndn Grants, 3071
Prince Charitable Trusts District of Columbia Grants, 3080
Princeton Area Comm Fndn Greater Mercer Grants, 3081
Pulaski County Comm Fndn Grants, 3091
Rasmuson Fndn Grants, 3108
Rhode Island Fndn Grants, 3154
Richard and Helen DeVos Fndn Grants, 3157
Roy and Christine Sturgis Trust Grants, 3191
Rush County Comm Fndn Grants, 3200
Saint Luke's Fndn Grants, 3239
Saint Luke's Health Initiatives Grants, 3240
San Diego Women's Fndn Grants, 3259
Sarasota Memorial Healthcare Fndn Grants, 3264
Schurz Communications Fndn Grants, 3271
Scott County Comm Fndn Grants, 3273
Siebert Lutheran Fndn Grants, 3285
Simple Advise Education Center Grants, 3289
SOCFOC Catholic Ministries Grants, 3317
Sonoco Fndn Grants, 3347
Spencer County Comm Fndn Grants, 3358
St. Joseph Comm Health Fndn Improving Healthcare Access Grants, 3368
Strowd Roses Grants, 3388
Susan Mott Webb Charitable Trust Grants, 3412
Susan Vaughan Fndn Grants, 3413
Thompson Charitable Fndn Grants, 3425
Union Benevolent Association Grants, 3460
Unity Fndn Of LaPorte County Grants, 3467
USCM HIV/AIDS Prevention Grants, 3476
Vancouver Fndn Grants and Comm Initiatives Program, 3477
Vancouver Sun Children's Fund Grants, 3479
Vanderburgh Comm Fndn Grants, 3480
VHA Health Fndn Grants, 3495
W. C. Griffith Fndn Grants, 3505
Warrick County Comm Fndn Grants, 3519
William G. Gilmore Fndn Grants, 3537
Wilson-Wood Fndn Grants, 3542
Women's Fndn of California Grants, 3550
YSA Get Ur Good On Grants, 3555

Community Service Programs

2COBS Private Charitable Fndn Grants, 9
3M Company Health and Human Services Grants, 10
49ers Fndn Grants, 12
A/H Fndn Grants, 19
AAMC Caring for Comm Grants, 136
Abbott Fund Comm Vitality Grants, 177
Able To Serve Grants, 185
ACF Ethnic Comm Self-Help Grants, 200
ACF Preferred Communities Grants, 201
ACF Standing Announcement for Unaccompanied Alien Children Grants, 202
Adelaide Breed Bayrd Fndn Grants, 234
Agnes M. Lindsay Trust Grants, 263
Agway Fndn Grants, 265
AHFMR Health Research Full-Time Studentships, 280
Allyn Fndn Grants, 365
AMA Fndn Fund for Better Health Grants, 388
American Express Fndn Comm Service Grants, 435
Amerisure Insurance Comm Service Grants, 461
Andersen Corp Fndn, 470
Angels Baseball Fndn Grants, 473
Anheuser-Busch Fndn Grants, 474
Ann and Robert H. Lurie Family Fndn Grants, 475
Anthem Blue Cross and Blue Shield Grants, 488
Ashland Corp Contributions Grants, 586
AT&T Fndn Civic and Comm Service Grants, 658
Austin College Leadership Award, 668
Bailey Fndn Grants, 680
Ball Brothers Fndn General Grants, 683
Bank of America Charitable Fndn National Programs and Partners Grants, 689
Biogen Corp Giving Grants, 758
Birds Eye Foods Fndn Grants, 759
Birmingham Fndn Grants, 760
BJ's Charitable Fndn Grants, 761
Black River Falls Area Fndn Grants, 762
Blue Mountain Comm Fndn Grants, 769
Blumenthal Fndn Grants, 773
Bonfils-Stanton Fndn Grants, 779
Boston Globe Fndn Grants, 784
Caddock Fndn Grants, 828
Cailloux Fndn Grants, 829
California Comm Fndn Health Care Grants, 831
California Comm Fndn Human Development Grants, 832
Callaway Fndn Grants, 835
Caring Fndn Grants, 866
Carrie E. and Lena V. Glenn Fndn Grants, 882
Catholic Campaign for Human Development Comm Organizing Grants, 891
Central Okanagan Fndn Grants, 937
Charles Delmar Fndn Grants, 963
Charles H. Dater Fndn Grants, 966
Charlotte County (FL) Comm Fndn Grants, 973
CNCS Engaging Persons with Disabilities in National and Comm Service Grants, 1047
CNCS Next Generation Grants, 1049
Coleman Fndn Cancer Care Grants, 1055
Comm Fndn of Central Illinois Grants, 1101
Comm Fndn of Grant County Grants, 1104
Comm Fndn of Greater Flint Grants, 1107
Comm Fndn Of Greater Lafayette Grants, 1110
Comm Fndn of Howard County Grants, 1116
Comm Fndn of Madison and Jefferson County Grants and Scholarships, 1117
Comm Fndn of St. Joseph County Special Project Challenge Grants, 1126
Comm Fndn of Switzerland County Grants, 1127
Comm Fndn Silicon Valley Grants, 1133
Comm Technology Fndn of California Building Communities Through Technology Grants, 1136
ConocoPhillips Fndn Grants, 1144
Cruise Industry Charitable Fndn Grants, 1166
Cullen Fndn Grants, 1172
CVS Caremark Charitable Trust Grants, 1176
CVS Comm Grants, 1177
D. W. McMillan Fndn Grants, 1180
Dade Comm Fndn Comm AIDS Partnership Grants, 1184
Dairy Queen Corp Contributions Grants, 1187
Dale and Edna Walsh Fndn Grants, 1189
Dallas Mavericks Fndn Grants, 1190
Daviess County Comm Fndn Health Grants, 1203
Dearborn Comm Fndn County Progress Grants, 1211
Dennis and Phyllis Washington Fndn Grants, 1222
Do Something BR!CK Awards, 1287
Eastman Chemical Company Fndn Grants, 1362
Edina Realty Fndn Grants, 1369
Effie and Wofford Cain Fndn Grants, 1385
Emerson Charitable Trust Grants, 1412
Ensworth Charitable Fndn Grants, 1416
Entergy Comm Partnership Grants, 1417

Essex County Comm Fndn Discretionary Fund Grant, 1428
Ethel S. Abbott Charitable Fndn Grants, 1430
Eugene B. Casey Fndn Grants, 1433
Evan and Susan Bayh Fndn Grants, 1437
ExxonMobil Grants, 1442
Florida BRAIVE Fund of Dade Comm Fndn, 1512
Florida BRAIVE Fund of Gulf Coast Comm Fndn of Venice, 1513
Florida BRAIVE Fund of The Comm Fndn in Jacksonville, 1514
Floyd A. and Kathleen C. Cailloux Fndn Grants, 1516
Foster Fndn Grants, 1524
Frank G. & Freida K. Brotz Family Fndn Grants, 1552
Frist Fndn Grants, 1563
Georgiana Goddard Eaton Memorial Fund Grants, 1604
Geraldine R. Dodge Fndn Morris County Grants, 1605
Giving Sum Annual Grant, 1619
Godfrey Fndn Grants, 1631
Goodrich Corp Fndn Grants, 1638
Goodyear Tire Grants, 1639
Green Bay Packers Fndn Grants, 1660
Guidant Fndn Grants, 1674
Hagedorn Fund Grants, 1685
Harden Fndn Grants, 1693
Harold Simmons Fndn Grants, 1698
Harrison County Comm Fndn Grants, 1700
Health Fndn of Greater Cincinnati Grants, 1724
Healthcare Fndn for Orange County Grants, 1728
Helen K. and Arthur E. Johnson Fndn Grants, 1740
Helena Rubinstein Fndn Grants, 1743
Henrietta Tower Wurts Memorial Fndn Grants, 1745
Horace A. Kimball and S. Ella Kimball Fndn Grants, 1792
Ida Alice Ryan Charitable Trust Grants, 1836
Ireland Family Fndn Grants, 1865
Jacob and Hilda Blaustein Fndn Grants, 1881
James A. and Faith Knight Fndn Grants, 1884
James M. Cox Fndn of Georgia Grants, 1892
Jasper Fndn Newton County Grants, 1908
Jennings County Comm Fndn Grants, 1916
John W. Anderson Fndn Grants, 1949
Johnson County Comm Fndn Grants, 1955
Joseph Drown Fndn Grants, 1960
K21 Health Fndn Grants, 1976
King Pharmaceuticals Corp Contributions Grants, 2003
Knox County Comm Fndn Grants, 2009
L. W. Pierce Family Fndn Grants, 2019
LaGrange County Comm Fndn Grants, 2020
Legacy Fndn Grants, 2040
Liberty Bank Fndn Grants, 2053
Lucy Gooding Charitable Fndn Trust Grants, 2083
Madison County Comm Fndn Grants, 2098
Maxtor Corp Contributions Grants, 2136
McGregor Fund Grants, 2143
Mead Johnson Nutritionals Evansville-Area Organizations Grants, 2157
MedImmune Charitable Grants, 2166
MONY Fndn Grants, 2215
New York Life Fndn Grants, 2304
NMF Franklin C. McLean Award, 2829
NMF William and Charlotte Cadbury Award, 2841
North Carolina Comm Development Grants, 2858
North Central Health Services Grants, 2861
Northwestern Mutual Fndn Grants, 2870
NYC Managed Care Consumer Assistance Workshop Re-Design Grants, 2918
NYCT Grants for the Elderly, 2925
NYCT Technical Assistance Grants, 2929
OceanFirst Fndn Grants, 2933
Ohio County Comm Fndn Grants, 2938
Ohio County Comm Fndn Mini-Grants, 2939
OSI-Baltimore Special Opportunities Grants, 2972
PacifiCorp Fndn for Learning Grants, 2982
Peacock Fndn Grants, 3011
Perpetual Trust for Charitable Giving Grants, 3015
Pfizer Fndn Grants, 3025
Pike County Comm Fndn Grants, 3049
Polk Bros. Fndn Grants, 3066
Pott Fndn Grants, 3071
Powell Fndn Grants, 3073
Princeton Area Comm Fndn Greater Mercer Grants, 3081
Prudential Fndn Grants, 3087
Putnam County Comm Fndn Grants, 3093
Regence Fndn Access to Health Care Grants, 3138
Regence Fndn Health Care Comm Awareness and Engagement Grants, 3139
Regence Fndn Health Care Connections Grants, 3140
Regence Fndn Improving End-of-Life Grants, 3141
Regence Fndn Tools and Technology Grants, 3142
Rochester Area Fndn Grants, 3177
Roy and Christine Sturgis Trust Grants, 3191
RWJF Comm Health Leaders Awards, 3208
RWJF Local Funding Partnerships Grants, 3223
RWJF Vulnerable Populations Portfolio Grants, 3232
Salem Fndn Charitable Trust Grants, 3241
Salem Fndn Grants, 3242
SAMHSA Strategic Prevention Framework State Incentive Grants, 3248
San Antonio Area Fndn Grants, 3254
San Diego Women's Fndn Grants, 3259
Sasco Fndn Grants, 3265
Schering-Plough Fndn Comm Initiatives Grants, 3269
Shaw's Supermarkets Donations, 3280
SHF Reach—Connecting Communities and Youth for a Healthy Future Grants, 3283
Simpson Fund Grants, 3290
Sir Dorabji Tata Trust Grants for NGOs or Voluntary Organizations, 3291
SOCFOC Catholic Ministries Grants, 3317
Southwest Gas Corp Fndn Grants, 3352
St. Joseph Comm Health Fndn Improving Healthcare Access Grants, 3368
Stan and Sandy Checketts Fndn, 3373
Thompson Charitable Fndn Grants, 3425
Tri-County Electric People Fund Grants, 3436
Triangle Comm Fndn Donor-Advised Grants, 3437
U.S. Department of Education Special Education—National Activities—Parent Information Centers, 3450
Until There's a Cure Fndn Grants, 3471
US Airways Comm Fndn Grants, 3473
US Trust Corp Fndn Grants, 3475
Vanderburgh Comm Fndn Grants, 3480
W.K. Kellogg Fndn Healthy Kids Grants, 3507
Wal-Mart Fndn Comm Grants, 3513
Warrick County Comm Fndn Grants, 3519
Washington Post Contributions Grants, 3520
Wilkins Family Fndn Grants, 3536
Wilson-Wood Fndn Grants, 3542
Winston-Salem Fndn Competitive Grants, 3544
Winston-Salem Fndn Stokes County Grants, 3546
Women's Fndn of California Grants, 3550
YSA Get Ur Good On Grants, 3555
YSA UnitedHealth Heroes Service Learning Grants, 3556

Comparative Government
Canada-U.S. Fulbright New Century Scholars Grants, 846
Canada-U.S. Fulbright Senior Specialists Grants, 847
Fulbright Alumni Initiatives Awards Grants, 1566
Fulbright Distinguished Chairs Grants, 1567
Fulbright New Century Scholars Grants, 1570
Fulbright Specialists Grants, 1571
Fulbright Traditional Scholar Program in Europe and Eurasia, 1572
Fulbright Traditional Scholar Program in Sub-Saharan Africa, 1573
Fulbright Traditional Scholar Program in the East Asia/Pacific Region, 1574
Fulbright Traditional Scholar Program in the Near East and North Africa Region, 1575
Fulbright Traditional Scholar Program in the South and Central Asia Region, 1576
Fulbright Traditional Scholar Program in the Western Hemisphere, 1577

Compensatory Education
Comm Fndn Silicon Valley Grants, 1133
DHHS Health Professions Preparatory Scholarship Program for Indians, 1257
William T. Grant Fndn Research Grants, 3541

Complementary Medicine
NCCAM Ruth L. Kirschstein National Research Service Awards for Postdoctoral Training in Complementary and Alternative Medicine, 2266

Complex Systems
James S. McDonnell Fndn Complex Systems Collaborative Activity Awards, 1897

Compulsive Behavior
Obsessive-Compulsive Fndn Research Awards, 2931

Computation
James S. McDonnell Fndn Complex Systems Collaborative Activity Awards, 1897

Computer Education/Literacy
Atkinson Fndn International Grants, 661
Bodman Fndn Grants, 776
Chestnut Hill Charitable Fndn, Inc Grants, 987
Farmers Insurance Group of Companies Grants, 1455
Polaroid Fund Grants, 3065
Verizon Fndn Maryland Grants, 3487
Verizon Fndn New York Grants, 3488
Verizon Fndn Northeast Region Grants, 3489
Verizon Fndn Pennsylvania Grants, 3490
Verizon Fndn Vermont Grants, 3491
Verizon Fndn Virginia Grants, 3492

Computer Engineering
Claude Worthington Benedum Fndn Grants, 1033

Computer Grants
Alice Tweed Tuohy Fndn Grants, 357
Armstrong McDonald Fndn Grants, 537
Atherton Family Fndn Grants, 659
Bill and Melinda Gates Fndn Grants, 756
Central Carolina Comm Fndn Comm Impact Grants, 936
Chatlos Fndn Grants, 977
DaimlerChrysler Corp Fund Grants, 1186
Dell Fndn Healthy Communities, Literate Communities, and Connected Communities Grants, 1217
E.L. Wiegand Fndn Grants, 1361
Grand Haven Area Comm Fndn Grants, 1644
Pasadena Fndn Average Grants, 2994
Paul E. and Klare N. Reinhold Fndn Grants, 2999
Polaroid Fund Grants, 3065
Puerto Rico Comm Fndn Grants, 3090
Weingart Fndn Grants, 3524

Computer Science
AACR Team Science Award, 89
Alcatel-Lucent Technologies Corp Contributions Grants, 332
Alfred P. Sloan Fndn Research Fellowships, 353
BWF Career Awards at the Scientific Interface, 819
Canada Graduate Scholarships and NSERC Postgraduate Scholarships, 845
Fndn for Science and Disability Grant Program for Physically Disabled Students in the Sciences, 1532
NHGRI Mentored Research Scientist Development Award, 2315
NIGMS Fellowships in Quantitative Biology, 2610
NIGMS Predoctoral Training in Bioinformatics and Computation Biology Grants, 2625
NIH Exploratory Centers for Alternative Medicine Research Grants, 2663
NIH Exploratory Innovations in Biomedical Computational Science and Technology Grants, 2664
NIH Innovations in Biomedical Computational Science and Technology Grants, 2679

NIH Innovations in Biomedical Computational Science and Technology Initiative Grants for SBIR, 2680
NIH Innovations in Biomedical Computational Science and Technology Initiative Grants for STTR, 2681
NIH Mechanisms Underlying Individual Variations in Drug Responses, 2685
NIMH Curriculum Development Award in Neuroinformatics Research and Analysis, 2754
NLM Academic Research Enhancement Awards, 2814
NLM Research Project Grants, 2825
North Carolina GlaxoSmithKline Fndn Grants, 2860
NSF Behavioral Neurosciences Research Grants, 2876
NSF Chemistry Research Experiences for Undergraduates, 2883
Rockwell International Corp Trust Grants, 3183
University of California President's Postdoctoral Fellowships, 3469

Computer Simulation/Modeling
Ethical Research Grants and Fellowships, 1431
NIGMS Predoctoral Training in Bioinformatics and Computation Biology Grants, 2625

Computer Software
Alice Tweed Tuohy Fndn Grants, 357
Chestnut Hill Charitable Fndn, Inc Grants, 987
Millipore/Charles P. Schaufus Parenteral-Processing Technology Research Grant, 2204

Computer Systems Analysis
NIGMS Predoctoral Training in Bioinformatics and Computation Biology Grants, 2625

Computer Technology
John R. Oishei Fndn Grants, 1944
Microsoft Research Cell Phone as a Platform for Healthcare Grants, 2195
NIGMS Integrative and Collaborative Approaches to Research Grants, 2615
NIH Exploratory Innovations in Biomedical Computational Science and Technology Grants, 2664
NIH Innovations in Biomedical Computational Science and Technology Grants, 2679
NIH Innovations in Biomedical Computational Science and Technology Initiative Grants for SBIR, 2680
NIH Innovations in Biomedical Computational Science and Technology Initiative Grants for STTR, 2681
NLM Academic Research Enhancement Awards, 2814
Olin Corp Charitable Trust Grants, 2943
Society for Imaging Informatics in Medicine Emeritus Mentor Grants, 3320
Society for Imaging Informatics in Medicine Micro Grants, 3321
Society for Imaging Informatics in Medicine Research Grants, 3322
Society for Imaging Informatics in Medicine Small Grant for Product Support Development, 3323
Society for Imaging Informatics in Medicine Small Training Grants, 3324
Verizon Fndn Maryland Grants, 3487
Verizon Fndn New York Grants, 3488
Verizon Fndn Northeast Region Grants, 3489
Verizon Fndn Pennsylvania Grants, 3490
Verizon Fndn Vermont Grants, 3491
Verizon Fndn Virginia Grants, 3492

Computer-Aided Instruction
Dell Fndn Healthy Communities, Literate Communities, and Connected Communities Grants, 1217
Leonsis Fndn Grants, 2045

Conferences
Alzheimer's Association Conference Grants, 385
ASHA Minority Student Leadership Program Awards, 570
ASHA Research Mentoring-Pair Travel Award, 572
ASHA Student Research Travel Award, 573
ASHA Students Preparing for Academic & Research Careers Award, 574
CCFF Small Conference Grants, 896
FDA Scientific Conferences Grants, 1463
Komen Greater NYC Conference Grants, 2012
Komen Greater NYC Small Grants, 2013
NIDDK Traditional Conference Grants, 2589
Potts Memorial Fndn Grants, 3072
RCPSC National Specialty Society Annual Meeting Grants, 3126
South Madison Comm Fndn Grants, 3349
Topeka Comm Fndn Kansas Blood Services Scholarships, 3429

Conferences, Travel to
AACAP Systems of Care Special Program Scholarships, 54
ASHA Minority Student Leadership Program Awards, 570
ASHA Research Mentoring-Pair Travel Award, 572
ASHA Student Research Travel Award, 573
ASHA Students Preparing for Academic & Research Careers Award, 574
ASM Millis-Colwell Postgraduate Travel Grant, 608
ASM-UNESCO Leadership Grant for International Educators, 626
NCIC Canadian Cancer Society Travel Award for Senior Level PhD Students, 2283
NIDDK Traditional Conference Grants, 2589
RCPSC National Specialty Society Annual Meeting Grants, 3126
St. Joseph Comm Health Fndn Schneider Fellowships, 3370
Topeka Comm Fndn Kansas Blood Services Scholarships, 3429

Conflict/Dispute Resolution
Allstate Corp Giving Grants, 363
Allstate Corp Hometown Commitment Grants, 364
American-Scandinavian Fndn Visiting Lectureship Grants, 460
FCNY Union Square Awards, 1461
Harry Frank Guggenheim Fndn Research Grants, 1704
Mary Owen Borden Fndn Grants, 2121
Pajaro Valley Comm Health Grants, 2985

Connective Tissue
NIAMS High Risk Arthritis and Musculoskeletal and Skin Diseases Research, 2470

Conservation
Columbus Fndn Competitive Grants, 1066
ConocoPhillips Fndn Grants, 1144
Prospect Burma Scholarships, 3085

Conservation, Agriculture
Bullitt Fndn Grants, 809
Clarence E. Heller Charitable Fndn Grants, 1022
CLIF Bar Family Fndn Grants, 1040
Dean Foods Comm Involvement Grants, 1209
Jessie Smith Noyes Fndn Grants, 1920
Joyce Fndn Grants, 1969

Conservation, Natural Resources
Abel Fndn Grants, 181
Allen P. and Josephine B. Green Fndn Grants, 361
Amgen Fndn Grants, 467
Archer Daniels Midland Fndn Grants, 525
Ashland Corp Contributions Grants, 586
Australian Academy of Science Grants, 670
Batchelor Fndn Grants, 701
Bella Vista Fndn Grants, 740
Boeing Company Contributions Grants, 777
Bullitt Fndn Grants, 809
Carls Fndn Grants, 876
Carpenter Fndn Grants, 881
Central Okanagan Fndn Grants, 937
Champlin Fndns Grants, 960
Chicago Tribune's Corp Contributions Grants, 991
Clarence E. Heller Charitable Fndn Grants, 1022
CLIF Bar Family Fndn Grants, 1040
Coeta and Donald Barker Fndn Grants, 1054
Collins Fndn Grants, 1058
Columbus Fndn Mary Eleanor Morris Fund Grants, 1069
Comm Fndn Of Greater Lafayette Grants, 1110
Comm Fndn of Santa Cruz County Grants, 1122
Crestlea Fndn Grants, 1159
Cyrus Eaton Fndn Grants, 1178
Donald and Sylvia Robinson Family Fndn Grants, 1310
Dorrance Family Fndn Grants, 1323
Evan and Susan Bayh Fndn Grants, 1437
FIC International Cooperative Biodiversity Groups Grants, 1487
Field Fndn of Illinois Grants, 1499
Ford Motor Company Fund Grants, 1522
Frank Stanley Beveridge Fndn Grants, 1553
Frey Fndn Grants, 1562
George B. Storer Fndn Grants, 1596
George Frederick Jewett Fndn Grants, 1599
Giving Sum Annual Grant, 1619
Greater Milwaukee Fndn Grants, 1653
Harry A. and Margaret D. Towsley Fndn Grants, 1701
Henry J. Kaiser Family Fndn Grants, 1748
J.W. Kieckhefer Fndn Grants, 1878
Jane's Trust Grants, 1904
Jessie B. Cox Charitable Trust Grants, 1918
Jessie Ball Dupont Fund Grants, 1919
Joyce Fndn Grants, 1969
KeySpan Fndn Grants, 1995
Kraft Cares US Grants, 2017
Lindbergh Grants, 2059
M.E. Raker Fndn Grants, 2094
Maine Comm Fndn Grants, 2099
Margaret L. Wendt Fndn Grants, 2104
Mark and Catherine Winkler Fndn Grants, 2112
Mary Owen Borden Fndn Grants, 2121
McLean Contributionship Grants, 2147
Meyer Memorial Trust Emergency Grants, 2178
Meyer Memorial Trust Grassroots Grants, 2179
Meyer Memorial Trust Operating Funds Grants, 2180
Meyer Memorial Trust Responsive Grants, 2181
Miguel Aleman Fndn Grants, 2197
Nelda C. and H.J. Lutcher Stark Fndn Grants, 2301
Nina Mason Pulliam Charitable Trust Grants, 2776
Ogden Codman Trust Grants, 2937
Olin Corp Charitable Trust Grants, 2943
Oscar Rennebohm Fndn Grants, 2963
Palm Beach and Martin Counties Grants, 2986
Plum Creek Fndn Grants, 3062
Posey Comm Fndn Grants, 3068
Prudential Fndn Grants, 3087
Pulte Homes Corp Contributions, 3092
Rajiv Gandhi Fndn Grants, 3104
Richard and Rhoda Goldman Fund Grants, 3158
Rohm and Haas Company Grants, 3185
Simpson Fund Grants, 3290
Sulzberger Fndn Grants, 3399
Susan Vaughan Fndn Grants, 3413
Wal-Mart Fndn Comm Grants, 3513

Consumer Behavior
Bodman Fndn Grants, 776
Cass County Comm Fndn Grants, 887

Consumer Education/Information
NYC Managed Care Consumer Assistance Workshop Re-Design Grants, 2918

Consumer Sciences
AAFCS International Graduate Fellowships, 109
AAFCS National Graduate Fellowships, 110
AAFCS National Undergraduate Scholarships, 111

Consumer Services
California Wellness Fndn Work and Health Grants, 834
EPA Children's Health Protection Grants, 1420
Jacob and Valeria Langeloth Fndn Grants, 1882

Contraceptives
Lalor Fndn Postdoctoral Research Grants, 2021
NIAID HIV Prevention Trial Units Grants, 2453

Control Systems
NIH National Occupational Research Agenda Grants, 2696
NSF Chemical, Biochemical, and Biotechnology Systems Research Grants, 2882

Cooperatives
Alexander von Humboldt Fndn Institutional Academic Cooperation Grants, 346

Corrosion
Millipore/Charles P. Schaufus Parenteral-Processing Technology Research Grant, 2204

Cosmetic Science
Society of Cosmetic Chemists Allan B. Black Award Sponsored by Presperse, 3328
Society of Cosmetic Chemists Award Sponsored by McIntyre Group, Ltd., 3329
Society of Cosmetic Chemists Award Sponsored by The HallStar Company, 3330
Society of Cosmetic Chemists Chapter Best Speaker Award, 3331
Society of Cosmetic Chemists Chapter Merit Award, 3332
Society of Cosmetic Chemists Frontier of Science Award, 3333
Society of Cosmetic Chemists Hans Schaeffer Award, 3334
Society of Cosmetic Chemists Joseph P. Ciaudelli Award, 3335
Society of Cosmetic Chemists Keynote Award Lecture Sponsored by Ruger Chemical Corp, 3336
Society of Cosmetic Chemists Literature Award, 3337
Society of Cosmetic Chemists Maison G. de Navarre Medal, 3338
Society of Cosmetic Chemists Merit Award, 3339
Society of Cosmetic Chemists Robert A. Kramer Lifetime Service Award, 3340
Society of Cosmetic Chemists Shaw Mudge Award, 3341
Society of Cosmetic Chemists Student Poster Awards, 3342
Society of Cosmetic Chemists Young Scientist Awards, 3343

Cosmology
Brinson Fndn Grants, 794
Gruber Fndn International Prizes, 1672

Costume
Mars Fndn Grants, 2114

Counseling/Guidance
CDC Hepatitis Education for Inmates and Correctional Staff Grants, 911
Comm Fndn for Southern Arizona Grants, 1095
DHHS Health Careers Opportunity Grants, 1253
DHHS Health Centers Grants for Residents of Public Housing, 1254
Edina Realty Fndn Grants, 1369
EF Behavioral Sciences Student Fellowships, 1379
Eric Berne Fund for the Future Grants, 1426
Florida BRAIVE Fund of Gulf Coast Comm Fndn of Venice, 1513
Florida BRAIVE Fund of The Comm Fndn in Jacksonville, 1514
Greater Worcester Comm Fndn Discretionary Grants, 1658
HRSA Ryan White HIV Early Intervention Services Grants, 1811
Hudson Webber Fndn Grants, 1813
Independence Comm Fndn Comm Quality of Life Grant, 1849
Mary Owen Borden Fndn Grants, 2121
NIDA Behavioral Therapies Development Grants, 2499
PacifiCare Fndn Grants, 2981
Ruth H. and Warren A. Ellsworth Fndn Grants, 3203
Seabury Fndn Grants, 3274
Vermont Comm Fndn Grants, 3493
Z. Smith Reynolds Fndn Small Grants, 3557

Crafts
Ruth Mott Fndn Grants, 3204

Craniofacial Anomalies
DHHS Oral Health Promotion Research Across the Lifespan, 1269
FACES Assistance Grants, 1444
Max Bell Fndn Grants, 2134
NIDCR Clinical Trial Pilot Grant, 2533
NIDCR Clinical Trial Planning Grant, 2534
NIDCR International Collaborative Oral Health Research Planning Grant, 2536
NIH Mechanisms of Orofacial Pain: Anatomy, Genomics, and Proteomics, 2684

Creative Writing
McKesson Fndn Grants, 2145

Crime Control
Cemala Fndn Grants, 933
Colorado Springs Comm Trust Fund Grants, 1061
DOJ Gang-Free Schools and Communities Intervention Grants, 1303
PacifiCare Fndn Grants, 2981

Crime Prevention
Baptist Comm Ministries Grants, 691
Beazley Fndn Grants, 730
BJ's Charitable Fndn Grants, 761
Clarcor Fndn Grants, 1021
ConocoPhillips Fndn Grants, 1144
Constantin Fndn Grants, 1145
Cornerstone Fndn of Northeastern Wisconsin Grants, 1152
Daphne Seybolt Culpeper Memorial Fndn Grants, 1201
Elliot Fndn Inc Grants, 1402
Farmers Insurance Group of Companies Grants, 1455
Frank Stanley Beveridge Fndn Grants, 1553
G.N. Wilcox Trust Grants, 1581
Hudson Webber Fndn Grants, 1813
Joseph H. and Florence A. Roblee Fndn Grants, 1961
Kahuku Comm Fund, 1977
Knox County Comm Fndn Grants, 2009
Ordean Fndn Grants, 2952
Perry County Comm Fndn Grants, 3016
Pike County Comm Fndn Grants, 3049
Plough Fndn Grants, 3061
Plum Creek Fndn Grants, 3062
Posey Comm Fndn Grants, 3068
R.C. Baker Fndn Grants, 3098
Sid W. Richardson Fndn Grants, 3284
Sonoco Fndn Grants, 3347

Crime Victims
Burton G. Bettingen Grants, 813
Carrie E. and Lena V. Glenn Fndn Grants, 882
Winston-Salem Fndn Victim Assistance Grants, 3547

Criminal Behavior
Cass County Comm Fndn Grants, 887
John R. Oishei Fndn Grants, 1944
Ordean Fndn Grants, 2952

Criminal Justice
Baptist Comm Ministries Grants, 691
Bernard F. and Alva B. Gimbel Fndn Grants, 747
Carroll County Comm Fndn Grants, 885
Chicago Comm Trust Grants, 989
Coastal Comm Fndn of South Carolina Grants, 1051
Comm Fndn of Howard County Grants, 1116
Daisy Marquis Jones Fndn Grants, 1188
Good Samaritan Inc Grants, 1637
Henry County Comm Fndn Grants, 1747
Margaret L. Wendt Fndn Grants, 2104
Marion I. and Henry J. Knott Fndn Grants, 2109
Meyer Fndn Grants, 2177
Ms. Fndn for Women Grants, 2222
Public Welfare Fndn Grants, 3089
Puerto Rico Comm Fndn Grants, 3090
Texas Commission on the Arts Arts Respond Project Grants, 3420
Vulcan Materials Company Fndn Grants, 3504

Crisis Counseling
Actors Fund Social Services and Financial Assistance, 225
Barr Fund Grants, 697
D. W. McMillan Fndn Grants, 1180
Duchossois Family Fndn Grants, 1337
Edwards Memorial Trust Grant, 1375
Ordean Fndn Grants, 2952
Perry County Comm Fndn Grants, 3016
Pike County Comm Fndn Grants, 3049
SAG Motion Picture Players Welfare Fund Grants, 3238
Spencer County Comm Fndn Grants, 3358
Vanderburgh Comm Fndn Grants, 3480
Warrick County Comm Fndn Grants, 3519

Critical Care Medicine
AACN Clinical Inquiry Fund Grants, 56
AACN Clinical Practice Grants, 57
AACN Critical Care Grants, 58
AACN End of Life/Palliative Care Small Projects Grants, 59
AACN Evidence-Based Clinical Practice Grants, 60
AACN Mentorship Grant, 61
AACN Physio-Control Small Projects Grants, 62
AACN-Edwards Lifesciences Nurse-Driven Clinical Practice Outcomes Grants, 63
AACN-Philips Medical Systems Clinical Outcomes Grants, 64
AACN-Sigma Theta Tau Critical Care Grant, 65
Baptist Comm Ministries Grants, 691
CDC National Training Information and Exchange Program, 920
Chest Fndn Eli Lilly and Company Distinguished Scholar in Critical Care Medicine Award, 983
Clarian Health Critical / Progressive Care Internships, 1023
DHHS Maternal and Child Health Research and Training Programs Grants, 1264
Duke University Adult Cardiothoracic Anesthesia and Critical Care Medicine Fellowships, 1340
Duke University Pediatric Anesthesiology Fellowship, 1347
E.L. Wiegand Fndn Grants, 1361
Herman Goldman Fndn Grants, 1753
HRSA Emergency Medical Services for Children Grants, 1804
Lowe Fndn Grants, 2067
National Emergency Medicine Association Grants, 2252
Questar Corp Contributions Grants, 3097
Stewart Huston Charitable Trust Grants, 3384
STTI Emergency Nurses Association Fndn Grant, 3390
STTI Environment of Elder Care Nursing Research Grants, 3391

Criticism
NLM Grants for Scholarly Works in Biomedicine and Health, 2818

Croatia
OSI European Commission Internships for Young Roma Graduates, 2965

Crohns Disease
Partnership for Cures Two Years To Cures Grants, 2992

Cross-Cultural Studies
eBay Fndn Comm Grants, 1363

Cryogenics
NIH Technologies to Improve the Utility of Animal Models Research Grants, 2735

Crystallography
NIGMS Pilot Projects for the Protein Structure Initiative (Structural Genomics), 2624
NIH Protein Structure Initiative (Structural Genomics) Research Grants, 2704
NIH Protein Structure Initiative (Structural Genomics)—SBIR/STTR GRANTS, 2705
NSF Small Business Innovation Research Grants, 2893

Cubans
American Sociological Association Minority Fellowships, 458

Culinary Arts
Adolph Coors Fndn Grants, 238
Carl B. and Florence E. King Fndn Grants, 869

Culteral Outreach Programs
Comm Fndn of Greenville-Greenville Women Giving Grants, 1115

Cultual Diversity
Lillian S. Wells Fndn Grants, 2056

Cultural Activities/Programs
2 Depot Square Ipswich Charitable Fndn Grants, 7
49ers Fndn Grants, 12
A. Gary Anderson Family Fndn Grants, 17
A.O. Smith Comm Grants, 18
Aaron Fndn (Massachusetts) Grants, 174
Abell-Hanger Fndn Grants, 183
Abington Fndn Grants, 184
Achelis and Bodman Fndns Grants, 206
Adelaide Breed Bayrd Fndn Grants, 234
Adobe Comm Investment Grants, 237
AEC Trust Grants, 242
AEGON Transamerica Fndn Grants, 243
African American Fund of New Jersey Grants, 260
Agnes Gund Fndn Grants, 262
Ahmanson Fndn Grants, 303
Air Products and Chemicals Grants, 319
Alabama Power Fndn Grants, 321
Aladdin Industries Fndn Grants, 322
Alaska Airlines Corp Giving Grants, 323
Alaska Airlines Fndn Grants, 324
Albert Pick Jr. Fund Grants, 328
Alberto Culver Corp Contributions Grants, 329
Albuquerque Comm Fndn Grants, 331
Alcatel-Lucent Technologies Fndn Grants, 333
Alcoa Fndn Grants, 334
Allegheny Technologies Charitable Trust, 359
Amarillo Area/Harrington Fndns Grants, 410
Andersen Fndn Grants, 471
Anheuser-Busch Fndn Grants, 474
Ann Arbor Area Comm Fndn Grants, 476
Ann Peppers Fndn Grants, 478
AON Fndn Grants, 491
AptarGroup Fndn Grants, 522
Aratani Fndn Grants, 523
Archer Daniels Midland Fndn Grants, 525
Argyros Fndn Grants, 527
Arie and Ida Crown Memorial Grants, 528
Arizona Cardinals Grants, 529
Arizona Public Service Corp Giving Grants, 531
Arkansas Comm Fndn Grants, 533
Armstrong McDonald Fndn Grants, 537
ArvinMeritor Grants, 544
ASHA Multicultural Activities Projects Grants, 571
Ashland Corp Contributions Grants, 586
Atherton Family Fndn Grants, 659
Atlanta Fndn Grants, 662
Bacon Family Fndn Grants, 679
Ball Brothers Fndn General Grants, 683
Ball Brothers Fndn Grants, 684
Barberton Comm Fndn Grants, 693
Barker Welfare Fndn Grants, 695
Barra Fndn Project Grants, 699
Batts Fndn Grants, 704
BCBSNC Fndn Grants, 725
Bechtel Group Fndn Building Positive Comm Relationships Grants, 731
Beckley Area Fndn Grants, 732
Belk Fndn Grants, 739
Ben B. Cheney Fndn Grants, 741
Benton Comm Fndn Grants, 743
Benton County Fndn Grants, 744
Berks County Comm Fndn Grants, 745
Bernard and Audre Rapoport Fndn Grants, 746
Berrien Comm Fndn Grants, 749
Bertha Russ Lytel Fndn Grants, 751
Besser Fndn Grants, 752
Blackford County Comm Fndn Grants, 763
Blue Grass Comm Fndn Grants, 768
Blue River Comm Fndn Grants, 770
Blum-Kovler Fndn Grants, 772
Bodenwein Public Benevolent Fndn Grants, 775
Bodman Fndn Grants, 776
Boeing Company Contributions Grants, 777
Boettcher Fndn Grants, 778
Boston Fndn Grants, 783
Bradley Turner Fndn Grants, 789
Brown County Comm Fndn Grants, 807
Burlington Northern Santa Fe Fndn Grants, 812
C.R. Bard Fndn Grants, 825
C.W. Titus Fndn Grants, 826
Cailloux Fndn Grants, 829
Cambridge Comm Fndn Grants, 837
Carl and Eloise Pohlad Family Fndn Grants, 867
Carl and Lily Pforzheimer Fndn Grants, 868
Carl B. and Florence E. King Fndn Grants, 869
Carl C. Icahn Fndn Grants, 870
Carolyn Fndn Grants, 880
Carroll County Comm Fndn Grants, 885
Cemala Fndn Grants, 933
Central Carolina Comm Fndn Comm Impact Grants, 936
Central Okanagan Fndn Grants, 937
Cessna Fndn Grants, 938
Charles M. Bair Family Trust Grants, 972
Charlotte County (FL) Comm Fndn Grants, 973
Chestnut Hill Charitable Fndn, Inc Grants, 987
Chicago Board of Trade Fndn Grants, 988
Chicago Tribune's Corp Contributions Grants, 991
Chiles Fndn Grants, 1003
Christy-Houston Fndn Grants, 1008
CICF Legacy Fund Comm Fndn Grants, 1010
CIGNA Fndn Grants, 1011
Cinergy Fndn Grants, 1013
Citizens Bank Mid-Atlantic Charitable Fndn Grants, 1015
Clarcor Fndn Grants, 1021
Clark County Comm Fndn Grants, 1028
Clark Fndn Grants, 1029
Clark-Winchcole Fndn Grants, 1030
Cleveland Browns Fndn Grants, 1036
CNA Fndn Grants, 1046
Coastal Comm Fndn of South Carolina Grants, 1051
Cockrell Fndn Grants, 1053
Collins Fndn Grants, 1058
Colorado Interstate Gas Grants, 1060
Columbus Fndn Robert E. and Genevieve B. Schaefer Fund Grants, 1070
Comer Fndn Grants, 1072
Comerica Charitable Fndn Grants, 1073
Comm Fndn Alliance City of Evansville Endowment Fund Grants, 1089
Comm Fndn for Southeastern Michigan Grants, 1094
Comm Fndn of Bartholomew County Heritage Fund Grants, 1096
Comm Fndn of Bartholomew County James A. Henderson Award for Fund-Raising, 1097
Comm Fndn of Bloomington and Monroe County Grants, 1098
Comm Fndn of Boone County Grants, 1099
Comm Fndn of Greater Birmingham Grants, 1106
Comm Fndn of Greater Fort Wayne: Comm Endowment & Clarke Endowment Fund Grants, 1108
Comm Fndn of Greater Greensboro Grants, 1109
Comm Fndn of Greater Tampa Grants, 1112
Comm Fndn of Howard County Grants, 1116
Comm Fndn of Mount Vernon and Knox County Grants, 1119
Comm Fndn of Muncie and Delaware County Grants, 1120
Comm Fndn of Randolph County Grants, 1121
Comm Fndn of South Puget Sound Grants, 1124
Comm Fndn of Southeastern Connecticut Grants, 1125
Comm Fndn of Western North Carolina Grants, 1132
ConAgra Foods Fndn Grants, 1140
Connecticut Comm Fndn Grants, 1141
Connelly Fndn Grants, 1143
Constantin Fndn Grants, 1145
Constellation Energy Group and Baltimore Gas and Electric Corp Contributions, 1146
Consumers Energy Fndn, 1147
Cooke Fndn Grants, 1148
Cooper Industries Fndn Grants, 1150
Cornerstone Fndn of Northeastern Wisconsin Grants, 1152
Cowles Charitable Trust Grants, 1155
Cranston Fndn Grants, 1158
CSX Corp Contributions Grants, 1169
Cullen Fndn Grants, 1172
Cultural Society of Filipino Americans Grants, 1173
Cyrus Eaton Fndn Grants, 1178
DaimlerChrysler Corp Fund Grants, 1186
Dairy Queen Corp Contributions Grants, 1187
Dana Brown Charitable Trust Grants, 1194
Dana Corp Fndn Grants, 1196
Dayton Power and Light Fndn Grants, 1205
Denver Fndn Comm Grants, 1227
Dr. Scholl Fndn Grants, 1329
Dunspaugh-Dalton Fndn Grants, 1351
DuPage Comm Fndn Grants, 1352
Eastman Chemical Company Fndn Grants, 1362
Eberly Fndn Grants, 1364
Edward S. Moore Fndn Grants, 1374
Edwin S. Webster Fndn Grants, 1376
Elkhart County Comm Fndn Grants, 1401
Elmer L. and Eleanor J. Andersen Fndn Grants, 1406
Emerson Charitable Trust Grants, 1412
Entergy Comm Partnership Grants, 1417
Erie Comm Fndn Grants, 1427
Essex County Comm Fndn Discretionary Fund Grant, 1428
Evjue Fndn Grants, 1439
Fargo-Moorhead Area Fndn Grants, 1454
Farmers Insurance Group of Companies Grants, 1455
Ferree Fndn Grants, 1486
Fidelity Fndn Grants, 1498
Field Fndn of Illinois Grants, 1499
Fireman's Fund Fndn Grants, 1504
FirstEnergy Fndn Comm Grants, 1505
Fishman Family Fndn Grants, 1510
Floyd A. and Kathleen C. Cailloux Fndn Grants, 1516
Fluor Fndn Grants, 1517
Fondren Fndn Grants, 1520
Fndn Northwest Grants, 1537
Francis L. Abreu Charitable Trust Grants, 1549
Frank E. and Seba B. Payne Fndn Grants, 1551
Fremont Area Comm Fndn Grants, 1561
Fuji Film Grants, 1565
Fulton County Comm Fndn Grants, 1579
G.N. Wilcox Trust Grants, 1581
Gebbie Fndn Grants, 1585
General Mills Fndn Grants, 1590
General Motors Fndn Grants Support Program, 1591
George Frederick Jewett Fndn Grants, 1599
Georgia Power Fndn Grants, 1603
Gertrude and William C. Wardlaw Fund Grants, 1607
Giving Sum Annual Grant, 1619
Glendale Comm Fndn Grants, 1626
Golden State Warriors Fndn Grants, 1633

Goodrich Corp Fndn Grants, 1638
Goodyear Tire Grants, 1639
Grand Haven Area Comm Fndn Grants, 1644
Grand Rapids Comm Fndn Grants, 1647
Greater Bridgeport Area Fndn Comm Impact Grants, 1650
Greater Green Bay Comm Fndn Grants, 1652
Greater Milwaukee Fndn Grants, 1653
Greater New Orleans Fndn Grants, 1654
Greater Tacoma Comm Fndn Grants, 1656
Greater Worcester Comm Fndn Discretionary Grants, 1658
Grundy Fndn Grants, 1673
Gulf Coast Comm Fndn Grants, 1676
H.J. Heinz Company Fndn Grants, 1682
Hannaford Charitable Fndn Grants, 1692
Harley Davidson Fndn Grants, 1694
Harrison County Comm Fndn Grants, 1700
Hearst Fndn and William Randolph Hearst Fndn Grants, 1730
Helen K. and Arthur E. Johnson Fndn Grants, 1740
High Meadow Fndn Grants, 1768
Hill Crest Fndn Grants, 1773
Hill Fndn Grants, 1774
Hillman Fndn Grants, 1775
Hillsdale Fund Grants, 1778
Hoblitzelle Fndn Grants, 1783
Holland/Zeeland Comm Fndn Grants, 1786
Homer Fndn Grants, 1789
Honeywell Fndn Grants, 1791
Houston Endowment Grants, 1797
Howard and Bush Fndn Grants, 1798
Hugh J. Andersen Fndn Grants, 1814
Humana Fndn Grants, 1818
Huntington County Comm Fndn Grants, 1823
Idaho Comm Fndn Eastern Region Competitive Grants, 1837
Idaho Power Company Corp Contributions, 1838
Impact 100 Grants, 1843
J.M. Long Fndn Grants, 1877
J.W. Kieckhefer Fndn Grants, 1878
Jane's Trust Grants, 1904
Jasper Fndn Jasper County Grants, 1907
Jessie Ball Dupont Fund Grants, 1919
Jewish Comm Fndn of Greater Los Angeles Grants, 1921
John Ben Snow Memorial Trust Grants, 1928
John Deere Fndn Grants, 1929
John H. and Wilhelmina D. Harland Charitable Fndn Grants, 1933
John J. Leidy Fndn Grants, 1936
John R. Oishei Fndn Grants, 1944
Johnson Controls Fndn Grants, 1954
Joyce Fndn Grants, 1969
Katharine Matthies Fndn Grants, 1982
Katherine John Murphy Fndn Grants, 1983
Kenneth T. and Eileen L. Norris Fndn Grants, 1989
Key Fndn Grants, 1994
King Pharmaceuticals Corp Contributions Grants, 2003
Land O'Lakes Fndn Mid-Atlantic Grants, 2027
Legacy Fndn Grants, 2040
Lincoln Financial Group Fndn Grants, 2058
Lockheed Martin Philanthropic Grants, 2062
Lowell Berry Fndn Grants, 2069
Lubbock Area Fndn Grants, 2079
Lynde and Harry Bradley Fndn Grants, 2089
Lynde and Harry Bradley Fndn Prizes: Bradley Prizes, 2090
Mabel Y. Hughes Charitable Trust Grants, 2097
Madison County Comm Fndn Grants, 2098
Marcia and Otto Koehler Fndn Grants, 2103
Margaret T. Morris Fndn Grants, 2105
Marion I. and Henry J. Knott Fndn Grants, 2109
Mars Fndn Grants, 2114
Mary Owen Borden Fndn Grants, 2121
Mary S. and David C. Corbin Fndn Grants, 2122
Max and Victoria Dreyfus Fndn Grants, 2133
Maxon Charitable Fndn Grants, 2135
Maxtor Corp Contributions Grants, 2136
McInerny Fndn Grants, 2144
McKesson Fndn Grants, 2145
Meadows Fndn Grants, 2161
Miami County Comm Fndn Operation Round Up Grants, 2188
Middlesex Savings Charitable Fndn Grants, 2196
Millipore Fndn Grants, 2203
Monfort Family Fndn Grants, 2213
New York Life Fndn Grants, 2304
Nicholas H. Noyes Jr. Memorial Fndn Grants, 2497
Nina Mason Pulliam Charitable Trust Grants, 2776
Noble County Comm Fndn Grants, 2848
Nordson Corp Fndn Grants, 2851
Northeast Utilities Fndn Grants, 2863
Northern New York Comm Fndn Grants, 2864
Northern Trust Company Charitable Trust and Corp Giving Program, 2865
Ogden Codman Trust Grants, 2937
Oleonda Jameson Trust Grants, 2941
Perkins Charitable Fndn Grants, 3014
Philadelphia Fndn Organizational Effectiveness Grants, 3029
Phoenix Suns Charities Grants, 3030
Piper Jaffray Companies Building Strong Communities Grants, 3053
Pittsburgh Fndn Comm Fund Grants, 3054
Plum Creek Fndn Grants, 3062
Polk Bros. Fndn Grants, 3066
Prince Charitable Trusts Chicago Grants, 3079
Principal Financial Group Fndn Grants, 3082
Procter and Gamble Fund Grants, 3083
Prudential Fndn Grants, 3087
Puerto Rico Comm Fndn Grants, 3090
R.C. Baker Fndn Grants, 3098
Rainbow Endowment Grants, 3102
Ralphs Food 4 Less Fndn Grants, 3106
Rasmuson Fndn Grants, 3108
Rich Fndn Grants, 3156
Richard and Rhoda Goldman Fund Grants, 3158
Richard and Susan Smith Family Fndn Grants, 3159
Richard King Mellon Fndn Grants, 3161
Robert B McMillen Fndn Grants, 3169
Robins Fndn Grants, 3175
Rochester Area Comm Fndn Grants, 3176
Rochester Area Fndn Grants, 3177
Rockefeller Brothers Fund Peace and Security Grants, 3179
Rockefeller Fndn Grants, 3181
Rockwell Collins Charitable Contributions, 3182
Rockwell International Corp Trust Grants, 3183
Rollin M. Gerstacker Fndn Grants, 3186
S. Livingston Mather Charitable Trust Grants, 3235
Salem Fndn Grants, 3242
San Antonio Area Fndn Grants, 3254
Sarah Scaife Fndn Grants, 3263
Schering-Plough Fndn Comm Initiatives Grants, 3269
Schurz Communications Fndn Grants, 3271
Scott County Comm Fndn Grants, 3273
Seabury Fndn Grants, 3274
Self Fndn Grants, 3277
Sonoco Fndn Grants, 3347
Sosland Fndn Grants, 3348
Southwest Florida Comm Fndn Competitive Grants, 3351
Southwest Gas Corp Fndn Grants, 3352
Spencer County Comm Fndn Grants, 3358
Sprague Fndn Grants, 3359
Square D Fndn Grants, 3361
Starr Fndn Grants, 3377
Stewart Huston Charitable Trust Grants, 3384
Sunderland Fndn Grants, 3400
Thomas C. Ackerman Fndn Grants, 3423
U.S. Department of Education 21st Century Comm Learning Centers, 3445
United Technologies Corp Grants, 3466
US Airways Comm Contributions, 3472
US Airways Comm Fndn Grants, 3473
US Trust Corp Fndn Grants, 3475
Vancouver Fndn Grants and Comm Initiatives Program, 3477
Vectren Fndn Grants, 3485
Wachovia Fndn Grants, 3511
Walt Disney Company Fndn Grants, 3516
Wells County Fndn Grants, 3527
Western Indiana Comm Fndn Grants, 3528
Wilkins Family Fndn Grants, 3536
Winston-Salem Fndn Competitive Grants, 3544
Z. Smith Reynolds Fndn Small Grants, 3557

Cultural Diversity

ACF Preferred Communities Grants, 201
Alcoa Fndn Grants, 334
American Society on Aging NOMA Award for Excellence in Multicultural Aging, 457
ASHA Multicultural Activities Projects Grants, 571
AT&T Fndn Civic and Comm Service Grants, 658
AVDF Health Care Grants, 673
Breast Cancer Fund Grants, 790
California Endowment CommunitiesFirst Grants, 833
Cargill Citizenship Fund-Corp Giving Grants, 865
Comm Fndn of Greater Greensboro Grants, 1109
Comm Fndn of Howard County Grants, 1116
Cultural Society of Filipino Americans Grants, 1173
DHHS HIV Demonstration Program for Children, Adolescents, and Women, 1262
Fndn for the Carolinas Grants, 1535
Henry County Comm Fndn Grants, 1747
Joyce Fndn Grants, 1969
Lesbian Health Fund Grants, 2046
Medtronic Fndn Health Care Grants, 2169
NIH Studies of Ethical, Legal, and Social Implications of Research into Human Genetic Variation Grants, 2731
Noble County Comm Fndn Grants, 2848
Philadelphia Fndn Organizational Effectiveness Grants, 3029
Pittsburgh Fndn Comm Fund Grants, 3054
Portland General Electric Fndn Grants, 3067
Seabury Fndn Grants, 3274
Vancouver Fndn Grants and Comm Initiatives Program, 3477

Cultural Heritage Preservation

Central Okanagan Fndn Grants, 937
Charlotte County (FL) Comm Fndn Grants, 973
Comm Fndn of Howard County Grants, 1116
Cultural Society of Filipino Americans Grants, 1173
Giving Sum Annual Grant, 1619
Hawaii Comm Fndn Reverend Takie Okumura Family Grants, 1717
Homer Fndn Grants, 1789
Infinity Fndn Grants, 1854
Jasper Fndn Jasper County Grants, 1907
Meyer Fndn Grants, 2177
OSI-Baltimore Special Opportunities Grants, 2972
Schering-Plough Fndn Comm Initiatives Grants, 3269
Winston-Salem Fndn Stokes County Grants, 3546

Cultural Identity

Cultural Society of Filipino Americans Grants, 1173
Homer Fndn Grants, 1789

Cultural Outreach

2 Depot Square Ipswich Charitable Fndn Grants, 7
3M Fndn Grants, 11
Abney Fndn Grants, 187
Agnes Gund Fndn Grants, 262
Alcatel-Lucent Technologies Corp Contributions Grants, 332
Alexander & Baldwin Fndn Hawaiian and Pacific Island Grants, 338
Alexander & Baldwin Fndn Mainland Grants, 339
Anheuser-Busch Fndn Grants, 474
Annie Sinclair Knudsen Memorial Fund/Kaua'i Comm Grants, 480
Avon Products Fndn Grants, 675
Ball Brothers Fndn General Grants, 683
Ball Brothers Fndn Grants, 684
Barnes Group Fndn Grants, 696
Baxter International Fndn Grants, 705

Benton County Fndn Grants, 744
Biogen Corp Giving Grants, 758
Bridgestone/Firestone Trust Fund Grants, 792
Carl B. and Florence E. King Fndn Grants, 869
Columbus Fndn Robert E. and Genevieve B. Schaefer Fund Grants, 1070
Comer Fndn Grants, 1072
Comm Fndn of Greater New Britain Grants, 1111
Comm Fndn of the Eastern Shore Comm Needs Grants, 1129
Cullen Fndn Grants, 1172
Cultural Society of Filipino Americans Grants, 1173
Dade Comm Fndn Grants, 1185
Delta Air Lines Fndn Grants, 1220
Edward Bangs Kelley and Elza Kelley Fndn Grants, 1373
Eisner Fndn Grants, 1387
El Paso Corp Fndn Grants, 1389
Eugene and Agnes E. Meyer Fndn Grants, 1432
Evjue Fndn Grants, 1439
Fairfield County Comm Fndn Grants, 1446
Fallon OrNda Comm Health Fund Grants, 1449
Federal Express Corp Contributions Program, 1483
Fishman Family Fndn Grants, 1510
Fred Baldwin Memorial Fndn Grants, 1556
Fulbright International Education Administrators Seminar Grants, 1569
Greater Worcester Comm Fndn Jeppson Memorial Fund for Brookfield Grants, 1659
Gulf Coast Comm of Venice Fndn Grants, 1677
H.A. and Mary K. Chapman Charitable Trust Grants, 1681
H.J. Heinz Company Fndn Grants, 1682
Harry Bramhall Gilbert Charitable Trust Grants, 1703
Hartford Fndn Regular Grants, 1711
Hawaii Comm Fndn West Hawaii Fund Grants, 1718
Heckscher Fndn for Children Grants, 1732
Henry & Ruth Blaustein Rosenberg Fndn Grants, 1746
Hershey Company Grants, 1754
Highmark Corp Giving Grants, 1769
Hilton Head Island Fndn Grants, 1779
Homer Fndn Grants, 1789
Horizons Comm Issues Grants, 1794
Humana Fndn Grants, 1818
Hut Fndn Grants, 1827
Infinity Fndn Grants, 1854
Irvin Stern Fndn Grants, 1866
Irving S. Gilmore Fndn Grants, 1867
Jackson County Comm Fndn Unrestricted Grants, 1879
Jacob G. Schmidlapp Trust Grants, 1883
James Ford Bell Fndn Grants, 1885
James S. Copley Fndn Grants, 1895
JELD-WEN Fndn Grants, 1914
Jewish Women's Fndn of New York Grants, 1924
Joseph H. and Florence A. Roblee Fndn Grants, 1961
Kahuku Comm Fund, 1977
Ludwick Family Fndn Grants, 2084
M.B. and Edna Zale Fndn Grants, 2093
M.J. Murdock Charitable Trust Grants, 2095
Maxtor Corp Contributions Grants, 2136
OSI-Baltimore Special Opportunities Grants, 2972
Pinellas County Grants, 3050
Richard and Susan Smith Family Fndn Grants, 3159
Salem Fndn Charitable Trust Grants, 3241
Southbury Comm Trust Fund, 3350
Trull Fndn Grants, 3441
Union Benevolent Association Grants, 3460

Cultural Programs/Activities

Allen P. and Josephine B. Green Fndn Grants, 361
Audrey and Sydney Irmas Charitable Fndn Grants, 665
Cass County Comm Fndn Grants, 887
Charles H. Dater Fndn Grants, 966
Chesapeake Corp Fndn Grants, 982
Comm Impact Fund, 1135
Cudd Fndn Grants, 1171
Fred L. Emerson Fndn Grants, 1557
Genuardi Family Fndn Grants, 1594
GlaxoSmithKline Corp Grants, 1623
Greater Cincinnati Fndn Priority and Small Projects/Capacity-Building Grants, 1651
Henry & Ruth Blaustein Rosenberg Fndn Grants, 1746
Hudson Webber Fndn Grants, 1813
Kraft Cares International Grants, 2016
Liberty Bank Fndn Grants, 2053
Meyer Fndn Grants, 2177
Northrop Grumman Corp Grants, 2866
Palm Beach and Martin Counties Grants, 2986
Pfizer Fndn Grants, 3025
Prince Charitable Trusts District of Columbia Grants, 3080
Riley Fndn Grants, 3165
Shell Oil Company Fndn Grants, 3281

Curriculum Development

A.O. Smith Comm Grants, 18
Adobe Comm Investment Grants, 237
Amgen Fndn Grants, 467
Bernard F. and Alva B. Gimbel Fndn Grants, 747
C.R. Bard Fndn Grants, 825
Cambridge Comm Fndn Grants, 837
Carnahan-Jackson Fndn Grants, 878
Crail-Johnson Fndn Grants, 1157
Ford Motor Company Fund Grants, 1522
GlaxoSmithKline Corp Grants, 1623
Huntington Beach Police Officers Fndn Grants, 1821
Jennings County Comm Fndn Grants, 1916
Josiah Macy Jr. Fndn Grants, 1966
Joyce Fndn Grants, 1969
King Pharmaceuticals Corp Contributions Grants, 2003
Louis R. Cappelli Fndn Grants, 2066
Lynde and Harry Bradley Fndn Grants, 2089
Lynde and Harry Bradley Fndn Prizes: Bradley Prizes, 2090
Meadows Fndn Grants, 2161
NIGMS Initiative for Minority Students: Bridges to the Doctoral Degree, 2613
NIGMS Minority Access to Research Careers Program, 2620
NIH School-based Interventions to Prevent Obesity, 2725
NIMH Curriculum Development Award in Neuroinformatics Research and Analysis, 2754
Paul and Mary Haas Fndn Contributions and Student Scholarships, 2997
Pfizer Fndn Grants, 3025
Polk Bros. Fndn Grants, 3066
Procter and Gamble Fund Grants, 3083
Pulte Homes Corp Contributions, 3092
Rathmann Family Fndn Grants, 3109
South Madison Comm Fndn Grants, 3349
STTI/ATI Educational Assessment Nursing Research Grants, 3397
Tellabs Fndn Grants, 3418
Vancouver Fndn Grants and Comm Initiatives Program, 3477
Vectren Fndn Grants, 3485
Western Indiana Comm Fndn Grants, 3528

Cystic Fibrosis

CCFF Clinic Incentive Grants, 892
CCFF Fellowships, 893
CCFF Research Grants, 894
CCFF Scholarships, 895
CCFF Small Conference Grants, 896
CCFF Studentships, 897
CCFF Summer Studentship, 898
CCFF Transplant Center Incentive Grants, 899
CCFF Visiting Scientist Awards, 900
CFF Clinical Research Grants, 942
CFF First- and Second-Year Clinical Fellowships, 943
CFF Leroy Matthews Physician-Scientist Awards, 944
CFF Pilot and Feasibility Awards, 945
CFF Postdoctoral Research Fellowships, 946
CFF Research Grants, 947
CFF Student Traineeships, 948
CFF Therapeutics Development Program, 949
CFF Third-Year Clinical Fellowships, 950
CFF-NIH Funding Grants, 951
Cystic Fibrosis Research Grants, 1179
Fndn of CVPH April LaValley Fund Grants, 1538
Harry Shwachman Clinical Investigator Award, 1707
Parker B. Francis Fellowships in Pulmonary Research, 2989

Cytoskeleton

NSF Cell Systems Cluster Grants, 2881

Dairy Products

National Dairy Promotion and Research Board Scholarships, 2251

Dance

AAHPERD Ruth Abernathy Presidential Scholarships, 128
Adaptec Fndn Grants, 232
Agnes Gund Fndn Grants, 262
Bodman Fndn Grants, 776
Carnahan-Jackson Fndn Grants, 878
Chicago Comm Trust Grants, 989
Comm Fndn of Western North Carolina Grants, 1132
Cooke Fndn Grants, 1148
Flinn Fndn Grants Programs, 1511
Kenneth T. and Eileen L. Norris Fndn Grants, 1989
Procter and Gamble Fund Grants, 3083
Puerto Rico Comm Fndn Grants, 3090
Ruth Mott Fndn Grants, 3204
Sid W. Richardson Fndn Grants, 3284
Southbury Comm Trust Fund, 3350

Dance Education

AAHPERD Ruth Abernathy Presidential Scholarships, 128

Data Analysis

NCI Academic-Industrial Partnerships for Development and Validation of In Vivo Imaging Systems and Methods for Cancer Investigations, 2268
NCI Application and Use of Transformative Emerging Technologies in Cancer Research, 2269
NEI Research Grant For Secondary Data Analysis Grants, 2296
NICHD Clinical Trial Planning Grants for Pediatric Rehabilitation, 2483
NIH Genetic Susceptibility and Variability of Human Malformations Research Grants, 2669
NIH Genetics of Neurobehavioral Disorders in Existing Samples Grants, 2670
NIMH Short Courses in Neuroinformatics, 2769
NSF Doctoral Dissertation Improvement Grants in the Directorate for Biological Sciences, 2884

Data Processing

NIH Exploratory Centers for Alternative Medicine Research Grants, 2663

Databases

NEI Research Grant For Secondary Data Analysis Grants, 2296
NIDDK Ancillary Studies of Kidney Disease Accessing Information from Clinical Trials, Epidemiological Studies, and Databases Grants, 2540
NIMH Core Support Program for Mental Health/AIDS Research Grants, 2753
NLM Internet Connection for Medical Institutions Grants, 2820
NLM Research Project Grants, 2825

Day Care

Bernard F. and Alva B. Gimbel Fndn Grants, 747
Carnegie Corp of New York Grants, 879
FCD Child Development Grants, 1458
Florida BRAIVE Fund of Dade Comm Fndn, 1512
Florida BRAIVE Fund of Gulf Coast Comm Fndn of Venice, 1513

Florida BRAIVE Fund of The Comm Fndn in Jacksonville, 1514
Hasbro Children's Fund, 1714
Josephine S. Gumbiner Fndn Grants, 1965
Ken W. Davis Fndn Grants, 1987
Knox County Comm Fndn Grants, 2009
Mary Owen Borden Fndn Grants, 2121
Michael and Susan Dell Fndn Grants, 2189
Perry County Comm Fndn Grants, 3016
Pike County Comm Fndn Grants, 3049
Posey Comm Fndn Grants, 3068
Spencer County Comm Fndn Grants, 3358
U.S. Department of Education 21st Century Comm Learning Centers, 3445
Vanderburgh Comm Fndn Grants, 3480

Death/Mortality
AAHPM Hospice and Palliative Medicine Fellowships, 132
Cardiac Arrhythmias Research and Education Fndn Research Grants, 863
CDC Injury Prevention and Control Research and State and Comm Based Programs, 914
CIGNA Fndn Grants, 1011
DHHS Health Centers Grants for Residents of Public Housing, 1254
DHHS Maternal and Child Health Projects Grants, 1263
FIC International Malaria Research Training Program Award, 1488
Greenwall Fndn Bioethics Grants, 1665
HRSA Eliminating Disparities in Perinatal Health Grants, 1803
LSA Specialized Center of Research Grants, 2077
NIA Health Behaviors and Aging Grants, 2408
NICHD Population Research Grants, 2490
NICHD Socioeconomic Status and Health Across the Life Course, 2495
NIDA National Drug Abuse Treatment Clinical Trials Network, 2510
NIH Collaborations for Advanced Strategies in Complication of HIV Infection, 2651
NIMH Socioeconomic Status and Health Across the Life Course, 2772
NINR Management of Symptoms at the End of Life Grants, 2796
NINR Quality of Life for Individuals at the End of Life Grants, 2802
Quantum Corp Snap Server Grants, 3095
United Cerebral Palsy Research Grants, 3462

Decision Sciences
AHFMR Population Health Investigator Awards, 292
Jane Beattie Memorial Scholarship, 1901
NLM Research Project Grants, 2825

Defense Technology
AAAS Science & Technology Policy Fellowships - National Defense & Global Security, 29

Demography
James S. McDonnell Fndn Complex Systems Collaborative Activity Awards, 1897
NIA Sociobehavorial Data Analysis and Archiving in Aging, 2434
NICHD Population Research Grants, 2490

Dental Education
ADA Fndn Dental Education Grants, 228
Alpha Omega Fndn Grants, 366
DHHS Grants for Dental Public Health, 1251
DHHS Health Careers Opportunity Grants, 1253
Fndn for Science and Disability Grant Program for Physically Disabled Students in the Sciences, 1532
HHMI Physician-Scientist Early Career Award, 1762
HHMI-NIH Cloister Research Scholars Program, 1765
HRB Clinical Research Training Fellowships, 1800
HRSA Health Professions Scholarships for Disadvantaged Students, 1807
Jewish Fndn for Education of Women Scholarships for Emigres in the Health Professions, 1922
Margoes Fndn Grants, 2106
NYAM David E. Rogers Fellowships, 2911
PAHO/WHO Fellowships, 2984
Pajaro Valley Comm Health Grants, 2985
RWJF Pipeline, Profession and Practice: Comm-Based Dental Education Grants, 3228
RWJF Summer Medical and Dental Education Program, 3231

Dental Health and Hygiene
Aetna Fndn Regional Comm Health Grants, 249
Alexander Eastman Fndn Grants, 341
Alpha Omega Fndn Grants, 366
Campbell Hoffman Fndn Grants, 840
Dental Laboratory Technology Scholarships, 1223
DHHS Oral Health Promotion Research Across the Lifespan, 1269
Grotto Fndn Project Grants, 1671
Health Fndn of Greater Indianapolis Grants, 1725
Henrietta Tower Wurts Memorial Fndn Grants, 1745
Jenkins Fndn: Improving the Health of Greater Richmond Grants, 1915
Nelda C. and H.J. Lutcher Stark Fndn Grants, 2301
NIDCR Clinical Trial Pilot Grant, 2533
NIDCR Clinical Trial Planning Grant, 2534
NIH Ruth L. Kirschstein National Research Service Awards for Individual Postdoctoral Fellows, 2719
NLM Manufacturing Processes of Medical, Dental, and Biological Technologies Grants, 2822
NYAM David E. Rogers Fellowships, 2911
Pajaro Valley Comm Health Grants, 2985
Pew Charitable Trusts Children & Youth Grants, 3020
Ruth Eleanor Bamberger and John Ernest Bamberger Memorial Fndn Grants, 3202
Saint Luke's Health Initiatives Grants, 3240
St. Joseph Comm Health Fndn Improving Healthcare Access Grants, 3368

Dental Health Education
Alpha Omega Fndn Grants, 366
Baxter International Fndn Grants, 705
Dental Teaching and Research Fellowships, 1224
HHMI Physician-Scientist Early Career Award, 1762
NYAM David E. Rogers Fellowships, 2911

Dentistry
ADA Fndn Dental Literature Grants, 229
AHFMR Clinical Fellowships, 269
Alpha Omega Fndn Grants, 366
Canadian Dental Research Fndn Award, 848
Canadian Friends of Hebrew University Research and Study Grants, 850
Dental Teaching and Research Fellowships, 1224
DHHS Geriatric Training for Physicians and Dentists Grants, 1250
DHHS Native American Health Service Loan Repayment Awards, 1267
DHHS Oral Health Promotion Research Across the Lifespan, 1269
DHHS Public Health Students Traineeships and Other Graduate Public Health Programs, 1277
HRB Postdoctoral Research Fellowships, 1802
Implant Dentistry Research and Education Fndn Grants, 1844
MHRC Postdoctoral Research Fellowships, 2187
NIA Mentored Clinical Scientist Research Career Development Awards, 2417
NYAM David E. Rogers Fellowships, 2911
PhRMA Fndn Health Outcomes Pre-Doctoral Fellowships, 3032
PhRMA Fndn Paul Calabresi Medical Student Research Fellowship, 3039
Special Olympics Health Professions Student Grants, 3355

Depression
AACAP Klingenstein Third Generation Fndn Award for Research in Depression or Suicide, 42
Aetna Fndn Quality of Care Grants for Depression, 246
Aetna Fndn Regional Comm Health Grants, 249
EF Behavioral Sciences Student Fellowships, 1379
Eli Lilly & Company Welcome Back Awards, 1391
Horizon Fndn for New Jersey Grants, 1793
Metrowest Comm Health Care Fndn Grants, 2176
NARSAD Distinguished Investigator Award, 2246
NARSAD Independent Investigator Award, 2247
NIDA Medications Development for Cannabis-Related Disorder, 2506
NIH Genetics of Neurobehavioral Disorders in Existing Samples Grants, 2670
NIMH Early Identification and Treatment of Mental Disorders in Children and Adolescents Grants, 2756
NINR Management of Symptoms at the End of Life Grants, 2796
NINR Quality of Life for Individuals at the End of Life Grants, 2802
Wellmark Fndn Grants, 3526

Dermatology
American Academy of Dermatology Camp Discovery Scholarships, 412
Carl J. Herzog Fndn Grants, 872
Dermatology Clinical Career Development Awards, 1235
Dermatology Fndn Grants, 1236
Dermatology Postdoctoral Research Fellowships, 1237
Dermatology Research Career Development Awards, 1238
MRC Career Establishment Grants, 2221
National Psoriasis Fndn Research Grants, 2259
Orentreich Fndn for the Advancement of Science Grants, 2959
Skin Cancer Fndn Research Grants, 3298
Society for Investigative Dermatology Career Development Award, 3325

Developing/Underdeveloped Nations
American Jewish World Service Grants, 437
Bill and Melinda Gates Fndn Grants, 756
FIC International Cooperative Biodiversity Groups Grants, 1487
FIC International Research and Training in Population and Health Grants, 1489
FIC International Research Scientist Development Award, 1491
FIC International Training and Research in Emerging Infectious Diseases Grants, 1492
FIC International Training and Research in Environmental and Occupational Health, 1493
FIC/NIH AIDS International Training and Research Program, 1496
FIC/ORMH Minority International Research Training Grants, 1497
Harold Simmons Fndn Grants, 1698
International Oncology Nursing Fellowships, 1862
John Deere Fndn Grants, 1929
Liliane Fndn Grants, 2055
MAP International Medical Fellowships, 2101
Pfizer Fndn Grants, 3025
Sir Dorabji Tata Trust Grants for NGOs or Voluntary Organizations, 3291
Takemi Program in International Health Research and Advanced Training Fellowships, 3416
UICC American Cancer Society International Fellowships for Beginning Investigators, 3455

Developmental Psychology
NSF Social Psychology Research Grants, 2894
Olfactory Research Fund Grants, 2942

Developmentally Disabled
Catherine Kennedy Home Fndn Grants, 890
Columbus Fndn Traditional Grants, 1071
CVS Comm Grants, 1177
DHHS Developmental Disabilities University Affiliated Programs Project Grants, 1248

Dr. Scholl Fndn Grants, 1329
H & R Fndn Grants, 1679
John Merck Fund Grants, 1940
John Merck Scholars Awards, 1941
John W. Anderson Fndn Grants, 1949
Leadership in Education in Neurodevelopmental Disabilities Postdoctoral Fellowships, 2037
Lucy Gooding Charitable Fndn Trust Grants, 2083
NIH Rett Syndrome: Genetics, Pathophysiology, and Biomarkers Research Grants, 2715
North Carolina GlaxoSmithKline Fndn Grants, 2860
Peter and Elizabeth C. Tower Fndn Comm Grants, 3018
Robert and Joan Dircks Fndn Grants, 3167
Simple Advise Education Center Grants, 3289
Spencer County Comm Fndn Grants, 3358
Strowd Roses Grants, 3388
United Cerebral Palsy Research Grants, 3462

Diabetes
Abbott Fund Access to Health Care Grants, 176
Abbott Fund Science and Medical Innovation Grants, 179
Aetna Fndn Regional Comm Health Grants, 249
Balfe Family Fndn Grants, 682
Chestnut Hill Charitable Fndn, Inc Grants, 987
Dietetic Outcomes Research Study Grants, 1285
Dorothy Rider Pool Health Care Grants, 1322
Fairlawn Fndn Grants, 1447
Gerber Fndn Grants, 1606
Gheens Fndn Grants, 1610
Greenwall Fndn Bioethics Grants, 1665
Hawaii Comm Fndn Health Education and Research Grants, 1716
Henry & Ruth Blaustein Rosenberg Fndn Grants, 1746
Horizon Fndn for New Jersey Grants, 1793
JDF Career Development Awards, 1910
Johnson & Johnson Comm Health Care Grants, 1951
Larry L. Hillblom Fndn Grants, 2031
M. Bastian Family Fndn Grants, 2092
NEI Innovative Patient Outreach Programs And Ocular Screening Technologies To Improve Detection Of Diabetic Retinopathy Grants, 2294
NHLBI Improving Heart Failure Disease Management Grants, 2338
NIDCR Oral Microbiology/Immunology of Type 1 Diabetes, 2537
NIDDK Collaborative Interdisciplinary Team Science in Diabetes, Endocrinology and Metabolic Diseases Grants, 2547
NIDDK Development of Disease Biomarkers Grants, 2549
NIDDK Diabetes Research Centers, 2551
NIDDK Diabetes, Endocrinology, and Metabolic Diseases NRSAs—Individual, 2552
NIDDK Education Grants, 2554
NIDDK Enhancing Zebrafish Research with Research Tools and Techniques, 2556
NIDDK Identifying and Reducing Diabetes and Obesity Related Health Disparities within Healthcare Systems, 2561
NIDDK Insulin Signaling and Receptor Cross Talk Grants, 2562
NIDDK Mentored Research Scientist Development Award, 2565
NIDDK Multi-Center Clinical Study Cooperative Agreements, 2566
NIDDK Multi-Center Clinical Study Implementation Planning Grants, 2567
NIDDK Neurobiology of Diabetic Complications Grants, 2568
NIDDK Non-Invasive Methods for Diagnosis and Progression of Diabetes, Kidney, Urological, Hematological and Digestive Diseases, 2572
NIDDK Pancreatic Development and Regeneration Grants: Toward Cellular Therapies for Diabetes, 2573
NIDDK Pilot and Feasibility Clinical Research Grants in Diabetes, Endocrine and Metabolic Diseases, 2574
NIDDK Planning Grants For Translational Research For The Prevention And Control Of Diabetes And Obesity, 2577
NIDDK Proteomics: Diabetes, Obesity, And Endocrine, Digestive, Kidney, Urologic, And Hematologic Diseases, 2578
NIDDK Race/Ethnic Disparities in the Incidence of Diabetes Complications, 2579
NIDDK Role of Gastrointestinal Surgical Procedures in Amelioration of Obesity-Related Insulin Resistance and Diabetes Independent of Weight Loss, 2582
NIDDK Secondary Analyses in Obesity, Diabetes and Digestive and Kidney Diseases Grants, 2583
NIDDK Seeding Collaborative Interdisciplinary Team Science in Diabetes, Endocrinology and Metabolic Diseases Grants, 2584
NIDDK Small Business Innovation Research to Develop New Therapeutics and Monitoring Technologies for Type 1 Diabetes (T1D)—Towards an Artificial Pancreas, 2586
NIDDK Small Grant Program for K08/K23 Recipients, 2587
NIDDK Small Grants for Underrepresented Minority Scientists in Diabetes and Digestive and Kidney Diseases, 2588
NIDDK Translational Research for the Prevention and Control of Diabetes and Obesity, 2591
NIDDK Type 2 Diabetes in the Pediatric Population Research Grants, 2593
NIGMS Short Courses on Mathematical, Statistical, and Computational Tools for Studying Biological Systems, 2629
NIH Enhancing Adherence to Diabetes Self-Management Behaviors, 2659
NIH Fine Mapping and Function of Genes for Type 1 Diabetes Grants, 2667
NIH Nonhuman Primate Immune Tolerance Cooperative Study Group Grants, 2699
NINR Diabetes Self-Management in Minority Populations Grants, 2795
OneSight Research Fndn Block Grants, 2944
Partnership for Cures Two Years To Cures Grants, 2992
Pittsburgh Fndn Medical Research Grants, 3055
Premera CARES Grants, 3074
Richard and Susan Smith Family Fndn Grants, 3159
Smith Family New Investigator Awards, 3299
Take Care to Learn: Teaching Clinical Care Management Grants, 3415
Wellmark Fndn Grants, 3526

Diabetic Retinopathy
NEI Innovative Patient Outreach Programs And Ocular Screening Technologies To Improve Detection Of Diabetic Retinopathy Grants, 2294

Diagnosis, Medical
Alexander and Margaret Stewart Trust Grants, 340
ALVRE Casselberry Award, 374
ALVRE Grant, 375
ALVRE Seymour R. Cohen Award, 376
ASM Scherago-Rubin Award, 617
CDC Research, Treatment, and Education Programs on Lyme Disease in the United States Cooperative Agreements, 927
Children's Cardiomyopathy Fndn Research Grants, 1002
DOE Medical Applications and Measurement Science Grants, 1301
Emma B. Howe Memorial Fndn Grants, 1415
FIC International Training and Research in Emerging Infectious Diseases Grants, 1492
FIC International Training and Research in Environmental and Occupational Health, 1493
HRSA Geriatric Education Centers, 1805
HRSA Ryan White HIV Early Intervention Services Grants, 1811
International Cancer Technology Transfer Fellowships, 1858
NCI Exploratory Grants for Behavioral Research in Cancer Control, 2274
NEI Innovative Patient Outreach Programs And Ocular Screening Technologies To Improve Detection Of Diabetic Retinopathy Grants, 2294
NIA Alzheimer's Disease Core Centers Grants, 2395
NIAMS/NICHD Deep Infections of Total Joint Replacements, 2481
NIDCD Neurobiology and Genetics of Autism Grants, 2526
NIDCR HIV/AIDS Associated Oral Viral Infections, 2535
NIH Collaborations for Advanced Strategies in Complication of HIV Infection, 2651
NIH Genetics of Neurobehavioral Disorders in Existing Samples Grants, 2670
NIH SBIR/STTR Study and Control of Microbial Biofilms Research Grants, 2724
NIH Urinary Incontinence Treatment Network, 2738
Partnership for Cures Two Years To Cures Grants, 2992
Susan G. Komen Breast Cancer Fndn Basic, Clinical, and Translational Research Grants, 3407
UICC American Cancer Society International Fellowships for Beginning Investigators, 3455
US CRDF Leishmaniasis: Collaborative Research Opportunities in North Africa and the Middle East, 3474

Dietary Foods
Institute for Agriculture and Trade Policy Food and Society Fellowships, 1856
NCI Diet, Epigenetic Events, and Cancer Prevention Grants, 2272
NCI Improving Diet and Physical Activity Assessment Grants, 2275
NHLBI Targeted Approaches to Weight Control for Young Adults Grants, 2387
NIH Dietary Supplement Research Centers: Botanicals Grants, 2654

Dietary Supplements
NIH Dietary Supplement Research Centers: Botanicals Grants, 2654

Dietetics/Nutrition
RWJF Healthy Eating Research Grants, 3218

Digestive Diseases and Disorders
ASGE Don Wilson Award, 565
ASGE Endoscopic Research Awards, 566
ASGE Endoscopic Research Career Development Awards, 567
ASGE Given Capsule Endoscopy Research Award, 568
CFF First- and Second-Year Clinical Fellowships, 943
CFF Postdoctoral Research Fellowships, 946
CFF Research Grants, 947
CFF Third-Year Clinical Fellowships, 950
Crohn's Disease and Colitis Research Fellowships, 1164
Crohn's Disease and Ulcerative Colitis Senior Research Grants, 1165
FDHN Bridging Grants, 1464
FDHN Centocor International Research Fellowship in Gastrointestinal Inflammation & Immunology, 1465
FDHN Designated Research Award in Geriatric Gastroenterology, 1467
FDHN Designated Research Award in Research Related to Pancreatitis, 1468
FDHN Fellow Abstract Prizes, 1469
FDHN Fellowship to Faculty Transition Awards, 1470
FDHN Graduate Student Awards, 1472
FDHN Jon I. Isenberg International Research Scholar Award, 1473
FDHN June & Donald O. Castell MD, Esophageal Clinical Research Award, 1474
FDHN Moti L. & Kamla Rustgi International Travel Awards, 1475

FDHN Non-Career Research Awards, 1476
FDHN Student Abstract Prizes, 1479
FDHN Student Research Fellowships, 1480
FDHN TAP Endowed Designated Research Award in Acid-Related Diseases, 1481
June Allyson Fndn Research Fellowships, 1972
NFID New Investigator Matching Grants, 2310
NIDDK Education Grants, 2554
NIDDK Enhancing Zebrafish Research with Research Tools and Techniques, 2556
NIDDK Intestinal Failure, Short Gut Syndrome and Small Bowel Transplantation Grants, 2563
NIDDK Intestinal Stem Cell Consortium Grants, 2564
NIDDK Mentored Research Scientist Development Award, 2565
NIDDK Multi-Center Clinical Study Cooperative Agreements, 2566
NIDDK Multi-Center Clinical Study Implementation Planning Grants, 2567
NIDDK Non-Invasive Methods for Diagnosis and Progression of Diabetes, Kidney, Urological, Hematological and Digestive Diseases, 2572
NIDDK Pilot and Feasibility Clinical Research Studies in Digestive Diseases and Nutrition, 2576
NIDDK Proteomics: Diabetes, Obesity, And Endocrine, Digestive, Kidney, Urologic, And Hematologic Diseases, 2578
NIDDK Secondary Analyses in Obesity, Diabetes and Digestive and Kidney Diseases Grants, 2583
NIDDK Silvio O. Conte Digestive Diseases Research Core Centers Grants, 2585
NIDDK Small Grant Program for K08/K23 Recipients, 2587
NIDDK Small Grants for Underrepresented Minority Scientists in Diabetes and Digestive and Kidney Diseases, 2588
NIGMS Short Courses on Mathematical, Statistical, and Computational Tools for Studying Biological Systems, 2629
Thrasher Research Fund Grants, 3426

Digestive System
ASGE Endoscopic Research Awards, 566
ASGE Endoscopic Research Career Development Awards, 567
ASGE Given Capsule Endoscopy Research Award, 568
FDHN Centocor International Research Fellowship in Gastrointestinal Inflammation & Immunology, 1465
FDHN Designated Research Award in Geriatric Gastroenterology, 1467
FDHN Fellow Abstract Prizes, 1469
FDHN June & Donald O. Castell MD, Esophageal Clinical Research Award, 1474
FDHN Moti L. & Kamla Rustgi International Travel Awards, 1475
FDHN Non-Career Research Awards, 1476
FDHN TAP Endowed Designated Research Award in Acid-Related Diseases, 1481
Millipore/Charles P. Schaufus Parenteral-Processing Technology Research Grant, 2204
NIDDK Development of Disease Biomarkers Grants, 2549
NIDDK Intestinal Failure, Short Gut Syndrome and Small Bowel Transplantation Grants, 2563
NIDDK Pilot and Feasibility Clinical Research Studies in Digestive Diseases and Nutrition, 2576
NIDDK Secondary Analyses in Obesity, Diabetes and Digestive and Kidney Diseases Grants, 2583
NIDDK Silvio O. Conte Digestive Diseases Research Core Centers Grants, 2585

Disabled
AAPD Henry B. Betts Award, 169
AAPD Paul G. Hearne Leadership Award, 170
Abell-Hanger Fndn Grants, 183
Able To Serve Grants, 185
Able Trust Vocational Rehabilitation Grants for Individuals, 186
AEGON Transamerica Fndn Grants, 243
Aetna Fndn Health Grants in Connecticut, 244
Alberto Culver Corp Contributions Grants, 329
Albuquerque Comm Fndn Grants, 331
Alexander and Margaret Stewart Trust Grants, 340
Ann Jackson Family Fndn Grants, 477
Ann Peppers Fndn Grants, 478
Annunziata Sanguinetti Fndn Grants, 481
Armstrong McDonald Fndn Grants, 537
ASHFndn Graduate Student Scholarships for Minority Students, 578
ASHFndn Graduate Student with a Disability Scholarship, 579
Atkinson Fndn International Grants, 661
Baxter International Fndn Grants, 705
Berrien Comm Fndn Grants, 749
Boston Fndn Grants, 783
Callaway Golf Company Fndn Grants, 836
Carl W. and Carrie Mae Joslyn Trust Grants, 873
Carls Fndn Grants, 876
Carnahan-Jackson Fndn Grants, 878
Carrie E. and Lena V. Glenn Fndn Grants, 882
Carrie Estelle Doheny Fndn Grants, 883
Catherine Kennedy Home Fndn Grants, 890
CDC Injury Prevention and Control Research and State and Comm Based Programs, 914
CDC Using Genetic Information to Prevent Disease and Improve Health Research Grants, 932
Cessna Fndn Grants, 938
Champ-A Champion Fur Kids Grants, 959
Charles Delmar Fndn Grants, 963
Chatlos Fndn Grants, 977
CHCF Grants, 979
Children's Trust Fund of Oregon Grants, 1001
Clark-Winchcole Fndn Grants, 1030
CNA Fndn Grants, 1046
CNCS Engaging Persons with Disabilities in National and Comm Service Grants, 1047
Collins Fndn Grants, 1058
Columbus Fndn Traditional Grants, 1071
Comm Fndn of Greater Birmingham Grants, 1106
Cooper Industries Fndn Grants, 1150
Cornerstone Fndn of Northeastern Wisconsin Grants, 1152
D. W. McMillan Fndn Grants, 1180
Dammann Fund Grants, 1192
Daniels Fund Grants, 1200
Daphne Seybolt Culpeper Memorial Fndn Grants, 1201
Denver Broncos Charities Fund Grants, 1226
Dept of Ed Rehabilitation Training Grants, 1229
Dept of Ed Special Education—Personnel Development to Improve Services and Results for Children with Disabilities, 1231
Dept of Ed Special Education—Studies and Evaluations, 1232
Dept of Ed Special Education—Technical Assistance and Dissemination to Improve Services and Results for Children with Disabilities, 1233
Dept of Ed Special Education-National Activities-Technology and Media Services for Individuals with Disabilities, 1234
Disable American Veterans Charitable Grants, 1286
Dolan Fndn Grants, 1306
Dorothea Haus Ross Fndn Grants, 1320
Edwards Memorial Trust Grants, 1375
Effie and Wofford Cain Fndn Grants, 1385
Eisner Fndn Grants, 1387
El Paso Comm Fndn Grants, 1388
Emma B. Howe Memorial Fndn Grants, 1415
Eva L. and Joseph M. Bruening Fndn Grants, 1436
Fisa Fndn Grants, 1506
Foellinger Fndn Grants, 1519
Fndn for Science and Disability Grant Program for Physically Disabled Students in the Sciences, 1532
Fourjay Fndn Grants, 1544
Gheens Fndn Grants, 1610
Giving in Action Society Children & Youth with Special Needs Grants, 1617
Giving in Action Society Family Independence Grants, 1618
Glendale Comm Fndn Grants, 1626
Greater Milwaukee Fndn Grants, 1653
Green Bay Packers Fndn Grants, 1660
Grundy Fndn Grants, 1673
Gulf Coast Comm Fndn Grants, 1676
Gulf Coast Comm of Venice Fndn Grants, 1677
Hackett Fndn Grants, 1684
Harry Kramer Memorial Fund Grants, 1705
Harry S. Black and Allon Fuller Fund, 1706
Hasbro Children's Fund, 1714
Hearst Fndn and William Randolph Hearst Fndn Grants, 1730
Helen Steiner Rice Fndn Grants, 1742
HHK Employment Grants, 1755
Hilda and Preston Davis Fndn Grants, 1772
Hill Fndn Grants, 1774
Hoblitzelle Fndn Grants, 1783
Horace A. Kimball and S. Ella Kimball Fndn Grants, 1792
Howe Fndn of North Carolina Grants, 1799
HRSA Geriatric Education Centers, 1805
Ireland Family Fndn Grants, 1865
J. Walton Bissell Fndn Grants, 1872
J.W. Kieckhefer Fndn Grants, 1878
Jacob and Valeria Langeloth Fndn Grants, 1882
James Ford Bell Fndn Grants, 1885
Janirve Fndn Grants, 1905
Jay and Rose Phillips Family Fndn Grants, 1909
John H. and Wilhelmina D. Harland Charitable Fndn Grants, 1933
John H. Wellons Fndn Grants, 1934
John I. Smith Charities Grants, 1935
John J. Leidy Fndn Grants, 1936
John W. Alden Trust Grants, 1947
Joseph P. Kennedy Jr. Fndn Grants, 1962
Josiah W. and Bessie H. Kline Fndn Grants, 1967
Ken W. Davis Fndn Grants, 1987
Kenneth T. and Eileen L. Norris Fndn Grants, 1989
Lands' End Corp Giving Program, 2030
Liliane Fndn Grants, 2055
Lucy Gooding Charitable Fndn Trust, 2082
Ludwick Family Fndn Grants, 2084
M.E. Raker Fndn Grants, 2094
M.J. Murdock Charitable Trust Grants, 2095
Mabel H. Flory Charitable Trust Grants, 2096
Manuel D. and Rhoda Mayerson Fndn Grants, 2100
Margaret L. Wendt Fndn Grants, 2104
Mary Allen Lindsey Branan Fndn Grants, 2116
Maxtor Corp Contributions Grants, 2136
May and Stanley Smith Trust Grants, 2137
Medicaid Infrastructure Grant Program to Support Employment of People with Disabilities, 2163
Medtronic Fndn Health Care Grants, 2169
Military Ex-Prisoners of War Fndn Grants, 2201
Ms. Fndn for Women Grants, 2222
National City Corp Contributions Grants, 2250
National Heart Fndn of New Zealand Grants, 2255
Newman's Own Inc Grants, 2306
NIAID Allergy, Immunology, Transplantation, Infectious Diseases, and AIDS NRSAs—Individual, 2450
NIAID Therapeutics Research on AIDS-Associated Opportunistic Infections, 2465
NIAMS Research on Musculoskeletal Fitness and Sports Medicine Grants, 2476
NICHD Medical Rehabilitation Research, 2487
NICHD Research on Musculoskeletal Fitness and Sports Medicine Grants, 2492
NICHD Socioeconomic Status and Health Across the Life Course, 2495
NIH Mechanisms Underlying Secondary Conditions in Mobility Disorders, 2686
NIH Urinary Incontinence Treatment Network, 2738
NIMH Socioeconomic Status and Health Across the Life Course, 2772
Nina Mason Pulliam Charitable Trust Grants, 2776
NINR Research on Musculoskeletal Fitness and Sports Medicine Grants, 2803
Northrop Grumman Corp Grants, 2866
NSF Biomedical Engineering and Engineering Healthcare Grants, 2879

NYCT Children and Youth with Disabilities Grants, 2923
Ordean Fndn Grants, 2952
OUT Fund for Lesbian and Gay Liberation Grants, 2978
Pasadena Fndn Average Grants, 2994
Paul Balint Charitable Trust Grants, 2998
Peabody Fndn Grants, 3010
Peacock Fndn Grants, 3011
Pittsburgh Fndn Comm Fund Grants, 3054
Polaroid Fund Grants, 3065
R.C. Baker Fndn Grants, 3098
Rajiv Gandhi Fndn Grants, 3104
Rayonier Fndn Grants, 3111
Rehab Therapy Fndn Grants, 3146
Rockwell International Corp Trust Grants, 3183
Roeher Institute Research Grants, 3184
S. Mark Taper Fndn Grants, 3236
Salem Fndn Grants, 3242
San Francisco Fndn Disability Rights Advocate Fund Emergency Grants, 3261
Schurz Communications Fndn Grants, 3271
Seabury Fndn Grants, 3274
Sheltering Arms Fund Grants, 3282
Sid W. Richardson Fndn Grants, 3284
Simple Advise Education Center Grants, 3289
Sir Halley Stewart Trust Grants, 3293
Special Olympics Health Professions Student Grants, 3355
Special People in Need Grants, 3356
Special People in Need Scholarships, 3357
Starr Fndn Grants, 3377
Steelcase Fndn Grants, 3379
Strowd Roses Grants, 3388
Taproot Fndn Capacity-Building Service Grants, 3417
U.S. Department of Education 21st Century Comm Learning Centers, 3445
U.S. Department of Education Rehabilitation Engineering Research Centers Grants, 3447
U.S. Department of Education Rehabilitation Research Training Centers, 3448
U.S. Department of Education Rehabilitation Training—Rehabilitation Continuing Education Programs—Institute on Rehabilitation Issues, 3449
U.S. Department of Education Special Education—National Activities—Parent Information Centers, 3450
U.S. Department of Education Vocational Rehabilitation Services Projects for American Indians with Disabilities Grants, 3452
Union Benevolent Association Grants, 3460
Union County Comm Fndn Grants, 3461
United Cerebral Palsy Research Grants, 3462
Vancouver Sun Children's Fund Grants, 3479
Washington Post Contributions Grants, 3520
Weingart Fndn Grants, 3524
Westinghouse Charitable Giving Grants, 3530
Wilson-Wood Fndn Grants, 3542
Women's Fndn of California Grants, 3550

Disabled (Target Groups)
Autodesk Comm Relations Grants, 671
Catherine Holmes Wilkins Fndn Grants, 889
Chiron Fndn Comm Grants, 1004
Hanna Andersson Children's Fndn Grants, 1691
HHK Employment Grants, 1755
Partners for Youth with Disabilities Grants, 2990
Rosalynn Carter Institute John and Betty Pope Fellowships, 3189
Verizon Fndn Maryland Grants, 3487
Verizon Fndn New York Grants, 3488
Verizon Fndn Northeast Region Grants, 3489
Verizon Fndn Pennsylvania Grants, 3490
Verizon Fndn Vermont Grants, 3491
Verizon Fndn Virginia Grants, 3492
William G. Kelley Fndn Grants, 3538

Disabled Student Support
Able Trust Vocational Rehabilitation Grants for Individuals, 186
ASHFndn Graduate Student Scholarships, 577
Champ-A Champion Fur Kids Grants, 959
CVS All Kids Can Grants, 1175
CVS Comm Grants, 1177
Florida High School/High Tech Project Grants, 1515
Lettie Pate Whitehead Fndn Grants, 2049
Marriott Fndn for People with Disabilities Bridges Grants, 2113
NIH NRSAs Predoctoral Fellowship Awards for Students with Disabilities, 2701
Peacock Fndn Grants, 3011
Special People in Need Scholarships, 3357

Disabled, Accessibility for
AAPD Henry B. Betts Award, 169
AAPD Paul G. Hearne Leadership Award, 170
Adolph Coors Fndn Grants, 238
Challenged Athletes Fndn Grants, 958
CVS Comm Grants, 1177
Giving in Action Society Children & Youth with Special Needs Grants, 1617
Giving in Action Society Family Independence Grants, 1618
HHK Employment Grants, 1755
Hugh J. Andersen Fndn Grants, 1814
Jay and Rose Phillips Family Fndn Grants, 1909
Multiple Sclerosis Fndn Brighter Tomorrow Grants, 2228
NIDRR Field-Initiated Projects, 2594
NYCT Children and Youth with Disabilities Grants, 2923
Robins Fndn Grants, 3175
Sheltering Arms Fund Grants, 3282
U.S. Department of Education Rehabilitation Engineering Research Centers Grants, 3447

Disabled, Education
Charles Lafitte Fndn Grants, 970
Jay and Rose Phillips Family Fndn Grants, 1909

Disabled, Higher Education
Greenspun Family Fndn Grants, 1664

Disadvantaged (Economically)
ACF Standing Announcement for Unaccompanied Alien Children Grants, 202
Achelis and Bodman Fndns Grants, 206
Ahmanson Fndn Grants, 303
Alberto Culver Corp Contributions Grants, 329
Albuquerque Comm Fndn Grants, 331
Allegis Group Fndn Grants, 360
Anschutz Family Fndn Grants, 486
Ansell, Zaro, Grimm & Aaron Fndn Grants, 487
ARCO Fndn Education Grants, 526
Atkinson Fndn International Grants, 661
Austin-Bailey Health and Wellness Fndn Grants, 669
Batchelor Fndn Grants, 701
BCBS of Massachusetts Catalyst Fund Grants, 708
BCBSM Comm Health Matching Grants, 715
Bernard and Audre Rapoport Fndn Grants, 746
Brinson Fndn Grants, 794
Callaway Golf Company Fndn Grants, 836
Carl B. and Florence E. King Fndn Grants, 869
Carls Fndn Grants, 876
Carolyn Fndn Grants, 880
Carrie E. and Lena V. Glenn Fndn Grants, 882
Catherine Holmes Wilkins Fndn Grants, 889
Catholic Campaign for Human Development Comm Organizing Grants, 891
Cessna Fndn Grants, 938
Charles Delmar Fndn Grants, 963
Charles H. Dater Fndn Grants, 966
CIT Corp Giving Grants, 1014
Claude Pepper Fndn Grants, 1032
CNA Fndn Grants, 1046
Commonweal Fndn Comm Assistance Grants, 1075
Commonweal Fndn Grants, 1076
Comm Fndn of Broward Grants, 1100
Comm Fndn of Greater Birmingham Grants, 1106
Comm Fndn of Greenville Hollingsworth Funds Program/Project Grants, 1114
Comm Fndn of Southeastern Connecticut Grants, 1125
Constantin Fndn Grants, 1145
Cooper Industries Fndn Grants, 1150
Cornerstone Fndn of Northeastern Wisconsin Grants, 1152
Crail-Johnson Fndn Grants, 1157
CVS All Kids Can Grants, 1175
CVS Comm Grants, 1177
D. W. McMillan Fndn Grants, 1180
Danellie Fndn Grants, 1198
Daniels Fund Grants, 1200
Daphne Seybolt Culpeper Memorial Fndn Grants, 1201
Dennis and Phyllis Washington Fndn Grants, 1222
Edina Realty Fndn Grants, 1369
Eisner Fndn Grants, 1387
Elsie Lee Garthwaite Memorial Fndn Grants, 1403
Flinn Fndn Grants Programs, 1511
Fourjay Fndn Grants, 1544
Georgiana Goddard Eaton Memorial Fund Grants, 1604
Global Fund for Children Grants, 1629
H.J. Heinz Company Fndn Grants, 1682
Hanna Andersson Children's Fndn Grants, 1691
Harold and Arlene Schnitzer CARE Fndn Grants, 1697
Harry S. Black and Allon Fuller Fund, 1706
Hasbro Children's Fund, 1714
Henrietta Tower Wurts Memorial Fndn Grants, 1745
Horace A. Kimball and S. Ella Kimball Fndn Grants, 1792
Howard and Bush Fndn Grants, 1798
Indiana Minority Teacher/Special Services Scholarships, 1852
Ittleson Fndn AIDS Grants, 1869
James Ford Bell Fndn Grants, 1885
James H. Cummings Fndn Grants, 1888
Jane Bradley Pettit Fndn Grants, 1902
Jane's Trust Grants, 1904
Janirve Fndn Grants, 1905
Jerome and Mildred Paddock Fndn Grants, 1917
Jessie B. Cox Charitable Trust Grants, 1918
Jim Moran Fndn Grants, 1925
John P. Murphy Fndn Grants, 1943
Joseph H. and Florence A. Roblee Fndn Grants, 1961
Josephine G. Russell Trust Grants, 1963
Kahuku Comm Fund, 1977
King Pharmaceuticals Corp Contributions Grants, 2003
Lands' End Corp Giving Program, 2030
Liberty Bank Fndn Grants, 2053
Long Island Comm Fndn Grants, 2063
Lucy Gooding Charitable Fndn Trust, 2082
Lucy Gooding Charitable Fndn Trust Grants, 2083
Margaret L. Wendt Fndn Grants, 2104
Mary Allen Lindsey Branan Fndn Grants, 2116
Mary Owen Borden Fndn Grants, 2121
Mattel Children's Fndn Grants, 2130
Mattel International Grants, 2131
Maxtor Corp Contributions Grants, 2136
May and Stanley Smith Trust Grants, 2137
Middlesex Savings Charitable Fndn Grants, 2196
Milagro Fndn Grants, 2198
Minneapolis Fndn Comm Grants, 2206
Morton K. and Jane Blaustein Fndn Grants, 2218
Nelda C. and H.J. Lutcher Stark Fndn Grants, 2301
Nicholas H. Noyes Jr. Memorial Fndn Grants, 2497
NIH Undergraduate Scholarships, 2737
Northern Trust Company Charitable Trust and Corp Giving Program, 2865
Northwestern Mutual Fndn Grants, 2870
NYC Managed Care Consumer Assistance Workshop Re-Design Grants, 2918
Oleonda Jameson Trust Grants, 2941
Ordean Fndn Grants, 2952
Peacock Fndn Grants, 3011
PeyBack Fndn Grants, 3022
Pfizer Fndn Grants, 3025
Plum Creek Fndn Grants, 3062

Powell Fndn Grants, 3073
Prince Charitable Trusts District of Columbia Grants, 3080
Prudential Fndn Grants, 3087
Public Welfare Fndn Grants, 3089
Raskob Fndn for Catholic Activities Grants, 3107
Rayonier Fndn Grants, 3111
Rhode Island Fndn Grants, 3154
Richard and Susan Smith Family Fndn Grants, 3159
Robert and Joan Dircks Fndn Grants, 3167
Robert B McMillen Fndn Grants, 3169
Rockefeller Fndn Grants, 3181
Roy and Christine Sturgis Trust Grants, 3191
RWJF Vulnerable Populations Portfolio Grants, 3232
S. Mark Taper Fndn Grants, 3236
Sheltering Arms Fund Grants, 3282
Sir Dorabji Tata Trust Grants for NGOs or Voluntary Organizations, 3291
Sir Dorabji Tata Trust Individual Medical Grants, 3292
Southwire Company Grants, 3353
Special People in Need Scholarships, 3357
Stark Comm Fndn Women's Fund Grants, 3376
Starr Fndn Grants, 3377
Steelcase Fndn Grants, 3379
Strowd Roses Grants, 3388
Thompson Charitable Fndn Grants, 3425
Trull Fndn Grants, 3441
Union Benevolent Association Grants, 3460
Vanderburgh Comm Fndn Grants, 3480
Volkswagen of America Corp Contributions Grants, 3503
Western Union Fndn Grants, 3529
Westinghouse Charitable Giving Grants, 3530
William H. Hannon Fndn Grants, 3540
Wilson-Wood Fndn Grants, 3542
Women's Fndn of California Comm Action Fund, 3549
Women's Fndn of California Grants, 3550

Disaster Relief
Albertson's Charitable Giving Grants, 330
Alice Tweed Tuohy Fndn Grants, 357
Allstate Corp Giving Grants, 363
Allstate Corp Hometown Commitment Grants, 364
Anheuser-Busch Fndn Grants, 474
AT&T Fndn Civic and Comm Service Grants, 658
Avon Products Fndn Grants, 675
Beazley Fndn Grants, 730
Becton Dickinson and Company Grants, 736
Bill and Melinda Gates Fndn Grants, 756
BJ's Charitable Fndn Grants, 761
Boeing Company Contributions Grants, 777
California Endowment CommunitiesFirst Grants, 833
Cargill Citizenship Fund-Corp Giving Grants, 865
Carnegie Corp of New York Grants, 879
Coca-Cola Fndn Grants, 1052
Constellation Energy Group and Baltimore Gas and Electric Corp Contributions, 1146
Cultural Society of Filipino Americans Grants, 1173
ExxonMobil Grants, 1442
Farmers Insurance Group of Companies Grants, 1455
Federal Express Corp Contributions Program, 1483
Greater New Orleans Fndn Grants, 1654
Gulf Coast Comm Fndn Grants, 1676
H. Schaffer Fndn Grants, 1680
Harry Kramer Memorial Fund Grants, 1705
HHMI Grants and Fellowships Programs, 1759
Home Building Industry Disaster Relief Fund, 1787
Humana Fndn Grants, 1818
Jessie Ball Dupont Fund Grants, 1919
Jewish Comm Fndn of Greater Los Angeles Grants, 1921
John Deere Fndn Grants, 1929
Kimberly-Clark Comm Grants, 2001
Lawrence Fndn Grants, 2034
M.J. Murdock Charitable Trust Grants, 2095
Mary Allen Lindsey Branan Fndn Grants, 2116
May Department Stores Charitable Contribution Grants, 2138
Noble County Comm Fndn Grants, 2848
Office Depot Fndn Grants, 2936
Perry County Comm Fndn Grants, 3016
Pfizer Fndn Grants, 3025
Pike County Comm Fndn Grants, 3049
Posey Comm Fndn Grants, 3068
Procter and Gamble Fund Grants, 3083
Public Welfare Fndn Grants, 3089
Ralphs Food 4 Less Fndn Grants, 3106
Richard and Rhoda Goldman Fund Grants, 3158
Rockefeller Fndn Grants, 3181
Schering-Plough Fndn Health Grants, 3270
Seneca Foods Fndn Grants, 3278
Spencer County Comm Fndn Grants, 3358
Susan G. Komen Breast Cancer Fndn Hurricane Relief Grants, 3409
Thompson Charitable Fndn Grants, 3425
Vanderburgh Comm Fndn Grants, 3480
VHA Health Fndn Grants, 3495
Warrick County Comm Fndn Grants, 3519

Disasters
Duke Energy Fndn Grants, 1339
Francis T. & Louise T. Nichols Fndn Grants, 1550
Harry Kramer Memorial Fund Grants, 1705
Hormel Foods Charitable Trust Grants, 1795
NIA Behavioral and Social Research Grants on Disasters and Health, 2401
Rohm and Haas Company Grants, 3185

Discrimination
Allstate Corp Giving Grants, 363
Allstate Corp Hometown Commitment Grants, 364
Georgia Power Fndn Grants, 1603
Otto Bremer Fndn Grants, 2977
San Diego Fndn for Change Grants, 3255
Waitt Family Fndn Grants, 3512

Disease, Chronic
NIH Self-Management Strategies Across Chronic Diseases Grants, 2726

Diseases
Affymetrix Corp Contributions Grants, 258
Albertson's Charitable Giving Grants, 330
Batchelor Fndn Grants, 701
HHMI Med into Grad Initiative Grants, 1761
Premera CARES Grants, 3074
Samueli Institute Scientific Research Grants, 3253

Distance Learning
Alfred P. Sloan Fndn Research Fellowships, 353
Chatlos Fndn Grants, 977
DOA Distance Learning and Telemedicine Grant Program, 1288
Doris Duke Charitable Fndn Clinical Scientist Development Award, 1316
Henry & Ruth Blaustein Rosenberg Fndn Grants, 1746
Hillsdale Fund Grants, 1778

Diversity
Bernard Van Leer Fndn Grants, 748
Boeing Company Contributions Grants, 777
Sisters of Mercy of North Carolina Fndn Grants, 3295
Stewart Huston Charitable Trust Grants, 3384
Volkswagen of America Corp Contributions Grants, 3503

DNA
Children's Medical Research Institute Grants, 1000
Elizabeth Glaser Pediatric AIDS Fndn Pediatric HIV Vaccine Research Grants, 1395
Innovative Technology Development Awards, 1855
NIAID HIV Vaccine Research and Design—Program Project Grants, 2455
NIH Genetic Architecture of Complex Phenotypes, 2668
NIH Studies of Ethical, Legal, and Social Implications of Research into Human Genetic Variation Grants, 2731
Osteogenesis Imperfecta Fndn Research Grants, 2975

Documentaries
Connecticut Comm Fndn Grants, 1141

Domestic Abuse
Fisa Fndn Grants, 1506
Hilton Head Island Fndn Grants, 1779
Hugh J. Andersen Fndn Grants, 1814
Jane Bradley Pettit Fndn Grants, 1902
Lewis Preston Fund for Girls Education Grants, 2052
Verizon Fndn Maryland Grants, 3487
Verizon Fndn New York Grants, 3488
Verizon Fndn Northeast Region Grants, 3489
Verizon Fndn Pennsylvania Grants, 3490
Verizon Fndn Vermont Grants, 3491
Verizon Fndn Virginia Grants, 3492

Domestic Violence
Adaptec Fndn Grants, 232
Andersen Fndn Grants, 471
Atherton Family Fndn Grants, 659
Austin-Bailey Health and Wellness Fndn Grants, 669
Baxter International Fndn Grants, 705
Blue Shield of California Grants, 771
Boston Jewish Comm Women's Fund Grants, 785
Bush Fndn Health & Human Services Grants, 814
Cambridge Comm Fndn Grants, 837
Carlisle Fndn Grants, 874
Carrie E. and Lena V. Glenn Fndn Grants, 882
Catherine Kennedy Home Fndn Grants, 890
Children's Trust Fund of Oregon Grants, 1001
Colorado Springs Comm Trust Fund Grants, 1061
Commission on Religion in Appalachia Grants, 1074
Comm Fndn of Broward Grants, 1100
Crail-Johnson Fndn Grants, 1157
Dallas Women's Fndn Grants, 1191
Dammann Fund Grants, 1192
Dennis and Phyllis Washington Fndn Grants, 1222
Detroit Lions Charities Grants, 1241
Edina Realty Fndn Grants, 1369
Faye McBeath Fndn Grants, 1456
Fremont Area Comm Fndn Grants, 1561
Greater Tacoma Comm Fndn Ryan Alan Hade Endowment Fund, 1657
Greater Worcester Comm Fndn Discretionary Grants, 1658
Hancock County Comm Fndn Grants, 1690
Hanna Andersson Children's Fndn Grants, 1691
Harry Frank Guggenheim Fndn Research Grants, 1704
Health Fndn of Greater Indianapolis Grants, 1725
Jacob and Valeria Langeloth Fndn Grants, 1882
James R. Dougherty Jr. Fndn Grants, 1894
Jim Moran Fndn Grants, 1925
Kahuku Comm Fund, 1977
Kraft Cares International Grants, 2016
Lesbian Health Fund Grants, 2046
Mary Kay Ash Charitable Fndn Grants, 2120
Metrowest Comm Health Care Fndn Grants, 2176
Meyer Fndn Grants, 2177
Michael and Susan Dell Fndn Grants, 2189
Morris and Gwendolyn Cafritz Fndn Grants, 2217
Ms. Fndn for Women Grants, 2222
NNEDVF/Altria Doors of Hope Program, 2847
Northern Trust Company Charitable Trust and Corp Giving Program, 2865
PacifiCorp Fndn for Learning Grants, 2982
Piper Jaffray Companies Building Strong Communities Grants, 3053
Posey Comm Fndn Womens Fund Grants, 3069
Quantum Fndn Grants, 3096
Reynolds and Reynolds Associate Fndn Grants, 3152
Robin Hood Fndn Grants, 3174
S. Mark Taper Fndn Grants, 3236

Drama
Herman Goldman Fndn Grants, 1753

Dramatic/Theater Arts
Adaptec Fndn Grants, 232
Alcatel-Lucent Technologies Fndn Grants, 333
Axe-Houghton Fndn Grants, 678

Blanche and Irving Laurie Fndn Grants, 764
Clarcor Fndn Grants, 1021
Comm Fndn for Greater New Haven Grants, 1091
F.M. Kirby Fndn Grants, 1443
Fndn Northwest Grants, 1537
Grundy Fndn Grants, 1673
High Meadow Fndn Grants, 1768
Kenneth T. and Eileen L. Norris Fndn Grants, 1989
Meyer Memorial Trust Emergency Grants, 2178
Meyer Memorial Trust Grassroots Grants, 2179
Meyer Memorial Trust Operating Funds Grants, 2180
Meyer Memorial Trust Responsive Grants, 2181
Procter and Gamble Fund Grants, 3083
Rich Fndn Grants, 3156
US Trust Corp Fndn Grants, 3475
Walt Disney Company Fndn Grants, 3516

Dropouts
Adaptec Fndn Grants, 232
Coca-Cola Fndn Grants, 1052
Joseph Drown Fndn Grants, 1960
Piedmont Natural Gas Grants, 3048
Wachovia Fndn Grants, 3511

Drug Design
FIC International Cooperative Biodiversity Groups Grants, 1487
NIA Alzheimer's Disease Drug Development Grants, 2396
NIH Impact of HAART on HIV/CNS Disease, 2676

Drug Education
Alcatel-Lucent Technologies Fndn Grants, 333
Comer Fndn Grants, 1072
Dept of Ed Safe and Drug-Free Schools and Communities State Grants, 1230
King Pharmaceuticals Corp Contributions Grants, 2003
NIDA Pilot and Feasibility Studies in Preparation for Drug Abuse Prevention Trials, 2513
NYCT Girls and Young Women Grants, 2924
NYCT Substance Abuse Grants, 2928
OSI Harm Reduction and Drug Use Grants, 2966
OSI-Baltimore Tackling Drug Addiction Grants, 2973

Drug Metabolism
ASPET Bernard B. Brodie Award in Drug Metabolism, 639
NIH Mechanisms Underlying Individual Variations in Drug Responses, 2685

Drug Testing
NIA Alzheimer's Disease Drug Development Grants, 2396
NIA Grants for Alzheimer's Disease Drug Discovery, 2406
NIDDK Development of Assays for High-Throughput Drug Screening Grants, 2548

Drugs/Drug Abuse
AACAP Jeanne Spurlock Research Fellowship in Substance Abuse and Addiction for Minority Medical Students, 40
Adaptec Fndn Grants, 232
African American Fund of New Jersey Grants, 260
Aladdin Industries Fndn Grants, 322
Alliance Healthcare Fndn Grants, 362
amfAR Fellowships, 462
amfAR Global Initiatives Grants, 463
amfAR Mathilde Krim Fellowships in Basic Biomedical Research, 464
amfAR Public Policy Grants, 465
amfAR Research Grants, 466
Andersen Fndn Grants, 471
Assurant Fndn Grants, 654
Audrey and Sydney Irmas Charitable Fndn Grants, 665
Barberton Comm Fndn Grants, 693
Battle Creek Comm Fndn Grants, 703
Benton Comm Fndn Grants, 743
Berks County Comm Fndn Grants, 745
Blackford County Comm Fndn Grants, 763
Blue River Comm Fndn Grants, 770
Bodman Fndn Grants, 776
Brown County Comm Fndn Grants, 807
Cambridge Comm Fndn Grants, 837
Carnahan-Jackson Fndn Grants, 878
Carpenter Fndn Grants, 881
Carrie E. and Lena V. Glenn Fndn Grants, 882
Cass County Comm Fndn Grants, 887
CDC Intervention Epidemiologic Research Studies of HIV/AIDS, 915
CDC Technology Translation and Transfer of Effective HIV Behavioral Interventions, 931
Cleo Fndn Grants, 1035
Colorado Springs Comm Trust Fund Grants, 1061
Comer Fndn Grants, 1072
Comm Fndn for Southern Arizona Grants, 1095
Comm Fndn of Bartholomew County Heritage Fund Grants, 1096
Comm Fndn of Bartholomew County James A. Henderson Award for Fund-Raising, 1097
Comm Fndn of Boone County Grants, 1099
Comm Fndn of Broward Grants, 1100
Comm Fndn of Greater Birmingham Grants, 1106
Comm Fndn of Greater Fort Wayne: Comm Endowment & Clarke Endowment Fund Grants, 1108
ConocoPhillips Fndn Grants, 1144
Constantin Fndn Grants, 1145
Cornerstone Fndn of Northeastern Wisconsin Grants, 1152
D.F. Halton Fndn Grants, 1181
Danellie Fndn Grants, 1198
Daniels Fund Grants, 1200
Delaware Comm Fndn-Youth Philanthropy Board for Kent County, 1216
Dennis and Phyllis Washington Fndn Grants, 1222
Dept of Ed Safe and Drug-Free Schools and Communities State Grants, 1230
DeRoy Testamentary Fndn Grants, 1239
DOJ Mental Health and Juvenile Justice, 1304
DPA Promoting Policy Change Advocacy Grants, 1324
eBay Fndn Comm Grants, 1363
EIF Comm Grants, 1386
Eva L. and Joseph M. Bruening Fndn Grants, 1436
FAR Fund, 1453
Farmers Insurance Group of Companies Grants, 1455
Florida BRAIVE Fund of Dade Comm Fndn, 1512
Florida BRAIVE Fund of Gulf Coast Comm Fndn of Venice, 1513
Florida BRAIVE Fund of The Comm Fndn in Jacksonville, 1514
Fndn for a Healthy Kentucky Grants, 1527
Fourjay Fndn Grants, 1544
Frances and John L. Loeb Family Fund Grants, 1546
GEICO Public Service Awards, 1586
Greater Worcester Comm Fndn Discretionary Grants, 1658
Harry Frank Guggenheim Fndn Research Grants, 1704
Hasbro Children's Fund, 1714
Health Fndn of Greater Cincinnati Grants, 1724
Johnson & Johnson Corp Contributions Grants, 1952
Joseph Drown Fndn Grants, 1960
Joseph H. and Florence A. Roblee Fndn Grants, 1961
Kahuku Comm Fund, 1977
Kalamazoo Fndn Grants, 1979
Kathryne Beynon Fndn Grants, 1984
L. W. Pierce Family Fndn Grants, 2019
Lesbian Health Fund Grants, 2046
Lester Ray Fleming Scholarships, 2048
Lillian S. Wells Fndn Grants, 2056
Lucile Horton Howe and Mitchell B. Howe Fndn Grants, 2081
Margaret L. Wendt Fndn Grants, 2104
Mary Owen Borden Fndn Grants, 2121
MDBD Basic Research Grants, 2152
Moses Cone-Wesley Long Comm Health Fndn Grants, 2219
Newman's Own Inc Grants, 2306
NIAAA Mechanisms of Alcohol and Drug-Induced Pancreatitis Grants, 2444
NIDA Behavioral Science Track Awards for Rapid Transition, 2498
NIDA Behavioral Therapies Development Grants, 2499
NIDA Clinical Research Education Programs in Drug Abuse and Addiction, 2500
NIDA Cutting-Edge Basic Research Awards, 2501
NIDA Drug Abuse Dissertation Research: Epidemiology, Prevention, Treatment, Services, and Women and Gender Differences, 2502
NIDA Drug Addiction Neuroscience Research Grants, 2503
NIDA HIV Drug Therapy for HIV Users: Access, Adherence, Effectiveness, 2504
NIDA International Studies on Drug Abuse and HIV/AIDS, 2505
NIDA Medications Development for Cannabis-Related Disorder, 2506
NIDA Mentored Clinical Scientist Research Career Development Awards, 2507
NIDA Microarray-Based Research on Drug Abuse, 2508
NIDA Minority Institutions Drug Abuse Research Development Program (MIDARP) Grants, 2509
NIDA National Drug Abuse Treatment Clinical Trials Network, 2510
NIDA Origins and Pathways to Drug Abuse Research Grants, 2512
NIDA Pilot and Feasibility Studies in Preparation for Drug Abuse Prevention Trials, 2513
NIDA Role of Limbic System and Brain Ontogeny in Drug Abuse Research Grants, 2514
NIDA Senior Scientist Award, 2515
NIDA Transition from Drug Abuse to Drug Addiction, 2516
NIH Exploratory/Development Grants for Mental Health Intervention Research, 2665
NIH NRSAs for Individual Predoctoral Fellowships, 2700
NIH Research on Sleep and Sleep Disorders, 2713
NIMH Early Identification and Treatment of Mental Disorders in Children and Adolescents Grants, 2756
NIMH HIV/AIDS, Severe Mental Illness, and Homelessness Research Grants, 2757
Northern Trust Company Charitable Trust and Corp Giving Program, 2865
NYCT Substance Abuse Grants, 2928
Oakland Fund for Children and Youth Grants, 2930
Olin Corp Charitable Trust Grants, 2943
Ordean Fndn Grants, 2952
OSI Harm Reduction and Drug Use Grants, 2966
PacifiCorp Fndn for Learning Grants, 2982
Pajaro Valley Comm Health Grants, 2985
Pasadena Fndn Average Grants, 2994
Peter and Elizabeth C. Tower Fndn Comm Grants, 3018
Phoenix Suns Charities Grants, 3030
Puerto Rico Comm Fndn Grants, 3090
Quantum Corp Snap Server Grants, 3095
Questar Corp Contributions Grants, 3097
Rayonier Fndn Grants, 3111
RWJF New Jersey Health Initiatives Grants, 3225
SAMHSA Campus Suicide Prevention Grants, 3244
SAMHSA Conference Grants, 3246
SAMHSA Drug Free Communities Support Grants, 3247
SAMHSA Strategic Prevention Framework State Incentive Grants, 3248
Seabury Fndn Grants, 3274
Sid W. Richardson Fndn Grants, 3284
Southbury Comm Trust Fund, 3350
Stewart Huston Charitable Trust Grants, 3384
Tides Fndn Syringe Access Fund, 3427
Triangle Comm Fndn Shaver-Hitchings Scholarship, 3438
Trull Fndn Grants, 3441

Dwarfism
Human Growth Fndn Small Grants, 1816

Dysautonomia
Dysautonomia Research Grants, 1353

Dyslexia
Good Samaritan Inc Grants, 1637

Early Childhood Education
Express Scripts Fndn Grants, 1441
Fndn for the Carolinas Grants, 1535
Hanna Andersson Children's Fndn Grants, 1691
Harry A. and Margaret D. Towsley Fndn Grants, 1701
McGregor Fund Grants, 2143
Michael and Susan Dell Fndn Grants, 2189
PacifiCorp Fndn for Learning Grants, 2982
Paul G. Allen Family Fndn Grants, 3000
Taproot Fndn Capacity-Building Service Grants, 3417

Earth Sciences
DOE Environmental Remediation Grants, 1297

Eating Disorders
Hilda and Preston Davis Fndn Grants, 1772
NEDA/AED Charron Family Research Grant, 2289
NEDA/AED Joan Wismer Research Grant, 2290
NEDA/AED Tampa Bay Eating Disorders Task Force Award, 2291
NIH Genetics of Neurobehavioral Disorders in Existing Samples Grants, 2670

Ecology
Beirne Carter Fndn Grants, 737
Carnahan-Jackson Fndn Grants, 878
Clarence E. Heller Charitable Fndn Grants, 1022
Coastal Comm Fndn of South Carolina Grants, 1051
NIH Ecology of Infectious Diseases, 2656
NSF Doctoral Dissertation Improvement Grants in the Directorate for Biological Sciences, 2884
Piedmont Natural Gas Grants, 3048
Prospect Burma Scholarships, 3085
Prudential Fndn Grants, 3087

Economic Development
A/H Fndn Grants, 19
Air Products and Chemicals Grants, 319
Alabama Power Fndn Grants, 321
Alcatel-Lucent Technologies Fndn Grants, 333
Allstate Corp Giving Grants, 363
Allstate Corp Hometown Commitment Grants, 364
Amador Comm Fndn Grants, 409
American Jewish World Service Grants, 437
AMI Semiconductors Corp Grants, 468
Arkansas Comm Fndn Arkansas Black Hall of Fame Grants, 532
Bacon Family Fndn Grants, 679
Barberton Comm Fndn Grants, 693
Berks County Comm Fndn Grants, 745
Bodman Fndn Grants, 776
Boeing Company Contributions Grants, 777
Carl and Eloise Pohlad Family Fndn Grants, 867
Carlisle Fndn Grants, 874
Carnegie Corp of New York Grants, 879
CharityWorks Grants, 961
Charles M. and Mary D. Grant Fndn Grants, 971
CIT Corp Giving Grants, 1014
Claude Worthington Benedum Fndn Grants, 1033
Columbus Fndn Robert E. and Genevieve B. Schaefer Fund Grants, 1070
Comerica Charitable Fndn Grants, 1073
Comm Fndn for Southeastern Michigan Grants, 1094
Comm Fndn of Grant County Grants, 1104
Comm Fndn of Greater New Britain Grants, 1111
Comm Fndn of Muncie and Delaware County Grants, 1120
Comm Fndn of Santa Cruz County Grants, 1122
Comm Fndn of Wabash County Grants, 1131
Comm Technology Fndn of California Building Communities Through Technology Grants, 1136
CSRA Comm Fndn Grants, 1168
Dade Comm Fndn Grants, 1185
Daywood Fndn Grants, 1206
Denver Fndn Comm Grants, 1227
Duke Energy Fndn Grants, 1339
eBay Fndn Comm Grants, 1363
El Paso Comm Fndn Grants, 1388
Erie Comm Fndn Grants, 1427
Fayette County Fndn Grants, 1457
Ferree Fndn Grants, 1486
FIC International Cooperative Biodiversity Groups Grants, 1487
Fndn for the Mid-South Grants, 1536
Frances W. Emerson Fndn Grants, 1548
Frist Fndn Grants, 1563
Gheens Fndn Grants, 1610
Greater New Orleans Fndn Grants, 1654
Greater Tacoma Comm Fndn Grants, 1656
Grotto Fndn Project Grants, 1671
Gulf Coast Comm of Venice Fndn Grants, 1677
Harvest Fndn Grants, 1713
Hawaii Comm Fndn West Hawaii Fund Grants, 1718
Helen Bader Fndn Grants, 1738
Holland/Zeeland Comm Fndn Grants, 1786
Hormel Fndn Grants, 1796
Howard and Bush Fndn Grants, 1798
Hudson Webber Fndn Grants, 1813
Humboldt Area Fndn Technical Assistance Program Grants, 1819
Huntington National Bank Comm Affairs Grants, 1824
Hut Fndn Grants, 1827
i2 Fndn Grants, 1829
J.L. Bedsole Fndn Grants, 1876
Jackson County Comm Fndn Unrestricted Grants, 1879
Janirve Fndn Grants, 1905
Jennings County Comm Fndn Grants, 1916
Jewish Women's Fndn of New York Grants, 1924
John Deere Fndn Grants, 1929
Joyce Fndn Grants, 1969
Kalamazoo Fndn Grants, 1979
King Pharmaceuticals Corp Contributions Grants, 2003
Liberty Bank Fndn Grants, 2053
Lincoln Financial Group Fndn Grants, 2058
Long Island Comm Fndn Grants, 2063
Lynde and Harry Bradley Fndn Grants, 2089
Lynde and Harry Bradley Fndn Prizes: Bradley Prizes, 2090
M.J. Murdock Charitable Trust Grants, 2095
Madison County Comm Fndn Grants, 2098
Maine Comm Fndn Grants, 2099
Maxon Charitable Fndn Grants, 2135
Miguel Aleman Fndn Grants, 2197
Minneapolis Fndn Comm Grants, 2206
Morris and Gwendolyn Cafritz Fndn Grants, 2217
Morton K. and Jane Blaustein Fndn Grants, 2218
National City Corp Contributions Grants, 2250
Northeast Utilities Fndn Grants, 2863
Northwest Minnesota Fndn Women's Fund Grants, 2869
NYCT Girls and Young Women Grants, 2924
OSI-Baltimore Special Opportunities Grants, 2972
Owen County Comm Fndn Grants, 2979
Paul Ogle Fndn Grants, 3003
Philadelphia Fndn Organizational Effectiveness Grants, 3029
Piedmont Natural Gas Grants, 3048
Pittsburgh Fndn Comm Fund Grants, 3054
Plough Fndn Grants, 3061
Polaroid Fund Grants, 3065
Prince Charitable Trusts District of Columbia Grants, 3080
Princeton Area Comm Fndn Greater Mercer Grants, 3081
Procter and Gamble Fund Grants, 3083
Progress Energy Fndn Grants, 3084
Public Welfare Fndn Grants, 3089
Puerto Rico Comm Fndn Grants, 3090
Pulaski County Comm Fndn Grants, 3091
Putnam County Comm Fndn Grants, 3093
Rhode Island Fndn Grants, 3154
Richard King Mellon Fndn Grants, 3161
Riley Fndn Grants, 3165
Robert F. Stoico / FIRSTFED Charitable Fndn Grants, 3171
Rockefeller Fndn Grants, 3181
S. Mark Taper Fndn Grants, 3236
San Diego Fndn for Change Grants, 3255
Simpson Fund Grants, 3290
Sisters of Saint Joseph Charitable Fund Grants, 3296
Sonoco Fndn Grants, 3347
Southbury Comm Trust Fund, 3350
Texas Commission on the Arts Arts Respond Project Grants, 3420
Thomas and Dorothy Leavey Fndn Grants, 3422
Union County Comm Fndn Grants, 3461
Vulcan Materials Company Fndn Grants, 3504
W.K. Kellogg Fndn Healthy Kids Grants, 3507
Waitt Family Fndn Grants, 3512
Wal-Mart Fndn Comm Grants, 3513
Westinghouse Charitable Giving Grants, 3530
Wilkins Family Fndn Grants, 3536
Women's Fndn of California Comm Action Fund, 3549
Women's Fndn of California Grants, 3550
YSA Get Ur Good On Grants, 3555
Z. Smith Reynolds Fndn Small Grants, 3557

Economic Justice
Otto Bremer Fndn Grants, 2977

Economic Self-Sufficiency
Abington Fndn Grants, 184
ACF Ethnic Comm Self-Help Grants, 200
ACF Preferred Communities Grants, 201
Adolph Coors Fndn Grants, 238
Atkinson Fndn International Grants, 661
Battle Creek Comm Fndn Grants, 703
Boeing Company Contributions Grants, 777
Citizens Bank Mid-Atlantic Charitable Fndn Grants, 1015
Comm Fndn Silicon Valley Grants, 1133
Emma B. Howe Memorial Fndn Grants, 1415
FCD Child Development Grants, 1458
FCNY Union Square Awards, 1461
Fndn for the Carolinas Grants, 1535
Graco Fndn Grants, 1642
Hearst Fndn and William Randolph Hearst Fndn Grants, 1730
Kahuku Comm Fund, 1977
Key Fndn Grants, 1994
Pinellas County Grants, 3050
Polaroid Fund Grants, 3065
Retirement Research Fndn General Grants, 3150
Robins Fndn Grants, 3175
Samuel S. Johnson Fndn Grants, 3251
Seabury Fndn Grants, 3274
U.S. Department of Education Rehabilitation Research Training Centers, 3448
US Trust Corp Fndn Grants, 3475
Wachovia Fndn Grants, 3511

Economic Stimulus
NIH Recovery Act Limited Competition: Academic Research Enhancement Awards, 2707
NIH Recovery Act Limited Competition: Biomedical Research, Development, and Growth to Spur the Acceleration of New Technologies (BRDG-SPAN) Pilot Grants, 2708
NIH Recovery Act Limited Competition: Small Business Catalyst Awards for Accelerating Innovative Research Grants, 2710
NIH Recovery Act Limited Competition: Supporting New Faculty Recruitment to Enhance Research Resources through Biomedical Research Core Centers Grants, 2711

Economically Disadvantaged
Josephine Goodyear Fndn Grants, 1964
Sisters of Mercy of North Carolina Fndn Grants, 3295
Sisters of St. Joseph Healthcare Fndn Grants, 3297
Stewart Huston Charitable Trust Grants, 3384

Economics
AHFMR Population Health Investigator Awards, 292
Alfred P. Sloan Fndn Research Fellowships, 353
AT&T Fndn Civic and Comm Service Grants, 658
Canada-U.S. Fulbright New Century Scholars Grants, 846
Canada-U.S. Fulbright Senior Specialists Grants, 847
Canadian Friends of Hebrew University Research and Study Grants, 850
Carnegie Corp of New York Grants, 879
Charles G. Koch Charitable Fndn Grants, 965
Deland Fellowships in Health Care and Society, 1214
Dr. Scholl Fndn Grants, 1329
EF Behavioral Sciences Student Fellowships, 1379
ExxonMobil Grants, 1442
Fairfield County Comm Fndn Grants, 1446
Ford Motor Company Fund Grants, 1522
Fulbright Alumni Initiatives Awards Grants, 1566
Fulbright Distinguished Chairs Grants, 1567
Fulbright New Century Scholars Grants, 1570
Fulbright Specialists Grants, 1571
Fulbright Traditional Scholar Program in Europe and Eurasia, 1572
Fulbright Traditional Scholar Program in Sub-Saharan Africa, 1573
Fulbright Traditional Scholar Program in the East Asia/Pacific Region, 1574
Fulbright Traditional Scholar Program in the Near East and North Africa Region, 1575
Fulbright Traditional Scholar Program in the South and Central Asia Region, 1576
Fulbright Traditional Scholar Program in the Western Hemisphere, 1577
George S. and Dolores Dore Eccles Fndn Grants, 1602
James S. McDonnell Fndn Complex Systems Collaborative Activity Awards, 1897
NCI/NIDA Transdisciplinary Tobacco Use Research Centers Grants, 2280
New York Life Fndn Grants, 2304
NFID Advanced Vaccinology Course Travel Grant, 2307
NIA Healthy Aging through Behavioral Economic Analyses of Situations Grants, 2409
NIA Sociobehavorial Data Analysis and Archiving in Aging, 2434
PhRMA Fndn Health Outcomes Post Doctoral Fellowships, 3031
PhRMA Fndn Informatics Post Doctoral Fellowships, 3036
Prospect Burma Scholarships, 3085
Prudential Fndn Grants, 3087
Rajiv Gandhi Fndn Grants, 3104
Rayonier Fndn Grants, 3111
RSC Thomas W. Eadie Medal, 3199
RWJF Investigator Awards in Health Policy Research, 3220
Takemi Program in International Health Research and Advanced Training Fellowships, 3416

Economics Education
3M Fndn Grants, 11
Air Products and Chemicals Grants, 319
Alcoa Fndn Grants, 334
Allstate Corp Giving Grants, 363
Allstate Corp Hometown Commitment Grants, 364
Coca-Cola Fndn Grants, 1052
FMC Fndn Grants, 1518
J.L. Bedsole Fndn Grants, 1876
Procter and Gamble Fund Grants, 3083
Sid W. Richardson Fndn Grants, 3284

Editing
AMA Virtual Mentor Theme Issue Editor Grants, 400

Education
1104 Fndn Grants, 3
1675 Fndn Grants, 4
1976 Fndn Grants, 5
2 Depot Square Ipswich Charitable Fndn Grants, 7
49ers Fndn Grants, 12
A Friend's Fndn Trust Grants, 13
A Fund for Women Grants, 14
AAP Resident Initiative Fund Grants, 167
Aaron & Cecile Goldman Family Fndn Grants, 171
Abbott Fund Comm Vitality Grants, 177
Abbott Fund Global AIDS Care Grants, 178
Abington Fndn Grants, 184
Able To Serve Grants, 185
Abney Fndn Grants, 187
Abramson Family Fndn Grants, 188
ACE Charitable Fndn Grants, 199
ACF Ethnic Comm Self-Help Grants, 200
Achelis and Bodman Fndns Grants, 206
Adams County Fndn Grants - Pennsylvania, 231
Adelaide Breed Bayrd Fndn Grants, 234
Administaff Comm Affairs Grants, 235
Administration on Aging Senior Medicare Patrol Project Grants, 236
Adobe Comm Investment Grants, 237
Advanced Micro Devices Comm Affairs Grants, 239
AEGON Transamerica Fndn Grants, 243
Aetna Fndn Voice Of Conscience Award, 252
AFG Industries Grants, 259
African American Fund of New Jersey Grants, 260
Agnes B. Hunt Trust Grants, 261
Agnes Gund Fndn Grants, 262
Agnes M. Lindsay Trust Grants, 263
Ahn Family Fndn Grants, 304
Air Products and Chemicals Grants, 319
Aladdin Industries Fndn Grants, 322
Alaska Airlines Corp Giving Grants, 323
Alaska Airlines Fndn Grants, 324
Albert and Margaret Alkek Fndn Grants, 326
Albert Pick Jr. Fund Grants, 328
Albertson's Charitable Giving Grants, 330
Albuquerque Comm Fndn Grants, 331
Alcatel-Lucent Technologies Corp Contributions Grants, 332
Alcoa Fndn Grants, 334
Alcon Fndn Grants, 336
Alex Brown and Sons Charitable Fndn Grants, 337
Alexander & Baldwin Fndn Hawaiian and Pacific Island Grants, 338
Alexander & Baldwin Fndn Mainland Grants, 339
Alice Tweed Tuohy Fndn Grants, 357
Allegan County Comm Fndn Grants, 358
Allegheny Technologies Charitable Trust, 359
Allegis Group Fndn Grants, 360
Allen P. and Josephine B. Green Fndn Grants, 361
Altman Fndn Health Care Grants, 372
AMA-MSS Chapter Involvement Grants, 401
AMA-MSS Government Relations Advocacy Fellowship, 403
AMA-MSS Government Relations Internship Programs, 404
AMA-RFS and AMA Fndn Medical Student & Resident/Fellow Elective-Medicine & the Media, 406
AMA-RFS Legislative Awareness Internships, 407
Amador Comm Fndn Grants, 409
Amarillo Area/Harrington Fndns Grants, 410
AMD Corp Contributions Grants, 411
American Electric Power Grants, 434
American Jewish World Service Grants, 437
American Schlafhorst Fndn Grants, 454
Amerisure Insurance Comm Service Grants, 461
Amgen Fndn Grants, 467
Andersen Corp Fndn, 470
Andersen Fndn Grants, 471
Angels Baseball Fndn Grants, 473
Anheuser-Busch Fndn Grants, 474
Ann Arbor Area Comm Fndn Grants, 476
Ann Peppers Fndn Grants, 478
Annenberg Fndn Grants, 479
Annie Sinclair Knudsen Memorial Fund/Kaua'i Comm Grants, 480
Anthony R. Abraham Fndn Grants, 490
AON Fndn Grants, 491
APF Call for Proposals, 505
APF Typical or Troubled School Mental Health Education Grants, 510
AptarGroup Fndn Grants, 522
Aratani Fndn Grants, 523
Arcadia Fndn Grants, 524
ARCO Fndn Education Grants, 526
Arie and Ida Crown Memorial Grants, 528
Arizona Cardinals Grants, 529
Arizona Diamondbacks Charities Grants, 530
Arizona Public Service Corp Giving Grants, 531
Arkansas Comm Fndn Arkansas Black Hall of Fame Grants, 532
Arkansas Comm Fndn Grants, 533
ARS Fndn Grants, 538
Arthritis Fndn of Australia Grants, 541
Arthur and Rochelle Belfer Fndn Grants, 542
ArvinMeritor Grants, 544
ASCO State Affiliate Grants, 547
ASCO Comparative Effectiveness Research Professorship in Breast Cancer, 553
ASCO Translational Research Professorships, 561
ASHA Multicultural Activities Projects Grants, 571
Ashland Corp Contributions Grants, 586
ASM Undergraduate Research Fellowship, 622
Assisi Fndn Grants, 653
Assurant Health Fndn Grants, 655
AT&T Excelerator, 657
AT&T Fndn Civic and Comm Service Grants, 658
Atherton Family Fndn Grants, 659
Athwin Fndn Grants, 660
Atkinson Fndn International Grants, 661
Atlanta Fndn Grants, 662
Aurora Fndn Grants, 667
Austin College Leadership Award, 668
Australian Academy of Science Grants, 670
Autodesk Comm Relations Grants, 671
Axe-Houghton Fndn Grants, 678
Bacon Family Fndn Grants, 679
Balfe Family Fndn Grants, 682
Ball Brothers Fndn General Grants, 683
Bank of America Client Fndn Grants, 690
Baptist Comm Ministries Grants, 691
Barberton Comm Fndn Grants, 693
Barker Fndn Grants, 694
Barker Welfare Fndn Grants, 695
Barra Fndn Comm Fund Grants, 698
Barra Fndn Project Grants, 699
Batchelor Fndn Grants, 701
Baton Rouge Area Fndn Grants, 702
Batts Fndn Grants, 704
BCBSM Fndn Student Award Program, 721
Beazley Fndn Grants, 730
Bechtel Group Fndn Building Positive Comm Relationships Grants, 731
Beckley Area Fndn Grants, 732
Beckman Coulter Comm Relations Grants, 733
Beirne Carter Fndn Grants, 737
Ben B. Cheney Fndn Grants, 741
Benton County Fndn Grants, 744
Berks County Comm Fndn Grants, 745
Bernard and Audre Rapoport Fndn Grants, 746
Bernard F. and Alva B. Gimbel Fndn Grants, 747
Berrien Comm Fndn Grants, 749
Besser Fndn Grants, 752
BHHS Legacy Fndn Grants, 753
BibleLands Grants, 754
Bill and Melinda Gates Fndn Grants, 756
Biogen Corp Giving Grants, 758
Birds Eye Foods Fndn Grants, 759
BJ's Charitable Fndn Grants, 761
Blanche and Irving Laurie Fndn Grants, 764
Blanche and Julian Robertson Family Fndn Grants, 765
Blowitz-Ridgeway Fndn Early Childhood Development Research Award, 766
Blowitz-Ridgeway Fndn Grants, 767
Blue Grass Comm Fndn Grants, 768
Bob and Delores Hope Charitable Fndn Grants, 774
Boettcher Fndn Grants, 778
Booth-Bricker Fund Grants, 780
Boston Globe Fndn Grants, 784

Boston Jewish Comm Women's Fund Grants, 785
Bradley Turner Fndn Grants, 789
Bridgestone/Firestone Trust Fund Grants, 792
Bright Family Fndn Grants, 793
Brinson Fndn Grants, 794
Bristol-Myers Squibb Fndn Health Education Grants, 798
Brook J. Lenfest Fndn Grants, 804
Burden Trust Grants, 810
Burton G. Bettingen Grants, 813
Business Bank of Nevada Comm Grants, 817
Byron W. and Alice L. Lockwood Fndn Grants, 824
C.R. Bard Fndn Grants, 825
Cailloux Fndn Grants, 829
Callaway Fndn Grants, 835
Callaway Golf Company Fndn Grants, 836
Cambridge Comm Fndn Grants, 837
Canada-U.S. Fulbright New Century Scholars Grants, 846
Canada-U.S. Fulbright Senior Specialists Grants, 847
Capital Region Comm Fndn Grants, 862
Cardinal Health Fndn Grants, 864
Cargill Citizenship Fund-Corp Giving Grants, 865
Caring Fndn Grants, 866
Carl and Eloise Pohlad Family Fndn Grants, 867
Carl and Lily Pforzheimer Fndn Grants, 868
Carl B. and Florence E. King Fndn Grants, 869
Carl C. Icahn Fndn Grants, 870
Carl Gellert and Celia Berta Gellert Fndn Grants, 871
Carl W. and Carrie Mae Joslyn Trust Grants, 873
Carnahan-Jackson Fndn Grants, 878
Carolyn Fndn Grants, 880
Carpenter Fndn Grants, 881
Carrie E. and Lena V. Glenn Fndn Grants, 882
Carrier Corp Contributions Grants, 884
Carroll County Comm Fndn Grants, 885
Cass County Comm Fndn Grants, 887
Central Carolina Comm Fndn Comm Impact Grants, 936
Central Okanagan Fndn Grants, 937
Cessna Fndn Grants, 938
CFFVR Opportunity Grants, 952
Champlin Fndns Grants, 960
CharityWorks Grants, 961
Charles Delmar Fndn Grants, 963
Charles H. Dater Fndn Grants, 966
Charles H. Revson Fndn Grants, 969
Charles Lafitte Fndn Grants, 970
Charles M. and Mary D. Grant Fndn Grants, 971
Charlotte County (FL) Comm Fndn Grants, 973
Chase Paymentech Corp Giving Grants, 975
Chazen Fndn Grants, 978
Chesapeake Corp Fndn Grants, 982
Chestnut Hill Charitable Fndn, Inc Grants, 987
Chicago Comm Trust Grants, 989
Chicago Tribune's Corp Contributions Grants, 991
Chiron Fndn Comm Grants, 1004
Christy-Houston Fndn Grants, 1008
Chula Vista Charitable Fndn Grants, 1009
CICF Legacy Fund Comm Fndn Grants, 1010
CIT Corp Giving Grants, 1014
Citizens Bank Mid-Atlantic Charitable Fndn Grants, 1015
Clarcor Fndn Grants, 1021
Clarence E. Heller Charitable Fndn Grants, 1022
Clarian Health Scholarships for LPNs, 1026
Clark County Comm Fndn Grants, 1028
Clark Fndn Grants, 1029
Claude Worthington Benedum Fndn Grants, 1033
Clay Fndn Grants, 1034
CNA Fndn Grants, 1046
CNCS Foster Grandparent Projects Grants, 1048
CNCS Next Generation Grants, 1049
Coastal Bend Comm Fndn Grants, 1050
Coastal Comm Fndn of South Carolina Grants, 1051
Coca-Cola Fndn Grants, 1052
Collins C. Diboll Private Fndn Grants, 1057
Colonel Stanley R. McNeil Fndn Grants, 1059
Columbus Fndn Competitive Grants, 1066
Columbus Fndn Mary Eleanor Morris Fund Grants, 1069
Columbus Fndn Traditional Grants, 1071
Comerica Charitable Fndn Grants, 1073
Commonweal Fndn Grants, 1076
Comm Fndn Alliance City of Evansville Endowment Fund Grants, 1089
Comm Fndn for Greater Buffalo Grants, 1090
Comm Fndn for Greater New Haven Grants, 1091
Comm Fndn for Monterey County Grants, 1092
Comm Fndn for Muskegon County Grants, 1093
Comm Fndn for Southeastern Michigan Grants, 1094
Comm Fndn for Southern Arizona Grants, 1095
Comm Fndn of Broward Grants, 1100
Comm Fndn of Champaign County Grants, 1102
Comm Fndn of Crawford County Grants and Scholarships, 1103
Comm Fndn of Grant County Grants, 1104
Comm Fndn of Greater Birmingham Grants, 1106
Comm Fndn of Greater Flint Grants, 1107
Comm Fndn Of Greater Lafayette Grants, 1110
Comm Fndn of Greater New Britain Grants, 1111
Comm Fndn of Greater Tampa Grants, 1112
Comm Fndn of Greenville Comm Enrichment Grants, 1113
Comm Fndn of Greenville Hollingsworth Funds Program/Project Grants, 1114
Comm Fndn of Greenville-Greenville Women Giving Grants, 1115
Comm Fndn of Howard County Grants, 1116
Comm Fndn of Madison and Jefferson County Grants and Scholarships, 1117
Comm Fndn of Mount Vernon and Knox County Grants, 1119
Comm Fndn of Muncie and Delaware County Grants, 1120
Comm Fndn of Randolph County Grants, 1121
Comm Fndn of Santa Cruz County Grants, 1122
Comm Fndn of South Alabama Grants, 1123
Comm Fndn of South Puget Sound Grants, 1124
Comm Fndn of Southeastern Connecticut Grants, 1125
Comm Fndn of St. Joseph County Special Project Challenge Grants, 1126
Comm Fndn of Switzerland County Grants, 1127
Comm Fndn of Tampa Bay Grants, 1128
Comm Fndn of the Ozarks Grants, 1130
Comm Fndn of Wabash County Grants, 1131
Comm Fndn of Western North Carolina Grants, 1132
ConAgra Foods Fndn Grants, 1140
Connecticut Comm Fndn Grants, 1141
Consumers Energy Fndn, 1147
Cooke Fndn Grants, 1148
Cooper Industries Fndn Grants, 1150
Cornerstone Fndn of Northeastern Wisconsin Grants, 1152
Covenant Fndn Grants, 1153
Cowles Charitable Trust Grants, 1155
Cranston Fndn Grants, 1158
Cruise Industry Charitable Fndn Grants, 1166
CSRA Comm Fndn Grants, 1168
CSX Corp Contributions Grants, 1169
Cudd Fndn Grants, 1171
Cullen Fndn Grants, 1172
Cultural Society of Filipino Americans Grants, 1173
CUNA Mutual Group Fndn, 1174
CVS Caremark Charitable Trust Grants, 1176
CVS Comm Grants, 1177
Cyrus Eaton Fndn Grants, 1178
D.F. Halton Fndn Grants, 1181
D.V. and Ida J. McEachern Charitable Trust Grants, 1182
DAAD Research Stays for University Academics and Scientists, 1183
Dade Comm Fndn Grants, 1185
DaimlerChrysler Corp Fund Grants, 1186
Dairy Queen Corp Contributions Grants, 1187
Dallas Mavericks Fndn Grants, 1190
Dammann Fund Grants, 1192
Dana Corp Fndn Grants, 1196
Dana Fndn Science and Health Grants, 1197
Danellie Fndn Grants, 1198
Daniels Fund Grants, 1200
Daphne Seybolt Culpeper Memorial Fndn Grants, 1201
Davis Family Fndn Grants, 1204
Deaconess Comm Fndn Grants, 1207
Dean Foods Comm Involvement Grants, 1209
Dearborn Comm Fndn City of Lawrenceburg Comm Grants, 1210
Dearborn Comm Fndn County Progress Grants, 1211
Del E. Webb Fndn Grants, 1213
Delaware Comm Fndn Grants, 1215
Delaware Comm Fndn-Youth Philanthropy Board for Kent County, 1216
Dell Fndn Open Grants, 1218
Delta Air Lines Fndn Grants, 1220
DeMatteis Family Fndn Grants, 1221
Denver Broncos Charities Fund Grants, 1226
Denver Fndn Comm Grants, 1227
Dept of Ed Safe and Drug-Free Schools and Communities State Grants, 1230
Dept of Ed Special Education—Personnel Development to Improve Services and Results for Children with Disabilities, 1231
DeRoy Testamentary Fndn Grants, 1239
Detroit Lions Charities Grants, 1241
DHHS Health Centers Grants for Residents of Public Housing, 1254
Dickson Fndn Grants, 1284
DOJ Gang-Free Schools and Communities Intervention Grants, 1303
Dolan Fndn Grants, 1306
Dole Food Company Charitable Contributions, 1307
Dominion Educational Partnership Grant, 1308
Dora Roberts Fndn Grants, 1311
Doris and Victor Day Fndn Grants, 1313
Dorothy Hooper Beattie Fndn Grants, 1321
Dorrance Family Fndn Grants, 1323
Dr. Leon Bromberg Charitable Trust Fund Grants, 1328
Drs. Bruce and Lee Fndn Grants, 1333
Dubois County Comm Fndn Grants, 1336
Duke Energy Fndn Grants, 1339
Duneland Health Council InCorpd Grants, 1350
DuPage Comm Fndn Grants, 1352
Dyson Fndn Mid-Hudson Valley General Operating Support Grants, 1354
E.L. Wiegand Fndn Grants, 1361
Eastman Chemical Company Fndn Grants, 1362
eBay Fndn Comm Grants, 1363
Eberly Fndn Grants, 1364
Eckerd Corp Fndn Grants, 1366
Eddie C. and Sylvia Brown Family Fndn Grants, 1367
Eden Hall Fndn Grants, 1368
Edna G. Kynett Memorial Fndn Grants, 1370
EDS Fndn Grants, 1371
Educational Fndn of America Grants, 1372
Edward Bangs Kelley and Elza Kelley Fndn Grants, 1373
Edward S. Moore Fndn Grants, 1374
Edwin S. Webster Fndn Grants, 1376
Edyth Bush Charitable Fndn Grants, 1378
EIF Comm Grants, 1386
El Paso Comm Fndn Grants, 1388
El Paso Corp Fndn Grants, 1389
El Pomar Fndn Awards and Grants, 1390
Elkhart County Comm Fndn Grants, 1401
Elmer L. and Eleanor J. Andersen Fndn Grants, 1406
Elsie Lee Garthwaite Memorial Fndn Grants, 1408
Emerson Electric Company Contributions Grants, 1413
Emma B. Howe Memorial Fndn Grants, 1415
Ensworth Charitable Fndn Grants, 1416
Entergy Comm Partnership Grants, 1417
Erie Comm Fndn Grants, 1427
Essex County Comm Fndn Discretionary Fund Grant, 1428
Estee Lauder Grants, 1429
Eugene and Agnes E. Meyer Fndn Grants, 1432
Eugene M. Lang Fndn Grants, 1434
Eugene McDermott Fndn Grants, 1435

Evan and Susan Bayh Fndn Grants, 1437
Evanston Comm Fndn Grants, 1438
Ewing Halsell Fndn Grants, 1440
Express Scripts Fndn Grants, 1441
ExxonMobil Grants, 1442
F.M. Kirby Fndn Grants, 1443
Fairfield County Comm Fndn Grants, 1446
FAR Fund, 1453
Fargo-Moorhead Area Fndn Grants, 1454
Farmers Insurance Group of Companies Grants, 1455
Faye McBeath Fndn Grants, 1456
Fayette County Fndn Grants, 1457
FCD Child Development Grants, 1458
Federal Express Corp Contributions Program, 1483
Ferree Fndn Grants, 1486
Fidelity Fndn Grants, 1498
Fifth Third Fndn Grants, 1501
Fireman's Fund Fndn Grants, 1504
FirstEnergy Fndn Comm Grants, 1505
Fishman Family Fndn Grants, 1510
Fishman Family Fndn Grants, 1510
Florida BRAIVE Fund of Dade Comm Fndn, 1512
Florida BRAIVE Fund of Gulf Coast Comm Fndn of Venice, 1513
Florida BRAIVE Fund of The Comm Fndn in Jacksonville, 1514
Floyd A. and Kathleen C. Cailloux Fndn Grants, 1516
Fluor Fndn Grants, 1517
FMC Fndn Grants, 1518
Foellinger Fndn Grants, 1519
Fondren Fndn Grants, 1520
Ford Motor Company Fund Grants, 1522
Forrest C. Lattner Fndn Grants, 1523
Foster Fndn Grants, 1524
Fndn Northwest Grants, 1537
Fourjay Fndn Grants, 1544
Frances and John L. Loeb Family Fund Grants, 1546
Frances W. Emerson Fndn Grants, 1548
Francis T. & Louise T. Nichols Fndn Grants, 1550
Frank E. and Seba B. Payne Fndn Grants, 1551
Frank Stanley Beveridge Fndn Grants, 1553
Franklin County Comm Fndn Grants, 1554
Fraser-Parker Fndn Grants, 1555
Fred Baldwin Memorial Fndn Grants, 1556
Freddie Mac Fndn Grants, 1558
Fremont Area Comm Fndn Grants, 1561
Fritz B. Burns Fndn Grants, 1564
Fuji Film Grants, 1565
Fulbright Alumni Initiatives Awards Grants, 1566
Fulbright Distinguished Chairs Grants, 1567
Fulbright International Education Administrators Seminar Grants, 1569
Fulbright New Century Scholars Grants, 1570
Fulbright Specialists Grants, 1571
Fulbright Traditional Scholar Program in Europe and Eurasia, 1572
Fulbright Traditional Scholar Program in Sub-Saharan Africa, 1573
Fulbright Traditional Scholar Program in the East Asia/Pacific Region, 1574
Fulbright Traditional Scholar Program in the Near East and North Africa Region, 1575
Fulbright Traditional Scholar Program in the South and Central Asia Region, 1576
Fulbright Traditional Scholar Program in the Western Hemisphere, 1577
Fuller E. Callaway Fndn Grants, 1578
G.N. Wilcox Trust Grants, 1581
Gebbie Fndn Grants, 1585
GEICO Public Service Awards, 1586
Genentech Corp Charitable Contributions Grants, 1588
General Mills Fndn Grants, 1590
General Motors Fndn Grants Support Program, 1591
Genesis Fndn Grants, 1593
Genuardi Family Fndn Grants, 1594
George and Ruth Bradford Fndn Grants, 1595
George B. Storer Fndn Grants, 1596
George Family Fndn Grants, 1598
George Frederick Jewett Fndn Grants, 1599
George Kress Fndn Grants, 1601
Georgia Power Fndn Grants, 1603
Georgiana Goddard Eaton Memorial Fund Grants, 1604
Gerber Fndn Grants, 1606
Gertrude and William C. Wardlaw Fund Grants, 1607
Gheens Fndn Grants, 1610
Gibson Fndn Grants, 1612
Gilroy and Lillian P. Roberts Charitable Fndn Grants, 1614
Ginn Fndn Grants, 1616
Giving Sum Annual Grant, 1619
GlaxoSmithKline Corp Grants, 1623
Glazer Family Fndn Grants, 1625
Glendale Comm Fndn Grants, 1626
Global Fund for Children Grants, 1629
Godfrey Fndn Grants, 1631
Golden State Warriors Fndn Grants, 1633
Goodrich Corp Fndn Grants, 1638
Goodyear Tire Grants, 1639
Graco Fndn Grants, 1642
Grand Haven Area Comm Fndn Grants, 1644
Grand Rapids Comm Fndn Grants, 1647
Great-West Life Grants, 1649
Greater Bridgeport Area Fndn Comm Impact Grants, 1650
Greater Cincinnati Fndn Priority and Small Projects/Capacity-Building Grants, 1651
Greater Green Bay Comm Fndn Grants, 1652
Greater Milwaukee Fndn Grants, 1653
Greater New Orleans Fndn Grants, 1654
Greater Saint Louis Comm Fndn Grants, 1655
Greater Tacoma Comm Fndn Grants, 1656
Greater Worcester Comm Fndn Discretionary Grants, 1658
Greater Worcester Comm Fndn Jeppson Memorial Fund for Brookfield Grants, 1659
Green Bay Packers Fndn Grants, 1660
Green Fndn Grants, 1661
Greene County Fndn Grants, 1662
Gregory L. Gibson Charitable Fndn Grants, 1668
Griffin Family Fndn Grants, 1669
Grotto Fndn Project Grants, 1671
Guidant Fndn Grants, 1674
Guitar Center Music Fndn Grants, 1675
Gulf Coast Comm Fndn Grants, 1676
Gulf Coast Comm of Venice Fndn Grants, 1677
H & R Fndn Grants, 1679
H.A. and Mary K. Chapman Charitable Trust Grants, 1681
H.J. Heinz Company Fndn Grants, 1682
Hagedorn Fund Grants, 1685
Hall-Perrine Fndn Grants, 1686
Halliburton Fndn Grants, 1687
Hallmark Corp Fndn Grants, 1688
Hannaford Charitable Fndn Grants, 1692
Harold Alfond Fndn Grants, 1695
Harold and Arlene Schnitzer CARE Fndn Grants, 1697
Harris and Eliza Kempner Fund Grants, 1699
Harry A. and Margaret D. Towsley Fndn Grants, 1701
Harry Bramhall Gilbert Charitable Trust Grants, 1703
Hartford Courant Fndn Grants, 1710
Hartford Fndn Regular Grants, 1711
Harvest Fndn Grants, 1713
Hawaii Comm Fndn West Hawaii Fund Grants, 1718
Hawn Fndn Grants, 1719
Hearst Fndn and William Randolph Hearst Fndn Grants, 1730
Heckscher Fndn for Children Grants, 1732
Hedco Fndn Grants, 1733
Helen Bader Fndn Grants, 1738
Helen K. and Arthur E. Johnson Fndn Grants, 1740
Helena Rubinstein Fndn Grants, 1743
Henrietta Tower Wurts Memorial Fndn Grants, 1745
Henry & Ruth Blaustein Rosenberg Fndn Grants, 1746
Henry County Comm Fndn Grants, 1747
Herman Goldman Fndn Grants, 1753
HHMI Biomedical Research Grants for International Scientists in Canada and Latin America, 1756
HHMI Biomedical Research Grants for International Scientists in the Baltics, Central and Eastern Europe, Russia, and Ukraine, 1757
HHMI Biomedical Research Grants for International Scientists: Infectious Diseases and Parasitology, 1758
Highmark Corp Giving Grants, 1769
Highmark Healthy High 5, 1770
Hilda and Preston Davis Fndn Grants, 1772
Hillman Fndn Grants, 1775
Hillsdale County Comm General Adult Fndn Grants, 1777
Hillsdale Fund Grants, 1778
Hilton Head Island Fndn Grants, 1779
Hilton Hotels Corp Giving Grants, 1780
Hirtzel Memorial Fndn Grants, 1781
Hoblitzelle Fndn Grants, 1783
Hoglund Fndn Grants, 1785
Holland/Zeeland Comm Fndn Grants, 1786
HomeBanc Fndn Grants, 1788
Homer Fndn Grants, 1789
Honda of America Manufacturing Fndn Grants, 1790
Honeywell Fndn Grants, 1791
Horace A. Kimball and S. Ella Kimball Fndn Grants, 1792
Hormel Foods Charitable Trust Grants, 1795
Hormel Fndn Grants, 1796
Howard and Bush Fndn Grants, 1798
Howe Fndn of North Carolina Grants, 1799
Hudson Webber Fndn Grants, 1813
Human Growth Fndn Small Grants, 1816
Huntington Beach Police Officers Fndn Grants, 1821
Huntington Clinical Fndn Grants, 1822
Huntington County Comm Fndn Grants, 1823
Huntington National Bank Comm Affairs Grants, 1824
Hut Fndn Grants, 1827
i2 Fndn Grants, 1829
Idaho Comm Fndn Eastern Region Competitive Grants, 1837
Idaho Power Company Corp Contributions, 1838
Ignacio Martin-Baro Fund for Mental Health and Human Rights Grants, 1839
Impact 100 Grants, 1843
Inasmuch Fndn Grants, 1845
Ireland Family Fndn Grants, 1865
Irvin Stern Fndn Grants, 1866
Irving S. Gilmore Fndn Grants, 1867
Isabel Allende Fndn Esperanza Grants, 1868
Ittleson Fndn Mental Health Grants, 1870
J.E. and L.E. Mabee Fndn Grants, 1875
J.W. Kieckhefer Fndn Grants, 1878
Jackson County Comm Fndn Unrestricted Grants, 1879
Jacob and Hilda Blaustein Fndn Grants, 1881
Jacob and Valeria Langeloth Fndn Grants, 1882
Jacob G. Schmidlapp Trust Grants, 1883
James A. and Faith Knight Fndn Grants, 1884
James Ford Bell Fndn Grants, 1885
James G.K. McClure Educational and Development Fund Grants, 1886
James J. and Angelia M. Harris Fndn Grants, 1890
James M. Cox Fndn of Georgia Grants, 1892
James S. Copley Fndn Grants, 1895
Jane Bradley Pettit Fndn Grants, 1902
Jane's Trust Grants, 1904
Jasper Fndn Jasper County Grants, 1907
Jasper Fndn Newton County Grants, 1908
Jay and Rose Phillips Family Fndn Grants, 1909
Jean and Louis Dreyfus Fndn Grants, 1911
Jeffress Research Grants, 1913
JELD-WEN Fndn Grants, 1914
Jennings County Comm Fndn Grants, 1916
Jessie B. Cox Charitable Trust Grants, 1918
Jessie Ball Dupont Fund Grants, 1919
Jewish Comm Fndn of Greater Los Angeles Grants, 1921
Jewish Women's Fndn of New York Grants, 1924

Jim Moran Fndn Grants, 1925
JM Fndn Grants, 1926
Joe W. and Dorothy Dorsett Brown Fndn Grants, 1927
John Deere Fndn Grants, 1929
John G. Duncan Trust Grants, 1931
John G. Martin Fndn Grants, 1932
John Jewett and Helen Chandler Garland Fndn Grants, 1937
John Lord Knight Fndn Grants, 1938
John P. McGovern Fndn Grants, 1942
John R. Oishei Fndn Grants, 1944
John Stauffer Charitable Trust Grants, 1946
John W. Alden Trust Grants, 1947
John W. and Anna H. Hanes Fndn Grants, 1948
Johns Manville Fund Grants, 1950
Johnson & Johnson Corp Contributions Grants, 1952
Joseph Drown Fndn Grants, 1960
Josephine G. Russell Trust Grants, 1963
Josephine S. Gumbiner Fndn Grants, 1965
Josiah W. and Bessie H. Kline Fndn Grants, 1967
Journal Gazette Fndn Grants, 1968
Joyce Fndn Grants, 1969
Julia Temple Davis Brown Fndn Grants, 1971
K and F Baxter Family Fndn Grants, 1973
Kahuku Comm Fund, 1977
Kalamazoo Fndn Grants, 1979
Kathryne Beynon Fndn Grants, 1984
Kavli Fndn Research Grants, 1985
Kelvin and Eleanor Smith Fndn Grants, 1986
Kenny's Kids Grants, 1990
Kettering Family Fndn Grants, 1991
Kevin P. and Sydney B. Knight Family Fndn Grants, 1993
KeySpan Fndn Grants, 1995
King Pharmaceuticals Corp Contributions Grants, 2003
Knight Family Charitable and Educational Fndn Grants, 2007
Knox County Comm Fndn Grants, 2009
Kosciusko County Comm Fndn Grants, 2015
Kraft Cares US Grants, 2017
LaGrange County Comm Fndn Grants, 2020
Land O'Lakes Fndn Mid-Atlantic Grants, 2027
Lands' End Corp Giving Program, 2030
Laura B. Vogler Fndn Grants, 2032
Lawrence Fndn Grants, 2034
Leahi Fund, 2038
Legacy Fndn Grants, 2040
Leo Goodwin Fndn Grants, 2043
Leonsis Fndn Grants, 2045
Lewis Preston Fund for Girls Education Grants, 2052
Liberty Bank Fndn Grants, 2053
Lincoln Financial Group Fndn Grants, 2058
Long Island Comm Fndn Grants, 2063
Louis Calder Fndn Grants, 2065
Lowell Area Comm Fund Grants, 2068
Lowell Berry Fndn Grants, 2069
Lucile Horton Howe and Mitchell B. Howe Fndn Grants, 2081
Lucy Gooding Charitable Fndn Trust Grants, 2083
Ludwick Family Fndn Grants, 2084
Lynde and Harry Bradley Fndn Grants, 2089
Lynde and Harry Bradley Fndn Prizes: Bradley Prizes, 2090
M.B. and Edna Zale Fndn Grants, 2093
M.E. Raker Fndn Grants, 2094
M.J. Murdock Charitable Trust Grants, 2095
Mabel Y. Hughes Charitable Trust Grants, 2097
Maine Comm Fndn Grants, 2099
Manuel D. and Rhoda Mayerson Fndn Grants, 2100
MAPFRE Fndn for Medicine Grants, 2102
Marcia and Otto Koehler Fndn Grants, 2103
Margaret L. Wendt Fndn Grants, 2104
Marion Park Deaver and Harry Gilbert Deaver Fndn Grants, 2110
Mark and Catherine Winkler Fndn Grants, 2112
Mars Fndn Grants, 2114
Marshall Field's Comm Grants, 2115
Mary Owen Borden Fndn Grants, 2121
Matilda R. Wilson Fund Grants, 2128
Mattel Children's Fndn Grants, 2130
Mattel International Grants, 2131
Max and Victoria Dreyfus Fndn Grants, 2133
Max Bell Fndn Grants, 2134
Maxtor Corp Contributions Grants, 2136
May and Stanley Smith Trust Grants, 2137
May Department Stores Charitable Contribution Grants, 2138
McCarthy Family Fndn Grants, 2141
McCombs Fndn Grants, 2142
McGregor Fund Grants, 2143
McInerny Fndn Grants, 2144
McKesson Fndn Grants, 2145
McLean Contributionship Grants, 2147
McMillen Fndn Grants, 2148
McMurry Fndn Grants, 2149
Mead Johnson Nutritionals Evansville-Area Organizations Grants, 2157
Mead Johnson Nutritionals Medical Education Grants, 2158
Mead Witter Fndn Grants, 2160
Meadows Fndn Grants, 2161
Medtronic Fndn Full Life Patient Partnership Program—Heart Rescue Grants, 2168
Mericos Fndn Grants, 2172
Meyer Memorial Trust Emergency Grants, 2178
Meyer Memorial Trust Grassroots Grants, 2179
Meyer Memorial Trust Operating Funds Grants, 2180
Meyer Memorial Trust Responsive Grants, 2181
Miami County Comm Fndn Operation Round Up Grants, 2188
Michael and Susan Dell Fndn Grants, 2189
Middlesex Savings Charitable Fndn Grants, 2196
Miguel Aleman Fndn Grants, 2197
Milagro Fndn Grants, 2198
Miriam and Peter Haas Fund Grants, 2208
Monfort Family Fndn Grants, 2213
Morris and Gwendolyn Cafritz Fndn Grants, 2217
Morton K. and Jane Blaustein Fndn Grants, 2218
Mount Zion Health Fund Grants, 2220
National City Corp Contributions Grants, 2250
Nelda C. and H.J. Lutcher Stark Fndn Grants, 2301
New York University Steinhardt School of Education Fellowships, 2305
Newman's Own Inc Grants, 2306
NIH Academic Career Awards, 2634
NIH School-based Interventions to Prevent Obesity, 2725
NIH Undergraduate Scholarships, 2737
NIMH Short Courses in Neuroinformatics, 2769
Nina Mason Pulliam Charitable Trust Grants, 2776
Noble County Comm Fndn Grants, 2848
Nordson Corp Fndn Grants, 2851
North Carolina Comm Fndn Grants, 2859
North Carolina GlaxoSmithKline Fndn Grants, 2860
North Central Health Services Grants, 2861
North Georgia Comm Fndn Grants, 2862
Northeast Utilities Fndn Grants, 2863
Northern New York Comm Fndn Grants, 2864
Northern Trust Company Charitable Trust and Corp Giving Program, 2865
Northrop Grumman Newport News Grants, 2867
Northwest Minnesota Fndn Women's Fund Grants, 2869
Northwestern Mutual Fndn Grants, 2870
Northwood University/Alden B. Dow Creativity Center Summer Residency Program, 2871
Norwin S. and Elizabeth N. Bean Fndn Grants, 2872
NYCT AIDS/HIV Grants, 2919
NYCT Girls and Young Women Grants, 2924
NYCT Substance Abuse Grants, 2928
OceanFirst Fndn Grants, 2933
Oceanside Charitable Fndn Grants, 2934
Office Depot Corp Comm Grants, 2935
Office Depot Fndn Grants, 2936
Ohio County Comm Fndn Grants, 2938
Ohio County Comm Fndn Mini-Grants, 2939
Ohio Learning Network Grants, 2940
Oleonda Jameson Trust Grants, 2941
OneStar Fndn AmeriCorps Grants, 2945
Ordean Fndn Grants, 2952
OSI European Commission Internships for Young Roma Graduates, 2965
OSI-Baltimore Special Opportunities Grants, 2972
OSI-Baltimore Tackling Drug Addiction Grants, 2973
Owen County Comm Fndn Grants, 2979
PacifiCorp Fndn for Learning Grants, 2982
Palm Beach and Martin Counties Grants, 2986
Paul and Mary Haas Fndn Contributions and Student Scholarships, 2997
Paul G. Allen Family Fndn Grants, 3000
Paul G. Duke Fndn Grants, 3001
Paul Ogle Fndn Grants, 3003
Peabody Fndn Grants, 3010
Peacock Fndn Grants, 3011
Perkins Charitable Fndn Grants, 3014
Perpetual Trust for Charitable Giving Grants, 3015
Perry County Comm Fndn Grants, 3016
Pew Charitable Trusts Children & Youth Grants, 3020
Pfizer Fndn Grants, 3025
Philadelphia Fndn Organizational Effectiveness Grants, 3029
Piedmont Natural Gas Grants, 3048
Pike County Comm Fndn Grants, 3049
Pinellas County Grants, 3050
Pioneer Hi-Bred Comm Grants, 3051
Pittsburgh Fndn Comm Fund Grants, 3054
Plough Fndn Grants, 3061
PMI Fndn Grants, 3063
PNC Charitable Trust and Fndn Grants, 3064
Polk Bros. Fndn Grants, 3066
Portland General Electric Fndn Grants, 3067
Posey Comm Fndn Grants, 3068
Powell Fndn Grants, 3073
Presbyterian Health Fndn Bridge, Seed and Equipment Grants, 3075
Priddy Fndn Grants, 3077
Pride Fndn Grants and Scholarships, 3078
Prince Charitable Trusts Chicago Grants, 3079
Princeton Area Comm Fndn Greater Mercer Grants, 3081
Principal Financial Group Fndn Grants, 3082
Progress Energy Fndn Grants, 3084
Prospect Burma Scholarships, 3085
Prudential Fndn Grants, 3087
Puerto Rico Comm Fndn Grants, 3090
Pulaski County Comm Fndn Grants, 3091
Putnam County Comm Fndn Grants, 3093
Quantum Fndn Grants, 3096
Questar Corp Contributions Grants, 3097
R.C. Baker Fndn Grants, 3098
Rajiv Gandhi Fndn Grants, 3104
Ralphs Food 4 Less Fndn Grants, 3106
Rasmuson Fndn Grants, 3108
Rathmann Family Fndn Grants, 3109
Raymond John Wean Fndn Grants, 3110
Rayonier Fndn Grants, 3111
Regenstrief General Internal Medicine - General Pediatrics Research Fellowship Program, 3144
Rehabilitation Nursing Fndn Research Grants, 3147
Retirement Research Fndn General Grants, 3150
RGK Fndn Grants, 3153
Rhode Island Fndn Grants, 3154
Richard and Helen DeVos Fndn Grants, 3157
Richard and Rhoda Goldman Fund Grants, 3158
Richard and Susan Smith Family Fndn Grants, 3159
Richard King Mellon Fndn Grants, 3161
Riley Fndn Grants, 3165
Ripley County Comm Fndn Grants, 3166
Robert and Joan Dircks Fndn Grants, 3167
Robert F. Stoico / FIRSTFED Charitable Fndn Grants, 3171
Robin Hood Fndn Grants, 3174
Robins Fndn Grants, 3175
Rochester Area Comm Fndn Grants, 3176
Rochester Area Fndn Grants, 3177
Rockefeller Brothers Fund Peace and Security Grants, 3179

Rockefeller Brothers Fund Pivotal Places Grants: South Africa, 3180
Rockwell Collins Charitable Contributions, 3182
Rockwell International Corp Trust Grants, 3183
Rohm and Haas Company Grants, 3185
Rollin M. Gerstacker Fndn Grants, 3186
Rosalynn Carter Institute John and Betty Pope Fellowships, 3189
Rosalynn Carter Institute Mattie J. T. Stepanek Caregiving Scholarships, 3190
Roy and Christine Sturgis Trust Grants, 3191
Roy J. Carver Charitable Trust Medical and Science Research Grants, 3192
RRF General Grants, 3193
RSC McNeil Medal for the Public Awareness of Science, 3198
Rush County Comm Fndn Grants, 3200
Ruth H. and Warren A. Ellsworth Fndn Grants, 3203
RWJF Jobs to Careers: Promoting Work-Based Learning for Quality Care - Research Grants, 3221
S. Livingston Mather Charitable Trust Grants, 3235
S. Livingston Mather Charitable Trust Grants, 3235
S. Mark Taper Fndn Grants, 3236
S.H. Cowell Fndn Grants, 3237
Salem Fndn Charitable Trust Grants, 3241
Salisbury Comm Fndn Grants, 3243
Samuel Freeman Charitable Trust Grants, 3249
Samuel S. Johnson Fndn Grants, 3251
San Diego Fndn for Change Grants, 3255
San Diego Women's Fndn Grants, 3259
San Francisco Fndn Comm Health Grants, 3260
Sarah Scaife Fndn Grants, 3263
Sasco Fndn Grants, 3265
Schurz Communications Fndn Grants, 3271
Scott County Comm Fndn Grants, 3273
Seabury Fndn Grants, 3274
Seattle Fndn Grants, 3276
Self Fndn Grants, 3277
Seneca Foods Fndn Grants, 3278
Shell Oil Company Fndn Grants, 3281
Siebert Lutheran Fndn Grants, 3285
Simmons Fndn Grants, 3287
Simpson Fund Grants, 3290
Sir Dorabji Tata Trust Grants for NGOs or Voluntary Organizations, 3291
Sir Halley Stewart Trust Grants, 3293
Sisters of Mercy of North Carolina Fndn Grants, 3295
Snee Reinhardt Charitable Fndn Grants, 3300
SNM PDEF Mickey Williams Minority Student Scholarships, 3302
SNMTS Clinical Advancement Scholarships, 3309
SNMTS Paul Cole Scholarships, 3312
SOCFOC Reducing Health & Educational Disparities in the Central Neighborhood Grants, 3318
Sosland Fndn Grants, 3348
South Madison Comm Fndn Grants, 3349
Southbury Comm Trust Fund, 3350
Southwest Florida Comm Fndn Competitive Grants, 3351
Southwest Gas Corp Fndn Grants, 3352
Southwire Company Grants, 3353
Special People in Need Grants, 3356
Spencer County Comm Fndn Grants, 3358
Sprague Fndn Grants, 3359
Springs Close Fndn Grants, 3360
Square D Fndn Grants, 3361
St. Joseph Comm Health Fndn Burn Care and Prevention Grants, 3367
St. Joseph Comm Health Fndn Improving Healthcare Access Grants, 3368
Stark Comm Fndn Women's Fund Grants, 3376
Steelcase Fndn Grants, 3379
Steele-Reese Fndn Grants, 3380
Steuben County Comm Fndn Grants, 3383
Stewart Huston Charitable Trust Grants, 3384
Strowd Roses Grants, 3388
Sulzberger Fndn Grants, 3399
Support Our Aging Religious Grants, 3406
Susan Mott Webb Charitable Trust Grants, 3412
Susan Vaughan Fndn Grants, 3413
Taproot Fndn Capacity-Building Service Grants, 3417
Tellabs Fndn Grants, 3418
Texas Commission on the Arts Arts Respond Project Grants, 3420
Thomas C. Ackerman Fndn Grants, 3423
Thompson Charitable Fndn Grants, 3425
Tifa Fndn Grants, 3428
Toro Fndn Grants, 3431
Triangle Comm Fndn Donor-Advised Grants, 3437
Triangle Comm Fndn Shaver-Hitchings Scholarship, 3438
Trull Fndn Grants, 3441
TWS Fndn Grants, 3443
U.S. Department of Education Erma Byrd Scholarships, 3446
U.S. Department of Education Rehabilitation Training—Rehabilitation Continuing Education Programs—Institute on Rehabilitation Issues, 3449
Union Benevolent Association Grants, 3460
United Technologies Corp Grants, 3466
Unity Fndn Of LaPorte County Grants, 3467
US Airways Comm Fndn Grants, 3473
Vancouver Fndn Grants and Comm Initiatives Program, 3477
Vanderburgh Comm Fndn Grants, 3480
VDH Emergency Medical Services Training Fund, 3483
Verizon Fndn Maryland Grants, 3487
Verizon Fndn New York Grants, 3488
Verizon Fndn Northeast Region Grants, 3489
Verizon Fndn Pennsylvania Grants, 3490
Verizon Fndn Vermont Grants, 3491
Verizon Fndn Virginia Grants, 3492
Vermont Comm Fndn Grants, 3493
Virginia W. Kettering Fndn Grants, 3502
Vulcan Materials Company Fndn Grants, 3504
W. C. Griffith Fndn Grants, 3505
W. Clarke Swanson, Jr. Fndn Grants, 3506
W.K. Kellogg Fndn Secure Families Grants, 3508
Wabash Valley Comm Fndn Grants, 3510
Wachovia Fndn Grants, 3511
Wal-Mart Fndn Comm Grants, 3513
Wal-Mart State Giving Grants, 3514
Wallace H. Coulter Fndn Grants, 3515
Warrick County Comm Fndn Grants, 3519
Washington Post Contributions Grants, 3520
Wayne and Gladys Valley Fndn Grants, 3522
Weatherwax Fndn Grants, 3523
Wells County Fndn Grants, 3527
Western Indiana Comm Fndn Grants, 3528
Western Union Fndn Grants, 3529
Westinghouse Charitable Giving Grants, 3530
WHO Fndn General Grants, 3534
Wilkins Family Fndn Grants, 3536
William G. McGowan Charitable Fund Grants, 3539
William H. Hannon Fndn Grants, 3540
Wilson-Wood Fndn Grants, 3542
Winifred & Harry B. Allen Fndn Grants, 3543
Winston-Salem Fndn Competitive Grants, 3544
Winston-Salem Fndn Elkin/Tri-County Grants, 3545
Winston-Salem Fndn Stokes County Grants, 3546
Women's Fndn of California Grants, 3550
Woodward Fund Grants, 3552
YSA Get Ur Good On Grants, 3555
Z. Smith Reynolds Fndn Small Grants, 3557

Education and Work

Brook J. Lenfest Fndn Grants, 804
SNMTS Outstanding Educator Awards, 3310
Vectren Fndn Grants, 3485

Education Reform

Anheuser-Busch Fndn Grants, 474
Bernard F. and Alva B. Gimbel Fndn Grants, 747
Bodman Fndn Grants, 776
Boeing Company Contributions Grants, 777
Carnegie Corp of New York Grants, 879
ExxonMobil Grants, 1442
Frances and John L. Loeb Family Fund Grants, 1546
J.C. Penney Company Grants, 1874
Joseph Drown Fndn Grants, 1960
Joseph H. and Florence A. Roblee Fndn Grants, 1961
Joyce Fndn Grants, 1969
K and F Baxter Family Fndn Grants, 1973
Minneapolis Fndn Comm Grants, 2206
Portland General Electric Fndn Grants, 3067
Prince Charitable Trusts Chicago Grants, 3079

Educational Administration

CFPC Fellowships, 955
Meadows Fndn Grants, 2161
Progress Energy Fndn Grants, 3084

Educational Evaluation/Assessment

A.O. Smith Comm Grants, 18
RCPSC Royal College Fellowship for Studies in Medical Education, 3127

Educational Finance

Allstate Corp Giving Grants, 363
Allstate Corp Hometown Commitment Grants, 364

Educational Instruction Programs

ASM International Fellowship for Latin America and the Caribbean, 601
ASM International Fellowships for Asia and Africa, 602
AT&T Excelerator, 657
Bayer Clinical Scholarship Award, 706
BCBSM Fndn Student Award Program, 721
Carroll County Comm Fndn Grants, 885
Charles H. Dater Fndn Grants, 966
Independence Blue Cross Nursing Internships, 1848
San Diego Women's Fndn Grants, 3259
VDH Rescue Squad Assistance Fund Grants, 3484
Warrick County Comm Fndn Grants, 3519

Educational Planning/Policy

Achelis and Bodman Fndns Grants, 206
Bristol-Myers Squibb Fndn Health Education Grants, 798
Charles G. Koch Charitable Fndn Grants, 965
K and F Baxter Family Fndn Grants, 1973

Educational Programs

Allstate Corp Giving Grants, 363
Allstate Corp Hometown Commitment Grants, 364
Blowitz-Ridgeway Fndn Early Childhood Development Research Award, 766
Comm Fndn of Morgan County Grants and Scholarships, 1118
Schering-Plough Fndn Health Grants, 3270

Educational Psychology

Helen McWilliam Memorial Scholarship, 1741
Ittleson Fndn Mental Health Grants, 1870
RCPSC Royal College Fellowship for Studies in Medical Education, 3127

Educational Technology

Alcatel-Lucent Technologies Fndn Grants, 333
AT&T Excelerator, 657
Bill and Melinda Gates Fndn Grants, 756
Brook J. Lenfest Fndn Grants, 804
Dept of Ed Special Education-National Activities-Technology and Media Services for Individuals with Disabilities, 1234
DOA Distance Learning and Telemedicine Grant Program, 1288
Green Fndn Grants, 1661
Hilda and Preston Davis Fndn Grants, 1772
Jessie Ball Dupont Fund Grants, 1919
Leonsis Fndn Grants, 2045
RCPSC Royal College Fellowship for Studies in Medical Education, 3127

Educational Testing/Measurement

NBME Stemmler Medical Education Research Fund Grants, 2263

Educational/Public Television
Air Products and Chemicals Grants, 319
Andersen Fndn Grants, 471
ConocoPhillips Fndn Grants, 1144
Farmers Insurance Group of Companies Grants, 1455
John Ben Snow Memorial Trust Grants, 1928

Egypt
Fulbright Traditional Scholar Program in the Near East and North Africa Region, 1575

Elder Abuse
Administration on Aging Senior Medicare Patrol Project Grants, 236
Peacock Fndn Grants, 3011
Reynolds and Reynolds Associate Fndn Grants, 3152

Elderly
Administration on Aging Senior Medicare Patrol Project Grants, 236
Agnes M. Lindsay Trust Grants, 263
Aladdin Industries Fndn Grants, 322
Allen P. and Josephine B. Green Fndn Grants, 361
American Schlafhorst Fndn Grants, 454
AMI Semiconductors Corp Grants, 468
Ann Arbor Area Comm Fndn Grants, 476
Ann Peppers Fndn Grants, 478
Anschutz Family Fndn Grants, 486
Arkell Hall Fndn Grants, 534
Arthur and Rochelle Belfer Fndn Grants, 542
Atkinson Fndn International Grants, 661
Avon Products Fndn Grants, 675
Bailey Fndn Grants, 680
Barberton Comm Fndn Grants, 693
BCBSM Claude Pepper Award, 714
BCBSM Corp Contributions Grants, 716
BCBSNC Fndn Grants, 725
Ben B. Cheney Fndn Grants, 741
Bender Fndn Grants, 742
Berrien Comm Fndn Grants, 749
Bertha Russ Lytel Fndn Grants, 751
Birmingham Fndn Grants, 760
Blanche and Irving Laurie Fndn Grants, 764
Boston Fndn Grants, 783
Brookdale Fndn National Group Respite and Early Memory Loss Grants, 806
Burden Trust Grants, 810
Bushrod H. Campbell and Adah F. Hall Charity Fund Grants, 816
Caleb C. and Julia W. Dula Educational and Charitable Fndn Grants, 830
California Endowment CommunitiesFirst Grants, 833
Callaway Fndn Grants, 835
Callaway Golf Company Fndn Grants, 836
Cambridge Comm Fndn Grants, 837
Carl W. and Carrie Mae Joslyn Trust Grants, 873
Carrie E. and Lena V. Glenn Fndn Grants, 882
Carrie Estelle Doheny Fndn Grants, 883
Carroll County Comm Fndn Grants, 885
Catherine Kennedy Home Fndn Grants, 890
CFPC Research and Education Fndn Grants, 956
Charles H. Farnsworth Trust Grants, 967
Chatlos Fndn Grants, 977
CNA Fndn Grants, 1046
Columbus Fndn Allen Eiry Fund Grants, 1064
Columbus Fndn J. Floyd Dixon Memorial Fund Grants, 1068
Commonwealth Fund Harkness Fellowships in Health Care Policy and Practice, 1079
Commonwealth Fund Quality of Care for Frail Elders Grants, 1083
Comm Fndn of Grant County Grants, 1104
Comm Fndn of Madison and Jefferson County Grants and Scholarships, 1117
Comm Fndn of Santa Cruz County Grants, 1122
Comm Fndn of the Ozarks Grants, 1130
Comprehensive Health Education Fndn Grants, 1139
Cooke Fndn Grants, 1148
Daisy Marquis Jones Fndn Grants, 1188
Danellie Fndn Grants, 1198
Daniels Fund Grants, 1200
Dennis and Phyllis Washington Fndn Grants, 1222
Dr. Scholl Fndn Grants, 1329
Edwin W. and Catherine M. Davis Fndn Grants, 1377
Eisner Fndn Grants, 1387
Elisabeth Severance Prentiss Fndn Grants, 1392
Eva L. and Joseph M. Bruening Fndn Grants, 1436
Fan Fox and Leslie R. Samuels Fndn Grants, 1451
Fannie E. Rippel Fndn Grants, 1452
Faye McBeath Fndn Grants, 1456
Fireman's Fund Fndn Grants, 1504
Foellinger Fndn Grants, 1519
Fndn for the Carolinas Grants, 1535
Fourjay Fndn Grants, 1544
Frances and John L. Loeb Family Fund Grants, 1546
G.N. Wilcox Trust Grants, 1581
Grundy Fndn Grants, 1673
Gulf Coast Comm of Venice Fndn Grants, 1677
Hackett Fndn Grants, 1684
Hagedorn Fund Grants, 1685
Harden Fndn Grants, 1693
Harry Kramer Memorial Fund Grants, 1705
Health Canada National Seniors Independence Grants, 1722
Health Fndn of Greater Indianapolis Grants, 1725
Hearst Fndn and William Randolph Hearst Fndn Grants, 1730
Helen Steiner Rice Fndn Grants, 1742
Henry County Comm Fndn Grants, 1747
Hilda and Preston Davis Fndn Grants, 1772
Hill Crest Fndn Grants, 1773
Hill Fndn Grants, 1774
Hoglund Fndn Grants, 1785
Holland/Zeeland Comm Fndn Grants, 1786
Hugh J. Andersen Fndn Grants, 1814
J. Walton Bissell Fndn Grants, 1872
Jacob G. Schmidlapp Trust Grants, 1883
Jane Bradley Pettit Fndn Grants, 1902
Janirve Fndn Grants, 1905
Jay and Rose Phillips Family Fndn Grants, 1909
Jean and Louis Dreyfus Fndn Grants, 1911
Jewish Fund Grants, 1923
John Edward Fowler Memorial Fndn Grants, 1930
John G. Martin Fndn Grants, 1932
John H. Wellons Fndn Grants, 1934
John W. Anderson Fndn Grants, 1949
Kaiser Permanente Cares for Communities Grants, 1978
Katharine Matthies Fndn Grants, 1982
Kimberly-Clark Comm Grants, 2001
Laura B. Vogler Fndn Grants, 2032
Legacy Fndn Grants, 2040
Lettie Pate Whitehead Fndn Grants, 2049
Long Island Comm Fndn Grants, 2063
Lowell Berry Fndn Grants, 2069
Mary Black Fndn Grants, 2118
Maxtor Corp Contributions Grants, 2136
May and Stanley Smith Trust Grants, 2137
Medtronic Fndn Health Care Grants, 2169
Mericos Fndn Grants, 2172
Metro Health Fndn Grants, 2175
Metrowest Comm Health Care Fndn Grants, 2176
Military Ex-Prisoners of War Fndn Grants, 2201
NCI Stages of Breast Development: Normal to Metastatic Disease Grants, 2278
Newman's Own Inc Grants, 2306
NIAMS Exploratory Developmental Grants for Multidisciplinary Clinical Studies of Sarcopenia, 2469
NIH Mechanisms Underlying Individual Variations in Drug Responses, 2685
NIH National Occupational Research Agenda Grants, 2696
NIH Roybal Centers for Translational Research on Aging, 2717
NIMH Interventions Infrastructure Program Research Grants, 2760
Nina Mason Pulliam Charitable Trust Grants, 2776
Nuffield Fndn Africa Grants, 2898
Nuffield Fndn Law and Society Grants, 2900
Nuffield Fndn Open Door Grants, 2902
Nuffield Fndn Small Grants, 2903
OUT Fund for Lesbian and Gay Liberation Grants, 2978
PacifiCare Fndn Grants, 2981
PacifiCorp Fndn for Learning Grants, 2982
Pasadena Fndn Average Grants, 2994
Paul and Mary Haas Fndn Contributions and Student Scholarships, 2997
Paul Balint Charitable Trust Grants, 2998
Piedmont Natural Gas Grants, 3048
Pinellas County Grants, 3050
Plum Creek Fndn Grants, 3062
Powell Fndn Grants, 3073
Prudential Fndn Grants, 3087
Public Welfare Fndn Grants, 3089
Puerto Rico Comm Fndn Grants, 3090
Quantum Fndn Grants, 3096
R.C. Baker Fndn Grants, 3098
Retirement Research Fndn General Grants, 3150
Reynolds and Reynolds Associate Fndn Grants, 3152
Richard and Rhoda Goldman Fund Grants, 3158
Robert P. & Clara I. Milton Fund for Senior Housing, 3172
Rochester Area Comm Fndn Grants, 3176
Rollin M. Gerstacker Fndn Grants, 3186
Rosalynn Carter Institute John and Betty Pope Fellowships, 3189
RRF General Grants, 3193
RRF Organizational Capacity Building Grants, 3194
Salisbury Comm Fndn Grants, 3243
Sid W. Richardson Fndn Grants, 3284
Sir Halley Stewart Trust Grants, 3293
Sisters of Mercy of North Carolina Fndn Grants, 3295
Sisters of Saint Joseph Charitable Fund Grants, 3296
Southwest Gas Corp Fndn Grants, 3352
Stewart Huston Charitable Trust Grants, 3384
STTI Environment of Elder Care Nursing Research Grants, 3391
Support Our Aging Religious Grants, 3406
Taproot Fndn Capacity-Building Service Grants, 3417
Thelma Doelger Charitable Trust Grants, 3421
Topfer Family Fndn Grants, 3430
Trull Fndn Grants, 3441
Union Benevolent Association Grants, 3460
Westinghouse Charitable Giving Grants, 3530
William H. Hannon Fndn Grants, 3540
Winston-Salem Fndn Competitive Grants, 3544

Electoral Systems
Baptist Comm Ministries Grants, 691
Carnegie Corp of New York Grants, 879

Electric Power
DOL Occupational Safety and Health—Susan Harwood Training Grants, 1305

Electronics/Electrical Engineering
NSF-NIST Interaction in Chemistry, Materials Research, Molecular Biosciences, Bioengineering, and Chemical Engineering, 2897

Electrophysiology
Cardiac Arrhythmias Research and Education Fndn Research Grants, 863
Duke University Clinical Cardiac Electrophysiology Fellowships, 1342
Heart Rhythm Society Fellowships, 1731
Mayo Fndn Multidisciplinary Training in Digestive Diseases Research Grants, 2140
NIGMS Molecular Pharmacology of Anesthetic Action Research Grants, 2621

Elementary Education
3M Fndn Grants, 11
A.O. Smith Comm Grants, 18
AEC Trust Grants, 242
Affymetrix Corp Contributions Grants, 258
Ahmanson Fndn Grants, 303
Alabama Power Fndn Grants, 321

Alcatel-Lucent Technologies Fndn Grants, 333
AMD Corp Contributions Grants, 411
American Electric Power Grants, 434
Andersen Fndn Grants, 471
Archer Daniels Midland Fndn Grants, 525
Arkema Fndn Science Teachers Program, 535
Armstrong McDonald Fndn Grants, 537
Ball Brothers Fndn Grants, 684
Benton County Fndn Grants, 744
Bernard and Audre Rapoport Fndn Grants, 746
Berrien Comm Fndn Grants, 749
Bertha Russ Lytel Fndn Grants, 751
Bill and Melinda Gates Fndn Grants, 756
Boeing Company Contributions Grants, 777
Booth-Bricker Fund Grants, 780
Boston Fndn Grants, 783
Bristol-Myers Squibb Fndn Health Education Grants, 798
Burlington Industries Fndn Grants, 811
Callaway Fndn Grants, 835
Carnegie Corp of New York Grants, 879
Carrie E. and Lena V. Glenn Fndn Grants, 882
Carrie Estelle Doheny Fndn Grants, 883
Carroll County Comm Fndn Grants, 885
Cass County Comm Fndn Grants, 887
CDC School Health Programs to Prevent the Spread of HIV Cooperative Agreements, 928
Charles Lafitte Fndn Grants, 970
Chesapeake Corp Fndn Grants, 982
Chicago Comm Trust Grants, 989
Cinergy Fndn Grants, 1013
Clarence E. Heller Charitable Fndn Grants, 1022
Coca-Cola Fndn Grants, 1052
Colorado Interstate Gas Grants, 1060
Colorado Springs Comm Trust Fund Grants, 1061
Columbus Fndn J. Floyd Dixon Memorial Fund Grants, 1068
Commonweal Fndn Comm Assistance Grants, 1075
Commonweal Fndn Grants, 1076
Comm Fndn for Greater Buffalo Grants, 1090
Comm Fndn of Central Illinois Grants, 1101
Comm Fndn Silicon Valley Grants, 1133
Connelly Fndn Grants, 1143
Cullen Fndn Grants, 1172
CVS All Kids Can Grants, 1175
CVS Comm Grants, 1177
DaimlerChrysler Corp Fund Grants, 1186
Daniels Fund Grants, 1200
Dean Foods Comm Involvement Grants, 1209
Dennis and Phyllis Washington Fndn Grants, 1222
Dominion Educational Partnership Grant, 1308
Dr. Scholl Fndn Grants, 1329
Duke Energy Fndn Grants, 1339
Dunspaugh-Dalton Fndn Grants, 1351
Effie and Wofford Cain Fndn Grants, 1385
Eisner Fndn Grants, 1387
Elizabeth McGraw Fndn Grants, 1399
Entergy Comm Partnership Grants, 1417
Eugene McDermott Fndn Grants, 1435
Ferree Fndn Grants, 1486
Field Fndn of Illinois Grants, 1499
Fisher Fndn Grants, 1508
Floyd A. and Kathleen C. Cailloux Fndn Grants, 1516
Frances and John L. Loeb Family Fund Grants, 1546
Frances L. and Edwin L. Cummings Memorial Fund Grants, 1547
Francis T. & Louise T. Nichols Fndn Grants, 1550
GenCorp Fndn Grants, 1587
General Mills Fndn Grants, 1590
George F. Baker Trust Grants, 1597
George Frederick Jewett Fndn Grants, 1599
Goodrich Corp Fndn Grants, 1638
Halliburton Fndn Grants, 1687
Harold Alfond Fndn Grants, 1695
Hedco Fndn Grants, 1733
Houston Endowment Grants, 1797
Hutton Fndn Grants, 1828
J.C. Penney Company Grants, 1874
J.L. Bedsole Fndn Grants, 1876
John P. Murphy Fndn Grants, 1943
Joyce Fndn Grants, 1969
Katharine Matthies Fndn Grants, 1982
KeySpan Fndn Grants, 1995
Leonsis Fndn Grants, 2045
Lockheed Martin Philanthropic Grants, 2062
Lowell Berry Fndn Grants, 2069
Lubbock Area Fndn Grants, 2079
Marion I. and Henry J. Knott Fndn Grants, 2109
Mead Johnson Nutritionals Evansville-Area Organizations Grants, 2157
Meadows Fndn Grants, 2161
Medtronic Fndn Health Care Grants, 2169
Morton K. and Jane Blaustein Fndn Grants, 2218
Newman's Own Inc Grants, 2306
Nicholas H. Noyes Jr. Memorial Fndn Grants, 2497
Nordson Corp Fndn Grants, 2851
Northrop Grumman Corp Grants, 2866
Northrop Grumman Newport News Grants, 2867
Oracle Corp Contributions Grants, 2951
PacifiCare Fndn Grants, 2981
Pew Charitable Trusts Children & Youth Grants, 3020
Pfizer Fndn Grants, 3025
Phoenix Suns Charities Grants, 3030
Pioneer Hi-Bred Comm Grants, 3051
Piper Jaffray Companies Building Strong Communities Grants, 3053
Plough Fndn Grants, 3061
Portland General Electric Fndn Grants, 3067
Powell Fndn Grants, 3073
Procter and Gamble Fund Grants, 3083
Progress Energy Fndn Grants, 3084
Quantum Fndn Grants, 3096
Rajiv Gandhi Fndn Grants, 3104
Raskob Fndn for Catholic Activities Grants, 3107
Richard and Susan Smith Family Fndn Grants, 3159
Rockefeller Brothers Fund Pivotal Places Grants: South Africa, 3180
Ruth Eleanor Bamberger and John Ernest Bamberger Memorial Fndn Grants, 3202
San Francisco Fndn Comm Health Grants, 3260
Seneca Foods Fndn Grants, 3278
Sid W. Richardson Fndn Grants, 3284
Southwest Gas Corp Fndn Grants, 3352
Strowd Roses Grants, 3388
Taproot Fndn Capacity-Building Service Grants, 3417
Temple-Inland Fndn Grants, 3419
Trull Fndn Grants, 3441
U.S. Department of Education 21st Century Comm Learning Centers, 3445
Union County Comm Fndn Grants, 3461
Westinghouse Charitable Giving Grants, 3530
WHO Fndn General Grants, 3534

Emergency Preparedness

ORISE Postgraduate Research Participation at the Agency for Toxic Substances and Disease Registry, 2960
South Madison Comm Fndn Grants, 3349
U.S. Lacrosse EAD Grants, 3453

Emergency Programs

Alcatel-Lucent Technologies Fndn Grants, 333
Alexander Fndn Cancer, Catastrophic Illness and Injury Grants, 342
Bill and Melinda Gates Fndn Grants, 756
BJ's Charitable Fndn Grants, 761
Blowitz-Ridgeway Fndn Grants, 767
Children Affected by AIDS Fndn Family Assistance Emergency Fund Grants, 996
Comm Fndn of Mount Vernon and Knox County Grants, 1119
Cooper Industries Fndn Grants, 1150
DHHS Emergency Medical Services for Children Program, 1249
Global Fund for Children Grants, 1629
Idaho Comm Fndn Eastern Region Competitive Grants, 1837
Jane's Trust Grants, 1904
McGregor Fund Grants, 2143
McKesson Fndn Grants, 2145
Prince Charitable Trusts District of Columbia Grants, 3080

Emergency Services

Actors Fund Social Services and Financial Assistance, 225
AGS Dennis W. Jahnigen Career Development Scholars Awards, 264
Alexander Fndn Cancer, Catastrophic Illness and Injury Grants, 342
Barberton Comm Fndn Grants, 693
Burlington Industries Fndn Grants, 811
Carpenter Fndn Grants, 881
Carrier Corp Contributions Grants, 884
Comm Fndn for Southeastern Michigan Grants, 1094
Comm Fndn of Crawford County Grants and Scholarships, 1103
Comm Fndn of Greater Birmingham Grants, 1106
DHHS Emergency Medical Services for Children Program, 1249
Fayette County Fndn Grants, 1457
Florida BRAIVE Fund of Dade Comm Fndn, 1512
Florida BRAIVE Fund of Gulf Coast Comm Fndn of Venice, 1513
Florida BRAIVE Fund of The Comm Fndn in Jacksonville, 1514
General Mills Fndn Grants, 1590
Gulf Coast Comm of Venice Fndn Grants, 1677
Huntington Beach Police Officers Fndn Grants, 1821
Indiana AIDS Fund Grants, 1851
Morris and Gwendolyn Cafritz Fndn Grants, 2217
Prince Charitable Trusts Chicago Grants, 3079
Raskob Fndn for Catholic Activities Grants, 3107
Rhode Island Fndn Grants, 3154
Rhode Island Fndn Grants, 3154
SAG Motion Picture Players Welfare Fund Grants, 3238
San Francisco Fndn Disability Rights Advocate Fund Emergency Grants, 3261
U.S. Lacrosse EAD Grants, 3453
VDH Emergency Medical Services Training Fund, 3483

Emission Control

HEI Grants, 1734

Emotion

NIMH Basic and Translational Research in Emotion Grants, 2746

Emotional/Mental Health

Advancing Colorado's Mental Health Care Project Grants, 240
Bella Vista Fndn Grants, 740
Gerber Fndn Grants, 1606
Hasbro Children's Fund, 1714
Illinois Children's Healthcare Fndn Grants, 1842
Long Island Comm Fndn Grants, 2063
Taproot Fndn Capacity-Building Service Grants, 3417

Emotionally Disturbed, Education

DHHS Comprehensive Comm Mental Health Services Grants for Children with Serious Emotional Disturbances, 1247
Greater Tacoma Comm Fndn Ryan Alan Hade Endowment Fund, 1657

Employment Opportunity Programs

A Fund for Women Grants, 14
Able Trust Vocational Rehabilitation Grants for Individuals, 186
Achelis and Bodman Fndns Grants, 206
AT&T Fndn Civic and Comm Service Grants, 658
Bernard and Audre Rapoport Fndn Grants, 746
Bernard F. and Alva B. Gimbel Fndn Grants, 747
Boston Fndn Grants, 783
Bush Fndn Health & Human Services Grants, 814
Chicago Comm Trust Grants, 989
Chiron Fndn Comm Grants, 1004
Comm Fndn of Howard County Grants, 1116

Connecticut Comm Fndn Grants, 1141
Crail-Johnson Fndn Grants, 1157
Cruise Industry Charitable Fndn Grants, 1166
Duke Energy Fndn Grants, 1339
FAR Fund, 1453
Fisa Fndn Grants, 1506
Fndn for the Mid-South Grants, 1536
Frank Stanley Beveridge Fndn Grants, 1553
Georgiana Goddard Eaton Memorial Fund Grants, 1604
Graco Fndn Grants, 1642
Henry County Comm Fndn Grants, 1747
HHK Employment Grants, 1755
Johnson & Johnson Corp Contributions Grants, 1952
Joyce Fndn Grants, 1969
King Pharmaceuticals Corp Contributions Grants, 2003
Marriott Fndn for People with Disabilities Bridges Grants, 2113
Medicaid Infrastructure Grant Program to Support Employment of People with Disabilities, 2163
Ms. Fndn for Women Grants, 2222
National City Corp Contributions Grants, 2250
NIDRR Field-Initiated Projects, 2594
Northern Trust Company Charitable Trust and Corp Giving Program, 2865
Northrop Grumman Corp Grants, 2866
Perry County Comm Fndn Grants, 3016
Prudential Fndn Grants, 3087
Richard King Mellon Fndn Grants, 3161
Richard M. Fairbanks Fndn Grants, 3162
Robert F. Stoico / FIRSTFED Charitable Fndn Grants, 3171
S. Mark Taper Fndn Grants, 3236
Starr Fndn Grants, 3377
U.S. Department of Education Vocational Rehabilitation Services Projects for American Indians with Disabilities Grants, 3452
Verizon Fndn Maryland Grants, 3487
Verizon Fndn New York Grants, 3488
Verizon Fndn Northeast Region Grants, 3489
Verizon Fndn Pennsylvania Grants, 3490
Verizon Fndn Vermont Grants, 3491
Verizon Fndn Virginia Grants, 3492
Warrick County Comm Fndn Grants, 3519

End of Life/Palliative Care
AACN End of Life/Palliative Care Small Projects Grants, 59
Aetna Fndn Quality of Care Grants, 245
Aetna Fndn Regional Comm Health Grants, 249

Endocrine Disorders
NIDDK Development of Disease Biomarkers Grants, 2549

Endocrinology
AHAF National Glaucoma Research Grants, 268
AMA Fndn Seed Grants for Research, 398
Fndn for Medical Research Grants, 1528
Genentech Corp Charitable Contributions Grants, 1588
NIDDK Co-Activators and Co-Repressors in Gene Expression Grants, 2546
NIDDK Collaborative Interdisciplinary Team Science in Diabetes, Endocrinology and Metabolic Diseases Grants, 2547
NIDDK Diabetes, Endocrinology, and Metabolic Diseases NRSAs—Individual, 2552
NIDDK Endoscopic Clinical Research Grants In Pancreatic And Biliary Diseases, 2555
NIDDK Pilot and Feasibility Clinical Research Grants in Diabetes, Endocrine and Metabolic Diseases, 2574
NIDDK Proteomics: Diabetes, Obesity, And Endocrine, Digestive, Kidney, Urologic, And Hematologic Diseases, 2578
NIDDK Seeding Collaborative Interdisciplinary Team Science in Diabetes, Endocrinology and Metabolic Diseases Grants, 2584
NIDDK Small Grants for Underrepresented Minority Scientists in Diabetes and Digestive and Kidney Diseases, 2588
NIDDK Translational Research for the Prevention and Control of Diabetes and Obesity, 2591
NIEHS Biological Response to Environmental Health Hazards Research Grants, 2596
NIH Biobehavioral Pain Research Grants, 2638
NIH Endocrine Disruptors: Epidemiologic Approaches Grants, 2658
Orentreich Fndn for the Advancement of Science Grants, 2959

Energy
Canada Graduate Scholarships and NSERC Postgraduate Scholarships, 845
Cass County Comm Fndn Grants, 887
Clarence E. Heller Charitable Fndn Grants, 1022
DOE Environmental Remediation Grants, 1297
DOE Health Effects and Life Sciences Research Grants, 1298
DOE Medical Applications and Measurement Science Grants, 1301
General Motors Fndn Grants Support Program, 1591
NSF-NIST Interaction in Chemistry, Materials Research, Molecular Biosciences, Bioengineering, and Chemical Engineering, 2897

Energy Conservation
Bullitt Fndn Grants, 809
Rohm and Haas Company Grants, 3185

Engineering
AAAS Science & Technology Policy Fellowships - National Defense & Global Security, 29
AACR Team Science Award, 89
Alcatel-Lucent Technologies Corp Contributions Grants, 332
Alfred P. Sloan Fndn Research Fellowships, 353
ARCO Fndn Education Grants, 526
ArvinMeritor Grants, 544
Award in Separations Science and Technology, 677
Beckman Young Investigators Grants, 735
BWF Career Awards at the Scientific Interface, 819
Canada Graduate Scholarships and NSERC Postgraduate Scholarships, 845
Canada-U.S. Fulbright New Century Scholars Grants, 846
Canada-U.S. Fulbright Senior Specialists Grants, 847
CDC Injury Control Research Centers Grants, 913
Chateaubriand Exact Sciences, Engineering, and Medicine Research Scholarships, 976
Comm Fndn of Greater Flint Grants, 1107
DAAD Research Stays for University Academics and Scientists, 1183
FIC International Training and Research in Environmental and Occupational Health, 1493
Fluor Fndn Grants, 1517
Fndn for Science and Disability Grant Program for Physically Disabled Students in the Sciences, 1532
Fulbright Alumni Initiatives Awards Grants, 1566
Fulbright Distinguished Chairs Grants, 1567
Fulbright New Century Scholars Grants, 1570
Fulbright Specialists Grants, 1571
Fulbright Traditional Scholar Program in Europe and Eurasia, 1572
Fulbright Traditional Scholar Program in Sub-Saharan Africa, 1573
Fulbright Traditional Scholar Program in the East Asia/Pacific Region, 1574
Fulbright Traditional Scholar Program in the Near East and North Africa Region, 1575
Fulbright Traditional Scholar Program in the South and Central Asia Region, 1576
Fulbright Traditional Scholar Program in the Western Hemisphere, 1577
HHMI-NIBIB Interfaces Initiative Grants, 1764
Matsumae International Fndn Grants, 2129
Meadows Fndn Grants, 2161
Millipore Fndn Grants, 2203
Minority Doctoral Fellowships in Science and Engineering, 2207
NHGRI Mentored Research Scientist Development Award, 2315
NIGMS Fellowships in Quantitative Biology, 2610
NIGMS Supplements for the Study of Complex Biological Systems, 2630
NIMH Curriculum Development Award in Neuroinformatics Research and Analysis, 2754
Northwood University/Alden B. Dow Creativity Center Summer Residency Program, 2871
NSERC Brockhouse Canada Prize for Interdisciplinary Research in Science and Engineering Grant, 2873
NSF Alan T. Waterman Award, 2874
NSF Chemical, Biochemical, and Biotechnology Systems Research Grants, 2882
NSF Emerging Frontiers in Research and Innovation Grants, 2885
NSF Grant Opportunities for Academic Liaison with Industry, 2887
NSF Presidential Early Career Awards for Scientists and Engineers (PECASE) Grants, 2892
NSF Small Business Innovation Research Grants, 2893
Prospect Burma Scholarships, 3085
Rayonier Fndn Grants, 3111
Rockwell International Corp Trust Grants, 3183
Roy and Christine Sturgis Trust Grants, 3191
RSC Thomas W. Eadie Medal, 3199
Society of Cosmetic Chemists Allan B. Black Award Sponsored by Presperse, 3328
Society of Cosmetic Chemists Award Sponsored by McIntyre Group, Ltd., 3329
Society of Cosmetic Chemists Award Sponsored by The HallStar Company, 3330
Society of Cosmetic Chemists Chapter Best Speaker Award, 3331
Society of Cosmetic Chemists Chapter Merit Award, 3332
Society of Cosmetic Chemists Frontier of Science Award, 3333
Society of Cosmetic Chemists Hans Schaeffer Award, 3334
Society of Cosmetic Chemists Joseph P. Ciaudelli Award, 3335
Society of Cosmetic Chemists Keynote Award Lecture Sponsored by Ruger Chemical Corp, 3336
Society of Cosmetic Chemists Literature Award, 3337
Society of Cosmetic Chemists Maison G. de Navarre Medal, 3338
Society of Cosmetic Chemists Merit Award, 3339
Society of Cosmetic Chemists Robert A. Kramer Lifetime Service Award, 3340
Society of Cosmetic Chemists Shaw Mudge Award, 3341
Society of Cosmetic Chemists Student Poster Awards, 3342
Society of Cosmetic Chemists Young Scientist Awards, 3343
University of California President's Postdoctoral Fellowships, 3469
Wallace H. Coulter Fndn Grants, 3515
Wayne and Gladys Valley Fndn Grants, 3522

Engineering Education
3M Fndn Grants, 11
Advanced Micro Devices Comm Affairs Grants, 239
Alcatel-Lucent Technologies Fndn Grants, 333
Alcoa Fndn Grants, 334
AMD Corp Contributions Grants, 411
ArvinMeritor Grants, 544
DaimlerChrysler Corp Fund Grants, 1186
Dayton Power and Light Fndn Grants, 1205
Emerson Charitable Trust Grants, 1412
FMC Fndn Grants, 1518
Ford Motor Company Fund Grants, 1522
Goodrich Corp Fndn Grants, 1638
HHMI Med into Grad Initiative Grants, 1761

NIGMS Minority Access to Research Careers Ancillary Training Activities Grants, 2619
Northrop Grumman Corp Grants, 2866
Northrop Grumman Newport News Grants, 2867
PAHO/WHO Fellowships, 2984
Rockwell Collins Charitable Contributions, 3182
Rollin M. Gerstacker Fndn Grants, 3186
Tellabs Fndn Grants, 3418
United Technologies Corp Grants, 3466
Wallace H. Coulter Fndn Grants, 3515

English as a Second Language
ACF Supplemental Services for Recently Arrived Refugees Grants, 203

Enteral Nutrition
ASPEN C. Richard Fleming Grant, 629
ASPEN Douglas Wilmore Grant, 630
ASPEN Dudrick Research Scholar Award, 631
ASPEN Harry M. Vars Award, 632
ASPEN Maurice Shils Grant, 633
ASPEN Norman Yoshimura Grant, 634
ASPEN Nutrition Research Grants, 635
ASPEN Scientific Abstracts Awards for Papers or Posters, 636
ASPEN Scientific Abstracts Promising Investigator Awards, 637

Entertainment Industry
Actors Fund Social Services and Financial Assistance, 225
SAG Motion Picture Players Welfare Fund Grants, 3238

Entrepreneurship
Achelis and Bodman Fndns Grants, 206
Allstate Corp Giving Grants, 363
Allstate Corp Hometown Commitment Grants, 364
Bodman Fndn Grants, 776
Echoing Green Fellowships, 1365
JM Fndn Grants, 1926
Minneapolis Fndn Comm Grants, 2206
Monfort Family Fndn Grants, 2213

Environment
DuPage Comm Fndn Grants, 1352
El Paso Corp Fndn Grants, 1389
El Pomar Fndn Awards and Grants, 1390
Erie Comm Fndn Grants, 1427
Fairfield County Comm Fndn Grants, 1446
Fuji Film Grants, 1565
Grand Haven Area Comm Fndn Grants, 1644
Greater Cincinnati Fndn Priority and Small Projects/ Capacity-Building Grants, 1651
H.A. and Mary K. Chapman Charitable Trust Grants, 1681
John W. and Anna H. Hanes Fndn Grants, 1948
Putnam County Comm Fndn Grants, 3093
Rohm and Haas Company Grants, 3185

Environment & Conservation
Dean Foods Comm Involvement Grants, 1209
Rohm and Haas Company Grants, 3185

Environmental Biology
NSF Doctoral Dissertation Improvement Grants in the Directorate for Biological Sciences, 2884

Environmental Design
Vancouver Fndn Grants and Comm Initiatives Program, 3477

Environmental Education
A Friend's Fndn Trust Grants, 13
Abbott Fund Comm Vitality Grants, 177
Administaff Comm Affairs Grants, 235
AEC Trust Grants, 242
Ahn Family Fndn Grants, 304
Alaska Airlines Corp Giving Grants, 323
Alaska Airlines Fndn Grants, 324
Alexander & Baldwin Fndn Hawaiian and Pacific Island Grants, 338
Alexander & Baldwin Fndn Mainland Grants, 339
Alpine Winter Fndn Grants, 368
Amador Comm Fndn Grants, 409
Barker Welfare Fndn Grants, 695
Beldon Fund Grants, 738
Blumenthal Fndn Grants, 773
Boeing Company Contributions Grants, 777
Bullitt Fndn Grants, 809
Cargill Citizenship Fund-Corp Giving Grants, 865
Carls Fndn Grants, 876
Carrier Corp Contributions Grants, 884
Clarence E. Heller Charitable Fndn Grants, 1022
Comm Fndn of Grant County Scholarships, 1105
CSX Corp Contributions Grants, 1169
Dean Foods Comm Involvement Grants, 1209
Del E. Webb Fndn Grants, 1213
Duke Energy Fndn Grants, 1339
Fargo-Moorhead Area Fndn Grants, 1454
Gamble Fndn Grants, 1582
George and Ruth Bradford Fndn Grants, 1595
Hilton Head Island Fndn Grants, 1779
Honda of America Manufacturing Fndn Grants, 1790
Jessie Ball Dupont Fund Grants, 1919
KeySpan Fndn Grants, 1995
Knox County Comm Fndn Grants, 2009
Lawrence S. Huntington Fund Grants, 2035
Lester E. Yeager Charitable Trust B Grants, 2047
Olin Corp Charitable Trust Grants, 2943
Oracle Corp Contributions Grants, 2951
Perry County Comm Fndn Grants, 3016
Pike County Comm Fndn Grants, 3049
Rohm and Haas Company Grants, 3185
Schering-Plough Fndn Comm Initiatives Grants, 3269
Scott County Comm Fndn Grants, 3273
Seabury Fndn Grants, 3274
Spencer County Comm Fndn Grants, 3358
Vancouver Fndn Grants and Comm Initiatives Program, 3477
Vulcan Materials Company Fndn Grants, 3504
Winifred & Harry B. Allen Fndn Grants, 3543

Environmental Effects
Alfred P. Sloan Fndn Research Fellowships, 353
Award for Creative Advances in Environmental Science and Technology, 676
Carrier Corp Contributions Grants, 884
Clarence E. Heller Charitable Fndn Grants, 1022
DHHS Neurodevelopmental Test Methods Research Grants, 1268
DOE Medical Applications and Measurement Science Grants, 1301
Duke Energy Fndn Grants, 1339
EPA Children's Health Protection Grants, 1420
Gerber Fndn Grants, 1606
Max Bell Fndn Grants, 2134
MDBD Basic Research Grants, 2152
NIEHS Environmental Justice: Partnerships for Communication, 2598
NIEHS Superfund Hazardous Substances Basic Research and Education Grants, 2607
NIH Ecology of Infectious Diseases, 2656
NIH Endocrine Disruptors: Epidemiologic Approaches Grants, 2658
NIH Genetic Susceptibility and Variability of Human Malformations Research Grants, 2669
NIH Xenobiotics and Cell Death/Injury in Neurodegenerative Disease Research Grants, 2739
NSF Chemistry Research Experiences for Undergraduates, 2883
NSF-NIST Interaction in Chemistry, Materials Research, Molecular Biosciences, Bioengineering, and Chemical Engineering, 2897

Environmental Engineering
FIC International Training and Research in Environmental and Occupational Health, 1493
NIEHS Superfund Hazardous Substances Basic Research and Education Grants, 2607

Environmental Health
AAOHN Fndn Experienced Researcher Grants, 153
AAOHN Fndn New Investigator Researcher Grants, 154
AAOHN Fndn Professional Development Scholarships, 155
Administaff Comm Affairs Grants, 235
AEC Trust Grants, 242
Ahn Family Fndn Grants, 304
Alaska Airlines Corp Giving Grants, 323
Alaska Airlines Fndn Grants, 324
Alcatel-Lucent Technologies Corp Contributions Grants, 332
Alexander & Baldwin Fndn Hawaiian and Pacific Island Grants, 338
Alexander & Baldwin Fndn Mainland Grants, 339
Alliance Healthcare Fndn Grants, 362
Ashland Corp Contributions Grants, 586
Beldon Fund Grants, 738
California Wellness Fndn Work and Health Grants, 834
Canada Graduate Scholarships and NSERC Postgraduate Scholarships, 845
Chicago Comm Trust Grants, 989
Comm Fndn of Morgan County Grants and Scholarships, 1118
Comm Fndn of Santa Cruz County Grants, 1122
Comm Fndn of Switzerland County Grants, 1127
Comm Toolbox for Children's Environmental Health Grants, 1137
DHHS Public Health Students Traineeships and Other Graduate Public Health Programs, 1277
DOE Environmental Remediation Grants, 1297
DOE Health Effects and Life Sciences Research Grants, 1298
Donald and Sylvia Robinson Family Fndn Grants, 1310
Duncan L. Gordon Fellowships, 1349
EPA Baseline Assessment of Risks of Exposure to Lead Poisoning of Native American Children, 1419
EPA Children's Health Protection Grants, 1420
EPA Lead Awareness Outreach for Native American Tribes, 1421
FIC International Training and Research in Environmental and Occupational Health, 1493
Health Fndn of Greater Cincinnati Grants, 1724
HEI Grants, 1734
Heineman Fndn for Research, Education, Charitable and Scientific Purposes, 1735
Houston Endowment Grants, 1797
Jessie B. Cox Charitable Trust Grants, 1918
Lawrence S. Huntington Fund Grants, 2035
NIDCD Mentored Research Scientist Development Award, 2523
NIEHS Applied Toxicological Research and Testing Grants, 2595
NIEHS Biological Response to Environmental Health Hazards Research Grants, 2596
NIEHS Carcinogenicity of Drinking Water Disinfection By-Products, 2597
NIEHS Independent Scientist Award, 2601
NIEHS Mentored Clinical Scientist Research Career Development Awards, 2602
NIEHS Mentored Research Scientist Development Award, 2603
NIEHS Small Business Innovation Research Grants, 2605
NIEHS Structure-Function Relationships of Environmentally Relevant Genetic Variants Research Grants, 2606
NIEHS Superfund Hazardous Substances Basic Research and Education Grants, 2607
NIEHS/NINDS Role of the Environment in Parkinson's Disease, 2608
NIH Mechanisms Underlying Individual Variations in Drug Responses, 2685
NIH National Occupational Research Agenda Grants, 2696
ORISE Postgraduate Research Participation at the National Center for Toxicological Research, 2961

Parker B. Francis Fellowships in Pulmonary Research, 2989
Pioneer Hi-Bred Comm Grants, 3051
Powell Fndn Grants, 3073
Prince Charitable Trusts District of Columbia Grants, 3080
Rayonier Fndn Grants, 3111
San Diego Fndn for Change Grants, 3255
San Francisco Fndn Comm Health Grants, 3260
Schering-Plough Fndn Comm Initiatives Grants, 3269
Seattle Fndn Grants, 3276
Sunflower Fndn Walking Trails Grants, 3403
Taproot Fndn Capacity-Building Service Grants, 3417
Thrasher Research Fund Grants, 3426
Vancouver Fndn Grants and Comm Initiatives Program, 3477
Winifred & Harry B. Allen Fndn Grants, 3543
Women's Fndn of California Comm Action Fund, 3549

Environmental Issues
Hillsdale County Comm General Adult Fndn Grants, 1777

Environmental Law
Bullitt Fndn Grants, 809
Jessie Smith Noyes Fndn Grants, 1920

Environmental Planning/Policy
A Friend's Fndn Trust Grants, 13
Achelis and Bodman Fndns Grants, 206
Beldon Fund Grants, 738
Clarence E. Heller Charitable Fndn Grants, 1022
CLIF Bar Family Fndn Grants, 1040
Honda of America Manufacturing Fndn Grants, 1790
OSI-Baltimore Special Opportunities Grants, 2972
Prince Charitable Trusts Chicago Grants, 3079
SSHRC Research/Creation Grants in Fine Arts, 3364

Environmental Programs
1675 Fndn Grants, 4
3M Fndn Grants, 11
Abbott Fund Comm Vitality Grants, 177
Abel Fndn Grants, 181
Abell-Hanger Fndn Grants, 183
ACE Charitable Fndn Grants, 199
Adam Richter Charitable Trust Grants, 230
Administaff Comm Affairs Grants, 235
AEC Trust Grants, 242
Ahn Family Fndn Grants, 304
Air Products and Chemicals Grants, 319
Alaska Airlines Corp Giving Grants, 323
Alaska Airlines Fndn Grants, 324
Albuquerque Comm Fndn Grants, 331
Alcoa Fndn Grants, 334
Alexander & Baldwin Fndn Hawaiian and Pacific Island Grants, 338
Alexander & Baldwin Fndn Mainland Grants, 339
Allegan County Comm Fndn Grants, 358
Allen P. and Josephine B. Green Fndn Grants, 361
Alpine Winter Fndn Grants, 368
Amador Comm Fndn Grants, 409
American Electric Power Grants, 434
Amgen Fndn Grants, 467
Anheuser-Busch Fndn Grants, 474
Ann Arbor Area Comm Fndn Grants, 476
Arizona Public Service Corp Giving Grants, 531
Arkansas Comm Fndn Grants, 533
Armstrong McDonald Fndn Grants, 537
Ashland Corp Contributions Grants, 586
AT&T Fndn Civic and Comm Service Grants, 658
Atherton Family Fndn Grants, 659
Autodesk Comm Relations Grants, 671
Autzen Fndn Grants, 672
Bacon Family Fndn Grants, 679
Ball Brothers Fndn General Grants, 683
Batchelor Fndn Grants, 701
Baton Rouge Area Fndn Grants, 702
Beazley Fndn Grants, 730
Beldon Fund Grants, 738
Bella Vista Fndn Grants, 740
Bender Fndn Grants, 742
Berks County Comm Fndn Grants, 745
Bernard F. and Alva B. Gimbel Fndn Grants, 747
Berrien Comm Fndn Grants, 749
Blanche and Julian Robertson Family Fndn Grants, 765
Bodenwein Public Benevolent Fndn Grants, 775
Bodman Fndn Grants, 776
Boeing Company Contributions Grants, 777
Borkee-Hagley Fndn Grants, 781
Boston Fndn Grants, 783
Boston Globe Fndn Grants, 784
Brian G. Dyson Fndn Grants, 791
Bridgestone/Firestone Trust Fund Grants, 792
Bullitt Fndn Grants, 809
Burton G. Bettingen Grants, 813
Cambridge Comm Fndn Grants, 837
Capital Region Comm Fndn Grants, 862
Carl and Eloise Pohlad Family Fndn Grants, 867
Carolyn Fndn Grants, 880
Carrie E. and Lena V. Glenn Fndn Grants, 882
Carrier Corp Contributions Grants, 884
Cass County Comm Fndn Grants, 887
CDC Research, Treatment, and Education Programs on Lyme Disease in the United States Cooperative Agreements, 927
Cessna Fndn Grants, 938
CFFVR Opportunity Grants, 952
Charles Delmar Fndn Grants, 963
Charlotte County (FL) Comm Fndn Grants, 973
Cinergy Fndn Grants, 1013
Citizens Bank Mid-Atlantic Charitable Fndn Grants, 1015
Clarence E. Heller Charitable Fndn Grants, 1022
Clark Fndn Grants, 1029
Claude Worthington Benedum Fndn Grants, 1033
CLIF Bar Family Fndn Grants, 1040
CNCS Next Generation Grants, 1049
Coastal Comm Fndn of South Carolina Grants, 1051
Colorado Interstate Gas Grants, 1060
Comm Fndn for Monterey County Grants, 1092
Comm Fndn for Muskegon County Grants, 1093
Comm Fndn for Southeastern Michigan Grants, 1094
Comm Fndn for Southern Arizona Grants, 1095
Comm Fndn of Champaign County Grants, 1102
Comm Fndn of Crawford County Grants and Scholarships, 1103
Comm Fndn of Greater Birmingham Grants, 1106
Comm Fndn of Greater Flint Grants, 1107
Comm Fndn of Greater Greensboro Grants, 1109
Comm Fndn Of Greater Lafayette Grants, 1110
Comm Fndn of Greater Tampa Grants, 1112
Comm Fndn of Greenville Comm Enrichment Grants, 1113
Comm Fndn of Greenville-Greenville Women Giving Grants, 1115
Comm Fndn of Morgan County Grants and Scholarships, 1118
Comm Fndn of Mount Vernon and Knox County Grants, 1119
Comm Fndn of Randolph County Grants, 1121
Comm Fndn of Santa Cruz County Grants, 1122
Comm Fndn of South Puget Sound Grants, 1124
Comm Fndn of Southeastern Connecticut Grants, 1125
Comm Fndn of St. Joseph County Special Project Challenge Grants, 1126
Comm Fndn of Tampa Bay Grants, 1128
Comm Fndn of the Eastern Shore Comm Needs Grants, 1129
Comm Fndn of Wabash County Grants, 1131
Comm Fndn of Western North Carolina Grants, 1132
Connecticut Comm Fndn Grants, 1141
Constellation Energy Group and Baltimore Gas and Electric Corp Contributions, 1146
Consumers Energy Fndn, 1147
Cooke Fndn Grants, 1148
Cooper Industries Fndn Grants, 1150
Coors Brewing Corp Contributions Grants, 1151
Cowles Charitable Trust Grants, 1155
Cruise Industry Charitable Fndn Grants, 1166
CSRA Comm Fndn Grants, 1168
Dade Comm Fndn Grants, 1185
DaimlerChrysler Corp Fund Grants, 1186
Dana Corp Fndn Grants, 1196
Dearborn Comm Fndn County Progress Grants, 1211
Delaware Comm Fndn Grants, 1215
Do Something BR!CK Awards, 1287
Dole Food Company Charitable Contributions, 1307
Donald and Sylvia Robinson Family Fndn Grants, 1310
Dorothy Hooper Beattie Fndn Grants, 1321
Dorrance Family Fndn Grants, 1323
Dr. Scholl Fndn Grants, 1329
Drs. Bruce and Lee Fndn Grants, 1333
Dubois County Comm Fndn Grants, 1336
Duke Energy Fndn Grants, 1339
E.J. Grassmann Trust Grants, 1360
eBay Fndn Comm Grants, 1363
Edward Bangs Kelley and Elza Kelley Fndn Grants, 1373
Edwin W. and Catherine M. Davis Fndn Grants, 1377
EIF Comm Grants, 1386
El Paso Comm Fndn Grants, 1388
Elliot Fndn Inc Grants, 1402
Elmer L. and Eleanor J. Andersen Fndn Grants, 1406
Ensworth Charitable Fndn Grants, 1416
EPA Children's Health Protection Grants, 1420
EPA Lead Awareness Outreach for Native American Tribes, 1421
Essex County Comm Fndn Discretionary Fund Grant, 1428
Estee Lauder Grants, 1429
Evjue Fndn Grants, 1439
Ewing Halsell Fndn Grants, 1440
ExxonMobil Grants, 1442
Ferree Fndn Grants, 1486
Field Fndn of Illinois Grants, 1499
FirstEnergy Fndn Comm Grants, 1505
Forrest C. Lattner Fndn Grants, 1523
Foster Fndn Grants, 1524
Frances and John L. Loeb Family Fund Grants, 1546
Franklin County Comm Fndn Grants, 1554
Fulton County Comm Fndn Grants, 1579
G.N. Wilcox Trust Grants, 1581
GenCorp Fndn Grants, 1587
General Motors Fndn Grants Support Program, 1591
George and Ruth Bradford Fndn Grants, 1595
George F. Baker Trust Grants, 1597
Georgia Power Fndn Grants, 1603
Gibson Fndn Grants, 1612
Giving Sum Annual Grant, 1619
Good Samaritan Inc Grants, 1637
Grand Rapids Comm Fndn Grants, 1647
Greater Bridgeport Area Fndn Comm Impact Grants, 1650
Greater Green Bay Comm Fndn Grants, 1652
Greater New Orleans Fndn Grants, 1654
Greater Saint Louis Comm Fndn Grants, 1655
Greater Tacoma Comm Fndn Grants, 1656
Greater Worcester Comm Fndn Discretionary Grants, 1658
Greenfield Fndn of Maine Grants, 1663
Gulf Coast Comm of Venice Fndn Grants, 1677
Hancock County Comm Fndn Grants, 1690
Hannaford Charitable Fndn Grants, 1692
Harley Davidson Fndn Grants, 1694
Harrison County Comm Fndn Grants, 1700
Hawaii Comm Fndn West Hawaii Fund Grants, 1718
HEI Grants, 1734
Heineman Fndn for Research, Education, Charitable and Scientific Purposes, 1735
Henry J. Kaiser Family Fndn Grants, 1748
Hershey Company Grants, 1754
High Meadow Fndn Grants, 1768
Hillman Fndn Grants, 1775
Hoblitzelle Fndn Grants, 1783
Holland/Zeeland Comm Fndn Grants, 1786
Homer Fndn Grants, 1789
Honda of America Manufacturing Fndn Grants, 1790
Horace A. Kimball and S. Ella Kimball Fndn Grants, 1792

Houston Endowment Grants, 1797
Hudson Webber Fndn Grants, 1813
Huntington County Comm Fndn Grants, 1823
i2 Fndn Grants, 1829
Idaho Power Company Corp Contributions, 1838
Impact 100 Grants, 1843
Inasmuch Fndn Grants, 1845
Jackson County Comm Fndn Unrestricted Grants, 1879
James A. and Faith Knight Fndn Grants, 1884
James Ford Bell Fndn Grants, 1885
James M. Cox Fndn of Georgia Grants, 1892
Jane's Trust Grants, 1904
Janirve Fndn Grants, 1905
Jennings County Comm Fndn Grants, 1916
Jessie B. Cox Charitable Trust Grants, 1918
Jessie Smith Noyes Fndn Grants, 1920
John Merck Fund Grants, 1940
John W. and Anna H. Hanes Fndn Grants, 1948
Katharine Matthies Fndn Grants, 1982
Kavli Fndn Research Grants, 1985
Kelvin and Eleanor Smith Fndn Grants, 1986
Kenneth T. and Eileen L. Norris Fndn Grants, 1989
Kettering Family Fndn Grants, 1991
Kettering Fund Grants, 1992
KeySpan Fndn Grants, 1995
Knox County Comm Fndn Grants, 2009
Kosciusko County Comm Fndn Grants, 2015
Kraft Cares US Grants, 2017
LaGrange County Comm Fndn Grants, 2020
Lands' End Corp Giving Program, 2030
Lawrence Fndn Grants, 2034
Lawrence S. Huntington Fund Grants, 2035
Legacy Fndn Grants, 2040
Long Island Comm Fndn Grants, 2063
Louis Calder Fndn Grants, 2065
Lowell Area Comm Fund Grants, 2068
Lubrizol Fndn Grants, 2080
M.E. Raker Fndn Grants, 2094
Maine Comm Fndn Grants, 2099
Margaret T. Morris Fndn Grants, 2105
Marion Park Deaver and Harry Gilbert Deaver Fndn Grants, 2110
Mark and Catherine Winkler Fndn Grants, 2112
Mars Fndn Grants, 2114
Mary Owen Borden Fndn Grants, 2121
Maxon Charitable Fndn Grants, 2135
McInerny Fndn Grants, 2144
McKesson Fndn Grants, 2145
McKnight Fndn Grants, 2146
McLean Contributionship Grants, 2147
Mead Witter Fndn Grants, 2160
Meyer Memorial Trust Emergency Grants, 2178
Meyer Memorial Trust Grassroots Grants, 2179
Meyer Memorial Trust Operating Funds Grants, 2180
Meyer Memorial Trust Responsive Grants, 2181
Miami County Comm Fndn Operation Round Up Grants, 2188
Miguel Aleman Fndn Grants, 2197
Miriam and Peter Haas Fund Grants, 2208
Morris and Gwendolyn Cafritz Fndn Grants, 2217
Nelda C. and H.J. Lutcher Stark Fndn Grants, 2301
Nina Mason Pulliam Charitable Trust Grants, 2776
North Carolina Comm Development Grants, 2858
North Carolina Comm Fndn Grants, 2859
North Georgia Comm Fndn Grants, 2862
Northeast Utilities Fndn Grants, 2863
Northrop Grumman Corp Grants, 2866
Ogden Codman Trust Grants, 2937
Oracle Corp Contributions Grants, 2951
Oscar Rennebohm Fndn Grants, 2963
OSI-Baltimore Special Opportunities Grants, 2972
Owen County Comm Fndn Grants, 2979
PacifiCorp Fndn for Learning Grants, 2982
Palm Beach and Martin Counties Grants, 2986
Paul G. Allen Family Fndn Grants, 3000
Peacock Fndn Grants, 3011
Perkins Charitable Fndn Grants, 3014
Perry County Comm Fndn Grants, 3016
Philadelphia Fndn Organizational Effectiveness Grants, 3029
Piedmont Natural Gas Grants, 3048
Pinellas County Grants, 3050
Pioneer Hi-Bred Comm Grants, 3051
Pittsburgh Fndn Comm Fund Grants, 3054
Plum Creek Fndn Grants, 3062
Portland General Electric Fndn Grants, 3067
Posey Comm Fndn Grants, 3068
Powell Fndn Grants, 3073
Prince Charitable Trusts Chicago Grants, 3079
Prince Charitable Trusts District of Columbia Grants, 3080
Princeton Area Comm Fndn Greater Mercer Grants, 3081
Principal Financial Group Fndn Grants, 3082
Procter and Gamble Fund Grants, 3083
Progress Energy Fndn Grants, 3084
Public Welfare Fndn Grants, 3089
Pulaski County Comm Fndn Grants, 3091
Rajiv Gandhi Fndn Grants, 3104
Rathmann Family Fndn Grants, 3109
Rayonier Fndn Grants, 3111
Rhode Island Fndn Grants, 3154
Rice Fndn Grants, 3155
Richard and Rhoda Goldman Fund Grants, 3158
Richard King Mellon Fndn Grants, 3161
Riley Fndn Grants, 3165
Ripley County Comm Fndn Grants, 3166
Robins Fndn Grants, 3175
Rochester Area Comm Fndn Grants, 3176
Rollin M. Gerstacker Fndn Grants, 3186
S. Livingston Mather Charitable Trust Grants, 3235
S. Mark Taper Fndn Grants, 3236
S.H. Cowell Fndn Grants, 3237
Salem Fndn Grants, 3242
Salisbury Comm Fndn Grants, 3243
Samuel S. Johnson Fndn Grants, 3251
San Diego Fndn for Change Grants, 3255
San Diego Women's Fndn Grants, 3259
San Francisco Fndn Comm Health Grants, 3260
Sasco Fndn Grants, 3265
Schering-Plough Fndn Comm Initiatives Grants, 3269
Scott County Comm Fndn Grants, 3273
Seabury Fndn Grants, 3274
Seattle Fndn Grants, 3276
Shaw's Supermarkets Donations, 3280
Shell Oil Company Fndn Grants, 3281
Simpson Fund Grants, 3290
Sisters of Saint Joseph Charitable Fund Grants, 3296
Snee Reinhardt Charitable Fndn Grants, 3300
Southwest Florida Comm Fndn Competitive Grants, 3351
Southwest Gas Corp Fndn Grants, 3352
Spencer County Comm Fndn Grants, 3358
SSHRC Research/Creation Grants in Fine Arts, 3364
Steelcase Fndn Grants, 3379
Steuben County Comm Fndn Grants, 3383
Stewart Huston Charitable Trust Grants, 3384
Strowd Roses Grants, 3388
Sulzberger Fndn Grants, 3399
Sunflower Fndn Walking Trails Grants, 3403
Susan Vaughan Fndn Grants, 3413
Taproot Fndn Capacity-Building Service Grants, 3417
Tellabs Fndn Grants, 3418
Thompson Charitable Fndn Grants, 3425
Toro Fndn Grants, 3431
Triangle Comm Fndn Donor-Advised Grants, 3437
Trull Fndn Grants, 3441
Union Benevolent Association Grants, 3460
United Technologies Corp Grants, 3466
Unity Fndn Of LaPorte County Grants, 3467
Vancouver Fndn Grants and Comm Initiatives Program, 3477
Vanderburgh Comm Fndn Grants, 3480
Vermont Comm Fndn Grants, 3493
Virginia W. Kettering Fndn Grants, 3502
Vulcan Materials Company Fndn Grants, 3504
W. C. Griffith Fndn Grants, 3505
Wal-Mart Fndn Comm Grants, 3513
Wal-Mart State Giving Grants, 3514
Warrick County Comm Fndn Grants, 3519
Westinghouse Charitable Giving Grants, 3530
Winifred & Harry B. Allen Fndn Grants, 3543
Winston-Salem Fndn Stokes County Grants, 3546
Women's Fndn of California Comm Action Fund, 3549
Women's Fndn of California Grants, 3550
YSA Get Ur Good On Grants, 3555
Z. Smith Reynolds Fndn Small Grants, 3557

Environmental Studies

American-Scandinavian Fndn Visiting Lectureship Grants, 460
Annie Sinclair Knudsen Memorial Fund/Kaua'i Comm Grants, 480
Canada-U.S. Fulbright New Century Scholars Grants, 846
Canada-U.S. Fulbright Senior Specialists Grants, 847
Collins Fndn Grants, 1058
Duke Energy Fndn Grants, 1339
Fred Baldwin Memorial Fndn Grants, 1556
Fulbright Alumni Initiatives Awards Grants, 1566
Fulbright Distinguished Chairs Grants, 1567
Fulbright New Century Scholars Grants, 1570
Fulbright Specialists Grants, 1571
Fulbright Traditional Scholar Program in Europe and Eurasia, 1572
Fulbright Traditional Scholar Program in Sub-Saharan Africa, 1573
Fulbright Traditional Scholar Program in the East Asia/Pacific Region, 1574
Fulbright Traditional Scholar Program in the Near East and North Africa Region, 1575
Fulbright Traditional Scholar Program in the South and Central Asia Region, 1576
Fulbright Traditional Scholar Program in the Western Hemisphere, 1577
Lawrence S. Huntington Fund Grants, 2035
NIEHS Environmental Justice: Partnerships for Communication, 2598
NIH Low Birthweight in Minority Populations Research Grants, 2683
Norwin S. and Elizabeth N. Bean Fndn Grants, 2872
NSF-NIST Interaction in Chemistry, Materials Research, Molecular Biosciences, Bioengineering, and Chemical Engineering, 2897
Olin Corp Charitable Trust Grants, 2943
Richard and Rhoda Goldman Fund Grants, 3158
Society for the Arts in Healthcare Environmental Arts Research Grant, 3327
Southbury Comm Trust Fund, 3350
SSHRC Research/Creation Grants in Fine Arts, 3364
Starr Fndn Grants, 3377
Trull Fndn Grants, 3441
U.S. Department of Education United States-Russia Program: Improving Research and Educational Activities in Higher Education, 3451
Weingart Fndn Grants, 3524

Enzymology

NIDDK Development of Assays for High-Throughput Drug Screening Grants, 2548
NSF Biomolecular Systems Cluster Grants, 2880

Epidemiology

AACR Career Development Awards for Pediatric Cancer Research, 70
AACR Judah Folkman Career Development Award for Anti-Angiogenesis Research, 79
AACR Outstanding Investigator Award for Breast Cancer Research, 84
AACR-American Cancer Society Award for Research Excellence in Cancer Epidemiology and Prevention, 91
AACR Basic Cancer Research Fellowships , 107
ACS Mentored Research Scholar Grant in Applied and Clinical Research, 217
AHAF Alzheimer's Disease Research Grants, 266
AHFMR Health Research Career Renewal Awards, 279
AHFMR Population Health Investigator Awards, 292

AMSSM Fndn Research Grants, 469
ASM-PAHO Infectious Diseases Epidemiology and Surveillance Fellowships, 625
Bristol-Myers Squibb Fndn Global HIV/AIDS Initiative Grants, 796
Bristol-Myers Squibb Virology and Oncology M.D. Research Fellowships, 802
Cancer Research UK Fellowships, 858
CDC Emerging Infectious Diseases Fellowships Program, 908
CDC Epidemiology and Laboratory Capacity Infectious Diseases Grants, 909
CDC Intervention Epidemiologic Research Studies of HIV/AIDS, 915
CDC Research, Treatment, and Education Programs on Lyme Disease in the United States Cooperative Agreements, 927
DHHS AIDS Project Grants, 1245
DHHS Public Health Students Traineeships and Other Graduate Public Health Programs, 1277
Elizabeth Glaser Pediatric AIDS Fndn Two-Year International Scholar Award, 1396
Ethical Research Grants and Fellowships, 1431
Fellowships in Infectious Diseases, 1485
FIC International Research Scientist Development Award, 1491
FIC International Training and Research in Emerging Infectious Diseases Grants, 1492
FIC International Training and Research in Environmental and Occupational Health, 1493
HRB Health Services Research Fellowships, 1801
HRB Postdoctoral Research Fellowships, 1802
IARC Expertise Transfer Fellowship, 1831
IARC Postdoctoral Fellowships for Training in Cancer Research, 1832
IARC Visiting Scientist Award for Senior Scientists, 1833
International Cancer Technology Transfer Fellowships, 1858
James S. McDonnell Fndn Complex Systems Collaborative Activity Awards, 1897
Landon Fndn-AACR Innovator Award for International Collaboration, 2028
Landon Fndn-AACR Innovator Award for Cancer Prevention Research, 2029
LSA Translational Research Grants, 2078
NCI Basic Cancer Research in Cancer Health Disparities Grants, 2271
NCI Stages of Breast Development: Normal to Metastatic Disease Grants, 2278
NCI/NIDA Transdisciplinary Tobacco Use Research Centers Grants, 2280
NCIC Terry Fox Postdoctoral Research Fellowships, 2285
NEI Clinical Study Planning Grant, 2292
NEI Clinical Vision Research Development Award, 2293
NFID New Investigator Matching Grants, 2310
NFID Postdoctoral Fellowships in Emerging Infectious Diseases, 2312
NHLBI National Research Service Award Programs in Cardiovascular Epidemiology and Biostatistics, 2357
NIA/NIEHS Biomedical Epidemiologic and Intervention Studies Planning Grants, 2441
NIDA Mentored Clinical Scientist Research Career Development Awards, 2507
NIDA Senior Scientist Award, 2515
NIDA Transition from Drug Abuse to Drug Addiction, 2516
NIDCR HIV/AIDS Associated Oral Viral Infections, 2535
NIDCR International Collaborative Oral Health Research Planning Grant, 2536
NIDDK Type 2 Diabetes in the Pediatric Population Research Grants, 2593
NIGMS/NIDCR Evolution of Infectious Diseases Research Grants, 2633
NIH Endocrine Disruptors: Epidemiologic Approaches Grants, 2658
NIH Genetic Susceptibility and Variability of Human Malformations Research Grants, 2669
NIH Mechanisms Underlying Individual Variations in Drug Responses, 2685
NIH Molecular Epidemiology of Prostate Carcinogenesis Grants, 2691
NIH Multidisciplinary Approach for Research on Oral Complications of HIV Infection, 2694
NIH Pathological Gambling: Basic, Clinical, and Services Research Grants, 2702
NIH Rett Syndrome: Genetics, Pathophysiology, and Biomarkers Research Grants, 2715
NIH Transitional Career Development Award in Women's Health Research, 2736
NIH/EPA Mechanistic-Based Cancer Risk Assessment Methods Research Grants, 2741
NIMH HIV/AIDS, Severe Mental Illness, and Homelessness Research Grants, 2757
NINR Aging Women and Breast Cancer Grants, 2789
NYAM Mary and David Hoar Fellowship, 2916
Pancreatic Cancer Action Network-AACR Fellowship, 2987
Pancreatic Cancer Action Network-AACR Pathway to Leadership Grants, 2988
RWJF Young Epidemiology Scholars Competition, 3233
Simone and Cino del Duca Grand Prix Awards, 3288
Susan G. Komen Breast Cancer Fndn Basic, Clinical, and Translational Research Grants, 3407
Susan G. Komen Breast Cancer Fndn Postdoctoral Fellowships, 3411
TSA Research Grant Awards, 3442
UICC American Cancer Society International Fellowships for Beginning Investigators, 3455
UK Fndn for the Study of Infant Deaths Grants, 3459
US CRDF Leishmaniasis: Collaborative Research Opportunities in North Africa and the Middle East, 3474

Epilepsy
ASPET Epilepsy Research Award for Outstanding Contributions to the Pharmacology of Antiepileptic Drugs, 641
EF Behavioral Sciences Student Fellowships, 1379
EF Health Sciences Student Fellowships, 1380
EF Making a Difference Award, 1381
EF Postdoctoral Research Training Fellowships, 1382
EF Predoctoral Research Training Fellowship, 1383
EF Research and Training Fellowships for Clinicians, 1384
Epilepsy Postdoctoral and Clinical Research Fellowships, 1422
Epilepsy Research Fndn New Therapy Grants, 1423
F.M. Kirby Fndn Grants, 1443
Klingenstein Neuroscience Fellowships, 2005
NIA Symptom Management for Chronic Neurological Conditions Research Grants, 2436
NICHD Symptom Management for Chronic Neurological Conditions Research Grants, 2496
NIDCD Symptom Management for Chronic Neurological Conditions Research Grants, 2532
NIH Research on Sleep and Sleep Disorders, 2713
NINDS Symptom Management for Chronic Neurological Conditions Research Grants, 2787
NINR Symptom Management for Chronic Neurological Conditions Research Grants, 2805
Partnership for Pediatric Epilepsy Research Grants, 2993
Pfizer Fndn Epilepsy Scholarship Award, 3024
Savoy Fndn Post-Doctoral and Clinical Research Fellowships, 3266
Savoy Fndn Research Grants, 3267
Savoy Fndn Studentships, 3268

Episcopal Church
Barra Fndn Project Grants, 699
Booth-Bricker Fund Grants, 780
Effie and Wofford Cain Fndn Grants, 1385
Robert E. and Evelyn McKee Fndn Grants, 3170

Equal Educational Opportunity
Air Products and Chemicals Grants, 319
Allstate Corp Giving Grants, 363
Allstate Corp Hometown Commitment Grants, 364
DaimlerChrysler Corp Fund Grants, 1186
Frances and John L. Loeb Family Fund Grants, 1546

Equal Employment Opportunity
Air Products and Chemicals Grants, 319
Allstate Corp Giving Grants, 363
Allstate Corp Hometown Commitment Grants, 364
DaimlerChrysler Corp Fund Grants, 1186

Equine Studies
Max Bell Fndn Grants, 2134

Equipment/Instrumentation
AHFMR Major Equipment Grants, 285
AMA Fndn Worldscopes Program, 399
Boeing Company Contributions Grants, 777
Cancer Research UK Grants, 859
Chatlos Fndn Grants, 977
Collins Fndn Grants, 1058
Covenant Fndn Grants, 1153
DOE Medical Applications and Measurement Science Grants, 1301
Dr. Scholl Fndn Grants, 1329
E.L. Wiegand Fndn Grants, 1361
Fritz B. Burns Fndn Grants, 1564
Gladys Brooks Fndn Grants, 1620
Hill Fndn Grants, 1774
Homer Fndn Grants, 1789
International Spinal Research Trust Grants, 1863
Jennings County Comm Fndn Grants, 1916
Ludwick Family Fndn Grants, 2084
NIGMS Integrative and Collaborative Approaches to Research Grants, 2615
Norwin S. and Elizabeth N. Bean Fndn Grants, 2872
NSF Doctoral Dissertation Improvement Grants in the Directorate for Biological Sciences, 2884
NSF Instrument Development for Biological Research, 2888
Potts Memorial Fndn Grants, 3072
Prudential Fndn Grants, 3087
RSC Thomas W. Eadie Medal, 3199
Saint Luke's Health Initiatives Grants, 3240
Schering-Plough Fndn Health Grants, 3270
South Madison Comm Fndn Grants, 3349
Square D Fndn Grants, 3361
St. Joseph Comm Health Fndn Burn Care and Prevention Grants, 3367
St. Joseph Comm Health Fndn Improving Healthcare Access Grants, 3368
St. Joseph Comm Health Fndn Pfeiffer Fund Grants, 3369
VDH Rescue Squad Assistance Fund Grants, 3484

Erythropoiesis
NIDDK Erythropoiesis: Components and Mechanisms Grants, 2558

Ethics
Alice Tweed Tuohy Fndn Grants, 357
Cargill Citizenship Fund-Corp Giving Grants, 865
Comm Fndn of Greater Flint Grants, 1107
DOE Health Effects and Life Sciences Research Grants, 1298
Graco Fndn Grants, 1642
James Hervey Johnson Charitable Educational Trust Grants, 1889
National Dairy Promotion and Research Board Scholarships, 2251
NFID Advanced Vaccinology Course Travel Grant, 2307
NIH Ethical Issues in Human Studies Research Grants, 2661
NIH Research On Ethical Issues In Human Subjects Research, 2712
Sarah Scaife Fndn Grants, 3263

Ethics/Values in Science and Technology
Affymetrix Corp Contributions Grants, 258
DOE Human Genome Program—Ethical, Legal, and Social Implications, 1299
RSC Abbyann D. Lynch Medal in Bioethics, 3195

Ethnology
Fyssen Fndn Postdoctoral Study Grants, 1580

Etiology
AACR Gertrude Elion Cancer Research Award, 76
Alzheimer's Association Everyday Technologies for Alzheimer Care Research Grants, 377
Alzheimer's Association Mentored New Investigator Research Grants to Promote Diversity, 379
Alzheimer's Association Molecular Imaging Grants, 380
Alzheimer's Association New Investigator Research Grants to Promote Diversity, 382
Alzheimer's Association Senator Mark Hatfield Award, 383
Alzheimer's Association Zenith Fellows Awards, 384
Alzheimer's Association Conference Grants, 385
IARC Expertise Transfer Fellowship, 1831
IARC Postdoctoral Fellowships for Training in Cancer Research, 1832
IARC Visiting Scientist Award for Senior Scientists, 1833
MDBD Basic Research Grants, 2152
NIA Alzheimer's Disease Core Centers Grants, 2395
NIH Genetic Susceptibility and Variability of Human Malformations Research Grants, 2669
NIH Xenobiotics and Cell Death/Injury in Neurodegenerative Disease Research Grants, 2739
NYAM Edward N. Gibbs Memorial Lecture and Award in Nephrology, 2912

Europe
Charles Delmar Fndn Grants, 963
Fulbright Traditional Scholar Program in Europe and Eurasia, 1572

Europe, Central
ASM-UNESCO Leadership Grant for International Educators, 626
Hamlet Trust Grants, 1689
UICC American Cancer Society International Fellowships for Beginning Investigators, 3455

Europe, Eastern
ASM-UNESCO Leadership Grant for International Educators, 626
Fulbright Traditional Scholar Program in Europe and Eurasia, 1572
Hamlet Trust Grants, 1689
International Oncology Nursing Fellowships, 1862
UICC American Cancer Society International Fellowships for Beginning Investigators, 3455

Evolutionary Biology
Alfred P. Sloan Fndn Research Fellowships, 353
NIGMS/NIDCR Evolution of Infectious Diseases Research Grants, 2633
NSF Doctoral Dissertation Improvement Grants in the Directorate for Biological Sciences, 2884
NSF Genes and Genome Systems Cluster Grants, 2886
NSF Systematic Biology and Biodiversity Inventories Grants, 2895

Exercise
Air Products and Chemicals Grants, 319
BCBSNC Fndn Grants, 725
Gebbie Fndn Grants, 1585
General Mills Champions for Healthy Kids Grants, 1589
Healthcare Fndn for Orange County Grants, 1728
Highmark Healthy High 5, 1770
NCI Improving Diet and Physical Activity Assessment Grants, 2275
NIAMS High Risk Arthritis and Musculoskeletal and Skin Diseases Research, 2470
NIAMS Research on Musculoskeletal Fitness and Sports Medicine Grants, 2476
NICHD Research on Musculoskeletal Fitness and Sports Medicine Grants, 2492
NINR Research on Musculoskeletal Fitness and Sports Medicine Grants, 2803
Paso del Norte Health Fndn Grants, 2995
United Methodist Health Ministry Fund Grants, 3465

Exhibitions, Collections, Performances
Greater Worcester Comm Fndn Jeppson Memorial Fund for Brookfield Grants, 1659
Principal Financial Group Fndn Grants, 3082

Eye Diseases
1976 Fndn Grants, 5
AHAF Macular Degeneration Research Grants, 267
Alice C. A. Sibley Fund Grants, 355
Columbus Fndn Competitive Grants, 1066
Compass Bank Fndn Grants, 1138
Donald and Sylvia Robinson Family Fndn Grants, 1310
E.A. Baker Fndn for the Prevention of Blindness Grants, 1357
E.L. Wiegand Fndn Grants, 1361
Fairlawn Fndn Grants, 1447
Fight for Sight Research Grants, 1502
Fight for Sight Research Grants and Fellowships, 1503
Glaucoma Fndn Grants, 1621
Glaucoma Research Pilot Project Grants, 1622
Larry L. Hillblom Fndn Grants, 2031
NEI Innovative Patient Outreach Programs And Ocular Screening Technologies To Improve Detection Of Diabetic Retinopathy Grants, 2294
NEI Scholars Program, 2298
NEI Translational Research Program On Therapy For Visual Disorders, 2299
OneSight Research Fndn Block Grants, 2944

Faculty Development
Beckman Young Investigators Grants, 735
BWF Institutional Program Unifying Population and Laboratory Based Sciences, 822
Carpenter Fndn Grants, 881
Dermatology Clinical Career Development Awards, 1235
Harold Amos Medical Faculty Development Program, 1696
HHMI/EMBO Start-up Grants for Central Europe, 1766
Humboldt Area Fndn Technical Assistance Program Grants, 1819
McGregor Fund Grants, 2143
MRC Career Establishment Grants, 2221
NHLBI Mentored Career Award For Faculty At Minority Institutions, 2346
PhRMA Fndn Health Outcomes Post Doctoral Fellowships, 3031
PhRMA Fndn Pharmaceutics Research Starter Grants, 3042
RCPSC Faculty Development Grants, 3117
Richard M. Fairbanks Fndn Grants, 3162
RWJF Generalist Physician Faculty Scholars, 3212
RWJF Harold Amos Medical Faculty Development Scholars, 3213
SNM Molecular Imaging Research Grant For Junior Medical Faculty, 3301
SNM Postdoctoral Molecular Imaging Scholar Grants, 3305

Familial Abuse
Adaptec Fndn Grants, 232
Ahmanson Fndn Grants, 303
California Endowment CommunitiesFirst Grants, 833
Comm Fndn of Broward Grants, 1100
Quantum Fndn Grants, 3096

Families
3M Fndn Grants, 11
ACF Ethnic Comm Self-Help Grants, 200
ACF Preferred Communities Grants, 201
Achelis and Bodman Fndns Grants, 206
ACS Pilot and Exploratory Projects in Palliative Care of Cancer Patients and Their Families Grants, 219
Actors Fund Social Services and Financial Assistance, 225
Acushnet Fndn Grants, 226
Adaptec Fndn Grants, 232
African American Fund of New Jersey Grants, 260
Agnes M. Lindsay Trust Grants, 263
Alcatel-Lucent Technologies Fndn Grants, 333
Alexander Eastman Fndn Grants, 341
Andersen Fndn Grants, 471
Anschutz Family Fndn Grants, 486
AptarGroup Fndn Grants, 522
Arizona Cardinals Grants, 529
Arizona Diamondbacks Charities Grants, 530
AT&T Fndn Civic and Comm Service Grants, 658
Atlanta Fndn Grants, 662
Auburn Fndn Grants, 664
Bank of America Client Fndn Grants, 690
Barberton Comm Fndn Grants, 693
Barker Welfare Fndn Grants, 695
Battle Creek Comm Fndn Grants, 703
Benton Comm Fndn Grants, 743
Berrien Comm Fndn Grants, 749
BJ's Charitable Fndn Grants, 761
Blackford County Comm Fndn Grants, 763
Blanche and Julian Robertson Family Fndn Grants, 765
Blue River Comm Fndn Grants, 770
Blumenthal Fndn Grants, 773
Bodenwein Public Benevolent Fndn Grants, 775
Bodman Fndn Grants, 776
Booth-Bricker Fund Grants, 780
Borkee-Hagley Fndn Grants, 781
Boston Fndn Grants, 783
Boston Globe Fndn Grants, 784
Bradley Turner Fndn Grants, 789
Brookdale Fndn Leadership in Aging Fellowships, 805
Brookdale Fndn National Group Respite and Early Memory Loss Grants, 806
Brown County Comm Fndn Grants, 807
Burlington Industries Fndn Grants, 811
Bush Fndn Health & Human Services Grants, 814
Cailloux Fndn Grants, 829
California Endowment CommunitiesFirst Grants, 833
Cargill Citizenship Fund-Corp Giving Grants, 865
Carlisle Fndn Grants, 874
Carpenter Fndn Grants, 881
Catherine Kennedy Home Fndn Grants, 890
Cemala Fndn Grants, 933
Central Carolina Comm Fndn Comm Impact Grants, 936
Central Okanagan Fndn Grants, 937
CharityWorks Grants, 961
Children's Trust Fund of Oregon Grants, 1001
Citizens Bank Mid-Atlantic Charitable Fndn Grants, 1015
Claude Worthington Benedum Fndn Grants, 1033
Clay Fndn Grants, 1034
Cleo Fndn Grants, 1035
Columbus Fndn Traditional Grants, 1071
Comer Fndn Grants, 1072
Comm Fndn for Greater Buffalo Grants, 1090
Comm Fndn of Bartholomew County Heritage Fund Grants, 1096
Comm Fndn of Bartholomew County James A. Henderson Award for Fund-Raising, 1097
Comm Fndn of Boone County Grants, 1099
Comm Fndn of Broward Grants, 1100
Comm Fndn of Central Illinois Grants, 1101
Comm Fndn of Greater Fort Wayne: Comm Endowment & Clarke Endowment Fund Grants, 1108
Comm Fndn of Greenville Comm Enrichment Grants, 1113

Comm Fndn of Greenville Hollingsworth Funds Program/Project Grants, 1114
Comm Fndn of Southeastern Connecticut Grants, 1125
Comm Impact Fund, 1135
Compass Bank Fndn Grants, 1138
Connecticut Comm Fndn Grants, 1141
Constantin Fndn Grants, 1145
Crail-Johnson Fndn Grants, 1157
CSRA Comm Fndn Grants, 1168
CSX Corp Contributions Grants, 1169
D.F. Halton Fndn Grants, 1181
Dairy Queen Corp Contributions Grants, 1187
Dammann Fund Grants, 1192
Daywood Fndn Grants, 1206
Delta Air Lines Fndn Grants, 1220
Dennis and Phyllis Washington Fndn Grants, 1222
Dept of Ed Special Education—Technical Assistance and Dissemination to Improve Services and Results for Children with Disabilities, 1233
DHHS Abandoned Infants Assistance Grants, 1242
DHHS Adolescent Family Life Demonstration Projects, 1243
DHHS Comprehensive Comm Mental Health Services Grants for Children with Serious Emotional Disturbances, 1247
DHHS HIV Demonstration Program for Children, Adolescents, and Women, 1262
DHHS Maternal and Child Health Research and Training Programs Grants, 1264
Donald and Sylvia Robinson Family Fndn Grants, 1310
Edina Realty Fndn Grants, 1369
Educational Fndn of America Grants, 1372
EIF Comm Grants, 1386
Eisner Fndn Grants, 1387
El Paso Comm Fndn Grants, 1388
Elsie Lee Garthwaite Memorial Fndn Grants, 1408
Emma B. Howe Memorial Fndn Grants, 1415
Entergy Comm Partnership Grants, 1417
EPA Children's Health Protection Grants, 1420
Eugene and Agnes E. Meyer Fndn Grants, 1432
Evanston Comm Fndn Grants, 1438
Express Scripts Fndn Grants, 1441
Fairfield County Comm Fndn Grants, 1446
Farmers Insurance Group of Companies Grants, 1455
FCD Child Development Grants, 1458
FCNY Union Square Awards, 1461
Fidelity Fndn Grants, 1498
Fifth Third Fndn Grants, 1501
Fisher House Fndn Newman's Own Awards, 1509
Florida BRAIVE Fund of Dade Comm Fndn, 1512
Florida BRAIVE Fund of Gulf Coast Comm Fndn of Venice, 1513
Florida BRAIVE Fund of The Comm Fndn in Jacksonville, 1514
Floyd A. and Kathleen C. Cailloux Fndn Grants, 1516
Foellinger Fndn Grants, 1519
Fndn for Seacoast Health Grants, 1533
Fndn for the Carolinas Grants, 1535
Fndn of CVPH Chelsea's Rainbow Fund Grants, 1539
Frey Fndn Grants, 1562
G.N. Wilcox Trust Grants, 1581
Gebbie Fndn Grants, 1585
General Mills Fndn Grants, 1590
George and Ruth Bradford Fndn Grants, 1595
George Kress Fndn Grants, 1601
Georgiana Goddard Eaton Memorial Fund Grants, 1604
Glazer Family Fndn Grants, 1625
Grand Rapids Comm Fndn Grants, 1647
H.J. Heinz Company Fndn Grants, 1682
Hagedorn Fund Grants, 1685
Harden Fndn Grants, 1693
Harold and Arlene Schnitzer CARE Fndn Grants, 1697
Harry Frank Guggenheim Fndn Research Grants, 1704
Hartford Courant Fndn Grants, 1710
Hasbro Children's Fund, 1714
Health Fndn of Greater Indianapolis Grants, 1725
Heckscher Fndn for Children Grants, 1732
Helen Bader Fndn Grants, 1738
Helen Steiner Rice Fndn Grants, 1742
Henrietta Tower Wurts Memorial Fndn Grants, 1745
Horizons Comm Issues Grants, 1794
Howard and Bush Fndn Grants, 1798
Hugh J. Andersen Fndn Grants, 1814
Hut Fndn Grants, 1827
Hutton Fndn Grants, 1828
Impact 100 Grants, 1843
J.C. Penney Company Grants, 1874
Jacob and Hilda Blaustein Fndn Grants, 1881
Jacob and Valeria Langeloth Fndn Grants, 1882
Jacob G. Schmidlapp Trust Grants, 1883
James A. and Faith Knight Fndn Grants, 1884
James M. Cox Fndn of Georgia Grants, 1892
James R. Dougherty Jr. Fndn Grants, 1894
Jane Bradley Pettit Fndn Grants, 1902
Janirve Fndn Grants, 1905
Jay and Rose Phillips Family Fndn Grants, 1909
Jim Moran Fndn Grants, 1925
John P. McGovern Fndn Grants, 1942
Johnson & Johnson Corp Contributions Grants, 1952
Josiah Macy Jr. Fndn Grants, 1966
Kahuku Comm Fund, 1977
Kalamazoo Fndn Grants, 1979
Kansas Health Fndn Grants, 1980
Kimberly-Clark Comm Grants, 2001
Lands' End Corp Giving Program, 2030
Lesbian Health Fund Grants, 2046
Louis Calder Fndn Grants, 2065
Lucile Horton Howe and Mitchell B. Howe Fndn Grants, 2081
M.B. and Edna Zale Fndn Grants, 2093
Margaret T. Morris Fndn Grants, 2105
Marshall Field's Comm Grants, 2115
Mary Owen Borden Fndn Grants, 2121
McGregor Fund Grants, 2143
McKesson Fndn Grants, 2145
McKnight Fndn Grants, 2146
Metrowest Comm Health Care Fndn Grants, 2176
Minneapolis Fndn Comm Grants, 2206
Miriam and Peter Haas Fund Grants, 2208
Morris and Gwendolyn Cafritz Fndn Grants, 2217
NAPNAP Fndn Graduate Student Research Grant, 2236
Newman's Own Inc Grants, 2306
NIA Multicenter Study on Exceptional Survival in Families: The Long Life Family Study Grants, 2420
NIA Symptom Management for Chronic Neurological Conditions Research Grants, 2436
NICHD Population Research Grants, 2490
NICHD Symptom Management for Chronic Neurological Conditions Research Grants, 2496
Nicholas H. Noyes Jr. Memorial Fndn Grants, 2497
NIDCD Symptom Management for Chronic Neurological Conditions Research Grants, 2532
NIDRR Field-Initiated Projects, 2594
NIH Supplements to Promote Reentry into Biomedical and Behavioral Research Careers, 2733
NIMH/NIDA Children's Services Grants, 2775
Nina Mason Pulliam Charitable Trust Grants, 2776
NINDS Symptom Management for Chronic Neurological Conditions Research Grants, 2787
NINR Symptom Management for Chronic Neurological Conditions Research Grants, 2805
Northwestern Mutual Fndn Grants, 2870
Nuffield Fndn Children and Families Grants, 2899
NYCT Girls and Young Women Grants, 2924
NYCT Substance Abuse Grants, 2928
Ohio County Comm Fndn Grants, 2938
Ohio County Comm Fndn Mini-Grants, 2939
Oleonda Jameson Trust Grants, 2941
Ordean Fndn Grants, 2952
PacifiCare Fndn Grants, 2981
Paul and Mary Haas Fndn Contributions and Student Scholarships, 2997
Paul G. Duke Fndn Grants, 3001
Perpetual Trust for Charitable Giving Grants, 3015
Peter and Elizabeth C. Tower Fndn Comm Grants, 3018
Philadelphia Fndn Organizational Effectiveness Grants, 3029
Phoenix Suns Charities Grants, 3030
Piper Jaffray Companies Building Strong Communities Grants, 3053
Pittsburgh Fndn Comm Fund Grants, 3054
Plough Fndn Grants, 3061
Polk Bros. Fndn Grants, 3066
Portland General Electric Fndn Grants, 3067
Posey Comm Fndn Womens Fund Grants, 3069
Pride Fndn Grants and Scholarships, 3078
Prince Charitable Trusts District of Columbia Grants, 3080
Prudential Fndn Grants, 3087
Rainbow Endowment Grants, 3102
Raymond John Wean Fndn Grants, 3110
Rayonier Fndn Grants, 3111
Rhode Island Fndn Grants, 3154
Richard and Helen DeVos Fndn Grants, 3157
Richard King Mellon Fndn Grants, 3161
Robins Fndn Grants, 3175
Rochester Area Comm Fndn Grants, 3176
Rosalynn Carter Institute Georgia Caregiver of the Year Awards, 3188
Ruth H. and Warren A. Ellsworth Fndn Grants, 3203
S. Livingston Mather Charitable Trust Grants, 3235
S. Mark Taper Fndn Grants, 3236
S.H. Cowell Fndn Grants, 3237
Scott County Comm Fndn Grants, 3273
Seabury Fndn Grants, 3274
Simmons Fndn Grants, 3287
Sisters of Saint Joseph Charitable Fund Grants, 3296
Southwire Company Grants, 3353
Taproot Fndn Capacity-Building Service Grants, 3417
Thompson Charitable Fndn Grants, 3425
U.S. Department of Education Special Education—National Activities—Parent Information Centers, 3450
Vancouver Fndn Grants and Comm Initiatives Program, 3477
Viking Children's Fund Grants, 3497
Volkswagen of America Corp Contributions Grants, 3503
Vulcan Materials Company Fndn Grants, 3504
W.K. Kellogg Fndn Secure Families Grants, 3508
Waitt Family Fndn Grants, 3512
Wal-Mart Fndn Comm Grants, 3513
Wayne and Gladys Valley Fndn Grants, 3522
William G. Gilmore Fndn Grants, 3537
Women's Fndn of California Comm Action Fund, 3549

Family Planning
Allyn Fndn Grants, 365
Atkinson Fndn International Grants, 661
Cowles Charitable Trust Grants, 1155
DHHS Adolescent Family Life Demonstration Projects, 1243
Donald and Sylvia Robinson Family Fndn Grants, 1310
Frances and John L. Loeb Family Fund Grants, 1546
Health Fndn of Greater Indianapolis Grants, 1725
Huber Fndn Grants, 1812
J.W. Kieckhefer Fndn Grants, 1878
Jacob and Hilda Blaustein Fndn Grants, 1881
James Ford Bell Fndn Grants, 1885
Mary Owen Borden Fndn Grants, 2121
NICHD Population Research Grants, 2490
Pasadena Fndn Average Grants, 2994
Perkins Charitable Fndn Grants, 3014
Richard and Rhoda Goldman Fund Grants, 3158
Robert Sterling Clark Fndn Reproductive Rights and Health Grants, 3173
S. Livingston Mather Charitable Trust Grants, 3235
S.H. Cowell Fndn Grants, 3237
Saint Luke's Health Initiatives Grants, 3240
Samuel S. Johnson Fndn Grants, 3251
Seabury Fndn Grants, 3274
Susan Vaughan Fndn Grants, 3413
Union Benevolent Association Grants, 3460
W. C. Griffith Fndn Grants, 3505
Women's Fndn of California Grants, 3550

Family Practice
AAFP Fndn Health Literacy State Grants, 112
AAFP Fndn Joint Grants, 113
AAFP Fndn Pfizer Teacher Development Awards, 114
AAFP Fndn Wyeth Immunization Awards, 115
AAFP Research Stimulation Grants, 116
ACS Cancer Control Career Development Awards for Primary Care Physicians, 209
CFPC Family Medicine Resident Leadership Awards, 953
CFPC Family Physician of the Year Award, 954
CFPC Fellowships, 955
CFPC Research and Education Fndn Grants, 956
CFPC Special Recognition Awards, 957
DHHS Geriatric Training for Physicians and Dentists Grants, 1250
DHHS National Health Service Corps Loan Repayment Awards, 1265
Dorothy Rider Pool Health Care Grants, 1322
Josiah Macy Jr. Fndn Grants, 1966
Pfizer/AAFP Fndn Visiting Professorship Program in Family Medicine, 3027
Regenstrief Geriatrics Fellowship, 3143

Family, Social Services
Sunderland Fndn Grants, 3400

Family/Marriage Counseling
DHHS Promoting Safe and Stable Families Grants, 1276
Florida BRAIVE Fund of Dade Comm Fndn, 1512
Florida BRAIVE Fund of Gulf Coast Comm Fndn of Venice, 1513
Florida BRAIVE Fund of The Comm Fndn in Jacksonville, 1514
NIDA Behavioral Therapies Development Grants, 2499

Farm and Ranch Management
Pajaro Valley Comm Health Grants, 2985
Pioneer Hi-Bred Comm Grants, 3051

Fatigue/Fracture
NIA Bioenergetics, Fatigability, and Activity Limitations in Aging, 2402
NIA Transdisciplinary Research on Fatigue and Fatigability in Aging Grants, 2438

Federal Government
APA Congressional Fellowships, 492
APSA Congressional Fellowships Health and Aging Policy Fellows Program, 514
APSA Robert Wood Johnson Fndn Health Policy Fellowships, 515
GEICO Public Service Awards, 1586
Pittsburgh Fndn Comm Fund Grants, 3054

Fellowship Programs, General
AACAP Jeanne Spurlock Research Fellowship in Substance Abuse and Addiction for Minority Medical Students, 40
AACAP Summer Medical Student Fellowships, 53
AACAP-NIDA K12 Career Development Awards, 55
AACR Centennial Pre-doctoral Fellowships in Cancer Research, 72
AACR-Colorectal Cancer Coalition Fellows Grant, 92
AFAR Medical Student Training in Aging Research Program, 255
AHRQ Individual Awards for Postdoctoral Fellows Ruth L. Kirschstein National Research Service Awards, 314
Alexander von Humboldt Fndn Georg Forster Fellowships for Experienced Researchers, 344
Alexander von Humboldt Fndn Georg Forster Fellowships for Postdoctoral Researchers, 345
AMA-MSS Government Relations Advocacy Fellowship, 403
American Academy of Nursing Claire M. Fagin Fellowships, 415
American College of Surgeons Australia and New Zealand Chapter Travelling Fellowships, 423
American College of Surgeons Nizar N. Oweida, MD, FACS, Scholarships, 430
American College of Surgeons Wound Care Management Award, 433
APSA Congressional Fellowships Health and Aging Policy Fellows Program, 514
APSA Robert Wood Johnson Fndn Health Policy Fellowships, 515
ASCO Long-Term International Fellowships, 556
ASM Congressional Science Fellowships, 590
ASM International Fellowship for Latin America and the Caribbean, 601
ASM International Fellowships for Asia and Africa, 602
ASM Microbiology Undergraduate Research Fellowship, 607
ASM Robert D. Watkins Graduate Research Fellowship, 614
ASM Undergraduate Research Fellowship, 622
ASM-PAHO Infectious Diseases Epidemiology and Surveillance Fellowships, 625
ASM/CCID Fellowships, 627
ASPO Fellowships, 651
Brookdale Fndn Leadership in Aging Fellowships, 805
Carrier Corp Contributions Grants, 884
Charles H. Revson Fndn Grants, 969
CLA Physiotherapy Cardio-Respiratory Society Fellowships, 1020
CMAP Physician Advocacy Fellowship, 1043
Duke University Adult Cardiothoracic Anesthesia and Critical Care Medicine Fellowships, 1340
Duke University Ambulatory and Regional Anesthesia Fellowships, 1341
Duke University Clinical Cardiac Electrophysiology Fellowships, 1342
Duke University Hyperbaric Center Fellowships, 1343
Duke University Interventional Cardiology Fellowships, 1344
Duke University Obstetric Anesthesia Fellowships, 1345
Duke University Pain Management Fellowships, 1346
Duke University Pediatric Anesthesiology Fellowship, 1347
Duke University Postdoctoral Research Fellowships in Aging, 1348
EMBO Long-Term Fellowships, 1410
EMBO Short-Term Fellowships, 1411
Fritz B. Burns Fndn Grants, 1564
Lynde and Harry Bradley Fndn Grants, 2089
Lynde and Harry Bradley Fndn Prizes: Bradley Prizes, 2090
MAP International Medical Fellowships, 2101
Marine Biological Laboratory Summer Research Fellowships, 2108
Mead Johnson Nutritionals Scholarships, 2159
MedImmune Charitable Grants, 2166
MGFA Post-Doctoral Research Fellowships, 2183
MGFA Student Fellowships, 2184
NCCAM Ruth L. Kirschstein National Research Service Awards for Postdoctoral Training in Complementary and Alternative Medicine, 2266
NFID John P. Utz Medical Mycology Postdoctoral Fellowship, 2309
NFID Nosocomial Infection Research and Training Postdoctoral Fellowship, 2311
NHLBI Individual Predoctoral Fellowships to Promote Diversity in Health-Related Research, 2341
NHLBI National Research Service Awards for Senior Fellowships, 2358
NIH National Research Service Awards—Senior Fellows, 2697
NIH Ruth L. Kirschstein National Research Service Awards for Individual Senior Fellows, 2718
NIH Ruth L. Kirschstein National Research Service Awards for Individual Predoctoral Fellowships to Promote Diversity in Health-Related Research, 2721
NIH Ruth L. Kirschstein National Research Service Awards for Individual Predoctoral MD/PhD and Other Dual Doctoral Degree Fellows, 2722
NINR Ruth L. Kirschstein National Research Service Award for Individual Predoctoral Fellows in Nursing Research, 2804
NMF General Electric Medical Scholars Fellowships, 2830
Northwood University/Alden B. Dow Creativity Center Summer Residency Program, 2871
NSF Postdoctoral Research Fellowships in Biology, 2891
Pancreatic Cancer Action Network-AACR Fellowship, 2987
PDF Postdoctoral Fellowships for Basic Scientists, 3006
PDF Postdoctoral Fellowships for Neurologists, 3007
PDF Summer Fellowships, 3008
PDF-AANF Clinician-Scientist Development Awards, 3009
PhRMA Fndn Health Outcomes Pre-Doctoral Fellowships, 3032
PhRMA Fndn Health Outcomes Sabbatical Fellowships, 3034
PhRMA Fndn Informatics Sabbatical Fellowships, 3035
PhRMA Fndn Paul Calabresi Medical Student Research Fellowship, 3039
Potts Memorial Fndn Grants, 3072
Regenstrief Geriatrics Fellowship, 3143
Regenstrief General Internal Medicine - General Pediatrics Research Fellowship Program, 3144
Rhode Island Fndn Grants, 3154
RWJF Clinical Scholars Grants, 3207
RWJF Executive Nurse Fellowships, 3210
RWJF Generalist Physician Faculty Scholars, 3212
RWJF Health & Society Scholars, 3214
RWJF Ladder to Leadership: Developing the Next Generation of Comm Health Leaders Fellowships, 3222
RWJF Scholars in Health Policy Research Fellowships, 3229
Siragusa Fndn Health Services & Medical Research Grants, 3294
SRC Medical Research Grants, 3362
St. Joseph Comm Health Fndn Schneider Fellowships, 3370
Stroke Association Clinical Fellowships, 3386
UCLA/RAND Corp Post-Doctoral Fellowships, 3454

Fermentation
NSF Chemical, Biochemical, and Biotechnology Systems Research Grants, 2882

Fetus Research
Elizabeth Glaser Pediatric AIDS Fndn International Leadership Awards, 1393
Elizabeth Glaser Pediatric AIDS Fndn Operations Research Grants, 1394
Elizabeth Glaser Pediatric AIDS Fndn Two-Year International Scholar Award, 1396
MRC Career Establishment Grants, 2221
NIH Research on Sleep and Sleep Disorders, 2713

Film Production
Canada-U.S. Fulbright New Century Scholars Grants, 846
Canada-U.S. Fulbright Senior Specialists Grants, 847
Comm Fndn of Greater Greensboro Grants, 1109
Fulbright Alumni Initiatives Awards Grants, 1566
Fulbright Distinguished Chairs Grants, 1567
Fulbright New Century Scholars Grants, 1570
Fulbright Specialists Grants, 1571
Fulbright Traditional Scholar Program in Europe and Eurasia, 1572
Fulbright Traditional Scholar Program in Sub-Saharan Africa, 1573
Fulbright Traditional Scholar Program in the East Asia/Pacific Region, 1574

Fulbright Traditional Scholar Program in the Near East and North Africa Region, 1575
Fulbright Traditional Scholar Program in the South and Central Asia Region, 1576
Fulbright Traditional Scholar Program in the Western Hemisphere, 1577
NLM Grants for Scholarly Works in Biomedicine and Health, 2818

Finance
Alcatel-Lucent Technologies Corp Contributions Grants, 332
John R. Oishei Fndn Grants, 1944
Lincoln Financial Group Fndn Grants, 2058
Paul and Mary Haas Fndn Contributions and Student Scholarships, 2997

Financial Aid (Scholarships and Loans)
ASM Robert D. Watkins Graduate Research Fellowship, 614
Indiana Minority Teacher/Special Services Scholarships, 1852
Indiana Nursing Scholarships, 1853
John H. Wellons Fndn Grants, 1934
K21 Health Fndn Cancer Care Fund Grants, 1975

Financial Education
Key Fndn Grants, 1994
New York Life Fndn Grants, 2304

Fine Arts
Abell-Hanger Fndn Grants, 183
Berks County Comm Fndn Grants, 745
Bodenwein Public Benevolent Fndn Grants, 775
E.L. Wiegand Fndn Grants, 1361
Gilroy and Lillian P. Roberts Charitable Fndn Grants, 1614
Harry and Grace Steele Fndn Grants, 1702
Puerto Rico Comm Fndn Grants, 3090
R.C. Baker Fndn Grants, 3098

Fire Prevention
Burlington Northern Santa Fe Fndn Grants, 812
DOL Occupational Safety and Health—Susan Harwood Training Grants, 1305
Francis T. & Louise T. Nichols Fndn Grants, 1550
GEICO Public Service Awards, 1586
Seneca Foods Fndn Grants, 3278
Thompson Charitable Fndn Grants, 3425

Fish and Fisheries
RSC Thomas W. Eadie Medal, 3199
Thrasher Research Fund Grants, 3426

Fitness
Anthem Blue Cross and Blue Shield School Nurse Grants, 489
BCBSNC Fndn Fit Together Grants, 724
BCBSNC Fndn Grants, 725
Boeing Company Contributions Grants, 777
Fndn for a Healthy Kentucky Grants, 1527
GoGirlGo! Ambassador Team Awards, 1632
Hanna Andersson Children's Fndn Grants, 1691
King Pharmaceuticals Corp Contributions Grants, 2003
Mary Black Fndn Grants, 2118
Medtronic Fndn Fitness and Nutrition Grants, 2167
Moses Cone-Wesley Long Comm Health Fndn Grants, 2219
Ruth Mott Fndn Grants, 3204

Folk/Ethnic Arts
Comm Fndn of Western North Carolina Grants, 1132

Folklore and Mythology
Canada-U.S. Fulbright New Century Scholars Grants, 846
Canada-U.S. Fulbright Senior Specialists Grants, 847
Fulbright Alumni Initiatives Awards Grants, 1566
Fulbright Distinguished Chairs Grants, 1567
Fulbright New Century Scholars Grants, 1570
Fulbright Specialists Grants, 1571
Fulbright Traditional Scholar Program in Europe and Eurasia, 1572
Fulbright Traditional Scholar Program in Sub-Saharan Africa, 1573
Fulbright Traditional Scholar Program in the East Asia/Pacific Region, 1574
Fulbright Traditional Scholar Program in the Near East and North Africa Region, 1575
Fulbright Traditional Scholar Program in the South and Central Asia Region, 1576
Fulbright Traditional Scholar Program in the Western Hemisphere, 1577

Food Analysis
DOA National Integrated Food Safety Initiative, 1289

Food Banks
Anthony R. Abraham Fndn Grants, 490
Batchelor Fndn Grants, 701
Bildner Family Fndn Grants, 755
Catherine Kennedy Home Fndn Grants, 890
Cessna Fndn Grants, 938
Daphne Seybolt Culpeper Memorial Fndn Grants, 1201
Denver Fndn Comm Grants, 1227
Edina Realty Fndn Grants, 1369
Frank Stanley Beveridge Fndn Grants, 1553
Green Bay Packers Fndn Grants, 1660
Independence Comm Fndn Comm Quality of Life Grant, 1849
Kenneth T. and Eileen L. Norris Fndn Grants, 1989
Lincoln Financial Group Fndn Grants, 2058
Newman's Own Inc Grants, 2306
Northwestern Mutual Fndn Grants, 2870
Ordean Fndn Grants, 2952
Pott Fndn Grants, 3071
Procter and Gamble Fund Grants, 3083
Samuel S. Johnson Fndn Grants, 3251
Shaw's Supermarkets Donations, 3280
Stewart Huston Charitable Trust Grants, 3384
Vancouver Fndn Grants and Comm Initiatives Program, 3477

Food Consumption
Anthem Blue Cross and Blue Shield School Nurse Grants, 489
Coca-Cola Fndn Grants, 1052
General Mills Champions for Healthy Kids Grants, 1589
Kraft Cares US Grants, 2017

Food Distribution
Albertson's Charitable Giving Grants, 330
Bacon Family Fndn Grants, 679
Benton Comm Fndn Grants, 743
Blackford County Comm Fndn Grants, 763
Blue River Comm Fndn Grants, 770
Brown County Comm Fndn Grants, 807
Catherine Kennedy Home Fndn Grants, 890
Chicago Comm Trust Grants, 989
Clark Fndn Grants, 1029
CNCS Foster Grandparent Projects Grants, 1048
Commission on Religion in Appalachia Grants, 1074
Comm Fndn of Bartholomew County Heritage Fund Grants, 1096
Comm Fndn of Bartholomew County James A. Henderson Award for Fund-Raising, 1097
Comm Fndn of Boone County Grants, 1099
Comm Fndn of Greater Fort Wayne: Comm Endowment & Clarke Endowment Fund Grants, 1108
DeRoy Testamentary Fndn Grants, 1239
Donald and Sylvia Robinson Family Fndn Grants, 1310
Doris and Victor Day Fndn Grants, 1313
General Mills Fndn Grants, 1590
Harden Fndn Grants, 1693
John Edward Fowler Memorial Fndn Grants, 1930
John G. Martin Fndn Grants, 1932
Ken W. Davis Fndn Grants, 1987
McGregor Fund Grants, 2143
NYCT Grants for the Elderly, 2925
PacifiCare Fndn Grants, 2981
Prince Charitable Trusts District of Columbia Grants, 3080
Rockefeller Fndn Grants, 3181
Sid W. Richardson Fndn Grants, 3284
Starr Fndn Grants, 3377
Thomas C. Ackerman Fndn Grants, 3423
Tri-County Electric People Fund Grants, 3436
W.K. Kellogg Fndn Healthy Kids Grants, 3507

Food Engineering
NSF-NIST Interaction in Chemistry, Materials Research, Molecular Biosciences, Bioengineering, and Chemical Engineering, 2897

Food Management
Adolph Coors Fndn Grants, 238

Food Preparation
CDC National Programs That Build the Capacity of Schools To Prevent Foodborne Illness Through Coordinated School Health Programs, 919

Food Processing
CDC National Programs That Build the Capacity of Schools To Prevent Foodborne Illness Through Coordinated School Health Programs, 919
Institute for Agriculture and Trade Policy Food and Society Fellowships, 1856
NSF Chemical, Biochemical, and Biotechnology Systems Research Grants, 2882

Food Safety
BCBS of Minnesota Healthy Together Grants, 712
CDC National Programs That Build the Capacity of Schools To Prevent Foodborne Illness Through Coordinated School Health Programs, 919
Dean Foods Comm Involvement Grants, 1209
DOA National Integrated Food Safety Initiative, 1289
NSF Chemical, Biochemical, and Biotechnology Systems Research Grants, 2882

Food Sciences
Canada Graduate Scholarships and NSERC Postgraduate Scholarships, 845
Coca-Cola Fndn Grants, 1052
Food, Pharmaceutical, and Bioengineering Division Award in Chemical Engineering, 1521

Food Service Industry
Roy and Christine Sturgis Trust Grants, 3191

Food Technology
CLIF Bar Family Fndn Grants, 1040
Food, Pharmaceutical, and Bioengineering Division Award in Chemical Engineering, 1521
Stephen S. Chang Award, 3382

Foods
AAAAI Research Award Grants, 25
CDC National Programs That Build the Capacity of Schools To Prevent Foodborne Illness Through Coordinated School Health Programs, 919
CLIF Bar Family Fndn Grants, 1040
Columbus Fndn Traditional Grants, 1071
Dean Foods Comm Involvement Grants, 1209
Institute for Agriculture and Trade Policy Food and Society Fellowships, 1856
Seneca Foods Fndn Grants, 3278
Simmons Fndn Grants, 3287
Soy Health Research Program Incentive Awards, 3354

Football
Arizona Cardinals Grants, 529
Green Bay Packers Fndn Grants, 1660
Viking Children's Fund Grants, 3497

Forest Products Industry
Simpson Fund Grants, 3290

Forestry Management
Comm Fndn of Western North Carolina Grants, 1132
RSC Thomas W. Eadie Medal, 3199

Forests and Woodlands
Canada Graduate Scholarships and NSERC Postgraduate Scholarships, 845
Eugene B. Casey Fndn Grants, 1433
Simpson Fund Grants, 3290

Fossil Fuels
Joyce Fndn Grants, 1969

Foster Care
Comm Fndn of Broward Grants, 1100
Educational Fndn of America Grants, 1372
Eisner Fndn Grants, 1387
i2 Fndn Grants, 1829
Michael and Susan Dell Fndn Grants, 2189
Pew Charitable Trusts Children & Youth Grants, 3020
Taproot Fndn Capacity-Building Service Grants, 3417

Fruits
DOA National Integrated Food Safety Initiative, 1289

Fund-Raising
Aetna Fndn Sponsorships Grants in Connecticut, 251
North Carolina Biotechnology Center Grantsmanship Training Grants, 2853

Gambling
Boyd Gaming Corp Contributions Program, 788
NIH Pathological Gambling: Basic, Clinical, and Services Research Grants, 2702

Gangs
ACF Standing Announcement for Unaccompanied Alien Children Grants, 202
DOJ Gang-Free Schools and Communities Intervention Grants, 1303
eBay Fndn Comm Grants, 1363
FAR Fund, 1453

Gastroenterology
ASGE / ConMed Award for Outstanding Manuscript by a Fellow/Resident, 564
ASGE Don Wilson Award, 565
ASGE Endoscopic Research Awards, 566
ASGE Endoscopic Research Career Development Awards, 567
ASGE Given Capsule Endoscopy Research Award, 568
CFF First- and Second-Year Clinical Fellowships, 943
Elizabeth Glaser Pediatric AIDS Fndn International Leadership Awards, 1393
Elizabeth Glaser Pediatric AIDS Fndn Operations Research Grants, 1394
Elizabeth Glaser Pediatric AIDS Fndn Two-Year International Scholar Award, 1396
FDHN Bridging Grants, 1464
FDHN Centocor International Research Fellowship in Gastrointestinal Inflammation & Immunology, 1465
FDHN Designated Outcomes Award in Geriatric Gastroenterology, 1466
FDHN Designated Research Award in Geriatric Gastroenterology, 1467
FDHN Designated Research Award in Research Related to Pancreatitis, 1468
FDHN Fellow Abstract Prizes, 1469
FDHN Fellowship to Faculty Transition Awards, 1470
FDHN Funderburg Research Scholar Award in Gastric Biology Related to Cancer, 1471
FDHN Graduate Student Awards, 1472
FDHN Jon I. Isenberg International Research Scholar Award, 1473
FDHN June & Donald O. Castell MD, Esophageal Clinical Research Award, 1474
FDHN Moti L. & Kamla Rustgi International Travel Awards, 1475
FDHN Non-Career Research Awards, 1476
FDHN Non-Career Research Grants, 1477
FDHN Research Scholar Awards, 1478
FDHN Student Research Fellowships, 1480
FDHN TAP Endowed Designated Research Award in Acid-Related Diseases, 1481
FDHN Translational Research Awards, 1482
Mayo Fndn Multidisciplinary Training in Digestive Diseases Research Grants, 2140
NFID New Investigator Matching Grants, 2310
Rett Syndrome Research Fndn Grants, 3151

Gender Equity
Cambridge Comm Fndn Grants, 837
Dallas Women's Fndn Grants, 1191
OUT Fund for Lesbian and Gay Liberation Grants, 2978
Women's Fndn of California Grants, 3550

Gene Regulation
NIDDK Co-Activators and Co-Repressors in Gene Expression Grants, 2546

Gene Therapy
ACGT Investigators Grants, 204

Genetic Counseling
DHHS Maternal and Child Health Projects Grants, 1263

Genetic Manipulation
Hunter's Hope Fndn Grants, 1820

Genetics
AFAR CART Fund Grants, 254
AFAR Research Grants, 257
Affymetrix Corp Contributions Grants, 258
Barth Syndrome Fndn Research Grants, 700
Cancer Treatment Research Fndn Clinical Investigation Grants, 861
Cardiac Arrhythmias Research and Education Fndn Research Grants, 863
CDC Using Genetic Information to Prevent Disease and Improve Health Research Grants, 932
Charles H. Hood Fndn Child Health Research Grants, 968
Dana Fndn Science and Health Grants, 1197
Deafness Research Fndn Research Grants, 1208
Del E. Webb Fndn Grants, 1213
DOE Human Genome Program—Ethical, Legal, and Social Implications, 1299
Dr. John T. Macdonald Fndn Grants, 1327
Dr. Scholl Fndn Grants, 1329
EF Predoctoral Research Training Fellowship, 1383
Elizabeth Glaser Pediatric AIDS Fndn International Leadership Awards, 1393
Elizabeth Glaser Pediatric AIDS Fndn Operations Research Grants, 1394
Elizabeth Glaser Pediatric AIDS Fndn Two-Year International Scholar Award, 1396
ExxonMobil Grants, 1442
Fannie E. Rippel Fndn Grants, 1452
Fragile X Syndrome Postdoctoral Research Fellowships Program, 1545
Glaucoma Research Pilot Project Grants, 1622
Gruber Fndn International Prizes, 1672
Hawaii Comm Fndn Health Education and Research Grants, 1716
Hereditary Disease Fndn John J. Wasmuth Postdoctoral Fellowships, 1750
Hereditary Disease Fndn Lieberman Award, 1751
Hereditary Disease Fndn Research Grants, 1752
Jackson Laboratory Postdoctoral Research Training Program, 1880
Leland McSpadden Memorial Fund for Medical and Scientific Research Grants, 2041
LRF New Investigator Leukemia Research Grants, 2070
MDBD Basic Research Grants, 2152
MDBD Research Grants and Basil O'Connor Starter Scholar Award Program, 2153
Milton Wexler Postdoctoral Fellowships, 2205
MRC Career Establishment Grants, 2221
National MPS Society Grants, 2257
NCI/NIDA Transdisciplinary Tobacco Use Research Centers Grants, 2280
NEI Clinical Vision Research Development Award, 2293
NFX Patient-Oriented Research Grants, 2313
NFX Summer Research Fellowships, 2314
NHGRI Mentored Research Scientist Development Award, 2315
NHLBI Pediatric Cardiac Genomics Consortium Grants, 2364
NIA Effects of Gene-Social Environment Interplay on Health and Behavior in Later Life Grants, 2404
NIA Nathan Shock Centers of Excellence in Basic Biology of Aging Grants, 2421
NIAID Preparedness against Illegitimate Use of Bacterial Pathogens, 2461
NICHD Innovative Therapies and Clinical Studies for Screenable Disorders Grants, 2485
NIDA Microarray-Based Research on Drug Abuse, 2508
NIDCD Mentored Research Scientist Development Award, 2523
NIDCD Neurobiology and Genetics of Autism Grants, 2526
NIDCR International Collaborative Oral Health Research Planning Grant, 2536
NIDDK Cell-Specific Delineation of Prostate and Genitourinary Development, 2545
NIDDK Co-Activators and Co-Repressors in Gene Expression Grants, 2546
NIDDK Erythroid Lineage Molecular Toolbox Grants, 2557
NIDDK Race/Ethnic Disparities in the Incidence of Diabetes Complications, 2579
NIEHS Biological Response to Environmental Health Hazards Research Grants, 2596
NIEHS Carcinogenicity of Drinking Water Disinfection By-Products, 2597
NIEHS Structure-Function Relationships of Environmentally Relevant Genetic Variants Research Grants, 2606
NIEHS/NINDS Role of the Environment in Parkinson's Disease, 2608
NIGMS Fellowships in Quantitative Biology, 2610
NIGMS Integrative and Collaborative Approaches to Research Grants, 2615
NIGMS Pharmacogenomics Research Network Grants, 2623
NIGMS Predoctoral Training in Bioinformatics and Computation Biology Grants, 2625
NIGMS Short Courses on Mathematical and Statistical Tools for the Study of Complex Phenotypes and Complex Systems, 2628
NIGMS Short Courses on Mathematical, Statistical, and Computational Tools for Studying Biological Systems, 2629
NIH Biobehavioral Pain Research Grants, 2638
NIH Fine Mapping and Function of Genes for Type 1 Diabetes Grants, 2667
NIH Genetic Architecture of Complex Phenotypes, 2668
NIH Genetic Susceptibility and Variability of Human Malformations Research Grants, 2669
NIH Genetics of Neurobehavioral Disorders in Existing Samples Grants, 2670
NIH Individual Postdoctoral Fellowships in Genomics and Related ELSI Topics, 2678
NIH Mechanisms Underlying Individual Variations in Drug Responses, 2685
NIH Molecular Epidemiology of Prostate Carcinogenesis Grants, 2691

NIH Mouse Mutagenesis and Phenotyping: Developmental Defects Research Grants, 2692
NIH National Occupational Research Agenda Grants, 2696
NIH Pathological Gambling: Basic, Clinical, and Services Research Grants, 2702
NIH Rett Syndrome: Genetics, Pathophysiology, and Biomarkers Research Grants, 2715
NIH Studies of Ethical, Legal, and Social Implications of Research into Human Genetic Variation Grants, 2731
NIH Xenobiotics and Cell Death/Injury in Neurodegenerative Disease Research Grants, 2739
NIMH Behavior Genetics in Adulthood and Old Age Research Grants, 2747
NIMH Short Courses on Mathematical and Statistical Tools for the Study of Complex Phenotypes and Complex Systems, 2770
NINR Opportunities in Genetics and Nursing Research Grants, 2801
NINR/NHGRI Nursing and Genetics Research Individual Postdoctoral and Senior Fellowships, 2806
NIOSH Occupational Safety and Health Research and Demonstration Grants, 2807
NSF Genes and Genome Systems Cluster Grants, 2886
Osteogenesis Imperfecta Fndn Research Grants, 2975
Parker B. Francis Fellowships in Pulmonary Research, 2989
PhRMA Fndn Informatics Sabbatical Fellowships, 3035
Rett Syndrome Research Fndn Grants, 3151
Searle Scholars Grants, 3275
Sigrid Juselius Fndn Grants, 3286
Starr Fndn Grants, 3377
Susan G. Komen Breast Cancer Fndn Basic, Clinical, and Translational Research Grants, 3407
Tourette Syndrome Association Post-Doc Fellowships, 3432
Tourette Syndrome Association Research Grants, 3433
TSA Research Grant Awards, 3442
US CRDF Leishmaniasis: Collaborative Research Opportunities in North Africa and the Middle East, 3474

Genetics, Molecular
GPP Charles E. Culpeper Fndn Biomedical Pilot Projects Initiative Grants, 1641
IARC Expertise Transfer Fellowship, 1831
IARC Postdoctoral Fellowships for Training in Cancer Research, 1832
IARC Visiting Scientist Award for Senior Scientists, 1833
NIDCD Molecular and Cellular Pathology of the Human Auditory and Vestibular Systems Grants, 2525
NIDDK Co-Activators and Co-Repressors in Gene Expression Grants, 2546
NIDDK Erythroid Lineage Molecular Toolbox Grants, 2557
NIGMS/NIDCR Evolution of Infectious Diseases Research Grants, 2633
NIH Biobehavioral Pain Research Grants, 2638
NIH Fine Mapping and Function of Genes for Type 1 Diabetes Grants, 2667
NIH New Directions in Pain Research Grants, 2698
NSF Animal Developmental Mechanisms Grants, 2875
NSF Genes and Genome Systems Cluster Grants, 2886

Genomics
PhRMA Fndn Informatics Sabbatical Fellowships, 3035

Geochemistry
NIEHS Superfund Hazardous Substances Basic Research and Education Grants, 2607

Geography
Canada Graduate Scholarships and NSERC Postgraduate Scholarships, 845
Canada-U.S. Fulbright New Century Scholars Grants, 846
Canada-U.S. Fulbright Senior Specialists Grants, 847
Detroit Lions Charities Grants, 1241
Fulbright Alumni Initiatives Awards Grants, 1566
Fulbright Distinguished Chairs Grants, 1567
Fulbright New Century Scholars Grants, 1570
Fulbright Specialists Grants, 1571
Fulbright Traditional Scholar Program in Europe and Eurasia, 1572
Fulbright Traditional Scholar Program in Sub-Saharan Africa, 1573
Fulbright Traditional Scholar Program in the East Asia/Pacific Region, 1574
Fulbright Traditional Scholar Program in the Near East and North Africa Region, 1575
Fulbright Traditional Scholar Program in the South and Central Asia Region, 1576
Fulbright Traditional Scholar Program in the Western Hemisphere, 1577

Geology
Award in Separations Science and Technology, 677
Canada Graduate Scholarships and NSERC Postgraduate Scholarships, 845
NIEHS Superfund Hazardous Substances Basic Research and Education Grants, 2607
Weingart Fndn Grants, 3524

Geophysics
Brinson Fndn Grants, 794
NIEHS Superfund Hazardous Substances Basic Research and Education Grants, 2607

Geriatric Oncology
ASCO Career Development Award, 551
ASCO State Affiliate Grants, 560
ASCO Young Investigator Award, 562
ASCO/UICC International Cancer Technology Transfer (ICRETT) Fellowships, 563

Geriatrics
AFAR Medical Student Training in Aging Research Program, 255
AGS Dennis W. Jahnigen Career Development Scholars Awards, 264
AHRQ Independent Scientist Award, 313
American Academy of Nursing Building Academic Geriatric Nursing Capacity Scholarships, 414
American Academy of Nursing Claire M. Fagin Fellowships, 415
American Academy of Nursing Mayday Fund Grants, 416
American Academy of Nursing MBA Scholarships, 417
Chest Fndn Geriatric Development Research Awards, 984
DHHS Geriatric Training for Physicians and Dentists Grants, 1250
DHHS Health Professions Training in Geriatrics Grants, 1259
Ellison Medical Fndn/AFAR Julie Martin Mid-Career Award in Aging Research, 1403
Ellison Medical Fndn/AFAR Postdoctoral Fellows in Aging Research Program, 1404
FDHN Designated Outcomes Award in Geriatric Gastroenterology, 1466
FDHN Designated Research Award in Geriatric Gastroenterology, 1467
Greenwall Fndn Bioethics Grants, 1665
Hartford Aging and Health Program Awards, 1709
Hartford Geriatrics Health Outcomes Research Scholars Program, 1712
Healthcare Fndn of New Jersey Grants, 1729
HRSA Geriatric Education Centers, 1805
HRSA Physician Assistant Training, 1810
Jenkins Fndn: Improving the Health of Greater Richmond Grants, 1915
Leonard and Helen R. Stulman Charitable Fndn Grants, 2044
NIA Health Behaviors and Aging Grants, 2408
NIA/NIEHS Biomedical Epidemiologic and Intervention Studies Planning Grants, 2441
OSI Palliative Cancer Care Grants, 2970
RCPSC Balfour M. Mount Visiting Professorship in Palliative Medicine, 3112
Regenstrief General Internal Medicine - General Pediatrics Research Fellowship Program, 3144

German Studies
Fulbright German Studies Seminar Grants, 1568
Fulbright International Education Administrators Seminar Grants, 1569

Germany
DAAD Research Stays for University Academics and Scientists, 1183
Fulbright German Studies Seminar Grants, 1568
Fulbright International Education Administrators Seminar Grants, 1569

Gerontology
Mount Zion Health Fund Grants, 2220
Postdoctoral Research Fellowships in Gerontological Public Health, 3070

Gifted/Talented Education
CNA Fndn Grants, 1046
Ford Motor Company Fund Grants, 1522
Lynde and Harry Bradley Fndn Grants, 2089
Lynde and Harry Bradley Fndn Prizes: Bradley Prizes, 2090

Girls
Dallas Women's Fndn Grants, 1191
Fisa Fndn Grants, 1506
GoGirlGo! Ambassador Team Awards, 1632
Jewish Women's Fndn of New York Grants, 1924
Lewis Preston Fund for Girls Education Grants, 2052
Mattel International Grants, 2131
Women's Fndn of California Comm Action Fund, 3549
Women's Fndn of California Grants, 3550

Glaucoma
AHAF National Glaucoma Research Grants, 268
Columbus Fndn Ann Ellis Fund Grants, 1065
Columbus Fndn Competitive Grants, 1066
Glaucoma Fndn Grants, 1621
Glaucoma Research Pilot Project Grants, 1622
NYAM Lewis Rudin Glaucoma Grants, 2915

Globalization
Boeing Company Contributions Grants, 777
Public Welfare Fndn Grants, 3089

Glomerular Disease
NIDDK Grants for Basic Research in Glomerular Diseases, 2560

Governance
Rockefeller Brothers Fund Peace and Security Grants, 3179

Government
Arlington Comm Fndn Grants, 536
ASM Congressional Science Fellowships, 590
AT&T Fndn Civic and Comm Service Grants, 658
Baptist Comm Ministries Grants, 691
Bernard and Audre Rapoport Fndn Grants, 746
Carl and Lily Pforzheimer Fndn Grants, 868
Carnegie Corp of New York Grants, 879
Castle Rock Fndn Grants, 888
Effie and Wofford Cain Fndn Grants, 1385
Eugene B. Casey Fndn Grants, 1433
James S. McDonnell Fndn Complex Systems Collaborative Activity Awards, 1897
Margaret L. Wendt Fndn Grants, 2104

Rajiv Gandhi Fndn Grants, 3104
Rockefeller Brothers Fund Peace and Security Grants, 3179
RWJF Bridging the Gap: Research Informing Practice and Policy for Healthy Youth Behavior, 3205
Sprague Fndn Grants, 3359

Government Studies
APA Congressional Fellowships, 492
APSA Congressional Fellowships Health and Aging Policy Fellows Program, 514
APSA Robert Wood Johnson Fndn Health Policy Fellowships, 515

Governmental Functions
ConocoPhillips Fndn Grants, 1144
Henry J. Kaiser Family Fndn Grants, 1748
Jacob and Hilda Blaustein Fndn Grants, 1881
Sosland Fndn Grants, 3348

Graphics
Ruth Mott Fndn Grants, 3204

Grassroots Leadership
Families USA Wellstone Fellowship for Social Justice, 1450
FCNY Union Square Awards, 1461
John Edward Fowler Memorial Fndn Grants, 1930
Meyer Fndn Grants, 2177
Sisters of Saint Joseph Charitable Fund Grants, 3296

Great Lakes
Joyce Fndn Grants, 1969
Max Bell Fndn Grants, 2134

Grief
Comm Fndn for Southeastern Michigan Grants, 1094
Dell Fndn Open Grants, 1218

Growth Factors
Human Growth Fndn Small Grants, 1816
NIH Receptors and Signaling in Bone in Health and Disease, 2706

Gun Control
Joyce Fndn Grants, 1969
Richard and Rhoda Goldman Fund Grants, 3158

Hair Diseases
Dermatology Research Career Development Awards, 1238

Hansen's Disease
Heiser Leprosy and Tuberculosis Research Postdoctoral Fellowships, 1736
Heiser Leprosy Research Grants, 1737
HRSA Hansen's Disease National Ambulatory Care Grants, 1806

Hawaiian Natives
AMA Fndn Minority Scholars Awards, 395

Hazardous Waste Disposal/Clean-Up
NIEHS Hazardous Materials Worker Health and Safety Training Grants, 2599
NIEHS Hazmat Training at Doe Nuclear Weapons Complex Grants, 2600
NIEHS SBIR E-Learning for HAZMAT and Emergency Response Grants, 2604
NIEHS Superfund Hazardous Substances Basic Research and Education Grants, 2607

Hazardous Wastes
DHHS Neurodevelopmental Test Methods Research Grants, 1268
DOE Medical Applications and Measurement Science Grants, 1301
Jessie Smith Noyes Fndn Grants, 1920
Joyce Fndn Grants, 1969
NIEHS Hazardous Materials Worker Health and Safety Training Grants, 2599
NIEHS Hazmat Training at Doe Nuclear Weapons Complex Grants, 2600
NIEHS SBIR E-Learning for HAZMAT and Emergency Response Grants, 2604
NIEHS Superfund Hazardous Substances Basic Research and Education Grants, 2607
San Diego Fndn for Change Grants, 3255
U.S. Department of Education Erma Byrd Scholarships, 3446

Head Injury
AHNS Alando J. Ballantyne Resident Research Pilot Grant, 305
AHNS Pilot Grant, 306
AHNS/AAO-HNSF Surgeon Scientist Combined Award, 307
AHNS/AAO-HNSF Young Investigator Combined Award, 308

Headaches
National Headache Fndn Research Grants, 2253
National Headache Fndn Seymour Diamond Clinical Fellowship in Headache Education, 2254

Health
1675 Fndn Grants, 4
3M Fndn Grants, 11
AIG American General Corp Grants, 316
Albert and Margaret Alkek Fndn Grants, 326
Allegis Group Fndn Grants, 360
American Electric Power Grants, 434
Amerisure Insurance Comm Service Grants, 461
Arkansas Comm Fndn Arkansas Black Hall of Fame Grants, 532
ASHFndn New Century Scholars Program Doctoral Scholarships, 580
ASHFndn New Century Scholars Research Grant, 581
ASHFndn Research Grant for New Investigators, 582
Austin College Leadership Award, 668
Autodesk Comm Relations Grants, 671
Cailloux Fndn Grants, 829
Cailloux Fndn Grants, 829
CFFVR Opportunity Grants, 952
Charles M. and Mary D. Grant Fndn Grants, 971
Columbus Fndn Competitive Grants, 1066
Comm Fndn of South Puget Sound Grants, 1124
CSX Corp Contributions Grants, 1169
D.V. and Ida J. McEachern Charitable Trust Grants, 1182
Daisy Marquis Jones Fndn Grants, 1188
Dale and Edna Walsh Fndn Grants, 1189
Edyth Bush Charitable Fndn Grants, 1378
El Paso Corp Fndn Grants, 1389
El Pomar Fndn Awards and Grants, 1390
Eugene and Agnes E. Meyer Fndn Grants, 1432
Faye McBeath Fndn Grants, 1456
Federal Express Corp Contributions Program, 1483
Fifth Third Fndn Grants, 1501
Fndn for the Carolinas Grants, 1535
Freddie Mac Fndn Grants, 1558
Genentech Corp Charitable Contributions Grants, 1588
Grand Haven Area Comm Fndn Grants, 1644
Halliburton Fndn Grants, 1687
Harold and Arlene Schnitzer CARE Fndn Grants, 1697
Harrison County Comm Fndn Grants, 1700
Harry S. Black and Allon Fuller Fund, 1706
Hilda and Preston Davis Fndn Grants, 1772
Hillsdale County Comm General Adult Fndn Grants, 1777
J.E. and L.E. Mabee Fndn Grants, 1875
Jane Bradley Pettit Fndn Grants, 1902
Kluge Center David B. Larson Fellowship in Health and Spirituality, 2006
Lindbergh Grants, 2059
Lowell Area Comm Fund Grants, 2068
Marion Park Deaver and Harry Gilbert Deaver Fndn Grants, 2110
Marshall Field's Comm Grants, 2115
Mary Baker Eddy Library Summer Research Fellowships, 2117
Massage Therapy Research Grants, 2127
Mattel International Grants, 2131
McMurry Fndn Grants, 2149
Meyer Fndn Grants, 2177
Nelda C. and H.J. Lutcher Stark Fndn Grants, 2301
NIH Building Interdisciplinary Research Careers in Women's Health Grants, 2644
OneStar Fndn AmeriCorps Grants, 2945
PMI Fndn Grants, 3063
Public Welfare Fndn Grants, 3089
Pulte Homes Corp Contributions, 3092
Rohm and Haas Company Grants, 3185
Snee Reinhardt Charitable Fndn Grants, 3300
Taproot Fndn Capacity-Building Service Grants, 3417
Tifa Fndn Grants, 3428
Toro Fndn Grants, 3431

Health Agencies
Beckman Coulter Comm Relations Grants, 733

Health and Health Services
Business Bank of Nevada Comm Grants, 817
Doris Duke Charitable Fndn Operations Research on AIDS Care and Treatment in Africa Grants, 1319
Johnson and Johnson / SAH Arts and Healing Grants, 1953
Office Depot Corp Comm Grants, 2935
Rosalynn Carter Institute John and Betty Pope Fellowships, 3189
Stewart Huston Charitable Trust Grants, 3384
TWS Fndn Grants, 3443
Until There's a Cure Fndn Grants, 3471

Health and Safety Education
AAHPERD Ruth Abernathy Presidential Scholarships, 128
ACE Charitable Fndn Grants, 199
Alexander and Margaret Stewart Trust Grants, 340
Alexis Gregory Fndn Grants, 349
Avon Fndn Breast Care Fund Grants, 674
BCBSNC Fndn Grants, 725
Becton Dickinson and Company Grants, 736
BJ's Charitable Fndn Grants, 761
Breast Cancer Fund Grants, 790
CDC Hepatitis Education for Inmates and Correctional Staff Grants, 911
CDC National Poison Prevention and Control Grants, 918
CDC Oral Diseases Prevention and Oral Health Promotion Grants, 921
CDC Public Health Conference Support Grant Program, 926
CDC Research, Treatment, and Education Programs on Lyme Disease in the United States Cooperative Agreements, 927
CDC School Health Programs to Prevent the Spread of HIV Cooperative Agreements, 928
CDC Technology Translation and Transfer of Effective HIV Behavioral Interventions, 931
Champ-A Champion Fur Kids Grants, 959
Charles Lafitte Fndn Grants, 970
CJ Fndn for SIDS Support Services Grants, 1017
CLIF Bar Family Fndn Grants, 1040
Comm Campus Partnerships for Health Fellowships, 1087
Daviess County Comm Fndn Health Grants, 1203
Dearborn Comm Fndn City of Lawrenceburg Comm Grants, 1210
Dorothy Rider Pool Health Care Grants, 1322
Dr. John T. Macdonald Fndn Grants, 1327
Edina Realty Fndn Grants, 1369
EPA Baseline Assessment of Risks of Exposure to Lead Poisoning of Native American Children, 1419
EPA Lead Awareness Outreach for Native American Tribes, 1421

Fairlawn Fndn Grants, 1447
Fndn for Seacoast Health Grants, 1533
Fndn for Spirituality and Medicine Grants, 1534
Frances and John L. Loeb Family Fund Grants, 1546
Good Samaritan Fndn Inc Grants, 1636
Health Fndn of Greater Cincinnati Grants, 1724
Health Fndn of Southern Florida Responsive Grants, 1726
Healthcare Fndn of New Jersey Grants, 1729
Horizon Fndn for New Jersey Grants, 1793
International Cancer Technology Transfer Fellowships, 1858
John P. McGovern Fndn Grants, 1942
John S. Dunn Research Fndn Grants and Chairs, 1945
Johnson & Johnson Corp Contributions Grants, 1952
Johnson County Comm Fndn Grants, 1955
Kansas Health Fndn Grants, 1980
KFC Allied Health Research Grants, 1996
Knight Family Charitable and Educational Fndn Grants, 2007
Mary Black Fndn Grants, 2118
Max Bell Fndn Grants, 2134
MedImmune Charitable Grants, 2166
Medtronic Fndn Full Life Patient Partnership Program—Heart Rescue Grants, 2168
Medtronic Fndn Health Care Grants, 2169
NAPNAP Fndn Shourd Parks Immunization Project Small Grants, 2243
National Blood Fndn Research Grant Program, 2249
NLM Understanding and Promoting Health Literacy Research Grants, 2827
ORISE Postgraduate Research Participation at the Agency for Toxic Substances and Disease Registry, 2960
OUT Fund for Lesbian and Gay Liberation Grants, 2978
Phoenix Suns Charities Grants, 3030
Posey Comm Fndn Womens Fund Grants, 3069
RWJF Jobs to Careers: Promoting Work-Based Learning for Quality Care - Research Grants, 3221
Saint Luke's Health Initiatives Grants, 3240
Shaw's Supermarkets Donations, 3280
Sisters of St. Joseph Healthcare Fndn Grants, 3297
SOCFOC Reducing Health & Educational Disparities in the Central Neighborhood Grants, 3318
Susan G. Komen Breast Cancer Fndn Breast Health, Breast Cancer Education, and Outreach Programs Grants, 3408
Tellabs Fndn Grants, 3418
Tylenol Scholarship, 3444
U.S. Department of Education 21st Century Comm Learning Centers, 3445
Warrick County Comm Fndn Grants, 3519

Health Care

100 Mile Man Fndn Grants, 2
1104 Fndn Grants, 3
1st Touch Fndn Grants, 6
2 Depot Square Ipswich Charitable Fndn Grants, 7
3M Company Health and Human Services Grants, 10
49ers Fndn Grants, 12
A Friend's Fndn Trust Grants, 13
A/H Fndn Grants, 19
AACAP Jeanne Spurlock Research Fellowship in Substance Abuse and Addiction for Minority Medical Students, 40
AACAP Summer Medical Student Fellowships, 53
AACR Scholar-in-Training Awards, 87
AACR Scholar-in-Training Awards - Special Conferences, 88
AAFA Investigator Research Grants, 108
AAMC Award for Distinguished Research, 135
AAMC David E. Rogers Award, 137
AAMC Herbert W. Nickens Award, 138
AAMC Herbert W. Nickens Medical Student Scholarships, 140
AAMC Humanism in Medicine Award, 141
AAP Comm Access To Child Health Implementation Grants, 158
AAP Resident Initiative Fund Grants, 167
Aaron & Freda Glickman Fndn Grants, 172
Aaron Fndn (California) Grants, 173
Aaron Fndn (Massachusetts) Grants, 174
Abbott Fund Access to Health Care Grants, 176
Abbott Fund Comm Vitality Grants, 177
Abbott Fund Global AIDS Care Grants, 178
Abbott Fund Science and Medical Innovation Grants, 179
Abell Fndn Health and Human Services Grants, 182
Abington Fndn Grants, 184
Able To Serve Grants, 185
Abney Fndn Grants, 187
Abramson Family Fndn Grants, 188
ACAAI Fndn Research Grants, 189
AcademyHealth Alice S. Hersh New Investigator Awards, 190
AcademyHealth Alice S. Hersh Student Scholarships, 191
AcademyHealth Awards, 192
AcademyHealth Nemours Child Health Services Research Awards, 194
AcademyHealth PHSR Interest Group Student Scholarships, 195
AcademyHealth PHSR Research Article of the Year Awards, 196
ACGT Young Investigator Grants, 205
Achelis and Bodman Fndns Grants, 206
ACS Pilot and Exploratory Projects in Palliative Care of Cancer Patients and Their Families Grants, 219
Acushnet Fndn Grants, 226
Adam Richter Charitable Trust Grants, 230
Adams County Fndn Grants - Pennsylvania, 231
Addison H. Gibson Fndn Medical Grants, 233
Adelaide Breed Bayrd Fndn Grants, 234
Administaff Comm Affairs Grants, 235
Adolph Coors Fndn Grants, 238
Advanced Micro Devices Comm Affairs Grants, 239
AEC Trust Grants, 242
AEGON Transamerica Fndn Grants, 243
Aetna Fndn Health Grants in Connecticut, 244
Aetna Fndn Quality of Care Grants, 245
Aetna Fndn Quality of Care Grants for Depression, 246
Aetna Fndn Quality of Care Grants for End of Life Care, 247
Aetna Fndn Regional Comm Health General Support Grants, 248
Aetna Fndn Regional Comm Health Outreach Grants, 250
Aetna Fndn Sponsorships Grants in Connecticut, 251
Aetna Fndn Voice Of Conscience Award, 252
AFG Industries Grants, 259
African American Fund of New Jersey Grants, 260
Agnes Gund Fndn Grants, 262
Agnes M. Lindsay Trust Grants, 263
AHFMR Comm Support Grants, 271
AHFMR Major Equipment Grants, 285
Ahmanson Fndn Grants, 303
AHRF Regular Research Grants, 311
Air Products and Chemicals Grants, 319
Alabama Power Fndn Grants, 321
Aladdin Industries Fndn Grants, 322
Albany Medical Center Prize in Medicine and Biomedical Research, 325
Albert Pick Jr. Fund Grants, 328
Alberto Culver Corp Contributions Grants, 329
Albertson's Charitable Giving Grants, 330
Albuquerque Comm Fndn Grants, 331
Alcatel-Lucent Technologies Corp Contributions Grants, 332
Alcatel-Lucent Technologies Fndn Grants, 333
Alcoa Fndn Grants, 334
Alcohol Misuse and Alcoholism Research Grants, 335
Alexander Fndn Cancer, Catastrophic Illness and Injury Grants, 342
Alexander Fndn Insurance Continuation Grants, 343
Alice C. A. Sibley Fund Grants, 355
Alice Tweed Tuohy Fndn Grants, 357
Allegan County Comm Fndn Grants, 358
Allegheny Technologies Charitable Trust, 359
ALSAM Fndn Grants, 369
Altman Fndn Health Care Grants, 372
AMA Fndn Dr. Nathan Davis International Awards in Medicine, 387
AMA Fndn Health Literacy Grants, 389
AMA Fndn Healthy Communities/Healthy America Grants, 390
AMA Fndn Jack B. McConnell, MD Awards for Excellence in Volunteerism, 391
AMA Fndn Jordan Fieldman, MD, Awards, 393
AMA Fndn Leadership Awards, 394
AMA Fndn Pride in the Profession Grants, 397
AMA Fndn Worldscopes Program, 399
AMA Virtual Mentor Theme Issue Editor Grants, 400
AMA-MSS Chapter Involvement Grants, 401
AMA-MSS Chapter of the Year Award, 402
AMA-MSS Research Poster Award, 405
AMA-RFS and AMA Fndn Medical Student & Resident/Fellow Elective-Medicine & the Media, 406
AMA-RFS Legislative Awareness Internships, 407
AMA-WPC Joan F. Giambalvo Memorial Scholarships, 408
Amador Comm Fndn Grants, 409
Amarillo Area/Harrington Fndns Grants, 410
American Express Fndn Comm Service Grants, 435
American Jewish World Service Grants, 437
American Schlafhorst Fndn Grants, 454
American-Italian Cancer Fndn Fellowships, 459
American-Scandinavian Fndn Visiting Lectureship Grants, 460
Andersen Corp Fndn, 470
Andersen Fndn Grants, 471
Angels Baseball Fndn Grants, 473
Anheuser-Busch Fndn Grants, 474
Ann and Robert H. Lurie Family Fndn Grants, 475
Ann Jackson Family Fndn Grants, 477
Ann Peppers Fndn Grants, 478
Annie Sinclair Knudsen Memorial Fund/Kaua'i Comm Grants, 480
Annunziata Sanguinetti Fndn Grants, 481
Anschutz Family Fndn Grants, 486
Anthem Blue Cross and Blue Shield Grants, 488
APF Disaster Recovery Fund for Psychiatrists, 506
AptarGroup Fndn Grants, 522
Aratani Fndn Grants, 523
Arcadia Fndn Grants, 524
Argyros Fndn Grants, 527
Arie and Ida Crown Memorial Grants, 528
Arizona Cardinals Grants, 529
Arizona Diamondbacks Charities Grants, 530
Arizona Public Service Corp Giving Grants, 531
Arkell Hall Fndn Grants, 534
Arlington Comm Fndn Grants, 536
Armstrong McDonald Fndn Grants, 537
ARS Fndn Grants, 538
Arthritis Fndn of Australia Grants, 541
ArvinMeritor Fndn Health Grants, 543
ArvinMeritor Grants, 544
Assisi Fndn Grants, 653
Assurant Health Fndn Grants, 655
AT&T Fndn Civic and Comm Service Grants, 658
Atherton Family Fndn Grants, 659
Athwin Fndn Grants, 660
Atlanta Fndn Grants, 662
Aurora Fndn Grants, 667
Austin-Bailey Health and Wellness Fndn Grants, 669
Autzen Fndn Grants, 672
Bacon Family Fndn Grants, 679
Bailey Fndn Grants, 680
Balfe Family Fndn Grants, 682
Ball Brothers Fndn Grants, 684
Banfi Vintners Fndn Grants, 687
Bank of America Charitable Fndn National Programs and Partners Grants, 689
Baptist-Trinity Lutheran Legacy Fndn Grants, 692
Barberton Comm Fndn Grants, 693
Barker Fndn Grants, 694

Barker Welfare Fndn Grants, 695
Barra Fndn Comm Fund Grants, 698
Barra Fndn Project Grants, 699
Barth Syndrome Fndn Research Grants, 700
Batchelor Fndn Grants, 701
Baton Rouge Area Fndn Grants, 702
Battle Creek Comm Fndn Grants, 703
Baxter International Fndn Grants, 705
BCBS of Massachusetts Catalyst Fund Grants, 708
BCBS of Massachusetts Fndn Grants, 709
BCBS of Massachusetts Health Coverage Fellowships, 710
BCBS of Minnesota Growing Up Healthy Grants, 711
BCBS of Minnesota Healthy Together Grants, 712
BCBSM Claude Pepper Award, 714
BCBSM Comm Health Matching Grants, 715
BCBSM Corp Contributions Grants, 716
BCBSM Fndn Excellence in Research Awards for Students, 717
BCBSM Fndn Physician Investigator Research Awards, 718
BCBSM Fndn Primary and Clinical Prevention Grants, 719
BCBSM Fndn Proposal Development Awards, 720
BCBSM Fndn Student Award Program, 721
BCBSM Frank J. McDevitt, DO, Excellence in Research Awards, 722
BCBSM Investigator-Initiated Research Grants, 723
Beazley Fndn Grants, 730
Bechtel Group Fndn Building Positive Comm Relationships Grants, 731
Beckley Area Fndn Grants, 732
Becton Dickinson and Company Grants, 736
Beirne Carter Fndn Grants, 737
Ben B. Cheney Fndn Grants, 741
Bender Fndn Grants, 742
Benton County Fndn Grants, 744
Berks County Comm Fndn Grants, 745
Bernard and Audre Rapoport Fndn Grants, 746
Berrien Comm Fndn Grants, 749
Bert W. Martin Fndn Grants, 750
Besser Fndn Grants, 752
BHHS Legacy Fndn Grants, 753
Bildner Family Fndn Grants, 755
Bill and Melinda Gates Fndn Grants, 756
Binney and Smith Comm Grants, 757
Biogen Corp Giving Grants, 758
Birds Eye Foods Fndn Grants, 759
Birmingham Fndn Grants, 760
Blanche and Irving Laurie Fndn Grants, 764
Blanche and Julian Robertson Family Fndn Grants, 765
Blowitz-Ridgeway Fndn Early Childhood Development Research Award, 766
Blowitz-Ridgeway Fndn Grants, 767
Blue Grass Comm Fndn Grants, 768
Blue Mountain Comm Fndn Grants, 769
Blue Shield of California Grants, 771
Blum-Kovler Fndn Grants, 772
Bob and Delores Hope Charitable Fndn Grants, 774
Bodenwein Public Benevolent Fndn Grants, 775
Bodman Fndn Grants, 776
Boeing Company Contributions Grants, 777
Boettcher Fndn Grants, 778
Booth-Bricker Fund Grants, 780
Bosque Fndn Grants, 782
Boston Fndn Grants, 783
Boston Globe Fndn Grants, 784
Boston Jewish Comm Women's Fund Grants, 785
Boyd Gaming Corp Contributions Program, 788
Bradley Turner Fndn Grants, 789
Brian G. Dyson Fndn Grants, 791
Bridgestone/Firestone Trust Fund Grants, 792
Bright Family Fndn Grants, 793
Bristol-Myers Squibb Fndn Health Disparities Grants, 797
Bristol-Myers Squibb Fndn Health Education Grants, 798
Bristol-Myers Squibb Fndn Product Donations Grants, 799
Bristol-Myers Squibb Fndn Women's Health Grants, 800
Bristol-Myers Squibb Patient Assistance Program, 801
Broad Fndn IBD Research Grants, 803
Brook J. Lenfest Fndn Grants, 804
Burlington Industries Fndn Grants, 811
Burlington Northern Santa Fe Fndn Grants, 812
Bush Fndn Health & Human Services Grants, 814
Bush Fndn Medical Fellowships, 815
Bushrod H. Campbell and Adah F. Hall Charity Fund Grants, 816
Byron W. and Alice L. Lockwood Fndn Grants, 824
C.R. Bard Fndn Grants, 825
Caleb C. and Julia W. Dula Educational and Charitable Fndn Grants, 830
California Comm Fndn Health Care Grants, 831
Callaway Fndn Grants, 835
Callaway Golf Company Fndn Grants, 836
Cambridge Comm Fndn Grants, 837
Camp-Younts Fndn Grants, 838
Campbell Hoffman Fndn Grants, 840
Canadian Nurses Fndn Study Awards, 852
Capital Region Comm Fndn Grants, 862
Cardinal Health Fndn Grants, 864
Caring Fndn Grants, 866
Carl and Eloise Pohlad Family Fndn Grants, 867
Carl and Lily Pforzheimer Fndn Grants, 868
Carl C. Icahn Fndn Grants, 870
Carl Gellert and Celia Berta Gellert Fndn Grants, 871
Carl W. and Carrie Mae Joslyn Trust Grants, 873
Carls Fndn Grants, 876
Carlsbad Charitable Fndn Grants, 877
Carolyn Fndn Grants, 880
Carpenter Fndn Grants, 881
Carrie Estelle Doheny Fndn Grants, 883
Carrier Corp Contributions Grants, 884
Carroll County Comm Fndn Grants, 885
Carylon Fndn Grants, 886
Catherine Kennedy Home Fndn Grants, 890
CDC Cancer Prevention and Control Programs, 903
CDC Cooperative Agreement for Partnership to Enhance Public Health Informatics, 905
CDC Cooperative Agreement for the Development, Operation, and Evaluation of an Entertainment Education Program, 906
CDC National Breast and Cervical Cancer Early Detection Program, 917
Cemala Fndn Grants, 933
Center for Science in the Public Interest Internships, 935
Central Carolina Comm Fndn Comm Impact Grants, 936
Central Okanagan Fndn Grants, 937
CF Clinical Research Trainee Awards, 940
Champlin Fndns Grants, 960
CharityWorks Grants, 961
Charles A. Frueauff Fndn Grants, 962
Charles Delmar Fndn Grants, 963
Charles H. Dater Fndn Grants, 966
Charles H. Farnsworth Trust Grants, 967
Charles Lafitte Fndn Grants, 970
Charlotte County (FL) Comm Fndn Grants, 973
Chase Paymentech Corp Giving Grants, 975
Chatlos Fndn Grants, 977
Chesapeake Corp Fndn Grants, 982
Chicago Board of Trade Fndn Grants, 988
Chicago Tribune's Corp Contributions Grants, 991
Chicago White Metal Charitable Fndn Grants, 992
Children Affected by AIDS Fndn Domestic Grants, 995
Children Affected by AIDS Fndn Family Assistance Emergency Fund Grants, 996
Children's Brain Tumor Fndn Research Grants, 998
Christopher Reeve Paralysis Fndn Quality of Life and Health Promotions Grants, 1007
Christy-Houston Fndn Grants, 1008
Chula Vista Charitable Fndn Grants, 1009
CICF Legacy Fund Comm Fndn Grants, 1010
CIGNA Fndn Grants, 1011
Cinergy Fndn Grants, 1013
CIT Corp Giving Grants, 1014
Citizens Bank Mid-Atlantic Charitable Fndn Grants, 1015
Clarcor Fndn Grants, 1021
Clarence E. Heller Charitable Fndn Grants, 1022
Clark County Comm Fndn Grants, 1028
Clark Fndn Grants, 1029
Clark-Winchcole Fndn Grants, 1030
Claude Bennett Family Fndn Grants, 1031
Claude Worthington Benedum Fndn Grants, 1033
Clay Fndn Grants, 1034
Cleo Fndn Grants, 1035
CLIF Bar Family Fndn Grants, 1040
CNA Fndn Grants, 1046
CNCS Foster Grandparent Projects Grants, 1048
Coastal Comm Fndn of South Carolina Grants, 1051
Coca-Cola Fndn Grants, 1052
Cockrell Fndn Grants, 1053
Coeta and Donald Barker Fndn Grants, 1054
Coleman Fndn Cancer Care Grants, 1055
Colin Higgins Fndn Grants, 1056
Collins C. Diboll Private Fndn Grants, 1057
Collins Fndn Grants, 1058
Colonel Stanley R. McNeil Fndn Grants, 1059
Colorado Interstate Gas Grants, 1060
Colorado Springs Comm Trust Fund Grants, 1061
Colorado Trust Grants, 1062
Columbus Fndn Allen Eiry Fund Grants, 1064
Columbus Fndn Ann Ellis Fund Grants, 1065
Columbus Fndn Estrich Fund Grants, 1067
Columbus Fndn J. Floyd Dixon Memorial Fund Grants, 1068
Columbus Fndn Mary Eleanor Morris Fund Grants, 1069
Columbus Fndn Robert E. and Genevieve B. Schaefer Fund Grants, 1070
Columbus Fndn Traditional Grants, 1071
Comer Fndn Grants, 1072
Comerica Charitable Fndn Grants, 1073
Commission on Religion in Appalachia Grants, 1074
Commonweal Fndn Comm Assistance Grants, 1075
Commonweal Fndn Grants, 1076
Commonwealth Fund Affordable Health Insurance Grants, 1077
Commonwealth Fund Australian-American Health Policy Fellowships, 1078
Commonwealth Fund Health Care Quality Improvement and Efficiency Grants, 1080
Commonwealth Fund Patient-Centered Coordinated Care Grants, 1081
Commonwealth Fund Payment System Reform Grants, 1082
Commonwealth Fund Quality of Care for Frail Elders Grants, 1083
Commonwealth Fund Small Grants, 1084
Commonwealth Fund State High Performance Health Systems Grants, 1085
Comm Campus Partnerships for Health Fellowships, 1087
Comm Fndn Alliance City of Evansville Endowment Fund Grants, 1089
Comm Fndn for Greater Buffalo Grants, 1090
Comm Fndn for Greater New Haven Grants, 1091
Comm Fndn for Monterey County Grants, 1092
Comm Fndn for Muskegon County Grants, 1093
Comm Fndn for Southeastern Michigan Grants, 1094
Comm Fndn for Southern Arizona Grants, 1095
Comm Fndn of Bloomington and Monroe County Grants, 1098
Comm Fndn of Broward Grants, 1100
Comm Fndn of Central Illinois Grants, 1101
Comm Fndn of Champaign County Grants, 1102
Comm Fndn of Crawford County Grants and Scholarships, 1103
Comm Fndn of Greater Birmingham Grants, 1106
Comm Fndn of Greater Flint Grants, 1107
Comm Fndn of Greater Greensboro Grants, 1109
Comm Fndn of Greater New Britain Grants, 1111
Comm Fndn of Greater Tampa Grants, 1112

Comm Fndn of Greenville Comm Enrichment Grants, 1113
Comm Fndn of Greenville Hollingsworth Funds Program/Project Grants, 1114
Comm Fndn of Greenville-Greenville Women Giving Grants, 1115
Comm Fndn of Howard County Grants, 1116
Comm Fndn of Madison and Jefferson County Grants and Scholarships, 1117
Comm Fndn of Morgan County Grants and Scholarships, 1118
Comm Fndn of Mount Vernon and Knox County Grants, 1119
Comm Fndn of Randolph County Grants, 1121
Comm Fndn of South Alabama Grants, 1123
Comm Fndn of Southeastern Connecticut Grants, 1125
Comm Fndn of Switzerland County Grants, 1127
Comm Fndn of Tampa Bay Grants, 1128
Comm Fndn of the Eastern Shore Comm Needs Grants, 1129
Comm Fndn of the Ozarks Grants, 1130
Comm Fndn of Wabash County Grants, 1131
Comm Fndn of Western North Carolina Grants, 1132
Comm Fndn Silicon Valley Grants, 1133
Comm Health Scholars Program Fellowships, 1134
Comm Technology Fndn of California Building Communities Through Technology Grants, 1136
Compass Bank Fndn Grants, 1138
Comprehensive Health Education Fndn Grants, 1139
ConAgra Foods Fndn Grants, 1140
Connecticut Health Fndn Health Initiative Grants, 1142
Connelly Fndn Grants, 1143
Constantin Fndn Grants, 1145
Constellation Energy Group and Baltimore Gas and Electric Corp Contributions, 1146
Cooke Fndn Grants, 1148
Cooper Industries Fndn Grants, 1150
Cornerstone Fndn of Northeastern Wisconsin Grants, 1152
Covenant Fndn Grants, 1153
Covenant Matters Fndn Grants, 1154
Crail-Johnson Fndn Grants, 1157
Cranston Fndn Grants, 1158
Crestlea Fndn Grants, 1159
CRH Fndn Grants, 1160
CSRA Comm Fndn Grants, 1168
Cudd Fndn Grants, 1171
Cullen Fndn Grants, 1172
CVS Caremark Charitable Trust Grants, 1176
Cyrus Eaton Fndn Grants, 1178
D. W. McMillan Fndn Grants, 1180
Dade Comm Fndn Grants, 1185
DaimlerChrysler Corp Fund Grants, 1186
Dairy Queen Corp Contributions Grants, 1187
Dallas Mavericks Fndn Grants, 1190
Dana Brown Charitable Trust Grants, 1194
Dana Corp Fndn Grants, 1196
Dana Fndn Science and Health Grants, 1197
Danellie Fndn Grants, 1198
David Geffen Fndn Grants, 1202
Daviess County Comm Fndn Health Grants, 1203
Davis Family Fndn Grants, 1204
Dayton Power and Light Fndn Grants, 1205
Daywood Fndn Grants, 1206
Deaconess Comm Fndn Grants, 1207
Dean Foods Comm Involvement Grants, 1209
Dearborn Comm Fndn County Progress Grants, 1211
Delaware Comm Fndn Grants, 1215
Delaware Comm Fndn-Youth Philanthropy Board for Kent County, 1216
Dell Fndn Open Grants, 1218
Delta Air Lines Fndn Grants, 1220
DeMatteis Family Fndn Grants, 1221
Dennis and Phyllis Washington Fndn Grants, 1222
Denton A. Cooley Fndn Grants, 1225
Denver Fndn Comm Grants, 1227
DeRoy Testamentary Fndn Grants, 1239
Detroit Lions Charities Grants, 1241
DHHS Adolescent Family Life Demonstration Projects, 1243
DHHS Emergency Medical Services for Children Program, 1249
DHHS Health Care Systems Cost and Access Research and Development Grants, 1252
DHHS Health Centers Grants for Residents of Public Housing, 1254
DHHS Healthy Tomorrows Partnership for Children, 1261
DHHS Oral Health Promotion Research Across the Lifespan, 1269
DHHS Technical and Non-Financial Assistance to Health Centers, 1280
DHHS Thimerosal Pharmacokinetics: Assessment of the Distribution, Metabolism, and Excretion, 1281
Dickson Fndn Grants, 1284
Do Something BR!CK Awards, 1287
Dolan Fndn Grants, 1306
Dole Food Company Charitable Contributions, 1307
Donaghue Practical Benefit Initiatives Grants, 1309
Dora Roberts Fndn Grants, 1311
Doris and Victor Day Fndn Grants, 1313
Doris and Victor Day Fndn Grants, 1313
Doris Duke Charitable Fndn Clinical Interfaces Award Program, 1314
Dorothea Haus Ross Fndn Grants, 1320
Dorothy Hooper Beattie Fndn Grants, 1321
Dorothy Rider Pool Health Care Grants, 1322
Dorrance Family Fndn Grants, 1323
Dr. Bob and Jean Smith Fndn Grants, 1325
Dr. John T. Macdonald Fndn Grants, 1327
Dr. Leon Bromberg Charitable Trust Fund Grants, 1328
Dreitzer Fndn Grants, 1332
Dubois County Comm Fndn Grants, 1336
Duke Endowment Health Care Grants, 1338
Duke Energy Fndn Grants, 1339
Duke University Pain Management Fellowships, 1346
Duneland Health Council InCorpd Grants, 1350
Dunspaugh-Dalton Fndn Grants, 1351
DuPage Comm Fndn Grants, 1352
Dyson Fndn Mid-Hudson Valley General Operating Support Grants, 1354
E.J. Grassmann Trust Grants, 1360
Eckerd Corp Fndn Grants, 1366
Eddie C. and Sylvia Brown Family Fndn Grants, 1367
Eden Hall Fndn Grants, 1368
EDS Fndn Grants, 1371
Educational Fndn of America Grants, 1372
Edward Bangs Kelley and Elza Kelley Fndn Grants, 1373
Edwards Memorial Trust Grants, 1375
Effie and Wofford Cain Fndn Grants, 1385
El Paso Comm Fndn Grants, 1388
Elisabeth Severance Prentiss Fndn Grants, 1392
Elizabeth Morse Genius Charitable Trust Grants, 1400
Elkhart County Comm Fndn Grants, 1401
Elsie Lee Garthwaite Memorial Fndn Grants, 1408
Emerson Electric Company Contributions Grants, 1413
Ensworth Charitable Fndn Grants, 1416
Entergy Corp Open Grants for Healthy Families, 1418
Erie Comm Fndn Grants, 1427
Estee Lauder Grants, 1429
Ethel S. Abbott Charitable Fndn Grants, 1430
Eugene M. Lang Fndn Grants, 1434
Eugene McDermott Fndn Grants, 1435
Evanston Comm Fndn Grants, 1438
Ewing Halsell Fndn Grants, 1440
Express Scripts Fndn Grants, 1441
ExxonMobil Grants, 1442
F.M. Kirby Fndn Grants, 1443
Fairfield County Comm Fndn Grants, 1446
Fairlawn Fndn Grants, 1447
Fairview Lutheran Fndn Grants, 1448
Families USA Wellstone Fellowship for Social Justice, 1450
Fan Fox and Leslie R. Samuels Fndn Grants, 1451
Fargo-Moorhead Area Fndn Grants, 1454
Farmers Insurance Group of Companies Grants, 1455
Fayette County Fndn Grants, 1457
Ferree Fndn Grants, 1486
FIC International Research and Training in Population and Health Grants, 1489
FIC International Research Scientist Development Award, 1491
FIC/ORMH Minority International Research Training Grants, 1497
Fidelity Fndn Grants, 1498
Field Fndn of Illinois Grants, 1499
FirstEnergy Fndn Comm Grants, 1505
Fisa Fndn Grants, 1506
Fisher Fndn Grants, 1508
Fisher House Fndn Newman's Own Awards, 1509
Flinn Fndn Grants Programs, 1511
Floyd A. and Kathleen C. Cailloux Fndn Grants, 1516
Fluor Fndn Grants, 1517
FMC Fndn Grants, 1518
Foellinger Fndn Grants, 1519
Fondren Fndn Grants, 1520
Ford Motor Company Fund Grants, 1522
Forrest C. Lattner Fndn Grants, 1523
Foster Fndn Grants, 1524
Fndn for Seacoast Health Grants, 1533
Fndn for Spirituality and Medicine Grants, 1534
Fndn for the Mid-South Grants, 1536
Fndn of CVPH April LaValley Fund Grants, 1538
Fndn of CVPH Melissa Lahtinen-Penfield Organ Donor Fund Grants, 1540
Fndn of CVPH Rabin Fund Grants, 1541
Fndn of CVPH Roger Senecal Endowment Fund Grants, 1542
Fndn of CVPH Travel Fund Grants, 1543
Fourjay Fndn Grants, 1544
Frances and John L. Loeb Family Fund Grants, 1546
Frances L. and Edwin L. Cummings Memorial Fund Grants, 1547
Frances W. Emerson Fndn Grants, 1548
Francis L. Abreu Charitable Trust Grants, 1549
Francis T. & Louise T. Nichols Fndn Grants, 1550
Frank Stanley Beveridge Fndn Grants, 1553
Franklin County Comm Fndn Grants, 1554
Fremont Area Comm Fndn Grants, 1561
Frist Fndn Grants, 1563
Fuji Film Grants, 1565
Fuller E. Callaway Fndn Grants, 1578
Fulton County Comm Fndn Grants, 1579
G.N. Wilcox Trust Grants, 1581
Gebbie Fndn Grants, 1585
GenCorp Fndn Grants, 1587
General Mills Fndn Grants, 1590
General Motors Fndn Grants Support Program, 1591
General Service Fndn Reproductive Health and Rights Grants, 1592
Genesis Fndn Grants, 1593
Genuardi Family Fndn Grants, 1594
George Family Fndn Grants, 1598
George Frederick Jewett Fndn Grants, 1599
George H. Hitchings New Investigator Award in Health Research, 1600
George Kress Fndn Grants, 1601
Georgia Power Fndn Grants, 1603
Gertrude and William C. Wardlaw Fund Grants, 1607
Gertrude B. Elion Mentored Medical Student Research Awards, 1608
Gertrude E. Skelly Charitable Fndn Grants, 1609
Gheens Fndn Grants, 1610
Giant Eagle Fndn Grants, 1611
Gibson Fndn Grants, 1612
Gill Fndn - Gay and Lesbian Fund Grants, 1613
Gilroy and Lillian P. Roberts Charitable Fndn Grants, 1614
Ginn Fndn Grants, 1616
Giving in Action Society Children & Youth with Special Needs Grants, 1617
Giving in Action Society Family Independence Grants, 1618
GlaxoSmithKline Corp Grants, 1623
Glendale Comm Fndn Grants, 1626

Goddess Scholars Grants, 1630
Godfrey Fndn Grants, 1631
Golden State Warriors Fndn Grants, 1633
Good Samaritan Fndn Inc Grants, 1636
Goodrich Corp Fndn Grants, 1638
Grand Rapids Comm Fndn Grants, 1647
Greater Bridgeport Area Fndn Comm Impact Grants, 1650
Greater Cincinnati Fndn Priority and Small Projects/Capacity-Building Grants, 1651
Greater Green Bay Comm Fndn Grants, 1652
Greater Milwaukee Fndn Grants, 1653
Greater Saint Louis Comm Fndn Grants, 1655
Greater Tacoma Comm Fndn Grants, 1656
Greater Tacoma Comm Fndn Ryan Alan Hade Endowment Fund, 1657
Greater Worcester Comm Fndn Discretionary Grants, 1658
Green Bay Packers Fndn Grants, 1660
Green Fndn Grants, 1661
Greene County Fndn Grants, 1662
Greenfield Fndn of Maine Grants, 1663
Gregory B. Davis Fndn Grants, 1666
Gregory L. Gibson Charitable Fndn Grants, 1668
Griffin Family Fndn Grants, 1669
Griffin Fndn Grants, 1670
Grotto Fndn Project Grants, 1671
Grundy Fndn Grants, 1673
Guidant Fndn Grants, 1674
Gulf Coast Comm Fndn Grants, 1676
Gulf Coast Comm of Venice Fndn Grants, 1677
Guy's and St. Thomas' Charity Grants, 1678
H & R Fndn Grants, 1679
H. Schaffer Fndn Grants, 1680
H.A. and Mary K. Chapman Charitable Trust Grants, 1681
H.J. Heinz Company Fndn Grants, 1682
Hagedorn Fund Grants, 1685
Hall-Perrine Fndn Grants, 1686
Hallmark Corp Fndn Grants, 1688
Hancock County Comm Fndn Grants, 1690
Harley Davidson Fndn Grants, 1694
Harold Alfond Fndn Grants, 1695
Harold Simmons Fndn Grants, 1698
Harris and Eliza Kempner Fund Grants, 1699
Harry S. Black and Allon Fuller Fund, 1706
Harry Sudakoff Fndn Grants, 1708
Hartford Courant Fndn Grants, 1710
Hartford Fndn Regular Grants, 1711
Hartford Geriatrics Health Outcomes Research Scholars Program, 1712
Harvest Fndn Grants, 1713
Hawaii Comm Fndn Reverend Takie Okumura Family Grants, 1717
Hawaii Comm Fndn West Hawaii Fund Grants, 1718
Hawn Fndn Grants, 1719
HCA Fndn Grants, 1721
Health Fndn of Greater Indianapolis Grants, 1725
Health Fndn of Southern Florida Responsive Grants, 1726
Healthcare Fndn of New Jersey Grants, 1729
Hearst Fndn and William Randolph Hearst Fndn Grants, 1730
Heckscher Fndn for Children Grants, 1732
Hedco Fndn Grants, 1733
HEI Grants, 1734
Heineman Fndn for Research, Education, Charitable and Scientific Purposes, 1735
Helen K. and Arthur E. Johnson Fndn Grants, 1740
Helen Steiner Rice Fndn Grants, 1742
Helena Rubinstein Fndn Grants, 1743
Hendrick Fndn for Children Grants, 1744
Henry County Comm Fndn Grants, 1747
Herman Goldman Fndn Grants, 1753
Hershey Company Grants, 1754
HHMI Biomedical Research Grants for International Scientists in Canada and Latin America, 1756
HHMI Biomedical Research Grants for International Scientists in the Baltics, Central and Eastern Europe, Russia, and Ukraine, 1757
HHMI Biomedical Research Grants for International Scientists: Infectious Diseases and Parasitology, 1758
HHMI Med into Grad Initiative Grants, 1761
High Meadow Fndn Grants, 1768
Highmark Corp Giving Grants, 1769
Highmark Healthy High 5, 1770
Hill Crest Fndn Grants, 1773
Hill Fndn Grants, 1774
Hillman Fndn Grants, 1775
Hillsdale Fund Grants, 1778
Hilton Head Island Fndn Grants, 1779
Hilton Hotels Corp Giving Grants, 1780
Hirtzel Memorial Fndn Grants, 1781
Hoblitzelle Fndn Grants, 1783
Holland/Zeeland Comm Fndn Grants, 1786
Homer Fndn Grants, 1789
Honda of America Manufacturing Fndn Grants, 1790
Honeywell Fndn Grants, 1791
Horace A. Kimball and S. Ella Kimball Fndn Grants, 1792
Horizon Fndn for New Jersey Grants, 1793
Hormel Foods Charitable Trust Grants, 1795
Hormel Fndn Grants, 1796
Houston Endowment Grants, 1797
Howard and Bush Fndn Grants, 1798
Hugh J. Andersen Fndn Grants, 1814
Huntington Beach Police Officers Fndn Grants, 1821
Huntington Clinical Fndn Grants, 1822
Huntington County Comm Fndn Grants, 1823
Huntington National Bank Comm Affairs Grants, 1824
Hut Fndn Grants, 1827
Hutton Fndn Grants, 1828
Idaho Comm Fndn Eastern Region Competitive Grants, 1837
Idaho Power Company Corp Contributions, 1838
IHS Native American and Alaskan Native Health Research Centers, 1840
Illinois Children's Healthcare Fndn Grants, 1842
Inasmuch Fndn Grants, 1845
Independence Blue Cross Charitable Medical Care Grants, 1846
IOM Gustav O. Lienhard Award, 1864
Irvin Stern Fndn Grants, 1866
Irving S. Gilmore Fndn Grants, 1867
Isabel Allende Fndn Esperanza Grants, 1868
J.C. Penney Company Grants, 1874
J.L. Bedsole Fndn Grants, 1876
J.W. Kieckhefer Fndn Grants, 1878
Jackson County Comm Fndn Unrestricted Grants, 1879
Jacob and Hilda Blaustein Fndn Grants, 1881
Jacob and Valeria Langeloth Fndn Grants, 1882
Jacob G. Schmidlapp Trust Grants, 1883
James Ford Bell Fndn Grants, 1885
James Graham Brown Fndn Grants, 1887
James J. and Angelia M. Harris Fndn Grants, 1890
James M. Collins Fndn Grants, 1891
James M. Cox Fndn of Georgia Grants, 1892
James R. Dougherty Jr. Fndn Grants, 1894
James S. Copley Fndn Grants, 1895
Janirve Fndn Grants, 1905
Jay and Rose Phillips Family Fndn Grants, 1909
Jean and Louis Dreyfus Fndn Grants, 1911
JELD-WEN Fndn Grants, 1914
Jenkins Fndn: Improving the Health of Greater Richmond Grants, 1915
Jennings County Comm Fndn Grants, 1916
Jerome and Mildred Paddock Fndn Grants, 1917
Jessie B. Cox Charitable Trust Grants, 1918
Jessie Ball Dupont Fund Grants, 1919
Jewish Fund Grants, 1923
John Deere Fndn Grants, 1929
John Edward Fowler Memorial Fndn Grants, 1930
John G. Duncan Trust Grants, 1931
John G. Martin Fndn Grants, 1932
John H. Wellons Fndn Grants, 1934
John J. Leidy Fndn Grants, 1936
John Jewett and Helen Chandler Garland Fndn Grants, 1937
John Lord Knight Fndn Grants, 1938
John P. McGovern Fndn Grants, 1942
John P. Murphy Fndn Grants, 1943
John R. Oishei Fndn Grants, 1944
John S. Dunn Research Fndn Grants and Chairs, 1945
John W. Alden Trust Grants, 1947
John W. and Anna H. Hanes Fndn Grants, 1948
John W. Anderson Fndn Grants, 1949
Johns Manville Fund Grants, 1950
Johnson & Johnson Corp Contributions Grants, 1952
Johnson and Johnson / SAH Arts and Healing Grants, 1953
Johnson Controls Fndn Grants, 1954
Johnson County Comm Fndn Grants, 1955
Joseph Drown Fndn Grants, 1960
Josephine G. Russell Trust Grants, 1963
Josephine S. Gumbiner Fndn Grants, 1965
Julia Temple Davis Brown Fndn Grants, 1971
K and F Baxter Family Fndn Grants, 1973
K. M. Hunter Charitable Fndn Social Welfare Grants, 1974
K21 Health Fndn Grants, 1976
Kahuku Comm Fund, 1977
Kaiser Permanente Cares for Communities Grants, 1978
Kalamazoo Fndn Grants, 1979
Kate B. Reynolds Charitable Trust Health Care Grants, 1981
Katharine Matthies Fndn Grants, 1982
Katherine John Murphy Fndn Grants, 1983
Kelvin and Eleanor Smith Fndn Grants, 1986
Ken W. Davis Fndn Grants, 1987
Kendrick Fndn Grants, 1988
Kettering Family Fndn Grants, 1991
KeySpan Fndn Grants, 1995
King Pharmaceuticals Corp Contributions Grants, 2003
Knight Family Charitable and Educational Fndn Grants, 2007
Kosair Charities Grants, 2014
L. W. Pierce Family Fndn Grants, 2019
Lance Armstrong Fndn Comm Grants, 2025
Lance Armstrong Fndn Research Grants, 2026
Land O'Lakes Fndn Mid-Atlantic Grants, 2027
Lands' End Corp Giving Program, 2030
Laura B. Vogler Fndn Grants, 2032
Lawrence Fndn Grants, 2034
Leadership in Education in Neurodevelopmental Disabilities Postdoctoral Fellowships, 2037
Leonsis Fndn Grants, 2045
Lester E. Yeager Charitable Trust B Grants, 2047
Leukemia and Lymphoma Society Research Grants, 2051
Liberty Bank Fndn Grants, 2053
Little Life Fndn Grants, 2060
Lockheed Martin Philanthropic Grants, 2062
Louis Calder Fndn Grants, 2065
Louis R. Cappelli Fndn Grants, 2066
Lowe Fndn Grants, 2067
Lowell Berry Fndn Grants, 2069
Lubrizol Fndn Grants, 2080
Ludwick Family Fndn Grants, 2084
Lymphoma Research Fndn Fellowships, 2087
M-A-C AIDS Fund Grants, 2091
M. Bastian Family Fndn Grants, 2092
M.B. and Edna Zale Fndn Grants, 2093
Mabel H. Flory Charitable Trust Grants, 2096
Mabel Y. Hughes Charitable Trust Grants, 2097
Maine Comm Fndn Grants, 2099
MAP International Medical Fellowships, 2101
MAPFRE Fndn for Medicine Grants, 2102
Margaret L. Wendt Fndn Grants, 2104
Marion I. and Henry J. Knott Fndn Grants, 2109
Mark and Catherine Winkler Fndn Grants, 2112
Mars Fndn Grants, 2114
Mary Owen Borden Fndn Grants, 2121
Mary S. and David C. Corbin Fndn Grants, 2122
Mattel Children's Fndn Grants, 2130
Max A. Adler Charitable Fndn Grants, 2132

Max and Victoria Dreyfus Fndn Grants, 2133
Max Bell Fndn Grants, 2134
Maxon Charitable Fndn Grants, 2135
Maxtor Corp Contributions Grants, 2136
McGregor Fund Grants, 2143
McInerny Fndn Grants, 2144
McLean Contributionship Grants, 2147
McMillen Fndn Grants, 2148
Mead Johnson Nutritionals Charitable Giving Grants, 2156
Mead Witter Fndn Grants, 2160
Meadows Fndn Grants, 2161
Medical/Nursing Education, Research, and Health Care Exchanges with Taiwan, 2165
Meriden Fndn Grants, 2173
Mesothelioma Applied Research Fndn Grants, 2174
Metro Health Fndn Grants, 2175
Metrowest Comm Health Care Fndn Grants, 2176
Meyer Memorial Trust Emergency Grants, 2178
Meyer Memorial Trust Grassroots Grants, 2179
Meyer Memorial Trust Operating Funds Grants, 2180
Meyer Memorial Trust Responsive Grants, 2181
Middlesex Savings Charitable Fndn Grants, 2196
Miguel Aleman Fndn Grants, 2197
Milagro Fndn Grants, 2198
Miles of Hope Breast Cancer Fndn Grants, 2199
Military Ex-Prisoners of War Fndn Grants, 2201
Military Ex-Prisoners of War Fndn Grants, 2201
Millipore Fndn Grants, 2203
Miriam and Peter Haas Fund Grants, 2208
Monfort Family Fndn Grants, 2213
Moses Cone-Wesley Long Comm Health Fndn Grants, 2219
NAPNAP Fndn Elaine Gelman Scholarship, 2235
NAPNAP Fndn Innovative Health Care Small Grant, 2237
NAPNAP Fndn McNeil Grant-in-Aid, 2238
NAPNAP Fndn McNeil PNP Scholarships, 2239
NAPNAP Fndn McNeil Rural and Underserved Scholarships, 2240
NAPNAP Fndn Nursing Research Grants, 2241
NAPNAP Fndn Reckitt Benckiser Student Scholarship, 2242
NAPNAP Fndn Shourd Parks Immunization Project Small Grants, 2243
NAPNAP Fndn Wyeth Pediatric Immunization Grant, 2244
National City Corp Contributions Grants, 2250
National Patient Safety Fndn Patient Safety Research Grants, 2258
Nell Warren Elkin and William Simpson Elkin Fndn, 2302
Newman's Own Inc Grants, 2306
NIAID Integrated Preclinical/Clinical AIDS Vaccine Development Grants, 2457
NICHD Socioeconomic Status and Health Across the Life Course, 2495
Nicholas H. Noyes Jr. Memorial Fndn Grants, 2497
NIDDK Race/Ethnic Disparities in the Incidence of Diabetes Complications, 2579
NIDDK Research Grants on Improving Health Care for Obese Patients, 2581
NIEHS Environmental Justice: Partnerships for Communication, 2598
NIH Exceptional, Unconventional Research Enabling Knowledge Acceleration (EUREKA) Grants, 2662
NIH National Centers for Neurofibromatosis Research, 2695
NIH National Research Service Awards—Senior Fellows, 2697
NIH Research Project Grants, 2714
NIH School-based Interventions to Prevent Obesity, 2725
NIH Studies of Ethical, Legal, and Social Implications of Research into Human Genetic Variation Grants, 2731
NIHCM Fndn Health Care Print Journalism Awards, 2742
NIHCM Fndn Health Care Research Awards, 2743
NIHCM Fndn Health Care Television and Radio Journalism Awards, 2744
NIMH Interventions Infrastructure Program Research Grants, 2760
NIMH Socioeconomic Status and Health Across the Life Course, 2772
NIMH/NIDA Children's Services Grants, 2775
Nina Mason Pulliam Charitable Trust Grants, 2776
NINR Mentored Research Scientist Development Award, 2798
Noble County Comm Fndn Grants, 2848
NORD Roscoe Brady Lysosomal Storage Disease Fellowships, 2850
Nordson Corp Fndn Grants, 2851
North Carolina Comm Development Grants, 2858
North Carolina Comm Fndn Grants, 2859
North Carolina GlaxoSmithKline Fndn Grants, 2860
North Central Health Services Grants, 2861
Northeast Utilities Fndn Grants, 2863
Northern New York Comm Fndn Grants, 2864
Northern Trust Company Charitable Trust and Corp Giving Program, 2865
Northrop Grumman Newport News Grants, 2867
Northwestern Mutual Fndn Grants, 2870
Northwood University/Alden B. Dow Creativity Center Summer Residency Program, 2871
Norwin S. and Elizabeth N. Bean Fndn Grants, 2872
Nuffield Fndn Africa Grants, 2898
Nuffield Fndn Law and Society Grants, 2900
Nuffield Fndn Small Grants, 2903
NWHF Health Advocacy Small Grants, 2905
NWHF Kaiser Permanente Comm Fund Grants, 2906
NWHF Mark O. Hatfield Research Fellowship, 2907
NYAM Brock Lecture, Award and Visiting Professorship in Pediatrics, 2909
NYC Managed Care Consumer Assistance Workshop Re-Design Grants, 2918
NYCT AIDS/HIV Grants, 2919
NYCT Blindness and Visual Disabilities Grants, 2921
NYCT Children and Youth with Disabilities Grants, 2923
NYCT Girls and Young Women Grants, 2924
NYCT Grants for the Elderly, 2925
NYCT Health Services, Systems, and Policies Grants, 2926
NYCT Mental Health and Mental Retardation Grants, 2927
Oceanside Charitable Fndn Grants, 2934
Ogden Codman Trust Grants, 2937
Ohio County Comm Fndn Grants, 2938
Ohio County Comm Fndn Mini-Grants, 2939
Oleonda Jameson Trust Grants, 2941
Olin Corp Charitable Trust Grants, 2943
Ordean Fndn Grants, 2952
Oscar Rennebohm Fndn Grants, 2963
OSI Access to Essential Medicines Grants, 2964
OSI Integrating Health and Legal Services Grants, 2968
OSI Mental Health Grants, 2969
OSI-Baltimore Special Opportunities Grants, 2972
Owen County Comm Fndn Grants, 2979
PacifiCare Fndn Grants, 2981
PacifiCorp Fndn for Learning Grants, 2982
Pajaro Valley Comm Health Grants, 2985
Palm Beach and Martin Counties Grants, 2986
Partnership for Pediatric Epilepsy Research Grants, 2993
Patron Saints Fndn Grants, 2996
Paul and Mary Haas Fndn Contributions and Student Scholarships, 2997
Paul E. and Klare N. Reinhold Fndn Grants, 2999
Paul Ogle Fndn Grants, 3003
Peabody Fndn Grants, 3010
Peacock Fndn Grants, 3011
Pediatric Brain Tumor Research Grants, 3012
Perkins Charitable Fndn Grants, 3014
Perpetual Trust for Charitable Giving Grants, 3015
Perry County Comm Fndn Grants, 3016
Pfizer Fndn Grants, 3025
Pfizer Fndn Health Literacy Grants, 3026
Philadelphia Fndn Organizational Effectiveness Grants, 3029
PhRMA Fndn Health Outcomes Research Starter Grants, 3033
PhRMA Fndn Health Outcomes Sabbatical Fellowships, 3034
Piedmont Natural Gas Grants, 3048
Pike County Comm Fndn Grants, 3049
Pittsburgh Fndn Comm Fund Grants, 3054
Plough Fndn Grants, 3061
Polk Bros. Fndn Grants, 3066
Posey Comm Fndn Grants, 3068
Posey Comm Fndn Womens Fund Grants, 3069
Potts Memorial Fndn Grants, 3072
Powell Fndn Grants, 3073
Presbyterian Health Fndn Bridge, Seed and Equipment Grants, 3075
Priddy Fndn Grants, 3077
Pride Fndn Grants and Scholarships, 3078
Prince Charitable Trusts Chicago Grants, 3079
Principal Financial Group Fndn Grants, 3082
Procter and Gamble Fund Grants, 3083
Prostate Cancer Fndn Research Grants, 3086
Prudential Fndn Grants, 3087
Puerto Rico Comm Fndn Grants, 3090
Pulaski County Comm Fndn Grants, 3091
Putnam County Comm Fndn Grants, 3093
Quality Health Fndn Grants, 3094
Quantum Fndn Grants, 3096
Questar Corp Contributions Grants, 3097
R.C. Baker Fndn Grants, 3098
RACGP Cardiovascular Research Grants in General Practice, 3099
Rainbow Endowment Grants, 3102
Rajiv Gandhi Fndn Grants, 3104
Ralphs Food 4 Less Fndn Grants, 3106
Raskob Fndn for Catholic Activities Grants, 3107
Rasmuson Fndn Grants, 3108
Rathmann Family Fndn Grants, 3109
Rayonier Fndn Grants, 3111
RCPSC Detweiler Traveling Fellowships, 3114
RCPSC James H. Graham Award of Merit, 3119
RCPSC Teasdale-Corti Humanitarian Award, 3131
Regence Fndn Access to Health Care Grants, 3138
Regence Fndn Health Care Comm Awareness and Engagement Grants, 3139
Regence Fndn Health Care Connections Grants, 3140
Regence Fndn Improving End-of-Life Grants, 3141
Regence Fndn Tools and Technology Grants, 3142
Regenstrief General Internal Medicine - General Pediatrics Research Fellowship Program, 3144
Rehabilitation Nursing Fndn Research Grants, 3147
Retirement Research Fndn General Grants, 3150
Reynolds and Reynolds Associate Fndn Grants, 3152
Rhode Island Fndn Grants, 3154
Richard and Helen DeVos Fndn Grants, 3157
Richard and Rhoda Goldman Fund Grants, 3158
Richard and Susan Smith Family Fndn Grants, 3159
Richard E. Griffin Family Fndn Grants, 3160
Richard King Mellon Fndn Grants, 3161
Richard M. Fairbanks Fndn Grants, 3162
Richmond Eye and Ear Fund Grants, 3164
Riley Fndn Grants, 3165
Ripley County Comm Fndn Grants, 3166
Robert and Joan Dircks Fndn Grants, 3167
Robert E. and Evelyn McKee Fndn Grants, 3170
Rochester Area Comm Fndn Grants, 3176
Rochester Area Fndn Grants, 3177
Rockefeller Brothers Fund Peace and Security Grants, 3179
Rockefeller Fndn Grants, 3181
Rockwell Collins Charitable Contributions, 3182
Rockwell International Corp Trust Grants, 3183
Rollin M. Gerstacker Fndn Grants, 3186
Rosalynn Carter Institute Mattie J. T. Stepanek Caregiving Scholarships, 3190
Roy and Christine Sturgis Trust Grants, 3191
RSC Thomas W. Eadie Medal, 3199
Rush County Comm Fndn Grants, 3200

Russell Berrie Fndn Grants, 3201
Ruth Eleanor Bamberger and John Ernest Bamberger Memorial Fndn Grants, 3202
Ruth H. and Warren A. Ellsworth Fndn Grants, 3203
RWJF Comm Health Leaders Awards, 3208
RWJF Evaluating Innovations in Nursing Education Grants, 3209
RWJF Executive Nurse Fellowships, 3210
RWJF Health & Society Scholars, 3214
RWJF Health Care Costs: Research to Inform Policy Grants, 3215
RWJF Health Impact Project Grants, 3216
RWJF Jobs to Careers: Promoting Work-Based Learning for Quality Care - Research Grants, 3221
RWJF Local Funding Partnerships Grants, 3223
RWJF Pioneer Portfolio Grants, 3227
RWJF Scholars in Health Policy Research Fellowships, 3229
RWJF State Coverage Initiatives Grants, 3230
RWJF Summer Medical and Dental Education Program, 3231
RWJF Vulnerable Populations Portfolio Grants, 3232
S. Livingston Mather Charitable Trust Grants, 3235
S. Mark Taper Fndn Grants, 3236
S. Mark Taper Fndn Grants, 3236
Saint Luke's Fndn Grants, 3239
Salem Fndn Grants, 3242
Samuel S. Johnson Fndn Grants, 3251
Samueli Institute Scientific Research Grants, 3253
San Antonio Area Fndn Grants, 3254
San Diego Fndn Health & Human Services Grants, 3256
San Diego Fndn Paradise Valley Hospital Comm Fund Grants, 3257
San Francisco Fndn Comm Health Grants, 3260
Sandler Program for Asthma Research Grants, 3262
Sarah Scaife Fndn Grants, 3263
Sarasota Memorial Healthcare Fndn Grants, 3264
Sasco Fndn Grants, 3265
Savoy Fndn Research Grants, 3267
Schering-Plough Fndn Health Grants, 3270
Schurz Communications Fndn Grants, 3271
Scott County Comm Fndn Grants, 3273
Seattle Fndn Grants, 3276
Self Fndn Grants, 3277
Seneca Foods Fndn Grants, 3278
Shell Oil Company Fndn Grants, 3281
Sheltering Arms Fund Grants, 3282
Siebert Lutheran Fndn Grants, 3285
Siebert Lutheran Fndn Grants, 3285
Simmons Fndn Grants, 3287
Simple Advise Education Center Grants, 3289
Simpson Fund Grants, 3290
Sir Dorabji Tata Trust Grants for NGOs or Voluntary Organizations, 3291
Sir Dorabji Tata Trust Individual Medical Grants, 3292
Sir Halley Stewart Trust Grants, 3293
Siragusa Fndn Health Services & Medical Research Grants, 3294
Sisters of Mercy of North Carolina Fndn Grants, 3295
Sisters of Saint Joseph Charitable Fund Grants, 3296
SOCFOC Catholic Ministries Grants, 3317
Society for the Arts in Healthcare Consulting Grants, 3326
Solo Cup Fndn Grants, 3346
Sonoco Fndn Grants, 3347
Sosland Fndn Grants, 3348
South Madison Comm Fndn Grants, 3349
Southbury Comm Trust Fund, 3350
Southwest Florida Comm Fndn Competitive Grants, 3351
Southwest Gas Corp Fndn Grants, 3352
Southwire Company Grants, 3353
Special People in Need Grants, 3356
Spencer County Comm Fndn Grants, 3358
Sprague Fndn Grants, 3359
Springs Close Fndn Grants, 3360
SSRC HIV/AIDS and Public Health Policy Research in Africa Fellowships, 3365
St. Joseph Comm Health Fndn Burn Care and Prevention Grants, 3367
St. Joseph Comm Health Fndn Pfeiffer Fund Grants, 3369
St. Joseph Comm Health Fndn Schneider Fellowships, 3370
Stan and Sandy Checketts Fndn, 3373
Starr Fndn Grants, 3377
Steelcase Fndn Grants, 3379
Steele-Reese Fndn Grants, 3380
Stephen Bechtel Fund Preventive Healthcare and Selected Research Grants, 3381
Steuben County Comm Fndn Grants, 3383
Stewart Huston Charitable Trust Grants, 3384
Strowd Roses Grants, 3388
STTI/Council for the Advancement of Nursing Science Grants, 3398
Sulzberger Fndn Grants, 3399
Sunderland Fndn Grants, 3400
Sunflower Fndn Bridge Grants, 3401
Sunflower Fndn Capacity Building Grants, 3402
Sunflower Fndn Walking Trails Grants, 3403
Sunshine Natural Wellbeing Fndn Grants, 3404
Support Our Aging Religious Grants, 3406
Susan Mott Webb Charitable Trust Grants, 3412
Susan Vaughan Fndn Grants, 3413
Take Care to Learn: Teaching Clinical Care Management Grants, 3415
Takemi Program in International Health Research and Advanced Training Fellowships, 3416
Tellabs Fndn Grants, 3418
Temple-Inland Fndn Grants, 3419
Thomas and Dorothy Leavey Fndn Grants, 3422
Thomas C. Ackerman Fndn Grants, 3423
Thompson Charitable Fndn Grants, 3425
Triangle Comm Fndn Donor-Advised Grants, 3437
TWS Fndn Grants, 3443
Tylenol Scholarship, 3444
U.S. Department of Education 21st Century Comm Learning Centers, 3445
UCLA / RAND Corp Post-Doctoral Fellowships, 3454
Union Benevolent Association Grants, 3460
Union Benevolent Association Grants, 3460
Union County Comm Fndn Grants, 3461
United Methodist Church Global AIDS Fund Grants, 3463
United Methodist Health Ministry Fund Grants, 3465
United Technologies Corp Grants, 3466
Unity Fndn Of LaPorte County Grants, 3467
Until There's a Cure Fndn Grants, 3471
US Airways Comm Fndn Grants, 3473
Vancouver Fndn Grants and Comm Initiatives Program, 3477
Vancouver Fndn Public Health Bursary Package, 3478
Vancouver Sun Children's Fund Grants, 3479
Vanderburgh Comm Fndn Grants, 3480
Varian Medical Systems Grants, 3481
Verizon Fndn Health Care and Accessibility Grants, 3486
Vermont Comm Fndn Grants, 3493
VHA Health Fndn Grants, 3495
Virginia W. Kettering Fndn Grants, 3502
Volkswagen of America Corp Contributions Grants, 3503
Vulcan Materials Company Fndn Grants, 3504
W. C. Griffith Fndn Grants, 3505
W. Clarke Swanson, Jr. Fndn Grants, 3506
W.K. Kellogg Fndn Secure Families Grants, 3508
Wabash Valley Comm Fndn Grants, 3510
Wachovia Fndn Grants, 3511
Waitt Family Fndn Grants, 3512
Wal-Mart Fndn Comm Grants, 3513
Wal-Mart State Giving Grants, 3514
Wallace H. Coulter Fndn Grants, 3515
Warren Alpert Fndn Prize, 3518
Warrick County Comm Fndn Grants, 3519
Washington Post Contributions Grants, 3520
Wayne and Gladys Valley Fndn Grants, 3522
Weatherwax Fndn Grants, 3523
Weingart Fndn Grants, 3524
Welborn Baptist Fndn Grants, 3525
Wellmark Fndn Grants, 3526
Wells County Fndn Grants, 3527
Western Indiana Comm Fndn Grants, 3528
Western Union Fndn Grants, 3529
WHO Fndn General Grants, 3534
Wilhelm Sander Fndn Grants, 3535
Wilkins Family Fndn Grants, 3536
William G. Gilmore Fndn Grants, 3537
William G. McGowan Charitable Fund Grants, 3539
William H. Hannon Fndn Grants, 3540
William T. Grant Fndn Research Grants, 3541
Wilson-Wood Fndn Grants, 3542
Winifred & Harry B. Allen Fndn Grants, 3543
Winston-Salem Fndn Competitive Grants, 3544
Winston-Salem Fndn Elkin/Tri-County Grants, 3545
Winston-Salem Fndn Stokes County Grants, 3546
Women's Fndn of California Grants, 3550
YSA Get Ur Good On Grants, 3555

Health Care Access

1104 Fndn Grants, 3
1976 Fndn Grants, 5
2 Depot Square Ipswich Charitable Fndn Grants, 7
3M Company Health and Human Services Grants, 10
A Friend's Fndn Trust Grants, 13
AAP Comm Access To Child Health Advocacy Training Grants, 157
AAP Comm Access To Child Health Implementation Grants, 158
AAP Comm Access to Child Health Planning Grants, 159
AAP Comm Access To Child Health Residency Training Grants, 160
AAP Comm Access To Child Health Resident Grants, 161
AAP Leonard P. Rome Comm Access to Child Health Visiting Professorships, 164
AAP Resident Initiative Fund Grants, 167
Abbott Fund Comm Vitality Grants, 177
Abell Fndn Health and Human Services Grants, 182
ACF Supplemental Services for Recently Arrived Refugees Grants, 203
Achelis and Bodman Fndns Grants, 206
Adam Richter Charitable Trust Grants, 230
Addison H. Gibson Fndn Medical Grants, 233
Administration on Aging Senior Medicare Patrol Project Grants, 236
Aetna Fndn Health Grants in Connecticut, 244
Agnes M. Lindsay Trust Grants, 263
Alexander Eastman Fndn Grants, 341
Alice C. A. Sibley Fund Grants, 355
Alliance Healthcare Fndn Grants, 362
AMA Fndn Fund for Better Health Grants, 388
AMA Fndn Healthy Communities/Healthy America Grants, 390
American Express Fndn Comm Service Grants, 435
Angels Baseball Fndn Grants, 473
Anheuser-Busch Fndn Grants, 474
APF Awards for Advancing Minority Mental Health, 504
APF Disaster Recovery Fund for Psychiatrists, 506
Assurant Health Fndn Grants, 655
AT&T Fndn Civic and Comm Service Grants, 658
Autzen Fndn Grants, 672
Balfe Family Fndn Grants, 682
Bank of America Charitable Fndn National Programs and Partners Grants, 689
Baptist Comm Ministries Grants, 691
Baptist-Trinity Lutheran Legacy Fndn Grants, 692
Barra Fndn Comm Fund Grants, 698
Baxter International Fndn Grants, 705
BCBS of Massachusetts Catalyst Fund Grants, 708
BCBS of Massachusetts Fndn Grants, 709
BCBS of Minnesota Growing Up Healthy Grants, 711
BCBSM Comm Health Matching Grants, 715
BCBSM Fndn Physician Investigator Research Awards, 718

BCBSM Investigator-Initiated Research Grants, 723
BCBSNC Fndn Grants, 725
Benton County Fndn Grants, 744
BHHS Legacy Fndn Grants, 753
Blue Shield of California Grants, 771
Breast Cancer Fund Grants, 790
Brian G. Dyson Fndn Grants, 791
Bristol-Myers Squibb Fndn Product Donations Grants, 799
Bristol-Myers Squibb Patient Assistance Program, 801
Bush Fndn Health & Human Services Grants, 814
California Comm Fndn Health Care Grants, 831
California Endowment CommunitiesFirst Grants, 833
California Wellness Fndn Work and Health Grants, 834
Cardinal Health Fndn Grants, 864
Cargill Citizenship Fund-Corp Giving Grants, 865
Carl B. and Florence E. King Fndn Grants, 869
Charlotte County (FL) Comm Fndn Grants, 973
CHCF Grants, 979
Christopher Reeve Paralysis Fndn Individual Research Grants, 1006
Claude Worthington Benedum Fndn Grants, 1033
Colorado Trust Grants, 1062
Columbus Fndn Allen Eiry Fund Grants, 1064
Columbus Fndn Estrich Fund Grants, 1067
Columbus Fndn J. Floyd Dixon Memorial Fund Grants, 1068
Columbus Fndn Mary Eleanor Morris Fund Grants, 1069
Comerica Charitable Fndn Grants, 1073
Comm Fndn of Greater Birmingham Grants, 1106
Comm Impact Fund, 1135
Connecticut Health Fndn Health Initiative Grants, 1142
Covenant Fndn Grants, 1153
CVS Comm Grants, 1177
D. W. McMillan Fndn Grants, 1180
Dana Brown Charitable Trust Grants, 1194
Daviess County Comm Fndn Health Grants, 1203
Deland Fellowships in Health Care and Society, 1214
DHHS Rural Telemedicine Grants, 1279
Dorothy Hooper Beattie Fndn Grants, 1321
Duke Endowment Health Care Grants, 1338
Edina Realty Fndn Grants, 1369
Eisner Fndn Grants, 1387
Emerson Electric Company Contributions Grants, 1413
FCD Child Development Grants, 1458
Flinn Fndn Grants Programs, 1511
Fndn for a Healthy Kentucky Grants, 1527
Fndn of CVPH Melissa Lahtinen-Penfield Organ Donor Fund Grants, 1540
Fndn of CVPH Rabin Fund Grants, 1541
Fndn of CVPH Roger Senecal Endowment Fund Grants, 1542
Fndn of CVPH Travel Fund Grants, 1543
Frances W. Emerson Fndn Grants, 1548
General Service Fndn Reproductive Health and Rights Grants, 1592
Gerber Fndn Grants, 1606
Gibson Fndn Grants, 1612
GlaxoSmithKline Corp Grants, 1623
Good Samaritan Fndn Inc Grants, 1636
Great-West Life Grants, 1649
Gregory B. Davis Fndn Grants, 1666
Gregory L. Gibson Charitable Fndn Grants, 1668
Guy's and St. Thomas' Charity Grants, 1678
Harold and Arlene Schnitzer CARE Fndn Grants, 1697
Harry S. Black and Allon Fuller Fund, 1706
Harry Sudakoff Fndn Grants, 1708
Harvest Fndn Grants, 1713
Health Fndn of Southern Florida Responsive Grants, 1726
Healthcare Fndn for Orange County Grants, 1728
Healthcare Fndn of New Jersey Grants, 1729
Henry J. Kaiser Family Fndn Grants, 1748
Huntington Clinical Fndn Grants, 1822
Huntington County Comm Fndn Grants, 1823
Independence Blue Cross Charitable Medical Care Grants, 1846
James M. Cox Fndn of Georgia Grants, 1892
Jerome and Mildred Paddock Fndn Grants, 1917
Jewish Fund Grants, 1923
John M. Lloyd Fndn Grants, 1939
Johnson & Johnson Comm Health Care Grants, 1951
Johnson & Johnson Corp Contributions Grants, 1952
Joseph Drown Fndn Grants, 1960
Kaiser Permanente Cares for Communities Grants, 1978
Kendrick Fndn Grants, 1988
Kenneth T. and Eileen L. Norris Fndn Grants, 1989
Mattel Children's Fndn Grants, 2130
Mattel International Grants, 2131
Maxtor Corp Contributions Grants, 2136
Mead Johnson Nutritionals Charitable Giving Grants, 2156
Metrowest Comm Health Care Fndn Grants, 2176
Michael and Susan Dell Fndn Grants, 2189
Morris and Gwendolyn Cafritz Fndn Grants, 2217
Moses Cone-Wesley Long Comm Health Fndn Grants, 2219
Mount Zion Health Fund Grants, 2220
NAPNAP Fndn Innovative Health Care Small Grant, 2237
NAPNAP Fndn McNeil Grant-in-Aid, 2238
NIDA HIV Drug Therapy for HIV Users: Access, Adherence, Effectiveness, 2504
Northern Trust Company Charitable Trust and Corp Giving Program, 2865
Northwest Airlines KidCares Medical Travel Assistance, 2868
NYCT AIDS/HIV Grants, 2919
NYCT Blindness and Visual Disabilities Grants, 2921
NYCT Children and Youth with Disabilities Grants, 2923
NYCT Grants for the Elderly, 2925
NYCT Health Services, Systems, and Policies Grants, 2926
NYCT Mental Health and Mental Retardation Grants, 2927
Ohio County Comm Fndn Grants, 2938
Ohio County Comm Fndn Mini-Grants, 2939
OSI Mental Health Grants, 2969
OSI-Baltimore Special Opportunities Grants, 2972
OSI-Baltimore Tackling Drug Addiction Grants, 2973
Otto Bremer Fndn Grants, 2977
PacifiCare Fndn Grants, 2981
Paul G. Allen Family Fndn Grants, 3000
Quantum Corp Snap Server Grants, 3095
Rainbow Endowment Grants, 3102
Raymond John Wean Fndn Grants, 3110
Regence Fndn Access to Health Care Grants, 3138
Regence Fndn Health Care Comm Awareness and Engagement Grants, 3139
Regence Fndn Health Care Connections Grants, 3140
Regence Fndn Improving End-of-Life Grants, 3141
Regence Fndn Tools and Technology Grants, 3142
Reynolds and Reynolds Associate Fndn Grants, 3152
Robert F. Stoico / FIRSTFED Charitable Fndn Grants, 3171
Robert Sterling Clark Fndn Reproductive Rights and Health Grants, 3173
Rockefeller Fndn Grants, 3181
RWJF Evaluating Innovations in Nursing Education Grants, 3209
RWJF Finding Answers: Disparities Research for Change Grants, 3211
RWJF Health Care Costs: Research to Inform Policy Grants, 3215
RWJF Investigator Awards in Health Policy Research, 3220
RWJF Local Funding Partnerships Grants, 3223
RWJF New Jersey Health Initiatives Grants, 3225
RWJF Partners Investing in Nursing's Future Grants, 3226
RWJF Pioneer Portfolio Grants, 3227
RWJF State Coverage Initiatives Grants, 3230
RWJF Vulnerable Populations Portfolio Grants, 3232
SAG Motion Picture Players Welfare Fund Grants, 3238
Saint Luke's Fndn Grants, 3239
San Diego Fndn Paradise Valley Hospital Comm Fund Grants, 3257
San Francisco Fndn Comm Health Grants, 3260
Sheltering Arms Fund Grants, 3282
Sir Dorabji Tata Trust Grants for NGOs or Voluntary Organizations, 3291
Siragusa Fndn Health Services & Medical Research Grants, 3294
Sisters of St. Joseph Healthcare Fndn Grants, 3297
Solo Cup Fndn Grants, 3346
Stephen Bechtel Fund Preventive Healthcare and Selected Research Grants, 3381
Topfer Family Fndn Grants, 3430
UCLA / RAND Corp Post-Doctoral Fellowships, 3454
United Methodist Health Ministry Fund Grants, 3465
Verizon Fndn Health Care and Accessibility Grants, 3486
W.K. Kellogg Fndn Secure Families Grants, 3508
Wal-Mart State Giving Grants, 3514
Welborn Baptist Fndn Grants, 3525
WHO Fndn General Grants, 3534
Women's Fndn of California Grants, 3550

Health Care Administration

Aaron & Freda Glickman Fndn Grants, 172
American Academy of Nursing Building Academic Geriatric Nursing Capacity Scholarships, 414
AUPHA Baxter International Fndn Prize for Health Services Research, 666
Beckman Coulter Comm Relations Grants, 733
Bush Fndn Medical Fellowships, 815
Byron W. and Alice L. Lockwood Fndn Grants, 824
Canada-U.S. Fulbright New Century Scholars Grants, 846
Canada-U.S. Fulbright Senior Specialists Grants, 847
CMS Historically Black Colleges and Universities Health Services Research Grants, 1044
Commonwealth Fund Payment System Reform Grants, 1082
Comm Health Scholars Program Fellowships, 1134
Covenant Matters Fndn Grants, 1154
Deland Fellowships in Health Care and Society, 1214
DHHS Professional Nurse Traineeships Program, 1274
DHHS Public Health Students Traineeships and Other Graduate Public Health Programs, 1277
DHHS Technical and Non-Financial Assistance to Health Centers, 1280
Duke Endowment Health Care Grants, 1338
E. Rhodes and Leona B. Carpenter Fndn Grants, 1356
FACHE Albert W. Dent Scholarships, 1445
Fulbright Alumni Initiatives Awards Grants, 1566
Fulbright Distinguished Chairs Grants, 1567
Fulbright New Century Scholars Grants, 1570
Fulbright Specialists Grants, 1571
Fulbright Traditional Scholar Program in Europe and Eurasia, 1572
Fulbright Traditional Scholar Program in Sub-Saharan Africa, 1573
Fulbright Traditional Scholar Program in the East Asia/Pacific Region, 1574
Fulbright Traditional Scholar Program in the Near East and North Africa Region, 1575
Fulbright Traditional Scholar Program in the South and Central Asia Region, 1576
Fulbright Traditional Scholar Program in the Western Hemisphere, 1577
Guy's and St. Thomas' Charity Grants, 1678
Hartford Aging and Health Program Awards, 1709
Health Care Financing Research, Demonstrations, and Evaluations Grants, 1723
Health Management Scholarships and Grants for Minorities, 1727
Henry J. Kaiser Family Fndn Grants, 1748
International Fellowships in Medical Education, 1861

Leadership in Education in Neurodevelopmental Disabilities Postdoctoral Fellowships, 2037
Mayday Fund Grants, 2139
NAPNAP Fndn Nursing Research Grants, 2241
National Blood Fndn Research Grant Program, 2249
NYCT Health Services, Systems, and Policies Grants, 2926
OREF/AAOS Clinical Research Training Fellowship, 2958
OSI-Baltimore Tackling Drug Addiction Grants, 2973
Richard P. Covert Scholarship, 3163
RWJF Health Policy Fellowships, 3217
Takemi Program in International Health Research and Advanced Training Fellowships, 3416
UCLA / RAND Corp Post-Doctoral Fellowships, 3454

Health Care Assessment
AACAP Jeanne Spurlock Research Fellowship in Substance Abuse and Addiction for Minority Medical Students, 40
AACAP Summer Medical Student Fellowships, 53
Alexander Eastman Fndn Grants, 341
APF Disaster Recovery Fund for Psychiatrists, 506
CHCF Grants, 979
Commonwealth Fund Harkness Fellowships in Health Care Policy and Practice, 1079
Commonwealth Fund Health Care Quality Improvement and Efficiency Grants, 1080
Deland Fellowships in Health Care and Society, 1214
Duke Endowment Health Care Grants, 1338
Guy's and St. Thomas' Charity Grants, 1678
Hartford Aging and Health Program Awards, 1709
Illinois Children's Healthcare Fndn Grants, 1842
Johnson & Johnson Comm Health Care Grants, 1951
Kansas Health Fndn Grants, 1980
National Patient Safety Fndn Patient Safety Research Grants, 2258
NYCT Children and Youth with Disabilities Grants, 2923
NYCT Health Services, Systems, and Policies Grants, 2926
RWJF Evaluating Innovations in Nursing Education Grants, 3209
UCLA / RAND Corp Post-Doctoral Fellowships, 3454

Health Care Economics
AMI Semiconductors Corp Grants, 468
CDC Antimicrobial Resistance in Hospital-Acquired Infections Among Intensive Care Unit Patients, 902
CHCF Grants, 979
Duke Endowment Health Care Grants, 1338
Elsa U. Pardee Fndn Grants, 1407
Fndn for Seacoast Health Grants, 1533
Good Samaritan Fndn Inc Grants, 1636
Guy's and St. Thomas' Charity Grants, 1678
Hartford Aging and Health Program Awards, 1709
HRB Health Services Research Fellowships, 1801
Kendrick Fndn Grants, 1988
National Patient Safety Fndn Patient Safety Research Grants, 2258
NIH Economic Studies in Cancer Prevention, Screening, and Care, 2657
NIMH Interventions Infrastructure Program Research Grants, 2760
Northern Trust Company Charitable Trust and Corp Giving Program, 2865
Pfizer Fndn Health Literacy Grants, 3026
PhRMA Fndn Health Outcomes Research Starter Grants, 3033
RWJF Health Care Costs: Research to Inform Policy Grants, 3215
RWJF State Coverage Initiatives Grants, 3230
SOCFOC Reducing Health & Educational Disparities in the Central Neighborhood Grants, 3318
UCLA / RAND Corp Post-Doctoral Fellowships, 3454

Health Care Financing
Aetna Fndn Regional Comm Health General Support Grants, 248
Alliance Healthcare Fndn Grants, 362
AUPHA Baxter International Fndn Prize for Health Services Research, 666
Baptist-Trinity Lutheran Legacy Fndn Grants, 692
BCBS of Massachusetts Catalyst Fund Grants, 708
BCBSM Investigator-Initiated Research Grants, 723
California Comm Fndn Health Care Grants, 831
CHCF Health Care Affordability Grants, 980
Deland Fellowships in Health Care and Society, 1214
DHHS National Health Service Corps Loan Repayment Awards, 1265
DHHS Native American Health Service Loan Repayment Awards, 1267
Duke Endowment Health Care Grants, 1338
Guy's and St. Thomas' Charity Grants, 1678
Hartford Aging and Health Program Awards, 1709
Health Care Financing Research, Demonstrations, and Evaluations Grants, 1723
NYCT AIDS/HIV Grants, 2919
RWJF Changes in Health Care Financing and Organization Grants, 3206
RWJF State Coverage Initiatives Grants, 3230
Sarasota Memorial Healthcare Fndn Grants, 3264
UCLA / RAND Corp Post-Doctoral Fellowships, 3454

Health Care Personnel
Connecticut Health Fndn Initiative Grants, 1142

Health Care Promotion
Saint Luke's Fndn Grants, 3239

Health Delivery Services
Cardinal Health Fndn Grants, 864

Health Disparities
OBSSR Behavioral and Social Science Research on Understanding and Reducing Health Disparities Grants, 2932

Health Education
Aetna Fndn Regional Comm Health Grants, 249
Anthem Blue Cross and Blue Shield Grants, 488
APF Disaster Recovery Fund for Psychiatrists, 506
Austin-Bailey Health and Wellness Fndn Grants, 669
Baxter International Fndn Grants, 705
BCBSNC Fndn Grants, 725
Blowitz-Ridgeway Fndn Early Childhood Development Research Award, 766
CampusRN/AACN Nursing Scholarship Fund, 841
Carlos and Marguerite Mason Trust Grants, 875
Chiron Fndn Comm Grants, 1004
Comprehensive Health Education Fndn Grants, 1139
Express Scripts Fndn Grants, 1441
Fndn for a Healthy Kentucky Grants, 1527
Global Fund for Children Grants, 1629
Great-West Life Grants, 1649
Hogg Fndn for Mental Health Grants, 1784
HomeBanc Fndn Grants, 1788
Indiana AIDS Fund Grants, 1851
John M. Lloyd Fndn Grants, 1939
Key Fndn Grants, 1994
M-A-C AIDS Fund Grants, 2091
McCarthy Family Fndn Grants, 2141
Moses Cone-Wesley Long Comm Health Fndn Grants, 2219
NAPNAP Fndn Innovative Health Care Small Grant, 2237
NAPNAP Fndn McNeil Grant-in-Aid, 2238
NAPNAP Fndn Nursing Research Grants, 2241
NAPNAP Fndn Wyeth Pediatric Immunization Grant, 2244
NIH Undergraduate Scholarships, 2737
PhRMA Fndn Health Outcomes Sabbatical Fellowships, 3034
Richmond Eye and Ear Fund Grants, 3164
Rosalynn Carter Institute John and Betty Pope Fellowships, 3189
Special Olympics Health Professions Student Grants, 3355
Sunshine Natural Wellbeing Fndn Grants, 3404
Varian Medical Systems Grants, 3481
Viking Children's Fund Grants, 3497
Women of the ELCA Opportunity Scholarships for Lutheran Laywomen, 3548

Health Facilities Studies
NYCT Health Services, Systems, and Policies Grants, 2926
RWJF Evaluating Innovations in Nursing Education Grants, 3209
UCLA / RAND Corp Post-Doctoral Fellowships, 3454

Health Insurance
AAP Comm Access To Child Health Advocacy Training Grants, 157
AAP Comm Access to Child Health Planning Grants, 159
AAP Comm Access To Child Health Residency Training Grants, 160
AAP Comm Access To Child Health Resident Grants, 161
AAP Leonard P. Rome Comm Access to Child Health Visiting Professorships, 164
Alliance Healthcare Fndn Grants, 362
AMA Fndn Fund for Better Health Grants, 388
Austin-Bailey Health and Wellness Fndn Grants, 669
BCBS of Massachusetts Catalyst Fund Grants, 708
BCBS of Massachusetts Fndn Grants, 709
BCBSNC Fndn Grants, 725
Blue Shield of California Grants, 771
California Wellness Fndn Work and Health Grants, 834
CDC National Training Information and Exchange Program, 920
CHCF Grants, 979
CHCF Local Coverage Expansion Initiative, 981
CMS Research and Demonstration Grants, 1045
Commonwealth Fund Payment System Reform Grants, 1082
Commonwealth Fund Small Grants, 1084
Deland Fellowships in Health Care and Society, 1214
Edwards Memorial Trust Grants, 1375
Families USA Wellstone Fellowship for Social Justice, 1450
Fndn for a Healthy Kentucky Grants, 1527
Health Fndn of Greater Cincinnati Grants, 1724
Kaiser Permanente Cares for Communities Grants, 1978
Medicaid/SCHIP Eligibility Pilots, 2164
Michael and Susan Dell Fndn Grants, 2189
NIH Cancer Surveillance Using Health Claims-Based Data System Grants, 2645
NYC Managed Care Consumer Assistance Workshop Re-Design Grants, 2918
Prince Charitable Trusts Chicago Grants, 3079
Quantum Corp Snap Server Grants, 3095
Quantum Fndn Grants, 3096
Rehab Therapy Fndn Grants, 3146
RWJF Health Care Costs: Research to Inform Policy Grants, 3215
RWJF Investigator Awards in Health Policy Research, 3220
RWJF State Coverage Initiatives Grants, 3230
RWJF Summer Medical and Dental Education Program, 3231
UCLA/RAND Corp Post-Doctoral Fellowships, 3454

Health Massage Therapy
Massage Therapy Research Grants, 2127

Health Personnel/Professions
BCBSM Fndn Student Award Program, 721
Comm Fndn Of Greater Lafayette Grants, 1110
NHLBI Short-Term Research Education Program to Increase Diversity in Health-Related Research, 2383

Prince Charitable Trusts Chicago Grants, 3079
RWJF Generalist Physician Faculty Scholars, 3212
RWJF Harold Amos Medical Faculty Development Scholars, 3213
Special Olympics Health Professions Student Grants, 3355
Topeka Comm Fndn Kansas Blood Services Scholarships, 3429

Health Planning/Policy

3M Company Health and Human Services Grants, 10
AAP Comm Access To Child Health Advocacy Training Grants, 157
AAP Comm Access to Child Health Planning Grants, 159
AAP Comm Access To Child Health Residency Training Grants, 160
AAP Comm Access To Child Health Resident Grants, 161
AAP Leonard P. Rome Comm Access to Child Health Visiting Professorships, 164
AcademyHealth Alice S. Hersh New Investigator Awards, 190
AcademyHealth Alice S. Hersh Student Scholarships, 191
AcademyHealth HSR Impact Awards, 193
AcademyHealth PHSR Interest Group Student Scholarships, 195
ACS Research Scholar Grants for Health Services and Health Policy Research, 222
AHFMR Clinical Investigator Awards, 270
AHFMR Infrastructure Funding Grants, 283
AHFMR Personnel Funding Grants, 290
AHFMR Scholar Awards, 295
AHFMR Scientist Awards, 296
AHFMR Senior Investigator Awards, 297
AHFMR Senior Scholar Awards, 299
APF Jeanne Spurlock Congressional Fellowships, 509
AUPHA Baxter International Fndn Prize for Health Services Research, 666
BCBSM Fndn Excellence in Research Awards for Students, 717
BCBSM Fndn Student Award Program, 721
BCBSM Frank J. McDevitt, DO, Excellence in Research Awards, 722
Becton Dickinson and Company Grants, 736
Blue Shield of California Grants, 771
California Wellness Fndn Work & Health Grants, 834
Canadian Fndn for Dietetic Research Awards, 849
CDC Epidemiology and Laboratory Capacity Infectious Diseases Grants, 909
CHCF Grants, 979
Chiron Fndn Comm Grants, 1004
Colorado Trust Grants, 1062
Commonwealth Fund Affordable Health Insurance Grants, 1077
Commonwealth Fund Australian-American Health Policy Fellowships, 1078
Commonwealth Fund Harkness Fellowships in Health Care Policy and Practice, 1079
Commonwealth Fund Health Care Quality Improvement and Efficiency Grants, 1080
Commonwealth Fund Patient-Centered Coordinated Care Grants, 1081
Commonwealth Fund Payment System Reform Grants, 1082
Commonwealth Fund Small Grants, 1084
Commonwealth Fund State High Performance Health Systems Grants, 1085
Commonwealth Fund/Harvard University Fellowship in Minority Health Policy, 1086
Covenant Matters Fndn Grants, 1154
DHHS Public Health Students Traineeships and Other Graduate Public Health Programs, 1277
Doris Duke Charitable Fndn Operations Research on AIDS Care and Treatment in Africa Grants, 1319
Entergy Corp Open Grants for Healthy Families, 1418
Fndn for a Healthy Kentucky Grants, 1527
General Service Fndn Reproductive Health and Rights Grants, 1592
Greenwall Fndn Bioethics Grants, 1665
Harry S. Black and Allon Fuller Fund, 1706
Health Care Financing Research, Demonstrations, and Evaluations Grants, 1723
Henry J. Kaiser Family Fndn Grants, 1748
HHMI Grants and Fellowships Programs, 1759
John M. Lloyd Fndn Grants, 1939
Kansas Health Fndn Grants, 1980
Lester Ray Fleming Scholarships, 2048
Mayday Fund Grants, 2139
NCI/NIDA Transdisciplinary Tobacco Use Research Centers Grants, 2280
New York Life Fndn Grants, 2304
NIH Economic Studies in Cancer Prevention, Screening, and Care, 2657
NYCT Girls and Young Women Grants, 2924
NYCT Health Services, Systems, and Policies Grants, 2926
NYCT Mental Health and Mental Retardation Grants, 2927
OSI Integrating Health and Legal Services Grants, 2968
OSI-Baltimore Special Opportunities Grants, 2972
OSI-Baltimore Tackling Drug Addiction Grants, 2973
OUT Fund for Lesbian and Gay Liberation Grants, 2978
Pfizer Fndn Health Literacy Grants, 3026
Rainbow Endowment Grants, 3102
Robert Sterling Clark Fndn Reproductive Rights and Health Grants, 3173
RWJF Changes in Health Care Financing and Organization Grants, 3206
RWJF Evaluating Innovations in Nursing Education Grants, 3209
RWJF Health Policy Fellowships, 3217
RWJF Investigator Awards in Health Policy Research, 3220
RWJF Partners Investing in Nursing's Future Grants, 3226
RWJF State Coverage Initiatives Grants, 3230
Takemi Program in International Health Research and Advanced Training Fellowships, 3416
Tides Fndn Syringe Access Fund, 3427
UCLA/RAND Corp Post-Doctoral Fellowships, 3454
William T. Grant Fndn Research Grants, 3541

Health Policy/Planning

BCBS of Massachusetts Fndn Grants, 709
Families USA Wellstone Fellowship for Social Justice, 1450
Henry J. Kaiser Family Fndn Media Fellowships, 1749
Hogg Fndn for Mental Health Grants, 1784
KFF Barbara Jordan Health Policy Scholarships, 2000
Until There's a Cure Fndn Grants, 3471

Health Promotion

49ers Fndn Grants, 12
A-T Medical Research Fndn Grants, 16
AAFP Fndn Health Literacy State Grants, 112
AAFP Research Stimulation Grants, 116
AAMC Abraham Flexner Award, 133
AAMC David E. Rogers Award, 137
Abington Fndn Grants, 184
ACGT Young Investigator Grants, 205
Air Products and Chemicals Grants, 319
Albertson's Charitable Giving Grants, 330
Alexander Eastman Fndn Grants, 341
Allen P. and Josephine B. Green Fndn Grants, 361
AMA Fndn Health Literacy Grants, 389
American Academy of Dermatology Shade Structure Grants, 413
American Academy of Nursing Media Awards, 418
American-Italian Cancer Fndn Fellowships, 459
Anheuser-Busch Fndn Grants, 474
Ann Arbor Area Comm Fndn Grants, 476
Ann Peppers Fndn Grants, 478
Anthem Blue Cross and Blue Shield School Nurse Grants, 489
AON Fndn Grants, 491
APF Disaster Recovery Fund for Psychiatrists, 506
AptarGroup Fndn Grants, 522
Assurant Health Fndn Grants, 655
Atkinson Fndn International Grants, 661
Autzen Fndn Grants, 672
BCBSM Investigator-Initiated Research Grants, 723
BCBSNC Fndn Fit Together Grants, 724
BCBSNC Fndn Grants, 725
Beldon Fund Grants, 738
Bernard and Audre Rapoport Fndn Grants, 746
Bildner Family Fndn Grants, 755
Bill and Melinda Gates Fndn Grants, 756
Bullitt Fndn Grants, 809
California Endowment CommunitiesFirst Grants, 833
California Wellness Fndn Work and Health Grants, 834
Canadian Fndn for Dietetic Research Awards, 849
CDC Core Capacity Grants, 907
CDC Oral Diseases Prevention and Oral Health Promotion Grants, 921
CDC Preventive Health Services-Sexually Transmitted Diseases Control Grants, 923
CDC Promoting Prevention in Managed Care Cooperative Agreements, 925
CDC Public Health Conference Support Grant Program, 926
CDC Using Genetic Information to Prevent Disease and Improve Health Research Grants, 932
Center for Science in the Public Interest Internships, 935
CF Clinical Research Trainee Awards, 940
CFPC Fellowships, 955
Champ-A Champion Fur Kids Grants, 959
Charles H. Hood Fndn Child Health Research Grants, 968
Chase Paymentech Corp Giving Grants, 975
CHCF Grants, 979
Chicago Comm Trust Grants, 989
Christopher Reeve Paralysis Fndn Quality of Life and Health Promotions Grants, 1007
CMA Fndn Grants, 1042
CNCS Next Generation Grants, 1049
Colorado Trust Grants, 1062
Colorado Trust Partnerships for Health Initiative, 1063
Comprehensive Health Education Fndn Grants, 1139
Connecticut Comm Fndn Grants, 1141
Connecticut Health Fndn Health Initiative Grants, 1142
Daniel Mendelsohn New Investigator Award, 1199
DHHS AIDS Project Grants, 1245
DHHS Health Care Systems Cost and Access Research and Development Grants, 1252
DHHS Health Conference Support Program for Toxic Substances and Disease Registry, 1255
DHHS Health Promotion and Disease Prevention Research and Demonstration Centers Grants, 1260
DHHS Maternal and Child Health Research and Training Programs Grants, 1264
DHHS Oral Health Promotion Research Across the Lifespan, 1269
Dickson Fndn Grants, 1284
Dorothy Rider Pool Health Care Grants, 1322
EPA Lead Awareness Outreach for Native American Tribes, 1421
Essex County Comm Fndn Discretionary Fund Grant, 1428
Ewing Halsell Fndn Grants, 1440
Express Scripts Fndn Grants, 1441
Floyd A. and Kathleen C. Cailloux Fndn Grants, 1516
Fndn for a Healthy Kentucky Grants, 1527
General Mills Champions for Healthy Kids Grants, 1589
General Mills Fndn Grants, 1590
Gerber Fndn Grants, 1606
Glazer Family Fndn Grants, 1625
Great-West Life Grants, 1649
Harry S. Black and Allon Fuller Fund, 1706
Hartford Geriatrics Health Outcomes Research Scholars Program, 1712

Harvest Fndn Grants, 1713
Hasbro Children's Fund, 1714
Hawn Fndn Grants, 1719
HCA Fndn Grants, 1721
Health Canada National Seniors Independence Grants, 1722
Health Fndn of Greater Cincinnati Grants, 1724
Health Fndn of Greater Indianapolis Grants, 1725
Health Fndn of Southern Florida Responsive Grants, 1726
Healthcare Fndn for Orange County Grants, 1728
Henry & Ruth Blaustein Rosenberg Fndn Grants, 1746
Hirtzel Memorial Fndn Grants, 1781
Hogg Fndn for Mental Health Grants, 1784
HomeBanc Fndn Grants, 1788
Homer Fndn Grants, 1789
Horizon Fndn for New Jersey Grants, 1793
HRSA Physician Assistant Training, 1810
Institute for Agriculture and Trade Policy Food and Society Fellowships, 1856
Jacob and Hilda Blaustein Fndn Grants, 1881
James Hervey Johnson Charitable Educational Trust Grants, 1889
Jane's Trust Grants, 1904
Jessie B. Cox Charitable Trust Grants, 1918
Jewish Fund Grants, 1923
Jewish Women's Fndn of New York Grants, 1924
Joe W. and Dorothy Dorsett Brown Fndn Grants, 1927
John P. McGovern Fndn Grants, 1942
Johnson and Johnson / SAH Arts and Healing Grants, 1953
Josephine S. Gumbiner Fndn Grants, 1965
Kaiser Permanente Cares for Communities Grants, 1978
Kansas Health Fndn Grants, 1980
Lance Armstrong Fndn Comm Grants, 2025
Lewis Preston Fund for Girls Education Grants, 2052
Louis R. Cappelli Fndn Grants, 2066
M-A-C AIDS Fund Grants, 2091
Mary Black Fndn Grants, 2118
Mass Youth Against Tobacco Mini-Grants, 2123
Maxtor Corp Contributions Grants, 2136
McCarthy Family Fndn Grants, 2141
Mead Johnson Nutritionals Charitable Giving Grants, 2156
MedImmune Charitable Grants, 2166
Medtronic Fndn Health Care Grants, 2169
Metrowest Comm Health Care Fndn Grants, 2176
Michael and Susan Dell Fndn Grants, 2189
Morton K. and Jane Blaustein Fndn Grants, 2218
Moses Cone-Wesley Long Comm Health Fndn Grants, 2219
Mount Zion Health Fund Grants, 2220
Ms. Fndn for Women Grants, 2222
NAPNAP Fndn Innovative Health Care Small Grant, 2237
NAPNAP Fndn McNeil Grant-in-Aid, 2238
NAPNAP Fndn Nursing Research Grants, 2241
NCIC Terry Fox Research Studentships, 2286
NIA Health Behaviors and Aging Grants, 2408
NIDCD Health Promotion and Disease Prevention: Health Communication, Development, and Dissemination, 2521
NIDCR Clinical Trial Pilot Grant, 2533
NIH Exploratory Centers for Alternative Medicine Research Grants, 2663
NIH Health Promotion Among Racial and Ethnic Minority Males, 2671
NLM Understanding and Promoting Health Literacy Research Grants, 2827
Northrop Grumman Corp Grants, 2866
Nuffield Fndn Africa Grants, 2898
Nuffield Fndn Law and Society Grants, 2900
Nuffield Fndn Small Grants, 2903
ORISE Postgraduate Research Participation at the Agency for Toxic Substances and Disease Registry, 2960
PacifiCare Fndn Grants, 2981
Paso del Norte Health Fndn Grants, 2995
Pfizer Fndn Grants, 3025
Portland General Electric Fndn Grants, 3067
Premera CARES Grants, 3074
Prince Charitable Trusts District of Columbia Grants, 3080
Quantum Fndn Grants, 3096
Rainbow Endowment Grants, 3102
RGK Fndn Grants, 3153
Ruth Mott Fndn Grants, 3204
RWJF Health & Society Scholars, 3214
RWJF Healthy Eating Research Grants, 3218
RWJF Young Epidemiology Scholars Competition, 3233
Scott County Comm Fndn Grants, 3273
Sisters of Saint Joseph Charitable Fund Grants, 3296
Sisters of St. Joseph Healthcare Fndn Grants, 3297
Special Olympics Health Professions Student Grants, 3355
SSRC HIV/AIDS and Public Health Policy Research in Africa Fellowships, 3365
Sunflower Fndn Bridge Grants, 3401
Sunflower Fndn Capacity Building Grants, 3402
Sunflower Fndn Walking Trails Grants, 3403
Sunshine Natural Wellbeing Fndn Grants, 3404
Susan G. Komen Breast Cancer Fndn Breast Health, Breast Cancer Education, and Outreach Programs Grants, 3408
Tellabs Fndn Grants, 3418
Tides Fndn Syringe Access Fund, 3427
United Methodist Health Ministry Fund Grants, 3465
Varian Medical Systems Grants, 3481
VHA Health Fndn Grants, 3495
Wachovia Fndn Grants, 3511
Warren Alpert Fndn Prize, 3518
Welborn Baptist Fndn Grants, 3525
Wellmark Fndn Grants, 3526
Western Union Fndn Grants, 3529

Health Records

Comm Campus Partnerships for Health Fellowships, 1087
Regenstrief General Internal Medicine - General Pediatrics Research Fellowship Program, 3144

Health Research

AHFMR Clinical Investigator Awards, 270
AHFMR Infrastructure Funding Grants, 283
AHFMR Personnel Funding Grants, 290
AHFMR Scholar Awards, 295
AHFMR Scientist Awards, 296
AHFMR Senior Investigator Awards, 297
AHFMR Senior Scholar Awards, 299

Health Sciences

AAHPERD Ruth Abernathy Presidential Scholarships, 128
AAHPERD-AAHE Undergraduate Scholarships, 131
Dr. Sydney Segal Research Grants, 1331
Duke University Adult Cardiothoracic Anesthesia and Critical Care Medicine Fellowships, 1340
Duke University Ambulatory and Regional Anesthesia Fellowships, 1341
Duke University Clinical Cardiac Electrophysiology Fellowships, 1342
Duke University Hyperbaric Center Fellowships, 1343
Duke University Interventional Cardiology Fellowships, 1344
EF Health Sciences Student Fellowships, 1380
FIC International Research Fellowship Program, 1490
Harry A. and Margaret D. Towsley Fndn Grants, 1701
Hoglund Fndn Grants, 1785
HRB Postdoctoral Research Fellowships, 1802
NHLBI Research Supplements to Promote Diversity in Health-Related Research (Postdoctoral Individuals/New Independent Researchers), 2373
NHLBI Research Supplements to Promote Diversity in Health-Related Research for Established Investigators Who Become Disabled, 2374
NHLBI Research Supplements to Promote Diversity in Health-Related Research for Graduate Research Assistants, 2375
NHLBI Research Supplements to Promote Diversity in Health-Related Research for Individuals in Postdoctoral Training, 2376
NHLBI Research Supplements to Promote Diversity in Health-Related Research for Undergraduate Students, 2377
NIA Promoting Careers in Aging and Health Disparities Research Grants, 2427
NIGMS Initiative for Minority Students: Bridges to the Doctoral Degree, 2613
NIH Recovery Act Limited Competition: Building Sustainable Comm-Linked Infrastructure to Enable Health Science Research, 2709
NIH Research Project Grants, 2714
NLM Grants for Scholarly Works in Biomedicine and Health, 2818
NLM Research Project Grants, 2825
North Carolina GlaxoSmithKline Fndn Grants, 2860
NWHF Mark O. Hatfield Research Fellowship, 2907
NYCT Blindness and Visual Disabilities Grants, 2921
Regenstrief General Internal Medicine - General Pediatrics Research Fellowship Program, 3144
Religion and Health: Effects, Mechanisms, and Interpretation RFP, 3149
San Diego Women's Fndn Grants, 3259
Savoy Fndn Post-Doctoral and Clinical Research Fellowships, 3266
Savoy Fndn Studentships, 3268
Siragusa Fndn Health Services & Medical Research Grants, 3294
SRC Medical Research Grants, 3362
STTI Emergency Nurses Association Fndn Grant, 3390
STTI/Council for the Advancement of Nursing Science Grants, 3398
US CRDF Leishmaniasis: Collaborative Research Opportunities in North Africa and the Middle East, 3474

Health Services Delivery

3M Company Health and Human Services Grants, 10
A.O. Smith Comm Grants, 18
AAHPM Hospice and Palliative Medicine Fellowships, 132
Abbott Fund Access to Health Care Grants, 176
Abell Fndn Health and Human Services Grants, 182
Abell-Hanger Fndn Grants, 183
Abington Fndn Grants, 184
Able To Serve Grants, 185
AcademyHealth Alice S. Hersh New Investigator Awards, 190
AcademyHealth HSR Impact Awards, 193
Administration on Aging Senior Medicare Patrol Project Grants, 236
Advancing Colorado's Mental Health Care Project Grants, 240
Aetna Fndn Regional Comm Health Outreach Grants, 250
Agnes B. Hunt Trust Grants, 261
Albertson's Charitable Giving Grants, 330
Allen P. and Josephine B. Green Fndn Grants, 361
AMA Fndn Fund for Better Health Grants, 388
Amgen Fndn Grants, 467
Anthem Blue Cross and Blue Shield Grants, 488
APA Young Investigator Grant Program, 502
APF Awards for Advancing Minority Mental Health, 504
APF Disaster Recovery Fund for Psychiatrists, 506
APF Helping Hands Grants, 507
APhA Fndn Incentive Grants, 512
ArvinMeritor Grants, 544
Assurant Fndn Grants, 654
Auburn Fndn Grants, 664
AUPHA Baxter International Fndn Prize for Health Services Research, 666
Barth Syndrome Fndn Research Grants, 700
BCBS of Massachusetts Fndn Grants, 709

BCBS of Minnesota Growing Up Healthy Grants, 711
BCBSM Claude Pepper Award, 714
BCBSM Fndn Proposal Development Awards, 720
BCBSM Fndn Student Award Program, 721
BCBSM Frank J. McDevitt, DO, Excellence in Research Awards, 722
BCBSM Investigator-Initiated Research Grants, 723
BCBSNC Fndn Grants, 725
BJ's Charitable Fndn Grants, 761
Blue Shield of California Grants, 771
Burlington Industries Fndn Grants, 811
California Wellness Fndn Work and Health Grants, 834
Carl B. and Florence E. King Fndn Grants, 869
CF Clinical Research Trainee Awards, 940
Champ-A Champion Fur Kids Grants, 959
Charlotte County (FL) Comm Fndn Grants, 973
Chase Paymentech Corp Giving Grants, 975
Claude Worthington Benedum Fndn Grants, 1033
CMA Fndn Grants, 1042
CMS Historically Black Colleges and Universities Health Services Research Grants, 1044
CNCS Next Generation Grants, 1049
Colorado Trust Grants, 1062
Colorado Trust Partnerships for Health Initiative, 1063
Commonwealth Fund Harkness Fellowships in Health Care Policy and Practice, 1079
Commonwealth Fund Quality of Care for Frail Elders Grants, 1083
Comm Fndn of Grant County Grants, 1104
Comm Fndn of Greenville Hollingsworth Funds Program/Project Grants, 1114
Comm Fndn of Morgan County Grants and Scholarships, 1118
Comm Fndn of St. Joseph County Special Project Challenge Grants, 1126
Comm Health Scholars Program Fellowships, 1134
Comm Impact Fund, 1135
Connecticut Health Fndn Initiative Grants, 1142
Consumers Energy Fndn, 1147
Covenant Fndn Grants, 1153
CVS Comm Grants, 1177
Daviess County Comm Fndn Health Grants, 1203
Dearborn Comm Fndn City of Lawrenceburg Comm Grants, 1210
Del E. Webb Fndn Grants, 1213
Deland Fellowships in Health Care and Society, 1214
DeMatteis Family Fndn Grants, 1221
Dennis and Phyllis Washington Fndn Grants, 1222
DHHS AIDS and HIV Epidemiologic Research Studies Grants, 1244
DHHS Oral Health Promotion Research Across the Lifespan, 1269
DHHS Technical and Non-Financial Assistance to Health Centers, 1280
Dorothy Rider Pool Health Care Grants, 1322
Duke Endowment Health Care Grants, 1338
Eastman Chemical Company Fndn Grants, 1362
Edina Realty Fndn Grants, 1369
Emma B. Howe Memorial Fndn Grants, 1415
Entergy Corp Open Grants for Healthy Families, 1418
Ewing Halsell Fndn Grants, 1440
Fairlawn Fndn Grants, 1447
Fairview Lutheran Fndn Grants, 1448
Fallon OrNda Comm Health Fund Grants, 1449
FCNY Union Square Awards, 1461
Flinn Fndn Grants Programs, 1511
Fndn for a Healthy Kentucky Grants, 1527
Fndn for Spirituality and Medicine Grants, 1534
Frances and John L. Loeb Family Fund Grants, 1546
Genesis Fndn Grants, 1593
George Frederick Jewett Fndn Grants, 1599
Giving Sum Annual Grant, 1619
GlaxoSmithKline Fndn IMPACT Awards, 1624
Good Samaritan Fndn Inc Grants, 1636
Goodyear Tire Grants, 1639
GPP Charles E. Culpeper Fndn Biomedical Pilot Projects Initiative Grants, 1641
Greater Cincinnati Fndn Priority and Small Projects/ Capacity-Building Grants, 1651
Green Bay Packers Fndn Grants, 1660
Hagedorn Fund Grants, 1685
Hall-Perrine Fndn Grants, 1686
Hartford Aging and Health Program Awards, 1709
Hasbro Children's Fund, 1714
Hawaii Comm Fndn Health Education and Research Grants, 1716
Health Fndn of Greater Cincinnati Grants, 1724
Hedco Fndn Grants, 1733
Helen Steiner Rice Fndn Grants, 1742
Highmark Physician eHealth Collaborative Grants, 1771
Hirtzel Memorial Fndn Grants, 1781
Hoglund Fndn Grants, 1785
HomeBanc Fndn Grants, 1788
Honda of America Manufacturing Fndn Grants, 1790
Horace A. Kimball and S. Ella Kimball Fndn Grants, 1792
HRB Health Services Research Fellowships, 1801
HRSA Hansen's Disease National Ambulatory Care Grants, 1806
HRSA Ryan White HIV Early Intervention Services Grants, 1811
Idaho Comm Fndn Eastern Region Competitive Grants, 1837
Illinois Children's Healthcare Fndn Grants, 1842
IOM Gustav O. Lienhard Award, 1864
Jay and Rose Phillips Family Fndn Grants, 1909
Jessie B. Cox Charitable Trust Grants, 1918
Jewish Comm Fndn of Greater Los Angeles Grants, 1921
Jewish Fund Grants, 1923
Joe W. and Dorothy Dorsett Brown Fndn Grants, 1927
Johnson & Johnson Corp Contributions Grants, 1952
Johnson County Comm Fndn Grants, 1955
Josephine S. Gumbiner Fndn Grants, 1965
K. M. Hunter Charitable Fndn Social Welfare Grants, 1974
K21 Health Fndn Grants, 1976
Kaiser Permanente Cares for Communities Grants, 1978
Ken W. Davis Fndn Grants, 1987
Kendrick Fndn Grants, 1988
Key Fndn Grants, 1994
King Pharmaceuticals Corp Contributions Grants, 2003
Liberty Bank Fndn Grants, 2053
Lynde and Harry Bradley Fndn Grants, 2089
Lynde and Harry Bradley Fndn Prizes: Bradley Prizes, 2090
M-A-C AIDS Fund Grants, 2091
M.J. Murdock Charitable Trust Grants, 2095
Maxtor Corp Contributions Grants, 2136
May Department Stores Charitable Contribution Grants, 2138
Mayday Fund Grants, 2139
McKesson Fndn Grants, 2145
Mead Johnson Nutritionals Charitable Giving Grants, 2156
Medtronic Fndn Health Care Grants, 2169
Metrowest Comm Health Care Fndn Grants, 2176
Middlesex Savings Charitable Fndn Grants, 2196
Miles of Hope Breast Cancer Fndn Grants, 2199
Minneapolis Fndn Comm Grants, 2206
Moses Cone-Wesley Long Comm Health Fndn Grants, 2219
Mount Zion Health Fund Grants, 2220
NAPNAP Fndn Elaine Gelman Scholarship, 2235
NAPNAP Fndn Innovative Health Care Small Grant, 2237
NAPNAP Fndn McNeil Grant-in-Aid, 2238
NAPNAP Fndn McNeil PNP Scholarships, 2239
NAPNAP Fndn McNeil Rural and Underserved Scholarships, 2240
NAPNAP Fndn Nursing Research Grants, 2241
NAPNAP Fndn Reckitt Benckiser Student Scholarship, 2242
NAPNAP Fndn Wyeth Pediatric Immunization Grant, 2244
National Emergency Medicine Association Grants, 2252
NCI Exploratory Grants for Behavioral Research in Cancer Control, 2274
NIA Alzheimer's Disease Core Centers Grants, 2395
NIDA Drug Abuse Dissertation Research: Epidemiology, Prevention, Treatment, Services, and Women and Gender Differences, 2502
NIDA Minority Institutions Drug Abuse Research Development Program (MIDARP) Grants, 2509
NMF General Electric Medical Scholars Fellowships, 2830
North Central Health Services Grants, 2861
North Georgia Comm Fndn Grants, 2862
Northern Trust Company Charitable Trust and Corp Giving Program, 2865
NYAM Mary and David Hoar Fellowship, 2916
NYCT Children and Youth with Disabilities Grants, 2923
NYCT Girls and Young Women Grants, 2924
OREF/AAOS Clinical Research Training Fellowship, 2958
PacifiCorp Fndn for Learning Grants, 2982
Pasadena Fndn Average Grants, 2994
Paul G. Duke Fndn Grants, 3001
Perry County Comm Fndn Grants, 3016
Piedmont Natural Gas Grants, 3048
Premera CARES Grants, 3074
Priddy Fndn Grants, 3077
Prince Charitable Trusts District of Columbia Grants, 3080
Prostate Cancer Fndn Research Grants, 3086
Quality Health Fndn Grants, 3094
Quantum Corp Snap Server Grants, 3095
Quantum Fndn Grants, 3096
Rochester Area Comm Fndn Grants, 3176
Rockwell International Corp Trust Grants, 3183
Ruth Eleanor Bamberger and John Ernest Bamberger Memorial Fndn Grants, 3202
RWJF Changes in Health Care Financing and Organization Grants, 3206
RWJF Evaluating Innovations in Nursing Education Grants, 3209
RWJF Finding Answers: Disparities Research for Change Grants, 3211
RWJF Harold Amos Medical Faculty Development Scholars, 3213
RWJF Health Care Costs: Research to Inform Policy Grants, 3215
RWJF New Jersey Health Initiatives Grants, 3225
Salem Fndn Charitable Trust Grants, 3241
Salem Fndn Grants, 3242
Samuel Roberts Noble Fndn Grants, 3250
Samuel S. Johnson Fndn Grants, 3251
San Diego Fndn Health & Human Services Grants, 3256
San Diego Fndn Paradise Valley Hospital Comm Fund Grants, 3257
San Diego Women's Fndn Grants, 3259
San Francisco Fndn Comm Health Grants, 3260
Schering-Plough Fndn Health Grants, 3270
Shell Oil Company Fndn Grants, 3281
Simpson Fund Grants, 3290
Sir Dorabji Tata Trust Individual Medical Grants, 3292
Sisters of St. Joseph Healthcare Fndn Grants, 3297
SOCFOC Catholic Ministries Grants, 3317
Sonoco Fndn Grants, 3347
Square D Fndn Grants, 3361
Starr Fndn Grants, 3377
Sulzberger Fndn Grants, 3399
Sunflower Fndn Bridge Grants, 3401
Sunflower Fndn Capacity Building Grants, 3402
Sunflower Fndn Walking Trails Grants, 3403
Susan G. Komen Breast Cancer Fndn Hurricane Relief Grants, 3409
Temple-Inland Fndn Grants, 3419
Tides Fndn Syringe Access Fund, 3427
Tri-County Electric People Fund Grants, 3436
UCLA/RAND Corp Post-Doctoral Fellowships, 3454

United Methodist Church Global AIDS Fund Grants, 3463
United Methodist Health Ministry Fund Grants, 3465
US Airways Comm Contributions, 3472
Vancouver Fndn Grants and Comm Initiatives Program, 3477
VHA Health Fndn Grants, 3495
W.K. Kellogg Fndn Healthy Kids Grants, 3507
Wachovia Fndn Grants, 3511
Wal-Mart Fndn Comm Grants, 3513
Walt Disney Company Fndn Grants, 3516
Warren Alpert Fndn Prize, 3518
Warrick County Comm Fndn Grants, 3519
Western Union Fndn Grants, 3529
Women of the ELCA Opportunity Scholarships for Lutheran Laywomen, 3548

Health, Allied Fields
BCBSM Corp Contributions Grants, 716
Deland Fellowships in Health Care and Society, 1214
DHHS Health Professions Preparatory Scholarship Program for Indians, 1257
DHHS Health Professions Scholarship Program, 1258
DHHS National Health Service Corps Loan Repayment Awards, 1265
DHHS Native American Health Service Loan Repayment Awards, 1267
Elsie Lee Garthwaite Memorial Fndn Grants, 1408
FIC International Training and Research in Environmental and Occupational Health, 1493
Humana Fndn Grants, 1818
Impact 100 Grants, 1843
Jasper Fndn Jasper County Grants, 1907
Jasper Fndn Newton County Grants, 1908
Jennings County Comm Fndn Grants, 1916
John W. Anderson Fndn Grants, 1949
Johnson County Comm Fndn Grants, 1955
K21 Health Fndn Grants, 1976
KFC Allied Health Research Grants, 1996
Knight Family Charitable and Educational Fndn Grants, 2007
Kosciusko County Comm Fndn Grants, 2015
Legacy Fndn Grants, 2040
Lubbock Area Fndn Grants, 2079
National City Corp Contributions Grants, 2250
New York University Steinhardt School of Education Fellowships, 2305
Noble County Comm Fndn Grants, 2848
North Central Health Services Grants, 2861
Posey Comm Fndn Grants, 3068
Pulaski County Comm Fndn Grants, 3091
Schering-Plough Fndn Health Grants, 3270
Scott County Comm Fndn Grants, 3273

Healthy Lifestyles
AMA Fndn Fund for Better Health Grants, 388

Hearing
AHRF Eugene L. Derlacki, M.D. Research Grants, 309
AHRF Georgia Birtman Grant, 310
AHRF Wiley H. Harrison Memorial Research Award, 312
DHHS Universal Newborn Hearing Screening and Intervention, 1282
Marjorie C. Adams Charitable Trust Grants, 2111
NIDCD Clinical Trial Planning Grant, 2517
NIDCD Exploratory/Developmental Research Grants, 2520
NIDCD Minority Dissertation Research Grants in Human Communication, 2524
NIDCD Molecular & Cellular Pathology of the Human Auditory and Vestibular Systems Grants, 2525
Oticon Focus on People Awards, 2976

Hearing Impairments
AHRF Eugene L. Derlacki, M.D. Research Grants, 309
AHRF Georgia Birtman Grant, 310
AHRF Wiley H. Harrison Memorial Research Award, 312
ASHFndn Graduate Student International Scholarship, 576
ASHFndn Graduate Student Scholarships, 577
ASHFndn Graduate Student Scholarships for Minority Students, 578
ASHFndn Graduate Student with a Disability Scholarship, 579
Batchelor Fndn Grants, 701
Bushrod H. Campbell and Adah F. Hall Charity Fund Grants, 816
Carl W. and Carrie Mae Joslyn Trust Grants, 873
Carls Fndn Grants, 876
Charles Delmar Fndn Grants, 963
Columbus Fndn Competitive Grants, 1066
Danellie Fndn Grants, 1198
Deafness Research Fndn Research Grants, 1208
DHHS Universal Newborn Hearing Screening and Intervention, 1282
Kenny's Kids Grants, 1990
Lettie Pate Whitehead Fndn Grants, 2049
Mabel H. Flory Charitable Trust Grants, 2096
Marjorie C. Adams Charitable Trust Grants, 2111
NIDCD Exploratory/Developmental Research Grants, 2520
NIDCD Physiologic and Molecular Bases of Tinnitus Research Grants, 2527
NIDCD Program for Postdoctoral Research Training in Clinical Trials, 2528
NIDCD Research Core Centers, 2529
NIDCD Small Grants, 2531
NIH National Occupational Research Agenda Grants, 2696
Oticon Focus on People Awards, 2976
U.S. Department of Education Rehabilitation Training—Rehabilitation Continuing Education Programs—Institute on Rehabilitation Issues, 3449
Union County Comm Fndn Grants, 3461

Heart Disease
Edna G. Kynett Memorial Fndn Grants, 1370
Horizon Fndn for New Jersey Grants, 1793
NIH Sarcoidosis: Research into the Cause of Multi-Organ Disease and Clinical Strategies for Therapy Grants, 2723

Hematologic Diseases
NIDDK Education Grants, 2554

Hematologic System
NIDDK Development of Disease Biomarkers Grants, 2549

Hematology
Cooley's Anemia Research Fellowships, 1149
E.D.Thomas Fellowship, 1359
Jackson Laboratory Postdoctoral Research Training Program, 1880
Leukemia and Lymphoma Society Research Grants, 2051
National Blood Fndn Research Grants, 2249
NHLBI Blood Diseases and Resources Research Grants, 2322
NHLBI Minority Institution Research Scientist Development Award, 2354
NHLBI Minority Institutional Research Training Grants, 2355
NHLBI Short-Term Research Education Program to Increase Diversity in Health-Related Research, 2383
NHLBI Transfusion-Related Acute Lung Injury Basic Research Grants, 2389
NIDDK Non-Invasive Methods for Diagnosis and Progression of Diabetes, Kidney, Urological, Hematological and Digestive Diseases, 2572
NIDDK Proteomics: Diabetes, Obesity, & Endocrine, Digestive, Kidney, Urologic, And Hematologic Diseases, 2578
NIDDK Small Grants for Underrepresented Minority Scientists in Diabetes and Digestive and Kidney Diseases, 2588
NIH Bone and the Hematopoietic and Immune Systems Research Grants, 2643
NIH Mechanisms Underlying Individual Variations in Drug Responses, 2685
Topeka Comm Fndn Kansas Blood Services Scholarships, 3429

Hemophilia
Bayer Clinical Scholarship Award, 706
Bayer Hemophilia Caregivers Education Award, 707
CSL Behring Local Empowerment for Advocacy Development Grants, 1167

Hepatitis
Bristol-Myers Squibb Fndn Health Disparities Grants, 797
Bristol-Myers Squibb Virology and Oncology M.D. Research Fellowships, 802
CDC Hepatitis Education for Inmates and Correctional Staff Grants, 911
NFID New Investigator Matching Grants, 2310
NHLBI Blood Diseases and Resources Research Grants, 2322
NIAAA Hepatitis C Infection and Alcoholic Liver Disease, 2442
NIDA International Studies on Drug Abuse and HIV/AIDS, 2505
NIDDK Research Grants for Studies of Hepatitis C in the Setting of Renal Disease, 2580
NIH Collaborations for Advanced Strategies in Complication of HIV Infection, 2651
NIH Small Business Innovation Research: Animal Models of HCV Infection Research Grants, 2728
Pajaro Valley Comm Health Grants, 2985

Hepatology
Canadian Liver Fndn Grants, 851
CLF Fellowships, 1037
CLF Graduate Studentships, 1038
CLF Operating Grants, 1039
FDHN Non-Career Research Grants, 1477
FDHN Research Scholar Awards, 1478
FDHN Translational Research Awards, 1482

Hereditary Diseases and Disorders
Barth Syndrome Fndn Research Grants, 700
Children's Medical Research Institute Grants, 1000
Dysautonomia Research Grants, 1353
NHLBI Elucidating Nature's Solutions to Heart, Lung, and Blood Diseases and Sleep Disorder Processes Research Grants, 2333

Heritage Preservation
North Carolina Comm Fndn Grants, 2859

Herpesviruses
NIDCR HIV/AIDS Associated Oral Viral Infections, 2535
Sexually Transmitted Diseases Postdoctoral Fellowships, 3279

High School Education
Affymetrix Corp Contributions Grants, 258
American Electric Power Grants, 434
Chicago Comm Trust Grants, 989
Florida High School/High Tech Project Grants, 1515
Hutton Fndn Grants, 1828
J.C. Penney Company Grants, 1874
KeySpan Fndn Grants, 1995
Progress Energy Fndn Grants, 3084
Raskob Fndn for Catholic Activities Grants, 3107
Taproot Fndn Capacity-Building Service Grants, 3417
Westinghouse Charitable Giving Grants, 3530

Higher Education
3M Fndn Grants, 11
A. Gary Anderson Family Fndn Grants, 17

A/H Fndn Grants, 19
AAHPERD Ruth Abernathy Presidential Scholarships, 128
Aaron Fndn (Massachusetts) Grants, 174
AARP Fndn Gerontology Graduate Scholarships and Fellowships, 175
Abbott Fund Global AIDS Care Grants, 178
Abel Fndn Grants, 181
Abell-Hanger Fndn Grants, 183
Abney Fndn Grants, 187
Abramson Family Fndn Grants, 188
Achelis and Bodman Fndns Grants, 206
Adam Richter Charitable Trust Grants, 230
Adaptec Fndn Grants, 232
Adolph Coors Fndn Grants, 238
Advanced Micro Devices Comm Affairs Grants, 239
AEC Trust Grants, 242
Agnes Gund Fndn Grants, 262
Agnes M. Lindsay Trust Grants, 263
Ahmanson Fndn Grants, 303
Air Products and Chemicals Grants, 319
Alabama Power Fndn Grants, 321
Alberto Culver Corp Contributions Grants, 329
Albertson's Charitable Giving Grants, 330
Alexander Eastman Fndn Grants, 341
Allyn Fndn Grants, 365
ALSAM Fndn Grants, 369
Amarillo Area/Harrington Fndns Grants, 410
AMD Corp Contributions Grants, 411
Andersen Fndn Grants, 471
Ann Peppers Fndn Grants, 478
Annenberg Fndn Grants, 479
AptarGroup Fndn Grants, 522
Archer Daniels Midland Fndn Grants, 525
ARCO Fndn Education Grants, 526
Argyros Fndn Grants, 527
Arkell Hall Fndn Grants, 534
Armstrong McDonald Fndn Grants, 537
ARS Fndn Grants, 538
Arthur and Rochelle Belfer Fndn Grants, 542
ASCO Loan Repayment Grants, 555
ASHA Students Preparing for Academic & Research Careers Award, 574
Ashland Corp Contributions Grants, 586
Athwin Fndn Grants, 660
Atlanta Fndn Grants, 662
Atran Fndn Grants, 663
Auburn Fndn Grants, 664
Autzen Fndn Grants, 672
Bailey Fndn Grants, 680
Balfe Family Fndn Grants, 682
Ball Brothers Fndn Grants, 684
Banfi Vintners Fndn Grants, 687
Bank of America Charitable Fndn Anchor Institutions Grants, 688
Barnes Group Fndn Grants, 696
Barr Fund Grants, 697
Batchelor Fndn Grants, 701
Batts Fndn Grants, 704
Beazley Fndn Grants, 730
Becton Dickinson and Company Grants, 736
Belk Fndn Grants, 739
Ben B. Cheney Fndn Grants, 741
Bender Fndn Grants, 742
Bert W. Martin Fndn Grants, 750
Bertha Russ Lytel Fndn Grants, 751
Bill and Melinda Gates Fndn Grants, 756
Blue Mountain Comm Fndn Grants, 769
Blum-Kovler Fndn Grants, 772
Blumenthal Fndn Grants, 773
Boeing Company Contributions Grants, 777
Boettcher Fndn Grants, 778
Booth-Bricker Fund Grants, 780
Bosque Fndn Grants, 782
Bradley Turner Fndn Grants, 789
Bright Family Fndn Grants, 793
Bruce and Adele Greenfield Fndn Grants, 808
Burlington Industries Fndn Grants, 811
Burlington Northern Santa Fe Fndn Grants, 812
Byron W. and Alice L. Lockwood Fndn Grants, 824
C.R. Bard Fndn Grants, 825
Callaway Fndn Grants, 835
Camp-Younts Fndn Grants, 838
Cancer Research UK Grants, 859
Cargill Citizenship Fund-Corp Giving Grants, 865
Caring Fndn Grants, 866
Carl B. and Florence E. King Fndn Grants, 869
Carnahan-Jackson Fndn Grants, 878
Carnegie Corp of New York Grants, 879
Carylon Fndn Grants, 886
Cass County Comm Fndn Grants, 887
CCFF Fellowships, 893
CDC School Health Programs to Prevent the Spread of HIV Cooperative Agreements, 928
Cemala Fndn Grants, 933
Cessna Fndn Grants, 938
Champlin Fndns Grants, 960
Charles Delmar Fndn Grants, 963
Charles H. Revson Fndn Grants, 969
Charles M. Bair Family Trust Grants, 972
Chazen Fndn Grants, 978
Chesapeake Corp Fndn Grants, 982
Chicago Board of Trade Fndn Grants, 988
Chiles Fndn Grants, 1003
Chiron Fndn Comm Grants, 1004
CIGNA Fndn Grants, 1011
Cinergy Fndn Grants, 1013
Clark-Winchcole Fndn Grants, 1030
Claude Bennett Family Fndn Grants, 1031
Claude Worthington Benedum Fndn Grants, 1033
Clay Fndn Grants, 1034
Coca-Cola Fndn Grants, 1052
Cockrell Fndn Grants, 1053
Coeta and Donald Barker Fndn Grants, 1054
Collins C. Diboll Private Fndn Grants, 1057
Collins Fndn Grants, 1058
Colorado Interstate Gas Grants, 1060
Colorado Springs Comm Trust Fund Grants, 1061
Comm Fndn of Greater Birmingham Grants, 1106
Comm Fndn of Greater New Britain Grants, 1111
Comm Fndn of Howard County Grants, 1116
Comm Fndn of Madison and Jefferson County Grants and Scholarships, 1117
Comm Fndn of Wabash County Grants, 1131
Connelly Fndn Grants, 1143
ConocoPhillips Fndn Grants, 1144
Constantin Fndn Grants, 1145
Consumers Energy Fndn, 1147
Cooper Industries Fndn Grants, 1150
Coors Brewing Corp Contributions Grants, 1151
Cowles Charitable Trust Grants, 1155
Crestlea Fndn Grants, 1159
CSRA Comm Fndn Grants, 1168
Cullen Fndn Grants, 1172
DaimlerChrysler Corp Fund Grants, 1186
Daniels Fund Grants, 1200
Daphne Seybolt Culpeper Memorial Fndn Grants, 1201
Davis Family Fndn Grants, 1204
Daywood Fndn Grants, 1206
Dennis and Phyllis Washington Fndn Grants, 1222
Dept of Ed College Assistance Migrant Program, 1228
DeRoy Testamentary Fndn Grants, 1239
Dickson Fndn Grants, 1284
Dolan Fndn Grants, 1306
Dora Roberts Fndn Grants, 1311
Dorrance Family Fndn Grants, 1323
Dr. Bob and Jean Smith Fndn Grants, 1325
Duke Energy Fndn Grants, 1339
Duke University Interventional Cardiology Fellowships, 1344
Dunspaugh-Dalton Fndn Grants, 1351
E. Rhodes and Leona B. Carpenter Fndn Grants, 1356
E.J. Grassmann Trust Grants, 1360
E.L. Wiegand Fndn Grants, 1361
Eberly Fndn Grants, 1364
Eckerd Corp Fndn Grants, 1366
Eden Hall Fndn Grants, 1368
Edna G. Kynett Memorial Fndn Grants, 1370
EDS Fndn Grants, 1371
Edwin W. and Catherine M. Davis Fndn Grants, 1377
Elsie Lee Garthwaite Memorial Fndn Grants, 1408
Emerson Charitable Trust Grants, 1412
Ethel S. Abbott Charitable Fndn Grants, 1430
Eugene B. Casey Fndn Grants, 1433
Eugene M. Lang Fndn Grants, 1434
Eugene McDermott Fndn Grants, 1435
Eva L. and Joseph M. Bruening Fndn Grants, 1436
Evjue Fndn Grants, 1439
Feldman Fndn Grants, 1484
Ferree Fndn Grants, 1486
FirstEnergy Fndn Comm Grants, 1505
Fluor Fndn Grants, 1517
FMC Fndn Grants, 1518
Foellinger Fndn Grants, 1519
Fondren Fndn Grants, 1520
Foster Fndn Grants, 1524
Frances L. and Edwin L. Cummings Memorial Fund Grants, 1547
Francis L. Abreu Charitable Trust Grants, 1549
Frank G. and Freida K. Brotz Family Fndn Grants, 1552
Fraser-Parker Fndn Grants, 1555
Fred L. Emerson Fndn Grants, 1557
Frederick Gardner Cottrell Fndn Grants, 1560
Fritz B. Burns Fndn Grants, 1564
Fuller E. Callaway Fndn Grants, 1578
Gebbie Fndn Grants, 1585
GenCorp Fndn Grants, 1587
George and Ruth Bradford Fndn Grants, 1595
George B. Storer Fndn Grants, 1596
George F. Baker Trust Grants, 1597
George Family Fndn Grants, 1598
George Frederick Jewett Fndn Grants, 1599
George Kress Fndn Grants, 1601
George S. and Dolores Dore Eccles Fndn Grants, 1602
Georgia Power Fndn Grants, 1603
Gertrude and William C. Wardlaw Fund Grants, 1607
Gertrude E. Skelly Charitable Fndn Grants, 1609
Gheens Fndn Grants, 1610
Gilroy and Lillian P. Roberts Charitable Fndn Grants, 1614
Good Samaritan Inc Grants, 1637
Goodrich Corp Fndn Grants, 1638
Goodyear Tire Grants, 1639
Greater Cincinnati Fndn Priority and Small Projects/ Capacity-Building Grants, 1651
Greater Milwaukee Fndn Grants, 1653
Griffin Fndn Grants, 1670
H & R Fndn Grants, 1679
H. Schaffer Fndn Grants, 1680
Hall-Perrine Fndn Grants, 1686
Halliburton Fndn Grants, 1687
Harold Alfond Fndn Grants, 1695
Harold Simmons Fndn Grants, 1698
Harry and Grace Steele Fndn Grants, 1702
Harry Kramer Memorial Fund Grants, 1705
Harry Sudakoff Fndn Grants, 1708
Hedco Fndn Grants, 1733
HHMI Grants and Fellowships Programs, 1759
High Meadow Fndn Grants, 1768
Hill Crest Fndn Grants, 1773
Hill Fndn Grants, 1774
Hirtzel Memorial Fndn Grants, 1781
Homer Fndn Grants, 1789
Honeywell Fndn Grants, 1791
Hormel Fndn Grants, 1796
Houston Endowment Grants, 1797
Howe Fndn of North Carolina Grants, 1799
Huie-Dellmon Trust Grants, 1815
Human Source Fndn Grants, 1817
Humana Fndn Grants, 1818
Hutton Fndn Grants, 1828
Idaho Power Company Corp Contributions, 1838
J. Walton Bissell Fndn Grants, 1872
J.B. Reynolds Fndn Grants, 1873
J.C. Penney Company Grants, 1874
J.M. Long Fndn Grants, 1877

J.W. Kieckhefer Fndn Grants, 1878
Jacob and Hilda Blaustein Fndn Grants, 1881
James Ford Bell Fndn Grants, 1885
James G.K. McClure Educational and Development Fund Grants, 1886
James Graham Brown Fndn Grants, 1887
James Hervey Johnson Charitable Educational Trust Grants, 1889
James J. and Angelia M. Harris Fndn Grants, 1890
James M. Collins Fndn Grants, 1891
James R. Dougherty Jr. Fndn Grants, 1894
Janirve Fndn Grants, 1905
JELD-WEN Fndn Grants, 1914
Jennings County Comm Fndn Grants, 1916
Joe W. and Dorothy Dorsett Brown Fndn Grants, 1927
John Ben Snow Memorial Trust Grants, 1928
John Deere Fndn Grants, 1929
John H. and Wilhelmina D. Harland Charitable Fndn Grants, 1933
John I. Smith Charities Grants, 1935
John J. Leidy Fndn Grants, 1936
John Lord Knight Fndn Grants, 1938
John P. Murphy Fndn Grants, 1943
John R. Oishei Fndn Grants, 1944
John Stauffer Charitable Trust Grants, 1946
John W. Anderson Fndn Grants, 1949
Johnson & Johnson Corp Contributions Grants, 1952
Johnson Controls Fndn Grants, 1954
Joseph Alexander Fndn Grants, 1957
Josiah W. and Bessie H. Kline Fndn Grants, 1967
Journal Gazette Fndn Grants, 1968
Katherine John Murphy Fndn Grants, 1983
Kavli Fndn Research Grants, 1985
KeySpan Fndn Grants, 1995
L. W. Pierce Family Fndn Grants, 2019
Leonard and Helen R. Stulman Charitable Fndn Grants, 2044
Lester E. Yeager Charitable Trust B Grants, 2047
Lillian S. Wells Fndn Grants, 2056
Lockheed Martin Philanthropic Grants, 2062
Long Island Comm Fndn Grants, 2063
Lowe Fndn Grants, 2067
Lowell Berry Fndn Grants, 2069
Lubbock Area Fndn Grants, 2079
Lubrizol Fndn Grants, 2080
Lynde and Harry Bradley Fndn Grants, 2089
Lynde and Harry Bradley Fndn Prizes: Bradley Prizes, 2090
M. Bastian Family Fndn Grants, 2092
M.E. Raker Fndn Grants, 2094
M.J. Murdock Charitable Trust Grants, 2095
Madison County Comm Fndn Grants, 2098
Manuel D. and Rhoda Mayerson Fndn Grants, 2100
Margaret L. Wendt Fndn Grants, 2104
Margaret T. Morris Fndn Grants, 2105
Marion Park Deaver and Harry Gilbert Deaver Fndn Grants, 2110
Mark and Catherine Winkler Fndn Grants, 2112
Mary S. and David C. Corbin Fndn Grants, 2122
Matilda R. Wilson Fund Grants, 2128
Max A. Adler Charitable Fndn Grants, 2132
Maxon Charitable Fndn Grants, 2135
McCombs Fndn Grants, 2142
McGregor Fund Grants, 2143
MDBDF Agnes Higgins Award, 2155
Mead Witter Fndn Grants, 2160
Meriden Fndn Grants, 2173
Metro Health Fndn Grants, 2175
Meyer Memorial Trust Emergency Grants, 2178
Meyer Memorial Trust Grassroots Grants, 2179
Meyer Memorial Trust Responsive Grants, 2181
Military Ex-Prisoners of War Fndn Grants, 2201
Morton K. and Jane Blaustein Fndn Grants, 2218
Mount Zion Health Fund Grants, 2220
National City Corp Contributions Grants, 2250
National Starch and Chemical Fndn Grants, 2261
Nell Warren Elkin and William Simpson Elkin Fndn, 2302
Newman's Own Inc Grants, 2306
NIA Mentored Clinical Scientist Research Career Development Awards, 2417
Nicholas H. Noyes Jr. Memorial Fndn Grants, 2497
NIEHS Applied Toxicological Research and Testing Grants, 2595
NIGMS Initiative for Minority Students: Bridges to the Baccalaureate Degree, 2612
Nina Mason Pulliam Charitable Trust Grants, 2776
Nordson Corp Fndn Grants, 2851
North Carolina Comm Development Grants, 2858
Northrop Grumman Newport News Grants, 2867
Northwestern Mutual Fndn Grants, 2870
NSF Grant Opportunities for Academic Liaison with Industry, 2887
Ohio Learning Network Grants, 2940
Oleonda Jameson Trust Grants, 2941
Olin Corp Charitable Trust Grants, 2943
Oscar Rennebohm Fndn Grants, 2963
Otto Bremer Fndn Grants, 2977
Paul Ogle Fndn Grants, 3003
Perkins Charitable Fndn Grants, 3014
Perry County Comm Fndn Grants, 3016
Piedmont Natural Gas Grants, 3048
Pike County Comm Fndn Grants, 3049
Pioneer Hi-Bred Comm Grants, 3051
Piper Jaffray Companies Building Strong Communities Grants, 3053
Polaroid Fund Grants, 3065
Portland General Electric Fndn Grants, 3067
Posey Comm Fndn Grants, 3068
Pott Fndn Grants, 3071
Powell Fndn Grants, 3073
Princeton Area Comm Fndn Greater Mercer Grants, 3081
Pulaski County Comm Fndn Grants, 3091
Pulte Homes Corp Contributions, 3092
R.C. Baker Fndn Grants, 3098
RGK Fndn Grants, 3153
Rice Fndn Grants, 3155
Rich Fndn Grants, 3156
Richard and Susan Smith Family Fndn Grants, 3159
Richard E. Griffin Family Fndn Grants, 3160
Richard King Mellon Fndn Grants, 3161
Ripley County Comm Fndn Grants, 3166
Robert and Polly Dunn Fndn Grants, 3168
Robins Fndn Grants, 3175
Rockwell International Corp Trust Grants, 3183
Rollin M. Gerstacker Fndn Grants, 3186
Rush County Comm Fndn Grants, 3200
Russell Berrie Fndn Grants, 3201
Ruth H. and Warren A. Ellsworth Fndn Grants, 3203
RWJF Young Epidemiology Scholars Competition, 3233
Salem Fndn Grants, 3242
SAMHSA Campus Suicide Prevention Grants, 3244
Samuel Freeman Charitable Trust Grants, 3249
Samuel Roberts Noble Fndn Grants, 3250
San Antonio Area Fndn Grants, 3254
Schering-Plough Fndn Health Grants, 3270
Schurz Communications Fndn Grants, 3271
Scientific Communities Initiative Grants, 3272
Scott County Comm Fndn Grants, 3273
Shell Oil Company Fndn Grants, 3281
Sid W. Richardson Fndn Grants, 3284
Simmons Fndn Grants, 3287
SOCFOC Reducing Health & Educational Disparities in the Central Neighborhood Grants, 3318
Solo Cup Fndn Grants, 3346
Sonoco Fndn Grants, 3347
Sosland Fndn Grants, 3348
Southwest Gas Corp Fndn Grants, 3352
Special People in Need Scholarships, 3357
Square D Fndn Grants, 3361
St. Joseph Comm Health Fndn Schneider Fellowships, 3370
Starr Fndn Grants, 3377
Steelcase Fndn Grants, 3379
Steele-Reese Fndn Grants, 3380
Strowd Roses Grants, 3388
Sunderland Fndn Grants, 3400
Susan Mott Webb Charitable Trust Grants, 3412
Susan Vaughan Fndn Grants, 3413
Temple-Inland Fndn Grants, 3419
Thomas and Dorothy Leavey Fndn Grants, 3422
Thomas M. and Irene B. Kirbo Charitable Trust Grants, 3424
Thompson Charitable Fndn Grants, 3425
TWS Fndn Grants, 3443
U.S. Department of Education United States-Russia Program: Improving Research and Educational Activities in Higher Education, 3451
United Technologies Corp Grants, 3466
University of California President's Postdoctoral Fellowships, 3469
Vancouver Fndn Public Health Bursary Package, 3478
Vanderburgh Comm Fndn Grants, 3480
Vulcan Materials Company Fndn Grants, 3504
W. C. Griffith Fndn Grants, 3505
W.K. Kellogg Fndn Healthy Kids Grants, 3507
Walt Disney Company Fndn Grants, 3516
Wasie Fndn Grants, 3521
Wayne and Gladys Valley Fndn Grants, 3522
Weatherwax Fndn Grants, 3523
Weingart Fndn Grants, 3524
William G. Gilmore Fndn Grants, 3537

Higher Education, Private

A/H Fndn Grants, 19
Abell-Hanger Fndn Grants, 183
Bank of America Charitable Fndn Anchor Institutions Grants, 688
Burlington Northern Santa Fe Fndn Grants, 812
Charles A. Frueauff Fndn Grants, 962
Coca-Cola Fndn Grants, 1052
Dr. Scholl Fndn Grants, 1329
Goodyear Tire Grants, 1639
Hall-Perrine Fndn Grants, 1686
Kenneth T. and Eileen L. Norris Fndn Grants, 1989
McGregor Fund Grants, 2143
Nordson Corp Fndn Grants, 2851
Plum Creek Fndn Grants, 3062

Higher Education, Public

A/H Fndn Grants, 19
Bank of America Charitable Fndn Anchor Institutions Grants, 688
Goodyear Tire Grants, 1639
Plum Creek Fndn Grants, 3062

Hispanic Education

Carl and Lily Pforzheimer Fndn Grants, 868
General Motors Fndn Grants Support Program, 1591
Ildaura Murillo-Rohde Scholarships, 1841
John R. Oishei Fndn Grants, 1944
KFF Barbara Jordan Health Policy Scholarships, 2000
NHLBI Minority Institutional Research Training Grants, 2355
NMF Need-Based Scholarships, 2839
S.H. Cowell Fndn Grants, 3237

Hispanics

AMA Fndn Minority Scholars Awards, 395
American Sociological Association Minority Fellowships, 458
ASM Robert D. Watkins Graduate Research Fellowship, 614
AT&T Fndn Civic and Comm Service Grants, 658
Charles Delmar Fndn Grants, 963
DHHS AIDS and HIV Epidemiologic Research Studies Grants, 1244
DHHS Maternal and Child Health Projects Grants, 1263
Effie and Wofford Cain Fndn Grants, 1385
FDHN Student Research Fellowships, 1480
Fndn for the Carolinas Grants, 1535
Harold Amos Medical Faculty Development Program, 1696
Healthcare Fndn for Orange County Grants, 1728
Henry J. Kaiser Family Fndn Grants, 1748
Kalamazoo Fndn Grants, 1979

NIA Prostate Cancer Aging, Race, and Ethnicity Research Grants, 2428
NIMH Career Opportunities in Research Education and Training Honors High School Research Education Grant, 2748
NIMH Career Opportunities in Research Education and Training Honors Undergraduate Research Training Grant, 2749
NMF Franklin C. McLean Award, 2829
Philadelphia Fndn Organizational Effectiveness Grants, 3029
Strowd Roses Grants, 3388

Historic Preservation
Carls Fndn Grants, 876
Collins C. Diboll Private Fndn Grants, 1057
ConocoPhillips Fndn Grants, 1144
Ferree Fndn Grants, 1486
Forrest C. Lattner Fndn Grants, 1523
Fndn for the Carolinas Grants, 1535
George Kress Fndn Grants, 1601
Inasmuch Fndn Grants, 1845
Jane's Trust Grants, 1904
John W. and Anna H. Hanes Fndn Grants, 1948
Margaret L. Wendt Fndn Grants, 2104
McCombs Fndn Grants, 2142
PacifiCorp Fndn for Learning Grants, 2982

History
1675 Fndn Grants, 4
AAHN Grant for Historical Research, 126
AAHN Pre-Doctoral Research Grant, 127
AHFMR Population Health Investigator Awards, 292
Alice Fisher Society Fellowships, 356
Blanche and Irving Laurie Fndn Grants, 764
Canada-U.S. Fulbright New Century Scholars Grants, 846
Canada-U.S. Fulbright Senior Specialists Grants, 847
Charles Edison Fund Grants, 964
Charles G. Koch Charitable Fndn Grants, 965
Comm Fndn of Bloomington and Monroe County Grants, 1098
Cooke Fndn Grants, 1148
Doris and Victor Day Fndn Grants, 1313
E.J. Grassmann Trust Grants, 1360
Eugene McDermott Fndn Grants, 1435
ExxonMobil Grants, 1442
Fischelis Grants for Research in the History of American Pharmacy, 1507
Fulbright Alumni Initiatives Awards Grants, 1566
Fulbright Distinguished Chairs Grants, 1567
Fulbright New Century Scholars Grants, 1570
Fulbright Specialists Grants, 1571
Fulbright Traditional Scholar Program in Europe and Eurasia, 1572
Fulbright Traditional Scholar Program in Sub-Saharan Africa, 1573
Fulbright Traditional Scholar Program in the East Asia/Pacific Region, 1574
Fulbright Traditional Scholar Program in the Near East and North Africa Region, 1575
Fulbright Traditional Scholar Program in the South and Central Asia Region, 1576
Fulbright Traditional Scholar Program in the Western Hemisphere, 1577
Lawrence S. Huntington Fund Grants, 2035
Margaret L. Wendt Fndn Grants, 2104
Mary Baker Eddy Library Summer Research Fellowships, 2117
OceanFirst Fndn Grants, 2933
Rockefeller Archive Center Research Grants, 3178
Self Fndn Grants, 3277
Sid W. Richardson Fndn Grants, 3284
Vermont Comm Fndn Grants, 3493
Warrick County Comm Fndn Grants, 3519

HIV
25th Anniversary Fndn Grants, 8
Abbott Fund Science and Medical Innovation Grants, 179
AIDS Vaccine Advocacy Coalition Fund Grants, 315
Alexander Fndn Insurance Continuation Grants, 343
Alexis Gregory Fndn Grants, 349
Alliance Healthcare Fndn Grants, 362
Alternatives Research and Development Fndn Alternatives in Education Grants, 370
Alternatives Research and Development Fndn Grants, 371
AMA Fndn Seed Grants for Research, 398
American Psychiatric Association Minority Medical Student Fellowship in HIV Psychiatry, 444
ASM Merck Irving S. Sigal Memorial Awards, 606
ASM/CCID Fellowships, 627
Bernard Van Leer Fndn Grants, 748
Blowitz-Ridgeway Fndn Grants, 767
Bodenwein Public Benevolent Fndn Grants, 775
Bristol-Myers Squibb Fndn Global HIV/AIDS Initiative Grants, 796
Bristol-Myers Squibb Fndn Health Disparities Grants, 797
Bristol-Myers Squibb Virology and Oncology M.D. Research Fellowships, 802
Cable Positive's Tony Cox Comm Fund Grants, 827
Campbell Fndn HIV/AIDS Research Grants, 839
CDC Intervention Epidemiologic Research Studies of HIV/AIDS, 915
CDC Prevention Education & Access to Care Services for Persons Infected and Affected by HIV, 922
CDC School Health Programs to Prevent the Spread of HIV Cooperative Agreements, 928
CDC Technology Translation and Transfer of Effective HIV Behavioral Interventions, 931
Children Affected by AIDS Fndn Camp Network Grants, 994
Children Affected by AIDS Fndn Domestic Grants, 995
Children Affected by AIDS Fndn Family Assistance Emergency Fund Grants, 996
Colin Higgins Fndn Grants, 1056
Comm Fndn for Southern Arizona Grants, 1095
Comm Fndn of Broward Grants, 1100
Dallas Women's Fndn Grants, 1191
DHHS Abandoned Infants Assistance Grants, 1242
DHHS AIDS and HIV Epidemiologic Research Studies Grants, 1244
DHHS Health Care Systems Cost and Access Research and Development Grants, 1252
DHHS HIV Demonstration Program for Children, Adolescents, and Women, 1262
El Paso Comm Fndn Grants, 1388
Elizabeth Glaser Pediatric AIDS Fndn International Leadership Awards, 1393
Elizabeth Glaser Pediatric AIDS Fndn Operations Research Grants, 1394
Elizabeth Glaser Pediatric AIDS Fndn Pediatric HIV Vaccine Research Grants, 1395
Elizabeth Glaser Pediatric AIDS Fndn Two-Year International Scholar Award, 1396
Elizabeth Glaser Pediatric AIDS Fndn Two-Year Scholar Awards, 1397
Elizabeth Glaser Scientist Award, 1398
Fairlawn Fndn Grants, 1447
FCNY Union Square Awards, 1461
FIC/NIH AIDS International Training and Research Program, 1496
Frances L. and Edwin L. Cummings Memorial Fund Grants, 1547
Gates Global HIV/AIDS Vaccine Grants, 1583
Gill Fndn - Gay and Lesbian Fund Grants, 1613
Hagedorn Fund Grants, 1685
Health Fndn of Greater Indianapolis Grants, 1725
Henry J. Kaiser Family Fndn Grants, 1748
HIV/AIDS Research Training Fellowship, 1782
Horizon Fndn for New Jersey Grants, 1793
HRSA Ryan White HIV Early Intervention Services Grants, 1811
Indiana AIDS Fund Grants, 1851
Jessie Smith Noyes Fndn Grants, 1920
John M. Lloyd Fndn Grants, 1939
Johnson & Johnson Corp Contributions Grants, 1952
Johnson and Johnson / SAH Arts and Healing Grants, 1953
M-A-C AIDS Fund Grants, 2091
McCarthy Family Fndn Grants, 2141
NFID New Investigator Matching Grants, 2310
NHLBI Microbiome of the Lung and Respiratory Tract in HIV-Infected Individuals and HIV-Uninfected Controls, 2352
NIA AIDS and Aging: Behavioral Sciences Prevention Research Grants, 2394
NIA Medical Management of Older Patients with HIV/AIDS Grants, 2416
NIAID HIV Prevention Trial Units Grants, 2453
NIAID HIV Vaccine Clinical Trial Units Grants, 2454
NIAID HIV Vaccine Research and Design—Program Project Grants, 2455
NIAID Laboratory Methods to Assess Responses to HIV Vaccine Candidates Research Grants, 2458
NIAID Pediatric Clinical Trials Program for AIDS, 2460
NIAID Statistical Methods in HIV and AIDS Research Grants, 2464
NICHD Central Nervous System Effects of HIV Infection: Neurobiological, Neurovirological, and Neurobehavioral Studies Grants, 2482
NIDA Behavioral Science Track Awards for Rapid Transition, 2498
NIDA Drug Abuse Dissertation Research: Epidemiology, Prevention, Treatment, Services, and Women and Gender Differences, 2502
NIDA HIV Drug Therapy for HIV Users: Access, Adherence, Effectiveness, 2504
NIDA International Studies on Drug Abuse and HIV/AIDS, 2505
NIDA Minority Institutions Drug Abuse Research Development Program (MIDARP) Grants, 2509
NIDA Pilot and Feasibility Studies in Preparation for Drug Abuse Prevention Trials, 2513
NIDCR HIV/AIDS Associated Oral Viral Infections, 2535
NIDDK Transmission of Human Immunodeficiency Virus In Semen, 2592
NIH Centers for AIDS Research, 2647
NIH Collaborations for Advanced Strategies in Complication of HIV Infection, 2651
NIH Demographic Research on Sexual Behaviors Related to HIV, 2653
NIH Impact of HAART on HIV/CNS Disease, 2676
NIH Targeting Research Gaps in HIV Therapeutics Research Grants, 2734
NIMH AIDS and Aging: Behavioral Sciences Prevention Research Grants, 2745
NIMH Central Nervous System Effects of HIV Infection: Neurobiological, Neurovirological, and Neurobehavioral Studies Grants, 2751
NIMH Early Detection of HIV Grants, 2755
NIMH HIV/AIDS, Severe Mental Illness, and Homelessness Research Grants, 2757
NINDS Central Nervous System Effects of HIV Infection: Neurobiological, Neurovirological, and Neurobehavioral Studies Grants, 2777
NINDS Specialized Neuroscience Research on Health Disparity: HIV and the Nervous System, 2785
NINR AIDS and Aging: Behavioral Sciences Prevention Research Grants, 2790
NYCT AIDS/HIV Grants, 2919
NYCT Girls and Young Women Grants, 2924
OSI Harm Reduction and Drug Use Grants, 2966
OUT Fund for Lesbian and Gay Liberation Grants, 2978
Pfizer Fndn Grants, 3025
Questar Corp Contributions Grants, 3097
Rainbow Endowment Grants, 3102
Rockefeller Brothers Fund Pivotal Places Grants: South Africa, 3180
San Diego HIV Funding Collaborative Grants, 3258
Sexually Transmitted Diseases Postdoctoral Fellowships, 3279

SSRC HIV/AIDS and Public Health Policy Research in Africa Fellowships, 3365
Tides Fndn Syringe Access Fund, 3427
United Methodist Church Global AIDS Fund Grants, 3463
Until There's a Cure Fndn Grants, 3471
USCM HIV/AIDS Prevention Grants, 3476

Holistic Medicine
Samueli Institute Scientific Research Grants, 3253

Home Economics
AAFCS International Graduate Fellowships, 109
AAFCS National Graduate Fellowships, 110
AAFCS National Undergraduate Scholarships, 111

Homeland Security
CNCS Next Generation Grants, 1049

Homeless Shelters
Adaptec Fndn Grants, 232
BJ's Charitable Fndn Grants, 761
Carl B. and Florence E. King Fndn Grants, 869
Comm Fndn of Switzerland County Grants, 1127
Danellie Fndn Grants, 1198
Edina Realty Fndn Grants, 1369
Elsie Lee Garthwaite Memorial Fndn Grants, 1408
Georgiana Goddard Eaton Memorial Fund Grants, 1604
Henrietta Tower Wurts Memorial Fndn Grants, 1745
HomeBanc Fndn Grants, 1788
Horace A. Kimball and S. Ella Kimball Fndn Grants, 1792
John H. Wellons Fndn Grants, 1934
L. W. Pierce Family Fndn Grants, 2019
Northwestern Mutual Fndn Grants, 2870
NYCT Grants for the Elderly, 2925
Ordean Fndn Grants, 2952
Plough Fndn Grants, 3061
Sisters of St. Joseph Healthcare Fndn Grants, 3297
Stewart Huston Charitable Trust Grants, 3384
Strowd Roses Grants, 3388
Wilson-Wood Fndn Grants, 3542

Homelessness
ACE Charitable Fndn Grants, 199
ACF Standing Announcement for Unaccompanied Alien Children Grants, 202
African American Fund of New Jersey Grants, 260
Anschutz Family Fndn Grants, 486
Arizona Diamondbacks Charities Grants, 530
Assurant Fndn Grants, 654
Atkinson Fndn International Grants, 661
Audrey and Sydney Irmas Charitable Fndn Grants, 665
Barker Welfare Fndn Grants, 695
Baxter International Fndn Grants, 705
Berrien Comm Fndn Grants, 749
BJ's Charitable Fndn Grants, 761
Bodman Fndn Grants, 776
Boston Fndn Grants, 783
Carl B. and Florence E. King Fndn Grants, 869
Carlisle Fndn Grants, 874
Charles Delmar Fndn Grants, 963
Comer Fndn Grants, 1072
Comm Fndn Of Greater Lafayette Grants, 1110
Comm Fndn of Greenville Hollingsworth Funds Program/Project Grants, 1114
D. W. McMillan Fndn Grants, 1180
Dade Comm Fndn Grants, 1185
Danellie Fndn Grants, 1198
Daniels Fund Grants, 1200
Daphne Seybolt Culpeper Memorial Fndn Grants, 1201
David Geffen Fndn Grants, 1202
Delaware Comm Fndn Grants, 1215
Denver Broncos Charities Fund Grants, 1226
Denver Fndn Comm Grants, 1227
Dreitzer Fndn Grants, 1332
Edina Realty Fndn Grants, 1369
Effie and Wofford Cain Fndn Grants, 1385
El Pomar Fndn Awards and Grants, 1390
Elsie Lee Garthwaite Memorial Fndn Grants, 1408
Ensworth Charitable Fndn Grants, 1416
Eugene and Agnes E. Meyer Fndn Grants, 1432
Eugene M. Lang Fndn Grants, 1434
FAR Fund, 1453
Faye McBeath Fndn Grants, 1456
FCNY Union Square Awards, 1461
Fourjay Fndn Grants, 1544
Frances and John L. Loeb Family Fund Grants, 1546
Georgiana Goddard Eaton Memorial Fund Grants, 1604
Glendale Comm Fndn Grants, 1626
Great-West Life Grants, 1649
Greenspun Family Fndn Grants, 1664
Hanna Andersson Children's Fndn Grants, 1691
Hasbro Children's Fund, 1714
Hearst Fndn and William Randolph Hearst Fndn Grants, 1730
Helen Steiner Rice Fndn Grants, 1742
Henrietta Tower Wurts Memorial Fndn Grants, 1745
Horace A. Kimball and S. Ella Kimball Fndn Grants, 1792
Howard and Bush Fndn Grants, 1798
Jacob G. Schmidlapp Trust Grants, 1883
Joe W. and Dorothy Dorsett Brown Fndn Grants, 1927
John Edward Fowler Memorial Fndn Grants, 1930
John H. and Wilhelmina D. Harland Charitable Fndn Grants, 1933
Joseph H. and Florence A. Roblee Fndn Grants, 1961
Kalamazoo Fndn Grants, 1979
L. W. Pierce Family Fndn Grants, 2019
Lands' End Corp Giving Program, 2030
Laura B. Vogler Fndn Grants, 2032
Lucy Gooding Charitable Fndn Trust, 2082
Lucy Gooding Charitable Fndn Trust Grants, 2083
M.J. Murdock Charitable Trust Grants, 2095
Manuel D. and Rhoda Mayerson Fndn Grants, 2100
McCarthy Family Fndn Grants, 2141
Meyer Fndn Grants, 2177
Morris and Gwendolyn Cafritz Fndn Grants, 2217
Northern Trust Company Charitable Trust and Corp Giving Program, 2865
NYCT Girls and Young Women Grants, 2924
NYCT Grants for the Elderly, 2925
Ordean Fndn Grants, 2952
Peacock Fndn Grants, 3011
Perpetual Trust for Charitable Giving Grants, 3015
Pinellas County Grants, 3050
Plough Fndn Grants, 3061
Portland General Electric Fndn Grants, 3067
Princeton Area Comm Fndn Greater Mercer Grants, 3081
Puerto Rico Comm Fndn Grants, 3090
Quantum Fndn Grants, 3096
Reynolds and Reynolds Associate Fndn Grants, 3152
Rhode Island Fndn Grants, 3154
Rich Fndn Grants, 3156
Richard and Susan Smith Family Fndn Grants, 3159
Roy and Christine Sturgis Trust Grants, 3191
RWJF Local Funding Partnerships Grants, 3223
S. Mark Taper Fndn Grants, 3236
Saint Luke's Health Initiatives Grants, 3240
Sisters of St. Joseph Healthcare Fndn Grants, 3297
Strowd Roses Grants, 3388
Susan Mott Webb Charitable Trust Grants, 3412
Taproot Fndn Capacity-Building Service Grants, 3417
Thomas C. Ackerman Fndn Grants, 3423
Vancouver Fndn Grants and Comm Initiatives Program, 3477
W. C. Griffith Fndn Grants, 3505
Wilson-Wood Fndn Grants, 3542
Women's Fndn of California Grants, 3550

Homeownership
Faye McBeath Fndn Grants, 1456
OceanFirst Fndn Grants, 2933
PMI Fndn Grants, 3063

Homosexuals, Familial Abuse
San Diego Fndn for Change Grants, 3255

Homosexuals, Female
Alexander Fndn Cancer, Catastrophic Illness and Injury Grants, 342
Alexander Fndn Insurance Continuation Grants, 343
California Endowment CommunitiesFirst Grants, 833
Colin Higgins Fndn Grants, 1056
Comm Fndn of Santa Cruz County Grants, 1122
Gill Fndn - Gay and Lesbian Fund Grants, 1613
Grotto Fndn Project Grants, 1671
Henry J. Kaiser Family Fndn Grants, 1748
Horizons Comm Issues Grants, 1794
Lesbian Health Fund Grants, 2046
OUT Fund for Lesbian and Gay Liberation Grants, 2978
Pride Fndn Grants and Scholarships, 3078
Rainbow Endowment Grants, 3102
Women's Fndn of California Grants, 3550

Homosexuals, Male
Alexander Fndn Cancer, Catastrophic Illness and Injury Grants, 342
Alexander Fndn Insurance Continuation Grants, 343
California Endowment CommunitiesFirst Grants, 833
Colin Higgins Fndn Grants, 1056
Comm Fndn of Santa Cruz County Grants, 1122
David Geffen Fndn Grants, 1202
Gill Fndn - Gay and Lesbian Fund Grants, 1613
Grotto Fndn Project Grants, 1671
Henry J. Kaiser Family Fndn Grants, 1748
Horizons Comm Issues Grants, 1794
OUT Fund for Lesbian and Gay Liberation Grants, 2978
Pride Fndn Grants and Scholarships, 3078
Rainbow Endowment Grants, 3102
San Diego Fndn for Change Grants, 3255

Hormones
CRI Prostate Cancer Initiative Grants, 1163
NIDDK Co-Activators and Co-Repressors in Gene Expression Grants, 2546
NIH New Directions in Pain Research Grants, 2698
NIH Receptors and Signaling in Bone in Health and Disease, 2706

Horticulture
Bruce and Adele Greenfield Fndn Grants, 808
Comm Fndn for Greater New Haven Grants, 1091
Comm Fndn of Muncie and Delaware County Grants, 1120
Comm Fndn of Western North Carolina Grants, 1132
Hagedorn Fund Grants, 1685
Nina Mason Pulliam Charitable Trust Grants, 2776
Posey Comm Fndn Grants, 3068

Hospices
AAHPM Hospice and Palliative Medicine Fellowships, 132
Aetna Fndn Quality of Care Grants for End of Life Care, 247
Arizona Public Service Corp Giving Grants, 531
Bailey Fndn Grants, 680
Bertha Russ Lytel Fndn Grants, 751
Borkee-Hagley Fndn Grants, 781
Burlington Industries Fndn Grants, 811
C.W. Titus Fndn Grants, 826
Carl B. and Florence E. King Fndn Grants, 869
Carl W. and Carrie Mae Joslyn Trust Grants, 873
Cemala Fndn Grants, 933
Christy-Houston Fndn Grants, 1008
D. W. McMillan Fndn Grants, 1180
Danellie Fndn Grants, 1198
Dell Fndn Open Grants, 1218
Dunspaugh-Dalton Fndn Grants, 1351
E. Rhodes and Leona B. Carpenter Fndn Grants, 1356
Gregory L. Gibson Charitable Fndn Grants, 1668
Hancock County Comm Fndn Grants, 1690
J.W. Kieckhefer Fndn Grants, 1878
L. W. Pierce Family Fndn Grants, 2019
Lubrizol Fndn Grants, 2080
Lucy Gooding Charitable Fndn Trust, 2082

Lucy Gooding Charitable Fndn Trust Grants, 2083
Margaret L. Wendt Fndn Grants, 2104
Margaret T. Morris Fndn Grants, 2105
Olin Corp Charitable Trust Grants, 2943
OSI Palliative Cancer Care Grants, 2970
RCPSC Balfour M. Mount Visiting Professorship in Palliative Medicine, 3112
Samuel S. Johnson Fndn Grants, 3251
Stewart Huston Charitable Trust Grants, 3384
Thompson Charitable Fndn Grants, 3425

Hospital Administration
Advocate HealthCare Post Graduate Administrative Fellowship, 241

Hospitalized Patients
Carlos and Marguerite Mason Trust Grants, 875
CDC Antimicrobial Resistance in Hospital-Acquired Infections Among Intensive Care Unit Patients, 902
Presbyterian Patient Assistance Program, 3076

Hospitals
Abramson Family Fndn Grants, 188
Acushnet Fndn Grants, 226
Adam Richter Charitable Trust Grants, 230
Adelaide Breed Bayrd Fndn Grants, 234
Advocate HealthCare Post Graduate Administrative Fellowship, 241
Alcoa Fndn Grants, 334
Allyn Fndn Grants, 365
Ann Jackson Family Fndn Grants, 477
Anthony R. Abraham Fndn Grants, 490
Archer Daniels Midland Fndn Grants, 525
Arthur and Rochelle Belfer Fndn Grants, 542
Atran Fndn Grants, 663
Auburn Fndn Grants, 664
Audrey and Sydney Irmas Charitable Fndn Grants, 665
Bacon Family Fndn Grants, 679
Banfi Vintners Fndn Grants, 687
Bank of America Charitable Fndn Anchor Institutions Grants, 688
Barker Fndn Grants, 694
Batchelor Fndn Grants, 701
BCBS of Minnesota Healthy Together Grants, 712
Beckman Coulter Comm Relations Grants, 733
Belk Fndn Grants, 739
Bert W. Martin Fndn Grants, 750
Bertha Russ Lytel Fndn Grants, 751
BibleLands Grants, 754
Bildner Family Fndn Grants, 755
Blum-Kovler Fndn Grants, 772
Blumenthal Fndn Grants, 773
Bob and Delores Hope Charitable Fndn Grants, 774
Bodman Fndn Grants, 776
Boettcher Fndn Grants, 778
Burden Trust Grants, 810
Burlington Industries Fndn Grants, 811
Burlington Northern Santa Fe Fndn Grants, 812
Bushrod H. Campbell and Adah F. Hall Charity Fund Grants, 816
Byron W. and Alice L. Lockwood Fndn Grants, 824
C.W. Titus Fndn Grants, 826
Caddock Fndn Grants, 828
Callaway Fndn Grants, 835
Camp-Younts Fndn Grants, 838
Cancer Research UK Grants, 859
Caring Fndn Grants, 866
Carl and Lily Pforzheimer Fndn Grants, 868
Carl B. and Florence E. King Fndn Grants, 869
Carl Gellert and Celia Berta Gellert Fndn Grants, 871
Carl J. Herzog Fndn Grants, 872
Carls Fndn Grants, 876
Carnahan-Jackson Fndn Grants, 878
Carrie Estelle Doheny Fndn Grants, 883
Carylon Fndn Grants, 886
CCFF Fellowships, 893
Cessna Fndn Grants, 938
Champlin Fndns Grants, 960
Charles Delmar Fndn Grants, 963
Charles M. Bair Family Trust Grants, 972
Chazen Fndn Grants, 978
Chestnut Hill Charitable Fndn, Inc Grants, 987
Christy-Houston Fndn Grants, 1008
Clark Fndn Grants, 1029
Clark-Winchcole Fndn Grants, 1030
CMA Fndn Grants, 1042
Cockrell Fndn Grants, 1053
Coeta and Donald Barker Fndn Grants, 1054
Commonwealth Fund Small Grants, 1084
Comm Fndn of Howard County Grants, 1116
Comm Fndn of Mount Vernon and Knox County Grants, 1119
Connelly Fndn Grants, 1143
ConocoPhillips Fndn Grants, 1144
Constantin Fndn Grants, 1145
Constellation Energy Group and Baltimore Gas and Electric Corp Contributions, 1146
Cowles Charitable Trust Grants, 1155
Dairy Queen Corp Contributions Grants, 1187
Daphne Seybolt Culpeper Memorial Fndn Grants, 1201
Davis Family Fndn Grants, 1204
Deland Fellowships in Health Care and Society, 1214
Dennis and Phyllis Washington Fndn Grants, 1222
Denton A. Cooley Fndn Grants, 1225
DeRoy Testamentary Fndn Grants, 1239
Detroit Lions Charities Grants, 1241
Dolan Fndn Grants, 1306
Dora Roberts Fndn Grants, 1311
Dr. Leon Bromberg Charitable Trust Fund Grants, 1328
Dr. Scholl Fndn Grants, 1329
Dunspaugh-Dalton Fndn Grants, 1351
E.J. Grassmann Trust Grants, 1360
Eberly Fndn Grants, 1364
Eckerd Corp Fndn Grants, 1366
Eden Hall Fndn Grants, 1368
Edward S. Moore Fndn Grants, 1374
Edwards Memorial Trust Grants, 1375
Edwin S. Webster Fndn Grants, 1376
Effie and Wofford Cain Fndn Grants, 1385
Elisabeth Severance Prentiss Fndn Grants, 1392
Eugene B. Casey Fndn Grants, 1433
Eugene McDermott Fndn Grants, 1435
F.M. Kirby Fndn Grants, 1443
Fairview Lutheran Fndn Grants, 1448
Fannie E. Rippel Fndn Grants, 1452
FirstEnergy Fndn Comm Grants, 1505
FMC Fndn Grants, 1518
Ford Motor Company Fund Grants, 1522
Foster Fndn Grants, 1524
Foster G. McGaw Prize, 1525
Frances L. and Edwin L. Cummings Memorial Fund Grants, 1547
Francis T. & Louise T. Nichols Fndn Grants, 1550
Frank E. and Seba B. Payne Fndn Grants, 1551
Frank G. and Freida K. Brotz Family Fndn Grants, 1552
Fraser-Parker Fndn Grants, 1555
Fritz B. Burns Fndn Grants, 1564
Fuji Film Grants, 1565
G.N. Wilcox Trust Grants, 1581
Gebbie Fndn Grants, 1585
George B. Storer Fndn Grants, 1596
George F. Baker Trust Grants, 1597
George Kress Fndn Grants, 1601
George S. and Dolores Dore Eccles Fndn Grants, 1602
Gertrude and William C. Wardlaw Fund Grants, 1607
Gilroy and Lillian P. Roberts Charitable Fndn Grants, 1614
Gladys Brooks Fndn Grants, 1620
Goodrich Corp Fndn Grants, 1638
Greenwall Fndn Bioethics Grants, 1665
Gregory Family Fndn Grants (Florida), 1667
Griffin Family Fndn Grants, 1669
Grundy Fndn Grants, 1673
Harold Alfond Fndn Grants, 1695
Harry and Grace Steele Fndn Grants, 1702
Harry Bramhall Gilbert Charitable Trust Grants, 1703
Hartford Aging and Health Program Awards, 1709
Hawn Fndn Grants, 1719
Healthcare Fndn for Orange County Grants, 1728
Henry County Comm Fndn Grants, 1747
HHS Children's Hospitals Graduate Medical Education Payment Program, 1767
Hilda and Preston Davis Fndn Grants, 1772
Hoblitzelle Fndn Grants, 1783
HRSA Geriatric Education Centers, 1805
Hudson Webber Fndn Grants, 1813
Huie-Dellmon Trust Grants, 1815
J. Walton Bissell Fndn Grants, 1872
J.L. Bedsole Fndn Grants, 1876
Jacob and Hilda Blaustein Fndn Grants, 1881
Jacob and Valeria Langeloth Fndn Grants, 1882
James G.K. McClure Educational and Development Fund Grants, 1886
James H. Cummings Fndn Grants, 1888
James J. and Angelia M. Harris Fndn Grants, 1890
Janirve Fndn Grants, 1905
Joe W. and Dorothy Dorsett Brown Fndn Grants, 1927
John Jewett and Helen Chandler Garland Fndn Grants, 1937
John Lord Knight Fndn Grants, 1938
John S. Dunn Research Fndn Grants and Chairs, 1945
Joseph Alexander Fndn Grants, 1957
Josephine Goodyear Fndn Grants, 1964
Josiah W. and Bessie H. Kline Fndn Grants, 1967
Journal Gazette Fndn Grants, 1968
Katherine John Murphy Fndn Grants, 1983
Lawrence S. Huntington Fund Grants, 2035
Leo Goodwin Fndn Grants, 2043
Lillian S. Wells Fndn Grants, 2056
Louis Calder Fndn Grants, 2065
Lubbock Area Fndn Grants, 2079
Lubrizol Fndn Grants, 2080
Lucile Horton Howe and Mitchell B. Howe Fndn Grants, 2081
Mabel Y. Hughes Charitable Trust Grants, 2097
Margaret L. Wendt Fndn Grants, 2104
Mary S. and David C. Corbin Fndn Grants, 2122
Matilda R. Wilson Fund Grants, 2128
Max and Victoria Dreyfus Fndn Grants, 2133
Maxon Charitable Fndn Grants, 2135
Mayday Fund Grants, 2139
McGregor Fund Grants, 2143
McLean Contributionship Grants, 2147
Meadows Fndn Grants, 2161
Meriden Fndn Grants, 2173
Morton K. and Jane Blaustein Fndn Grants, 2218
National Starch and Chemical Fndn Grants, 2261
Nicholas H. Noyes Jr. Memorial Fndn Grants, 2497
NNEDVF/Altria Doors of Hope Program, 2847
North Carolina Comm Development Grants, 2858
North Central Health Services Grants, 2861
OceanFirst Fndn Grants, 2933
Olin Corp Charitable Trust Grants, 2943
Pasadena Fndn Average Grants, 2994
Peacock Fndn Grants, 3011
Piedmont Natural Gas Grants, 3048
Piper Jaffray Companies Building Strong Communities Grants, 3053
Plum Creek Fndn Grants, 3062
Pott Fndn Grants, 3071
Procter and Gamble Fund Grants, 3083
Questar Corp Contributions Grants, 3097
R.C. Baker Fndn Grants, 3098
Ralphs Food 4 Less Fndn Grants, 3106
Raskob Fndn for Catholic Activities Grants, 3107
Rayonier Fndn Grants, 3111
Rice Fndn Grants, 3155
Rich Fndn Grants, 3156
Richard and Susan Smith Family Fndn Grants, 3159
Robert E. and Evelyn McKee Fndn Grants, 3170
Robins Fndn Grants, 3175
Rockwell International Corp Trust Grants, 3183
Roy and Christine Sturgis Trust Grants, 3191
Russell Berrie Fndn Grants, 3201
Ruth Eleanor Bamberger and John Ernest Bamberger Memorial Fndn Grants, 3202
Ruth H. and Warren A. Ellsworth Fndn Grants, 3203
RWJF New Jersey Health Initiatives Grants, 3225

Saint Luke's Health Initiatives Grants, 3240
Salem Fndn Grants, 3242
Schering-Plough Fndn Health Grants, 3270
Scott County Comm Fndn Grants, 3273
Seabury Fndn Grants, 3274
Shell Oil Company Fndn Grants, 3281
Sid W. Richardson Fndn Grants, 3284
Solo Cup Fndn Grants, 3346
Sosland Fndn Grants, 3348
Sprague Fndn Grants, 3359
Starr Fndn Grants, 3377
Sulzberger Fndn Grants, 3399
Sunderland Fndn Grants, 3400
Tellabs Fndn Grants, 3418
Temple-Inland Fndn Grants, 3419
Thelma Doelger Charitable Trust Grants, 3421
Thomas and Dorothy Leavey Fndn Grants, 3422
Thomas M. and Irene B. Kirbo Charitable Trust Grants, 3424
Thompson Charitable Fndn Grants, 3425
W. C. Griffith Fndn Grants, 3505
Weingart Fndn Grants, 3524
William H. Hannon Fndn Grants, 3540
Winifred & Harry B. Allen Fndn Grants, 3543

Hotel and Restaurant Management
Coors Brewing Corp Contributions Grants, 1151

Housing
Adaptec Fndn Grants, 232
African American Fund of New Jersey Grants, 260
Alexander Fndn Cancer, Catastrophic Illness and Injury Grants, 342
AMD Corp Contributions Grants, 411
American Electric Power Grants, 434
Ann Arbor Area Comm Fndn Grants, 476
Ann Peppers Fndn Grants, 478
Arizona Cardinals Grants, 529
Arizona Diamondbacks Charities Grants, 530
Armstrong McDonald Fndn Grants, 537
Atlanta Fndn Grants, 662
Audrey and Sydney Irmas Charitable Fndn Grants, 665
Bacon Family Fndn Grants, 679
Batchelor Fndn Grants, 701
Beazley Fndn Grants, 730
Boston Fndn Grants, 783
Byron W. and Alice L. Lockwood Fndn Grants, 824
Cambridge Comm Fndn Grants, 837
Carl and Eloise Pohlad Family Fndn Grants, 867
Carl B. and Florence E. King Fndn Grants, 869
Carlisle Fndn Grants, 874
Carnahan-Jackson Fndn Grants, 878
Carpenter Fndn Grants, 881
Cemala Fndn Grants, 933
Cessna Fndn Grants, 938
Chicago Comm Trust Grants, 989
Children Affected by AIDS Fndn Family Assistance Emergency Fund Grants, 996
Citizens Bank Mid-Atlantic Charitable Fndn Grants, 1015
Claude Worthington Benedum Fndn Grants, 1033
Cleo Fndn Grants, 1035
Comerica Charitable Fndn Grants, 1073
Commission on Religion in Appalachia Grants, 1074
Comm Fndn AIDS Endowment Awards, 1088
Comm Fndn Alliance City of Evansville Endowment Fund Grants, 1089
Comm Fndn of Greater Birmingham Grants, 1106
Comm Fndn Of Greater Lafayette Grants, 1110
Comm Fndn of Western North Carolina Grants, 1132
Constantin Fndn Grants, 1145
Crestlea Fndn Grants, 1159
Danellie Fndn Grants, 1198
Delaware Comm Fndn Grants, 1215
Dennis and Phyllis Washington Fndn Grants, 1222
Denver Fndn Comm Grants, 1227
DHHS Health Centers Grants for Residents of Public Housing, 1254
Edwin W. and Catherine M. Davis Fndn Grants, 1377
Ensworth Charitable Fndn Grants, 1416
Eugene and Agnes E. Meyer Fndn Grants, 1432
Evanston Comm Fndn Grants, 1438
Fairfield County Comm Fndn Grants, 1446
Fisa Fndn Grants, 1506
Fisher Fndn Grants, 1508
Fourjay Fndn Grants, 1544
Frank Stanley Beveridge Fndn Grants, 1553
Frist Fndn Grants, 1563
George and Ruth Bradford Fndn Grants, 1595
Georgiana Goddard Eaton Memorial Fund Grants, 1604
Ginn Fndn Grants, 1616
Giving in Action Society Children & Youth with Special Needs Grants, 1617
Giving in Action Society Family Independence Grants, 1618
Greater Bridgeport Area Fndn Comm Impact Grants, 1650
Greater New Orleans Fndn Grants, 1654
Greater Worcester Comm Fndn Discretionary Grants, 1658
Gulf Coast Comm Fndn Grants, 1676
Gulf Coast Comm of Venice Fndn Grants, 1677
HCA Fndn Grants, 1721
Holland/Zeeland Comm Fndn Grants, 1786
Home Building Industry Disaster Relief Fund, 1787
HomeBanc Fndn Grants, 1788
Huntington National Bank Comm Affairs Grants, 1824
Idaho Power Company Corp Contributions, 1838
Jacob G. Schmidlapp Trust Grants, 1883
Janirve Fndn Grants, 1905
Joe W. and Dorothy Dorsett Brown Fndn Grants, 1927
John H. Wellons Fndn Grants, 1934
Joseph H. and Florence A. Roblee Fndn Grants, 1961
Josephine S. Gumbiner Fndn Grants, 1965
Kahuku Comm Fund, 1977
Kalamazoo Fndn Grants, 1979
Katharine Matthies Fndn Grants, 1982
Knox County Comm Fndn Grants, 2009
Liberty Bank Fndn Grants, 2053
Maine Comm Fndn Grants, 2099
Manuel D. and Rhoda Mayerson Fndn Grants, 2100
Mary Owen Borden Fndn Grants, 2121
Mary S. and David C. Corbin Fndn Grants, 2122
McGregor Fund Grants, 2143
Meyer Fndn Grants, 2177
Minneapolis Fndn Comm Grants, 2206
Morris and Gwendolyn Cafritz Fndn Grants, 2217
Newman's Own Inc Grants, 2306
Northeast Utilities Fndn Grants, 2863
Northwest Minnesota Fndn Women's Fund Grants, 2869
Northwestern Mutual Fndn Grants, 2870
NYCT Girls and Young Women Grants, 2924
OceanFirst Fndn Grants, 2933
Oleonda Jameson Trust Grants, 2941
Olin Corp Charitable Trust Grants, 2943
Ordean Fndn Grants, 2952
PacifiCare Fndn Grants, 2981
Paul G. Allen Family Fndn Grants, 3000
Peacock Fndn Grants, 3011
Perry County Comm Fndn Grants, 3016
Philadelphia Fndn Organizational Effectiveness Grants, 3029
Piedmont Natural Gas Grants, 3048
Pike County Comm Fndn Grants, 3049
Pinellas County Grants, 3050
Piper Jaffray Companies Building Strong Communities Grants, 3053
Pittsburgh Fndn Comm Fund Grants, 3054
Plough Fndn Grants, 3061
Polk Bros. Fndn Grants, 3066
Posey Comm Fndn Grants, 3068
Presbyterian Patient Assistance Program, 3076
Prince Charitable Trusts District of Columbia Grants, 3080
Princeton Area Comm Fndn Greater Mercer Grants, 3081
Puerto Rico Comm Fndn Grants, 3090
Ralphs Food 4 Less Fndn Grants, 3106
Rhode Island Fndn Grants, 3154
Robert F. Stoico / FIRSTFED Charitable Fndn Grants, 3171
Robert P. & Clara I. Milton Fund for Senior Housing, 3172
Robin Hood Fndn Grants, 3174
S. Mark Taper Fndn Grants, 3236
S.H. Cowell Fndn Grants, 3237
Salem Fndn Charitable Trust Grants, 3241
Sid W. Richardson Fndn Grants, 3284
Southbury Comm Trust Fund, 3350
Spencer County Comm Fndn Grants, 3358
Starr Fndn Grants, 3377
Taproot Fndn Capacity-Building Service Grants, 3417
Thompson Charitable Fndn Grants, 3425
Union Benevolent Association Grants, 3460
US Trust Corp Fndn Grants, 3475
Vancouver Fndn Grants and Comm Initiatives Program, 3477
Vanderburgh Comm Fndn Grants, 3480
Warrick County Comm Fndn Grants, 3519
Wilson-Wood Fndn Grants, 3542

Human Connectome
NIH Human Connectome Project Grants, 2673

Human Development
California Comm Fndn Human Development Grants, 832
Grammy Fndn Grants, 1643
Human Growth Fndn Small Grants, 1816
NICHD NRSAs—Institutional, 2489
NICHD Small Grants, 2494
NIDA Neurobiological and Behavioral Research on Nicotine and Tobacco Products, 2511
NIH Endocrine Disruptors: Epidemiologic Approaches Grants, 2658
NIH Genetic Susceptibility and Variability of Human Malformations Research Grants, 2669
NIH Research on Sleep and Sleep Disorders, 2713
NSF Behavioral Neurosciences Research Grants, 2876

Human Factors in Engineering
NLM Research Project Grants, 2825

Human Genome
AACR Team Science Award, 89
DOE Health Effects and Life Sciences Research Grants, 1298
DOE Human Genome Program—Ethical, Legal, and Social Implications, 1299
NHGRI Mentored Research Scientist Development Award, 2315
NHLBI Integrating Lung Genetics and Genomics in Human Populations Grants, 2342
NIGMS Pilot Projects for the Protein Structure Initiative (Structural Genomics), 2624
NIH Genetic Architecture of Complex Phenotypes, 2668
NIH Human Connectome Project Grants, 2673
NIH Individual Postdoctoral Fellowships in Genomics and Related ELSI Topics, 2678
NIH Protein Structure Initiative (Structural Genomics) Research Grants, 2704
NIH Protein Structure Initiative (Structural Genomics)—SBIR/STTR GRANTS, 2705
NIH Studies of Ethical, Legal, and Social Implications of Research into Human Genetic Variation Grants, 2731

Human Learning and Memory
Coca-Cola Fndn Grants, 1052
Helen Bader Fndn Grants, 1738
NICHD NRSAs—Individual, 2488
NICHD NRSAs—Institutional, 2489
NIDA Drug Addiction Neuroscience Research Grants, 2503

NIMH Central Nervous System Effects of HIV Infection: Neurobiological, Neurovirological, and Neurobehavioral Studies Grants, 2751
NSF Perception, Action & Cognition Research Grants, 2890
RCPSC Royal College Fellowship for Studies in Medical Education, 3127

Human Reproduction/Fertility
Bernard F. and Alva B. Gimbel Fndn Grants, 747
Donald and Sylvia Robinson Family Fndn Grants, 1310
Educational Fndn of America Grants, 1372
FIC Israeli Ministry of Health Postdoctoral Research Fellowships, 1494
General Service Fndn Reproductive Health and Rights Grants, 1592
Henry J. Kaiser Family Fndn Grants, 1748
Huber Fndn Grants, 1812
Jessie Smith Noyes Fndn Grants, 1920
NICHD Cooperative Specialized Infertility Research Centers, 2484
NICHD NRSAs—Individual, 2488
NICHD NRSAs—Institutional, 2489
NICHD Population Research Grants, 2490
NIEHS Biological Response to Environmental Health Hazards Research Grants, 2596
NIH Endocrine Disruptors: Epidemiologic Approaches Grants, 2658
Robert Sterling Clark Fndn Reproductive Rights and Health Grants, 3173
Susan Vaughan Fndn Grants, 3413
Women's Fndn of California Comm Action Fund, 3549

Human Rights
John M. Lloyd Fndn Grants, 1939
Prospect Burma Scholarships, 3085

Human Services
1675 Fndn Grants, 4
3M Fndn Grants, 11
Abbott Fund Global AIDS Care Grants, 178
Aetna Fndn Voice Of Conscience Award, 252
AIG American General Corp Grants, 316
American Electric Power Grants, 434
Arkansas Comm Fndn Grants, 533
Assisi Fndn Grants, 653
Autodesk Comm Relations Grants, 671
Batchelor Fndn Grants, 701
Blanche and Julian Robertson Family Fndn Grants, 765
Boeing Company Contributions Grants, 777
Business Bank of Nevada Comm Grants, 817
CFFVR Opportunity Grants, 952
Charles M. and Mary D. Grant Fndn Grants, 971
Charles M. Bair Family Trust Grants, 972
Chazen Fndn Grants, 978
Comm Fndn for Southeastern Michigan Grants, 1094
Comm Fndn of St. Joseph County Special Project Challenge Grants, 1126
Comm Impact Fund, 1135
Compass Bank Fndn Grants, 1138
Connelly Fndn Grants, 1143
ConocoPhillips Fndn Grants, 1144
CSRA Comm Fndn Grants, 1168
CSX Corp Contributions Grants, 1169
D.V. and Ida J. McEachern Charitable Trust Grants, 1182
Denver Fndn Comm Grants, 1227
Drs. Bruce and Lee Fndn Grants, 1333
Elizabeth Morse Genius Charitable Trust Grants, 1400
Federal Express Corp Contributions Program, 1483
Ferree Fndn Grants, 1486
Fifth Third Fndn Grants, 1501
Foster Fndn Grants, 1524
Genuardi Family Fndn Grants, 1594
George Kress Fndn Grants, 1601
Great-West Life Grants, 1649
Hackett Fndn Grants, 1684
Harold & Arlene Schnitzer CARE Fndn Grants, 1697
HCA Fndn Grants, 1721
Hilda and Preston Davis Fndn Grants, 1772
Hirtzel Memorial Fndn Grants, 1781
Hormel Fndn Grants, 1796
Human Source Fndn Grants, 1817
Hutton Fndn Grants, 1828
Irving S. Gilmore Fndn Grants, 1867
Jackson County Comm Fndn Unrestricted Grants, 1879
Jacob G. Schmidlapp Trust Grants, 1883
James Ford Bell Fndn Grants, 1885
James J. and Angelia M. Harris Fndn Grants, 1890
Jane's Trust Grants, 1904
John W. and Anna H. Hanes Fndn Grants, 1948
Josephine Goodyear Fndn Grants, 1964
Kettering Family Fndn Grants, 1991
Liberty Bank Fndn Grants, 2053
Lowell Area Comm Fund Grants, 2068
Margaret L. Wendt Fndn Grants, 2104
May Department Stores Charitable Contribution Grants, 2138
McMurry Fndn Grants, 2149
Oscar Rennebohm Fndn Grants, 2963
Paul G. Allen Family Fndn Grants, 3000
Piedmont Natural Gas Grants, 3048
PMI Fndn Grants, 3063
Priddy Fndn Grants, 3077
Pulte Homes Corp Contributions, 3092
Putnam County Comm Fndn Grants, 3093
Rohm and Haas Company Grants, 3185
Shell Oil Company Fndn Grants, 3281
Solo Cup Fndn Grants, 3346
Sosland Fndn Grants, 3348
Sprague Fndn Grants, 3359
Steelcase Fndn Grants, 3379
Stewart Huston Charitable Trust Grants, 3384
Toro Fndn Grants, 3431
TWS Fndn Grants, 3443
US Airways Comm Fndn Grants, 3473
Virginia W. Kettering Fndn Grants, 3502
Weatherwax Fndn Grants, 3523
Winston-Salem Fndn Competitive Grants, 3544

Human Subjects Policy
Alternatives Research and Development Fndn Alternatives in Education Grants, 370
Alternatives Research and Development Fndn Grants, 371
NIH Ethical Issues in Human Studies Research Grants, 2661
NIH Research On Ethical Issues In Human Subjects Research, 2712
NIMH Informed Consent in Research Grants, 2758
ONF Small Grants, 2947

Human/Civil Rights
Aetna Fndn Voice Of Conscience Award, 252
American Jewish World Service Grants, 437
Ford Motor Company Fund Grants, 1522
Global Fund for Children Grants, 1629
Jay and Rose Phillips Family Fndn Grants, 1909
Otto Bremer Fndn Grants, 2977

Humanities
AFG Industries Grants, 259
Ahmanson Fndn Grants, 303
Alex Brown and Sons Charitable Fndn Grants, 337
amfAR Fellowships, 462
amfAR Global Initiatives Grants, 463
amfAR Mathilde Krim Fellowships in Basic Biomedical Research, 464
amfAR Public Policy Grants, 465
amfAR Research Grants, 466
Arkansas Comm Fndn Grants, 533
Armstrong McDonald Fndn Grants, 537
Atherton Family Fndn Grants, 659
Athwin Fndn Grants, 660
Aurora Fndn Grants, 667
Avon Products Fndn Grants, 675
Banfi Vintners Fndn Grants, 687
Barra Fndn Comm Fund Grants, 698
Baton Rouge Area Fndn Grants, 702
Benton County Fndn Grants, 744
Berrien Comm Fndn Grants, 749
Blue Grass Comm Fndn Grants, 768
Boston Globe Fndn Grants, 784
Brookdale Fndn Leadership in Aging Fellowships, 805
Bush Fndn Health & Human Services Grants, 814
Caleb C. and Julia W. Dula Educational and Charitable Fndn Grants, 830
Callaway Fndn Grants, 835
Canada-U.S. Fulbright New Century Scholars Grants, 846
Canada-U.S. Fulbright Senior Specialists Grants, 847
Canadian Friends of Hebrew University Research and Study Grants, 850
Cass County Comm Fndn Grants, 887
Chestnut Hill Charitable Fndn, Inc Grants, 987
Chicago Comm Trust Grants, 989
Chula Vista Charitable Fndn Grants, 1009
Clark County Comm Fndn Grants, 1028
Columbus Fndn Competitive Grants, 1066
Comer Fndn Grants, 1072
Comm Fndn for Southern Arizona Grants, 1095
Comm Fndn of Central Illinois Grants, 1101
Comm Fndn of Champaign County Grants, 1102
Comm Fndn of Greater Birmingham Grants, 1106
Comm Fndn of Greater Flint Grants, 1107
Comm Fndn of Howard County Grants, 1116
Comm Fndn of Madison and Jefferson County Grants and Scholarships, 1117
Comm Fndn of Randolph County Grants, 1121
Comm Fndn of Santa Cruz County Grants, 1122
Comm Fndn Silicon Valley Grants, 1133
Connecticut Comm Fndn Grants, 1141
Cooke Fndn Grants, 1148
DAAD Research Stays for University Academics and Scientists, 1183
Delaware Comm Fndn Grants, 1215
Dubois County Comm Fndn Grants, 1336
El Paso Comm Fndn Grants, 1388
El Pomar Fndn Awards and Grants, 1390
F.M. Kirby Fndn Grants, 1443
Fairfield County Comm Fndn Grants, 1446
Foellinger Fndn Grants, 1519
Ford Motor Company Fund Grants, 1522
Forrest C. Lattner Fndn Grants, 1523
Fulbright Alumni Initiatives Awards Grants, 1566
Fulbright Distinguished Chairs Grants, 1567
Fulbright New Century Scholars Grants, 1570
Fulbright Specialists Grants, 1571
Fulbright Traditional Scholar Program in Europe and Eurasia, 1572
Fulbright Traditional Scholar Program in Sub-Saharan Africa, 1573
Fulbright Traditional Scholar Program in the East Asia/Pacific Region, 1574
Fulbright Traditional Scholar Program in the Near East and North Africa Region, 1575
Fulbright Traditional Scholar Program in the South and Central Asia Region, 1576
Fulbright Traditional Scholar Program in the Western Hemisphere, 1577
George Frederick Jewett Fndn Grants, 1599
Greenwall Fndn Bioethics Grants, 1665
Hallmark Corp Fndn Grants, 1688
Harold and Arlene Schnitzer CARE Fndn Grants, 1697
Honda of America Manufacturing Fndn Grants, 1790
Idaho Power Company Corp Contributions, 1838
J.B. Reynolds Fndn Grants, 1873
JELD-WEN Fndn Grants, 1914
John W. Anderson Fndn Grants, 1949
Johnson County Comm Fndn Grants, 1955
Joseph Drown Fndn Grants, 1960
Katharine Matthies Fndn Grants, 1982
Knox County Comm Fndn Grants, 2009
Land O'Lakes Fndn Mid-Atlantic Grants, 2027
Legacy Fndn Grants, 2040
Lester E. Yeager Charitable Trust B Grants, 2047
Lowell Berry Fndn Grants, 2069
Maxon Charitable Fndn Grants, 2135

McGregor Fund Grants, 2143
McMurry Fndn Grants, 2149
Meyer Memorial Trust Emergency Grants, 2178
Meyer Memorial Trust Grassroots Grants, 2179
Meyer Memorial Trust Operating Funds Grants, 2180
Meyer Memorial Trust Responsive Grants, 2181
Miami County Comm Fndn Operation Round Up Grants, 2188
Miguel Aleman Fndn Grants, 2197
Miriam and Peter Haas Fund Grants, 2208
Morris and Gwendolyn Cafritz Fndn Grants, 2217
Nelda C. and H.J. Lutcher Stark Fndn Grants, 2301
Noble County Comm Fndn Grants, 2848
Northrop Grumman Newport News Grants, 2867
Northwood University/Alden B. Dow Creativity Center Summer Residency Program, 2871
Norwin S. and Elizabeth N. Bean Fndn Grants, 2872
Oceanside Charitable Fndn Grants, 2934
OSI Supplementary Grant Program: Burma, 2971
Owen County Comm Fndn Grants, 2979
Paul Ogle Fndn Grants, 3003
Perry County Comm Fndn Grants, 3016
Pike County Comm Fndn Grants, 3049
Pittsburgh Fndn Comm Fund Grants, 3054
Pulaski County Comm Fndn Grants, 3091
Rajiv Gandhi Fndn Grants, 3104
Ripley County Comm Fndn Grants, 3166
Rush County Comm Fndn Grants, 3200
Snee Reinhardt Charitable Fndn Grants, 3300
South Madison Comm Fndn Grants, 3349
Spencer County Comm Fndn Grants, 3358
SSHRC Image, Text, Sound and Technology Grants, 3363
SSHRC Research/Creation Grants in Fine Arts, 3364
Steele-Reese Fndn Grants, 3380
Steuben County Comm Fndn Grants, 3383
Vanderburgh Comm Fndn Grants, 3480
Vermont Comm Fndn Grants, 3493
Vulcan Materials Company Fndn Grants, 3504
Warrick County Comm Fndn Grants, 3519

Humanities Education
Chatlos Fndn Grants, 977
Honda of America Manufacturing Fndn Grants, 1790
Northwood University/Alden B. Dow Creativity Center Summer Residency Program, 2871
SSHRC Image, Text, Sound and Technology Grants, 3363
SSHRC Research/Creation Grants in Fine Arts, 3364

Hunger
ACE Charitable Fndn Grants, 199
Albertson's Charitable Giving Grants, 330
American Electric Power Grants, 434
BJ's Charitable Fndn Grants, 761
Boston Jewish Comm Women's Fund Grants, 785
ConAgra Foods Fndn Grants, 1140
Coors Brewing Corp Contributions Grants, 1151
Denver Broncos Charities Fund Grants, 1226
Eugene and Agnes E. Meyer Fndn Grants, 1432
Farmers Insurance Group of Companies Grants, 1455
FCNY Union Square Awards, 1461
Fourjay Fndn Grants, 1544
John Deere Fndn Grants, 1929
John Edward Fowler Memorial Fndn Grants, 1930
Kraft Cares International Grants, 2016
Kraft Cares US Grants, 2017
Land O'Lakes Fndn Mid-Atlantic Grants, 2027
Meyer Fndn Grants, 2177
Northern Trust Company Charitable Trust and Corp Giving Program, 2865
NYCT Girls and Young Women Grants, 2924
Peacock Fndn Grants, 3011
Quantum Fndn Grants, 3096
R.C. Baker Fndn Grants, 3098
Robin Hood Fndn Grants, 3174
Rockefeller Fndn Grants, 3181
S. Mark Taper Fndn Grants, 3236
Shaw's Supermarkets Donations, 3280
Southbury Comm Trust Fund, 3350

Huntington's Disease
Hereditary Disease Fndn John J. Wasmuth Postdoctoral Fellowships, 1750
Hereditary Disease Fndn Lieberman Award, 1751
Hereditary Disease Fndn Research Grants, 1752
Huntington's Disease Society of America Research Fellowships, 1825
Huntington's Disease Society of America Research Grants, 1826
Milton Wexler Postdoctoral Fellowships, 2205

Hyperglycemia
NHLBI Hyperglycemic Exacerbation of Ischemia/Reperfusion Injury after Ischemic Insult Grants, 2335

Hyperparathyroidism
NIH Receptors and Signaling in Bone in Health and Disease, 2706

Hypersensitivity
NHLBI Hypersensitivity Pneumonitis – Grants for Early Identification and Mechanisms of Disease, 2336

Hypertension
NHLBI Improving Heart Failure Disease Management Grants, 2338
NHLBI Research Grants on the Relationship Between Hypertension and Inflammation, 2371
Premera CARES Grants, 3074

Ileitis
Crohn's Disease and Colitis Research Fellowships, 1164
Crohn's Disease and Ulcerative Colitis Senior Research Grants, 1165

Illegal Aliens
San Diego Fndn for Change Grants, 3255

Immigrants
ACF Preferred Communities Grants, 201
ACF Supplemental Services for Recently Arrived Refugees Grants, 203
Boston Fndn Grants, 783
Dallas Women's Fndn Grants, 1191
Eugene and Agnes E. Meyer Fndn Grants, 1432
Grotto Fndn Project Grants, 1671
Henry J. Kaiser Family Fndn Grants, 1748
Jewish Fndn for Education of Women Scholarships for Emigres in the Health Professions, 1922
Margaret L. Wendt Fndn Grants, 2104
Meyer Fndn Grants, 2177
Minneapolis Fndn Comm Grants, 2206
NYC Managed Care Consumer Assistance Workshop Re-Design Grants, 2918
RWJF Local Funding Partnerships Grants, 3223
San Diego Fndn for Change Grants, 3255
Strowd Roses Grants, 3388
Taproot Fndn Capacity-Building Service Grants, 3417

Immune System
ASM Abbott Laboratories Award in Clinical and Diagnostic Immunology, 587
Dana Clinical Hypotheses Program in Brain and Immuno-Imaging Research Grants, 1195
Elizabeth Glaser Pediatric AIDS Fndn International Leadership Awards, 1393
Elizabeth Glaser Pediatric AIDS Fndn Operations Research Grants, 1394
Elizabeth Glaser Pediatric AIDS Fndn Pediatric HIV Vaccine Research Grants, 1395
Elizabeth Glaser Pediatric AIDS Fndn Two-Year International Scholar Award, 1396
NHLBI Developmental Origins of Altered Lung Physiology and Immune Function Grants, 2332
NHLBI Pathogenesis And Treatment of Lymphedema And Lymphatic Diseases Grants, 2362
NIAID HIV Vaccine Research and Design—Program Project Grants, 2455
NIH Bone and the Hematopoietic and Immune Systems Research Grants, 2643
Sunshine Natural Wellbeing Fndn Grants, 3404
Whitehall Fndn Neurobiology Research Grants, 3533

Immune System Disorders
DHHS Priority Health Conditions Studies Initiative, 1273
Fairlawn Fndn Grants, 1447
HRSA Ryan White HIV Early Intervention Services Grants, 1811
NHLBI Pathogenesis And Treatment of Lymphedema And Lymphatic Diseases Grants, 2362
NIAID Allergy, Immunology, and Transplantation Program Research Grants, 2449
NIH Bone and the Hematopoietic and Immune Systems Research Grants, 2643
NIH Hyperaccelerated Award/Mechanisms in Immunomodulation Trials, 2675
Sunshine Natural Wellbeing Fndn Grants, 3404

Immunization Programs
BCBS of Minnesota Healthy Together Grants, 712
Chiron Fndn Comm Grants, 1004
NAPNAP Fndn Shourd Parks Immunization Project Small Grants, 2243
NAPNAP Fndn Wyeth Pediatric Immunization Grant, 2244
Premera CARES Grants, 3074
Western Union Fndn Grants, 3529

Immunogenetics
National Psoriasis Fndn Research Grants, 2259

Immunology
AAAAI / Schering Allergy/Immunology Fellowship of Excellence Training Awards, 20
AAAAI Allergy, Asthma and Immunology Education and Research Trust Allied Health Travel Grants, 21
AAAAI Allergy, Asthma and Immunology Education and Research Trust Clinical Research Grants, 22
AAAAI Allergy, Asthma and Immunology Education and Research Trust Faculty Development Award, 23
AAAAI STAR Grants, 26
AAAAI Summer Clinical Research Fellowship Medical Student Grants, 27
AAAAI Summer Research Fellowship Medical Student Grants, 28
AAO-HNSF Health Services Research Grants, 147
AAO-HNSF Maureen Hannley Research Training Awards, 148
AAO-HNSF Percy Memorial Research Award, 149
AAO-HNSF Rande H. Lazar Health Services Research Grant, 150
AAO-HNSF Resident Research Awards, 151
AAOA Fndn/AAO-HNSF Combined Research Grants, 152
AFAR Research Grants, 257
ASM Eli Lilly and Company Research Award, 594
ASM TREK Diagnostic ABMM/ABMLI Professional Recognition Award, 621
CRI Clinical Investigator Award in Cancer Immunology, 1161
CRI Postdoctoral Fellowships, 1162
Dana Fndn Science and Health Grants, 1197
Deafness Research Fndn Research Grants, 1208
FDHN Fellowship to Faculty Transition Awards, 1470
Fndn for Medical Research Grants, 1528
Gates Global HIV/AIDS Vaccine Grants, 1583
Hawaii Comm Fndn Health Education and Research Grants, 1716
HIV/AIDS Research Training Fellowship, 1782
Jackson Laboratory Postdoctoral Research Training Program, 1880
LRF New Investigator Leukemia Research Grants, 2070

Marine Biological Laboratory Summer Research Fellowships, 2108
Mayo Fndn Multidisciplinary Training in Digestive Diseases Research Grants, 2140
National Blood Fndn Research Grant Program, 2249
NCI Technologies and Software to Support Integrative Cancer Biology Research Grants, 2279
NFID Advanced Vaccinology Course Travel Grant, 2307
NIAAA Hepatitis C Infection and Alcoholic Liver Disease, 2442
NIAID Allergy, Immunology, and Transplantation Program Research Grants, 2449
NIAID Allergy, Immunology, Transplantation, Infectious Diseases, and AIDS NRSAs—Individual, 2450
NIAID Enhancing Vaccine-Elicited Protective Immunity in Malaria Research Grants, 2452
NIAID Preparedness against Illegitimate Use of Bacterial Pathogens, 2461
NIAMS Skin Diseases Research Core Centers Grants, 2478
NIDCR HIV/AIDS Associated Oral Viral Infections, 2535
NIDCR Oral Microbiology/Immunology of Type 1 Diabetes, 2537
NIGMS Molecular Pharmacology of Anesthetic Action Research Grants, 2621
NIGMS/NIDCR Evolution of Infectious Diseases Research Grants, 2633
NIH Biobehavioral Pain Research Grants, 2638
NIH Hyperaccelerated Award/Mechanisms in Immunomodulation Trials, 2675
NIH Impact of HAART on HIV/CNS Disease, 2676
NIH Nonhuman Primate Immune Tolerance Cooperative Study Group Grants, 2699
NIH Role of Microglia in Normal and Abnormal Immune Responses of the Nervous System, 2716
NIH Ruth L. Kirschstein National Research Service Awards for Individual Postdoctoral Fellows, 2719
NIH Small Business Innovation Research: Animal Models of HCV Infection Research Grants, 2728
NIH Targeting Research Gaps in HIV Therapeutics Research Grants, 2734
NIMH Central Nervous System Effects of HIV Infection: Neurobiological, Neurovirological, and Neurobehavioral Studies Grants, 2751
Rett Syndrome Research Fndn Grants, 3151
Searle Scholars Grants, 3275
Stanley Fndn Schizophrenia and Bipolar Disorder Research Grants, 3375
UK Fndn for the Study of Infant Deaths Grants, 3459
US CRDF Leishmaniasis: Collaborative Research Opportunities in North Africa and the Middle East, 3474

Immunopathology
AAAAI Research Award Grants, 25
National Psoriasis Fndn Research Grants, 2259

Immunotherapy
Cancer Treatment Research Fndn Clinical Investigation Grants, 861
CRI Prostate Cancer Initiative Grants, 1163

Independent Living Programs
Arizona Public Service Corp Giving Grants, 531
Dept of Ed Rehabilitation Training Grants, 1229
John Edward Fowler Memorial Fndn Grants, 1930
Margoes Fndn Grants, 2106
Robert P. & Clara I. Milton Fund for Senior Housing, 3172
S. Mark Taper Fndn Grants, 3236
Sisters of Saint Joseph Charitable Fund Grants, 3296
U.S. Department of Education Rehabilitation Research Training Centers, 3448

India
Fulbright Traditional Scholar Program in the Near East and North Africa Region, 1575
OSI Access to Essential Medicines Grants, 2964
Rajiv Gandhi Fndn Grants, 3104
Sir Dorabji Tata Trust Grants for NGOs or Voluntary Organizations, 3291
Sir Dorabji Tata Trust Individual Medical Grants, 3292

Indigenous Cultures
Bernard Van Leer Fndn Grants, 748

Indonesia
OSI Indonesia Project Grants, 2967
Tifa Fndn Grants, 3428

Industrial Engineering
Canada Graduate Scholarships and NSERC Postgraduate Scholarships, 845
NSF-NIST Interaction in Chemistry, Materials Research, Molecular Biosciences, Bioengineering, and Chemical Engineering, 2897
U.S. Department of Education Erma Byrd Scholarships, 3446

Industrial Hygiene
FIC International Training and Research in Environmental and Occupational Health, 1493
U.S. Department of Education Erma Byrd Scholarships, 3446

Industry
Duke Energy Fndn Grants, 1339
ExxonMobil Grants, 1442
Millipore Fndn Grants, 2203
NCI/NIDA Transdisciplinary Tobacco Use Research Centers Grants, 2280
NIEHS Applied Toxicological Research and Testing Grants, 2595
Northern Trust Company Charitable Trust and Corp Giving Program, 2865
NSF Grant Opportunities for Academic Liaison with Industry, 2887
RSC Thomas W. Eadie Medal, 3199

Infants
AAP Nutrition Award, 165
CIGNA Fndn Grants, 1011
CNCS Foster Grandparent Projects Grants, 1048
Comm Fndn of Crawford County Grants and Scholarships, 1103
DHHS Abandoned Infants Assistance Grants, 1242
DHHS Health Centers Grants for Residents of Public Housing, 1254
DHHS Maternal and Child Health Projects Grants, 1263
DHHS Universal Newborn Hearing Screening and Intervention, 1282
Duke University Pediatric Anesthesiology Fellowship, 1347
Elizabeth Glaser Pediatric AIDS Fndn International Leadership Awards, 1393
Elizabeth Glaser Pediatric AIDS Fndn Operations Research Grants, 1394
Elizabeth Glaser Pediatric AIDS Fndn Pediatric HIV Vaccine Research Grants, 1395
Elizabeth Glaser Pediatric AIDS Fndn Two-Year International Scholar Award, 1396
Fndn for Seacoast Health Grants, 1533
Gerber Fndn Grants, 1606
Health Fndn of Greater Indianapolis Grants, 1725
HRSA Eliminating Disparities in Perinatal Health Grants, 1803
Johnson & Johnson Comm Health Care Grants, 1951
Lowell Berry Fndn Grants, 2069
NICHD NRSAs—Individual, 2488
NICHD NRSAs—Institutional, 2489
NIH Research on Sleep and Sleep Disorders, 2713
Oakland Fund for Children and Youth Grants, 2930
RWJF Local Funding Partnerships Grants, 3223
UK Fndn for the Study of Infant Deaths Grants, 3459
United Cerebral Palsy Research Grants, 3462

Infectious Diseases/Agents
Alliance Healthcare Fndn Grants, 362
ASM Merck Irving S. Sigal Memorial Awards, 606
ASM Siemens Healthcare Diagnostics Young Investigator Award, 618
ASM-PAHO Infectious Diseases Epidemiology and Surveillance Fellowships, 625
ASM/CCID Fellowships, 627
CDC Antimicrobial Resistance in Hospital-Acquired Infections Among Intensive Care Unit Patients, 902
CDC Cooperative Agreement for Continuing Enhanced National Surveillance for Prion Diseases in the United States, 904
CDC Emerging Infectious Diseases Fellowships, 908
CDC Epidemiology and Laboratory Capacity Infectious Diseases Grants, 909
CDC Evaluation of the Use of Rapid Testing For Influenza in Outpatient Medical Settings, 910
Chiron Fndn Comm Grants, 1004
Duncan L. Gordon Fellowships, 1349
Elizabeth Glaser Pediatric AIDS Fndn International Leadership Awards, 1393
Elizabeth Glaser Pediatric AIDS Fndn Operations Research Grants, 1394
Elizabeth Glaser Pediatric AIDS Fndn Two-Year International Scholar Award, 1396
Fellowships in Infectious Diseases, 1485
FIC International Cooperative Biodiversity Groups Grants, 1487
FIC International Research Scientist Development Award, 1491
FIC International Training and Research in Emerging Infectious Diseases Grants, 1492
Marine Biological Laboratory Summer Research Fellowships, 2108
MDBD Basic Research Grants, 2152
National Blood Fndn Research Grant Program, 2249
NFID New Investigator Matching Grants, 2310
NFID Nosocomial Infection Research and Training Postdoctoral Fellowship, 2311
NFID Postdoctoral Fellowships in Emerging Infectious Diseases, 2312
NHLBI Hypersensitivity Pneumonitis – Grants for Early Identification and Mechanisms of Disease, 2336
NIAID Allergy, Immunology, Transplantation, Infectious Diseases, and AIDS NRSAs—Individual, 2450
NIAID Challenge Grants: Joint Ventures in Biomedicine and Biotechnology, 2451
NIAID Independent Scientist Award, 2456
NIAID Microbiology and Infectious Diseases Research Grants and Contracts, 2459
NIAID Research Scholar Development Award, 2462
NIAID Small Business Innovation Research Advanced Technology Grants, 2463
NIAID Therapeutics Research on AIDS-Associated Opportunistic Infections, 2465
NIAMS/NICHD Deep Infections of Total Joint Replacements, 2481
NIDCR HIV/AIDS Associated Oral Viral Infections, 2535
NIGMS/NIDCR Evolution of Infectious Diseases Research Grants, 2633
NIH Ecology of Infectious Diseases, 2656
NIH SBIR/STTR Study and Control of Microbial Biofilms Research Grants, 2724
Pfizer Fndn Grants, 3025
Thrasher Research Fund Grants, 3426
UK Fndn for the Study of Infant Deaths Grants, 3459

Inflammation
AAAAI Summer Clinical Research Fellowship Medical Student Grants, 27
AAAAI Summer Research Fellowship Medical Student Grants, 28
Broad Fndn IBD Research Grants, 803
NHLBI Research Grants on the Relationship Between Hypertension and Inflammation, 2371

Informatics
NLM Limited Competition for Continuation of Biomedical Informatics/Bioinformatics Resource Grants, 2821
PhRMA Fndn Informatics Sabbatical Fellowships, 3035

Information Dissemination
CDC Cooperative Agreement for Partnership to Enhance Public Health Informatics, 905
Fndn for Seacoast Health Grants, 1533
Healthcare Fndn for Orange County Grants, 1728
NIMH Mental Health Dissemination Research Grants, 2762
NLM Informatics Conference Grants, 2819
NLM Research Project Grants, 2825
SAMHSA Conference Grants, 3246

Information Science Education
U.S. Department of Education Erma Byrd Scholarships, 3446

Information Science/Systems
Canada Graduate Scholarships and NSERC Postgraduate Scholarships, 845
DaimlerChrysler Corp Fund Grants, 1186
DOE Health Effects and Life Sciences Research Grants, 1298
NIGMS Predoctoral Training in Bioinformatics and Computation Biology Grants, 2625
NLM Internet Connection for Medical Institutions Grants, 2820
NLM Research Project Grants, 2825
Sarah Scaife Fndn Grants, 3263
Scientific Communities Initiative Grants, 3272
U.S. Department of Education Erma Byrd Scholarships, 3446

Injury
CDC Injury Control Research Centers Grants, 913
CDC Injury Prevention and Control Research and State and Comm Based Programs, 914
CDC National Training Information and Exchange Program, 920
CDC Oral Diseases Prevention and Oral Health Promotion Grants, 921
DOL Occupational Safety and Health—Susan Harwood Training Grants, 1305
Dorothea Haus Ross Fndn Grants, 1320
FIC International Training and Research in Environmental and Occupational Health, 1493
Moses Cone-Wesley Long Comm Health Fndn Grants, 2219
National Patient Safety Fndn Patient Safety Research Grants, 2258
NIAMS High Risk Arthritis and Musculoskeletal and Skin Diseases Research, 2470
NIEHS Biological Response to Environmental Health Hazards Research Grants, 2596
NIH National Occupational Research Agenda Grants, 2696
NIOSH Occupational Safety and Health Research and Demonstration Grants, 2807
Quantum Fndn Grants, 3096

Inner Cities
Adolph Coors Fndn Grants, 238
Arie and Ida Crown Memorial Grants, 528
Comm Fndn for Greater Buffalo Grants, 1090
Detroit Lions Charities Grants, 1241
Millipore Fndn Grants, 2203
Nina Mason Pulliam Charitable Trust Grants, 2776
Northern Trust Company Charitable Trust and Corp Giving Program, 2865
Prudential Fndn Grants, 3087
Saint Luke's Fndn Grants, 3239
US Trust Corp Fndn Grants, 3475

Instructional Materials and Practices
CDC Hepatitis Education for Inmates and Correctional Staff Grants, 911

Instrumentation, Medical
NHLBI Cardiac Translational Research Implementation Grants, 2324

Instrumentation, Scientific
NSF Instrument Development for Biological Research, 2888
NSF Major Research Instrumentation Program Grants, 2889

Insurance/Actuarial Science
New York Life Fndn Grants, 2304
Starr Fndn Grants, 3377

Intellectual Freedom
Chicago Tribune's Corp Contributions Grants, 991

International Education/Training
Alexander von Humboldt Fndn Research Fellowships for Experienced Researchers, 347
Alexander von Humboldt Fndn Research Fellowships for Postdoctoral Researchers, 348
Amarillo Area/Harrington Fndns Grants, 410
ASM International Fellowship for Latin America and the Caribbean, 601
ASM International Fellowships for Asia and Africa, 602
ASM International Professorship for Latin America, 603
ASM International Professorships for Asia and Africa, 604
ASM Millis-Colwell Postgraduate Travel Grant, 608
ASM-PAHO Infectious Diseases Epidemiology and Surveillance Fellowships, 625
ASM-UNESCO Leadership Grant for International Educators, 626
Australian Academy of Science Grants, 670
Cancer Society of New Zealand Grants, 860
Coca-Cola Fndn Grants, 1052
DAAD Research Stays for University Academics and Scientists, 1183
FIC International Research and Training in Population and Health Grants, 1489
FIC International Training and Research in Emerging Infectious Diseases Grants, 1492
FIC International Training and Research in Environmental and Occupational Health, 1493
FIC/ORMH Minority International Research Training Grants, 1497
HHMI Physician-Scientist Early Career Award, 1762
HHMI-NIH Cloister Research Scholars, 1765
International Fellowships in Medical Education, 1861
National Heart Fndn of New Zealand Grants, 2255
OSI European Commission Internships for Young Roma Graduates, 2965
PAHO-ASM International Professorship for Latin America, 2983
PAHO/WHO Fellowships, 2984
Susan G. Komen Breast Cancer Fndn Postdoctoral Fellowships, 3411
U.S. Department of Education United States-Russia Program: Improving Research and Educational Activities in Higher Education, 3451
Whitaker International Fellows and Scholars Program, 3532
Women of the ELCA Opportunity Scholarships for Lutheran Laywomen, 3548

International Exchange Programs
Albuquerque Comm Fndn Grants, 331
American College of Surgeons International Guest Scholarships, 429
ASM Millis-Colwell Postgraduate Travel Grant, 608
Chateaubriand Exact Sciences, Engineering, and Medicine Research Scholarships, 976
Coca-Cola Fndn Grants, 1052
International Cancer Technology Transfer Fellowships, 1858
Medical/Nursing Education, Research, and Health Care Exchanges with Taiwan, 2165
U.S. Department of Education United States-Russia Program: Improving Research and Educational Activities in Higher Education, 3451

International Grants
Pediatric Brain Tumor Research Grants, 3012

International Organizations
Alexander von Humboldt Fndn Institutional Academic Cooperation Grants, 346
Harry Kramer Memorial Fund Grants, 1705

International Planning/Policy
John Merck Fund Grants, 1940
Lynde and Harry Bradley Fndn Grants, 2089
Lynde and Harry Bradley Fndn Prizes: Bradley Prizes, 2090

International Programs
AFAR Paul Beeson Career Development Awards in Aging Research for the Island of Ireland, 256
Alcatel-Lucent Technologies Corp Contributions Grants, 332
Alcoa Fndn Grants, 334
Alexander von Humboldt Fndn Georg Forster Fellowships for Experienced Researchers, 344
Alexander von Humboldt Fndn Georg Forster Fellowships for Postdoctoral Researchers, 345
American Jewish World Service Grants, 437
Archer Daniels Midland Fndn Grants, 525
ASCO International Development and Education Awards, 554
ASCO Long-Term International Fellowships, 556
ASM GlaxoSmithKline International Member of the Year Award, 599
Atkinson Fndn International Grants, 661
Atran Fndn Grants, 663
Banfi Vintners Fndn Grants, 687
Baxter International Fndn Grants, 705
Beatrice Laing Trust Grants, 729
Bechtel Group Fndn Building Positive Comm Relationships Grants, 731
Becton Dickinson and Company Grants, 736
Besser Fndn Grants, 752
Bill and Melinda Gates Fndn Grants, 756
Boston Jewish Comm Women's Fund Grants, 785
Bristol-Myers Squibb Fndn Health Disparities Grants, 797
Broad Fndn IBD Research Grants, 803
Burden Trust Grants, 810
Caddock Fndn Grants, 828
Cargill Citizenship Fund-Corp Giving Grants, 865
Carylon Fndn Grants, 886
Charles Delmar Fndn Grants, 963
Chase Paymentech Corp Giving Grants, 975
Chatlos Fndn Grants, 977
Chesapeake Corp Fndn Grants, 982
CIGNA Fndn Grants, 1011
Commonwealth Fund Australian-American Health Policy Fellowships, 1078
ConAgra Foods Fndn Grants, 1140
ConocoPhillips Fndn Grants, 1144
Cystic Fibrosis Research Grants, 1179
Danellie Fndn Grants, 1198
Dental Teaching and Research Fellowships, 1224
DOD Multidisciplinary Postdoctoral Award for Breast Cancer Research, 1295
Doreen Kronick Scholarship, 1312
Duke University Clinical Cardiac Electrophysiology Fellowships, 1342
Duke University Interventional Cardiology Fellowships, 1344
Elizabeth Glaser Scientist Award, 1398
FIC International Research Fellowships, 1490
FIC International Research Scientist Development Award, 1491

Fndn for Medical Research Grants, 1528
Hamlet Trust Grants, 1689
Harold Simmons Fndn Grants, 1698
Helen Bader Fndn Grants, 1738
Henry J. Kaiser Family Fndn Grants, 1748
Hershey Company Grants, 1754
Honeywell Fndn Grants, 1791
i2 Fndn Grants, 1829
Jacob and Hilda Blaustein Fndn Grants, 1881
James H. Cummings Fndn Grants, 1888
Japan Heart Fndn Grants, 1906
John Deere Fndn Grants, 1929
Johnson and Johnson / SAH Arts and Healing Grants, 1953
Kiwanis International Fndn Grants, 2004
Landon Fndn-AACR Innovator Award for International Collaboration, 2028
Lawrence Fndn Grants, 2034
Ludwick Family Fndn Grants, 2084
Lustgarten Fndn for Pancreatic Cancer Research Grants, 2086
Mead Johnson Nutritionals Charitable Giving Grants, 2156
Mead Johnson Nutritionals Medical Education Grants, 2158
MGFA Post-Doctoral Research Fellowships, 2183
MGFA Student Fellowships, 2184
National Lottery Comm Fund Grants, 2256
NIA Research Grants on Chemical Senses: Neurotransmitters and Neuromodulators, 2430
NIDA International Studies on Drug Abuse and HIV/AIDS, 2505
NIDCR International Collaborative Oral Health Research Planning Grant, 2536
Nuffield Fndn Africa Grants, 2898
Nuffield Fndn Law and Society Grants, 2900
Nuffield Fndn Small Grants, 2903
Paul Balint Charitable Trust Grants, 2998
PDF International Research Grants, 3005
Pfizer Fndn Grants, 3025
Potts Memorial Fndn Grants, 3072
Procter and Gamble Fund Grants, 3083
Rett Syndrome Research Fndn Grants, 3151
Rockefeller Archive Center Research Grants, 3178
Rockefeller Fndn Grants, 3181
Rockwell Collins Charitable Contributions, 3182
Rosalinde and Arthur Gilbert Fndn/AFAR New Investigator Awards in Alzheimer's Disease, 3187
Russell Berrie Fndn Grants, 3201
Savoy Fndn Post-Doctoral and Clinical Research Fellowships, 3266
Savoy Fndn Research Grants, 3267
Savoy Fndn Studentships, 3268
Sigrid Juselius Fndn Grants, 3286
SNM Postdoctoral Molecular Imaging Scholar Grants, 3305
SNM/ Covidien Seed Grant in Molecular Imaging/ Nuclear Medicine Research, 3308
Trull Fndn Grants, 3441
UK Fndn for the Study of Infant Deaths Grants, 3459
United Technologies Corp Grants, 3466
W.K. Kellogg Fndn Healthy Kids Grants, 3507

International Relations
AAAS Science & Technology Policy Fellowships - National Defense & Global Security, 29
Alexander von Humboldt Fndn Institutional Academic Cooperation Grants, 346
American College of Surgeons International Guest Scholarships, 429
Archer Daniels Midland Fndn Grants, 525
Arie and Ida Crown Memorial Grants, 528
Coca-Cola Fndn Grants, 1052
Donald and Sylvia Robinson Family Fndn Grants, 1310
Eugene McDermott Fndn Grants, 1435
George F. Baker Trust Grants, 1597
Harry Kramer Memorial Fund Grants, 1705
Max Bell Fndn Grants, 2134
Miguel Aleman Fndn Grants, 2197
Rajiv Gandhi Fndn Grants, 3104
Starr Fndn Grants, 3377
U.S. Department of Education United States-Russia Program: Improving Research and Educational Activities in Higher Education, 3451

International Students
OSI European Commission Internships for Young Roma Graduates, 2965

International Studies
AAP International Travel Grants, 162
Alexander von Humboldt Fndn Research Fellowships for Experienced Researchers, 347
Coca-Cola Fndn Grants, 1052
DAAD Research Stays for University Academics and Scientists, 1183
OSI European Commission Internships for Young Roma Graduates, 2965
SRC Medical Research Grants, 3362

International Trade and Finance
Archer Daniels Midland Fndn Grants, 525
Starr Fndn Grants, 3377

Internet
Bill and Melinda Gates Fndn Grants, 756
EDS Fndn Grants, 1371
Leonsis Fndn Grants, 2045
NLM Internet Connection for Medical Institutions Grants, 2820
RSC Thomas W. Eadie Medal, 3199
Scientific Communities Initiative Grants, 3272
Verizon Fndn Maryland Grants, 3487
Verizon Fndn New York Grants, 3488
Verizon Fndn Northeast Region Grants, 3489
Verizon Fndn Pennsylvania Grants, 3490
Verizon Fndn Vermont Grants, 3491
Verizon Fndn Virginia Grants, 3492

Internship Programs
AFAR Medical Student Training in Aging Research Program, 255
AMA-MSS Government Relations Internship Programs, 404
Independence Blue Cross Nursing Internships, 1848
Strowd Roses Grants, 3388
Susan Mott Webb Charitable Trust Grants, 3412

Intervention Programs
Bodman Fndn Grants, 776
Cambridge Comm Fndn Grants, 837
CDC Injury Control Research Centers Grants, 913
Comm Fndn Silicon Valley Grants, 1133
Dept of Ed Special Education—Personnel Development to Improve Services and Results for Children with Disabilities, 1231
DHHS Universal Newborn Hearing Screening and Intervention, 1282
DOJ Gang-Free Schools and Communities Intervention Grants, 1303
Hasbro Children's Fund, 1714
NIH Biobehavioral Research for Effective Sleep, 2639
NIH National Occupational Research Agenda Grants, 2696
NIH New Directions in Pain Research Grants, 2698
NIH Pathological Gambling: Basic, Clinical, and Services Research Grants, 2702
NIMH HIV/AIDS, Severe Mental Illness, and Homelessness Research Grants, 2757
NIMH Pilot Effectiveness Trials for Mental Disorders Grants, 2766
SAMHSA Conference Grants, 3246
William T. Grant Fndn Research Grants, 3541

Inventions
Lemelson-MIT Lifetime Achievement Award, 2042

Isotope/Radiation Technology
DSO Radiation Biodosimetry Grants, 1335

Israel
Abramson Family Fndn Grants, 188
Atran Fndn Grants, 663
Boston Jewish Comm Women's Fund Grants, 785
Canadian Friends of Hebrew University Research and Study Grants, 850
Chazen Fndn Grants, 978
Donald and Sylvia Robinson Family Fndn Grants, 1310
Feldman Fndn Grants, 1484
FIC Israeli Ministry of Health Postdoctoral Research Fellowships, 1494
Fishman Family Fndn Grants, 1510
Harry Kramer Memorial Fund Grants, 1705
Helen Bader Fndn Grants, 1738
Jacob and Hilda Blaustein Fndn Grants, 1881
Russell Berrie Fndn Grants, 3201

Japan
Fulbright International Education Administrators Seminar Grants, 1569

Japanese Americans
California Endowment CommunitiesFirst Grants, 833

Japanese Art
Fulbright International Education Administrators Seminar Grants, 1569

Jewish Services
100 Mile Man Fndn Grants, 2
A/H Fndn Grants, 19
Aaron & Cecile Goldman Family Fndn Grants, 171
Aaron & Freda Glickman Fndn Grants, 172
Aaron Fndn (Massachusetts) Grants, 174
Abramson Family Fndn Grants, 188
Adolph Coors Fndn Grants, 238
Albuquerque Comm Fndn Grants, 331
Alexis Gregory Fndn Grants, 349
Ansell, Zaro, Grimm & Aaron Fndn Grants, 487
Archer Daniels Midland Fndn Grants, 525
Arie and Ida Crown Memorial Grants, 528
Arthur and Rochelle Belfer Fndn Grants, 542
Atran Fndn Grants, 663
Audrey and Sydney Irmas Charitable Fndn Grants, 665
Barr Fund Grants, 697
Bender Fndn Grants, 742
Bildner Family Fndn Grants, 755
Blanche and Irving Laurie Fndn Grants, 764
Blumenthal Fndn Grants, 773
Boettcher Fndn Grants, 778
Boston Jewish Comm Women's Fund Grants, 785
Caddock Fndn Grants, 828
Carl C. Icahn Fndn Grants, 870
Charles H. Revson Fndn Grants, 969
Chazen Fndn Grants, 978
CRH Fndn Grants, 1160
David Geffen Fndn Grants, 1202
Donald and Sylvia Robinson Family Fndn Grants, 1310
Feldman Fndn Grants, 1484
Fishman Family Fndn Grants, 1510
Giant Eagle Fndn Grants, 1611
Gilroy and Lillian P. Roberts Charitable Fndn Grants, 1614
Greenspun Family Fndn Grants, 1664
H. Schaffer Fndn Grants, 1680
Harold and Arlene Schnitzer CARE Fndn Grants, 1697
Harry Kramer Memorial Fund Grants, 1705
Healthcare Fndn of New Jersey Grants, 1729
Howard and Bush Fndn Grants, 1798
Irvin Stern Fndn Grants, 1866
Jacob and Hilda Blaustein Fndn Grants, 1881
Jewish Comm Fndn of Greater Los Angeles Grants, 1921
Jewish Fndn for Education of Women Scholarships for Emigres in the Health Professions, 1922
Jewish Fund Grants, 1923
Jewish Women's Fndn of New York Grants, 1924
John J. Leidy Fndn Grants, 1936

Joseph Alexander Fndn Grants, 1957
Manuel D. and Rhoda Mayerson Fndn Grants, 2100
Max A. Adler Charitable Fndn Grants, 2132
Michael and Susan Dell Fndn Grants, 2189
Morton K. and Jane Blaustein Fndn Grants, 2218
Mount Zion Health Fund Grants, 2220
New York University Steinhardt School of Education Fellowships, 2305
Paul Balint Charitable Trust Grants, 2998
Sosland Fndn Grants, 3348

Jewish Studies
Aaron & Cecile Goldman Family Fndn Grants, 171
Aaron & Freda Glickman Fndn Grants, 172
Alexis Gregory Fndn Grants, 349
Ansell, Zaro, Grimm & Aaron Fndn Grants, 487
Arthur and Rochelle Belfer Fndn Grants, 542
Atran Fndn Grants, 663
Barr Fund Grants, 697
Blanche and Irving Laurie Fndn Grants, 764
Blumenthal Fndn Grants, 773
Fishman Family Fndn Grants, 1510
Helen Bader Fndn Grants, 1738
Howard and Bush Fndn Grants, 1798
Irvin Stern Fndn Grants, 1866
Jewish Women's Fndn of New York Grants, 1924
M.B. and Edna Zale Fndn Grants, 2093
Meadows Fndn Grants, 2161
Richard and Rhoda Goldman Fund Grants, 3158
Russell Berrie Fndn Grants, 3201

Job Training Programs
3M Fndn Grants, 11
ACF Supplemental Services for Recently Arrived Refugees Grants, 203
Achelis and Bodman Fndns Grants, 206
Adaptec Fndn Grants, 232
AMD Corp Contributions Grants, 411
Anschutz Family Fndn Grants, 486
AT&T Excelerator, 657
Bernard and Audre Rapoport Fndn Grants, 746
Bodman Fndn Grants, 776
Boeing Company Contributions Grants, 777
Cass County Comm Fndn Grants, 887
Chiron Fndn Comm Grants, 1004
Citizens Bank Mid-Atlantic Charitable Fndn Grants, 1015
Comer Fndn Grants, 1072
Coors Brewing Corp Contributions Grants, 1151
DaimlerChrysler Corp Fund Grants, 1186
Dallas Women's Fndn Grants, 1191
eBay Fndn Comm Grants, 1363
Fairfield County Comm Fndn Grants, 1446
Fndn for the Carolinas Grants, 1535
General Mills Fndn Grants, 1590
Global Fund for Children Grants, 1629
Heineman Fndn for Research, Education, Charitable and Scientific Purposes, 1735
Highmark Corp Giving Grants, 1769
Houston Endowment Grants, 1797
John Edward Fowler Memorial Fndn Grants, 1930
John Merck Fund Grants, 1940
Johnson & Johnson Corp Contributions Grants, 1952
Katharine Matthies Fndn Grants, 1982
Kenny's Kids Grants, 1990
Liberty Bank Fndn Grants, 2053
M.B. and Edna Zale Fndn Grants, 2093
McGregor Fund Grants, 2143
Middlesex Savings Charitable Fndn Grants, 2196
Minneapolis Fndn Comm Grants, 2206
Northeast Utilities Fndn Grants, 2863
Northern Trust Company Charitable Trust and Corp Giving Program, 2865
OceanFirst Fndn Grants, 2933
PacifiCare Fndn Grants, 2981
Piedmont Natural Gas Grants, 3048
Pinellas County Grants, 3050
Piper Jaffray Companies Building Strong Communities Grants, 3053
Polk Bros. Fndn Grants, 3066
Portland General Electric Fndn Grants, 3067
Procter and Gamble Fund Grants, 3083
Richard King Mellon Fndn Grants, 3161
Robin Hood Fndn Grants, 3174
Rockefeller Fndn Grants, 3181
S.H. Cowell Fndn Grants, 3237
Starr Fndn Grants, 3377
Taproot Fndn Capacity-Building Service Grants, 3417
Topfer Family Fndn Grants, 3430
U.S. Department of Education 21st Century Comm Learning Centers, 3445
Verizon Fndn Maryland Grants, 3487
Verizon Fndn New York Grants, 3488
Verizon Fndn Northeast Region Grants, 3489
Verizon Fndn Pennsylvania Grants, 3490
Verizon Fndn Vermont Grants, 3491
Verizon Fndn Virginia Grants, 3492
Waitt Family Fndn Grants, 3512
Wal-Mart State Giving Grants, 3514

Journalism
AcademyHealth PHSR Research Article of the Year Awards, 196
AMA Virtual Mentor Theme Issue Editor Grants, 400
American Academy of Nursing Media Awards, 418
APSA Congressional Fellowships Health and Aging Policy Fellows Program, 514
APSA Robert Wood Johnson Fndn Health Policy Fellowships, 515
BCBS of Massachusetts Health Coverage Fellowships, 710
Canada-U.S. Fulbright New Century Scholars Grants, 846
Canada-U.S. Fulbright Senior Specialists Grants, 847
Chicago Tribune's Corp Contributions Grants, 991
Fulbright Alumni Initiatives Awards Grants, 1566
Fulbright Distinguished Chairs Grants, 1567
Fulbright New Century Scholars Grants, 1570
Fulbright Specialists Grants, 1571
Fulbright Traditional Scholar Program in Europe and Eurasia, 1572
Fulbright Traditional Scholar Program in Sub-Saharan Africa, 1573
Fulbright Traditional Scholar Program in the East Asia/Pacific Region, 1574
Fulbright Traditional Scholar Program in the Near East and North Africa Region, 1575
Fulbright Traditional Scholar Program in the South and Central Asia Region, 1576
Fulbright Traditional Scholar Program in the Western Hemisphere, 1577
IWMF Public Health Fellowship, 1871
James M. Cox Fndn of Georgia Grants, 1892
John Ben Snow Memorial Trust Grants, 1928
Johnson F. Hammond Memorial Scholarship, 1956
Knight Public Health Journalism Fellowships at CDC, 2008
Mary Baker Eddy Library Summer Research Fellowships, 2117
NIHCM Fndn Health Care Print Journalism Awards, 2742
NIHCM Fndn Health Care Television and Radio Journalism Awards, 2744
NMF National Medical Association Awards for Medical Journalism, 2836
Prudential Fndn Grants, 3087

Junior and Community Colleges
Comm Fndn of Western North Carolina Grants, 1132
FirstEnergy Fndn Comm Grants, 1505
Halliburton Fndn Grants, 1687
J.M. Long Fndn Grants, 1877
James G.K. McClure Educational and Development Fund Grants, 1886
NIGMS Initiative for Minority Students: Bridges to the Baccalaureate Degree, 2612

Junior High School Education
Eisner Fndn Grants, 1387

Justice
Nuffield Fndn Africa Grants, 2898
Tifa Fndn Grants, 3428

Juvenile Delinquency
Barker Welfare Fndn Grants, 695
Beazley Fndn Grants, 730
Boston Fndn Grants, 783
Cambridge Comm Fndn Grants, 837
Connecticut Comm Fndn Grants, 1141
DOJ Gang-Free Schools and Communities Intervention Grants, 1303
DOJ Mental Health and Juvenile Justice, 1304
G.N. Wilcox Trust Grants, 1581
Green Fndn Grants, 1661
Mary Owen Borden Fndn Grants, 2121
McKesson Fndn Grants, 2145

Juvenile Law
Chicago Comm Trust Grants, 989
DOJ Mental Health and Juvenile Justice, 1304
NYCT Girls and Young Women Grants, 2924

Kazakhstan
Fulbright Traditional Scholar Program in the South and Central Asia Region, 1576

Kenya
OSI Access to Essential Medicines Grants, 2964

Kidney Cancer
ASCO Career Development Award, 551
ASCO Young Investigator Award, 562
ASCO/UICC International Cancer Technology Transfer (ICRETT) Fellowships, 563

Kidney Diseases and Disorders
Andersen Fndn Grants, 471
Collins C. Diboll Private Fndn Grants, 1057
DHHS Priority Health Conditions Studies Initiative, 1273
Henry & Ruth Blaustein Rosenberg Fndn Grants, 1746
KFC Allied Health Research Grants, 1996
KFC Biomedical Fellowships, 1997
KFC Biomedical Research Grants, 1998
NIA Renal Function and Chronic Kidney Disease in Aging Grants, 2429
NIDDK Advances in Polycystic Kidney Disease Grants, 2539
NIDDK Ancillary Studies of Kidney Disease Accessing Information from Clinical Trials, Epidemiological Studies, and Databases Grants, 2540
NIDDK Calcium Oxalate Stone Diseases Grants, 2544
NIDDK Development of Disease Biomarkers Grants, 2549
NIDDK Education Grants, 2554
NIDDK Enhancing Zebrafish Research with Research Tools and Techniques, 2556
NIDDK Mentored Research Scientist Development Award, 2565
NIDDK Multi-Center Clinical Study Cooperative Agreements, 2566
NIDDK Multi-Center Clinical Study Implementation Planning Grants, 2567
NIDDK Non-Invasive Methods for Diagnosis and Progression of Diabetes, Kidney, Urological, Hematological and Digestive Diseases, 2572
NIDDK Pilot and Feasibility Clinical Research Grants in Kidney or Urologic Diseases, 2575
NIDDK Proteomics: Diabetes, Obesity, And Endocrine, Digestive, Kidney, Urologic, And Hematologic Diseases, 2578
NIDDK Research Grants for Studies of Hepatitis C in the Setting of Renal Disease, 2580
NIDDK Secondary Analyses in Obesity, Diabetes and Digestive and Kidney Diseases Grants, 2583
NIDDK Small Grant Program for K08/K23 Recipients, 2587

NIDDK Small Grants for Underrepresented Minority Scientists in Diabetes and Digestive and Kidney Diseases, 2588
NIDDK Training in Clinical Investigation in Kidney and Urology Grants, 2590
NIEHS Biological Response to Environmental Health Hazards Research Grants, 2596
NIGMS Short Courses on Mathematical, Statistical, and Computational Tools for Studying Biological Systems, 2629
NIH Nonhuman Primate Immune Tolerance Cooperative Study Group Grants, 2699
NIH Sarcoidosis: Research into the Cause of Multi-Organ Disease and Clinical Strategies for Therapy Grants, 2723
NKF Clinical Scientist Awards, 2809
NKF Franklin McDonald/Fresenius Medical Care Clinical Research Grants, 2810
NKF Professional Councils Research Grants, 2811
NKF Research Fellowships, 2812
NKF Young Investigator Grants, 2813
NYAM Edward N. Gibbs Memorial Lecture and Award in Nephrology, 2912
Oxalosis and Hyperoxaluria Fndn Grants, 2980
PKD Fndn Lillian Kaplan International Prize for the Advancement in the Understanding of Polycystic Kidney Disease, 3056
PKD Fndn Research Grants, 3057

Kinesiology
Canada Graduate Scholarships and NSERC Postgraduate Scholarships, 845

Knowledge Acceleration
NLM Exceptional, Unconventional Research Grants Enabling Knowledge Acceleration, 2815

Korea
Fulbright International Education Administrators Seminar Grants, 1569

Kosovo
OSI European Commission Internships for Young Roma Graduates, 2965

Kyrgyz Republic
Fulbright Traditional Scholar Program in the South and Central Asia Region, 1576

Labor Law
Global Fund for Children Grants, 1629

Labor Relations
Ms. Fndn for Women Grants, 2222
NIEHS Applied Toxicological Research and Testing Grants, 2595

Land Management
Bella Vista Fndn Grants, 740
Champlin Fndns Grants, 960
Richard King Mellon Fndn Grants, 3161
Samuel S. Johnson Fndn Grants, 3251

Land Pollution
San Diego Fndn for Change Grants, 3255

Land Use Planning/Policy
Comm Fndn for Southeastern Michigan Grants, 1094
Emma B. Howe Memorial Fndn Grants, 1415
KeySpan Fndn Grants, 1995
NIEHS Mentored Clinical Scientist Research Career Development Awards, 2602
Pioneer Hi-Bred Comm Grants, 3051

Language
NIDCD Clinical Trial Planning Grant, 2517
NIDCD Exploratory Research: Feasibility Pilot Studies Grants, 2519
NIDCD Exploratory/Developmental Research Grants, 2520
NIDCD Minority Dissertation Research Grants in Human Communication, 2524
NIDCD Program for Postdoctoral Research Training in Clinical Trials, 2528

Language Acquisition and Development
ASHFndn Student Research Grants in Early Childhood Language Development, 585
NIDCD Small Grants, 2531

Laryngology
ALVRE Casselberry Award, 374
ALVRE Grant, 375
ALVRE Seymour R. Cohen Award, 376

Latin America
ASM-UNESCO Leadership Grant for International Educators, 626
Atkinson Fndn International Grants, 661
Charles Delmar Fndn Grants, 963

Law
AHFMR Population Health Investigator Awards, 292
AMA-MSS Government Relations Advocacy Fellowship, 403
AMA-MSS Government Relations Internship Programs, 404
AMA-RFS Legislative Awareness Internships, 407
Bush Fndn Health & Human Services Grants, 814
Canada-U.S. Fulbright New Century Scholars Grants, 846
Canada-U.S. Fulbright Senior Specialists Grants, 847
Compass Bank Fndn Grants, 1138
Deland Fellowships in Health Care and Society, 1214
DOE Health Effects and Life Sciences Research Grants, 1298
E.L. Wiegand Fndn Grants, 1361
Eugene and Agnes E. Meyer Fndn Grants, 1432
Fulbright Alumni Initiatives Awards Grants, 1566
Fulbright Distinguished Chairs Grants, 1567
Fulbright New Century Scholars Grants, 1570
Fulbright Specialists Grants, 1571
Fulbright Traditional Scholar Program in Europe and Eurasia, 1572
Fulbright Traditional Scholar Program in Sub-Saharan Africa, 1573
Fulbright Traditional Scholar Program in the East Asia/Pacific Region, 1574
Fulbright Traditional Scholar Program in the Near East and North Africa Region, 1575
Fulbright Traditional Scholar Program in the South and Central Asia Region, 1576
Fulbright Traditional Scholar Program in the Western Hemisphere, 1577
John Ben Snow Memorial Trust Grants, 1928
Meyer Fndn Grants, 2177
NIH Individual Postdoctoral Fellowships in Genomics and Related ELSI Topics, 2678
NIH Studies of Ethical, Legal, and Social Implications of Research into Human Genetic Variation Grants, 2731
Prudential Fndn Grants, 3087
Rajiv Gandhi Fndn Grants, 3104
Special Olympics Health Professions Student Grants, 3355
Takemi Program in International Health Research and Advanced Training Fellowships, 3416
Tifa Fndn Grants, 3428
Triangle Comm Fndn Donor-Advised Grants, 3437
Vulcan Materials Company Fndn Grants, 3504

Law Enforcement
Baptist Comm Ministries Grants, 691
Burlington Northern Santa Fe Fndn Grants, 812
Cass County Comm Fndn Grants, 887
Cemala Fndn Grants, 933
Colorado Springs Comm Trust Fund Grants, 1061
Hudson Webber Fndn Grants, 1813
Kenneth T. and Eileen L. Norris Fndn Grants, 1989
Ms. Fndn for Women Grants, 2222

Leadership
AACR Margaret Foti Award for Leadership and Extraordinary Achievements in Cancer Research, 81
AACR-Minorities in Cancer Research Jane Cooke Wright Lectureship Awards, 99
AAOHN Fndn New Investigator Researcher Grants, 154
AAOHN Fndn Professional Development Scholarships, 155
AAPD Paul G. Hearne Leadership Award, 170
African American Fund of New Jersey Grants, 260
AMA-MSS Government Relations Advocacy Fellowship, 403
AMA-MSS Government Relations Internship Programs, 404
American College of Surgeons Resident and Associate Society (RAS-ACS) Leadership Scholarships, 431
ASHA Minority Student Leadership Program Awards, 570
ASM bioMerieux Sonnenwirth Award for Leadership in Clinical Microbiology, 589
ASM Gen-Probe Joseph Public Health Award, 597
ASM GlaxoSmithKline International Member of the Year Award, 599
ASM TREK Diagnostic ABMM/ABMLI Professional Recognition Award, 621
Austin College Leadership Award, 668
Bodman Fndn Grants, 776
Boeing Company Contributions Grants, 777
Bullitt Fndn Grants, 809
Carroll County Comm Fndn Grants, 885
Cass County Comm Fndn Grants, 887
Castle Rock Fndn Grants, 888
CDC Oral Diseases Prevention and Oral Health Promotion Grants, 921
Central Carolina Comm Fndn Comm Impact Grants, 936
CFPC Fellowships, 955
Charles Lafitte Fndn Grants, 970
Chicago Comm Trust Grants, 989
Comm Fndn of Howard County Grants, 1116
Constellation Energy Group and Baltimore Gas and Electric Corp Contributions, 1146
Cowles Charitable Trust Grants, 1155
CPhA Centennial Award, 1156
Dallas Mavericks Fndn Grants, 1190
Dorothy Rider Pool Health Care Grants, 1322
Duke Energy Fndn Grants, 1339
Educational Fndn of America Grants, 1372
FCD Child Development Grants, 1458
FIC International Training and Research in Emerging Infectious Diseases Grants, 1492
Frist Fndn Grants, 1563
George Family Fndn Grants, 1598
Grotto Fndn Project Grants, 1671
Heineman Fndn for Research, Education, Charitable and Scientific Purposes, 1735
Hutton Fndn Grants, 1828
Jewish Women's Fndn of New York Grants, 1924
John Edward Fowler Memorial Fndn Grants, 1930
John M. Lloyd Fndn Grants, 1939
Johnson & Johnson Corp Contributions Grants, 1952
Lubrizol Fndn Grants, 2080
Marshall Field's Comm Grants, 2115
MLA Lois Ann Colaianni Award for Excellence and Achievement in Hospital Librarianship, 2210
Ms. Fndn for Women Grants, 2222
National Dairy Promotion and Research Board Scholarships, 2251
NIH Academic Career Awards, 2634
NMF Franklin C. McLean Award, 2829
NMF Hugh J. Andersen Memorial Scholarship, 2832
NMF Metropolitan Life Fndn Awards Program for Academic Excellence in Medicine, 2835
NMF National Medical Association Awards for Medical Journalism, 2836
NMF National Medical Association Emerging Scholar Awards, 2837
NMF Ralph W. Ellison Prize, 2840
NMF William and Charlotte Cadbury Award, 2841

Nordson Corp Fndn Grants, 2851
Northwest Minnesota Fndn Women's Fund Grants, 2869
NSF Presidential Early Career Awards for Scientists and Engineers (PECASE) Grants, 2892
PeyBack Fndn Grants, 3022
Philadelphia Fndn Organizational Effectiveness Grants, 3029
Portland General Electric Fndn Grants, 3067
Progress Energy Fndn Grants, 3084
Prudential Fndn Grants, 3087
RCPSC James H. Graham Award of Merit, 3119
Rhode Island Fndn Grants, 3154
Rockefeller Brothers Fund Peace and Security Grants, 3179
RWJF Comm Health Leaders Awards, 3208
RWJF Executive Nurse Fellowships, 3210
RWJF Health Policy Fellowships, 3217
RWJF Ladder to Leadership: Developing the Next Generation of Comm Health Leaders Fellowships, 3222
Tifa Fndn Grants, 3428
W.K. Kellogg Fndn Healthy Kids Grants, 3507
Women's Fndn of California Grants, 3550

Learning Disabilities
AACAP Pilot Research Award for Learning Disabilities, Supported by the Elaine Schlosser Lewis Fund, 46
AACAP Sidney Berman Award for the School-Based Study and Intervention for Learning Disorders and Mental Ilness, 51
Comm Fndn of Grant County Grants, 1104
CVS All Kids Can Grants, 1175
Learning and Behavioral Disorders Research Grants, 2039

Learning Disabled, Education for
Comm Fndn of Grant County Grants, 1104
Doreen Kronick Scholarship, 1312
Educational Fndn of America Grants, 1372

Legal Education
Canadian Friends of Hebrew University Research and Study Grants, 850
Center for Science in the Public Interest Internships, 935
Hearst Fndn and William Randolph Hearst Fndn Grants, 1730

Legal Services
Bodenwein Public Benevolent Fndn Grants, 775
David Geffen Fndn Grants, 1202
Georgiana Goddard Eaton Memorial Fund Grants, 1604
Howard and Bush Fndn Grants, 1798
Margaret L. Wendt Fndn Grants, 2104
Morris and Gwendolyn Cafritz Fndn Grants, 2217
NNEDVF/Altria Doors of Hope Program, 2847
OSI Integrating Health and Legal Services Grants, 2968
Otto Bremer Fndn Grants, 2977
Perry County Comm Fndn Grants, 3016
Rhode Island Fndn Grants, 3154
SAG Motion Picture Players Welfare Fund Grants, 3238
Southbury Comm Trust Fund, 3350

Legal Systems
Carrier Corp Contributions Grants, 884

Leukemia
ACGT Investigators Grants, 204
AMA Fndn Seed Grants for Research, 398
Angel Kiss Fndn Grants, 472
Children's Leukemia Research Association Research Grants, 999
Children's Medical Research Institute Grants, 1000
E.D.Thomas Fellowship, 1359
Leukaemia Research Fund Grants, 2050
Leukemia and Lymphoma Society Research Grants, 2051
Louis R. Cappelli Fndn Grants, 2066
LRF New Investigator Leukemia Research Grants, 2070
LRF Physician-Scientist Postdoctoral Fellowships, 2071
LRF Postdoctoral Fellowships, 2072
LSA Fellowships, 2073
LSA Scholar Award for Clinical Research, 2074
LSA Scholar Awards, 2075
LSA Special Fellowships, 2076
LSA Specialized Center of Research Grants, 2077
LSA Translational Research Grants, 2078
NCIC Canadian Cancer Society Research Grants, 2282
NYCT Biomedical Research Grants, 2920
Ryan Gibson Fndn Grants, 3234

Libraries
Ahmanson Fndn Grants, 303
Air Products and Chemicals Grants, 319
Alcatel-Lucent Technologies Fndn Grants, 333
Alexis Gregory Fndn Grants, 349
Andersen Fndn Grants, 471
Auburn Fndn Grants, 664
Bertha Russ Lytel Fndn Grants, 751
Bill and Melinda Gates Fndn Grants, 756
Bodenwein Public Benevolent Fndn Grants, 775
Boettcher Fndn Grants, 778
Booth-Bricker Fund Grants, 780
Brinson Fndn Grants, 794
Burlington Northern Santa Fe Fndn Grants, 812
Caleb C. and Julia W. Dula Educational and Charitable Fndn Grants, 830
Callaway Fndn Grants, 835
Carl and Lily Pforzheimer Fndn Grants, 868
Carnahan-Jackson Fndn Grants, 878
Champlin Fndns Grants, 960
Chicago Board of Trade Fndn Grants, 988
Clarcor Fndn Grants, 1021
Comm Fndn of Randolph County Grants, 1121
Comm Fndn of Southeastern Connecticut Grants, 1125
Constantin Fndn Grants, 1145
Cooper Industries Fndn Grants, 1150
Faye McBeath Fndn Grants, 1456
George Kress Fndn Grants, 1601
Gladys Brooks Fndn Grants, 1620
Green Bay Packers Fndn Grants, 1660
H. Schaffer Fndn Grants, 1680
Hall-Perrine Fndn Grants, 1686
Harry Bramhall Gilbert Charitable Trust Grants, 1703
High Meadow Fndn Grants, 1768
Huie-Dellmon Trust Grants, 1815
Idaho Comm Fndn Eastern Region Competitive Grants, 1837
J.L. Bedsole Fndn Grants, 1876
James G.K. McClure Educational and Development Fund Grants, 1886
John Ben Snow Memorial Trust Grants, 1928
Louis Calder Fndn Grants, 2065
Margaret L. Wendt Fndn Grants, 2104
McLean Contributionship Grants, 2147
NLM Internet Connection for Medical Institutions Grants, 2820
Portland General Electric Fndn Grants, 3067
Posey Comm Fndn Grants, 3068
Procter and Gamble Fund Grants, 3083
Rayonier Fndn Grants, 3111
Rice Fndn Grants, 3155
Rochester Area Comm Fndn Grants, 3176
Roy and Christine Sturgis Trust Grants, 3191
Scientific Communities Initiative Grants, 3272
Susan Vaughan Fndn Grants, 3413
Thomas M. and Irene B. Kirbo Charitable Trust Grants, 3424
W. C. Griffith Fndn Grants, 3505
William H. Hannon Fndn Grants, 3540

Libraries, Academic
Humana Fndn Grants, 1818
John Deere Fndn Grants, 1929
Kelvin and Eleanor Smith Fndn Grants, 1986
Richard King Mellon Fndn Grants, 3161
Roy J. Carver Charitable Trust Medical and Science Research Grants, 3192
Starr Fndn Grants, 3377
Wayne and Gladys Valley Fndn Grants, 3522

Libraries, Medical
ASM USFCC/J. Roger Porter Award, 623
MLA Ida and George Eliot Prize, 2209
MLA Lois Ann Colaianni Award for Excellence and Achievement in Hospital Librarianship, 2210
NLM Exploratory/Developmental Grants, 2816
NLM Grants for Scholarly Works in Biomedicine and Health, 2818

Libraries, Public
Adelaide Breed Bayrd Fndn Grants, 234
Champlin Fndns Grants, 960
John G. Martin Fndn Grants, 1932
Louis R. Cappelli Fndn Grants, 2066
Milagro Fndn Grants, 2198
Piedmont Natural Gas Grants, 3048

Library Automation
Clarcor Fndn Grants, 1021
MLA Ida and George Eliot Prize, 2209

Library Science
Alexis Gregory Fndn Grants, 349
Canada-U.S. Fulbright New Century Scholars Grants, 846
Canada-U.S. Fulbright Senior Specialists Grants, 847
Canadian Friends of Hebrew University Research and Study Grants, 850
Fulbright Alumni Initiatives Awards Grants, 1566
Fulbright Distinguished Chairs Grants, 1567
Fulbright New Century Scholars Grants, 1570
Fulbright Specialists Grants, 1571
Fulbright Traditional Scholar Program in Europe and Eurasia, 1572
Fulbright Traditional Scholar Program in Sub-Saharan Africa, 1573
Fulbright Traditional Scholar Program in the East Asia/Pacific Region, 1574
Fulbright Traditional Scholar Program in the Near East and North Africa Region, 1575
Fulbright Traditional Scholar Program in the South and Central Asia Region, 1576
Fulbright Traditional Scholar Program in the Western Hemisphere, 1577
Margaret L. Wendt Fndn Grants, 2104
Roy and Christine Sturgis Trust Grants, 3191
W. C. Griffith Fndn Grants, 3505

Life Sciences
Beckman Young Investigators Grants, 735
DOE Health Effects and Life Sciences Research Grants, 1298
HHMI Grants and Fellowships Programs, 1759
Homer Fndn Grants, 1789
Kavli Fndn Research Grants, 1985
Life Sciences Research Fndn Postdoctoral Fellowships, 2054
NSF Biomedical Engineering and Engineering Healthcare Grants, 2879
NSF Chemical, Biochemical, and Biotechnology Systems Research Grants, 2882
ONR Human Performance Division Research Grants, 2948
RSC Thomas W. Eadie Medal, 3199
Whitehall Fndn Neurobiology Research Grants, 3533

Life Skills Training
Cargill Citizenship Fund-Corp Giving Grants, 865
Coors Brewing Corp Contributions Grants, 1151
Cruise Industry Charitable Fndn Grants, 1166
Global Fund for Children Grants, 1629

Linguistics/Philology
Canada-U.S. Fulbright New Century Scholars Grants, 846
Canada-U.S. Fulbright Senior Specialists Grants, 847
Fulbright Alumni Initiatives Awards Grants, 1566
Fulbright Distinguished Chairs Grants, 1567
Fulbright New Century Scholars Grants, 1570
Fulbright Specialists Grants, 1571
Fulbright Traditional Scholar Program in Europe and Eurasia, 1572
Fulbright Traditional Scholar Program in Sub-Saharan Africa, 1573
Fulbright Traditional Scholar Program in the East Asia/Pacific Region, 1574
Fulbright Traditional Scholar Program in the Near East and North Africa Region, 1575
Fulbright Traditional Scholar Program in the South and Central Asia Region, 1576
Fulbright Traditional Scholar Program in the Western Hemisphere, 1577
NLM Research Project Grants, 2825

Lipids
NIH Structural Biology of Membrane Proteins Grants, 2730
Robert B McMillen Fndn Grants, 3169

Literacy
AAFP Fndn Health Literacy State Grants, 112
Ahmanson Fndn Grants, 303
Alcatel-Lucent Technologies Fndn Grants, 333
Allen P. and Josephine B. Green Fndn Grants, 361
Allyn Fndn Grants, 365
AMD Corp Contributions Grants, 411
Amgen Fndn Grants, 467
Anschutz Family Fndn Grants, 486
Arizona Cardinals Grants, 529
Arizona Diamondbacks Charities Grants, 530
Arkell Hall Fndn Grants, 534
Arlington Comm Fndn Grants, 536
Ashland Corp Contributions Grants, 586
Assisi Fndn Grants, 653
Atkinson Fndn International Grants, 661
Atlanta Fndn Grants, 662
Auburn Fndn Grants, 664
Bacon Family Fndn Grants, 679
Ball Brothers Fndn Grants, 684
Barker Welfare Fndn Grants, 695
Battle Creek Comm Fndn Grants, 703
Benton Comm Fndn Grants, 743
Berrien Comm Fndn Grants, 749
Blackford County Comm Fndn Grants, 763
Blue Mountain Comm Fndn Grants, 769
Blue River Comm Fndn Grants, 770
Bodenwein Public Benevolent Fndn Grants, 775
Bodman Fndn Grants, 776
Boettcher Fndn Grants, 778
Booth-Bricker Fund Grants, 780
Boston Fndn Grants, 783
Boston Globe Fndn Grants, 784
Brinson Fndn Grants, 794
Brown County Comm Fndn Grants, 807
Carl and Lily Pforzheimer Fndn Grants, 868
Cass County Comm Fndn Grants, 887
Cemala Fndn Grants, 933
Charles Lafitte Fndn Grants, 970
Charles M. and Mary D. Grant Fndn Grants, 971
Chicago Board of Trade Fndn Grants, 988
Chicago Comm Trust Grants, 989
CIGNA Fndn Grants, 1011
Colorado Springs Comm Trust Fund Grants, 1061
Comerica Charitable Fndn Grants, 1073
Commonweal Fndn Grants, 1076
Comm Fndn Alliance City of Evansville Endowment Fund Grants, 1089
Comm Fndn of Bartholomew County Heritage Fund Grants, 1096
Comm Fndn of Bartholomew County James A. Henderson Award for Fund-Raising, 1097
Comm Fndn of Boone County Grants, 1099
Comm Fndn of Broward Grants, 1100
Comm Fndn of Central Illinois Grants, 1101
Comm Fndn of Grant County Grants, 1104
Comm Fndn of Greater Birmingham Grants, 1106
Comm Fndn of Greater Fort Wayne: Comm Endowment & Clarke Endowment Fund Grants, 1108
Comm Fndn of Greenville Hollingsworth Funds Program/Project Grants, 1114
Comm Fndn of Western North Carolina Grants, 1132
Cooper Industries Fndn Grants, 1150
Coors Brewing Corp Contributions Grants, 1151
Cornerstone Fndn of Northeastern Wisconsin Grants, 1152
Cowles Charitable Trust Grants, 1155
Crail-Johnson Fndn Grants, 1157
Cruise Industry Charitable Fndn Grants, 1166
CVS All Kids Can Grants, 1175
Dayton Power and Light Fndn Grants, 1205
Deaconess Comm Fndn Grants, 1207
Dell Fndn Healthy Communities, Literate Communities, and Connected Communities Grants, 1217
Delta Air Lines Fndn Grants, 1220
Edyth Bush Charitable Fndn Grants, 1378
EIF Comm Grants, 1386
Entergy Comm Partnership Grants, 1417
Evjue Fndn Grants, 1439
Farmers Insurance Group of Companies Grants, 1455
Faye McBeath Fndn Grants, 1456
Field Fndn of Illinois Grants, 1499
Fourjay Fndn Grants, 1544
Frances L. and Edwin L. Cummings Memorial Fund Grants, 1547
G.N. Wilcox Trust Grants, 1581
GenCorp Fndn Grants, 1587
General Mills Fndn Grants, 1590
GlaxoSmithKline Corp Grants, 1623
Green Bay Packers Fndn Grants, 1660
Hallmark Corp Fndn Grants, 1688
Hanna Andersson Children's Fndn Grants, 1691
Harold Simmons Fndn Grants, 1698
Harvest Fndn Grants, 1713
Hasbro Children's Fund, 1714
Hearst Fndn and William Randolph Hearst Fndn Grants, 1730
Helen Steiner Rice Fndn Grants, 1742
Henry & Ruth Blaustein Rosenberg Fndn Grants, 1746
Highmark Corp Giving Grants, 1769
Hilda and Preston Davis Fndn Grants, 1772
Houston Endowment Grants, 1797
Howard and Bush Fndn Grants, 1798
Hugh J. Andersen Fndn Grants, 1814
Humana Fndn Grants, 1818
i2 Fndn Grants, 1829
Irvin Stern Fndn Grants, 1866
James A. and Faith Knight Fndn Grants, 1884
James S. Copley Fndn Grants, 1895
Jean and Louis Dreyfus Fndn Grants, 1911
Jim Moran Fndn Grants, 1925
John Edward Fowler Memorial Fndn Grants, 1930
John H. and Wilhelmina D. Harland Charitable Fndn Grants, 1933
John I. Smith Charities Grants, 1935
John P. McGovern Fndn Grants, 1942
Joseph H. and Florence A. Roblee Fndn Grants, 1961
Kraft Cares International Grants, 2016
Lincoln Financial Group Fndn Grants, 2058
Louis Calder Fndn Grants, 2065
Lubrizol Fndn Grants, 2080
Mattel Children's Fndn Grants, 2130
Mattel International Grants, 2131
Milagro Fndn Grants, 2198
New York Life Fndn Grants, 2304
Newman's Own Inc Grants, 2306
NLM Understanding and Promoting Health Literacy Research Grants, 2827
Nordson Corp Fndn Grants, 2851
Northern Trust Company Charitable Trust and Corp Giving Program, 2865
OceanFirst Fndn Grants, 2933
PacifiCare Fndn Grants, 2981
Paul and Mary Haas Fndn Contributions and Student Scholarships, 2997
Pfizer Fndn Health Literacy Grants, 3026
Rajiv Gandhi Fndn Grants, 3104
Reynolds and Reynolds Associate Fndn Grants, 3152
RGK Fndn Grants, 3153
Richard and Rhoda Goldman Fund Grants, 3158
Samuel S. Johnson Fndn Grants, 3251
San Antonio Area Fndn Grants, 3254
Self Fndn Grants, 3277
Southbury Comm Trust Fund, 3350
Starr Fndn Grants, 3377
U.S. Department of Education 21st Century Comm Learning Centers, 3445
Verizon Fndn Maryland Grants, 3487
Verizon Fndn New York Grants, 3488
Verizon Fndn Northeast Region Grants, 3489
Verizon Fndn Pennsylvania Grants, 3490
Verizon Fndn Vermont Grants, 3491
Verizon Fndn Virginia Grants, 3492
Vulcan Materials Company Fndn Grants, 3504
Wachovia Fndn Grants, 3511
Wal-Mart Fndn Comm Grants, 3513
Western Union Fndn Grants, 3529
Wilson-Wood Fndn Grants, 3542

Literary Arts
Marion Park Deaver and Harry Gilbert Deaver Fndn Grants, 2110
Society for the Arts in Healthcare Consulting Grants, 3326
Strowd Roses Grants, 3388

Literature
ADA Fndn Dental Literature Grants, 229
Albert and Margaret Alkek Fndn Grants, 326
Canada-U.S. Fulbright New Century Scholars Grants, 846
Canada-U.S. Fulbright Senior Specialists Grants, 847
Fulbright Alumni Initiatives Awards Grants, 1566
Fulbright Distinguished Chairs Grants, 1567
Fulbright New Century Scholars Grants, 1570
Fulbright Specialists Grants, 1571
Fulbright Traditional Scholar Program in Europe and Eurasia, 1572
Fulbright Traditional Scholar Program in Sub-Saharan Africa, 1573
Fulbright Traditional Scholar Program in the East Asia/Pacific Region, 1574
Fulbright Traditional Scholar Program in the Near East and North Africa Region, 1575
Fulbright Traditional Scholar Program in the South and Central Asia Region, 1576
Fulbright Traditional Scholar Program in the Western Hemisphere, 1577
Heineman Fndn for Research, Education, Charitable and Scientific Purposes, 1735
Hoblitzelle Fndn Grants, 1783
Jeffress Research Grants, 1913
Josiah W. and Bessie H. Kline Fndn Grants, 1967
Larry L. Hillblom Fndn Grants, 2031
McKesson Fndn Grants, 2145
Milagro Fndn Grants, 2198
Northwood University/Alden B. Dow Creativity Center Summer Residency Program, 2871
Paul G. Allen Family Fndn Grants, 3000
Samuel Freeman Charitable Trust Grants, 3249

Liver Diseases and Disorders
Canadian Liver Fndn Grants, 851
CLF Fellowships, 1037
CLF Graduate Studentships, 1038
CLF Operating Grants, 1039
DHHS Priority Health Conditions Studies Initiative, 1273
FDHN Fellowship to Faculty Transition Awards, 1470
FDHN Graduate Student Awards, 1472

FDHN Moti L. & Kamla Rustgi International Travel Awards, 1475
FDHN Research Scholar Awards, 1478
NIAAA Hepatitis C Infection and Alcoholic Liver Disease, 2442
NIAAA Mechanisms of Alcohol-Induced Hepatic Fibrosis Research Grants, 2445
NIDDK Development of Disease Biomarkers Grants, 2549
NIDDK Developmental Biology and Regeneration of the Liver Grants, 2550
NIDDK New Technologies for Liver Disease SBIR, 2570
NIDDK New Technologies for Liver Disease STTR, 2571
NIH Small Business Innovation Research: Animal Models of HCV Infection Research Grants, 2728
NLM New Technologies for Liver Disease Grants, 2823

Local Government
Lynde and Harry Bradley Fndn Grants, 2089
Lynde and Harry Bradley Fndn Prizes: Bradley Prizes, 2090
NIEHS Applied Toxicological Research and Testing Grants, 2595

Local History
Beirne Carter Fndn Grants, 737

Long-Term Care
Blanche and Irving Laurie Fndn Grants, 764
NINR Acute and Chronic Care During Mechanical Ventilation Research Grants, 2788
Prudential Fndn Grants, 3087
Retirement Research Fndn General Grants, 3150
Russell Berrie Fndn Grants, 3201

Lung Disease
NIH Sarcoidosis: Research into the Cause of Multi-Organ Disease and Clinical Strategies for Therapy Grants, 2723

Lupus
Gina Finzi Memorial Student Summer Fellowship, 1615
Lupus Fndn of America Research Grants, 2085
NIAMS High Risk Arthritis and Musculoskeletal and Skin Diseases Research, 2470
NIAMS Specialized Centers of Research in Osteoarthritis and Systemic Lupus Erythematosus, 2479
Partnership for Cures Two Years To Cures Grants, 2992

Lyme Disease
CDC Research, Treatment, and Education Programs on Lyme Disease in the United States Cooperative Agreements, 927

Lymphatic System
LSA Specialized Center of Research Grants, 2077
NHLBI Lymphatic Biology in Health and Disease Grants, 2345
NHLBI Pathogenesis And Treatment of Lymphedema And Lymphatic Diseases Grants, 2362

Lymphoma
ACGT Investigators Grants, 204
Leukemia & Lymphoma Society Research Grants, 2051

Macedonia
OSI European Commission Internships for Young Roma Graduates, 2965

Malaria
United Methodist Church Malaria Control Grants, 3464

Malaysia
OSI Access to Essential Medicines Grants, 2964

Mammalogy
Lalor Fndn Postdoctoral Research Grants, 2021

Managed Care
Bush Fndn Medical Fellowships, 815
CDC Promoting Prevention in Managed Care Cooperative Agreements, 925
CHCF Grants, 979
CMS Research and Demonstration Grants, 1045
Fallon OrNda Comm Health Fund Grants, 1449
NIH Cancer Surveillance Using Health Claims-Based Data System Grants, 2645

Management
Benton Comm Fndn Grants, 743
Blackford County Comm Fndn Grants, 763
Blue River Comm Fndn Grants, 770
Brown County Comm Fndn Grants, 807
CJ Fndn for SIDS Support Services Grants, 1017
Comm Fndn of Bartholomew County Heritage Fund Grants, 1096
Comm Fndn of Bartholomew County James A. Henderson Award for Fund-Raising, 1097
Comm Fndn of Boone County Grants, 1099
Comm Fndn of Greater Fort Wayne: Comm Endowment & Clarke Endowment Fund Grants, 1108
Greater Bridgeport Area Fndn Comm Impact Grants, 1650
HRB Health Services Research Fellowships, 1801
Richard and Helen DeVos Fndn Grants, 3157
Richard King Mellon Fndn Grants, 3161
Takemi Program in International Health Research and Advanced Training Fellowships, 3416
VDH Rescue Squad Assistance Fund Grants, 3484

Management Information Systems
Richard P. Covert Scholarship, 3163

Management Policy/Planning
Comm Fndn of Santa Cruz County Grants, 1122

Management Sciences
AAFCS International Graduate Fellowships, 109
AAFCS National Graduate Fellowships, 110
AAFCS National Undergraduate Scholarships, 111
C.R. Bard Fndn Grants, 825
DaimlerChrysler Corp Fund Grants, 1186
General Motors Fndn Grants Support Program, 1591
Johnson & Johnson Corp Contributions Grants, 1952
Pfizer Fndn Health Literacy Grants, 3026

Manufacturing
Indiana 21st Century Research and Technology Fund Awards, 1850
NSF Chemical, Biochemical, and Biotechnology Systems Research Grants, 2882

Manufacturing Processes
NSF Chemistry Research Experiences for Undergraduates, 2883

Manufacturing Processes (Industrial Engineering)
NSF-NIST Interaction in Chemistry, Materials Research, Molecular Biosciences, Bioengineering, and Chemical Engineering, 2897

Manuscripts/Books/Music Scores
ASHA Advancing Academic-Research Careers Award, 569
H. Schaffer Fndn Grants, 1680

Marijuana
Marijuana Policy Project Grants, 2107
NIDA Drug Abuse Dissertation Research: Epidemiology, Prevention, Treatment, Services, and Women and Gender Differences, 2502
NIDA Medications Development for Cannabis-Related Disorder, 2506

Marine Resources
Coastal Comm Fndn of South Carolina Grants, 1051
Richard and Rhoda Goldman Fund Grants, 3158
Vancouver Fndn Grants and Comm Initiatives Program, 3477

Marine Sciences
Frederick Gardner Cottrell Fndn Grants, 1560
Margaret T. Morris Fndn Grants, 2105
Marine Biological Laboratory Summer Research Fellowships, 2108
ONR Human Performance Division Research Grants, 2948

Marketing
National Dairy Promotion and Research Board Scholarships, 2251
NCI/NIDA Transdisciplinary Tobacco Use Research Centers Grants, 2280

Marketing/Public Relations
Humboldt Area Fndn Technical Assistance Program Grants, 1819

Mass Communication
OSI Indonesia Project Grants, 2967
Tifa Fndn Grants, 3428

Mass Media
American Academy of Nursing Media Awards, 418
Chicago Board of Trade Fndn Grants, 988
Gill Fndn - Gay and Lesbian Fund Grants, 1613
OSI Indonesia Project Grants, 2967
Tifa Fndn Grants, 3428

Mass Spectrometry
Ethical Research Grants and Fellowships, 1431

Massage Therapy
Massage Therapy Fndn Comm Service Grants, 2124
Massage Therapy Fndn Practitioner Case Report Contest, 2125
Massage Therapy Fndn Research Grants, 2126

Materials Acquisition (Books, Tapes, etc.)
Vancouver Fndn Grants and Comm Initiatives Program, 3477

Materials Sciences
Canada Graduate Scholarships and NSERC Postgraduate Scholarships, 845
HHMI-NIBIB Interfaces Initiative Grants, 1764
Millipore/Charles P. Schaufus Parenteral-Processing Technology Research Grant, 2204
NSF Major Research Instrumentation Grants, 2889
NSF-NIST Interaction in Chemistry, Materials Research, Molecular Biosciences, Bioengineering, and Chemical Engineering, 2897
ONR Human Performance Division Research Grants, 2948

Materials, Metals/Alloys
NSF Small Business Innovation Research Grants, 2893

Materials, Processing and Finishing
NSF-NIST Interaction in Chemistry, Materials Research, Molecular Biosciences, Bioengineering, and Chemical Engineering, 2897

Maternal/Child Health
MDBDF Agnes Higgins Award, 2155

Mathematics
Alcatel-Lucent Technologies Corp Contributions Grants, 332
Alfred P. Sloan Fndn Research Fellowships, 353
BWF Career Awards at the Scientific Interface, 819
Canada Graduate Scholarships and NSERC Postgraduate Scholarships, 845

Canada-U.S. Fulbright New Century Scholars Grants, 846
Canada-U.S. Fulbright Senior Specialists Grants, 847
Comm Fndn of Greater Flint Grants, 1107
Duke Energy Fndn Grants, 1339
Ethical Research Grants and Fellowships, 1431
Fluor Fndn Grants, 1517
Fndn for Science and Disability Grant Program for Physically Disabled Students in the Sciences, 1532
Fulbright Alumni Initiatives Awards Grants, 1566
Fulbright Distinguished Chairs Grants, 1567
Fulbright New Century Scholars Grants, 1570
Fulbright Specialists Grants, 1571
Fulbright Traditional Scholar Program in Europe and Eurasia, 1572
Fulbright Traditional Scholar Program in Sub-Saharan Africa, 1573
Fulbright Traditional Scholar Program in the East Asia/Pacific Region, 1574
Fulbright Traditional Scholar Program in the Near East and North Africa Region, 1575
Fulbright Traditional Scholar Program in the South and Central Asia Region, 1576
Fulbright Traditional Scholar Program in the Western Hemisphere, 1577
Gladys Brooks Fndn Grants, 1620
Grand Rapids Comm Fndn Grants, 1647
HHMI-NIBIB Interfaces Initiative Grants, 1764
NHGRI Mentored Research Scientist Development Award, 2315
NIGMS Fellowships in Quantitative Biology, 2610
NIGMS MARC Undergraduate Student Training in Academic Research (U-STAR) Program, 2617
NIGMS Short Courses on Mathematical and Statistical Tools for the Study of Complex Phenotypes and Complex Systems, 2628
NIGMS Short Courses on Mathematical, Statistical, and Computational Tools for Studying Biological Systems, 2629
NIGMS Supplements for the Study of Complex Biological Systems, 2630
NIGMS/NIDCR Evolution of Infectious Diseases Research Grants, 2633
NIH Genetic Susceptibility and Variability of Human Malformations Research Grants, 2669
NIMH Curriculum Development Award in Neuroinformatics Research and Analysis, 2754
NIMH Quantitative Approaches to the Analysis of Complex Biological Systems, 2767
NIMH Short Courses on Mathematical and Statistical Tools for the Study of Complex Phenotypes and Complex Systems, 2770
North Carolina GlaxoSmithKline Fndn Grants, 2860
NSF Alan T. Waterman Award, 2874
Simone and Cino del Duca Grand Prix Awards, 3288
University of California President's Postdoctoral Fellowships, 3469

Mathematics Education
3M Fndn Grants, 11
Affymetrix Corp Contributions Grants, 258
Alcoa Fndn Grants, 334
Alfred P. Sloan Fndn History of Science and Technology Grants, 352
AMD Corp Contributions Grants, 411
American Electric Power Grants, 434
ARCO Fndn Education Grants, 526
Baptist Comm Ministries Grants, 691
Chiron Fndn Comm Grants, 1004
Comm Fndn of Grant County Scholarships, 1105
Dell Fndn Healthy Communities, Literate Communities, and Connected Communities Grants, 1217
Dominion Educational Partnership Grant, 1308
Emily Davie and Joseph S. Kornfeld Fndn Grants, 1414
Ford Motor Company Fund Grants, 1522
Goodrich Corp Fndn Grants, 1638
Houston Endowment Grants, 1797
Joyce Fndn Grants, 1969
Lockheed Martin Philanthropic Grants, 2062
MfA Newton Fellowships, 2182
NIGMS Minority Access to Research Careers Ancillary Training Activities Grants, 2619
Oracle Corp Contributions Grants, 2951
Progress Energy Fndn Grants, 3084
Rathmann Family Fndn Grants, 3109
RGK Fndn Grants, 3153
Rockwell Collins Charitable Contributions, 3182
Rohm and Haas Company Grants, 3185
Tellabs Fndn Grants, 3418
United Technologies Corp Grants, 3466
Westinghouse Charitable Giving Grants, 3530

Mathematics, Applied
Alfred P. Sloan Fndn Research Fellowships, 353
Canada Graduate Scholarships and NSERC Postgraduate Scholarships, 845
NIGMS Predoctoral Training in Bioinformatics and Computation Biology Grants, 2625

Mechanical Engineering
Lubrizol Fndn Grants, 2080

Media
BCBS of Massachusetts Health Coverage Fellowships, 710
New York University Steinhardt School of Education Fellowships, 2305

Media Arts
Dept of Ed Special Education-National Activities-Technology and Media Services for Individuals with Disabilities, 1234
Grand Rapids Area Comm Fndn Grants, 1645
Grand Rapids Area Comm Fndn Nashwauk Area Endowment Fund Grants, 1646
Pittsburgh Fndn Comm Fund Grants, 3054
Ruth Mott Fndn Grants, 3204

Medical Pharmacy
Schering-Plough Fndn Health Grants, 3270

Medical Devices Engineering
ORISE Postgraduate Research Program at the Center for Devices and Radiological Health, 2962

Medical Education
AACAP Child and Adolescent Psychiatry Teaching Scholarships, 31
AACAP Jeanne Spurlock Research Fellowship in Substance Abuse and Addiction for Minority Medical Students, 40
AACAP Summer Medical Student Fellowships, 53
AAFP Fndn Health Literacy State Grants, 112
AAFP Fndn Pfizer Teacher Development Awards, 114
AAFP Fndn Wyeth Immunization Awards, 115
AAFP Research Stimulation Grants, 116
AAMC Abraham Flexner Award, 133
AAMC Alpha Omega Alpha Robert J. Glaser Distinguished Teacher Awards, 134
AAMC Caring for Comm Grants, 136
AAMC Herbert W. Nickens Award, 138
AAMC Herbert W. Nickens Faculty Fellowship, 139
AAMC Herbert W. Nickens Medical Student Scholarships, 140
AAMC Humanism in Medicine Award, 141
AAO-HNS Medical Student Research Prize, 144
AAP Resident Research Grants, 168
ACS Cancer Control Career Development Awards for Primary Care Physicians, 209
ACS Doctoral Degree Scholarships in Cancer Nursing, 211
ACS Doctoral Training Grants in Oncology Social Work, 213
ACS Graduate Scholarships in Cancer Nursing Practice, 214
ACS Physician Training Awards in Preventive Medicine, 218
Advocate HealthCare Post Graduate Administrative Fellowship, 241
Allyn Fndn Grants, 365
AMA Fndn Arthur N. Wilson, MD, Scholarship, 386
AMA Fndn Joan F. Giambalvo Memorial Scholarships, 392
AMA Fndn Physicians of Tomorrow Scholarships, 396
American College of Surgeons Co-Sponsored K08/K23 NIH Supplement Awards, 424
American College of Surgeons Health Policy Scholarships, 427
American College of Surgeons Health Policy Scholarships for General Surgeons, 428
American College of Surgeons International Guest Scholarships, 429
American College of Surgeons Resident Research Scholarships, 432
APA Young Investigator Grant Program, 502
APF Helping Hands Grants, 507
Arkell Hall Fndn Grants, 534
ASCO International Development and Education Awards, 554
Australian Academy of Science Grants, 670
AVDF Health Care Grants, 673
Booth-Bricker Fund Grants, 780
Bright Family Fndn Grants, 793
Bush Fndn Medical Fellowships, 815
BWF Ad Hoc Grants, 818
BWF Career Awards for Medical Scientists, 820
C.R. Bard Fndn Grants, 825
California Wellness Fndn Work and Health Grants, 834
Canadian Patient Safety Institute Patient Safety Studentships, 854
Canadian Patient Safety Institute Research Grants, 855
Cancer Research UK Grants, 859
Carl J. Herzog Fndn Grants, 872
Catherine Holmes Wilkins Fndn Grants, 889
Center for Science in the Public Interest Internships, 935
Clarian Health Critical / Progressive Care Internships, 1023
Clarian Health Multi-Specialty Internships, 1024
Clarian Health OR Internships, 1025
Clarian Health Student Nurse Extern Scholarships, 1027
CLF Operating Grants, 1039
Clowes ACS/AAST/NIGMS Jointly Sponsored Mentored Clinical Scientist Development Award, 1041
CMAP Physician Advocacy Fellowship, 1043
Cowles Charitable Trust Grants, 1155
Daphne Seybolt Culpeper Memorial Fndn Grants, 1201
Deafness Research Fndn Research Grants, 1208
DeBakey Medical Fndn Fellowships and Scholarships, 1212
Denton A. Cooley Fndn Grants, 1225
DHHS Health Careers Opportunity Grants, 1253
DHHS Health Education and Training Centers Project Grants, 1256
DHHS Health Professions Preparatory Scholarship Program for Indians, 1257
DHHS Health Professions Scholarship Program, 1258
DHHS National Health Service Corps Loan Repayment Awards, 1265
DHHS Native American Health Service Loan Repayment Awards, 1267
DHHS Preventive Medicine, 1271
DHHS Residency Training in Family Practice, General Internal Medicine, or General Pediatrics Grants, 1278
Doris Duke Charitable Fndn Clinical Research Fellowships for Medical Students, 1315
Dr. Bob and Jean Smith Fndn Grants, 1325
Dr. Scholl Fndn Grants, 1329
Drs. Bruce and Lee Fndn Grants, 1333
Duke University Adult Cardiothoracic Anesthesia and Critical Care Medicine Fellowships, 1340
Duke University Ambulatory and Regional Anesthesia Fellowships, 1341

Duke University Clinical Cardiac Electrophysiology Fellowships, 1342
Duke University Hyperbaric Center Fellowships, 1343
Duke University Interventional Cardiology Fellowships, 1344
Duke University Obstetric Anesthesia Fellowships, 1345
Duke University Pain Management Fellowships, 1346
Duke University Pediatric Anesthesiology Fellowship, 1347
EF Health Sciences Student Fellowships, 1380
Effie and Wofford Cain Fndn Grants, 1385
Elisabeth Severance Prentiss Fndn Grants, 1392
Flinn Fndn Grants Programs, 1511
FMC Fndn Grants, 1518
Fndn for Physical Therapy Mary McMillan Doctoral Scholarships, 1529
Fndn for Physical Therapy Research Grants, 1530
Fndn for Science and Disability Grant Program for Physically Disabled Students in the Sciences, 1532
Goldman Philanthropic Partnerships Program, 1635
Good Samaritan Fndn Inc Grants, 1636
Harry A. and Margaret D. Towsley Fndn Grants, 1701
Hawaii Comm Fndn Health Education and Research Grants, 1716
Health Fndn of Greater Indianapolis Grants, 1725
Healthcare Fndn of New Jersey Grants, 1729
Herman Goldman Fndn Grants, 1753
HHMI Biomedical Research Grants for International Scientists in Canada and Latin America, 1756
HHMI Biomedical Research Grants for International Scientists in the Baltics, Central and Eastern Europe, Russia, and Ukraine, 1757
HHMI Biomedical Research Grants for International Scientists: Infectious Diseases and Parasitology, 1758
HHMI Med into Grad Initiative Grants, 1761
HHMI Physician-Scientist Early Career Award, 1762
HHMI Research Training Fellowships, 1763
HHMI-NIH Cloister Research Scholars Program, 1765
HHS Children's Hospitals Graduate Medical Education Payment Program, 1767
HRB Clinical Research Training Fellowships, 1800
HRSA Geriatric Education Centers, 1805
HRSA Health Professions Scholarships for Disadvantaged Students, 1807
HRSA Nurse Anesthetist Traineeships Program, 1808
HRSA Physician Assistant Training, 1810
Institute of Human Values in Health Care Interdisciplinary Fellowships, 1857
International Fellowships in Medical Education, 1861
J.W. Kieckhefer Fndn Grants, 1878
James H. Cummings Fndn Grants, 1888
James M. Collins Fndn Grants, 1891
Jewish Fndn for Education of Women Scholarships for Emigres in the Health Professions, 1922
John I. Smith Charities Grants, 1935
John S. Dunn Research Fndn Grants and Chairs, 1945
Johnson F. Hammond Memorial Scholarship, 1956
Joseph Collins Fndn Grants, 1959
Josiah Macy Jr. Fndn Grants, 1966
Kaiser Permanente Cares for Communities Grants, 1978
KFC Nephrology and Urology Scholarships, 1999
Lester Ray Fleming Scholarships, 2048
Lettie Pate Whitehead Fndn Grants, 2049
Lubbock Area Fndn Grants, 2079
Mead Johnson Nutritionals Medical Education Grants, 2158
Mead Johnson Nutritionals Scholarships, 2159
Measey Fndn Medical Education Grants, 2162
Medical/Nursing Education, Research, and Health Care Exchanges with Taiwan, 2165
MHRC Graduate Studentships, 2185
NBME Stemmler Medical Education Research Fund Grants, 2263
New York Life Fndn Grants, 2304
NHLBI Short-Term Research Education to Increase Diversity in Health-Related Research, 2383
NIGMS Institutional Research and Academic Career Development Award, 2614
NIH Complementary and Alternative Medicine Postdoctoral Training Grants, 2652
NLM Internet Connection for Medical Institutions Grants, 2820
NMF Aura E. Severinghaus Award, 2828
NMF Franklin C. McLean Award, 2829
NMF General Electric Medical Scholars Fellowships, 2830
NMF Henry G. Halladay Awards, 2831
NMF Hugh J. Andersen Memorial Scholarship, 2832
NMF Irving Graef Memorial Scholarship, 2833
NMF Mary Ball Carrera Scholarship, 2834
NMF Metropolitan Life Fndn Awards Program for Academic Excellence in Medicine, 2835
NMF National Medical Association Awards for Medical Journalism, 2836
NMF National Medical Association Emerging Scholar Awards, 2837
NMF National Medical Association Patti LaBelle Award, 2838
NMF Need-Based Scholarships, 2839
NMF Ralph W. Ellison Prize, 2840
NMF William and Charlotte Cadbury Award, 2841
Nuffield Fndn Africa Grants, 2898
Nuffield Fndn Law and Society Grants, 2900
Nuffield Fndn Small Grants, 2903
NYAM David E. Rogers Fellowships, 2911
Ohio Learning Network Grants, 2940
PAHO/WHO Fellowships, 2984
Partnership for Cures Charles E. Culpeper Scholarships in Medical Science, 2991
Paso del Norte Health Fndn Grants, 2995
Pfizer/AAFP Fndn Visiting Professorship Program in Family Medicine, 3027
PhRMA Fndn Informatics Pre Doctoral Fellowships, 3037
Potts Memorial Fndn Grants, 3072
Presbyterian Health Fndn Bridge, Seed and Equipment Grants, 3075
Rathmann Family Fndn Grants, 3109
RCPSC Canadian Research Awards for Specialty Residents (Medicine, Surgery), 3113
RCPSC Duncan Graham Award, 3115
RCPSC Faculty Development Grants, 3117
RCPSC International Traveling Fellowship, 3118
RCPSC Janes Visiting Professorship in Surgery, 3120
RCPSC Kilborn Memorial Visiting Professorship, 3121
RCPSC McLaughlin-Gallie Visiting Professorship, 3123
RCPSC Medical Education Research Grants, 3124
RCPSC Medical Education Traveling Fellowships, 3125
RCPSC National Specialty Society Annual Meeting Grants, 3126
RCPSC Royal College Fellowship for Studies in Medical Education, 3127
RCPSC Royal College Medal Award in Medicine, 3128
RCPSC Royal College Medal Award in Surgery, 3129
RCPSC Royal College Visiting Professorships in Medical Research, 3130
RCPSC Traineeships, 3132
RCPSC Wightman Visiting Professorship in Medicine, 3134
RCPSC/AMS CanMEDs Research and Development Grants, 3135
RCPSC/AMS Donald Richards Wilson Award, 3136
Regenstrief Geriatrics Fellowship, 3143
Regenstrief General Internal Medicine - General Pediatrics Research Fellowship Program, 3144
Regenstrief Master Of Science In Clinical Research/CITE Program, 3145
Rice Fndn Grants, 3155
Ruth Eleanor Bamberger and John Ernest Bamberger Memorial Fndn Grants, 3202
RWJF Clinical Scholars Grants, 3207
RWJF Generalist Physician Faculty Scholars, 3212
RWJF Harold Amos Medical Faculty Development Scholars, 3213
RWJF Summer Medical and Dental Education Program, 3231
Saint Luke's Health Initiatives Grants, 3240
Samueli Fndn Health Grants, 3252
San Antonio Area Fndn Grants, 3254
Schering-Plough Fndn Health Grants, 3270
SNM Student Fellowship Awards, 3306
Society for Imaging Informatics in Medicine Emeritus Mentor Grants, 3320
Society for Imaging Informatics in Medicine Micro Grants, 3321
Society for Imaging Informatics in Medicine Research Grants, 3322
Society for Imaging Informatics in Medicine Small Grant for Product Support Development, 3323
Society for Imaging Informatics in Medicine Small Training Grants, 3324
Special Olympics Health Professions Student Grants, 3355
Starr Fndn Grants, 3377
Vancouver Fndn Public Health Bursary Package, 3478
VDH Emergency Medical Services Training Fund, 3483
VDH Rescue Squad Assistance Fund Grants, 3484
Viets Medical Student Myasthenia Gravis Research Fellowships, 3496
Virginia Tuition Assistance Grant Program, 3501

Medical Ethics

AAMC Herbert W. Nickens Award, 138
Deland Fellowships in Health Care and Society, 1214
Greenwall Fndn Bioethics Grants, 1665
Hastings Center International Visiting Scholars Program, 1715
HHMI Grants and Fellowships Programs, 1759
NIH Individual Postdoctoral Fellowships in Genomics and Related ELSI Topics, 2678
NIH Studies of Ethical, Legal, and Social Implications of Research into Human Genetic Variation Grants, 2731
NIMH Informed Consent in Research Grants, 2758
NINR Acute and Chronic Care During Mechanical Ventilation Research Grants, 2788
NINR Opportunities in Genetics and Nursing Research Grants, 2801
Pfizer Fndn Health Literacy Grants, 3026
RCPSC KJR Wightman Award for Scholarship in Ethics, 3122
Regenstrief Geriatrics Fellowship, 3143
RSC Abbyann D. Lynch Medal in Bioethics, 3195
Sir Halley Stewart Trust Grants, 3293

Medical Informatics

AHIMA Dissertation Assistance Grants, 300
AHIMA Faculty Development Stipends, 301
AHIMA Grant-In-Aid Research Grants, 302
Fannie E. Rippel Fndn Grants, 1452
Fndn for Seacoast Health Grants, 1533
Healthcare Fndn for Orange County Grants, 1728
MLA Ida and George Eliot Prize, 2209
NEI Ruth L. Kirschstein National Research Service Award Short-Term Institutional Research Training Grants, 2297
NHGRI Mentored Research Scientist Development Award, 2315
NIGMS Predoctoral Training in Bioinformatics and Computation Biology Grants, 2625
NIH Human Brain Project (Neuroinformatics) Phase I & II, 2672
NIMH Curriculum Development Award in Neuroinformatics Research and Analysis, 2754
NIMH Short Courses in Neuroinformatics, 2769
NLM Exploratory/Developmental Grants, 2816
NLM Grants for Scholarly Works in Biomedicine and Health, 2818
NLM Internet Connection for Medical Institutions Grants, 2820
NLM Research Project Grants, 2825

NSF Postdoctoral Research Fellowships in Biology, 2891
ORISE Postgraduate Research Participation at the Agency for Toxic Substances and Disease Registry, 2960
PhRMA Fndn Informatics Sabbatical Fellowships, 3035
PhRMA Fndn Informatics Postdoctoral Fellowships, 3036
PhRMA Fndn Informatics Pre Doctoral Fellowships, 3037
PhRMA Fndn Informatics Research Starter Grants, 3038
PhRMA Fndn Pharmacology/Toxicology Post Doctoral Fellowships, 3044
PhRMA Fndn Pharmacology/Toxicology Sabbatical Fellowships, 3047
Regenstrief Geriatrics Fellowship, 3143
Regenstrief General Internal Medicine - General Pediatrics Research Fellowship Program, 3144
Regenstrief Master Of Science In Clinical Research/ CITE Program, 3145
Richard P. Covert Scholarship, 3163
Society for Imaging Informatics in Medicine Emeritus Mentor Grants, 3320
Society for Imaging Informatics in Medicine Micro Grants, 3321
Society for Imaging Informatics in Medicine Research Grants, 3322
Society for Imaging Informatics in Medicine Small Grant for Product Support Development, 3323
Society for Imaging Informatics in Medicine Small Training Grants, 3324

Medical Physics
A Social Corp Grants, 15
NIGMS Support of Competitive Research Pilot Project Awards, 2631
NIGMS Support of Competitive Research Research Advancement Awards, 2632

Medical Programs
AACAP Child and Adolescent Psychiatry Teaching Scholarships, 31
AAP Comm Access To Child Health Implementation Grants, 158
AAP Legislative Conference Scholarships, 163
Addison H. Gibson Fndn Medical Grants, 233
Advocate HealthCare Post Graduate Administrative Fellowship, 241
American Medical Association Awards, 440
Baptist-Trinity Lutheran Legacy Fndn Grants, 692
Baton Rouge Area Fndn Grants, 702
Blowitz-Ridgeway Fndn Early Childhood Development Research Award, 766
Bristol-Myers Squibb Fndn Product Donations Grants, 799
BWF Ad Hoc Grants, 818
BWF Career Awards for Medical Scientists, 820
Carroll County Comm Fndn Grants, 885
CDC Evaluation of the Use of Rapid Testing For Influenza in Outpatient Medical Settings, 910
Comm Fndn AIDS Endowment Awards, 1088
ConocoPhillips Fndn Grants, 1144
Cultural Society of Filipino Americans Grants, 1173
Denton A. Cooley Fndn Grants, 1225
DHHS Emergency Medical Services for Children Program, 1249
Edna G. Kynett Memorial Fndn Grants, 1370
George S. and Dolores Dore Eccles Fndn Grants, 1602
Goldman Philanthropic Partnerships Program, 1635
Huntington Beach Police Officers Fndn Grants, 1821
Independence Blue Cross Charitable Medical Care Grants, 1846
Independence Blue Cross Nursing Internships, 1848
James M. Collins Fndn Grants, 1891
John Edward Fowler Memorial Fndn Grants, 1930
Marcia and Otto Koehler Fndn Grants, 2103
Mead Johnson Nutritionals Medical Education Grants, 2158
Miami County Comm Fndn Operation Round Up Grants, 2188
Nelda C. and H.J. Lutcher Stark Fndn Grants, 2301
NIGMS Support of Competitive Research Pilot Project Awards, 2631
NIGMS Support of Competitive Research Research Advancement Awards, 2632
Pittsburgh Fndn Medical Research Grants, 3055
Posey Comm Fndn Grants, 3068
Rayonier Fndn Grants, 3111
RCPSC Events, Speakers and Visiting Professors Grants, 3116
RCPSC National Specialty Society Annual Meeting Grants, 3126
RCPSC Royal College Medal Award in Medicine, 3128
RCPSC Royal College Visiting Professorships in Medical Research, 3130
RCPSC Traineeships, 3132
RCPSC Wightman Visiting Professorship in Medicine, 3134
RCPSC/AMS CanMEDs Research and Development Grants, 3135
Regenstrief Geriatrics Fellowship, 3143
Robert and Joan Dircks Fndn Grants, 3167
Robert B McMillen Fndn Grants, 3169
RWJF Generalist Physician Faculty Scholars, 3212
RWJF Harold Amos Medical Faculty Development Scholars, 3213
Samueli Fndn Health Grants, 3252
Sarasota Memorial Healthcare Fndn Grants, 3264
Seabury Fndn Grants, 3274
SOCFOC Catholic Ministries Grants, 3317
SRC Medical Research Grants, 3362
St. Joseph Comm Health Fndn Burn Care and Prevention Grants, 3367
St. Joseph Comm Health Fndn Improving Healthcare Access Grants, 3368
STTI/ATI Educational Assessment Nursing Research Grants, 3397
Vancouver Fndn Grants and Comm Initiatives Program, 3477
Volkswagen of America Corp Contributions Grants, 3503

Medical Research
Australian Academy of Science Grants, 670
Blowitz-Ridgeway Fndn Early Childhood Development Research Award, 766
Carlos and Marguerite Mason Trust Grants, 875
Hirtzel Memorial Fndn Grants, 1781

Medical Sciences
ASHFndn New Century Scholars Program Doctoral Scholarships, 580
ASHFndn New Century Scholars Research Grant, 581
ASHFndn Research Grant for New Investigators, 582

Medical Technology
A Social Corp Grants, 15
Deland Fellowships in Health Care and Society, 1214
DHHS Emergency Medical Services for Children Program, 1249
DHHS Rural Telemedicine Grants, 1279
DOA Distance Learning and Telemedicine Grant Program, 1288
DOE Medical Applications and Measurement Science Grants, 1301
Highmark Physician eHealth Collaborative Grants, 1771
Independence Blue Cross Charitable Medical Care Grants, 1846
Mead Johnson Nutritionals Medical Education Grants, 2158
NCCAM Translational Tools for Clinical Studies of CAM Interventions Grants, 2267
NCI Academic-Industrial Partnerships for Development and Validation of In Vivo Imaging Systems and Methods for Cancer Investigations, 2268
NCI Application and Use of Transformative Emerging Technologies in Cancer Research, 2269
NHLBI Improving Heart Failure Disease Management Grants, 2338
NIGMS Support of Competitive Research Pilot Project Awards, 2631
NIGMS Support of Competitive Research Research Advancement Awards, 2632
NIH Bioengineering Nanotechnology Initiative, 2640
NIH Individual Postdoctoral Fellowships in Genomics and Related ELSI Topics, 2678
NLM Manufacturing Processes of Medical, Dental, and Biological Technologies Grants, 2822
RCPSC/AMS CanMEDs Research and Development Grants, 3135
Regenstrief General Internal Medicine - General Pediatrics Research Fellowship Program, 3144
Regenstrief Master Of Science In Clinical Research/ CITE Program, 3145
Samueli Fndn Health Grants, 3252
STTI Joan K. Stout RN Research Grants, 3392
Topeka Comm Fndn Kansas Blood Services Scholarships, 3429

Medical/Diagnostics Imaging
A Social Corp Grants, 15
NCCAM Translational Tools for Clinical Studies of CAM Interventions Grants, 2267
NCI/NIDA Transdisciplinary Tobacco Use Research Centers Grants, 2280
NIH New Directions in Pain Research Grants, 2698
NINDS Cerebral Radiobiology and Neuroimaging of Brain Tumors Research Grants, 2778
Regenstrief General Internal Medicine - General Pediatrics Research Fellowship Program, 3144
Samueli Fndn Health Grants, 3252
SNM Molecular Imaging Research Grant For Junior Medical Faculty, 3301
SNM Postdoctoral Molecular Imaging Scholar Grants, 3305

Medicinal Chemistry
Alfred Burger Award in Medicinal Chemistry, 351
Beckman Scholars Grants, 734
E.B. Hershberg Award for Important Discoveries in Medicinally Active Substances, 1358

Medicine
Ahmanson Fndn Grants, 303
Award in Separations Science and Technology, 677
Blowitz-Ridgeway Fndn Early Childhood Development Research Award, 766
Elisabeth Severance Prentiss Fndn Grants, 1392
HHMI Biomedical Research Grants for International Scientists in Canada and Latin America, 1756
HHMI Biomedical Research Grants for International Scientists in the Baltics, Central and Eastern Europe, Russia, and Ukraine, 1757
HHMI Biomedical Research Grants for International Scientists: Infectious Diseases and Parasitology, 1758
HHMI Med into Grad Initiative Grants, 1761
JELD-WEN Fndn Grants, 1914
OSI Access to Essential Medicines Grants, 2964
Pfizer Fndn Grants, 3025

Medicine, History of
AIHP Sonnedecker Visiting Scholar Grants, 317
AIHP Thesis Support Grants, 318
Lillian Sholtis Brunner Summer Fellowships for Historical Research in Nursing, 2057
NLM Grants for Scholarly Works in Biomedicine and Health, 2818
NYAM Student Essay Grants, 2917
RSC Jason A. Hannah Medal, 3196

Medicine, Internal
AAHPM Hospice and Palliative Medicine Fellowships, 132
ACS Cancer Control Career Development Awards for Primary Care Physicians, 209

Alex Brown and Sons Charitable Fndn Grants, 337
American Philosophical Society Daland Fellowships in Clinical Investigation, 441
ARS Fndn Grants, 538
Bonfils-Stanton Fndn Grants, 779
CFF First- and Second-Year Clinical Fellowships, 943
CFF Leroy Matthews Physician-Scientist Awards, 944
CMAP Physician Advocacy Fellowship, 1043
DHHS Geriatric Training for Physicians and Dentists Grants, 1250
DHHS Residency Training in Family Practice, General Internal Medicine, or General Pediatrics Grants, 1278
EF Research and Training Fellowships for Clinicians, 1384
Fellowships in Infectious Diseases, 1485
Hartford Aging and Health Program Awards, 1709
NCCAM Translational Tools for Clinical Studies of CAM Interventions Grants, 2267
NIA Diversity in Medication Use and Outcomes in Aging Populations Grants, 2403
RCPSC Canadian Research Awards for Specialty Residents (Medicine, Surgery), 3113
RCPSC Royal College Medal Award in Medicine, 3128
Regenstrief Geriatrics Fellowship, 3143
Regenstrief General Internal Medicine - General Pediatrics Research Fellowship Program, 3144

Medicine, Palliative
RCPSC Balfour M. Mount Visiting Professorship in Palliative Medicine, 3112

Membrane Structure/Function
NIH Structural Biology of Membrane Proteins Grants, 2730

Membranes
NIGMS Molecular Pharmacology of Anesthetic Action Research Grants, 2621
NSF Cell Systems Cluster Grants, 2881

Men
Charles Delmar Fndn Grants, 963
NIAAA Hepatitis C Infection and Alcoholic Liver Disease, 2442
NIH New Directions in Pain Research Grants, 2698
Prudential Fndn Grants, 3087

Menopause
AFAR Research Grants, 257

Mental Disorders
AACAP Rieger Service Program Award for Excellence, 49
AACAP Sidney Berman Award for the School-Based Study and Intervention for Learning Disorders and Mental Ilness, 51
Able To Serve Grants, 185
Adolph Coors Fndn Grants, 238
Alexander and Margaret Stewart Trust Grants, 340
Annunziata Sanguinetti Fndn Grants, 481
APF Alexander Gralnick, MD, Award for Research in Schizophrenia, 503
APF Awards for Advancing Minority Mental Health, 504
APF Call for Proposals, 505
APF Disaster Recovery Fund for Psychiatrists, 506
APF James H. Scully Jr., M.D., Educational Fund Grants, 508
APF Jeanne Spurlock Congressional Fellowships, 509
APF Typical or Troubled School Mental Health Education Grants, 510
Auburn Fndn Grants, 664
Catherine Holmes Wilkins Fndn Grants, 889
Collins Fndn Grants, 1058
Comm Fndn for Southern Arizona Grants, 1095
Dammann Fund Grants, 1192
Danellie Fndn Grants, 1198
Della Martin Fndn Grants, 1219
Eli Lilly & Company Welcome Back Awards, 1391
Erie Comm Fndn Grants, 1427
Eva L. and Joseph M. Bruening Fndn Grants, 1436
Fairlawn Fndn Grants, 1447
FIC International Cooperative Biodiversity Groups Grants, 1487
FIC International Research Scientist Development Award, 1491
Health Fndn of Greater Cincinnati Grants, 1724
Hogg Fndn for Mental Health Grants, 1784
Howe Fndn of North Carolina Grants, 1799
James H. Cummings Fndn Grants, 1888
John W. Alden Trust Grants, 1947
Leonard and Helen R. Stulman Charitable Fndn Grants, 2044
Lincoln Financial Group Fndn Grants, 2058
Margoes Fndn Grants, 2106
NARSAD Distinguished Investigator Award, 2246
NARSAD Independent Investigator Award, 2247
NFX Patient-Oriented Research Grants, 2313
NFX Summer Research Fellowships, 2314
NIEHS Small Business Innovation Research Grants, 2605
NIH Exploratory/Development Grants for Mental Health Intervention Research, 2665
NIH Genetics of Neurobehavioral Disorders in Existing Samples Grants, 2670
NIH Mechanisms Underlying Individual Variations in Drug Responses, 2685
NIMH Collaborative R01s for Clinical Studies of Mental Disorders, 2752
NIMH Early Identification and Treatment of Mental Disorders in Children and Adolescents Grants, 2756
NIMH HIV/AIDS, Severe Mental Illness, and Homelessness Research Grants, 2757
NIMH Interventions Infrastructure Program Research Grants, 2760
NIMH National Research Service Awards—Individual, 2764
NIMH Pilot Effectiveness Trials for Mental Disorders Grants, 2766
NIMH Silvio O. Conte Centers for Neuroscience Research Grants, 2771
Nina Mason Pulliam Charitable Trust Grants, 2776
NNEDVF/Altria Doors of Hope Program, 2847
NYCT Mental Health and Mental Retardation Grants, 2927
Obsessive-Compulsive Fndn Research Awards, 2931
Peter and Elizabeth C. Tower Fndn Comm Grants, 3018
Robert and Joan Dircks Fndn Grants, 3167
Rollin M. Gerstacker Fndn Grants, 3186
Rosalynn Carter Institute John and Betty Pope Fellowships, 3189
SAMHSA Campus Suicide Prevention Grants, 3244
SAMHSA Conference Grants, 3246
Simple Advise Education Center Grants, 3289
Strowd Roses Grants, 3388
Union County Comm Fndn Grants, 3461
Vancouver Sun Children's Fund Grants, 3479

Mental Health
AACAP Sidney Berman Award for the School-Based Study and Intervention for Learning Disorders and Mental Ilness, 51
Abbott Fund Science and Medical Innovation Grants, 179
Able Trust Vocational Rehabilitation Grants for Individuals, 186
Advancing Colorado's Mental Health Care Project Grants, 240
Allen P. and Josephine B. Green Fndn Grants, 361
Alliance Healthcare Fndn Grants, 362
American Sociological Association Minority Fellowships, 458
Andersen Fndn Grants, 471
AON Fndn Grants, 491
APF Alexander Gralnick, MD, Award for Research in Schizophrenia, 503
APF Awards for Advancing Minority Mental Health, 504
APF Call for Proposals, 505
APF Disaster Recovery Fund for Psychiatrists, 506
APF Helping Hands Grants, 507
APF James H. Scully Jr., M.D., Educational Fund Grants, 508
APF Jeanne Spurlock Congressional Fellowships, 509
APF Typical or Troubled School Mental Health Education Grants, 510
Arizona Diamondbacks Charities Grants, 530
ASA Metlife Fndn MindAlert Awards, 545
Barr Fund Grants, 697
Baxter International Fndn Grants, 705
BCBS of Massachusetts Fndn Grants, 709
Blackford County Comm Fndn Grants, 763
Blowitz-Ridgeway Fndn Early Childhood Development Research Award, 766
Bodenwein Public Benevolent Fndn Grants, 775
Boyd Gaming Corp Contributions Program, 788
Brookdale Fndn National Group Respite and Early Memory Loss Grants, 806
Burton G. Bettingen Grants, 813
Bush Fndn Health & Human Services Grants, 814
California Endowment CommunitiesFirst Grants, 833
Callaway Golf Company Fndn Grants, 836
Campbell Hoffman Fndn Grants, 840
Cass County Comm Fndn Grants, 887
Chicago Board of Trade Fndn Grants, 988
Children Affected by AIDS Fndn Domestic Grants, 995
Colorado Springs Comm Trust Fund Grants, 1061
Comm Fndn for Southeastern Michigan Grants, 1094
Comm Fndn of Broward Grants, 1100
Comm Fndn of Grant County Grants, 1104
Comm Fndn Of Greater Lafayette Grants, 1110
Comprehensive Health Education Fndn Grants, 1139
Connecticut Comm Fndn Grants, 1141
Connecticut Health Fndn Health Initiative Grants, 1142
Cornerstone Fndn of Northeastern Wisconsin Grants, 1152
D. W. McMillan Fndn Grants, 1180
Dammann Fund Grants, 1192
Daniels Fund Grants, 1200
DHHS Adolescent Family Life Demonstration Projects, 1243
DHHS Comprehensive Comm Mental Health Services Grants for Children with Serious Emotional Disturbances, 1247
DOJ Mental Health and Juvenile Justice, 1304
Dolan Fndn Grants, 1306
Duchossois Family Fndn Grants, 1337
eBay Fndn Comm Grants, 1363
Edwards Memorial Trust Grants, 1375
Edwin W. and Catherine M. Davis Fndn Grants, 1377
EF Behavioral Sciences Student Fellowships, 1379
Eisner Fndn Grants, 1387
Eli Lilly & Company Welcome Back Awards, 1391
Eugene and Agnes E. Meyer Fndn Grants, 1432
Evjue Fndn Grants, 1439
Fairlawn Fndn Grants, 1447
FAR Fund, 1453
Faye McBeath Fndn Grants, 1456
Florida BRAIVE Fund of Dade Comm Fndn, 1512
Florida BRAIVE Fund of Gulf Coast Comm Fndn of Venice, 1513
Florida BRAIVE Fund of The Comm Fndn in Jacksonville, 1514
Fndn for a Healthy Kentucky Grants, 1527
Fndn for Seacoast Health Grants, 1533
Fourjay Fndn Grants, 1544
Frank Stanley Beveridge Fndn Grants, 1553
Frey Fndn Grants, 1562
Gheens Fndn Grants, 1610
Greater Bridgeport Area Fndn Comm Impact Grants, 1650
Greater Tacoma Comm Fndn Ryan Alan Hade Endowment Fund, 1657
Gulf Coast Comm of Venice Fndn Grants, 1677

Hamlet Trust Grants, 1689
Hanna Andersson Children's Fndn Grants, 1691
Hasbro Children's Fund, 1714
Hawaii Comm Fndn Health Education and Research Grants, 1716
HCA Fndn Grants, 1721
HCA Fndn Grants, 1721
Hearst Fndn and William Randolph Hearst Fndn Grants, 1730
Hilton Head Island Fndn Grants, 1779
HIV/AIDS Research Training Fellowship, 1782
Hogg Fndn for Mental Health Grants, 1784
Ignacio Martin-Baro Fund for Mental Health and Human Rights Grants, 1839
Irvin Stern Fndn Grants, 1866
Ittleson Fndn Mental Health Grants, 1870
Jacob and Hilda Blaustein Fndn Grants, 1881
Jane Bradley Pettit Fndn Grants, 1902
Jewish Women's Fndn of New York Grants, 1924
Leo Goodwin Fndn Grants, 2043
Leonard and Helen R. Stulman Charitable Fndn Grants, 2044
Lesbian Health Fund Grants, 2046
M.J. Murdock Charitable Trust Grants, 2095
Margaret L. Wendt Fndn Grants, 2104
Margaret T. Morris Fndn Grants, 2105
Massage Therapy Research Grants, 2127
Mattel Children's Fndn Grants, 2130
Mattel International Grants, 2131
McCarthy Family Fndn Grants, 2141
Medtronic Fndn Health Care Grants, 2169
Meyer Fndn Grants, 2177
Morris and Gwendolyn Cafritz Fndn Grants, 2217
Morton K. and Jane Blaustein Fndn Grants, 2218
Moses Cone-Wesley Long Comm Health Fndn Grants, 2219
NICHD Socioeconomic Status and Health Across the Life Course, 2495
NIH Exploratory/Development Grants for Mental Health Intervention Research, 2665
NIH NRSAs for Individual Predoctoral Fellowships, 2700
NIH Research on Sleep and Sleep Disorders, 2713
NIMH Career Opportunities in Research Education and Training Honors High School Research Education Grant, 2748
NIMH Career Opportunities in Research Education and Training Honors Undergraduate Research Training Grant, 2749
NIMH Core Support Program for Mental Health/ AIDS Research Grants, 2753
NIMH Informed Consent in Research Grants, 2758
NIMH Interdisciplinary Behavioral Science Centers for Mental Health, 2759
NIMH Mental Health Dissemination Research Grants, 2762
NIMH Minority Research Infrastructure Support Grants, 2763
NIMH National Research Service Awards—Individual, 2764
NIMH New Minority Faculty Scientist Development Award, 2765
NIMH Risk Factors for Psychopathology Using Existing Data Sets Grants, 2768
NIMH Short Courses on Mathematical and Statistical Tools for the Study of Complex Phenotypes and Complex Systems, 2770
NIMH Silvio O. Conte Centers for Neuroscience Research Grants, 2771
NIMH Socioeconomic Status and Health Across the Life Course, 2772
NIMH Supplements for Underrepresented Minorities, 2773
NIMH Therapeutic Effectiveness Protocol Development Grants, 2774
NIMH/NIDA Children's Services Grants, 2775
Northern Trust Company Charitable Trust and Corp Giving Program, 2865
NYCT Girls and Young Women Grants, 2924
NYCT Mental Health and Mental Retardation Grants, 2927
Ordean Fndn Grants, 2952
OSI Mental Health Grants, 2969
PacifiCare Fndn Grants, 2981
Pasadena Fndn Average Grants, 2994
Perry County Comm Fndn Grants, 3016
Peter & Elizabeth C. Tower Fndn Comm Grants, 3018
Pike County Comm Fndn Grants, 3049
Posey Comm Fndn Grants, 3068
Posey Comm Fndn Womens Fund Grants, 3069
Quantum Corp Snap Server Grants, 3095
Rainbow Endowment Grants, 3102
Rayonier Fndn Grants, 3111
Retirement Research Fndn General Grants, 3150
Robert E. and Evelyn McKee Fndn Grants, 3170
Rosalynn Carter Institute Mattie J. T. Stepanek Caregiving Scholarships, 3190
SAMHSA Campus Suicide Prevention Grants, 3244
SAMHSA Child Mental Health Initiative Grants, 3245
SAMHSA Conference Grants, 3246
SAMHSA Drug Free Communities Support Grants, 3247
SAMHSA Strategic Prevention Framework State Incentive Grants, 3248
Seabury Fndn Grants, 3274
Simone and Cino del Duca Grand Prix Awards, 3288
Sisters of St. Joseph Healthcare Fndn Grants, 3297
Society of Neuroscience Minority Fellowships, 3345
Southbury Comm Trust Fund, 3350
Spencer County Comm Fndn Grants, 3358
St. Joseph Comm Health Fndn Improving Healthcare Access Grants, 3368
Staglin Family Music Festival NARSAD Schizophrenia Research Award, 3372
Staunton Farm Fndn Grants, 3378
Vanderburgh Comm Fndn Grants, 3480
Warrick County Comm Fndn Grants, 3519
William T. Grant Fndn Research Grants, 3541

Mental Retardation

Able To Serve Grants, 185
Benton Comm Fndn Grants, 743
Blue River Comm Fndn Grants, 770
Brown County Comm Fndn Grants, 807
Comm Fndn of Bartholomew County Heritage Fund Grants, 1096
Comm Fndn of Bartholomew County James A. Henderson Award for Fund-Raising, 1097
Comm Fndn of Boone County Grants, 1099
Comm Fndn of Greater Fort Wayne: Comm Endowment & Clarke Endowment Fund Grants, 1108
Dept of Ed Rehabilitation Training Grants, 1229
Duncan L. Gordon Fellowships, 1349
Fragile X Syndrome Postdoctoral Research Fellowships Program, 1545
John W. Alden Trust Grants, 1947
Joseph P. Kennedy Jr. Fndn Grants, 1962
Mental Retardation Distinguished Research Award, 2171
NFX Patient-Oriented Research Grants, 2313
NFX Summer Research Fellowships, 2314
NICHD NRSAs—Individual, 2488
NICHD NRSAs—Institutional, 2489
NYCT Mental Health and Mental Retardation Grants, 2927
Roeher Institute Research Grants, 3184
Simple Advise Education Center Grants, 3289

Mentoring Programs

AACN Mentorship Grant, 61
AAMC Humanism in Medicine Award, 141
American Psychiatric Association Minority Medical Student Summer Mentoring Program, 446
ASCO Comparative Effectiveness Research Professorship in Breast Cancer, 553
ASCO International Development and Education Awards, 554
ASCO Translational Research Professorships, 561
ASHA Advancing Academic-Research Careers Award, 569
ASHA Research Mentoring-Pair Travel Award, 572
ASHA Students Preparing for Academic & Research Careers Award, 574
ASM D.C. White Research and Mentoring Award, 592
ASM Roche Diagnostics Alice C. Evans Award, 615
Boeing Company Contributions Grants, 777
CMA Fndn Grants, 1042
Coca-Cola Fndn Grants, 1052
Comm Fndn of Grant County Grants, 1104
Cooper Industries Fndn Grants, 1150
Cruise Industry Charitable Fndn Grants, 1166
DOD Multidisciplinary Postdoctoral Award for Breast Cancer Research, 1295
eBay Fndn Comm Grants, 1363
Farmers Insurance Group of Companies Grants, 1455
Fisa Fndn Grants, 1506
Greater Milwaukee Fndn Grants, 1653
Hanna Andersson Children's Fndn Grants, 1691
Highmark Corp Giving Grants, 1769
John Edward Fowler Memorial Fndn Grants, 1930
Kansas Health Fndn Grants, 1980
Leonsis Fndn Grants, 2045
Liberty Bank Fndn Grants, 2053
Mericos Fndn Grants, 2172
NCI Mentored Career Development Award to Promote Diversity, 2276
NEI Mentored Clinical Scientist Development Program Award (K12), 2295
NHLBI Mentored Career Award for Faculty at Minority Institutions, 2347
NHLBI Mentored Career Development Award to Promote Faculty Diversity/Re-Entry in Biomedical Research, 2348
NHLBI Mentored Quantitative Research Career Development Awards, 2351
NIA Mentored Clinical Scientist Research Career Development Awards, 2417
NIDA International Studies on Drug Abuse and HIV/AIDS, 2505
NIDDK Mentored Research Scientist Development Award, 2565
NIGMS Initiative for Minority Students: Bridges to the Doctoral Degree, 2613
NIH Mentored Clinical Scientist Development Award, 2687
NSF Undergraduate Research and Mentoring in the Biological Sciences, 2896
Partners for Youth with Disabilities Grants, 2990
Prudential Fndn Grants, 3087
Society for Imaging Informatics in Medicine Emeritus Mentor Grants, 3320
Society of Neuroscience Minority Fellowships, 3345
Vancouver Fndn Grants and Comm Initiatives Program, 3477
Weingart Fndn Grants, 3524

Metabolic Diseases

Astellas Fndn Research Grants, 656
CFF Postdoctoral Research Fellowships, 946
CFF Research Grants, 947
Leland McSpadden Memorial Fund for Medical and Scientific Research Grants, 2041
MDA Neuromuscular Disease Research Grants, 2151
NIDDK Collaborative Interdisciplinary Team Science in Diabetes, Endocrinology and Metabolic Diseases Grants, 2547
NIDDK Diabetes, Endocrinology, and Metabolic Diseases NRSAs—Individual, 2552
NIDDK Pilot and Feasibility Clinical Research Grants in Diabetes, Endocrine and Metabolic Diseases, 2574
NIDDK Seeding Collaborative Interdisciplinary Team Science in Diabetes, Endocrinology and Metabolic Diseases Grants, 2584
NIDDK Translational Research for the Prevention and Control of Diabetes and Obesity, 2591

Metabolic Disorders
NIDDK Development of Disease Biomarkers Grants, 2549

Metabolism
AFAR Research Grants, 257
Astellas Fndn Research Grants, 656
Beckman Young Investigators Grants, 735
CFF Postdoctoral Research Fellowships, 946
CFF Research Grants, 947
Dietetic Outcomes Research Study Grants, 1285
Helen Hay Whitney Fndn Postdoctoral Research Fellowships, 1739
NCI Application of Metabolomics for Translational and Biological Research Grants, 2270
NIAMS Exploratory Developmental Grants for Multidisciplinary Clinical Studies of Sarcopenia, 2469
NIDDK Collaborative Interdisciplinary Team Science in Diabetes, Endocrinology and Metabolic Diseases Grants, 2547
NIDDK Diet Composition and Energy Balance Grants, 2553
NIDDK Race/Ethnic Disparities in the Incidence of Diabetes Complications, 2579
NIDDK Small Grants for Underrepresented Minority Scientists in Diabetes and Digestive and Kidney Diseases, 2588
NIDDK Type 2 Diabetes in the Pediatric Population Research Grants, 2593
NIEHS Applied Toxicological Research and Testing Grants, 2595
NSF Biomolecular Systems Cluster Grants, 2880
NSF Chemical, Biochemical, and Biotechnology Systems Research Grants, 2882

Metallurgy
Canada Graduate Scholarships and NSERC Postgraduate Scholarships, 845

Meteorology
Canada Graduate Scholarships and NSERC Postgraduate Scholarships, 845

Methodist Church
Barra Fndn Project Grants, 699
Bradley Turner Fndn Grants, 789
Danellie Fndn Grants, 1198
Effie and Wofford Cain Fndn Grants, 1385
United Methodist Church Global AIDS Fund Grants, 3463
United Methodist Church Malaria Control Grants, 3464
United Methodist Health Ministry Fund Grants, 3465

Mexico
Fulbright Traditional Scholar Program in the Western Hemisphere, 1577

Microbiology
Abbott-ASM Lifetime Achievement Award, 180
ASM BD Award for Research in Clinical Microbiology, 588
ASM bioMerieux Sonnenwirth Award for Leadership in Clinical Microbiology, 589
ASM Congressional Science Fellowships, 590
ASM Corp Activities Student Travel Grants, 591
ASM D.C. White Research and Mentoring Award, 592
ASM Early-Career Faculty Travel Award, 593
ASM Eli Lilly and Company Research Award, 594
ASM Faculty Ehancement Program -Travel Awards, 595
ASM Founders Distinguished Service Award, 596
ASM Gen-Probe Joseph Public Health Award, 597
ASM General Meeting Minority Travel Grants, 598
ASM GlaxoSmithKline International Member of the Year Award, 599
ASM Intel Awards, 600
ASM International Fellowship for Latin America and the Caribbean, 601
ASM International Fellowships for Asia and Africa, 602
ASM International Professorship for Latin America, 603
ASM International Professorships for Asia and Africa, 604
ASM Merck Irving S. Sigal Memorial Awards, 606
ASM Microbiology Undergraduate Research Fellowship, 607
ASM Millis-Colwell Postgraduate Travel Grant, 608
ASM Procter & Gamble Award in Applied and Environmental Microbiology, 609
ASM Promega Biotechnology Research Award, 610
ASM Public Communications Award, 611
ASM Raymond W. Sarber Awards, 612
ASM Richard and Mary Finkelstein Travel Grant, 613
ASM Robert D. Watkins Graduate Research Fellowship, 614
ASM Roche Diagnostics Alice C. Evans Award, 615
ASM sanofi-aventis ICAAC Award, 616
ASM Scherago-Rubin Award, 617
ASM Siemens Healthcare Diagnostics Young Investigator Award, 618
ASM Student and Post Doctoral Fellow Travel Grants, 619
ASM Student Travel Grants, 620
ASM TREK Diagnostic ABMM/ABMLI Professional Recognition Award, 621
ASM Undergraduate Research Fellowship, 622
ASM USFCC/J. Roger Porter Award, 623
ASM William A Hinton Research Training Award, 624
ASM-PAHO Infectious Diseases Epidemiology and Surveillance Fellowships, 625
ASM-UNESCO Leadership Grant for International Educators, 626
ASM/CCID Fellowships, 627
ASMCUE/GM Travel Assistance Grants, 628
CDC Antimicrobial Resistance in Hospital-Acquired Infections Among Intensive Care Unit Patients, 902
DOE Health Effects and Life Sciences Research Grants, 1298
LRF New Investigator Leukemia Research Grants, 2070
NFID Colin L. Powell Minority Postdoctoral Fellowship in Tropical Disease Research, 2308
NFID New Investigator Matching Grants, 2310
NIAID Microbiology and Infectious Diseases Research Grants and Contracts, 2459
NIDCR HIV/AIDS Associated Oral Viral Infections, 2535
NIDCR Oral Microbiology/Immunology of Type 1 Diabetes, 2537
NIGMS/NIDCR Evolution of Infectious Diseases Research Grants, 2633
NIH Ruth L. Kirschstein National Research Service Awards for Individual Postdoctoral Fellows, 2719
NIH SBIR/STTR Study and Control of Microbial Biofilms Research Grants, 2724
NSF Animal Developmental Mechanisms Grants, 2875
NSF Cell Systems Cluster Grants, 2881
NSF Chemical, Biochemical, and Biotechnology Systems Research Grants, 2882
NSF Genes and Genome Systems Cluster Grants, 2886
PAHO-ASM International Professorship for Latin America, 2983

Microbiome
NHLBI Microbiome of the Lung and Respiratory Tract in HIV-Infected Individuals and HIV-Uninfected Controls, 2352

Microscopy
Beckman Young Investigators Grants, 735

Middle School Education
American Electric Power Grants, 434
Bill and Melinda Gates Fndn Grants, 756
Carnegie Corp of New York Grants, 879
DaimlerChrysler Corp Fund Grants, 1186
Fndn for the Mid-South Grants, 1536
Hutton Fndn Grants, 1828
J.C. Penney Company Grants, 1874
KeySpan Fndn Grants, 1995
New York Life Fndn Grants, 2304
Progress Energy Fndn Grants, 3084
Raskob Fndn for Catholic Activities Grants, 3107
Taproot Fndn Capacity-Building Service Grants, 3417

Midwifery
DHHS National Health Service Corps Loan Repayment Awards, 1265
Hazel Corbin/Maternity Center Association Grant for Evidence-Based Midwifery Care, 1720
Virginia Department of Health Nurse Practitioner/Nurse Midwife Scholarships, 3500

Migrant Labor
Charles Delmar Fndn Grants, 963

Migrants
Dept of Ed College Assistance Migrant Program, 1228
Farmers Insurance Group of Companies Grants, 1455

Migration
NICHD Population Research Grants, 2490

Military Sciences
Fisher House Fndn Newman's Own Awards, 1509
Military Medical Research and Development Grants, 2202

Military Training
Florida BRAIVE Fund of Dade Comm Fndn, 1512
Florida BRAIVE Fund of Gulf Coast Comm Fndn of Venice, 1513
Florida BRAIVE Fund of The Comm Fndn in Jacksonville, 1514

Mineralogy
U.S. Department of Education Erma Byrd Scholarships, 3446

Mining
U.S. Department of Education Erma Byrd Scholarships, 3446

Ministry
Joseph and Luella Abell Charitable Trust Scholarships, 1958

Minorities
AACR Minority Scholar in Cancer Research Awards, 82
AACR Minority-Serving Institution Faculty Scholar in Cancer Research Awards, 83
AACR-Minorities in Cancer Research Jane Cooke Wright Lectureship Awards, 99
AAMC Herbert W. Nickens Faculty Fellowship, 139
AAMC Herbert W. Nickens Medical Student Scholarships, 140
Adolph Coors Fndn Grants, 238
Alberto Culver Corp Contributions Grants, 329
Alfred P. Sloan Fndn Research Fellowships, 353
ALSAM Fndn Grants, 369
American Sociological Association Minority Fellowships, 458
Anheuser-Busch Fndn Grants, 474
APF Awards for Advancing Minority Mental Health, 504
APF Jeanne Spurlock Congressional Fellowships, 509
Archer Daniels Midland Fndn Grants, 525
Arlington Comm Fndn Grants, 536
Armstrong McDonald Fndn Grants, 537
ASCO Loan Repayment Grants, 555
ASCO Medical Student Rotation Grants, 557
ASCO Resident Travel Awards, 559

ASM General Meeting Minority Travel Grants, 598
ASM Microbiology Undergraduate Research Fellowship, 607
ASM William A Hinton Research Training Award, 624
Avon Products Fndn Grants, 675
Benton Comm Fndn Grants, 743
Blue River Comm Fndn Grants, 770
Bodenwein Public Benevolent Fndn Grants, 775
Boston Fndn Grants, 783
Boyd Gaming Corp Contributions Program, 788
Breast Cancer Fund Grants, 790
Brown County Comm Fndn Grants, 807
Carnegie Corp of New York Grants, 879
CDC Minority Health Statistics Dissertation Research Grants, 916
Charles Delmar Fndn Grants, 963
Chicago Board of Trade Fndn Grants, 988
CNA Fndn Grants, 1046
Colorado Interstate Gas Grants, 1060
Comm Fndn of Bartholomew County Heritage Fund Grants, 1096
Comm Fndn of Bartholomew County James A. Henderson Award for Fund-Raising, 1097
Comm Fndn of Boone County Grants, 1099
Comm Fndn of Greater Fort Wayne: Comm Endowment & Clarke Endowment Fund Grants, 1108
Comm Toolbox for Children's Environmental Health Grants, 1137
ConocoPhillips Fndn Grants, 1144
Daphne Seybolt Culpeper Memorial Fndn Grants, 1201
DHHS Health Centers Grants for Residents of Public Housing, 1254
DHHS Maternal and Child Health Projects Grants, 1263
Dr. Stanley Pearle Scholarships, 1330
Edwin S. Webster Fndn Grants, 1376
Eugene M. Lang Fndn Grants, 1434
Eugene McDermott Fndn Grants, 1435
ExxonMobil Grants, 1442
Farmers Insurance Group of Companies Grants, 1455
FDHN Student Research Fellowships, 1480
Fireman's Fund Fndn Grants, 1504
Ford Motor Company Fund Grants, 1522
General Service Fndn Reproductive Health and Rights Grants, 1592
Grotto Fndn Project Grants, 1671
H.J. Heinz Company Fndn Grants, 1682
Harold Amos Medical Faculty Development Program, 1696
Health Fndn of Greater Indianapolis Grants, 1725
Hearst Fndn and William Randolph Hearst Fndn Grants, 1730
Helen Steiner Rice Fndn Grants, 1742
HIV/AIDS Research Training Fellowship, 1782
Jacob G. Schmidlapp Trust Grants, 1883
James Ford Bell Fndn Grants, 1885
Janirve Fndn Grants, 1905
John P. Murphy Fndn Grants, 1943
Joseph H. and Florence A. Roblee Fndn Grants, 1961
Katharine Matthies Fndn Grants, 1982
MONY Fndn Grants, 2215
National City Corp Contributions Grants, 2250
NCI/NIDA Transdisciplinary Tobacco Use Research Centers Grants, 2280
NFID Colin L. Powell Minority Postdoctoral Fellowship in Tropical Disease Research, 2308
NHLBI Individual Predoctoral Fellowships to Promote Diversity in Health-Related Research, 2341
NHLBI Research Supplements to Promote Diversity in Health-Related Research (Postdoctoral Individuals/New Independent Researchers), 2373
NHLBI Research Supplements to Promote Diversity in Health-Related Research for Established Investigators Who Become Disabled, 2374
NHLBI Research Supplements to Promote Diversity in Health-Related Research for Graduate Research Assistants, 2375
NHLBI Research Supplements to Promote Diversity in Health-Related Research for Individuals in Postdoctoral Training, 2376
NHLBI Research Supplements to Promote Diversity in Health-Related Research for Undergraduate Students, 2377
NIAAA Hepatitis C Infection and Alcoholic Liver Disease, 2442
NIAID Allergy, Immunology, Transplantation, Infectious Diseases, and AIDS NRSAs—Individual, 2450
NIAID Therapeutics Research on AIDS-Associated Opportunistic Infections, 2465
NIDA National Drug Abuse Treatment Clinical Trials Network, 2510
NIDA Neurobiological and Behavioral Research on Nicotine and Tobacco Products, 2511
NIDDK Small Grants for Underrepresented Minority Scientists in Diabetes and Digestive and Kidney Diseases, 2588
NIEHS Small Business Innovation Research Grants, 2605
NIGMS Mentored Clinical Scientist Research Career Development Awards, 2618
NIH Enhancing Adherence to Diabetes Self-Management Behaviors, 2659
NIH Health Promotion Among Racial and Ethnic Minority Males, 2671
NIH Low Birthweight in Minority Populations Research Grants, 2683
NIH National Occupational Research Agenda Grants, 2696
NIH Studies of Ethical, Legal, and Social Implications of Research into Human Genetic Variation Grants, 2731
NIH Urinary Incontinence Treatment Network, 2738
NIMH New Minority Faculty Scientist Development Award, 2765
NIMH Supplements for Underrepresented Minorities, 2773
NINR Diabetes Self-Management in Minority Populations Grants, 2795
NMF Franklin C. McLean Award, 2829
NMF General Electric Medical Scholars Fellowships, 2830
NNEDVF/Altria Doors of Hope Program, 2847
NSF BIO Minority Postdoctoral Research Fellowships, 2877
NSF Postdoc Research Fellowships in Biology, 2891
NSF Undergraduate Research and Mentoring in the Biological Sciences, 2896
Portland General Electric Fndn Grants, 3067
Powell Fndn Grants, 3073
Prudential Fndn Grants, 3087
Rayonier Fndn Grants, 3111
Rhode Island Fndn Grants, 3154
Richard and Susan Smith Family Fndn Grants, 3159
RWJF Finding Answers: Disparities Research for Change Grants, 3211
RWJF Harold Amos Medical Faculty Development Scholars, 3213
Shell Oil Company Fndn Grants, 3281
SNM PDEF Mickey Williams Minority Student Scholarships, 3302
Steelcase Fndn Grants, 3379
Volkswagen of America Corp Contributions Grants, 3503
Vulcan Materials Company Fndn Grants, 3504
W. C. Griffith Fndn Grants, 3505
Westinghouse Charitable Giving Grants, 3530
Wilson-Wood Fndn Grants, 3542
Winston-Salem Fndn Stokes County Grants, 3546
Women's Fndn of California Grants, 3550
Z. Smith Reynolds Fndn Small Grants, 3557

Minority Education

3M Fndn Grants, 11
AACAP Jeanne Spurlock Minority Medical Student Clinical Fellowship in Child and Adolescent Psychiatry, 39
AAMC Herbert W. Nickens Faculty Fellowship, 139
AAMC Herbert W. Nickens Medical Student Scholarships, 140
Air Products and Chemicals Grants, 319
Alcoa Fndn Grants, 334
American Psychiatric Association Minority Fellowships Program, 443
Andersen Fndn Grants, 471
Anheuser-Busch Fndn Grants, 474
APF Jeanne Spurlock Congressional Fellowships, 509
ARCO Fndn Education Grants, 526
ASHFndn Graduate Student Scholarships, 577
ASHFndn Graduate Student Scholarships for Minority Students, 578
ASM Robert D. Watkins Graduate Research Fellowship, 614
Chiron Fndn Comm Grants, 1004
CIGNA Fndn Grants, 1011
CMS Historically Black Colleges and Universities Health Services Research Grants, 1044
Coca-Cola Fndn Grants, 1052
Constellation Energy Group and Baltimore Gas and Electric Corp Contributions, 1146
Cruise Industry Charitable Fndn Grants, 1166
DaimlerChrysler Corp Fund Grants, 1186
FACHE Albert W. Dent Scholarships, 1445
FIC/ORMH Minority International Research Training Grants, 1497
FMC Fndn Grants, 1518
Graco Fndn Grants, 1642
Health Management Scholarships and Grants for Minorities, 1727
HRSA Health Professions Scholarships for Disadvantaged Students, 1807
HRSA Nursing Education Opportunities for the Disadvantaged Project Grants, 1809
Indiana Minority Teacher/Special Services Scholarships, 1852
Johnson & Johnson Corp Contributions Grants, 1952
Josiah Macy Jr. Fndn Grants, 1966
KFF Barbara Jordan Health Policy Scholarships, 2000
Margoes Fndn Grants, 2106
Marine Biological Laboratory Summer Research Fellowships, 2108
Millipore Fndn Grants, 2203
Minority Doctoral Fellowships in Science and Engineering, 2207
NHLBI Mentored Career Award For Faculty At Minority Institutions, 2346
NHLBI Minority Institution Research Scientist Development Award, 2354
NHLBI Minority Institutional Research Training Grants, 2355
NHLBI Short-Term Research Education Program to Increase Diversity in Health-Related Research, 2383
NIA Minority Dissertation Research Grants in Aging, 2419
NIDCD Minority Dissertation Research Grants in Human Communication, 2524
NIGMS Initiative for Minority Students: Bridges to the Baccalaureate Degree, 2612
NIGMS Initiative for Minority Students: Bridges to the Doctoral Degree, 2613
NIGMS Institutional Research and Academic Career Development Award, 2614
NIGMS MARC Undergraduate Student Training in Academic Research (U-STAR) Program, 2617
NIGMS Minority Access to Research Careers Ancillary Training Activities Grants, 2619
NIGMS Minority Access to Research Careers Program, 2620
NIH Health Promotion Among Racial and Ethnic Minority Males, 2671
NIH Predoctoral Fellowship Awards for Minority Students, 2703
NIMH Career Opportunities in Research Education and Training Honors High School Research Education Grant, 2748

NIMH Career Opportunities in Research Education and Training Honors Undergraduate Research Training Grant, 2749
NMF Aura E. Severinghaus Award, 2828
NMF General Electric Medical Scholars Fellowships, 2830
NMF Henry G. Halladay Awards, 2831
NMF Hugh J. Andersen Memorial Scholarship, 2832
NMF Irving Graef Memorial Scholarship, 2833
NMF Mary Ball Carrera Scholarship, 2834
NMF Metropolitan Life Fndn Awards Program for Academic Excellence in Medicine, 2835
NMF National Medical Association Awards for Medical Journalism, 2836
NMF National Medical Association Emerging Scholar Awards, 2837
NMF National Medical Association Patti LaBelle Award, 2838
NMF Need-Based Scholarships, 2839
NMF Ralph W. Ellison Prize, 2840
NMF William and Charlotte Cadbury Award, 2841
Northern Trust Company Charitable Trust and Corp Giving Program, 2865
Northrop Grumman Newport News Grants, 2867
NSF Undergraduate Research and Mentoring in the Biological Sciences, 2896
Oracle Corp Contributions Grants, 2951
Polaroid Fund Grants, 3065
RGK Fndn Grants, 3153
RWJF Summer Medical and Dental Education Program, 3231

Minority Employment
Chicago Tribune's Corp Contributions Grants, 991

Minority Health
Aetna Fndn Quality of Care Grants, 245
AHRQ Independent Scientist Award, 313
Anheuser-Busch Fndn Grants, 474
APF Awards for Advancing Minority Mental Health, 504
APF Disaster Recovery Fund for Psychiatrists, 506
Avon Fndn Breast Care Fund Grants, 674
BCBS of Massachusetts Fndn Grants, 709
BCBSNC Fndn Grants, 725
California Endowment CommunitiesFirst Grants, 833
Commonwealth Fund Harkness Fellowships in Health Care Policy and Practice, 1079
Commonwealth Fund/Harvard University Fellowship in Minority Health Policy, 1086
Connecticut Health Fndn Health Initiative Grants, 1142
DHHS AIDS and HIV Epidemiologic Research Studies Grants, 1244
DHHS Maternal and Child Health Research and Training Programs Grants, 1264
Henry J. Kaiser Family Fndn Grants, 1748
HIV/AIDS Research Training Fellowship, 1782
NIDDK Race/Ethnic Disparities in the Incidence of Diabetes Complications, 2579
NIGMS Initiative for Minority Students: Bridges to the Baccalaureate Degree, 2612
NMF General Electric Medical Scholars Fellowships, 2830
Portland General Electric Fndn Grants, 3067
RWJF Finding Answers: Disparities Research for Change Grants, 3211
RWJF Health Impact Project Grants, 3216

Minority Schools
Alcoa Fndn Grants, 334
Allyn Fndn Grants, 365
Coca-Cola Fndn Grants, 1052
DHHS Maternal and Child Health Projects Grants, 1263
FIC/ORMH Minority International Research Training Grants, 1497
NHLBI Minority Institution Research Scientist Development Award, 2354
NHLBI Minority Institutional Research Training Grants, 2355
NIDA Minority Institutions Drug Abuse Research Development Program (MIDARP) Grants, 2509
NIEHS Mentored Research Scientist Development Award, 2603
NIGMS Institutional Research and Academic Career Development Award, 2614
NIMH Career Opportunities in Research Education and Training Honors Undergraduate Research Training Grant, 2749
NIMH Minority Research Infrastructure Support Grants, 2763
NINDS Specialized Neuroscience Research Programs on Health Disparity: HIV and the Nervous System, 2785
NINR Mentored Research Scientist Development Award, 2798
Procter and Gamble Fund Grants, 3083

Minority/Woman-Owned Business
NSF Small Business Innovation Research Grants, 2893

Molecular Probes
Eppendorf & Science Prize for Neurobiology, 1424
NIH Solicitation of Assays for High Throughput Screening in the Molecular Libraries Probe Production Centers Network, 2729
NINDS Optimization of Small Molecule Probes for the Nervous System Grants, 2780
NINDS Optimization of Small Molecule Probes for the Nervous System Grants, 2781
NINDS Optimization of Small Molecule Probes for the Nervous System Grants, 2782

Montenegro
OSI European Commission Internships for Young Roma Graduates, 2965

Morphology
NSF Systematic Biology and Biodiversity Inventories Grants, 2895

Multi-Organ Diseases
NHLBI Sarcoidosis: Research Grants into the Cause of Multi-Organ Disease and Clinical Strategies for Therapy, 2382

Multiculturalism
American-Scandinavian Fndn Visiting Lectureship Grants, 460

Multiple Myeloma
ASCO Career Development Award, 551
ASCO Young Investigator Award, 562
ASCO/UICC International Cancer Technology Transfer (ICRETT) Fellowships, 563

Multiple Sclerosis
Compass Bank Fndn Grants, 1138
Henry & Ruth Blaustein Rosenberg Fndn Grants, 1746
MSSC Career Development Awards, 2224
MSSC Postdoctoral Fellowships, 2225
MSSC Research Grants, 2226
MSSC Research Studentships, 2227
Multiple Sclerosis Fndn Brighter Tomorrow Grants, 2228
NIA Symptom Management for Chronic Neurological Conditions Research Grants, 2436
NICHD Symptom Management for Chronic Neurological Conditions Research Grants, 2496
NIDCD Symptom Management for Chronic Neurological Conditions Research Grants, 2532
NINDS Symptom Management for Chronic Neurological Conditions Research Grants, 2787
NINR Symptom Management for Chronic Neurological Conditions Research Grants, 2805
NMSS Daniel Haughton Senior Faculty Awards, 2842
NMSS Harry Weaver Neuroscience Scholar Awards, 2843
NMSS Research Grants, 2844
NMSS Scholarships, 2845
NMSS Sylvia Lawry Physician Fellowships, 2846
Pittsburgh Fndn Medical Research Grants, 3055

Muscular Dystrophy
Doris and Victor Day Fndn Grants, 1313
MDA Neuromuscular Disease Research Grants, 2151
NIAMS High Risk Arthritis and Musculoskeletal and Skin Diseases Research, 2470
NIAMS Pathogenesis and Therapy of the Muscular Dystrophies Research Grants, 2474
NINDS Pathogenesis and Therapy of the Muscular Dystrophies Research Grants, 2783

Musculoskeletal Disorders
NIAMS Clinical Trial Planning Grants, 2466
NIAMS Collaborative Arthritis and Musculoskeletal and Skin Diseases Science Award, 2467
NIAMS Core Centers for Musculoskeletal Disorders Grants, 2468
NIAMS Exploratory Developmental Grants for Multidisciplinary Clinical Studies of Sarcopenia, 2469
NIAMS High Risk Arthritis and Musculoskeletal and Skin Diseases Research, 2470
NIAMS Mechanisms of Chondroprotection Research Grants, 2472
NIAMS Specialized Centers of Research in Osteoporosis, Rheumatoid Arthritis, and Scleroderma, 2480
NIAMS/NICHD Deep Infections of Total Joint Replacements, 2481
NIH Human Models and Markers of Skeletal Aging Grants, 2674
Osteogenesis Imperfecta Fndn Research Grants, 2975

Musculoskeletal System
Dystonia Medical Research Grants and Fellowships, 1355
Musculoskeletal Rehabilitation Fellowships, 2229
NIA Significance of Sarcopenia in Old Age Grants, 2433
NIAMS Research on Musculoskeletal Fitness and Sports Medicine Grants, 2476
NIAMS Significance of Sarcopenia in Old Age Grants, 2477
NICHD Research on Musculoskeletal Fitness and Sports Medicine Grants, 2492
NINR Research on Musculoskeletal Fitness and Sports Medicine Grants, 2803
NIOSH Occupational Safety and Health Research and Demonstration Grants, 2807

Museums
AEGON Transamerica Fndn Grants, 243
Agnes Gund Fndn Grants, 262
Air Products and Chemicals Grants, 319
Albuquerque Comm Fndn Grants, 331
Alexis Gregory Fndn Grants, 349
Aratani Fndn Grants, 523
Arthur and Rochelle Belfer Fndn Grants, 542
Auburn Fndn Grants, 664
Ball Brothers Fndn Grants, 684
Bank of America Charitable Fndn Anchor Institutions Grants, 688
Barra Fndn Project Grants, 699
Batchelor Fndn Grants, 701
Bender Fndn Grants, 742
Berrien Comm Fndn Grants, 749
Bertha Russ Lytel Fndn Grants, 751
Booth-Bricker Fund Grants, 780
Bruce and Adele Greenfield Fndn Grants, 808
Burlington Industries Fndn Grants, 811
Burlington Northern Santa Fe Fndn Grants, 812
Byron W. and Alice L. Lockwood Fndn Grants, 824
Caleb C. and Julia W. Dula Educational and Charitable Fndn Grants, 830
Carl Gellert and Celia Berta Gellert Fndn Grants, 871
Carylon Fndn Grants, 886

Cessna Fndn Grants, 938
Charles M. Bair Family Trust Grants, 972
Chazen Fndn Grants, 978
Chestnut Hill Charitable Fndn, Inc Grants, 987
Chicago Board of Trade Fndn Grants, 988
Cockrell Fndn Grants, 1053
Collins C. Diboll Private Fndn Grants, 1057
Colorado Springs Comm Trust Fund Grants, 1061
Comm Fndn Alliance City of Evansville Endowment Fund Grants, 1089
Comm Fndn of Southeastern Connecticut Grants, 1125
Connecticut Comm Fndn Grants, 1141
Constantin Fndn Grants, 1145
Cooper Industries Fndn Grants, 1150
Cowles Charitable Trust Grants, 1155
David Geffen Fndn Grants, 1202
Daywood Fndn Grants, 1206
DeRoy Testamentary Fndn Grants, 1239
Doris and Victor Day Fndn Grants, 1313
Dorrance Family Fndn Grants, 1323
Dr. Scholl Fndn Grants, 1329
E. Rhodes and Leona B. Carpenter Fndn Grants, 1356
Edward S. Moore Fndn Grants, 1374
Elizabeth McGraw Fndn Grants, 1399
Eugene McDermott Fndn Grants, 1435
ExxonMobil Grants, 1442
FirstEnergy Fndn Comm Grants, 1505
Greater Green Bay Comm Fndn Grants, 1652
Greater Worcester Comm Fndn Discretionary Grants, 1658
Harold & Arlene Schnitzer CARE Fndn Grants, 1697
High Meadow Fndn Grants, 1768
Hillman Fndn Grants, 1775
Hudson Webber Fndn Grants, 1813
Hugh J. Andersen Fndn Grants, 1814
Huie-Dellmon Trust Grants, 1815
Idaho Power Company Corp Contributions, 1838
Jessie Ball Dupont Fund Grants, 1919
John H. and Wilhelmina D. Harland Charitable Fndn Grants, 1933
Joseph Alexander Fndn Grants, 1957
Kalamazoo Fndn Grants, 1979
Kenneth T. and Eileen L. Norris Fndn Grants, 1989
King Pharmaceuticals Corp Contributions Grants, 2003
Louis Calder Fndn Grants, 2065
Lubbock Area Fndn Grants, 2079
Lubrizol Fndn Grants, 2080
Mabel Y. Hughes Charitable Trust Grants, 2097
Marcia and Otto Koehler Fndn Grants, 2103
Margaret L. Wendt Fndn Grants, 2104
Maxon Charitable Fndn Grants, 2135
McLean Contributionship Grants, 2147
Morris and Gwendolyn Cafritz Fndn Grants, 2217
National City Corp Contributions Grants, 2250
Nicholas H. Noyes Jr. Memorial Fndn Grants, 2497
OceanFirst Fndn Grants, 2933
Perkins Charitable Fndn Grants, 3014
Piedmont Natural Gas Grants, 3048
R.C. Baker Fndn Grants, 3098
Richard and Susan Smith Family Fndn Grants, 3159
Samuel S. Johnson Fndn Grants, 3251
Schurz Communications Fndn Grants, 3271
Sid W. Richardson Fndn Grants, 3284
Sunderland Fndn Grants, 3400
Susan Vaughan Fndn Grants, 3413
Temple-Inland Fndn Grants, 3419
Thelma Doelger Charitable Trust Grants, 3421
Vermont Comm Fndn Grants, 3493
W. C. Griffith Fndn Grants, 3505
Weatherwax Fndn Grants, 3523
William G. Gilmore Fndn Grants, 3537

Music
Adaptec Fndn Grants, 232
Agnes Gund Fndn Grants, 262
Alexis Gregory Fndn Grants, 349
Auburn Fndn Grants, 664
Barberton Comm Fndn Grants, 693
Berks County Comm Fndn Grants, 745
Blanche and Irving Laurie Fndn Grants, 764
Canada-U.S. Fulbright New Century Scholars Grants, 846
Canada-U.S. Fulbright Senior Specialists Grants, 847
Chazen Fndn Grants, 978
Clarence E. Heller Charitable Fndn Grants, 1022
Comm Fndn of Bloomington and Monroe County Grants, 1098
Comm Fndn of Mount Vernon and Knox County Grants, 1119
Cudd Fndn Grants, 1171
DAAD Research Stays for University Academics and Scientists, 1183
Edwin W. and Catherine M. Davis Fndn Grants, 1377
Ensworth Charitable Fndn Grants, 1416
FirstEnergy Fndn Comm Grants, 1505
Fndn Northwest Grants, 1537
Frist Fndn Grants, 1563
Fulbright Alumni Initiatives Awards Grants, 1566
Fulbright Distinguished Chairs Grants, 1567
Fulbright New Century Scholars Grants, 1570
Fulbright Specialists Grants, 1571
Fulbright Traditional Scholar Program in Europe and Eurasia, 1572
Fulbright Traditional Scholar Program in Sub-Saharan Africa, 1573
Fulbright Traditional Scholar Program in the East Asia/Pacific Region, 1574
Fulbright Traditional Scholar Program in the Near East and North Africa Region, 1575
Fulbright Traditional Scholar Program in the South and Central Asia Region, 1576
Fulbright Traditional Scholar Program in the Western Hemisphere, 1577
Gibson Fndn Grants, 1612
Grammy Fndn Grants, 1643
Grand Rapids Area Comm Fndn Grants, 1645
Grand Rapids Area Comm Fndn Nashwauk Area Endowment Fund Grants, 1646
Greater Milwaukee Fndn Grants, 1653
Guitar Center Music Fndn Grants, 1675
High Meadow Fndn Grants, 1768
Idaho Comm Fndn Eastern Region Competitive Grants, 1837
John Ben Snow Memorial Trust Grants, 1928
Long Island Comm Fndn Grants, 2063
M. Bastian Family Fndn Grants, 2092
Margaret T. Morris Fndn Grants, 2105
New York University Steinhardt School of Education Fellowships, 2305
Procter and Gamble Fund Grants, 3083
Rollin M. Gerstacker Fndn Grants, 3186
Ruth Mott Fndn Grants, 3204
Sosland Fndn Grants, 3348
Walt Disney Company Fndn Grants, 3516

Music Appreciation
Paul E. and Klare N. Reinhold Fndn Grants, 2999

Music Education
Cemala Fndn Grants, 933
Clarence E. Heller Charitable Fndn Grants, 1022
Gibson Fndn Grants, 1612
Grand Rapids Area Comm Fndn Grants, 1645
Grand Rapids Area Comm Fndn Nashwauk Area Endowment Fund Grants, 1646
Guitar Center Music Fndn Grants, 1675
Heineman Fndn for Research, Education, Charitable and Scientific Purposes, 1735
Milagro Fndn Grants, 2198
Paul E. and Klare N. Reinhold Fndn Grants, 2999
Portland General Electric Fndn Grants, 3067
Southbury Comm Trust Fund, 3350

Music Therapy
Guitar Center Music Fndn Grants, 1675

Music, Vocal
Bonfils-Stanton Fndn Grants, 779
Meyer Memorial Trust Emergency Grants, 2178
Meyer Memorial Trust Grassroots Grants, 2179
Meyer Memorial Trust Responsive Grants, 2181
Pasadena Fndn Average Grants, 2994

Musical Instruments
Gibson Fndn Grants, 1612
Guitar Center Music Fndn Grants, 1675

Mutagenics
NHLBI Elucidating Nature's Solutions to Heart, Lung, and Blood Diseases and Sleep Disorder Processes Research Grants, 2333
NIEHS Biological Response to Environmental Health Hazards Research Grants, 2596
NIH Mouse Mutagenesis and Phenotyping: Developmental Defects Research Grants, 2692
NIH Mouse Mutagenesis and Phenotyping: Nervous System and Behavior Research Grants, 2693

Myasthenia Gravis
MDA Neuromuscular Disease Research Grants, 2151
MGFA Post-Doctoral Research Fellowships, 2183
MGFA Student Fellowships, 2184
Osserman-Sosin Postdoctoral Myasthenia Gravis Research Fellowships, 2974

Mycology
NFID John P. Utz Medical Mycology Postdoctoral Fellowship, 2309
NIAID Microbiology and Infectious Diseases Research Grants and Contracts, 2459

Myeloma
Leukemia and Lymphoma Society Research Grants, 2051

National Disease Organizations
Alcatel-Lucent Technologies Fndn Grants, 333
Archer Daniels Midland Fndn Grants, 525
ArvinMeritor Fndn Health Grants, 543
Lockheed Martin Philanthropic Grants, 2062

National Planning/Policy
AMA-MSS Government Relations Internship Programs, 404

National Security
AAAS Science & Technology Policy Fellowships - National Defense & Global Security, 29
Carnegie Corp of New York Grants, 879
Florida BRAIVE Fund of Dade Comm Fndn, 1512
Florida BRAIVE Fund of Gulf Coast Comm Fndn of Venice, 1513
Florida BRAIVE Fund of The Comm Fndn in Jacksonville, 1514

Native American Education
Burlington Northern Santa Fe Fndn Grants, 812
DHHS Health Professions Preparatory Scholarship Program for Indians, 1257
Dorothea Haus Ross Fndn Grants, 1320
General Motors Fndn Grants Support Program, 1591
John R. Oishei Fndn Grants, 1944
KFF Barbara Jordan Health Policy Scholarships, 2000
NHLBI Minority Institutional Research Training Grants, 2355
NIDA Minority Institutions Drug Abuse Research Development Program (MIDARP) Grants, 2509
NMF Mary Ball Carrera Scholarship, 2834
NMF Need-Based Scholarships, 2839
U.S. Department of Education Rehabilitation Training—Rehabilitation Continuing Education Programs—Institute on Rehabilitation Issues, 3449

Native Americans
Administration on Aging Senior Medicare Patrol Project Grants, 236
AMA Fndn Minority Scholars Awards, 395
American Sociological Association Minority Fellowships, 458

amfAR Fellowships, 462
amfAR Global Initiatives Grants, 463
amfAR Mathilde Krim Fellowships in Basic Biomedical Research, 464
amfAR Public Policy Grants, 465
amfAR Research Grants, 466
ASM Robert D. Watkins Graduate Research Fellowship, 614
CDC Increasing Breast and Cervical Cancer Screening Services for Urban American Indian/ Alaska Native Women, 912
Charles Delmar Fndn Grants, 963
DHHS AIDS and HIV Epidemiologic Research Studies Grants, 1244
DHHS Emergency Medical Services for Children Program, 1249
DHHS Health Professions Scholarship Program, 1258
DHHS Maternal and Child Health Projects Grants, 1263
DHHS Native American Health Service Loan Repayment Awards, 1267
EPA Baseline Assessment of Risks of Exposure to Lead Poisoning of Native American Children, 1419
EPA Lead Awareness Outreach for Native American Tribes, 1421
FDHN Student Research Fellowships, 1480
Grotto Fndn Project Grants, 1671
Harold Amos Medical Faculty Development Program, 1696
IHS Native American and Alaskan Native Health Research Centers, 1840
Lotus 88 Fndn for Women and Children Grants, 2064
NIMH Career Opportunities in Research Education and Training Honors High School Research Education Grant, 2748
NIMH Career Opportunities in Research Education and Training Honors Undergraduate Research Training Grant, 2749
NMF Franklin C. McLean Award, 2829
SNM PDEF Mickey Williams Minority Student Scholarships, 3302
U.S. Department of Education Vocational Rehabilitation Services Projects for American Indians with Disabilities Grants, 3452

Natural History
NIDDK Type 2 Diabetes in the Pediatric Population Research Grants, 2593

Natural Products
Dean Foods Comm Involvement Grants, 1209

Natural Resources
Ahn Family Fndn Grants, 304
Beirne Carter Fndn Grants, 737
Cessna Fndn Grants, 938
Charles Delmar Fndn Grants, 963
Comm Fndn of Greater Birmingham Grants, 1106
Dorrance Family Fndn Grants, 1323
Duke Energy Fndn Grants, 1339
Elliot Fndn Inc Grants, 1402
Gulf Coast Comm of Venice Fndn Grants, 1677
High Meadow Fndn Grants, 1768
Hoblitzelle Fndn Grants, 1783
Horace A. Kimball and S. Ella Kimball Fndn Grants, 1792
James Ford Bell Fndn Grants, 1885
Janirve Fndn Grants, 1905
John W. and Anna H. Hanes Fndn Grants, 1948
Knox County Comm Fndn Grants, 2009
Kosciusko County Comm Fndn Grants, 2015
Maxon Charitable Fndn Grants, 2135
Owen County Comm Fndn Grants, 2979
Perkins Charitable Fndn Grants, 3014
Pinellas County Grants, 3050
Posey Comm Fndn Grants, 3068
Pulaski County Comm Fndn Grants, 3091
Rhode Island Fndn Grants, 3154
Ripley County Comm Fndn Grants, 3166
Samuel S. Johnson Fndn Grants, 3251
Seabury Fndn Grants, 3274
Sir Dorabji Tata Trust Grants for NGOs or Voluntary Organizations, 3291
Spencer County Comm Fndn Grants, 3358
Texas Commission on the Arts Arts Respond Project Grants, 3420
Triangle Comm Fndn Donor-Advised Grants, 3437
Vancouver Fndn Grants and Comm Initiatives Program, 3477
Vanderburgh Comm Fndn Grants, 3480

Natural Sciences
Bank of America Client Fndn Grants, 690
Charles A. Frueauff Fndn Grants, 962
Cockrell Fndn Grants, 1053
DAAD Research Stays for University Academics and Scientists, 1183
Harry Frank Guggenheim Fndn Research Grants, 1704
Matsumae International Fndn Grants, 2129

Nature Centers
Boston Fndn Grants, 783
Lubrizol Fndn Grants, 2080

Naval Sciences
DOL Occupational Safety and Health—Susan Harwood Training Grants, 1305
ONR Human Performance Division Research Grants, 2948

Naval Technology
ONR Human Performance Division Research Grants, 2948

Neighborhoods
Allstate Corp Giving Grants, 363
Allstate Corp Hometown Commitment Grants, 364
Beckley Area Fndn Grants, 732
Bernard and Audre Rapoport Fndn Grants, 746
Bill and Melinda Gates Fndn Grants, 756
Carnegie Corp of New York Grants, 879
Chestnut Hill Charitable Fndn, Inc Grants, 987
CIT Corp Giving Grants, 1014
Citizens Bank Mid-Atlantic Charitable Fndn Grants, 1015
Columbus Fndn Competitive Grants, 1066
Comm Fndn for Monterey County Grants, 1092
Comm Fndn for Southeastern Michigan Grants, 1094
Comm Fndn of Muncie and Delaware County Grants, 1120
Comm Fndn Silicon Valley Grants, 1133
Cooper Industries Fndn Grants, 1150
Crail-Johnson Fndn Grants, 1157
CSRA Comm Fndn Grants, 1168
DOJ Gang-Free Schools and Communities Intervention Grants, 1303
Erie Comm Fndn Grants, 1427
Farmers Insurance Group of Companies Grants, 1455
Frances L. and Edwin L. Cummings Memorial Fund Grants, 1547
Graco Fndn Grants, 1642
Greater Milwaukee Fndn Grants, 1653
Greater Worcester Comm Fndn Discretionary Grants, 1658
Hannaford Charitable Fndn Grants, 1692
Hasbro Children's Fund, 1714
Helen Bader Fndn Grants, 1738
Hirtzel Memorial Fndn Grants, 1781
Independence Comm Fndn Comm Quality of Life Grant, 1849
Liberty Bank Fndn Grants, 2053
Lynde and Harry Bradley Fndn Grants, 2089
Lynde and Harry Bradley Fndn Prizes: Bradley Prizes, 2090
Meyer Fndn Grants, 2177
Nordson Corp Fndn Grants, 2851
Northern Trust Company Charitable Trust and Corp Giving Program, 2865
Paul and Mary Haas Fndn Contributions and Student Scholarships, 2997
Polaroid Fund Grants, 3065
Prudential Fndn Grants, 3087
Ralphs Food 4 Less Fndn Grants, 3106
Ruth Mott Fndn Grants, 3204
RWJF New Jersey Health Initiatives Grants, 3225
San Diego Fndn for Change Grants, 3255

Nepal
Fulbright Traditional Scholar Program in the South and Central Asia Region, 1576

Nephrology
Canadian Liver Fndn Grants, 851
Fndn for Medical Research Grants, 1528
KFC Biomedical Research Grants, 1998
KFC Nephrology and Urology Scholarships, 1999
NIDDK Training in Clinical Investigation in Kidney and Urology Grants, 2590
NKF Research Fellowships, 2812
NKF Young Investigator Grants, 2813
NYAM Edward N. Gibbs Memorial Lecture and Award in Nephrology, 2912
PKD Fndn Lillian Kaplan International Prize for the Advancement in the Understanding of Polycystic Kidney Disease, 3056

Nervous System
Elizabeth Glaser Pediatric AIDS Fndn International Leadership Awards, 1393
Elizabeth Glaser Pediatric AIDS Fndn Operations Research Grants, 1394
Elizabeth Glaser Pediatric AIDS Fndn Two-Year International Scholar Award, 1396
NICHD Central Nervous System Effects of HIV Infection: Neurobiological, Neurovirological, and Neurobehavioral Studies Grants, 2482
NIDA Drug Addiction Neuroscience Research Grants, 2503
NIDA Role of Limbic System and Brain Ontogeny in Drug Abuse Research Grants, 2514
NIH Impact of HAART on HIV/CNS Disease, 2676
NIH Mouse Mutagenesis and Phenotyping: Nervous System and Behavior Research Grants, 2693
NIH Role of Microglia in Normal and Abnormal Immune Responses of the Nervous System, 2716
NINDS Central Nervous System Effects of HIV Infection: Neurobiological, Neurovirological, and Neurobehavioral Studies Grants, 2777
NINDS Cerebral Radiobiology and Neuroimaging of Brain Tumors Research Grants, 2778
NINDS Optimization of Small Molecule Probes for the Nervous System Grants, 2780
NINDS Optimization of Small Molecule Probes for the Nervous System Grants, 2781
NINDS Optimization of Small Molecule Probes for the Nervous System Grants, 2782
NINDS Specialized Neuroscience Research Programs on Health Disparity: HIV and the Nervous System, 2785
NSF Behavioral Neurosciences Research Grants, 2876
Simone and Cino del Duca Grand Prix Awards, 3288
United Cerebral Palsy Research Grants, 3462

Networking (Computers)
NLM Exploratory/Developmental Grants, 2816

Neuroanatomy
EF Postdoctoral Research Training Fellowships, 1382
NIDDK Neuroimaging in Obesity Research Grants, 2569
TSA Research Grant Awards, 3442

Neurobiology
AFAR Research Grants, 257
AHAF Alzheimer's Disease Research Grants, 266
Alfred P. Sloan Fndn History of Science and Technology Grants, 352
ASHA Research Mentoring-Pair Travel Award, 572
Eppendorf & Science Prize for Neurobiology, 1424
Fndn for Medical Research Grants, 1528

Fyssen Fndn Postdoctoral Study Grants, 1580
Grass Fndn Marine Biological Laboratory Fellowships, 1648
Hereditary Disease Fndn John J. Wasmuth Postdoctoral Fellowships, 1750
Hereditary Disease Fndn Lieberman Award, 1751
Hereditary Disease Fndn Research Grants, 1752
Hunter's Hope Fndn Grants, 1820
John Merck Scholars Awards, 1941
Marine Biological Laboratory Summer Research Fellowships, 2108
Milton Wexler Postdoctoral Fellowships, 2205
NHLBI Exploratory Studies in the Neurobiology of Pain in Sickle Cell Disease, 2334
NIA Role of Nuclear Receptors in Tissue and Organismal Aging Grants, 2432
NICHD Central Nervous System Effects of HIV Infection: Neurobiological, Neurovirological, and Neurobehavioral Studies Grants, 2482
NIDA Drug Addiction Neuroscience Research Grants, 2503
NIDA Neurobiological and Behavioral Research on Nicotine and Tobacco Products, 2511
NIDCD Neurobiology and Genetics of Autism Grants, 2526
NIDDK Neurobiology of Diabetic Complications Grants, 2568
NIH Research on Sleep and Sleep Disorders, 2713
NIH Rett Syndrome: Genetics, Pathophysiology, and Biomarkers Research Grants, 2715
NIMH Central Nervous System Effects of HIV Infection: Neurobiological, Neurovirological, and Neurobehavioral Studies Grants, 2751
NINDS Central Nervous System Effects of HIV Infection: Neurobiological, Neurovirological, and Neurobehavioral Studies Grants, 2777
NINDS Cerebral Radiobiology and Neuroimaging of Brain Tumors Research Grants, 2778
NSF Behavioral Neurosciences Research Grants, 2876
Whitehall Fndn Neurobiology Research Grants, 3533

Neurochemistry

NIEHS/NINDS Role of the Environment in Parkinson's Disease, 2608
NIH Xenobiotics and Cell Death/Injury in Neurodegenerative Disease Research Grants, 2739

Neuroendocrinology

Charles H. Hood Fndn Child Health Research Grants, 968
NSF Behavioral Neurosciences Research Grants, 2876

Neurological Disorders

AMA Fndn Seed Grants for Research, 398
Christopher Reeve Paralysis Fndn Individual Research Grants, 1006
Dana Fndn Science and Health Grants, 1197
Fairlawn Fndn Grants, 1447
John Merck Scholars Awards, 1941
Judith and Jean Pape Adams Charitable Fndn ALS Grants, 1970
Larry L. Hillblom Fndn Grants, 2031
NIA Symptom Management for Chronic Neurological Conditions Research Grants, 2436
NICHD Symptom Management for Chronic Neurological Conditions Research Grants, 2496
NIDCD Symptom Management for Chronic Neurological Conditions Research Grants, 2532
NIEHS Biological Response to Environmental Health Hazards Research Grants, 2596
NIEHS Small Business Innovation Research Grants, 2605
NIH Research on Sleep and Sleep Disorders, 2713
NIH Xenobiotics and Cell Death/Injury in Neurodegenerative Disease Research Grants, 2739
NINDS Support of Scientific Meetings as Cooperative Agreements, 2786
NINDS Symptom Management for Chronic Neurological Conditions Research Grants, 2787
NINR Symptom Management for Chronic Neurological Conditions Research Grants, 2805
PDF Summer Fellowships, 3008
Pittsburgh Fndn Medical Research Grants, 3055

Neurology

American Philosophical Society Daland Fellowships in Clinical Investigation, 441
ANS Neurotology Fellows Award, 482
ANS Nicholas Torok Vestibular Award, 483
ANS Trainee Award, 484
ANS/AAO-HNSF Herbert Silverstein Otology and Neurotology Research Award, 485
DHHS Geriatric Training for Physicians and Dentists Grants, 1250
DHHS Neurodevelopmental Test Methods Research Grants, 1268
DHHS Priority Health Conditions Studies Initiative, 1273
EF Research and Training Fellowships for Clinicians, 1384
Joseph Collins Fndn Grants, 1959
MDBD Research Grants and Basil O'Connor Starter Scholar Award Program, 2153
MNI Jeanne Timmins Fellowships, 2212
NIA Role of Nuclear Receptors in Tissue and Organismal Aging Grants, 2432
NICHD Central Nervous System Effects of HIV Infection: Neurobiological, Neurovirological, and Neurobehavioral Studies Grants, 2482
NIDDK Neurobiology of Diabetic Complications Grants, 2568
NIH Biobehavioral Pain Research Grants, 2638
NIH Genetics of Neurobehavioral Disorders in Existing Samples Grants, 2670
NIH Impact of HAART on HIV/CNS Disease, 2676
NIMH Central Nervous System Effects of HIV Infection: Neurobiological, Neurovirological, and Neurobehavioral Studies Grants, 2751
NINDS Central Nervous System Effects of HIV Infection: Neurobiological, Neurovirological, and Neurobehavioral Studies Grants, 2777
NINDS Support of Scientific Meetings as Cooperative Agreements, 2786
NYAM Charles A. Elsberg Fellowship, 2910
PDF Postdoctoral Fellowships for Neurologists, 3007
Rett Syndrome Research Fndn Grants, 3151
TSA Research Grant Awards, 3442
United Cerebral Palsy Research Grants, 3462

Neuromuscular Disorders

Human Growth Fndn Small Grants, 1816
Judith and Jean Pape Adams Charitable Fndn ALS Grants, 1970
MDA Development Grant, 2150
MDA Neuromuscular Disease Research Grants, 2151
MGFA Post-Doctoral Research Fellowships, 2183
MGFA Student Fellowships, 2184
NAF Fellowships, 2230
NAF Kyle Bryant Translational Research Award, 2231
NAF Research Grants, 2232
NAF Young Investigator Awards, 2233
Osserman-Sosin Postdoctoral Myasthenia Gravis Research Fellowships, 2974
Viets Medical Student Myasthenia Gravis Research Fellowships, 3496

Neuropharmacology

Grass Fndn Marine Biological Laboratory Fellowships, 1648
NIDA Drug Addiction Neuroscience Research Grants, 2503

Neurophysiology

Grass Fndn Marine Biological Laboratory Fellowships, 1648
Learning and Behavioral Disorders Research Grants, 2039
TSA Research Grant Awards, 3442

Neuroscience

Alfred P. Sloan Fndn Research Fellowships, 353
Children's Medical Research Institute Grants, 1000
Dana Fndn Science and Health Grants, 1197
Deafness Research Fndn Research Grants, 1208
Dorothy Rider Pool Health Care Grants, 1322
EF Predoctoral Research Training Fellowship, 1383
Fndn for Psychocultural Research Postdoctoral Fellowships, 1531
Grass Fndn Marine Biological Laboratory Fellowships, 1648
Gruber Fndn International Prizes, 1672
HIV/AIDS Research Training Fellowship, 1782
Klingenstein Neuroscience Fellowships, 2005
Marine Biological Laboratory Summer Research Fellowships, 2108
MNI Jeanne Timmins Fellowships, 2212
NCI/NIDA Transdisciplinary Tobacco Use Research Centers Grants, 2280
NIA Vulnerable Dendrites and Synapses in Aging and Alzheimer's Disease Grants, 2440
NIDA Drug Addiction Neuroscience Research Grants, 2503
NIDA Microarray-Based Research on Drug Abuse, 2508
NIDA Minority Institutions Drug Abuse Research Development Program (MIDARP) Grants, 2509
NIGMS Molecular Pharmacology of Anesthetic Action Research Grants, 2621
NIGMS Predoctoral Training in Bioinformatics and Computation Biology Grants, 2625
NIH Human Brain Project Phase I & II, 2672
NIH Mouse Mutagenesis and Phenotyping: Nervous System and Behavior Research Grants, 2693
NIH Pathological Gambling: Basic, Clinical, and Services Research Grants, 2702
NIH Research on Sleep and Sleep Disorders, 2713
NIMH Curriculum Development Award in Neuroinformatics Research and Analysis, 2754
NIMH HIV/AIDS, Severe Mental Illness, and Homelessness Research Grants, 2757
NIMH Interdisciplinary Behavioral Science Centers for Mental Health, 2759
NIMH Jointly Sponsored Ruth L. Kirschstein National Research Service Award Institutional Predoctoral Training Program in the Neurosciences, 2761
NIMH Minority Research Infrastructure Support Grants, 2763
NIMH Quantitative Approaches to the Analysis of Complex Biological Systems, 2767
NIMH Short Courses in Neuroinformatics, 2769
NIMH Silvio O. Conte Centers for Neuroscience Research Grants, 2771
NINDS Specialized Neuroscience Research Programs on Health Disparity: HIV and the Nervous System, 2785
NMSS Harry Weaver Neuroscience Scholar Awards, 2843
NSF Behavioral Neurosciences Research Grants, 2876
Oracle Corp Contributions Grants, 2951
Rosalinde and Arthur Gilbert Fndn/AFAR New Investigator Awards in Alzheimer's Disease, 3187
Searle Scholars Grants, 3275
Smith Family New Investigator Awards, 3299
Society of Neuroscience Minority Fellowships, 3345

Neurosurgery

AANS Neurosurgery Research and Education Fndn Young Clinician Investigator Award, 142
AANS Neurosurgery Research and Education Fndn/ Spine Section Young Clinician Investigator Award, 143
American College of Surgeons and The Triological Society Clinical Scientist Development Awards, 422
American College of Surgeons Resident and Associate Society (RAS-ACS) Leadership Scholarships, 431
EF Research and Training Fellowships for Clinicians, 1384
MNI Jeanne Timmins Fellowships, 2212

Neurotology
ANS Neurotology Fellows Award, 482
ANS Nicholas Torok Vestibular Award, 483
ANS Trainee Award, 484

Neurotransmitters
EF Health Sciences Student Fellowships, 1380
NIA Research Grants on Chemical Senses: Neurotransmitters and Neuromodulators, 2430
NIDCD Research Grants on Chemical Senses: Neurotransmitters and Neuromodulators, 2530

New Independent States
Hamlet Trust Grants, 1689

New Zealand
American College of Surgeons Australia and New Zealand Chapter Travelling Fellowships, 423

Noise Pollution
San Diego Fndn for Change Grants, 3255

Nonfiction
CFPC Special Recognition Awards, 957
NLM Grants for Scholarly Works in Biomedicine and Health, 2818
Quantum Corp Snap Server Grants, 3095

Nonprofit Organizations
Altman Fndn Health Care Grants, 372
Battle Creek Comm Fndn Grants, 703
Chicago Comm Trust Grants, 989
Comm Fndn for Southeastern Michigan Grants, 1094
Comm Fndn of Broward Grants, 1100
Comm Fndn of Grant County Grants, 1104
Comm Fndn of Morgan County Grants and Scholarships, 1118
Comm Fndn of St. Joseph County Special Project Challenge Grants, 1126
Denver Fndn Comm Grants, 1227
Dyson Fndn Mid-Hudson Valley General Operating Support Grants, 1354
Frey Fndn Grants, 1562
Frist Fndn Grants, 1563
Great-West Life Grants, 1649
Greater Green Bay Comm Fndn Grants, 1652
Greater New Orleans Fndn Grants, 1654
Helen Bader Fndn Grants, 1738
Hilton Head Island Fndn Grants, 1779
Jessie Smith Noyes Fndn Grants, 1920
M.J. Murdock Charitable Trust Grants, 2095
Maine Comm Fndn Grants, 2099
Meyer Fndn Grants, 2177
Middlesex Savings Charitable Fndn Grants, 2196
Morris and Gwendolyn Cafritz Fndn Grants, 2217
Nina Mason Pulliam Charitable Trust Grants, 2776
NWHF Health Advocacy Small Grants, 2905
NWHF Kaiser Permanente Comm Fund Grants, 2906
Otto Bremer Fndn Grants, 2977
Rhode Island Fndn Grants, 3154
Richard King Mellon Fndn Grants, 3161
Rockefeller Archive Center Research Grants, 3178
RRF Organizational Capacity Building Grants, 3194
San Francisco Fndn Comm Health Grants, 3260
Shaw's Supermarkets Donations, 3280
Verizon Fndn Virginia Grants, 3492
Z. Smith Reynolds Fndn Small Grants, 3557

Nuclear Medicine
SNM PDEF Mickey Williams Minority Student Scholarships, 3302
SNM Pilot Research Grants, 3303
SNM Pilot Research Grants in Nuclear Medicine/ Molecular Imaging, 3304
SNM Student Fellowship Awards, 3306
SNM Tetalman Memorial Young Investigator Awards, 3307
SNM/ Covidien Seed Grant in Molecular Imaging/ Nuclear Medicine Research, 3308
SNMTS Clinical Advancement Scholarships, 3309
SNMTS Outstanding Educator Awards, 3310
SNMTS Outstanding Technologist Awards, 3311
SNMTS Paul Cole Scholarships, 3312

Nuclear Receptors
NIA Role of Nuclear Receptors in Tissue and Organismal Aging Grants, 2432

Nuclear Sciences
Canada Graduate Scholarships and NSERC Postgraduate Scholarships, 845

Nuclear Weapons
DOE Environmental Remediation Grants, 1297
NIEHS Hazmat Training at Doe Nuclear Weapons Complex Grants, 2600

Nuclear/Radioactive Waste Disposal
NIEHS Hazmat Training at Doe Nuclear Weapons Complex Grants, 2600

Nucleic Acids
NSF Biomolecular Systems Cluster Grants, 2880

Nurse Practitioners
AACN Clinical Inquiry Fund Grants, 56
AACN End of Life/Palliative Care Small Projects Grants, 59
AACN-Sigma Theta Tau Critical Care Grant, 65
NAPNAP Fndn Elaine Gelman Scholarship, 2235
NAPNAP Fndn McNeil PNP Scholarships, 2239
NAPNAP Fndn McNeil Rural and Underserved Scholarships, 2240
NAPNAP Fndn Nursing Research Grants, 2241
NAPNAP Fndn Reckitt Benckiser Student Scholarship, 2242

Nursing
AACN Clinical Practice Grants, 57
AACN Critical Care Grants, 58
AACN Evidence-Based Clinical Practice Grants, 60
AACN Mentorship Grant, 61
AACN Physio-Control Small Projects Grants, 62
AACN-Edwards Lifesciences Nurse-Driven Clinical Practice Outcomes Grants, 63
AACN-Philips Medical Systems Clinical Outcomes Grants, 64
AAHN Grant for Historical Research, 126
AAHN Pre-Doctoral Research Grant, 127
Abington Fndn Grants, 184
ACS Doctoral Scholarships in Cancer Nursing, 212
Alice Fisher Society Fellowships, 356
American Academy of Nursing Building Academic Geriatric Nursing Capacity Scholarships, 414
American Academy of Nursing Claire M. Fagin Fellowships, 415
American Academy of Nursing Mayday Fund Grants, 416
American Academy of Nursing MBA Scholarships, 417
American Academy of Nursing Media Awards, 418
Anthem Blue Cross and Blue Shield School Nurse Grants, 489
ASPEN C. Richard Fleming Grant, 629
ASPEN Douglas Wilmore Grant, 630
ASPEN Maurice Shils Grant, 633
ASPEN Norman Yoshimura Grant, 634
ASPEN Nutrition Research Grants, 635
AVDF Health Care Grants, 673
Brookdale Fndn Leadership in Aging Fellowships, 805
CampusRN/AACN Nursing Scholarship Fund, 841
Canadian Nurses Fndn Study Awards, 852
Christy-Houston Fndn Grants, 1008
CLA Nurses Respiratory Society Fellowships, 1018
CLA Nurses Respiratory Society Nursing Research Grants, 1019
Clarian Health Scholarships for LPNs, 1026
Deland Fellowships in Health Care and Society, 1214
DHHS National Health Service Corps Loan Repayment Awards, 1265
DHHS Native American Indian Health Service Loan Repayment Awards, 1267
DHHS Professional Nurse Traineeships Program, 1274
Dr. Sydney Segal Research Grants, 1331
EF Behavioral Sciences Student Fellowships, 1379
EF Predoctoral Research Training Fellowship, 1383
Hazel Corbin/Maternity Center Association Grant for Evidence-Based Midwifery Care, 1720
HRSA Nurse Anesthetist Traineeships Program, 1808
HRSA Nursing Education Opportunities for the Disadvantaged Project Grants, 1809
Independence Blue Cross Nurse Scholars Program, 1847
Independence Blue Cross Nursing Internships, 1848
Indiana Nursing Scholarships, 1853
International Oncology Nursing Fellowships, 1862
Jenkins Fndn: Improving the Health of Greater Richmond Grants, 1915
Joseph and Luella Abell Charitable Trust Scholarships, 1958
Kaiser Permanente Cares for Communities Grants, 1978
L. A. Hollinger Respiratory Therapy and Nursing Scholarships, 2018
Leadership in Education in Neurodevelopmental Disabilities Postdoctoral Fellowships, 2037
Lillian Sholtis Brunner Summer Fellowships for Historical Research in Nursing, 2057
Mayday Fund Grants, 2139
MDBDF Agnes Higgins Award, 2155
Medical/Nursing Education, Research, and Health Care Exchanges with Taiwan, 2165
NAPNAP Fndn Innovative Health Care Small Grant, 2237
NAPNAP Fndn McNeil Grant-in-Aid, 2238
NAPNAP Fndn Nursing Research Grants, 2241
NCI Stages of Breast Development: Normal to Metastatic Disease Grants, 2278
NFID New Investigator Matching Grants, 2310
NINR Acute and Chronic Care During Mechanical Ventilation Research Grants, 2788
NINR Aging Women and Breast Cancer Grants, 2789
NINR Career Transition Award, 2791
NINR Clinical Trials: Collaborations for Nursing Research, 2794
NINR Mentored Research Scientist Development Award, 2798
NINR Nursing National Research Service Awards—Individuals, 2799
NINR Nursing Research Exploratory Center Grants, 2800
NINR Opportunities in Genetics and Nursing Research Grants, 2801
NINR Ruth L. Kirschstein National Research Service Award for Individual Predoctoral Fellows in Nursing Research, 2804
NINR/NHGRI Nursing and Genetics Research Individual Postdoctoral and Senior Fellowships, 2806
NWHF Partners Investing in Nursing's Future Grants, 2908
ONF Small Grants, 2947
ONS Major Research Grants, 2949
Pfizer Fndn Health Literacy Grants, 3026
PhRMA Fndn Health Outcomes Post Doctoral Fellowships, 3031
Prospect Burma Scholarships, 3085
Rehabilitation Nursing Fndn Research Grants, 3147
RWJF Executive Nurse Fellowships, 3210
RWJF Interdisciplinary Nursing Quality Research Initiative, 3219
RWJF New Careers in Nursing Scholarships, 3224
RWJF Partners Investing in Nursing's Future Grants, 3226
RWJF Summer Medical and Dental Education Program, 3231
Sid W. Richardson Fndn Grants, 3284
Special Olympics Health Professions Student Grants, 3355

STTI Doris Bloch Research Awards, 3389
STTI Emergency Nurses Association Fndn Grant, 3390
STTI Environment of Elder Care Nursing Research Grants, 3391
STTI Joan K. Stout RN Research Grants, 3392
STTI National League for Nursing Grants, 3393
STTI Rosemary Berkel Crisp Research Awards, 3394
STTI Small Grants, 3395
STTI Virginia Henderson Clinical Research Grants, 3396
STTI/Council for the Advancement of Nursing Science Grants, 3398
Trinity Lutheran School of Nursing Alumnae Scholarships, 3439
University of Calgary Nursing Alumni Scholarship, 3468
VDH Commonwealth of Virginia Nurse Educator Scholarships, 3482
Virginia Department of Health Mary Marshall Nursing Scholarships for Licensed Practical Nurses, 3498
Virginia Department of Health Mary Marshall Nursing Scholarships for Registered Nurses, 3499
Virginia Department of Health Nurse Practitioner/ Nurse Midwife Scholarships, 3500

Nursing Education
AAOHN Fndn Experienced Researcher Grants, 153
AAOHN Fndn New Investigator Researcher Grants, 154
AAOHN Fndn Professional Development Scholarships, 155
Abell-Hanger Fndn Grants, 183
Ahmanson Fndn Grants, 303
American Academy of Nursing Building Academic Geriatric Nursing Capacity Scholarships, 414
American Academy of Nursing Claire M. Fagin Fellowships, 415
American Academy of Nursing Mayday Fund Grants, 416
American Academy of Nursing MBA Scholarships, 417
Bertha Russ Lytel Fndn Grants, 751
Burlington Industries Fndn Grants, 811
CampusRN/AACN Nursing Scholarship Fund, 841
Clarian Health OR Internships, 1025
Clarian Health Scholarships for LPNs, 1026
Clarian Health Student Nurse Extern Scholarships, 1027
Daphne Seybolt Culpeper Memorial Fndn Grants, 1201
DHHS Health Professions Training in Geriatrics Grants, 1259
DHHS Professional Nurse Traineeships, 1274
Dr. Scholl Fndn Grants, 1329
E. Rhodes and Leona B. Carpenter Fndn Grants, 1356
Effie and Wofford Cain Fndn Grants, 1385
Health Fndn of Greater Indianapolis Grants, 1725
HRSA Health Professions Scholarships for Disadvantaged Students, 1807
HRSA Nurse Anesthetist Traineeships Program, 1808
HRSA Nursing Education Opportunities for the Disadvantaged Project Grants, 1809
Ildaura Murillo-Rohde Scholarships, 1841
Independence Blue Cross Nurse Scholars, 1847
Independence Blue Cross Nursing Internships, 1848
Indiana Nursing Scholarships, 1853
Jewish Fndn for Education of Women Scholarships for Emigres in the Health Professions, 1922
Joseph and Luella Abell Charitable Trust Scholarships, 1958
Josiah Macy Jr. Fndn Grants, 1966
L. A. Hollinger Respiratory Therapy and Nursing Scholarships, 2018
Leadership in Education in Neurodevelopmental Disabilities Postdoctoral Fellowships, 2037
Lettie Pate Whitehead Fndn Grants, 2049
Lubbock Area Fndn Grants, 2079
MDBDF Agnes Higgins Award, 2155
Medical/Nursing Education, Research, and Health Care Exchanges with Taiwan, 2165
NAPNAP Fndn Elaine Gelman Scholarship, 2235
NAPNAP Fndn Graduate Student Research Grant, 2236
NAPNAP Fndn McNeil PNP Scholarships, 2239
NAPNAP Fndn McNeil Rural and Underserved Scholarships, 2240
NAPNAP Fndn Nursing Research Grants, 2241
NAPNAP Fndn Reckitt Benckiser Student Scholarship, 2242
National Student Nurses' Association Fndn Scholarship Program, 2262
NBNA Lauranne Sams Scholarships, 2264
New York University Steinhardt School of Education Fellowships, 2305
NHLBI Short-Term Research Education Program to Increase Diversity in Health-Related Research, 2383
NIA Mentored Clinical Scientist Research Career Development Awards, 2417
NINR Nursing Research Exploratory Center Grants, 2800
NINR Ruth L. Kirschstein National Research Service Award for Individual Predoctoral Fellows in Nursing Research, 2804
ONF Career Development Awards, 2946
ONF Small Grants, 2947
ONS Scholarships, 2950
PAHO/WHO Fellowships, 2984
Rehabilitation Nursing Fndn Research Grants, 3147
Rehabilitation Nursing Fndn Scholarships, 3148
Ruth Eleanor Bamberger and John Ernest Bamberger Memorial Fndn Grants, 3202
RWJF Executive Nurse Fellowships, 3210
RWJF New Careers in Nursing Scholarships, 3224
RWJF Partners Investing in Nursing's Future Grants, 3226
Saint Luke's Health Initiatives Grants, 3240
Samuel S. Johnson Fndn Grants, 3251
San Antonio Area Fndn Grants, 3254
Stroke Association Allied Health Professional Research Bursaries, 3385
STTI Joan K. Stout RN Research Grants, 3392
STTI National League for Nursing Grants, 3393
STTI/ATI Educational Assessment Nursing Research Grants, 3397
Trinity Lutheran School of Nursing Alumnae Scholarships, 3439
VDH Commonwealth of Virginia Nurse Educator Scholarships, 3482
Virginia Department of Health Mary Marshall Nursing Scholarships for Licensed Practical Nurses, 3498
Virginia Department of Health Mary Marshall Nursing Scholarships for Registered Nurses, 3499
Virginia Department of Health Nurse Practitioner/ Nurse Midwife Scholarships, 3500

Nursing Homes
Arkell Hall Fndn Grants, 534
Burden Trust Grants, 810
CHCF Grants, 979
Health Care Financing Research, Demonstrations, and Evaluations Grants, 1723
HRSA Geriatric Education Centers, 1805
Jacob and Valeria Langeloth Fndn Grants, 1882
McLean Contributionship Grants, 2147
Robert P. & Clara I. Milton Fund for Senior Housing, 3172

Nutrition
Albertson's Charitable Giving Grants, 330
Assurant Fndn Grants, 654
Bristol-Myers Squibb/Meade Johnson Award for Distinguished Achievement in Nutrition Research, 795
Kraft Cares International Grants, 2016
MDBDF Agnes Higgins Award, 2155
Moses Cone-Wesley Long Comm Health Fndn Grants, 2219
Ruth Mott Fndn Grants, 3204

Nutrition and Physical Fitness
AMA Fndn Fund for Better Health Grants, 388

Nutrition Education
Abbott Fund Access to Health Care Grants, 176
Abbott Fund Science and Medical Innovation Grants, 179
ASPEN C. Richard Fleming Grant, 629
ASPEN Douglas Wilmore Grant, 630
ASPEN Dudrick Research Scholar Award, 631
ASPEN Harry M. Vars Award, 632
ASPEN Maurice Shils Grant, 633
ASPEN Norman Yoshimura Grant, 634
ASPEN Nutrition Research Grants, 635
ASPEN Scientific Abstracts Awards for Papers or Posters, 636
ASPEN Scientific Abstracts Promising Investigator Awards, 637
BCBS of Minnesota Healthy Together Grants, 712
BCBSM Building Healthy Communities Engaging Elementary Schools and Comm Partners Grants, 713
Coca-Cola Fndn Grants, 1052
Fargo-Moorhead Area Fndn Grants, 1454
Fndn for Seacoast Health Grants, 1533
General Mills Champions for Healthy Kids Grants, 1589
Great-West Life Grants, 1649
Greater Bridgeport Area Fndn Comm Impact Grants, 1650
Highmark Healthy High 5, 1770
Leadership in Education in Neurodevelopmental Disabilities Postdoctoral Fellowships, 2037
Perry County Comm Fndn Grants, 3016
Posey Comm Fndn Grants, 3068
Posey Comm Fndn Womens Fund Grants, 3069
Shaw's Supermarkets Donations, 3280
U.S. Department of Education 21st Century Comm Learning Centers, 3445
Vancouver Fndn Grants and Comm Initiatives Program, 3477
Wilson-Wood Fndn Grants, 3542

Nutrition/Dietetics
AAFCS International Graduate Fellowships, 109
AAFCS National Graduate Fellowships, 110
AAFCS National Undergraduate Scholarships, 111
AAP Nutrition Award, 165
Abbott Fund Science and Medical Innovation Grants, 179
Administration on Aging Senior Medicare Patrol Project Grants, 236
AFAR Research Grants, 257
ASPEN C. Richard Fleming Grant, 629
ASPEN Douglas Wilmore Grant, 630
ASPEN Dudrick Research Scholar Award, 631
ASPEN Harry M. Vars Award, 632
ASPEN Maurice Shils Grant, 633
ASPEN Norman Yoshimura Grant, 634
ASPEN Nutrition Research Grants, 635
ASPEN Scientific Abstracts Awards for Papers or Posters, 636
ASPEN Scientific Abstracts Promising Investigator Awards, 637
Beazley Fndn Grants, 730
Boeing Company Contributions Grants, 777
Boston Fndn Grants, 783
Bristol-Myers Squibb Fndn Health Disparities Grants, 797
Canadian Fndn for Dietetic Research Awards, 849
Cancer Treatment Research Fndn Clinical Investigation Grants, 861
Center for Science in Public Interest Internships, 935
Charles H. Farnsworth Trust Grants, 967
Child Nutrition Fndn School Comm Kitchens Grants, 993
Christy-Houston Fndn Grants, 1008
ConAgra Foods Fndn Grants, 1140
Connecticut Health Fndn Health Initiative Grants, 1142

Denver Fndn Comm Grants, 1227
DHHS Adolescent Family Life Demonstration Projects, 1243
DHHS Public Health Students Traineeships and Other Graduate Public Health Programs, 1277
Dietetic Outcomes Research Study Grants, 1285
Dole Food Company Charitable Contributions, 1307
Duncan L. Gordon Fellowships, 1349
EF Health Sciences Student Fellowships, 1380
Elizabeth Glaser Pediatric AIDS Fndn International Leadership Awards, 1393
Elizabeth Glaser Pediatric AIDS Fndn Operations Research Grants, 1394
Elizabeth Glaser Pediatric AIDS Fndn Two-Year International Scholar Award, 1396
FDHN Bridging Grants, 1464
FDHN Jon I. Isenberg International Research Scholar Award, 1473
FDHN Student Research Fellowships, 1480
Fndn for a Healthy Kentucky Grants, 1527
General Mills Champions for Healthy Kids Grants, 1589
General Mills Fndn Grants, 1590
Gerber Fndn Grants, 1606
H.J. Heinz Company Fndn Grants, 1682
Health Fndn of Greater Indianapolis Grants, 1725
Healthcare Fndn for Orange County Grants, 1728
Human Growth Fndn Small Grants, 1816
Leadership in Education in Neurodevelopmental Disabilities Postdoctoral Fellowships, 2037
MDBD Basic Research Grants, 2152
Medtronic Fndn Fitness and Nutrition Grants, 2167
National 4-H Healthy Lifestyles Grants, 2248
NCI Technologies and Software to Support Integrative Cancer Biology Research Grants, 2279
NHLBI Nutrition and Diet in the Causation, Prevention, and Management of Heart Failure Research Grants, 2361
NIA Malnutrition in Older Persons Research Grants, 2413
NICHD NRSAs—Individual, 2488
NICHD NRSAs—Institutional, 2489
NIDDK Diet Composition and Energy Balance Grants, 2553
NIDDK Pilot and Feasibility Clinical Research Studies in Digestive Diseases and Nutrition, 2576
NIDDK Research Grants on Improving Health Care for Obese Patients, 2581
NIDDK Small Grants for Underrepresented Minority Scientists in Diabetes and Digestive and Kidney Diseases, 2588
NIH Centers for Dietary Supplements Research: Botanicals, 2648
NIH Exploratory Centers for Alternative Medicine Research Grants, 2663
Paso del Norte Health Fndn Grants, 2995
Paul G. Allen Family Fndn Grants, 3000
Sheltering Arms Fund Grants, 3282
Soy Health Research Program Incentive Awards, 3354
Susan G. Komen Breast Cancer Fndn Basic, Clinical, and Translational Research Grants, 3407
Thrasher Research Fund Grants, 3426
United Methodist Health Ministry Fund Grants, 3465
Western Union Fndn Grants, 3529

Nutritional Diseases and Disorders

Abbott Fund Science and Medical Innovation Grants, 179
ASPEN C. Richard Fleming Grant, 629
ASPEN Douglas Wilmore Grant, 630
ASPEN Dudrick Research Scholar Award, 631
ASPEN Harry M. Vars Award, 632
ASPEN Maurice Shils Grant, 633
ASPEN Norman Yoshimura Grant, 634
ASPEN Nutrition Research Grants, 635
ASPEN Scientific Abstracts Awards for Papers or Posters, 636
ASPEN Scientific Abstracts Promising Investigator Awards, 637
FDHN Bridging Grants, 1464
FDHN Fellow Abstract Prizes, 1469
FDHN Graduate Student Awards, 1472
FDHN Jon I. Isenberg International Research Scholar Award, 1473
Leadership in Education in Neurodevelopmental Disabilities Postdoctoral Fellowships, 2037
NIDDK Exploratory/Developmental Clinical Research Grants in Obesity, 2559
NIDDK Pilot and Feasibility Clinical Research Studies in Digestive Diseases and Nutrition, 2576

Obesity

Anthem Blue Cross and Blue Shield School Nurse Grants, 489
Charles H. Hood Fndn Child Health Research Grants, 968
Dietetic Outcomes Research Study Grants, 1285
Gerber Fndn Grants, 1606
Healthcare Fndn for Orange County Grants, 1728
Horizon Fndn for New Jersey Grants, 1793
Institute for Agriculture and Trade Policy Food and Society Fellowships, 1856
Johnson & Johnson Comm Health Care Grants, 1951
Moses Cone-Wesley Long Comm Health Fndn Grants, 2219
National 4-H Healthy Lifestyles Grants, 2248
NHLBI Bioengineering and Obesity Grants, 2318
NHLBI Bioengineering Approaches to Energy Balance and Obesity Grants for SBIR, 2319
NHLBI Bioengineering Approaches to Energy Balance and Obesity Grants for STTR, 2320
NHLBI Childhood Obesity Prevention and Treatment Research Consortium Grants, 2328
NHLBI Targeted Approaches to Weight Control for Young Adults Grants, 2387
NHLBI Translating Basic Behavioral and Social Science Discoveries into Interventions to Reduce Obesity: Centers for Behavioral Intervention Development Grants, 2390
NIDDK Development of Disease Biomarkers Grants, 2549
NIDDK Education Grants, 2554
NIDDK Exploratory/Developmental Clinical Research Grants in Obesity, 2559
NIDDK Identifying and Reducing Diabetes and Obesity Related Health Disparities within Healthcare Systems, 2561
NIDDK Neuroimaging in Obesity Research Grants, 2569
NIDDK Planning Grants For Translational Research For The Prevention And Control Of Diabetes And Obesity, 2577
NIDDK Proteomics: Diabetes, Obesity, And Endocrine, Digestive, Kidney, Urologic, And Hematologic Diseases, 2578
NIDDK Research Grants on Improving Health Care for Obese Patients, 2581
NIDDK Role of Gastrointestinal Surgical Procedures in Amelioration of Obesity-Related Insulin Resistance and Diabetes Independent of Weight Loss, 2582
NIH School-based Interventions to Prevent Obesity, 2725
Northwestern Mutual Fndn Grants, 2870
Pajaro Valley Comm Health Grants, 2985
RWJF Healthy Eating Research Grants, 3218
YSA UnitedHealth Heroes Service Learning Grants, 3556

Obstetrics-Gynecology

ACOG History of American Obstetrics and Gynecology Fellowship, 207
ACS Cancer Control Career Development Awards for Primary Care Physicians, 209
Blanche and Irving Laurie Fndn Grants, 764
Charles H. Hood Fndn Child Health Research Grants, 968
DHHS Geriatric Training for Physicians and Dentists Grants, 1250
DHHS National Health Service Corps Loan Repayment Awards, 1265
Duke University Obstetric Anesthesia Fellowships, 1345
Fairlawn Fndn Grants, 1447
John S. Dunn Research Fndn Grants and Chairs, 1945

Occupational Health and Safety

AAOHN Fndn Experienced Researcher Grants, 153
AAOHN Fndn New Investigator Researcher Grants, 154
AAOHN Fndn Professional Development Scholarships, 155
California Wellness Fndn Work and Health Grants, 834
DHHS Public Health Students Traineeships and Other Graduate Public Health Programs, 1277
DOL Occupational Safety and Health—Susan Harwood Training Grants, 1305
FIC International Training and Research in Environmental and Occupational Health, 1493
Leadership in Education in Neurodevelopmental Disabilities Postdoctoral Fellowships, 2037
Ms. Fndn for Women Grants, 2222
NIAMS High Risk Arthritis and Musculoskeletal and Skin Diseases Research, 2470
NIEHS Superfund Hazardous Substances Basic Research and Education Grants, 2607
NIH Endocrine Disruptors: Epidemiologic Approaches Grants, 2658
NIH National Occupational Research Agenda Grants, 2696
NIOSH Occupational Safety and Health Research and Demonstration Grants, 2807
Pioneer Hi-Bred Comm Grants, 3051
U.S. Department of Education Erma Byrd Scholarships, 3446

Oceanography

Canada Graduate Scholarships and NSERC Postgraduate Scholarships, 845
Lindbergh Grants, 2059
Richard and Rhoda Goldman Fund Grants, 3158

Odontology

SRC Medical Research Grants, 3362

Olfaction

NIA Research Grants on Chemical Senses: Neurotransmitters and Neuromodulators, 2430
NIDCD Clinical Trial Planning Grant, 2517
NIDCD Exploratory Research: Feasibility Pilot Studies Grants, 2519
NIDCD Exploratory/Developmental Research Grants, 2520
NIDCD Minority Dissertation Research Grants in Human Communication, 2524
NIDCD Program for Postdoctoral Research Training in Clinical Trials, 2528
NIDCD Research Grants on Chemical Senses: Neurotransmitters and Neuromodulators, 2530
NIDCD Small Grants, 2531
Olfactory Research Fund Grants, 2942

Oncology

AACR Clinical and Translational Research Fellowships, 73
Abbott Fund Science and Medical Innovation Grants, 179
ACS Master's Training Grants in Clinical Oncology Social Work, 208
ACS Doctoral Training Grants in Oncology Social Work, 213
ACS Research Scholar Grants in Basic, Preclinical, Clinical and Epidemiology Research, 223
AHNS Alando J. Ballantyne Resident Research Pilot Grant, 305
AHNS Pilot Grant, 306
AHNS/AAO-HNSF Surgeon Scientist Combined Award, 307

AHNS/AAO-HNSF Young Investigator Combined Award, 308
AMA Fndn Seed Grants for Research, 398
Ann and Robert H. Lurie Family Fndn Grants, 475
ASCO Improving Cancer Care Grants, 546
ASCO State Affiliate Grants, 547
ASCO Advanced Clinical Research Award in Colorectal Cancer, 548
ASCO Advanced Clinical Research Awards in Breast Cancer, 549
ASCO Advanced Clinical Research Awards in Sarcoma, 550
ASCO Career Development Award, 551
ASCO Comm Oncology Research Grants, 552
ASCO Comparative Effectiveness Research Professorship in Breast Cancer, 553
ASCO International Development and Education Awards, 554
ASCO Loan Repayment Grants, 555
ASCO Long-Term International Fellowships, 556
ASCO Medical Student Rotation Grants, 557
ASCO Merit Awards, 558
ASCO Resident Travel Awards, 559
ASCO State Affiliate Grants, 560
ASCO Translational Research Professorships, 561
ASCO Young Investigator Award, 562
ASCO/UICC International Cancer Technology Transfer (ICRETT) Fellowships, 563
Bristol-Myers Squibb Virology and Oncology M.D. Research Fellowships, 802
C.R. Bard Fndn Grants, 825
Cancer Treatment Research Fndn Clinical Investigation Grants, 861
Genentech Corp Charitable Contributions Grants, 1588
International Oncology Nursing Fellowships, 1862
NCI Technologies and Software to Support Integrative Cancer Biology Research Grants, 2279
NCIC Terry Fox Postdoctoral Research Fellowships, 2285
ONF Career Development Awards, 2946
ONF Small Grants, 2947
ONS Major Research Grants, 2949
ONS Scholarships, 2950
STTI Rosemary Berkel Crisp Research Awards, 3394
UICC American Cancer Society International Fellowships for Beginning Investigators, 3455
UICC International Cancer Technology Transfer (ICRETT) Fellowships, 3456
UICC Raisa Gorbachev Memorial International Cancer Fellowships, 3457

Opera/Musical Theater
Adaptec Fndn Grants, 232
Bonfils-Stanton Fndn Grants, 779
Boston Fndn Grants, 783
Comm Fndn for Greater Buffalo Grants, 1090
Edward S. Moore Fndn Grants, 1374
Elizabeth McGraw Fndn Grants, 1399
George Frederick Jewett Fndn Grants, 1599
Mabel Y. Hughes Charitable Trust Grants, 2097
Rollin M. Gerstacker Fndn Grants, 3186

Operations Research
AHFMR Population Health Investigator Awards, 292

Ophthalmology
AGS Dennis W. Jahnigen Career Development Scholars Awards, 264
AHAF National Glaucoma Research Grants, 268
Alcon Fndn Grants, 336
Alice C. A. Sibley Fund Grants, 355
Dr. Stanley Pearle Scholarships, 1330
E.A. Baker Fndn for the Prevention of Blindness Grants, 1357
Fight for Sight Research Grants and Fellowships, 1503
Frederick Gardner Cottrell Fndn Grants, 1560
Joseph Alexander Fndn Grants, 1957
NEI Clinical Vision Research Development Award, 2293
NEI Vision Research Core Grants, 2300
OneSight Research Fndn Block Grants, 2944
Richmond Eye and Ear Fund Grants, 3164

Optometry
Alice C. A. Sibley Fund Grants, 355
Canadian Optometric Education Trust Fund Grants, 853
DHHS Health Careers Opportunity Grants, 1253
Dr. Stanley Pearle Scholarships, 1330
HRSA Health Professions Scholarships for Disadvantaged Students, 1807
OneSight Research Fndn Block Grants, 2944
Special Olympics Health Professions Student Grants, 3355

Oral Diseases
CDC Oral Diseases Prevention and Oral Health Promotion Grants, 921
DHHS Oral Health Promotion Research Across the Lifespan, 1269
NIDCR Clinical Trial Pilot Grant, 2533
NIDCR Clinical Trial Planning Grant, 2534
NIDCR HIV/AIDS Associated Oral Viral Infections, 2535
NIDCR Oral Microbiology/Immunology of Type 1 Diabetes, 2537
NIH Cancer Surveillance Using Health Claims-Based Data System Grants, 2645
NIH Economic Studies in Cancer Prevention, Screening, and Care, 2657
NIH Epidemiological and Behavioral Research in Oral Health, 2660

Oral Health and Hygiene
Aetna Fndn Regional Comm Health Grants, 249
CDC Oral Diseases Prevention and Oral Health Promotion Grants, 921
Connecticut Health Fndn Health Initiative Grants, 1142
DHHS Oral Health Promotion Research Across the Lifespan, 1269
Illinois Children's Healthcare Fndn Grants, 1842
NIDCR International Collaborative Oral Health Research Planning Grant, 2536
NIH Epidemiological and Behavioral Research in Oral Health, 2660
NIH Mechanisms of Orofacial Pain: Anatomy, Genomics, and Proteomics, 2684
Pajaro Valley Comm Health Grants, 2985
United Methodist Health Ministry Fund Grants, 3465

Oral-Motor Disorders
NIDCD Communicative Competence of Users of Augmentative and Alternative Communication Systems Research Grants, 2518

Orchestras
Ahmanson Fndn Grants, 303
Alcatel-Lucent Technologies Fndn Grants, 333
Barr Fund Grants, 697
Clarence E. Heller Charitable Fndn Grants, 1022
Claude Worthington Benedum Fndn Grants, 1033
Comm Fndn Alliance City of Evansville Endowment Fund Grants, 1089
Comm Fndn of the Ozarks Grants, 1130
Constantin Fndn Grants, 1145
El Paso Comm Fndn Grants, 1388
Fremont Area Comm Fndn Grants, 1561
Griffin Fndn Grants, 1670
Hearst Fndn and William Randolph Hearst Fndn Grants, 1730
Howard and Bush Fndn Grants, 1798
Kenneth T. and Eileen L. Norris Fndn Grants, 1989
Lubbock Area Fndn Grants, 2079
Salisbury Comm Fndn Grants, 3243
San Antonio Area Fndn Grants, 3254
Sid W. Richardson Fndn Grants, 3284
Walt Disney Company Fndn Grants, 3516

Organ Transplants
Carlos and Marguerite Mason Trust Grants, 875
CCFF Transplant Center Incentive Grants, 899
Fndn of CVPH Melissa Lahtinen-Penfield Organ Donor Fund Grants, 1540
NHLBI Blood Diseases and Resources Research Grants, 2322
NIAID Allergy, Immunology, and Transplantation Program Research Grants, 2449
NIAID Allergy, Immunology, Transplantation, Infectious Diseases, and AIDS NRSAs—Individual, 2450
NIH Hyperaccelerated Award/Mechanisms in Immunomodulation Trials, 2675
ONF Small Grants, 2947
Robert B McMillen Fndn Grants, 3169
Sid W. Richardson Fndn Grants, 3284

Organizational Development
NWHF Health Advocacy Small Grants, 2905
NWHF Kaiser Permanente Comm Fund Grants, 2906
Otto Bremer Fndn Grants, 2977

Organizational Theory and Behavior
Charles G. Koch Charitable Fndn Grants, 965
Jane Beattie Memorial Scholarship, 1901
NIH National Occupational Research Agenda Grants, 2696

Orphan Products
FDA Orphan Products Clinical Studies Grants, 1462

Orthopedics
AGS Dennis W. Jahnigen Career Development Scholars Awards, 264
El Paso Comm Fndn Grants, 1388
John S. Dunn Research Fndn Grants and Chairs, 1945
Musculoskeletal Rehabilitation Fellowships, 2229
NIAMS High Risk Arthritis and Musculoskeletal and Skin Diseases Research, 2470
OREF Educational Awards, 2953
OREF Orthopedic Career Development Awards, 2954
OREF Orthopedic Resident Research Awards, 2955
OREF Prospective Clinical Research Proposal Grants, 2956
OREF Research Grants, 2957
OREF/AAOS Clinical Research Training Fellowship, 2958
Osteogenesis Imperfecta Fndn Research Grants, 2975
Rett Syndrome Research Fndn Grants, 3151

Osteopathic Medicine
DHHS Health Careers Opportunity Grants, 1253
DHHS Health Education and Training Centers Project Grants, 1256
DHHS National Health Service Corps Loan Repayment Awards, 1265
DHHS Native American Health Service Loan Repayment Awards, 1267
Heart Rhythm Society Fellowships, 1731
HRSA Health Professions Scholarships for Disadvantaged Students, 1807
New Jersey Osteopathic Education Fndn Scholarships, 2303
NMF Need-Based Scholarships, 2839

Osteoporosis
Fairlawn Fndn Grants, 1447
NIAMS High Risk Arthritis and Musculoskeletal and Skin Diseases Research, 2470
NIAMS Specialized Centers of Research in Osteoporosis, Rheumatoid Arthritis, and Scleroderma, 2480
NIH Human Models and Markers of Skeletal Aging Grants, 2674
NIH Receptors and Signaling in Bone in Health and Disease, 2706
Premera CARES Grants, 3074

Otolaryngic Allergies
AAO-HNSF Health Services Research Grants, 147
AAO-HNSF Maureen Hannley Research Training Awards, 148
AAO-HNSF Percy Memorial Research Award, 149
AAO-HNSF Rande H. Lazar Health Services Research Grant, 150
AAO-HNSF Resident Research Awards, 151
AAOA Fndn/AAO-HNSF Combined Research Grants, 152

Otolaryngology
AAO-HNS Medical Student Research Prize, 144
AAO-HNS Resident Research Prizes, 145
AAO-HNSF CORE Research Grants, 146
ASPO Daiichi Innovative Technology Grant, 650
ASPO Fellowships, 651
ASPO Research Grants, 652
Richmond Eye and Ear Fund Grants, 3164
Triological Society Research Career Development Awards, 3440
Xoran Technologies Resident Research Grant, 3554

Otology
AHRF Eugene L. Derlacki, M.D. Research Grants, 309
AHRF Georgia Birtman Grant, 310
AHRF Wiley H. Harrison Memorial Research Award, 312
ANS Neurotology Fellows Award, 482
ANS Nicholas Torok Vestibular Award, 483
ANS Trainee Award, 484
ANS/AAO-HNSF Herbert Silverstein Otology and Neurotology Research Award, 485
Deafness Research Fndn Research Grants, 1208
Oticon Focus on People Awards, 2976
Triological Society Research Career Development Awards, 3440

Outpatient Care
CDC Evaluation of the Use of Rapid Testing For Influenza in Outpatient Medical Settings, 910
Erie Comm Fndn Grants, 1427

Ovarian Cancer
ASCO Career Development Award, 551
ASCO Young Investigator Award, 562
ASCO/UICC International Cancer Technology Transfer (ICRETT) Fellowships, 563

Pacific Islanders
American Sociological Association Minority Fellowships, 458
ASM Robert D. Watkins Graduate Research Fellowship, 614
FDHN Student Research Fellowships, 1480
Fulbright Traditional Scholar Program in the East Asia/Pacific Region, 1574
Max Bell Fndn Grants, 2134
NHLBI Minority Institutional Research Training Grants, 2355
NIMH Career Opportunities in Research Education and Training Honors High School Research Education Grant, 2748
NIMH Career Opportunities in Research Education and Training Honors Undergraduate Research Training Grant, 2749
SNM PDEF Mickey Williams Minority Student Scholarships, 3302

Pain
AAHPM Hospice and Palliative Medicine Fellowships, 132
APhA Fndn Incentive Grants, 512
Duke University Pain Management Fellowships, 1346
Duke University Pediatric Anesthesiology Fellowship, 1347
IAFF Burn Fndn Research Grants, 1830
Mayday Fund Grants, 2139
Musculoskeletal Rehabilitation Fellowships, 2229
NIA Mechanisms, Measurement, and Management of Pain in Aging: from Molecular to Clinical, 2415
NIDA Drug Addiction Neuroscience Research Grants, 2503
NIH Biobehavioral Pain Research Grants, 2638
NIH Mechanisms Underlying Secondary Conditions in Mobility Disorders, 2686
NIH New Directions in Pain Research Grants, 2698
NINR Management of Symptoms at the End of Life Grants, 2796
NINR Mechanisms, Models, Measurement, & Management in Pain Research Grants, 2797
NINR Quality of Life for Individuals at the End of Life Grants, 2802

Paleontology
Fyssen Fndn Postdoctoral Study Grants, 1580
NSF Systematic Biology and Biodiversity Inventories Grants, 2895

Pancreas
AACR-FNAB Fellows Grant for Translational Pancreatic Cancer Research, 94
AACR-Pancreatic Cancer Action Network Career Development Award for Pancreatic Cancer Research, 102
AACR-Pancreatic Cancer Action Network Innovative Grants, 103
FDHN Designated Research Award in Research Related to Pancreatitis, 1468
FDHN Graduate Student Awards, 1472
NIAAA Mechanisms of Alcohol and Drug-Induced Pancreatitis Grants, 2444
NIDDK Pancreatic Development and Regeneration Grants: Toward Cellular Therapies for Diabetes, 2573
NIDDK Small Business Innovation Research to Develop New Therapeutics and Monitoring Technologies for Type 1 Diabetes (T1D)—Towards an Artificial Pancreas, 2586

Pancreatic Cancer
ASCO Career Development Award, 551
ASCO Young Investigator Award, 562
ASCO/UICC International Cancer Technology Transfer (ICRETT) Fellowships, 563

Parasitology
ASM/CCID Fellowships, 627
BWF Ad Hoc Grants, 818
BWF Investigators in the Pathogenesis of Infectious Disease, 823
FIC International Malaria Research Training Program Award, 1488
NFID New Investigator Matching Grants, 2310
NIAID Microbiology and Infectious Diseases Research Grants and Contracts, 2459
US CRDF Leishmaniasis: Collaborative Research Opportunities in North Africa and the Middle East, 3474

Parent Education
A Fund for Women Grants, 14
Bender Fndn Grants, 742
Bodman Fndn Grants, 776
CDC School Health Programs to Prevent the Spread of HIV Cooperative Agreements, 928
Children's Trust Fund of Oregon Grants, 1001
Comm Fndn for Southern Arizona Grants, 1095
Comprehensive Health Education Fndn Grants, 1139
Connecticut Comm Fndn Grants, 1141
DHHS Adolescent Family Life Demonstration Projects, 1243
FCD Child Development Grants, 1458
Gerber Fndn Grants, 1606
Mary Black Fndn Grants, 2118
National Emergency Medicine Association Grants, 2252
Philadelphia Fndn Organizational Effectiveness Grants, 3029
Piper Jaffray Companies Building Strong Communities Grants, 3053
San Diego Fndn for Change Grants, 3255
Southbury Comm Trust Fund, 3350
U.S. Department of Education 21st Century Comm Learning Centers, 3445
U.S. Department of Education Special Education—National Activities—Parent Information Centers, 3450

Parent Involvement
Bella Vista Fndn Grants, 740
Bernard F. and Alva B. Gimbel Fndn Grants, 747
Bernard Van Leer Fndn Grants, 748
Bodman Fndn Grants, 776
Comm Fndn of Broward Grants, 1100
Fndn for the Carolinas Grants, 1535
GenCorp Fndn Grants, 1587
Healthcare Fndn for Orange County Grants, 1728
Kimberly-Clark Comm Grants, 2001
Northern Trust Company Charitable Trust and Corp Giving Program, 2865
Prince Charitable Trusts Chicago Grants, 3079
Pulaski County Comm Fndn Grants, 3091
Vancouver Fndn Grants and Comm Initiatives Program, 3477

Parenteral Nutrition
ASPEN C. Richard Fleming Grant, 629
ASPEN Douglas Wilmore Grant, 630
ASPEN Dudrick Research Scholar Award, 631
ASPEN Harry M. Vars Award, 632
ASPEN Maurice Shils Grant, 633
ASPEN Norman Yoshimura Grant, 634
ASPEN Nutrition Research Grants, 635
ASPEN Scientific Abstracts Awards for Papers or Posters, 636
ASPEN Scientific Abstracts Promising Investigator Awards, 637

Parenting Education
3M Fndn Grants, 11

Parkinson's Disease
Fairlawn Fndn Grants, 1447
Michael J. Fox Fndn Clinical Discovery Grants, 2190
Michael J. Fox Fndn for Parkinson's Research LEAPS Program, 2191
Michael J. Fox Fndn Parkinson's Cell Line Research Grants, 2192
NIA Symptom Management for Chronic Neurological Conditions Research Grants, 2436
NICHD Symptom Management for Chronic Neurological Conditions Research Grants, 2496
NIDCD Symptom Management for Chronic Neurological Conditions Research Grants, 2532
NIEHS/NINDS Role of the Environment in Parkinson's Disease, 2608
NIH Xenobiotics and Cell Death/Injury in Neurodegenerative Disease Research Grants, 2739
NINDS Symptom Management for Chronic Neurological Conditions Research Grants, 2787
NINR Symptom Management for Chronic Neurological Conditions Research Grants, 2805
Partnership for Cures Two Years To Cures Grants, 2992
PDF International Research Grants, 3005
PDF Postdoctoral Fellowships for Basic Scientists, 3006
PDF Postdoctoral Fellowships for Neurologists, 3007
PDF Summer Fellowships, 3008
PDF-AANF Clinician-Scientist Development Awards, 3009
PSG Mentored Clinical Research Awards, 3088

Parks
Bacon Family Fndn Grants, 679
Blackford County Comm Fndn Grants, 763
Cinergy Fndn Grants, 1013
Comm Fndn of Bloomington and Monroe County Grants, 1098

Comm Fndn of Crawford County Grants and Scholarships, 1103
Comm Fndn of Grant County Grants, 1104
Comm Fndn of Muncie and Delaware County Grants, 1120
Comm Fndn of St. Joseph County Special Project Challenge Grants, 1126
Comm Fndn of the Ozarks Grants, 1130
ConocoPhillips Fndn Grants, 1144
Del E. Webb Fndn Grants, 1213
Knox County Comm Fndn Grants, 2009
Lincoln Financial Group Fndn Grants, 2058
Lubrizol Fndn Grants, 2080
Perry County Comm Fndn Grants, 3016
Pike County Comm Fndn Grants, 3049
Prince Charitable Trusts Chicago Grants, 3079
Pulaski County Comm Fndn Grants, 3091

Pathogenesis
AHNS Alando J. Ballantyne Resident Research Pilot Grant, 305
AHNS Pilot Grant, 306
AHNS/AAO-HNSF Surgeon Scientist Combined Award, 307
AHNS/AAO-HNSF Young Investigator Combined Award, 308
ALVRE Casselberry Award, 374
ALVRE Grant, 375
ALVRE Seymour R. Cohen Award, 376
Alzheimer's Association Everyday Technologies for Alzheimer Care Research Grants, 377
Alzheimer's Association Mentored New Investigator Research Grants to Promote Diversity, 379
Alzheimer's Association Molecular Imaging Grants, 380
Alzheimer's Association New Investigator Research Grants to Promote Diversity, 382
Alzheimer's Association Senator Mark Hatfield Award, 383
Alzheimer's Association Zenith Fellows Awards, 384
Alzheimer's Association Conference Grants, 385
ASM Maurice Hilleman/Merck Award, 605
BWF Ad Hoc Grants, 818
BWF Investigators in the Pathogenesis of Infectious Disease, 823
DSO Controlling Pathogen Evolution Workshop Grants, 1334
Elizabeth Glaser Pediatric AIDS Fndn International Leadership Awards, 1393
Elizabeth Glaser Pediatric AIDS Fndn Operations Research Grants, 1394
Elizabeth Glaser Pediatric AIDS Fndn Two-Year International Scholar Award, 1396
NIA Alzheimer's Disease Core Centers Grants, 2395
NIAAA Hepatitis C Infection and Alcoholic Liver Disease, 2442
NIAID Preparedness against Illegitimate Use of Bacterial Pathogens, 2461
NIAMS Molecular Pathogenesis and New Interventions in Scleroderma, 2473
NIDCR HIV/AIDS Associated Oral Viral Infections, 2535
NIH Collaborations for Advanced Strategies in Complication of HIV Infection, 2651
NIH Hyperaccelerated Award/Mechanisms in Immunomodulation Trials, 2675
NIH Small Business Innovation Research: Animal Models of HCV Infection Research Grants, 2728
Tourette Syndrome Association Post-Doc Fellowships, 3432
Tourette Syndrome Association Research Grants, 3433

Pathology
AHAF Alzheimer's Disease Research Grants, 266
CIIT Postdoctoral Fellowships, 1012
Deafness Research Fndn Research Grants, 1208
Joseph Drown Fndn Grants, 1960
Marine Biological Laboratory Summer Research Fellowships, 2108
NIDCR HIV/AIDS Associated Oral Viral Infections, 2535
NIH Impact of HAART on HIV/CNS Disease, 2676
NIH Midcareer Investigator Award in Mouse Pathobiology Research Grants, 2690
NIH Multidisciplinary Approach for Research on Oral Complications of HIV Infection, 2694
NIH Xenobiotics and Cell Death/Injury in Neurodegenerative Disease Research Grants, 2739
NYAM Edward N. Gibbs Memorial Lecture and Award in Nephrology, 2912
PhRMA Fndn Pharmacology/Toxicology Post Doctoral Fellowships, 3044
PhRMA Fndn Pharmacology/Toxicology Sabbatical Fellowships, 3047
Simone and Cino del Duca Grand Prix Awards, 3288
UICC Raisa Gorbachev Memorial International Cancer Fellowships, 3457
UK Fndn for the Study of Infant Deaths Grants, 3459

Pathophysiology
AHNS Alando J. Ballantyne Resident Research Pilot Grant, 305
AHNS Pilot Grant, 306
AHNS/AAO-HNSF Surgeon Scientist Combined Award, 307
AHNS/AAO-HNSF Young Investigator Combined Award, 308
ALVRE Casselberry Award, 374
ALVRE Grant, 375
ALVRE Seymour R. Cohen Award, 376
CFF Clinical Research Grants, 942
NIAMS/NICHD Deep Infections of Total Joint Replacements, 2481
NIDDK Type 2 Diabetes in the Pediatric Population Research Grants, 2593
NIH Human Models and Markers of Skeletal Aging Grants, 2674
NIH National Occupational Research Agenda Grants, 2696
NIH Rett Syndrome: Genetics, Pathophysiology, and Biomarkers Research Grants, 2715
Tourette Syndrome Association Post-Doc Fellowships, 3432
Tourette Syndrome Association Research Grants, 3433

Patient Care and Education
AACN Physio-Control Small Projects Grants, 62
AAFP Fndn Joint Grants, 113
AMA Fndn Health Literacy Grants, 389
AMSSM Fndn Research Grants, 469
APA Young Investigator Grant Program, 502
AVDF Health Care Grants, 673
Becton Dickinson and Company Grants, 736
BWF Clinical Scientist Awards in Translational Research, 821
BWF Institutional Program Unifying Population and Laboratory Based Sciences, 822
Canadian Patient Safety Institute Patient Safety Studentships, 854
Carlos and Marguerite Mason Trust Grants, 875
CCFF Clinic Incentive Grants, 892
CLF Operating Grants, 1039
DHHS Project Grants for Renovation or Construction of Nonacute Health Care Facilities, 1275
EF Research and Training Fellowships for Clinicians, 1384
Fairlawn Fndn Grants, 1447
FIC International Training and Research in Emerging Infectious Diseases Grants, 1492
Greenwall Fndn Bioethics Grants, 1665
Healthcare Fndn of New Jersey Grants, 1729
HRSA Geriatric Education Centers, 1805
Institute of Human Values in Health Care Interdisciplinary Fellowships, 1857
Jacob and Valeria Langeloth Fndn Grants, 1882
KFC Allied Health Research Grants, 1996
McCarthy Family Fndn Grants, 2141
Medtronic Fndn Health Care Grants, 2169
National Emergency Medicine Association Grants, 2252
National Patient Safety Fndn Patient Safety Research Grants, 2258
NHLBI Mentored Patient-Oriented Research Career Development Awards, 2350
NIH Enhancing Adherence to Diabetes Self-Management Behaviors, 2659
NIH Mentored Patient-Oriented Research Career Development Award, 2688
NINR Acute and Chronic Care During Mechanical Ventilation Research Grants, 2788
NINR Management of Symptoms at the End of Life Grants, 2796
NINR Nursing Research Exploratory Center Grants, 2800
NINR Quality of Life for Individuals at the End of Life Grants, 2802
Pfizer Fndn Health Literacy Grants, 3026
PhRMA Fndn Health Outcomes Research Starter Grants, 3033
Presbyterian Patient Assistance Program, 3076
Rathmann Family Fndn Grants, 3109
STTI Environment of Elder Care Nursing Research Grants, 3391

Patient/Physician Relationship
AMA Fndn Health Literacy Grants, 389
AVDF Health Care Grants, 673
Jacob and Valeria Langeloth Fndn Grants, 1882
NHLBI Midcareer Investigator Award in Patient-Oriented Research, 2353

Peace
Lewis Preston Fund for Girls Education Grants, 2052

Peace/Disarmament
Donald and Sylvia Robinson Family Fndn Grants, 1310
Jewish Comm Fndn of Greater Los Angeles Grants, 1921
S.H. Cowell Fndn Grants, 3237

Pediatrics
1976 Fndn Grants, 5
AACAP Robert Cancro Academic Leadership Award, 50
AACR Career Development Awards for Pediatric Cancer Research, 70
AAP Anne E. Dyson Child Advocacy Awards, 156
AAP Comm Access To Child Health Advocacy Training Grants, 157
AAP Comm Access To Child Health Implementation Grants, 158
AAP Comm Access to Child Health Planning Grants, 159
AAP Comm Access To Child Health Residency Training Grants, 160
AAP Comm Access To Child Health Resident Grants, 161
AAP Legislative Conference Scholarships, 163
AAP Leonard P. Rome Comm Access to Child Health Visiting Professorships, 164
AAP Nutrition Award, 165
AAP Resident Initiative Fund Grants, 167
AAP Resident Research Grants, 168
AcademyHealth Nemours Child Health Services Research Awards, 194
ACS Cancer Control Career Development Awards for Primary Care Physicians, 209
Alexander and Margaret Stewart Trust Grants, 340
American Philosophical Society Daland Fellowships in Clinical Investigation, 441
APA Young Investigator Grant Program, 502
ASPO Daiichi Innovative Technology Grant, 650
ASPO Fellowships, 651
ASPO Research Grants, 652
Blowitz-Ridgeway Fndn Grants, 767
CFF First- and Second-Year Clinical Fellowships, 943
CFF Leroy Matthews Physician-Scientist Awards, 944

Charles H. Hood Fndn Child Health Research Grants, 968
Children's Brain Tumor Fndn Research Grants, 998
Children's Medical Research Institute Grants, 1000
Children's Cardiomyopathy Fndn Research Grants, 1002
DHHS Adolescent Family Life Demonstration Projects, 1243
DHHS National Health Service Corps Loan Repayment Awards, 1265
DHHS Residency Training in Family Practice, General Internal Medicine, or General Pediatrics Grants, 1278
Duncan L. Gordon Fellowships, 1349
EF Research and Training Fellowships for Clinicians, 1384
Elizabeth Glaser Pediatric AIDS Fndn International Leadership Awards, 1393
Elizabeth Glaser Pediatric AIDS Fndn Operations Research Grants, 1394
Elizabeth Glaser Pediatric AIDS Fndn Pediatric HIV Vaccine Research Grants, 1395
Elizabeth Glaser Pediatric AIDS Fndn Two-Year International Scholar Award, 1396
Elizabeth Glaser Pediatric AIDS Fndn Two-Year Scholar Awards, 1397
Elizabeth Glaser Scientist Award, 1398
Fellowships in Infectious Diseases, 1485
Fuji Film Grants, 1565
Gerber Fndn Grants, 1606
Health Fndn of Greater Indianapolis Grants, 1725
Hearst Fndn and William Randolph Hearst Fndn Grants, 1730
HHS Children's Hospitals Graduate Medical Education Payment Program, 1767
HRSA Emergency Medical Services for Children Grants, 1804
Leadership in Education in Neurodevelopmental Disabilities Postdoctoral Fellowships, 2037
Lowe Fndn Grants, 2067
M. Bastian Family Fndn Grants, 2092
Mary S. and David C. Corbin Fndn Grants, 2122
Mayday Fund Grants, 2139
MedImmune Charitable Grants, 2166
NAPNAP Fndn Elaine Gelman Scholarship, 2235
NAPNAP Fndn Graduate Student Research Grant, 2236
NAPNAP Fndn Innovative Health Care Small Grant, 2237
NAPNAP Fndn McNeil Grant-in-Aid, 2238
NAPNAP Fndn McNeil PNP Scholarships, 2239
NAPNAP Fndn McNeil Rural and Underserved Scholarships, 2240
NAPNAP Fndn Nursing Research Grants, 2241
NAPNAP Fndn Reckitt Benckiser Student Scholarship, 2242
NHLBI Pediatric Cardiac Genomics Consortium Grants, 2364
NIAID HIV Prevention Trial Units Grants, 2453
NIAID HIV Vaccine Clinical Trial Units Grants, 2454
NIAID Pediatric Clinical Trials Program for AIDS, 2460
NIAMS Mechanisms of Chondroprotection Research Grants, 2472
NICHD Clinical Trial Planning Grants for Pediatric Rehabilitation, 2483
NIDCD Neurobiology and Genetics of Autism Grants, 2526
NIDDK Planning Grants For Translational Research For The Prevention And Control Of Diabetes And Obesity, 2577
NIDDK Type 2 Diabetes in the Pediatric Population Research Grants, 2593
NYAM Brock Lecture, Award and Visiting Professorship in Pediatrics, 2909
OneSight Research Fndn Block Grants, 2944
Partnership for Pediatric Epilepsy Research Grants, 2993
Peabody Fndn Grants, 3010
Pediatric Brain Tumor Research Grants, 3012
Pediatric Cancer Research Fndn Grants, 3013
Regenstrief General Internal Medicine - General Pediatrics Research Fellowship Program, 3144
Saint Luke's Health Initiatives Grants, 3240
STTI Rosemary Berkel Crisp Research Awards, 3394
Thrasher Research Fund Grants, 3426

Penology/Correctional Institutions and Procedures

Baptist Comm Ministries Grants, 691
Caddock Fndn Grants, 828
Cambridge Comm Fndn Grants, 837
CDC Hepatitis Education for Inmates and Correctional Staff Grants, 911
Fndn for the Carolinas Grants, 1535

Peptides

NIAAA Peptide Regulation of Alcohol Intake, 2447
Ralph F. Hirschmann Award in Peptide Chemistry, 3105

Performance Art

George S. and Dolores Dore Eccles Fndn Grants, 1602
Southbury Comm Trust Fund, 3350

Performing Arts

Adaptec Fndn Grants, 232
AEGON Transamerica Fndn Grants, 243
Agnes Gund Fndn Grants, 262
Aladdin Industries Fndn Grants, 322
Alcatel-Lucent Technologies Fndn Grants, 333
Alexis Gregory Fndn Grants, 349
Amgen Fndn Grants, 467
AMI Semiconductors Corp Grants, 468
Andersen Fndn Grants, 471
Arizona Public Service Corp Giving Grants, 531
Arlington Comm Fndn Grants, 536
Atlanta Fndn Grants, 662
Autzen Fndn Grants, 672
Avon Products Fndn Grants, 675
Bildner Family Fndn Grants, 755
Blue Mountain Comm Fndn Grants, 769
Bodenwein Public Benevolent Fndn Grants, 775
Boeing Company Contributions Grants, 777
Booth-Bricker Fund Grants, 780
Bruce and Adele Greenfield Fndn Grants, 808
Burlington Northern Santa Fe Fndn Grants, 812
Carl and Lily Pforzheimer Fndn Grants, 868
Carnahan-Jackson Fndn Grants, 878
Cass County Comm Fndn Grants, 887
Cemala Fndn Grants, 933
Charles Delmar Fndn Grants, 963
Charles M. Bair Family Trust Grants, 972
Colorado Springs Comm Trust Fund Grants, 1061
Compass Bank Fndn Grants, 1138
Connecticut Comm Fndn Grants, 1141
ConocoPhillips Fndn Grants, 1144
Cowles Charitable Trust Grants, 1155
Cudd Fndn Grants, 1171
Cullen Fndn Grants, 1172
D.F. Halton Fndn Grants, 1181
Davis Family Fndn Grants, 1204
Delta Air Lines Fndn Grants, 1220
DeMatteis Family Fndn Grants, 1221
DeRoy Testamentary Fndn Grants, 1239
Donald and Sylvia Robinson Family Fndn Grants, 1310
E. Rhodes and Leona B. Carpenter Fndn Grants, 1356
EIF Comm Grants, 1386
Elizabeth McGraw Fndn Grants, 1399
Elizabeth Morse Genius Charitable Trust Grants, 1400
Eugene B. Casey Fndn Grants, 1433
Eugene M. Lang Fndn Grants, 1434
Fan Fox and Leslie R. Samuels Fndn Grants, 1451
FirstEnergy Fndn Comm Grants, 1505
Flinn Fndn Grants Programs, 1511
G.N. Wilcox Trust Grants, 1581
General Mills Fndn Grants, 1590
Georgia Power Fndn Grants, 1603
Giant Eagle Fndn Grants, 1611
Grand Rapids Area Comm Fndn Grants, 1645
Grand Rapids Area Comm Fndn Nashwauk Area Endowment Fund Grants, 1646
Griffin Fndn Grants, 1670
Herman Goldman Fndn Grants, 1753
High Meadow Fndn Grants, 1768
Howard and Bush Fndn Grants, 1798
James M. Cox Fndn of Georgia Grants, 1892
James S. Copley Fndn Grants, 1895
John I. Smith Charities Grants, 1935
Kelvin and Eleanor Smith Fndn Grants, 1986
King Pharmaceuticals Corp Contributions Grants, 2003
Kraft Cares International Grants, 2016
Lubrizol Fndn Grants, 2080
Lucile Horton Howe and Mitchell B. Howe Fndn Grants, 2081
Mabel Y. Hughes Charitable Trust Grants, 2097
Margaret L. Wendt Fndn Grants, 2104
McKesson Fndn Grants, 2145
McLean Contributionship Grants, 2147
Morris and Gwendolyn Cafritz Fndn Grants, 2217
Nicholas H. Noyes Jr. Memorial Fndn Grants, 2497
Northwestern Mutual Fndn Grants, 2870
PacifiCorp Fndn for Learning Grants, 2982
Paul G. Allen Family Fndn Grants, 3000
Piedmont Natural Gas Grants, 3048
Powell Fndn Grants, 3073
Principal Financial Group Fndn Grants, 3082
Rainbow Fund Grants, 3103
Rayonier Fndn Grants, 3111
Rhode Island Fndn Grants, 3154
Rich Fndn Grants, 3156
Schurz Communications Fndn Grants, 3271
Sid W. Richardson Fndn Grants, 3284
Society for the Arts in Healthcare Consulting Grants, 3326
Sosland Fndn Grants, 3348
Sprague Fndn Grants, 3359
Temple-Inland Fndn Grants, 3419
W. C. Griffith Fndn Grants, 3505
William G. Gilmore Fndn Grants, 3537
Winifred & Harry B. Allen Fndn Grants, 3543

Perinatal Disorders

Charles H. Hood Fndn Child Health Research Grants, 968
HRSA Eliminating Disparities in Perinatal Health Grants, 1803
NIEHS Applied Toxicological Research and Testing Grants, 2595
United Cerebral Palsy Research Grants, 3462

Periodontal Disorders

ADA Fndn Dental Literature Grants, 229
Pajaro Valley Comm Health Grants, 2985

Periodontics

DHHS Oral Health Promotion Research Across the Lifespan, 1269

Personnel Training and Development

AHFMR Personnel Funding Grants, 290
Charlotte County (FL) Comm Fndn Grants, 973
Children Affected by AIDS Fndn Camp Network Grants, 994
Claude Worthington Benedum Fndn Grants, 1033
Dept of Ed Special Education—Personnel Development to Improve Services and Results for Children with Disabilities, 1231
FIC/NIH AIDS International Training and Research Program, 1496

Pesticides

Clarence E. Heller Charitable Fndn Grants, 1022

Petroleum Science

ExxonMobil Grants, 1442
NSF-NIST Interaction in Chemistry, Materials Research, Molecular Biosciences, Bioengineering, and Chemical Engineering, 2897

Pharmaceuticals

American Chemical Society GCI Pharmaceutical Roundtable Research Grants, 420
APhA Fndn Incentive Grants, 512
Campbell Hoffman Fndn Grants, 840
Food, Pharmaceutical, and Bioengineering Division Award in Chemical Engineering, 1521
Hawaii Comm Fndn Health Education and Research Grants, 1716
Millipore/Charles P. Schaufus Parenteral-Processing Technology Research Grant, 2204
NIAID Challenge Grants: Joint Ventures in Biomedicine and Biotechnology, 2451
NSF Chemistry Research Experiences for Undergraduates, 2883
PhRMA Fndn Health Outcomes Post Doctoral Fellowships, 3031
PhRMA Fndn Health Outcomes Research Starter Grants, 3033
PhRMA Fndn Informatics Post Doctoral Fellowships, 3036
PhRMA Fndn Pharmaceutics Postdoctoral Fellowships, 3040
PhRMA Fndn Pharmaceutics Pre Doctoral Fellowships, 3041
PhRMA Fndn Pharmaceutics Research Starter Grants, 3042
PhRMA Fndn Pharmaceutics Sabbatical Fellowships, 3043
Society of Cosmetic Chemists Allan B. Black Award Sponsored by Presperse, 3328
Society of Cosmetic Chemists Award Sponsored by McIntyre Group, Ltd., 3329
Society of Cosmetic Chemists Award Sponsored by The HallStar Company, 3330
Society of Cosmetic Chemists Chapter Best Speaker Award, 3331
Society of Cosmetic Chemists Chapter Merit Award, 3332
Society of Cosmetic Chemists Frontier of Science Award, 3333
Society of Cosmetic Chemists Hans Schaeffer Award, 3334
Society of Cosmetic Chemists Joseph P. Ciaudelli Award, 3335
Society of Cosmetic Chemists Keynote Award Lecture Sponsored by Ruger Chemical Corp, 3336
Society of Cosmetic Chemists Literature Award, 3337
Society of Cosmetic Chemists Maison G. de Navarre Medal, 3338
Society of Cosmetic Chemists Merit Award, 3339
Society of Cosmetic Chemists Robert A. Kramer Lifetime Service Award, 3340
Society of Cosmetic Chemists Shaw Mudge Award, 3341
Society of Cosmetic Chemists Student Poster Awards, 3342
Society of Cosmetic Chemists Young Scientist Awards, 3343
SRC Medical Research Grants, 3362
Staney Fndn Treatment Trials for Schizophrenia and Bipolar Disorder, 3374

Pharmacogenomics

NIGMS Pharmacogenomics Research Network Grants, 2623

Pharmacology

AAAAI Summer Clinical Research Fellowship Medical Student Grants, 27
AAAAI Summer Research Fellowship Medical Student Grants, 28
AHAF Alzheimer's Disease Research Grants, 266
AHAF National Glaucoma Research Grants, 268
APhA Fndn Incentive Grants, 512
ASM sanofi-aventis ICAAC Award, 616
ASPEN C. Richard Fleming Grant, 629
ASPEN Douglas Wilmore Grant, 630
ASPEN Maurice Shils Grant, 633
ASPEN Norman Yoshimura Grant, 634
ASPEN Nutrition Research Grants, 635
ASPET Benedict R. Lucchesi Award in Cardiac Pharmacology, 638
ASPET Bernard B. Brodie Award in Drug Metabolism, 639
ASPET Division for Drug Metabolism Early Career Achievement Award, 640
ASPET Epilepsy Research Award for Outstanding Contributions to the Pharmacology of Antiepileptic Drugs, 641
ASPET Goodman and Gilman Award in Drug Receptor Pharmacology, 642
ASPET John J. Abel Award in Pharmacology, 643
ASPET Julius Axelrod Award in Pharmacology, 644
ASPET P. B. Dews Lifetime Achievement Award for Research in Behavioral Pharmacology, 645
ASPET Paul M. Vanhoutte Award, 646
ASPET Torald Sollmann Award in Pharmacology, 647
ASPET Travel Awards, 648
ASPET-Astellas Awards in Translational Pharmacology, 649
Astellas Fndn Research Grants, 656
CDC Epidemiology and Laboratory Capacity Infectious Diseases Grants, 909
Dermatology Clinical Career Development Awards, 1235
DHHS Thimerosal Pharmacokinetics: Assessment of the Distribution, Metabolism, and Excretion, 1281
Duncan L. Gordon Fellowships, 1349
EF Health Sciences Student Fellowships, 1380
EF Predoctoral Research Training Fellowship, 1383
Ethical Research Grants and Fellowships, 1431
FDA Orphan Products Clinical Studies Grants, 1462
FDA Scientific Conferences Grants, 1463
FIC International Cooperative Biodiversity Groups Grants, 1487
FIC/NIH AIDS International Training and Research Program, 1496
Fragile X Syndrome Postdoctoral Research Fellowships Program, 1545
GPP Charles E. Culpeper Fndn Biomedical Pilot Projects Initiative Grants, 1641
Hartford Aging and Health Program Awards, 1709
Mayday Fund Grants, 2139
Millipore/Charles P. Schaufus Parenteral-Processing Technology Research Grant, 2204
NCI/NIDA Transdisciplinary Tobacco Use Research Centers Grants, 2280
NIAAA Peptide Regulation of Alcohol Intake, 2447
NIAID Microbiology and Infectious Diseases Research Grants and Contracts, 2459
NIDA Drug Addiction Neuroscience Research Grants, 2503
NIDA HIV Drug Therapy for HIV Users: Access, Adherence, Effectiveness, 2504
NIDA Mentored Clinical Scientist Research Career Development Awards, 2507
NIDA Microarray-Based Research on Drug Abuse, 2508
NIDA National Drug Abuse Treatment Clinical Trials Network, 2510
NIDA Senior Scientist Award, 2515
NIGMS Fellowships in Quantitative Biology, 2610
NIGMS Individual Postdoctoral NRSA Fellowships in Clinical Pharmacology, 2611
NIGMS Integrative and Collaborative Approaches to Research Grants, 2615
NIGMS Mentored Clinical Scientist Research Career Development Awards, 2618
NIGMS Molecular Pharmacology of Anesthetic Action Research Grants, 2621
NIGMS Pharmacogenomics Research Network Grants, 2623
NIH Alzheimer's Disease Clinical Trial Planning Grant, 2636
NIH Exploratory Centers for Alternative Medicine Research Grants, 2663
NIH Exploratory/Development Grants for Mental Health Intervention Research, 2665
NIH Impact of HAART on HIV/CNS Disease, 2676
NIH Mechanisms Underlying Individual Variations in Drug Responses, 2685
NIH Multidisciplinary Approach for Research on Oral Complications of HIV Infection, 2694
NIH Ruth L. Kirschstein National Research Service Awards for Individual Postdoctoral Fellows, 2719
NIH Targeting Research Gaps in HIV Therapeutics Research Grants, 2734
Pharmacia-ASPET Award for Experimental Therapeutics, 3028
PhRMA Fndn Health Outcomes Post Doctoral Fellowships, 3031
PhRMA Fndn Health Outcomes Pre-Doctoral Fellowships, 3032
PhRMA Fndn Health Outcomes Research Starter Grants, 3033
PhRMA Fndn Informatics Sabbatical Fellowships, 3035
PhRMA Fndn Informatics Post Doctoral Fellowships, 3036
PhRMA Fndn Informatics Pre Doctoral Fellowships, 3037
PhRMA Fndn Informatics Research Starter Grants, 3038
PhRMA Fndn Paul Calabresi Medical Student Research Fellowship, 3039
PhRMA Fndn Pharmaceutics Postdoctoral Fellowships, 3040
PhRMA Fndn Pharmaceutics Research Starter Grants, 3042
PhRMA Fndn Pharmaceutics Sabbatical Fellowships, 3043
PhRMA Fndn Pharmacology/Toxicology Post Doctoral Fellowships, 3044
PhRMA Fndn Pharmacology/Toxicology Pre Doctoral Fellowships, 3045
PhRMA Fndn Pharmacology/Toxicology Research Starter Grants, 3046
PhRMA Fndn Pharmacology/Toxicology Sabbatical Fellowships, 3047
Rett Syndrome Research Fndn Grants, 3151
Searle Scholars Grants, 3275
Sigrid Juselius Fndn Grants, 3286
Simone and Cino del Duca Grand Prix Awards, 3288
Staney Fndn Treatment Trials for Schizophrenia and Bipolar Disorder, 3374
TSA Research Grant Awards, 3442

Pharmacy

AIHP Sonnedecker Visiting Scholar Grants, 317
AIHP Thesis Support Grants, 318
Canadian Friends of Hebrew University Research and Study Grants, 850
EF Predoctoral Research Training Fellowship, 1383
Fischelis Grants for Research in the History of American Pharmacy, 1507
J.M. Long Fndn Grants, 1877
Pfizer Fndn Health Literacy Grants, 3026
PhRMA Fndn Informatics Pre Doctoral Fellowships, 3037

Pharmacy Education

Amarillo Area/Harrington Fndns Grants, 410
CPhA Centennial Award, 1156
DHHS Health Careers Opportunity Grants, 1253
HRSA Health Professions Scholarships for Disadvantaged Students, 1807
Jewish Fndn for Education of Women Scholarships for Emigres in the Health Professions, 1922
North Carolina GlaxoSmithKline Fndn Grants, 2860
Schering-Plough Fndn Health Grants, 3270

Philanthropy

Annunziata Sanguinetti Fndn Grants, 481
Ashland Corp Contributions Grants, 586
Beazley Fndn Grants, 730
Berrien Comm Fndn Grants, 749
Carl Gellert and Celia Berta Gellert Fndn Grants, 871
Chestnut Hill Charitable Fndn, Inc Grants, 987

Clark Fndn Grants, 1029
Columbus Fndn Competitive Grants, 1066
Comm Fndn for Greater Buffalo Grants, 1090
Comm Fndn for Monterey County Grants, 1092
Comm Fndn of Greater Flint Grants, 1107
Comm Fndn of Muncie and Delaware County Grants, 1120
Comm Fndn of Southeastern Connecticut Grants, 1125
Comm Fndn Silicon Valley Grants, 1133
Compass Bank Fndn Grants, 1138
DaimlerChrysler Corp Fund Grants, 1186
Estee Lauder Grants, 1429
Fargo-Moorhead Area Fndn Grants, 1454
Fndn Northwest Grants, 1537
Frey Fndn Grants, 1562
Giant Eagle Fndn Grants, 1611
Hillsdale County Comm General Adult Fndn Grants, 1777
Hoblitzelle Fndn Grants, 1783
Jeffress Research Grants, 1913
Josiah W. and Bessie H. Kline Fndn Grants, 1967
Lewis Preston Fund for Girls Education Grants, 2052
Mary S. and David C. Corbin Fndn Grants, 2122
McCombs Fndn Grants, 2142
National Lottery Comm Fund Grants, 2256
Newman's Own Inc Grants, 2306
Paul and Mary Haas Fndn Contributions and Student Scholarships, 2997
Pittsburgh Fndn Comm Fund Grants, 3054
Rochester Area Comm Fndn Grants, 3176
Rockefeller Archive Center Research Grants, 3178
Samuel Freeman Charitable Trust Grants, 3249
Stewart Huston Charitable Trust Grants, 3384

Philosophy
AHFMR Population Health Investigator Awards, 292
Charles G. Koch Charitable Fndn Grants, 965
Heart Rhythm Society Fellowships, 1731
James Hervey Johnson Charitable Educational Trust Grants, 1889

Photography
Polaroid Fund Grants, 3065
Ruth Mott Fndn Grants, 3204

Physical Education
AAHPERD Ruth Abernathy Presidential Scholarships, 128
BCBSM Building Healthy Communities Engaging Elementary Schools and Comm Partners Grants, 713
Homer Fndn Grants, 1789
Women's Sports Fndn Grants, 3551

Physical Growth/Retardation
Able To Serve Grants, 185
Columbus Fndn Traditional Grants, 1071
Human Growth Fndn Small Grants, 1816
Vancouver Sun Children's Fund Grants, 3479
WHAS Crusade for Children Grants, 3531

Physical Medicine and Rehabilitation
AAPD Henry B. Betts Award, 169
AGS Dennis W. Jahnigen Career Development Scholars Awards, 264
Annunziata Sanguinetti Fndn Grants, 481
DHHS Geriatric Training for Physicians and Dentists Grants, 1250
Disable American Veterans Charitable Grants, 1286
GEICO Public Service Awards, 1586
IATA Research Grants, 1834
IATA Scholarships, 1835
Jacob and Valeria Langeloth Fndn Grants, 1882
Leadership in Education in Neurodevelopmental Disabilities Postdoctoral Fellowships, 2037
Musculoskeletal Rehabilitation Fellowships, 2229
NICHD Small Grants, 2494
Special Olympics Health Professions Student Grants, 3355
WHAS Crusade for Children Grants, 3531

Physical Sciences
AAAS Science & Technology Policy Fellowships - National Defense & Global Security, 29
BWF Career Awards at the Scientific Interface, 819
Canada-U.S. Fulbright New Century Scholars Grants, 846
Canada-U.S. Fulbright Senior Specialists Grants, 847
DOE Environmental Remediation Grants, 1297
DOE Medical Applications and Measurement Science Grants, 1301
Eppley Fndn Postdoctoral Grants, 1425
Fulbright Alumni Initiatives Awards Grants, 1566
Fulbright Distinguished Chairs Grants, 1567
Fulbright New Century Scholars Grants, 1570
Fulbright Specialists Grants, 1571
Fulbright Traditional Scholar Program in Europe and Eurasia, 1572
Fulbright Traditional Scholar Program in Sub-Saharan Africa, 1573
Fulbright Traditional Scholar Program in the East Asia/Pacific Region, 1574
Fulbright Traditional Scholar Program in the Near East and North Africa Region, 1575
Fulbright Traditional Scholar Program in the South and Central Asia Region, 1576
Fulbright Traditional Scholar Program in the Western Hemisphere, 1577
HHMI-NIBIB Interfaces Initiative Grants, 1764
Marion I. and Henry J. Knott Fndn Grants, 2109
Minority Doctoral Fellowships in Science and Engineering, 2207
North Carolina GlaxoSmithKline Fndn Grants, 2860
NSF Alan T. Waterman Award, 2874
Society of Cosmetic Chemists Allan B. Black Award Sponsored by Presperse, 3328
Society of Cosmetic Chemists Award Sponsored by McIntyre Group, Ltd., 3329
Society of Cosmetic Chemists Award Sponsored by The HallStar Company, 3330
Society of Cosmetic Chemists Chapter Best Speaker Award, 3331
Society of Cosmetic Chemists Chapter Merit Award, 3332
Society of Cosmetic Chemists Frontier of Science Award, 3333
Society of Cosmetic Chemists Hans Schaeffer Award, 3334
Society of Cosmetic Chemists Joseph P. Ciaudelli Award, 3335
Society of Cosmetic Chemists Keynote Award Lecture Sponsored by Ruger Chemical Corp, 3336
Society of Cosmetic Chemists Literature Award, 3337
Society of Cosmetic Chemists Maison G. de Navarre Medal, 3338
Society of Cosmetic Chemists Merit Award, 3339
Society of Cosmetic Chemists Robert A. Kramer Lifetime Service Award, 3340
Society of Cosmetic Chemists Shaw Mudge Award, 3341
Society of Cosmetic Chemists Student Poster Awards, 3342
Society of Cosmetic Chemists Young Scientist Awards, 3343
University of California President's Postdoctoral Fellowships, 3469

Physics
AACR Team Science Award, 89
Alcatel-Lucent Technologies Corp Contributions Grants, 332
Alfred P. Sloan Fndn History of Science and Technology Grants, 352
Alfred P. Sloan Fndn Research Fellowships, 353
BWF Career Awards at the Scientific Interface, 819
Canada Graduate Scholarships and NSERC Postgraduate Scholarships, 845
Canada-U.S. Fulbright New Century Scholars Grants, 846
Canada-U.S. Fulbright Senior Specialists Grants, 847
Fulbright Alumni Initiatives Awards Grants, 1566
Fulbright Distinguished Chairs Grants, 1567
Fulbright New Century Scholars Grants, 1570
Fulbright Specialists Grants, 1571
Fulbright Traditional Scholar Program in Europe and Eurasia, 1572
Fulbright Traditional Scholar Program in Sub-Saharan Africa, 1573
Fulbright Traditional Scholar Program in the East Asia/Pacific Region, 1574
Fulbright Traditional Scholar Program in the Near East and North Africa Region, 1575
Fulbright Traditional Scholar Program in the South and Central Asia Region, 1576
Fulbright Traditional Scholar Program in the Western Hemisphere, 1577
HHMI-NIBIB Interfaces Initiative Grants, 1764
Marion I. and Henry J. Knott Fndn Grants, 2109
NHGRI Mentored Research Scientist Development Award, 2315
NIGMS Fellowships in Quantitative Biology, 2610
NIGMS Supplements for the Study of Complex Biological Systems, 2630
NIMH Curriculum Development Award in Neuroinformatics Research and Analysis, 2754
Northwood University/Alden B. Dow Creativity Center Summer Residency Program, 2871
NSF Biological Physics (BP), 2878
Weingart Fndn Grants, 3524

Physiology
AAAAI Summer Clinical Research Fellowship Medical Student Grants, 27
AAAAI Summer Research Fellowship Medical Student Grants, 28
AHAF Alzheimer's Disease Research Grants, 266
AHAF National Glaucoma Research Grants, 268
Deafness Research Fndn Research Grants, 1208
EF Predoctoral Research Training Fellowship, 1383
Lalor Fndn Postdoctoral Research Grants, 2021
Marine Biological Laboratory Summer Research Fellowships, 2108
NIGMS Fellowships in Quantitative Biology, 2610
NIGMS Integrative and Collaborative Approaches to Research Grants, 2615
NIH Biobehavioral Research for Effective Sleep, 2639
Rett Syndrome Research Fndn Grants, 3151

Physiology, Human
Mayo Fndn Multidisciplinary Training in Digestive Diseases Research Grants, 2140
NIEHS Biological Response to Environmental Health Hazards Research Grants, 2596

Plant Diseases/Pathology
NIGMS/NIDCR Evolution of Infectious Diseases Research Grants, 2633

Plant Genetics
Pioneer Hi-Bred Society Fellowships, 3052

Plant Sciences
Janirve Fndn Grants, 1905
NSF Animal Developmental Mechanisms Grants, 2875
NSF Cell Systems Cluster Grants, 2881
Pioneer Hi-Bred Society Fellowships, 3052
Samuel Roberts Noble Fndn Grants, 3250

Plastic Surgery
AAFPRS Ben Shuster Memorial Award, 117
AAFPRS Bernstein Grant, 118
AAFPRS Fellowships, 119
AAFPRS Investigator Development Grant, 120
AAFPRS John Orlando Roe Award, 122
AAFPRS Leslie Bernstein Resident Research Grants, 123
AAFPRS Residency Travel Awards, 124
AAFPRS Sir Harold Delf Gillies Award, 125
Plastic Surgery Educational Fndn Basic Research Grants, 3058

Plastic Surgery Educational Fndn Research Fellowship Grants, 3059
Plastic Surgery Educational Fndn/AAO-HNSF Combined Grant, 3060

Playgrounds
American Academy of Dermatology Shade Structure Grants, 413
Hasbro Children's Fund, 1714
Paul E. and Klare N. Reinhold Fndn Grants, 2999

Pneumonitis
NHLBI Hypersensitivity Pneumonitis – Grants for Early Identification and Mechanisms of Disease, 2336

Podiatry
DHHS Health Careers Opportunity Grants, 1253
DHHS National Health Service Corps Scholarships Program, 1266
DHHS Podiatric Primary Care Residency Training Grants, 1270
HRSA Health Professions Scholarships for Disadvantaged Students, 1807
Special Olympics Health Professions Student Grants, 3355

Poetry
Axe-Houghton Fndn Grants, 678

Poison Control
CDC National Poison Prevention and Control Grants, 918
Comm Toolbox for Children's Environmental Health Grants, 1137

Political Behavior
Bernard and Audre Rapoport Fndn Grants, 746
Carnegie Corp of New York Grants, 879
Harry Frank Guggenheim Fndn Research Grants, 1704
Ignacio Martin-Baro Fund for Mental Health and Human Rights Grants, 1839
RWJF Investigator Awards in Health Policy Research, 3220

Political Economics
Charles G. Koch Charitable Fndn Grants, 965

Political Science
AHFMR Population Health Investigator Awards, 292
Canada-U.S. Fulbright New Century Scholars Grants, 846
Canada-U.S. Fulbright Senior Specialists Grants, 847
Charles G. Koch Charitable Fndn Grants, 965
Coca-Cola Fndn Grants, 1052
EF Behavioral Sciences Student Fellowships, 1379
Fulbright Alumni Initiatives Awards Grants, 1566
Fulbright Distinguished Chairs Grants, 1567
Fulbright New Century Scholars Grants, 1570
Fulbright Specialists Grants, 1571
Fulbright Traditional Scholar Program in Europe and Eurasia, 1572
Fulbright Traditional Scholar Program in Sub-Saharan Africa, 1573
Fulbright Traditional Scholar Program in the East Asia/Pacific Region, 1574
Fulbright Traditional Scholar Program in the Near East and North Africa Region, 1575
Fulbright Traditional Scholar Program in the South and Central Asia Region, 1576
Fulbright Traditional Scholar Program in the Western Hemisphere, 1577
Margaret L. Wendt Fndn Grants, 2104
NFID Advanced Vaccinology Course Travel Grant, 2307

Pollution
Gamble Fndn Grants, 1582
HEI Grants, 1734

Polymer Science
Beckman Young Investigators Grants, 735

Population Biology
NIGMS Predoctoral Training in Bioinformatics and Computation Biology Grants, 2625
NIGMS/NIDCR Evolution of Infectious Diseases Research Grants, 2633

Population Control
Bushrod H. Campbell and Adah F. Hall Charity Fund Grants, 816
General Service Fndn Reproductive Health and Rights Grants, 1592
Harry and Grace Steele Fndn Grants, 1702
Huber Fndn Grants, 1812
S.H. Cowell Fndn Grants, 3237

Population Studies
AHFMR Population Health Investigator Awards, 292
CDC Minority Health Statistics Dissertation Research Grants, 916
CDC Using Genetic Information to Prevent Disease and Improve Health Research Grants, 932
FIC International Research and Training in Population and Health Grants, 1489
George Frederick Jewett Fndn Grants, 1599
NCI Academic-Industrial Partnerships for Development and Validation of In Vivo Imaging Systems & Methods for Cancer Investigations, 2268
NCI Application and Use of Transformative Emerging Technologies in Cancer Research, 2269
NICHD NRSAs—Individual, 2488
NICHD NRSAs—Institutional, 2489
NICHD Population Research Grants, 2490
NICHD Small Grants, 2494
NIH Genetic Susceptibility and Variability of Human Malformations Research Grants, 2669
NIH Genetics of Neurobehavioral Disorders in Existing Samples Grants, 2670
NIH Molecular Epidemiology of Prostate Carcinogenesis Grants, 2691
NIMH Interventions Infrastructure Program Research Grants, 2760
NINR Clinical Trials: Collaborations for Nursing Research, 2794
Richard and Rhoda Goldman Fund Grants, 3158
Takemi Program in International Health Research and Advanced Training Fellowships, 3416

Poverty and the Poor
ACE Charitable Fndn Grants, 199
Achelis and Bodman Fndns Grants, 206
Alice Tweed Tuohy Fndn Grants, 357
Alliance Healthcare Fndn Grants, 362
Ann Arbor Area Comm Fndn Grants, 476
Arizona Diamondbacks Charities Grants, 530
Avon Fndn Breast Care Fund Grants, 674
Barberton Comm Fndn Grants, 693
Beatrice Laing Trust Grants, 729
Bill and Melinda Gates Fndn Grants, 756
Birmingham Fndn Grants, 760
Breast Cancer Fund Grants, 790
Burden Trust Grants, 810
Carnegie Corp of New York Grants, 879
Carrie Estelle Doheny Fndn Grants, 883
Catholic Campaign for Human Development Comm Organizing Grants, 891
CharityWorks Grants, 961
Chestnut Hill Charitable Fndn, Inc Grants, 987
CNCS Foster Grandparent Projects Grants, 1048
Comm Fndn for Greater Buffalo Grants, 1090
Comm Fndn of Greater Flint Grants, 1107
Comm Fndn of Greenville Hollingsworth Funds Program/Project Grants, 1114
Comm Toolbox for Children's Environmental Health Grants, 1137
Connelly Fndn Grants, 1143
CRH Fndn Grants, 1160
Danellie Fndn Grants, 1198
Deland Fellowships in Health Care and Society, 1214
Eden Hall Fndn Grants, 1368
Educational Fndn of America Grants, 1372
Edyth Bush Charitable Fndn Grants, 1378
Emma B. Howe Memorial Fndn Grants, 1415
Farmers Insurance Group of Companies Grants, 1455
Foster G. McGaw Prize, 1525
General Service Fndn Reproductive Health and Rights Grants, 1592
Gertrude E. Skelly Charitable Fndn Grants, 1609
Ginn Fndn Grants, 1616
Good Samaritan Fndn Inc Grants, 1636
Greater Milwaukee Fndn Grants, 1653
Greater Worcester Comm Fndn Discretionary Grants, 1658
Gulf Coast Comm of Venice Fndn Grants, 1677
Hasbro Children's Fund, 1714
Health Fndn of Greater Cincinnati Grants, 1724
Healthcare Fndn for Orange County Grants, 1728
Hearst Fndn and William Randolph Hearst Fndn Grants, 1730
Henry J. Kaiser Family Fndn Grants, 1748
Hilda and Preston Davis Fndn Grants, 1772
Independence Blue Cross Charitable Medical Care Grants, 1846
Irvin Stern Fndn Grants, 1866
J.L. Bedsole Fndn Grants, 1876
Jacob G. Schmidlapp Trust Grants, 1883
Jenkins Fndn: Improving the Health of Greater Richmond Grants, 1915
Jessie Ball Dupont Fund Grants, 1919
John Edward Fowler Memorial Fndn Grants, 1930
Josephine Goodyear Fndn Grants, 1964
Joyce Fndn Grants, 1969
Kahuku Comm Fund, 1977
Kraft Cares International Grants, 2016
Kraft Cares US Grants, 2017
Lynde and Harry Bradley Fndn Grants, 2089
Lynde and Harry Bradley Fndn Prizes: Bradley Prizes, 2090
MAP International Medical Fellowships, 2101
Marion Park Deaver and Harry Gilbert Deaver Fndn Grants, 2110
Medtronic Fndn Health Care Grants, 2169
Ms. Fndn for Women Grants, 2222
National Lottery Comm Fund Grants, 2256
Northern Trust Company Charitable Trust and Corp Giving Program, 2865
OUT Fund for Lesbian and Gay Liberation Grants, 2978
Paso del Norte Health Fndn Grants, 2995
Pittsburgh Fndn Comm Fund Grants, 3054
S.H. Cowell Fndn Grants, 3237
Seattle Fndn Grants, 3276
Sir Dorabji Tata Trust Grants for NGOs or Voluntary Organizations, 3291
Starr Fndn Grants, 3377
Stewart Huston Charitable Trust Grants, 3384
W.K. Kellogg Fndn Healthy Kids Grants, 3507
W.K. Kellogg Fndn Secure Families Grants, 3508
Washington Post Contributions Grants, 3520
William G. McGowan Charitable Fund Grants, 3539
YSA Get Ur Good On Grants, 3555

Pregnancy
Alliance Healthcare Fndn Grants, 362
Bill and Melinda Gates Fndn Grants, 756
DHHS Health Centers Grants for Residents of Public Housing, 1254
General Service Fndn Reproductive Health and Rights Grants, 1592
NHLBI Prematurity and Respiratory Outcomes Program Grants, 2366
NIAID Pediatric Clinical Trials Program for AIDS, 2460
NICHD NRSAs—Individual, 2488
NICHD NRSAs—Institutional, 2489
NIH Low Birthweight in Minority Populations Research Grants, 2683
NIH Research on Sleep and Sleep Disorders, 2713

Premature Births
NHLBI Prematurity and Respiratory Outcomes Program Grants, 2366

Presbyterian Church
Barra Fndn Project Grants, 699
Booth-Bricker Fund Grants, 780
Bradley Turner Fndn Grants, 789
Effie and Wofford Cain Fndn Grants, 1385

Preschool Education
Alabama Power Fndn Grants, 321
American Electric Power Grants, 434
Arizona Diamondbacks Charities Grants, 530
Benton Comm Fndn Grants, 743
Bernard and Audre Rapoport Fndn Grants, 746
Blackford County Comm Fndn Grants, 763
Blue River Comm Fndn Grants, 770
Bodenwein Public Benevolent Fndn Grants, 775
Booth-Bricker Fund Grants, 780
Boston Fndn Grants, 783
Brown County Comm Fndn Grants, 807
Carnegie Corp of New York Grants, 879
Cass County Comm Fndn Grants, 887
Chestnut Hill Charitable Fndn, Inc Grants, 987
CNCS Foster Grandparent Projects Grants, 1048
Comm Fndn Alliance City of Evansville Endowment Fund Grants, 1089
Comm Fndn of Bartholomew County Heritage Fund Grants, 1096
Comm Fndn of Bartholomew County James A. Henderson Award for Fund-Raising, 1097
Comm Fndn of Boone County Grants, 1099
Comm Fndn of Greater Fort Wayne: Comm Endowment & Clarke Endowment Fund Grants, 1108
Comm Fndn of Greenville Comm Enrichment Grants, 1113
Comm Fndn of Greenville Hollingsworth Funds Program/Project Grants, 1114
Constellation Energy Group and Baltimore Gas and Electric Corp Contributions, 1146
Cowles Charitable Trust Grants, 1155
Effie and Wofford Cain Fndn Grants, 1385
Eugene M. Lang Fndn Grants, 1434
FCD Child Development Grants, 1458
Fisher Fndn Grants, 1508
Fndn for the Carolinas Grants, 1535
Frances and John L. Loeb Family Fund Grants, 1546
Helen Steiner Rice Fndn Grants, 1742
J.C. Penney Company Grants, 1874
John Edward Fowler Memorial Fndn Grants, 1930
Johnson & Johnson Corp Contributions Grants, 1952
Laura B. Vogler Fndn Grants, 2032
Miriam and Peter Haas Fund Grants, 2208
Phoenix Suns Charities Grants, 3030
Portland General Electric Fndn Grants, 3067
Quantum Fndn Grants, 3096
San Antonio Area Fndn Grants, 3254
Sid W. Richardson Fndn Grants, 3284

Preservation and Restoration
Boeing Company Contributions Grants, 777
Carls Fndn Grants, 876
Grammy Fndn Grants, 1643
North Carolina Comm Development Grants, 2858
Palm Beach and Martin Counties Grants, 2986
Stewart Huston Charitable Trust Grants, 3384

Preventive Care
Express Scripts Fndn Grants, 1441

Preventive Dentistry
Pajaro Valley Comm Health Grants, 2985

Preventive Medicine
Alexander and Margaret Stewart Trust Grants, 340
ALVRE Casselberry Award, 374
ALVRE Grant, 375
ALVRE Seymour R. Cohen Award, 376
Alzheimer's Association Everyday Technologies for Alzheimer Care Research Grants, 377
Alzheimer's Association Mentored New Investigator Research Grants to Promote Diversity, 379
Alzheimer's Association Molecular Imaging Grants, 380
Alzheimer's Association New Investigator Research Grants to Promote Diversity, 382
Alzheimer's Association Senator Mark Hatfield Award, 383
Alzheimer's Association Zenith Fellows Awards, 384
Alzheimer's Association Conference Grants, 385
Banfi Vintners Fndn Grants, 687
Baptist Comm Ministries Grants, 691
Battle Creek Comm Fndn Grants, 703
BCBSM Fndn Primary and Clinical Prevention Grants, 719
Bill and Melinda Gates Fndn Grants, 756
California Endowment CommunitiesFirst Grants, 833
California Wellness Fndn Work and Health Grants, 834
Cardiac Arrhythmias Research and Education Fndn Research Grants, 863
CDC Core Capacity Grants, 907
CDC Emerging Infectious Diseases Fellowships Program, 908
CDC Hepatitis Education for Inmates and Correctional Staff Grants, 911
CDC Injury Prevention and Control Research and State and Comm Based Programs, 914
CDC Oral Diseases Prevention and Oral Health Promotion Grants, 921
CDC Promoting Prevention in Managed Care Cooperative Agreements, 925
CDC Public Health Conference Support Grant Program, 926
CDC Research, Treatment, and Education Programs on Lyme Disease in the United States Cooperative Agreements, 927
CDC Technology Translation and Transfer of Effective HIV Behavioral Interventions, 931
CDC Using Genetic Information to Prevent Disease and Improve Health Research Grants, 932
CMA Fndn Grants, 1042
Comm Fndn AIDS Endowment Awards, 1088
Daniel Mendelsohn New Investigator Award, 1199
DHHS Adolescent Family Life Demonstration Projects, 1243
DHHS AIDS and HIV Epidemiologic Research Studies Grants, 1244
DHHS Health Care Systems Cost and Access Research and Development Grants, 1252
DHHS Health Conference Support Program for Toxic Substances and Disease Registry, 1255
DHHS Health Promotion and Disease Prevention Research and Demonstration Centers Grants, 1260
DHHS Preventive Medicine, 1271
DHHS Public Health Students Traineeships and Other Graduate Public Health Programs, 1277
Dr. John T. Macdonald Fndn Grants, 1327
E.A. Baker Fndn for the Prevention of Blindness Grants, 1357
Eden Hall Fndn Grants, 1368
Edwards Memorial Trust Grants, 1375
Emma B. Howe Memorial Fndn Grants, 1415
Fannie E. Rippel Fndn Grants, 1452
FIC International Training and Research in Emerging Infectious Diseases Grants, 1492
FIC International Training and Research in Environmental and Occupational Health, 1493
Fndn for Seacoast Health Grants, 1533
Frances and John L. Loeb Family Fund Grants, 1546
General Mills Fndn Grants, 1590
Good Samaritan Fndn Inc Grants, 1636
Health Fndn of Southern Florida Responsive Grants, 1726
Healthcare Fndn for Orange County Grants, 1728
HRSA Geriatric Education Centers, 1805
HRSA Physician Assistant Training, 1810
Ignacio Martin-Baro Fund for Mental Health and Human Rights Grants, 1839
Independence Comm Fndn Comm Quality of Life Grant, 1849
Johnson & Johnson Corp Contributions Grants, 1952
Kansas Health Fndn Grants, 1980
Leahi Fund, 2038
Mary Black Fndn Grants, 2118
Max Bell Fndn Grants, 2134
Medtronic Fndn Health Care Grants, 2169
NCI/NIDA Transdisciplinary Tobacco Use Research Centers Grants, 2280
NIA Health Behaviors and Aging Grants, 2408
NIAAA Mechanisms of Alcohol-Induced Hepatic Fibrosis Research Grants, 2445
NIAID HIV Prevention Trial Units Grants, 2453
NIDA Drug Addiction Neuroscience Research Grants, 2503
NIDA Mentored Clinical Scientist Research Career Development Awards, 2507
NIDA Senior Scientist Award, 2515
NIDCD Health Promotion and Disease Prevention: Health Communication, Development, and Dissemination, 2521
NIDCR Clinical Trial Pilot Grant, 2533
NIDCR HIV/AIDS Associated Oral Viral Infections, 2535
NIDCR International Collaborative Oral Health Research Planning Grant, 2536
NIDDK Type 2 Diabetes in the Pediatric Population Research Grants, 2593
NIGMS/NIDCR Evolution of Infectious Diseases Research Grants, 2633
NIH Collaborations for Advanced Strategies in Complication of HIV Infection, 2651
NIH Exploratory/Development Grants for Mental Health Intervention Research, 2665
NIH Genetic Susceptibility and Variability of Human Malformations Research Grants, 2669
NIH Human Models and Markers of Skeletal Aging Grants, 2674
NIH SBIR/STTR Study and Control of Microbial Biofilms Research Grants, 2724
NIH Transitional Career Development Award in Women's Health Research, 2736
NIMH Early Detection of HIV Grants, 2755
NIMH Interventions Infrastructure Program Research Grants, 2760
NIOSH Occupational Safety and Health Research and Demonstration Grants, 2807
OUT Fund for Lesbian & Gay Liberation Grants, 2978
Paso del Norte Health Fndn Grants, 2995
Pfizer Fndn Grants, 3025
Premera CARES Grants, 3074
SAMHSA Conference Grants, 3246
Self Fndn Grants, 3277
Sid W. Richardson Fndn Grants, 3284
Sisters of Saint Joseph Charitable Fund Grants, 3296
United Cerebral Palsy Research Grants, 3462
USCM HIV/AIDS Prevention Grants, 3476
Wilhelm Sander Fndn Grants, 3535

Primary Care Services
ACS Cancer Control Career Development Awards for Primary Care Physicians, 209
CVS Comm Grants, 1177
DHHS Adolescent Family Life Demonstration Projects, 1243
DHHS Health Centers Grants for Residents of Public Housing, 1254
DHHS HIV Demonstration Program for Children, Adolescents, and Women, 1262
DHHS Primary Medical Care National Research Service Awards, 1272
DHHS Technical and Non-Financial Assistance to Health Centers, 1280
Good Samaritan Fndn Inc Grants, 1636
Health Fndn of Greater Cincinnati Grants, 1724
Health Fndn of Southern Florida Responsive Grants, 1726

HRSA Physician Assistant Training, 1810
Josiah Macy Jr. Fndn Grants, 1966
Kansas Health Fndn Grants, 1980
Mayday Fund Grants, 2139
NCI/NIDA Transdisciplinary Tobacco Use Research Centers Grants, 2280
RWJF New Jersey Health Initiatives Grants, 3225
W.K. Kellogg Fndn Healthy Kids Grants, 3507

Primatology
NIH Nonhuman Primate Immune Tolerance Cooperative Study Group Grants, 2699
Whitehall Fndn Neurobiology Research Grants, 3533

Print Media
APSA Congressional Fellowships Health and Aging Policy Fellows Program, 514
APSA Robert Wood Johnson Fndn Health Policy Fellowships, 515
Henry J. Kaiser Family Fndn Grants, 1748

Prion Disease
CDC Cooperative Agreement for Continuing Enhanced National Surveillance for Prion Diseases in the United States, 904

Prison Reform
Bernard F. and Alva B. Gimbel Fndn Grants, 747

Prisoners
Achelis and Bodman Fndns Grants, 206
CDC Hepatitis Education for Inmates and Correctional Staff Grants, 911
Jacob and Valeria Langeloth Fndn Grants, 1882

Private and Parochial Education
Bailey Fndn Grants, 680
Boettcher Fndn Grants, 778
Coca-Cola Fndn Grants, 1052
Commission on Religion in Appalachia Grants, 1074
Comm Fndn for Greater Buffalo Grants, 1090
ConocoPhillips Fndn Grants, 1144
Dr. Scholl Fndn Grants, 1329
Eugene B. Casey Fndn Grants, 1433
Frank G. and Freida K. Brotz Family Fndn Grants, 1552
George F. Baker Trust Grants, 1597
Kenneth T. and Eileen L. Norris Fndn Grants, 1989
Lubbock Area Fndn Grants, 2079
Lubrizol Fndn Grants, 2080
Lynde and Harry Bradley Fndn Grants, 2089
Lynde and Harry Bradley Fndn Prizes: Bradley Prizes, 2090
Marion I. and Henry J. Knott Fndn Grants, 2109
Marion Park Deaver and Harry Gilbert Deaver Fndn Grants, 2110
PacifiCorp Fndn for Learning Grants, 2982
Piper Jaffray Companies Building Strong Communities Grants, 3053
Richard King Mellon Fndn Grants, 3161
Russell Berrie Fndn Grants, 3201
S.H. Cowell Fndn Grants, 3237
Sunderland Fndn Grants, 3400
Wachovia Fndn Grants, 3511

Problem Solving
NSF Grant Opportunities for Academic Liaison with Industry, 2887
NSF Perception, Action & Cognition Research Grants, 2890
US Trust Corp Fndn Grants, 3475

Process Development Engineering
NSF Chemical, Biochemical, and Biotechnology Systems Research Grants, 2882

Process Simulation and Control
NSF-NIST Interaction in Chemistry, Materials Research, Molecular Biosciences, Bioengineering, and Chemical Engineering, 2897

Production/Operations Management
NSF Grant Opportunities for Academic Liaison with Industry, 2887

Professional Associations
ASHA Minority Student Leadership Program Awards, 570
Cemala Fndn Grants, 933
Scientific Communities Initiative Grants, 3272

Program Evaluation
Dept of Ed Special Education—Studies and Evaluations, 1232
RCPSC Royal College Fellowship for Studies in Medical Education, 3127
South Madison Comm Fndn Grants, 3349

Prostate Gland
CRI Prostate Cancer Initiative Grants, 1163
NIA Prostate Cancer Aging, Race, and Ethnicity Research Grants, 2428
NIDDK Cell-Specific Delineation of Prostate and Genitourinary Development, 2545
NIH Biology, Development, and Progression of Malignant Prostate Disease Research Grants, 2641
NIH Molecular Epidemiology of Prostate Carcinogenesis Grants, 2691
Soy Health Research Program Incentive Awards, 3354
William G. McGowan Charitable Fund Grants, 3539

Prosthetic Devices
NIAMS/NICHD Deep Infections of Total Joint Replacements, 2481
U.S. Department of Education Rehabilitation Engineering Research Centers Grants, 3447

Protein Pathways
NCRR Networks and Pathways Collaborative Research Projects Grants, 2287

Proteins and Macromolecules
DOE Health Effects and Life Sciences Research Grants, 1298
Elizabeth Glaser Pediatric AIDS Fndn Pediatric HIV Vaccine Research Grants, 1395
NCRR Networks and Pathways Collaborative Research Projects Grants, 2287
NHLBI Protein Interactions Governing Membrane Transport in Pulmonary Health and Disease Grants, 2369
NIGMS Molecular Pharmacology of Anesthetic Action Research Grants, 2621
NIGMS Pilot Projects for the Protein Structure Initiative (Structural Genomics), 2624
NIH Mechanisms Underlying Individual Variations in Drug Responses, 2685
NIH Protein Structure Initiative (Structural Genomics) Research Grants, 2704
NIH Protein Structure Initiative (Structural Genomics)—SBIR/STTR GRANTS, 2705
NIH Structural Biology of Membrane Proteins Grants, 2730
NSF Biomolecular Systems Cluster Grants, 2880

Protestant Church
Atherton Family Fndn Grants, 659
Camp-Younts Fndn Grants, 838
Charles Delmar Fndn Grants, 963
Collins C. Diboll Private Fndn Grants, 1057
Dora Roberts Fndn Grants, 1311
E. Rhodes and Leona B. Carpenter Fndn Grants, 1356
G.N. Wilcox Trust Grants, 1581
Huie-Dellmon Trust Grants, 1815
Stewart Huston Charitable Trust Grants, 3384

Psychiatry
AACAP Beatrix A. Hamburg Award for the Best New Research Poster by a Child and Adolescent Psychiatry Resident, 30
AACAP Child and Adolescent Psychiatry Teaching Scholarships, 31
AACAP Educational Outreach Program for Child and Adolescent Psychiatry Residents, 33
AACAP Educational Outreach Program for General Psychiatry Residents, 34
AACAP Elaine Schlosser Lewis Award for Research on Attention-Deficit Disorder, 35
AACAP George Tarjan Award for Contributions in Developmental Disabilities, 36
AACAP Irving Philips Award for Prevention, 37
AACAP Jeanne Spurlock Lecture and Award on Diversity and Culture, 38
AACAP Klingenstein Third Generation Fndn Award for Research in Depression or Suicide, 42
AACAP Norbert and Charlotte Rieger Award for Scientific Achievement, 43
AACAP Norbert and Charlotte Rieger Psychodynamic Psychotherapy Award, 44
AACAP Pilot Research Award for Learning Disabilities, Supported by the Elaine Schlosser Lewis Fund, 46
AACAP Rieger Service Program Award for Excellence, 49
AACAP Robert Cancro Academic Leadership Award, 50
AACAP Sidney Berman Award for the School-Based Study and Intervention for Learning Disorders and Mental Ilness, 51
AACAP Simon Wile Leadership in Consultation Award, 52
American Philosophical Society Daland Fellowships in Clinical Investigation, 441
American Psychiatric Association Award for Research in Psychiatry, 442
American Psychiatric Association Minority Fellowships Program, 443
American Psychiatric Association Minority Medical Student Fellowship in HIV Psychiatry, 444
American Psychiatric Association Minority Medical Student Summer Externship in Addiction Psychiatry, 445
American Psychiatric Association Minority Medical Student Summer Mentoring Program, 446
American Psychiatric Association Program for Minority Research Training in Psychiatry, 447
American Psychiatric Association Research Colloquium for Junior Investigators, 448
American Psychiatric Association Travel Scholarships for Minority Medical Students, 449
American Psychiatric Association/AstraZeneca Young Minds in Psychiatry International Awards, 450
American Psychiatric Association/Bristol-Myers Squibb Fellowships in Public Psychiatry, 451
American Psychiatric Association/Janssen Resident Psychiatric Research Scholars, 452
American Psychiatric Association/Merck Co. Early Academic Career Research Award, 453
APF Alexander Gralnick, MD, Award for Research in Schizophrenia, 503
APF Awards for Advancing Minority Mental Health, 504
APF Call for Proposals, 505
APF Disaster Recovery Fund for Psychiatrists, 506
APF James H. Scully Jr., M.D., Educational Fund Grants, 508
APF Jeanne Spurlock Congressional Fellowships, 509
APF Typical or Troubled School Mental Health Education Grants, 510
APSAA Fellowships, 516
APSAA Fndn Grants, 517
APSAA Mini-Career Grants, 518
APSAA Research Grants, 519
APSAA Small Beginning Scholar Pre-Investigation Grants, 520
APSAA Small Beginning Scholar Visiting and Consulting Grants, 521
Baltimore Washington Center Adult Psychoanalysis Fellowships, 685

Baltimore Washington Center Child Psychotherapy Fellowships, 686
Blowitz-Ridgeway Fndn Grants, 767
Boston Psychoanalytic Society and Institute Fellowship in Child Psychoanalytic Psychotherapy, 786
Boston Psychoanalytic Society and Institute Fellowship in Psychoanalytic Psychotherapy, 787
Chicago Institute for Psychoanalysis Fellowships, 990
DHHS Geriatric Training for Physicians and Dentists Grants, 1250
EF Research and Training Fellowships for Clinicians, 1384
Fndn for Psychocultural Research Postdoctoral Fellowships, 1531
Joseph Collins Fndn Grants, 1959
Michigan Psychoanalytic Institute and Society SATA Grants, 2193
Michigan Psychoanalytic Institute and Society Scholarships, 2194
NIMH HIV/AIDS, Severe Mental Illness, and Homelessness Research Grants, 2757
SOBP A.E. Bennett Research Award, 3313
SOBP Travel Fellowships, 3315
SOBP Ziskind-Somerfeld Research Awards, 3316
TSA Research Grant Awards, 3442

Psychodynamics
AACAP Norbert and Charlotte Rieger Psychodynamic Psychotherapy Award, 44
APSAA Fellowships, 516
FAR Fund, 1453
NIH Low Birthweight in Minority Populations Research Grants, 2683

Psychology
AHFMR Population Health Investigator Awards, 292
American Fndn for Suicide Prevention Grants, 436
APA Congressional Fellowships, 492
APA Culture of Service in the Psychological Sciences Award, 493
APA Dissertation Research Awards, 494
APA Distinguished Scientific Award for Early Career Contribution to Psychology, 495
APA Distinguished Scientific Award for the Applications of Psychology, 496
APA Distinguished Scientific Contribution Award, 497
APA Distinguished Service to Psychological Science Award, 498
APA Meritorious Research Service Commendation, 499
APA Scientific Conferences Grants, 500
APA Travel Awards, 501
APF/COGDOP Graduate Research Scholarships in Psychology, 511
APSAA Fellowships, 516
APSAA Fndn Grants, 517
APSAA Mini-Career Grants, 518
APSAA Research Grants, 519
APSAA Small Beginning Scholar Pre-Investigation Grants, 520
APSAA Small Beginning Scholar Visiting and Consulting Grants, 521
Baltimore Washington Center Adult Psychoanalysis Fellowships, 685
Baltimore Washington Center Child Psychotherapy Fellowships, 686
Blowitz-Ridgeway Fndn Grants, 767
Boston Psychoanalytic Society and Institute Fellowship in Child Psychoanalytic Psychotherapy, 786
Boston Psychoanalytic Society and Institute Fellowship in Psychoanalytic Psychotherapy, 787
Canada Graduate Scholarships and NSERC Postgraduate Scholarships, 845
Canada-U.S. Fulbright New Century Scholars Grants, 846
Canada-U.S. Fulbright Senior Specialists Grants, 847
Chicago Institute for Psychoanalysis Fellowships, 990
Dr. Sydney Segal Research Grants, 1331
Edward Bangs Kelley and Elza Kelley Fndn Grants, 1373
EF Behavioral Sciences Student Fellowships, 1379
EF Predoctoral Research Training Fellowship, 1383
Field Psychology Research Grants, 1500
Fndn for Psychocultural Research Postdoctoral Fellowships, 1531
Fulbright Alumni Initiatives Awards Grants, 1566
Fulbright Distinguished Chairs Grants, 1567
Fulbright New Century Scholars Grants, 1570
Fulbright Specialists Grants, 1571
Fulbright Traditional Scholar Program in Europe and Eurasia, 1572
Fulbright Traditional Scholar Program in Sub-Saharan Africa, 1573
Fulbright Traditional Scholar Program in the East Asia/Pacific Region, 1574
Fulbright Traditional Scholar Program in the Near East and North Africa Region, 1575
Fulbright Traditional Scholar Program in the South and Central Asia Region, 1576
Fulbright Traditional Scholar Program in the Western Hemisphere, 1577
Fyssen Fndn Postdoctoral Study Grants, 1580
HIV/AIDS Research Training Fellowship, 1782
HRSA Health Professions Scholarships for Disadvantaged Students, 1807
Human Growth Fndn Small Grants, 1816
James McKeen Cattell Fund Fellowships, 1893
Leadership in Education in Neurodevelopmental Disabilities Postdoctoral Fellowships, 2037
Michigan Psychoanalytic Institute and Society SATA Grants, 2193
Michigan Psychoanalytic Institute and Society Scholarships, 2194
NCIC Canadian Cancer Society Research Grants, 2282
New York University Steinhardt School of Education Fellowships, 2305
NIH Biobehavioral Research for Effective Sleep, 2639
NIH Impact of HAART on HIV/CNS Disease, 2676
NSF Social Psychology Research Grants, 2894
TSA Research Grant Awards, 3442
UICC American Cancer Society International Fellowships for Beginning Investigators, 3455
University of Georgia Counseling and Psychological Services Postdoctoral Fellowship, 3470

Psychology Education
APF/COGDOP Graduate Research Scholarships in Psychology, 511
Blowitz-Ridgeway Fndn Early Childhood Development Research Award, 766
University of Georgia Counseling and Psychological Services Postdoctoral Fellowship, 3470

Psychology of Aging
NIA Health Behaviors and Aging Grants, 2408

Psychopathology
NIH Pathological Gambling: Basic, Clinical, and Services Research Grants, 2702
NIMH Risk Factors for Psychopathology Using Existing Data Sets Grants, 2768

Psychotherapy
AACAP Norbert and Charlotte Rieger Psychodynamic Psychotherapy Award, 44
APSAA Fndn Grants, 517
APSAA Mini-Career Grants, 518
APSAA Research Grants, 519
APSAA Small Beginning Scholar Pre-Investigation Grants, 520
APSAA Small Beginning Scholar Visiting and Consulting Grants, 521
Baltimore Washington Center Adult Psychoanalysis Fellowships, 685
Baltimore Washington Center Child Psychotherapy Fellowships, 686
Boston Psychoanalytic Society & Institute Fellowship in Child Psychoanalytic Psychotherapy, 786
Boston Psychoanalytic Society and Institute Fellowship in Psychoanalytic Psychotherapy, 787
Chicago Institute for Psychoanalysis Fellowships, 990
Eric Berne Fund for the Future Grants, 1426
Michigan Psychoanalytic Institute and Society SATA Grants, 2193
Michigan Psychoanalytic Institute and Society Scholarships, 2194
NIA Mechanisms Underlying the Links between Psychosocial Stress, Aging, the Brain and the Body Grants, 2414
NIDA Behavioral Therapies Development Grants, 2499

Public Administration
APSA Congressional Fellowships Health and Aging Policy Fellows Program, 514
APSA Robert Wood Johnson Fndn Health Policy Fellowships, 515
Arlington Comm Fndn Grants, 536
Canada-U.S. Fulbright New Century Scholars Grants, 846
Canada-U.S. Fulbright Senior Specialists Grants, 847
Carpenter Fndn Grants, 881
Commonwealth Fund/Harvard University Fellowship in Minority Health Policy, 1086
Effie and Wofford Cain Fndn Grants, 1385
Fulbright Alumni Initiatives Awards Grants, 1566
Fulbright Distinguished Chairs Grants, 1567
Fulbright New Century Scholars Grants, 1570
Fulbright Specialists Grants, 1571
Fulbright Traditional Scholar Program in Europe and Eurasia, 1572
Fulbright Traditional Scholar Program in Sub-Saharan Africa, 1573
Fulbright Traditional Scholar Program in the East Asia/Pacific Region, 1574
Fulbright Traditional Scholar Program in the Near East and North Africa Region, 1575
Fulbright Traditional Scholar Program in the South and Central Asia Region, 1576
Fulbright Traditional Scholar Program in the Western Hemisphere, 1577
Prospect Burma Scholarships, 3085
S. Mark Taper Fndn Grants, 3236
Sosland Fndn Grants, 3348
Special Olympics Health Professions Student Grants, 3355
Sprague Fndn Grants, 3359

Public Affairs
AFG Industries Grants, 259
Allegheny Technologies Charitable Trust, 359
Armstrong McDonald Fndn Grants, 537
Axe-Houghton Fndn Grants, 678
Banfi Vintners Fndn Grants, 687
Battle Creek Comm Fndn Grants, 703
Bernard and Audre Rapoport Fndn Grants, 746
Berrien Comm Fndn Grants, 749
Blue Grass Comm Fndn Grants, 768
Burlington Northern Santa Fe Fndn Grants, 812
Carl and Lily Pforzheimer Fndn Grants, 868
Carpenter Fndn Grants, 881
Clark County Comm Fndn Grants, 1028
Crestlea Fndn Grants, 1159
CSRA Comm Fndn Grants, 1168
Cullen Fndn Grants, 1172
Cyrus Eaton Fndn Grants, 1178
Daisy Marquis Jones Fndn Grants, 1188
Emerson Electric Company Contributions Grants, 1413
Eugene McDermott Fndn Grants, 1435
F.M. Kirby Fndn Grants, 1443
Field Fndn of Illinois Grants, 1499
FirstEnergy Fndn Comm Grants, 1505
Fluor Fndn Grants, 1517
FMC Fndn Grants, 1518
Howard and Bush Fndn Grants, 1798
Idaho Comm Fndn Eastern Region Competitive Grants, 1837
John Merck Fund Grants, 1940
Katharine Matthies Fndn Grants, 1982

Land O'Lakes Fndn Mid-Atlantic Grants, 2027
Lockheed Martin Philanthropic Grants, 2062
Lynde and Harry Bradley Fndn Grants, 2089
Lynde and Harry Bradley Fndn Prizes: Bradley Prizes, 2090
Margaret L. Wendt Fndn Grants, 2104
Meadows Fndn Grants, 2161
Miriam and Peter Haas Fund Grants, 2208
National City Corp Contributions Grants, 2250
New York Life Fndn Grants, 2304
Noble County Comm Fndn Grants, 2848
Paul E. and Klare N. Reinhold Fndn Grants, 2999
Pike County Comm Fndn Grants, 3049
Prudential Fndn Grants, 3087
Putnam County Comm Fndn Grants, 3093
Rajiv Gandhi Fndn Grants, 3104
Salisbury Comm Fndn Grants, 3243
Samuel Roberts Noble Fndn Grants, 3250
Sarah Scaife Fndn Grants, 3263
Shell Oil Company Fndn Grants, 3281
Starr Fndn Grants, 3377
Steelcase Fndn Grants, 3379
Vanderburgh Comm Fndn Grants, 3480
Vermont Comm Fndn Grants, 3493
Warrick County Comm Fndn Grants, 3519
Winston-Salem Fndn Competitive Grants, 3544
Z. Smith Reynolds Fndn Small Grants, 3557

Public Broadcasting
Air Products and Chemicals Grants, 319
Andersen Fndn Grants, 471
ASM Public Communications Award, 611
Comm Fndn of Western North Carolina Grants, 1132
ConocoPhillips Fndn Grants, 1144
Cooper Industries Fndn Grants, 1150
Foellinger Fndn Grants, 1519
G.N. Wilcox Trust Grants, 1581
Lubrizol Fndn Grants, 2080
Piedmont Natural Gas Grants, 3048
Rasmuson Fndn Grants, 3108

Public Education
ConocoPhillips Fndn Grants, 1144
ConocoPhillips Fndn Grants, 1144
DPA Promoting Policy Change Advocacy Grants, 1324
Express Scripts Fndn Grants, 1441
HomeBanc Fndn Grants, 1788
John P. Murphy Fndn Grants, 1943
Komen Greater NYC Clinical Trials Enrollment Grants, 2010
Komen Greater NYC Comm Breast Health Grants, 2011
Komen Greater NYC Conference Grants, 2012
Minneapolis Fndn Comm Grants, 2206
PacifiCorp Fndn for Learning Grants, 2982
Stewart Huston Charitable Trust Grants, 3384
Taproot Fndn Capacity-Building Service Grants, 3417

Public Health
AcademyHealth PHSR Research Article of the Year Awards, 196
AHFMR Clinical Investigator Awards, 270
AHFMR Infrastructure Funding Grants, 283
AHFMR Personnel Funding Grants, 290
AHFMR Scholar Awards, 295
AHFMR Scientist Awards, 296
AHFMR Senior Investigator Awards, 297
AHFMR Senior Scholar Awards, 299
AMA Fndn Fund for Better Health Grants, 388
AMA Fndn Pride in the Profession Grants, 397
AMA-MSS Government Relations Advocacy Fellowship, 403
AMA-MSS Government Relations Internship Programs, 404
APF Awards for Advancing Minority Mental Health, 504
APF Disaster Recovery Fund for Psychiatrists, 506
ASM Congressional Science Fellowships, 590
ASM Gen-Probe Joseph Public Health Award, 597
ASM Public Communications Award, 611
ASM/CCID Fellowships, 627
AUPHA Baxter International Fndn Prize for Health Services Research, 666
Baxter International Fndn Grants, 705
BCBS of Minnesota Healthy Together Grants, 712
BCBSM Frank J. McDevitt, DO, Excellence in Research Awards, 722
BCBSNC Fndn Fit Together Grants, 724
Bill and Melinda Gates Fndn Grants, 756
Brinson Fndn Grants, 794
California Wellness Fndn Work and Health Grants, 834
Canada-U.S. Fulbright New Century Scholars Grants, 846
Canada-U.S. Fulbright Senior Specialists Grants, 847
Cass County Comm Fndn Grants, 887
CDC Cooperative Agreement for the Development, Operation, and Evaluation of an Entertainment Education Program, 906
CDC Emerging Infectious Diseases Fellowships Program, 908
CDC Epidemiology and Laboratory Capacity Infectious Diseases Grants, 909
CDC Injury Control Research Centers Grants, 913
CDC National Training Information and Exchange Program, 920
CDC Public Health Conference Support Grant Program, 926
CDC Technology Translation and Transfer of Effective HIV Behavioral Interventions, 931
Center for Alternatives to Animal Testing Grants, 934
CHCF Grants, 979
Colorado Trust Partnerships for Health Initiative, 1063
Commonwealth Fund Small Grants, 1084
Commonwealth Fund/Harvard University Fellowship in Minority Health Policy, 1086
Comm Health Scholars Program Fellowships, 1134
Cruise Industry Charitable Fndn Grants, 1166
Deaconess Comm Fndn Grants, 1207
DeRoy Testamentary Fndn Grants, 1239
DHHS AIDS and HIV Epidemiologic Research Studies Grants, 1244
DHHS Grants for Dental Public Health, 1251
DHHS Health Careers Opportunity Grants, 1253
DHHS Maternal and Child Health Research and Training Programs Grants, 1264
DHHS National Health Service Corps Loan Repayment Awards, 1265
DHHS Preventive Medicine, 1271
DHHS Priority Health Conditions Studies Initiative, 1273
DHHS Public Health Students Traineeships and Other Graduate Public Health Programs, 1277
E. Rhodes and Leona B. Carpenter Fndn Grants, 1356
FIC International Training and Research in Emerging Infectious Diseases Grants, 1492
Fndn for Seacoast Health Grants, 1533
Frances and John L. Loeb Family Fund Grants, 1546
Fred L. Emerson Fndn Grants, 1557
Fulbright Alumni Initiatives Awards Grants, 1566
Fulbright Distinguished Chairs Grants, 1567
Fulbright New Century Scholars Grants, 1570
Fulbright Specialists Grants, 1571
Fulbright Traditional Scholar Program in Europe and Eurasia, 1572
Fulbright Traditional Scholar Program in Sub-Saharan Africa, 1573
Fulbright Traditional Scholar Program in the East Asia/Pacific Region, 1574
Fulbright Traditional Scholar Program in the Near East and North Africa Region, 1575
Fulbright Traditional Scholar Program in the South and Central Asia Region, 1576
Fulbright Traditional Scholar Program in the Western Hemisphere, 1577
Greater Worcester Comm Fndn Jeppson Memorial Fund for Brookfield Grants, 1659
Henry J. Kaiser Family Fndn Grants, 1748
HRB Health Services Research Fellowships, 1801
HRSA Health Professions Scholarships for Disadvantaged Students, 1807
International Fellowships in Medical Education, 1861
IWMF Public Health Fellowship, 1871
Jane's Trust Grants, 1904
Johnson & Johnson Comm Health Care Grants, 1951
Joyce Fndn Grants, 1969
Kaiser Permanente Cares for Communities Grants, 1978
Kansas Health Fndn Grants, 1980
Knight Public Health Journalism Fellowships at CDC, 2008
Knox County Comm Fndn Grants, 2009
M-A-C AIDS Fund Grants, 2091
McCarthy Family Fndn Grants, 2141
Morris and Gwendolyn Cafritz Fndn Grants, 2217
NCI/NIDA Transdisciplinary Tobacco Use Research Centers Grants, 2280
NIA Mentored Clinical Scientist Research Career Development Awards, 2417
NIAID Challenge Grants: Joint Ventures in Biomedicine and Biotechnology, 2451
NIDA Minority Institutions Drug Abuse Research Development Program (MIDARP) Grants, 2509
NIDCD Health Promotion and Disease Prevention: Health Communication, Development, and Dissemination, 2521
NIEHS Superfund Hazardous Substances Basic Research and Education Grants, 2607
NIMH Interventions Infrastructure Program Research Grants, 2760
NIMH Pilot Effectiveness Trials for Mental Disorders Grants, 2766
NIMH Therapeutic Effectiveness Protocol Development Grants, 2774
Northwestern Mutual Fndn Grants, 2870
NYAM Student Essay Grants, 2917
ORISE Postgraduate Research Participation at the Agency for Toxic Substances and Disease Registry, 2960
PAHO/WHO Fellowships, 2984
Pfizer Fndn Grants, 3025
Pfizer Fndn Health Literacy Grants, 3026
PhRMA Fndn Health Outcomes Post Doctoral Fellowships, 3031
Postdoctoral Research Fellowships in Gerontological Public Health, 3070
Premera CARES Grants, 3074
Prospect Burma Scholarships, 3085
RWJF Comm Health Leaders Awards, 3208
RWJF Pioneer Portfolio Grants, 3227
RWJF Summer Medical and Dental Education Program, 3231
RWJF Young Epidemiology Scholars Competition, 3233
Saint Luke's Health Initiatives Grants, 3240
Samueli Institute Scientific Research Grants, 3253
San Francisco Fndn Comm Health Grants, 3260
Siragusa Fndn Health Services & Medical Research Grants, 3294
Special Olympics Health Professions Student Grants, 3355
Steelcase Fndn Grants, 3379
Susan G. Komen Breast Cancer Fndn Postdoctoral Fellowships, 3411
Takemi Program in International Health Research and Advanced Training Fellowships, 3416
Texas Commission on the Arts Arts Respond Project Grants, 3420
United Methodist Church Malaria Control Grants, 3464
Vancouver Fndn Public Health Bursary Package, 3478
Vanderburgh Comm Fndn Grants, 3480
Wal-Mart State Giving Grants, 3514

Public Planning/Policy
Able Trust Vocational Rehabilitation Grants for Individuals, 186
Achelis and Bodman Fndns Grants, 206

AMA-MSS Government Relations Advocacy Fellowship, 403
American-Scandinavian Fndn Visiting Lectureship Grants, 460
amfAR Fellowships, 462
amfAR Global Initiatives Grants, 463
amfAR Mathilde Krim Fellowships in Basic Biomedical Research, 464
amfAR Public Policy Grants, 465
amfAR Research Grants, 466
APA Congressional Fellowships, 492
Assurant Health Fndn Grants, 655
AT&T Fndn Civic and Comm Service Grants, 658
Austin College Leadership Award, 668
Bernard F. and Alva B. Gimbel Fndn Grants, 747
Carnegie Corp of New York Grants, 879
Charles G. Koch Charitable Fndn Grants, 965
Charles H. Revson Fndn Grants, 969
CIGNA Fndn Grants, 1011
Claude Pepper Fndn Grants, 1032
Commonwealth Fund Patient-Centered Coordinated Care Grants, 1081
Comm Fndn of Mount Vernon and Knox County Grants, 1119
Comm Fndn of Southeastern Connecticut Grants, 1125
Deland Fellowships in Health Care and Society, 1214
DPA Promoting Policy Change Advocacy Grants, 1324
E.L. Wiegand Fndn Grants, 1361
Eberly Fndn Grants, 1364
Emma B. Howe Memorial Fndn Grants, 1415
ExxonMobil Grants, 1442
F.M. Kirby Fndn Grants, 1443
FCD Child Development Grants, 1458
Ferree Fndn Grants, 1486
Frances and John L. Loeb Family Fund Grants, 1546
General Motors Fndn Grants Support Program, 1591
Gill Fndn - Gay and Lesbian Fund Grants, 1613
Hilton Hotels Corp Giving Grants, 1780
J.W. Kieckhefer Fndn Grants, 1878
Jacob and Hilda Blaustein Fndn Grants, 1881
JM Fndn Grants, 1926
Joseph P. Kennedy Jr. Fndn Grants, 1962
Joyce Fndn Grants, 1969
Kaiser Permanente Cares for Communities Grants, 1978
Lester Ray Fleming Scholarships, 2048
Lynde and Harry Bradley Fndn Grants, 2089
Lynde and Harry Bradley Fndn Prizes: Bradley Prizes, 2090
Marijuana Policy Project Grants, 2107
Max Bell Fndn Grants, 2134
Millipore Fndn Grants, 2203
Minneapolis Fndn Comm Grants, 2206
Miriam and Peter Haas Fund Grants, 2208
Ms. Fndn for Women Grants, 2222
Nordson Corp Fndn Grants, 2851
Oleonda Jameson Trust Grants, 2941
Piedmont Natural Gas Grants, 3048
Pittsburgh Fndn Comm Fund Grants, 3054
Procter and Gamble Fund Grants, 3083
Richard and Helen DeVos Fndn Grants, 3157
RRF General Grants, 3193
Sarah Scaife Fndn Grants, 3263
TWS Fndn Grants, 3443
Women's Fndn of California Comm Action Fund, 3549
Z. Smith Reynolds Fndn Small Grants, 3557

Public Relations
Carrier Corp Contributions Grants, 884

Public Safety
CNCS Next Generation Grants, 1049
OneStar Fndn AmeriCorps Grants, 2945
Westinghouse Charitable Giving Grants, 3530

Public Safety Law
AMA Fndn Fund for Better Health Grants, 388
Baptist Comm Ministries Grants, 691
Perry County Comm Fndn Grants, 3016
Pike County Comm Fndn Grants, 3049
Posey Comm Fndn Grants, 3068
Texas Commission on the Arts Arts Respond Project Grants, 3420

Publication
ASHA Advancing Academic-Research Careers Award, 569
ASHA Student Research Travel Award, 573
CDC Promoting Prevention in Managed Care Cooperative Agreements, 925
Lynde and Harry Bradley Fndn Grants, 2089
Lynde and Harry Bradley Fndn Prizes: Bradley Prizes, 2090
MLA Lois Ann Colaianni Award for Excellence and Achievement in Hospital Librarianship, 2210
NLM Exploratory/Developmental Grants, 2816
NLM Grants for Scholarly Works in Biomedicine and Health, 2818
Potts Memorial Fndn Grants, 3072
RSC Jason A. Hannah Medal, 3196
South Madison Comm Fndn Grants, 3349

Publication Education
Bullitt Fndn Grants, 809

Publishing, Electronic
NLM Grants for Scholarly Works in Biomedicine and Health, 2818
Scientific Communities Initiative Grants, 3272

Puerto Ricans
American Sociological Association Minority Fellowships, 458
Harold Amos Medical Faculty Development Program, 1696
NMF Franklin C. McLean Award, 2829
NMF Need-Based Scholarships, 2839

Pulmonary Diseases
AMA Fndn Seed Grants for Research, 398
CFF First- and Second-Year Clinical Fellowships, 943
CFF Postdoctoral Research Fellowships, 946
CFF Research Grants, 947
CFF Third-Year Clinical Fellowships, 950
Chest Fndn Grant in Venous Thromboembolism, 985
Chestnut Hill Charitable Fndn, Inc Grants, 987
CLA Nurses Respiratory Society Fellowships, 1018
CLA Nurses Respiratory Society Nursing Research Grants, 1019
Duke University Adult Cardiothoracic Anesthesia and Critical Care Medicine Fellowships, 1340
Genentech Corp Charitable Contributions Grants, 1588
Hawaii Comm Fndn Health Education and Research Grants, 1716
Jacob and Valeria Langeloth Fndn Grants, 1882
LAM Fndn Established Investigator Awards, 2022
LAM Fndn Pilot Project Awards, 2023
LAM Fndn Research Grants, 2024
Leahi Fund, 2038
M. Bastian Family Fndn Grants, 2092
NHLBI Ancillary Studies in Clinical Trials, 2317
NHLBI Career Transition Award, 2326
NHLBI Circadian-Coupled Cellular Function in Heart, Lung, and Blood Tissue Grants, 2330
NHLBI Developmental Origins of Altered Lung Physiology and Immune Function Grants, 2332
NHLBI Elucidating Nature's Solutions to Heart, Lung, and Blood Diseases and Sleep Disorder Processes Research Grants, 2333
NHLBI Integrating Lung Genetics and Genomics in Human Populations Grants, 2342
NHLBI Mentored Career Award For Faculty At Minority Institutions, 2346
NHLBI Minority Institution Research Scientist Development Award, 2354
NHLBI Minority Institutional Research Training Grants, 2355
NHLBI Nutrition and Diet in the Causation, Prevention, and Management of Heart Failure Research Grants, 2361
NHLBI Phase II Clinical Trials of Novel Therapies for Lung Diseases, 2365
NHLBI Protein Interactions Governing Membrane Transport in Pulmonary Health and Disease Grants, 2369
NHLBI Ruth L. Kirschstein National Research Service Awards for Individual Predoctoral MD/PhD Fellows, 2381
NHLBI Short-Term Research Education Program to Increase Diversity in Health-Related Research, 2383
NHLBI Stress Management Interventions to Reduce Risk of Coronary Artery Disease, 2384
NHLBI Translational Programs in Lung Diseases, 2391
NIH Mechanisms Underlying Individual Variations in Drug Responses, 2685
NIH National Occupational Research Agenda Grants, 2696
NIH Research on Sleep and Sleep Disorders, 2713
Parker B. Francis Fellowships in Pulmonary Research, 2989

Quality of Life
Allen P. and Josephine B. Green Fndn Grants, 361
Business Bank of Nevada Comm Grants, 817
CharityWorks Grants, 961
CSL Behring Local Empowerment for Advocacy Development Grants, 1167
Dennis and Phyllis Washington Fndn Grants, 1222
FCNY Union Square Awards, 1461
Fifth Third Fndn Grants, 1501
Foster Fndn Grants, 1524
Hall-Perrine Fndn Grants, 1686
Harry S. Black and Allon Fuller Fund, 1706
HHK Employment Grants, 1755
Hilton Head Island Fndn Grants, 1779
Horizon Fndn for New Jersey Grants, 1793
Jim Moran Fndn Grants, 1925
Ken W. Davis Fndn Grants, 1987
Key Fndn Grants, 1994
Middlesex Savings Charitable Fndn Grants, 2196
Payless ShoeSource Fndn Grants, 3004
Ruth Mott Fndn Grants, 3204
Wachovia Fndn Grants, 3511
Westinghouse Charitable Giving Grants, 3530

Quality/Product Control
U.S. Department of Education Erma Byrd Scholarships, 3446

Racism/Race Relations
Allstate Corp Giving Grants, 363
Allstate Corp Hometown Commitment Grants, 364
Cowles Charitable Trust Grants, 1155
Fndn for the Carolinas Grants, 1535
Georgia Power Fndn Grants, 1603
Joseph H. and Florence A. Roblee Fndn Grants, 1961
Meadows Fndn Grants, 2161
NEI Ruth L. Kirschstein National Research Service Award Short-Term Institutional Research Training Grants, 2297
OUT Fund for Lesbian & Gay Liberation Grants, 2978
Palm Beach and Martin Counties Grants, 2986
Pittsburgh Fndn Comm Fund Grants, 3054
RWJF Finding Answers: Disparities Research for Change Grants, 3211
San Diego Fndn for Change Grants, 3255

Radiation
DOE Health Effects and Life Sciences Research Grants, 1298
DOE Low Dose Radiation Research Program, 1300
DOE Medical Applications and Measurement Science Grants, 1301
DSO Radiation Biodosimetry Grants, 1335
NCIC Canadian Cancer Society Research Grants, 2282

Radiation Effects
American Academy of Dermatology Shade Structure Grants, 413
DOE Low Dose Radiation Research Program, 1300
DSO Radiation Biodosimetry Grants, 1335
MDBD Basic Research Grants, 2152
NINDS Cerebral Radiobiology and Neuroimaging of Brain Tumors Research Grants, 2778
ORISE Postgraduate Research Program at the Center for Devices and Radiological Health, 2962

Radiation Instrumentation
DSO Radiation Biodosimetry Grants, 1335

Radio
Albert Pick Jr. Fund Grants, 328
American Academy of Nursing Media Awards, 418
Andersen Fndn Grants, 471
Comm Fndn of Crawford County Grants and Scholarships, 1103
G.N. Wilcox Trust Grants, 1581
Gill Fndn - Gay and Lesbian Fund Grants, 1613

Radiology
Ethical Research Grants and Fellowships, 1431
NIGMS Pilot Projects for the Protein Structure Initiative (Structural Genomics), 2624
Society for Imaging Informatics in Medicine Emeritus Mentor Grants, 3320
Society for Imaging Informatics in Medicine Micro Grants, 3321
Society for Imaging Informatics in Medicine Research Grants, 3322
Society for Imaging Informatics in Medicine Small Grant for Product Support Development, 3323
Society for Imaging Informatics in Medicine Small Training Grants, 3324

Radiotherapy
NINDS Cerebral Radiobiology and Neuroimaging of Brain Tumors Research Grants, 2778

Reading
Atkinson Fndn International Grants, 661
Barker Welfare Fndn Grants, 695
Bodenwein Public Benevolent Fndn Grants, 775
Boettcher Fndn Grants, 778
Boston Fndn Grants, 783
Colorado Springs Comm Trust Fund Grants, 1061
Howard and Bush Fndn Grants, 1798
Kalamazoo Fndn Grants, 1979
Louis Calder Fndn Grants, 2065
Marshall Field's Comm Grants, 2115
NSF Perception, Action & Cognition Research Grants, 2890

Reading Education
Arlington Comm Fndn Grants, 536
Baptist Comm Ministries Grants, 691
DaimlerChrysler Corp Fund Grants, 1186
Emily Davie and Joseph S. Kornfeld Fndn Grants, 1414

Recombinant DNA
NIGMS Molecular Pharmacology of Anesthetic Action Research Grants, 2621
NSF Chemical, Biochemical, and Biotechnology Systems Research Grants, 2882

Reconstructive Surgery
AAFPRS Ben Shuster Memorial Award, 117
AAFPRS Bernstein Grant, 118
AAFPRS Fellowships, 119
AAFPRS Investigator Development Grant, 120
AAFPRS John Orlando Roe Award, 122
AAFPRS Leslie Bernstein Resident Research Grants, 123
AAFPRS Residency Travel Awards, 124
AAFPRS Sir Harold Delf Gillies Award, 125
Plastic Surgery Educational Fndn Basic Research Grants, 3058
Plastic Surgery Educational Fndn Research Fellowship Grants, 3059
Plastic Surgery Educational Fndn/AAO-HNSF Combined Grant, 3060

Recreation and Leisure
African American Fund of New Jersey Grants, 260
Alice Tweed Tuohy Fndn Grants, 357
Amador Comm Fndn Grants, 409
American Academy of Dermatology Camp Discovery Scholarships, 412
Aratani Fndn Grants, 523
Argyros Fndn Grants, 527
Armstrong McDonald Fndn Grants, 537
Atlanta Fndn Grants, 662
Bacon Family Fndn Grants, 679
Balance Bar Sports Individual/Team Grants, 681
Beazley Fndn Grants, 730
Beckley Area Fndn Grants, 732
Blanche and Julian Robertson Family Fndn Grants, 765
Boston Fndn Grants, 783
C.R. Bard Fndn Grants, 825
Carls Fndn Grants, 876
Carrie Estelle Doheny Fndn Grants, 883
Carrier Corp Contributions Grants, 884
Cass County Comm Fndn Grants, 887
Children Affected by AIDS Fndn Domestic Grants, 995
Comm Fndn for Southern Arizona Grants, 1095
Comm Fndn of Crawford County Grants and Scholarships, 1103
Comm Fndn of Mount Vernon and Knox County Grants, 1119
Comm Fndn of South Alabama Grants, 1123
Comm Fndn of St. Joseph County Special Project Challenge Grants, 1126
Comm Fndn of Wabash County Grants, 1131
Dubois County Comm Fndn Grants, 1336
Emma B. Howe Memorial Fndn Grants, 1415
Fargo-Moorhead Area Fndn Grants, 1454
Foellinger Fndn Grants, 1519
Frank Stanley Beveridge Fndn Grants, 1553
Fulton County Comm Fndn Grants, 1579
George Kress Fndn Grants, 1601
Glazer Family Fndn Grants, 1625
Grand Haven Area Comm Fndn Grants, 1644
Grand Rapids Comm Fndn Grants, 1647
Greater Bridgeport Area Fndn Comm Impact Grants, 1650
Greater Worcester Comm Fndn Jeppson Memorial Fund for Brookfield Grants, 1659
Harrison County Comm Fndn Grants, 1700
Hasbro Children's Fund, 1714
Heckscher Fndn for Children Grants, 1732
Holland/Zeeland Comm Fndn Grants, 1786
Idaho Comm Fndn Eastern Region Competitive Grants, 1837
Impact 100 Grants, 1843
James S. Copley Fndn Grants, 1895
Josephine S. Gumbiner Fndn Grants, 1965
Kahuku Comm Fund, 1977
Knox County Comm Fndn Grants, 2009
Kosciusko County Comm Fndn Grants, 2015
LaGrange County Comm Fndn Grants, 2020
Lowell Area Comm Fund Grants, 2068
Lubrizol Fndn Grants, 2080
M-A-C AIDS Fund Grants, 2091
Maxon Charitable Fndn Grants, 2135
McKesson Fndn Grants, 2145
McMillen Fndn Grants, 2148
Miami County Comm Fndn Operation Round Up Grants, 2188
Owen County Comm Fndn Grants, 2979
Perry County Comm Fndn Grants, 3016
Phoenix Suns Charities Grants, 3030
Pike County Comm Fndn Grants, 3049
Posey Comm Fndn Grants, 3068
Pride Fndn Grants and Scholarships, 3078
Principal Financial Group Fndn Grants, 3082
Putnam County Comm Fndn Grants, 3093
Ralphs Food 4 Less Fndn Grants, 3106
Rayonier Fndn Grants, 3111
Rochester Area Fndn Grants, 3177
Sarah Scaife Fndn Grants, 3263
Scott County Comm Fndn Grants, 3273
Seabury Fndn Grants, 3274
Seneca Foods Fndn Grants, 3278
Southbury Comm Trust Fund, 3350
Spencer County Comm Fndn Grants, 3358
Springs Close Fndn Grants, 3360
Steuben County Comm Fndn Grants, 3383
Strowd Roses Grants, 3388
U.S. Department of Education 21st Century Comm Learning Centers, 3445
Vanderburgh Comm Fndn Grants, 3480
Warrick County Comm Fndn Grants, 3519
Winston-Salem Fndn Competitive Grants, 3544
Winston-Salem Fndn Stokes County Grants, 3546

Recreation and Leisure Studies
Huntington County Comm Fndn Grants, 1823

Reference Materials
ASM USFCC/J. Roger Porter Award, 623
NLM Grants for Scholarly Works in Biomedicine and Health, 2818

Refugees
ACF Ethnic Comm Self-Help Grants, 200
ACF Preferred Communities Grants, 201
ACF Standing Announcement for Unaccompanied Alien Children Grants, 202
ACF Supplemental Services for Recently Arrived Refugees Grants, 203
Atkinson Fndn International Grants, 661
Blumenthal Fndn Grants, 773
Dallas Women's Fndn Grants, 1191
Grotto Fndn Project Grants, 1671
Jacob and Valeria Langeloth Fndn Grants, 1882
Minneapolis Fndn Comm Grants, 2206
San Diego Fndn for Change Grants, 3255

Regional Planning/Policy
Bill and Melinda Gates Fndn Grants, 756
Canada-U.S. Fulbright New Century Scholars Grants, 846
Canada-U.S. Fulbright Senior Specialists Grants, 847
Carpenter Fndn Grants, 881
Dorothy Rider Pool Health Care Grants, 1322
Fndn for the Carolinas Grants, 1535
Fulbright Alumni Initiatives Awards Grants, 1566
Fulbright Distinguished Chairs Grants, 1567
Fulbright New Century Scholars Grants, 1570
Fulbright Specialists Grants, 1571
Fulbright Traditional Scholar Program in Europe and Eurasia, 1572
Fulbright Traditional Scholar Program in Sub-Saharan Africa, 1573
Fulbright Traditional Scholar Program in the East Asia/Pacific Region, 1574
Fulbright Traditional Scholar Program in the Near East and North Africa Region, 1575
Fulbright Traditional Scholar Program in the South and Central Asia Region, 1576
Fulbright Traditional Scholar Program in the Western Hemisphere, 1577
Lockheed Martin Philanthropic Grants, 2062

Rehabilitation/Therapy
Alberto Culver Corp Contributions Grants, 329
Bodman Fndn Grants, 776
Cailloux Fndn Grants, 829
Carl W. and Carrie Mae Joslyn Trust Grants, 873
Chicago Board of Trade Fndn Grants, 988
Comm Fndn for Southern Arizona Grants, 1095
Dammann Fund Grants, 1192
Dolan Fndn Grants, 1306
Dr. John T. Macdonald Fndn Grants, 1327
Henry County Comm Fndn Grants, 1747
IAFF Burn Fndn Research Grants, 1830

John W. Alden Trust Grants, 1947
Kathryne Beynon Fndn Grants, 1984
Lubrizol Fndn Grants, 2080
NIA Health Behaviors and Aging Grants, 2408
NICHD Clinical Trial Planning Grants for Pediatric Rehabilitation, 2483
NICHD Medical Rehabilitation Research, 2487
NIDA Behavioral Therapies Development Grants, 2499
NIDRR Field-Initiated Projects, 2594
NIH Exploratory Centers for Alternative Medicine Research Grants, 2663
NIMH Interventions Infrastructure Program Research Grants, 2760
NYCT Girls and Young Women Grants, 2924
Ordean Fndn Grants, 2952
Peabody Fndn Grants, 3010
Phoenix Suns Charities Grants, 3030
Potts Memorial Fndn Grants, 3072
Raskob Fndn for Catholic Activities Grants, 3107
Robert B McMillen Fndn Grants, 3169
Robert E. and Evelyn McKee Fndn Grants, 3170
Russell Berrie Fndn Grants, 3201
U.S. Department of Education Rehabilitation Engineering Research Centers Grants, 3447

Rehabilitation/Therapy, Emotional/Social
Dept of Ed Rehabilitation Training Grants, 1229
Fourjay Fndn Grants, 1544
Liliane Fndn Grants, 2055
Lincoln Financial Group Fndn Grants, 2058
Margoes Fndn Grants, 2106
Military Ex-Prisoners of War Fndn Grants, 2201
NIDA Behavioral Therapies Development Grants, 2499
NIH Exploratory/Development Grants for Mental Health Intervention Research, 2665
Perry County Comm Fndn Grants, 3016
Posey Comm Fndn Grants, 3068
Robert B McMillen Fndn Grants, 3169
Robert E. and Evelyn McKee Fndn Grants, 3170
Seabury Fndn Grants, 3274
Vanderburgh Comm Fndn Grants, 3480

Rehabilitation/Therapy, Occupational/Vocational
Able Trust Vocational Rehabilitation Grants for Individuals, 186
Achelis and Bodman Fndns Grants, 206
Dept of Ed Rehabilitation Training Grants, 1229
EF Behavioral Sciences Student Fellowships, 1379
Jewish Fndn for Education of Women Scholarships for Emigres in the Health Professions, 1922
Lincoln Financial Group Fndn Grants, 2058
U.S. Department of Education Rehabilitation Research Training Centers, 3448
U.S. Department of Education Vocational Rehabilitation Services Projects for American Indians with Disabilities Grants, 3452

Rehabilitation/Therapy, Physical
AAPD Henry B. Betts Award, 169
Fndn for Physical Therapy Mary McMillan Doctoral Scholarships, 1529
Fndn for Physical Therapy Research Grants, 1530
Jewish Fndn for Education of Women Scholarships for Emigres in the Health Professions, 1922
Liliane Fndn Grants, 2055
NIH Urinary Incontinence Treatment Network, 2738
Robert B McMillen Fndn Grants, 3169
Seabury Fndn Grants, 3274

Religion
1104 Fndn Grants, 3
A Friend's Fndn Trust Grants, 13
Aaron Fndn (Massachusetts) Grants, 174
Abel Fndn Grants, 181
Abell-Hanger Fndn Grants, 183
Able To Serve Grants, 185
Abramson Family Fndn Grants, 188
Adams County Fndn Grants - Pennsylvania, 231
Adolph Coors Fndn Grants, 238
Ahmanson Fndn Grants, 303
Ahn Family Fndn Grants, 304
Albert and Margaret Alkek Fndn Grants, 326
Alcoa Fndn Grants, 334
ALSAM Fndn Grants, 369
Andersen Fndn Grants, 471
Anschutz Family Fndn Grants, 486
Anthony R. Abraham Fndn Grants, 490
Aratani Fndn Grants, 523
Archer Daniels Midland Fndn Grants, 525
Argyros Fndn Grants, 527
Arkansas Comm Fndn Grants, 533
Arkell Hall Fndn Grants, 534
Armstrong McDonald Fndn Grants, 537
Atherton Family Fndn Grants, 659
Audrey and Sydney Irmas Charitable Fndn Grants, 665
Bacon Family Fndn Grants, 679
Bailey Fndn Grants, 680
Banfi Vintners Fndn Grants, 687
Barra Fndn Project Grants, 699
Baton Rouge Area Fndn Grants, 702
Beatrice Laing Trust Grants, 729
Beazley Fndn Grants, 730
Belk Fndn Grants, 739
Bender Fndn Grants, 742
Besser Fndn Grants, 752
BibleLands Grants, 754
Blumenthal Fndn Grants, 773
Bodenwein Public Benevolent Fndn Grants, 775
Bodman Fndn Grants, 776
Borkee-Hagley Fndn Grants, 781
Bradley Turner Fndn Grants, 789
Bright Family Fndn Grants, 793
Bruce and Adele Greenfield Fndn Grants, 808
Burden Trust Grants, 810
Burton G. Bettingen Grants, 813
Byron W. and Alice L. Lockwood Fndn Grants, 824
Caddock Fndn Grants, 828
Caleb C. and Julia W. Dula Educational and Charitable Fndn Grants, 830
Callaway Fndn Grants, 835
Carl Gellert and Celia Berta Gellert Fndn Grants, 871
Carrie Estelle Doheny Fndn Grants, 883
Carylon Fndn Grants, 886
Castle Rock Fndn Grants, 888
Chatlos Fndn Grants, 977
Chiles Fndn Grants, 1003
Citizens Bank Mid-Atlantic Charitable Fndn Grants, 1015
Clark-Winchcole Fndn Grants, 1030
Claude Bennett Family Fndn Grants, 1031
Coastal Comm Fndn of South Carolina Grants, 1051
Collins Fndn Grants, 1058
Commission on Religion in Appalachia Grants, 1074
Comm Fndn of Greenville Comm Enrichment Grants, 1113
Comm Fndn of Greenville Hollingsworth Funds Program/Project Grants, 1114
Comm Fndn of Madison and Jefferson County Grants and Scholarships, 1117
Comm Fndn of Mount Vernon and Knox County Grants, 1119
Connelly Fndn Grants, 1143
Constellation Energy Group and Baltimore Gas and Electric Corp Contributions, 1146
CRH Fndn Grants, 1160
Dade Comm Fndn Grants, 1185
DaimlerChrysler Corp Fund Grants, 1186
Danellie Fndn Grants, 1198
Daywood Fndn Grants, 1206
Deaconess Comm Fndn Grants, 1207
Donald and Sylvia Robinson Family Fndn Grants, 1310
Dora Roberts Fndn Grants, 1311
Dorothy Hooper Beattie Fndn Grants, 1321
Dr. Scholl Fndn Grants, 1329
Edward S. Moore Fndn Grants, 1374
Edwin W. and Catherine M. Davis Fndn Grants, 1377
Effie and Wofford Cain Fndn Grants, 1385
Elliot Fndn Inc Grants, 1402
Emily Davie and Joseph S. Kornfeld Fndn Grants, 1414
Ensworth Charitable Fndn Grants, 1416
Eugene B. Casey Fndn Grants, 1433
Evjue Fndn Grants, 1439
F.M. Kirby Fndn Grants, 1443
Fndn for Spirituality and Medicine Grants, 1534
Fndn for the Carolinas Grants, 1535
Frank G. & Freida K. Brotz Family Fndn Grants, 1552
Frank Stanley Beveridge Fndn Grants, 1553
Franklin County Comm Fndn Grants, 1554
Fraser-Parker Fndn Grants, 1555
Frist Fndn Grants, 1563
Fritz B. Burns Fndn Grants, 1564
Fuller E. Callaway Fndn Grants, 1578
George F. Baker Trust Grants, 1597
George Family Fndn Grants, 1598
George Frederick Jewett Fndn Grants, 1599
George Kress Fndn Grants, 1601
Giant Eagle Fndn Grants, 1611
Gilroy and Lillian P. Roberts Charitable Fndn Grants, 1614
Glendale Comm Fndn Grants, 1626
Great-West Life Grants, 1649
Greater Saint Louis Comm Fndn Grants, 1655
Greater Worcester Comm Fndn Discretionary Grants, 1658
Gregory Family Fndn Grants (Florida), 1667
Griffin Family Fndn Grants, 1669
Hackett Fndn Grants, 1684
Harold Simmons Fndn Grants, 1698
Harry and Grace Steele Fndn Grants, 1702
Harry Frank Guggenheim Fndn Research Grants, 1704
Hearst Fndn and William Randolph Hearst Fndn Grants, 1730
Hedco Fndn Grants, 1733
Helen Bader Fndn Grants, 1738
Hillsdale Fund Grants, 1778
Ida Alice Ryan Charitable Trust Grants, 1836
J.C. Penney Company Grants, 1874
J.E. and L.E. Mabee Fndn Grants, 1875
Jacob and Hilda Blaustein Fndn Grants, 1881
James Hervey Johnson Charitable Educational Trust Grants, 1889
James J. and Angelia M. Harris Fndn Grants, 1890
James M. Collins Fndn Grants, 1891
Jessie Ball Dupont Fund Grants, 1919
Jewish Women's Fndn of New York Grants, 1924
Joe W. and Dorothy Dorsett Brown Fndn Grants, 1927
John G. Duncan Trust Grants, 1931
John H. and Wilhelmina D. Harland Charitable Fndn Grants, 1933
John J. Leidy Fndn Grants, 1936
John P. Murphy Fndn Grants, 1943
Joseph H. and Florence A. Roblee Fndn Grants, 1961
Katharine Matthies Fndn Grants, 1982
King Pharmaceuticals Corp Contributions Grants, 2003
Kluge Center David B. Larson Fellowship in Health and Spirituality, 2006
Knight Family Charitable and Educational Fndn Grants, 2007
Larry L. Hillblom Fndn Grants, 2031
Louis Calder Fndn Grants, 2065
Lowell Berry Fndn Grants, 2069
Lubbock Area Fndn Grants, 2079
Lucile Horton Howe and Mitchell B. Howe Fndn Grants, 2081
M. Bastian Family Fndn Grants, 2092
Margaret L. Wendt Fndn Grants, 2104
Marion I. and Henry J. Knott Fndn Grants, 2109
Marion Park Deaver and Harry Gilbert Deaver Fndn Grants, 2110
Maxon Charitable Fndn Grants, 2135
McMurry Fndn Grants, 2149
Meriden Fndn Grants, 2173
Nell Warren Elkin and William Simpson Elkin Fndn, 2302
North Carolina Comm Development Grants, 2858
North Carolina Comm Fndn Grants, 2859
North Georgia Comm Fndn Grants, 2862
Paul and Mary Haas Fndn Contributions and Student Scholarships, 2997

Paul E. and Klare N. Reinhold Fndn Grants, 2999
Perkins Charitable Fndn Grants, 3014
Pittsburgh Fndn Comm Fund Grants, 3054
PNC Charitable Trust and Fndn Grants, 3064
Polk Bros. Fndn Grants, 3066
R.C. Baker Fndn Grants, 3098
Rainbow Fund Grants, 3103
Religion and Health: Effects, Mechanisms, and Interpretation RFP, 3149
Richard and Helen DeVos Fndn Grants, 3157
Robert E. and Evelyn McKee Fndn Grants, 3170
Robins Fndn Grants, 3175
Roy J. Carver Charitable Trust Medical and Science Research Grants, 3192
Rush County Comm Fndn Grants, 3200
Russell Berrie Fndn Grants, 3201
S.H. Cowell Fndn Grants, 3237
Salem Fndn Grants, 3242
Salisbury Comm Fndn Grants, 3243
Siebert Lutheran Fndn Grants, 3285
Sir Halley Stewart Trust Grants, 3293
Sisters of St. Joseph Healthcare Fndn Grants, 3297
SOCFOC Catholic Ministries Grants, 3317
Solo Cup Fndn Grants, 3346
Southwire Company Grants, 3353
Stewart Huston Charitable Trust Grants, 3384
Sunderland Fndn Grants, 3400
Support Our Aging Religious Grants, 3406
Susan Mott Webb Charitable Trust Grants, 3412
Thomas and Dorothy Leavey Fndn Grants, 3422
Thomas M. and Irene B. Kirbo Charitable Trust Grants, 3424
Thompson Charitable Fndn Grants, 3425
Trull Fndn Grants, 3441
Vancouver Fndn Grants and Comm Initiatives Program, 3477
W. C. Griffith Fndn Grants, 3505
Wabash Valley Comm Fndn Grants, 3510
Wayne and Gladys Valley Fndn Grants, 3522
Weingart Fndn Grants, 3524
William H. Hannon Fndn Grants, 3540
Woodward Fund Grants, 3552

Religious Programs
Dale and Edna Walsh Fndn Grants, 1189
Gheens Fndn Grants, 1610
Hagedorn Fund Grants, 1685
Irvin Stern Fndn Grants, 1866

Religious Studies
Able To Serve Grants, 185
Andersen Fndn Grants, 471
Bailey Fndn Grants, 680
Blumenthal Fndn Grants, 773
Boettcher Fndn Grants, 778
Booth-Bricker Fund Grants, 780
Chatlos Fndn Grants, 977
Cockrell Fndn Grants, 1053
Comm Fndn of Grant County Grants, 1104
Comm Fndn of Grant County Scholarships, 1105
E. Rhodes and Leona B. Carpenter Fndn Grants, 1356
FirstEnergy Fndn Comm Grants, 1505
Frank G. and Freida K. Brotz Family Fndn Grants, 1552
Hedco Fndn Grants, 1733
John I. Smith Charities Grants, 1935
Mary Baker Eddy Library Summer Research Fellowships, 2117
Nell Warren Elkin and William Simpson Elkin Fndn, 2302
Rainbow Fund Grants, 3103
Richard and Helen DeVos Fndn Grants, 3157
Russell Berrie Fndn Grants, 3201
Siebert Lutheran Fndn Grants, 3285

Religious Welfare Programs
Able To Serve Grants, 185
Adams County Fndn Grants - Pennsylvania, 231
Bob and Delores Hope Charitable Fndn Grants, 774
Byron W. and Alice L. Lockwood Fndn Grants, 824
Carrie E. and Lena V. Glenn Fndn Grants, 882
Claude Bennett Family Fndn Grants, 1031
Ensworth Charitable Fndn Grants, 1416
Greenspun Family Fndn Grants, 1664
Gregory Family Fndn Grants (Florida), 1667
Harry Kramer Memorial Fund Grants, 1705
Ida Alice Ryan Charitable Trust Grants, 1836
Meriden Fndn Grants, 2173
Richard and Helen DeVos Fndn Grants, 3157
Solo Cup Fndn Grants, 3346
St. Joseph Comm Health Fndn Improving Healthcare Access Grants, 3368
Triangle Comm Fndn Donor-Advised Grants, 3437
Vancouver Fndn Grants and Comm Initiatives Program, 3477
W. C. Griffith Fndn Grants, 3505
Women of the ELCA Opportunity Scholarships for Lutheran Laywomen, 3548

Remedial Education
Amgen Fndn Grants, 467

Renewable Energy Sources
Carolyn Fndn Grants, 880

Repetitive Motion Disorders
NIAMS Repetitive Motion Disorders Research Grants, 2475
NICHD Repetitive Motion Disorders Research Grants, 2491
NINDS Repetitive Motion Disorders Research Grants, 2784
NIOSH Repetitive Motion Disorders Research Grants, 2808

Reproduction
Public Welfare Fndn Grants, 3089

Reproductive Disorders
CIIT Postdoctoral Fellowships, 1012
DHHS Priority Health Conditions Studies Initiative, 1273
NIEHS Applied Toxicological Research and Testing Grants, 2595
NIEHS Biological Response to Environmental Health Hazards Research Grants, 2596

Reproductive Rights
Lewis Preston Fund for Girls Education Grants, 2052

Research Participation
A-T Medical Research Fndn Grants, 16
AACR Award for Outstanding Achievement in Cancer Research, 67
AACR Clinical and Translational Research Fellowships, 73
AACR Minority-Serving Institution Faculty Scholar in Cancer Research Awards, 83
AACR Richard and Hinda Rosenthal Memorial Awards, 86
AACR-FNAB Fellows Grant for Translational Pancreatic Cancer Research, 93
AACR-Minorities in Cancer Research Jane Cooke Wright Lectureship Awards, 99
AACR-National Brain Tumor Fndn Fellows Grant, 100
AACR-Women in Cancer Research Charlotte Friend Memorial Lectureship Awards, 106
AACR Basic Cancer Research Fellowships , 107
ACS Doctoral Training Grants in Oncology Social Work, 213
ACS Physician Training Awards in Preventive Medicine, 218
AFAR Medical Student Training in Aging Research Program, 255
AFAR Paul Beeson Career Development Awards in Aging Research for the Island of Ireland, 256
AHFMR Health Research Full-Time Studentships, 280
AHRF Regular Research Grants, 311
Alexander Eastman Fndn Grants, 341
AMA-MSS Research Poster Award, 405
AMA-WPC Joan F. Giambalvo Memorial Scholarships, 408
ASHFndn Clinical Research Grants, 575
ASM Abbott Laboratories Award in Clinical and Diagnostic Immunology, 587
ASM BD Award for Research in Clinical Microbiology, 588
ASM D.C. White Research and Mentoring Award, 592
ASM Eli Lilly and Company Research Award, 594
ASM Merck Irving S. Sigal Memorial Awards, 606
ASM Microbiology Undergraduate Research Fellowship, 607
ASM Procter & Gamble Award in Applied and Environmental Microbiology, 609
ASM Promega Biotechnology Research Award, 610
ASM Raymond W. Sarber Awards, 612
ASM Robert D. Watkins Graduate Research Fellowship, 614
ASM sanofi-aventis ICAAC Award, 616
ASM Siemens Healthcare Diagnostics Young Investigator Award, 618
ASM Undergraduate Research Fellowship, 622
ASM William Hinton Research Training Award, 624
ASM-PAHO Infectious Diseases Epidemiology and Surveillance Fellowships, 625
ASM/CCID Fellowships, 627
BCBSM Fndn Excellence in Research Awards for Students, 717
BCBSM Fndn Physician Investigator Research Awards, 718
BCBSM Fndn Primary and Clinical Prevention Grants, 719
Carrier Corp Contributions Grants, 884
Comm Campus Partnerships for Health Fellowships, 1087
Cruise Industry Charitable Fndn Grants, 1166
DHHS Oral Health Promotion Research Across the Lifespan, 1269
Duke University Adult Cardiothoracic Anesthesia and Critical Care Medicine Fellowships, 1340
Duke University Ambulatory and Regional Anesthesia Fellowships, 1341
Duke University Clinical Cardiac Electrophysiology Fellowships, 1342
Duke University Hyperbaric Center Fellowships, 1343
Duke University Interventional Cardiology Fellowships, 1344
Duke University Obstetric Anesthesia Fellowships, 1345
Duke University Pain Management Fellowships, 1346
Duke University Postdoctoral Research Fellowships in Aging, 1348
Ellison Medical Fndn/AFAR Julie Martin Mid-Career Award in Aging Research, 1403
George H. Hitchings New Investigator Award in Health Research, 1600
Gertrude B. Elion Mentored Medical Student Research Awards, 1608
Gill Fndn - Gay and Lesbian Fund Grants, 1613
Goldman Philanthropic Partnerships Program, 1635
Hawaii Comm Fndn Health Education and Research Grants, 1716
Hoglund Fndn Grants, 1785
HomeBanc Fndn Grants, 1788
Ireland Family Fndn Grants, 1865
John G. Duncan Trust Grants, 1931
John W. Anderson Fndn Grants, 1949
Lymphoma Research Fndn Fellowships, 2087
Mabel H. Flory Charitable Trust Grants, 2096
MGFA Post-Doctoral Research Fellowships, 2183
MGFA Student Fellowships, 2184
NEI Mentored Clinical Scientist Development Program Award (K12), 2295
NEI Research Grant For Secondary Data Analysis Grants, 2296
NEI Ruth L. Kirschstein National Research Service Award Short-Term Institutional Research Training Grants, 2297

Nelda C. and H.J. Lutcher Stark Fndn Grants, 2301
NHLBI Independent Scientist Award, 2339
NHLBI Research Supplements to Promote Diversity in Health-Related Research (Postdoctoral Individuals/New Independent Researchers), 2373
NHLBI Research Supplements to Promote Diversity in Health-Related Research for Established Investigators Who Become Disabled, 2374
NHLBI Research Supplements to Promote Diversity in Health-Related Research for Graduate Research Assistants, 2375
NHLBI Research Supplements to Promote Diversity in Health-Related Research for Individuals in Postdoctoral Training, 2376
NHLBI Research Supplements to Promote Diversity in Health-Related Research for Undergraduate Students, 2377
NIA Independent Scientist Award, 2412
NIH Exploratory/Developmental Research Grant, 2666
NYAM Edward N. Gibbs Memorial Lecture and Award in Nephrology, 2912
NYCT Blood Disease Research Grants, 2922
Pancreatic Cancer Action Network-AACR Fellowship, 2987
Pancreatic Cancer Action Network-AACR Pathway to Leadership Grants, 2988
PDF International Research Grants, 3005
PDF Postdoctoral Fellowships for Neurologists, 3007
Peacock Fndn Grants, 3011
Perpetual Trust for Charitable Giving Grants, 3015
Pittsburgh Fndn Comm Fund Grants, 3054
Pittsburgh Fndn Medical Research Grants, 3055
Pott Fndn Grants, 3071
Potts Memorial Fndn Grants, 3072
R.C. Baker Fndn Grants, 3098
Regenstrief General Internal Medicine - General Pediatrics Research Fellowship Program, 3144
Regenstrief Master Of Science In Clinical Research/CITE Program, 3145
Retirement Research Fndn General Grants, 3150
Robert B McMillen Fndn Grants, 3169
Rockefeller Archive Center Research Grants, 3178
Rosalinde and Arthur Gilbert Fndn/AFAR New Investigator Awards in Alzheimer's Disease, 3187
RWJF Scholars in Health Policy Research Fellowships, 3229
Savoy Fndn Post-Doctoral and Clinical Research Fellowships, 3266
Savoy Fndn Research Grants, 3267
Sigrid Juselius Fndn Grants, 3286
SNM Molecular Imaging Research Grant For Junior Medical Faculty, 3301
SNM Pilot Research Grants, 3303
SNM Pilot Research Grants in Nuclear Medicine/Molecular Imaging, 3304
SNM Postdoctoral Molecular Imaging Scholar Grants, 3305
SNM Student Fellowship Awards, 3306
SNM Tetalman Memorial Young Investigator Awards, 3307
SNM/ Covidien Seed Grant in Molecular Imaging/Nuclear Medicine Research, 3308
STTI Doris Bloch Research Awards, 3389
STTI Emergency Nurses Association Fndn Grant, 3390
STTI Environment of Elder Care Nursing Research Grants, 3391
STTI Joan K. Stout RN Research Grants, 3392
STTI National League for Nursing Grants, 3393
STTI Rosemary Berkel Crisp Research Awards, 3394
STTI Small Grants, 3395
STTI Virginia Henderson Clinical Research Grants, 3396
STTI/ATI Educational Assessment Nursing Research Grants, 3397
STTI/Council for the Advancement of Nursing Science Grants, 3398
Vancouver Fndn Grants and Comm Initiatives Program, 3477
W. C. Griffith Fndn Grants, 3505
Women's Fndn of California Grants, 3550

Research Resources (Health/Safety/Medical)

John W. Anderson Fndn Grants, 1949
NEI Research Grant For Secondary Data Analysis Grants, 2296
NSERC Brockhouse Canada Prize for Interdisciplinary Research in Science and Engineering Grant, 2873
Pittsburgh Fndn Medical Research Grants, 3055
Regenstrief Geriatrics Fellowship, 3143
Regenstrief General Internal Medicine - General Pediatrics Research Fellowship Program, 3144
RWJF Jobs to Careers: Promoting Work-Based Learning for Quality Care - Research Grants, 3221

Respiratory Diseases

CF Clinical Research Trainee Awards, 940
CLA Nurses Respiratory Society Fellowships, 1018
CLA Nurses Respiratory Society Nursing Research Grants, 1019
DHHS Priority Health Conditions Studies Initiative, 1273
DOL Occupational Safety and Health—Susan Harwood Training Grants, 1305
Fairlawn Fndn Grants, 1447
NFID New Investigator Matching Grants, 2310
NHLBI Ancillary Studies in Clinical Trials, 2317
NHLBI Developmental Origins of Altered Lung Physiology and Immune Function Grants, 2332
NHLBI Hypersensitivity Pneumonitis – Grants for Early Identification and Mechanisms of Disease, 2336
NHLBI Microbiome of the Lung and Respiratory Tract in HIV-Infected Individuals and HIV-Uninfected Controls, 2352
NHLBI Phase II Clinical Trials of Novel Therapies for Lung Diseases, 2365
NHLBI Prematurity and Respiratory Outcomes Program Grants, 2366
NHLBI Right Heart Function in Health and Chronic Lung Diseases Grants, 2378
NHLBI Ruth L. Kirschstein National Research Service Awards for Individual Predoctoral MD/PhD Fellows, 2381
NHLBI Transfusion-Related Acute Lung Injury Basic Research Grants, 2389
NHLBI Translational Programs in Lung Diseases, 2391
NIAID Allergy, Immunology, and Transplantation Program Research Grants, 2449
NIEHS Biological Response to Environmental Health Hazards Research Grants, 2596
NIEHS Small Business Innovation Research Grants, 2605
Thrasher Research Fund Grants, 3426

Respiratory System

L. A. Hollinger Respiratory Therapy and Nursing Scholarships, 2018
NHLBI Microbiome of the Lung and Respiratory Tract in HIV-Infected Individuals and HIV-Uninfected Controls, 2352
NHLBI Prematurity and Respiratory Outcomes Program Grants, 2366
Trinity Lutheran School of Nursing Alumnae Scholarships, 3439

Restoration and Preservation

Albuquerque Comm Fndn Grants, 331
Andersen Fndn Grants, 471
Auburn Fndn Grants, 664
Barberton Comm Fndn Grants, 693
Berrien Comm Fndn Grants, 749
Blue Mountain Comm Fndn Grants, 769
Booth-Bricker Fund Grants, 780
Champlin Fndns Grants, 960
Charles Edison Fund Grants, 964
Charlotte County (FL) Comm Fndn Grants, 973
CLIF Bar Family Fndn Grants, 1040
Comm Fndn Alliance City of Evansville Endowment Fund Grants, 1089
Comm Fndn for Monterey County Grants, 1092
Cudd Fndn Grants, 1171
D.F. Halton Fndn Grants, 1181
E. Rhodes and Leona B. Carpenter Fndn Grants, 1356
Fayette County Fndn Grants, 1457
FirstEnergy Fndn Comm Grants, 1505
George Frederick Jewett Fndn Grants, 1599
Greater Green Bay Comm Fndn Grants, 1652
Greater Milwaukee Fndn Grants, 1653
Grundy Fndn Grants, 1673
High Meadow Fndn Grants, 1768
Hoblitzelle Fndn Grants, 1783
Holland/Zeeland Comm Fndn Grants, 1786
Jane's Trust Grants, 1904
Jasper Fndn Jasper County Grants, 1907
Jennings County Comm Fndn Grants, 1916
Jessie Ball Dupont Fund Grants, 1919
Legacy Fndn Grants, 2040
M.E. Raker Fndn Grants, 2094
Mars Fndn Grants, 2114
Mary Black Fndn Grants, 2118
McLean Contributionship Grants, 2147
North Carolina Comm Fndn Grants, 2859
Norwin S. and Elizabeth N. Bean Fndn Grants, 2872
Ogden Codman Trust Grants, 2937
Perkins Charitable Fndn Grants, 3014
S.H. Cowell Fndn Grants, 3237
Salisbury Comm Fndn Grants, 3243
Samuel Freeman Charitable Trust Grants, 3249
Samuel Roberts Noble Fndn Grants, 3250
Sosland Fndn Grants, 3348
Southwest Florida Comm Fndn Competitive Grants, 3351

Restoration and Preservation, Structural/Architectural

Benton Comm Fndn Grants, 743
Blackford County Comm Fndn Grants, 763
Blue River Comm Fndn Grants, 770
Brown County Comm Fndn Grants, 807
Caleb C. and Julia W. Dula Educational and Charitable Fndn Grants, 830
Comm Fndn for Greater New Haven Grants, 1091
Comm Fndn of Bartholomew County Heritage Fund Grants, 1096
Comm Fndn of Bartholomew County James A. Henderson Award for Fund-Raising, 1097
Comm Fndn of Boone County Grants, 1099
Comm Fndn of Greater Fort Wayne: Comm Endowment & Clarke Endowment Fund Grants, 1108
Delaware Comm Fndn Grants, 1215
Grand Rapids Comm Fndn Grants, 1647
Rhode Island Fndn Grants, 3154
Ripley County Comm Fndn Grants, 3166
Trull Fndn Grants, 3441

Retirement

Prudential Fndn Grants, 3087
Robert P. & Clara I. Milton Fund for Senior Housing, 3172
RRF General Grants, 3193

Rheumatic Diseases

AF Doctoral Dissertation Award for Arthritis Health Professionals, 253
AMA Fndn Seed Grants for Research, 398
NIAMS High Risk Arthritis and Musculoskeletal and Skin Diseases Research, 2470
NIAMS Mechanisms of Chondroprotection Research Grants, 2472
NIAMS Specialized Centers of Research in Osteoporosis, Rheumatoid Arthritis, and Scleroderma, 2480
Nuffield Fndn Oliver Bird Rheumatism Grants, 2901

Rheumatology
AF Doctoral Dissertation Award for Arthritis Health Professionals, 253
American College of Rheumatology Fellows-in-Training Travel Scholarships, 421
Nuffield Fndn Oliver Bird Rheumatism Grants, 2901

Rhinology
AAO-HNSF Health Services Research Grants, 147
AAO-HNSF Maureen Hannley Research Training Awards, 148
AAO-HNSF Percy Memorial Research Award, 149
AAO-HNSF Rande H. Lazar Health Services Research Grant, 150
AAO-HNSF Resident Research Awards, 151
AAOA Fndn/AAO-HNSF Combined Research Grants, 152
ALVRE Casselberry Award, 374
ALVRE Grant, 375
ALVRE Seymour R. Cohen Award, 376
ARS New Investigator Award, 539
ARS Resident Research Grants, 540

Risk Factors/Analysis
Award for Creative Advances in Environmental Science and Technology, 676
CDC Technology Translation and Transfer of Effective HIV Behavioral Interventions, 931
CDC Using Genetic Information to Prevent Disease and Improve Health Research Grants, 932
DOE Low Dose Radiation Research Program, 1300
Glaucoma Research Pilot Project Grants, 1622
NIDDK Race/Ethnic Disparities in the Incidence of Diabetes Complications, 2579
NIH National Occupational Research Agenda Grants, 2696
NIH/EPA Mechanistic-Based Cancer Risk Assessment Methods Research Grants, 2741
NIMH HIV/AIDS, Severe Mental Illness, and Homelessness Research Grants, 2757
NIMH Risk Factors for Psychopathology Using Existing Data Sets Grants, 2768
NIOSH Occupational Safety and Health Research and Demonstration Grants, 2807

Romania
OSI European Commission Internships for Young Roma Graduates, 2965

Runaway Youth
Burton G. Bettingen Grants, 813
ConocoPhillips Fndn Grants, 1144
Denver Fndn Comm Grants, 1227
McCarthy Family Fndn Grants, 2141

Rural Areas
Agnes M. Lindsay Trust Grants, 263
Agway Fndn Grants, 265
BCBS of Minnesota Growing Up Healthy Grants, 711
Colin Higgins Fndn Grants, 1056
Dean Foods Comm Involvement Grants, 1209
Greenwall Fndn Bioethics Grants, 1665
Health Canada National Seniors Independence Grants, 1722
J.L. Bedsole Fndn Grants, 1876
James G.K. McClure Educational and Development Fund Grants, 1886
Land O'Lakes Fndn Mid-Atlantic Grants, 2027
OUT Fund for Lesbian & Gay Liberation Grants, 2978
Rochester Area Comm Fndn Grants, 3176
Samuel S. Johnson Fndn Grants, 3251
Steele-Reese Fndn Grants, 3380
W.K. Kellogg Fndn Healthy Kids Grants, 3507

Rural Education
Coastal Comm Fndn of South Carolina Grants, 1051
DOA Distance Learning and Telemedicine Grant Program, 1288
U.S. Department of Education 21st Century Comm Learning Centers, 3445

Rural Health Care
Agway Fndn Grants, 265
CFPC Research and Education Fndn Grants, 956
Claude Worthington Benedum Fndn Grants, 1033
DHHS Rural Telemedicine Grants, 1279
DOA Distance Learning and Telemedicine Grant Program, 1288
Fannie E. Rippel Fndn Grants, 1452
Jenkins Fndn: Improving the Health of Greater Richmond Grants, 1915
Kansas Health Fndn Grants, 1980
Pioneer Hi-Bred Comm Grants, 3051
Rajiv Gandhi Fndn Grants, 3104
RWJF Local Funding Partnerships Grants, 3223

Russia
Carnegie Corp of New York Grants, 879
U.S. Department of Education United States-Russia Program: Improving Research and Educational Activities in Higher Education, 3451

Safety
Air Products and Chemicals Grants, 319
Alcatel-Lucent Technologies Fndn Grants, 333
Allstate Corp Giving Grants, 363
Allstate Corp Hometown Commitment Grants, 364
Alpine Winter Fndn Grants, 368
AMD Corp Contributions Grants, 411
American Academy of Dermatology Shade Structure Grants, 413
American Electric Power Grants, 434
Beazley Fndn Grants, 730
BJ's Charitable Fndn Grants, 761
Canadian Patient Safety Institute Patient Safety Studentships, 854
Canadian Patient Safety Institute Research Grants, 855
Caring Fndn Grants, 866
Cooper Industries Fndn Grants, 1150
DaimlerChrysler Corp Fund Grants, 1186
Detroit Lions Charities Grants, 1241
Duke Energy Fndn Grants, 1339
EPA Children's Health Protection Grants, 1420
Farmers Insurance Group of Companies Grants, 1455
Faye McBeath Fndn Grants, 1456
Federal Express Corp Contributions Program, 1483
Ford Motor Company Fund Grants, 1522
Frank Stanley Beveridge Fndn Grants, 1553
GEICO Public Service Awards, 1586
General Mills Fndn Grants, 1590
Glazer Family Fndn Grants, 1625
Goodyear Tire Grants, 1639
Greater Worcester Comm Fndn Jeppson Memorial Fund for Brookfield Grants, 1659
Gulf Coast Comm of Venice Fndn Grants, 1677
Harrison County Comm Fndn Grants, 1700
Harvest Fndn Grants, 1713
Huntington County Comm Fndn Grants, 1823
John Deere Fndn Grants, 1929
Michael and Susan Dell Fndn Grants, 2189
Ms. Fndn for Women Grants, 2222
National Patient Safety Fndn Patient Safety Research Grants, 2258
NNEDVF/Altria Doors of Hope Program, 2847
Noble County Comm Fndn Grants, 2848
Olin Corp Charitable Trust Grants, 2943
PacifiCorp Fndn for Learning Grants, 2982
Pioneer Hi-Bred Comm Grants, 3051
Rohm and Haas Company Grants, 3185
William G. McGowan Charitable Fund Grants, 3539

Safety Engineering
FIC International Training and Research in Environmental and Occupational Health, 1493

Sarcoidosis
NHLBI Sarcoidosis: Research Grants into the Cause of Multi-Organ Disease and Clinical Strategies for Therapy, 2382
NIH Sarcoidosis: Research into the Cause of Multi-Organ Disease and Clinical Strategies for Therapy Grants, 2723

Sarcoma
ASCO Career Development Award, 551
ASCO Young Investigator Award, 562
ASCO/UICC International Cancer Technology Transfer (ICRETT) Fellowships, 563

Schizophrenia
American Psychiatric Association/AstraZeneca Young Minds in Psychiatry International Awards, 450
American Psychiatric Association/Merck Co. Early Academic Career Research Award, 453
APF Alexander Gralnick, MD, Award for Research in Schizophrenia, 503
NARSAD Distinguished Investigator Award, 2246
NARSAD Independent Investigator Award, 2247
NIH Genetics of Neurobehavioral Disorders in Existing Samples Grants, 2670
NIMH Collaborative R01s for Clinical Studies of Mental Disorders, 2752
NIMH Early Identification and Treatment of Mental Disorders in Children and Adolescents Grants, 2756
Staglin Family Music Festival NARSAD Schizophrenia Research Award, 3372
Staney Fndn Treatment Trials for Schizophrenia and Bipolar Disorder, 3374
Wasie Fndn Grants, 3521

Scholarship Programs, General
AAHPERD Ruth Abernathy Presidential Scholarships, 128
AAHPERD-AAHE Barbara A. Cooley Scholarships, 129
AAHPERD-AAHE Delbert Oberteuffer Scholarships, 130
AAHPERD-AAHE Undergraduate Scholarships, 131
AAP Legislative Conference Scholarships, 163
Abell-Hanger Fndn Grants, 183
Abney Fndn Grants, 187
AcademyHealth Alice S. Hersh Student Scholarships, 191
AcademyHealth PHSR Interest Group Student Scholarships, 195
Achelis and Bodman Fndns Grants, 206
Agnes M. Lindsay Trust Grants, 263
Aladdin Industries Fndn Grants, 322
Albuquerque Comm Fndn Grants, 331
Alpha Omega Fndn Grants, 366
AMA Fndn Arthur N. Wilson, MD, Scholarship, 386
AMA Fndn Joan F. Giambalvo Memorial Scholarships, 392
AMA Fndn Minority Scholars Awards, 395
AMA Fndn Physicians of Tomorrow Scholarships, 396
AMA-WPC Joan F. Giambalvo Memorial Scholarships, 408
Amarillo Area/Harrington Fndns Grants, 410
American College of Surgeons Health Policy Scholarships, 427
American College of Surgeons Health Policy Scholarships for General Surgeons, 428
Arkansas Comm Fndn Grants, 533
Arlington Comm Fndn Grants, 536
ASM BD Award for Research in Clinical Microbiology, 588
ASM bioMerieux Sonnenwirth Award for Leadership in Clinical Microbiology, 589
ASM D.C. White Research and Mentoring Award, 592
ASM Eli Lilly and Company Research Award, 594
ASM Gen-Probe Joseph Public Health Award, 597
ASM Maurice Hilleman/Merck Award, 605
ASM Merck Irving S. Sigal Memorial Awards, 606
ASM Procter & Gamble Award in Applied and Environmental Microbiology, 609
ASM Promega Biotechnology Research Award, 610

ASM Public Communications Award, 611
ASM Raymond W. Sarber Awards, 612
ASM sanofi-aventis ICAAC Award, 616
ASM Scherago-Rubin Award, 617
ASM Siemens Healthcare Diagnostics Young Investigator Award, 618
ASM USFCC/J. Roger Porter Award, 623
ASM William A Hinton Research Training Award, 624
Bailey Fndn Grants, 680
Barberton Comm Fndn Grants, 693
Baton Rouge Area Fndn Grants, 702
Batts Fndn Grants, 704
Benton Comm Fndn Grants, 743
Blackford County Comm Fndn Grants, 763
Blue Mountain Comm Fndn Grants, 769
Boettcher Fndn Grants, 778
Brook J. Lenfest Fndn Grants, 804
Burlington Industries Fndn Grants, 811
Burlington Northern Santa Fe Fndn Grants, 812
Carnahan-Jackson Fndn Grants, 878
Carpenter Fndn Grants, 881
Carrier Corp Contributions Grants, 884
Carroll County Comm Fndn Grants, 885
Cetana Educational Fndn Scholarships, 939
Champlin Fndns Grants, 960
Chiles Fndn Grants, 1003
Christy-Houston Fndn Grants, 1008
Clarian Health Critical / Progressive Care Internships, 1023
Clarian Health Multi-Specialty Internships, 1024
Clarian Health OR Internships, 1025
Clarian Health Scholarships for LPNs, 1026
Clarian Health Student Nurse Extern Scholarships, 1027
Coca-Cola Fndn Grants, 1052
Comerica Charitable Fndn Grants, 1073
Comm Fndn for Greater Buffalo Grants, 1090
Comm Fndn for Southeastern Michigan Grants, 1094
Comm Fndn of Bloomington and Monroe County Grants, 1098
Comm Fndn of Central Illinois Grants, 1101
Comm Fndn of Crawford County Grants and Scholarships, 1103
Comm Fndn of Grant County Scholarships, 1105
Comm Fndn of Greater Greensboro Grants, 1109
Comm Fndn of Greater New Britain Grants, 1111
Comm Fndn of Howard County Grants, 1116
Comm Fndn of Madison and Jefferson County Grants and Scholarships, 1117
Comm Fndn of Morgan County Grants and Scholarships, 1118
Comm Fndn of Mount Vernon and Knox County Grants, 1119
Comm Fndn of Muncie and Delaware County Grants, 1120
Comm Fndn of Randolph County Grants, 1121
Comm Fndn of South Puget Sound Grants, 1124
Comm Fndn Silicon Valley Grants, 1133
Cooper Industries Fndn Grants, 1150
CSRA Comm Fndn Grants, 1168
DAAD Research Stays for University Academics and Scientists, 1183
Danellie Fndn Grants, 1198
Daphne Seybolt Culpeper Memorial Fndn Grants, 1201
Dr. Courtney W. Shropshire Scholarship Grant, 1326
Dr. Stanley Pearle Scholarships, 1330
Dubois County Comm Fndn Grants, 1336
Duke Energy Fndn Grants, 1339
Fairfield County Comm Fndn Grants, 1446
Farmers Insurance Group of Companies Grants, 1455
Flinn Fndn Grants Programs, 1511
FMC Fndn Grants, 1518
Fourjay Fndn Grants, 1544
Frances and John L. Loeb Family Fund Grants, 1546
Franklin County Comm Fndn Grants, 1554
Fritz B. Burns Fndn Grants, 1564
General Mills Fndn Grants, 1590
George Family Fndn Grants, 1598
Gertrude E. Skelly Charitable Fndn Grants, 1609
Gladys Brooks Fndn Grants, 1620
Greater New Orleans Fndn Grants, 1654
Greater Saint Louis Comm Fndn Grants, 1655
Green Bay Packers Fndn Grants, 1660
Griffin Fndn Grants, 1670
Gulf Coast Comm Fndn Grants, 1676
Gulf Coast Comm of Venice Fndn Grants, 1677
Hannaford Charitable Fndn Grants, 1692
Harold Simmons Fndn Grants, 1698
Harry and Grace Steele Fndn Grants, 1702
Harry Bramhall Gilbert Charitable Trust Grants, 1703
Harry Kramer Memorial Fund Grants, 1705
Hearst Fndn and William Randolph Hearst Fndn Grants, 1730
Henry County Comm Fndn Grants, 1747
High Meadow Fndn Grants, 1768
Hirtzel Memorial Fndn Grants, 1781
Hoglund Fndn Grants, 1785
Holland/Zeeland Comm Fndn Grants, 1786
HomeBanc Fndn Grants, 1788
Homer Fndn Grants, 1789
Honeywell Fndn Grants, 1791
Hormel Foods Charitable Trust Grants, 1795
HRSA Health Professions Scholarships for Disadvantaged Students, 1807
Huie-Dellmon Trust Grants, 1815
Humana Fndn Grants, 1818
i2 Fndn Grants, 1829
IATA Scholarships, 1835
Idaho Power Company Corp Contributions, 1838
Indiana Minority Teacher/Special Services Scholarships, 1852
Indiana Nursing Scholarships, 1853
Isabel Allende Fndn Esperanza Grants, 1868
J.E. and L.E. Mabee Fndn Grants, 1875
J.L. Bedsole Fndn Grants, 1876
Jacob G. Schmidlapp Trust Grants, 1883
James G.K. McClure Educational and Development Fund Grants, 1886
James Graham Brown Fndn Grants, 1887
JELD-WEN Fndn Grants, 1914
John J. Leidy Fndn Grants, 1936
John Jewett and Helen Chandler Garland Fndn Grants, 1937
John R. Oishei Fndn Grants, 1944
John W. Anderson Fndn Grants, 1949
Johnson Controls Fndn Grants, 1954
Joseph Alexander Fndn Grants, 1957
Joseph and Luella Abell Charitable Trust Scholarships, 1958
Josephine G. Russell Trust Grants, 1963
Kettering Fund Grants, 1992
L. A. Hollinger Respiratory Therapy and Nursing Scholarships, 2018
Lester Ray Fleming Scholarships, 2048
Lillian S. Wells Fndn Grants, 2056
Louis Calder Fndn Grants, 2065
Lubbock Area Fndn Grants, 2079
Lubrizol Fndn Grants, 2080
Lynde and Harry Bradley Fndn Grants, 2089
Lynde and Harry Bradley Fndn Prizes: Bradley Prizes, 2090
M. Bastian Family Fndn Grants, 2092
Madison County Comm Fndn Grants, 2098
Maine Comm Fndn Grants, 2099
Margoes Fndn Grants, 2106
Maxon Charitable Fndn Grants, 2135
McInerny Fndn Grants, 2144
Mead Johnson Nutritionals Scholarships, 2159
Mead Witter Fndn Grants, 2160
Meadows Fndn Grants, 2161
Military Ex-Prisoners of War Fndn Grants, 2201
NAPNAP Fndn Elaine Gelman Scholarship, 2235
NAPNAP Fndn McNeil PNP Scholarships, 2239
NAPNAP Fndn McNeil Rural and Underserved Scholarships, 2240
Nelda C. and H.J. Lutcher Stark Fndn Grants, 2301
New York Life Fndn Grants, 2304
NIH Undergraduate Scholarships, 2737
NMF Hugh J. Andersen Memorial Scholarship, 2832
NMF Irving Graef Memorial Scholarship, 2833
NMF Mary Ball Carrera Scholarship, 2834
NMSS Scholarships, 2845
North Carolina Comm Fndn Grants, 2859
Oleonda Jameson Trust Grants, 2941
Ordean Fndn Grants, 2952
Paul and Mary Haas Fndn Contributions and Student Scholarships, 2997
Pfizer Fndn Epilepsy Scholarship Award, 3024
Pott Fndn Grants, 3071
Potts Memorial Fndn Grants, 3072
Prospect Burma Scholarships, 3085
Rathmann Family Fndn Grants, 3109
Regenstrief Master Of Science In Clinical Research/CITE Program, 3145
Rehabilitation Nursing Fndn Scholarships, 3148
Rhode Island Fndn Grants, 3154
Roy and Christine Sturgis Trust Grants, 3191
Roy J. Carver Charitable Trust Medical and Science Research Grants, 3192
Rush County Comm Fndn Grants, 3200
Ruth Eleanor Bamberger and John Ernest Bamberger Memorial Fndn Grants, 3202
RWJF New Careers in Nursing Scholarships, 3224
RWJF Young Epidemiology Scholars Competition, 3233
S. Livingston Mather Charitable Trust Grants, 3235
Samuel S. Johnson Fndn Grants, 3251
Seabury Fndn Grants, 3274
Seattle Fndn Grants, 3276
Seneca Foods Fndn Grants, 3278
Simmons Fndn Grants, 3287
SNM PDEF Mickey Williams Minority Student Scholarships, 3302
SNMTS Clinical Advancement Scholarships, 3309
SNMTS Paul Cole Scholarships, 3312
Square D Fndn Grants, 3361
Starr Fndn Grants, 3377
Strowd Roses Grants, 3388
Temple-Inland Fndn Grants, 3419
Thomas and Dorothy Leavey Fndn Grants, 3422
Thompson Charitable Fndn Grants, 3425
Trinity Lutheran School of Nursing Alumnae Scholarships, 3439
Trull Fndn Grants, 3441
U.S. Department of Education Erma Byrd Scholarships, 3446
VDH Commonwealth of Virginia Nurse Educator Scholarships, 3482
Virginia Department of Health Mary Marshall Nursing Scholarships for Licensed Practical Nurses, 3498
Virginia Department of Health Mary Marshall Nursing Scholarships for Registered Nurses, 3499
Virginia Department of Health Nurse Practitioner/Nurse Midwife Scholarships, 3500
Vulcan Materials Company Fndn Grants, 3504
Walt Disney Company Fndn Grants, 3516
Wasie Fndn Grants, 3521
Wells County Fndn Grants, 3527
William G. Gilmore Fndn Grants, 3537
William G. McGowan Charitable Fund Grants, 3539
Women of the ELCA Opportunity Scholarships for Lutheran Laywomen, 3548
Women's Sports Fndn Grants, 3551
Z. Smith Reynolds Fndn Small Grants, 3557

School Dental Programs

Healthcare Fndn of New Jersey Grants, 1729
Pajaro Valley Comm Health Grants, 2985

School Food Programs

CDC National Programs That Build the Capacity of Schools To Prevent Foodborne Illness Through Coordinated School Health Programs, 919

School Health Programs

Anthem Blue Cross and Blue Shield School Nurse Grants, 489

CDC National Programs That Build the Capacity of Schools To Prevent Foodborne Illness Through Coordinated School Health Programs, 919
DHHS Oral Health Promotion Research Across the Lifespan, 1269
Dr. John T. Macdonald Fndn Grants, 1327
Fairlawn Fndn Grants, 1447
Health Fndn of Greater Cincinnati Grants, 1724
Healthcare Fndn of New Jersey Grants, 1729
McKesson Fndn Grants, 2145

School-to-Work Transition
CNCS Engaging Persons with Disabilities in National and Comm Service Grants, 1047
Crail-Johnson Fndn Grants, 1157
Denver Fndn Comm Grants, 1227
Liberty Bank Fndn Grants, 2053
Polaroid Fund Grants, 3065
Rohm and Haas Company Grants, 3185
S.H. Cowell Fndn Grants, 3237
Vectren Fndn Grants, 3485
Verizon Fndn Maryland Grants, 3487
Verizon Fndn New York Grants, 3488
Verizon Fndn Northeast Region Grants, 3489
Verizon Fndn Pennsylvania Grants, 3490
Verizon Fndn Vermont Grants, 3491
Verizon Fndn Virginia Grants, 3492

Science
AAAS Science & Technology Policy Fellowships - National Defense & Global Security, 29
AHRQ Independent Scientist Award, 313
Albert and Margaret Alkek Fndn Grants, 326
Alcoa Fndn Grants, 334
Alex Brown and Sons Charitable Fndn Grants, 337
Alfred P. Sloan Fndn History of Science and Technology Grants, 352
Alfred P. Sloan Fndn Research Fellowships, 353
Alfred W. Bressler Prize in Vision Science, 354
Alton Ochsner Award, 373
American Schlafhorst Fndn Grants, 454
Angels Baseball Fndn Grants, 473
ARCO Fndn Education Grants, 526
Arizona Cardinals Grants, 529
Arkema Fndn Science Teachers Program, 535
Armstrong McDonald Fndn Grants, 537
ArvinMeritor Grants, 544
ASM bioMerieux Sonnenwirth Award for Leadership in Clinical Microbiology, 589
ASM Intel Awards, 600
Australian Academy of Science Grants, 670
Banfi Vintners Fndn Grants, 687
Bonfils-Stanton Fndn Grants, 779
Brinson Fndn Grants, 794
BWF Ad Hoc Grants, 818
BWF Career Awards for Medical Scientists, 820
Canada Graduate Scholarships and NSERC Postgraduate Scholarships, 845
Canada-U.S. Fulbright New Century Scholars Grants, 846
Canada-U.S. Fulbright Senior Specialists Grants, 847
Canadian Friends of Hebrew University Research and Study Grants, 850
Carl Gellert and Celia Berta Gellert Fndn Grants, 871
Carylon Fndn Grants, 886
Chateaubriand Exact Sciences, Engineering, and Medicine Research Scholarships, 976
Comm Fndn of Greater Flint Grants, 1107
Cyrus Eaton Fndn Grants, 1178
DAAD Research Stays for University Academics and Scientists, 1183
DaimlerChrysler Corp Fund Grants, 1186
Dana Fndn Science and Health Grants, 1197
Dolan Fndn Grants, 1306
Duke Energy Fndn Grants, 1339
E.L. Wiegand Fndn Grants, 1361
Elisabeth Severance Prentiss Fndn Grants, 1392
EMBO Installation Grants, 1409
Eppley Fndn Postdoctoral Grants, 1425
FDA Scientific Conferences Grants, 1463
FIC International Research Scientist Development Award, 1491
FIC International Training and Research in Emerging Infectious Diseases Grants, 1492
Fluor Fndn Grants, 1517
Fndn for Science and Disability Grant Program for Physically Disabled Students in the Sciences, 1532
Frank Stanley Beveridge Fndn Grants, 1553
Frederick Gardner Cottrell Fndn Grants, 1560
Fulbright Alumni Initiatives Awards Grants, 1566
Fulbright Distinguished Chairs Grants, 1567
Fulbright German Studies Seminar Grants, 1568
Fulbright New Century Scholars Grants, 1570
Fulbright Specialists Grants, 1571
Fulbright Traditional Scholar Program in Europe and Eurasia, 1572
Fulbright Traditional Scholar Program in Sub-Saharan Africa, 1573
Fulbright Traditional Scholar Program in the East Asia/Pacific Region, 1574
Fulbright Traditional Scholar Program in the Near East and North Africa Region, 1575
Fulbright Traditional Scholar Program in the South and Central Asia Region, 1576
Fulbright Traditional Scholar Program in the Western Hemisphere, 1577
Genentech Corp Charitable Contributions Grants, 1588
Gladys Brooks Fndn Grants, 1620
Grand Rapids Comm Fndn Grants, 1647
Green Fndn Grants, 1661
Heart Rhythm Society Fellowships, 1731
Heineman Fndn for Research, Education, Charitable and Scientific Purposes, 1735
Hoblitzelle Fndn Grants, 1783
i2 Fndn Grants, 1829
Idaho Comm Fndn Eastern Region Competitive Grants, 1837
Jeffress Research Grants, 1913
Josiah W. and Bessie H. Kline Fndn Grants, 1967
Kavli Fndn Research Grants, 1985
Kenneth T. and Eileen L. Norris Fndn Grants, 1989
Land O'Lakes Fndn Mid-Atlantic Grants, 2027
Lowell Berry Fndn Grants, 2069
M.J. Murdock Charitable Trust Grants, 2095
MAPFRE Fndn for Medicine Grants, 2102
Marion Park Deaver and Harry Gilbert Deaver Fndn Grants, 2110
Mary Ingraham Bunting Institute Biomedical Research Fellowships, 2119
Matsumae International Fndn Grants, 2129
McCarthy Family Fndn Grants, 2141
McGregor Fund Grants, 2143
Meadows Fndn Grants, 2161
Miguel Aleman Fndn Grants, 2197
Minority Doctoral Fellowships in Science and Engineering, 2207
NIGMS Support of Competitive Research Pilot Project Awards, 2631
NIGMS Support of Competitive Research Research Advancement Awards, 2632
NIH Academic Career Awards, 2634
NIH Independent Scientist Award, 2677
NIH Mentored Clinical Scientist Development Award, 2687
NIH Mentored Research Scientist Development Awards, 2689
NIH National Research Service Awards—Senior Fellows, 2697
NIH Senior Scientist Award, 2727
NIMH Career Opportunities in Research Education and Training Honors Undergraduate Research Training Grant, 2749
NIMH New Minority Faculty Scientist Development Award, 2765
North Carolina GlaxoSmithKline Fndn Grants, 2860
Northwood University/Alden B. Dow Creativity Center Summer Residency Program, 2871
NSERC Brockhouse Canada Prize for Interdisciplinary Research in Science and Engineering Grant, 2873
NSF Presidential Early Career Awards for Scientists and Engineers (PECASE) Grants, 2892
NSF Small Business Innovation Research Grants, 2893
Nuffield Fndn Africa Grants, 2898
Nuffield Fndn Law and Society Grants, 2900
Nuffield Fndn Small Grants, 2903
Phoenix Suns Charities Grants, 3030
Prospect Burma Scholarships, 3085
Puerto Rico Comm Fndn Grants, 3090
R.C. Baker Fndn Grants, 3098
Rajiv Gandhi Fndn Grants, 3104
Rayonier Fndn Grants, 3111
Richard and Rhoda Goldman Fund Grants, 3158
Robins Fndn Grants, 3175
Rockefeller Fndn Grants, 3181
Roy J. Carver Charitable Trust Medical and Science Research Grants, 3192
RSC McNeil Medal for the Public Awareness of Science, 3198
RSC Thomas W. Eadie Medal, 3199
Russell Berrie Fndn Grants, 3201
Samuel Freeman Charitable Trust Grants, 3249
San Diego Women's Fndn Grants, 3259
Sarah Scaife Fndn Grants, 3263
Scientific Communities Initiative Grants, 3272
Sid W. Richardson Fndn Grants, 3284
Wallace H. Coulter Fndn Grants, 3515
Wayne and Gladys Valley Fndn Grants, 3522

Science and Technology
ASM Congressional Science Fellowships, 590
ASM Intel Awards, 600
ASM International Fellowship for Latin America and the Caribbean, 601
ASM International Professorship for Latin America, 603
ASM International Professorships for Asia and Africa, 604
ASM Public Communications Award, 611
Autodesk Comm Relations Grants, 671
Beckman Coulter Comm Relations Grants, 733
Duke Energy Fndn Grants, 1339
NSF Biological Physics (BP), 2878
NSF Emerging Frontiers in Research and Innovation Grants, 2885
PAHO-ASM International Professorship for Latin America, 2983
Paul G. Allen Family Fndn Grants, 3000
Rohm and Haas Company Grants, 3185
Roy and Christine Sturgis Trust Grants, 3191
STTI National League for Nursing Grants, 3393

Science Education
3M Fndn Grants, 11
Abbott Fund Global AIDS Care Grants, 178
Abell-Hanger Fndn Grants, 183
Affymetrix Corp Contributions Grants, 258
Alcoa Fndn Grants, 334
Alfred P. Sloan Fndn History of Science and Technology Grants, 352
AMD Corp Contributions Grants, 411
American Electric Power Grants, 434
Amgen Fndn Grants, 467
Arkema Fndn Science Teachers Program, 535
ArvinMeritor Grants, 544
Baptist Comm Ministries Grants, 691
Beckman Coulter Comm Relations Grants, 733
Bodman Fndn Grants, 776
Charles Edison Fund Grants, 964
Chicago Board of Trade Fndn Grants, 988
Chiron Fndn Comm Grants, 1004
Comm Fndn of Grant County Scholarships, 1105
DaimlerChrysler Corp Fund Grants, 1186
Dell Fndn Healthy Communities, Literate Communities, and Connected Communities Grants, 1217

Dominion Educational Partnership Grant, 1308
Emily Davie and Joseph S. Kornfeld Fndn Grants, 1414
Ford Motor Company Fund Grants, 1522
Genentech Corp Charitable Contributions Grants, 1588
Goodrich Corp Fndn Grants, 1638
Heineman Fndn for Research, Education, Charitable and Scientific Purposes, 1735
HHMI Biomedical Research Grants for International Scientists in Canada and Latin America, 1756
HHMI Biomedical Research Grants for International Scientists in the Baltics, Central and Eastern Europe, Russia, and Ukraine, 1757
HHMI Biomedical Research Grants for International Scientists: Infectious Diseases and Parasitology, 1758
HHMI Grants and Fellowships Programs, 1759
HHMI Med into Grad Initiative Grants, 1761
HHMI-NIBIB Interfaces Initiative Grants, 1764
Houston Endowment Grants, 1797
Joyce Fndn Grants, 1969
Lockheed Martin Philanthropic Grants, 2062
McCarthy Family Fndn Grants, 2141
MedImmune Charitable Grants, 2166
Medtronic Fndn Health Care Grants, 2169
NIGMS Minority Access to Research Careers Program, 2620
NIMH Career Opportunities in Research Education and Training Honors High School Research Education Grant, 2748
Northrop Grumman Newport News Grants, 2867
Northwood University/Alden B. Dow Creativity Center Summer Residency Program, 2871
Olin Corp Charitable Trust Grants, 2943
Oracle Corp Contributions Grants, 2951
Pfizer Fndn Grants, 3025
Pittsburgh Fndn Comm Fund Grants, 3054
Progress Energy Fndn Grants, 3084
Rathmann Family Fndn Grants, 3109
RGK Fndn Grants, 3153
Rockwell Collins Charitable Contributions, 3182
Rohm and Haas Company Grants, 3185
RSC McNeil Medal for the Public Awareness of Science, 3198
Schering-Plough Fndn Health Grants, 3270
Tellabs Fndn Grants, 3418
United Technologies Corp Grants, 3466
Wallace H. Coulter Fndn Grants, 3515
Weatherwax Fndn Grants, 3523
Westinghouse Charitable Giving Grants, 3530

Science Planning/Policy

Alfred P. Sloan Fndn Research Fellowships, 353

Scleroderma

NIAMS Molecular Pathogenesis and New Interventions in Scleroderma, 2473
NIAMS Specialized Centers of Research in Osteoporosis, Rheumatoid Arthritis, and Scleroderma, 2480

Secondary Education

3M Fndn Grants, 11
A Fund for Women Grants, 14
A.O. Smith Comm Grants, 18
Adolph Coors Fndn Grants, 238
AEGON Transamerica Fndn Grants, 243
Ahmanson Fndn Grants, 303
Alabama Power Fndn Grants, 321
Alcatel-Lucent Technologies Fndn Grants, 333
Alcoa Fndn Grants, 334
AMD Corp Contributions Grants, 411
Andersen Fndn Grants, 471
Ann Jackson Family Fndn Grants, 477
Archer Daniels Midland Fndn Grants, 525
ARCO Fndn Education Grants, 526
Armstrong McDonald Fndn Grants, 537
Auburn Fndn Grants, 664
Ball Brothers Fndn Grants, 684
Benton County Fndn Grants, 744
Berrien Comm Fndn Grants, 749
Bill and Melinda Gates Fndn Grants, 756
Boeing Company Contributions Grants, 777
Boettcher Fndn Grants, 778
Booth-Bricker Fund Grants, 780
Boston Fndn Grants, 783
Bristol-Myers Squibb Fndn Health Education Grants, 798
Burlington Industries Fndn Grants, 811
Callaway Fndn Grants, 835
Camp-Younts Fndn Grants, 838
Carl and Lily Pforzheimer Fndn Grants, 868
Carnegie Corp of New York Grants, 879
Carrie E. and Lena V. Glenn Fndn Grants, 882
Carrie Estelle Doheny Fndn Grants, 883
Carroll County Comm Fndn Grants, 885
Cass County Comm Fndn Grants, 887
CDC School Health Programs to Prevent the Spread of HIV Cooperative Agreements, 928
Chesapeake Corp Fndn Grants, 982
CIGNA Fndn Grants, 1011
Cinergy Fndn Grants, 1013
Clarence E. Heller Charitable Fndn Grants, 1022
CMS Historically Black Colleges and Universities Health Services Research Grants, 1044
Coca-Cola Fndn Grants, 1052
Coeta and Donald Barker Fndn Grants, 1054
Colorado Interstate Gas Grants, 1060
Commonweal Fndn Comm Assistance Grants, 1075
Comm Fndn of Central Illinois Grants, 1101
Comm Fndn of Grant County Grants, 1104
Comm Fndn of Howard County Grants, 1116
Comm Fndn Silicon Valley Grants, 1133
Connelly Fndn Grants, 1143
Constantin Fndn Grants, 1145
Cowles Charitable Trust Grants, 1155
Crail-Johnson Fndn Grants, 1157
Crestlea Fndn Grants, 1159
Cullen Fndn Grants, 1172
CVS All Kids Can Grants, 1175
DaimlerChrysler Corp Fund Grants, 1186
Dean Foods Comm Involvement Grants, 1209
Dennis and Phyllis Washington Fndn Grants, 1222
Dept of Ed College Assistance Migrant Program, 1228
Dickson Fndn Grants, 1284
Dominion Educational Partnership Grant, 1308
Dr. Scholl Fndn Grants, 1329
Duke Energy Fndn Grants, 1339
Dunspaugh-Dalton Fndn Grants, 1351
E.J. Grassmann Trust Grants, 1360
Effie and Wofford Cain Fndn Grants, 1385
Eisner Fndn Grants, 1387
Elizabeth McGraw Fndn Grants, 1399
Eugene McDermott Fndn Grants, 1435
Eva L. and Joseph M. Bruening Fndn Grants, 1436
Ferree Fndn Grants, 1486
Field Fndn of Illinois Grants, 1499
FirstEnergy Fndn Comm Grants, 1505
Fondren Fndn Grants, 1520
Frances and John L. Loeb Family Fund Grants, 1546
Frances L. and Edwin L. Cummings Memorial Fund Grants, 1547
Francis L. Abreu Charitable Trust Grants, 1549
Francis T. & Louise T. Nichols Fndn Grants, 1550
GenCorp Fndn Grants, 1587
General Mills Fndn Grants, 1590
George F. Baker Trust Grants, 1597
George Frederick Jewett Fndn Grants, 1599
Goodrich Corp Fndn Grants, 1638
Greater Milwaukee Fndn Grants, 1653
Greenwall Fndn Bioethics Grants, 1665
Halliburton Fndn Grants, 1687
Harold Alfond Fndn Grants, 1695
Harrison County Comm Fndn Grants, 1700
Harry and Grace Steele Fndn Grants, 1702
Hearst Fndn and William Randolph Hearst Fndn Grants, 1730
Hedco Fndn Grants, 1733
HHMI Grants and Fellowships Programs, 1759
Horace A. Kimball and S. Ella Kimball Fndn Grants, 1792
Houston Endowment Grants, 1797
Howe Fndn of North Carolina Grants, 1799
Huie-Dellmon Trust Grants, 1815
Hutton Fndn Grants, 1828
Idaho Power Company Corp Contributions, 1838
J. Walton Bissell Fndn Grants, 1872
J.L. Bedsole Fndn Grants, 1876
Janirve Fndn Grants, 1905
John H. Wellons Fndn Grants, 1934
John P. Murphy Fndn Grants, 1943
Joyce Fndn Grants, 1969
Katharine Matthies Fndn Grants, 1982
Kenneth T. and Eileen L. Norris Fndn Grants, 1989
Lockheed Martin Philanthropic Grants, 2062
Louis R. Cappelli Fndn Grants, 2066
Lowell Berry Fndn Grants, 2069
Lubbock Area Fndn Grants, 2079
Lubrizol Fndn Grants, 2080
Marion I. and Henry J. Knott Fndn Grants, 2109
McCarthy Family Fndn Grants, 2141
Mead Johnson Nutritionals Evansville-Area Organizations Grants, 2157
Mead Witter Fndn Grants, 2160
Medtronic Fndn Health Care Grants, 2169
Military Ex-Prisoners of War Fndn Grants, 2201
Morton K. and Jane Blaustein Fndn Grants, 2218
Newman's Own Inc Grants, 2306
Nicholas H. Noyes Jr. Memorial Fndn Grants, 2497
NIMH Career Opportunities in Research Education and Training Honors High School Research Education Grant, 2748
Nina Mason Pulliam Charitable Trust Grants, 2776
Nordson Corp Fndn Grants, 2851
Northrop Grumman Corp Grants, 2866
Northrop Grumman Newport News Grants, 2867
Oracle Corp Contributions Grants, 2951
PacifiCare Fndn Grants, 2981
Pew Charitable Trusts Children & Youth Grants, 3020
Pfizer Fndn Grants, 3025
Phoenix Suns Charities Grants, 3030
Pioneer Hi-Bred Comm Grants, 3051
Piper Jaffray Companies Building Strong Communities Grants, 3053
Portland General Electric Fndn Grants, 3067
Procter and Gamble Fund Grants, 3083
Quantum Fndn Grants, 3096
Richard and Susan Smith Family Fndn Grants, 3159
Ruth Eleanor Bamberger and John Ernest Bamberger Memorial Fndn Grants, 3202
RWJF Young Epidemiology Scholars Competition, 3233
Salem Fndn Grants, 3242
Samuel Freeman Charitable Trust Grants, 3249
Schering-Plough Fndn Health Grants, 3270
Scott County Comm Fndn Grants, 3273
Seabury Fndn Grants, 3274
Seneca Foods Fndn Grants, 3278
Sid W. Richardson Fndn Grants, 3284
Sonoco Fndn Grants, 3347
Sosland Fndn Grants, 3348
Southwest Gas Corp Fndn Grants, 3352
Sprague Fndn Grants, 3359
Strowd Roses Grants, 3388
Susan Vaughan Fndn Grants, 3413
Temple-Inland Fndn Grants, 3419
Thomas and Dorothy Leavey Fndn Grants, 3422
Trull Fndn Grants, 3441
U.S. Department of Education 21st Century Comm Learning Centers, 3445
Union County Comm Fndn Grants, 3461
W. C. Griffith Fndn Grants, 3505
Wal-Mart Fndn Comm Grants, 3513
Weingart Fndn Grants, 3524
Westinghouse Charitable Giving Grants, 3530
Z. Smith Reynolds Fndn Small Grants, 3557

Security

Henry J. Kaiser Family Fndn Grants, 1748
Otto Bremer Fndn Grants, 2977
Public Welfare Fndn Grants, 3089

Rockefeller Brothers Fund Peace and Security Grants, 3179

Seminars
Alaska Airlines Fndn Grants, 324
Greater Worcester Comm Fndn Jeppson Memorial Fund for Brookfield Grants, 1659
Potts Memorial Fndn Grants, 3072
St. Joseph Comm Health Fndn Schneider Fellowships, 3370

Senile Dementia
AHAF Alzheimer's Disease Research Grants, 266
Alzheimer's Association Everyday Technologies for Alzheimer Care Research Grants, 377
Alzheimer's Association Investigator-Initiated Research Grants, 378
Alzheimer's Association Mentored New Investigator Research Grants to Promote Diversity, 379
Alzheimer's Association Molecular Imaging Grants, 380
Alzheimer's Association New Investigator Research Grants, 381
Alzheimer's Association New Investigator Research Grants to Promote Diversity, 382
Alzheimer's Association Senator Mark Hatfield Award, 383
Alzheimer's Association Zenith Fellows Awards, 384
Alzheimer's Association Conference Grants, 385
Helen Bader Fndn Grants, 1738

Senior Citizen Programs and Services
Arkell Hall Fndn Grants, 534
California Endowment CommunitiesFirst Grants, 833
Carlsbad Charitable Fndn Grants, 877
Comm Fndn for Southeastern Michigan Grants, 1094
Comm Fndn of Grant County Grants, 1104
ConocoPhillips Fndn Grants, 1144
Eisner Fndn Grants, 1387
Glendale Comm Fndn Grants, 1626
Helen K. and Arthur E. Johnson Fndn Grants, 1740
Kansas Health Fndn Grants, 1980
Morris and Gwendolyn Cafritz Fndn Grants, 2217
Robert P. & Clara I. Milton Fund for Senior Housing, 3172
Scott County Comm Fndn Grants, 3273

Sensing Devices and Transducers
NSF Biomedical Engineering and Engineering Healthcare Grants, 2879
NSF Chemical, Biochemical, and Biotechnology Systems Research Grants, 2882
ONR Human Performance Division Research Grants, 2948

Sensory System
DHHS Neurodevelopmental Test Methods Research Grants, 1268
NIA Research Grants on Chemical Senses: Neurotransmitters and Neuromodulators, 2430
NIDA Drug Addiction Neuroscience Research Grants, 2503
NIDCD Research Grants on Chemical Senses: Neurotransmitters and Neuromodulators, 2530
NIDCD Small Grants, 2531
NSF Behavioral Neurosciences Research Grants, 2876
Whitehall Fndn Neurobiology Research Grants, 3533

Separation Process
NSF Chemical, Biochemical, and Biotechnology Systems Research Grants, 2882

Serbia
OSI European Commission Internships for Young Roma Graduates, 2965

Serology
Orentreich Fndn for the Advancement of Science Grants, 2959

Service Delivery Programs
Able To Serve Grants, 185
Administration on Aging Senior Medicare Patrol Project Grants, 236
AMD Corp Contributions Grants, 411
APA Meritorious Research Service Commendation, 499
Bernard and Audre Rapoport Fndn Grants, 746
Chase Paymentech Corp Giving Grants, 975
CMS Research and Demonstration Grants, 1045
Comm Fndn of Broward Grants, 1100
Comm Fndn of Santa Cruz County Grants, 1122
Consumers Energy Fndn, 1147
DOJ Mental Health and Juvenile Justice, 1304
Eugene McDermott Fndn Grants, 1435
Fallon OrNda Comm Health Fund Grants, 1449
Ferree Fndn Grants, 1486
Gertrude E. Skelly Charitable Fndn Grants, 1609
Goodrich Corp Fndn Grants, 1638
Guidant Fndn Grants, 1674
Hasbro Children's Fund, 1714
Health Care Financing Research, Demonstrations, and Evaluations Grants, 1723
Health Fndn of Southern Florida Responsive Grants, 1726
Hogg Fndn for Mental Health Grants, 1784
Howard and Bush Fndn Grants, 1798
Ittleson Fndn AIDS Grants, 1869
Jenkins Fndn: Improving the Health of Greater Richmond Grants, 1915
Jerome and Mildred Paddock Fndn Grants, 1917
JM Fndn Grants, 1926
Kraft Cares US Grants, 2017
LaGrange County Comm Fndn Grants, 2020
Louis R. Cappelli Fndn Grants, 2066
Mary Allen Lindsey Branan Fndn Grants, 2116
NHLBI National Research Service Awards for Senior Fellowships, 2358
NIMH HIV/AIDS, Severe Mental Illness, and Homelessness Research Grants, 2757
Richard and Susan Smith Family Fndn Grants, 3159
Robert and Joan Dircks Fndn Grants, 3167
Robert E. and Evelyn McKee Fndn Grants, 3170
Tri-County Electric People Fund Grants, 3436
US Trust Corp Fndn Grants, 3475
Women of the ELCA Opportunity Scholarships for Lutheran Laywomen, 3548
YSA UnitedHealth Heroes Service Learning Grants, 3556

Sex Differences
Jeanne Humphrey Block Dissertation Award, 1912

Sex Education
DHHS Adolescent Family Life Demonstration Projects, 1243
Ittleson Fndn AIDS Grants, 1869
NIH Demographic Research on Sexual Behaviors Related to HIV, 2653

Sex Roles
NIDA Neurobiological and Behavioral Research on Nicotine and Tobacco Products, 2511
NIH Pathological Gambling: Basic, Clinical, and Services Research Grants, 2702

Sexual Abuse
Baxter International Fndn Grants, 705
Burton G. Bettingen Grants, 813
Comm Fndn for Southern Arizona Grants, 1095
Educational Fndn of America Grants, 1372
Global Fund for Children Grants, 1629
Greater Tacoma Comm Fndn Ryan Alan Hade Endowment Fund, 1657
Lewis Preston Fund for Girls Education Grants, 2052
Ms. Fndn for Women Grants, 2222

Sexual Behavior
amfAR Fellowships, 462
amfAR Global Initiatives Grants, 463
amfAR Mathilde Krim Fellowships in Basic Biomedical Research, 464
amfAR Public Policy Grants, 465
amfAR Research Grants, 466
CDC Technology Translation and Transfer of Effective HIV Behavioral Interventions, 931
DHHS Adolescent Family Life Demonstration Projects, 1243
Moses Cone-Wesley Long Comm Health Fndn Grants, 2219
NIH Demographic Research on Sexual Behaviors Related to HIV, 2653
NIMH HIV/AIDS, Severe Mental Illness, and Homelessness Research Grants, 2757
Pride Fndn Grants and Scholarships, 3078
Ruth Mott Fndn Grants, 3204
SSSS Student Research Grants, 3366

Sexually Transmitted Diseases
ASM/CCID Fellowships, 627
CDC Preventive Health Services-Sexually Transmitted Diseases Control Grants, 923
CDC Sexually Transmitted Diseases Research, Demonstration, Public Information, and Education Grants, 929
CDC Technology Translation and Transfer of Effective HIV Behavioral Interventions, 931
DHHS Adolescent Family Life Demonstration Projects, 1243
Ittleson Fndn AIDS Grants, 1869
Kate B. Reynolds Charitable Trust Health Care Grants, 1981
Moses Cone-Wesley Long Comm Health Fndn Grants, 2219
NFID New Investigator Matching Grants, 2310
NIAID HIV Prevention Trial Units Grants, 2453
NICHD Population Research Grants, 2490
NIH Demographic Research on Sexual Behaviors Related to HIV, 2653
Sexually Transmitted Diseases Postdoctoral Fellowships, 3279

Shade
American Academy of Dermatology Shade Structure Grants, 413

Shelters
ACF Standing Announcement for Unaccompanied Alien Children Grants, 202
Blowitz-Ridgeway Fndn Grants, 767
Cemala Fndn Grants, 933
Columbus Fndn Traditional Grants, 1071
Comer Fndn Grants, 1072
Comm Fndn of Bloomington and Monroe County Grants, 1098
Constantin Fndn Grants, 1145
Dallas Women's Fndn Grants, 1191
Dennis and Phyllis Washington Fndn Grants, 1222
Doris and Victor Day Fndn Grants, 1313
Edina Realty Fndn Grants, 1369
HomeBanc Fndn Grants, 1788
Jacob G. Schmidlapp Trust Grants, 1883
Kalamazoo Fndn Grants, 1979
Ken W. Davis Fndn Grants, 1987
Laura B. Vogler Fndn Grants, 2032
Lincoln Financial Group Fndn Grants, 2058
NNEDVF/Altria Doors of Hope Program, 2847
Oleonda Jameson Trust Grants, 2941
Otto Bremer Fndn Grants, 2977
Posey Comm Fndn Grants, 3068
S. Mark Taper Fndn Grants, 3236
Samuel S. Johnson Fndn Grants, 3251
Spencer County Comm Fndn Grants, 3358
Thompson Charitable Fndn Grants, 3425
Tri-County Electric People Fund Grants, 3436
Vancouver Fndn Grants and Comm Initiatives Program, 3477
Vanderburgh Comm Fndn Grants, 3480
Warrick County Comm Fndn Grants, 3519

Sickle Cell Disease
NHLBI Exploratory Studies in the Neurobiology of Pain in Sickle Cell Disease, 2334

Single-Parent Families
Arkell Hall Fndn Grants, 534
Austin-Bailey Health and Wellness Fndn Grants, 669
Crail-Johnson Fndn Grants, 1157
Eugene M. Lang Fndn Grants, 1434
Harden Fndn Grants, 1693

Skin Diseases
American Academy of Dermatology Camp Discovery Scholarships, 412
Center for Alternatives to Animal Testing Grants, 934
Dermatology Fndn Grants, 1236
Dermatology Postdoctoral Research Fellowships, 1237
Dermatology Research Career Development Awards, 1238
Gina Finzi Memorial Student Summer Fellowship, 1615
Lupus Fndn of America Research Grants, 2085
National Psoriasis Fndn Research Grants, 2259
NIAMS Clinical Trial Planning Grants, 2466
NIAMS High Risk Arthritis and Musculoskeletal and Skin Diseases Research, 2470
NIAMS Skin Diseases Research Core Centers Grants, 2478
Skin Cancer Fndn Research Grants, 3298
Society for Investigative Dermatology Career Development Award, 3325

Sleep
Narcolepsy Network Seed Grants, 2245
NIDA Drug Addiction Neuroscience Research Grants, 2503
NIH Biobehavioral Research for Effective Sleep, 2639

Sleep Disorders
American Psychiatric Association/Merck Co. Early Academic Career Research Award, 453
Narcolepsy Network Seed Grants, 2245
National Sleep Fndn Pickwick Postdoctoral Fellowship, 2260
NHLBI Elucidating Nature's Solutions to Heart, Lung, and Blood Diseases and Sleep Disorder Processes Research Grants, 2333
NHLBI Mentored Career Award For Faculty At Minority Institutions, 2346
NHLBI Minority Institution Research Scientist Development Award, 2354
NHLBI Minority Institutional Research Training Grants, 2355
NHLBI Short-Term Research Education Program to Increase Diversity in Health-Related Research, 2383
NIH Biobehavioral Research for Effective Sleep, 2639
NIH Research on Sleep and Sleep Disorders, 2713

Small Businesses
Indiana 21st Century Research and Technology Fund Awards, 1850
NCI Academic-Industrial Partnerships for Development and Validation of In Vivo Imaging Systems and Methods for Cancer Investigations, 2268
NHLBI Bioengineering Approaches to Energy Balance and Obesity Grants for SBIR, 2319
NHLBI Bioengineering Approaches to Energy Balance and Obesity Grants for STTR, 2320
NIAID Small Business Innovation Research Advanced Technology Grants, 2463
NIEHS Small Business Innovation Research Grants, 2605
NIH Recovery Act Limited Competition: Small Business Catalyst Awards for Accelerating Innovative Research Grants, 2710
NIH Small Business Innovation Research: Animal Models of HCV Infection Research Grants, 2728
NIH Technologies to Improve the Utility of Animal Models Research Grants, 2735
NSF Small Business Innovation Research Grants, 2893

Smoking
APPEAL Social Justice and Tobacco Control Grants, 513
BCBS of Minnesota Healthy Together Grants, 712
CDC Program to Prevent Smoking Among Urban Youth, 924
NCI/NIDA Transdisciplinary Tobacco Use Research Centers Grants, 2280
Thrasher Research Fund Grants, 3426

Smoking Behavior
Alton Ochsner Award, 373
American Legacy Fndn Small Innovative Grants, 439
APPEAL Social Justice and Tobacco Control Grants, 513
BCBS of Minnesota Healthy Together Grants, 712
CDC Program to Prevent Smoking Among Urban Youth, 924
Christine O. Gregoire Youth/Young Adult Award for Outstanding Use of Tobacco Industry Documents, 1005
Comm Fndn for Southeastern Michigan Grants, 1094
CTCRI Idea Grants, 1170
Fndn for a Healthy Kentucky Grants, 1527
Health Fndn of Greater Indianapolis Grants, 1725
Hillsdale County Comm Fndn Healthy Senior/Healthy Youth Fund Grants, 1776
Moses Cone-Wesley Long Comm Health Fndn Grants, 2219
NCI/NIDA Transdisciplinary Tobacco Use Research Centers Grants, 2280
Premera CARES Grants, 3074
Sybil G. Jacobs Award for Outstanding Use of Tobacco Industry Documents, 3414
Thrasher Research Fund Grants, 3426
TRDRP California Research Awards, 3434

Social Change
Aetna Fndn Voice Of Conscience Award, 252
Colin Higgins Fndn Grants, 1056
Comm Fndn of Broward Grants, 1100
Comm Technology Fndn of California Building Communities Through Technology Grants, 1136
Echoing Green Fellowships, 1365
Educational Fndn of America Grants, 1372
Families USA Wellstone Fellowship for Social Justice, 1450
FCNY Union Square Awards, 1461
Frey Fndn Grants, 1562
Ittleson Fndn Mental Health Grants, 1870
Jay and Rose Phillips Family Fndn Grants, 1909
John M. Lloyd Fndn Grants, 1939
Lewis Preston Fund for Girls Education Grants, 2052
Minneapolis Fndn Comm Grants, 2206
Ms. Fndn for Women Grants, 2222
Paul G. Allen Family Fndn Grants, 3000
San Diego Fndn for Change Grants, 3255
Women's Fndn of California Comm Action Fund, 3549

Social Psychology
NSF Social Psychology Research Grants, 2894
Olfactory Research Fund Grants, 2942

Social Science Education
Blowitz-Ridgeway Fndn Early Childhood Development Research Award, 766
SSHRC Image, Text, Sound and Technology Grants, 3363
SSHRC Research/Creation Grants in Fine Arts, 3364

Social Sciences
AAAS Science & Technology Policy Fellowships - National Defense & Global Security, 29
Alzheimer's Association Investigator-Initiated Research Grants, 378
amfAR Fellowships, 462
amfAR Global Initiatives Grants, 463
amfAR Mathilde Krim Fellowships in Basic Biomedical Research, 464
amfAR Public Policy Grants, 465
amfAR Research Grants, 466
APA Congressional Fellowships, 492
Banfi Vintners Fndn Grants, 687
Blowitz-Ridgeway Fndn Early Childhood Development Research Award, 766
Blowitz-Ridgeway Fndn Grants, 767
Brookdale Fndn Leadership in Aging Fellowships, 805
Canada-U.S. Fulbright New Century Scholars Grants, 846
Canada-U.S. Fulbright Senior Specialists Grants, 847
Canadian Friends of Hebrew University Research and Study Grants, 850
Comm Fndn of Wabash County Grants, 1131
DAAD Research Stays for University Academics and Scientists, 1183
Duke University Postdoctoral Research Fellowships in Aging, 1348
Fulbright Alumni Initiatives Awards Grants, 1566
Fulbright Distinguished Chairs Grants, 1567
Fulbright New Century Scholars Grants, 1570
Fulbright Specialists Grants, 1571
Fulbright Traditional Scholar Program in Europe and Eurasia, 1572
Fulbright Traditional Scholar Program in Sub-Saharan Africa, 1573
Fulbright Traditional Scholar Program in the East Asia/Pacific Region, 1574
Fulbright Traditional Scholar Program in the Near East and North Africa Region, 1575
Fulbright Traditional Scholar Program in the South and Central Asia Region, 1576
Fulbright Traditional Scholar Program in the Western Hemisphere, 1577
Fyssen Fndn Postdoctoral Study Grants, 1580
Harry Frank Guggenheim Fndn Research Grants, 1704
Health Fndn of Greater Cincinnati Grants, 1724
HRB Health Services Research Fellowships, 1801
John Ben Snow Memorial Trust Grants, 1928
John Lord Knight Fndn Grants, 1938
McGregor Fund Grants, 2143
National Lottery Comm Fund Grants, 2256
NCI Stages of Breast Development: Normal to Metastatic Disease Grants, 2278
NFID Advanced Vaccinology Course Travel Grant, 2307
NHLBI Translating Basic Behavioral and Social Science Discoveries into Interventions to Reduce Obesity: Centers for Behavioral Intervention Development Grants, 2390
NIA Behavioral and Social Research Grants on Disasters and Health, 2401
NIDA Behavioral Science Track Awards for Rapid Transition, 2498
NIDA Minority Institutions Drug Abuse Research Development Program (MIDARP) Grants, 2509
NIDA Neurobiological and Behavioral Research on Nicotine and Tobacco Products, 2511
NIH Career Development Awards: Child Abuse and Neglect Research, 2646
NIH Pathological Gambling: Basic, Clinical, and Services Research Grants, 2702
NIMH Supplements for Underrepresented Minorities, 2773
NINR Aging Women and Breast Cancer Grants, 2789
NSF Alan T. Waterman Award, 2874
Nuffield Fndn Africa Grants, 2898
Nuffield Fndn Law and Society Grants, 2900
Nuffield Fndn Small Grants, 2903
OBSSR Behavioral and Social Science Research on Understanding and Reducing Health Disparities Grants, 2932
Oleonda Jameson Trust Grants, 2941
OSI Supplementary Grant Program: Burma, 2971
Savoy Fndn Studentships, 3268
SSHRC Image, Text, Sound and Technology Grants, 3363

SSHRC Research/Creation Grants in Fine Arts, 3364
Takemi Program in International Health Research and Advanced Training Fellowships, 3416

Social Services
100 Mile Man Fndn Grants, 2
A Friend's Fndn Trust Grants, 13
A. Gary Anderson Family Fndn Grants, 17
A.O. Smith Comm Grants, 18
A/H Fndn Grants, 19
Aaron Fndn (California) Grants, 173
Aaron Fndn (Massachusetts) Grants, 174
Abbott Fund Comm Vitality Grants, 177
Abel Fndn Grants, 181
Able To Serve Grants, 185
Abney Fndn Grants, 187
Abramson Family Fndn Grants, 188
ACF Ethnic Comm Self-Help Grants, 200
ACF Preferred Communities Grants, 201
ACF Standing Announcement for Unaccompanied Alien Children Grants, 202
ACF Supplemental Services for Recently Arrived Refugees Grants, 203
Administaff Comm Affairs Grants, 235
Advanced Micro Devices Comm Affairs Grants, 239
AEC Trust Grants, 242
AEGON Transamerica Fndn Grants, 243
AFG Industries Grants, 259
Ahmanson Fndn Grants, 303
Air Products and Chemicals Grants, 319
Alabama Power Fndn Grants, 321
Aladdin Industries Fndn Grants, 322
Albert Pick Jr. Fund Grants, 328
Alberto Culver Corp Contributions Grants, 329
Albertson's Charitable Giving Grants, 330
Albuquerque Comm Fndn Grants, 331
Alcatel-Lucent Technologies Fndn Grants, 333
Alcoa Fndn Grants, 334
Alexander & Baldwin Fndn Hawaiian and Pacific Island Grants, 338
Alexander & Baldwin Fndn Mainland Grants, 339
Alexander Eastman Fndn Grants, 341
Allegheny Technologies Charitable Trust, 359
Allyn Fndn Grants, 365
ALSAM Fndn Grants, 369
Amador Comm Fndn Grants, 409
Amarillo Area/Harrington Fndns Grants, 410
Amgen Fndn Grants, 467
AMI Semiconductors Corp Grants, 468
Andersen Fndn Grants, 471
Anheuser-Busch Fndn Grants, 474
Ann Arbor Area Comm Fndn Grants, 476
Ann Peppers Fndn Grants, 478
Anthony R. Abraham Fndn Grants, 490
Archer Daniels Midland Fndn Grants, 525
Argyros Fndn Grants, 527
Arizona Cardinals Grants, 529
Arizona Public Service Corp Giving Grants, 531
Arkansas Comm Fndn Grants, 533
Armstrong McDonald Fndn Grants, 537
ARS Fndn Grants, 538
AT&T Fndn Civic and Comm Service Grants, 658
Atherton Family Fndn Grants, 659
Atkinson Fndn International Grants, 661
Atlanta Fndn Grants, 662
Auburn Fndn Grants, 664
Aurora Fndn Grants, 667
Autzen Fndn Grants, 672
Bailey Fndn Grants, 680
Balfe Family Fndn Grants, 682
Ball Brothers Fndn General Grants, 683
Ball Brothers Fndn General Grants, 683
Ball Brothers Fndn Grants, 684
Bank of America Client Fndn Grants, 690
Barberton Comm Fndn Grants, 693
Barker Fndn Grants, 694
Barker Welfare Fndn Grants, 695
Barr Fund Grants, 697
Barra Fndn Comm Fund Grants, 698
Barra Fndn Project Grants, 699
Batchelor Fndn Grants, 701
Baton Rouge Area Fndn Grants, 702
Battle Creek Comm Fndn Grants, 703
Batts Fndn Grants, 704
Baxter International Fndn Grants, 705
Beazley Fndn Grants, 730
Bechtel Group Fndn Building Positive Comm Relationships Grants, 731
Becton Dickinson and Company Grants, 736
Ben B. Cheney Fndn Grants, 741
Bender Fndn Grants, 742
Benton Comm Fndn Grants, 743
Berks County Comm Fndn Grants, 745
Bernard F. and Alva B. Gimbel Fndn Grants, 747
Besser Fndn Grants, 752
Blackford County Comm Fndn Grants, 763
Blanche and Irving Laurie Fndn Grants, 764
Blanche and Julian Robertson Family Fndn Grants, 765
Blue Grass Comm Fndn Grants, 768
Blue Mountain Comm Fndn Grants, 769
Blue River Comm Fndn Grants, 770
Blum-Kovler Fndn Grants, 772
Blumenthal Fndn Grants, 773
Bob and Delores Hope Charitable Fndn Grants, 774
Bodenwein Public Benevolent Fndn Grants, 775
Bodman Fndn Grants, 776
Boeing Company Contributions Grants, 777
Boettcher Fndn Grants, 778
Booth-Bricker Fund Grants, 780
Borkee-Hagley Fndn Grants, 781
Bosque Fndn Grants, 782
Boston Fndn Grants, 783
Bridgestone/Firestone Trust Fund Grants, 792
Bright Family Fndn Grants, 793
Brookdale Fndn National Group Respite and Early Memory Loss Grants, 806
Brown County Comm Fndn Grants, 807
Burlington Industries Fndn Grants, 811
Burlington Northern Santa Fe Fndn Grants, 812
Burton G. Bettingen Grants, 813
C.W. Titus Fndn Grants, 826
Cambridge Comm Fndn Grants, 837
Camp-Younts Fndn Grants, 838
Carl and Eloise Pohlad Family Fndn Grants, 867
Carl B. and Florence E. King Fndn Grants, 869
Carolyn Fndn Grants, 880
Carpenter Fndn Grants, 881
Carrie E. and Lena V. Glenn Fndn Grants, 882
Cass County Comm Fndn Grants, 887
Catherine Kennedy Home Fndn Grants, 890
Central Carolina Comm Fndn Comm Impact Grants, 936
Cessna Fndn Grants, 938
Champlin Fndns Grants, 960
Charles A. Frueauff Fndn Grants, 962
Charles Delmar Fndn Grants, 963
Charles M. Bair Family Trust Grants, 972
Charlotte County (FL) Comm Fndn Grants, 973
Chase Paymentech Corp Giving Grants, 975
Chatlos Fndn Grants, 977
Chestnut Hill Charitable Fndn, Inc Grants, 987
CIGNA Fndn Grants, 1011
Cinergy Fndn Grants, 1013
Clarcor Fndn Grants, 1021
Clark County Comm Fndn Grants, 1028
Claude Worthington Benedum Fndn Grants, 1033
CNA Fndn Grants, 1046
CNCS Foster Grandparent Projects Grants, 1048
Coastal Comm Fndn of South Carolina Grants, 1051
Cockrell Fndn Grants, 1053
Coeta and Donald Barker Fndn Grants, 1054
Collins Fndn Grants, 1058
Colorado Interstate Gas Grants, 1060
Colorado Springs Comm Trust Fund Grants, 1061
Columbus Fndn Competitive Grants, 1066
Columbus Fndn J. Floyd Dixon Memorial Fund Grants, 1068
Columbus Fndn Mary Eleanor Morris Fund Grants, 1069
Columbus Fndn Traditional Grants, 1071
Comer Fndn Grants, 1072
Comerica Charitable Fndn Grants, 1073
Commission on Religion in Appalachia Grants, 1074
Comm Fndn Alliance City of Evansville Endowment Fund Grants, 1089
Comm Fndn for Greater New Haven Grants, 1091
Comm Fndn for Monterey County Grants, 1092
Comm Fndn for Muskegon County Grants, 1093
Comm Fndn for Southeastern Michigan Grants, 1094
Comm Fndn for Southern Arizona Grants, 1095
Comm Fndn of Bartholomew County Heritage Fund Grants, 1096
Comm Fndn of Bartholomew County James A. Henderson Award for Fund-Raising, 1097
Comm Fndn of Bloomington and Monroe County Grants, 1098
Comm Fndn of Boone County Grants, 1099
Comm Fndn of Central Illinois Grants, 1101
Comm Fndn of Champaign County Grants, 1102
Comm Fndn of Greater Birmingham Grants, 1106
Comm Fndn of Greater Flint Grants, 1107
Comm Fndn of Greater Fort Wayne: Comm Endowment & Clarke Endowment Fund Grants, 1108
Comm Fndn of Greater Greensboro Grants, 1109
Comm Fndn of Greater New Britain Grants, 1111
Comm Fndn of Greater Tampa Grants, 1112
Comm Fndn of Greenville Comm Enrichment Grants, 1113
Comm Fndn of Greenville Hollingsworth Funds Program/Project Grants, 1114
Comm Fndn of Greenville-Greenville Women Giving Grants, 1115
Comm Fndn of Mount Vernon and Knox County Grants, 1119
Comm Fndn of Santa Cruz County Grants, 1122
Comm Fndn of South Alabama Grants, 1123
Comm Fndn of Southeastern Connecticut Grants, 1125
Comm Fndn of Tampa Bay Grants, 1128
Comm Fndn of Wabash County Grants, 1131
Comm Fndn of Western North Carolina Grants, 1132
Comm Fndn Silicon Valley Grants, 1133
ConAgra Foods Fndn Grants, 1140
Connelly Fndn Grants, 1143
ConocoPhillips Fndn Grants, 1144
Constantin Fndn Grants, 1145
Constellation Energy Group and Baltimore Gas and Electric Corp Contributions, 1146
Consumers Energy Fndn, 1147
Cooke Fndn Grants, 1148
Cooper Industries Fndn Grants, 1150
Cornerstone Fndn of Northeastern Wisconsin Grants, 1152
Cowles Charitable Trust Grants, 1155
Crail-Johnson Fndn Grants, 1157
Cranston Fndn Grants, 1158
Crestlea Fndn Grants, 1159
CRH Fndn Grants, 1160
CSX Corp Contributions Grants, 1169
Cultural Society of Filipino Americans Grants, 1173
CUNA Mutual Group Fndn, 1174
Cyrus Eaton Fndn Grants, 1178
D. W. McMillan Fndn Grants, 1180
D.F. Halton Fndn Grants, 1181
Dade Comm Fndn Grants, 1185
DaimlerChrysler Corp Fund Grants, 1186
Dana Corp Fndn Grants, 1196
Danellie Fndn Grants, 1198
Dayton Power and Light Fndn Grants, 1205
Daywood Fndn Grants, 1206
Dearborn Comm Fndn County Progress Grants, 1211
Delaware Comm Fndn Grants, 1215
Delaware Comm Fndn-Youth Philanthropy Board for Kent County, 1216
Dell Fndn Open Grants, 1218
Delta Air Lines Fndn Grants, 1220
DeMatteis Family Fndn Grants, 1221
Denver Fndn Comm Grants, 1227
DeRoy Testamentary Fndn Grants, 1239
Detroit Lions Charities Grants, 1241

DHHS Adolescent Family Life Demonstration Projects, 1243
DHHS Health Centers Grants for Residents of Public Housing, 1254
DHHS HIV Demonstration Program for Children, Adolescents, and Women, 1262
Donald and Sylvia Robinson Family Fndn Grants, 1310
Dorrance Family Fndn Grants, 1323
Dr. Scholl Fndn Grants, 1329
Duchossois Family Fndn Grants, 1337
Duke Energy Fndn Grants, 1339
Dunspaugh-Dalton Fndn Grants, 1351
E.J. Grassmann Trust Grants, 1360
Eden Hall Fndn Grants, 1368
Edina Realty Fndn Grants, 1369
Edwards Memorial Trust Grants, 1375
Edwin W. and Catherine M. Davis Fndn Grants, 1377
EIF Comm Grants, 1386
Eisner Fndn Grants, 1387
El Paso Comm Fndn Grants, 1388
Elkhart County Comm Fndn Grants, 1401
Emerson Charitable Trust Grants, 1412
Ensworth Charitable Fndn Grants, 1416
Erie Comm Fndn Grants, 1427
Estee Lauder Grants, 1429
Eugene M. Lang Fndn Grants, 1434
Evan and Susan Bayh Fndn Grants, 1437
Evjue Fndn Grants, 1439
F.M. Kirby Fndn Grants, 1443
Fargo-Moorhead Area Fndn Grants, 1454
Farmers Insurance Group of Companies Grants, 1455
Feldman Fndn Grants, 1484
Field Fndn of Illinois Grants, 1499
Fireman's Fund Fndn Grants, 1504
FirstEnergy Fndn Comm Grants, 1505
Fisher Fndn Grants, 1508
Flinn Fndn Grants Programs, 1511
Fluor Fndn Grants, 1517
FMC Fndn Grants, 1518
Foellinger Fndn Grants, 1519
Fondren Fndn Grants, 1520
Ford Motor Company Fund Grants, 1522
Forrest C. Lattner Fndn Grants, 1523
Fndn for the Mid-South Grants, 1536
Fndn Northwest Grants, 1537
Fourjay Fndn Grants, 1544
Frances L. and Edwin L. Cummings Memorial Fund Grants, 1547
Frank Stanley Beveridge Fndn Grants, 1553
Fred L. Emerson Fndn Grants, 1557
Fremont Area Comm Fndn Grants, 1561
Frist Fndn Grants, 1563
Fritz B. Burns Fndn Grants, 1564
Fuji Film Grants, 1565
Fuller E. Callaway Fndn Grants, 1578
G.N. Wilcox Trust Grants, 1581
GenCorp Fndn Grants, 1587
George and Ruth Bradford Fndn Grants, 1595
George F. Baker Trust Grants, 1597
George Frederick Jewett Fndn Grants, 1599
Georgiana Goddard Eaton Memorial Fund Grants, 1604
Gill Fndn - Gay and Lesbian Fund Grants, 1613
Giving Sum Annual Grant, 1619
Glendale Comm Fndn Grants, 1626
Graco Fndn Grants, 1642
Grand Haven Area Comm Fndn Grants, 1644
Grand Rapids Comm Fndn Grants, 1647
Greater Bridgeport Area Fndn Comm Impact Grants, 1650
Greater Cincinnati Fndn Priority and Small Projects/ Capacity-Building Grants, 1651
Greater Green Bay Comm Fndn Grants, 1652
Greater Milwaukee Fndn Grants, 1653
Greater Saint Louis Comm Fndn Grants, 1655
Greater Tacoma Comm Fndn Grants, 1656
Greater Worcester Comm Fndn Discretionary Grants, 1658
Green Bay Packers Fndn Grants, 1660
Green Fndn Grants, 1661
Grotto Fndn Project Grants, 1671
Gulf Coast Comm Fndn Grants, 1676
H & R Fndn Grants, 1679
H. Schaffer Fndn Grants, 1680
H.J. Heinz Company Fndn Grants, 1682
Hall-Perrine Fndn Grants, 1686
Halliburton Fndn Grants, 1687
Hallmark Corp Fndn Grants, 1688
Hannaford Charitable Fndn Grants, 1692
Harden Fndn Grants, 1693
Harold and Arlene Schnitzer CARE Fndn Grants, 1697
Harold Simmons Fndn Grants, 1698
Harris and Eliza Kempner Fund Grants, 1699
Harry A. and Margaret D. Towsley Fndn Grants, 1701
Harry Kramer Memorial Fund Grants, 1705
Harry Sudakoff Fndn Grants, 1708
Hartford Aging and Health Program Awards, 1709
Hartford Courant Fndn Grants, 1710
Hartford Fndn Regular Grants, 1711
Hawn Fndn Grants, 1719
Health Fndn of Greater Indianapolis Grants, 1725
Hearst Fndn and William Randolph Hearst Fndn Grants, 1730
Helen K. and Arthur E. Johnson Fndn Grants, 1740
Henrietta Tower Wurts Memorial Fndn Grants, 1745
Hershey Company Grants, 1754
High Meadow Fndn Grants, 1768
Highmark Corp Giving Grants, 1769
Hill Fndn Grants, 1774
Hillman Fndn Grants, 1775
Hoblitzelle Fndn Grants, 1783
Hoglund Fndn Grants, 1785
Holland/Zeeland Comm Fndn Grants, 1786
Homer Fndn Grants, 1789
Honeywell Fndn Grants, 1791
Horace A. Kimball and S. Ella Kimball Fndn Grants, 1792
Houston Endowment Grants, 1797
Howard and Bush Fndn Grants, 1798
Howe Fndn of North Carolina Grants, 1799
HRSA Ryan White HIV Early Intervention Services Grants, 1811
Huie-Dellmon Trust Grants, 1815
Humana Fndn Grants, 1818
Huntington National Bank Comm Affairs Grants, 1824
Hutton Fndn Grants, 1828
Ireland Family Fndn Grants, 1865
J.B. Reynolds Fndn Grants, 1873
J.C. Penney Company Grants, 1874
J.E. and L.E. Mabee Fndn Grants, 1875
J.L. Bedsole Fndn Grants, 1876
J.M. Long Fndn Grants, 1877
J.W. Kieckhefer Fndn Grants, 1878
Jacob G. Schmidlapp Trust Grants, 1883
James Graham Brown Fndn Grants, 1887
James H. Cummings Fndn Grants, 1888
James J. and Angelia M. Harris Fndn Grants, 1890
James M. Collins Fndn Grants, 1891
James R. Dougherty Jr. Fndn Grants, 1894
James S. Copley Fndn Grants, 1895
Janirve Fndn Grants, 1905
Jean and Louis Dreyfus Fndn Grants, 1911
Jerome and Mildred Paddock Fndn Grants, 1917
Jessie Ball Dupont Fund Grants, 1919
Jewish Comm Fndn of Greater Los Angeles Grants, 1921
John Deere Fndn Grants, 1929
John Edward Fowler Memorial Fndn Grants, 1930
John G. Duncan Trust Grants, 1931
John G. Martin Fndn Grants, 1932
John H. and Wilhelmina D. Harland Charitable Fndn Grants, 1933
John I. Smith Charities Grants, 1935
John J. Leidy Fndn Grants, 1936
John Jewett and Helen Chandler Garland Fndn Grants, 1937
John P. McGovern Fndn Grants, 1942
John P. Murphy Fndn Grants, 1943
John R. Oishei Fndn Grants, 1944
Johns Manville Fund Grants, 1950
Johnson Controls Fndn Grants, 1954
Joseph Alexander Fndn Grants, 1957
Joseph Drown Fndn Grants, 1960
Josephine G. Russell Trust Grants, 1963
Josiah W. and Bessie H. Kline Fndn Grants, 1967
Journal Gazette Fndn Grants, 1968
K. M. Hunter Charitable Fndn Social Welfare Grants, 1974
Kahuku Comm Fund, 1977
Katharine Matthies Fndn Grants, 1982
Knight Family Charitable and Educational Fndn Grants, 2007
Kraft Cares US Grants, 2017
L. W. Pierce Family Fndn Grants, 2019
Land O'Lakes Fndn Mid-Atlantic Grants, 2027
Lands' End Corp Giving Program, 2030
Laura B. Vogler Fndn Grants, 2032
Lawrence S. Huntington Fund Grants, 2035
Lillian S. Wells Fndn Grants, 2056
Lincoln Financial Group Fndn Grants, 2058
Lockheed Martin Philanthropic Grants, 2062
Louis Calder Fndn Grants, 2065
Lowell Berry Fndn Grants, 2069
Lubbock Area Fndn Grants, 2079
Lubrizol Fndn Grants, 2080
Lucile Horton Howe and Mitchell B. Howe Fndn Grants, 2081
Lucy Gooding Charitable Fndn Trust Grants, 2083
Lynde and Harry Bradley Fndn Grants, 2089
Lynde and Harry Bradley Fndn Prizes: Bradley Prizes, 2090
M. Bastian Family Fndn Grants, 2092
M.B. and Edna Zale Fndn Grants, 2093
M.E. Raker Fndn Grants, 2094
Mabel Y. Hughes Charitable Trust Grants, 2097
Maine Comm Fndn Grants, 2099
MAPFRE Fndn for Medicine Grants, 2102
Marcia and Otto Koehler Fndn Grants, 2103
Margaret T. Morris Fndn Grants, 2105
Mark and Catherine Winkler Fndn Grants, 2112
Mars Fndn Grants, 2114
Mary Allen Lindsey Branan Fndn Grants, 2116
Mary S. and David C. Corbin Fndn Grants, 2122
Matilda R. Wilson Fund Grants, 2128
Maxtor Corp Contributions Grants, 2136
May and Stanley Smith Trust Grants, 2137
McInerny Fndn Grants, 2144
McKesson Fndn Grants, 2145
Mead Johnson Nutritionals Evansville-Area Organizations Grants, 2157
Mead Witter Fndn Grants, 2160
Meadows Fndn Grants, 2161
Meriden Fndn Grants, 2173
Metro Health Fndn Grants, 2175
Meyer Memorial Trust Emergency Grants, 2178
Meyer Memorial Trust Grassroots Grants, 2179
Meyer Memorial Trust Operating Funds Grants, 2180
Meyer Memorial Trust Responsive Grants, 2181
Miguel Aleman Fndn Grants, 2197
Millipore Fndn Grants, 2203
Miriam and Peter Haas Fund Grants, 2208
Morton K. and Jane Blaustein Fndn Grants, 2218
Nelda C. and H.J. Lutcher Stark Fndn Grants, 2301
Newman's Own Inc Grants, 2306
Nicholas H. Noyes Jr. Memorial Fndn Grants, 2497
Nordson Corp Fndn Grants, 2851
North Carolina Comm Development Grants, 2858
North Carolina Comm Fndn Grants, 2859
Northeast Utilities Fndn Grants, 2863
Northern New York Comm Fndn Grants, 2864
Northern Trust Company Charitable Trust and Corp Giving Program, 2865
Northrop Grumman Corp Grants, 2866
Northrop Grumman Newport News Grants, 2867
Northwestern Mutual Fndn Grants, 2870
Norwin S. and Elizabeth N. Bean Fndn Grants, 2872
Nuffield Fndn Africa Grants, 2898
Nuffield Fndn Law and Society Grants, 2900
Nuffield Fndn Open Door Grants, 2902

Nuffield Fndn Small Grants, 2903
NYCT Girls and Young Women Grants, 2924
Ogden Codman Trust Grants, 2937
Oleonda Jameson Trust Grants, 2941
Ordean Fndn Grants, 2952
Owen County Comm Fndn Grants, 2979
PacifiCare Fndn Grants, 2981
PacifiCorp Fndn for Learning Grants, 2982
Paul Balint Charitable Trust Grants, 2998
Paul G. Duke Fndn Grants, 3001
Peacock Fndn Grants, 3011
Perpetual Trust for Charitable Giving Grants, 3015
Pew Charitable Trusts Children & Youth Grants, 3020
Philadelphia Fndn Organizational Effectiveness Grants, 3029
Phoenix Suns Charities Grants, 3030
Pinellas County Grants, 3050
Pittsburgh Fndn Comm Fund Grants, 3054
Plough Fndn Grants, 3061
PNC Charitable Trust and Fndn Grants, 3064
Polk Bros. Fndn Grants, 3066
Pott Fndn Grants, 3071
Powell Fndn Grants, 3073
Pride Fndn Grants and Scholarships, 3078
Principal Financial Group Fndn Grants, 3082
Procter and Gamble Fund Grants, 3083
Questar Corp Contributions Grants, 3097
R.C. Baker Fndn Grants, 3098
Rajiv Gandhi Fndn Grants, 3104
Raskob Fndn for Catholic Activities Grants, 3107
Rasmuson Fndn Grants, 3108
Rayonier Fndn Grants, 3111
Regence Fndn Access to Health Care Grants, 3138
Regence Fndn Health Care Comm Awareness and Engagement Grants, 3139
Regence Fndn Health Care Connections Grants, 3140
Regence Fndn Improving End-of-Life Grants, 3141
Regence Fndn Tools and Technology Grants, 3142
Rhode Island Fndn Grants, 3154
Rich Fndn Grants, 3156
Richard and Helen DeVos Fndn Grants, 3157
Richard E. Griffin Family Fndn Grants, 3160
Richard King Mellon Fndn Grants, 3161
Ripley County Comm Fndn Grants, 3166
Robert and Joan Dircks Fndn Grants, 3167
Robins Fndn Grants, 3175
Rochester Area Comm Fndn Grants, 3176
Rockwell International Corp Trust Grants, 3183
Roeher Institute Research Grants, 3184
Rollin M. Gerstacker Fndn Grants, 3186
RRF General Grants, 3193
Russell Berrie Fndn Grants, 3201
S. Livingston Mather Charitable Trust Grants, 3235
S.H. Cowell Fndn Grants, 3237
Salisbury Comm Fndn Grants, 3243
Samuel S. Johnson Fndn Grants, 3251
San Antonio Area Fndn Grants, 3254
San Diego Fndn Health & Human Services Grants, 3256
Self Fndn Grants, 3277
Sid W. Richardson Fndn Grants, 3284
Siebert Lutheran Fndn Grants, 3285
Sir Halley Stewart Trust Grants, 3293
Sisters of Mercy of North Carolina Fndn Grants, 3295
Sisters of Saint Joseph Charitable Fund Grants, 3296
Sosland Fndn Grants, 3348
Southwest Florida Comm Fndn Competitive Grants, 3351
Southwest Gas Corp Fndn Grants, 3352
Sprague Fndn Grants, 3359
Starr Fndn Grants, 3377
Steele-Reese Fndn Grants, 3380
Stewart Huston Charitable Trust Grants, 3384
Susan Mott Webb Charitable Trust Grants, 3412
Tellabs Fndn Grants, 3418
Thomas and Dorothy Leavey Fndn Grants, 3422
Thomas C. Ackerman Fndn Grants, 3423
Thompson Charitable Fndn Grants, 3425
Topfer Family Fndn Grants, 3430
Triangle Comm Fndn Donor-Advised Grants, 3437
Trull Fndn Grants, 3441
TWS Fndn Grants, 3443
U.S. Department of Education 21st Century Comm Learning Centers, 3445
Union Benevolent Association Grants, 3460
United Technologies Corp Grants, 3466
US Airways Comm Contributions, 3472
Vancouver Fndn Grants and Comm Initiatives Program, 3477
Vermont Comm Fndn Grants, 3493
Vulcan Materials Company Fndn Grants, 3504
Wabash Valley Comm Fndn Grants, 3510
Wachovia Fndn Grants, 3511
Washington Post Contributions Grants, 3520
Wayne and Gladys Valley Fndn Grants, 3522
Weatherwax Fndn Grants, 3523
Weingart Fndn Grants, 3524
WHO Fndn General Grants, 3534
William G. Gilmore Fndn Grants, 3537
Wilson-Wood Fndn Grants, 3542
Winston-Salem Fndn Competitive Grants, 3544
YSA Get Ur Good On Grants, 3555
Z. Smith Reynolds Fndn Small Grants, 3557

Social Services Delivery

Aaron Fndn (Massachusetts) Grants, 174
Abbott Fund Comm Vitality Grants, 177
Abel Fndn Grants, 181
Able To Serve Grants, 185
African American Fund of New Jersey Grants, 260
Agnes B. Hunt Trust Grants, 261
Albert and Margaret Alkek Fndn Grants, 326
Alexander & Baldwin Fndn Hawaiian and Pacific Island Grants, 338
Alexander & Baldwin Fndn Mainland Grants, 339
Allegan County Comm Fndn Grants, 358
American Schlafhorst Fndn Grants, 454
Andersen Corp Fndn, 470
Anheuser-Busch Fndn Grants, 474
Ann Peppers Fndn Grants, 478
AptarGroup Fndn Grants, 522
Arlington Comm Fndn Grants, 536
ArvinMeritor Grants, 544
Aurora Fndn Grants, 667
Autzen Fndn Grants, 672
Bacon Family Fndn Grants, 679
Balfe Family Fndn Grants, 682
Barra Fndn Comm Fund Grants, 698
Bernard and Audre Rapoport Fndn Grants, 746
Bernard F. and Alva B. Gimbel Fndn Grants, 747
Boston Jewish Comm Women's Fund Grants, 785
Byron W. and Alice L. Lockwood Fndn Grants, 824
C.W. Titus Fndn Grants, 826
Catherine Holmes Wilkins Fndn Grants, 889
Charles Lafitte Fndn Grants, 970
Charlotte County (FL) Comm Fndn Grants, 973
Chase Paymentech Corp Giving Grants, 975
Chiron Fndn Comm Grants, 1004
CICF Legacy Fund Comm Fndn Grants, 1010
CIT Corp Giving Grants, 1014
Columbus Fndn Mary Eleanor Morris Fund Grants, 1069
Comm Fndn of South Puget Sound Grants, 1124
Comm Fndn of St. Joseph County Special Project Challenge Grants, 1126
CSRA Comm Fndn Grants, 1168
Cudd Fndn Grants, 1171
Cultural Society of Filipino Americans Grants, 1173
Dairy Queen Corp Contributions Grants, 1187
Deaconess Comm Fndn Grants, 1207
Dell Fndn Healthy Communities, Literate Communities, and Connected Communities Grants, 1217
DeMatteis Family Fndn Grants, 1221
Dennis and Phyllis Washington Fndn Grants, 1222
DeRoy Testamentary Fndn Grants, 1239
DHL Charitable Shipment Support, 1283
Donald and Sylvia Robinson Family Fndn Grants, 1310
Dora Roberts Fndn Grants, 1311
Dr. Leon Bromberg Charitable Trust Fund Grants, 1328
Dreitzer Fndn Grants, 1332
Drs. Bruce and Lee Fndn Grants, 1333
DuPage Comm Fndn Grants, 1352
Eastman Chemical Company Fndn Grants, 1362
EDS Fndn Grants, 1371
Eva L. and Joseph M. Bruening Fndn Grants, 1436
Evan and Susan Bayh Fndn Grants, 1437
Ewing Halsell Fndn Grants, 1440
Foster Fndn Grants, 1524
Fndn for the Carolinas Grants, 1535
Francis L. Abreu Charitable Trust Grants, 1549
George B. Storer Fndn Grants, 1596
Gilroy and Lillian P. Roberts Charitable Fndn Grants, 1614
Goodyear Tire Grants, 1639
Greater Cincinnati Fndn Priority and Small Projects/ Capacity-Building Grants, 1651
Hagedorn Fund Grants, 1685
Hall-Perrine Fndn Grants, 1686
Harold Alfond Fndn Grants, 1695
Harrison County Comm Fndn Grants, 1700
Harvest Fndn Grants, 1713
Hasbro Children's Fund, 1714
Hawn Fndn Grants, 1719
Heckscher Fndn for Children Grants, 1732
Hillsdale Fund Grants, 1778
Hirtzel Memorial Fndn Grants, 1781
Homer Fndn Grants, 1789
Howard and Bush Fndn Grants, 1798
Hugh J. Andersen Fndn Grants, 1814
Ida Alice Ryan Charitable Trust Grants, 1836
Ittleson Fndn Mental Health Grants, 1870
James M. Collins Fndn Grants, 1891
Jay and Rose Phillips Family Fndn Grants, 1909
Jerome and Mildred Paddock Fndn Grants, 1917
Joe W. and Dorothy Dorsett Brown Fndn Grants, 1927
K. M. Hunter Charitable Fndn Social Welfare Grants, 1974
Ken W. Davis Fndn Grants, 1987
Kettering Family Fndn Grants, 1991
Key Fndn Grants, 1994
KeySpan Fndn Grants, 1995
King Pharmaceuticals Corp Contributions Grants, 2003
Ludwick Family Fndn Grants, 2084
M-A-C AIDS Fund Grants, 2091
Marion I. and Henry J. Knott Fndn Grants, 2109
Mark and Catherine Winkler Fndn Grants, 2112
Mary Allen Lindsey Branan Fndn Grants, 2116
Max and Victoria Dreyfus Fndn Grants, 2133
Maxtor Corp Contributions Grants, 2136
May and Stanley Smith Trust Grants, 2137
Meriden Fndn Grants, 2173
North Georgia Comm Fndn Grants, 2862
Oscar Rennebohm Fndn Grants, 2963
Palm Beach and Martin Counties Grants, 2986
Pew Charitable Trusts Children & Youth Grants, 3020
Polk Bros. Fndn Grants, 3066
Powell Fndn Grants, 3073
Priddy Fndn Grants, 3077
Prince Charitable Trusts Chicago Grants, 3079
Rasmuson Fndn Grants, 3108
Rayonier Fndn Grants, 3111
Regence Fndn Access to Health Care Grants, 3138
Regence Fndn Health Care Comm Awareness and Engagement Grants, 3139
Regence Fndn Health Care Connections Grants, 3140
Regence Fndn Improving End-of-Life Grants, 3141
Regence Fndn Tools and Technology Grants, 3142
Richard and Susan Smith Family Fndn Grants, 3159
San Diego Fndn Health & Human Services Grants, 3256
San Francisco Fndn Comm Health Grants, 3260
Shell Oil Company Fndn Grants, 3281
Sisters of Mercy of North Carolina Fndn Grants, 3295
Sisters of St. Joseph Healthcare Fndn Grants, 3297
Sonoco Fndn Grants, 3347
Southwest Gas Corp Fndn Grants, 3352

Square D Fndn Grants, 3361
Sulzberger Fndn Grants, 3399
Support Our Aging Religious Grants, 3406
Taproot Fndn Capacity-Building Service Grants, 3417
Trull Fndn Grants, 3441
TWS Fndn Grants, 3443
United Methodist Health Ministry Fund Grants, 3465
US Airways Comm Contributions, 3472
Virginia W. Kettering Fndn Grants, 3502
Volkswagen of America Corp Contributions Grants, 3503
Western Union Fndn Grants, 3529
Westinghouse Charitable Giving Grants, 3530
WHO Fndn General Grants, 3534
William H. Hannon Fndn Grants, 3540
Woodward Fund Grants, 3552

Social Services: Health Care
Daphne Seybolt Culpeper Memorial Fndn Grants, 1201
Horizons Comm Issues Grants, 1794

Social Services: Women
Rochester Area Fndn Grants, 3177

Social Services: Youth Programs
Greater New Orleans Fndn Grants, 1654

Social Stratification/Mobility
NICHD Socioeconomic Status and Health Across the Life Course, 2495
NIH Studies of Ethical, Legal, and Social Implications of Research into Human Genetic Variation Grants, 2731
NIMH Socioeconomic Status and Health Across the Life Course, 2772
OUT Fund for Lesbian and Gay Liberation Grants, 2978
RWJF Investigator Awards in Health Policy Research, 3220

Social Work
ACS Doctoral Training Grants in Oncology Social Work, 213
APSAA Fellowships, 516
Canada-U.S. Fulbright New Century Scholars Grants, 846
Canada-U.S. Fulbright Senior Specialists Grants, 847
Deland Fellowships in Health Care and Society, 1214
EF Behavioral Sciences Student Fellowships, 1379
Fulbright Alumni Initiatives Awards Grants, 1566
Fulbright Distinguished Chairs Grants, 1567
Fulbright New Century Scholars Grants, 1570
Fulbright Specialists Grants, 1571
Fulbright Traditional Scholar Program in Europe and Eurasia, 1572
Fulbright Traditional Scholar Program in Sub-Saharan Africa, 1573
Fulbright Traditional Scholar Program in the East Asia/Pacific Region, 1574
Fulbright Traditional Scholar Program in the Near East and North Africa Region, 1575
Fulbright Traditional Scholar Program in the South and Central Asia Region, 1576
Fulbright Traditional Scholar Program in the Western Hemisphere, 1577
Leadership in Education in Neurodevelopmental Disabilities Postdoctoral Fellowships, 2037
Pfizer Fndn Health Literacy Grants, 3026

Social Work Education
ACS Master's Training Grants in Clinical Oncology Social Work, 208
Leadership in Education in Neurodevelopmental Disabilities Postdoctoral Fellowships, 2037

Sociology
AAO-HNSF Rande H. Lazar Health Services Research Grant, 150
AHFMR Population Health Investigator Awards, 292
American Fndn for Suicide Prevention Grants, 436
American Sociological Association Minority Fellowships, 458
Canada-U.S. Fulbright New Century Scholars Grants, 846
Canada-U.S. Fulbright Senior Specialists Grants, 847
Dr. Sydney Segal Research Grants, 1331
Edward Bangs Kelley & Elza Kelley Fndn Grants, 1373
EF Behavioral Sciences Student Fellowships, 1379
Fulbright Alumni Initiatives Awards Grants, 1566
Fulbright Distinguished Chairs Grants, 1567
Fulbright New Century Scholars Grants, 1570
Fulbright Specialists Grants, 1571
Fulbright Traditional Scholar Program in Europe and Eurasia, 1572
Fulbright Traditional Scholar Program in Sub-Saharan Africa, 1573
Fulbright Traditional Scholar Program in the East Asia/Pacific Region, 1574
Fulbright Traditional Scholar Program in the Near East and North Africa Region, 1575
Fulbright Traditional Scholar Program in the South and Central Asia Region, 1576
Fulbright Traditional Scholar Program in the Western Hemisphere, 1577
NIH Biobehavioral Research for Effective Sleep, 2639
NIH Enhancing Adherence to Diabetes Self-Management Behaviors, 2659

Solid Waste Disposal
Estee Lauder Grants, 1429

South Africa
OSI Access to Essential Medicines Grants, 2964

South America
Fulbright Traditional Scholar Program in the Western Hemisphere, 1577

Space Sciences
Canada Graduate Scholarships and NSERC Postgraduate Scholarships, 845
GenCorp Fndn Grants, 1587
Kansas Health Fndn Grants, 1980
NIH Biomedical Research on the International Space Station, 2642

Spain
Good Samaritan Inc Grants, 1637

Special Education
Air Products and Chemicals Grants, 319
Andersen Fndn Grants, 471
Annunziata Sanguinetti Fndn Grants, 481
Becton Dickinson and Company Grants, 736
Carroll County Comm Fndn Grants, 885
CVS Comm Grants, 1177
Dept of Ed Special Education—Personnel Development to Improve Services and Results for Children with Disabilities, 1231
Dept of Ed Special Education—Studies and Evaluations, 1232
Dept of Ed Special Education—Technical Assistance and Dissemination to Improve Services and Results for Children with Disabilities, 1233
Dept of Ed Special Education-National Activities-Technology and Media Services for Individuals with Disabilities, 1234
Doreen Kronick Scholarship, 1312
Hasbro Children's Fund, 1714
Henry County Comm Fndn Grants, 1747
Indiana Minority Teacher/Special Services Scholarships, 1852
Scott County Comm Fndn Grants, 3273
Stewart Huston Charitable Trust Grants, 3384
U.S. Department of Education Rehabilitation Training—Rehabilitation Continuing Education Programs—Institute on Rehabilitation Issues, 3449
U.S. Department of Education Special Education—National Activities—Parent Information Centers, 3450

Spectroscopy
EF Postdoctoral Research Training Fellowships, 1382

Speech
Axe-Houghton Fndn Grants, 678
Claude Pepper Fndn Grants, 1032
NIDCD Clinical Trial Planning Grant, 2517
NIDCD Exploratory/Developmental Research Grants, 2520
NIDCD Minority Dissertation Research Grants in Human Communication, 2524

Speech Pathology
ASHA Multicultural Activities Projects Grants, 571
ASHA Student Research Travel Award, 573
ASHFndn Graduate Student International Scholarship, 576
ASHFndn Graduate Student Scholarships, 577
ASHFndn Graduate Student Scholarships for Minority Students, 578
ASHFndn Graduate Student with a Disability Scholarship, 579
ASHFndn New Century Scholars Program Doctoral Scholarships, 580
ASHFndn Research Grant for New Investigators, 582
ASHFndn Research Grant in Speech Science, 583
Deafness Research Fndn Research Grants, 1208
Leadership in Education in Neurodevelopmental Disabilities Postdoctoral Fellowships, 2037
Mabel H. Flory Charitable Trust Grants, 2096
NIDCD Small Grants, 2531

Speech Therapy
ASHA Multicultural Activities Projects Grants, 571
Axe-Houghton Fndn Grants, 678
Mabel H. Flory Charitable Trust Grants, 2096

Speech/Communication Education
Axe-Houghton Fndn Grants, 678
Comm Fndn of Grant County Scholarships, 1105
Mabel H. Flory Charitable Trust Grants, 2096

Spinal Cord Injury
Christopher Reeve Paralysis Fndn Individual Research Grants, 1006
Christopher Reeve Paralysis Fndn Quality of Life and Health Promotions Grants, 1007
Detroit Lions Charities Grants, 1241
International Spinal Research Trust Grants, 1863
NIA Symptom Management for Chronic Neurological Conditions Research Grants, 2436
NICHD Symptom Management for Chronic Neurological Conditions Research Grants, 2496
NIDCD Symptom Management for Chronic Neurological Conditions Research Grants, 2532
NINDS Symptom Management for Chronic Neurological Conditions Research Grants, 2787
NINR Symptom Management for Chronic Neurological Conditions Research Grants, 2805
NIOSH Occupational Safety and Health Research and Demonstration Grants, 2807

Sports
AMSSM Fndn Research Grants, 469
Angels Baseball Fndn Grants, 473
Balance Bar Sports Individual/Team Grants, 681
Barberton Comm Fndn Grants, 693
Bert W. Martin Fndn Grants, 750
Carl and Eloise Pohlad Family Fndn Grants, 867
Carl C. Icahn Fndn Grants, 870
Challenged Athletes Fndn Grants, 958
Children Affected by AIDS Fndn Domestic Grants, 995
Chiles Fndn Grants, 1003
Collins C. Diboll Private Fndn Grants, 1057
Comm Fndn of Grant County Scholarships, 1105
Comm Fndn of the Ozarks Grants, 1130
Daniels Fund Grants, 1200
Denver Broncos Charities Fund Grants, 1226
Detroit Lions Charities Grants, 1241

El Pomar Fndn Awards and Grants, 1390
General Mills Champions for Healthy Kids Grants, 1589
George Kress Fndn Grants, 1601
GoGirlGo! Ambassador Team Awards, 1632
Greater Worcester Comm Fndn Jeppson Memorial Fund for Brookfield Grants, 1659
Gregory L. Gibson Charitable Fndn Grants, 1668
Grotto Fndn Project Grants, 1671
Helen Bader Fndn Grants, 1738
Henrietta Tower Wurts Memorial Fndn Grants, 1745
Homer Fndn Grants, 1789
IATA Research Grants, 1834
IATA Scholarships, 1835
Jewish Women's Fndn of New York Grants, 1924
Kenny's Kids Grants, 1990
Kevin P. and Sydney Knight Family Fndn Grants, 1993
Knox County Comm Fndn Grants, 2009
Louis R. Cappelli Fndn Grants, 2066
Marion I. and Henry J. Knott Fndn Grants, 2109
McCombs Fndn Grants, 2142
Newman's Own Inc Grants, 2306
NIAMS High Risk Arthritis and Musculoskeletal and Skin Diseases Research, 2470
NIAMS Research on Musculoskeletal Fitness and Sports Medicine Grants, 2476
NICHD Research on Musculoskeletal Fitness and Sports Medicine Grants, 2492
NINR Research on Musculoskeletal Fitness and Sports Medicine Grants, 2803
Paul E. and Klare N. Reinhold Fndn Grants, 2999
Perry County Comm Fndn Grants, 3016
Posey Comm Fndn Grants, 3068
Richard and Helen DeVos Fndn Grants, 3157
Seneca Foods Fndn Grants, 3278
U.S. Lacrosse EAD Grants, 3453

Sports Medicine
AMSSM Fndn Research Grants, 469
Angels Baseball Fndn Grants, 473
IATA Research Grants, 1834
IATA Scholarships, 1835
Musculoskeletal Rehabilitation Fellowships, 2229
U.S. Lacrosse EAD Grants, 3453

Sri Lanka
Fulbright Traditional Scholar Program in the South and Central Asia Region, 1576

State Government
CDC Core Capacity Grants, 907
Lynde and Harry Bradley Fndn Grants, 2089
Lynde and Harry Bradley Fndn Prizes: Bradley Prizes, 2090
NIEHS Applied Toxicological Research and Testing Grants, 2595

Statistics
Canada Graduate Scholarships and NSERC Postgraduate Scholarships, 845
NEI Clinical Vision Research Development Award, 2293
NHGRI Mentored Research Scientist Development Award, 2315
NIAID Statistical Methods in HIV and AIDS Research Grants, 2464
NIGMS Predoctoral Training in Bioinformatics and Computation Biology Grants, 2625
NIGMS Short Courses on Mathematical and Statistical Tools for the Study of Complex Phenotypes and Complex Systems, 2628
NIGMS Short Courses on Mathematical, Statistical, and Computational Tools for Studying Biological Systems, 2629
NIH Genetic Susceptibility and Variability of Human Malformations Research Grants, 2669
NIH Mechanisms Underlying Individual Variations in Drug Responses, 2685
NIMH Core Support Program for Mental Health/AIDS Research Grants, 2753
NIMH Short Courses on Mathematical and Statistical Tools for the Study of Complex Phenotypes and Complex Systems, 2770
RCPSC Royal College Fellowship for Studies in Medical Education, 3127
UK Fndn for the Study of Infant Deaths Grants, 3459

Stem Cell Transplantation
Michael J. Fox Fndn Parkinson's Cell Line Research Grants, 2192
NCRR Novel Approaches to Enhance Animal Stem Cell Research, 2288
NHLBI Career Enhancement Awards for Stem Cell Research, 2325
NIDDK Intestinal Stem Cell Consortium Grants, 2564
NIH Hyperaccelerated Award/Mechanisms in Immunomodulation Trials, 2675

Storytelling
Ruth Mott Fndn Grants, 3204

Strategic Planning
Humboldt Area Fndn Technical Assistance Program Grants, 1819

Stress
NHLBI Stress Management Interventions to Reduce Risk of Coronary Artery Disease, 2384
NIA Aging, Oxidative Stress and Cell Death Grants, 2393
NIA Mechanisms Underlying the Links between Psychosocial Stress, Aging, the Brain and the Body Grants, 2414

Stroke
Goddess Scholars Grants, 1630
National Emergency Medicine Association Grants, 2252
National Heart Fndn of New Zealand Grants, 2255
NIA Symptom Management for Chronic Neurological Conditions Research Grants, 2436
NICHD Symptom Management for Chronic Neurological Conditions Research Grants, 2496
NIDCD Symptom Management for Chronic Neurological Conditions Research Grants, 2532
NIH Research on Sleep and Sleep Disorders, 2713
NINDS Support of Scientific Meetings as Cooperative Agreements, 2786
NINDS Symptom Management for Chronic Neurological Conditions Research Grants, 2787
NINR Clinical Interventions for Managing the Symptoms of Stroke Research Grants, 2793
NINR Symptom Management for Chronic Neurological Conditions Research Grants, 2805
Premera CARES Grants, 3074
Stroke Association Allied Health Professional Research Bursaries, 3385
Stroke Association Clinical Fellowships, 3386
Stroke Association Research Project Grants, 3387

Substance Abuse
Children's Trust Fund of Oregon Grants, 1001
Gamble Fndn Grants, 1582
Hearst Fndn and William Randolph Hearst Fndn Grants, 1730
Hoblitzelle Fndn Grants, 1783
Steelcase Fndn Grants, 3379

Sudden Infant Death Syndrome
CJ Fndn for SIDS Express Grants, 1016
CJ Fndn for SIDS Support Services Grants, 1017
Dr. Sydney Segal Research Grants, 1331
MDBD Research Grants and Basil O'Connor Starter Scholar Award Program, 2153
UK Fndn for the Study of Infant Deaths Grants, 3459

Suicide
AACAP Klingenstein Third Generation Fndn Award for Research in Depression or Suicide, 42
American Fndn for Suicide Prevention Grants, 436
Metrowest Comm Health Care Fndn Grants, 2176
NARSAD Distinguished Investigator Award, 2246
NARSAD Independent Investigator Award, 2247
SAMHSA Campus Suicide Prevention Grants, 3244

Suicide Prevention
AACAP Klingenstein Third Generation Fndn Award for Research in Depression or Suicide, 42
American Fndn for Suicide Prevention Grants, 436
CDC Suicide Prevention Research Center, 930
Florida BRAIVE Fund of Dade Comm Fndn, 1512
Florida BRAIVE Fund of Gulf Coast Comm Fndn of Venice, 1513
Florida BRAIVE Fund of The Comm Fndn in Jacksonville, 1514
Metrowest Comm Health Care Fndn Grants, 2176

Supportive Housing Programs
Charles H. Farnsworth Trust Grants, 967
Home Building Industry Disaster Relief Fund, 1787
SAG Motion Picture Players Welfare Fund Grants, 3238

Surgery
AAFPRS Bernstein Grant, 118
AAFPRS Fellowships, 119
AAFPRS Investigator Development Grant, 120
AAFPRS Ira J. Tresley Research Award, 121
AAFPRS John Orlando Roe Award, 122
AAFPRS Leslie Bernstein Resident Research Grants, 123
AAFPRS Residency Travel Awards, 124
AAFPRS Sir Harold Delf Gillies Award, 125
AANS Neurosurgery Research and Education Fndn Young Clinician Investigator Award, 142
AANS Neurosurgery Research and Education Fndn/Spine Section Young Clinician Investigator Award, 143
AAO-HNS Medical Student Research Prize, 144
AAO-HNS Resident Research Prizes, 145
AAO-HNSF CORE Research Grants, 146
AAO-HNSF Health Services Research Grants, 147
AAO-HNSF Maureen Hannley Research Training Awards, 148
AAO-HNSF Percy Memorial Research Award, 149
AAO-HNSF Rande H. Lazar Health Services Research Grant, 150
AAO-HNSF Resident Research Awards, 151
AAOA Fndn/AAO-HNSF Combined Research Grants, 152
AGS Dennis W. Jahnigen Career Development Scholars Awards, 264
AHAF Alzheimer's Disease Research Grants, 266
AHNS Alando J. Ballantyne Resident Research Pilot Grant, 305
AHNS Pilot Grant, 306
AHNS/AAO-HNSF Surgeon Scientist Combined Award, 307
AHNS/AAO-HNSF Young Investigator Combined Award, 308
American College of Surgeons and The Triological Society Clinical Scientist Development Awards, 422
American College of Surgeons Co-Sponsored K08/K23 NIH Supplement Awards, 424
American College of Surgeons Faculty Career Development Award for Neurological Surgeons, 425
American College of Surgeons Faculty Research Fellowships, 426
American College of Surgeons Health Policy Scholarships, 427
American College of Surgeons Health Policy Scholarships for General Surgeons, 428
American College of Surgeons International Guest Scholarships, 429
American College of Surgeons Nizar N. Oweida, MD, FACS, Scholarships, 430
American College of Surgeons Resident and Associate Society (RAS-ACS) Leadership Scholarships, 431
American College of Surgeons Resident Research Scholarships, 432

American College of Surgeons Wound Care Management Award, 433
American Philosophical Society Daland Fellowships in Clinical Investigation, 441
Carlos and Marguerite Mason Trust Grants, 875
Charles H. Hood Fndn Child Health Research Grants, 968
Clark Fndn Grants, 1029
Clowes ACS/AAST/NIGMS Jointly Sponsored Mentored Clinical Scientist Development Award, 1041
Denton A. Cooley Fndn Grants, 1225
E.L. Wiegand Fndn Grants, 1361
EF Behavioral Sciences Student Fellowships, 1379
Fellowships in Infectious Diseases, 1485
International College of Surgeons Grants and Scholarships, 1859
Mark and Catherine Winkler Fndn Grants, 2112
NIH Urinary Incontinence Treatment Network, 2738
NYAM Charles A. Elsberg Fellowship, 2910
OREF Orthopedic Career Development Awards, 2954
OREF Orthopedic Resident Research Awards, 2955
OREF Research Grants, 2957
Pfizer Fndn Grants, 3025
RCPSC Canadian Research Awards for Specialty Residents (Medicine, Surgery), 3113
RCPSC Detweiler Traveling Fellowships, 3114
RCPSC Janes Visiting Professorship in Surgery, 3120
RCPSC McLaughlin-Gallie Visiting Professorship, 3123
RCPSC Royal College Medal Award in Surgery, 3129
RCPSC Walter C. MacKenzie Fellowship in Surgery, 3133
Richmond Eye and Ear Fund Grants, 3164
Triological Society Research Career Development Awards, 3440
United Cerebral Palsy Research Grants, 3462
Xoran Technologies Resident Research Grant, 3554

Sustainable Development
American Jewish World Service Grants, 437
Boeing Company Contributions Grants, 777
Charlotte County (FL) Comm Fndn Grants, 973
Clarence E. Heller Charitable Fndn Grants, 1022
CLIF Bar Family Fndn Grants, 1040
Jessie Smith Noyes Fndn Grants, 1920
Pulte Homes Corp Contributions, 3092
Rockefeller Brothers Fund Peace and Security Grants, 3179
Shaw's Supermarkets Donations, 3280

Sweden
FIC Swedish Medical Research Council Fellowships, 1495

Symposiums
FDHN Non-Career Research Awards, 1476

Systems Theory
LSA Translational Research Grants, 2078
RSC Thomas W. Eadie Medal, 3199

Taiwan
Medical/Nursing Education, Research, and Health Care Exchanges with Taiwan, 2165

Tajikistan
Fulbright Traditional Scholar Program in the South and Central Asia Region, 1576

Taste
NIA Research Grants on Chemical Senses: Neurotransmitters and Neuromodulators, 2430
NIDCD Clinical Trial Planning Grant, 2517
NIDCD Exploratory Research: Feasibility Pilot Studies Grants, 2519
NIDCD Exploratory/Developmental Research Grants, 2520
NIDCD Minority Dissertation Research Grants in Human Communication, 2524
NIDCD Program for Postdoctoral Research Training in Clinical Trials, 2528
NIDCD Research Grants on Chemical Senses: Neurotransmitters and Neuromodulators, 2530
NIDCD Small Grants, 2531

Taxonomy, Animal
NSF Systematic Biology and Biodiversity Inventories Grants, 2895

Taxonomy, Plant
NSF Systematic Biology and Biodiversity Inventories Grants, 2895

Teacher Certification
DaimlerChrysler Corp Fund Grants, 1186
MfA Newton Fellowships, 2182

Teacher Education
Abell-Hanger Fndn Grants, 183
AMD Corp Contributions Grants, 411
ASHA Advancing Academic-Research Careers Award, 569
Benton County Fndn Grants, 744
Carnegie Corp of New York Grants, 879
Chiron Fndn Comm Grants, 1004
Clarence E. Heller Charitable Fndn Grants, 1022
Claude Worthington Benedum Fndn Grants, 1033
Doreen Kronick Scholarship, 1312
Fritz B. Burns Fndn Grants, 1564
GenCorp Fndn Grants, 1587
Houston Endowment Grants, 1797
Indiana Minority Teacher/Special Services Scholarships, 1852
Jewish Women's Fndn of New York Grants, 1924
Johnson & Johnson Corp Contributions Grants, 1952
Joseph H. and Florence A. Roblee Fndn Grants, 1961
Marion Park Deaver and Harry Gilbert Deaver Fndn Grants, 2110
Meadows Fndn Grants, 2161
MfA Newton Fellowships, 2182
Moses Cone-Wesley Long Comm Health Fndn Grants, 2219
Ohio Learning Network Grants, 2940
Procter and Gamble Fund Grants, 3083
Progress Energy Fndn Grants, 3084
Union County Comm Fndn Grants, 3461

Teacher Education, Inservice
Benton County Fndn Grants, 744
Bill and Melinda Gates Fndn Grants, 756
Coca-Cola Fndn Grants, 1052
eBay Fndn Comm Grants, 1363
Flinn Fndn Grants Programs, 1511

Technological Change
James S. McDonnell Fndn Complex Systems Collaborative Activity Awards, 1897

Technology
Alfred P. Sloan Fndn History of Science and Technology Grants, 352
ArvinMeritor Grants, 544
AT&T Excelerator, 657
AT&T Fndn Civic and Comm Service Grants, 658
Award for Creative Advances in Environmental Science and Technology, 676
Award in Separations Science and Technology, 677
Barberton Comm Fndn Grants, 693
Bill and Melinda Gates Fndn Grants, 756
Comm Fndn for Southeastern Michigan Grants, 1094
Comm Fndn of Broward Grants, 1100
Comm Fndn of Crawford County Grants and Scholarships, 1103
Comm Technology Fndn of California Building Communities Through Technology Grants, 1136
Crail-Johnson Fndn Grants, 1157
Dell Fndn Healthy Communities, Literate Communities, and Connected Communities Grants, 1217
DOE Health Effects and Life Sciences Research Grants, 1298
Dolan Fndn Grants, 1306
EDS Fndn Grants, 1371
Ford Motor Company Fund Grants, 1522
Fndn for Science and Disability Grant Program for Physically Disabled Students in the Sciences, 1532
Frist Fndn Grants, 1563
i2 Fndn Grants, 1829
Indiana 21st Century Research and Technology Fund Awards, 1850
Innovative Technology Development Awards, 1855
Jessie Ball Dupont Fund Grants, 1919
Jim Moran Fndn Grants, 1925
John R. Oishei Fndn Grants, 1944
Leonsis Fndn Grants, 2045
Lindbergh Grants, 2059
Lowell Berry Fndn Grants, 2069
MAPFRE Fndn for Medicine Grants, 2102
Matsumae International Fndn Grants, 2129
Meadows Fndn Grants, 2161
Mericos Fndn Grants, 2172
Meyer Memorial Trust Emergency Grants, 2178
Meyer Memorial Trust Grassroots Grants, 2179
Meyer Memorial Trust Responsive Grants, 2181
Miguel Aleman Fndn Grants, 2197
Monfort Family Fndn Grants, 2213
National Dairy Promotion and Research Board Scholarships, 2251
NHGRI Mentored Research Scientist Development Award, 2315
NIAID Small Business Innovation Research Advanced Technology Grants, 2463
NIEHS SBIR E-Learning for HAZMAT and Emergency Response Grants, 2604
NIH Enhancing Adherence to Diabetes Self-Management Behaviors, 2659
NIH Human Brain Project Phase I & II, 2672
NIH Recovery Act Limited Competition: Academic Research Enhancement Awards, 2707
NIH Recovery Act Limited Competition: Biomedical Research, Development, and Growth to Spur the Acceleration of New Technologies (BRDG-SPAN) Pilot Grants, 2708
NIH Recovery Act Limited Competition: Small Business Catalyst Awards for Accelerating Innovative Research Grants, 2710
NIH Recovery Act Limited Competition: Supporting New Faculty Recruitment to Enhance Research Resources through Biomedical Research Core Centers Grants, 2711
NIH Technologies to Improve the Utility of Animal Models Research Grants, 2735
NIMH Silvio O. Conte Centers for Neuroscience Research Grants, 2771
NLM Informatics Conference Grants, 2819
North Carolina Biotechnology Center Technology Enhancement Grants, 2856
NSF Small Business Innovation Research Grants, 2893
Ohio Learning Network Grants, 2940
Pittsburgh Fndn Comm Fund Grants, 3054
Puerto Rico Comm Fndn Grants, 3090
Rajiv Gandhi Fndn Grants, 3104
Rayonier Fndn Grants, 3111
Rockefeller Fndn Grants, 3181
Rockwell International Corp Trust Grants, 3183
San Diego Women's Fndn Grants, 3259
Scientific Communities Initiative Grants, 3272
Tellabs Fndn Grants, 3418
Verizon Fndn Maryland Grants, 3487
Verizon Fndn New York Grants, 3488
Verizon Fndn Northeast Region Grants, 3489
Verizon Fndn Pennsylvania Grants, 3490
Verizon Fndn Vermont Grants, 3491
Verizon Fndn Virginia Grants, 3492
Waitt Family Fndn Grants, 3512

Technology Education
American Electric Power Grants, 434
ArvinMeritor Grants, 544

AT&T Excelerator, 657
Boeing Company Contributions Grants, 777
Charles Edison Fund Grants, 964
Charles Lafitte Fndn Grants, 970
Chicago Board of Trade Fndn Grants, 988
Comm Technology Fndn of California Building Communities Through Technology Grants, 1136
Kenny's Kids Grants, 1990
Medtronic Fndn Health Care Grants, 2169
Microsoft Research Cell Phone as a Platform for Healthcare Grants, 2195
Northrop Grumman Corp Grants, 2866
Ohio Learning Network Grants, 2940
Olin Corp Charitable Trust Grants, 2943
Oracle Corp Contributions Grants, 2951
Procter and Gamble Fund Grants, 3083
RGK Fndn Grants, 3153
Verizon Fndn Maryland Grants, 3487
Verizon Fndn New York Grants, 3488
Verizon Fndn Northeast Region Grants, 3489
Verizon Fndn Pennsylvania Grants, 3490
Verizon Fndn Vermont Grants, 3491
Verizon Fndn Virginia Grants, 3492
Wayne and Gladys Valley Fndn Grants, 3522

Technology Planning/Policy
Gill Fndn - Gay and Lesbian Fund Grants, 1613

Technology Transfer
Boeing Company Contributions Grants, 777
CDC Technology Translation and Transfer of Effective HIV Behavioral Interventions, 931
Indiana 21st Century Research and Technology Fund Awards, 1850
International Cancer Technology Transfer Fellowships, 1858
NCI Academic-Industrial Partnerships for Development and Validation of In Vivo Imaging Systems and Methods for Cancer Investigations, 2268
NHLBI Bioengineering Approaches to Energy Balance and Obesity Grants for STTR, 2320
U.S. Department of Education Rehabilitation Engineering Research Centers Grants, 3447

Teen Pregnancy
African American Fund of New Jersey Grants, 260
California Wellness Fndn Work and Health Grants, 834
Comm Fndn of Western North Carolina Grants, 1132
DHHS Adolescent Family Life Demonstration Projects, 1243
Fisa Fndn Grants, 1506
Health Fndn of Greater Indianapolis Grants, 1725
Joseph Drown Fndn Grants, 1960
Moses Cone-Wesley Long Comm Health Fndn Grants, 2219
Northern Trust Company Charitable Trust and Corp Giving Program, 2865
Philadelphia Fndn Organizational Effectiveness Grants, 3029
Prince Charitable Trusts Chicago Grants, 3079
Thompson Charitable Fndn Grants, 3425

Telecommunications
DHHS Rural Telemedicine Grants, 1279
DOA Distance Learning and Telemedicine Grant Program, 1288

Telemedicine
DOA Distance Learning and Telemedicine Grant Program, 1288

Television
American Academy of Nursing Media Awards, 418
CDC Cooperative Agreement for the Development, Operation, and Evaluation of an Entertainment Education Program, 906

Teratology
CIIT Postdoctoral Fellowships, 1012

Terminally Ill
Columbus Fndn Estrich Fund Grants, 1067

Terrorism
Harry Kramer Memorial Fund Grants, 1705
NIAID Preparedness against Illegitimate Use of Bacterial Pathogens, 2461

Thailand
OSI Access to Essential Medicines Grants, 2964

Theater
Bildner Family Fndn Grants, 755
Idaho Power Company Corp Contributions, 1838
Ruth Mott Fndn Grants, 3204

Theology
AHFMR Population Health Investigator Awards, 292
Atherton Family Fndn Grants, 659
Boettcher Fndn Grants, 778
Booth-Bricker Fund Grants, 780
E. Rhodes and Leona B. Carpenter Fndn Grants, 1356
FirstEnergy Fndn Comm Grants, 1505
Hedco Fndn Grants, 1733
John I. Smith Charities Grants, 1935
Rainbow Fund Grants, 3103

Therapy Evaluation
Baltimore Washington Center Adult Psychoanalysis Fellowships, 685
Baltimore Washington Center Child Psychotherapy Fellowships, 686
Boston Psychoanalytic Society and Institute Fellowship in Child Psychoanalytic Psychotherapy, 786
Boston Psychoanalytic Society and Institute Fellowship in Psychoanalytic Psychotherapy, 787
Chicago Institute for Psychoanalysis Fellowships, 990
Michigan Psychoanalytic Institute and Society SATA Grants, 2193
Michigan Psychoanalytic Institute and Society Scholarships, 2194
NHLBI Airway Smooth Muscle Function and Targeted Therapeutics in Human Asthma Grants, 2316
NICHD Innovative Therapies and Clinical Studies for Screenable Disorders Grants, 2485

Therapy/Rehabilitation
ASHFndn New Century Scholars Program Doctoral Scholarships, 580
ASHFndn New Century Scholars Research Grant, 581
ASHFndn Research Grant for New Investigators, 582
ASHFndn Student Research Grants in Audiology, 584

Thoracic Medicine
AGS Dennis W. Jahnigen Career Development Scholars Awards, 264

Tissue
NIA Role of Nuclear Receptors in Tissue and Organismal Aging Grants, 2432

Tissue Culture
Ethical Research Grants and Fellowships, 1431
NSF Biomedical Engineering and Engineering Healthcare Grants, 2879

Tobacco
American Legacy Fndn National Calls for Proposals Grants, 438
American Legacy Fndn Small Innovative Grants, 439
APPEAL Social Justice and Tobacco Control Grants, 513
BCBS of Minnesota Healthy Together Grants, 712
CDC Oral Diseases Prevention and Oral Health Promotion Grants, 921
Christine O. Gregoire Youth/Young Adult Award for Outstanding Use of Tobacco Industry Documents, 1005
Comm Fndn for Southeastern Michigan Grants, 1094
CTCRI Idea Grants, 1170
Health Fndn of Greater Indianapolis Grants, 1725
Hillsdale County Comm Fndn Healthy Senior/Healthy Youth Fund Grants, 1776
Mass Youth Against Tobacco Mini-Grants, 2123
NCI/NIDA Transdisciplinary Tobacco Use Research Centers Grants, 2280
NIDA Drug Abuse Dissertation Research: Epidemiology, Prevention, Treatment, Services, and Women and Gender Differences, 2502
NIDA Neurobiological and Behavioral Research on Nicotine and Tobacco Products, 2511
NIH Mechanisms Underlying Individual Variations in Drug Responses, 2685
Sybil G. Jacobs Award for Outstanding Use of Tobacco Industry Documents, 3414
Thrasher Research Fund Grants, 3426
TRDRP California Research Awards, 3434
TRDRP Exploratory/Developmental Research Awards, 3435

Tourette Syndrome
NIH Genetics of Neurobehavioral Disorders in Existing Samples Grants, 2670
Tourette Syndrome Association Post-Doc Fellowships, 3432
Tourette Syndrome Association Research Grants, 3433
TSA Research Grant Awards, 3442

Tourism
Principal Financial Group Fndn Grants, 3082

Toxic Substances
Beldon Fund Grants, 738
Bullitt Fndn Grants, 809
Clarence E. Heller Charitable Fndn Grants, 1022

Toxicology
ASM sanofi-aventis ICAAC Award, 616
Canada Graduate Scholarships and NSERC Postgraduate Scholarships, 845
Center for Alternatives to Animal Testing Grants, 934
CIIT Postdoctoral Fellowships, 1012
DHHS Health Conference Support Program for Toxic Substances and Disease Registry, 1255
DHHS Neurodevelopmental Test Methods Research Grants, 1268
DHHS Priority Health Conditions Studies Initiative, 1273
FIC International Training and Research in Environmental and Occupational Health, 1493
NIEHS Applied Toxicological Research and Testing Grants, 2595
NIEHS Small Business Innovation Research Grants, 2605
ORISE Postgraduate Research Participation at the Agency for Toxic Substances and Disease Registry, 2960
ORISE Postgraduate Research Participation at the National Center for Toxicological Research, 2961
PhRMA Fndn Health Outcomes Post Doctoral Fellowships, 3031
PhRMA Fndn Health Outcomes Research Starter Grants, 3033
PhRMA Fndn Informatics Post Doctoral Fellowships, 3036
PhRMA Fndn Pharmacology/Toxicology Post Doctoral Fellowships, 3044
PhRMA Fndn Pharmacology/Toxicology Pre Doctoral Fellowships, 3045
PhRMA Fndn Pharmacology/Toxicology Research Starter Grants, 3046
PhRMA Fndn Pharmacology/Toxicology Sabbatical Fellowships, 3047

Training and Development
Able Trust Vocational Rehabilitation Grants for Individuals, 186
Alberto Culver Corp Contributions Grants, 329
Boeing Company Contributions Grants, 777
Burden Trust Grants, 810
CDC Hepatitis Education for Inmates and Correctional Staff Grants, 911
CDC National Training Information and Exchange Program, 920
CDC Promoting Prevention in Managed Care Cooperative Agreements, 925
Clarian Health Critical / Progressive Care Internships, 1023
Clarian Health Multi-Specialty Internships, 1024
Clarian Health OR Internships, 1025
Cruise Industry Charitable Fndn Grants, 1166
DHHS Maternal and Child Health Research and Training Programs Grants, 1264
DHHS Technical and Non-Financial Assistance to Health Centers, 1280
DOL Occupational Safety and Health—Susan Harwood Training Grants, 1305
FIC International Research and Training in Population and Health Grants, 1489
FIC International Training and Research in Emerging Infectious Diseases Grants, 1492
Fndn for Spirituality and Medicine Grants, 1534
Good Samaritan Fndn Inc Grants, 1636
Greater Milwaukee Fndn Grants, 1653
Hartford Aging and Health Program Awards, 1709
HRSA Geriatric Education Centers, 1805
IHS Native American and Alaskan Native Health Research Centers, 1840
Jacob and Hilda Blaustein Fndn Grants, 1881
Joyce Fndn Grants, 1969
MAP International Medical Fellowships, 2101
Medtronic Fndn Full Life Patient Partnership Program—Heart Rescue Grants, 2168
National Patient Safety Fndn Patient Safety Research Grants, 2258
NEI Ruth L. Kirschstein National Research Service Award Short-Term Institutional Research Training Grants, 2297
NIDA Behavioral Therapies Development Grants, 2499
NIDCD Mentored Research Scientist Development Award, 2523
NIMH Career Opportunities in Research Education and Training Honors High School Research Education Grant, 2748
NNEDVF/Altria Doors of Hope Program, 2847
Prudential Fndn Grants, 3087
Raskob Fndn for Catholic Activities Grants, 3107
Regenstrief Geriatrics Fellowship, 3143
RRF General Grants, 3193
Saint Luke's Health Initiatives Grants, 3240
Scott County Comm Fndn Grants, 3273
South Madison Comm Fndn Grants, 3349
U.S. Department of Education Rehabilitation Research Training Centers, 3448
VDH Emergency Medical Services Training Fund, 3483

Transfusion Medicine
National Blood Fndn Research Grant Program, 2249
NHLBI Blood Diseases and Resources Research Grants, 2322
NHLBI Immunomodulatory, Inflammatory, and Vasoregulatory Properties of Transfused Red Blood Cell Units as a Function of Preparation and Storage Grants, 2337
NHLBI Mentored Career Award For Faculty At Minority Institutions, 2346

Translation
NCI Application of Metabolomics for Translational and Biological Research Grants, 2270

Transplantation Immunology
National Blood Fndn Research Grants, 2249
NIH Nonhuman Primate Immune Tolerance Cooperative Study Group Grants, 2699

Transportation
Able To Serve Grants, 185
Barberton Comm Fndn Grants, 693
Bullitt Fndn Grants, 809
CNCS Foster Grandparent Projects Grants, 1048
Comm Fndn of Greater Birmingham Grants, 1106
Fallon OrNda Comm Health Fund Grants, 1449
Farmers Insurance Group of Companies Grants, 1455
Foellinger Fndn Grants, 1519
Giving in Action Society Children & Youth with Special Needs Grants, 1617
Giving in Action Society Family Independence Grants, 1618
Helen Steiner Rice Fndn Grants, 1742
Joyce Fndn Grants, 1969
Rochester Area Comm Fndn Grants, 3176
Samuel Freeman Charitable Trust Grants, 3249
US Airways Comm Contributions, 3472

Trauma
CDC Injury Prevention and Control Research and State and Comm Based Programs, 914
CDC National Training Information and Exchange Program, 920
Comm Fndn for Southeastern Michigan Grants, 1094
HRSA Emergency Medical Services for Children Grants, 1804
National Emergency Medicine Association Grants, 2252
NIGMS Fellowships in Quantitative Biology, 2610
NIGMS Mentored Clinical Scientist Research Career Development Awards, 2618
Quantum Fndn Grants, 3096

Travel
AAAAI Allergy, Asthma and Immunology Education and Research Trust Allied Health Travel Grants, 21
AACAP Educational Outreach Program for Child and Adolescent Psychiatry Residents, 33
AACAP Educational Outreach Program for General Psychiatry Residents, 34
AACAP Systems of Care Special Program Scholarships, 54
AACR Brigid G. Leventhal Scholar in Cancer Research Awards, 69
AACR Minority Scholar in Cancer Research Awards, 82
AACR Scholar-in-Training Awards, 87
AACR Scholar-in-Training Awards - Special Conferences, 88
AACR Thomas J. Bardos Science Education Awards, 90
AACR-GlaxoSmithKline Clinical Cancer Research Scholar Awards, 98
AACR-NCI International Investigator Opportunity Grants, 101
AACR-WICR Scholar Awards, 105
AAP International Travel Grants, 162
AAP Program Delegate Awards, 166
AcademyHealth Alice S. Hersh Student Scholarships, 191
AcademyHealth Awards, 192
AHFMR Comm Support Grants, 271
AIHP Sonnedecker Visiting Scholar Grants, 317
AMA Fndn Jordan Fieldman, MD, Awards, 393
AMA Fndn Leadership Awards, 394
AMA Fndn Pride in the Profession Grants, 397
AMA Virtual Mentor Theme Issue Editor Grants, 400
AMA-MSS Research Poster Award, 405
AMA-WPC Joan F. Giambalvo Memorial Scholarships, 408
American College of Rheumatology Fellows-in-Training Travel Scholarships, 421
American College of Surgeons Australia and New Zealand Chapter Travelling Fellowships, 423
American College of Surgeons Nizar N. Oweida, MD, FACS, Scholarships, 430
American Psychiatric Association Travel Scholarships for Minority Medical Students, 449
ASCO Merit Awards, 558
ASCO Resident Travel Awards, 559
ASM Corp Activities Program Student Travel Grants, 591
ASM Early-Career Faculty Travel Award, 593
ASM Faculty Ehancement Program -Travel Awards, 595
ASM Founders Distinguished Service Award, 596
ASM General Meeting Minority Travel Grants, 598
ASM GlaxoSmithKline International Member of the Year Award, 599
ASM Richard and Mary Finkelstein Travel Grant, 613
ASM Roche Diagnostics Alice C. Evans Award, 615
ASM Student and Post Doctoral Fellow Travel Grants, 619
ASM Student Travel Grants, 620
ASM TREK Diagnostic ABMM/ABMLI Professional Recognition Award, 621
ASM Undergraduate Research Fellowship, 622
ASMCUE/GM Travel Assistance Grants, 628
ASPET Travel Awards, 648
FDHN Moti L. & Kamla Rustgi International Travel Awards, 1475
FDHN Non-Career Research Awards, 1476
Fndn of CVPH Travel Fund Grants, 1543
Jane Beattie Memorial Scholarship, 1901
Komen Greater NYC Small Grants, 2013
MAP International Medical Fellowships, 2101
Mead Johnson Nutritionals Scholarships, 2159
NAPNAP Fndn McNeil Grant-in-Aid, 2238
NAPNAP Fndn Reckitt Benckiser Student Scholarship, 2242
Northwest Airlines KidCares Medical Travel Assistance, 2868
Pinellas County Grants, 3050
Sigrid Juselius Fndn Grants, 3286
SOBP International Travel Fellowships, 3314
SOBP Travel Fellowships, 3315
SRC Medical Research Grants, 3362
St. Joseph Comm Health Fndn Schneider Fellowships, 3370
UICC International Cancer Technology Transfer (ICRETT) Fellowships, 3456
UICC Raisa Gorbachev Memorial International Cancer Fellowships, 3457

Tropical Medicine
NFID Colin L. Powell Minority Postdoctoral Fellowship in Tropical Disease Research, 2308
NFID New Investigator Matching Grants, 2310
Sir Halley Stewart Trust Grants, 3293

Tuberculosis
Alliance Healthcare Fndn Grants, 362
FIC/NIH AIDS International Training and Research Program, 1496
Heiser Leprosy and Tuberculosis Research Postdoctoral Fellowships, 1736
Heiser Leprosy Research Grants, 1737
NFID New Investigator Matching Grants, 2310
NIAID Challenge Grants: Joint Ventures in Biomedicine and Biotechnology, 2451
NIDA International Studies on Drug Abuse and HIV/AIDS, 2505
NYCT Biomedical Research Grants, 2920
Potts Memorial Fndn Grants, 3072

Tumor Immunology
Children's Brain Tumor Fndn Research Grants, 993
CRI Postdoctoral Fellowships, 1162
NIH Molecular Epidemiology of Prostate Carcinogenesis Grants, 2691

Undergraduate Education
AAHPERD Ruth Abernathy Presidential Scholarships, 128
Flinn Fndn Grants Programs, 1511
HHMI Grants and Fellowships Programs, 1759

NBME Stemmler Medical Education Research Fund Grants, 2263
NHLBI Research Supplements to Promote Diversity in Health-Related Research for Undergraduate Students, 2377
NIMH Career Opportunities in Research Education and Training Honors Undergraduate Research Training Grant, 2749
North Carolina GlaxoSmithKline Fndn Grants, 2860
NSF Undergraduate Research and Mentoring in the Biological Sciences, 2896
RWJF Summer Medical and Dental Education Program, 3231
U.S. Department of Education Erma Byrd Scholarships, 3446

University/Industry Cooperative Activities
American Chemical Society GCI Pharmaceutical Roundtable Research Grants, 420
Bank of America Charitable Fndn Anchor Institutions Grants, 688
Innovative Technology Development Awards, 1855
NSF Grant Opportunities for Academic Liaison with Industry, 2887

Urban Affairs
Audrey and Sydney Irmas Charitable Fndn Grants, 665
Charles H. Revson Fndn Grants, 969
Columbus Fndn Competitive Grants, 1066
Comm Fndn for Muskegon County Grants, 1093
Comm Fndn of Champaign County Grants, 1102
Comm Fndn of St. Joseph County Special Project Challenge Grants, 1126
Howard and Bush Fndn Grants, 1798
Nordson Corp Fndn Grants, 2851
Pittsburgh Fndn Comm Fund Grants, 3054
Prudential Fndn Grants, 3087
US Trust Corp Fndn Grants, 3475

Urban Areas
Bodman Fndn Grants, 776
CDC Program to Prevent Smoking Among Urban Youth, 924
Commonwealth Fund Harkness Fellowships in Health Care Policy and Practice, 1079
Comm Toolbox for Children's Environmental Health Grants, 1137
CUNA Mutual Group Fndn, 1174
E.L. Wiegand Fndn Grants, 1361
Elmer L. and Eleanor J. Andersen Fndn Grants, 1406
Hasbro Children's Fund, 1714
Hudson Webber Fndn Grants, 1813
Irvin Stern Fndn Grants, 1866
Joyce Fndn Grants, 1969
Lynde and Harry Bradley Fndn Grants, 2089
Lynde and Harry Bradley Fndn Prizes: Bradley Prizes, 2090
Rajiv Gandhi Fndn Grants, 3104
Richard King Mellon Fndn Grants, 3161
Walt Disney Company Fndn Grants, 3516
William G. McGowan Charitable Fund Grants, 3539

Urban Education
Carnegie Corp of New York Grants, 879
Frances and John L. Loeb Family Fund Grants, 1546
Joyce Fndn Grants, 1969
U.S. Department of Education 21st Century Comm Learning Centers, 3445

Urban Planning/Policy
Air Products and Chemicals Grants, 319
Canada-U.S. Fulbright New Century Scholars Grants, 846
Canada-U.S. Fulbright Senior Specialists Grants, 847
Comm Fndn for Muskegon County Grants, 1093
FMC Fndn Grants, 1518
Fulbright Alumni Initiatives Awards Grants, 1566
Fulbright Distinguished Chairs Grants, 1567
Fulbright New Century Scholars Grants, 1570
Fulbright Specialists Grants, 1571
Fulbright Traditional Scholar Program in Europe and Eurasia, 1572
Fulbright Traditional Scholar Program in Sub-Saharan Africa, 1573
Fulbright Traditional Scholar Program in the East Asia/Pacific Region, 1574
Fulbright Traditional Scholar Program in the Near East and North Africa Region, 1575
Fulbright Traditional Scholar Program in the South and Central Asia Region, 1576
Fulbright Traditional Scholar Program in the Western Hemisphere, 1577

Urinary Tract
NIDDK Basic Research Grants in the Bladder and Lower Urinary Tract, 2543

Urogenital System
NIDDK Cell-Specific Delineation of Prostate and Genitourinary Development, 2545
NIH Urinary Incontinence Treatment Network, 2738

Urological Tract Disease
NIDDK Development of Disease Biomarkers Grants, 2549
NIDDK Education Grants, 2554

Urology
AGS Dennis W. Jahnigen Career Development Scholars Awards, 264
C.R. Bard Fndn Grants, 825
June Allyson Fndn Research Fellowships, 1972
KFC Allied Health Research Grants, 1996
KFC Biomedical Fellowships, 1997
KFC Biomedical Research Grants, 1998
KFC Nephrology and Urology Scholarships, 1999
NIDDK Basic and Clinical Studies of Congenital Urinary Tract Obstruction Grants, 2542
NIDDK Non-Invasive Methods for Diagnosis and Progression of Diabetes, Kidney, Urological, Hematological and Digestive Diseases, 2572
NIDDK Pilot and Feasibility Clinical Research Grants in Kidney or Urologic Diseases, 2575
NIDDK Proteomics: Diabetes, Obesity, And Endocrine, Digestive, Kidney, Urologic, And Hematologic Diseases, 2578
NIDDK Small Grants for Underrepresented Minority Scientists in Diabetes and Digestive and Kidney Diseases, 2588
NIDDK Training in Clinical Investigation in Kidney and Urology Grants, 2590
NIH Urinary Incontinence Treatment Network, 2738
NKF Research Fellowships, 2812
NKF Young Investigator Grants, 2813
NYAM Edwin Beer Research Fellowship, 2913
NYAM Ferdinand C. Valentine Fellowship, 2914

Utilities
Actors Fund Social Services and Financial Assistance, 225
Alexander Fndn Cancer, Catastrophic Illness and Injury Grants, 342
Barberton Comm Fndn Grants, 693
Children Affected by AIDS Fndn Family Assistance Emergency Fund Grants, 996
Presbyterian Patient Assistance Program, 3076

Uzbekistan
Fulbright Traditional Scholar Program in the South and Central Asia Region, 1576

Vaccines
Alternatives Research and Development Fndn Alternatives in Education Grants, 370
Alternatives Research and Development Fndn Grants, 371
ASM Maurice Hilleman/Merck Award, 605
CDC Epidemiology and Laboratory Capacity Infectious Diseases Grants, 909
Chiron Fndn Comm Grants, 1004
DOI Biological Resource Division Brucellosis Program, 1302
Elizabeth Glaser Pediatric AIDS Fndn International Leadership Awards, 1393
Elizabeth Glaser Pediatric AIDS Fndn Operations Research Grants, 1394
Elizabeth Glaser Pediatric AIDS Fndn Pediatric HIV Vaccine Research Grants, 1395
Elizabeth Glaser Pediatric AIDS Fndn Two-Year International Scholar Award, 1396
Gates Global HIV/AIDS Vaccine Grants, 1583
NFID Advanced Vaccinology Course Travel Grant, 2307
NIAID Challenge Grants: Joint Ventures in Biomedicine and Biotechnology, 2451
NIAID Enhancing Vaccine-Elicited Protective Immunity in Malaria Research Grants, 2452
NIAID HIV Prevention Trial Units Grants, 2453
NIAID HIV Vaccine Clinical Trial Units Grants, 2454
NIAID HIV Vaccine Research and Design—Program Project Grants, 2455
NIAID Integrated Preclinical/Clinical AIDS Vaccine Development Grants, 2457
NIAID Laboratory Methods to Assess Responses to HIV Vaccine Candidates Research Grants, 2458
NIH Small Business Innovation Research: Animal Models of HCV Infection Research Grants, 2728
Thrasher Research Fund Grants, 3426
Until There's a Cure Fndn Grants, 3471

Values/Moral Education
Cargill Citizenship Fund-Corp Giving Grants, 865
Institute of Human Values in Health Care Interdisciplinary Fellowships, 1857

Vegetables
DOA National Integrated Food Safety Initiative, 1289

Venereal Diseases
DHHS Adolescent Family Life Demonstration Projects, 1243

Vestibular System
NIDCD Clinical Trial Planning Grant, 2517
NIDCD Exploratory Research: Feasibility Pilot Studies Grants, 2519
NIDCD Exploratory/Developmental Research Grants, 2520
NIDCD Minority Dissertation Research Grants in Human Communication, 2524
NIDCD Molecular and Cellular Pathology of the Human Auditory and Vestibular Systems Grants, 2525
NIDCD Program for Postdoctoral Research Training in Clinical Trials, 2528
NIDCD Small Grants, 2531

Veterans
Balfe Family Fndn Grants, 682
Charles Delmar Fndn Grants, 963
CNCS Engaging Persons with Disabilities in National and Comm Service Grants, 1047
Disable American Veterans Charitable Grants, 1286
Military Ex-Prisoners of War Fndn Grants, 2201

Veterinary Medicine
ACVIM Fndn Clinical Investigation Grants, 227
Bodman Fndn Grants, 776
DHHS Health Careers Opportunity Grants, 1253
Jackson Laboratory Postdoctoral Research Training Program, 1880
Max Bell Fndn Grants, 2134
MHRC Postdoctoral Research Fellowships, 2187
NIGMS/NIDCR Evolution of Infectious Diseases Research Grants, 2633
NIH Midcareer Investigator Award in Mouse Pathobiology Research Grants, 2690
Posey Comm Fndn Grants, 3068

Veterinary Medicine Education
HRSA Health Professions Scholarships for Disadvantaged Students, 1807
NHLBI Short-Term Research Education Program to Increase Diversity in Health-Related Research, 2383
PAHO/WHO Fellowships, 2984
Pet Care Trust Sue Busch Memorial Award, 3017

Violence
Ahmanson Fndn Grants, 303
Chicago Comm Trust Grants, 989
Joyce Fndn Grants, 1969
Pajaro Valley Comm Health Grants, 2985
Waitt Family Fndn Grants, 3512

Violence in Schools
49ers Fndn Grants, 12
DHHS Maternal and Child Health Research and Training Programs Grants, 1264
DOJ Gang-Free Schools and Communities Intervention Grants, 1303
FAR Fund, 1453
Pajaro Valley Comm Health Grants, 2985

Violence Prevention
AMA Fndn Fund for Better Health Grants, 388
Pajaro Valley Comm Health Grants, 2985

Violent Behavior
49ers Fndn Grants, 12
Alliance Healthcare Fndn Grants, 362
Allstate Corp Giving Grants, 363
Allstate Corp Hometown Commitment Grants, 364
California Endowment CommunitiesFirst Grants, 833
California Wellness Fndn Work & Health Grants, 834
Carlisle Fndn Grants, 874
CDC Injury Prevention and Control Research and State and Comm Based Programs, 914
Chicago Comm Trust Grants, 989
FAR Fund, 1453
Greater Tacoma Comm Fndn Ryan Alan Hade Endowment Fund, 1657
Harry Frank Guggenheim Fndn Research Grants, 1704
Hasbro Children's Fund, 1714
Ignacio Martin-Baro Fund for Mental Health and Human Rights Grants, 1839
Isabel Allende Fndn Esperanza Grants, 1868
Jewish Women's Fndn of New York Grants, 1924
Joseph Drown Fndn Grants, 1960
Joseph H. and Florence A. Roblee Fndn Grants, 1961
Joyce Fndn Grants, 1969
Lewis Preston Fund for Girls Education Grants, 2052
Meadows Fndn Grants, 2161
Ms. Fndn for Women Grants, 2222
Oakland Fund for Children and Youth Grants, 2930
Pajaro Valley Comm Health Grants, 2985
Quantum Fndn Grants, 3096
Richard and Rhoda Goldman Fund Grants, 3158
San Diego Fndn for Change Grants, 3255
Sisters of St. Joseph Healthcare Fndn Grants, 3297
Sonoco Fndn Grants, 3347
Women's Fndn of California Grants, 3550

Violent Crime
Allstate Corp Giving Grants, 363
Allstate Corp Hometown Commitment Grants, 364
FAR Fund, 1453
Plough Fndn Grants, 3061

Viral Studies
CDC Evaluation of the Use of Rapid Testing For Influenza in Outpatient Medical Settings, 910
NIAID Microbiology and Infectious Diseases Research Grants and Contracts, 2459

Virology
ASM/CCID Fellowships, 627
Bristol-Myers Squibb Fndn Global HIV/AIDS Initiative Grants, 796
Bristol-Myers Squibb Virology and Oncology M.D. Research Fellowships, 802
LRF New Investigator Leukemia Research Grants, 2070
NIAAA Hepatitis C Infection and Alcoholic Liver Disease, 2442
NICHD Central Nervous System Effects of HIV Infection: Neurobiological, Neurovirological, and Neurobehavioral Studies Grants, 2482
NIDCR HIV/AIDS Associated Oral Viral Infections, 2535
NIH Impact of HAART on HIV/CNS Disease, 2676
NIH Multidisciplinary Approach for Research on Oral Complications of HIV Infection, 2694
NIH Small Business Innovation Research: Animal Models of HCV Infection Research Grants, 2728
NINDS Central Nervous System Effects of HIV Infection: Neurobiological, Neurovirological, and Neurobehavioral Studies Grants, 2777
NSF Genes and Genome Systems Cluster Grants, 2886

Vision
1st Touch Fndn Grants, 6
Alcon Fndn Grants, 336
Alfred W. Bressler Prize in Vision Science, 354
Andersen Fndn Grants, 471
Canadian Optometric Education Trust Fund Grants, 853
Dr. Stanley Pearle Scholarships, 1330
Fight for Sight Research Grants and Fellowships, 1503
Fndn Fighting Blindness Marjorie Carr Adams Women's Career Development Awards, 1526
Hawaii Comm Fndn Health Education and Research Grants, 1716
NEI Mentored Clinical Scientist Development Program Award (K12), 2295
NEI Scholars Program, 2298
NEI Translational Research Program On Therapy For Visual Disorders, 2299
NEI Vision Research Core Grants, 2300
Nina Mason Pulliam Charitable Trust Grants, 2776
NYCT Blindness and Visual Disabilities Grants, 2921
OneSight Research Fndn Block Grants, 2944

Visual Arts
Amgen Fndn Grants, 467
Booth-Bricker Fund Grants, 780
Chestnut Hill Charitable Fndn, Inc Grants, 987
Colorado Springs Comm Trust Fund Grants, 1061
ConocoPhillips Fndn Grants, 1144
DAAD Research Stays for University Academics and Scientists, 1183
Delta Air Lines Fndn Grants, 1220
Flinn Fndn Grants Programs, 1511
General Mills Fndn Grants, 1590
George S. and Dolores Dore Eccles Fndn Grants, 1602
Georgia Power Fndn Grants, 1603
Grand Rapids Area Comm Fndn Grants, 1645
Grand Rapids Area Comm Fndn Nashwauk Area Endowment Fund Grants, 1646
James M. Cox Fndn of Georgia Grants, 1892
Kelvin and Eleanor Smith Fndn Grants, 1986
King Pharmaceuticals Corp Contributions Grants, 2003
Kraft Cares International Grants, 2016
Margaret L. Wendt Fndn Grants, 2104
PacifiCorp Fndn for Learning Grants, 2982
Paul G. Allen Family Fndn Grants, 3000
Piedmont Natural Gas Grants, 3048
Powell Fndn Grants, 3073
Procter and Gamble Fund Grants, 3083
Sid W. Richardson Fndn Grants, 3284
Society for the Arts in Healthcare Consulting Grants, 3326
Winifred & Harry B. Allen Fndn Grants, 3543

Visual Impairments
AHAF National Glaucoma Research Grants, 268
Alfred W. Bressler Prize in Vision Science, 354
Armstrong McDonald Fndn Grants, 537
Atran Fndn Grants, 663
Bushrod H. Campbell and Adah F. Hall Charity Fund Grants, 816
Carl W. and Carrie Mae Joslyn Trust Grants, 873
Charles Delmar Fndn Grants, 963
Chicago Board of Trade Fndn Grants, 988
Comm Fndn of Grant County Scholarships, 1105
Cornerstone Fndn of Northeastern Wisconsin Grants, 1152
Donald and Sylvia Robinson Family Fndn Grants, 1310
Dr. Stanley Pearle Scholarships, 1330
E.A. Baker Fndn for the Prevention of Blindness Grants, 1357
Fight for Sight Research Grants and Fellowships, 1503
Fndn Fighting Blindness Marjorie Carr Adams Women's Career Development Awards, 1526
Hagedorn Fund Grants, 1685
J. Walton Bissell Fndn Grants, 1872
John W. Alden Trust Grants, 1947
Josiah W. and Bessie H. Kline Fndn Grants, 1967
Lavelle Fund for the Blind Grants, 2033
Lettie Pate Whitehead Fndn Grants, 2049
Mabel H. Flory Charitable Trust Grants, 2096
Marjorie C. Adams Charitable Trust Grants, 2111
May and Stanley Smith Trust Grants, 2137
NEI Clinical Vision Research Development Award, 2293
NEI Scholars Program, 2298
NEI Translational Research Program On Therapy For Visual Disorders, 2299
Nina Mason Pulliam Charitable Trust Grants, 2776
NYCT Blindness and Visual Disabilities Grants, 2921
OneSight Research Fndn Block Grants, 2944
Pfizer Fndn Grants, 3025
Philadelphia Fndn Organizational Effectiveness Grants, 3029
Reader's Digest Partners for Sight Fndn Grants, 3137
S. Mark Taper Fndn Grants, 3236
Starr Fndn Grants, 3377
U.S. Department of Education Rehabilitation Training—Rehabilitation Continuing Education Programs—Institute on Rehabilitation Issues, 3449
Union County Comm Fndn Grants, 3461

Vocational Counseling
Achelis and Bodman Fndns Grants, 206
DHHS Adolescent Family Life Demonstration Projects, 1243
Graco Fndn Grants, 1642

Vocational/Technical Education
Besser Fndn Grants, 752
Burlington Industries Fndn Grants, 811
Cass County Comm Fndn Grants, 887
Clay Fndn Grants, 1034
Constantin Fndn Grants, 1145
Cooper Industries Fndn Grants, 1150
Crail-Johnson Fndn Grants, 1157
D.F. Halton Fndn Grants, 1181
DaimlerChrysler Corp Fund Grants, 1186
Duke Energy Fndn Grants, 1339
FirstEnergy Fndn Comm Grants, 1505
Frances L. and Edwin L. Cummings Memorial Fund Grants, 1547
Gamble Fndn Grants, 1582
Graco Fndn Grants, 1642
Heckscher Fndn for Children Grants, 1732
Irvin Stern Fndn Grants, 1866
Paul and Mary Haas Fndn Contributions and Student Scholarships, 2997
Principal Financial Group Fndn Grants, 3082
Richard King Mellon Fndn Grants, 3161
Samuel S. Johnson Fndn Grants, 3251
Seabury Fndn Grants, 3274
U.S. Department of Education Rehabilitation Research Training Centers, 3448
United Technologies Corp Grants, 3466
Wal-Mart State Giving Grants, 3514

Volunteerism
AIG American General Corp Grants, 316
Compass Bank Fndn Grants, 1138
McCombs Fndn Grants, 2142

Volunteers
ACE Charitable Fndn Grants, 199
Agway Fndn Grants, 265
AMA Fndn Jack B. McConnell, MD Awards for Excellence in Volunteerism, 391
Ann Arbor Area Comm Fndn Grants, 476
Anschutz Family Fndn Grants, 486
ASM Founders Distinguished Service Award, 596
BCBS of Minnesota Healthy Together Grants, 712
Benton Comm Fndn Grants, 743
Blackford County Comm Fndn Grants, 763
Blue River Comm Fndn Grants, 770
Bodman Fndn Grants, 776
Brown County Comm Fndn Grants, 807
Cambridge Comm Fndn Grants, 837
CharityWorks Grants, 961
Charles G. Koch Charitable Fndn Grants, 965
CNCS Foster Grandparent Projects Grants, 1048
CNCS Next Generation Grants, 1049
Colorado Interstate Gas Grants, 1060
Comerica Charitable Fndn Grants, 1073
Comm Fndn for Southeastern Michigan Grants, 1094
Comm Fndn of Bartholomew County Heritage Fund Grants, 1096
Comm Fndn of Bartholomew County James A. Henderson Award for Fund-Raising, 1097
Comm Fndn of Boone County Grants, 1099
Comm Fndn of Greater Fort Wayne: Comm Endowment & Clarke Endowment Fund Grants, 1108
Comm Fndn of Greenville Comm Enrichment Grants, 1113
Cooper Industries Fndn Grants, 1150
Coors Brewing Corp Contributions Grants, 1151
Dell Fndn Open Grants, 1218
eBay Fndn Comm Grants, 1363
Express Scripts Fndn Grants, 1441
Fargo-Moorhead Area Fndn Grants, 1454
Fidelity Fndn Grants, 1498
G.N. Wilcox Trust Grants, 1581
Giant Eagle Fndn Grants, 1611
Great-West Life Grants, 1649
Gulf Coast Comm of Venice Fndn Grants, 1677
Harden Fndn Grants, 1693
Helen Steiner Rice Fndn Grants, 1742
Hormel Foods Charitable Trust Grants, 1795
J.C. Penney Company Grants, 1874
Jessie Ball Dupont Fund Grants, 1919
John Ben Snow Memorial Trust Grants, 1928
Johns Manville Fund Grants, 1950
Lillian S. Wells Fndn Grants, 2056
Lockheed Martin Philanthropic Grants, 2062
MONY Fndn Grants, 2215
Nordson Corp Fndn Grants, 2851
North Carolina GlaxoSmithKline Fndn Grants, 2860
Olin Corp Charitable Trust Grants, 2943
Portland General Electric Fndn Grants, 3067
Princeton Area Comm Fndn Greater Mercer Grants, 3081
Procter and Gamble Fund Grants, 3083
Prudential Fndn Grants, 3087
Rayonier Fndn Grants, 3111
Rhode Island Fndn Grants, 3154
Rohm and Haas Company Grants, 3185
Sisters of Mercy of North Carolina Fndn Grants, 3295
Sisters of Saint Joseph Charitable Fund Grants, 3296
Taproot Fndn Capacity-Building Service Grants, 3417
Triangle Comm Fndn Donor-Advised Grants, 3437
Union Benevolent Association Grants, 3460
W.K. Kellogg Fndn Healthy Kids Grants, 3507
YSA UnitedHealth Heroes Service Learning Grants, 3556

Voter Educational Programs
Farmers Insurance Group of Companies Grants, 1455

Waste Management/Fossil Energy
Lindbergh Grants, 2059
Rohm and Haas Company Grants, 3185

Water Pollution
Beldon Fund Grants, 738
Heineman Fndn for Research, Education, Charitable and Scientific Purposes, 1735
Joyce Fndn Grants, 1969
Rohm and Haas Company Grants, 3185
San Diego Fndn for Change Grants, 3255
Takemi Program in International Health Research and Advanced Training Fellowships, 3416

Water Resources
1675 Fndn Grants, 4
Beldon Fund Grants, 738
Bella Vista Fndn Grants, 740
Bullitt Fndn Grants, 809
Carolyn Fndn Grants, 880
Comm Fndn for Muskegon County Grants, 1093
Gebbie Fndn Grants, 1585
Greater Milwaukee Fndn Grants, 1653
Pioneer Hi-Bred Comm Grants, 3051
Progress Energy Fndn Grants, 3084
Thompson Charitable Fndn Grants, 3425
W.K. Kellogg Fndn Healthy Kids Grants, 3507

Water Resources, Environmental Impacts
Bella Vista Fndn Grants, 740

Water Resources, Management/Planning
Lindbergh Grants, 2059

Water Supply
Land O'Lakes Fndn Mid-Atlantic Grants, 2027
Thrasher Research Fund Grants, 3426

Water Treatment
NIEHS Carcinogenicity of Drinking Water Disinfection By-Products, 2597

Weapons
AAAS Science & Technology Policy Fellowships - National Defense & Global Security, 29

Welding
DOL Occupational Safety and Health—Susan Harwood Training Grants, 1305

Welfare Reform
Public Welfare Fndn Grants, 3089

Welfare-to-Work Programs
Benton County Fndn Grants, 744
Cessna Fndn Grants, 938
D. W. McMillan Fndn Grants, 1180
Joyce Fndn Grants, 1969
Prudential Fndn Grants, 3087
Verizon Fndn Maryland Grants, 3487
Verizon Fndn New York Grants, 3488
Verizon Fndn Northeast Region Grants, 3489
Verizon Fndn Pennsylvania Grants, 3490
Verizon Fndn Vermont Grants, 3491
Verizon Fndn Virginia Grants, 3492

Wellness
Hillsdale County Comm General Adult Fndn Grants, 1777
Samueli Institute Scientific Research Grants, 3253

Wetlands
Bella Vista Fndn Grants, 740

Wildlife
Banfi Vintners Fndn Grants, 687
Batchelor Fndn Grants, 701
Bullitt Fndn Grants, 809
Cambridge Comm Fndn Grants, 837
Chicago Board of Trade Fndn Grants, 988
Chicago White Metal Charitable Fndn Grants, 992
Collins Fndn Grants, 1058
Comm Fndn of Greater Tampa Grants, 1112
Cruise Industry Charitable Fndn Grants, 1166
DOI Biological Resource Division Brucellosis Program, 1302
Donald and Sylvia Robinson Family Fndn Grants, 1310
ExxonMobil Grants, 1442
George and Ruth Bradford Fndn Grants, 1595
Gulf Coast Comm of Venice Fndn Grants, 1677
J.M. Long Fndn Grants, 1877
James Ford Bell Fndn Grants, 1885
James M. Cox Fndn of Georgia Grants, 1892
James S. Copley Fndn Grants, 1895
Knox County Comm Fndn Grants, 2009
Lawrence Fndn Grants, 2034
Lindbergh Grants, 2059
M. Bastian Family Fndn Grants, 2092
Mars Fndn Grants, 2114
Meyer Memorial Trust Emergency Grants, 2178
Meyer Memorial Trust Grassroots Grants, 2179
Meyer Memorial Trust Responsive Grants, 2181
Newman's Own Inc Grants, 2306
Nina Mason Pulliam Charitable Trust Grants, 2776
Olin Corp Charitable Trust Grants, 2943
Oracle Corp Contributions Grants, 2951
Perkins Charitable Fndn Grants, 3014
Perry County Comm Fndn Grants, 3016
Pike County Comm Fndn Grants, 3049
Posey Comm Fndn Grants, 3068
Richard King Mellon Fndn Grants, 3161
Spencer County Comm Fndn Grants, 3358
Susan Mott Webb Charitable Trust Grants, 3412
Trull Fndn Grants, 3441
Vanderburgh Comm Fndn Grants, 3480
Warrick County Comm Fndn Grants, 3519
Winifred & Harry B. Allen Fndn Grants, 3543

Wine and Grape Industry
Society of Medical Friends of Wine Research Award, 3344

Women
A Fund for Women Grants, 14
AACR-WICR Scholar Awards, 105
ACE Charitable Fndn Grants, 199
AEC Trust Grants, 242
Alberto Culver Corp Contributions Grants, 329
Alfred P. Sloan Fndn Research Fellowships, 353
Allstate Corp Giving Grants, 363
Allstate Corp Hometown Commitment Grants, 364
AMA Fndn Joan F. Giambalvo Memorial Scholarships, 392
AMA-WPC Joan F. Giambalvo Memorial Scholarships, 408
American Jewish World Service Grants, 437
American Legacy Fndn National Calls for Proposals Grants, 438
Archer Daniels Midland Fndn Grants, 525
Arkell Hall Fndn Grants, 534
Armstrong McDonald Fndn Grants, 537
Arthur and Rochelle Belfer Fndn Grants, 542
ASM Roche Diagnostics Alice C. Evans Award, 615
Atran Fndn Grants, 663
Avon Products Fndn Grants, 675
Bodenwein Public Benevolent Fndn Grants, 775
Boston Fndn Grants, 783
Boston Jewish Comm Women's Fund Grants, 785
Cambridge Comm Fndn Grants, 837
Carnegie Corp of New York Grants, 879
Carrie E. and Lena V. Glenn Fndn Grants, 882
Catherine Holmes Wilkins Fndn Grants, 889
Charles Delmar Fndn Grants, 963
CNA Fndn Grants, 1046
Commission on Religion in Appalachia Grants, 1074
Comm Fndn of Crawford County Grants and Scholarships, 1103
ConocoPhillips Fndn Grants, 1144
Cowles Charitable Trust Grants, 1155
Daisy Marquis Jones Fndn Grants, 1188

Dallas Women's Fndn Grants, 1191
Daphne Seybolt Culpeper Memorial Fndn Grants, 1201
Dennis and Phyllis Washington Fndn Grants, 1222
Eckerd Corp Fndn Grants, 1366
EF Making a Difference Award, 1381
Elisabeth Severance Prentiss Fndn Grants, 1392
ExxonMobil Grants, 1442
Fisa Fndn Grants, 1506
Fndn for the Carolinas Grants, 1535
Fourjay Fndn Grants, 1544
General Service Fndn Reproductive Health and Rights Grants, 1592
George Family Fndn Grants, 1598
Georgia Power Fndn Grants, 1603
Goddess Scholars Grants, 1630
Greater Worcester Comm Fndn Discretionary Grants, 1658
H.J. Heinz Company Fndn Grants, 1682
Health Canada National Seniors Independence Grants, 1722
Health Fndn of Greater Indianapolis Grants, 1725
Heineman Fndn for Research, Education, Charitable and Scientific Purposes, 1735
Helen Steiner Rice Fndn Grants, 1742
Helena Rubinstein Fndn Grants, 1743
Henrietta Tower Wurts Memorial Fndn Grants, 1745
Isabel Allende Fndn Esperanza Grants, 1868
IWMF Public Health Fellowship, 1871
James A. and Faith Knight Fndn Grants, 1884
James Ford Bell Fndn Grants, 1885
James R. Dougherty Jr. Fndn Grants, 1894
Jane Bradley Pettit Fndn Grants, 1902
Jean and Louis Dreyfus Fndn Grants, 1911
Jeanne Humphrey Block Dissertation Award, 1912
Jewish Women's Fndn of New York Grants, 1924
Joseph H. and Florence A. Roblee Fndn Grants, 1961
Josephine Goodyear Fndn Grants, 1964
Josephine S. Gumbiner Fndn Grants, 1965
Katharine Matthies Fndn Grants, 1982
Kosciusko County Comm Fndn Grants, 2015
Laura B. Vogler Fndn Grants, 2032
Lewis Preston Fund for Girls Education Grants, 2052
Long Island Comm Fndn Grants, 2063
Lotus 88 Fndn for Women and Children Grants, 2064
Lowell Berry Fndn Grants, 2069
Mary Baker Eddy Library Summer Research Fellowships, 2117
Mary Ingraham Bunting Institute Biomedical Research Fellowships, 2119
Mary Kay Ash Charitable Fndn Grants, 2120
Metro Health Fndn Grants, 2175
Ms. Fndn for Women Grants, 2222
Ms. Fndn Women and AIDS Fund Grants, 2223
National City Corp Contributions Grants, 2250
NIAID Therapeutics Research on AIDS-Associated Opportunistic Infections, 2465
NIDA Drug Abuse Dissertation Research: Epidemiology, Prevention, Treatment, Services, and Women and Gender Differences, 2502
NIGMS Mentored Clinical Scientist Research Career Development Awards, 2618
Nina Mason Pulliam Charitable Trust Grants, 2776
NMF Mary Ball Carrera Scholarship, 2834
North Carolina Comm Fndn Grants, 2859
NYCT Girls and Young Women Grants, 2924
Olin Corp Charitable Trust Grants, 2943
Peacock Fndn Grants, 3011
Perpetual Trust for Charitable Giving Grants, 3015
Posey Comm Fndn Womens Fund Grants, 3069
Pott Fndn Grants, 3071
Rajiv Gandhi Fndn Grants, 3104
Rayonier Fndn Grants, 3111
Rochester Area Comm Fndn Grants, 3176
S. Mark Taper Fndn Grants, 3236
San Diego Fndn for Change Grants, 3255
Simmons Fndn Grants, 3287
Sisters of Mercy of North Carolina Fndn Grants, 3295
Southwest Gas Corp Fndn Grants, 3352
Stark Comm Fndn Women's Fund Grants, 3376
Strowd Roses Grants, 3388
Vulcan Materials Company Fndn Grants, 3504
Weingart Fndn Grants, 3524
WHO Fndn General Grants, 3534
Wilson-Wood Fndn Grants, 3542
Women's Fndn of California Comm Action Fund, 3549
Women's Fndn of California Grants, 3550
Women's Sports Fndn Grants, 3551
WWNFF Dissertation Grants in Women's Health, 3553
Z. Smith Reynolds Fndn Small Grants, 3557

Women's Education
A Fund for Women Grants, 14
Alcatel-Lucent Technologies Corp Contributions Grants, 332
AMA Fndn Joan F. Giambalvo Memorial Scholarships, 392
Avon Products Fndn Grants, 675
Boston Jewish Comm Women's Fund Grants, 785
Heineman Fndn for Research, Education, Charitable and Scientific Purposes, 1735
James A. and Faith Knight Fndn Grants, 1884
Jeanne Humphrey Block Dissertation Award, 1912
Jewish Fndn for Education of Women Scholarships for Emigres in the Health Professions, 1922
Jewish Women's Fndn of New York Grants, 1924
Lettie Pate Whitehead Fndn Grants, 2049
Ms. Fndn for Women Grants, 2222
Posey Comm Fndn Womens Fund Grants, 3069
RGK Fndn Grants, 3153
Stark Comm Fndn Women's Fund Grants, 3376
WHO Fndn General Grants, 3534
Women of the ELCA Opportunity Scholarships for Lutheran Laywomen, 3548
Women's Sports Fndn Grants, 3551

Women's Employment
Anschutz Family Fndn Grants, 486
Avon Products Fndn Grants, 675
Comm Fndn of Greater Flint Grants, 1107
Lewis Preston Fund for Girls Education Grants, 2052
Ms. Fndn for Women Grants, 2222
Pasadena Fndn Average Grants, 2994
Posey Comm Fndn Womens Fund Grants, 3069
Stark Comm Fndn Women's Fund Grants, 3376

Women's Health
A Fund for Women Grants, 14
Alliance Healthcare Fndn Grants, 362
American Legacy Fndn National Calls for Proposals Grants, 438
Avon Fndn Breast Care Fund Grants, 674
Avon Products Fndn Grants, 675
Bill and Melinda Gates Fndn Grants, 756
Blanche and Irving Laurie Fndn Grants, 764
Boston Jewish Comm Women's Fund Grants, 785
Breast Cancer Fund Grants, 790
Bristol-Myers Squibb Fndn Women's Health Grants, 800
California Endowment CommunitiesFirst Grants, 833
California Wellness Fndn Work and Health Grants, 834
CDC Increasing Breast and Cervical Cancer Screening Services for Urban American Indian/Alaska Native Women, 912
CF Clinical Research Trainee Awards, 940
DHHS HIV Demonstration Program for Children, Adolescents, and Women, 1262
DHHS Maternal and Child Health Research and Training Programs Grants, 1264
Duke University Obstetric Anesthesia Fellowships, 1345
Fannie E. Rippel Fndn Grants, 1452
Fisa Fndn Grants, 1506
Fndn for Seacoast Health Grants, 1533
Goddess Scholars Grants, 1630
James A. and Faith Knight Fndn Grants, 1884
Jewish Women's Fndn of New York Grants, 1924
Johnson & Johnson Comm Health Care Grants, 1951
Kate B. Reynolds Charitable Trust Health Care Grants, 1981
Lesbian Health Fund Grants, 2046
Lewis Preston Fund for Girls Education Grants, 2052
Lillian S. Wells Fndn Grants, 2056
Lowe Fndn Grants, 2067
Mary Kay Ash Charitable Fndn Grants, 2120
Ms. Fndn for Women Grants, 2222
Ms. Fndn Women and AIDS Fund Grants, 2223
NCI Stages of Breast Development: Normal to Metastatic Disease Grants, 2278
NCIC Canadian Breast Cancer Research Initiative Grants, 2281
NIAAA Hepatitis C Infection and Alcoholic Liver Disease, 2442
NIDA National Drug Abuse Treatment Clinical Trials Network, 2510
NIH Building Interdisciplinary Research Careers in Women's Health Grants, 2644
NIH New Directions in Pain Research Grants, 2698
NIH Transitional Career Development Award in Women's Health Research, 2736
NIH Urinary Incontinence Treatment Network, 2738
NINR Aging Women and Breast Cancer Grants, 2789
Posey Comm Fndn Womens Fund Grants, 3069
Pride Fndn Grants and Scholarships, 3078
Stark Comm Fndn Women's Fund Grants, 3376
STTI Rosemary Berkel Crisp Research Awards, 3394
Susan G. Komen Breast Cancer Fndn Basic, Clinical, and Translational Research Grants, 3407
Susan G. Komen Breast Cancer Fndn Interdisciplinary Fellowships, 3410
Susan G. Komen Breast Cancer Fndn Postdoctoral Fellowships, 3411
WHO Fndn General Grants, 3534
Women's Sports Fndn Grants, 3551
WWNFF Dissertation Grants in Women's Health, 3553

Women's Rights
Lewis Preston Fund for Girls Education Grants, 2052

Women's Studies
AMA-WPC Joan F. Giambalvo Memorial Scholarships, 408
Gruber Fndn International Prizes, 1672
Jeanne Humphrey Block Dissertation Award, 1912
Stark Comm Fndn Women's Fund Grants, 3376

Workforce Development
Boeing Company Contributions Grants, 777
Comm Fndn for Southeastern Michigan Grants, 1094
Harry S. Black and Allon Fuller Fund, 1706
Key Fndn Grants, 1994
King Pharmaceuticals Corp Contributions Grants, 2003
NWHF Partners Investing in Nursing's Future Grants, 2908

Workshops
Pfizer/AAFP Fndn Visiting Professorship Program in Family Medicine, 3027

Wound Healing
IAFF Burn Fndn Research Grants, 1830
Plastic Surgery Educational Fndn Basic Research Grants, 3058

Writing/Composition Education
Baptist Comm Ministries Grants, 691
Emily Davie and Joseph S. Kornfeld Fndn Grants, 1414
Houston Endowment Grants, 1797
Kalamazoo Fndn Grants, 1979

Youth and Education
Henry & Ruth Blaustein Rosenberg Fndn Grants, 1746

Youth Programs
3M Fndn Grants, 11
Aaron Fndn (Massachusetts) Grants, 174

Abell-Hanger Fndn Grants, 183
Acushnet Fndn Grants, 226
Adaptec Fndn Grants, 232
Adelaide Breed Bayrd Fndn Grants, 234
Adolph Coors Fndn Grants, 238
African American Fund of New Jersey Grants, 260
Agway Fndn Grants, 265
Ahmanson Fndn Grants, 303
Aladdin Industries Fndn Grants, 322
Albert Pick Jr. Fund Grants, 328
Alberto Culver Corp Contributions Grants, 329
Albertson's Charitable Giving Grants, 330
Alcatel-Lucent Technologies Fndn Grants, 333
Alice Tweed Tuohy Fndn Grants, 357
Allegan County Comm Fndn Grants, 358
Alliance Healthcare Fndn Grants, 362
Allyn Fndn Grants, 365
Andersen Corp Fndn, 470
Ann and Robert H. Lurie Family Fndn Grants, 475
Ann Arbor Area Comm Fndn Grants, 476
Annenberg Fndn Grants, 479
Anschutz Family Fndn Grants, 486
Anthony R. Abraham Fndn Grants, 490
Archer Daniels Midland Fndn Grants, 525
Arizona Diamondbacks Charities Grants, 530
Arkansas Comm Fndn Arkansas Black Hall of Fame Grants, 532
Arkema Fndn Science Teachers Program, 535
Armstrong McDonald Fndn Grants, 537
AT&T Fndn Civic and Comm Service Grants, 658
Atkinson Fndn International Grants, 661
Atlanta Fndn Grants, 662
Autzen Fndn Grants, 672
Bacon Family Fndn Grants, 679
Bailey Fndn Grants, 680
Barker Welfare Fndn Grants, 695
Batchelor Fndn Grants, 701
Beazley Fndn Grants, 730
Beirne Carter Fndn Grants, 737
Belk Fndn Grants, 739
Ben B. Cheney Fndn Grants, 741
Bender Fndn Grants, 742
Benton Comm Fndn Grants, 743
Benton County Fndn Grants, 744
Berks County Comm Fndn Grants, 745
Berrien Comm Fndn Grants, 749
Birds Eye Foods Fndn Grants, 759
Birmingham Fndn Grants, 760
Blackford County Comm Fndn Grants, 763
Blanche and Julian Robertson Family Fndn Grants, 765
Blue River Comm Fndn Grants, 770
Blumenthal Fndn Grants, 773
Bodenwein Public Benevolent Fndn Grants, 775
Bodman Fndn Grants, 776
Boston Fndn Grants, 783
Boston Globe Fndn Grants, 784
Brown County Comm Fndn Grants, 807
Bullitt Fndn Grants, 809
Burlington Industries Fndn Grants, 811
Bush Fndn Health & Human Services Grants, 814
C.R. Bard Fndn Grants, 825
Caddock Fndn Grants, 828
Callaway Golf Company Fndn Grants, 836
Camp-Younts Fndn Grants, 838
Cardinal Health Fndn Grants, 864
Cargill Citizenship Fund-Corp Giving Grants, 865
Carl and Eloise Pohlad Family Fndn Grants, 867
Carl and Lily Pforzheimer Fndn Grants, 868
Carl B. and Florence E. King Fndn Grants, 869
Carnahan-Jackson Fndn Grants, 878
Carnegie Corp of New York Grants, 879
Carrie E. and Lena V. Glenn Fndn Grants, 882
Carrier Corp Contributions Grants, 884
Carroll County Comm Fndn Grants, 885
CDC Program to Prevent Smoking Among Urban Youth, 924
Cessna Fndn Grants, 938
Champlin Fndns Grants, 960
Charles M. Bair Family Trust Grants, 972
Chestnut Hill Charitable Fndn, Inc Grants, 987
Chicago Tribune's Corp Contributions Grants, 991
Chicago White Metal Charitable Fndn Grants, 992
Christine O. Gregoire Youth/Young Adult Award for Outstanding Use of Tobacco Industry Documents, 1005
Cinergy Fndn Grants, 1013
Clarcor Fndn Grants, 1021
Clark Fndn Grants, 1029
Clark-Winchcole Fndn Grants, 1030
Clay Fndn Grants, 1034
CLIF Bar Family Fndn Grants, 1040
CNA Fndn Grants, 1046
CNCS Engaging Persons with Disabilities in National and Comm Service Grants, 1047
Coca-Cola Fndn Grants, 1052
Cockrell Fndn Grants, 1053
Collins C. Diboll Private Fndn Grants, 1057
Collins Fndn Grants, 1058
Colonel Stanley R. McNeil Fndn Grants, 1059
Colorado Interstate Gas Grants, 1060
Colorado Springs Comm Trust Fund Grants, 1061
Comm Fndn of Bartholomew County Heritage Fund Grants, 1096
Comm Fndn of Bartholomew County James A. Henderson Award for Fund-Raising, 1097
Comm Fndn of Boone County Grants, 1099
Comm Fndn of Champaign County Grants, 1102
Comm Fndn of Crawford County Grants and Scholarships, 1103
Comm Fndn of Grant County Grants, 1104
Comm Fndn of Greater Fort Wayne: Comm Endowment & Clarke Endowment Fund Grants, 1108
Comm Fndn of Greater Tampa Grants, 1112
Comm Fndn of Howard County Grants, 1116
Comm Fndn of Madison and Jefferson County Grants and Scholarships, 1117
Comm Fndn of Morgan County Grants and Scholarships, 1118
Comm Fndn of Mount Vernon and Knox County Grants, 1119
Comm Fndn of Randolph County Grants, 1121
Comm Fndn of Santa Cruz County Grants, 1122
Comm Fndn of Southeastern Connecticut Grants, 1125
Comm Fndn of St. Joseph County Special Project Challenge Grants, 1126
Comm Fndn of Switzerland County Grants, 1127
Comm Fndn of the Ozarks Grants, 1130
Comm Fndn Silicon Valley Grants, 1133
Comm Impact Fund, 1135
Connecticut Comm Fndn Grants, 1141
ConocoPhillips Fndn Grants, 1144
Constantin Fndn Grants, 1145
Cooke Fndn Grants, 1148
Cooper Industries Fndn Grants, 1150
Cornerstone Fndn of Northeastern Wisconsin Grants, 1152
Cowles Charitable Trust Grants, 1155
Cruise Industry Charitable Fndn Grants, 1166
Cudd Fndn Grants, 1171
D. W. McMillan Fndn Grants, 1180
D.F. Halton Fndn Grants, 1181
Dade Comm Fndn Grants, 1185
Dairy Queen Corp Contributions Grants, 1187
Dallas Women's Fndn Grants, 1191
Dana Brown Charitable Trust Grants, 1194
Dana Corp Fndn Grants, 1196
Daniels Fund Grants, 1200
Daphne Seybolt Culpeper Memorial Fndn Grants, 1201
Daywood Fndn Grants, 1206
Dearborn Comm Fndn City of Lawrenceburg Comm Grants, 1210
Delaware Comm Fndn-Youth Philanthropy Board for Kent County, 1216
Delta Air Lines Fndn Grants, 1220
Dennis and Phyllis Washington Fndn Grants, 1222
Denver Broncos Charities Fund Grants, 1226
DeRoy Testamentary Fndn Grants, 1239
Detroit Lions Charities Grants, 1241
Dickson Fndn Grants, 1284
Do Something BR!CK Awards, 1287
Dreitzer Fndn Grants, 1332
Dubois County Comm Fndn Grants, 1336
Dunspaugh-Dalton Fndn Grants, 1351
Eberly Fndn Grants, 1364
Edward S. Moore Fndn Grants, 1374
Edwin S. Webster Fndn Grants, 1376
Edwin W. and Catherine M. Davis Fndn Grants, 1377
EIF Comm Grants, 1386
Eisner Fndn Grants, 1387
El Paso Comm Fndn Grants, 1388
Elsie Lee Garthwaite Memorial Fndn Grants, 1408
Emerson Charitable Trust Grants, 1412
Ensworth Charitable Fndn Grants, 1416
Essex County Comm Fndn Discretionary Fund Grant, 1428
Evjue Fndn Grants, 1439
Ewing Halsell Fndn Grants, 1440
F.M. Kirby Fndn Grants, 1443
Fargo-Moorhead Area Fndn Grants, 1454
Farmers Insurance Group of Companies Grants, 1455
Fayette County Fndn Grants, 1457
FCNY Union Square Awards, 1461
Ferree Fndn Grants, 1486
Field Fndn of Illinois Grants, 1499
Fireman's Fund Fndn Grants, 1504
FirstEnergy Fndn Comm Grants, 1505
Foellinger Fndn Grants, 1519
Fondren Fndn Grants, 1520
Ford Motor Company Fund Grants, 1522
Fndn for the Carolinas Grants, 1535
Francis T. & Louise T. Nichols Fndn Grants, 1550
Frank G. and Freida K. Brotz Family Fndn Grants, 1552
Frank Stanley Beveridge Fndn Grants, 1553
Frist Fndn Grants, 1563
Fuller E. Callaway Fndn Grants, 1578
G.N. Wilcox Trust Grants, 1581
General Mills Champions for Healthy Kids Grants, 1589
George B. Storer Fndn Grants, 1596
Gertrude and William C. Wardlaw Fund Grants, 1607
Glazer Family Fndn Grants, 1625
Glendale Comm Fndn Grants, 1626
Godfrey Fndn Grants, 1631
Graco Fndn Grants, 1642
Grand Haven Area Comm Fndn Grants, 1644
Grand Rapids Comm Fndn Grants, 1647
Greater Milwaukee Fndn Grants, 1653
Greater Tacoma Comm Fndn Grants, 1656
Greater Tacoma Comm Fndn Ryan Alan Hade Endowment Fund, 1657
Greater Worcester Comm Fndn Discretionary Grants, 1658
Green Bay Packers Fndn Grants, 1660
Green Fndn Grants, 1661
Grotto Fndn Project Grants, 1671
H.J. Heinz Company Fndn Grants, 1682
Hancock County Comm Fndn Grants, 1690
Harden Fndn Grants, 1693
Harold and Arlene Schnitzer CARE Fndn Grants, 1697
Harold Simmons Fndn Grants, 1698
Harris and Eliza Kempner Fund Grants, 1699
Harry and Grace Steele Fndn Grants, 1702
Harry Bramhall Gilbert Charitable Trust Grants, 1703
Hartford Courant Fndn Grants, 1710
Hawaii Comm Fndn Reverend Takie Okumura Family Grants, 1717
HCA Fndn Grants, 1721
Healthcare Fndn for Orange County Grants, 1728
Hearst Fndn and William Randolph Hearst Fndn Grants, 1730
Hedco Fndn Grants, 1733
Helen K. and Arthur E. Johnson Fndn Grants, 1740
Helena Rubinstein Fndn Grants, 1743
Henrietta Tower Wurts Memorial Fndn Grants, 1745
Henry & Ruth Blaustein Rosenberg Fndn Grants, 1746
Hill Crest Fndn Grants, 1773

Hill Fndn Grants, 1774
Hillman Fndn Grants, 1775
Hilton Hotels Corp Giving Grants, 1780
Hoglund Fndn Grants, 1785
Holland/Zeeland Comm Fndn Grants, 1786
Honeywell Fndn Grants, 1791
Horace A. Kimball and S. Ella Kimball Fndn Grants, 1792
Howard and Bush Fndn Grants, 1798
Humana Fndn Grants, 1818
Hut Fndn Grants, 1827
Hutton Fndn Grants, 1828
i2 Fndn Grants, 1829
J. Walton Bissell Fndn Grants, 1872
J.M. Long Fndn Grants, 1877
J.W. Kieckhefer Fndn Grants, 1878
James Graham Brown Fndn Grants, 1887
James J. and Angelia M. Harris Fndn Grants, 1890
James S. Copley Fndn Grants, 1895
Janirve Fndn Grants, 1905
Jean and Louis Dreyfus Fndn Grants, 1911
JELD-WEN Fndn Grants, 1914
John Edward Fowler Memorial Fndn Grants, 1930
John G. Martin Fndn Grants, 1932
John H. and Wilhelmina D. Harland Charitable Fndn Grants, 1933
John Jewett and Helen Chandler Garland Fndn Grants, 1937
John W. and Anna H. Hanes Fndn Grants, 1948
John W. Anderson Fndn Grants, 1949
Joseph H. and Florence A. Roblee Fndn Grants, 1961
Josephine G. Russell Trust Grants, 1963
Josephine Goodyear Fndn Grants, 1964
Josiah W. and Bessie H. Kline Fndn Grants, 1967
Katharine Matthies Fndn Grants, 1982
Katherine John Murphy Fndn Grants, 1983
Kenneth T. and Eileen L. Norris Fndn Grants, 1989
King Pharmaceuticals Corp Contributions Grants, 2003
Knox County Comm Fndn Grants, 2009
Kosciusko County Comm Fndn Grants, 2015
L. W. Pierce Family Fndn Grants, 2019
LaGrange County Comm Fndn Grants, 2020
Land O'Lakes Fndn Mid-Atlantic Grants, 2027
Legacy Fndn Grants, 2040
Leo Goodwin Fndn Grants, 2043
Liberty Bank Fndn Grants, 2053
Lillian S. Wells Fndn Grants, 2056
Louis Calder Fndn Grants, 2065
Louis R. Cappelli Fndn Grants, 2066
Lowell Berry Fndn Grants, 2069
Lubrizol Fndn Grants, 2080
Lucile Horton Howe and Mitchell B. Howe Fndn Grants, 2081
Lucy Gooding Charitable Fndn Trust Grants, 2083
M.E. Raker Fndn Grants, 2094
M.J. Murdock Charitable Trust Grants, 2095
Mabel Y. Hughes Charitable Trust Grants, 2097
Maine Comm Fndn Grants, 2099
Margoes Fndn Grants, 2106
Marshall Field's Comm Grants, 2115
Mary Owen Borden Fndn Grants, 2121
Mary S. and David C. Corbin Fndn Grants, 2122
Matilda R. Wilson Fund Grants, 2128
Max and Victoria Dreyfus Fndn Grants, 2133
Maxon Charitable Fndn Grants, 2135
McCombs Fndn Grants, 2142
McGregor Fund Grants, 2143
McInerny Fndn Grants, 2144
McKesson Fndn Grants, 2145
McLean Contributionship Grants, 2147
McMillen Fndn Grants, 2148
Mead Witter Fndn Grants, 2160
Mericos Fndn Grants, 2172
Meriden Fndn Grants, 2173
Meyer Memorial Trust Emergency Grants, 2178
Meyer Memorial Trust Grassroots Grants, 2179
Meyer Memorial Trust Responsive Grants, 2181
Michael and Susan Dell Fndn Grants, 2189
Millipore Fndn Grants, 2203
Minneapolis Fndn Comm Grants, 2206
MONY Fndn Grants, 2215
New York Life Fndn Grants, 2304
Nicholas H. Noyes Jr. Memorial Fndn Grants, 2497
Noble County Comm Fndn Grants, 2848
North Carolina Comm Fndn Grants, 2859
Northrop Grumman Newport News Grants, 2867
Northwestern Mutual Fndn Grants, 2870
NYCT Girls and Young Women Grants, 2924
Oakland Fund for Children and Youth Grants, 2930
OceanFirst Fndn Grants, 2933
Oleonda Jameson Trust Grants, 2941
Olin Corp Charitable Trust Grants, 2943
Ordean Fndn Grants, 2952
PacifiCare Fndn Grants, 2981
PacifiCorp Fndn for Learning Grants, 2982
Partners for Youth with Disabilities Grants, 2990
Pasadena Fndn Average Grants, 2994
Paul G. Allen Family Fndn Grants, 3000
Peacock Fndn Grants, 3011
Perkins Charitable Fndn Grants, 3014
Perpetual Trust for Charitable Giving Grants, 3015
Perry County Comm Fndn Grants, 3016
PeyBack Fndn Grants, 3022
Piedmont Natural Gas Grants, 3048
Pike County Comm Fndn Grants, 3049
Piper Jaffray Companies Building Strong Communities Grants, 3053
Plough Fndn Grants, 3061
Plum Creek Fndn Grants, 3062
PMI Fndn Grants, 3063
Polk Bros. Fndn Grants, 3066
Posey Comm Fndn Grants, 3068
Posey Comm Fndn Womens Fund Grants, 3069
Pott Fndn Grants, 3071
Priddy Fndn Grants, 3077
Pride Fndn Grants and Scholarships, 3078
Prince Charitable Trusts District of Columbia Grants, 3080
Procter and Gamble Fund Grants, 3083
Prudential Fndn Grants, 3087
R.C. Baker Fndn Grants, 3098
Ralphs Food 4 Less Fndn Grants, 3106
Raskob Fndn for Catholic Activities Grants, 3107
Rhode Island Fndn Grants, 3154
Rice Fndn Grants, 3155
Rich Fndn Grants, 3156
Richard and Rhoda Goldman Fund Grants, 3158
Richard King Mellon Fndn Grants, 3161
Robert and Polly Dunn Fndn Grants, 3168
Robert B McMillen Fndn Grants, 3169
Robert E. and Evelyn McKee Fndn Grants, 3170
Rochester Area Fndn Grants, 3177
Rockwell Collins Charitable Contributions, 3182
Rockwell International Corp Trust Grants, 3183
Rohm and Haas Company Grants, 3185
Rollin M. Gerstacker Fndn Grants, 3186
Roy J. Carver Charitable Trust Medical and Science Research Grants, 3192
Rush County Comm Fndn Grants, 3200
Russell Berrie Fndn Grants, 3201
Ruth Eleanor Bamberger and John Ernest Bamberger Memorial Fndn Grants, 3202
S. Livingston Mather Charitable Trust Grants, 3235
Salisbury Comm Fndn Grants, 3243
SAMHSA Strategic Prevention Framework State Incentive Grants, 3248
Samuel S. Johnson Fndn Grants, 3251
San Diego Fndn for Change Grants, 3255
Schurz Communications Fndn Grants, 3271
Scott County Comm Fndn Grants, 3273
Seabury Fndn Grants, 3274
Self Fndn Grants, 3277
Seneca Foods Fndn Grants, 3278
Sid W. Richardson Fndn Grants, 3284
Snee Reinhardt Charitable Fndn Grants, 3300
Sonoco Fndn Grants, 3347
Southbury Comm Trust Fund, 3350
Southwest Gas Corp Fndn Grants, 3352
Spencer County Comm Fndn Grants, 3358
Strowd Roses Grants, 3388
Sunderland Fndn Grants, 3400
Susan Mott Webb Charitable Trust Grants, 3412
Thomas C. Ackerman Fndn Grants, 3423
Thomas M. and Irene B. Kirbo Charitable Trust Grants, 3424
Thompson Charitable Fndn Grants, 3425
Trull Fndn Grants, 3441
Union Benevolent Association Grants, 3460
Until There's a Cure Fndn Grants, 3471
US Trust Corp Fndn Grants, 3475
Vancouver Fndn Grants and Comm Initiatives Program, 3477
Vanderburgh Comm Fndn Grants, 3480
Vulcan Materials Company Fndn Grants, 3504
W.K. Kellogg Fndn Healthy Kids Grants, 3507
Wal-Mart Fndn Comm Grants, 3513
Walt Disney Company Fndn Grants, 3516
Warrick County Comm Fndn Grants, 3519
Wayne and Gladys Valley Fndn Grants, 3522
William G. Gilmore Fndn Grants, 3537
William T. Grant Fndn Research Grants, 3541
Wilson-Wood Fndn Grants, 3542
Women's Fndn of California Grants, 3550
YSA Get Ur Good On Grants, 3555

Youth Violence

Alliance Healthcare Fndn Grants, 362
FAR Fund, 1453
Gamble Fndn Grants, 1582
i2 Fndn Grants, 1829
Kansas Health Fndn Grants, 1980
Mary Black Fndn Grants, 2118
Ordean Fndn Grants, 2952
William G. McGowan Charitable Fund Grants, 3539
William T. Grant Fndn Research Grants, 3541

Zoology

Cessna Fndn Grants, 938
DeRoy Testamentary Fndn Grants, 1239
ExxonMobil Grants, 1442
FirstEnergy Fndn Comm Grants, 1505
Katherine John Murphy Fndn Grants, 1983
Oscar Rennebohm Fndn Grants, 2963
Perry County Comm Fndn Grants, 3016
Pike County Comm Fndn Grants, 3049
Posey Comm Fndn Grants, 3068
Procter and Gamble Fund Grants, 3083
Spencer County Comm Fndn Grants, 3358
Thelma Doelger Charitable Trust Grants, 3421
Vanderburgh Comm Fndn Grants, 3480
Warrick County Comm Fndn Grants, 3519

Program Type Index

NOTE: Numbers refer to entry numbers

Adult Basic Education
ACE Charitable Fndn Grants, 199
Achelis and Bodman Fndns Grants, 206
Ahmanson Fndn Grants, 303
Allyn Fndn Grants, 365
Arkell Hall Fndn Grants, 534
Arlington Comm Fndn Grants, 536
Atlanta Fndn Grants, 662
Auburn Fndn Grants, 664
Ball Brothers Fndn General Grants, 683
Ball Brothers Fndn Grants, 684
Battle Creek Comm Fndn Grants, 703
Benton Comm Fndn Grants, 743
Benton County Fndn Grants, 744
Blackford County Comm Fndn Grants, 763
Blue Mountain Comm Fndn Grants, 769
Blue River Comm Fndn Grants, 770
Bodenwein Public Benevolent Fndn Grants, 775
Boettcher Fndn Grants, 778
Booth-Bricker Fund Grants, 780
Boston Fndn Grants, 783
Boston Globe Fndn Grants, 784
Bridgestone/Firestone Trust Fund Grants, 792
Brook J. Lenfest Fndn Grants, 804
Brown County Comm Fndn Grants, 807
Carl and Lily Pforzheimer Fndn Grants, 868
Carrie Estelle Doheny Fndn Grants, 883
Cass County Comm Fndn Grants, 887
Catholic Campaign for Human Development (CCHD) Comm Organizing Grants, 891
Cemala Fndn Grants, 933
Charlotte County (FL) Comm Fndn Grants, 973
Chicago Board of Trade Fndn Grants, 988
CIGNA Fndn Grants, 1011
Coastal Bend Comm Fndn Grants, 1050
Colorado Springs Comm Trust Fund Grants, 1061
Columbus Fndn Competitive Grants, 1066
Comm Fndn of Bartholomew County Heritage Fund Grants, 1096
Comm Fndn of Boone County Grants, 1099
Comm Fndn of Central Illinois Grants, 1101
Comm Fndn of Greater Fort Wayne: Comm Endowment & Clarke Endowment Fund Grants, 1108
Comm Fndn of Greater New Britain Grants, 1111
Comm Fndn of Southeastern Connecticut Grants, 1125
Constantin Fndn Grants, 1145
Coors Brewing Corp Contributions Grants, 1151
Cornerstone Fndn of Northeastern Wisconsin Grants, 1152
Cowles Charitable Trust Grants, 1155
Daisy Marquis Jones Fndn Grants, 1188
Dayton Power and Light Fndn Grants, 1205
Dean Foods Comm Involvement Grants, 1209
Dr. Scholl Fndn Grants, 1329
El Pomar Fndn Awards and Grants, 1390
Evjue Fndn Grants, 1439
FAR Fund, 1453
Field Fndn of Illinois Grants, 1499
Frances L. and Edwin L. Cummings Memorial Fund Grants, 1547
G.N. Wilcox Trust Grants, 1581
Goodrich Corporation Fndn Grants, 1638
Green Fndn Grants, 1661
Gulf Coast Comm of Venice Fndn Grants, 1677
Hallmark Corp Fndn Grants, 1688
Harold Simmons Fndn Grants, 1698
Harris and Eliza Kempner Fund Grants, 1699
Helen Steiner Rice Fndn Grants, 1742
Hoblitzelle Fndn Grants, 1783
Howard and Bush Fndn Grants, 1798
Idaho Power Company Corp Contributions, 1838
James A. and Faith Knight Fndn Grants, 1884
James Ford Bell Fndn Grants, 1885
James S. Copley Fndn Grants, 1895
Jane Bradley Pettit Fndn Grants, 1902
John H. and Wilhelmina D. Harland Charitable Fndn Grants, 1933
John I. Smith Charities Grants, 1935
Joseph H. and Florence A. Roblee Fndn Grants, 1961
KeySpan Fndn Grants, 1995
Kraft Cares International Grants, 2016
Liberty Bank Fndn Grants, 2053
Lubrizol Fndn Grants, 2080
Maine Comm Fndn Grants, 2099
McCarthy Family Fndn Grants, 2141
Middlesex Savings Charitable Fndn Grants, 2196
Nina Mason Pulliam Charitable Trust Grants, 2776
Palm Beach and Martin Counties Grants, 2986
Paul and Mary Haas Fndn Contributions and Student Scholarships, 2997
Piper Jaffray Companies Building Strong Communities Grants, 3053
Polaroid Fund Grants, 3065
Portland General Electric Fndn Grants, 3067
Princeton Area Comm Fndn Greater Mercer Grants, 3081
Principal Financial Group Fndn Grants, 3082
Putnam County Comm Fndn Grants, 3093
Richard and Rhoda Goldman Fund Grants, 3158
San Antonio Area Fndn Grants, 3254
SOCFOC Reducing Health & Educational Disparities in the Central Neighborhood Grants, 3318
Texas Commission on the Arts Arts Respond Project Grants, 3420
U.S. Department of Education Rehabilitation Training--Rehabilitation Continuing Education Programs (RCEP)--Institute on Rehabilitation Issues (IRI), 3449
Vectren Fndn Grants, 3485
Verizon Fndn New York Grants, 3488
Verizon Fndn Virginia Grants, 3492
Wabash Valley Comm Fndn Grants, 3510
Wal-Mart Fndn Comm Grants, 3513
WHO Fndn General Grants, 3534
Wilson-Wood Fndn Grants, 3542

Adult/Family Literacy Training
AAFP Fndn Health Literacy State Grants, 112
Able Trust Vocational Rehabilitation Grants for Individuals, 186
ACE Charitable Fndn Grants, 199
Achelis and Bodman Fndns Grants, 206
Ahmanson Fndn Grants, 303
Alcatel-Lucent Technologies Fndn Grants, 333
Allyn Fndn Grants, 365
Altman Fndn Health Care Grants, 372
Amador Comm Fndn Grants, 409
Amgen Fndn Grants, 467
Andersen Corp Fndn, 470
Annenberg Fndn Grants, 479
Anschutz Family Fndn Grants, 486
Arizona Cardinals Grants, 529
Arkell Hall Fndn Grants, 534
Arlington Comm Fndn Grants, 536
ASHA Multicultural Activities Projects Grants, 571
Assisi Fndn Grants, 653
Atkinson Fndn International Grants, 661
Atlanta Fndn Grants, 662
Auburn Fndn Grants, 664
Bacon Family Fndn Grants, 679
Ball Brothers Fndn General Grants, 683
Ball Brothers Fndn Grants, 684
Barra Fndn Comm Fund Grants, 698
Battle Creek Comm Fndn Grants, 703
Beazley Fndn Grants, 730
Benton Comm Fndn Grants, 743
Blackford County Comm Fndn Grants, 763
Blue Mountain Comm Fndn Grants, 769
Blue River Comm Fndn Grants, 770
Bodenwein Public Benevolent Fndn Grants, 775
Bodman Fndn Grants, 776
Boettcher Fndn Grants, 778
Booth-Bricker Fund Grants, 780
Boston Fndn Grants, 783
Boston Globe Fndn Grants, 784
Brown County Comm Fndn Grants, 807
Carl and Lily Pforzheimer Fndn Grants, 868
Carl B. and Florence E. King Fndn Grants, 869
Carrie Estelle Doheny Fndn Grants, 883
Cass County Comm Fndn Grants, 887
Cemala Fndn Grants, 933
Central Okanagan Fndn Grants, 937
Charles Delmar Fndn Grants, 963
Charlotte County (FL) Comm Fndn Grants, 973
Chicago Board of Trade Fndn Grants, 988
CIGNA Fndn Grants, 1011
Coastal Bend Comm Fndn Grants, 1050
Colorado Springs Comm Trust Fund Grants, 1061
Columbus Fndn Competitive Grants, 1066
Comerica Charitable Fndn Grants, 1073
Comm Fndn of Bartholomew County Heritage Fund Grants, 1096
Comm Fndn of Boone County Grants, 1099
Comm Fndn of Broward Grants, 1100
Comm Fndn of Central Illinois Grants, 1101
Comm Fndn of Crawford County Grants and Scholarships, 1103
Comm Fndn of Grant County Grants, 1104
Comm Fndn of Greater Birmingham Grants, 1106
Comm Fndn of Greater Fort Wayne: Comm Endowment & Clarke Endowment Fund Grants, 1108
Comm Fndn of Greenville Hollingsworth Funds Program/Project Grants, 1114
Comm Fndn of Southeastern Connecticut Grants, 1125
Comm Fndn Silicon Valley Grants, 1133
Cooper Industries Fndn Grants, 1150
Coors Brewing Corp Contributions Grants, 1151
Cornerstone Fndn of Northeastern Wisconsin Grants, 1152
Cowles Charitable Trust Grants, 1155
Crail-Johnson Fndn Grants, 1157
Cruise Industry Charitable Fndn Grants, 1166
Daisy Marquis Jones Fndn Grants, 1188
Dallas Women's Fndn Grants, 1191
Danellie Fndn Grants, 1198
Dayton Power and Light Fndn Grants, 1205
Deaconess Comm Fndn Grants, 1207
Delta Air Lines Fndn Grants, 1220
Denver Fndn Comm Grants, 1227
Dr. Scholl Fndn Grants, 1329
Duke Energy Fndn Grants, 1339
EIF Comm Grants, 1386
Entergy Comm Partnership Grants, 1417
Eugene and Agnes E. Meyer Fndn Grants, 1432
Evjue Fndn Grants, 1439
Farmers Insurance Group of Companies Grants, 1455
Field Fndn of Illinois Grants, 1499
Fisher Fndn Grants, 1508
Fourjay Fndn Grants, 1544
Frances L. and Edwin L. Cummings Memorial Fund Grants, 1547
G.N. Wilcox Trust Grants, 1581
GenCorp Fndn Grants, 1587
Genuardi Family Fndn Grants, 1594
Gibson Fndn Grants, 1612
Greater New Orleans Fndn Grants, 1654
Green Bay Packers Fndn Grants, 1660
Hallmark Corp Fndn Grants, 1688
Harold Simmons Fndn Grants, 1698
Harris and Eliza Kempner Fund Grants, 1699
Harry S. Black and Allon Fuller Fund, 1706
Harvest Fndn Grants, 1713
Hasbro Children's Fund, 1714
Hearst Fndn and William Randolph Hearst Fndn Grants, 1730
Helen Bader Fndn Grants, 1738
Helen Steiner Rice Fndn Grants, 1742

Henry and Ruth Blaustein Rosenberg Fndn Grants, 1746
Highmark Corp Giving Grants, 1769
Hilda and Preston Davis Fndn Grants, 1772
Hoblitzelle Fndn Grants, 1783
Hoglund Fndn Grants, 1785
Howard and Bush Fndn Grants, 1798
Humana Fndn Grants, 1818
Irvin Stern Fndn Grants, 1866
James A. and Faith Knight Fndn Grants, 1884
James S. Copley Fndn Grants, 1895
Jean and Louis Dreyfus Fndn Grants, 1911
Jessie Ball Dupont Fund Grants, 1919
Jim Moran Fndn Grants, 1925
John Edward Fowler Memorial Fndn Grants, 1930
John H. and Wilhelmina D. Harland Charitable Fndn Grants, 1933
John I. Smith Charities Grants, 1935
John Merck Fund Grants, 1940
John P. McGovern Fndn Grants, 1942
Joseph H. and Florence A. Roblee Fndn Grants, 1961
Knight Family Charitable and Educational Fndn Grants, 2007
Kraft Cares International Grants, 2016
Louis Calder Fndn Grants, 2065
Lubrizol Fndn Grants, 2080
Marshall Field's Comm Grants, 2115
May Department Stores Charitable Contribution Grants, 2138
Montgomery County Comm Fndn Grants, 2214
Morris and Gwendolyn Cafritz Fndn Grants, 2217
New York Life Fndn Grants, 2304
Newman's Own Inc Grants, 2306
NLM Understanding and Promoting Health Literacy Research Grants, 2827
Nordson Corporation Fndn Grants, 2851
Northern Trust Company Charitable Trust and Corp Giving Program, 2865
PacifiCare Fndn Grants, 2981
Palm Beach and Martin Counties Grants, 2986
Paul and Mary Haas Fndn Contributions and Student Scholarships, 2997
Pew Charitable Trusts Children and Youth Grants, 3020
Polaroid Fund Grants, 3065
Principal Financial Group Fndn Grants, 3082
Reynolds and Reynolds Associate Fndn Grants, 3152
RGK Fndn Grants, 3153
Richard and Rhoda Goldman Fund Grants, 3158
Rochester Area Comm Fndn Grants, 3176
Samuel S. Johnson Fndn Grants, 3251
San Antonio Area Fndn Grants, 3254
San Diego Women's Fndn Grants, 3259
Seattle Fndn Grants, 3276
SOCFOC Reducing Health & Educational Disparities in the Central Neighborhood Grants, 3318
Southbury Comm Trust Fund, 3350
Stark Comm Fndn Women's Fund Grants, 3376
Strowd Roses Grants, 3388
US Airways Comm Contributions, 3472
Vectren Fndn Grants, 3485
Verizon Fndn Maryland Grants, 3487
Verizon Fndn New York Grants, 3488
Verizon Fndn Northeast Region Grants, 3489
Verizon Fndn Pennsylvania Grants, 3490
Verizon Fndn Vermont Grants, 3491
Verizon Fndn Virginia Grants, 3492
Vulcan Materials Company Fndn Grants, 3504
Wabash Valley Comm Fndn Grants, 3510
Wachovia Fndn Grants, 3511
Wal-Mart Fndn Comm Grants, 3513
Western Union Fndn Grants, 3529
WHO Fndn General Grants, 3534
Wilson-Wood Fndn Grants, 3542
Winston-Salem Fndn Stokes County Grants, 3546

Awards/Prizes

AAAAI Phoenix Program Award, 24
AACAP Beatrix A. Hamburg Award for the Best New Research Poster by a Child and Adolescent Psychiatry Resident, 30
AACAP Elaine Schlosser Lewis Award for Research on Attention-Deficit Disorder, 35
AACAP George Tarjan Award for Contributions in Developmental Disabilities, 36
AACAP Irving Philips Award for Prevention, 37
AACAP Jeanne Spurlock Lecture and Award on Diversity and Culture, 38
AACAP Klingenstein Third Generation Fndn Award for Research in Depression or Suicide, 42
AACAP Norbert and Charlotte Rieger Award for Scientific Achievement, 43
AACAP Norbert and Charlotte Rieger Psychodynamic Psychotherapy Award, 44
AACAP Pilot Research Awards, Supported by Eli Lilly and Company, 47
AACAP Rieger Service Program Award for Excellence, 49
AACAP Robert Cancro Academic Leadership Award, 50
AACAP Sidney Berman Award for the School-Based Study and Intervention for Learning Disorders and Mental Ilness, 51
AACAP Simon Wile Leadership in Consultation Award, 52
AACR Award for Lifetime Achievement in Cancer Research, 66
AACR Award for Outstanding Achievement in Cancer Research, 67
AACR Award for Outstanding Achievement in Chemistry in Cancer Research, 68
AACR G.H.A. Clowes Memorial Award, 75
AACR Joseph H. Burchenal Memorial Award, 78
AACR Margaret Foti Award for Leadership and Extraordinary Achievements in Cancer Research, 81
AACR Outstanding Investigator Award for Breast Cancer Research, 84
AACR Princess Takamatsu Memorial Lectureship, 85
AACR Richard and Hinda Rosenthal Memorial Awards, 86
AACR Scholar-in-Training Awards, 87
AACR Scholar-in-Training Awards - Special Conferences, 88
AACR Team Science Award, 89
AACR-American Cancer Society Award for Research Excellence in Cancer Epidemiology and Prevention, 91
AACR-Minorities in Cancer Research Jane Cooke Wright Lectureship Awards, 99
AACR-Prevent Cancer Fndn Award for Excellence in Cancer Prevention Research, 104
AACR-Women in Cancer Research Charlotte Friend Memorial Lectureship Awards, 106
AAFP Fndn Wyeth Immunization Awards, 115
AAFPRS Ben Shuster Memorial Award, 117
AAFPRS Bernstein Grant, 118
AAFPRS Ira J. Tresley Research Award, 121
AAFPRS John Orlando Roe Award, 122
AAFPRS Leslie Bernstein Resident Research Grants, 123
AAFPRS Residency Travel Awards, 124
AAFPRS Sir Harold Delf Gillies Award, 125
AAMC Abraham Flexner Award, 133
AAMC Alpha Omega Alpha Robert J. Glaser Distinguished Teacher Awards, 134
AAMC Award for Distinguished Research, 135
AAMC David E. Rogers Award, 137
AAMC Herbert W. Nickens Award, 138
AAMC Humanism in Medicine Award, 141
AAO-HNS Medical Student Research Prize, 144
AAO-HNS Resident Research Prizes, 145
AAP Anne E. Dyson Child Advocacy Awards, 156
AAP Nutrition Award, 165
AAPD Henry B. Betts Award, 169
AAPD Paul G. Hearne Leadership Award, 170
Abbott-ASM Lifetime Achievement Award, 180
AcademyHealth Alice S. Hersh New Investigator Awards, 190
AcademyHealth Awards, 192
AcademyHealth HSR Impact Awards, 193
AcademyHealth Nemours Child Health Services Research Awards, 194
AcademyHealth PHSR Research Article of the Year Awards, 196
ACS Doctoral Training Grants in Oncology Social Work, 213
ACS Physician Training Awards in Preventive Medicine, 218
Aetna Fndn Voice Of Conscience Award, 252
AFAR Medical Student Training in Aging Research Program, 255
AHFMR Comm Support Program Grants, 271
AHFMR Research Prize, 294
Albany Medical Center Prize in Medicine and Biomedical Research, 325
Alfred Bader Award in BioInorganic or BioOrganic Chemistry, 350
Alfred Burger Award in Medicinal Chemistry, 351
Alfred W. Bressler Prize in Vision Science, 354
Alton Ochsner Award, 373
ALVRE Casselberry Award, 374
ALVRE Seymour R. Cohen Award, 376
AMA Fndn Dr. Nathan Davis International Awards in Medicine, 387
AMA Fndn Jordan Fieldman, MD, Awards, 393
AMA Fndn Leadership Awards, 394
AMA Fndn Pride in the Profession Grants, 397
AMA-MSS Chapter of the Year (COTY) Award, 402
AMA-MSS Research Poster Award, 405
American Academy of Nursing Media Awards, 418
American Chemical Society Claude S. Hudson Awards, 419
American Medical Association Awards, 440
American Psychiatric Association Award for Research in Psychiatry, 442
American Psychiatric Association/AstraZeneca Young Minds in Psychiatry International Awards, 450
American Society on Aging Mental Health and Aging Awards, 456
American Society on Aging NOMA Award for Excellence in Multicultural Aging, 457
ANS Neurotology Fellows Award, 482
ANS Nicholas Torok Vestibular Award, 483
ANS Trainee Award, 484
APA Culture of Service in the Psychological Sciences Award, 493
APA Distinguished Scientific Award for Early Career Contribution to Psychology, 495
APA Distinguished Scientific Award for the Applications of Psychology, 496
APA Distinguished Scientific Contribution Award, 497
APA Distinguished Service to Psychological Science Award, 498
APA Meritorious Research Service Commendation, 499
APF Alexander Gralnick, MD, Award for Research in Schizophrenia, 503
APF Awards for Advancing Minority Mental Health, 504
ASA Metlife Fndn MindAlert Awards, 545
ASCO Comm Oncology Research Grants, 552
ASGE / ConMed Award for Outstanding Manuscript by a Fellow/Resident, 564
ASGE Don Wilson Award, 565
ASHA Advancing Academic-Research Careers (AARC) Award, 569
ASHA Minority Student Leadership Program Awards, 570
ASHA Research Mentoring-Pair Travel Award, 572
ASHA Student Research Travel Award, 573
ASHA Students Preparing for Academic & Research Careers (SPARC) Award, 574

ASM Abbott Laboratories Award in Clinical and Diagnostic Immunology, 587
ASM BD Award for Research in Clinical Microbiology, 588
ASM bioMerieux Sonnenwirth Award for Leadership in Clinical Microbiology, 589
ASM D.C. White Research and Mentoring Award, 592
ASM Eli Lilly and Company Research Award, 594
ASM Founders Distinguished Service Award, 596
ASM Gen-Probe Joseph Public Health Award, 597
ASM GlaxoSmithKline International Member of the Year Award, 599
ASM Intel Awards, 600
ASM Maurice Hilleman/Merck Award, 605
ASM Merck Irving S. Sigal Memorial Awards, 606
ASM Procter & Gamble Award in Applied and Environmental Microbiology, 609
ASM Promega Biotechnology Research Award, 610
ASM Public Communications Award, 611
ASM Raymond W. Sarber Awards, 612
ASM Richard and Mary Finkelstein Travel Grant, 613
ASM Roche Diagnostics Alice C. Evans Award, 615
ASM sanofi-aventis ICAAC Award, 616
ASM Scherago-Rubin Award, 617
ASM Siemens Healthcare Diagnostics Young Investigator Award, 618
ASM TREK Diagnostic ABMM/ABMLI Professional Recognition Award, 621
ASM USFCC/J. Roger Porter Award, 623
ASM William A Hinton Research Training Award, 624
ASPEN Dudrick Research Scholar Award, 631
ASPEN Harry M. Vars Award, 632
ASPEN Scientific Abstracts Awards for Papers or Posters, 636
ASPET Benedict R. Lucchesi Award in Cardiac Pharmacology, 638
ASPET Bernard B. Brodie Award in Drug Metabolism, 639
ASPET Division for Drug Metabolism Early Career Achievement Award, 640
ASPET Epilepsy Research Award for Outstanding Contributions to the Pharmacology of Antiepileptic Drugs, 641
ASPET Goodman and Gilman Award in Drug Receptor Pharmacology, 642
ASPET John J. Abel Award in Pharmacology, 643
ASPET Julius Axelrod Award in Pharmacology, 644
ASPET P. B. Dews Lifetime Achievement Award for Research in Behavioral Pharmacology, 645
ASPET Paul M. Vanhoutte Award, 646
ASPET Torald Sollmann Award in Pharmacology, 647
AUPHA Baxter International Fndn Prize for Health Services Research, 666
Austin College Leadership Award, 668
Award for Creative Advances in Environmental Science and Technology, 676
Award in Separations Science and Technology, 677
BCBSM Claude Pepper Award, 714
BCBSM Fndn Excellence in Research Awards for Students, 717
BCBSM Fndn Proposal Development Awards, 720
BCBSM Frank J. McDevitt, DO, Excellence in Research Awards, 722
Bristol-Myers Squibb / Meade Johnson Award for Distinguished Achievement in Nutrition Research, 795
Canadian Dental Research Fndn Award, 848
CFPC Family Physician of the Year Award, 954
CFPC Special Recognition Awards, 957
Christine O. Gregoire Youth/Young Adult Award for Outstanding Use of Tobacco Industry Documents, 1005
Claude Pepper Fndn Grants, 1032
Comm Fndn AIDS Endowment Awards, 1088
Comm Fndn of Bartholomew County James A. Henderson Award for Fund-Raising, 1097
Daniel Mendelsohn New Investigator Award, 1199
Do Something BR!CK Awards, 1287
E.B. Hershberg Award for Important Discoveries in Medicinally Active Substances, 1358
EF Making a Difference Award, 1381
El Pomar Fndn Awards and Grants, 1390
Eli Lilly & Company Welcome Back Awards, 1391
Eppendorf & Science Prize for Neurobiology, 1424
FCER Chiropractic Research Grants, 1459
FCNY Union Square Awards, 1461
FDHN Designated Outcomes Award in Geriatric Gastroenterology, 1466
FDHN Designated Research Award in Research Related to Pancreatitis, 1468
FDHN Fellow Abstract Prizes, 1469
FDHN Funderburg Research Scholar Award in Gastric Biology Related to Cancer, 1471
FDHN Graduate Student Awards, 1472
FDHN Jon I. Isenberg International Research Scholar Award, 1473
FDHN Moti L. & Kamla Rustgi International Travel Awards, 1475
FDHN Research Scholar Awards, 1478
FDHN Student Abstract Prizes, 1479
Food, Pharmaceutical, and Bioengineering Division Award in Chemical Engineering, 1521
Foster G. McGaw Prize, 1525
Fndn for Medical Research Grants, 1528
Frederic Stanley Kipping Award in Silicon Chemistry, 1559
GE & Science Prize for Young Life Scientists, 1584
GEICO Public Service Awards, 1586
GlaxoSmithKline Corp Grants, 1623
GlaxoSmithKline Fndn IMPACT Awards, 1624
Google Grants Beta, 1640
Gruber Fndn International Prizes, 1672
H.R. Lissner Award, 1683
Hereditary Disease Fndn Lieberman Award, 1751
IOM Gustav O. Lienhard Award, 1864
Jewish Comm Fndn of Greater Los Angeles Grants, 1921
Landon Fndn-AACR Innovator Award for International Collaboration, 2028
Landon Fndn-AACR Innovator Award for Cancer Prevention Research, 2029
Layne Beachley Aim For The Stars Fndn Grants, 2036
Lemelson-MIT Lifetime Achievement Award, 2042
Lynde and Harry Bradley Fndn Prizes: Bradley Prizes, 2090
MAPFRE Fndn for Medicine Grants, 2102
Massage Therapy Fndn Practitioner Case Report Contest, 2125
MDBD Research Prize in Developmental Biology, 2154
Mental Retardation Distinguished Research Award, 2171
Miguel Aleman Fndn Grants, 2197
MLA Ida and George Eliot Prize, 2209
MLA Lois Ann Colaianni Award for Excellence and Achievement in Hospital Librarianship, 2210
National Dairy Promotion and Research Board Scholarships, 2251
NHLBI Career Transition Award, 2326
NIA Mentored Clinical Scientist Research Career Development Awards, 2417
NIH Senior Scientist Award, 2727
NIH Transitional Career Development Award in Women's Health Research, 2736
NIHCM Fndn Health Care Print Journalism Awards, 2742
NIHCM Fndn Health Care Research Awards, 2743
NIHCM Fndn Health Care Television and Radio Journalism Awards, 2744
NINR Career Transition Award, 2791
NKF Clinical Scientist Awards, 2809
NMF Aura E. Severinghaus Award, 2828
NMF Franklin C. McLean Award, 2829
NMF Henry G. Halladay Awards, 2831
NMF National Medical Association Awards for Medical Journalism, 2836
NMF National Medical Association Emerging Scholar Awards, 2837
NMF National Medical Association Patti LaBelle Award, 2838
NMF Ralph W. Ellison Prize, 2840
NMF William and Charlotte Cadbury Award, 2841
NMSS Daniel Haughton Senior Faculty Awards, 2842
NSERC Brockhouse Canada Prize for Interdisciplinary Research in Science and Engineering Grant, 2873
NSF Alan T. Waterman Award, 2874
NSF Systematic Biology and Biodiversity Inventories Grants, 2895
NYAM Brock Lecture, Award and Visiting Professorship in Pediatrics, 2909
NYAM Edward N. Gibbs Memorial Lecture and Award in Nephrology, 2912
NYAM Lewis Rudin Glaucoma Grants, 2915
NYAM Student Essay Grants, 2917
Oticon Focus on People Awards, 2976
Paul Marks Prizes for Cancer Research, 3002
Pet Care Trust Sue Busch Memorial Award, 3017
Pezcoller Fndn-AACR International Award for Cancer Research, 3023
Pharmacia-ASPET Award for Experimental Therapeutics, 3028
Portland General Electric Fndn Grants, 3067
Prince Charitable Trusts Chicago Grants, 3079
RACGP National Asthma Council Research Award, 3100
Rajiv Gandhi Fndn Grants, 3104
Ralph F. Hirschmann Award in Peptide Chemistry, 3105
RCPSC Canadian Research Awards for Specialty Residents (Medicine, Surgery), 3113
RCPSC Duncan Graham Award, 3115
RCPSC James H. Graham Award of Merit, 3119
RCPSC KJR Wightman Award for Scholarship in Ethics, 3122
RCPSC Royal College Medal Award in Medicine, 3128
RCPSC Royal College Medal Award in Surgery, 3129
RCPSC Teasdale-Corti Humanitarian Award, 3131
RCPSC/AMS Donald Richards Wilson Award, 3136
Rosalynn Carter Institute Georgia Caregiver of the Year Awards, 3188
RSC Abbyann D. Lynch Medal in Bioethics, 3195
RSC Jason A. Hannah Medal, 3196
RSC McLaughlin Medal, 3197
RSC McNeil Medal for the Public Awareness of Science, 3198
RSC Thomas W. Eadie Medal, 3199
RWJF Comm Health Leaders Awards, 3208
RWJF Young Epidemiology Scholars (YES) Competition, 3233
Simone and Cino del Duca Grand Prix Awards, 3288
SNM Tetalman Memorial Young Investigator Awards, 3307
SNMTS Outstanding Educator Awards, 3310
SNMTS Outstanding Technologist Awards, 3311
SOBP A.E. Bennett Research Award, 3313
SOBP Ziskind-Somerfeld Research Awards, 3316
Society of Cosmetic Chemists Allan B. Black Award Sponsored by Presperse, 3328
Society of Cosmetic Chemists Award Sponsored by McIntyre Group, Ltd., 3329
Society of Cosmetic Chemists Award Sponsored by The HallStar Company, 3330
Society of Cosmetic Chemists Chapter Best Speaker Award, 3331
Society of Cosmetic Chemists Chapter Merit Award, 3332

Society of Cosmetic Chemists Frontier of Science Award, 3333
Society of Cosmetic Chemists Hans Schaeffer Award, 3334
Society of Cosmetic Chemists Joseph P. Ciaudelli Award, 3335
Society of Cosmetic Chemists Keynote Award Lecture Sponsored by Ruger Chemical Corporation, 3336
Society of Cosmetic Chemists Literature Award, 3337
Society of Cosmetic Chemists Maison G. de Navarre Medal, 3338
Society of Cosmetic Chemists Merit Award, 3339
Society of Cosmetic Chemists Robert A. Kramer Lifetime Service Award, 3340
Society of Cosmetic Chemists Shaw Mudge Award, 3341
Society of Cosmetic Chemists Student Poster Awards, 3342
Society of Cosmetic Chemists Young Scientist Awards, 3343
Stephen S. Chang Award, 3382
Supelco AOCS Research Award, 3405
Sybil G. Jacobs Award for Outstanding Use of Tobacco Industry Documents, 3414
TRDRP California Research Awards, 3434
TRDRP Exploratory/Developmental Research Awards, 3435
Walter Nicolai Prize in Biomedical Gerontology, 3517
Warren Alpert Fndn Prize, 3518

Basic Research

1 in 9: Long Island Breast Cancer Action Coalition Grants, 1
100 Mile Man Fndn Grants, 2
1976 Fndn Grants, 5
1st Touch Fndn Grants, 6
25th Anniversary Fndn Grants, 8
A Friend's Fndn Trust Grants, 13
A Social Corporation Grants, 15
A-T Medical Research Fndn Grants, 16
A.O. Smith Comm Grants, 18
AAAAI Allergy, Asthma and Immunology Education and Research Trust (ART) Clinical Research Grants, 22
AAAAI Allergy, Asthma and Immunology Education and Research Trust (ART) Faculty Development Award, 23
AAAAI Phoenix Program Award, 24
AAAAI Research Award Grants, 25
AAAAI Summer Clinical Research Fellowship Medical Student Grants, 27
AACAP Beatrix A. Hamburg Award for the Best New Research Poster by a Child and Adolescent Psychiatry Resident, 30
AACAP Congressional Fellowships, 32
AACAP Educational Outreach Program for General Psychiatry Residents, 34
AACAP Elaine Schlosser Lewis Award for Research on Attention-Deficit Disorder, 35
AACAP George Tarjan Award for Contributions in Developmental Disabilities, 36
AACAP Irving Philips Award for Prevention, 37
AACAP Jeanne Spurlock Lecture and Award on Diversity and Culture, 38
AACAP Jeanne Spurlock Minority Medical Student Clinical Fellowship in Child and Adolescent Psychiatry, 39
AACAP Jeanne Spurlock Research Fellowship in Substance Abuse and Addiction for Minority Medical Students, 40
AACAP Junior Investigator Awards, 41
AACAP Klingenstein Third Generation Fndn Award for Research in Depression or Suicide, 42
AACAP Norbert and Charlotte Rieger Psychodynamic Psychotherapy Award, 44
AACAP Pilot Research Award for Attention-Deficit Disorder, Supported by the Elaine Schlosser Lewis Fund, 45
AACAP Pilot Research Award for Learning Disabilities, Supported by the Elaine Schlosser Lewis Fund, 46
AACAP Pilot Research Awards, Supported by Eli Lilly and Company, 47
AACAP Quest for the Test Bipolar Disorder Pilot Research Award, 48
AACAP Rieger Service Program Award for Excellence, 49
AACAP Robert Cancro Academic Leadership Award, 50
AACAP Sidney Berman Award for the School-Based Study and Intervention for Learning Disorders and Mental Ilness, 51
AACAP Summer Medical Student Fellowships, 53
AACAP-NIDA K12 Career Development Awards, 55
AACN Clinical Inquiry Fund Grants, 56
AACN Clinical Practice Grants, 57
AACN Critical Care Grants, 58
AACN End of Life/Palliative Care Small Projects Grants, 59
AACN Evidence-Based Clinical Practice Grants, 60
AACN Physio-Control Small Projects Grants, 62
AACN-Edwards Lifesciences Nurse-Driven Clinical Practice Outcomes Grants, 63
AACN-Philips Medical Systems Clinical Outcomes Grants, 64
AACN-Sigma Theta Tau Critical Care Grant, 65
AACR Award for Lifetime Achievement in Cancer Research, 66
AACR Award for Outstanding Achievement in Cancer Research, 67
AACR Award for Outstanding Achievement in Chemistry in Cancer Research, 68
AACR Brigid G. Leventhal Scholar in Cancer Research Awards, 69
AACR Career Development Awards for Pediatric Cancer Research, 70
AACR Centennial Postdoctoral Fellowships in Cancer Research, 71
AACR Centennial Pre-doctoral Fellowships in Cancer Research, 72
AACR Fellows Grants, 74
AACR Henry Shepard Bladder Cancer Research Grants, 77
AACR Joseph H. Burchenal Memorial Award, 78
AACR Judah Folkman Career Development Award for Anti-Angiogenesis Research, 79
AACR Kirk A. Landon and Dorothy P. Landon Fndn Prizes, 80
AACR Margaret Foti Award for Leadership and Extraordinary Achievements in Cancer Research, 81
AACR Minority Scholar in Cancer Research Awards, 82
AACR Minority-Serving Institution Faculty Scholar in Cancer Research Awards, 83
AACR Outstanding Investigator Award for Breast Cancer Research, 84
AACR Richard and Hinda Rosenthal Memorial Awards, 86
AACR Team Science Award, 89
AACR Thomas J. Bardos Science Education Awards, 90
AACR-American Cancer Society Award for Research Excellence in Cancer Epidemiology and Prevention, 91
AACR-Colorectal Cancer Coalition Fellows Grant, 92
AACR-FNAB Fellows Grant for Translational Pancreatic Cancer Research, 93
AACR-FNAB Fellows Grant for Translational Pancreatic Cancer Research, 94
AACR-FNAB Fndn Career Development Award for Translational Cancer Research, 95
AACR-Genentech BioOncology Career Development Award for Cancer Research on the HER Family Pathway, 96
AACR-Genentech BioOncology Fellowship for Cancer Research in Angiogenesis, 97
AACR-Minorities in Cancer Research Jane Cooke Wright Lectureship Awards, 99
AACR-National Brain Tumor Fndn Fellows Grant, 100
AACR-NCI International Investigator Opportunity Grants, 101
AACR-Pancreatic Cancer Action Network Career Development Award for Pancreatic Cancer Research, 102
AACR-Pancreatic Cancer Action Network Innovative Grants, 103
AACR-Prevent Cancer Fndn Award for Excellence in Cancer Prevention Research, 104
AACR-Women in Cancer Research Charlotte Friend Memorial Lectureship Awards, 106
AACR Basic Cancer Research Fellowships , 107
AAFA Investigator Research Grants, 108
AAFP Fndn Joint Grants, 113
AAFP Fndn Wyeth Immunization Awards, 115
AAFP Research Stimulation Grants, 116
AAFPRS Bernstein Grant, 118
AAFPRS Fellowships, 119
AAFPRS Investigator Development Grant, 120
AAFPRS Leslie Bernstein Resident Research Grants, 123
AAHN Grant for Historical Research, 126
AAHN Pre-Doctoral Research Grant, 127
AAMC Award for Distinguished Research, 135
AANS Neurosurgery Research and Education Fndn/Spine Section Young Clinician Investigator Award, 143
AAO-HNS Medical Student Research Prize, 144
AAO-HNS Resident Research Prizes, 145
AAO-HNSF CORE Research Grants, 146
AAO-HNSF Health Services Research Grants, 147
AAO-HNSF Maureen Hannley Research Training Awards, 148
AAO-HNSF Percy Memorial Research Award, 149
AAO-HNSF Rande H. Lazar Health Services Research Grant, 150
AAO-HNSF Resident Research Awards, 151
AAOA Fndn/AAO-HNSF Combined Research Grants, 152
AAOHN Fndn Experienced Researcher Grants, 153
AAOHN Fndn New Investigator Researcher Grants, 154
Abbott Fund Access to Health Care Grants, 176
Abbott Fund Global AIDS Care Grants, 178
Abbott Fund Science and Medical Innovation Grants, 179
ACAAI Fndn Research Grants, 189
AcademyHealth HSR Impact Awards, 193
ACGT Investigators Grants, 204
ACGT Young Investigator Grants, 205
Achelis and Bodman Fndns Grants, 206
ACS Clinical Research Professor Grants, 210
ACS Doctoral Training Grants in Oncology Social Work, 213
ACS Institutional Research Grants, 215
ACS Mentored Research Scholar Grant in Applied and Clinical Research, 217
ACS Physician Training Awards in Preventive Medicine, 218
ACS Pilot and Exploratory Projects in Palliative Care of Cancer Patients and Their Families Grants, 219
ACS Research Professor Grants, 221
ACS Research Scholar Grants for Health Services and Health Policy Research, 222
ACS Research Scholar Grants in Basic, Preclinical, Clinical and Epidemiology Research, 223
ACS Research Scholar Grants in Psychosocial and Behavioral and Cancer Control Research, 224
ACVIM Fndn Clinical Investigation Grants, 227

ADA Fndn Dental Literature Grants, 229
Adam Richter Charitable Trust Grants, 230
Adams County Fndn Grants - Pennsylvania, 231
Adaptec Fndn Grants, 232
Administration on Aging Senior Medicare Patrol Project Grants, 236
AFAR CART Fund Grants, 254
AFAR Paul Beeson Career Development Awards in Aging Research for the Island of Ireland, 256
AFAR Research Grants, 257
Affymetrix Corp Contributions Grants, 258
AHAF Alzheimer's Disease Research Grants, 266
AHAF Macular Degeneration Research Grants, 267
AHAF National Glaucoma Research Grants, 268
AHFMR Clinical Fellowships, 269
AHFMR Clinical Investigator Awards, 270
AHFMR Comm Support Program Grants, 271
AHFMR Dr. Lionel E. McLeod Health Research Scholarship, 272
AHFMR Establishment and Independent Establishment Grants, 273
AHFMR Fast-Track Studentships and Fellowships, 274
AHFMR Forefront Internship Program Grants, 275
AHFMR Full-Time M.D./Ph.D. Studentships, 277
AHFMR Full-Time Studentships, 278
AHFMR Health Research Career Renewal Awards, 279
AHFMR Health Research Full-Time Studentships, 280
AHFMR Health Research Fund Grants, 281
AHFMR Heritage Summer Studentships, 282
AHFMR Infrastructure Funding Grants, 283
AHFMR Interdisciplinary Team Grants, 284
AHFMR Major Equipment Grants, 285
AHFMR Medical or Health Scholars Investigator Grants, 286
AHFMR Medical or Health Scientist Awards, 287
AHFMR Part-Time Studentships, 289
AHFMR Personnel Funding Grants, 290
AHFMR Polaris Awards, 291
AHFMR Population Health Investigator (PHI) Awards, 292
AHFMR Proposals for Special Initiatives, 293
AHFMR Research Prize, 294
AHFMR Scholar Awards, 295
AHFMR Scientist Awards, 296
AHFMR Senior Investigator Awards, 297
AHFMR Senior Medical or Health Scholars Investigator Grants, 298
AHFMR Senior Scholar Awards, 299
AHIMA Dissertation Assistance Grants, 300
AHIMA Faculty Development Stipends, 301
AHIMA Grant-In-Aid Research Grants, 302
AHNS Alando J. Ballantyne Resident Research Pilot Grant, 305
AHNS Pilot Grant, 306
AHNS/AAO-HNSF Surgeon Scientist Combined Award, 307
AHNS/AAO-HNSF Young Investigator Combined Award, 308
AHRF Eugene L. Derlacki, M.D. Research Grants, 309
AHRF Georgia Birtman Grant, 310
AHRF Regular Research Grants, 311
AHRF Wiley H. Harrison Memorial Research Award, 312
AHRQ Independent Scientist Award, 313
AHRQ Individual Awards for Postdoctoral Fellows Ruth L. Kirschstein National Research Service Awards (NRSA), 314
AIHP Sonnedecker Visiting Scholar Grants, 317
AJCC Cancer Staging Grants, 320
Albany Medical Center Prize in Medicine and Biomedical Research, 325
Albert and Margaret Alkek Fndn Grants, 326
Albert and Mary Lasker Fndn Awards, 327
Alcoa Fndn Grants, 334
Alcohol Misuse and Alcoholism Research Grants, 335
Alexander and Margaret Stewart Trust Grants, 340
Alexander von Humboldt Fndn Georg Forster Fellowships for Experienced Researchers, 344
Alexander von Humboldt Fndn Georg Forster Fellowships for Postdoctoral Researchers, 345
Alexander von Humboldt Fndn Institutional Academic Cooperation Grants, 346
Alexander von Humboldt Fndn Research Fellowships for Experienced Researchers, 347
Alexander von Humboldt Fndn Research Fellowships for Postdoctoral Researchers, 348
Alfred P. Sloan Fndn History of Science and Technology Grants, 352
Alfred P. Sloan Fndn Research Fellowships, 353
Alfred W. Bressler Prize in Vision Science, 354
Allyn Fndn Grants, 365
Alpha Omega Fndn Grants, 366
Alpha Research Fndn Grants, 367
ALSAM Fndn Grants, 369
Alternatives Research and Development Fndn Alternatives in Education Grants, 370
Alternatives Research and Development Fndn Grants, 371
Alton Ochsner Award, 373
ALVRE Grant, 375
Alzheimer's Association Everyday Technologies for Alzheimer Care (ETAC) Research Grants, 377
Alzheimer's Association Investigator-Initiated Research Grants, 378
Alzheimer's Association Mentored New Investigator Research Grants to Promote Diversity, 379
Alzheimer's Association Molecular Imaging Grants, 380
Alzheimer's Association New Investigator Research Grants, 381
Alzheimer's Association New Investigator Research Grants to Promote Diversity, 382
Alzheimer's Association Senator Mark Hatfield Award, 383
Alzheimer's Association Zenith Fellows Awards, 384
AMA Fndn Joan F. Giambalvo Memorial Scholarships, 392
AMA Fndn Seed Grants for Research, 398
AMA-WPC Joan F. Giambalvo Memorial Scholarships, 408
Amarillo Area/Harrington Fndns Grants, 410
American Academy of Nursing Building Academic Geriatric Nursing Capacity (BAGNC) Scholarships, 414
American Academy of Nursing Claire M. Fagin Fellowships, 415
American Academy of Nursing Mayday Fund Grants, 416
American Chemical Society GCI Pharmaceutical Roundtable Research Grants, 420
American College of Rheumatology Fellows-in-Training Travel Scholarships, 421
American College of Surgeons and The Triological Society Clinical Scientist Development Awards, 422
American College of Surgeons Australia and New Zealand Chapter Travelling Fellowships, 423
American College of Surgeons Co-Sponsored K08/K23 NIH Supplement Awards, 424
American College of Surgeons Faculty Research Fellowships, 426
American College of Surgeons Nizar N. Oweida, MD, FACS, Scholarships, 430
American College of Surgeons Wound Care Management Award, 433
American Fndn for Suicide Prevention Grants, 436
American Legacy Fndn National Calls for Proposals Grants, 438
American Legacy Fndn Small Innovative Grants, 439
American Psychiatric Association Award for Research in Psychiatry, 442
American Psychiatric Association Minority Medical Student Fellowship in HIV Psychiatry, 444
American Psychiatric Association Minority Medical Student Summer Externship in Addiction Psychiatry, 445
American Psychiatric Association Minority Medical Student Summer Mentoring Program, 446
American Psychiatric Association Program for Minority Research Training in Psychiatry (PMRTP), 447
American Psychiatric Association Research Colloquium for Junior Investigators, 448
American Psychiatric Association/AstraZeneca Young Minds in Psychiatry International Awards, 450
American Psychiatric Association/Janssen Resident Psychiatric Research Scholars, 452
American Psychiatric Association/Merck Co. Early Academic Career Research Award, 453
American Schlafhorst Fndn Grants, 454
American Society on Aging Graduate Student Research Award, 455
American Sociological Association Minority Fellowships, 458
American-Italian Cancer Fndn Fellowships, 459
amfAR Fellowships, 462
amfAR Mathilde Krim Fellowships in Basic Biomedical Research, 464
amfAR Research Grants, 466
Amgen Fndn Grants, 467
AMI Semiconductors Corp Grants, 468
AMSSM Fndn Research Grants, 469
Angels Baseball Fndn Grants, 473
Ann and Robert H. Lurie Family Fndn Grants, 475
Ann Arbor Area Comm Fndn Grants, 476
Ann Peppers Fndn Grants, 478
ANS Neurotology Fellows Award, 482
ANS/AAO-HNSF Herbert Silverstein Otology and Neurotology Research Award, 485
Anthem Blue Cross and Blue Shield School Nurse Grants, 489
Anthony R. Abraham Fndn Grants, 490
APA Culture of Service in the Psychological Sciences Award, 493
APA Distinguished Scientific Award for Early Career Contribution to Psychology, 495
APA Distinguished Scientific Award for the Applications of Psychology, 496
APA Distinguished Scientific Contribution Award, 497
APA Distinguished Service to Psychological Science Award, 498
APA Young Investigator Grants, 502
APF Call for Proposals, 505
APF James H. Scully Jr., M.D., Educational Fund Grants, 508
APF Jeanne Spurlock Congressional Fellowships, 509
APSAA Fellowships, 516
APSAA Mini-Career Grants, 518
APSAA Research Grants, 519
APSAA Small Beginning Scholar Pre-Investigation Grants, 520
APSAA Small Beginning Scholar Visiting and Consulting Grants, 521
Arcadia Fndn Grants, 524
Arie and Ida Crown Memorial Grants, 528
Arizona Cardinals Grants, 529
Arizona Public Service Corp Giving Program Grants, 531
ARS New Investigator Award, 539
ARS Resident Research Grants, 540
Arthritis Fndn of Australia Grants, 541
ArvinMeritor Fndn Health Grants, 543
ASCO Improving Cancer Care Grants, 546
ASCO Advanced Clinical Research Award in Colorectal Cancer, 548
ASCO Advanced Clinical Research Awards in Breast Cancer, 549

ASCO Advanced Clinical Research Awards in Sarcoma, 550
ASCO Career Development Award, 551
ASCO Comm Oncology Research Grants, 552
ASCO Comparative Effectiveness Research Professorship (CERP) in Breast Cancer, 553
ASCO International Development and Education Awards (IDEA), 554
ASCO Merit Awards, 558
ASCO Translational Research Professorships, 561
ASCO Young Investigator Award, 562
ASCO/UICC International Cancer Technology Transfer (ICRETT) Fellowships, 563
ASGE / ConMed Award for Outstanding Manuscript by a Fellow/Resident, 564
ASGE Don Wilson Award, 565
ASGE Endoscopic Research Awards, 566
ASGE Endoscopic Research Career Development Awards, 567
ASGE Given Capsule Endoscopy Research Award, 568
ASHA Advancing Academic-Research Careers (AARC) Award, 569
ASHA Research Mentoring-Pair Travel Award, 572
ASHA Student Research Travel Award, 573
ASHA Students Preparing for Academic & Research Careers (SPARC) Award, 574
ASHFndn Clinical Research Grants, 575
ASHFndn New Century Scholars Program Doctoral Scholarships, 580
ASHFndn New Century Scholars Research Grant, 581
ASHFndn Research Grant for New Investigators, 582
ASHFndn Research Grant in Speech Science, 583
ASHFndn Student Research Grants in Audiology, 584
ASHFndn Student Research Grants in Early Childhood Language Development, 585
ASM Abbott Laboratories Award in Clinical and Diagnostic Immunology, 587
ASM International Fellowship for Latin America and the Caribbean, 601
ASM Microbiology Undergraduate Research Fellowship, 607
ASM Millis-Colwell Postgraduate Travel Grant, 608
ASM Robert D. Watkins Graduate Research Fellowship, 614
ASM Undergraduate Research Fellowship, 622
ASM-PAHO Infectious Diseases Epidemiology and Surveillance Fellowships, 625
ASM-UNESCO Leadership Grant for International Educators, 626
ASM/CCID Fellowships, 627
ASPEN C. Richard Fleming Grant, 629
ASPEN Douglas Wilmore Grant, 630
ASPEN Maurice Shils Grant, 633
ASPEN Norman Yoshimura Grant, 634
ASPEN Nutrition Research Grants, 635
ASPET Bernard B. Brodie Award in Drug Metabolism, 639
ASPET Division for Drug Metabolism Early Career Achievement Award, 640
ASPET Epilepsy Research Award for Outstanding Contributions to the Pharmacology of Antiepileptic Drugs, 641
ASPET P. B. Dews Lifetime Achievement Award for Research in Behavioral Pharmacology, 645
ASPET Paul M. Vanhoutte Award, 646
ASPET Torald Sollmann Award in Pharmacology, 647
ASPET-Astellas Awards in Translational Pharmacology, 649
ASPO Daiichi Innovative Technology Grant, 650
ASPO Fellowships, 651
ASPO Research Grants, 652
Assisi Fndn Grants, 653
Assurant Health Fndn Grants, 655
Astellas Fndn Research Grants, 656
Atran Fndn Grants, 663
Australian Academy of Science Grants, 670
AVDF Health Care Grants, 673
Avon Fndn Breast Care Fund Grants, 674
Award for Creative Advances in Environmental Science and Technology, 676
Award in Separations Science and Technology, 677
Ball Brothers Fndn Grants, 684
Baltimore Washington Center Adult Psychoanalysis Fellowships, 685
Baltimore Washington Center Child Psychotherapy Fellowships, 686
Barra Fndn Project Grants, 699
Barth Syndrome Fndn Research Grants, 700
Batchelor Fndn Grants, 701
Baxter International Fndn Grants, 705
BCBS of Massachusetts Fndn Grants, 709
BCBSM Fndn Physician Investigator Research Awards, 718
BCBSM Fndn Primary and Clinical Prevention Grants, 719
BCBSM Fndn Student Award Program, 721
BCBSM Frank J. McDevitt, DO, Excellence in Research Awards, 722
BCBSM Investigator-Initiated Research Program Grants, 723
BCBSNC Fndn Grants, 725
BCRF Research Grants, 726
BCRF-AACR Grants for Translational Breast Cancer Research, 727
Beckman Coulter Comm Relations Grants, 733
Beckman Scholars Program Grants, 734
Beckman Young Investigators Program Grants, 735
Becton Dickinson and Company Grants, 736
Berks County Comm Fndn Grants, 745
Blowitz-Ridgeway Fndn Early Childhood Development Research Award, 766
Blowitz-Ridgeway Fndn Grants, 767
Blue Shield of California Grants, 771
Bodenwein Public Benevolent Fndn Grants, 775
Bodman Fndn Grants, 776
Booth-Bricker Fund Grants, 780
Bosque Fndn Grants, 782
Boston Psychoanalytic Society and Institute Fellowship in Child Psychoanalytic Psychotherapy, 786
Boston Psychoanalytic Society and Institute Fellowship in Psychoanalytic Psychotherapy, 787
Breast Cancer Fund Grants, 790
Bridgestone/Firestone Trust Fund Grants, 792
Bright Family Fndn Grants, 793
Brinson Fndn Grants, 794
Bristol-Myers Squibb Fndn Global HIV/AIDS Initiative Grants, 796
Bristol-Myers Squibb Fndn Health Disparities Grants, 797
Bristol-Myers Squibb Fndn Women's Health Grants, 800
Bristol-Myers Squibb Virology and Oncology M.D. Research Fellowships, 802
Broad Fndn IBD Research Grants, 803
Brookdale Fndn Leadership in Aging Fellowships, 805
Burden Trust Grants, 810
Burton G. Bettingen Grants, 813
Bushrod H. Campbell and Adah F. Hall Charity Fund Grants, 816
BWF Ad Hoc Grants, 818
BWF Career Awards at the Scientific Interface, 819
BWF Institutional Program Unifying Population and Laboratory Based Sciences, 822
BWF Investigators in the Pathogenesis of Infectious Disease, 823
Byron W. and Alice L. Lockwood Fndn Grants, 824
Campbell Fndn HIV/AIDS Research Grants, 839
CAN Autism Treatment-Related Study Awards, 842
CAN Pilot Research Projects, 843
CAN Young Investigator Awards, 844
Canada Graduate Scholarships (CGS) and NSERC Postgraduate Scholarships (PGS), 845
Canadian Fndn for Dietetic Research Awards, 849
Canadian Liver Fndn Grants, 851
Canadian Optometric Education Trust Fund Grants, 853
Canadian Patient Safety Institute (CPSI) Research Grants, 855
Cancer Research UK Grants, 859
Cancer Society of New Zealand Grants, 860
Cancer Treatment Research Fndn Clinical Investigation Grants, 861
Cargill Citizenship Fund-Corp Giving Grants, 865
Carl and Eloise Pohlad Family Fndn Grants, 867
Carl Gellert and Celia Berta Gellert Fndn Grants, 871
Carl J. Herzog Fndn Grants, 872
Carnegie Corporation of New York Grants, 879
Carrier Corporation Contributions Grants, 884
Castle Rock Fndn Grants, 888
Catherine Holmes Wilkins Fndn Grants, 889
CCFF Clinic Incentive Grants, 892
CCFF Research Grants, 894
CCFF Small Conference Grants, 896
CCFF Studentships, 897
CCFF Summer Studentship, 898
CCFF Visiting Scientist Awards, 900
CDC Evidence-Based Laboratory Medicine: Quality/Performance Measure Evaluation, 901
CDC Antimicrobial Resistance in Hospital-Acquired Infections Among Intensive Care Unit Patients, 902
CDC Cancer Prevention and Control Programs, 903
CDC Cooperative Agreement for Continuing Enhanced National Surveillance for Prion Diseases in the United States, 904
CDC Cooperative Agreement for the Development, Operation, and Evaluation of an Entertainment Education Program, 906
CDC Core Capacity Program Grants, 907
CDC Evaluation of the Use of Rapid Testing For Influenza in Outpatient Medical Settings, 910
CDC Injury Prevention and Control Research and State and Comm Based Programs, 914
CDC Intervention Epidemiologic Research Studies of HIV/AIDS, 915
CDC National Breast and Cervical Cancer Early Detection Program, 917
CDC National Programs That Build the Capacity of Schools To Prevent Foodborne Illness Through Coordinated School Health Programs, 919
CDC National Training Information and Exchange Program, 920
CDC Promoting Prevention in Managed Care Cooperative Agreements, 925
CDC Public Health Conference Support Grants, 926
CDC Sexually Transmitted Diseases Research, Demonstration, Public Information, and Education Grants, 929
CDC Technology Translation and Transfer of Effective HIV Behavioral Interventions, 931
CDC Using Genetic Information to Prevent Disease and Improve Health Research Grants, 932
Center for Alternatives to Animal Testing Grants, 934
CF Clinical Research Trainee Awards, 940
CF Roger C. Bone Award for Advances in End-of-Life Care, 941
CFF Clinical Research Grants, 942
CFF Pilot and Feasibility Awards, 945
CFF Research Grants, 947
CFF Therapeutics Development Program, 949
CFF-NIH Funding Grants, 951
CFPC Research and Education Fndn Grants, 956
Champ-A Champion Fur Kids Grants, 959
Charles Edison Fund Grants, 964
Charles G. Koch Charitable Fndn Grants, 965

Charles H. Farnsworth Trust Grants, 967
Charles H. Hood Fndn Child Health Research Grants, 968
Charles H. Revson Fndn Grants, 969
Charles Lafitte Fndn Grants, 970
Charlotte Geyer Fndn Cancer Research Grants, 974
CHCF Grants, 979
Chest Fndn Eli Lilly and Company Distinguished Scholar in Critical Care Medicine Award, 983
Chest Fndn Geriatric Development Research Awards, 984
Chest Fndn Grant in Venous Thromboembolism, 985
Chest Fndn/LUNGevity Fndn Clinical Research in Lung Cancer Grants, 986
Chestnut Hill Charitable Fndn, Inc Grants, 987
Chicago Board of Trade Fndn Grants, 988
Chicago Institute for Psychoanalysis Fellowships, 990
Children's Brain Tumor Fndn Research Grants, 998
Children's Leukemia Research Association Research Grants, 999
Children's Medical Research Institute Grants, 1000
Children's Cardiomyopathy Fndn Research Grants, 1002
Chiles Fndn Grants, 1003
Chiron Fndn Comm Grants, 1004
Christine O. Gregoire Youth/Young Adult Award for Outstanding Use of Tobacco Industry Documents, 1005
Christopher Reeve Paralysis Fndn Individual Research Grants, 1006
Christopher Reeve Paralysis Fndn Quality of Life and Health Promotions Grants, 1007
CLA Nurses Respiratory Society Nursing Research Grants, 1019
Clarence E. Heller Charitable Fndn Grants, 1022
Clark Fndn Grants, 1029
Claude Pepper Fndn Grants, 1032
CLF Fellowships, 1037
CLF Operating Grants, 1039
Clowes ACS/AAST/NIGMS Jointly Sponsored Mentored Clinical Scientist Development Award, 1041
CMA Fndn Grants, 1042
CMS Historically Black Colleges and Universities (HBCU) Health Services Research Grants, 1044
CMS Research and Demonstration Grants, 1045
Coeta and Donald Barker Fndn Grants, 1054
Coleman Fndn Cancer Care Grants, 1055
Colonel Stanley R. McNeil Fndn Grants, 1059
Columbus Fndn Ann Ellis Fund Grants, 1065
Commonweal Fndn Comm Assistance Grants, 1075
Commonweal Fndn Grants, 1076
Commonwealth Fund Affordable Health Insurance Grants, 1077
Commonwealth Fund Australian-American Health Policy Fellowships, 1078
Commonwealth Fund Harkness Fellowships in Health Care Policy and Practice, 1079
Commonwealth Fund Health Care Quality Improvement and Efficiency Grants, 1080
Commonwealth Fund Payment System Reform Grants, 1082
Commonwealth Fund Quality of Care for Frail Elders Grants, 1083
Commonwealth Fund Small Grants, 1084
Commonwealth Fund State High Performance Health Systems Grants, 1085
Comm Campus Partnerships for Health Fellowships, 1087
Comm Fndn AIDS Endowment Awards, 1088
Comm Fndn for Greater Buffalo Grants, 1090
Comm Fndn for Muskegon County Grants, 1093
Comm Fndn for Southern Arizona Grants, 1095
Comm Fndn of Broward Grants, 1100
Comm Fndn of Mount Vernon and Knox County Grants, 1119
Cooley's Anemia Research Fellowships, 1149
Coors Brewing Corp Contributions Grants, 1151
Cowles Charitable Trust Grants, 1155
CRI Clinical Investigator Award in Cancer Immunology, 1161
CRI Prostate Cancer Initiative Grants, 1163
Crohn's Disease and Ulcerative Colitis Senior Research Grants, 1165
CTCRI Idea Grants, 1170
Cudd Fndn Grants, 1171
Cystic Fibrosis Research Grants, 1179
D.F. Halton Fndn Grants, 1181
DAAD Research Stays for University Academics and Scientists, 1183
Dana Clinical Hypotheses Program in Brain and Immuno-Imaging Research Grants, 1195
Dana Fndn Science and Health Grants, 1197
Daniel Mendelsohn New Investigator Award, 1199
Davis Family Fndn Grants, 1204
Daywood Fndn Grants, 1206
Deafness Research Fndn Research Grants, 1208
Del E. Webb Fndn Grants, 1213
Della Martin Fndn Grants, 1219
DeMatteis Family Fndn Grants, 1221
Denton A. Cooley Fndn Grants, 1225
Dermatology Fndn Grants, 1236
Detroit Lions Charities Grants, 1241
DHHS AIDS and HIV Epidemiologic Research Studies Grants, 1244
DHHS Emergency Medical Services for Children (EMSC) Program, 1249
DHHS Health Care Systems Cost and Access Research and Development Grants, 1252
DHHS Neurodevelopmental Test Methods Research Grants, 1268
DHHS Oral Health Promotion Research Across the Lifespan, 1269
DHHS Primary Medical Care National Research Service Awards (NRSA), 1272
DHHS Priority Health Conditions Studies Initiative, 1273
DHHS Promoting Safe and Stable Families Grants, 1276
DHHS Universal Newborn Hearing Screening and Intervention, 1282
Dietetic Outcomes Research Study Grants, 1285
DOA National Integrated Food Safety Initiative, 1289
DOD Clinical Translational Research Grants, 1291
DOD Era of Hope Scholar Award, 1292
DOD HBCU/MI Partnership Training Award, 1293
DOD Idea Award for Breast Cancer Research, 1294
DOD Multidisciplinary Postdoctoral Award for Breast Cancer Research, 1295
DOD Predoctoral Traineeship in Breast Cancer Research, 1296
DOE Environmental Remediation Grants, 1297
DOE Health Effects and Life Sciences Research Grants, 1298
DOE Human Genome Program--Ethical, Legal, and Social Implications, 1299
DOE Low Dose Radiation Research Program, 1300
DOE Medical Applications and Measurement Science Grants, 1301
DOI Biological Resource Division Brucellosis Program, 1302
DOJ Mental Health and Juvenile Justice, 1304
Donaghue Practical Benefit Initiatives Grants, 1309
Donald and Sylvia Robinson Family Fndn Grants, 1310
Doris Duke Charitable Fndn Clinical Interfaces Award Program, 1314
Doris Duke Charitable Fndn Clinical Research Fellowships for Medical Students, 1315
Doris Duke Charitable Fndn Clinical Scientist Development Award, 1316
Doris Duke Charitable Fndn Clinical Scientist Development Award (CSDA) Bridge Grants, 1317
Doris Duke Charitable Fndn Distinguished Clinical Scientist Award Program, 1318
Doris Duke Charitable Fndn Operations Research on AIDS Care and Treatment in Africa (ORACTA) Grants, 1319
Dorothea Haus Ross Fndn Grants, 1320
Dorothy Rider Pool Health Care Grants, 1322
Dr. Bob and Jean Smith Fndn Grants, 1325
Drs. Bruce and Lee Fndn Grants, 1333
DSO Controlling Pathogen Evolution Workshop Grants, 1334
DSO Radiation Biodosimetry (RaBiD) Grants, 1335
Duchossois Family Fndn Grants, 1337
Duke Endowment Health Care Grants, 1338
Duke Energy Fndn Grants, 1339
Duke University Ambulatory and Regional Anesthesia Fellowships, 1341
Duke University Clinical Cardiac Electrophysiology Fellowships, 1342
Duke University Hyperbaric Center Fellowships, 1343
Duke University Interventional Cardiology Fellowships, 1344
Duke University Obstetric Anesthesia Fellowships, 1345
Duke University Pain Management Fellowships, 1346
Duke University Postdoctoral Research Fellowships in Aging, 1348
Dysautonomia Research Grants, 1353
E.D.Thomas Fellowship, 1359
Eberly Fndn Grants, 1364
Educational Fndn of America Grants, 1372
Edward Bangs Kelley and Elza Kelley Fndn Grants, 1373
Edward S. Moore Fndn Grants, 1374
Edwin S. Webster Fndn Grants, 1376
Edwin W. and Catherine M. Davis Fndn Grants, 1377
EF Predoctoral Research Training Fellowship, 1383
EIF Comm Grants, 1386
Elisabeth Severance Prentiss Fndn Grants, 1392
Elizabeth Glaser Pediatric AIDS Fndn International Leadership Awards, 1393
Elizabeth Glaser Pediatric AIDS Fndn Operations Research Grants, 1394
Elizabeth Glaser Pediatric AIDS Fndn Pediatric HIV Vaccine Research Grants, 1395
Elizabeth Glaser Pediatric AIDS Fndn Two-Year Scholar Awards, 1397
Elizabeth Glaser Scientist Award, 1398
Elizabeth McGraw Fndn Grants, 1399
Ellison Medical Fndn/AFAR Julie Martin Mid-Career Award in Aging Research, 1403
Ellison Medical Fndn/AFAR Postdoctoral Fellows in Aging Research Program, 1404
Ellison Medical Fndn/AFAR Senior Postdoctoral Fellows Research Program, 1405
Elmer L. and Eleanor J. Andersen Fndn Grants, 1406
Elsa U. Pardee Fndn Grants, 1407
EMBO Installation Grants, 1409
Emerson Charitable Trust Grants, 1412
EPA Baseline Assessment of Risks of Exposure to Lead Poisoning of Native American Children, 1419
EPA Lead Awareness Outreach for Native American Tribes, 1421
Epilepsy Research Fndn New Therapy Grants, 1423
Eppendorf & Science Prize for Neurobiology, 1424
Eppley Fndn Postdoctoral Grants, 1425
Eric Berne Fund for the Future Grants, 1426
Ethical Research Grants and Fellowships, 1431
Eugene McDermott Fndn Grants, 1435
Ewing Halsell Fndn Grants, 1440
F.M. Kirby Fndn Grants, 1443
Fairlawn Fndn Grants, 1447
FAR Fund, 1453
Farmers Insurance Group of Companies Grants, 1455
FCD Child Development Grants, 1458
FCER Chiropractic Research Grants, 1459

FCER Research Grants and Fellowships, 1460
FDA Orphan Products Clinical Studies Grants, 1462
FDHN Bridging Grants, 1464
FDHN Centocor International Research Fellowship in Gastrointestinal Inflammation & Immunology, 1465
FDHN Designated Outcomes Award in Geriatric Gastroenterology, 1466
FDHN Designated Research Award in Geriatric Gastroenterology, 1467
FDHN Designated Research Award in Research Related to Pancreatitis, 1468
FDHN Fellow Abstract Prizes, 1469
FDHN Funderburg Research Scholar Award in Gastric Biology Related to Cancer, 1471
FDHN Graduate Student Awards, 1472
FDHN Jon I. Isenberg International Research Scholar Award, 1473
FDHN June & Donald O. Castell MD, Esophageal Clinical Research Award, 1474
FDHN Moti L. & Kamla Rustgi International Travel Awards, 1475
FDHN Non-Career Research Awards, 1476
FDHN Non-Career Research Grants, 1477
FDHN Research Scholar Awards, 1478
FDHN TAP Endowed Designated Research Award in Acid-Related Diseases, 1481
FDHN Translational Research Awards, 1482
Feldman Fndn Grants, 1484
FIC International Cooperative Biodiversity Groups Grants, 1487
FIC International Research Scientist Development Award, 1491
FIC/NIH AIDS International Training and Research Program, 1496
FIC/ORMH Minority International Research Training Grants, 1497
Fidelity Fndn Grants, 1498
Field Psychology Research Grants, 1500
Fight for Sight Research Grants, 1502
Fight for Sight Research Grants and Fellowships, 1503
Fischelis Grants for Research in the History of American Pharmacy, 1507
Fishman Family Fndn Grants, 1510
Flinn Fndn Grantss, 1511
Forrest C. Lattner Fndn Grants, 1523
Fndn Fighting Blindness Marjorie Carr Adams Women's Career Development Awards, 1526
Fndn for Medical Research Grants, 1528
Fndn for Physical Therapy Research Grants, 1530
Fndn for Psychocultural Research Postdoctoral Fellowships, 1531
Fndn for Seacoast Health Grants, 1533
Fndn for the Carolinas Grants, 1535
Frank Stanley Beveridge Fndn Grants, 1553
Fraser-Parker Fndn Grants, 1555
Frederick Gardner Cottrell Fndn Grants, 1560
Fritz B. Burns Fndn Grants, 1564
Fulbright Alumni Initiatives Awards Program Grants, 1566
Fulbright New Century Scholars (NCS) Program Grants, 1570
Fyssen Fndn Postdoctoral Study Grants, 1580
Gates Global HIV/AIDS Vaccine Grants, 1583
GE & Science Prize for Young Life Scientists, 1584
Gebbie Fndn Grants, 1585
General Motors Fndn Grants Support Program, 1591
George B. Storer Fndn Grants, 1596
George Frederick Jewett Fndn Grants, 1599
George H. Hitchings New Investigator Award in Health Research, 1600
George Kress Fndn Grants, 1601
George S. and Dolores Dore Eccles Fndn Grants, 1602
Georgia Power Fndn Grants, 1603
Gerber Fndn Grants, 1606
Gertrude B. Elion Mentored Medical Student Research Awards, 1608
Gill Fndn - Gay and Lesbian Fund Grants, 1613
Glaucoma Fndn Grants, 1621
Glaucoma Research Pilot Project Grants, 1622
Glenn/AFAR Breakthroughs in Gerontology Awards, 1627
Glenn/AFAR Research Grants for Postdoctoral Fellows, 1628
Goddess Scholars Grants, 1630
Goldhirsh Fndn Brain Tumor Research Grants, 1634
Goldman Philanthropic Partnerships Program, 1635
GPP Charles E. Culpeper Fndn Biomedical Pilot Projects Initiative Grants, 1641
Grammy Fndn Grants, 1643
Green Fndn Grants, 1661
Greenspun Family Fndn Grants, 1664
Greenwall Fndn Bioethics Grants, 1665
Harold Simmons Fndn Grants, 1698
Harris and Eliza Kempner Fund Grants, 1699
Harry A. and Margaret D. Towsley Fndn Grants, 1701
Harry Frank Guggenheim Fndn Research Grants, 1704
Hartford Aging and Health Program Awards, 1709
Hartford Geriatrics Health Outcomes Research Scholars Program, 1712
Hawaii Comm Fndn Health Education and Research Grants, 1716
Hawn Fndn Grants, 1719
Health Care Financing Research, Demonstrations, and Evaluations Grants, 1723
Health Fndn of Southern Florida Responsive Grants, 1726
Healthcare Fndn of New Jersey Grants, 1729
HEI Grants, 1734
Heineman Fndn for Research, Education, Charitable and Scientific Purposes, 1735
Heiser Leprosy Research Grants, 1737
Helen Bader Fndn Grants, 1738
Hendrick Fndn for Children Grants, 1744
Hereditary Disease Fndn Lieberman Award, 1751
Hereditary Disease Fndn Research Grants, 1752
HHMI Biomedical Research Grants for International Scientists in Canada and Latin America, 1756
HHMI Biomedical Research Grants for International Scientists in the Baltics, Central and Eastern Europe, Russia, and Ukraine, 1757
HHMI Biomedical Research Grants for International Scientists: Infectious Diseases and Parasitology, 1758
HHMI Grants and Fellowships Programs, 1759
HHMI International Research Scholars Program, 1760
HHMI Med into Grad Initiative Grants, 1761
HHMI Physician-Scientist Early Career Award, 1762
HHMI-NIBIB Interfaces Initiative Grants, 1764
HHMI-NIH Cloister Research Scholars Program, 1765
HHMI/EMBO Start-up Grants for Central Europe, 1766
HHS Children's Hospitals Graduate Medical Education Payment Program, 1767
Hilda and Preston Davis Fndn Grants, 1772
Hill Crest Fndn Grants, 1773
Hirtzel Memorial Fndn Grants, 1781
Hoglund Fndn Grants, 1785
HomeBanc Fndn Grants, 1788
Hormel Fndn Grants, 1796
HRSA Eliminating Disparities in Perinatal Health Grants, 1803
HRSA Geriatric Education Centers, 1805
HRSA Hansen's Disease National Ambulatory Care Program Grants, 1806
Huie-Dellmon Trust Grants, 1815
Human Growth Fndn Small Grants, 1816
Hunter's Hope Fndn Grants, 1820
Huntington's Disease Society of America Research Grants, 1826
IAFF Burn Fndn Research Grants, 1830
IARC Expertise Transfer Fellowship, 1831
IARC Postdoctoral Fellowships for Training in Cancer Research, 1832
IARC Visiting Scientist Award for Senior Scientists, 1833
IATA Research Grants, 1834
Ignacio Martin-Baro Fund for Mental Health and Human Rights Grants, 1839
IHS Native American and Alaskan Native Health Research Centers, 1840
Impact 100 Grants, 1843
Implant Dentistry Research and Education Fndn Grants, 1844
Indiana 21st Century Research and Technology Fund Awards, 1850
Infinity Fndn Grants, 1854
Innovative Technology Development Award Program, 1855
International College of Surgeons Grants and Scholarships, 1859
International Essential Tremor Fndn Grants, 1860
International Spinal Research Trust Grants, 1863
Ireland Family Fndn Grants, 1865
Ittleson Fndn AIDS Grants, 1869
Ittleson Fndn Mental Health Grants, 1870
J.B. Reynolds Fndn Grants, 1873
J.W. Kieckhefer Fndn Grants, 1878
Jacob and Hilda Blaustein Fndn Grants, 1881
Jacob and Valeria Langeloth Fndn Grants, 1882
James H. Cummings Fndn Grants, 1888
James M. Collins Fndn Grants, 1891
James R. Dougherty Jr. Fndn Grants, 1894
James S. McDonnell Fndn Brain Cancer Research Collaborative Activity Awards, 1896
James S. McDonnell Fndn Complex Systems Collaborative Activity Awards, 1897
James S. McDonnell Fndn Research Grants, 1898
James S. McDonnell Fndn Scholar Awards, 1899
James S. McDonnell Fndn Understanding Human Cognition Awards, 1900
Jane Beattie Memorial Scholarship, 1901
Japan Heart Fndn Grants, 1906
Jeffress Research Grants, 1913
Jessie Ball Dupont Fund Grants, 1919
Jewish Women's Fndn of New York Grants, 1924
JM Fndn Grants, 1926
Joe W. and Dorothy Dorsett Brown Fndn Grants, 1927
John Deere Fndn Grants, 1929
John Merck Scholars Awards, 1941
John P. McGovern Fndn Grants, 1942
John S. Dunn Research Fndn Grants and Chairs, 1945
John W. Alden Trust Grants, 1947
Johnson & Johnson Corp Contributions Grants, 1952
Joseph Alexander Fndn Grants, 1957
Josephine Goodyear Fndn Grants, 1964
Josiah W. and Bessie H. Kline Fndn Grants, 1967
Joyce Fndn Grants, 1969
Judith and Jean Pape Adams Charitable Fndn ALS Grants, 1970
June Allyson Fndn Research Fellowships, 1972
Kavli Fndn Research Grants, 1985
Kenneth T. and Eileen L. Norris Fndn Grants, 1989
Kettering Fund Grants, 1992
Kevin P. and Sydney B. Knight Family Fndn Grants, 1993
KFC Allied Health Research Grants, 1996
KFC Biomedical Research Grants, 1998
KFC Nephrology and Urology Scholarships, 1999
Kimmel Scholar Award, 2002
Komen Greater NYC Clinical Trials Enrollment Grants, 2010
Komen Greater NYC Comm Breast Health Grants, 2011

Komen Greater NYC Conference Grants, 2012
Lalor Fndn Postdoctoral Research Grants, 2021
LAM Fndn Established Investigator Awards, 2022
LAM Fndn Pilot Project Awards, 2023
LAM Fndn Research Grants, 2024
Lance Armstrong Fndn Research Grants, 2026
Larry L. Hillblom Fndn Grants, 2031
Laura B. Vogler Fndn Grants, 2032
Lawrence S. Huntington Fund Grants, 2035
Leadership in Education in Neurodevelopmental Disabilities Postdoctoral Fellowships, 2037
Leahi Fund, 2038
Learning and Behavioral Disorders Research Grants, 2039
Leland McSpadden Memorial Fund for Medical and Scientific Research Grants, 2041
Leo Goodwin Fndn Grants, 2043
Lesbian Health Fund Grants, 2046
Leukemia and Lymphoma Society Research Grants, 2051
Lillian S. Wells Fndn Grants, 2056
Lindbergh Grants, 2059
Little Life Fndn Grants, 2060
Littlefield-AACR Grants in Metastatic Colon Cancer Research, 2061
LRF New Investigator Leukemia Research Grants, 2070
LSA Translational Research Program Grants, 2078
Lubbock Area Fndn Grants, 2079
Lubrizol Fndn Grants, 2080
Lucile Horton Howe and Mitchell B. Howe Fndn Grants, 2081
Lupus Fndn of America Research Grants, 2085
Lustgarten Fndn for Pancreatic Cancer Research Grants, 2086
Lymphoma Research Fndn Fellowships, 2087
Lymphoma Research Fndn Grants, 2088
Lynde and Harry Bradley Fndn Grants, 2089
M. Bastian Family Fndn Grants, 2092
M.J. Murdock Charitable Trust Grants, 2095
Mabel H. Flory Charitable Trust Grants, 2096
Mabel Y. Hughes Charitable Trust Grants, 2097
Marcia and Otto Koehler Fndn Grants, 2103
Margaret L. Wendt Fndn Grants, 2104
Margaret T. Morris Fndn Grants, 2105
Margoes Fndn Grants, 2106
Marijuana Policy Project Grants, 2107
Marjorie C. Adams Charitable Trust Grants, 2111
Mark and Catherine Winkler Fndn Grants, 2112
Marshall Field's Comm Grants, 2115
Mary Kay Ash Charitable Fndn Grants, 2120
Mary S. and David C. Corbin Fndn Grants, 2122
Massage Therapy Fndn Practitioner Case Report Contest, 2125
Massage Therapy Fndn Research Grants, 2126
Massage Therapy Research Grants, 2127
Matilda R. Wilson Fund Grants, 2128
Mattel Children's Fndn Grants, 2130
Mattel International Grants, 2131
Max and Victoria Dreyfus Fndn Grants, 2133
Max Bell Fndn Grants, 2134
McCarthy Family Fndn Grants, 2141
McCombs Fndn Grants, 2142
McGregor Fund Grants, 2143
McLean Contributionship Grants, 2147
MDA Development Grant, 2150
MDA Neuromuscular Disease Research Grants, 2151
MDBD Basic Research Grants, 2152
MDBD Research Grants and Basil O'Connor Starter Scholar Award Program, 2153
MDBD Research Prize in Developmental Biology, 2154
Mead Johnson Nutritionals Medical Education Grants, 2158
Mead Johnson Nutritionals Scholarships, 2159
Meadows Fndn Grants, 2161
Medicaid Infrastructure Grants to Support Employment of People with Disabilities, 2163
MedImmune Charitable Grants, 2166
Melanoma Research Fndn Grants, 2170
Mericos Fndn Grants, 2172
Mesothelioma Applied Research Fndn Grants, 2174
Meyer Memorial Trust Operating Funds Grants, 2180
Meyer Memorial Trust Responsive Grants, 2181
MGFA Post-Doctoral Research Fellowships, 2183
MGFA Student Fellowships, 2184
Michael J. Fox Fndn Clinical Discovery Grants, 2190
Michael J. Fox Fndn for Parkinson's Research LEAPS Program, 2191
Michael J. Fox Fndn Parkinson's Cell Line Research Grants, 2192
Microsoft Research Cell Phone as a Platform for Healthcare Grants, 2195
Miguel Aleman Fndn Grants, 2197
Milheim Fndn Cancer Research Grants, 2200
Military Medical Research and Development Grants, 2202
Millipore Fndn Grants, 2203
Millipore/Charles P. Schaufus Parenteral-Processing Technology Research Grant, 2204
MMRF Research Grants, 2211
MNI Jeanne Timmins Fellowships, 2212
Monfort Family Fndn Grants, 2213
Morgan Adams Fndn Grants, 2216
Morton K. and Jane Blaustein Fndn Grants, 2218
Mount Zion Health Fund Grants, 2220
MSSC Research Grants, 2226
NAF Kyle Bryant Translational Research Award, 2231
NAF Research Grants, 2232
NAF Young Investigator Awards, 2233
NAPNAP Fndn Graduate Student Research Grant, 2236
NAPNAP Fndn Nursing Research Grants, 2241
Narcolepsy Network Seed Grants, 2245
NARSAD Distinguished Investigator Award, 2246
NARSAD Independent Investigator Award, 2247
National Blood Fndn Research Grants, 2249
National Emergency Medicine Association Grants, 2252
National Headache Fndn Research Grants, 2253
National Headache Fndn Seymour Diamond Clinical Fellowship in Headache Education, 2254
National Heart Fndn of New Zealand Grants, 2255
National Lottery Comm Fund Grants, 2256
National MPS Society Grants, 2257
National Patient Safety Fndn Patient Safety Research Grants, 2258
National Psoriasis Fndn Research Grants, 2259
National Sleep Fndn Pickwick Postdoctoral Fellowship, 2260
NBME Stemmler Medical Education Research Fund Grants, 2263
NCCAM Exploratory Developmental Grants for Complementary and Alternative Medicine (CAM) Studies of Humans, 2265
NCCAM Translational Tools for Clinical Studies of CAM Interventions Grants, 2267
NCI Academic-Industrial Partnerships for Development and Validation of In Vivo Imaging Systems and Methods for Cancer Investigations, 2268
NCI Application and Use of Transformative Emerging Technologies in Cancer Research, 2269
NCI Application of Metabolomics for Translational and Biological Research Grants, 2270
NCI Basic Cancer Research in Cancer Health Disparities Grants, 2271
NCI Diet, Epigenetic Events, and Cancer Prevention Grants, 2272
NCI Engineered Isogenic Cell Lines with Relevant Cancer Targets Research Grants, 2273
NCI Exploratory Grants for Behavioral Research in Cancer Control, 2274
NCI Improving Diet and Physical Activity Assessment Grants, 2275
NCI Mentored Career Development Award to Promote Diversity, 2276
NCI Ruth L. Kirschstein National Research Service Award (NRSA) Institutional Research Training Grants, 2277
NCI Stages of Breast Development: Normal to Metastatic Disease Grants, 2278
NCIC Canadian Cancer Society Research Grants, 2282
NCRR Networks and Pathways Collaborative Research Projects Grants, 2287
NCRR Novel Approaches to Enhance Animal Stem Cell Research, 2288
NEDA/AED Charron Family Research Grant, 2289
NEDA/AED Joan Wismer Research Grant, 2290
NEDA/AED Tampa Bay Eating Disorders Task Force Award, 2291
NEI Clinical Study Planning Grant, 2292
NEI Clinical Vision Research Development Award, 2293
NEI Research Grant For Secondary Data Analysis Grants, 2296
NEI Ruth L. Kirschstein National Research Service Award Short-Term Institutional Research Training Grants, 2297
NEI Translational Research Program On Therapy For Visual Disorders, 2299
NEI Vision Research Core Grants, 2300
Nell Warren Elkin and William Simpson Elkin Fndn, 2302
NFID Advanced Vaccinology Course Travel Grant, 2307
NFX Patient-Oriented Research Grants, 2313
NHGRI Mentored Research Scientist Development Award, 2315
NHLBI Airway Smooth Muscle Function and Targeted Therapeutics in Human Asthma Grants, 2316
NHLBI Ancillary Studies in Clinical Trials, 2317
NHLBI Bioengineering and Obesity Grants, 2318
NHLBI Bioengineering Approaches to Energy Balance and Obesity Grants for SBIR, 2319
NHLBI Bioengineering Approaches to Energy Balance and Obesity Grants for STTR, 2320
NHLBI Biomedical Research Training Program for Individuals from Underrepresented Groups, 2321
NHLBI Blood Diseases and Resources Research Grants, 2322
NHLBI Cardiac Development Consortium Grants, 2323
NHLBI Career Enhancement Awards for Stem Cell Research, 2325
NHLBI Career Transition Award, 2326
NHLBI Characterizing the Blood Stem Cell Niche Grants, 2327
NHLBI Childhood Obesity Prevention and Treatment Research Consortium Grants, 2328
NHLBI Childhood Obesity Prevention and Treatment Research Coordinating Unit Grants, 2329
NHLBI Circadian-Coupled Cellular Function in Heart, Lung, and Blood Tissue Grants, 2330
NHLBI Clinical Centers for the NHLBI Asthma Network (AsthmaNet) Grants, 2331
NHLBI Developmental Origins of Altered Lung Physiology and Immune Function Grants, 2332
NHLBI Elucidating Nature's Solutions to Heart, Lung, and Blood Diseases and Sleep Disorder Processes Research Grants, 2333
NHLBI Exploratory Studies in the Neurobiology of Pain in Sickle Cell Disease, 2334
NHLBI Hyperglycemic Exacerbation of Ischemia/Reperfusion Injury after Ischemic Insult Grants, 2335
NHLBI Hypersensitivity Pneumonitis – Grants for Early Identification and Mechanisms of Disease, 2336
NHLBI Immunomodulatory, Inflammatory, and Vasoregulatory Properties of Transfused Red

Blood Cell Units as a Function of Preparation and Storage Grants, 2337
NHLBI Improving Heart Failure Disease Management Grants, 2338
NHLBI Independent Scientist Award, 2339
NHLBI Individual Postdoctoral National Research Service Awards, 2340
NHLBI Individual Predoctoral Fellowships to Promote Diversity in Health-Related Research, 2341
NHLBI Integrating Lung Genetics and Genomics in Human Populations Grants, 2342
NHLBI Intramural Research Training Awards, 2343
NHLBI Investigator Initiated Multi-Site Clinical Trials, 2344
NHLBI Lymphatic Biology in Health and Disease Grants, 2345
NHLBI Mentored Career Award for Faculty at Minority Institutions, 2347
NHLBI Mentored Career Development Award to Promote Faculty Diversity/Re-Entry in Biomedical Research, 2348
NHLBI Mentored Clinical Scientist Research Career Development Awards, 2349
NHLBI Mentored Patient-Oriented Research Career Development Awards, 2350
NHLBI Mentored Quantitative Research Career Development Awards, 2351
NHLBI Microbiome of the Lung and Respiratory Tract in HIV-Infected Individuals and HIV-Uninfected Controls, 2352
NHLBI Midcareer Investigator Award in Patient-Oriented Research, 2353
NHLBI Minority Institution Research Scientist Development Award, 2354
NHLBI Multidisciplinary Translational Research in Critical Care Grants, 2356
NHLBI National Research Service Awards for Senior Fellowships, 2358
NHLBI New Approaches to Arrhythmia Detection and Treatment Grants for SBIR, 2359
NHLBI New Approaches to Arrhythmia Detection and Treatment Grants for STTR, 2360
NHLBI Nutrition and Diet in the Causation, Prevention, and Management of Heart Failure Research Grants, 2361
NHLBI Pathogenesis And Treatment Of Lymphedema And Lymphatic Diseases Grants, 2362
NHLBI Pathway to Independence Award, 2363
NHLBI Pediatric Cardiac Genomics Consortium Grants, 2364
NHLBI Phase II Clinical Trials of Novel Therapies for Lung Diseases, 2365
NHLBI Prematurity and Respiratory Outcomes Program (PROP) Grants, 2366
NHLBI Progenitor Cell Biology Consortium Administrative Coordinating Center Grants, 2367
NHLBI Progenitor Cell Biology Consortium Research Hubs, 2368
NHLBI Protein Interactions Governing Membrane Transport in Pulmonary Health and Disease Grants, 2369
NHLBI Research Demonstration and Dissemination Grants, 2370
NHLBI Research Grants on the Relationship Between Hypertension and Inflammation, 2371
NHLBI Research on the Role of Cardiomyocyte Mitochondria in Heart Disease: An Integrated Approach, 2372
NHLBI Research Supplements to Promote Diversity in Health-Related Research (Postdoctoral Individuals/New Independent Researchers), 2373
NHLBI Research Supplements to Promote Diversity in Health-Related Research for Established Investigators Who Become Disabled, 2374
NHLBI Research Supplements to Promote Diversity in Health-Related Research for Graduate Research Assistants, 2375
NHLBI Research Supplements to Promote Diversity in Health-Related Research for Individuals in Postdoctoral Training, 2376
NHLBI Research Supplements to Promote Diversity in Health-Related Research for Undergraduate Students, 2377
NHLBI Right Heart Function in Health and Chronic Lung Diseases Grants, 2378
NHLBI Ruth L. Kirschstein National Research Service Award (NRSA) Institutional Research Training Grants, 2379
NHLBI Ruth L. Kirschstein National Research Service Award Short-Term Institutional Research Training Grants, 2380
NHLBI Sarcoidosis: Research Grants into the Cause of Multi-Organ Disease and Clinical Strategies for Therapy, 2382
NHLBI Stress Management Interventions to Reduce Risk of Coronary Artery Disease, 2384
NHLBI Summer Institute for Training in Biostatistics II, 2385
NHLBI Summer Internship Program in Biomedical Research, 2386
NHLBI Targeted Approaches to Weight Control for Young Adults Grants, 2387
NHLBI Targeting Calcium Regulatory Molecules for Arrhythmia Prevention Grants, 2388
NHLBI Transfusion-Related Acute Lung Injury (TRALI) Basic Research Grants, 2389
NHLBI Translating Basic Behavioral and Social Science Discoveries into Interventions to Reduce Obesity: Centers for Behavioral Intervention Development Grants, 2390
NHLBI Translational Programs in Lung Diseases, 2391
NIA Aging Research Dissertation Awards to Increase Diversity, 2392
NIA Aging, Oxidative Stress and Cell Death Grants, 2393
NIA AIDS and Aging: Behavioral Sciences Prevention Research Grants, 2394
NIA Alzheimer's Disease Core Centers Grants, 2395
NIA Alzheimer's Disease Drug Development Program Grants, 2396
NIA Alzheimer's Disease Pilot Clinical Trials, 2397
NIA Alzheimer's Disease Research Centers Grants, 2398
NIA Archiving and Development of Socialbehavioral Datasets in Aging Related Studies Grants, 2399
NIA Awards to Support Research on the Biology of Aging in Invertebrates Grants, 2400
NIA Behavioral and Social Research Grants on Disasters and Health, 2401
NIA Bioenergetics, Fatigability, and Activity Limitations in Aging, 2402
NIA Diversity in Medication Use and Outcomes in Aging Populations Grants, 2403
NIA Effects of Gene-Social Environment Interplay on Health and Behavior in Later Life Grants, 2404
NIA Factors Affecting Cognitive Function in Adults with Down Syndrome Grants, 2405
NIA Grants for Alzheimer's Disease Drug Discovery, 2406
NIA Harmonization of Longitudinal Cross-National Surveys of Aging Grants, 2407
NIA Health Behaviors and Aging Grants, 2408
NIA Healthy Aging through Behavioral Economic Analyses of Situations Grants, 2409
NIA Higher-Order Cognitive Functioning and Aging Grants, 2410
NIA Human Biospecimen Resources for Aging Research Grants, 2411
NIA Independent Scientist Award, 2412
NIA Malnutrition in Older Persons Research Grants, 2413
NIA Mechanisms Underlying the Links between Psychosocial Stress, Aging, the Brain and the Body Grants, 2414
NIA Mechanisms, Measurement, and Management of Pain in Aging: from Molecular to Clinical, 2415
NIA Medical Management of Older Patients with HIV/AIDS Grants, 2416
NIA Mentored Clinical Scientist Research Career Development Awards, 2417
NIA Minority Dissertation Research Grants in Aging, 2419
NIA Multicenter Study on Exceptional Survival in Families: The Long Life Family Study (LLFS) Grants, 2420
NIA NRSAs--Institutional Training Awards, 2423
NIA Paul Beeson Career Development Awards in Aging, 2424
NIA Postdoctoral Training in Research on Aging in Canada, 2426
NIA Promoting Careers in Aging and Health Disparities Research Grants, 2427
NIA Prostate Cancer Aging, Race, and Ethnicity Research Grants, 2428
NIA Renal Function and Chronic Kidney Disease in Aging Grants, 2429
NIA Research Grants on Chemical Senses: Neurotransmitters and Neuromodulators, 2430
NIA Role of Apolipoprotein E, Lipoprotein Receptors and CNS Lipid Homeostasis in Brain Aging and Alzheimer's Disease, 2431
NIA Role of Nuclear Receptors in Tissue and Organismal Aging Grants, 2432
NIA Significance of Sarcopenia in Old Age Grants, 2433
NIA Sociobehavorial Data Analysis and Archiving in Aging, 2434
NIA Symptom Management for Chronic Neurological Conditions Research Grants, 2436
NIA Thyroid in Aging Grants, 2437
NIA Transdisciplinary Research on Fatigue and Fatigability in Aging Grants, 2438
NIA Translational Research at the Aging/Cancer Interface (TRACI) Grants, 2439
NIA Vulnerable Dendrites and Synapses in Aging and Alzheimer's Disease Grants, 2440
NIA/NIEHS Biomedical Epidemiologic and Intervention Studies Planning Grants, 2441
NIAAA Hepatitis C Infection and Alcoholic Liver Disease, 2442
NIAAA Independent Scientist Award, 2443
NIAAA Mechanisms of Alcohol and Drug-Induced Pancreatitis Grants, 2444
NIAAA Mechanisms of Alcohol-Induced Hepatic Fibrosis Research Grants, 2445
NIAAA Mentored Clinical Scientist Research Career Development Awards, 2446
NIAAA Peptide Regulation of Alcohol Intake, 2447
NIAAA Secondary Analysis of Existing Health Services Data Sets Grants, 2448
NIAID Allergy, Immunology, Transplantation, Infectious Diseases, and AIDS NRSAs--Individual, 2450
NIAID Challenge Grants: Joint Ventures in Biomedicine and Biotechnology, 2451
NIAID Enhancing Vaccine-Elicited Protective Immunity in Malaria Research Grants, 2452
NIAID HIV Prevention Trial Units Grants, 2453
NIAID HIV Vaccine Clinical Trial Units Grants, 2454
NIAID HIV Vaccine Research and Design--Program Project Grants, 2455
NIAID Independent Scientist Award, 2456
NIAID Integrated Preclinical/Clinical AIDS Vaccine Development Grants, 2457
NIAID Laboratory Methods to Assess Responses to HIV Vaccine Candidates Research Grants, 2458

NIAID Microbiology and Infectious Diseases Research Grants and Contracts, 2459
NIAID Pediatric Clinical Trials Program for AIDS, 2460
NIAID Preparedness against Illegitimate Use of Bacterial Pathogens, 2461
NIAID Small Business Innovation Research Advanced Technology Grants, 2463
NIAID Statistical Methods in HIV and AIDS Research Grants, 2464
NIAID Therapeutics Research on AIDS-Associated Opportunistic Infections, 2465
NIAMS Clinical Trial Planning Grants, 2466
NIAMS Exploratory Developmental Grants for Multidisciplinary Clinical Studies of Sarcopenia, 2469
NIAMS High Risk Arthritis and Musculoskeletal and Skin Diseases Research, 2470
NIAMS Low-Back Pain and Common Spinal Disorders Research Grants, 2471
NIAMS Mechanisms of Chondroprotection Research Grants, 2472
NIAMS Molecular Pathogenesis and New Interventions in Scleroderma, 2473
NIAMS Pathogenesis and Therapy of the Muscular Dystrophies Research Grants, 2474
NIAMS Repetitive Motion Disorders Research Grants, 2475
NIAMS Research on Musculoskeletal Fitness and Sports Medicine Grants, 2476
NIAMS Significance of Sarcopenia in Old Age Grants, 2477
NIAMS/NICHD Deep Infections of Total Joint Replacements, 2481
NICHD Central Nervous System Effects of HIV Infection: Neurobiological, Neurovirological, and Neurobehavioral Studies Grants, 2482
NICHD Cooperative Specialized Infertility Research Centers, 2484
NICHD Innovative Therapies and Clinical Studies for Screenable Disorders Grants, 2485
NICHD Low-Back Pain and Common Spinal Disorders Research Grants, 2486
NICHD Medical Rehabilitation Research, 2487
NICHD NRSAs--Individual, 2488
NICHD NRSAs--Institutional, 2489
NICHD Repetitive Motion Disorders Research Grants, 2491
NICHD Research on Musculoskeletal Fitness and Sports Medicine Grants, 2492
NICHD Ruth L. Kirschstein National Research Service Award (NRSA) Institutional Predoctoral Training Program in Systems Biology of Developmental Biology & Birth Defects, 2493
NICHD Small Grants, 2494
NICHD Socioeconomic Status and Health Across the Life Course, 2495
NICHD Symptom Management for Chronic Neurological Conditions Research Grants, 2496
NIDA Behavioral Science Track Awards for Rapid Transition, 2498
NIDA Behavioral Therapies Development Program Grants, 2499
NIDA Clinical Research Education Programs in Drug Abuse and Addiction, 2500
NIDA Cutting-Edge Basic Research Awards (CEBRA), 2501
NIDA Drug Abuse Dissertation Research: Epidemiology, Prevention, Treatment, Services, and Women and Gender Differences, 2502
NIDA Drug Addiction Neuroscience Research Grants, 2503
NIDA HIV Drug Therapy for HIV Users: Access, Adherence, Effectiveness, 2504
NIDA International Studies on Drug Abuse and HIV/AIDS, 2505
NIDA Medications Development for Cannabis-Related Disorder, 2506
NIDA Microarray-Based Research on Drug Abuse, 2508
NIDA National Drug Abuse Treatment Clinical Trials Network, 2510
NIDA Neurobiological and Behavioral Research on Nicotine and Tobacco Products, 2511
NIDA Origins and Pathways to Drug Abuse Research Grants, 2512
NIDA Pilot and Feasibility Studies in Preparation for Drug Abuse Prevention Trials, 2513
NIDA Role of Limbic System and Brain Ontogeny in Drug Abuse Research Grants, 2514
NIDA Transition from Drug Abuse to Drug Addiction, 2516
NIDCD Clinical Trial Planning Grant, 2517
NIDCD Communicative Competence of Users of Augmentative and Alternative Communication Systems Research Grants, 2518
NIDCD Exploratory Research: Feasibility Pilot Studies Grants, 2519
NIDCD Exploratory/Developmental Research Grants, 2520
NIDCD Health Promotion and Disease Prevention: Health Communication, Development, and Dissemination, 2521
NIDCD Mentored Clinical Scientist Research Career Development Award, 2522
NIDCD Mentored Research Scientist Development Award, 2523
NIDCD Molecular and Cellular Pathology of the Human Auditory and Vestibular Systems Grants, 2525
NIDCD Neurobiology and Genetics of Autism Grants, 2526
NIDCD Physiologic and Molecular Bases of Tinnitus Research Grants, 2527
NIDCD Program for Postdoctoral Research Training in Clinical Trials, 2528
NIDCD Research Grants on Chemical Senses: Neurotransmitters and Neuromodulators, 2530
NIDCD Small Grants, 2531
NIDCD Symptom Management for Chronic Neurological Conditions Research Grants, 2532
NIDCR Clinical Trial Pilot Grant, 2533
NIDCR Clinical Trial Planning Grant, 2534
NIDCR HIV/AIDS Associated Oral Viral Infections, 2535
NIDCR International Collaborative Oral Health Research Planning Grant, 2536
NIDCR Oral Microbiology/Immunology of Type 1 Diabetes, 2537
NIDCR Priorities in Behavioral Research in Cancer Prevention and Control Grants, 2538
NIDDK Advances in Polycystic Kidney Disease Grants, 2539
NIDDK Ancillary Studies of Kidney Disease Accessing Information from Clinical Trials, Epidemiological Studies, and Databases Grants, 2540
NIDDK Ancillary Studies to Major Ongoing NIDDK and NHLBI Clinical Research Studies, 2541
NIDDK Basic and Clinical Studies of Congenital Urinary Tract Obstruction Grants, 2542
NIDDK Basic Research Grants in the Bladder and Lower Urinary Tract, 2543
NIDDK Calcium Oxalate Stone Diseases Grants, 2544
NIDDK Cell-Specific Delineation of Prostate and Genitourinary Development, 2545
NIDDK Co-Activators and Co-Repressors in Gene Expression Grants, 2546
NIDDK Collaborative Interdisciplinary Team Science in Diabetes, Endocrinology and Metabolic Diseases Grants, 2547
NIDDK Development of Assays for High-Throughput Drug Screening Grants, 2548
NIDDK Development of Disease Biomarkers Grants, 2549
NIDDK Developmental Biology and Regeneration of the Liver Grants, 2550
NIDDK Diabetes Research Centers, 2551
NIDDK Diabetes, Endocrinology, and Metabolic Diseases NRSAs--Individual, 2552
NIDDK Diet Composition and Energy Balance Grants, 2553
NIDDK Education Program Grants, 2554
NIDDK Endoscopic Clinical Research Grants In Pancreatic And Biliary Diseases, 2555
NIDDK Enhancing Zebrafish Research with Research Tools and Techniques, 2556
NIDDK Erythroid Lineage Molecular Toolbox Grants, 2557
NIDDK Erythropoiesis: Components and Mechanisms Grants, 2558
NIDDK Exploratory/Developmental Clinical Research Grants in Obesity, 2559
NIDDK Grants for Basic Research in Glomerular Diseases, 2560
NIDDK Identifying and Reducing Diabetes and Obesity Related Health Disparities within Healthcare Systems, 2561
NIDDK Insulin Signaling and Receptor Cross Talk Grants, 2562
NIDDK Intestinal Failure, Short Gut Syndrome and Small Bowel Transplantation Grants, 2563
NIDDK Intestinal Stem Cell Consortium Grants, 2564
NIDDK Mentored Research Scientist Development Award, 2565
NIDDK Multi-Center Clinical Study Cooperative Agreements, 2566
NIDDK Multi-Center Clinical Study Implementation Planning Grants, 2567
NIDDK Neurobiology of Diabetic Complications Grants, 2568
NIDDK Neuroimaging in Obesity Research Grants, 2569
NIDDK New Technologies for Liver Disease SBIR, 2570
NIDDK New Technologies for Liver Disease STTR, 2571
NIDDK Non-Invasive Methods for Diagnosis and Progression of Diabetes, Kidney, Urological, Hematological and Digestive Diseases, 2572
NIDDK Pancreatic Development and Regeneration Grants: Toward Cellular Therapies for Diabetes, 2573
NIDDK Pilot and Feasibility Clinical Research Grants in Diabetes, Endocrine and Metabolic Diseases, 2574
NIDDK Pilot and Feasibility Clinical Research Grants in Kidney or Urologic Diseases, 2575
NIDDK Pilot and Feasibility Clinical Research Studies in Digestive Diseases and Nutrition, 2576
NIDDK Planning Grants For Translational Research For The Prevention And Control Of Diabetes And Obesity, 2577
NIDDK Proteomics: Diabetes, Obesity, And Endocrine, Digestive, Kidney, Urologic, And Hematologic Diseases, 2578
NIDDK Race/Ethnic Disparities in the Incidence of Diabetes Complications, 2579
NIDDK Research Grants for Studies of Hepatitis C in the Setting of Renal Disease, 2580
NIDDK Research Grants on Improving Health Care for Obese Patients, 2581
NIDDK Role of Gastrointestinal Surgical Procedures in Amelioration of Obesity-Related Insulin Resistance and Diabetes Independent of Weight Loss, 2582
NIDDK Secondary Analyses in Obesity, Diabetes and Digestive and Kidney Diseases Grants, 2583
NIDDK Seeding Collaborative Interdisciplinary Team Science in Diabetes, Endocrinology and Metabolic Diseases Grants, 2584
NIDDK Silvio O. Conte Digestive Diseases Research Core Centers Grants, 2585
NIDDK Small Business Innovation Research to Develop New Therapeutics and Monitoring Technologies for Type 1 Diabetes (T1D)--Towards an Artificial Pancreas (SBIR), 2586

NIDDK Small Grants for K08/K23 Recipients, 2587
NIDDK Small Grants for Underrepresented Minority Scientists in Diabetes and Digestive and Kidney Diseases, 2588
NIDDK Traditional Conference Grants, 2589
NIDDK Training in Clinical Investigation in Kidney and Urology Grants, 2590
NIDDK Translational Research for the Prevention and Control of Diabetes and Obesity, 2591
NIDDK Transmission of Human Immunodeficiency Virus (HIV) In Semen, 2592
NIDDK Type 2 Diabetes in the Pediatric Population Research Grants, 2593
NIDRR Field-Initiated Projects, 2594
NIEHS Applied Toxicological Research and Testing Grants, 2595
NIEHS Biological Response to Environmental Health Hazards Research Grants, 2596
NIEHS Carcinogenicity of Drinking Water Disinfection By-Products, 2597
NIEHS Environmental Justice: Partnerships for Communication, 2598
NIEHS Hazardous Materials Worker Health and Safety Training Grants, 2599
NIEHS Hazmat Training at Doe Nuclear Weapons Complex Grants, 2600
NIEHS Independent Scientist Award, 2601
NIEHS SBIR E-Learning for HAZMAT and Emergency Response Grants, 2604
NIEHS Small Business Innovation Research (SBIR) Program Grants, 2605
NIEHS Structure-Function Relationships of Environmentally Relevant Genetic Variants Research Grants, 2606
NIEHS/NINDS Role of the Environment in Parkinson's Disease, 2608
NIGMS Exploratory Studies for High Risk/High Impact Research Grants, 2609
NIGMS Fellowships in Quantitative Biology, 2610
NIGMS Individual Postdoctoral NRSA Fellowships in Clinical Pharmacology, 2611
NIGMS Institutional Research and Academic Career Development Award, 2614
NIGMS Integrative and Collaborative Approaches to Research Grants, 2615
NIGMS Large-Scale Collaborative Project Awards, 2616
NIGMS Mentored Clinical Scientist Research Career Development Awards, 2618
NIGMS Molecular Pharmacology of Anesthetic Action Research Grants, 2621
NIGMS Pharmacogenomics Research Network Grants, 2623
NIGMS Pilot Projects for the Protein Structure Initiative (Structural Genomics), 2624
NIGMS Quantitative Approaches to the Analysis of Complex Biological Systems, 2626
NIGMS Ruth L. Kirschstein National Research Service Awards for Individual Predoctoral Fellows in PharmD/PhD Grants, 2627
NIGMS Short Courses on Mathematical, Statistical, and Computational Tools for Studying Biological Systems, 2629
NIGMS Supplements for the Study of Complex Biological Systems, 2630
NIGMS Support of Competitive Research (SCORE) Pilot Project Awards, 2631
NIGMS Support of Competitive Research (SCORE) Research Advancement Awards, 2632
NIGMS/NIDCR Evolution of Infectious Diseases Research Grants, 2633
NIH Academic Research Enhancement Awards (AREA), 2635
NIH Alzheimer's Disease Clinical Trial Planning Grant, 2636
NIH Autism and Autism Spectrum Disorders Research, 2637
NIH Biobehavioral Pain Research Grants, 2638
NIH Biobehavioral Research for Effective Sleep, 2639
NIH Bioengineering Nanotechnology Initiative, 2640
NIH Biology, Development, and Progression of Malignant Prostate Disease Research Grants, 2641
NIH Biomedical Research on the International Space Station, 2642
NIH Bone and the Hematopoietic and Immune Systems Research Grants, 2643
NIH Building Interdisciplinary Research Careers in Women's Health Grants, 2644
NIH Cancer Surveillance Using Health Claims-Based Data System Grants, 2645
NIH Career Development Awards: Child Abuse and Neglect Research, 2646
NIH Centers for AIDS Research (CFARs), 2647
NIH Clinical Bioethics Postdoctoral Fellowships, 2649
NIH Collaborations for Advanced Strategies in Complication of HIV Infection, 2651
NIH Complementary and Alternative Medicine Postdoctoral Training Grants, 2652
NIH Demographic Research on Sexual Behaviors Related to HIV, 2653
NIH Dietary Supplement Research Centers: Botanicals Grants, 2654
NIH Earth-Based Research Relevant to the Space Environment, 2655
NIH Ecology of Infectious Diseases, 2656
NIH Economic Studies in Cancer Prevention, Screening, and Care, 2657
NIH Endocrine Disruptors: Epidemiologic Approaches Grants, 2658
NIH Enhancing Adherence to Diabetes Self-Management Behaviors, 2659
NIH Epidemiological and Behavioral Research in Oral Health, 2660
NIH Ethical Issues in Human Studies Research Grants, 2661
NIH Exceptional, Unconventional Research Enabling Knowledge Acceleration (EUREKA) Grants, 2662
NIH Exploratory Centers for Alternative Medicine Research Grants, 2663
NIH Exploratory Innovations in Biomedical Computational Science and Technology (BISTI) Grants, 2664
NIH Exploratory/Development Grants for Mental Health Intervention Research, 2665
NIH Exploratory/Developmental Research Grant, 2666
NIH Fine Mapping and Function of Genes for Type 1 Diabetes Grants, 2667
NIH Genetic Architecture of Complex Phenotypes, 2668
NIH Genetic Susceptibility and Variability of Human Malformations Research Grants, 2669
NIH Health Promotion Among Racial and Ethnic Minority Males, 2671
NIH Human Brain Project (Neuroinformatics) Phase I & II, 2672
NIH Human Connectome Project Grants, 2673
NIH Human Models and Markers of Skeletal Aging Grants, 2674
NIH Hyperaccelerated Award/Mechanisms in Immunomodulation Trials, 2675
NIH Impact of HAART on HIV/CNS Disease, 2676
NIH Independent Scientist Award, 2677
NIH Individual Postdoctoral Fellowships in Genomics and Related ELSI Topics, 2678
NIH Innovations in Biomedical Computational Science and Technology Grants, 2679
NIH Innovations in Biomedical Computational Science and Technology Initiative Grants for SBIR, 2680
NIH Innovations in Biomedical Computational Science and Technology Initiative Grants for STTR, 2681
NIH Investigator-Initiated Interactive Research Project Grants, 2682
NIH Low Birthweight in Minority Populations Research Grants, 2683
NIH Mechanisms of Orofacial Pain: Anatomy, Genomics, and Proteomics, 2684
NIH Mechanisms Underlying Individual Variations in Drug Responses, 2685
NIH Mechanisms Underlying Secondary Conditions in Mobility Disorders, 2686
NIH Mentored Patient-Oriented Research Career Development Award, 2688
NIH Mentored Research Scientist Development Awards, 2689
NIH Midcareer Investigator Award in Mouse Pathobiology Research Grants, 2690
NIH Molecular Epidemiology of Prostate Carcinogenesis Grants, 2691
NIH Mouse Mutagenesis and Phenotyping: Developmental Defects Research Grants, 2692
NIH Mouse Mutagenesis and Phenotyping: Nervous System and Behavior Research Grants, 2693
NIH Multidisciplinary Approach for Research on Oral Complications of HIV Infection, 2694
NIH National Centers for Neurofibromatosis Research, 2695
NIH National Occupational Research Agenda Grants, 2696
NIH National Research Service Awards--Senior Fellows, 2697
NIH New Directions in Pain Research Grants, 2698
NIH Nonhuman Primate Immune Tolerance Cooperative Study Group Grants, 2699
NIH NRSAs for Individual Predoctoral Fellowships, 2700
NIH NRSAs Predoctoral Fellowship Awards for Students with Disabilities, 2701
NIH Pathological Gambling: Basic, Clinical, and Services Research Grants, 2702
NIH Predoctoral Fellowship Awards for Minority Students, 2703
NIH Protein Structure Initiative (Structural Genomics) Research Grants, 2704
NIH Protein Structure Initiative (Structural Genomics)--SBIR/STTR GRANTS, 2705
NIH Receptors and Signaling in Bone in Health and Disease, 2706
NIH Recovery Act Limited Competition: Academic Research Enhancement Awards, 2707
NIH Recovery Act Limited Competition: Biomedical Research, Development, and Growth to Spur the Acceleration of New Technologies (BRDG-SPAN) Pilot Program Grants, 2708
NIH Recovery Act Limited Competition: Building Sustainable Comm-Linked Infrastructure to Enable Health Science Research, 2709
NIH Recovery Act Limited Competition: Small Business Catalyst Awards for Accelerating Innovative Research Grants, 2710
NIH Recovery Act Limited Competition: Supporting New Faculty Recruitment to Enhance Research Resources through Biomedical Research Core Centers Grants, 2711
NIH Research On Ethical Issues In Human Subjects Research, 2712
NIH Research on Sleep and Sleep Disorders, 2713
NIH Research Project Grants, 2714
NIH Rett Syndrome: Genetics, Pathophysiology, and Biomarkers Research Grants, 2715
NIH Role of Microglia in Normal and Abnormal Immune Responses of the Nervous System, 2716
NIH Roybal Centers for Translational Research on Aging, 2717

NIH Ruth L. Kirschstein National Research Service Awards (NRSA) for Individual Senior Fellows, 2718
NIH Ruth L. Kirschstein National Research Service Awards for Individual Predoctoral Fellows, 2720
NIH Ruth L. Kirschstein National Research Service Awards for Individual Predoctoral Fellowships to Promote Diversity in Health-Related Research, 2721
NIH Ruth L. Kirschstein National Research Service Awards for Individual Predoctoral MD/PhD and Other Dual Doctoral Degree Fellows, 2722
NIH Sarcoidosis: Research into the Cause of Multi-Organ Disease and Clinical Strategies for Therapy Grants, 2723
NIH SBIR/STTR Study and Control of Microbial Biofilms Research Grants, 2724
NIH School-based Interventions to Prevent Obesity, 2725
NIH Self-Management Strategies Across Chronic Diseases Grants, 2726
NIH Senior Scientist Award, 2727
NIH Small Business Innovation Research (SBIR): Animal Models of HCV Infection Research Grants, 2728
NIH Solicitation of Assays for High Throughput Screening (HTS) in the Molecular Libraries Probe Production Centers Network (MLPCN), 2729
NIH Structural Biology of Membrane Proteins Grants, 2730
NIH Studies of Ethical, Legal, and Social Implications of Research into Human Genetic Variation Grants, 2731
NIH Summer Internship Program in Biomedical Research, 2732
NIH Supplements to Promote Reentry into Biomedical and Behavioral Research Careers, 2733
NIH Targeting Research Gaps in HIV Therapeutics Research Grants, 2734
NIH Technologies to Improve the Utility of Animal Models Research Grants, 2735
NIH Transitional Career Development Award in Women's Health Research, 2736
NIH Urinary Incontinence Treatment Network, 2738
NIH Xenobiotics and Cell Death/Injury in Neurodegenerative Disease Research Grants, 2739
NIH Zebrafish as an Animal Model for Development and Disease Research Grants, 2740
NIH/EPA Mechanistic-Based Cancer Risk Assessment Methods Research Grants, 2741
NIMH AIDS and Aging: Behavioral Sciences Prevention Research Grants, 2745
NIMH Basic and Translational Research in Emotion Grants, 2746
NIMH Behavior Genetics in Adulthood and Old Age Research Grants, 2747
NIMH Career Opportunities in Research (COR) Education and Training Honors High School Research Education Grant, 2748
NIMH Career Opportunities in Research (COR) Education and Training Honors Undergraduate Research Training Grant, 2749
NIMH Central Nervous System Effects of HIV Infection: Neurobiological, Neurovirological, and Neurobehavioral Studies Grants, 2751
NIMH Collaborative R01s for Clinical Studies of Mental Disorders, 2752
NIMH Core Support Program for Mental Health/AIDS Research Grants, 2753
NIMH Curriculum Development Award in Neuroinformatics Research and Analysis, 2754
NIMH Early Detection of HIV Grants, 2755
NIMH Early Identification and Treatment of Mental Disorders in Children and Adolescents Grants, 2756
NIMH HIV/AIDS, Severe Mental Illness, and Homelessness Research Grants, 2757
NIMH Informed Consent in Research Grants, 2758
NIMH Interdisciplinary Behavioral Science Centers for Mental Health, 2759
NIMH Interventions Infrastructure Program Research Grants, 2760
NIMH Jointly Sponsored Ruth L. Kirschstein National Research Service Award Institutional Predoctoral Training Program in the Neurosciences, 2761
NIMH Mental Health Dissemination Research Grants, 2762
NIMH New Minority Faculty Scientist Development Award, 2765
NIMH Quantitative Approaches to the Analysis of Complex Biological Systems, 2767
NIMH Short Courses in Neuroinformatics, 2769
NIMH Socioeconomic Status and Health Across the Life Course, 2772
NIMH Supplements for Underrepresented Minorities, 2773
NIMH/NIDA Children's Services Program Grants, 2775
NINDS Central Nervous System Effects of HIV Infection: Neurobiological, Neurovirological, and Neurobehavioral Studies Grants, 2777
NINDS Cerebral Radiobiology and Neuroimaging of Brain Tumors Research Grants, 2778
NINDS Low-Back Pain and Common Spinal Disorders Research Grants, 2779
NINDS Optimization of Small Molecule Probes for the Nervous System (SBIR) Grants, 2780
NINDS Optimization of Small Molecule Probes for the Nervous System (STTR) Grants, 2781
NINDS Optimization of Small Molecule Probes for the Nervous System Grants, 2782
NINDS Pathogenesis and Therapy of the Muscular Dystrophies Research Grants, 2783
NINDS Repetitive Motion Disorders Research Grants, 2784
NINDS Specialized Neuroscience Research Programs (SNRP) on Health Disparity: HIV and the Nervous System, 2785
NINDS Support of Scientific Meetings as Cooperative Agreements, 2786
NINDS Symptom Management for Chronic Neurological Conditions Research Grants, 2787
NINR Acute and Chronic Care During Mechanical Ventilation Research Grants, 2788
NINR Aging Women and Breast Cancer Grants, 2789
NINR AIDS and Aging: Behavioral Sciences Prevention Research Grants, 2790
NINR Career Transition Award, 2791
NINR Chronic Illness Self-Management in Children and Adolescents Grants, 2792
NINR Clinical Interventions for Managing the Symptoms of Stroke Research Grants, 2793
NINR Clinical Trials: Collaborations for Nursing Research, 2794
NINR Diabetes Self-Management in Minority Populations Grants, 2795
NINR Management of Symptoms at the End of Life Grants, 2796
NINR Mechanisms, Models, Measurement, & Management in Pain Research Grants, 2797
NINR Mentored Research Scientist Development Award, 2798
NINR Nursing National Research Service Awards (NRSA)--Individuals, 2799
NINR Nursing Research Exploratory Center Grants, 2800
NINR Quality of Life for Individuals at the End of Life Grants, 2802
NINR Research on Musculoskeletal Fitness and Sports Medicine Grants, 2803
NINR Ruth L. Kirschstein National Research Service Award (NRSA) for Individual Predoctoral Fellows in Nursing Research, 2804
NINR Symptom Management for Chronic Neurological Conditions Research Grants, 2805
NIOSH Occupational Safety and Health Research and Demonstration Grants, 2807
NIOSH Repetitive Motion Disorders Research Grants, 2808
NKF Clinical Scientist Awards, 2809
NKF Franklin McDonald/Fresenius Medical Care Clinical Research Grants, 2810
NKF Professional Councils Research Grants, 2811
NKF Research Fellowships, 2812
NKF Young Investigator Grants, 2813
NLM Academic Research Enhancement Awards (AREA), 2814
NLM Exceptional, Unconventional Research Grants Enabling Knowledge Acceleration, 2815
NLM Exploratory/Developmental Grants, 2816
NLM Express Research Grants in Biomedical Informatics and Bioinformatics, 2817
NLM Grants for Scholarly Works in Biomedicine and Health, 2818
NLM Limited Competition for Continuation of Biomedical Informatics/Bioinformatics Resource Grants, 2821
NLM Manufacturing Processes of Medical, Dental, and Biological Technologies (SBIR) Grants, 2822
NLM New Technologies for Liver Disease Grants, 2823
NLM Predictive Multiscale Models of the Physiome in Health and Disease Grants, 2824
NLM Research Project Grants, 2825
NLM Research Supplements to Promote Reentry in Health-Related Research, 2826
NMF General Electric Medical Scholars Fellowships, 2830
NMF National Medical Association Awards for Medical Journalism, 2836
NMF Ralph W. Ellison Prize, 2840
NMSS Research Grants, 2844
NORD Orphan Diseases Research Grants, 2849
NORD Roscoe Brady Lysosomal Storage Disease Fellowships, 2850
Northwestern Mutual Fndn Grants, 2870
NSF Alan T. Waterman Award, 2874
NSF Animal Developmental Mechanisms Grants, 2875
NSF Behavioral Neurosciences Research Grants, 2876
NSF Biological Physics (BP), 2878
NSF Biomedical Engineering and Engineering Healthcare Grants, 2879
NSF Biomolecular Systems Cluster Grants, 2880
NSF Cell Systems Cluster Grants, 2881
NSF Chemical, Biochemical, and Biotechnology Systems Research Grants, 2882
NSF Chemistry Research Experiences for Undergraduates (REU), 2883
NSF Doctoral Dissertation Improvement Grants in the Directorate for Biological Sciences (DDIG), 2884
NSF Emerging Frontiers in Research and Innovation (EFRI) Grants, 2885
NSF Genes and Genome Systems Cluster Grants, 2886
NSF Perception, Action & Cognition Research Grants, 2890
NSF Postdoctoral Research Fellowships in Biology (PRFB), 2891
NSF Presidential Early Career Awards for Scientists and Engineers (PECASE) Grants, 2892
NSF Small Business Innovation Research (SBIR) Grants, 2893
NSF Social Psychology Research Grants, 2894
NSF Systematic Biology and Biodiversity Inventories Grants, 2895
NSF Undergraduate Research and Mentoring in the Biological Sciences (URM), 2896

NSF-NIST Interaction in Chemistry, Materials Research, Molecular Biosciences, Bioengineering, and Chemical Engineering, 2897
Nuffield Fndn Children and Families Grants, 2899
Nuffield Fndn Law and Society Grants, 2900
Nuffield Fndn Oliver Bird Rheumatism Program Grants, 2901
Nuffield Fndn Open Door Grants, 2902
Nuffield Fndn Small Grants, 2903
NWHF Comm-Based Participatory Research Grants, 2904
NWHF Mark O. Hatfield Research Fellowship, 2907
NYAM Charles A. Elsberg Fellowship, 2910
NYAM David E. Rogers Fellowships, 2911
NYAM Edward N. Gibbs Memorial Lecture and Award in Nephrology, 2912
NYAM Edwin Beer Research Fellowship, 2913
NYAM Ferdinand C. Valentine Fellowship, 2914
NYAM Mary and David Hoar Fellowship, 2916
NYCT Biomedical Research Grants, 2920
NYCT Blood Disease Research Grants, 2922
Obsessive-Compulsive Fndn Research Awards, 2931
OBSSR Behavioral and Social Science Research on Understanding and Reducing Health Disparities Grants, 2932
Ohio Learning Network Grants, 2940
Olfactory Research Fund Grants, 2942
Olin Corporation Charitable Trust Grants, 2943
OneSight Research Fndn Block Grants, 2944
ONF Small Grants, 2947
ONR Human Performance Division Research Grants, 2948
ONS Major Research Grants, 2949
Oracle Corp Contributions Grants, 2951
OREF Educational Awards, 2953
OREF Orthopedic Resident Research Awards, 2955
OREF Prospective Clinical Research Proposal Grants, 2956
OREF Research Grants, 2957
Orentreich Fndn for the Advancement of Science Grants, 2959
Oscar Rennebohm Fndn Grants, 2963
OSI Harm Reduction and Drug Use Grants, 2966
OSI Integrating Health and Legal Services Grants, 2968
Osteogenesis Imperfecta Fndn Research Grants, 2975
Oxalosis and Hyperoxaluria Fndn Grants, 2980
PacifiCorp Fndn for Learning Grants, 2982
Pancreatic Cancer Action Network-AACR Fellowship , 2987
Pancreatic Cancer Action Network-AACR Pathway to Leadership Grants, 2988
Partnership for Cures Charles E. Culpeper Scholarships in Medical Science, 2991
Partnership for Cures Two Years To Cures Grants, 2992
Partnership for Pediatric Epilepsy Research Grants, 2993
Patron Saints Fndn Grants, 2996
Paul G. Allen Family Fndn Grants, 3000
PDF International Research Grants, 3005
Peabody Fndn Grants, 3010
Peacock Fndn Grants, 3011
Pediatric Brain Tumor Research Grants, 3012
Pediatric Cancer Research Fndn Grants, 3013
Perpetual Trust for Charitable Giving Grants, 3015
Pew Charitable Trusts Biomedical Research Grants, 3019
Pezcoller Fndn-AACR International Award for Cancer Research, 3023
Pfizer Fndn Grants, 3025
Pfizer Fndn Health Literacy Grants, 3026
PhRMA Fndn Health Outcomes Post Doctoral Fellowships, 3031
PhRMA Fndn Health Outcomes Pre-Doctoral Fellowships, 3032
PhRMA Fndn Health Outcomes Research Starter Grants, 3033
PhRMA Fndn Health Outcomes Sabbatical Fellowships, 3034
PhRMA Fndn Informatics Sabbatical Fellowships, 3035
PhRMA Fndn Informatics Research Starter Grants, 3038
PhRMA Fndn Paul Calabresi Medical Student Research Fellowship, 3039
PhRMA Fndn Pharmaceutics Postdoctoral Fellowships, 3040
PhRMA Fndn Pharmaceutics Pre Doctoral Fellowships, 3041
PhRMA Fndn Pharmaceutics Research Starter Grants, 3042
PhRMA Fndn Pharmaceutics Sabbatical Fellowships, 3043
PhRMA Fndn Pharmacology/Toxicology Post Doctoral Fellowships, 3044
PhRMA Fndn Pharmacology/Toxicology Pre Doctoral Fellowships, 3045
PhRMA Fndn Pharmacology/Toxicology Research Starter Grants, 3046
PhRMA Fndn Pharmacology/Toxicology Sabbatical Fellowships, 3047
Pioneer Hi-Bred Society Fellowships, 3052
Pittsburgh Fndn Medical Research Grants, 3055
PKD Fndn Lillian Kaplan International Prize for the Advancement in the Understanding of Polycystic Kidney Disease, 3056
PKD Fndn Research Grants, 3057
Plastic Surgery Educational Fndn Basic Research Grants, 3058
Plastic Surgery Educational Fndn Research Fellowship Grants, 3059
Plastic Surgery Educational Fndn/AAO-HNSF Combined Grant, 3060
Potts Memorial Fndn Grants, 3072
Presbyterian Health Fndn Bridge, Seed and Equipment Grants, 3075
Prostate Cancer Fndn Research Grants, 3086
Prudential Fndn Grants, 3087
Puerto Rico Comm Fndn Grants, 3090
R.C. Baker Fndn Grants, 3098
RACGP Cardiovascular Research Grants in General Practice, 3099
RACGP Vicki Kotsirilos Integrative Medicine Grants, 3101
Rajiv Gandhi Fndn Grants, 3104
Rathmann Family Fndn Grants, 3109
Rayonier Fndn Grants, 3111
RCPSC Medical Education Research Grants, 3124
RCPSC Royal College Visiting Professorships in Medical Research, 3130
RCPSC/AMS CanMEDs Research and Development Grants, 3135
Regenstrief Geriatrics Fellowship, 3143
Regenstrief General Internal Medicine - General Pediatrics Research Fellowship Program, 3144
Regenstrief Master Of Science In Clinical Research/CITE Program, 3145
Rehabilitation Nursing Fndn Research Grants, 3147
Religion and Health: Effects, Mechanisms, and Interpretation RFP, 3149
Rett Syndrome Research Fndn Grants, 3151
RGK Fndn Grants, 3153
Rich Fndn Grants, 3156
Richard and Susan Smith Family Fndn Grants, 3159
Robert B McMillen Fndn Grants, 3169
Robert E. and Evelyn McKee Fndn Grants, 3170
Robert Sterling Clark Fndn Reproductive Rights and Health Grants, 3173
Rockefeller Archive Center Research Grants, 3178
Rockefeller Fndn Grants, 3181
Rockwell International Corp Trust Grants, 3183
Roeher Institute Research Grants, 3184
Rohm and Haas Company Grants, 3185
Rosalinde and Arthur Gilbert Fndn/AFAR New Investigator Awards in Alzheimer's Disease, 3187
Roy and Christine Sturgis Trust Grants, 3191
Roy J. Carver Charitable Trust Medical and Science Research Grants, 3192
RRF General Program Grants, 3193
RSC Abbyann D. Lynch Medal in Bioethics, 3195
RSC Jason A. Hannah Medal, 3196
RSC McLaughlin Medal, 3197
Russell Berrie Fndn Grants, 3201
RWJF Bridging the Gap: Research Informing Practice and Policy for Healthy Youth Behavior, 3205
RWJF Changes in Health Care Financing and Organization Grants, 3206
RWJF Clinical Scholars Program Grants, 3207
RWJF Evaluating Innovations in Nursing Education Grants, 3209
RWJF Executive Nurse Fellowships, 3210
RWJF Finding Answers: Disparities Research for Change Grants, 3211
RWJF Generalist Physician Faculty Scholars, 3212
RWJF Harold Amos Medical Faculty Development Scholars, 3213
RWJF Health & Society Scholars, 3214
RWJF Health Care Costs: Research to Inform Policy Grants, 3215
RWJF Health Impact Project Grants, 3216
RWJF Health Policy Fellowships, 3217
RWJF Healthy Eating Research Grants, 3218
RWJF Interdisciplinary Nursing Quality Research Initiative, 3219
RWJF Investigator Awards in Health Policy Research, 3220
RWJF Jobs to Careers: Promoting Work-Based Learning for Quality Care - Research Grants, 3221
RWJF Partners Investing in Nursing's Future Grants, 3226
RWJF Pioneer Portfolio Grants, 3227
RWJF Scholars in Health Policy Research Fellowships, 3229
RWJF State Coverage Initiatives Grants, 3230
RWJF Young Epidemiology Scholars (YES) Competition, 3233
Ryan Gibson Fndn Grants, 3234
S. Mark Taper Fndn Grants, 3236
Saint Luke's Fndn Grants, 3239
Samuel Freeman Charitable Trust Grants, 3249
Samuel Roberts Noble Fndn Grants, 3250
Samueli Fndn Health Grants, 3252
Samueli Institute Scientific Research Grants, 3253
San Antonio Area Fndn Grants, 3254
Sandler Program for Asthma Research Grants, 3262
Sarah Scaife Fndn Grants, 3263
Sarasota Memorial Healthcare Fndn Grants, 3264
Savoy Fndn Post-Doctoral and Clinical Research Fellowships, 3266
Savoy Fndn Research Grants, 3267
Savoy Fndn Studentships, 3268
Scientific Communities Initiative Grants, 3272
Self Fndn Grants, 3277
Sid W. Richardson Fndn Grants, 3284
Sigrid Juselius Fndn Grants, 3286
Simone and Cino del Duca Grand Prix Awards, 3288
Simpson Fund Grants, 3290
Sir Halley Stewart Trust Grants, 3293
Siragusa Fndn Health Services & Medical Research Grants, 3294
Skin Cancer Fndn Research Grants, 3298
Smith Family New Investigator Awards, 3299
SNM Molecular Imaging Research Grant For Junior Medical Faculty, 3301
SNM Pilot Research Grants, 3303
SNM Pilot Research Grants in Nuclear Medicine/Molecular Imaging, 3304
SNM Postdoctoral Molecular Imaging Scholar Grants, 3305

SNM Tetalman Memorial Young Investigator Awards, 3307
SNM/ Covidien Seed Grant in Molecular Imaging/ Nuclear Medicine Research, 3308
SOBP A.E. Bennett Research Award, 3313
Society for Biomedical Screening Small Grants, 3319
Society for Imaging Informatics in Medicine (SIIM) Emeritus Mentor Grants, 3320
Society for Imaging Informatics in Medicine (SIIM) Micro Grants, 3321
Society for Imaging Informatics in Medicine (SIIM) Research Grants, 3322
Society for Imaging Informatics in Medicine (SIIM) Small Grant for Product Support Development, 3323
Society for Imaging Informatics in Medicine (SIIM) Small Training Grants, 3324
Society for the Arts in Healthcare Environmental Arts Research Grant, 3327
Society of Medical Friends of Wine Research Award, 3344
Southwest Gas Corporation Fndn Grants, 3352
Soy Health Research Program Incentive Awards, 3354
SRC Medical Research Grants, 3362
SSHRC Image, Text, Sound and Technology (ITST) Grants, 3363
SSHRC Research/Creation Grants in Fine Arts, 3364
SSRC HIV/AIDS and Public Health Policy Research in Africa Fellowships, 3365
Stackner Family Fndn Grants, 3371
Staglin Family Music Festival NARSAD Schizophrenia Research Award, 3372
Staney Fndn Treatment Trials for Schizophrenia and Bipolar Disorder, 3374
Stanley Fndn Schizophrenia and Bipolar Disorder Research Grants, 3375
Starr Fndn Grants, 3377
Stephen Bechtel Fund Preventive Healthcare and Selected Research Grants, 3381
Stroke Association Allied Health Professional Research Bursaries, 3385
Stroke Association Clinical Fellowships, 3386
Stroke Association Research Project Grants, 3387
STTI Doris Bloch Research Awards, 3389
STTI Emergency Nurses Association Fndn Grant, 3390
STTI Environment of Elder Care Nursing Research Grants, 3391
STTI Joan K. Stout RN Research Grants, 3392
STTI National League for Nursing Grants, 3393
STTI Rosemary Berkel Crisp Research Awards, 3394
STTI Small Grants, 3395
STTI Virginia Henderson Clinical Research Grants, 3396
STTI/ATI Educational Assessment Nursing Research Grants, 3397
STTI/Council for the Advancement of Nursing Science Grants, 3398
Sunshine Natural Wellbeing Fndn Grants, 3404
Susan G. Komen Breast Cancer Fndn Basic, Clinical, and Translational Research Grants, 3407
Sybil G. Jacobs Award for Outstanding Use of Tobacco Industry Documents, 3414
Tellabs Fndn Grants, 3418
Temple-Inland Fndn Grants, 3419
Thomas and Dorothy Leavey Fndn Grants, 3422
Thompson Charitable Fndn Grants, 3425
Thrasher Research Fund Grants, 3426
Tourette Syndrome Association Post-Doc Fellowships, 3432
Tourette Syndrome Association Research Grants, 3433
TRDRP California Research Awards, 3434
TRDRP Exploratory/Developmental Research Awards, 3435
Triological Society Research Career Development Awards, 3440
TSA Research Grant Awards, 3442
TWS Fndn Grants, 3443
U.S. Department of Education Rehabilitation Engineering Research Centers Grants, 3447
U.S. Department of Education Rehabilitation Research Training Centers (RRTCs), 3448
U.S. Department of Education United States-Russia Program: Improving Research and Educational Activities in Higher Education, 3451
UCLA / RAND Corporation Post-Doctoral Fellowships, 3454
UICC American Cancer Society International Fellowships for Beginning Investigators, 3455
UICC International Cancer Technology Transfer (ICRETT) Fellowships, 3456
UICC Yamagiwa-Yoshida Memorial International Cancer Study Grants, 3458
UK Fndn for the Study of Infant Deaths Grants, 3459
United Cerebral Palsy Research Grants, 3462
Until There's a Cure Fndn Grants, 3471
US CRDF Leishmaniasis: Collaborative Research Opportunities in North Africa and the Middle East, 3474
Vancouver Fndn Grants and Comm Initiatives Program, 3477
VFW Ladies Auxiliary Cancer Research Postdoctoral Fellowships, 3494
Viking Children's Fund Grants, 3497
Virginia W. Kettering Fndn Grants, 3502
Volkswagen of America Corp Contributions Grants, 3503
Vulcan Materials Company Fndn Grants, 3504
W.W. Smith Charitable Trust Grants for Medical Research in Cancer, AIDS, and Heart Disease, 3509
Wallace H. Coulter Fndn Grants, 3515
Wasie Fndn Grants, 3521
Wayne and Gladys Valley Fndn Grants, 3522
Whitaker International Fellows and Scholars Program, 3532
Whitehall Fndn Neurobiology Research Grants, 3533
Wilhelm Sander Fndn Grants, 3535
William G. McGowan Charitable Fund Grants, 3539
William H. Hannon Fndn Grants, 3540
William T. Grant Fndn Research Grants, 3541
Xoran Technologies Resident Research Grant, 3554

Building Construction and/or Renovation

A.O. Smith Comm Grants, 18
Abel Fndn Grants, 181
Abell-Hanger Fndn Grants, 183
Abington Fndn Grants, 184
Acushnet Fndn Grants, 226
Adams County Fndn Grants - Pennsylvania, 231
Adelaide Breed Bayrd Fndn Grants, 234
Adolph Coors Fndn Grants, 238
AEC Trust Grants, 242
Agnes M. Lindsay Trust Grants, 263
Ahmanson Fndn Grants, 303
Air Products and Chemicals Grants, 319
Alabama Power Fndn Grants, 321
Albertson's Charitable Giving Grants, 330
Alcoa Fndn Grants, 334
Alex Brown and Sons Charitable Fndn Grants, 337
Alexander & Baldwin Fndn Hawaiian and Pacific Island Grants, 338
Alexander & Baldwin Fndn Mainland Grants, 339
Alice Tweed Tuohy Fndn Grants, 357
Allegan County Comm Fndn Grants, 358
Allegheny Technologies Charitable Trust, 359
Allen P. and Josephine B. Green Fndn Grants, 361
Allyn Fndn Grants, 365
American Schlafhorst Fndn Grants, 454
Andersen Fndn Grants, 471
Anheuser-Busch Fndn Grants, 474
Ann Jackson Family Fndn Grants, 477
Ann Peppers Fndn Grants, 478
Annenberg Fndn Grants, 479
Anthony R. Abraham Fndn Grants, 490
APF Disaster Recovery Fund for Psychiatrists, 506
Aratani Fndn Grants, 523
Arcadia Fndn Grants, 524
Arie and Ida Crown Memorial Grants, 528
Arkell Hall Fndn Grants, 534
Armstrong McDonald Fndn Grants, 537
Assisi Fndn Grants, 653
Atherton Family Fndn Grants, 659
Atlanta Fndn Grants, 662
Auburn Fndn Grants, 664
Autzen Fndn Grants, 672
AVDF Health Care Grants, 673
Bacon Family Fndn Grants, 679
Bailey Fndn Grants, 680
Ball Brothers Fndn Grants, 684
Bank of America Charitable Fndn Anchor Institutions Grants, 688
Barker Fndn Grants, 694
Barker Welfare Fndn Grants, 695
Barra Fndn Project Grants, 699
Battle Creek Comm Fndn Grants, 703
Batts Fndn Grants, 704
Beazley Fndn Grants, 730
Beckley Area Fndn Grants, 732
Becton Dickinson and Company Grants, 736
Belk Fndn Grants, 739
Bender Fndn Grants, 742
Benton Comm Fndn Grants, 743
Berrien Comm Fndn Grants, 749
Bertha Russ Lytel Fndn Grants, 751
Besser Fndn Grants, 752
Bill and Melinda Gates Fndn Grants, 756
Blackford County Comm Fndn Grants, 763
Blanche and Irving Laurie Fndn Grants, 764
Blanche and Julian Robertson Family Fndn Grants, 765
Blowitz-Ridgeway Fndn Early Childhood Development Research Award, 766
Blue Grass Comm Fndn Grants, 768
Blue Mountain Comm Fndn Grants, 769
Blue River Comm Fndn Grants, 770
Blumenthal Fndn Grants, 773
Bob and Delores Hope Charitable Fndn Grants, 774
Bodenwein Public Benevolent Fndn Grants, 775
Bodman Fndn Grants, 776
Boeing Company Contributions Program Grants, 777
Boettcher Fndn Grants, 778
Booth-Bricker Fund Grants, 780
Borkee-Hagley Fndn Grants, 781
Bosque Fndn Grants, 782
Boston Globe Fndn Grants, 784
Bright Family Fndn Grants, 793
Burlington Industries Fndn Grants, 811
Burlington Northern Santa Fe Fndn Grants, 812
Burton G. Bettingen Grants, 813
Bushrod H. Campbell and Adah F. Hall Charity Fund Grants, 816
Byron W. and Alice L. Lockwood Fndn Grants, 824
C.R. Bard Fndn Grants, 825
C.W. Titus Fndn Grants, 826
Cailloux Fndn Grants, 829
Callaway Fndn Grants, 835
Cambridge Comm Fndn Grants, 837
Capital Region Comm Fndn Grants, 862
Cargill Citizenship Fund-Corp Giving Grants, 865
Carl and Eloise Pohlad Family Fndn Grants, 867
Carl C. Icahn Fndn Grants, 870
Carl Gellert and Celia Berta Gellert Fndn Grants, 871
Carl W. and Carrie Mae Joslyn Trust Grants, 873
Carlos and Marguerite Mason Trust Grants, 875
Carls Fndn Grants, 876
Carnahan-Jackson Fndn Grants, 878
Carolyn Fndn Grants, 880

Carrie E. and Lena V. Glenn Fndn Grants, 882
Carrie Estelle Doheny Fndn Grants, 883
Cemala Fndn Grants, 933
Cessna Fndn Grants, 938
Champlin Fndns Grants, 960
Charles A. Frueauff Fndn Grants, 962
Charles Delmar Fndn Grants, 963
Charles H. Farnsworth Trust Grants, 967
Charles M. and Mary D. Grant Fndn Grants, 971
Chatlos Fndn Grants, 977
Chazen Fndn Grants, 978
Chestnut Hill Charitable Fndn, Inc Grants, 987
Chiles Fndn Grants, 1003
Christy-Houston Fndn Grants, 1008
Citizens Bank Mid-Atlantic Charitable Fndn Grants, 1015
Clark County Comm Fndn Grants, 1028
Clark Fndn Grants, 1029
Clark-Winchcole Fndn Grants, 1030
Claude Worthington Benedum Fndn Grants, 1033
Clay Fndn Grants, 1034
Coastal Comm Fndn of South Carolina Grants, 1051
Cockrell Fndn Grants, 1053
Coeta and Donald Barker Fndn Grants, 1054
Collins C. Diboll Private Fndn Grants, 1057
Collins Fndn Grants, 1058
Colonel Stanley R. McNeil Fndn Grants, 1059
Colorado Springs Comm Trust Fund Grants, 1061
Columbus Fndn Competitive Grants, 1066
Comm Fndn Alliance City of Evansville Endowment Fund Grants, 1089
Comm Fndn for Greater Buffalo Grants, 1090
Comm Fndn for Greater New Haven Grants, 1091
Comm Fndn for Monterey County Grants, 1092
Comm Fndn for Muskegon County Grants, 1093
Comm Fndn for Southern Arizona Grants, 1095
Comm Fndn of Bartholomew County Heritage Fund Grants, 1096
Comm Fndn of Bloomington and Monroe County Grants, 1098
Comm Fndn of Boone County Grants, 1099
Comm Fndn of Broward Grants, 1100
Comm Fndn of Champaign County Grants, 1102
Comm Fndn of Greater Birmingham Grants, 1106
Comm Fndn of Greater Flint Grants, 1107
Comm Fndn of Greater Fort Wayne: Comm Endowment & Clarke Endowment Fund Grants, 1108
Comm Fndn of Greater New Britain Grants, 1111
Comm Fndn of Mount Vernon and Knox County Grants, 1119
Comm Fndn of Muncie and Delaware County Grants, 1120
Comm Fndn of South Alabama Grants, 1123
Comm Fndn of Southeastern Connecticut Grants, 1125
Comm Fndn of Wabash County Grants, 1131
ConAgra Foods Fndn Grants, 1140
Connecticut Comm Fndn Grants, 1141
ConocoPhillips Fndn Grants, 1144
Constantin Fndn Grants, 1145
Constellation Energy Group and Baltimore Gas and Electric Corp Contributions, 1146
Consumers Energy Fndn, 1147
Cooke Fndn Grants, 1148
Cooper Industries Fndn Grants, 1150
Cornerstone Fndn of Northeastern Wisconsin Grants, 1152
Cowles Charitable Trust Grants, 1155
Crail-Johnson Fndn Grants, 1157
Crestlea Fndn Grants, 1159
Cudd Fndn Grants, 1171
Cullen Fndn Grants, 1172
CVS Comm Grants, 1177
D.V. and Ida J. McEachern Charitable Trust Grants, 1182
DaimlerChrysler Corporation Fund Grants, 1186
Daisy Marquis Jones Fndn Grants, 1188
Dana Corporation Fndn Grants, 1196
Danellie Fndn Grants, 1198
Daphne Seybolt Culpeper Memorial Fndn Grants, 1201
Daywood Fndn Grants, 1206
Del E. Webb Fndn Grants, 1213
Delaware Comm Fndn Grants, 1215
DeMatteis Family Fndn Grants, 1221
Dennis and Phyllis Washington Fndn Grants, 1222
Denver Fndn Comm Grants, 1227
DeRoy Testamentary Fndn Grants, 1239
DHHS Project Grants for Renovation or Construction of Nonacute Health Care Facilities, 1275
Dolan Fndn Grants, 1306
Donald and Sylvia Robinson Family Fndn Grants, 1310
Doris and Victor Day Fndn Grants, 1313
Dorothea Haus Ross Fndn Grants, 1320
Dr. Bob and Jean Smith Fndn Grants, 1325
Dr. John T. Macdonald Fndn Grants, 1327
Dr. Leon Bromberg Charitable Trust Fund Grants, 1328
Drs. Bruce and Lee Fndn Grants, 1333
Duke Energy Fndn Grants, 1339
E.J. Grassmann Trust Grants, 1360
E.L. Wiegand Fndn Grants, 1361
Eastman Chemical Company Fndn Grants, 1362
Eberly Fndn Grants, 1364
Edward S. Moore Fndn Grants, 1374
Edwards Memorial Trust Grants, 1375
Edwin S. Webster Fndn Grants, 1376
Edyth Bush Charitable Fndn Grants, 1378
Effie and Wofford Cain Fndn Grants, 1385
Eisner Fndn Grants, 1387
El Paso Corp Fndn Grants, 1389
El Pomar Fndn Awards and Grants, 1390
Elisabeth Severance Prentiss Fndn Grants, 1392
Elmer L. and Eleanor J. Andersen Fndn Grants, 1406
Erie Comm Fndn Grants, 1427
Eugene and Agnes E. Meyer Fndn Grants, 1432
Eugene B. Casey Fndn Grants, 1433
Eugene McDermott Fndn Grants, 1435
Eva L. and Joseph M. Bruening Fndn Grants, 1436
Ewing Halsell Fndn Grants, 1440
Fairfield County Comm Fndn Grants, 1446
Fallon OrNda Comm Health Fund Grants, 1449
Fan Fox and Leslie R. Samuels Fndn Grants, 1451
Fannie E. Rippel Fndn Grants, 1452
Fargo-Moorhead Area Fndn Grants, 1454
Faye McBeath Fndn Grants, 1456
Fayette County Fndn Grants, 1457
Feldman Fndn Grants, 1484
Fidelity Fndn Grants, 1498
Field Fndn of Illinois Grants, 1499
Fifth Third Fndn Grants, 1501
FirstEnergy Fndn Comm Grants, 1505
Fisa Fndn Grants, 1506
Fluor Fndn Grants, 1517
FMC Fndn Grants, 1518
Foellinger Fndn Grants, 1519
Ford Motor Company Fund Grants, 1522
Foster Fndn Grants, 1524
Fndn for the Carolinas Grants, 1535
Fndn Northwest Grants, 1537
Francis L. Abreu Charitable Trust Grants, 1549
Frank E. and Seba B. Payne Fndn Grants, 1551
Frank G. and Freida K. Brotz Family Fndn Grants, 1552
Fred L. Emerson Fndn Grants, 1557
Frey Fndn Grants, 1562
Fritz B. Burns Fndn Grants, 1564
Fuller E. Callaway Fndn Grants, 1578
G.N. Wilcox Trust Grants, 1581
Gebbie Fndn Grants, 1585
GenCorp Fndn Grants, 1587
General Motors Fndn Grants Support Program, 1591
Genesis Fndn Grants, 1593
George B. Storer Fndn Grants, 1596
George Frederick Jewett Fndn Grants, 1599
George Kress Fndn Grants, 1601
George S. and Dolores Dore Eccles Fndn Grants, 1602
Gheens Fndn Grants, 1610
Gilroy and Lillian P. Roberts Charitable Fndn Grants, 1614
Giving in Action Society Children & Youth with Special Needs Grants, 1617
Giving in Action Society Family Independence Grants, 1618
Gladys Brooks Fndn Grants, 1620
Goodrich Corporation Fndn Grants, 1638
Graco Fndn Grants, 1642
Greater New Orleans Fndn Grants, 1654
Greater Saint Louis Comm Fndn Grants, 1655
Greater Tacoma Comm Fndn Grants, 1656
Greater Worcester Comm Fndn Jeppson Memorial Fund for Brookfield Grants, 1659
Grundy Fndn Grants, 1673
Gulf Coast Comm of Venice Fndn Grants, 1677
Guy's and St. Thomas' Charity Grants, 1678
H & R Fndn Grants, 1679
H.A. and Mary K. Chapman Charitable Trust Grants, 1681
Hall-Perrine Fndn Grants, 1686
Harden Fndn Grants, 1693
Harold Alfond Fndn Grants, 1695
Harold and Arlene Schnitzer CARE Fndn Grants, 1697
Harold Simmons Fndn Grants, 1698
Harris and Eliza Kempner Fund Grants, 1699
Harry A. and Margaret D. Towsley Fndn Grants, 1701
Harry and Grace Steele Fndn Grants, 1702
Harry Bramhall Gilbert Charitable Trust Grants, 1703
Harry Kramer Memorial Fund Grants, 1705
Hartford Fndn Regular Grants, 1711
Harvest Fndn Grants, 1713
Health Fndn of Greater Indianapolis Grants, 1725
Hedco Fndn Grants, 1733
Helen Bader Fndn Grants, 1738
Herman Goldman Fndn Grants, 1753
High Meadow Fndn Grants, 1768
Hill Crest Fndn Grants, 1773
Hillman Fndn Grants, 1775
Hirtzel Memorial Fndn Grants, 1781
Hoblitzelle Fndn Grants, 1783
Hoglund Fndn Grants, 1785
Home Building Industry Disaster Relief Fund, 1787
Honeywell Fndn Grants, 1791
Horace A. Kimball and S. Ella Kimball Fndn Grants, 1792
Hormel Fndn Grants, 1796
Howard and Bush Fndn Grants, 1798
Hudson Webber Fndn Grants, 1813
Huie-Dellmon Trust Grants, 1815
Huntington County Comm Fndn Grants, 1823
Idaho Power Company Corp Contributions, 1838
Inasmuch Fndn Grants, 1845
Independence Comm Fndn Comm Quality of Life Grant, 1849
J.B. Reynolds Fndn Grants, 1873
J.E. and L.E. Mabee Fndn Grants, 1875
J.W. Kieckhefer Fndn Grants, 1878
Jacob and Hilda Blaustein Fndn Grants, 1881
James A. and Faith Knight Fndn Grants, 1884
James Graham Brown Fndn Grants, 1887
James H. Cummings Fndn Grants, 1888
James J. and Angelia M. Harris Fndn Grants, 1890
James M. Cox Fndn of Georgia Grants, 1892
James R. Dougherty Jr. Fndn Grants, 1894
James S. Copley Fndn Grants, 1895
Jane's Trust Grants, 1904
Janirve Fndn Grants, 1905
Jay and Rose Phillips Family Fndn Grants, 1909
JELD-WEN Fndn Grants, 1914
Jenkins Fndn: Improving the Health of Greater Richmond Grants, 1915

Jennings County Comm Fndn Grants, 1916
Jessie Ball Dupont Fund Grants, 1919
Jewish Comm Fndn of Greater Los Angeles Grants, 1921
John Ben Snow Memorial Trust Grants, 1928
John Deere Fndn Grants, 1929
John Edward Fowler Memorial Fndn Grants, 1930
John G. Duncan Trust Grants, 1931
John G. Martin Fndn Grants, 1932
John H. and Wilhelmina D. Harland Charitable Fndn Grants, 1933
John J. Leidy Fndn Grants, 1936
John Jewett and Helen Chandler Garland Fndn Grants, 1937
John Stauffer Charitable Trust Grants, 1946
John W. and Anna H. Hanes Fndn Grants, 1948
Johnson and Johnson / SAH Arts and Healing Grants, 1953
Joseph Alexander Fndn Grants, 1957
Joseph H. and Florence A. Roblee Fndn Grants, 1961
Josephine Goodyear Fndn Grants, 1964
Josiah W. and Bessie H. Kline Fndn Grants, 1967
Kalamazoo Fndn Grants, 1979
Katherine John Murphy Fndn Grants, 1983
Kathryne Beynon Fndn Grants, 1984
Kelvin and Eleanor Smith Fndn Grants, 1986
Kenneth T. and Eileen L. Norris Fndn Grants, 1989
Kenny's Kids Grants, 1990
Key Fndn Grants, 1994
KFC Allied Health Research Grants, 1996
L. W. Pierce Family Fndn Grants, 2019
Land O'Lakes Fndn Mid-Atlantic Grants, 2027
Larry L. Hillblom Fndn Grants, 2031
Lavelle Fund for the Blind Grants, 2033
Lillian S. Wells Fndn Grants, 2056
Lowe Fndn Grants, 2067
Lubbock Area Fndn Grants, 2079
Lubrizol Fndn Grants, 2080
Lucy Gooding Charitable Fndn Trust, 2082
Lucy Gooding Charitable Fndn Trust Grants, 2083
Ludwick Family Fndn Grants, 2084
M.E. Raker Fndn Grants, 2094
M.J. Murdock Charitable Trust Grants, 2095
Mabel Y. Hughes Charitable Trust Grants, 2097
Manuel D. and Rhoda Mayerson Fndn Grants, 2100
Marcia and Otto Koehler Fndn Grants, 2103
Margaret T. Morris Fndn Grants, 2105
Marion I. and Henry J. Knott Fndn Grants, 2109
Marion Park Deaver and Harry Gilbert Deaver Fndn Grants, 2110
Mark and Catherine Winkler Fndn Grants, 2112
Mars Fndn Grants, 2114
Mary Black Fndn Grants, 2118
Mary S. and David C. Corbin Fndn Grants, 2122
Matilda R. Wilson Fund Grants, 2128
Max A. Adler Charitable Fndn Grants, 2132
McGregor Fund Grants, 2143
McInerny Fndn Grants, 2144
McLean Contributionship Grants, 2147
McMillen Fndn Grants, 2148
McMurry Fndn Grants, 2149
Mead Witter Fndn Grants, 2160
Meadows Fndn Grants, 2161
Mericos Fndn Grants, 2172
Meyer Fndn Grants, 2177
Meyer Memorial Trust Grassroots Grants, 2179
Meyer Memorial Trust Operating Funds Grants, 2180
Meyer Memorial Trust Responsive Grants, 2181
Minneapolis Fndn Comm Grants, 2206
Miriam and Peter Haas Fund Grants, 2208
Montgomery County Comm Fndn Grants, 2214
Morton K. and Jane Blaustein Fndn Grants, 2218
National City Corporation Contributions Grants, 2250
National Emergency Medicine Association Grants, 2252
National Lottery Comm Fund Grants, 2256
NCI Technologies and Software to Support Integrative Cancer Biology Research (SBIR) Grants, 2279
New York Life Fndn Grants, 2304
Nina Mason Pulliam Charitable Trust Grants, 2776
Noble County Comm Fndn Grants, 2848
Nordson Corporation Fndn Grants, 2851
North Carolina Biotechnology Centers of Innovation Grants, 2857
North Carolina Comm Development Grants, 2858
Northern New York Comm Fndn Grants, 2864
Northern Trust Company Charitable Trust and Corp Giving Program, 2865
Northwestern Mutual Fndn Grants, 2870
Norwin S. and Elizabeth N. Bean Fndn Grants, 2872
Oleonda Jameson Trust Grants, 2941
Olin Corporation Charitable Trust Grants, 2943
Oscar Rennebohm Fndn Grants, 2963
OSI-Baltimore Special Opportunities Program Grants, 2972
Otto Bremer Fndn Grants, 2977
Pasadena Fndn Average Grants, 2994
Patron Saints Fndn Grants, 2996
Paul and Mary Haas Fndn Contributions and Student Scholarships, 2997
Paul E. and Klare N. Reinhold Fndn Grants, 2999
Paul Ogle Fndn Grants, 3003
Pfizer Fndn Grants, 3025
Phoenix Suns Charities Grants, 3030
Pioneer Hi-Bred Comm Grants, 3051
Piper Jaffray Companies Building Strong Communities Grants, 3053
Pittsburgh Fndn Comm Fund Grants, 3054
Plough Fndn Grants, 3061
Polaroid Fund Grants, 3065
Potts Memorial Fndn Grants, 3072
Prince Charitable Trusts Chicago Grants, 3079
Prince Charitable Trusts District of Columbia Grants, 3080
Principal Financial Group Fndn Grants, 3082
Procter and Gamble Fund Grants, 3083
Progress Energy Fndn Grants, 3084
Prudential Fndn Grants, 3087
Public Welfare Fndn Grants, 3089
Pulte Homes Corp Contributions, 3092
Quantum Corporation Snap Server Grants, 3095
Quantum Fndn Grants, 3096
R.C. Baker Fndn Grants, 3098
Raskob Fndn for Catholic Activities Grants, 3107
Rasmuson Fndn Grants, 3108
Rayonier Fndn Grants, 3111
Rhode Island Fndn Grants, 3154
Rich Fndn Grants, 3156
Richard and Helen DeVos Fndn Grants, 3157
Richard King Mellon Fndn Grants, 3161
Riley Fndn Grants, 3165
Robert P. & Clara I. Milton Fund for Senior Housing, 3172
Robins Fndn Grants, 3175
Rochester Area Comm Fndn Grants, 3176
Rockwell International Corp Trust Grants, 3183
Rollin M. Gerstacker Fndn Grants, 3186
Roy and Christine Sturgis Trust Grants, 3191
Roy J. Carver Charitable Trust Medical and Science Research Grants, 3192
Rush County Comm Fndn Grants, 3200
Russell Berrie Fndn Grants, 3201
Ruth H. and Warren A. Ellsworth Fndn Grants, 3203
S. Livingston Mather Charitable Trust Grants, 3235
S. Mark Taper Fndn Grants, 3236
S.H. Cowell Fndn Grants, 3237
Salem Fndn Grants, 3242
Samuel Roberts Noble Fndn Grants, 3250
Samuel S. Johnson Fndn Grants, 3251
San Antonio Area Fndn Grants, 3254
Schering-Plough Fndn Comm Initiatives Grants, 3269
Seabury Fndn Grants, 3274
Seneca Foods Fndn Grants, 3278
Sid W. Richardson Fndn Grants, 3284
Siebert Lutheran Fndn Grants, 3285
Simmons Fndn Grants, 3287
Simpson Fund Grants, 3290
Sisters of Mercy of North Carolina Fndn Grants, 3295
Solo Cup Fndn Grants, 3346
Sosland Fndn Grants, 3348
Southbury Comm Trust Fund, 3350
Southwest Gas Corporation Fndn Grants, 3352
Spencer County Comm Fndn Grants, 3358
Stackner Family Fndn Grants, 3371
Starr Fndn Grants, 3377
Steuben County Comm Fndn Grants, 3383
Stewart Huston Charitable Trust Grants, 3384
Strowd Roses Grants, 3388
Sulzberger Fndn Grants, 3399
Sunderland Fndn Grants, 3400
Sunflower Fndn Walking Trails Grants, 3403
Support Our Aging Religious (SOAR) Grants, 3406
Susan G. Komen Breast Cancer Fndn Hurricane Relief Grants, 3409
Susan Mott Webb Charitable Trust Grants, 3412
Susan Vaughan Fndn Grants, 3413
Tellabs Fndn Grants, 3418
Thompson Charitable Fndn Grants, 3425
Triangle Comm Fndn Donor-Advised Grants, 3437
United Technologies Corporation Grants, 3466
US Airways Comm Fndn Grants, 3473
US Trust Corporation Fndn Grants, 3475
W. C. Griffith Fndn Grants, 3505
Wachovia Fndn Grants, 3511
Warrick County Comm Fndn Grants, 3519
Wayne and Gladys Valley Fndn Grants, 3522
Weatherwax Fndn Grants, 3523
Weingart Fndn Grants, 3524
Wells County Fndn Grants, 3527
William G. Gilmore Fndn Grants, 3537
William G. McGowan Charitable Fund Grants, 3539
William H. Hannon Fndn Grants, 3540
Wilson-Wood Fndn Grants, 3542
Winston-Salem Fndn Competitive Grants, 3544
Woodward Fund Grants, 3552
Z. Smith Reynolds Fndn Small Grants, 3557

Capital Campaigns

A. Gary Anderson Family Fndn Grants, 17
Aaron Fndn (Massachusetts) Grants, 174
Abbott Fund Global AIDS Care Grants, 178
Abel Fndn Grants, 181
Abell-Hanger Fndn Grants, 183
ACGT Investigators Grants, 204
Achelis and Bodman Fndns Grants, 206
Acushnet Fndn Grants, 226
Adams County Fndn Grants - Pennsylvania, 231
Adelaide Breed Bayrd Fndn Grants, 234
AEC Trust Grants, 242
Agnes M. Lindsay Trust Grants, 263
Ahmanson Fndn Grants, 303
Air Products and Chemicals Grants, 319
Alabama Power Fndn Grants, 321
Alberto Culver Corp Contributions Grants, 329
Alcoa Fndn Grants, 334
Alex Brown and Sons Charitable Fndn Grants, 337
Alexander & Baldwin Fndn Hawaiian and Pacific Island Grants, 338
Alexander & Baldwin Fndn Mainland Grants, 339
Alexander Eastman Fndn Grants, 341
Alice Tweed Tuohy Fndn Grants, 357
Allen P. and Josephine B. Green Fndn Grants, 361
Allyn Fndn Grants, 365
American Electric Power Grants, 434
American Schlafhorst Fndn Grants, 454
Amgen Fndn Grants, 467
Angels Baseball Fndn Grants, 473
Anheuser-Busch Fndn Grants, 474

Ann Jackson Family Fndn Grants, 477
Ann Peppers Fndn Grants, 478
Aratani Fndn Grants, 523
Arcadia Fndn Grants, 524
Arie and Ida Crown Memorial Grants, 528
Arizona Public Service Corp Giving Program Grants, 531
Arkell Hall Fndn Grants, 534
Armstrong McDonald Fndn Grants, 537
Assurant Health Fndn Grants, 655
Atherton Family Fndn Grants, 659
Athwin Fndn Grants, 660
Atran Fndn Grants, 663
Auburn Fndn Grants, 664
AVDF Health Care Grants, 673
Avon Products Fndn Grants, 675
Bacon Family Fndn Grants, 679
Bailey Fndn Grants, 680
Ball Brothers Fndn General Grants, 683
Ball Brothers Fndn Grants, 684
Barker Fndn Grants, 694
Barker Welfare Fndn Grants, 695
Barra Fndn Project Grants, 699
Batchelor Fndn Grants, 701
Baton Rouge Area Fndn Grants, 702
Batts Fndn Grants, 704
Beazley Fndn Grants, 730
Ben B. Cheney Fndn Grants, 741
Bender Fndn Grants, 742
Benton Comm Fndn Grants, 743
Berks County Comm Fndn Grants, 745
Berrien Comm Fndn Grants, 749
Besser Fndn Grants, 752
Bill and Melinda Gates Fndn Grants, 756
Binney and Smith Comm Grants, 757
Blanche and Irving Laurie Fndn Grants, 764
Blanche and Julian Robertson Family Fndn Grants, 765
Blowitz-Ridgeway Fndn Early Childhood Development Research Award, 766
Blowitz-Ridgeway Fndn Grants, 767
Blue Mountain Comm Fndn Grants, 769
Blue River Comm Fndn Grants, 770
Bodenwein Public Benevolent Fndn Grants, 775
Boeing Company Contributions Program Grants, 777
Boettcher Fndn Grants, 778
Bonfils-Stanton Fndn Grants, 779
Booth-Bricker Fund Grants, 780
Borkee-Hagley Fndn Grants, 781
Bosque Fndn Grants, 782
Bradley Turner Fndn Grants, 789
Brown County Comm Fndn Grants, 807
Burlington Industries Fndn Grants, 811
Burlington Northern Santa Fe Fndn Grants, 812
Burton G. Bettingen Grants, 813
Byron W. and Alice L. Lockwood Fndn Grants, 824
Cailloux Fndn Grants, 829
Callaway Fndn Grants, 835
Cargill Citizenship Fund-Corp Giving Grants, 865
Carl and Eloise Pohlad Family Fndn Grants, 867
Carl and Lily Pforzheimer Fndn Grants, 868
Carl B. and Florence E. King Fndn Grants, 869
Carl C. Icahn Fndn Grants, 870
Carl Gellert and Celia Berta Gellert Fndn Grants, 871
Carl W. and Carrie Mae Joslyn Trust Grants, 873
Carlisle Fndn Grants, 874
Carls Fndn Grants, 876
Carnahan-Jackson Fndn Grants, 878
Carpenter Fndn Grants, 881
Carrie Estelle Doheny Fndn Grants, 883
Carrier Corporation Contributions Grants, 884
Cemala Fndn Grants, 933
Cessna Fndn Grants, 938
Champlin Fndns Grants, 960
Charles A. Frueauff Fndn Grants, 962
Charles Delmar Fndn Grants, 963
Charles H. Revson Fndn Grants, 969
Charles M. and Mary D. Grant Fndn Grants, 971
Chatlos Fndn Grants, 977
Chazen Fndn Grants, 978
Chesapeake Corporation Fndn Grants, 982
Chestnut Hill Charitable Fndn, Inc Grants, 987
Chicago Board of Trade Fndn Grants, 988
Clarcor Fndn Grants, 1021
Clark Fndn Grants, 1029
Claude Worthington Benedum Fndn Grants, 1033
Coastal Comm Fndn of South Carolina Grants, 1051
Coca-Cola Fndn Grants, 1052
Cockrell Fndn Grants, 1053
Collins C. Diboll Private Fndn Grants, 1057
Colonel Stanley R. McNeil Fndn Grants, 1059
Colorado Interstate Gas Grants, 1060
Colorado Springs Comm Trust Fund Grants, 1061
Columbus Fndn Competitive Grants, 1066
Comm Fndn for Greater Buffalo Grants, 1090
Comm Fndn for Monterey County Grants, 1092
Comm Fndn for Muskegon County Grants, 1093
Comm Fndn of Bartholomew County Heritage Fund Grants, 1096
Comm Fndn of Boone County Grants, 1099
Comm Fndn of Central Illinois Grants, 1101
Comm Fndn of Greater Birmingham Grants, 1106
Comm Fndn of Greater Flint Grants, 1107
Comm Fndn of Greater Fort Wayne: Comm Endowment & Clarke Endowment Fund Grants, 1108
Comm Fndn Of Greater Lafayette Grants, 1110
Comm Fndn of Greater New Britain Grants, 1111
Comm Fndn of Greenville Hollingsworth Funds Program/Project Grants, 1114
Comm Fndn of Mount Vernon and Knox County Grants, 1119
Comm Fndn of South Alabama Grants, 1123
Comm Fndn of St. Joseph County Special Project Challenge Grants, 1126
Compass Bank Fndn Grants, 1138
Connecticut Comm Fndn Grants, 1141
Connelly Fndn Grants, 1143
Constantin Fndn Grants, 1145
Constellation Energy Group and Baltimore Gas and Electric Corp Contributions, 1146
Consumers Energy Fndn, 1147
Cooke Fndn Grants, 1148
Cooper Industries Fndn Grants, 1150
Cornerstone Fndn of Northeastern Wisconsin Grants, 1152
Cowles Charitable Trust Grants, 1155
Crail-Johnson Fndn Grants, 1157
Crestlea Fndn Grants, 1159
CRI Clinical Investigator Award in Cancer Immunology, 1161
CSRA Comm Fndn Grants, 1168
Cudd Fndn Grants, 1171
Cullen Fndn Grants, 1172
D.F. Halton Fndn Grants, 1181
Dale and Edna Walsh Fndn Grants, 1189
Dana Corporation Fndn Grants, 1196
Danellie Fndn Grants, 1198
Daphne Seybolt Culpeper Memorial Fndn Grants, 1201
David Geffen Fndn Grants, 1202
Daywood Fndn Grants, 1206
Deaconess Comm Fndn Grants, 1207
Delaware Comm Fndn Grants, 1215
Della Martin Fndn Grants, 1219
DeMatteis Family Fndn Grants, 1221
Denton A. Cooley Fndn Grants, 1225
Dolan Fndn Grants, 1306
Donald and Sylvia Robinson Family Fndn Grants, 1310
Dorrance Family Fndn Grants, 1323
Dr. Bob and Jean Smith Fndn Grants, 1325
Dr. Leon Bromberg Charitable Trust Fund Grants, 1328
Drs. Bruce and Lee Fndn Grants, 1333
Duchossois Family Fndn Grants, 1337
Duke Energy Fndn Grants, 1339
Dunspaugh-Dalton Fndn Grants, 1351
DuPage Comm Fndn Grants, 1352
E. Rhodes and Leona B. Carpenter Fndn Grants, 1356
E.J. Grassmann Trust Grants, 1360
Eastman Chemical Company Fndn Grants, 1362
Eden Hall Fndn Grants, 1368
Edward S. Moore Fndn Grants, 1374
Edwards Memorial Trust Grants, 1375
Edwin S. Webster Fndn Grants, 1376
Edwin W. and Catherine M. Davis Fndn Grants, 1377
Edyth Bush Charitable Fndn Grants, 1378
Effie and Wofford Cain Fndn Grants, 1385
Eisner Fndn Grants, 1387
Elisabeth Severance Prentiss Fndn Grants, 1392
Elmer L. and Eleanor J. Andersen Fndn Grants, 1406
Erie Comm Fndn Grants, 1427
Eugene and Agnes E. Meyer Fndn Grants, 1432
Eugene McDermott Fndn Grants, 1435
Eva L. and Joseph M. Bruening Fndn Grants, 1436
Evjue Fndn Grants, 1439
Ewing Halsell Fndn Grants, 1440
Fallon OrNda Comm Health Fund Grants, 1449
Fargo-Moorhead Area Fndn Grants, 1454
Faye McBeath Fndn Grants, 1456
Ferree Fndn Grants, 1486
Fidelity Fndn Grants, 1498
Field Fndn of Illinois Grants, 1499
FirstEnergy Fndn Comm Grants, 1505
Fisa Fndn Grants, 1506
Fluor Fndn Grants, 1517
FMC Fndn Grants, 1518
Foellinger Fndn Grants, 1519
Fndn Northwest Grants, 1537
Fourjay Fndn Grants, 1544
Francis L. Abreu Charitable Trust Grants, 1549
Frank Stanley Beveridge Fndn Grants, 1553
Franklin County Comm Fndn Grants, 1554
Fraser-Parker Fndn Grants, 1555
Fred Baldwin Memorial Fndn Grants, 1556
Fred L. Emerson Fndn Grants, 1557
Freddie Mac Fndn Grants, 1558
Frederick Gardner Cottrell Fndn Grants, 1560
Frist Fndn Grants, 1563
Fritz B. Burns Fndn Grants, 1564
Fuller E. Callaway Fndn Grants, 1578
G.N. Wilcox Trust Grants, 1581
Gebbie Fndn Grants, 1585
GenCorp Fndn Grants, 1587
General Mills Fndn Grants, 1590
Genesis Fndn Grants, 1593
Genuardi Family Fndn Grants, 1594
George B. Storer Fndn Grants, 1596
George Kress Fndn Grants, 1601
George S. and Dolores Dore Eccles Fndn Grants, 1602
Georgia Power Fndn Grants, 1603
Gheens Fndn Grants, 1610
Gill Fndn - Gay and Lesbian Fund Grants, 1613
Gilroy and Lillian P. Roberts Charitable Fndn Grants, 1614
Giving in Action Society Children & Youth with Special Needs Grants, 1617
Giving in Action Society Family Independence Grants, 1618
Gladys Brooks Fndn Grants, 1620
Goodrich Corporation Fndn Grants, 1638
Graco Fndn Grants, 1642
Grand Haven Area Comm Fndn Grants, 1644
Grand Rapids Comm Fndn Grants, 1647
Greater New Orleans Fndn Grants, 1654
Greater Tacoma Comm Fndn Grants, 1656
Greater Worcester Comm Fndn Jeppson Memorial Fund for Brookfield Grants, 1659
Grundy Fndn Grants, 1673
Guy's and St. Thomas' Charity Grants, 1678
H & R Fndn Grants, 1679
H. Schaffer Fndn Grants, 1680
H.A. and Mary K. Chapman Charitable Trust Grants, 1681

Hagedorn Fund Grants, 1685
Hall-Perrine Fndn Grants, 1686
Hallmark Corp Fndn Grants, 1688
Hannaford Charitable Fndn Grants, 1692
Harold and Arlene Schnitzer CARE Fndn Grants, 1697
Harold Simmons Fndn Grants, 1698
Harris and Eliza Kempner Fund Grants, 1699
Harry A. and Margaret D. Towsley Fndn Grants, 1701
Harry and Grace Steele Fndn Grants, 1702
Harry Bramhall Gilbert Charitable Trust Grants, 1703
Harry Kramer Memorial Fund Grants, 1705
Hartford Courant Fndn Grants, 1710
Hartford Fndn Regular Grants, 1711
HCA Fndn Grants, 1721
Hearst Fndn and William Randolph Hearst Fndn Grants, 1730
Heckscher Fndn for Children Grants, 1732
Hedco Fndn Grants, 1733
Helen Bader Fndn Grants, 1738
Helen K. and Arthur E. Johnson Fndn Grants, 1740
Hershey Company Grants, 1754
High Meadow Fndn Grants, 1768
Hill Crest Fndn Grants, 1773
Hillman Fndn Grants, 1775
Hirtzel Memorial Fndn Grants, 1781
Hoglund Fndn Grants, 1785
Holland/Zeeland Comm Fndn Grants, 1786
Horace A. Kimball and S. Ella Kimball Fndn Grants, 1792
Hormel Fndn Grants, 1796
Houston Endowment Grants, 1797
Hudson Webber Fndn Grants, 1813
Hugh J. Andersen Fndn Grants, 1814
Huie-Dellmon Trust Grants, 1815
Huntington County Comm Fndn Grants, 1823
Ida Alice Ryan Charitable Trust Grants, 1836
Idaho Power Company Corp Contributions, 1838
Impact 100 Grants, 1843
Inasmuch Fndn Grants, 1845
Independence Comm Fndn Comm Quality of Life Grant, 1849
Irving S. Gilmore Fndn Grants, 1867
J.B. Reynolds Fndn Grants, 1873
Jackson County Comm Fndn Unrestricted Grants, 1879
Jacob G. Schmidlapp Trust Grants, 1883
James A. and Faith Knight Fndn Grants, 1884
James Graham Brown Fndn Grants, 1887
James H. Cummings Fndn Grants, 1888
James J. and Angelia M. Harris Fndn Grants, 1890
James M. Cox Fndn of Georgia Grants, 1892
James R. Dougherty Jr. Fndn Grants, 1894
James S. Copley Fndn Grants, 1895
Jane's Trust Grants, 1904
Janirve Fndn Grants, 1905
Jay and Rose Phillips Family Fndn Grants, 1909
JELD-WEN Fndn Grants, 1914
Jenkins Fndn: Improving the Health of Greater Richmond Grants, 1915
Jessie Ball Dupont Fund Grants, 1919
Jewish Comm Fndn of Greater Los Angeles Grants, 1921
John G. Martin Fndn Grants, 1932
John H. and Wilhelmina D. Harland Charitable Fndn Grants, 1933
John I. Smith Charities Grants, 1935
John Jewett and Helen Chandler Garland Fndn Grants, 1937
John R. Oishei Fndn Grants, 1944
John Stauffer Charitable Trust Grants, 1946
John W. and Anna H. Hanes Fndn Grants, 1948
John W. Anderson Fndn Grants, 1949
Joseph Alexander Fndn Grants, 1957
Joseph H. and Florence A. Roblee Fndn Grants, 1961
Josephine Goodyear Fndn Grants, 1964
Josiah W. and Bessie H. Kline Fndn Grants, 1967
Journal Gazette Fndn Grants, 1968
Kalamazoo Fndn Grants, 1979
Kansas Health Fndn Grants, 1980
Katherine John Murphy Fndn Grants, 1983
Kathryne Beynon Fndn Grants, 1984
Kelvin and Eleanor Smith Fndn Grants, 1986
Kenneth T. and Eileen L. Norris Fndn Grants, 1989
Kenny's Kids Grants, 1990
Kettering Fund Grants, 1992
L. W. Pierce Family Fndn Grants, 2019
Land O'Lakes Fndn Mid-Atlantic Grants, 2027
Larry L. Hillblom Fndn Grants, 2031
Lavelle Fund for the Blind Grants, 2033
Lillian S. Wells Fndn Grants, 2056
Lowe Fndn Grants, 2067
Lubbock Area Fndn Grants, 2079
Lubrizol Fndn Grants, 2080
Lucy Gooding Charitable Fndn Trust, 2082
Lucy Gooding Charitable Fndn Trust Grants, 2083
Lynde and Harry Bradley Fndn Grants, 2089
M.E. Raker Fndn Grants, 2094
Mabel Y. Hughes Charitable Trust Grants, 2097
Margaret T. Morris Fndn Grants, 2105
Marion I. and Henry J. Knott Fndn Grants, 2109
Mark and Catherine Winkler Fndn Grants, 2112
Mars Fndn Grants, 2114
Mary Owen Borden Fndn Grants, 2121
Matilda R. Wilson Fund Grants, 2128
Max A. Adler Charitable Fndn Grants, 2132
McGregor Fund Grants, 2143
McInerny Fndn Grants, 2144
McLean Contributionship Grants, 2147
McMillen Fndn Grants, 2148
McMurry Fndn Grants, 2149
Mead Witter Fndn Grants, 2160
Meadows Fndn Grants, 2161
Measey Fndn Medical Education Grants, 2162
Meyer Fndn Grants, 2177
Michael and Susan Dell Fndn Grants, 2189
Minneapolis Fndn Comm Grants, 2206
Miriam and Peter Haas Fund Grants, 2208
National City Corporation Contributions Grants, 2250
Nicholas H. Noyes Jr. Memorial Fndn Grants, 2497
Nina Mason Pulliam Charitable Trust Grants, 2776
Noble County Comm Fndn Grants, 2848
Nordson Corporation Fndn Grants, 2851
North Carolina Comm Development Grants, 2858
North Carolina Comm Fndn Grants, 2859
North Central Health Services Grants, 2861
Northern New York Comm Fndn Grants, 2864
Northern Trust Company Charitable Trust and Corp Giving Program, 2865
Northwestern Mutual Fndn Grants, 2870
Norwin S. and Elizabeth N. Bean Fndn Grants, 2872
Oleonda Jameson Trust Grants, 2941
Otto Bremer Fndn Grants, 2977
Owen County Comm Fndn Grants, 2979
Paul E. and Klare N. Reinhold Fndn Grants, 2999
Phoenix Suns Charities Grants, 3030
Pinellas County Grants, 3050
Piper Jaffray Companies Building Strong Communities Grants, 3053
Plough Fndn Grants, 3061
Polaroid Fund Grants, 3065
Powell Fndn Grants, 3073
Presbyterian Health Fndn Bridge, Seed and Equipment Grants, 3075
Pride Fndn Grants and Scholarships, 3078
Principal Financial Group Fndn Grants, 3082
Prudential Fndn Grants, 3087
Pulte Homes Corp Contributions, 3092
R.C. Baker Fndn Grants, 3098
Rasmuson Fndn Grants, 3108
Rathmann Family Fndn Grants, 3109
Rayonier Fndn Grants, 3111
Rhode Island Fndn Grants, 3154
Richard and Helen DeVos Fndn Grants, 3157
Richard and Rhoda Goldman Fund Grants, 3158
Richard and Susan Smith Family Fndn Grants, 3159
Robert and Polly Dunn Fndn Grants, 3168
Robert F. Stoico / FIRSTFED Charitable Fndn Grants, 3171
Robins Fndn Grants, 3175
Rockwell International Corp Trust Grants, 3183
Roy and Christine Sturgis Trust Grants, 3191
Ruth Eleanor Bamberger and John Ernest Bamberger Memorial Fndn Grants, 3202
S. Livingston Mather Charitable Trust Grants, 3235
S. Mark Taper Fndn Grants, 3236
Salem Fndn Grants, 3242
Samuel Roberts Noble Fndn Grants, 3250
Sasco Fndn Grants, 3265
Schering-Plough Fndn Comm Initiatives Grants, 3269
Schering-Plough Fndn Health Grants, 3270
Schurz Communications Fndn Grants, 3271
Seattle Fndn Grants, 3276
Self Fndn Grants, 3277
Sid W. Richardson Fndn Grants, 3284
Sisters of Mercy of North Carolina Fndn Grants, 3295
Solo Cup Fndn Grants, 3346
Sosland Fndn Grants, 3348
Southwest Gas Corporation Fndn Grants, 3352
Square D Fndn Grants, 3361
St. Joseph Comm Health Fndn Burn Care and Prevention Grants, 3367
St. Joseph Comm Health Fndn Pfeiffer Fund Grants, 3369
Stackner Family Fndn Grants, 3371
Starr Fndn Grants, 3377
Steelcase Fndn Grants, 3379
Steele-Reese Fndn Grants, 3380
Stewart Huston Charitable Trust Grants, 3384
Strowd Roses Grants, 3388
Sunderland Fndn Grants, 3400
Support Our Aging Religious (SOAR) Grants, 3406
Susan Mott Webb Charitable Trust Grants, 3412
Susan Vaughan Fndn Grants, 3413
Thompson Charitable Fndn Grants, 3425
Until There's a Cure Fndn Grants, 3471
US Airways Comm Fndn Grants, 3473
US Trust Corporation Fndn Grants, 3475
Vulcan Materials Company Fndn Grants, 3504
W. C. Griffith Fndn Grants, 3505
W.K. Kellogg Fndn Healthy Kids Grants, 3507
Wachovia Fndn Grants, 3511
Walt Disney Company Fndn Grants, 3516
Wasie Fndn Grants, 3521
Wayne and Gladys Valley Fndn Grants, 3522
Weatherwax Fndn Grants, 3523
Weingart Fndn Grants, 3524
William G. Gilmore Fndn Grants, 3537
Wilson-Wood Fndn Grants, 3542
Winston-Salem Fndn Competitive Grants, 3544
Winston-Salem Fndn Elkin/Tri-County Grants, 3545
Woodward Fund Grants, 3552

Centers: Research/Demonstration/Service

AAAS Science & Technology Policy Fellowships - National Defense & Global Security, 29
ACF Ethnic Comm Self-Help Grants, 200
ACF Preferred Communities Grants, 201
ACF Standing Announcement for Unaccompanied Alien Children Grants, 202
ACF Supplemental Services for Recently Arrived Refugees Grants, 203
Administration on Aging Senior Medicare Patrol Project Grants, 236
AMA Fndn Fund for Better Health Grants, 388
ASCO State Affiliate Grants, 560
Bank of America Charitable Fndn Anchor Institutions Grants, 688
Bearemy's Kennel Pals Grants, 728
Bildner Family Fndn Grants, 755
Cambridge Comm Fndn Grants, 837
Catholic Campaign for Human Development (CCHD) Comm Organizing Grants, 891

CCFF Transplant Center Incentive Grants, 899
CDC Evidence-Based Laboratory Medicine: Quality/Performance Measure Evaluation, 901
CDC Cooperative Agreement for Continuing Enhanced National Surveillance for Prion Diseases in the United States, 904
CDC Cooperative Agreement for Partnership to Enhance Public Health Informatics, 905
CDC Emerging Infectious Diseases Fellowships Program, 908
CDC Epidemiology and Laboratory Capacity Infectious Diseases Program Grants, 909
CDC Evaluation of the Use of Rapid Testing For Influenza in Outpatient Medical Settings, 910
CDC Injury Control Research Centers Grants, 913
CDC National Poison Prevention and Control Program Grants, 918
CDC National Training Information and Exchange Program, 920
CDC Suicide Prevention Research Center, 930
Champ-A Champion Fur Kids Grants, 959
Chicago Tribune's Corp Contributions Grants, 991
Children's Advocacy Center Grants, 997
CMS Historically Black Colleges and Universities (HBCU) Health Services Research Grants, 1044
CMS Research and Demonstration Grants, 1045
Collins C. Diboll Private Fndn Grants, 1057
ConocoPhillips Fndn Grants, 1144
Dallas Women's Fndn Grants, 1191
DHHS Developmental Disabilities University Affiliated Programs Project Grants, 1248
DHHS Health Centers Grants for Residents of Public Housing, 1254
DHHS Health Education and Training Centers Project Grants, 1256
DHHS Health Professions Training in Geriatrics Grants, 1259
DHHS Health Promotion and Disease Prevention Research and Demonstration Centers Grants, 1260
DHHS Technical and Non-Financial Assistance to Health Centers, 1280
DOD Breast Cancer Center of Excellence Award, 1290
Dr. John T. Macdonald Fndn Grants, 1327
Duke Endowment Health Care Grants, 1338
Dystonia Medical Research Grants and Fellowships, 1355
EMBO Installation Grants, 1409
Evjue Fndn Grants, 1439
Hartford Aging and Health Program Awards, 1709
Health Fndn of Greater Indianapolis Grants, 1725
Health Fndn of Southern Florida Responsive Grants, 1726
HRSA Geriatric Education Centers, 1805
HRSA Hansen's Disease National Ambulatory Care Program Grants, 1806
Hudson Webber Fndn Grants, 1813
IAFF Burn Fndn Research Grants, 1830
IHS Native American and Alaskan Native Health Research Centers, 1840
John Merck Fund Grants, 1940
John W. and Anna H. Hanes Fndn Grants, 1948
Joseph P. Kennedy Jr. Fndn Grants, 1962
Josephine Goodyear Fndn Grants, 1964
LSA Specialized Center of Research Grants, 2077
Lucy Gooding Charitable Fndn Trust, 2082
Margaret L. Wendt Fndn Grants, 2104
Max Bell Fndn Grants, 2134
Miles of Hope Breast Cancer Fndn Grants, 2199
NCI/NIDA Transdisciplinary Tobacco Use Research Centers Grants, 2280
NEI Mentored Clinical Scientist Development Program Award (K12), 2295
NHLBI Multidisciplinary Translational Research in Critical Care Grants, 2356
NIA Alzheimer's Disease Core Centers Grants, 2395
NIA Nathan Shock Centers of Excellence in Basic Biology of Aging Grants, 2421
NIAMS Collaborative Arthritis and Musculoskeletal and Skin Diseases Science Award, 2467
NIAMS Core Centers for Musculoskeletal Disorders Grants, 2468
NIAMS Skin Diseases Research Core Centers Grants, 2478
NIAMS Specialized Centers of Research in Osteoarthritis and Systemic Lupus Erythematosus, 2479
NIAMS Specialized Centers of Research in Osteoporosis, Rheumatoid Arthritis, and Scleroderma, 2480
NICHD Cooperative Specialized Infertility Research Centers, 2484
NICHD Population Research Grants, 2490
NIDCD Research Core Centers, 2529
NIDDK Diabetes Research Centers, 2551
NIDDK Multi-Center Clinical Study Cooperative Agreements, 2566
NIDDK Multi-Center Clinical Study Implementation Planning Grants, 2567
NIDDK Pilot and Feasibility Clinical Research Grants in Kidney or Urologic Diseases, 2575
NIDDK Pilot and Feasibility Clinical Research Studies in Digestive Diseases and Nutrition, 2576
NIDDK Race/Ethnic Disparities in the Incidence of Diabetes Complications, 2579
NIDDK Seeding Collaborative Interdisciplinary Team Science in Diabetes, Endocrinology and Metabolic Diseases Grants, 2584
NIGMS Pilot Projects for the Protein Structure Initiative (Structural Genomics), 2624
NIH Biology, Development, and Progression of Malignant Prostate Disease Research Grants, 2641
NIH Centers for AIDS Research (CFARs), 2647
NIH Centers for Dietary Supplements Research: Botanicals, 2648
NIH Exploratory Centers for Alternative Medicine Research Grants, 2663
NIH Mouse Mutagenesis and Phenotyping: Developmental Defects Research Grants, 2692
NIH Mouse Mutagenesis and Phenotyping: Nervous System and Behavior Research Grants, 2693
NIH National Centers for Neurofibromatosis Research, 2695
NIH National Occupational Research Agenda Grants, 2696
NIH Nonhuman Primate Immune Tolerance Cooperative Study Group Grants, 2699
NIMH Centers for AIDS Research (CFARs), 2750
NIMH Core Support Program for Mental Health/AIDS Research Grants, 2753
NIMH Interdisciplinary Behavioral Science Centers for Mental Health, 2759
NIMH Silvio O. Conte Centers for Neuroscience Research Grants, 2771
NNEDVF/Altria Doors of Hope Program, 2847
North Carolina Biotechnology Centers of Innovation Grants, 2857
NSERC Brockhouse Canada Prize for Interdisciplinary Research in Science and Engineering Grant, 2873
NSF Emerging Frontiers in Research and Innovation (EFRI) Grants, 2885
NSF Major Research Instrumentation Program (MRI) Grants, 2889
OSI-Baltimore Tackling Drug Addiction Grants, 2973
Portland General Electric Fndn Grants, 3067
Rockefeller Brothers Fund Peace and Security Grants, 3179
Rockwell International Corp Trust Grants, 3183
RWJF Clinical Scholars Program Grants, 3207
RWJF State Coverage Initiatives Grants, 3230
Salem Fndn Charitable Trust Grants, 3241
Samueli Fndn Health Grants, 3252
San Diego Women's Fndn Grants, 3259
Schering-Plough Fndn Health Grants, 3270
Sisters of Mercy of North Carolina Fndn Grants, 3295
Sisters of St. Joseph Healthcare Fndn Grants, 3297
Southwest Florida Comm Fndn Competitive Grants, 3351
Sprague Fndn Grants, 3359
Stewart Huston Charitable Trust Grants, 3384
TWS Fndn Grants, 3443
U.S. Department of Education 21st Century Comm Learning Centers, 3445
U.S. Department of Education Rehabilitation Engineering Research Centers Grants, 3447
U.S. Department of Education Rehabilitation Research Training Centers (RRTCs), 3448
U.S. Department of Education Special Education--National Activities--Parent Information Centers, 3450
UCLA / RAND Corporation Post-Doctoral Fellowships, 3454
Until There's a Cure Fndn Grants, 3471
Weatherwax Fndn Grants, 3523
Weingart Fndn Grants, 3524

Citizenship Instruction

AT&T Fndn Civic and Comm Service Program Grants, 658
Atkinson Fndn International Grants, 661
Axe-Houghton Fndn Grants, 678
Brinson Fndn Grants, 794
Catholic Campaign for Human Development (CCHD) Comm Organizing Grants, 891
Harvest Fndn Grants, 1713
John Edward Fowler Memorial Fndn Grants, 1930
Kraft Cares US Grants, 2017
Lynde and Harry Bradley Fndn Grants, 2089
Miles of Hope Breast Cancer Fndn Grants, 2199

Community Development

100 Mile Man Fndn Grants, 2
2 Depot Square Ipswich Charitable Fndn Grants, 7
3M Company Health and Human Services Grants, 10
3M Fndn Grants, 11
A Friend's Fndn Trust Grants, 13
A Fund for Women Grants, 14
A.O. Smith Comm Grants, 18
A/H Fndn Grants, 19
AAP Comm Access To Child Health (CATCH) Implementation Grants, 158
AAP Resident Initiative Fund Grants, 167
Aaron & Cecile Goldman Family Fndn Grants, 171
Aaron & Freda Glickman Fndn Grants, 172
Aaron Fndn (California) Grants, 173
Aaron Fndn (Massachusetts) Grants, 174
Abbott Fund Access to Health Care Grants, 176
Abbott Fund Comm Vitality Grants, 177
Abbott Fund Global AIDS Care Grants, 178
Abbott Fund Science and Medical Innovation Grants, 179
Abel Fndn Grants, 181
Abell Fndn Health and Human Services Grants, 182
Abell-Hanger Fndn Grants, 183
Abington Fndn Grants, 184
Able To Serve Grants, 185
Able Trust Vocational Rehabilitation Grants for Individuals, 186
Abney Fndn Grants, 187
ACE Charitable Fndn Grants, 199
ACF Ethnic Comm Self-Help Grants, 200
ACF Preferred Communities Grants, 201
ACF Standing Announcement for Unaccompanied Alien Children Grants, 202
ACF Supplemental Services for Recently Arrived Refugees Grants, 203
Achelis and Bodman Fndns Grants, 206
Actors Fund Social Services and Financial Assistance, 225
Acushnet Fndn Grants, 226
Adam Richter Charitable Trust Grants, 230
Administaff Comm Affairs Grants, 235

Adobe Comm Investment Grants, 237
Adolph Coors Fndn Grants, 238
Advanced Micro Devices Comm Affairs Grants, 239
AEC Trust Grants, 242
AEGON Transamerica Fndn Grants, 243
Aetna Fndn Health Grants in Connecticut, 244
Aetna Fndn Quality of Care Grants for Depression, 246
Aetna Fndn Quality of Care Grants for End of Life Care, 247
Aetna Fndn Regional Comm Health General Support Grants, 248
Aetna Fndn Regional Comm Health Outreach Grants, 250
Aetna Fndn Sponsorships Grants in Connecticut, 251
AFG Industries Grants, 259
African American Fund of New Jersey Grants, 260
Agnes M. Lindsay Trust Grants, 263
Agway Fndn Grants, 265
AHFMR Comm Support Program Grants, 271
Ahmanson Fndn Grants, 303
Ahn Family Fndn Grants, 304
AIG American General Corporation Grants, 316
Air Products and Chemicals Grants, 319
Alabama Power Fndn Grants, 321
Alaska Airlines Corp Giving Grants, 323
Alaska Airlines Fndn Grants, 324
Albert and Margaret Alkek Fndn Grants, 326
Albert Pick Jr. Fund Grants, 328
Alberto Culver Corp Contributions Grants, 329
Albertson's Charitable Giving Grants, 330
Albuquerque Comm Fndn Grants, 331
Alcatel-Lucent Technologies Corp Contributions Grants, 332
Alcatel-Lucent Technologies Fndn Grants, 333
Alcoa Fndn Grants, 334
Alcon Fndn Grants, 336
Alexander & Baldwin Fndn Hawaiian and Pacific Island Grants, 338
Alexander & Baldwin Fndn Mainland Grants, 339
Alexander and Margaret Stewart Trust Grants, 340
Alexander Eastman Fndn Grants, 341
Alexander Fndn Cancer, Catastrophic Illness and Injury Grants, 342
Alexis Gregory Fndn Grants, 349
Alice C. A. Sibley Fund Grants, 355
Alice Tweed Tuohy Fndn Grants, 357
Allegan County Comm Fndn Grants, 358
Allegheny Technologies Charitable Trust, 359
Allen P. and Josephine B. Green Fndn Grants, 361
Allstate Corp Giving Grants, 363
Allstate Corp Hometown Commitment Grants, 364
Allyn Fndn Grants, 365
ALSAM Fndn Grants, 369
Altman Fndn Health Care Grants, 372
AMA Fndn Fund for Better Health Grants, 388
AMA Fndn Healthy Communities/Healthy America Grants, 390
AMA Fndn Jack B. McConnell, MD Awards for Excellence in Volunteerism, 391
AMA-MSS Chapter Involvement Grants, 401
Amador Comm Fndn Grants, 409
Amarillo Area/Harrington Fndns Grants, 410
AMD Corp Contributions Grants, 411
American Academy of Dermatology Shade Structure Grants, 413
American Express Fndn Comm Service Grants, 435
American Jewish World Service Grants, 437
American Schlafhorst Fndn Grants, 454
amfAR Global Initiatives Grants, 463
amfAR Public Policy Grants, 465
Amgen Fndn Grants, 467
AMI Semiconductors Corp Grants, 468
Andersen Corp Fndn, 470
Angels Baseball Fndn Grants, 473
Anheuser-Busch Fndn Grants, 474
Ann and Robert H. Lurie Family Fndn Grants, 475
Ann Arbor Area Comm Fndn Grants, 476
Annie Sinclair Knudsen Memorial Fund/Kaua'i Comm Grants, 480
Annunziata Sanguinetti Fndn Grants, 481
Ansell, Zaro, Grimm & Aaron Fndn Grants, 487
APSAA Fndn Grants, 517
Arcadia Fndn Grants, 524
Archer Daniels Midland Fndn Grants, 525
Argyros Fndn Grants, 527
Arizona Cardinals Grants, 529
Arizona Diamondbacks Charities Grants, 530
Arizona Public Service Corp Giving Program Grants, 531
Arkansas Comm Fndn Arkansas Black Hall of Fame Grants, 532
Arkansas Comm Fndn Grants, 533
Arkell Hall Fndn Grants, 534
Arlington Comm Fndn Grants, 536
Armstrong McDonald Fndn Grants, 537
ArvinMeritor Fndn Health Grants, 543
ArvinMeritor Grants, 544
ASCO State Affiliate Grants, 547
Ashland Corp Contributions Grants, 586
Assisi Fndn Grants, 653
Assurant Fndn Grants, 654
Assurant Health Fndn Grants, 655
AT&T Excelerator, 657
AT&T Fndn Civic and Comm Service Program Grants, 658
Atherton Family Fndn Grants, 659
Athwin Fndn Grants, 660
Atkinson Fndn International Grants, 661
Atlanta Fndn Grants, 662
Auburn Fndn Grants, 664
Audrey and Sydney Irmas Charitable Fndn Grants, 665
Aurora Fndn Grants, 667
Autodesk Comm Relations Grants, 671
Bacon Family Fndn Grants, 679
Bailey Fndn Grants, 680
Balance Bar Sports Individual/Team Grants, 681
Balfe Family Fndn Grants, 682
Ball Brothers Fndn General Grants, 683
Ball Brothers Fndn Grants, 684
Banfi Vintners Fndn Grants, 687
Bank of America Charitable Fndn Anchor Institutions Grants, 688
Bank of America Charitable Fndn National Programs and Partners Grants, 689
Bank of America Client Fndn Grants, 690
Baptist Comm Ministries Grants, 691
Baptist-Trinity Lutheran Legacy Fndn Grants, 692
Barberton Comm Fndn Grants, 693
Barker Fndn Grants, 694
Barker Welfare Fndn Grants, 695
Barnes Group Fndn Grants, 696
Barr Fund Grants, 697
Barra Fndn Comm Fund Grants, 698
Barra Fndn Project Grants, 699
Batchelor Fndn Grants, 701
Baton Rouge Area Fndn Grants, 702
Battle Creek Comm Fndn Grants, 703
Batts Fndn Grants, 704
Baxter International Fndn Grants, 705
BCBS of Massachusetts Fndn Grants, 709
BCBS of Minnesota Growing Up Healthy Grants, 711
BCBS of Minnesota Healthy Together Grants, 712
BCBSM Building Healthy Communities Engaging Elementary Schools and Comm Partners Grants, 713
BCBSM Comm Health Matching Grants, 715
BCBSM Corp Contributions Grants, 716
BCBSNC Fndn Grants, 725
Bearemy's Kennel Pals Grants, 728
Beazley Fndn Grants, 730
Bechtel Group Fndn Building Positive Comm Relationships Grants, 731
Beckley Area Fndn Grants, 732
Beirne Carter Fndn Grants, 737
Beldon Fund Grants, 738
Ben B. Cheney Fndn Grants, 741
Bender Fndn Grants, 742
Benton Comm Fndn Grants, 743
Benton County Fndn Grants, 744
Berks County Comm Fndn Grants, 745
Bernard and Audre Rapoport Fndn Grants, 746
Berrien Comm Fndn Grants, 749
Besser Fndn Grants, 752
BHHS Legacy Fndn Grants, 753
Bill and Melinda Gates Fndn Grants, 756
Biogen Corp Giving Grants, 758
Birds Eye Foods Fndn Grants, 759
Birmingham Fndn Grants, 760
BJ's Charitable Fndn Grants, 761
Black River Falls Area Fndn Grants, 762
Blackford County Comm Fndn Grants, 763
Blanche and Irving Laurie Fndn Grants, 764
Blanche and Julian Robertson Family Fndn Grants, 765
Blue Grass Comm Fndn Grants, 768
Blue Mountain Comm Fndn Grants, 769
Blue River Comm Fndn Grants, 770
Blum-Kovler Fndn Grants, 772
Blumenthal Fndn Grants, 773
Bodenwein Public Benevolent Fndn Grants, 775
Bodman Fndn Grants, 776
Boeing Company Contributions Program Grants, 777
Boettcher Fndn Grants, 778
Bonfils-Stanton Fndn Grants, 779
Boston Fndn Grants, 783
Boston Globe Fndn Grants, 784
Boyd Gaming Corporation Contributions Program, 788
Bradley Turner Fndn Grants, 789
Brian G. Dyson Fndn Grants, 791
Bridgestone/Firestone Trust Fund Grants, 792
Bright Family Fndn Grants, 793
Bristol-Myers Squibb Fndn Health Disparities Grants, 797
Bristol-Myers Squibb Fndn Product Donations Grants, 799
Brook J. Lenfest Fndn Grants, 804
Brookdale Fndn National Group Respite and Early Memory Loss Program Grants, 806
Brown County Comm Fndn Grants, 807
Bruce and Adele Greenfield Fndn Grants, 808
Burlington Industries Fndn Grants, 811
Burlington Northern Santa Fe Fndn Grants, 812
Burton G. Bettingen Grants, 813
Bush Fndn Health & Human Services Grants, 814
Bush Fndn Medical Fellowships, 815
Bushrod H. Campbell and Adah F. Hall Charity Fund Grants, 816
Business Bank of Nevada Comm Grants, 817
C.R. Bard Fndn Grants, 825
C.W. Titus Fndn Grants, 826
Cable Positive's Tony Cox Comm Fund Grants, 827
Caddock Fndn Grants, 828
Caleb C. and Julia W. Dula Educational and Charitable Fndn Grants, 830
California Comm Fndn Health Care Grants, 831
California Comm Fndn Human Development Grants, 832
California Endowment CommunitiesFirst Grants, 833
Callaway Fndn Grants, 835
Callaway Golf Company Fndn Grants, 836
Cambridge Comm Fndn Grants, 837
Camp-Younts Fndn Grants, 838
Campbell Hoffman Fndn Grants, 840
Capital Region Comm Fndn Grants, 862
Cargill Citizenship Fund-Corp Giving Grants, 865
Caring Fndn Grants, 866
Carl and Eloise Pohlad Family Fndn Grants, 867
Carl and Lily Pforzheimer Fndn Grants, 868
Carl B. and Florence E. King Fndn Grants, 869
Carl C. Icahn Fndn Grants, 870
Carl Gellert and Celia Berta Gellert Fndn Grants, 871

Carl W. and Carrie Mae Joslyn Trust Grants, 873
Carlisle Fndn Grants, 874
Carlsbad Charitable Fndn Grants, 877
Carnahan-Jackson Fndn Grants, 878
Carnegie Corporation of New York Grants, 879
Carolyn Fndn Grants, 880
Carpenter Fndn Grants, 881
Carrie E. and Lena V. Glenn Fndn Grants, 882
Carrier Corporation Contributions Grants, 884
Carroll County Comm Fndn Grants, 885
Cass County Comm Fndn Grants, 887
Catherine Kennedy Home Fndn Grants, 890
Catholic Campaign for Human Development (CCHD) Comm Organizing Grants, 891
CDC National Poison Prevention and Control Program Grants, 918
Cemala Fndn Grants, 933
Central Carolina Comm Fndn Comm Impact Grants, 936
Central Okanagan Fndn Grants, 937
Cessna Fndn Grants, 938
Champ-A Champion Fur Kids Grants, 959
Champlin Fndns Grants, 960
CharityWorks Grants, 961
Charles A. Frueauff Fndn Grants, 962
Charles Delmar Fndn Grants, 963
Charles G. Koch Charitable Fndn Grants, 965
Charles H. Dater Fndn Grants, 966
Charles H. Farnsworth Trust Grants, 967
Charles H. Revson Fndn Grants, 969
Charles M. and Mary D. Grant Fndn Grants, 971
Charles M. Bair Family Trust Grants, 972
Charlotte County (FL) Comm Fndn Grants, 973
Chatlos Fndn Grants, 977
CHCF Grants, 979
Chesapeake Corporation Fndn Grants, 982
Chicago Board of Trade Fndn Grants, 988
Chicago Comm Trust Grants, 989
Chicago Tribune's Corp Contributions Grants, 991
Chicago White Metal Charitable Fndn Grants, 992
Children Affected by AIDS Fndn Camp Network Grants, 994
Children Affected by AIDS Fndn Domestic Grants, 995
Children Affected by AIDS Fndn Family Assistance Emergency Fund Grants, 996
Chiles Fndn Grants, 1003
Christy-Houston Fndn Grants, 1008
Chula Vista Charitable Fndn Grants, 1009
CICF Legacy Fund Comm Fndn Grants, 1010
Cinergy Fndn Grants, 1013
CIT Corp Giving Grants, 1014
Citizens Bank Mid-Atlantic Charitable Fndn Grants, 1015
Clarcor Fndn Grants, 1021
Clarence E. Heller Charitable Fndn Grants, 1022
Clark County Comm Fndn Grants, 1028
Clark Fndn Grants, 1029
Clark-Winchcole Fndn Grants, 1030
Claude Bennett Family Fndn Grants, 1031
Claude Worthington Benedum Fndn Grants, 1033
Clay Fndn Grants, 1034
Cleo Fndn Grants, 1035
CLIF Bar Family Fndn Grants, 1040
CMA Fndn Grants, 1042
CNA Fndn Grants, 1046
CNCS Foster Grandparent Projects Grants, 1048
CNCS Next Generation Grants, 1049
Coastal Bend Comm Fndn Grants, 1050
Coastal Comm Fndn of South Carolina Grants, 1051
Cockrell Fndn Grants, 1053
Coeta and Donald Barker Fndn Grants, 1054
Coleman Fndn Cancer Care Grants, 1055
Collins C. Diboll Private Fndn Grants, 1057
Collins Fndn Grants, 1058
Colonel Stanley R. McNeil Fndn Grants, 1059
Colorado Interstate Gas Grants, 1060
Colorado Springs Comm Trust Fund Grants, 1061
Colorado Trust Grants, 1062
Columbus Fndn Competitive Grants, 1066
Columbus Fndn Robert E. and Genevieve B. Schaefer Fund Grants, 1070
Columbus Fndn Traditional Grants, 1071
Comerica Charitable Fndn Grants, 1073
Commission on Religion in Appalachia Grants, 1074
Commonweal Fndn Grants, 1076
Commonwealth Fund Patient-Centered Coordinated Care Program Grants, 1081
Comm Fndn AIDS Endowment Awards, 1088
Comm Fndn Alliance City of Evansville Endowment Fund Grants, 1089
Comm Fndn for Greater Buffalo Grants, 1090
Comm Fndn for Greater New Haven Grants, 1091
Comm Fndn for Monterey County Grants, 1092
Comm Fndn for Muskegon County Grants, 1093
Comm Fndn for Southeastern Michigan Grants, 1094
Comm Fndn for Southern Arizona Grants, 1095
Comm Fndn of Bartholomew County Heritage Fund Grants, 1096
Comm Fndn of Bloomington and Monroe County Grants, 1098
Comm Fndn of Boone County Grants, 1099
Comm Fndn of Broward Grants, 1100
Comm Fndn of Central Illinois Grants, 1101
Comm Fndn of Champaign County Grants, 1102
Comm Fndn of Crawford County Grants and Scholarships, 1103
Comm Fndn of Grant County Grants, 1104
Comm Fndn of Greater Birmingham Grants, 1106
Comm Fndn of Greater Flint Grants, 1107
Comm Fndn of Greater Fort Wayne: Comm Endowment & Clarke Endowment Fund Grants, 1108
Comm Fndn of Greater Greensboro Grants, 1109
Comm Fndn Of Greater Lafayette Grants, 1110
Comm Fndn of Greater New Britain Grants, 1111
Comm Fndn of Greater Tampa Grants, 1112
Comm Fndn of Greenville Comm Enrichment Grants, 1113
Comm Fndn of Greenville Hollingsworth Funds Program/Project Grants, 1114
Comm Fndn of Greenville-Greenville Women Giving Grants, 1115
Comm Fndn of Howard County Grants, 1116
Comm Fndn of Morgan County Grants and Scholarships, 1118
Comm Fndn of Mount Vernon and Knox County Grants, 1119
Comm Fndn of Muncie and Delaware County Grants, 1120
Comm Fndn of Randolph County Grants, 1121
Comm Fndn of Santa Cruz County Grants, 1122
Comm Fndn of South Alabama Grants, 1123
Comm Fndn of South Puget Sound Grants, 1124
Comm Fndn of Southeastern Connecticut Grants, 1125
Comm Fndn of St. Joseph County Special Project Challenge Grants, 1126
Comm Fndn of Switzerland County Grants, 1127
Comm Fndn of Tampa Bay Grants, 1128
Comm Fndn of the Eastern Shore Comm Needs Grants, 1129
Comm Fndn of the Ozarks Grants, 1130
Comm Fndn of Western North Carolina Grants, 1132
Comm Fndn Silicon Valley Grants, 1133
Comm Impact Fund, 1135
Comm Technology Fndn of California Building Communities Through Technology Grants, 1136
ConAgra Foods Fndn Grants, 1140
Connecticut Comm Fndn Grants, 1141
Connelly Fndn Grants, 1143
ConocoPhillips Fndn Grants, 1144
Constantin Fndn Grants, 1145
Constellation Energy Group and Baltimore Gas and Electric Corp Contributions, 1146
Consumers Energy Fndn, 1147
Cooke Fndn Grants, 1148
Cooper Industries Fndn Grants, 1150
Coors Brewing Corp Contributions Grants, 1151
Cornerstone Fndn of Northeastern Wisconsin Grants, 1152
Covenant Fndn Grants (Iowa), 1153
Crail-Johnson Fndn Grants, 1157
Cranston Fndn Grants, 1158
Cruise Industry Charitable Fndn Grants, 1166
CSL Behring Local Empowerment for Advocacy Development (LEAD) Grants, 1167
CSRA Comm Fndn Grants, 1168
CSX Corp Contributions Grants, 1169
Cullen Fndn Grants, 1172
Cultural Society of Filipino Americans Grants, 1173
CUNA Mutual Group Fndn, 1174
CVS All Kids Can Grants, 1175
CVS Caremark Charitable Trust Grants, 1176
CVS Comm Grants, 1177
Cyrus Eaton Fndn Grants, 1178
D. W. McMillan Fndn Grants, 1180
D.F. Halton Fndn Grants, 1181
Dade Comm Fndn Comm AIDS Partnership Grants, 1184
Dade Comm Fndn Grants, 1185
DaimlerChrysler Corporation Fund Grants, 1186
Daisy Marquis Jones Fndn Grants, 1188
Dale and Edna Walsh Fndn Grants, 1189
Dallas Mavericks Fndn Grants, 1190
Dallas Women's Fndn Grants, 1191
Dammann Fund Grants, 1192
Dana Brown Charitable Trust Grants, 1194
Dana Corporation Fndn Grants, 1196
Danellie Fndn Grants, 1198
Daniels Fund Grants, 1200
Daphne Seybolt Culpeper Memorial Fndn Grants, 1201
David Geffen Fndn Grants, 1202
Daviess County Comm Fndn Health Grants, 1203
Dayton Power and Light Fndn Grants, 1205
Daywood Fndn Grants, 1206
Deaconess Comm Fndn Grants, 1207
Dean Foods Comm Involvement Grants, 1209
Dearborn Comm Fndn City of Lawrenceburg Comm Grants, 1210
Dearborn Comm Fndn County Progress Grants, 1211
Delaware Comm Fndn Grants, 1215
Delaware Comm Fndn-Youth Philanthropy Board for Kent County, 1216
Dell Fndn Healthy Communities, Literate Communities, and Connected Communities Grants, 1217
Dell Fndn Open Grants, 1218
Delta Air Lines Fndn Grants, 1220
DeMatteis Family Fndn Grants, 1221
Dennis and Phyllis Washington Fndn Grants, 1222
Denver Broncos Charities Fund Grants, 1226
Denver Fndn Comm Grants, 1227
Dept of Ed Safe and Drug-Free Schools and Communities State Grants, 1230
DeRoy Testamentary Fndn Grants, 1239
Detlef Schrempf Fndn Grants, 1240
Detroit Lions Charities Grants, 1241
DHHS Abandoned Infants Assistance Grants, 1242
DHHS AIDS Project Grants, 1245
DHHS Comprehensive Comm Mental Health Services Grants for Children with Serious Emotional Disturbances, 1247
DHHS Emergency Medical Services for Children (EMSC) Program, 1249
DHHS Healthy Tomorrows Partnership for Children, 1261
Do Something BR!CK Awards, 1287
DOA Distance Learning and Telemedicine Grants, 1288
DOJ Gang-Free Schools and Communities Intervention Grants, 1303
Dole Food Company Charitable Contributions, 1307
Dora Roberts Fndn Grants, 1311
Doris and Victor Day Fndn Grants, 1313
Dorothea Haus Ross Fndn Grants, 1320

Dorothy Rider Pool Health Care Grants, 1322
Dorrance Family Fndn Grants, 1323
DPA Promoting Policy Change Advocacy Grants, 1324
Dr. John T. Macdonald Fndn Grants, 1327
Dr. Scholl Fndn Grants, 1329
Drs. Bruce and Lee Fndn Grants, 1333
Dubois County Comm Fndn Grants, 1336
Duke Energy Fndn Grants, 1339
Duneland Health Council InCorpd Grants, 1350
Dunspaugh-Dalton Fndn Grants, 1351
DuPage Comm Fndn Grants, 1352
E. Rhodes and Leona B. Carpenter Fndn Grants, 1356
E.J. Grassmann Trust Grants, 1360
E.L. Wiegand Fndn Grants, 1361
Eastman Chemical Company Fndn Grants, 1362
eBay Fndn Comm Grants, 1363
Eberly Fndn Grants, 1364
Eddie C. and Sylvia Brown Family Fndn Grants, 1367
Eden Hall Fndn Grants, 1368
Edina Realty Fndn Grants, 1369
Edward Bangs Kelley and Elza Kelley Fndn Grants, 1373
Edward S. Moore Fndn Grants, 1374
Edwards Memorial Trust Grants, 1375
Edwin S. Webster Fndn Grants, 1376
Edyth Bush Charitable Fndn Grants, 1378
Effie and Wofford Cain Fndn Grants, 1385
EIF Comm Grants, 1386
Eisner Fndn Grants, 1387
El Paso Comm Fndn Grants, 1388
El Paso Corp Fndn Grants, 1389
El Pomar Fndn Awards and Grants, 1390
Elkhart County Comm Fndn Grants, 1401
Elliot Fndn Inc Grants, 1402
Elmer L. and Eleanor J. Andersen Fndn Grants, 1406
Elsie Lee Garthwaite Memorial Fndn Grants, 1408
Emily Davie and Joseph S. Kornfeld Fndn Grants, 1414
Emma B. Howe Memorial Fndn Grants, 1415
Ensworth Charitable Fndn Grants, 1416
Entergy Comm Partnership Grants, 1417
Entergy Corporation Open Grants for Healthy Families, 1418
EPA Children's Health Protection Grants, 1420
Erie Comm Fndn Grants, 1427
Essex County Comm Fndn Discretionary Fund Grant, 1428
Ethel S. Abbott Charitable Fndn Grants, 1430
Eugene and Agnes E. Meyer Fndn Grants, 1432
Eugene M. Lang Fndn Grants, 1434
Eva L. and Joseph M. Bruening Fndn Grants, 1436
Evan and Susan Bayh Fndn Grants, 1437
Evanston Comm Fndn Grants, 1438
Evjue Fndn Grants, 1439
ExxonMobil Grants, 1442
F.M. Kirby Fndn Grants, 1443
Fairfield County Comm Fndn Grants, 1446
Fairview Lutheran Fndn Grants, 1448
Fallon OrNda Comm Health Fund Grants, 1449
Fan Fox and Leslie R. Samuels Fndn Grants, 1451
FAR Fund, 1453
Fargo-Moorhead Area Fndn Grants, 1454
Farmers Insurance Group of Companies Grants, 1455
Faye McBeath Fndn Grants, 1456
Fayette County Fndn Grants, 1457
FCNY Union Square Awards, 1461
Federal Express Corp Contributions Program, 1483
Feldman Fndn Grants, 1484
Ferree Fndn Grants, 1486
Fidelity Fndn Grants, 1498
Field Fndn of Illinois Grants, 1499
Fifth Third Fndn Grants, 1501
FirstEnergy Fndn Comm Grants, 1505
Fisher Fndn Grants, 1508
Fisher House Fndn Newman's Own Awards, 1509
Flinn Fndn Grantss, 1511
Florida BRAIVE Fund of Dade Comm Fndn, 1512
Florida BRAIVE Fund of Gulf Coast Comm Fndn of Venice, 1513
Florida BRAIVE Fund of The Comm Fndn in Jacksonville, 1514
Floyd A. and Kathleen C. Cailloux Fndn Grants, 1516
Fluor Fndn Grants, 1517
FMC Fndn Grants, 1518
Foellinger Fndn Grants, 1519
Fondren Fndn Grants, 1520
Ford Motor Company Fund Grants, 1522
Forrest C. Lattner Fndn Grants, 1523
Foster Fndn Grants, 1524
Foster G. McGaw Prize, 1525
Fndn for Seacoast Health Grants, 1533
Fndn for the Carolinas Grants, 1535
Fndn for the Mid-South Grants, 1536
Fndn Northwest Grants, 1537
Fndn of CVPH Rabin Fund Grants, 1541
Fndn of CVPH Roger Senecal Endowment Fund Grants, 1542
Fourjay Fndn Grants, 1544
Frances and John L. Loeb Family Fund Grants, 1546
Frances L. and Edwin L. Cummings Memorial Fund Grants, 1547
Frances W. Emerson Fndn Grants, 1548
Francis L. Abreu Charitable Trust Grants, 1549
Francis T. & Louise T. Nichols Fndn Grants, 1550
Frank G. and Freida K. Brotz Family Fndn Grants, 1552
Frank Stanley Beveridge Fndn Grants, 1553
Franklin County Comm Fndn Grants, 1554
Fred Baldwin Memorial Fndn Grants, 1556
Fred L. Emerson Fndn Grants, 1557
Freddie Mac Fndn Grants, 1558
Fremont Area Comm Fndn Grants, 1561
Frey Fndn Grants, 1562
Frist Fndn Grants, 1563
Fritz B. Burns Fndn Grants, 1564
Fuller E. Callaway Fndn Grants, 1578
Fulton County Comm Fndn Grants, 1579
Gebbie Fndn Grants, 1585
GenCorp Fndn Grants, 1587
Genentech Corp Charitable Contributions Grants, 1588
General Mills Fndn Grants, 1590
General Motors Fndn Grants Support Program, 1591
General Service Fndn Reproductive Health and Rights Grants, 1592
Genuardi Family Fndn Grants, 1594
George and Ruth Bradford Fndn Grants, 1595
George F. Baker Trust Grants, 1597
George Family Fndn Grants, 1598
George Frederick Jewett Fndn Grants, 1599
George S. and Dolores Dore Eccles Fndn Grants, 1602
Georgia Power Fndn Grants, 1603
Georgiana Goddard Eaton Memorial Fund Grants, 1604
Geraldine R. Dodge Fndn Morris County Grants, 1605
Gertrude and William C. Wardlaw Fund Grants, 1607
Gertrude E. Skelly Charitable Fndn Grants, 1609
Gheens Fndn Grants, 1610
Giant Eagle Fndn Grants, 1611
Gibson Fndn Grants, 1612
Gill Fndn - Gay and Lesbian Fund Grants, 1613
Ginn Fndn Grants, 1616
Giving Sum Annual Grant, 1619
Gladys Brooks Fndn Grants, 1620
GlaxoSmithKline Corp Grants, 1623
Glazer Family Fndn Grants, 1625
Glendale Comm Fndn Grants, 1626
Global Fund for Children Grants, 1629
Godfrey Fndn Grants, 1631
GoGirlGo! Ambassador Team Awards, 1632
Golden State Warriors Fndn Grants, 1633
Goodrich Corporation Fndn Grants, 1638
Goodyear Tire Grants, 1639
Graco Fndn Grants, 1642
Grand Haven Area Comm Fndn Grants, 1644
Grand Rapids Area Comm Fndn Grants, 1645
Grand Rapids Area Comm Fndn Nashwauk Area Endowment Fund Grants, 1646
Grand Rapids Comm Fndn Grants, 1647
Great-West Life Grants, 1649
Greater Bridgeport Area Fndn Comm Impact Grants, 1650
Greater Cincinnati Fndn Priority and Small Projects/Capacity-Building Grants, 1651
Greater Green Bay Comm Fndn Grants, 1652
Greater Milwaukee Fndn Grants, 1653
Greater New Orleans Fndn Grants, 1654
Greater Saint Louis Comm Fndn Grants, 1655
Greater Tacoma Comm Fndn Grants, 1656
Greater Worcester Comm Fndn Discretionary Grants, 1658
Greater Worcester Comm Fndn Jeppson Memorial Fund for Brookfield Grants, 1659
Green Bay Packers Fndn Grants, 1660
Greene County Fndn Grants, 1662
Greenwall Fndn Bioethics Grants, 1665
Gregory B. Davis Fndn Grants, 1666
Grotto Fndn Project Grants, 1671
Grundy Fndn Grants, 1673
Gulf Coast Comm Fndn Grants, 1676
Gulf Coast Comm of Venice Fndn Grants, 1677
H & R Fndn Grants, 1679
H. Schaffer Fndn Grants, 1680
H.A. and Mary K. Chapman Charitable Trust Grants, 1681
H.J. Heinz Company Fndn Grants, 1682
Hackett Fndn Grants, 1684
Hagedorn Fund Grants, 1685
Hallmark Corp Fndn Grants, 1688
Hancock County Comm Fndn Grants, 1690
Hannaford Charitable Fndn Grants, 1692
Harden Fndn Grants, 1693
Harley Davidson Fndn Grants, 1694
Harold Alfond Fndn Grants, 1695
Harold and Arlene Schnitzer CARE Fndn Grants, 1697
Harold Simmons Fndn Grants, 1698
Harris and Eliza Kempner Fund Grants, 1699
Harrison County Comm Fndn Grants, 1700
Harry and Grace Steele Fndn Grants, 1702
Harry Bramhall Gilbert Charitable Trust Grants, 1703
Harry Kramer Memorial Fund Grants, 1705
Harry S. Black and Allon Fuller Fund, 1706
Harry Sudakoff Fndn Grants, 1708
Hartford Aging and Health Program Awards, 1709
Hartford Courant Fndn Grants, 1710
Hartford Fndn Regular Grants, 1711
Harvest Fndn Grants, 1713
Hasbro Children's Fund, 1714
Hawaii Comm Fndn Reverend Takie Okumura Family Grants, 1717
Hawaii Comm Fndn West Hawaii Fund Grants, 1718
Health Canada National Seniors Independence Program Grants, 1722
Health Fndn of Greater Cincinnati Grants, 1724
Health Fndn of Greater Indianapolis Grants, 1725
Health Fndn of Southern Florida Responsive Grants, 1726
Healthcare Fndn for Orange County Grants, 1728
Healthcare Fndn of New Jersey Grants, 1729
Hearst Fndn and William Randolph Hearst Fndn Grants, 1730
Helen Bader Fndn Grants, 1738
Helen K. and Arthur E. Johnson Fndn Grants, 1740
Helen Steiner Rice Fndn Grants, 1742
Helena Rubinstein Fndn Grants, 1743
Hendrick Fndn for Children Grants, 1744
Henrietta Tower Wurts Memorial Fndn Grants, 1745
Henry and Ruth Blaustein Rosenberg Fndn Grants, 1746
Henry J. Kaiser Family Fndn Grants, 1748

Herman Goldman Fndn Grants, 1753
Hershey Company Grants, 1754
High Meadow Fndn Grants, 1768
Highmark Corp Giving Grants, 1769
Hilda and Preston Davis Fndn Grants, 1772
Hill Crest Fndn Grants, 1773
Hill Fndn Grants, 1774
Hillman Fndn Grants, 1775
Hillsdale County Comm Fndn Healthy Senior/ Healthy Youth Fund Grants, 1776
Hillsdale County Comm General Adult Fndn Grants, 1777
Hilton Head Island Fndn Grants, 1779
Hilton Hotels Corp Giving Program Grants, 1780
Hirtzel Memorial Fndn Grants, 1781
Hoblitzelle Fndn Grants, 1783
Hogg Fndn for Mental Health Grants, 1784
Hoglund Fndn Grants, 1785
Holland/Zeeland Comm Fndn Grants, 1786
Home Building Industry Disaster Relief Fund, 1787
HomeBanc Fndn Grants, 1788
Homer Fndn Grants, 1789
Honda of America Manufacturing Fndn Grants, 1790
Honeywell Fndn Grants, 1791
Horace A. Kimball and S. Ella Kimball Fndn Grants, 1792
Horizon Fndn for New Jersey Grants, 1793
Horizons Comm Issues Grants, 1794
Houston Endowment Grants, 1797
Howard and Bush Fndn Grants, 1798
Howe Fndn of North Carolina Grants, 1799
HRSA Ryan White HIV Early Intervention Services Grants, 1811
Huber Fndn Grants, 1812
Hudson Webber Fndn Grants, 1813
Hugh J. Andersen Fndn Grants, 1814
Huie-Dellmon Trust Grants, 1815
Human Source Fndn Grants, 1817
Humana Fndn Grants, 1818
Humboldt Area Fndn Technical Assistance Program (TAP) Grants, 1819
Huntington Beach Police Officers Fndn Grants, 1821
Huntington Clinical Fndn Grants, 1822
Huntington County Comm Fndn Grants, 1823
Hut Fndn Grants, 1827
Hutton Fndn Grants, 1828
Ida Alice Ryan Charitable Trust Grants, 1836
Idaho Comm Fndn Eastern Region Competitive Grants, 1837
Idaho Power Company Corp Contributions, 1838
Impact 100 Grants, 1843
Inasmuch Fndn Grants, 1845
Independence Blue Cross Charitable Medical Care Grants, 1846
Independence Comm Fndn Comm Quality of Life Grant, 1849
Indiana 21st Century Research and Technology Fund Awards, 1850
Indiana AIDS Fund Grants, 1851
Ireland Family Fndn Grants, 1865
Irvin Stern Fndn Grants, 1866
Irving S. Gilmore Fndn Grants, 1867
Isabel Allende Fndn Esperanza Grants, 1868
Ittleson Fndn AIDS Grants, 1869
Ittleson Fndn Mental Health Grants, 1870
J. Walton Bissell Fndn Grants, 1872
J.B. Reynolds Fndn Grants, 1873
J.C. Penney Company Grants, 1874
J.E. and L.E. Mabee Fndn Grants, 1875
J.L. Bedsole Fndn Grants, 1876
J.M. Long Fndn Grants, 1877
J.W. Kieckhefer Fndn Grants, 1878
Jackson County Comm Fndn Unrestricted Grants, 1879
Jacob and Hilda Blaustein Fndn Grants, 1881
Jacob G. Schmidlapp Trust Grants, 1883
James A. and Faith Knight Fndn Grants, 1884
James Ford Bell Fndn Grants, 1885
James G.K. McClure Educational and Development Fund Grants, 1886
James Graham Brown Fndn Grants, 1887
James J. and Angelia M. Harris Fndn Grants, 1890
James M. Collins Fndn Grants, 1891
James M. Cox Fndn of Georgia Grants, 1892
James R. Dougherty Jr. Fndn Grants, 1894
James S. Copley Fndn Grants, 1895
Jane Bradley Pettit Fndn Grants, 1902
Jane's Trust Grants, 1904
Janirve Fndn Grants, 1905
Jasper Fndn Jasper County Grants, 1907
Jasper Fndn Newton County Grants, 1908
Jean and Louis Dreyfus Fndn Grants, 1911
JELD-WEN Fndn Grants, 1914
Jenkins Fndn: Improving the Health of Greater Richmond Grants, 1915
Jennings County Comm Fndn Grants, 1916
Jerome and Mildred Paddock Fndn Grants, 1917
Jessie B. Cox Charitable Trust Grants, 1918
Jessie Ball Dupont Fund Grants, 1919
Jessie Smith Noyes Fndn Grants, 1920
Jewish Comm Fndn of Greater Los Angeles Grants, 1921
Jewish Fund Grants, 1923
Jim Moran Fndn Grants, 1925
JM Fndn Grants, 1926
Joe W. and Dorothy Dorsett Brown Fndn Grants, 1927
John Ben Snow Memorial Trust Grants, 1928
John Deere Fndn Grants, 1929
John Edward Fowler Memorial Fndn Grants, 1930
John G. Duncan Trust Grants, 1931
John H. and Wilhelmina D. Harland Charitable Fndn Grants, 1933
John H. Wellons Fndn Grants, 1934
John I. Smith Charities Grants, 1935
John J. Leidy Fndn Grants, 1936
John Jewett and Helen Chandler Garland Fndn Grants, 1937
John Lord Knight Fndn Grants, 1938
John Merck Fund Grants, 1940
John P. McGovern Fndn Grants, 1942
John R. Oishei Fndn Grants, 1944
John Stauffer Charitable Trust Grants, 1946
John W. Alden Trust Grants, 1947
John W. and Anna H. Hanes Fndn Grants, 1948
John W. Anderson Fndn Grants, 1949
Johns Manville Fund Grants, 1950
Johnson Controls Fndn Grants, 1954
Johnson County Comm Fndn Grants, 1955
Joseph Drown Fndn Grants, 1960
Joseph H. and Florence A. Roblee Fndn Grants, 1961
Joseph P. Kennedy Jr. Fndn Grants, 1962
Josephine G. Russell Trust Grants, 1963
Josephine Goodyear Fndn Grants, 1964
Josiah W. and Bessie H. Kline Fndn Grants, 1967
Journal Gazette Fndn Grants, 1968
Joyce Fndn Grants, 1969
K. M. Hunter Charitable Fndn Social Welfare Grants, 1974
K21 Health Fndn Cancer Care Fund Grants, 1975
K21 Health Fndn Grants, 1976
Kahuku Comm Fund, 1977
Kalamazoo Fndn Grants, 1979
Kansas Health Fndn Grants, 1980
Kate B. Reynolds Charitable Trust Health Care Grants, 1981
Katharine Matthies Fndn Grants, 1982
Kathryne Beynon Fndn Grants, 1984
Kelvin and Eleanor Smith Fndn Grants, 1986
Kendrick Fndn Grants, 1988
Kenny's Kids Grants, 1990
Kettering Fund Grants, 1992
Kevin P. and Sydney B. Knight Family Fndn Grants, 1993
Key Fndn Grants, 1994
KeySpan Fndn Grants, 1995
Kimberly-Clark Comm Grants, 2001
Knox County Comm Fndn Grants, 2009
Komen Greater NYC Comm Breast Health Grants, 2011
Kosair Charities Grants, 2014
Kosciusko County Comm Fndn Grants, 2015
L. W. Pierce Family Fndn Grants, 2019
LaGrange County Comm Fndn Grants, 2020
Land O'Lakes Fndn Mid-Atlantic Grants, 2027
Lands' End Corp Giving Program, 2030
Laura B. Vogler Fndn Grants, 2032
Lawrence Fndn Grants, 2034
Legacy Fndn Grants, 2040
Leonard and Helen R. Stulman Charitable Fndn Grants, 2044
Lester E. Yeager Charitable Trust B Grants, 2047
Lettie Pate Whitehead Fndn Grants, 2049
Lewis Preston Fund for Girls Education Grants, 2052
Liberty Bank Fndn Grants, 2053
Lillian S. Wells Fndn Grants, 2056
Lincoln Financial Group Fndn Grants, 2058
Long Island Comm Fndn Grants, 2063
Lotus 88 Fndn for Women and Children Grants, 2064
Louis Calder Fndn Grants, 2065
Lowe Fndn Grants, 2067
Lowell Area Comm Fund Grants, 2068
Lowell Berry Fndn Grants, 2069
Lubbock Area Fndn Grants, 2079
Lubrizol Fndn Grants, 2080
Lucile Horton Howe and Mitchell B. Howe Fndn Grants, 2081
Lucy Gooding Charitable Fndn Trust, 2082
Lucy Gooding Charitable Fndn Trust Grants, 2083
Lynde and Harry Bradley Fndn Grants, 2089
M. Bastian Family Fndn Grants, 2092
M.B. and Edna Zale Fndn Grants, 2093
M.E. Raker Fndn Grants, 2094
M.J. Murdock Charitable Trust Grants, 2095
Madison County Comm Fndn Grants, 2098
Maine Comm Fndn Grants, 2099
Manuel D. and Rhoda Mayerson Fndn Grants, 2100
Marcia and Otto Koehler Fndn Grants, 2103
Margaret L. Wendt Fndn Grants, 2104
Marijuana Policy Project Grants, 2107
Mark and Catherine Winkler Fndn Grants, 2112
Mars Fndn Grants, 2114
Mary Black Fndn Grants, 2118
Mary Owen Borden Fndn Grants, 2121
Mary S. and David C. Corbin Fndn Grants, 2122
Mass Youth Against Tobacco Mini-Grants, 2123
Massage Therapy Fndn Comm Service Grants, 2124
Maxon Charitable Fndn Grants, 2135
Maxtor Corp Contributions Grants, 2136
McCarthy Family Fndn Grants, 2141
McGregor Fund Grants, 2143
McInerny Fndn Grants, 2144
McKesson Fndn Grants, 2145
McKnight Fndn Grants, 2146
Mead Johnson Nutritionals Charitable Giving Grants, 2156
Mead Johnson Nutritionals Evansville-Area Organizations Grants, 2157
Mead Johnson Nutritionals Medical Education Grants, 2158
Mead Witter Fndn Grants, 2160
Meadows Fndn Grants, 2161
Medicaid/SCHIP Eligibility Pilots, 2164
MedImmune Charitable Grants, 2166
Medtronic Fndn Full Life Patient Partnership Program--Heart Rescue Grants, 2168
Mericos Fndn Grants, 2172
Meriden Fndn Grants, 2173
Metro Health Fndn Grants, 2175
Metrowest Comm Health Care Fndn Grants, 2176
Meyer Memorial Trust Emergency Grants, 2178
Meyer Memorial Trust Grassroots Grants, 2179
Meyer Memorial Trust Operating Funds Grants, 2180
Meyer Memorial Trust Responsive Grants, 2181
Miami County Comm Fndn Operation Round Up Grants, 2188
Middlesex Savings Charitable Fndn Grants, 2196
Miguel Aleman Fndn Grants, 2197

Military Ex-Prisoners of War Fndn Grants, 2201
Millipore Fndn Grants, 2203
Minneapolis Fndn Comm Grants, 2206
Miriam and Peter Haas Fund Grants, 2208
Monfort Family Fndn Grants, 2213
Montgomery County Comm Fndn Grants, 2214
MONY Fndn Grants, 2215
Morris and Gwendolyn Cafritz Fndn Grants, 2217
Morton K. and Jane Blaustein Fndn Grants, 2218
Ms. Fndn for Women Grants, 2222
National City Corporation Contributions Grants, 2250
National Lottery Comm Fund Grants, 2256
NEI Innovative Patient Outreach Programs And Ocular Screening Technologies To Improve Detection Of Diabetic Retinopathy Grants, 2294
Nelda C. and H.J. Lutcher Stark Fndn Grants, 2301
New York Life Fndn Grants, 2304
Nicholas H. Noyes Jr. Memorial Fndn Grants, 2497
NIH Exploratory Innovations in Biomedical Computational Science and Technology (BISTI) Grants, 2664
NIH Innovations in Biomedical Computational Science and Technology Grants, 2679
NIH Recovery Act Limited Competition: Building Sustainable Comm-Linked Infrastructure to Enable Health Science Research, 2709
Nina Mason Pulliam Charitable Trust Grants, 2776
NLM Understanding and Promoting Health Literacy Research Grants, 2827
NNEDVF/Altria Doors of Hope Program, 2847
Noble County Comm Fndn Grants, 2848
Nordson Corporation Fndn Grants, 2851
North Carolina Biotechnology Center Event Sponsorship Grants, 2852
North Carolina Biotechnology Center Meeting Grants, 2854
North Carolina Biotechnology Center Regional Development Grants, 2855
North Carolina Comm Development Grants, 2858
North Carolina Comm Fndn Grants, 2859
North Carolina GlaxoSmithKline Fndn Grants, 2860
North Central Health Services Grants, 2861
North Georgia Comm Fndn Grants, 2862
Northeast Utilities Fndn Grants, 2863
Northern New York Comm Fndn Grants, 2864
Northern Trust Company Charitable Trust and Corp Giving Program, 2865
Northrop Grumman Newport News Grants, 2867
Northwest Airlines KidCares Medical Travel Assistance, 2868
Northwest Minnesota Fndn Women's Fund Grants, 2869
Northwestern Mutual Fndn Grants, 2870
Norwin S. and Elizabeth N. Bean Fndn Grants, 2872
NSERC Brockhouse Canada Prize for Interdisciplinary Research in Science and Engineering Grant, 2873
Nuffield Fndn Africa Program Grants, 2898
Nuffield Fndn Children and Families Grants, 2899
Nuffield Fndn Small Grants, 2903
NWHF Comm-Based Participatory Research Grants, 2904
NWHF Health Advocacy Small Grants, 2905
NWHF Kaiser Permanente Comm Fund Grants, 2906
NWHF Partners Investing in Nursing's Future Grants, 2908
NYCT AIDS/HIV Grants, 2919
NYCT Children and Youth with Disabilities Grants, 2923
NYCT Girls and Young Women Grants, 2924
NYCT Grants for the Elderly, 2925
NYCT Health Services, Systems, and Policies Grants, 2926
NYCT Mental Health and Mental Retardation Grants, 2927
NYCT Technical Assistance Grants, 2929
Oakland Fund for Children and Youth Grants, 2930
OceanFirst Fndn Grants, 2933
Oceanside Charitable Fndn Grants, 2934
Office Depot Fndn Grants, 2936
Ogden Codman Trust Grants, 2937
Ohio County Comm Fndn Grants, 2938
Ohio County Comm Fndn Mini-Grants, 2939
Oleonda Jameson Trust Grants, 2941
Olin Corporation Charitable Trust Grants, 2943
OneStar Fndn AmeriCorps Grants, 2945
Oracle Corp Contributions Grants, 2951
Ordean Fndn Grants, 2952
OSI Harm Reduction and Drug Use Grants, 2966
OSI Indonesia Project Grants, 2967
OSI Integrating Health and Legal Services Grants, 2968
OSI Mental Health Grants, 2969
OSI Palliative Cancer Care Grants, 2970
OSI-Baltimore Special Opportunities Program Grants, 2972
OSI-Baltimore Tackling Drug Addiction Grants, 2973
Otto Bremer Fndn Grants, 2977
Owen County Comm Fndn Grants, 2979
PacifiCare Fndn Grants, 2981
PacifiCorp Fndn for Learning Grants, 2982
Pajaro Valley Comm Health Grants, 2985
Palm Beach and Martin Counties Grants, 2986
Pasadena Fndn Average Grants, 2994
Paso del Norte Health Fndn Grants, 2995
Patron Saints Fndn Grants, 2996
Paul and Mary Haas Fndn Contributions and Student Scholarships, 2997
Paul E. and Klare N. Reinhold Fndn Grants, 2999
Paul G. Duke Fndn Grants, 3001
Paul Ogle Fndn Grants, 3003
Payless ShoeSource Fndn Grants, 3004
Peacock Fndn Grants, 3011
Perkins Charitable Fndn Grants, 3014
Perpetual Trust for Charitable Giving Grants, 3015
Perry County Comm Fndn Grants, 3016
Pet Care Trust Sue Busch Memorial Award, 3017
Pew Charitable Trusts Children and Youth Grants, 3020
Pfizer Fndn Grants, 3025
Philadelphia Fndn Organizational Effectiveness Grants, 3029
Phoenix Suns Charities Grants, 3030
Piedmont Natural Gas Grants, 3048
Pike County Comm Fndn Grants, 3049
Pinellas County Grants, 3050
Pioneer Hi-Bred Comm Grants, 3051
Piper Jaffray Companies Building Strong Communities Grants, 3053
Pittsburgh Fndn Comm Fund Grants, 3054
Plough Fndn Grants, 3061
Plum Creek Fndn Grants, 3062
PMI Fndn Grants, 3063
PNC Charitable Trust and Fndn Grants, 3064
Polaroid Fund Grants, 3065
Polk Bros. Fndn Grants, 3066
Portland General Electric Fndn Grants, 3067
Posey Comm Fndn Grants, 3068
Posey Comm Fndn Womens Fund Grants, 3069
Pott Fndn Grants, 3071
Powell Fndn Grants, 3073
Presbyterian Health Fndn Bridge, Seed and Equipment Grants, 3075
Presbyterian Patient Assistance Program, 3076
Pride Fndn Grants and Scholarships, 3078
Prince Charitable Trusts Chicago Grants, 3079
Prince Charitable Trusts District of Columbia Grants, 3080
Princeton Area Comm Fndn Greater Mercer Grants, 3081
Principal Financial Group Fndn Grants, 3082
Procter and Gamble Fund Grants, 3083
Progress Energy Fndn Grants, 3084
Prudential Fndn Grants, 3087
Public Welfare Fndn Grants, 3089
Puerto Rico Comm Fndn Grants, 3090
Pulaski County Comm Fndn Grants, 3091
Pulte Homes Corp Contributions, 3092
Putnam County Comm Fndn Grants, 3093
Quantum Corporation Snap Server Grants, 3095
Quantum Fndn Grants, 3096
Questar Corp Contributions Grants, 3097
R.C. Baker Fndn Grants, 3098
Rainbow Endowment Grants, 3102
Rainbow Fund Grants, 3103
Ralphs Food 4 Less Fndn Grants, 3106
Rathmann Family Fndn Grants, 3109
Raymond John Wean Fndn Grants, 3110
Rayonier Fndn Grants, 3111
Regence Fndn Access to Health Care Grants, 3138
Regence Fndn Health Care Comm Awareness and Engagement Grants, 3139
Regence Fndn Health Care Connections Grants, 3140
Regence Fndn Improving End-of-Life Grants, 3141
Regence Fndn Tools and Technology Grants, 3142
Retirement Research Fndn General Program Grants, 3150
Reynolds and Reynolds Associate Fndn Grants, 3152
Rhode Island Fndn Grants, 3154
Rice Fndn Grants, 3155
Rich Fndn Grants, 3156
Richard and Helen DeVos Fndn Grants, 3157
Richard and Rhoda Goldman Fund Grants, 3158
Richard and Susan Smith Family Fndn Grants, 3159
Richard M. Fairbanks Fndn Grants, 3162
Richmond Eye and Ear Fund Grants, 3164
Riley Fndn Grants, 3165
Ripley County Comm Fndn Grants, 3166
Robert and Joan Dircks Fndn Grants, 3167
Robert and Polly Dunn Fndn Grants, 3168
Robert B McMillen Fndn Grants, 3169
Robert F. Stoico / FIRSTFED Charitable Fndn Grants, 3171
Robert P. & Clara I. Milton Fund for Senior Housing, 3172
Robert Sterling Clark Fndn Reproductive Rights and Health Grants, 3173
Robin Hood Fndn Grants, 3174
Robins Fndn Grants, 3175
Rochester Area Comm Fndn Grants, 3176
Rochester Area Fndn Grants, 3177
Rockefeller Brothers Fund Peace and Security Grants, 3179
Rockefeller Fndn Grants, 3181
Rockwell International Corp Trust Grants, 3183
Rohm and Haas Company Grants, 3185
Rollin M. Gerstacker Fndn Grants, 3186
Roy and Christine Sturgis Trust Grants, 3191
RRF General Program Grants, 3193
Rush County Comm Fndn Grants, 3200
Russell Berrie Fndn Grants, 3201
Ruth Eleanor Bamberger and John Ernest Bamberger Memorial Fndn Grants, 3202
Ruth H. and Warren A. Ellsworth Fndn Grants, 3203
Ruth Mott Fndn Grants, 3204
RWJF Comm Health Leaders Awards, 3208
RWJF Health Care Costs: Research to Inform Policy Grants, 3215
RWJF Health Policy Fellowships, 3217
RWJF Healthy Eating Research Grants, 3218
RWJF Investigator Awards in Health Policy Research, 3220
RWJF Ladder to Leadership: Developing the Next Generation of Comm Health Leaders Fellowships, 3222
RWJF Local Funding Partnerships Program Grants, 3223
RWJF New Jersey Health Initiatives Grants, 3225
RWJF Partners Investing in Nursing's Future Grants, 3226
RWJF Pioneer Portfolio Grants, 3227
RWJF Pipeline, Profession and Practice: Comm-Based Dental Education Grants, 3228
RWJF State Coverage Initiatives Grants, 3230

RWJF Vulnerable Populations Portfolio Grants, 3232
S. Mark Taper Fndn Grants, 3236
S.H. Cowell Fndn Grants, 3237
SAG Motion Picture Players Welfare Fund Grants, 3238
Saint Luke's Fndn Grants, 3239
Saint Luke's Health Initiatives Grants, 3240
Salem Fndn Charitable Trust Grants, 3241
Salisbury Comm Fndn Grants, 3243
SAMHSA Child Mental Health Initiative (CMHI) Grants, 3245
SAMHSA Drug Free Communities Support Program Grants, 3247
SAMHSA Strategic Prevention Framework State Incentive Grants, 3248
Samuel S. Johnson Fndn Grants, 3251
San Antonio Area Fndn Grants, 3254
San Diego Fndn for Change Grants, 3255
San Diego Fndn Health & Human Services Grants, 3256
San Diego Fndn Paradise Valley Hospital Comm Fund Grants, 3257
San Diego HIV Funding Collaborative (SDHFC) Grants, 3258
San Diego Women's Fndn Grants, 3259
San Francisco Fndn Comm Health Grants, 3260
Sarah Scaife Fndn Grants, 3263
Sarasota Memorial Healthcare Fndn Grants, 3264
Sasco Fndn Grants, 3265
Schering-Plough Fndn Comm Initiatives Grants, 3269
Schering-Plough Fndn Health Grants, 3270
Schurz Communications Fndn Grants, 3271
Scott County Comm Fndn Grants, 3273
Seabury Fndn Grants, 3274
Seattle Fndn Grants, 3276
Self Fndn Grants, 3277
Seneca Foods Fndn Grants, 3278
Shaw's Supermarkets Donations, 3280
Shell Oil Company Fndn Grants, 3281
Sheltering Arms Fund Grants, 3282
Sid W. Richardson Fndn Grants, 3284
Siebert Lutheran Fndn Grants, 3285
Simmons Fndn Grants, 3287
Simple Advise Education Center Grants, 3289
Simpson Fund Grants, 3290
Sir Dorabji Tata Trust Grants for NGOs or Voluntary Organizations, 3291
Siragusa Fndn Health Services & Medical Research Grants, 3294
Sisters of Mercy of North Carolina Fndn Grants, 3295
Sisters of Saint Joseph Charitable Fund Grants, 3296
Sisters of St. Joseph Healthcare Fndn Grants, 3297
Snee Reinhardt Charitable Fndn Grants, 3300
SOCFOC Catholic Ministries Grants, 3317
SOCFOC Reducing Health & Educational Disparities in the Central Neighborhood Grants, 3318
Society for the Arts in Healthcare Consulting Grants, 3326
Society for the Arts in Healthcare Environmental Arts Research Grant, 3327
Solo Cup Fndn Grants, 3346
Sonoco Fndn Grants, 3347
Sosland Fndn Grants, 3348
South Madison Comm Fndn Grants, 3349
Southbury Comm Trust Fund, 3350
Southwest Florida Comm Fndn Competitive Grants, 3351
Southwest Gas Corporation Fndn Grants, 3352
Southwire Company Grants, 3353
Spencer County Comm Fndn Grants, 3358
Sprague Fndn Grants, 3359
Springs Close Fndn Grants, 3360
Square D Fndn Grants, 3361
St. Joseph Comm Health Fndn Improving Healthcare Access Grants, 3368
Stark Comm Fndn Women's Fund Grants, 3376
Starr Fndn Grants, 3377
Steelcase Fndn Grants, 3379
Steele-Reese Fndn Grants, 3380
Stephen Bechtel Fund Preventive Healthcare and Selected Research Grants, 3381
Steuben County Comm Fndn Grants, 3383
Stewart Huston Charitable Trust Grants, 3384
Strowd Roses Grants, 3388
Sulzberger Fndn Grants, 3399
Sunderland Fndn Grants, 3400
Sunflower Fndn Capacity Building Grants, 3402
Sunflower Fndn Walking Trails Grants, 3403
Susan Mott Webb Charitable Trust Grants, 3412
Susan Vaughan Fndn Grants, 3413
Taproot Fndn Capacity-Building Service Grants, 3417
Temple-Inland Fndn Grants, 3419
Texas Commission on the Arts Arts Respond Project Grants, 3420
Thelma Doelger Charitable Trust Grants, 3421
Thomas C. Ackerman Fndn Grants, 3423
Thomas M. and Irene B. Kirbo Charitable Trust Grants, 3424
Thompson Charitable Fndn Grants, 3425
Tides Fndn Syringe Access Fund, 3427
Tifa Fndn Grants, 3428
Topeka Comm Fndn Kansas Blood Services Scholarships, 3429
Toro Fndn Grants, 3431
Triangle Comm Fndn Donor-Advised Grants, 3437
Triangle Comm Fndn Shaver-Hitchings Scholarship, 3438
Trull Fndn Grants, 3441
TWS Fndn Grants, 3443
U.S. Department of Education 21st Century Comm Learning Centers, 3445
U.S. Department of Education Rehabilitation Training--Rehabilitation Continuing Education Programs (RCEP)--Institute on Rehabilitation Issues (IRI), 3449
U.S. Department of Education Special Education--National Activities--Parent Information Centers, 3450
U.S. Department of Education Vocational Rehabilitation Services Projects for American Indians with Disabilities Grants, 3452
Union Benevolent Association Grants, 3460
Union County Comm Fndn Grants, 3461
United Methodist Church Malaria Control Grants, 3464
United Technologies Corporation Grants, 3466
Unity Fndn Of LaPorte County Grants, 3467
Until There's a Cure Fndn Grants, 3471
US Airways Comm Contributions, 3472
US Airways Comm Fndn Grants, 3473
US Trust Corporation Fndn Grants, 3475
USCM HIV/AIDS Prevention Grants, 3476
Vancouver Fndn Grants and Comm Initiatives Program, 3477
Vancouver Sun Children's Fund Grants, 3479
Vanderburgh Comm Fndn Grants, 3480
Vectren Fndn Grants, 3485
Verizon Fndn Health Care and Accessibility Grants, 3486
Verizon Fndn Maryland Grants, 3487
Verizon Fndn New York Grants, 3488
Verizon Fndn Northeast Region Grants, 3489
Verizon Fndn Pennsylvania Grants, 3490
Verizon Fndn Vermont Grants, 3491
Verizon Fndn Virginia Grants, 3492
Vermont Comm Fndn Grants, 3493
Virginia W. Kettering Fndn Grants, 3502
Volkswagen of America Corp Contributions Grants, 3503
Vulcan Materials Company Fndn Grants, 3504
W.K. Kellogg Fndn Healthy Kids Grants, 3507
W.K. Kellogg Fndn Secure Families Grants, 3508
Wabash Valley Comm Fndn Grants, 3510
Wachovia Fndn Grants, 3511
Waitt Family Fndn Grants, 3512
Wal-Mart Fndn Comm Grants, 3513
Wal-Mart State Giving Program Grants, 3514
Walt Disney Company Fndn Grants, 3516
Warrick County Comm Fndn Grants, 3519
Washington Post Contributions Program Grants, 3520
Wayne and Gladys Valley Fndn Grants, 3522
Weatherwax Fndn Grants, 3523
Weingart Fndn Grants, 3524
Welborn Baptist Fndn Grants, 3525
Wellmark Fndn Grants, 3526
Wells County Fndn Grants, 3527
Western Indiana Comm Fndn Grants, 3528
Westinghouse Charitable Giving Grants, 3530
WHAS Crusade for Children Grants, 3531
WHO Fndn General Grants, 3534
Wilkins Family Fndn Grants, 3536
William G. Gilmore Fndn Grants, 3537
William G. McGowan Charitable Fund Grants, 3539
Wilson-Wood Fndn Grants, 3542
Winston-Salem Fndn Competitive Grants, 3544
Winston-Salem Fndn Elkin/Tri-County Grants, 3545
Winston-Salem Fndn Stokes County Grants, 3546
Women's Fndn of California Comm Action Fund, 3549
Women's Fndn of California Grants, 3550
YSA Get Ur Good On Grants, 3555
YSA UnitedHealth Heroes Service Learning Grants, 3556
Z. Smith Reynolds Fndn Small Grants, 3557

Consulting/Visiting Personnel

AAAS Science & Technology Policy Fellowships - National Defense & Global Security, 29
AAP Leonard P. Rome Comm Access to Child Health (CATCH) Visiting Professorships, 164
Abbott Fund Access to Health Care Grants, 176
Abbott Fund Global AIDS Care Grants, 178
Able To Serve Grants, 185
AHFMR Personnel Funding Grants, 290
American College of Surgeons International Guest Scholarships, 429
American-Scandinavian Fndn Visiting Lectureship Grants, 460
APhA Fndn Incentive Grants, 512
APSAA Small Beginning Scholar Visiting and Consulting Grants, 521
ASM International Professorship for Latin America, 603
ASM International Professorships for Asia and Africa, 604
Assurant Health Fndn Grants, 655
Avon Products Fndn Grants, 675
Beckley Area Fndn Grants, 732
Bodenwein Public Benevolent Fndn Grants, 775
CFPC Family Medicine Resident Leadership Awards, 953
Clarence E. Heller Charitable Fndn Grants, 1022
Claude Pepper Fndn Grants, 1032
Claude Worthington Benedum Fndn Grants, 1033
Columbus Fndn Traditional Grants, 1071
Comm Fndn for Greater Buffalo Grants, 1090
Comm Fndn for Greater New Haven Grants, 1091
Comm Fndn for Monterey County Grants, 1092
Comm Fndn for Muskegon County Grants, 1093
Comm Fndn for Southern Arizona Grants, 1095
Comm Fndn of Champaign County Grants, 1102
Comm Fndn of Greater Fort Wayne: Comm Endowment & Clarke Endowment Fund Grants, 1108
Comm Fndn Silicon Valley Grants, 1133
Connecticut Comm Fndn Grants, 1141
D. W. McMillan Fndn Grants, 1180
Dade Comm Fndn Comm AIDS Partnership Grants, 1184
Delaware Comm Fndn-Youth Philanthropy Board for Kent County, 1216
DHHS Chiropractic Demonstration Project Grants, 1246

Drs. Bruce and Lee Fndn Grants, 1333
Eddie C. and Sylvia Brown Family Fndn Grants, 1367
Edina Realty Fndn Grants, 1369
Eisner Fndn Grants, 1387
Emily Davie and Joseph S. Kornfeld Fndn Grants, 1414
Eugene and Agnes E. Meyer Fndn Grants, 1432
Families USA Wellstone Fellowship for Social Justice, 1450
FCER Chiropractic Research Grants, 1459
Florida BRAIVE Fund of Dade Comm Fndn, 1512
Florida BRAIVE Fund of Gulf Coast Comm Fndn of Venice, 1513
Florida BRAIVE Fund of The Comm Fndn in Jacksonville, 1514
Foellinger Fndn Grants, 1519
Frances L. and Edwin L. Cummings Memorial Fund Grants, 1547
Grass Fndn Marine Biological Laboratory Fellowships, 1648
Hastings Center International Visiting Scholars Program, 1715
Hawaii Comm Fndn Health Education and Research Grants, 1716
Helen Steiner Rice Fndn Grants, 1742
Hogg Fndn for Mental Health Grants, 1784
Jennings County Comm Fndn Grants, 1916
Jessie Ball Dupont Fund Grants, 1919
John G. Martin Fndn Grants, 1932
KFF Barbara Jordan Health Policy Scholars Program, 2000
Knight Public Health Journalism Fellowships at CDC, 2008
Mary Baker Eddy Library Summer Research Fellowships, 2117
Meadows Fndn Grants, 2161
Montgomery County Comm Fndn Grants, 2214
NCI Technologies and Software to Support Integrative Cancer Biology Research (SBIR) Grants, 2279
NIGMS Minority Access to Research Careers (MARC) Program, 2620
Noble County Comm Fndn Grants, 2848
North Carolina Biotechnology Center Grantsmanship Training Grants, 2853
North Carolina Comm Fndn Grants, 2859
Northwood University/Alden B. Dow Creativity Center Summer Residency Program, 2871
Ordean Fndn Grants, 2952
OREF Educational Awards, 2953
PAHO-ASM International Professorship for Latin America, 2983
Pfizer/AAFP Fndn Visiting Professorship Program in Family Medicine, 3027
PhRMA Fndn Health Outcomes Sabbatical Fellowships, 3034
Pike County Comm Fndn Grants, 3049
Pinellas County Grants, 3050
Pittsburgh Fndn Comm Fund Grants, 3054
Prudential Fndn Grants, 3087
Puerto Rico Comm Fndn Grants, 3090
RCPSC Events, Speakers and Visiting Professors Grants, 3116
RCPSC McLaughlin-Gallie Visiting Professorship, 3123
RCPSC Royal College Visiting Professorships in Medical Research, 3130
RCPSC Walter C. MacKenzie Fellowship in Surgery, 3133
RCPSC Wightman Visiting Professorship in Medicine, 3134
Rhode Island Fndn Grants, 3154
Rochester Area Comm Fndn Grants, 3176
RWJF Local Funding Partnerships Program Grants, 3223
Samuel S. Johnson Fndn Grants, 3251
Seabury Fndn Grants, 3274
Shell Oil Company Fndn Grants, 3281
Society for the Arts in Healthcare Consulting Grants, 3326
St. Joseph Comm Health Fndn Schneider Fellowships, 3370
Texas Commission on the Arts Arts Respond Project Grants, 3420
US CRDF Leishmaniasis: Collaborative Research Opportunities in North Africa and the Middle East, 3474

Cultural Outreach

3M Fndn Grants, 11
A Friend's Fndn Trust Grants, 13
A. Gary Anderson Family Fndn Grants, 17
A.O. Smith Comm Grants, 18
Aaron Fndn (Massachusetts) Grants, 174
Abbott Fund Comm Vitality Grants, 177
Abell-Hanger Fndn Grants, 183
Abington Fndn Grants, 184
Achelis and Bodman Fndns Grants, 206
Adaptec Fndn Grants, 232
Adelaide Breed Bayrd Fndn Grants, 234
Advanced Micro Devices Comm Affairs Grants, 239
AEC Trust Grants, 242
AFG Industries Grants, 259
African American Fund of New Jersey Grants, 260
Agnes Gund Fndn Grants, 262
Agway Fndn Grants, 265
Ahmanson Fndn Grants, 303
Ahn Family Fndn Grants, 304
AIG American General Corporation Grants, 316
Air Products and Chemicals Grants, 319
Aladdin Industries Fndn Grants, 322
Albert and Margaret Alkek Fndn Grants, 326
Albert Pick Jr. Fund Grants, 328
Alberto Culver Corp Contributions Grants, 329
Albertson's Charitable Giving Grants, 330
Albuquerque Comm Fndn Grants, 331
Alcatel-Lucent Technologies Corp Contributions Grants, 332
Alcatel-Lucent Technologies Fndn Grants, 333
Alexander & Baldwin Fndn Hawaiian and Pacific Island Grants, 338
Alexander & Baldwin Fndn Mainland Grants, 339
Allen P. and Josephine B. Green Fndn Grants, 361
Allstate Corp Hometown Commitment Grants, 364
Altman Fndn Health Care Grants, 372
Amador Comm Fndn Grants, 409
Amgen Fndn Grants, 467
Anheuser-Busch Fndn Grants, 474
Ann Peppers Fndn Grants, 478
Annenberg Fndn Grants, 479
Annie Sinclair Knudsen Memorial Fund/Kaua'i Comm Grants, 480
Anschutz Family Fndn Grants, 486
AON Fndn Grants, 491
Aratani Fndn Grants, 523
Arcadia Fndn Grants, 524
Archer Daniels Midland Fndn Grants, 525
Argyros Fndn Grants, 527
Arie and Ida Crown Memorial Grants, 528
Arizona Cardinals Grants, 529
Arizona Public Service Corp Giving Program Grants, 531
Arkansas Comm Fndn Grants, 533
Armstrong McDonald Fndn Grants, 537
ARS Fndn Grants, 538
ArvinMeritor Grants, 544
ASHA Multicultural Activities Projects Grants, 571
Ashland Corp Contributions Grants, 586
Assisi Fndn Grants, 653
Assurant Health Fndn Grants, 655
AT&T Fndn Civic and Comm Service Program Grants, 658
Atherton Family Fndn Grants, 659
Athwin Fndn Grants, 660
Atlanta Fndn Grants, 662
Auburn Fndn Grants, 664
Audrey and Sydney Irmas Charitable Fndn Grants, 665
Aurora Fndn Grants, 667
Autzen Fndn Grants, 672
Avon Products Fndn Grants, 675
Axe-Houghton Fndn Grants, 678
Bacon Family Fndn Grants, 679
Bailey Fndn Grants, 680
Ball Brothers Fndn Grants, 684
Banfi Vintners Fndn Grants, 687
Bank of America Client Fndn Grants, 690
Barberton Comm Fndn Grants, 693
Barker Welfare Fndn Grants, 695
Barnes Group Fndn Grants, 696
Barr Fund Grants, 697
Barra Fndn Comm Fund Grants, 698
Barra Fndn Project Grants, 699
Batchelor Fndn Grants, 701
Baton Rouge Area Fndn Grants, 702
Battle Creek Comm Fndn Grants, 703
Batts Fndn Grants, 704
Baxter International Fndn Grants, 705
BCBS of Minnesota Healthy Together Grants, 712
BCBSNC Fndn Grants, 725
Bechtel Group Fndn Building Positive Comm Relationships Grants, 731
Beckley Area Fndn Grants, 732
Belk Fndn Grants, 739
Benton County Fndn Grants, 744
Berks County Comm Fndn Grants, 745
Bernard and Audre Rapoport Fndn Grants, 746
Berrien Comm Fndn Grants, 749
Besser Fndn Grants, 752
Bildner Family Fndn Grants, 755
Binney and Smith Comm Grants, 757
Biogen Corp Giving Grants, 758
Blanche and Irving Laurie Fndn Grants, 764
Blanche and Julian Robertson Family Fndn Grants, 765
Blue Grass Comm Fndn Grants, 768
Blue Mountain Comm Fndn Grants, 769
Blum-Kovler Fndn Grants, 772
Bob and Delores Hope Charitable Fndn Grants, 774
Bodenwein Public Benevolent Fndn Grants, 775
Bodman Fndn Grants, 776
Boeing Company Contributions Program Grants, 777
Boettcher Fndn Grants, 778
Bonfils-Stanton Fndn Grants, 779
Booth-Bricker Fund Grants, 780
Boston Fndn Grants, 783
Boston Globe Fndn Grants, 784
Boston Jewish Comm Women's Fund Grants, 785
Bradley Turner Fndn Grants, 789
Bridgestone/Firestone Trust Fund Grants, 792
Burlington Industries Fndn Grants, 811
Burlington Northern Santa Fe Fndn Grants, 812
Business Bank of Nevada Comm Grants, 817
Byron W. and Alice L. Lockwood Fndn Grants, 824
C.R. Bard Fndn Grants, 825
Caleb C. and Julia W. Dula Educational and Charitable Fndn Grants, 830
Cambridge Comm Fndn Grants, 837
Campbell Hoffman Fndn Grants, 840
Canada-U.S. Fulbright New Century Scholars Program Grants, 846
Canada-U.S. Fulbright Senior Specialists Program Grants, 847
Carl and Eloise Pohlad Family Fndn Grants, 867
Carl and Lily Pforzheimer Fndn Grants, 868
Carl B. and Florence E. King Fndn Grants, 869
Carl C. Icahn Fndn Grants, 870
Carl Gellert and Celia Berta Gellert Fndn Grants, 871
Carnegie Corporation of New York Grants, 879
Carolyn Fndn Grants, 880
Carpenter Fndn Grants, 881
Carroll County Comm Fndn Grants, 885
Cemala Fndn Grants, 933
Central Carolina Comm Fndn Comm Impact Grants, 936
Central Okanagan Fndn Grants, 937
Cessna Fndn Grants, 938

CFFVR Opportunity Grants, 952
Champlin Fndns Grants, 960
Charles H. Dater Fndn Grants, 966
Charles Lafitte Fndn Grants, 970
Charles M. Bair Family Trust Grants, 972
Charlotte County (FL) Comm Fndn Grants, 973
Chatlos Fndn Grants, 977
Chazen Fndn Grants, 978
Chesapeake Corporation Fndn Grants, 982
Chicago Board of Trade Fndn Grants, 988
Chicago Comm Trust Grants, 989
Chicago Tribune's Corp Contributions Grants, 991
Chiles Fndn Grants, 1003
Christy-Houston Fndn Grants, 1008
CICF Legacy Fund Comm Fndn Grants, 1010
CIGNA Fndn Grants, 1011
Cinergy Fndn Grants, 1013
Citizens Bank Mid-Atlantic Charitable Fndn Grants, 1015
Clarcor Fndn Grants, 1021
Clarence E. Heller Charitable Fndn Grants, 1022
Clark-Winchcole Fndn Grants, 1030
Cleveland Browns Fndn Grants, 1036
CNA Fndn Grants, 1046
Coastal Bend Comm Fndn Grants, 1050
Coastal Comm Fndn of South Carolina Grants, 1051
Coca-Cola Fndn Grants, 1052
Cockrell Fndn Grants, 1053
Collins Fndn Grants, 1058
Colorado Springs Comm Trust Fund Grants, 1061
Columbus Fndn Competitive Grants, 1066
Comer Fndn Grants, 1072
Comerica Charitable Fndn Grants, 1073
Comm Fndn Alliance City of Evansville Endowment Fund Grants, 1089
Comm Fndn for Monterey County Grants, 1092
Comm Fndn for Muskegon County Grants, 1093
Comm Fndn for Southeastern Michigan Grants, 1094
Comm Fndn for Southern Arizona Grants, 1095
Comm Fndn of Bartholomew County Heritage Fund Grants, 1096
Comm Fndn of Bloomington and Monroe County Grants, 1098
Comm Fndn of Broward Grants, 1100
Comm Fndn of Central Illinois Grants, 1101
Comm Fndn of Champaign County Grants, 1102
Comm Fndn of Grant County Grants, 1104
Comm Fndn of Greater Birmingham Grants, 1106
Comm Fndn of Greater Flint Grants, 1107
Comm Fndn of Greater Fort Wayne: Comm Endowment & Clarke Endowment Fund Grants, 1108
Comm Fndn of Greater Greensboro Grants, 1109
Comm Fndn of Greater Tampa Grants, 1112
Comm Fndn of Greenville Hollingsworth Funds Program/Project Grants, 1114
Comm Fndn of Greenville-Greenville Women Giving Grants, 1115
Comm Fndn of Howard County Grants, 1116
Comm Fndn of Morgan County Grants and Scholarships, 1118
Comm Fndn of Mount Vernon and Knox County Grants, 1119
Comm Fndn of Muncie and Delaware County Grants, 1120
Comm Fndn of Randolph County Grants, 1121
Comm Fndn of Santa Cruz County Grants, 1122
Comm Fndn of South Alabama Grants, 1123
Comm Fndn of South Puget Sound Grants, 1124
Comm Fndn of Southeastern Connecticut Grants, 1125
Comm Fndn of the Eastern Shore Comm Needs Grants, 1129
Comm Fndn of Western North Carolina Grants, 1132
Comm Fndn Silicon Valley Grants, 1133
Comm Impact Fund, 1135
ConAgra Foods Fndn Grants, 1140
Connecticut Comm Fndn Grants, 1141
Connelly Fndn Grants, 1143
ConocoPhillips Fndn Grants, 1144
Constantin Fndn Grants, 1145
Constellation Energy Group and Baltimore Gas and Electric Corp Contributions, 1146
Consumers Energy Fndn, 1147
Cooke Fndn Grants, 1148
Cooper Industries Fndn Grants, 1150
Cornerstone Fndn of Northeastern Wisconsin Grants, 1152
Cowles Charitable Trust Grants, 1155
Cranston Fndn Grants, 1158
CSRA Comm Fndn Grants, 1168
CSX Corp Contributions Grants, 1169
Cudd Fndn Grants, 1171
Cullen Fndn Grants, 1172
Cultural Society of Filipino Americans Grants, 1173
CUNA Mutual Group Fndn, 1174
Cyrus Eaton Fndn Grants, 1178
D.F. Halton Fndn Grants, 1181
Dade Comm Fndn Grants, 1185
Dairy Queen Corp Contributions Grants, 1187
Dale and Edna Walsh Fndn Grants, 1189
Dana Brown Charitable Trust Grants, 1194
Davis Family Fndn Grants, 1204
Dayton Power and Light Fndn Grants, 1205
Daywood Fndn Grants, 1206
Delaware Comm Fndn Grants, 1215
Delaware Comm Fndn-Youth Philanthropy Board for Kent County, 1216
DeMatteis Family Fndn Grants, 1221
Denver Broncos Charities Fund Grants, 1226
Denver Fndn Comm Grants, 1227
DeRoy Testamentary Fndn Grants, 1239
Dole Food Company Charitable Contributions, 1307
Donald and Sylvia Robinson Family Fndn Grants, 1310
Dorothy Rider Pool Health Care Grants, 1322
Dorrance Family Fndn Grants, 1323
Dr. Bob and Jean Smith Fndn Grants, 1325
Dr. Leon Bromberg Charitable Trust Fund Grants, 1328
Dr. Scholl Fndn Grants, 1329
Drs. Bruce and Lee Fndn Grants, 1333
Dunspaugh-Dalton Fndn Grants, 1351
DuPage Comm Fndn Grants, 1352
E. Rhodes and Leona B. Carpenter Fndn Grants, 1356
E.L. Wiegand Fndn Grants, 1361
Eastman Chemical Company Fndn Grants, 1362
Eberly Fndn Grants, 1364
Eddie C. and Sylvia Brown Family Fndn Grants, 1367
Eden Hall Fndn Grants, 1368
Edina Realty Fndn Grants, 1369
Educational Fndn of America Grants, 1372
Edward Bangs Kelley and Elza Kelley Fndn Grants, 1373
Edward S. Moore Fndn Grants, 1374
Edwin S. Webster Fndn Grants, 1376
Edwin W. and Catherine M. Davis Fndn Grants, 1377
Edyth Bush Charitable Fndn Grants, 1378
Eisner Fndn Grants, 1387
El Paso Comm Fndn Grants, 1388
El Pomar Fndn Awards and Grants, 1390
Elizabeth Morse Genius Charitable Trust Grants, 1400
Elkhart County Comm Fndn Grants, 1401
Elmer L. and Eleanor J. Andersen Fndn Grants, 1406
Emerson Charitable Trust Grants, 1412
Emily Davie and Joseph S. Kornfeld Fndn Grants, 1414
Emma B. Howe Memorial Fndn Grants, 1415
Entergy Comm Partnership Grants, 1417
Erie Comm Fndn Grants, 1427
Essex County Comm Fndn Discretionary Fund Grant, 1428
Estee Lauder Grants, 1429
Eugene and Agnes E. Meyer Fndn Grants, 1432
Eugene M. Lang Fndn Grants, 1434
Evanston Comm Fndn Grants, 1438
Evjue Fndn Grants, 1439
ExxonMobil Grants, 1442
F.M. Kirby Fndn Grants, 1443
Fallon OrNda Comm Health Fund Grants, 1449
Fargo-Moorhead Area Fndn Grants, 1454
Farmers Insurance Group of Companies Grants, 1455
Faye McBeath Fndn Grants, 1456
FCNY Union Square Awards, 1461
Federal Express Corp Contributions Program, 1483
Ferree Fndn Grants, 1486
Field Fndn of Illinois Grants, 1499
Fireman's Fund Fndn Grants, 1504
Fishman Family Fndn Grants, 1510
Flinn Fndn Grantss, 1511
Florida BRAIVE Fund of Dade Comm Fndn, 1512
Floyd A. and Kathleen C. Cailloux Fndn Grants, 1516
Fluor Fndn Grants, 1517
Foellinger Fndn Grants, 1519
Fondren Fndn Grants, 1520
Ford Motor Company Fund Grants, 1522
Forrest C. Lattner Fndn Grants, 1523
Foster Fndn Grants, 1524
Fndn for the Carolinas Grants, 1535
Fndn Northwest Grants, 1537
Francis L. Abreu Charitable Trust Grants, 1549
Francis T. & Louise T. Nichols Fndn Grants, 1550
Frank Stanley Beveridge Fndn Grants, 1553
Fred Baldwin Memorial Fndn Grants, 1556
Fred L. Emerson Fndn Grants, 1557
Fremont Area Comm Fndn Grants, 1561
Fuji Film Grants, 1565
Fulbright Alumni Initiatives Awards Program Grants, 1566
Fulbright Distinguished Chairs Program Grants, 1567
Fulbright German Studies Seminar Grants, 1568
Fulbright International Education Administrators (IEA) Seminar Program Grants, 1569
Fulbright New Century Scholars (NCS) Program Grants, 1570
Fulbright Specialists Program Grants, 1571
Fulbright Traditional Scholar Program in Europe and Eurasia, 1572
Fulbright Traditional Scholar Program in Sub-Saharan Africa, 1573
Fulbright Traditional Scholar Program in the East Asia/Pacific Region, 1574
Fulbright Traditional Scholar Program in the Near East and North Africa Region, 1575
Fulbright Traditional Scholar Program in the South and Central Asia Region, 1576
Fulbright Traditional Scholar Program in the Western Hemisphere, 1577
G.N. Wilcox Trust Grants, 1581
Gebbie Fndn Grants, 1585
GenCorp Fndn Grants, 1587
General Mills Fndn Grants, 1590
General Motors Fndn Grants Support Program, 1591
Genesis Fndn Grants, 1593
Genuardi Family Fndn Grants, 1594
George and Ruth Bradford Fndn Grants, 1595
George B. Storer Fndn Grants, 1596
George Family Fndn Grants, 1598
George Frederick Jewett Fndn Grants, 1599
George Kress Fndn Grants, 1601
George S. and Dolores Dore Eccles Fndn Grants, 1602
Georgia Power Fndn Grants, 1603
Gertrude and William C. Wardlaw Fund Grants, 1607
Giant Eagle Fndn Grants, 1611
Gibson Fndn Grants, 1612
Gill Fndn - Gay and Lesbian Fund Grants, 1613
Gilroy and Lillian P. Roberts Charitable Fndn Grants, 1614
GlaxoSmithKline Corp Grants, 1623
Glendale Comm Fndn Grants, 1626
Golden State Warriors Fndn Grants, 1633

Goodrich Corporation Fndn Grants, 1638
Goodyear Tire Grants, 1639
Grammy Fndn Grants, 1643
Grand Rapids Area Comm Fndn Grants, 1645
Grand Rapids Area Comm Fndn Nashwauk Area Endowment Fund Grants, 1646
Greater Bridgeport Area Fndn Comm Impact Grants, 1650
Greater Cincinnati Fndn Priority and Small Projects/Capacity-Building Grants, 1651
Greater Green Bay Comm Fndn Grants, 1652
Greater Milwaukee Fndn Grants, 1653
Greater New Orleans Fndn Grants, 1654
Greater Saint Louis Comm Fndn Grants, 1655
Greater Tacoma Comm Fndn Grants, 1656
Greater Worcester Comm Fndn Discretionary Grants, 1658
Greater Worcester Comm Fndn Jeppson Memorial Fund for Brookfield Grants, 1659
Green Bay Packers Fndn Grants, 1660
Green Fndn Grants, 1661
Grundy Fndn Grants, 1673
Gulf Coast Comm Fndn Grants, 1676
Gulf Coast Comm of Venice Fndn Grants, 1677
H & R Fndn Grants, 1679
H.A. and Mary K. Chapman Charitable Trust Grants, 1681
H.J. Heinz Company Fndn Grants, 1682
Halliburton Fndn Grants, 1687
Hallmark Corp Fndn Grants, 1688
Hanna Andersson Children's Fndn Grants, 1691
Harden Fndn Grants, 1693
Harley Davidson Fndn Grants, 1694
Harold Alfond Fndn Grants, 1695
Harold and Arlene Schnitzer CARE Fndn Grants, 1697
Harold Simmons Fndn Grants, 1698
Harris and Eliza Kempner Fund Grants, 1699
Harrison County Comm Fndn Grants, 1700
Harry Bramhall Gilbert Charitable Trust Grants, 1703
Hartford Fndn Regular Grants, 1711
Hawaii Comm Fndn Reverend Takie Okumura Family Grants, 1717
Hawaii Comm Fndn West Hawaii Fund Grants, 1718
Hawn Fndn Grants, 1719
HCA Fndn Grants, 1721
Hearst Fndn and William Randolph Hearst Fndn Grants, 1730
Heckscher Fndn for Children Grants, 1732
Heineman Fndn for Research, Education, Charitable and Scientific Purposes, 1735
Helen Bader Fndn Grants, 1738
Helen K. and Arthur E. Johnson Fndn Grants, 1740
Helena Rubinstein Fndn Grants, 1743
Henrietta Tower Wurts Memorial Fndn Grants, 1745
Henry and Ruth Blaustein Rosenberg Fndn Grants, 1746
Herman Goldman Fndn Grants, 1753
Hershey Company Grants, 1754
Highmark Corp Giving Grants, 1769
Hill Crest Fndn Grants, 1773
Hill Fndn Grants, 1774
Hillman Fndn Grants, 1775
Hillsdale County Comm General Adult Fndn Grants, 1777
Hillsdale Fund Grants, 1778
Hilton Head Island Fndn Grants, 1779
Hoblitzelle Fndn Grants, 1783
Hoglund Fndn Grants, 1785
Holland/Zeeland Comm Fndn Grants, 1786
Homer Fndn Grants, 1789
Honda of America Manufacturing Fndn Grants, 1790
Honeywell Fndn Grants, 1791
Horace A. Kimball and S. Ella Kimball Fndn Grants, 1792
Horizon Fndn for New Jersey Grants, 1793
Horizons Comm Issues Grants, 1794
Houston Endowment Grants, 1797
Howard and Bush Fndn Grants, 1798
Hudson Webber Fndn Grants, 1813
Hugh J. Andersen Fndn Grants, 1814
Huie-Dellmon Trust Grants, 1815
Humana Fndn Grants, 1818
Huntington National Bank Comm Affairs Grants, 1824
Hut Fndn Grants, 1827
Hutton Fndn Grants, 1828
Idaho Comm Fndn Eastern Region Competitive Grants, 1837
Idaho Power Company Corp Contributions, 1838
Impact 100 Grants, 1843
Inasmuch Fndn Grants, 1845
Infinity Fndn Grants, 1854
Irvin Stern Fndn Grants, 1866
Irving S. Gilmore Fndn Grants, 1867
J. Walton Bissell Fndn Grants, 1872
J.B. Reynolds Fndn Grants, 1873
J.C. Penney Company Grants, 1874
J.L. Bedsole Fndn Grants, 1876
J.M. Long Fndn Grants, 1877
Jackson County Comm Fndn Unrestricted Grants, 1879
Jacob G. Schmidlapp Trust Grants, 1883
James Ford Bell Fndn Grants, 1885
James G.K. McClure Educational and Development Fund Grants, 1886
James Graham Brown Fndn Grants, 1887
James J. and Angelia M. Harris Fndn Grants, 1890
James M. Collins Fndn Grants, 1891
James M. Cox Fndn of Georgia Grants, 1892
James S. Copley Fndn Grants, 1895
Jane Bradley Pettit Fndn Grants, 1902
Jane's Trust Grants, 1904
Jay and Rose Phillips Family Fndn Grants, 1909
Jean and Louis Dreyfus Fndn Grants, 1911
JELD-WEN Fndn Grants, 1914
Jessie B. Cox Charitable Trust Grants, 1918
Jessie Ball Dupont Fund Grants, 1919
Jewish Women's Fndn of New York Grants, 1924
Jim Moran Fndn Grants, 1925
John Ben Snow Memorial Trust Grants, 1928
John Deere Fndn Grants, 1929
John I. Smith Charities Grants, 1935
John J. Leidy Fndn Grants, 1936
John P. Murphy Fndn Grants, 1943
John R. Oishei Fndn Grants, 1944
John W. and Anna H. Hanes Fndn Grants, 1948
Johns Manville Fund Grants, 1950
Johnson and Johnson / SAH Arts and Healing Grants, 1953
Joseph Drown Fndn Grants, 1960
Joseph H. and Florence A. Roblee Fndn Grants, 1961
Joyce Fndn Grants, 1969
Kahuku Comm Fund, 1977
Katharine Matthies Fndn Grants, 1982
Kelvin and Eleanor Smith Fndn Grants, 1986
Kenneth T. and Eileen L. Norris Fndn Grants, 1989
Kettering Family Fndn Grants, 1991
Key Fndn Grants, 1994
KeySpan Fndn Grants, 1995
King Pharmaceuticals Corp Contributions Grants, 2003
Kraft Cares International Grants, 2016
Kraft Cares US Grants, 2017
L. W. Pierce Family Fndn Grants, 2019
Land O'Lakes Fndn Mid-Atlantic Grants, 2027
Larry L. Hillblom Fndn Grants, 2031
Legacy Fndn Grants, 2040
Liberty Bank Fndn Grants, 2053
Lillian S. Wells Fndn Grants, 2056
Lincoln Financial Group Fndn Grants, 2058
Lindbergh Grants, 2059
Lockheed Martin Philanthropic Grants, 2062
Lotus 88 Fndn for Women and Children Grants, 2064
Louis Calder Fndn Grants, 2065
Lowell Area Comm Fund Grants, 2068
Lubrizol Fndn Grants, 2080
Ludwick Family Fndn Grants, 2084
Lynde and Harry Bradley Fndn Grants, 2089
M. Bastian Family Fndn Grants, 2092
M.J. Murdock Charitable Trust Grants, 2095
Mabel Y. Hughes Charitable Trust Grants, 2097
Madison County Comm Fndn Grants, 2098
Maine Comm Fndn Grants, 2099
Manuel D. and Rhoda Mayerson Fndn Grants, 2100
Marcia and Otto Koehler Fndn Grants, 2103
Margaret T. Morris Fndn Grants, 2105
Marion I. and Henry J. Knott Fndn Grants, 2109
Mars Fndn Grants, 2114
Marshall Field's Comm Grants, 2115
Mary Baker Eddy Library Summer Research Fellowships, 2117
Mary Owen Borden Fndn Grants, 2121
Matilda R. Wilson Fund Grants, 2128
Mattel Children's Fndn Grants, 2130
Max A. Adler Charitable Fndn Grants, 2132
Max and Victoria Dreyfus Fndn Grants, 2133
Maxon Charitable Fndn Grants, 2135
Maxtor Corp Contributions Grants, 2136
May Department Stores Charitable Contribution Grants, 2138
McInerny Fndn Grants, 2144
McKesson Fndn Grants, 2145
McKnight Fndn Grants, 2146
McLean Contributionship Grants, 2147
McMurry Fndn Grants, 2149
Mead Johnson Nutritionals Evansville-Area Organizations Grants, 2157
Mead Witter Fndn Grants, 2160
Meadows Fndn Grants, 2161
Mericos Fndn Grants, 2172
Meriden Fndn Grants, 2173
Meyer Memorial Trust Grassroots Grants, 2179
Meyer Memorial Trust Responsive Grants, 2181
Miami County Comm Fndn Operation Round Up Grants, 2188
Middlesex Savings Charitable Fndn Grants, 2196
Miguel Aleman Fndn Grants, 2197
Milagro Fndn Grants, 2198
Millipore Fndn Grants, 2203
Miriam and Peter Haas Fund Grants, 2208
Monfort Family Fndn Grants, 2213
Morris and Gwendolyn Cafritz Fndn Grants, 2217
New York Life Fndn Grants, 2304
Newman's Own Inc Grants, 2306
Nicholas H. Noyes Jr. Memorial Fndn Grants, 2497
Noble County Comm Fndn Grants, 2848
Nordson Corporation Fndn Grants, 2851
North Carolina Comm Fndn Grants, 2859
North Georgia Comm Fndn Grants, 2862
Northeast Utilities Fndn Grants, 2863
Northern Trust Company Charitable Trust and Corp Giving Program, 2865
Northrop Grumman Corporation Grants, 2866
Northrop Grumman Newport News Grants, 2867
Northwestern Mutual Fndn Grants, 2870
Norwin S. and Elizabeth N. Bean Fndn Grants, 2872
Nuffield Fndn Africa Program Grants, 2898
Ogden Codman Trust Grants, 2937
Oleonda Jameson Trust Grants, 2941
Ordean Fndn Grants, 2952
OSI-Baltimore Special Opportunities Grants, 2972
Otto Bremer Fndn Grants, 2977
Palm Beach and Martin Counties Grants, 2986
Paul and Mary Haas Fndn Contributions and Student Scholarships, 2997
Paul E. and Klare N. Reinhold Fndn Grants, 2999
Paul G. Allen Family Fndn Grants, 3000
Perkins Charitable Fndn Grants, 3014
Pfizer Fndn Grants, 3025
Philadelphia Fndn Organizational Effectiveness Grants, 3029
Phoenix Suns Charities Grants, 3030
Piedmont Natural Gas Grants, 3048
Pittsburgh Fndn Comm Fund Grants, 3054
Plum Creek Fndn Grants, 3062
PMI Fndn Grants, 3063

Polk Bros. Fndn Grants, 3066
Portland General Electric Fndn Grants, 3067
Posey Comm Fndn Womens Fund Grants, 3069
Powell Fndn Grants, 3073
Priddy Fndn Grants, 3077
Pride Fndn Grants and Scholarships, 3078
Prince Charitable Trusts Chicago Grants, 3079
Prince Charitable Trusts District of Columbia Grants, 3080
Principal Financial Group Fndn Grants, 3082
Procter and Gamble Fund Grants, 3083
Prudential Fndn Grants, 3087
Puerto Rico Comm Fndn Grants, 3090
Putnam County Comm Fndn Grants, 3093
R.C. Baker Fndn Grants, 3098
Rajiv Gandhi Fndn Grants, 3104
Ralphs Food 4 Less Fndn Grants, 3106
Rasmuson Fndn Grants, 3108
Rathmann Family Fndn Grants, 3109
Regence Fndn Access to Health Care Grants, 3138
Rhode Island Fndn Grants, 3154
Rice Fndn Grants, 3155
Rich Fndn Grants, 3156
Richard and Rhoda Goldman Fund Grants, 3158
Richard and Susan Smith Family Fndn Grants, 3159
Richard King Mellon Fndn Grants, 3161
Riley Fndn Grants, 3165
Robert B McMillen Fndn Grants, 3169
Robert F. Stoico / FIRSTFED Charitable Fndn Grants, 3171
Rochester Area Comm Fndn Grants, 3176
Rochester Area Fndn Grants, 3177
Rockefeller Brothers Fund Peace and Security Grants, 3179
Rockefeller Fndn Grants, 3181
Rockwell International Corp Trust Grants, 3183
Rohm and Haas Company Grants, 3185
Rollin M. Gerstacker Fndn Grants, 3186
Ruth Mott Fndn Grants, 3204
S. Mark Taper Fndn Grants, 3236
Salem Fndn Charitable Trust Grants, 3241
Salisbury Comm Fndn Grants, 3243
Samuel S. Johnson Fndn Grants, 3251
San Antonio Area Fndn Grants, 3254
San Diego Fndn for Change Grants, 3255
San Diego Women's Fndn Grants, 3259
Sarah Scaife Fndn Grants, 3263
Sasco Fndn Grants, 3265
Schering-Plough Fndn Comm Initiatives Grants, 3269
Scott County Comm Fndn Grants, 3273
Siebert Lutheran Fndn Grants, 3285
Simmons Fndn Grants, 3287
Simpson Fund Grants, 3290
SOCFOC Catholic Ministries Grants, 3317
Sonoco Fndn Grants, 3347
Sosland Fndn Grants, 3348
Southbury Comm Trust Fund, 3350
Southwest Florida Comm Fndn Competitive Grants, 3351
Spencer County Comm Fndn Grants, 3358
Sprague Fndn Grants, 3359
Square D Fndn Grants, 3361
Starr Fndn Grants, 3377
Steelcase Fndn Grants, 3379
Stewart Huston Charitable Trust Grants, 3384
Sulzberger Fndn Grants, 3399
Susan Mott Webb Charitable Trust Grants, 3412
Temple-Inland Fndn Grants, 3419
Texas Commission on the Arts Arts Respond Project Grants, 3420
Thomas C. Ackerman Fndn Grants, 3423
Thompson Charitable Fndn Grants, 3425
Toro Fndn Grants, 3431
Triangle Comm Fndn Donor-Advised Grants, 3437
Trull Fndn Grants, 3441
TWS Fndn Grants, 3443
U.S. Department of Education United States-Russia Program: Improving Research and Educational Activities in Higher Education, 3451
United Technologies Corporation Grants, 3466
US Trust Corporation Fndn Grants, 3475
Vancouver Fndn Grants and Comm Initiatives Program, 3477
Virginia W. Kettering Fndn Grants, 3502
Wachovia Fndn Grants, 3511
Waitt Family Fndn Grants, 3512
Walt Disney Company Fndn Grants, 3516
Washington Post Contributions Program Grants, 3520
Weatherwax Fndn Grants, 3523
Weingart Fndn Grants, 3524
Western Indiana Comm Fndn Grants, 3528
Westinghouse Charitable Giving Grants, 3530
Wilkins Family Fndn Grants, 3536
William G. Gilmore Fndn Grants, 3537
Winston-Salem Fndn Competitive Grants, 3544
Winston-Salem Fndn Stokes County Grants, 3546
Women's Fndn of California Grants, 3550
Z. Smith Reynolds Fndn Small Grants, 3557

Curriculum Development/Teacher Training

3M Fndn Grants, 11
A Fund for Women Grants, 14
Abbott Fund Science and Medical Innovation Grants, 179
Advanced Micro Devices Comm Affairs Grants, 239
Affymetrix Corp Contributions Grants, 258
Albertson's Charitable Giving Grants, 330
AMD Corp Contributions Grants, 411
American Electric Power Grants, 434
Amgen Fndn Grants, 467
Angels Baseball Fndn Grants, 473
Annenberg Fndn Grants, 479
APF Typical or Troubled School Mental Health Education Grants, 510
Aratani Fndn Grants, 523
Arkema Fndn Science Teachers Program, 535
ASHA Advancing Academic-Research Careers (AARC) Award, 569
Ball Brothers Fndn Grants, 684
Barra Fndn Comm Fund Grants, 698
Benton Comm Fndn Grants, 743
Bernard and Audre Rapoport Fndn Grants, 746
Blackford County Comm Fndn Grants, 763
Blanche and Julian Robertson Family Fndn Grants, 765
Blue River Comm Fndn Grants, 770
Boeing Company Contributions Program Grants, 777
Bonfils-Stanton Fndn Grants, 779
Bristol-Myers Squibb Fndn Health Education Grants, 798
Brown County Comm Fndn Grants, 807
Cambridge Comm Fndn Grants, 837
Carnahan-Jackson Fndn Grants, 878
Carnegie Corporation of New York Grants, 879
Carolyn Fndn Grants, 880
Carrie Estelle Doheny Fndn Grants, 883
Chestnut Hill Charitable Fndn, Inc Grants, 987
Chicago Comm Trust Grants, 989
Chiron Fndn Comm Grants, 1004
Clarence E. Heller Charitable Fndn Grants, 1022
Clark County Comm Fndn Grants, 1028
Coca-Cola Fndn Grants, 1052
Comm Fndn Alliance City of Evansville Endowment Fund Grants, 1089
Comm Fndn of Bartholomew County Heritage Fund Grants, 1096
Comm Fndn of Boone County Grants, 1099
Comm Fndn of Greater Birmingham Grants, 1106
Comm Fndn of Wabash County Grants, 1131
Comprehensive Health Education Fndn Grants, 1139
ConocoPhillips Fndn Grants, 1144
Crail-Johnson Fndn Grants, 1157
Cudd Fndn Grants, 1171
Dean Foods Comm Involvement Grants, 1209
Dubois County Comm Fndn Grants, 1336
eBay Fndn Comm Grants, 1363
Eddie C. and Sylvia Brown Family Fndn Grants, 1367
Effie and Wofford Cain Fndn Grants, 1385
Emily Davie and Joseph S. Kornfeld Fndn Grants, 1414
Eugene McDermott Fndn Grants, 1435
ExxonMobil Grants, 1442
Faye McBeath Fndn Grants, 1456
Field Fndn of Illinois Grants, 1499
Ford Motor Company Fund Grants, 1522
Fndn for the Mid-South Grants, 1536
Frank Stanley Beveridge Fndn Grants, 1553
GenCorp Fndn Grants, 1587
Genuardi Family Fndn Grants, 1594
Gheens Fndn Grants, 1610
Gibson Fndn Grants, 1612
Goodrich Corporation Fndn Grants, 1638
Grand Rapids Area Comm Fndn Grants, 1645
Grand Rapids Area Comm Fndn Nashwauk Area Endowment Fund Grants, 1646
Greater Tacoma Comm Fndn Ryan Alan Hade Endowment Fund, 1657
Greater Worcester Comm Fndn Jeppson Memorial Fund for Brookfield Grants, 1659
Heineman Fndn for Research, Education, Charitable and Scientific Purposes, 1735
Highmark Healthy High 5, 1770
Hillsdale County Comm General Adult Fndn Grants, 1777
Hoglund Fndn Grants, 1785
Honda of America Manufacturing Fndn Grants, 1790
Hormel Fndn Grants, 1796
Huntington Beach Police Officers Fndn Grants, 1821
Huntington County Comm Fndn Grants, 1823
J.C. Penney Company Grants, 1874
James R. Dougherty Jr. Fndn Grants, 1894
Jennings County Comm Fndn Grants, 1916
Jessie Ball Dupont Fund Grants, 1919
Jewish Women's Fndn of New York Grants, 1924
Joe W. and Dorothy Dorsett Brown Fndn Grants, 1927
John Jewett and Helen Chandler Garland Fndn Grants, 1937
John P. McGovern Fndn Grants, 1942
Joseph Alexander Fndn Grants, 1957
Joseph H. and Florence A. Roblee Fndn Grants, 1961
Josephine Goodyear Fndn Grants, 1964
Josiah W. and Bessie H. Kline Fndn Grants, 1967
Joyce Fndn Grants, 1969
K and F Baxter Family Fndn Grants, 1973
King Pharmaceuticals Corp Contributions Grants, 2003
Knight Family Charitable and Educational Fndn Grants, 2007
Louis R. Cappelli Fndn Grants, 2066
Lubbock Area Fndn Grants, 2079
Marion Park Deaver and Harry Gilbert Deaver Fndn Grants, 2110
Mattel Children's Fndn Grants, 2130
Mead Johnson Nutritionals Evansville-Area Organizations Grants, 2157
Mead Johnson Nutritionals Medical Education Grants, 2158
Meadows Fndn Grants, 2161
Meyer Memorial Trust Responsive Grants, 2181
MfA Newton Fellowships, 2182
Miriam and Peter Haas Fund Grants, 2208
Montgomery County Comm Fndn Grants, 2214
Moses Cone-Wesley Long Comm Health Fndn Grants, 2219
New York Life Fndn Grants, 2304
NIH School-based Interventions to Prevent Obesity, 2725
Office Depot Fndn Grants, 2936
OSI-Baltimore Special Opportunities Program Grants, 2972
Paul and Mary Haas Fndn Contributions and Student Scholarships, 2997

Pew Charitable Trusts Children and Youth Grants, 3020
Pfizer Fndn Grants, 3025
Polk Bros. Fndn Grants, 3066
Portland General Electric Fndn Grants, 3067
Procter and Gamble Fund Grants, 3083
Rathmann Family Fndn Grants, 3109
Richard and Susan Smith Family Fndn Grants, 3159
San Diego Women's Fndn Grants, 3259
Seabury Fndn Grants, 3274
Shell Oil Company Fndn Grants, 3281
South Madison Comm Fndn Grants, 3349
Strowd Roses Grants, 3388
STTI/ATI Educational Assessment Nursing Research Grants, 3397
Tellabs Fndn Grants, 3418
Union County Comm Fndn Grants, 3461
Vancouver Fndn Grants and Comm Initiatives Program, 3477
Vectren Fndn Grants, 3485
Verizon Fndn Maryland Grants, 3487
Verizon Fndn Vermont Grants, 3491
Verizon Fndn Virginia Grants, 3492
Wabash Valley Comm Fndn Grants, 3510
Wal-Mart Fndn Comm Grants, 3513
Weatherwax Fndn Grants, 3523
Weingart Fndn Grants, 3524
Western Indiana Comm Fndn Grants, 3528
Winston-Salem Fndn Elkin/Tri-County Grants, 3545
Winston-Salem Fndn Stokes County Grants, 3546
YSA UnitedHealth Heroes Service Learning Grants, 3556

Demonstration Grants
Aetna Fndn Quality of Care Grants for Depression, 246
American Legacy Fndn Small Innovative Grants, 439
amfAR Public Policy Grants, 465
Barra Fndn Project Grants, 699
Berks County Comm Fndn Grants, 745
Bullitt Fndn Grants, 809
Campbell Hoffman Fndn Grants, 840
Carlisle Fndn Grants, 874
CDC Evidence-Based Laboratory Medicine: Quality/Performance Measure Evaluation, 901
CDC Oral Diseases Prevention and Oral Health Promotion Grants, 921
CDC Research, Treatment, and Education Programs on Lyme Disease in the United States Cooperative Agreements, 927
CDC Sexually Transmitted Diseases Research, Demonstration, Public Information, and Education Grants, 929
Children's Cardiomyopathy Fndn Research Grants, 1002
Columbus Fndn Competitive Grants, 1066
Commonwealth Fund Patient-Centered Coordinated Care Program Grants, 1081
Commonwealth Fund Quality of Care for Frail Elders Grants, 1083
Comm Fndn of Greater Fort Wayne: Comm Endowment & Clarke Endowment Fund Grants, 1108
Comm Fndn of South Alabama Grants, 1123
Comm Fndn of Western North Carolina Grants, 1132
Denver Fndn Comm Grants, 1227
DHHS Adolescent Family Life Demonstration Projects, 1243
DHHS Chiropractic Demonstration Project Grants, 1246
DHHS Developmental Disabilities University Affiliated Programs Project Grants, 1248
DHHS Emergency Medical Services for Children (EMSC) Program, 1249
DHHS Health Promotion and Disease Prevention Research and Demonstration Centers Grants, 1260
DHHS HIV Demonstration Program for Children, Adolescents, and Women, 1262
DHHS Maternal and Child Health Research and Training Programs Grants, 1264
DHHS Oral Health Promotion Research Across the Lifespan, 1269
DHHS Rural Telemedicine Grants, 1279
Educational Fndn of America Grants, 1372
FCER Chiropractic Research Grants, 1459
FDA Orphan Products Clinical Studies Grants, 1462
Health Care Financing Research, Demonstrations, and Evaluations Grants, 1723
Health Fndn of Greater Cincinnati Grants, 1724
Henry J. Kaiser Family Fndn Grants, 1748
Ittleson Fndn AIDS Grants, 1869
Ittleson Fndn Mental Health Grants, 1870
James S. McDonnell Fndn Complex Systems Collaborative Activity Awards, 1897
James S. McDonnell Fndn Scholar Awards, 1899
Joyce Fndn Grants, 1969
Mayday Fund Grants, 2139
National Psoriasis Fndn Research Grants, 2259
NIGMS Short Courses on Mathematical, Statistical, and Computational Tools for Studying Biological Systems, 2629
NIH National Occupational Research Agenda Grants, 2696
NIMH Mental Health Dissemination Research Grants, 2762
NIOSH Occupational Safety and Health Research and Demonstration Grants, 2807
NLM Exploratory/Developmental Grants, 2816
PhRMA Fndn Health Outcomes Research Starter Grants, 3033
Pittsburgh Fndn Comm Fund Grants, 3054
Plough Fndn Grants, 3061
Principal Financial Group Fndn Grants, 3082
RRF General Program Grants, 3193
RWJF Changes in Health Care Financing and Organization Grants, 3206
RWJF New Jersey Health Initiatives Grants, 3225
RWJF State Coverage Initiatives Grants, 3230
Saint Luke's Health Initiatives Grants, 3240
SAMHSA Campus Suicide Prevention Grants, 3244
Self Fndn Grants, 3277
Skin Cancer Fndn Research Grants, 3298
Unity Fndn Of LaPorte County Grants, 3467

Development (Institutional/Departmental)
AAAAI / Schering Allergy/Immunology Fellowship of Excellence Training Awards, 20
AEGON Transamerica Fndn Grants, 243
Aetna Fndn Quality of Care Grants for Depression, 246
AHFMR Polaris Awards, 291
Albuquerque Comm Fndn Grants, 331
AMA Fndn Seed Grants for Research, 398
amfAR Global Initiatives Grants, 463
Anheuser-Busch Fndn Grants, 474
Ann and Robert H. Lurie Family Fndn Grants, 475
Ann Arbor Area Comm Fndn Grants, 476
AptarGroup Fndn Grants, 522
ASCO State Affiliate Grants, 560
ASHA Multicultural Activities Projects Grants, 571
Assisi Fndn Grants, 653
AT&T Excelerator, 657
Ball Brothers Fndn General Grants, 683
Bank of America Charitable Fndn Anchor Institutions Grants, 688
Baxter International Fndn Grants, 705
BCBS of Massachusetts Catalyst Fund Grants, 708
BCBS of Minnesota Healthy Together Grants, 712
BCBSNC Fndn Grants, 725
Bernard Van Leer Fndn Grants, 748
Blowitz-Ridgeway Fndn Early Childhood Development Research Award, 766
Bonfils-Stanton Fndn Grants, 779
Boyd Gaming Corporation Contributions Program, 788
Burlington Industries Fndn Grants, 811
Bush Fndn Health & Human Services Grants, 814
California Wellness Fndn Work and Health Program Grants, 834
Cambridge Comm Fndn Grants, 837
Caring Fndn Grants, 866
Carl C. Icahn Fndn Grants, 870
Carnegie Corporation of New York Grants, 879
Carolyn Fndn Grants, 880
CDC Epidemiology and Laboratory Capacity Infectious Diseases Program Grants, 909
CFF Pilot and Feasibility Awards, 945
CFF Therapeutics Development Program, 949
Charles M. Bair Family Trust Grants, 972
Charlotte County (FL) Comm Fndn Grants, 973
CHCF Grants, 979
Chicago Comm Trust Grants, 989
Children Affected by AIDS Fndn Camp Network Grants, 994
CLIF Bar Family Fndn Grants, 1040
Colorado Trust Partnerships for Health Initiative, 1063
Comm Fndn of Broward Grants, 1100
Comm Fndn of Santa Cruz County Grants, 1122
Comm Fndn of St. Joseph County Special Project Challenge Grants, 1126
Comm Technology Fndn of California Building Communities Through Technology Grants, 1136
Comm Toolbox for Children's Environmental Health Grants, 1137
Covenant Matters Fndn Grants, 1154
CSL Behring Local Empowerment for Advocacy Development (LEAD) Grants, 1167
Dallas Women's Fndn Grants, 1191
Daphne Seybolt Culpeper Memorial Fndn Grants, 1201
DHHS Grants for Dental Public Health, 1251
DHHS Health Care Systems Cost and Access Research and Development Grants, 1252
DOD HBCU/MI Partnership Training Award, 1293
DOJ Gang-Free Schools and Communities Intervention Grants, 1303
Doris Duke Charitable Fndn Operations Research on AIDS Care and Treatment in Africa (ORACTA) Grants, 1319
Dubois County Comm Fndn Grants, 1336
Duke Endowment Health Care Grants, 1338
Dystonia Medical Research Grants and Fellowships, 1355
Edward Bangs Kelley and Elza Kelley Fndn Grants, 1373
Evjue Fndn Grants, 1439
Fannie E. Rippel Fndn Grants, 1452
Farmers Insurance Group of Companies Grants, 1455
Feldman Fndn Grants, 1484
FIC International Malaria Research Training Program Award, 1488
Fidelity Fndn Grants, 1498
Fifth Third Fndn Grants, 1501
Fisa Fndn Grants, 1506
Fndn for the Carolinas Grants, 1535
Frist Fndn Grants, 1563
Ginn Fndn Grants, 1616
Good Samaritan Fndn Inc Grants, 1636
Grand Rapids Comm Fndn Grants, 1647
Greater Cincinnati Fndn Priority and Small Projects/Capacity-Building Grants, 1651
Greater Saint Louis Comm Fndn Grants, 1655
Guy's and St. Thomas' Charity Grants, 1678
Harry A. and Margaret D. Towsley Fndn Grants, 1701
Harry Kramer Memorial Fund Grants, 1705
Harvest Fndn Grants, 1713
Health Fndn of Southern Florida Responsive Grants, 1726
Hilton Head Island Fndn Grants, 1779
Hilton Hotels Corp Giving Program Grants, 1780
Hudson Webber Fndn Grants, 1813
Humboldt Area Fndn Technical Assistance Program (TAP) Grants, 1819
Indiana 21st Century Research and Technology Fund Awards, 1850

Jacob and Valeria Langeloth Fndn Grants, 1882
James Ford Bell Fndn Grants, 1885
Jay and Rose Phillips Family Fndn Grants, 1909
Jessie Ball Dupont Fund Grants, 1919
Jewish Comm Fndn of Greater Los Angeles Grants, 1921
John J. Leidy Fndn Grants, 1936
John Merck Fund Grants, 1940
John W. and Anna H. Hanes Fndn Grants, 1948
Johnson and Johnson / SAH Arts and Healing Grants, 1953
Johnson Controls Fndn Grants, 1954
Lettie Pate Whitehead Fndn Grants, 2049
Long Island Comm Fndn Grants, 2063
Lucy Gooding Charitable Fndn Trust Grants, 2083
Maine Comm Fndn Grants, 2099
Max Bell Fndn Grants, 2134
McMurry Fndn Grants, 2149
Mead Johnson Nutritionals Charitable Giving Grants, 2156
Metrowest Comm Health Care Fndn Grants, 2176
Middlesex Savings Charitable Fndn Grants, 2196
Miles of Hope Breast Cancer Fndn Grants, 2199
Moses Cone-Wesley Long Comm Health Fndn Grants, 2219
NIAMS Mechanisms of Chondroprotection Research Grants, 2472
NIDA Clinical Research Education Programs in Drug Abuse and Addiction, 2500
NIDA Minority Institutions Drug Abuse Research Development Program (MIDARP) Grants, 2509
NIDCD Physiologic and Molecular Bases of Tinnitus Research Grants, 2527
NIH Biology, Development, and Progression of Malignant Prostate Disease Research Grants, 2641
NIH Genetics of Neurobehavioral Disorders in Existing Samples Grants, 2670
NIH Mouse Mutagenesis and Phenotyping: Developmental Defects Research Grants, 2692
NIH Mouse Mutagenesis and Phenotyping: Nervous System and Behavior Research Grants, 2693
NIMH Minority Research Infrastructure Support Program Grants, 2763
NIMH Pilot Effectiveness Trials for Mental Disorders Grants, 2766
NIMH Risk Factors for Psychopathology Using Existing Data Sets Grants, 2768
NIMH Therapeutic Effectiveness Protocol Development Program Grants, 2774
Noble County Comm Fndn Grants, 2848
North Carolina Biotechnology Center Regional Development Grants, 2855
North Carolina Biotechnology Center Technology Enhancement Grants, 2856
North Carolina Biotechnology Centers of Innovation Grants, 2857
North Georgia Comm Fndn Grants, 2862
NSF Chemistry Research Experiences for Undergraduates (REU), 2883
NSF Undergraduate Research and Mentoring in the Biological Sciences (URM), 2896
NWHF Partners Investing in Nursing's Future Grants, 2908
Otto Bremer Fndn Grants, 2977
Pajaro Valley Comm Health Grants, 2985
Peter and Elizabeth C. Tower Fndn Comm Grants, 3018
Pfizer/AAFP Fndn Visiting Professorship Program in Family Medicine, 3027
Philadelphia Fndn Organizational Effectiveness Grants, 3029
Pittsburgh Fndn Comm Fund Grants, 3054
Portland General Electric Fndn Grants, 3067
Pride Fndn Grants and Scholarships, 3078
Prince Charitable Trusts Chicago Grants, 3079
Prince Charitable Trusts District of Columbia Grants, 3080
Progress Energy Fndn Grants, 3084
Rhode Island Fndn Grants, 3154
Rockwell International Corp Trust Grants, 3183
Rohm and Haas Company Grants, 3185
RRF Organizational Capacity Building Grants, 3194
Ruth Mott Fndn Grants, 3204
RWJF Partners Investing in Nursing's Future Grants, 3226
RWJF Vulnerable Populations Portfolio Grants, 3232
Saint Luke's Health Initiatives Grants, 3240
Salem Fndn Grants, 3242
Schering-Plough Fndn Health Grants, 3270
SHF Reach--Connecting Communities and Youth for a Healthy Future Grants, 3283
Sisters of Mercy of North Carolina Fndn Grants, 3295
Sisters of St. Joseph Healthcare Fndn Grants, 3297
Solo Cup Fndn Grants, 3346
Sosland Fndn Grants, 3348
Sprague Fndn Grants, 3359
Starr Fndn Grants, 3377
Stewart Huston Charitable Trust Grants, 3384
Strowd Roses Grants, 3388
Sunflower Fndn Bridge Grants, 3401
Sunflower Fndn Capacity Building Grants, 3402
Susan Mott Webb Charitable Trust Grants, 3412
Taproot Fndn Capacity-Building Service Grants, 3417
Trull Fndn Grants, 3441
TWS Fndn Grants, 3443
U.S. Department of Education 21st Century Comm Learning Centers, 3445
U.S. Department of Education Rehabilitation Research Training Centers (RRTCs), 3448
U.S. Department of Education Rehabilitation Training--Rehabilitation Continuing Education Programs (RCEP)--Institute on Rehabilitation Issues (IRI), 3449
U.S. Department of Education Vocational Rehabilitation Services Projects for American Indians with Disabilities Grants, 3452
Until There's a Cure Fndn Grants, 3471
Vancouver Fndn Grants and Comm Initiatives Program, 3477
Waitt Family Fndn Grants, 3512
Wal-Mart State Giving Program Grants, 3514
Wasie Fndn Grants, 3521
Weatherwax Fndn Grants, 3523
Women's Fndn of California Grants, 3550
Z. Smith Reynolds Fndn Small Grants, 3557

Dissertation/Thesis Research Support

AAHN Pre-Doctoral Research Grant, 127
AF Doctoral Dissertation Award for Arthritis Health Professionals, 253
AHIMA Dissertation Assistance Grants, 300
AIHP Thesis Support Grants, 318
APA Dissertation Research Awards, 494
CDC Minority Health Statistics Dissertation Research Grants, 916
Dale and Edna Walsh Fndn Grants, 1189
FDHN Graduate Student Awards, 1472
Jeanne Humphrey Block Dissertation Award, 1912
NIA Aging Research Dissertation Awards to Increase Diversity, 2392
NIA Minority Dissertation Research Grants in Aging, 2419
NIDCD Minority Dissertation Research Grants in Human Communication, 2524
NSF Doctoral Dissertation Improvement Grants in the Directorate for Biological Sciences, 2884
ONF Small Grants, 2947
PhRMA Fndn Health Outcomes Post Doctoral Fellowships, 3031
PhRMA Fndn Health Outcomes Pre-Doctoral Fellowships, 3032
PhRMA Fndn Informatics Pre Doctoral Fellowships, 3037
PhRMA Fndn Pharmaceutics Pre Doctoral Fellowships, 3041
WWNFF Dissertation Grants in Women's Health, 3553

Educational Programs

1104 Fndn Grants, 3
1675 Fndn Grants, 4
2 Depot Square Ipswich Charitable Fndn Grants, 7
3M Company Health and Human Services Grants, 10
3M Fndn Grants, 11
49ers Fndn Grants, 12
A Friend's Fndn Trust Grants, 13
A Fund for Women Grants, 14
A. Gary Anderson Family Fndn Grants, 17
A.O. Smith Comm Grants, 18
AACAP Child and Adolescent Psychiatry (CAP) Teaching Scholarships, 31
AAFA Investigator Research Grants, 108
AAFP Fndn Health Literacy State Grants, 112
AAFP Fndn Pfizer Teacher Development Awards, 114
AAFP Fndn Wyeth Immunization Awards, 115
AAHN Pre-Doctoral Research Grant, 127
AAHPERD Ruth Abernathy Presidential Scholarships, 128
AAHPERD-AAHE Barbara A. Cooley Scholarships, 129
AAHPERD-AAHE Delbert Oberteuffer Scholarships, 130
AAHPERD-AAHE Undergraduate Scholarships, 131
AAHPM Hospice and Palliative Medicine Fellowships, 132
AAMC Alpha Omega Alpha Robert J. Glaser Distinguished Teacher Awards, 134
AAMC Caring for Comm Grants, 136
AAMC Herbert W. Nickens Faculty Fellowship, 139
AAMC Herbert W. Nickens Medical Student Scholarships, 140
AAP Resident Initiative Fund Grants, 167
Aaron & Cecile Goldman Family Fndn Grants, 171
Aaron Fndn (Massachusetts) Grants, 174
Abbott Fund Access to Health Care Grants, 176
Abbott Fund Comm Vitality Grants, 177
Abbott Fund Global AIDS Care Grants, 178
Abbott Fund Science and Medical Innovation Grants, 179
Abel Fndn Grants, 181
Abell-Hanger Fndn Grants, 183
Abington Fndn Grants, 184
Able To Serve Grants, 185
Abney Fndn Grants, 187
Abramson Family Fndn Grants, 188
ACE Charitable Fndn Grants, 199
ACF Ethnic Comm Self-Help Grants, 200
ACF Supplemental Services for Recently Arrived Refugees Grants, 203
Achelis and Bodman Fndns Grants, 206
ACOG History of American Obstetrics and Gynecology Fellowship, 207
ACS Doctoral Degree Scholarships in Cancer Nursing, 211
ACS Graduate Scholarships in Cancer Nursing Practice, 214
Actors Fund Social Services and Financial Assistance, 225
ACVIM Fndn Clinical Investigation Grants, 227
ADA Fndn Dental Education Grants, 228
Adam Richter Charitable Trust Grants, 230
Adaptec Fndn Grants, 232
Adelaide Breed Bayrd Fndn Grants, 234
Administaff Comm Affairs Grants, 235
Administration on Aging Senior Medicare Patrol Project Grants, 236
Adobe Comm Investment Grants, 237
Adolph Coors Fndn Grants, 238
Advanced Micro Devices Comm Affairs Grants, 239
AEC Trust Grants, 242
AEGON Transamerica Fndn Grants, 243
Affymetrix Corp Contributions Grants, 258
AFG Industries Grants, 259
African American Fund of New Jersey Grants, 260
Agnes B. Hunt Trust Grants, 261

Agnes Gund Fndn Grants, 262
Agnes M. Lindsay Trust Grants, 263
Agway Fndn Grants, 265
AHFMR Comm Support Program Grants, 271
AHIMA Grant-In-Aid Research Grants, 302
Ahmanson Fndn Grants, 303
Ahn Family Fndn Grants, 304
AIDS Vaccine Advocacy Coalition (AVAC) Fund Grants, 315
AIG American General Corporation Grants, 316
Air Products and Chemicals Grants, 319
Alaska Airlines Corp Giving Grants, 323
Alaska Airlines Fndn Grants, 324
Albert and Margaret Alkek Fndn Grants, 326
Albert Pick Jr. Fund Grants, 328
Alberto Culver Corp Contributions Grants, 329
Albertson's Charitable Giving Grants, 330
Albuquerque Comm Fndn Grants, 331
Alcatel-Lucent Technologies Corp Contributions Grants, 332
Alcatel-Lucent Technologies Fndn Grants, 333
Alcoa Fndn Grants, 334
Alcohol Misuse and Alcoholism Research Grants, 335
Alcon Fndn Grants, 336
Alexander & Baldwin Fndn Hawaiian and Pacific Island Grants, 338
Alexander & Baldwin Fndn Mainland Grants, 339
Alexander and Margaret Stewart Trust Grants, 340
Alexander Eastman Fndn Grants, 341
Alexis Gregory Fndn Grants, 349
Allegan County Comm Fndn Grants, 358
Allegheny Technologies Charitable Trust, 359
Allegis Group Fndn Grants, 360
Allen P. and Josephine B. Green Fndn Grants, 361
Alliance Healthcare Fndn Grants, 362
Allstate Corp Giving Grants, 363
Allstate Corp Hometown Commitment Grants, 364
Allyn Fndn Grants, 365
Alpha Omega Fndn Grants, 366
Altman Fndn Health Care Grants, 372
AMA Fndn Arthur N. Wilson, MD, Scholarship, 386
AMA Fndn Fund for Better Health Grants, 388
AMA Fndn Joan F. Giambalvo Memorial Scholarships, 392
AMA Fndn Minority Scholars Awards, 395
AMA Fndn Physicians of Tomorrow Scholarships, 396
AMA-MSS Chapter Involvement Grants, 401
AMA-MSS Government Relations Advocacy Fellowship, 403
AMA-RFS and AMA Fndn Medical Student & Resident/Fellow Elective-Medicine & the Media, 406
AMA-RFS Legislative Awareness Internships, 407
Amador Comm Fndn Grants, 409
AMD Corp Contributions Grants, 411
American Academy of Nursing Building Academic Geriatric Nursing Capacity (BAGNC) Scholarships, 414
American Academy of Nursing Claire M. Fagin Fellowships, 415
American Academy of Nursing MBA Scholarships, 417
American Chemical Society GCI Pharmaceutical Roundtable Research Grants, 420
American College of Surgeons and The Triological Society Clinical Scientist Development Awards, 422
American College of Surgeons Resident and Associate Society (RAS-ACS) Leadership Scholarships, 431
American Electric Power Grants, 434
American Jewish World Service Grants, 437
American Legacy Fndn National Calls for Proposals Grants, 438
American Psychiatric Association/Merck Co. Early Academic Career Research Award, 453
American Society on Aging Graduate Student Research Award, 455
American-Italian Cancer Fndn Fellowships, 459
American-Scandinavian Fndn Visiting Lectureship Grants, 460
Amerisure Insurance Comm Service Grants, 461
AMI Semiconductors Corp Grants, 468
Andersen Corp Fndn, 470
Andersen Fndn Grants, 471
Angels Baseball Fndn Grants, 473
Anheuser-Busch Fndn Grants, 474
Ann and Robert H. Lurie Family Fndn Grants, 475
Ann Arbor Area Comm Fndn Grants, 476
Annenberg Fndn Grants, 479
Annie Sinclair Knudsen Memorial Fund/Kaua'i Comm Grants, 480
Annunziata Sanguinetti Fndn Grants, 481
Anschutz Family Fndn Grants, 486
Anthem Blue Cross and Blue Shield Grants, 488
Anthem Blue Cross and Blue Shield School Nurse Grants, 489
Anthony R. Abraham Fndn Grants, 490
AON Fndn Grants, 491
APF Call for Proposals, 505
APF Helping Hands Grants, 507
APF James H. Scully Jr., M.D., Educational Fund Grants, 508
APF Jeanne Spurlock Congressional Fellowships, 509
APF Typical or Troubled School Mental Health Education Grants, 510
APF/COGDOP Graduate Research Scholarships in Psychology, 511
APSAA Fndn Grants, 517
APSAA Mini-Career Grants, 518
APSAA Small Beginning Scholar Pre-Investigation Grants, 520
APSAA Small Beginning Scholar Visiting and Consulting Grants, 521
Aratani Fndn Grants, 523
Arcadia Fndn Grants, 524
Archer Daniels Midland Fndn Grants, 525
ARCO Fndn Education Grants, 526
Arie and Ida Crown Memorial Grants, 528
Arizona Cardinals Grants, 529
Arizona Diamondbacks Charities Grants, 530
Arizona Public Service Corp Giving Program Grants, 531
Arkansas Comm Fndn Arkansas Black Hall of Fame Grants, 532
Arkansas Comm Fndn Grants, 533
Arkell Hall Fndn Grants, 534
Arkema Fndn Science Teachers Program, 535
Arlington Comm Fndn Grants, 536
Armstrong McDonald Fndn Grants, 537
ARS Fndn Grants, 538
Arthritis Fndn of Australia Grants, 541
Arthur and Rochelle Belfer Fndn Grants, 542
ArvinMeritor Grants, 544
ASCO State Affiliate Grants, 547
ASCO Career Development Award, 551
ASCO Comparative Effectiveness Research Professorship (CERP) in Breast Cancer, 553
ASCO International Development and Education Awards (IDEA), 554
ASCO Loan Repayment Grants, 555
ASCO Long-Term International Fellowships, 556
ASCO Medical Student Rotation Grants, 557
ASHA Advancing Academic-Research Careers (AARC) Award, 569
ASHA Minority Student Leadership Program Awards, 570
ASHA Multicultural Activities Projects Grants, 571
ASHA Research Mentoring-Pair Travel Award, 572
ASHA Student Research Travel Award, 573
ASHA Students Preparing for Academic & Research Careers (SPARC) Award, 574
ASHFndn New Century Scholars Program Doctoral Scholarships, 580
Ashland Corp Contributions Grants, 586
ASM International Fellowships for Asia and Africa, 602
ASM International Professorship for Latin America, 603
ASM International Professorships for Asia and Africa, 604
ASM Robert D. Watkins Graduate Research Fellowship, 614
Assisi Fndn Grants, 653
Assurant Fndn Grants, 654
Assurant Health Fndn Grants, 655
AT&T Excelerator, 657
AT&T Fndn Civic and Comm Service Program Grants, 658
Atherton Family Fndn Grants, 659
Athwin Fndn Grants, 660
Atkinson Fndn International Grants, 661
Atlanta Fndn Grants, 662
Atran Fndn Grants, 663
Auburn Fndn Grants, 664
Audrey and Sydney Irmas Charitable Fndn Grants, 665
Aurora Fndn Grants, 667
Austin-Bailey Health and Wellness Fndn Grants, 669
Australian Academy of Science Grants, 670
Autodesk Comm Relations Grants, 671
Autzen Fndn Grants, 672
AVDF Health Care Grants, 673
Axe-Houghton Fndn Grants, 678
Bacon Family Fndn Grants, 679
Bailey Fndn Grants, 680
Balfe Family Fndn Grants, 682
Ball Brothers Fndn Grants, 684
Banfi Vintners Fndn Grants, 687
Bank of America Client Fndn Grants, 690
Baptist Comm Ministries Grants, 691
Barberton Comm Fndn Grants, 693
Barker Fndn Grants, 694
Barker Welfare Fndn Grants, 695
Barnes Group Fndn Grants, 696
Barr Fund Grants, 697
Barra Fndn Comm Fund Grants, 698
Barra Fndn Project Grants, 699
Batchelor Fndn Grants, 701
Baton Rouge Area Fndn Grants, 702
Battle Creek Comm Fndn Grants, 703
Batts Fndn Grants, 704
Baxter International Fndn Grants, 705
Bayer Clinical Scholarship Award, 706
Bayer Hemophilia Caregivers Education Award, 707
BCBS of Minnesota Growing Up Healthy Grants, 711
BCBS of Minnesota Healthy Together Grants, 712
BCBSM Building Healthy Communities Engaging Elementary Schools and Comm Partners Grants, 713
BCBSM Fndn Student Award Program, 721
BCBSNC Fndn Grants, 725
Bearemy's Kennel Pals Grants, 728
Beazley Fndn Grants, 730
Bechtel Group Fndn Building Positive Comm Relationships Grants, 731
Beckley Area Fndn Grants, 732
Beckman Coulter Comm Relations Grants, 733
Beirne Carter Fndn Grants, 737
Belk Fndn Grants, 739
Ben B. Cheney Fndn Grants, 741
Bender Fndn Grants, 742
Benton Comm Fndn Grants, 743
Benton County Fndn Grants, 744
Berks County Comm Fndn Grants, 745
Bernard and Audre Rapoport Fndn Grants, 746
Bernard F. and Alva B. Gimbel Fndn Grants, 747
Berrien Comm Fndn Grants, 749
Bert W. Martin Fndn Grants, 750
Besser Fndn Grants, 752
Bill and Melinda Gates Fndn Grants, 756
Binney and Smith Comm Grants, 757
Biogen Corp Giving Grants, 758
Birds Eye Foods Fndn Grants, 759

BJ's Charitable Fndn Grants, 761
Black River Falls Area Fndn Grants, 762
Blackford County Comm Fndn Grants, 763
Blanche and Irving Laurie Fndn Grants, 764
Blanche and Julian Robertson Family Fndn Grants, 765
Blowitz-Ridgeway Fndn Early Childhood Development Research Award, 766
Blue Mountain Comm Fndn Grants, 769
Blue River Comm Fndn Grants, 770
Blue Shield of California Grants, 771
Blum-Kovler Fndn Grants, 772
Blumenthal Fndn Grants, 773
Bob and Delores Hope Charitable Fndn Grants, 774
Bodenwein Public Benevolent Fndn Grants, 775
Bodman Fndn Grants, 776
Boeing Company Contributions Program Grants, 777
Boettcher Fndn Grants, 778
Booth-Bricker Fund Grants, 780
Bosque Fndn Grants, 782
Boston Fndn Grants, 783
Boston Globe Fndn Grants, 784
Boston Jewish Comm Women's Fund Grants, 785
Boyd Gaming Corporation Contributions Program, 788
Bradley Turner Fndn Grants, 789
Brian G. Dyson Fndn Grants, 791
Bridgestone/Firestone Trust Fund Grants, 792
Bright Family Fndn Grants, 793
Brinson Fndn Grants, 794
Bristol-Myers Squibb Fndn Global HIV/AIDS Initiative Grants, 796
Bristol-Myers Squibb Fndn Health Disparities Grants, 797
Bristol-Myers Squibb Fndn Health Education Grants, 798
Bristol-Myers Squibb Fndn Women's Health Grants, 800
Brook J. Lenfest Fndn Grants, 804
Brown County Comm Fndn Grants, 807
Bruce and Adele Greenfield Fndn Grants, 808
Bullitt Fndn Grants, 809
Burlington Industries Fndn Grants, 811
Burlington Northern Santa Fe Fndn Grants, 812
Burton G. Bettingen Grants, 813
Bush Fndn Health & Human Services Grants, 814
Business Bank of Nevada Comm Grants, 817
BWF Ad Hoc Grants, 818
BWF Career Awards for Medical Scientists (CAMS), 820
Byron W. and Alice L. Lockwood Fndn Grants, 824
Cable Positive's Tony Cox Comm Fund Grants, 827
Caddock Fndn Grants, 828
California Wellness Fndn Work and Health Program Grants, 834
Callaway Fndn Grants, 835
Callaway Golf Company Fndn Grants, 836
Cambridge Comm Fndn Grants, 837
Camp-Younts Fndn Grants, 838
CampusRN/AACN Nursing Scholarship Fund, 841
Canada Graduate Scholarships (CGS) and NSERC Postgraduate Scholarships (PGS), 845
Canada-U.S. Fulbright New Century Scholars Program Grants, 846
Canada-U.S. Fulbright Senior Specialists Program Grants, 847
Canadian Optometric Education Trust Fund Grants, 853
Canadian Patient Safety Institute (CPSI) Patient Safety Studentships, 854
Capital Region Comm Fndn Grants, 862
Cardiac Arrhythmias Research and Education Fndn Research Grants, 863
Cardinal Health Fndn Grants, 864
Cargill Citizenship Fund-Corp Giving Grants, 865
Caring Fndn Grants, 866
Carl and Eloise Pohlad Family Fndn Grants, 867
Carl and Lily Pforzheimer Fndn Grants, 868
Carl B. and Florence E. King Fndn Grants, 869
Carls Fndn Grants, 876
Carnegie Corporation of New York Grants, 879
Carolyn Fndn Grants, 880
Carpenter Fndn Grants, 881
Carrie E. and Lena V. Glenn Fndn Grants, 882
Carrie Estelle Doheny Fndn Grants, 883
Carrier Corporation Contributions Grants, 884
Carroll County Comm Fndn Grants, 885
Carylon Fndn Grants, 886
Cass County Comm Fndn Grants, 887
Castle Rock Fndn Grants, 888
Catherine Holmes Wilkins Fndn Grants, 889
Catholic Campaign for Human Development (CCHD) Comm Organizing Grants, 891
CDC Cooperative Agreement for Partnership to Enhance Public Health Informatics, 905
CDC Cooperative Agreement for the Development, Operation, and Evaluation of an Entertainment Education Program, 906
CDC Hepatitis Education for Inmates and Correctional Staff Program Grants, 911
CDC National Poison Prevention and Control Program Grants, 918
CDC Oral Diseases Prevention and Oral Health Promotion Grants, 921
CDC Prevention Education and Access to Care Services for Persons Infected and Affected by HIV, 922
CDC School Health Programs to Prevent the Spread of HIV Cooperative Agreements, 928
Cemala Fndn Grants, 933
Central Carolina Comm Fndn Comm Impact Grants, 936
Central Okanagan Fndn Grants, 937
Cessna Fndn Grants, 938
Cetana Educational Fndn Scholarships, 939
CFFVR Opportunity Grants, 952
Champ-A Champion Fur Kids Grants, 959
Champlin Fndns Grants, 960
CharityWorks Grants, 961
Charles A. Frueauff Fndn Grants, 962
Charles Delmar Fndn Grants, 963
Charles Edison Fund Grants, 964
Charles H. Dater Fndn Grants, 966
Charles H. Revson Fndn Grants, 969
Charles Lafitte Fndn Grants, 970
Charles M. and Mary D. Grant Fndn Grants, 971
Charles M. Bair Family Trust Grants, 972
Charlotte County (FL) Comm Fndn Grants, 973
Chase Paymentech Corp Giving Grants, 975
Chatlos Fndn Grants, 977
Chazen Fndn Grants, 978
Chesapeake Corporation Fndn Grants, 982
Chestnut Hill Charitable Fndn, Inc Grants, 987
Chicago Board of Trade Fndn Grants, 988
Chicago Comm Trust Grants, 989
Chicago Tribune's Corp Contributions Grants, 991
Child Nutrition Fndn School Comm Kitchens Grants, 993
Chiles Fndn Grants, 1003
Chiron Fndn Comm Grants, 1004
Christopher Reeve Paralysis Fndn Quality of Life and Health Promotions Grants, 1007
Christy-Houston Fndn Grants, 1008
Chula Vista Charitable Fndn Grants, 1009
CICF Legacy Fund Comm Fndn Grants, 1010
CIGNA Fndn Grants, 1011
CIT Corp Giving Grants, 1014
Citizens Bank Mid-Atlantic Charitable Fndn Grants, 1015
Clarcor Fndn Grants, 1021
Clarence E. Heller Charitable Fndn Grants, 1022
Clarian Health Critical / Progressive Care Internships, 1023
Clarian Health Multi-Specialty Internships, 1024
Clarian Health OR Internships, 1025
Clark County Comm Fndn Grants, 1028
Clark Fndn Grants, 1029
Clark-Winchcole Fndn Grants, 1030
Claude Bennett Family Fndn Grants, 1031
Claude Pepper Fndn Grants, 1032
Claude Worthington Benedum Fndn Grants, 1033
Clay Fndn Grants, 1034
Cleveland Browns Fndn Grants, 1036
CMA Fndn Grants, 1042
CNA Fndn Grants, 1046
CNCS Next Generation Grants, 1049
Coastal Bend Comm Fndn Grants, 1050
Coastal Comm Fndn of South Carolina Grants, 1051
Coca-Cola Fndn Grants, 1052
Cockrell Fndn Grants, 1053
Coeta and Donald Barker Fndn Grants, 1054
Colin Higgins Fndn Grants, 1056
Collins C. Diboll Private Fndn Grants, 1057
Colorado Interstate Gas Grants, 1060
Colorado Springs Comm Trust Fund Grants, 1061
Columbus Fndn Competitive Grants, 1066
Columbus Fndn J. Floyd Dixon Memorial Fund Grants, 1068
Columbus Fndn Mary Eleanor Morris Fund Grants, 1069
Columbus Fndn Traditional Grants, 1071
Comer Fndn Grants, 1072
Comerica Charitable Fndn Grants, 1073
Commission on Religion in Appalachia Grants, 1074
Commonweal Fndn Comm Assistance Grants, 1075
Commonweal Fndn Grants, 1076
Commonwealth Fund/Harvard University Fellowship in Minority Health Policy, 1086
Comm Fndn AIDS Endowment Awards, 1088
Comm Fndn Alliance City of Evansville Endowment Fund Grants, 1089
Comm Fndn for Greater Buffalo Grants, 1090
Comm Fndn for Greater New Haven Grants, 1091
Comm Fndn for Monterey County Grants, 1092
Comm Fndn for Muskegon County Grants, 1093
Comm Fndn for Southeastern Michigan Grants, 1094
Comm Fndn for Southern Arizona Grants, 1095
Comm Fndn of Bartholomew County Heritage Fund Grants, 1096
Comm Fndn of Bloomington and Monroe County Grants, 1098
Comm Fndn of Boone County Grants, 1099
Comm Fndn of Broward Grants, 1100
Comm Fndn of Central Illinois Grants, 1101
Comm Fndn of Champaign County Grants, 1102
Comm Fndn of Crawford County Grants and Scholarships, 1103
Comm Fndn of Grant County Grants, 1104
Comm Fndn of Grant County Scholarships, 1105
Comm Fndn of Greater Birmingham Grants, 1106
Comm Fndn of Greater Flint Grants, 1107
Comm Fndn of Greater Fort Wayne: Comm Endowment & Clarke Endowment Fund Grants, 1108
Comm Fndn of Greater New Britain Grants, 1111
Comm Fndn of Greater Tampa Grants, 1112
Comm Fndn of Greenville Hollingsworth Funds Program/Project Grants, 1114
Comm Fndn of Greenville-Greenville Women Giving Grants, 1115
Comm Fndn of Howard County Grants, 1116
Comm Fndn of Morgan County Grants and Scholarships, 1118
Comm Fndn of Mount Vernon and Knox County Grants, 1119
Comm Fndn of Muncie and Delaware County Grants, 1120
Comm Fndn of Randolph County Grants, 1121
Comm Fndn of Santa Cruz County Grants, 1122
Comm Fndn of South Alabama Grants, 1123
Comm Fndn of South Puget Sound Grants, 1124
Comm Fndn of Southeastern Connecticut Grants, 1125
Comm Fndn of St. Joseph County Special Project Challenge Grants, 1126

Comm Fndn of Switzerland County Grants, 1127
Comm Fndn of Tampa Bay Grants, 1128
Comm Fndn of Western North Carolina Grants, 1132
Comm Fndn Silicon Valley Grants, 1133
Comm Impact Fund, 1135
Comm Technology Fndn of California Building Communities Through Technology Grants, 1136
Comprehensive Health Education Fndn Grants, 1139
ConAgra Foods Fndn Grants, 1140
Connecticut Comm Fndn Grants, 1141
Connelly Fndn Grants, 1143
ConocoPhillips Fndn Grants, 1144
Constantin Fndn Grants, 1145
Constellation Energy Group and Baltimore Gas and Electric Corp Contributions, 1146
Consumers Energy Fndn, 1147
Cooper Industries Fndn Grants, 1150
Coors Brewing Corp Contributions Grants, 1151
Cornerstone Fndn of Northeastern Wisconsin Grants, 1152
Covenant Fndn Grants (Iowa), 1153
Cowles Charitable Trust Grants, 1155
Crail-Johnson Fndn Grants, 1157
Cranston Fndn Grants, 1158
Cruise Industry Charitable Fndn Grants, 1166
CSRA Comm Fndn Grants, 1168
CSX Corp Contributions Grants, 1169
Cudd Fndn Grants, 1171
Cullen Fndn Grants, 1172
Cultural Society of Filipino Americans Grants, 1173
CUNA Mutual Group Fndn, 1174
CVS All Kids Can Grants, 1175
CVS Caremark Charitable Trust Grants, 1176
CVS Comm Grants, 1177
Cyrus Eaton Fndn Grants, 1178
D.F. Halton Fndn Grants, 1181
D.V. and Ida J. McEachern Charitable Trust Grants, 1182
DAAD Research Stays for University Academics and Scientists, 1183
Dade Comm Fndn Comm AIDS Partnership Grants, 1184
Dade Comm Fndn Grants, 1185
Dairy Queen Corp Contributions Grants, 1187
Daisy Marquis Jones Fndn Grants, 1188
Dale and Edna Walsh Fndn Grants, 1189
Dallas Mavericks Fndn Grants, 1190
Dallas Women's Fndn Grants, 1191
Dammann Fund Grants, 1192
Dana Fndn Science and Health Grants, 1197
Daniel Mendelsohn New Investigator Award, 1199
Daniels Fund Grants, 1200
Daphne Seybolt Culpeper Memorial Fndn Grants, 1201
Davis Family Fndn Grants, 1204
Dayton Power and Light Fndn Grants, 1205
Daywood Fndn Grants, 1206
Deaconess Comm Fndn Grants, 1207
Dean Foods Comm Involvement Grants, 1209
Dearborn Comm Fndn County Progress Grants, 1211
Del E. Webb Fndn Grants, 1213
Delaware Comm Fndn Grants, 1215
Delaware Comm Fndn-Youth Philanthropy Board for Kent County, 1216
Dell Fndn Healthy Communities, Literate Communities, and Connected Communities Grants, 1217
Dell Fndn Open Grants, 1218
Delta Air Lines Fndn Grants, 1220
DeMatteis Family Fndn Grants, 1221
Dennis and Phyllis Washington Fndn Grants, 1222
Denver Broncos Charities Fund Grants, 1226
Dept of Ed College Assistance MiGrants (CAMP), 1228
Dept of Ed Safe and Drug-Free Schools and Communities State Grants, 1230
Dept of Ed Special Education--Personnel Development to Improve Services and Results for Children with Disabilities, 1231
Dept of Ed Special Education--Studies and Evaluations, 1232
Dept of Ed Special Education--Technical Assistance and Dissemination to Improve Services and Results for Children with Disabilities, 1233
Dept of Ed Special Education-National Activities-Technology and Media Services for Individuals with Disabilities, 1234
DeRoy Testamentary Fndn Grants, 1239
Detroit Lions Charities Grants, 1241
Dickson Fndn Grants, 1284
Do Something BR!CK Awards, 1287
DOA Distance Learning and Telemedicine Grants, 1288
DOD HBCU/MI Partnership Training Award, 1293
Dole Food Company Charitable Contributions, 1307
Dominion Educational Partnership Grant, 1308
Dora Roberts Fndn Grants, 1311
Doris and Victor Day Fndn Grants, 1313
Dorothea Haus Ross Fndn Grants, 1320
Dorothy Hooper Beattie Fndn Grants, 1321
Dorothy Rider Pool Health Care Grants, 1322
Dorrance Family Fndn Grants, 1323
DPA Promoting Policy Change Advocacy Grants, 1324
Dr. Leon Bromberg Charitable Trust Fund Grants, 1328
Drs. Bruce and Lee Fndn Grants, 1333
Dubois County Comm Fndn Grants, 1336
Duke Energy Fndn Grants, 1339
Duke University Adult Cardiothoracic Anesthesia and Critical Care Medicine Fellowships, 1340
Duke University Ambulatory and Regional Anesthesia Fellowships, 1341
Duke University Clinical Cardiac Electrophysiology Fellowships, 1342
Duke University Hyperbaric Center Fellowships, 1343
Duke University Interventional Cardiology Fellowships, 1344
Duke University Obstetric Anesthesia Fellowships, 1345
Duke University Pain Management Fellowships, 1346
Duke University Pediatric Anesthesiology Fellowship, 1347
Duneland Health Council InCorpd Grants, 1350
Dunspaugh-Dalton Fndn Grants, 1351
DuPage Comm Fndn Grants, 1352
E. Rhodes and Leona B. Carpenter Fndn Grants, 1356
E.J. Grassmann Trust Grants, 1360
E.L. Wiegand Fndn Grants, 1361
Eastman Chemical Company Fndn Grants, 1362
eBay Fndn Comm Grants, 1363
Eberly Fndn Grants, 1364
Eckerd Corporation Fndn Grants, 1366
Eddie C. and Sylvia Brown Family Fndn Grants, 1367
Eden Hall Fndn Grants, 1368
Edina Realty Fndn Grants, 1369
Edna G. Kynett Memorial Fndn Grants, 1370
EDS Fndn Grants, 1371
Educational Fndn of America Grants, 1372
Edward Bangs Kelley and Elza Kelley Fndn Grants, 1373
Edward S. Moore Fndn Grants, 1374
Edwin S. Webster Fndn Grants, 1376
Edwin W. and Catherine M. Davis Fndn Grants, 1377
Edyth Bush Charitable Fndn Grants, 1378
Effie and Wofford Cain Fndn Grants, 1385
EIF Comm Grants, 1386
Eisner Fndn Grants, 1387
El Paso Comm Fndn Grants, 1388
El Paso Corp Fndn Grants, 1389
El Pomar Fndn Awards and Grants, 1390
Elizabeth McGraw Fndn Grants, 1399
Elkhart County Comm Fndn Grants, 1401
Elliot Fndn Inc Grants, 1402
Elmer L. and Eleanor J. Andersen Fndn Grants, 1406
Elsie Lee Garthwaite Memorial Fndn Grants, 1408
Emerson Charitable Trust Grants, 1412
Emily Davie and Joseph S. Kornfeld Fndn Grants, 1414
Emma B. Howe Memorial Fndn Grants, 1415
Ensworth Charitable Fndn Grants, 1416
Entergy Comm Partnership Grants, 1417
EPA Children's Health Protection Grants, 1420
Erie Comm Fndn Grants, 1427
Essex County Comm Fndn Discretionary Fund Grant, 1428
Estee Lauder Grants, 1429
Ethel S. Abbott Charitable Fndn Grants, 1430
Eugene and Agnes E. Meyer Fndn Grants, 1432
Eugene B. Casey Fndn Grants, 1433
Eugene M. Lang Fndn Grants, 1434
Eugene McDermott Fndn Grants, 1435
Eva L. and Joseph M. Bruening Fndn Grants, 1436
Evan and Susan Bayh Fndn Grants, 1437
Evanston Comm Fndn Grants, 1438
Evjue Fndn Grants, 1439
Express Scripts Fndn Grants, 1441
F.M. Kirby Fndn Grants, 1443
Fairfield County Comm Fndn Grants, 1446
Fairlawn Fndn Grants, 1447
FAR Fund, 1453
Fargo-Moorhead Area Fndn Grants, 1454
Farmers Insurance Group of Companies Grants, 1455
Faye McBeath Fndn Grants, 1456
Fayette County Fndn Grants, 1457
FCNY Union Square Awards, 1461
Federal Express Corp Contributions Program, 1483
Feldman Fndn Grants, 1484
Ferree Fndn Grants, 1486
FIC/ORMH Minority International Research Training Grants, 1497
Fidelity Fndn Grants, 1498
Field Fndn of Illinois Grants, 1499
Fifth Third Fndn Grants, 1501
Fireman's Fund Fndn Grants, 1504
FirstEnergy Fndn Comm Grants, 1505
Fisher Fndn Grants, 1508
Fishman Family Fndn Grants, 1510
Florida BRAIVE Fund of Dade Comm Fndn, 1512
Florida BRAIVE Fund of Gulf Coast Comm Fndn of Venice, 1513
Florida BRAIVE Fund of The Comm Fndn in Jacksonville, 1514
Florida High School/High Tech Project Grants, 1515
Floyd A. and Kathleen C. Cailloux Fndn Grants, 1516
Fluor Fndn Grants, 1517
FMC Fndn Grants, 1518
Foellinger Fndn Grants, 1519
Fondren Fndn Grants, 1520
Ford Motor Company Fund Grants, 1522
Forrest C. Lattner Fndn Grants, 1523
Foster Fndn Grants, 1524
Fndn for Science and Disability Grants for Physically Disabled Students in the Sciences, 1532
Fndn for Seacoast Health Grants, 1533
Fndn for Spirituality and Medicine Grants, 1534
Fndn for the Mid-South Grants, 1536
Fndn Northwest Grants, 1537
Fourjay Fndn Grants, 1544
Frances and John L. Loeb Family Fund Grants, 1546
Frances L. and Edwin L. Cummings Memorial Fund Grants, 1547
Frances W. Emerson Fndn Grants, 1548
Francis L. Abreu Charitable Trust Grants, 1549
Francis T. & Louise T. Nichols Fndn Grants, 1550

Frank E. and Seba B. Payne Fndn Grants, 1551
Frank G. and Freida K. Brotz Family Fndn Grants, 1552
Frank Stanley Beveridge Fndn Grants, 1553
Franklin County Comm Fndn Grants, 1554
Fraser-Parker Fndn Grants, 1555
Fred Baldwin Memorial Fndn Grants, 1556
Fred L. Emerson Fndn Grants, 1557
Freddie Mac Fndn Grants, 1558
Frederick Gardner Cottrell Fndn Grants, 1560
Fremont Area Comm Fndn Grants, 1561
Fritz B. Burns Fndn Grants, 1564
Fuji Film Grants, 1565
Fulbright Alumni Initiatives Awards Program Grants, 1566
Fulbright Distinguished Chairs Program Grants, 1567
Fulbright German Studies Seminar Grants, 1568
Fulbright International Education Administrators (IEA) Seminar Program Grants, 1569
Fulbright Specialists Program Grants, 1571
Fulbright Traditional Scholar Program in Europe and Eurasia, 1572
Fulbright Traditional Scholar Program in Sub-Saharan Africa, 1573
Fulbright Traditional Scholar Program in the East Asia/Pacific Region, 1574
Fulbright Traditional Scholar Program in the Near East and North Africa Region, 1575
Fulbright Traditional Scholar Program in the South and Central Asia Region, 1576
Fulbright Traditional Scholar Program in the Western Hemisphere, 1577
Fulton County Comm Fndn Grants, 1579
G.N. Wilcox Trust Grants, 1581
Gamble Fndn Grants, 1582
Gebbie Fndn Grants, 1585
GEICO Public Service Awards, 1586
GenCorp Fndn Grants, 1587
Genentech Corp Charitable Contributions Grants, 1588
General Mills Champions for Healthy Kids Grants, 1589
General Mills Fndn Grants, 1590
General Motors Fndn Grants Support Program, 1591
Genesis Fndn Grants, 1593
Genuardi Family Fndn Grants, 1594
George and Ruth Bradford Fndn Grants, 1595
George B. Storer Fndn Grants, 1596
George F. Baker Trust Grants, 1597
George Family Fndn Grants, 1598
George Frederick Jewett Fndn Grants, 1599
George H. Hitchings New Investigator Award in Health Research, 1600
George Kress Fndn Grants, 1601
George S. and Dolores Dore Eccles Fndn Grants, 1602
Georgia Power Fndn Grants, 1603
Georgiana Goddard Eaton Memorial Fund Grants, 1604
Gertrude and William C. Wardlaw Fund Grants, 1607
Gertrude E. Skelly Charitable Fndn Grants, 1609
Gheens Fndn Grants, 1610
Giant Eagle Fndn Grants, 1611
Gibson Fndn Grants, 1612
Gill Fndn - Gay and Lesbian Fund Grants, 1613
Gilroy and Lillian P. Roberts Charitable Fndn Grants, 1614
Ginn Fndn Grants, 1616
Giving Sum Annual Grant, 1619
Gladys Brooks Fndn Grants, 1620
GlaxoSmithKline Corp Grants, 1623
Glazer Family Fndn Grants, 1625
Glendale Comm Fndn Grants, 1626
Global Fund for Children Grants, 1629
Godfrey Fndn Grants, 1631
GoGirlGo! Ambassador Team Awards, 1632
Golden State Warriors Fndn Grants, 1633
Good Samaritan Inc Grants, 1637
Goodrich Corporation Fndn Grants, 1638
Goodyear Tire Grants, 1639
Graco Fndn Grants, 1642
Grand Haven Area Comm Fndn Grants, 1644
Grand Rapids Area Comm Fndn Grants, 1645
Grand Rapids Area Comm Fndn Nashwauk Area Endowment Fund Grants, 1646
Grand Rapids Comm Fndn Grants, 1647
Grass Fndn Marine Biological Laboratory Fellowships, 1648
Great-West Life Grants, 1649
Greater Bridgeport Area Fndn Comm Impact Grants, 1650
Greater Cincinnati Fndn Priority and Small Projects/Capacity-Building Grants, 1651
Greater Green Bay Comm Fndn Grants, 1652
Greater Milwaukee Fndn Grants, 1653
Greater New Orleans Fndn Grants, 1654
Greater Saint Louis Comm Fndn Grants, 1655
Greater Tacoma Comm Fndn Grants, 1656
Greater Tacoma Comm Fndn Ryan Alan Hade Endowment Fund, 1657
Greater Worcester Comm Fndn Discretionary Grants, 1658
Greater Worcester Comm Fndn Jeppson Memorial Fund for Brookfield Grants, 1659
Green Bay Packers Fndn Grants, 1660
Green Fndn Grants, 1661
Greene County Fndn Grants, 1662
Greenspun Family Fndn Grants, 1664
Grotto Fndn Project Grants, 1671
Guidant Fndn Grants, 1674
Guitar Center Music Fndn Grants, 1675
Gulf Coast Comm Fndn Grants, 1676
Gulf Coast Comm of Venice Fndn Grants, 1677
H & R Fndn Grants, 1679
H.A. and Mary K. Chapman Charitable Trust Grants, 1681
H.J. Heinz Company Fndn Grants, 1682
Hackett Fndn Grants, 1684
Hagedorn Fund Grants, 1685
Halliburton Fndn Grants, 1687
Hallmark Corp Fndn Grants, 1688
Hancock County Comm Fndn Grants, 1690
Hanna Andersson Children's Fndn Grants, 1691
Hannaford Charitable Fndn Grants, 1692
Harley Davidson Fndn Grants, 1694
Harold Alfond Fndn Grants, 1695
Harold and Arlene Schnitzer CARE Fndn Grants, 1697
Harris and Eliza Kempner Fund Grants, 1699
Harrison County Comm Fndn Grants, 1700
Harry Bramhall Gilbert Charitable Trust Grants, 1703
Harry S. Black and Allon Fuller Fund, 1706
Harry Sudakoff Fndn Grants, 1708
Hartford Courant Fndn Grants, 1710
Hartford Fndn Regular Grants, 1711
Harvest Fndn Grants, 1713
Hasbro Children's Fund, 1714
Hawaii Comm Fndn Health Education and Research Grants, 1716
Hawaii Comm Fndn Reverend Takie Okumura Family Grants, 1717
Hawaii Comm Fndn West Hawaii Fund Grants, 1718
Hawn Fndn Grants, 1719
HCA Fndn Grants, 1721
Health Fndn of Greater Cincinnati Grants, 1724
Health Fndn of Southern Florida Responsive Grants, 1726
Healthcare Fndn of New Jersey Grants, 1729
Hearst Fndn and William Randolph Hearst Fndn Grants, 1730
Heckscher Fndn for Children Grants, 1732
Hedco Fndn Grants, 1733
Heineman Fndn for Research, Education, Charitable and Scientific Purposes, 1735
Helen Bader Fndn Grants, 1738
Helen K. and Arthur E. Johnson Fndn Grants, 1740
Helen Steiner Rice Fndn Grants, 1742
Helena Rubinstein Fndn Grants, 1743
Hendrick Fndn for Children Grants, 1744
Henrietta Tower Wurts Memorial Fndn Grants, 1745
Henry and Ruth Blaustein Rosenberg Fndn Grants, 1746
Henry J. Kaiser Family Fndn Media Fellowships, 1749
Hershey Company Grants, 1754
HHMI Biomedical Research Grants for International Scientists in Canada and Latin America, 1756
HHMI Biomedical Research Grants for International Scientists in the Baltics, Central and Eastern Europe, Russia, and Ukraine, 1757
HHMI Grants and Fellowships Programs, 1759
HHMI Med into Grad Initiative Grants, 1761
HHMI-NIBIB Interfaces Initiative Grants, 1764
High Meadow Fndn Grants, 1768
Highmark Corp Giving Grants, 1769
Highmark Healthy High 5, 1770
Hilda and Preston Davis Fndn Grants, 1772
Hill Crest Fndn Grants, 1773
Hillman Fndn Grants, 1775
Hillsdale County Comm Fndn Healthy Senior/Healthy Youth Fund Grants, 1776
Hillsdale County Comm General Adult Fndn Grants, 1777
Hillsdale Fund Grants, 1778
Hilton Head Island Fndn Grants, 1779
Hilton Hotels Corp Giving Program Grants, 1780
Hirtzel Memorial Fndn Grants, 1781
Hoblitzelle Fndn Grants, 1783
Hogg Fndn for Mental Health Grants, 1784
Hoglund Fndn Grants, 1785
Holland/Zeeland Comm Fndn Grants, 1786
Home Building Industry Disaster Relief Fund, 1787
HomeBanc Fndn Grants, 1788
Homer Fndn Grants, 1789
Honda of America Manufacturing Fndn Grants, 1790
Horace A. Kimball and S. Ella Kimball Fndn Grants, 1792
Houston Endowment Grants, 1797
Howard and Bush Fndn Grants, 1798
Howe Fndn of North Carolina Grants, 1799
HRSA Nursing Education Opportunities for the Disadvantaged Project Grants, 1809
Huber Fndn Grants, 1812
Hudson Webber Fndn Grants, 1813
Hugh J. Andersen Fndn Grants, 1814
Huie-Dellmon Trust Grants, 1815
Human Source Fndn Grants, 1817
Humana Fndn Grants, 1818
Huntington Beach Police Officers Fndn Grants, 1821
Huntington Clinical Fndn Grants, 1822
Huntington County Comm Fndn Grants, 1823
Huntington National Bank Comm Affairs Grants, 1824
Hut Fndn Grants, 1827
Hutton Fndn Grants, 1828
i2 Fndn Grants, 1829
Ida Alice Ryan Charitable Trust Grants, 1836
Idaho Comm Fndn Eastern Region Competitive Grants, 1837
Idaho Power Company Corp Contributions, 1838
Ignacio Martin-Baro Fund for Mental Health and Human Rights Grants, 1839
Impact 100 Grants, 1843
Inasmuch Fndn Grants, 1845
Independence Blue Cross Nurse Scholars Program, 1847
Independence Blue Cross Nursing Internships, 1848
Independence Comm Fndn Comm Quality of Life Grant, 1849
Indiana AIDS Fund Grants, 1851
Infinity Fndn Grants, 1854
Ireland Family Fndn Grants, 1865
Irvin Stern Fndn Grants, 1866

Irving S. Gilmore Fndn Grants, 1867
Isabel Allende Fndn Esperanza Grants, 1868
Ittleson Fndn AIDS Grants, 1869
Ittleson Fndn Mental Health Grants, 1870
J. Walton Bissell Fndn Grants, 1872
J.B. Reynolds Fndn Grants, 1873
J.C. Penney Company Grants, 1874
J.E. and L.E. Mabee Fndn Grants, 1875
J.L. Bedsole Fndn Grants, 1876
J.M. Long Fndn Grants, 1877
Jackson County Comm Fndn Unrestricted Grants, 1879
Jacob and Hilda Blaustein Fndn Grants, 1881
Jacob and Valeria Langeloth Fndn Grants, 1882
Jacob G. Schmidlapp Trust Grants, 1883
James A. and Faith Knight Fndn Grants, 1884
James Ford Bell Fndn Grants, 1885
James Graham Brown Fndn Grants, 1887
James H. Cummings Fndn Grants, 1888
James J. and Angelia M. Harris Fndn Grants, 1890
James M. Collins Fndn Grants, 1891
James M. Cox Fndn of Georgia Grants, 1892
James S. Copley Fndn Grants, 1895
Jane Bradley Pettit Fndn Grants, 1902
Jane's Trust Grants, 1904
Janirve Fndn Grants, 1905
Jay and Rose Phillips Family Fndn Grants, 1909
Jean and Louis Dreyfus Fndn Grants, 1911
JELD-WEN Fndn Grants, 1914
Jenkins Fndn: Improving the Health of Greater Richmond Grants, 1915
Jennings County Comm Fndn Grants, 1916
Jessie B. Cox Charitable Trust Grants, 1918
Jessie Ball Dupont Fund Grants, 1919
Jewish Women's Fndn of New York Grants, 1924
Jim Moran Fndn Grants, 1925
JM Fndn Grants, 1926
Joe W. and Dorothy Dorsett Brown Fndn Grants, 1927
John Deere Fndn Grants, 1929
John Edward Fowler Memorial Fndn Grants, 1930
John G. Duncan Trust Grants, 1931
John H. and Wilhelmina D. Harland Charitable Fndn Grants, 1933
John I. Smith Charities Grants, 1935
John J. Leidy Fndn Grants, 1936
John Jewett and Helen Chandler Garland Fndn Grants, 1937
John Lord Knight Fndn Grants, 1938
John M. Lloyd Fndn Grants, 1939
John Merck Fund Grants, 1940
John P. McGovern Fndn Grants, 1942
John P. Murphy Fndn Grants, 1943
John R. Oishei Fndn Grants, 1944
John W. Alden Trust Grants, 1947
John W. and Anna H. Hanes Fndn Grants, 1948
John W. Anderson Fndn Grants, 1949
Johns Manville Fund Grants, 1950
Johnson & Johnson Corp Contributions Grants, 1952
Johnson Controls Fndn Grants, 1954
Joseph Alexander Fndn Grants, 1957
Joseph Collins Fndn Grants, 1959
Joseph Drown Fndn Grants, 1960
Joseph H. and Florence A. Roblee Fndn Grants, 1961
Josephine G. Russell Trust Grants, 1963
Josephine Goodyear Fndn Grants, 1964
Josephine S. Gumbiner Fndn Grants, 1965
Josiah Macy Jr. Fndn Grants, 1966
Josiah W. and Bessie H. Kline Fndn Grants, 1967
Journal Gazette Fndn Grants, 1968
Joyce Fndn Grants, 1969
Julia Temple Davis Brown Fndn Grants, 1971
K and F Baxter Family Fndn Grants, 1973
K. M. Hunter Charitable Fndn Social Welfare Grants, 1974
Kahuku Comm Fund, 1977
Kaiser Permanente Cares for Communities Grants, 1978
Kalamazoo Fndn Grants, 1979
Katharine Matthies Fndn Grants, 1982
Kathryne Beynon Fndn Grants, 1984
Kavli Fndn Research Grants, 1985
Kelvin and Eleanor Smith Fndn Grants, 1986
Kendrick Fndn Grants, 1988
Kenneth T. and Eileen L. Norris Fndn Grants, 1989
Kettering Family Fndn Grants, 1991
Kevin P. and Sydney B. Knight Family Fndn Grants, 1993
KeySpan Fndn Grants, 1995
KFF Barbara Jordan Health Policy Scholars Program, 2000
Kimberly-Clark Comm Grants, 2001
King Pharmaceuticals Corp Contributions Grants, 2003
Kluge Center David B. Larson Fellowship in Health and Spirituality, 2006
Knight Family Charitable and Educational Fndn Grants, 2007
Knight Public Health Journalism Fellowships at CDC, 2008
Knox County Comm Fndn Grants, 2009
Komen Greater NYC Clinical Trials Enrollment Grants, 2010
Komen Greater NYC Comm Breast Health Grants, 2011
Kosciusko County Comm Fndn Grants, 2015
Kraft Cares International Grants, 2016
Kraft Cares US Grants, 2017
L. W. Pierce Family Fndn Grants, 2019
LaGrange County Comm Fndn Grants, 2020
Lalor Fndn Postdoctoral Research Grants, 2021
Lance Armstrong Fndn Comm Grants, 2025
Land O'Lakes Fndn Mid-Atlantic Grants, 2027
Lands' End Corp Giving Program, 2030
Larry L. Hillblom Fndn Grants, 2031
Laura B. Vogler Fndn Grants, 2032
Lawrence Fndn Grants, 2034
Leahi Fund, 2038
Legacy Fndn Grants, 2040
Leo Goodwin Fndn Grants, 2043
Leonard and Helen R. Stulman Charitable Fndn Grants, 2044
Leonsis Fndn Grants, 2045
Lester E. Yeager Charitable Trust B Grants, 2047
Lester Ray Fleming Scholarships, 2048
Lewis Preston Fund for Girls Education Grants, 2052
Liberty Bank Fndn Grants, 2053
Lincoln Financial Group Fndn Grants, 2058
Lockheed Martin Philanthropic Grants, 2062
Long Island Comm Fndn Grants, 2063
Louis Calder Fndn Grants, 2065
Louis R. Cappelli Fndn Grants, 2066
Lowe Fndn Grants, 2067
Lowell Area Comm Fund Grants, 2068
Lubbock Area Fndn Grants, 2079
Lubrizol Fndn Grants, 2080
Lucile Horton Howe and Mitchell B. Howe Fndn Grants, 2081
Lucy Gooding Charitable Fndn Trust, 2082
Lucy Gooding Charitable Fndn Trust Grants, 2083
Lynde and Harry Bradley Fndn Grants, 2089
M-A-C AIDS Fund Grants, 2091
M. Bastian Family Fndn Grants, 2092
M.B. and Edna Zale Fndn Grants, 2093
M.E. Raker Fndn Grants, 2094
M.J. Murdock Charitable Trust Grants, 2095
Mabel Y. Hughes Charitable Trust Grants, 2097
Madison County Comm Fndn Grants, 2098
Maine Comm Fndn Grants, 2099
Manuel D. and Rhoda Mayerson Fndn Grants, 2100
MAPFRE Fndn for Medicine Grants, 2102
Marcia and Otto Koehler Fndn Grants, 2103
Margaret L. Wendt Fndn Grants, 2104
Margaret T. Morris Fndn Grants, 2105
Margoes Fndn Grants, 2106
Marion I. and Henry J. Knott Fndn Grants, 2109
Marion Park Deaver and Harry Gilbert Deaver Fndn Grants, 2110
Mark and Catherine Winkler Fndn Grants, 2112
Mars Fndn Grants, 2114
Marshall Field's Comm Grants, 2115
Mary Baker Eddy Library Summer Research Fellowships, 2117
Mary Black Fndn Grants, 2118
Mary Owen Borden Fndn Grants, 2121
Mary S. and David C. Corbin Fndn Grants, 2122
Mass Youth Against Tobacco Mini-Grants, 2123
Matilda R. Wilson Fund Grants, 2128
Matsumae International Fndn Grants, 2129
Mattel Children's Fndn Grants, 2130
Mattel International Grants, 2131
Max and Victoria Dreyfus Fndn Grants, 2133
Maxon Charitable Fndn Grants, 2135
Maxtor Corp Contributions Grants, 2136
May and Stanley Smith Trust Grants, 2137
May Department Stores Charitable Contribution Grants, 2138
McCarthy Family Fndn Grants, 2141
McCombs Fndn Grants, 2142
McGregor Fund Grants, 2143
McInerny Fndn Grants, 2144
McKesson Fndn Grants, 2145
McLean Contributionship Grants, 2147
McMillen Fndn Grants, 2148
McMurry Fndn Grants, 2149
MDBDF Agnes Higgins Award, 2155
Mead Johnson Nutritionals Evansville-Area Organizations Grants, 2157
Mead Johnson Nutritionals Medical Education Grants, 2158
Mead Witter Fndn Grants, 2160
Meadows Fndn Grants, 2161
MedImmune Charitable Grants, 2166
Medtronic Fndn Fitness and Nutrition Grants, 2167
Medtronic Fndn Full Life Patient Partnership Program--Heart Rescue Grants, 2168
Medtronic Fndn Health Care Grants, 2169
Mericos Fndn Grants, 2172
Meriden Fndn Grants, 2173
Metro Health Fndn Grants, 2175
Metrowest Comm Health Care Fndn Grants, 2176
Meyer Memorial Trust Grassroots Grants, 2179
Meyer Memorial Trust Operating Funds Grants, 2180
Meyer Memorial Trust Responsive Grants, 2181
MfA Newton Fellowships, 2182
MGFA Post-Doctoral Research Fellowships, 2183
MHRC Graduate Studentships, 2185
Miami County Comm Fndn Operation Round Up Grants, 2188
Michael and Susan Dell Fndn Grants, 2189
Middlesex Savings Charitable Fndn Grants, 2196
Miguel Aleman Fndn Grants, 2197
Milagro Fndn Grants, 2198
Miles of Hope Breast Cancer Fndn Grants, 2199
Military Ex-Prisoners of War Fndn Grants, 2201
Millipore Fndn Grants, 2203
Minneapolis Fndn Comm Grants, 2206
Miriam and Peter Haas Fund Grants, 2208
MMRF Research Grants, 2211
Montgomery County Comm Fndn Grants, 2214
MONY Fndn Grants, 2215
Morris and Gwendolyn Cafritz Fndn Grants, 2217
Moses Cone-Wesley Long Comm Health Fndn Grants, 2219
Mount Zion Health Fund Grants, 2220
Ms. Fndn for Women Grants, 2222
NAPNAP Fndn Elaine Gelman Scholarship, 2235
NAPNAP Fndn Graduate Student Research Grant, 2236
NAPNAP Fndn McNeil PNP Scholarships, 2239
NAPNAP Fndn McNeil Rural and Underserved Scholarships, 2240
NAPNAP Fndn Shourd Parks Immunization Project Small Grants, 2243
NAPNAP Fndn Wyeth Pediatric Immunization Grant, 2244
National 4-H Healthy Lifestyles Grants, 2248

National City Corporation Contributions Grants, 2250
National Starch and Chemical Fndn Grants, 2261
NBNA Lauranne Sams Scholarships, 2264
Nelda C. and H.J. Lutcher Stark Fndn Grants, 2301
New York Life Fndn Grants, 2304
Newman's Own Inc Grants, 2306
NFX Summer Research Fellowships, 2314
NHLBI Individual Postdoctoral National Research Service Awards, 2340
NHLBI Research Supplements to Promote Diversity in Health-Related Research for Graduate Research Assistants, 2375
NHLBI Research Supplements to Promote Diversity in Health-Related Research for Undergraduate Students, 2377
Nicholas H. Noyes Jr. Memorial Fndn Grants, 2497
NIDA Clinical Research Education Programs in Drug Abuse and Addiction, 2500
NIEHS Hazardous Materials Worker Health and Safety Training Grants, 2599
NIEHS Hazmat Training at Doe Nuclear Weapons Complex Grants, 2600
NIEHS SBIR E-Learning for HAZMAT and Emergency Response Grants, 2604
NIH Academic Research Enhancement Awards (AREA), 2635
NIH Clinical Bioethics Postdoctoral Fellowships, 2649
NIH Clinical Bioethics Predoctoral Fellowships, 2650
NIH Midcareer Investigator Award in Mouse Pathobiology Research Grants, 2690
NIH School-based Interventions to Prevent Obesity, 2725
NIH Summer Internship Program in Biomedical Research, 2732
NIH Undergraduate Scholarships, 2737
NIMH Career Opportunities in Research (COR) Education and Training Honors High School Research Education Grant, 2748
NIMH Career Opportunities in Research (COR) Education and Training Honors Undergraduate Research Training Grant, 2749
NIMH Jointly Sponsored Ruth L. Kirschstein National Research Service Award Institutional Predoctoral Training Program in the Neurosciences, 2761
NLM Understanding and Promoting Health Literacy Research Grants, 2827
NMF General Electric Medical Scholars Fellowships, 2830
NMF National Medical Association Awards for Medical Journalism, 2836
NMF National Medical Association Emerging Scholar Awards, 2837
NMF National Medical Association Patti LaBelle Award, 2838
NMF William and Charlotte Cadbury Award, 2841
NMSS Scholarships, 2845
NNEDVF/Altria Doors of Hope Program, 2847
Noble County Comm Fndn Grants, 2848
Nordson Corporation Fndn Grants, 2851
North Carolina Biotechnology Center Event Sponsorship Grants, 2852
North Carolina Comm Development Grants, 2858
North Carolina Comm Fndn Grants, 2859
North Carolina GlaxoSmithKline Fndn Grants, 2860
North Central Health Services Grants, 2861
North Georgia Comm Fndn Grants, 2862
Northeast Utilities Fndn Grants, 2863
Northern New York Comm Fndn Grants, 2864
Northern Trust Company Charitable Trust and Corp Giving Program, 2865
Northrop Grumman Corporation Grants, 2866
Northrop Grumman Newport News Grants, 2867
Northwest Minnesota Fndn Women's Fund Grants, 2869
Northwestern Mutual Fndn Grants, 2870
Norwin S. and Elizabeth N. Bean Fndn Grants, 2872
NSF Chemistry Research Experiences for Undergraduates (REU), 2883
NSF Instrument Development for Biological Research (IDBR), 2888
NSF Postdoctoral Research Fellowships in Biology (PRFB), 2891
NSF Presidential Early Career Awards for Scientists and Engineers (PECASE) Grants, 2892
NSF Undergraduate Research and Mentoring in the Biological Sciences (URM), 2896
Nuffield Fndn Africa Program Grants, 2898
NYCT AIDS/HIV Grants, 2919
NYCT Girls and Young Women Grants, 2924
NYCT Substance Abuse Grants, 2928
OceanFirst Fndn Grants, 2933
Oceanside Charitable Fndn Grants, 2934
Office Depot Corporation Comm Grants, 2935
Office Depot Fndn Grants, 2936
Ohio County Comm Fndn Grants, 2938
Ohio County Comm Fndn Mini-Grants, 2939
Ohio Learning Network Grants, 2940
Oleonda Jameson Trust Grants, 2941
Olin Corporation Charitable Trust Grants, 2943
OneSight Research Fndn Block Grants, 2944
Oracle Corp Contributions Grants, 2951
Ordean Fndn Grants, 2952
OREF Educational Awards, 2953
Oscar Rennebohm Fndn Grants, 2963
OSI European Commission Internships for Young Roma Graduates, 2965
OSI Supplementary Grants: Burma, 2971
OSI-Baltimore Special Opportunities Program Grants, 2972
OSI-Baltimore Tackling Drug Addiction Grants, 2973
Otto Bremer Fndn Grants, 2977
Owen County Comm Fndn Grants, 2979
PacifiCare Fndn Grants, 2981
PacifiCorp Fndn for Learning Grants, 2982
Palm Beach and Martin Counties Grants, 2986
Partnership for Cures Charles E. Culpeper Scholarships in Medical Science, 2991
Paso del Norte Health Fndn Grants, 2995
Paul and Mary Haas Fndn Contributions and Student Scholarships, 2997
Paul E. and Klare N. Reinhold Fndn Grants, 2999
Paul G. Allen Family Fndn Grants, 3000
Paul G. Duke Fndn Grants, 3001
Paul Ogle Fndn Grants, 3003
Peacock Fndn Grants, 3011
Perkins Charitable Fndn Grants, 3014
Perpetual Trust for Charitable Giving Grants, 3015
Perry County Comm Fndn Grants, 3016
Pew Charitable Trusts Children and Youth Grants, 3020
PeyBack Fndn Grants, 3022
Pfizer Fndn Grants, 3025
Pfizer Fndn Health Literacy Grants, 3026
Pfizer/AAFP Fndn Visiting Professorship Program in Family Medicine, 3027
Philadelphia Fndn Organizational Effectiveness Grants, 3029
Phoenix Suns Charities Grants, 3030
PhRMA Fndn Informatics Sabbatical Fellowships, 3035
PhRMA Fndn Informatics Pre Doctoral Fellowships, 3037
PhRMA Fndn Informatics Research Starter Grants, 3038
PhRMA Fndn Paul Calabresi Medical Student Research Fellowship, 3039
PhRMA Fndn Pharmaceutics Postdoctoral Fellowships, 3040
PhRMA Fndn Pharmaceutics Pre Doctoral Fellowships, 3041
PhRMA Fndn Pharmaceutics Research Starter Grants, 3042
PhRMA Fndn Pharmaceutics Sabbatical Fellowships, 3043
PhRMA Fndn Pharmacology/Toxicology Sabbatical Fellowships, 3047
Piedmont Natural Gas Grants, 3048
Pike County Comm Fndn Grants, 3049
Pinellas County Grants, 3050
Pioneer Hi-Bred Comm Grants, 3051
Pittsburgh Fndn Comm Fund Grants, 3054
Plough Fndn Grants, 3061
Plum Creek Fndn Grants, 3062
PMI Fndn Grants, 3063
PNC Charitable Trust and Fndn Grants, 3064
Polaroid Fund Grants, 3065
Polk Bros. Fndn Grants, 3066
Portland General Electric Fndn Grants, 3067
Posey Comm Fndn Grants, 3068
Posey Comm Fndn Womens Fund Grants, 3069
Postdoctoral Research Fellowships in Gerontological Public Health, 3070
Pott Fndn Grants, 3071
Potts Memorial Fndn Grants, 3072
Powell Fndn Grants, 3073
Presbyterian Health Fndn Bridge, Seed and Equipment Grants, 3075
Priddy Fndn Grants, 3077
Pride Fndn Grants and Scholarships, 3078
Prince Charitable Trusts Chicago Grants, 3079
Prince Charitable Trusts District of Columbia Grants, 3080
Princeton Area Comm Fndn Greater Mercer Grants, 3081
Principal Financial Group Fndn Grants, 3082
Procter and Gamble Fund Grants, 3083
Progress Energy Fndn Grants, 3084
Prudential Fndn Grants, 3087
PSG Mentored Clinical Research Awards, 3088
Puerto Rico Comm Fndn Grants, 3090
Pulaski County Comm Fndn Grants, 3091
Pulte Homes Corp Contributions, 3092
Putnam County Comm Fndn Grants, 3093
Quantum Fndn Grants, 3096
Questar Corp Contributions Grants, 3097
R.C. Baker Fndn Grants, 3098
Rainbow Fund Grants, 3103
Rajiv Gandhi Fndn Grants, 3104
Ralphs Food 4 Less Fndn Grants, 3106
Raskob Fndn for Catholic Activities Grants, 3107
Rasmuson Fndn Grants, 3108
Rathmann Family Fndn Grants, 3109
Raymond John Wean Fndn Grants, 3110
RCPSC Balfour M. Mount Visiting Professorship in Palliative Medicine, 3112
RCPSC Events, Speakers and Visiting Professors Grants, 3116
RCPSC Janes Visiting Professorship in Surgery, 3120
RCPSC Kilborn Memorial Visiting Professorship, 3121
RCPSC McLaughlin-Gallie Visiting Professorship, 3123
RCPSC Medical Education Research Grants, 3124
RCPSC Traineeships, 3132
RCPSC Wightman Visiting Professorship in Medicine, 3134
Regence Fndn Health Care Comm Awareness and Engagement Grants, 3139
Regence Fndn Improving End-of-Life Grants, 3141
Rehabilitation Nursing Fndn Scholarships, 3148
Retirement Research Fndn General Program Grants, 3150
Reynolds and Reynolds Associate Fndn Grants, 3152
RGK Fndn Grants, 3153
Rhode Island Fndn Grants, 3154
Rice Fndn Grants, 3155
Rich Fndn Grants, 3156
Richard and Susan Smith Family Fndn Grants, 3159
Richard King Mellon Fndn Grants, 3161
Richmond Eye and Ear Fund Grants, 3164
Riley Fndn Grants, 3165
Ripley County Comm Fndn Grants, 3166
Robert and Joan Dircks Fndn Grants, 3167
Robert and Polly Dunn Fndn Grants, 3168

Robert E. and Evelyn McKee Fndn Grants, 3170
Robert P. & Clara I. Milton Fund for Senior Housing, 3172
Robin Hood Fndn Grants, 3174
Robins Fndn Grants, 3175
Rochester Area Comm Fndn Grants, 3176
Rochester Area Fndn Grants, 3177
Rockefeller Brothers Fund Pivotal Places Grants: South Africa, 3180
Rockwell Collins Charitable Contributions, 3182
Rohm and Haas Company Grants, 3185
Rosalynn Carter Institute John and Betty Pope Fellowships, 3189
Rosalynn Carter Institute Mattie J. T. Stepanek Caregiving Scholarships, 3190
Roy and Christine Sturgis Trust Grants, 3191
RRF General Program Grants, 3193
RSC McNeil Medal for the Public Awareness of Science, 3198
Rush County Comm Fndn Grants, 3200
Russell Berrie Fndn Grants, 3201
Ruth Eleanor Bamberger and John Ernest Bamberger Memorial Fndn Grants, 3202
Ruth H. and Warren A. Ellsworth Fndn Grants, 3203
RWJF Clinical Scholars Program Grants, 3207
RWJF Executive Nurse Fellowships, 3210
RWJF Health & Society Scholars, 3214
RWJF Jobs to Careers: Promoting Work-Based Learning for Quality Care - Research Grants, 3221
RWJF Ladder to Leadership: Developing the Next Generation of Comm Health Leaders Fellowships, 3222
RWJF New Careers in Nursing Scholarships, 3224
RWJF Partners Investing in Nursing's Future Grants, 3226
RWJF Pipeline, Profession and Practice: Comm-Based Dental Education Grants, 3228
RWJF Summer Medical and Dental Education Program (SMDEP), 3231
RWJF Young Epidemiology Scholars (YES) Competition, 3233
S. Mark Taper Fndn Grants, 3236
S.H. Cowell Fndn Grants, 3237
Salem Fndn Charitable Trust Grants, 3241
Salisbury Comm Fndn Grants, 3243
Samuel Freeman Charitable Trust Grants, 3249
Samuel Roberts Noble Fndn Grants, 3250
Samuel S. Johnson Fndn Grants, 3251
Samueli Fndn Health Grants, 3252
San Antonio Area Fndn Grants, 3254
San Diego Fndn for Change Grants, 3255
San Diego HIV Funding Collaborative (SDHFC) Grants, 3258
San Diego Women's Fndn Grants, 3259
San Francisco Fndn Comm Health Grants, 3260
Sarah Scaife Fndn Grants, 3263
Sasco Fndn Grants, 3265
Schering-Plough Fndn Health Grants, 3270
Scientific Communities Initiative Grants, 3272
Scott County Comm Fndn Grants, 3273
Seabury Fndn Grants, 3274
Seattle Fndn Grants, 3276
Self Fndn Grants, 3277
Seneca Foods Fndn Grants, 3278
Shaw's Supermarkets Donations, 3280
Shell Oil Company Fndn Grants, 3281
Sheltering Arms Fund Grants, 3282
Sid W. Richardson Fndn Grants, 3284
Siebert Lutheran Fndn Grants, 3285
Simmons Fndn Grants, 3287
Simpson Fund Grants, 3290
Sir Dorabji Tata Trust Grants for NGOs or Voluntary Organizations, 3291
Sir Halley Stewart Trust Grants, 3293
Sisters of Mercy of North Carolina Fndn Grants, 3295
Sisters of St. Joseph Healthcare Fndn Grants, 3297
Snee Reinhardt Charitable Fndn Grants, 3300
SNM PDEF Mickey Williams Minority Student Scholarships, 3302
SNMTS Paul Cole Scholarships, 3312
SOCFOC Reducing Health & Educational Disparities in the Central Neighborhood Grants, 3318
Society for Imaging Informatics in Medicine (SIIM) Emeritus Mentor Grants, 3320
Society for Imaging Informatics in Medicine (SIIM) Micro Grants, 3321
Society for Imaging Informatics in Medicine (SIIM) Research Grants, 3322
Society for Imaging Informatics in Medicine (SIIM) Small Training Grants, 3324
Sonoco Fndn Grants, 3347
Sosland Fndn Grants, 3348
South Madison Comm Fndn Grants, 3349
Southbury Comm Trust Fund, 3350
Southwest Florida Comm Fndn Competitive Grants, 3351
Southwire Company Grants, 3353
Special Olympics Health Professions Student Grants, 3355
Special People in Need Grants, 3356
Spencer County Comm Fndn Grants, 3358
Springs Close Fndn Grants, 3360
Square D Fndn Grants, 3361
SSRC HIV/AIDS and Public Health Policy Research in Africa Fellowships, 3365
St. Joseph Comm Health Fndn Burn Care and Prevention Grants, 3367
St. Joseph Comm Health Fndn Schneider Fellowships, 3370
Stark Comm Fndn Women's Fund Grants, 3376
Staunton Farm Fndn Grants, 3378
Steelcase Fndn Grants, 3379
Steele-Reese Fndn Grants, 3380
Steuben County Comm Fndn Grants, 3383
Stewart Huston Charitable Trust Grants, 3384
Strowd Roses Grants, 3388
Sulzberger Fndn Grants, 3399
Sunderland Fndn Grants, 3400
Sunshine Natural Wellbeing Fndn Grants, 3404
Support Our Aging Religious (SOAR) Grants, 3406
Susan G. Komen Breast Cancer Fndn Interdisciplinary Fellowships, 3410
Susan Mott Webb Charitable Trust Grants, 3412
Susan Vaughan Fndn Grants, 3413
Take Care to Learn: Teaching Clinical Care Management Grants, 3415
Taproot Fndn Capacity-Building Service Grants, 3417
Tellabs Fndn Grants, 3418
Temple-Inland Fndn Grants, 3419
Texas Commission on the Arts Arts Respond Project Grants, 3420
Thomas and Dorothy Leavey Fndn Grants, 3422
Thomas C. Ackerman Fndn Grants, 3423
Thompson Charitable Fndn Grants, 3425
Tifa Fndn Grants, 3428
Topeka Comm Fndn Kansas Blood Services Scholarships, 3429
Toro Fndn Grants, 3431
Triangle Comm Fndn Donor-Advised Grants, 3437
Triangle Comm Fndn Shaver-Hitchings Scholarship, 3438
Trull Fndn Grants, 3441
TWS Fndn Grants, 3443
Tylenol Scholarship, 3444
U.S. Department of Education 21st Century Comm Learning Centers, 3445
U.S. Department of Education Erma Byrd Scholarships, 3446
U.S. Department of Education Rehabilitation Engineering Research Centers Grants, 3447
U.S. Department of Education Rehabilitation Research Training Centers (RRTCs), 3448
U.S. Department of Education Rehabilitation Training--Rehabilitation Continuing Education Programs (RCEP)--Institute on Rehabilitation Issues (IRI), 3449
U.S. Department of Education Special Education--National Activities--Parent Information Centers, 3450
U.S. Department of Education United States-Russia Program: Improving Research and Educational Activities in Higher Education, 3451
U.S. Department of Education Vocational Rehabilitation Services Projects for American Indians with Disabilities Grants, 3452
UCLA / RAND Corporation Post-Doctoral Fellowships, 3454
Union Benevolent Association Grants, 3460
Union County Comm Fndn Grants, 3461
United Methodist Church Global AIDS Fund Grants, 3463
United Technologies Corporation Grants, 3466
Unity Fndn Of LaPorte County Grants, 3467
Until There's a Cure Fndn Grants, 3471
US Airways Comm Contributions, 3472
US Airways Comm Fndn Grants, 3473
US Trust Corporation Fndn Grants, 3475
Vancouver Fndn Grants and Comm Initiatives Program, 3477
Vancouver Fndn Public Health Bursary Package, 3478
Vanderburgh Comm Fndn Grants, 3480
Varian Medical Systems Grants, 3481
VDH Commonwealth of Virginia Nurse Educator Scholarships, 3482
VDH Emergency Medical Services Training Fund (EMSTF), 3483
Vectren Fndn Grants, 3485
Verizon Fndn Maryland Grants, 3487
Verizon Fndn New York Grants, 3488
Verizon Fndn Northeast Region Grants, 3489
Verizon Fndn Pennsylvania Grants, 3490
Verizon Fndn Vermont Grants, 3491
Verizon Fndn Virginia Grants, 3492
Vermont Comm Fndn Grants, 3493
Viets Medical Student Myasthenia Gravis Research Fellowships, 3496
Viking Children's Fund Grants, 3497
Virginia Department of Health Mary Marshall Nursing Scholarships for Licensed Practical Nurses, 3498
Virginia Department of Health Mary Marshall Nursing Scholarships for Registered Nurses, 3499
Virginia Department of Health Nurse Practitioner/ Nurse Midwife Scholarships, 3500
Virginia W. Kettering Fndn Grants, 3502
Volkswagen of America Corp Contributions Grants, 3503
Vulcan Materials Company Fndn Grants, 3504
W.K. Kellogg Fndn Healthy Kids Grants, 3507
W.K. Kellogg Fndn Secure Families Grants, 3508
Wabash Valley Comm Fndn Grants, 3510
Wachovia Fndn Grants, 3511
Wal-Mart Fndn Comm Grants, 3513
Wal-Mart State Giving Program Grants, 3514
Wallace H. Coulter Fndn Grants, 3515
Walt Disney Company Fndn Grants, 3516
Warrick County Comm Fndn Grants, 3519
Washington Post Contributions Program Grants, 3520
Wayne and Gladys Valley Fndn Grants, 3522
Weatherwax Fndn Grants, 3523
Weingart Fndn Grants, 3524
Wells County Fndn Grants, 3527
Western Indiana Comm Fndn Grants, 3528
Western Union Fndn Grants, 3529
Westinghouse Charitable Giving Grants, 3530
WHO Fndn General Grants, 3534
Wilkins Family Fndn Grants, 3536
William G. Gilmore Fndn Grants, 3537
William G. McGowan Charitable Fund Grants, 3539
William H. Hannon Fndn Grants, 3540
William T. Grant Fndn Research Grants, 3541
Wilson-Wood Fndn Grants, 3542

Winifred & Harry B. Allen Fndn Grants, 3543
Winston-Salem Fndn Competitive Grants, 3544
Winston-Salem Fndn Elkin/Tri-County Grants, 3545
Winston-Salem Fndn Stokes County Grants, 3546
Women of the ELCA Opportunity Scholarships for Lutheran Laywomen, 3548
Women's Fndn of California Grants, 3550
Women's Sports Fndn Grants, 3551
Woodward Fund Grants, 3552
YSA Get Ur Good On Grants, 3555
YSA UnitedHealth Heroes Service Learning Grants, 3556
Z. Smith Reynolds Fndn Small Grants, 3557

Emergency Programs
Able Trust Vocational Rehabilitation Grants for Individuals, 186
Actors Fund Social Services and Financial Assistance, 225
Acushnet Fndn Grants, 226
Adaptec Fndn Grants, 232
Alcatel-Lucent Technologies Fndn Grants, 333
American Express Fndn Comm Service Grants, 435
Anheuser-Busch Fndn Grants, 474
Auburn Fndn Grants, 664
Avon Products Fndn Grants, 675
Becton Dickinson and Company Grants, 736
Blanche and Julian Robertson Family Fndn Grants, 765
Blowitz-Ridgeway Fndn Grants, 767
Boeing Company Contributions Program Grants, 777
Borkee-Hagley Fndn Grants, 781
Byron W. and Alice L. Lockwood Fndn Grants, 824
Cargill Citizenship Fund-Corp Giving Grants, 865
Carpenter Fndn Grants, 881
Central Okanagan Fndn Grants, 937
Children Affected by AIDS Fndn Family Assistance Emergency Fund Grants, 996
Coastal Comm Fndn of South Carolina Grants, 1051
Cockrell Fndn Grants, 1053
Comm Fndn for Monterey County Grants, 1092
Comm Fndn for Muskegon County Grants, 1093
Comm Fndn for Southeastern Michigan Grants, 1094
Comm Fndn of Crawford County Grants and Scholarships, 1103
Comm Fndn of Greater Birmingham Grants, 1106
Comm Fndn of Greater Fort Wayne: Comm Endowment & Clarke Endowment Fund Grants, 1108
Comm Fndn of Mount Vernon and Knox County Grants, 1119
Comm Fndn of Southeastern Connecticut Grants, 1125
Connelly Fndn Grants, 1143
Cornerstone Fndn of Northeastern Wisconsin Grants, 1152
Cruise Industry Charitable Fndn Grants, 1166
Cudd Fndn Grants, 1171
Cullen Fndn Grants, 1172
Dana Corporation Fndn Grants, 1196
Daywood Fndn Grants, 1206
Donald and Sylvia Robinson Family Fndn Grants, 1310
Doris and Victor Day Fndn Grants, 1313
Doris Duke Charitable Fndn Operations Research on AIDS Care and Treatment in Africa (ORACTA) Grants, 1319
Drs. Bruce and Lee Fndn Grants, 1333
Edyth Bush Charitable Fndn Grants, 1378
Erie Comm Fndn Grants, 1427
Florida BRAIVE Fund of Gulf Coast Comm Fndn of Venice, 1513
Frank Stanley Beveridge Fndn Grants, 1553
Fred L. Emerson Fndn Grants, 1557
George Kress Fndn Grants, 1601
Gill Fndn - Gay and Lesbian Fund Grants, 1613
Greater New Orleans Fndn Grants, 1654
Gulf Coast Comm Fndn Grants, 1676
Gulf Coast Comm of Venice Fndn Grants, 1677
Harold and Arlene Schnitzer CARE Fndn Grants, 1697
Henrietta Tower Wurts Memorial Fndn Grants, 1745
High Meadow Fndn Grants, 1768
Hoglund Fndn Grants, 1785
Home Building Industry Disaster Relief Fund, 1787
Humana Fndn Grants, 1818
Indiana AIDS Fund Grants, 1851
James Graham Brown Fndn Grants, 1887
Jane's Trust Grants, 1904
John Deere Fndn Grants, 1929
John G. Duncan Trust Grants, 1931
John I. Smith Charities Grants, 1935
John Jewett and Helen Chandler Garland Fndn Grants, 1937
John P. McGovern Fndn Grants, 1942
John W. and Anna H. Hanes Fndn Grants, 1948
Johns Manville Fund Grants, 1950
Josephine G. Russell Trust Grants, 1963
Josiah W. and Bessie H. Kline Fndn Grants, 1967
Kalamazoo Fndn Grants, 1979
McMurry Fndn Grants, 2149
Morris and Gwendolyn Cafritz Fndn Grants, 2217
Nordson Corporation Fndn Grants, 2851
Northwest Airlines KidCares Medical Travel Assistance, 2868
Northwestern Mutual Fndn Grants, 2870
Office Depot Fndn Grants, 2936
Oleonda Jameson Trust Grants, 2941
Prince Charitable Trusts District of Columbia Grants, 3080
Public Welfare Fndn Grants, 3089
Rhode Island Fndn Grants, 3154
Richard and Rhoda Goldman Fund Grants, 3158
S. Livingston Mather Charitable Trust Grants, 3235
SAG Motion Picture Players Welfare Fund Grants, 3238
Samuel S. Johnson Fndn Grants, 3251
San Francisco Fndn Disability Rights Advocate Fund Emergency Grants, 3261
Seneca Foods Fndn Grants, 3278
Susan G. Komen Breast Cancer Fndn Hurricane Relief Grants, 3409
Texas Commission on the Arts Arts Respond Project Grants, 3420
VHA Health Fndn Grants, 3495
Wal-Mart Fndn Comm Grants, 3513
Western Union Fndn Grants, 3529
Winston-Salem Fndn Victim Assistance Grants, 3547

Environmental Programs
1675 Fndn Grants, 4
3M Fndn Grants, 11
Abbott Fund Comm Vitality Grants, 177
Abel Fndn Grants, 181
Abell-Hanger Fndn Grants, 183
ACE Charitable Fndn Grants, 199
Achelis and Bodman Fndns Grants, 206
ACS Doctoral Training Grants in Oncology Social Work, 213
Administaff Comm Affairs Grants, 235
Adobe Comm Investment Grants, 237
Ahn Family Fndn Grants, 304
Air Products and Chemicals Grants, 319
Alaska Airlines Corp Giving Grants, 323
Alaska Airlines Fndn Grants, 324
Albert Pick Jr. Fund Grants, 328
Albuquerque Comm Fndn Grants, 331
Alcatel-Lucent Technologies Corp Contributions Grants, 332
Alcoa Fndn Grants, 334
Alexander & Baldwin Fndn Hawaiian and Pacific Island Grants, 338
Alexander & Baldwin Fndn Mainland Grants, 339
Allegan County Comm Fndn Grants, 358
Allen P. and Josephine B. Green Fndn Grants, 361
Allstate Corp Giving Grants, 363
Allstate Corp Hometown Commitment Grants, 364
Alpine Winter Fndn Grants, 368
ALSAM Fndn Grants, 369
Amador Comm Fndn Grants, 409
American Chemical Society GCI Pharmaceutical Roundtable Research Grants, 420
American College of Surgeons International Guest Scholarships, 429
American Electric Power Grants, 434
American Psychiatric Association Minority Medical Student Summer Externship in Addiction Psychiatry, 445
Amgen Fndn Grants, 467
Angels Baseball Fndn Grants, 473
Anheuser-Busch Fndn Grants, 474
Ann Arbor Area Comm Fndn Grants, 476
Annie Sinclair Knudsen Memorial Fund/Kaua'i Comm Grants, 480
Arcadia Fndn Grants, 524
Archer Daniels Midland Fndn Grants, 525
Arizona Public Service Corp Giving Program Grants, 531
Arkansas Comm Fndn Grants, 533
Ashland Corp Contributions Grants, 586
AT&T Fndn Civic and Comm Service Program Grants, 658
Atherton Family Fndn Grants, 659
Atkinson Fndn International Grants, 661
Autodesk Comm Relations Grants, 671
Autzen Fndn Grants, 672
Bacon Family Fndn Grants, 679
Ball Brothers Fndn General Grants, 683
Banfi Vintners Fndn Grants, 687
Barker Welfare Fndn Grants, 695
Barra Fndn Comm Fund Grants, 698
Batchelor Fndn Grants, 701
Baton Rouge Area Fndn Grants, 702
BCBS of Minnesota Growing Up Healthy Grants, 711
BCBS of Minnesota Healthy Together Grants, 712
Beazley Fndn Grants, 730
Beirne Carter Fndn Grants, 737
Beldon Fund Grants, 738
Belk Fndn Grants, 739
Bella Vista Fndn Grants, 740
Bender Fndn Grants, 742
Benton Comm Fndn Grants, 743
Benton County Fndn Grants, 744
Berks County Comm Fndn Grants, 745
Bernard F. and Alva B. Gimbel Fndn Grants, 747
Blackford County Comm Fndn Grants, 763
Blanche and Julian Robertson Family Fndn Grants, 765
Blue Mountain Comm Fndn Grants, 769
Blue River Comm Fndn Grants, 770
Blumenthal Fndn Grants, 773
Bodenwein Public Benevolent Fndn Grants, 775
Bodman Fndn Grants, 776
Boeing Company Contributions Program Grants, 777
Boston Fndn Grants, 783
Boyd Gaming Corporation Contributions Program, 788
Brian G. Dyson Fndn Grants, 791
Bridgestone/Firestone Trust Fund Grants, 792
Brown County Comm Fndn Grants, 807
Bruce and Adele Greenfield Fndn Grants, 808
Bullitt Fndn Grants, 809
Burlington Northern Santa Fe Fndn Grants, 812
Burton G. Bettingen Grants, 813
California Wellness Fndn Work and Health Program Grants, 834
Cambridge Comm Fndn Grants, 837
Capital Region Comm Fndn Grants, 862
Cargill Citizenship Fund-Corp Giving Grants, 865
Carl and Eloise Pohlad Family Fndn Grants, 867
Carls Fndn Grants, 876
Carolyn Fndn Grants, 880
Carpenter Fndn Grants, 881
Carrie E. and Lena V. Glenn Fndn Grants, 882
Carrier Corporation Contributions Grants, 884

Cass County Comm Fndn Grants, 887
CDC Research, Treatment, and Education Programs on Lyme Disease in the United States Cooperative Agreements, 927
Central Okanagan Fndn Grants, 937
Cessna Fndn Grants, 938
CFFVR Opportunity Grants, 952
Champlin Fndns Grants, 960
Charles Delmar Fndn Grants, 963
Charles G. Koch Charitable Fndn Grants, 965
Charlotte County (FL) Comm Fndn Grants, 973
Chicago Board of Trade Fndn Grants, 988
Chicago Comm Trust Grants, 989
Chula Vista Charitable Fndn Grants, 1009
Cinergy Fndn Grants, 1013
Citizens Bank Mid-Atlantic Charitable Fndn Grants, 1015
Clarence E. Heller Charitable Fndn Grants, 1022
Clark County Comm Fndn Grants, 1028
Clark Fndn Grants, 1029
Claude Worthington Benedum Fndn Grants, 1033
CLIF Bar Family Fndn Grants, 1040
CNCS Next Generation Grants, 1049
Coastal Comm Fndn of South Carolina Grants, 1051
Coca-Cola Fndn Grants, 1052
Coeta and Donald Barker Fndn Grants, 1054
Collins Fndn Grants, 1058
Colorado Interstate Gas Grants, 1060
Columbus Fndn Competitive Grants, 1066
Columbus Fndn Mary Eleanor Morris Fund Grants, 1069
Comm Fndn Alliance City of Evansville Endowment Fund Grants, 1089
Comm Fndn for Greater New Haven Grants, 1091
Comm Fndn for Monterey County Grants, 1092
Comm Fndn for Muskegon County Grants, 1093
Comm Fndn for Southeastern Michigan Grants, 1094
Comm Fndn of Bartholomew County Heritage Fund Grants, 1096
Comm Fndn of Boone County Grants, 1099
Comm Fndn of Champaign County Grants, 1102
Comm Fndn of Crawford County Grants and Scholarships, 1103
Comm Fndn of Grant County Grants, 1104
Comm Fndn of Grant County Scholarships, 1105
Comm Fndn of Greater Birmingham Grants, 1106
Comm Fndn of Greater Flint Grants, 1107
Comm Fndn of Greater Greensboro Grants, 1109
Comm Fndn of Greater Tampa Grants, 1112
Comm Fndn of Greenville-Greenville Women Giving Grants, 1115
Comm Fndn of Morgan County Grants and Scholarships, 1118
Comm Fndn of Mount Vernon and Knox County Grants, 1119
Comm Fndn of Muncie and Delaware County Grants, 1120
Comm Fndn of Randolph County Grants, 1121
Comm Fndn of Santa Cruz County Grants, 1122
Comm Fndn of South Alabama Grants, 1123
Comm Fndn of South Puget Sound Grants, 1124
Comm Fndn of Southeastern Connecticut Grants, 1125
Comm Fndn of Switzerland County Grants, 1127
Comm Fndn of Tampa Bay Grants, 1128
Comm Fndn of the Eastern Shore Comm Needs Grants, 1129
Comm Fndn of Western North Carolina Grants, 1132
Comm Fndn Silicon Valley Grants, 1133
Connecticut Comm Fndn Grants, 1141
ConocoPhillips Fndn Grants, 1144
Constellation Energy Group and Baltimore Gas and Electric Corp Contributions, 1146
Cooke Fndn Grants, 1148
Cooper Industries Fndn Grants, 1150
Coors Brewing Corp Contributions Grants, 1151
Cowles Charitable Trust Grants, 1155
Cranston Fndn Grants, 1158
Cruise Industry Charitable Fndn Grants, 1166
CSRA Comm Fndn Grants, 1168
CSX Corp Contributions Grants, 1169
Cudd Fndn Grants, 1171
Cyrus Eaton Fndn Grants, 1178
Dade Comm Fndn Grants, 1185
DaimlerChrysler Corporation Fund Grants, 1186
Dana Corporation Fndn Grants, 1196
Dean Foods Comm Involvement Grants, 1209
Dearborn Comm Fndn County Progress Grants, 1211
Delaware Comm Fndn Grants, 1215
Do Something BR!CK Awards, 1287
Dole Food Company Charitable Contributions, 1307
Dorothy Hooper Beattie Fndn Grants, 1321
Dr. Scholl Fndn Grants, 1329
Drs. Bruce and Lee Fndn Grants, 1333
Dubois County Comm Fndn Grants, 1336
Duke Energy Fndn Grants, 1339
E.J. Grassmann Trust Grants, 1360
eBay Fndn Comm Grants, 1363
Educational Fndn of America Grants, 1372
Edward Bangs Kelley and Elza Kelley Fndn Grants, 1373
Edwin W. and Catherine M. Davis Fndn Grants, 1377
EIF Comm Grants, 1386
El Paso Comm Fndn Grants, 1388
El Pomar Fndn Awards and Grants, 1390
Elliot Fndn Inc Grants, 1402
Elmer L. and Eleanor J. Andersen Fndn Grants, 1406
Ensworth Charitable Fndn Grants, 1416
EPA Baseline Assessment of Risks of Exposure to Lead Poisoning of Native American Children, 1419
EPA Children's Health Protection Grants, 1420
EPA Lead Awareness Outreach for Native American Tribes, 1421
Erie Comm Fndn Grants, 1427
Essex County Comm Fndn Discretionary Fund Grant, 1428
Estee Lauder Grants, 1429
Eugene B. Casey Fndn Grants, 1433
Evjue Fndn Grants, 1439
Ewing Halsell Fndn Grants, 1440
ExxonMobil Grants, 1442
Fairfield County Comm Fndn Grants, 1446
FCNY Union Square Awards, 1461
Ferree Fndn Grants, 1486
FirstEnergy Fndn Comm Grants, 1505
Forrest C. Lattner Fndn Grants, 1523
Frances and John L. Loeb Family Fund Grants, 1546
Francis T. & Louise T. Nichols Fndn Grants, 1550
Frank Stanley Beveridge Fndn Grants, 1553
Franklin County Comm Fndn Grants, 1554
Fred Baldwin Memorial Fndn Grants, 1556
Frey Fndn Grants, 1562
Fulbright German Studies Seminar Grants, 1568
Fulton County Comm Fndn Grants, 1579
G.N. Wilcox Trust Grants, 1581
Gamble Fndn Grants, 1582
General Motors Fndn Grants Support Program, 1591
Genuardi Family Fndn Grants, 1594
George and Ruth Bradford Fndn Grants, 1595
George B. Storer Fndn Grants, 1596
George F. Baker Trust Grants, 1597
George Frederick Jewett Fndn Grants, 1599
George S. and Dolores Dore Eccles Fndn Grants, 1602
Georgia Power Fndn Grants, 1603
Gerber Fndn Grants, 1606
Giving Sum Annual Grant, 1619
Good Samaritan Inc Grants, 1637
Goodrich Corporation Fndn Grants, 1638
Grand Haven Area Comm Fndn Grants, 1644
Grand Rapids Area Comm Fndn Nashwauk Area Endowment Fund Grants, 1646
Grand Rapids Comm Fndn Grants, 1647
Greater Bridgeport Area Fndn Comm Impact Grants, 1650
Greater Cincinnati Fndn Priority and Small Projects/Capacity-Building Grants, 1651
Greater Green Bay Comm Fndn Grants, 1652
Greater Milwaukee Fndn Grants, 1653
Greater New Orleans Fndn Grants, 1654
Greater Saint Louis Comm Fndn Grants, 1655
Greater Tacoma Comm Fndn Grants, 1656
Greater Worcester Comm Fndn Discretionary Grants, 1658
H.A. and Mary K. Chapman Charitable Trust Grants, 1681
Hancock County Comm Fndn Grants, 1690
Hannaford Charitable Fndn Grants, 1692
Harrison County Comm Fndn Grants, 1700
Harry A. and Margaret D. Towsley Fndn Grants, 1701
Hawaii Comm Fndn West Hawaii Fund Grants, 1718
HEI Grants, 1734
Heineman Fndn for Research, Education, Charitable and Scientific Purposes, 1735
Henry J. Kaiser Family Fndn Grants, 1748
Hershey Company Grants, 1754
High Meadow Fndn Grants, 1768
Hillman Fndn Grants, 1775
Hillsdale County Comm General Adult Fndn Grants, 1777
Hilton Head Island Fndn Grants, 1779
Hoblitzelle Fndn Grants, 1783
Holland/Zeeland Comm Fndn Grants, 1786
Homer Fndn Grants, 1789
Honda of America Manufacturing Fndn Grants, 1790
Horace A. Kimball and S. Ella Kimball Fndn Grants, 1792
Houston Endowment Grants, 1797
Huntington County Comm Fndn Grants, 1823
Idaho Power Company Corp Contributions, 1838
Impact 100 Grants, 1843
Inasmuch Fndn Grants, 1845
J.C. Penney Company Grants, 1874
J.W. Kieckhefer Fndn Grants, 1878
Jackson County Comm Fndn Unrestricted Grants, 1879
James Ford Bell Fndn Grants, 1885
James M. Cox Fndn of Georgia Grants, 1892
James S. Copley Fndn Grants, 1895
Jane's Trust Grants, 1904
Janirve Fndn Grants, 1905
Jennings County Comm Fndn Grants, 1916
Jessie B. Cox Charitable Trust Grants, 1918
Jessie Smith Noyes Fndn Grants, 1920
John Deere Fndn Grants, 1929
John W. and Anna H. Hanes Fndn Grants, 1948
Joyce Fndn Grants, 1969
Kalamazoo Fndn Grants, 1979
Kavli Fndn Research Grants, 1985
Kelvin and Eleanor Smith Fndn Grants, 1986
Kettering Family Fndn Grants, 1991
Kettering Fund Grants, 1992
KeySpan Fndn Grants, 1995
Knox County Comm Fndn Grants, 2009
Kosciusko County Comm Fndn Grants, 2015
Kraft Cares US Grants, 2017
LaGrange County Comm Fndn Grants, 2020
Land O'Lakes Fndn Mid-Atlantic Grants, 2027
Lands' End Corp Giving Program, 2030
Lawrence S. Huntington Fund Grants, 2035
Legacy Fndn Grants, 2040
Lester E. Yeager Charitable Trust B Grants, 2047
Lewis Preston Fund for Girls Education Grants, 2052
Lincoln Financial Group Fndn Grants, 2058
Lindbergh Grants, 2059
Long Island Comm Fndn Grants, 2063
Louis Calder Fndn Grants, 2065
Lowell Area Comm Fund Grants, 2068
Lubrizol Fndn Grants, 2080
Lynde and Harry Bradley Fndn Grants, 2089
M.E. Raker Fndn Grants, 2094
Maine Comm Fndn Grants, 2099
Margaret L. Wendt Fndn Grants, 2104

Margaret T. Morris Fndn Grants, 2105
Marion Park Deaver and Harry Gilbert Deaver Fndn Grants, 2110
Mark and Catherine Winkler Fndn Grants, 2112
Mars Fndn Grants, 2114
Mary Owen Borden Fndn Grants, 2121
Maxon Charitable Fndn Grants, 2135
McInerny Fndn Grants, 2144
McKesson Fndn Grants, 2145
McKnight Fndn Grants, 2146
McLean Contributionship Grants, 2147
Mead Johnson Nutritionals Evansville-Area Organizations Grants, 2157
Mead Witter Fndn Grants, 2160
Meyer Memorial Trust Grassroots Grants, 2179
Meyer Memorial Trust Operating Funds Grants, 2180
Meyer Memorial Trust Responsive Grants, 2181
Miami County Comm Fndn Operation Round Up Grants, 2188
Miguel Aleman Fndn Grants, 2197
Miriam and Peter Haas Fund Grants, 2208
Montgomery County Comm Fndn Grants, 2214
Morris and Gwendolyn Cafritz Fndn Grants, 2217
Nelda C. and H.J. Lutcher Stark Fndn Grants, 2301
NIEHS Hazardous Materials Worker Health and Safety Training Grants, 2599
NIEHS Hazmat Training at Doe Nuclear Weapons Complex Grants, 2600
NIEHS SBIR E-Learning for HAZMAT and Emergency Response Grants, 2604
NIH National Occupational Research Agenda Grants, 2696
Nina Mason Pulliam Charitable Trust Grants, 2776
North Carolina Comm Fndn Grants, 2859
North Georgia Comm Fndn Grants, 2862
Northeast Utilities Fndn Grants, 2863
Northrop Grumman Corporation Grants, 2866
Norwin S. and Elizabeth N. Bean Fndn Grants, 2872
Ogden Codman Trust Grants, 2937
Ohio County Comm Fndn Grants, 2938
Ohio County Comm Fndn Mini-Grants, 2939
Olin Corporation Charitable Trust Grants, 2943
Oracle Corp Contributions Grants, 2951
Oscar Rennebohm Fndn Grants, 2963
OSI-Baltimore Special Opportunities Program Grants, 2972
Otto Bremer Fndn Grants, 2977
Owen County Comm Fndn Grants, 2979
PacifiCorp Fndn for Learning Grants, 2982
Palm Beach and Martin Counties Grants, 2986
Paul G. Allen Family Fndn Grants, 3000
Peacock Fndn Grants, 3011
Perkins Charitable Fndn Grants, 3014
Perry County Comm Fndn Grants, 3016
Piedmont Natural Gas Grants, 3048
Pike County Comm Fndn Grants, 3049
Pinellas County Grants, 3050
Pioneer Hi-Bred Comm Grants, 3051
Pittsburgh Fndn Comm Fund Grants, 3054
Plum Creek Fndn Grants, 3062
Portland General Electric Fndn Grants, 3067
Posey Comm Fndn Grants, 3068
Powell Fndn Grants, 3073
Prince Charitable Trusts Chicago Grants, 3079
Prince Charitable Trusts District of Columbia Grants, 3080
Princeton Area Comm Fndn Greater Mercer Grants, 3081
Principal Financial Group Fndn Grants, 3082
Procter and Gamble Fund Grants, 3083
Progress Energy Fndn Grants, 3084
Prudential Fndn Grants, 3087
Public Welfare Fndn Grants, 3089
Pulaski County Comm Fndn Grants, 3091
Pulte Homes Corp Contributions, 3092
Putnam County Comm Fndn Grants, 3093
Rajiv Gandhi Fndn Grants, 3104
Rathmann Family Fndn Grants, 3109
Rhode Island Fndn Grants, 3154
Rice Fndn Grants, 3155
Richard and Rhoda Goldman Fund Grants, 3158
Richard King Mellon Fndn Grants, 3161
Riley Fndn Grants, 3165
Ripley County Comm Fndn Grants, 3166
Rochester Area Comm Fndn Grants, 3176
Rohm and Haas Company Grants, 3185
Ruth Eleanor Bamberger and John Ernest Bamberger Memorial Fndn Grants, 3202
S. Livingston Mather Charitable Trust Grants, 3235
S. Mark Taper Fndn Grants, 3236
Salisbury Comm Fndn Grants, 3243
Samuel S. Johnson Fndn Grants, 3251
San Diego Fndn for Change Grants, 3255
Sasco Fndn Grants, 3265
Schering-Plough Fndn Comm Initiatives Grants, 3269
Scott County Comm Fndn Grants, 3273
Seabury Fndn Grants, 3274
Seattle Fndn Grants, 3276
Shaw's Supermarkets Donations, 3280
Shell Oil Company Fndn Grants, 3281
Simpson Fund Grants, 3290
Sir Dorabji Tata Trust Grants for NGOs or Voluntary Organizations, 3291
Snee Reinhardt Charitable Fndn Grants, 3300
Southbury Comm Trust Fund, 3350
Southwest Florida Comm Fndn Competitive Grants, 3351
Spencer County Comm Fndn Grants, 3358
Springs Close Fndn Grants, 3360
SSHRC Research/Creation Grants in Fine Arts, 3364
Steelcase Fndn Grants, 3379
Steuben County Comm Fndn Grants, 3383
Strowd Roses Grants, 3388
Sulzberger Fndn Grants, 3399
Sunderland Fndn Grants, 3400
Sunflower Fndn Walking Trails Grants, 3403
Susan Mott Webb Charitable Trust Grants, 3412
Susan Vaughan Fndn Grants, 3413
Taproot Fndn Capacity-Building Service Grants, 3417
Tellabs Fndn Grants, 3418
Texas Commission on the Arts Arts Respond Project Grants, 3420
Thompson Charitable Fndn Grants, 3425
Toro Fndn Grants, 3431
Triangle Comm Fndn Donor-Advised Grants, 3437
Trull Fndn Grants, 3441
U.S. Department of Education United States-Russia Program: Improving Research and Educational Activities in Higher Education, 3451
Union Benevolent Association Grants, 3460
United Technologies Corporation Grants, 3466
Unity Fndn Of LaPorte County Grants, 3467
Vancouver Fndn Grants and Comm Initiatives Program, 3477
Vanderburgh Comm Fndn Grants, 3480
Vermont Comm Fndn Grants, 3493
Virginia W. Kettering Fndn Grants, 3502
Vulcan Materials Company Fndn Grants, 3504
Wal-Mart Fndn Comm Grants, 3513
Wal-Mart State Giving Program Grants, 3514
Warrick County Comm Fndn Grants, 3519
Western Indiana Comm Fndn Grants, 3528
Westinghouse Charitable Giving Grants, 3530
Winifred & Harry B. Allen Fndn Grants, 3543
Winston-Salem Fndn Stokes County Grants, 3546
Women's Fndn of California Grants, 3550
YSA Get Ur Good On Grants, 3555
Z. Smith Reynolds Fndn Small Grants, 3557

Exhibitions, Collections, Performances, Video/ Film Production

3M Fndn Grants, 11
Aaron Fndn (Massachusetts) Grants, 174
Abell-Hanger Fndn Grants, 183
Adaptec Fndn Grants, 232
Agnes Gund Fndn Grants, 262
Alaska Airlines Fndn Grants, 324
Alcatel-Lucent Technologies Fndn Grants, 333
AMA-RFS and AMA Fndn Medical Student & Resident/Fellow Elective-Medicine & the Media, 406
Bacon Family Fndn Grants, 679
Ball Brothers Fndn General Grants, 683
Bank of America Client Fndn Grants, 690
Benton Comm Fndn Grants, 743
Blackford County Comm Fndn Grants, 763
Blanche and Julian Robertson Family Fndn Grants, 765
Blue Mountain Comm Fndn Grants, 769
Blue River Comm Fndn Grants, 770
Boeing Company Contributions Program Grants, 777
Bonfils-Stanton Fndn Grants, 779
Cable Positive's Tony Cox Comm Fund Grants, 827
Carl and Lily Pforzheimer Fndn Grants, 868
CFFVR Opportunity Grants, 952
Charles M. Bair Family Trust Grants, 972
Coca-Cola Fndn Grants, 1052
Collins Fndn Grants, 1058
Comm Fndn of Crawford County Grants and Scholarships, 1103
Comm Fndn of Southeastern Connecticut Grants, 1125
Comm Fndn of Western North Carolina Grants, 1132
Cowles Charitable Trust Grants, 1155
CSRA Comm Fndn Grants, 1168
D.F. Halton Fndn Grants, 1181
Donald and Sylvia Robinson Family Fndn Grants, 1310
Dorrance Family Fndn Grants, 1323
Dr. Leon Bromberg Charitable Trust Fund Grants, 1328
Drs. Bruce and Lee Fndn Grants, 1333
Eddie C. and Sylvia Brown Family Fndn Grants, 1367
Edyth Bush Charitable Fndn Grants, 1378
Elizabeth McGraw Fndn Grants, 1399
Elmer L. and Eleanor J. Andersen Fndn Grants, 1406
FCNY Union Square Awards, 1461
Fifth Third Fndn Grants, 1501
Flinn Fndn Grantss, 1511
Foster Fndn Grants, 1524
George B. Storer Fndn Grants, 1596
George S. and Dolores Dore Eccles Fndn Grants, 1602
Gilroy and Lillian P. Roberts Charitable Fndn Grants, 1614
Global Fund for Children Grants, 1629
Goodrich Corporation Fndn Grants, 1638
Grand Rapids Area Comm Fndn Grants, 1645
Greater Worcester Comm Fndn Jeppson Memorial Fund for Brookfield Grants, 1659
Green Fndn Grants, 1661
Health Fndn of Greater Indianapolis Grants, 1725
Honda of America Manufacturing Fndn Grants, 1790
Horizons Comm Issues Grants, 1794
Jewish Women's Fndn of New York Grants, 1924
Johnson and Johnson / SAH Arts and Healing Grants, 1953
Key Fndn Grants, 1994
Kraft Cares US Grants, 2017
Maine Comm Fndn Grants, 2099
Margaret L. Wendt Fndn Grants, 2104
Marion Park Deaver and Harry Gilbert Deaver Fndn Grants, 2110
Mary Baker Eddy Library Summer Research Fellowships, 2117
McCombs Fndn Grants, 2142
McMurry Fndn Grants, 2149
Meriden Fndn Grants, 2173
Newman's Own Inc Grants, 2306
Northeast Utilities Fndn Grants, 2863
Palm Beach and Martin Counties Grants, 2986

Paul G. Allen Family Fndn Grants, 3000
Piedmont Natural Gas Grants, 3048
Rasmuson Fndn Grants, 3108
Richard and Rhoda Goldman Fund Grants, 3158
Robert F. Stoico / FIRSTFED Charitable Fndn Grants, 3171
Rockwell Collins Charitable Contributions, 3182
Rohm and Haas Company Grants, 3185
Ruth Mott Fndn Grants, 3204
Samuel Freeman Charitable Trust Grants, 3249
San Diego Fndn for Change Grants, 3255
Schurz Communications Fndn Grants, 3271
Snee Reinhardt Charitable Fndn Grants, 3300
Southbury Comm Trust Fund, 3350
Stewart Huston Charitable Trust Grants, 3384
Toro Fndn Grants, 3431
United Technologies Corporation Grants, 3466
Winston-Salem Fndn Competitive Grants, 3544

Faculty/Professional Development
AAAAI Research Award Grants, 25
AACN Physio-Control Small Projects Grants, 62
AACR Career Development Awards for Pediatric Cancer Research, 70
AACR Gertrude Elion Cancer Research Award, 76
AACR Judah Folkman Career Development Award for Anti-Angiogenesis Research, 79
AAFP Fndn Pfizer Teacher Development Awards, 114
AANS Neurosurgery Research and Education Fndn Young Clinician Investigator Award, 142
Able Trust Vocational Rehabilitation Grants for Individuals, 186
ACS Cancer Control Career Development Awards for Primary Care Physicians, 209
ACS MEN2 Thyroid Cancer Professorship Grants, 216
AFAR Paul Beeson Career Development Awards in Aging Research for the Island of Ireland, 256
AGS Dennis W. Jahnigen Career Development Scholars Awards, 264
AHFMR Clinical Investigator Awards, 270
AHFMR Interdisciplinary Team Grants, 284
AHFMR Medical or Health Scholars Investigator Grants, 286
AHFMR Medical or Health Scientist Awards, 287
AHFMR Research Prize, 294
AHFMR Senior Medical or Health Scholars Investigator Grants, 298
AHIMA Faculty Development Stipends, 301
AIHP Sonnedecker Visiting Scholar Grants, 317
Alexander von Humboldt Fndn Research Fellowships for Experienced Researchers, 347
Alexander von Humboldt Fndn Research Fellowships for Postdoctoral Researchers, 348
Alfred P. Sloan Fndn Research Fellowships, 353
AMA Fndn Leadership Awards, 394
American College of Surgeons Faculty Career Development Award for Neurological Surgeons, 425
American Psychiatric Association/AstraZeneca Young Minds in Psychiatry International Awards, 450
AMI Semiconductors Corp Grants, 468
Anheuser-Busch Fndn Grants, 474
Annenberg Fndn Grants, 479
ASCO Career Development Award, 551
ASCO Comparative Effectiveness Research Professorship (CERP) in Breast Cancer, 553
ASCO International Development and Education Awards (IDEA), 554
ASCO Translational Research Professorships, 561
ASHA Research Mentoring-Pair Travel Award, 572
ASHA Students Preparing for Academic & Research Careers (SPARC) Award, 574
Assisi Fndn Grants, 653
Ball Brothers Fndn General Grants, 683
Ball Brothers Fndn Grants, 684
Baxter International Fndn Grants, 705
Beckman Young Investigators Program Grants, 735
Boeing Company Contributions Program Grants, 777
Boyd Gaming Corporation Contributions Program, 788
Brookdale Fndn Leadership in Aging Fellowships, 805
Bush Fndn Medical Fellowships, 815
BWF Career Awards at the Scientific Interface, 819
BWF Clinical Scientist Awards in Translational Research, 821
BWF Institutional Program Unifying Population and Laboratory Based Sciences, 822
Byron W. and Alice L. Lockwood Fndn Grants, 824
Canada-U.S. Fulbright New Century Scholars Program Grants, 846
Canada-U.S. Fulbright Senior Specialists Program Grants, 847
Canadian Optometric Education Trust Fund Grants, 853
Cardiac Arrhythmias Research and Education Fndn Research Grants, 863
Carl and Lily Pforzheimer Fndn Grants, 868
Carl B. and Florence E. King Fndn Grants, 869
Carpenter Fndn Grants, 881
Carrie Estelle Doheny Fndn Grants, 883
Carrier Corporation Contributions Grants, 884
CDC Technology Translation and Transfer of Effective HIV Behavioral Interventions, 931
CFF Leroy Matthews Physician-Scientist Awards, 944
CFF Research Grants, 947
Charlotte County (FL) Comm Fndn Grants, 973
Chazen Fndn Grants, 978
Chicago Comm Trust Grants, 989
Chiron Fndn Comm Grants, 1004
Clarence E. Heller Charitable Fndn Grants, 1022
Claude Worthington Benedum Fndn Grants, 1033
Clowes ACS/AAST/NIGMS Jointly Sponsored Mentored Clinical Scientist Development Award, 1041
Cockrell Fndn Grants, 1053
Columbus Fndn Competitive Grants, 1066
Comm Fndn for Muskegon County Grants, 1093
Comm Fndn of Greater Birmingham Grants, 1106
Comm Fndn of Greater New Britain Grants, 1111
Cowles Charitable Trust Grants, 1155
Della Martin Fndn Grants, 1219
Denton A. Cooley Fndn Grants, 1225
Dept of Ed Special Education--Personnel Development to Improve Services and Results for Children with Disabilities, 1231
Dept of Ed Special Education--Technical Assistance and Dissemination to Improve Services and Results for Children with Disabilities, 1233
Dermatology Clinical Career Development Awards, 1235
Dermatology Research Career Development Awards, 1238
Dr. Leon Bromberg Charitable Trust Fund Grants, 1328
Drs. Bruce and Lee Fndn Grants, 1333
Dubois County Comm Fndn Grants, 1336
Dunspaugh-Dalton Fndn Grants, 1351
Eberly Fndn Grants, 1364
Edwin S. Webster Fndn Grants, 1376
Effie and Wofford Cain Fndn Grants, 1385
Elizabeth Glaser Pediatric AIDS Fndn Two-Year International Scholar Award, 1396
Emily Davie and Joseph S. Kornfeld Fndn Grants, 1414
Eugene M. Lang Fndn Grants, 1434
Eugene McDermott Fndn Grants, 1435
Evjue Fndn Grants, 1439
FDHN Fellowship to Faculty Transition Awards, 1470
FDHN Research Scholar Awards, 1478
Fndn for the Mid-South Grants, 1536
Frances L. and Edwin L. Cummings Memorial Fund Grants, 1547
Fritz B. Burns Fndn Grants, 1564
Fulbright Distinguished Chairs Program Grants, 1567
Fulbright International Education Administrators (IEA) Seminar Program Grants, 1569
Fulbright New Century Scholars (NCS) Program Grants, 1570
Fulbright Specialists Program Grants, 1571
Fulbright Traditional Scholar Program in Europe and Eurasia, 1572
Fulbright Traditional Scholar Program in Sub-Saharan Africa, 1573
Fulbright Traditional Scholar Program in the East Asia/Pacific Region, 1574
Fulbright Traditional Scholar Program in the Near East and North Africa Region, 1575
Fulbright Traditional Scholar Program in the South and Central Asia Region, 1576
Fulbright Traditional Scholar Program in the Western Hemisphere, 1577
George Kress Fndn Grants, 1601
George S. and Dolores Dore Eccles Fndn Grants, 1602
Gilroy and Lillian P. Roberts Charitable Fndn Grants, 1614
Good Samaritan Inc Grants, 1637
Harry A. and Margaret D. Towsley Fndn Grants, 1701
Harry Shwachman Clinical Investigator Award, 1707
Hartford Aging and Health Program Awards, 1709
Health Fndn of Greater Indianapolis Grants, 1725
HHMI/EMBO Start-up Grants for Central Europe, 1766
Hill Crest Fndn Grants, 1773
Hillman Fndn Grants, 1775
Humboldt Area Fndn Technical Assistance Program (TAP) Grants, 1819
Independence Blue Cross Charitable Medical Care Grants, 1846
J.M. Long Fndn Grants, 1877
Jacob and Hilda Blaustein Fndn Grants, 1881
James McKeen Cattell Fund Fellowships, 1893
James R. Dougherty Jr. Fndn Grants, 1894
JDF Career Development Awards, 1910
Jessie Ball Dupont Fund Grants, 1919
John P. McGovern Fndn Grants, 1942
John S. Dunn Research Fndn Grants and Chairs, 1945
Johnson & Johnson Corp Contributions Grants, 1952
Joseph Alexander Fndn Grants, 1957
Josiah Macy Jr. Fndn Grants, 1966
Kenneth T. and Eileen L. Norris Fndn Grants, 1989
Kosciusko County Comm Fndn Grants, 2015
Landon Fndn-AACR Innovator Award for International Collaboration, 2028
Lowe Fndn Grants, 2067
LSA Scholar Award for Clinical Research, 2074
Lynde and Harry Bradley Fndn Grants, 2089
M.B. and Edna Zale Fndn Grants, 2093
Maine Comm Fndn Grants, 2099
Mark and Catherine Winkler Fndn Grants, 2112
Mary Kay Ash Charitable Fndn Grants, 2120
Mead Johnson Nutritionals Medical Education Grants, 2158
Mead Witter Fndn Grants, 2160
Meadows Fndn Grants, 2161
Measey Fndn Medical Education Grants, 2162
MfA Newton Fellowships, 2182
MRC Career Establishment Grants, 2221
MSSC Career Development Awards, 2224
NCI Mentored Career Development Award to Promote Diversity, 2276
NCIC Canadian Breast Cancer Research Initiative Grants, 2281
NFID New Investigator Matching Grants, 2310
NHGRI Mentored Research Scientist Development Award, 2315
NHLBI Mentored Career Award For Faculty At Minority Institutions, 2346
NHLBI Minority Institution Research Scientist Development Award, 2354

NHLBI Minority Institutional Research Training Program Grants, 2355
NIA Independent Scientist Award, 2412
NIA Mentored Research Scientist Development Award, 2418
NIA Paul Beeson Career Development Awards in Aging, 2424
NIA Pilot Research Grants, 2425
NIAAA Independent Scientist Award, 2443
NIAID Research Scholar Development Award, 2462
NIDA Mentored Clinical Scientist Research Career Development Awards, 2507
NIDA Minority Institutions Drug Abuse Research Development Program (MIDARP) Grants, 2509
NIDA Senior Scientist Award, 2515
NIDCD Mentored Clinical Scientist Research Career Development Award, 2522
NIEHS Independent Scientist Award, 2601
NIEHS Mentored Clinical Scientist Research Career Development Awards, 2602
NIEHS Mentored Research Scientist Development Award, 2603
NIGMS Initiative for Minority Students: Bridges to the Baccalaureate Degree, 2612
NIGMS Initiative for Minority Students: Bridges to the Doctoral Degree, 2613
NIGMS Mentored Clinical Scientist Research Career Development Awards, 2618
NIGMS Minority Access to Research Careers (MARC) Ancillary Training Activities Grants, 2619
NIGMS Minority Access to Research Careers (MARC) Program, 2620
NIGMS MORE Faculty Development Awards, 2622
NIGMS Short Courses on Mathematical and Statistical Tools for the Study of Complex Phenotypes and Complex Systems, 2628
NIH Academic Career Awards, 2634
NIH Mentored Clinical Scientist Development Award, 2687
NIMH Minority Research Infrastructure Support Program Grants, 2763
NIMH Short Courses on Mathematical and Statistical Tools for the Study of Complex Phenotypes and Complex Systems, 2770
NINR Mentored Research Scientist Development Award, 2798
NINR Opportunities in Genetics and Nursing Research Grants, 2801
NKF Research Fellowships, 2812
NKF Young Investigator Grants, 2813
Noble County Comm Fndn Grants, 2848
North Carolina Biotechnology Center Grantsmanship Training Grants, 2853
North Carolina Biotechnology Center Regional Development Grants, 2855
North Carolina GlaxoSmithKline Fndn Grants, 2860
NSF Postdoctoral Research Fellowships in Biology (PRFB), 2891
NSF Presidential Early Career Awards for Scientists and Engineers (PECASE) Grants, 2892
NSF Undergraduate Research and Mentoring in the Biological Sciences (URM), 2896
ONF Career Development Awards, 2946
OREF Orthopedic Career Development Awards, 2954
Pancreatic Cancer Action Network-AACR Pathway to Leadership Grants, 2988
PDF-AANF Clinician-Scientist Development Awards, 3009
Philadelphia Fndn Organizational Effectiveness Grants, 3029
PhRMA Fndn Health Outcomes Post Doctoral Fellowships, 3031
PhRMA Fndn Informatics Sabbatical Fellowships, 3035
PhRMA Fndn Informatics Post Doctoral Fellowships, 3036
PhRMA Fndn Informatics Research Starter Grants, 3038
PhRMA Fndn Pharmaceutics Postdoctoral Fellowships, 3040
PhRMA Fndn Pharmaceutics Research Starter Grants, 3042
PhRMA Fndn Pharmaceutics Sabbatical Fellowships, 3043
PhRMA Fndn Pharmacology/Toxicology Post Doctoral Fellowships, 3044
PhRMA Fndn Pharmacology/Toxicology Pre Doctoral Fellowships, 3045
PhRMA Fndn Pharmacology/Toxicology Research Starter Grants, 3046
PhRMA Fndn Pharmacology/Toxicology Sabbatical Fellowships, 3047
Presbyterian Health Fndn Bridge, Seed and Equipment Grants, 3075
Prince Charitable Trusts District of Columbia Grants, 3080
PSG Mentored Clinical Research Awards, 3088
Puerto Rico Comm Fndn Grants, 3090
Pulaski County Comm Fndn Grants, 3091
Pulte Homes Corp Contributions, 3092
RCPSC Faculty Development Grants, 3117
Rhode Island Fndn Grants, 3154
Robert P. & Clara I. Milton Fund for Senior Housing, 3172
Rohm and Haas Company Grants, 3185
Roy J. Carver Charitable Trust Medical and Science Research Grants, 3192
RRF General Program Grants, 3193
RRF Organizational Capacity Building Grants, 3194
RWJF Clinical Scholars Program Grants, 3207
RWJF Executive Nurse Fellowships, 3210
RWJF Generalist Physician Faculty Scholars, 3212
RWJF Harold Amos Medical Faculty Development Scholars, 3213
San Antonio Area Fndn Grants, 3254
Schering-Plough Fndn Health Grants, 3270
Searle Scholars Program Grants, 3275
SNM Molecular Imaging Research Grant For Junior Medical Faculty, 3301
SNM Postdoctoral Molecular Imaging Scholar Grants, 3305
Society for Investigative Dermatology Career Development Award, 3325
Square D Fndn Grants, 3361
SSHRC Research/Creation Grants in Fine Arts, 3364
St. Joseph Comm Health Fndn Burn Care and Prevention Grants, 3367
St. Joseph Comm Health Fndn Improving Healthcare Access Grants, 3368
Steele-Reese Fndn Grants, 3380
Susan G. Komen Breast Cancer Fndn Interdisciplinary Fellowships, 3410
Topeka Comm Fndn Kansas Blood Services Scholarships, 3429
UICC Yamagiwa-Yoshida Memorial International Cancer Study Grants, 3458
Union County Comm Fndn Grants, 3461
Vancouver Fndn Grants and Comm Initiatives Program, 3477
VDH Rescue Squad Assistance Fund Grants, 3484
Wayne and Gladys Valley Fndn Grants, 3522
Weingart Fndn Grants, 3524

Fellowships

3M Fndn Grants, 11
AAAAI Summer Clinical Research Fellowship Medical Student Grants, 27
AAAAI Summer Research Fellowship Medical Student Grants, 28
AAAS Science & Technology Policy Fellowships - National Defense & Global Security, 29
AACAP Congressional Fellowships, 32
AACAP Jeanne Spurlock Minority Medical Student Clinical Fellowship in Child and Adolescent Psychiatry, 39
AACAP Jeanne Spurlock Research Fellowship in Substance Abuse and Addiction for Minority Medical Students, 40
AACAP Pilot Research Awards, Supported by Eli Lilly and Company, 47
AACAP Summer Medical Student Fellowships, 53
AACAP-NIDA K12 Career Development Awards, 55
AACR Centennial Postdoctoral Fellowships in Cancer Research, 71
AACR Centennial Pre-doctoral Fellowships in Cancer Research, 72
AACR Clinical and Translational Research Fellowships, 73
AACR Fellows Grants, 74
AACR-Colorectal Cancer Coalition Fellows Grant, 92
AACR-FNAB Fellows Grant for Translational Pancreatic Cancer Research, 94
AACR-Genentech BioOncology Fellowship for Cancer Research in Angiogenesis, 97
AACR-National Brain Tumor Fndn Fellows Grant, 100
AACR Basic Cancer Research Fellowships , 107
AAFA Investigator Research Grants, 108
AAFCS International Graduate Fellowships, 109
AAFCS National Graduate Fellowships, 110
AAFPRS Fellowships, 119
AAHPM Hospice and Palliative Medicine Fellowships, 132
AAMC Herbert W. Nickens Faculty Fellowship, 139
AARP Fndn Gerontology Graduate Scholarships and Fellowships, 175
Abbott Fund Science and Medical Innovation Grants, 179
Abell-Hanger Fndn Grants, 183
Abney Fndn Grants, 187
ACAAI Fndn Research Grants, 189
ACOG History of American Obstetrics and Gynecology Fellowship, 207
ACS Postdoctoral Fellowships, 220
Advocate HealthCare Post Graduate Administrative Fellowship, 241
AFAR Medical Student Training in Aging Research Program, 255
AHFMR Clinical Fellowships, 269
AHFMR Fast-Track Studentships and Fellowships, 274
AHFMR Full-Time Fellowships, 276
AHFMR Health Research Career Renewal Awards, 279
AHFMR Part-Time Fellowships, 288
AHRQ Individual Awards for Postdoctoral Fellows Ruth L. Kirschstein National Research Service Awards (NRSA), 314
Alexander von Humboldt Fndn Georg Forster Fellowships for Experienced Researchers, 344
Alexander von Humboldt Fndn Georg Forster Fellowships for Postdoctoral Researchers, 345
Alexander von Humboldt Fndn Research Fellowships for Postdoctoral Researchers, 348
Alfred P. Sloan Fndn History of Science and Technology Grants, 352
Alfred P. Sloan Fndn Research Fellowships, 353
Alzheimer's Association Zenith Fellows Awards, 384
AMA Fndn Joan F. Giambalvo Memorial Scholarships, 392
AMA-MSS Government Relations Advocacy Fellowship, 403
American Academy of Nursing Claire M. Fagin Fellowships, 415
American College of Surgeons Faculty Research Fellowships, 426
American College of Surgeons Nizar N. Oweida, MD, FACS, Scholarships, 430
American College of Surgeons Wound Care Management Award, 433
American Fndn for Suicide Prevention Grants, 436
American Philosophical Society Daland Fellowships in Clinical Investigation, 441

American Psychiatric Association Minority Fellowships Program, 443
American Psychiatric Association Minority Medical Student Fellowship in HIV Psychiatry, 444
American Psychiatric Association/Bristol-Myers Squibb Fellowships in Public Psychiatry, 451
American Sociological Association Minority Fellowships, 458
American-Italian Cancer Fndn Fellowships, 459
amfAR Fellowships, 462
amfAR Mathilde Krim Fellowships in Basic Biomedical Research, 464
amfAR Research Grants, 466
APA Congressional Fellowships, 492
APF Jeanne Spurlock Congressional Fellowships, 509
APSA Congressional Fellowships Health and Aging Policy Fellows Program, 514
APSA Robert Wood Johnson Fndn Health Policy Fellowships, 515
APSAA Fellowships, 516
Aratani Fndn Grants, 523
Arie and Ida Crown Memorial Grants, 528
Arthur and Rochelle Belfer Fndn Grants, 542
ArvinMeritor Fndn Health Grants, 543
ASCO Long-Term International Fellowships, 556
ASCO/UICC International Cancer Technology Transfer (ICRETT) Fellowships, 563
ASM Congressional Science Fellowships, 590
ASM International Fellowship for Latin America and the Caribbean, 601
ASM International Fellowships for Asia and Africa, 602
ASM Microbiology Undergraduate Research Fellowship, 607
ASM Robert D. Watkins Graduate Research Fellowship, 614
ASM Undergraduate Research Fellowship, 622
ASM-PAHO Infectious Diseases Epidemiology and Surveillance Fellowships, 625
ASM/CCID Fellowships, 627
ASPO Fellowships, 651
Australian Academy of Science Grants, 670
Ball Brothers Fndn Grants, 684
Baltimore Washington Center Adult Psychoanalysis Fellowships, 685
Baltimore Washington Center Child Psychotherapy Fellowships, 686
BCBS of Massachusetts Health Coverage Fellowships, 710
Blumenthal Fndn Grants, 773
Bodman Fndn Grants, 776
Boeing Company Contributions Program Grants, 777
Boston Psychoanalytic Society and Institute Fellowship in Child Psychoanalytic Psychotherapy, 786
Boston Psychoanalytic Society and Institute Fellowship in Psychoanalytic Psychotherapy, 787
Bristol-Myers Squibb Virology and Oncology M.D. Research Fellowships, 802
Brookdale Fndn Leadership in Aging Fellowships, 805
BWF Institutional Program Unifying Population and Laboratory Based Sciences, 822
Caddock Fndn Grants, 828
Canadian Liver Fndn Grants, 851
Cancer Research Postdoctoral Fellowships for Basic and Physician Scientists, 856
Cancer Research Society Fellowships and Grants, 857
Cancer Research UK Fellowships, 858
Cancer Research UK Grants, 859
Cancer Society of New Zealand Grants, 860
Carl and Lily Pforzheimer Fndn Grants, 868
Carrier Corporation Contributions Grants, 884
Carroll County Comm Fndn Grants, 885
CCFF Fellowships, 893
Cemala Fndn Grants, 933
CFF First- and Second-Year Clinical Fellowships, 943
CFF Postdoctoral Research Fellowships, 946
CFF Third-Year Clinical Fellowships, 950
CFPC Fellowships, 955
Charles H. Revson Fndn Grants, 969
Chicago Institute for Psychoanalysis Fellowships, 990
Christopher Reeve Paralysis Fndn Individual Research Grants, 1006
CIGNA Fndn Grants, 1011
CIIT Postdoctoral Fellowships, 1012
CLA Nurses Respiratory Society Fellowships, 1018
CLA Physiotherapy Cardio-Respiratory Society Fellowships, 1020
CMAP Physician Advocacy Fellowship, 1043
Coastal Bend Comm Fndn Grants, 1050
Coca-Cola Fndn Grants, 1052
Commonwealth Fund Australian-American Health Policy Fellowships, 1078
Commonwealth Fund Harkness Fellowships in Health Care Policy and Practice, 1079
Commonwealth Fund/Harvard University Fellowship in Minority Health Policy, 1086
Comm Fndn for Southern Arizona Grants, 1095
Comm Health Scholars Program Fellowships, 1134
Comm Technology Fndn of California Building Communities Through Technology Grants, 1136
Cooley's Anemia Research Fellowships, 1149
CRI Postdoctoral Fellowships, 1162
Crohn's Disease and Colitis Research Fellowships, 1164
Damon Runyon Cancer Fndn Fellowships, 1193
DeBakey Medical Fndn Fellowships and Scholarships, 1212
Deland Fellowships in Health Care and Society, 1214
Della Martin Fndn Grants, 1219
Dental Teaching and Research Fellowships, 1224
Dermatology Postdoctoral Research Fellowships, 1237
Doris Duke Charitable Fndn Clinical Research Fellowships for Medical Students, 1315
Dr. Sydney Segal Research Grants, 1331
Duke University Adult Cardiothoracic Anesthesia and Critical Care Medicine Fellowships, 1340
Duke University Ambulatory and Regional Anesthesia Fellowships, 1341
Duke University Clinical Cardiac Electrophysiology Fellowships, 1342
Duke University Hyperbaric Center Fellowships, 1343
Duke University Interventional Cardiology Fellowships, 1344
Duke University Obstetric Anesthesia Fellowships, 1345
Duke University Pain Management Fellowships, 1346
Duke University Pediatric Anesthesiology Fellowship, 1347
Duke University Postdoctoral Research Fellowships in Aging, 1348
Duncan L. Gordon Fellowships, 1349
E.A. Baker Fndn for the Prevention of Blindness Grants, 1357
Echoing Green Fellowships, 1365
Edwin S. Webster Fndn Grants, 1376
Edwin W. and Catherine M. Davis Fndn Grants, 1377
EF Behavioral Sciences Student Fellowships, 1379
EF Health Sciences Student Fellowships, 1380
EF Postdoctoral Research Training Fellowships, 1382
EF Research and Training Fellowships for Clinicians, 1384
Effie and Wofford Cain Fndn Grants, 1385
Epilepsy Postdoctoral and Clinical Research Fellowships, 1422
Ethical Research Grants and Fellowships, 1431
Eugene M. Lang Fndn Grants, 1434
Families USA Wellstone Fellowship for Social Justice, 1450
FCER Chiropractic Research Grants, 1459
FCER Research Grants and Fellowships, 1460
FDHN Centocor International Research Fellowship in Gastrointestinal Inflammation & Immunology, 1465
FDHN Student Research Fellowships, 1480
Fellowships in Infectious Diseases, 1485
Fight for Sight Research Grants and Fellowships, 1503
Fragile X Syndrome Postdoctoral Research Fellowships Program, 1545
Fritz B. Burns Fndn Grants, 1564
Fulbright Traditional Scholar Program in the East Asia/Pacific Region, 1574
Fulbright Traditional Scholar Program in the Near East and North Africa Region, 1575
Fulbright Traditional Scholar Program in the Western Hemisphere, 1577
Gertrude E. Skelly Charitable Fndn Grants, 1609
Gilroy and Lillian P. Roberts Charitable Fndn Grants, 1614
Gina Finzi Memorial Student Summer Fellowship, 1615
Grass Fndn Marine Biological Laboratory Fellowships, 1648
H. Schaffer Fndn Grants, 1680
H.A. and Mary K. Chapman Charitable Trust Grants, 1681
Harold Amos Medical Faculty Development Program, 1696
Heart Rhythm Society Fellowships, 1731
Heiser Leprosy and Tuberculosis Research Postdoctoral Fellowships, 1736
Heiser Leprosy Research Grants, 1737
Helen Hay Whitney Fndn Postdoctoral Research Fellowships, 1739
Henry J. Kaiser Family Fndn Media Fellowships, 1749
Hereditary Disease Fndn John J. Wasmuth Postdoctoral Fellowships, 1750
Hereditary Disease Fndn Research Grants, 1752
Herman Goldman Fndn Grants, 1753
HHMI Grants and Fellowships Programs, 1759
HHMI Research Training Fellowships, 1763
Hirtzel Memorial Fndn Grants, 1781
HIV/AIDS Research Training Fellowship, 1782
Honeywell Fndn Grants, 1791
HRB Clinical Research Training Fellowships, 1800
HRB Health Services Research Fellowships, 1801
HRB Postdoctoral Research Fellowships, 1802
Hunter's Hope Fndn Grants, 1820
Huntington's Disease Society of America Research Fellowships, 1825
IARC Expertise Transfer Fellowship, 1831
IARC Postdoctoral Fellowships for Training in Cancer Research, 1832
Institute for Agriculture and Trade Policy Food and Society Fellowships, 1856
Institute of Human Values in Health Care Interdisciplinary Fellowships, 1857
International Cancer Technology Transfer Fellowships, 1858
International Fellowships in Medical Education, 1861
International Oncology Nursing Fellowships, 1862
IWMF Public Health Fellowship, 1871
Jackson Laboratory Postdoctoral Research Training Program, 1880
James McKeen Cattell Fund Fellowships, 1893
Jane Coffin Childs Memorial Fund for Medical Research Fellowships, 1903
Jeffress Research Grants, 1913
John Deere Fndn Grants, 1929
John Merck Scholars Awards, 1941
John Stauffer Charitable Trust Grants, 1946
Johnson & Johnson Corp Contributions Grants, 1952
K and F Baxter Family Fndn Grants, 1973
Kansas Health Fndn Grants, 1980
KFC Allied Health Research Grants, 1996
KFC Biomedical Fellowships, 1997
Klingenstein Neuroscience Fellowships, 2005
Kluge Center David B. Larson Fellowship in Health and Spirituality, 2006

Knight Public Health Journalism Fellowships at CDC, 2008
Lalor Fndn Postdoctoral Research Grants, 2021
Larry L. Hillblom Fndn Grants, 2031
Leadership in Education in Neurodevelopmental Disabilities Postdoctoral Fellowships, 2037
Learning and Behavioral Disorders Research Grants, 2039
Leukaemia Research Fund Grants, 2050
Life Sciences Research Fndn Postdoctoral Fellowships, 2054
Lillian Sholtis Brunner Summer Fellowships for Historical Research in Nursing, 2057
LRF New Investigator Leukemia Research Grants, 2070
LRF Physician-Scientist Postdoctoral Fellowships, 2071
LRF Postdoctoral Fellowships, 2072
LSA Fellowships, 2073
LSA Special Fellowships, 2076
Lubrizol Fndn Grants, 2080
Lymphoma Research Fndn Grants, 2088
Lynde and Harry Bradley Fndn Grants, 2089
MAP International Medical Fellowships, 2101
MAPFRE Fndn for Medicine Grants, 2102
Marine Biological Laboratory Summer Research Fellowships, 2108
Mark and Catherine Winkler Fndn Grants, 2112
Mary Baker Eddy Library Summer Research Fellowships, 2117
Mary Ingraham Bunting Institute Biomedical Research Fellowships, 2119
Matsumae International Fndn Grants, 2129
Mayo Fndn Multidisciplinary Training in Digestive Diseases Research Grants, 2140
Mead Johnson Nutritionals Scholarships, 2159
Meadows Fndn Grants, 2161
Measey Fndn Medical Education Grants, 2162
MedImmune Charitable Grants, 2166
Medtronic Fndn Health Care Grants, 2169
Mericos Fndn Grants, 2172
MfA Newton Fellowships, 2182
MGFA Post-Doctoral Research Fellowships, 2183
MGFA Student Fellowships, 2184
MHRC Postdoctoral Research Fellowships, 2187
Michigan Psychoanalytic Institute and Society Scholarships, 2194
Milton Wexler Postdoctoral Fellowships, 2205
Minority Doctoral Fellowships in Science and Engineering, 2207
MNI Jeanne Timmins Fellowships, 2212
Morris and Gwendolyn Cafritz Fndn Grants, 2217
MSSC Postdoctoral Fellowships, 2225
Musculoskeletal Rehabilitation Fellowships, 2229
NAF Fellowships, 2230
National Headache Fndn Seymour Diamond Clinical Fellowship in Headache Education, 2254
National Heart Fndn of New Zealand Grants, 2255
National MPS Society Grants, 2257
National Sleep Fndn Pickwick Postdoctoral Fellowship, 2260
NCCAM Ruth L. Kirschstein National Research Service Awards for Postdoctoral Training in Complementary and Alternative Medicine, 2266
NCIC Terry Fox Postdoctoral Research Fellowships, 2285
New York University Steinhardt School of Education Fellowships, 2305
NFID Colin L. Powell Minority Postdoctoral Fellowship in Tropical Disease Research, 2308
NFID John P. Utz Medical Mycology Postdoctoral Fellowship, 2309
NFID Nosocomial Infection Research and Training Postdoctoral Fellowship, 2311
NFID Postdoctoral Fellowships in Emerging Infectious Diseases, 2312
NFX Summer Research Fellowships, 2314
NHLBI Individual Predoctoral Fellowships to Promote Diversity in Health-Related Research, 2341
NHLBI Ruth L. Kirschstein National Research Service Awards for Individual Predoctoral MD/PhD Fellows, 2381
NIA NRSAs--Individual Postdoctoral Fellowships, 2422
NIGMS Fellowships in Quantitative Biology, 2610
NIGMS Individual Postdoctoral NRSA Fellowships in Clinical Pharmacology, 2611
NIGMS Minority Access to Research Careers (MARC) Program, 2620
NIGMS Ruth L. Kirschstein National Research Service Awards for Individual Predoctoral Fellows in PharmD/PhD Grants, 2627
NIH Clinical Bioethics Postdoctoral Fellowships, 2649
NIH Clinical Bioethics Predoctoral Fellowships, 2650
NIH Individual Postdoctoral Fellowships in Genomics and Related ELSI Topics, 2678
NIH National Research Service Awards--Senior Fellows, 2697
NIH Ruth L. Kirschstein National Research Service Awards (NRSA) for Individual Senior Fellows, 2718
NIH Ruth L. Kirschstein National Research Service Awards for Individual Postdoctoral Fellows, 2719
NIH Ruth L. Kirschstein National Research Service Awards for Individual Predoctoral Fellows, 2720
NIH Ruth L. Kirschstein National Research Service Awards for Individual Predoctoral Fellowships to Promote Diversity in Health-Related Research, 2721
NIH Ruth L. Kirschstein National Research Service Awards for Individual Predoctoral MD/PhD and Other Dual Doctoral Degree Fellows, 2722
NINR Ruth L. Kirschstein National Research Service Award (NRSA) for Individual Predoctoral Fellows in Nursing Research, 2804
NINR/NHGRI Nursing and Genetics Research Individual Postdoctoral and Senior Fellowships, 2806
NKF Research Fellowships, 2812
NMF General Electric Medical Scholars Fellowships, 2830
NMSS Sylvia Lawry Physician Fellowships, 2846
NORD Roscoe Brady Lysosomal Storage Disease Fellowships, 2850
Northwood University/Alden B. Dow Creativity Center Summer Residency Program, 2871
NSF BIO Minority Postdoctoral Research Fellowships, 2877
NSF Grant Opportunities for Academic Liaison with Industry (GOALI), 2887
NSF Postdoctoral Research Fellowships in Biology (PRFB), 2891
Nuffield Fndn Law and Society Grants, 2900
NWHF Mark O. Hatfield Research Fellowship, 2907
NYAM Charles A. Elsberg Fellowship, 2910
NYAM David E. Rogers Fellowships, 2911
NYAM Edwin Beer Research Fellowship, 2913
NYAM Ferdinand C. Valentine Fellowship, 2914
NYAM Mary and David Hoar Fellowship, 2916
Olin Corporation Charitable Trust Grants, 2943
OREF/AAOS Clinical Research Training Fellowship, 2958
ORISE Postgraduate Research Participation at the Agency for Toxic Substances and Disease Registry, 2960
ORISE Postgraduate Research Participation at the National Center for Toxicological Research, 2961
ORISE Postgraduate Research Program at the Center for Devices and Radiological Health, 2962
Osserman-Sosin Postdoctoral Myasthenia Gravis Research Fellowships, 2974
Osteogenesis Imperfecta Fndn Research Grants, 2975
PAHO/WHO Fellowships, 2984
Pancreatic Cancer Action Network-AACR Fellowship , 2987
Pancreatic Cancer Action Network-AACR Pathway to Leadership Grants, 2988
Parker B. Francis Fellowships in Pulmonary Research, 2989
PDF Postdoctoral Fellowships for Basic Scientists, 3006
PDF Postdoctoral Fellowships for Neurologists, 3007
PDF Summer Fellowships, 3008
PDF-AANF Clinician-Scientist Development Awards, 3009
Pew Charitable Trusts Biomedical Research Grants, 3019
Pew Scholars in the Biomedical Sciences, 3021
PhRMA Fndn Health Outcomes Post Doctoral Fellowships, 3031
PhRMA Fndn Health Outcomes Pre-Doctoral Fellowships, 3032
PhRMA Fndn Health Outcomes Sabbatical Fellowships, 3034
PhRMA Fndn Informatics Sabbatical Fellowships, 3035
PhRMA Fndn Informatics Post Doctoral Fellowships, 3036
PhRMA Fndn Informatics Pre Doctoral Fellowships, 3037
PhRMA Fndn Paul Calabresi Medical Student Research Fellowship, 3039
PhRMA Fndn Pharmaceutics Postdoctoral Fellowships, 3040
PhRMA Fndn Pharmaceutics Pre Doctoral Fellowships, 3041
PhRMA Fndn Pharmaceutics Sabbatical Fellowships, 3043
PhRMA Fndn Pharmacology/Toxicology Post Doctoral Fellowships, 3044
PhRMA Fndn Pharmacology/Toxicology Pre Doctoral Fellowships, 3045
PhRMA Fndn Pharmacology/Toxicology Sabbatical Fellowships, 3047
Pioneer Hi-Bred Society Fellowships, 3052
Plastic Surgery Educational Fndn Research Fellowship Grants, 3059
Polaroid Fund Grants, 3065
Postdoctoral Research Fellowships in Gerontological Public Health, 3070
Potts Memorial Fndn Grants, 3072
PSG Mentored Clinical Research Awards, 3088
R.C. Baker Fndn Grants, 3098
Rajiv Gandhi Fndn Grants, 3104
Rathmann Family Fndn Grants, 3109
RCPSC International Traveling Fellowship, 3118
RCPSC Medical Education Traveling Fellowships, 3125
RCPSC Royal College Fellowship for Studies in Medical Education, 3127
Regenstrief Geriatrics Fellowship, 3143
Regenstrief General Internal Medicine - General Pediatrics Research Fellowship Program, 3144
Rett Syndrome Research Fndn Grants, 3151
Rhode Island Fndn Grants, 3154
Rosalynn Carter Institute John and Betty Pope Fellowships, 3189
Roy J. Carver Charitable Trust Medical and Science Research Grants, 3192
RWJF Clinical Scholars Program Grants, 3207
RWJF Executive Nurse Fellowships, 3210
RWJF Generalist Physician Faculty Scholars, 3212
RWJF Harold Amos Medical Faculty Development Scholars, 3213
RWJF Health & Society Scholars, 3214
RWJF Health Policy Fellowships, 3217
RWJF Investigator Awards in Health Policy Research, 3220
RWJF Ladder to Leadership: Developing the Next Generation of Comm Health Leaders Fellowships, 3222

RWJF Scholars in Health Policy Research Fellowships, 3229
Sarah Scaife Fndn Grants, 3263
Savoy Fndn Post-Doctoral and Clinical Research Fellowships, 3266
Sexually Transmitted Diseases Postdoctoral Fellowships, 3279
Shell Oil Company Fndn Grants, 3281
Siragusa Fndn Health Services & Medical Research Grants, 3294
SNM Student Fellowship Awards, 3306
Society of Neuroscience Minority Fellowships, 3345
SRC Medical Research Grants, 3362
SSRC HIV/AIDS and Public Health Policy Research in Africa Fellowships, 3365
St. Joseph Comm Health Fndn Schneider Fellowships, 3370
Stroke Association Clinical Fellowships, 3386
Susan G. Komen Breast Cancer Fndn Interdisciplinary Fellowships, 3410
Susan G. Komen Breast Cancer Fndn Postdoctoral Fellowships, 3411
Takemi Program in International Health Research and Advanced Training Fellowships, 3416
Tourette Syndrome Association Post-Doc Fellowships, 3432
TSA Research Grant Awards, 3442
UCLA / RAND Corporation Post-Doctoral Fellowships, 3454
UICC American Cancer Society International Fellowships for Beginning Investigators, 3455
UICC International Cancer Technology Transfer (ICRETT) Fellowships, 3456
University of California President's Postdoctoral Fellowships, 3469
University of Georgia Counseling and Psychological Services Postdoctoral Fellowship, 3470
VFW Ladies Auxiliary Cancer Research Postdoctoral Fellowships, 3494
Viets Medical Student Myasthenia Gravis Research Fellowships, 3496
Vulcan Materials Company Fndn Grants, 3504
Walt Disney Company Fndn Grants, 3516
Whitaker International Fellows and Scholars Program, 3532

General Operating Support
1104 Fndn Grants, 3
2COBS Private Charitable Fndn Grants, 9
A/H Fndn Grants, 19
Abbott Fund Access to Health Care Grants, 176
Abbott Fund Comm Vitality Grants, 177
Abbott Fund Global AIDS Care Grants, 178
Abbott Fund Science and Medical Innovation Grants, 179
Abel Fndn Grants, 181
Abell Fndn Health and Human Services Grants, 182
Abell-Hanger Fndn Grants, 183
Able To Serve Grants, 185
ACF Preferred Communities Grants, 201
ACF Standing Announcement for Unaccompanied Alien Children Grants, 202
ACF Supplemental Services for Recently Arrived Refugees Grants, 203
Achelis and Bodman Fndns Grants, 206
Actors Fund Social Services and Financial Assistance, 225
Adam Richter Charitable Trust Grants, 230
Adams County Fndn Grants - Pennsylvania, 231
Adolph Coors Fndn Grants, 238
AEC Trust Grants, 242
AEGON Transamerica Fndn Grants, 243
Aetna Fndn Regional Comm Health General Support Grants, 248
AFG Industries Grants, 259
African American Fund of New Jersey Grants, 260
Agnes Gund Fndn Grants, 262
AHFMR Establishment and Independent Establishment Grants, 273
Air Products and Chemicals Grants, 319
Alabama Power Fndn Grants, 321
Aladdin Industries Fndn Grants, 322
Alaska Airlines Corp Giving Grants, 323
Albert Pick Jr. Fund Grants, 328
Alberto Culver Corp Contributions Grants, 329
Albertson's Charitable Giving Grants, 330
Albuquerque Comm Fndn Grants, 331
Alcatel-Lucent Technologies Fndn Grants, 333
Alcoa Fndn Grants, 334
Alcon Fndn Grants, 336
Alex Brown and Sons Charitable Fndn Grants, 337
Alexander & Baldwin Fndn Hawaiian and Pacific Island Grants, 338
Alexander & Baldwin Fndn Mainland Grants, 339
Allegheny Technologies Charitable Trust, 359
Alpine Winter Fndn Grants, 368
AMA Fndn Healthy Communities/Healthy America Grants, 390
Amador Comm Fndn Grants, 409
American Express Fndn Comm Service Grants, 435
American Schlafhorst Fndn Grants, 454
Amgen Fndn Grants, 467
AMI Semiconductors Corp Grants, 468
Andersen Corp Fndn, 470
Andersen Fndn Grants, 471
Anheuser-Busch Fndn Grants, 474
Ann Jackson Family Fndn Grants, 477
Ann Peppers Fndn Grants, 478
Anschutz Family Fndn Grants, 486
Anthony R. Abraham Fndn Grants, 490
APF Disaster Recovery Fund for Psychiatrists, 506
Aratani Fndn Grants, 523
Arcadia Fndn Grants, 524
ARCO Fndn Education Grants, 526
Arie and Ida Crown Memorial Grants, 528
Arizona Diamondbacks Charities Grants, 530
Arizona Public Service Corp Giving Program Grants, 531
Arkell Hall Fndn Grants, 534
Arlington Comm Fndn Grants, 536
Armstrong McDonald Fndn Grants, 537
ARS Fndn Grants, 538
Arthur and Rochelle Belfer Fndn Grants, 542
ASCO State Affiliate Grants, 560
Assurant Fndn Grants, 654
Atherton Family Fndn Grants, 659
Athwin Fndn Grants, 660
Atkinson Fndn International Grants, 661
Atlanta Fndn Grants, 662
Atran Fndn Grants, 663
Auburn Fndn Grants, 664
Audrey and Sydney Irmas Charitable Fndn Grants, 665
Avon Products Fndn Grants, 675
Bacon Family Fndn Grants, 679
Bailey Fndn Grants, 680
Balfe Family Fndn Grants, 682
Ball Brothers Fndn General Grants, 683
Ball Brothers Fndn Grants, 684
Banfi Vintners Fndn Grants, 687
Bank of America Charitable Fndn Anchor Institutions Grants, 688
Bank of America Charitable Fndn National Programs and Partners Grants, 689
Bank of America Client Fndn Grants, 690
Baptist-Trinity Lutheran Legacy Fndn Grants, 692
Barker Fndn Grants, 694
Barker Welfare Fndn Grants, 695
Barr Fund Grants, 697
Batchelor Fndn Grants, 701
Batts Fndn Grants, 704
BCBS of Minnesota Growing Up Healthy Grants, 711
BCBS of Minnesota Healthy Together Grants, 712
BCBSM Fndn Primary and Clinical Prevention Grants, 719
Bearemy's Kennel Pals Grants, 728
Beazley Fndn Grants, 730
Bechtel Group Fndn Building Positive Comm Relationships Grants, 731
Beldon Fund Grants, 738
Belk Fndn Grants, 739
Bender Fndn Grants, 742
Berks County Comm Fndn Grants, 745
Berrien Comm Fndn Grants, 749
Bertha Russ Lytel Fndn Grants, 751
Besser Fndn Grants, 752
Bildner Family Fndn Grants, 755
Bill and Melinda Gates Fndn Grants, 756
Blackford County Comm Fndn Grants, 763
Blanche and Julian Robertson Family Fndn Grants, 765
Blowitz-Ridgeway Fndn Grants, 767
Blue Mountain Comm Fndn Grants, 769
Blum-Kovler Fndn Grants, 772
Blumenthal Fndn Grants, 773
Bodman Fndn Grants, 776
Boettcher Fndn Grants, 778
Bonfils-Stanton Fndn Grants, 779
Borkee-Hagley Fndn Grants, 781
Boston Fndn Grants, 783
Boston Globe Fndn Grants, 784
Boyd Gaming Corporation Contributions Program, 788
Bradley Turner Fndn Grants, 789
Bright Family Fndn Grants, 793
Bristol-Myers Squibb Fndn Health Disparities Grants, 797
Brookdale Fndn National Group Respite and Early Memory Loss Program Grants, 806
Bruce and Adele Greenfield Fndn Grants, 808
Bullitt Fndn Grants, 809
Burlington Northern Santa Fe Fndn Grants, 812
Burton G. Bettingen Grants, 813
Bush Fndn Health & Human Services Grants, 814
Bushrod H. Campbell and Adah F. Hall Charity Fund Grants, 816
Byron W. and Alice L. Lockwood Fndn Grants, 824
C.R. Bard Fndn Grants, 825
C.W. Titus Fndn Grants, 826
Caddock Fndn Grants, 828
Cailloux Fndn Grants, 829
Caleb C. and Julia W. Dula Educational and Charitable Fndn Grants, 830
California Comm Fndn Health Care Grants, 831
California Wellness Fndn Work and Health Program Grants, 834
Callaway Fndn Grants, 835
Callaway Golf Company Fndn Grants, 836
Cambridge Comm Fndn Grants, 837
Camp-Younts Fndn Grants, 838
Campbell Hoffman Fndn Grants, 840
Cargill Citizenship Fund-Corp Giving Grants, 865
Caring Fndn Grants, 866
Carl and Eloise Pohlad Family Fndn Grants, 867
Carl C. Icahn Fndn Grants, 870
Carl Gellert and Celia Berta Gellert Fndn Grants, 871
Carl J. Herzog Fndn Grants, 872
Carl W. and Carrie Mae Joslyn Trust Grants, 873
Carnahan-Jackson Fndn Grants, 878
Carnegie Corporation of New York Grants, 879
Carolyn Fndn Grants, 880
Carpenter Fndn Grants, 881
Carrie E. and Lena V. Glenn Fndn Grants, 882
Carrie Estelle Doheny Fndn Grants, 883
Carrier Corporation Contributions Grants, 884
Carylon Fndn Grants, 886
Castle Rock Fndn Grants, 888
CDC Cooperative Agreement for Continuing Enhanced National Surveillance for Prion Diseases in the United States, 904
CDC Increasing Breast and Cervical Cancer Screening Services for Urban American Indian/Alaska Native Women, 912
Cemala Fndn Grants, 933
Champ-A Champion Fur Kids Grants, 959

Charles A. Frueauff Fndn Grants, 962
Charles Delmar Fndn Grants, 963
Charles G. Koch Charitable Fndn Grants, 965
Charles H. Farnsworth Trust Grants, 967
Charles M. and Mary D. Grant Fndn Grants, 971
Charles M. Bair Family Trust Grants, 972
Charlotte County (FL) Comm Fndn Grants, 973
Chatlos Fndn Grants, 977
Chazen Fndn Grants, 978
Chestnut Hill Charitable Fndn, Inc Grants, 987
Chicago Board of Trade Fndn Grants, 988
Chicago Comm Trust Grants, 989
Chicago Tribune's Corp Contributions Grants, 991
Chiles Fndn Grants, 1003
CIGNA Fndn Grants, 1011
Clarcor Fndn Grants, 1021
Clarence E. Heller Charitable Fndn Grants, 1022
Clark Fndn Grants, 1029
Clark-Winchcole Fndn Grants, 1030
Claude Bennett Family Fndn Grants, 1031
Claude Worthington Benedum Fndn Grants, 1033
CMA Fndn Grants, 1042
CNA Fndn Grants, 1046
CNCS Foster Grandparent Projects Grants, 1048
Coastal Bend Comm Fndn Grants, 1050
Coastal Comm Fndn of South Carolina Grants, 1051
Coca-Cola Fndn Grants, 1052
Coeta and Donald Barker Fndn Grants, 1054
Coleman Fndn Cancer Care Grants, 1055
Colin Higgins Fndn Grants, 1056
Collins C. Diboll Private Fndn Grants, 1057
Collins Fndn Grants, 1058
Colorado Interstate Gas Grants, 1060
Colorado Springs Comm Trust Fund Grants, 1061
Colorado Trust Grants, 1062
Columbus Fndn Estrich Fund Grants, 1067
Columbus Fndn Mary Eleanor Morris Fund Grants, 1069
Columbus Fndn Traditional Grants, 1071
Comer Fndn Grants, 1072
Commission on Religion in Appalachia Grants, 1074
Comm Fndn for Greater Buffalo Grants, 1090
Comm Fndn for Greater New Haven Grants, 1091
Comm Fndn for Monterey County Grants, 1092
Comm Fndn for Southeastern Michigan Grants, 1094
Comm Fndn for Southern Arizona Grants, 1095
Comm Fndn of Bartholomew County Heritage Fund Grants, 1096
Comm Fndn of Central Illinois Grants, 1101
Comm Fndn of Grant County Grants, 1104
Comm Fndn of Greater Birmingham Grants, 1106
Comm Fndn of Greater Flint Grants, 1107
Comm Fndn of Greater Greensboro Grants, 1109
Comm Fndn of Greenville Hollingsworth Funds Program/Project Grants, 1114
Comm Fndn of Madison and Jefferson County Grants and Scholarships, 1117
Comm Fndn of Muncie and Delaware County Grants, 1120
Comm Fndn of South Alabama Grants, 1123
Comm Fndn of South Puget Sound Grants, 1124
Comm Fndn of St. Joseph County Special Project Challenge Grants, 1126
Comm Fndn of Switzerland County Grants, 1127
Comm Fndn of the Ozarks Grants, 1130
Comm Fndn of Wabash County Grants, 1131
Comm Fndn Silicon Valley Grants, 1133
Compass Bank Fndn Grants, 1138
Comprehensive Health Education Fndn Grants, 1139
ConAgra Foods Fndn Grants, 1140
Connelly Fndn Grants, 1143
ConocoPhillips Fndn Grants, 1144
Constellation Energy Group and Baltimore Gas and Electric Corp Contributions, 1146
Consumers Energy Fndn, 1147
Cooke Fndn Grants, 1148
Cooper Industries Fndn Grants, 1150
Cornerstone Fndn of Northeastern Wisconsin Grants, 1152
Cowles Charitable Trust Grants, 1155
Crail-Johnson Fndn Grants, 1157
Cranston Fndn Grants, 1158
Crestlea Fndn Grants, 1159
CRH Fndn Grants, 1160
Cullen Fndn Grants, 1172
D. W. McMillan Fndn Grants, 1180
D.F. Halton Fndn Grants, 1181
Dade Comm Fndn Comm AIDS Partnership Grants, 1184
Dade Comm Fndn Grants, 1185
DaimlerChrysler Corporation Fund Grants, 1186
Dale and Edna Walsh Fndn Grants, 1189
Dallas Women's Fndn Grants, 1191
Dana Corporation Fndn Grants, 1196
Danellie Fndn Grants, 1198
Daphne Seybolt Culpeper Memorial Fndn Grants, 1201
David Geffen Fndn Grants, 1202
Dayton Power and Light Fndn Grants, 1205
Daywood Fndn Grants, 1206
Deaconess Comm Fndn Grants, 1207
Denton A. Cooley Fndn Grants, 1225
DeRoy Testamentary Fndn Grants, 1239
DHHS Oral Health Promotion Research Across the Lifespan, 1269
DHHS Thimerosal Pharmacokinetics: Assessment of the Distribution, Metabolism, and Excretion, 1281
DHL Charitable Shipment Support, 1283
Dolan Fndn Grants, 1306
Donald and Sylvia Robinson Family Fndn Grants, 1310
Dora Roberts Fndn Grants, 1311
Doris and Victor Day Fndn Grants, 1313
Dorothy Hooper Beattie Fndn Grants, 1321
Dorrance Family Fndn Grants, 1323
DPA Promoting Policy Change Advocacy Grants, 1324
Dr. Bob and Jean Smith Fndn Grants, 1325
Dreitzer Fndn Grants, 1332
Dubois County Comm Fndn Grants, 1336
Duchossois Family Fndn Grants, 1337
Duke Endowment Health Care Grants, 1338
Duke Energy Fndn Grants, 1339
Dunspaugh-Dalton Fndn Grants, 1351
Dyson Fndn Mid-Hudson Valley General Operating Support Grants, 1354
eBay Fndn Comm Grants, 1363
Edina Realty Fndn Grants, 1369
Edward S. Moore Fndn Grants, 1374
Edwards Memorial Trust Grants, 1375
Edwin S. Webster Fndn Grants, 1376
Edwin W. and Catherine M. Davis Fndn Grants, 1377
Effie and Wofford Cain Fndn Grants, 1385
Eisner Fndn Grants, 1387
El Paso Comm Fndn Grants, 1388
El Pomar Fndn Awards and Grants, 1390
Elisabeth Severance Prentiss Fndn Grants, 1392
Elizabeth Morse Genius Charitable Trust Grants, 1400
Elliot Fndn Inc Grants, 1402
Elmer L. and Eleanor J. Andersen Fndn Grants, 1406
Elsie Lee Garthwaite Memorial Fndn Grants, 1408
EMBO Installation Grants, 1409
Emerson Charitable Trust Grants, 1412
Emerson Electric Company Contributions Grants, 1413
Emma B. Howe Memorial Fndn Grants, 1415
Essex County Comm Fndn Discretionary Fund Grant, 1428
Ethel S. Abbott Charitable Fndn Grants, 1430
Eugene and Agnes E. Meyer Fndn Grants, 1432
Eugene B. Casey Fndn Grants, 1433
Eugene M. Lang Fndn Grants, 1434
Eugene McDermott Fndn Grants, 1435
Fairfield County Comm Fndn Grants, 1446
Fallon OrNda Comm Health Fund Grants, 1449
Fan Fox and Leslie R. Samuels Fndn Grants, 1451
Fannie E. Rippel Fndn Grants, 1452
Faye McBeath Fndn Grants, 1456
Feldman Fndn Grants, 1484
Ferree Fndn Grants, 1486
Field Fndn of Illinois Grants, 1499
FirstEnergy Fndn Comm Grants, 1505
Fisa Fndn Grants, 1506
Fisher Fndn Grants, 1508
Florida BRAIVE Fund of Dade Comm Fndn, 1512
Florida BRAIVE Fund of Gulf Coast Comm Fndn of Venice, 1513
Florida BRAIVE Fund of The Comm Fndn in Jacksonville, 1514
Fluor Fndn Grants, 1517
FMC Fndn Grants, 1518
Foellinger Fndn Grants, 1519
Fondren Fndn Grants, 1520
Ford Motor Company Fund Grants, 1522
Foster Fndn Grants, 1524
Fndn Northwest Grants, 1537
Fourjay Fndn Grants, 1544
Frances W. Emerson Fndn Grants, 1548
Francis L. Abreu Charitable Trust Grants, 1549
Francis T. & Louise T. Nichols Fndn Grants, 1550
Frank E. and Seba B. Payne Fndn Grants, 1551
Frank G. and Freida K. Brotz Family Fndn Grants, 1552
Frank Stanley Beveridge Fndn Grants, 1553
Franklin County Comm Fndn Grants, 1554
Fraser-Parker Fndn Grants, 1555
Freddie Mac Fndn Grants, 1558
Fremont Area Comm Fndn Grants, 1561
Frist Fndn Grants, 1563
Fuller E. Callaway Fndn Grants, 1578
G.N. Wilcox Trust Grants, 1581
Gebbie Fndn Grants, 1585
GenCorp Fndn Grants, 1587
Genentech Corp Charitable Contributions Grants, 1588
General Mills Fndn Grants, 1590
General Motors Fndn Grants Support Program, 1591
Genesis Fndn Grants, 1593
Genuardi Family Fndn Grants, 1594
George and Ruth Bradford Fndn Grants, 1595
George B. Storer Fndn Grants, 1596
George F. Baker Trust Grants, 1597
George Frederick Jewett Fndn Grants, 1599
George S. and Dolores Dore Eccles Fndn Grants, 1602
Georgiana Goddard Eaton Memorial Fund Grants, 1604
Geraldine R. Dodge Fndn Morris County Grants, 1605
Gertrude and William C. Wardlaw Fund Grants, 1607
Gheens Fndn Grants, 1610
Gibson Fndn Grants, 1612
Gilroy and Lillian P. Roberts Charitable Fndn Grants, 1614
Ginn Fndn Grants, 1616
Global Fund for Children Grants, 1629
Godfrey Fndn Grants, 1631
Good Samaritan Inc Grants, 1637
Goodrich Corporation Fndn Grants, 1638
Google Grants Beta, 1640
Grand Rapids Area Comm Fndn Grants, 1645
Grand Rapids Area Comm Fndn Nashwauk Area Endowment Fund Grants, 1646
Greater Tacoma Comm Fndn Grants, 1656
Greater Worcester Comm Fndn Jeppson Memorial Fund for Brookfield Grants, 1659
Greene County Fndn Grants, 1662
Greenfield Fndn of Maine Grants, 1663
Gregory B. Davis Fndn Grants, 1666
Gregory L. Gibson Charitable Fndn Grants, 1668
Griffin Family Fndn Grants, 1669
Griffin Fndn Grants, 1670
Grotto Fndn Project Grants, 1671
Grundy Fndn Grants, 1673
Gulf Coast Comm of Venice Fndn Grants, 1677

Guy's and St. Thomas' Charity Grants, 1678
H & R Fndn Grants, 1679
H. Schaffer Fndn Grants, 1680
H.A. and Mary K. Chapman Charitable Trust Grants, 1681
H.J. Heinz Company Fndn Grants, 1682
Hagedorn Fund Grants, 1685
Halliburton Fndn Grants, 1687
Hallmark Corp Fndn Grants, 1688
Hannaford Charitable Fndn Grants, 1692
Harden Fndn Grants, 1693
Harold and Arlene Schnitzer CARE Fndn Grants, 1697
Harold Simmons Fndn Grants, 1698
Harris and Eliza Kempner Fund Grants, 1699
Harry and Grace Steele Fndn Grants, 1702
Harry Bramhall Gilbert Charitable Trust Grants, 1703
Harry S. Black and Allon Fuller Fund, 1706
Hartford Aging and Health Program Awards, 1709
Hartford Fndn Regular Grants, 1711
Harvest Fndn Grants, 1713
Hawaii Comm Fndn Health Education and Research Grants, 1716
HCA Fndn Grants, 1721
Health Fndn of Greater Indianapolis Grants, 1725
Health Fndn of Southern Florida Responsive Grants, 1726
Hearst Fndn and William Randolph Hearst Fndn Grants, 1730
Heckscher Fndn for Children Grants, 1732
Helen Bader Fndn Grants, 1738
Helen K. and Arthur E. Johnson Fndn Grants, 1740
Helen Steiner Rice Fndn Grants, 1742
Helena Rubinstein Fndn Grants, 1743
Henrietta Tower Wurts Memorial Fndn Grants, 1745
Henry J. Kaiser Family Fndn Grants, 1748
Herman Goldman Fndn Grants, 1753
HHK Employment Grants, 1755
High Meadow Fndn Grants, 1768
Hillman Fndn Grants, 1775
Hillsdale County Comm Fndn Healthy Senior/Healthy Youth Fund Grants, 1776
Hirtzel Memorial Fndn Grants, 1781
Hoglund Fndn Grants, 1785
Honeywell Fndn Grants, 1791
Horace A. Kimball and S. Ella Kimball Fndn Grants, 1792
Horizon Fndn for New Jersey Grants, 1793
Horizons Comm Issues Grants, 1794
Hormel Foods Charitable Trust Grants, 1795
Hormel Fndn Grants, 1796
Howe Fndn of North Carolina Grants, 1799
Huber Fndn Grants, 1812
Hudson Webber Fndn Grants, 1813
Hugh J. Andersen Fndn Grants, 1814
Huie-Dellmon Trust Grants, 1815
Human Source Fndn Grants, 1817
Huntington Clinical Fndn Grants, 1822
Idaho Power Company Corp Contributions, 1838
Independence Blue Cross Charitable Medical Care Grants, 1846
Independence Comm Fndn Comm Quality of Life Grant, 1849
Indiana 21st Century Research and Technology Fund Awards, 1850
Irvin Stern Fndn Grants, 1866
Irving S. Gilmore Fndn Grants, 1867
Ittleson Fndn Mental Health Grants, 1870
J. Walton Bissell Fndn Grants, 1872
J.B. Reynolds Fndn Grants, 1873
J.W. Kieckhefer Fndn Grants, 1878
Jacob and Hilda Blaustein Fndn Grants, 1881
James A. and Faith Knight Fndn Grants, 1884
James Ford Bell Fndn Grants, 1885
James R. Dougherty Jr. Fndn Grants, 1894
Jane's Trust Grants, 1904
Jean and Louis Dreyfus Fndn Grants, 1911
JELD-WEN Fndn Grants, 1914
Jenkins Fndn: Improving the Health of Greater Richmond Grants, 1915
Jessie Ball Dupont Fund Grants, 1919
Jessie Smith Noyes Fndn Grants, 1920
Jewish Fund Grants, 1923
Joe W. and Dorothy Dorsett Brown Fndn Grants, 1927
John Deere Fndn Grants, 1929
John Edward Fowler Memorial Fndn Grants, 1930
John H. and Wilhelmina D. Harland Charitable Fndn Grants, 1933
John I. Smith Charities Grants, 1935
John J. Leidy Fndn Grants, 1936
John Jewett and Helen Chandler Garland Fndn Grants, 1937
John P. McGovern Fndn Grants, 1942
John W. Anderson Fndn Grants, 1949
Johns Manville Fund Grants, 1950
Johnson & Johnson Corp Contributions Grants, 1952
Joseph Alexander Fndn Grants, 1957
Joseph Drown Fndn Grants, 1960
Joseph H. and Florence A. Roblee Fndn Grants, 1961
Josephine G. Russell Trust Grants, 1963
Josephine S. Gumbiner Fndn Grants, 1965
Journal Gazette Fndn Grants, 1968
Joyce Fndn Grants, 1969
K and F Baxter Family Fndn Grants, 1973
K. M. Hunter Charitable Fndn Social Welfare Grants, 1974
K21 Health Fndn Cancer Care Fund Grants, 1975
Kalamazoo Fndn Grants, 1979
Kansas Health Fndn Grants, 1980
Kate B. Reynolds Charitable Trust Health Care Grants, 1981
Katharine Matthies Fndn Grants, 1982
Kathryne Beynon Fndn Grants, 1984
Kelvin and Eleanor Smith Fndn Grants, 1986
Kenneth T. and Eileen L. Norris Fndn Grants, 1989
Kenny's Kids Grants, 1990
KFC Allied Health Research Grants, 1996
KFC Biomedical Research Grants, 1998
L. W. Pierce Family Fndn Grants, 2019
Land O'Lakes Fndn Mid-Atlantic Grants, 2027
Lavelle Fund for the Blind Grants, 2033
Leo Goodwin Fndn Grants, 2043
Lester E. Yeager Charitable Trust B Grants, 2047
Lewis Preston Fund for Girls Education Grants, 2052
Lillian S. Wells Fndn Grants, 2056
Louis Calder Fndn Grants, 2065
Lowe Fndn Grants, 2067
Lowell Berry Fndn Grants, 2069
Lubbock Area Fndn Grants, 2079
Lubrizol Fndn Grants, 2080
Lucile Horton Howe and Mitchell B. Howe Fndn Grants, 2081
Lucy Gooding Charitable Fndn Trust, 2082
M. Bastian Family Fndn Grants, 2092
M.B. and Edna Zale Fndn Grants, 2093
M.E. Raker Fndn Grants, 2094
Mabel Y. Hughes Charitable Trust Grants, 2097
Madison County Comm Fndn Grants, 2098
Maine Comm Fndn Grants, 2099
Manuel D. and Rhoda Mayerson Fndn Grants, 2100
Marcia and Otto Koehler Fndn Grants, 2103
Margaret T. Morris Fndn Grants, 2105
Margoes Fndn Grants, 2106
Marion I. and Henry J. Knott Fndn Grants, 2109
Mark and Catherine Winkler Fndn Grants, 2112
Mars Fndn Grants, 2114
Mary Black Fndn Grants, 2118
Mary Owen Borden Fndn Grants, 2121
Matilda R. Wilson Fund Grants, 2128
Mattel International Grants, 2131
Max A. Adler Charitable Fndn Grants, 2132
Maxon Charitable Fndn Grants, 2135
May and Stanley Smith Trust Grants, 2137
McGregor Fund Grants, 2143
McInerny Fndn Grants, 2144
McKesson Fndn Grants, 2145
McKnight Fndn Grants, 2146
McMurry Fndn Grants, 2149
Mead Johnson Nutritionals Charitable Giving Grants, 2156
Mead Witter Fndn Grants, 2160
Meadows Fndn Grants, 2161
Medtronic Fndn Full Life Patient Partnership Program--Heart Rescue Grants, 2168
Meriden Fndn Grants, 2173
Metro Health Fndn Grants, 2175
Meyer Memorial Trust Emergency Grants, 2178
Meyer Memorial Trust Grassroots Grants, 2179
Meyer Memorial Trust Operating Funds Grants, 2180
Meyer Memorial Trust Responsive Grants, 2181
MHRC Operating Grants, 2186
Michael and Susan Dell Fndn Grants, 2189
Miles of Hope Breast Cancer Fndn Grants, 2199
Millipore Fndn Grants, 2203
Minneapolis Fndn Comm Grants, 2206
Miriam and Peter Haas Fund Grants, 2208
Monfort Family Fndn Grants, 2213
Montgomery County Comm Fndn Grants, 2214
MONY Fndn Grants, 2215
Morris and Gwendolyn Cafritz Fndn Grants, 2217
Moses Cone-Wesley Long Comm Health Fndn Grants, 2219
Ms. Fndn for Women Grants, 2222
Ms. Fndn Women and AIDS Fund Grants, 2223
National Starch and Chemical Fndn Grants, 2261
NCI Technologies and Software to Support Integrative Cancer Biology Research (SBIR) Grants, 2279
New York Life Fndn Grants, 2304
Newman's Own Inc Grants, 2306
Nicholas H. Noyes Jr. Memorial Fndn Grants, 2497
NIDA Clinical Research Education Programs in Drug Abuse and Addiction, 2500
NIH Biology, Development, and Progression of Malignant Prostate Disease Research Grants, 2641
NIMH New Minority Faculty Scientist Development Award, 2765
Nina Mason Pulliam Charitable Trust Grants, 2776
NNEDVF/Altria Doors of Hope Program, 2847
Noble County Comm Fndn Grants, 2848
Nordson Corporation Fndn Grants, 2851
North Carolina Comm Development Grants, 2858
North Carolina GlaxoSmithKline Fndn Grants, 2860
Northern Trust Company Charitable Trust and Corp Giving Program, 2865
Northwestern Mutual Fndn Grants, 2870
Norwin S. and Elizabeth N. Bean Fndn Grants, 2872
NSF Presidential Early Career Awards for Scientists and Engineers (PECASE) Grants, 2892
NYCT AIDS/HIV Grants, 2919
NYCT Blood Disease Research Grants, 2922
NYCT Girls and Young Women Grants, 2924
NYCT Health Services, Systems, and Policies Grants, 2926
Olin Corporation Charitable Trust Grants, 2943
Ordean Fndn Grants, 2952
Otto Bremer Fndn Grants, 2977
Owen County Comm Fndn Grants, 2979
PacifiCare Fndn Grants, 2981
Pajaro Valley Comm Health Grants, 2985
Paul and Mary Haas Fndn Contributions and Student Scholarships, 2997
Paul E. and Klare N. Reinhold Fndn Grants, 2999
Perpetual Trust for Charitable Giving Grants, 3015
Pfizer Fndn Grants, 3025
Philadelphia Fndn Organizational Effectiveness Grants, 3029
Phoenix Suns Charities Grants, 3030
Pinellas County Grants, 3050
Pioneer Hi-Bred Comm Grants, 3051
Piper Jaffray Companies Building Strong Communities Grants, 3053
Polaroid Fund Grants, 3065
Portland General Electric Fndn Grants, 3067

Powell Fndn Grants, 3073
Pride Fndn Grants and Scholarships, 3078
Prince Charitable Trusts Chicago Grants, 3079
Prince Charitable Trusts District of Columbia Grants, 3080
Principal Financial Group Fndn Grants, 3082
Procter and Gamble Fund Grants, 3083
Progress Energy Fndn Grants, 3084
Prudential Fndn Grants, 3087
Public Welfare Fndn Grants, 3089
Putnam County Comm Fndn Grants, 3093
R.C. Baker Fndn Grants, 3098
Ralphs Food 4 Less Fndn Grants, 3106
Raskob Fndn for Catholic Activities Grants, 3107
Rathmann Family Fndn Grants, 3109
Rayonier Fndn Grants, 3111
Rhode Island Fndn Grants, 3154
Rice Fndn Grants, 3155
Rich Fndn Grants, 3156
Richard and Helen DeVos Fndn Grants, 3157
Richard and Rhoda Goldman Fund Grants, 3158
Richard and Susan Smith Family Fndn Grants, 3159
Richard E. Griffin Family Fndn Grants, 3160
Richard King Mellon Fndn Grants, 3161
Riley Fndn Grants, 3165
Ripley County Comm Fndn Grants, 3166
Robert and Polly Dunn Fndn Grants, 3168
Robert B McMillen Fndn Grants, 3169
Robins Fndn Grants, 3175
Rochester Area Comm Fndn Grants, 3176
Rockefeller Brothers Fund Pivotal Places Grants: South Africa, 3180
Rockwell International Corp Trust Grants, 3183
Roy and Christine Sturgis Trust Grants, 3191
RRF General Program Grants, 3193
RRF Organizational Capacity Building Grants, 3194
Russell Berrie Fndn Grants, 3201
Ruth Eleanor Bamberger and John Ernest Bamberger Memorial Fndn Grants, 3202
Ruth H. and Warren A. Ellsworth Fndn Grants, 3203
Ruth Mott Fndn Grants, 3204
RWJF Partners Investing in Nursing's Future Grants, 3226
RWJF State Coverage Initiatives Grants, 3230
S. Livingston Mather Charitable Trust Grants, 3235
S. Mark Taper Fndn Grants, 3236
S.H. Cowell Fndn Grants, 3237
Salem Fndn Charitable Trust Grants, 3241
Salem Fndn Grants, 3242
Samuel Freeman Charitable Trust Grants, 3249
Samuel S. Johnson Fndn Grants, 3251
San Antonio Area Fndn Grants, 3254
San Diego HIV Funding Collaborative (SDHFC) Grants, 3258
San Diego Women's Fndn Grants, 3259
San Francisco Fndn Comm Health Grants, 3260
Sarah Scaife Fndn Grants, 3263
Sasco Fndn Grants, 3265
Schering-Plough Fndn Comm Initiatives Grants, 3269
Schering-Plough Fndn Health Grants, 3270
Schurz Communications Fndn Grants, 3271
Seneca Foods Fndn Grants, 3278
Sheltering Arms Fund Grants, 3282
Sid W. Richardson Fndn Grants, 3284
Siebert Lutheran Fndn Grants, 3285
Simmons Fndn Grants, 3287
Simpson Fund Grants, 3290
Sisters of Mercy of North Carolina Fndn Grants, 3295
Sisters of St. Joseph Healthcare Fndn Grants, 3297
SOCFOC Catholic Ministries Grants, 3317
SOCFOC Reducing Health & Educational Disparities in the Central Neighborhood Grants, 3318
Solo Cup Fndn Grants, 3346
Sonoco Fndn Grants, 3347
Sosland Fndn Grants, 3348
Southwest Gas Corporation Fndn Grants, 3352
Sprague Fndn Grants, 3359
Square D Fndn Grants, 3361
St. Joseph Comm Health Fndn Improving Healthcare Access Grants, 3368
Stackner Family Fndn Grants, 3371
Stan and Sandy Checketts Fndn, 3373
Starr Fndn Grants, 3377
Staunton Farm Fndn Grants, 3378
Steelcase Fndn Grants, 3379
Steele-Reese Fndn Grants, 3380
Stewart Huston Charitable Trust Grants, 3384
Strowd Roses Grants, 3388
Sulzberger Fndn Grants, 3399
Susan Mott Webb Charitable Trust Grants, 3412
Susan Vaughan Fndn Grants, 3413
Temple-Inland Fndn Grants, 3419
Texas Commission on the Arts Arts Respond Project Grants, 3420
Thelma Doelger Charitable Trust Grants, 3421
Thomas and Dorothy Leavey Fndn Grants, 3422
Thomas C. Ackerman Fndn Grants, 3423
Thompson Charitable Fndn Grants, 3425
Triangle Comm Fndn Donor-Advised Grants, 3437
TWS Fndn Grants, 3443
Until There's a Cure Fndn Grants, 3471
US Trust Corporation Fndn Grants, 3475
VDH Rescue Squad Assistance Fund Grants, 3484
Vulcan Materials Company Fndn Grants, 3504
W. C. Griffith Fndn Grants, 3505
W. Clarke Swanson, Jr. Fndn Grants, 3506
W.W. Smith Charitable Trust Grants for Medical Research in Cancer, AIDS, and Heart Disease, 3509
Wachovia Fndn Grants, 3511
Walt Disney Company Fndn Grants, 3516
Washington Post Contributions Program Grants, 3520
Wayne and Gladys Valley Fndn Grants, 3522
Weatherwax Fndn Grants, 3523
Wells County Fndn Grants, 3527
WHAS Crusade for Children Grants, 3531
Whitehall Fndn Neurobiology Research Grants, 3533
William G. Gilmore Fndn Grants, 3537
William G. McGowan Charitable Fund Grants, 3539
Wilson-Wood Fndn Grants, 3542
Winifred & Harry B. Allen Fndn Grants, 3543
Women's Fndn of California Comm Action Fund, 3549
Women's Fndn of California Grants, 3550
YSA Get Ur Good On Grants, 3555
Z. Smith Reynolds Fndn Small Grants, 3557

Graduate Assistantships

Abbott Fund Science and Medical Innovation Grants, 179
ASHA Minority Student Leadership Program Awards, 570
Evjue Fndn Grants, 1439
GE & Science Prize for Young Life Scientists, 1584
Health Management Scholarships and Grants for Minorities, 1727
NAPNAP Fndn Graduate Student Research Grant, 2236
NCIC Terry Fox Research Studentships, 2286
NHLBI Research Supplements to Promote Diversity in Health-Related Research for Graduate Research Assistants, 2375
SSSS Student Research Grants, 3366
Vancouver Fndn Grants and Comm Initiatives Program, 3477

International Exchange Programs

Alexander von Humboldt Fndn Institutional Academic Cooperation Grants, 346
American College of Surgeons International Guest Scholarships, 429
Aratani Fndn Grants, 523
ASM International Fellowship for Latin America and the Caribbean, 601
ASM International Fellowships for Asia and Africa, 602
ASM Millis-Colwell Postgraduate Travel Grant, 608
Canada-U.S. Fulbright Senior Specialists Program Grants, 847
Chateaubriand Exact Sciences, Engineering, and Medicine Research Scholarships, 976
Coca-Cola Fndn Grants, 1052
FIC International Research and Training in Population and Health Grants, 1489
FIC International Research Fellowships, 1490
FIC Israeli Ministry of Health Postdoctoral Research Fellowships, 1494
FIC Swedish Medical Research Council Fellowships, 1495
Fulbright Alumni Initiatives Awards Program Grants, 1566
Fulbright Distinguished Chairs Program Grants, 1567
Fulbright German Studies Seminar Grants, 1568
Fulbright Specialists Program Grants, 1571
Fulbright Traditional Scholar Program in Europe and Eurasia, 1572
Fulbright Traditional Scholar Program in Sub-Saharan Africa, 1573
Fulbright Traditional Scholar Program in the East Asia/Pacific Region, 1574
Fulbright Traditional Scholar Program in the Near East and North Africa Region, 1575
Fulbright Traditional Scholar Program in the South and Central Asia Region, 1576
Fulbright Traditional Scholar Program in the Western Hemisphere, 1577
Hastings Center International Visiting Scholars Program, 1715
International Cancer Technology Transfer Fellowships, 1858
International Oncology Nursing Fellowships, 1862
Matsumae International Fndn Grants, 2129
Medical/Nursing Education, Research, and Health Care Exchanges with Taiwan, 2165
Nuffield Fndn Open Door Grants, 2902
RCPSC Kilborn Memorial Visiting Professorship, 3121
U.S. Department of Education United States-Russia Program: Improving Research and Educational Activities in Higher Education, 3451
UICC American Cancer Society International Fellowships for Beginning Investigators, 3455

International Grants

A-T Medical Research Fndn Grants, 16
AAAS Science & Technology Policy Fellowships - National Defense & Global Security, 29
AACR Gertrude Elion Cancer Research Award, 76
AACR Kirk A. Landon and Dorothy P. Landon Fndn Prizes, 80
AAFCS International Graduate Fellowships, 109
Abbott Fund Global AIDS Care Grants, 178
Abbott-ASM Lifetime Achievement Award, 180
ACGT Young Investigator Grants, 205
AFAR Paul Beeson Career Development Awards in Aging Research for the Island of Ireland, 256
AHFMR Infrastructure Funding Grants, 283
AHFMR Polaris Awards, 291
AHFMR Proposals for Special Initiatives, 293
Air Products and Chemicals Grants, 319
AJCC Cancer Staging Grants, 320
Albany Medical Center Prize in Medicine and Biomedical Research, 325
Albert and Mary Lasker Fndn Awards, 327
Alcatel-Lucent Technologies Corp Contributions Grants, 332
Alcoa Fndn Grants, 334
Alcohol Misuse and Alcoholism Research Grants, 335
Alexander von Humboldt Fndn Georg Forster Fellowships for Experienced Researchers, 344
Alexander von Humboldt Fndn Georg Forster Fellowships for Postdoctoral Researchers, 345

Alexander von Humboldt Fndn Research Fellowships for Experienced Researchers, 347
Alexander von Humboldt Fndn Research Fellowships for Postdoctoral Researchers, 348
Alternatives Research and Development Fndn Alternatives in Education Grants, 370
Alternatives Research and Development Fndn Grants, 371
Alzheimer's Association Investigator-Initiated Research Grants, 378
Alzheimer's Association New Investigator Research Grants, 381
Amarillo Area/Harrington Fndns Grants, 410
AMD Corp Contributions Grants, 411
American Jewish World Service Grants, 437
American Philosophical Society Daland Fellowships in Clinical Investigation, 441
American Psychiatric Association/AstraZeneca Young Minds in Psychiatry International Awards, 450
American-Italian Cancer Fndn Fellowships, 459
American-Scandinavian Fndn Visiting Lectureship Grants, 460
amfAR Global Initiatives Grants, 463
amfAR Research Grants, 466
Amgen Fndn Grants, 467
AON Fndn Grants, 491
Archer Daniels Midland Fndn Grants, 525
Arthritis Fndn of Australia Grants, 541
ASCO International Development and Education Awards (IDEA), 554
ASGE Don Wilson Award, 565
ASGE Endoscopic Research Awards, 566
ASGE Given Capsule Endoscopy Research Award, 568
ASHFndn Graduate Student International Scholarship, 576
ASM International Fellowships for Asia and Africa, 602
ASM Millis-Colwell Postgraduate Travel Grant, 608
ASM-PAHO Infectious Diseases Epidemiology and Surveillance Fellowships, 625
ASM-UNESCO Leadership Grant for International Educators, 626
ASPET Paul M. Vanhoutte Award, 646
Atkinson Fndn International Grants, 661
Atran Fndn Grants, 663
AUPHA Baxter International Fndn Prize for Health Services Research, 666
Australian Academy of Science Grants, 670
Avon Fndn Breast Care Fund Grants, 674
Avon Products Fndn Grants, 675
Banfi Vintners Fndn Grants, 687
Barth Syndrome Fndn Research Grants, 700
Baxter International Fndn Grants, 705
Bayer Hemophilia Caregivers Education Award, 707
Beatrice Laing Trust Grants, 729
Beckman Young Investigators Program Grants, 735
Becton Dickinson and Company Grants, 736
Bernard Van Leer Fndn Grants, 748
Besser Fndn Grants, 752
BibleLands Grants, 754
Bill and Melinda Gates Fndn Grants, 756
Boston Jewish Comm Women's Fund Grants, 785
Bristol-Myers Squibb Fndn Global HIV/AIDS Initiative Grants, 796
Bristol-Myers Squibb Fndn Health Disparities Grants, 797
Bristol-Myers Squibb Fndn Product Donations Grants, 799
Burden Trust Grants, 810
BWF Career Awards at the Scientific Interface, 819
BWF Clinical Scientist Awards in Translational Research, 821
BWF Institutional Program Unifying Population and Laboratory Based Sciences, 822
Caddock Fndn Grants, 828
Canada Graduate Scholarships (CGS) and NSERC Postgraduate Scholarships (PGS), 845
Canada-U.S. Fulbright New Century Scholars Program Grants, 846
Canada-U.S. Fulbright Senior Specialists Program Grants, 847
Canadian Dental Research Fndn Award, 848
Canadian Fndn for Dietetic Research Awards, 849
Canadian Friends of Hebrew University Research and Study Grants, 850
Canadian Liver Fndn Grants, 851
Canadian Nurses Fndn Study Awards, 852
Canadian Optometric Education Trust Fund Grants, 853
Cancer Research UK Fellowships, 858
Cancer Research UK Grants, 859
Cancer Society of New Zealand Grants, 860
Cargill Citizenship Fund-Corp Giving Grants, 865
Carnegie Corporation of New York Grants, 879
Carylon Fndn Grants, 886
CCFF Clinic Incentive Grants, 892
CCFF Fellowships, 893
CCFF Research Grants, 894
CCFF Scholarships, 895
CCFF Studentships, 897
CCFF Transplant Center Incentive Grants, 899
Central Okanagan Fndn Grants, 937
Cetana Educational Fndn Scholarships, 939
Charles Delmar Fndn Grants, 963
Charles H. Revson Fndn Grants, 969
Chase Paymentech Corp Giving Grants, 975
Chateaubriand Exact Sciences, Engineering, and Medicine Research Scholarships, 976
Chatlos Fndn Grants, 977
Chazen Fndn Grants, 978
Chesapeake Corporation Fndn Grants, 982
Children's Cardiomyopathy Fndn Research Grants, 1002
Chiles Fndn Grants, 1003
Christopher Reeve Paralysis Fndn Individual Research Grants, 1006
Christopher Reeve Paralysis Fndn Quality of Life and Health Promotions Grants, 1007
CIGNA Fndn Grants, 1011
CLA Nurses Respiratory Society Fellowships, 1018
CLA Nurses Respiratory Society Nursing Research Grants, 1019
CLA Physiotherapy Cardio-Respiratory Society Fellowships, 1020
CLF Fellowships, 1037
CLF Graduate Studentships, 1038
CLF Operating Grants, 1039
Coca-Cola Fndn Grants, 1052
Commonwealth Fund Harkness Fellowships in Health Care Policy and Practice, 1079
Commonwealth Fund Small Grants, 1084
ConAgra Foods Fndn Grants, 1140
ConocoPhillips Fndn Grants, 1144
Cooper Industries Fndn Grants, 1150
CPhA Centennial Award, 1156
CRI Clinical Investigator Award in Cancer Immunology, 1161
CRI Postdoctoral Fellowships, 1162
CTCRI Idea Grants, 1170
Cultural Society of Filipino Americans Grants, 1173
Cystic Fibrosis Research Grants, 1179
Dale and Edna Walsh Fndn Grants, 1189
Danellie Fndn Grants, 1198
Dental Teaching and Research Fellowships, 1224
DOD Breast Cancer Center of Excellence Award, 1290
DOD Clinical Translational Research Grants, 1291
DOD Era of Hope Scholar Award, 1292
DOD Idea Award for Breast Cancer Research, 1294
DOD Multidisciplinary Postdoctoral Award for Breast Cancer Research, 1295
DOD Predoctoral Traineeship in Breast Cancer Research, 1296
Doreen Kronick Scholarship, 1312
Doris Duke Charitable Fndn Operations Research on AIDS Care and Treatment in Africa (ORACTA) Grants, 1319
Dr. Courtney W. Shropshire Scholarship Grant, 1326
Duke University Adult Cardiothoracic Anesthesia and Critical Care Medicine Fellowships, 1340
Duke University Clinical Cardiac Electrophysiology Fellowships, 1342
Duke University Interventional Cardiology Fellowships, 1344
Duncan L. Gordon Fellowships, 1349
E.A. Baker Fndn for the Prevention of Blindness Grants, 1357
E.D.Thomas Fellowship, 1359
eBay Fndn Comm Grants, 1363
Echoing Green Fellowships, 1365
Elizabeth Glaser Pediatric AIDS Fndn International Leadership Awards, 1393
Elizabeth Glaser Pediatric AIDS Fndn Operations Research Grants, 1394
Elizabeth Glaser Pediatric AIDS Fndn Pediatric HIV Vaccine Research Grants, 1395
Elizabeth Glaser Scientist Award, 1398
EMBO Installation Grants, 1409
EMBO Long-Term Fellowships, 1410
EMBO Short-Term Fellowships, 1411
Eppley Fndn Postdoctoral Grants, 1425
Ethical Research Grants and Fellowships, 1431
ExxonMobil Grants, 1442
FDHN Moti L. & Kamla Rustgi International Travel Awards, 1475
Federal Express Corp Contributions Program, 1483
Feldman Fndn Grants, 1484
FIC International Cooperative Biodiversity Groups Grants, 1487
FIC International Malaria Research Training Program Award, 1488
FIC International Research and Training in Population and Health Grants, 1489
FIC International Research Fellowships, 1490
FIC International Research Scientist Development Award, 1491
FIC International Training and Research in Emerging Infectious Diseases Grants, 1492
FIC International Training and Research in Environmental and Occupational Health, 1493
FIC Israeli Ministry of Health Postdoctoral Research Fellowships, 1494
FIC Swedish Medical Research Council Fellowships, 1495
FIC/NIH AIDS International Training and Research Program, 1496
FIC/ORMH Minority International Research Training Grants, 1497
Fight for Sight Research Grants, 1502
Fight for Sight Research Grants and Fellowships, 1503
Fishman Family Fndn Grants, 1510
Fluor Fndn Grants, 1517
FMC Fndn Grants, 1518
Fndn for Medical Research Grants, 1528
Fulbright Alumni Initiatives Awards Grants, 1566
Fulbright Distinguished Chairs Grants, 1567
Fulbright German Studies Seminar Grants, 1568
Fulbright International Education Administrators (IEA) Seminar Program Grants, 1569
Fulbright New Century Scholars (NCS) Program Grants, 1570
Fulbright Specialists Program Grants, 1571
Fulbright Traditional Scholar Program in Europe and Eurasia, 1572
Fulbright Traditional Scholar Program in Sub-Saharan Africa, 1573
Fulbright Traditional Scholar Program in the East Asia/Pacific Region, 1574
Fulbright Traditional Scholar Program in the Near East and North Africa Region, 1575
Fulbright Traditional Scholar Program in the South and Central Asia Region, 1576
Fulbright Traditional Scholar Program in the Western Hemisphere, 1577
Fyssen Fndn Postdoctoral Study Grants, 1580
Gates Global HIV/AIDS Vaccine Grants, 1583

GE & Science Prize for Young Life Scientists, 1584
Genesis Fndn Grants, 1593
George F. Baker Trust Grants, 1597
Gerber Fndn Grants, 1606
Glaucoma Fndn Grants, 1621
Global Fund for Children Grants, 1629
Grass Fndn Marine Biological Laboratory Fellowships, 1648
Gruber Fndn International Prizes, 1672
Hamlet Trust Grants, 1689
Harold Simmons Fndn Grants, 1698
Hastings Center International Visiting Scholars Program, 1715
Health Canada National Seniors Independence Program Grants, 1722
Hedco Fndn Grants, 1733
Heiser Leprosy and Tuberculosis Research Postdoctoral Fellowships, 1736
Helen Bader Fndn Grants, 1738
Helen Hay Whitney Fndn Postdoctoral Research Fellowships, 1739
Henry J. Kaiser Family Fndn Grants, 1748
Hershey Company Grants, 1754
HHMI Grants and Fellowships Programs, 1759
HHMI International Research Scholars Program, 1760
HHMI/EMBO Start-up Grants for Central Europe, 1766
Honeywell Fndn Grants, 1791
HRB Clinical Research Training Fellowships, 1800
HRB Health Services Research Fellowships, 1801
HRB Postdoctoral Research Fellowships, 1802
IARC Postdoctoral Fellowships for Training in Cancer Research, 1832
International Cancer Technology Transfer Fellowships, 1858
International College of Surgeons Grants and Scholarships, 1859
International Essential Tremor Fndn Grants, 1860
International Fellowships in Medical Education, 1861
International Oncology Nursing Fellowships, 1862
International Spinal Research Trust Grants, 1863
Isabel Allende Fndn Esperanza Grants, 1868
IWMF Public Health Fellowship, 1871
Jacob and Hilda Blaustein Fndn Grants, 1881
James H. Cummings Fndn Grants, 1888
James S. McDonnell Fndn Research Grants, 1898
Jane Coffin Childs Memorial Fund for Medical Research Fellowships, 1903
Japan Heart Fndn Grants, 1906
Jewish Women's Fndn of New York Grants, 1924
John Deere Fndn Grants, 1929
Johns Manville Fund Grants, 1950
Johnson & Johnson Comm Health Care Program Grants, 1951
Johnson & Johnson Corp Contributions Grants, 1952
Johnson and Johnson / SAH Arts and Healing Grants, 1953
KFC Allied Health Research Grants, 1996
KFC Biomedical Fellowships, 1997
KFC Biomedical Research Grants, 1998
KFC Nephrology and Urology Scholarships, 1999
Kiwanis International Fndn Grants, 2004
Kraft Cares International Grants, 2016
LAM Fndn Established Investigator Awards, 2022
LAM Fndn Research Grants, 2024
Lance Armstrong Fndn Research Grants, 2026
Landon Fndn-AACR Innovator Award for International Collaboration, 2028
Leukaemia Research Fund Grants, 2050
Lewis Preston Fund for Girls Education Grants, 2052
Life Sciences Research Fndn Postdoctoral Fellowships, 2054
Liliane Fndn Grants, 2055
Lindbergh Grants, 2059
LRF New Investigator Leukemia Research Grants, 2070
LSA Translational Research Program Grants, 2078
Ludwick Family Fndn Grants, 2084
Lustgarten Fndn for Pancreatic Cancer Research Grants, 2086
Lymphoma Research Fndn Grants, 2088
M-A-C AIDS Fund Grants, 2091
Manuel D. and Rhoda Mayerson Fndn Grants, 2100
MAP International Medical Fellowships, 2101
MAPFRE Fndn for Medicine Grants, 2102
Mary Kay Ash Charitable Fndn Grants, 2120
Matsumae International Fndn Grants, 2129
Mattel International Grants, 2131
Max Bell Fndn Grants, 2134
McKnight Fndn Grants, 2146
Mead Johnson Nutritionals Charitable Giving Grants, 2156
Mead Johnson Nutritionals Medical Education Grants, 2158
Medical/Nursing Education, Research, and Health Care Exchanges with Taiwan, 2165
Mesothelioma Applied Research Fndn Grants, 2174
MGFA Post-Doctoral Research Fellowships, 2183
Michael J. Fox Fndn Clinical Discovery Grants, 2190
Miguel Aleman Fndn Grants, 2197
Milagro Fndn Grants, 2198
Millipore Fndn Grants, 2203
MRC Career Establishment Grants, 2221
MSSC Research Grants, 2226
National Heart Fndn of New Zealand Grants, 2255
National Lottery Comm Fund Grants, 2256
NCI/NIDA Transdisciplinary Tobacco Use Research Centers Grants, 2280
NCIC Canadian Breast Cancer Research Initiative Grants, 2281
NCIC Canadian Cancer Society Research Grants, 2282
NCIC Canadian Cancer Society Travel Award for Senior Level PhD Students, 2283
NCIC Terry Fox Postdoctoral Research Fellowships, 2285
NCIC Terry Fox Research Studentships, 2286
NHLBI Elucidating Nature's Solutions to Heart, Lung, and Blood Diseases and Sleep Disorder Processes Research Grants, 2333
NIA Malnutrition in Older Persons Research Grants, 2413
NIA Research Grants on Chemical Senses: Neurotransmitters and Neuromodulators, 2430
NIA Symptom Management for Chronic Neurological Conditions Research Grants, 2436
NIA/NIEHS Biomedical Epidemiologic and Intervention Studies Planning Grants, 2441
NIAAA Hepatitis C Infection and Alcoholic Liver Disease, 2442
NIAAA Mechanisms of Alcohol-Induced Hepatic Fibrosis Research Grants, 2445
NIAAA Peptide Regulation of Alcohol Intake, 2447
NIAID Enhancing Vaccine-Elicited Protective Immunity in Malaria Research Grants, 2452
NIAID HIV Prevention Trial Units Grants, 2453
NIAID HIV Vaccine Clinical Trial Units Grants, 2454
NIAID HIV Vaccine Research and Design-- Program Project Grants, 2455
NIAID Laboratory Methods to Assess Responses to HIV Vaccine Candidates Research Grants, 2458
NIAID Statistical Methods in HIV and AIDS Research Grants, 2464
NIAID Therapeutics Research on AIDS-Associated Opportunistic Infections, 2465
NIAMS Mechanisms of Chondroprotection Research Grants, 2472
NIAMS Pathogenesis and Therapy of the Muscular Dystrophies Research Grants, 2474
NICHD Socioeconomic Status and Health Across the Life Course, 2495
NICHD Symptom Management for Chronic Neurological Conditions Research Grants, 2496
NIDA Behavioral Therapies Development Program Grants, 2499
NIDA Drug Addiction Neuroscience Research Grants, 2503
NIDA International Studies on Drug Abuse and HIV/AIDS, 2505
NIDA Role of Limbic System and Brain Ontogeny in Drug Abuse Research Grants, 2514
NIDCD Health Promotion and Disease Prevention: Health Communication, Development, and Dissemination, 2521
NIDCD Symptom Management for Chronic Neurological Conditions Research Grants, 2532
NIDCR Clinical Trial Pilot Grant, 2533
NIDCR Clinical Trial Planning Grant, 2534
NIDCR International Collaborative Oral Health Research Planning Grant, 2536
NIDDK Co-Activators and Co-Repressors in Gene Expression Grants, 2546
NIDDK Neurobiology of Diabetic Complications Grants, 2568
NIEHS Structure-Function Relationships of Environmentally Relevant Genetic Variants Research Grants, 2606
NIEHS/NINDS Role of the Environment in Parkinson's Disease, 2608
NIGMS Institutional Research and Academic Career Development Award, 2614
NIGMS Large-Scale Collaborative Project Awards, 2616
NIGMS Quantitative Approaches to the Analysis of Complex Biological Systems, 2626
NIGMS Supplements for the Study of Complex Biological Systems, 2630
NIGMS/NIDCR Evolution of Infectious Diseases Research Grants, 2633
NIH Alzheimer's Disease Clinical Trial Planning Grant, 2636
NIH Biobehavioral Pain Research Grants, 2638
NIH Biology, Development, and Progression of Malignant Prostate Disease Research Grants, 2641
NIH Bone and the Hematopoietic and Immune Systems Research Grants, 2643
NIH Cancer Surveillance Using Health Claims-Based Data System Grants, 2645
NIH Centers for Dietary Supplements Research: Botanicals, 2648
NIH Ethical Issues in Human Studies Research Grants, 2661
NIH Exploratory/Development Grants for Mental Health Intervention Research, 2665
NIH Genetic Architecture of Complex Phenotypes, 2668
NIH Genetic Susceptibility and Variability of Human Malformations Research Grants, 2669
NIH Human Brain Project (Neuroinformatics) Phase I & II, 2672
NIH Low Birthweight in Minority Populations Research Grants, 2683
NIH Mechanisms Underlying Individual Variations in Drug Responses, 2685
NIH Molecular Epidemiology of Prostate Carcinogenesis Grants, 2691
NIH National Occupational Research Agenda Grants, 2696
NIH New Directions in Pain Research Grants, 2698
NIH Pathological Gambling: Basic, Clinical, and Services Research Grants, 2702
NIH Protein Structure Initiative (Structural Genomics) Research Grants, 2704
NIH Structural Biology of Membrane Proteins Grants, 2730
NIH Studies of Ethical, Legal, and Social Implications of Research into Human Genetic Variation Grants, 2731
NIH Targeting Research Gaps in HIV Therapeutics Research Grants, 2734
NIH Xenobiotics and Cell Death/Injury in Neurodegenerative Disease Research Grants, 2739

NIH Zebrafish as an Animal Model for Development and Disease Research Grants, 2740
NIH/EPA Mechanistic-Based Cancer Risk Assessment Methods Research Grants, 2741
NIMH Behavior Genetics in Adulthood and Old Age Research Grants, 2747
NIMH Collaborative R01s for Clinical Studies of Mental Disorders, 2752
NIMH Early Identification and Treatment of Mental Disorders in Children and Adolescents Grants, 2756
NIMH HIV/AIDS, Severe Mental Illness, and Homelessness Research Grants, 2757
NIMH Mental Health Dissemination Research Grants, 2762
NIMH Quantitative Approaches to the Analysis of Complex Biological Systems, 2767
NIMH Risk Factors for Psychopathology Using Existing Data Sets Grants, 2768
NIMH Socioeconomic Status and Health Across the Life Course, 2772
NIMH/NIDA Children's Services Program Grants, 2775
NINDS Cerebral Radiobiology and Neuroimaging of Brain Tumors Research Grants, 2778
NINDS Pathogenesis and Therapy of the Muscular Dystrophies Research Grants, 2783
NINDS Symptom Management for Chronic Neurological Conditions Research Grants, 2787
NINR Acute and Chronic Care During Mechanical Ventilation Research Grants, 2788
NINR Clinical Interventions for Managing the Symptoms of Stroke Research Grants, 2793
NINR Management of Symptoms at the End of Life Grants, 2796
NINR Quality of Life for Individuals at the End of Life Grants, 2802
NINR Symptom Management for Chronic Neurological Conditions Research Grants, 2805
Northwood University/Alden B. Dow Creativity Center Summer Residency Program, 2871
NSERC Brockhouse Canada Prize for Interdisciplinary Research in Science and Engineering Grant, 2873
Nuffield Fndn Children and Families Grants, 2899
Nuffield Fndn Law and Society Grants, 2900
Nuffield Fndn Small Grants, 2903
Olin Corporation Charitable Trust Grants, 2943
OREF Orthopedic Career Development Awards, 2954
OREF Orthopedic Resident Research Awards, 2955
OREF Research Grants, 2957
OREF/AAOS Clinical Research Training Fellowship, 2958
OSI Access to Essential Medicines Grants, 2964
OSI European Commission Internships for Young Roma Graduates, 2965
OSI Indonesia Project Grants, 2967
OSI Integrating Health and Legal Services Grants, 2968
OSI Mental Health Grants, 2969
OSI Palliative Cancer Care Grants, 2970
OSI Supplementary Grants: Burma, 2971
PAHO-ASM International Professorship for Latin America, 2983
PAHO/WHO Fellowships, 2984
Parker B. Francis Fellowships in Pulmonary Research, 2989
Paul Balint Charitable Trust Grants, 2998
PDF International Research Grants, 3005
Pediatric Brain Tumor Research Grants, 3012
Pfizer Fndn Grants, 3025
PKD Fndn Lillian Kaplan International Prize for the Advancement in the Understanding of Polycystic Kidney Disease, 3056
Potts Memorial Fndn Grants, 3072
Prospect Burma Scholarships, 3085
Public Welfare Fndn Grants, 3089
Puerto Rico Comm Fndn Grants, 3090
Rajiv Gandhi Fndn Grants, 3104
Raskob Fndn for Catholic Activities Grants, 3107
RCPSC Detweiler Traveling Fellowships, 3114
RCPSC International Traveling Fellowship, 3118
RCPSC Medical Education Traveling Fellowships, 3125
RCPSC Royal College Fellowship for Studies in Medical Education, 3127
RCPSC Walter C. MacKenzie Fellowship in Surgery, 3133
Rett Syndrome Research Fndn Grants, 3151
Richard and Rhoda Goldman Fund Grants, 3158
Rockefeller Archive Center Research Grants, 3178
Rockefeller Brothers Fund Peace and Security Grants, 3179
Rockefeller Brothers Fund Pivotal Places Grants: South Africa, 3180
Rockefeller Fndn Grants, 3181
Rockwell Collins Charitable Contributions, 3182
Rohm and Haas Company Grants, 3185
Rosalinde and Arthur Gilbert Fndn/AFAR New Investigator Awards in Alzheimer's Disease, 3187
RSC Abbyann D. Lynch Medal in Bioethics, 3195
RSC Jason A. Hannah Medal, 3196
RSC McLaughlin Medal, 3197
RSC McNeil Medal for the Public Awareness of Science, 3198
RSC Thomas W. Eadie Medal, 3199
Russell Berrie Fndn Grants, 3201
Sigrid Juselius Fndn Grants, 3286
Simone and Cino del Duca Grand Prix Awards, 3288
Sir Dorabji Tata Trust Grants for NGOs or Voluntary Organizations, 3291
Sir Halley Stewart Trust Grants, 3293
SNM Postdoctoral Molecular Imaging Scholar Grants, 3305
SNM Student Fellowship Awards, 3306
SNM/ Covidien Seed Grant in Molecular Imaging/ Nuclear Medicine Research, 3308
SOBP A.E. Bennett Research Award, 3313
Special Olympics Health Professions Student Grants, 3355
SRC Medical Research Grants, 3362
SSHRC Image, Text, Sound and Technology (ITST) Grants, 3363
SSHRC Research/Creation Grants in Fine Arts, 3364
Starr Fndn Grants, 3377
Steelcase Fndn Grants, 3379
Susan G. Komen Breast Cancer Fndn Postdoctoral Fellowships, 3411
Takemi Program in International Health Research and Advanced Training Fellowships, 3416
Thrasher Research Fund Grants, 3426
Tifa Fndn Grants, 3428
Trull Fndn Grants, 3441
U.S. Department of Education United States-Russia Program: Improving Research and Educational Activities in Higher Education, 3451
UICC American Cancer Society International Fellowships for Beginning Investigators, 3455
UICC International Cancer Technology Transfer (ICRETT) Fellowships, 3456
UICC Yamagiwa-Yoshida Memorial International Cancer Study Grants, 3458
UK Fndn for the Study of Infant Deaths Grants, 3459
United Methodist Church Malaria Control Grants, 3464
United Technologies Corporation Grants, 3466
W.K. Kellogg Fndn Healthy Kids Grants, 3507
Warren Alpert Fndn Prize, 3518
Whitaker International Fellows and Scholars Program, 3532
Wilhelm Sander Fndn Grants, 3535
YSA Get Ur Good On Grants, 3555

Job Training/Adult Vocational Programs

3M Fndn Grants, 11
A Fund for Women Grants, 14
Able Trust Vocational Rehabilitation Grants for Individuals, 186
ACE Charitable Fndn Grants, 199
ACF Supplemental Services for Recently Arrived Refugees Grants, 203
Achelis and Bodman Fndns Grants, 206
Actors Fund Social Services and Financial Assistance, 225
Adaptec Fndn Grants, 232
Alaska Airlines Fndn Grants, 324
Alcoa Fndn Grants, 334
Allstate Corp Giving Grants, 363
AMD Corp Contributions Grants, 411
Anschutz Family Fndn Grants, 486
ARCO Fndn Education Grants, 526
ASHA Students Preparing for Academic & Research Careers (SPARC) Award, 574
Ashland Corp Contributions Grants, 586
Assisi Fndn Grants, 653
Assurant Health Fndn Grants, 655
AT&T Excelerator, 657
AT&T Fndn Civic and Comm Service Program Grants, 658
Atkinson Fndn International Grants, 661
Benton Comm Fndn Grants, 743
Berks County Comm Fndn Grants, 745
Bernard and Audre Rapoport Fndn Grants, 746
Bernard F. and Alva B. Gimbel Fndn Grants, 747
Blue River Comm Fndn Grants, 770
Boeing Company Contributions Program Grants, 777
Boston Fndn Grants, 783
Boston Jewish Comm Women's Fund Grants, 785
Bridgestone/Firestone Trust Fund Grants, 792
Brown County Comm Fndn Grants, 807
Burlington Industries Fndn Grants, 811
Bush Fndn Health & Human Services Grants, 814
Cargill Citizenship Fund-Corp Giving Grants, 865
Carrie Estelle Doheny Fndn Grants, 883
Catholic Campaign for Human Development (CCHD) Comm Organizing Grants, 891
Charlotte County (FL) Comm Fndn Grants, 973
Chiron Fndn Comm Grants, 1004
Citizens Bank Mid-Atlantic Charitable Fndn Grants, 1015
Clark Fndn Grants, 1029
Clay Fndn Grants, 1034
Cleveland Browns Fndn Grants, 1036
Comer Fndn Grants, 1072
Comm Fndn of Bartholomew County Heritage Fund Grants, 1096
Comm Fndn of Broward Grants, 1100
Comm Fndn of Grant County Grants, 1104
Coors Brewing Corp Contributions Grants, 1151
Cruise Industry Charitable Fndn Grants, 1166
DaimlerChrysler Corporation Fund Grants, 1186
Dallas Women's Fndn Grants, 1191
Denver Fndn Comm Grants, 1227
Duke Energy Fndn Grants, 1339
eBay Fndn Comm Grants, 1363
Evjue Fndn Grants, 1439
Faye McBeath Fndn Grants, 1456
Field Fndn of Illinois Grants, 1499
Fisher Fndn Grants, 1508
Ford Motor Company Fund Grants, 1522
Fndn for the Carolinas Grants, 1535
Frances L. and Edwin L. Cummings Memorial Fund Grants, 1547
George Family Fndn Grants, 1598
Greater Milwaukee Fndn Grants, 1653
Gulf Coast Comm of Venice Fndn Grants, 1677
Hallmark Corp Fndn Grants, 1688
Harry S. Black and Allon Fuller Fund, 1706
Harvest Fndn Grants, 1713
Helen Bader Fndn Grants, 1738
HHK Employment Grants, 1755
Highmark Corp Giving Grants, 1769
Hudson Webber Fndn Grants, 1813
Irvin Stern Fndn Grants, 1866
Isabel Allende Fndn Esperanza Grants, 1868
Jane Bradley Pettit Fndn Grants, 1902

Jewish Comm Fndn of Greater Los Angeles Grants, 1921
JM Fndn Grants, 1926
John Edward Fowler Memorial Fndn Grants, 1930
John Merck Fund Grants, 1940
Johnson & Johnson Corp Contributions Grants, 1952
Joyce Fndn Grants, 1969
K. M. Hunter Charitable Fndn Social Welfare Grants, 1974
Katharine Matthies Fndn Grants, 1982
King Pharmaceuticals Corp Contributions Grants, 2003
Liberty Bank Fndn Grants, 2053
M.B. and Edna Zale Fndn Grants, 2093
McGregor Fund Grants, 2143
McKnight Fndn Grants, 2146
Middlesex Savings Charitable Fndn Grants, 2196
Montgomery County Comm Fndn Grants, 2214
Morris and Gwendolyn Cafritz Fndn Grants, 2217
Ms. Fndn for Women Grants, 2222
NNEDVF/Altria Doors of Hope Program, 2847
Northeast Utilities Fndn Grants, 2863
Northern Trust Company Charitable Trust and Corp Giving Program, 2865
Northrop Grumman Corporation Grants, 2866
OceanFirst Fndn Grants, 2933
PacifiCare Fndn Grants, 2981
Palm Beach and Martin Counties Grants, 2986
Paul and Mary Haas Fndn Contributions and Student Scholarships, 2997
Perry County Comm Fndn Grants, 3016
Piedmont Natural Gas Grants, 3048
Piper Jaffray Companies Building Strong Communities Grants, 3053
Polk Bros. Fndn Grants, 3066
Portland General Electric Fndn Grants, 3067
Principal Financial Group Fndn Grants, 3082
Public Welfare Fndn Grants, 3089
Pulaski County Comm Fndn Grants, 3091
Rasmuson Fndn Grants, 3108
Richard King Mellon Fndn Grants, 3161
Robert P. & Clara I. Milton Fund for Senior Housing, 3172
Robin Hood Fndn Grants, 3174
Rockefeller Fndn Grants, 3181
RWJF Jobs to Careers: Promoting Work-Based Learning for Quality Care - Research Grants, 3221
S. Mark Taper Fndn Grants, 3236
SAG Motion Picture Players Welfare Fund Grants, 3238
Samuel S. Johnson Fndn Grants, 3251
Seneca Foods Fndn Grants, 3278
Sid W. Richardson Fndn Grants, 3284
Starr Fndn Grants, 3377
Taproot Fndn Capacity-Building Service Grants, 3417
Topfer Family Fndn Grants, 3430
U.S. Department of Education Rehabilitation Research Training Centers (RRTCs), 3448
U.S. Department of Education Vocational Rehabilitation Services Projects for American Indians with Disabilities Grants, 3452
Vectren Fndn Grants, 3485
Verizon Fndn Maryland Grants, 3487
Verizon Fndn New York Grants, 3488
Verizon Fndn Pennsylvania Grants, 3490
Waitt Family Fndn Grants, 3512
Wal-Mart Fndn Comm Grants, 3513
Wal-Mart State Giving Program Grants, 3514

Matching/Challenge Funds

3M Fndn Grants, 11
A.O. Smith Comm Grants, 18
Abbott Fund Global AIDS Care Grants, 178
Abell-Hanger Fndn Grants, 183
ACE Charitable Fndn Grants, 199
Adaptec Fndn Grants, 232
AEC Trust Grants, 242
AEGON Transamerica Fndn Grants, 243
Aetna Fndn Sponsorships Grants in Connecticut, 251
Ahmanson Fndn Grants, 303
AIG American General Corporation Grants, 316
Air Products and Chemicals Grants, 319
Alabama Power Fndn Grants, 321
Alberto Culver Corp Contributions Grants, 329
Albertson's Charitable Giving Grants, 330
Alcoa Fndn Grants, 334
Alice Tweed Tuohy Fndn Grants, 357
Allegan County Comm Fndn Grants, 358
Allegheny Technologies Charitable Trust, 359
Allen P. and Josephine B. Green Fndn Grants, 361
Allstate Corp Giving Grants, 363
Allstate Corp Hometown Commitment Grants, 364
Allyn Fndn Grants, 365
Amarillo Area/Harrington Fndns Grants, 410
AMI Semiconductors Corp Grants, 468
Anheuser-Busch Fndn Grants, 474
Ann Arbor Area Comm Fndn Grants, 476
Ann Peppers Fndn Grants, 478
ARCO Fndn Education Grants, 526
Arie and Ida Crown Memorial Grants, 528
Arizona Public Service Corp Giving Program Grants, 531
Arkell Hall Fndn Grants, 534
Ashland Corp Contributions Grants, 586
Assurant Health Fndn Grants, 655
Atherton Family Fndn Grants, 659
Atran Fndn Grants, 663
Autzen Fndn Grants, 672
Avon Products Fndn Grants, 675
Bailey Fndn Grants, 680
Ball Brothers Fndn Grants, 684
Barker Welfare Fndn Grants, 695
Barra Fndn Project Grants, 699
Batchelor Fndn Grants, 701
Baton Rouge Area Fndn Grants, 702
Battle Creek Comm Fndn Grants, 703
Batts Fndn Grants, 704
Baxter International Fndn Grants, 705
BCBSM Comm Health Matching Grants, 715
Beckley Area Fndn Grants, 732
Becton Dickinson and Company Grants, 736
Bender Fndn Grants, 742
Benton Comm Fndn Grants, 743
Bernard and Audre Rapoport Fndn Grants, 746
Bertha Russ Lytel Fndn Grants, 751
Besser Fndn Grants, 752
Blackford County Comm Fndn Grants, 763
Blanche and Julian Robertson Family Fndn Grants, 765
Blue Grass Comm Fndn Grants, 768
Blue River Comm Fndn Grants, 770
Blumenthal Fndn Grants, 773
Bodenwein Public Benevolent Fndn Grants, 775
Bodman Fndn Grants, 776
Boeing Company Contributions Program Grants, 777
Boettcher Fndn Grants, 778
Boston Fndn Grants, 783
Bridgestone/Firestone Trust Fund Grants, 792
Bristol-Myers Squibb Fndn Health Disparities Grants, 797
Bullitt Fndn Grants, 809
Burlington Industries Fndn Grants, 811
Burlington Northern Santa Fe Fndn Grants, 812
Burton G. Bettingen Grants, 813
C.R. Bard Fndn Grants, 825
Cailloux Fndn Grants, 829
Callaway Fndn Grants, 835
Callaway Golf Company Fndn Grants, 836
Cardinal Health Fndn Grants, 864
Cargill Citizenship Fund-Corp Giving Grants, 865
Carl and Lily Pforzheimer Fndn Grants, 868
Carl C. Icahn Fndn Grants, 870
Carlisle Fndn Grants, 874
Carlos and Marguerite Mason Trust Grants, 875
Carnahan-Jackson Fndn Grants, 878
Carpenter Fndn Grants, 881
Carrie E. and Lena V. Glenn Fndn Grants, 882
Carrie Estelle Doheny Fndn Grants, 883
Cass County Comm Fndn Grants, 887
Catholic Campaign for Human Development (CCHD) Comm Organizing Grants, 891
CDC Public Health Conference Support Grants, 926
Cemala Fndn Grants, 933
Central Carolina Comm Fndn Comm Impact Grants, 936
Cessna Fndn Grants, 938
CFF Therapeutics Development Program, 949
Charles A. Frueauff Fndn Grants, 962
Charles H. Revson Fndn Grants, 969
Chatlos Fndn Grants, 977
CHCF Local Coverage Expansion Initiative, 981
Chesapeake Corporation Fndn Grants, 982
Chestnut Hill Charitable Fndn, Inc Grants, 987
Chicago Tribune's Corp Contributions Grants, 991
Christy-Houston Fndn Grants, 1008
CIGNA Fndn Grants, 1011
Claude Worthington Benedum Fndn Grants, 1033
Clay Fndn Grants, 1034
CNA Fndn Grants, 1046
Coca-Cola Fndn Grants, 1052
Cockrell Fndn Grants, 1053
Collins Fndn Grants, 1058
Colonel Stanley R. McNeil Fndn Grants, 1059
Columbus Fndn Competitive Grants, 1066
Commonwealth Fund Small Grants, 1084
Comm Fndn for Greater Buffalo Grants, 1090
Comm Fndn for Greater New Haven Grants, 1091
Comm Fndn for Monterey County Grants, 1092
Comm Fndn for Muskegon County Grants, 1093
Comm Fndn for Southern Arizona Grants, 1095
Comm Fndn of Bartholomew County Heritage Fund Grants, 1096
Comm Fndn of Boone County Grants, 1099
Comm Fndn of Greater Birmingham Grants, 1106
Comm Fndn of Greater Fort Wayne: Comm Endowment & Clarke Endowment Fund Grants, 1108
Comm Fndn Of Greater Lafayette Grants, 1110
Comm Fndn of Greater Tampa Grants, 1112
Comm Fndn of Greenville Comm Enrichment Grants, 1113
Comm Fndn of Greenville-Greenville Women Giving Grants, 1115
Comm Fndn of Mount Vernon and Knox County Grants, 1119
Comm Fndn of Muncie and Delaware County Grants, 1120
Comm Fndn of South Alabama Grants, 1123
Comm Fndn of South Puget Sound Grants, 1124
Comm Fndn of St. Joseph County Special Project Challenge Grants, 1126
Comm Fndn of the Ozarks Grants, 1130
Comm Fndn of Wabash County Grants, 1131
Comm Fndn Silicon Valley Grants, 1133
Comm Technology Fndn of California Building Communities Through Technology Grants, 1136
Compass Bank Fndn Grants, 1138
ConAgra Foods Fndn Grants, 1140
Connecticut Comm Fndn Grants, 1141
Connelly Fndn Grants, 1143
ConocoPhillips Fndn Grants, 1144
Constantin Fndn Grants, 1145
Cooke Fndn Grants, 1148
Cooper Industries Fndn Grants, 1150
Cornerstone Fndn of Northeastern Wisconsin Grants, 1152
Cowles Charitable Trust Grants, 1155
Cranston Fndn Grants, 1158
CSRA Comm Fndn Grants, 1168
DaimlerChrysler Corporation Fund Grants, 1186
Dale and Edna Walsh Fndn Grants, 1189
Dana Corporation Fndn Grants, 1196
Dana Fndn Science and Health Grants, 1197
Daniels Fund Grants, 1200
Daphne Seybolt Culpeper Memorial Fndn Grants, 1201

Daywood Fndn Grants, 1206
Della Martin Fndn Grants, 1219
DHHS Adolescent Family Life Demonstration Projects, 1243
DHHS Healthy Tomorrows Partnership for Children, 1261
DOL Occupational Safety and Health--Susan Harwood Training Grants, 1305
Dolan Fndn Grants, 1306
Dorothea Haus Ross Fndn Grants, 1320
Dr. Bob and Jean Smith Fndn Grants, 1325
Dr. John T. Macdonald Fndn Grants, 1327
Drs. Bruce and Lee Fndn Grants, 1333
Duchossois Family Fndn Grants, 1337
Duke Energy Fndn Grants, 1339
Dunspaugh-Dalton Fndn Grants, 1351
DuPage Comm Fndn Grants, 1352
Eberly Fndn Grants, 1364
Educational Fndn of America Grants, 1372
Edward Bangs Kelley and Elza Kelley Fndn Grants, 1373
Edward S. Moore Fndn Grants, 1374
Edwin S. Webster Fndn Grants, 1376
Edyth Bush Charitable Fndn Grants, 1378
Effie and Wofford Cain Fndn Grants, 1385
Eisner Fndn Grants, 1387
El Paso Comm Fndn Grants, 1388
Elizabeth Morse Genius Charitable Trust Grants, 1400
Elkhart County Comm Fndn Grants, 1401
Emerson Charitable Trust Grants, 1412
Emily Davie and Joseph S. Kornfeld Fndn Grants, 1414
Ensworth Charitable Fndn Grants, 1416
Erie Comm Fndn Grants, 1427
Eugene McDermott Fndn Grants, 1435
Ewing Halsell Fndn Grants, 1440
ExxonMobil Grants, 1442
Fairfield County Comm Fndn Grants, 1446
Fannie E. Rippel Fndn Grants, 1452
Farmers Insurance Group of Companies Grants, 1455
Fayette County Fndn Grants, 1457
FCER Chiropractic Research Grants, 1459
Federal Express Corp Contributions Program, 1483
Fidelity Fndn Grants, 1498
Field Fndn of Illinois Grants, 1499
Fireman's Fund Fndn Grants, 1504
FirstEnergy Fndn Comm Grants, 1505
Fluor Fndn Grants, 1517
FMC Fndn Grants, 1518
Foellinger Fndn Grants, 1519
Foster Fndn Grants, 1524
Fndn for Physical Therapy Research Grants, 1530
Fndn for Seacoast Health Grants, 1533
Fndn for Spirituality and Medicine Grants, 1534
Fndn for the Carolinas Grants, 1535
Fndn Northwest Grants, 1537
Frances L. and Edwin L. Cummings Memorial Fund Grants, 1547
Francis L. Abreu Charitable Trust Grants, 1549
Franklin County Comm Fndn Grants, 1554
Fred L. Emerson Fndn Grants, 1557
Frey Fndn Grants, 1562
Fuller E. Callaway Fndn Grants, 1578
G.N. Wilcox Trust Grants, 1581
Gebbie Fndn Grants, 1585
GenCorp Fndn Grants, 1587
Genentech Corp Charitable Contributions Grants, 1588
General Mills Fndn Grants, 1590
George B. Storer Fndn Grants, 1596
George F. Baker Trust Grants, 1597
George Frederick Jewett Fndn Grants, 1599
George S. and Dolores Dore Eccles Fndn Grants, 1602
Georgia Power Fndn Grants, 1603
Gertrude E. Skelly Charitable Fndn Grants, 1609
Goldman Philanthropic Partnerships Program, 1635
Goodrich Corporation Fndn Grants, 1638
Graco Fndn Grants, 1642
Grand Haven Area Comm Fndn Grants, 1644
Grand Rapids Area Comm Fndn Grants, 1645
Grand Rapids Area Comm Fndn Nashwauk Area Endowment Fund Grants, 1646
Grand Rapids Comm Fndn Grants, 1647
Great-West Life Grants, 1649
Greater Cincinnati Fndn Priority and Small Projects/Capacity-Building Grants, 1651
Greater Worcester Comm Fndn Discretionary Grants, 1658
Gulf Coast Comm Fndn Grants, 1676
H & R Fndn Grants, 1679
H.A. and Mary K. Chapman Charitable Trust Grants, 1681
Hall-Perrine Fndn Grants, 1686
Halliburton Fndn Grants, 1687
Harden Fndn Grants, 1693
Harold and Arlene Schnitzer CARE Fndn Grants, 1697
Harris and Eliza Kempner Fund Grants, 1699
Harry A. and Margaret D. Towsley Fndn Grants, 1701
Harry and Grace Steele Fndn Grants, 1702
Hartford Courant Fndn Grants, 1710
Hartford Fndn Regular Grants, 1711
Health Fndn of Greater Indianapolis Grants, 1725
Hedco Fndn Grants, 1733
HHK Employment Grants, 1755
High Meadow Fndn Grants, 1768
Hill Crest Fndn Grants, 1773
Hill Fndn Grants, 1774
Holland/Zeeland Comm Fndn Grants, 1786
Honda of America Manufacturing Fndn Grants, 1790
Honeywell Fndn Grants, 1791
Horace A. Kimball and S. Ella Kimball Fndn Grants, 1792
Hormel Foods Charitable Trust Grants, 1795
Howard and Bush Fndn Grants, 1798
Hugh J. Andersen Fndn Grants, 1814
Huie-Dellmon Trust Grants, 1815
Humana Fndn Grants, 1818
Hutton Fndn Grants, 1828
Idaho Power Company Corp Contributions, 1838
Indiana 21st Century Research and Technology Fund Awards, 1850
J.W. Kieckhefer Fndn Grants, 1878
James H. Cummings Fndn Grants, 1888
James J. and Angelia M. Harris Fndn Grants, 1890
James McKeen Cattell Fund Fellowships, 1893
James R. Dougherty Jr. Fndn Grants, 1894
James S. Copley Fndn Grants, 1895
Jane's Trust Grants, 1904
Jean and Louis Dreyfus Fndn Grants, 1911
JELD-WEN Fndn Grants, 1914
Jennings County Comm Fndn Grants, 1916
Jessie Ball Dupont Fund Grants, 1919
Jewish Comm Fndn of Greater Los Angeles Grants, 1921
JM Fndn Grants, 1926
John Ben Snow Memorial Trust Grants, 1928
John Deere Fndn Grants, 1929
John G. Martin Fndn Grants, 1932
John Jewett and Helen Chandler Garland Fndn Grants, 1937
John P. McGovern Fndn Grants, 1942
John R. Oishei Fndn Grants, 1944
John Stauffer Charitable Trust Grants, 1946
John W. Alden Trust Grants, 1947
John W. and Anna H. Hanes Fndn Grants, 1948
Joseph Drown Fndn Grants, 1960
Josephine Goodyear Fndn Grants, 1964
Josiah W. and Bessie H. Kline Fndn Grants, 1967
Kalamazoo Fndn Grants, 1979
Kenneth T. and Eileen L. Norris Fndn Grants, 1989
KeySpan Fndn Grants, 1995
Land O'Lakes Fndn Mid-Atlantic Grants, 2027
Lillian S. Wells Fndn Grants, 2056
Louis Calder Fndn Grants, 2065
Lubbock Area Fndn Grants, 2079
Lubrizol Fndn Grants, 2080
Lynde and Harry Bradley Fndn Grants, 2089
M.E. Raker Fndn Grants, 2094
Maine Comm Fndn Grants, 2099
Manuel D. and Rhoda Mayerson Fndn Grants, 2100
Margaret T. Morris Fndn Grants, 2105
Margoes Fndn Grants, 2106
Marion I. and Henry J. Knott Fndn Grants, 2109
Mark and Catherine Winkler Fndn Grants, 2112
Mary Owen Borden Fndn Grants, 2121
Mary S. and David C. Corbin Fndn Grants, 2122
Matilda R. Wilson Fund Grants, 2128
Max Bell Fndn Grants, 2134
McCarthy Family Fndn Grants, 2141
McGregor Fund Grants, 2143
McKesson Fndn Grants, 2145
McMillen Fndn Grants, 2148
Mead Witter Fndn Grants, 2160
Meadows Fndn Grants, 2161
Medtronic Fndn Health Care Grants, 2169
Mericos Fndn Grants, 2172
Metro Health Fndn Grants, 2175
Meyer Memorial Trust Grassroots Grants, 2179
Meyer Memorial Trust Responsive Grants, 2181
Millipore Fndn Grants, 2203
Miriam and Peter Haas Fund Grants, 2208
MONY Fndn Grants, 2215
Morris and Gwendolyn Cafritz Fndn Grants, 2217
National Starch and Chemical Fndn Grants, 2261
Nelda C. and H.J. Lutcher Stark Fndn Grants, 2301
New York Life Fndn Grants, 2304
NFID New Investigator Matching Grants, 2310
Nina Mason Pulliam Charitable Trust Grants, 2776
Noble County Comm Fndn Grants, 2848
Nordson Corporation Fndn Grants, 2851
North Carolina Comm Development Grants, 2858
Northwestern Mutual Fndn Grants, 2870
NSF BIO Minority Postdoctoral Research Fellowships, 2877
NSF Grant Opportunities for Academic Liaison with Industry (GOALI), 2887
NWHF Partners Investing in Nursing's Future Grants, 2908
Ordean Fndn Grants, 2952
Otto Bremer Fndn Grants, 2977
Pasadena Fndn Average Grants, 2994
Patron Saints Fndn Grants, 2996
Paul and Mary Haas Fndn Contributions and Student Scholarships, 2997
Paul E. and Klare N. Reinhold Fndn Grants, 2999
Paul G. Duke Fndn Grants, 3001
PeyBack Fndn Grants, 3022
Philadelphia Fndn Organizational Effectiveness Grants, 3029
Phoenix Suns Charities Grants, 3030
PhRMA Fndn Health Outcomes Sabbatical Fellowships, 3034
PhRMA Fndn Informatics Sabbatical Fellowships, 3035
PhRMA Fndn Pharmaceutics Sabbatical Fellowships, 3043
PhRMA Fndn Pharmacology/Toxicology Sabbatical Fellowships, 3047
Piper Jaffray Companies Building Strong Communities Grants, 3053
Plough Fndn Grants, 3061
Polaroid Fund Grants, 3065
Principal Financial Group Fndn Grants, 3082
Progress Energy Fndn Grants, 3084
Prudential Fndn Grants, 3087
Public Welfare Fndn Grants, 3089
Puerto Rico Comm Fndn Grants, 3090
Pulaski County Comm Fndn Grants, 3091
Putnam County Comm Fndn Grants, 3093
Quantum Fndn Grants, 3096
R.C. Baker Fndn Grants, 3098
Raskob Fndn for Catholic Activities Grants, 3107
Rasmuson Fndn Grants, 3108
Rathmann Family Fndn Grants, 3109
Rayonier Fndn Grants, 3111

Rhode Island Fndn Grants, 3154
Richard and Helen DeVos Fndn Grants, 3157
Richard King Mellon Fndn Grants, 3161
Ripley County Comm Fndn Grants, 3166
Rochester Area Fndn Grants, 3177
Rockwell International Corp Trust Grants, 3183
Rohm and Haas Company Grants, 3185
Roy and Christine Sturgis Trust Grants, 3191
Roy J. Carver Charitable Trust Medical and Science Research Grants, 3192
RRF General Program Grants, 3193
Rush County Comm Fndn Grants, 3200
RWJF Executive Nurse Fellowships, 3210
RWJF Local Funding Partnerships Program Grants, 3223
RWJF Partners Investing in Nursing's Future Grants, 3226
S. Mark Taper Fndn Grants, 3236
Samuel Roberts Noble Fndn Grants, 3250
Samuel S. Johnson Fndn Grants, 3251
San Diego Women's Fndn Grants, 3259
Sarah Scaife Fndn Grants, 3263
Schering-Plough Fndn Health Grants, 3270
Scott County Comm Fndn Grants, 3273
Self Fndn Grants, 3277
Shell Oil Company Fndn Grants, 3281
Sid W. Richardson Fndn Grants, 3284
Sisters of St. Joseph Healthcare Fndn Grants, 3297
Sonoco Fndn Grants, 3347
Sosland Fndn Grants, 3348
South Madison Comm Fndn Grants, 3349
Southwest Florida Comm Fndn Competitive Grants, 3351
Sprague Fndn Grants, 3359
Square D Fndn Grants, 3361
SSHRC Research/Creation Grants in Fine Arts, 3364
St. Joseph Comm Health Fndn Improving Healthcare Access Grants, 3368
Steelcase Fndn Grants, 3379
Steele-Reese Fndn Grants, 3380
Steuben County Comm Fndn Grants, 3383
Stewart Huston Charitable Trust Grants, 3384
Strowd Roses Grants, 3388
Sunderland Fndn Grants, 3400
Susan Vaughan Fndn Grants, 3413
Temple-Inland Fndn Grants, 3419
Texas Commission on the Arts Arts Respond Project Grants, 3420
Thomas C. Ackerman Fndn Grants, 3423
Trull Fndn Grants, 3441
United Technologies Corporation Grants, 3466
US Trust Corporation Fndn Grants, 3475
Varian Medical Systems Grants, 3481
VDH Rescue Squad Assistance Fund Grants, 3484
Verizon Fndn Virginia Grants, 3492
Vulcan Materials Company Fndn Grants, 3504
W.W. Smith Charitable Trust Grants for Medical Research in Cancer, AIDS, and Heart Disease, 3509
Wachovia Fndn Grants, 3511
Walt Disney Company Fndn Grants, 3516
Washington Post Contributions Program Grants, 3520
Wasie Fndn Grants, 3521
Wayne and Gladys Valley Fndn Grants, 3522
Weatherwax Fndn Grants, 3523
Weingart Fndn Grants, 3524
Wells County Fndn Grants, 3527
William G. McGowan Charitable Fund Grants, 3539
Winston-Salem Fndn Competitive Grants, 3544
Z. Smith Reynolds Fndn Small Grants, 3557

Materials/Equipment Acquisition (Computers, Books, Videos, etc.)

AACN Clinical Inquiry Fund Grants, 56
AACN End of Life/Palliative Care Small Projects Grants, 59
AACN Physio-Control Small Projects Grants, 62
AACN-Edwards Lifesciences Nurse-Driven Clinical Practice Outcomes Grants, 63
Abell-Hanger Fndn Grants, 183
Abington Fndn Grants, 184
Able To Serve Grants, 185
Able Trust Vocational Rehabilitation Grants for Individuals, 186
ACGT Investigators Grants, 204
Achelis and Bodman Fndns Grants, 206
Acushnet Fndn Grants, 226
Adams County Fndn Grants - Pennsylvania, 231
Adelaide Breed Bayrd Fndn Grants, 234
Administaff Comm Affairs Grants, 235
AEC Trust Grants, 242
Agnes M. Lindsay Trust Grants, 263
AHFMR Establishment and Independent Establishment Grants, 273
AHFMR Major Equipment Grants, 285
Ahmanson Fndn Grants, 303
AIDS Vaccine Advocacy Coalition (AVAC) Fund Grants, 315
Air Products and Chemicals Grants, 319
Alex Brown and Sons Charitable Fndn Grants, 337
Alexander and Margaret Stewart Trust Grants, 340
Alfred P. Sloan Fndn History of Science and Technology Grants, 352
Alice Tweed Tuohy Fndn Grants, 357
Allegan County Comm Fndn Grants, 358
Allegheny Technologies Charitable Trust, 359
Allen P. and Josephine B. Green Fndn Grants, 361
Allyn Fndn Grants, 365
AMA Fndn Worldscopes Program, 399
American Academy of Dermatology Shade Structure Grants, 413
American Schlafhorst Fndn Grants, 454
Amgen Fndn Grants, 467
Andersen Fndn Grants, 471
Anheuser-Busch Fndn Grants, 474
Ann Arbor Area Comm Fndn Grants, 476
Arcadia Fndn Grants, 524
ARCO Fndn Education Grants, 526
Arie and Ida Crown Memorial Grants, 528
Arkell Hall Fndn Grants, 534
Armstrong McDonald Fndn Grants, 537
ASCO State Affiliate Grants, 547
ASHFndn Research Grant in Speech Science, 583
Assisi Fndn Grants, 653
AT&T Excelerator, 657
AT&T Fndn Civic and Comm Service Program Grants, 658
Atherton Family Fndn Grants, 659
Atlanta Fndn Grants, 662
Auburn Fndn Grants, 664
Aurora Fndn Grants, 667
AVDF Health Care Grants, 673
Bailey Fndn Grants, 680
Balance Bar Sports Individual/Team Grants, 681
Ball Brothers Fndn General Grants, 683
Barker Welfare Fndn Grants, 695
Barnes Group Fndn Grants, 696
Battle Creek Comm Fndn Grants, 703
BCBSM Fndn Primary and Clinical Prevention Grants, 719
BCBSNC Fndn Grants, 725
Bearemy's Kennel Pals Grants, 728
Beazley Fndn Grants, 730
Beckley Area Fndn Grants, 732
Ben B. Cheney Fndn Grants, 741
Benton Comm Fndn Grants, 743
Bill and Melinda Gates Fndn Grants, 756
Blackford County Comm Fndn Grants, 763
Blanche and Irving Laurie Fndn Grants, 764
Blanche and Julian Robertson Family Fndn Grants, 765
Blowitz-Ridgeway Fndn Early Childhood Development Research Award, 766
Blue Grass Comm Fndn Grants, 768
Blue River Comm Fndn Grants, 770
Blumenthal Fndn Grants, 773
Bodenwein Public Benevolent Fndn Grants, 775
Bodman Fndn Grants, 776
Boeing Company Contributions Program Grants, 777
Boettcher Fndn Grants, 778
Booth-Bricker Fund Grants, 780
Borkee-Hagley Fndn Grants, 781
Bosque Fndn Grants, 782
Boston Globe Fndn Grants, 784
Brown County Comm Fndn Grants, 807
Bushrod H. Campbell and Adah F. Hall Charity Fund Grants, 816
Byron W. and Alice L. Lockwood Fndn Grants, 824
C.W. Titus Fndn Grants, 826
Cailloux Fndn Grants, 829
California Endowment CommunitiesFirst Grants, 833
Callaway Fndn Grants, 835
Cambridge Comm Fndn Grants, 837
Campbell Hoffman Fndn Grants, 840
Cancer Research UK Grants, 859
Capital Region Comm Fndn Grants, 862
Cargill Citizenship Fund-Corp Giving Grants, 865
Carl Gellert and Celia Berta Gellert Fndn Grants, 871
Carl W. and Carrie Mae Joslyn Trust Grants, 873
Carlos and Marguerite Mason Trust Grants, 875
Carls Fndn Grants, 876
Carnahan-Jackson Fndn Grants, 878
Carpenter Fndn Grants, 881
Carrie E. and Lena V. Glenn Fndn Grants, 882
Carrie Estelle Doheny Fndn Grants, 883
CCFF Research Grants, 894
Cemala Fndn Grants, 933
Central Carolina Comm Fndn Comm Impact Grants, 936
Central Okanagan Fndn Grants, 937
Cessna Fndn Grants, 938
Challenged Athletes Fndn Grants, 958
Champ-A Champion Fur Kids Grants, 959
Champlin Fndns Grants, 960
Charles A. Frueauff Fndn Grants, 962
Charles H. Dater Fndn Grants, 966
Charles H. Farnsworth Trust Grants, 967
Chatlos Fndn Grants, 977
Chestnut Hill Charitable Fndn, Inc Grants, 987
Children Affected by AIDS Fndn Family Assistance Emergency Fund Grants, 996
Chiles Fndn Grants, 1003
Christy-Houston Fndn Grants, 1008
Clark County Comm Fndn Grants, 1028
Clark Fndn Grants, 1029
Claude Worthington Benedum Fndn Grants, 1033
CNA Fndn Grants, 1046
CNCS Foster Grandparent Projects Grants, 1048
Coastal Bend Comm Fndn Grants, 1050
Coeta and Donald Barker Fndn Grants, 1054
Collins Fndn Grants, 1058
Colorado Interstate Gas Grants, 1060
Colorado Springs Comm Trust Fund Grants, 1061
Comerica Charitable Fndn Grants, 1073
Comm Fndn for Greater Buffalo Grants, 1090
Comm Fndn for Greater New Haven Grants, 1091
Comm Fndn for Monterey County Grants, 1092
Comm Fndn for Muskegon County Grants, 1093
Comm Fndn for Southern Arizona Grants, 1095
Comm Fndn of Bartholomew County Heritage Fund Grants, 1096
Comm Fndn of Bloomington and Monroe County Grants, 1098
Comm Fndn of Boone County Grants, 1099
Comm Fndn of Broward Grants, 1100
Comm Fndn of Central Illinois Grants, 1101
Comm Fndn of Champaign County Grants, 1102
Comm Fndn of Greater Birmingham Grants, 1106
Comm Fndn of Greater Fort Wayne: Comm Endowment & Clarke Endowment Fund Grants, 1108
Comm Fndn of Greater Tampa Grants, 1112
Comm Fndn of Greenville-Greenville Women Giving Grants, 1115

Comm Fndn of Mount Vernon and Knox County Grants, 1119
Comm Fndn of Muncie and Delaware County Grants, 1120
Comm Fndn of South Puget Sound Grants, 1124
Comm Fndn of Southeastern Connecticut Grants, 1125
Comm Fndn of Wabash County Grants, 1131
Connecticut Comm Fndn Grants, 1141
Connelly Fndn Grants, 1143
ConocoPhillips Fndn Grants, 1144
Constantin Fndn Grants, 1145
Constellation Energy Group and Baltimore Gas and Electric Corp Contributions, 1146
Consumers Energy Fndn, 1147
Coors Brewing Corp Contributions Grants, 1151
Cornerstone Fndn of Northeastern Wisconsin Grants, 1152
Covenant Fndn Grants (Iowa), 1153
Cowles Charitable Trust Grants, 1155
Crail-Johnson Fndn Grants, 1157
Crestlea Fndn Grants, 1159
CSRA Comm Fndn Grants, 1168
Cudd Fndn Grants, 1171
Cullen Fndn Grants, 1172
D.V. and Ida J. McEachern Charitable Trust Grants, 1182
Dade Comm Fndn Comm AIDS Partnership Grants, 1184
DaimlerChrysler Corporation Fund Grants, 1186
Daisy Marquis Jones Fndn Grants, 1188
Dallas Women's Fndn Grants, 1191
Dana Corporation Fndn Grants, 1196
Daphne Seybolt Culpeper Memorial Fndn Grants, 1201
Daywood Fndn Grants, 1206
Deaconess Comm Fndn Grants, 1207
Delaware Comm Fndn Grants, 1215
Dell Fndn Healthy Communities, Literate Communities, and Connected Communities Grants, 1217
DeMatteis Family Fndn Grants, 1221
Denver Fndn Comm Grants, 1227
DHHS Health Care Systems Cost and Access Research and Development Grants, 1252
DOD Idea Award for Breast Cancer Research, 1294
DOJ Gang-Free Schools and Communities Intervention Grants, 1303
Dolan Fndn Grants, 1306
Doris and Victor Day Fndn Grants, 1313
Dorothea Haus Ross Fndn Grants, 1320
Dr. Leon Bromberg Charitable Trust Fund Grants, 1328
Drs. Bruce and Lee Fndn Grants, 1333
Dubois County Comm Fndn Grants, 1336
E. Rhodes and Leona B. Carpenter Fndn Grants, 1356
E.D.Thomas Fellowship, 1359
E.J. Grassmann Trust Grants, 1360
E.L. Wiegand Fndn Grants, 1361
Eastman Chemical Company Fndn Grants, 1362
EDS Fndn Grants, 1371
Edward S. Moore Fndn Grants, 1374
Edwards Memorial Trust Grants, 1375
Edwin S. Webster Fndn Grants, 1376
Edyth Bush Charitable Fndn Grants, 1378
Effie and Wofford Cain Fndn Grants, 1385
Eisner Fndn Grants, 1387
El Paso Comm Fndn Grants, 1388
El Pomar Fndn Awards and Grants, 1390
Elisabeth Severance Prentiss Fndn Grants, 1392
Ellison Medical Fndn/AFAR Postdoctoral Fellows in Aging Research Program, 1404
Erie Comm Fndn Grants, 1427
Eugene B. Casey Fndn Grants, 1433
Eugene McDermott Fndn Grants, 1435
Eva L. and Joseph M. Bruening Fndn Grants, 1436
Evjue Fndn Grants, 1439
Ewing Halsell Fndn Grants, 1440
ExxonMobil Grants, 1442
F.M. Kirby Fndn Grants, 1443
Fairfield County Comm Fndn Grants, 1446
Fan Fox and Leslie R. Samuels Fndn Grants, 1451
Fannie E. Rippel Fndn Grants, 1452
Faye McBeath Fndn Grants, 1456
Field Fndn of Illinois Grants, 1499
FirstEnergy Fndn Comm Grants, 1505
Fisa Fndn Grants, 1506
FMC Fndn Grants, 1518
Foellinger Fndn Grants, 1519
Ford Motor Company Fund Grants, 1522
Fndn for Medical Research Grants, 1528
Fndn for Seacoast Health Grants, 1533
Fndn for the Carolinas Grants, 1535
Francis L. Abreu Charitable Trust Grants, 1549
Frank E. and Seba B. Payne Fndn Grants, 1551
Frank G. and Freida K. Brotz Family Fndn Grants, 1552
Frank Stanley Beveridge Fndn Grants, 1553
Frey Fndn Grants, 1562
Frist Fndn Grants, 1563
Fritz B. Burns Fndn Grants, 1564
Fuller E. Callaway Fndn Grants, 1578
G.N. Wilcox Trust Grants, 1581
Gamble Fndn Grants, 1582
Gebbie Fndn Grants, 1585
General Motors Fndn Grants Support Program, 1591
Genesis Fndn Grants, 1593
George Frederick Jewett Fndn Grants, 1599
George Kress Fndn Grants, 1601
Giving in Action Society Children & Youth with Special Needs Grants, 1617
Giving in Action Society Family Independence Grants, 1618
Gladys Brooks Fndn Grants, 1620
Graco Fndn Grants, 1642
Grand Rapids Comm Fndn Grants, 1647
Greater New Orleans Fndn Grants, 1654
Greater Saint Louis Comm Fndn Grants, 1655
Greater Tacoma Comm Fndn Grants, 1656
Greater Worcester Comm Fndn Jeppson Memorial Fund for Brookfield Grants, 1659
Green Bay Packers Fndn Grants, 1660
Grundy Fndn Grants, 1673
Guitar Center Music Fndn Grants, 1675
Gulf Coast Comm of Venice Fndn Grants, 1677
H & R Fndn Grants, 1679
Hackett Fndn Grants, 1684
Harold and Arlene Schnitzer CARE Fndn Grants, 1697
Harris and Eliza Kempner Fund Grants, 1699
Harrison County Comm Fndn Grants, 1700
Harry and Grace Steele Fndn Grants, 1702
Hartford Fndn Regular Grants, 1711
Harvest Fndn Grants, 1713
Hawaii Comm Fndn Health Education and Research Grants, 1716
Health Fndn of Greater Indianapolis Grants, 1725
Heckscher Fndn for Children Grants, 1732
Helen Bader Fndn Grants, 1738
Henrietta Tower Wurts Memorial Fndn Grants, 1745
HHK Employment Grants, 1755
High Meadow Fndn Grants, 1768
Highmark Physician eHealth Collaborative Grants, 1771
Hill Crest Fndn Grants, 1773
Hill Fndn Grants, 1774
Hillman Fndn Grants, 1775
Hirtzel Memorial Fndn Grants, 1781
Homer Fndn Grants, 1789
Honeywell Fndn Grants, 1791
Hormel Fndn Grants, 1796
Howard and Bush Fndn Grants, 1798
Hudson Webber Fndn Grants, 1813
Huie-Dellmon Trust Grants, 1815
Huntington Clinical Fndn Grants, 1822
Idaho Power Company Corp Contributions, 1838
Independence Blue Cross Charitable Medical Care Grants, 1846
International Spinal Research Trust Grants, 1863
Irvin Stern Fndn Grants, 1866
J.B. Reynolds Fndn Grants, 1873
J.M. Long Fndn Grants, 1877
J.W. Kieckhefer Fndn Grants, 1878
Jacob and Hilda Blaustein Fndn Grants, 1881
Jacob G. Schmidlapp Trust Grants, 1883
James Graham Brown Fndn Grants, 1887
James Hervey Johnson Charitable Educational Trust Grants, 1889
James S. Copley Fndn Grants, 1895
Janirve Fndn Grants, 1905
Jay and Rose Phillips Family Fndn Grants, 1909
JELD-WEN Fndn Grants, 1914
Jenkins Fndn: Improving the Health of Greater Richmond Grants, 1915
Jennings County Comm Fndn Grants, 1916
Jessie Ball Dupont Fund Grants, 1919
Jewish Comm Fndn of Greater Los Angeles Grants, 1921
John Ben Snow Memorial Trust Grants, 1928
John G. Duncan Trust Grants, 1931
John H. and Wilhelmina D. Harland Charitable Fndn Grants, 1933
John J. Leidy Fndn Grants, 1936
John Jewett and Helen Chandler Garland Fndn Grants, 1937
John P. Murphy Fndn Grants, 1943
John S. Dunn Research Fndn Grants and Chairs, 1945
John W. and Anna H. Hanes Fndn Grants, 1948
Joseph Alexander Fndn Grants, 1957
Joseph H. and Florence A. Roblee Fndn Grants, 1961
Josephine Goodyear Fndn Grants, 1964
Josiah W. and Bessie H. Kline Fndn Grants, 1967
Katherine John Murphy Fndn Grants, 1983
Kelvin and Eleanor Smith Fndn Grants, 1986
Kenneth T. and Eileen L. Norris Fndn Grants, 1989
KFC Allied Health Research Grants, 1996
KFC Biomedical Research Grants, 1998
Land O'Lakes Fndn Mid-Atlantic Grants, 2027
Lavelle Fund for the Blind Grants, 2033
Lubbock Area Fndn Grants, 2079
Lubrizol Fndn Grants, 2080
Lucy Gooding Charitable Fndn Trust, 2082
Lucy Gooding Charitable Fndn Trust Grants, 2083
Ludwick Family Fndn Grants, 2084
Lynde and Harry Bradley Fndn Grants, 2089
M.J. Murdock Charitable Trust Grants, 2095
Mabel Y. Hughes Charitable Trust Grants, 2097
Maine Comm Fndn Grants, 2099
Marcia and Otto Koehler Fndn Grants, 2103
Margaret L. Wendt Fndn Grants, 2104
Marion I. and Henry J. Knott Fndn Grants, 2109
Marion Park Deaver and Harry Gilbert Deaver Fndn Grants, 2110
Mark and Catherine Winkler Fndn Grants, 2112
Mars Fndn Grants, 2114
Mary Black Fndn Grants, 2118
Mary Owen Borden Fndn Grants, 2121
Mary S. and David C. Corbin Fndn Grants, 2122
Matilda R. Wilson Fund Grants, 2128
Max A. Adler Charitable Fndn Grants, 2132
Maxon Charitable Fndn Grants, 2135
Maxtor Corp Contributions Grants, 2136
McGregor Fund Grants, 2143
McInerny Fndn Grants, 2144
McKesson Fndn Grants, 2145
McKnight Fndn Grants, 2146
McLean Contributionship Grants, 2147
Mead Witter Fndn Grants, 2160
Meadows Fndn Grants, 2161
Mericos Fndn Grants, 2172
Metro Health Fndn Grants, 2175
Meyer Fndn Grants, 2177
Meyer Memorial Trust Grassroots Grants, 2179
Meyer Memorial Trust Responsive Grants, 2181
MHRC Operating Grants, 2186
Milagro Fndn Grants, 2198
Millipore/Charles P. Schaufus Parenteral-Processing Technology Research Grant, 2204

Minneapolis Fndn Comm Grants, 2206
Miriam and Peter Haas Fund Grants, 2208
Montgomery County Comm Fndn Grants, 2214
Morris and Gwendolyn Cafritz Fndn Grants, 2217
MSSC Research Grants, 2226
Multiple Sclerosis Fndn Brighter Tomorrow Grants, 2228
National City Corporation Contributions Grants, 2250
National Emergency Medicine Association Grants, 2252
NCI Technologies and Software to Support Integrative Cancer Biology Research (SBIR) Grants, 2279
NCIC Canadian Cancer Society Research Grants, 2282
NCIC Equipment Grants, 2284
NHLBI Cardiac Translational Research Implementation Program Grants, 2324
NIAID Allergy, Immunology, and Transplantation Program Research Grants, 2449
NIGMS Minority Access to Research Careers Ancillary Training Activities Grants, 2619
NLM Internet Connection for Medical Institutions Grants, 2820
Noble County Comm Fndn Grants, 2848
Nordson Corporation Fndn Grants, 2851
North Carolina Comm Development Grants, 2858
North Central Health Services Grants, 2861
Northern Trust Company Charitable Trust and Corp Giving Program, 2865
Norwin S. and Elizabeth N. Bean Fndn Grants, 2872
NSF Instrument Development for Biological Research (IDBR), 2888
NSF-NIST Interaction in Chemistry, Materials Research, Molecular Biosciences, Bioengineering, and Chemical Engineering, 2897
NYCT Blood Disease Research Grants, 2922
NYCT Technical Assistance Grants, 2929
Oleonda Jameson Trust Grants, 2941
Olin Corporation Charitable Trust Grants, 2943
OneSight Research Fndn Block Grants, 2944
Oscar Rennebohm Fndn Grants, 2963
Pasadena Fndn Average Grants, 2994
Patron Saints Fndn Grants, 2996
Paul and Mary Haas Fndn Contributions and Student Scholarships, 2997
Paul E. and Klare N. Reinhold Fndn Grants, 2999
Paul Ogle Fndn Grants, 3003
Pew Charitable Trusts Children and Youth Grants, 3020
Pfizer Fndn Grants, 3025
Pinellas County Grants, 3050
Pioneer Hi-Bred Comm Grants, 3051
Pittsburgh Fndn Comm Fund Grants, 3054
Plum Creek Fndn Grants, 3062
Polaroid Fund Grants, 3065
Portland General Electric Fndn Grants, 3067
Posey Comm Fndn Womens Fund Grants, 3069
Potts Memorial Fndn Grants, 3072
Presbyterian Health Fndn Bridge, Seed and Equipment Grants, 3075
Prince Charitable Trusts Chicago Grants, 3079
Prince Charitable Trusts District of Columbia Grants, 3080
Principal Financial Group Fndn Grants, 3082
Progress Energy Fndn Grants, 3084
Prudential Fndn Grants, 3087
R.C. Baker Fndn Grants, 3098
Raskob Fndn for Catholic Activities Grants, 3107
Rasmuson Fndn Grants, 3108
Rathmann Family Fndn Grants, 3109
Rayonier Fndn Grants, 3111
Rett Syndrome Research Fndn Grants, 3151
Rhode Island Fndn Grants, 3154
Rich Fndn Grants, 3156
Richard and Susan Smith Family Fndn Grants, 3159
Ripley County Comm Fndn Grants, 3166
Robins Fndn Grants, 3175
Rochester Area Comm Fndn Grants, 3176
Rochester Area Fndn Grants, 3177
Roy and Christine Sturgis Trust Grants, 3191
Rush County Comm Fndn Grants, 3200
Russell Berrie Fndn Grants, 3201
Ruth Eleanor Bamberger and John Ernest Bamberger Memorial Fndn Grants, 3202
Ruth H. and Warren A. Ellsworth Fndn Grants, 3203
RWJF Partners Investing in Nursing's Future Grants, 3226
Saint Luke's Health Initiatives Grants, 3240
Samuel S. Johnson Fndn Grants, 3251
San Antonio Area Fndn Grants, 3254
Sarah Scaife Fndn Grants, 3263
Schering-Plough Fndn Health Grants, 3270
Seabury Fndn Grants, 3274
Sheltering Arms Fund Grants, 3282
SHF Reach--Connecting Communities and Youth for a Healthy Future Grants, 3283
Sid W. Richardson Fndn Grants, 3284
Siebert Lutheran Fndn Grants, 3285
Simmons Fndn Grants, 3287
Simpson Fund Grants, 3290
Sisters of Mercy of North Carolina Fndn Grants, 3295
Sisters of St. Joseph Healthcare Fndn Grants, 3297
SOCFOC Catholic Ministries Grants, 3317
Solo Cup Fndn Grants, 3346
Sosland Fndn Grants, 3348
Square D Fndn Grants, 3361
St. Joseph Comm Health Fndn Burn Care and Prevention Grants, 3367
St. Joseph Comm Health Fndn Improving Healthcare Access Grants, 3368
St. Joseph Comm Health Fndn Pfeiffer Fund Grants, 3369
Stackner Family Fndn Grants, 3371
Starr Fndn Grants, 3377
Steele-Reese Fndn Grants, 3380
Stewart Huston Charitable Trust Grants, 3384
Strowd Roses Grants, 3388
Sunderland Fndn Grants, 3400
Support Our Aging Religious (SOAR) Grants, 3406
Susan G. Komen Breast Cancer Fndn Hurricane Relief Grants, 3409
Susan Mott Webb Charitable Trust Grants, 3412
Tri-County Electric People Fund Grants, 3436
Trull Fndn Grants, 3441
U.S. Department of Education Rehabilitation Engineering Research Centers Grants, 3447
U.S. Lacrosse EAD Grants, 3453
United Methodist Church Malaria Control Grants, 3464
Until There's a Cure Fndn Grants, 3471
US Airways Comm Fndn Grants, 3473
Vancouver Fndn Grants and Comm Initiatives Program, 3477
VDH Rescue Squad Assistance Fund Grants, 3484
Vectren Fndn Grants, 3485
Verizon Fndn Health Care and Accessibility Grants, 3486
Waitt Family Fndn Grants, 3512
Wasie Fndn Grants, 3521
Weatherwax Fndn Grants, 3523
Weingart Fndn Grants, 3524
Wells County Fndn Grants, 3527
Western Indiana Comm Fndn Grants, 3528
Whitehall Fndn Neurobiology Research Grants, 3533
William G. Gilmore Fndn Grants, 3537
William G. McGowan Charitable Fund Grants, 3539
Wilson-Wood Fndn Grants, 3542
Woodward Fund Grants, 3552
YSA Get Ur Good On Grants, 3555
Z. Smith Reynolds Fndn Small Grants, 3557

Preservation/Restoration

Abell-Hanger Fndn Grants, 183
Albuquerque Comm Fndn Grants, 331
Andersen Fndn Grants, 471
Annenberg Fndn Grants, 479
Anschutz Family Fndn Grants, 486
APA Distinguished Service to Psychological Science Award, 498
Ashland Corp Contributions Grants, 586
Ball Brothers Fndn General Grants, 683
Bank of America Client Fndn Grants, 690
Barker Welfare Fndn Grants, 695
Batchelor Fndn Grants, 701
Blue Mountain Comm Fndn Grants, 769
Blue River Comm Fndn Grants, 770
Booth-Bricker Fund Grants, 780
Callaway Fndn Grants, 835
Cessna Fndn Grants, 938
Champlin Fndns Grants, 960
Charles Edison Fund Grants, 964
Charlotte County (FL) Comm Fndn Grants, 973
Chula Vista Charitable Fndn Grants, 1009
Clarence E. Heller Charitable Fndn Grants, 1022
CLIF Bar Family Fndn Grants, 1040
Comm Fndn Alliance City of Evansville Endowment Fund Grants, 1089
Comm Fndn for Greater Buffalo Grants, 1090
Comm Fndn for Monterey County Grants, 1092
Comm Fndn of Crawford County Grants and Scholarships, 1103
Comm Fndn of Grant County Grants, 1104
Comm Fndn of Greater Tampa Grants, 1112
Comm Fndn of Western North Carolina Grants, 1132
ConocoPhillips Fndn Grants, 1144
Consumers Energy Fndn, 1147
Cudd Fndn Grants, 1171
D.F. Halton Fndn Grants, 1181
E. Rhodes and Leona B. Carpenter Fndn Grants, 1356
Edwin S. Webster Fndn Grants, 1376
El Pomar Fndn Awards and Grants, 1390
ExxonMobil Grants, 1442
Fargo-Moorhead Area Fndn Grants, 1454
Ferree Fndn Grants, 1486
Forrest C. Lattner Fndn Grants, 1523
Fndn for the Carolinas Grants, 1535
George Kress Fndn Grants, 1601
Geraldine R. Dodge Fndn Morris County Grants, 1605
Grammy Fndn Grants, 1643
Greater Green Bay Comm Fndn Grants, 1652
Greater Milwaukee Fndn Grants, 1653
Greater Tacoma Comm Fndn Grants, 1656
Harrison County Comm Fndn Grants, 1700
High Meadow Fndn Grants, 1768
Hoblitzelle Fndn Grants, 1783
Holland/Zeeland Comm Fndn Grants, 1786
Huntington County Comm Fndn Grants, 1823
J.W. Kieckhefer Fndn Grants, 1878
Jennings County Comm Fndn Grants, 1916
John Ben Snow Memorial Trust Grants, 1928
John J. Leidy Fndn Grants, 1936
John W. and Anna H. Hanes Fndn Grants, 1948
Knox County Comm Fndn Grants, 2009
Lawrence S. Huntington Fund Grants, 2035
Legacy Fndn Grants, 2040
M.E. Raker Fndn Grants, 2094
Maine Comm Fndn Grants, 2099
Marcia and Otto Koehler Fndn Grants, 2103
Margaret L. Wendt Fndn Grants, 2104
Mars Fndn Grants, 2114
Mary Black Fndn Grants, 2118
McCombs Fndn Grants, 2142
McLean Contributionship Grants, 2147
Nina Mason Pulliam Charitable Trust Grants, 2776
North Carolina Comm Fndn Grants, 2859
Ogden Codman Trust Grants, 2937
OSI-Baltimore Special Opportunities Program Grants, 2972
PacifiCorp Fndn for Learning Grants, 2982
Palm Beach and Martin Counties Grants, 2986
Pasadena Fndn Average Grants, 2994
Perkins Charitable Fndn Grants, 3014

Posey Comm Fndn Grants, 3068
Prince Charitable Trusts Chicago Grants, 3079
Prince Charitable Trusts District of Columbia Grants, 3080
Putnam County Comm Fndn Grants, 3093
Rhode Island Fndn Grants, 3154
Ripley County Comm Fndn Grants, 3166
Salem Fndn Charitable Trust Grants, 3241
Salisbury Comm Fndn Grants, 3243
Samuel Freeman Charitable Trust Grants, 3249
Schering-Plough Fndn Comm Initiatives Grants, 3269
Simpson Fund Grants, 3290
Southwest Florida Comm Fndn Competitive Grants, 3351
Spencer County Comm Fndn Grants, 3358
Stewart Huston Charitable Trust Grants, 3384
Trull Fndn Grants, 3441
Vermont Comm Fndn Grants, 3493
Western Indiana Comm Fndn Grants, 3528
Winston-Salem Fndn Stokes County Grants, 3546

Publishing/Editing/Translating
AACN Clinical Inquiry Fund Grants, 56
AACN End of Life/Palliative Care Small Projects Grants, 59
AACN Physio-Control Small Projects Grants, 62
AACN-Edwards Lifesciences Nurse-Driven Clinical Practice Outcomes Grants, 63
AEC Trust Grants, 242
Ahn Family Fndn Grants, 304
Albuquerque Comm Fndn Grants, 331
AMA Virtual Mentor Theme Issue Editor Grants, 400
Ann Arbor Area Comm Fndn Grants, 476
ASCO State Affiliate Grants, 547
ASHA Advancing Academic-Research Careers (AARC) Award, 569
ASHA Student Research Travel Award, 573
Atran Fndn Grants, 663
Ball Brothers Fndn Grants, 684
Battle Creek Comm Fndn Grants, 703
Bodenwein Public Benevolent Fndn Grants, 775
Bodman Fndn Grants, 776
Carl and Lily Pforzheimer Fndn Grants, 868
Carl Gellert and Celia Berta Gellert Fndn Grants, 871
Chatlos Fndn Grants, 977
Chicago Tribune's Corp Contributions Grants, 991
Christine O. Gregoire Youth/Young Adult Award for Outstanding Use of Tobacco Industry Documents, 1005
Clarence E. Heller Charitable Fndn Grants, 1022
Coastal Comm Fndn of South Carolina Grants, 1051
Columbus Fndn Competitive Grants, 1066
Comm Fndn for Muskegon County Grants, 1093
Comm Fndn for Southern Arizona Grants, 1095
Comm Fndn of Champaign County Grants, 1102
Comm Fndn of Greater Birmingham Grants, 1106
Comm Fndn of Southeastern Connecticut Grants, 1125
Connecticut Comm Fndn Grants, 1141
DHHS Developmental Disabilities University Affiliated Programs Project Grants, 1248
Elmer L. and Eleanor J. Andersen Fndn Grants, 1406
Ewing Halsell Fndn Grants, 1440
Frank Stanley Beveridge Fndn Grants, 1553
General Motors Fndn Grants Support Program, 1591
Hartford Aging and Health Program Awards, 1709
Henry J. Kaiser Family Fndn Media Fellowships, 1749
HHMI International Research Scholars Program, 1760
Hill Crest Fndn Grants, 1773
Huber Fndn Grants, 1812
J.B. Reynolds Fndn Grants, 1873
Jessie Ball Dupont Fund Grants, 1919
Jewish Women's Fndn of New York Grants, 1924
JM Fndn Grants, 1926
John P. McGovern Fndn Grants, 1942
Josephine G. Russell Trust Grants, 1963
Lubbock Area Fndn Grants, 2079
Lynde and Harry Bradley Fndn Grants, 2089
McLean Contributionship Grants, 2147
Meadows Fndn Grants, 2161
MHRC Operating Grants, 2186
National Headache Fndn Seymour Diamond Clinical Fellowship in Headache Education, 2254
NIGMS Minority Access to Research Careers (MARC) Ancillary Training Activities Grants, 2619
NIHCM Fndn Health Care Print Journalism Awards, 2742
NLM Grants for Scholarly Works in Biomedicine and Health, 2818
Olin Corporation Charitable Trust Grants, 2943
Polaroid Fund Grants, 3065
Potts Memorial Fndn Grants, 3072
Puerto Rico Comm Fndn Grants, 3090
Rochester Area Comm Fndn Grants, 3176
RSC Jason A. Hannah Medal, 3196
Sarah Scaife Fndn Grants, 3263
Shell Oil Company Fndn Grants, 3281
Sid W. Richardson Fndn Grants, 3284
South Madison Comm Fndn Grants, 3349
Susan Mott Webb Charitable Trust Grants, 3412
Whitehall Fndn Neurobiology Research Grants, 3533
Women's Fndn of California Comm Action Fund, 3549

Religious Programs
100 Mile Man Fndn Grants, 2
1104 Fndn Grants, 3
A Friend's Fndn Trust Grants, 13
A/H Fndn Grants, 19
Aaron & Cecile Goldman Family Fndn Grants, 171
Aaron & Freda Glickman Fndn Grants, 172
Aaron Fndn (Massachusetts) Grants, 174
Abel Fndn Grants, 181
Abell-Hanger Fndn Grants, 183
Able To Serve Grants, 185
Abramson Family Fndn Grants, 188
Achelis and Bodman Fndns Grants, 206
Adaptec Fndn Grants, 232
Adolph Coors Fndn Grants, 238
Aetna Fndn Regional Comm Health Grants, 249
Ahmanson Fndn Grants, 303
Alabama Power Fndn Grants, 321
Albert and Margaret Alkek Fndn Grants, 326
Albertson's Charitable Giving Grants, 330
Albuquerque Comm Fndn Grants, 331
Alcoa Fndn Grants, 334
Allyn Fndn Grants, 365
ALSAM Fndn Grants, 369
American Jewish World Service Grants, 437
Andersen Fndn Grants, 471
Anheuser-Busch Fndn Grants, 474
Ann Arbor Area Comm Fndn Grants, 476
Anschutz Family Fndn Grants, 486
Ansell, Zaro, Grimm & Aaron Fndn Grants, 487
Anthony R. Abraham Fndn Grants, 490
Aratani Fndn Grants, 523
Arcadia Fndn Grants, 524
Archer Daniels Midland Fndn Grants, 525
Argyros Fndn Grants, 527
Arie and Ida Crown Memorial Grants, 528
Arkansas Comm Fndn Grants, 533
Arkell Hall Fndn Grants, 534
Arlington Comm Fndn Grants, 536
Armstrong McDonald Fndn Grants, 537
Arthur and Rochelle Belfer Fndn Grants, 542
ArvinMeritor Grants, 544
Ashland Corp Contributions Grants, 586
Assisi Fndn Grants, 653
Atherton Family Fndn Grants, 659
Athwin Fndn Grants, 660
Atkinson Fndn International Grants, 661
Atran Fndn Grants, 663
Audrey and Sydney Irmas Charitable Fndn Grants, 665
AVDF Health Care Grants, 673
Bacon Family Fndn Grants, 679
Bailey Fndn Grants, 680
Banfi Vintners Fndn Grants, 687
Baptist Comm Ministries Grants, 691
Barr Fund Grants, 697
Barra Fndn Project Grants, 699
Baton Rouge Area Fndn Grants, 702
BCBS of Massachusetts Fndn Grants, 709
BCBS of Minnesota Growing Up Healthy Grants, 711
BCBS of Minnesota Healthy Together Grants, 712
Beatrice Laing Trust Grants, 729
Beazley Fndn Grants, 730
Beldon Fund Grants, 738
Belk Fndn Grants, 739
Bender Fndn Grants, 742
Benton County Fndn Grants, 744
Bernard and Audre Rapoport Fndn Grants, 746
Besser Fndn Grants, 752
BibleLands Grants, 754
Bildner Family Fndn Grants, 755
Bill and Melinda Gates Fndn Grants, 756
Biogen Corp Giving Grants, 758
Blanche and Irving Laurie Fndn Grants, 764
Blowitz-Ridgeway Fndn Early Childhood Development Research Award, 766
Blowitz-Ridgeway Fndn Grants, 767
Blue Shield of California Grants, 771
Blumenthal Fndn Grants, 773
Bob and Delores Hope Charitable Fndn Grants, 774
Bodenwein Public Benevolent Fndn Grants, 775
Bodman Fndn Grants, 776
Boettcher Fndn Grants, 778
Booth-Bricker Fund Grants, 780
Borkee-Hagley Fndn Grants, 781
Boston Fndn Grants, 783
Boston Jewish Comm Women's Fund Grants, 785
Bradley Turner Fndn Grants, 789
Bright Family Fndn Grants, 793
Bristol-Myers Squibb Fndn Health Disparities Grants, 797
Burden Trust Grants, 810
Burton G. Bettingen Grants, 813
Byron W. and Alice L. Lockwood Fndn Grants, 824
Caddock Fndn Grants, 828
Caleb C. and Julia W. Dula Educational and Charitable Fndn Grants, 830
Callaway Fndn Grants, 835
Callaway Golf Company Fndn Grants, 836
Cambridge Comm Fndn Grants, 837
Camp-Younts Fndn Grants, 838
Campbell Hoffman Fndn Grants, 840
Cargill Citizenship Fund-Corp Giving Grants, 865
Carl C. Icahn Fndn Grants, 870
Carl Gellert and Celia Berta Gellert Fndn Grants, 871
Carnahan-Jackson Fndn Grants, 878
Carolyn Fndn Grants, 880
Carrie E. and Lena V. Glenn Fndn Grants, 882
Carrie Estelle Doheny Fndn Grants, 883
Carylon Fndn Grants, 886
Castle Rock Fndn Grants, 888
Catherine Kennedy Home Fndn Grants, 890
Catholic Campaign for Human Development (CCHD) Comm Organizing Grants, 891
Central Okanagan Fndn Grants, 937
Champlin Fndns Grants, 960
Charles Delmar Fndn Grants, 963
Charles H. Revson Fndn Grants, 969
Chatlos Fndn Grants, 977
Chazen Fndn Grants, 978
Chicago Comm Trust Grants, 989
Chiles Fndn Grants, 1003
CIT Corp Giving Grants, 1014

Citizens Bank Mid-Atlantic Charitable Fndn Grants, 1015
Clark-Winchcole Fndn Grants, 1030
Claude Worthington Benedum Fndn Grants, 1033
Cleveland Browns Fndn Grants, 1036
CNA Fndn Grants, 1046
CNCS Foster Grandparent Projects Grants, 1048
CNCS Next Generation Grants, 1049
Coastal Comm Fndn of South Carolina Grants, 1051
Coca-Cola Fndn Grants, 1052
Cockrell Fndn Grants, 1053
Coeta and Donald Barker Fndn Grants, 1054
Colin Higgins Fndn Grants, 1056
Collins C. Diboll Private Fndn Grants, 1057
Collins Fndn Grants, 1058
Columbus Fndn Competitive Grants, 1066
Commission on Religion in Appalachia Grants, 1074
Commonwealth Fund Small Grants, 1084
Comm Fndn for Greater Buffalo Grants, 1090
Comm Fndn for Greater New Haven Grants, 1091
Comm Fndn for Monterey County Grants, 1092
Comm Fndn for Muskegon County Grants, 1093
Comm Fndn for Southeastern Michigan Grants, 1094
Comm Fndn of Central Illinois Grants, 1101
Comm Fndn of Champaign County Grants, 1102
Comm Fndn of Crawford County Grants and Scholarships, 1103
Comm Fndn of Grant County Grants, 1104
Comm Fndn of Grant County Scholarships, 1105
Comm Fndn of Greater Flint Grants, 1107
Comm Fndn of Greater Fort Wayne: Comm Endowment & Clarke Endowment Fund Grants, 1108
Comm Fndn of Greenville Hollingsworth Funds Program/Project Grants, 1114
Comm Fndn of Mount Vernon and Knox County Grants, 1119
Comm Fndn of Muncie and Delaware County Grants, 1120
ConAgra Foods Fndn Grants, 1140
Connecticut Health Fndn Health Initiative Grants, 1142
Connelly Fndn Grants, 1143
ConocoPhillips Fndn Grants, 1144
Constellation Energy Group and Baltimore Gas and Electric Corp Contributions, 1146
CRH Fndn Grants, 1160
CSRA Comm Fndn Grants, 1168
CUNA Mutual Group Fndn, 1174
Dade Comm Fndn Grants, 1185
DaimlerChrysler Corporation Fund Grants, 1186
Danellie Fndn Grants, 1198
David Geffen Fndn Grants, 1202
Daywood Fndn Grants, 1206
Delaware Comm Fndn Grants, 1215
Dennis and Phyllis Washington Fndn Grants, 1222
DHL Charitable Shipment Support, 1283
Donald and Sylvia Robinson Family Fndn Grants, 1310
Dora Roberts Fndn Grants, 1311
Dorothy Hooper Beattie Fndn Grants, 1321
Dorrance Family Fndn Grants, 1323
Dr. Scholl Fndn Grants, 1329
E. Rhodes and Leona B. Carpenter Fndn Grants, 1356
eBay Fndn Comm Grants, 1363
Eden Hall Fndn Grants, 1368
Edward S. Moore Fndn Grants, 1374
Edwin W. and Catherine M. Davis Fndn Grants, 1377
Edyth Bush Charitable Fndn Grants, 1378
Effie and Wofford Cain Fndn Grants, 1385
El Paso Comm Fndn Grants, 1388
El Pomar Fndn Awards and Grants, 1390
Elliot Fndn Inc Grants, 1402
Emily Davie and Joseph S. Kornfeld Fndn Grants, 1414
Entergy Comm Partnership Grants, 1417
Essex County Comm Fndn Discretionary Fund Grant, 1428
Eugene and Agnes E. Meyer Fndn Grants, 1432
Eugene B. Casey Fndn Grants, 1433
Evjue Fndn Grants, 1439
F.M. Kirby Fndn Grants, 1443
Feldman Fndn Grants, 1484
FirstEnergy Fndn Comm Grants, 1505
Fishman Family Fndn Grants, 1510
Floyd A. and Kathleen C. Cailloux Fndn Grants, 1516
Fndn for a Healthy Kentucky Grants, 1527
Fndn for Spirituality and Medicine Grants, 1534
Fndn for the Carolinas Grants, 1535
Fndn Northwest Grants, 1537
Frank G. and Freida K. Brotz Family Fndn Grants, 1552
Frank Stanley Beveridge Fndn Grants, 1553
Franklin County Comm Fndn Grants, 1554
Fraser-Parker Fndn Grants, 1555
Fred L. Emerson Fndn Grants, 1557
Frist Fndn Grants, 1563
Fritz B. Burns Fndn Grants, 1564
Fuller E. Callaway Fndn Grants, 1578
G.N. Wilcox Trust Grants, 1581
George F. Baker Trust Grants, 1597
George Family Fndn Grants, 1598
George Frederick Jewett Fndn Grants, 1599
George Kress Fndn Grants, 1601
Gertrude E. Skelly Charitable Fndn Grants, 1609
Gheens Fndn Grants, 1610
Giant Eagle Fndn Grants, 1611
Gilroy and Lillian P. Roberts Charitable Fndn Grants, 1614
Ginn Fndn Grants, 1616
Glendale Comm Fndn Grants, 1626
Golden State Warriors Fndn Grants, 1633
Great-West Life Grants, 1649
Greater Cincinnati Fndn Priority and Small Projects/Capacity-Building Grants, 1651
Greater Saint Louis Comm Fndn Grants, 1655
Greater Tacoma Comm Fndn Grants, 1656
Greater Worcester Comm Fndn Discretionary Grants, 1658
Green Bay Packers Fndn Grants, 1660
Greenspun Family Fndn Grants, 1664
Gregory Family Fndn Grants (Florida), 1667
Guy's and St. Thomas' Charity Grants, 1678
H. Schaffer Fndn Grants, 1680
Hackett Fndn Grants, 1684
Hagedorn Fund Grants, 1685
Harden Fndn Grants, 1693
Harold and Arlene Schnitzer CARE Fndn Grants, 1697
Harold Simmons Fndn Grants, 1698
Harrison County Comm Fndn Grants, 1700
Harry and Grace Steele Fndn Grants, 1702
Harry Frank Guggenheim Fndn Research Grants, 1704
Harry Kramer Memorial Fund Grants, 1705
Hawaii Comm Fndn Reverend Takie Okumura Family Grants, 1717
HCA Fndn Grants, 1721
Healthcare Fndn for Orange County Grants, 1728
Healthcare Fndn of New Jersey Grants, 1729
Hearst Fndn and William Randolph Hearst Fndn Grants, 1730
Hedco Fndn Grants, 1733
Helen Bader Fndn Grants, 1738
Helen Steiner Rice Fndn Grants, 1742
Hilda and Preston Davis Fndn Grants, 1772
Hillsdale Fund Grants, 1778
Hilton Hotels Corp Giving Program Grants, 1780
Howe Fndn of North Carolina Grants, 1799
Huie-Dellmon Trust Grants, 1815
Ida Alice Ryan Charitable Trust Grants, 1836
Infinity Fndn Grants, 1854
Irvin Stern Fndn Grants, 1866
J.C. Penney Company Grants, 1874
J.E. and L.E. Mabee Fndn Grants, 1875
Jacob and Hilda Blaustein Fndn Grants, 1881
James Hervey Johnson Charitable Educational Trust Grants, 1889
James J. and Angelia M. Harris Fndn Grants, 1890
James M. Collins Fndn Grants, 1891
Jessie Ball Dupont Fund Grants, 1919
Jewish Comm Fndn of Greater Los Angeles Grants, 1921
Jewish Fndn for Education of Women Scholarships for Emigres in the Health Professions, 1922
Jewish Fund Grants, 1923
Jewish Women's Fndn of New York Grants, 1924
Joe W. and Dorothy Dorsett Brown Fndn Grants, 1927
John Edward Fowler Memorial Fndn Grants, 1930
John G. Duncan Trust Grants, 1931
John H. and Wilhelmina D. Harland Charitable Fndn Grants, 1933
John I. Smith Charities Grants, 1935
John P. Murphy Fndn Grants, 1943
Johns Manville Fund Grants, 1950
Joseph Alexander Fndn Grants, 1957
Joseph and Luella Abell Charitable Trust Scholarships, 1958
Joseph H. and Florence A. Roblee Fndn Grants, 1961
Joyce Fndn Grants, 1969
Kaiser Permanente Cares for Communities Grants, 1978
Kalamazoo Fndn Grants, 1979
Katharine Matthies Fndn Grants, 1982
Ken W. Davis Fndn Grants, 1987
Kevin P. and Sydney B. Knight Family Fndn Grants, 1993
Kimberly-Clark Comm Grants, 2001
King Pharmaceuticals Corp Contributions Grants, 2003
Kluge Center David B. Larson Fellowship in Health and Spirituality, 2006
Knight Family Charitable and Educational Fndn Grants, 2007
Kraft Cares US Grants, 2017
Lands' End Corp Giving Program, 2030
Larry L. Hillblom Fndn Grants, 2031
Lettie Pate Whitehead Fndn Grants, 2049
Liberty Bank Fndn Grants, 2053
Lockheed Martin Philanthropic Grants, 2062
Louis Calder Fndn Grants, 2065
Lowell Berry Fndn Grants, 2069
Lubbock Area Fndn Grants, 2079
Lucile Horton Howe and Mitchell B. Howe Fndn Grants, 2081
Lynde and Harry Bradley Fndn Grants, 2089
M. Bastian Family Fndn Grants, 2092
M.J. Murdock Charitable Trust Grants, 2095
Maine Comm Fndn Grants, 2099
Manuel D. and Rhoda Mayerson Fndn Grants, 2100
Margaret L. Wendt Fndn Grants, 2104
Marion I. and Henry J. Knott Fndn Grants, 2109
Marion Park Deaver and Harry Gilbert Deaver Fndn Grants, 2110
Mary Allen Lindsey Branan Fndn Grants, 2116
Mary Baker Eddy Library Summer Research Fellowships, 2117
Mary Black Fndn Grants, 2118
Max A. Adler Charitable Fndn Grants, 2132
Maxon Charitable Fndn Grants, 2135
McKesson Fndn Grants, 2145
McKnight Fndn Grants, 2146
McMurry Fndn Grants, 2149
Mead Johnson Nutritionals Evansville-Area Organizations Grants, 2157
Mead Witter Fndn Grants, 2160
Medtronic Fndn Full Life Patient Partnership Program--Heart Rescue Grants, 2168
Meriden Fndn Grants, 2173
Morris and Gwendolyn Cafritz Fndn Grants, 2217
Morton K. and Jane Blaustein Fndn Grants, 2218
Moses Cone-Wesley Long Comm Health Fndn Grants, 2219

Mount Zion Health Fund Grants, 2220
Nell Warren Elkin and William Simpson Elkin Fndn, 2302
New York University Steinhardt School of Education Fellowships, 2305
Nina Mason Pulliam Charitable Trust Grants, 2776
North Carolina Comm Development Grants, 2858
North Carolina Comm Fndn Grants, 2859
North Georgia Comm Fndn Grants, 2862
Otto Bremer Fndn Grants, 2977
PacifiCare Fndn Grants, 2981
PacifiCorp Fndn for Learning Grants, 2982
Palm Beach and Martin Counties Grants, 2986
Partners for Youth with Disabilities Grants, 2990
Paul and Mary Haas Fndn Contributions and Student Scholarships, 2997
Paul Balint Charitable Trust Grants, 2998
Paul E. and Klare N. Reinhold Fndn Grants, 2999
Perkins Charitable Fndn Grants, 3014
Perpetual Trust for Charitable Giving Grants, 3015
Pfizer Fndn Grants, 3025
Philadelphia Fndn Organizational Effectiveness Grants, 3029
Pittsburgh Fndn Comm Fund Grants, 3054
PNC Charitable Trust and Fndn Grants, 3064
Polk Bros. Fndn Grants, 3066
Powell Fndn Grants, 3073
Premera CARES Grants, 3074
Priddy Fndn Grants, 3077
Procter and Gamble Fund Grants, 3083
Public Welfare Fndn Grants, 3089
Quality Health Fndn Grants, 3094
R.C. Baker Fndn Grants, 3098
Rainbow Endowment Grants, 3102
Raskob Fndn for Catholic Activities Grants, 3107
Rasmuson Fndn Grants, 3108
Rathmann Family Fndn Grants, 3109
Religion and Health: Effects, Mechanisms, and Interpretation RFP, 3149
RGK Fndn Grants, 3153
Richard and Helen DeVos Fndn Grants, 3157
Richard and Rhoda Goldman Fund Grants, 3158
Richard King Mellon Fndn Grants, 3161
Robert E. and Evelyn McKee Fndn Grants, 3170
Robins Fndn Grants, 3175
Rockwell Collins Charitable Contributions, 3182
Rockwell International Corp Trust Grants, 3183
Rollin M. Gerstacker Fndn Grants, 3186
Roy J. Carver Charitable Trust Medical and Science Research Grants, 3192
RRF Organizational Capacity Building Grants, 3194
Russell Berrie Fndn Grants, 3201
RWJF Local Funding Partnerships Program Grants, 3223
S.H. Cowell Fndn Grants, 3237
Saint Luke's Fndn Grants, 3239
Salisbury Comm Fndn Grants, 3243
San Antonio Area Fndn Grants, 3254
San Diego Fndn for Change Grants, 3255
Siebert Lutheran Fndn Grants, 3285
Sir Halley Stewart Trust Grants, 3293
Sisters of Saint Joseph Charitable Fund Grants, 3296
Sisters of St. Joseph Healthcare Fndn Grants, 3297
SOCFOC Catholic Ministries Grants, 3317
SOCFOC Reducing Health & Educational Disparities in the Central Neighborhood Grants, 3318
Solo Cup Fndn Grants, 3346
Sosland Fndn Grants, 3348
Southwire Company Grants, 3353
Square D Fndn Grants, 3361
St. Joseph Comm Health Fndn Improving Healthcare Access Grants, 3368
Stan and Sandy Checketts Fndn, 3373
Stewart Huston Charitable Trust Grants, 3384
Strowd Roses Grants, 3388
Sunderland Fndn Grants, 3400
Support Our Aging Religious (SOAR) Grants, 3406
Susan Mott Webb Charitable Trust Grants, 3412
Temple-Inland Fndn Grants, 3419
Thomas and Dorothy Leavey Fndn Grants, 3422
Thomas C. Ackerman Fndn Grants, 3423
Thomas M. and Irene B. Kirbo Charitable Trust Grants, 3424
Thompson Charitable Fndn Grants, 3425
Triangle Comm Fndn Donor-Advised Grants, 3437
Trull Fndn Grants, 3441
United Methodist Church Global AIDS Fund Grants, 3463
United Methodist Church Malaria Control Grants, 3464
United Methodist Health Ministry Fund Grants, 3465
United Technologies Corporation Grants, 3466
Vancouver Fndn Grants and Comm Initiatives Program, 3477
W.K. Kellogg Fndn Secure Families Grants, 3508
Wabash Valley Comm Fndn Grants, 3510
Wachovia Fndn Grants, 3511
Washington Post Contributions Program Grants, 3520
Wasie Fndn Grants, 3521
Wayne and Gladys Valley Fndn Grants, 3522
Welborn Baptist Fndn Grants, 3525
William H. Hannon Fndn Grants, 3540
Women of the ELCA Opportunity Scholarships for Lutheran Laywomen, 3548
Woodward Fund Grants, 3552

Scholarships

A.O. Smith Comm Grants, 18
AACAP Child and Adolescent Psychiatry (CAP) Teaching Scholarships, 31
AAFCS National Undergraduate Scholarships, 111
AAHPERD Ruth Abernathy Presidential Scholarships, 128
AAHPERD-AAHE Barbara A. Cooley Scholarships, 129
AAHPERD-AAHE Delbert Oberteuffer Scholarships, 130
AAHPERD-AAHE Undergraduate Scholarships, 131
AAMC Herbert W. Nickens Medical Student Scholarships, 140
AAOHN Fndn Professional Development Scholarships, 155
AAP Resident Research Grants, 168
AARP Fndn Gerontology Graduate Scholarships and Fellowships, 175
Abbott Fund Science and Medical Innovation Grants, 179
Abell-Hanger Fndn Grants, 183
Abramson Family Fndn Grants, 188
AcademyHealth Alice S. Hersh Student Scholarships, 191
AcademyHealth PHSR Interest Group Student Scholarships, 195
ACS Doctoral Degree Scholarships in Cancer Nursing, 211
ACS Doctoral Scholarships in Cancer Nursing, 212
ACS Graduate Scholarships in Cancer Nursing Practice, 214
Acushnet Fndn Grants, 226
Adams County Fndn Grants - Pennsylvania, 231
Adaptec Fndn Grants, 232
Adelaide Breed Bayrd Fndn Grants, 234
Agnes M. Lindsay Trust Grants, 263
AHFMR Dr. Lionel E. McLeod Health Research Scholarship, 272
AHFMR Full-Time M.D./Ph.D. Studentships, 277
AHFMR Full-Time Studentships, 278
AHFMR Health Research Full-Time Studentships, 280
AHFMR Heritage Summer Studentships, 282
AHFMR Part-Time Studentships, 289
Ahmanson Fndn Grants, 303
Alabama Power Fndn Grants, 321
Aladdin Industries Fndn Grants, 322
Albert and Margaret Alkek Fndn Grants, 326
Albuquerque Comm Fndn Grants, 331
Alcatel-Lucent Technologies Fndn Grants, 333
Alcoa Fndn Grants, 334
Alex Brown and Sons Charitable Fndn Grants, 337
Alexis Gregory Fndn Grants, 349
Alice Fisher Society Fellowships, 356
Alice Tweed Tuohy Fndn Grants, 357
Allyn Fndn Grants, 365
Alpha Omega Fndn Grants, 366
Alpine Winter Fndn Grants, 368
ALSAM Fndn Grants, 369
AMA Fndn Arthur N. Wilson, MD, Scholarship, 386
AMA Fndn Joan F. Giambalvo Memorial Scholarships, 392
AMA Fndn Minority Scholars Awards, 395
AMA Fndn Physicians of Tomorrow Scholarships, 396
AMA-WPC Joan F. Giambalvo Memorial Scholarships, 408
American Academy of Dermatology Camp Discovery Scholarships, 412
American Academy of Nursing Building Academic Geriatric Nursing Capacity (BAGNC) Scholarships, 414
American Academy of Nursing Mayday Fund Grants, 416
American Academy of Nursing MBA Scholarships, 417
American College of Surgeons and The Triological Society Clinical Scientist Development Awards, 422
American College of Surgeons Health Policy Scholarships, 427
American College of Surgeons Health Policy Scholarships for General Surgeons, 428
American College of Surgeons Resident Research Scholarships, 432
American Psychiatric Association Travel Scholarships for Minority Medical Students, 449
American Schlafhorst Fndn Grants, 454
AMI Semiconductors Corp Grants, 468
Angels Baseball Fndn Grants, 473
Anheuser-Busch Fndn Grants, 474
Ann Arbor Area Comm Fndn Grants, 476
Ann Peppers Fndn Grants, 478
APF/COGDOP Graduate Research Scholarships in Psychology, 511
Aratani Fndn Grants, 523
Arcadia Fndn Grants, 524
ARCO Fndn Education Grants, 526
Argyros Fndn Grants, 527
Arie and Ida Crown Memorial Grants, 528
Arkansas Comm Fndn Grants, 533
Arkell Hall Fndn Grants, 534
Arlington Comm Fndn Grants, 536
ASHA Minority Student Leadership Program Awards, 570
ASHA Students Preparing for Academic & Research Careers (SPARC) Award, 574
ASHFndn Graduate Student International Scholarship, 576
ASHFndn Graduate Student Scholarships, 577
ASHFndn Graduate Student Scholarships for Minority Students, 578
ASHFndn Graduate Student with a Disability Scholarship, 579
ASHFndn New Century Scholars Program Doctoral Scholarships, 580
ASHFndn Student Research Grants in Early Childhood Language Development, 585
Assurant Fndn Grants, 654
Assurant Health Fndn Grants, 655
Atherton Family Fndn Grants, 659
Atkinson Fndn International Grants, 661
Atran Fndn Grants, 663
Australian Academy of Science Grants, 670
Avon Products Fndn Grants, 675
Bailey Fndn Grants, 680
Barberton Comm Fndn Grants, 693

Baton Rouge Area Fndn Grants, 702
Battle Creek Comm Fndn Grants, 703
Batts Fndn Grants, 704
Bayer Clinical Scholarship Award, 706
Beazley Fndn Grants, 730
Beckley Area Fndn Grants, 732
Beckman Scholars Program Grants, 734
Becton Dickinson and Company Grants, 736
Ben B. Cheney Fndn Grants, 741
Bender Fndn Grants, 742
Benton Comm Fndn Grants, 743
Berks County Comm Fndn Grants, 745
Bernard and Audre Rapoport Fndn Grants, 746
Bertha Russ Lytel Fndn Grants, 751
Besser Fndn Grants, 752
Blackford County Comm Fndn Grants, 763
Blanche and Irving Laurie Fndn Grants, 764
Blowitz-Ridgeway Fndn Early Childhood Development Research Award, 766
Blue Grass Comm Fndn Grants, 768
Blue Mountain Comm Fndn Grants, 769
Bodenwein Public Benevolent Fndn Grants, 775
Bodman Fndn Grants, 776
Boeing Company Contributions Program Grants, 777
Bright Family Fndn Grants, 793
Brook J. Lenfest Fndn Grants, 804
Burlington Northern Santa Fe Fndn Grants, 812
C.R. Bard Fndn Grants, 825
California Wellness Fndn Work and Health Program Grants, 834
Callaway Fndn Grants, 835
Cambridge Comm Fndn Grants, 837
CampusRN/AACN Nursing Scholarship Fund, 841
Canada Graduate Scholarships (CGS) and NSERC Postgraduate Scholarships (PGS), 845
Canadian Friends of Hebrew University Research and Study Grants, 850
Canadian Nurses Fndn Study Awards, 852
Cargill Citizenship Fund-Corp Giving Grants, 865
Carl and Eloise Pohlad Family Fndn Grants, 867
Carl and Lily Pforzheimer Fndn Grants, 868
Carl Gellert and Celia Berta Gellert Fndn Grants, 871
Carl J. Herzog Fndn Grants, 872
Carnahan-Jackson Fndn Grants, 878
Carolyn Fndn Grants, 880
Carpenter Fndn Grants, 881
Carrie Estelle Doheny Fndn Grants, 883
Carrier Corporation Contributions Grants, 884
Carroll County Comm Fndn Grants, 885
CCFF Scholarships, 895
Cemala Fndn Grants, 933
Central Carolina Comm Fndn Comm Impact Grants, 936
Central Okanagan Fndn Grants, 937
Cessna Fndn Grants, 938
Cetana Educational Fndn Scholarships, 939
CFPC Research and Education Fndn Grants, 956
Champlin Fndns Grants, 960
Charles A. Frueauff Fndn Grants, 962
Charles Delmar Fndn Grants, 963
Charles G. Koch Charitable Fndn Grants, 965
Chateaubriand Exact Sciences, Engineering, and Medicine Research Scholarships, 976
Chatlos Fndn Grants, 977
Chazen Fndn Grants, 978
Chesapeake Corporation Fndn Grants, 982
Chicago White Metal Charitable Fndn Grants, 992
Children's Medical Research Institute Grants, 1000
Chiles Fndn Grants, 1003
Christy-Houston Fndn Grants, 1008
CICF Legacy Fund Comm Fndn Grants, 1010
CIGNA Fndn Grants, 1011
Clarence E. Heller Charitable Fndn Grants, 1022
Clarian Health Scholarships for LPNs, 1026
Clarian Health Student Nurse Extern Scholarships, 1027
Clark Fndn Grants, 1029
Claude Pepper Fndn Grants, 1032
CLF Graduate Studentships, 1038
Coastal Bend Comm Fndn Grants, 1050
Coastal Comm Fndn of South Carolina Grants, 1051
Coca-Cola Fndn Grants, 1052
Coeta and Donald Barker Fndn Grants, 1054
Colin Higgins Fndn Grants, 1056
Collins Fndn Grants, 1058
Colorado Interstate Gas Grants, 1060
Columbus Fndn Competitive Grants, 1066
Comerica Charitable Fndn Grants, 1073
Comm Fndn for Greater Buffalo Grants, 1090
Comm Fndn for Greater New Haven Grants, 1091
Comm Fndn for Muskegon County Grants, 1093
Comm Fndn for Southeastern Michigan Grants, 1094
Comm Fndn for Southern Arizona Grants, 1095
Comm Fndn of Bartholomew County Heritage Fund Grants, 1096
Comm Fndn of Bloomington and Monroe County Grants, 1098
Comm Fndn of Central Illinois Grants, 1101
Comm Fndn of Champaign County Grants, 1102
Comm Fndn of Crawford County Grants and Scholarships, 1103
Comm Fndn of Grant County Scholarships, 1105
Comm Fndn of Greater Flint Grants, 1107
Comm Fndn of Greater Fort Wayne: Comm Endowment & Clarke Endowment Fund Grants, 1108
Comm Fndn of Greater Greensboro Grants, 1109
Comm Fndn of Greater New Britain Grants, 1111
Comm Fndn of Madison and Jefferson County Grants and Scholarships, 1117
Comm Fndn of Morgan County Grants and Scholarships, 1118
Comm Fndn of Mount Vernon and Knox County Grants, 1119
Comm Fndn of Muncie and Delaware County Grants, 1120
Comm Fndn of Randolph County Grants, 1121
Comm Fndn of South Alabama Grants, 1123
Comm Fndn of South Puget Sound Grants, 1124
Comm Fndn of the Ozarks Grants, 1130
Comm Fndn of Wabash County Grants, 1131
Comm Fndn of Western North Carolina Grants, 1132
Comm Fndn Silicon Valley Grants, 1133
Compass Bank Fndn Grants, 1138
Connecticut Comm Fndn Grants, 1141
Connecticut Health Fndn Health Initiative Grants, 1142
Constellation Energy Group and Baltimore Gas and Electric Corp Contributions, 1146
Cooper Industries Fndn Grants, 1150
Cranston Fndn Grants, 1158
Cruise Industry Charitable Fndn Grants, 1166
CSRA Comm Fndn Grants, 1168
Cudd Fndn Grants, 1171
Cultural Society of Filipino Americans Grants, 1173
D.F. Halton Fndn Grants, 1181
DAAD Research Stays for University Academics and Scientists, 1183
DaimlerChrysler Corporation Fund Grants, 1186
Danellie Fndn Grants, 1198
Daphne Seybolt Culpeper Memorial Fndn Grants, 1201
DeBakey Medical Fndn Fellowships and Scholarships, 1212
Dennis and Phyllis Washington Fndn Grants, 1222
Dental Laboratory Technology Scholarships, 1223
DeRoy Testamentary Fndn Grants, 1239
DHHS Health Professions Preparatory Scholarship Program for Indians, 1257
DHHS Health Professions Scholarship Program, 1258
DHHS National Health Service Corps Loan Repayment Awards, 1265
DHHS National Health Service Corps Scholarships Program, 1266
DHHS Native American Health Service Loan Repayment Awards, 1267
DHHS Preventive Medicine, 1271
Do Something BR!CK Awards, 1287
Doreen Kronick Scholarship, 1312
Doris and Victor Day Fndn Grants, 1313
Dr. Bob and Jean Smith Fndn Grants, 1325
Dr. Courtney W. Shropshire Scholarship Grant, 1326
Dr. Leon Bromberg Charitable Trust Fund Grants, 1328
Dr. Stanley Pearle Scholarships, 1330
Dubois County Comm Fndn Grants, 1336
Duke Energy Fndn Grants, 1339
DuPage Comm Fndn Grants, 1352
eBay Fndn Comm Grants, 1363
Eden Hall Fndn Grants, 1368
Edward Bangs Kelley and Elza Kelley Fndn Grants, 1373
Edward S. Moore Fndn Grants, 1374
Edwin S. Webster Fndn Grants, 1376
Edwin W. and Catherine M. Davis Fndn Grants, 1377
Effie and Wofford Cain Fndn Grants, 1385
El Paso Comm Fndn Grants, 1388
Elizabeth Glaser Pediatric AIDS Fndn Two-Year Scholar Awards, 1397
Emerson Charitable Trust Grants, 1412
Emerson Electric Company Contributions Grants, 1413
Erie Comm Fndn Grants, 1427
Eugene B. Casey Fndn Grants, 1433
Eugene M. Lang Fndn Grants, 1434
Eugene McDermott Fndn Grants, 1435
Evan and Susan Bayh Fndn Grants, 1437
Evjue Fndn Grants, 1439
FACHE Albert W. Dent Scholarships, 1445
Fairfield County Comm Fndn Grants, 1446
Farmers Insurance Group of Companies Grants, 1455
FDHN Jon I. Isenberg International Research Scholar Award, 1473
Feldman Fndn Grants, 1484
Fishman Family Fndn Grants, 1510
Flinn Fndn Grantss, 1511
Fluor Fndn Grants, 1517
FMC Fndn Grants, 1518
Fndn for Physical Therapy Mary McMillan Doctoral Scholarships, 1529
Fndn for Science and Disability Grants for Physically Disabled Students in the Sciences, 1532
Fndn for Seacoast Health Grants, 1533
Fndn for the Carolinas Grants, 1535
Frances and John L. Loeb Family Fund Grants, 1546
Fred L. Emerson Fndn Grants, 1557
Fritz B. Burns Fndn Grants, 1564
Fuller E. Callaway Fndn Grants, 1578
G.N. Wilcox Trust Grants, 1581
Genuardi Family Fndn Grants, 1594
George and Ruth Bradford Fndn Grants, 1595
George Family Fndn Grants, 1598
George Kress Fndn Grants, 1601
George S. and Dolores Dore Eccles Fndn Grants, 1602
Gertrude B. Elion Mentored Medical Student Research Awards, 1608
Gertrude E. Skelly Charitable Fndn Grants, 1609
Giant Eagle Fndn Grants, 1611
Gilroy and Lillian P. Roberts Charitable Fndn Grants, 1614
Gladys Brooks Fndn Grants, 1620
Glendale Comm Fndn Grants, 1626
Global Fund for Children Grants, 1629
Graco Fndn Grants, 1642
Grand Haven Area Comm Fndn Grants, 1644
Greater New Orleans Fndn Grants, 1654
Greater Saint Louis Comm Fndn Grants, 1655
Greater Worcester Comm Fndn Discretionary Grants, 1658
Green Bay Packers Fndn Grants, 1660
Griffin Fndn Grants, 1670
Gulf Coast Comm Fndn Grants, 1676
Gulf Coast Comm of Venice Fndn Grants, 1677
H & R Fndn Grants, 1679

H. Schaffer Fndn Grants, 1680
H.A. and Mary K. Chapman Charitable Trust Grants, 1681
Hannaford Charitable Fndn Grants, 1692
Harold and Arlene Schnitzer CARE Fndn Grants, 1697
Harrison County Comm Fndn Grants, 1700
Harry and Grace Steele Fndn Grants, 1702
Harry Bramhall Gilbert Charitable Trust Grants, 1703
Harry Kramer Memorial Fund Grants, 1705
Hazel Corbin/Maternity Center Association Grant for Evidence-Based Midwifery Care, 1720
Health Management Scholarships and Grants for Minorities, 1727
Hearst Fndn and William Randolph Hearst Fndn Grants, 1730
Helen Bader Fndn Grants, 1738
Helen McWilliam Memorial Scholarship, 1741
Helena Rubinstein Fndn Grants, 1743
Herman Goldman Fndn Grants, 1753
High Meadow Fndn Grants, 1768
Hill Crest Fndn Grants, 1773
Hill Fndn Grants, 1774
Hillsdale County Comm General Adult Fndn Grants, 1777
Hirtzel Memorial Fndn Grants, 1781
HomeBanc Fndn Grants, 1788
Homer Fndn Grants, 1789
Honeywell Fndn Grants, 1791
Hormel Foods Charitable Trust Grants, 1795
Hormel Fndn Grants, 1796
Houston Endowment Grants, 1797
HRSA Health Professions Scholarships for Disadvantaged Students, 1807
HRSA Nursing Education Opportunities for the Disadvantaged Project Grants, 1809
Huie-Dellmon Trust Grants, 1815
Humana Fndn Grants, 1818
Huntington County Comm Fndn Grants, 1823
IATA Scholarships, 1835
Ildaura Murillo-Rohde Scholarships, 1841
Independence Blue Cross Nurse Scholars, 1847
Indiana Minority Teacher/Special Services Scholarships, 1852
Indiana Nursing Scholarships, 1853
International College of Surgeons Grants and Scholarships, 1859
Isabel Allende Fndn Esperanza Grants, 1868
J.C. Penney Company Grants, 1874
J.E. and L.E. Mabee Fndn Grants, 1875
J.L. Bedsole Fndn Grants, 1876
Jacob and Hilda Blaustein Fndn Grants, 1881
James G.K. McClure Educational and Development Fund Grants, 1886
James Graham Brown Fndn Grants, 1887
James J. and Angelia M. Harris Fndn Grants, 1890
James R. Dougherty Jr. Fndn Grants, 1894
James S. Copley Fndn Grants, 1895
Jane Beattie Memorial Scholarship, 1901
JELD-WEN Fndn Grants, 1914
Jewish Fndn for Education of Women Scholarships for Emigres in the Health Professions, 1922
Joe W. and Dorothy Dorsett Brown Fndn Grants, 1927
John Ben Snow Memorial Trust Grants, 1928
John Deere Fndn Grants, 1929
John H. and Wilhelmina D. Harland Charitable Fndn Grants, 1933
John I. Smith Charities Grants, 1935
John J. Leidy Fndn Grants, 1936
John Jewett and Helen Chandler Garland Fndn Grants, 1937
John P. McGovern Fndn Grants, 1942
John Stauffer Charitable Trust Grants, 1946
John W. Anderson Fndn Grants, 1949
Johns Manville Fund Grants, 1950
Johnson Controls Fndn Grants, 1954
Johnson F. Hammond Memorial Scholarship, 1956
Joseph Alexander Fndn Grants, 1957
Joseph and Luella Abell Charitable Trust Scholarships, 1958
Joseph Collins Fndn Grants, 1959
Joseph Drown Fndn Grants, 1960
Josephine G. Russell Trust Grants, 1963
Josiah W. and Bessie H. Kline Fndn Grants, 1967
Julia Temple Davis Brown Fndn Grants, 1971
K and F Baxter Family Fndn Grants, 1973
Kaiser Permanente Cares for Communities Grants, 1978
Kalamazoo Fndn Grants, 1979
Kathryne Beynon Fndn Grants, 1984
Kenneth T. and Eileen L. Norris Fndn Grants, 1989
Kettering Fund Grants, 1992
KFC Allied Health Research Grants, 1996
L. A. Hollinger Respiratory Therapy and Nursing Scholarships, 2018
Leo Goodwin Fndn Grants, 2043
Leonsis Fndn Grants, 2045
Lester Ray Fleming Scholarships, 2048
Lettie Pate Whitehead Fndn Grants, 2049
Lillian S. Wells Fndn Grants, 2056
Lincoln Financial Group Fndn Grants, 2058
Louis Calder Fndn Grants, 2065
Lowell Berry Fndn Grants, 2069
LSA Scholar Awards, 2075
Lubbock Area Fndn Grants, 2079
Lubrizol Fndn Grants, 2080
Lynde and Harry Bradley Fndn Grants, 2089
M. Bastian Family Fndn Grants, 2092
Madison County Comm Fndn Grants, 2098
Maine Comm Fndn Grants, 2099
MAPFRE Fndn for Medicine Grants, 2102
Margaret T. Morris Fndn Grants, 2105
Margoes Fndn Grants, 2106
Marion Park Deaver and Harry Gilbert Deaver Fndn Grants, 2110
Mars Fndn Grants, 2114
Matilda R. Wilson Fund Grants, 2128
Matsumae International Fndn Grants, 2129
Maxon Charitable Fndn Grants, 2135
May and Stanley Smith Trust Grants, 2137
McInerny Fndn Grants, 2144
McKesson Fndn Grants, 2145
McLean Contributionship Grants, 2147
MDBDF Agnes Higgins Award, 2155
Mead Johnson Nutritionals Scholarships, 2159
Mead Witter Fndn Grants, 2160
Meadows Fndn Grants, 2161
Measey Fndn Medical Education Grants, 2162
Medtronic Fndn Health Care Grants, 2169
Meriden Fndn Grants, 2173
Metro Health Fndn Grants, 2175
MHRC Graduate Studentships, 2185
Michael and Susan Dell Fndn Grants, 2189
Michigan Psychoanalytic Institute and Society Scholarships, 2194
Military Ex-Prisoners of War Fndn Grants, 2201
Minority Doctoral Fellowships in Science and Engineering, 2207
MONY Fndn Grants, 2215
Morris and Gwendolyn Cafritz Fndn Grants, 2217
NAPNAP Fndn Elaine Gelman Scholarship, 2235
NAPNAP Fndn McNeil PNP Scholarships, 2239
NAPNAP Fndn McNeil Rural and Underserved Scholarships, 2240
NAPNAP Fndn Nursing Research Grants, 2241
National Starch and Chemical Fndn Grants, 2261
National Student Nurses' Association Fndn Scholarship Program, 2262
NBNA Lauranne Sams Scholarships, 2264
New Jersey Osteopathic Education Fndn Scholarships, 2303
New York Life Fndn Grants, 2304
Nicholas H. Noyes Jr. Memorial Fndn Grants, 2497
NIH Undergraduate Scholarships, 2737
NMF Aura E. Severinghaus Award, 2828
NMF Henry G. Halladay Awards, 2831
NMF Hugh J. Andersen Memorial Scholarship, 2832
NMF Irving Graef Memorial Scholarship, 2833
NMF Mary Ball Carrera Scholarship, 2834
NMF Metropolitan Life Fndn Awards Program for Academic Excellence in Medicine, 2835
NMF National Medical Association Emerging Scholar Awards, 2837
NMF National Medical Association Patti LaBelle Award, 2838
NMF Need-Based Scholarships, 2839
NMSS Harry Weaver Neuroscience Scholar Awards, 2843
NMSS Scholarships, 2845
Nordson Corporation Fndn Grants, 2851
North Carolina Comm Fndn Grants, 2859
North Carolina GlaxoSmithKline Fndn Grants, 2860
North Georgia Comm Fndn Grants, 2862
Northwestern Mutual Fndn Grants, 2870
Oleonda Jameson Trust Grants, 2941
Olin Corporation Charitable Trust Grants, 2943
ONS Scholarships, 2950
Ordean Fndn Grants, 2952
OSI Supplementary Grants: Burma, 2971
Partnership for Cures Charles E. Culpeper Scholarships in Medical Science, 2991
Paso del Norte Health Fndn Grants, 2995
Paul and Mary Haas Fndn Contributions and Student Scholarships, 2997
Pfizer Fndn Epilepsy Scholarship Award, 3024
Piper Jaffray Companies Building Strong Communities Grants, 3053
Portland General Electric Fndn Grants, 3067
Pott Fndn Grants, 3071
Potts Memorial Fndn Grants, 3072
Pride Fndn Grants and Scholarships, 3078
Principal Financial Group Fndn Grants, 3082
Progress Energy Fndn Grants, 3084
Prudential Fndn Grants, 3087
Pulte Homes Corp Contributions, 3092
Putnam County Comm Fndn Grants, 3093
R.C. Baker Fndn Grants, 3098
Rajiv Gandhi Fndn Grants, 3104
Rathmann Family Fndn Grants, 3109
Rayonier Fndn Grants, 3111
Regenstrief Master Of Science In Clinical Research/CITE Program, 3145
Rehabilitation Nursing Fndn Scholarships, 3148
Rhode Island Fndn Grants, 3154
Richard P. Covert Scholarship, 3163
Robert and Polly Dunn Fndn Grants, 3168
Robert E. and Evelyn McKee Fndn Grants, 3170
Rockwell International Corp Trust Grants, 3183
Rosalynn Carter Institute Mattie J. T. Stepanek Caregiving Scholarships, 3190
Roy and Christine Sturgis Trust Grants, 3191
Roy J. Carver Charitable Trust Medical and Science Research Grants, 3192
Rush County Comm Fndn Grants, 3200
Ruth Eleanor Bamberger and John Ernest Bamberger Memorial Fndn Grants, 3202
RWJF New Careers in Nursing Scholarships, 3224
RWJF Summer Medical and Dental Education Program (SMDEP), 3231
RWJF Young Epidemiology Scholars (YES) Competition, 3233
S. Livingston Mather Charitable Trust Grants, 3235
S. Mark Taper Fndn Grants, 3236
Samuel S. Johnson Fndn Grants, 3251
San Antonio Area Fndn Grants, 3254
Schering-Plough Fndn Health Grants, 3270
Seabury Fndn Grants, 3274
Searle Scholars Program Grants, 3275
Seattle Fndn Grants, 3276
Seneca Foods Fndn Grants, 3278
Shell Oil Company Fndn Grants, 3281
Simmons Fndn Grants, 3287
SNM PDEF Mickey Williams Minority Student Scholarships, 3302
SNMTS Clinical Advancement Scholarships, 3309
SNMTS Paul Cole Scholarships, 3312
Solo Cup Fndn Grants, 3346
Special People in Need Scholarships, 3357

Square D Fndn Grants, 3361
Starr Fndn Grants, 3377
Steele-Reese Fndn Grants, 3380
Strowd Roses Grants, 3388
Sulzberger Fndn Grants, 3399
Temple-Inland Fndn Grants, 3419
Thomas and Dorothy Leavey Fndn Grants, 3422
Thomas C. Ackerman Fndn Grants, 3423
Thompson Charitable Fndn Grants, 3425
Topeka Comm Fndn Kansas Blood Services Scholarships, 3429
Trinity Lutheran School of Nursing Alumnae Scholarships, 3439
Trull Fndn Grants, 3441
TWS Fndn Grants, 3443
Tylenol Scholarship, 3444
U.S. Department of Education Erma Byrd Scholarships, 3446
University of Calgary Nursing Alumni Scholarship, 3468
VDH Commonwealth of Virginia Nurse Educator Scholarships, 3482
Virginia Department of Health Mary Marshall Nursing Scholarships for Licensed Practical Nurses, 3498
Virginia Department of Health Mary Marshall Nursing Scholarships for Registered Nurses, 3499
Virginia Department of Health Nurse Practitioner/ Nurse Midwife Scholarships, 3500
Virginia Tuition Assistance Grants, 3501
Vulcan Materials Company Fndn Grants, 3504
W.W. Smith Charitable Trust Grants for Medical Research in Cancer, AIDS, and Heart Disease, 3509
Wabash Valley Comm Fndn Grants, 3510
Wachovia Fndn Grants, 3511
Walt Disney Company Fndn Grants, 3516
Wasie Fndn Grants, 3521
Wayne and Gladys Valley Fndn Grants, 3522
Weatherwax Fndn Grants, 3523
Wells County Fndn Grants, 3527
William G. Gilmore Fndn Grants, 3537
William G. McGowan Charitable Fund Grants, 3539
Winston-Salem Fndn Competitive Grants, 3544
Women of the ELCA Opportunity Scholarships for Lutheran Laywomen, 3548
Women's Sports Fndn Grants, 3551
Z. Smith Reynolds Fndn Small Grants, 3557

Seed Grants

100 Mile Man Fndn Grants, 2
A Friend's Fndn Trust Grants, 13
A-T Medical Research Fndn Grants, 16
AAFPRS Bernstein Grant, 118
Abbott Fund Comm Vitality Grants, 177
Abell-Hanger Fndn Grants, 183
ACS Institutional Research Grants, 215
Acushnet Fndn Grants, 226
Adams County Fndn Grants - Pennsylvania, 231
Adelaide Breed Bayrd Fndn Grants, 234
Adolph Coors Fndn Grants, 238
AFAR CART Fund Grants, 254
Agnes M. Lindsay Trust Grants, 263
Ahmanson Fndn Grants, 303
Air Products and Chemicals Grants, 319
Alabama Power Fndn Grants, 321
Aladdin Industries Fndn Grants, 322
Albuquerque Comm Fndn Grants, 331
Alcoa Fndn Grants, 334
Alcon Fndn Grants, 336
Alexander and Margaret Stewart Trust Grants, 340
Allen P. and Josephine B. Green Fndn Grants, 361
Alliance Healthcare Fndn Grants, 362
Allstate Corp Giving Grants, 363
Allstate Corp Hometown Commitment Grants, 364
Allyn Fndn Grants, 365
Alpha Omega Fndn Grants, 366
AMA Fndn Fund for Better Health Grants, 388
AMA Fndn Seed Grants for Research, 398
AMA-WPC Joan F. Giambalvo Memorial Scholarships, 408
Amador Comm Fndn Grants, 409
American Fndn for Suicide Prevention Grants, 436
American Legacy Fndn National Calls for Proposals Grants, 438
American Schlafhorst Fndn Grants, 454
amfAR Research Grants, 466
Andersen Fndn Grants, 471
Angels Baseball Fndn Grants, 473
Ann Arbor Area Comm Fndn Grants, 476
Annenberg Fndn Grants, 479
Anschutz Family Fndn Grants, 486
APF Disaster Recovery Fund for Psychiatrists, 506
APhA Fndn Incentive Grants, 512
Aratani Fndn Grants, 523
ARCO Fndn Education Grants, 526
Arkansas Comm Fndn Grants, 533
Arkell Hall Fndn Grants, 534
Arlington Comm Fndn Grants, 536
AT&T Fndn Civic and Comm Service Program Grants, 658
Atherton Family Fndn Grants, 659
Atlanta Fndn Grants, 662
Atran Fndn Grants, 663
Autzen Fndn Grants, 672
Axe-Houghton Fndn Grants, 678
Bacon Family Fndn Grants, 679
Ball Brothers Fndn General Grants, 683
Ball Brothers Fndn Grants, 684
Bank of America Charitable Fndn Anchor Institutions Grants, 688
Barker Welfare Fndn Grants, 695
Barra Fndn Comm Fund Grants, 698
Barra Fndn Project Grants, 699
Barth Syndrome Fndn Research Grants, 700
Baton Rouge Area Fndn Grants, 702
Battle Creek Comm Fndn Grants, 703
Baxter International Fndn Grants, 705
BCBS of Minnesota Healthy Together Grants, 712
BCBSM Fndn Physician Investigator Research Awards, 718
Beckley Area Fndn Grants, 732
Becton Dickinson and Company Grants, 736
Beldon Fund Grants, 738
Bender Fndn Grants, 742
Berks County Comm Fndn Grants, 745
Bertha Russ Lytel Fndn Grants, 751
Blue Grass Comm Fndn Grants, 768
Blue Mountain Comm Fndn Grants, 769
Blue River Comm Fndn Grants, 770
Blumenthal Fndn Grants, 773
Bodenwein Public Benevolent Fndn Grants, 775
Bodman Fndn Grants, 776
Boeing Company Contributions Program Grants, 777
Boettcher Fndn Grants, 778
Boston Fndn Grants, 783
Brookdale Fndn National Group Respite and Early Memory Loss Program Grants, 806
Bullitt Fndn Grants, 809
Bushrod H. Campbell and Adah F. Hall Charity Fund Grants, 816
California Comm Fndn Human Development Grants, 832
Cambridge Comm Fndn Grants, 837
Cancer Research Society Fellowships and Grants, 857
Capital Region Comm Fndn Grants, 862
Carl and Lily Pforzheimer Fndn Grants, 868
Carlisle Fndn Grants, 874
Carlos and Marguerite Mason Trust Grants, 875
Carls Fndn Grants, 876
Carnahan-Jackson Fndn Grants, 878
Carpenter Fndn Grants, 881
Carrie E. and Lena V. Glenn Fndn Grants, 882
Carrie Estelle Doheny Fndn Grants, 883
Catholic Campaign for Human Development (CCHD) Comm Organizing Grants, 891
Cemala Fndn Grants, 933
Central Carolina Comm Fndn Comm Impact Grants, 936
Central Okanagan Fndn Grants, 937
CFPC Research and Education Fndn Grants, 956
Charles Delmar Fndn Grants, 963
Charles Edison Fund Grants, 964
Charles G. Koch Charitable Fndn Grants, 965
Charles H. Farnsworth Trust Grants, 967
Charles H. Hood Fndn Child Health Research Grants, 968
Charlotte County (FL) Comm Fndn Grants, 973
Chestnut Hill Charitable Fndn, Inc Grants, 987
Child Nutrition Fndn School Comm Kitchens Grants, 993
Children's Leukemia Research Association Research Grants, 999
Children's Medical Research Institute Grants, 1000
Children's Cardiomyopathy Fndn Research Grants, 1002
Clarence E. Heller Charitable Fndn Grants, 1022
Clark County Comm Fndn Grants, 1028
Clark Fndn Grants, 1029
Claude Worthington Benedum Fndn Grants, 1033
Clay Fndn Grants, 1034
CLF Operating Grants, 1039
CNCS Next Generation Grants, 1049
Coastal Bend Comm Fndn Grants, 1050
Coastal Comm Fndn of South Carolina Grants, 1051
Collins C. Diboll Private Fndn Grants, 1057
Colorado Springs Comm Trust Fund Grants, 1061
Columbus Fndn Competitive Grants, 1066
Columbus Fndn Traditional Grants, 1071
Comm Fndn Alliance City of Evansville Endowment Fund Grants, 1089
Comm Fndn for Greater Buffalo Grants, 1090
Comm Fndn for Greater New Haven Grants, 1091
Comm Fndn for Monterey County Grants, 1092
Comm Fndn for Muskegon County Grants, 1093
Comm Fndn for Southeastern Michigan Grants, 1094
Comm Fndn for Southern Arizona Grants, 1095
Comm Fndn of Bartholomew County Heritage Fund Grants, 1096
Comm Fndn of Bloomington and Monroe County Grants, 1098
Comm Fndn of Boone County Grants, 1099
Comm Fndn of Central Illinois Grants, 1101
Comm Fndn of Greater Birmingham Grants, 1106
Comm Fndn of Greater Flint Grants, 1107
Comm Fndn of Greater Fort Wayne: Comm Endowment & Clarke Endowment Fund Grants, 1108
Comm Fndn of Greater Greensboro Grants, 1109
Comm Fndn of Howard County Grants, 1116
Comm Fndn of Mount Vernon and Knox County Grants, 1119
Comm Fndn of Muncie and Delaware County Grants, 1120
Comm Fndn of Randolph County Grants, 1121
Comm Fndn of South Alabama Grants, 1123
Comm Fndn of Southeastern Connecticut Grants, 1125
Comm Fndn of Tampa Bay Grants, 1128
Comm Fndn of the Eastern Shore Comm Needs Grants, 1129
Comm Fndn of the Ozarks Grants, 1130
Comm Fndn of Wabash County Grants, 1131
Comm Fndn of Western North Carolina Grants, 1132
Comm Fndn Silicon Valley Grants, 1133
Connecticut Comm Fndn Grants, 1141
Cooke Fndn Grants, 1148
Cooper Industries Fndn Grants, 1150
Cowles Charitable Trust Grants, 1155
CSRA Comm Fndn Grants, 1168
Dana Corporation Fndn Grants, 1196
Daywood Fndn Grants, 1206
Deafness Research Fndn Research Grants, 1208
DHHS Developmental Disabilities University Affiliated Programs Project Grants, 1248
Doris and Victor Day Fndn Grants, 1313
Dorothea Haus Ross Fndn Grants, 1320
Dr. John T. Macdonald Fndn Grants, 1327

Drs. Bruce and Lee Fndn Grants, 1333
Echoing Green Fellowships, 1365
Eddie C. and Sylvia Brown Family Fndn Grants, 1367
Educational Fndn of America Grants, 1372
Edward Bangs Kelley and Elza Kelley Fndn Grants, 1373
Edward S. Moore Fndn Grants, 1374
Edyth Bush Charitable Fndn Grants, 1378
EF Predoctoral Research Training Fellowship, 1383
Effie and Wofford Cain Fndn Grants, 1385
Eisner Fndn Grants, 1387
El Paso Comm Fndn Grants, 1388
El Pomar Fndn Awards and Grants, 1390
Elisabeth Severance Prentiss Fndn Grants, 1392
Elizabeth Morse Genius Charitable Trust Grants, 1400
Elmer L. and Eleanor J. Andersen Fndn Grants, 1406
Emily Davie and Joseph S. Kornfeld Fndn Grants, 1414
Emma B. Howe Memorial Fndn Grants, 1415
Ensworth Charitable Fndn Grants, 1416
Epilepsy Research Fndn New Therapy Grants, 1423
Eppley Fndn Postdoctoral Grants, 1425
Erie Comm Fndn Grants, 1427
Essex County Comm Fndn Discretionary Fund Grant, 1428
Eugene and Agnes E. Meyer Fndn Grants, 1432
Eugene M. Lang Fndn Grants, 1434
Eugene McDermott Fndn Grants, 1435
Eva L. and Joseph M. Bruening Fndn Grants, 1436
Evan and Susan Bayh Fndn Grants, 1437
Evanston Comm Fndn Grants, 1438
Evjue Fndn Grants, 1439
Ewing Halsell Fndn Grants, 1440
F.M. Kirby Fndn Grants, 1443
Fargo-Moorhead Area Fndn Grants, 1454
Federal Express Corp Contributions Program, 1483
Field Fndn of Illinois Grants, 1499
Flinn Fndn Grantss, 1511
Foellinger Fndn Grants, 1519
Fondren Fndn Grants, 1520
Fndn for Seacoast Health Grants, 1533
Fndn for the Carolinas Grants, 1535
Fndn Northwest Grants, 1537
Frances L. and Edwin L. Cummings Memorial Fund Grants, 1547
Francis L. Abreu Charitable Trust Grants, 1549
Frank Stanley Beveridge Fndn Grants, 1553
Frey Fndn Grants, 1562
Fulton County Comm Fndn Grants, 1579
G.N. Wilcox Trust Grants, 1581
Gebbie Fndn Grants, 1585
General Motors Fndn Grants Support Program, 1591
George Frederick Jewett Fndn Grants, 1599
George H. Hitchings New Investigator Award in Health Research, 1600
Georgiana Goddard Eaton Memorial Fund Grants, 1604
GlaxoSmithKline Corp Grants, 1623
Good Samaritan Inc Grants, 1637
Grand Haven Area Comm Fndn Grants, 1644
Grand Rapids Comm Fndn Grants, 1647
Greater Saint Louis Comm Fndn Grants, 1655
Greater Tacoma Comm Fndn Grants, 1656
Greater Worcester Comm Fndn Discretionary Grants, 1658
H. Schaffer Fndn Grants, 1680
Harold Simmons Fndn Grants, 1698
Harris and Eliza Kempner Fund Grants, 1699
Harry A. and Margaret D. Towsley Fndn Grants, 1701
Harry Kramer Memorial Fund Grants, 1705
Hartford Courant Fndn Grants, 1710
Hartford Fndn Regular Grants, 1711
Hasbro Children's Fund, 1714
Health Fndn of Greater Indianapolis Grants, 1725
Heineman Fndn for Research, Education, Charitable and Scientific Purposes, 1735
Helen Steiner Rice Fndn Grants, 1742
Henrietta Tower Wurts Memorial Fndn Grants, 1745
Hereditary Disease Fndn Research Grants, 1752
Herman Goldman Fndn Grants, 1753
Hill Crest Fndn Grants, 1773
Hilton Head Island Fndn Grants, 1779
Holland/Zeeland Comm Fndn Grants, 1786
Horace A. Kimball and S. Ella Kimball Fndn Grants, 1792
Howard and Bush Fndn Grants, 1798
Huber Fndn Grants, 1812
Hunter's Hope Fndn Grants, 1820
Huntington's Disease Society of America Research Grants, 1826
Idaho Comm Fndn Eastern Region Competitive Grants, 1837
Impact 100 Grants, 1843
Implant Dentistry Research and Education Fndn Grants, 1844
Indiana 21st Century Research and Technology Fund Awards, 1850
Innovative Technology Development Award Program, 1855
Ittleson Fndn AIDS Grants, 1869
Ittleson Fndn Mental Health Grants, 1870
J. Walton Bissell Fndn Grants, 1872
Jackson County Comm Fndn Unrestricted Grants, 1879
Jacob G. Schmidlapp Trust Grants, 1883
James Ford Bell Fndn Grants, 1885
James H. Cummings Fndn Grants, 1888
James J. and Angelia M. Harris Fndn Grants, 1890
James R. Dougherty Jr. Fndn Grants, 1894
JELD-WEN Fndn Grants, 1914
Jessie Ball Dupont Fund Grants, 1919
Jewish Comm Fndn of Greater Los Angeles Grants, 1921
Jewish Fund Grants, 1923
JM Fndn Grants, 1926
John Ben Snow Memorial Trust Grants, 1928
John Deere Fndn Grants, 1929
John G. Duncan Trust Grants, 1931
John Merck Fund Grants, 1940
John P. Murphy Fndn Grants, 1943
John W. Alden Trust Grants, 1947
John W. and Anna H. Hanes Fndn Grants, 1948
Johns Manville Fund Grants, 1950
Johnson County Comm Fndn Grants, 1955
Joseph Drown Fndn Grants, 1960
Joseph P. Kennedy Jr. Fndn Grants, 1962
Josephine Goodyear Fndn Grants, 1964
Kalamazoo Fndn Grants, 1979
Kate B. Reynolds Charitable Trust Health Care Grants, 1981
Katharine Matthies Fndn Grants, 1982
Katherine John Murphy Fndn Grants, 1983
Kenny's Kids Grants, 1990
Kettering Fund Grants, 1992
Komen Greater NYC Small Grants, 2013
Kosciusko County Comm Fndn Grants, 2015
LAM Fndn Research Grants, 2024
Land O'Lakes Fndn Mid-Atlantic Grants, 2027
Laura B. Vogler Fndn Grants, 2032
Layne Beachley Aim For The Stars Fndn Grants, 2036
Lubbock Area Fndn Grants, 2079
Lucy Gooding Charitable Fndn Trust, 2082
M.B. and Edna Zale Fndn Grants, 2093
Mabel Y. Hughes Charitable Trust Grants, 2097
Maine Comm Fndn Grants, 2099
Manuel D. and Rhoda Mayerson Fndn Grants, 2100
Margoes Fndn Grants, 2106
Marion I. and Henry J. Knott Fndn Grants, 2109
Mark and Catherine Winkler Fndn Grants, 2112
Mary Owen Borden Fndn Grants, 2121
Mass Youth Against Tobacco Mini-Grants, 2123
Max Bell Fndn Grants, 2134
McCarthy Family Fndn Grants, 2141
McGregor Fund Grants, 2143
McInerny Fndn Grants, 2144
McKesson Fndn Grants, 2145
McLean Contributionship Grants, 2147
McMurry Fndn Grants, 2149
Mead Witter Fndn Grants, 2160
Meadows Fndn Grants, 2161
Medtronic Fndn Health Care Grants, 2169
Metro Health Fndn Grants, 2175
Meyer Memorial Trust Grassroots Grants, 2179
Meyer Memorial Trust Responsive Grants, 2181
Morris and Gwendolyn Cafritz Fndn Grants, 2217
NAF Research Grants, 2232
Nancy R. Gelman Fndn Breast Cancer Seed Grants, 2234
Narcolepsy Network Seed Grants, 2245
National Psoriasis Fndn Research Grants, 2259
NIH Genetics of Neurobehavioral Disorders in Existing Samples Grants, 2670
NIMH Pilot Effectiveness Trials for Mental Disorders Grants, 2766
NIMH Therapeutic Effectiveness Protocol Development Program Grants, 2774
Nina Mason Pulliam Charitable Trust Grants, 2776
Noble County Comm Fndn Grants, 2848
NORD Orphan Diseases Research Grants, 2849
Nordson Corporation Fndn Grants, 2851
North Carolina GlaxoSmithKline Fndn Grants, 2860
North Georgia Comm Fndn Grants, 2862
Northern New York Comm Fndn Grants, 2864
Northwest Minnesota Fndn Women's Fund Grants, 2869
NWHF Health Advocacy Small Grants, 2905
Olin Corporation Charitable Trust Grants, 2943
OREF Research Grants, 2957
Osteogenesis Imperfecta Fndn Research Grants, 2975
PacifiCare Fndn Grants, 2981
Palm Beach and Martin Counties Grants, 2986
Partners for Youth with Disabilities Grants, 2990
Patron Saints Fndn Grants, 2996
Paul and Mary Haas Fndn Contributions and Student Scholarships, 2997
Paul E. and Klare N. Reinhold Fndn Grants, 2999
Philadelphia Fndn Organizational Effectiveness Grants, 3029
PhRMA Fndn Health Outcomes Research Starter Grants, 3033
PhRMA Fndn Informatics Research Starter Grants, 3038
PhRMA Fndn Pharmaceutics Research Starter Grants, 3042
PhRMA Fndn Pharmacology/Toxicology Research Starter Grants, 3046
Pioneer Hi-Bred Comm Grants, 3051
Plastic Surgery Educational Fndn Basic Research Grants, 3058
Plough Fndn Grants, 3061
Polaroid Fund Grants, 3065
Portland General Electric Fndn Grants, 3067
Potts Memorial Fndn Grants, 3072
Pride Fndn Grants and Scholarships, 3078
Principal Financial Group Fndn Grants, 3082
Prudential Fndn Grants, 3087
Public Welfare Fndn Grants, 3089
Quantum Fndn Grants, 3096
Raskob Fndn for Catholic Activities Grants, 3107
Rathmann Family Fndn Grants, 3109
Rayonier Fndn Grants, 3111
Rhode Island Fndn Grants, 3154
Richard and Helen DeVos Fndn Grants, 3157
Richard and Rhoda Goldman Fund Grants, 3158
Richard and Susan Smith Family Fndn Grants, 3159
Richard King Mellon Fndn Grants, 3161
Ripley County Comm Fndn Grants, 3166
Rochester Area Comm Fndn Grants, 3176
Rohm and Haas Company Grants, 3185
Roy J. Carver Charitable Trust Medical and Science Research Grants, 3192
Ruth H. and Warren A. Ellsworth Fndn Grants, 3203
S. Livingston Mather Charitable Trust Grants, 3235
S. Mark Taper Fndn Grants, 3236
Salem Fndn Charitable Trust Grants, 3241

Samuel Freeman Charitable Trust Grants, 3249
Samuel S. Johnson Fndn Grants, 3251
San Antonio Area Fndn Grants, 3254
San Diego Women's Fndn Grants, 3259
San Francisco Fndn Comm Health Grants, 3260
Sarah Scaife Fndn Grants, 3263
Schering-Plough Fndn Health Grants, 3270
Scott County Comm Fndn Grants, 3273
Seabury Fndn Grants, 3274
Sid W. Richardson Fndn Grants, 3284
Siebert Lutheran Fndn Grants, 3285
Sisters of Mercy of North Carolina Fndn Grants, 3295
Sisters of St. Joseph Healthcare Fndn Grants, 3297
SNM/ Covidien Seed Grant in Molecular Imaging/ Nuclear Medicine Research, 3308
Society for Biomedical Screening Small Grants, 3319
Sosland Fndn Grants, 3348
St. Joseph Comm Health Fndn Improving Healthcare Access Grants, 3368
Stewart Huston Charitable Trust Grants, 3384
Strowd Roses Grants, 3388
Thomas C. Ackerman Fndn Grants, 3423
U.S. Lacrosse EAD Grants, 3453
Union County Comm Fndn Grants, 3461
Unity Fndn Of LaPorte County Grants, 3467
Verizon Fndn Vermont Grants, 3491
Virginia W. Kettering Fndn Grants, 3502
Vulcan Materials Company Fndn Grants, 3504
W.K. Kellogg Fndn Secure Families Grants, 3508
Wachovia Fndn Grants, 3511
Weingart Fndn Grants, 3524
Wells County Fndn Grants, 3527
William G. McGowan Charitable Fund Grants, 3539
Winston-Salem Fndn Competitive Grants, 3544
Z. Smith Reynolds Fndn Small Grants, 3557

Service Delivery Programs

1 in 9: Long Island Breast Cancer Action Coalition Grants, 1
1104 Fndn Grants, 3
1976 Fndn Grants, 5
2 Depot Square Ipswich Charitable Fndn Grants, 7
2COBS Private Charitable Fndn Grants, 9
3M Fndn Grants, 11
49ers Fndn Grants, 12
A Friend's Fndn Trust Grants, 13
A Fund for Women Grants, 14
A. Gary Anderson Family Fndn Grants, 17
A.O. Smith Comm Grants, 18
AAHPERD Ruth Abernathy Presidential Scholarships, 128
AAHPM Hospice and Palliative Medicine Fellowships, 132
AAMC Caring for Comm Grants, 136
AAP Comm Access To Child Health (CATCH) Advocacy Training Grants, 157
AAP Comm Access To Child Health (CATCH) Implementation Grants, 158
AAP Comm Access to Child Health (CATCH) Planning Grants, 159
AAP Comm Access To Child Health (CATCH) Residency Training Grants, 160
AAP Comm Access To Child Health (CATCH) Resident Grants, 161
AAP Leonard P. Rome Comm Access to Child Health (CATCH) Visiting Professorships, 164
AAP Resident Initiative Fund Grants, 167
Aaron & Freda Glickman Fndn Grants, 172
Aaron Fndn (California) Grants, 173
Aaron Fndn (Massachusetts) Grants, 174
Abbott Fund Access to Health Care Grants, 176
Abbott Fund Comm Vitality Grants, 177
Abbott Fund Global AIDS Care Grants, 178
Abbott Fund Science and Medical Innovation Grants, 179
Abel Fndn Grants, 181
Abell Fndn Health and Human Services Grants, 182
Abell-Hanger Fndn Grants, 183
Abington Fndn Grants, 184
Able To Serve Grants, 185
Able Trust Vocational Rehabilitation Grants for Individuals, 186
Abramson Family Fndn Grants, 188
ACE Charitable Fndn Grants, 199
ACF Ethnic Comm Self-Help Grants, 200
ACF Preferred Communities Grants, 201
ACF Standing Announcement for Unaccompanied Alien Children Grants, 202
ACF Supplemental Services for Recently Arrived Refugees Grants, 203
Achelis and Bodman Fndns Grants, 206
Acushnet Fndn Grants, 226
Adam Richter Charitable Trust Grants, 230
Adaptec Fndn Grants, 232
Addison H. Gibson Fndn Medical Grants, 233
Adelaide Breed Bayrd Fndn Grants, 234
Administaff Comm Affairs Grants, 235
Administration on Aging Senior Medicare Patrol Project Grants, 236
Adobe Comm Investment Grants, 237
Adolph Coors Fndn Grants, 238
Advanced Micro Devices Comm Affairs Grants, 239
Advancing Colorado's Mental Health Care Project Grants, 240
Advocate HealthCare Post Graduate Administrative Fellowship, 241
AEC Trust Grants, 242
AEGON Transamerica Fndn Grants, 243
Aetna Fndn Health Grants in Connecticut, 244
Aetna Fndn Quality of Care Grants for Depression, 246
Aetna Fndn Quality of Care Grants for End of Life Care, 247
Aetna Fndn Regional Comm Health Grants, 249
Aetna Fndn Regional Comm Health Outreach Grants, 250
AFG Industries Grants, 259
African American Fund of New Jersey Grants, 260
Agnes B. Hunt Trust Grants, 261
Agnes M. Lindsay Trust Grants, 263
Agway Fndn Grants, 265
Ahmanson Fndn Grants, 303
Ahn Family Fndn Grants, 304
AIDS Vaccine Advocacy Coalition (AVAC) Fund Grants, 315
AIG American General Corporation Grants, 316
Air Products and Chemicals Grants, 319
Aladdin Industries Fndn Grants, 322
Alaska Airlines Corp Giving Grants, 323
Alaska Airlines Fndn Grants, 324
Albert and Margaret Alkek Fndn Grants, 326
Albert Pick Jr. Fund Grants, 328
Alberto Culver Corp Contributions Grants, 329
Albertson's Charitable Giving Grants, 330
Albuquerque Comm Fndn Grants, 331
Alcatel-Lucent Technologies Corp Contributions Grants, 332
Alcatel-Lucent Technologies Fndn Grants, 333
Alcoa Fndn Grants, 334
Alexander & Baldwin Fndn Hawaiian and Pacific Island Grants, 338
Alexander & Baldwin Fndn Mainland Grants, 339
Alexander and Margaret Stewart Trust Grants, 340
Alexander Eastman Fndn Grants, 341
Alexander Fndn Cancer, Catastrophic Illness and Injury Grants, 342
Alexander Fndn Insurance Continuation Grants, 343
Alice C. A. Sibley Fund Grants, 355
Allegan County Comm Fndn Grants, 358
Allegheny Technologies Charitable Trust, 359
Allegis Group Fndn Grants, 360
Allen P. and Josephine B. Green Fndn Grants, 361
Alliance Healthcare Fndn Grants, 362
Allstate Corp Giving Grants, 363
Allstate Corp Hometown Commitment Grants, 364
Allyn Fndn Grants, 365
ALSAM Fndn Grants, 369
AMA Fndn Fund for Better Health Grants, 388
AMA Fndn Health Literacy Grants, 389
AMA Fndn Healthy Communities/Healthy America Grants, 390
AMA Fndn Seed Grants for Research, 398
Amador Comm Fndn Grants, 409
Amarillo Area/Harrington Fndns Grants, 410
AMD Corp Contributions Grants, 411
American Academy of Dermatology Camp Discovery Scholarships, 412
American Electric Power Grants, 434
American Express Fndn Comm Service Grants, 435
American Jewish World Service Grants, 437
American Legacy Fndn National Calls for Proposals Grants, 438
Amerisure Insurance Comm Service Grants, 461
amfAR Global Initiatives Grants, 463
Amgen Fndn Grants, 467
AMI Semiconductors Corp Grants, 468
Andersen Fndn Grants, 471
Angel Kiss Fndn Grants, 472
Angels Baseball Fndn Grants, 473
Anheuser-Busch Fndn Grants, 474
Ann and Robert H. Lurie Family Fndn Grants, 475
Ann Arbor Area Comm Fndn Grants, 476
Ann Peppers Fndn Grants, 478
Annie Sinclair Knudsen Memorial Fund/Kaua'i Comm Grants, 480
Annunziata Sanguinetti Fndn Grants, 481
Ansell, Zaro, Grimm & Aaron Fndn Grants, 487
Anthem Blue Cross and Blue Shield Grants, 488
Anthony R. Abraham Fndn Grants, 490
AON Fndn Grants, 491
APA Culture of Service in the Psychological Sciences Award, 493
APA Meritorious Research Service Commendation, 499
APF Call for Proposals, 505
APF Disaster Recovery Fund for Psychiatrists, 506
APF Helping Hands Grants, 507
APhA Fndn Incentive Grants, 512
APPEAL Social Justice and Tobacco Control Grants, 513
APSAA Fndn Grants, 517
Aratani Fndn Grants, 523
Arcadia Fndn Grants, 524
Archer Daniels Midland Fndn Grants, 525
ARCO Fndn Education Grants, 526
Argyros Fndn Grants, 527
Arie and Ida Crown Memorial Grants, 528
Arizona Cardinals Grants, 529
Arizona Diamondbacks Charities Grants, 530
Arkansas Comm Fndn Arkansas Black Hall of Fame Grants, 532
Arkansas Comm Fndn Grants, 533
Arkell Hall Fndn Grants, 534
Arlington Comm Fndn Grants, 536
Armstrong McDonald Fndn Grants, 537
ARS Fndn Grants, 538
Arthur and Rochelle Belfer Fndn Grants, 542
ArvinMeritor Fndn Health Grants, 543
ArvinMeritor Grants, 544
ASCO State Affiliate Grants, 560
ASHA Advancing Academic-Research Careers (AARC) Award, 569
ASHA Multicultural Activities Projects Grants, 571
Ashland Corp Contributions Grants, 586
Assisi Fndn Grants, 653
Assurant Fndn Grants, 654
AT&T Excelerator, 657
AT&T Fndn Civic and Comm Service Program Grants, 658
Atherton Family Fndn Grants, 659
Athwin Fndn Grants, 660
Atkinson Fndn International Grants, 661
Atlanta Fndn Grants, 662
Atran Fndn Grants, 663
Auburn Fndn Grants, 664
Audrey and Sydney Irmas Charitable Fndn Grants, 665

Austin-Bailey Health and Wellness Fndn Grants, 669
Autodesk Comm Relations Grants, 671
Autzen Fndn Grants, 672
AVDF Health Care Grants, 673
Avon Fndn Breast Care Fund Grants, 674
Avon Products Fndn Grants, 675
Bailey Fndn Grants, 680
Balfe Family Fndn Grants, 682
Ball Brothers Fndn Grants, 684
Banfi Vintners Fndn Grants, 687
Bank of America Charitable Fndn National Programs and Partners Grants, 689
Bank of America Client Fndn Grants, 690
Baptist Comm Ministries Grants, 691
Baptist-Trinity Lutheran Legacy Fndn Grants, 692
Barberton Comm Fndn Grants, 693
Barker Fndn Grants, 694
Barker Welfare Fndn Grants, 695
Barr Fund Grants, 697
Barra Fndn Comm Fund Grants, 698
Barra Fndn Project Grants, 699
Batchelor Fndn Grants, 701
Baton Rouge Area Fndn Grants, 702
Battle Creek Comm Fndn Grants, 703
Baxter International Fndn Grants, 705
BCBS of Massachusetts Catalyst Fund Grants, 708
BCBS of Massachusetts Fndn Grants, 709
BCBS of Minnesota Growing Up Healthy Grants, 711
BCBS of Minnesota Healthy Together Grants, 712
BCBSM Claude Pepper Award, 714
BCBSM Fndn Proposal Development Awards, 720
BCBSNC Fndn Fit Together Grants, 724
BCBSNC Fndn Grants, 725
Bearemy's Kennel Pals Grants, 728
Beazley Fndn Grants, 730
Beckley Area Fndn Grants, 732
Becton Dickinson and Company Grants, 736
Belk Fndn Grants, 739
Ben B. Cheney Fndn Grants, 741
Bender Fndn Grants, 742
Benton Comm Fndn Grants, 743
Benton County Fndn Grants, 744
Berks County Comm Fndn Grants, 745
Bernard and Audre Rapoport Fndn Grants, 746
Bernard F. and Alva B. Gimbel Fndn Grants, 747
Bernard Van Leer Fndn Grants, 748
Besser Fndn Grants, 752
BHHS Legacy Fndn Grants, 753
BibleLands Grants, 754
Bildner Family Fndn Grants, 755
Bill and Melinda Gates Fndn Grants, 756
Biogen Corp Giving Grants, 758
Birmingham Fndn Grants, 760
BJ's Charitable Fndn Grants, 761
Black River Falls Area Fndn Grants, 762
Blackford County Comm Fndn Grants, 763
Blanche and Irving Laurie Fndn Grants, 764
Blowitz-Ridgeway Fndn Grants, 767
Blue Grass Comm Fndn Grants, 768
Blue Mountain Comm Fndn Grants, 769
Blue River Comm Fndn Grants, 770
Blue Shield of California Grants, 771
Blum-Kovler Fndn Grants, 772
Blumenthal Fndn Grants, 773
Bodenwein Public Benevolent Fndn Grants, 775
Bodman Fndn Grants, 776
Boettcher Fndn Grants, 778
Booth-Bricker Fund Grants, 780
Boston Fndn Grants, 783
Boston Globe Fndn Grants, 784
Boston Jewish Comm Women's Fund Grants, 785
Bradley Turner Fndn Grants, 789
Brian G. Dyson Fndn Grants, 791
Bridgestone/Firestone Trust Fund Grants, 792
Bright Family Fndn Grants, 793
Bristol-Myers Squibb Fndn Global HIV/AIDS Initiative Grants, 796
Bristol-Myers Squibb Fndn Health Disparities Grants, 797
Bristol-Myers Squibb Fndn Women's Health Grants, 800
Bristol-Myers Squibb Patient Assistance Program, 801
Brookdale Fndn Leadership in Aging Fellowships, 805
Brown County Comm Fndn Grants, 807
Burden Trust Grants, 810
Burlington Northern Santa Fe Fndn Grants, 812
Burton G. Bettingen Grants, 813
Bush Fndn Health & Human Services Grants, 814
Bushrod H. Campbell and Adah F. Hall Charity Fund Grants, 816
Business Bank of Nevada Comm Grants, 817
Byron W. and Alice L. Lockwood Fndn Grants, 824
C.R. Bard Fndn Grants, 825
C.W. Titus Fndn Grants, 826
Cable Positive's Tony Cox Comm Fund Grants, 827
Caddock Fndn Grants, 828
Caleb C. and Julia W. Dula Educational and Charitable Fndn Grants, 830
California Comm Fndn Health Care Grants, 831
California Comm Fndn Human Development Grants, 832
California Endowment CommunitiesFirst Grants, 833
California Wellness Fndn Work and Health Program Grants, 834
Callaway Golf Company Fndn Grants, 836
Cambridge Comm Fndn Grants, 837
Camp-Younts Fndn Grants, 838
Campbell Hoffman Fndn Grants, 840
Canadian Optometric Education Trust Fund Grants, 853
Cardinal Health Fndn Grants, 864
Cargill Citizenship Fund-Corp Giving Grants, 865
Carl and Eloise Pohlad Family Fndn Grants, 867
Carl C. Icahn Fndn Grants, 870
Carl W. and Carrie Mae Joslyn Trust Grants, 873
Carlisle Fndn Grants, 874
Carlos and Marguerite Mason Trust Grants, 875
Carlsbad Charitable Fndn Grants, 877
Carnahan-Jackson Fndn Grants, 878
Carolyn Fndn Grants, 880
Carpenter Fndn Grants, 881
Cass County Comm Fndn Grants, 887
Catherine Holmes Wilkins Fndn Grants, 889
Catherine Kennedy Home Fndn Grants, 890
Catholic Campaign for Human Development (CCHD) Comm Organizing Grants, 891
CDC Evaluation of the Use of Rapid Testing For Influenza in Outpatient Medical Settings, 910
CDC Increasing Breast and Cervical Cancer Screening Services for Urban American Indian/Alaska Native Women, 912
CDC Preventive Health Services-Sexually Transmitted Diseases Control Grants, 923
CDC Program to Prevent Smoking Among Urban Youth, 924
Cemala Fndn Grants, 933
Central Carolina Comm Fndn Comm Impact Grants, 936
Cessna Fndn Grants, 938
CFFVR Opportunity Grants, 952
Champ-A Champion Fur Kids Grants, 959
Champlin Fndns Grants, 960
CharityWorks Grants, 961
Charles A. Frueauff Fndn Grants, 962
Charles G. Koch Charitable Fndn Grants, 965
Charles H. Dater Fndn Grants, 966
Charles H. Farnsworth Trust Grants, 967
Charles Lafitte Fndn Grants, 970
Charles M. and Mary D. Grant Fndn Grants, 971
Charles M. Bair Family Trust Grants, 972
Charlotte County (FL) Comm Fndn Grants, 973
Chase Paymentech Corp Giving Grants, 975
Chatlos Fndn Grants, 977
Chazen Fndn Grants, 978
CHCF Grants, 979
CHCF Local Coverage Expansion Initiative, 981
Chesapeake Corporation Fndn Grants, 982
Chestnut Hill Charitable Fndn, Inc Grants, 987
Chicago Comm Trust Grants, 989
Chicago White Metal Charitable Fndn Grants, 992
Children Affected by AIDS Fndn Camp Network Grants, 994
Children Affected by AIDS Fndn Domestic Grants, 995
Children Affected by AIDS Fndn Family Assistance Emergency Fund Grants, 996
Children's Trust Fund of Oregon Grants, 1001
Chiron Fndn Comm Grants, 1004
Christy-Houston Fndn Grants, 1008
Chula Vista Charitable Fndn Grants, 1009
CICF Legacy Fund Comm Fndn Grants, 1010
CIGNA Fndn Grants, 1011
Cinergy Fndn Grants, 1013
CIT Corp Giving Grants, 1014
Citizens Bank Mid-Atlantic Charitable Fndn Grants, 1015
CJ Fndn for SIDS Express Grants, 1016
CJ Fndn for SIDS Support Services Grants, 1017
Clarcor Fndn Grants, 1021
Clarence E. Heller Charitable Fndn Grants, 1022
Clark County Comm Fndn Grants, 1028
Clark Fndn Grants, 1029
Clark-Winchcole Fndn Grants, 1030
Claude Bennett Family Fndn Grants, 1031
Claude Worthington Benedum Fndn Grants, 1033
Clay Fndn Grants, 1034
Cleo Fndn Grants, 1035
Cleveland Browns Fndn Grants, 1036
CLIF Bar Family Fndn Grants, 1040
CMA Fndn Grants, 1042
CMS Research and Demonstration Grants, 1045
CNA Fndn Grants, 1046
CNCS Engaging Persons with Disabilities in National and Comm Service Grants, 1047
CNCS Foster Grandparent Projects Grants, 1048
CNCS Next Generation Grants, 1049
Coastal Bend Comm Fndn Grants, 1050
Coastal Comm Fndn of South Carolina Grants, 1051
Cockrell Fndn Grants, 1053
Colin Higgins Fndn Grants, 1056
Collins Fndn Grants, 1058
Colorado Interstate Gas Grants, 1060
Colorado Springs Comm Trust Fund Grants, 1061
Colorado Trust Partnerships for Health Initiative, 1063
Columbus Fndn Allen Eiry Fund Grants, 1064
Columbus Fndn Competitive Grants, 1066
Columbus Fndn Estrich Fund Grants, 1067
Columbus Fndn J. Floyd Dixon Memorial Fund Grants, 1068
Columbus Fndn Mary Eleanor Morris Fund Grants, 1069
Columbus Fndn Robert E. and Genevieve B. Schaefer Fund Grants, 1070
Columbus Fndn Traditional Grants, 1071
Comer Fndn Grants, 1072
Comerica Charitable Fndn Grants, 1073
Commission on Religion in Appalachia Grants, 1074
Commonweal Fndn Comm Assistance Grants, 1075
Commonweal Fndn Grants, 1076
Commonwealth Fund Small Grants, 1084
Comm Fndn AIDS Endowment Awards, 1088
Comm Fndn Alliance City of Evansville Endowment Fund Grants, 1089
Comm Fndn for Greater New Haven Grants, 1091
Comm Fndn for Monterey County Grants, 1092
Comm Fndn for Muskegon County Grants, 1093
Comm Fndn for Southeastern Michigan Grants, 1094
Comm Fndn for Southern Arizona Grants, 1095
Comm Fndn of Bartholomew County Heritage Fund Grants, 1096
Comm Fndn of Bloomington and Monroe County Grants, 1098

Comm Fndn of Boone County Grants, 1099
Comm Fndn of Broward Grants, 1100
Comm Fndn of Central Illinois Grants, 1101
Comm Fndn of Champaign County Grants, 1102
Comm Fndn of Grant County Grants, 1104
Comm Fndn of Greater Birmingham Grants, 1106
Comm Fndn of Greater Flint Grants, 1107
Comm Fndn of Greater Fort Wayne: Comm Endowment & Clarke Endowment Fund Grants, 1108
Comm Fndn of Greater Greensboro Grants, 1109
Comm Fndn of Greater Tampa Grants, 1112
Comm Fndn of Greenville Hollingsworth Funds Program/Project Grants, 1114
Comm Fndn of Morgan County Grants and Scholarships, 1118
Comm Fndn of Mount Vernon and Knox County Grants, 1119
Comm Fndn of Muncie and Delaware County Grants, 1120
Comm Fndn of Santa Cruz County Grants, 1122
Comm Fndn of South Puget Sound Grants, 1124
Comm Fndn of Southeastern Connecticut Grants, 1125
Comm Fndn of St. Joseph County Special Project Challenge Grants, 1126
Comm Fndn of Western North Carolina Grants, 1132
Comm Fndn Silicon Valley Grants, 1133
Comm Impact Fund, 1135
Comm Technology Fndn of California Building Communities Through Technology Grants, 1136
Comm Toolbox for Children's Environmental Health Grants, 1137
Comprehensive Health Education Fndn Grants, 1139
ConAgra Foods Fndn Grants, 1140
Connecticut Comm Fndn Grants, 1141
Connecticut Health Fndn Health Initiative Grants, 1142
Connelly Fndn Grants, 1143
ConocoPhillips Fndn Grants, 1144
Constantin Fndn Grants, 1145
Constellation Energy Group and Baltimore Gas and Electric Corp Contributions, 1146
Consumers Energy Fndn, 1147
Cooke Fndn Grants, 1148
Cooper Industries Fndn Grants, 1150
Coors Brewing Corp Contributions Grants, 1151
Cornerstone Fndn of Northeastern Wisconsin Grants, 1152
Covenant Matters Fndn Grants, 1154
Cowles Charitable Trust Grants, 1155
Crail-Johnson Fndn Grants, 1157
Cranston Fndn Grants, 1158
CRH Fndn Grants, 1160
Cruise Industry Charitable Fndn Grants, 1166
CSL Behring Local Empowerment for Advocacy Development (LEAD) Grants, 1167
CSRA Comm Fndn Grants, 1168
CSX Corp Contributions Grants, 1169
Cudd Fndn Grants, 1171
Cullen Fndn Grants, 1172
Cultural Society of Filipino Americans Grants, 1173
CUNA Mutual Group Fndn, 1174
CVS All Kids Can Grants, 1175
CVS Caremark Charitable Trust Grants, 1176
CVS Comm Grants, 1177
Cyrus Eaton Fndn Grants, 1178
D.F. Halton Fndn Grants, 1181
D.V. and Ida J. McEachern Charitable Trust Grants, 1182
DaimlerChrysler Corporation Fund Grants, 1186
Dairy Queen Corp Contributions Grants, 1187
Dallas Mavericks Fndn Grants, 1190
Dammann Fund Grants, 1192
Dana Brown Charitable Trust Grants, 1194
Daniels Fund Grants, 1200
Daphne Seybolt Culpeper Memorial Fndn Grants, 1201
David Geffen Fndn Grants, 1202
Daviess County Comm Fndn Health Grants, 1203
Dayton Power and Light Fndn Grants, 1205
Daywood Fndn Grants, 1206
Deaconess Comm Fndn Grants, 1207
Dean Foods Comm Involvement Grants, 1209
Delaware Comm Fndn Grants, 1215
Dell Fndn Open Grants, 1218
Delta Air Lines Fndn Grants, 1220
DeMatteis Family Fndn Grants, 1221
Dennis and Phyllis Washington Fndn Grants, 1222
Denver Broncos Charities Fund Grants, 1226
Denver Fndn Comm Grants, 1227
DeRoy Testamentary Fndn Grants, 1239
Detlef Schrempf Fndn Grants, 1240
Detroit Lions Charities Grants, 1241
DHHS Abandoned Infants Assistance Grants, 1242
DHHS Adolescent Family Life Demonstration Projects, 1243
DHHS AIDS Project Grants, 1245
DHHS Comprehensive Comm Mental Health Services Grants for Children with Serious Emotional Disturbances, 1247
DHHS Maternal and Child Health Projects Grants, 1263
DHHS Oral Health Promotion Research Across the Lifespan, 1269
DHHS Rural Telemedicine Grants, 1279
Dickson Fndn Grants, 1284
Disable American Veterans Charitable Grants, 1286
Do Something BR!CK Awards, 1287
DOA Distance Learning and Telemedicine Grants, 1288
DOJ Gang-Free Schools and Communities Intervention Grants, 1303
Dolan Fndn Grants, 1306
Dole Food Company Charitable Contributions, 1307
Dominion Educational Partnership Grant, 1308
Donald and Sylvia Robinson Family Fndn Grants, 1310
Dora Roberts Fndn Grants, 1311
Doris and Victor Day Fndn Grants, 1313
Doris Duke Charitable Fndn Operations Research on AIDS Care and Treatment in Africa (ORACTA) Grants, 1319
Dorothy Hooper Beattie Fndn Grants, 1321
Dorothy Rider Pool Health Care Grants, 1322
Dorrance Family Fndn Grants, 1323
Dr. Bob and Jean Smith Fndn Grants, 1325
Dr. John T. Macdonald Fndn Grants, 1327
Dr. Scholl Fndn Grants, 1329
Dreitzer Fndn Grants, 1332
Drs. Bruce and Lee Fndn Grants, 1333
Duke Endowment Health Care Grants, 1338
Dunspaugh-Dalton Fndn Grants, 1351
DuPage Comm Fndn Grants, 1352
E. Rhodes and Leona B. Carpenter Fndn Grants, 1356
E.J. Grassmann Trust Grants, 1360
Eastman Chemical Company Fndn Grants, 1362
Eckerd Corporation Fndn Grants, 1366
Eddie C. and Sylvia Brown Family Fndn Grants, 1367
Eden Hall Fndn Grants, 1368
Edina Realty Fndn Grants, 1369
EDS Fndn Grants, 1371
Edward Bangs Kelley and Elza Kelley Fndn Grants, 1373
Edward S. Moore Fndn Grants, 1374
Edwards Memorial Trust Grants, 1375
Edwin W. and Catherine M. Davis Fndn Grants, 1377
Edyth Bush Charitable Fndn Grants, 1378
Effie and Wofford Cain Fndn Grants, 1385
EIF Comm Grants, 1386
Eisner Fndn Grants, 1387
El Paso Comm Fndn Grants, 1388
El Pomar Fndn Awards and Grants, 1390
Elizabeth Morse Genius Charitable Trust Grants, 1400
Elkhart County Comm Fndn Grants, 1401
Elmer L. and Eleanor J. Andersen Fndn Grants, 1406
Elsa U. Pardee Fndn Grants, 1407
Emerson Charitable Trust Grants, 1412
Emily Davie and Joseph S. Kornfeld Fndn Grants, 1414
Emma B. Howe Memorial Fndn Grants, 1415
Entergy Comm Partnership Grants, 1417
Entergy Corporation Open Grants for Healthy Families, 1418
EPA Children's Health Protection Grants, 1420
Erie Comm Fndn Grants, 1427
Essex County Comm Fndn Discretionary Fund Grant, 1428
Estee Lauder Grants, 1429
Ethel S. Abbott Charitable Fndn Grants, 1430
Eugene and Agnes E. Meyer Fndn Grants, 1432
Eugene M. Lang Fndn Grants, 1434
Eva L. and Joseph M. Bruening Fndn Grants, 1436
Evan and Susan Bayh Fndn Grants, 1437
Evanston Comm Fndn Grants, 1438
Express Scripts Fndn Grants, 1441
ExxonMobil Grants, 1442
F.M. Kirby Fndn Grants, 1443
Fairfield County Comm Fndn Grants, 1446
Fairlawn Fndn Grants, 1447
Fairview Lutheran Fndn Grants, 1448
Fallon OrNda Comm Health Fund Grants, 1449
Fan Fox and Leslie R. Samuels Fndn Grants, 1451
Fannie E. Rippel Fndn Grants, 1452
FAR Fund, 1453
Fargo-Moorhead Area Fndn Grants, 1454
Farmers Insurance Group of Companies Grants, 1455
Faye McBeath Fndn Grants, 1456
FCD Child Development Grants, 1458
FCNY Union Square Awards, 1461
Federal Express Corp Contributions Program, 1483
Feldman Fndn Grants, 1484
Ferree Fndn Grants, 1486
Fidelity Fndn Grants, 1498
Field Fndn of Illinois Grants, 1499
Fifth Third Fndn Grants, 1501
Fireman's Fund Fndn Grants, 1504
FirstEnergy Fndn Comm Grants, 1505
Fisher Fndn Grants, 1508
Flinn Fndn Grantss, 1511
Floyd A. and Kathleen C. Cailloux Fndn Grants, 1516
Foellinger Fndn Grants, 1519
Fondren Fndn Grants, 1520
Ford Motor Company Fund Grants, 1522
Forrest C. Lattner Fndn Grants, 1523
Fndn for a Healthy Kentucky Grants, 1527
Fndn for Seacoast Health Grants, 1533
Fndn for the Carolinas Grants, 1535
Fndn Northwest Grants, 1537
Fndn of CVPH April LaValley Fund Grants, 1538
Fndn of CVPH Chelsea's Rainbow Fund Grants, 1539
Fndn of CVPH Melissa Lahtinen-Penfield Organ Donor Fund Grants, 1540
Fndn of CVPH Rabin Fund Grants, 1541
Fndn of CVPH Roger Senecal Endowment Fund Grants, 1542
Fourjay Fndn Grants, 1544
Frances and John L. Loeb Family Fund Grants, 1546
Frances L. and Edwin L. Cummings Memorial Fund Grants, 1547
Francis L. Abreu Charitable Trust Grants, 1549
Francis T. & Louise T. Nichols Fndn Grants, 1550
Frank E. and Seba B. Payne Fndn Grants, 1551
Frank G. and Freida K. Brotz Family Fndn Grants, 1552
Frank Stanley Beveridge Fndn Grants, 1553
Fred Baldwin Memorial Fndn Grants, 1556
Fred L. Emerson Fndn Grants, 1557
Freddie Mac Fndn Grants, 1558
Fremont Area Comm Fndn Grants, 1561
Frey Fndn Grants, 1562
Frist Fndn Grants, 1563
Fuji Film Grants, 1565

Fuller E. Callaway Fndn Grants, 1578
G.N. Wilcox Trust Grants, 1581
Gebbie Fndn Grants, 1585
GEICO Public Service Awards, 1586
GenCorp Fndn Grants, 1587
Genentech Corp Charitable Contributions Grants, 1588
General Mills Champions for Healthy Kids Grants, 1589
General Mills Fndn Grants, 1590
Genuardi Family Fndn Grants, 1594
George and Ruth Bradford Fndn Grants, 1595
George B. Storer Fndn Grants, 1596
George F. Baker Trust Grants, 1597
George Family Fndn Grants, 1598
George Frederick Jewett Fndn Grants, 1599
George Kress Fndn Grants, 1601
Georgia Power Fndn Grants, 1603
Georgiana Goddard Eaton Memorial Fund Grants, 1604
Gerber Fndn Grants, 1606
Gheens Fndn Grants, 1610
Gibson Fndn Grants, 1612
Gill Fndn - Gay and Lesbian Fund Grants, 1613
Gilroy and Lillian P. Roberts Charitable Fndn Grants, 1614
Ginn Fndn Grants, 1616
Giving Sum Annual Grant, 1619
GlaxoSmithKline Corp Grants, 1623
Glazer Family Fndn Grants, 1625
Glendale Comm Fndn Grants, 1626
Global Fund for Children Grants, 1629
Godfrey Fndn Grants, 1631
GoGirlGo! Ambassador Team Awards, 1632
Golden State Warriors Fndn Grants, 1633
Good Samaritan Fndn Inc Grants, 1636
Goodrich Corporation Fndn Grants, 1638
Goodyear Tire Grants, 1639
Graco Fndn Grants, 1642
Grand Rapids Area Comm Fndn Grants, 1645
Grand Rapids Area Comm Fndn Nashwauk Area Endowment Fund Grants, 1646
Grand Rapids Comm Fndn Grants, 1647
Great-West Life Grants, 1649
Greater Bridgeport Area Fndn Comm Impact Grants, 1650
Greater Cincinnati Fndn Priority and Small Projects/Capacity-Building Grants, 1651
Greater Green Bay Comm Fndn Grants, 1652
Greater Milwaukee Fndn Grants, 1653
Greater New Orleans Fndn Grants, 1654
Greater Saint Louis Comm Fndn Grants, 1655
Greater Tacoma Comm Fndn Grants, 1656
Greater Tacoma Comm Fndn Ryan Alan Hade Endowment Fund, 1657
Greater Worcester Comm Fndn Discretionary Grants, 1658
Green Bay Packers Fndn Grants, 1660
Green Fndn Grants, 1661
Greenspun Family Fndn Grants, 1664
Greenwall Fndn Bioethics Grants, 1665
Gregory Family Fndn Grants (Florida), 1667
Griffin Fndn Grants, 1670
Grotto Fndn Project Grants, 1671
Grundy Fndn Grants, 1673
Guidant Fndn Grants, 1674
Guitar Center Music Fndn Grants, 1675
Gulf Coast Comm Fndn Grants, 1676
Gulf Coast Comm of Venice Fndn Grants, 1677
Guy's and St. Thomas' Charity Grants, 1678
H & R Fndn Grants, 1679
H. Schaffer Fndn Grants, 1680
H.A. and Mary K. Chapman Charitable Trust Grants, 1681
H.J. Heinz Company Fndn Grants, 1682
Hackett Fndn Grants, 1684
Hagedorn Fund Grants, 1685
Halliburton Fndn Grants, 1687
Hallmark Corp Fndn Grants, 1688
Hanna Andersson Children's Fndn Grants, 1691
Hannaford Charitable Fndn Grants, 1692
Harden Fndn Grants, 1693
Harley Davidson Fndn Grants, 1694
Harold Alfond Fndn Grants, 1695
Harold and Arlene Schnitzer CARE Fndn Grants, 1697
Harold Simmons Fndn Grants, 1698
Harris and Eliza Kempner Fund Grants, 1699
Harrison County Comm Fndn Grants, 1700
Harry Sudakoff Fndn Grants, 1708
Hartford Aging and Health Program Awards, 1709
Hartford Fndn Regular Grants, 1711
Harvest Fndn Grants, 1713
Hasbro Children's Fund, 1714
Hawaii Comm Fndn Reverend Takie Okumura Family Grants, 1717
Hawaii Comm Fndn West Hawaii Fund Grants, 1718
Hawn Fndn Grants, 1719
HCA Fndn Grants, 1721
Health Canada National Seniors Independence Program Grants, 1722
Health Fndn of Greater Cincinnati Grants, 1724
Health Fndn of Greater Indianapolis Grants, 1725
Health Fndn of Southern Florida Responsive Grants, 1726
Healthcare Fndn for Orange County Grants, 1728
Healthcare Fndn of New Jersey Grants, 1729
Hearst Fndn and William Randolph Hearst Fndn Grants, 1730
Heckscher Fndn for Children Grants, 1732
Helen Bader Fndn Grants, 1738
Helen K. and Arthur E. Johnson Fndn Grants, 1740
Helen Steiner Rice Fndn Grants, 1742
Helena Rubinstein Fndn Grants, 1743
Hendrick Fndn for Children Grants, 1744
Henry and Ruth Blaustein Rosenberg Fndn Grants, 1746
Henry J. Kaiser Family Fndn Grants, 1748
Herman Goldman Fndn Grants, 1753
Hershey Company Grants, 1754
HHK Employment Grants, 1755
Highmark Corp Giving Grants, 1769
Hill Crest Fndn Grants, 1773
Hill Fndn Grants, 1774
Hillman Fndn Grants, 1775
Hillsdale County Comm Fndn Healthy Senior/ Healthy Youth Fund Grants, 1776
Hillsdale County Comm General Adult Fndn Grants, 1777
Hillsdale Fund Grants, 1778
Hilton Head Island Fndn Grants, 1779
Hilton Hotels Corp Giving Program Grants, 1780
Hirtzel Memorial Fndn Grants, 1781
Hoblitzelle Fndn Grants, 1783
Hogg Fndn for Mental Health Grants, 1784
Hoglund Fndn Grants, 1785
Holland/Zeeland Comm Fndn Grants, 1786
Home Building Industry Disaster Relief Fund, 1787
HomeBanc Fndn Grants, 1788
Homer Fndn Grants, 1789
Honda of America Manufacturing Fndn Grants, 1790
Honeywell Fndn Grants, 1791
Horizon Fndn for New Jersey Grants, 1793
Horizons Comm Issues Grants, 1794
Houston Endowment Grants, 1797
Howard and Bush Fndn Grants, 1798
HRSA Emergency Medical Services for Children Grants, 1804
HRSA Ryan White HIV Early Intervention Services Grants, 1811
Huber Fndn Grants, 1812
Hudson Webber Fndn Grants, 1813
Hugh J. Andersen Fndn Grants, 1814
Huie-Dellmon Trust Grants, 1815
Human Source Fndn Grants, 1817
Humana Fndn Grants, 1818
Huntington Beach Police Officers Fndn Grants, 1821
Huntington County Comm Fndn Grants, 1823
Huntington National Bank Comm Affairs Grants, 1824
Hut Fndn Grants, 1827
Hutton Fndn Grants, 1828
IATA Research Grants, 1834
Ida Alice Ryan Charitable Trust Grants, 1836
Idaho Comm Fndn Eastern Region Competitive Grants, 1837
Idaho Power Company Corp Contributions, 1838
Ignacio Martin-Baro Fund for Mental Health and Human Rights Grants, 1839
Illinois Children's Healthcare Fndn Grants, 1842
Inasmuch Fndn Grants, 1845
Independence Blue Cross Charitable Medical Care Grants, 1846
Independence Comm Fndn Comm Quality of Life Grant, 1849
Indiana AIDS Fund Grants, 1851
IOM Gustav O. Lienhard Award, 1864
Irvin Stern Fndn Grants, 1866
Irving S. Gilmore Fndn Grants, 1867
Isabel Allende Fndn Esperanza Grants, 1868
Ittleson Fndn AIDS Grants, 1869
Ittleson Fndn Mental Health Grants, 1870
J. Walton Bissell Fndn Grants, 1872
J.B. Reynolds Fndn Grants, 1873
J.C. Penney Company Grants, 1874
J.E. and L.E. Mabee Fndn Grants, 1875
J.L. Bedsole Fndn Grants, 1876
J.M. Long Fndn Grants, 1877
J.W. Kieckhefer Fndn Grants, 1878
Jackson County Comm Fndn Unrestricted Grants, 1879
Jacob and Hilda Blaustein Fndn Grants, 1881
Jacob and Valeria Langeloth Fndn Grants, 1882
Jacob G. Schmidlapp Trust Grants, 1883
James A. and Faith Knight Fndn Grants, 1884
James Ford Bell Fndn Grants, 1885
James M. Collins Fndn Grants, 1891
James M. Cox Fndn of Georgia Grants, 1892
James S. Copley Fndn Grants, 1895
Jane Bradley Pettit Fndn Grants, 1902
Jane's Trust Grants, 1904
Jay and Rose Phillips Family Fndn Grants, 1909
Jean and Louis Dreyfus Fndn Grants, 1911
JELD-WEN Fndn Grants, 1914
Jenkins Fndn: Improving the Health of Greater Richmond Grants, 1915
Jerome and Mildred Paddock Fndn Grants, 1917
Jessie Ball Dupont Fund Grants, 1919
Jewish Comm Fndn of Greater Los Angeles Grants, 1921
Jewish Fund Grants, 1923
Jewish Women's Fndn of New York Grants, 1924
Jim Moran Fndn Grants, 1925
JM Fndn Grants, 1926
Joe W. and Dorothy Dorsett Brown Fndn Grants, 1927
John Deere Fndn Grants, 1929
John Edward Fowler Memorial Fndn Grants, 1930
John J. Leidy Fndn Grants, 1936
John Lord Knight Fndn Grants, 1938
John Merck Fund Grants, 1940
John P. Murphy Fndn Grants, 1943
John R. Oishei Fndn Grants, 1944
John W. and Anna H. Hanes Fndn Grants, 1948
Johns Manville Fund Grants, 1950
Johnson & Johnson Comm Health Care Program Grants, 1951
Johnson & Johnson Corp Contributions Grants, 1952
Johnson and Johnson / SAH Arts and Healing Grants, 1953
Johnson Controls Fndn Grants, 1954
Joseph H. and Florence A. Roblee Fndn Grants, 1961
Joseph P. Kennedy Jr. Fndn Grants, 1962
Josephine Goodyear Fndn Grants, 1964
Josephine S. Gumbiner Fndn Grants, 1965
Josiah W. and Bessie H. Kline Fndn Grants, 1967
Joyce Fndn Grants, 1969
K. M. Hunter Charitable Fndn Social Welfare Grants, 1974
Kahuku Comm Fund, 1977

Kaiser Permanente Cares for Communities Grants, 1978
Kalamazoo Fndn Grants, 1979
Kansas Health Fndn Grants, 1980
Kate B. Reynolds Charitable Trust Health Care Grants, 1981
Katharine Matthies Fndn Grants, 1982
Kathryne Beynon Fndn Grants, 1984
Kelvin and Eleanor Smith Fndn Grants, 1986
Ken W. Davis Fndn Grants, 1987
Kendrick Fndn Grants, 1988
Kenneth T. and Eileen L. Norris Fndn Grants, 1989
Kenny's Kids Grants, 1990
Kettering Family Fndn Grants, 1991
Kettering Fund Grants, 1992
Key Fndn Grants, 1994
KeySpan Fndn Grants, 1995
KFC Allied Health Research Grants, 1996
Kimberly-Clark Comm Grants, 2001
King Pharmaceuticals Corp Contributions Grants, 2003
Kiwanis International Fndn Grants, 2004
Knight Family Charitable and Educational Fndn Grants, 2007
Kraft Cares International Grants, 2016
Kraft Cares US Grants, 2017
L. W. Pierce Family Fndn Grants, 2019
LaGrange County Comm Fndn Grants, 2020
Lance Armstrong Fndn Comm Grants, 2025
Land O'Lakes Fndn Mid-Atlantic Grants, 2027
Lands' End Corp Giving Program, 2030
Larry L. Hillblom Fndn Grants, 2031
Laura B. Vogler Fndn Grants, 2032
Leo Goodwin Fndn Grants, 2043
Leonard and Helen R. Stulman Charitable Fndn Grants, 2044
Leonsis Fndn Grants, 2045
Lester Ray Fleming Scholarships, 2048
Lettie Pate Whitehead Fndn Grants, 2049
Liberty Bank Fndn Grants, 2053
Liliane Fndn Grants, 2055
Lincoln Financial Group Fndn Grants, 2058
Little Life Fndn Grants, 2060
Lockheed Martin Philanthropic Grants, 2062
Louis Calder Fndn Grants, 2065
Louis R. Cappelli Fndn Grants, 2066
Lowe Fndn Grants, 2067
Lowell Area Comm Fund Grants, 2068
Lowell Berry Fndn Grants, 2069
Lubbock Area Fndn Grants, 2079
Lucile Horton Howe and Mitchell B. Howe Fndn Grants, 2081
Lucy Gooding Charitable Fndn Trust, 2082
Ludwick Family Fndn Grants, 2084
Lynde and Harry Bradley Fndn Grants, 2089
M-A-C AIDS Fund Grants, 2091
M. Bastian Family Fndn Grants, 2092
M.B. and Edna Zale Fndn Grants, 2093
M.E. Raker Fndn Grants, 2094
Mabel Y. Hughes Charitable Trust Grants, 2097
Maine Comm Fndn Grants, 2099
Manuel D. and Rhoda Mayerson Fndn Grants, 2100
MAP International Medical Fellowships, 2101
Marcia and Otto Koehler Fndn Grants, 2103
Margaret L. Wendt Fndn Grants, 2104
Margaret T. Morris Fndn Grants, 2105
Marion I. and Henry J. Knott Fndn Grants, 2109
Marion Park Deaver and Harry Gilbert Deaver Fndn Grants, 2110
Mark and Catherine Winkler Fndn Grants, 2112
Marriott Fndn for People with Disabilities Bridges Program Grants, 2113
Mars Fndn Grants, 2114
Mary Allen Lindsey Branan Fndn Grants, 2116
Mary Black Fndn Grants, 2118
Mary Owen Borden Fndn Grants, 2121
Mary S. and David C. Corbin Fndn Grants, 2122
Mass Youth Against Tobacco Mini-Grants, 2123
Massage Therapy Fndn Comm Service Grants, 2124
Matilda R. Wilson Fund Grants, 2128
Mattel Children's Fndn Grants, 2130
Mattel International Grants, 2131
Max and Victoria Dreyfus Fndn Grants, 2133
Max Bell Fndn Grants, 2134
Maxtor Corp Contributions Grants, 2136
May and Stanley Smith Trust Grants, 2137
May Department Stores Charitable Contribution Grants, 2138
Mayday Fund Grants, 2139
McCarthy Family Fndn Grants, 2141
McCombs Fndn Grants, 2142
McGregor Fund Grants, 2143
McInerny Fndn Grants, 2144
McKnight Fndn Grants, 2146
McLean Contributionship Grants, 2147
McMurry Fndn Grants, 2149
Mead Johnson Nutritionals Charitable Giving Grants, 2156
Mead Johnson Nutritionals Evansville-Area Organizations Grants, 2157
Mead Johnson Nutritionals Medical Education Grants, 2158
Mead Witter Fndn Grants, 2160
Meadows Fndn Grants, 2161
MedImmune Charitable Grants, 2166
Medtronic Fndn Health Care Grants, 2169
Meriden Fndn Grants, 2173
Metro Health Fndn Grants, 2175
Metrowest Comm Health Care Fndn Grants, 2176
Meyer Memorial Trust Emergency Grants, 2178
Meyer Memorial Trust Grassroots Grants, 2179
Meyer Memorial Trust Responsive Grants, 2181
Michael and Susan Dell Fndn Grants, 2189
Middlesex Savings Charitable Fndn Grants, 2196
Miguel Aleman Fndn Grants, 2197
Miles of Hope Breast Cancer Fndn Grants, 2199
Millipore Fndn Grants, 2203
Minneapolis Fndn Comm Grants, 2206
Miriam and Peter Haas Fund Grants, 2208
Montgomery County Comm Fndn Grants, 2214
MONY Fndn Grants, 2215
Morris and Gwendolyn Cafritz Fndn Grants, 2217
Moses Cone-Wesley Long Comm Health Fndn Grants, 2219
Mount Zion Health Fund Grants, 2220
Ms. Fndn for Women Grants, 2222
NAPNAP Fndn Innovative Health Care Small Grant, 2237
NAPNAP Fndn McNeil Grant-in-Aid, 2238
NAPNAP Fndn Nursing Research Grants, 2241
NAPNAP Fndn Shourd Parks Immunization Project Small Grants, 2243
NAPNAP Fndn Wyeth Pediatric Immunization Grant, 2244
National Emergency Medicine Association Grants, 2252
National Starch and Chemical Fndn Grants, 2261
Nelda C. and H.J. Lutcher Stark Fndn Grants, 2301
Nell Warren Elkin and William Simpson Elkin Fndn, 2302
Newman's Own Inc Grants, 2306
NHLBI National Research Service Awards for Senior Fellowships, 2358
Nicholas H. Noyes Jr. Memorial Fndn Grants, 2497
Nina Mason Pulliam Charitable Trust Grants, 2776
NMF General Electric Medical Scholars Fellowships, 2830
Nordson Corporation Fndn Grants, 2851
North Carolina Comm Development Grants, 2858
North Carolina Comm Fndn Grants, 2859
North Carolina GlaxoSmithKline Fndn Grants, 2860
North Georgia Comm Fndn Grants, 2862
Northeast Utilities Fndn Grants, 2863
Northern New York Comm Fndn Grants, 2864
Northern Trust Company Charitable Trust and Corp Giving Program, 2865
Northrop Grumman Corporation Grants, 2866
Northrop Grumman Newport News Grants, 2867
Northwest Minnesota Fndn Women's Fund Grants, 2869
Northwestern Mutual Fndn Grants, 2870
Norwin S. and Elizabeth N. Bean Fndn Grants, 2872
NSF Chemistry Research Experiences for Undergraduates (REU), 2883
NSF Emerging Frontiers in Research and Innovation (EFRI) Grants, 2885
NSF Instrument Development for Biological Research (IDBR), 2888
NYC Managed Care Consumer Assistance Workshop Re-Design Grants, 2918
NYCT AIDS/HIV Grants, 2919
NYCT Blindness and Visual Disabilities Grants, 2921
NYCT Children and Youth with Disabilities Grants, 2923
NYCT Girls and Young Women Grants, 2924
NYCT Grants for the Elderly, 2925
NYCT Health Services, Systems, and Policies Grants, 2926
NYCT Mental Health and Mental Retardation Grants, 2927
NYCT Substance Abuse Grants, 2928
NYCT Technical Assistance Grants, 2929
Oakland Fund for Children and Youth Grants, 2930
OceanFirst Fndn Grants, 2933
Office Depot Corporation Comm Grants, 2935
Office Depot Fndn Grants, 2936
Ogden Codman Trust Grants, 2937
Ohio County Comm Fndn Grants, 2938
Ohio County Comm Fndn Mini-Grants, 2939
Oleonda Jameson Trust Grants, 2941
Olin Corporation Charitable Trust Grants, 2943
OneSight Research Fndn Block Grants, 2944
OneStar Fndn AmeriCorps Grants, 2945
Ordean Fndn Grants, 2952
Oscar Rennebohm Fndn Grants, 2963
OSI Access to Essential Medicines Grants, 2964
OSI Harm Reduction and Drug Use Grants, 2966
OSI Indonesia Project Grants, 2967
OSI Palliative Cancer Care Grants, 2970
OSI-Baltimore Special Opportunities Program Grants, 2972
OSI-Baltimore Tackling Drug Addiction Grants, 2973
Otto Bremer Fndn Grants, 2977
OUT Fund for Lesbian and Gay Liberation Grants, 2978
PacifiCare Fndn Grants, 2981
PacifiCorp Fndn for Learning Grants, 2982
Pajaro Valley Comm Health Grants, 2985
Palm Beach and Martin Counties Grants, 2986
Partners for Youth with Disabilities Grants, 2990
Pasadena Fndn Average Grants, 2994
Paso del Norte Health Fndn Grants, 2995
Patron Saints Fndn Grants, 2996
Paul and Mary Haas Fndn Contributions and Student Scholarships, 2997
Paul Balint Charitable Trust Grants, 2998
Paul G. Allen Family Fndn Grants, 3000
Paul G. Duke Fndn Grants, 3001
Peabody Fndn Grants, 3010
Peter and Elizabeth C. Tower Fndn Comm Grants, 3018
Pew Charitable Trusts Children and Youth Grants, 3020
PeyBack Fndn Grants, 3022
Pfizer Fndn Grants, 3025
Pfizer/AAFP Fndn Visiting Professorship Program in Family Medicine, 3027
Philadelphia Fndn Organizational Effectiveness Grants, 3029
Phoenix Suns Charities Grants, 3030
Piedmont Natural Gas Grants, 3048
Pinellas County Grants, 3050
Pioneer Hi-Bred Comm Grants, 3051
Piper Jaffray Companies Building Strong Communities Grants, 3053

Pittsburgh Fndn Comm Fund Grants, 3054
Plough Fndn Grants, 3061
Plum Creek Fndn Grants, 3062
PMI Fndn Grants, 3063
Polk Bros. Fndn Grants, 3066
Portland General Electric Fndn Grants, 3067
Premera CARES Grants, 3074
Priddy Fndn Grants, 3077
Pride Fndn Grants and Scholarships, 3078
Prince Charitable Trusts Chicago Grants, 3079
Prince Charitable Trusts District of Columbia Grants, 3080
Princeton Area Comm Fndn Greater Mercer Grants, 3081
Principal Financial Group Fndn Grants, 3082
Procter and Gamble Fund Grants, 3083
Progress Energy Fndn Grants, 3084
Prudential Fndn Grants, 3087
Public Welfare Fndn Grants, 3089
Puerto Rico Comm Fndn Grants, 3090
Pulte Homes Corp Contributions, 3092
Putnam County Comm Fndn Grants, 3093
Quality Health Fndn Grants, 3094
Quantum Corporation Snap Server Grants, 3095
Quantum Fndn Grants, 3096
Questar Corp Contributions Grants, 3097
R.C. Baker Fndn Grants, 3098
Rainbow Fund Grants, 3103
Ralphs Food 4 Less Fndn Grants, 3106
Raskob Fndn for Catholic Activities Grants, 3107
Rasmuson Fndn Grants, 3108
Rathmann Family Fndn Grants, 3109
Raymond John Wean Fndn Grants, 3110
Reader's Digest Partners for Sight Fndn Grants, 3137
Regence Fndn Access to Health Care Grants, 3138
Regence Fndn Health Care Comm Awareness and Engagement Grants, 3139
Regence Fndn Health Care Connections Grants, 3140
Regence Fndn Improving End-of-Life Grants, 3141
Regence Fndn Tools and Technology Grants, 3142
Rehab Therapy Fndn Grants, 3146
Reynolds and Reynolds Associate Fndn Grants, 3152
RGK Fndn Grants, 3153
Rhode Island Fndn Grants, 3154
Rice Fndn Grants, 3155
Rich Fndn Grants, 3156
Richard and Helen DeVos Fndn Grants, 3157
Richard and Rhoda Goldman Fund Grants, 3158
Richard and Susan Smith Family Fndn Grants, 3159
Richard King Mellon Fndn Grants, 3161
Richmond Eye and Ear Fund Grants, 3164
Riley Fndn Grants, 3165
Robert and Joan Dircks Fndn Grants, 3167
Robert and Polly Dunn Fndn Grants, 3168
Robert E. and Evelyn McKee Fndn Grants, 3170
Robert P. & Clara I. Milton Fund for Senior Housing, 3172
Robin Hood Fndn Grants, 3174
Robins Fndn Grants, 3175
Rochester Area Comm Fndn Grants, 3176
Rochester Area Fndn Grants, 3177
Rockefeller Brothers Fund Pivotal Places Grants: South Africa, 3180
Rockefeller Fndn Grants, 3181
Rockwell Collins Charitable Contributions, 3182
Rockwell International Corp Trust Grants, 3183
Rohm and Haas Company Grants, 3185
Rollin M. Gerstacker Fndn Grants, 3186
Rosalynn Carter Institute Georgia Caregiver of the Year Awards, 3188
Rosalynn Carter Institute John and Betty Pope Fellowships, 3189
RRF General Program Grants, 3193
RRF Organizational Capacity Building Grants, 3194
RSC McNeil Medal for the Public Awareness of Science, 3198
Russell Berrie Fndn Grants, 3201
Ruth Eleanor Bamberger and John Ernest Bamberger Memorial Fndn Grants, 3202
Ruth H. and Warren A. Ellsworth Fndn Grants, 3203
Ruth Mott Fndn Grants, 3204
RWJF Comm Health Leaders Awards, 3208
RWJF Finding Answers: Disparities Research for Change Grants, 3211
RWJF Generalist Physician Faculty Scholars, 3212
RWJF Harold Amos Medical Faculty Development Scholars, 3213
RWJF Local Funding Partnerships Program Grants, 3223
RWJF New Jersey Health Initiatives Grants, 3225
RWJF Pioneer Portfolio Grants, 3227
RWJF State Coverage Initiatives Grants, 3230
RWJF Vulnerable Populations Portfolio Grants, 3232
S. Mark Taper Fndn Grants, 3236
Saint Luke's Fndn Grants, 3239
Saint Luke's Health Initiatives Grants, 3240
Salem Fndn Charitable Trust Grants, 3241
Salem Fndn Grants, 3242
Salisbury Comm Fndn Grants, 3243
SAMHSA Campus Suicide Prevention Grants, 3244
SAMHSA Child Mental Health Initiative (CMHI) Grants, 3245
Samuel S. Johnson Fndn Grants, 3251
Samueli Fndn Health Grants, 3252
San Antonio Area Fndn Grants, 3254
San Diego Fndn for Change Grants, 3255
San Diego Fndn Health & Human Services Grants, 3256
San Diego Fndn Paradise Valley Hospital Comm Fund Grants, 3257
San Diego HIV Funding Collaborative (SDHFC) Grants, 3258
San Diego Women's Fndn Grants, 3259
San Francisco Fndn Comm Health Grants, 3260
San Francisco Fndn Disability Rights Advocate Fund Emergency Grants, 3261
Schering-Plough Fndn Comm Initiatives Grants, 3269
Schering-Plough Fndn Health Grants, 3270
Seattle Fndn Grants, 3276
Self Fndn Grants, 3277
Shaw's Supermarkets Donations, 3280
Shell Oil Company Fndn Grants, 3281
Sheltering Arms Fund Grants, 3282
SHF Reach--Connecting Communities and Youth for a Healthy Future Grants, 3283
Sid W. Richardson Fndn Grants, 3284
Siebert Lutheran Fndn Grants, 3285
Simmons Fndn Grants, 3287
Simpson Fund Grants, 3290
Sir Dorabji Tata Trust Grants for NGOs or Voluntary Organizations, 3291
Sir Dorabji Tata Trust Individual Medical Grants, 3292
Sisters of Mercy of North Carolina Fndn Grants, 3295
Sisters of Saint Joseph Charitable Fund Grants, 3296
Sisters of St. Joseph Healthcare Fndn Grants, 3297
Solo Cup Fndn Grants, 3346
Sonoco Fndn Grants, 3347
Sosland Fndn Grants, 3348
Southbury Comm Trust Fund, 3350
Southwest Florida Comm Fndn Competitive Grants, 3351
Southwire Company Grants, 3353
Special People in Need Grants, 3356
Square D Fndn Grants, 3361
Stackner Family Fndn Grants, 3371
Stan and Sandy Checketts Fndn, 3373
Starr Fndn Grants, 3377
Staunton Farm Fndn Grants, 3378
Steelcase Fndn Grants, 3379
Steele-Reese Fndn Grants, 3380
Stewart Huston Charitable Trust Grants, 3384
Sulzberger Fndn Grants, 3399
Sunflower Fndn Bridge Grants, 3401
Sunflower Fndn Capacity Building Grants, 3402
Sunflower Fndn Walking Trails Grants, 3403
Sunshine Natural Wellbeing Fndn Grants, 3404
Support Our Aging Religious (SOAR) Grants, 3406
Susan G. Komen Breast Cancer Fndn Breast Health, Breast Cancer Education, and Outreach Programs Grants, 3408
Susan G. Komen Breast Cancer Fndn Hurricane Relief Grants, 3409
Taproot Fndn Capacity-Building Service Grants, 3417
Tellabs Fndn Grants, 3418
Temple-Inland Fndn Grants, 3419
Thelma Doelger Charitable Trust Grants, 3421
Thomas C. Ackerman Fndn Grants, 3423
Thomas M. and Irene B. Kirbo Charitable Trust Grants, 3424
Thompson Charitable Fndn Grants, 3425
Tides Fndn Syringe Access Fund, 3427
Tifa Fndn Grants, 3428
Topfer Family Fndn Grants, 3430
Toro Fndn Grants, 3431
Tri-County Electric People Fund Grants, 3436
Triangle Comm Fndn Donor-Advised Grants, 3437
Trull Fndn Grants, 3441
TWS Fndn Grants, 3443
U.S. Department of Education 21st Century Comm Learning Centers, 3445
U.S. Department of Education Rehabilitation Engineering Research Centers Grants, 3447
U.S. Department of Education Rehabilitation Research Training Centers (RRTCs), 3448
U.S. Department of Education Rehabilitation Training--Rehabilitation Continuing Education Programs (RCEP)--Institute on Rehabilitation Issues (IRI), 3449
U.S. Department of Education Special Education--National Activities--Parent Information Centers, 3450
U.S. Department of Education Vocational Rehabilitation Services Projects for American Indians with Disabilities Grants, 3452
UCLA / RAND Corporation Post-Doctoral Fellowships, 3454
Union Benevolent Association Grants, 3460
United Methodist Church Global AIDS Fund Grants, 3463
United Methodist Church Malaria Control Grants, 3464
United Methodist Health Ministry Fund Grants, 3465
United Technologies Corporation Grants, 3466
Until There's a Cure Fndn Grants, 3471
US Airways Comm Contributions, 3472
US Airways Comm Fndn Grants, 3473
US Trust Corporation Fndn Grants, 3475
Vancouver Fndn Grants and Comm Initiatives Program, 3477
Varian Medical Systems Grants, 3481
Vectren Fndn Grants, 3485
Verizon Fndn Health Care and Accessibility Grants, 3486
Verizon Fndn New York Grants, 3488
Verizon Fndn Northeast Region Grants, 3489
Verizon Fndn Virginia Grants, 3492
VHA Health Fndn Grants, 3495
Viking Children's Fund Grants, 3497
Virginia W. Kettering Fndn Grants, 3502
Volkswagen of America Corp Contributions Grants, 3503
Vulcan Materials Company Fndn Grants, 3504
W.K. Kellogg Fndn Healthy Kids Grants, 3507
Wabash Valley Comm Fndn Grants, 3510
Wachovia Fndn Grants, 3511
Waitt Family Fndn Grants, 3512
Wal-Mart Fndn Comm Grants, 3513
Wal-Mart State Giving Program Grants, 3514
Walt Disney Company Fndn Grants, 3516
Washington Post Contributions Program Grants, 3520

Wayne and Gladys Valley Fndn Grants, 3522
Weingart Fndn Grants, 3524
Welborn Baptist Fndn Grants, 3525
Wellmark Fndn Grants, 3526
Western Indiana Comm Fndn Grants, 3528
Western Union Fndn Grants, 3529
Westinghouse Charitable Giving Grants, 3530
WHAS Crusade for Children Grants, 3531
WHO Fndn General Grants, 3534
Wilkins Family Fndn Grants, 3536
William G. Kelley Fndn Grants, 3538
William G. McGowan Charitable Fund Grants, 3539
Wilson-Wood Fndn Grants, 3542
Winston-Salem Fndn Competitive Grants, 3544
Winston-Salem Fndn Elkin/Tri-County Grants, 3545
Winston-Salem Fndn Stokes County Grants, 3546
Winston-Salem Fndn Victim Assistance Grants, 3547
Women's Fndn of California Grants, 3550
Woodward Fund Grants, 3552
YSA Get Ur Good On Grants, 3555
YSA UnitedHealth Heroes Service Learning Grants, 3556
Z. Smith Reynolds Fndn Small Grants, 3557

Symposiums, Conferences, Workshops, Seminars
AACAP Systems of Care Special Program Scholarships, 54
AACR Scholar-in-Training Awards - Special Conferences, 88
AAP Comm Access To Child Health (CATCH) Advocacy Training Grants, 157
AcademyHealth Alice S. Hersh Student Scholarships, 191
AcademyHealth Awards, 192
AcademyHealth PHSR Interest Group Student Scholarships, 195
Alaska Airlines Fndn Grants, 324
Alcoa Fndn Grants, 334
Alfred P. Sloan Fndn History of Science and Technology Grants, 352
Allen P. and Josephine B. Green Fndn Grants, 361
Alzheimer's Association Conference Grants, 385
AMA Fndn Dr. Nathan Davis International Awards in Medicine, 387
AMA Fndn Jack B. McConnell, MD Awards for Excellence in Volunteerism, 391
AMA Fndn Jordan Fieldman, MD, Awards, 393
AMA Fndn Leadership Awards, 394
AMA Fndn Pride in the Profession Grants, 397
AMA-MSS Chapter Involvement Grants, 401
American College of Rheumatology Fellows-in-Training Travel Scholarships, 421
American College of Surgeons Nizar N. Oweida, MD, FACS, Scholarships, 430
American College of Surgeons Resident and Associate Society (RAS-ACS) Leadership Scholarships, 431
AMI Semiconductors Corp Grants, 468
Ann Arbor Area Comm Fndn Grants, 476
APA Scientific Conferences Grants, 500
Aratani Fndn Grants, 523
Archer Daniels Midland Fndn Grants, 525
Arizona Public Service Corp Giving Program Grants, 531
ASCO State Affiliate Grants, 547
ASHA Minority Student Leadership Program Awards, 570
ASHA Research Mentoring-Pair Travel Award, 572
ASHA Student Research Travel Award, 573
ASHA Students Preparing for Academic & Research Careers (SPARC) Award, 574
ASM Millis-Colwell Postgraduate Travel Grant, 608
ASM-UNESCO Leadership Grant for International Educators, 626
Atran Fndn Grants, 663
Avon Fndn Breast Care Fund Grants, 674
Ball Brothers Fndn Grants, 684
Battle Creek Comm Fndn Grants, 703
Berks County Comm Fndn Grants, 745
Blanche and Julian Robertson Family Fndn Grants, 765
Bodenwein Public Benevolent Fndn Grants, 775
Bodman Fndn Grants, 776
Boeing Company Contributions Program Grants, 777
Bullitt Fndn Grants, 809
Caddock Fndn Grants, 828
Canadian Patient Safety Institute (CPSI) Patient Safety Studentships, 854
Cancer Research UK Grants, 859
CDC Cooperative Agreement for the Development, Operation, and Evaluation of an Entertainment Education Program, 906
CDC Public Health Conference Support Grants, 926
Charles Delmar Fndn Grants, 963
Charles G. Koch Charitable Fndn Grants, 965
Charles Lafitte Fndn Grants, 970
CIGNA Fndn Grants, 1011
Claude Worthington Benedum Fndn Grants, 1033
Comm Fndn for Greater Buffalo Grants, 1090
Comm Fndn for Muskegon County Grants, 1093
Comm Fndn of Muncie and Delaware County Grants, 1120
Comm Fndn of Southeastern Connecticut Grants, 1125
Comm Fndn of Western North Carolina Grants, 1132
Comm Toolbox for Children's Environmental Health Grants, 1137
Connecticut Comm Fndn Grants, 1141
Constellation Energy Group and Baltimore Gas and Electric Corp Contributions, 1146
CPhA Centennial Award, 1156
Dallas Women's Fndn Grants, 1191
Denver Fndn Comm Grants, 1227
DHHS Health Conference Support Program for Toxic Substances and Disease Registry, 1255
Dr. Leon Bromberg Charitable Trust Fund Grants, 1328
DSO Controlling Pathogen Evolution Workshop Grants, 1334
Dubois County Comm Fndn Grants, 1336
Elizabeth Glaser Pediatric AIDS Fndn International Leadership Awards, 1393
Eugene M. Lang Fndn Grants, 1434
Evanston Comm Fndn Grants, 1438
Faye McBeath Fndn Grants, 1456
Fayette County Fndn Grants, 1457
FCER Chiropractic Research Grants, 1459
FDA Scientific Conferences Grants, 1463
FDHN Non-Career Research Awards, 1476
Foellinger Fndn Grants, 1519
Fulbright German Studies Seminar Grants, 1568
Fulton County Comm Fndn Grants, 1579
Gill Fndn - Gay and Lesbian Fund Grants, 1613
Greater Saint Louis Comm Fndn Grants, 1655
Greater Worcester Comm Fndn Jeppson Memorial Fund for Brookfield Grants, 1659
Halliburton Fndn Grants, 1687
Hartford Aging and Health Program Awards, 1709
Health Fndn of Greater Indianapolis Grants, 1725
Helen Bader Fndn Grants, 1738
J.W. Kieckhefer Fndn Grants, 1878
Jewish Comm Fndn of Greater Los Angeles Grants, 1921
Jewish Women's Fndn of New York Grants, 1924
John P. McGovern Fndn Grants, 1942
Joseph Alexander Fndn Grants, 1957
Kaiser Permanente Cares for Communities Grants, 1978
Komen Greater NYC Conference Grants, 2012
Komen Greater NYC Small Grants, 2013
Landon Fndn-AACR Innovator Award for International Collaboration, 2028
Lewis Preston Fund for Girls Education Grants, 2052
Lillian S. Wells Fndn Grants, 2056
Lowell Berry Fndn Grants, 2069
Lynde and Harry Bradley Fndn Grants, 2089
Maine Comm Fndn Grants, 2099
Manuel D. and Rhoda Mayerson Fndn Grants, 2100
Mark and Catherine Winkler Fndn Grants, 2112
Mary Black Fndn Grants, 2118
McLean Contributionship Grants, 2147
Meadows Fndn Grants, 2161
Michigan Psychoanalytic Institute and Society SATA Grants, 2193
NAPNAP Fndn McNeil Grant-in-Aid, 2238
NAPNAP Fndn Reckitt Benckiser Student Scholarship, 2242
NAPNAP Fndn Wyeth Pediatric Immunization Grant, 2244
NIA Support of Scientific Meetings as Cooperative Agreements, 2435
NIDDK Traditional Conference Grants, 2589
NIGMS Minority Access to Research Careers Ancillary Training Activities Grants, 2619
NIGMS Short Courses on Mathematical and Statistical Tools for the Study of Complex Phenotypes and Complex Systems, 2628
NIH Individual Postdoctoral Fellowships in Genomics and Related ELSI Topics, 2678
NIMH Short Courses on Mathematical and Statistical Tools for the Study of Complex Phenotypes and Complex Systems, 2770
NINDS Support of Scientific Meetings as Cooperative Agreements, 2786
NLM Informatics Conference Grants, 2819
Noble County Comm Fndn Grants, 2848
North Carolina Biotechnology Center Event Sponsorship Grants, 2852
North Carolina Biotechnology Center Grantsmanship Training Grants, 2853
North Carolina Biotechnology Center Meeting Grants, 2854
North Carolina Comm Fndn Grants, 2859
North Carolina GlaxoSmithKline Fndn Grants, 2860
NYAM Brock Lecture, Award and Visiting Professorship in Pediatrics, 2909
Olin Corporation Charitable Trust Grants, 2943
OREF Educational Awards, 2953
Palm Beach and Martin Counties Grants, 2986
Pfizer/AAFP Fndn Visiting Professorship Program in Family Medicine, 3027
Pinellas County Grants, 3050
Potts Memorial Fndn Grants, 3072
Principal Financial Group Fndn Grants, 3082
Progress Energy Fndn Grants, 3084
Prudential Fndn Grants, 3087
Puerto Rico Comm Fndn Grants, 3090
Quantum Corporation Snap Server Grants, 3095
Raskob Fndn for Catholic Activities Grants, 3107
Rathmann Family Fndn Grants, 3109
RCPSC Balfour M. Mount Visiting Professorship in Palliative Medicine, 3112
RCPSC Events, Speakers and Visiting Professors Grants, 3116
RCPSC National Specialty Society Annual Meeting Grants, 3126
RGK Fndn Grants, 3153
Rhode Island Fndn Grants, 3154
Rochester Area Comm Fndn Grants, 3176
Rochester Area Fndn Grants, 3177
Rockwell International Corp Trust Grants, 3183
RRF Organizational Capacity Building Grants, 3194
RWJF Changes in Health Care Financing and Organization Grants, 3206
RWJF Local Funding Partnerships Program Grants, 3223
RWJF Partners Investing in Nursing's Future Grants, 3226
RWJF Summer Medical and Dental Education Program (SMDEP), 3231
SAMHSA Conference Grants, 3246
San Antonio Area Fndn Grants, 3254
Sarah Scaife Fndn Grants, 3263
Sid W. Richardson Fndn Grants, 3284
South Madison Comm Fndn Grants, 3349

St. Joseph Comm Health Fndn Schneider Fellowships, 3370
Strowd Roses Grants, 3388
Topeka Comm Fndn Kansas Blood Services Scholarships, 3429
Wasie Fndn Grants, 3521
Weatherwax Fndn Grants, 3523
Z. Smith Reynolds Fndn Small Grants, 3557

Technical Assistance

AAAS Science & Technology Policy Fellowships - National Defense & Global Security, 29
Abbott Fund Access to Health Care Grants, 176
Abbott Fund Global AIDS Care Grants, 178
AEC Trust Grants, 242
African American Fund of New Jersey Grants, 260
Albert Pick Jr. Fund Grants, 328
Albuquerque Comm Fndn Grants, 331
Allstate Corp Giving Grants, 363
Altman Fndn Health Care Grants, 372
AMA-RFS and AMA Fndn Medical Student & Resident/Fellow Elective-Medicine & the Media, 406
Amador Comm Fndn Grants, 409
Anschutz Family Fndn Grants, 486
ARCO Fndn Education Grants, 526
Arie and Ida Crown Memorial Grants, 528
Arlington Comm Fndn Grants, 536
Assisi Fndn Grants, 653
Atkinson Fndn International Grants, 661
Avon Products Fndn Grants, 675
Ball Brothers Fndn Grants, 684
BCBS of Massachusetts Fndn Grants, 709
BCBSM Fndn Proposal Development Awards, 720
BCBSNC Fndn Fit Together Grants, 724
Beldon Fund Grants, 738
Blanche and Julian Robertson Family Fndn Grants, 765
Blue River Comm Fndn Grants, 770
Boeing Company Contributions Program Grants, 777
Boston Fndn Grants, 783
Bullitt Fndn Grants, 809
Burlington Industries Fndn Grants, 811
Cailloux Fndn Grants, 829
Cambridge Comm Fndn Grants, 837
Canadian Patient Safety Institute (CPSI) Patient Safety Studentships, 854
Carpenter Fndn Grants, 881
Cass County Comm Fndn Grants, 887
CDC Epidemiology and Laboratory Capacity Infectious Diseases Program Grants, 909
CDC School Health Programs to Prevent the Spread of HIV Cooperative Agreements, 928
CDC Technology Translation and Transfer of Effective HIV Behavioral Interventions, 931
Charles H. Farnsworth Trust Grants, 967
CHCF Local Coverage Expansion Initiative, 981
Children's Advocacy Center Grants, 997
Clarence E. Heller Charitable Fndn Grants, 1022
Clark Fndn Grants, 1029
CNCS Foster Grandparent Projects Grants, 1048
Coastal Comm Fndn of South Carolina Grants, 1051
Colorado Trust Partnerships for Health Initiative, 1063
Columbus Fndn Competitive Grants, 1066
Columbus Fndn Traditional Grants, 1071
Comm Fndn Alliance City of Evansville Endowment Fund Grants, 1089
Comm Fndn for Greater Buffalo Grants, 1090
Comm Fndn for Greater New Haven Grants, 1091
Comm Fndn for Monterey County Grants, 1092
Comm Fndn for Southeastern Michigan Grants, 1094
Comm Fndn for Southern Arizona Grants, 1095
Comm Fndn of Boone County Grants, 1099
Comm Fndn of Greater Flint Grants, 1107
Comm Fndn of Greater Fort Wayne: Comm Endowment & Clarke Endowment Fund Grants, 1108
Comm Fndn of Muncie and Delaware County Grants, 1120
Comm Fndn of Santa Cruz County Grants, 1122
Comm Fndn of Southeastern Connecticut Grants, 1125
Comm Fndn of the Ozarks Grants, 1130
Comm Fndn of Wabash County Grants, 1131
Comm Fndn of Western North Carolina Grants, 1132
Comm Fndn Silicon Valley Grants, 1133
Connecticut Comm Fndn Grants, 1141
ConocoPhillips Fndn Grants, 1144
Consumers Energy Fndn, 1147
Cooke Fndn Grants, 1148
Covenant Matters Fndn Grants, 1154
Crail-Johnson Fndn Grants, 1157
CRI Clinical Investigator Award in Cancer Immunology, 1161
Daisy Marquis Jones Fndn Grants, 1188
Dallas Women's Fndn Grants, 1191
Dept of Ed Special Education--Technical Assistance and Dissemination to Improve Services and Results for Children with Disabilities, 1233
DHHS Maternal and Child Health Projects Grants, 1263
DHHS Technical and Non-Financial Assistance to Health Centers, 1280
Dorothea Haus Ross Fndn Grants, 1320
Echoing Green Fellowships, 1365
Edina Realty Fndn Grants, 1369
Educational Fndn of America Grants, 1372
Edward Bangs Kelley and Elza Kelley Fndn Grants, 1373
Edyth Bush Charitable Fndn Grants, 1378
El Paso Comm Fndn Grants, 1388
Elizabeth Morse Genius Charitable Trust Grants, 1400
Elkhart County Comm Fndn Grants, 1401
Elmer L. and Eleanor J. Andersen Fndn Grants, 1406
Elsie Lee Garthwaite Memorial Fndn Grants, 1408
Ensworth Charitable Fndn Grants, 1416
Eugene and Agnes E. Meyer Fndn Grants, 1432
Ewing Halsell Fndn Grants, 1440
Fairfield County Comm Fndn Grants, 1446
Fan Fox and Leslie R. Samuels Fndn Grants, 1451
Fargo-Moorhead Area Fndn Grants, 1454
Fidelity Fndn Grants, 1498
Field Fndn of Illinois Grants, 1499
Florida BRAIVE Fund of Dade Comm Fndn, 1512
Florida BRAIVE Fund of Gulf Coast Comm Fndn of Venice, 1513
Florida BRAIVE Fund of The Comm Fndn in Jacksonville, 1514
Fluor Fndn Grants, 1517
Frances L. and Edwin L. Cummings Memorial Fund Grants, 1547
Frank Stanley Beveridge Fndn Grants, 1553
Frey Fndn Grants, 1562
General Motors Fndn Grants Support Program, 1591
George Frederick Jewett Fndn Grants, 1599
Greater Tacoma Comm Fndn Grants, 1656
Greater Worcester Comm Fndn Discretionary Grants, 1658
Gulf Coast Comm Fndn Grants, 1676
Health Fndn of Greater Indianapolis Grants, 1725
Hill Crest Fndn Grants, 1773
Humboldt Area Fndn Technical Assistance Program (TAP) Grants, 1819
Jacob G. Schmidlapp Trust Grants, 1883
James R. Dougherty Jr. Fndn Grants, 1894
JM Fndn Grants, 1926
Joseph H. and Florence A. Roblee Fndn Grants, 1961
Josephine Goodyear Fndn Grants, 1964
Joyce Fndn Grants, 1969
Kalamazoo Fndn Grants, 1979
Kansas Health Fndn Grants, 1980
L. W. Pierce Family Fndn Grants, 2019
Maine Comm Fndn Grants, 2099
Manuel D. and Rhoda Mayerson Fndn Grants, 2100
McMurry Fndn Grants, 2149
Minneapolis Fndn Comm Grants, 2206
Miriam and Peter Haas Fund Grants, 2208
Montgomery County Comm Fndn Grants, 2214
Moses Cone-Wesley Long Comm Health Fndn Grants, 2219
Ms. Fndn Women and AIDS Fund Grants, 2223
NIDDK Small Business Innovation Research to Develop New Therapeutics and Monitoring Technologies for Type 1 Diabetes (T1D)--Towards an Artificial Pancreas (SBIR), 2586
NIEHS SBIR E-Learning for HAZMAT and Emergency Response Grants, 2604
NIGMS Minority Access to Research Careers (MARC) Ancillary Training Activities Grants, 2619
NIH Exploratory Centers for Alternative Medicine Research Grants, 2663
Nordson Corporation Fndn Grants, 2851
North Carolina Biotechnology Center Technology Enhancement Grants, 2856
NWHF Health Advocacy Small Grants, 2905
NYCT Technical Assistance Grants, 2929
OSI Mental Health Grants, 2969
OSI Palliative Cancer Care Grants, 2970
Pfizer/AAFP Fndn Visiting Professorship Program in Family Medicine, 3027
Philadelphia Fndn Organizational Effectiveness Grants, 3029
Portland General Electric Fndn Grants, 3067
Prudential Fndn Grants, 3087
Puerto Rico Comm Fndn Grants, 3090
Putnam County Comm Fndn Grants, 3093
Rainbow Fund Grants, 3103
RCPSC Balfour M. Mount Visiting Professorship in Palliative Medicine, 3112
RCPSC Janes Visiting Professorship in Surgery, 3120
RCPSC Kilborn Memorial Visiting Professorship, 3121
Rett Syndrome Research Fndn Grants, 3151
Rhode Island Fndn Grants, 3154
Rich Fndn Grants, 3156
Rochester Area Comm Fndn Grants, 3176
RRF Organizational Capacity Building Grants, 3194
SAG Motion Picture Players Welfare Fund Grants, 3238
San Diego Fndn for Change Grants, 3255
Seabury Fndn Grants, 3274
Solo Cup Fndn Grants, 3346
Sosland Fndn Grants, 3348
South Madison Comm Fndn Grants, 3349
St. Joseph Comm Health Fndn Burn Care and Prevention Grants, 3367
St. Joseph Comm Health Fndn Improving Healthcare Access Grants, 3368
Stewart Huston Charitable Trust Grants, 3384
Susan Mott Webb Charitable Trust Grants, 3412
U.S. Department of Education Rehabilitation Training--Rehabilitation Continuing Education Programs (RCEP)--Institute on Rehabilitation Issues (IRI), 3449
Until There's a Cure Fndn Grants, 3471
Vancouver Fndn Grants and Comm Initiatives Program, 3477
Verizon Fndn Vermont Grants, 3491
Weatherwax Fndn Grants, 3523
Western Indiana Comm Fndn Grants, 3528
William G. Gilmore Fndn Grants, 3537

Training Programs/Internships

AAAAI / Schering Allergy/Immunology Fellowship of Excellence Training Awards, 20
AACAP Child and Adolescent Psychiatry (CAP) Teaching Scholarships, 31
AACN Mentorship Grant, 61
AAP Comm Access To Child Health (CATCH) Advocacy Training Grants, 157
AAP Comm Access To Child Health (CATCH) Residency Training Grants, 160

ACCP Anticoagulation Training Program Grants, 197
ACCP Heart Failure Training Program Grants, 198
Achelis and Bodman Fndns Grants, 206
ACS Master's Training Grants in Clinical Oncology Social Work, 208
ACS Physician Training Awards in Preventive Medicine, 218
AFAR Medical Student Training in Aging Research Program, 255
AHFMR Forefront Internship Program Grants, 275
AHFMR Personnel Funding Grants, 290
AHIMA Faculty Development Stipends, 301
AHNS/AAO-HNSF Surgeon Scientist Combined Award, 307
AHNS/AAO-HNSF Young Investigator Combined Award, 308
AMA-MSS Government Relations Internship Programs, 404
AMA-RFS Legislative Awareness Internships, 407
AMD Corp Contributions Grants, 411
American Psychiatric Association Minority Medical Student Summer Externship in Addiction Psychiatry, 445
American Psychiatric Association Minority Medical Student Summer Mentoring Program, 446
American Psychiatric Association/Janssen Resident Psychiatric Research Scholars, 452
American-Scandinavian Fndn Visiting Lectureship Grants, 460
Anschutz Family Fndn Grants, 486
ASGE Endoscopic Research Awards, 566
ASHA Research Mentoring-Pair Travel Award, 572
ASHA Students Preparing for Academic & Research Careers (SPARC) Award, 574
AT&T Excelerator, 657
Atkinson Fndn International Grants, 661
BCBS of Minnesota Growing Up Healthy Grants, 711
BCBS of Minnesota Healthy Together Grants, 712
Blowitz-Ridgeway Fndn Grants, 767
Canada-U.S. Fulbright New Century Scholars Program Grants, 846
Canadian Patient Safety Institute (CPSI) Patient Safety Studentships, 854
Cancer Research Postdoctoral Fellowships for Basic and Physician Scientists, 856
Carl and Lily Pforzheimer Fndn Grants, 868
Carrie Estelle Doheny Fndn Grants, 883
Carrier Corporation Contributions Grants, 884
CDC Preventive Health Services-Sexually Transmitted Diseases Control Grants, 923
Center for Science in the Public Interest Internships, 935
CFF Student Traineeships, 948
CFPC Research and Education Fndn Grants, 956
Challenged Athletes Fndn Grants, 958
Charles A. Frueauff Fndn Grants, 962
Charles Delmar Fndn Grants, 963
Charles H. Revson Fndn Grants, 969
Children's Advocacy Center Grants, 997
CIIT Postdoctoral Fellowships, 1012
Clarian Health Critical / Progressive Care Internships, 1023
Clarian Health Multi-Specialty Internships, 1024
Clarian Health OR Internships, 1025
Collins Fndn Grants, 1058
Columbus Fndn Competitive Grants, 1066
Comm Fndn for Greater Buffalo Grants, 1090
Cruise Industry Charitable Fndn Grants, 1166
Dept of Ed College Assistance MiGrants (CAMP), 1228
Dept of Ed Rehabilitation Training Grants, 1229
DHHS Adolescent Family Life Demonstration Projects, 1243
DHHS Developmental Disabilities University Affiliated Programs Project Grants, 1248
DHHS Geriatric Training for Physicians and Dentists Grants, 1250
DHHS Grants for Dental Public Health, 1251
DHHS Health Careers Opportunity Program Grants, 1253
DHHS Health Professions Training in Geriatrics Grants, 1259
DHHS Maternal and Child Health Research and Training Programs Grants, 1264
DHHS Podiatric Primary Care Residency Training Grants, 1270
DHHS Preventive Medicine, 1271
DHHS Professional Nurse Traineeships, 1274
DHHS Public Health Students Traineeships and Other Graduate Public Health Programs, 1277
DHHS Residency Training in Family Practice, General Internal Medicine, or General Pediatrics Grants, 1278
DHHS Technical and Non-Financial Assistance to Health Centers, 1280
DOD HBCU/MI Partnership Training Award, 1293
DOD Predoctoral Traineeship in Breast Cancer Research, 1296
DOJ Gang-Free Schools and Communities Intervention Grants, 1303
DOL Occupational Safety and Health--Susan Harwood Training Grants, 1305
Dr. John T. Macdonald Fndn Grants, 1327
E.L. Wiegand Fndn Grants, 1361
Educational Fndn of America Grants, 1372
Edward S. Moore Fndn Grants, 1374
Edwin S. Webster Fndn Grants, 1376
Effie and Wofford Cain Fndn Grants, 1385
Elizabeth Glaser Pediatric AIDS Fndn Two-Year Scholar Awards, 1397
Eugene M. Lang Fndn Grants, 1434
Evjue Fndn Grants, 1439
Faye McBeath Fndn Grants, 1456
FCD Child Development Grants, 1458
FIC International Training and Research in Emerging Infectious Diseases Grants, 1492
FIC International Training and Research in Environmental and Occupational Health, 1493
Fndn for Seacoast Health Grants, 1533
Fred L. Emerson Fndn Grants, 1557
Frist Fndn Grants, 1563
Fulbright Alumni Initiatives Awards Program Grants, 1566
Fulbright International Education Administrators (IEA) Seminar Program Grants, 1569
Fulbright New Century Scholars (NCS) Program Grants, 1570
Fulbright Traditional Scholar Program in the Near East and North Africa Region, 1575
Genesis Fndn Grants, 1593
George Family Fndn Grants, 1598
Green Bay Packers Fndn Grants, 1660
Hearst Fndn and William Randolph Hearst Fndn Grants, 1730
Henry J. Kaiser Family Fndn Media Fellowships, 1749
HHK Employment Grants, 1755
Hogg Fndn for Mental Health Grants, 1784
Holland/Zeeland Comm Fndn Grants, 1786
HRSA Nurse Anesthetist Traineeships, 1808
HRSA Physician Assistant Training, 1810
Independence Blue Cross Nursing Internships, 1848
Jewish Comm Fndn of Greater Los Angeles Grants, 1921
JM Fndn Grants, 1926
John Merck Fund Grants, 1940
Johnson & Johnson Corp Contributions Grants, 1952
Lynde and Harry Bradley Fndn Grants, 2089
Marriott Fndn for People with Disabilities Bridges Program Grants, 2113
Max and Victoria Dreyfus Fndn Grants, 2133
McLean Contributionship Grants, 2147
Mead Johnson Nutritionals Scholarships, 2159
Meadows Fndn Grants, 2161
Montgomery County Comm Fndn Grants, 2214
MSSC Research Studentships, 2227
National Emergency Medicine Association Grants, 2252
NEI Ruth L. Kirschstein National Research Service Award Short-Term Institutional Research Training Grants, 2297
NEI Scholars Program, 2298
NHLBI Minority Institution Research Scientist Development Award, 2354
NHLBI Minority Institutional Research Training Program Grants, 2355
NHLBI National Research Service Award Programs in Cardiovascular Epidemiology and Biostatistics, 2357
NHLBI Short-Term Research Education Program to Increase Diversity in Health-Related Research, 2383
NIDDK Mentored Research Scientist Development Award, 2565
NIDDK Training in Clinical Investigation in Kidney and Urology Grants, 2590
NIEHS Superfund Hazardous Substances Basic Research and Education Grants, 2607
NIGMS Individual Postdoctoral NRSA Fellowships in Clinical Pharmacology, 2611
NIGMS MARC Undergraduate Student Training in Academic Research (U-STAR) Program, 2617
NIGMS Predoctoral Training in Bioinformatics and Computation Biology Grants, 2625
NIH Midcareer Investigator Award in Mouse Pathobiology Research Grants, 2690
NIH Summer Internship Program in Biomedical Research, 2732
NIMH National Research Service Awards (NRSA)--Individual, 2764
NLM Exploratory/Developmental Grants, 2815
NNEDVF/Altria Doors of Hope Program, 2847
Olin Corporation Charitable Trust Grants, 2943
OSI European Commission Internships for Young Roma Graduates, 2965
Otto Bremer Fndn Grants, 2977
Pfizer Fndn Grants, 3025
PhRMA Fndn Health Outcomes Pre-Doctoral Fellowships, 3032
Polaroid Fund Grants, 3065
Principal Financial Group Fndn Grants, 3082
Progress Energy Fndn Grants, 3084
Prudential Fndn Grants, 3087
Raskob Fndn for Catholic Activities Grants, 3107
Rathmann Family Fndn Grants, 3109
RCPSC Janes Visiting Professorship in Surgery, 3120
RCPSC Kilborn Memorial Visiting Professorship, 3121
RCPSC Traineeships, 3132
Regenstrief Geriatrics Fellowship, 3143
Regenstrief General Internal Medicine - General Pediatrics Research Fellowship Program, 3144
Regenstrief Master Of Science In Clinical Research/CITE Program, 3145
Ruth Eleanor Bamberger and John Ernest Bamberger Memorial Fndn Grants, 3202
RWJF Clinical Scholars Program Grants, 3207
RWJF Executive Nurse Fellowships, 3210
Saint Luke's Health Initiatives Grants, 3240
Savoy Fndn Studentships, 3268
SHF Reach--Connecting Communities and Youth for a Healthy Future Grants, 3283
Society for Imaging Informatics in Medicine (SIIM) Small Training Grants, 3324
Society of Neuroscience Minority Fellowships, 3345
Strowd Roses Grants, 3388
Susan Mott Webb Charitable Trust Grants, 3412
Vectren Fndn Grants, 3485
Verizon Fndn New York Grants, 3488
Wal-Mart State Giving Program Grants, 3514
Weingart Fndn Grants, 3524

Travel Grants

AAAAI Allergy, Asthma and Immunology Education and Research Trust (ART) Allied Health Travel Grants, 21
AAAAI STAR Program Grants, 26

AACAP Educational Outreach Program for Child and Adolescent Psychiatry Residents, 33
AACAP Educational Outreach Program for General Psychiatry Residents, 34
AACAP Systems of Care Special Program Scholarships, 54
AACR Brigid G. Leventhal Scholar in Cancer Research Awards, 69
AACR Gertrude Elion Cancer Research Award, 76
AACR Minority Scholar in Cancer Research Awards, 82
AACR Minority-Serving Institution Faculty Scholar in Cancer Research Awards, 83
AACR Scholar-in-Training Awards, 87
AACR Scholar-in-Training Awards - Special Conferences, 88
AACR Thomas J. Bardos Science Education Awards, 90
AACR-GlaxoSmithKline Clinical Cancer Research Scholar Awards, 98
AACR-NCI International Investigator Opportunity Grants, 101
AACR-WICR Scholar Awards, 105
AAFPRS Residency Travel Awards, 124
AAP Anne E. Dyson Child Advocacy Awards, 156
AAP International Travel Grants, 162
AAP Program Delegate Awards, 166
Abbott-ASM Lifetime Achievement Award, 180
AcademyHealth Alice S. Hersh Student Scholarships, 191
AcademyHealth Awards, 192
AcademyHealth PHSR Interest Group Student Scholarships, 195
ACCP Anticoagulation Training Program Grants, 197
ACCP Heart Failure Training Program Grants, 198
AIHP Sonnedecker Visiting Scholar Grants, 317
AMA Fndn Dr. Nathan Davis International Awards in Medicine, 387
AMA Fndn Jack B. McConnell, MD Awards for Excellence in Volunteerism, 391
AMA Fndn Jordan Fieldman, MD, Awards, 393
AMA Fndn Leadership Awards, 394
AMA Fndn Pride in the Profession Grants, 397
AMA Virtual Mentor Theme Issue Editor Grants, 400
AMA-MSS Research Poster Award, 405
AMA-WPC Joan F. Giambalvo Memorial Scholarships, 408
Amarillo Area/Harrington Fndns Grants, 410
American Academy of Dermatology Camp Discovery Scholarships, 412
American College of Rheumatology Fellows-in-Training Travel Scholarships, 421
American College of Surgeons Australia and New Zealand Chapter Travelling Fellowships, 423
American College of Surgeons Nizar N. Oweida, MD, FACS, Scholarships, 430
American Psychiatric Association Travel Scholarships for Minority Medical Students, 449
amfAR Research Grants, 466
APA Travel Awards, 501
ASCO Merit Awards, 558
ASCO Resident Travel Awards, 559
ASGE Don Wilson Award, 565
ASHA Minority Student Leadership Program Awards, 570
ASHA Research Mentoring-Pair Travel Award, 572
ASHA Student Research Travel Award, 573
ASHA Students Preparing for Academic & Research Careers (SPARC) Award, 574
ASHFndn Research Grant in Speech Science, 583
ASM Corp Activities Program Student Travel Grants, 591
ASM Early-Career Faculty Travel Award, 593
ASM Faculty Ehancement Program -Travel Awards, 595
ASM Founders Distinguished Service Award, 596
ASM General Meeting Minority Travel Grants, 598
ASM GlaxoSmithKline International Member of the Year Award, 599
ASM International Professorship for Latin America, 603
ASM International Professorships for Asia and Africa, 604
ASM Millis-Colwell Postgraduate Travel Grant, 608
ASM Richard and Mary Finkelstein Travel Grant, 613
ASM Roche Diagnostics Alice C. Evans Award, 615
ASM Student and Post Doctoral Fellow Travel Grants, 619
ASM Student Travel Grants, 620
ASM TREK Diagnostic ABMM/ABMLI Professional Recognition Award, 621
ASM-UNESCO Leadership Grant for International Educators, 626
ASMCUE/GM Travel Assistance Grants, 628
ASPEN Scientific Abstracts Awards for Papers or Posters, 636
ASPEN Scientific Abstracts Promising Investigator Awards, 637
ASPET Travel Awards, 648
Australian Academy of Science Grants, 670
Bush Fndn Medical Fellowships, 815
Canada-U.S. Fulbright Senior Specialists Program Grants, 847
Canadian Friends of Hebrew University Research and Study Grants, 850
Cancer Research UK Grants, 859
Cancer Society of New Zealand Grants, 860
CCFF Visiting Scientist Awards, 900
CDC Public Health Conference Support Grants, 926
CNCS Foster Grandparent Projects Grants, 1048
DHHS Chiropractic Demonstration Project Grants, 1246
DHHS Health Care Systems Cost and Access Research and Development Grants, 1252
DHHS Thimerosal Pharmacokinetics: Assessment of the Distribution, Metabolism, and Excretion, 1281
DOD Idea Award for Breast Cancer Research, 1294
Elizabeth Glaser Pediatric AIDS Fndn International Leadership Awards, 1393
Elizabeth Glaser Pediatric AIDS Fndn Two-Year Scholar Awards, 1397
Epilepsy Research Fndn New Therapy Grants, 1423
FACES Assistance Grants, 1444
FDHN Moti L. & Kamla Rustgi International Travel Awards, 1475
FDHN Non-Career Research Awards, 1476
Fndn for Medical Research Grants, 1528
Fndn of CVPH Travel Fund Grants, 1543
Fulbright Alumni Initiatives Awards Program Grants, 1566
Fulbright Distinguished Chairs Grants, 1567
Fulbright German Studies Seminar Grants, 1568
Fulbright International Education Administrators (IEA) Seminar Program Grants, 1569
Fulbright Specialists Program Grants, 1571
Fulbright Traditional Scholar Program in Europe and Eurasia, 1572
Fulbright Traditional Scholar Program in Sub-Saharan Africa, 1573
Fulbright Traditional Scholar Program in the East Asia/Pacific Region, 1574
Fulbright Traditional Scholar Program in the South and Central Asia Region, 1576
Fulbright Traditional Scholar Program in the Western Hemisphere, 1577
Fulton County Comm Fndn Grants, 1579
Grass Fndn Marine Biological Laboratory Fellowships, 1648
Heart Rhythm Society Fellowships, 1731
Henry J. Kaiser Family Fndn Media Fellowships, 1749
International Cancer Technology Transfer Fellowships, 1858
International Fellowships in Medical Education, 1861
International Oncology Nursing Fellowships, 1862
IWMF Public Health Fellowship, 1871
Jane Beattie Memorial Scholarship, 1901
KFC Allied Health Research Grants, 1996
KFC Biomedical Research Grants, 1998
Komen Greater NYC Small Grants, 2013
Lewis Preston Fund for Girls Education Grants, 2052
MAP International Medical Fellowships, 2101
Matsumae International Fndn Grants, 2129
Medical/Nursing Education, Research, and Health Care Exchanges with Taiwan, 2165
Michigan Psychoanalytic Institute and Society SATA Grants, 2193
NAPNAP Fndn McNeil Grant-in-Aid, 2238
NAPNAP Fndn Reckitt Benckiser Student Scholarship, 2242
NCI Technologies and Software to Support Integrative Cancer Biology Research (SBIR) Grants, 2279
NCIC Canadian Cancer Society Research Grants, 2282
NCIC Canadian Cancer Society Travel Award for Senior Level PhD Students, 2283
NFID Advanced Vaccinology Course Travel Grant, 2307
NFID John P. Utz Medical Mycology Postdoctoral Fellowship, 2309
NFID Nosocomial Infection Research and Training Postdoctoral Fellowship, 2311
NIDDK Traditional Conference Grants, 2589
NIGMS Minority Access to Research Careers Ancillary Training Activities Grants, 2619
Northwest Airlines KidCares Medical Travel Assistance, 2868
NSF BIO Minority Postdoctoral Research Fellowships, 2877
NSF Grant Opportunities for Academic Liaison with Industry (GOALI), 2887
NSF-NIST Interaction in Chemistry, Materials Research, Molecular Biosciences, Bioengineering, and Chemical Engineering, 2897
NYAM Edward N. Gibbs Memorial Lecture and Award in Nephrology, 2912
ONS Scholarships, 2950
OSI Supplementary Grants: Burma, 2971
PAHO-ASM International Professorship for Latin America, 2983
Pinellas County Grants, 3050
RCPSC Balfour M. Mount Visiting Professorship in Palliative Medicine, 3112
RCPSC Detweiler Traveling Fellowships, 3114
RCPSC Janes Visiting Professorship in Surgery, 3120
RCPSC Kilborn Memorial Visiting Professorship, 3121
RCPSC McLaughlin-Gallie Visiting Professorship, 3123
RCPSC National Specialty Society Annual Meeting Grants, 3126
RCPSC Royal College Visiting Professorships in Medical Research, 3130
RCPSC Wightman Visiting Professorship in Medicine, 3134
Rett Syndrome Research Fndn Grants, 3151
Rockefeller Archive Center Research Grants, 3178
RWJF Summer Medical and Dental Education Program (SMDEP), 3231
Sigrid Juselius Fndn Grants, 3286
SOBP International Travel Fellowships, 3314
SOBP Travel Fellowships, 3315
Society of Neuroscience Minority Fellowships, 3345
SRC Medical Research Grants, 3362
St. Joseph Comm Health Fndn Schneider Fellowships, 3370
Topeka Comm Fndn Kansas Blood Services Scholarships, 3429
UICC American Cancer Society International Fellowships for Beginning Investigators, 3455
UICC International Cancer Technology Transfer (ICRETT) Fellowships, 3456
UICC Yamagiwa-Yoshida Memorial International Cancer Study Grants, 3458

US Airways Comm Contributions, 3472
US CRDF Leishmaniasis: Collaborative Research Opportunities in North Africa and the Middle East, 3474
Whitaker International Fellows and Scholars Program, 3532
Whitehall Fndn Neurobiology Research Grants, 3533

Vocational Education
Achelis and Bodman Fndns Grants, 206
AMD Corp Contributions Grants, 411
ArvinMeritor Grants, 544
AT&T Excelerator, 657
Bush Fndn Health & Human Services Grants, 814
Carrier Corporation Contributions Grants, 884
Charlotte County (FL) Comm Fndn Grants, 973
Claude Pepper Fndn Grants, 1032
Cleveland Browns Fndn Grants, 1036
Comm Fndn of Grant County Scholarships, 1105
ConocoPhillips Fndn Grants, 1144
Consumers Energy Fndn, 1147
Crail-Johnson Fndn Grants, 1157
D.F. Halton Fndn Grants, 1181
Danellie Fndn Grants, 1198
Duke Energy Fndn Grants, 1339
Gamble Fndn Grants, 1582
Goodrich Corporation Fndn Grants, 1638
Gulf Coast Comm of Venice Fndn Grants, 1677
Harvest Fndn Grants, 1713
Irvin Stern Fndn Grants, 1866
Jane Bradley Pettit Fndn Grants, 1902
John Merck Fund Grants, 1940
Northrop Grumman Corporation Grants, 2866
RWJF Jobs to Careers: Promoting Work-Based Learning for Quality Care - Research Grants, 3221
Samuel S. Johnson Fndn Grants, 3251
Seabury Fndn Grants, 3274
TWS Fndn Grants, 3443
U.S. Department of Education Rehabilitation Research Training Centers (RRTCs), 3448
U.S. Department of Education Vocational Rehabilitation Services Projects for American Indians with Disabilities Grants, 3452
Vancouver Fndn Grants and Comm Initiatives Program, 3477
Vectren Fndn Grants, 3485
Verizon Fndn Pennsylvania Grants, 3490
Wal-Mart Fndn Comm Grants, 3513
Wal-Mart State Giving Program Grants, 3514
Women of the ELCA Opportunity Scholars

Geographic Index

Note: This index lists grants for which applicants must be residents of or located in a specific geographic area. Numbers refer to entry numbers.

United States

Alabama

3M Company Health and Human Services Grants, 10
3M Foundation Grants, 11
ACF Ethnic Community Self-Help Grants, 200
ACF Preferred Communities Grants, 201
ACF Standing Announcement for Unaccompanied Alien Children Grants, 202
ACF Supplemental Services for Recently Arrived Refugees Grants, 203
Actors Fund Social Services and Financial Assistance, 225
Alabama Power Foundation Grants, 321
American College of Surgeons and The Triological Society Clinical Scientist Development Awards, 422
Arkema Foundation Science Teachers Program, 535
ASHA Advancing Academic-Research Careers (AARC) Award, 569
ASHA Minority Student Leadership Program Awards, 570
ASHA Multicultural Activities Projects Grants, 571
ASHA Research Mentoring-Pair Travel Award, 572
ASHA Student Research Travel Award, 573
ASHA Students Preparing for Academic & Research Careers (SPARC) Award, 574
ASM Millis-Colwell Postgraduate Travel Grant, 608
AT&T Excelerator, 657
Bearemy's Kennel Pals Grants, 728
Belk Foundation Grants, 739
Bridgestone/Firestone Trust Fund Grants, 792
Cable Positive's Tony Cox Community Fund Grants, 827
Caring Foundation Grants, 866
Carrier Corporation Contributions Grants, 884
CDC Injury Control Research Centers Grants, 913
Champ-A Champion Fur Kids Grants, 959
Charles A. Frueauff Foundation Grants, 962
Children Affected by AIDS Foundation Camp Network Grants, 994
Children Affected by AIDS Foundation Family Assistance Emergency Fund Grants, 996
CLIF Bar Family Foundation Grants, 1040
Community Foundation of Greater Birmingham Grants, 1106
Community Foundation of South Alabama Grants, 1123
Compass Bank Foundation Grants, 1138
Cooper Industries Foundation Grants, 1150
CSX Corporate Contributions Grants, 1169
D. W. McMillan Foundation Grants, 1180
Dean Foods Community Involvement Grants, 1209
DHHS Healthy Tomorrows Partnership for Children, 1261
Do Something BR!CK Awards, 1287
Dr. Stanley Pearle Scholarships, 1330
El Paso Corporate Foundation Grants, 1389
GenCorp Foundation Grants, 1587
GoGirlGo! Ambassador Team Awards, 1632
Guitar Center Music Foundation Grants, 1675
Harley Davidson Foundation Grants, 1694
Harry Kramer Memorial Fund Grants, 1705
Hill Crest Foundation Grants, 1773
IAFF Burn Foundation Research Grants, 1830
J.L. Bedsole Foundation Grants, 1876
John Merck Fund Grants, 1940
John Merck Scholars Awards, 1941
Johnson & Johnson Community Health Care Program Grants, 1951
Kimberly-Clark Community Grants, 2001
Lettie Pate Whitehead Foundation Grants, 2049
Multiple Sclerosis Foundation Brighter Tomorrow Grants, 2228
NEI Mentored Clinical Scientist Development Program Award (K12), 2295
NMF Franklin C. McLean Award, 2829
NMF General Electric Medical Scholars Fellowships, 2830
NMF Henry G. Halladay Awards, 2831
NMF Mary Ball Carrera Scholarship, 2834
NMF National Medical Association Awards for Medical Journalism, 2836
NMF National Medical Association Emerging Scholar Awards, 2837
NMF National Medical Association Patti LaBelle Award, 2838
NMF Need-Based Scholarships, 2839
NMF Ralph W. Ellison Prize, 2840
NMF William and Charlotte Cadbury Award, 2841
NSF Major Research Instrumentation Program (MRI) Grants, 2889
OneSight Research Foundation Block Grants, 2944
Pfizer/AAFP Foundation Visiting Professorship Program in Family Medicine, 3027
Plum Creek Foundation Grants, 3062
Rosalinde and Arthur Gilbert Foundation/AFAR New Investigator Awards in Alzheimer's Disease, 3187
Southwire Company Grants, 3353
Steelcase Foundation Grants, 3379
Susan Mott Webb Charitable Trust Grants, 3412
Tylenol Scholarship, 3444
U.S. Department of Education Erma Byrd Scholarships, 3446
U.S. Department of Education United States-Russia Program: Improving Research and Educational Activities in Higher Education, 3451
US CRDF Leishmaniasis: Collaborative Research Opportunities in North Africa and the Middle East, 3474
Vulcan Materials Company Foundation Grants, 3504
Wal-Mart Foundation Community Grants, 3513
Wal-Mart State Giving Program Grants, 3514
Woodward Fund Grants, 3552
YSA UnitedHealth Heroes Service Learning Grants, 3556

Alaska

3M Company Health and Human Services Grants, 10
3M Foundation Grants, 11
ACF Ethnic Community Self-Help Grants, 200
ACF Preferred Communities Grants, 201
ACF Standing Announcement for Unaccompanied Alien Children Grants, 202
ACF Supplemental Services for Recently Arrived Refugees Grants, 203
Actors Fund Social Services and Financial Assistance, 225
Alaska Airlines Corporate Giving Grants, 323
Alaska Airlines Foundation Grants, 324
AMA Foundation Arthur N. Wilson, MD, Scholarship, 386
American College of Surgeons and The Triological Society Clinical Scientist Development Awards, 422
ARCO Foundation Education Grants, 526
ASHA Advancing Academic-Research Careers (AARC) Award, 569
ASHA Minority Student Leadership Program Awards, 570
ASHA Multicultural Activities Projects Grants, 571
ASHA Research Mentoring-Pair Travel Award, 572
ASHA Student Research Travel Award, 573
ASHA Students Preparing for Academic & Research Careers (SPARC) Award, 574
ASM Millis-Colwell Postgraduate Travel Grant, 608
Bearemy's Kennel Pals Grants, 728
Bullitt Foundation Grants, 809
Cable Positive's Tony Cox Community Fund Grants, 827
CDC Injury Control Research Centers Grants, 913
Champ-A Champion Fur Kids Grants, 959
Children Affected by AIDS Foundation Camp Network Grants, 994
Children Affected by AIDS Foundation Family Assistance Emergency Fund Grants, 996
CLIF Bar Family Foundation Grants, 1040
ConocoPhillips Foundation Grants, 1144
Do Something BR!CK Awards, 1287
Dr. Stanley Pearle Scholarships, 1330
Fluor Foundation Grants, 1517
Foster Foundation Grants, 1524
GoGirlGo! Ambassador Team Awards, 1632
Guitar Center Music Foundation Grants, 1675
Harry Kramer Memorial Fund Grants, 1705
Homer Foundation Grants, 1789
IAFF Burn Foundation Research Grants, 1830
John Merck Fund Grants, 1940
John Merck Scholars Awards, 1941
M.J. Murdock Charitable Trust Grants, 2095
Multiple Sclerosis Foundation Brighter Tomorrow Grants, 2228
NEI Mentored Clinical Scientist Development Program Award (K12), 2295
NMF Franklin C. McLean Award, 2829
NMF General Electric Medical Scholars Fellowships, 2830
NMF Henry G. Halladay Awards, 2831
NMF Mary Ball Carrera Scholarship, 2834
NMF National Medical Association Awards for Medical Journalism, 2836
NMF National Medical Association Emerging Scholar Awards, 2837
NMF National Medical Association Patti LaBelle Award, 2838
NMF Need-Based Scholarships, 2839
NMF Ralph W. Ellison Prize, 2840
NMF William and Charlotte Cadbury Award, 2841
NSF Major Research Instrumentation Program (MRI) Grants, 2889
OneSight Research Foundation Block Grants, 2944
Paul G. Allen Family Foundation Grants, 3000
Pfizer/AAFP Foundation Visiting Professorship Program in Family Medicine, 3027
Premera CARES Grants, 3074
Pride Foundation Grants and Scholarships, 3078
Rasmuson Foundation Grants, 3108
Robert B McMillen Foundation Grants, 3169
Rosalinde and Arthur Gilbert Foundation/AFAR New Investigator Awards in Alzheimer's Disease, 3187
Tylenol Scholarship, 3444
U.S. Department of Education Erma Byrd Scholarships, 3446
U.S. Department of Education United States-Russia Program: Improving Research and Educational Activities in Higher Education, 3451
US CRDF Leishmaniasis: Collaborative Research Opportunities in North Africa and the Middle East, 3474
Wal-Mart Foundation Community Grants, 3513
Wal-Mart State Giving Program Grants, 3514

Arizona

Abbott Fund Access to Health Care Grants, 176
Abbott Fund Community Vitality Grants, 177
Abbott Fund Global AIDS Care Grants, 178
Abbott Fund Science and Medical Innovation Grants, 179
ACE Charitable Foundation Grants, 199
ACF Ethnic Community Self-Help Grants, 200
ACF Preferred Communities Grants, 201
ACF Standing Announcement for Unaccompanied Alien Children Grants, 202
ACF Supplemental Services for Recently Arrived Refugees Grants, 203
Actors Fund Social Services and Financial Assistance, 225
Albertson's Charitable Giving Grants, 330
American College of Surgeons and The Triological Society Clinical Scientist Development Awards, 422

ARCO Foundation Education Grants, 526
Arizona Cardinals Grants, 529
Arizona Diamondbacks Charities Grants, 530
Arizona Public Service Corporate Giving Program Grants, 531
ASHA Advancing Academic-Research Careers (AARC) Award, 569
ASHA Minority Student Leadership Program Awards, 570
ASHA Multicultural Activities Projects Grants, 571
ASHA Research Mentoring-Pair Travel Award, 572
ASHA Student Research Travel Award, 573
ASHA Students Preparing for Academic & Research Careers (SPARC) Award, 574
ASM Millis-Colwell Postgraduate Travel Grant, 608
Bearemy's Kennel Pals Grants, 728
Bechtel Group Foundation Building Positive Community Relationships Grants, 731
Bert W. Martin Foundation Grants, 750
BHHS Legacy Foundation Grants, 753
Cable Positive's Tony Cox Community Fund Grants, 827
Carrier Corporation Contributions Grants, 884
CDC Injury Control Research Centers Grants, 913
Champ-A Champion Fur Kids Grants, 959
Chase Paymentech Corporate Giving Grants, 975
Children Affected by AIDS Foundation Camp Network Grants, 994
Children Affected by AIDS Foundation Family Assistance Emergency Fund Grants, 996
CLIF Bar Family Foundation Grants, 1040
Comerica Charitable Foundation Grants, 1073
Community Foundation for Southern Arizona Grants, 1095
Compass Bank Foundation Grants, 1138
Del E. Webb Foundation Grants, 1213
Do Something BR!CK Awards, 1287
Dorrance Family Foundation Grants, 1323
Dr. Stanley Pearle Scholarships, 1330
E.L. Wiegand Foundation Grants, 1361
Flinn Foundation Grants Programs, 1511
FMC Foundation Grants, 1518
General Mills Foundation Grants, 1590
GoGirlGo! Ambassador Team Awards, 1632
Guitar Center Music Foundation Grants, 1675
Harry Kramer Memorial Fund Grants, 1705
Honeywell Foundation Grants, 1791
Humana Foundation Grants, 1818
IAFF Burn Foundation Research Grants, 1830
John Merck Fund Grants, 1940
John Merck Scholars Awards, 1941
Kevin P. and Sydney B. Knight Family Foundation Grants, 1993
Margaret T. Morris Foundation Grants, 2105
Multiple Sclerosis Foundation Brighter Tomorrow Grants, 2228
NEI Mentored Clinical Scientist Development Program Award (K12), 2295
Nina Mason Pulliam Charitable Trust Grants, 2776
NMF Franklin C. McLean Award, 2829
NMF General Electric Medical Scholars Fellowships, 2830
NMF Henry G. Halladay Awards, 2831
NMF Mary Ball Carrera Scholarship, 2834
NMF National Medical Association Awards for Medical Journalism, 2836
NMF National Medical Association Emerging Scholar Awards, 2837
NMF National Medical Association Patti LaBelle Award, 2838
NMF Need-Based Scholarships, 2839
NMF Ralph W. Ellison Prize, 2840
NMF William and Charlotte Cadbury Award, 2841
NSF Major Research Instrumentation Program (MRI) Grants, 2889
OneSight Research Foundation Block Grants, 2944
PacifiCare Foundation Grants, 2981
Pfizer/AAFP Foundation Visiting Professorship Program in Family Medicine, 3027
Phoenix Suns Charities Grants, 3030
Piper Jaffray Companies Building Strong Communities Grants, 3053
Prudential Foundation Grants, 3087
Rosalinde and Arthur Gilbert Foundation/AFAR New Investigator Awards in Alzheimer's Disease, 3187
Saint Luke's Health Initiatives Grants, 3240
Southwest Gas Corporation Foundation Grants, 3352
Susan G. Komen Breast Cancer Foundation Breast Health, Breast Cancer Education, and Outreach Programs Grants, 3408
Tylenol Scholarship, 3444
U.S. Department of Education Erma Byrd Scholarships, 3446
U.S. Department of Education United States-Russia Program: Improving Research and Educational Activities in Higher Education, 3451
US Airways Community Contributions, 3472
US Airways Community Foundation Grants, 3473
US CRDF Leishmaniasis: Collaborative Research Opportunities in North Africa and the Middle East, 3474
Vulcan Materials Company Foundation Grants, 3504
Wal-Mart Foundation Community Grants, 3513
Wal-Mart State Giving Program Grants, 3514
YSA UnitedHealth Heroes Service Learning Grants, 3556

Arkansas

3M Company Health and Human Services Grants, 10
3M Foundation Grants, 11
ACE Charitable Foundation Grants, 199
ACF Ethnic Community Self-Help Grants, 200
ACF Preferred Communities Grants, 201
ACF Standing Announcement for Unaccompanied Alien Children Grants, 202
ACF Supplemental Services for Recently Arrived Refugees Grants, 203
Actors Fund Social Services and Financial Assistance, 225
AEGON Transamerica Foundation Grants, 243
Albertson's Charitable Giving Grants, 330
American College of Surgeons and The Triological Society Clinical Scientist Development Awards, 422
American Electric Power Grants, 434
Arkansas Community Foundation Arkansas Black Hall of Fame Grants, 532
Arkansas Community Foundation Grants, 533
ASHA Advancing Academic-Research Careers (AARC) Award, 569
ASHA Minority Student Leadership Program Awards, 570
ASHA Multicultural Activities Projects Grants, 571
ASHA Research Mentoring-Pair Travel Award, 572
ASHA Student Research Travel Award, 573
ASHA Students Preparing for Academic & Research Careers (SPARC) Award, 574
ASM Millis-Colwell Postgraduate Travel Grant, 608
AT&T Excelerator, 657
Bearemy's Kennel Pals Grants, 728
Belk Foundation Grants, 739
Bridgestone/Firestone Trust Fund Grants, 792
Cable Positive's Tony Cox Community Fund Grants, 827
Carl B. and Florence E. King Foundation Grants, 869
CDC Injury Control Research Centers Grants, 913
Champ-A Champion Fur Kids Grants, 959
Charles A. Frueauff Foundation Grants, 962
Children Affected by AIDS Foundation Camp Network Grants, 994
Children Affected by AIDS Foundation Family Assistance Emergency Fund Grants, 996
CLIF Bar Family Foundation Grants, 1040
Do Something BR!CK Awards, 1287
Dr. Stanley Pearle Scholarships, 1330
Entergy Community Partnership Grants, 1417
Entergy Corporation Open Grants for Healthy Families, 1418
Foundation for the Mid-South Grants, 1536
GenCorp Foundation Grants, 1587
General Mills Foundation Grants, 1590
GoGirlGo! Ambassador Team Awards, 1632
Guitar Center Music Foundation Grants, 1675
H.A. and Mary K. Chapman Charitable Trust Grants, 1681
Harry Kramer Memorial Fund Grants, 1705
IAFF Burn Foundation Research Grants, 1830
J.E. and L.E. Mabee Foundation Grants, 1875
John Merck Fund Grants, 1940
John Merck Scholars Awards, 1941
Johnson & Johnson Community Health Care Program Grants, 1951
Kimberly-Clark Community Grants, 2001
Multiple Sclerosis Foundation Brighter Tomorrow Grants, 2228
NEI Mentored Clinical Scientist Development Program Award (K12), 2295
NMF Franklin C. McLean Award, 2829
NMF General Electric Medical Scholars Fellowships, 2830
NMF Henry G. Halladay Awards, 2831
NMF Mary Ball Carrera Scholarship, 2834
NMF National Medical Association Awards for Medical Journalism, 2836
NMF National Medical Association Emerging Scholar Awards, 2837
NMF National Medical Association Patti LaBelle Award, 2838
NMF Need-Based Scholarships, 2839
NMF Ralph W. Ellison Prize, 2840
NMF William and Charlotte Cadbury Award, 2841
NSF Major Research Instrumentation Program (MRI) Grants, 2889
OneSight Research Foundation Block Grants, 2944
Pfizer/AAFP Foundation Visiting Professorship Program in Family Medicine, 3027
Piper Jaffray Companies Building Strong Communities Grants, 3053
Plum Creek Foundation Grants, 3062
Rosalinde and Arthur Gilbert Foundation/AFAR New Investigator Awards in Alzheimer's Disease, 3187
Roy and Christine Sturgis Trust Grants, 3191
Southwire Company Grants, 3353
Sunderland Foundation Grants, 3400
Tylenol Scholarship, 3444
U.S. Department of Education Erma Byrd Scholarships, 3446
U.S. Department of Education United States-Russia Program: Improving Research and Educational Activities in Higher Education, 3451
US CRDF Leishmaniasis: Collaborative Research Opportunities in North Africa and the Middle East, 3474
Vulcan Materials Company Foundation Grants, 3504
Wal-Mart Foundation Community Grants, 3513
Wal-Mart State Giving Program Grants, 3514

California

1st Touch Foundation Grants, 6
3M Company Health and Human Services Grants, 10
3M Foundation Grants, 11
49ers Foundation Grants, 12
A. Gary Anderson Family Foundation Grants, 17
A/H Foundation Grants, 19
Aaron Foundation (California) Grants, 173
Abbott Fund Access to Health Care Grants, 176
Abbott Fund Community Vitality Grants, 177
Abbott Fund Global AIDS Care Grants, 178
Abbott Fund Science and Medical Innovation Grants, 179
ACE Charitable Foundation Grants, 199
ACF Ethnic Community Self-Help Grants, 200
ACF Preferred Communities Grants, 201
ACF Standing Announcement for Unaccompanied Alien Children Grants, 202
ACF Supplemental Services for Recently Arrived Refugees Grants, 203

Actors Fund Social Services and Financial Assistance, 225
Adobe Community Investment Grants, 237
Advanced Micro Devices Community Affairs Grants, 239
AEGON Transamerica Foundation Grants, 243
Ahmanson Foundation Grants, 303
Albertson's Charitable Giving Grants, 330
Alice Tweed Tuohy Foundation Grants Program, 357
Alliance Healthcare Foundation Grants, 362
Alpine Winter Foundation Grants, 368
Amador Community Foundation Grants, 409
American College of Surgeons and The Triological Society Clinical Scientist Development Awards, 422
Angels Baseball Foundation Grants, 473
Anheuser-Busch Foundation Grants, 474
Ann Jackson Family Foundation Grants, 477
Ann Peppers Foundation Grants, 478
Annunziata Sanguinetti Foundation Grants, 481
Aratani Foundation Grants, 523
ARCO Foundation Education Grants, 526
Argyros Foundation Grants Program, 527
ASHA Advancing Academic-Research Careers (AARC) Award, 569
ASHA Minority Student Leadership Program Awards, 570
ASHA Multicultural Activities Projects Grants, 571
ASHA Research Mentoring-Pair Travel Award, 572
ASHA Student Research Travel Award, 573
ASHA Students Preparing for Academic & Research Careers (SPARC) Award, 574
ASM Millis-Colwell Postgraduate Travel Grant, 608
AT&T Excelerator, 657
Atkinson Foundation International Grants, 661
Audrey and Sydney Irmas Charitable Foundation Grants, 665
Bearemy's Kennel Pals Grants, 728
Bechtel Group Foundation Building Positive Community Relationships Grants, 731
Bella Vista Foundation Grants, 740
Ben B. Cheney Foundation Grants, 741
Bertha Russ Lytel Foundation Grants, 751
Biogen Corporate Giving Grants, 758
Blue Shield of California Grants, 771
Bob and Delores Hope Charitable Foundation Grants, 774
Bright Family Foundation Grants, 793
Burton G. Bettingen Grants, 813
C.R. Bard Foundation Grants, 825
Cable Positive's Tony Cox Community Fund Grants, 827
California Community Foundation Health Care Grants, 831
California Community Foundation Human Development Grants, 832
California Endowment CommunitiesFirst Grants, 833
California Wellness Foundation Work and Health Program Grants, 834
Callaway Golf Company Foundation Grants, 836
Carl Gellert and Celia Berta Gellert Foundation Grants, 871
Carlsbad Charitable Foundation Grants, 877
Carrie Estelle Doheny Foundation Grants, 883
CDC Cancer Prevention and Control Programs, 903
CDC Injury Control Research Centers Grants, 913
Champ-A Champion Fur Kids Grants, 959
CHCF Grants, 979
Children Affected by AIDS Foundation Camp Network Grants, 994
Children Affected by AIDS Foundation Family Assistance Emergency Fund Grants, 996
Chiles Foundation Grants, 1003
Chiron Foundation Community Grants, 1004
Chula Vista Charitable Foundation Grants, 1009
Clarence E. Heller Charitable Foundation Grants, 1022
Cleo Foundation Grants, 1035
CLIF Bar Family Foundation Grants, 1040
Coeta and Donald Barker Foundation Grants, 1054
Comerica Charitable Foundation Grants, 1073
Community Foundation for Monterey County Grants, 1092
Community Foundation of Santa Cruz County Grants, 1122
Community Foundation Silicon Valley Grants, 1133
Community Technology Foundation of California Building Communities Through Technology Grants, 1136
ConAgra Foods Foundation Grants, 1140
ConocoPhillips Foundation Grants, 1144
Crail-Johnson Foundation Grants, 1157
David Geffen Foundation Grants, 1202
Dean Foods Community Involvement Grants, 1209
Del E. Webb Foundation Grants, 1213
Della Martin Foundation Grants, 1219
Do Something BR!CK Awards, 1287
Dr. Stanley Pearle Scholarships, 1330
Dunspaugh-Dalton Foundation Grants, 1351
E.L. Wiegand Foundation Grants, 1361
eBay Foundation Community Grants, 1363
EDS Foundation Grants, 1371
EIF Community Grants, 1386
Eisner Foundation Grants, 1387
Fireman's Fund Foundation Grants, 1504
Fluor Foundation Grants, 1517
FMC Foundation Grants, 1518
Fritz B. Burns Foundation Grants, 1564
Gamble Foundation Grants, 1582
GenCorp Foundation Grants, 1587
Genentech Corporate Charitable Contributions Grants, 1588
General Mills Foundation Grants, 1590
George and Ruth Bradford Foundation Grants, 1595
George Frederick Jewett Foundation Grants Program, 1599
Glendale Community Foundation Grants, 1626
GoGirlGo! Ambassador Team Awards, 1632
Golden State Warriors Foundation Grants, 1633
Guitar Center Music Foundation Grants, 1675
Harden Foundation Grants, 1693
Harry and Grace Steele Foundation Grants, 1702
Harry Kramer Memorial Fund Grants, 1705
Healthcare Foundation for Orange County Grants, 1728
Hedco Foundation Grants, 1733
Horizons Community Issues Grants, 1794
Hormel Foods Charitable Trust Grants, 1795
Humboldt Area Foundation Technical Assistance Program (TAP) Grants, 1819
Huntington Beach Police Officers Foundation Grants, 1821
Hut Foundation Grants, 1827
Hutton Foundation Grants, 1828
IAFF Burn Foundation Research Grants, 1830
Ireland Family Foundation Grants, 1865
Isabel Allende Foundation Esperanza Grants, 1868
J.M. Long Foundation Grants, 1877
James S. Copley Foundation Grants, 1895
Jewish Community Foundation of Greater Los Angeles Grants, 1921
John Jewett and Helen Chandler Garland Foundation Grants, 1937
John Merck Fund Grants, 1940
John Merck Scholars Awards, 1941
John Stauffer Charitable Trust Grants, 1946
Johnson & Johnson Community Health Care Program Grants, 1951
Joseph Drown Foundation Grants, 1960
Josephine S. Gumbiner Foundation Grants, 1965
Kathryne Beynon Foundation Grants, 1984
Kenneth T. and Eileen L. Norris Foundation Grants, 1989
Kimberly-Clark Community Grants, 2001
Lowell Berry Foundation Grants, 2069
Lucile Horton Howe and Mitchell B. Howe Foundation Grants, 2081
Margoes Foundation Grants, 2106
Marriott Foundation for People with Disabilities Bridges Program Grants, 2113
Maxtor Corporate Contributions Grants, 2136
McCarthy Family Foundation Grants, 2141
Mericos Foundation Grants, 2172
Miriam and Peter Haas Fund Grants, 2208
Mount Zion Health Fund Grants, 2220
Multiple Sclerosis Foundation Brighter Tomorrow Grants, 2228
NEI Mentored Clinical Scientist Development Program Award (K12), 2295
NMF Franklin C. McLean Award, 2829
NMF General Electric Medical Scholars Fellowships, 2830
NMF Henry G. Halladay Awards, 2831
NMF Mary Ball Carrera Scholarship, 2834
NMF National Medical Association Awards for Medical Journalism, 2836
NMF National Medical Association Emerging Scholar Awards, 2837
NMF National Medical Association Patti LaBelle Award, 2838
NMF Need-Based Scholarships, 2839
NMF Ralph W. Ellison Prize, 2840
NMF William and Charlotte Cadbury Award, 2841
Nordson Corporation Foundation Grants, 2851
NSF Major Research Instrumentation Program (MRI) Grants, 2889
Oakland Fund for Children and Youth Grants, 2930
Oceanside Charitable Foundation Grants, 2934
OneSight Research Foundation Block Grants, 2944
PacifiCare Foundation Grants, 2981
PacifiCorp Foundation for Learning Grants, 2982
Pajaro Valley Community Health Grants, 2985
Pasadena Foundation Average Grants, 2994
Patron Saints Foundation Grants, 2996
Pfizer/AAFP Foundation Visiting Professorship Program in Family Medicine, 3027
Piper Jaffray Companies Building Strong Communities Grants, 3053
Prudential Foundation Grants, 3087
Quantum Corporation Snap Server Grants, 3095
Ralphs Food 4 Less Foundation Grants, 3106
Rathmann Family Foundation Grants, 3109
Richard and Rhoda Goldman Fund Grants, 3158
Rosalinde and Arthur Gilbert Foundation/AFAR New Investigator Awards in Alzheimer's Disease, 3187
S. Mark Taper Foundation Grants, 3236
S.H. Cowell Foundation Grants, 3237
San Diego Foundation Health & Human Services Grants, 3256
San Diego Foundation Paradise Valley Hospital Community Fund Grants, 3257
San Diego HIV Funding Collaborative (SDHFC) Grants, 3258
San Diego Women's Foundation Grants, 3259
San Francisco Foundation Community Health Grants, 3260
San Francisco Foundation Disability Rights Advocate Fund Emergency Grants, 3261
SHF Reach--Connecting Communities and Youth for a Healthy Future Grants, 3283
Simpson Fund Grants, 3290
Sisters of St. Joseph Healthcare Foundation Grants, 3297
Southwest Gas Corporation Foundation Grants, 3352
Steelcase Foundation Grants, 3379
Stephen Bechtel Fund Preventive Healthcare and Selected Research Grants, 3381
Taproot Foundation Capacity-Building Service Grants, 3417
Thelma Doelger Charitable Trust Grants, 3421
Thomas and Dorothy Leavey Foundation Grants, 3422
Thomas C. Ackerman Foundation Grants, 3423
Toro Foundation Grants, 3431
TRDRP California Research Awards, 3434

Tylenol Scholarship, 3444
U.S. Department of Education Erma Byrd Scholarships, 3446
U.S. Department of Education United States-Russia Program: Improving Research and Educational Activities in Higher Education, 3451
US CRDF Leishmaniasis: Collaborative Research Opportunities in North Africa and the Middle East, 3474
US Trust Corporation Foundation Grants, 3475
Vulcan Materials Company Foundation Grants, 3504
Waitt Family Foundation Grants, 3512
Wal-Mart Foundation Community Grants, 3513
Wal-Mart State Giving Program Grants, 3514
Walt Disney Company Foundation Grants, 3516
Wayne and Gladys Valley Foundation Grants, 3522
Weingart Foundation Grants, 3524
William G. Gilmore Foundation Grants, 3537
William G. McGowan Charitable Fund Grants, 3539
William H. Hannon Foundation Grants, 3540
Winifred & Harry B. Allen Foundation Grants, 3543
Women's Foundation of California Community Action Fund, 3549
Women's Foundation of California Grants, 3550
YSA UnitedHealth Heroes Service Learning Grants, 3556

Colorado
ACE Charitable Foundation Grants, 199
ACF Ethnic Community Self-Help Grants, 200
ACF Preferred Communities Grants, 201
ACF Standing Announcement for Unaccompanied Alien Children Grants, 202
ACF Supplemental Services for Recently Arrived Refugees Grants, 203
Actors Fund Social Services and Financial Assistance, 225
Adolph Coors Foundation Grants, 238
Advancing Colorado's Mental Health Care Project Grants, 240
AEC Trust Grants, 242
Albertson's Charitable Giving Grants, 330
Alexander Foundation Cancer, Catastrophic Illness and Injury Grants, 342
Alexander Foundation Insurance Continuation Grants, 343
American College of Surgeons and The Triological Society Clinical Scientist Development Awards, 422
Anheuser-Busch Foundation Grants, 474
Anschutz Family Foundation Grants, 486
Anthem Blue Cross and Blue Shield Grants, 488
ARCO Foundation Education Grants, 526
ASHA Advancing Academic-Research Careers (AARC) Award, 569
ASHA Minority Student Leadership Program Awards, 570
ASHA Multicultural Activities Projects Grants, 571
ASHA Research Mentoring-Pair Travel Award, 572
ASHA Student Research Travel Award, 573
ASHA Students Preparing for Academic & Research Careers (SPARC) Award, 574
ASM Millis-Colwell Postgraduate Travel Grant, 608
Bacon Family Foundation Grants, 679
Bearemy's Kennel Pals Grants, 728
Boettcher Foundation Grants, 778
Bonfils-Stanton Foundation Grants, 779
Bridgestone/Firestone Trust Fund Grants, 792
Cable Positive's Tony Cox Community Fund Grants, 827
Carl W. and Carrie Mae Joslyn Trust Grants, 873
Champ-A Champion Fur Kids Grants, 959
Charles A. Frueauff Foundation Grants, 962
Children Affected by AIDS Foundation Camp Network Grants, 994
Children Affected by AIDS Foundation Family Assistance Emergency Fund Grants, 996
CLIF Bar Family Foundation Grants, 1040
Colorado Interstate Gas Grants, 1060
Colorado Springs Community Trust Fund Grants, 1061
Colorado Trust Grants, 1062
Colorado Trust Partnerships for Health Initiative, 1063
Compass Bank Foundation Grants, 1138
ConAgra Foods Foundation Grants, 1140
Coors Brewing Corporate Contributions Grants, 1151
D.F. Halton Foundation Grants, 1181
Daniels Fund Grants, 1200
Dean Foods Community Involvement Grants, 1209
Denver Broncos Charities Fund Grants, 1226
Denver Foundation Community Grants, 1227
Do Something BR!CK Awards, 1287
Dr. Stanley Pearle Scholarships, 1330
EDS Foundation Grants, 1371
El Paso Corporate Foundation Grants, 1389
El Pomar Foundation Awards and Grants, 1390
Gill Foundation - Gay and Lesbian Fund Grants, 1613
GoGirlGo! Ambassador Team Awards, 1632
Griffin Foundation Grants, 1670
Guitar Center Music Foundation Grants, 1675
Harry Kramer Memorial Fund Grants, 1705
Helen K. and Arthur E. Johnson Foundation Grants, 1740
Hill Foundation Grants, 1774
Humana Foundation Grants, 1818
IAFF Burn Foundation Research Grants, 1830
Inasmuch Foundation Grants, 1845
John G. Duncan Trust Grants, 1931
John Merck Fund Grants, 1940
John Merck Scholars Awards, 1941
Johns Manville Fund Grants, 1950
Mabel Y. Hughes Charitable Trust Grants, 2097
Maxtor Corporate Contributions Grants, 2136
Monfort Family Foundation Grants, 2213
Multiple Sclerosis Foundation Brighter Tomorrow Grants, 2228
NEI Mentored Clinical Scientist Development Program Award (K12), 2295
NMF Franklin C. McLean Award, 2829
NMF General Electric Medical Scholars Fellowships, 2830
NMF Henry G. Halladay Awards, 2831
NMF Mary Ball Carrera Scholarship, 2834
NMF National Medical Association Awards for Medical Journalism, 2836
NMF National Medical Association Emerging Scholar Awards, 2837
NMF National Medical Association Patti LaBelle Award, 2838
NMF Need-Based Scholarships, 2839
NMF Ralph W. Ellison Prize, 2840
NMF William and Charlotte Cadbury Award, 2841
NSF Major Research Instrumentation Program (MRI) Grants, 2889
OneSight Research Foundation Block Grants, 2944
PacifiCare Foundation Grants, 2981
Pfizer/AAFP Foundation Visiting Professorship Program in Family Medicine, 3027
Piper Jaffray Companies Building Strong Communities Grants, 3053
Questar Corporate Contributions Grants, 3097
Rosalinde and Arthur Gilbert Foundation/AFAR New Investigator Awards in Alzheimer's Disease, 3187
Tylenol Scholarship, 3444
U.S. Department of Education Erma Byrd Scholarships, 3446
U.S. Department of Education United States-Russia Program: Improving Research and Educational Activities in Higher Education, 3451
US CRDF Leishmaniasis: Collaborative Research Opportunities in North Africa and the Middle East, 3474
Wal-Mart Foundation Community Grants, 3513
Wal-Mart State Giving Program Grants, 3514
Western Union Foundation Grants, 3529
William G. Gilmore Foundation Grants, 3537
YSA UnitedHealth Heroes Service Learning Grants, 3556

Connecticut
3M Company Health and Human Services Grants, 10
3M Foundation Grants, 11
Aaron Foundation (Massachusetts) Grants, 174
ACE Charitable Foundation Grants, 199
ACF Ethnic Community Self-Help Grants, 200
ACF Preferred Communities Grants, 201
ACF Standing Announcement for Unaccompanied Alien Children Grants, 202
ACF Supplemental Services for Recently Arrived Refugees Grants, 203
Actors Fund Social Services and Financial Assistance, 225
Aetna Foundation Health Grants in Connecticut, 244
Aetna Foundation Sponsorships Grants in Connecticut, 251
Ahn Family Foundation Grants, 304
American College of Surgeons and The Triological Society Clinical Scientist Development Awards, 422
Anthem Blue Cross and Blue Shield Grants, 488
ARS Foundation Grants, 538
ASHA Advancing Academic-Research Careers (AARC) Award, 569
ASHA Minority Student Leadership Program Awards, 570
ASHA Multicultural Activities Projects Grants, 571
ASHA Research Mentoring-Pair Travel Award, 572
ASHA Student Research Travel Award, 573
ASHA Students Preparing for Academic & Research Careers (SPARC) Award, 574
ASM Millis-Colwell Postgraduate Travel Grant, 608
AT&T Excelerator, 657
Barnes Group Foundation Grants, 696
Bearemy's Kennel Pals Grants, 728
BJ's Charitable Foundation Grants, 761
Bodenwein Public Benevolent Foundation Grants, 775
Bridgestone/Firestone Trust Fund Grants, 792
Bristol-Myers Squibb Foundation Health Disparities Grants, 797
Cable Positive's Tony Cox Community Fund Grants, 827
Carl J. Herzog Foundation Grants, 872
Carlisle Foundation Grants, 874
Carolyn Foundation Grants, 880
Carrier Corporation Contributions Grants, 884
Champ-A Champion Fur Kids Grants, 959
Charles A. Frueauff Foundation Grants, 962
Charles H. Hood Foundation Child Health Research Grants, 968
Children Affected by AIDS Foundation Camp Network Grants, 994
Children Affected by AIDS Foundation Family Assistance Emergency Fund Grants, 996
CLIF Bar Family Foundation Grants, 1040
Community Foundation for Greater New Haven Grants, 1091
Community Foundation of Greater New Britain Grants, 1111
Community Foundation of Southeastern Connecticut Grants, 1125
Connecticut Community Foundation Grants, 1141
Connecticut Health Foundation Health Initiative Grants, 1142
CSX Corporate Contributions Grants, 1169
Dammann Fund Grants, 1192
Daphne Seybolt Culpeper Memorial Foundation Grants, 1201
Dean Foods Community Involvement Grants, 1209
Do Something BR!CK Awards, 1287
Dominion Educational Partnership Grant, 1308
Dr. Stanley Pearle Scholarships, 1330
Edward S. Moore Foundation Grants, 1374

Ensworth Charitable Foundation Grants, 1416
Fairfield County Community Foundation Grants, 1446
Fisher Foundation Grants, 1508
Gladys Brooks Foundation Grants, 1620
GoGirlGo! Ambassador Team Awards, 1632
Greater Bridgeport Area Foundation Community Impact Grants, 1650
Guitar Center Music Foundation Grants, 1675
Hallmark Corporate Foundation Grants, 1688
Harry Kramer Memorial Fund Grants, 1705
Hartford Courant Foundation Grants, 1710
Hartford Foundation Regular Grants, 1711
IAFF Burn Foundation Research Grants, 1830
J. Walton Bissell Foundation Grants, 1872
Jessie B. Cox Charitable Trust Grants, 1918
John G. Martin Foundation Grants, 1932
John Merck Fund Grants, 1940
John Merck Scholars Awards, 1941
Katharine Matthies Foundation Grants, 1982
Kimberly-Clark Community Grants, 2001
Lincoln Financial Group Foundation Grants, 2058
Meriden Foundation Grants, 2173
Multiple Sclerosis Foundation Brighter Tomorrow Grants, 2228
NEI Mentored Clinical Scientist Development Program Award (K12), 2295
NMF Franklin C. McLean Award, 2829
NMF General Electric Medical Scholars Fellowships, 2830
NMF Henry G. Halladay Awards, 2831
NMF Mary Ball Carrera Scholarship, 2834
NMF National Medical Association Awards for Medical Journalism, 2836
NMF National Medical Association Emerging Scholar Awards, 2837
NMF National Medical Association Patti LaBelle Award, 2838
NMF Need-Based Scholarships, 2839
NMF Ralph W. Ellison Prize, 2840
NMF William and Charlotte Cadbury Award, 2841
Northeast Utilities Foundation Grants, 2863
NSF Major Research Instrumentation Program (MRI) Grants, 2889
OneSight Research Foundation Block Grants, 2944
Pfizer/AAFP Foundation Visiting Professorship Program in Family Medicine, 3027
Rosalinde and Arthur Gilbert Foundation/AFAR New Investigator Awards in Alzheimer's Disease, 3187
Sasco Foundation Grants, 3265
Shaw's Supermarkets Donations, 3280
Southbury Community Trust Fund, 3350
TWS Foundation Grants, 3443
Tylenol Scholarship, 3444
U.S. Department of Education Erma Byrd Scholarships, 3446
U.S. Department of Education United States-Russia Program: Improving Research and Educational Activities in Higher Education, 3451
US CRDF Leishmaniasis: Collaborative Research Opportunities in North Africa and the Middle East, 3474
US Trust Corporation Foundation Grants, 3475
Wal-Mart Foundation Community Grants, 3513
Wal-Mart State Giving Program Grants, 3514

Delaware

ACE Charitable Foundation Grants, 199
ACF Ethnic Community Self-Help Grants, 200
ACF Preferred Communities Grants, 201
ACF Standing Announcement for Unaccompanied Alien Children Grants, 202
ACF Supplemental Services for Recently Arrived Refugees Grants, 203
Actors Fund Social Services and Financial Assistance, 225
Albertson's Charitable Giving Grants, 330
American College of Surgeons and The Triological Society Clinical Scientist Development Awards, 422
ASHA Advancing Academic-Research Careers (AARC) Award, 569
ASHA Minority Student Leadership Program Awards, 570
ASHA Multicultural Activities Projects Grants, 571
ASHA Research Mentoring-Pair Travel Award, 572
ASHA Student Research Travel Award, 573
ASHA Students Preparing for Academic & Research Careers (SPARC) Award, 574
ASM Millis-Colwell Postgraduate Travel Grant, 608
Bearemy's Kennel Pals Grants, 728
BJ's Charitable Foundation Grants, 761
Borkee-Hagley Foundation Grants, 781
Brook J. Lenfest Foundation Grants, 804
Cable Positive's Tony Cox Community Fund Grants, 827
CDC Injury Control Research Centers Grants, 913
Champ-A Champion Fur Kids Grants, 959
Charles A. Frueauff Foundation Grants, 962
Children Affected by AIDS Foundation Camp Network Grants, 994
Children Affected by AIDS Foundation Family Assistance Emergency Fund Grants, 996
CLIF Bar Family Foundation Grants, 1040
Crestlea Foundation Grants, 1159
CSX Corporate Contributions Grants, 1169
Delaware Community Foundation Grants, 1215
Delaware Community Foundation-Youth Philanthropy Board for Kent County, 1216
DHHS Healthy Tomorrows Partnership for Children, 1261
Do Something BR!CK Awards, 1287
Dr. Stanley Pearle Scholarships, 1330
FMC Foundation Grants, 1518
Gladys Brooks Foundation Grants, 1620
GoGirlGo! Ambassador Team Awards, 1632
Guitar Center Music Foundation Grants, 1675
Harry Kramer Memorial Fund Grants, 1705
IAFF Burn Foundation Research Grants, 1830
John Merck Fund Grants, 1940
John Merck Scholars Awards, 1941
Multiple Sclerosis Foundation Brighter Tomorrow Grants, 2228
NEI Mentored Clinical Scientist Development Program Award (K12), 2295
NMF Franklin C. McLean Award, 2829
NMF General Electric Medical Scholars Fellowships, 2830
NMF Henry G. Halladay Awards, 2831
NMF Mary Ball Carrera Scholarship, 2834
NMF National Medical Association Awards for Medical Journalism, 2836
NMF National Medical Association Emerging Scholar Awards, 2837
NMF National Medical Association Patti LaBelle Award, 2838
NMF Need-Based Scholarships, 2839
NMF Ralph W. Ellison Prize, 2840
NMF William and Charlotte Cadbury Award, 2841
NSF Major Research Instrumentation Program (MRI) Grants, 2889
OneSight Research Foundation Block Grants, 2944
Pfizer/AAFP Foundation Visiting Professorship Program in Family Medicine, 3027
PNC Charitable Trust and Foundation Grants, 3064
Principal Financial Group Foundation Grants, 3082
Rosalinde and Arthur Gilbert Foundation/AFAR New Investigator Awards in Alzheimer's Disease, 3187
Tylenol Scholarship, 3444
U.S. Department of Education Erma Byrd Scholarships, 3446
U.S. Department of Education United States-Russia Program: Improving Research and Educational Activities in Higher Education, 3451
US CRDF Leishmaniasis: Collaborative Research Opportunities in North Africa and the Middle East, 3474
US Trust Corporation Foundation Grants, 3475
Wal-Mart Foundation Community Grants, 3513
Wal-Mart State Giving Program Grants, 3514

District of Columbia

Aaron & Cecile Goldman Family Foundation Grants, 171
ACE Charitable Foundation Grants, 199
ACF Ethnic Community Self-Help Grants, 200
ACF Preferred Communities Grants, 201
ACF Standing Announcement for Unaccompanied Alien Children Grants, 202
ACF Supplemental Services for Recently Arrived Refugees Grants, 203
Actors Fund Social Services and Financial Assistance, 225
Alexander and Margaret Stewart Trust Grants, 340
American College of Surgeons and The Triological Society Clinical Scientist Development Awards, 422
ASHA Advancing Academic-Research Careers (AARC) Award, 569
ASHA Minority Student Leadership Program Awards, 570
ASHA Multicultural Activities Projects Grants, 571
ASHA Research Mentoring-Pair Travel Award, 572
ASHA Student Research Travel Award, 573
ASHA Students Preparing for Academic & Research Careers (SPARC) Award, 574
ASM Millis-Colwell Postgraduate Travel Grant, 608
Bearemy's Kennel Pals Grants, 728
Bender Foundation Grants, 742
Cable Positive's Tony Cox Community Fund Grants, 827
CDC Injury Control Research Centers Grants, 913
Champ-A Champion Fur Kids Grants, 959
CharityWorks Grants, 961
Charles A. Frueauff Foundation Grants, 962
Charles Delmar Foundation Grants, 963
Children Affected by AIDS Foundation Camp Network Grants, 994
Children Affected by AIDS Foundation Family Assistance Emergency Fund Grants, 996
Clark-Winchcole Foundation Grants, 1030
CLIF Bar Family Foundation Grants, 1040
Commonweal Foundation Community Assistance Grants, 1075
Commonweal Foundation Grants, 1076
Do Something BR!CK Awards, 1287
Dr. Stanley Pearle Scholarships, 1330
E.L. Wiegand Foundation Grants, 1361
Eugene and Agnes E. Meyer Foundation Grants, 1432
Eugene B. Casey Foundation Grants, 1433
Freddie Mac Foundation Grants, 1558
Genesis Foundation Grants, 1593
Ginn Foundation Grants, 1616
GoGirlGo! Ambassador Team Awards, 1632
Guitar Center Music Foundation Grants, 1675
Harry Kramer Memorial Fund Grants, 1705
IAFF Burn Foundation Research Grants, 1830
John Edward Fowler Memorial Foundation Grants, 1930
John Merck Fund Grants, 1940
John Merck Scholars Awards, 1941
Leonsis Foundation Grants, 2045
Mabel H. Flory Charitable Trust Grants, 2096
Marriott Foundation for People with Disabilities Bridges Program Grants, 2113
Morris and Gwendolyn Cafritz Foundation Grants, 2217
Multiple Sclerosis Foundation Brighter Tomorrow Grants, 2228
NEI Mentored Clinical Scientist Development Program Award (K12), 2295
NMF Franklin C. McLean Award, 2829

NMF General Electric Medical Scholars Fellowships, 2830
NMF Henry G. Halladay Awards, 2831
NMF Mary Ball Carrera Scholarship, 2834
NMF National Medical Association Awards for Medical Journalism, 2836
NMF National Medical Association Emerging Scholar Awards, 2837
NMF National Medical Association Patti LaBelle Award, 2838
NMF Need-Based Scholarships, 2839
NMF Ralph W. Ellison Prize, 2840
NMF William and Charlotte Cadbury Award, 2841
NSF Major Research Instrumentation Program (MRI) Grants, 2889
OneSight Research Foundation Block Grants, 2944
Pfizer/AAFP Foundation Visiting Professorship Program in Family Medicine, 3027
Prince Charitable Trusts District of Columbia Grants, 3080
Quality Health Foundation Grants, 3094
Rosalinde and Arthur Gilbert Foundation/AFAR New Investigator Awards in Alzheimer's Disease, 3187
Tylenol Scholarship, 3444
U.S. Department of Education Erma Byrd Scholarships, 3446
U.S. Department of Education Rehabilitation Training--Rehabilitation Continuing Education Programs (RCEP)--Institute on Rehabilitation Issues (IRI), 3449
U.S. Department of Education United States-Russia Program: Improving Research and Educational Activities in Higher Education, 3451
US Airways Community Contributions, 3472
US CRDF Leishmaniasis: Collaborative Research Opportunities in North Africa and the Middle East, 3474
US Trust Corporation Foundation Grants, 3475
Wal-Mart Foundation Community Grants, 3513
Wal-Mart State Giving Program Grants, 3514
William G. McGowan Charitable Fund Grants, 3539
Winifred & Harry B. Allen Foundation Grants, 3543

Florida

A Friend's Foundation Trust Grants, 13
Able Trust Vocational Rehabilitation Grants for Individuals, 186
ACE Charitable Foundation Grants, 199
ACF Ethnic Community Self-Help Grants, 200
ACF Preferred Communities Grants, 201
ACF Standing Announcement for Unaccompanied Alien Children Grants, 202
ACF Supplemental Services for Recently Arrived Refugees Grants, 203
Actors Fund Social Services and Financial Assistance, 225
AEC Trust Grants, 242
Albertson's Charitable Giving Grants, 330
American College of Surgeons and The Triological Society Clinical Scientist Development Awards, 422
Anheuser-Busch Foundation Grants, 474
ASHA Advancing Academic-Research Careers (AARC) Award, 569
ASHA Minority Student Leadership Program Awards, 570
ASHA Multicultural Activities Projects Grants, 571
ASHA Research Mentoring-Pair Travel Award, 572
ASHA Student Research Travel Award, 573
ASHA Students Preparing for Academic & Research Careers (SPARC) Award, 574
ASM Millis-Colwell Postgraduate Travel Grant, 608
AT&T Excelerator, 657
Bank of America Client Foundation Grants, 690
Batchelor Foundation Grants, 701
Bearemy's Kennel Pals Grants, 728
Beldon Fund Grants, 738
Belk Foundation Grants, 739
Bert W. Martin Foundation Grants, 750
BJ's Charitable Foundation Grants, 761
Bridgestone/Firestone Trust Fund Grants, 792
Bruce and Adele Greenfield Foundation Grants, 808
Cable Positive's Tony Cox Community Fund Grants, 827
Camp-Younts Foundation Grants, 838
CDC Cancer Prevention and Control Programs, 903
CDC Injury Control Research Centers Grants, 913
Champ-A Champion Fur Kids Grants, 959
Charles A. Frueauff Foundation Grants, 962
Charlotte County (FL) Community Foundation Grants, 973
Chase Paymentech Corporate Giving Grants, 975
Children Affected by AIDS Foundation Camp Network Grants, 994
Children Affected by AIDS Foundation Family Assistance Emergency Fund Grants, 996
CLIF Bar Family Foundation Grants, 1040
Comerica Charitable Foundation Grants, 1073
Community Foundation of Broward Grants, 1100
Community Foundation of Greater Tampa Grants, 1112
Community Foundation of Tampa Bay Grants, 1128
Compass Bank Foundation Grants, 1138
Cowles Charitable Trust Grants, 1155
CSX Corporate Contributions Grants, 1169
D. W. McMillan Foundation Grants, 1180
Dade Community Foundation Community AIDS Partnership Grants, 1184
Dade Community Foundation Grants, 1185
Daphne Seybolt Culpeper Memorial Foundation Grants, 1201
Dean Foods Community Involvement Grants, 1209
DHHS Healthy Tomorrows Partnership for Children, 1261
Do Something BR!CK Awards, 1287
Dr. John T. Macdonald Foundation Grants, 1327
Dr. Stanley Pearle Scholarships, 1330
Dunspaugh-Dalton Foundation Grants, 1351
Edyth Bush Charitable Foundation Grants, 1378
Elizabeth McGraw Foundation Grants, 1399
Fifth Third Foundation Grants, 1501
Florida BRAIVE Fund of Dade Community Foundation, 1512
Florida BRAIVE Fund of Gulf Coast Community Foundation of Venice, 1513
Florida BRAIVE Fund of The Community Foundation in Jacksonville, 1514
Florida High School/High Tech Project Grants, 1515
FMC Foundation Grants, 1518
Forrest C. Lattner Foundation Grants, 1523
Genesis Foundation Grants, 1593
Gladys Brooks Foundation Grants, 1620
Glazer Family Foundation Grants, 1625
GoGirlGo! Ambassador Team Awards, 1632
Gregory Family Foundation Grants (Florida), 1667
Guitar Center Music Foundation Grants, 1675
Gulf Coast Community of Venice Foundation Grants, 1677
Harold Alfond Foundation Grants, 1695
Harry Kramer Memorial Fund Grants, 1705
Harry Sudakoff Foundation Grants, 1708
Health Foundation of Southern Florida Responsive Grants, 1726
HomeBanc Foundation Grants, 1788
Honeywell Foundation Grants, 1791
Humana Foundation Grants, 1818
IAFF Burn Foundation Research Grants, 1830
Jane's Trust Grants, 1904
Jim Moran Foundation Grants, 1925
John Lord Knight Foundation Grants, 1938
John Merck Fund Grants, 1940
John Merck Scholars Awards, 1941
Johnson & Johnson Community Health Care Program Grants, 1951
Joseph H. and Florence A. Roblee Foundation Grants, 1961
L. W. Pierce Family Foundation Grants, 2019
Leo Goodwin Foundation Grants, 2043
Lettie Pate Whitehead Foundation Grants, 2049
Lillian S. Wells Foundation Grants, 2056
Lucy Gooding Charitable Foundation Trust, 2082
Lucy Gooding Charitable Foundation Trust Grants, 2083
M.B. and Edna Zale Foundation Grants, 2093
Marion Park Deaver and Harry Gilbert Deaver Foundation Grants, 2110
Multiple Sclerosis Foundation Brighter Tomorrow Grants, 2228
NEI Mentored Clinical Scientist Development Program Award (K12), 2295
NMF Franklin C. McLean Award, 2829
NMF General Electric Medical Scholars Fellowships, 2830
NMF Henry G. Halladay Awards, 2831
NMF Mary Ball Carrera Scholarship, 2834
NMF National Medical Association Awards for Medical Journalism, 2836
NMF National Medical Association Emerging Scholar Awards, 2837
NMF National Medical Association Patti LaBelle Award, 2838
NMF Need-Based Scholarships, 2839
NMF Ralph W. Ellison Prize, 2840
NMF William and Charlotte Cadbury Award, 2841
NSF Major Research Instrumentation Program (MRI) Grants, 2889
OneSight Research Foundation Block Grants, 2944
Palm Beach and Martin Counties Grants, 2986
Paul E. and Klare N. Reinhold Foundation Grants, 2999
Peacock Foundation Grants, 3011
Pfizer/AAFP Foundation Visiting Professorship Program in Family Medicine, 3027
Pinellas County Grants, 3050
Plum Creek Foundation Grants, 3062
Progress Energy Foundation Grants, 3084
Prudential Foundation Grants, 3087
Quantum Foundation Grants, 3096
Rainbow Fund Grants, 3103
Rayonier Foundation Grants, 3111
Richard and Helen DeVos Foundation Grants, 3157
Rosalinde and Arthur Gilbert Foundation/AFAR New Investigator Awards in Alzheimer's Disease, 3187
RRF General Program Grants, 3193
Salem Foundation Grants, 3242
Sarasota Memorial Healthcare Foundation Grants, 3264
Southwest Florida Community Foundation Competitive Grants, 3351
Sunshine Natural Wellbeing Foundation Grants, 3404
Thomas M. and Irene B. Kirbo Charitable Trust Grants, 3424
Tylenol Scholarship, 3444
U.S. Department of Education Erma Byrd Scholarships, 3446
U.S. Department of Education United States-Russia Program: Improving Research and Educational Activities in Higher Education, 3451
US CRDF Leishmaniasis: Collaborative Research Opportunities in North Africa and the Middle East, 3474
US Trust Corporation Foundation Grants, 3475
Vulcan Materials Company Foundation Grants, 3504
Wal-Mart Foundation Community Grants, 3513
Wal-Mart State Giving Program Grants, 3514
Walt Disney Company Foundation Grants, 3516
Wasie Foundation Grants, 3521
Western Union Foundation Grants, 3529
Wilson-Wood Foundation Grants, 3542
Woodward Fund Grants, 3552
YSA UnitedHealth Heroes Service Learning Grants, 3556

Georgia
3M Company Health and Human Services Grants, 10
3M Foundation Grants, 11
ACE Charitable Foundation Grants, 199
ACF Ethnic Community Self-Help Grants, 200
ACF Preferred Communities Grants, 201
ACF Standing Announcement for Unaccompanied Alien Children Grants, 202
ACF Supplemental Services for Recently Arrived Refugees Grants, 203
Actors Fund Social Services and Financial Assistance, 225
AEC Trust Grants, 242
AEGON Transamerica Foundation Grants, 243
Agnes B. Hunt Trust Grants, 261
Albertson's Charitable Giving Grants, 330
American College of Surgeons and The Triological Society Clinical Scientist Development Awards, 422
Anheuser-Busch Foundation Grants, 474
ASHA Advancing Academic-Research Careers (AARC) Award, 569
ASHA Minority Student Leadership Program Awards, 570
ASHA Multicultural Activities Projects Grants, 571
ASHA Research Mentoring-Pair Travel Award, 572
ASHA Student Research Travel Award, 573
ASHA Students Preparing for Academic & Research Careers (SPARC) Award, 574
ASM Millis-Colwell Postgraduate Travel Grant, 608
AT&T Excelerator, 657
Atlanta Foundation Grants, 662
Bearemy's Kennel Pals Grants, 728
Belk Foundation Grants, 739
BJ's Charitable Foundation Grants, 761
Bradley Turner Foundation Grants, 789
Brian G. Dyson Foundation Grants, 791
Cable Positive's Tony Cox Community Fund Grants, 827
Callaway Foundation Grants, 835
Camp-Younts Foundation Grants, 838
Carlos and Marguerite Mason Trust Grants, 875
Carrier Corporation Contributions Grants, 884
CDC Injury Control Research Centers Grants, 913
Champ-A Champion Fur Kids Grants, 959
Charles A. Frueauff Foundation Grants, 962
Children Affected by AIDS Foundation Camp Network Grants, 994
Children Affected by AIDS Foundation Family Assistance Emergency Fund Grants, 996
CLIF Bar Family Foundation Grants, 1040
Cooper Industries Foundation Grants, 1150
CSRA Community Foundation Grants, 1168
CSX Corporate Contributions Grants, 1169
Dean Foods Community Involvement Grants, 1209
DHHS Healthy Tomorrows Partnership for Children, 1261
Do Something BR!CK Awards, 1287
Dr. Stanley Pearle Scholarships, 1330
E.J. Grassmann Trust Grants, 1360
EDS Foundation Grants, 1371
Forrest C. Lattner Foundation Grants, 1523
Francis L. Abreu Charitable Trust Grants, 1549
Fraser-Parker Foundation Grants, 1555
Fuller E. Callaway Foundation Grants, 1578
General Mills Foundation Grants, 1590
Georgia Power Foundation Grants, 1603
Gertrude and William C. Wardlaw Fund Grants, 1607
GoGirlGo! Ambassador Team Awards, 1632
Guitar Center Music Foundation Grants, 1675
Hallmark Corporate Foundation Grants, 1688
Harry Kramer Memorial Fund Grants, 1705
HomeBanc Foundation Grants, 1788
Hormel Foods Charitable Trust Grants, 1795
Humana Foundation Grants, 1818
IAFF Burn Foundation Research Grants, 1830
Ida Alice Ryan Charitable Trust Grants, 1836
James J. and Angelia M. Harris Foundation Grants, 1890
John Deere Foundation Grants, 1929
John H. and Wilhelmina D. Harland Charitable Foundation Grants, 1933
John Merck Fund Grants, 1940
John Merck Scholars Awards, 1941
Katherine John Murphy Foundation Grants, 1983
Kimberly-Clark Community Grants, 2001
Lettie Pate Whitehead Foundation Grants, 2049
Marriott Foundation for People with Disabilities Bridges Program Grants, 2113
Multiple Sclerosis Foundation Brighter Tomorrow Grants, 2228
National Starch and Chemical Foundation Grants, 2261
NEI Mentored Clinical Scientist Development Program Award (K12), 2295
NMF Franklin C. McLean Award, 2829
NMF General Electric Medical Scholars Fellowships, 2830
NMF Henry G. Halladay Awards, 2831
NMF Mary Ball Carrera Scholarship, 2834
NMF National Medical Association Awards for Medical Journalism, 2836
NMF National Medical Association Emerging Scholar Awards, 2837
NMF National Medical Association Patti LaBelle Award, 2838
NMF Need-Based Scholarships, 2839
NMF Ralph W. Ellison Prize, 2840
NMF William and Charlotte Cadbury Award, 2841
Nordson Corporation Foundation Grants, 2851
North Georgia Community Foundation Grants, 2862
NSF Major Research Instrumentation Program (MRI) Grants, 2889
OneSight Research Foundation Block Grants, 2944
Pfizer/AAFP Foundation Visiting Professorship Program in Family Medicine, 3027
Plum Creek Foundation Grants, 3062
Prudential Foundation Grants, 3087
Rainbow Fund Grants, 3103
Rayonier Foundation Grants, 3111
Rich Foundation Grants, 3156
Robert and Polly Dunn Foundation Grants, 3168
Rosalinde and Arthur Gilbert Foundation/AFAR New Investigator Awards in Alzheimer's Disease, 3187
Rosalynn Carter Institute Georgia Caregiver of the Year Awards, 3188
Southwire Company Grants, 3353
Steele-Reese Foundation Grants, 3380
Stewart Huston Charitable Trust Grants, 3384
Thomas M. and Irene B. Kirbo Charitable Trust Grants, 3424
Tylenol Scholarship, 3444
U.S. Department of Education Erma Byrd Scholarships, 3446
U.S. Department of Education United States-Russia Program: Improving Research and Educational Activities in Higher Education, 3451
US CRDF Leishmaniasis: Collaborative Research Opportunities in North Africa and the Middle East, 3474
Vulcan Materials Company Foundation Grants, 3504
Wal-Mart Foundation Community Grants, 3513
Wal-Mart State Giving Program Grants, 3514
Winifred & Harry B. Allen Foundation Grants, 3543
Woodward Fund Grants, 3552

Guam
ACF Ethnic Community Self-Help Grants, 200
ACF Preferred Communities Grants, 201
ACF Standing Announcement for Unaccompanied Alien Children Grants, 202
ACF Supplemental Services for Recently Arrived Refugees Grants, 203
American College of Surgeons and The Triological Society Clinical Scientist Development Awards, 422
ASHA Advancing Academic-Research Careers (AARC) Award, 569
ASHA Minority Student Leadership Program Awards, 570
ASHA Multicultural Activities Projects Grants, 571
ASHA Research Mentoring-Pair Travel Award, 572
ASHA Student Research Travel Award, 573
ASHA Students Preparing for Academic & Research Careers (SPARC) Award, 574
Bearemy's Kennel Pals Grants, 728
Champ-A Champion Fur Kids Grants, 959
CLIF Bar Family Foundation Grants, 1040
GoGirlGo! Ambassador Team Awards, 1632
Harry Kramer Memorial Fund Grants, 1705
John Merck Scholars Awards, 1941
NEI Mentored Clinical Scientist Development Program Award (K12), 2295
NSF Major Research Instrumentation Program (MRI) Grants, 2889
Rosalinde and Arthur Gilbert Foundation/AFAR New Investigator Awards in Alzheimer's Disease, 3187
U.S. Department of Education Erma Byrd Scholarships, 3446
U.S. Department of Education United States-Russia Program: Improving Research and Educational Activities in Higher Education, 3451
US CRDF Leishmaniasis: Collaborative Research Opportunities in North Africa and the Middle East, 3474

Hawaii
3M Company Health and Human Services Grants, 10
3M Foundation Grants, 11
ACE Charitable Foundation Grants, 199
ACF Ethnic Community Self-Help Grants, 200
ACF Preferred Communities Grants, 201
ACF Standing Announcement for Unaccompanied Alien Children Grants, 202
ACF Supplemental Services for Recently Arrived Refugees Grants, 203
Actors Fund Social Services and Financial Assistance, 225
Alexander & Baldwin Foundation Hawaiian and Pacific Island Grants, 338
American College of Surgeons and The Triological Society Clinical Scientist Development Awards, 422
Annie Sinclair Knudsen Memorial Fund/Kaua'i Community Grants Program, 480
ASHA Advancing Academic-Research Careers (AARC) Award, 569
ASHA Minority Student Leadership Program Awards, 570
ASHA Multicultural Activities Projects Grants, 571
ASHA Research Mentoring-Pair Travel Award, 572
ASHA Student Research Travel Award, 573
ASHA Students Preparing for Academic & Research Careers (SPARC) Award, 574
ASM Millis-Colwell Postgraduate Travel Grant, 608
Atherton Family Foundation Grants, 659
Bearemy's Kennel Pals Grants, 728
Boyd Gaming Corporation Contributions Program, 788
Cable Positive's Tony Cox Community Fund Grants, 827
CDC Injury Control Research Centers Grants, 913
Champ-A Champion Fur Kids Grants, 959
Children Affected by AIDS Foundation Camp Network Grants, 994
Children Affected by AIDS Foundation Family Assistance Emergency Fund Grants, 996
CLIF Bar Family Foundation Grants, 1040
Cooke Foundation Grants, 1148
Dean Foods Community Involvement Grants, 1209
DHHS Healthy Tomorrows Partnership for Children, 1261
Do Something BR!CK Awards, 1287
Dr. Stanley Pearle Scholarships, 1330
Fred Baldwin Memorial Foundation Grants, 1556

G.N. Wilcox Trust Grants, 1581
GoGirlGo! Ambassador Team Awards, 1632
Guitar Center Music Foundation Grants, 1675
Harry Kramer Memorial Fund Grants, 1705
Hawaii Community Foundation Health Education and Research Grants, 1716
Hawaii Community Foundation Reverend Takie Okumura Family Grants, 1717
Hawaii Community Foundation West Hawaii Fund Grants, 1718
Hershey Company Grants, 1754
IAFF Burn Foundation Research Grants, 1830
J.M. Long Foundation Grants, 1877
John Merck Fund Grants, 1940
John Merck Scholars Awards, 1941
Julia Temple Davis Brown Foundation Grants, 1971
Kahuku Community Fund, 1977
Leahi Fund, 2038
McInerny Foundation Grants, 2144
Multiple Sclerosis Foundation Brighter Tomorrow Grants, 2228
NEI Mentored Clinical Scientist Development Program Award (K12), 2295
NMF Franklin C. McLean Award, 2829
NMF General Electric Medical Scholars Fellowships, 2830
NMF Henry G. Halladay Awards, 2831
NMF Mary Ball Carrera Scholarship, 2834
NMF National Medical Association Awards for Medical Journalism, 2836
NMF National Medical Association Emerging Scholar Awards, 2837
NMF National Medical Association Patti LaBelle Award, 2838
NMF Need-Based Scholarships, 2839
NMF Ralph W. Ellison Prize, 2840
NMF William and Charlotte Cadbury Award, 2841
NSF Major Research Instrumentation Program (MRI) Grants, 2889
OneSight Research Foundation Block Grants, 2944
Pfizer/AAFP Foundation Visiting Professorship Program in Family Medicine, 3027
Rosalinde and Arthur Gilbert Foundation/AFAR New Investigator Awards in Alzheimer's Disease, 3187
Tylenol Scholarship, 3444
U.S. Department of Education Erma Byrd Scholarships, 3446
U.S. Department of Education United States-Russia Program: Improving Research and Educational Activities in Higher Education, 3451
US CRDF Leishmaniasis: Collaborative Research Opportunities in North Africa and the Middle East, 3474
Wal-Mart Foundation Community Grants, 3513
Wal-Mart State Giving Program Grants, 3514

Idaho

ACF Ethnic Community Self-Help Grants, 200
ACF Preferred Communities Grants, 201
ACF Standing Announcement for Unaccompanied Alien Children Grants, 202
ACF Supplemental Services for Recently Arrived Refugees Grants, 203
Actors Fund Social Services and Financial Assistance, 225
Albertson's Charitable Giving Grants, 330
American College of Surgeons and The Triological Society Clinical Scientist Development Awards, 422
ASHA Advancing Academic-Research Careers (AARC) Award, 569
ASHA Minority Student Leadership Program Awards, 570
ASHA Multicultural Activities Projects Grants, 571
ASHA Research Mentoring-Pair Travel Award, 572
ASHA Student Research Travel Award, 573
ASHA Students Preparing for Academic & Research Careers (SPARC) Award, 574
ASM Millis-Colwell Postgraduate Travel Grant, 608
Bearemy's Kennel Pals Grants, 728
Bullitt Foundation Grants, 809
Cable Positive's Tony Cox Community Fund Grants, 827
CDC Injury Control Research Centers Grants, 913
Champ-A Champion Fur Kids Grants, 959
Children Affected by AIDS Foundation Camp Network Grants, 994
Children Affected by AIDS Foundation Family Assistance Emergency Fund Grants, 996
CLIF Bar Family Foundation Grants, 1040
Dean Foods Community Involvement Grants, 1209
Dell Foundation Open Grants, 1218
DHHS Healthy Tomorrows Partnership for Children, 1261
Do Something BR!CK Awards, 1287
Dr. Stanley Pearle Scholarships, 1330
E.L. Wiegand Foundation Grants, 1361
Foster Foundation Grants, 1524
Foundation Northwest Grants, 1537
GoGirlGo! Ambassador Team Awards, 1632
Guitar Center Music Foundation Grants, 1675
Harry Kramer Memorial Fund Grants, 1705
IAFF Burn Foundation Research Grants, 1830
Idaho Community Foundation Eastern Region Competitive Grants, 1837
Idaho Power Company Corporate Contributions, 1838
John Merck Fund Grants, 1940
John Merck Scholars Awards, 1941
Kimberly-Clark Community Grants, 2001
M.J. Murdock Charitable Trust Grants, 2095
Multiple Sclerosis Foundation Brighter Tomorrow Grants, 2228
NEI Mentored Clinical Scientist Development Program Award (K12), 2295
NMF Franklin C. McLean Award, 2829
NMF General Electric Medical Scholars Fellowships, 2830
NMF Henry G. Halladay Awards, 2831
NMF Mary Ball Carrera Scholarship, 2834
NMF National Medical Association Awards for Medical Journalism, 2836
NMF National Medical Association Emerging Scholar Awards, 2837
NMF National Medical Association Patti LaBelle Award, 2838
NMF Need-Based Scholarships, 2839
NMF Ralph W. Ellison Prize, 2840
NMF William and Charlotte Cadbury Award, 2841
NSF Major Research Instrumentation Program (MRI) Grants, 2889
OneSight Research Foundation Block Grants, 2944
PacifiCorp Foundation for Learning Grants, 2982
Paul G. Allen Family Foundation Grants, 3000
Pfizer/AAFP Foundation Visiting Professorship Program in Family Medicine, 3027
Piper Jaffray Companies Building Strong Communities Grants, 3053
Plum Creek Foundation Grants, 3062
Pride Foundation Grants and Scholarships, 3078
Regence Foundation Access to Health Care Grants, 3138
Regence Foundation Health Care Community Awareness and Engagement Grants, 3139
Regence Foundation Health Care Connections Grants, 3140
Regence Foundation Improving End-of-Life Grants, 3141
Regence Foundation Tools and Technology Grants, 3142
Rosalinde and Arthur Gilbert Foundation/AFAR New Investigator Awards in Alzheimer's Disease, 3187
Steele-Reese Foundation Grants, 3380
Sunderland Foundation Grants, 3400
Tylenol Scholarship, 3444
U.S. Department of Education Erma Byrd Scholarships, 3446
U.S. Department of Education United States-Russia Program: Improving Research and Educational Activities in Higher Education, 3451
US CRDF Leishmaniasis: Collaborative Research Opportunities in North Africa and the Middle East, 3474
Wal-Mart Foundation Community Grants, 3513
Wal-Mart State Giving Program Grants, 3514

Illinois

3M Company Health and Human Services Grants, 10
3M Foundation Grants, 11
Abbott Fund Access to Health Care Grants, 176
Abbott Fund Community Vitality Grants, 177
Abbott Fund Global AIDS Care Grants, 178
Abbott Fund Science and Medical Innovation Grants, 179
ACE Charitable Foundation Grants, 199
ACF Ethnic Community Self-Help Grants, 200
ACF Preferred Communities Grants, 201
ACF Standing Announcement for Unaccompanied Alien Children Grants, 202
ACF Supplemental Services for Recently Arrived Refugees Grants, 203
Actors Fund Social Services and Financial Assistance, 225
Albert Pick Jr. Fund Grants, 328
Albertson's Charitable Giving Grants, 330
Allstate Corporate Hometown Commitment Grants, 364
American College of Surgeons and The Triological Society Clinical Scientist Development Awards, 422
Ann and Robert H. Lurie Family Foundation Grants, 475
AptarGroup Foundation Grants, 522
Arie and Ida Crown Memorial Grants, 528
ASHA Advancing Academic-Research Careers (AARC) Award, 569
ASHA Minority Student Leadership Program Awards, 570
ASHA Multicultural Activities Projects Grants, 571
ASHA Research Mentoring-Pair Travel Award, 572
ASHA Student Research Travel Award, 573
ASHA Students Preparing for Academic & Research Careers (SPARC) Award, 574
ASM Millis-Colwell Postgraduate Travel Grant, 608
AT&T Excelerator, 657
Aurora Foundation Grants, 667
Barr Fund Grants, 697
Baxter International Foundation Grants, 705
Bearemy's Kennel Pals Grants, 728
Blowitz-Ridgeway Foundation Grants, 767
Blum-Kovler Foundation Grants, 772
Boyd Gaming Corporation Contributions Program, 788
Bridgestone/Firestone Trust Fund Grants, 792
Cable Positive's Tony Cox Community Fund Grants, 827
Carrier Corporation Contributions Grants, 884
CDC Injury Control Research Centers Grants, 913
Champ-A Champion Fur Kids Grants, 959
Charles A. Frueauff Foundation Grants, 962
Chicago Board of Trade Foundation Grants, 988
Chicago Community Trust Grants, 989
Chicago Tribune's Corporate Contributions Grants, 991
Chicago White Metal Charitable Foundation Grants, 992
Children Affected by AIDS Foundation Camp Network Grants, 994
Children Affected by AIDS Foundation Family Assistance Emergency Fund Grants, 996
Clarcor Foundation Grants, 1021
CLIF Bar Family Foundation Grants, 1040
CNA Foundation Grants, 1046
Coleman Foundation Cancer Care Grants, 1055
Colonel Stanley R. McNeil Foundation Grants, 1059
Comer Foundation Grants, 1072

Community Foundation of Central Illinois Grants, 1101
Community Foundation of Champaign County Grants, 1102
ConAgra Foods Foundation Grants, 1140
ConocoPhillips Foundation Grants, 1144
Cooper Industries Foundation Grants, 1150
CSX Corporate Contributions Grants, 1169
Dean Foods Community Involvement Grants, 1209
Do Something BR!CK Awards, 1287
Doris and Victor Day Foundation Grants, 1313
Dr. Stanley Pearle Scholarships, 1330
Duchossois Family Foundation Grants, 1337
DuPage Community Foundation Grants, 1352
EDS Foundation Grants, 1371
Elizabeth Morse Genius Charitable Trust Grants, 1400
Evanston Community Foundation Grants, 1438
Field Foundation of Illinois Grants, 1499
Fifth Third Foundation Grants, 1501
FMC Foundation Grants, 1518
Frank E. and Seba B. Payne Foundation Grants, 1551
General Mills Foundation Grants, 1590
Ginn Foundation Grants, 1616
Gladys Brooks Foundation Grants, 1620
GoGirlGo! Ambassador Team Awards, 1632
Greater Saint Louis Community Foundation Grants, 1655
Guitar Center Music Foundation Grants, 1675
Hallmark Corporate Foundation Grants, 1688
Harry Kramer Memorial Fund Grants, 1705
Harry S. Black and Allon Fuller Fund, 1706
Hershey Company Grants, 1754
Honeywell Foundation Grants, 1791
Hormel Foods Charitable Trust Grants, 1795
Humana Foundation Grants, 1818
IAFF Burn Foundation Research Grants, 1830
IATA Research Grants, 1834
IATA Scholarships, 1835
James S. Copley Foundation Grants, 1895
John Deere Foundation Grants, 1929
John Merck Fund Grants, 1940
John Merck Scholars Awards, 1941
Joseph H. and Florence A. Roblee Foundation Grants, 1961
Joyce Foundation Grants, 1969
Kenny's Kids Grants, 1990
Lillian S. Wells Foundation Grants, 2056
Lincoln Financial Group Foundation Grants, 2058
Marriott Foundation for People with Disabilities Bridges Program Grants, 2113
Multiple Sclerosis Foundation Brighter Tomorrow Grants, 2228
National City Corporation Contributions Grants, 2250
National Starch and Chemical Foundation Grants, 2261
NEI Mentored Clinical Scientist Development Program Award (K12), 2295
NMF Franklin C. McLean Award, 2829
NMF General Electric Medical Scholars Fellowships, 2830
NMF Henry G. Halladay Awards, 2831
NMF Mary Ball Carrera Scholarship, 2834
NMF National Medical Association Awards for Medical Journalism, 2836
NMF National Medical Association Emerging Scholar Awards, 2837
NMF National Medical Association Patti LaBelle Award, 2838
NMF Need-Based Scholarships, 2839
NMF Ralph W. Ellison Prize, 2840
NMF William and Charlotte Cadbury Award, 2841
Northern Trust Company Charitable Trust and Corporate Giving Program, 2865
NSF Major Research Instrumentation Program (MRI) Grants, 2889
OneSight Research Foundation Block Grants, 2944
Pfizer/AAFP Foundation Visiting Professorship Program in Family Medicine, 3027
Piper Jaffray Companies Building Strong Communities Grants, 3053
Polk Bros. Foundation Grants, 3066
Prince Charitable Trusts Chicago Grants, 3079
Rice Foundation Grants, 3155
Rosalinde and Arthur Gilbert Foundation/AFAR New Investigator Awards in Alzheimer's Disease, 3187
Roy J. Carver Charitable Trust Medical and Science Research Grants, 3192
RRF General Program Grants, 3193
RRF Organizational Capacity Building Grants, 3194
Seabury Foundation Grants, 3274
Siragusa Foundation Health Services & Medical Research Grants, 3294
Solo Cup Foundation Grants, 3346
Southwire Company Grants, 3353
Square D Foundation Grants, 3361
Topfer Family Foundation Grants, 3430
Tylenol Scholarship, 3444
U.S. Department of Education Erma Byrd Scholarships, 3446
U.S. Department of Education United States-Russia Program: Improving Research and Educational Activities in Higher Education, 3451
US CRDF Leishmaniasis: Collaborative Research Opportunities in North Africa and the Middle East, 3474
Vulcan Materials Company Foundation Grants, 3504
Wal-Mart Foundation Community Grants, 3513
Wal-Mart State Giving Program Grants, 3514
Welborn Baptist Foundation Grants, 3525
William G. McGowan Charitable Fund Grants, 3539
YSA UnitedHealth Heroes Service Learning Grants, 3556

Indiana

3M Company Health and Human Services Grants, 10
3M Foundation Grants, 11
ACE Charitable Foundation Grants, 199
ACF Ethnic Community Self-Help Grants, 200
ACF Preferred Communities Grants, 201
ACF Standing Announcement for Unaccompanied Alien Children Grants, 202
ACF Supplemental Services for Recently Arrived Refugees Grants, 203
Actors Fund Social Services and Financial Assistance, 225
Albertson's Charitable Giving Grants, 330
Allstate Corporate Hometown Commitment Grants, 364
American College of Surgeons and The Triological Society Clinical Scientist Development Awards, 422
American Electric Power Grants, 434
Anthem Blue Cross and Blue Shield Grants, 488
Anthem Blue Cross and Blue Shield School Nurse Grants, 489
ASHA Advancing Academic-Research Careers (AARC) Award, 569
ASHA Minority Student Leadership Program Awards, 570
ASHA Multicultural Activities Projects Grants, 571
ASHA Research Mentoring-Pair Travel Award, 572
ASHA Student Research Travel Award, 573
ASHA Students Preparing for Academic & Research Careers (SPARC) Award, 574
ASM Millis-Colwell Postgraduate Travel Grant, 608
AT&T Excelerator, 657
Ball Brothers Foundation General Grants, 683
Ball Brothers Foundation Grants, 684
Barker Welfare Foundation Grants, 695
Bearemy's Kennel Pals Grants, 728
Benton Community Foundation Grants, 743
Blackford County Community Foundation Grants, 763
Blue River Community Foundation Grants, 770
Boyd Gaming Corporation Contributions Program, 788
Bridgestone/Firestone Trust Fund Grants, 792
Bristol-Myers Squibb Foundation Health Disparities Grants, 797
Brown County Community Foundation Grants, 807
Cable Positive's Tony Cox Community Fund Grants, 827
Carrier Corporation Contributions Grants, 884
Carroll County Community Foundation Grants, 885
Cass County Community Foundation Grants, 887
CDC Injury Control Research Centers Grants, 913
Champ-A Champion Fur Kids Grants, 959
Charles A. Frueauff Foundation Grants, 962
Charles H. Dater Foundation Grants, 966
Children Affected by AIDS Foundation Camp Network Grants, 994
Children Affected by AIDS Foundation Family Assistance Emergency Fund Grants, 996
CICF Legacy Fund Community Foundation Grants, 1010
Cinergy Foundation Grants, 1013
Clarian Health Critical / Progressive Care Internships, 1023
Clarian Health Multi-Specialty Internships, 1024
Clarian Health OR Internships, 1025
Clarian Health Scholarships for LPNs, 1026
Clarian Health Student Nurse Extern Scholarships, 1027
CLIF Bar Family Foundation Grants, 1040
Community Foundation Alliance City of Evansville Endowment Fund Grants, 1089
Community Foundation of Bartholomew County Heritage Fund Grants, 1096
Community Foundation of Bartholomew County James A. Henderson Award for Fund-Raising, 1097
Community Foundation of Bloomington and Monroe County Grants, 1098
Community Foundation of Boone County Grants, 1099
Community Foundation of Crawford County Grants and Scholarships, 1103
Community Foundation of Grant County Grants, 1104
Community Foundation of Grant County Scholarships, 1105
Community Foundation of Greater Fort Wayne: Community Endowment & Clarke Endowment Fund Grants, 1108
Community Foundation Of Greater Lafayette Grants, 1110
Community Foundation of Howard County Grants, 1116
Community Foundation of Madison and Jefferson County Grants and Scholarships, 1117
Community Foundation of Morgan County Grants and Scholarships, 1118
Community Foundation of Muncie and Delaware County Grants, 1120
Community Foundation of Randolph County Grants, 1121
Community Foundation of St. Joseph County Special Project Challenge Grants, 1126
Community Foundation of Switzerland County Grants, 1127
Community Foundation of Wabash County Grants, 1131
CSX Corporate Contributions Grants, 1169
Daviess County Community Foundation Health Grants, 1203
Dean Foods Community Involvement Grants, 1209
Dearborn Community Foundation City of Lawrenceburg Community Grants, 1210
Dearborn Community Foundation County Progress Grants, 1211
DHHS Healthy Tomorrows Partnership for Children, 1261

Do Something BR!CK Awards, 1287
Dr. Stanley Pearle Scholarships, 1330
Dubois County Community Foundation Grants, 1336
Duke Energy Foundation Grants, 1339
Duneland Health Council Incorporated Grants, 1350
Elkhart County Community Foundation Grants, 1401
Elliot Foundation Inc Grants, 1402
Evan and Susan Bayh Foundation Grants, 1437
Fayette County Foundation Grants, 1457
Fifth Third Foundation Grants, 1501
Foellinger Foundation Grants, 1519
Franklin County Community Foundation Grants, 1554
Fulton County Community Foundation Grants, 1579
General Mills Foundation Grants, 1590
Giving Sum Annual Grant, 1619
Gladys Brooks Foundation Grants, 1620
GoGirlGo! Ambassador Team Awards, 1632
Greater Cincinnati Foundation Priority and Small Projects/Capacity-Building Grants, 1651
Greene County Foundation Grants, 1662
Gregory L. Gibson Charitable Foundation Grants, 1668
Guitar Center Music Foundation Grants, 1675
Hancock County Community Foundation Grants, 1690
Harrison County Community Foundation Grants, 1700
Harry Kramer Memorial Fund Grants, 1705
Health Foundation of Greater Cincinnati Grants, 1724
Health Foundation of Greater Indianapolis Grants, 1725
Henry County Community Foundation Grants, 1747
Humana Foundation Grants, 1818
Huntington County Community Foundation Grants, 1823
Huntington National Bank Community Affairs Grants, 1824
IAFF Burn Foundation Research Grants, 1830
Impact 100 Grants, 1843
Indiana 21st Century Research and Technology Fund Awards, 1850
Indiana AIDS Fund Grants, 1851
Indiana Minority Teacher/Special Services Scholarships, 1852
Indiana Nursing Scholarships, 1853
Jacob G. Schmidlapp Trust Grants, 1883
Jasper Foundation Jasper County Grants, 1907
Jasper Foundation Newton County Grants, 1908
Jennings County Community Foundation Grants, 1916
John Merck Fund Grants, 1940
John Merck Scholars Awards, 1941
John W. Anderson Foundation Grants, 1949
Johnson County Community Foundation Grants, 1955
Joseph and Luella Abell Charitable Trust Scholarships, 1958
Journal Gazette Foundation Grants, 1968
Joyce Foundation Grants, 1969
K21 Health Foundation Cancer Care Fund Grants, 1975
K21 Health Foundation Grants, 1976
Kendrick Foundation Grants, 1988
Knox County Community Foundation Grants, 2009
Kosair Charities Grants, 2014
Kosciusko County Community Foundation Grants, 2015
LaGrange County Community Foundation Grants, 2020
Legacy Foundation Grants, 2040
Lester E. Yeager Charitable Trust B Grants, 2047
Lincoln Financial Group Foundation Grants, 2058
M.E. Raker Foundation Grants, 2094
Madison County Community Foundation Grants, 2098
Maxon Charitable Foundation Grants, 2135
McMillen Foundation Grants, 2148
Mead Johnson Nutritionals Evansville-Area Organizations Grants, 2157
Miami County Community Foundation Operation Round Up Grants, 2188
Montgomery County Community Foundation Grants, 2214
Multiple Sclerosis Foundation Brighter Tomorrow Grants, 2228
National City Corporation Contributions Grants, 2250
National Starch and Chemical Foundation Grants, 2261
NEI Mentored Clinical Scientist Development Program Award (K12), 2295
Nicholas H. Noyes Jr. Memorial Foundation Grants, 2497
Nina Mason Pulliam Charitable Trust Grants, 2776
NMF Franklin C. McLean Award, 2829
NMF General Electric Medical Scholars Fellowships, 2830
NMF Henry G. Halladay Awards, 2831
NMF Mary Ball Carrera Scholarship, 2834
NMF National Medical Association Awards for Medical Journalism, 2836
NMF National Medical Association Emerging Scholar Awards, 2837
NMF National Medical Association Patti LaBelle Award, 2838
NMF Need-Based Scholarships, 2839
NMF Ralph W. Ellison Prize, 2840
NMF William and Charlotte Cadbury Award, 2841
Noble County Community Foundation Grants, 2848
North Central Health Services Grants, 2861
NSF Major Research Instrumentation Program (MRI) Grants, 2889
Ohio County Community Foundation Grants, 2938
Ohio County Community Foundation Mini-Grants, 2939
OneSight Research Foundation Block Grants, 2944
Owen County Community Foundation Grants, 2979
Paul Ogle Foundation Grants, 3003
Perry County Community Foundation Grants, 3016
PeyBack Foundation Grants, 3022
Pfizer/AAFP Foundation Visiting Professorship Program in Family Medicine, 3027
Pike County Community Foundation Grants, 3049
PNC Charitable Trust and Foundation Grants, 3064
Posey Community Foundation Grants, 3068
Posey Community Foundation Womens Fund Grants, 3069
Pulaski County Community Foundation Grants, 3091
Putnam County Community Foundation Grants, 3093
Richard M. Fairbanks Foundation Grants, 3162
Ripley County Community Foundation Grants, 3166
Robert P. & Clara I. Milton Fund for Senior Housing, 3172
Rosalinde and Arthur Gilbert Foundation/AFAR New Investigator Awards in Alzheimer's Disease, 3187
RRF General Program Grants, 3193
Rush County Community Foundation Grants, 3200
Schurz Communications Foundation Grants, 3271
Scott County Community Foundation Grants, 3273
South Madison Community Foundation Grants, 3349
Spencer County Community Foundation Grants, 3358
Square D Foundation Grants, 3361
St. Joseph Community Health Foundation Burn Care and Prevention Grants, 3367
St. Joseph Community Health Foundation Improving Healthcare Access Grants, 3368
St. Joseph Community Health Foundation Pfeiffer Fund Grants, 3369
St. Joseph Community Health Foundation Schneider Fellowships, 3370
Steuben County Community Foundation Grants, 3383
Tylenol Scholarship, 3444
U.S. Department of Education Erma Byrd Scholarships, 3446
U.S. Department of Education United States-Russia Program: Improving Research and Educational Activities in Higher Education, 3451
Unity Foundation Of LaPorte County Grants, 3467
US CRDF Leishmaniasis: Collaborative Research Opportunities in North Africa and the Middle East, 3474
Vanderburgh Community Foundation Grants, 3480
Vectren Foundation Grants, 3485
Vulcan Materials Company Foundation Grants, 3504
W. C. Griffith Foundation Grants, 3505
Wabash Valley Community Foundation Grants, 3510
Wal-Mart Foundation Community Grants, 3513
Wal-Mart State Giving Program Grants, 3514
Warrick County Community Foundation Grants, 3519
Welborn Baptist Foundation Grants, 3525
Wells County Foundation Grants, 3527
Western Indiana Community Foundation Grants, 3528
WHAS Crusade for Children Grants, 3531
YSA UnitedHealth Heroes Service Learning Grants, 3556

Iowa

3M Company Health and Human Services Grants, 10
3M Foundation Grants, 11
ACF Ethnic Community Self-Help Grants, 200
ACF Preferred Communities Grants, 201
ACF Standing Announcement for Unaccompanied Alien Children Grants, 202
ACF Supplemental Services for Recently Arrived Refugees Grants, 203
Actors Fund Social Services and Financial Assistance, 225
AEGON Transamerica Foundation Grants, 243
Albertson's Charitable Giving Grants, 330
American College of Surgeons and The Triological Society Clinical Scientist Development Awards, 422
Andersen Corporate Foundation, 470
ASHA Advancing Academic-Research Careers (AARC) Award, 569
ASHA Minority Student Leadership Program Awards, 570
ASHA Multicultural Activities Projects Grants, 571
ASHA Research Mentoring-Pair Travel Award, 572
ASHA Student Research Travel Award, 573
ASHA Students Preparing for Academic & Research Careers (SPARC) Award, 574
ASM Millis-Colwell Postgraduate Travel Grant, 608
Bearemy's Kennel Pals Grants, 728
Bridgestone/Firestone Trust Fund Grants, 792
Cable Positive's Tony Cox Community Fund Grants, 827
Champ-A Champion Fur Kids Grants, 959
Children Affected by AIDS Foundation Camp Network Grants, 994
Children Affected by AIDS Foundation Family Assistance Emergency Fund Grants, 996
CLIF Bar Family Foundation Grants, 1040
Covenant Foundation Grants (Iowa), 1153
CUNA Mutual Group Foundation, 1174
DHHS Healthy Tomorrows Partnership for Children, 1261
Do Something BR!CK Awards, 1287
Doris and Victor Day Foundation Grants, 1313
Dr. Stanley Pearle Scholarships, 1330
General Mills Foundation Grants, 1590

GoGirlGo! Ambassador Team Awards, 1632
Guitar Center Music Foundation Grants, 1675
Hall-Perrine Foundation Grants, 1686
Harry Kramer Memorial Fund Grants, 1705
Hormel Foods Charitable Trust Grants, 1795
IAFF Burn Foundation Research Grants, 1830
John Deere Foundation Grants, 1929
John Merck Fund Grants, 1940
John Merck Scholars Awards, 1941
Joyce Foundation Grants, 1969
Multiple Sclerosis Foundation Brighter Tomorrow Grants, 2228
NEI Mentored Clinical Scientist Development Program Award (K12), 2295
NMF Franklin C. McLean Award, 2829
NMF General Electric Medical Scholars Fellowships, 2830
NMF Henry G. Halladay Awards, 2831
NMF Mary Ball Carrera Scholarship, 2834
NMF National Medical Association Awards for Medical Journalism, 2836
NMF National Medical Association Emerging Scholar Awards, 2837
NMF National Medical Association Patti LaBelle Award, 2838
NMF Need-Based Scholarships, 2839
NMF Ralph W. Ellison Prize, 2840
NMF William and Charlotte Cadbury Award, 2841
NSF Major Research Instrumentation Program (MRI) Grants, 2889
OneSight Research Foundation Block Grants, 2944
Pfizer/AAFP Foundation Visiting Professorship Program in Family Medicine, 3027
Piper Jaffray Companies Building Strong Communities Grants, 3053
Principal Financial Group Foundation Grants, 3082
Rosalinde and Arthur Gilbert Foundation/AFAR New Investigator Awards in Alzheimer's Disease, 3187
Roy J. Carver Charitable Trust Medical and Science Research Grants, 3192
RRF General Program Grants, 3193
Square D Foundation Grants, 3361
Sunderland Foundation Grants, 3400
Tylenol Scholarship, 3444
U.S. Department of Education Erma Byrd Scholarships, 3446
U.S. Department of Education United States-Russia Program: Improving Research and Educational Activities in Higher Education, 3451
US CRDF Leishmaniasis: Collaborative Research Opportunities in North Africa and the Middle East, 3474
Viking Children's Fund Grants, 3497
Vulcan Materials Company Foundation Grants, 3504
Waitt Family Foundation Grants, 3512
Wal-Mart Foundation Community Grants, 3513
Wal-Mart State Giving Program Grants, 3514
Wellmark Foundation Grants, 3526

Kansas

Abbott Fund Access to Health Care Grants, 176
Abbott Fund Community Vitality Grants, 177
Abbott Fund Global AIDS Care Grants, 178
Abbott Fund Science and Medical Innovation Grants, 179
ACE Charitable Foundation Grants, 199
ACF Ethnic Community Self-Help Grants, 200
ACF Preferred Communities Grants, 201
ACF Standing Announcement for Unaccompanied Alien Children Grants, 202
ACF Supplemental Services for Recently Arrived Refugees Grants, 203
Actors Fund Social Services and Financial Assistance, 225
Albertson's Charitable Giving Grants, 330
American College of Surgeons and The Triological Society Clinical Scientist Development Awards, 422
ASHA Advancing Academic-Research Careers (AARC) Award, 569
ASHA Minority Student Leadership Program Awards, 570
ASHA Multicultural Activities Projects Grants, 571
ASHA Research Mentoring-Pair Travel Award, 572
ASHA Student Research Travel Award, 573
ASHA Students Preparing for Academic & Research Careers (SPARC) Award, 574
ASM Millis-Colwell Postgraduate Travel Grant, 608
AT&T Excelerator, 657
Bearemy's Kennel Pals Grants, 728
Cable Positive's Tony Cox Community Fund Grants, 827
Champ-A Champion Fur Kids Grants, 959
Charles A. Frueauff Foundation Grants, 962
Children Affected by AIDS Foundation Camp Network Grants, 994
Children Affected by AIDS Foundation Family Assistance Emergency Fund Grants, 996
CLIF Bar Family Foundation Grants, 1040
DHHS Healthy Tomorrows Partnership for Children, 1261
Do Something BR!CK Awards, 1287
Dr. Stanley Pearle Scholarships, 1330
Forrest C. Lattner Foundation Grants, 1523
GoGirlGo! Ambassador Team Awards, 1632
Guitar Center Music Foundation Grants, 1675
H & R Foundation Grants, 1679
Hallmark Corporate Foundation Grants, 1688
Harry Kramer Memorial Fund Grants, 1705
Hormel Foods Charitable Trust Grants, 1795
Humana Foundation Grants, 1818
IAFF Burn Foundation Research Grants, 1830
J.E. and L.E. Mabee Foundation Grants, 1875
John Deere Foundation Grants, 1929
John Merck Fund Grants, 1940
John Merck Scholars Awards, 1941
Kansas Health Foundation Grants, 1980
Multiple Sclerosis Foundation Brighter Tomorrow Grants, 2228
NEI Mentored Clinical Scientist Development Program Award (K12), 2295
NMF Franklin C. McLean Award, 2829
NMF General Electric Medical Scholars Fellowships, 2830
NMF Henry G. Halladay Awards, 2831
NMF Mary Ball Carrera Scholarship, 2834
NMF National Medical Association Awards for Medical Journalism, 2836
NMF National Medical Association Emerging Scholar Awards, 2837
NMF National Medical Association Patti LaBelle Award, 2838
NMF Need-Based Scholarships, 2839
NMF Ralph W. Ellison Prize, 2840
NMF William and Charlotte Cadbury Award, 2841
NSF Major Research Instrumentation Program (MRI) Grants, 2889
OneSight Research Foundation Block Grants, 2944
Pfizer/AAFP Foundation Visiting Professorship Program in Family Medicine, 3027
Piper Jaffray Companies Building Strong Communities Grants, 3053
Rosalinde and Arthur Gilbert Foundation/AFAR New Investigator Awards in Alzheimer's Disease, 3187
Sosland Foundation Grants, 3348
Sunderland Foundation Grants, 3400
Sunflower Foundation Bridge Grants, 3401
Sunflower Foundation Capacity Building Grants, 3402
Sunflower Foundation Walking Trails Grants, 3403
Topeka Community Foundation Kansas Blood Services Scholarships, 3429
Tylenol Scholarship, 3444
U.S. Department of Education Erma Byrd Scholarships, 3446
U.S. Department of Education United States-Russia Program: Improving Research and Educational Activities in Higher Education, 3451
US CRDF Leishmaniasis: Collaborative Research Opportunities in North Africa and the Middle East, 3474
Vulcan Materials Company Foundation Grants, 3504
Wal-Mart Foundation Community Grants, 3513
Wal-Mart State Giving Program Grants, 3514

Kentucky

3M Company Health and Human Services Grants, 10
3M Foundation Grants, 11
ACF Ethnic Community Self-Help Grants, 200
ACF Preferred Communities Grants, 201
ACF Standing Announcement for Unaccompanied Alien Children Grants, 202
ACF Supplemental Services for Recently Arrived Refugees Grants, 203
Actors Fund Social Services and Financial Assistance, 225
AEGON Transamerica Foundation Grants, 243
American College of Surgeons and The Triological Society Clinical Scientist Development Awards, 422
American Electric Power Grants, 434
Anthem Blue Cross and Blue Shield Grants, 488
Anthem Blue Cross and Blue Shield School Nurse Grants, 489
Arkema Foundation Science Teachers Program, 535
ASHA Advancing Academic-Research Careers (AARC) Award, 569
ASHA Minority Student Leadership Program Awards, 570
ASHA Multicultural Activities Projects Grants, 571
ASHA Research Mentoring-Pair Travel Award, 572
ASHA Student Research Travel Award, 573
ASHA Students Preparing for Academic & Research Careers (SPARC) Award, 574
Ashland Corporate Contributions Grants, 586
ASM Millis-Colwell Postgraduate Travel Grant, 608
AT&T Excelerator, 657
Bearemy's Kennel Pals Grants, 728
Belk Foundation Grants, 739
Blue Grass Community Foundation Grants, 768
Bridgestone/Firestone Trust Fund Grants, 792
Cable Positive's Tony Cox Community Fund Grants, 827
CDC Injury Control Research Centers Grants, 913
Champ-A Champion Fur Kids Grants, 959
Charles A. Frueauff Foundation Grants, 962
Charles H. Dater Foundation Grants, 966
Children Affected by AIDS Foundation Camp Network Grants, 994
Children Affected by AIDS Foundation Family Assistance Emergency Fund Grants, 996
Cinergy Foundation Grants, 1013
Clarcor Foundation Grants, 1021
Clark County Community Foundation Grants, 1028
CLIF Bar Family Foundation Grants, 1040
CSX Corporate Contributions Grants, 1169
Dean Foods Community Involvement Grants, 1209
Do Something BR!CK Awards, 1287
Dr. Stanley Pearle Scholarships, 1330
Duke Energy Foundation Grants, 1339
Fidelity Foundation Grants, 1498
Fifth Third Foundation Grants, 1501
Gheens Foundation Grants, 1610
GoGirlGo! Ambassador Team Awards, 1632
Good Samaritan Foundation Inc Grants, 1636
Greater Cincinnati Foundation Priority and Small Projects/Capacity-Building Grants, 1651
Guitar Center Music Foundation Grants, 1675
Harry Kramer Memorial Fund Grants, 1705
Health Foundation of Greater Cincinnati Grants, 1724
Humana Foundation Grants, 1818
Huntington National Bank Community Affairs Grants, 1824
IAFF Burn Foundation Research Grants, 1830

Impact 100 Grants, 1843
Jacob G. Schmidlapp Trust Grants, 1883
James Graham Brown Foundation Grants, 1887
John Merck Fund Grants, 1940
John Merck Scholars Awards, 1941
Kimberly-Clark Community Grants, 2001
Kosair Charities Grants, 2014
Lester E. Yeager Charitable Trust B Grants, 2047
Multiple Sclerosis Foundation Brighter Tomorrow Grants, 2228
National City Corporation Contributions Grants, 2250
NEI Mentored Clinical Scientist Development Program Award (K12), 2295
NMF Franklin C. McLean Award, 2829
NMF General Electric Medical Scholars Fellowships, 2830
NMF Henry G. Halladay Awards, 2831
NMF Mary Ball Carrera Scholarship, 2834
NMF National Medical Association Awards for Medical Journalism, 2836
NMF National Medical Association Emerging Scholar Awards, 2837
NMF National Medical Association Patti LaBelle Award, 2838
NMF Need-Based Scholarships, 2839
NMF Ralph W. Ellison Prize, 2840
NMF William and Charlotte Cadbury Award, 2841
NSF Major Research Instrumentation Program (MRI) Grants, 2889
OneSight Research Foundation Block Grants, 2944
Paul Ogle Foundation Grants, 3003
Pfizer/AAFP Foundation Visiting Professorship Program in Family Medicine, 3027
Piper Jaffray Companies Building Strong Communities Grants, 3053
PNC Charitable Trust and Foundation Grants, 3064
Rainbow Fund Grants, 3103
Rosalinde and Arthur Gilbert Foundation/AFAR New Investigator Awards in Alzheimer's Disease, 3187
RRF General Program Grants, 3193
Southwire Company Grants, 3353
Square D Foundation Grants, 3361
Steele-Reese Foundation Grants, 3380
Thompson Charitable Foundation Grants, 3425
Tylenol Scholarship, 3444
U.S. Department of Education Erma Byrd Scholarships, 3446
U.S. Department of Education United States-Russia Program: Improving Research and Educational Activities in Higher Education, 3451
US CRDF Leishmaniasis: Collaborative Research Opportunities in North Africa and the Middle East, 3474
Vulcan Materials Company Foundation Grants, 3504
Wal-Mart Foundation Community Grants, 3513
Wal-Mart State Giving Program Grants, 3514
Welborn Baptist Foundation Grants, 3525
WHAS Crusade for Children Grants, 3531

Louisiana

ACE Charitable Foundation Grants, 199
ACF Ethnic Community Self-Help Grants, 200
ACF Preferred Communities Grants, 201
ACF Standing Announcement for Unaccompanied Alien Children Grants, 202
ACF Supplemental Services for Recently Arrived Refugees Grants, 203
Actors Fund Social Services and Financial Assistance, 225
Albertson's Charitable Giving Grants, 330
American College of Surgeons and The Triological Society Clinical Scientist Development Awards, 422
American Electric Power Grants, 434
ASHA Advancing Academic-Research Careers (AARC) Award, 569
ASHA Minority Student Leadership Program Awards, 570
ASHA Multicultural Activities Projects Grants, 571
ASHA Research Mentoring-Pair Travel Award, 572
ASHA Student Research Travel Award, 573
ASHA Students Preparing for Academic & Research Careers (SPARC) Award, 574
ASM Millis-Colwell Postgraduate Travel Grant, 608
AT&T Excelerator, 657
Baptist Community Ministries Grants, 691
Baton Rouge Area Foundation Grants, 702
Bearemy's Kennel Pals Grants, 728
Belk Foundation Grants, 739
Booth-Bricker Fund Grants, 780
Boyd Gaming Corporation Contributions Program, 788
Bridgestone/Firestone Trust Fund Grants, 792
Cable Positive's Tony Cox Community Fund Grants, 827
CDC Injury Control Research Centers Grants, 913
Champ-A Champion Fur Kids Grants, 959
Charles A. Frueauff Foundation Grants, 962
Children Affected by AIDS Foundation Camp Network Grants, 994
Children Affected by AIDS Foundation Family Assistance Emergency Fund Grants, 996
CLIF Bar Family Foundation Grants, 1040
Collins C. Diboll Private Foundation Grants, 1057
ConocoPhillips Foundation Grants, 1144
CSX Corporate Contributions Grants, 1169
Cudd Foundation Grants, 1171
Dean Foods Community Involvement Grants, 1209
DHHS Healthy Tomorrows Partnership for Children, 1261
Do Something BR!CK Awards, 1287
Dr. Stanley Pearle Scholarships, 1330
Entergy Community Partnership Grants, 1417
Entergy Corporation Open Grants for Healthy Families, 1418
Fluor Foundation Grants, 1517
FMC Foundation Grants, 1518
Foundation for the Mid-South Grants, 1536
Gheens Foundation Grants, 1610
Gladys Brooks Foundation Grants, 1620
GoGirlGo! Ambassador Team Awards, 1632
Greater New Orleans Foundation Grants, 1654
Guitar Center Music Foundation Grants, 1675
Harry Kramer Memorial Fund Grants, 1705
Huie-Dellmon Trust Grants, 1815
Humana Foundation Grants, 1818
IAFF Burn Foundation Research Grants, 1830
Joe W. and Dorothy Dorsett Brown Foundation Grants, 1927
John Deere Foundation Grants, 1929
John Merck Fund Grants, 1940
John Merck Scholars Awards, 1941
Lettie Pate Whitehead Foundation Grants, 2049
Multiple Sclerosis Foundation Brighter Tomorrow Grants, 2228
NEI Mentored Clinical Scientist Development Program Award (K12), 2295
NMF Franklin C. McLean Award, 2829
NMF General Electric Medical Scholars Fellowships, 2830
NMF Henry G. Halladay Awards, 2831
NMF Mary Ball Carrera Scholarship, 2834
NMF National Medical Association Awards for Medical Journalism, 2836
NMF National Medical Association Emerging Scholar Awards, 2837
NMF National Medical Association Patti LaBelle Award, 2838
NMF Need-Based Scholarships, 2839
NMF Ralph W. Ellison Prize, 2840
NMF William and Charlotte Cadbury Award, 2841
NSF Major Research Instrumentation Program (MRI) Grants, 2889
OneSight Research Foundation Block Grants, 2944
PeyBack Foundation Grants, 3022
Pfizer/AAFP Foundation Visiting Professorship Program in Family Medicine, 3027
Plum Creek Foundation Grants, 3062
Rosalinde and Arthur Gilbert Foundation/AFAR New Investigator Awards in Alzheimer's Disease, 3187
Tylenol Scholarship, 3444
U.S. Department of Education Erma Byrd Scholarships, 3446
U.S. Department of Education United States-Russia Program: Improving Research and Educational Activities in Higher Education, 3451
US CRDF Leishmaniasis: Collaborative Research Opportunities in North Africa and the Middle East, 3474
Vulcan Materials Company Foundation Grants, 3504
Wal-Mart Foundation Community Grants, 3513
Wal-Mart State Giving Program Grants, 3514

Maine

ACF Ethnic Community Self-Help Grants, 200
ACF Preferred Communities Grants, 201
ACF Standing Announcement for Unaccompanied Alien Children Grants, 202
ACF Supplemental Services for Recently Arrived Refugees Grants, 203
Actors Fund Social Services and Financial Assistance, 225
Agnes M. Lindsay Trust Grants, 263
Albertson's Charitable Giving Grants, 330
American College of Surgeons and The Triological Society Clinical Scientist Development Awards, 422
Anthem Blue Cross and Blue Shield Grants, 488
ASHA Advancing Academic-Research Careers (AARC) Award, 569
ASHA Minority Student Leadership Program Awards, 570
ASHA Multicultural Activities Projects Grants, 571
ASHA Research Mentoring-Pair Travel Award, 572
ASHA Student Research Travel Award, 573
ASHA Students Preparing for Academic & Research Careers (SPARC) Award, 574
ASM Millis-Colwell Postgraduate Travel Grant, 608
Barnes Group Foundation Grants, 696
Bearemy's Kennel Pals Grants, 728
BJ's Charitable Foundation Grants, 761
Cable Positive's Tony Cox Community Fund Grants, 827
Carlisle Foundation Grants, 874
Champ-A Champion Fur Kids Grants, 959
Charles A. Frueauff Foundation Grants, 962
Charles H. Hood Foundation Child Health Research Grants, 968
Children Affected by AIDS Foundation Camp Network Grants, 994
Children Affected by AIDS Foundation Family Assistance Emergency Fund Grants, 996
CLIF Bar Family Foundation Grants, 1040
Davis Family Foundation Grants, 1204
Dean Foods Community Involvement Grants, 1209
DHHS Healthy Tomorrows Partnership for Children, 1261
Do Something BR!CK Awards, 1287
Dr. Stanley Pearle Scholarships, 1330
FMC Foundation Grants, 1518
Foundation for Seacoast Health Grants, 1533
Frances W. Emerson Foundation Grants, 1548
Francis T. & Louise T. Nichols Foundation Grants, 1550
Frederick Gardner Cottrell Foundation Grants, 1560
Gladys Brooks Foundation Grants, 1620
GoGirlGo! Ambassador Team Awards, 1632
Greenfield Foundation of Maine Grants, 1663
Guitar Center Music Foundation Grants, 1675
Hannaford Charitable Foundation Grants, 1692
Harold Alfond Foundation Grants, 1695
Harry Kramer Memorial Fund Grants, 1705
IAFF Burn Foundation Research Grants, 1830
Jane's Trust Grants, 1904

Jessie B. Cox Charitable Trust Grants, 1918
John Merck Fund Grants, 1940
John Merck Scholars Awards, 1941
Maine Community Foundation Grants, 2099
Multiple Sclerosis Foundation Brighter Tomorrow Grants, 2228
NEI Mentored Clinical Scientist Development Program Award (K12), 2295
NMF Franklin C. McLean Award, 2829
NMF General Electric Medical Scholars Fellowships, 2830
NMF Henry G. Halladay Awards, 2831
NMF Mary Ball Carrera Scholarship, 2834
NMF National Medical Association Awards for Medical Journalism, 2836
NMF National Medical Association Emerging Scholar Awards, 2837
NMF National Medical Association Patti LaBelle Award, 2838
NMF Need-Based Scholarships, 2839
NMF Ralph W. Ellison Prize, 2840
NMF William and Charlotte Cadbury Award, 2841
NSF Major Research Instrumentation Program (MRI) Grants, 2889
OneSight Research Foundation Block Grants, 2944
Pfizer/AAFP Foundation Visiting Professorship Program in Family Medicine, 3027
Plum Creek Foundation Grants, 3062
Rosalinde and Arthur Gilbert Foundation/AFAR New Investigator Awards in Alzheimer's Disease, 3187
Salem Foundation Grants, 3242
Sasco Foundation Grants, 3265
Shaw's Supermarkets Donations, 3280
Simmons Foundation Grants, 3287
Tylenol Scholarship, 3444
U.S. Department of Education Erma Byrd Scholarships, 3446
U.S. Department of Education United States-Russia Program: Improving Research and Educational Activities in Higher Education, 3451
US CRDF Leishmaniasis: Collaborative Research Opportunities in North Africa and the Middle East, 3474
Wal-Mart Foundation Community Grants, 3513
Wal-Mart State Giving Program Grants, 3514

Maryland
Abell Foundation Health and Human Services Grants, 182
ACE Charitable Foundation Grants, 199
ACF Ethnic Community Self-Help Grants, 200
ACF Preferred Communities Grants, 201
ACF Standing Announcement for Unaccompanied Alien Children Grants, 202
ACF Supplemental Services for Recently Arrived Refugees Grants, 203
Actors Fund Social Services and Financial Assistance, 225
AEGON Transamerica Foundation Grants, 243
Albertson's Charitable Giving Grants, 330
Alex Brown and Sons Charitable Foundation Grants, 337
Alpha Research Foundation Grants, 367
American College of Surgeons and The Triological Society Clinical Scientist Development Awards, 422
ASHA Advancing Academic-Research Careers (AARC) Award, 569
ASHA Minority Student Leadership Program Awards, 570
ASHA Multicultural Activities Projects Grants, 571
ASHA Research Mentoring-Pair Travel Award, 572
ASHA Student Research Travel Award, 573
ASHA Students Preparing for Academic & Research Careers (SPARC) Award, 574
ASM Millis-Colwell Postgraduate Travel Grant, 608
Bearemy's Kennel Pals Grants, 728
Bechtel Group Foundation Building Positive Community Relationships Grants, 731
Belk Foundation Grants, 739
Bender Foundation Grants, 742
BJ's Charitable Foundation Grants, 761
Cable Positive's Tony Cox Community Fund Grants, 827
CDC Injury Control Research Centers Grants, 913
Champ-A Champion Fur Kids Grants, 959
Charles A. Frueauff Foundation Grants, 962
Charles Delmar Foundation Grants, 963
Chase Paymentech Corporate Giving Grants, 975
Children Affected by AIDS Foundation Camp Network Grants, 994
Children Affected by AIDS Foundation Family Assistance Emergency Fund Grants, 996
CLIF Bar Family Foundation Grants, 1040
Commonweal Foundation Community Assistance Grants, 1075
Commonweal Foundation Grants, 1076
Community Foundation of the Eastern Shore Community Needs Grants, 1129
CSX Corporate Contributions Grants, 1169
Danellie Foundation Grants, 1198
Dean Foods Community Involvement Grants, 1209
DHHS Healthy Tomorrows Partnership for Children, 1261
Do Something BR!CK Awards, 1287
Dominion Educational Partnership Grant, 1308
Dr. Stanley Pearle Scholarships, 1330
Eddie C. and Sylvia Brown Family Foundation Grants, 1367
Eugene and Agnes E. Meyer Foundation Grants, 1432
Eugene B. Casey Foundation Grants, 1433
FMC Foundation Grants, 1518
Freddie Mac Foundation Grants, 1558
Frederick Gardner Cottrell Foundation Grants, 1560
General Mills Foundation Grants, 1590
Gladys Brooks Foundation Grants, 1620
GoGirlGo! Ambassador Team Awards, 1632
Guitar Center Music Foundation Grants, 1675
Harry Kramer Memorial Fund Grants, 1705
Henry and Ruth Blaustein Rosenberg Foundation Grants, 1746
IAFF Burn Foundation Research Grants, 1830
Jacob and Hilda Blaustein Foundation Grants, 1881
John Edward Fowler Memorial Foundation Grants, 1930
John J. Leidy Foundation Grants, 1936
John Merck Fund Grants, 1940
John Merck Scholars Awards, 1941
Land O'Lakes Foundation Mid-Atlantic Grants Program, 2027
Leonsis Foundation Grants, 2045
Mabel H. Flory Charitable Trust Grants, 2096
Marion I. and Henry J. Knott Foundation Grants Program, 2109
Marjorie C. Adams Charitable Trust Grants, 2111
Marriott Foundation for People with Disabilities Bridges Program Grants, 2113
Morris and Gwendolyn Cafritz Foundation Grants, 2217
Morton K. and Jane Blaustein Foundation Grants, 2218
Multiple Sclerosis Foundation Brighter Tomorrow Grants, 2228
NEI Mentored Clinical Scientist Development Program Award (K12), 2295
NMF Franklin C. McLean Award, 2829
NMF General Electric Medical Scholars Fellowships, 2830
NMF Henry G. Halladay Awards, 2831
NMF Mary Ball Carrera Scholarship, 2834
NMF National Medical Association Awards for Medical Journalism, 2836
NMF National Medical Association Emerging Scholar Awards, 2837
NMF National Medical Association Patti LaBelle Award, 2838
NMF Need-Based Scholarships, 2839
NMF Ralph W. Ellison Prize, 2840
NMF William and Charlotte Cadbury Award, 2841
NSF Major Research Instrumentation Program (MRI) Grants, 2889
OneSight Research Foundation Block Grants, 2944
OSI-Baltimore Special Opportunities Program Grants, 2972
OSI-Baltimore Tackling Drug Addiction Grants, 2973
Pfizer/AAFP Foundation Visiting Professorship Program in Family Medicine, 3027
PNC Charitable Trust and Foundation Grants, 3064
Quality Health Foundation Grants, 3094
Rathmann Family Foundation Grants, 3109
Rosalinde and Arthur Gilbert Foundation/AFAR New Investigator Awards in Alzheimer's Disease, 3187
Tylenol Scholarship, 3444
U.S. Department of Education Erma Byrd Scholarships, 3446
U.S. Department of Education United States-Russia Program: Improving Research and Educational Activities in Higher Education, 3451
US CRDF Leishmaniasis: Collaborative Research Opportunities in North Africa and the Middle East, 3474
Verizon Foundation Maryland Grants, 3487
Vulcan Materials Company Foundation Grants, 3504
Wal-Mart Foundation Community Grants, 3513
Wal-Mart State Giving Program Grants, 3514
YSA UnitedHealth Heroes Service Learning Grants, 3556

Massachusetts
1675 Foundation Grants, 4
2 Depot Square Ipswich Charitable Foundation Grants, 7
3M Company Health and Human Services Grants, 10
3M Foundation Grants, 11
Aaron Foundation (Massachusetts) Grants, 174
Abbott Fund Access to Health Care Grants, 176
Abbott Fund Community Vitality Grants, 177
Abbott Fund Global AIDS Care Grants, 178
Abbott Fund Science and Medical Innovation Grants, 179
ACE Charitable Foundation Grants, 199
ACF Ethnic Community Self-Help Grants, 200
ACF Preferred Communities Grants, 201
ACF Standing Announcement for Unaccompanied Alien Children Grants, 202
ACF Supplemental Services for Recently Arrived Refugees Grants, 203
Actors Fund Social Services and Financial Assistance, 225
Acushnet Foundation Grants, 226
Adelaide Breed Bayrd Foundation Grants, 234
AEC Trust Grants, 242
Agnes M. Lindsay Trust Grants, 263
Ahn Family Foundation Grants, 304
Albertson's Charitable Giving Grants, 330
Alice C. A. Sibley Fund Grants, 355
American College of Surgeons and The Triological Society Clinical Scientist Development Awards, 422
ASHA Advancing Academic-Research Careers (AARC) Award, 569
ASHA Minority Student Leadership Program Awards, 570
ASHA Multicultural Activities Projects Grants, 571
ASHA Research Mentoring-Pair Travel Award, 572
ASHA Student Research Travel Award, 573
ASHA Students Preparing for Academic & Research Careers (SPARC) Award, 574
ASM Millis-Colwell Postgraduate Travel Grant, 608
Auburn Foundation Grants, 664
Banfi Vintners Foundation Grants, 687
Barnes Group Foundation Grants, 696
BCBS of Massachusetts Foundation Grants, 709
Bearemy's Kennel Pals Grants, 728

Biogen Corporate Giving Grants, 758
BJ's Charitable Foundation Grants, 761
Boston Foundation Grants, 783
Boston Globe Foundation Grants, 784
Boston Jewish Community Women's Fund Grants, 785
Bristol-Myers Squibb Foundation Health Disparities Grants, 797
Bushrod H. Campbell and Adah F. Hall Charity Fund Grants, 816
C.R. Bard Foundation Grants, 825
Cable Positive's Tony Cox Community Fund Grants, 827
Cambridge Community Foundation Grants, 837
Carlisle Foundation Grants, 874
Champ-A Champion Fur Kids Grants, 959
Charles A. Frueauff Foundation Grants, 962
Charles H. Hood Foundation Child Health Research Grants, 968
Chestnut Hill Charitable Foundation, Inc Grants, 987
Children Affected by AIDS Foundation Camp Network Grants, 994
Children Affected by AIDS Foundation Family Assistance Emergency Fund Grants, 996
CLIF Bar Family Foundation Grants, 1040
Cranston Foundation Grants, 1158
CSX Corporate Contributions Grants, 1169
Dean Foods Community Involvement Grants, 1209
DHHS Healthy Tomorrows Partnership for Children, 1261
Do Something BR!CK Awards, 1287
Dominion Educational Partnership Grant, 1308
Dr. Stanley Pearle Scholarships, 1330
Edward Bangs Kelley and Elza Kelley Foundation Grants, 1373
Edwin S. Webster Foundation Grants, 1376
Elizabeth McGraw Foundation Grants, 1399
Entergy Corporation Open Grants for Healthy Families, 1418
Essex County Community Foundation Discretionary Fund Grant, 1428
Fairlawn Foundation Grants, 1447
Fallon OrNda Community Health Fund Grants, 1449
Fidelity Foundation Grants, 1498
Frances W. Emerson Foundation Grants, 1548
Frank Stanley Beveridge Foundation Grants, 1553
Frederick Gardner Cottrell Foundation Grants, 1560
General Mills Foundation Grants, 1590
Georgiana Goddard Eaton Memorial Fund Grants, 1604
Gladys Brooks Foundation Grants, 1620
GoGirlGo! Ambassador Team Awards, 1632
Greater Worcester Community Foundation Discretionary Grants, 1658
Greater Worcester Community Foundation Jeppson Memorial Fund for Brookfield Grants, 1659
Guitar Center Music Foundation Grants, 1675
Hannaford Charitable Foundation Grants, 1692
Harry Kramer Memorial Fund Grants, 1705
Hasbro Children's Fund, 1714
High Meadow Foundation Grants, 1768
IAFF Burn Foundation Research Grants, 1830
J. Walton Bissell Foundation Grants, 1872
Jane's Trust Grants, 1904
Jessie B. Cox Charitable Trust Grants, 1918
John Merck Fund Grants, 1940
John Merck Scholars Awards, 1941
John W. Alden Trust Grants, 1947
Johnson & Johnson Community Health Care Program Grants, 1951
Josephine G. Russell Trust Grants, 1963
KeySpan Foundation Grants, 1995
Mass Youth Against Tobacco Mini-Grants, 2123
Maxtor Corporate Contributions Grants, 2136
Metrowest Community Health Care Foundation Grants, 2176
Middlesex Savings Charitable Foundation Grants, 2196
Multiple Sclerosis Foundation Brighter Tomorrow Grants, 2228
NEI Mentored Clinical Scientist Development Program Award (K12), 2295
NMF Franklin C. McLean Award, 2829
NMF General Electric Medical Scholars Fellowships, 2830
NMF Henry G. Halladay Awards, 2831
NMF Mary Ball Carrera Scholarship, 2834
NMF National Medical Association Awards for Medical Journalism, 2836
NMF National Medical Association Emerging Scholar Awards, 2837
NMF National Medical Association Patti LaBelle Award, 2838
NMF Need-Based Scholarships, 2839
NMF Ralph W. Ellison Prize, 2840
NMF William and Charlotte Cadbury Award, 2841
Nordson Corporation Foundation Grants, 2851
Northeast Utilities Foundation Grants, 2863
NSF Major Research Instrumentation Program (MRI) Grants, 2889
OneSight Research Foundation Block Grants, 2944
Peabody Foundation Grants, 3010
Perpetual Trust for Charitable Giving Grants, 3015
Peter and Elizabeth C. Tower Foundation Community Grants, 3018
Pfizer/AAFP Foundation Visiting Professorship Program in Family Medicine, 3027
Polaroid Fund Grants Program, 3065
Richard and Susan Smith Family Foundation Grants, 3159
Robert F. Stoico / FIRSTFED Charitable Foundation Grants, 3171
Rosalinde and Arthur Gilbert Foundation/AFAR New Investigator Awards in Alzheimer's Disease, 3187
Ruth H. and Warren A. Ellsworth Foundation Grants, 3203
Shaw's Supermarkets Donations, 3280
Smith Family New Investigator Awards, 3299
Sprague Foundation Grants Program, 3359
Tylenol Scholarship, 3444
U.S. Department of Education Erma Byrd Scholarships, 3446
U.S. Department of Education United States-Russia Program: Improving Research and Educational Activities in Higher Education, 3451
US Airways Community Contributions, 3472
US CRDF Leishmaniasis: Collaborative Research Opportunities in North Africa and the Middle East, 3474
Verizon Foundation Northeast Region Grants, 3489
Wal-Mart Foundation Community Grants, 3513
Wal-Mart State Giving Program Grants, 3514
William G. Kelley Foundation Grants, 3538
Winifred & Harry B. Allen Foundation Grants, 3543

Michigan

3M Company Health and Human Services Grants, 10
3M Foundation Grants, 11
Abbott Fund Access to Health Care Grants, 176
Abbott Fund Community Vitality Grants, 177
Abbott Fund Global AIDS Care Grants, 178
Abbott Fund Science and Medical Innovation Grants, 179
ACE Charitable Foundation Grants, 199
ACF Ethnic Community Self-Help Grants, 200
ACF Preferred Communities Grants, 201
ACF Standing Announcement for Unaccompanied Alien Children Grants, 202
ACF Supplemental Services for Recently Arrived Refugees Grants, 203
Actors Fund Social Services and Financial Assistance, 225
Albertson's Charitable Giving Grants, 330
Allegan County Community Foundation Grants, 358
American College of Surgeons and The Triological Society Clinical Scientist Development Awards, 422
American Electric Power Grants, 434
Ann and Robert H. Lurie Family Foundation Grants, 475
Ann Arbor Area Community Foundation Grants, 476
Arkema Foundation Science Teachers Program, 535
ASHA Advancing Academic-Research Careers (AARC) Award, 569
ASHA Minority Student Leadership Program Awards, 570
ASHA Multicultural Activities Projects Grants, 571
ASHA Research Mentoring-Pair Travel Award, 572
ASHA Student Research Travel Award, 573
ASHA Students Preparing for Academic & Research Careers (SPARC) Award, 574
ASM Millis-Colwell Postgraduate Travel Grant, 608
AT&T Excelerator, 657
Battle Creek Community Foundation Grants, 703
Batts Foundation Grants, 704
BCBSM Building Healthy Communities Engaging Elementary Schools and Community Partners Grants, 713
BCBSM Claude Pepper Award, 714
BCBSM Community Health Matching Grants, 715
BCBSM Corporate Contributions Grants, 716
BCBSM Foundation Excellence in Research Awards for Students, 717
BCBSM Foundation Physician Investigator Research Awards, 718
BCBSM Foundation Primary and Clinical Prevention Grants, 719
BCBSM Foundation Proposal Development Awards, 720
BCBSM Foundation Student Award Program, 721
BCBSM Frank J. McDevitt, DO, Excellence in Research Awards, 722
BCBSM Investigator-Initiated Research Program Grants, 723
Bearemy's Kennel Pals Grants, 728
Beldon Fund Grants, 738
Berrien Community Foundation Grants, 749
Besser Foundation Grants, 752
Birds Eye Foods Foundation Grants, 759
Bridgestone/Firestone Trust Fund Grants, 792
Cable Positive's Tony Cox Community Fund Grants, 827
Capital Region Community Foundation Grants, 862
Carls Foundation Grants, 876
Carrier Corporation Contributions Grants, 884
CDC Injury Control Research Centers Grants, 913
Champ-A Champion Fur Kids Grants, 959
Children Affected by AIDS Foundation Camp Network Grants, 994
Children Affected by AIDS Foundation Family Assistance Emergency Fund Grants, 996
CLIF Bar Family Foundation Grants, 1040
Comerica Charitable Foundation Grants, 1073
Community Foundation for Muskegon County Grants, 1093
Community Foundation for Southeastern Michigan Grants, 1094
Community Foundation of Greater Flint Grants, 1107
Consumers Energy Foundation, 1147
CSX Corporate Contributions Grants, 1169
Dean Foods Community Involvement Grants, 1209
DeRoy Testamentary Foundation Grants, 1239
Detroit Lions Charities Grants, 1241
Do Something BR!CK Awards, 1287
Dr. Stanley Pearle Scholarships, 1330
EDS Foundation Grants, 1371
Entergy Corporation Open Grants for Healthy Families, 1418
Fifth Third Foundation Grants, 1501
Fremont Area Community Foundation Grants, 1561
Frey Foundation Grants, 1562
General Mills Foundation Grants, 1590

GoGirlGo! Ambassador Team Awards, 1632
Grand Haven Area Community Foundation Grants, 1644
Grand Rapids Community Foundation Grants, 1647
Guitar Center Music Foundation Grants, 1675
Harry A. and Margaret D. Towsley Foundation Grants, 1701
Harry Kramer Memorial Fund Grants, 1705
Hillsdale County Community Foundation Healthy Senior/Healthy Youth Fund Grants, 1776
Hillsdale County Community General Adult Foundation Grants, 1777
Holland/Zeeland Community Foundation Grants, 1786
Hudson Webber Foundation Grants, 1813
Humana Foundation Grants, 1818
Huntington National Bank Community Affairs Grants, 1824
IAFF Burn Foundation Research Grants, 1830
Irving S. Gilmore Foundation Grants, 1867
Jackson County Community Foundation Unrestricted Grants, 1879
Jacob G. Schmidlapp Trust Grants, 1883
James A. and Faith Knight Foundation Grants, 1884
Jewish Fund Grants, 1923
John Merck Fund Grants, 1940
John Merck Scholars Awards, 1941
Joyce Foundation Grants, 1969
Kalamazoo Foundation Grants, 1979
Kimberly-Clark Community Grants, 2001
Matilda R. Wilson Fund Grants, 2128
McGregor Fund Grants, 2143
Metro Health Foundation Grants, 2175
Multiple Sclerosis Foundation Brighter Tomorrow Grants, 2228
National City Corporation Contributions Grants, 2250
NEI Mentored Clinical Scientist Development Program Award (K12), 2295
NMF Franklin C. McLean Award, 2829
NMF General Electric Medical Scholars Fellowships, 2830
NMF Henry G. Halladay Awards, 2831
NMF Mary Ball Carrera Scholarship, 2834
NMF National Medical Association Awards for Medical Journalism, 2836
NMF National Medical Association Emerging Scholar Awards, 2837
NMF National Medical Association Patti LaBelle Award, 2838
NMF Need-Based Scholarships, 2839
NMF Ralph W. Ellison Prize, 2840
NMF William and Charlotte Cadbury Award, 2841
NSF Major Research Instrumentation Program (MRI) Grants, 2889
OneSight Research Foundation Block Grants, 2944
Pfizer/AAFP Foundation Visiting Professorship Program in Family Medicine, 3027
Richard and Helen DeVos Foundation Grants, 3157
Rollin M. Gerstacker Foundation Grants Program, 3186
Rosalinde and Arthur Gilbert Foundation/AFAR New Investigator Awards in Alzheimer's Disease, 3187
Steelcase Foundation Grants, 3379
Tri-County Electric People Fund Grants, 3436
Tylenol Scholarship, 3444
U.S. Department of Education Erma Byrd Scholarships, 3446
U.S. Department of Education United States-Russia Program: Improving Research and Educational Activities in Higher Education, 3451
US CRDF Leishmaniasis: Collaborative Research Opportunities in North Africa and the Middle East, 3474
Wal-Mart Foundation Community Grants, 3513
Wal-Mart State Giving Program Grants, 3514
Weatherwax Foundation Grants, 3523

Minnesota
3M Company Health and Human Services Grants, 10
3M Foundation Grants, 11
ACE Charitable Foundation Grants, 199
ACF Ethnic Community Self-Help Grants, 200
ACF Preferred Communities Grants, 201
ACF Standing Announcement for Unaccompanied Alien Children Grants, 202
ACF Supplemental Services for Recently Arrived Refugees Grants, 203
Actors Fund Social Services and Financial Assistance, 225
Albertson's Charitable Giving Grants, 330
American College of Surgeons and The Triological Society Clinical Scientist Development Awards, 422
Andersen Corporate Foundation, 470
Arkema Foundation Science Teachers Program, 535
ASHA Advancing Academic-Research Careers (AARC) Award, 569
ASHA Minority Student Leadership Program Awards, 570
ASHA Multicultural Activities Projects Grants, 571
ASHA Research Mentoring-Pair Travel Award, 572
ASHA Student Research Travel Award, 573
ASHA Students Preparing for Academic & Research Careers (SPARC) Award, 574
ASM Millis-Colwell Postgraduate Travel Grant, 608
Athwin Foundation Grants, 660
BCBS of Minnesota Growing Up Healthy Grants, 711
BCBS of Minnesota Healthy Together Grants, 712
Bearemy's Kennel Pals Grants, 728
Beldon Fund Grants, 738
Birds Eye Foods Foundation Grants, 759
Bridgestone/Firestone Trust Fund Grants, 792
Bush Foundation Health & Human Services Grants, 814
Bush Foundation Medical Fellowships, 815
Cable Positive's Tony Cox Community Fund Grants, 827
Carl and Eloise Pohlad Family Foundation Grants, 867
Carolyn Foundation Grants, 880
CDC Injury Control Research Centers Grants, 913
Champ-A Champion Fur Kids Grants, 959
Children Affected by AIDS Foundation Camp Network Grants, 994
Children Affected by AIDS Foundation Family Assistance Emergency Fund Grants, 996
CLIF Bar Family Foundation Grants, 1040
ConAgra Foods Foundation Grants, 1140
Dairy Queen Corporate Contributions Grants, 1187
Dean Foods Community Involvement Grants, 1209
Do Something BR!CK Awards, 1287
Dr. Stanley Pearle Scholarships, 1330
Edina Realty Foundation Grants, 1369
Edwards Memorial Trust Grants, 1375
Elmer L. and Eleanor J. Andersen Foundation Grants, 1406
Emma B. Howe Memorial Foundation Grants, 1415
Fargo-Moorhead Area Foundation Grants, 1454
General Mills Foundation Grants, 1590
George Family Foundation Grants, 1598
Ginn Foundation Grants, 1616
GoGirlGo! Ambassador Team Awards, 1632
Graco Foundation Grants, 1642
Grand Rapids Area Community Foundation Grants, 1645
Grand Rapids Area Community Foundation Nashwauk Area Endowment Fund Grants, 1646
Grotto Foundation Project Grants, 1671
Guitar Center Music Foundation Grants, 1675
Harry Kramer Memorial Fund Grants, 1705
Honeywell Foundation Grants, 1791
Hormel Foods Charitable Trust Grants, 1795
Hormel Foundation Grants, 1796
Hugh J. Andersen Foundation Grants, 1814
IAFF Burn Foundation Research Grants, 1830
James Ford Bell Foundation Grants, 1885
Jay and Rose Phillips Family Foundation Grants, 1909
John Merck Fund Grants, 1940
John Merck Scholars Awards, 1941
Joyce Foundation Grants, 1969
Marion Park Deaver and Harry Gilbert Deaver Foundation Grants, 2110
Medtronic Foundation Fitness and Nutrition Grants, 2167
Medtronic Foundation Health Care Grants, 2169
Minneapolis Foundation Community Grants, 2206
Multiple Sclerosis Foundation Brighter Tomorrow Grants, 2228
NEI Mentored Clinical Scientist Development Program Award (K12), 2295
NMF Franklin C. McLean Award, 2829
NMF General Electric Medical Scholars Fellowships, 2830
NMF Henry G. Halladay Awards, 2831
NMF Hugh J. Andersen Memorial Scholarship, 2832
NMF Mary Ball Carrera Scholarship, 2834
NMF National Medical Association Awards for Medical Journalism, 2836
NMF National Medical Association Emerging Scholar Awards, 2837
NMF National Medical Association Patti LaBelle Award, 2838
NMF Need-Based Scholarships, 2839
NMF Ralph W. Ellison Prize, 2840
NMF William and Charlotte Cadbury Award, 2841
Northwest Minnesota Foundation Women's Fund Grants, 2869
NSF Major Research Instrumentation Program (MRI) Grants, 2889
OneSight Research Foundation Block Grants, 2944
Ordean Foundation Grants, 2952
Otto Bremer Foundation Grants, 2977
Pfizer/AAFP Foundation Visiting Professorship Program in Family Medicine, 3027
Piper Jaffray Companies Building Strong Communities Grants, 3053
Prudential Foundation Grants, 3087
Rathmann Family Foundation Grants, 3109
Rochester Area Foundation Grants, 3177
Rosalinde and Arthur Gilbert Foundation/AFAR New Investigator Awards in Alzheimer's Disease, 3187
Salem Foundation Grants, 3242
Toro Foundation Grants, 3431
Tylenol Scholarship, 3444
U.S. Department of Education Erma Byrd Scholarships, 3446
U.S. Department of Education United States-Russia Program: Improving Research and Educational Activities in Higher Education, 3451
US CRDF Leishmaniasis: Collaborative Research Opportunities in North Africa and the Middle East, 3474
US Trust Corporation Foundation Grants, 3475
Viking Children's Fund Grants, 3497
Wal-Mart Foundation Community Grants, 3513
Wal-Mart State Giving Program Grants, 3514
Wasie Foundation Grants, 3521

Mississippi
ACF Ethnic Community Self-Help Grants, 200
ACF Preferred Communities Grants, 201
ACF Standing Announcement for Unaccompanied Alien Children Grants, 202
ACF Supplemental Services for Recently Arrived Refugees Grants, 203
Actors Fund Social Services and Financial Assistance, 225
Albertson's Charitable Giving Grants, 330
American College of Surgeons and The Triological Society Clinical Scientist Development Awards, 422
ASHA Advancing Academic-Research Careers (AARC) Award, 569

ASHA Minority Student Leadership Program Awards, 570
ASHA Multicultural Activities Projects Grants, 571
ASHA Research Mentoring-Pair Travel Award, 572
ASHA Student Research Travel Award, 573
ASHA Students Preparing for Academic & Research Careers (SPARC) Award, 574
ASM Millis-Colwell Postgraduate Travel Grant, 608
AT&T Excelerator, 657
Bearemy's Kennel Pals Grants, 728
Belk Foundation Grants, 739
Boyd Gaming Corporation Contributions Program, 788
Bridgestone/Firestone Trust Fund Grants, 792
Cable Positive's Tony Cox Community Fund Grants, 827
CDC Injury Control Research Centers Grants, 913
Champ-A Champion Fur Kids Grants, 959
Charles A. Frueauff Foundation Grants, 962
Children Affected by AIDS Foundation Camp Network Grants, 994
Children Affected by AIDS Foundation Family Assistance Emergency Fund Grants, 996
CLIF Bar Family Foundation Grants, 1040
Commission on Religion in Appalachia Grants, 1074
CSX Corporate Contributions Grants, 1169
DHHS Healthy Tomorrows Partnership for Children, 1261
Do Something BR!CK Awards, 1287
Dr. Stanley Pearle Scholarships, 1330
Entergy Community Partnership Grants, 1417
Entergy Corporation Open Grants for Healthy Families, 1418
Foundation for the Mid-South Grants, 1536
GoGirlGo! Ambassador Team Awards, 1632
Guitar Center Music Foundation Grants, 1675
Gulf Coast Community Foundation Grants, 1676
Harry Kramer Memorial Fund Grants, 1705
IAFF Burn Foundation Research Grants, 1830
Joe W. and Dorothy Dorsett Brown Foundation Grants, 1927
John Merck Fund Grants, 1940
John Merck Scholars Awards, 1941
Kimberly-Clark Community Grants, 2001
Lettie Pate Whitehead Foundation Grants, 2049
Multiple Sclerosis Foundation Brighter Tomorrow Grants, 2228
NEI Mentored Clinical Scientist Development Program Award (K12), 2295
NMF Franklin C. McLean Award, 2829
NMF General Electric Medical Scholars Fellowships, 2830
NMF Henry G. Halladay Awards, 2831
NMF Mary Ball Carrera Scholarship, 2834
NMF National Medical Association Awards for Medical Journalism, 2836
NMF National Medical Association Emerging Scholar Awards, 2837
NMF National Medical Association Patti LaBelle Award, 2838
NMF Need-Based Scholarships, 2839
NMF Ralph W. Ellison Prize, 2840
NMF William and Charlotte Cadbury Award, 2841
NSF Major Research Instrumentation Program (MRI) Grants, 2889
OneSight Research Foundation Block Grants, 2944
Pfizer/AAFP Foundation Visiting Professorship Program in Family Medicine, 3027
Plum Creek Foundation Grants, 3062
Rainbow Fund Grants, 3103
Riley Foundation Grants, 3165
Rosalinde and Arthur Gilbert Foundation/AFAR New Investigator Awards in Alzheimer's Disease, 3187
Southwire Company Grants, 3353
Toro Foundation Grants, 3431
Tylenol Scholarship, 3444
U.S. Department of Education Erma Byrd Scholarships, 3446
U.S. Department of Education United States-Russia Program: Improving Research and Educational Activities in Higher Education, 3451
US CRDF Leishmaniasis: Collaborative Research Opportunities in North Africa and the Middle East, 3474
Vulcan Materials Company Foundation Grants, 3504
Wal-Mart Foundation Community Grants, 3513
Wal-Mart State Giving Program Grants, 3514

Missouri

3M Company Health and Human Services Grants, 10
3M Foundation Grants, 11
ACF Ethnic Community Self-Help Grants, 200
ACF Preferred Communities Grants, 201
ACF Standing Announcement for Unaccompanied Alien Children Grants, 202
ACF Supplemental Services for Recently Arrived Refugees Grants, 203
Actors Fund Social Services and Financial Assistance, 225
Albertson's Charitable Giving Grants, 330
Allen P. and Josephine B. Green Foundation Grants, 361
American College of Surgeons and The Triological Society Clinical Scientist Development Awards, 422
Anheuser-Busch Foundation Grants, 474
Anthem Blue Cross and Blue Shield Grants, 488
ASHA Advancing Academic-Research Careers (AARC) Award, 569
ASHA Minority Student Leadership Program Awards, 570
ASHA Multicultural Activities Projects Grants, 571
ASHA Research Mentoring-Pair Travel Award, 572
ASHA Student Research Travel Award, 573
ASHA Students Preparing for Academic & Research Careers (SPARC) Award, 574
ASM Millis-Colwell Postgraduate Travel Grant, 608
AT&T Excelerator, 657
Baptist-Trinity Lutheran Legacy Foundation Grants, 692
Bearemy's Kennel Pals Grants, 728
C.W. Titus Foundation Grants, 826
Cable Positive's Tony Cox Community Fund Grants, 827
Champ-A Champion Fur Kids Grants, 959
Charles A. Frueauff Foundation Grants, 962
Children Affected by AIDS Foundation Camp Network Grants, 994
Children Affected by AIDS Foundation Family Assistance Emergency Fund Grants, 996
CLIF Bar Family Foundation Grants, 1040
Community Foundation of the Ozarks Grants, 1130
Cooper Industries Foundation Grants, 1150
Dana Brown Charitable Trust Grants, 1194
DHHS Healthy Tomorrows Partnership for Children, 1261
Do Something BR!CK Awards, 1287
Dr. Stanley Pearle Scholarships, 1330
FMC Foundation Grants, 1518
General Mills Foundation Grants, 1590
GoGirlGo! Ambassador Team Awards, 1632
Guitar Center Music Foundation Grants, 1675
H & R Foundation Grants, 1679
Hallmark Corporate Foundation Grants, 1688
Harley Davidson Foundation Grants, 1694
Harry Kramer Memorial Fund Grants, 1705
IAFF Burn Foundation Research Grants, 1830
J.B. Reynolds Foundation Grants, 1873
J.E. and L.E. Mabee Foundation Grants, 1875
John Deere Foundation Grants, 1929
John Merck Fund Grants, 1940
John Merck Scholars Awards, 1941
Joseph H. and Florence A. Roblee Foundation Grants, 1961
Multiple Sclerosis Foundation Brighter Tomorrow Grants, 2228
National City Corporation Contributions Grants, 2250
National Starch and Chemical Foundation Grants, 2261
NEI Mentored Clinical Scientist Development Program Award (K12), 2295
NMF Franklin C. McLean Award, 2829
NMF General Electric Medical Scholars Fellowships, 2830
NMF Henry G. Halladay Awards, 2831
NMF Mary Ball Carrera Scholarship, 2834
NMF National Medical Association Awards for Medical Journalism, 2836
NMF National Medical Association Emerging Scholar Awards, 2837
NMF National Medical Association Patti LaBelle Award, 2838
NMF Need-Based Scholarships, 2839
NMF Ralph W. Ellison Prize, 2840
NMF William and Charlotte Cadbury Award, 2841
NSF Major Research Instrumentation Program (MRI) Grants, 2889
OneSight Research Foundation Block Grants, 2944
Pfizer/AAFP Foundation Visiting Professorship Program in Family Medicine, 3027
Piper Jaffray Companies Building Strong Communities Grants, 3053
Pott Foundation Grants, 3071
Rosalinde and Arthur Gilbert Foundation/AFAR New Investigator Awards in Alzheimer's Disease, 3187
RRF General Program Grants, 3193
Sosland Foundation Grants, 3348
Sunderland Foundation Grants, 3400
Tylenol Scholarship, 3444
U.S. Department of Education Erma Byrd Scholarships, 3446
U.S. Department of Education United States-Russia Program: Improving Research and Educational Activities in Higher Education, 3451
US CRDF Leishmaniasis: Collaborative Research Opportunities in North Africa and the Middle East, 3474
Vulcan Materials Company Foundation Grants, 3504
Wal-Mart Foundation Community Grants, 3513
Wal-Mart State Giving Program Grants, 3514
William G. McGowan Charitable Fund Grants, 3539

Montana

ACF Ethnic Community Self-Help Grants, 200
ACF Preferred Communities Grants, 201
ACF Standing Announcement for Unaccompanied Alien Children Grants, 202
ACF Supplemental Services for Recently Arrived Refugees Grants, 203
Actors Fund Social Services and Financial Assistance, 225
Albertson's Charitable Giving Grants, 330
American College of Surgeons and The Triological Society Clinical Scientist Development Awards, 422
ASHA Advancing Academic-Research Careers (AARC) Award, 569
ASHA Minority Student Leadership Program Awards, 570
ASHA Multicultural Activities Projects Grants, 571
ASHA Research Mentoring-Pair Travel Award, 572
ASHA Student Research Travel Award, 573
ASHA Students Preparing for Academic & Research Careers (SPARC) Award, 574
ASM Millis-Colwell Postgraduate Travel Grant, 608
Athwin Foundation Grants, 660
Bearemy's Kennel Pals Grants, 728
Bullitt Foundation Grants, 809
Cable Positive's Tony Cox Community Fund Grants, 827
Champ-A Champion Fur Kids Grants, 959
Charles M. Bair Family Trust Grants, 972
Children Affected by AIDS Foundation Camp Network Grants, 994

Children Affected by AIDS Foundation Family Assistance Emergency Fund Grants, 996
CLIF Bar Family Foundation Grants, 1040
ConocoPhillips Foundation Grants, 1144
Dean Foods Community Involvement Grants, 1209
Dennis and Phyllis Washington Foundation Grants, 1222
DHHS Healthy Tomorrows Partnership for Children, 1261
Do Something BR!CK Awards, 1287
Dr. Stanley Pearle Scholarships, 1330
Foster Foundation Grants, 1524
General Mills Foundation Grants, 1590
GoGirlGo! Ambassador Team Awards, 1632
Guitar Center Music Foundation Grants, 1675
Harry Kramer Memorial Fund Grants, 1705
IAFF Burn Foundation Research Grants, 1830
John Merck Fund Grants, 1940
John Merck Scholars Awards, 1941
M.J. Murdock Charitable Trust Grants, 2095
Multiple Sclerosis Foundation Brighter Tomorrow Grants, 2228
NEI Mentored Clinical Scientist Development Program Award (K12), 2295
NMF Franklin C. McLean Award, 2829
NMF General Electric Medical Scholars Fellowships, 2830
NMF Henry G. Halladay Awards, 2831
NMF Mary Ball Carrera Scholarship, 2834
NMF National Medical Association Awards for Medical Journalism, 2836
NMF National Medical Association Emerging Scholar Awards, 2837
NMF National Medical Association Patti LaBelle Award, 2838
NMF Need-Based Scholarships, 2839
NMF Ralph W. Ellison Prize, 2840
NMF William and Charlotte Cadbury Award, 2841
NSF Major Research Instrumentation Program (MRI) Grants, 2889
OneSight Research Foundation Block Grants, 2944
Paul G. Allen Family Foundation Grants, 3000
Pfizer/AAFP Foundation Visiting Professorship Program in Family Medicine, 3027
Piper Jaffray Companies Building Strong Communities Grants, 3053
Plum Creek Foundation Grants, 3062
Pride Foundation Grants and Scholarships, 3078
Rosalinde and Arthur Gilbert Foundation/AFAR New Investigator Awards in Alzheimer's Disease, 3187
Steele-Reese Foundation Grants, 3380
Sunderland Foundation Grants, 3400
Tylenol Scholarship, 3444
U.S. Department of Education Erma Byrd Scholarships, 3446
U.S. Department of Education United States-Russia Program: Improving Research and Educational Activities in Higher Education, 3451
US CRDF Leishmaniasis: Collaborative Research Opportunities in North Africa and the Middle East, 3474
Wal-Mart Foundation Community Grants, 3513
Wal-Mart State Giving Program Grants, 3514

Nebraska

3M Company Health and Human Services Grants, 10
3M Foundation Grants, 11
Abel Foundation Grants, 181
ACF Ethnic Community Self-Help Grants, 200
ACF Preferred Communities Grants, 201
ACF Standing Announcement for Unaccompanied Alien Children Grants, 202
ACF Supplemental Services for Recently Arrived Refugees Grants, 203
Actors Fund Social Services and Financial Assistance, 225
Albertson's Charitable Giving Grants, 330
American College of Surgeons and The Triological Society Clinical Scientist Development Awards, 422
ASHA Advancing Academic-Research Careers (AARC) Award, 569
ASHA Minority Student Leadership Program Awards, 570
ASHA Multicultural Activities Projects Grants, 571
ASHA Research Mentoring-Pair Travel Award, 572
ASHA Student Research Travel Award, 573
ASHA Students Preparing for Academic & Research Careers (SPARC) Award, 574
ASM Millis-Colwell Postgraduate Travel Grant, 608
Bearemy's Kennel Pals Grants, 728
Cable Positive's Tony Cox Community Fund Grants, 827
Champ-A Champion Fur Kids Grants, 959
Charles A. Frueauff Foundation Grants, 962
Children Affected by AIDS Foundation Camp Network Grants, 994
Children Affected by AIDS Foundation Family Assistance Emergency Fund Grants, 996
Clarcor Foundation Grants, 1021
CLIF Bar Family Foundation Grants, 1040
ConAgra Foods Foundation Grants, 1140
Dean Foods Community Involvement Grants, 1209
Do Something BR!CK Awards, 1287
Dr. Stanley Pearle Scholarships, 1330
Ethel S. Abbott Charitable Foundation Grants, 1430
GoGirlGo! Ambassador Team Awards, 1632
Guitar Center Music Foundation Grants, 1675
Harry Kramer Memorial Fund Grants, 1705
Hormel Foods Charitable Trust Grants, 1795
IAFF Burn Foundation Research Grants, 1830
John Merck Fund Grants, 1940
John Merck Scholars Awards, 1941
Lincoln Financial Group Foundation Grants, 2058
Multiple Sclerosis Foundation Brighter Tomorrow Grants, 2228
NEI Mentored Clinical Scientist Development Program Award (K12), 2295
NMF Franklin C. McLean Award, 2829
NMF General Electric Medical Scholars Fellowships, 2830
NMF Henry G. Halladay Awards, 2831
NMF Mary Ball Carrera Scholarship, 2834
NMF National Medical Association Awards for Medical Journalism, 2836
NMF National Medical Association Emerging Scholar Awards, 2837
NMF National Medical Association Patti LaBelle Award, 2838
NMF Need-Based Scholarships, 2839
NMF Ralph W. Ellison Prize, 2840
NMF William and Charlotte Cadbury Award, 2841
NSF Major Research Instrumentation Program (MRI) Grants, 2889
OneSight Research Foundation Block Grants, 2944
Pfizer/AAFP Foundation Visiting Professorship Program in Family Medicine, 3027
Piper Jaffray Companies Building Strong Communities Grants, 3053
Principal Financial Group Foundation Grants, 3082
Rosalinde and Arthur Gilbert Foundation/AFAR New Investigator Awards in Alzheimer's Disease, 3187
Square D Foundation Grants, 3361
Sunderland Foundation Grants, 3400
Toro Foundation Grants, 3431
Tylenol Scholarship, 3444
U.S. Department of Education Erma Byrd Scholarships, 3446
U.S. Department of Education United States-Russia Program: Improving Research and Educational Activities in Higher Education, 3451
US CRDF Leishmaniasis: Collaborative Research Opportunities in North Africa and the Middle East, 3474
Waitt Family Foundation Grants, 3512
Wal-Mart Foundation Community Grants, 3513
Wal-Mart State Giving Program Grants, 3514
Western Union Foundation Grants, 3529

Nevada

ACE Charitable Foundation Grants, 199
ACF Ethnic Community Self-Help Grants, 200
ACF Preferred Communities Grants, 201
ACF Standing Announcement for Unaccompanied Alien Children Grants, 202
ACF Supplemental Services for Recently Arrived Refugees Grants, 203
Actors Fund Social Services and Financial Assistance, 225
Albertson's Charitable Giving Grants, 330
American College of Surgeons and The Triological Society Clinical Scientist Development Awards, 422
Anthem Blue Cross and Blue Shield Grants, 488
ARCO Foundation Education Grants, 526
ASHA Advancing Academic-Research Careers (AARC) Award, 569
ASHA Minority Student Leadership Program Awards, 570
ASHA Multicultural Activities Projects Grants, 571
ASHA Research Mentoring-Pair Travel Award, 572
ASHA Student Research Travel Award, 573
ASHA Students Preparing for Academic & Research Careers (SPARC) Award, 574
ASM Millis-Colwell Postgraduate Travel Grant, 608
AT&T Excelerator, 657
Bearemy's Kennel Pals Grants, 728
Boyd Gaming Corporation Contributions Program, 788
Bridgestone/Firestone Trust Fund Grants, 792
Business Bank of Nevada Community Grants, 817
Cable Positive's Tony Cox Community Fund Grants, 827
Carrier Corporation Contributions Grants, 884
CDC Injury Control Research Centers Grants, 913
Champ-A Champion Fur Kids Grants, 959
Children Affected by AIDS Foundation Camp Network Grants, 994
Children Affected by AIDS Foundation Family Assistance Emergency Fund Grants, 996
CLIF Bar Family Foundation Grants, 1040
Dean Foods Community Involvement Grants, 1209
Del E. Webb Foundation Grants, 1213
DHHS Healthy Tomorrows Partnership for Children, 1261
Do Something BR!CK Awards, 1287
Dr. Stanley Pearle Scholarships, 1330
E.L. Wiegand Foundation Grants, 1361
GoGirlGo! Ambassador Team Awards, 1632
Greenspun Family Foundation Grants, 1664
Guitar Center Music Foundation Grants, 1675
Harry Kramer Memorial Fund Grants, 1705
IAFF Burn Foundation Research Grants, 1830
John Merck Fund Grants, 1940
John Merck Scholars Awards, 1941
Multiple Sclerosis Foundation Brighter Tomorrow Grants, 2228
NEI Mentored Clinical Scientist Development Program Award (K12), 2295
NMF Franklin C. McLean Award, 2829
NMF General Electric Medical Scholars Fellowships, 2830
NMF Henry G. Halladay Awards, 2831
NMF Mary Ball Carrera Scholarship, 2834
NMF National Medical Association Awards for Medical Journalism, 2836
NMF National Medical Association Emerging Scholar Awards, 2837
NMF National Medical Association Patti LaBelle Award, 2838
NMF Need-Based Scholarships, 2839
NMF Ralph W. Ellison Prize, 2840
NMF William and Charlotte Cadbury Award, 2841
NSF Major Research Instrumentation Program (MRI) Grants, 2889

OneSight Research Foundation Block Grants, 2944
PacifiCare Foundation Grants, 2981
Pfizer/AAFP Foundation Visiting Professorship Program in Family Medicine, 3027
Piper Jaffray Companies Building Strong Communities Grants, 3053
Rosalinde and Arthur Gilbert Foundation/AFAR New Investigator Awards in Alzheimer's Disease, 3187
Southwest Gas Corporation Foundation Grants, 3352
Tylenol Scholarship, 3444
U.S. Department of Education Erma Byrd Scholarships, 3446
U.S. Department of Education United States-Russia Program: Improving Research and Educational Activities in Higher Education, 3451
US Airways Community Contributions, 3472
US CRDF Leishmaniasis: Collaborative Research Opportunities in North Africa and the Middle East, 3474
Wal-Mart Foundation Community Grants, 3513
Wal-Mart State Giving Program Grants, 3514

New Hampshire
ACF Ethnic Community Self-Help Grants, 200
ACF Preferred Communities Grants, 201
ACF Standing Announcement for Unaccompanied Alien Children Grants, 202
ACF Supplemental Services for Recently Arrived Refugees Grants, 203
Actors Fund Social Services and Financial Assistance, 225
Agnes M. Lindsay Trust Grants, 263
Albertson's Charitable Giving Grants, 330
Alexander Eastman Foundation Grants, 341
American College of Surgeons and The Triological Society Clinical Scientist Development Awards, 422
Anheuser-Busch Foundation Grants, 474
Anthem Blue Cross and Blue Shield Grants, 488
ASHA Advancing Academic-Research Careers (AARC) Award, 569
ASHA Minority Student Leadership Program Awards, 570
ASHA Multicultural Activities Projects Grants, 571
ASHA Research Mentoring-Pair Travel Award, 572
ASHA Student Research Travel Award, 573
ASHA Students Preparing for Academic & Research Careers (SPARC) Award, 574
ASM Millis-Colwell Postgraduate Travel Grant, 608
Barker Foundation Grants, 694
Barnes Group Foundation Grants, 696
Bearemy's Kennel Pals Grants, 728
BJ's Charitable Foundation Grants, 761
Cable Positive's Tony Cox Community Fund Grants, 827
Carlisle Foundation Grants, 874
Champ-A Champion Fur Kids Grants, 959
Charles A. Frueauff Foundation Grants, 962
Charles H. Hood Foundation Child Health Research Grants, 968
Chase Paymentech Corporate Giving Grants, 975
Children Affected by AIDS Foundation Camp Network Grants, 994
Children Affected by AIDS Foundation Family Assistance Emergency Fund Grants, 996
CLIF Bar Family Foundation Grants, 1040
DHHS Healthy Tomorrows Partnership for Children, 1261
Do Something BR!CK Awards, 1287
Dr. Stanley Pearle Scholarships, 1330
Entergy Corporation Open Grants for Healthy Families, 1418
Fidelity Foundation Grants, 1498
Foundation for Seacoast Health Grants, 1533
Gladys Brooks Foundation Grants, 1620
GoGirlGo! Ambassador Team Awards, 1632
Guitar Center Music Foundation Grants, 1675
Hannaford Charitable Foundation Grants, 1692
Harry Kramer Memorial Fund Grants, 1705
IAFF Burn Foundation Research Grants, 1830
J. Walton Bissell Foundation Grants, 1872
Jane's Trust Grants, 1904
Jessie B. Cox Charitable Trust Grants, 1918
John Merck Fund Grants, 1940
John Merck Scholars Awards, 1941
KeySpan Foundation Grants, 1995
Lincoln Financial Group Foundation Grants, 2058
Multiple Sclerosis Foundation Brighter Tomorrow Grants, 2228
NEI Mentored Clinical Scientist Development Program Award (K12), 2295
NMF Franklin C. McLean Award, 2829
NMF General Electric Medical Scholars Fellowships, 2830
NMF Henry G. Halladay Awards, 2831
NMF Mary Ball Carrera Scholarship, 2834
NMF National Medical Association Awards for Medical Journalism, 2836
NMF National Medical Association Emerging Scholar Awards, 2837
NMF National Medical Association Patti LaBelle Award, 2838
NMF Need-Based Scholarships, 2839
NMF Ralph W. Ellison Prize, 2840
NMF William and Charlotte Cadbury Award, 2841
Northeast Utilities Foundation Grants, 2863
Norwin S. and Elizabeth N. Bean Foundation Grants, 2872
NSF Major Research Instrumentation Program (MRI) Grants, 2889
Oleonda Jameson Trust Grants, 2941
OneSight Research Foundation Block Grants, 2944
Pfizer/AAFP Foundation Visiting Professorship Program in Family Medicine, 3027
Rosalinde and Arthur Gilbert Foundation/AFAR New Investigator Awards in Alzheimer's Disease, 3187
Shaw's Supermarkets Donations, 3280
Tylenol Scholarship, 3444
U.S. Department of Education Erma Byrd Scholarships, 3446
U.S. Department of Education United States-Russia Program: Improving Research and Educational Activities in Higher Education, 3451
US CRDF Leishmaniasis: Collaborative Research Opportunities in North Africa and the Middle East, 3474
Wal-Mart Foundation Community Grants, 3513
Wal-Mart State Giving Program Grants, 3514

New Jersey
1 in 9: Long Island Breast Cancer Action Coalition Grants, 1
3M Company Health and Human Services Grants, 10
Abbott Fund Access to Health Care Grants, 176
Abbott Fund Community Vitality Grants, 177
Abbott Fund Global AIDS Care Grants, 178
Abbott Fund Science and Medical Innovation Grants, 179
ACE Charitable Foundation Grants, 199
ACF Ethnic Community Self-Help Grants, 200
ACF Preferred Communities Grants, 201
ACF Standing Announcement for Unaccompanied Alien Children Grants, 202
ACF Supplemental Services for Recently Arrived Refugees Grants, 203
Achelis and Bodman Foundations Grants, 206
Actors Fund Social Services and Financial Assistance, 225
African American Fund of New Jersey Grants, 260
Albertson's Charitable Giving Grants, 330
American College of Surgeons and The Triological Society Clinical Scientist Development Awards, 422
Anheuser-Busch Foundation Grants, 474
Ansell, Zaro, Grimm & Aaron Foundation Grants, 487
Arkema Foundation Science Teachers Program, 535
ASHA Advancing Academic-Research Careers (AARC) Award, 569
ASHA Minority Student Leadership Program Awards, 570
ASHA Multicultural Activities Projects Grants, 571
ASHA Research Mentoring-Pair Travel Award, 572
ASHA Student Research Travel Award, 573
ASHA Students Preparing for Academic & Research Careers (SPARC) Award, 574
ASM Millis-Colwell Postgraduate Travel Grant, 608
Bearemy's Kennel Pals Grants, 728
Bildner Family Foundation Grants, 755
BJ's Charitable Foundation Grants, 761
Blanche and Irving Laurie Foundation Grants, 764
Bodman Foundation Grants Program, 776
Boyd Gaming Corporation Contributions Program, 788
Bristol-Myers Squibb Foundation Health Disparities Grants, 797
Brook J. Lenfest Foundation Grants, 804
C.R. Bard Foundation Grants, 825
Cable Positive's Tony Cox Community Fund Grants, 827
Carl C. Icahn Foundation Grants, 870
CDC Injury Control Research Centers Grants, 913
Champ-A Champion Fur Kids Grants, 959
Charles A. Frueauff Foundation Grants, 962
Children Affected by AIDS Foundation Camp Network Grants, 994
Children Affected by AIDS Foundation Family Assistance Emergency Fund Grants, 996
CLIF Bar Family Foundation Grants, 1040
ConocoPhillips Foundation Grants, 1144
CSX Corporate Contributions Grants, 1169
Danellie Foundation Grants, 1198
Dean Foods Community Involvement Grants, 1209
DHHS Healthy Tomorrows Partnership for Children, 1261
Do Something BR!CK Awards, 1287
Dr. Stanley Pearle Scholarships, 1330
F.M. Kirby Foundation Grants, 1443
FirstEnergy Foundation Community Grants, 1505
Fluor Foundation Grants, 1517
FMC Foundation Grants, 1518
Frances L. and Edwin L. Cummings Memorial Fund Grants, 1547
General Mills Foundation Grants, 1590
Geraldine R. Dodge Foundation Morris County Grants, 1605
Gladys Brooks Foundation Grants, 1620
GoGirlGo! Ambassador Team Awards, 1632
Guitar Center Music Foundation Grants, 1675
Hackett Foundation Grants, 1684
Harry Kramer Memorial Fund Grants, 1705
Healthcare Foundation of New Jersey Grants, 1729
HHK Employment Grants, 1755
Horizon Foundation for New Jersey Grants, 1793
IAFF Burn Foundation Research Grants, 1830
Independence Community Foundation Community Quality of Life Grant, 1849
John Merck Fund Grants, 1940
John Merck Scholars Awards, 1941
Johnson & Johnson Community Health Care Program Grants, 1951
Land O'Lakes Foundation Mid-Atlantic Grants Program, 2027
Little Life Foundation Grants, 2060
Mary Owen Borden Foundation Grants, 2121
Multiple Sclerosis Foundation Brighter Tomorrow Grants, 2228
National Starch and Chemical Foundation Grants, 2261
NEI Mentored Clinical Scientist Development Program Award (K12), 2295
New Jersey Osteopathic Education Foundation Scholarships, 2303
NMF Franklin C. McLean Award, 2829
NMF General Electric Medical Scholars Fellowships, 2830
NMF Henry G. Halladay Awards, 2831

NMF Mary Ball Carrera Scholarship, 2834
NMF National Medical Association Awards for Medical Journalism, 2836
NMF National Medical Association Emerging Scholar Awards, 2837
NMF National Medical Association Patti LaBelle Award, 2838
NMF Need-Based Scholarships, 2839
NMF Ralph W. Ellison Prize, 2840
NMF William and Charlotte Cadbury Award, 2841
NSF Major Research Instrumentation Program (MRI) Grants, 2889
OceanFirst Foundation Grants, 2933
OneSight Research Foundation Block Grants, 2944
Pfizer/AAFP Foundation Visiting Professorship Program in Family Medicine, 3027
PNC Charitable Trust and Foundation Grants, 3064
Princeton Area Community Foundation Greater Mercer Grants, 3081
Prudential Foundation Grants, 3087
Rosalinde and Arthur Gilbert Foundation/AFAR New Investigator Awards in Alzheimer's Disease, 3187
Russell Berrie Foundation Grants, 3201
RWJF New Jersey Health Initiatives Grants, 3225
Tylenol Scholarship, 3444
U.S. Department of Education Erma Byrd Scholarships, 3446
U.S. Department of Education United States-Russia Program: Improving Research and Educational Activities in Higher Education, 3451
US CRDF Leishmaniasis: Collaborative Research Opportunities in North Africa and the Middle East, 3474
US Trust Corporation Foundation Grants, 3475
W.W. Smith Charitable Trust Grants for Medical Research in Cancer, AIDS, and Heart Disease, 3509
Wal-Mart Foundation Community Grants, 3513
Wal-Mart State Giving Program Grants, 3514
YSA UnitedHealth Heroes Service Learning Grants, 3556

New Mexico

ACF Ethnic Community Self-Help Grants, 200
ACF Preferred Communities Grants, 201
ACF Standing Announcement for Unaccompanied Alien Children Grants, 202
ACF Supplemental Services for Recently Arrived Refugees Grants, 203
Actors Fund Social Services and Financial Assistance, 225
Albertson's Charitable Giving Grants, 330
Albuquerque Community Foundation Grants, 331
American College of Surgeons and The Triological Society Clinical Scientist Development Awards, 422
ASHA Advancing Academic-Research Careers (AARC) Award, 569
ASHA Minority Student Leadership Program Awards, 570
ASHA Multicultural Activities Projects Grants, 571
ASHA Research Mentoring-Pair Travel Award, 572
ASHA Student Research Travel Award, 573
ASHA Students Preparing for Academic & Research Careers (SPARC) Award, 574
ASM Millis-Colwell Postgraduate Travel Grant, 608
Bearemy's Kennel Pals Grants, 728
Cable Positive's Tony Cox Community Fund Grants, 827
CDC Injury Control Research Centers Grants, 913
Champ-A Champion Fur Kids Grants, 959
Charles A. Frueauff Foundation Grants, 962
Children Affected by AIDS Foundation Camp Network Grants, 994
Children Affected by AIDS Foundation Family Assistance Emergency Fund Grants, 996
CLIF Bar Family Foundation Grants, 1040
Compass Bank Foundation Grants, 1138
Cudd Foundation Grants, 1171
Daniels Fund Grants, 1200
Dean Foods Community Involvement Grants, 1209
Do Something BR!CK Awards, 1287
Dr. Stanley Pearle Scholarships, 1330
GenCorp Foundation Grants, 1587
General Mills Foundation Grants, 1590
GoGirlGo! Ambassador Team Awards, 1632
Guitar Center Music Foundation Grants, 1675
Harry Kramer Memorial Fund Grants, 1705
Honeywell Foundation Grants, 1791
IAFF Burn Foundation Research Grants, 1830
J.E. and L.E. Mabee Foundation Grants, 1875
John Merck Fund Grants, 1940
John Merck Scholars Awards, 1941
Multiple Sclerosis Foundation Brighter Tomorrow Grants, 2228
NEI Mentored Clinical Scientist Development Program Award (K12), 2295
NMF Franklin C. McLean Award, 2829
NMF General Electric Medical Scholars Fellowships, 2830
NMF Henry G. Halladay Awards, 2831
NMF Mary Ball Carrera Scholarship, 2834
NMF National Medical Association Awards for Medical Journalism, 2836
NMF National Medical Association Emerging Scholar Awards, 2837
NMF National Medical Association Patti LaBelle Award, 2838
NMF Need-Based Scholarships, 2839
NMF Ralph W. Ellison Prize, 2840
NMF William and Charlotte Cadbury Award, 2841
NSF Major Research Instrumentation Program (MRI) Grants, 2889
OneSight Research Foundation Block Grants, 2944
Pfizer/AAFP Foundation Visiting Professorship Program in Family Medicine, 3027
Rosalinde and Arthur Gilbert Foundation/AFAR New Investigator Awards in Alzheimer's Disease, 3187
Tylenol Scholarship, 3444
U.S. Department of Education Erma Byrd Scholarships, 3446
U.S. Department of Education United States-Russia Program: Improving Research and Educational Activities in Higher Education, 3451
US CRDF Leishmaniasis: Collaborative Research Opportunities in North Africa and the Middle East, 3474
Vulcan Materials Company Foundation Grants, 3504
Wal-Mart Foundation Community Grants, 3513
Wal-Mart State Giving Program Grants, 3514

New York

1 in 9: Long Island Breast Cancer Action Coalition Grants, 1
100 Mile Man Foundation Grants, 2
3M Company Health and Human Services Grants, 10
3M Foundation Grants, 11
Aaron & Freda Glickman Foundation Grants, 172
Abbott Fund Access to Health Care Grants, 176
Abbott Fund Community Vitality Grants, 177
Abbott Fund Global AIDS Care Grants, 178
Abbott Fund Science and Medical Innovation Grants, 179
ACE Charitable Foundation Grants, 199
ACF Ethnic Community Self-Help Grants, 200
ACF Preferred Communities Grants, 201
ACF Standing Announcement for Unaccompanied Alien Children Grants, 202
ACF Supplemental Services for Recently Arrived Refugees Grants, 203
Achelis and Bodman Foundations Grants, 206
Actors Fund Social Services and Financial Assistance, 225
AEGON Transamerica Foundation Grants, 243
Agnes Gund Foundation Grants, 262
Ahn Family Foundation Grants, 304
Alexis Gregory Foundation Grants, 349
Allyn Foundation Grants, 365
Altman Foundation Health Care Grants, 372
American College of Surgeons and The Triological Society Clinical Scientist Development Awards, 422
Anheuser-Busch Foundation Grants, 474
Arkell Hall Foundation Grants, 534
Arkema Foundation Science Teachers Program, 535
ARS Foundation Grants, 538
Arthur and Rochelle Belfer Foundation Grants, 542
ASHA Advancing Academic-Research Careers (AARC) Award, 569
ASHA Minority Student Leadership Program Awards, 570
ASHA Multicultural Activities Projects Grants, 571
ASHA Research Mentoring-Pair Travel Award, 572
ASHA Student Research Travel Award, 573
ASHA Students Preparing for Academic & Research Careers (SPARC) Award, 574
ASM Millis-Colwell Postgraduate Travel Grant, 608
Assurant Foundation Grants, 654
Axe-Houghton Foundation Grants, 678
Banfi Vintners Foundation Grants, 687
Barker Welfare Foundation Grants, 695
Bearemy's Kennel Pals Grants, 728
Bernard F. and Alva B. Gimbel Foundation Grants, 747
Bildner Family Foundation Grants, 755
Birds Eye Foods Foundation Grants, 759
BJ's Charitable Foundation Grants, 761
Bodman Foundation Grants Program, 776
Bristol-Myers Squibb Foundation Health Disparities Grants, 797
Cable Positive's Tony Cox Community Fund Grants, 827
Carl C. Icahn Foundation Grants, 870
Carnahan-Jackson Foundation Grants, 878
Carrier Corporation Contributions Grants, 884
CDC Cancer Prevention and Control Programs, 903
CDC Injury Control Research Centers Grants, 913
Champ-A Champion Fur Kids Grants, 959
Charles A. Frueauff Foundation Grants, 962
Children Affected by AIDS Foundation Camp Network Grants, 994
Children Affected by AIDS Foundation Family Assistance Emergency Fund Grants, 996
Clark Foundation Grants, 1029
CLIF Bar Family Foundation Grants, 1040
Community Foundation for Greater Buffalo Grants, 1090
Cooper Industries Foundation Grants, 1150
Cowles Charitable Trust Grants, 1155
Cranston Foundation Grants, 1158
CSX Corporate Contributions Grants, 1169
Daisy Marquis Jones Foundation Grants, 1188
Dammann Fund Grants, 1192
David Geffen Foundation Grants, 1202
Dean Foods Community Involvement Grants, 1209
DeMatteis Family Foundation Grants, 1221
Do Something BR!CK Awards, 1287
Dolan Foundation Grants, 1306
Dr. Stanley Pearle Scholarships, 1330
Dreitzer Foundation Grants, 1332
Dyson Foundation Mid-Hudson Valley General Operating Support Grants, 1354
E.L. Wiegand Foundation Grants, 1361
Edward S. Moore Foundation Grants, 1374
Elizabeth McGraw Foundation Grants, 1399
Entergy Corporation Open Grants for Healthy Families, 1418
Eugene M. Lang Foundation Grants, 1434
Fan Fox and Leslie R. Samuels Foundation Grants Program, 1451
FAR Fund, 1453
FCNY Union Square Awards, 1461
Feldman Foundation Grants Program, 1484
Fidelity Foundation Grants, 1498
Fluor Foundation Grants, 1517
FMC Foundation Grants, 1518

Foundation of CVPH April LaValley Fund Grants, 1538
Foundation of CVPH Chelsea's Rainbow Fund Grants, 1539
Foundation of CVPH Melissa Lahtinen-Penfield Organ Donor Fund Grants, 1540
Foundation of CVPH Rabin Fund Grants, 1541
Foundation of CVPH Roger Senecal Endowment Fund Grants, 1542
Foundation of CVPH Travel Fund Grants, 1543
Frances L. and Edwin L. Cummings Memorial Fund Grants, 1547
Fred L. Emerson Foundation Grants, 1557
Gebbie Foundation Grants, 1585
General Mills Foundation Grants, 1590
Genesis Foundation Grants, 1593
Gladys Brooks Foundation Grants, 1620
GoGirlGo! Ambassador Team Awards, 1632
Gregory Family Foundation Grants (Florida), 1667
Griffin Family Foundation Grants, 1669
Guitar Center Music Foundation Grants, 1675
H. Schaffer Foundation Grants, 1680
Hackett Foundation Grants, 1684
Hagedorn Fund Grants, 1685
Hannaford Charitable Foundation Grants, 1692
Harry Kramer Memorial Fund Grants, 1705
Harry S. Black and Allon Fuller Fund, 1706
Heckscher Foundation for Children Grants, 1732
Helena Rubinstein Foundation Grants, 1743
Herman Goldman Foundation Grants, 1753
Hirtzel Memorial Foundation Grants, 1781
Howard and Bush Foundation Grants, 1798
IAFF Burn Foundation Research Grants, 1830
Independence Community Foundation Community Quality of Life Grant, 1849
Innovative Technology Development Award Program, 1855
Jacob and Valeria Langeloth Foundation Grants, 1882
James H. Cummings Foundation Grants, 1888
Jean and Louis Dreyfus Foundation Grants, 1911
Jewish Foundation for Education of Women Scholarships for Emigres in the Health Professions, 1922
Jewish Women's Foundation of New York Grants, 1924
John Merck Fund Grants, 1940
John Merck Scholars Awards, 1941
John R. Oishei Foundation Grants, 1944
Joseph Alexander Foundation Grants, 1957
Josephine Goodyear Foundation Grants, 1964
KeySpan Foundation Grants, 1995
Komen Greater NYC Clinical Trials Enrollment Grants, 2010
Komen Greater NYC Community Breast Health Grants, 2011
Komen Greater NYC Conference Grants, 2012
Komen Greater NYC Small Grants Program, 2013
Land O'Lakes Foundation Mid-Atlantic Grants Program, 2027
Laura B. Vogler Foundation Grants, 2032
Lawrence S. Huntington Fund Grants, 2035
Long Island Community Foundation Grants, 2063
Louis Calder Foundation Grants, 2065
Louis R. Cappelli Foundation Grants, 2066
M.B. and Edna Zale Foundation Grants, 2093
Margaret L. Wendt Foundation Grants, 2104
Marjorie C. Adams Charitable Trust Grants, 2111
Max A. Adler Charitable Foundation Grants, 2132
MfA Newton Fellowships, 2182
Miles of Hope Breast Cancer Foundation Grants, 2199
Morton K. and Jane Blaustein Foundation Grants, 2218
Multiple Sclerosis Foundation Brighter Tomorrow Grants, 2228
NEI Mentored Clinical Scientist Development Program Award (K12), 2295
NMF Aura E. Severinghaus Award, 2828
NMF Franklin C. McLean Award, 2829
NMF General Electric Medical Scholars Fellowships, 2830
NMF Henry G. Halladay Awards, 2831
NMF Mary Ball Carrera Scholarship, 2834
NMF National Medical Association Awards for Medical Journalism, 2836
NMF National Medical Association Emerging Scholar Awards, 2837
NMF National Medical Association Patti LaBelle Award, 2838
NMF Need-Based Scholarships, 2839
NMF Ralph W. Ellison Prize, 2840
NMF William and Charlotte Cadbury Award, 2841
Northern New York Community Foundation Grants, 2864
NSF Major Research Instrumentation Program (MRI) Grants, 2889
NYCT AIDS/HIV Grants, 2919
NYCT Biomedical Research Grants, 2920
NYCT Blindness and Visual Disabilities Grants, 2921
NYCT Blood Disease Research Grants, 2922
NYCT Children and Youth with Disabilities Grants, 2923
NYCT Girls and Young Women Grants, 2924
NYCT Grants for the Elderly, 2925
NYCT Health Services, Systems, and Policies Grants, 2926
NYCT Mental Health and Mental Retardation Grants, 2927
NYCT Substance Abuse Grants, 2928
NYCT Technical Assistance Grants, 2929
OneSight Research Foundation Block Grants, 2944
Peter and Elizabeth C. Tower Foundation Community Grants, 3018
Pfizer/AAFP Foundation Visiting Professorship Program in Family Medicine, 3027
Robin Hood Foundation Grants, 3174
Rochester Area Community Foundation Grants, 3176
Rosalinde and Arthur Gilbert Foundation/AFAR New Investigator Awards in Alzheimer's Disease, 3187
Russell Berrie Foundation Grants, 3201
SAG Motion Picture Players Welfare Fund Grants, 3238
Sasco Foundation Grants, 3265
Sprague Foundation Grants Program, 3359
Taproot Foundation Capacity-Building Service Grants, 3417
TWS Foundation Grants, 3443
Tylenol Scholarship, 3444
U.S. Department of Education Erma Byrd Scholarships, 3446
U.S. Department of Education United States-Russia Program: Improving Research and Educational Activities in Higher Education, 3451
US Airways Community Contributions, 3472
US CRDF Leishmaniasis: Collaborative Research Opportunities in North Africa and the Middle East, 3474
US Trust Corporation Foundation Grants, 3475
Verizon Foundation New York Grants, 3488
Wal-Mart Foundation Community Grants, 3513
Wal-Mart State Giving Program Grants, 3514
Walt Disney Company Foundation Grants, 3516
Western Union Foundation Grants, 3529
William G. McGowan Charitable Fund Grants, 3539
Winifred & Harry B. Allen Foundation Grants, 3543
YSA UnitedHealth Heroes Service Learning Grants, 3556

North Carolina

Abbott Fund Access to Health Care Grants, 176
Abbott Fund Community Vitality Grants, 177
Abbott Fund Global AIDS Care Grants, 178
Abbott Fund Science and Medical Innovation Grants, 179
Able To Serve Grants, 185
ACE Charitable Foundation Grants, 199
ACF Ethnic Community Self-Help Grants, 200
ACF Preferred Communities Grants, 201
ACF Standing Announcement for Unaccompanied Alien Children Grants, 202
ACF Supplemental Services for Recently Arrived Refugees Grants, 203
Actors Fund Social Services and Financial Assistance, 225
AEGON Transamerica Foundation Grants, 243
American College of Surgeons and The Triological Society Clinical Scientist Development Awards, 422
American Schlafhorst Foundation Grants, 454
ASHA Advancing Academic-Research Careers (AARC) Award, 569
ASHA Minority Student Leadership Program Awards, 570
ASHA Multicultural Activities Projects Grants, 571
ASHA Research Mentoring-Pair Travel Award, 572
ASHA Student Research Travel Award, 573
ASHA Students Preparing for Academic & Research Careers (SPARC) Award, 574
ASM Millis-Colwell Postgraduate Travel Grant, 608
AT&T Excelerator, 657
BCBSNC Foundation Fit Together Grants, 724
BCBSNC Foundation Grants, 725
Bearemy's Kennel Pals Grants, 728
Beldon Fund Grants, 738
Belk Foundation Grants, 739
Biogen Corporate Giving Grants, 758
BJ's Charitable Foundation Grants, 761
Blanche and Julian Robertson Family Foundation Grants, 765
Blumenthal Foundation Grants, 773
Bridgestone/Firestone Trust Fund Grants, 792
Burlington Industries Foundation Grants, 811
Cable Positive's Tony Cox Community Fund Grants, 827
Camp-Younts Foundation Grants, 838
Carrie E. and Lena V. Glenn Foundation Grants, 882
Carrier Corporation Contributions Grants, 884
Catherine Kennedy Home Foundation Grants, 890
CDC Injury Control Research Centers Grants, 913
Cemala Foundation Grants, 933
Champ-A Champion Fur Kids Grants, 959
Charles A. Frueauff Foundation Grants, 962
Children Affected by AIDS Foundation Camp Network Grants, 994
Children Affected by AIDS Foundation Family Assistance Emergency Fund Grants, 996
Clarcor Foundation Grants, 1021
CLIF Bar Family Foundation Grants, 1040
Community Foundation of Greater Greensboro Grants, 1109
Community Foundation of Western North Carolina Grants, 1132
Cooper Industries Foundation Grants, 1150
CSX Corporate Contributions Grants, 1169
D.F. Halton Foundation Grants, 1181
Dean Foods Community Involvement Grants, 1209
DHHS Healthy Tomorrows Partnership for Children, 1261
Dickson Foundation Grants, 1284
Do Something BR!CK Awards, 1287
Dominion Educational Partnership Grant, 1308
Dr. Stanley Pearle Scholarships, 1330
Duke Endowment Health Care Grants, 1338
Duke Energy Foundation Grants, 1339
Dunspaugh-Dalton Foundation Grants, 1351
F.M. Kirby Foundation Grants, 1443
Fluor Foundation Grants, 1517
FMC Foundation Grants, 1518
Foundation for the Carolinas Grants, 1535
George H. Hitchings New Investigator Award in Health Research, 1600
Gertrude B. Elion Mentored Medical Student Research Awards, 1608

GoGirlGo! Ambassador Team Awards, 1632
Guitar Center Music Foundation Grants, 1675
Harry Kramer Memorial Fund Grants, 1705
Hillsdale Fund Grants, 1778
Howe Foundation of North Carolina Grants, 1799
IAFF Burn Foundation Research Grants, 1830
Ireland Family Foundation Grants, 1865
James G.K. McClure Educational and Development Fund Grants, 1886
James H. Cummings Foundation Grants, 1888
James J. and Angelia M. Harris Foundation Grants, 1890
Janirve Foundation Grants, 1905
John Deere Foundation Grants, 1929
John H. Wellons Foundation Grants, 1934
John Merck Fund Grants, 1940
John Merck Scholars Awards, 1941
John W. and Anna H. Hanes Foundation Grants, 1948
Kate B. Reynolds Charitable Trust Health Care Grants, 1981
Kimberly-Clark Community Grants, 2001
Lester Ray Fleming Scholarships, 2048
Lettie Pate Whitehead Foundation Grants, 2049
Lincoln Financial Group Foundation Grants, 2058
Moses Cone-Wesley Long Community Health Foundation Grants, 2219
Multiple Sclerosis Foundation Brighter Tomorrow Grants, 2228
National Starch and Chemical Foundation Grants, 2261
NEI Mentored Clinical Scientist Development Program Award (K12), 2295
NMF Franklin C. McLean Award, 2829
NMF General Electric Medical Scholars Fellowships, 2830
NMF Henry G. Halladay Awards, 2831
NMF Mary Ball Carrera Scholarship, 2834
NMF National Medical Association Awards for Medical Journalism, 2836
NMF National Medical Association Emerging Scholar Awards, 2837
NMF National Medical Association Patti LaBelle Award, 2838
NMF Need-Based Scholarships, 2839
NMF Ralph W. Ellison Prize, 2840
NMF William and Charlotte Cadbury Award, 2841
North Carolina Biotechnology Center Event Sponsorship Grants, 2852
North Carolina Biotechnology Center Grantsmanship Training Grants, 2853
North Carolina Biotechnology Center Meeting Grants, 2854
North Carolina Biotechnology Center Regional Development Grants, 2855
North Carolina Biotechnology Center Technology Enhancement Grants, 2856
North Carolina Biotechnology Centers of Innovation Grants, 2857
North Carolina Community Development Grants, 2858
North Carolina Community Foundation Grants, 2859
North Carolina GlaxoSmithKline Foundation Grants, 2860
NSF Major Research Instrumentation Program (MRI) Grants, 2889
OneSight Research Foundation Block Grants, 2944
Pfizer/AAFP Foundation Visiting Professorship Program in Family Medicine, 3027
Piedmont Natural Gas Grants, 3048
Plum Creek Foundation Grants, 3062
Progress Energy Foundation Grants, 3084
Rehab Therapy Foundation Grants, 3146
Rosalinde and Arthur Gilbert Foundation/AFAR New Investigator Awards in Alzheimer's Disease, 3187
Salisbury Community Foundation Grants, 3243
Simple Advise Education Center Grants, 3289
Sisters of Mercy of North Carolina Foundation Grants, 3295
Square D Foundation Grants, 3361
Steele-Reese Foundation Grants, 3380
Strowd Roses Grants, 3388
Triangle Community Foundation Donor-Advised Grants, 3437
Triangle Community Foundation Shaver-Hitchings Scholarship, 3438
Tylenol Scholarship, 3444
U.S. Department of Education Erma Byrd Scholarships, 3446
U.S. Department of Education United States-Russia Program: Improving Research and Educational Activities in Higher Education, 3451
Union County Community Foundation Grants, 3461
US Airways Community Contributions, 3472
US Airways Community Foundation Grants, 3473
US CRDF Leishmaniasis: Collaborative Research Opportunities in North Africa and the Middle East, 3474
US Trust Corporation Foundation Grants, 3475
Vulcan Materials Company Foundation Grants, 3504
Wal-Mart Foundation Community Grants, 3513
Wal-Mart State Giving Program Grants, 3514
Winston-Salem Foundation Competitive Grants, 3544
Winston-Salem Foundation Elkin/Tri-County Grants, 3545
Winston-Salem Foundation Stokes County Grants, 3546
Winston-Salem Foundation Victim Assistance Grants, 3547
Woodward Fund Grants, 3552
YSA UnitedHealth Heroes Service Learning Grants, 3556
Z. Smith Reynolds Foundation Small Grants, 3557

North Dakota

ACF Ethnic Community Self-Help Grants, 200
ACF Preferred Communities Grants, 201
ACF Standing Announcement for Unaccompanied Alien Children Grants, 202
ACF Supplemental Services for Recently Arrived Refugees Grants, 203
Actors Fund Social Services and Financial Assistance, 225
Albertson's Charitable Giving Grants, 330
American College of Surgeons and The Triological Society Clinical Scientist Development Awards, 422
ASHA Advancing Academic-Research Careers (AARC) Award, 569
ASHA Minority Student Leadership Program Awards, 570
ASHA Multicultural Activities Projects Grants, 571
ASHA Research Mentoring-Pair Travel Award, 572
ASHA Student Research Travel Award, 573
ASHA Students Preparing for Academic & Research Careers (SPARC) Award, 574
ASM Millis-Colwell Postgraduate Travel Grant, 608
Bearemy's Kennel Pals Grants, 728
Bush Foundation Health & Human Services Grants, 814
Bush Foundation Medical Fellowships, 815
Cable Positive's Tony Cox Community Fund Grants, 827
Champ-A Champion Fur Kids Grants, 959
Children Affected by AIDS Foundation Camp Network Grants, 994
Children Affected by AIDS Foundation Family Assistance Emergency Fund Grants, 996
CLIF Bar Family Foundation Grants, 1040
Dean Foods Community Involvement Grants, 1209
DHHS Healthy Tomorrows Partnership for Children, 1261
Do Something BR!CK Awards, 1287
Dr. Stanley Pearle Scholarships, 1330
Fargo-Moorhead Area Foundation Grants, 1454
GoGirlGo! Ambassador Team Awards, 1632
Guitar Center Music Foundation Grants, 1675
Harry Kramer Memorial Fund Grants, 1705
IAFF Burn Foundation Research Grants, 1830
John Merck Fund Grants, 1940
John Merck Scholars Awards, 1941
Multiple Sclerosis Foundation Brighter Tomorrow Grants, 2228
NEI Mentored Clinical Scientist Development Program Award (K12), 2295
NMF Franklin C. McLean Award, 2829
NMF General Electric Medical Scholars Fellowships, 2830
NMF Henry G. Halladay Awards, 2831
NMF Mary Ball Carrera Scholarship, 2834
NMF National Medical Association Awards for Medical Journalism, 2836
NMF National Medical Association Emerging Scholar Awards, 2837
NMF National Medical Association Patti LaBelle Award, 2838
NMF Need-Based Scholarships, 2839
NMF Ralph W. Ellison Prize, 2840
NMF William and Charlotte Cadbury Award, 2841
NSF Major Research Instrumentation Program (MRI) Grants, 2889
OneSight Research Foundation Block Grants, 2944
Otto Bremer Foundation Grants, 2977
Pfizer/AAFP Foundation Visiting Professorship Program in Family Medicine, 3027
Piper Jaffray Companies Building Strong Communities Grants, 3053
Rosalinde and Arthur Gilbert Foundation/AFAR New Investigator Awards in Alzheimer's Disease, 3187
Tylenol Scholarship, 3444
U.S. Department of Education Erma Byrd Scholarships, 3446
U.S. Department of Education United States-Russia Program: Improving Research and Educational Activities in Higher Education, 3451
US CRDF Leishmaniasis: Collaborative Research Opportunities in North Africa and the Middle East, 3474
Viking Children's Fund Grants, 3497
Wal-Mart Foundation Community Grants, 3513
Wal-Mart State Giving Program Grants, 3514

Ohio

3M Company Health and Human Services Grants, 10
3M Foundation Grants, 11
Abbott Fund Access to Health Care Grants, 176
Abbott Fund Community Vitality Grants, 177
Abbott Fund Global AIDS Care Grants, 178
Abbott Fund Science and Medical Innovation Grants, 179
Abington Foundation Grants, 184
ACE Charitable Foundation Grants, 199
ACF Ethnic Community Self-Help Grants, 200
ACF Preferred Communities Grants, 201
ACF Standing Announcement for Unaccompanied Alien Children Grants, 202
ACF Supplemental Services for Recently Arrived Refugees Grants, 203
Actors Fund Social Services and Financial Assistance, 225
American College of Surgeons and The Triological Society Clinical Scientist Development Awards, 422
American Electric Power Grants, 434
Anheuser-Busch Foundation Grants, 474
Anthem Blue Cross and Blue Shield Grants, 488
Anthem Blue Cross and Blue Shield School Nurse Grants, 489
ASHA Advancing Academic-Research Careers (AARC) Award, 569
ASHA Minority Student Leadership Program Awards, 570
ASHA Multicultural Activities Projects Grants, 571
ASHA Research Mentoring-Pair Travel Award, 572

ASHA Student Research Travel Award, 573
ASHA Students Preparing for Academic & Research Careers (SPARC) Award, 574
Ashland Corporate Contributions Grants, 586
ASM Millis-Colwell Postgraduate Travel Grant, 608
AT&T Excelerator, 657
Austin-Bailey Health and Wellness Foundation Grants, 669
Barberton Community Foundation Grants, 693
Bearemy's Kennel Pals Grants, 728
BJ's Charitable Foundation Grants, 761
Bridgestone/Firestone Trust Fund Grants, 792
Cable Positive's Tony Cox Community Fund Grants, 827
CDC Injury Control Research Centers Grants, 913
Champ-A Champion Fur Kids Grants, 959
Charles H. Dater Foundation Grants, 966
Chase Paymentech Corporate Giving Grants, 975
Children Affected by AIDS Foundation Camp Network Grants, 994
Children Affected by AIDS Foundation Family Assistance Emergency Fund Grants, 996
Cinergy Foundation Grants, 1013
Clarcor Foundation Grants, 1021
Cleveland Browns Foundation Grants, 1036
CLIF Bar Family Foundation Grants, 1040
CMA Foundation Grants, 1042
Columbus Foundation Allen Eiry Fund Grants, 1064
Columbus Foundation Competitive Grants, 1066
Columbus Foundation Estrich Fund Grants, 1067
Columbus Foundation J. Floyd Dixon Memorial Fund Grants, 1068
Columbus Foundation Mary Eleanor Morris Fund Grants, 1069
Columbus Foundation Robert E. and Genevieve B. Schaefer Fund Grants, 1070
Columbus Foundation Traditional Grants, 1071
Community Foundation of Mount Vernon and Knox County Grants, 1119
CSX Corporate Contributions Grants, 1169
Cyrus Eaton Foundation Grants, 1178
Dayton Power and Light Foundation Grants, 1205
Deaconess Community Foundation Grants, 1207
Dean Foods Community Involvement Grants, 1209
Do Something BR!CK Awards, 1287
Dominion Educational Partnership Grant, 1308
Dr. Stanley Pearle Scholarships, 1330
Duke Energy Foundation Grants, 1339
Elisabeth Severance Prentiss Foundation Grants Program, 1392
Eva L. and Joseph M. Bruening Foundation Grants, 1436
Fairview Lutheran Foundation Grants, 1448
Fidelity Foundation Grants, 1498
Fifth Third Foundation Grants, 1501
FirstEnergy Foundation Community Grants, 1505
General Mills Foundation Grants, 1590
Giant Eagle Foundation Grants, 1611
Ginn Foundation Grants, 1616
Gladys Brooks Foundation Grants, 1620
GoGirlGo! Ambassador Team Awards, 1632
Graco Foundation Grants, 1642
Greater Cincinnati Foundation Priority and Small Projects/Capacity-Building Grants, 1651
Guitar Center Music Foundation Grants, 1675
Harry Kramer Memorial Fund Grants, 1705
Health Foundation of Greater Cincinnati Grants, 1724
Helen Steiner Rice Foundation Grants, 1742
Honda of America Manufacturing Foundation Grants, 1790
Humana Foundation Grants, 1818
Huntington National Bank Community Affairs Grants, 1824
IAFF Burn Foundation Research Grants, 1830
Impact 100 Grants, 1843
Jacob G. Schmidlapp Trust Grants, 1883
James S. Copley Foundation Grants, 1895
John Lord Knight Foundation Grants, 1938
John Merck Fund Grants, 1940
John Merck Scholars Awards, 1941
John P. Murphy Foundation Grants, 1943
Johnson & Johnson Community Health Care Program Grants, 1951
Joyce Foundation Grants, 1969
Kelvin and Eleanor Smith Foundation Grants, 1986
Kettering Fund Grants, 1992
Kimberly-Clark Community Grants, 2001
Lubrizol Foundation Grants Program, 2080
Mary S. and David C. Corbin Foundation Grants, 2122
Multiple Sclerosis Foundation Brighter Tomorrow Grants, 2228
National City Corp Contributions Grants, 2250
NEI Mentored Clinical Scientist Development Program Award (K12), 2295
NMF Franklin C. McLean Award, 2829
NMF General Electric Medical Scholars Fellowships, 2830
NMF Henry G. Halladay Awards, 2831
NMF Mary Ball Carrera Scholarship, 2834
NMF National Medical Association Awards for Medical Journalism, 2836
NMF National Medical Association Emerging Scholar Awards, 2837
NMF National Medical Association Patti LaBelle Award, 2838
NMF Need-Based Scholarships, 2839
NMF Ralph W. Ellison Prize, 2840
NMF William and Charlotte Cadbury Award, 2841
Nordson Corporation Foundation Grants, 2851
NSF Major Research Instrumentation Program (MRI) Grants, 2889
Ohio Learning Network Grants, 2940
OneSight Research Foundation Block Grants, 2944
Paul G. Duke Foundation Grants, 3001
Pfizer/AAFP Foundation Visiting Professorship Program in Family Medicine, 3027
Piper Jaffray Companies Building Strong Communities Grants, 3053
PNC Charitable Trust and Foundation Grants, 3064
Raymond John Wean Foundation Grants, 3110
Reynolds and Reynolds Associate Foundation Grants, 3152
Rollin M. Gerstacker Foundation Grants Program, 3186
Rosalinde and Arthur Gilbert Foundation/AFAR New Investigator Awards in Alzheimer's Disease, 3187
S. Livingston Mather Charitable Trust Grants, 3235
Saint Luke's Foundation Grants, 3239
Sisters of Saint Joseph Charitable Fund Grants, 3296
SOCFOC Catholic Ministries Grants, 3317
SOCFOC Reducing Health & Educational Disparities in the Central Neighborhood Grants, 3318
Stark Community Foundation Women's Fund Grants, 3376
Tylenol Scholarship, 3444
U.S. Department of Education Erma Byrd Scholarships, 3446
U.S. Department of Education United States-Russia Program: Improving Research and Educational Activities in Higher Education, 3451
US CRDF Leishmaniasis: Collaborative Research Opportunities in North Africa and the Middle East, 3474
Virginia W. Kettering Foundation Grants, 3502
Wal-Mart Foundation Community Grants, 3513
Wal-Mart State Giving Program Grants, 3514
YSA UnitedHealth Heroes Service Learning Grants, 3556

Oklahoma

ACF Ethnic Community Self-Help Grants, 200
ACF Preferred Communities Grants, 201
ACF Standing Announcement for Unaccompanied Alien Children Grants, 202
ACF Supplemental Services for Recently Arrived Refugees Grants, 203
Actors Fund Social Services and Financial Assistance, 225
Albertson's Charitable Giving Grants, 330
American College of Surgeons and The Triological Society Clinical Scientist Development Awards, 422
American Electric Power Grants, 434
ASHA Advancing Academic-Research Careers (AARC) Award, 569
ASHA Minority Student Leadership Program Awards, 570
ASHA Multicultural Activities Projects Grants, 571
ASHA Research Mentoring-Pair Travel Award, 572
ASHA Student Research Travel Award, 573
ASHA Students Preparing for Academic & Research Careers (SPARC) Award, 574
ASM Millis-Colwell Postgraduate Travel Grant, 608
AT&T Excelerator, 657
Bearemy's Kennel Pals Grants, 728
C.W. Titus Foundation Grants, 826
Cable Positive's Tony Cox Community Fund Grants, 827
CDC Injury Control Research Centers Grants, 913
Champ-A Champion Fur Kids Grants, 959
Charles A. Frueauff Foundation Grants, 962
Children Affected by AIDS Foundation Camp Network Grants, 994
Children Affected by AIDS Foundation Family Assistance Emergency Fund Grants, 996
Clarcor Foundation Grants, 1021
CLIF Bar Family Foundation Grants, 1040
ConocoPhillips Foundation Grants, 1144
Dean Foods Community Involvement Grants, 1209
Do Something BR!CK Awards, 1287
Dr. Stanley Pearle Scholarships, 1330
General Mills Foundation Grants, 1590
GoGirlGo! Ambassador Team Awards, 1632
Guitar Center Music Foundation Grants, 1675
H.A. and Mary K. Chapman Charitable Trust Grants, 1681
Harry Kramer Memorial Fund Grants, 1705
IAFF Burn Foundation Research Grants, 1830
Inasmuch Foundation Grants, 1845
J.E. and L.E. Mabee Foundation Grants, 1875
John Merck Fund Grants, 1940
John Merck Scholars Awards, 1941
Kimberly-Clark Community Grants, 2001
Multiple Sclerosis Foundation Brighter Tomorrow Grants, 2228
NEI Mentored Clinical Scientist Development Program Award (K12), 2295
NMF Franklin C. McLean Award, 2829
NMF General Electric Medical Scholars Fellowships, 2830
NMF Henry G. Halladay Awards, 2831
NMF Mary Ball Carrera Scholarship, 2834
NMF National Medical Association Awards for Medical Journalism, 2836
NMF National Medical Association Emerging Scholar Awards, 2837
NMF National Medical Association Patti LaBelle Award, 2838
NMF Need-Based Scholarships, 2839
NMF Ralph W. Ellison Prize, 2840
NMF William and Charlotte Cadbury Award, 2841
NSF Major Research Instrumentation Program (MRI) Grants, 2889
OneSight Research Foundation Block Grants, 2944
PacifiCare Foundation Grants, 2981
Pfizer/AAFP Foundation Visiting Professorship Program in Family Medicine, 3027
Plum Creek Foundation Grants, 3062
Presbyterian Health Foundation Bridge, Seed and Equipment Grants, 3075
Priddy Foundation Grants, 3077
Questar Corporate Contributions Grants, 3097

Rosalinde and Arthur Gilbert Foundation/AFAR New Investigator Awards in Alzheimer's Disease, 3187
Tylenol Scholarship, 3444
U.S. Department of Education Erma Byrd Scholarships, 3446
U.S. Department of Education United States-Russia Program: Improving Research and Educational Activities in Higher Education, 3451
US CRDF Leishmaniasis: Collaborative Research Opportunities in North Africa and the Middle East, 3474
Wal-Mart Foundation Community Grants, 3513
Wal-Mart State Giving Program Grants, 3514

Oregon
ACE Charitable Foundation Grants, 199
ACF Ethnic Community Self-Help Grants, 200
ACF Preferred Communities Grants, 201
ACF Standing Announcement for Unaccompanied Alien Children Grants, 202
ACF Supplemental Services for Recently Arrived Refugees Grants, 203
Actors Fund Social Services and Financial Assistance, 225
Albertson's Charitable Giving Grants, 330
American College of Surgeons and The Triological Society Clinical Scientist Development Awards, 422
ASHA Advancing Academic-Research Careers (AARC) Award, 569
ASHA Minority Student Leadership Program Awards, 570
ASHA Multicultural Activities Projects Grants, 571
ASHA Research Mentoring-Pair Travel Award, 572
ASHA Student Research Travel Award, 573
ASHA Students Preparing for Academic & Research Careers (SPARC) Award, 574
ASM Millis-Colwell Postgraduate Travel Grant, 608
Autzen Foundation Grants, 672
Bearemy's Kennel Pals Grants, 728
Bella Vista Foundation Grants, 740
Ben B. Cheney Foundation Grants, 741
Benton County Foundation Grants, 744
Blue Mountain Community Foundation Grants, 769
Bullitt Foundation Grants, 809
Cable Positive's Tony Cox Community Fund Grants, 827
Carpenter Foundation Grants, 881
CDC Injury Control Research Centers Grants, 913
Champ-A Champion Fur Kids Grants, 959
Children Affected by AIDS Foundation Camp Network Grants, 994
Children Affected by AIDS Foundation Family Assistance Emergency Fund Grants, 996
Chiles Foundation Grants, 1003
CLIF Bar Family Foundation Grants, 1040
Coeta and Donald Barker Foundation Grants, 1054
Collins Foundation Grants, 1058
Dell Foundation Open Grants, 1218
Do Something BR!CK Awards, 1287
Dr. Stanley Pearle Scholarships, 1330
E.L. Wiegand Foundation Grants, 1361
Foster Foundation Grants, 1524
GoGirlGo! Ambassador Team Awards, 1632
Guitar Center Music Foundation Grants, 1675
Harold and Arlene Schnitzer CARE Foundation Grants, 1697
Harry Kramer Memorial Fund Grants, 1705
IAFF Burn Foundation Research Grants, 1830
Idaho Power Company Corporate Contributions, 1838
John Merck Fund Grants, 1940
John Merck Scholars Awards, 1941
M.B. and Edna Zale Foundation Grants, 2093
M.J. Murdock Charitable Trust Grants, 2095
Meyer Memorial Trust Emergency Grants, 2178
Meyer Memorial Trust Grassroots Grants, 2179
Meyer Memorial Trust Operating Funds Grants, 2180
Meyer Memorial Trust Responsive Grants, 2181
Multiple Sclerosis Foundation Brighter Tomorrow Grants, 2228
NEI Mentored Clinical Scientist Development Program Award (K12), 2295
NMF Franklin C. McLean Award, 2829
NMF General Electric Medical Scholars Fellowships, 2830
NMF Henry G. Halladay Awards, 2831
NMF Mary Ball Carrera Scholarship, 2834
NMF National Medical Association Awards for Medical Journalism, 2836
NMF National Medical Association Emerging Scholar Awards, 2837
NMF National Medical Association Patti LaBelle Award, 2838
NMF Need-Based Scholarships, 2839
NMF Ralph W. Ellison Prize, 2840
NMF William and Charlotte Cadbury Award, 2841
NSF Major Research Instrumentation Program (MRI) Grants, 2889
NWHF Community-Based Participatory Research Grants, 2904
NWHF Kaiser Permanente Community Fund Grants, 2906
OneSight Research Foundation Block Grants, 2944
PacifiCare Foundation Grants, 2981
PacifiCorp Foundation for Learning Grants, 2982
Paul G. Allen Family Foundation Grants, 3000
Pfizer/AAFP Foundation Visiting Professorship Program in Family Medicine, 3027
Piper Jaffray Companies Building Strong Communities Grants, 3053
Plum Creek Foundation Grants, 3062
Portland General Electric Foundation Grants, 3067
Premera CARES Grants, 3074
Pride Foundation Grants and Scholarships, 3078
Regence Foundation Access to Health Care Grants, 3138
Regence Foundation Health Care Community Awareness and Engagement Grants, 3139
Regence Foundation Health Care Connections Grants, 3140
Regence Foundation Improving End-of-Life Grants, 3141
Regence Foundation Tools and Technology Grants, 3142
Rosalinde and Arthur Gilbert Foundation/AFAR New Investigator Awards in Alzheimer's Disease, 3187
Salem Foundation Charitable Trust Grants, 3241
Samuel S. Johnson Foundation Grants, 3251
Simpson Fund Grants, 3290
Sunderland Foundation Grants, 3400
Tylenol Scholarship, 3444
U.S. Department of Education Erma Byrd Scholarships, 3446
U.S. Department of Education United States-Russia Program: Improving Research and Educational Activities in Higher Education, 3451
US CRDF Leishmaniasis: Collaborative Research Opportunities in North Africa and the Middle East, 3474
US Trust Corporation Foundation Grants, 3475
Wal-Mart Foundation Community Grants, 3513
Wal-Mart State Giving Program Grants, 3514
William G. Gilmore Foundation Grants, 3537

Pennsylvania
1 in 9: Long Island Breast Cancer Action Coalition Grants, 1
1675 Foundation Grants, 4
1976 Foundation Grants, 5
ACE Charitable Foundation Grants, 199
ACF Ethnic Community Self-Help Grants, 200
ACF Preferred Communities Grants, 201
ACF Standing Announcement for Unaccompanied Alien Children Grants, 202
ACF Supplemental Services for Recently Arrived Refugees Grants, 203
Actors Fund Social Services and Financial Assistance, 225
Adams County Foundation Grants - Pennsylvania, 231
Addison H. Gibson Foundation Medical Grants, 233
AEGON Transamerica Foundation Grants, 243
Albertson's Charitable Giving Grants, 330
Allegheny Technologies Charitable Trust, 359
American College of Surgeons and The Triological Society Clinical Scientist Development Awards, 422
Arcadia Foundation Grants, 524
Arkema Foundation Science Teachers Program, 535
ASHA Advancing Academic-Research Careers (AARC) Award, 569
ASHA Minority Student Leadership Program Awards, 570
ASHA Multicultural Activities Projects Grants, 571
ASHA Research Mentoring-Pair Travel Award, 572
ASHA Student Research Travel Award, 573
ASHA Students Preparing for Academic & Research Careers (SPARC) Award, 574
ASM Millis-Colwell Postgraduate Travel Grant, 608
Barra Foundation Community Fund Grants, 698
Barra Foundation Project Grants, 699
Bearemy's Kennel Pals Grants, 728
Berks County Community Foundation Grants, 745
Binney and Smith Community Grants, 757
Birds Eye Foods Foundation Grants, 759
Birmingham Foundation Grants, 760
BJ's Charitable Foundation Grants, 761
Bridgestone/Firestone Trust Fund Grants, 792
Brook J. Lenfest Foundation Grants, 804
Bruce and Adele Greenfield Foundation Grants, 808
Cable Positive's Tony Cox Community Fund Grants, 827
CDC Injury Control Research Centers Grants, 913
Champ-A Champion Fur Kids Grants, 959
Charles A. Frueauff Foundation Grants, 962
Children Affected by AIDS Foundation Camp Network Grants, 994
Children Affected by AIDS Foundation Family Assistance Emergency Fund Grants, 996
Chiron Foundation Community Grants, 1004
Clarcor Foundation Grants, 1021
Claude Worthington Benedum Foundation Grants, 1033
CLIF Bar Family Foundation Grants, 1040
Connelly Foundation Grants, 1143
ConocoPhillips Foundation Grants, 1144
CSX Corporate Contributions Grants, 1169
Dean Foods Community Involvement Grants, 1209
Do Something BR!CK Awards, 1287
Dominion Educational Partnership Grant, 1308
Donald and Sylvia Robinson Family Foundation Grants, 1310
Dorothy Rider Pool Health Care Grants, 1322
Dr. Stanley Pearle Scholarships, 1330
Eastman Chemical Company Foundation Grants, 1362
Eberly Foundation Grants, 1364
Eden Hall Foundation Grants, 1368
Edna G. Kynett Memorial Foundation Grants, 1370
Elsie Lee Garthwaite Memorial Foundation Grants, 1408
Erie Community Foundation Grants, 1427
Eugene M. Lang Foundation Grants, 1434
F.M. Kirby Foundation Grants, 1443
Ferree Foundation Grants, 1486
FirstEnergy Foundation Community Grants, 1505
Fisa Foundation Grants, 1506
Fluor Foundation Grants, 1517
FMC Foundation Grants, 1518
Fourjay Foundation Grants, 1544
Frank E. and Seba B. Payne Foundation Grants, 1551
General Mills Foundation Grants, 1590
Genuardi Family Foundation Grants, 1594
Giant Eagle Foundation Grants, 1611

Gilroy and Lillian P. Roberts Charitable Foundation Grants, 1614
Gladys Brooks Foundation Grants, 1620
GlaxoSmithKline Corporate Grants, 1623
GlaxoSmithKline Foundation IMPACT Awards, 1624
GoGirlGo! Ambassador Team Awards, 1632
Grundy Foundation Grants, 1673
Guitar Center Music Foundation Grants, 1675
H.J. Heinz Company Foundation Grants, 1682
Hackett Foundation Grants, 1684
Harley Davidson Foundation Grants, 1694
Harry Kramer Memorial Fund Grants, 1705
Henrietta Tower Wurts Memorial Foundation Grants, 1745
Hershey Company Grants, 1754
Highmark Corporate Giving Grants, 1769
Highmark Healthy High 5, 1770
Highmark Physician eHealth Collaborative Grants, 1771
Hillman Foundation Grants, 1775
Hirtzel Memorial Foundation Grants, 1781
IAFF Burn Foundation Research Grants, 1830
Independence Blue Cross Charitable Medical Care Grants, 1846
Independence Blue Cross Nurse Scholars Program, 1847
Independence Blue Cross Nursing Internships, 1848
John Merck Fund Grants, 1940
John Merck Scholars Awards, 1941
Josiah W. and Bessie H. Kline Foundation Grants, 1967
Kimberly-Clark Community Grants, 2001
L. W. Pierce Family Foundation Grants, 2019
Land O'Lakes Foundation Mid-Atlantic Grants Program, 2027
Lincoln Financial Group Foundation Grants, 2058
Marriott Foundation for People with Disabilities Bridges Program Grants, 2113
Measey Foundation Medical Education Grants, 2162
Multiple Sclerosis Foundation Brighter Tomorrow Grants, 2228
National City Corporation Contributions Grants, 2250
National Starch and Chemical Foundation Grants, 2261
NEI Mentored Clinical Scientist Development Program Award (K12), 2295
NMF Franklin C. McLean Award, 2829
NMF General Electric Medical Scholars Fellowships, 2830
NMF Henry G. Halladay Awards, 2831
NMF Mary Ball Carrera Scholarship, 2834
NMF National Medical Association Awards for Medical Journalism, 2836
NMF National Medical Association Emerging Scholar Awards, 2837
NMF National Medical Association Patti LaBelle Award, 2838
NMF Need-Based Scholarships, 2839
NMF Ralph W. Ellison Prize, 2840
NMF William and Charlotte Cadbury Award, 2841
NSF Major Research Instrumentation Program (MRI) Grants, 2889
OneSight Research Foundation Block Grants, 2944
Pfizer/AAFP Foundation Visiting Professorship Program in Family Medicine, 3027
Philadelphia Foundation Organizational Effectiveness Grants, 3029
Pittsburgh Foundation Community Fund Grants, 3054
Pittsburgh Foundation Medical Research Grants, 3055
Plum Creek Foundation Grants, 3062
PNC Charitable Trust and Foundation Grants, 3064
Prudential Foundation Grants, 3087
Rathmann Family Foundation Grants, 3109
Raymond John Wean Foundation Grants, 3110
Richard King Mellon Foundation Grants, 3161
Rosalinde and Arthur Gilbert Foundation/AFAR New Investigator Awards in Alzheimer's Disease, 3187
Staunton Farm Foundation Grants, 3378
Stewart Huston Charitable Trust Grants, 3384
Tylenol Scholarship, 3444
U.S. Department of Education Erma Byrd Scholarships, 3446
U.S. Department of Education United States-Russia Program: Improving Research and Educational Activities in Higher Education, 3451
Union Benevolent Association Grants, 3460
US Airways Community Contributions, 3472
US Airways Community Foundation Grants, 3473
US CRDF Leishmaniasis: Collaborative Research Opportunities in North Africa and the Middle East, 3474
US Trust Corporation Foundation Grants, 3475
Verizon Foundation Pennsylvania Grants, 3490
Vulcan Materials Company Foundation Grants, 3504
Wal-Mart Foundation Community Grants, 3513
Wal-Mart State Giving Program Grants, 3514
William G. McGowan Charitable Fund Grants, 3539
YSA UnitedHealth Heroes Service Learning Grants, 3556

Puerto Rico

Abbott Fund Access to Health Care Grants, 176
Abbott Fund Community Vitality Grants, 177
Abbott Fund Global AIDS Care Grants, 178
Abbott Fund Science and Medical Innovation Grants, 179
ACE Charitable Foundation Grants, 199
ACF Ethnic Community Self-Help Grants, 200
ACF Preferred Communities Grants, 201
ACF Standing Announcement for Unaccompanied Alien Children Grants, 202
ACF Supplemental Services for Recently Arrived Refugees Grants, 203
American College of Surgeons and The Triological Society Clinical Scientist Development Awards, 422
ASHA Advancing Academic-Research Careers (AARC) Award, 569
ASHA Minority Student Leadership Program Awards, 570
ASHA Multicultural Activities Projects Grants, 571
ASHA Research Mentoring-Pair Travel Award, 572
ASHA Student Research Travel Award, 573
ASHA Students Preparing for Academic & Research Careers (SPARC) Award, 574
ASM Millis-Colwell Postgraduate Travel Grant, 608
Bearemy's Kennel Pals Grants, 728
Champ-A Champion Fur Kids Grants, 959
Children Affected by AIDS Foundation Family Assistance Emergency Fund Grants, 996
CLIF Bar Family Foundation Grants, 1040
GoGirlGo! Ambassador Team Awards, 1632
Guitar Center Music Foundation Grants, 1675
Harry Kramer Memorial Fund Grants, 1705
John Merck Scholars Awards, 1941
NEI Mentored Clinical Scientist Development Program Award (K12), 2295
NMF Franklin C. McLean Award, 2829
NMF General Electric Medical Scholars Fellowships, 2830
NMF Henry G. Halladay Awards, 2831
NMF Mary Ball Carrera Scholarship, 2834
NMF National Medical Association Awards for Medical Journalism, 2836
NMF National Medical Association Emerging Scholar Awards, 2837
NMF National Medical Association Patti LaBelle Award, 2838
NMF Need-Based Scholarships, 2839
NMF Ralph W. Ellison Prize, 2840
NMF William and Charlotte Cadbury Award, 2841
NSF Major Research Instrumentation Program (MRI) Grants, 2889
Puerto Rico Community Foundation Grants, 3090
Rosalinde and Arthur Gilbert Foundation/AFAR New Investigator Awards in Alzheimer's Disease, 3187
U.S. Department of Education Erma Byrd Scholarships, 3446
U.S. Department of Education Rehabilitation Training--Rehabilitation Continuing Education Programs (RCEP)--Institute on Rehabilitation Issues (IRI), 3449
U.S. Department of Education United States-Russia Program: Improving Research and Educational Activities in Higher Education, 3451
US CRDF Leishmaniasis: Collaborative Research Opportunities in North Africa and the Middle East, 3474
Wal-Mart Foundation Community Grants, 3513

Rhode Island

Aaron Foundation (Massachusetts) Grants, 174
ACF Ethnic Community Self-Help Grants, 200
ACF Preferred Communities Grants, 201
ACF Standing Announcement for Unaccompanied Alien Children Grants, 202
ACF Supplemental Services for Recently Arrived Refugees Grants, 203
Actors Fund Social Services and Financial Assistance, 225
American College of Surgeons and The Triological Society Clinical Scientist Development Awards, 422
ASHA Advancing Academic-Research Careers (AARC) Award, 569
ASHA Minority Student Leadership Program Awards, 570
ASHA Multicultural Activities Projects Grants, 571
ASHA Research Mentoring-Pair Travel Award, 572
ASHA Student Research Travel Award, 573
ASHA Students Preparing for Academic & Research Careers (SPARC) Award, 574
ASM Millis-Colwell Postgraduate Travel Grant, 608
Barnes Group Foundation Grants, 696
Bearemy's Kennel Pals Grants, 728
BJ's Charitable Foundation Grants, 761
Cable Positive's Tony Cox Community Fund Grants, 827
Carlisle Foundation Grants, 874
CDC Cancer Prevention and Control Programs, 903
Champ-A Champion Fur Kids Grants, 959
Champlin Foundations Grants, 960
Charles A. Frueauff Foundation Grants, 962
Charles H. Hood Foundation Child Health Research Grants, 968
Children Affected by AIDS Foundation Camp Network Grants, 994
Children Affected by AIDS Foundation Family Assistance Emergency Fund Grants, 996
Citizens Bank Mid-Atlantic Charitable Foundation Grants, 1015
CLIF Bar Family Foundation Grants, 1040
Cranston Foundation Grants, 1158
Do Something BR!CK Awards, 1287
Dominion Educational Partnership Grant, 1308
Dora Roberts Foundation Grants, 1311
Dr. Stanley Pearle Scholarships, 1330
Fidelity Foundation Grants, 1498
Forrest C. Lattner Foundation Grants, 1523
Gladys Brooks Foundation Grants, 1620
GoGirlGo! Ambassador Team Awards, 1632
Guitar Center Music Foundation Grants, 1675
Harry Kramer Memorial Fund Grants, 1705
Hasbro Children's Fund, 1714
Horace A. Kimball and S. Ella Kimball Foundation Grants, 1792
IAFF Burn Foundation Research Grants, 1830
Jessie B. Cox Charitable Trust Grants, 1918
John Merck Fund Grants, 1940
John Merck Scholars Awards, 1941

Multiple Sclerosis Foundation Brighter Tomorrow Grants, 2228
NEI Mentored Clinical Scientist Development Program Award (K12), 2295
NMF Franklin C. McLean Award, 2829
NMF General Electric Medical Scholars Fellowships, 2830
NMF Henry G. Halladay Awards, 2831
NMF Mary Ball Carrera Scholarship, 2834
NMF National Medical Association Awards for Medical Journalism, 2836
NMF National Medical Association Emerging Scholar Awards, 2837
NMF National Medical Association Patti LaBelle Award, 2838
NMF Need-Based Scholarships, 2839
NMF Ralph W. Ellison Prize, 2840
NMF William and Charlotte Cadbury Award, 2841
Nordson Corporation Foundation Grants, 2851
NSF Major Research Instrumentation Program (MRI) Grants, 2889
OneSight Research Foundation Block Grants, 2944
Pfizer/AAFP Foundation Visiting Professorship Program in Family Medicine, 3027
Rhode Island Foundation Grants, 3154
Robert F. Stoico / FIRSTFED Charitable Foundation Grants, 3171
Rosalinde and Arthur Gilbert Foundation/AFAR New Investigator Awards in Alzheimer's Disease, 3187
Shaw's Supermarkets Donations, 3280
TWS Foundation Grants, 3443
Tylenol Scholarship, 3444
U.S. Department of Education Erma Byrd Scholarships, 3446
U.S. Department of Education United States-Russia Program: Improving Research and Educational Activities in Higher Education, 3451
US CRDF Leishmaniasis: Collaborative Research Opportunities in North Africa and the Middle East, 3474
Verizon Foundation Northeast Region Grants, 3489
Wal-Mart Foundation Community Grants, 3513
Wal-Mart State Giving Program Grants, 3514

South Carolina

3M Company Health and Human Services Grants, 10
3M Foundation Grants, 11
Abney Foundation Grants, 187
ACE Charitable Foundation Grants, 199
ACF Ethnic Community Self-Help Grants, 200
ACF Preferred Communities Grants, 201
ACF Standing Announcement for Unaccompanied Alien Children Grants, 202
ACF Supplemental Services for Recently Arrived Refugees Grants, 203
Actors Fund Social Services and Financial Assistance, 225
American College of Surgeons and The Triological Society Clinical Scientist Development Awards, 422
ASHA Advancing Academic-Research Careers (AARC) Award, 569
ASHA Minority Student Leadership Program Awards, 570
ASHA Multicultural Activities Projects Grants, 571
ASHA Research Mentoring-Pair Travel Award, 572
ASHA Student Research Travel Award, 573
ASHA Students Preparing for Academic & Research Careers (SPARC) Award, 574
ASM Millis-Colwell Postgraduate Travel Grant, 608
AT&T Excelerator, 657
Bailey Foundation Grants, 680
Bearemy's Kennel Pals Grants, 728
Belk Foundation Grants, 739
BJ's Charitable Foundation Grants, 761
Bridgestone/Firestone Trust Fund Grants, 792
Burlington Industries Foundation Grants, 811
Cable Positive's Tony Cox Community Fund Grants, 827
Carrier Corporation Contributions Grants, 884
CDC Injury Control Research Centers Grants, 913
Central Carolina Community Foundation Community Impact Grants, 936
Champ-A Champion Fur Kids Grants, 959
Charles A. Frueauff Foundation Grants, 962
Children Affected by AIDS Foundation Camp Network Grants, 994
Children Affected by AIDS Foundation Family Assistance Emergency Fund Grants, 996
CLIF Bar Family Foundation Grants, 1040
Coastal Community Foundation of South Carolina Grants, 1051
Community Foundation of Greenville Community Enrichment Grants, 1113
Community Foundation of Greenville Hollingsworth Funds Program/Project Grants, 1114
Community Foundation of Greenville-Greenville Women Giving Grants, 1115
Cooper Industries Foundation Grants, 1150
CSX Corporate Contributions Grants, 1169
Dean Foods Community Involvement Grants, 1209
DHHS Healthy Tomorrows Partnership for Children, 1261
Do Something BR!CK Awards, 1287
Dorothy Hooper Beattie Foundation Grants, 1321
Dr. Stanley Pearle Scholarships, 1330
Drs. Bruce and Lee Foundation Grants, 1333
Duke Endowment Health Care Grants, 1338
Duke Energy Foundation Grants, 1339
Eastman Chemical Company Foundation Grants, 1362
Fluor Foundation Grants, 1517
Foundation for the Carolinas Grants, 1535
GoGirlGo! Ambassador Team Awards, 1632
Guitar Center Music Foundation Grants, 1675
Harry Kramer Memorial Fund Grants, 1705
Hilton Head Island Foundation Grants, 1779
IAFF Burn Foundation Research Grants, 1830
John I. Smith Charities Grants, 1935
John Merck Fund Grants, 1940
John Merck Scholars Awards, 1941
Kimberly-Clark Community Grants, 2001
Lettie Pate Whitehead Foundation Grants, 2049
Mary Black Foundation Grants, 2118
Multiple Sclerosis Foundation Brighter Tomorrow Grants, 2228
National Starch and Chemical Foundation Grants, 2261
NEI Mentored Clinical Scientist Development Program Award (K12), 2295
NMF Franklin C. McLean Award, 2829
NMF General Electric Medical Scholars Fellowships, 2830
NMF Henry G. Halladay Awards, 2831
NMF Mary Ball Carrera Scholarship, 2834
NMF National Medical Association Awards for Medical Journalism, 2836
NMF National Medical Association Emerging Scholar Awards, 2837
NMF National Medical Association Patti LaBelle Award, 2838
NMF Need-Based Scholarships, 2839
NMF Ralph W. Ellison Prize, 2840
NMF William and Charlotte Cadbury Award, 2841
NSF Major Research Instrumentation Program (MRI) Grants, 2889
OneSight Research Foundation Block Grants, 2944
Pfizer/AAFP Foundation Visiting Professorship Program in Family Medicine, 3027
Piedmont Natural Gas Grants, 3048
Plum Creek Foundation Grants, 3062
Progress Energy Foundation Grants, 3084
Rosalinde and Arthur Gilbert Foundation/AFAR New Investigator Awards in Alzheimer's Disease, 3187
Self Foundation Grants, 3277
Sisters of Mercy of North Carolina Foundation Grants, 3295
Sonoco Foundation Grants, 3347
Springs Close Foundation Grants, 3360
Tylenol Scholarship, 3444
U.S. Department of Education Erma Byrd Scholarships, 3446
U.S. Department of Education United States-Russia Program: Improving Research and Educational Activities in Higher Education, 3451
US CRDF Leishmaniasis: Collaborative Research Opportunities in North Africa and the Middle East, 3474
Vulcan Materials Company Foundation Grants, 3504
Wal-Mart Foundation Community Grants, 3513
Wal-Mart State Giving Program Grants, 3514
Woodward Fund Grants, 3552
YSA UnitedHealth Heroes Service Learning Grants, 3556

South Dakota

3M Company Health and Human Services Grants, 10
3M Foundation Grants, 11
ACF Ethnic Community Self-Help Grants, 200
ACF Preferred Communities Grants, 201
ACF Standing Announcement for Unaccompanied Alien Children Grants, 202
ACF Supplemental Services for Recently Arrived Refugees Grants, 203
Actors Fund Social Services and Financial Assistance, 225
Albertson's Charitable Giving Grants, 330
American College of Surgeons and The Triological Society Clinical Scientist Development Awards, 422
ASHA Advancing Academic-Research Careers (AARC) Award, 569
ASHA Minority Student Leadership Program Awards, 570
ASHA Multicultural Activities Projects Grants, 571
ASHA Research Mentoring-Pair Travel Award, 572
ASHA Student Research Travel Award, 573
ASHA Students Preparing for Academic & Research Careers (SPARC) Award, 574
ASM Millis-Colwell Postgraduate Travel Grant, 608
Bearemy's Kennel Pals Grants, 728
Bush Foundation Health & Human Services Grants, 814
Bush Foundation Medical Fellowships, 815
Cable Positive's Tony Cox Community Fund Grants, 827
Champ-A Champion Fur Kids Grants, 959
Charles A. Frueauff Foundation Grants, 962
Children Affected by AIDS Foundation Camp Network Grants, 994
Children Affected by AIDS Foundation Family Assistance Emergency Fund Grants, 996
CLIF Bar Family Foundation Grants, 1040
Dean Foods Community Involvement Grants, 1209
Do Something BR!CK Awards, 1287
Dr. Stanley Pearle Scholarships, 1330
GoGirlGo! Ambassador Team Awards, 1632
Graco Foundation Grants, 1642
Guitar Center Music Foundation Grants, 1675
Harry Kramer Memorial Fund Grants, 1705
IAFF Burn Foundation Research Grants, 1830
John Merck Fund Grants, 1940
John Merck Scholars Awards, 1941
Multiple Sclerosis Foundation Brighter Tomorrow Grants, 2228
NEI Mentored Clinical Scientist Development Program Award (K12), 2295
NMF Franklin C. McLean Award, 2829
NMF General Electric Medical Scholars Fellowships, 2830
NMF Henry G. Halladay Awards, 2831
NMF Mary Ball Carrera Scholarship, 2834
NMF National Medical Association Awards for Medical Journalism, 2836
NMF National Medical Association Emerging Scholar Awards, 2837

NMF National Medical Association Patti LaBelle Award, 2838
NMF Need-Based Scholarships, 2839
NMF Ralph W. Ellison Prize, 2840
NMF William and Charlotte Cadbury Award, 2841
NSF Major Research Instrumentation Program (MRI) Grants, 2889
OneSight Research Foundation Block Grants, 2944
Pfizer/AAFP Foundation Visiting Professorship Program in Family Medicine, 3027
Piper Jaffray Companies Building Strong Communities Grants, 3053
Rosalinde and Arthur Gilbert Foundation/AFAR New Investigator Awards in Alzheimer's Disease, 3187
Tylenol Scholarship, 3444
U.S. Department of Education Erma Byrd Scholarships, 3446
U.S. Department of Education United States-Russia Program: Improving Research and Educational Activities in Higher Education, 3451
US CRDF Leishmaniasis: Collaborative Research Opportunities in North Africa and the Middle East, 3474
Viking Children's Fund Grants, 3497
Waitt Family Foundation Grants, 3512
Wal-Mart Foundation Community Grants, 3513
Wal-Mart State Giving Program Grants, 3514
Wellmark Foundation Grants, 3526

Tennessee

ACF Ethnic Community Self-Help Grants, 200
ACF Preferred Communities Grants, 201
ACF Standing Announcement for Unaccompanied Alien Children Grants, 202
ACF Supplemental Services for Recently Arrived Refugees Grants, 203
Actors Fund Social Services and Financial Assistance, 225
AFG Industries Grants, 259
Aladdin Industries Foundation Grants, 322
Albertson's Charitable Giving Grants, 330
American College of Surgeons and The Triological Society Clinical Scientist Development Awards, 422
American Electric Power Grants, 434
Arkema Foundation Science Teachers Program, 535
ASHA Advancing Academic-Research Careers (AARC) Award, 569
ASHA Minority Student Leadership Program Awards, 570
ASHA Multicultural Activities Projects Grants, 571
ASHA Research Mentoring-Pair Travel Award, 572
ASHA Student Research Travel Award, 573
ASHA Students Preparing for Academic & Research Careers (SPARC) Award, 574
ASM Millis-Colwell Postgraduate Travel Grant, 608
Assisi Foundation Grants, 653
AT&T Excelerator, 657
Bearemy's Kennel Pals Grants, 728
Bechtel Group Foundation Building Positive Community Relationships Grants, 731
Belk Foundation Grants, 739
Bridgestone/Firestone Trust Fund Grants, 792
Cable Positive's Tony Cox Community Fund Grants, 827
Carrier Corporation Contributions Grants, 884
CDC Cancer Prevention and Control Programs, 903
CDC Injury Control Research Centers Grants, 913
Champ-A Champion Fur Kids Grants, 959
Charles A. Frueauff Foundation Grants, 962
Children Affected by AIDS Foundation Camp Network Grants, 994
Children Affected by AIDS Foundation Family Assistance Emergency Fund Grants, 996
Christy-Houston Foundation Grants, 1008
CLIF Bar Family Foundation Grants, 1040
Coors Brewing Corporate Contributions Grants, 1151
CSX Corporate Contributions Grants, 1169
Dean Foods Community Involvement Grants, 1209
Dell Foundation Healthy Communities, Literate Communities, and Connected Communities Grants, 1217
Dell Foundation Open Grants, 1218
Do Something BR!CK Awards, 1287
Dr. Stanley Pearle Scholarships, 1330
Eastman Chemical Company Foundation Grants, 1362
Fifth Third Foundation Grants, 1501
Fluor Foundation Grants, 1517
FMC Foundation Grants, 1518
Frist Foundation Grants, 1563
GenCorp Foundation Grants, 1587
General Mills Foundation Grants, 1590
Gladys Brooks Foundation Grants, 1620
GoGirlGo! Ambassador Team Awards, 1632
Guitar Center Music Foundation Grants, 1675
Harry Kramer Memorial Fund Grants, 1705
HCA Foundation Grants, 1721
Hershey Company Grants, 1754
Humana Foundation Grants, 1818
IAFF Burn Foundation Research Grants, 1830
John Deere Foundation Grants, 1929
John Merck Fund Grants, 1940
John Merck Scholars Awards, 1941
Johns Manville Fund Grants, 1950
Kimberly-Clark Community Grants, 2001
King Pharmaceuticals Corporate Contributions Grants, 2003
Lettie Pate Whitehead Foundation Grants, 2049
Multiple Sclerosis Foundation Brighter Tomorrow Grants, 2228
National Starch & Chemical Found Grants, 2261
NEI Mentored Clinical Scientist Development Program Award (K12), 2295
NMF Franklin C. McLean Award, 2829
NMF General Electric Medical Scholars Fellowships, 2830
NMF Henry G. Halladay Awards, 2831
NMF Mary Ball Carrera Scholarship, 2834
NMF National Medical Association Awards for Medical Journalism, 2836
NMF National Medical Association Emerging Scholar Awards, 2837
NMF National Medical Association Patti LaBelle Award, 2838
NMF Need-Based Scholarships, 2839
NMF Ralph W. Ellison Prize, 2840
NMF William and Charlotte Cadbury Award, 2841
NSF Major Research Instrumentation Program (MRI) Grants, 2889
OneSight Research Foundation Block Grants, 2944
PeyBack Foundation Grants, 3022
Pfizer/AAFP Foundation Visiting Professorship Program in Family Medicine, 3027
Piedmont Natural Gas Grants, 3048
Piper Jaffray Companies Building Strong Communities Grants, 3053
Plough Foundation Grants, 3061
Rosalinde and Arthur Gilbert Foundation/AFAR New Investigator Awards in Alzheimer's Disease, 3187
Square D Foundation Grants, 3361
Thompson Charitable Foundation Grants, 3425
Tylenol Scholarship, 3444
U.S. Department of Education Erma Byrd Scholarships, 3446
U.S. Department of Education United States-Russia Program: Improving Research and Educational Activities in Higher Education, 3451
US CRDF Leishmaniasis: Collaborative Research Opportunities in North Africa and the Middle East, 3474
Vulcan Materials Company Foundation Grants, 3504
Wal-Mart Foundation Community Grants, 3513
Wal-Mart State Giving Program Grants, 3514
Woodward Fund Grants, 3552
YSA UnitedHealth Heroes Service Learning Grants, 3556

Texas

3M Company Health and Human Services Grants, 10
3M Foundation Grants, 11
Abbott Fund Access to Health Care Grants, 176
Abbott Fund Community Vitality Grants, 177
Abbott Fund Global AIDS Care Grants, 178
Abbott Fund Science and Medical Innovation Grants, 179
Abell-Hanger Foundation Grants, 183
ACE Charitable Foundation Grants, 199
ACF Ethnic Community Self-Help Grants, 200
ACF Preferred Communities Grants, 201
ACF Standing Announcement for Unaccompanied Alien Children Grants, 202
ACF Supplemental Services for Recently Arrived Refugees Grants, 203
Actors Fund Social Services and Financial Assistance, 225
Advanced Micro Devices Community Affairs Grants, 239
AEGON Transamerica Foundation Grants, 243
Albert and Margaret Alkek Foundation Grants, 326
Albertson's Charitable Giving Grants, 330
Amarillo Area/Harrington Foundations Grants, 410
American College of Surgeons and The Triological Society Clinical Scientist Development Awards, 422
American Electric Power Grants, 434
Anheuser-Busch Foundation Grants, 474
ARCO Foundation Education Grants, 526
Arkema Foundation Science Teachers Program, 535
ASHA Advancing Academic-Research Careers (AARC) Award, 569
ASHA Minority Student Leadership Program Awards, 570
ASHA Multicultural Activities Projects Grants, 571
ASHA Research Mentoring-Pair Travel Award, 572
ASHA Student Research Travel Award, 573
ASHA Students Preparing for Academic & Research Careers (SPARC) Award, 574
ASM Millis-Colwell Postgraduate Travel Grant, 608
AT&T Excelerator, 657
Bearemy's Kennel Pals Grants, 728
Bechtel Group Foundation Building Positive Community Relationships Grants, 731
Belk Foundation Grants, 739
Bernard and Audre Rapoport Foundation Grants, 746
Bob and Delores Hope Charitable Foundation Grants, 774
Bosque Foundation Grants, 782
Bridgestone/Firestone Trust Fund Grants, 792
Cable Positive's Tony Cox Community Fund Grants, 827
Carl B. and Florence E. King Foundation Grants, 869
Carrier Corporation Contributions Grants, 884
CDC Injury Control Research Centers Grants, 913
Champ-A Champion Fur Kids Grants, 959
Charles A. Frueauff Foundation Grants, 962
Chase Paymentech Corporate Giving Grants, 975
Children Affected by AIDS Foundation Camp Network Grants, 994
Children Affected by AIDS Foundation Family Assistance Emergency Fund Grants, 996
CLIF Bar Family Foundation Grants, 1040
Coastal Bend Community Foundation Grants, 1050
Cockrell Foundation Grants, 1053
Comerica Charitable Foundation Grants, 1073
Compass Bank Foundation Grants, 1138
ConocoPhillips Foundation Grants, 1144
Constantin Foundation Grants, 1145
Cooper Industries Foundation Grants, 1150
Cullen Foundation Grants, 1172
Dallas Mavericks Foundation Grants, 1190
Dallas Women's Foundation Grants, 1191
Dean Foods Community Involvement Grants, 1209
Dell Foundation Healthy Communities, Literate Communities, and Connected Communities Grants, 1217

Dell Foundation Open Grants, 1218
Denton A. Cooley Foundation Grants, 1225
DHHS Healthy Tomorrows Partnership for Children, 1261
Do Something BR!CK Awards, 1287
Dominion Educational Partnership Grant, 1308
Dr. Bob and Jean Smith Foundation Grants, 1325
Dr. Stanley Pearle Scholarships, 1330
Eastman Chemical Company Foundation Grants, 1362
EDS Foundation Grants, 1371
Effie and Wofford Cain Foundation Grants, 1385
El Paso Community Foundation Grants, 1388
El Paso Corporate Foundation Grants, 1389
Entergy Community Partnership Grants, 1417
Entergy Corporation Open Grants for Healthy Families, 1418
Eugene McDermott Foundation Grants, 1435
Ewing Halsell Foundation Grants, 1440
Feldman Foundation Grants Program, 1484
Fidelity Foundation Grants, 1498
Fluor Foundation Grants, 1517
FMC Foundation Grants, 1518
Fondren Foundation Grants, 1520
Forrest C. Lattner Foundation Grants, 1523
Frederick Gardner Cottrell Foundation Grants, 1560
GoGirlGo! Ambassador Team Awards, 1632
Guitar Center Music Foundation Grants, 1675
H.A. and Mary K. Chapman Charitable Trust Grants, 1681
Halliburton Foundation Grants, 1687
Hallmark Corporate Foundation Grants, 1688
Harold Simmons Foundation Grants, 1698
Harris and Eliza Kempner Fund Grants, 1699
Harry Kramer Memorial Fund Grants, 1705
Hawn Foundation Grants, 1719
Hoblitzelle Foundation Grants, 1783
Hogg Foundation for Mental Health Grants, 1784
Hoglund Foundation Grants, 1785
Houston Endowment Grants, 1797
Human Source Foundation Grants, 1817
Humana Foundation Grants, 1818
IAFF Burn Foundation Research Grants, 1830
J.E. and L.E. Mabee Foundation Grants, 1875
James M. Collins Foundation Grants, 1891
James R. Dougherty Jr. Foundation Grants, 1894
John Merck Fund Grants, 1940
John Merck Scholars Awards, 1941
John P. McGovern Foundation Grants, 1942
John S. Dunn Research Foundation Grants and Chairs, 1945
Ken W. Davis Foundation Grants, 1987
Kimberly-Clark Community Grants, 2001
Lowe Foundation Grants, 2067
Lubbock Area Foundation Grants, 2079
Lubrizol Foundation Grants Program, 2080
M.B. and Edna Zale Foundation Grants, 2093
Marcia and Otto Koehler Foundation Grants, 2103
McCombs Foundation Grants, 2142
Meadows Foundation Grants, 2161
Michael and Susan Dell Foundation Grants, 2189
Multiple Sclerosis Foundation Brighter Tomorrow Grants, 2228
NEI Mentored Clinical Scientist Development Program Award (K12), 2295
NMF Franklin C. McLean Award, 2829
NMF General Electric Medical Scholars Fellowships, 2830
NMF Henry G. Halladay Awards, 2831
NMF Mary Ball Carrera Scholarship, 2834
NMF National Medical Association Awards for Medical Journalism, 2836
NMF National Medical Association Emerging Scholar Awards, 2837
NMF National Medical Association Patti LaBelle Award, 2838
NMF Need-Based Scholarships, 2839
NMF Ralph W. Ellison Prize, 2840
NMF William and Charlotte Cadbury Award, 2841
NSF Major Research Instrumentation Program (MRI) Grants, 2889
OneSight Research Foundation Block Grants, 2944
PacifiCare Foundation Grants, 2981
Paso del Norte Health Foundation Grants, 2995
Paul and Mary Haas Foundation Contributions and Student Scholarships, 2997
Pfizer/AAFP Foundation Visiting Professorship Program in Family Medicine, 3027
Plum Creek Foundation Grants, 3062
Powell Foundation Grants, 3073
Priddy Foundation Grants, 3077
Prudential Foundation Grants, 3087
Rainbow Fund Grants, 3103
Robert E. and Evelyn McKee Foundation Grants, 3170
Rosalinde and Arthur Gilbert Foundation/AFAR New Investigator Awards in Alzheimer's Disease, 3187
Roy and Christine Sturgis Trust Grants, 3191
San Antonio Area Foundation Grants, 3254
Sid W. Richardson Foundation Grants, 3284
Southwire Company Grants, 3353
Square D Foundation Grants, 3361
Steele-Reese Foundation Grants, 3380
Susan Vaughan Foundation Grants, 3413
Texas Commission on the Arts Arts Respond Project Grants, 3420
Topfer Family Foundation Grants, 3430
Toro Foundation Grants, 3431
TWS Foundation Grants, 3443
Tylenol Scholarship, 3444
U.S. Department of Education Erma Byrd Scholarships, 3446
U.S. Department of Education United States-Russia Program: Improving Research and Educational Activities in Higher Education, 3451
US CRDF Leishmaniasis: Collaborative Research Opportunities in North Africa and the Middle East, 3474
US Trust Corporation Foundation Grants, 3475
Vulcan Materials Company Foundation Grants, 3504
Wal-Mart Foundation Community Grants, 3513
Wal-Mart State Giving Program Grants, 3514
Western Union Foundation Grants, 3529

US Virgin Islands

ACF Ethnic Community Self-Help Grants, 200
ACF Preferred Communities Grants, 201
ACF Standing Announcement for Unaccompanied Alien Children Grants, 202
ACF Supplemental Services for Recently Arrived Refugees Grants, 203
American College of Surgeons and The Triological Society Clinical Scientist Development Awards, 422
ASHA Advancing Academic-Research Careers (AARC) Award, 569
ASHA Minority Student Leadership Program Awards, 570
ASHA Multicultural Activities Projects Grants, 571
ASHA Research Mentoring-Pair Travel Award, 572
ASHA Student Research Travel Award, 573
ASHA Students Preparing for Academic & Research Careers (SPARC) Award, 574
Bearemy's Kennel Pals Grants, 728
Champ-A Champion Fur Kids Grants, 959
CLIF Bar Family Foundation Grants, 1040
GoGirlGo! Ambassador Team Awards, 1632
Harry Kramer Memorial Fund Grants, 1705
John Merck Scholars Awards, 1941
NEI Mentored Clinical Scientist Development Program Award (K12), 2295
NSF Major Research Instrumentation Program (MRI) Grants, 2889
Rosalinde and Arthur Gilbert Foundation/AFAR New Investigator Awards in Alzheimer's Disease, 3187
U.S. Department of Education Erma Byrd Scholarships, 3446
U.S. Department of Education Rehabilitation Training--Rehabilitation Continuing Education Programs (RCEP)--Institute on Rehabilitation Issues (IRI), 3449
U.S. Department of Education United States-Russia Program: Improving Research and Educational Activities in Higher Education, 3451
US CRDF Leishmaniasis: Collaborative Research Opportunities in North Africa and the Middle East, 3474

Utah

3M Company Health and Human Services Grants, 10
3M Foundation Grants, 11
Abbott Fund Access to Health Care Grants, 176
Abbott Fund Community Vitality Grants, 177
Abbott Fund Global AIDS Care Grants, 178
Abbott Fund Science and Medical Innovation Grants, 179
ACF Ethnic Community Self-Help Grants, 200
ACF Preferred Communities Grants, 201
ACF Standing Announcement for Unaccompanied Alien Children Grants, 202
ACF Supplemental Services for Recently Arrived Refugees Grants, 203
Actors Fund Social Services and Financial Assistance, 225
Albertson's Charitable Giving Grants, 330
American College of Surgeons and The Triological Society Clinical Scientist Development Awards, 422
ASHA Advancing Academic-Research Careers (AARC) Award, 569
ASHA Minority Student Leadership Program Awards, 570
ASHA Multicultural Activities Projects Grants, 571
ASHA Research Mentoring-Pair Travel Award, 572
ASHA Student Research Travel Award, 573
ASHA Students Preparing for Academic & Research Careers (SPARC) Award, 574
ASM Millis-Colwell Postgraduate Travel Grant, 608
Bearemy's Kennel Pals Grants, 728
Bridgestone/Firestone Trust Fund Grants, 792
Cable Positive's Tony Cox Community Fund Grants, 827
Champ-A Champion Fur Kids Grants, 959
Children Affected by AIDS Foundation Camp Network Grants, 994
Children Affected by AIDS Foundation Family Assistance Emergency Fund Grants, 996
CLIF Bar Family Foundation Grants, 1040
Daniels Fund Grants, 1200
Dean Foods Community Involvement Grants, 1209
Do Something BR!CK Awards, 1287
Dr. Stanley Pearle Scholarships, 1330
E.L. Wiegand Foundation Grants, 1361
eBay Foundation Community Grants, 1363
Fidelity Foundation Grants, 1498
GenCorp Foundation Grants, 1587
George S. and Dolores Dore Eccles Foundation Grants, 1602
GoGirlGo! Ambassador Team Awards, 1632
Guitar Center Music Foundation Grants, 1675
Harry Kramer Memorial Fund Grants, 1705
Humana Foundation Grants, 1818
IAFF Burn Foundation Research Grants, 1830
John Merck Fund Grants, 1940
John Merck Scholars Awards, 1941
Kimberly-Clark Community Grants, 2001
Multiple Sclerosis Foundation Brighter Tomorrow Grants, 2228
NEI Mentored Clinical Scientist Development Program Award (K12), 2295
NMF Franklin C. McLean Award, 2829
NMF General Electric Medical Scholars Fellowships, 2830
NMF Henry G. Halladay Awards, 2831
NMF Mary Ball Carrera Scholarship, 2834
NMF National Medical Association Awards for Medical Journalism, 2836

NMF National Medical Association Emerging Scholar Awards, 2837
NMF National Medical Association Patti LaBelle Award, 2838
NMF Need-Based Scholarships, 2839
NMF Ralph W. Ellison Prize, 2840
NMF William and Charlotte Cadbury Award, 2841
NSF Major Research Instrumentation Program (MRI) Grants, 2889
OneSight Research Foundation Block Grants, 2944
PacifiCorp Foundation for Learning Grants, 2982
Pfizer/AAFP Foundation Visiting Professorship Program in Family Medicine, 3027
Piper Jaffray Companies Building Strong Communities Grants, 3053
Questar Corporate Contributions Grants, 3097
Regence Foundation Access to Health Care Grants, 3138
Regence Foundation Health Care Community Awareness and Engagement Grants, 3139
Regence Foundation Health Care Connections Grants, 3140
Regence Foundation Improving End-of-Life Grants, 3141
Regence Foundation Tools and Technology Grants, 3142
Rosalinde and Arthur Gilbert Foundation/AFAR New Investigator Awards in Alzheimer's Disease, 3187
Ruth Eleanor Bamberger and John Ernest Bamberger Memorial Foundation Grants, 3202
Southwire Company Grants, 3353
Stan and Sandy Checketts Foundation, 3373
Sunderland Foundation Grants, 3400
Tylenol Scholarship, 3444
U.S. Department of Education Erma Byrd Scholarships, 3446
U.S. Department of Education United States-Russia Program: Improving Research and Educational Activities in Higher Education, 3451
US CRDF Leishmaniasis: Collaborative Research Opportunities in North Africa and the Middle East, 3474
Wal-Mart Foundation Community Grants, 3513
Wal-Mart State Giving Program Grants, 3514

Vermont

ACF Ethnic Community Self-Help Grants, 200
ACF Preferred Communities Grants, 201
ACF Standing Announcement for Unaccompanied Alien Children Grants, 202
ACF Supplemental Services for Recently Arrived Refugees Grants, 203
Actors Fund Social Services and Financial Assistance, 225
Agnes M. Lindsay Trust Grants, 263
Albertson's Charitable Giving Grants, 330
American College of Surgeons and The Triological Society Clinical Scientist Development Awards, 422
ASHA Advancing Academic-Research Careers (AARC) Award, 569
ASHA Minority Student Leadership Program Awards, 570
ASHA Multicultural Activities Projects Grants, 571
ASHA Research Mentoring-Pair Travel Award, 572
ASHA Student Research Travel Award, 573
ASHA Students Preparing for Academic & Research Careers (SPARC) Award, 574
ASM Millis-Colwell Postgraduate Travel Grant, 608
Barnes Group Foundation Grants, 696
Bearemy's Kennel Pals Grants, 728
Cable Positive's Tony Cox Community Fund Grants, 827
Carlisle Foundation Grants, 874
Champ-A Champion Fur Kids Grants, 959
Charles A. Frueauff Foundation Grants, 962
Charles H. Hood Foundation Child Health Research Grants, 968
Children Affected by AIDS Foundation Camp Network Grants, 994
Children Affected by AIDS Foundation Family Assistance Emergency Fund Grants, 996
CLIF Bar Family Foundation Grants, 1040
Do Something BR!CK Awards, 1287
Dr. Stanley Pearle Scholarships, 1330
Entergy Corporation Open Grants for Healthy Families, 1418
Gladys Brooks Foundation Grants, 1620
GoGirlGo! Ambassador Team Awards, 1632
Guitar Center Music Foundation Grants, 1675
Hannaford Charitable Foundation Grants, 1692
Harry Kramer Memorial Fund Grants, 1705
IAFF Burn Foundation Research Grants, 1830
J. Walton Bissell Foundation Grants, 1872
Jane's Trust Grants, 1904
Jessie B. Cox Charitable Trust Grants, 1918
John Merck Fund Grants, 1940
John Merck Scholars Awards, 1941
Multiple Sclerosis Foundation Brighter Tomorrow Grants, 2228
NEI Mentored Clinical Scientist Development Program Award (K12), 2295
NMF Franklin C. McLean Award, 2829
NMF General Electric Medical Scholars Fellowships, 2830
NMF Henry G. Halladay Awards, 2831
NMF Mary Ball Carrera Scholarship, 2834
NMF National Medical Association Awards for Medical Journalism, 2836
NMF National Medical Association Emerging Scholar Awards, 2837
NMF National Medical Association Patti LaBelle Award, 2838
NMF Need-Based Scholarships, 2839
NMF Ralph W. Ellison Prize, 2840
NMF William and Charlotte Cadbury Award, 2841
NSF Major Research Instrumentation Program (MRI) Grants, 2889
OneSight Research Foundation Block Grants, 2944
Pfizer/AAFP Foundation Visiting Professorship Program in Family Medicine, 3027
Rosalinde and Arthur Gilbert Foundation/AFAR New Investigator Awards in Alzheimer's Disease, 3187
Shaw's Supermarkets Donations, 3280
Tylenol Scholarship, 3444
U.S. Department of Education Erma Byrd Scholarships, 3446
U.S. Department of Education United States-Russia Program: Improving Research and Educational Activities in Higher Education, 3451
US CRDF Leishmaniasis: Collaborative Research Opportunities in North Africa and the Middle East, 3474
Verizon Foundation Vermont Grants, 3491
Vermont Community Foundation Grants, 3493
Wal-Mart Foundation Community Grants, 3513
Wal-Mart State Giving Program Grants, 3514

Virginia

Abbott Fund Access to Health Care Grants, 176
Abbott Fund Community Vitality Grants, 177
Abbott Fund Global AIDS Care Grants, 178
Abbott Fund Science and Medical Innovation Grants, 179
ACE Charitable Foundation Grants, 199
ACF Ethnic Community Self-Help Grants, 200
ACF Preferred Communities Grants, 201
ACF Standing Announcement for Unaccompanied Alien Children Grants, 202
ACF Supplemental Services for Recently Arrived Refugees Grants, 203
Actors Fund Social Services and Financial Assistance, 225
American College of Surgeons and The Triological Society Clinical Scientist Development Awards, 422
American Electric Power Grants, 434
Andersen Corporate Foundation, 470
Anheuser-Busch Foundation Grants, 474
Anthem Blue Cross and Blue Shield Grants, 488
Arlington Community Foundation Grants, 536
ASHA Advancing Academic-Research Careers (AARC) Award, 569
ASHA Minority Student Leadership Program Awards, 570
ASHA Multicultural Activities Projects Grants, 571
ASHA Research Mentoring-Pair Travel Award, 572
ASHA Student Research Travel Award, 573
ASHA Students Preparing for Academic & Research Careers (SPARC) Award, 574
ASM Millis-Colwell Postgraduate Travel Grant, 608
Bearemy's Kennel Pals Grants, 728
Beazley Foundation Grants, 730
Bechtel Group Foundation Building Positive Community Relationships Grants, 731
Beirne Carter Foundation Grants, 737
Belk Foundation Grants, 739
BJ's Charitable Foundation Grants, 761
Burlington Industries Foundation Grants, 811
Cable Positive's Tony Cox Community Fund Grants, 827
Camp-Younts Foundation Grants, 838
Campbell Hoffman Foundation Grants, 840
CDC Injury Control Research Centers Grants, 913
Champ-A Champion Fur Kids Grants, 959
Charles A. Frueauff Foundation Grants, 962
Charles Delmar Foundation Grants, 963
Children Affected by AIDS Foundation Camp Network Grants, 994
Children Affected by AIDS Foundation Family Assistance Emergency Fund Grants, 996
CLIF Bar Family Foundation Grants, 1040
Commonweal Foundation Community Assistance Grants, 1075
Commonweal Foundation Grants, 1076
Community Foundation AIDS Endowment Awards, 1088
Coors Brewing Corporate Contributions Grants, 1151
CSX Corporate Contributions Grants, 1169
Dammann Fund Grants, 1192
Dean Foods Community Involvement Grants, 1209
Do Something BR!CK Awards, 1287
Dominion Educational Partnership Grant, 1303
Dr. Stanley Pearle Scholarships, 1330
EDS Foundation Grants, 1371
Eugene and Agnes E. Meyer Foundation Grants, 1432
Fluor Foundation Grants, 1517
Freddie Mac Foundation Grants, 1558
GenCorp Foundation Grants, 1587
GoGirlGo! Ambassador Team Awards, 1632
Guitar Center Music Foundation Grants, 1675
Harry Bramhall Gilbert Charitable Trust Grants, 1703
Harry Kramer Memorial Fund Grants, 1705
Harvest Foundation Grants, 1713
Hershey Company Grants, 1754
Hut Foundation Grants, 1827
IAFF Burn Foundation Research Grants, 1830
Jeffress Research Grants, 1913
Jenkins Foundation: Improving the Health of Greater Richmond Grants, 1915
John Edward Fowler Memorial Foundation Grants, 1930
John Merck Fund Grants, 1940
John Merck Scholars Awards, 1941
Land O'Lakes Foundation Mid-Atlantic Grants Program, 2027
Leonsis Foundation Grants, 2045
Lettie Pate Whitehead Foundation Grants, 2049
Morris and Gwendolyn Cafritz Foundation Grants, 2217
Multiple Sclerosis Foundation Brighter Tomorrow Grants, 2228
NEI Mentored Clinical Scientist Development Program Award (K12), 2295

NMF Franklin C. McLean Award, 2829
NMF General Electric Medical Scholars Fellowships, 2830
NMF Henry G. Halladay Awards, 2831
NMF Mary Ball Carrera Scholarship, 2834
NMF National Medical Association Awards for Medical Journalism, 2836
NMF National Medical Association Emerging Scholar Awards, 2837
NMF National Medical Association Patti LaBelle Award, 2838
NMF Need-Based Scholarships, 2839
NMF Ralph W. Ellison Prize, 2840
NMF William and Charlotte Cadbury Award, 2841
NSF Major Research Instrumentation Program (MRI) Grants, 2889
OneSight Research Foundation Block Grants, 2944
Pfizer/AAFP Foundation Visiting Professorship Program in Family Medicine, 3027
Plum Creek Foundation Grants, 3062
Richmond Eye and Ear Fund Grants, 3164
Robins Foundation Grants, 3175
Rosalinde and Arthur Gilbert Foundation/AFAR New Investigator Awards in Alzheimer's Disease, 3187
Sheltering Arms Fund Grants, 3282
Thompson Charitable Foundation Grants, 3425
Tylenol Scholarship, 3444
U.S. Department of Education Erma Byrd Scholarships, 3446
U.S. Department of Education United States-Russia Program: Improving Research and Educational Activities in Higher Education, 3451
US CRDF Leishmaniasis: Collaborative Research Opportunities in North Africa and the Middle East, 3474
US Trust Corporation Foundation Grants, 3475
VDH Commonwealth of Virginia Nurse Educator Scholarships, 3482
VDH Emergency Medical Services Training Fund (EMSTF), 3483
VDH Rescue Squad Assistance Fund Grants, 3484
Verizon Foundation Virginia Grants, 3492
Virginia Department of Health Mary Marshall Nursing Scholarships for Licensed Practical Nurses, 3498
Virginia Department of Health Mary Marshall Nursing Scholarships for Registered Nurses, 3499
Virginia Department of Health Nurse Practitioner/Nurse Midwife Scholarships, 3500
Virginia Tuition Assistance Grant Program, 3501
Vulcan Materials Company Foundation Grants, 3504
Wal-Mart Foundation Community Grants, 3513
Wal-Mart State Giving Program Grants, 3514
William G. McGowan Charitable Fund Grants, 3539

Washington
ACE Charitable Foundation Grants, 199
ACF Ethnic Community Self-Help Grants, 200
ACF Preferred Communities Grants, 201
ACF Standing Announcement for Unaccompanied Alien Children Grants, 202
ACF Supplemental Services for Recently Arrived Refugees Grants, 203
Actors Fund Social Services and Financial Assistance, 225
Adobe Community Investment Grants, 237
Alaska Airlines Corporate Giving Grants, 323
Alaska Airlines Foundation Grants, 324
Albertson's Charitable Giving Grants, 330
American College of Surgeons and The Triological Society Clinical Scientist Development Awards, 422
ARCO Foundation Education Grants, 526
ASHA Advancing Academic-Research Careers (AARC) Award, 569
ASHA Minority Student Leadership Program Awards, 570
ASHA Multicultural Activities Projects Grants, 571
ASHA Research Mentoring-Pair Travel Award, 572
ASHA Student Research Travel Award, 573
ASHA Students Preparing for Academic & Research Careers (SPARC) Award, 574
ASM Millis-Colwell Postgraduate Travel Grant, 608
Bearemy's Kennel Pals Grants, 728
Bechtel Group Foundation Building Positive Community Relationships Grants, 731
Ben B. Cheney Foundation Grants, 741
Birds Eye Foods Foundation Grants, 759
Blue Mountain Community Foundation Grants, 769
Bullitt Foundation Grants, 809
Cable Positive's Tony Cox Community Fund Grants, 827
CDC Injury Control Research Centers Grants, 913
Champ-A Champion Fur Kids Grants, 959
Children Affected by AIDS Foundation Camp Network Grants, 994
Children Affected by AIDS Foundation Family Assistance Emergency Fund Grants, 996
Chiron Foundation Community Grants, 1004
CLIF Bar Family Foundation Grants, 1040
Community Foundation of South Puget Sound Grants, 1124
Comprehensive Health Education Foundation Grants, 1139
ConocoPhillips Foundation Grants, 1144
D.V. and Ida J. McEachern Charitable Trust Grants, 1182
Do Something BR!CK Awards, 1287
Dr. Stanley Pearle Scholarships, 1330
E.L. Wiegand Foundation Grants, 1361
Edwin W. and Catherine M. Davis Foundation Grants, 1377
Fluor Foundation Grants, 1517
Foster Foundation Grants, 1524
Foundation Northwest Grants, 1537
GenCorp Foundation Grants, 1587
George Frederick Jewett Foundation Grants Program, 1599
GoGirlGo! Ambassador Team Awards, 1632
Greater Tacoma Community Foundation Grants, 1656
Greater Tacoma Community Foundation Ryan Alan Hade Endowment Fund, 1657
Guitar Center Music Foundation Grants, 1675
Harold and Arlene Schnitzer CARE Foundation Grants, 1697
Harry Kramer Memorial Fund Grants, 1705
Hasbro Children's Fund, 1714
IAFF Burn Foundation Research Grants, 1830
John Merck Fund Grants, 1940
John Merck Scholars Awards, 1941
Kimberly-Clark Community Grants, 2001
M.J. Murdock Charitable Trust Grants, 2095
Meyer Memorial Trust Emergency Grants, 2178
Meyer Memorial Trust Grassroots Grants, 2179
Meyer Memorial Trust Operating Funds Grants, 2180
Meyer Memorial Trust Responsive Grants, 2181
Multiple Sclerosis Foundation Brighter Tomorrow Grants, 2228
NEI Mentored Clinical Scientist Development Program Award (K12), 2295
NMF Franklin C. McLean Award, 2829
NMF General Electric Medical Scholars Fellowships, 2830
NMF Henry G. Halladay Awards, 2831
NMF Mary Ball Carrera Scholarship, 2834
NMF National Medical Association Awards for Medical Journalism, 2836
NMF National Medical Association Emerging Scholar Awards, 2837
NMF National Medical Association Patti LaBelle Award, 2838
NMF Need-Based Scholarships, 2839
NMF Ralph W. Ellison Prize, 2840
NMF William and Charlotte Cadbury Award, 2841
NSF Major Research Instrumentation Program (MRI) Grants, 2889
NWHF Community-Based Participatory Research Grants, 2904
NWHF Kaiser Permanente Community Fund Grants, 2906
OneSight Research Foundation Block Grants, 2944
PacifiCare Foundation Grants, 2981
PacifiCorp Foundation for Learning Grants, 2982
Paul G. Allen Family Foundation Grants, 3000
Pfizer/AAFP Foundation Visiting Professorship Program in Family Medicine, 3027
Piper Jaffray Companies Building Strong Communities Grants, 3053
Plum Creek Foundation Grants, 3062
PNC Charitable Trust and Foundation Grants, 3064
Premera CARES Grants, 3074
Pride Foundation Grants and Scholarships, 3078
Principal Financial Group Foundation Grants, 3082
Rathmann Family Foundation Grants, 3109
Rayonier Foundation Grants, 3111
Regence Foundation Access to Health Care Grants, 3138
Regence Foundation Health Care Community Awareness and Engagement Grants, 3139
Regence Foundation Health Care Connections Grants, 3140
Regence Foundation Improving End-of-Life Grants, 3141
Regence Foundation Tools and Technology Grants, 3142
Robert B McMillen Foundation Grants, 3169
Rosalinde and Arthur Gilbert Foundation/AFAR New Investigator Awards in Alzheimer's Disease, 3187
Samuel S. Johnson Foundation Grants, 3251
Seattle Foundation Grants, 3276
Simpson Fund Grants, 3290
Sunderland Foundation Grants, 3400
Tylenol Scholarship, 3444
U.S. Department of Education Erma Byrd Scholarships, 3446
U.S. Department of Education United States-Russia Program: Improving Research and Educational Activities in Higher Education, 3451
US CRDF Leishmaniasis: Collaborative Research Opportunities in North Africa and the Middle East, 3474
Wal-Mart Foundation Community Grants, 3513
Wal-Mart State Giving Program Grants, 3514

West Virginia
ACF Ethnic Community Self-Help Grants, 200
ACF Preferred Communities Grants, 201
ACF Standing Announcement for Unaccompanied Alien Children Grants, 202
ACF Supplemental Services for Recently Arrived Refugees Grants, 203
Actors Fund Social Services and Financial Assistance, 225
American College of Surgeons and The Triological Society Clinical Scientist Development Awards, 422
American Electric Power Grants, 434
ASHA Advancing Academic-Research Careers (AARC) Award, 569
ASHA Minority Student Leadership Program Awards, 570
ASHA Multicultural Activities Projects Grants, 571
ASHA Research Mentoring-Pair Travel Award, 572
ASHA Student Research Travel Award, 573
ASHA Students Preparing for Academic & Research Careers (SPARC) Award, 574
Ashland Corporate Contributions Grants, 586
ASM Millis-Colwell Postgraduate Travel Grant, 608
Bearemy's Kennel Pals Grants, 728
Beckley Area Foundation Grants, 732
Belk Foundation Grants, 739
Cable Positive's Tony Cox Community Fund Grants, 827
CDC Injury Control Research Centers Grants, 913

Champ-A Champion Fur Kids Grants, 959
Charles A. Frueauff Foundation Grants, 962
Charles Delmar Foundation Grants, 963
Children Affected by AIDS Foundation Camp Network Grants, 994
Children Affected by AIDS Foundation Family Assistance Emergency Fund Grants, 996
Claude Worthington Benedum Foundation Grants, 1033
Clay Foundation Grants, 1034
CLIF Bar Family Foundation Grants, 1040
CSX Corporate Contributions Grants, 1169
Daywood Foundation Grants, 1206
DHHS Healthy Tomorrows Partnership for Children, 1261
Do Something BR!CK Awards, 1287
Dominion Educational Partnership Grant, 1308
Dr. Stanley Pearle Scholarships, 1330
Fifth Third Foundation Grants, 1501
FMC Foundation Grants, 1518
GoGirlGo! Ambassador Team Awards, 1632
Guitar Center Music Foundation Grants, 1675
Harry Kramer Memorial Fund Grants, 1705
Huntington Clinical Foundation Grants, 1822
Huntington National Bank Community Affairs Grants, 1824
IAFF Burn Foundation Research Grants, 1830
John Merck Fund Grants, 1940
John Merck Scholars Awards, 1941
Multiple Sclerosis Foundation Brighter Tomorrow Grants, 2228
NEI Mentored Clinical Scientist Development Program Award (K12), 2295
NMF Franklin C. McLean Award, 2829
NMF General Electric Medical Scholars Fellowships, 2830
NMF Henry G. Halladay Awards, 2831
NMF Mary Ball Carrera Scholarship, 2834
NMF National Medical Association Awards for Medical Journalism, 2836
NMF National Medical Association Emerging Scholar Awards, 2837
NMF National Medical Association Patti LaBelle Award, 2838
NMF Need-Based Scholarships, 2839
NMF Ralph W. Ellison Prize, 2840
NMF William and Charlotte Cadbury Award, 2841
NSF Major Research Instrumentation Program (MRI) Grants, 2889
OneSight Research Foundation Block Grants, 2944
Pfizer/AAFP Foundation Visiting Professorship Program in Family Medicine, 3027
Plum Creek Foundation Grants, 3062
Rosalinde and Arthur Gilbert Foundation/AFAR New Investigator Awards in Alzheimer's Disease, 3187
Sisters of Saint Joseph Charitable Fund Grants, 3296
Tylenol Scholarship, 3444
U.S. Department of Education Erma Byrd Scholarships, 3446
U.S. Department of Education United States-Russia Program: Improving Research and Educational Activities in Higher Education, 3451
US CRDF Leishmaniasis: Collaborative Research Opportunities in North Africa and the Middle East, 3474
Wal-Mart Foundation Community Grants, 3513
Wal-Mart State Giving Program Grants, 3514

Wisconsin

3M Company Health and Human Services Grants, 10
3M Foundation Grants, 11
A Fund for Women Grants, 14
A Social Corporation Grants, 15
ACF Ethnic Community Self-Help Grants, 200
ACF Preferred Communities Grants, 201
ACF Standing Announcement for Unaccompanied Alien Children Grants, 202
ACF Supplemental Services for Recently Arrived Refugees Grants, 203
Actors Fund Social Services and Financial Assistance, 225
AEC Trust Grants, 242
Albertson's Charitable Giving Grants, 330
American College of Surgeons and The Triological Society Clinical Scientist Development Awards, 422
Andersen Corporate Foundation, 470
Anthem Blue Cross and Blue Shield Grants, 488
ASHA Advancing Academic-Research Careers (AARC) Award, 569
ASHA Minority Student Leadership Program Awards, 570
ASHA Multicultural Activities Projects Grants, 571
ASHA Research Mentoring-Pair Travel Award, 572
ASHA Student Research Travel Award, 573
ASHA Students Preparing for Academic & Research Careers (SPARC) Award, 574
ASM Millis-Colwell Postgraduate Travel Grant, 608
Assurant Health Foundation Grants, 655
AT&T Excelerator, 657
Bearemy's Kennel Pals Grants, 728
Beldon Fund Grants, 738
Birds Eye Foods Foundation Grants, 759
Black River Falls Area Foundation Grants, 762
Bridgestone/Firestone Trust Fund Grants, 792
Cable Positive's Tony Cox Community Fund Grants, 827
CDC Injury Control Research Centers Grants, 913
CFFVR Opportunity Grants, 952
Champ-A Champion Fur Kids Grants, 959
Children Affected by AIDS Foundation Camp Network Grants, 994
Children Affected by AIDS Foundation Family Assistance Emergency Fund Grants, 996
CLIF Bar Family Foundation Grants, 1040
ConAgra Foods Foundation Grants, 1140
Cooper Industries Foundation Grants, 1150
Cornerstone Foundation of Northeastern Wisconsin Grants, 1152
Dean Foods Community Involvement Grants, 1209
DHHS Healthy Tomorrows Partnership for Children, 1261
Do Something BR!CK Awards, 1287
Dr. Stanley Pearle Scholarships, 1330
Evjue Foundation Grants, 1439
Faye McBeath Foundation Grants, 1456
Frank G. and Freida K. Brotz Family Foundation Grants, 1552
General Mills Foundation Grants, 1590
George Kress Foundation Grants, 1601
Godfrey Foundation Grants, 1631
GoGirlGo! Ambassador Team Awards, 1632
Greater Green Bay Community Foundation Grants, 1652
Greater Milwaukee Foundation Grants, 1653
Green Bay Packers Foundation Grants, 1660
Guitar Center Music Foundation Grants, 1675
Harley Davidson Foundation Grants, 1694
Harry Kramer Memorial Fund Grants, 1705
Helen Bader Foundation Grants, 1738
Hormel Foods Charitable Trust Grants, 1795
Hugh J. Andersen Foundation Grants, 1814
Humana Foundation Grants, 1818
IAFF Burn Foundation Research Grants, 1830
Jane Bradley Pettit Foundation Grants, 1902
John Deere Foundation Grants, 1929
John Merck Fund Grants, 1940
John Merck Scholars Awards, 1941
Joyce Foundation Grants, 1969
Kimberly-Clark Community Grants, 2001
Marion Park Deaver and Harry Gilbert Deaver Foundation Grants, 2110
Mead Witter Foundation Grants, 2160
Multiple Sclerosis Foundation Brighter Tomorrow Grants, 2228
NEI Mentored Clinical Scientist Development Program Award (K12), 2295
NMF Franklin C. McLean Award, 2829
NMF General Electric Medical Scholars Fellowships, 2830
NMF Henry G. Halladay Awards, 2831
NMF Mary Ball Carrera Scholarship, 2834
NMF National Medical Association Awards for Medical Journalism, 2836
NMF National Medical Association Emerging Scholar Awards, 2837
NMF National Medical Association Patti LaBelle Award, 2838
NMF Need-Based Scholarships, 2839
NMF Ralph W. Ellison Prize, 2840
NMF William and Charlotte Cadbury Award, 2841
Northwestern Mutual Foundation Grants, 2870
NSF Major Research Instrumentation Program (MRI) Grants, 2889
OneSight Research Foundation Block Grants, 2944
Oscar Rennebohm Foundation Grants, 2963
Otto Bremer Foundation Grants, 2977
Pfizer/AAFP Foundation Visiting Professorship Program in Family Medicine, 3027
Piper Jaffray Companies Building Strong Communities Grants, 3053
Plum Creek Foundation Grants, 3062
Rosalinde and Arthur Gilbert Foundation/AFAR New Investigator Awards in Alzheimer's Disease, 3187
RRF General Program Grants, 3193
Siebert Lutheran Foundation Grants, 3285
Square D Foundation Grants, 3361
Stackner Family Foundation Grants, 3371
Toro Foundation Grants, 3431
Tylenol Scholarship, 3444
U.S. Department of Education Erma Byrd Scholarships, 3446
U.S. Department of Education United States-Russia Program: Improving Research and Educational Activities in Higher Education, 3451
US CRDF Leishmaniasis: Collaborative Research Opportunities in North Africa and the Middle East, 3474
Viking Children's Fund Grants, 3497
Vulcan Materials Company Foundation Grants, 3504
Wal-Mart Foundation Community Grants, 3513
Wal-Mart State Giving Program Grants, 3514

Wyoming

ACF Ethnic Community Self-Help Grants, 200
ACF Preferred Communities Grants, 201
ACF Standing Announcement for Unaccompanied Alien Children Grants, 202
ACF Supplemental Services for Recently Arrived Refugees Grants, 203
Actors Fund Social Services and Financial Assistance, 225
Albertson's Charitable Giving Grants, 330
American College of Surgeons and The Triological Society Clinical Scientist Development Awards, 422
ASHA Advancing Academic-Research Careers (AARC) Award, 569
ASHA Minority Student Leadership Program Awards, 570
ASHA Multicultural Activities Projects Grants, 571
ASHA Research Mentoring-Pair Travel Award, 572
ASHA Student Research Travel Award, 573
ASHA Students Preparing for Academic & Research Careers (SPARC) Award, 574
ASM Millis-Colwell Postgraduate Travel Grant, 608
Bearemy's Kennel Pals Grants, 728
Cable Positive's Tony Cox Community Fund Grants, 827
Champ-A Champion Fur Kids Grants, 959
Children Affected by AIDS Foundation Camp Network Grants, 994
Children Affected by AIDS Foundation Family Assistance Emergency Fund Grants, 996
CLIF Bar Family Foundation Grants, 1040
Daniels Fund Grants, 1200

DHHS Healthy Tomorrows Partnership for Children, 1261
Do Something BR!CK Awards, 1287
Dr. Stanley Pearle Scholarships, 1330
FMC Foundation Grants, 1518
GoGirlGo! Ambassador Team Awards, 1632
Griffin Foundation Grants, 1670
Guitar Center Music Foundation Grants, 1675
Harry Kramer Memorial Fund Grants, 1705
Hill Foundation Grants, 1774
IAFF Burn Foundation Research Grants, 1830
John Merck Fund Grants, 1940
John Merck Scholars Awards, 1941
Multiple Sclerosis Foundation Brighter Tomorrow Grants, 2228
NEI Mentored Clinical Scientist Development Program Award (K12), 2295
NMF Franklin C. McLean Award, 2829
NMF General Electric Medical Scholars Fellowships, 2830
NMF Henry G. Halladay Awards, 2831
NMF Mary Ball Carrera Scholarship, 2834
NMF National Medical Association Awards for Medical Journalism, 2836
NMF National Medical Association Emerging Scholar Awards, 2837
NMF National Medical Association Patti LaBelle Award, 2838
NMF Need-Based Scholarships, 2839
NMF Ralph W. Ellison Prize, 2840
NMF William and Charlotte Cadbury Award, 2841
NSF Major Research Instrumentation Program (MRI) Grants, 2889
OneSight Research Foundation Block Grants, 2944
PacifiCorp Foundation for Learning Grants, 2982
Pfizer/AAFP Foundation Visiting Professorship Program in Family Medicine, 3027
Piper Jaffray Companies Building Strong Communities Grants, 3053
Questar Corporate Contributions Grants, 3097
Rosalinde and Arthur Gilbert Foundation/AFAR New Investigator Awards in Alzheimer's Disease, 3187
Steele-Reese Foundation Grants, 3380
Tylenol Scholarship, 3444
U.S. Department of Education Erma Byrd Scholarships, 3446
U.S. Department of Education United States-Russia Program: Improving Research and Educational Activities in Higher Education, 3451
US CRDF Leishmaniasis: Collaborative Research Opportunities in North Africa and the Middle East, 3474
Wal-Mart Foundation Community Grants, 3513
Wal-Mart State Giving Program Grants, 3514

Outside the United States

Canada

Adobe Community Investment Grants, 237
AHFMR Clinical Fellowships, 269
AHFMR Clinical Investigator Awards, 270
AHFMR Community Support Program Grants, 271
AHFMR Dr. Lionel E. McLeod Health Research Scholarship, 272
AHFMR Establishment and Independent Establishment Grants, 273
AHFMR Fast-Track Studentships and Fellowships, 274
AHFMR Forefront Internship Program Grants, 275
AHFMR Full-Time Fellowships, 276
AHFMR Full-Time M.D./Ph.D. Studentships, 277
AHFMR Full-Time Studentships, 278
AHFMR Health Research Career Renewal Awards, 279
AHFMR Health Research Full-Time Studentships, 280
AHFMR Health Research Fund Grants, 281
AHFMR Heritage Summer Studentships, 282
AHFMR Infrastructure Funding Grants, 283
AHFMR Interdisciplinary Team Grants, 284
AHFMR Major Equipment Grants, 285
AHFMR Medical or Health Scholars Investigator Grants, 286
AHFMR Medical or Health Scientist Awards, 287
AHFMR Part-Time Fellowships, 288
AHFMR Part-Time Studentships, 289
AHFMR Personnel Funding Grants, 290
AHFMR Polaris Awards, 291
AHFMR Population Health Investigator (PHI) Awards, 292
AHFMR Proposals for Special Initiatives, 293
AHFMR Research Prize, 294
AHFMR Scholar Awards, 295
AHFMR Scientist Awards, 296
AHFMR Senior Investigator Awards, 297
AHFMR Senior Medical or Health Scholars Investigator Grants, 298
AHFMR Senior Scholar Awards, 299
Alaska Airlines Corporate Giving Grants, 323
Alfred P. Sloan Foundation Research Fellowships, 353
Andersen Corporate Foundation, 470
ASM-UNESCO Leadership Grant for International Educators, 626
Baxter International Foundation Grants, 705
Bearemy's Kennel Pals Grants, 728
Bechtel Group Foundation Building Positive Community Relationships Grants, 731
Bullitt Foundation Grants, 809
BWF Investigators in the Pathogenesis of Infectious Disease, 823
Canada Graduate Scholarships (CGS) and NSERC Postgraduate Scholarships (PGS), 845
Canada-U.S. Fulbright New Century Scholars Program Grants, 846
Canada-U.S. Fulbright Senior Specialists Program Grants, 847
Canadian Dental Research Foundation Award, 848
Canadian Foundation for Dietetic Research Awards, 849
Canadian Friends of Hebrew University Research and Study Grants, 850
Canadian Liver Foundation Grants, 851
Canadian Nurses Foundation Study Awards, 852
Canadian Optometric Education Trust Fund Grants, 853
Canadian Patient Safety Institute (CPSI) Patient Safety Studentships, 854
Canadian Patient Safety Institute (CPSI) Research Grants, 855
Cancer Research Society Fellowships and Grants, 857
CCFF Clinic Incentive Grants, 892
CCFF Research Grants, 894
CCFF Scholarships, 895
CCFF Small Conference Grants, 896
CCFF Studentships, 897
CCFF Summer Studentship, 898
CCFF Transplant Center Incentive Grants, 899
Central Okanagan Foundation Grants, 937
CFPC Family Medicine Resident Leadership Awards, 953
CFPC Family Physician of the Year Award, 954
CFPC Fellowships, 955
CFPC Research and Education Foundation Grants, 956
CFPC Special Recognition Awards, 957
Champ-A Champion Fur Kids Grants, 959
Chase Paymentech Corporate Giving Grants, 975
Children's Cardiomyopathy Foundation Research Grants, 1002
CLA Nurses Respiratory Society Fellowships, 1018
CLA Nurses Respiratory Society Nursing Research Grants, 1019
CLA Physiotherapy Cardio-Respiratory Society Fellowships, 1020
CLF Fellowships, 1037
CLF Graduate Studentships, 1038
CLF Operating Grants, 1039
CPhA Centennial Award, 1156
CTCRI Idea Grants, 1170
Dental Teaching and Research Fellowships, 1224
Doreen Kronick Scholarship, 1312
E.A. Baker Foundation for the Prevention of Blindness Grants, 1357
Epilepsy Postdoctoral and Clinical Research Fellowships, 1422
Fidelity Foundation Grants, 1498
Fluor Foundation Grants, 1517
FMC Foundation Grants, 1518
Fulbright Traditional Scholar Program in the Western Hemisphere, 1577
Giving in Action Society Children & Youth with Special Needs Grants, 1617
Giving in Action Society Family Independence Grants, 1618
Health Canada National Seniors Independence Program Grants, 1722
Helen McWilliam Memorial Scholarship, 1741
IAFF Burn Foundation Research Grants, 1830
James H. Cummings Foundation Grants, 1888
John Deere Foundation Grants, 1929
Johns Manville Fund Grants, 1950
Johnson and Johnson / SAH Arts and Healing Grants, 1953
Joyce Foundation Grants, 1969
K. M. Hunter Charitable Foundation Social Welfare Grants, 1974
KFC Allied Health Research Grants, 1996
KFC Biomedical Fellowships, 1997
KFC Biomedical Research Grants, 1998
KFC Nephrology and Urology Scholarships, 1999
Max Bell Foundation Grants, 2134
MHRC Operating Grants, 2186
MSSC Career Development Awards, 2224
MSSC Research Grants, 2226
MSSC Research Studentships, 2227
NCIC Canadian Breast Cancer Research Initiative Grants, 2281
NCIC Canadian Cancer Society Research Grants, 2282
NCIC Canadian Cancer Society Travel Award for Senior Level PhD Students, 2283
NCIC Terry Fox Postdoctoral Research Fellowships, 2285
NCIC Terry Fox Research Studentships, 2286
Nelda C. and H.J. Lutcher Stark Foundation Grants, 2301
NSERC Brockhouse Canada Prize for Interdisciplinary Research in Science and Engineering Grant, 2873
Pediatric Brain Tumor Research Grants, 3012
RCPSC Balfour M. Mount Visiting Professorship in Palliative Medicine, 3112
RCPSC Canadian Research Awards for Specialty Residents (Medicine, Surgery), 3113
RCPSC Detweiler Traveling Fellowships, 3114
RCPSC Duncan Graham Award, 3115
RCPSC Events, Speakers and Visiting Professors Grants, 3116
RCPSC Faculty Development Grants, 3117
RCPSC International Traveling Fellowship, 3118
RCPSC James H. Graham Award of Merit, 3119
RCPSC Janes Visiting Professorship in Surgery, 3120
RCPSC Kilborn Memorial Visiting Professorship, 3121
RCPSC KJR Wightman Award for Scholarship in Ethics, 3122
RCPSC Medical Education Research Grants, 3124
RCPSC Medical Education Traveling Fellowships, 3125
RCPSC National Specialty Society Annual Meeting Grants, 3126
RCPSC Royal College Fellowship for Studies in Medical Education, 3127
RCPSC Royal College Medal Award in Medicine, 3128

RCPSC Royal College Medal Award in Surgery, 3129
RCPSC Royal College Visiting Professorships in Medical Research, 3130
RCPSC Teasdale-Corti Humanitarian Award, 3131
RCPSC Traineeships, 3132
RCPSC Walter C. MacKenzie Fellowship in Surgery, 3133
RCPSC Wightman Visiting Professorship in Medicine, 3134
RCPSC/AMS CanMEDs Research and Development Grants, 3135
RCPSC/AMS Donald Richards Wilson Award, 3136
RSC Abbyann D. Lynch Medal in Bioethics, 3195
RSC Jason A. Hannah Medal, 3196
RSC McLaughlin Medal, 3197
RSC McNeil Medal for the Public Awareness of Science, 3198
RSC Thomas W. Eadie Medal, 3199
Savoy Foundation Post-Doctoral and Clinical Research Fellowships, 3266
Savoy Foundation Research Grants, 3267
Savoy Foundation Studentships, 3268
SSHRC Image, Text, Sound and Technology (ITST) Grants, 3363
SSHRC Research/Creation Grants in Fine Arts, 3364
Steelcase Foundation Grants, 3379
University of Calgary Nursing Alumni Scholarship, 3468
Vancouver Foundation Grants and Community Initiatives Program, 3477
Vancouver Foundation Public Health Bursary Package, 3478
Vancouver Sun Children's Fund Grants, 3479

Africa
ASM-UNESCO Leadership Grant for International Educators, 626
Beatrice Laing Trust Grants, 729
Cargill Citizenship Fund-Corporate Giving Grants, 865
Fulbright Traditional Scholar Program in Sub-Saharan Africa, 1573
Fulbright Traditional Scholar Program in the Near East and North Africa Region, 1575
Nuffield Foundation Africa Program Grants, 2898
Rockefeller Brothers Fund Pivotal Places Grants: South Africa, 3180
SSRC HIV/AIDS and Public Health Policy Research in Africa Fellowships, 3365

Argentina
ASM-UNESCO Leadership Grant for International Educators, 626
Fulbright Traditional Scholar Program in the Western Hemisphere, 1577

Asia
Advanced Micro Devices Community Affairs Grants, 239
ASM-UNESCO Leadership Grant for International Educators, 626
Baxter International Foundation Grants, 705
Fluor Foundation Grants, 1517
Fulbright Traditional Scholar Program in the East Asia/Pacific Region, 1574
Sir Dorabji Tata Trust Grants for NGOs or Voluntary Organizations, 3291

Australia
ASM-UNESCO Leadership Grant for International Educators, 626
Australian Academy of Science Grants, 670
Baxter International Foundation Grants, 705
Bechtel Group Foundation Building Positive Community Relationships Grants, 731
Fluor Foundation Grants, 1517
Fulbright Traditional Scholar Program in the East Asia/Pacific Region, 1574
Layne Beachley Aim For The Stars Foundation Grants, 2036
Pediatric Brain Tumor Research Grants, 3012
RACGP Cardiovascular Research Grants in General Practice, 3099
RACGP National Asthma Council Research Award, 3100
RACGP Vicki Kotsirilos Integrative Medicine Grants, 3101

Belgium
ASM-UNESCO Leadership Grant for International Educators, 626
Fluor Foundation Grants, 1517

Bolivia
ASM-PAHO Infectious Diseases Epidemiology and Surveillance Fellowships, 625
ASM-UNESCO Leadership Grant for International Educators, 626
Fulbright Traditional Scholar Program in the Western Hemisphere, 1577

Brazil
ASM-UNESCO Leadership Grant for International Educators, 626
Bechtel Group Foundation Building Positive Community Relationships Grants, 731
Fulbright Traditional Scholar Program in the Western Hemisphere, 1577
Hershey Company Grants, 1754
John Deere Foundation Grants, 1929

Bulgaria
ASM-UNESCO Leadership Grant for International Educators, 626

Caribbean
ASM International Fellowship for Latin America and the Caribbean, 601
ASM-UNESCO Leadership Grant for International Educators, 626
Atkinson Foundation International Grants, 661
Fluor Foundation Grants, 1517
Fulbright Traditional Scholar Program in the Western Hemisphere, 1577

Central America
ASM-UNESCO Leadership Grant for International Educators, 626
Atkinson Foundation International Grants, 661
Fulbright Traditional Scholar Program in the Western Hemisphere, 1577

China
ASM-UNESCO Leadership Grant for International Educators, 626
Bechtel Group Foundation Building Positive Community Relationships Grants, 731
Fluor Foundation Grants, 1517
Fulbright Traditional Scholar Program in the East Asia/Pacific Region, 1574
Hershey Company Grants, 1754

Colombia
ASM-PAHO Infectious Diseases Epidemiology and Surveillance Fellowships, 625
ASM-UNESCO Leadership Grant for International Educators, 626
Fulbright Traditional Scholar Program in the Western Hemisphere, 1577
Genesis Foundation Grants, 1593

Czech Republic
ASM-UNESCO Leadership Grant for International Educators, 626
EMBO Installation Grants, 1409
HHMI Biomedical Research Grants for International Scientists in the Baltics, Central and Eastern Europe, Russia, and Ukraine, 1757

Ecuador
ASM-PAHO Infectious Diseases Epidemiology and Surveillance Fellowships, 625
ASM-UNESCO Leadership Grant for International Educators, 626
Fulbright Traditional Scholar Program in the Western Hemisphere, 1577

Estonia
ASM-UNESCO Leadership Grant for International Educators, 626
EMBO Installation Grants, 1409

Germany
Advanced Micro Devices Community Affairs Grants, 239
ASM-UNESCO Leadership Grant for International Educators, 626
Chiles Foundation Grants, 1003
EMBO Long-Term Fellowships, 1410
EMBO Short-Term Fellowships, 1411
Fulbright German Studies Seminar Grants, 1568
Wilhelm Sander Foundation Grants, 3535

Hungary
ASM-UNESCO Leadership Grant for International Educators, 626
EMBO Installation Grants, 1409
HHMI Biomedical Research Grants for International Scientists in the Baltics, Central and Eastern Europe, Russia, and Ukraine, 1757

Israel
ASM-UNESCO Leadership Grant for International Educators, 626
Boston Jewish Community Women's Fund Grants, 785
David Geffen Foundation Grants, 1202
Fulbright Traditional Scholar Program in the Near East and North Africa Region, 1575
Harry Kramer Memorial Fund Grants, 1705
Rosalinde and Arthur Gilbert Foundation/AFAR New Investigator Awards in Alzheimer's Disease, 3187
Russell Berrie Foundation Grants, 3201

Japan
ASM-UNESCO Leadership Grant for International Educators, 626
Bechtel Group Foundation Building Positive Community Relationships Grants, 731
Fluor Foundation Grants, 1517
Fulbright Traditional Scholar Program in the East Asia/Pacific Region, 1574
Japan Heart Foundation Grants, 1906

Kazakhstan
ASM-UNESCO Leadership Grant for International Educators, 626
Fulbright Traditional Scholar Program in the South and Central Asia Region, 1576

Kyrgyzstan
ASM-UNESCO Leadership Grant for International Educators, 626

Marshall Islands
ASM-UNESCO Leadership Grant for International Educators, 626

Mexico
Alaska Airlines Corporate Giving Grants, 323
ASM-UNESCO Leadership Grant for International Educators, 626
Atkinson Foundation International Grants, 661
Baxter International Foundation Grants, 705

Fluor Foundation Grants, 1517
Fulbright Traditional Scholar Program in the Western Hemisphere, 1577
Hershey Company Grants, 1754
Steelcase Foundation Grants, 3379

Micronesia
ASM-UNESCO Leadership Grant for International Educators, 626

New Independent States
ASM-UNESCO Leadership Grant for International Educators, 626

New Zealand
ASM-UNESCO Leadership Grant for International Educators, 626
Cancer Society of New Zealand Grants, 860
Fluor Foundation Grants, 1517
Fulbright Traditional Scholar Program in the East Asia/Pacific Region, 1574
National Heart Foundation of New Zealand Grants, 2255

Northern Mariana Islands
ASM-UNESCO Leadership Grant for International Educators, 626

Peru
ASM-PAHO Infectious Diseases Epidemiology and Surveillance Fellowships, 625
ASM-UNESCO Leadership Grant for International Educators, 626
Bechtel Group Foundation Building Positive Community Relationships Grants, 731
Fluor Foundation Grants, 1517
Fulbright Traditional Scholar Program in the Western Hemisphere, 1577

Philippines
ASM-UNESCO Leadership Grant for International Educators, 626
Bechtel Group Foundation Building Positive Community Relationships Grants, 731
Fluor Foundation Grants, 1517
Fulbright Traditional Scholar Program in the East Asia/Pacific Region, 1574

Poland
ASM-UNESCO Leadership Grant for International Educators, 626
Bechtel Group Foundation Building Positive Community Relationships Grants, 731
EMBO Installation Grants, 1409
Fluor Foundation Grants, 1517

Republic of Palau
ASM-UNESCO Leadership Grant for International Educators, 626

Romania
ASM-UNESCO Leadership Grant for International Educators, 626

Russia
ASM-UNESCO Leadership Grant for International Educators, 626
Bechtel Group Foundation Building Positive Community Relationships Grants, 731
Fluor Foundation Grants, 1517
HHMI Biomedical Research Grants for International Scientists in the Baltics, Central and Eastern Europe, Russia, and Ukraine, 1757
U.S. Department of Education United States-Russia Program: Improving Research and Educational Activities in Higher Education, 3451

Scandinavia
ASM-UNESCO Leadership Grant for International Educators, 626

Slovakia
ASM-UNESCO Leadership Grant for International Educators, 626

Slovenia
ASM-UNESCO Leadership Grant for International Educators, 626

South America
ASM International Fellowship for Latin America and the Caribbean, 601
ASM-PAHO Infectious Diseases Epidemiology and Surveillance Fellowships, 625
ASM-UNESCO Leadership Grant for International Educators, 626
Charles Delmar Foundation Grants, 963

Sweden
ASM-UNESCO Leadership Grant for International Educators, 626
Wilhelm Sander Foundation Grants, 3535

Ukraine
ASM-UNESCO Leadership Grant for International Educators, 626
HHMI Biomedical Research Grants for International Scientists in the Baltics, Central and Eastern Europe, Russia, and Ukraine, 1757

United Kingdom
ASM-UNESCO Leadership Grant for International Educators, 626
Beatrice Laing Trust Grants, 729
Bechtel Group Foundation Building Positive Community Relationships Grants, 731
Cancer Research UK Grants, 859
Commonwealth Fund Harkness Fellowships in Health Care Policy and Practice, 1079
Cooper Industries Foundation Grants, 1150
Fight for Sight Research Grants, 1502
Fluor Foundation Grants, 1517
Guy's and St. Thomas' Charity Grants, 1678
Leukaemia Research Fund Grants, 2050
Lincoln Financial Group Foundation Grants, 2058
MRC Career Establishment Grants, 2221
Nuffield Foundation Africa Program Grants, 2898
Nuffield Foundation Children and Families Grants, 2899
Nuffield Foundation Law and Society Grants, 2900
Nuffield Foundation Oliver Bird Rheumatism Program Grants, 2901
Nuffield Foundation Open Door Grants, 2902
Nuffield Foundation Small Grants, 2903
Stroke Association Allied Health Professional Research Bursaries, 3385
Stroke Association Clinical Fellowships, 3386
Stroke Association Research Project Grants, 3387
UK Foundation for the Study of Infant Deaths Grants, 3459

Uzbekistan
ASM-UNESCO Leadership Grant for International Educators, 626
Fulbright Traditional Scholar Program in the Near East and North Africa Region, 1575
Fulbright Traditional Scholar Program in the South and Central Asia Region, 1576

Venezuela
ASM-UNESCO Leadership Grant for International Educators, 626
Fluor Foundation Grants, 1517
Fulbright Traditional Scholar Program in the Western Hemisphere, 1577

www.ingramcontent.com/pod-product-compliance
Lightning Source LLC
LaVergne TN
LVHW082000200926
848481LV00010B/2774